NATHAN AND OSKI'S
HEMATOLOGY OF INFANCY AND CHILDHOOD

Edition: 7

NATHAN AND OSKI'S
HEMATOLOGY OF INFANCY AND CHILDHOOD

Edition: **7**

Stuart H. Orkin, MD
David G. Nathan Professor of Pediatrics
Harvard Medical School
Chief, Department of Pediatric Oncology
Dana-Farber Cancer Institute
Investigator, Howard Hughes Medical Institute
Boston, Massachusetts

David G. Nathan, MD
Robert A. Stranahan Distinguished Professor of
    Pediatrics
Harvard Medical School
Physician-in-Chief Emeritus
Children's Hospital Boston
President Emeritus, Dana-Farber Cancer Institute
Boston, Massachusetts

David Ginsburg, MD
James V. Neel Distinguished University Professor
Departments of Internal Medicine and Human
    Genetics
Investigator, Howard Hughes Medical Institute
University of Michigan Medical School
Ann Arbor, Michigan

A. Thomas Look, MD
Professor of Pediatrics
Harvard Medical School
Department of Pediatric Oncology
Dana-Farber Cancer Institute
Boston, Massachusetts

David E. Fisher, MD, PhD
Professor of Pediatrics
Wigglesworth Professor of Dermatology
Harvard Medical School
Chief, Department of Dermatology
Massachusetts General Hospital
Boston, Massachusetts

Samuel E. Lux IV, MD
Robert A. Stranahan Professor of Pediatrics
Harvard Medical School
Chief Emeritus, Division of Hematology/Oncology
Children's Hospital Boston
Boston, Massachusetts

Managing Editor: *Cathryn J. Lantigua*

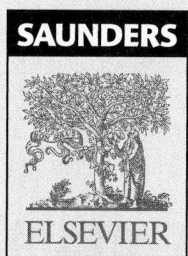

SAUNDERS

ELSEVIER

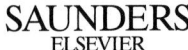

SAUNDERS
ELSEVIER

1600 John F. Kennedy Blvd.
Suite 1800
Philadelphia, PA 19103-2899

NATHAN AND OSKI'S HEMATOLOGY OF INFANCY AND
CHILDHOOD, 7TH EDITION

ISBN: 978-1-4160-3430-8

Library of Congress Cataloging-in-Publication Data
Nathan and Oski's hematology of infancy and childhood.—7th ed. / edited by Stuart H. Orkin . . . [et al.].
    p. ; cm.
   Includes bibliographical references and index.
   ISBN 978-1-4160-3430-8
   1. Pediatric hematology.   2. Neonatal hematology.   I. Nathan, David G.   II. Orkin, Stuart H.   III. Title: Hematology of infancy and childhood.
   [DNLM: 1. Hematologic Diseases.   2. Child.   3. Infant.   WS 300 N274 2009]
RJ411.N37 2009
618.92'15—dc22

2008018555

Acquisitions Editor: Dolores Meloni
Developmental Editor: Ann Anderson
Publishing Services Manager: Frank Polizzano
Senior Project Manager: Robin E. Hayward
Design Direction: Karen O'Keefe-Owens
Marketing Manager: William Veltre

Printed in Canada.

Last digit is the print number: 9   8   7   6   5   4   3   2   1

Contributors

Nancy C. Andrews, MD, PhD

Professor of Pediatrics, Professor of Pharmacology and Cancer Biology, and Dean and Vice-Chancellor for Academic Affairs, Duke University School of Medicine, Durham, North Carolina

Disorders of Iron Metabolism and Sideroblastic Anemia

Ida Annunziata, PhD

Postdoctoral Fellow, Department of Genetics and Tumor Cell Biology, St. Jude Children's Research Hospital, Memphis, Tennessee

Storage Diseases of the Reticuloendothelial System

Alessandra d'Azzo, PhD

Affiliated Professor of Anatomy and Neurobiology, University of Tennessee Health Science Center; Member and Endowed Chair, Department of Genetics and Tumor Cell Biology, St. Jude Children's Research Hospital, Memphis, Tennessee

Storage Diseases of the Reticuloendothelial System

Kenneth A. Bauer, MD

Professor of Medicine, Harvard Medical School; Director, Thrombosis Clinical Research, Beth Israel Deaconess Medical Center, Boston, Massachusetts

Rare Hereditary Coagulation Factor Abnormalities; Inherited Disorders of Thrombosis and Fibrinolysis

Mark J. Bergeron, MD

Fellow, Neonatal-Perinatal Medicine, Department of Pediatrics, University of Minnesota Medical School; University of Minnesota Children's Hospital, Fairview, Minneapolis, Minnesota

Disorders of Bilirubin Metabolism

Monica Bessler, MD, PhD

Professor of Internal Medicine, Division of Hematology, Professor of Molecular Biology and Pharmacology, Washington University School of Medicine, St. Louis, Missouri

Inherited Bone Marrow Failure Syndromes

Barbara Bierer, MD

Professor of Medicine (Pediatrics), Harvard Medical School; Senior Vice President, Research, and Director, Center for Faculty Development and Diversity, Brigham and Women's Hospital, Boston, Massachusetts

The Immune Response

Francisco A. Bonilla, MD, PhD

Assistant Professor of Pediatrics, Harvard Medical School; Director, Clinical Immunology Program, Children's Hospital Boston, Boston, Massachusetts

Primary Immunodeficiency Diseases

Erik Bonten, PhD

Associate Scientist, Department of Genetics and Tumor Cell Biology, St. Jude Children's Research Hospital, Memphis, Tennessee

Storage Diseases of the Reticuloendothelial System

Carlo Brugnara, MD

Professor of Pathology, Harvard Medical School; Director, Hematology Laboratory, Department of Laboratory Medicine, Children's Hospital Boston, Boston, Massachusetts

The Neonatal Erythrocyte and Its Disorders; Diagnostic Approach to the Anemic Patient; Reference Values in Infancy and Childhood

Kathleen Brummel-Ziedens, PhD

Associate Professor of Biochemistry, University of Vermont College of Medicine, Colchester, Vermont

Blood Coagulation

H. Franklin Bunn, MD

Professor of Medicine, Harvard Medical School; Physician, Brigham and Women's Hospital, Boston, Massachusetts

Hemoglobins: Normal and Abnormal

Alan B. Cantor, MD, PhD

Assistant Professor of Pediatrics, Harvard Medical School; Assistant in Medicine, Children's Hospital Boston, Dana-Farber Cancer Institute, Boston, Massachusetts

Developmental Hemostasis: Relevance to Newborns and Infants

Melody J. Cunningham, MD

Assistant Professor of Pediatrics, Harvard Medical School; Division of Hematology/Oncology, Children's Hospital Boston, Boston, Massachusetts

The Thalassemias

Mary C. Dinauer, MD, PhD

Nora Letzter Professor of Pediatrics and Professor of Microbiology/Immunology and Medical and Molecular Gentetics, Indiana University School of Medicine; Pediatric Hematology/Oncology, Riley Hospital for Children, Indianapolis, Indiana

The Phagocyte System and Disorders of Granulopoiesis and Granulocyte Function

Jorge Di Paola, MD

Associate Professor of Pediatrics, University of Iowa Carver College of Medicine; Director, Hemophilia Treatment Center, University of Iowa Children's Hospital, Iowa City, Iowa

Hemophilia and von Willebrand Disease

George J. Dover, MD

Professor and Director of Pediatrics, Johns Hopkins University School of Medicine; Pediatrician-in-Chief, Johns Hopkins Hospital, Baltimore, Maryland

Sickle Cell Disease

Christine Duncan, MD

Instructor, Harvard Medical School; Outpatient Clinical Director HSCT, Dana-Farber Cancer Institute, Boston, Massachusetts

Principles of Bone Marrow and Stem Cell Transplantation

R. Alan B. Ezekowitz, MBChB, DPhil

Department of Pediatrics, Harvard Medical School, Boston, Massachusetts; Merck Research Laboratories, Rahway, New Jersey

Hematologic Manifestations of Systemic Diseases

Mark D. Fleming, MD, DPhil

Associate Professor of Pathology, Harvard Medical School; Interim Pathologist-in-Chief, Department of Pathology, Children's Hospital Boston, Boston, Massachusetts

Disorders of Iron Metabolism and Sideroblastic Anemia

David F. Friedman, MD

Clinical Assistant Professor of Pediatrics, University of Pennsylvania College of Medicine; Associate Medical Director, Transfusion Service, Children's Hospital of Philadelphia, Philadelphia, Pennsylvania

Transfusion Medicine

Raif S. Geha, MD

James L. Gamble Professor of Pediatrics, Harvard Medical School; Chief, Division of Immunology, Children's Hospital Boston, Boston, Massachusetts

Primary Immunodeficiency Diseases

Joan Cox Gill, MD

Professor of Pediatrics and Medicine, Medical College of Wisconsin; Director, Comprehensive Center for Bleeding Disorders, Blood Center of Wisconsin, Milwaukee, Wisconsin

Hemophilia and von Willebrand Disease

Neil A. Goldenberg, MD, PhD

Assistant Professor of Pediatrics and Medicine and Associate Director of Mountain States Regional Hemophilia and Thrombosis Center, University of Colorado at Denver; Co-Director, Thrombosis and Stroke Programs, The Children's Hospital, Colorado, Aurora, Colorado

Acquired Disorders of Hemostasis

Glenn R. Gourley, MD

Professor of Pediatrics and Research Director, Pediatric Gastroenterology, University of Minnesota Medical School; University of Minnesota Children's Hospital, Fairview, Minneapolis, Minnesota

Disorders of Bilirubin Metabolism

Rachael F. Grace, MD

Instructor in Pediatrics, Harvard Medical School; Pediatric Hematology/Oncology, Dana-Farber Cancer Institute, Children's Hospital Boston, Boston, Massachusetts

Disorders of the Red Cell Membrane

W. Nicholas Haining, BM, BCh

Assistant Professor of Pediatrics, Harvard Medical School; Staff Physician, Dana-Farber Cancer Institute, Children's Hospital Boston, Boston, Massachusetts

Principles of Bone Marrow and Stem Cell Transplantation

Katherine Amberson Hajjar, MD

Brine Family Professor of Cell and Developmental Biology and Professor of Pediatrics, Weill Cornell Medical College; Attending Pediatrician, New York-Presbyterian Hospital, New York, New York

The Molecular Basis of Fibrinolysis

Matthew Heeney, MD

Instructor in Pediatrics, Harvard Medical School; Director, Pediatric Sickle Cell Program, Children's Hospital Boston, Boston, Massachusetts

Sickle Cell Disease

Grace Kao, MD

Instructor in Pathology, Harvard Medical School; Assistant Medical Director, Connell & O'Reilly Families Cell Manipulation Core Facility, Dana-Farber Cancer Institute, Boston, Massachusetts

Transfusion Medicine

Richard M. Kaufman, MD

Assistant Professor of Pathology, Harvard Medical School; Medical Director, Adult Transfusion Service, Brigham and Women's Hospital, Boston, Massachusetts

Transfusion Medicine

Edwin H. Kolodny, MD

Bernard A. and Charlotte Marden Professor and Chair, Department of Neurology, New York University School of Medicine; Attending Neurologist, Langone Medical Center and The Bellevue Hospital Center, New York, New York

Storage Diseases of the Reticuloendothelial System

James P. Kushner, MD

M. M. Wintrobe Distinguished Professor of Medicine, Department of Internal Medicine, Division of Hematology, University of Utah School of Medicine; Chief, Division of Hematology, University Hospital, Salt Lake City, Utah

The Porphyrias

Dominic P. Kwiatkowski, FRCP, FRCPCH, FMedSci

Medical Research Council Professor, Wellcome Trust Centre for Human Genetics; University Department of Paediatrics, John Radcliffe Hospital, Oxford, United Kingdom

Hematologic Manifestations of Systemic Diseases in Children of the Developing World

Michele P. Lambert, MD

Assistant Professor of Pediatrics, University of Pennsylvania College of Medicine; Attending Physician, Division of Hematology, Children's Hospital of Philadelphia, Philadelphia, Pennsylvania

Inherited Platelet Disorders

Leslie E. Lehmann, MD

Assistant Professor of Pediatrics, Harvard Medical School; Clinical Director, Pediatric Hematopoietic Stem Cell Transplant, Dana-Farber Cancer Institute, Children's Hospital Boston, Boston, Massachusetts

Principles of Bone Marrow and Stem Cell Transplantation

Helen G. Liley, MB, ChB

Senior Lecturer in Pediatrics and Child Health, University of Queensland School of Medicine; Senior Staff Specialist, Neonatology, Mater Mothers' Hospital, South Brisbane, Queensland, Australia

Immune Hemolytic Disease of the Newborn

Daniel C. Link, MD

Associate Professor of Internal Medicine, Division of Oncology, Washington University School of Medicine, St. Louis, Missouri

Inherited Bone Marrow Failure Syndromes

Jeanne M. Lusher, MD

Distinguished Professor of Pediatrics, Wayne State University School of Medicine; Director, Hemostasis Program, Co-Director, Division of Hematology-Oncology, Children's Hospital of Michigan, Detroit, Michigan

Clinical and Laboratory Approach to the Patient with Bleeding

Samuel E. Lux IV, MD

Robert A. Stranahan Professor of Pediatrics, Harvard Medical School; Chief Emeritus, Division of Hematology/Oncology, Children's Hospital Boston, Boston, Massachusetts

Disorders of the Red Cell Membrane

Lucio Luzzatto, MD, PhD

Professor of Hematology, University of Florence Medical School; Attending Physician, University Hospital, Careggi; Scientific Director, Istituto Toscano Tumori, Firenze, Italy

Glucose-6-Phosphate Dehydrogenase Deficiency

Kenneth G. Mann, PhD

Professor of Biochemistry and Medicine, University of Vermont College of Medicine, Colchester, Vermont

Blood Coagulation

Philip J. Mason, PhD

Professor of Internal Medicine, Division of Hematology, Professor of Genetics, Washington University School of Medicine, St. Louis, Missouri

Inherited Bone Marrow Failure Syndromes

William C. Mentzer, Jr., MD

Professor Emeritus, Department of Pediatrics, University of California, San Francisco, School of Medicine; Attending Hematologist, University of California Hospitals, San Francisco, California

Pyruvate Kinase Deficiency and Disorders of Glycolysis

Robert R. Montgomery, MD

Professor of Pediatric Hematology, Medical College of Wisconsin; Senior Investigator, Blood Research Institute of BloodCenter of Wisconsin; Staff Physician, Children's Hospital of Wisconsin, Children's Hospital Research Institute, Milwaukee, Wisconsin

Hemophilia and von Willebrand Disease

Ronald L. Nagel, MD

Irving D. Karpas Professor of Medicine, Professor of Physiology and Biophysics, and Head, Division of Hematology, Albert Einstein College of Medicine; Director, Bronx Comprehensive Sickle Cell Center, Montefiore Medical Center, Bronx, New York

Hemoglobins: Normal and Abnormal

David G. Nathan, MD

Robert A. Stranahan Distinguished Professor of Pediatrics and Professor of Medicine, Harvard Medical School; Physician-in-Chief Emeritus, Children's Hospital Boston; President Emeritus, Dana-Farber Cancer Institute, Boston, Massachusetts

Pediatric Hematology in Historical Perspective; Acquired Aplastic Anemia and Pure Red Cell Aplasia; Diagnostic Approach to the Anemic Patient; The Thalassemias

Peter E. Newburger, MD

Ali and John Pierce Professor of Pediatric Hematology/Oncology, University of Massachusetts Medical School; Director, Pediatric Hematology/Oncology, UMass/Memorial Medical Center, Worcester, Massachusetts

The Phagocyte System and Disorders of Granulopoiesis and Granulocyte Function

Debra K. Newman, PhD

Assistant Professor of Pharmacology and Microbiology, Medical College of Wisconsin; Associate Investigator, Blood Research Institute, Blood Center of Wisconsin, Milwaukee, Wisconsin

Platelets and the Vessel Wall

Peter J. Newman, PhD

Professor of Pharmacology and Cellular Biology, Medical College of Wisconsin; Vice President for Research, Blood Research Institute, Blood Center of Wisconsin, Milwaukee, Wisconsin

Platelets and the Vessel Wall

Stuart H. Orkin, MD

David G. Nathan Professor of Pediatrics, Harvard Medical School; Chief, Department of Pediatric Oncology, Dana-Farber Cancer Institute; Investigator, Howard Hughes Medical Institute, Boston, Massachusetts

The Thalassemias

Frank A. Oski, MD*

Distinguished Service Professor, Johns Hopkins University School of Medicine, Baltimore, Maryland

Diagnostic Approach to the Anemic Patient

Sung-Yun Pai, MD

Assistant Professor of Pediatrics, Harvard Medical School; Staff Physician, Dana-Farber Cancer Institute; Attending in Medicine, Children's Hospital Boston, Boston, Massachusetts

The Immune Response

John D. Phillips, PhD

Associate Professor of Medicine, Department of Internal Medicine, Division of Hematology, University of Utah School of Medicine, Salt Lake City, Utah

The Porphyrias

Steven W. Pipe, MD

Associate Professor of Pediatrics and Communicable Diseases, University of Michigan Medical School, Ann Arbor, Michigan

Acquired Disorders of Hemostasis

Orah S. Platt, MD

Professor of Pediatrics, Harvard Medical School; Director, Department of Laboratory Medicine, Children's Hospital Boston, Boston, Massachusetts

The Neonatal Erythrocyte and Its Disorders

Vincenzo Poggi, MD

Professor of Pediatric Hematology and Oncology, Federico II University; Chief, Division of Hematology-Oncology, Pediatric Oncology, Pausilipon Hospital, Naples, Italy

Glucose-6-Phosphate Dehydrogenase Deficiency

Mortimer Poncz, MD

Professor of Pediatrics, University of Pennsylvania College of Medicine; Chief, Division of Hematology, Children's Hospital of Philadelphia, Philadelphia, Pennsylvania

Inherited Platelet Disorders

Madhvi Rajpurkar, MD

Assistant Professor of Pediatrics, Wayne State University School of Medicine; Associate Hematologist, Children's Hospital of Michigan, Detroit, Michigan

Clinical and Laboratory Approach to the Patient with Bleeding

*Deceased.

David J. Roberts, MB, MRCP, MRCPath

Professor of Haematology, National Blood Service, University of Oxford; John Radcliffe Hospital, Oxford, United Kingdom

Hematologic Manifestations of Systemic Diseases in Children of the Developing World

David S. Rosenblatt, MDCM

Professor and Chair, Department of Human Genetics, McGill University; Director, Division of Medical Genetics, McGill University Medical Centre, Montreal, Quebec, Canada

Megaloblastic Anemia

Vijay G. Sankaran, MS, MPhil

Harvard Medical School; Division of Hematology/Oncology, Children's Hospital Boston, Boston, Massachusetts

The Thalassemias

Akiko Shimamura, MD, PhD

Associate Professor of Pediatrics, University of Washington School of Medicine; Children's Hospital and Regional Medical Center, Fred Hutchinson Cancer Research Center, Seattle, Washington

Acquired Aplastic Anemia and Pure Red Cell Aplasia

Colin A. Sieff, MB, BCh

Associate Professor of Pediatrics, Harvard Medical School; Senior Associate in Medicine, Pediatric Hematology/Oncology, Children's Hospital, Boston, Massachusetts

Anatomy and Physiology of Hematopoiesis

Leslie Silberstein, MD

Professor of Pathology, Harvard Medical School; Director, Joint Program in Transfusion Medicine; Director, Center for Human Cell Therapy, Children's Hospital Boston, Brigham and Women's Hospital, Dana-Farber Cancer Institute, Boston, Massachusetts

Transfusion Medicine

Steven R. Sloan, MD, PhD

Assistant Professor of Pathology, Harvard Medical School; Medical Director, Blood Bank, Children's Hospital Boston, Boston, Massachusetts

Transfusion Medicine

Christina K. Ullrich, MD, MPH

Instructor in Pediatrics, Harvard Medical School; Staff Physician, Pediatric Hematology/Oncology and Pediatric Palliative Care, Dana-Farber Cancer Institute, Children's Hospital Boston, Boston, Massachusetts

Disorders of Iron Metabolism and Sideroblastic Anemia

Russell E. Ware, MD, PhD

Lemuel Diggs Endowed Chair of Sickle Cell Disease, Department of Hematology, St. Jude Children's Research Hospital, Memphis, Tennessee

Autoimmune Hemolytic Anemia

David Watkins, PhD

Research Associate, Department of Human Genetics, McGill University, Montreal, Quebec, Canada

Megaloblastic Anemia

David J. Weatherall, MD

Regius Professor of Medicine Emeritus and Former Director of the Weatherall Institute of Molecular Medicine, University of Oxford, Oxford, United Kingdom

Hematologic Manifestations of Systemic Diseases in Children of the Developing World

V. Michael Whitehead, MDCM

Cole Professor Emeritus, Department of Pediatrics, Faculty of Medicine, McGill University; Former Director of Hematology, Department of Pediatrics, Montreal Children's Hospital of the McGill University Health Centre, Quebec, Canada

Megaloblastic Anemia

David B. Wilson, MD, PhD

Associate Professor of Pediatrics and Molecular Biology and Pharmacology, Washington University School of Medicine; St. Louis Children's Hospital, St. Louis, Missouri

Inherited Bone Marrow Failure Syndromes; Acquired Platelet Defects

Leonard I. Zon, MD

Grousbeck Professor of Pediatrics, Harvard Medical School; Stem Cell Program and Division of Hematology/Oncology, Children's Hospital of Boston and Dana-Farber Cancer Institute; Investigator, Howard Hughes Medical Institute, Boston, Massachusetts

Anatomy and Physiology of Hematopoiesis

Wolf W. Zuelzer, MD*

Emeritus Professor of Pediatric Research, Wayne State University School of Medicine; Emeritus Director of Laboratories and Hematologist-in-Chief, Children's Hospital of Michigan, Detroit, Michigan; Emeritus Director, Division of Blood Diseases and Resources, National Heart, Lung, and Blood Institute, National Institutes of Health, Bethesda, Maryland

Pediatric Hematology in Historical Perspective

---

*Deceased.

Preface

On behalf of all the editors, I welcome you to the seventh edition of *Nathan and Oski's Hematology of Infancy and Childhood*. For more than 30 years this textbook has served as the premier resource for students, clinical fellows, investigators, and practitioners in the field of pediatric hematology. From its inception, David Nathan and Frank Oski sought to relate pathophysiology to the hematologic diseases afflicting children. Their goal was to stimulate bench-to-bedside and bedside-to-bench activities to understand and then treat pediatric hematological disorders. What was not envisioned in those early days was how rapidly the basic biology and genetics underlying the field would develop. With each new edition, the text and the roster of editors have grown. We take this as a healthy sign. So much has been learned in this timeframe that has contributed to improved care of children with hematologic disorders.

The seventh edition of *Hematology of Infancy and Childhood* represents a further evolution of the life of this organic textbook. We have recruited Sam Lux to join us as an editor in order to incorporate his remarkable insights and vision to the current edition. In prior editions we drew the boundary for the scope of the textbook to encompass hematology *per se*, both nonmalignant and malignant, despite the reality that we, and others, train clinical fellows in pediatric hematology *and* oncology. For several editions we provided superficial coverage of pediatric oncology with a single chapter on solid tumors. In the sixth edition, on the urging of Tom Look, an insightful investigator of childhood malignancies, we eliminated this chapter. Though beautifully done by Arnold Altman, it could never fully capture the increasing knowledge base and breadth of pediatric oncology. Reflecting on this history and the extraordinary progress in cancer biology and genetics, we chose to create an entirely new volume devoted to pediatric oncology. Going forward, we present our readers with parallel textbooks: *Hematology of Infancy and Childhood* and *Oncology of Infancy and Childhood*.

To meet the daunting challenge of bringing forward a new oncology volume, we invited David Fisher, an extraordinary cancer biologist, physician, and cellist, to join Tom Look as editors for this venture. The goal, as before, has been to join basic pathophysiology and clinical medicine at the hip. The creation of the Oncology volume necessitated moving the chapters on malignant hematology, including the leukemias, from *Hematology of Infancy and Childhood*. We hope that readers find the new volume as useful and perhaps as inspiring as prior editions of Nathan and Oski. Launching a new venture is never without some missteps. We welcome feedback from our readers on the extent to which these new developments meet the needs of students, investigators, and clinicians in the field. After all, the success of *Hematology of Infancy and Childhood* and *Oncology of Infancy and Childhood* cannot be measured in numbers of pages or volumes sold. We will be pleased only if these textbooks provide students, fellows, and faculty with the knowledge and inspiration to move the frontier of pediatric hematology and oncology forward and reduce the burden of disease on children.

This seventh edition of *Hematology of Infancy and Childhood* has truly been a team effort. I thank the other editors for their dedication to this project. We are grateful to the authors of each chapter for their contributions. Our efforts, however, would be futile if it were not for the hard work, patience, and guidance of our editors at Elsevier, Dolores Meloni and Ann Ruzycka Anderson, and our managing editor, Cathy Lantigua. We appreciate everything they have done.

Finally, we want to express our deep gratitude to those who trained us in academic medicine. This is a glorious field that we have mightily enjoyed. In many ways, this book is our expression of appreciation to them.

Stuart H. Orkin, MD

Contents

Acronyms

A

A2, annexin 2
AABB, American Association of Blood Banks
AAE, acquired angioedema
AAV, adeno-associated virus
ABC, ATP-binding cassette transporter superfamily
ABO, ABO(H) blood group system
ABP, actin-binding protein
ACS, acute chest syndrome
ACE, angiotensin-converting enzyme
ACTH, adrenocorticotropic hormone, adrenocorticotropin
AD, anauxetic dysplasia, autosomal dominant
ADA, adenosine deaminase
ADAD, ADA deficiency
ADC, apparent diffusion coefficient
ADCC, antibody-dependent cellular toxicity
AdoCbl, adenosylcobalamin, 5′-deoxyadenosylcobalamin
AdoHcy, *S*-adenosylhomocysteine
AdoMet, *S*-adenosylmethionine
ADP, adenosine diphosphate, ALA-D deficiency porphyria
ADPase, adenosine diphosphatase
AE1, anion exchange protein 1 (band 3 protein of the red cell membrane)
AFP, α-fetoprotein
AGLT, acidified glycerol lysis test
AGM, aorta-gonad-mesonephros
aGVHD, acute graft-versus-host disease
AHA, acute hemolytic anemia
AHSP, α-hemoglobin–stabilizing protein
AICAR, amino-4-imidazolecarboxamide ribonucleotide
AICD, activation-induced cell death
AID, activation-induced cytidine deaminase, activation-induced deaminase
AIDS, acquired immunodeficiency virus
AIHA, autoimmune hemolytic anemia
AIN, autoimmune neutropenia
AIP, acute intermittent porphyria
AIRE, autoimmune regulator
AK, adenylate kinase
ALA, δ-aminolevulinic acid
ALA-D, δ-aminolevulinic acid dehydratase
ALA-S, δ-aminolevulinic acid synthase
ALD, adrenoleukodystrophy
ALG, antilymphocyte globulin
ALL, acute lymphoblastic leukemia, acute lymphocytic leukemia
ALPS, autoimmune lymphoproliferative syndrome

AMKL, acute megakaryoblastic leukemia
AML, acute myelogenous leukemia, acute myeloid leukemia
AMT, amegakaryocytic thrombocytopenia
ANC, absolute neutrophil count
ANCA, antineutrophil cytoplasmic antibody
α₂-AP, α_2-antiplasmin
APA, antiphospholipid antibody
APC, activated protein C, adenomatous polyposis coli, antigen-presenting cell
APECED, autoimmune polyendocrinopathy–candidiasis–ectodermal dystrophy
APRCA, acquired pure red cell aplasia
APRIL, α-proliferation–inducing ligand
APS-1, autoimmune polyglandular syndrome type 1
APTT, activated partial thromboplastin time
AQP1, aquaporin-1
AR, autosomal recessive
Ara-C, cytosine arabinoside
ARSB, arylsulfatase B
ARTUS, amegakaryocytic thrombocytopenia with radioulnar synostosis
ASBMT, American Society for Blood and Marrow transplantation
ASCO, American Society of Clinical Oncology
ASH, American Society of Hematology
ASM, acid sphingomyelinase
AT, antithrombin, ataxia-telangiectasia
ATG, antithymocyte globulin
ATIII, antithrombin III
ATP, adenosine triphosphate
ATPase, adenosine triphosphatase
ATRUS, amegakaryocytic thrombocytopenia with radioulnar synostosis
AVN, avascular necrosis
AVWS, acquired von Willebrand's syndrome

B

BACT, BCNU (carmustine), Ara-C (cytarabine), cyclophosphamide, 6-thioguanine
BAEP, brainstem auditory evoked potential
BAFF, B-cell–activating factor
BAL, bronchoalveolar lavage
BCAM, basal cell adhesion molecule
BCG, bacille Calmette-Guérin
BCNU, carmustine
BCR, B-cell receptor
BEAM, BCNU (carmustine), etoposide, Ara-C (cytarabine), melphalan
BFU-E, burst-forming unit–erythrocyte
BFU-Meg, burst-forming unit–megakaryocyte
bHLH, basic helix-loop-helix

BLNK, B-cell linker protein
BM, bone marrow
BMD, bone mineral density
BMF, bone marrow failure
BMP, bone morphogenetic protein
BMT, bone marrow transplantation
BPGM, 2,3-bisphosphoglycerate mutase
BPI, bactericidal/permeability-increasing protein
BrdU, bromodeoxyuridine
BrOb, bronchiolitis obliterans
BSP, bromsulfophthalein
BSS, Bernard-Soulier syndrome
BT, bleeding time
Btk, Bruton's tyrosine kinase
BU, Bethesda units, busulfan
BUGT, bilirubin UDP-glucuronyltransferase
bZIP, basic region–leucine zipper domain

C

CADP, collagen/adenosine diphosphate
CAFC, cobblestone area–forming cell
CAIV, carbonic anhydrase IV
CaM, calmodulin
cAMP, cyclic adenosine monophosphate
CAMT, congenital amegakaryocytic thrombocytopenia
CAR, Central African Republic
CAT, calibrated automated thrombography
CBB, cord blood bank
C4bBP, C4b-binding protein
CBF, core-binding factor
CBP, cyclophosphamide, BCNU (carmustine), cisplatin
CBV, cyclophosphamide, BCNU (carmustine), VP-16 (etoposide)
CCG, Children's Cancer Study Group
CCI, corrected count increment
CDA, congenital dyserythropoietic anemia
CDP, CCAAT displacement protein, cytidine diphosphate
CDR3, complementarity-determining region 3
C/EBPα, CCAAT/enhancer-binding protein α
CEP, congenital erythropoietic porphyria
CEPI, collagen/epinephrine
CFC, colony-forming cell
CFC-Eo, eosinophil colony-forming cell
CFU-C, colony-forming unit in culture
CFU-E, colony-forming unit–erythrocyte
CFU-Eo, colony-forming unit–eosinophil
CFU-GEMM, colony-forming unit–multipotent (granulocyte, erythrocyte, macrophage, megakaryocyte)
CFU-GM, colony-forming unit–granulocyte-macrophage
CFU-Meg, colony-forming unit–megakaryocyte
CFU-S, colony-forming unit–spleen
CGD, chronic granulomatous disease
cGMP, current good manufacturing practice, cyclic guanosine monophosphate

CGP, circulatory granulocyte pool
cGVHD, chronic graft-versus-disease
CH, calponin homology domain
CHH, cartilage-hair hypoplasia
CHO, Chinese hamster ovary
CHr, reticulocyte hemoglobin content
CHS, Chédiak-Higashi syndrome
CIITA, class II *trans*-activator
C1-INH, C1 esterase inhibitor
CIS, cytokine-inducible SH2-containing protein
CLC, Charcot-Leyden crystal
CLIA, Clinical Laboratory Improvement Amendment
CLL, chronic lymphocytic leukemia
CLN-1, neuronal ceroid lipofuscinosis type 1
CLP, common lymphoid progenitor
CMC, chronic mucocutaneous candidiasis
CML, chronic myelocytic leukemia
cMOAT, canalicular multispecific organic anion transporter
CMP, common myeloid progenitor, cytidine monophosphate
CMV, cytomegalovirus
CN, Crigler-Najjar syndrome, type I (CNI) or type II (CNII)
CNCbl, cyanocobalamin
CNS, central nervous system
CNSHA, congenital nonspherocytic hemolytic anemia
CNTF, ciliary neurotrophic factor
CO, carbon monoxide
CoA, coenzyme A
COG, Children's Oncology Group
COX-2, cyclooxygenase-2
CPD, citrate-phosphate-dextrose
CPDA-1, citrate-phosphate-dextrose-adenosine
CPO, coproporphyrinogen oxidase
CR, complete remission
CR2, complement receptor 2
CRAC, calcium release–activated calcium
CREG, cross-reactive group
CRF, chronic renal failure
CRIg, complement receptor of the immunoglobulin superfamily
CRM, cross-reacting material
CRT, catheter-related thrombosis
CSF, cerebrospinal fluid, colony-stimulating factor
c-SMAC, central supramolecular activation cluster
CSSCD, Cooperative Study of Sickle Cell Disease
CSVT, cerebral sinovenous thrombosis
CT, closure time, computed tomography
CT-1, cardiotropin-1
CTD, C-terminal domain
CTLA-4, cytotoxic T-lymphocyte antigen 4
CTP, cytidine triphosphate
CVID, common variable immunodeficiency
CVS, chorionic villus sampling
CXCR4, CXC chemokine receptor 4
CY, cyclophosphamide

D

DAF, decay accelerating factor
DAG, diacylglycerol
DAT, direct antibody test, direct antiglobulin test
dATP, deoxyadenosine triphosphatase
DBA, Diamond-Blackfan anemia
DC, dyskeratosis congenita
DCE, downstream core element
DCLRE1C, DNA cross-link repair enzyme 1C
DDAVP, 1-deamino-8-D-arginine vasopressin
DEB, diepoxybutane
DFS, disease-free survival
DGS, DiGeorge's syndrome
dGTP, deoxyguanosine triphosphatase
DHAP, dihydroxyacetone phosphate
DHF, dengue hemorrhagic fever, 7,8-dihydrofolate
DHR 123, dihydroxyrhodamine 123
DIC, disseminated intravascular coagulation
DIDMOAD, diabetes insipidus, diabetes mellitus, optic atrophy, and deafness
DIDS, 4,4′-diisothiocyanostilbene-2,2′-disulfonate (anion channel inhibitor)
DJS, Dubin-Johnson syndrome
DLI, donor lymphocyte infusion
DMS, demarcation membrane system
DMSO, dimethyl sulfoxide
DMT1, divalent metal transporter 1
2,3-DPG, 2,3-diphosphoglycerate
DPT, diphtheria and tetanus toxoids and pertussis
DRESS, drug rash with eosinophilia and systemic symptoms (syndrome)
dRTA, distal renal tubular acidosis
DRVVT, dilute Russell viper venom time
DS, Down syndrome
DS-AMKL, Down syndrome–acute megakaryoblastic leukemia
DSS, dengue shock syndrome
DS-TMD, Down syndrome–transient myeloproliferative disorder
DTB, ditaurobilirubin
dTMP, thymidylate (deoxythymidine monophosphate)
DTS, dense tubular system
DVT, deep venous thrombosis
DWI, diffusion-weighted magnetic resonance (MR) imaging

E

EA, early antigen
EBA140, *Plasmodium falciparum* erythrocyte binding antigen 140
EBMT, European Group for Blood and Marrow Transplantation
EBP, elastin-binding protein
EBV, Epstein-Barr virus
EC, Enzyme Commission
ECLT, euglobulin clot lysis time
ECMO, extracorporeal membrane oxygenation

EDA-ID, anhidrotic ectodermal dysplasia with immunodeficiency
EDAMS, encephaloduroarteriomyosynangiosis
EDTA, ethylenediaminetetraacetic acid
EFS, event-free survival
EGA, estimated gestational age
EGF, epidermal growth factor
EGFR, epidermal growth factor receptor
EHEC, enterohemorrhagic *Escherichia coli*
EKLF, erythroid Krüppel-like factor
EM, extramedullary
eNOS, endothelial nitric oxide synthase
EPCR, endothelial cell protein C receptor
EPEC, enteropathogenic *Escherichia coli*
EPO, erythropoietin
EpoR, erythropoietin receptor
EPP, erythropoietic protoporphyria
ER, endoplasmic reticulum
ERGIC-53, endoplasmic reticulum–Golgi intermediate compartment, 53 kilodalton protein
ERT, enzyme replacement therapy
ES, embryonic stem
ESC, embryonic stem cell
ESL-1, E-selectin ligand-1

F

FA, Fanconi's anemia
FAAP, Fanconi's anemia–associated protein
FAB, French-American-British (staging)
FACS, fluorescence-activated cell sorting
FACT, Foundation for the Accreditation of Cell Therapy
FAD, flavin adenine dinucleotide
FAH, fumarylacetoacetate hydrolase
FAICAR, formamido-4-imidazolecarboxamide ribonucleotide
FBN, fibronectin
FCP, F-cell production (locus)
FcR, Fc receptor
FDA, Food and Drug Administration
FDC, follicular dendritic cell
FDP, familial platelet deficiency, fibrin(ogen) degradation product, fructose 6-diphosphate
FECH, ferrochelatase
FEIBA, factor eight inhibitor–bypassing activity
Fe-SIH, ferric salicylaldehyde-isonicotinyl-hydrazone
FFP, fresh frozen plasma
FGAR, formylglycinamide ribonucleotide
FGF, fibroblast growth factor
fH, factor H
fI, factor I
FIGlu, formiminoglutamic acid
FISH, fluorescence in situ hybridization
FL, ligand for the Flks/Flt3 receptor
FLAER, fluorescent aerolysin
FLAIR, fluid-attenuated inversion recovery
FOG-1, friend of GATA-1
FPA, fibrinopeptide A

FPB, fibrinopeptide A
F-PCT, familial porphyria cutanea tarda
FRAP, fluorescence recovery after photobleaching
FSGS, focal sclerosing glomerulosclerosis
FTCD, formiminotransferase-cyclodeaminase
5-FU, 5-fluorouracil

G

GABA, γ-aminobutyric acid
GAG, glycosaminoglycan
β-gal, β-D-galactosidase
GalNAc-T, N-acetylgalactosaminyltransferase
GALNS, N-acetylgalactosamine-6-sulfatase
GAP, GTPase-activating protein
GAR, glycinamide ribonucleotide
GAS, IFN-γ–activated sequence
GAT, granulocyte agglutination test
GBS, Guillain-Barré syndrome
GC, germinal center
G-CSF, granulocyte colony-stimulating factor
G-CSFR, granulocyte colony-stimulating factor receptor
GDF, growth and differentiation factor
GDP, guanosine diphosphate
GFR, glomerular filtration rate
GH, growth hormone
GI, gastrointestinal
GIF, gastric intrinsic factor
GIFT, granulocyte immunofluorescence test
GITMO, Gruppo Italiano Trapianti di Midollo Osseo
GlcNAc, N-acetylglucosamine
Glu-Plg, glutamic acid plasminogen
GluR1, glutamate receptor type 1
G$_{M2}$A, G$_{M2}$ activator protein
GM-CSF, granulocyte-macrophage colony-stimulating factor
GMP, granulocyte/monocyte precursor, guanosine monophosphate
GNPT, UDP-N-acetylglucosamine:lysosomal-enzyme N-acetylglucosamine-1-phosphotransferase
GnRH, gonadotropin-releasing hormone
GPA, glycophorin A
GPB, glycophorin B
GPC, glycophorin C
GPCR, G protein–coupled receptor
GPD, glycophorin D
G3PD, glyceraldehyde-3-phosphate dehydrogenase
G6PD, glucose-6-phosphate dehydrogenase
GPE, glycophorin E
GPI, glucose phosphate isomerase, glycosylphosphatidylinositol
GPIb, glycoprotein Ib
GPS, gray platelet syndrome
GRF, guanine nucleotide–releasing factor
GS, Gilbert's syndrome, Griscelli's syndrome
GSCbl, glutathionylcobalamin
GSH, reduced glutathione

GSK3, glycogen synthase kinase 3
GSL, glycosphingolipid
GSSG, oxidized glutathione
GSHPX, glutathione peroxidase
GST, glutathione-S-transferase
GT, Glanzmann's thrombasthenia
GTP, guanosine triphosphate
GTPase, guanosine triphosphatase
GVHD, graft-versus-host disease
GVL, graft versus leukemia

H

HAART, highly active antiretroviral therapy
HABA, 2(4′-hydroxyazobenzene) benzoic acid
HAE, hereditary angioedema
Hb, hemoglobin
HB, Heinz body
HbF, fetal hemoglobin
HBV, hepatitis B virus
HC, homocysteine
4-HC, 4-hydroperoxycyclophosphamide
HCP, hereditary coproporphyria, hematopoietic cell phosphatase
HCV, hepatitis C virus
HD, Hodgkin's disease
HDN, hemolytic disease of the fetus and newborn, hemorrhagic disease of the newborn
HDW, hemoglobin distribution width
HE, hereditary elliptocytosis
HELLP, hemolytic anemia, elevated liver enzymes, low platelet count
HEMPAS, hereditary erythroblastic multinuclearity with a positive acidified serum lysis test
HEP, hepatoerythropoietic porphyria
HES, Hairy and Enhancer of Split, hypereosinophilic syndrome
HETE, 15(S)-hydroxyeicosatetraenoic acid
Hex-A, hexosaminidase A
Hex-B, hexosaminidase B
HGF, hematopoietic growth factor, hepatocyte growth factor
HGFR, hematopoietic growth factor receptor
HHS, Hoyeraal-Hreidarsson syndrome
HHV-6, human herpesvirus 6
HiB, *H. influenzae* type B
HIDA, hepatobiliary iminodiacetic acid
HIES, hyper-IgE syndrome, hyperimmunoglobulin E syndrome
HIF-1, hypoxia-inducible factor 1
HIT, heparin-induced thrombocytopenia
HITTS, HIT with thrombosis syndrome
HIV, human immunodeficiency virus
HK, hexokinase
HLA, human leukocyte antigen
HLH, hemophagocytic lymphohistiocytosis
HMB, hydroxymethylbilane
HMGB1, high–molecular group box 1 protein
HMP, hexose monophosphate

HMS, hyperreactive malarial splenomegaly
HMWK, high-molecular-weight kininogen
HNE, hydroxynonenal
hnRNA, heterogeneous nuclear RNA
HO, heme oxygenase
H$_2$O$_2$, hydrogen peroxide
H$_2$OCbl, aquocobalamin
holo-HC, holohaptocorrin
holo-TC, holotranscobalamin
HOX, homeobox transcription factor
HPA-1a, human platelet antigen 1a
HPC, hematopoietic progenitor cell
HPCHA, high-phosphatidylcholine hemolytic anemia
HPFH, hereditary persistence of fetal hemoglobin
HPLC, high-performance liquid chromatography, high-pressure liquid chromatography
HPP, hereditary pyropoikilocytosis
HPP-CFCs, high–proliferative potential colony-forming cells
HPRT, hypoxanthine phosphoribosyltransferase
HPS, Hermansky-Pudlak syndrome
HPV, human papillomavirus
HR, homologous recombination
HRE, hypoxia response element
HRI, heme-regulated inhibitor kinase
HRM, heme regulatory motif
HS, hereditary spherocytosis, hypersensitivity site
HSC, hematopoietic stem cell
HSCT, hematopoietic stem cell transplantation
HSP, heat shock protein, Henoch-Schönlein purpura
5-HT, 5′-hydroxytryptamine (serotonin)
HTLV, human T-cell leukemia/lymphoma virus, human T-cell lymphotropic virus
HUS, hemolytic-uremic syndrome
HUVEC, human umbilical vein endothelial cell

I

IAP, integrin-associated protein or CD47
IAS, ischemic arterial stroke
IBMFS, inherited bone marrow failure syndrome
IBMTR, International Bone Marrow Transplant Registry
ICAM, intercellular adhesion molecule
ICD-9, International Classification of Diseases, 9th revision
ICG, indocyanine green
ICH, intracranial hemorrhage
ICN, intracellular domain of Notch
ICOS, inducible costimulator, inducible T-cell costimulator
ICOSL, inducible costimulator ligand
IDO, indolamine 2,3-dioxygenase
IDS, iduronate 2-sulfatase
IDUA, α-L-iduronidase
IFAR, International Fanconi Anemia Registry
IFN-γ, interferon-γ
IGAD, IgA deficiency

IGF-I, insulin-like growth factor I
IgG, immunoglobulin G
IκB, inhibitor of NF-κB
IKK, IκB kinase
IL-1RA, IL-1 receptor antagonist
IL-2, interleukin-2
IL-6R, interleukin-6 receptor
IMP, inosine 5′-monophosphate, intramembrane particle
iNOS, inducible nitric oxide synthase
INR, international normalized ratio
IP, isoprostenoid
IP$_3$, inositol 1,4,5-triphosphate
IPEX, immune dysregulation, polyendocrinopathy, enteropathy, X-linked (syndrome)
IPH, idiopathic pulmonary hemosiderosis
IPT, intraperitoneal fetal transfusion
IRAG, IP$_3$ receptor–associated cGMP
IRAK-4, interleukin-1 receptor–associated kinase 4
IRE, iron response element, iron responsive element
IRF, interferon regulatory factor
IRIDA, iron-refractory iron deficiency anemia
IRP, IRE-binding protein, iron regulatory protein
ISBT, International Society for Blood Transfusion
ISC, irreversibly sickled cell
ISHAGE, International Society for Hematotherapy and Graft Engineering
ISI, International Sensitivity Index
ISP, intermediate single positive
ISRE, interferon-stimulated response element
IST, immunosuppressive therapy
ISTH, International Society on Thrombosis and Hemostasis
ITAM, immunoreceptor tyrosine–based activation motif, immunoreceptor tyrosine activation motif
ITIM, immunoreceptor tyrosine–based inhibitory motif, immunoreceptor tyrosine activation motif
ITP, immune thrombocytopenia purpura
IVIG, intravenous immune serum globulin, intravenous immunoglobulin
IVS, intervening sequence (intron)
IVT, intravascular transfusion

J

JAK, Janus kinase
JAM-1, junctional adhesion molecule 1
JMML, juvenile myelomonocytic leukemia

K

KCC, K$^+$-Cl$^-$ cotransporter
K_d, dissociation constant
KD, Kostmann's disease, kyphomelic dysplasia
KEYY, lysine–glutamic acid–tyrosine-tyrosine
KIR, killer cell immunoglobulin-like receptor
KL, Klotho (gene)
K_m, Michaelis constant
KTLS, c-Kit$^+$, Thy-1^{lo}, Lin$^-$, Sca-1$^+$ cell
KSS, Kearns-Sayre syndrome

L

LA, lupus anticoagulant

LAD I, leukocyte adhesion deficiency (type I)

LAMP-3, lysosome-associated membrane protein 3

LAT, linker for activation of T cells

LCAT, lecithin-cholesterol acyltransferase

LCL, large cell lymphoma

LCR, locus control region

LDH, lactate dehydrogenase

LDL, low-density lipoprotein

LEF-1, lymphoid enhancer–binding factor 1

LELY, low-expression allele Lyon

LEPRA, low-expression allele Prague

LFA-3, lymphocyte function antigen 3

LGL, large granular lymphocyte leukemia

LHRF, luteinizing hormone–releasing factor

LIF, leukemia inhibitory factor

LIFR, leukemia inhibitory factor receptor

LIR, leukocyte immunoglobulin-like receptor

LJP, localized juvenile periodontitis

LMWH, low-molecular-weight heparin

LMWK, low-molecular-weight kininogen

LPS, lipopolysaccharide

LRP, lipoprotein receptor–related protein

LRRC8, leucine-rich repeat–containing 8

LSD, lysosomal storage disease

LSP1, lymphocyte-specific protein 1

LTB$_4$, leukotriene B$_4$

LTC-IC, long-term culture–initiating cell

LTR-HSCs, long-term–reconstituting hematopoietic stem cells

LW, Landsteiner-Weiner glycoprotein

Lyso-PC, lysophosphatidylcholine

Lys-Plg, lysine plasminogen

LYST, lysosomal trafficking regulator

M

MAGUK, membrane-associated guanylate kinase

MAP, mitogen-activated protein

MAPK, mitogen-activated protein kinase

MARCKS, myristoylated alanine-rich C kinase substrate

MASP, MBL-associated serine protease

MBD, membrane binding domain

MBL, mannose-binding lectin

MBP, major basic protein

MCH, mean corpuscular hemoglobin

MCHC, mean corpuscular hemoglobin concentration

MCP, membrane cofactor protein

MCP-1, monocyte chemotactic protein 1

MCV, mean cell volume, mean corpuscular volume

MCV4, meningococcal conjugate vaccine

MDCK, Madin-Darby canine kidney (cells)

MDS, myelodysplastic syndrome

MDWH, metaphyseal dysplasia without hypotrichosis

MeCbl, methylcobalamin

MEK, MAPK kinase

MELAS, mitochondrial myopathy, encephalopathy, lactic acidosis, and stroke-like episodes

MEP, megakaryocyte, erythroid, and basophil (lineage); megakaryocyte/erythroid precursor

Met-Hb, methemoglobin

5-methyl-THF, 5-methyltetrahydrofolate

α$_2$-MG, α$_2$-macroglobulin

MGF, myelomonocytic growth factor

MGP, marginating granulocyte pool

MGSA, melanoma growth stimulatory activity

mHA, minor histocompatibility antigen

MHA, May-Hegglin anomaly

MHC, major histocompatibility complex

MIBG, metaiodobenzylguanidine

micro-PET, micro–positron emission tomography

MIDAS, metal ion–dependent adhesion site

MIM, Mendelian Inheritance in Man

MIP-1α, macrophage inflammatory protein 1α

MLASA, mitochondrial myopathy with lactic acidosis and sideroblastic anemia

MLL, mixed-lineage leukemia

MMC, mitomycin C

MMF, mycophenolate mofetil

MMP-25, the membrane-associated metalloproteinase leukolysin

MoAb, monoclonal antibody

M6P, mannose 6-phosphate

MPGM, monophosphoglycerate mutase

Mpl, ligand for the myeloproliferative ligand receptor

MPO, myeloperoxidase

MPS, Montreal platelet syndrome, mucopolysaccharidosis

MPSV4, meningococcal polysaccharide vaccine

MPV, mean platelet volume

M$_r$, molecular weight

MRA, magnetic resonance angiography

MRI, magnetic resonance imaging

MRC, Medical Research Council

mRNP, messenger ribonucleoprotein

MRP2, multidrug resistance–associated protein 2 (a.k.a. ABCC2, cMOAT)

MSCV, murine stem cell virus

MSMD, mendelian susceptibility to mycobacterial diseases

MSP1, *Plasmodium falciparum* merozoite surface protein 1

MTD, maximum tolerated dose

mtDNA, mitochondrial DNA

mTEC, medullary thymic epithelial cell

MTHFR, methylenetetrahydrofolate reductase, methylene-THF reductase

mTOR, mammalian target of rapamycin

MTP, microsomal triglyceride transfer protein

MVB, multivesicular body

MWC, Monod, Wyman, and Changeaux (model of cooperativity)

MYHIIA, myosin heavy chain IIA

N

NAD, nicotinamide adenine dinucleotide

NAD 47/89, neutrophil actin dysfunction with 47- and 89-kd protein abnormalities

NADH, reduced nicotinamide adenine dinucleotide

NADP, nicotinamide adenine dinucleotide phosphate

NADPH, reduced nicotinamide adenine dinucleotide phosphate

NAIT, neonatal alloimmune thrombocytopenia

NAT, nucleic acid testing

NATP, neonatal alloimmune thrombocytopenic purpura

NB-DGJ, *N*-butyldeoxygalactonojirimycin

NBS, Nijmegen's breakage syndrome

NBT, nitroblue tetrazolium

NDPase, nucleoside diphosphatase

NE, neutrophil elastase

NEMO, NF-κB essential modulator

NET, neutrophil extracellular trap

NF-1, neurofibromatosis type 1

NF-AT, nuclear factor of activated T cells

NF-κB, nuclear factor κB

NGAL, neutrophil gelatinase–associated lipocalin

NH, neonatal hemochromatosis

NHANES, National Health and Nutrition Examination Survey

NHEJ, nonhomologous end joining

NHL, non-Hodgkin's lymphoma

NHLBI, National Heart, Lung, and Blood Institute

NICU, neonatal intensive care unit

NIH, National Institutes of Health

NK, natural killer (cell)

NMDP, National Marrow Donor Program

NMR, nuclear magnetic resonance

NNJ, neonatal jaundice

NPD-C, Niemann-Pick disease type C

Nrf-1, nuclear regulatory factor 1

NRTI, nucleoside reverse transcriptase inhibitors

NS, Noonan's syndrome

NTD, neural tube defect

NO, nitric oxide

NOD, nonobese diabetic

NOS, nitric oxide synthase

NOX, NAD(P)H oxidase

NSAID, nonsteroidal anti-inflammatory drug

NuMA, nuclear mitotic apparatus (protein)

O

OATP, organic acid–transporting polypeptide

OCA, oral contraceptive agent

OCS, open canalicular system

OF, osmotic fragility

OHCbl, hydroxycobalamin

OMIM, Online Mendelian Inheritance in Man

OPSI, overwhelming postsplenectomy infection

OS, Omenn's syndrome

OSM, oncostatin M

OSMR, oncostatin M receptor

P

PA, phosphatidic acid

PAF, platelet-activating factor

PAGE, polyacrylamide gel electrophoresis

PAI-1, plasminogen activator inhibitor 1

PAIgG, platelet-associated IgG

PALS, periarterial (or periarteriolar) lymphoid sheath

PAMP, pathogen-associated molecular pattern

PANDAS, pediatric autoimmune neuropsychiatric disorders associated with streptococcal infections

PAR, protease-activated receptor

PAS, periodic acid–Schiff

PBG, porphobilinogen

PBG-D, porphobilinogen deaminase

PBREM, phenobarbital-responsive enhancer module

PBSC, peripheral blood stem cell

PC, phosphatidylcholine

PCC, prothrombin complex concentrate

PCFT, proton-coupled folate transporter

PCH, paroxysmal cold hemoglobinuria

PCP, *Pneumocystis carinii* pneumonia

PCR, polymerase chain reaction

PCT, porphyria cutanea tarda

PCV, polycythemia vera

PCV7, 7-valent pneumococcal polysaccharide vaccine

PCV23, 23-valent pneumococcal polysaccharide vaccine

PD-1, programmed death 1

PDGF, platelet-derived growth factor

PE, phosphatidylethanolamine, pulmonary embolism

PEBP2, polyomavirus enhancer–binding protein 2

PECAM-1, platelet–endothelial cell adhesion molecule 1

PEG, polyethylene glycol

PEG-MGDF, pegylated megakaryocyte growth and development factor

PF4, platelet factor 4

PFA-100, Platelet Functional Analyzer 100

PFK, phosphofructokinase

PFT, pulmonary function test

PGC-1α, peroxisomal proliferator–activated cofactor 1α

PGD, preimplantation genetic diagnosis

6-PGD, 6-phosphogluconate dehydrogenase

PGI$_2$, prostaglandin I$_2$ (prostacyclin)

PGK, phosphoglycerate kinase

PH, Pleckstrin homology

PHA, phytohemagglutinin

PHT, primary hypertension

P$_i$, inorganic phosphate

PI, phosphatidylinositol

PIG-A, phosphatidylinositol glycan class A (gene: *PIGA*)

PI3K, phosphatidylinositol 3′-kinase

PIP, phosphatidylinositol 4-phosphate

PIP$_2$, phosphatidylinositol 4,5-bisphosphate

PIP$_3$, phosphatidylinositol 3,4,5-triphosphate

PIT, plasma iron turnover

PIVKA, protein induced by vitamin K antagonists

PK, pyruvate kinase

PKA, protein kinase A

PKB, protein kinase B

PKC, protein kinase C

PKG, protein kinase G

PKR, protein kinase regulated by RNA

PLCγ2, phospholipase Cγ2

PLP, pyridoxal 5-phosphate

PLTP, phospholipid transfer protein

PMN, polymorphonuclear neutrophil

PMPS, Pearson's marrow-pancreas syndrome

PN, parenteral nutrition

P-5′-N, pyrimidine-5′-nucleotidase

PN2/APP, protease nexin-2/amyloid β-protein precursor

PNET, primary neuroectodermal tumor

PNH, paroxysmal nocturnal hemoglobinuria

PNP, purine nucleoside phosphorylase

PNPD, purine nucleoside phosphorylase deficiency

PPCA, protective protein cathepsin A

PPO, protoporphyrinogen oxidase

PPP, platelet-poor plasma

PR, partial remission

PRCA, pure red cell aplasia

PROWESS, Protein C Worldwide Evaluation in Severe Sepsis (trial)

PRP, platelet-rich plasma

PRPP, 5-phosphoribosylpyrophosphate

PRR, pattern recognition receptor

PS, Pearson's marrow-pancreas syndrome, phosphatidylserine

PSD95, postsynaptic density protein of 95 kd

PSGL-1, P-selectin glycoprotein ligand-1

p-SMAC, peripheral central supramolecular activation cluster

PT, prothrombin time

PTH, parathyroid hormone

PTK, phosphotyrosine kinase

PTP, post-transfusion purpura

PTS, post-thrombotic syndrome

PTT, partial thromboplastin time

R

RA, refractory anemia

RAD, recombinase-activating gene

RAEB, refractory anemia with an excess of blasts

RAEBIT (RAEB-T), RAEB in transformation

RAG, recombination-activating gene

RANTES, regulated on activation, normal T cell expressed and secreted

RARS, refractory anemia with ringed sideroblasts

RBC, red blood cell

RDA, recommended dietary allowance

RDS, respiratory distress syndrome

RDW, red cell distribution width, red cell volume distribution width

RFC, reduced folate carrier

RFLP, restriction fragment length polymorphism

rFVIIa, recombinant activated factor VII

RGD, arginine, glycine, aspartic acid

Rh, rhesus

RhAG, Rh-associated glycoprotein

rhG-CSF, recombinant human granulocyte colony-stimulating factor

r-HuEPO, rhEPO, rHuEPO, recombinant human erythropoietin

RIAM, Rap1$_{GTP}$-interacting adaptor molecule

RMRP, RNase mitochondrial RNA processing

rNAPc2, recombinant nematode anticoagulant protein c2

RNP, ribonucleoprotein

RPA, replication protein A

RPL, ribosomal protein of the large ribosomal subunit

RPS, ribosomal protein of the small ribosomal subunit

RPS19, ribosomal protein S19

rRNA, ribosomal RNA

RS, Rotor's syndrome

RSC, reversibly sickled cell

RSP-2, ring surface protein 2

RTA, renal tubular acidosis

RTK, receptor tyrosine kinase

rVIIa, recombinant factor VIIa

RVT, renal vein thrombosis

S

SAA, severe aplastic anemia

SABD, spectrin-actin binding domain

SAGE, serial analysis of gene expression

SAO, Southeast Asian ovalocytosis

SAP, SLAM-associated protein

SBDS, Shwachman-Bodian-Diamond syndrome

Sca-1, stem cell antigen 1

SCD, sickle cell disease

SCDSC, subacute combined degeneration of the spinal cord

SCF, stem cell factor

SCID, severe combined immunodeficiency

SCN, severe congenital neutropenia

SCNIR, Severe Chronic Neutropenia International Registry

SCT, stem cell transplantation

SDF-1, stromal cell–derived factor 1

SDS, Shwachman-Diamond syndrome, sodium dodecyl sulfate

SDS-PAGE, sodium dodecyl sulfate–polyacrylamide gel electrophoresis

SERCA, sarcoplasmic/endoplasmic reticulum Ca^{2+}-ATPase

SGD, specific (secondary) granule deficiency

SH2, Src homology domain 2

SHD, sex hormone–binding domain

SH2D1A, SH2-containing protein 1A, Src homology 2 domain–containing protein

Shh, Sonic hedgehog

SHIP1, SH2 domain–containing inositol 5′-phosphatase 1

SHP-2, SH2 domain–containing protein tyrosine phosphatase-2

sIgM, surface IgM

SIV, simian immunodeficiency virus

SLAM, signaling lymphocyte activation molecule

SLC4A, solute carrier family 4A

SLE, systemic lupus erythematosus

SLP3, stomatin-like protein 3

SLP76, SH2 domain–containing leukocyte protein of 76 kd

SM, sphingomyelin

SMD, spondylometaphyseal dysplasia

Smo, Smoothened receptor

SNARE, soluble N-ethylmaleimide–sensitive attachment protein receptor

snoRNA, small nucleolar RNA

SNP, single nucleotide polymorphism

SOCbl, sulfitocobalamin

SOCS, suppressor of cytokine signaling

SOS, sinusoidal obstruction syndrome, son of sevenless (protein)

S-PCT, sporadic porphyria cutanea tarda

SPD, storage pool deficiency

sPLA2, secretory phospholipase A_2

SQUID, superconducting quantum interference device

SRC, SCID-reconstituting cell

SRT, substrate reduction therapy

SSCP, single-strand conformation polymorphism

SSP, stage-selector protein

STAT, signal transducer and activator of transcription

sTfR, serum transferrin receptor

STOP, Stroke Prevention Trial in Sickle Cell Anemia

STR-HSC, short-term–reconstituting hematopoietic stem cell

Stx, Shiga-like toxin

SUMF1, sulfatase-modifying factor

SVC, superior vena cava

T

TACI, transmembrane activator and calcium modulator and cyclophilin ligand interactor

TAFI, thrombin-activatable fibrinolysis inhibitor

T-ALL, T-cell acute lymphoblastic leukemia

T antigen, Thomsen-Friedenreich cryptoantigen

TAP1 or TAP2, transporter associated with antigen processing 1 or 2

TAR, thrombocytopenia with absent radii

TAT, thrombin-antithrombin complex

TBI, total body irradiation

TBP, TATA-binding protein

TCD, transcranial Doppler

TCDD, 2,3,7,8-tetrachlorodibenzo-p-dioxin

TCR, T-cell antigen receptor, T-cell receptor

TCT, thrombin clotting time

TD, thymus dependent (antigen)

TdT, terminal deoxyribonucleotidyl transferase

TE, thromboembolism

TEC, transient erythroblastopenia of childhood

TEG, thromboelastography

TERT, telomerase reverse transcriptase

TF, tissue factor

TFPI, tissue factor pathway inhibitor

TGA, thrombin generation assay

TGF-β, transforming growth factor β

THF, 5,6,7,8-tetrahydrofolate

THI, transient hypogammaglobulinemia of infancy

TI, thymus independent (antigen)

TIA, transient ischemic attack

TIBC, total iron-binding capacity

TIPS, intrahepatic portosystemic shunting

TKI, tyrosine kinase inhibitor

TLR2, Toll-like receptor 2

TLS, translesion synthesis

TLT-1, TREM cells–like transcript-1

TM, tropomyosin

TM8, transmembrane domain 8

TMD, transient myeloproliferative disorder

TOF, time-of-flight (imaging)

TMod, tropomodulin

7-TMS, seven-transmembrane–spanning domain

TNF-α, tumor necrosis factor-α

tPA, tissue plasminogen activator

TPH, transplacental hemorrhage

TPI, triose phosphate isomerase

TPN, total parenteral nutrition

TPO, thrombopoietin

TPOR, thrombopoietin receptor

TPR, tetratricopeptide repeat

TQM, total quality management

TRAF, TNF receptor–associated factor

TRALI, transfusion-related acute lung injury

TRAP, Trial to Reduce Alloimmunization to Platelets

TREC, T-cell receptor excision circle, T-cell receptor gene excision circle

TREM, triggering receptor expressed on myeloid cells

TfR, transferrin receptor

TRMA, thiamine-responsive megaloblastic anemia

tRNA, transfer RNA

TSB, total serum bilirubin

TSH, thyroid-stimulating hormone

TSLP, thymic stromal thymopoietin

TT, thrombin time

TTP, thrombotic thrombocytopenic purpura

TTTS, twin-to-twin transfusion syndrome

TXA₂, thromboxane A_2

U

UCB, umbilical cord blood

UDP, uridine diphosphate

UDPG, uridine diphosphate glucose

UDPGA, uridine diphosphate glucuronic acid

UDPNAG, uridine diphosphate N-acetylglucosamine

UGT1A1, UDP glucuronosyltransferase 1A1 gene

ULVWF, unusually large VWF

UMP, uridine monophosphate
UNG, uracil nucleoside glycosylase
uPA, urokinase plasminogen activator
uPAR, uPA receptor
UPR, unfolded protein response
URO-D, uroporphyrinogen decarboxylase
URO3-S, uroporphyrinogen III synthase
UTP, uridine triphosphate
UV, ultraviolet

V

VACTERL, vertebral abnormalities, anal atresia, cardiac abnormalities, tracheoesophageal fistula, and/or esophageal atresia, renal agenesis and dysplasia, and limb defects
VASP, vasodilator-stimulated phosphoprotein
VATER, vertebral defects, imperforate anus, tracheoesophageal fistula, and radial and renal dysplasia
VCA, viral capsid antigen
VCAM-1, vascular cell adhesion molecule 1
VDRL, Venereal Disease Research Laboratory
VEGF, vascular endothelial growth factor
VHL, von Hippel-Lindau (protein)
VK, vitamin K
VK1, phylloquinone
VK2, menaquinone
VKDB, vitamin K–dependent bleeding
VKDP, vitamin K–dependent protein
VKOR, vitamin K 2,3-epoxide reductase
VLA-4, very late antigen 4
VLDL, very-low-density lipoproteins
VOD, veno-occlusive disease
VP, variegate porphyria
VP-16, etoposide
VTE, venous thromboembolism
V/Q, ventilation-perfusion

VWD, von Willebrand disease
VWF, von Willebrand factor
VWF:Ag, von Willebrand factor antigen
VWF:CB, collagen-binding assay for von Willebrand factor
VWFpp, von Willebrand factor propeptide
VWF:RCo, VWF activity by ristocetin cofactor assay

W

WAS, Wiskott-Aldrich syndrome
WASP, Wiskott-Aldrich syndrome protein
WBC, white blood cell
WHIM, warts, hypogammaglobulinemia, infections, myelokathexis (syndrome)
WIP, WASP-interacting protein
WNV, West Nile virus
WRK, Woodward's reagent K
WSXWS, Trp-Ser-Xaa-Trp-Ser

X

X-CGD, X-linked chronic granulomatous disease
XHIM, X-linked immunodeficiency with normal or elevated IgM
XLA, X-linked agammaglobulinemia
XLPD, X-linked lymphoproliferative disease
XLSA, X-linked sideroblastic anemia
XLSA/A, X-linked sideroblastic anemia with ataxia
XPD, xeroderma pigmentosum disease
XRT, x-ray therapy
XSCID, X-linked severe combined immunodeficiency

Y

YTRF, tyrosine-threonine-arginine-phenylalanine (sequence)

Z

ZAP-70, TCR{zeta}–associated protein of 70 kd
ZPI, protein Z–dependent protease inhibitor

I History

Pediatric Hematology in Historical Perspective

1 Pediatric Hematology in Historical Perspective

Wolf W. Zuelzer and David G. Nathan

Wolf W. Zuelzer, who died on March 19, 1987, at the age of 77, wrote the history of pediatric hematology for the first edition of this book. We reprint it here in his memory.

As a subspecialty of pediatrics and a sine qua non of the modern teaching institution, pediatric hematology is a latecomer, naturally enough, for diseases of the blood were a minor problem—one is tempted to say a mere hobby of a few inquisitive and farseeing minds—compared with the great challenges of infectious and nutritional disorders that faced the pioneers of pediatrics. As a serious concern of investigators, however, pediatric hematology is as old as scientific pediatrics as a whole, though its early history is too closely interwoven with that of general hematology to be traced separately. Its tools as well as its basic concepts came largely from internal medicine and from the experimental sciences, and one needs only to mention such names as Ehrlich, Metchnikoff, Landsteiner, Chauffard, Downey, Minot, Castle, Whipple, and Wintrobe to appreciate the magnitude of this debt.

The discoveries of these and many other men were applied to the special problems of infancy and childhood by investigators who, with few exceptions, were pediatricians with diverse interests rather than hematologists with a specialized background. This is true even of those whose names are familiar through eponymic usage, such as von Jaksch, Lederer, Cooley, Blackfan, and Fanconi. Those who labored patiently in the vineyards without stumbling on a buried syndrome are mostly forgotten, though it is among them that one finds the first true pediatric hematologists. A case in point is that of Heinrich Lehndorff, who grew up in the Vienna of von Pirquet and Escherich and devoted his life to the study of both normal and abnormal hematologic conditions in childhood, publishing his first paper at the age of 29 in 1906 and his last at

the age of 86 in 1963. His interest was in the blood of the newborn, in the anemias of infancy, and in leukemia. Like that of most of his contemporaries, his work was almost entirely descriptive, but he was a good morphologist and clinical observer. Lehndorff was forced to leave Vienna in 1939 at the age of 63, found temporary shelter in Birmingham with Leonard Parsons (then the leading figure in pediatric hematology in England), came to the United States during World War II, and ended his career as an octogenarian with an honorary appointment at the New York Medical College. *Sic transit gloria mundi.*

From the very beginning, the unique blood picture of the newborn received special attention. In one of the oldest hematologic texts, *Du Sang et de ses Altérations Anatomiques*, published in Paris in 1889, Hayem—known to this day as the inventor of Hayem's solution but deserving to be remembered for more important contributions—discussed the blood at birth in great detail, giving the number of red and white corpuscles and platelets on the basis of his own counts; describing macrocytosis, anisocytosis, and a tendency toward spherocytosis; and attributing the high hemoglobin level of the newborn to hyperactivity of the bone marrow. The title of a paper by E. Schiff in the *Jahrbuch für Kinderheilkunde* in 1892, "Newer contributions to the hematology of the neonate, with special reference to the time of ligation of the umbilical cord," implies the existence of earlier studies and anticipates those of Windle and his associates some 50 years later.

The hematology of the neonate remained a cardinal concern of investigators for many decades. Progress was slow, perhaps in part because of the tediousness of the methods used and in part because of variables in obstetric and pediatric practice and differences in the timing of observations. Schiff himself, working successively in Prague and Budapest, found hemoglobin levels on the first day after birth to average 104 per cent in one city and 144 per cent in the other. Much controversy arose over normal values because the early workers did not come to grips with the problems of individual variation and frequency distribution. A German author, H. Flesch,[1] wrote despairingly in 1909, "The differences in the hemoglobin values of different observers according to the ages of the children are so considerable that one is really in no position to give definite normal figures." It was difficult, moreover, to draw a line between normal and abnormal conditions. ABO hemolytic disease, for example, was unknown until 1944, when Halbrecht[2] in Hadera recognized the relationship between "icterus praecox" and incompatibility of the major blood groups of mother and child. Prior to the studies of Lippman[3] in 1924, on the other hand, the transient normoblastemia of normal full-term infants was considered pathologic, although Neumann[4] had observed it in 1871 and König[5] had written about it in 1910. Supravital staining, introduced by Ehrlich in 1880, was not used until 1925, when Friedländer and Wiedemer,[6] writing in the *American Journal of Diseases of Children*—then the only major pediatric journal in the United States—reported reticulocytosis as a regular feature of neonatal blood. Although it was known by then that reticulocytes were young cell forms, the belief still prevailed that the high hemoglobin level at birth was due solely to hemoconcentration rather than to active erythropoiesis, as postulated by Hayem.

Conversely, the postnatal drop in hemoglobin concentration was taken as evidence of accelerated hemolysis, which in turn was held by some to be the cause of physiologic jaundice. That puzzling phenomenon was long thought to signify the entry of bile into the blood as a result of temporary mechanical obstruction by a mucous plug in the common bile duct or a "desquamative catarrh" of the small radicles, or liver damage from bacterial toxins from the recently colonized intestine of the newborn. The noted Finnish neonatologist Ylppö,[7] however, had demonstrated increased bilirubin levels in the cord blood as early as 1913 and had concluded that icterus neonatorum was due to a "functional inferiority" of the liver. All theories involving the regurgitation of bile became untenable in 1922, when Erwin Schiff and E. Färber,[8] pupils of the renowned Adalbert Czerny, showed that "during the period of bilirubinemia only the indirect van den Bergh reaction is positive." The alternative that the jaundice was due to increased blood destruction, however, could not be proved. Summarizing the argument in 1928, the Viennese pediatric hematologist Eugene Stransky[9] wrote, "Although the morphologic stigmata of a hemolytic icterus (i.e., spherocytosis) are lacking and the red blood counts do not permit a firm explanation, a hematogenous origin of icterus neonatorum nevertheless seems likely. Why destruction of red corpuscles takes place is still an unsolved question."

One must sympathize with these early investigators who formulated the alternatives clearly enough but could not solve the riddle of neonatal jaundice with the means at their disposal. To them icterus meant either regurgitation of bile or increased destruction of blood. Hemolysis seemed indeed a plausible explanation for the combination of bilirubinemia of the indirect variety with a falling hemoglobin level and a regenerative blood picture, all the more because mild forms of hemolytic disease were undoubtedly included in studies of infants presumed to be normal. The life span of fetal—or, for that matter, adult—red cells remained an unknown quantity, even after Winifred Ashby in 1919 had measured it in adults, using the differential agglutination technique, as the range of 30 to 100 days reported by her was too great to be of practical value. This was also true of the blood volume of the newborn, which William Palmer Lucas and B. F. Dearing[10] of San Francisco had actually attempted to measure in the same year, using the brilliant vital red dilution method. They obtained a range of values from 107 to 195 mL per kg of body weight, almost twice that found in 1950 by Mollison and his associates[11] with a method combining isotope and dye dilution. The mere fact that they concerned themselves with such questions in 1919 puts them ahead of their pediatric contemporaries. Neither of the first two books devoted specifically to pediatric hematology, that of Ferruccio Zibordi of Modena, *Ematologia Infantile Normale e Patologica*,[12] which appeared in 1925, and that of Baar and Stransky of Vienna, *Die Klinische Hämatologie des Kindesalters*,[1] published in 1928, mentioned blood volume or red cell survival. The name of Lucas deserves recognition in any survey of pediatric hematology, for, apart from looking after patients with blood diseases in the Children's Department of the University of California before such specialization had become accepted elsewhere, he was an enterprising and thoughtful investigator. His chapters on blood in *Abt's Pediatrics* of 1924, written with E. C. Fleischner,[13] are outstanding in their emphasis on physiologic processes, clarity of thought, and absence of semantic claptrap, and in these respects are superior to the two works just cited.

As for the solution to the puzzle of neonatal jaundice, the functional inferiority of the liver postulated so long ago by Ylppö could not be defined, of course, until Hijmans van den Bergh's two pigments had been identified as free and glucuronide-conjugated bilirubin by the independent studies of Billing and Lathe,[14] Schmid,[15] and Talafant[16] in 1956. The results of the preceding demonstration of the role of uridine diphosphate glucuronic acid (UDPGA) as a glucuronide donor by Dutton[17] and others could be applied to bilirubin, and the enzymatic reactions involved in the conjugation process could be investigated as a function of hepatic maturation by Brown and co-workers.[18]

Traditionally, the history of pediatric hematology begins in 1889 with von Jaksch's report[19] on the condition that bears his name, which he designated *anemia pseudoleucaemica infantum*. By an irony of fate, not only the term but the very syndrome has long since vanished from the horizon, although in its day it had an enormous vogue and was considered by some to be the anemia of infancy *par excellence.* In 1891, the condition was described independently by Hayem[20] and his compatriot Luzet,[21] so that their names were also attached to it. The clinical picture was overshadowed by severe nutritional disturbances, wasting, diarrhea, rickets, and, as a rule, chronic infections of the respiratory tract, otitis media, pyoderma, and the like. The findings suggestive of leukemia were marked splenomegaly, anemia, and that which later hematologists would call a leukemoid reaction, characterized by leukocytosis and immature granulocytes. It was Luzet who noted the normoblastemia that led to the use of the term "erythroblastic anemia," until that term was temporarily pre-empted by Cooley for the anemia that he described. At that time, the combination of splenomegaly and leukocytosis meant leukemia, and von Jaksch's paper was therefore a distinct step forward, though its essence was the simple observation that some of the patients survived, a remarkable fact in itself given their general condition and the paucity of therapeutic means then available.

Von Jaksch was not a hematologist, and except for a follow-up report in 1890, he made no further contributions to the understanding of the disease that made him famous. He practiced pediatrics in Prague, then the capital of the Austrian province of Bohemia, and held an appointment at the Charles University, where, as a legendary octogenarian, he was pointed out to this writer in 1934, a tall aristocratic figure with a massive white head who bore his fame with a casual elegance reminiscent of the old Hapsburg Empire. The riddle of von Jaksch's anemia was never properly solved. It was at one time common in central Europe and in France, less so in England, and still less so in the United States. Its disappearance paralleled the gradual improvement in child health and care. As Lehndorff[22] wrote many years afterward in an almost nostalgic epitaph on the extinct entity, it had been "a poor people's disease." In truth, it was not an entity at all but a convenient diagnostic wastebasket, though an interesting one. The contemporaries finally agreed that it was a nonspecific response of the infantile organism to the horrendous combinations of infectious and nutritional insults that were so common at the time and so difficult to sort out.

More lasting and far more important, of course, was the contribution made to pediatric hematology—and indeed to medical science as a whole—by Thomas B. Cooley of Detroit in 1925,[23] when he salvaged from this wastebasket the distinct entity now known as thalassemia. He soon abandoned his original designation of "erythroblastic anemia," for he realized that the conspicuous normoblastemia that had first attracted his attention was neither a specific nor a central feature of the disorder, and in his later publications he emphasized the fragmentation and shape anomalies of the red cells and the paucity and uneven distribution of the hemoglobin. He did not know, of course, that the ultimate distur-

bance was one of hemoglobin, let alone β chain synthesis, but he came to conceive of the disease as a fundamental disorder of hematopoiesis and was fully aware of its genetic nature from the beginning. He himself had originally proposed a recessive mode of inheritance, anticipating the classic study of Valentine and Neel of 1944.[24] Strangely enough, he failed to investigate the seemingly normal parents and siblings of the propositi. Later, unverified reports of hereditary transmission of the disorder by a single affected parent seemed to militate against a recessive mode and left him uncertain.

Cooley was, in any case, profoundly interested in the genetic aspects of the anemias and was in this respect far ahead of most contemporary hematologists. He corresponded with geneticists, used such terms as "heterozygote" for humans at a time when their use was still largely restricted to plants and *Drosophila*, and for years pondered the then wholly puzzling relationship between "sicklemia" and sickle cell anemia. He reported the first instance of sickle cell disease (which this writer later had occasion to identify as a case of sickle-thalassemia) in a Greek family.[25] He also proposed an X-linked mode of inheritance, backed by pedigree studies over five generations, for a familial hypochromic anemia in a kindred first described by him[26] and later restudied by Rundles and Falls[27] at Ann Arbor, Michigan. In accepting the term "Mediterranean anemia," which Whipple had suggested at a time when the known cases were restricted to Italian and Greek families, Cooley[28] made an interesting and prophetic reservation: "We are not inclined," he wrote in 1932, "to lay great stress on the limitation of this or any similar disease to a particular race. We have found that sickle cell anemia, formerly supposed to be peculiar to Negroes, occurs in Greeks, and it seems likely to us that any disease in which there is a hereditary element, as presumably there is in this disease, is limited more by locality and association than by race."

The style is as characteristic of the man as the thought. Cooley was articulate, well educated—he spoke or at least read four languages and maintained a global correspondence—and highly intelligent. He came from a family of distinguished jurists, the only one to eschew the law and enter the medical profession. Born in Ann Arbor, the son of a future justice of the Michigan Supreme Court, he obtained his degree in medicine at the University of Michigan, worked for 3 years in "clinical chemistry," interned at Boston City Hospital, spent a year visiting clinics in Germany, returned to Boston for prolonged training in contagious diseases, and then was appointed Assistant Professor of Hygiene at his alma mater. Except for a stint with the Children's Bureau of the American Red Cross during World War I, he remained in Michigan for the rest of his life, first as a practicing pediatrician and, after the death of Raymond Hoobler in 1936, as a professor of pediatrics in Detroit. Throughout these years he was closely associated with The Children's Hospital of Michigan, whose pediatrician-in-chief he ultimately became.

As mentioned, Cooley had no formal training in hematology and very little technical help. He and his faithful associate of many years, Pearl Lee, examined blood smears, roentgenograms, and, of course, the patients themselves, making sketchy notes on index cards and keeping the bulk of their observations in their heads. His equipment consisted of a monocular microscope of ancient vintage, a staining rack, a rather small card file, and—in an otherwise vacant room upstairs intended for the affairs of the Child Research Council of the American Academy of Pediatrics—a couch on which he took siestas and did much of his thinking. His daughter Emily, a gifted and artistic young woman, made the beautiful camera lucida and freehand drawings with which he illustrated his papers. She also chauffeured him about town, went to the library for him, and accompanied him to meetings. His home in Detroit's "Indian Village" and his garden, professionally landscaped by Emily, were oases of good taste. He owned a cottage on the coast of Maine where he spent his summers. He loved music, knew his wines, enjoyed good food, and was an excellent conversationalist. He knew how to live.

At times, his penchant for conversation got him into trouble. Old-time Detroiters recall the story of his house call to a well-to-do family whose child had contracted an undiagnosed illness. As a social acquaintance Dr. Cooley was led into the living room, offered refreshments, and asked his opinion on some topic of current interest. A lively discussion ensued, at the end of which the doctor, having forgotten the original purpose of his visit, grabbed his hat and coat and was out of the house before the astonished parents could remind him of the patient upstairs.

Cooley's influence extended well beyond the field of hematology. His was the conception behind a series of studies on the chemical composition of the red cell stroma carried out in the 1930s by Erickson and associates in the laboratories of Icie Macy Hoobler of the Children's Fund of Michigan, which earned high praise from Eric Ponder. He was one of the founders of the Academy of Pediatrics and, long before the time was ripe, saw the role of pediatrics in terms of preventive medicine. Politically he was a liberal, scientifically a radical, personally a patrician. Combined with a rather haughty expression, an irrepressible wit, and an utter lack of reverence for established authority, these traits were bound to earn him enmities on the part of town and gown alike, but his enemies respected and his friends admired him. He was well ahead of his time, a lucid thinker and a giant in the history of pediatric hematology.

An entirely different personality was George Guest, for many years one of the mainstays of the Children's Hospital Research Foundation in Cincinnati, whose contributions were equally important, if less spectacular. Guest was as much a physiologist as a hematologist, interested in the basic aspects of blood during growth, a stickler for precise measurements, a patient investigator who set himself longterm goals and took a systematic approach to reaching them. The meticulous studies he conducted between 1932 and 1942 on the hemoglobin levels, red blood counts, and packed cell volumes of a large group of infants and young children of widely different social and economic backgrounds are a model of intelligent and purposeful data-gathering, the purpose being both physiologic and clinical. In the face of the rather arbitrary definitions and therapeutic practices then prevailing, Guest set out to ascertain the range of normal variation and to delineate optimal values against hypoferric states. Such data were badly needed then and have remained valid to this day. In serial studies[29] involving, among other things, intrafamily and twin comparisons, he showed convincingly that a fall of the mean corpuscular volume (MCV) and mean corpuscular hemoglobin (MCH) in the presence of seemingly adequate hemoglobin levels could be reversed or altogether prevented by the administration of iron and is therefore a sensitive indicator of an incipient deficiency state rather than a physiologic phenomenon. He concluded that iron deficiency anemia was far more common among infants than had been previously thought, and advocated the general use of prophylactic measures. His earlier observations on glycolysis and the rise of inorganic phosphorus levels in stored blood[30] and his joint observations with Sam Rapoport[31] on the role of the pH in the breakdown of diphosphoglycerate were milestones in the understanding of red cell metabolism. He also made significant contributions to the knowledge of the osmometric properties of erythrocytes,[32] both normal and abnormal, devising a method that was, typically, both practical and precise and permitted simultaneous determinations of hemolysis and red cell volume at each stage of the procedure.

Apart from these accomplishments, George Guest was a delightful friend and, with the help of his wife, a perfect host, so that the house on Dana Avenue in Cincinnati became a kind of unofficial headquarters for the entertainment of the many visitors to the Children's Hospital. Here they were offered the vin d'honneur from a well-stocked wine cellar decorated with frescoes by an artist friend—the owners' pride and the first and last stop for the visitor—and here they would find good conversation, interesting people, and exquisite cuisine. The Guests were passionate Francophiles, and the cooking was French, unless a keg of oysters had just arrived from the East to be prepared in endless variations, or unless Jesse, the houseman, more friend than butler, just happened to have shot—illegally, of course—a fat squirrel from one of the magnificent old trees in the garden. George, a short, stocky, quiet-spoken man, understood the art of good fellowship, but the soul of the house and its social genius was his wife "M.L.," a handsome woman with red hair who had a passion for poetry and a gift for conversation. They had met in Europe after World War I as young and idealistic members of the Hoover Relief team, were drawn together by their love for all things French, and remained deeply devoted to one another. A large part of every summer was spent in France visiting friends, traveling through the countryside, and sampling wines. George Guest was the only American member of the French Pediatric Society, a fact in which he took greater pride than in all his other achievements, and though his French accent left much to be desired, he liked to attend meetings and even present papers in such delightful places as Bordeaux, Lyon, and Paris. When M.L. died about 1964, the house was sold and an era passed.

It would be instructive to trace in detail the thinking of earlier observers concerning the iron deficiency anemia of infancy, to whose definition Guest made such a solid contribution, but which remained an object of controversy, confusion, and neglect for generations of pediatricians. Although Bunge had proposed an essentially correct explanation as early as 1889, the nature of the most common anemia of infancy eluded investigators for many years. The reasons for this paradox are enlightening. One was the belief that not only mild anemia but also hypochromasia was a physiologic phenomenon. "That the hemoglobin content suffers more than the red blood count," Heinrich Baar wrote in 1928,[33] "is surely a purposeful mechanism, for the same quantity of hemoglobin can serve its function better when it is distributed over a larger number of red corpuscles." More important, no doubt, is the fact that among the clinic patients on whom most studies were conducted, pure iron deficiency anemia was rare. In the face of the multiple ailments to which such patients were prone, failure to respond to iron alone was common, and it was easy to draw erroneous conclusions from therapeutic trials. Conversely, of course, a rise of the hemoglobin level following the administration of iron was just as uncritically taken as proof of its efficacy on the principle of *post hoc propter hoc*, though it was believed that iron was a bone marrow "stimulant" rather than a specific substance effective only when correcting or preventing a deficiency.

Much of the problem was semantic in nature. Whereas French pediatricians described iron-responsive hypochromic anemia in infants as "chlorose du jeune âge" or "chlorose alimentaire," most German and Austrian authors rejected this concept, if only because "chlorosis occurs only during puberty and only in females." The highly influential Czerny, in particular, set the clock back by stating categorically that an entire group of alimentary anemias existed that could be influenced by diet but in which iron was utterly ineffective. Baar wrote: "If it appears, a priori, unjustified to group together, and attribute to direct or indirect lack of iron, anemias of the most diverse origin solely because they are all hypochromic, fail to show nucleated red cells in the peripheral blood and lack splenomegaly, the notion of chlorosis of alimentary origin was definitely refuted by Czerny's findings." If this was to pour the baby out with the bathwater, Baar retreated from his a prioristic position to the extent of recognizing a "pseudochlorosis infantum," or infantile iron deficiency anemia, as an "etiologically uniform type to be separated from the rest of the alimentary anemias

of infancy." This was rare, however, he asserted, in comparison with "the overwhelming majority [which] remains uninfluenced by iron administration, though nevertheless improved or cured by appropriate changes in diet." In reading such statements, one must remember that even fresh air and sunshine were still considered essential adjuncts to the treatment of anemia. Moreover, no less an authority than Haldane[34] had asserted earlier that "recovery affords no ground for assuming that iron is built up into hemoglobin," and that "in typical cases [of chlorosis] the curative factor of iron salts must be exercised otherwise than simply in building up the hemoglobin." Haldane went on to say that "The essential process in the cure of chlorosis is the reduction in the volume of the plasma [sic]." In addition, the notion of toxic hemolysis due to the fatty acids in cow's milk and especially in goat's milk had a prolonged vogue on the Continent, where "cow's milk anemia" and "goat's milk anemia" were accepted entities.

Related to the semantic difficulties was the problem of classification. Ever since Hayem had introduced the color index in 1877, hypochromasia had been used to characterize certain anemias. It was soon apparent that most anemias of older infants were of this type, but the difficulty of relating morphologic criteria to pathogenetic mechanisms and of recognizing in turn that different etiologic factors could operate through identical pathways proved too much. Not until the work of Minot and Castle established the characteristic response of hemoglobin and reticulocytes to specific hematinics, and Wintrobe put the morphologic classification on the firm basis of red cell measurements, did pediatric hematologists gradually abandon terms such as "alimentary-infectious" anemia. In 1936, Hugh Josephs[35] still used this term as a common denominator that, to him, included deficient hemoglobin formation, deficient erythropoiesis and deficient stimulation of erythropoiesis, deficient maturation (the "erythroblastoses"), and blood destruction. Such usage, apart from the vagueness of the etiologic concept, was bound to delay both the understanding of the pathogenesis and the development of a workable classification of the anemias. It was an internist who said that "the infant bleeds into its own increasing blood volume," and the importance of the hemoglobin mass at birth was not appreciated until later. When Blackfan and Diamond's *Atlas of the Blood in Children* finally appeared in 1944,[36] it used Wintrobe's classification and described the principal anemia of infancy under the title "iron deficiency anemia."

One cannot leave the subject of iron deficiency without reference to Hugh Josephs, a strange figure, and in his day an authority in the field of American pediatric hematology. It is remarkable that this should have been the case, for he published little and confined his work primarily to the relationship between iron metabolism and anemia in infancy. His chapters on diseases of the blood in Holt and McIntosh's textbook were excellent, but his mind had a somewhat pedantic cast and a tendency to look for profound meanings underneath simple facts. His forte was a thorough knowledge of the literature, which he analyzed in erudite but unconscionably lengthy reviews, complete with foreword, statement of scope and purpose, introduction, presentation of fundamental concepts, summary, table of contents, and a bibliography that in one instance exceeded 750 titles. He was Associate Professor of Pediatrics in Dr. Park's department at Johns Hopkins University and published mostly in the *Johns Hopkins Bulletin*. His manner and appearance were those of a college professor or a don—mild, pleasant, serious, single-minded, a slight, gray-haired man who smoked a pipe, wore soft collars and a velvet jacket with elbow patches, and received his visitors in a drab office in the old Harriet Lane Home cluttered with books, magazines, and reprints.

By means of a curious logic, Josephs came to the unshakable conclusion that the hypochromic iron deficiency anemia of infants was not due to depletion of iron but to its diversion to unknown sites by unknown mechanisms.[37] He based this hypothesis on theoretical calculations that proved that an anemic baby of 18 months should have an excess of 200 mg of unused iron—other than the necessary tissue iron—somewhere in his body; ergo the baby suffered from "iron deficiency without depletion." This hypothetical baby, Josephs said, "is starving in the midst of plenty. Give this baby a small amount of iron by mouth and he will utilize it avidly for hemoglobin formation, and may as a result use even more than he was given." In the absence of infection, the unavailability of iron might be due, he thought, to hormonal, histotrophic, or even emotional factors. But in 1956, 3 years after these speculations, Philip Sturgeon[38] calculated on the basis of the same data that had been available to Josephs that a seemingly normal newborn could easily have a hemoglobin mass low enough to account for severe anemia in later infancy, reflecting the expansion of the blood volume with growth. Earlier, Bruce Chown[39] of Winnipeg had documented the occurrence of massive transplacental hemorrhage. Soon afterward, Kleihauer and Betke[40] devised their ingenious method for demonstrating fetal cells in maternal blood by the acid elution technique. Subsequent studies by Cohen, Zuelzer, and associates[41] and others showed that moderate and repeated fetal bleeds were not at all rare. A mechanism for depriving the fetus of hemoglobin iron without necessarily causing overt anemia at birth but capable of explaining the later development of iron deficiency in the absence of further blood loss seemed to offer a simpler solution than the tortuous hypothesis of "iron deficiency without depletion." The modern age had arrived.

Their semantic difficulties did not keep the earlier pediatricians from devising eminently practical methods of treatment, as exemplified by the story of pediatric transfusion therapy. The technical problems of transfusing infants were overcome in various ways. In 1915, Helmholz of the Mayo Clinic advocated the use of the superior sagittal sinus, and in 1925 Hart of the Sick Children's Hospital of Toronto used this route for the first exchange transfusion ever given for "icterus gravis."[42] Though his patient recovered, exchange transfusion was not again used for this indication until Wallerstein revived it in 1946 on the grounds that "the removal of most of the Rh-positive cells and of the circulating antibody shortly after birth prevents the incidence of the more severe pathological and physiological changes." Wallerstein,[43] then Director of the Erythroblastosis Fetalis Clinic of the Jewish Memorial Hospital in New York, had used the sagittal sinus for most of his cases, but stated that "the umbilical vessels should be an excellent route for both the withdrawal and replacement procedures," with the strange proviso that they could be used "only if the decision to perform the substitution is made before birth...." J. B. Sidbury,[44] a pediatrician at the Babies' Hospital in Wrightsville, North Carolina, in a little-noticed report had described a simple transfusion via the umbilical vein in the case of a bleeding newborn in 1923. It was Diamond[45] who later established the umbilical route as the safest and simplest for exchange transfusion in hemolytic disease and who, with Allen and Vaughan,[46] was the first to recognize that the prevention of kernicterus was the main rationale of the procedure. It is interesting to recall that exsanguination transfusion through the fontanelle or the femoral vein was used on a large scale at the Sick Children's Hospital in Toronto for the treatment of burns, erysipelas, and other conditions since 1921. This procedure was introduced by Bruce Robertson, who in 1916 during the campaign in France had observed two soldiers recover from severe carbon monoxide poisoning after venesections followed by transfusions. By March of 1924, when Robertson was already dead, 501 exsanguination transfusions had been performed at the Sick Children's Hospital.[47]

In the late 1950s there was a small flurry of papers reporting successful transfusions by the intraperitoneal route. This subject had been thoroughly explored in two studies, one experimental,[48] the other clinical,[49] in 1923 by a young pediatric resident in Minneapolis, David Siperstein, whose concise and accurate summary read as follows: "1. The intraperitoneal transfusion of citrated blood is a therapeutic procedure of possible merit. 2. It can apparently be utilized in cases in which transfusion is indicated, when other routes are unavailable." The author documented the effective reabsorption of the transfused cells not only with serial red counts and hemoglobin determinations but also with photomicrographs showing the dual population of hypochromic recipient and normochromic donor cells. In his review of the literature, he found that intraperitoneal transfusion was first used by Ponfick of Berlin in 1875, and that Hayem in 1884 had performed ingenious experiments involving cross transfusions of dog and rabbit blood in order to prove absorption from the peritoneal cavity. Although technical progress has since made the procedure obsolete, Siperstein's work deserves to be rescued from oblivion, if only to show that there is nothing new under the sun. He recognized a potential need, defined the problem, and solved it with an enviable economy of means (and words).

Passing mention should also be made of the use of bone marrow transfusions as a means of side-stepping technical difficulties in transfusing infants, especially for the general pediatrician with little practice in "needle-work." The method had its day in England and particularly in Denmark, where Heinild[50] in 1947 described the experience of 4 years, during which 686 blood transfusions were given via the bone marrow without a single mishap. He stated that the risk of osteomyelitis was limited to patients receiving continuous infusions. One hesitates to argue with success and realizes that, in places and under conditions in which the required skills or supplies are lacking, it is better to apply unorthodox methods than to let a baby die for lack of blood.

A less desirable development that took place in the late 1920s and continued until the early 1940s was the practice of giving newborn infants intramuscular injections of adult blood as a prophylactic measure against hemorrhagic disease of the newborn. During those years, according to recollections provided by James L. Wilson, who for many years was Dr. Blackfan's right arm at The Children's Hospital in Boston, hemorrhagic disease was becoming so great a problem that this practice seemed justified. The blood was given without typing or cross-matching, and the procedure undoubtedly was responsible for a significant number of sensitizations against the Rh factor that did not come to light until these infants had grown up (and the Rh factor had meanwhile been discovered). The subsequent decline in hemorrhagic disease of the newborn coincided with both the introduction of vitamin K and a significant improvement in obstetric practices. Since the condition has now become rare and its definition was always vague and without clear distinction between traumatic hemorrhages and those primarily attributable to a coagulation difficulty, the mystery of its upsurge and the reasons for its virtual disappearance have never become quite clear.

If pediatricians proved resourceful in the matter of blood transfusions, it must be said that they showed little innovative spirit in certain other respects. It is a curious fact that the study of the bone marrow in children was neglected, especially in the United States, long after its usefulness had been amply demonstrated in adults. Thus Cooley, for example, never looked at anything but the peripheral blood, and Blackfan and Diamond's otherwise exhaustive *Atlas* of 1944 appeared without a single illustration of bone marrow. This writer remembers visiting a major pediatric center on the East Coast about 1946 and being shown half a dozen patients on the wards suspected of having leukemia and awaiting surgical biopsies—to be performed when and if they stopped bleeding. His own interest in the cytology of the bone marrow, which led to the recognition of megaloblastic anemia of infancy and its reversal by folic acid,[51] had been stimulated by many "curb-stone" discussions with Lawrence Berman, a

student of Downey and himself an outstanding morphologist. It should be noted that Amato of Naples, Italy,[52] gave an excellent description of infantile megaloblastic anemia independently in the same year as Zuelzer and Ogden,[51] though he did not have folic acid at his disposal and concluded from the response to potent liver extract that he was dealing with true pernicious anemia or at least with a temporary deficiency of intrinsic factor. An even earlier report by Veeneklaas of Holland[53] had the misfortune of being prevented from reaching readers abroad because of World War II.

This is the place to pay tribute to the memory of Katsuji Kato, pupil and associate of Downey, a superb morphologist and illustrator, who was the first student of the infantile bone marrow in the United States. In 1937, Kato[54] published a definitive study based on bone marrow aspirations in 51 normal infants and children. He commented on the lymphocytosis in the younger subjects and gave the myeloid-erythroid ratios for the various ages. He also illustrated the diagnostic value of the procedure by citing a case of leukemia and one of Niemann-Pick disease. Kato was on the staff of Bobs Roberts Memorial Hospital in Chicago and often made the long trek to the North Side to participate in Dr. Brennemann's grand rounds at the Children's Memorial Hospital. One remembers him, a jolly, round-faced, smiling figure reminiscent of the Hotei-Sama statuettes of his native Japan, a rapid speaker with an atrocious accent but interesting ideas, showing off his delicate colored drawings with as much aesthetic pleasure as scientific pride and at the same time implying by his self-deprecating manner that it was all quite simple and hardly worth the honorable listener's attention. World War II put an end to his career. He returned to Japan and was lost from sight.

Perhaps it was Kato's unfortunate choice of the sternum as the site for diagnostic punctures, making the procedure unnecessarily difficult and unpleasant in pediatric practice, that kept others from emulating him. American authors virtually ignored Kato's work, except for the enterprising Peter Vogel at Mount Sinai Hospital in New York, whose study with Frank Bassen[55] in 1939 covered 113 examples of diverse conditions, including leukemia, Gaucher's disease, and metastatic neuroblastoma, illustrated with excellent photomicrographs. In Europe, and especially in Switzerland under the influence of Rohr and Moeschlin, pediatric hematologists were more curious. Zürich, where Naegeli had created a strong tradition, had already become a mecca of Continental hematology. Writing in 1937, Guido Fanconi[56] declared: "The painstaking exploration of every case [of unexplained anemia] with old and new methods, which include bone marrow puncture, handled at the Zürich [Children's] Clinic with consummate skill by my Oberarzt, Dozent Willi, promises to uncover new, sharply defined entities." In the short span between 1935 and 1938, H. Willi[57] published four excellent studies on the bone marrow in thrombocytopenic purpura, leukemia, and various anemias of childhood. Fanconi had the satisfaction of seeing his prophecy fulfilled, in part by his next Oberarzt, Conrad Gasser. In addition to megaloblastic anemia of infancy, a whole series of conditions came to light or were clarified by bone marrow studies, among them the acute erythroblastopenia described in 1949 by Gasser[58]; chronic benign neutropenia, also studied by Gasser[59] and later by Zuelzer and Bajoghli[60]; Kostmann's infantile genetic agranulocytosis[61]; "myelokathexis"[62] or "ineffective granulopoiesis"[63]; and the aplastic and hypoplastic anemias.

Hematology occupied a special place among Fanconi's far-flung interests, and in giving encouragement and support to his associates—in this respect not unlike Blackfan—he contributed as much to progress in this field as he had done earlier with the recognition of the anemia that bears his name.[64] A tall, handsome man, every inch the professor yet gracious and outgoing, capable of charming an audience in six languages, a lively and eclectic spirit, Fanconi was a superb clinician and an excellent organizer to whom pediatric hematology owes much. With Fanconi one must rank his colleague in Bern, Glanzmann,[65] whose report in 1918 on "hereditary hemorrhagic thrombasthenia" as a condition characterized by prolonged bleeding time and poor clot retraction in the presence of a normal platelet count opened the era of platelet function studies. Glanzmann postulated the existence of a platelet factor specifically involved in clot retraction. He contributed greatly to the knowledge of the various purpuras. The term "anaphylactoid purpura" stems from his studies[66] and was based partly on clinical observations and similarities with human serum sickness and partly on his interpretation of Hayem's findings in dogs injected intravenously with bovine serum.

Conrad Gasser, one of the ablest and most productive pediatric hematologists in Europe, deserves more than passing mention in this narrative. Apart from his discovery of acute erythroblastopenia—known until then only from the report of Owren[67] as a complication of congenital spherocytosis—and his study of chronic neutropenia, he added greatly to our knowledge of hemolytic anemias in childhood. His monograph *Die Hämolytischen Syndrome des Kindesalters*,[68] which appeared in 1951, ranks in quality if not in scope with Dacie's well-known book. In 1948, in a paper with Grumbach,[69] Gasser described spherocytosis as a feature of ABO hemolytic disease. In the same year he gave a detailed report of anemia with spontaneous Heinz body formation in a premature infant,[70] a condition then unknown except for a brief note by Willi. In his book, and in subsequent publications, he added a large compilation of case material, described the detailed morphologic picture of the abnormal red cells—which were identical with the "pyknocytes" later observed in full-term infants by Tuffy, Brown, and Zuelzer,[71] but which he called more graphically "ruptured eggshells"—and determined their incidence in the blood of normal premature infants. He coined the term "hemolytic-uremic syndrome," being among the first to recognize that condition.

One reports with regret that so fruitful a career was disrupted by the exigencies of an academic system that, at the time at least, provided insufficient "room at the top" and effectively eliminated key people upon the retirement of their chief (unless they happened to be chosen to succeed him). Such a system was, and to a large extent still is, in force in Switzerland and elsewhere on the Continent. Fanconi's retirement from the Kinderspital in Zürich almost automatically entailed that of his Oberarzt Gasser. The latter, a modest man with a quiet sense of humor and a gemütlich Alemannic temperament, maintained his interest in hematology, which came to include the treatment of childhood leukemia, but he did so as a practicing pediatrician in a private office. Similar reasons prematurely ended the academic career of Sansone in Genoa, author of a book on favism and one of the most promising pediatric hematologists in Italy.

It is manifestly impossible in the allotted space to do justice to, or even name, all those who contributed to the evolution of pediatric hematology. Among European workers one would like to dwell on the achievements of Sir Leonard Parsons of Birmingham, England, the Grand Old Man of British pediatric hematology, founder of a veritable school that attracted students from many countries, including the United States. Parsons was an original thinker who refused to accept the confused semantics of childhood anemias and created his own system along pathophysiologic lines. He was the first to recognize, in 1933, the hemolytic nature of erythroblastosis fetalis and to defend that concept[72] even against the authority of Castle and Minot. These men, along with Diamond, Blackfan and Baty, Josephs, and others, regarded erythroblastosis fetalis as a defect of hematopoiesis in a class with Cooley's anemia and other "erythroblastoses." One would like to describe the achievements of Parson's associates, Hawksley and Lightwood; of Cathie, Gairdner, Walker, Hardisty, and so many other British colleagues of Lichtenstein in Sweden—an early student of the anemia of prematurity, which he was the first to call physiologic and to separate from the later phase of iron deficiency; of his compatriots Wallgren and Vahlquist; of Plum in Copenhagen, the discoverer of vitamin K and originator of the thesis of a temporary deficiency of this substance as the cause of hemorrhagic disease of the newborn; of van Crefeld of Amsterdam, a pioneer in the study of coagulation factors in the newborn; of Betke, then in Tübingen, who with Kleihauer developed the acid elution technique for the demonstration of fetal hemoglobin in individual cells and who later, in Munich, made his department into a strong base of pediatric hematology; of Jonxis in Leyden, an imaginative investigator, who among other things organized a comparative study of the incidence of sickling in Curaçao and Dutch Guiana (now Surinam) to test Allison's hypothesis of the selective effect of malaria on two genetically similar populations exposed for centuries to different risks of the infection.

To return closer to home, credit must be given to James M. Baty as a member, with Blackfan and Diamond, of the triumvirate at Children's Hospital, Boston, that set the pattern for the development of pediatric hematology in the United States. Their collaborative effort resulted in, among other things, the recognition that hydrops fetalis, icterus gravis, and hemolytic anemia of the newborn, in spite of the differences in their clinical manifestations, were etiologically related conditions.[73] This was truly a breakthrough in the understanding of hemolytic disease. After Baty moved to the Floating Hospital and Blackfan died an untimely death, Diamond emerged as the American pediatric hematologist *par excellence*. His role cannot be described solely in terms of his publications, which are too numerous to be listed here. He became the mentor of a whole generation of pediatric hematologists who later held, and in most instances still hold, key positions in teaching institutions throughout the United States. Directly or indirectly we all owe him a debt of gratitude, even those of us who from time to time disagreed with some of his ideas. This writer vividly remembers his first meeting with Dr. Diamond, when as a lowly intern in 1935 he consulted him in connection with a case of Cooley's anemia, then an unheard-of rarity in the small New England hospital where he served. This writer made the pilgrimage to Children's Hospital—which under Blackfan was forbidden territory to those who were not graduates of Harvard, Yale, Columbia, or Johns Hopkins—with some trepidation. His fears were not allayed when he laid eyes on Dr. Diamond, rather fierce-looking in a dark, Assyrian sort of way. But Diamond proved to be a gracious consultant, willing to discuss the case at hand without condescension or conceit with an insignificant beginner, to listen to the history and examine the blood films, and above all to confirm the beginner's diagnosis. Over the years, hundreds of colleagues and young would-be hematologists came to appreciate "L.K.'s" kindness and unfailing courtesy. Of his numerous contributions one need mention here only the "Diamond-Blackfan" syndrome of hypoplastic anemia[74]; the studies on the nature, diagnostics, and treatment of hemolytic disease; and the *Atlas*, an outstanding achievement for its day, which was his work rather than Blackfan's. But perhaps even more important was the guidance and encouragement he provided for pediatric hematologists of the next generation, of whom—at the risk of being selective—we can name here only a few: Fred ("Hal") Allen, Park Gerald, Frank Oski, N. T. Shahidi, Victor Vaughan, and William Zinkham.

Less influential, though no less respected, was the late Carl Smith of New York. His book, *Blood Diseases of Infancy and Childhood*,[75] was the first of its kind in the United States and for many years served as the major reference work in the field. Smith's most important contribution was the description of infectious lymphocytosis, an essentially asymptomatic condition associated with a blood picture reminiscent of that of whooping cough (or chronic lymphocytic leukemia), endemic and probably of viral origin. He took a great interest in thalassemia and established a model outpatient transfusion service at The New York Hospital. Carl Smith was a modest and generous man, always willing to praise and give credit, even when credit was not due. Through his untiring efforts, Cornell became one of the important centers of pediatric hematology on the East Coast.

The prime mover in the field on the West Coast was Philip Sturgeon, who created the hematology service at the Children's Hospital of Los Angeles. He emerged about 1950 as an independent investigator interested in the study of the infantile bone marrow. His research provided quantitative measurements, then badly needed,[76] and stimulated the diagnostic use of bone marrow aspiration. A great traveller and sportsman in private life, Sturgeon combined in his work the elements of common sense and scientific curiosity, establishing the outstanding hematology clinic that was later carried on by his successor, Dennis Hammond. In the midst of a productive career, Sturgeon surprised his friends and colleagues by retiring to Zermatt in Switzerland, but skiing and hiking even in the most glorious of landscapes was not enough to fill his existence, and after a few years he returned to his work, and California.

The fact that a major pediatric teaching institution in the United States (or in many European countries, for that matter) today is almost unthinkable without a pediatric hematologist reflects the influence of a few model institutions in the post–World War II era. We have noted the importance of a Diamond "school" of pediatric hematology. During this same critical era, the only other center of comparable importance was the Hematology Service at the Children's Hospital of Michigan in Detroit, which this writer was privileged to direct, and which over a quarter of a century turned out well over 100 fellows, many of them today directing services of their own in the United States and abroad, among them Audrey Brown, Flossie Cohen, Eugene Kaplan, Sanford Leikin, Jeanne Lusher, and William A. Newton. The work of this group includes contributions to the knowledge of ABO hemolytic disease, fetal-maternal hemorrhage, immune hemolytic anemia, the hemoglobinopathies, purpura and other bleeding disorders, and the therapy of childhood leukemia. The creation some time ago of a subspecialty board in pediatric hematology, whether or not it serves a practical purpose, is a sure indication that among Boston, Detroit, Los Angeles and San Francisco, New York, and more recently New Haven, Cincinnati and Syracuse, Minneapolis and Memphis, and Seattle and Houston, a sufficiency of man- (and woman-) power exists to provide service, teaching, and research at a high level of excellence today and in the future.

Throughout its history, pediatric hematology has benefited from the advances of adult hematology, and in fact some of its major achievements rest on contributions made by scientists in other fields (e.g., immunology, chemistry, genetics, and physiology). A striking example is the history of hemolytic disease of the newborn. In

1938, Ruth Darrow, a pathologist who had a deep personal interest in the subject, having experienced a series of stillbirths, reflected on the pathogenesis of what was then called erythroblastosis fetalis.[77] Assembling all of the then known facts, notably the sparing of the first child, the involvement of all or most children born after the first afflicted baby, and the range of clinical and hematologic manifestations, she discarded all the current theories and concluded that the disease could be explained only as the result of maternal sensitization to an as yet unknown fetal antigen—a splendid example of the value of intelligent speculation.

Within 3 years Darrow's hypothesis was confirmed, and the Rh factor, described in a brief communication by Landsteiner and Wiener[78] in 1940, was identified as the offending antigen. Wiener,[79] and independently Levine,[80] observed transfusion reactions after administration of ABO-compatible blood that could be attributed to Rh antibodies. It was Levine, observing such a reaction in a woman who had received no prior transfusions[81] but had received blood from her husband after delivering a stillborn fetus, who recognized the relationship between the Rh factor and hemolytic disease of the newborn.[82] He showed that mothers of affected infants possessed antibodies that reacted with most random blood samples and with blood samples of their husbands and children but not with each other's. Gentle, unassertive, and scholarly, Levine characteristically sought the opinions of those experienced in neonatal pathology before publishing his revolutionary conclusion. This writer remembers Levine's visit to his laboratory in Detroit in this connection, which took place sometime in 1941. Bubbling with excitement yet reluctant to overturn established dogma and aware that he was venturing into uncharted seas, Levine was visibly reassured when his attention was called to Ruth Darrow's paper in the *Archives of Pathology*. But the serologic evidence was conclusive in itself, and the paper Levine and his associates published the same year bore the title "The role of isoimmunization in the pathogenesis of erythroblastosis." Levine had been an associate of Landsteiner at the Rockefeller Institute, but by this time he had withdrawn from that prestigious institution and was working at a hospital in Elizabeth, New Jersey, a modest, unpretentious man, content to pursue his research in any setting. When this writer first knew him, he was a devoted paterfamilias, amateur pianist, and bridge player. After the death of his wife he moved to New York City and continued his work at the Sloan-Kettering Institute, where he remains active to this day. The scope and the fruitfulness of his investigations, which extend from fetal-maternal isoimmunization to the relationship between blood group and cancer antibodies, have made him one of the most creative scientists of our time.

The names of Levine and Alexander Wiener were antithetically linked for the generation that witnessed their ascent, largely because both had been associates of Landsteiner and both contributed enormously to the knowledge of immunohematology and of human genetics, but above all because their views often clashed. This was confusing for the bystanders but in no way detracts from the achievements of each man. Wiener's role in the technical and conceptual understanding of hemolytic disease, both Rh and ABO, cannot be underestimated, but his obsession with nomenclature, his tendency to pile hypothesis upon hypothesis, usually without bothering to inform the reader that he was discarding pieces from the bottom without toppling the edifice, and most of all his imperviousness to the needs of clinicians unfamiliar with the mysteries of blood group immunology isolated him from the mainstream of clinical investigation. Of Wiener's enormous output—by 1954, when the theory of Rh isoimmunization was essentially complete, he had published more than 333 papers, and a typical Wiener bibliography might contain 60 references by A. S. Wiener (with or without et al.)—the contributions relevant to pediatric and obstetric practice were above all those dealing with the "blocking" Rh antibodies,[83] which he discovered and named "univalent," recognizing that they alone could pass the placental barrier and cause disease in the fetus.[84] He was one of the pioneers of exchange transfusion[85] and personally performed the procedure countless times at the Brooklyn Jewish Hospital, but his technique involving transection of the radial artery and the use of heparinized blood did not gain general acceptance. Less reticent to invade the domain of the clinician and the clinical pathologist than his rival Levine, he proposed ingenious but purely speculative theories of the pathophysiology of hemolytic disease that did not stand the test of time and tended to detract from his brilliant achievements in his proper field of blood group immunology. Personally a likable, friendly, unassuming man, he was always in the thick of a battle in which he was his own worst enemy.

Rh hemolytic disease has become a rarity. Within the life span of one generation the condition was defined, its etiology and pathogenesis identified, effective treatment devised, and a program of prophylaxis instituted that prevents maternal sensitization and has virtually eliminated the disease. This crowning achievement rests on the work of two teams of investigators working independently in Britain and the United States: Clarke and Finn in Liverpool,[86] and Freda, Gorman, Pollack, and their associates in New York.[87] Starting from different theoretical premises, both groups, by 1967, had demonstrated the effectiveness of passive isoimmunization of previously unsensitized mothers by means of a potent anti-Rh gamma globulin. The story of the conquest of hemolytic disease of the newborn is matched by few other chapters in the history of medicine.

The modern era of leukemia therapy begins in the 1940s with the work of Sidney Farber,[88] then pathologist at Children's Hospital of Boston and the leading pediatric pathologist in the United States and indeed the world, who in 1948 developed the concept of cancer chemotherapy. Farber had the good fortune of finding, in Subarov of Lederle Laboratories, a chemist able to give him the "antifol" compounds he needed, but the idea of disrupting the growth of malignant cells with antimetabolites was his, and he pursued and promoted it with single-minded energy. It led him to the creation of the Children's Cancer Research Foundation and to the organization of a vast program of clinical and fundamental research that in turn gave rise to the nationwide collaborative studies sponsored by the National Cancer Institute and to the efforts of countless institutions and individuals the world over. Although married to a charming woman of great artistic talent, and the father of gifted and lively children, Farber was a man of almost monastic dedication to his work, a magnificent hermit who spent day and night in his rather resplendent cell in the Jimmy Fund building planning new approaches, an indefatigable optimist who was convinced from the beginning that a cure for leukemia would come forth and who did much to bring it nearer.

It is a little known irony of fate that Farber's concept of antimetabolite therapy evolved as the result of a faulty—or at least doubtful—observation, namely the impression that the administration of folic acid accelerated the growth of leukemic cells in the bone marrow. This writer became privy to this information because it was he who, during a visit to Boston in 1946, showed his former chief slides of aspirated bone marrow from leukemic children. Farber, hitherto strictly a "tissue pathologist," became very interested in the cytologic method and switched from surgical biopsies to needle aspirations. At that time folic acid had just become available, and in view of its striking effects on the bone marrow in megaloblastic anemia, Farber decided to investigate its effects on leukemia. From sequential examinations he gained the—probably erroneous—impression that the administration of folic acid per os led to more rapid growth of the leukemic cell population. It seems unlikely that the difference, if any, between treated and untreated patients was real, given the pitfalls of quantitating the cellular elements of aspirated bone marrow, but correct or not, the observation gave rise to the idea of using folic acid antagonists, of which aminopterin was the first, and the era of cancer chemotherapy had begun.

Shortly afterward, in 1949, new ground was broken in another field. In that year, by coincidence, two papers bearing on the same subject from different angles appeared within a few months of each other; they were destined to revolutionize the study of what became known as the "hemoglobinopathies." One was the report of Linus Pauling, Harvey Itano, and their co-workers[89] identifying sickle hemoglobin as a discrete protein separable by electrophoresis from normal hemoglobin, and characterizing sickle cell anemia as a "molecular disease." The other was James V. Neel's study of the genetics of sickle cell anemia and the sickle trait, establishing the former as the homozygous and the latter as the heterozygous state for the sickling gene.[90] The findings of the two reports meshed and became the fountainhead of a veritable flood of investigations leading to the discovery

of other hemoglobinopathies and enormously widening the scope of human genetics. The next major achievement was Vernon Ingram's demonstration, by means of the "fingerprinting" of hemoglobin fragments obtained by tryptic digestion, that sickle hemoglobin differs from normal adult hemoglobin (HbA) only in the replacement of a single amino acid among the more than 300 components of the half-molecule, and his subsequent identification of the abnormality as the substitution of a valine for a glutamic acid residue.[91,92] Since then, abnormalities in the amino acid sequence of the hemoglobin molecule (for the most part involving β chain mutations) have been found in hundreds of variants, and amino acid sequencing has become a basic tool of molecular genetics.

Following the identification of point mutations affecting the amino acid skeleton of globin molecules as the basis of sickling and other hemoglobinopathies, it seemed logical to search for similar structural anomalies of hemoglobin in thalassemia and, when none were found, to postulate "silent" mutations (i.e., amino acid substitutions that did not alter the electrophoretic behavior of the hemoglobin, but inhibited the rate of its synthesis).[93] While this hypothesis proved to be incorrect, it implied the valid assumption that, in analogy to the known structural mutants, the abnormality would be specific for either the α or β chain synthesis. This assumption was made explicit in 1959 by Ingram and Stretton,[94] when they postulated two classes of thalassemia, α- and β-thalassemias, corresponding to the α and β chain variants, respectively, of the hemoglobinopathies proper. This concept proved to be extraordinarily fruitful. It soon became apparent that the thalassemias constitute a highly heterogeneous group of disorders, and that these disorders generally can be classified as either α- or β-thalassemias. Following the development of a method for separating α and β (as well as γ and δ) chains by Weatherall and co-workers,[95] it became possible—by means of incorporating radioactive amino acids into the hemoglobin of reticulocytes in vitro—to determine the rate of synthesis of these chains directly and to identify α- and β-thalassemias as disorders of globin chain production of one or the other type. A new explosion of knowledge began with the demonstrations by Nienhuis and Anderson,[96] and Benz and Forget[97] of reduced β chain synthesis by β messenger RNA from β-thalassemic patients, measured in a cell-free heterologous system. The emphasis now shifted to the investigation of quantitative and qualitative defects of mRNA. As additional new techniques became available—e.g., the use of DNA polymerase (reverse transcriptase) to make complementary DNA from mRNA templates, the mapping of DNA sequences by means of restriction endonucleases, and the cloning of DNA fragments—it was possible to identify coding, transcription, translation, and many other defects in the genetic machinery of both α- and β-thalassemic cells. This writer cannot trace the ramifications of this work, which is still ongoing and is discussed elsewhere in this book, nor would I presume to select the names of the investigators from among the many—in the United States, Great Britain, Greece, Thailand, and many other countries—who deserve special recognition. Suffice it to say that the elucidation of the defects in the various forms of thalassemia constitutes one of the great triumphs of biomedical and genetic research. The hoped-for conquest of these disorders surely will come from the application of this knowledge.

In yet another field, that of the enzymopathies, the red cell proved to be an almost inexhaustible source of information of equal interest to the hematologist and the geneticist. The point of departure was the 1956 report of Carson and associates[98] of a deficiency of glucose-6-phosphate dehydrogenase (G-6-PD) in primaquine-sensitive erythrocytes. Not only did this prove to be the explanation for the acute severe hemolytic anemia seen in certain adults who had received the antimalarial drug but, as shown within 2 years by Zinkham and Childs,[99] it also accounted for the then common hemolytic anemia associated with naphthalene poisoning in infants and young children (described in 1949 by this writer and Leonard Apt[100]), as well as for the previously mysterious hemolysis associated with favism, elucidated by Sansone in Genoa.[101] Through the investigations of Kirkman and co-workers[102] and those of Marks and associates,[103] it was soon apparent that G-6-PD deficiency is genetically as heterogeneous (and geographically as widespread) as are the thalassemias. Of special interest to the pediatric hematologist and to the neonatologist are the numerous reports of an association of G-6-PD deficiency and neonatal hyperbilirubinemia in certain Mediterranean and African countries, as well as in China. In addition to the many mutants of G-6-PD, all under the control of genes located on the X chromosome, other defects of the pentose pathway inherited as autosomal recessives were found, but these proved to be rare and chiefly of theoretical interest. Of greater importance for the understanding of the hereditary nonspherocytic hemolytic anemias was the discovery of a whole series of defects in the glycolytic pathway, beginning with pyruvate kinase deficiency, by Tanaka and Valentine and their co-workers.[104] Here too, an association with severe neonatal hyperbilirubinemia was observed. Here too, a high degree of genetic polymorphism soon became apparent. Today, when the well-equipped pediatric hematology laboratory must be able to perform a whole range of red cell enzyme studies as a matter of course, it seems strange that less than a generation ago the entire field of the enzymopathies was *terra incognita*.

The same can be said for several other areas of hematology that are today considered essential, but that were hardly dreamed of a few decades ago. One example is cellular immunity. During much of this writer's early career the thymus was a wholly mysterious organ, "status thymico-lymphaticus" was a widely accepted entity (and an indication for the ill-founded practice of "prophylactic" irradiation), and the different classes and functions of lymphocytes, T and B cells, and helper, suppressor,

and killer cells were unknown. Similarly, immunologic tolerance, self-recognition and graft-versus-host disease, the HLA system, and the importance of these observations for bone marrow transplantation (and transplantation in general) are now such well-established concepts that it is easy to forget how recently they were elaborated. Still another example involves the origin of the various lines of blood cells. The existence of a common ancestral cell in the bone marrow, which earlier generations of hematologists so heatedly debated for so many years, was not established until the 1960s, when morphologic arguments suddenly became irrelevant in the face of Till and McCulloch's[105] demonstration of pluripotential colony-forming cells, and the subsequent studies of these and many other workers elucidating the conditions of amplification and differentiation of these precursors. A comparable quantum jump occurred in the field of blood coagulation. Only those who had to deal with the horrendous problems of hemophiliacs in the days before cryoprecipitates and factor VIII (and IX) concentrates made replacement therapy and home care possible can truly appreciate the magnitude of this progress.

It cannot be our purpose here to give a complete overview of our subject. To do so would require a book of its own and duplicate much of the information contained in the following chapters. From what has been said it is clear that pediatric hematology has come into its own. After a prolonged infancy beset by semantic and morphologic woes, it has moved out of the descriptive and empirical phase into an era of functional and physiologic concepts well beyond the fondest dreams of the pioneers. In the process, it has again become part of the mainstream of hematology, yet preserved its identity and its impetus. It seems fitting that this text, which represents the sum of current knowledge, should begin with an account of this evolution and a tribute to those who brought it about, the men and women who did the best they could with the tools available to them and on whose work the new generation is building.

ADDENDUM

Wolf Zeulzer's history of pediatric hematology has graced the pages of this textbook since its inception, and the editors of this, the seventh edition, see no reason to alter it in any way. Zeulzer knew many of the individuals who began our field, and he described them and their contributions with consummate skill. Since Zeulzer's exposition, Howard Pearson, who also knew many of the main actors, has provided a more up-to-date history from the perspective of an active clinical investigator and teacher of the discipline.[106]

However, neither Zeulzer nor Pearson were given enough space to describe the impact of the genetics revolution of the 1960s and 1970s on all of pediatrics and particularly on pediatric hematology and oncology. The tools that made the enormous recent advances in our field possible were fashioned 40 years ago by basic scientists and first applied in globin genetics. Our burgeoning field has its present roots in the remarkable tumor virus program at Indiana University, where Luria, Dulbecco, and students such as Watson and Temin probed the human genome. The discovery of reverse transcriptase by Temin and Baltimore and of restriction enzymes by Nathans and Smith gave clinical investigators their first ability to attack the globin genes, discover the molecular basis of the disorders of hemoglobin, and develop prenatal diagnostics that could reduce disease incidence. Shortly thereafter and particularly after the discovery of polymerase chain reaction by Kary Mullis in the mid-1980s, the mysteries of the leukemias and the sarcomas began to be resolved and the complexities of the coagulopathies and disorders of immunity clarified. Pediatric hematology/oncology is now a discipline in full spate. However, its depth measurements have largely been made possible by basic molecular genetics laboratories.

All of this discovery and application through the science of clinical trial and outcome analysis has been of huge benefit to pediatrics and to patients and families, but the rate of change in our field has necessitated a marked alteration in our approach to training. In Pearson's history, attention is paid to the development of clinical board examinations, which are new creations of the past 25 years, but training programs that have as their primary goal achievement of a passing score on a long quiz make very little contribution to the growth and development of pediatric hematology and oncology. The real task is to create a clinically strong physician who has equally strong skills in biology, epidemiology, behavioral science, or biostatistics. These multiple demands strain trainees and trainers alike. The stress on trainees has been the subject of in-depth analysis by the National Institutes of Health (NIH), the agency most responsible for biomedical research training in the United States.[107] Although the NIH has made inroads on the problem,[108] the fact remains that the length of time necessary to train a fully qualified pediatric hematologist/oncologist who can make an intellectual contribution to the field is dauntingly long, and the training can never stop because the biologic rules of the road are ever changing. As Pearson emphasizes the complexity forces specialists to become subspecialists and even sub-sub-specialists.

All this growth of knowledge demands that pediatric hematologists/oncologists learn to work in teams and value each others' contributions. Training programs must instill a cooperative attitude while still retaining that necessary drive on the part of investigators and full-time clinicians to be considered the very best in their fields. That competitive spirit drives any intellectual effort, but it must be tempered with the realization that the skills of others may be sorely needed in the clinic or in wet and dry laboratories.

Zeulzer and Pearson give us reason to be very proud of the history of pediatric hematology and oncology. This textbook is written to help others to contribute to that fascinating history. The editors take satisfaction from knowing that some of the readers of this edition will do exactly that.

REFERENCES

1. Flesch H, quoted by Baar H, Stransky E. Die Klinische Hämatologie des Kindesalters. Leipzig, Germany, Franz Deuticke, 1928.
2. Halbrecht I. Role of hemo-agglutinins anti-A and anti-B in pathogenesis of the newborn (icterus neonatorum praecox). Am J Dis Child. 1964;45:1.
3. Lippman HS. A morphologic and quantitative study of the blood corpuscles in the new-born period. Am J Dis Child. 1924;27:473.
4. Neumann NA, quoted by Baar H, Stransky E. Die Klinische Hämatologie des Kindesalters. Leipzig, Germany, Franz Deuticke, 1928.
5. König H. Die Blutbefunde bei Neugeborenen. Folia Haematol (Leipz). 1910;9:278.
6. Friedländer A, Wiedemer C, quoted by Baar H, Stransky E. Die Klinische Hämatologie des Kindesalters. Leipzig, Germany, Franz Deuticke, 1928.
7. Ylppö A. Icterus neonatorum. Z Kinderheilk. 1913; 9:208.
8. Schiff E, Färber E. Beitrag zur Lehre des Icterus Neonatorum. Jb Kinderheilk. 1922;97:245.
9. Stransky E. In Baar H, Stransky E (eds). Die Klinische Hämatologie des Kindesalters. Leipzig, Germany, Franz Deuticke, 1928.
10. Lucas WP, Dearing BF. Blood volume in infants estimated by the vital dye method. Am J Dis Child. 1921;21:96.
11. Mollison PL, Veall N, Cutbush M. Red cell volume and plasma volume in newborn infants. Arch Dis Child. 1950; 25:242-253.
12. Zibordi F. Ematologia Infantile Normale e Patologica. Milano, Italy, Istituto Editoriale Scientifico, 1925.
13. Lucas WP, Fleischner EC. In Abt IA (ed). Pediatrics. Philadelphia, WB Saunders, 1924, p 406.
14. Billing BH, Lathe GH. The excretion of bilirubin as an ester glucuronide, giving the direct van den Bergh reaction. Biochem J. 1956;63:68.
15. Schmid R. Direct-reacting bilirubin, bilirubin glucuronide in serum, bile and urine. Science. 1956;124:76.
16. Talafant E. On the nature of direct and indirect bilirubin. V. The presence of glucuronic acid in the direct bile pigment. Chem Listy. 1956;50:1329.
17. Dutton GJ. Uridine-diphosphate-glucuronic acid and ester glucuronide synthesis. Biochemistry 1955;60: XIX.
18. Brown AK, Zuelzer WW. Studies on the neonatal development of the glucuronide conjugating system. J Clin Invest. 1958;37:332-340.
19. von Jaksch R, quoted by Baar H, Stransky E. Die Klinische Hämatologie des Kindesalters. Leipzig, Germany, Franz Deuticke, 1928.
20. Hayem G, quoted by Baar H, Stransky E. Die Klinische Hämatologie des Kindesalters. Leipzig, Germany, Franz Deuticke, 1928.
21. Luzet C. Etude sur L'Anémie de la Premiére Enfance et sur l'Anémie Enfantile Pseudoleucémique. Thése de Paris, 1891.

22. Lehndorff H. Jaksch-Hayem anaemia pseudoleucaemica infantum. Helv Paediatr Acta. 1963;18:1.

23. Cooley TB, Lee P. Series of cases of splenomegaly in children with anemia and peculiar bone changes. Trans Am Pediatr Soc. 1925;37:29.

24. Valentine WN, Neel JV. Hematologic and genetic study of the transmission of thalassemia (Cooley's anemia: Mediterranean anemia). Arch Intern Med. 1944;74:185.

25. Cooley TB, Lee P. Sickle cell anemia in a Greek family. Am J Dis Child. 1929;38:103.

26. Cooley TB. A severe type of hereditary anemia with elliptocytosis. Am J Med Sci. 1945;209:561.

27. Rundles LW, Falls HF. Hereditary (sex-linked) anemia. Am J Med Sci. 1946;211:641.

28. Cooley TB, Lee P. Erythroblastic anemia, additional comments. Am J Dis Child. 1932;43:705.

29. Guest GM. Hypoferric Anemia in Infancy. Symposium on Nutrition, Robert Gould Research Foundation, Cincinnati, OH, 1947.

30. Guest GM. Studies of blood glycolysis: sugar and phosphorus relationships during glycolysis in normal blood. J Clin Invest. 1932;11:555.

31. Guest GM, Rapoport S. Organic acid–soluble phosphorus compounds of the blood. Physiol Rev. 1941;21:410.

32. Guest GM. Osmometric behavior of normal and abnormal human erythrocytes. Blood. 1948;3:541.

33. Baar H. Die Anämien. In Baar H, Stransky E (eds). Die Klinische Hämatologie des Kindesalters. Leipzig, Germany, Franz Deuticke, 1928.

34. Haldane and Smith, quoted by Lucas WP, Fleischner EC. In Abt IA (ed). Pediatrics. Philadelphia, WB Saunders, 1924, pp 406-623.

35. Josephs HW. Anaemia of infancy and early childhood. Medicine (Baltimore). 1936;15:307.

36. Blackfan KD, Diamond LK. Atlas of the Blood in Children. New York, The Commonwealth Fund, 1944.

37. Josephs HW. Iron metabolism and the hypochromic anemia of infancy. Medicine (Baltimore). 1953;22:125.

38. Sturgeon P. Iron metabolism: a review. Pediatrics. 1956; 18:267.

39. Chown B. Anaemia in a newborn due to the fetus bleeding into the mother's circulation: proof of the bleeding. Lancet. 1954;1:1213.

40. Kleihauer E, Betke K. Praktische Anwendung des Nachweises von Hb F—haltigen Zellen in fixierten Blutausstrichen. Internist. 1960;6:292.

41. Cohen F, Zuelzer WW, Gustafson DC, Evans MM. Mechanisms of isoimmunization. I. The transplacental passage of fetal erythrocytes in homospecific pregnancies. Blood. 1964;23:621-646.

42. Hart AP. Familial icterus gravis of the newborn and its treatment. Can Med Assoc. 1925;15:1008.

43. Wallerstein H. Erythroblastosis foetalis and its treatment. Lancet. 1946;2:922.

44. Sidbury JB. Transfusion through the umbilical vein in hemorrhage of the newborn. Am J Dis Child. 1923; 25:290.

45. Diamond LK, Allen FH, Thomas WO. Erythroblastosis fetalis. VII. Treatment with exchange transfusion. N Engl J Med. 1951;244:39-49.

46. Allen FH, Diamond LK, Vaughan VC. Erythroblastosis fetalis. VI. Prevention of kernicterus. AMA Am J Dis Child. 1950;80:779-791.

47. Robertson B. Exsanguination-transfusion: a new therapeutic measure in the treatment of severe toxemias. Arch Surg. 1924;9:1.

48. Siperstein DM, Sansby TM. Intraperitoneal transfusion with citrated blood: an experimental study. Am J Dis Child. 1923;25:107.

49. Siperstein DM. Intraperitoneal transfusion with citrated blood: a clinical study. Am J Dis Child. 1923;25:203.

50. Heinild S, Søndergaard T, et al. Bone marrow infusion in childhood. J Pediatr. 1947;30:400.

51. Zuelzer WW, Ogden F. Megaloblastic anemia in infancy. Am J Dis Child. 1946;71:211.

52. Amato M. Rilievi anamnesto-clinici_._._. su 25 casi di anemie ipercromiche megaloblastiche osservate in bambini della prima infanzia. Pediatria. 1946;54:71.

53. Veeneklaas GMH. Über Megalozytäre Mangelanämien bei Kleinkindern. Folia Haematol (Leipz). 1940;65:203.

54. Kato K. Sternal marrow puncture in infants. Am J Dis Child. 1937;54:209.

55. Vogel P, Bassen FA. Sternal marrow of children in normal and in pathologic states. Am J Dis Child. 1939;57:246.

56. Fanconi G. Die primären Anämien und Erythroblastosen im Kindesalter. Monatsschr Kinderheilkd. 1937;68:129.

57. Willi H, quoted by Rohr K. Das Menschliche Knochenmark. Stuttgart, Germany, Georg Thieme Verlag, 1949.

58. Gasser C. Akute Erythroblastopenie. Helv Paediatr Acta. 1949;4:107.

59. Gasser C. Die Pathogenese der essentiellen chronischen Granulocytopenie. Helv Paediatr Acta. 1952;7:426.

60. Zuelzer WW, Bajoghli M. Chronic granulocytopenia in childhood. Blood. 1964;23:359.

61. Kostmann R. Infantile genetic agranulocytosis (agranulocytosis infantilis hereditaria). A new recessive lethal disease in man. Acta Paediatr. 1956;45(Suppl 105):1.

62. Zuelzer WW. "Myelokathexis"—a new form of chronic granulocytopenia. Report of a case. N Engl J Med. 1964;270:699.

63. Krill CE, Smith HD, Mauer AM. Chronic idiopathic granulocytopenia. N Engl J Med. 1964;270:973-979.

64. Fanconi F. Familiäre infantile perniciosa-artige Anämie (Perniziöses Blutbild und Konstitution). Jb Kinderheilk. 1927;117:257.

65. Glanzmann E. Hereditäre hämorrhagische Thrombasthenie. Jb Kinderheilk. 1918;88:113.

66. Glanzmann E. Die Konzeption der anaphylaktoiden Purpura. Jb Kinderheilk. 1920;91:371.

67. Owren PA. Congenital hemolytic jaundice. The pathogenesis of the "hemolytic crisis." Blood. 1948;3:231.

68. Gasser C. Die Hämolytischen Syndrome des Kindesalters. Stuttgart, Germany, Georg Thieme Verlag, 1951.

69. Grumbach A, Gasser C. ABO-Inkompatibilitäten und Morbus Hemolyticus Neonatorum. Helv Paediatr Acta. 1948;3:447.

70. Gasser C, Karrer J. Deletäre hämolytische Anämie mit "Spontan-Innen-Körper" Bildung bei Frühgeburten. Helv Paediatr Acta. 1948;3:387.

71. Tuffy P, Brown AK, Zuelzer WW. Infantile pyknocytosis; a common erythrocyte abnormality of the first trimester. AMA J Dis Child. 1959;98:227-241.

72. Parsons LG. The haemolytic anaemias of childhood. Lancet. 1938;2:1395.

73. Diamond LK, Blackfan FD, et al. Erythroblastosis foetalis and its association with universal edema of the fetus,

icterus gravis neonatorum and anemia of the newborn. J Pediatr. 1932;1:269.

74. Diamond LK, Blackfan KD. Hypoplastic anemia. Am J Dis Child. 1938;54:464.

75. Smith CH. Blood Diseases of Infancy and Childhood. 2nd ed. St Louis, CV Mosby, 1966.

76. Sturgeon P. Volumetric and microscopic pattern of bone marrow in normal infants and children. II. Cytologic pattern. Pediatrics. 1951;7:642.

77. Darrow RR. Icterus gravis neonatorum. An examination of etiologic considerations. Arch Pathol. 1938;25:378.

78. Landsteiner K, Wiener AS. An agglutinable factor in human blood recognized by human sera for rhesus blood. Proc Soc Exp Biol Med. 1940;43:223.

79. Wiener AS, Peters HR. Hemolytic reactions following transfusions of blood of the homologous group with 3 cases in which the same agglutinogen was responsible. Ann Intern Med. 1946;13:2306.

80. Levine P, Katzin EM, et al. Atypical warm isoagglutinins. Proc Soc Exp Biol Med. 1940;45:346.

81. Levine P, Katzin EM, et al. Isoimmunization in pregnancy, its possible bearing on the etiology of erythroblastosis fetalis. JAMA. 1941;116:825.

82. Levine P, Burnham L, et al. The role of isoimmunization in the pathogenesis of erythroblastosis fetalis. Am J Obstet Gynecol. 1941;42:825.

83. Wiener AS. A new test (blocking test) for Rh sensitization. Proc Soc Exp Biol Med. 1944;56:173.

84. Wiener AS. Pathogenesis of congenital hemolytic disease (erythroblastosis fetalis) I. Theoretic considerations. Am J Dis Child. 1946;71:14.

85. Wiener AS, Wexler IB. The use of heparin in performing exchange transfusions in newborn infants. J Lab Clin Med. 1946;31:1016.

86. Clarke CA. Prevention of Rh hemolytic disease. Br Med J. 1967;4:7.

87. Freda VJ, Gorman JG, Pollack W, et al. Prevention of Rh isoimmunization. Progress report of the clinical trial in mothers. JAMA. 1967;199:390-394.

88. Farber S, Diamond LK, et al. Temporary remissions in acute leukemia in children produced by folic acid antagonist, 4-aminopteroylglutamic acid (aminopterin). N Engl J Med. 1948;238:787.

89. Pauling L, Itano AH, et al. Sickle cell anemia, a molecular disease. Science. 1949;110:543.

90. Neel JV. The inheritance of sickle cell anemia. Science. 1949;110:64.

91. Ingram VM. A specific chemical difference between the globins of normal human and sickle cell anaemia haemoglobin. Nature. 1956;178:792.

92. Ingram VM. The chemical difference between normal human and sickle cell anaemia haemoglobins. Conference on Hemoglobin. Publication No. 557, National Academy of Sciences–National Research Council, 1958, pp 233-238.

93. Itano HA. The human hemoglobins: their properties and genetic control. Adv Protein Chem. 1957;12:216.

94. Ingram VM, Stretton AOW. Genetic basis of the thalassaemia diseases. Nature. 1959;184:1903.

95. Weatherall DJ, Clegg JB, Naughton MA. Globin synthesis in thalassaemia. Nature. 1965;208:1061-1065.

96. Nienhuis AW, Anderson WF. Isolation and translation of hemoglobin messenger RNA from thalassemia, sickle cell anemia, and normal human reticulocytes. J Clin Invest. 1971;50:2458.

97. Benz EJ, Forget BC. Defect in messenger RNA for human hemoglobin synthesis in beta thalassemia. J Clin Invest. 1971;50:2755.

98. Carson PE, Flanagan CL, et al. Enzymatic deficiency in primaquine-sensitive erythrocytes. Science. 1956;124:484.

99. Zinkham WH, Childs B. A defect of glutathione metabolism in erythrocytes from patients with a naphthalene-induced hemolytic anemia. Pediatrics. 1958;22:461.

100. Zuelzer WW, Apt L. Acute hemolytic anemia due to naphthalene poisoning, a clinical and experimental study. JAMA. 1949;141:185.

101. Sansone G, Piga AM, et al. Favismo. Torino, Italy, Minerva Medica, 1958.

102. Kirkman HN, Riley HD, Crowell BB. Different enzymic expressions of mutants of human glucose-6-phosphate dehydrogenase. Proc Natl Acad Sci U S A. 1960;46:938-944.

103. Marks PA, Szeinberg A, Banks J. Erythrocyte glucose 6-phosphate dehydrogenase of normal and mutant subjects: properties of the purified enzymes. J Biol Chem. 1961;236:10-17.

104. Tanaka KR, Valentine WN, Miwa S. Pyruvate kinase (PK) deficiency hereditary nonspherocytic hemolytic anaemia. Blood. 1962;19:267-295.

105. Till JE, McCulloch EA. Direct measurement of the radiation sensitivity of normal mouse bone marrow cells. Radiat Res. 1961;14:213.

106. Pearson HA. History of pediatric hematology oncology. Pediatr Res. 2002;52:979-992.

107. Nathan DG. The several Cs of translational clinical research. J Clin Invest. 2005;115:795-797.

108. Nathan DG, Wilson JD. Clinical research and the NIH—a report card. N Engl J Med. 2003;349:1860-1865.

II Neonatal Hematology

2

The Neonatal Erythrocyte and Its Disorders

Carlo Brugnara and Orah S. Platt

THE NEONATAL ERYTHROCYTE

At no other time in the life of a patient is the physician confronted with as many diagnostic considerations in the interpretation of apparent disturbances in the erythrocyte as during the neonatal period.

The erythrocytes produced by the human fetus are fundamentally different from those produced by older infants and children. These cells possess different membrane properties, different hemoglobins, a unique metabolic profile, and a much shorter red cell life span. In a variety of pathologic conditions, erythrocytes bearing some of the properties of fetal erythrocytes again appear in the circulation. A better understanding of the factors that regulate fetal erythropoiesis and a precise definition of the fetal erythrocyte may eventually result in the development of a unifying hypothesis that explains these acquired disorders of erythropoiesis. Interpretation of hematologic abnormalities in neonates is confounded by the interactions of genetics, acquired disease in the neonate, and maternal factors with the gestationally related peculiarities of the fetal erythrocyte.

Development of Erythropoiesis

Hematopoiesis in the embryo and fetus can be divided into three periods conceptually: mesoblastic, hepatic, and myeloid (see also Chapter 6).[1-3] All blood cells are derived from embryonic connective tissue—the mesenchyme—and blood formation can first be detected by the 14th day of gestation. Isolated foci of erythropoiesis can be observed throughout the extraembryonic mesoblastic tissue in the area vasculosa of the yolk sac at 3 to 4 weeks after conception. Blood islands in the yolk sac differentiate in two directions. Peripheral cells in the islands form the walls of the first blood vessels, whereas the centrally located cells become the primitive blood cells, or hematocytoblasts.[4,5] The hemangioblast has been shown to be a common precursor for both blood and endothelial cells.[6,7] This three-stage migration of hematopoietic precursors from an initial vascular-mesoblastic area to a definitive erythropoietic organ via an intermediate stage seems to be conserved ontogenically, even between mammals and zebra fish.[8]

The first blood cells produced by the embryo belong to the red cell series. Two distinct generations of erythrocytes can be observed in the developing embryo. Red cells arise as a result of either primitive megaloblastic erythropoiesis or definitive normoblastic erythropoiesis. Both megaloblasts and normoblasts apparently derive from similar-appearing hematocytoblasts and develop through roughly similar but morphologically distinct series of erythroblasts. In the very early embryo, red cells arise from primitive erythroblasts. These cells were termed "megaloblasts" by Ehrlich because of their resemblance to the erythroid precursors found in patients with pernicious anemia.[9] Megaloblasts are large cells with abundant polychromatophilic cytoplasm, and they possess a nucleus in which fine chromatin is widely dispersed. Megaloblasts give rise to large, irregularly shaped, somewhat hypochromic erythrocytes that can be seen in circulating blood 4 to 5 weeks after conception. The primitive erythroblasts arise primarily from intravascular sites; as development continues, these cells are gradually replaced by smaller cells of the definitive or normoblastic series.

Normoblastic erythropoiesis begins at about the 6th gestational week, and enucleated macrocytes enter the circulation by the 8th week; by the 10th week of development, normoblastic erythropoiesis accounts for more than 90% of the circulating erythrocytic cells. Maturation of normoblastic erythroid cells resembles that seen in postnatal life, and these cells give rise to enucleated erythrocytes and are primarily extravascular.

By about the fifth to sixth week of gestation, blood formation begins in the liver. In the period between the 5th and 10th weeks, the liver undergoes a substantial increase in size, with an associated increase in the total nucleated cell count from 2.3×10^6 to 1.7×10^8 cells.[10] The fetal liver appears to be a site of pure erythropoiesis, and during the third to fifth months of gestation, erythroid precursors represent approximately 50% of the total nucleated cells of this organ.[11] Migration of pluripotent cells and early progenitors via the bloodstream is probably responsible for the transition from yolk sac to liver.[10] However, more recently it has been proposed that circulating stem cells and progenitors do not derive from the yolk sac but from an intraembryonic site, the so-called aorta-gonad-mesonephros (AGM) region.[12,13] This is supported by the fact that stem cells derived from the yolk sac can produce transient primitive hematopoiesis but cannot reconstitute definitive hematopoiesis[14,15] (Fig. 2-1).

The liver is the chief organ of hematopoiesis from the third to the sixth fetal month and continues to produce formed elements into the first postnatal week (Fig. 2-2). During the third fetal month, hematopoiesis can also be detected in the spleen and thymus and, shortly afterward, in the lymph nodes. Blood cell formation can still be observed in the spleen during the first week of postnatal life.

Fukuda used electron microscopy to examine the characteristics of hepatic hematopoiesis in 26 human embryos and fetuses from 26 days after conception to 30 weeks of gestation.[16] The development of hepatic hematopoiesis appeared to correlate closely with histologic development of the liver. In the earliest stages of hepatic hematopoiesis, undifferentiated mononuclear cells, presumably stem cells, were present in the intercellular spaces of hepatocytes. With maturation of the fetus, the number of erythroid cells in the hepatic parenchyma increased, and stem cells diminished in number and eventually disappeared. These stem cells were exclusively observed in the extravascular spaces and were thought to derive from the septum transversum.

Erythropoietic progenitors from the livers of fetuses studied between 13 and 23 weeks of gestation appear to

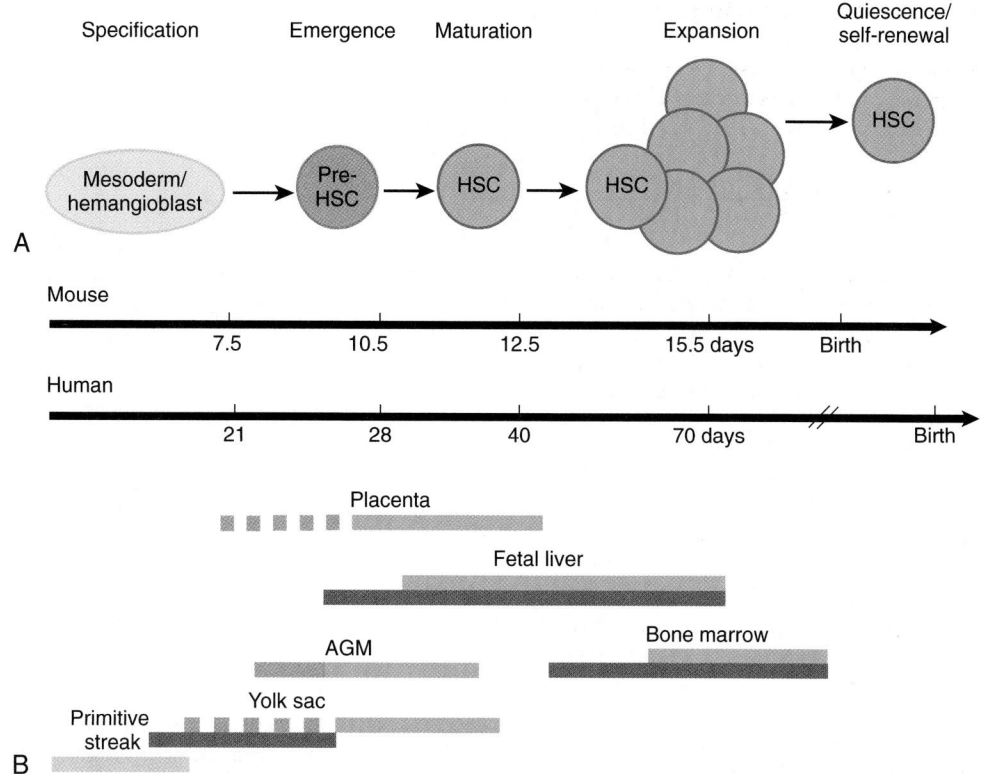

FIGURE 2-1. Establishment of definitive hematopoietic stem cell (HSC) pools in mouse and human embryos. **A,** Hematopoietic development starts as specification of primitive streak mesoderm (yellow) into hematopoietic and vascular fates. Nascent HSCs undergo a maturation process (blue) that allows them to engraft, survive, and self-renew in future hematopoietic niches. Subsequently, fetal HSCs expand rapidly, after which a steady state is established in which HSCs reside in a relatively quiescent state in the bone marrow. **B,** Ages at which mouse and human hematopoietic sites are active. *Yellow bars,* mesoderm; *red bars,* active hematopoietic differentiation; *orange bars,* HSC genesis; *blue bars,* presence of functional adult-type HSCs. *Broken orange bars* for the yolk sac and placenta indicate that de novo HSC genesis has not been experimentally proven. AGM, aorta-gonad-mesonephros. *(Redrawn from Mikkola HKA, Orkin SH. The journey of developing hematopoietic stem cells. Development. 2006; 133:3733-3744.)*

be more sensitive to humoral stimuli—colony-forming units–erythrocyte (CFU-E) for erythropoietin (EPO) and burst-forming units–erythrocyte (BFU-E) for burst-promoting activity—than progenitors from adult bone marrow do.[17] Large numbers of multipotent and committed (erythroid and granulocytic-monocytic) progenitor cells have been found in blood obtained by fetoscopy at 12 to 19 weeks of gestation.[12,18] These fetal progenitor cells are more sensitive than adult progenitor cells grown under the same conditions to appropriate stimuli, presumably as a consequence of intrinsic differences in the progenitor cells of fetal origin.[19,20] Functional and genetic differences between fetal and adult stem cells indicate that the hematopoietic stem cell is not an invariable cell type.[21]

The myeloid period of hematopoiesis commences during the fourth to fifth fetal month and becomes quantitatively important by the sixth fetal month. During the last 3 months of gestation, the bone marrow is the chief site of blood cell formation. Marrow cellularity becomes maximal at about the 30th gestational week, although the volume of marrow occupied by hematopoietic tissue continues to increase until term.[21] A summary of the time of

first appearance of the different blood cells in the various fetal hematopoietic organs, based on the observations of Kelemen and associates from an analysis of 190 fetuses and embryos, is provided in Table 2-1.[22]

Cord blood is rich in bone marrow progenitor cells and contains multipotential cell lines: granulocyte-erythroid-monocyte-macrophage (CFU-GEMM), erythroid (BFU-E), and granulocyte-macrophage (CFU-GM).[23] The frequency of circulating CFU-GM from the 23rd week of gestation to full term is consistently high and provides evidence that CFU-GM is produced in the yolk sac, as well as at other hematopoietic sites.[24] The frequency of BFU-E is highest at midgestation, with values being 3-fold greater than those for cord blood and 10-fold greater than those for adult bone marrow.[25] CD34+ circulating progenitors also peak at the second trimester and fall thereafter, with an inverse relationship with gestational age noted between 24 and 40 weeks.[26,27] Table 2-2 shows a comparison of circulating hematopoietic progenitors at different gestational ages.[18]

The in vitro behavior of progenitor cells obtained from umbilical cord blood is substantially different from that of progenitor cells in the bone marrow of adults. In

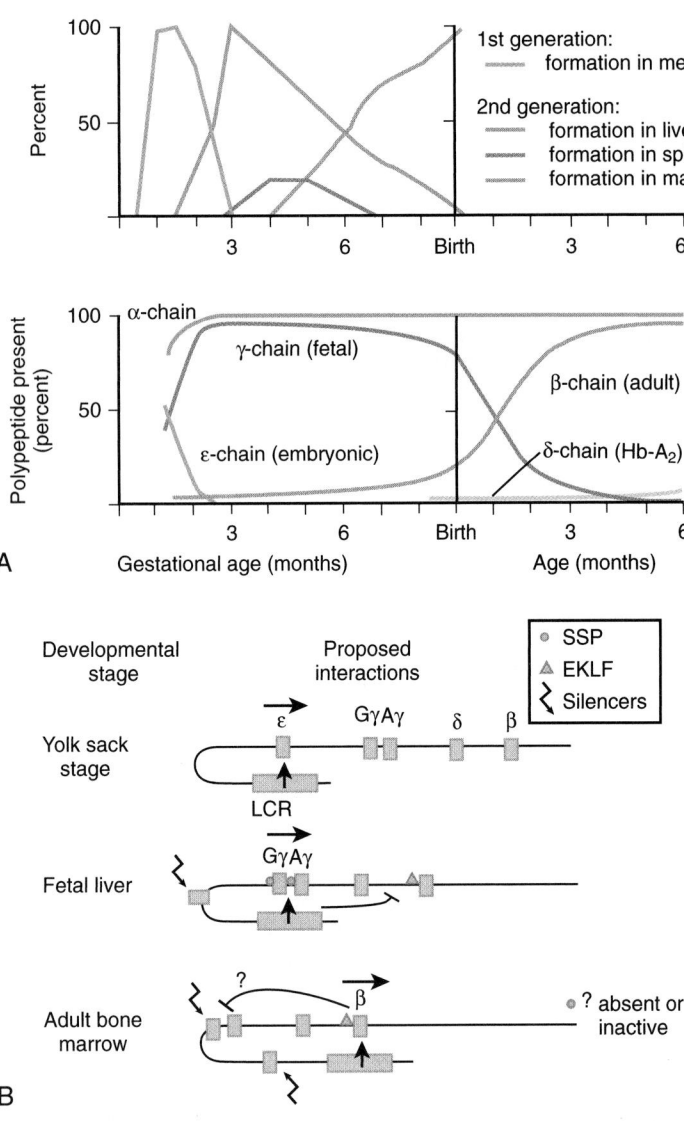

FIGURE 2-2. A, Hematopoietic sites and development of different globin chains during fetal life and early infancy. **B,** Globin gene switching in the human β-globin gene cluster. Some of the postulated interactions at each developmental stage of the human are indicated. *Arcs* ending in *oblique lines* are meant to depict competitive interactions. In the fetal liver stage, interaction of the β-globin genes with the locus control region (LCR) prevents β-globin expression despite the presence of EKLF, a β-globin gene–specific activator. In adult bone marrow erythroid cells, interaction of the β-globin gene with the LCR may facilitate shutoff of the β-globin gene (as indicated by ?). Though not established, EKLF is shown bound to the β-globin promoter at the fetal stage to emphasize that transcription of β-globin genes prevails even in its presence. The status of the stage-selector protein (SSP) complex, as well as the postulated embryonic/fetal-specific subunit in adult cells, is unknown (as shown at the *bottom*). It is likely that SSP is present at the yolk sac stage. If such is the case, interactions between the β-globin gene and the LCR presumably are dominant for β-globin expression. (*A, After Knoll W, Pingel E. Der Gang der Erythropoese beim menschlichen Embryo. Acta Haematol. 1949;2:369-380, with permission of Karger, Basel; and Huehns ER, Dance N, Beaven GH, et al. Human embryonic hemoglobins. Symp Quant Biol. 1964;29: 327-331. B, Redrawn from Orkin SH. Regulation of globin gene expression in erythroid cells. Eur J Biochem. 1995;231:271-281.)*

TABLE 2-1   First Appearance of Different Blood Cell Types in Hematopoietic Organs and in Circulating Blood, Given by Fertilization Age in Weeks

	Extraembryonic*	Liver	Thymus	Spleen	Lymph Nodes	Bone Marrow	Blood
Primitive erythroblasts	3-4	5	—	8	—	—	3-4
Definitive erythroblasts	6-7†	5	10	8	11	8-9	6-7
Granulocytes	3-4‡	5	10	8	12	8-9	7-8
Monocytes (classic)	—	?	—	11	12-13	11	7-8
Histiocytes, macrophages	3-4	5	10	8	11	8-9	3-4
Megakaryocytes, platelets	5†	5	—	11	—	8-9	6-7
Lymphocytes	6	6	8	8	9-12	10-12	7-9
Mast cells§	—	—	—	—	—	—	—

*Yolk sac, chorion, allantois, and body stalk.
†From circulating blood?
‡Maternal origin is possible.
§Bone marrow was the only site where substantial amounts of mast cells were distinguished.
From Kelemen E, Calvo W, Filedner TM. Atlas of Human Hemopoietic Development. Berlin, Springer-Verlag, 1979.

TABLE 2-2	Hematopoietic Progenitors Circulating in Fetal Blood			
Median Gestational Age (Range)	**CFU-GEMM Total**	**CFU-GM**	**BFU-E**	**Number of Progenitors ($\times 10^3$/mL)***
10^{+0} weeks (7^{+6}-13^{+1})	10.5 ± 1.3	3.3 ± 0.4	5.4 ± 0.8	19.2 ± 2.1
15^{+0} weeks (14^{+5}-20^{+0})	$32.5 \pm 15.7^{\dagger}$	$31.4 \pm 12.0^{\ddagger}$	$19.7 \pm 12.6^{\dagger}$	$83.6 \pm 31.3^{\ddagger}$
39^{+0} weeks (38^{+0}-40^{+0})	5.6 ± 0.7	9.7 ± 5.7	$11.1 \pm 2.1^{\dagger}$	26.4 ± 5.6

*Mean ± SEM.
[†]$P < .01$ in comparing mean ± SEM with the first trimester.
[‡]$P < .0001$ in comparing mean ± SEM with the first trimester.
BFU-E, burst-forming unit–erythrocyte; CFU-GEMM, colony-forming unit–granulocyte, erythrocyte, macrophage, megakaryocyte; CFU-GM, colony-forming unit–granulocyte-macrophage.
From Campagnoli C, Fisk NM, Overton T, et al. Circulating hematopoietic progenitor cells in first trimester fetal blood. Blood. 2000;95:1967-1972.

contrast to adult progenitors, which require the presence of multiple growth factors, fetal progenitors can mature in vitro with no growth factors present or with the addition of only one. Recombinant human erythropoietin (r-HuEPO),[28,29] interleukin-6,[30] interleukin-9,[31] and interleukin-11[32] are active as single agents in fetal but not adult progenitors. It has been shown that in vitro cultures of CD34+ fetal hematopoietic progenitors produce hematopoietic factors such as granulocyte-macrophage colony-stimulating factor (GM-CSF) and interleukin-3, which can sustain their growth factor–independent proliferation.[33] Exit from the G_0/G_1 phase of the cell cycle in response to stem cell factor is also accelerated in umbilical cord blood CD34+ cells.[34]

Adult hematopoietic stem cells are mostly quiescent, whereas fetal ones cycle at a higher rate.[35] An intrinsically regulated master switch takes place 3 to 4 weeks after birth (in mice) and facilitates the change from "fetal" to the "adult" type of hematopoietic stem cells.[36-38]

The number of hematopoietic progenitors in cord blood is in the range of the requirements for successful engraftment by bone marrow cells.[23] Although the average cord blood collection contains only 14% of the nucleated cells present in an autologous bone marrow collection, it contains 91.6% of the CFU-GM colonies, 24% of the CFU-GEMM colonies, and 29% of the BFU-E colonies.[23] Studies of long-term culture–initiating cells have indicated that the number of putative stem cells in cord blood is comparable to that of allogeneic bone marrow or peripheral stem cell collections.[39]

Human umbilical cord blood has been used successfully for hematopoietic reconstitution in patients with Fanconi's anemia,[40] aplastic anemia, X-linked lymphoproliferative disease, sickle cell anemia, leukemia, immune deficiency, genetic and metabolic diseases (e.g., Hunter's syndrome),[41,42] and severe hemoglobin E–β-thalassemia disease.[43-46] For recent reviews, see Ballen and Symthe and colleagues.[47,48] The clinical use of umbilical cord blood may be expanded based on evidence of the presence of vascular/endothelial progenitor cells.[49]

After birth, the amount of marrow tissue continues to grow, with no apparent increase in cellular concentration. The only way for an infant to increase cell production is to effect a more rapid turnover of cells or to increase the volume of hematopoietic tissue. This increase in tissue produces the marrow expansion that is most readily observed in the calvaria.

An increasing role for EPO is observed during the hepatic and myeloid phases of erythropoiesis. EPO is detectable in the cord blood of nonanemic premature infants in quantities that are comparable to or greater than those in the blood of normal adults.[50] Fetal erythropoiesis is only partially influenced by maternal factors and is primarily under control of the fetus. In the mouse, suppression of maternal erythropoiesis by hypertransfusion does not suppress fetal erythropoiesis,[51] nor does stimulation of maternal EPO production result in stimulation of fetal red cell production; these findings indicate that EPO is incapable of crossing the placenta.[52] The exact site of EPO production in the fetus is unknown, but the liver is a probable candidate. In other animal species, nephrectomy of the fetus does not influence EPO production or the erythropoietic response to stress such as bleeding.[53]

The development of hematopoiesis is controlled by the effect of growth factors on cell proliferation and activation of lineage-specific genes by transcription factors (nuclear regulators).[2,54] Some genes, such as *Scl/Tal1* (stem cell leukemia protein) and *Klf6*, are crucial for the embryonal development of both endothelial and hematopoietic cells.[55-57] The divergence of hematopoietic stem cells from their hemangioblastic precursor is accompanied first by the expression of CD41 (GBIIb, a megakaryocytic/platelet marker in adult hematopoiesis) and c-kit and then by the panhematopoietic marker CD45.[58] Some other genes, such as *Notch1*, and growth factors, such as hepatocyte growth factor (HGF) and bone morphogenic protein (BMP), are essential for early hematopoietic development but may not be required for definitive hematopoiesis.[59-63] Others, such as *Runx1*, *AML1/EVI1*, and other members of the AML1-CBFβ transcription factor complex, and genes crucial for the erythropoietic microenvironment, such as *paladin*, are essential for the establishment of definitive erythropoiesis.[64-66]

For each cell lineage, cell-specific transcription depends on critical DNA-binding motifs in promoters or enhancers. Differentiation in the erythroid series depends on the presence of GATA- and AP-1/NFE2-binding proteins, as well as the transcription factors TAL1/SCL, EKLF, RBTN2, GATA-1, and GATA-2.[54,67-70]

A *GATA1* mutation has been shown to be responsible for a form of familial dyserythropoietic anemia and thrombocytopenia.[71] Other mutations have been described in newborns with Down syndrome and in a case of congenital erythropoietic porphyria.[72,73]

STAT5 is a latent cytoplasmic transcription factor, which after activation of the EPO receptor, binds to phosphorylated tyrosines on the receptor and itself becomes tyrosine-phosphorylated.[74,75] This process results in STAT5 dimerization and translocation to the nucleus, where it initiates transcription of target genes. STAT5 is critical during fetal erythropoiesis.[75] Mice mutant for both isoforms of STAT5 (STAT5A and STAT5B) show a profound alteration in fetal (definitive) erythropoiesis.[76] Fetal liver cells give rise to fewer erythroid colonies, and a marked increase in apoptosis is seen in vitro. [76] The fetal anemia of STAT5a$^{-/-}$5b$^{-/-}$ mice seems to resolve in 50% of adults, but adult mice are deficient in generating high erythropoietic rates in response to stress.[77] STAT5a$^{-/-}$5b$^{-/-}$ hematopoietic tissue shows a dramatic increase in early erythroblast numbers, but these cells fail to progress in differentiation.[77] The effects seen in the STAT5a$^{-/-}$5b$^{-/-}$ mice are mostly mediated by decreased expression of bcl-x$_L$, which is a crucial determinant of early erythroblast survival and plays a major role in fetal erythroid development and response to stress.[78] Thus, both STAT5 and bcl-x$_L$ seem to be crucial not only for fetal hematopoietic development but also for response to erythropoietic stress in adulthood.

Erythroid progenitors found in the liver, bone marrow, or peripheral blood of the fetus appear to produce identical quantities of fetal hemoglobin (HbF).[79] Fetal erythropoiesis results in the orderly evolution of a series of different hemoglobins. Developmentally, there is embryonic, fetal, and adult hemoglobin (Table 2-3). Globin genes are arranged in order of expression in the α- and β-globin clusters and are selectively activated and silenced at the various stages of erythroid development. Distal, *cis*-regulatory elements in the β-globin–like cluster are contained in the locus control region (LCR), which consists of four hypersensitivity sites[80]; additional *cis*-regulatory downstream core elements (DCEs) have also been described.[81] Figure 2-1 presents some of the postulated interactions involved in gene switching for the human β-globin gene cluster.

The first globin chains to be produced are the ε chains, which appear to be similar to β chains in certain aspects of their structural sequences.[82] Before other chains begin to form, these unpaired globin chains may form tetramers (ε$_4$) that result in the presence of hemoglobin Gower-1 (Hb Gower-1). Almost immediately thereafter, α- and ζ-chain production begins, and Hb Gower-2 (α$_2$ε$_2$) and Hb Portland (ζ$_2$γ$_2$) are formed. Early γ-chain formation also results in the presence of HbF (α$_2$γ$_2$). By the time that the fetus has a crown-rump length of about 16 mm (about 37 days of gestation), Hb Gower-1 and Gower-2 constitute 42% and 24% of the total hemoglobin, respectively, with HbF accounting for the remainder.[83] At a crown-rump length of about 30 mm, HbF represents 50% of the total hemoglobin, and at a length of 50 mm it is responsible for more than 90% of the hemoglobin. Very small quantities of HbA begin to be found at 6 to 8 weeks of gestation.

Although Hb Portland may constitute as much as 20% of the hemoglobin at 10 weeks of gestation, only trace amounts are normally present at birth. The ζ chain is quite similar to the α chain in its amino acid sequences.[84] Studies of steady-state liver messenger ribonucleic acid (mRNA) globin levels in human embryos (gestational age, 10 to 25 weeks) indicate that levels of globin proteins are regulated by the relative amount of each globin mRNA.[85] Studies on the physiologic properties of embryonal hemoglobin will be facilitated by their recent expression in a transgenic mouse model.[86]

The absolute rate of synthesis of hemoglobin or formation of red cells during fetal life is difficult to estimate because neither the absolute increase in circulating hemoglobin or red cells nor the absolute rate of destruction is known. The absolute rate of production of red cells at birth, however, can be estimated fairly well. A value of 2.5% to 3.0% per day of the circulating red cell mass, or about 4.5 mL/day in a 3.5-kg infant, can be calculated by determining the relative number of circulating reticulocytes and the in vitro mean life span of reticulocytes obtained from cord blood.[87] A very similar figure was obtained by analysis of the distribution kinetics of radioiron in plasma and red cells (Fig. 2-3).[88]

The intrinsic stability of embryonic, fetal, and adult hemoglobin differs by 3 orders of magnitude, with subunit interface strength increasing from the embryonic to the fetal to the adult types. These differences may play a role in determining the life span of the three cell types.[89]

Measurement of circulating red cell volume in newborn infants at various gestational ages, as shown in Figure 2-4, demonstrated an increase in red cell mass of about 1.5% per day.[90] Assuming a mean life span of these cells of 45 to 70 days (discussed later in this chapter), these data show a production rate of 3.6% to 4.2% per

TABLE 2-3	Globin Chain Development	
Stage	**Hemoglobin**	**Composition**
Embryo	Gower 1	ε$_4$ or ζ$_2$ε$_2$
Embryo	Gower 2	α$_2$ε$_2$
Embryo	Portland	ζ$_2$γ$_2$
Embryo	Fetal	α$_2$γ$_2$
Fetus	Fetal	α$_2$γ$_2$
Fetus	A	α$_2$β$_2$
Adult	A	α$_2$β$_2$
Adult	A$_2$	α$_2$δ$_2$
Adult	F	α$_2$γ$_2$

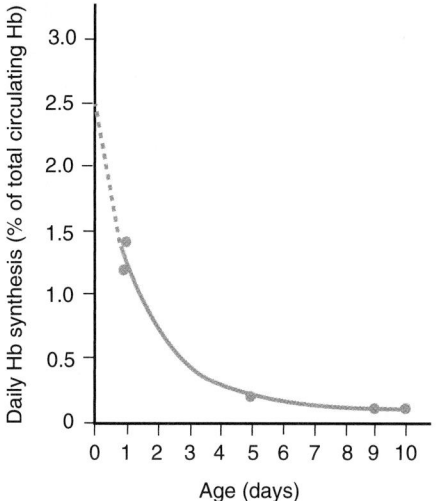

FIGURE 2-3. Relative rate of hemoglobin (Hb) synthesis at birth and during the first 10 days of life. *(Redrawn from Garby L, Sjölin S, Vuille JC. Studies on erythro-kinetics in infancy. III. Plasma disappearance and red-cell uptake of radio-active iron injected intravenously. Acta Paediatr. 1963;52:537-553.)*

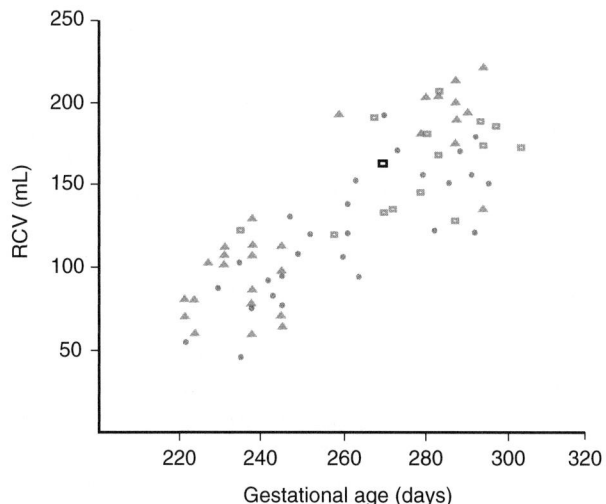

FIGURE 2-4. Circulating red blood cell mass in newborn infants in relation to gestational age. *Circles,* by the ⁵¹Cr-dilution method; *triangles* and *squares,* from plasma volume measurements. *(Redrawn from Bratteby LE. Studies on erythro-kinetics in infancy. X. Red cell volume of newborn infants in relation to gestational age. Acta Paediatr Scand. 1968;57:132-136.)*

day of red cell volume 2 months before term and a rate of 2.5% to 3.5% per day of red cell volume at term. The combined data therefore indicate very strongly that the rate of red cell production during the latter part of fetal life is quite high—about threefold to fivefold that of a normal adult subject. This finding is in agreement with the well-established facts that at the same period of development, all the bones are filled with red marrow, the concentration of red cell precursors per unit volume of marrow is markedly increased,[91-93] and the number of erythroid and granulocyte-monocyte progenitors in cord blood is greater than that in normal adult blood.[94]

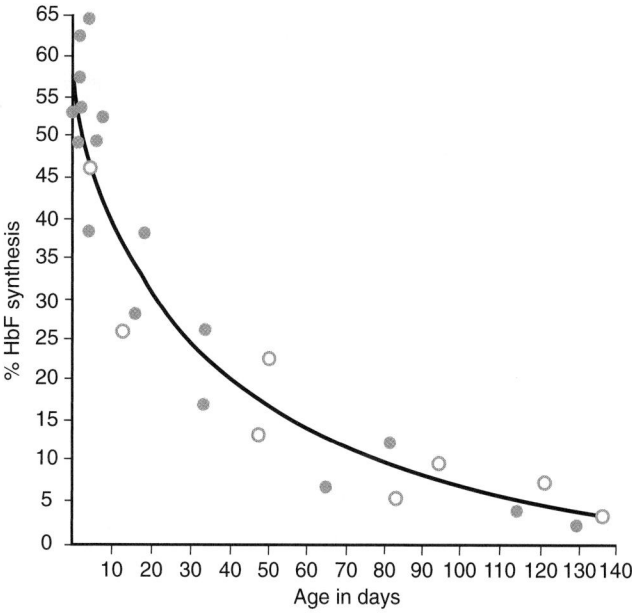

FIGURE 2-5. Time course of the relative synthesis of hemoglobin F (HbF) in normal infants during the first 140 days of life. *Closed circles,* radioiron method; *open circles,* reticulocyte method. *(Redrawn from Garby L, Sjölin S, Vuille JC. Studies on erythro-kinetics in infancy. II. The relative rate of synthesis of haemoglobin F and haemoglobin A during the first months of life. Acta Paediatr. 1962;51:245-254.)*

Erythropoiesis after Birth

The rate of hemoglobin synthesis and red cell production decreases dramatically during the first few days after delivery. Production of red cells (or hemoglobin) decreases by a factor of 2 to 3 during the first few days after birth and by a factor of about 10 during the first week of life. This sudden and marked decrease in red cell production is undoubtedly initiated by the equally sudden increase in tissue oxygen level that takes place at birth, as reflected by the virtual disappearance of EPO in plasma.[95] At the time of birth, between 55% and 65% of total hemoglobin synthesis consists of HbF.[96] Thereafter, synthesis of HbF decreases much more rapidly than that of HbA; the time course is shown in Figure 2-5. The switch from HbF to HbA is delayed in infants of diabetic mothers,[97] in those with metabolic diseases characterized by an inability to metabolize propionic acid,[98] and in infants with chronic bronchopulmonary dysplasia.[99] Synthesis of HbF can also be "reactivated" in severe cases of anemia of prematurity.[100] The rate of production of red cells (and of hemoglobin), which reaches a minimum during the second week of life, increases during the following months and reaches a maximum, at about 3 months of age, of approximately 2 mL of packed red cells per day, or about 2% of the circulating red cell mass per day.

Life Span of the Erythrocyte

The life span of erythrocytes obtained from term infants is somewhat shorter than that of red cells from adults,

TABLE 2-4   Reported ^{51}Cr Survival Data

Authors	No. of Cases	Range (Days)	Average (Days)
TERM INFANTS			
Hollingsworth	6	13-23	18.2
Giblett	10	—	20.0
Foconi and Sjölin	10	17-25	22.8
Vest	8	20-27	23.5
Gilardi and Miescher	3	21-26	23.5
Kaplan and Hsu	14	21-35	26.8
Total	51	13-35	23.3
PREMATURE INFANTS			
Foconi and Sjölin	6	10-18	15.8
Kaplan and Hsu	11	9-26	17.8
Vest	7	15-19	16.0
Gilardi and Miescher	7	15-19	16.1
Total	31	9-26	16.6

From Pearson HA. Life-span of the fetal red blood cell. J Pediatr. 1967;70:166-171.

whereas the life span of red cells obtained from premature infants is considerably shorter. The more immature the infant, the greater the degree of reduction in life span.

Because of their relative simplicity, studies using ^{51}Cr have been performed most extensively. The results of numerous investigators are summarized in Table 2-4.[101] These data indicate that the mean ^{51}Cr half-life of erythrocytes from term infants is 23.3 days (range, 13 to 35 days), whereas the mean value for red cells from premature infants is 16.6 days (range, 9 to 26 days). Conversion of these fetal red cell life spans for term infants from ^{51}Cr half-life to true red cell survival indicates an actual life span of approximately 60 to 70 days. Similar calculations for the red cells of premature infants yield values of 35 to 50 days.

Wranne, using the carbon monoxide technique, found that 1.5% of term infants' red cell mass was broken down daily during the first week of life.[96] Wranne concluded that the life span of most erythrocytes formed during the late fetal and early neonatal period is only 90 days. Equations derived from accumulated data led Bratteby and Garby to the conclusion that the mean life span of cells produced during the last 60 days of fetal life was between 45 and 70 days and that the life span frequency was skewed, with a majority of the cells dying before the mean life span was achieved.[102]

No unifying hypothesis has been presented to explain why the red cells produced in fetal life have a shortened life span. Landaw and Guancial demonstrated a similar shortening of the life span of erythrocytes obtained from the fetal rat.[103] In their studies, the decrease in life span correlated with red cell rigidity, as reflected by red cell filtration studies.[104] These observations suggest that alterations in membrane function and increased susceptibility to mechanical damage may ultimately be responsible for the decreased life span of fetal erythrocytes.[105]

Unique Characteristics of the Neonatal Erythrocyte

The Red Cell Membrane

Simple clinical laboratory studies, as well as sophisticated biochemical procedures, have provided evidence that the red cell membrane of fetal erythrocytes differs from that of its adult counterpart.

The red cells from normal newborns are slightly more resistant to osmotic lysis than those of adults are.[106] A minor population of cells with increased osmotic fragility is also present; however, these cells appear to be selectively destroyed within the first several days after birth.[101] The mechanical fragility of cord blood red cells is likewise increased. Neonatal reticulocytes are composed of mostly motile R1 reticulocytes,[107] which have been shown to be capable of performing receptor-mediated endocytosis.[108] Neonatal red cells have greater total and membrane-associated myosin content than adult red cells do[109]; possibly, this increased content is a remnant of these cells' motile machinery.

Figure 2-6 presents flow cytometric measurements of cell volume and hemoglobin concentration in neonatal red cells versus adult red cells. Measurements of reticulocyte indices in neonatal and adult blood are also presented. Neonatal red cells have a larger volume and lower hemoglobin concentration than adult cells do.[110] Neonatal reticulocytes also have a larger volume and lower hemoglobin concentration than adult reticulocytes do. Macrocytosis is more prominent in premature newborns and appears to decrease with gestational age, probably as spleen function matures and assumes a greater role in red cell membrane remodeling. Spleen function and remodeling are major determinants of the decrease in cell volume observed when reticulocytes become mature erythrocytes. The difference in volume between reticulo-

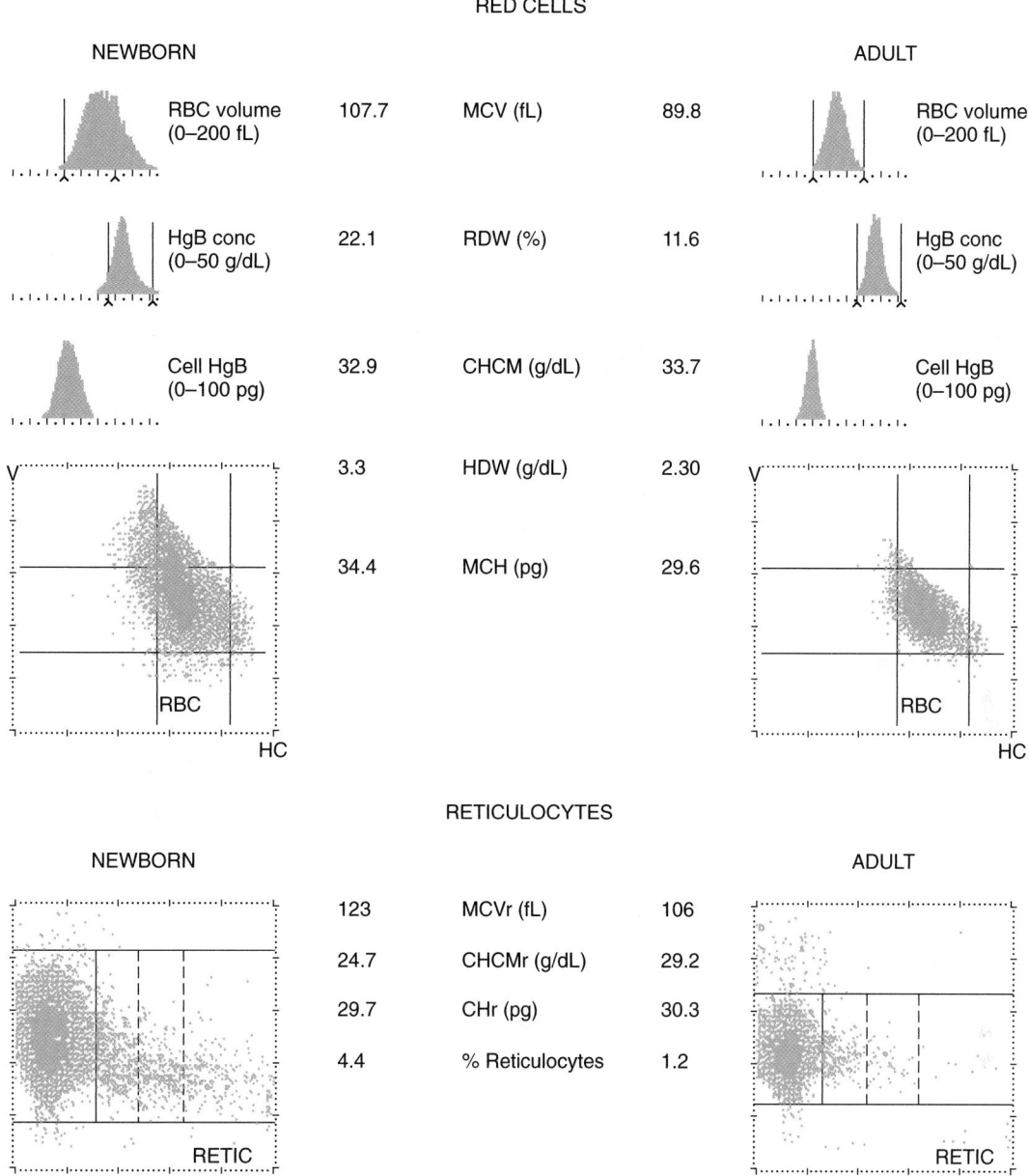

FIGURE 2-6. Red blood cell (RBC) and reticulocyte (RETIC) indices in neonatal and adult blood. **Top,** Histograms for RBC volume, RBC hemoglobin (Hb) concentration, and RBC Hb content obtained in a newborn (*left*) and an adult (*right*). **Bottom,** Reticulocyte analysis of newborn and adult RBC. The staining intensity of reticulocytes (x-axis) is plotted against the cell Hb concentration (y-axis). CHCM, cell hemoglobin concentration, mean; CHCMr, reticulocyte CHCM; CHr, reticulocyte cell hemoglobin content; HDW, hemoglobin distribution width; MCH, mean corpuscular hemoglobin; MCV, mean corpuscular volume; MCVr, reticulocyte MCV; RDW, RBC distribution width.

cytes and erythrocytes is greatly reduced in blood from premature newborns, another indication of reduced spleen function.[110]

The red cells of normal newborns also appear different by conventional light microscopy, interference phase microscopy, and electron microscopy. Zipursky and co-workers, via careful analysis of wet preparations suspended in 0.2% glutaraldehyde, observed that 78% of erythrocytes from adults appeared as biconcave discs and 18% as "bowl" forms; in contrast, only 43% of cells from term infants appeared as discs and 40% as bowl forms.[111] In addition, only up to 3% of cells from normal adults

appeared as assorted spherocytes and poikilocytes of various types, whereas up to 14% of cells from term infants showed these morphologic distortions.

In premature infants, the departure from normal adult cells was even more marked. In these infants, 40% of the cells were discs, 30% were bowls, and 27% displayed a variety of morphologic disturbances (Fig. 2-7). The high frequency of dysmorphology in hematologically normal neonates creates great difficulty in diagnosing specific disorders of the red cell at birth. When the dysmorphology is severe, the condition is sometimes called "infantile pyknocytosis." In this usually transient disor-

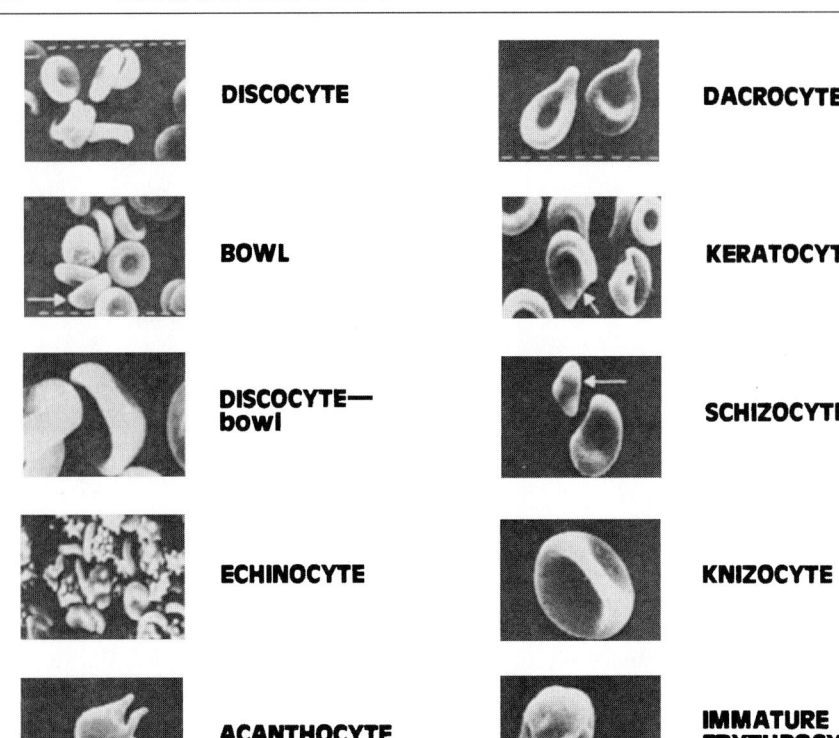

FIGURE 2-7. Variety of morphologic erythrocyte abnormalities observed in premature infants, term infants, and normal adults. *(Photomicrographs courtesy of Zipursky, Brown, and Brown. Adapted from Zipursky A, Brown E, Palko J, Brown EJ. The erythrocyte differential count in newborn infants. Am J Pediatr Hematol Oncol. 1983;5:45-51.)*

THE ERYTHROCYTE DIFFERENTIAL COUNT
(Median and 5% to 95% range)

Cell Type	Premature Infant	Term Infant	Normal Adult
Discocyte	39.5 (18-57)	43 (18-62)	78 (42-94)
Bowl	29.0 (13-53)	40 (14-58)	18 (4-50)
Discocyte–bowl	3.0 (0-10)	2 (0-5)	2 (0-4)
Spherocyte	0.0 (0-3)	0 (0-1)	0 (0-0)
Echinocyte	5.5 (1-23)	1 (0-4)	0 (0-3)
Acanthocyte	0.0 (0-2)	1 (0-2)	0 (0-1)
Dacrocyte	1.0 (0-5)	1 (0-3)	0 (0-1)
Keratocyte	3.0 (0-7)	2 (0-5)	0 (0-1)
Schizocyte	2.0 (0-5)	0 (0-2)	0 (0-1)
Knizocyte	3.0 (0-11)	3 (0-8)	1 (0-5)
Immature erythrocyte	1.0 (0-6)	0 (0-2)	0 (0-0)

der, red cell life span is even shorter than normal,[112] and the disorder may represent a neonatal form of hereditary ovalocytosis (see Chapter 15). Using interference phase microscopy, Holroyde and associates[113] observed that the red cells from both premature and term infants displayed the "pocked" appearance that was first noted by Nathan and Gunn in splenectomized patients with thalassemia.[114] These surface alterations are believed to reflect the presence of vacuoles and internal structures just below the red cell membrane. They were observed in greatest number among the most immature infants. Similar surface abnormalities are seen in patients without spleens and in those with sickle cell hemoglobinopathies with reduced splenic function.[113,115] The presence of these red cell "pocks" is presumed to reflect impaired splenic function in the immature infant but may also be a reflection of the tendency of fetal erythrocytes for increased vesicle formation, which overwhelms the clearance capacity of the spleen.[116,117]

Examination of fetal red cells by electron microscopy also reveals the presence of vacuoles and internal structures just below the cell membrane.[118,119] Freeze-etching and transmission electron microscopy of fetal erythrocyte membranes indicate that the protoplasmic fracture faces have 24% more intramembrane particles than do those of adult cells and that the number of particles on exoplasmic fracture faces exceeds that of the adult by 45%.[120]

The membrane of fetal erythrocytes also appears to be more fluid than that of adult cells. Both ferritin-labeled anti-A antibodies[119] and concanavalin A[121] are taken up by endocytosis in the mature erythrocytes of newborn infants but not by cells from normal adults. This unique phenomenon does not appear to be the result of differences in lipid viscosity of the membrane.[122]

When compared with adult cells, the erythrocyte membrane of the newborn has more binding sites for insulin,[123] more insulin-like growth factor,[124] and more prolactin[125]; however, it has fewer digoxin receptor sites[126] and reduced membrane acetylcholinesterase.[127,128] Membrane proteins from both premature and term infants are indistinguishable from those of normal adults when solubilized in sodium dodecyl sulfate and analyzed with polyacrylamide gel electrophoresis.[121,126]

The red cells of the cord blood of full-term infants contain increased quantities of total lipid, lipid phosphorus, and cholesterol per cell, although the percentage of total lipid composed of lipid phosphorus and cholesterol is similar to that found in adults.[129] These erythrocytes have a greater percentage of their phospholipid as sphingomyelin and a lesser proportion as lecithin. Phospholipid fatty acid patterns in cord blood erythrocytes show a greater percentage of palmitic, stearic, arachidonic, and combined 22- and 24-carbon fatty acids and a lesser proportion of oleic and linoleic acid. The cells are much more prone to lipid peroxidation on oxidant challenge,[130,131] which may contribute to their removal from the circulation after birth. It is likely that the relative hyposplenism of the neonate contributes to these membrane alterations. Erythrocytes of babies born to mothers with gestational diabetes have reduced choline phosphoglycerides and reduced total ω-6 and ω-3 fatty acids.[132]

From an immunologic perspective, the erythrocyte membrane of the newborn is also different from that of the adult. At birth, the Lewis system of absorbed serum antigens is incompletely expressed, partly because the receptor sites of the membrane are weak or absent. In the ABO system, the A antigen, particularly the A_1 antigen, and the B antigen sites are weakly expressed, and in the Ii system, the I antigen is either weak or absent. Other weakly expressed antigens are Sd^a, P1, Lu^a, Lu^b, Yt^a, Xg, and Vel.[133]

The cells are less permeable to the nonelectrolytes glycerol and thiourea[134]; they display reduced potassium influx via the Na^+,K^+-adenosine triphosphatase (ATPase) and Na^+,K^+,Cl^- cotransport systems[135] and altered kinetics of glucose transfer[136]; and they are prone to acid lysis.[137] The number of Na^+-K^+ pumps, estimated from ouabain binding, is greater in premature infants than in term infants.[138] The chloride and bicarbonate transport systems of fetal and adult red cells are similar.[139]

The filtration rate of red blood cells from preterm and term infants is lower than that of adults.[140-142] This decreased filterability may be a manifestation of the larger size of erythrocytes from newborns rather than their different lipid composition.

Metabolism of Erythrocytes of the Newborn Infant (Box 2-1)

Enzymes of the Embden-Meyerhof Pathway

Numerous investigators are in agreement that the activity of the enzymes phosphoglycerate kinase and enolase in the red cells of newborn infants is much more intense than would be anticipated from their young cell age.[128,143-147] The activity of the enzymes glyceraldehyde-3-phosphate dehydrogenase and glucose phosphate isomerase is also probably significantly greater than would be anticipated from cell age.[145]

The activity of phosphofructokinase (PFK), a rate-controlling enzyme in glycolysis, has repeatedly been found to be lower than normal in the red cells of newborn infants.[144,145,148] The decreased PFK activity may reflect the accelerated decay of an unstable enzyme. Travis and Garvin fractionated cord blood red cells into cohorts of varying cell age and compared them with adult red cells fractionated in similar fashion.[149] The rate of decline in pyruvate kinase activity was essentially the same in neonates and adults, whereas PFK activity in cord erythrocytes decreased at a significantly greater rate than it did in adult erythrocytes.

Studies of Vora and Piomelli have provided a clear understanding of the nature of PFK in fetal erythrocytes.[150] They found that human muscle PFK and liver PFK are homotetramers, each of which is composed of identical subunits, which they termed "M_4" and "L_4." Study of adult erythrocytes revealed the presence of three heterotetramers—M_3L, M_2L_2, and ML_3. Analysis of cord blood erythrocytes revealed the presence of the three heterotetramers in adult erythrocytes; the L_4 isoenzyme was also identified. The presence of the liver homotetramer in fetal erythrocytes may be responsible for the decreased PFK stability observed by Travis and Garvin.[149]

Differences in the distribution of other red cell isoenzymes have also been described. Hemolysates normally contain two isoenzymes of hexokinase, types I and III. Holmes and co-workers found that in the cells of a newborn infant, type II hexokinase was the predominant isoenzyme.[151] Schröter and Tillman, in contrast, observed that type I predominated, although the predominance of type I was not characteristic of young cells in general but was a unique feature of the red cells of newborn infants.[152] Chen and associates also observed differences in the distribution of hexokinase isoenzymes obtained from first-trimester and midtrimester fetuses.[153]

Enolase exists as multiple isoenzymes in erythrocytes as well, and the distribution of enolase isoenzymes appears to be a unique characteristic of fetal erythrocytes.[154]

Chen and associates studied a total of 26 enzyme patterns in hemolysates prepared from 11 fetuses ranging

Box 2-1 **Metabolic Characteristics of the Erythrocytes of Newborns**

CARBOHYDRATE METABOLISM

Glucose consumption increased

Galactose more completely used as substrate both under normal circumstances and for reduction of methemoglobin*

Decreased activity of the sorbitol pathway*

Decreased triokinase activity*

GLYCOLYTIC ENZYMES

Increased activity of hexokinase, phosphoglucose isomerase,* aldolase, glyceraldehyde 3-phosphate,* phosphoglycerate kinase,* phosphoglycerate mutase, enolase,* pyruvate kinase, lactate dehydrogenase, glucose-6-phosphate dehydrogenase, 6-phosphogluconate dehydrogenase, galactokinase, and galactose 1-phosphate uridyltransferase

Decreased activity of phosphofructokinase*

Different distribution of hexokinase isoenzymes*

NONGLYCOLYTIC ENZYMES

Increased activity of aspartate transaminase and glutathione reductase

Decreased activity of NADP-dependent methemoglobin reductase,* catalase,* glutathione peroxidase, superoxide dismutase, carbonic anhydrase,* adenylate kinase,* and glutathione synthetase*

Presence of α-glycerol-3-phosphate dehydrogenase*

ATP AND PHOSPHATE METABOLISM

Decreased phosphate uptake,* slower incorporation into ATP and 2,3-diphosphoglycerate*

Accelerated decline of 2,3-diphosphoglycerate on red blood cell incubation*

Increased ATP and 2,3-diphosphoglycerate levels

Accelerated decline of ATP during brief incubation

STORAGE CHARACTERISTICS

Increased potassium efflux and greater degrees of hemolysis during short periods of storage

More rapid assumption of altered morphologic forms on storage or incubation*

MEMBRANE

Decreased ouabain-sensitive Na^+,K^+-ATPase*; decreased ouabain-resistant potassium influx*

Decreased permeability to glycerol and thiourea*

Decreased membrane deformability*

Increased sphingomyelin, decreased lecithin content of stromal phospholipids

Decreased content of linoleic acid*

Increased lipid phosphorus and cholesterol per cell

Greater affinity for glucose*

Increased number of insulin, insulin-like growth factor, and prolactin binding sites

Increased membrane-associated myosin

Reduced membrane acetylcholinesterase activity

OTHER

Increased methemoglobin content*

Increased affinity of hemoglobin for oxygen*

Glutathione instability*

Increased tendency for Heinz body formation in the presence of oxidant compounds*

---

*Appears to be a unique characteristic of the newborn's erythrocytes and not merely a function of the presence of young red blood cells. ATP, adenosine triphosphate; ATPase, adenosine triphosphatase; NADP, nicotinamide adenine dinucleotide phosphate.

---

in gestational age from 65 to 138 days.[153] Six enzymes—enolase, guanylate kinase, lactate dehydrogenase, nucleoside phosphorylase, PFK, and the previously mentioned hexokinase—showed differences in the staining intensity of certain isoenzyme zones as compared with adult controls. The fetal red cell zymograms contained the mitochondrial forms of isocitric dehydrogenase and aspartate transaminase, as well as more definite zones of phosphoglucomutase type 3.

Glucose Consumption

Glucose consumption by the erythrocytes of both term and premature infants has generally been found to be greater than that observed in the cells of normal adults.[155,156] This would be anticipated in view of the fact that young red cells consume more glucose. However, when the cells from infants are compared with adult cell populations of similar young age, their rate of glucose consumption appears to be less than would be expected.[155]

Circumstantial evidence suggests that the relative deficiency of PFK may be responsible for this relative impairment in glycolysis. All strategies designed to maximize PFK activity produce far greater augmentation of glucose consumption in the cells of neonates. Incubation of cells at high phosphate concentration causes the cells of both premature and term infants to consume glucose at rates commensurate with their age.[157] Increasing the pH of the incubation medium produces a much greater increase in red cell glucose consumption in cells from newborn infants.[155] Analysis of glycolytic intermediates reveals that as pH increases, there is a decrease in levels of glucose 6-phosphate and fructose 6-phosphate and an increase in the concentration of fructose 1,6-diphosphate, glyceraldehyde 3-phosphate, dihydroxyacetone phosphate, and 2,3-diphosphoglycerate (2,3,-DPG). All these changes are consistent with activation of PFK. It would appear that this pH-induced augmentation of PFK obscures the relative deficiency that is manifested as lower than expected glucose consumption at pH 7.4.

Further evidence that the relative deficiency of PFK may play the major role in depressing glucose consumption in the newborn comes from the incubation of neonatal red cells with methylene blue, 10^{-6} mol. At this concentration of methylene blue, 90% of glucose consumption proceeds via the pentose phosphate pathway, which bypasses the PFK step. Incubation of red cells from newborn infants in the presence of methylene blue produces a far greater acceleration of glycolysis than observed either in the red cells of normal adults or in those of subjects with reticulocytosis.[158]

Finally, when one examines the oldest cells from the cord blood of newborn infants, the profound PFK deficiency that was previously described is found to be associated with a marked decrease in glucose consumption and a pattern of glycolytic intermediates that suggests a relative block in glycolysis at this step.

2,3-Diphosphoglycerate Metabolism

When the red cells of infants and adults are incubated under identical conditions, the concentration of 2,3-DPG declines far more rapidly in the erythrocytes of newborns than in those of adults.[133-134] Various postulates have been advanced to explain this 2,3-DPG instability. Zipursky and co-workers presented evidence to suggest that a relative block in glycolysis, proximal to the formation of glyceraldehyde 3-phosphate, was responsible for the failure to maintain 2,3-DPG levels.[159] Trueworthy and Lowman proposed that the instability of 2,3-DPG was the result of an accelerated rate of hydrolysis as a consequence of increased 2,3-DPG phosphatase activity.[160] The 2,3-DPG content of normal fetal red cells is greater than that of adult cells and is further increased in anemic fetuses, possibly as a consequence of the relative preponderance of PFK activity over pyruvate kinase activity.[161]

The Pentose Phosphate Pathway and Response to Oxidant-Induced Injury

Oxidative stress induced by the formation of O_2, H_2O_2, or related species is handled within the red cell by the combined activities of the hexose monophosphate shunt (in which reduced nicotinamide adenine dinucleotide phosphate [NADPH] is generated), glutathione peroxidase, catalase, and superoxide dismutase. There is general agreement that the red cells from newborn infants are more susceptible to oxidant-induced injury than adult cells are and that this susceptibility is greater in very-low-birth-weight infants [128,162-164]

Fetal hemoglobin is more prone than adult hemoglobin to denaturation; however, there is no relationship between the fetal hemoglobin content of the cell and the tendency to form Heinz bodies. The pentose phosphate pathway in the cells of both term and premature infants is intact and responds appropriately to oxidant-induced stimulation.[158,165] The cell content of glutathione is normal in neonatal erythrocytes.[166] The activity of glutathione peroxidase is decreased in comparison to that of adult cells[167,168]; however, metabolic studies have failed to demonstrate a convincing direct relationship between this relative deficiency and vulnerability to oxidant.[140,144] Decreased levels of reduced glutathione and increased levels of oxidized glutathione have been found in patients with retinopathy of prematurity.[169] Erythrocytes from extremely-low-birth-weight infants exhibit a marked reduction in the 6-phosphogluconate dehydrogenase (6PGD)/glucose-6-phosphate dehydrogenase (G6PD) ratio, glutathione peroxidase, methemoglobin (Met-Hb) reductase, and catalase.[128] A slight decrease in superoxide dismutase activity has been observed in fetal red cells.[170] The relative deficiencies of glutathione peroxidase and catalase may act in concert with plasma factors to produce this metabolic handicap.[171,172] Vitamin E plays a crucial role in limiting membrane lipid auto-oxidation. Vitamin E deficiency has been observed in the plasma of full-term and premature newborns.[173]

G6PD activity is increased in cord/neonatal blood,[144,148,158,174] whereas 6PGD activity is similar in neonatal and adult blood.[144,175] In fetal and extremely-low-birth-weight infant cells, 6PGD activity is markedly reduced[128,176]; the associated reduction in the 6PGD/G6PD ratio has been proposed as a marker of developmental immaturity of erythrocytes.[128,147]

Suggestions that other factors are implicated come from observations that the red cells of newborn infants, when compared with those of adults, have a decreased number of membrane SH groups,[177] that the membranes isolated from them contain more residual hemoglobin and form Heinz bodies faster,[178] and that after the transfusion of adult cells into newborn infants, these cells also appear to be more prone to the development of Heinz bodies.[179,180]

The red cells from newborn infants, like other young red cells, consume more oxygen and produce more hydrogen peroxide than the red cells of adults do.[181,182]

HEMATOLOGIC VALUES AT BIRTH

Several variables influence the interpretation of what might be considered normal values for hemoglobin, hematocrit, red cell indices, and reticulocyte count at the time of birth and during the early weeks of life. These variables include the gestational age of the infant, the conduct of labor and treatment of the umbilical vessels, the site of sampling, and the time of sampling. The Appendix of this text contains a series of tables describing representative norms that have appeared in the literature. A few of these norms are highlighted in the following discussion to illustrate pertinent points.

Site of Sampling

Capillary samples obtained by skin prick, generally from the heel or toe, have a higher hemoglobin concentration than simultaneously collected venous samples do. During the first hours of life, this difference averages approximately 3.5 g/dL, as is illustrated in Figure 2-8.[183] In some instances the capillary hemoglobin–venous hemoglobin difference may exceed 10 g/dL.[184]

The clinical importance of the site of sampling was illustrated by Moe in a study of 54 infants with erythroblastosis fetalis.[184] Simultaneously obtained cord blood and capillary samples were compared. In this study, 41 infants eventually required exchange transfusion for hyperbilirubinemia. Of these 41 infants, 25 were found to be anemic based on determinations performed on cord blood samples, whereas only 14 could be considered anemic on the basis of the results of capillary sample analysis.

In virtually all infants, the capillary-to-venous hematocrit ratio is greater than 1.00. The greatest ratios, often in excess of 1.20, are observed in infants born before 30 weeks of gestation, infants with arterial blood pH values below 7.20, infants with hypotension, and infants with a red cell mass of less than 35 mL/kg.[185] In other words, capillary hemoglobin values are falsely elevated in the sickest infants. These are the same infants in whom accurate determination of the hemoglobin concentration is most important for clinical management. The capillary-to-venous hematocrit ratio gradually decreases with increasing gestational age.[185] Infants born between 26 and 30 weeks of gestation have a mean ratio of 1.21; infants born at 31 to 32 weeks, 1.12; infants born at 33 to 35 weeks, 1.16; and infants born between 36 and 41 weeks, 1.12. By the fifth day of life, the capillary-to-venous difference has decreased in healthy infants, and capillary samples may have a hematocrit that is only 2.5% higher when blood is obtained by deep stick from a well-warmed heel.

Several studies have shown that venipuncture is as effective and less painful than heel blood collections.[186]

The use of automated incision devices for heel sticks should be encouraged because they reduce the number of sticks needed and induce less bruising and inflammation.[187] Pain and stress are associated with the heel prick procedure,[188,189] as well as some rare but severe permanent sequelae.[190] The use of topical anesthetics reduces the pain associated with drawing blood in infants,[191,192] although Met-Hb levels may be transiently increased if prilocaine is used.[193]

Treatment of the Umbilical Vessels

At birth, the volume of blood of the infant may be increased by as much as 61% if the placental vessels are allowed to empty completely before the cord is clamped.[194,195] It has been estimated that the placental vessels contain 75 to 125 mL of blood at birth—or a quarter to a third of the fetal blood volume. Under normal circumstances, about a quarter of placental transfusion takes place within 15 seconds of birth and half by the end of the first minute. The ratio of blood in the neonatal and placental circulations has been found to average 67:33 at birth, 80:20 at 1 minute, and 87:13 at the end of placental transfusion.[195]

The umbilical arteries generally constrict shortly after birth, so no blood flows from the infant to the mother; however, the umbilical vein remains dilated and permits blood to flow in the direction of gravity. Infants held below the level of the placenta continue to gain blood; infants held above the placenta may bleed into it.[196] Yao and co-workers demonstrated that hydrostatic pressure, produced by placing the infant 40 cm below the mother's introitus, hastened placental transfusion to virtual completion in 30 seconds.[195] In infants delivered at term by cesarean section, maximal placental transfusion is achieved within 40 seconds after birth; however, net blood flow reverses, with blood traveling from the infant back to the placenta, if clamping is delayed for longer than 40 seconds.[197] A recent controlled study has shown that delayed cord clamping significantly increases

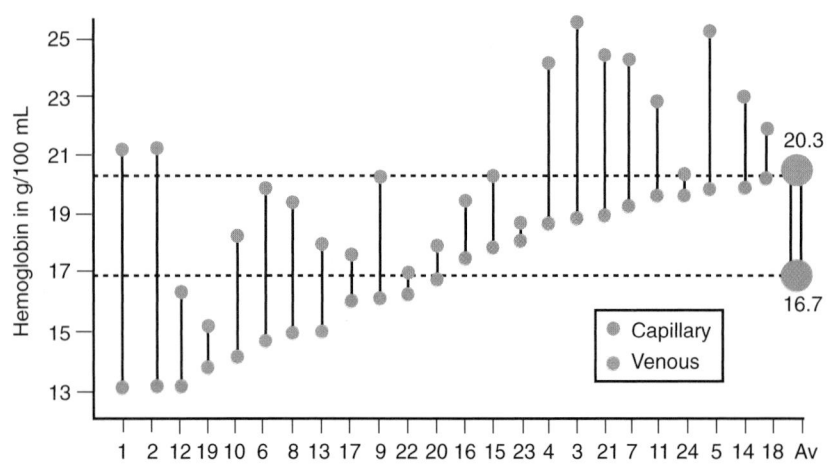

FIGURE 2-8. Simultaneous capillary and venous hemoglobin determinations in 24 newborn infants. Av, average. (*Redrawn from Oettinger L, Mills WB. Simultaneous capillary and venous hemoglobin determinations in newborn infants. J Pediatr. 1949;35:362-365.*)

the hematocrit and reduces the incidence of neonatal anemia with no harmful effects.[198]

The effects of placental transfusion on the total blood volume of the infant show wide variability, partially because of the techniques used and the time at which the samples were taken. During the first hours after birth, plasma apparently leaves the circulation. It seems that the greater the placental transfusion, the greater the plasma loss. Thus, by the third day of life, there are only small differences in total blood volume, regardless of the method of cord clamping. Usher and associates found that infants with delayed cord clamping had an average blood volume of 93 mL/kg at an age of 72 hours; infants with immediate cord clamping had a blood volume of 82 mL/kg.[194] Although the total blood volume may be only slightly altered by the timing of cord clamping, more significant differences can be observed in red cell mass or hemoglobin concentration. In the study of Usher and colleagues, infants with delayed cord clamping had an average red cell mass of 49 mL/kg at 72 hours of age as compared with only 31 mL/kg in infants with immediate cord clamping.[194] The results of other investigators are listed in Table 2-5.[199-201]

Infants with delayed cord clamping tend to have higher hemoglobin values during the first week of life than do those whose clamping was not delayed. A reduced volume of red blood cells is associated with increased mortality in premature infants with respiratory distress syndrome.[202] Thus, delayed cord clamping could be particularly indicated for premature births. Studies have shown that delayed cord clamping in premature infants is associated with a significant reduction in transfusion requirements and improved outcome, but not with a reduced incidence of periventricular/intraventricular hemorrhage.[201,203-205]

There have been reports of circulatory overload and congestive cardiac failure in the setting of delayed cord clamping. "Symptomatic neonatal plethora" was observed in eight premature and three full-term infants.[206] Radiologic findings of volume overload and reduced left ventricular performance have been reported in infants with delayed cord clamping.[207,208] For cesarean section, a delay of 3 minutes in cord clamping has been associated with signs of respiratory and metabolic acidosis (reduced oxygen tension and pH and elevated plasma lactate levels), thus indicating that earlier clamping may be preferable in this setting.[209]

Blood Volume

Both blood volume and red cell mass are influenced by the treatment of the cord vessels and by the clinical condition of the infant. Shortly after birth, the blood volume of term infants may range from 50 to 100 mL/kg, with the mean value being 85 mL/kg.[194,210,211] As previously discussed, blood volume in infants with early cord clamping averages 78 mL/kg at 30 minutes of age, in contrast to a value of 98.6 mL/kg in infants with cords that were clamped late. By 72 hours of age, these differences are not as great; infants with early clamping have an average blood volume of 82 mL/kg, whereas those with late clamping have an average of 93 mL/kg.

The blood volume of premature infants ranges from 89 to 105 mL/kg during the first few days of life.[212,213] This increased blood volume is primarily the result of an increase in plasma volume, with the total red cell volume per kilogram of body weight being quite similar to that of term infants. Plasma volume decreases with increasing gestational age, except in infants with intrauterine growth retardation.[214]

For infants born at term, blood volumes are approximately 73 to 77 mL/kg by 1 month of life.[215,216]

Reduced blood volume and decreased red cell mass are frequently observed in infants with hyaline mem-

TABLE 2-5	Effect of Cord Clamping on Hematocrit and Hemoglobin Concentration at Various Times after Delivery				
	EARLY CLAMPING		**DELAYED CLAMPING**		
Reference	Hb (g/dL)	Hct (%)	Hb (g/dL)	Hct (%)	Time of Study
Phillips (1941)	15.6	—	19.3	—	20-30 hr
Marsh et al. (1948)	17.4	—	20.8	—	3rd day
Colozzi (1954)	14.7	—	17.3	—	72 hr
Lanzkowsky (1960)	18.1	—	19.7	—	72-96 hr
	11.1	—	11.1	—	3 mo
Linderkamp et al. (1992)[199]	—	48 ± 4	—	50 ± 4	At birth
	—	47 ± 5	—	63 ± 5	2 hr
	—	43 ± 6	—	59 ± 5	24 hr
	—	44 ± 5	—	59 ± 6	120 hr
Nelle and Zilow (1993)[200]	—	48 ± 6	—	58 ± 6	2 hr
	—	44 ± 5	—	56 ± 7	24 hr
	—	44 ± 5	—	54 ± 8	5 days
Kinmond et al. (1993)[201]	—	50.9 ± 4.5	—	56.4 ± 4.8	Not standardized

Hb, hemoglobin; Hct, hematocrit.

brane disease and in newborns delivered with a tight nuchal cord.[217,218] Approximately 16% of infants born with a nuchal cord are anemic in the neonatal period.[219] Infants born after late intrauterine asphyxia tend to have a greater blood volume and red cell mass.[218]

Hemoglobin, Hematocrit, Red Cell Count, and Red Cell and Reticulocyte Indices

Representative values for these hematologic measurements are presented in Tables 2-6 to 2-9. Hemoglobin values increase gradually until approximately 32 to 33 weeks of gestation and remain relatively constant until term. Mean corpuscular volume (MCV) and the mean reticulocyte count decline continuously during the course of gestation. Hematologic values from normal fetuses with gestational ages between 18 to 30 weeks reflect this trend.[220]

In healthy term infants, no measurable decrease in hemoglobin values occurs during the first week of life (see Fig. 2-9); in contrast, in infants born weighing less than 1500 g but of appropriate weight for gestational age, the hemoglobin concentration may decrease by as much as 1.0 to 1.5 g/dL during this interval (Fig. 2-10).

Considerable differences are seen in the peripheral blood cell counts and indices of infants born in developing countries. A study carried out by Tchernia's group in 199 newborns in Bamako (Mali) indicated that 32% were anemic (hemoglobin level <13 g/dL).[221] When compared with a control group of French newborns, the Bamako group had lower hemoglobin levels (13.9 ± 2.0 g/dL versus 15.1 ± 1.4 g/dL), lower mean corpuscular hemoglobin (MCH) levels (32.9 ± 3.0 pg versus 35 ± 1.9 pg), lower serum ferritin levels (97.5 µg/L versus 135 µg/L, geometric means), and lower erythrocyte ferritin levels (244.7 attogram [ag] per cell versus 348 ag per cell, geometric means). These differences cannot be explained by hemoglobinopathies, malaria, or folate deficiency, and they are probably due to iron deficiency. However, in developed countries, there seems to be very little difference in neonatal hemoglobin, erythrocyte zinc protoporphyrin, and cord blood serum ferritin levels between neonates born to iron-deficient and iron-replete mothers.[222]

FETAL ANEMIA

Improved diagnostic and therapeutic techniques have made early identification and treatment of anemia in the fetus possible. The experience gained in the in utero treatment of hemolytic diseases of the fetus has been applied to a wide spectrum of pathologic conditions.[223] Normal fetal hematologic values are also available

TABLE 2-6	Hematologic Values for Normal Cord Blood		
Parameter	**Mean**	**SD**	***n***
Hb (g/dL)	15.9	1.86	28
Hct (%)	50.2	6.9	18
RBC count ($\times 10^6$/mm^3)	4.64	0.68	18
MCV (fL)	110	5.05	28
MCH (pg)	34.6	1.5	18
MCHC (g/dL)	31.9	1.13	18
CHCM (g/dL)	30.9	1.78	26
% Hypochromic (MCHC <28 g/dL)	12.7	12.9	18
% Hyperchromic (MCHC >41 g/dL)	0.97	0.74	28
% Microcytic (MCV <61 fL)	0.73	0.3	18
% Macrocytic (MCV >120 fL)	22.5	8.41	18
RETICULOCYTES			
%	3.69	0.95	27
MCVr (fL)	125	8.6	25
CHCMr (g/dL)	27.1	1.95	17
CHr (pg)	32.9	3.1	17

CHCM, cell hemoglobin concentration, mean; CHCMr, reticulocyte CHCM; CHr, reticulocyte cell hemoglobin content; Hb, hemoglobin; Hct, hematocrit; MCH, mean corpuscular hemoglobin; MCHC, mean corpuscular hemoglobin concentration; MCV, mean corpuscular volume; MCVr, reticulocyte MCV; RBC, red blood cell.

Values obtained with an ADVIA 120 hematology analyzer (Bayer Diagnostics, Tarrytown, NY) in neonates delivered at term with weight greater than 2500 g. These data were kindly provided by Drs. Gil Tchernia and Therese Cynober, Laboratoire d'Hematologie, Centre Hospitalier de Bicetre, Bicetre, France.

TABLE 2-7	Normal Hematologic Values during the First 2 Weeks of Life in Term Infant				
	Cord Blood	**Day 1**	**Day 3**	**Day 7**	**Day 14**
Hb (g/dL)	16.8	18.4	17.8	17.0	16.8
Hct (%)	53.0	58.0	55.0	54.0	52.0
RBC count ($\times 10^6$/mm^3)	5.25	5.8	5.6	5.2	5.1
MCV (fL)	107.0	108.0	99.0	98.0	96.0
MCH (pg)	34.0	35.0	33.0	32.5	31.5
MCHC (g/dL)	31.7	32.5	33.0	33.0	33.0
Reticulocytes (%)	3-7	3-7	1-3	0-1	0-1
Nucleated RBCs/(mm^3)	500.0	200.0	0-5	0	0
Platelets (1000/mm^3)	290.0	192.0	213.0	248.0	252.0

Hb, hemoglobin; Hct, hematocrit; MCH, mean corpuscular hemoglobin; MCHC, mean corpuscular hemoglobin concentration; MCV, mean corpuscular volume; RBC, red blood cell.

TABLE 2-8   Red Blood Cell Values on the First Postnatal Day

	GESTATIONAL AGE (WEEKS)							
	24-25 (7)*	26-27 (11)	28-29 (7)	30-31 (25)	32-33 (23)	34-35 (23)	36-37 (20)	Term (19)
RBC count (×10⁶/mm³)	4.65 ± 0.43†	4.73 ± 0.45	4.62 ± 0.75	4.79 ± 0.74	5.0 ± 0.76	5.09 ± 0.5	5.27 ± 0.68	5.14 ± 0.7
Hb (g/dL)	19.4 ± 1.5	19.0 ± 2.5	19.3 ± 1.8	19.1 ± 2.2	18.5 ± 2.0	19.6 ± 2.1	19.2 ± 1.7	19.3 ± 2.2
Hct (%)	63 ± 4	62 ± 8	60 ± 7	60 ± 8	60 ± 8	61 ± 7	64 ± 7	61 ± 7.4
MCV (fL)	135 ± 0.2	132 ± 14.4	131 ± 13.5	127 ± 12.7	123 ± 15.7	122 ± 10.0	121 ± 12.5	119 ± 9.4
Reticulocytes (%)	6.0 ± 0.5	9.6 ± 3.2	7.5 ± 2.5	5.8 ± 2.0	5.0 ± 1.9	3.9 ± 1.6	4.2 ± 1.8	3.2 ± 1.4
Weight (g)	725 ± 185	993 ± 194	1174 ± 128	1450 ± 232	1816 ± 192	1957 ± 291	2245 ± 213	—

*Number of infants listed in parentheses.
†Mean values ± SD.
Hb, hemoglobin; Hct, hematocrit; MCV, mean corpuscular volume; RBC, red blood cell.
From Zaizov R, Matoth Y. Red cell values on the first postnatal day during the last 16 weeks of gestation. Am J Hematol. 1976;1:275-278. Copyright © 1976 Wiley-Liss. Reprinted by permission of Wiley-Liss, A Division of John Wiley and Sons, Inc.

TABLE 2-9   Normal Hematologic Values during the First 12 Weeks of Life in Term Infants

Age	No. of Cases	Hb (g/dL) ± 1 SD	RBC (×10⁶/mm³) ± 1 SD	Hct (%) ± 1 SD	MCV (fL) ± 1 SD	MCHC (g/dL) ± 1 SD	Reticulocytes (%) ± 1 SD
DAYS							
1	19	19.0 ± 2.2	5.14 ± 0.7	61 ± 7.4	119 ± 9.4	31.6 ± 1.9	3.2 ± 1.4
2	19	19.0 ± 1.9	5.15 ± 0.8	60 ± 6.4	115 ± 7.0	31.6 ± 1.4	3.2 ± 1.3
3	19	18.7 ± 3.4	5.11 ± 0.7	62 ± 9.3	116 ± 5.3	31.1 ± 2.8	2.8 ± 1.7
4	10	18.6 ± 2.1	5.00 ± 0.6	57 ± 8.1	114 ± 7.5	32.6 ± 1.5	1.8 ± 1.1
5	12	17.6 ± 1.1	4.97 ± 0.4	57 ± 7.3	114 ± 8.9	30.9 ± 2.2	1.2 ± 0.2
6	15	17.4 ± 2.2	5.00 ± 0.7	54 ± 7.2	113 ± 10.0	32.2 ± 1.6	0.6 ± 0.2
7	12	17.9 ± 2.5	4.86 ± 0.6	56 ± 9.4	118 ± 11.2	32.0 ± 1.6	0.5 ± 0.4
WEEKS							
1-2	32	17.3 ± 2.3	4.80 ± 0.8	54 ± 8.3	112 ± 19.0	32.1 ± 2.9	0.5 ± 0.3
2-3	11	15.6 ± 2.6	4.20 ± 0.6	46 ± 7.3	111 ± 8.2	33.9 ± 1.9	0.8 ± 0.6
3-4	17	14.2 ± 2.1	4.00 ± 0.6	43 ± 5.7	105 ± 7.5	33.5 ± 1.6	0.6 ± 0.3
4-5	15	12.7 ± 1.6	3.60 ± 0.4	36 ± 4.8	101 ± 8.1	34.9 ± 1.6	0.9 ± 0.8
5-6	10	11.9 ± 1.5	3.55 ± 0.2	36 ± 6.2	102 ± 10.2	34.1 ± 2.9	1.0 ± 0.7
6-7	10	12.0 ± 1.5	3.40 ± 0.4	36 ± 4.8	105 ± 12.0	33.8 ± 2.3	1.2 ± 0.7
7-8	17	11.1 ± 1.1	3.40 ± 0.4	33 ± 3.7	100 ± 13.0	33.7 ± 2.6	1.5 ± 0.7
8-9	13	10.7 ± 0.9	3.40 ± 0.5	31 ± 2.5	93 ± 12.0	34.1 ± 2.2	1.8 ± 1.0
9-10	12	11.2 ± 0.9	3.60 ± 0.3	32 ± 2.7	91 ± 9.3	34.3 ± 2.9	1.2 ± 0.6
10-11	11	11.4 ± 0.9	3.70 ± 0.4	34 ± 2.1	91 ± 7.7	33.2 ± 2.4	1.2 ± 0.7
11-12	13	11.3 ± 0.9	3.70 ± 0.3	33 ± 3.3	88 ± 7.9	34.8 ± 2.2	0.7 ± 0.3

Hb, hemoglobin; Hct, hematocrit; MCHC, mean corpuscular hemoglobin concentration; MCV, mean corpuscular volume; RBC, red blood cell; SD, standard deviation.
From Matoth Y, Zaizov R, Varsano I. Postnatal changes in some red cell parameters. Acta Paediatr Scand. 1971;60:317-323.

as a consequence of the development of percutaneous umbilical blood sampling and prenatal diagnosis (see Table 2-10).[220] There is evidence that intravascular transfusion to treat anemia in fetuses with immune hydrops results in high survival rates and favorable long-term neuropsychological outcomes.[224]

A substantial proportion of cases of nonimmune fetal hydrops are due to chromosomal abnormalities and thus are not treatable presently.[225,226] Fetuses with hydrops fetalis and anemia have characteristic sonographic abnormalities (thickened placenta, less pleural effusion, less marked edema); these abnormalities aid in the distinction of infants with hydrops fetalis but without anemia from those with anemia.[227] In growth-restricted fetuses,

Doppler studies of the middle cerebral artery and umbilical artery showed significant anemia-related changes, although their predictive accuracy was not high enough to justify clinical use.[228-230] In Rh-alloimmunized pregnancies, Doppler ultrasonography is more sensitive and accurate than amniocentesis in predicting severe fetal anemia.[231,232]

The major causes of treatable fetal anemia are listed in Box 2-2. Most of them are related to hemolytic disease of the fetus, hemoglobinopathies, or severe red cell enzyme defects.[233]

Cases of severe fetal anemia caused by acquired maternal chronic pure red cell aplasia[234] or congenital type I dyserythropoietic anemia[235] have been described.

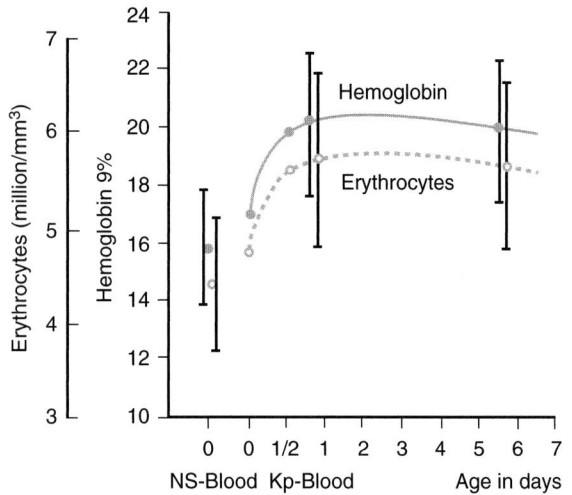

FIGURE 2-9. Hemoglobin concentration and red cell count in cord and venous blood in normal infants during the first week of life. Kp-Blood, capillary blood; NS-Blood, cord blood. *(After Künzer W. In Kepp R, Oehlert G [eds]. Blutbildung und Blutumsatz beim Feter und Neugeboreren. Stuttgart, Germany, Ferdinand Enke, 1962, p 4.)*

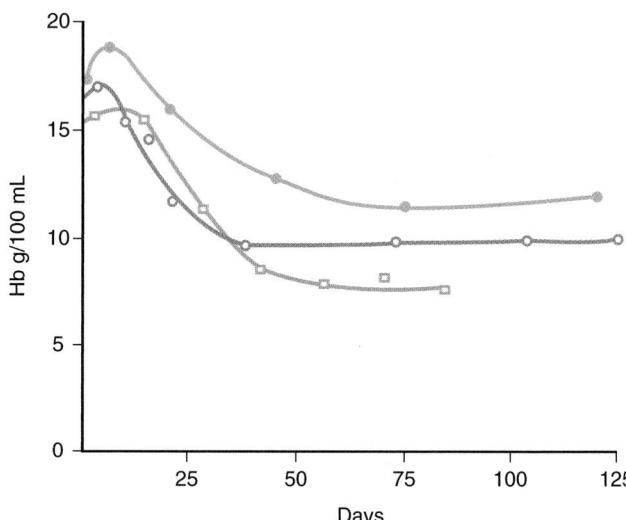

FIGURE 2-10. Hemoglobin concentration in infants of different degree of maturation at birth. *Filled circles,* full-term infants; *open circles,* premature infants with birth weights of 1200 to 2350 g; *squares,* premature infants with birth weights less than 1200 g.

TABLE 2-10   Evolution of Hematologic Values of 163 Fetuses during Pregnancy*

Week of Gestation	Hb (g/dL)	Hct (%)	RBC (×10⁹/L)	MCV (fL)	RDW (%)	MCH (pg)
18-20 (*n* = 25)	11.47 ± 0.78	35.86 ± 3.29	2.66 ± 0.29	133.92 ± 8.83	20.64 ± 2.28	43.14 ± 2.71
21-22 (*n* = 55)	12.28 ± 0.89	38.53 ± 3.21	2.96 ± 0.26	130.06 ± 6.17	20.15 ± 1.92	41.39 ± 3.32
23-25 (*n* = 61)	12.40 ± 0.77	38.59 ± 2.41	3.06 ± 0.26	126.19 ± 6.23	19.29 ± 1.62	40.48 ± 2.88
26-30 (*n* = 22)	13.35 ± 1.17	41.54 ± 3.31	3.52 ± 0.32	118.17 ± 5.75	18.35 ± 1.67	37.94 ± 3.67

*Data ± SD. Studies performed with a Coulter Hematology Analyzer, model S-PLUS II.

Hb, hemoglobin; Hct, hematocrit; MCH, mean corpuscular hemoglobin; MCV, mean corpuscular volume; RBC, red blood cell; RDW, RBC distribution width; SD, standard deviation.

Modified from Forestier F, Daffos F, Galacteros F, et al. Hematological values of 163 normal fetuses between 18 and 30 weeks of gestation. Pediatr Res. 1986;20:342-346.

Box 2-2   Fetal Anemia Treatable by Intrauterine Transfusion

IMMUNE

Hemolytic disease of the fetus

NONIMMUNE

Hemolytic: hemoglobinopathies (e.g., α-thalassemia [four-gene deletion]), G6PD deficiency
Nonhemolytic: acquired chronic pure red cell aplasia

OTHER

Severe antepartum fetomaternal hemorrhage
Twin-to-twin transfusion syndrome
Cystic hygroma with hydrops fetalis
Placenta chorioangioma
Intrauterine parvovirus B19 infection
Malaria

G6PD, glucose-6-phosphate dehydrogenase.

However, other pathologic conditions have been associated with anemia during the fetal period, such as hydrops fetalis in combination with either cystic hygroma[236] or placental chorioangioma,[237] parvovirus B19 infection,[238-243] cytomegalovirus infection,[244] and malaria.[245] Rarely, congenital mesoblastic nephroma can induce marked prenatal hematuria and hemorrhagic shock.[246] For a more comprehensive list of causes, management, and outcome of nonimmune hydrops fetalis, see elsewhere.[247-250]

Drug-induced cases of fetal anemia have also been described, such as after antiretroviral therapy during pregnancy[251,252] and in association with mycophenolate therapy.[253]

Severe chronic anemia in the prenatal period may result in cutaneous manifestations called "blueberry muffin baby"[254]; these expressions of cutaneous hematopoiesis need to be distinguished from neoplastic diseases and from the angioedema seen in neonates with parvovirus B19 maternal infection.[255,256]

ANEMIA IN THE NEONATE

Anemia present at birth or appearing during the first week of life can be broadly classified into three major categories: anemia as a result of blood loss, anemia as a result of a hemolytic process, or anemia secondary to less than normal red cell production. Many of the disorders producing a hemolytic process are discussed in greater detail in other sections of this text (see Chapters 3, 15, 16, and 17 and Section VI).

Anemias that are unique to the newborn and not the result of isoimmunization are the focus of the following discussion. The reader is encouraged to consult other monographs in which the primary focus is anemia in the newborn period.[257-268]

BLOOD LOSS AS A CAUSE OF ANEMIA

Blood loss resulting in anemia may occur prenatally, at the time of delivery, or in the first few days of life. Blood loss may be the result of occult hemorrhage before birth, obstetric accidents, internal hemorrhage, or excessive blood sampling by physicians.

The multiple causes of blood loss in the newborn period are listed in Box 2-3. Faxelius and associates estimated the red cell volume in 259 infants admitted to a high-risk unit in an attempt to determine which clinical events were frequently associated with a reduction in red cell mass.[218] Low red cell volume was frequently associated with a maternal history of vaginal bleeding, with placenta previa or abruptio placentae, with nonelective cesarean section, and with deliveries complicated by cord compression. Asphyxiated infants (Apgar score of 6 or less at 1 minute) often had low red cell volume. An early central venous hematocrit below 45% correlated with low red cell volume, but a normal or even high early hematocrit did not exclude the possibility that the infant was hypovolemic. Infants with a mean arterial pressure of less than 30 mm Hg and infants in whom the hematocrit fell by more than 10% during the first 6 hours of life were also frequently found to have reduced red cell mass. These findings serve to underscore the fact that much of the anemia in early life is the result of obstetric factors that produce blood loss in the infant.

Occult Hemorrhage before Birth

Occult hemorrhage before birth may be caused by bleeding of the fetus into the maternal circulation or by bleeding of one fetus into another when multiple fetuses are present.

Fetal-to-Maternal Hemorrhage

In approximately 50% of all pregnancies, some fetal cells can be demonstrated in the maternal circulation.[269] Nucleated fetal erythrocytes can be detected in the maternal circulation as early as the fifth gestational

---

Box 2-3   Types of Hemorrhage in the Newborn

OCCULT HEMORRHAGE BEFORE BIRTH

Fetomaternal
Abdominal or multiple trauma
Amniocentesis in the third trimester
After external cephalic version
Placental tumors
Spontaneous

Twin to Twin
Velamentous cord insertion
"Stuck twin" phenomenon

OBSTETRIC ACCIDENTS, MALFORMATION OF THE PLACENTA AND CORD

Rupture of a normal umbilical cord (precipitous delivery, entanglement)
Hematoma of the cord or placenta
Rupture of an abnormal umbilical cord (varices, aneurysm)
Rupture of anomalous vessels (aberrant vessels, velamentous insertion; communicating vessels in a multilobed placenta)
Intrauterine manipulation★
Manual removal of the placenta★
Cesarean section★
Incision of the placenta during cesarean section
Placenta previa★
Abruptio placentae★

INTERNAL HEMORRHAGE

Intracranial
Giant cephalohematoma, caput succedaneum
Retroperitoneal
Ruptured liver
Ruptured spleen

★Defined by the American College of Obstetrics and Gynecology as conditions associated with high risk for the development of fetomaternal hemorrhage of 30 mL or greater. Additional high-risk conditions are antepartum fetal death and antepartum bleeding.

---

week,[270] and substantial progress has been made in recent years to isolate these cells for prenatal diagnosis of genetic disease.[271-273] Fetal DNA is also present in maternal plasma and is another possible source of fetal genetic material for diagnostic testing.[274-276]

The estimated volume of fetal blood present in the maternal circulation is less than 2 mL in 98% of pregnancies.[277] Fetal-to-maternal hemorrhage of 30 mL or greater is observed in 3 in 1000 women, and it is most common after traumatic diagnostic amniocentesis or external cephalic version before delivery. A study of 30,944 Rh-negative mothers showed that 1 in 1146 had fetal bleeding of at least 80 mL whereas 1 in 2813 had bleeding of 150 mL or greater.[278] Risk factors for fetal-to-maternal bleeding are summarized in Box 2-3. Trau-

TABLE 2-11 Characteristics of Acute and Chronic Blood Loss in the Newborn

Characteristics	Acute Blood Loss	Chronic Blood Loss
Clinical	Acute distress; pallor; shallow, rapid, and often irregular respiration; tachycardia; weak or absent peripheral pulses; low or absent blood pressure; no hepatosplenomegaly	Marked pallor disproportionate to evidence of distress; on occasion, signs of congestive heart failure may be present, including hepatomegaly
Venous pressure	Low	Normal or elevated
LABORATORY VALUES		
Hb concentration	May be normal initially, then drops quickly during first 24 hr of life	Low at birth
RBC morphology	Normochromic and macrocytic	Hypochromic and microcytic; anisocytosis and poikilocytosis
Serum iron level	Normal at birth	Low at birth
Course	Prompt treatment of anemia and shock necessary to prevent death	Generally uneventful
Treatment	Intravenous fluids and whole blood; iron therapy later	Iron therapy; packed RBCs may be necessary on occasion

Hb, hemoglobin; RBC, red blood cell.

matic injury to the mother during pregnancy (e.g., injury secondary to motor vehicle accidents, falls, abdominal trauma),[279] third-trimester amniocentesis, placental abnormalities (abruptio placentae and placental tumors),[280] and manual removal of the placenta have also been associated with fetal-to-maternal hemorrhage.[277]

The clinical manifestations of fetal-to-maternal hemorrhage depend on the volume of hemorrhage and the rapidity with which it has occurred. If the hemorrhage has been prolonged or repeated during the course of the pregnancy, the anemia develops slowly and the fetus has an opportunity for hemodynamic compensation. Such an infant may manifest only pallor at birth. After acute hemorrhage, just before delivery, the infant may be pale and sluggish, have gasping respirations, and exhibit signs of circulatory shock. The typical physical findings and laboratory data that are useful in distinguishing the acute and chronic forms of fetal-to-maternal blood loss are described in Table 2-11.

The degree of anemia is quite variable. Usually, the hemoglobin value is less than 12 g/dL before signs and symptoms of anemia can be recognized by the physician. Hemoglobin values as low as 3 to 4 g/dL have been recorded in infants who were born alive and survived. If the hemorrhage has been acute, particularly when hypovolemic shock is present, the hemoglobin value may not reflect the magnitude of the blood loss. In such instances, several hours may elapse before hemodilution occurs and the magnitude of the hemorrhage is appreciated. In general, acute loss of 20% of blood volume is sufficient to produce signs of shock and is reflected in a decrease in hemoglobin levels within 3 hours of the event.

Examination of a peripheral blood smear provides useful diagnostic information. In acute hemorrhage, the red cells appear normochromic and normocytic, whereas in chronic hemorrhage, the cells are generally hypochromic and microcytic.

In anemia that is a direct result of fetal-to-maternal hemorrhage, the Coombs test yields a negative result, and the infants are not jaundiced. Infants with anemia secondary to blood loss generally have much lower bilirubin values throughout the neonatal period as a consequence of their reduced red cell mass.

The diagnosis of fetomaternal hemorrhage of sufficient magnitude to result in anemia at birth can be made with certainty only through demonstration of the presence of fetal cells in the maternal circulation. Techniques for demonstrating these cells include differential agglutination, mixed agglutination, fluorescent antibody techniques, and the acid elution method of staining for cells containing fetal hemoglobin.

The Kleihauer-Betke technique of acid elution is the simplest of these methods and the one most commonly used for detection of fetal cells,[281,282] although its value in monitoring patients at risk has been questioned.[283] The test is based on the resistance of fetal hemoglobin to elution from the intact cell in an acid medium. The acid elution technique can be relied on with certainty for diagnosis only when other conditions capable of producing elevations in maternal fetal hemoglobin levels are absent. Interpretation of this visual test shows considerable interobserver and interhospital variation, with up to 500% differences[284] for certain conditions, including maternal thalassemia minor, sickle cell anemia, hereditary persistence of fetal hemoglobin, and in some normal women, pregnancy-induced increase in fetal hemoglobin production. In such circumstances, other techniques based on differential agglutination should be used.[285] In addition, flow cytometry has been shown to be an acceptable alternative to the acid elution test for detection of fetomaternal hemorrhage.[286] However, most of the flow cytometry tests are designed to quantify D-positive fetal cells in D-negative mothers and are not applicable to D-positive mothers.[287,288]

The diagnosis of fetomaternal hemorrhage may be missed in situations in which the mother and infant are incompatible for the ABO blood group system. In such instances, the infant's A or B cells are rapidly cleared from the maternal circulation by maternal anti-A or anti-B antibodies and are not available for staining. A presumptive diagnosis may be made by demonstration of either marked erythrophagocytosis in smears of the maternal buffy coat or an increase in maternal immune anti-A or anti-B titer in the weeks after delivery.

Twin-to-Twin Transfusion Syndrome

This form of hemorrhage is observed only in monozygotic multiple births with monochorial placentas. In approximately 70% of monozygotic twin pregnancies, a monochorial placenta exists.[289] The incidence of twin-to-twin transfusion syndrome (TTTS) in pregnancies in which a monochorial placenta is present has been estimated to be 13% to 33% in one study[290] and 6.2% in another.[291] Velamentous cord insertion is associated with an increased risk for TTTS, possibly as a result of compression force, which reduces blood flow to one twin.[292] This blood exchange can produce anemia in the donor and polycythemia in the recipient and is associated with a characteristic twin oligohydramnios-polyhydramnios sequence except in rare cases.[293] When significant transfer of blood has occurred, the difference in hemoglobin concentration between the twins exceeds 5.0 g/dL. This is in contrast to a maximal discrepancy of 3.3 g/dL in cord blood hemoglobin in dizygotic twins. The survival rate of fetuses with TTTS diagnosed before the 28th week of gestation varies between 21% and 50%.[290,294,295] Clinical characteristics, diagnostic modalities, and the possible therapeutic role of amniocentesis and cordocentesis with fetal transfusion in reducing the high perinatal mortality associated with this syndrome have been reviewed.[291,295-298] Laser ablation of the chorionic plate vessels at the intertwin membrane has been shown to improve the survival of at least one of the two fetuses and reduce neurologic complication when compared with serial removal of a large volume of amniotic fluid.[299-301]

Congestive heart failure may develop in the anemic infant, whereas the plethoric twin may have symptoms and signs of hyperviscosity syndrome, disseminated intravascular coagulation, and hyperbilirubinemia.[302] Rarely, hydrops fetalis may develop if TTTS occurs early in the pregnancy.[303]

The hemorrhage may be acute or chronic. In a review of 482 twin pairs by Tan and associates, 35 pairs were found to have TTTS.[304] They pointed out how the difference in weight of the twins could be used to establish the timing of the hemorrhage. When the weight difference exceeded 20% of the weight of the larger twin, the transfusion was chronic and the smaller infant was invariably the donor. The anemic smaller twin displayed reticulocytosis. When the difference in the weight of the twins did not exceed 20% of the weight of the larger twin, the larger twin was the donor in almost 50% of all instances. In these presumably acute transfusions, significant reticulocytosis was not observed in the anemic donor. Although hemoglobin values of the recipient were increased equally with both acute and chronic transfusion, the donor twin in the chronic transfusion group was found to be more anemic than the donor in the acute transfusion group. These findings support and extend the original proposal of Klebe and Ingomar, who suggested these two types of transfusion on the basis of a review of previously documented cases.[305]

Obstetric Accidents and Malformations of the Placenta and Cord

The normal umbilical cord may rupture during precipitous deliveries. The cord may also rupture during a normal delivery when it is unusually short or entangled around the fetus or when traction is applied to the infant with forceps.[306]

Other abnormalities of the umbilical cord that predispose to hemorrhage and the development of anemia in the infant include vascular abnormalities such as umbilical venous tortuosity and arterial aneurysm. Inflammation of the cord can weaken vessels and predispose them to rupture.

Velamentous insertion of the umbilical cord is observed in approximately 1% of all pregnancies. It appears to be most common in twin pregnancies and in pregnancies accompanied by low-lying placentas. It is estimated that 1% to 2% of pregnancies associated with velamentous insertion of the cord result in fetal blood loss.[306] The perinatal death rate in such circumstances ranges from 58% to 80%, with many of the infants being stillborn. Approximately 12% of these infants who are born alive will be anemic.

The placenta may be inadvertently incised during cesarean section, with the incision producing fetal hemorrhage.[307] As previously mentioned, placenta previa or abruptio placentae often results in fetal hemorrhage.[308] In women with late third-trimester bleeding, the physician may anticipate the birth of an anemic infant by examining vaginal blood for the presence of fetal erythrocytes with the acid elution technique of Kleihauer and Betke.[309]

Internal Hemorrhage

When internal hemorrhage takes place in the newborn, it may not be recognized until shock has occurred.

Anemia that appears in the first 24 to 72 hours after birth and is not associated with jaundice is commonly due to internal hemorrhage. It is well recognized that traumatic deliveries may result in subdural or subarachnoid hemorrhage of sufficient magnitude to result in anemia. Cephalohematomas may be of giant size and result in anemia.[310]

Blood loss into the subaponeurotic area of the scalp tends to be greater than that observed with cephalohematomas. The bleeding is not confined by periosteal attachments and thus is not limited to an area overlying a single skull bone. A subaponeurotic hemorrhage usually extends through the soft tissue of the scalp and covers the entire calvaria. Blood loss in this area can result in exsanguination.[311] Pachman observed a hemoglobin value of 2.2 g/dL in an infant 48 hours of age in whom massive hemorrhage into the scalp had occurred.[312] This form of hemorrhage most commonly occurs after difficult deliveries or vacuum extraction.[313] It also appears with vitamin K deficiency and may be more frequent in African American infants than in those of other ethnicity. Examination of the infant reveals a boggy edema of the head extending into the frontal region and to the nape of the neck. The edema, which may have bluish coloration, obscures the fontanelles and swells the eyelids. The infant may be in shock. Robinson and Rossiter have developed a formula for predicting the volume of blood loss in this condition.[311] For each centimeter of increase in head circumference above that expected, a 38-mL loss of blood has occurred. When the products of red cell breakdown are absorbed from these entrapped hemorrhages, hyperbilirubinemia may develop.[314]

Breech deliveries may be associated with hemorrhage into the adrenal glands, kidneys, spleen, or retroperitoneal area. Blood loss of this type should be suspected in infants found to be anemic during the first few days of life after a traumatic delivery. Hemorrhage into the adrenal glands may also be observed after any difficult delivery or after the birth of a large infant. In adrenal hemorrhage, the clinical picture may include sudden collapse, cyanosis, limpness, jaundice, irregular respirations, elevated or subnormal temperatures, and the presence of a flank mass accompanied by bluish discoloration of the overlying skin.

Rupture of the liver, with resultant anemia, appears to occur more frequently than clinically appreciated. In stillbirths and neonatal deaths, the incidence of hepatic hemorrhage found at autopsy ranges from 1.2% to 5.6%.[315] In approximately half of the cases reviewed by Henderson, the hemorrhage was subcapsular only; in the remainder, the capsule had ruptured, and free blood was present in the peritoneal cavity.[316]

An infant with a ruptured liver generally appears to be well for 24 to 48 hours and then suddenly goes into shock. The moment of onset of shock appears to coincide with the time when the gradually increasing hematoma finally ruptures the hepatic capsule and causes hemoperitoneum. At this time the upper part of the abdomen may appear distended, and often a mass contiguous with the liver is palpable. Shifting dullness can be demonstrated on abdominal percussion. Flat films of the abdomen taken with the patient in both the erect and supine positions frequently confirm the presence of free fluid in the abdomen. Paracentesis, performed with the infant in the lateral position, reveals free blood in the abdomen.

The prognosis is poor, but infants have been saved after multiple blood transfusions and prompt surgical repair of the laceration.

Splenic rupture may also occur after a difficult delivery or as a result of the extreme distention of the spleen that often accompanies severe erythroblastosis fetalis.[317,318] The physician should always suspect rupture of the spleen with associated hemorrhage when at the time of exchange transfusion, an anemic and hydropic infant with erythroblastosis fetalis is found to have decreased rather than increased venous pressure. Rupture of the spleen may also occur during the exchange transfusion.

Splenic rupture occurs, though uncommonly, in healthy infants born after seemingly normal deliveries.[319] Many of these infants are of large size. Pallor, abdominal distention, scrotal swelling, and radiographic evidence of peritoneal effusion without free air should alert the physician to the presence of splenic rupture.

Other less common causes of neonatal bleeding include maternal treatment with antiepileptic drugs during pregnancy associated with vitamin K deficiency,[320] neonatal adenovirus infection,[321] fetal cytomegalovirus infection,[322] hemangiomas of the gastrointestinal tract, and hemangioendotheliomas of the skin.[323,324]

Bleeding into the ventricles and subarachnoid space can also produce significant anemia. Intraventricular hemorrhage may occur in half of all infants with birth weights of less than 1500 g and with even greater frequency when the mother has ingested aspirin in the week before birth of the infant.[325] In many of these infants, no neurologic symptoms are present, and the hemorrhage is recognized on computed tomography of the head.[326]

Anemia Caused by Drawing Blood for Laboratory Analysis

A major cause of anemia in critically ill neonates treated in neonatal intensive care units (NICUs) is frequent blood drawing for laboratory analysis. In very-low-birth-weight infants (<1500 g), a 1-mL blood draw represents 1% or more of the total blood volume (Fig. 2-11). In neonates weighing less than 1500 g, blood drawings during the first 4 weeks of hospitalization may range from 5% to 45% of the calculated total blood volume.[327] A study of 60 very-low-birth-weight infants (560 to 1450 g) showed an average of 4.8 punctures per day per infant, with a mean blood loss for diagnostic sampling of 50.3 mL/kg per 28-day period (range, 7 to 142 mL).[328] Increased blood loss was associated with increased number of transfusions. There is also evidence that the volume of blood drawn for laboratory tests may exceed the actual laboratory requirement for the tests ordered by almost 20%.[329] Another study showed lower blood loss (13.6 mL/kg), with the most frequently ordered tests being glucose, sodium, and potassium.[330]

Various approaches for limiting the amount of blood drawn for laboratory tests include the following:

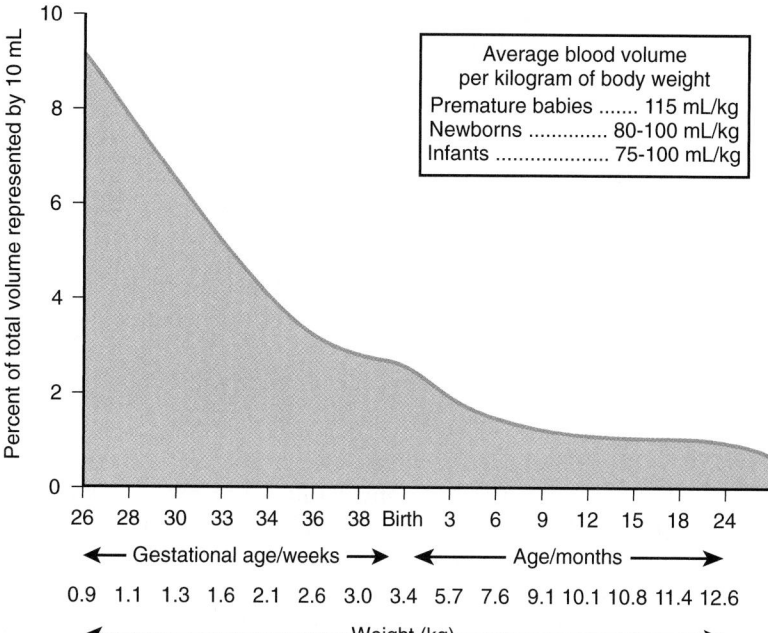

FIGURE 2-11. Average blood volume per kilogram of body weight. *(Redrawn from Werner M. Microtechniques for the Clinical Laboratory. New York, John Wiley & Sons, 1976, p 2. Reprinted by permission of John Wiley & Sons, Inc.)*

1. Reducing the amount of blood discarded from central venous lines before blood is obtained for culture. It has been shown that discarding only 0.3 mL in infants and 1.0 mL in children does not affect the accuracy of central venous line cultures.[331]
2. Use of micromethods that reduce blood loss from peripheral arterial catheters during sampling.[332]
3. Use of a closed method that allows return of the initial sample drawn to clear a line to the patient. This technique has been shown to reduce blood loss as a result of diagnostic sampling, even in adult patients.[333,334]
4. Reducing the amount of blood drawn in excess of that needed for the analytic procedure (25% of the blood removed in NICU settings is in excess of the analytic need).[327] Phlebotomy overdraw is more prominent in the most critically ill infants and is greater when syringes are used.[329]
5. Reducing the need for blood drawing through the use of transcutaneous monitoring techniques (40% of the blood drawn in an NICU setting is for analysis of blood gases and electrolytes).[327]

Recognition of Infants with Blood Loss

The clinical manifestations of hemorrhage are dependent on the site of bleeding, the extent of the hemorrhage, and whether the blood loss is acute or chronic. Features useful in distinguishing infants with acute and chronic blood loss at the time of delivery are described in Table 2-11. Asphyxiated infants may also display pallor. Features that aid in distinguishing an infant with asphyxia from an infant with acute blood loss are presented in Box 2-4. In all circumstances associated with late third-trimester bleeding, multiple births, cesarean section, a nuchal cord, any form of cord compression, or a difficult delivery, a hemoglobin determination should be obtained promptly

in the infant. Even when the first value is normal, a repeat hemoglobin determination should be performed 6 to 12 hours after birth.

ANEMIA AS A RESULT OF A HEMOLYTIC PROCESS

A *hemolytic process* is generally defined as a pathologic process that results in shortening of the normal red cell

---

Box 2-4 Differential Diagnosis of Pallor in the Newborn

ASPHYXIA

Respiratory findings: retractions, response to oxygen, cyanosis
Moribund appearance
Bradycardia
Stable hemoglobin

ACUTE SEVERE BLOOD LOSS

Decrease in venous and arterial pressure
Rapid shallow respirations
Acyanotic
Tachycardia
Drop in hemoglobin

HEMOLYTIC DISEASE

Hepatosplenomegaly, jaundice
Positive result on the Coombs test
Anemia

Adapted from Kirkman HN, Riley HD Jr. Posthemorrhagic anemia and shock in the newborn due to hemorrhage during delivery: Report of 8 cases. Pediatrics. 1959;24:97-105. Copyright American Academy of Pediatrics, 1959.

life span of 120 days. For neonates, a different definition that recognizes that the normal red cell life span of term infants is only 60 to 80 days (and may be as short as 20 to 30 days in infants born at 30 to 32 weeks of gestation) must be used. A hemolytic process during the neonatal period is usually manifested by one of the following combinations of clinical and laboratory findings:

1. A persistent increase in the reticulocyte count, with or without an abnormally low hemoglobin concentration in the absence of current or previous hemorrhage
2. A rapidly declining hemoglobin concentration without an increase in the reticulocyte count in the absence of hemorrhage

Most infants with hemolytic anemia have accompanying hyperbilirubinemia; however, in the majority of infants in whom the bilirubin level exceeds 12 mg/dL, an increase in red cell destruction, as reflected by an increase in blood carboxyhemoglobin levels, cannot be demonstrated.[335] Approximately 30% of infants with an increase in carboxyhemoglobin levels have maximum bilirubin values of less than 8 mg/dL. The major causes of a shortened red cell life span in the neonatal period are listed in Box 2-5. Only the most salient features of the hereditary hemolytic anemias that are manifested in the neonatal period are discussed in this section. Extensive descriptions of these disorders appear in other portions of the text.

Hemoglobinopathies

Clinically significant hemoglobinopathies in the newborn may be categorized, as in older children, as defects in structure or defects in synthesis (thalassemic syndromes). Because of the rapid evolutionary changes that occur in the fetus and newborn with respect to globin chain synthesis, a unique situation exists. Certain hereditary defects of hemoglobin may be seen at this age; some of these defects spontaneously resolve (e.g., γ-chain defects), whereas other defects, clinically inapparent at birth, produce problems at a later age (e.g., β-chain disorders). Other defects that might be thought to be similar in their clinical manifestations throughout life, such as α-chain defects, may in fact act differently in the newborn period when paired with a γ chain rather than with a β chain.

Defects in Hemoglobin Structure

α-Chain Structural Defects

When α-chain variants of hemoglobin occur, they are present in significant concentration at birth because the α chain is common to all forms of hemoglobin present at birth. In contrast, β-chain variants such as HbS become quantitatively significant only as β-chain synthesis replaces γ-chain production during the first months after birth. When the amino acid alteration is in the α chain, the concentration of abnormal hemoglobin will remain

Box 2-5	Causes of a Hemolytic Process in the Neonatal Period

Immune
  Rh incompatibility
  ABO incompatibility
  Minor blood group incompatibility
  Maternal autoimmune hemolytic anemia
  Drug-induced hemolytic anemia
Infection
  Bacterial sepsis
  Congenital infections
  Syphilis
  Malaria
  Cytomegalovirus
  Adenovirus
  Rubella
  Toxoplasmosis
  Disseminated herpes
Disseminated intravascular coagulation
Macroangiopathic and microangiopathic anemia
  Cavernous hemangioma or hemangioendothelioma
  Large vessel thrombi
  Renal artery stenosis
  Severe coarctation of the aorta
Galactosemia
Prolonged or recurrent metabolic or respiratory acidosis
Hereditary disorders of the red cell membrane
  Hereditary spherocytosis
  Hereditary elliptocytosis
  Hereditary stomatocytosis
  Hereditary xerocytosis
  Other rare membrane disorders
Pyknocytosis
Red cell enzyme deficiencies
G6PD deficiency, pyruvate kinase deficiency, 5′-nucleotidase deficiency, glucose phosphate isomerase deficiency
α-Thalassemia syndromes
α-Chain structural abnormalities
γ-Thalassemia syndromes
γ-Chain structural abnormalities

G6PD, glucose-6-phosphate dehydrogenase.

fairly constant during infancy and adulthood; however, during infancy, the abnormal hemoglobin will be present primarily in a fetal form ($\alpha_2^x \gamma_2$), with a lesser amount in the adult form ($\alpha_2^x \beta_2$). An example of this is the HbD St. Louis trait ($\alpha_2^{Asn68 \rightarrow Lys} \beta_2$), in which the total concentration of abnormal hemoglobin ($\alpha_2^x \gamma_2 + \alpha_2^x \beta_2$) was found to be 27% in neonates, as opposed to an average of 28% HbD in the heterozygous state in adults.[336]

Fortunately, most α-chain mutations do not cause clinically significant disorders in adults, and the same situation appears to exist in newborns. Most infants with α-chain mutations are detected only as part of routine neonatal screening programs. Occasionally, the fetal form of an α-chain mutation is clinically more significant than the adult form of the mutation. Neonates with Hb Hasharon ($\alpha_2^{Asp14 \rightarrow His}\beta_2$) are an example of this phenomenon. Hb Hasharon is mildly unstable; unstable mutant hemoglobins have a greater tendency to dissociate into subunits, and this increased dissociation leads to hemolysis. HbF is less stable than HbA, presumably as a result of a 10-fold greater affinity between α and β chains than between α and γ chains. As a mildly unstable hemoglobin, the interaction between Hasharon α chains and normal β chains must be minimally decreased, but the interaction between Hasharon α chains and γ chains in the fetal form of Hb Hasharon would be expected to be considerably less and result in an even more unstable form of the α-chain variant. Levine and co-workers described a 965-g newborn who was heterozygous for Hb Hasharon.[337] This infant manifested a hemolytic anemia that resolved coincidentally with the transition from the fetal to the adult form of Hb Hasharon trait at several months of age.

β-Chain Structural Defects

β-Chain mutations generally produce no clinical symptomatology in the newborn period. This does not mean that chain variants are never a problem in the neonate, nor does it mean that these variants cannot be easily detected in the laboratory.

Although HbA usually constitutes less than 30% of the normal hemoglobin at birth, it is possible that the amount may, under certain circumstances, be far greater. Because the γ- to β-chain switchover begins at about 32 weeks' gestation, any disorder that causes the fetus to destroy its existing red cell population will result in replacement with red cells that have a markedly different HbF/HbA ratio at the time of delivery. Fetomaternal blood group incompatibility and intrauterine blood loss may, for example, unmask a β-chain defect earlier than it might otherwise be detected.

Sickle cell hemoglobinopathies are the most commonly encountered β-chain variants in the newborn period. Several cases of homozygous sickle cell disease have been seen clinically in neonates. In patients with homozygous sickle cell disease, the HbS concentration at birth is usually about 20%.

In infants in whom sickle cell anemia has been diagnosed in the first 30 days of life because of some specific symptomatology, the most frequent findings are jaundice, fever, pallor, respiratory distress, and abdominal distention. Hyperbilirubinemia appears to be more common in newborns with sickle cell anemia.[338] Hegyi and co-workers described a full-term newborn in whom abdominal distention developed during the first day of life.[339] The cord bilirubin value was 3.1 mg/dL, the hemoglobin level was 12.7 g/dL, and the reticulocyte count was 13.3%. No evidence of G6PD deficiency or blood group incompatibility was found, but hemoglobin electrophoresis demonstrated 20% HbS and 80% HbF. The child rapidly improved but was later found dead in her crib on the fifth day of life. Postmortem examination revealed

sickle cells in multiple organs and histopathologic findings consistent with widespread vaso-occlusion, including multifocal enterocolitis.

Of special concern is the problem of "iatrogenic" sickle cell crisis—exchange transfusion of neonates with respiratory distress syndrome with the use of blood from apparently healthy donors who happen to have sickle cell trait.[340] Such transfusions can produce death in hypoxic infants.

γ-Chain Structural Defects

Table 2-12 lists the most commonly observed γ-chain structural hemoglobinopathies. These variants are quite interesting because they represent disorders that spontaneously resolve as γ-chain production diminishes. Concentrations of these hemoglobin variants in cord blood average 10% to 20% of the total hemoglobin and appear to represent the heterozygous state of these γ-chain hemoglobinopathies.[336] The structural γ-chain defects are not generally associated with any hematologic disturbances and are usually found during newborn screening programs. HbF Poole is an exception to this rule. HbF Poole is an unstable hemoglobin that is manifested as a Heinz body hemolytic anemia during the first weeks of life.[341]

Defects in Hemoglobin Synthesis

In newborn infants, defects in hemoglobin synthesis create a greater variety of thalassemia syndromes than may occur at any other time of life. Newborns may demonstrate all varieties of α-thalassemia, β-thalassemia, γ-thalassemia, or δ-thalassemia, or any combination of these types.

α-Thalassemia Syndromes in the Neonate

In the newborn period, hemolytic disease secondary to thalassemia has invariably been associated with homozygous α-thalassemia. A large spectrum of α-thalassemia syndromes may be observed in the newborn period.

Silent Carrier (One-Gene Defect). Thus far, no observations have been made of this disorder in the neonatal period. This entity would be suspected only if a parent were known to be a silent carrier.

α-Thalassemia Trait (Two-Gene Defect). Although the α-thalassemia syndromes have been described for more than 20 years, the heterozygous state (trait) has been difficult to identify because of the mild hematologic changes that accompany this disorder. Older children and adults may demonstrate a very mild anemia and microcytosis in the presence of normal hemoglobin electrophoresis. The diagnosis is more easily made in the neonatal period than at any other time of life because of two unique occurrences. First, microcytosis is observed in the cord blood of newborns with α-thalassemia trait. Because other causes of microcytosis are rare at this age, infants who are born with a low MCV are more likely to

TABLE 2-12   γ-Chain Hemoglobinopathies: $^G\gamma$ or $^A\gamma$

Hb Name	Residue/Substitution	% Total Hb	% Total HbF	Notes
$^G\gamma$				
F-Malaysia	1 Gly → Cys	12.8	18.8	
F-Meinohama	5 Glu → Gly	10.0		
F-Aukland	7 Asp → Asn	19	22.5	
F-Albaicin	8 Lys → Glu or Gln	29		
F-Catalonia	15 Trp → Arg	45.5	51.5	
F-Melbourne	16 Gly → Arg	26	29	
F-Saskatoon	21 Glu → Lys	16.2	23.3	
F-Urumqi	22 Asp → Gly	21.5		
F-Granada	22 Asp → Val	22		
F-Cosenza	25 Gly → Glu	22.4		
F-Oakland	26 Glu → Lys	32		
F-Austell	40 Arg → Lys	27		
F-Lodz	44 Ser → Arg	37.1		
F-Kingston	55 Met → Arg	21		
F-Sacromonte	59 Lys → Gln	25		
F-Emirates	59 Lys → Glu	37		
F-M-Osaka	63 His → Tyr			Decreased O_2 affinity, methemoglobinemia
F-Brooklyn	66 Lys → Gln	23		
F-Kennestone	77 His → Arg	25.3	30.7	
F-Marietta	80 Asp → Asn	12.4	16.2	
F-Columbus-GA	94 Asp → Asn	30.5		
F-La Grange	101 Glu → Lys	14.0		Increased O_2 affinity, mildly unstable
F-Malta-I	117 His → Arg			
F-Carlton	121 Glu → Lys	26		
F-Port Royal	125 Glu → Ala	14-16		
F-Onoda	146 His → Tyr	26.4	35	Increased O_2 affinity
$^A\gamma$				
F-Macedonia-I	2 His → Gln	15		
F-Texas-I	5 Glu → Lys	12		Increased acetylation (3-fold)
F-Pordenone	6 Glu → Gln	5.7	8.6	
F-Calluna	12 Thr → Arg	8.7	10.8	
F-Kuala Lumpur	22 Asp → Gly	11		
F-Pendergrass	36 Pro → Arg	6.7	8.5	
F-Bonaire-GA	39 Gln → Arg	8.3	9.8	
F-Beech Island	53 Ala → Asp	15-16		
F-Jamaica	61 Lys → Glu	11-15		
F-Iawata	72 Gly → Arg	11		
F-Sardinia	75 Ile → Thr	15		
F-Damman	79 Asp → Asn	6.9	13.1	
F-Victoria Jubilee	80 Asp → Tyr	7.0		
F-Hull	121 Glu → Lys	7-9		

have α-thalassemia trait than any other disease. Second, α-thalassemia in newborns is associated with the presence of Hb Bart's (γ_4), which is easily identified.

Hemoglobin values in neonates with thalassemia trait are no different from those of normal neonates (range, 15.2 to 18.5 g/dL).[342] MCV is significantly lower (≈94 μm³) than that in normal term infants (106.4 ± 5.7 μm³). In addition, patients with the trait syndrome usually have an MCH of less than 29.3 pg. Determination of MCV and MCH appears to be an adequate screening test. The presence of Hb Bart's is the confirmatory finding.

Hemoglobin H Disease. This disorder appears to caused by the inheritance of a three-gene deletion that results in sufficient α/β + γ-chain imbalance to result in the presence of large quantities of Hb Bart's (γ_4) and some HbH (β_4) in the newborn period. After the first few months of life, the Hb Bart's disappears, and the only remaining abnormal hemoglobin is HbH.

Infants born with HbH disease have higher levels of Hb Bart's in their cord blood than do normal infants or individuals with α-thalassemia trait; however, they have lower levels than homozygous infants with hydrops fetalis do. Unlike infants with α-thalassemia trait, infants with HbH disease are born with significant anemia. Microcytosis is present.[343] The hemolytic process may contribute to a somewhat increased incidence of neonatal jaundice.

Hydrops Fetalis. This four-gene deletion disease results in death of the affected fetus. Because of the virtual absence of α-chain synthesis, affected infants are born with Hb Bart's only (occasionally, however, some Hb Portland may be found). The peripheral blood smear demonstrates marked hypochromia, poikilocytosis, and target cells. This disorder must be distinguished from other causes of hydrops fetalis with severe anemia. A negative result on the Coombs test and the demonstration of intracellular crystals of Hb Bart's with supravital staining rapidly confirm the high probability of the homozygous state as the correct diagnosis. If death does not occur in utero, it occurs within minutes after birth. Although infants with hydrops fetalis have been reported to have cord hemoglobin values as high as 11 g/dL, the usual levels are much lower.[344] Oxygen delivery is severely impaired even when hemoglobin levels are greater because of the profound leftward shift of the oxyhemoglobin dissociation curve for Hb Bart's. There is a possible association between homozygous α-thalassemia and hypospadias.[345,346] When this disorder is detected in utero, the fetus may be salvaged with intrauterine transfusion and maintained by a postdelivery transfusion program.[347,348] Prevention of severe forms of α-thalassemia and hydrops fetalis can be achieved with prenatal testing and counseling.[349]

β-Thalassemias

In the β-thalassemia syndromes (both trait and homozygous states), the disorders become apparent only after 2 or 3 months of age. In β-thalassemia minor, hematologic findings at birth are entirely normal, with microcytosis being noted later in the first 6 months of life. Similarly, in β-thalassemia major, no clinical findings are present initially; the first sign of any abnormality is the presence of nucleated red cells on smears or maintenance of high HbF concentrations. Any disorder that significantly alters the survival of fetal red cells (e.g., intrauterine blood loss or blood group incompatibility) could make the β-thalassemia syndromes clinically obvious at an earlier age.

Erlandson and Hilgartner recorded their observations of infants in whom thalassemia major was diagnosed during the first 3 months of life.[350] In four infants in whom the disease was diagnosed between 1 and 2 months of age, hemoglobin concentrations were abnormally low. Morphologic erythrocyte abnormalities were already present at 3 days of age in one infant who was also mildly anemic (hemoglobin level, 12.7 g/dL). The earliest morphologic abnormalities were similar to those found in the heterozygous state; however, by 2 months of age, the presence of marked numbers of normoblasts, consistent with homozygous thalassemia, was noted in all infants. Splenomegaly was not present in the one infant who was examined at birth but was apparent in all infants between 1 and 3 months of age. Fetal hemoglobin levels were elevated at 1 to 2 months of age. It would seem then that at least some manifestations of thalassemia major may be present at birth.

γ-Thalassemias

Theoretically, a decrease in γ-chain synthesis (γ-thalassemia) would produce symptoms in utero. Because there are multiple structural genes for γ-chain synthesis, the severity of γ-thalassemia would depend on the extent to which these genes are involved. The condition would be lethal if no γ chains were formed; if only one or two genes were involved, only slight hypochromia or, at most, a mild anemia would ensue. If the diagnosis were not established in the neonatal period, it would be missed because as β-chain synthesis replaces γ-chain synthesis, the red cell changes would disappear.[351]

Combinations of Thalassemia Syndromes

Kan and co-workers described a full-term infant who had hemolytic hypochromic anemia at birth associated with microcytosis and nucleated red cells on smear.[352] Neither HbH nor Hb Bart's was detected. Studies of globin chain synthesis in peripheral blood revealed a deficiency in the synthesis of γ and β chains. As the infant matured, the peripheral smear morphology improved and became identical to that of the subject's father, who had β-thalassemia trait. Since then, several such cases have been reported (see Chapter 20).

Methemoglobinemia in Neonates Treated with Nitric Oxide

Methemoglobinemia is discussed in detail in Chapter 18. A new form of drug-induced Met-Hb has special relevance for oxygen transport in neonates. Pulmonary vasoconstriction is characteristic of persistent pulmonary hypertension of the newborn and is frequently seen in neonatal respiratory distress syndromes. Inhaled nitric oxide (NO) acts as a potent vasodilator on the pulmonary vasculature, improves oxygenation, and lowers pulmonary vascular resistance.[353-358] A potentially serious side effect of the administration of NO is the oxidation of Fe^{2+} of hemoglobin to form Fe^{3+} and Met-Hb. This is usually transient but has been reported to be as high as 40%.[359] Detection of Met-Hb formation is particularly problematic in neonates because of the interference of HbF on determination of Met-Hb. Multiwavelength hemoglobin co-oximeters can provide reliable estimates of Met-Hb in samples with high HbF, although their reliability differs in different models.[360-362] It is advisable to monitor Met-Hb levels in all neonates treated with NO.

Methemoglobinemia in Neonates with Diarrhea

Diarrhea in neonates can be associated with methemoglobinemia, in some cases requiring infusion of methylene blue. Affected patients are usually seen in the first 1 to 3 months of life, frequently with failure to thrive, weight on admission below the 10th percentile, and formula-feeding.[363-365]

Hereditary Disorders of the Red Cell Membrane

Hereditary spherocytosis, hereditary elliptocytosis, hereditary stomatocytosis, and hereditary xerocytosis all may be manifested in the newborn period.[366] If hemolytic anemia is detected during evaluation for hyperbilirubinemia, a precise diagnosis is not generally established in most patients until they are older. It should also be kept in mind that genetic defects in bilirubin metabolism may be associated with hereditary disorders of the red cell membrane and lead to marked neonatal hyperbilirubinemia.[367]

In hereditary spherocytosis, the condition is diagnosed in only a third of patients during the first year of life. Neonates with hereditary spherocytosis have dehydrated erythrocytes with decreased membrane surface area and exhibit a sharp fall in hemoglobin (near-normal at birth) and reticulocyte counts during the first 20 days of life, with transfusion required in 75% of cases.[368] The reticulocyte response to the anemia is also blunted in the first year of life.[368] Two cases of severe neonatal anemia caused by hereditary spherocytosis and absence of the anion exchange protein band 3 have been reported.[369,370]

The classic morphologic abnormalities of patients with hereditary elliptocytosis may not be present during the first few weeks of life. Patients with the hemolytic form of hereditary elliptocytosis may display pyknocytes rather than elliptocytes early in life, and only after several months are the typical elliptocytes observed. These membrane disorders are described in detail in Chapter 15.

Hereditary xerocytosis (or dehydrated hereditary spherocytosis) is associated in some families with perinatal edema that resolves in a few weeks after birth. In other families it is associated with pseudohyperkalemia. Erythrocyte MCV and MCH are both increased, and the defect has been localized to 16q23-q24.[371,372]

Red Cell Enzyme Deficiencies

Inherited disorders of red cell metabolism may also be anticipated to produce hemolytic anemia early in life. The most common of these abnormalities are G6PD deficiency and pyruvate kinase deficiency.[266,373] These and other disorders of red cell metabolism are described in Chapters 16 and 17. G6PD deficiency may be associated with Gilbert's syndrome and lead to marked hyperbilirubinemia and jaundice.[374,375] Severe transfusion-dependent neonatal anemia accompanied at birth by jaundice, by pyropoikilocytosis, and in the first 3 to 4 years of life by rhabdomyolysis and hyperkalemia has been described in a patient with compound mutations for the erythrocyte/muscle enzyme aldolase A.[376]

Malaria

Although the pathophysiology of malaria-associated anemia is not fully understood,[377] it has been shown that congenital malaria and the presence of parasitemia at birth are strongly associated with neonatal anemia (hemoglobin <14 g/dL).[378-381]

Infantile Pyknocytosis

Infantile pyknocytosis, with pyknocytes defined as "distorted, irregular, densely stained erythrocytes, presenting with several to many spiny projections," has been shown to account for up to 10% of cases of otherwise unexplained neonatal hemolytic anemia and jaundice.[382] The proportion of pyknocytes varied from 4% to 23% in this series, whereas lower numbers have been described in full-term or premature infants.

Neonatal Cobalamin and Folate Deficiency

Both severe maternal dietary deficiency of cobalamin and folate and inherited errors in the absorption, transport, and metabolism of these two key metabolites have been associated with neonatal anemia.[383] In a normal pregnancy, plasma and red cell folate decrease and total plasma homocysteine levels increase without producing folate deficiency in the newborn.[384]

IMPAIRED RED BLOOD CELL PRODUCTION

Diamond-Blackfan syndrome (pure red cell anemia, erythrogenesis imperfecta, or chronic aregenerative anemia) is an uncommon condition characterized by failure of erythropoiesis but normal production of white blood cells and platelets (see Chapter 8).[385] The disease may affect more than red cell production because it is associated with pancytopenia, hypoplasia of the bone marrow, and reduced in vitro clonogenic potential.[386]

Two reviews of the subject suggest that as many as 25% of affected patients may be anemic at birth.[387,388] Hemoglobin values as low as 9.4 g/dL, accompanied by reticulocytopenia, have been observed during the first days of life.[389] There is no correlation between the various types of gene mutations described in this disease and clinical expression and severity.[390,391] However, the severity of the disease is greater in patients affected at a young age and born prematurely.[392] Congenital Diamond-Blackfan anemia may be missed if associated with other more common causes of fetal anemia, such as hemorrhage.[393]

Low birth weight occurs in approximately 10% of all affected patients, with about half of this group being small for gestational age. There appears to be a slight increase in the incidence of miscarriage, stillbirth, and complications of pregnancy in mothers who have given birth to infants with this syndrome.

Abnormalities that have been described include microcephaly, cleft palate, anomalies of the eye, web neck, and thumb deformity. A triphalangeal thumb, duplications of the thumb, and a bifid thumb have been reported in association with this syndrome.[394-396]

Another cause of impaired red cell production in the neonatal period is Pearson's syndrome.[397] This syndrome is characterized by vacuolization of bone marrow precursors, sideroblastic anemia, and exocrine pancreatic dysfunction.[398] It may be associated with Leigh's disease (subacute necrotizing encephalopathy)[399] or with Kearns-Sayre syndrome (bilateral ptosis and atypical retinitis pigmentosa).[400] A deletion in mitochondrial DNA has been found in Pearson's syndrome.[401-403] A case of pyridoxine-refractory congenital sideroblastic anemia with autosomal recessive inheritance has also been described.[404] Neonatal anemia with macrocytosis has been reported in some cases of cartilage-hair hypoplasia.[405]

Cases of congenital dyserythropoietic anemia (CDA) resulting in severe fetal and neonatal anemia have been described.[235,406] Anemia and early jaundice, with or without splenomegaly/hepatomegaly, accompany the bone abnormalities in almost all cases described thus far.[407,408] The reticulocyte count is characteristically lower than expected based on the degree of anemia. Pulmonary hypertension of the newborn has been shown to accompany CDA in neonates.[409]

Association with Gilbert's syndrome increases neonatal hyperbilirubinemia in CDA type II.[410]

Impaired red cell production resulting in anemia during the neonatal period may also be observed as a result of congenital infections such as rubella, cytomegalovirus, adenovirus, and human parvovirus.[411-413] Congenital leukemia, Down syndrome, and osteoporosis may likewise produce anemia during the early days of life as a result of inadequate erythropoiesis.

A DIAGNOSTIC APPROACH TO THE ANEMIC NEWBORN

In view of the great number of entities that may be responsible for anemia in the newborn period, a disciplined approach to diagnosis is essential. A detailed family and obstetric history should be obtained. The placenta should be examined whenever possible.

During physical examination of the infant, particular attention should be devoted to detection of congenital anomalies, stigmata of intrauterine infection, internal hemorrhage, and the presence of hepatosplenomegaly.

Initial laboratory studies should include a complete blood count, red cell indices, reticulocyte count, direct Coombs test, and examination of a well-prepared peripheral blood smear. Other useful simple procedures include a Heinz body preparation and performance of a "wet prep" of the infant's erythrocytes.

One approach that relies on the reticulocyte count and cellular indices in arriving at a diagnosis is illustrated

in Figure 2-12. This approach can be supplemented with specific diagnostic tests as indicated.

PHYSIOLOGIC ANEMIA OF PREMATURITY

The hemoglobin concentration of term infants normally decreases over the first weeks of life, and this is known as the "physiologic anemia of infancy." Infants who are born prematurely but are otherwise healthy experience a more exaggerated decrease in hemoglobin concentration (see the following paragraph), which has been termed the "physiologic anemia of prematurity."[414] Factors that influence the magnitude of this physiologic anemia include the nutritional status of the infant and a variety of complex adaptations to changes in oxygen availability.[415]

Cord hemoglobin values do not change significantly during the last trimester of pregnancy. After birth, the rapidity with which the hemoglobin level declines and the magnitude of the actual decrease vary directly with the degree of immaturity of the newborn. Although the nadir in hemoglobin concentration for normal full-term infants may be as low as 11.4 ± 0.9 g/dL by the age of 8 to 12 weeks, the average hemoglobin value observed by Schulman in premature infants weighing less than 1500 g was 8.0 g/dL at the age of 4 to 8 weeks.[414] These data are consistent with the normal data found by others.[416]

It is generally agreed that this fall in hemoglobin concentration results in greatest part from a decrease in red cell mass rather than a hemodilutional effect of an expanding plasma volume.[90] These changes occur at a time when the red cell survival of both term and premature infants is known to be shortened and when a striking decrease occurs in hematopoietic activity, as evidenced by a fall in the reticulocyte count and a decrease in marrow erythroid elements.

Cord blood analysis generally demonstrates elevated levels of EPO; these elevated levels are increased further in infants who experience transient hypoxemia at the time of delivery.[417,418] One notable exception is seen in neonates with severe isoimmunization treated by intrauterine transfusion, in whom severe anemia typically develops postnatally. The anemia is due to a combination of continued immune-mediated hemolysis and suppressed erythropoiesis. Serum EPO in these neonates surged transiently at birth but did not reach "appropriate" levels until the hemoglobin level decreased to below 5 g/dL.[419] Otherwise, infants born anemic demonstrate reticulocytosis. Increased erythropoiesis is generally seen in small-for-gestational-age infants who have experienced intrauterine hypoxia.[420] The anemia of prematurity rarely occurs in association with cyanotic congenital heart disease or respiratory insufficiency, which indicates that infants in the first few weeks of life can maintain higher oxygen-carrying capacity if the need arises. In premature infants, early neonatal anemia is an important predictor of mortality and neurologic sequelae.[421]

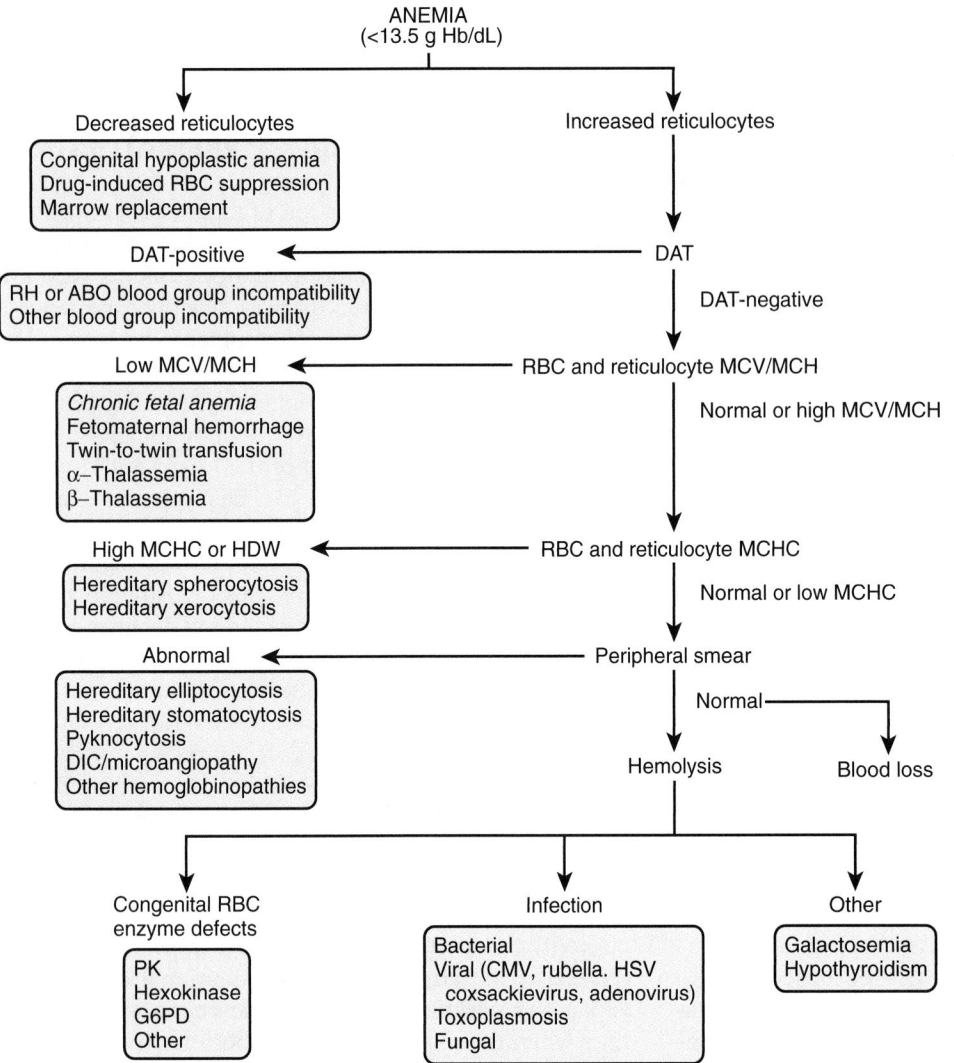

FIGURE 2-12. Diagnostic approach to anemia in the newborn. CMV, cytomegalovirus; DAT, direct antiglobulin test; DIC, disseminated intravascular coagulation; G6PD, glucose-6-phosphate dehydrogenase; HDW, hemoglobin distribution width; HSV, herpes simplex virus; MCHC, mean corpuscular hemoglobin concentration; MCV/MCH, mean corpuscular volume/mean corpuscular hemoglobin; PK, pyruvate kinase; RBC, red blood cell.

An important insight into the ability of preterm infants to adjust the hemoglobin level adequately to their own specific requirements may be noted if the hematologic status of infants who are born with widely varying hemoglobin concentrations is compared in the first few months of life. Differences in initial hemoglobin levels greatly affect the hemoglobin concentration in the weeks after birth. Infants with lower hemoglobin levels at birth achieve minimum hemoglobin values more rapidly, and their recovery phase occurs earlier than in infants born with higher hemoglobin levels.[415] It is interesting to note, however, that the minimum hemoglobin levels achieved are similar in infants born with widely discrepant hemoglobin values, thus suggesting that the signal for return of active erythropoiesis is roughly equivalent among infants.

Until recently it was not clear how infants, particularly premature infants, could tolerate large declines in hemoglobin concentration while at the same time provide sufficient supplies of oxygen to tissues. Adequate tissue oxygenation in the face of diminished oxygen-carrying capacity (lower hemoglobin concentration) can be accomplished only if oxygen demands are reduced or if one or more compensatory changes that are known to accompany anemia are observed. These responses include, in part, higher cardiac output, improved oxygen-unloading capacity, redistribution of blood flow, and greater oxygen extraction (a decrease in oxygen tension in mixed central venous blood). Apparently, only some of these responses occur.

Cardiac output does not change significantly between the end of the first week of life and 3 months of age. Although the oxygen content of blood (milliliters of oxygen carried per 100 mL of blood) decreases to its lowest level in the first 2 to 3 months of life, this reflects nothing more than the overall decline in hemoglobin concentration. The oxygen-unloading capacity of blood—that is, the actual quantity of oxygen that is theoretically capable of being delivered to tissues—is constantly increasing from the moment of birth, even as the hemoglobin level falls.[422] This increase in oxygen unloading results from a gradual rightward shift in the oxyhemoglobin dissociation curve as fetal hemoglobin levels decrease and the red cell 2,3-DPG level increases. The magnitude of this shift may have profound physiologic significance for both term and premature infants.

Recombinant Human Erythropoietin and the Anemia of Prematurity

In 1977, Stockman and associates observed EPO concentrations within or below the normal adult range in infants with the anemia of prematurity.[423] Very low levels for the degree of anemia have subsequently been observed and reported by others.[424,425] EPO levels in neonates of different weight at birth vary over a wide range, but they seem to reach a nadir between days 7 and 50 independent of weight at birth; this is followed by the nadir in hemoglobin concentration (between day 51 and 150).[426] These and other data indicate that the increase in EPO levels is insufficient for the degree of anemia when the neonates are compared with matched adults.[50,427]

Investigation of in vitro erythroid colony growth has demonstrated normal numbers of both circulating BFU-E[428] and bone marrow CFU-E[429] in the anemia of prematurity. Both classes of erythroid progenitors show normal EPO dose-response curves. Taken together, the findings of low serum EPO concentrations, relative bone marrow erythroid hypoplasia, and a normal EPO dose-response curve suggest that inadequate EPO production is a major factor in the genesis of anemia of prematurity.

The blunted EPO response to decreasing hemoglobin levels[312] may be a consequence of the incomplete switch from liver to kidney as the major source of EPO production in premature infants and the relative insensitivity of liver-controlled EPO production to hypoxia.[424] An additional factor may be related to a different clearance and volume of distribution of EPO in neonates that results in lower EPO levels.[430,431] The anemia of prematurity is also due to blood loss related to the shorter life span of neonatal erythrocytes and to the rapid growth observed in the first weeks of life, which is not accompanied by a parallel increase in red cell mass. Detailed reviews of the pathophysiology and treatment of anemia of prematurity have been published.[262-264,431,432]

The use of r-HuEPO reduces the need for transfusions in premature infants weighing more than 1000 g, a group that rarely undergoes transfusion.[432] r-HuEPO may not be as effective in reducing transfusion requirements when it is used in infants weighing less than 1000 g or in neonates requiring artificial ventilation.[433-435] In a large, double-blind, placebo-controlled trial, r-HuEPO was shown to reduce blood transfusion requirements in preterm infants (weight at birth, 924 ± 183 g).[436] Although the reduction in blood transfusions was statistically significant, use of r-HuEPO resulted in only a small increase in the number of untransfused infants (from 31% to 43%). This disappointing result could have been due to poor EPO responsiveness, variability in the r-HuEPO

dosages used, or inconsistency in providing supplemental iron for sustaining the enhanced erythropoiesis induced by r-HuEPO. A detailed cost analysis of the use of r-HuEPO for the anemia of prematurity has been published.[437] A meta-analysis of 21 clinical trials in which r-HuEPO was administered to premature neonates showed an average reduction of 11 mL/kg in red cell transfusion in neonates weighing less than 1000 g.[438] However, the large variability in published results does not permit r-HuEPO to be recommended as standard of care in this setting.[438] Early (first 2 weeks of life) use of r-HuEPO does not seem to reduce the number of transfusion in infants with birth weight less than 1250 g.[439] However, it lowers transfusion requirements in infants with birth weight lower than 800 g and phlebotomy losses of greater than 30 mL/kg.[439]

A potential advantage of the use of r-HuEPO in the anemia of prematurity is the associated right shift in the oxyhemoglobin dissociation curve, most likely secondary to the increased erythrocyte 2,3-DPG content.[440] The incidence of necrotizing enterocolitis is lower in very-low-birth-weight infants treated with r-HuEPO,[441] whereas neurodevelopmental outcomes are unaffected by r-HuEPO therapy.[442]

Studies in adult subjects have identified a functional iron deficiency in normal iron-replete subjects treated with r-HuEPO and oral iron.[443] Oral iron administration is insufficient for sustaining the increased marrow activity in the presence of r-HuEPO, and intravenous iron supplementation should always be considered for premature infants, possibly in association with vitamin E supplementation. In very-low-birth-weight premature infants, no measurable detriment in antioxidant defense could be shown in conjunction with oral iron supplementation therapy.[444] Use of intravenous iron together with r-HuEPO was associated with a greater hemoglobin and reticulocyte response in premature infants.[445]

Studies in adult patients have indicated that autologous donation is not cost-effective when compared with allogeneic blood transfusion, mostly as a consequence of the high cost of collecting and discarding units that are not used.[446] However, reduction of allogeneic blood use by means of autologous blood donation (and the use of r-HuEPO) may be a prudent practice to follow despite the associated additional cost.[447] Cost-benefit analysis does not indicate cost-effectiveness for the use of EPO in the neonatal setting,[448] but this conclusion is based on the high cost of the product (to reach a break-even point would require a 54% reduction in product cost) and the way it is currently packaged: a 2000-unit vial cannot be used more than once for the same patient, although it can be used for multiple patients on the same day. However, any vial-sharing practice should be carefully scrutinized, given the reports of *Serratia liquefaciens* sepsis from multiple use of single-use vials in adult dialysis centers.[449] Changes in r-HuEPO price and packaging could make r-HuEPO therapy more similar in cost to allogeneic blood transfusion. r-HuEPO is a remarkably safe drug. No significant side effects have been reported with its use, with the exception of the occurrence of seizures and blood pressure elevation when the circulating red cell mass is increased too rapidly. r-HuEPO has been shown to increase total bilirubin production in premature infants without inducing clinically significant jaundice.[450] Use of r-HuEPO in preterm infants does not affect the ratio of HbF to HbA.[451]

NEONATAL HYPERVISCOSITY

Neonates with hematocrit values in excess of 65% are at some risk for *hyperviscosity syndrome*, a condition that consists of hypoglycemia, central nervous system injury,[452] and hypocalcemia with elevated plasma calcitonin gene–related peptide levels.[453] Infants with polycythemic hyperviscosity should undergo careful isovolumic partial plasma exchange transfusion, especially when abnormal results are obtained on cerebral blood flow velocity studies.[454] Although there is good correlation between polycythemia and hyperviscosity, several infants with hyperviscosity syndrome have normal hematocrit values and can be identified only with the use of viscosity measurements.[455] Several risk factors for neonatal polycythemia and hyperviscosity have been identified, such as maternal insulin-dependent diabetes,[456,457] intrauterine growth retardation, perinatal asphyxia, twin-to-twin transfusion (recipient), delayed cord clamping, and Beckwith's syndrome.[458]

TRANSFUSIONS IN PREMATURE INFANTS

Red cell transfusion is discussed in Chapter 35; however, some of the problems unique to the neonatal setting are discussed in this section. For a more detailed discussion of issues related to neonatal red cell transfusion, consult recent publications.[263,459-463]

Decisions regarding the need for transfusion in low-birth-weight infants cannot be based on hemoglobin concentration or hematocrit alone. Wardrop and co-workers have demonstrated that "available oxygen" and not the absolute hemoglobin level most closely correlates with the presence of symptoms and signs of hypoxemia such as tachycardia, tachypnea, easy fatigability, and poor feeding in low-birth-weight infants.[464] Available oxygen is a reflection of the position of the oxyhemoglobin dissociation curve, the hemoglobin concentration, and arterial oxygen saturation. Nomograms that illustrate the importance of these factors in making decisions regarding transfusion have been prepared.[465] These nomograms are based on assumptions regarding cardiac output and oxygen consumption that have been derived from serial measurements in low-birth-weight infants.[466] An example of the importance of P_{50} and arterial oxygen saturation in making decisions regarding the hemoglobin required

TABLE 2-13	Hemoglobin Levels Required in Low-Birth-Weight Infants* to Maintain Central Venous Oxygen Tension of 30 mm Hg			
	ARTERIAL OXYGEN SATURATION (%)			
P_{50} (mm Hg)	**95**	**90**	**85**	**80**
20	10.0	13.0	20.0	>25.0
23	7.3	9.0	11.0	15.5
25	6.2	7.3	8.8	11.0
27	5.3	6.3	7.3	8.9

*Assumes a cardiac output of 250 mL/kg/min and an oxygen consumption of 6.5 mL/kg/min.

for maintaining central venous oxygen tension at 30 mm Hg is illustrated in Table 2-13.

As a general rule, hemoglobin values in otherwise healthy low-birth-weight infants should be maintained above 12 g/dL during the first 2 weeks of life. After that period, decisions regarding transfusion when determinations of "available oxygen" cannot be performed should be based on the infant's clinical condition. Factors to evaluate include the infant's weight gain, evidence of fatigue during feeding, tachycardia, tachypnea, and evidence of hypoxemia as reflected by an increase in blood lactic acid concentrations.[467] Although a study in premature infants has shown no relationship between hematocrit (values from 19% to 64%) and either heart or respiratory rates or the occurrence of bradycardia,[468] hematocrit still seems to be the best indicator of red cell mass in low-birth-weight infants.[469] Capillary whole blood lactate has been shown to have little value in transfusion decisions,[440,470] although plasma lactate levels decrease after transfusion.[440] In a study comparing "liberal" and "restrictive" hematocrit transfusion thresholds (46% versus 34% for tracheal incubation, 38% versus 28% for nasal continuous positive airway pressure or supplemental oxygen, and 30% versus 22% for neither), the "liberal" group received more transfusions without being exposed to more donors, whereas infants in the "restrictive" groups experienced more frequent major neurologic adverse events.[462] However, a recent study comparing two hemoglobin thresholds for transfusion (7 versus 9.5 g/dL, with target ranges of 8.5 to 9.5 g/dL versus 11 to 12 g/dL, respectively) showed that the 7.0-g/dL threshold was associated with decreased transfusion requirements and no worse adverse outcomes.[471,472]

Infants with cardiac or pulmonary disease that reduces arterial oxygen saturation may require hemoglobin concentrations of at least 16 to 17 g/dL for their oxygen requirements to be met adequately. No guidelines for neonatal transfusion have been clearly defined. It is common practice to transfuse neonates for the following reasons[473]:

1. Replacement of blood drawn for testing when cumulative blood loss reaches 5% or 10% of total blood volume
2. Maintenance of hematocrit greater than 40% in patients with severe respiratory distress or symptomatic heart disease
3. Maintenance of hematocrit greater than 30% in neonates with cardiopulmonary problems or growth failure

It has been estimated that more than 300,000 red blood cell transfusions are given annually to 38,000 premature neonates in the United States.[473] Most infants who weigh more than 1000 g do not receive transfusions in this country.[474] There has been a significant reduction in the prevalence of transfusions because of improved treatment and prevention of neonatal lung disease with surfactants, better ventilation, inhalation of NO, reduction in blood loss for analytic purposes, and less aggressive transfusion regimens. Neonatal transfusion practices in the United States have been studied in a national survey,[475,476] which indicated that a large number of institutions in the United States still perform unnecessary major antiglobulin crossmatches for neonatal transfusions. This practice leads to a greater amount of blood being drawn and thus more transfusions.

Standards issued by the American Association of Blood Banks require testing for ABO group and Rh type, as well as red cell antibody screening before the first transfusion. If the red cell antibody screen is negative, it is unnecessary to crossmatch red cells for the initial or subsequent transfusions. Repeat testing may be omitted for the remainder of the neonate's hospital admission. If a non–group O neonate is to receive non–group O red blood cells that are not compatible with the maternal ABO group, the initial sample should also be tested for passively acquired anti-A or anti-B immunoglobulin.[477]

Infants do not usually produce red cell–specific antibodies. Production of antibodies against white cells has been described, but its clinical significance is unclear.[478,479]

Traditionally, blood used for neonatal transfusion is less than 7 to 10 days old and is collected in anticoagulant citrate-phosphate-dextrose-adenine (CPDA) rather than in additive solutions, even though there is no good scientific evidence to support this practice with small-volume (10 mL/kg) red cell transfusions.[475,480,481] When transfused in small volumes (15 mL/kg), up to 42-day-old red cells in additive solutions are equivalent to fresh red cells in CPDA.[482] Use of specifically assigned units less than 14 days old and sterile connecting devices allows a reduction in donor exposure and has no adverse effects.[483] Exposure to different donors can be drastically reduced by the multiple use of a single unit of blood for a patient over a period of 35 to 42 days without affecting cost.[484-486]

Blood products with a low risk for cytomegalovirus (cytomegalovirus negative or leukodepleted red cells) should be used only for neonates with weight at birth of less than 1200 g who are cytomegalovirus negative or of unknown cytomegalovirus status.[487,488] Universal leukodepletion is now applied to all red cells collected in the United States.[489] Early immunostimulatory (increase in lymphocyte count) and late (day 14) immunosuppressive effects (increase in lymphocytes expressing CD45RA, CD3$^-$/CD16$^+$CD56, CD80, and CD3$^-$/DR) have been described in transfused very-low-birth-weight infants.[490]

Packed red cells should be adjusted to the desired hematocrit (60% to 79%) with normal saline or 5% albumin solution. However, a significant number of institutions still use fresh frozen plasma from the same donor or from a different donor for this purpose.[475] This practice is particularly widespread for exchange transfusions in which red cells reconstituted in fresh frozen plasma from different donors are used—that is, each neonate is exposed to two different donors. In some settings, partial exchange transfusion may be preferable to simple transfusion.[491] Use of a small-bore central venous line (1.90-French NeoPICC) may not be associated with significant hemolysis, at least based on in vitro data.[492]

A significant factor in determining different blood use in the neonatal setting is related to existing institutional practice. Comparison of blood use in two NICUs has revealed major differences in the percentage of patients transfused and the number of transfusions that cannot be accounted for by differences in disease severity.[493-495] Because no differences can be demonstrated in clinical outcome between high-transfusion and low-transfusion NICUs, implementation of guidelines on blood drawing, use of arterial catheters, and transfusion should result in a reduction in transfusion rates and associated complications and cost.

REFERENCES

1. Wintrobe MM. Clinical Hematology, 5th ed. Philadelphia, Lea & Febiger, 1961.
2. Orkin SH. Diversification of haematopoietic stem cells to specific lineages. Nat Rev Genet. 2000;1:57-64.
3. Mikkola HKA, Orkin SH. The journey of developing hematopoietic stem cells. Development. 2006;133:3733-3744.
4. Maximov AA. Relation of blood cells to connective tissue and endothelium. Physiol Rev. 1924;4:533.
5. Bloom W, Bartelmez GW. Hematopoiesis in young human embryos. Am J Anat. 1940;67:21-53.
6. Keller G. The hemangioblast. In Marshak D, Gardner R, Gottlieb D (eds). Stem Cell Biology. New York, Cold Spring Harbor Laboratory Press, 2001, pp 329-348.
7. Kennedy M, D'Souza SL, Lynch-Kattman M, et al. Development of the hemangioblast defines the onset of hematopoiesis in human ES cell differentiation cultures. Blood. 2007;109:2679-2687.
8. Jin H, Xu J, Wen Z. Migratory path of definitive hematopoietic stem/progenitor cells during zebrafish development. Blood. 2007;109:5208-5214.

9. Ehrlich P. De- und Regeneration roter Blutscheiben. Berhandl Gesellsch Charite Arzte. 1880.

10. Migliaccio G, Migliaccio AR, Petti S, et al. Human embryonic hemopoiesis. Kinetics of progenitors and precursors underlying the yolk sac–liver transformation. J Clin Invest. 1986;78:51-60.

11. Thomas DB, Yoffey JM. Human foetal haematopoiesis. II. Hepatic haematopoiesis in the human foetus. Br J Haematol. 1964;10:193-197.

12. Tavian M, Coulombel L, Luton D, et al. Aorta-associated CD34+ hematopoietic cells in the early human embryo. Blood. 1996;87:67-72.

13. Tavian M, Hallais MF, Péault B. Emergence of intraembryonic hematopoietic precursors in the pre-liver human embryo. Development. 1999;126:793-803.

14. Medvinsky AL, Dzierzak E. Definitive hematopoiesis is autonomously initiated by the AGM region. Cell. 1996;86:897-906.

15. Cumano A, Dieterlen-Lievre F, Godin I. Lymphoid potential, probed before circulation in mouse, is restricted to caudal intraembryonic splanchnopleura. Cell. 1996;86:907-916.

16. Fukuda T. Fetal hemopoiesis. II. Electron microscopic studies on human hepatic hemopoiesis. Virchows Arch B Zell Pathol. 1974;16:249-270.

17. Kimura N, Yamano Y, Nito Y, Yanase T. Erythroid progenitors in human fetal liver. Nippon Ketsueki Gakkai Zasshi. 1984;47:1235-1241.

18. Campagnoli C, Fisk NM, Overton T, et al. Circulating hematopoietic progenitor cells in first trimester fetal blood. Blood. 2000;95:1967-1972.

19. Linch DC, Knott LJ, Rodeck CH, Heuhns ER. Studies of circulating hemopoietic progenitor cells in human fetal blood. Blood. 1982;59:976-979.

20. Zauli G, Vitale M, Re MC, et al. In vitro growth of human fetal CD34+ cells in the presence of various combinations of recombinant cytokines under serum-free conditions. Br J Haematol. 1994;86:461-467.

21. Lansdorp PM. Developmental changes in the function of hematopoietic stem cells. Exp Hematol. 1995;23:187-191.

22. Kelemen E, Calvo W, Friedner TM. Atlas of Human Hemopoietic Development. Berlin, Springer-Verlag, 1979.

23. Broxmeyer HE, Douglas GW, Hangoc C, et al. Human umbilical cord blood as a potential source of transplantable hematopoietic stem/progenitor cells. Proc Natl Acad Sci U S A. 1989;86:3828-3832.

24. Liang DC, Ma SW, Lin-Chu M, Lan CC. Granulocyte/macrophage colony-forming units from cord blood of premature and full-term neonates: its role in ontogeny of human hematopoiesis. Pediatr Res. 1988;24:701-702.

25. Forestier F, Daffos F, Catherine N, et al. Developmental hematopoiesis in normal human fetal blood. Blood. 1991;77:2360-2363.

26. Murray NA, Roberts IAG. Circulating megakaryocytes and their progenitors (BFU-MK and CFU-MK) in term and pre-term neonates. Br J Haematol. 1995;89:41-46.

27. Shields LE, Andrews RG. Gestational age changes in circulating CD34+ hematopoietic stem/progenitor cells in fetal cord blood. Am J Obstet Gynecol. 1998;178:931-937.

28. Valtieri M, Gabbianelli M, Pelosi E, et al. Erythropoietin alone induces erythroid burst formation by human embryonic but not adult BFU-E in unicellular-serum-free culture. Blood. 1989;74:460-470.

29. Emerson S, Thomas S, Ferrara JL, Greenstein JL. Developmental regulation of erythropoiesis by hematopoietic growth factors: analysis of populations of BFU-E from bone marrow, peripheral blood, and fetal liver. Blood. 1989;74:49-55.

30. Gardner D, Liechty KW, Christensen RD. Effects of interleukin-6 on fetal hematopoietic progenitors. Blood. 1990;75:2150-2155.

31. Holbrook ST, Ohls RK, Schibler KR, et al. Effect of interleukin-9 on clonogenic maturation and cell-cycle status of fetal and adult hematopoietic progenitors. Blood. 1991;77:2129-2134.

32. Schibler KR, Yang YC, Christensen RD. Effect of interleukin-11 on cycling status and clonogenic maturation of fetal and adult hematopoietic progenitors. Blood. 1992;80:900-903.

33. Schibler KR, Li Y, Ohls RK, et al. Possible mechanisms accounting for the growth factor independence of hematopoietic progenitors from umbilical cord blood. Blood. 1994;84:3679-3684.

34. Traycoff CM, Abboud MR, Laver J, et al. Rapid exit from G_0/G_1 phases of cell cycle in response to stem cell factor confers on umbilical cord blood CD34+ cells an enhanced ex vivo expansion potential. Exp Hematol. 1994;22:1264-1272.

35. Williams DA, Xu H, Cancelas JA. Children are not little adults: just ask their hematopoietic stem cells. J Clin Invest. 2006;116:2593-2596.

36. Bowie MB, McKnight KD, Kent DG, et al. Hematopoietic stem cells proliferate until after birth and show a reversible phase-specific engraftment defect. J Clin Invest. 2006;116:2808-2816.

37. Bowie MB, Kent DG, Dykstra B, et al. Identification of a new intrinsically timed developmental checkpoint that reprograms key hematopoietic stem cell properties. Proc Natl Acad Sci U S A. 2007;104:5878-5882.

38. Melero-Martin JM, Khan ZA, Picard A, et al. In vivo vasculogenic potential of human blood-derived endothelial progenitor cells. Blood. 2007;109:4761-4768.

39. Pettengell R, Luft T, Henschler R, et al. Direct comparison by limiting dilution analysis of long-term culture–initiating cells in human bone marrow, umbilical cord blood, and blood stem cells. Blood. 1994;84:3653-3659.

40. Gluckman E, Broxmeyer HE, Auerbach AD, et al. Hematopoietic reconstitution in a patient with Fanconi's anemia by means of umbilical-cord blood from an HLA-identical sibling. N Engl J Med. 1989;321:1174-1178.

41. Gale RP. Cord-blood-cell transplantation—a real sleeper. N Engl J Med. 1995;332:392-394.

42. Wagner JE, Kerman NA, Broxmeyer HE, et al. Transplantation of umbilical cord blood in 50 patients: analysis of the registry data. Blood. 1994;84:395a.

43. Issaragrisil S, Visuthisakchai S, Suvatte V, et al. Brief report: transplantation of cord-blood stem cells into a patient with severe thalassemia. N Engl J Med. 1995;332:367-369.

44. Sirchia G, Rebulla P. Placental/umbilical cord blood transplantation. Haematologica. 1999;84:738-747.

45. Gluckman E, Locatelli F. Umbilical cord blood transplants. Curr Opin Hematol. 2000;7:353-357.

46. Hows JM. Status of umbilical cord blood transplantation in the year 2001. J Clin Pathol. 2001;54:428-434.

47. Ballen KK. New trends in umbilical cord blood transplantation. Blood. 2005;105:3786-3792.

48. Smythe J, Armitage S, McDonald D, et al. Directed sibling cord blood banking for transplantation: the 10-year experience in the National Blood Service in England. Stem Cells. 2007;25:2087-2093.

49. Nagano M, Yamashita T, Hamada H, et al. Identification of functional endothelial progenitor cells suitable for the treatment of ischemic tissue using human umbilical cord blood. Blood. 2007;110:151-160.

50. Halvorsen S. Plasma erythropoietin in cord blood during the first few weeks of life. Acta Paediatr Scand. 1963;52:425-435.

51. Matoth Y, Zaizov R. Regulation of erythropoiesis in the fetal rat. The Tel Aviv University Conference on Erythropoiesis. Petak Tikva, Israel. New York, Academic Press, 1970, p 24.

52. Jacobsen LO, Marks EK, Gaston EO. The effect of transfusion-induced polycythemia in the mother of the fetus. Blood. 1959;14:644-653.

53. Zanjani ED, Gidari AS, Peterson EN, et al. Humoral regulation of erythropoiesis in the foetus. In Comline KS, Cross KW, Davies GS (eds). Foetal and Neonatal Physiology. London, Cambridge University Press, 1973.

54. Orkin SH. Transcription factors and hematopoietic development. J Biol Chem. 1995;270:4955-4958.

55. Patterson LJ, Gering M, Patient R. Scl is required for dorsal aorta as well as blood formation in zebrafish embryos. Blood. 2005;105:3502-3511.

56. Matsumoto N, Kubo A, Liu H, et al. Developmental regulation of yolk sac hematopoiesis by Kruppel-like factor 6. Blood. 2006;107:1357-1365.

57. Goardon N, Schuh A, Hajar I, et al. Ectopic expression of TAL-1 protein in Ly-6E.1-htal-1 transgenic mice induces defects in B- and T-lymphoid differentiation. Blood. 2002;100:491-500.

58. Mikkola HKA, Fujiwara Y, Schlaeger TM, et al. Expression of CD41 marks the initiation of definitive hematopoiesis in the mouse embryo. Blood. 2003;101:508-516.

59. Hadland BK, Huppert SS, Kanungo J, et al. A requirement for Notch1 distinguishes 2 phases of definitive hematopoiesis during development. Blood. 2004;104:3097-3105.

60. Koibuchi N, Kaneda Y, Taniyama Y, et al. Essential role of HGF (hepatocyte growth factor) in blood formation in *Xenopus*. Blood. 2004;103:3320-3325.

61. Burns CE, Traver D, Mayhall E, et al. Hematopoietic stem cell fate is established by the Notch-Runx pathway. Genes Dev. 2005;19:2331-2342.

62. Schmerer M, Evans T. Primitive erythropoiesis is regulated by Smad-dependent signaling in postgastrulation mesoderm. Blood. 2003;102:3196-3205.

63. Delaney C, Varnum-Finney B, Aoyama K, et al. Dose-dependent effects of the Notch ligand Delta1 on ex vivo differentiation and in vivo marrow repopulating ability of cord blood cells. Blood. 2005;106:2693-2699.

64. Li Z, Chen MJ, Stacy T, Speck NA. Runx1 function in hematopoiesis is required in cells that express Tek. Blood. 2006;107:106-110.

65. Maki K, Yamagata T, Asai T, et al. Dysplastic definitive hematopoiesis in AML1/EVI1 knock-in embryos. Blood. 2005;106:2147-2155.

66. Liu X-S, Li X-H, Wang Y, et al. Disruption of palladin leads to defects in definitive erythropoiesis by interfering with erythroblastic island formation in mouse fetal liver. Blood. 2007;110:870-876.

67. Simon MC, Pevny L, Wiles MV, et al. Rescue of erythroid development in gene-targeted GATA-1-mouse embryonic stem cells. Nature Genet. 1992;1:92-98.

68. Perkins A, Sharpe AH, Orkin SH. Lethal beta-thalassemia in mice lacking the erythroid CACCC-transcription factor EKLF. Nature. 1995;375:318-322.

69. Gregory T, Yu C, Ma A, et al. GATA-1 and erythropoietin cooperate to promote erythroid cell survival by regulating bcl-xL expression. Blood. 1999;94:87-96.

70. Fujiwara Y, Chang AN, Williams AM, Orkin SH. Functional overlap of GATA-1 and GATA-2 in primitive hematopoietic development. Blood. 2004;103:583-585.

71. Nichols KE, Crispino JD, Poncz M, et al. Familial dyserythropoietic anaemia and thrombocytopenia due to an inherited mutation in GATA1. Nat Genet. 2000;24:266-270.

72. Pine SR, Guo Q, Yin C, et al. Incidence and clinical implications of GATA1 mutations in newborns with Down syndrome. Blood. 2007;110:2128-2131.

73. Phillips JD, Steensma DP, Pulsipher MA, et al. Congenital erythropoietic porphyria due to a mutation in GATA1: the first *trans*-acting mutation causative for a human porphyria. Blood. 2007;109:2618-2621.

74. Ward AC, Touw I, Yoshimura A. The Jak-Stat pathway in normal and perturbed hematopoiesis. Blood. 2000;95:19-29.

75. Bromberg J, Darnell JEJ. The role of STATs in transcriptional control and their impact on cellular function. Oncogene. 2000;19:2468-2473.

76. Socolovsky M, Fallon AEJ, Wang S, et al. Fetal anemia and apoptosis of red cell progenitors in Stat5a$^{-/-}$5b$^{-/-}$ mice: a direct role for Stat5 in bcl-XL induction. Cell. 1999;98:181-191.

77. Socolovsky M, Nam HS, Fleming MD, et al. Ineffective erythropoiesis in SAT5A$^{-/-}$5B$^{-/-}$ mice due to decreased survival of early erythroblasts. Blood. 2001;98:3261-3273.

78. Wagner KU, Claudio E, Rucker EB, et al. Conditional deletion of the BCl-x gene from erythroid cells results in hemolytic anemia and profound splenomegaly. Development. 2000;127:4949-4958.

79. Stamatoyannopoulos G, Rosenblum BB, Papayannopoulos T, et al. Hb F and Hb A production in erythroid cultures from human fetuses and neonates. Blood. 1979;54:440-450.

80. Orkin SH. Regulation of globin gene expression in erythroid cells. Eur J Biochem. 1995;231:271-281.

81. Lewis BA, Kim TK, Orkin SH. A downstream element in the human beta-globin promoter: evidence of extended sequence-specific transcription factor IID contacts. Proc Natl Acad Sci U S A. 2000;97:7172-7177.

82. Szelèngi JG, Hollán SR. Studies on the structure of human embryonic haemoglobin. Acta Biochim Biophys Acad Sci Hung. 1969;4:47-55.

83. Hecht F, Motulsky AG, Lemire RJ, Shepard TE. Predominance of hemoglobin Gower 1 in early human embryonic development. Science. 1966;152:91-92.

84. Kamuzora H, Lehmann H. Human embryonic haemoglobins including a comparison by homology of the human and chains. Nature. 1975;256:511-513.

85. Ley TJ, Maloney KA, Gordon JI, Schwartz AL. Globin gene expression in erythroid human fetal liver cells. J Clin Invest. 1989;83:1032-1038.

86. He Z, Russell JE. Expression, purification, and characterization of human hemoglobins Gower-1 (zeta$_2$epsilon$_2$), Gower-2 (alpha$_2$epsilon$_2$), and Portland-2 (zeta$_2$beta$_2$) assembled in complex transgenic-knockout mice. Blood. 2001;97:1099-1105.

87. Seip M. The reticulocyte level and the erythrocyte production judged from reticulocyte studies in newborn infants during the first week of life. Acta Paediatr. 1955; 44:355-369.

88. Garby L, Sjölin S, Vuille J-C. Studies on erythrokinetics in infancy. III. Plasma disappearance and red cell uptake of intravenously injected radioiron. Acta Paediatr. 1963; 52:537-553.

89. Manning LR, Russell JE, Padovan JC, et al. Human embryonic, fetal, and adult hemoglobins have different subunit interface strengths. Correlation with lifespan in the red cell. Protein Sci. 2007;16:1641-1658.

90. Bratteby LE. Studies on erythrokinetics in infancy. XI. The change in circulating red cell volume during the first five months of life. Acta Paediatr Scand. 1968;54:215-224.

91. Gairdner D, Marks J, Roscoe JE. Blood formation in infancy. Part II—normal erythropoiesis. Arch Dis Child. 1952;27:214-221.

92. Sturgeon P. Volumetric and microscopic pattern of bone marrow in normal infants and children. I. Volumetric pattern. Pediatrics. 1951;7:577-588.

93. Sturgeon P. Volumetric and microscopic pattern of bone marrow in normal infants and children. II. Cytologic pattern. Pediatrics. 1951;7:642-650.

94. Issaragrisil S. Correlation between hematopoietic progenitors and erythroblasts in cord blood. Am J Clin Pathol. 1983;80:865-867.

95. Mann DL, Sites MD, Donati RM, Gallagher NI. Erythropoietic stimulating activity during the first 90 days of life. Proc Soc Exp Biol Med. 1965;118:212-214.

96. Wranne L. Studies on erythrokinetics in infancy. Acta Paediatr Scand. 1967;56:381-390.

97. Perrine SP, Greene MF, Faller DV. Delay in the fetal globin switch in infants of diabetic mothers. N Engl J Med. 1985;312:334-338.

98. Little JA, Dempsey NJ, Tuchman M, Ginder GD. Metabolic persistence of fetal hemoglobin. Blood. 1995;85: 1712-1718.

99. Bard H, Prosmanne J. Elevated levels of fetal hemoglobin synthesis in infants with chronic bronchopulmonary dysplasia. Pediatrics. 1990;86:193-196.

100. Bard H, Lachance C, Widness JA, Gagnon C. The reactivation of fetal hemoglobin synthesis during anemia of prematurity. Pediatr Res. 1994;36:253-256.

101. Pearson HA. Life span of the fetal red blood cell. J Pediatr. 1967;70:166-171.

102. Bratteby E, Garby L. Development of Erythropoiesis: Infant Erythrokinetics. Philadelphia, WB Saunders, 1974.

103. Landaw SA, Guancial RL. Shortened survival of fetal erythrocytes in the rat. Pediatr Res. 1977;11:1155-1158.

104. Landaw SA. Decreased survival and altered membrane properties of red blood cells (RBC) in the newborn rat. Pediatr Res. 1978;12:395-398.

105. Meyburg J, Bohler T, Linderkamp O. Decreased mechanical stability of neonatal red cell membrane quantified by measurement of the elastic area compressibility modulus. Clin Hemorheol Microcirc. 2000;22:67-73.

106. Serrani RE, Alonso D, Corchs JL. States of stability/lysis in human fetal and adult red blood cells. Arch Intern Physiol Biochim. 1989;97:309-316.

107. Coulombel L, Tchernia G, Mohandas N. Human reticulocyte maturation and its relevance to erythropoietic stress. J Lab Clin Med. 1979;94:467-474.

108. Thatte HS, Schrier SL. Comparison of transferrin receptor B mediated endocytosis and drug-induced endocytosis in human neonatal and adult RBCs. Blood. 1988;72:1693-1700.

109. Colin FC, Schrier SL. Myosin content and distribution in human neonatal erythrocytes are different from adult erythrocytes. Blood. 1991;78:3052-3055.

110. Diagne I, Archambeaud MP, Diallo D, et al. Parametres erythocytaires et reserves en fer dans le sang du cordon. Arch Pediatrie. 1995;2:208-214.

111. Zipursky A, Brown E, Palko J, Brown EJ. The erythrocyte differential count in newborn infants. Am J Pediatr Hematol Oncol. 1983;5:45-51.

112. Maxwell DJ, Seshadri R, Rumpf DJ, Miller JM. Infantile pyknocytosis: a cause of intrauterine haemolysis in 2 siblings. Aust N Z J Obstet Gynaecol. 1983;23:182-185.

113. Holroyde CP, Oski FA, Gardner FH. The "pocked" erythrocyte. Red-cell surface alterations in reticuloendothelial immaturity of the neonate. N Engl J Med. 1969;281:516-520.

114. Nathan DG, Gunn RB. Thalassemia: the consequences of unbalanced hemoglobin synthesis. Am J Med. 1966;41: 815-830.

115. Pearson HA, Macintosh S, Rooks Y, et al. Interference phase microscopic enumeration of pitted RBC and splenic function in sickle cell anemia. Pediatr Res. 1978;12:471.

116. Sills RH, Tamburlin JH, Burrios NJ, et al. Formation of intracellular vesicles in neonatal and adult erythrocytes: evidence against the concept of neonatal hyposplenism. Pediatr Res. 1988;24:703-708.

117. Matovcik LM, Junga IG, Schrier SL. Drug-induced endocytosis of neonatal erythrocytes. Blood. 1985;65:1056-1063.

118. Dervichian D, Fournet C, Guinier A, Ponder E. Structure submicroscopique des globules rouges contenant des hemoglobines abnormales. Rev Hematol. 1952;7:567.

119. Haberman S, Blanton P, Martin J. Some observations on ABO antigen sites of the erythrocyte membranes of adults and newborn infants. J Immunol. 1967;98:150-160.

120. Kurantsin-Mills J, Lessin LS. Freeze-etching and biochemical analysis of human fetal erythrocyte membranes. Pediatr Res. 1984;18:1035-1041.

121. Schekman R, Singer SJ. Clustering and endocytosis of membrane receptors can be induced in mature erythrocytes of neonatal but not adult humans. Proc Natl Acad Sci U S A. 1976;73:4075-4079.

122. Kehry M, Yguerabid J, Singer SJ. Fluidity in the membranes of adult and neonatal human erythrocytes. Science. 1977;195:486-487.

123. Polychronakos C, Ruggere MD, Benjamin A, et al. The role of cell age in the difference in insulin binding between adult and cord erythrocytes. J Clin Endocrinol Metab. 1982;55:290-294.

124. Funakoshi T, Morikawa H, Ueda Y, Mochizuki M. [Insulin-like growth factor (IGF) receptor in human fetal erythrocytes and fetal rat liver.] Nippon Naibunpi Gakkai Zasshi. 1989;65:728-742.

125. Bellussi G, Muccioli G, Ghe C, Di Carlo R. Prolactin binding sites in human erythrocytes and lymphocytes. Life Sci. 1987;41:951-959.

126. Kearin M, Kelly JG, O'Malley K. Digoxin "receptors" in neonates: an explanation of less sensitivity to digoxin than in adults. Clin Pharmacol Ther. 1980;28:346-349.

127. Koekebakker M, Barr RD. Acetylcholinesterase in the human erythron. I. Cytochemistry. Am J Hematol. 1988;28:252-259.

128. Miyazono Y, Hirono A, Miyamoto Y, Miwa S. Erythrocyte enzyme activities in cord blood of extremely low-birth-weight infants. Am J Hematol. 1999;62:88-92.

129. Neerhout RC. Erythrocyte lipids in the neonate. Pediatr Res. 1968;2:172-178.

130. Younkin S, Oski FA, Barness LA. Observations on the mechanism of the hydrogen peroxide hemolysis test and its reversal with phenols. Am J Clin Nutr. 1971;24:7-13.

131. Hermle T, Shumilina E, Attanasio P, et al. Decreased cation channel activity and blunted channel-dependent eryptosis in neonatal erythrocytes. Am J Physiol Cell Physiol. 2006;291:C710-C717.

132. Min C, Lowy C, Ghebremeskel K, et al. Fetal erythrocyte membrane lipids modification: preliminary observation of an early sign of compromised insulin sensitivity in offspring of gestational diabetic women. Diabet Med. 2005;22:914-920.

133. Vengelen-Tyler V. Technical Manual, 13th ed. Bethesda, MD, American Association of Blood Banks, 1999.

134. Hollán SR, Szeleny JG, Breuer JH, et al. Structural and functional differences between human foetal and adult erythrocytes. Haematology. 1967;4:409.

135. Serrani RE, Venera G, Gioia IA, Corchs JL. Potassium influx in human neonatal red blood cells. Partition into its major components. Arch Intern Physiol Biochim. 1990;98:27-34.

136. Moore TJ, Hall N. Kinetics of glucose transfer in adult and fetal human erythrocytes. Pediatr Res. 1971;5:356-359.

137. Schettini F, Bratta A, Mautone A, Zizzadoro P. Acid lysis of red blood cells in normal children. Acta Paediatr Scand. 1971;60:17-21.

138. Matsuo Y, Inoue F, Yoshioka H, et al. Changes of erythrocyte ouabain maximum binding after birth in neonates in relation to erythrocyte sodium and potassium concentrations. Early Hum Dev. 1995;43:59-69.

139. Brahm J, Wimberley PD. Chloride and bicarbonate transport in fetal red cells. J Physiol. 1989;419:141-156.

140. Linderkamp O, Hammer BJ, Miller R. Filterability of erythrocytes and whole blood in preterm and full-term neonates and adults. Pediatr Res. 1986;20:1269-1273.

141. Colin FC, Gallois Y, Rapin D, et al. Impaired fetal erythrocyte's filterability: relationship with cell size, membrane fluidity, and membrane lipid composition. Blood. 1992;79:2148-2153.

142. Buonocore G, Berni S, Gioia D, Bracci R. Characteristics and functional properties of red cells during the first days of life. Biol Neonate. 1991;60:137-143.

143. Gross RT, Schroeder EA, Brownstein SA. Energy metabolism in the erythrocytes of premature infants compared to full-term newborn infants and adults. Blood. 1963;21:755-763.

144. Konrad PN, Valentine WN, Paglia DE. Enzymatic activities and glutathione content of erythrocytes in the newborn: comparison with red cells of older normal subjects and those with comparable reticulocytosis. Acta Haematol. 1972;48:193-201.

145. Oski FA. Red cell metabolism in the newborn infant. V. Glycolytic intermediates and glycolytic enzymes. Pediatrics. 1969;44:84-91.

146. Witt I, Herdan M, Künzer W. Vergleichende Untersuchungen von enzymaktivitäten in Reticulocyten-reichen und Reticlotyten-armen Fraktionen aus Neugeborenen- und Erwachsenenblut. Klin Wochenschr. 1968;46:149-151.

147. Lestas AN, Rodeck CH, White JM. Normal activities of glycolytic enzymes in the fetal erythrocytes. Br J Haematol. 1982;50:439-444.

148. Mohrenweiser HW, Fielek S, Wurzinger KH. Characteristics of enzymes of erythrocytes from newborn infant and adults: activity, thermostability, and electrophoretic profile as a function of cell age. Am J Hematol. 1981;11:125-136.

149. Travis SF, Garvin JH. In vivo lability of red cell phosphofructokinase in term infants: the possible molecular basis of the relative phosphofructokinase deficiency in neonatal red cells. Pediatr Res. 1977;11:1159-1161.

150. Vora S, Piomelli S. A fetal isozyme of phosphofructokinase in newborn erythrocytes. Pediatr Res. 1977;11:483.

151. Holmes EW, Malone JI, Winegrad AI, Oski FA. Hexokinase isoenzymes in human erythrocytes: association of type II with fetal hemoglobin. Science. 1967;156:646-648.

152. Schröter W, Tillman W. Hexokinase isoenzymes in human erythrocytes of adults and newborns. Biochem Biophys Res Commun. 1968;31:92-97.

153. Chen SH, Anderson JE, Gibblet ER, Stamatoyannopoulos G. Lysozyme patterns in erythrocytes from human fetuses. Am J Hematol. 1977;2:23-28.

154. Witt I, Witz D. Reinigung und Charakterisierung von Phosphopyruvatz-Hydratase (=Enolase; EC 4.2.1.11) aus Neugeborenen- und Erwachsenen-Erythrozyten. Hoppe Seylers Z Physiol Chem. 1970;351:1232-1240.

155. Oski FA, Smith CA. Effect of pH on glycolysis in the erythrocytes of the newborn infant. Proc Soc Pediatr Res. 1972:106 (abstract).

156. Witt I, Müller H, Künzer W. Vergleichende biochemische Untersuchunger an Erythrocyten aus Neugeborenen- und Erwachsenen-blut. Klin Wochenschr. 1967;45:262-264.

157. Bentley HP, Alford CA, Diseker M. Erythrocyte glucose consumption in the neonate. J Lab Clin Med. 1970;76:311-321.

158. Oski FA. Red cell metabolism in the premature infant. II. The pentose phosphate pathway. Pediatrics. 1967;39:689-695.

159. Zipursky A, LaRue T, Israels LG. The in vitro metabolism of erythrocytes from newborn infants. Can J Biochem Physiol. 1960;38:727-738.

160. Trueworthy R, Lowman JT. Intracellular control of 2,3-diphosphoglycerate concentration in fetal red cells. Proc Soc Pediatr Res. 1971:86 (abstract).

161. Lestas AN, Bellingham AJ, Nicolaides KH. Red cell glycolytic intermediates in normal, anemic and transfused human fetuses. Br J Haematol. 1989;73:387-391.

162. Jain SK. The neonatal erythrocyte and its oxidative susceptibility. Semin Hematol. 1989;26:286-300.

163. Shahal Y, Bauminger ER, Zmora E, et al. Oxidative stress in newborn erythrocytes. Pediatr Res. 1991;29:119-122.

164. Abbasi S, Ludomirski A, Bhutani VK, et al. Maternal and fetal plasma vitamin E to total lipid ratio and fetal RBC antioxidant function during gestational development. J Am Coll Nutr. 1990;9:314-319.

165. Glader BE, Conrad ME. Decreased glutathione peroxidase in neonatal erythrocytes: lack of relation to hydrogen peroxide metabolism. Pediatr Res. 1972;6:900-904.

166. Lestas AN, Rodeck CH. Normal glutathione content and some related enzyme activities in the fetal erythrocytes. Br J Haematol. 1984;57:695-702.

167. Gross RT, Bracci R, Rudolph N, et al. Hydrogen peroxide toxicity and detoxification in the erythrocytes of newborn infants. Blood. 1967;29:481-493.

168. Whaun JM, Oski FA. Relation of red blood cell glutathione peroxidase to neonatal jaundice. J Pediatr. 1970;76:555-560.

169. Papp A, Nemeth I, Karg E, Papp E. Glutathione status in retinopathy of prematurity. Free Radic Biol Med. 1999;27:738-743.

170. Aliakbar S, Brown PR, Bidwell D, Nicolaides KH. Human erythrocyte superoxide dismutase in adults, neonates, and normal, hypoxaemic, anaemic and chromosomally abnormal fetuses. Clin Biochem. 1993;26:109-115.

171. Agostoni A, Gerli GC, Beretta L, et al. Superoxide dismutase, catalase, and glutathione peroxidase activities in maternal and cord blood erythrocytes. J Clin Chem Clin Biochem. 1980;18:771-773.

172. Bracci R, Martini G, Buonocore G, et al. Changes in erythrocyte properties during the first hours of life: electron spin resonance of reacting sulfhydryl groups. Pediatr Res. 1988;24:391-395.

173. Hågå P, Lunde G. Selenium and vitamin E in cord blood from preterm and full-term infants. Acta Paediatr Scand. 1978;67:735-739.

174. Travis SF, Kumar SP, Paez PC, Delivoria-Papadopulos M. Red cell metabolic alterations in postnatal life in term infants: glycolytic enzymes and glucose-6-phosphate dehydrogenase. Pediatr Res. 1980;14:1349-1352.

175. Jansen G, Koenderman L, Rijksen G, et al. Characteristics of hexokinase, pyruvate kinase, and glucose-6-phosphate dehydrogenase during adult and neonatal reticulocyte maturation. Am J Hematol. 1985;20:203-215.

176. Vetrella M, Barthelmai W. Enzyme activities in the erythrocytes of human fetuses. I. Glucose-6-phosphate dehydrogenase, 6-phosphogluconic dehydrogenase and glutathione reductase. Z Kinderheilkd. 1971;110:99-103.

177. Schröter W, Bodemann H. Experimentally induced cation leaks of the red cell membrane. Biol Neonate. 1970;15:291-299.

178. Tillman W, Menke J, Schröter W. The formation of Heinz bodies in ghosts of human erythrocytes of adults and newborn infants. Klin Wochenschr. 1973;51:201-203.

179. Kleihauer E, Bernau A, Betke A, et al. Heinzkörperbildung in Neugeborenerythrozyten. 1. In-vitro-Studien über experimentelle Bedingungen und den Einfluss von Austauschtransfusionen. Acta Haematol. 1970;43:333-347.

180. Schröter W, Tillman W. Heinz body susceptibility of red cells and exchange transfusion. Acta Haematol. 1973;49:74-79.

181. Bracci R, Benedetti PA, Ciambellotti V. Hydrogen peroxide generation in the erythrocytes of newborn infants. Biol Neonate. 1970;15:135-141.

182. Lipschutz F, Lubin B, et al. Red cell oxygen consumption and hydrogen peroxide formation. Proc Soc Pediatr Res. 1972:1051 (abstract).

183. Oettinger L Jr, Mills WB. Simultaneous capillary and venous hemoglobin determinations in newborn infants. J Pediatr. 1949;35:362-365.

184. Moe PJ. Umbilical cord blood and capillary blood in the evaluation of anemia in erythroblastosis fetalis. Acta Paediatr Scand. 1967;56:391-394.

185. Linderkamp O, Versmold HT, Strohhacker I, et al. Capillary-venous hematocrit differences in newborn infants. I. Relationship to blood volume, peripheral blood flow, and acid-base parameters. Eur J Pediatr. 1977;127:9-14.

186. Larsson BA, Tannfeldt G, Lagercrantz H, Olsson GL. Venipuncture is more effective and less painful than heel lancing for blood tests in neonates. Pediatrics. 1998;101:882-886.

187. Vertanen H, Fellman V, Brommels M, Viinikka L. An automatic incision device for obtaining blood samples from the heels of preterm infants causes less damage than a conventional manual lancet. Arch Dis Child Fetal Neonatal Ed. 2001;84:F53-F55.

188. Lindh V, Wiklund U, Hakansson S. Heel lancing in term new-born infants: an evaluation of pain by frequency domain analysis of heart rate variability. Pain. 1999;80:143-148.

189. Eriksson M, Gradin M, Schollin J. Oral glucose and venepuncture reduce blood sampling pain in newborns. Early Hum Dev. 1999;55:211-218.

190. Abril Martin JC, Aguilar Rodriguez L, Albinana Cilveti J. Flatfoot and calcaneal deformity secondary to osteomyelitis after neonatal heel puncture. J Pediatr Orthop B. 1999;8:122-124.

191. Jain A, Rutter N. Does topical amethocaine gel reduce the pain of venepuncture in newborn infants? A randomised double blind controlled trial. Arch Dis Child Fetal Neonatal Ed. 2000;83:F207-F210.

192. Lindh V, Wiklund U, Hakansson S. Assessment of the effect of EMLA during venipuncture in the newborn by analysis of heart rate variability. Pain. 2000;86:247-254.

193. Brisman M, Ljung BM, Otterbom I, et al. Methaemoglobin formation after the use of EMLA cream in term neonates. Acta Paediatr. 1998;87:1191-1194.

194. Usher R, Shepard M, Lind J. The blood volume of the newborn infant and placental transfusion. Acta Paediatr Scand. 1963;52:497-512.

195. Yao AC, Lind J, Tiisala R, Michelsson K. Placental transfusion in the premature infant with observation on clinical course and outcome. Acta Paediatr Scand. 1969;58:561-566.

196. Gunther M. The transfer of blood between baby and placenta in the minutes after birth. Lancet. 1957;1:1277-1280.

197. Ogata ES, Kitterman JA, Kleinberg F, et al. The effect of time of cord clamping and maternal blood pressure on placental transfusion with cesarean section. Am J Obstet Gynecol. 1977;128:197-200.

198. Cernadas JMC, Carroli G, Pellegrini L, et al. The effect of timing of cord clamping on neonatal venous hematocrit values and clinical outcome at term: a randomized, controlled trial. Pediatrics. 2006;117:E779-E786.

199. Linderkamp O, Nelle M, Kraus M, Zilow EP. The effect of early and late cord clamping on blood viscosity and other hemorhealogical parameters in full-term neonates. Acta Paediatr. 1992;81:745-750.

200. Nelle M, Zilow EP, Kraus M, et al. the effect of Leboyer delivery on blood viscosity and other hemorheological parameters in term neonates. Am J Obstet Gynecol. 1993;169:189-193.

201. Kinmond S, Aitchison TC, Holland BM, et al. Umbilical cord clamping and preterm infants: a randomized trial. BMJ. 1993;306:172-175.

202. Usher RH, Saigal S, O'Neil A, et al. Estimation of red blood cell volume in premature infants with and without respiratory distress syndrome. Biol Neonate. 1975;26:241-248.

203. Hofmeyr GJ, Gobetz L, Bex PJ, et al. Periventricular/intraventricular hemorrhage following early and delayed umbilical cord clamping. A randomized controlled trial. Online J Curr Clin Trials. Doc. No. 110, Dec 29, 1993.

204. Rabe H, Wacker A, Hulskamp G, et al. A randomised controlled trial of delayed cord clamping in very low birth weight preterm infants. Eur J Pediatr. 2000;159:775-777.

205. Ibrahim HM, Krouskop RW, Lewis DF, Dhanireddy R. Placental transfusion: umbilical cord clamping and preterm infants. J Perinatol. 2000;20:351-354.

206. Saigal S, Usher RH. Symptomatic neonatal plethora. Biol Neonate. 1977;32:62-72.

207. Saigal S, Wilson R, Usher R. Radiological findings in symptomatic neonatal plethora resulting from placental transfusion. Radiology. 1977;125:185-188.

208. Yao AC, Lind J. Effect of early and late cord clamping on the systolic time intervals of the newborn infant. Acta Paediatr Scand. 1977;66:489-493.

209. Erkkola R, Kero P, Kanto J, et al. Delayed cord clamping in cesarean section with general anesthesia. Am J Perinatol. 1984;1:165-169.

210. Mollison PL, Veall N, Cutbush M. Red cell and plasma volume in newborn infants. Arch Dis Child. 1950;25:242-253.

211. Jegier W, MacLaurin J, Blankenship W, Lind J. Comparative study of blood volume estimation in the newborn infant using I 131–labeled human serum albumin (IHSA) and T-1824. Scand J Clin Lab Invest. 1964;16:125-132.

212. Usher R, Lind J. Blood volume of the newborn premature infant. Acta Paediatr Scand. 1965;54:419-431.

213. Sisson TRC, Lund CJ, Whalen LE, Telek A. The blood volume of infants. I. The full-term infant in the first year of life. J Pediatr. 1959;55:163-179.

214. Cassady G. Plasma volume studies in low birth weight infants. Pediatrics. 1966;38:1020-1027.

215. Russell SJM. Blood volume studies in healthy children. Arch Dis Child. 1949;24:88-98.

216. Brines JK, Gibson JG Jr, Kunkel P. Blood volume in normal infants and children. J Pediatr. 1941;18:447-457.

217. Brown E, Krouskop RW, McDonnell FE, Sweet AY. Blood volume and blood pressure in infants with respiratory distress. J Pediatr. 1975;87:1133-1138.

218. Faxelius G, Raye J, Gutberlet R, et al. Red cell volume measurements and acute blood loss in high risk newborn infants. J Pediatr. 1977;90:273-281.

219. Shepherd AJ, Richardson CJ, Brown JP. Nuchal cord as a cause of neonatal anemia. Am J Dis Child. 1985;139:71-73.

220. Forestier F, Daffos F, Galactèros F, et al. Hematological values of 163 normal fetuses between 18 and 30 weeks of gestation. Pediatr Res. 1986;20:342-346.

221. Dialio DH, Sidibe S. Prèvalence de l'anèmie du nouveau-nè au Mali. Cah Sante. 1994;4:341.

222. Harthoorn-Lasthuizen EJ, Lindemans J, Langenhuijsen MMAC. Does iron-deficient erythropoiesis in pregnancy influence fetal iron supply? Acta Obstet Gynecol Scand. 2001;80:392-396.

223. Abdel-Fattah SA, Carroll SG, Kyle PM, Soothill PW. The effect of fetal hydrops on the rate of fall of hemoglobin after fetal intravascular transfusion for red cell alloimmunization. Fetal Diagn Ther. 2000;15:262-266.

224. Harper DC, Swingle HM, Weiner CP, et al. Long-term neurodevelopmental outcome and brain volume after treatment for hydrops fetalis by in utero intravascular transfusion. Am J Obstet Gynecol. 2006;195:192-200.

225. Boyd PA, Keeling JW. Fetal hydrops. J Med Genet. 1992;29:91-97.

226. Horn LC, Faber R, Meiner A, et al. Greenberg dysplasia: first reported case with additional non-skeletal malformations and without consanguinity. Prenat Diagn. 2000;20:1008-1011.

227. Saltzman DH, Frigoletto FD, Harlow BL, et al. Sonographic evaluation of hydrops fetalis. Obstet Gynecol. 1989;74:106-111.

228. Makh DS, Harman CR, Baschat AA. Is Doppler prediction of anemia effective in the growth-restricted fetus? Ultrasound Obstet Gynecol. 2003;22:489-492.

229. Turan O, Makh D, Harman C, Baschat A. The value of multi-vessel Doppler in the prediction of complex hematologic abnormalities in fetal growth restriction (FGR). Am J Obstet Gynecol. 2006:S206 (abstract).

230. Collins CY, Ott WJ. Evaluating suspected fetal anemia with Doppler ultrasound. J Reprod Med. 2005;50:379-382.

231. Oepkes D, Seaward PG, Vandenbussche FPHA, et al. Doppler ultrasonography versus amniocentesis to predict fetal anemia. N Engl J Med. 2006;355:156-164.

232. Moise K. Diagnosing hemolytic disease of the fetus—time to put the needles away. N Engl J Med. 2006;355:192-194.

233. Ferreira P, Morais L, Costa R, et al. Hydrops fetalis associated with erythrocyte pyruvate kinase deficiency. Eur J Pediatr. 2000;159:481-482.

234. Oie BK, Hertel J, Seip M, et al. Hydrops foetalis in 3 infants of a mother with acquired chronic pure red cell aplasia. Transitory red cell aplasia in 1 of the infants. Scand J Haematol. 1984;33:466-470.

235. Parez N, Dommergues M, Zupan V, et al. Severe congenital dyserythropoietic anaemia type I: prenatal management, transfusion support and alpha-interferon therapy. Br J Haematol. 2000;110:420-423.

236. Rejjal AL, Nazer H. Resolution of cystic hygroma, hydrops fetalis, and fetal anemia. Am J Perinatol. 1993;10:455-459.

237. Hirata GI, Masaki DI, O'Toole M, et al. Color flow mapping and Doppler velocimetry in the diagnosis and management of a placental chorioangioma associated with non-immune fetal hydrops. Obstet Gynecol. 1993;81:850-852.

238. Panero C, Azzi A, Carbone C, et al. Fetoneonatal hydrops from human parvovirus B19. Case report. J Perinat Med. 1994;22:257-261.

239. Yaegashi N, Niinuma T, Chisaka H, et al. The incidence of, and factors leading to, parvovirus B19–related hydrops fetalis following maternal infection; report of 10 cases and meta-analysis. J Infect. 1998;37:28-35.

240. Essary LR, Vnencak-Jones CL, Manning SS, et al. Frequency of parvovirus B19 infection in nonimmune hydrops fetalis and utility of three diagnostic methods. Hum Pathol. 1998;29:696-701.

241. Rodis JF, Borgida AF, Wilson M, et al. Management of parvovirus infection in pregnancy and outcomes of hydrops: a survey of members of the Society of Perinatal Obstetricians. Am J Obstet Gynecol. 1998;179:985-988.

242. Forestier F, Tissot JD, Vial Y, et al. Haematological parameters of parvovirus B19 infection in 13 fetuses with hydrops foetalis. Br J Haematol. 1999;104:925-927.

243. Bousquet F, Segondy M, Faure JM, et al. B19 parvovirus–induced fetal hydrops: good outcome after intrauterine blood transfusion at 18 weeks of gestation. Fetal Diagn Ther. 2000;15:132-133.

244. Inoue T, Matsumura N, Fukuoka M, et al. Severe congenital cytomegalovirus infection with fetal hydrops in a cytomegalovirus-seropositive healthy woman. Eur J Obstet Gynecol Reprod Biol. 2001;95:184-186.

245. Brabin B. Fetal anemia in malarious areas: its causes and significance. Ann Trop Paediatr. 1992;12:303-310.

246. Willert JR, Feusner J, Beckwith JB. Congenital mesoblastic nephroma: a rare cause of perinatal anemia. J Pediatr. 1999;134:248.

247. Norton ME. Nonimmune hydrops fetalis. Semin Perinatol. 1994;18:321-332.

248. Lallemand AV, Doco-Fenzy M, Gaillard DA. Investigation of nonimmune hydrops fetalis: multidisciplinary studies are necessary for diagnosis—review of 94 cases. Pediatr Dev Pathol. 1999;2:432-439.

249. Nakayama H, Kukita J, Hikino S, et al. Long-term outcome of 51 liveborn neonates with non-immune hydrops fetalis. Acta Paediatr. 1999;88:24-28.

250. Wafelman LS, Pollock BH, Kreutzer J, et al. Nonimmune hydrops fetalis: fetal and neonatal outcome during 1983-1992. Biol Neonate. 1999;75:73-81.

251. Myers SADO, Torrente SMD, Hinthorn DMD, Clark PLMD. Life-threatening maternal and fetal macrocytic anemia from antiretroviral therapy. Obstet Gynecol. 2005;106:1189-1191.

252. European Collaborative Study. Exposure to antiretroviral therapy in utero or early life: the health of uninfected children born to HIV-infected women. J Acquir Immune Defic Syndr. 2003;32:380-387.

253. Tjeertes IF, Bastiaans DE, van Ganzewinkel CJ, Zegers SH. Neonatal anemia and hydrops fetalis after maternal mycophenolate mofetil use. J Perinatol. 2007;27:62-64.

254. Smets K, Van Aken S. Fetomaternal haemorrhage and prenatal intracranial bleeding: two more causes of blueberry muffin baby. Eur J Pediatr. 1998;157:932-934.

255. Sohan K, Carroll S, Byrne D, et al. Parvovirus as a differential diagnosis of hydrops fetalis in the first trimester. Fetal Diagn Ther. 2000;15:234-236.

256. Miyagawa S, Takahashi Y, Nagai A, et al. Angio-oedema in a neonate with IgG antibodies to parvovirus B19 following intrauterine parvovirus B19 infection. Br J Dermatol. 2000;143:428-430.

257. Lubin B. Neonatal anaemia secondary to blood loss. Clin Haematol. 1978;7:19-34.

258. Glader BE, Platt O. Haemolytic disorders of infancy. Clin Haematol. 1978;7:35-61.

259. Oski FA, Naiman JL. Hematologic Problems of the Newborn, 3rd ed. Philadelphia, WB Saunders, 1982.

260. Blanchette VS, Zipursky A. Assessment of anemia in newborn infants. Clin Perinatol. 1984;11:489-510.

261. Dickerman JD. Anemia in the newborn infant. Pediatr Rev. 1984;6:131.

262. Halperin DS. Use of recombinant erythropoietin in treatment of the anemia of prematurity. Am J Pediatr Hematol Oncol. 1991;13:351-363.

263. Dallman PR. Anemia of prematurity: the prospects for avoiding blood transfusions by treatment with recombinant human erythropoietin. Adv Pediatr. 1993;40:385-403.

264. Gallagher PG, Ehrenkranz RA. Erythropoietin therapy for anemia of prematurity. Clin Perinatol. 1993;20:169-191.

265. Kannourakis G. The biology of erythropoietin and its role in the anemia of prematurity. J Paediatr Child Health. 1994;30:293-295.

266. Pissard SMDP, de Montalembert MMD, Bachir DMD, et al. Pyruvate kinase (PK) deficiency in newborns: the pitfalls of diagnosis. J Pediatr. 2007;150:443-445.

267. Van Kamp IL, Klumper FJCM, Meerman RH, et al. Treatment of fetal anemia due to red-cell alloimmunization with intrauterine transfusions in the Netherlands, 1988-1999. Acta Obstet Gynecol Scand. 2004;83:731-737.

268. Laosombat V, Dissaneevate S, Wongchanchailert M, Satayasevana B. Neonatal anemia associated with Southeast Asian ovalocytosis. Int J Hematol. 2005;82:201-205.

269. Zipursky A, Hull A, White FD, Israels LG. Foetal erythrocytes in the maternal circulation. Lancet. 1959;1:451-452.

270. Gänshirt-Ahlert D, Börjesson-Stoll R, Burschyk M, et al. Detection of fetal trisomies 21 and 18 from maternal blood using triple gradient and magnetic cell sorting. Am J Reprod Immunol. 1993;30:194-201.

271. Geifman-Holtzman O, Blatman RN, Bianchi DW. Prenatal genetic diagnosis by isolation and analysis of fetal cells circulating in maternal blood. Semin Perinatol. 1994;18:366-375.

272. Bianchi DW. Fetal cells in the mother: from genetic diagnosis to diseases associated with fetal cell microchime-

rism. Eur J Obstet Gynecol Reprod Biol. 2000;92: 103-108.

273. Samura O, Sohda S, Johnson KL, et al. Diagnosis of trisomy 21 in fetal nucleated erythrocytes from maternal blood by use of short tandem repeat sequences. Clin Chem. 2001;47:1622-1626.

274. Pertl B, Bianchi DW. Fetal DNA in maternal plasma: emerging clinical applications. Obstet Gynecol. 2001;98: 483-490.

275. Bianchi DW, LeShane ES, Cowan JM. Large amounts of cell-free fetal DNA are present in amniotic fluid. Clin Chem. 2001;47:1867-1869.

276. Pertl B, Sekizawa A, Samura O, et al. Detection of male and female fetal DNA in maternal plasma by multiplex fluorescent polymerase chain reaction amplification of short tandem repeats. Hum Genet. 2000;106:45-49.

277. Sebring ES, Polesky HF. Fetomaternal hemorrhage: incidence, risk factors, time of occurrence, and clinical effects. Transfusion. 1990;30:344-357.

278. de Almeida V, Bowman JM. Massive fetomaternal hemorrhage: Manitoba experience. Obstet Gynecol. 1994;83: 323-328.

279. Pearlman MD, Tintinallli JE, Lorenz RP. A prospective controlled study of outcome after trauma during pregnancy. Am J Obstet Gynecol. 1990;162:1502-1507; discussion 1507-1510.

280. Duleba AJ, Miller D, Taylor G, Effer S. Expectant management of choriocarcinoma limited to placenta. Gynecol Oncol. 1992;44:277-280.

281. Kleihauer E, Hildegard B, Betke K. Demonstration von fetalem Hämoglobin in den Erythrocyten eines Blutausstrichs. Klin Wochenschr. 1957;35:637-638.

282. Boulos J, Andrini P, Haddad J, Villar CF. Fetomaternal hemorrhage: a series of 9 cases. Arch Pediatr. 1998;5: 1206-1210.

283. Dupre AR, Morrison JC, Martin JN Jr, et al. Clinical application of the Kleihauer-Betke test. J Reprod Med. 1993;38:621-624.

284. Duckett J, Constantine G. The Kleihauer technique: an accurate method of quantifying fetomaternal haemorrhage? Br J Obstet Gynaecol. 1997;104:845-846.

285. Patton WN, Nicholson GS, Sawers AH, et al. Assessment of fetal-maternal hemorrhage in mothers with hereditary persistence of fetal hemoglobin. J Clin Pathol. 1990;43: 728-731.

286. Bayliss KM, Kueck BD, Johnson ST, et al. Detecting fetomaternal hemorrhage: a comparison of five methods. Transfusion. 1991;31:303-307.

287. Greenwalt TJ, Dumaswala UJ, Domino MM. The quantification of fetomaternal hemorrhage by an enzyme-linked antibody test with glutaraldehyde fixation. Vox Sang. 1992;63:268-271.

288. Garratty G, Arndt P. Applications of flow cytometry to transfusion science. Transfusion. 1995;35:157-178.

289. Benirschke K. Accurate recording of twin placenta: a plea to the obstetrician. Obstet Gynecol. 1961;18:334-347.

290. Strong SJ, Comey G. The Placenta in Twin Pregnancy. New York, Pergamon Press, 1967.

291. Seng YC, Rajadurai VS. Twin-twin transfusion syndrome: a five year review. Arch Dis Child Fetal Neonatal Ed. 2000;83:F168-F170.

292. Fries MH, Goldstein RB, Kilpatrick SJ, et al. The role of velamentous cord insertion in the etiology of twin-twin transfusion syndrome. Obstet Gynecol. 1993;81:569-574.

293. Lopriore E, Middeldorp JM, Oepkes D, et al. Twin anemia-polycythemia sequence in two monochorionic twin pairs without oligo-polyhydramnios sequence. Placenta. 2007;28:47-51.

294. Gonsoulin W, Moise KJ Jr, Kirshon B, et al. Outcome of twin-twin transfusion diagnosed before 28 weeks of gestation. Obstet Gynecol. 1990;75:214-216.

295. Hayakawa M, Oshiro M, Mimura S, et al. Twin-to-twin transfusion syndrome with hydrops: a retrospective analysis of ten cases. Am J Perinatol. 1999;16:263-267.

296. Blickstein I. The twin-twin transfusion syndrome. Obstet Gynecol. 1990;75:714-722.

297. Bruner JP, Rosemond RL. Twin-to-twin transfusion syndrome: a subset of the twin oligohydramnios-polyhydramnios sequence. Am J Obstet Gynecol. 1993;169: 925-930.

298. Pinette MG, Pan Y, Pinette SG, Stubblefield PG. Treatment of twin-twin transfusion syndrome. Obstet Gynecol. 1993;82:841-846.

299. Fox C, Kilby M, Khan K. Contemporary treatments for twin-twin transfusion syndrome. Obstet Gynecol. 2005; 105:1469-1477.

300. Middeldorp JM, Sueters M, Lopriore E, et al. Fetoscopic laser surgery in 100 pregnancies with severe twin-to-twin transfusion syndrome in the Netherlands. Fetal Diagn Ther. 2007;22:190-194.

301. Lopriore E, Middeldorp JM, Oepkes D, et al. Residual anastomoses after fetoscopic laser surgery in twin-to-twin transfusion syndrome: frequency, associated risks and outcome. Placenta. 2007;28:204-208.

302. Pochedly C, Musiker S. Twin-to-twin transfusion syndrome. Postgrad Med. 1970;47:172-176.

303. Su RM, Yu CH, Chang CH, et alM. Prenatal diagnosis of twin-twin transfusion syndrome complicated with hydrops fetalis at 14 weeks of gestation. Int J Gynaecol Obstet. 2001;73:151-154.

304. Tan KL, Tan R, Tan SH, Tan AM. The twin transfusion syndrome. Clinical observations on 35 affected pairs. Clin Pediatr (Phila). 1979;18:111-114.

305. Klebe JG, Ingomar CJ. The fetoplacental circulation during parturition illustrated by the interfetal transfusion syndrome. Pediatrics. 1972;49:112-116.

306. Kirkman HN, Riley HD Jr. Posthemorrhagic anemia and shock in the newborn. A review. Pediatrics. 1959;24: 97-105.

307. Weiner AS. Diagnosis and treatment of anemia of the newborn caused by occult placental hemorrhage. Am J Obstet Gynecol. 1948;56:717-722.

308. Novak F. Posthemorrhagic shock in newborns during labor and after delivery. Acta Med Iugoslav. 1953;7:280.

309. Clayton EM, Pryor JA, Wierdsma JG, Whitacre FE. Fetal and maternal components of third-trimester obstetric hemorrhage. Obstet Gynecol. 1964;24:56-66.

310. Leonard S, Anthony B. Giant cephalohematoma of newborn. Am J Dis Child. 1961;101:170-173.

311. Robinson RJ, Rossiter MA. Massive subaponeurotic hemorrhage in babies of African origin. Arch Dis Child. 1968;43:684-687.

312. Pachman DJ. Massive hemorrhage in the scalp of the newborn infant. Hemorrhagic caput succedaneum. Pediatrics. 1962;29:907-910.

313. Florentino-Pineda I, Ezhuthachan SG, Sineni LG, Kumar SP. Subgaleal hemorrhage in the newborn infant associated with silicone elastomer vacuum extractor. J Perinatol. 1994;14:95-100.

314. Rausen AR, Diamond LK. Enclosed hemorrhage and neonatal jaundice. Am J Dis Child. 1961;101:164-169.

315. Potter EL. Fetal and neonatal deaths. A statistical analysis of 2000 autopsies. JAMA. 1940;115:996-1001.

316. Henderson JL. Hepatic hemorrhage in stillborn and newborn infants; clinical and pathological study of 47 cases. J Obstet Gynaecol Br Emp. 1941;48:377.

317. Erakalis AJ. Abdominal injury related to the trauma of birth. Pediatrics. 1967;39:421-424.

318. Philipsborn HF Jr, Traisman HS, Greer D Jr. Rupture of the spleen: a complication of erythroblastosis fetalis. N Engl J Med. 1955;252:159-162.

319. Leape LL, Bordy MD. Neonatal rupture of the spleen. Report of a case successfully treated after spontaneous cessation of hemorrhage. Pediatrics. 1971;47:101-104.

320. Yerby M. Epilepsy and pregnancy. New issues for an old disorder. Neurol Clin. 1993;4:777-786.

321. Abzug AJ, Levin MJ. Neonatal adenovirus infection: four patients and review of the literature. Pediatrics. 1991;87:890-896.

322. Hohlfeld P, Vial Y, Maillard-Brignon C, et al. Cytomegalovirus fetal infection: prenatal diagnosis. Obstet Gynecol. 1991;78:615-618.

323. Nader PR, Margolin F. Hemangioma causing gastrointestinal bleeding. Case report and review of the literature. Am J Dis Child. 1966;111:215-222.

324. Svane S. Foetal exsanguination from hemangioendothelioma of the skin. Acta Paediatr Scand. 1966;55:536-539.

325. Rumack CM, Guggenheim MA, Rumack BH, et al. Neonatal intracranial hemorrhage and maternal use of aspirin. Obstet Gynecol. 1981;58(Suppl):52S-56S.

326. Papile L, Burstein J, Burstein R, Koffler H. Incidence and evolution of subependymal and intraventricular hemorrhage: study of infants with birth weights less than 1500 grams. J Pediatr. 1978;92:529-534.

327. Nexo E, Christensen NC, Olesen H. Volume of blood removed for analytical purposes during hospitalization of low-birthweight infants. Clin Chem. 1981;27:759-761.

328. Obladen M, Sachsenweger M, Stahnke M. Blood sampling in very low birth weight infants receiving different levels of intensive care. Eur J Pediatr. 1988;147:399-404.

329. Lin JC, Strauss RG, Kulhavy JC, et al. Phlebotomy overdraw in the neonatal intensive care nursery. Pediatrics. 2000;106:E19.

330. Madsen LP, Rasmussen MK, Bjerregaard LL, et al. Impact of blood sampling in very preterm infants. Scand J Clin Lab Invest. 2000;60:125-132.

331. Shulman RJ, Phillips S, Laine L, et al. Volume of blood required to obtain central venous catheter blood cultures in infants and children. JPEN J Parenter Enteral Nutr. 1993;17:177-179.

332. Thorkelsson T, Hoath SB. Accurate micromethod of neonatal blood sampling from peripheral arterial catheters. J Perinatol. 1995;15:43-46.

333. Gleason E, Grossman S, Campbell C. Minimizing diagnostic blood loss in critically ill patients. Am J Crit Care. 1992;1:85-90.

334. Silver MJ, Li YH, Gragg LA, et al. Reduction of blood loss from diagnostic sampling in critically ill patients using a blood-conserving arterial line system. Chest. 1993;104:1711-1715.

335. Necheles TF, Rai US, Valaes T. The role of haemolysis in neonatal hyperbilirubinemia as reflected in carboxyhaemoglobin levels. Acta Paediatr Scand. 1976;65:361-367.

336. Minnich V, Cordonnier JK, Williams WJ, Moore CV. Alpha, beta and gamma hemoglobin polypeptide chains during the neonatal period with a description of a fetal form of hemoglobin D St. Louis. Blood. 1962;19:137-161.

337. Levine RL, Lincoln DR. Hemoglobin Hasharon in a premature infant with hemolytic anemia. Pediatr Res. 1975;9:7.

338. van Wijgerden JA. Clinical expression of sickle cell anemia in the newborn. South Med J. 1983;76:478-480.

339. Hegyi T, Delphin ES, Bank A, et al. Sickle cell anemia in the newborn. Pediatrics. 1977;60:213-216.

340. Veiga S, Varthianathan T. Massive intravascular sickling after exchange transfusion with sickle cell trait blood. Transfusion. 1963;3:387-391.

341. Lee-Potter JP, Deacon-Smith RA, Simpkiss MJ, et al. A new cause of hemolytic anemia in the newborn. J Clin Pathol. 1975;28:317-320.

342. Schmaier AH, Maurer HM, Johnston CL, Scott RB. Alpha thalassemia screening in neonates by mean corpuscular volume and mean corpuscular hemoglobin concentration. J Pediatr. 1973;83:794-797.

343. Koenig HM, Vedvidk TS, Dozy AM, et al. Prenatal diagnosis of hemoglobin H disease. J Pediatr. 1978;92:278-281.

344. Thumasathit B, Nondasuta A, Silpisornkosol S, et al. Hydrops fetalis associated with Bart's hemoglobin in northern Thailand. J Pediatr. 1968;73:132-138.

345. Fung TY, Kin LT, Kong LC, Keung LC. Homozygous alpha-thalassemia associated with hypospadias in three survivors. Am J Med Genet. 1999;82:225-227.

346. Dame C, Albers N, Hasan C, et al. Homozygous alpha-thalassaemia and hypospadias—common aetiology or incidental association? Long-term survival of Hb Bart's hydrops syndrome leads to new aspects for counselling of alpha-thalassaemic traits. Eur J Pediatr. 1999;158:217-220.

347. Beaudry MA, Ferguson DJ, Pearse K, et al. Survival of a hydropic infant with homozygous alpha-thalassemia-I. J Pediatr. 1986;108:713-716.

348. Bianchi DW, Beyer EC, Stark AR, et al. Normal long-term survival with alpha-thalassemia. J Pediatr. 1986;108:716-718.

349. Tongsong T, Wanapirak C, Sirivatanapa P, et al. Prenatal eradication of Hb Bart's hydrops fetalis. J Reprod Med. 2001;46:18-22.

350. Erlandson ME, Hilgartner M. Hemolytic disease in the neonatal period. J Pediatr. 1959;54:566-585.

351. Stamatoyannopoulos G. Gamma-thalassemia. Lancet. 1971;2:192-193.

352. Kan YW, Forget BG, Nathan DG. Gamma-beta thalassemia: a cause of hemolytic disease of the newborn. N Engl J Med. 1972;286:129-134.

353. Abman SH, Griebel JL, Parker DK, et al. Acute effect of inhaled nitric oxide in children with severe hypoxemic respiratory failure. J Pediatr. 1994;124:881-888.

354. Journois D, Pouard P, Mauriat P, et al. Inhaled nitric oxide as a therapy for pulmonary hypertension after operation for congenital heart defects. J Thorac Cardiovasc Surg. 1994;107:1129-1135.

355. Winberg P, Lundell BP, Gustafsson LE. Effect of inhaled nitric oxide on raised pulmonary vascular resistance in children with congenital heart disease. Br Heart J. 1994; 71:282-286.

356. Wessel DL, Adatia I, Van Marter LJ, et al. Improved oxygenation in a randomized trial of inhaled nitric oxide for persistent pulmonary hypertension of the newborn. Pediatrics. 1997;100(5):E7.

357. Roberts JD Jr, Fineman JR, Morin FC 3rd, et al. Inhaled nitric oxide and persistent pulmonary hypertension of the newborn. The Inhaled Nitric Oxide Study Group. N Engl J Med. 1997;336:605-610.

358. Banks BA, Seri I, Ischiropoulos H, et al. Changes in oxygenation with inhaled nitric oxide in severe bronchopulmonary dysplasia. Pediatrics. 1999;103:610-618.

359. Nakajima W, Ishida A, Arai H, Takada G. Methaemoglobinemia after inhalation of nitric oxide in infant with pulmonary hypertension. Lancet. 1997;350:1002-1003.

360. Speakman ED, Boyd JC, Bruns DE. Measurement of methemoglobin in neonatal samples containing fetal hemoglobin. Clin Chem. 1995;41:458-461.

361. Lynch PL, Bruns DE, Boyd JC, Savory J. Chiron 800 system CO-oximeter module overestimates methemoglobin concentrations in neonatal samples containing fetal hemoglobin. Clin Chem. 1998;44:1569-1570.

362. de Keijzer MH, Brandts R, Giesendorf BA. Comment on the overestimation of methemoglobin concentrations in neonatal samples with the Chiron 800 system CO-oximeter module. Clin Chem. 1999;45:1313-1314.

363. Lebby T, Roco JJ, Arcinue EL. Infantile methemoglobinemia associated with acute diarrheal illness. Am J Emerg Med. 1993;11:471-472.

364. Pollack ES, Pollack CV Jr. Incidence of subclinical methemoglobinemia in infants with diarrhea. Ann Emerg Med. 1994;24:652-656.

365. Hanukoglu A, Danon PN. Endogenous methemoglobinemia associated with diarrheal disease in infancy. J Pediatr Gastroenterol Nutr. 1996;23:1-7.

366. Ogburn PL Jr, Ramin KD, Danilenko-Dixon D, et al. In utero erythrocyte transfusion for fetal xerocytosis associated with severe anemia and non-immune hydrops fetalis. Am J Obstet Gynecol. 2001;185:238-239.

367. del Giudice EM, Perrotta S, Nobili B, et al. Coinheritance of Gilbert syndrome increases the risk for developing gallstones in patients with hereditary spherocytosis. Blood. 1999;94:2259-2262.

368. Delhommeau F, Cynober T, Schischmanoff PO, et al. Natural history of hereditary spherocytosis during the first year of life. Blood. 2000;95:393-397.

369. Ribeiro ML, Alloisio N, Almeida H, et al. Severe hereditary spherocytosis and distal renal tubular acidosis associated with the total absence of band 3. Blood. 2000;96: 1602-1604.

370. Perrotta S, Nigro V, Iolascon A, et al. Dominant hereditary spherocytosis due to band 3 Neapolis produces a life-threatening anemia at the homozygous state. Blood. 1998;92(Suppl):9a.

371. Grootenboer S, Schischmanoff PO, Cynober T, et al. A genetic syndrome associating dehydrated hereditary stomatocytosis, pseudohyperkalaemia and perinatal oedema. Br J Haematol. 1998;103:383-386.

372. Grootenboer S, Schischmanoff PO, Laurendeau I, et al. Pleiotropic syndrome of dehydrated hereditary stomatocytosis, pseudohyperkalemia, and perinatal edema maps to 16q23-q24. Blood. 2000;96:2599-2605.

373. Zanella A, Bianchi P, Fermo E, et al. Molecular characterization of the PK-LR gene in sixteen pyruvate kinase–deficient patients. Br J Haematol. 2001;113:43-48.

374. Iolascon A, Faienza MF, Perrotta S, et al. Gilbert's syndrome and jaundice in glucose-6-phosphate dehydrogenase deficient neonates. Haematologica. 1999;84: 99-102.

375. Iolascon A, Faienza MF, Giordani L, et al. Bilirubin levels in the acute hemolytic crisis of G6PD deficiency are related to Gilbert's syndrome. Eur J Haematol. 1999; 62:307-310.

376. Yao DC, Tolan DR, Murray MF, et al. Hemolytic anemia and severe rhabdomyolysis caused by compound heterozygous mutations of the gene for erythrocyte/muscle isozyme of aldolase, ALDOA(Arg303X/Cys338Tyr). Blood. 2004;103:2401-2403.

377. English M. Life-threatening severe malarial anaemia. Trans R Soc Trop Med Hyg. 2000;94:585-588.

378. Ndyomugyenyi R, Magnussen P. Chloroquine prophylaxis, iron/folic-acid supplementation or case management of malaria attacks in primigravidae in western Uganda: effects on congenital malaria and infant haemoglobin concentrations. Ann Trop Med Parasitol. 2000;94:759-768; discussion 769-770.

379. Viraraghavan R, Jantausch B. Congenital malaria: diagnosis and therapy. Clin Pediatr (Phila). 2000;39:66-67.

380. Brabin BJ, Premji Z, Verhoeff F. An analysis of anemia and child mortality. J Nutr. 2001;131:636S-645S; discussion 646S-648S.

381. Brabin BJ, Hakimi M, Pelletier D. An analysis of anemia and pregnancy-related maternal mortality. J Nutr. 2001;131:604S-614S; discussion 614S-615S.

382. Eyssette-Guerreau S, Bader-Meunier B, Garcon L, et al. Infantile pyknocytosis: a cause of haemolytic anaemia of the newborn. Br J Haematol. 2006;133:439-442.

383. Whitehead VM. Acquired and inherited disorders of cobalamin and folate in children. Br J Haematol. 2006;134: 125-136.

384. Milman N, Byg K-E, Hvas A-M, et al. Erythrocyte folate, plasma folate and plasma homocysteine during normal pregnancy and postpartum: a longitudinal study comprising 404 Danish women. Eur J Haematol. 2006;76: 200-205.

385. Sieff CA, Nisbet-Brown E, Nathan DG. Congenital bone marrow failure syndromes. Br J Haematol. 2000;111: 30-42.

386. Giri N, Kang E, Tisdale JF, et al. Clinical and laboratory evidence for a trilineage haematopoietic defect in patients with refractory Diamond-Blackfan anaemia. Br J Haematol. 2000;108:167-175.

387. Alter BP, Nathan DG. Red cell aplasia in children. Arch Dis Child. 1979;54:263-267.

388. Diamond LK, Wang WC, Alter BP. Congenital hypoplastic anemia. Adv Pediatr. 1976;22:349-378.

389. Diamond LK, Allen DM, Magill FB. Congenital (erythroid) hypoplastic anemia. Am J Dis Child. 1961;102: 149.

390. Willig TN, Draptchinskaia N, Dianzani I, et al. Mutations in ribosomal protein S19 gene and Diamond Blackfan anemia: wide variations in phenotypic expression. Blood. 1999;94:4294-4306.

391. Matsson H, Klar J, Draptchinskaia N, et al. Truncating ribosomal protein S19 mutations and variable clinical expression in Diamond-Blackfan anemia. Hum Genet. 1999;105:496-500.

392. Willig TN, Niemeyer CM, Leblanc T, et al. Identification of new prognosis factors from the clinical and epidemiologic analysis of a registry of 229 Diamond-Blackfan anemia patients. DBA group of Société d'Hématologie et d'Immunologie Pédiatrique (SHIP), Gesellshaft für Pädiatrische Onkologie und Hämatologie (GPOH), and the European Society for Pediatric Hematology and Immunology (ESPHI). Pediatr Res. 1999;46:553-561.

393. Beauchamp-Nicoud AMD, Da Costa LMD, Proust A, et al. Postmortem diagnosis of Diamond-Blackfan anemia. J Pediatr Hematol Oncol. 2004;26:847-848.

394. Da Costa L, Willig TN, Fixler J, et al. Diamond-Blackfan anemia. Curr Opin Pediatr. 2001;13:10-15.

395. Dianzani I, Garelli E, Ramenghi U. Diamond-Blackfan anaemia: an overview. Paediatr Drugs. 2000;2:345-355.

396. Willig TN, Gazda H, Sieff CA. Diamond-Blackfan anemia. Curr Opin Hematol. 2000;7:85-94.

397. Pearson HA, Lobel JS, Kocoshis SA, et al. A new syndrome of refractory sideroblastic anemia with vacuolization of marrow precursors and exocrine pancreatic dysfunction. J Pediatr. 1979;95:976-984.

398. Mayes C, Sweeney C, Savage JM, Loughrey CM. Pearson's syndrome: a multisystem disorder. Acta Paediatr. 2001;90:235-237.

399. Blatt J, Katerji A, Barmada M, et al. Pancytopenia and vacuolization of marrow precursors associated with necrotizing encephalopathy. Br J Haematol. 1994;86:207-209.

400. Simonsz HJ, Barlocher K, Rotig A. Kearns-Sayre's syndrome developing in a boy who survived Pearson's syndrome caused by mitochondrial DNA deletion. Doc Ophthalmol. 1992;82:73-79.

401. Rotig A, Colonna M, Bonnefont JP, et al. A 13-bp direct repeat in mitochondrial DNA promotes deletions in Pearson's syndrome. Lancet. 1989;1:250.

402. Lestienne P, Bataille N. Mitochondrial DNA alterations and genetic diseases: a review. Biomed Pharmacol. 1994;48:199-214.

403. Lacbawan F, Tifft CJ, Luban NL, et al. Clinical heterogeneity in mitochondrial DNA deletion disorders: a diagnostic challenge of Pearson syndrome. Am J Med Genet. 2000;95:266-268.

404. Jardine PE, Cotter PD, Johnson SA, et al. Pyridoxine-refractory congenital sideroblastic anemia with evidence for autosomal inheritance: exclusions of linkage to ALAS2 at Xp11.21 by polymorphism analysis. J Med Genet. 1994;31:213-218.

405. Mäkitie O, Rajantie J, Kaitila I. Anemia and macrocytosis—unrecognized features in cartilage-hair hypoplasia. Acta Paediatr. 1992;81:1026-1029.

406. Shalev H, Tamary H, Shaft D, et al. Neonatal manifestations of congenital dyserythropoietic anaemia. J Pediatr. 1997;131:95-97.

407. Bader-Meunier BMD, Leverger GMD, Tchernia GMD, et al. Clinical and laboratory manifestations of congenital dyserythropoietic anemia type I in a cohort of French children. J Pediatr Hematol Oncol. 2005;27:416-419.

408. Shalev HMD, Kapelushnik JMD, Moser AMD, et al. A comprehensive study of the neonatal manifestations of congenital dyserythropoietic anemia type I. J Pediatr Hematol Oncol. 2004;26:746-748.

409. Shalev HMD, Moser AMD, Kapelushnik JMD, et al. Congenital dyserythropoietic anemia type I presenting as persistent pulmonary hypertension of the newborn. J Pediatr. 2000;136:553-555.

410. Perrotta S, del Giudice EM, Carbone R, et al. Gilbert's syndrome accounts for the phenotypic variability of congenital dyserythropoietic anemia type II (CDA-II). J Pediatr. 2000;136:556-559.

411. Tugal O, Pallant B, Shehare KN, Jayabose S. Transient erythroblastopenia of the newborn caused by human parvovirus. Am J Pediatr Hematol Oncol. 1994;16:352-355.

412. Heegaard ED, Hasle H, Skibsted L, et al. Congenital anemia caused by parvovirus B19 infection. Pediatr Infect Dis J. 2000;19:1216-1218.

413. von Kaisenberg CS, Jonat W. Fetal parvovirus B19 infection. Ultrasound Obstetr Gynecol. 2001;18:280-288.

414. Schulman J. The anemia of prematurity. J Pediatr. 1959;54:633-672.

415. Stockman JA Jr. The anemia of prematurity and the decision when to transfuse. Adv Pediatr. 1983;30:191-219.

416. Melhorn DK, Gross S. Vitamin E–dependent anemia in the preterm infant. I. Effects of large doses of medicinal iron. J Pediatr. 1971;79:569-580.

417. Halvorsen S, Finne PH. Erythropoietin production in the human fetus and newborn. Ann N Y Acad Sci. 1968;149:576-577.

418. Rollins MD, Maxwell AP, Afrasiabi M, et al. Cord blood erythropoietin, pH, PaO_2 and hematocrit following caesarean section before labour. Biol Neonate. 1993;63:147-152.

419. Millard DD, Gidding SS, Socol ML, et al. Effect of intravascular, intrauterine transfusion on prenatal and postnatal hemolysis and erythropoiesis in severe fetal isoimmunization. J Pediatr. 1990;117:447-454.

420. Humbert JR, Abelson H, Hathaway WE, Battaglia FC. Polycythemia in small for gestational age infants. J Pediatr. 1969;75:812-819.

421. Sann L, Bourgeois J, Stephant A, Putet G. Outcome of 249 premature infants, less than 29 weeks gestational age. Arch Pediatr. 2001;8:250-258.

422. Cook CD, Brodie HR, Allen DW. Measurement of fetal hemoglobin in newborn infants. Correlation with gestational age and intrauterine hypoxia. Pediatrics. 1957;20:272-278.

423. Stockman JA, III, Garcia JF, Oski FA. The anemia of prematurity. Factors governing the erythropoietin response. N Engl J Med. 1977;296:647-650.

424. Brown MS, Phibb RH, Phibbs RH, Dallman PR. Decreased response of plasma immunoreactive erythropoietin to "available oxygen" in anemia of prematurity. J Pediatr. 1984;105:793-798.

425. Stockman JA 3rd, Graeber JE, Clark DA, et al. Anemia of prematurity. Determinants of erythropoietin response. J Pediatr. 1984;105:786-792.

426. Yamashita H, Kukita J, Ohga S, et al. Serum erythropoietin levels in term and preterm infants during the first year of life. Am J Pediatr Hematol Oncol. 1994;16:213-218.

427. Emmerson AJB, Westwood NB, Rackham RA, et al. Erythropoietin responsive progenitors in anemia of prematurity. Arch Dis Child. 1991;66:810-811.

428. Shannon KM, Naylor GS, Torkildson JC, et al. Circulating erythroid progenitors in the anemia of prematurity. N Engl J Med. 1987;317:728-733.

429. Rhondeau SM, Christensen RD, Ross MP, et al. Responsiveness to recombinant erythropoietin of marrow erythroid progenitors in infants with anemia of prematurity. J Pediatr. 1988;112:935-940.

430. Brown MS, Jones MA, Ohls RK, Christensen RD. Single-dose pharmacokinetics of recombinant human erythropoietin in preterm infants after intravenous and subcutaneous administration. J Pediatr. 1993;122:655-657.

431. Attias D. Pathophysiology and treatment of the anemia of prematurity. J Pediatr Hematol Oncol. 1995;17:13-18.

432. Meyer M, Meyer JH, Commerford A, et al. Recombinant human erythropoietin in the treatment of the anemia of prematurity: results of a double-blind, placebo-controlled study. Pediatrics. 1994;93:918-923.

433. Soubasi V, Kremenopoulos G, Diamandi E, et al. In which neonates does early recombinant human erythropoietin treatment prevent anemia of prematurity? Results of a randomized, controlled study. Pediatr Res. 1993;34:675-679.

434. Brown MS, Keith JF 3rd. Comparison between two and five doses a week of recombinant human erythropoietin for anemia of prematurity: a randomized trial. Pediatrics. 1999;104:210-215.

435. Reiter PD, Rosenberg AA, Valuck RJ. Factors associated with successful epoetin alfa therapy in premature infants. Ann Pharmacother. 2000;34:433-439.

436. Shannon KM, Keith JF 3rd, Mentzer WC, et al. Recombinant human erythropoietin stimulates erythropoiesis and reduces erythrocyte transfusions in very low birth weight preterm infants. Pediatrics. 1995;95:1-8.

437. Fain J, Hilsenrath P, Widness JA, et al. A cost analysis comparing erythropoietin and red cell transfusions in the treatment of anemia of prematurity. Transfusion. 1995;35:936-943.

438. Vamvakas EC, Strauss RG. Meta-analysis of controlled clinical trials studying the efficacy of rHuEPO in reducing blood transfusions in the anemia of prematurity. Transfusion. 2001;41:406-415.

439. Donato H, Vain N, Rendo P, et al. Effect of early versus late administration of human recombinant erythropoietin on transfusion requirements in premature infants: results of a randomized, placebo-controlled, multicenter trial. Pediatrics. 2000;105:1066-1072.

440. Soubasi V, Kremenopoulos G, Tsantali C, et al. Use of erythropoietin and its effects on blood lactate and 2,3-diphosphoglycerate in premature neonates. Biol Neonate. 2000;78:281-287.

441. Ledbetter DJ, Juul SE. Erythropoietin and the incidence of necrotizing enterocolitis in infants with very low birth weight. J Pediatr Surg. 2000;35:178-181; discussion 182.

442. Newton NR, Leonard CH, Piecuch RE, Phibbs RH. Neurodevelopmental outcome of prematurely born children treated with recombinant human erythropoietin in infancy. J Perinatol. 1999;19:403-406.

443. Brugnara C, Colella GM, Cremins J, et al. Effects of subcutaneous recombinant human erythropoietin in normal subjects: development of decreased reticulocyte hemoglobin content and iron-deficient erythropoiesis. J Lab Clin Med. 1994;123:660-667.

444. Friel J, Aziz K, Andrews W, Serfass R. Iron absorption and oxidant stress during erythropoietin therapy in very low birth weight premature infants: a cohort study. BMC Pediatr. 2005;5:29.

445. Widness JA, Serfass RE, Haiden N, et al. Erythrocyte iron incorporation but not absorption is increased by intravenous iron administration to erythropoietin-treated premature infants. J Nutr. 2006;136:1868-1873.

446. Etchason J, Petz L, Keeler E, et al. The cost effectiveness of preoperative autologous blood donations. N Engl J Med. 1995;332:719-724.

447. Rutherford CJ, Kaplan HS. Autologous blood donation—can we bank on it? N Engl J Med. 1995;332:740-742.

448. Shireman TI, Hilsenrath P, Strauss RG, et al. Recombinant human erythropoietin vs. transfusions in the treatment of anemia of prematurity. Arch Pediatr Adolesc Med. 1994;148:582-588.

449. Grohskopf LA, Roth VR, Feikin DR, et al. *Serratia liquefaciens* bloodstream infections from contamination of epoietin alfa at a hemodialysis center. N Engl J Med. 2001;344:1491-1497.

450. Baxter LM, Vreman HJ, Ball B, Stevenson DK. Recombinant human erythropoietin (r-HuEPO) increases total bilirubin production in premature infants. Clin Pediatr (Phila). 1995;34:213-217.

451. Bechensteen AG, Refsum HE, Halvorsen S, et al. Effects of recombinant human erythropoietin on fetal and adult hemoglobin in preterm infants. Pediatr Res. 1995;38:729-732.

452. Black VD, Lubchenco LO, Luckey DW, et al. Developmental and neurologic sequelae of neonatal hyperviscosity syndrome. Pediatrics. 1982;69:426-431.

453. Saggese G, Bertelloni S, Baroncelli GI, Cipolloni C. Elevated calcitonin gene–related peptide in polycythemic newborn infants. Acta Paediatr. 1992;81:966-968.

454. Bada HS, Korones SB, Pourcyrous M, et al. Asymptomatic syndrome of polycythemic hyperviscosity: effect of partial plasma exchange transfusion. J Pediatr. 1992;120:579-585.

455. Drew JH, Guaran RL, Grauer S, Hobbs JB. Cord whole blood hyperviscosity: measurement, definition, incidence and clinical features. J Paediatr Child Health. 1991;26:363-363.

456. Mimouni F, Miodovnik M, Siddiqi TA, et al. Neonatal polycythemia in infants of insulin-dependent diabetic mothers. Obstet Gynecol. 1986;68:370-372.

457. Piacquadio K, Hollingsworth DR, Murphy H. Effects of in-utero exposure to oral hypoglycemic drugs. Lancet. 1991;338:866-869.

458. Oh W. Neonatal polycythemia and hyperviscosity. Pediatr Clin North Am. 1986;33:523-532.

459. Sacher R, Luban NLC, Strauss RG. Current practice and guidelines for the transfusion of cellular blood components in the newborn. Transfus Med Rev. 1989;3:39-54.

460. Yu VY, Gan TE. Red cell transfusion in the preterm infant. J Paediatr Child Health. 1994;30:301-309.

461. Strauss RG. Controversies in the management of the anemia of prematurity using single-donor red blood cell

transfusions and/or recombinant human erythropoietin. Transfus Med Rev. 2006;20:34-44.

462. Bell EF, Strauss RG, Widness JA, et al. Randomized trial of liberal versus restrictive guidelines for red blood cell transfusion in preterm infants. Pediatrics. 2005;115:1685-1691.

463. Ohls RK. Transfusions in the preterm infant. NeoReviews. 2007;8:e377-386.

464. Wardrop CA, Holland BM, Veale KE, et al. Non physiological anemia of prematurity. Arch Dis Child. 1978;53:855-860.

465. Schneider AJ, Stockman JA III, Oski FA. Transfusion nomogram: an application of physiology to clinical decisions regarding the use of blood. Crit Care Med. 1981;9:469-473.

466. Stockman JA III, Levin E, Clark D, Graeber JE. O_2 consumption of premature infants in the first 10 weeks of life: Response to transfusion. Pediatr Res. 1979;13:442.

467. Izraeli S, Ben-Sira L, Harell D, et al. Lactic acid as a predictor for erythrocyte transfusion in healthy preterm infants with anemia of prematurity. J Pediatr. 1993;122:629-631.

468. Keyes WG, Donohue PK, Spivak JL, et al. Assessing the need for transfusion of premature infants and role of hematocrit, clinical signs, and erythropoietin level. Pediatrics. 1989;84:412-417.

469. Mock DM, Bell EF, Lankford GL, Widness JA. Hematocrit correlates well with circulating red blood cell volume in very low birth weight infants. Pediatr Res. 2001;50:525-531.

470. Frey B, Losa M. The value of capillary whole blood lactate for blood transfusion requirements in anaemia of prematurity. Intensive Care Med. 2001;27:222-227.

471. Lacroix J, Hebert PC, Hutchison JS, et al. Transfusion strategies for patients in pediatric intensive care units. N Engl J Med. 2007;356:1609-1619.

472. Corwin HL, Carson JL. Blood transfusion—when is more really less? N Engl J Med. 2007;356:1667-1669.

473. Strauss RG. Transfusion therapy in neonates. Am J Dis Child. 1991;145:904-911.

474. Strauss RG. Erythropoietin and neonatal anemia. N Engl J Med. 1994;330:1227-1228.

475. Levy GJ, Strauss RG, Hume H, et al. National survey of neonatal transfusion practices: I. Red blood cell therapy. Pediatrics. 1993;91:523-527.

476. Strauss RG, Levy GJ, Sotelo-Avila C, et al. National survey of neonatal transfusion practices: II. Blood component therapy. Pediatrics. 1993;91:530-536.

477. American Association of Blood Banks. Standards for Blood Banks and Transfusion Services, 20th ed. Bethesda, MD, American Association of Blood Banks, 2000.

478. Strauss RG, Cordle DG, Quijana J, Goeken NE. Comparing alloimmunization in preterm infants after transfusion of fresh unmodified versus stored leukocyte-reduced red blood cells. J Pediatr Hematol Oncol. 1999;21:224-230.

479. Strauss RG, Johnson K, Cress G, Cordle DG. Alloimmunization in preterm infants after repeated transfusions of WBC-reduced RBCs from the same donor. Transfusion. 2000;40:1463-1468.

480. Luban NL, Strauss RG, Hume HA. Commentary on the safety of red cells preserved in extended-storage media for neonatal transfusions. Transfusion. 1991;31:229-235.

481. Patten E, Robbins M, Vincent J, et al. Use of red blood cells older than five days for neonatal transfusion. J Perinatol. 1991;11:37-40.

482. Strauss RG, Burmeister LF, Johnson K, et alD. Feasibility and safety of AS-3 red blood cells for neonatal transfusions. J Pediatr. 2000;136:215-219.

483. Cook S, Gunter J, Wissel M. Effective use of a strategy using assigned red cell units to limit donor exposure for neonatal patients. Transfusion. 1993;33:379-383.

484. Liu EA, Mannino FL, Lane TA. Prospective randomized trial of the safety and efficacy of a limited donor exposure transfusion program for premature neonates. J Pediatr. 1994;125:92-96.

485. Strauss RG, Burmeister LF, Johnson K, et al. Randomized trial assessing the feasibility and safety of biologic parents as RBC donors for their preterm infants. Transfusion. 2000;40:450-456.

486. Hilsenrath P, Nemechek J, Widness JA, et al. Cost-effectiveness of a limited-donor blood program for neonatal red cell transfusions. Transfusion. 1999;39:938-943.

487. Strauss RG. Leukocyte-reduction to prevent transfusion-transmitted cytomegalovirus infections. Pediatr Transplant. 1999;3:19-22.

488. Luban NL, Manno C. Lack of difference in CMV transmission via the transfusion of filtered irradiated and non-filtered irradiated blood to newborn infants in an endemic area. Transfusion. 2000;40:387-389.

489. Thurer RL, Luban NL, AuBuchon JP, et al. Universal WBC reduction. Transfusion. 2000;40:751-752.

490. Wang-Rodriguez J, Fry E, Fiebig E, et al. Immune response to blood transfusion in very-low-birthweight infants. Transfusion. 2000;40:25-34.

491. Naulaers G, Barten S, Vanhole C, et al. Management of severe neonatal anemia due to fetomaternal transfusion. Am J Perinatol. 1999;16:193-196.

492. Wong EC, Schreiber S, Criss VR, et al. Feasibility of red blood cell transfusion through small bore central venous catheters used in neonates. Pediatr Crit Care Med. 2004;5:69-74.

493. Ringer SA, Richardson D, Sacher RA, et al. Blood utilization in neonatal intensive care. Blood. 1991;78:353a.

494. Ringer SA, Richardson DK, Sacher RA, et al. Variations in transfusion practice in neonatal intensive care. Pediatrics. 1998;101:194-200.

495. Bednarek FJ, Weisberger S, Richardson DK, et al. Variations in blood transfusions among newborn intensive care units. SNAP II Study Group. J Pediatr. 1998;133:601-607.

3

Immune Hemolytic Disease of the Newborn

Helen G. Liley

HISTORICAL ASPECTS

Whereas many serious complications of pregnancy were well known in antiquity, maternofetal blood group incompatibility was recognized more recently. Much of the understanding of the disease developed between the 1930s and 1970s, although since the late 1980s, the molecular basis of both Rh and other blood group genotypes and phenotypes has been revealed. Despite the spectacular appearance of a hydropic fetus and placenta and the drastic effect of recurrent perinatal death on family size and structure, only about 1 in 200 pregnancies in Occidental societies is vulnerable to complication by antibodies. Even without any effective treatment only about half the babies would die. Against the high perinatal mortality prevailing until the mid-20th century, deaths from hemolytic disease were of little statistical significance. Louyse Bourgeois, midwife to Marie de Medici, may have been the first (in 1609) to give an account of hemolytic disease of the fetus and newborn (HDN).[1] She described twins: the first was hydropic and died shortly after birth; the second initially appeared well but rapidly became jaundiced, then opisthotonic, and subsequently died.

The connection between "congenital anemia," icterus gravis, and hydrops fetalis was not recognized until 1932 despite detailed descriptions of each condition by pathologists. Diamond and co-workers[2] deduced that these conditions were variations on a common theme and coined the term *erythroblastosis fetalis* for disease characterized by hemolytic anemia, intramedullary and extramedullary erythropoiesis, and hepatosplenomegaly. Darrow, who had lost a baby of her own to kernicterus, correctly speculated in 1938 that the disease was caused by maternal antibodies to fetal antigens developed as a result of transplacental fetomaternal hemorrhage.[3] However, because she incorrectly concluded that the antibody was to fetal hemoglobin (HbF), much of the recognition for this remarkable insight was given to those who provided the evidence.

In 1939, Levine and Stetson linked a woman's severe transfusion reaction to her husband's blood with her recent delivery of a hydropic stillborn infant.[4] She was found to have an antibody that agglutinated her husband's red blood cells (RBCs). Levine postulated that she had become sensitized to an antigen that the fetus had inherited from its father.

In 1940, Landsteiner and Wiener[5] proposed the identity of the antigen by generating antibodies to rhesus monkey RBCs in guinea pigs and rabbits. The antisera agglutinated RBCs from 85% of whites. These people were designated rhesus (Rh) positive. The 15% whose RBCs did not agglutinate were Rh negative.

Levine and associates then used Landsteiner and Wiener's antiserum to show that Levine and Stetson's patient was Rh negative and her husband was Rh positive. Furthermore, her serum agglutinated the RBCs from Wiener and Landsteiner's Rh-positive but not their Rh-negative individuals.[6] The monkey RBC antigen and antibody (LW and anti-LW) are not the same as the human RhD antigen and antibody, but reactivity was linked to Rh status because LW is more strongly expressed on Rh-positive RBCs. Subsequent years saw rapid and dramatic progress, including recognition that immunoglobulin G (IgG) crossed the placenta and development of the Coombs test.[7] This test uses anti-human IgG antibodies to agglutinate IgG-labeled RBCs and remains important in the detection and management of HDN. Chown reported in 1954 that mothers could be sensitized by transplacental hemorrhage of fetal blood,[8] although until crossmatching for Rh groups became routine, transfusion for postpartum hemorrhage and other indications also contributed to the incidence of the disease. Chown's observation plus subsequent recognition that most sensitizing fetomaternal hemorrhages occurred at delivery, thus explaining why Rh HDN was mainly a disease of multipara, paved the way for the development of immunoprophylaxis. Since the late 1960s, RhD immunoglobulin has been available to treat Rh-negative mothers of Rh-positive infants at delivery to prevent Rh HDN.

These discoveries all contributed to understanding of the delicate balance in the immunology of pregnancy; the maternal immune system generally remains in a state of armed neutrality toward the fetus and its foreign antigens, which remain shielded by the trophoblast. Meanwhile, the advantages of maternal immunologic memory are conferred on the fetus and newborn via active transplacental passage of antibodies, thereby creating optimal conditions for awakening of the newborn's own adaptive immune system. However, if a maternal antibody develops to a self-antigen or a fetal antigen, fetal disease can result. Thus, when an Rh-negative woman exposed to Rh-positive RBCs develops anti-D IgG, the antibody traverses the placenta and can bind fetal D-positive RBCs and lead to their destruction. The subsequent fetal hemolysis can lead to icterus gravis, kernicterus, and hydrops fetalis.

For many problems of pregnancy, obscurity of the pathophysiology until recently often led to management that at best was symptomatic. In contrast, with hemolytic disease the genetic predilection, molecular mechanism, and rationale for treatment were rapidly deduced, which led to remarkable success in preventing the disease and mitigating its effects. Indeed, the history of prevention and management of Rh HDN includes a number of pivotal discoveries that have influenced the management of other diseases. These breakthroughs include exchange transfusion for neonatal treatment, development of screening programs for maternal blood group antibodies, strategies for managing early delivery to optimize neonatal outcomes, the use of amniocentesis for fetal diagnosis, the first example of intrauterine fetal treatment, and the development of one of the earliest and most successful forms of immunoprophylaxis using human antibodies. Subsequently, many of the successes of fetal and neonatal

TABLE 3-1		Incidence of Rh Allelic Combinations Expressed by the Fisher-Race and Wiener Nomenclature				
	NOMENCLATURE		**Expressed Alleles**	**FREQUENCY**[12]		
	Fisher-Race	Wiener		Whites	Blacks	Asians*
RhD positive	CDe	R_1	*RHD RHCe*	0.42	0.17	0.70
	cDE	R_2	*RHD RHcE*	0.14	0.11	0.21
	cDe	R_0	*RHD RHce*	0.04	0.44	0.03
	CDE	R_z	*RHD RHCE*	0.00	0.00	0.01
TOTAL				0.6	0.72	0.95
RhD negative†	cde	R	*RHce*	0.37	0.26	0.03
	Cde	r′	*RHCe*	0.02	0.02	0.02
	cdE	r″	*RHcE*	0.01	<0.01	<0.01
	CdE	R^y	*RHCE*	<0.01	<0.01	<0.01
TOTAL				0.4	0.28	0.05
Ratio of RhD-positive to RhD-negative phenotypes				0.84:0.16	0.92:0.08	0.99:<0.01

*The predominant reasons for failure to express RHD vary by racial group. RHD deletions predominate in whites, but other variants, such as partial deletions and RHD-RHCE recombinations, are more common in other populations.

†Rh negativity is more common in Indo-Asians.

treatment of Rh HDN have been extrapolated to HDN caused by other blood group antibodies and other problems of pregnancy.

Advances in molecular biology and biochemistry allowed identification of the Rh polypeptides in 1982 and Rh genes in 1991. Until these discoveries, controversy existed between two models to explain Rh genotype and phenotype relationships. Wiener and Wexler[9] proposed the existence of a single gene with multiple epitopic sites, whereas Fisher and Race[10,11] postulated that there were two closely linked genes encoding three pairs of Rh antigens: Dd, Cc, and Ee inherited in two sets of three (one set from each parent) (Table 3-1).[12] Both models have been shown to be partly correct, although like many disorders that were once thought to have been genetically simple and phenotypically diverse, the diversity of Rh genotype/phenotype relationships is much greater than previously envisaged.

THE Rh BLOOD GROUP SYSTEM

Biochemistry and Molecular Genetics

Although the incidence of Rh HDN has declined and the incidence of HDN secondary to other alloantibodies has increased, the Rh blood group system remains the most common cause of HDN (particularly severe HDN), especially in whites, for whom about one in seven conceptions involves an Rh-negative mother and an Rh-positive father. Individuals are classed as Rh positive or negative based on expression of the major D antigen on their RBCs; however, more than 50 other Rh antigens have been identified, the most commonly recognized of which in clinical practice are those designated D, C, c, E, and e. The Rh blood group system is the most complex blood group system in humans.[13,14]

After the landmark descriptions of the RhD protein in 1982,[15,16] non-D[17,18] and D complementary DNA

(cDNA) and genes were cloned in the early 1990s.[19,20] In most individuals the Rh blood group loci are the products of two very similar genes, one of which encodes CD240CE, the polypeptide that carries the Cc/Ee epitopes in combinations (Ce, ce, cE, or CE), and the other of which encodes CD240D, the D antigen polypeptide[14,21,22] (Table 3-2).[23] The two genes are separated by only 30 kilobases (kb) and are organized in opposite orientation on chromosome bands 1p36.2-p34. The small *SMP1* gene (a "small membrane protein" family member) lies between them. They share a very similar 10-exon structure, and their intronic sequences are also highly conserved. Their sequence identity strongly suggests that they evolved by duplication of an ancestral gene about 8 million years ago.[24] Worldwide, the Rh blood group system displays considerable polymorphism. A wide variety of both small and large mutations (including gene deletion and recombination to form hybrid *RHD-RHCE* products) and the effects of other modifying genes account for the diverse common and rare Rh phenotypes[25,26] (Table 3-3). Although some genotypic and phenotypic variants are confined to a single family, for others the incidence in various gene pools is much higher or unknown. This diversity mandates caution in the use of DNA-based clinical diagnostic approaches, especially when these approaches are applied to populations other than the ones in which they were piloted, but it may open the door for future individualization of prevention and therapy.[27,28]

The predicted product of the RhD messenger RNA is a 417–amino acid polypeptide with a molecular mass of 45,100. The D and Cc/Ee polypeptides have greater than 90% amino acid identity. Of the 32 to 37 amino acid substitutions that usually differ between the D and CE polypeptides, about a quarter are located in extracellular domains of the protein. Within RhCE, E/e specificity is conferred by a single amino acid substitution (P226A) encoded by exon 5 of the *RHCE* gene and found in the fourth extracellular loop. C/c specificity is

TABLE 3-2   Incidence of Common Rh Haplotypes

Gene	Allele	Translated Product	ALLELE FREQUENCY IN THE UNITED STATES (%)			
			Whites	Blacks	Native Americans	Asians
RHD	*RHD*	RhD polypeptide	61	97	99	99
	RHD deletion or silent	None	39	3	1	1
RHCE	*RHCe*	RhCe polypeptide	44	19	46	72
	RHcE	RhcE polypeptide	15	11	40	21
	RHce	Rhce polypeptide	41	70	8	6
	RHCE	RhCE polypeptide	0	0	6	1

From Huang CH. Blood Group Antigen Gene Mutation Database: Rh Blood Group System. HUGO Mutation Database Initiative, 2001. Available at http://www.bioc.aecom.yu.edu/bgmut/index.htm (accessed 2004).

TABLE 3-3   Examples of Variant Rh Phenotypes for Which a Corresponding Genotype Has Been Described to Illustrate the Diversity of the *RHD* Genotype

Category	Phenotype	Typical Mutations
Partial D	D^{II} to D^{VII} and others	Variety of point mutations and *RHD-RHCE* hybrids
Weak D	Weak D (D^u) types 1-16	Variety of point mutations leading to amino acid substitutions in the transmembrane or cytoplasmic domains
D negative (silent D or d)	D negative	Variety of mechanisms: *RHD* complete or partial deletion, *CE* hybrids, point mutations; some prevent transcription, but all prevent expression at the cell surface
CE variants	RN, E^{I-III}, VN, CX, C^W, etc.	Variety of hybrids and point mutations
CE silent	D.., D– and various others	Mostly *RHD-RHCE* hybrids
Rh deficiency states (no D or CE expression)	Rh$_{null}$ amorph	*RHCE* silent genes plus *RHD* deletion
	Rh$_{null}$ reg, Rh$_{null}$mod	*RHAG* mutations that prevent expression

associated with four amino acid differences: C16W encoded by exon 1 and I60L, S68N, and S103P all encoded by exon 2 of the *RHCE* gene.[29] Of these, the S103P substitution is the only extracellular substitution and is most important in determining antigenic reactivity.[14,29,30]

It has been well established for decades that no d antigen exists. RhD negativity is defined as the absence of RhD antigen, and its incidence is highest in the Basque population.[31] It has been suggested that peripatetic Basque traders and fishermen (or their ancestors) may have spread this genotype to other populations. In these European-descended populations in which Rh negativity is relatively common, most RhD-negative individuals are homozygous for an *RHD* gene deletion.[19,20] This mutation appears to have arisen because two highly homologous sequences (1463-bp "rhesus boxes") flank the *RHD* gene and provide the opportunity for unequal crossing over.[32] However, although Rh negativity is less common among them, other mechanisms for D negativity appear more commonly in other populations, such as individuals of African, Chinese, or Japanese ancestry.[33-35] These alternative mechanisms include partial deletion, recombination between *RHD* and *RHCE* genes, and point mutation. An Rh allele that comprises a pseudogene (*RHDΨ*) is prevalent among RhD-negative people of African ancestry, including approximately 66% in South Africa and about one in five RhD-seronegative African Americans.[35,36] *RHDΨ* is not expressed because of two inactivating mutations, a 37-bp duplication in exon 4 that causes a premature stop codon and a nonsense mutation (Y269X) in exon 6. Four characteristic single-nucleotide polymorphisms also occur in exons 4 and 5. Singleton and colleagues found that 15% of RhD-negative black South Africans carry a hybrid *RHD-CE-D* that also encodes an altered C antigen.[35]

The molecular basis of the D-positive phenotype is also intricate. Studies using site-directed mutagenesis, naturally occurring variants of *RHD*, and monoclonal antibodies or molecular modeling indicate that the D antigen is composed of at least 37 different, but overlapping epitopes,[25,37-41] some of which are missing in individuals who express partial D antigenicity. Most of the epitope clusters are located in exofacial loops 3, 4, and 6 of the D protein. RhD variants are discussed in more detail later.

The *RHD* and *RHCE* gene products are unique among blood group antigens in being nonglycosylated, palmitoylated integral membrane proteins (Fig. 3-1). Their 12 predicted helical transmembrane domains are connected by small extracellular and cytoplasmic loops. Their expression is confined to erythroid cells, whereas

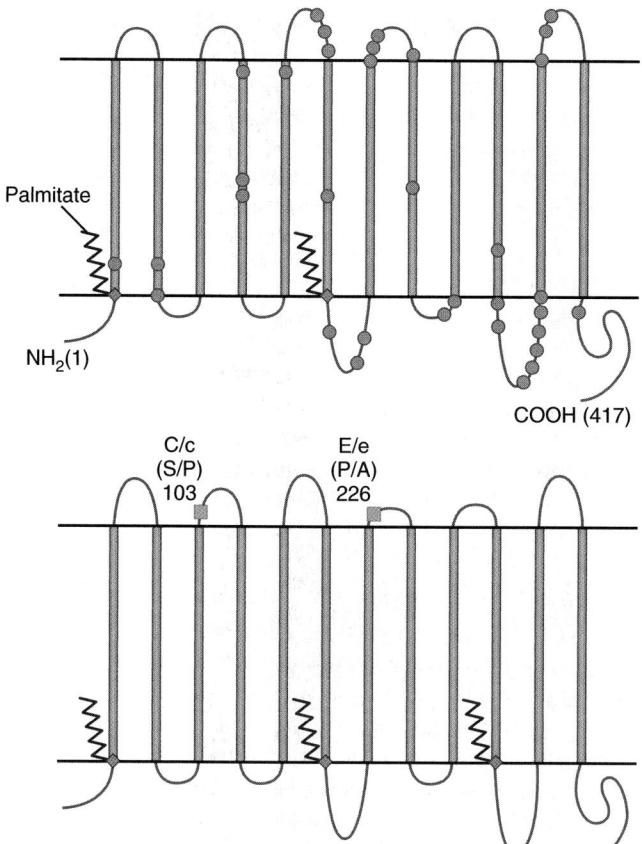

FIGURE 3-1. Diagram of the Rh peptides RhD (*top*) and RhCE (*bottom*) inserted in the cell membrane (*parallel horizontal lines*). The amino acid sequence of both proteins predicts 12 transmembrane domains. Neither is glycosylated, but RhD has two sites of palmitoylation (*zigzag lines*) and RhCE has three. D-specific amino acids are marked with *open circles*. The predicted position of most is in the transmembrane and cytoplasmic domains. E/e specificity appears to be conferred by a single proline-to-alanine amino acid substitution at residue 226 (P226A) encoded by exon 5 of the *RHCE* gene and C/c specificity by the S103P (serine 103 to proline) substitution encoded by exon 2. Four other amino acid differences are also associated with C/c polymorphism but do not appear to affect antigen characteristics: C16W encoded by exon 1 and I60L, S68N, and S103P all encoded by exon 2 of the *RHCE* gene.[29]

many other blood group antigens are present in many tissues. They are found in hetero-oligomeric complexes, the structure and function of which are still under investigation. In these oligomers, Rh antigens are found in association with a glycosylated membrane component that migrates diffusely on sodium dodecyl sulfate–polyacrylamide gel electrophoresis at approximately 45 to 75 kd.[15,16] This 409–amino acid glycoprotein, formerly known as Rh50 glycoprotein, is now designated Rh-associated glycoprotein (RhAG). It is about a third identical to RhD and RhCE and, putatively, has a similar configuration involving 12 helical membrane-spanning domains. Its gene has an exon-intron organization similar to that of *RHD* and *CE*; however, it maps to chromosome bands 6p21.1-p11. Its expression is also confined to erythroid cells.[42] Nonerythroid homologues (RhBG and RhCG) have been found in other tissues.[43] The Rh

complex was thought to comprise a tetramer of two RhD and/or CE subunits and two RhAG subunits[44]; however, more recently a model consisting of trimers of two RhAG subunits and either an RhD or CE or possibly two RhD or CE subunits with one RhAG has been supported by hydrophobic cluster analysis.[45]

Cartron[13] and Cartron and Colin[22] have reviewed the Rh deficiency states. Rare individuals with the Rh deficiency syndrome (Rh$_{null}$) lack expression of all or virtually all RhD, C/c, and E/e antigens. This recessive condition can result (in RhD-negative individuals) from homozygous silent mutations in the *RHCE* gene that appear to reduce cell surface expression of RhAG ("amorph type"). Homozygotes for mutations that prevent expression of RhAG have the more common "regulator type" or the Rh$_{null}$mod phenotype. Despite normal transcription of Rh genes, the proteins are not found at the cell surface.[46]

The functional significance of the Rh complex is indicated by the fact that Rh-deficient individuals have spherocytosis, stomatocytosis, and chronic hemolysis of varying severity. Their RBCs have altered ion transport and membrane composition and are partly or completely deficient in certain other membrane proteins, including RhAG, CD47, LW (Landsteiner-Wiener glycoprotein, or intercellular adhesion molecule 4 [ICAM-4]), GPB (glycophorin B, which confers the Ss blood group), and Duffy Fy5 (Duffy antigen receptor for chemokines). These deficiencies suggest that Rh proteins form complexes with RhAG and other proteins and that the complexes fail to form if components are missing.[13,47] There is also strong evidence for an interaction with the anion exchange protein (band 3) and linkage of the Rh complex to the spectrin-based RBC membrane skeleton, thus indicating a role in maintaining the biconcave disc shape of RBCs (Fig. 3-2).[47] Failure of this association may explain some of the dysfunction of Rh-deficient cells. However, many details of when, how, and why the Rh complexes form remain to be explained.

An additional functional role for components of the Rh complex is also suggested by their evolutionary conservation, particularly in regard to molecules similar to RhAG.[13,24,43] The probable function of these glycoproteins was suspected because of sequence identity between them and the yeast Mep proteins. This led to the discovery that RhAG and a second Rh-related glycoprotein, RhGK (normally expressed in kidney cells), rescue Mep-deficient mutant cells grown on media with low ammonium. These and related experiments suggested a role for Rh glycoproteins in ammonia or ammonium ion import and export across cell membranes.[48-51] However, more recent studies indicate that RhCE and RhD proteins lack the key residues essential for ammonium transport, and it has been proposed instead that Rh complexes in RBCs form CO_2 channels.[25,52,53] The diversity of abnormalities in Rh-deficient RBCs raises the possibility of ancillary functions.

In contrast to the common Rh-negative and very rare Rh deficiency states, weak and partial D phenotypes are

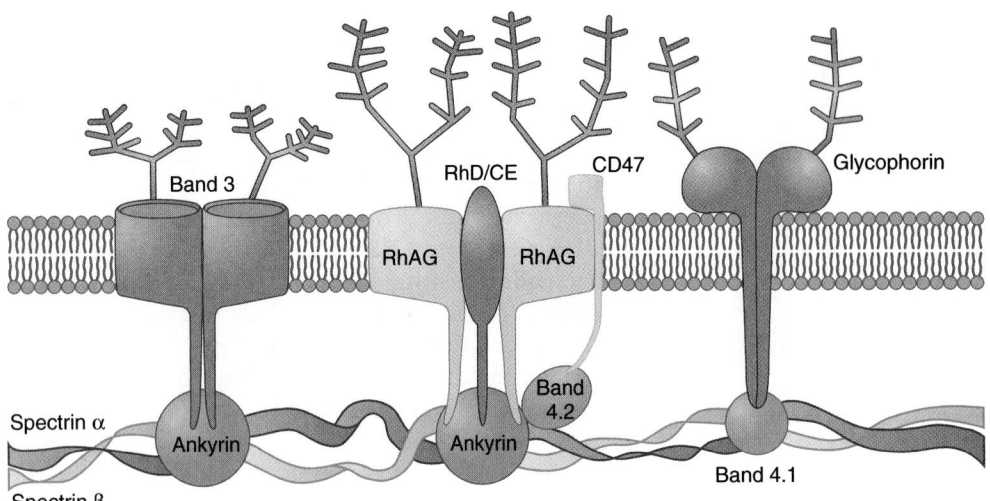

FIGURE 3-2. Diagram of the proposed Rh complex and its interactions. The trimer, composed of RhAG molecules and either RhCE molecules or RhD, interacts with other membrane proteins and with the cytoskeleton.

fairly common (e.g., 0.2% to 1% of populations of European ancestry) and are caused by *RHD* coding region alterations that affect the number and antibody-binding characteristics of RhD sites per cell. The term "partial D" has been used to describe RBCs that react with some monoclonal anti-D antibodies and not others, and their RhD proteins typically have one or more amino acid substitutions on or near the RBC surface or consist of RhD-RhCE hybrids. In contrast, "weak D" has been used for RBCs with a markedly reduced number of antigenic sites and in which one or more amino acid substitutions are found in regions that are presumed to be in or below the membrane and may interfere with the assembly of Rh complexes.[25,54] Most weak D individuals, especially those with types 1, 2, and 3, do not make anti-D. However, it has been recognized that there is overlap and some imprecision in allocation of these phenotypes, and the terms "aberrant D" or "D variant" have been proposed as collective terms for these plus the (very weak) D-elute phenotype[26,54-56] (see Table 3-3).

Because of variable antigenic potential and the potential to form antibodies to RhD, certain weak and partial D phenotypes are significant in transfusion therapy and pregnancy. Some individuals need to be regarded as RhD negative in pregnancy and as transfusion recipients (eligible for anti-D immunoprophylaxis and Rh-negative blood) but Rh positive as blood donors.[54,56,57] For example, if some blood donors with aberrant/variant D are regarded as D negative, their blood can cause alloimmunization of D-negative recipients. On some occasions, women with partial D (especially partial D[IV]) form anti-D antibodies capable of causing severe HDN if they carry a D-positive child,[58] or D-negative women can form antibodies if their babies have some types of aberrant/variant D. Some partial D phenotypes are also associated with distinct antigens.

The C antigen is most common in Southeast Asia, parts of South America, and the southern tip of Greenland, whereas the E antigen occurs most often in populations indigenous to parts of South America and Alaska.[31]

The genetics underlying the RhCc/Ee phenotypes also display more subtle variation than was once envisaged, and weak, partial, and variant antigen phenotypes have also been recognized. Internet databases are a good source of up-to-date information about the phenotype-genotype relationships for RhD and RhCE.[23,59]

RhD ALLOIMMUNIZATION

HDN is a disease of the fetus caused by a maternal response to pregnancy. As such, the pathogenesis can be considered in three stages: maternal alloimmunization, antibody transfer to the fetus, and fetal response.

Maternal Rh Sensitization

Maternal sensitization to Rh antigens can occur as a result of exposure to antigenically dissimilar fetal RBCs during pregnancy, as a result of therapeutic transfusion, or occasionally as a result of needle sharing.[60,61] Transfusion has become a rare cause of RhD sensitization because compatibility testing for RhD antigen has been routine practice for several decades. However, it accounts for a high proportion of sensitization to other blood group antigens, including RhCE, and among those with RhD and RhCE variants. Furthermore, the need for emergency transfusion of Rh-positive blood to Rh-negative women is likely to remain an occasional cause of sensitization to RhD in locations where the Rh-negative phenotype is rare and Rh-negative blood is scarce.

Exposure to fetal antigens remains the most common cause of maternal antibodies to RhD. Although Chown first described maternal Rh immunization occurring as a result of fetal transplacental hemorrhage (TPH), the test of Kleihauer and associates[62] in 1957 was needed to show the incidence, size, and timing of these events and to show that most maternal Rh sensitization occurs this way.[63] The test depends on the resistance of HbF to acid elution (Fig. 3-3) and can detect 1 fetal RBC in 200,000

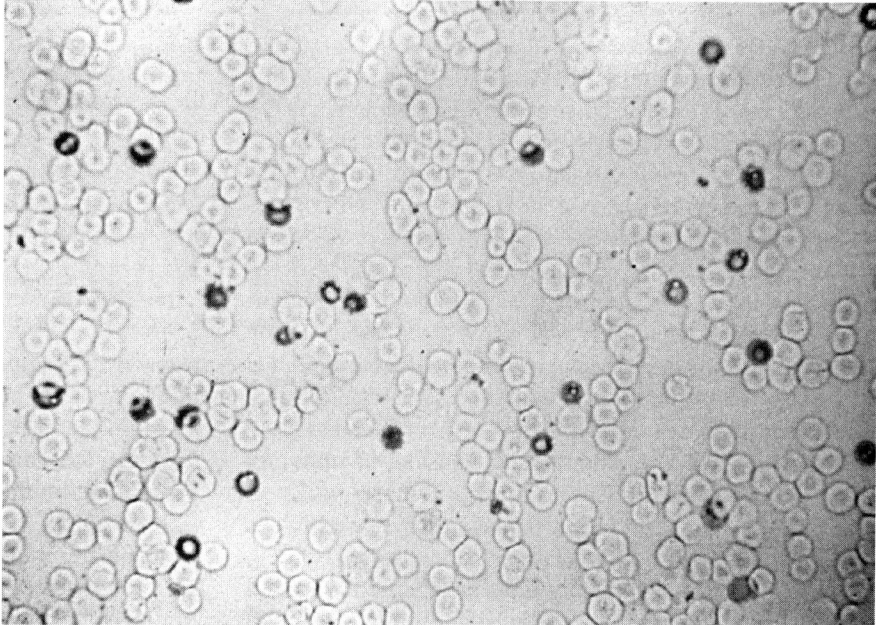

FIGURE 3-3. Acid elution technique of Kleihauer. Fetal red blood cells (RBCs) stain with eosin and appear dark. Adult RBCs do not stain and appear as ghosts. This maternal blood smear contained 11.2% fetal RBCs and represents transplacental hemorrhage of about 450 mL of blood. *(From Bowman JM. Hemolytic disease of the newborn. In Conn HF, Conn RB [eds]. Current Diagnosis 5. Philadelphia, WB Saunders, 1977, p 1103.)*

adult RBCs, which corresponds to a fraction of a milliliter in the circulating maternal blood volume. Bowman and colleagues[64] used this technique for two weekly tests in a group of 33 women and concluded that 76% had had experienced TPH. The incidence increased as pregnancy progressed: 3% had TPH in the first trimester, 12% in the second trimester, 45% in the third trimester, and 64% immediately after birth. However, acid elution studies must be interpreted with some caution because of rapid destruction of fetal cells when ABO incompatibility exists and because of natural variation and pregnancy-induced increases in expression of HbF among adults. Subsequently, using flow cytometric techniques and DNA amplification of fetal sequences, researchers have confirmed that some fetal cells can be detected in maternal blood during all trimesters of most pregnancies.[65,66] Because strategies for detection vary among studies and because of uncertainties about the persistence of various types of fetal cells in the maternal circulation, the volume and timing of this transplacental passage of fetal cells remain unclear. However, most of these "hemorrhages" are likely to be tiny. Delivery is the time of greatest risk for fetomaternal hemorrhage and for larger hemorrhages, especially when complications of delivery of the fetus or placenta occur.[66]

Larger TPHs are uncommon; the amount of fetal blood exceeds 2.5 mL in less than 1% of gestations and is greater than 30 mL in less than 0.25%.[66] However, certain obstetric situations increase the risk for significant TPH, including antepartum hemorrhage, pre-eclampsia, external version,[67] cesarean section,[68,69] and manual removal of the placenta.[70] Abdominal trauma and placental vascular malformations are additional, but uncommon causes. TPH occurs in about 2.5% to 8.4% of patients after amniocentesis,[71,72] but the risk after early-gestation chorionic villus sampling (CVS) is uncertain.[73]

The level of risk for sensitization as a result of first-trimester pregnancy loss is also uncertain and, in the case of spontaneous miscarriage, will depend on whether an embryo with circulating blood ever formed, but surgical evacuation of the uterus is thought to present a greater risk for TPH than medically induced or spontaneous evacuation is.[74] The Rh antigen may be expressed by about 38 days after conception,[75] early enough in gestation for early CVS or pregnancy loss to present a risk.

All studies have focused on fetal cells in the maternal bloodstream, which may have gained access across the placenta but in some situations could have been absorbed from the maternal peritoneum, but the responses to submucosal, subcutaneous, or intramuscular antigen presentation differ from those to intravascular presentation. Therefore, deposition of fetal RBCs in these sites could be more immunogenic than deposition via the intravascular route and could account for some of the propensity for Rh sensitization after invasive procedures. If this is the case, techniques such as those recommended to minimize exposure of the fetus to maternal blood[76] might be effective in reducing the risk for blood group sensitization.

The Nature of Rh Sensitization

Primary and Secondary Immune Responses

In most Rh-negative individuals, the primary immune response develops slowly. In experimental Rh immunization of male volunteers, antibody responses are typically detected at 8 to 9 weeks, although they can occur at any time from 4 weeks to 6 months. Hemolytic anemia caused by anti-D has been detected as early as 10 days after a massive Rh-incompatible transfusion in a previously unsensitized patient.[77] A primary, often weak IgM response will not affect the fetus, even if it occurs before delivery in a sensitizing pregnancy, because IgM anti-D does not cross the placenta. However, IgG anti-D production usually ensues, and if sensitization occurs early in pregnancy, there is the potential for continued antigenic challenge, which can account for the rare occurrence of HDN in the progeny of women during their first Rh-positive pregnancy.

After a primary response has been invoked, subsequent exposure to Rh-positive RBCs induces a rapid increase in anti-D IgG, which can cross the placenta and affect the fetus. Repeated exposure can progressively increase the titer and change the characteristics (including IgG subclass distribution) of the Rh antibody, thus increasing the severity of Rh hemolytic disease in successive pregnancies.

Dose of Rh Antigen Necessary to Produce Rh Sensitization

Experiments involving injection of Rh-positive blood into Rh-negative males show, not unexpectedly, that the likelihood of Rh sensitization depends on both the dose and repetition of exposure to the antigen.[78,79] A proportion of individuals are anergic to RhD, regardless of the dose and repetition of exposure ("nonresponders").[80] Secondary immune responses may occur after exposure to very small amounts of RhD-positive RBCs (as little as 0.03 mL).

Studies performed during and immediately after pregnancy using the Kleihauer technique indicated that if the volume of TPH was always less than 0.1 mL of RBCs, the prevalence of Rh sensitization detectable up to 6 months after delivery was 3%, whereas when volumes exceeded 0.4 mL, the prevalence was 22%.[78,79] Nevertheless, because in 75% to 80% of pregnancies the amount of TPH is always less than 0.1 mL, it is likely that either small or undetectable TPH or fetal cells deposited in other sites account for the majority of sensitization.

Incidence of Rh Sensitization

Rh sensitization has decreased markedly with the introduction of Rh immunoprophylaxis. In its absence, about 16% of Rh-negative women become sensitized in their first ABO-compatible Rh-positive pregnancy. Of these, about half have detectable anti-D 6 months after delivery, and in half a rapid secondary response is seen in the next susceptible pregnancy, thus indicating that primary sensitization had occurred previously.[78,81] If sensitization does not occur, the risk in a second D-positive, ABO-compatible pregnancy is similar. By the time that an Rh-negative woman has completed her fifth ABO-compatible, Rh-positive pregnancy, the probability that she will be Rh sensitized is about 50%.

As parity increases and the number of women capable of an Rh immune response diminishes because they have already become immunized, the proportion of the remainder whose systems mount a primary immune response decreases because of a greater residual number of "nonresponders." About 25% to 30% of D-negative women

are nonresponders in that they do not become Rh sensitized despite having many D-positive pregnancies; however, some may yet become Rh sensitized if they are exposed to a very large amount of Rh-positive blood. Immunologic tolerance can be induced by several different mechanisms and can depend on the context of antigen presentation to the immune system. It is not known which mechanisms of tolerance predominate in nonresponding Rh-negative women.

ABO incompatibility provides partial protection against Rh sensitization. Without anti-D immunoprophylaxis, it has been estimated that in whites, blood group A incompatibility between the mother and fetus reduces the risk for Rh sensitization by 90% and group B incompatibility by 55%.[82] Bowman[81] suggested that this partial protection is due to rapid intravascular hemolysis of the ABO-incompatible, D-positive RBCs, with sequestration of D-positive cells in the stroma of the liver (an organ with poor antibody-forming potential) rather than the spleen (the site of RBC sequestration when extravascular RBC destruction occurs). However, it is not clear whether the immune system remains naïve with respect to the Rh antigens or whether tolerance is induced in these instances. Although ABO incompatibility provides substantial protection against the primary Rh immune response, it provides no protection against the secondary Rh immune response[83,84] and should not influence the management of an already affected pregnancy. Maternal HLA type does not have any consistent effect on the risk for sensitization, although it may affect antibody titer and the severity of HDN.[85,86]

Other factors that influence the likelihood and severity of sensitization include fetal gender and fetal red cell phenotype, which affects the number and antigenicity of D antigen sites on fetal RBCs. For example, R1r (CDe/cde) cells, with only 9900 to 14,400 D antigen sites per cell, are less immunogenic than R2r (cDE/cde) cells, which have 14,000 to 16,000 sites.[87,88] The possibility that Rh-negative women were exposed to RhD during their own fetal life (the so-called "grandmother theory") has been considered, but the evidence from a case-control study is against it.[89] Nevertheless, convincing evidence of maternal-to-fetal hemorrhage has been found in other circumstances, and these events could explain the occasional presence of Rh antibodies in Rh-negative men and nulliparous women who have never had a transfusion.

Rh sensitization during pregnancy, once considered to be rare, occurred in about 1.8% of susceptible pregnancies in one study.[90] The proportion of all occurrences of Rh sensitization that are attributable to antenatal sensitization now varies among studies, depending on the application of antenatal immunoprophylaxis.

In summary, some general rules apply to Rh HDN. The probability of incompatible pregnancies is predictable from the Hardy-Weinberg genetic principles, but the impact of HDN on a population will also depend on typical family size and on careful management of obstetric complications.[91] The risk should be low when good blood bank procedures, parsimonious approaches to blood transfusion, effective screening of pregnant women, and evidence-based administration of Rh immunoprophylaxis are applied. The disease should be uncommon or mild in a woman's first incompatible pregnancy, and 50% of the infants of heterozygous fathers and sensitized mothers should be safe. However, as pointed out by Kinnock and Liley,[84] the striking feature of pregnancies in severely isoimmunized women is their clinical variability. Because these women have often become sensitized despite the predictions of conventional wisdom, their care requires astute and conscientiousness management to ensure satisfactory outcomes.

Prevention of Rh Sensitization

The background to prevention of Rh sensitization lies in the experiments of Von Dungern at the beginning of the 20th century.[92] He showed that serum from rabbits that had previously been injected with ox cells prevented the development of antibodies to ox cells in a second group of rabbits. The partial protective effect of ABO incompatibility also suggested that antibody-mediated destruction of fetal RBCs could prevent maternal Rh sensitization. Finn and co-workers[93] suggested a strategy of administering anti-D immunoprophylaxis, and it was put to the test almost simultaneously in New York[94] and Liverpool[95] and shortly thereafter in Winnipeg.[96] Because anti-RhD immunoglobulin was strikingly successful in preventing sensitization in males, clinical trials were then undertaken in which Rh-negative, unsensitized women were given anti-D intramuscularly after delivery of an Rh-positive infant.[96-98] The licensing of Rh immune globulin in 1968 profoundly influenced the prevalence of Rh sensitization. Despite its success, the exact mechanism of action of anti-D remains elusive.[99,100]

The level of evidence for the postpartum use of anti-D immunoprophylaxis is high. A recent systematic review collated data from six eligible trials involving more than 10,000 women in which postpartum anti-D prophylaxis was compared with no treatment or placebo.[101] The conclusion was that anti-D prophylaxis strikingly lowered the incidence of RhD alloimmunization 6 months after birth (relative risk, 0.04; 95% confidence interval, 0.02 to 0.06) and in a subsequent pregnancy (relative risk, 0.12; 95% confidence interval, 0.07 to 0.23). These benefits were seen regardless of the ABO status of the mother and baby when anti-D was given within 72 hours of birth. Higher doses (up to 200 µg) were more effective than lower doses (up to 50 µg) in preventing RhD alloimmunization in a subsequent pregnancy. The usual dose after full-term delivery in the United States and Canada is 300 µg (1500 IU), which will effectively suppress the immunizing potential of approximately 17 mL of RhD RBCs,[102] although lower doses are administered elsewhere with almost equivalent effectiveness. Postpartum prophylaxis is recommended whenever a D-positive

infant is born to an unsensitized D-negative mother.[103] Some guidelines also recommend anti-D if the infant is weak D positive.[57,103]

After postnatal immunoprophylaxis, the risk for RhD alloimmunization is between 1% and 2%. Administration of 100 µg (500 IU) of anti-D at 28 and 34 weeks' gestation to women in their first pregnancy can reduce this risk to about 0.2%.[104,105] Most current guidelines[57,106-109] therefore recommend routine administration of Rh immunoglobulin to all D-negative pregnant women in the early and mid third trimester unless the father of the fetus is known and can be shown conclusively to be Rh negative. This combined antenatal and postnatal prophylaxis will prevent 96% of cases of RhD isoimmunization.[103] Most guidelines are silent on the issue, but many transfusion services also recommend prophylaxis for weak D-positive women,[110] although more extensive serologic or genetic characterization can obviate the need for such prophylaxis in many cases.[54] Additional or earlier doses (depending on the timing and circumstances) for D-negative women who are not already sensitized and who abort, experience abdominal trauma, or are undergoing amniocentesis, CVS, or other relevant procedures may further reduce the risk for sensitization.[107,111,112] Small amounts of anti-D cross the placenta and cause a weakly positive antiglobulin test, but there are no apparent adverse effects on the infant.[113] It is important to note that the results of maternal antibody screening tests performed near term may be positive (albeit usually at low titer) after anti-D administration during pregnancy, but under the current guidelines these results should not preclude the postnatal administration of anti-D.

About 1 in 400 woman will have fetal-to-maternal TPH of greater than 30 mL of fetal blood at the time of delivery. Prevention of Rh sensitization in the presence of such a large dose of antigen requires prompt assessment (by the Kleihauer-Betke test or flow cytometry) and administration of a titrated dose of anti-D.[109] Pediatricians must be aware of this possibility and promptly notify their obstetric colleagues of any suspected anemia or blood loss in the newborn infant of an Rh-negative mother. Assessment of the magnitude of TPH is also recommended after pregnancy complications such as abdominal trauma.

Certain knowledge of Rh negativity in the biologic father of the fetus can obviate the need for antenatal immunoprophylaxis. However, this information should be established with a very high degree of certainty because of the potential for severe consequences in a future pregnancy in case of error.[109]

Reports from numerous countries have documented a reduction in RhD HDN as a result of anti-D immunoglobulin. Nevertheless, there is no room for complacency because 30% to 40% of the reduction in incidence of HDN over recent decades has been attributed to decreased family size rather than administration of anti-D.[114] Chavez and colleagues[115] noted that the incidence of Rh sensitization in the United States is three times the rate predicted if anti-D were always applied according to guidelines issued by the American College of Obstetricians and Gynecologists. Failure of the anti-D program to completely abolish RhD HDN can be partly attributed to noncompliance with guidelines. In addition, recommendations for additional doses during pregnancy have led to a scarcity of anti-D in some locations. These problems are even greater in poorer countries.[116] Giving donors booster doses consisting of carefully screened RhD-positive RBCs has been a necessity as the number of suitable sensitized donors decreases, but this practice requires extreme care to protect both the donor and eventual recipients. Distribution of the Rh-negative phenotype may increase as a result of migration. As with the use of any blood product, issues of safety cannot be disregarded.[117] All these forces threaten the supply of anti-D. Recombinant monoclonal or polyclonal preparations, which could in principle replace the current polyclonal anti-D and thereby resolve problems of availability and safety, have been under development in recent years. However, although monoclonal antibodies have significant diagnostic and research applications, they are not yet available for prophylaxis against sensitization.[118,119]

Overall, it is unlikely that the incidence of Rh HDN will ever return to the levels seen in previous generations, but it is also not likely to be abolished altogether.

Pathogenesis of Rh Hemolytic Disease

Erythropoiesis begins in the yolk sac by the third week of gestation, and Rh antigen is expressed by the sixth week. By 6 to 8 weeks' gestation, the liver replaces the yolk sac as the main site of RBC production. Normally, erythropoiesis then diminishes in the liver and takes place nearly entirely in the bone marrow by the late third trimester of pregnancy.[120]

Erythroblastosis is caused by coating of fetal RBCs with maternal IgG, which leads to their destruction. The subsequent fetal anemia stimulates erythropoiesis via the production of erythropoietin and other erythroid growth factors. When fetal marrow RBC production cannot keep up with RBC destruction, marked extramedullary erythropoiesis can be found in other organs, including the liver and in more severe cases also in the spleen, kidneys, skin, intestine, and adrenal glands. Hepatosplenomegaly is a hallmark of erythroblastosis fetalis. In the presence of erythroblastosis, immature nucleated RBCs, from normoblasts to early erythroblasts (Fig. 3-4), are poured into the circulation.

SEVERITY OF Rh HEMOLYTIC DISEASE

Degrees of Severity

For purposes of audit, research, and planning of treatment, degrees of severity of HDN have been used since the 1950s.

In general, fetuses and infants with mild HDN have had antibody-coated RBCs that yield positive results on a direct antiglobulin (Coombs) test, but they have no anemia or anemia that is well compensated for in utero and after birth and do not require exchange transfusion to prevent bilirubin toxicity. This group historically accounted for about half of affected fetuses. Nearly all survive and do well without invasive treatment.

Moderately affected fetuses are at risk for neural toxicity from bilirubin if they do not receive treatment. Historically, they are a group who routinely underwent exchange transfusion after birth. They are likely to have some signs of anemia in utero and ex utero but are not significantly acidotic or hydropic. Their peripheral blood typically shows polychromasia, anisocytosis, and reticulocytosis, although these conditions can be suppressed by intrauterine treatment. Maternal clearance copes with the products of hemolysis, and the fetus is usually born

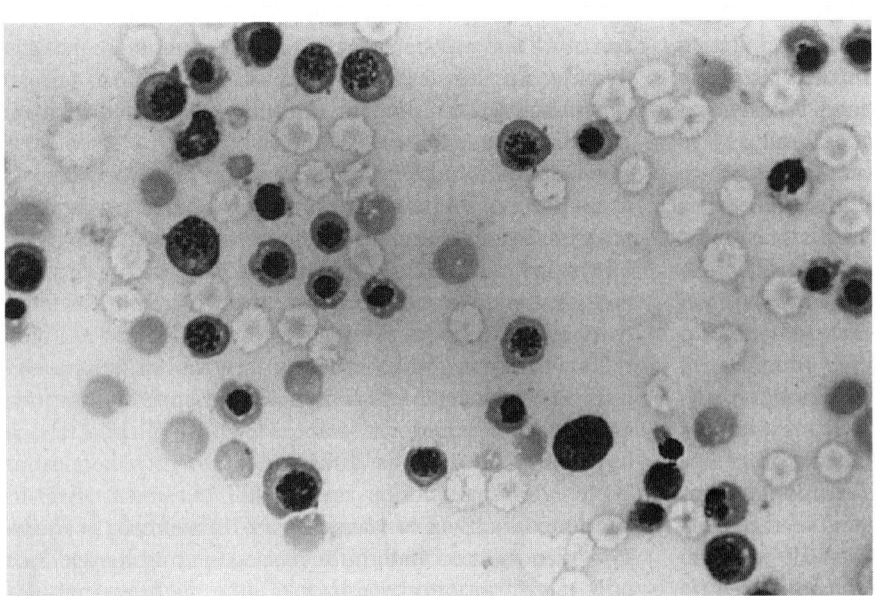

FIGURE 3-4. Cord blood from a baby with severe Rh erythroblastosis fetalis who required multiple fetal transfusions and exchange transfusions. The smear was treated by Kleihauer's technique with Wright staining. Note the adult donor ghost red blood cells (RBCs), dark fetal RBCs, and early fetal erythroid series consisting of erythroblasts through normoblasts. *(From Bowman JM. The management of Rh-isoimmunization. Obstet Gynecol. 1978;52:1. Reprinted with permission from The American College of Obstetricians and Gynecologists.)*

in good condition at or near term. This category historically represented about a third of fetuses. Moderately affected neonates do require vigilant neonatal management, including intensive phototherapy or exchange transfusion, to manage jaundice.

Severely affected fetuses have hydrops or hydrops is impending, and they would die before, during, or after birth unless managed intensively. Untreated, hydrops develops in half between 18 and 34 weeks' gestation and in the other half between 34 and 40 weeks' gestation. Polyhydramnios usually occurs early in the course or precedes the development of hydrops. Ascites and pleural and pericardial effusions develop. In infants with the most extreme conditions, compression hypoplasia of the lungs makes gas exchange after birth precarious.

When these categories of disease were first devised, severe fetal disease predicted severe neonatal disease. However, as fetal and neonatal management has been refined, the predictions must be updated, and the proportion of mildly and moderately affected neonates has risen. For example, some mildly anemic but not hydropic neonates who met previous criteria for exchange transfusion are now managed effectively with intensive phototherapy and would therefore be regarded as having mild rather than moderate disease. Similarly, a fetus with the early development of hydrops (severe fetal HDN) may respond well to one or more intrauterine transfusions and would therefore be born with mild neonatal disease and yet still have severe late anemia that is as much a consequence of hematopoietic suppression caused by effective intrauterine treatment as of hemolysis caused by the underlying disease. A suggested update to the working definitions that separates the criteria into epochs and includes a summary of implications for practice is given in Table 3-4.[121]

Pathogenesis of Hydrops

Hydrops in HDN was originally attributed to fetal heart failure, but other factors probably play a role (Fig. 3-5).[122] With severe hemolysis and progressively greater extra-medullary erythropoiesis, the hepatic architecture and circulation are distorted by the islets of erythropoiesis. It has been suggested that this alteration results in portal and umbilical venous obstruction and portal hypertension. Impairment of umbilical venous return would exacerbate the fetal tissue hypoxia caused by anemia and explain the placental edema that is usually seen in severe hydrops. The placental edema, by increasing the placental barrier to gas exchange, could then impair oxygen delivery even more. The theory that liver distortion and dysfunction are at least as important as heart failure in the pathogenesis of hydrops fetalis could explain why hydrops is not always accompanied by hypervolemia or even anemia.[122] Support for the suggestion that portal hypertension is present is provided by ultrasound assessment of waveforms in the portal venous system.[123]

Hypoalbuminemia is a common feature, but the mechanism has not been explained. It could be caused by a greater volume of distribution for albumin or reversion to α-fetoprotein expression rather than failure of hepatic synthesis.

The mechanisms that lead to hydrops remain poorly understood, both in anemic fetuses and in nonanemic fetuses with "nonimmune" hydrops. Various inflammatory mediators could play a role but have not been examined. Genes that are regulated by hypoxia include those for vascular endothelial growth factor and other molecules involved in capillary morphogenesis. Depending on the pattern of expression, these molecules can markedly affect capillary permeability and could also play a role.

Factors Affecting the Severity of Fetal/Neonatal Hemolytic Disease

If a sensitized mother is pregnant with an Rh-incompatible fetus, a number of factors influence the severity of disease in the fetus, including placental transfer of antibody, antibody characteristics, antigen characteristics, state of maturation of the fetal spleen, and resilience of fetal erythropoiesis.

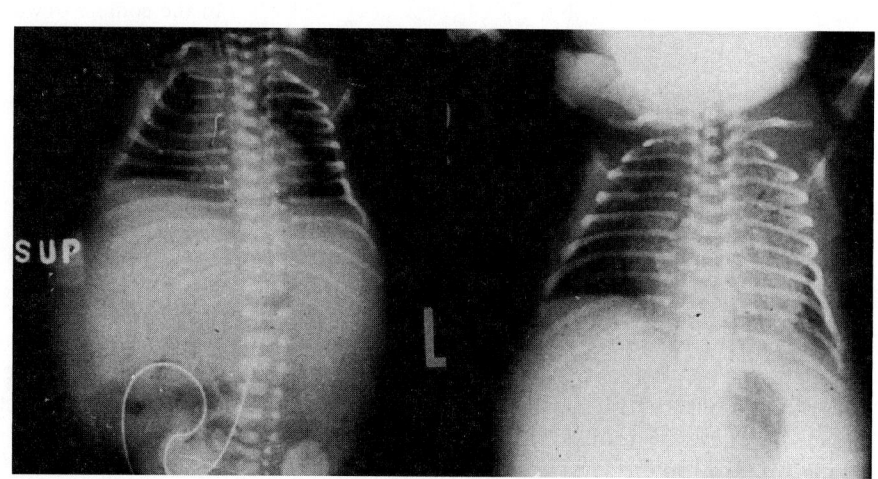

FIGURE 3-5. Radiograph of a hydropic newborn at birth and 6 hours later after exchange transfusion. Note the small size of the heart at the time of birth and the very marked increase in heart size and evidence of pulmonary congestion denoting heart failure 6 hours later. The fetus has extreme ascites. *(From Bowman JM. Blood-group incompatibilities. In Iffy L, Kaminetzky HA [eds]. Principles and Practice of Obstetrics and Perinatology. New York, John Wiley & Sons, 1981, p 1203. © Leslie Iffy, MD, Newark, NJ.)*

TABLE 3-4   Degrees of Severity of Rh Hemolytic Disease of the Fetus and Newborn

	Mild	Moderate	Severe
IN THE FETUS			
Historical proportion of Rh HDN before intrauterine therapy was available	≈50%	25-30%	20-25%
Probable history in previous siblings	No exchange	Exchange unless in utero treatment performed	Severe unless in utero treatment performed
Probable maternal anti-D titer	<1:64	>1:64	>1:64
Ultrasound abnormalities	None	Altered patterns of flow in fetal vessels	Signs of severe anemia (see Table 3-5), hydrops, portal hypertension, ascites and other effusions, polyhydramnios
IN THE NEONATE			
Clinical condition at birth	Normal	Mildly or moderately ill	Hydrops
Hemoglobin at birth	No anemia	Mild or moderate anemia; HgB >0.6 MoM for gestation	Severe, symptomatic anemia, HgB <0.6 MoM
Hemoglobin nadir	Transfusion not needed	At risk for symptomatic anemia	Risk of death unless transfusion performed
Bilirubin cord	<3.5 mg/dL (≈70 μmol/L)	>3.5 mg/dL (≈70 μmol/L)	>3.5 mg/dL (≈70 μmol/L)
Bilirubin peak	Term: <20 mg/dL (≈380 μmol/L) Premature: lower levels, depending on prematurity	Term: >20 mg/dL (≈380 μmol/L) Premature: lower levels, depending on prematurity	Rate of RBC destruction depends on (low) HgB; peak bilirubin is variable, toxicity increased
Phototherapy	If bilirubin increases faster than 0.4-0.5 mg/dL/hr; lower threshold for premature infants	If bilirubin increases faster than 0.4-0.5 mg/dL/hr; lower threshold for premature infants	Immediate, intensive, pending measurement of bilirubin increase
"Early" exchange	No	If rate of increase in bilirubin >0.8-1 mg/dL/hr; lower threshold for premature infants	Yes
"Late" exchange	If bilirubin > exchange level	If bilirubin ≥ exchange level	If bilirubin approaches exchange level
Heme oxygenase inhibition	Unnecessary—number needed to treat to avoid exchange will be high	In the context of well-designed clinical trials	In clinical trial to avert late exchange; unlikely to allow avoidance of early exchange
Intravenous immunoglobulin	Unnecessary—number needed to treat to avoid exchange will be high	In the context of well-designed clinical trials	In clinical trial to avert late exchange; unlikely to allow avoidance of early exchange
Phenobarbital	No	No	No clear benefit if optimal phototherapy performed
Erythropoietin for late anemia	No	In the context of well-designed clinical trials	In the context of well-designed clinical trials

HDN, hemolytic disease of the fetus and newborn; MoM, multiples of mean; RBC, red blood cell.
Modified from Peterec SM. Management of neonatal Rh disease. Clin Perinatol. 1995;22:561-592.

Transfer of Antibody to the Fetus

All four IgG subclasses are transported across the placenta via FcRn-mediated endocytosis and then exocytosis.[124-126] The fetal-to-maternal ratio for total IgG is approximately 0.4 at 28 weeks' gestation and increases to 1.4 at term,[127] but fetal levels of IgG1 are close to maternal levels by 17 to 20 weeks' gestation.[128] The efficiency of placental transport of antibody may be an important factor in the severity of Rh HDN, and reduced IgG transport can result in unexpectedly mild disease.[129]

Mechanism of Red Blood Cell Hemolysis

When anti-RBC antibodies bind complement and are present in high concentration (as with transfusion reactions to ABO-incompatible blood in adults), extravascular RBC destruction occurs and may cause a clinically severe reaction that includes hemoglobinemia, shock, and disseminated intravascular coagulopathy. Products of

RBC destruction are cleared predominantly by the liver.

When antibodies do not fix complement, as is typical with anti-D in the fetus and neonate,[130,131] the mechanisms of hemolysis are more subtle but, in the end, equally destructive. Three Fc receptor–mediated pathways have been implicated in the destruction of opsonized RBCs: direct phagocytosis, phagocytic damage leading to later lysis, and killer cell–mediated damage. When anti-D becomes concentrated on the membrane of RhD-positive RBCs, the RBCs adhere to macrophages and form rosettes, particularly in the red pulp of the spleen, where RBCs and macrophages come into close apposition. The phagocytic cell can then destroy the RBC or damage and deplete the membrane, thereby causing loss of RBC deformability. If the RBC escapes being consumed by the macrophage, its membrane is damaged and its osmotic fragility and likelihood of lysis are greater (Fig. 3-6).

Antibody-dependent cellular cytotoxicity (ADCC) probably also accounts for the destruction of some RBCs.[132] Large granular "K cells" (natural killer lymphocytes) or myeloid cells (polymorphonuclear leukocytes and monocytes) bind antibody-labeled cells and release lysosomal enzymes and perforin, which causes lysis.

Hemolysis also requires a competent system of phagocytic cells in the fetus. The clinical manifestations of the disease suggest that maturation is sufficient as early as the mid second trimester.

Antibody Specificity and Severity of Hemolytic Disease

Antigen characteristics, including details of antibody distribution, density, and structure, all affect the risk for HDN and have been reviewed by Hadley.[133] Antibodies with the potential to cause HDN generally recognize antigens restricted to erythroid cells (such as Rh antigens) rather than those with wider tissue distribution (such as A and B antigens, found on many cell types). The antigens must be expressed in the fetus and neonate. Thus, antibodies to Kell and Rh antigens, which are expressed early in fetal life, cause severe HDN, whereas antibodies to Lewis antigens, which are not synthesized in erythrocyte progenitors, never cause HDN. The circulating glycosphingolipids carrying the antigenic Le^a or Le^b epitopes generally adsorb to the erythrocyte membrane only during postnatal life. Lewis antibodies are also usually IgM. Lewis is the only human blood group system that has never been reported to cause HDN of any severity.

Antigen density is also an important factor. Within the Rh system, even in the presence of high maternal anti-D titer, fetuses with aberrant D phenotypes are unlikely to be severely affected. As might be expected, homozygotes for *RHD* appear to have higher D antigen density than heterozygotes do,[88] although this is not usually clinically relevant in Rh HDN because RhD-positive infants of RhD-negative mothers are obligate heterozygotes. The *RHCE* genotype also affects RhD antigen density, and in particular there seems to be higher expression of D when CE is deleted or underexpressed.[134,135] The density of several other antigens, including A and B and the Lutheran antigens,[136] is developmentally regulated, and antigen density on immature RBCs limits the severity of hemolysis.

Antigen structure may also play a role, with some antigens being more capable of promoting recognition of RBCs by phagocytic cells.

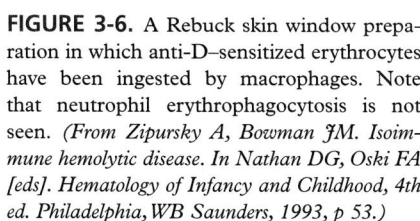

FIGURE 3-6. A Rebuck skin window preparation in which anti-D–sensitized erythrocytes have been ingested by macrophages. Note that neutrophil erythrophagocytosis is not seen. *(From Zipursky A, Bowman JM. Isoimmune hemolytic disease. In Nathan DG, Oski FA [eds]. Hematology of Infancy and Childhood, 4th ed. Philadelphia, WB Saunders, 1993, p 53.)*

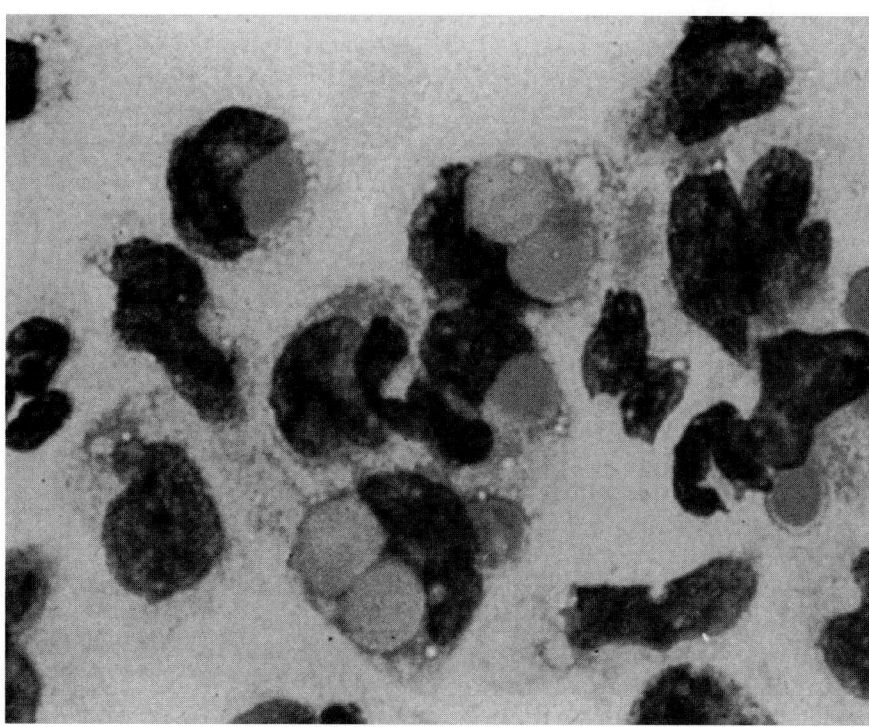

Antibody characteristics likewise play a role in determining the severity of HDN. IgG subclasses bind different classes of Fc receptors, although it has not yet been established conclusively which receptors are involved in RBC destruction in vivo. Fc receptor polymorphisms (analogous to an FcRII allele found in whites, which binds IgG2 very avidly and may play a role in ABO HDN) may yet be found to account for some of the heterogeneity of Rh HDN.[133]

Whereas anti-A and anti-B antibodies are predominantly IgG2, IgG1 and IgG3 anti-D antibodies tend to predominate in Rh-sensitized women.[137-140] They are often present in combination.

The capacity of RBC-bound IgG3 antibodies to bind to the Fc receptors of monocytes is greater than that of IgG1 antibodies. Threshold levels of antibody binding for rosette formation in vitro are approximately 1000 IgG3 or 2000 IgG1 molecules per RBC.[141] Both can promote phagocytosis, but their relative potencies depend on circumstances. IgG3 usually causes more efficient lysis by monocytes than IgG1 does.[142-144] Clearance of Rh-positive RBCs is caused by fewer molecules of IgG3 anti-D than of IgG1 anti-D.[145] However, the relationship of these factors to HDN is still unclear. Studies of maternal IgG subclasses do not indicate a clear relationship between subclass distribution and disease severity.[146]

HLA antibodies have been found in the sera of some women who have infants with mild HDN despite high anti-D antibody levels. The HLA antibodies may block antibody-antigen interactions on the macrophage membrane.[133]

ANTIBODY DETECTION

ABO and RhD typing plus antibody screening is recommended at the first prenatal visit in all pregnancies, including visits for elective abortion. A history of previous pregnancies and blood transfusions should also be elicited. If the blood group is D negative or weak D, another antibody screening is recommended at 24 to 28 weeks' gestation, before the administration of anti-D immunoprophylaxis. If an alloantibody is detected at low titer, screening is usually repeated at regular intervals to detect any increase. There are a variety of methods for assessing maternal antibodies, some that are better suited for screening methods and some that are more useful for predicting the severity of disease.[133]

Manual Methods

Rh-positive RBCs suspended in isotonic saline are agglutinated only by IgM anti-D because although IgG anti-D can bind to antigen, it cannot bridge the gap between RBCs suspended in saline. Therefore, a maternal serum sample containing only IgG anti-D does not agglutinate Rh-positive RBCs suspended in saline. The addition of albumin lowers the negative electrical potential of the RBC membrane, and IgG anti-D can then bridge the smaller gaps between the RBCs.[147] Because IgM anti-D also agglutinates Rh-positive RBCs suspended in albumin, if saline and albumin titers are similar, the albumin titer does not accurately assess IgG anti-D. Addition of dithiothreitol disrupts IgM sulfhydryl bonds and reveals the true IgG anti-D titer. Albumin methods have been surpassed but are described to clarify the earlier literature that refers to them.

Coombs' serum is an anti-human globulin produced by immunizing another species.[7] Rh-positive RBCs are incubated with the serum sample that is being tested for the presence of anti-D. If anti-D is present in the sample, it adheres to the Rh-positive RBC membrane. The RBCs are then washed to remove nonadherent human protein and suspended in Coombs' serum. If the RBCs are coated with anti-D, they are agglutinated by the antibodies to human immunoglobulin (positive test result). The reciprocal of the highest dilution of maternal serum that produces agglutination is the indirect antiglobulin titer.

Incubation of RBCs with enzymes such as papain, trypsin, and bromelin reduces the electrical potential of the RBC membrane and thus allows agglutination of Rh-positive cells by IgG anti-D, even in saline. Enzyme screening methods are the most sensitive manual techniques available for detecting Rh sensitization, but they detect many antibodies that have no clinical significance.[148]

These manual methods have the advantages of sensitivity and flexibility, but the correlation between antibody titer and disease severity is poor.

Automated Analysis

Autoanalyzer methods have been developed and refined for more efficient and reproducible detection and quantitation of Rh and other antibodies.[149-151] Autoanalyzer techniques are very sensitive, and the finding of an Rh antibody detected only by an autoanalyzer method does not necessarily indicate the presence of HDN or even true sensitization, especially if the titer is very low and stable. Gel and solid-phase assays have also been developed.[152-156] Rising titers indicate worsening disease and suggest the need for assessment of the fetus.

PREDICTION OF FETAL HEMOLYTIC DISEASE

Once sensitization is detected, subsequent investigative measures are required. To refine the estimation of risk, one or more of the following may need to be considered.

Determination of fetal blood type by

• Paternal blood typing
• Fetal blood typing

Prediction of the severity of disease by

- A history indicating the severity of HDN in previous infants
- Maternal antibody titers
- Cell-mediated maternal antibody functional assays
- Fetal ultrasound
- Amniotic fluid spectrophotometry
- Percutaneous fetal blood sampling

Determination of Fetal Blood Type

Paternal Blood Typing

In some instances, paternal blood typing can indicate that the baby has no risk for HDN. This situation occurs if the father is Rh negative and the mother was sensitized not by his offspring but by those of a previous partner or by transfusion. If the father is predicted to be Rh negative or heterozygous, the fetus may be completely unaffected regardless of the maternal antibody titer. In predominantly white populations, about 56% of Rh-positive individuals are heterozygous. It is important, however, to not place too much weight on heterozygosity when it is present. Half the offspring of a heterozygous father should be Rh negative, but to come reliably ($P = .95$) within 20% of this ideal state, it can be deduced statistically that each mother would have to have about 30 pregnancies.[84]

Historically, paternal genotype was estimated by determination of the father's RhCE type, in combination with information about the distribution of Rh phenotypes in different racial groups. Molecular genetic techniques now allow more direct determination of genotype and correlation with phenotype.

Fetal Blood Typing

Fetal Rh typing, either by traditional antigen typing or by genotyping via DNA amplification techniques, is becoming increasingly feasible and widespread. Although the need for it can be obviated if paternal homozygosity is certain, it can be an especially important technique if paternity is uncertain or the father is heterozygous.

Molecular methods are now used routinely and with high accuracy in many locations to detect fetal *RHD*, *RHCE*, *KEL*, *FY*, and *JK* genes in fetal DNA obtained by amniocentesis or from fetal cells or free DNA in maternal blood.[157-164] Cell-free fetal DNA, presumed to be from apoptotic syncytiotrophoblasts, is now most commonly used for amplification because unlike some fetal cells, it is cleared rapidly after delivery and therefore reflects only the current pregnancy.[165] These tests have the potential to reduce the need for assessment throughout the pregnancy, including the need for invasive tests, and to avert the need for administration of anti-D during some pregnancies. Single-cell preimplantation diagnosis has also been described.[166]

The genetic diversity of the Rh blood group system outlined in an earlier section of this chapter provides an important reminder to use caution in choosing primers that minimize false-positive and false-negative test results and to keep in mind the fact that genotype does not always obviously predict phenotype. The prevalence of *RHD-RHCE* hybrids and partially intact but functionally inert *RH* genes in certain populations can invalidate some tests designed for application in whites. The use of appropriate controls, amplification of several diagnostic sites, preferably checking the correlation between the parents' genotype and phenotype in parallel, and using the tests with a good understanding of the typical genotypes in the populations for which they were developed and to which they are being applied should minimize errors.[167,168] The need to have a good positive control for fetal DNA to identify false-negative results is critical. The *SRY* sequence can be used if the fetus is male, but more complicated comparison of multiple fetal and parental polymorphisms in other genes may be necessary if the fetus is female. Differential methylation of the maspin gene in fetal and maternal tissues recommends it as a universal positive control.[164,169]

Because *RHD* genotyping of amniotic and chorionic cells agrees with serologic and tissue typing,[157] CVS or amniocentesis can be used for typing of the fetus. However, the need to use these procedures should diminish as procedures involving fetal DNA from maternal blood become more widely available. If maternal blood samples are used for diagnosis, advantages include the fact that typing can be done early in pregnancy and that sample acquisition neither risks harming the fetus nor increases maternal exposure to fetal antigens.

Prediction of Severity of Disease

The relative roles of methods for assessing the severity of hemolytic disease in the fetus have changed in recent years.

Pregnancy History

Although it is usually true that the severity of HDN remains the same or increases during subsequent affected pregnancies, the disease sometimes becomes less severe. If a previous baby was hydropic, a subsequent affected fetus has a 90%, not a 100% chance of the development of hydrops. If hydrops is going to develop, it usually does so at the same gestation or earlier, but occasionally it develops later. In a first D-sensitized pregnancy with no previous history of HDN, there is an 8% to 10% probability that hydrops will develop. If a mother has had a previous fetus with hydrops and the father is heterozygous for the offending antigen, the fetus may be negative and completely unaffected or be positive and very severely affected, a dilemma that requires resolution, usually by fetal typing. Thus, though worth noting, there are a variety of situations in which a history of previous pregnancies is unreliable.

Maternal Antibody Titers

Although antibody titrations carried out in the same laboratory by the same experienced personnel using the same methods and test cells are reproducible and do give the physician some indication of risk, their predictive value is inadequate to guide invasive fetal treatment. The autoanalyzer technique provides somewhat better prediction of the severity of HDN than manual methods do, but the two approaches have not been compared rigorously. Hadley[133] has stated that although many laboratories can and should undertake screening for alloantibodies, antibody quantitation is best limited to regional centers with proven reliability. Ideally, these laboratories will also have programs auditing the outcomes of pregnancies in which antibodies have been detected. This can lead over time to the recognition of a critical titer, below which no cases of severe disease have occurred, and allow targeting of more extensive and invasive tests to those with titers above the threshold. However, the follow-up needed is laborious, is prone to ascertainment bias, and can threaten patient privacy. Generally, if the obstetric history is good, low titers ($\leq 1:16$ by manual methods or <5 IU/mL [1 μg/mL] by autoanalyzer) that increase slowly or not at all are reassuring and an indication for continued surveillance with antibody titers and ultrasound.

Although rising titers suggest increasing risk to the fetus, it has not been possible, even with autoanalyzer methods, to establish a titer above which the fetus must be sensitized,[170,171] and sometimes antibody levels increase significantly (but presumably nonspecifically) despite the presence of a compatible and therefore unaffected fetus. Nevertheless, in the presence of very high or rising titers, fetal assessment becomes urgent.

Maternal Antibody Functional Assays

Various functional assays that measure the ability of maternal antibody to promote interactions between RBCs and monocytes or K cells have been developed.[172] These assays include the monocyte monolayer assay,[173,174] the ADCC assay using lymphocytes[175] or monocytes,[176] and monocyte chemiluminescence.[141]

Each assay has its proponents, and their advantages and limitations have been reviewed.[133,174] Hadley and associates[153] compared monocyte chemiluminescence, K-cell lymphocyte ADCC, monocyte-macrophage ADCC, and a rosette assay using U937 cells. They found that monocyte chemiluminescence and monocyte ADCC functional assays predicted severity of disease better than rosette assay with U937 cells and K-lymphocyte ADCC did. Similarly, Zupanska and colleagues[140] found that the results of a monocyte-based assay (monocyte monolayer assay) correlated better with the clinical severity of hemolytic disease than did the results of rosette assays with lymphocytes. A survey of nine European laboratories that carried out functional assays on sera from mothers delivering babies with varying degrees of HDN revealed correct results as follows: ADCC (monocytes), 60%; ADCC (lymphocytes), 57%; chemiluminescence, 51%; and rosetting and phagocytosis with peripheral monocytes, 41% (with U937 cells or cultured macrophages, 32%).[177] However, a more recent report has cast doubt

on the ability of the monocyte-macrophage assay to predict the severity of HDN.[178]

Overall, when taken in conjunction with ultrasonography, consideration of the outcomes of previous pregnancies, and antibody quantitation, bioassays are somewhat useful in helping weigh the risks associated with invasive procedures in women with borderline levels of alloantibodies because they seem to be better in predicting mild rather than severe disease. However, there is no consensus that bioassays reduce the need for other forms of fetal assessment, and most published reports involve relatively small numbers of participants. These tests should be carried out in reference laboratories that perform them regularly and validate them carefully. Because they are measuring characteristics of the antibody, not the fetal antigen, bioassays are of no use in excluding an antigen-negative, unaffected fetus.

Amniotic Fluid Spectrophotometry

Bevis[179] showed that bilirubin could be found in the amniotic fluid of infants with HDN, and in 1961, Liley[180] plotted fetal outcomes by gestation and the results of amniotic fluid spectrophotometry, thus devising a prenatal test of the severity of fetal hemolytic disease that has only recently been surpassed as the standard method of assessing fetuses with hemolytic disease. Liley used the ΔOD_{450} reading (the deviation from linearity at 450 nm caused by the absorption spectrum of bilirubin) as a measurement of the amniotic fluid bilirubin level. Three zones of predicted severity of disease were defined (Fig 3-7). Readings in zone I indicated either no disease or no anemia at the time of testing but reflected a 10% chance that exchange transfusion would be needed. Readings in zone II indicated moderate disease that becomes more severe as readings approach the zone III boundary. Readings falling into very high zone II or zone III indicated severe disease. Hydrops was present or would develop within 7 to 10 days. When serial ΔOD_{450} measurements are taken, the overall accuracy of prediction of hemolytic disease with the amniotic fluid technique is 95%. Accuracy is higher in the third trimester than in the second trimester. Because the graphs were developed before intervention at earlier than 27 weeks' gestation was contemplated, zone boundaries in the second trimester were not defined. The Liley zone boundaries were subsequently modified by inclining them downward before 24 weeks' gestation because of the observation that ΔOD_{450} readings peak at 23 to 24 weeks' gestation in pregnancies unaffected by HDN.[181] The division lines for Queenan's chart are lower at all gestations than those of Liley's system. Although it was suggested that Queenan's modification could overestimate severity and lead to too many interventions,[182] others concluded that a more conservative approach was appropriate as safer and more effective intervention became available.[183] Monitoring with ultrasound and selective direct fetal blood sampling has markedly reduced the need for assessment by amniocentesis. Amniocentesis may be useful as

FIGURE 3-7. Superimposed Queenan and Liley charts of the deviation of absorbance at a wavelength of 450 nm (ΔOD_{450}) versus gestation. Liley's lines began at 27 weeks, and they were rectilinear when shown on a log-linear plot.[150] They were subsequently extrapolated back to 20 weeks.[151] Queenan's chart demonstrates that the lines should deflect downward in the early second trimester.[154] However, the division lines for Queenan's chart are lower at all gestations and may overestimate the risk in some fetuses. Current practice is to use fetal cerebral velicometry instead of or sometimes in addition to amniotic fluid results in determining the need and timing for intrauterine treatment. *(Redrawn from Scott F, Chan FY. Assessment of the clinical usefulness of the 'Queenan' chart versus the 'Liley' chart in predicting severity of rhesus iso-immunization. Prenat Diagn. 1998;18:1143-1148.)*

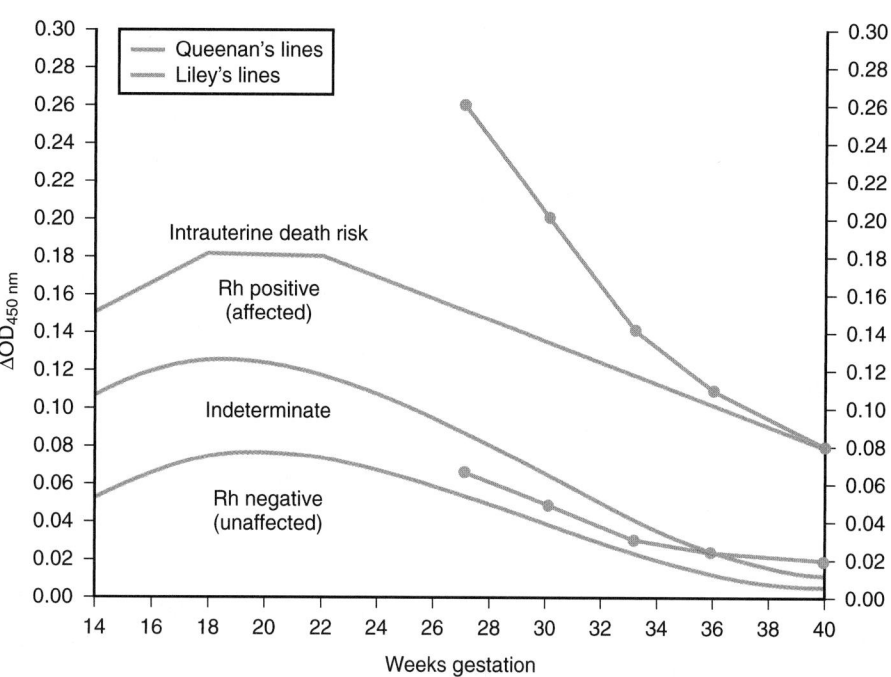

TABLE 3-5	Comparison of Test Characteristics for Peak Systolic Velocity in the MCA Measured via Doppler Ultrasonography and Amniotic Fluid ΔOD_{450} in Predicting Severe Fetal Anemia*		
Test	**Sensitivity[†]**	**Specificity[†]**	**Accuracy[†]**
MCA blood flow >1.5 MoM[189]	88 (78-94)	82 (73-89)	85 (79-90)
Amniotic fluid ΔOD_{450}			
Modified Liley chart—upper third of zone II or zone III[182]	76 (65-84)	77 (67-84)	76 (69-82)
Queenan chart—zone IV[181]	81 (71-88)	81 (72-88)	81 (75-86)

*Severe fetal anemia is defined as a hemoglobin level 5 SD or more below the mean for gestation.[192]
[†]Values are percentages (95% confidence interval).
MCA, middle cerebral artery; MoM, multiples of the median.

an adjunct to ultrasound to assess severity when factors such as fetal and placental position complicate fetal umbilical blood sampling.

Amniocentesis has risks, although ultrasound guidance has improved its safety and reliability considerably. Blood in amniotic fluid can obscure the 450-nm peak and thus make the fluid worthless for predicting the severity of hemolytic disease and complicate the determination of fetal genotype. Ultrasound guidance has reduced this risk from about 10% to 2.5%. Increases in antibody titer occur after some amniocenteses, although the risk is reported to be lower than that after umbilical blood sampling.[71,184]

Ultrasound Assessment

The development of obstetric ultrasonography in the late 1970s was a major advance in the management of maternal blood group isoimmunization. Ultrasound allows estimation of placental and hepatic size and determination of the presence or absence of polyhydramnios, edema, ascites, and other effusions. It has increased the safety of amniocentesis and intraperitoneal transfusion and is essential for umbilical blood sampling and intravascular fetal transfusions.

Although ultrasound was previously said to be of little use in assessing the severity of disease until hydrops had developed, assessment of flow velocity in major fetal vessels has now been shown by several groups to be very reliable in detecting significant fetal anemia. Middle cerebral artery velocimetry is the most extensively used assessment.[185-191] As with any critical test, responsible practitioners should audit outcomes and refine their judgments according to them, but when skills to perform it are available, ultrasound velocimetry has become the method of choice for monitoring women with blood group–sensitized pregnancies and for planning and timing invasive fetal sampling, fetal treatment, and delivery (Table 3-5).[192]

Percutaneous Fetal Blood Sampling

With the development of sophisticated ultrasound equipment and the availability of perinatologists skilled in its use, percutaneous fetal umbilical blood sampling became feasible in the mid-1980s.[193] This procedure allows direct diagnosis of fetal blood type, anemia, and acidosis and therefore provided the "gold standard" for diagnosis of fetal anemia against which the accuracy of other assessment techniques has been assessed. The procedure does carry with it a likelihood of fetal-to-maternal hemorrhage and a small risk of mortality.[193,194] Generally, it should be reserved for use when ultrasound (or amniocentesis) indicates moderately severe or severe disease with a probable need for intrauterine treatment. It is not usually indicated unless fetal treatment of severe anemia appears to be justified for continuation of the pregnancy and safe delivery. Fetal blood sampling may be possible as early as 18 weeks' gestation; it is generally feasible by 20 to 21 weeks' gestation. The preferred sampling site is the umbilical vein at its insertion into the placenta. For this reason, the procedure is technically easier to perform if the placenta is implanted on the anterior uterine wall.

MANAGEMENT OF MATERNAL ALLOIMMUNIZATION

Suppression of Alloimmunization

Since the mid-1940s, efforts have been made to suppress the strength of already developed maternal immune responses against fetal RBCs. Administration of Rh immune globulin, of great value in preventing Rh sensitization, has been shown to be ineffective in suppressing an established antibody response, no matter how weak, once it has begun.[195,196]

Two measures that have potential to reduce maternal antibody levels and ameliorate hemolytic disease are (1) intensive plasma exchange[197,198] and (2) the administration of nonspecific intravenous immune serum globulin (IVIG).[199-201] With intensive plasma exchange, alloantibody levels can be lowered by as much as 75% but tend to rebound, at times to levels higher than they were before.[202] Vascular access becomes difficult and IgG and albumin administration is needed. Plasma exchange is tedious, costly, and uncomfortable.[203] It may have a role in a mother with a fetus known to be susceptible to the antigen to which she is immunized and who has a previous history of hydrops at or before 24 to 26 weeks' gestation. However, the risk-to-benefit ratio remains insufficiently high to recommend it for routine management.

High-dose IVIG administration can also be effective in a severely alloimmunized pregnant woman, but its use should likewise be the subject of clinical audit and research. The mechanism of action has not been defined, but it could include inhibition of antibody synthesis or competitive blockade of receptor-mediated transfer across the placenta or binding sites on fetal immune cells. If IVIG therapy is considered, it should be used in the same situation as intensive plasma exchange, beginning at 10 to 12 weeks' gestation. Ongoing assessment of fetal disease remains essential because not all fetuses respond adequately. As a result of its cost, inconvenience, and side effects,[204] its use, like that of plasmapheresis, is reserved for fetal disease that is expected to be refractory to other therapy.[205]

Fetal Treatment

Induced Early Delivery

Premature delivery of fetuses with Rh HDN has been important in prevention of mortality since the late 1940s. With the introduction of amniotic fluid assessment in 1961, it became possible for the first time to predict which fetuses should be considered candidates for early delivery. Subsequent advances in perinatal and neonatal management of premature infants have had a major impact on survival. However, HDN is different from many other pregnancy complications in that intrauterine treatment has been effective in prolonging many gestations. As the effectiveness of fetal treatment has improved, particularly after the introduction of intravascular intrauterine transfusion, the need for premature delivery of infants with HDN has diminished. If premature delivery is required, antenatal betamethasone therapy should be given to the mother according to consensus guidelines. It is probable that infants with HDN have as much or more to gain from the use of this important preparation for extrauterine life than their gestation-matched peers with other fetal conditions do. A possible role for antenatal phenobarbital treatment to reduce the need for exchange transfusion of the neonate may warrant investigation in randomized controlled trials.[206]

Intrauterine Transfusion for Fetal Hemolytic Disease

In 1961, induced early delivery could not be undertaken before 31 to 32 weeks' gestation without the risk of prohibitive mortality from prematurity and severe Rh disease. Hydrops develops in 8% of fetuses before 32 weeks' gestation. In 1963, the introduction of intraperitoneal fetal transfusion (IPT) by Liley[207] completely altered the prognosis for these most severely affected of all fetuses (Fig. 3-8).

Since the beginning of the 20th century it was known that RBCs placed in the peritoneal cavity are absorbed and function normally. At one time, IPT was a preferred method for giving transfusions to children with thalassemia. It was abandoned in favor of vascular transfusions because of the severe discomfort that it caused. Absorption is via the subdiaphragmatic lymphatic lacunae, up the right lymphatic duct, and into the venous circulation. In the fetus, breathing movements are necessary for absorption to occur.[208] In the absence of hydrops, 10% to 12% of infused RBCs are absorbed daily. Ascites does not prevent absorption per se, although the rate of absorption in its presence is less predictable and the procedure is more risky. Rupture of membranes and spontaneous labor after IPT are also risks.

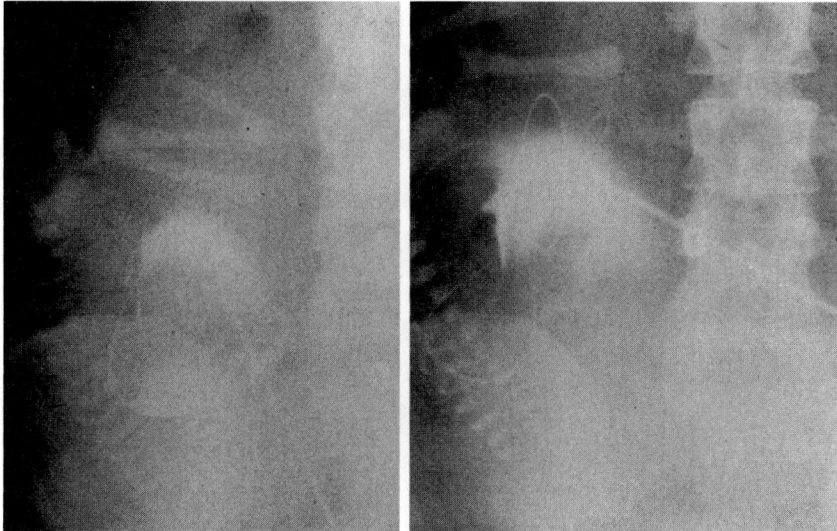

FIGURE 3-8. Hydrops fetalis at intraperitoneal fetal transfusion (IPT). Note the gross ascites at both the first and second IPTs. The fetus, hydropic at birth with a cord hemoglobin level of 9 g/100 mL (all donor RBCs), survived. *(From Bowman JM. Maternal blood group immunization. In Creasy RK, Resnik R [eds]. Maternal-Fetal Medicine: Principles and Practice, 2nd ed. Philadelphia, WB Saunders, 1989, p 636.)*

Although IPT was a major advance in the management of severe erythroblastosis fetalis, intravascular transfusion (IVT) has proved to be even more successful for most fetuses. The earliest attempts at direct IVT, either into a fetal or into a placental blood vessel approached via a hysterotomy incision, were made in the mid-1960s, but outcomes were poor because complications, including premature labor, almost invariably ensued.[209,210]

In 1981, Rodeck and co-workers[211] reported direct fetal transfusions through a fetoscope. Intracardiac transfusion has also been described,[212] but this method was soon superseded by percutaneous transfusion into umbilical vessels.[213-217] Under ultrasound guidance and local anesthesia, the tip of a 22- or 20-gauge spinal needle is introduced into an umbilical blood vessel, preferably the vein at its insertion into the placenta (Fig. 3-9). Fetal blood sampling usually precedes and follows the transfusion, and confirmation that the needle tip remains in the correct position can be obtained throughout the procedure by observing altered echoes in the vessel via ultrasonography.

There are a number of advantages of IVT over IPT. IVT allows direct diagnostic sampling at the onset and completion of the procedure. For skilled practitioners, the failure rate and procedure-related mortality are lower, especially in hydropic fetuses.[218,219] IVT allows larger transfusions and administration of platelets if needed.[216,220] It is effective in correcting anemia and its immediate physiologic consequences[221,222] and in reversing hydrops.[215] Survival and the neonatal condition were improved so rapidly by the introduction of IVT that just as with IPT before it, its merits have been determined by comparison with historical control data rather than prospective randomized studies. Comparison with historical control data may fail to take into account numerous other improvements in perinatal and neonatal care since the 1970s. However, babies with more severe disease respond to IVT, and they need less invasive and intensive neonatal care afterward. Undoubtedly, if an intrauterine procedure is necessary and IVT is feasible, it is the procedure of choice. Because of the rarity of severe disease, follow-up studies are limited, but they indicate that most survivors of both IPT and IVT have a good prognosis for neurologic development and general health.[223-228] Umbilical and inguinal hernias are reported to occur often after IPT.[227]

Despite the great advantages of IVT, there remain some situations in which IPT is necessary, including a fetus that is severely afflicted early in pregnancy, at a time when the cord vein is too small for successful venipuncture. In late pregnancy or with twin gestation, fetal size and position may preclude access to the umbilical vessels. IPT may also be necessary to "top up" an incomplete IVT if needle dislodgement or other immediate complications occur.

IVT and IPT can expose the mother to fetal cells, thereby raising her antibody titer and potentially worsening disease. As stated earlier, there is no benefit to giving anti-D antibody to already sensitized mothers. In the future, other methods of immunomodulation might prove beneficial to improve the safety of this aspect of treatment.

It has been recommended that both IPT and IVT be done in centers that perform at least 20 to 30 cordocenteses and 10 to 15 transfusions annually to maintain competence and allow adequate surveillance of outcomes.[229,230] Some perinatologists advocate the use of pancuronium before IVT to prevent fetal movement,[218] but others use it selectively or rarely. Transfusion volume should be optimized.[231,232] Complications include fetal bradycardia, cord hematoma, thrombosis or bleeding, rupture of membranes, infection, and premature labor.

Blood for Intrauterine Transfusion

No general guidelines have been published recently for many aspects of intrauterine transfusion. Although there

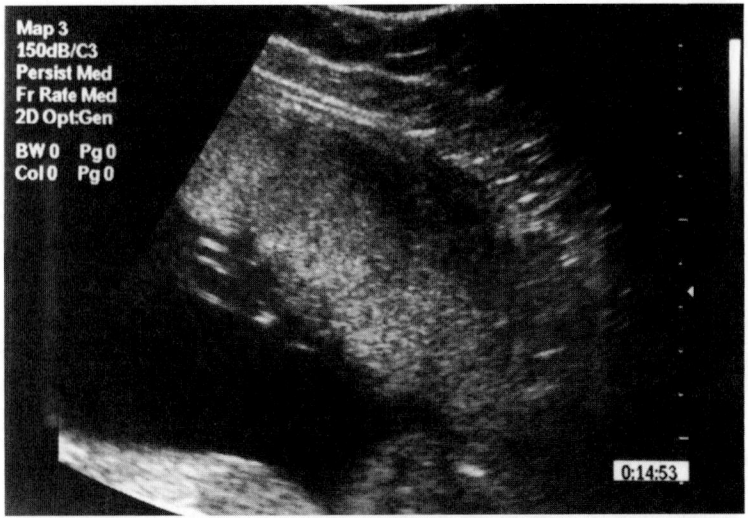

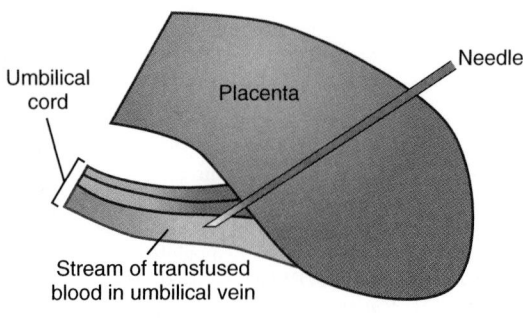

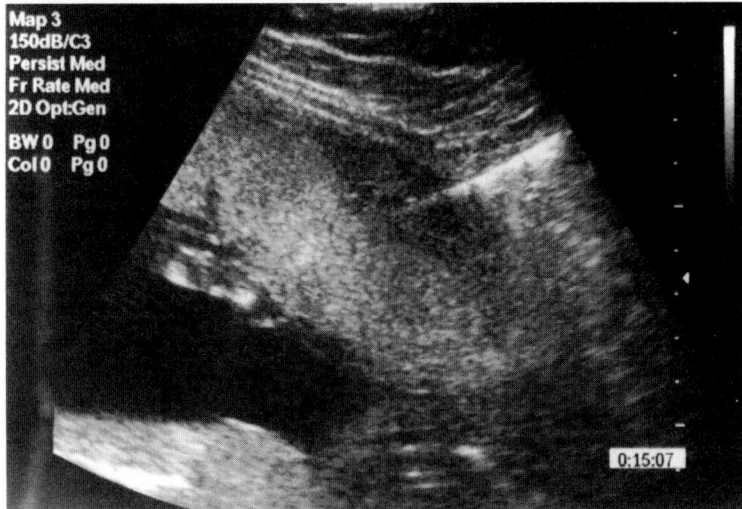

FIGURE 3-9. Real-time ultrasound view of intravascular transfusion via insertion of the umbilicus into the anterior surface of the placenta. The *bottom* panel shows a needle inserted (in this case through the placenta) into the umbilical vein. The intravascular transfusion in progress is shown by the echogenicity of the transfused blood in the umbilical vein.

have undoubtedly been advances in equipment design and blood banking techniques, reports of their application to intrauterine transfusion have not been published in peer-reviewed literature. By extrapolation from the results of neonatal transfusion therapy, it seems reasonable to propose that cytomegalovirus-negative packed RBCs be used for intrauterine transfusion. Cells should be as fresh as is compatible with careful screening and crossmatch against maternal blood and should be leukocyte depleted and irradiated. The risk for graft-versus-host disease is very low but not zero.[233,234] The use of Kell antigen–negative blood is optimal, if it is available.

Treatment of Neonates with Hemolytic Disease

General Measures

As a result of advances in antenatal assessment and treatment, the pediatrician often has the benefit of treating an infant with HDN whose condition is better and whose disease course is more predictable than those of infants with HDN in previous decades. Management of an infant

with severe hydrops fetalis remains difficult, and because the disease is now very uncommon, there is little opportunity for well-designed trials to test various approaches to management. Uncertainties include the role of antenatal drainage of pleural effusions and ascites, which resuscitation fluids and drugs to use, and when to perform top-up or exchange transfusion. Surfactant therapy may be necessary because of prematurity or surfactant inactivation.[235,236] Top-up transfusion may be useful for stabilization[122,237] because nearly all hydropic infants are severely anemic and some have low central venous pressure.

Even in a mildly affected infant, careful assessment and anticipatory management are required. A fetus that has coped well in the intrauterine environment and has not needed or has responded well to intrauterine treatment can still have significant problems with the transition to independent extrauterine life. Problems attributable to HDN, such as hyperinsulinemic hypoglycemia,[238] may be compounded by the problems of prematurity. The baby should be assessed promptly at birth and resuscitated if necessary. Physical examination may reveal hepatic and splenic enlargement and signs of anemia. Occasionally, stigmata resulting from accidents of intrauterine therapy are found.

Laboratory assessment should include a complete blood count, assessment of blood group and relevant antibodies, and baseline measurement of the bilirubin level so that the rate of increase in bilirubin can be calculated. In severely affected infants, liver function, acid-base balance, and coagulation profile should also be assessed. Cord blood can be useful for these tests but may provide misleading results unless the sample is obtained promptly. Many blood banks will not accept cord blood for crossmatch. In infants who have received multiple transfusions, assessment of iron status should be considered, especially if there is evidence of liver dysfunction.[239-241]

In regard to general care, breast-feeding should commence early in infants who are not deemed to be in imminent need of exchange transfusion. If mature and in good condition, the infant can be breast-fed while receiving phototherapy via a suitable fiberoptic blanket or spotlight. Although Rh antibodies are present in breast milk, particularly in colostrum, very little antibody is absorbed.[242] There is no evidence that forced fluid administration (beyond requirements for nutrition and compensation for any increased insensible loss) improves the outcome of the disease, and it is hazardous in premature infants and those with heart failure.

Folate is normally stored in the liver in late gestation, but reserves may be deficient in premature infants and depleted by ineffective erythropoiesis or by exchange transfusion, which replaces the infant's blood with adult blood that has a lower folate level.[243,244] Supplemental folic acid at a dose of 100 to 200 µg/day is recommended for several weeks. Vitamin B_{12} will usually be supplied in adequate amounts in breast milk (unless the mother has a deficiency), and supplemental iron is not only unnecessary but potentially hazardous.[239] Drugs that interfere with binding of bilirubin to albumin or with bilirubin metabolism should be avoided.

The use of phototherapy and other measures for hyperbilirubinemia is discussed in Chapter 4 and has been reviewed elsewhere.[245,246] The principles that we now apply in deciding when to begin and end phototherapy are little more than traditional rules of thumb. However, it seems clear that phototherapy is effective in preventing many exchange transfusions in infants with hemolysis.[247,248] Most guidelines still recommend lower thresholds for beginning phototherapy for HDN than for nonhemolytic jaundice, despite the improved condition of most of the infants with HDN whom we now treat. Intensive phototherapy is justified for infants with high or rapidly rising bilirubin levels. The risks and resource implications of phototherapy are low in comparison to those of exchange transfusion.

Phototherapy can be discontinued when serum bilirubin levels decrease or if the conjugated fraction of bilirubin increases substantially. Commonly, well near-term infants who have received intrauterine transfusions can be discharged at about a week of age. Conversely, many weeks of tertiary-level neonatal intensive care may be needed for premature, very anemic prehydropic or hydropic infants.

Administration of IVIG to prevent the need for exchange transfusion in HDN has been the subject of limited investigation.[249-252] These small studies used different IVIG preparations for different thresholds.[253] IVIG therapy deserves further investigation in selected infants, but there is not sufficient published evidence to recommend it outside of carefully conducted clinical trials.

Exchange Transfusion

Exchange transfusion originated in the 1920s in a procedure done via the anterior fontanelle. Refinements to the technique of "exsanguination transfusion" were introduced by Wallerstein and Wiener in 1946.[254,255] Generations of infants and pediatric residents should be grateful that Diamond pioneered the use of umbilical catheters[256] because Wiener's technique involved infusion of blood through a saphenous vein cutdown and drainage (after heparinization of the baby) via an incision in the radial artery at the wrist. A randomized controlled trial in 1952 confirmed that the technique could save lives and prevent kernicterus.[257]

During exchange transfusion, RBCs coated with antibody are replaced with RBCs negative for the antigen to which the mother is alloimmunized. Exchange transfusion corrects the anemia of a severely affected newborn, mitigates hyperbilirubinemia by removing the infant's hemolyzing erythrocytes and suppressing erythropoiesis, removes some of the already formed bilirubin, and depletes unbound anti-D antibody. Only modest amounts of the offending antibody are removed by exchange transfusion because unbound antibody is widely distributed in extracellular fluid, both within and outside the vascular compartment.

Exchange transfusion produces a significant drop in neutrophil levels, the functional significance of which is uncertain, but the initial neutropenia and subsequent "left shift" during rebound from it can certainly complicate the diagnosis of sepsis in the hours and days after exchange. A similar decrease in platelets is generally well tolerated, provided that the baby does not have thrombocytopenia or other coagulopathy before the exchange transfusion. Because a variety of coagulation defects increase the risk for intraventricular hemorrhage,[258] platelet therapy should be considered in sick and premature infants with thrombocytopenia.

Indications for Exchange Transfusion

Exchange transfusion is generally performed early for severe anemia or later when phototherapy and other conservative measures fail to control the bilirubin level. However, the exact thresholds at which it should be applied are controversial and warrant the development of contemporary guidelines. Traditional criteria for early exchange transfusion included a cord hemoglobin level less than 13 to 15 g/dL (130 to 150 g/L) and a cord serum bilirubin level greater than 60 to 130 μmol/L (3 to 7 mg/dL). However, Wennberg and colleagues[259] showed in 1978 that neither cord hematocrit nor bilirubin level had much value in predicting a postnatal increase in bilirubin level. They suggested using the criterion of rate of increase in bilirubin. Rates of increase of 8 to 13 μmol/L/hr, despite intensive phototherapy, indicate that exchange transfusion is likely to be needed. Improved antenatal treatment, phototherapy, and other supportive care has cast even these guidelines into doubt. Many neonatal intensive care units that have prompt blood bank support and the ability to perform exchange transfusion at short notice will delay exchange transfusion in babies who do not have symptomatic anemia until the risk associated with exchange transfusion is thought to approximate that of kernicterus. The decision process is clearly hampered by imprecise knowledge of where these risk boundaries lie. Jackson[260] recently estimated the risk of serious complications of exchange transfusion to be less than 1% in previously well infants and about 12% in ill infants. In a recent audit of 141 exchange transfusions over a period of 21 years in one center (69% of which were for immune hemolytic disease), there were no exchange transfusion–related deaths and only 14% had any transfusion-related complication.[261] In severely anemic hydropic babies, early exchange transfusion still seems warranted to improve oxygen transport. Peterec has suggested working guidelines.[121]

Free Bilirubin and Reserve Albumin Binding Studies

It appears that the level of free unconjugated bilirubin is the determining factor in the pathogenesis of bilirubin encephalopathy (kernicterus; see Chapter 4). Measurements of free bilirubin have not routinely influenced clinical practice in most centers, but some take the bilirubin-to-albumin ratio into account.[262]

Technique of Exchange Transfusion

The specific technical details of exchange transfusion are clearly set out elsewhere[263] and are discussed only briefly here. The safest location for catheter tips and whether it is better to use a single-catheter "push-pull" technique or a double-catheter continuous technique have not been determined conclusively. In practice, these decisions are often based on local tradition and on the number and type of catheters that can be inserted easily. The procedure should be conducted precisely and with meticulous attention to precautions against infection.

The blood should be ABO compatible and, for anti-D HDN, Rh negative. If the mother is alloimmunized to an antigen other than D, the blood should be missing that antigen. It should be crossmatch compatible with the mother's serum. Ideally, the blood should also be negative for Kell antigen (to avoid sensitizing the infant) and hemoglobin S (to avoid problems with filtration). If the initial exchange transfusion is carried out with group O blood, any further exchange transfusions should use group O blood. Otherwise, brisk hemolysis and jaundice secondary to ABO incompatibility may become a further complication. Graft-versus-host disease occurs rarely after exchange transfusion, but blood should be irradiated if possible, especially for premature infants. The question of whether to use whole blood or packed RBCs partially reconstituted with plasma or saline plus or minus platelets has not been subjected to rigorous study, but component therapy is widely used. Component therapy potentially exposes the infant to more donors and more risk of handling errors, but less risk of white blood cell–related complications. For very unusual antibodies or combinations of antibodies, RBCs may need to be transported over long distances. Occasionally, stored washed maternal RBCs must be used. In these circumstances, whole blood is unlikely to be available.

Depending on the local strategy for neonatal screening for metabolic and other diseases, it is strongly recommended that some of the blood from the first drawback be applied to a neonatal screening card. Otherwise, the diagnosis of some disorders such as galactosemia may be masked for some time to come. If any blood for serologic analysis or a DNA sample is needed for other diagnostic purposes such as congenital infection, it should also be collected at this time.

Aliquots of the infant's blood are removed and replaced with antigen-negative donor blood. In choosing a technique for transfusion, the practitioner should take into account the following considerations: the infant's tolerance of the metabolic, hemodynamic, and hematologic demands; the effectiveness of the procedure in treating anemia and preventing an increase in bilirubin level; and safe handling of the blood for transfusion. The size of aliquot should be chosen to take into account the tolerance of the infant and, if a single catheter is used, its dead space. Principles of calculus make it clear that the largest aliquots that the infant can tolerate will correct anemia most rapidly, but very rapid correction of anemia is not usually the prime objective. Allowing sufficient time for equilibration of bilirubin and antibody between the vascular and extravascular compartments is another concern, but with very long procedures there is the risk of clotted catheters and degradation of the donor blood. Generally, between 1.5 and 2 infant blood volumes are exchanged (130 to 170 mL/kg of body weight) over a 1- to 2-hour period.[264] A two–blood volume exchange transfusion removes approximately 90% of the affected RBCs of the infant, but the response is asymptotic rather than linear, and 70% removal occurs after the first blood volume has been exchanged. Only about 25% to 30% of total bilirubin is removed because it is sequestered in the extravascular and cellular compartments. A decrease of about 50% in the serum bilirubin level can be expected, but rapid rebound to about 75% of the pre-exchange level is typically seen.

Administration of albumin, 1 g/kg of body weight, before the exchange transfusion or addition of albumin, 4 to 6 g, to the blood used for exchange transfusion modestly increases the amount of bilirubin removed to about 35% of the total body bilirubin by drawing bilirubin into the vascular compartment. Caution is advised in administering albumin to a severely anemic infant because it may precipitate heart failure.

Many previous guidelines suggested routine administration of calcium gluconate. However, contemporary anticoagulants affect ionized calcium much less than the citrate-phosphate-dextrose used in years gone by does. Furthermore, most neonatal units now have immediate access to blood gas analyzers that also measure ionized calcium, electrolytes, and glucose in tiny samples. Periodic measurement of ionized calcium, electrolytes, glucose, and blood gas is therefore a reasonable alternative (e.g., every 30 minutes or earlier if the infant manifests any instability).

Complications of Exchange Transfusion

Complications of exchange transfusion include all those of simple transfusion plus a variety of others related to the large size of the transfusion, the catheters, and the technique.[260,261] As fewer procedures are being performed, experience with the procedure among neonatal and pediatric medical and nursing staff is declining. Furthermore, well infants who were previously given exchange transfusions are now being managed conservatively, whereas the sickest and most premature infants still require exchange transfusion. Thus, paradoxically, at a time when most transfusion therapy has never been safer, exchange transfusion has the potential become more hazardous, although improved monitoring and supervision may be compensating for these trends.[261]

Necrotizing enterocolitis is a potentially life-threatening hazard. The occurrence of necrotizing enterocolitis may be related to the technique. In the absence of evidence-based guidelines, effort should be made to prevent wide pressure and volume variations during exchange transfusion. Blood injection and withdrawal should be carried out smoothly, without undue haste. The use of blood products that are anti–T cryptantigen negative, prolongation of the interval until oral feeding is restarted, and the use of prophylactic antibiotics might also influence the risk for necrotizing enterocolitis, but there is no clear evidence for any of these practices in relation to exchange transfusion.

As discussed earlier for intrauterine transfusions, performance of exchange transfusions in neonatal intensive care units with experienced staff and with blood banks familiar with supplying neonates is likely to yield the best results for infants and the best hope of accumulating evidence to guide practice.

OTHER MATERNAL ALLOANTIBODIES CAUSING FETAL/NEONATAL HEMOLYTIC DISEASE

Alloantibodies Other Than A and B

Although reports from numerous geographic areas demonstrate the effectiveness of administration of anti-D IgG to prevent RhD alloimmunization, most find that Rh is still the blood group system causing most cases of HDN and that anti-D is still the most common single antibody causing severe HDN. Of non-D Rh antigens, anti-c is the next most important in causing clinically significant HDN. About half of anti-c antibodies are attributable to transfusion, and they are often present at low titer or the fetus is c negative. However, because anti-c can cause severe HDN or fetal death, careful assessment is warranted.[66] Anti-E is relatively common but seldom causes HDN. A variety of other non-D Rh antigens, such as anti-C, anti-e, and anti-Rh17, have also been reported to very occasionally cause moderate or severe HDN.[66] Rh antigens are not infrequently found in combination, such as anti-D plus -C, anti-D plus -E, or anti-c plus -ce. Often, one of the antibodies (e.g., anti-c) is present in higher titer and has the predominant influence on disease severity, but the combination adds to the complexity of finding suitable donors for intrauterine exchange or top-up transfusion.

There are at least 26 blood group systems with more than 900 alleles of 39 genes, and the molecules carrying these antigens are very diverse in structure, function, and tendency to cause HDN. The molecules include transporters and channels (e.g., Diego, Kidd, Colton, and Rh), receptors for pathogens (Duffy, P, and others) and for adhesion to other cells (e.g., Landsteiner-Wiener), enzymes (ABO, H, Lewis, P, and Kell), structural proteins (Ge), and complement receptors (Ch/Rg).[22]

As the incidence of RhD HDN has been decreasing, other blood group antibodies have assumed greater importance. Bowman[265] found that in Manitoba (population, 1 million), the mean annual occurrence of D alloimmunization in pregnant women dropped from 194 in 1962 through 1967 to 23 in 1989 through 1994. In the same two periods, the mean annual occurrence of detected non-D alloimmunization in pregnant women, excluding ABO alloimmunization, increased from 14 to 108. This rise was partially the result of increased screening of pregnant D-positive women. It also reflected a real increase in the occurrence of non-D alloimmunization because of the increased incidence of blood transfusion (transfused blood is generally crossmatched only for ABO and D). A summary of results of seven studies from the 1960s to 2000 is presented in Table 3-6.

There is marked international variation in the frequency and distribution of alloantibodies. For example, in Asian countries where RhD negativity is rare, so is anti-D. Lee and associates identified one case in 28,303 women in Hong Kong over a 5-year period, and Rh

TABLE 3-6   Antibody Occurrence in Seven Series

Antibody*	Polesky (1967)[298]	Queenan et al. (1969)[266]	Pepperell et al. (1977)[267]	Filbey et al. (1995)[268]	Geifman-Holtzman et al. (1997)[159]	Howard et al. (1998)[269]	Jovanovic-Szentic et al (2003)[270]
D	1864 (63.1)	304 (48.3)	958 (65.3)	159 (19.0)	101 (18.4)	100[†] (40.9)	200[†] (35)
E	80 (2.7)	34 (5.3)	69 (4.7)	51 (6.1)	77 (14. 0)	29 (11.9)	67 (11.6)
C	448 (15.2)	34 (5.3)	9 (0.6)	36 (4.3)	26 (4.7)	15 (6.1)	145 (25.2)
c	68 (2.3)	12 (1.9)	59 (4.0)	38 (4.5)	32 (5.8)	28 (8.6)	17 (3.0)
C^w	4 (0.14)	—	—	10 (1.2)	1 (0.2)	—	2 (0.3)
e	2 (0.07)	3 (0.4)	6 (0.04)	1 (0.1)	—	—	—
Kell	93 (3. 1)	30 (4.7)	34 (2.3)	48 (5.7)	121 (22)	42 (17.2)	—
Duffy	17 (0.6)	12 (1.9)	8 (0.5)	26 (3.1)	31 (5.6)	9 (3.6)	6 (0.9)
MNS	45 (1.5)	20 (3.1)	18 (1.2)	35 (4.2)	26 (4.7)	10 (4.1)	27 (4.7)
Kidd	7 (0.2)	7 (1.1)	2 (0.14)	10 (1.2)	8 (1.5)	10 (4.1)	4 (0.6)
Lutheran	—	3 (0.4)	—	13 (1.6)	7 (1.3)	—	—
P_1	27 (0.9)	15 (2.3)	129 (8.8)	48 (5.7)	1 (0.2)	—	9 (1.6)
Le^a, Le^b	94 (3.2)	51 (8.1)	174 (11.9)	241 (28.8)	113 (20.5)	NR	50 (8.7)
I	13 (0.4)	15 (2.3)	—	—	5 (0.9)	NR	—
Others	194 (6.6)	90 (14.3)	1 (0.07)	120 (14.4)	1 (0.2)	NR	49 (8.5)
Total antibodies	2956	630	1467	836	550	244[†]	576[†]
Blood samples	43,000	18,378	72,138	110,765	37,506	22,264	21,730
Time period	1960-1966 (7 yr)	1960-1967 (8 yr)	1965-1975 (10 yr)	1980-1991 (12 yr)	1993-1995 (2.5 yr)	1993-1994 (1 yr)	1995-2000 (4.5 yr)
Place	Minnesota	New York	Australia	Sweden	Central New York	Liverpool, UK	Croatia
D[‡]	43.3	16.5	1.3	1.4	2.6	4.5	9.2
E[‡]	1.9	1.9	1.0	0.5	2.0	1.3	3.1
C[‡]	11.3	1.9	0.1	0.3	0.7	0.7	6.7
c[‡]	1.6	0.7	0.8	0.3	0.8	1.3	0.8
Kell[‡]	2.2	1.6	0.5	0.4	3.2	1.9	0
Le^a, $Le^{b‡}$	2.2	2.8	2.4	2.2	3.2	NR	2.3

*Values are given as numbers (percentage of positive samples) of antibodies.
[†]Excludes women given anti-D during pregnancy.
[‡]Values are given as numbers of antibodies per 1000 samples.
NR, not reported.

antibodies accounted for only 27.3% overall. Anti-Mi, which recognizes an antigen in the MNS blood group system, was about twice as common, and although it caused no cases of severe HDN in this series, its potential to do so has been reported.[271]

The alloantibodies listed by Mollison and co-workers and Bowman as having been reported to cause HDN are listed in Table 3-7.[66,272] Of the multitude of antibodies implicated as causes of HDN, most are fortunately rare or rarely cause severe disease (Table 3-8). Some are the subject of single case reports.

There are various reasons why the incidence and severity of HDN differ from one blood group antigen system to another. In some cases it is because of the rarity of the offending antigen or the lack of it and the likelihood of incompatibility between parents being low. An example is the Colton blood group system, which comprises the high-incidence antigens Co_a and Co_3 found on aquaporin-1. Rare individuals lacking this aquaporin can produce antibodies that lead to severe HDN. In others, it is because of low levels of expression on the RBC surface. For this reason, maternal anti-I and anti-Lutheran

antibodies, even when present at high titer, usually do not cause HDN because of low cell surface expression of these antigens on fetal RBCs. Lutheran antigens are also widely distributed in endothelial cells.

Disease attributable to anti-Kell antibodies can be very severe. Maternal antibodies to KEL1 causing neonatal anemia were first described in 1945,[7] and the blood group system was named for the woman in whom the antibodies were found. Kell glycoprotein is an endopeptidase involved in the activation of endothelin,[273] and it is more properly regarded as a subunit of a larger protein because it is linked via a disulfide bond to the XK protein. Absence of XK can cause weak Kell expression and dysfunction of other organs (McLeod's syndrome). Null Kell alleles also occur. Redman and associates[273,274] reviewed the Kell blood group and summarized the low- and high-incidence antigens, about 25 of which have been described. They occur as variants of several epitopes. The most immunogenic antigen, KEL1, is second to RhD in its immunizing potential and occurs in about 9% of whites and 2% of blacks. It results from a point mutation causing a Thr193 (KEL2) to Met193 (KEL1)

TABLE 3-7	Non-ABO Alloantibodies Reported to Cause Hemolytic Disease	
	Any HDN	**Moderate or Severe HDN**
Within the Rh system	Anti-D, -c, -C, -C^w, -C^x, -e, -E, -E^w, -ce, -Ce^s, -Rh32, -Go^a, -Be^a, -Evans, -Rh17	Anti-D, -c, -C, -C^w, -C^x, -e, -E, -E^w, -ce, -Ce^s, -Rh32, -Go^a, -Be^a, -Evans, -Rh17
Outside the Rh system	Anti-LW, -K, -k, -Ku, -Kp^a, -Kp^b, -Js^a, -Js^b, -Fy^a, -Fy3, -Jk^a, -Jk^b, -M, -N, -S, -s, -U, -Vw, -Far, -M^v, -Mit, -Mt^a, -Mur, -Hil, -Hut, -En^a, -PP$_1$P^k, -Lu^a, -Lu^b, -Lu9, -Di^a, -Di^b, -Yt^a, -Yt^b, -Do^a, -Co^a, -Wr^a	Anti-LW, -K, -k, -Kp^a, -Jk^a, -Js^a, -Js^b, -Ku, -Fy^a, -M, -N, -S, -s, -U, -PP$_1$P^k, -Di^b, -Far
Antibodies to low-incidence antigens	Anti-Bi, -By, -Fr^a, -Good, -Sc2, -Rd, -Re^a, -Zd	Anti-Good, -Zd
Antibodies to high-incidence antigens	Anti-At^a, -Jr^a, -Lan, -Ge	Anti-Lan

HDN, hemolytic disease of the fetus and newborn.

Data from Klein HG, Anstee DJ. Haemolytic disease of the fetus and newborn. In Klein HG (ed). Mollison's Blood Transfusion in Clinical Medicine. Malden, MA, Blackwell, 2006, pp 496-545; and Bowman JM. Immune hemolytic disease. In Nathan DG, Orkin SH (eds). Nathan and Oski's Hematology of Infancy and Childhood, 5th ed. Philadelphia, WB Saunders, 1998.

TABLE 3-8	Severity of Hemolytic Disease in Manitoba over a 32-Year Period*				
Alloantibody Specificity	No. of Patients	Affected Patients (%)	No Treatment Required (%)	Phototherapy and/or Exchange Transfusion Required (%)	Hydropic or Hb <60 g/L (%)
D (19 yr)	566	257 (47)	51	30	19
E	633	162 (26)	89	11	—
c, cE	302	164 (54)	70	23	7
C, Ce, C^w, e	193	50 (36)	86	14	—
Kell	478	16 (3.3)	50	37	13
Kp^a	7	3 (43)	67	33	—
k	1	1 (100)	—	100	—
Fy^a	35	6 (17)	67	16	16
S	20	11 (55)	64	36	—

Hb, hemoglobin.

*From November 1, 1962, to October 31, 1994, except for anti-D (November 1, 1975, to October 31, 1994).

From Bowman JM. Immune hemolytic disease. In Nathan DG, Orkin SH (eds). Nathan and Oski's Hematology of Infancy and Childhood, 5th ed. Philadelphia, WB Saunders, 1998.

substitution, which in turn leads to loss of a glycosylation site. The other Kell phenotypes are also generally due to single-base substitutions, so genotyping is more straightforward than that in the Rh system.

Sensitization occurs most commonly as a result of unmatched blood transfusion but can arise during pregnancy. Although the number of incompatible pregnancies is lower for Kell than for RhD, the proportion of anti-KEL1–affected fetuses that are severely affected is thought to be 20% or greater.[275-278]

Kell antibodies, which recognize antigens expressed in early erythroid progenitors and at an early stage of erythropoiesis in fetal liver, appear to be capable of suppressing erythropoiesis.[279] This is the putative reason for the tendency for hydrops early in pregnancy seen in anti-Kell HDN. It has also been proposed as the reason why amniotic fluid spectrophotometry is not as reliable as in Rh hemolytic disease, although not all studies agree on this point.[275,280,281] Paternal typing followed, when necessary, by fetal genotyping and early, close monitoring by ultrasound is recommended in pregnancies complicated by anti-Kell antibodies.

Rarely, anti-Kp^a, -k, -Fy^a, -s, -S, -U, and occasionally other antibodies (see Table 3-8) have caused hemolytic disease severe enough to require intrauterine or postnatal treatment.[66,265] Bowman also reported that 34 pregnant non–D-alloimmunized women referred from outside Manitoba (a highly selected group with very severely affected fetuses drawn from a much greater population base) showed the following distribution of antibodies that produced HDN so severe that intrauterine treatment was required: anti-K (18 fetuses), -c (9 fetuses), -cE (2 fetuses), -k[34] (1 fetus), -Jk^a (1 fetus), -Fy^a (1 fetus), -CC^w (1 fetus), and -E (1 fetus). There are rare instances of other alloantibodies, usually benign ones, causing severe hemolytic disease (e.g., anti-Kp^b, anti-Di, and anti-M).

ABO Hemolytic Disease

ABO HDN behaves differently from HDN caused by either anti-D or other blood group antibodies. Anti-A and anti-B, which bind complement in adults, cause violent, life-threatening intravascular hemolysis after the transfusion of ABO-incompatible blood. Fetal ABO

HDN is usually much milder than HDN caused by D, c, K, and E. Although kernicterus may develop if a baby with ABO HDN is left untreated, hydrops rarely occurs, anemia is usually absent or moderate at birth, and late anemia is rare. There are rare reports of hydrops fetalis being due to ABO erythroblastosis.[282] It is possible that some of these involve other causes of increased ineffective erythropoiesis (such as RBC enzyme deficiency or α-thalassemia trait) or nonimmune hydrops superimposed on ABO HDN. Some but not all series have found that ABO antibodies are a more common cause of HDN (and severe HDN) in Southeast Asia, Africa, and Latin America for reasons that have yet to be determined.[66]

Several reasons have been proposed for the mildness of ABO HDN in comparison to HDN caused by other antibodies and to adult ABO hemolysis.[283] First, there are fewer A and B antigenic sites on the fetal RBC membrane,[284] and anti-A and anti-B do not bind complement on the fetal RBC membrane.[285] Second, anti-A and anti-B are often IgM, which does not cross the placenta, or IgG2, which plays a minor role in HDN.[286] Third, the small amounts of IgG anti-A and anti-B that do traverse the placenta have myriad antigenic sites both on tissues other than on RBCs and on secretions to which they may bind. Because there is very little antibody on the RBC, the result of the cord blood direct antiglobulin test in ABO hemolytic disease is usually only weakly positive and may be negative unless a sensitive test is used. Capillary blood taken at 2 or 3 days of age often yields a negative direct antiglobulin test result regardless of test sensitivity. In at least 25% of ABO-incompatible babies, cord blood RBCs give weakly positive results on the direct antiglobulin test at delivery, and an excess of babies with blood types A and B from mothers with blood type O become severely jaundiced.[287,288] The A- or B-incompatible infants of mothers with blood type A or B do not appear to be at increased risk for hemolysis or jaundice.[289]

In only a small fraction of A- or B-incompatible infants of O mothers does clinical evidence of HDN develop (early and severe jaundice).[288,290,291] One study found that only 0.07% of more than 88,000 infants required exchange transfusion for anti-A or -B HDN.[290] Nevertheless, ABO HDN continues to account for a significant proportion of infants with troublesome jaundice that necessitates prolongation of the hospital stay, readmission to the hospital, or home therapy. The same large study found that ABO incompatibility accounted for 5.5% of infants with jaundice.

Although anemia is rarely severe, mild hemolysis appears to be common. In a series of 1704 infants of blood group O mothers, infants with blood group A or B had significantly higher cord bilirubin and lower cord hemoglobin concentrations than did the babies with blood group O.[292] Blood films may show polychromasia, reticulocytosis, and prominent spherocytosis, which can be difficult at times to differentiate from hereditary spherocytosis.

Control of hyperbilirubinemia is usually the major issue in infants with ABO HDN, and thresholds for phototherapy and exchange transfusion are generally regarded as similar to those for Rh HDN. The risk for symptomatic late anemia in ABO HDN is very low. The risk for recurrence of jaundice attributable to anti-A or -B in future incompatible siblings is high, and mothers should be counseled accordingly.[293]

MANAGEMENT OF SPECIAL PROBLEMS

Syndrome of Hepatocellular Damage

Most infants with severe anemia and erythroblastosis, particularly those who are hydropic or prehydropic, show signs of obstructive jaundice. They have extreme hepatomegaly and evidence of biliary canalicular obstruction. Extreme or prolonged jaundice may develop in these infants, but with half or more of the total bilirubin being direct-acting conjugated bilirubin. The threshold for exchange transfusion in such infants is unclear and should be individualized. If hepatic damage is so severe that symptomatic coagulopathy has ensued, exchange transfusion (with appropriate components) may be necessary to remove activated clotting factors and degradation products and to replenish clotting factor levels.

Infants Who Have Undergone Fetal Transfusions

Assessment of infants who have undergone IVT or IPT does not differ from that of other babies with HDN. Because these infants are often delivered with few residual Rh-positive hemolyzing RBCs, their postdelivery management may be simple. Nevertheless, some require one or more exchange transfusions. When compared with those who received IPT, relatively few babies born after undergoing IVT require exchange transfusion. However, careful individual assessment is still required, and delivery in or near a center that can perform exchange transfusion is still advisable.

Follow-up Care of Infants with Hemolytic Disease

Regardless of whether an affected infant has required fetal transfusions or exchange transfusions, anemia is commonly seen in the first few weeks of life.[294] Hemoglobin levels should be checked at 7- to 14-day intervals until the infant is 8 to 12 weeks of age. The anemia is due to gradual loss of transfused Rh-negative RBCs and to failure of the infant's Rh-positive RBCs to replace them. This failure is initially due to hemolysis of any RBCs produced and to transient erythroblastopenia, which usually resolves spontaneously at about 6 to 8 weeks of age.

In the interim, if symptomatic anemia develops or if hemoglobin levels are falling rapidly toward symptomatic levels, a simple transfusion of 20 mL/kg of body weight of crossmatched, packed RBCs compatible with the infant's serum is administered. Iron supplementation is not indicated, but folic acid and, in some circumstances, vitamin B_{12} should be given.

Recombinant erythropoietin has been used with some success in the treatment of anemia of prematurity. Erythropoietin treatment for prevention of "late" anemia in infants with HDN has been tested in small trials.[295-297] A larger trial is needed to evaluate the role of erythropoietin in preventing the late anemia of HDN.

CONCLUSIONS

Advances in prevention of Rh sensitization and the management of immune HDN in the past 30 years have been dramatic. Statistics from all over the developed world have indicated that the prevalence of Rh sensitization in pregnant women has been reduced by more than 90%. The number of exchange transfusions has also decreased by more than 100-fold. In addition, the number of perinatal deaths caused by HDN has plummeted. However, for those still affected by anti-D or other significant antibodies, the disease burden remains significant.

Despite a recent explosion in knowledge about antigen presentation and provocation of the immune response in general, little detail at the molecular and cellular level is known about maternal sensitization to RhD. Better understanding of these events, together with the recent elucidation of the molecular genetics of RhD and other blood groups, is likely to provide new tools for prevention, diagnosis, and treatment.

REFERENCES

1. Bowman JM. RhD hemolytic disease of the newborn. N Engl J Med. 1998;339:1775-1777.
2. Diamond L, Blackfan K, Baty J. Erythroblastosis fetalis and its association with universal edema of the fetus, icterus gravis neonatorum and anemia of the newborn. J Pediatr. 1932;1:269.
3. Darrow R. Icterus gravis (erythroblastosis neonatorum). An examination of etiologic considerations. Arch Pathol. 1938;25:378.
4. Levine P, Stetson R. An unusual case of intra-group agglutination. JAMA. 1939;113:126.
5. Landsteiner K, Wiener A. An agglutinable factor in human blood recognised by immune sera for rhesus blood. Proc Soc Exp Biol Med. 1940;43:223.
6. Levine P, Katsin E, Burnham L. Isoimmunization in pregnancy: its possible bearing on the etiology of erythroblastosis fetalis. JAMA. 1941;116:825.
7. Coombs R, Mourant A, Race R. Detection of weak and "incomplete" Rh agglutinins: a new test. Lancet. 1945;2:15.
8. Chown B. Anemia from bleeding of the fetus into the mother's circulation. Lancet. 1954;1:1213.
9. Wiener A, Wexler I. Heredity of the Blood Groups. New York, Grune & Stratton, 1958.
10. Edwards AW. R. A. Fisher's 1943 unravelling of the Rhesus blood-group system. Genetics. 2007;175:471-476.
11. Race R. The Rh genotype and Fisher's theory. Blood. 1948;3:27.
12. Urbaniak SJ, Greiss MA. RhD haemolytic disease of the fetus and the newborn. Blood Rev. 2000;14:44-61.
13. Cartron JP. RH blood group system and molecular basis of Rh-deficiency. Baillieres Best Pract Res Clin Haematol. 1999;12:655-689.
14. Westhoff CM. The structure and function of the Rh antigen complex. Semin Hematol. 2007;44:42-50.
15. Gahmberg CG. Molecular identification of the human Rho (D) antigen. FEBS Lett. 1982;140:93-97.
16. Moore S, Woodrow CF, McClelland DB. Isolation of membrane components associated with human red cell antigens Rh(D), (c), (E) and Fy. Nature. 1982;295:529-531.
17. Avent ND, Ridgwell K, Tanner MJ, Anstee DJ. cDNA cloning of a 30 kDa erythrocyte membrane protein associated with Rh (Rhesus)-blood-group-antigen expression. Biochem J. 1990;271:821-825.
18. Cherif-Zahar B, Bloy C, Le Van Kim C, et al. Molecular cloning and protein structure of a human blood group Rh polypeptide. Proc Natl Acad Sci U S A. 1990;87:6243-6247.
19. Arce MA, Thompson ES, Wagner S, et al. Molecular cloning of RhD cDNA derived from a gene present in RhD-positive, but not RhD-negative individuals. Blood. 1993;82:651-655.
20. Le van Kim C, Mouro I, Cherif-Zahar B, et al. Molecular cloning and primary structure of the human blood group RhD polypeptide. Proc Natl Acad Sci U S A. 1992;89:10925-10929.
21. Avent ND, Reid ME. The Rh blood group system: a review. Blood. 2000;95:375-387.
22. Cartron JP, Colin Y. Structural and functional diversity of blood group antigens. Transfus Clin Biol. 2001;8:163-199.
23. Huang CH. Blood Group Antigen Gene Mutation Database; Rh Blood Group System. National Center for Biotechnology Information, 2005.
24. Matassi G, Cherif-Zahar B, Pesole G, et al. The members of the RH gene family (RH50 and RH30) followed different evolutionary pathways. J Mol Evol. 1999;48:151-159.
25. Avent ND, Madgett TE, Lee ZE, et al. Molecular biology of Rh proteins and relevance to molecular medicine. Exp Rev Mol Med. 2006;8(13):1-20.
26. Flegel WA. Molecular genetics of RH and its clinical application. Transfus Clin Biol. 2006;13:4-12.
27. Daniels G, Finning K, Martin P, Summers J. Fetal blood group genotyping: present and future. Ann NY Acad Sci. 2006;1075:88-95.
28. Gassner C, Doescher A, Drnovsek TD, et al. Presence of RHD in serologically D-, C/E+ individuals: a European multicenter study. Transfusion. 2005;45:527-538.

29. Mouro I, Colin Y, Cherif-Zahar B, et al. Molecular genetic basis of the human Rhesus blood group system. Nat Genet. 1993;5:62-65.

30. Simsek S, de Jong CA, Cuijpers HT, et al. Sequence analysis of cDNA derived from reticulocyte mRNAs coding for Rh polypeptides and demonstration of E/e and C/c polymorphisms. Vox Sang. 1994;67:203-209.

31. Mourant A, Kopec A, Domaniewska-Sobczak K. Distribution of Human Blood Groups and Other Polymorphisms, 2nd ed. London, Oxford University Press, 1976.

32. Wagner FF, Flegel WA. RHD gene deletion occurred in the Rhesus box. Blood. 2000;95:3662-3668.

33. Lan JC, Chen Q, Wu DL, et al. Genetic polymorphism of RhD-negative associated haplotypes in the Chinese. J Hum Genet. 2000;45:224-227.

34. Okuda H, Kawano M, Iwamoto S, et al. The RHD gene is highly detectable in RhD-negative Japanese donors. J Clin Invest. 1997;100:373-379.

35. Singleton BK, Green CA, Avent ND, et al. The presence of an RHD pseudogene containing a 37 base pair duplication and a nonsense mutation in Africans with the Rh D–negative blood group phenotype. Blood. 2000;95: 12-18.

36. Ekman GC, Billingsly R, Hessner MJ. Rh genotyping: avoiding false-negative and false-positive results among individuals of African ancestry. Am J Hematol. 2002;69: 34-40.

37. Avent ND, Jones JW, Liu W, et al. Molecular basis of the D variant phenotypes DNU and DII allows localization of critical amino acids required for expression of Rh D epitopes epD3, 4 and 9 to the sixth external domain of the Rh D protein. Br J Haematol. 1997;97:366-371.

38. Cartron JP. A molecular approach to the structure, polymorphism and function of blood groups. Transfus Clin Biol. 1996;3:181-210.

39. Jones J, Scott ML, Voak D. Monoclonal anti-D specificity and Rh D structure: criteria for selection of monoclonal anti-D reagents for routine typing of patients and donors. Transfus Med. 1995;5:171-184.

40. Liu W, Smythe JS, Scott ML, et al. Site-directed mutagenesis of the human D antigen: definition of D epitopes on the sixth external domain of the D protein expressed on K562 cells. Transfusion. 1999;39:17-25.

41. Urbaniak SJ. Alloimmunity to RhD in humans. Transfus Clin Biol. 2006;13:19-22.

42. Iwamoto S, Omi T, Yamasaki M, et al. Identification of 5′ flanking sequence of RH50 gene and the core region for erythroid-specific expression. Biochem Biophys Res Commun. 1998;243:233-240.

43. Liu Z, Chen Y, Mo R, et al. Characterization of human RhCG and mouse Rhcg as novel nonerythroid Rh glycoprotein homologues predominantly expressed in kidney and testis. J Biol Chem. 2000;275:25641-25651.

44. Eyers SA, Ridgwell K, Mawby WJ, Tanner MJ. Topology and organization of human Rh (rhesus) blood group–related polypeptides. J Biol Chem. 1994;269:6417-6423.

45. Callebaut I, Dulin F, Bertrand O, et al. Hydrophobic cluster analysis and modeling of the human Rh protein three-dimensional structures. Transfus Clin Biol. 2006; 13:70-84.

46. Huang CH, Cheng G, Liu Z, et al. Molecular basis for Rh(null) syndrome: identification of three new missense mutations in the Rh50 glycoprotein gene. Am J Hematol. 1999;62:25-32.

47. Nicolas V, Mouro-Chanteloup I, Lopez C, et al. Functional interaction between Rh proteins and the spectrin-based skeleton in erythroid and epithelial cells. Transfus Clin Biol. 2006;13:23-28.

48. Marini AM, Matassi G, Raynal V, et al. The human Rhesus-associated RhAG protein and a kidney homologue promote ammonium transport in yeast. Nat Genet. 2000;26:341-344.

49. Marini AM, Vissers S, Urrestarazu A, Andre B. Cloning and expression of the MEP1 gene encoding an ammonium transporter in *Saccharomyces cerevisiae*. EMBO J. 1994;13:3456-3463.

50. Westhoff CM, Ferreri-Jacobia M, Mak DO, Foskett JK. Identification of the erythrocyte Rh blood group glycoprotein as a mammalian ammonium transporter. J Biol Chem. 2002;277:12499-12502.

51. Liu Z, Peng J, Mo R, et al. Rh type B glycoprotein is a new member of the Rh superfamily and a putative ammonia transporter in mammals. J Biol Chem. 2001; 276:1424-1433.

52. Kustu S, Inwood W. Biological gas channels for NH_3 and CO_2: evidence that Rh (Rhesus) proteins are CO_2 channels. Transfus Clin Biol. 2006;13:103-110.

53. Soupene E, King N, Feild E, et al. Rhesus expression in a green alga is regulated by CO_2. Proc Natl Acad Sci U S A. 2002;99:7769-7773.

54. Flegel WA. How I manage donors and patients with a weak D phenotype. Curr Opin Hematol. 2006;13: 476-483.

55. Avent ND. Molecular biology of the Rh blood group system. J Pediatr Hematol Oncol. 2001;23:394-402.

56. Daniels G, Poole G, Poole J. Partial D and weak D: can they be distinguished? Transfus Med. 2007;17: 145-146.

57. Judd WJ. Guidelines for Prenatal and Perinatal Immunohematology. Bethesda, MD, American Association of Blood Banks/S Karger, 2005.

58. Prasad MR, Krugh D, Rossi KQ, O'Shaughnessy RW. Anti-D in Rh positive pregnancies. Am J Obstet Gynecol. 2006;195:1158-1162.

59. Flegel WA, Wagner FF. The Rhesus site. In Abteilung Blutgruppenserologie und Immunhämatologie. Baden, Germany, Institut für Klinische Transfusionsmedizin und Immungenetik Ulm, 2002.

60. Vontver LA. RH sensitization associated with drug use [letter]. JAMA. 1973;226:469.

61. Williamson I, Hofmeyr GJ, Crookes RL. Hemolytic disease of the newborn as an unusual consequence of drug abuse. A case report. J Reprod Med. 1990;35: 46-48.

62. Kleihauer E, Braun H, Betke K. Demonstration of fetal hemoglobin in erythrocytes of a blood smear. Klin Wochenschr. 1957;35:637-638.

63. Clarke CA. Prevention of RH haemolytic disease. A method based on the post-delivery injection of the mother with anti-D antibody. Vox Sang. 1966;11:641-655.

64. Bowman JM, Pollock JM, Penston LE. Fetomaternal transplacental hemorrhage during pregnancy and after delivery. Vox Sang. 1986;51:117-121.

65. Medearis AL, Hensleigh PA, Parks DR, Herzenberg LA. Detection of fetal erythrocytes in maternal blood post

partum with the fluorescence-activated cell sorter. Am J Obstet Gynecol. 1984;148:290-295.

66. Klein HG, Anstee DJ. Haemolytic disease of the fetus and newborn. In Klein HG (ed). Mollison's Blood Transfusion in Clinical Medicine. Malden, MA, Blackwell, 2006, pp 496-545.
67. Lau TK, Lo KW, Chan LY, et al. Cell-free fetal deoxyribonucleic acid in maternal circulation as a marker of fetal-maternal hemorrhage in patients undergoing external cephalic version near term. Am J Obstet Gynecol. 2000;183:712-716.
68. Feldman N, Skoll A, Sibai B. The incidence of significant fetomaternal hemorrhage in patients undergoing cesarean section. Am J Obstet Gynecol. 1990;163:855-858.
69. Harrison KL, Baker JW. Fetal-maternal macrotransfusion—a study of 400 postpartum women. Aust N Z J Obstet Gynaecol. 1978;18:176-178.
70. Lloyd LK, Miya F, Hebertson RM, et al. Intrapartum fetomaternal bleeding in Rh-negative women. Obstet Gynecol. 1980;56:285-288.
71. Bowman JM, Pollock JM. Transplacental fetal hemorrhage after amniocentesis. Obstet Gynecol. 1985;66:749-754.
72. Mennuti MT, Brummond W, Crombleholme WR, et al. Fetal-maternal bleeding associated with genetic amniocentesis. Obstet Gynecol. 1980;55:48-54.
73. Warren RC, Butler J, Morsman JM, et al. Does chorionic villus sampling cause fetomaternal haemorrhage? Lancet. 1985;1:691.
74. Fiala C, Fux M, Gemzell Danielsson K. Rh-prophylaxis in early abortion. Acta Obstet Gynecol Scand. 2003;82:892-903.
75. Bergstrom H, Nilsson LA, Nilsson L, Ryttinger L. Demonstration of Rh antigens in a 38-day-old fetus. Am J Obstet Gynecol. 1967;99:130-133.
76. Towers CV, Deveikis A, Asrat T, et al. A "bloodless cesarean section" and perinatal transmission of the human immunodeficiency virus. Am J Obstet Gynecol. 1998;179:708-714.
77. von Zabern I, Ehlers M, Grunwald U, et al. Release of mediators of systemic inflammatory response syndrome in the course of a severe delayed hemolytic transfusion reaction caused by anti-D. Transfusion. 1998;38:459-468.
78. Woodrow J. Rh immunization and its prevention. The immune response in the mother. In Jensen K, Killmann S (eds). Series Haematologica, vol 3. Copenhagen, Munksgaard, 1970.
79. Zipursky A, Israels LG. The pathogenesis and prevention of Rh immunization. Can Med Assoc J. 1967;97:1245-1257.
80. Klein HG, Anstee DJ. The Rh blood group system (and LW). In Klein HG (ed). Mollison's Blood Transfusion in Clinical Medicine. Malden, MA, Blackwell, 2006, pp 163-208.
81. Bowman JM. The prevention of Rh immunization. Transfus Med Rev. 1988;2:129-150.
82. Murray S, Knox EG, Walker W. Rhesus haemolytic disease of the newborn and the ABO groups. Vox Sang. 1965;10:6-31.
83. Bowman JM. Fetomaternal AB0 incompatibility and erythroblastosis fetalis. Vox Sang. 1986;50:104-106.
84. Kinnock S, Liley AW. The epidemiology of severe haemolytic disease of the newborn. N Z Med J. 1970;71:76-83.
85. Hilden JO, Gottvall T, Lindblom B. HLA phenotypes and severe Rh(D) immunization. Tissue Antigens. 1995;46:313-315.
86. Kruskall MS, Yunis EJ, Watson A, et al. Major histocompatibility complex markers and red cell antibodies to the Rh (D) antigen. Absence of association. Transfusion. 1990;30:15-19.
87. Murray S. The effect of Rh genotypes on severity in haemolytic disease of the newborn. Br J Haematol. 1957;3:143-152.
88. Rochna E, Hughes-Jones NC. The use of purified 125-I-labelled anti–gamma globulin in the determination of the number of D antigen sites on red cells of different phenotypes. Vox Sang. 1965;10:675-686.
89. Scott JR, Beer AE, Guy LR, et al. Pathogenesis of Rh immunization in primigravidas. Fetomaternal versus maternofetal bleeding. Obstet Gynecol. 1977;49:9-14.
90. Bowman JM, Chown B, Lewis M, Pollock JM. Rh isoimmunization during pregnancy: antenatal prophylaxis. Can Med Assoc J. 1978;118:623-627.
91. Joseph KS, Kramer MS. The decline in Rh hemolytic disease: should Rh prophylaxis get all the credit? Am J Public Health. 1998;88:209-215.
92. Von Dungern EF. Beiträge zur Immunitätslehr. Munch Med Wochenschr. 1900;47:677.
93. Finn R, Clarke CA, Donohoe WT, et al. Experimental studies on the prevention of Rh haemolytic disease. BMJ. 1961;1:1486-1490.
94. Freda VJ, Gorman JG, Pollack W. Successful prevention of experimental Rh sensitization in man with an anti-Rh gamma2-globulin antibody preparation: a preliminary report. Transfusion. 1964;4:26-32.
95. Clarke CA, Donohoe WT, McConnell RB, et al. Further experimental studies on the prevention of Rh haemolytic disease. BMJ. 1963;1:979-984.
96. Chown B, Bowman JM. Prevention of Rh immunization. Can Med Assoc J. 1969;100:303-304.
97. Prevention of Rh-haemolytic disease: results of the clinical trial. A combined study from centres in England and Baltimore. BMJ. 1966;2:907-914.
98. Pollack W, Gorman JG, Freda VJ, et al. Results of clinical trials of RhoGAM in women. Transfusion. 1968;8:151-153.
99. Kumpel BM. On the mechanism of tolerance to the Rh D antigen mediated by passive anti-D (Rh D prophylaxis). Immunol Lett. 2002;82:67-73.
100. Ware RE, Zimmerman SA. Anti-D: mechanisms of action. Semin Hematol. 1998;35(Suppl 1):14-22.
101. Crowther C, Middleton P. Anti-D administration after childbirth for preventing Rhesus alloimmunisation. Cochrane Database Syst Rev. 2000;2:CD000021.
102. Rho(D) Immune Globulin Intravenous (Human); Label. Rockville, MD, U.S. Food and Drug Administration, 2005.
103. DiGuiseppi C. Screening for D (Rh) incompatibility: recommendation statement. Guide to Preventive Services Report of the US Preventive Services Task Force. Rockville, MD, National Library of Medicine, 2004.
104. Crowther CA, Keirse MJ. Anti-D administration in pregnancy for preventing rhesus alloimmunisation. Cochrane Database Syst Rev. 2000;2:CD000020.
105. Jones ML, Wray J, Wight J, et al. A review of the clinical effectiveness of routine antenatal anti-D prophylaxis for

rhesus-negative women who are pregnant. Br J Obstet Gynaecol. 2004;111:892-902.

106. Consensus Conference on Anti-D Prophylaxis. Edinburgh, United Kingdom, 8-9 April 1997. Papers and abstracts. Br J Obstet Gynaecol. 1998;105(Suppl 18):iv, 1-44.

107. ACOG practice bulletin. Prevention of Rh D alloimmunization. Number 4, May 1999. Clinical management guidelines for obstetrician-gynecologists. ACOG. Int J Gynaecol Obstet. 1999;66:63-70.

108. Engelfriet CP, Reesink HW, Judd WJ, et al. Current status of immunoprophylaxis with anti-D immunoglobin. Vox Sang. 2003;85:328-337.

109. Hartwell EA. Use of Rh immune globulin: ASCP practice parameter. American Society of Clinical Pathologists. Am J Clin Pathol. 1998;110:281-292.

110. Domen RE. Policies and procedures related to weak D phenotype testing and Rh immune globulin administration. Results from supplementary questions to the Comprehensive Transfusion Medicine Survey of the College of American Pathologists. Arch Pathol Lab Med. 2000;124: 1118-1121.

111. Fung Kee Fung K, Eason E, Crane J, et al. Prevention of Rh alloimmunization. J Obstet Gynaecol Can. 2003;25: 765-773.

112. Parker J, Wray J, Gooch A, et al. Guidelines for the Use of Prophylactic Anti-D Immunoglobulin. London, British Committee for Standards in Haematology, 2006.

113. Maayan-Metzger A, Schwartz T, Sulkes J, Merlob P. Maternal anti-D prophylaxis during pregnancy does not cause neonatal haemolysis. Arch Dis Child Fetal Neonatal Ed. 2001;84:F60-F62.

114. Adams MM, Marks JS, Gustafson J, Oakley GP Jr. Rh hemolytic disease of the newborn: using incidence observations to evaluate the use of RH immune globulin. Am J Public Health. 1981;71:1031-1035.

115. Chavez GF, Mulinare J, Edmonds LD. Epidemiology of Rh hemolytic disease of the newborn in the United States. JAMA. 1991;265:3270-3274.

116. Zavala C, Salamanca F. Mothers at risk of alloimmunization to the Rh (D) antigen and availability of gammaglobulin at the Mexican Institute of Social Security. Arch Med Res. 1996;27:373-376.

117. Kenny-Walsh E. Clinical outcomes after hepatitis C infection from contaminated anti-D immune globulin. Irish Hepatology Research Group. N Engl J Med. 1999;340: 1228-1233.

118. Beliard R. Monoclonal anti-D antibodies to prevent alloimmunization: lessons from clinical trials. Transfus Clin Biol. 2006;13:58-64.

119. Scott ML, Voak D. Monoclonal antibodies to Rh D—development and uses. Vox Sang. 2000;78(Suppl 2): 79-82.

120. Ohls RK. Developmental erythropoiesis. In Polin RA, Fox WW, Abman S (eds). Fetal and Neonatal Physiology. Philadelphia, WB Saunders, 2004, pp 1397-420.

121. Peterec SM. Management of neonatal Rh disease. Clin Perinatol. 1995;22:561-592.

122. Phibbs RH, Johnson P, Tooley WH. Cardiorespiratory status of erythroblastotic newborn infants. II. Blood volume, hematocrit, and serum albumin concentration in relation to hydrops fetalis. Pediatrics. 1974;53:13-23.

123. d'Ancona RL, Rahman F, Ozcan T, et al. The effect of intravascular blood transfusion on the flow velocity wave-

form of the portal venous system of the anemic fetus. Ultrasound Obstet Gynecol. 1997;10:333-337.

124. Leach JL, Sedmak DD, Osborne JM, et al. Isolation from human placenta of the IgG transporter, FcRn, and localization to the syncytiotrophoblast: implications for maternal-fetal antibody transport. J Immunol. 1996;157: 3317-3322.

125. Pearse BM. Coated vesicles from human placenta carry ferritin, transferrin, and immunoglobulin G. Proc Natl Acad Sci U S A. 1982;79:451-455.

126. Story CM, Mikulska JE, Simister NE. A major histocompatibility complex class I–like Fc receptor cloned from human placenta: possible role in transfer of immunoglobulin G from mother to fetus. J Exp Med. 1994; 180:2377-2381.

127. Pitcher-Wilmott RW, Hindocha P, Wood CB. The placental transfer of IgG subclasses in human pregnancy. Clin Exp Immunol. 1980;41:303-308.

128. Malek A, Sager R, Kuhn P, et al. Evolution of maternofetal transport of immunoglobulins during human pregnancy. Am J Reprod Immunol. 1996;36:248-255.

129. Dooren MC, Engelfriet CP. Protection against Rh D–haemolytic disease of the newborn by a diminished transport of maternal IgG to the fetus. Vox Sang. 1993;65: 59-61.

130. Freedman J, Massey A, Chaplin H, Monroe MC. Assessment of complement binding by anti-D and anti-M antibodies employing labelled antiglobulin antibodies. Br J Haematol. 1980;45:309-318.

131. Poorkhorsandi ME, Gupte SC. Role of C1q in Rhesus haemolytic disease of the newborn. Indian J Med Res. 1996;104:208-212.

132. Urbaniak SJ. Lymphoid cell dependent (K-cell) lysis of human erythrocytes sensitized with Rhesus alloantibodies. Br J Haematol. 1976;33:409-413.

133. Hadley AG. A comparison of in vitro tests for predicting the severity of haemolytic disease of the fetus and newborn. Vox Sang. 1998;74(Suppl 2):375-383.

134. Contreras M, Armitage S, Daniels GL, Tippett P. Homozygous D. Vox Sang. 1979;36:81-84.

135. Hughes-Jones NC, Gardner B, Lincoln PJ. Observations of the number of available c, D, and E antigen sites on red cells. Vox Sang. 1971;21:210-216.

136. Novotny VM, Kanhai HH, Overbeeke MA, et al. Misleading results in the determination of haemolytic disease of the newborn using antibody titration and ADCC in a woman with anti-Lub. Vox Sang. 1992;62:49-52.

137. Frankowska K, Gorska B. IgG subclasses of anti-Rh antibodies in pregnant women. Arch Immunol Ther Exp (Warsz). 1978;26:1095-1100.

138. Parinaud J, Blanc M, Grandjean H, et al. IgG subclasses and Gm allotypes of anti-D antibodies during pregnancy: correlation with the gravity of the fetal disease. Am J Obstet Gynecol. 1985;151:1111-1115.

139. Pollock JM, Bowman JM. Anti-Rh(D) IgG subclasses and severity of Rh hemolytic disease of the newborn. Vox Sang. 1990;59:176-179.

140. Zupanska B, Brojer E, Richards Y, et al. Serological and immunological characteristics of maternal anti-Rh(D) antibodies in predicting the severity of haemolytic disease of the newborn. Vox Sang. 1989;56:247-253.

141. Hadley AG, Kumpel BM, Merry AH. The chemiluminescent response of human monocytes to red cells sensitized

with monoclonal anti-Rh(D) antibodies. Clin Lab Haematol. 1988;10:377-384.

142. Hadley AG, Kumpel BM, Leader K, et al. An in-vitro assessment of the functional activity of monoclonal anti-D. Clin Lab Haematol. 1989;11:47-54.

143. Hadley AG, Wilkes A, Goodrick J, et al. The ability of the chemiluminescence test to predict clinical outcome and the necessity for amniocenteses in pregnancies at risk of haemolytic disease of the newborn. Br J Obstet Gynaecol. 1998;105:231-234.

144. Kumpel BM, Hadley AG. Functional interactions of red cells sensitized by IgG1 and IgG3 human monoclonal anti-D with enzyme-modified human monocytes and FcR-bearing cell lines. Mol Immunol. 1990;27:247-256.

145. Thomson A, Contreras M, Gorick B, et al. Clearance of Rh D–positive red cells with monoclonal anti-D. Lancet. 1990;336:1147-1150.

146. Hadley AG, Kumpel BM. The role of Rh antibodies in haemolytic disease of the newborn. Baillieres Clin Haematol. 1993;6:423-444.

147. Lewis M, Chown B. A short albumin method for the demonstration of isohemagglutinins, particularly incomplete Rh antibodies. J Lab Clin Med. 1957;50:494-497.

148. Filbey D, Garner SF, Hadley AG, Shepard SL. Quantitative and functional assessment of anti-RhD: a comparative study of non-invasive methods in antenatal prediction of Rh hemolytic disease. Acta Obstet Gynecol Scand. 1996;75:102-107.

149. Lalezari P. A new method for detection of red blood cell antibodies. Transfusion. 1968;8:372-380.

150. Moore BP. Automation in the blood transfusion laboratory: I. Antibody detection and quantitation in the Technicon autoanalyzer. Can Med Assoc J. 1969;100:381-387.

151. Rosenfield RE, Szymanski IO, Haber GV, Kochwa S. Automated methods for the detection and measurement of hemagglutination. Bibl Haematol. 1965;23:985-991.

152. Alie-Daram SJ, Fournie A, Dugoujon JM. Gel test assay for IgG subclass detection by GM typing: application to hemolytic disease of the newborn. J Clin Lab Anal. 2000;14:1-4.

153. Hadley AG, Kumpel BM, Leader KA, et al. Correlation of serological, quantitative and cell-mediated functional assays of maternal alloantibodies with the severity of haemolytic disease of the newborn. Br J Haematol. 1991;77:221-228.

154. Hirvonen M, Tervonen S, Pirkola A, Sievers G. An enzyme-linked immunosorbent assay for the quantitative determination of anti-D in plasma samples and immunoglobulin preparations. Vox Sang. 1995;69:341-346.

155. Lambin P, Ahaded A, Debbia M, et al. An enzyme-linked immunosorbent assay for the quantitation of IgG anti-D and IgG subclasses in the sera of alloimmunized patients. Transfusion. 1998;38:252-261.

156. Weisbach V, Kohnhauser T, Zimmermann R, et al. Comparison of the performance of microtube column systems and solid-phase systems and the tube low-ionic-strength solution additive indirect antiglobulin test in the detection of red cell alloantibodies. Transfus Med. 2006;16:276-284.

157. Bennett PR, Le Van Kim C, Colin Y, et al. Prenatal determination of fetal RhD type by DNA amplification. N Engl J Med. 1993;329:607-610.

158. Faas BH, Maaskant-Van Wijk PA, von dem Borne AE, et al. The applicability of different PCR-based methods for fetal RHD and K1 genotyping: a prospective study. Prenat Diagn. 2000;20:453-458.

159. Geifman-Holtzman O, Wojtowycz M, Kosmas E, Artal R. Female alloimmunization with antibodies known to cause hemolytic disease. Obstet Gynecol. 1997;89:272-275.

160. Hessner MJ, McFarland JG, Endean DJ. Genotyping of KEL1 and KEL2 of the human Kell blood group system by the polymerase chain reaction with sequence-specific primers. Transfusion. 1996;36:495-499.

161. Lo YM, Hjelm NM, Fidler C, et al. Prenatal diagnosis of fetal RhD status by molecular analysis of maternal plasma. N Engl J Med. 1998;339:1734-1738.

162. Spence WC, Maddalena A, Demers DB, Bick DP. Molecular analysis of the RhD genotype in fetuses at risk for RhD hemolytic disease. Obstet Gynecol. 1995;85:296-298.

163. Spence WC, Potter P, Maddalena A, et al. DNA-based prenatal determination of the RhEe genotype. Obstet Gynecol. 1995;86:670-672.

164. Bianchi DW, Avent ND, Costa JM, van der Schoot CE. Noninvasive prenatal diagnosis of fetal Rhesus D: ready for Prime(r) Time. Obstet Gynecol. 2005;106:841-844.

165. Lo YM. Recent developments in fetal nucleic acids in maternal plasma: implications to noninvasive prenatal fetal blood group genotyping. Transfus Clin Biol. 2006;13:50-52.

166. Van den Veyver IB, Chong SS, Cota J, et al. Single-cell analysis of the RhD blood type for use in preimplantation diagnosis in the prevention of severe hemolytic disease of the newborn. Am J Obstet Gynecol. 1995;172:533-540.

167. Westhoff CM. Molecular testing for transfusion medicine. Curr Opin Hematol. 2006;13:471-475.

168. Allen RW, Ward S, Harris R. Prenatal genotyping for the RhD blood group antigen: considerations in developing an accurate test. Genet Test. 2000;4:377-381.

169. Chim SS, Tong YK, Chiu RW, et al. Detection of the placental epigenetic signature of the maspin gene in maternal plasma. Proc Natl Acad Sci U S A. 2005;102:14753-14758.

170. Bowell P, Wainscoat JS, Peto TE, Gunson HH. Maternal anti-D concentrations and outcome in rhesus haemolytic disease of the newborn. BMJ. 1982;285:327-329.

171. Harrison KL, Baker JW, Popper EI, Harden PA. Value of maternal anti-D concentration in predicting the outcome of Rh(D) haemolytic disease. Aust N Z J Obstet Gynaecol. 1984;24:6-8.

172. Hadley AG. In vitro assays to predict the severity of hemolytic disease of the newborn. Transfus Med Rev. 1995;9:302-313.

173. Nance SJ, Nelson JM, Horenstein J, et al. Monocyte monolayer assay: an efficient noninvasive technique for predicting the severity of hemolytic disease of the newborn. Am J Clin Pathol. 1989;92:89-92.

174. Zupanska B. Assays to predict the clinical significance of blood group antibodies. Curr Opin Hematol. 1998;5:412-416.

175. Urbaniak SJ, Greiss MA, Crawford RJ, Fergusson MJ. Prediction of the outcome of rhesus haemolytic disease of the newborn: additional information using an ADCC assay. Vox Sang. 1984;46:323-329.

176. Engelfriet CP, Brouwers HA, et al. Prognostic value of the ADCC with monocytes and maternal antibodies for haemolytic disease of the newborn. In XXIst Congress of the International Society of Hematol and XIXth Congress of the International Society of Blood Transfusion. Sydney, Australia, 1986, p 162.

177. Results of tests with different cellular bioassays in relation to severity of RhD haemolytic disease. Report from nine collaborating laboratories. Vox Sang. 1991;60: 225-229.

178. Moise KJ Jr, Perkins JT, Sosler SD, et al. The predictive value of maternal serum testing for detection of fetal anemia in red blood cell alloimmunization. Am J Obstet Gynecol. 1995;172:1003-1009.

179. Bevis DC. Blood pigments in haemolytic disease of the newborn. J Obstet Gynaecol Br Emp. 1956;63: 68-75.

180. Liley AW. Liquor amnii analysis in the management of the pregnancy complicated by rhesus sensitization. Am J Obstet Gynecol. 1961;82:1359-1370.

181. Queenan JT, Tomai TP, Ural SH, King JC. Deviation in amniotic fluid optical density at a wavelength of 450 nm in Rh-immunized pregnancies from 14 to 40 weeks' gestation: a proposal for clinical management. Am J Obstet Gynecol. 1993;168:1370-1376.

182. Spinnato JA, Clark AL, Ralston KK, et al. Hemolytic disease of the fetus: a comparison of the Queenan and extended Liley methods. Obstet Gynecol. 1998;92: 441-445.

183. Scott F, Chan FY. Assessment of the clinical usefulness of the 'Queenan' chart versus the 'Liley' chart in predicting severity of rhesus iso-immunization. Prenat Diagn. 1998;18:1143-1148.

184. Peddle LJ. Increase of antibody titer following amniocentesis. Am J Obstet Gynecol. 1968;100:567-569.

185. Bahado-Singh RO, Oz AU, Hsu C, et al. Middle cerebral artery Doppler velocimetric deceleration angle as a predictor of fetal anemia in Rh-alloimmunized fetuses without hydrops. Am J Obstet Gynecol. 2000;183: 746-751.

186. Oepkes D. Invasive versus non-invasive testing in red-cell alloimmunized pregnancies. Eur J Obstet Gynecol Reprod Biol. 2000;92:83-89.

187. Delle Chiaie L, Buck G, Grab D, Terinde R. Prediction of fetal anemia with Doppler measurement of the middle cerebral artery peak systolic velocity in pregnancies complicated by maternal blood group alloimmunization or parvovirus B19 infection. Ultrasound Obstet Gynecol. 2001;18:232-236.

188. Detti L, Oz U, Guney I, et al. Doppler ultrasound velocimetry for timing the second intrauterine transfusion in fetuses with anemia from red cell alloimmunization. Am J Obstet Gynecol. 2001;185:1048-1051.

189. Mari G, Deter RL, Carpenter RL, et al. Noninvasive diagnosis by Doppler ultrasonography of fetal anemia due to maternal red-cell alloimmunization. Collaborative group for Doppler assessment of the blood velocity in anemic fetuses. N Engl J Med. 2000;342:9-14.

190. Roberts AB, Mitchell JM, Lake Y, Pattison NS. Ultrasonographic surveillance in red blood cell alloimmunization. Am J Obstet Gynecol. 2001;184:1251-1255.

191. Teixeira JM, Duncan K, Letsky E, Fisk NM. Middle cerebral artery peak systolic velocity in the prediction of fetal anemia. Ultrasound Obstet Gynecol. 2000;15: 205-208.

192. Oepkes D, Seaward PG, Vandenbussche FP, et al. Doppler ultrasonography versus amniocentesis to predict fetal anemia. N Engl J Med. 2006;355:156-164.

193. Daffos F, Capella-Pavlovsky M, Forestier F. Fetal blood sampling during pregnancy with use of a needle guided by ultrasound: a study of 606 consecutive cases. Am J Obstet Gynecol. 1985;153:655-660.

194. Bowman JM, Pollock JM, Peterson LE, et al. Fetomaternal hemorrhage following funipuncture: increase in severity of maternal red-cell alloimmunization. Obstet Gynecol. 1994;84:839-843.

195. Bowman JM, Pollock JM. Reversal of Rh alloimmunization. Fact or fancy? Vox Sang. 1984;47:209-215.

196. de Silva M, Contreras M, Mollison PL. Failure of passively administered anti-Rh to prevent secondary Rh responses. Vox Sang. 1985;48:178-180.

197. Angela E, Robinson E, Tovey LA. Intensive plasma exchange in the management of severe Rh disease. Br J Haematol. 1980;45:621-631.

198. Graham-Pole J, Barr W, Willoughby ML. Continuous-flow plasmapheresis in management of severe rhesus disease. BMJ. 1977;1:1185-1188.

199. Berlin G, Selbing A, Ryden G. Rhesus haemolytic disease treated with high-dose intravenous immunoglobulin. Lancet. 1985;1:1153.

200. Gottvall T, Selbing A. Alloimmunization during pregnancy treated with high dose intravenous immunoglobulin. Effects on fetal hemoglobin concentration and anti-D concentrations in the mother and fetus. Acta Obstet Gynecol Scand. 1995;74:777-783.

201. Margulies M, Voto LS, Mathet E, Margulies M. High-dose intravenous IgG for the treatment of severe rhesus alloimmunization. Vox Sang 1991;61:181-189.

202. Barclay GR, Greiss MA, Urbaniak SJ. Adverse effect of plasma exchange on anti-D production in rhesus immunisation owing to removal of inhibitory factors. BMJ 1980;280:1569-1571.

203. Huntley B. Red cell antigens. The fetus as a patient. Lancet 2001;358(Suppl):S58.

204. Katz U, Achiron A, Sherer Y, Shoenfeld Y. Safety of intravenous immunoglobulin (IVIG) therapy. Autoimmunity reviews 2007;6:257-259.

205. Porter TF, Silver RM, Jackson GM, et al. Intravenous immune globulin in the management of severe Rh D hemolytic disease. Obstet Gynecol Surv 1997;52: 193-197.

206. Thomas JT, Muller P, Wilkinson C. Antenatal phenobarbital for reducing neonatal jaundice after red cell isoimmunization. Cochrane Database Syst Rev. 2007;2: CD005541.

207. Liley AW. Intrauterine transfusion of foetus in haemolytic disease. BMJ. 1963;2:1107-1109.

208. Menticoglou SM, Harman CR, Manning FA, Bowman JM. Intraperitoneal fetal transfusion: paralysis inhibits red cell absorption. Fetal Ther. 1987;2:154-159.

209. Adamsons K Jr, Freda VJ, James LS, Towell ME. Prenatal treatment of erythroblastosis fetalis following hysterotomy. Pediatrics. 1965;35:848-855.

210. Asensio SH, Figueroa-Longo JG, Pelegrina IA. Intrauterine exchange transfusion. Am J Obstet Gynecol. 1966;95: 1129-1133.

211. Rodeck CH, Kemp JR, Holman CA, et al. Direct intravascular fetal blood transfusion by fetoscopy in severe Rhesus isoimmunisation. Lancet. 1981;1:625-627.

212. Galligan BR, Cairns R, Schifano JV, et al. Preparation of packed red cells suitable for intravascular transfusion in utero. Transfusion. 1989;29:179-181.

213. Berkowitz RL, Chitkara U, Goldberg JD, et al. Intravascular transfusion in utero: the percutaneous approach. Am J Obstet Gynecol. 1986;154:622-623.

214. de Crespigny LC, Robinson HP, Quinn M, et al. Ultrasound-guided fetal blood transfusion for severe rhesus isoimmunization. Obstet Gynecol. 1985;66:529-532.

215. Grannum PA, Copel JA, Moya FR, et al. The reversal of hydrops fetalis by intravascular intrauterine transfusion in severe isoimmune fetal anemia. Am J Obstet Gynecol. 1988;158:914-919.

216. Harman CR, Bowman JM, Manning FA, Menticoglou SM. Intrauterine transfusion—intraperitoneal versus intravascular approach: a case-control comparison. Am J Obstet Gynecol. 1990;162:1053-1059.

217. Nicolaides KH, Soothill PW, Rodeck CH, Clewell W. Rh disease: intravascular fetal blood transfusion by cordocentesis. Fetal Ther. 1986;1:185-192.

218. Van Kamp IL, Klumper FJ, Oepkes D, et al. Complications of intrauterine intravascular transfusion for fetal anemia due to maternal red-cell alloimmunization. Am J Obstet Gynecol. 2005;192:171-177.

219. van Kamp IL, Klumper FJ, Bakkum RS, et al. The severity of immune fetal hydrops is predictive of fetal outcome after intrauterine treatment. Am J Obstet Gynecol. 2001;185:668-673.

220. Bennebroek Gravenhorst J. Management of serious alloimmunization in pregnancy. Vox Sang. 1988;55:1-8.

221. Moise KJ. Red blood cell alloimmunization in pregnancy. Semin Hematol. 2005;42:169-178.

222. Soothill PW, Lestas AN, Nicolaides KH, et al. 2,3-Diphosphoglycerate in normal, anaemic and transfused human fetuses. Clin Sci (Lond). 1988;74:527-530.

223. Doyle LW, Kelly EA, Rickards AL, et al. Sensorineural outcome at 2 years for survivors of erythroblastosis treated with fetal intravascular transfusions. Obstet Gynecol. 1993;81:931-935.

224. Hudon L, Moise KJ Jr, Hegemier SE, et al. Long-term neurodevelopmental outcome after intrauterine transfusion for the treatment of fetal hemolytic disease. Am J Obstet Gynecol. 1998;179:858-863.

225. Janssens HM, de Haan MJ, van Kamp IL, et al. Outcome for children treated with fetal intravascular transfusions because of severe blood group antagonism. J Pediatr. 1997;131:373-380.

226. Stewart G, Day RE, Del Priore C, et al. Developmental outcome after intravascular intrauterine transfusion for rhesus haemolytic disease. Arch Dis Child Fetal Neonatal Ed. 1994;70:F52-F53.

227. White CA, Goplerud CP, Kisker CT, et al. Intrauterine fetal transfusion, 1965-1976, with an assessment of the surviving children. Am J Obstet Gynecol. 1978;130:933-942.

228. Harper DC, Swingle HM, Weiner CP, et al. Long-term neurodevelopmental outcome and brain volume after treatment for hydrops fetalis by in utero intravascular transfusion. Am J Obstet Gynecol. 2006;195:192-200.

229. Anderson KC, Ness PM. Scientific Basis of Transfusion Medicine. Implications for Clinical Practice. Philadelphia, WB Saunders, 2000.

230. Murphy KW, Whitfield CR. Rhesus disease in this decade. Comtemp Rev Obstet Gynaecol. 1994;6:61.

231. Inglis SR, Lysikiewicz A, Sonnenblick AL, et al. Advantages of larger volume, less frequent intrauterine red blood cell transfusions for maternal red cell alloimmunization. Am J Perinatol. 1996;13:27-33.

232. Plecas DV, Chitkara U, Berkowitz GS, et al. Intrauterine intravascular transfusion for severe erythroblastosis fetalis: how much to transfuse? Obstet Gynecol. 1990;75:965-969.

233. Harte G, Payton D, Carmody F, et al. Graft versus host disease following intrauterine and exchange transfusions for rhesus haemolytic disease. Aust N Z J Obstet Gynaecol. 1997;37:319-322.

234. Naiman JL, Punnett HH, Lischner HW, et al. Possible graft-versus-host reaction after intrauterine transfusion for Rh erythroblastosis fetalis. N Engl J Med. 1969;281:697-701.

235. Amato M, Schurch S, Grunder R, et al. Influence of bilirubin on surface tension properties of lung surfactant. Arch Dis Child Fetal Neonatal Ed. 1996;75:F191-F196.

236. Phibbs RH, Johnson P, Kitterman JA, et al. Cardiorespiratory status of erythroblastotic infants. 1. Relationship of gestational age, severity of hemolytic diseases, and birth asphyxia to idiopathic respiratory distress syndrome and survival. Pediatrics. 1972;49:5-14.

237. Phibbs RH, Johnson P, Kitterman JA, et al. Cardiorespiratory status of erythroblastotic newborn infants: III. Intravascular pressures during the first hours of life. Pediatrics. 1976;58:484-493.

238. Barrett CT, Oliver TK Jr. Hypoglycemia and hyperinsulinism in infants with erythroblastosis fetalis. N Engl J Med. 1968;278:1260-1262.

239. Abbas A, Nicolaides K. Fetal serum ferritin and cobalamin in red blood cell isoimmunisation. Fetal Diagn Ther. 1995;10:297-300.

240. Lasker MR, Eddleman K, Toor AH. Neonatal hepatitis and excessive hepatic iron deposition following intrauterine blood transfusion. Am J Perinatol. 1995;12:14-17.

241. Sreenan C, Idikio HA, Osiovich H. Successful chelation therapy in a case of neonatal iron overload following intravascular intrauterine transfusion. J Perinatol. 2000;20:509-512.

242. Bowman JM. Gastrointestinal absorption of isohemagglutinin. Am J Dis Child. 1963;105:352-357.

243. Gallagher PG, Ehrenkranz RA. Nutritional anemias in infancy. Clin Perinatol. 1995;22:671-692.

244. Purugganan G, Leikin S, Gautier G. Folate metabolism in erythroid hyperplastic and hypoplastic states. Am J Dis Child. 1971;122:48-52.

245. Dennery PA, Seidman DS, Stevenson DK. Neonatal hyperbilirubinemia. N Engl J Med. 2001;344:581-590.

246. Mills JF, Tudehope D. Fibreoptic phototherapy for neonatal jaundice. Cochrane Database Syst Rev. 2001;1:CD002060.

247. Hansen TW. Acute management of extreme neonatal jaundice—the potential benefits of intensified phototherapy and interruption of enterohepatic bilirubin circulation. Acta Paediatr. 1997;86:843-846.

248. Valaes T, Koliopoulos C, Koltsidopoulos A. The impact of phototherapy in the management of neonatal hyperbilirubinemia: comparison of historical cohorts. Acta Paediatr. 1996;85:273-276.

249. Alpay F, Sarici SU, Okutan V, et al. High-dose intravenous immunoglobulin therapy in neonatal immune haemolytic jaundice. Acta Paediatr. 1999;88:216-219.

250. Dagoglu T, Ovali F, Samanci N, Bengisu E. High-dose intravenous immunoglobulin therapy for rhesus haemolytic disease. J Int Med Res. 1995;23:264-271.

251. Nasseri F, Mamouri GA, Babaei H. Intravenous immunoglobulin in ABO and Rh hemolytic diseases of newborn. Saudi Med J. 2006;27:1827-1830.

252. Rubo J, Albrecht K, Lasch P, et al. High-dose intravenous immune globulin therapy for hyperbilirubinemia caused by Rh hemolytic disease. J Pediatr. 1992;121: 93-97.

253. Alcock GS, Liley H. Immunoglobulin infusion for isoimmune haemolytic jaundice in neonates. Cochrane Database Syst Rev. 2002;3:CD003313.

254. Wallerstein H. Treatment of severe erythroblastosis by simultaneous removal and replacement of blood of the newborn infant. Science. 1946;103:583-584.

255. Wiener AS, Wexler IB. The use of heparin when performing exchange transfusions in newborn infants. J Lab Clin Med. 1946;31:1016-1017.

256. Diamond LK. Replacement transfusion as a treatment for erythroblastosis fetalis. Pediatrics. 1948;2:520-524.

257. Mollison PL, Walker W. Controlled trials of the treatment of haemolytic disease of the newborn. Lancet. 1952;1: 429-433.

258. Setzer ES, Webb IB, Wassenaar JW, et al. Platelet dysfunction and coagulopathy in intraventricular hemorrhage in the premature infant. J Pediatr. 1982;100:599-605.

259. Wennberg RP, Depp R, Heinrichs WL. Indications for early exchange transfusion in patients with erythroblastosis fetalis. J Pediatr. 1978;92:789-792.

260. Jackson JC. Adverse events associated with exchange transfusion in healthy and ill newborns. Pediatrics. 1997;99:E7.

261. Steiner LA, Bizzarro MJ, Ehrenkranz RA, Gallagher PG. A decline in the frequency of neonatal exchange transfusions and its effect on exchange-related morbidity and mortality. Pediatrics. 2007;120:27-32.

262. Management of hyperbilirubinemia in the newborn infant 35 or more weeks of gestation. Pediatrics. 2004;114: 297-316.

263. Ramasethu J. Exchange transfusions. In MacDonald M, Ramasethu J (eds). Atlas of Procedures in Neonatology. Philadelphia, Lippincott, Williams & Wilkins, 2007.

264. Thayyil S, Milligan DW. Single versus double volume exchange transfusion in jaundiced newborn infants. Cochrane Database Syst Rev. 2006;4:CD004592.

265. Bowman JM. Immune hemolytic disease. In Nathan DG, Orkin SH (eds). Nathan and Oski's Hematology of Infancy and Childhood, 5th ed. Philadelphia, WB Saunders, 1998.

266. Queenan JT, Smith BD, Haber JM, et al. Irregular antibodies in the obstetric patient. Obstet Gynecol. 1969;34: 767-771.

267. Pepperell RJ, Barrie JU, Fliegner JR. Significance of redcell irregular antibodies in the obstetric patient. Med J Aust. 1977;2:453-456.

268. Filbey D, Hanson U, Wesstrom G. The prevalence of red cell antibodies in pregnancy correlated to the outcome of the newborn: a 12 year study in central Sweden. Acta Obstet Gynecol Scand. 1995;74:687-692.

269. Howard H, Martlew V, McFadyen I, et al. Consequences for fetus and neonate of maternal red cell alloimmunisation. Arch Dis Child Fetal Neonatal Ed. 1998;78:F62-F66.

270. Jovanovic-Srzentic S, Djokic M, Tijanic N, et al. Antibodies detected in samples from 21,730 pregnant women. Immunohematology. 2003;19:89-92.

271. Lee CK, Ma ES, Tang M, et al. Prevalence and specificity of clinically significant red cell alloantibodies in Chinese women during pregnancy—a review of cases from 1997 to 2001. Transfus Med. 2003;13:227-231.

272. Bowman JM. Treatment options for the fetus with alloimmune hemolytic disease. Transfus Med Rev. 1990;4: 191-207.

273. Redman CM, Russo D, Lee S. Kell, Kx and the McLeod syndrome. Baillieres Best Pract Res Clin Haematol. 1999;12:621-635.

274. Lee S, Russo D, Redman CM. The Kell blood group system: Kell and XK membrane proteins. Semin Hematol. 2000;37:113-121.

275. Bowman JM, Pollock JM, Manning FA, et al. Maternal Kell blood group alloimmunization. Obstet Gynecol. 1992;79:239-244.

276. Caine ME, Mueller-Heubach E. Kell sensitization in pregnancy. Am J Obstet Gynecol. 1986;154:85-90.

277. Mayne KM, Bowell PJ, Pratt GA. The significance of anti-Kell sensitization in pregnancy. Clin Lab Haematol. 1990;12:379-385.

278. Grant SR, Kilby MD, Meer L, et al. The outcome of pregnancy in Kell alloimmunisation. Br J Obstet Gynaecol. 2000;107:481-485.

279. Vaughan JI, Manning M, Warwick RM, et al. Inhibition of erythroid progenitor cells by anti-Kell antibodies in fetal alloimmune anemia. N Engl J Med. 1998;338:798-803.

280. Babinszki A, Lapinski RH, Berkowitz RL. Prognostic factors and management in pregnancies complicated with severe Kell alloimmunization: experiences of the last 13 years. Am J Perinatol. 1998;15:695-701.

281. McKenna DS, Nagaraja HN, O'Shaughnessy R. Management of pregnancies complicated by anti-Kell isoimmunization. Obstet Gynecol. 1999;93:667-673.

282. McDonnell M, Hannam S, Devane SP. Hydrops fetalis due to ABO incompatibility. Arch Dis Child Fetal Neonatal Ed. 1998;78:F220-F221.

283. Grundbacher FJ. The etiology of ABO hemolytic disease of the newborn. Transfusion. 1980;20:563-568.

284. Romano EL, Mollison PL, Linares J. Number of B sites generated on group O red cells from adults and newborn infants. Vox Sang. 1978;34:14-17.

285. Brouwers HA, Overbeeke MA, Huiskes E, et al. Complement is not activated in ABO-haemolytic disease of the newborn. Br J Haematol. 1988;68:363-366.

286. Ukita M, Takahashi A, Nunotani T, et al. IgG subclasses of anti-A and anti-B antibodies bound to the cord red cells in ABO incompatible pregnancies. Vox Sang. 1989;56:181-186.

287. Feng CS, Wan CP, Lau J, et al. Incidence of ABO haemolytic disease of the newborn in a group of Hong Kong

babies with severe neonatal jaundice. J Paediatr Child Health. 1990;26:155-157.

288. Meberg A, Johansen KB. Screening for neonatal hyperbilirubinaemia and ABO alloimmunization at the time of testing for phenylketonuria and congenital hypothyreosis. Acta Paediatr. 1998;87:1269-1274.

289. Ozolek JA, Watchko JF, Mimouni F. Prevalence and lack of clinical significance of blood group incompatibility in mothers with blood type A or B. J Pediatr. 1994;125:87-91.

290. Guaran RL, Drew JH, Watkins AM. Jaundice: clinical practice in 88,000 liveborn infants. Aust N Z J Obstet Gynaecol. 1992;32:186-192.

291. Palmer DC, Drew JH. Jaundice: a 10 year review of 41,000 live born infants. Aust Paediatr J. 1983;19:86-89.

292. Desjardins L, Blajchman MA, Chintu C, et al. The spectrum of ABO hemolytic disease of the newborn infant. J Pediatr. 1979;95:447-449.

293. Katz MA, Kanto WP Jr, Korotkin JH. Recurrence rate of ABO hemolytic disease of the newborn. Obstet Gynecol. 1982;59:611-614.

294. al-Alaiyan S, al Omran A. Late hyporegenerative anemia in neonates with rhesus hemolytic disease. J Perinat Med. 1999;27:112-115.

295. Ohls RK, Wirkus PE, Christensen RD. Recombinant erythropoietin as treatment for the late hyporegenerative anemia of Rh hemolytic disease. Pediatrics. 1992;90:678-680.

296. Ovali F, Samanci N, Dagoglu T. Management of late anemia in Rhesus hemolytic disease: use of recombinant human erythropoietin (a pilot study). Pediatr Res. 1996;39:831-834.

297. Zuppa AA, Maragliano G, Scapillati ME, et al. Recombinant erythropoietin in the prevention of late anaemia in intrauterine transfused neonates with Rh-haemolytic disease. Fetal Diagn Ther. 1999;14:270-274.

298. Polesky HF. Blood group antibodies in prenatal sera. Results of screening 43,000 individuals. Minn Med. 1967;50:601-603.

4 Disorders of Bilirubin Metabolism

Mark J. Bergeron and Glenn R. Gourley

Elevation of serum bilirubin level is a common, if not universal finding during the first week of life and has been reviewed elsewhere.[1-3] It can be a transient phenomenon that will resolve spontaneously or can signify a serious or even potentially life-threatening condition. There are many causes of hyperbilirubinemia and related therapeutic and prognostic implications. Independent of the cause, elevated serum bilirubin levels can potentially be toxic to newborn infants. This chapter reviews perinatal bilirubin metabolism and addresses assessment, etiology, toxicity, and treatment of neonatal jaundice. Diseases in which there is a primary disorder in the metabolism of bilirubin are reviewed with regard to their clinical findings, pathophysiology, diagnosis, and treatment.

BILIRUBIN METABOLISM

Bilirubin Production and Transport

In 1864 Städeler used the term "bilirubin," derived from Latin (*bilis*, bile; *ruber*, red), for the red-colored bile pigment.[4] Bilirubin is formed from the degradation of heme-containing compounds (Fig. 4-1). The largest source for the production of bilirubin is hemoglobin. However, other heme-containing proteins are also degraded to bilirubin, including the cytochromes, catalases, tryptophan pyrrolase, and muscle myoglobin.[5]

Formation of bilirubin is initiated by cleavage of the tetrapyrrole ring of protoheme (protoporphyrin IX), which results in a linear tetrapyrrole (biliverdin). The first enzyme system and rate-limiting step in bilirubin synthesis is microsomal heme oxygenase (HO).[6] HO can be up-regulated threefold to fivefold in response to hemolysis. Two major forms of HO have been identified. HO1, the inducible form, is located in the spleen, liver, and bone marrow. HO2, the constitutive form, is located in the testes, central nervous system (CNS), vasculature, liver, kidney, and gut. HO results in the reduction of porphyrin iron (Fe^{III} to Fe^{II}) and hydroxylation of the α-methine ($=C—$) carbon. This α carbon is then oxidatively excised from the tetrapyrrole ring to yield carbon monoxide (CO). Such excision opens the ring structure and is associated with oxygenation of the two carbons adjacent to the site of cleavage. The cleaved α carbon is excreted as CO, which has numerous biologic effects, including neurotransmission, vasodilation, and mediation of apoptosis and anti-inflammatory processes. The iron released by HO can be reused by the body. The stereospecificity of the enzyme produces cleavage almost exclusively at the α carbon of the tetrapyrrole. This is unlike in vitro chemical oxidation, which results in cleavage at any of the four carbons (α, β, γ, and δ; see Fig. 4-1, structure 1) linking the four pyrrole rings and produces equimolar amount of the α, β, γ, and δ isomers.[7] HO produces a linear tetrapyrrole, biliverdin IXα. The IX designation is a result of Fischer and Orth's grouping of the protoporphyrin isomers, with group IX being the

physiologic source of bilirubin.[8] In utero, bilirubin IXβ is the first bile pigment seen and can be found in bile or meconium by 15 weeks' gestation.[9] Small amounts of bilirubin IXβ are also found in adult human bile.[10] The central (C-10) carbon on biliverdin IXα is then reduced from a methine to a methylene group ($—CH_2—$), thereby forming bilirubin IXα. This reaction is accomplished by the cytosolic enzyme biliverdin reductase.[11] The proximity of this enzyme results in very little biliverdin ever being present in the circulation. Bilirubin formation can be assessed by measurement of CO production.[12] Such assessments indicate that the daily rate of production of bilirubin is 6 to 8 mg/kg/24 hr in healthy term infants and 3 to 4 mg/kg/24 hr in healthy adults.[13,14] In mammals, 80% to 85% of the bilirubin produced daily originates from hemoglobin.[15] Degradation of hepatic and renal heme appears to account for most of the remainder and reflects the very rapid turnover of certain of these heme proteins. Although the precise fate of myoglobin heme is unknown, its turnover appears to be so slow that it is relatively insignificant.[16] Catabolism of hemoglobin occurs largely from the sequestration of erythrocytes at the end of their life span (120 days in adult humans, 90 days in newborns, 50 to 60 days in rats). A small fraction of newly synthesized hemoglobin is degraded in bone marrow. This process, termed "ineffective erythropoiesis," normally represents less than 3% of daily bilirubin production but may be substantially increased in persons with hemoglobinopathies, vitamin deficiencies, and heavy metal intoxication.[17-19] Infants produce more bilirubin per unit body weight because of their greater red blood cell (RBC) mass and shorter RBC life span. Additionally, hepatic heme proteins represent a larger fraction of total body weight in infants.

Although bilirubin has long been thought of solely as a waste product, data suggest that some mild degree of hyperbilirubinemia may be helpful because of the antioxidant capacity of bilirubin and its potential role as a free radical scavenger and cytoprotectant.[20] Although bilirubin crosses the placenta more easily than biliverdin does,[21] it is not clear what biologic advantage this offers.

Bilirubin is poorly soluble in aqueous solvents and thus requires biotransformation to more water-soluble derivatives for excretion from the body. This poor solubility is related to the structure of bilirubin.[22] Rather than being linear (structure 5, Fig. 4-1), bilirubin undergoes extensive internal hydrogen bonding (structure 4, Fig. 4-1). This extensive bonding occurs because the saturated middle carbon (C-10) permits the two halves of the bilirubin molecule to rotate such that the pyrrole nitrogens and lactam oxygen of one half form hydrogen bonds with the carboxyl groups of the propionic acid side chain on the other half. This shields the polar propionic acid side chains and makes bilirubin very nonpolar and lipophilic. The carbon-carbon double bonds at positions 4-5 and 15-16 can assume two different configurations (similar to "*cis*" and "*trans*"), depending on whether the

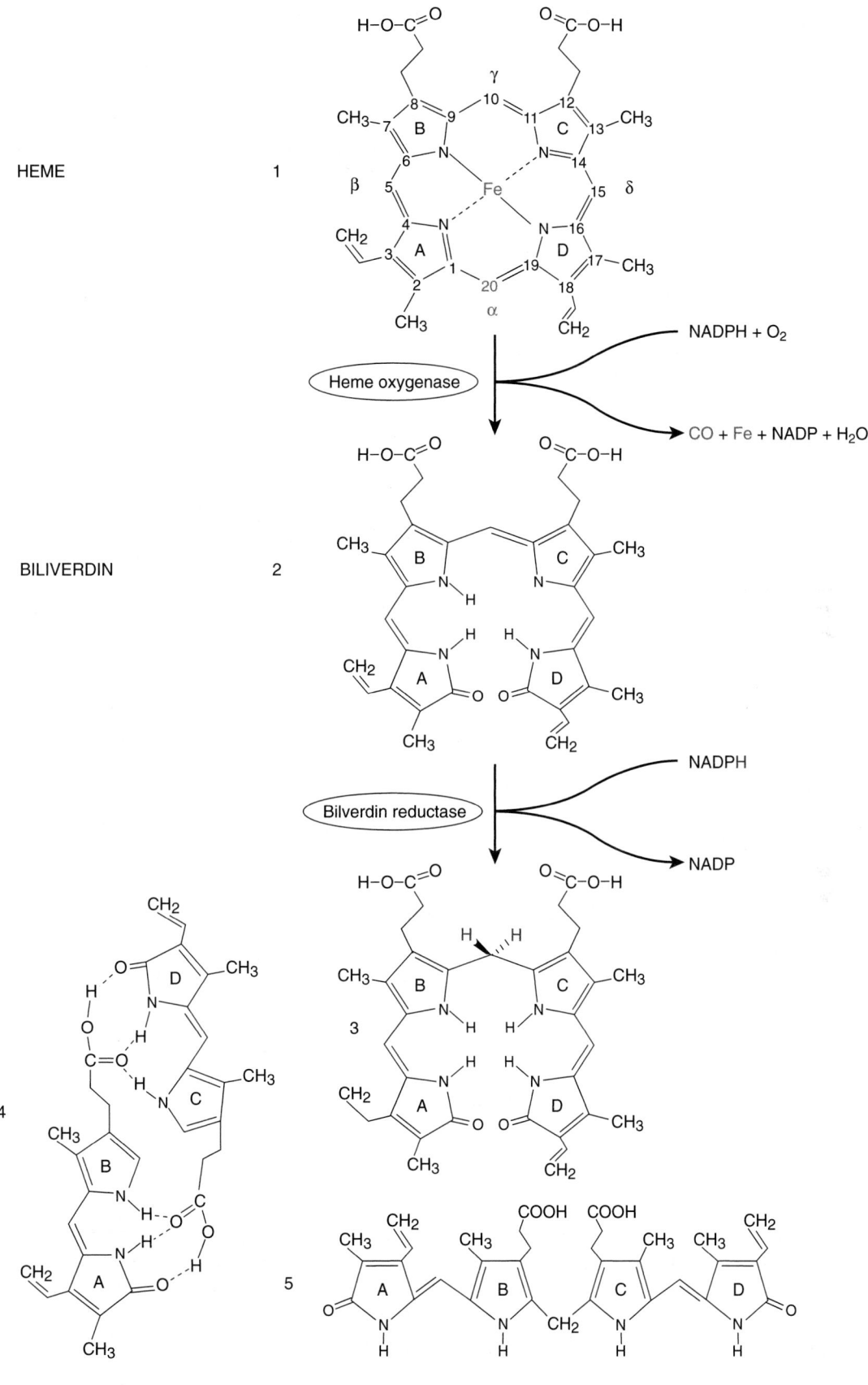

HEME   1

BILIVERDIN   2

NADPH + O₂

Heme oxygenase

CO + Fe + NADP + H₂O

NADPH

Bilverdin reductase

NADP

BILIRUBIN

FIGURE 4-1. Chemical structures depicting the conversion of heme to bilirubin. Bilirubin is frequently represented by any of the three structures (3 to 5) shown at the bottom. *(Redrawn from Gourley GR. Neonatal jaundice and disorders of bilirubin metabolism. In Suchy FJ, Sokol RJ, Balistreri WF [eds]. Liver Disease in Children, 3rd ed. New York, Cambridge University Press, 2007. Used with permission.)*

higher-priority atoms or groups (based on atomic number) are on the same (German: Z, *zusammen*, "together") or opposite (E, *entgegen*, "opposite") sides of the double bond. The naturally occurring form of bilirubin, 4Z,15Z-bilirubin IXα, can be represented by any of the three structures (3-5) depicted at the bottom of Figure 4-1. Knowledge of this stereochemistry is important in understanding phototherapy, which is discussed later.

Bilirubin's poor aqueous solubility necessitates a carrier molecule, albumin, for transport from sites of production in the reticuloendothelial system to the liver for excretion (Fig. 4-2).[23] Each albumin molecule possesses a single high-affinity ($K_a = 7 \times 10^7$ M^{-1}) binding site for one molecule of bilirubin.[24] A binding affinity of this magnitude implies that at normal serum bilirubin levels, all bilirubin will be transported to the liver bound to albumin, with negligible amounts free to diffuse into

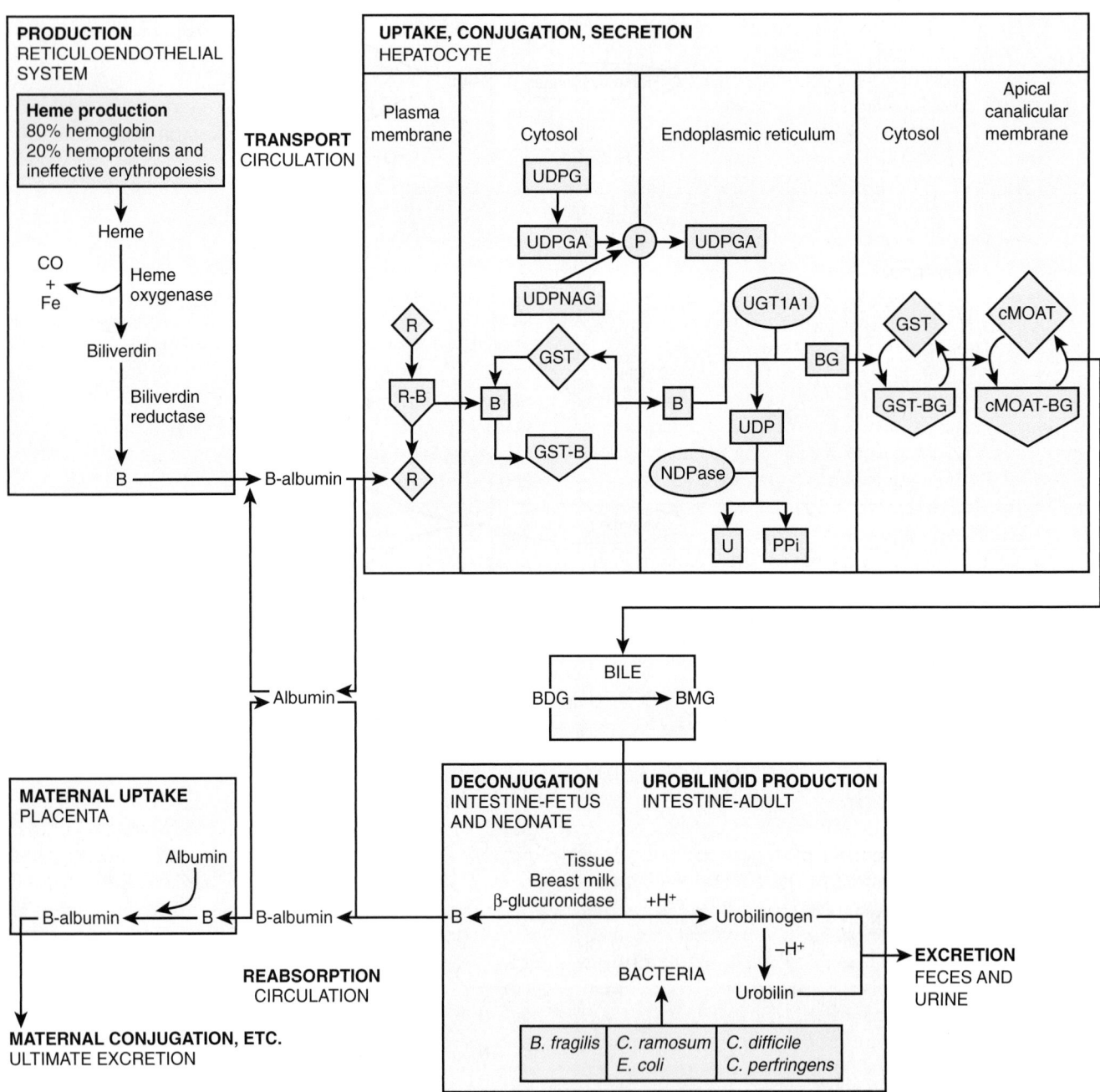

FIGURE 4-2. Schematic overview of bilirubin (B) metabolism in the fetus, neonate, and adult. BDG/BMG, bilirubin diglucuronide/monoglucuronide; BG, bilirubin glucuronide; cMOAT, canalicular multispecific organic anion transporter (also known as MRP2 or ABCC2); GST, glutathione-S-transferase (ligandin); NDPase, nucleoside diphosphatase; P, permease; PPi, inorganic pyrophosphate; R, membrane carrier; UDPG, uridine diphosphate glucose; UDPGA, uridine diphosphate glucuronic acid; UDPNAG, uridine diphosphate N-acetylglucosamine; UGT1A1, bilirubin glucuronosyltransferase. *(Redrawn from Gourley GR. Neonatal jaundice and disorders of bilirubin metabolism. In Suchy FJ, Sokol RJ, Balistreri WF [eds]. Liver Disease in Children, 3rd ed. New York, Cambridge University Press, 2007. Used with permission.)*

other tissues. Secondary binding sites of lesser affinity also exist on albumin. Albumin additionally serves as a carrier for other compounds such as xenobiotics and fatty acids. It is important to remember that albumin from each animal species has different binding characteristics for various ligands.[25]

Hepatic Uptake of Bilirubin

The structure of the liver is well suited for uptake of bilirubin by individual hepatocytes. Cords of hepatocytes are arranged radially such that adjacent sinusoids border all hepatocytes. Flow of blood through the sinusoids is slower than that through other capillary beds because it is generated by portal venous pressure rather than arterial pressure. Albumin-bound bilirubin easily passes from plasma into the tissue fluid space (space of Disse) between the endothelium and the hepatocyte because the sinusoidal endothelium of the liver lacks the basal laminae found in other organ capillary systems.[26] The pores of the endothelium allow direct contact with the plasma membrane of the hepatocyte.

A hepatocyte with a schematic illustration of bilirubin metabolism is shown in Figure 4-2. In the first step, bilirubin dissociates from its albumin carrier[27] and enters the hepatocyte via a membrane receptor-carrier that facilitates entry into the hepatocyte. Carrier-mediated transport into the hepatocyte has been demonstrated for several organic anions, including bilirubin, bromsulfophthalein (BSP), and indocyanine green (ICG),[28] although bilirubin has been shown to be able to pass through membranes by simple passive diffusion.[29] Evidence suggests that bilirubin, BSP, and ICG share the same hepatocyte receptor-carrier because they exhibit competitive inhibition when injected simultaneously. This finding cannot be explained by subsequent intrahepatic metabolism inasmuch as these anions are handled differently by the hepatocyte: bilirubin is conjugated with glucuronic acid in the endoplasmic reticulum (ER), BSP is conjugated with glutathione in the cytosol, and ICG is excreted directly without biotransformation. Data from rat hepatocytes suggest that the anion-binding receptor-carrier is a dimeric protein with a subunit molecular weight of 55,000.[30-32] Antibody studies confirm the expected location in the plasma membrane[31] and demonstrate blockage of uptake.[32] Organic anion–transporting polypeptide 2 (OATP2, recently named OATP1B1 under new nomenclature[33]) has shown high-affinity uptake of bilirubin in the presence of albumin and is a member of the OATP family, transporter symbol SLC21A.

Carrier-mediated transport of bilirubin into the hepatocyte is necessary because of differences in protein binding inside and outside the hepatocyte. Outside the hepatocyte, bilirubin is bound to albumin (affinity constant, $\approx 10^8$; concentration, 0.6 mM).[24] Inside the hepatocyte, bilirubin is bound to glutathione-S-transferase B (GST), historically known as ligandin or Y protein (affinity constant, $\approx 10^6$; concentration, 0.04 mM).[34,35] GST

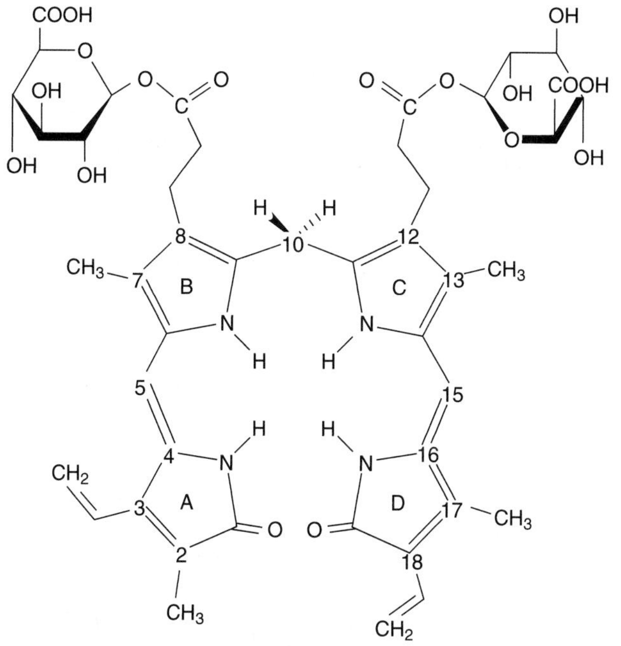

FIGURE 4-3. Bilirubin diglucuronide. In bilirubin monoglucuronide, only one propionic acid side chain (C-8 or C-12) is glucuronidated. *(Redrawn from Gourley GR. Neonatal jaundice and disorders of bilirubin metabolism. In Suchy FJ, Sokol RJ, Balistreri WF [eds]. Liver Disease in Children, 3rd ed. New York, Cambridge University Press, 2007. Used with permission.)*

constitutes a family of proteins that exhibit important functions both as enzymes and as intracellular binding proteins for nonsubstrate ligands such as bilirubin.[36] Carrier-mediated uptake helps generate a concentration gradient for bilirubin uptake despite the difference in affinity between albumin and GST. GST is important in the intracellular storage of bilirubin and bilirubin conjugates and reduces efflux from the hepatocyte back into plasma.[35]

Bilirubin Conjugation

Inside the hepatocyte, bilirubin is conjugated with glucuronic acid[37] within the ER (microsomes). The glucuronic acid donor is uridine diphosphate glucuronic acid (UDPGA). Conjugation results in an ester linkage formed with either or both of the propionic acid side chains on the B and C pyrrole rings of bilirubin (Fig. 4-3). The enzyme responsible for this esterification is bilirubin UDP-glucuronosyltransferase (BUGT; Online Mendelian Inheritance in Man★ [OMIM] 191740). BUGT is distinct from the other glucuronosyltransferase isoforms that catalyze the conjugation of thyroxine, steroids, bile acids, and xenobiotics.[38] BUGT is embedded in the lipid environment of the microsomal membrane, and perturbations of this environment greatly affect in vitro measurements of BUGT activity. Because BUGT

★Available at http://www.ncbi.nlm.nih.gov/Omim/.

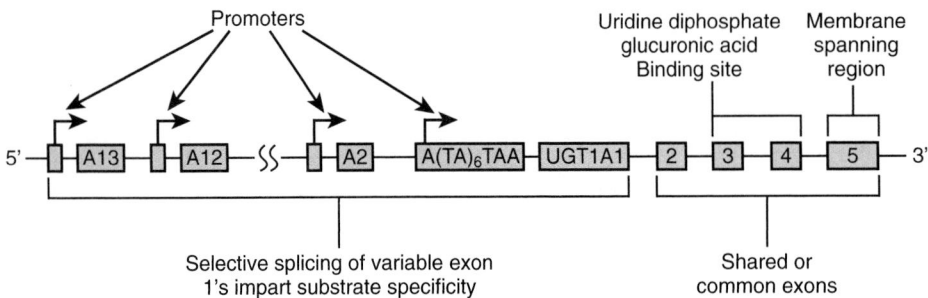

FIGURE 4-4. Human uridine diphosphate glucuronosyltransferase-1 gene (*UGT1*). UDPGA, uridine diphosphate glucuronic acid. (*Redrawn from Gourley GR. Neonatal jaundice and disorders of bilirubin metabolism. In Suchy FJ, Sokol RJ, Balistreri WF [eds]. Liver Disease in Children, 3rd ed. New York, Cambridge University Press, 2007. Used with permission.*)

is located on the interior of the ER, the existence of a permease has been hypothesized to facilitate transport of UDPGA from the cytosol across the lipid layers of the ER. The permease has been proposed because uridine diphosphate glucose (UDPG) is present in the cytosol in higher concentrations yet UDPGA serves as the preferred donor for bilirubin conjugation.[39] Uridine diphosphate *N*-acetylglucosamine (UDPNAG) is considered to be a natural regulator of BUGT[40] because UDPNAG increases in vitro BUGT activity threefold. The mechanism for such regulation is unknown and could possibly involve facilitation of the permease UDPGA transporter.[41] After providing glucuronic acid for conjugation, UDP is converted to uridine and inorganic pyrophosphate by a nucleoside diphosphatase that is also located on the interior of the ER[42] and prevents the reverse reaction.

The specific isoform responsible for bilirubin conjugation is UGT1A1 (trivial name, HUG-Br1, EC 2.4.1.17).[38] It is part of the UDP-glycosyltransferase superfamily of enzymes encoded by the *UGT* gene complex on chromosome 2 that is involved in the metabolism of many xenobiotic and endogenous substances. The *UGT1* gene encodes several isoforms and has a complex structure consisting of four common exons (2 to 5) and 13 variable exons encoding different isoforms (Fig. 4-4).[43,44] At least 30 different *UGT1* mutant alleles have been described that cause Gilbert's syndrome and Crigler-Najjar syndromes I and II.[45] UGT1A1 catalyzes the formation of both bilirubin monoglucuronides[46] but also metabolizes other hormones and drugs, so mutations could be involved in carcinogenesis and adverse drug reactions.[47] In normal adult humans the majority of bilirubin conjugates are excreted in bile as bilirubin diglucuronides ($\approx$80%)[48-53] (Fig. 4-5, middle panel). Lesser amounts of bilirubin monoglucuronides ($\approx$15%) are also excreted along with very small amounts of unconjugated bilirubin and other bilirubin conjugates (e.g., glucose, xylose, and mixed diesters). Because UGT1A1 activity is lower in infants than adults, the bile of infants contains less bilirubin diglucuronide and more bilirubin monoglucuronide (Fig. 4-6, middle panel).

Bilirubin Excretion

After conjugation, bilirubin conjugates are excreted against a concentration gradient from the hepatocyte through the canalicular membrane into bile. Data from purified canalicular membrane vesicles of rat liver suggest that transport of bilirubin diglucuronide through the canalicular membrane is carrier mediated, electrogenic, and stimulated by HCO_3^-.[54] Similar data also suggest that bilirubin glucuronides are transported across the canalicular membrane by both adenosine triphosphate (ATP)-dependent and membrane potential–dependent transport systems and that these systems are additive in normal rats.[55] The ATP-dependent transporter responsible for passage of bilirubin glucuronide from the hepatocyte through the canalicular membrane is the canalicular multispecific organic anion transporter (cMOAT). cMOAT is a member of the ATP-binding cassette (ABC) transporter superfamily; it is homologous to the multidrug resistance–associated protein (MRP2)[56,57] and is also known as ABCC2 because it is encoded by the *ABCC2* gene.[58] cMOAT/MRP2/ABCC2 is involved in ATP-dependent transport across the apical canalicular membrane of a variety of endogenous compounds and xenobiotics,[59] including both bilirubin monoglucuronide and diglucuronide.[60] cMOAT has previously been described as the non–bile acid organic anion transporter, the glutathione S-conjugate export pump, and the leukotriene export pump.[61] Genetic mutations in which these ABC transporters are altered cause diseases that include cystic fibrosis, hyperinsulinemia, adrenoleukodystrophy, multidrug resistance,[62] and as discussed later in this chapter, Dubin-Johnson syndrome. This mechanism can be saturated with increasing amounts of bilirubin or bilirubin conjugates.[63-65] Many other organic anions (e.g., BSP, ICG) share this same canalicular membrane excretion mechanism.[66] Simultaneous infusion of BSP and ICG will decrease the maximal canalicular excretion of bilirubin and vice versa.[67,68] The canalicular excretion mechanism for bilirubin and BSP is different from that for bile salts. Biliary excretion of conjugated bilirubin and BSP is decreased in individuals with Dubin-Johnson syndrome,[69] although bile salt excretion is not

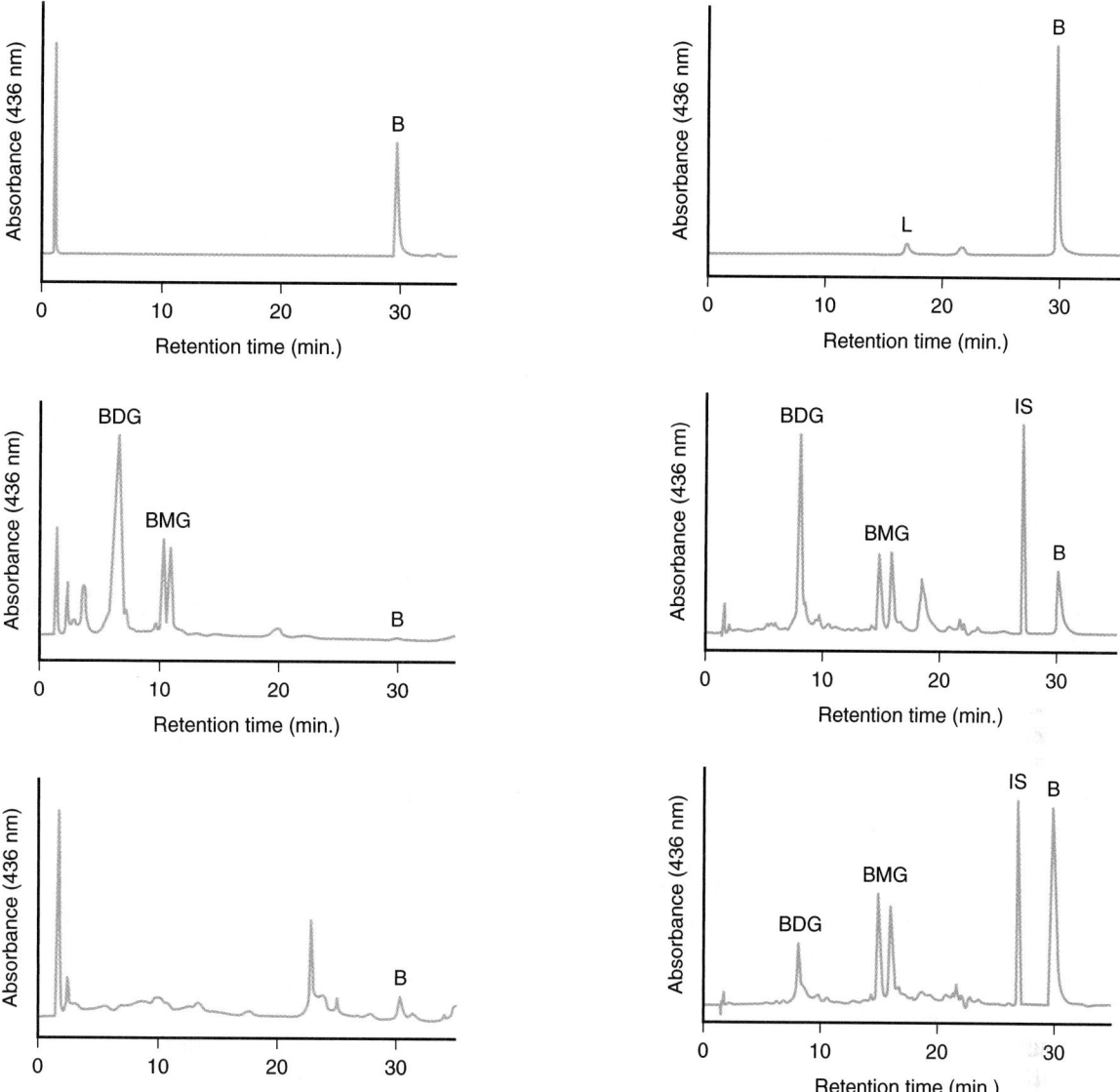

FIGURE 4-5. Bile pigment excretion in an adult human as assessed by high-performance liquid chromatography. Chromatograms represent analysis of serum (20 μL, *top*), duodenal bile (20 μL, *middle*), and stool extract (equivalent to 50 mg of wet stool, *bottom*) from a normal man. The scale of the y-axes varies. Serum bile pigments are almost all bilirubin. The bilirubin diglucuronide and monoglucuronide (BDG, BMG) that predominate over bilirubin (B) in adult bile are not present in adult feces because of metabolism by intestinal bacteria. *(Redrawn from Gourley GR. Neonatal jaundice and disorders of bilirubin metabolism. In Suchy FJ, Sokol RJ, Balistreri WF [eds]. Liver Disease in Children, 3rd ed. New York, Cambridge University Press, 2007. Used with permission.)*

FIGURE 4-6. Bile pigment excretion in a newborn human as assessed by high-performance liquid chromatography. Chromatograms represent analysis of serum (20 μL, *top*) from an infant receiving phototherapy in the first week of life and duodenal bile (20 μL, *middle*) and stool extract (equivalent to 50 mg of wet stool, *bottom*) from a normal full-term, formula-fed female infant on day 3 of life. Serum bile pigments include lumirubin (L). The scale of the y-axes varies. Neonates lack intestinal bacterial flora, and hence large quantities of bilirubin diglucuronide and monoglucuronide (BDG, BMG) and bilirubin (B) are present in feces. *(Redrawn from Gourley GR. Neonatal jaundice and disorders of bilirubin metabolism. In Suchy FJ, Sokol RJ, Balistreri WF [eds]. Liver Disease in Children, 3rd ed. New York, Cambridge University Press, 2007. Used with permission.)*

impaired. However, excretion of bile salts and bilirubin conjugates by the canalicular membrane is not completely independent because infusion of bile salts does increase the maximal excretion of bilirubin conjugates.[70] A similar effect in seen with phenobarbital.[71] Conversely, the maximal excretion of bilirubin conjugates can be decreased by cholestatic agents such as estrogens and anabolic steroids.[72,73]

Under normal conditions, there is evidence that bilirubin conjugates equilibrate across the sinusoidal mem-

brane of hepatocytes, thereby resulting in small amounts of bilirubin conjugates being present in the systemic circulation.[74-76] If hepatic glucuronidation of bilirubin is diminished (e.g., in the neonate), a decreased amount of bilirubin conjugates will be present in serum.[74,75,77] Data show that in full-term newborns there is an increase in the serum level of bilirubin diconjugates (0.55% ± 0.25% on days 2 to 4 increasing to 1.62% ± 0.99% on days 9 to 13), consistent with the maturation of bilirubin glucuronidation.[78] In contrast, in premature infants younger than 33 weeks' gestation, bilirubin diconjugates were very low and remained so, thus suggesting more severe immaturity of the glucuronidation process.

In many pathologic circumstances, bilirubin monoglucuronides and diglucuronides are not excreted from the hepatocyte fast enough to prevent significant reflux back into the circulation. The ensuing elevation in serum bilirubin conjugate levels results in transesterification of bilirubin glucuronide with an amino group on albumin and creation of a covalent bond between albumin and bilirubin.[79] This product is formed spontaneously and is known as delta bilirubin or bilirubin-albumin.[80] Similar nonenzymatic reactions have been demonstrated between albumin and various drugs.[79,81-83] Delta bilirubin is not formed in hyperbilirubinemic conditions unless the conjugated bilirubin fraction is elevated. Both delta bilirubin and bilirubin conjugates are direct reacting, which explains a situation that has long confounded clinicians. Direct bilirubin may continue to be elevated in patients who are otherwise recovering from a hepatic insult because the delta bilirubin formed lingers as a result of the long (≈20 days[84]) half-life of albumin.

Enterohepatic Circulation of Bilirubin

When bilirubin conjugates enter the intestinal lumen (see Fig. 4-2), several possibilities for further metabolism arise. In adults, the normal bacterial flora hydrogenate various carbon double bonds in bilirubin to produce assorted urobilinogens (Fig. 4-7). Subsequent oxidation of the middle (C-10) carbon produces the related urobilins. Because there are a large number of unsaturated bonds in bilirubin, many compounds are formed by reduction and oxidation of these bonds. This large family of related reduction-oxidation products of bilirubin is known as urobilinoids,[85] and they are excreted in feces and urine. Bacteria capable of producing urobilinoids include *Clostridium ramosum*,[86] *Escherichia coli*, *Bacteroides fragilis*,[87] *Clostridium perfringens*, and *Clostridium difficile*.[88] Conversion of bilirubin conjugates to urobilinoids is important because it blocks the intestinal absorption of bilirubin known as the enterohepatic circulation.[89,90] Neonates lack intestinal bacterial flora and are more likely to absorb bilirubin from the intestine. This difference in bile pigment excretion between adults and neonates is demonstrated by comparing Figures 4-5 and 4-6 (lower panels).

Bilirubin conjugates in the intestine can also act as substrate for either bacterial[91-93] or endogenous tissue[94] β-glucuronidase. This enzyme hydrolyzes glucuronic acid from bilirubin glucuronides. The unconjugated bilirubin produced is more rapidly absorbed from the intestine.[95] In the fetus, tissue β-glucuronidase is detectable by 12 weeks' gestation and is believed to play an important role in facilitating the intestinal absorption of bilirubin that enables it to be cleared via the placenta. After birth, increased intestinal β-glucuronidase can increase the neonate's likelihood of experiencing higher serum bilirubin levels.[96] The ability of endogenous tissue β-glucuronidase to deconjugate bilirubin glucuronides has been demonstrated in germ-free animals.[97] Breast milk can contain high levels of β-glucuronidase, and it has been suggested that this is one factor related to the higher jaundice levels seen in breast-fed infants.[98] Feeding specific nutritional ingredients that inhibit β-glucuronidase, such as hydrolyzed casein or L-aspartic acid,[99] has been shown to result in increased fecal bilirubin excretion and lower levels of jaundice.[100]

DIAGNOSIS OF HYPERBILIRUBINEMIA

Jaundice and icterus both refer to the yellow discoloration of tissues (skin, sclerae, etc.) caused by the deposition of bilirubin. "Jaundice," from the French *jaune*, means yellow. "Icterus" is derived from the Greek word for jaundice (*ikteros*). Jaundice is a sign that hyperbilirubinemia exists (i.e., total serum bilirubin greater than ≈1.4 mg/dL after 6 months of age; 1 mg/dL = 17 μmol/L). The degree of jaundice is directly related to the level of serum bilirubin and the amount of bilirubin deposited in extravascular tissues. Hypercarotenemia, occasionally mistaken for jaundice, can impart a yellow hue to the skin, but the sclerae remain white. There are many conditions associated with neonatal jaundice, some of which are so commonly recognized that they are termed "physiologic." Alternatively, jaundice can be a sign of severe disease.

Total Serum Bilirubin Measurements

Measurement of the total serum bilirubin concentration allows quantitation of jaundice. Such measurements are very common in the newborn nursery and in one study were made at least once in 61% of term newborn infants.[101] Two components of total serum bilirubin can be routinely measured in the clinical laboratory: conjugated bilirubin ("direct" reacting because in the Van den Bergh test, color development takes place directly without adding methanol) and unconjugated bilirubin ("indirect" fraction). Although the terms "direct" and "indirect" are often used equivalently with conjugated and unconjugated bilirubin, this is not quantitatively correct because the direct fraction includes both conjugated bilirubin and albumin-bound delta bilirubin.[102] Elevation of either of these fractions can result in jaundice. There is a long history of undesirable variability in the measurement of serum bilirubin fractions.[103,104] One problem is the ditaurobilirubin (DTB) content of standards sent by the College of American Pathologists.[104] DTB influences the result variably because of protein matrix differences related to the specific bilirubin measurement used. This has prompted the suggestion that standards should consist of human serum enriched solely with unconjugated bilirubin rather than bovine serum containing a mixture of unconjugated bilirubin and DTB.[105] The auto-

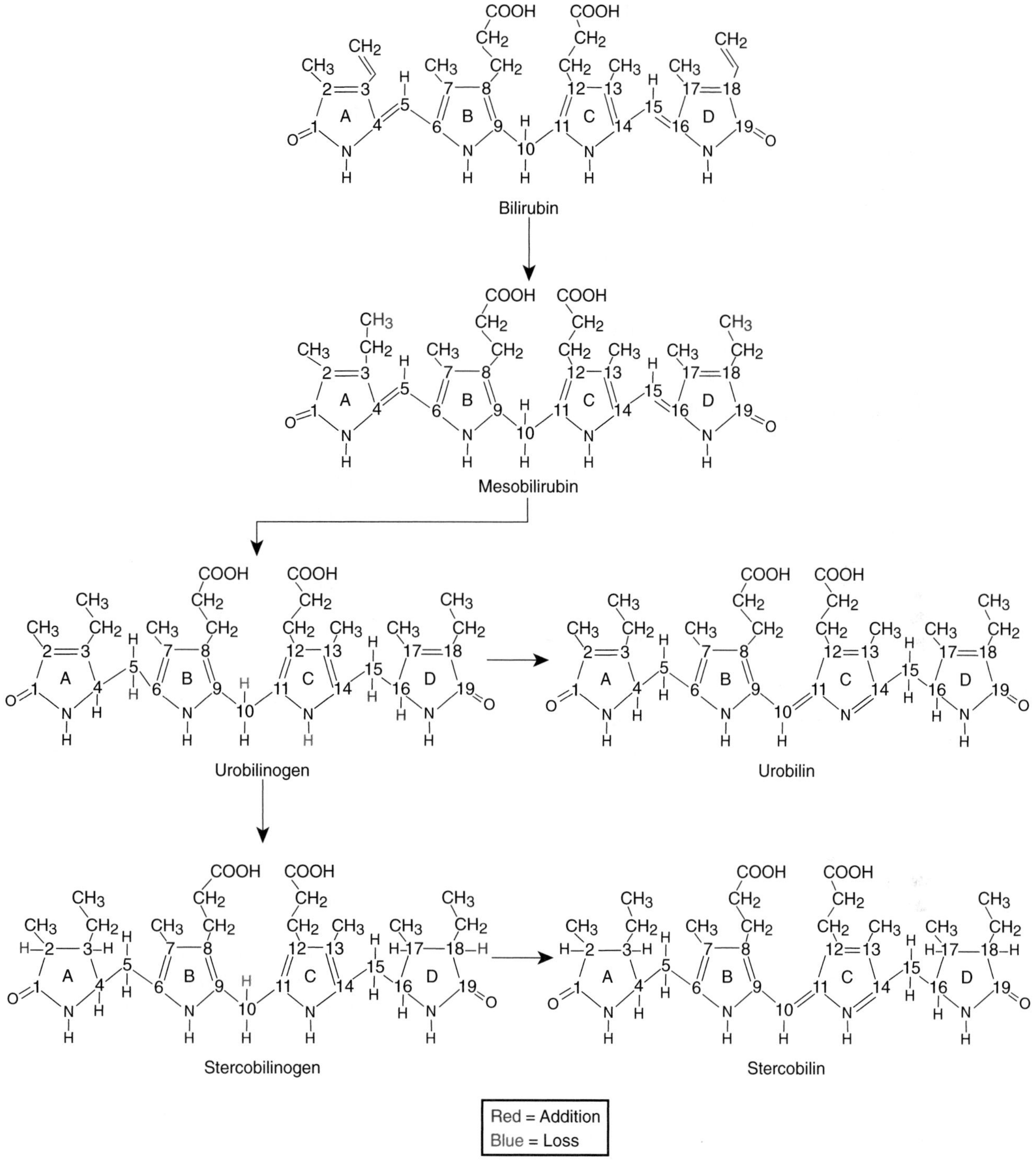

FIGURE 4-7. Reduction and oxidation of bilirubin to a family of related compounds known collectively as urobilinoids. Only several examples are given of this much larger family. *(Redrawn from Gourley GR. Neonatal jaundice and disorders of bilirubin metabolism. In Suchy FJ, Sokol RJ, Balistreri WF [eds]. Liver Disease in Children, 3rd ed. New York, Cambridge University Press, 2007. Used with permission.)*

mated laboratory methods now used to measure serum bilirubin have been reviewed elsewhere.[102,106-108] The Jendrassik-Grof procedure is the method of choice for measurement of total bilirubin, although this method also has problems.[109] When the total serum bilirubin level is high, factitious elevation of the direct fraction has been reported.[110] Three newer methods have been developed that can more accurately determine the various bilirubin fractions (unconjugated, monoconjugated, diconjugated, and albumin bound or delta): high-pressure liquid chromatography (HPLC),[111] multilayered slides,[112,113] and use of bilirubin oxidase.[114] HPLC analysis is superior and is used as the "gold standard,"[115,116] but it is too expensive and time consuming for the clinical laboratory.[102] HPLC analysis of serum from normal human neonates in the first 4 days of life[117] showed that unconjugated and conjugated bilirubin levels rose in parallel, with the conjugated fraction making up only 1.2% to 1.6% of the total pigment (3.6% in adults). Although the absolute concentration of conjugates was two to six times higher in neonates, only 20% were diconjugates (54% in adults). These sensitive HPLC data are consistent with the increased bilirubin production and relatively deficient glucuronidation seen in neonates. Analysis with automated multilayered slide technology (Johnson & Johnson—Vitros), used in many clinical laboratories, allows measurement of specific conjugated and unconjugated bilirubin fractions without the inclusion of delta bilirubin. Measurement of conjugated bilirubin provides an earlier indicator of relief from biliary cholestasis than measurement of direct bilirubin does because of the long half-life of delta bilirubin.[118] In a comparison of the bilirubin oxidase method it was concluded that determinations of total bilirubin in neonatal serum were not advanced by this method.[119]

Newer methods of total bilirubin measurement (Twin Beam, Ginevri, Rome; ABL 735, Radiometer, Copenhagen; Roche OMNI S, Roche Diagnostics, Graz, Austria) using nonenzymatic photochemical analysis offer the convenience of bilirubin quantitation outside a core laboratory setting (i.e., blood gas analyzer in the nursery) with a smaller blood sample than needed for traditional serum analysis. However, these measurements must be interpreted with caution because the instruments tend to underestimate the total bilirubin concentration when greater than 15 mg/dL.[120]

There are conflicting data regarding the accuracy of capillary versus venous serum bilirubin levels.[121,122] However, as Maisels has pointed out, the literature regarding kernicterus, phototherapy, and exchange transfusion is based on bilirubin measurements in capillary samples.[123]

Transcutaneous Bilirubinometry

Noninvasive methods of measuring jaundice levels have been shown to be useful in neonates. Current commercially available methods include the BiliCheck (Respironics, Pittsburgh)[115] and the Minolta/Hill-Rom Air-Shields Transcutaneous Jaundice Meter 103 (Air-Shields, Hatboro, PA).[124] The technique uses principles of reflectance spectrophotometry, has been validated against both HPLC and clinical laboratory measures,[115,116] and is advocated by the American Academy of Pediatrics.[125] Touching the skin with the device in a painless manner results immediately in point-of-care measurement of transcutaneous bilirubin. Significant transcutaneous bilirubin levels (e.g., >13 mg/dL) should prompt measurement of a serum or plasma bilirubin level. Some suggest that the yellow color of the skin is a better indicator of the risk for bilirubin-dependent brain damage than the serum bilirubin level is.[126] A less expensive[127] method useful in assessing jaundice[128,129] involves pressing a Plexiglas color chart against the baby's nose (Ingram icterometer, Thos. A. Ingram and Co., Ltd, Birmingham, England).

TOXICITY OF UNCONJUGATED HYPERBILIRUBINEMIA

Kernicterus

Reviews of neonatal bilirubin toxicity have been published elsewhere.[1,130,131] Kernicterus (German: *kern* = nucleus; Latin: *icterus* = yellow) is the neuropathologic finding associated with severe unconjugated hyperbilirubinemia and is named for the yellow staining of certain regions of the brain, particularly the basal ganglia, hippocampus, cerebellum, and nuclei of the floor of the fourth ventricle.[130,132] Acute clinical findings associated with kernicterus, termed acute bilirubin encephalopathy, include a sluggish Moro reflex, opisthotonos, retrocollis, hypotonia, vomiting, high-pitched cry, hyperpyrexia, seizures, gaze paresis ("setting sun sign"), oculogyric crisis, and death. Long-term findings (chronic bilirubin encephalopathy) include spasticity, choreoathetosis, dental enamel dysplasia of the deciduous teeth, and sensorineural hearing loss. Milder forms of bilirubin encephalopathy include cognitive dysfunction and learning disabilities.[133,134] In 17-year-old males, the risk of having an IQ score lower than 85 was found to be significantly higher in fullterm subjects with neonatal serum bilirubin levels above 20 mg/dL.[135] The mechanisms of bilirubin cytotoxicity are complex and have been reviewed elsewhere.[130,131,136-138] Although the neonatal period is the most common time for bilirubin-related brain damage, the neurotoxicity of bilirubin has also been documented in older children and adults with Crigler-Najjar syndrome type I.[139,140]

The absolute level of serum bilirubin has not been a good predictor of the risk for bilirubin encephalopathy. However, it has long been known that kernicterus is likely with serum unconjugated bilirubin levels greater than 30 mg/dL and unlikely with levels less than 20 mg/dL.[141-143] In one study, 90% of patients with a bilirubin level higher than 35 mg/dL either died or had cerebral palsy or physical retardation.[143] Alternatively, no developmental retardation was found in 129 infants with bilirubin levels less than 20 mg/dL. The albumin concentration is an important variable because of its high-affinity binding with bilirubin and because the ratio of bilirubin to albumin is a risk factor that has been included in the most recent American Academy of Pediatrics guidelines.[125] Drugs and organic anions also bind to albumin and can displace bilirubin, thereby increasing free bilirubin, which can diffuse into cells and cause toxicity.[144,145] The most notable example of this is kernicterus, which occurred with low bilirubin levels when sulfisoxazole was given to premature infants.[146] Walker has reviewed neonatal bilirubin toxicity and drug-induced bilirubin displacement.[136] In recent years there has been a re-emergence of kernicterus.[131] Although it has been acknowledged that total serum bilirubin may not be the most important factor related to risk, there are, at present, no other generally accepted tests (e.g., albumin saturation, reserve bilirubin binding capacity, or free bilirubin concentration) that are more helpful in identifying infants at risk for bilirubin encephalopathy. Recently, the basics of bilirubin-albumin binding and neonatal jaundice have been reviewed by Ahlfors and Wennberg.[147] Additionally, Ahlfors and colleagues have recently described how to use zone fluidics to measure free bilirubin and overcome some of the existing problems with measurement of unbound (free) bilirubin.[148] Wennberg and co-workers speculate that the enhanced sensitivity and specificity of newer methods of measurement of free bilirubin will establish an improved risk threshold for kernicterus and therefore reduce unnecessary aggressive intervention (i.e., exchange transfusion) and its associated cost and morbidity.[149]

Another approach aimed at measuring early changes in the CNS caused by bilirubin has assessed the use of brainstem auditory evoked potentials (BAEPs).[150,151] Abnormalities in BAEP have been demonstrated in jaundiced infants and were shown to improve after exchange transfusion.[152,153] Data have shown that even moderate hyperbilirubinemia (mean ± SD: 14.3 ± 2.8 mg/dL) affects the BAEP, specific components of the Brazelton Neonatal Behavioral Assessment Scale,[154] and cry characteristics.[155]

Another reported adverse effect of neonatal jaundice relates not to the CNS of a jaundiced infant but rather to the attitude of the infant's parents. Mothers of jaundiced infants more frequently exhibit behavior suggesting the "vulnerable child syndrome,"[156,157] including inappropriate visits to the physician because of unrealistic perceptions of illness, separation difficulty, and early termination of breast-feeding. Another study, however, showed that hyperbilirubinemia, phototherapy, or both during the neonatal period is not associated with impaired mother-child attachment after the first year of life.[158]

Nonpathologic Unconjugated Hyperbilirubinemia

Physiologic Jaundice

The term "physiologic jaundice" has been used to describe the frequently observed jaundice in otherwise completely normal neonates. However, physiologic jaundice is merely the result of a number of factors involving increased bilirubin production and decreased excretion.

Jaundice should always be considered a sign of possible disease and not routinely explained as physiologic. Specific characteristics of neonatal jaundice to be considered abnormal until proved otherwise include (1) the development of jaundice before 36 hours of age, (2) persistence beyond 10 days of age, (3) serum bilirubin greater than 12 mg/dL at any time, and (4) elevation of direct bilirubin (direct bilirubin >1.0 mg/dL if total bilirubin is less than 5 mg/dL or direct bilirubin >20% of total bilirubin if total bilirubin is greater than 5 mg/dL[159]).

The physiologic immaturity of premature infants is associated with both higher peak serum bilirubin levels and pathologic conditions.[160]

In general, infants are not jaundiced at the moment of birth because of the impressive ability of the placenta to clear bilirubin from the fetal circulation. However, within the next few days, elevated serum bilirubin levels (>1.4 mg/dL) will develop in most if not all infants, with clinical jaundice becoming evident when the total bilirubin level exceeds 2 to 5 mg/dL. As serum bilirubin rises, the skin becomes more jaundiced in a cephalocaudad manner.[161] Icterus is first observed in the face and progresses caudally to the palms and soles. Kramer found the following serum indirect bilirubin levels as jaundice progressed: head and neck—4 to 8 mg/dL; upper part of the trunk—5 to 12 mg/dL; lower part of the trunk and thighs—8 to 16 mg/dL; arms and lower part of the legs—11 to 18 mg/dL; and palms and soles—greater than 15 mg/dL.[162] Hence, when the bilirubin level was higher than 15 mg/dL, the entire body was icteric. However, darker skin tones can make jaundice difficult to estimate visually.[125] Jaundice is best observed by blanching the skin with gentle digital pressure under well-illuminated (white light) conditions. Visible jaundice develops in at least a third of infants. A combined analysis of several large studies involving thousands of infants during the first week of life showed that moderate jaundice (bilirubin >12 mg/dL) occurs in at least 12% of breast-fed infants and 4 percent of formula-fed infants whereas severe jaundice (>15 mg/dL) occurs in 2% and 0.3% of these respective feeding groups.[163]

There are a number of epidemiologic risk factors related to neonatal jaundice that have been reviewed elsewhere.[125,164-166] Risk factors include male gender, low birth weight, prematurity, polycythemia, certain ethnicities (Asian, Native American, Greek), maternal medications (e.g., oxytocin, promethazine hydrochloride), premature rupture of membranes, increased weight loss after birth, delayed passage of meconium, breast-feeding, and neonatal infection. Delivery with a vacuum extractor increases the risk for cephalohematoma and neonatal jaundice.[167] Data suggest that pancuronium is associated with an increased risk for hyperbilirubinemia.[168] A significant correlation has been found between the umbilical cord serum bilirubin level and subsequent hyperbilirubinemia.[169,170] The maternal serum bilirubin level at the time of delivery and the transplacental bilirubin gradient also correlate positively with neonatal serum bilirubin concentrations.[170] Factors associated with decreased neonatal bilirubin levels[125,171] include African race, exclusive formula feeding, gestational age of 41 weeks or older, maternal smoking, and certain drugs given to the mother (e.g., phenobarbital).

Breast-Feeding and Jaundice

Breast-feeding has clearly been identified as a factor related to neonatal jaundice,[163] and this subject has been reviewed elsewhere.[172,173] Breast-fed infants have been shown to have significantly higher serum bilirubin levels than formula-fed infants on each of the first 5 days of life,[174] and this unconjugated hyperbilirubinemia can persist for weeks[175] to months.[176,177] Jaundice during the first week of life is sometimes described as "breast-feeding jaundice" to differentiate it from "breast milk jaundice syndrome," which occurs after the first week of life.[178-180] The former is frequently associated with inadequate breast milk intake, whereas the latter generally occurs in otherwise thriving infants. There is probably overlap between these conditions and physiologic jaundice. Early reports linking breast milk and neonatal jaundice with a steroid (pregnane-3α,20β-diol) in some milk samples[181] have not been confirmed by more recent larger studies using more sensitive methods.[182] There are also conflicting data regarding efforts to attribute this jaundice to increased lipase activity in breast milk with resultant elevated levels of free fatty acids, which could inhibit hepatic glucuronosyltransferase.[183] It has been suggested that the enterohepatic circulation of bilirubin can be facilitated by the presence of β-glucuronidase[96,184] or some other substance in human milk.[185] Other factors possibly related to jaundice in breast-fed infants include caloric intake, fluid intake, weight loss, delayed passage of meconium, intestinal bacterial flora, and inhibition of bilirubin glucuronosyltransferase by an unidentified factor in the milk.[98] Lascari suggested that a healthy breast-fed infant with unconjugated hyperbilirubinemia, a normal hemoglobin concentration, reticulocyte count, and blood smear, no blood group incompatibility, and no other abnormalities on physical examination may be presumed to have early breast-feeding jaundice.[179] Because there is no specific laboratory test to confirm a diagnosis of breast milk jaundice, it is important to rule out treatable causes of jaundice before ascribing the hyperbilirubinemia to breast milk. Some infants with presumed breast milk jaundice exhibit elevated serum bile acid levels suggesting mild hepatic dysfunction or cholestasis,[186] although in general this is not the case. Breast-fed infants who are fed specific nutritional ingredients that inhibit β-glucuronidase,[99] such as L-aspartic acid, excrete more fecal bilirubin and have lower levels of jaundice[100] than do breast-fed infants who receive no supplements. No commercial preparations of these specific ingredients are presently available.

DISORDERS OF PATHOLOGIC UNCONJUGATED HYPERBILIRUBINEMIA

Disorders of Production

Isoimmunization

The most common cause of severe early jaundice is fetal-maternal blood group incompatibility with resulting isoimmunization. Maternal immunization develops when erythrocytes leak from the fetal to the maternal circulation. Fetal erythrocytes carrying different antigens are recognized as foreign by the maternal immune system, which forms antibodies against them (maternal sensitization). These antibodies (IgG immunoglobulins) cross the placental barrier into the fetal circulation and bind to fetal erythrocytes. In Rh incompatibility, sequestration plus destruction of the antibody-coated erythrocytes takes place in the reticuloendothelial system of the fetus. In ABO incompatibility, hemolysis is intravascular, complement mediated, and not usually as severe as in Rh disease.[187] Significant hemolysis can also result from incompatibilities between minor blood group antigens (e.g., Kell).[188] Although hemolysis is predominantly associated with elevation of unconjugated bilirubin, the conjugated fraction can also be elevated.[189] Any type of isoimmune hemolytic disease is a risk factor for kernicterus.[125]

Rh incompatibility problems do not usually develop until the second pregnancy; thus, prenatal blood typing and serial testing of Rh-negative mothers for the development of Rh antibodies provide important information to guide possible intrauterine care. If maternal Rh antibodies develop during pregnancy, potentially helpful measures include serial amniocentesis (with bilirubin measurement),[190,191] ultrasound assessment of the fetus,[192,193] intrauterine transfusion,[194,195] and premature delivery. The prophylactic administration of anti-D gamma globulin[196] has been most helpful in preventing Rh sensitization. A newborn infant with Rh incompatibility exhibits pallor, hepatosplenomegaly, and rapidly developing jaundice in the first hours of life. In severe cases the infant may be born with generalized edema (fetal hydrops). Laboratory findings in the neonate's blood include reticulocytosis, anemia, a positive direct Coombs test, and a rapidly rising serum bilirubin level. Conjugated hyperbilirubinemia is occasionally observed in Rh erythroblastosis, particularly when intrauterine transfusions have been administered.[117] It may be the result of exceeding the hepatic excretory capacity. Alternatively, cholestasis may also be caused by hepatic congestion from extramedullary erythropoiesis and heart failure or by tissue hypoxia from reduced hepatic blood flow and anemia.[197] In addition, cholestasis in infants with erythroblastosis fetalis may be exacerbated by secondary complications, including biliary obstruction, sepsis, and hepatic failure.[198]

Therapeutic intervention consisting of phototherapy and consideration of exchange transfusion should be initiated at lower serum bilirubin concentrations in infants with isoimmune hemolysis, and intravenous gamma globulin has been shown to reduce the need for exchange transfusions in infants with Rh and ABO hemolytic disease.[125] Serum bilirubin should be measured as frequently as every 4 hours to establish the rate of increase and to assess the effect of therapy. Exchange transfusions may be performed as emergency procedures in severe cases almost immediately after delivery to treat anemia and heart failure.

In contrast to Rh incompatibility, ABO incompatibility is usually clinically apparent with the first pregnancy.

ABO hemolytic disease is largely limited to blood group A or B infants born to group O mothers.[199] ABO hemolytic disease is relatively rare in type A or B mothers. Development of jaundice is not as rapid as with Rh disease, and a serum bilirubin level greater than 12 mg/dL on day 3 of life would be typical. Laboratory abnormalities include reticulocytosis (>10%) and a weakly positive direct Coombs test, although it is sometimes negative. Anti-A or anti-B antibodies may be seen in the serum of the newborn if examined within the first few days of life before they rapidly disappear. Spherocytes are the most prominent feature seen in a peripheral blood smear with ABO incompatibility.

Erythrocyte Enzymatic and Structural Defects

A number of specific abnormalities of RBCs can result in neonatal jaundice, including hemoglobinopathies and RBC membrane and enzyme defects. Hereditary spherocytosis is not usually a neonatal problem, but hemolytic crises can occur and be manifested as a rising bilirubin level and a falling hematocrit.[200] A family history of spherocytosis, anemia, or early gallstone disease (before 40 years of age) is helpful in suggesting this diagnosis. The characteristic spherocytes seen in the peripheral blood smear may be impossible to distinguish from those seen with ABO hemolytic disease. Other erythrocyte conditions associated with neonatal jaundice include drug-induced hemolysis, deficiencies of erythrocyte enzymes (glucose-6-phosphate dehydrogenase [G6PD] deficiency,[201,202] pyruvate kinase deficiency, and others), and hemolysis induced by vitamin K or bacteria. Recent studies of G6PD activity in African American neonates suggest that hemolysis is neither the predominate factor in the pathogenesis of hyperbilirubinemia nor predictive of hyperbilirubinemia by itself,[203] although African American male neonates may be at higher risk for hyperbilirubinemia, particularly if breast-fed and premature.[204] This emphasizes the important relationship between bilirubin excretion and serum bilirubin concentration.[205] α-Thalassemia can result in severe hemolysis and lethal hydrops fetalis.[206] β-Thalassemia may also be accompanied by hemolysis and severe neonatal hyperbilirubinemia.[207] A wide variety of clinical findings are associated with the thalassemias, from profound intrauterine hydrops and death, to mild neonatal jaundice and anemia, to no jaundice or anemia. Southeast Asian ovalocytosis has been associated with severe hyperbilirubinemia.[208] These RBC abnormalities are more likely to result in hyperbilirubinemia in the presence of Gilbert's syndrome, as described later in this chapter.

Drugs or other substances responsible for hemolysis can be passed to the fetus across the placenta or to the neonate via breast milk. Induction of labor with oxytocin has been shown to be associated with neonatal jaundice. There is a significant association between hyponatremia and jaundice in infants of mothers who received oxytocin to induce labor.[209,210] The vasopressin-like action of oxytocin prompts electrolyte and water transport such that erythrocytes swell and increased osmotic fragility and hyperbilirubinemia can result. Steroid administration at the initiation of oxytocin and 4 hours later may be helpful in preventing this hyperbilirubinemia.[211]

Infection

Bacterial sepsis increases bilirubin production through initiation of erythrocyte hemolysis or via endotoxin-mediated reduction of canalicular bile secretion resulting in a combination of conjugated and unconjugated hyperbilirubinemia. However, hyperbilirubinemia is rarely the only manifestation of bacteremia or sepsis,[212] and some data suggest that sepsis may result in lower peak levels of unconjugated bilirubin through consumption of bilirubin as an antioxidant in response to oxidant production by phagocytic cells.[213]

Sequestration

Extravascular blood within the body can be rapidly metabolized to bilirubin by tissue macrophages. Examples of this increased bilirubin production include cephalohematoma, ecchymoses, petechiae, and hemorrhage. Although the diagnosis can often be made on physical examination, occult intracranial, intestinal, or pulmonary hemorrhage can also produce hyperbilirubinemia. Similarly, swallowed blood can be converted to bilirubin by the HO of intestinal epithelium. From a red sample of bloody gastric contents, meconium, or stool, the Apt test can be used to distinguish blood of maternal or infant origin because of differences in alkali resistance between fetal and adult hemoglobin[214,215]; however, this test has low sensitivity and poor reproducibility, and an HPLC method has been shown to be superior.[216]

Polycythemia

Polycythemia can cause hyperbilirubinemia because the absolute increase in RBC mass results in elevated bilirubin production through normal rates of erythrocyte breakdown. A number of mechanisms may result in neonatal polycythemia (usually defined by a venipuncture hematocrit >65%), as reviewed by Werner.[217] Maternal-fetal transfusion during peripartum placental separation, a delay in umbilical cord clamping at birth, and twin-twin transfusion syndrome are all commonly encountered causes of polycythemia. Similarly, intrauterine hypoxia and maternal diseases such as diabetes mellitus can result in neonatal polycythemia. Therapy for symptomatic polycythemia is partial exchange transfusion, although therapy for asymptomatic polycythemia remains controversial.[218]

Disorders of Conjugation

The disorders described in this section, summarized in Tables 4-1 and 4-2, are those in which there is a primary abnormality in bilirubin metabolism without other liver disease.[219] The disorders can best be understood in the context of the normal pathway in which bilirubin is

TABLE 4-1	Comparison of Disorders of Unconjugated Hyperbilirubinemia		
	Gilbert's Syndrome	Crigler-Najjar Syndrome Type 1	Crigler-Najjar Syndrome Type 2
Prevalence	3%	Rare	Rare
Inheritance	Autosomal dominant or recessive	Autosomal recessive	Autosomal recessive, rarely dominant
Genetic defect	*UGT1A1* gene	*UGT1A1* gene	*UGT1A1* gene
Hepatocyte defect site	Microsomes ± plasma membrane	Microsomes	Microsomes
Deficient hepatocyte function	Glucuronidation ± uptake	Glucuronidation	Glucuronidation
BUGT activity	5-53% of controls	Severely decreased	2-23% of controls
Hepatocyte uptake	Decreased in 20-30%	Normal	Normal
Serum total bilirubin level (mg/dL)	0.8-4.3	15-45	8-25
Serum bilirubin decrease with phenobarbital (%)	70	0	77
HPLC SERUM BILIRUBIN COMPOSITION Normal (%)			
Unconjugated	92.6	98.8	≈100	99.1
Diglucuronide	6.2	1.1	0	0.6
Monoglucuronide	0.5	0	0	0
BILE BILIRUBIN CONJUGATES Normal (%)			
Diglucuronide	≈80	60	0 to trace	5-10
Monoglucuronide	≈15	30	Predominant if measurable	90-95
Other routine liver function tests	Normal	Normal	Normal
Prognosis	Benign	Kernicterus common	Occasional kernicterus

BUTG, bilirubin UDP-glucuronyltransferase; HPLC, high-pressure liquid chromatography.
From Suchy FJ, Sokol RJ, Balistreri WF (eds). Liver Disease in Children, 3rd ed. New York, Cambridge University Press, 2007. Used with permission.

TABLE 4-2	Comparison of Disorders of Conjugated Hyperbilirubinemia	
	Rotor's Syndrome	Dubin-Johnson Syndrome
Prevalence	Rare	Rare
Inheritance	Autosomal recessive	Autosomal recessive
Genetic defect	Unknown	*cMOAT/MRP2/ABCC2* gene
Hepatocyte defect site	GST	Apical canalicular membrane
Deficient hepatocyte function	Intracellular binding of bilirubin and conjugates	Canalicular secretion of bilirubin conjugates
Brown-black liver	No	Yes
Serum total bilirubin level (mg/dL)	2-7	1.5-6.0
Serum conjugated bilirubin (%)	>50	>50
Other routine liver function tests	Normal	Normal
Oral cholecystogram	Usually visualizes	Usually does not visualize
^{99m}Tc-HIDA cholescintigraphy		
Liver	Poor to no visualization	Intense, prolonged visualization
Gallbladder	Poor to no visualization	Delayed or nonvisualization
BSP clearance test	Serum BSP levels elevated (delayed clearance)	Serum BSP levels normal at 45 min but elevated at 90-120 min
ICG clearance test	Delayed clearance	Normal
Response to estrogens or pregnancy	No change	Increased jaundice
Total urinary coproporphyrin excretion (isomers I + III)	2.5-5.0 times increased	Normal
Urinary coproporphyrin isomer I composition (normal = 25%)	Usually <80% of total	>80% of total
Prognosis	Benign (asymptomatic)	Benign (occasional abdominal complaints—probably incidental)

BSP, bromsulfophthalein; GST, glutathione-S-transferase; HIDA, hepatobiliary iminodiacetic acid; ICG, indocyanine green.
From Suchy FJ, Sokol RJ, Balistreri WF (eds). Liver Disease in Children, 3rd ed. New York, Cambridge University Press, 2007. Used with permission.

cleared from the circulation (see Fig. 4-2). Defects in these metabolic steps are responsible for the disorders to be described in the final section of this chapter.

Gilbert's Syndrome

Clinical Findings

Gilbert's syndrome (GS, OMIM 143500) was first described in 1901 by Gilbert and Lereboullet.[220] It is characterized by a hereditary chronic or recurrent, mild unconjugated hyperbilirubinemia with otherwise normal liver function test results (for reviews see elsewhere[221-223]). The elevation in serum unconjugated bilirubin is variable and usually ranges from 1 to 4 mg/dL (1 mg/dL = 17 µmol/L). Frequently, patients are first identified when an elevated serum bilirubin level is found on screening blood chemistry or mild jaundice (perhaps only scleral icterus) is noted during a period of fasting associated with a nonspecific viral illness or religious activities.[224] Icteric plasma from a blood donor may suggest GS.[225] Alternatively, hyperbilirubinemia after liver transplantation may be a sign that the donor had GS.[226-229] GS is generally associated with no negative implications for health or longevity; however, a large variety of common symptoms have been reported by patients with GS,[230,231] including vertigo, headache, fatigue, abdominal pain, nausea, diarrhea, constipation, and loss of appetite. The possible relationship of these symptoms to GS was evaluated in a group of 2395 Swedish subjects.[232] The only symptom that was more common in GS was diarrhea in men aged 57 to 67 years. The authors suggested that this was most likely a type I error because of the large number of comparisons made and concluded that there was no higher prevalence of symptoms associated with GS. There are limited reports suggesting that GS is a risk factor for chronic fatigue syndrome.[233,234]

In two large surveys of normal individuals, approximately 3% had serum bilirubin levels greater than 1.0 mg/dL.[235,236] If the normal upper limit of serum bilirubin is defined as 1.4 mg/dL, there is a strong male preponderance (≈4:1). This finding might be related to the observation that females clear bilirubin better than males do.[237] GS may be inherited in either an autosomal dominant[238-241] or recessive[242] fashion.

Although GS is a congenital disorder, it rarely becomes clinically apparent until after puberty. The reasons for this are unknown but have been suggested to be related to the hormonal changes of puberty. Steroid hormones can suppress hepatic bilirubin clearance.[73] During pregnancy, increased estrogen levels are associated with impaired clearance of exogenous bilirubin.[243] Gonadectomy has been shown to alter BUGT activity.[244] Odell speculated that some infants with nonhemolytic neonatal jaundice are manifesting GS.[245] Use of genetic markers (see later) has allowed investigation of the role that GS plays in neonatal jaundice. Individuals carrying such markers have been shown to have a more rapid rise in their jaundice levels during the first 2 days of life,[246] a

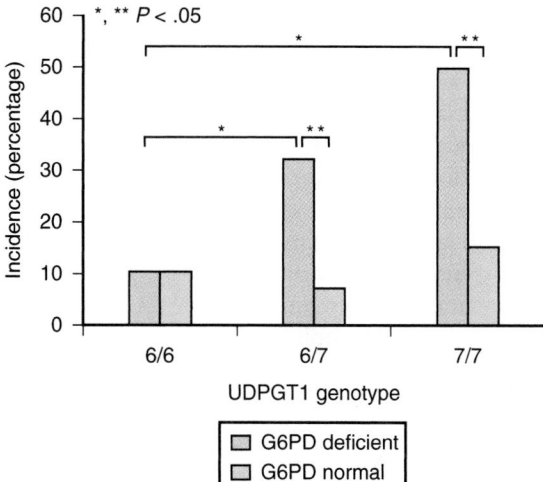

FIGURE 4-8. Incidence (percentage) of hyperbilirubinemia (serum total bilirubin ≥257 µmol/L = 15.1 mg/dL) in glucose-6-phosphate dehydrogenase (G6PD)-deficient neonates and normal controls, stratified for the three genotypes of the UGT1A1 promoter. *(Redrawn from Kaplan M, Renbaum P, Levy-Lahad E, et al. Gilbert syndrome and glucose-6-phosphate dehydrogenase deficiency: a dose-dependent genetic interaction crucial to neonatal hyperbilirubinemia. Proc Natl Acad Sci U S A 1997;94:12128-12132. Copyright © 1997, with permission from the National Academy of Sciences, U.S.A.)*

predisposition to prolonged or severe neonatal hyperbilirubinemia,[247-249] and variably increased jaundice when the GS polymorphism occurs with pyloric stenosis[250,251] or is coinherited with hematologic abnormalities such as G6PD deficiency,[205,252] β-thalassemia,[252-255] or hereditary spherocytosis.[256] Thus, studies from several different parts of the world indicate that GS, as detected by *UGT1A1* analysis, does play some role in neonatal jaundice. Kaplan and colleagues[205] noted in their study that neither G6PD deficiency nor the GS type UDPGT1 promoter polymorphism (also known as UGT1A1*28) alone increased the incidence of hyperbilirubinemia but that both in combination did (Fig. 4-8). They speculated that this gene interaction may serve as a paradigm of the interaction of benign genetic polymorphisms in the causation of disease; that is, it may take two genetic abnormalities to produce disease symptoms.

Pathophysiology

GS consists of a heterogeneous group of disorders, all of which share at least a 50% decrease in hepatic BUGT activity.[257-260] Based on plasma clearance of other organic anions (BSP and ICG) that share the same hepatocyte uptake receptor-carrier, there appear to be at least four subtypes of GS.[261,262] In GS type I, clearance of BSP and ICG is normal. In GS type II, BSP clearance is delayed but ICG clearance is normal. Because BSP uptake is normal in type II, the delayed clearance must be related to subsequent intrahepatic metabolism or canalicular excretion.[263] In GS type III, clearance of both BSP and ICG is delayed. The delay in the initial rate of disappearance from plasma suggests a defect in uptake at the hepatocyte plasma membrane.[263] Those with GS type IV have delayed uptake of ICG but not BSP. Thus, some individuals with GS have delayed uptake of bilirubin into the hepatocyte, others have delayed biotransformation, and others demonstrate both abnormalities.[53,264-266] Immunohistochemical staining for UDP-glucuronosyltransferase shows a clear reduction throughout the hepatic lobule in specimens from individuals with GS when compared with normal individualss.[267]

Elucidation of the structure of the *UGT1* gene, which encodes human bilirubin, phenol, and other UDP-glucuronosyltransferase isozymes,[268,269] led to the discovery of *UGT1A1* mutations or polymorphisms associated with GS. In white populations, the homozygous finding of an additional TA repeat in the promoter region of the so-called TATA box (i.e., [TA]$_7$TAA rather than [TA]$_6$TAA) of the *UGT1A1* gene has been shown to be a necessary, though not sufficient condition for GS.[270-272] Individuals who are heterozygous for seven TA repeats have significantly higher serum bilirubin levels than do those with the homozygous wild-type six repeats.[270] In Asian populations, the (TA)$_7$TAA mutation is relatively rare,[273] but several different *UGT1A1* mutations have been associated with GS.[241,274,275] These Asian mutations involve exon 1 of the *UGT1A1* gene rather than the TATA promoter region. One of the most common mutations in Asians, a Gly71Arg mutation in exon 1, has also linked GS and severe neonatal hyperbilirubinemia.[248] It has been reported that although the promoter TA repeat number and bilirubin level in whites have a strong positive correlation, in other ethnic groups (e.g., Africans, where two other variants, [TA]$_5$ and [TA]$_8$, have been identified) there is a negative correlation.[276] Rarely, the (TA)$_8$ variant has been reported in white individuals,[277] so the ethnic implications of these genetic polymorphisms of the *UGT1A1* gene require further analysis.

Although decreased hepatic BUGT activity is universal in GS, there is poor correlation between measured enzyme activity in the liver and the serum bilirubin level.[278] This may be explained by the increased bilirubin production associated with the decreased RBC half-life seen in as many as 40% of patients with GS.[240,266] Although early authors[258,260] concluded that there was little or no induction of BUGT after the administration of phenobarbital, more recent work has revealed that in fact, phenobarbital does increase UGT1A1 activity via a phenobarbital-responsive enhancer module (PBREM) of the *UGT1A1* promoter region[279] and that such polymorphisms could represent an additional risk factor for GS.[280]

Related to the decreased BUGT activity is the observation that duodenal bile from individuals with GS contains a decreased amount of bilirubin diglucuronides and an increased amount of bilirubin monoglucuronides in comparison to normal persons[50,53,260,281] (Fig. 4-9). This distribution is similar to that seen in infants.[282] Administration of phenobarbital has been shown to normalize the bile pigment profile in duodenal fluid,[53] lower plasma

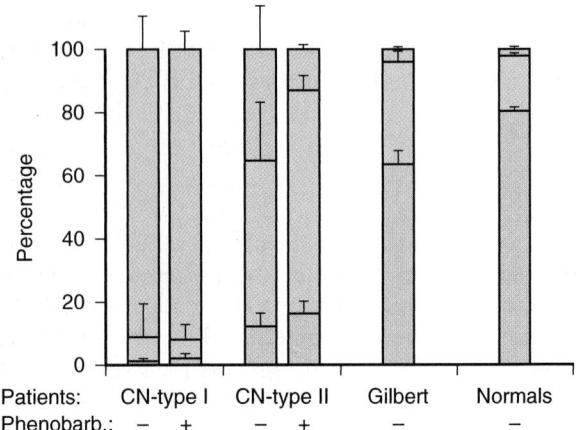

FIGURE 4-9. Bile pigment composition in bile from normal ($n = 8$), Crigler-Najjar (CN) type I ($n = 3$), CN type II ($n = 3$), and Gilbert's syndrome ($n = 16$) patients receiving (+) or not receiving (−) phenobarbital. The relative bile pigment composition is indicated in the vertical columns as a percentage of the total ± SD. Shading: red, unconjugated bilirubin; blue, bilirubin monoconjugate; green, bilirubin diconjugate. *(Redrawn from Sinaasappel M, Jansen PL. The differential diagnosis of Crigler-Najjar disease, types 1 and 2, by bile pigment analysis. Gastroenterology 1991;100:783-789. Copyright © 1991, with permission from the American Gastroenterological Association.)*

bilirubin levels, and increase hepatic clearance of bilirubin.[283,284] Clofibrate and glutethimide also normalize serum bilirubin concentrations but do not normalize the duodenal bile pigment profile.[285] In animals, clofibrate is an inducer of BUGT but does not affect BSP uptake or GST.[286] An additional unexplained phenomenon in GS is the exaggerated rise in serum bilirubin associated with fasting.[287-290] Even though normal individuals can double their serum bilirubin level in response to fasting, in GS a more pronounced rise occurs. This increase is not related to decreased hepatic blood flow because ICG clearance is not affected.[288] Although fasting can reduce BUGT activity[290] and increase HO (the enzyme responsible for bilirubin production) activity,[291] neither of these effects are believed to explain the fasting hyperbilirubinemia of GS.[283,292] The enhanced enterohepatic circulation of bilirubin is suggested to be a major factor in the pathogenesis of fasting-induced hyperbilirubinemia.[293] Intraluminal noncalorie food bulk can blunt the bilirubin rise.[294]

Diagnosis and Treatment

Generally, a diagnosis of GS can be made when there is mild, fluctuating unconjugated hyperbilirubinemia, the results of the other liver function tests are normal, and there is no hemolysis. Hemolysis can add confusion because it can result in similar findings and is not unusual in GS. Hence, other tests are sometimes used to aid in diagnosis.

One test frequently used to aid in diagnosing GS involves the intravenous administration of nicotinic acid (niacin) with assessment of the subsequent rise in serum bilirubin concentration.[295] Nicotinic acid is usually administered to adults in a dose of 50 mg[296-298] over a period of 30 seconds, although results were similar with 300-mg injections in one study.[299] Nonconjugated serum bilirubin is then measured every 30 to 60 minutes for the next 4 to 5 hours. Nicotinic acid produces a rise in serum unconjugated bilirubin in normal individuals and in those with GS. However, in GS the rise in bilirubin is higher and clearance is delayed longer than in normal people.[295,299-302] Nicotinic acid causes increased osmotic fragility and hemolysis of RBCs with sequestration in the spleen. Splenic HO is also induced, with rapid conversion of heme to bilirubin.[301] Nicotinic acid–induced hemolysis produces a rise in serum iron that is similar in healthy controls and those with GS.[302] Hence, the prolonged serum bilirubin levels are related to delayed hepatic clearance of bilirubin. Nicotinic acid infusion has been suggested to be a better method to diagnose GS than a 400-kcal fast because delayed bilirubin clearance was seen after the administration of nicotinic acid to GS subjects who otherwise had normal serum bilirubin levels.[296] The nicotinic acid test is not useful in differentiating GS from chronic liver disease because both groups showed positive tests.[303]

Rifampin, given to fasting or nonfasting adults in one oral dose of 900 mg, increases total serum bilirubin levels in normal individuals and those with GS, although there is an exaggerated rise in patients with GS (fasting: >1.9-mg/dL rise in bilirubin concentration 2 to 6 hours after rifampin; nonfasting: >1.5-mg/dL rise 4 to 6 hours after rifampin).[304] This exaggerated rise in serum bilirubin enabled differentiation of 10 normal individuals and 15 GS patients with high sensitivity and specificity. This finding could not be explained by hemolysis, although haptoglobin levels were significantly lower in GS patients, compatible with baseline hemolysis.

Another test suggested to aid in the diagnosis of GS involves fractionation of total serum bilirubin by alkaline methanolysis and thin-layer chromatography.[77,189] This test allows precise measurement of conjugated and unconjugated bilirubin levels. This approach has shown that in GS, approximately 6% of the total serum bilirubin is conjugated, as opposed to about 17% in normal persons and those with chronic hemolysis. Individuals with chronic persistent hepatitis had 28% of their total bilirubin present as conjugates. Fasting did not change the percentage of conjugates in GS despite the rise in total serum bilirubin concentration. An overlap of only three individuals was seen among the 77 with GS and 60 normal subjects.[189] Other studies support these findings.[305] In patients with GS, fractionation of total serum bilirubin by HPLC showed significantly decreased bilirubin monoglucuronides (1.1% versus 6.2% in normal individuals) and increased unconjugated bilirubin (98.8% versus 92.6% in normal individuals).[306]

Monaghan and associates[247] have suggested GS genetic screening for the *UGT1A1* TA repeat as a simple, useful additional test in the investigation of very prolonged neonatal jaundice in North American, African,

and European populations and for the Gly71Arg mutation in Asians. However, the value of such a genetic test cannot be fully determined until accurate data regarding the prevalence and penetrance of the GS genotype are known.[307] Thus, genetic testing for GS cannot be routinely recommended.[307]

GS has no significant negative implications regarding morbidity or mortality. In general, drug metabolism studies have revealed no major dangers,[305,308] although there appears to be an increased incidence of slow acetylators[309,310] and clearance of lorazepam is decreased 20% to 40%.[311] Concurrent genetic deficiencies in other xenobiotic pathways may put individuals with GS at increased risk for drug toxicity with compounds such as acetaminophen,[312,313] the cancer chemotherapeutic agents CPT-11 (irinotecan)[314] and TAS-103,[315] or the viral protease inhibitor indinavir.[219,316] For this reason, Bosma suggests that screening for GS is of clinical importance.[219] No specific treatment is necessary for GS, although phenobarbital has been shown to lower serum bilirubin levels in these patients.[317] If the well-documented antioxidant effect of bilirubin[318] provides a biologic advantage,[319] the mild hyperbilirubinemia of GS might actually be a significant benefit in patients with conditions such as vascular disease,[320,321] in which free radicals are involved in the pathogenesis. However, Bosma concluded that a selective advantage in GS because of the antioxidant capacity of bilirubin seems unlikely.[219]

Crigler-Najjar Syndrome Types I and II

In 1952, Crigler and Najjar described seven infants with congenital familial nonhemolytic jaundice in whom severe unconjugated hyperbilirubinemia developed shortly after birth, with death from kernicterus ensuing within months.[322] These infants were from three related families. The serum bilirubin concentration reached 25 to 35 mg/dL despite a lack of hemolytic disease. Other liver function test results were normal. Liver histology was normal except for the deposition of bile pigments. Subsequent reports documented that the main risk in patients with Crigler-Najjar syndrome (CN) is kernicterus.[1] An excellent review of the neurologic perspectives of CN has been published.[323] Although some patients survive into the second decade with normal development,[324] the possibility of kernicterus developing late is always a concern, even in adulthood.[325-328] Serum bilirubin levels vary from approximately 15 to 45 mg/dL.

In 1969, Arias and co-authors described a second, more frequent type of severe nonhemolytic hyperbilirubinemia.[329] The previous syndrome was termed Crigler-Najjar syndrome type I (CNI, OMIM 218800), whereas the new findings were termed Crigler-Najjar syndrome type II (CNII, OMIM 606785) or Arias' syndrome.[329] Hyperbilirubinemia is less severe in type II patients and varies from approximately 8 to 25 mg/dL. Hence, these individuals have a much lower incidence of kernicterus, but such damage does occur.[330,331]

Pathophysiology

Both CNI and CNII are generally inherited in an autosomal recessive manner, although one case of autosomal dominant inheritance of CNII has been reported.[332] CNI and CNII result from mutations in the *UGT* gene complex.[43] Patients with one normal allele demonstrate normal metabolism of bilirubin.[333] The genetic details determine the severity of clinical disease. In CNI there is complete absence of functional UGT1A1, whereas in CNII, UGT1A1 activity is markedly reduced.[334] In CNI, 18 of 23 mutations described in the *UGT1* gene are found in the common exons 2 to 5 (see Fig. 4-4) and thus affect many UGT1 enzymes.[43,335] Intronic mutations causing CNI have also been reported.[336] However, in CNII, four of nine known mutations are found in exon 1A1. There is some overlap in classification of mild CNII and GS (e.g., Gly71Arg) that relates to differences in definitions based on serum bilirubin levels.[43] The TATA box (TA)$_7$ repeat mutation found in GS can be seen along with other mutations resulting in either CNI or CNII.[337] In both CNI and CNII, assays of liver tissue from affected patients demonstrate negligible or very low BUGT activity.[50,51,260,326,329,338,339] Therefore, patients with these disorders experience a profound block in bilirubin excretion because they lack the ability to conjugate bilirubin with UDPGA. Thus, liver biopsy is not helpful in differentiating CNI and CNII. Study of resected livers from four patients with CNI after liver transplantation showed that there was heterogeneous glucuronidation of various substrates other than bilirubin.[340] Hence, several of the family of glucuronosyltransferase isoenzymes can be affected in the same patient. There is considerable overlap of hepatic BUGT activity between CNII and GS[260] (see Table 4-2).

In family studies of CNI patients,[341,342] partial deficiencies in the glucuronidation of salicylate and menthol have been found in siblings, parents, and grandparents. As a result, it has generally been accepted that this condition is inherited in an autosomal recessive manner.[341] In family studies of CNII patients, the original report by Arias and colleagues found abnormalities in glucuronidation (menthol) in only one parent, thus suggesting autosomal dominant inheritance. Subsequent studies of siblings or parents often found elevated serum bilirubin levels (1.2 to 4 mg/dL), delayed bilirubin clearance, and decreased hepatic BUGT activity, as would be seen in GS.[284,326,329,331,343,344] These findings in both parents[284,343] suggested that CNII may represent homozygous GS. However, if CNII were truly the homozygous form of GS, one would expect many more affected individuals because GS occurs in at least 3% of the population. Pertinent genetic data have been reviewed[337] and support the inheritance mode of CNII as autosomal recessive.

The major differentiating characteristic between CNI and CNII is the response to drugs that stimulate hyperplasia of the ER. When CNII patients received phenobarbital or diphenylhydantoin, there was a significant decline in the serum bilirubin level, increased hepatic clearance of radiolabeled bilirubin,[284,329,330,345-348] and increased biliary levels of bilirubin diglucuronides[50,331] (see Fig. 4-9). In a study of five CNII patients, the magnitude of the phenobarbital-induced decrease in serum bilirubin ranged from 2.1 to 12.1 mg/dL (27% to 72%), with prephenobarbital and postphenobarbital serum bilirubin levels ranging from 7.8 to 16.9 and 4.7 to 10.1 mg/dL, respectively.[50] Data from seven earlier studies[284,329,330,345-348] regarding the response of CNII patients to oral phenobarbital revealed that 11 females and 13 males had a total serum bilirubin level of 15.7 ± 13.8 mg/dL (mean ± SD) before the administration of phenobarbital. After doses ranging from 90 to 390 mg/day or, alternatively, 4 mg/kg/day, serum bilirubin decreased 12.0 ± 4.0 mg/dL (77% ± 13%). The lowest total serum bilirubin after phenobarbital therapy was 5.9 mg/dL. In contrast, CNI patients show neither a decrease in serum bilirubin nor significantly increased biliary bilirubin conjugates in response to drugs[50,325] (see Fig. 4-9). The response to phenobarbital is the criterion used to differentiate between these two disorders.[349] Bile analysis has also been suggested as another method to differentiate CNI and CNII.[50] In CNI, bile contains insignificant bilirubin conjugates (<10%), and unconjugated bilirubin predominates. In CNII, bile contains small amounts of bilirubin conjugates, and those present are predominantly bilirubin monoglucuronides (>60%).[260]

Two cousins with CN have been described with unique features that raise the possibility of a new variant of this syndrome (type III).[350] This new variant resembled CNI in that there was no biliary excretion of bilirubin diglucuronide or monoglucuronide. However, the type III patients did excrete monoglucoside and diglucoside conjugates of bilirubin. It has been speculated that type III patients lack the long proposed permease[41] that has been hypothesized to transport UDPGA to the luminal side of the ER where glucuronosyltransferase is located. This absence is suggested to force utilization of a very inefficient substrate for conjugation to bilirubin, UDPG.

Diagnosis and Treatment

Although CN can be diagnosed during the prenatal period,[351,352] evaluation of infants with CN more typically begins during the first days of life when serum bilirubin levels exceed 20 mg/dL. The conjugated fraction will not be elevated except possibly for the factitious elevation sometimes seen when the total serum bilirubin level is very high.[110] Evaluation of such infants will eliminate hemolysis, hypothyroidism, infection, and other more common causes of jaundice. Formula feedings will help identify infants with jaundice related to human milk. During this period of testing, the magnitude of the elevation in serum bilirubin will prompt the use of phototherapy to avoid kernicterus.[130] Exchange transfusion may be necessary. Yet despite these efforts, CN patients will have persistent jaundice. There is currently no widely available, simple clinical test to confirm a diagnosis of CN. CN can be excluded by finding significant amounts of bilirubin conjugates in neonatal stool if collected before the establishment of sufficient intestinal bacteria to convert bilirubin conjugates to urobilinoids.[1] HPLC analysis of duodenal bile will show that in CNI there are negligible bilirubin diglucuronides or monoglucuronides whereas in CNII these conjugates are present but in low concentration.[43,50] An easy method to collect such fluid for analysis involves use of the pediatric Enterotest capsule.[281] This approach to diagnosis is much less invasive than performing a liver biopsy to confirm negligible BUGT activity in an in vitro assay. The ratio of serum bilirubin conjugates (as determined by alkaline methanolysis with thin-layer chromatography) to total bilirubin, though abnormally low, does not allow differentiation of CN patients from those with GS.[189] Similar overlap occurs with HPLC fractionation of serum bilirubin conjugates.[306] DNA analysis can be very helpful in establishing the correct diagnosis,[353] and in the future it is expected that DNA array technology will allow rapid screening for known mutations.

A world registry of patients with CNI aimed at developing management guidelines has been published.[354] Phenobarbital (4 mg/kg/day in infants) should be used when there is concern about deficiency of BUGT. Within 48 hours, CNII patients can demonstrate a significant decrease in serum bilirubin levels (as detailed earlier) and increased biliary excretion of bilirubin diglucuronide and monoglucuronide,[51,331] whereas CNI patients will show no significant response. Occasionally, CNII patients do not respond to the first trial of phenobarbital therapy, but subsequent trials months later will demonstrate a significant decrease in serum bilirubin levels.[349] However, despite the decrease in serum bilirubin in response to phenobarbital, CNII patients will usually continue to manifest significant hyperbilirubinemia (approximately 5 to 15 mg/dL). Phototherapy for 6 to 12 hours daily has been the primary modality to keep serum bilirubin levels below 20 mg/dL during the first several months of life[355] because CNI patients can excrete all bilirubin photoisomers.[356] CNI patients will require lifelong treatment with phototherapy until more definitive therapy such as liver transplantation is available. Phototherapy has been found to be least intrusive when given at night, and improvements have been made in effectiveness and comfort.[357,358] Although phototherapy is very helpful in infancy, in adolescence, social inconvenience and compliance problems can increase the risk for kernicterus.[354]

Other therapeutic considerations involve the oral administration of binding agents such as agar, cholestyramine, or calcium phosphate.[359-362] These agents bind to bilirubin in the intestinal lumen as a result of phototherapy or through direct intestinal permeation.[363] They prevent the enterohepatic circulation of bilirubin. Problems associated with the use of cholestyramine include cost, taste, and concern about bile salt depletion and fat

malabsorption. Problems regarding agar include significant variation in bilirubin binding affinity among various preparations and batches.[326,359,364] During acute episodes of severe hyperbilirubinemia after the first year of life, plasmapheresis has been shown to rapidly decrease serum bilirubin levels.[326,365] Peritoneal dialysis and exchange transfusion have not been helpful in this setting.[325] Repeated intramuscular injections of tin-protoporphyrin, an HO inhibitor that blocks bilirubin formation, have been used in one CNI patient, with data suggesting a decreased need for phototherapy.[366] Two patients with CNI were treated with tin-mesoporphyrin to block bilirubin formation and also underwent daily phototherapy and intermittent plasmapheresis over a 400-day period.[367] Iron deficiency anemia believed to be due to the porphyrin therapy developed in these patients,[368] but tin-mesoporphyrin (stannsoporfin) (6 μmol/kg or 4.5 mg/kg)[369] is suggested to be a promising, though still experimental additional therapy for controlling episodes of acute, severe jaundice.[370] Drugs that bind to albumin and can potentially displace bilirubin should be avoided at all times.[371]

Because patients with CN have good hepatic function other than conjugating bilirubin, they are ideal candidates for auxiliary liver transplantation. This option has recently become clinically available.[372-374] More commonly, orthotopic liver transplantation has been performed,[375-382] and this represents the only true cure for the hyperbilirubinemia of CNI. Ideally, transplantation would be timed so that it precedes irreversible neurologic injury.[383,384] Transplantation of other BUGT-containing tissues (e.g., segments of the small intestine,[385,386] kidneys,[387] or hepatocytes[388]) remains experimental. Successful cloning of the gene responsible for bilirubin glucuronosyltransferase activity offers the hope of future gene therapy to correct this deficiency based on studies in Gunn rats, the congenitally jaundiced model for CNI.[383,389-391]

Disorders of Enterohepatic Circulation

Increased enterohepatic circulation of bilirubin is believed to be an important factor in neonatal jaundice. As previously reviewed, neonates are at risk for intestinal absorption of bilirubin because (1) their bile contains increased levels of bilirubin monoglucuronide, which allows easier conversion to bilirubin; (2) they have significant amounts of β-glucuronidase within the intestinal lumen that hydrolyzes bilirubin conjugates to bilirubin, which is then more easily absorbed from the intestine; (3) they lack the intestinal flora to convert bilirubin conjugates to urobilinoids; and (4) meconium, the intestinal contents accumulated during gestation, contains significant amounts of bilirubin.[392] Conditions that prolong passage of meconium (e.g., Hirschsprung's disease, meconium ileus, meconium plug syndrome) are associated with hyperbilirubinemia.[393,394] Earlier passage of meconium has been shown to be associated with lower serum bilirubin levels.[395,396] This may be facilitated by rectal temperature measurement during the neonatal period.[397] The enterohepatic circulation of bilirubin can be blocked by the enteral administration of compounds that bind bilirubin, such as agar,[89,359,364,398] charcoal,[399] and cholestyramine.[360]

Other Causes of Unconjugated Hyperbilirubinemia

Various hormones may cause the development of neonatal unconjugated hyperbilirubinemia. Congenital hypothyroidism can be accompanied by serum bilirubin levels higher than 12 mg/dL before the development of other clinical findings.[400] Prolonged jaundice is seen in a third of infants with congenital hypothyroidism.[401] Similarly, hypopituitarism and anencephaly may be associated with jaundice as a result of inadequate thyroxine, which is necessary for hepatic clearance of bilirubin.

Certain drugs may affect the metabolism of bilirubin and result in hyperbilirubinemia or displacement of bilirubin from albumin. Such displacement increases the risk for kernicterus and can be caused by sulfonamides,[402] moxalactam,[403] and ceftriaxone[404] (independent of its sludge-producing effect[405]). The popular Chinese herb Chuen-Lin, given to 28% to 51% of Chinese newborn infants, has been shown to have a significant effect in displacing bilirubin from albumin.[406] Pancuronium bromide[168] and chloral hydrate[407] have been suggested as causes of neonatal hyperbilirubinemia.

Infants of diabetic mothers have higher peak bilirubin levels and a greater frequency of hyperbilirubinemia than normal neonates do.[408] These patients have shown a positive correlation between total bilirubin and hematocrit, thus implicating polycythemia as a possible mechanism.[408] Other potential causes of this hyperbilirubinemia include prematurity, deficiency of substrate for glucuronidation (secondary to hypoglycemia), and poor hepatic perfusion (secondary to either respiratory distress, persistent fetal circulation, or cardiomyopathy).

The Lucey-Driscoll syndrome[409] consists of neonatal hyperbilirubinemia within families in whom there is in vitro inhibition of glucuronosyltransferase by both maternal and infant serum. It is presumed to be caused by gestational hormones.

Prematurity is frequently associated with unconjugated hyperbilirubinemia in the neonatal period. Hepatic UDP-glucuronosyltransferase activity is markedly decreased in premature infants and rises steadily from 30 weeks' gestation until reaching adult levels 14 weeks after birth.[410] In addition, there may be deficiencies in both uptake[411] and secretion.[412] Bilirubin clearance improves rapidly after birth.[413]

Hepatic hypoperfusion can result in neonatal jaundice. Inadequate perfusion of the hepatic sinusoids may not allow sufficient hepatocyte uptake and metabolism of bilirubin. Causes might include patent ductus venosus,[414] congestive heart failure, and portal vein thrombosis.

Box 4-1	Causes of Neonatal Hyperbilirubinemia

INCREASED PRODUCTION OF BILIRUBIN

Fetal-maternal blood group incompatibilities
Extravascular blood in body tissues
Polycythemia
Red blood cell abnormalities (hemoglobinopathies, membrane and enzyme defects)
Induction of labor

DECREASED EXCRETION OF BILIRUBIN

Increased enterohepatic circulation of bilirubin
Breast-feeding
Inborn errors of metabolism
Hormones and drugs
Prematurity
Hepatic hypoperfusion
Cholestatic syndromes
Obstruction of the biliary tree

COMBINED INCREASED PRODUCTION AND DECREASED EXCRETION OF BILIRUBIN

Sepsis
Intrauterine infection
Congenital cirrhosis

From Suchy FJ, Sokol RJ, Balistreri WF (eds). Liver Disease in Children, 3rd ed. New York, Cambridge University Press, 2007. Used with permission.

Other specific liver diseases, as listed in Box 4-1 and described elsewhere in this text, can result in neonatal jaundice.

MANAGEMENT AND TREATMENT OF UNCONJUGATED HYPERBILIRUBINEMIA

Phototherapy

In recent years, changes in perinatal care have made severe neonatal jaundice a larger problem, and there has been a re-emergence of kernicterus.[415-417] Possible reasons[417,418] include (1) early hospital discharge (before the extent of jaundice is known and signs of impending brain damage have appeared)[419]; (2) lack of adequate concern for the risks associated with severe jaundice in healthy term and near-term newborns[416]; (3) an increase in the incidence of breast-feeding[173]; (4) medical care cost constraints; (5) a paucity of educational materials to enable parents to participate in safeguarding their newborns; (6) limitations within health care systems in monitoring the outpatient progression of jaundice[420]; (7) difficulty estimating the degree of jaundice, particularly in dark-skinned infants[421]; and (8) demonstration of bilirubin being an antioxidant.[20] There are case reports of newborn infants who, following early hospital discharge, develop severe hyperbilirubinemia (30-40 mg/dL) at home and present with classic signs of kernicterus.[1,125,416,422-425] This has been reported in otherwise healthy breast-fed infants with no other identified cause of their jaundice.[426-428] Although early postpartum discharge has advantages, one disadvantage is the risk associated with the delayed diagnosis of severe hyperbilirubinemia. The American Academy of Pediatrics has recommended that infants discharged at younger than 48 hours of age be seen in follow-up within 48 hours of discharge.[429] Many physicians do not follow these recommendations[125,430] despite the serious impact that a short hospital stay has on a jaundiced newborn.[431] The Academy updated its 1994 guideline[432] for the management of hyperbilirubinemia in newborn infants in 2004.[125]

Jaundice can be caused by increased bilirubin production, decreased bilirubin excretion, or a combination of these mechanisms (see Box 4-1 for specific examples). An approach to the management of jaundice in the newborn nursery has been published elsewhere.[125] Although Newman and associates found that obtaining a direct bilirubin measurement was seldom helpful because of low yield and poor specificity,[433] others advocate early measurement of conjugated bilirubin as a population screening test that could lead to earlier diagnosis of neonatal liver disease.[434] Bhutani and colleagues advocated universal bilirubin measurement before hospital discharge to identify infants at risk for severe neonatal hyperbilirubinemia on the basis of a predischarge hour-specific total serum bilirubin measurement[435,436] (Fig. 4-10). Such universal predischarge screening is now recommended by the American Academy of Pediatrics[125] and has been shown in a recent study to reduce the incidence of significant hyperbilirubinemia and the rate of hospital readmission of infants for the treatment of jaundice.[437] Despite the large number of causes of neonatal jaundice, no cause of jaundice could be identified in nearly half of the infants evaluated during one study of 447 infants[101] and in a third of the infants in a kernicterus registry.[428]

Hyperbilirubinemia is the most frequent reason that infants are readmitted to the hospital in the first weeks of life.[419,438,439] Management of neonatal jaundice has been reviewed elsewhere[125] (Figs. 4-11 and 4-12). The most important step in treatment of jaundice is determination of the primary cause. However, independent of the cause of the jaundice, elevation of the serum unconjugated bilirubin fraction prompts concern about possible kernicterus. As previously reviewed,[136,145] when the unconjugated bilirubin fraction is elevated, care must be taken to avoid the administration of agents that bind to albumin and displace bilirubin, thereby promoting kernicterus. Although sulfonamides are historically the most well known bilirubin-displacing agents, drugs such as ceftriaxone and ibuprofen are also strong bilirubin displacers with a potential for inducing bilirubin encephalopathy.[404,440] Therapeutic options to lower unconjugated bilirubin levels include phototherapy, exchange transfusion, interruption of the enterohepatic circulation, enzyme induction, and alteration of breast-feeding. Research into these and other modalities continues actively. The outcome of rational therapeutic guidelines for unconjugated hyperbilirubinemia during the first 7 days of life has been published elsewhere.[441]

Phototherapy consists of irradiation of the jaundiced infant with light and has been reviewed.[442,443] Photon energy derived from light changes the structure of the bilirubin molecule in two ways (Fig. 4-13) that allow bilirubin to be excreted into bile or urine without the usual requirement for hepatic glucuronidation. One change involves a 180-degree rotation around the double bonds between either the A and B or the C and D rings[444] to convert the normal Z configuration to the E configuration. 4Z,15E-bilirubin is formed preferentially and can spontaneously reisomerize to native bilirubin. More

FIGURE 4-10. Risk designation of term and near-term well newborns based on their hour-specific serum bilirubin values. *(Redrawn from Bhutani VK, Johnson L, Sivieri EM. Predictive ability of a predischarge hour-specific serum bilirubin for subsequent significant hyperbilirubinemia in healthy term and near-term newborns. Pediatrics 1999;103:6-14. Reproduced with permission from Pediatrics 2004;114:297-316; Copyright © 2004 by the American Academy of Pediatrics.)*

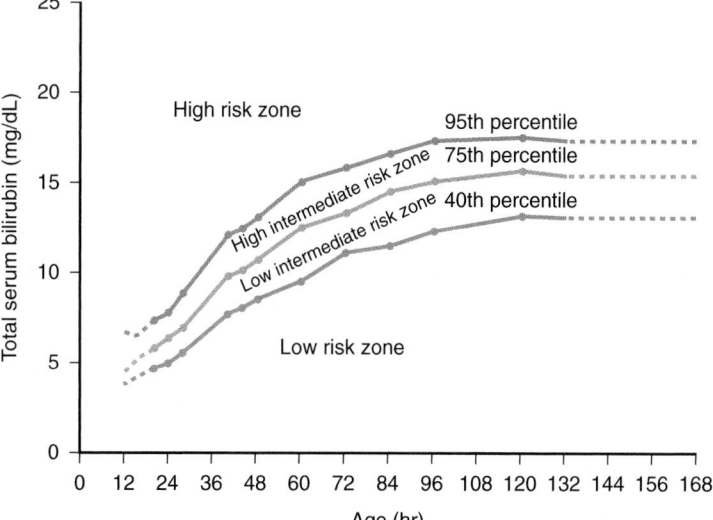

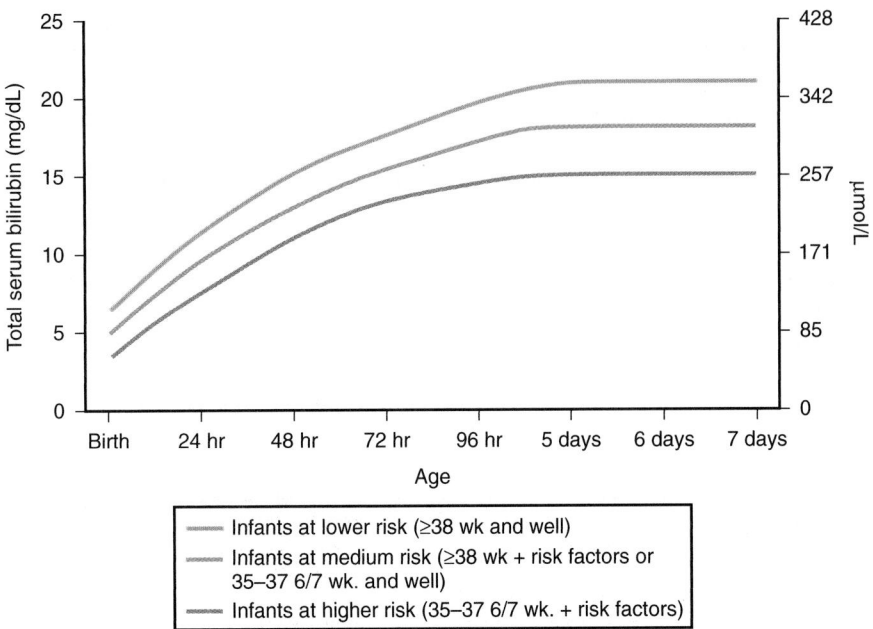

FIGURE 4-11. Guidelines for phototherapy in hospitalized infants of 35 or more weeks' gestation. These guidelines are based on limited evidence and the levels shown are approximations. The guidelines refer to the use of intensive phototherapy, which should be used when total serum bilirubin (TSB) exceeds the line indicated for each category. "Intensive phototherapy" implies irradiance in the blue-green spectrum (wavelengths of approximately 430 to 490 nm) of at least 30 µW/cm²/nm (measured at the infant's skin directly below the center of the phototherapy unit) and delivered to as much of the infant's surface area as possible. If TSB does not decrease or continues to rise in an infant who is undergoing intensive phototherapy, the presence of hemolysis is strongly suggested. In infants who receive phototherapy and have an elevated direct-reacting or conjugated bilirubin levels (cholestatic jaundice), the bronze-baby syndrome may develop. Total bilirubin should be used without subtracting direct-reacting or conjugated bilirubin. Risk factors include isoimmune hemolytic disease, glucose-6-phosphate dehydrogenase deficiency, asphyxia, significant lethargy, temperature instability, sepsis, acidosis, or albumin less than 3.0 g/dL. For well infants 35 to 37⁶/₇ weeks, TSB levels can be adjusted for intervention around the medium-risk line. It is an option to intervene at lower TSB levels for infants closer to 35 weeks and at higher TSB levels for those closer to 37⁶/₇ weeks. It is also an option to provide conventional phototherapy in the hospital or at home with TSB levels of 2 to 3 mg/dL (35 to 50 µmol/L) below those shown, but home phototherapy should not be used in any infant with risk factors. *(Reproduced with permission from Pediatrics 2004;114:297-316; Copyright © 2004 by the American Academy of Pediatrics.)*

importantly, a new seven-membered ring structure can be formed between rings A and B and result in "lumirubin"[445] or "cyclobilirubin"[446] via the 4E,15Z-isomer intermediate.[447] This isomerization interferes with the internal hydrogen bonding of native bilirubin and, by exposing the propionic acid groups, results in a more polar compound. Thus, the lumirubin and E-isomers can be excreted directly into bile. Lumirubin appears to be the major route by which bilirubin is eliminated via phototherapy.[448,449] The choice of light for phototherapy is a subject about which there are much conflicting data.[442] Special Blue light (or Super Blue, but not regular blue) appears to be better than white or green light, although white is less disturbing to nursery personnel.[450] New phototherapy devices using woven fiberoptic pads are currently available,[451] are effective (comparable to conventional phototherapy) and safe, eliminate the need for eye patches, and permit greater time for maternal-infant bonding.[452-454] Proposed guidelines for phototherapy have been published elsewhere.[455-457] In general, phototherapy is used to prevent serum bilirubin concentrations from reaching levels necessitating exchange transfusion (see

Fig. 4-12). Phototherapy is now frequently performed at home,[458,459] a practice accepted and recommended by the American Academy of Pediatrics.[125] Despite documented complications,[460-462] phototherapy is widely used and generally safe.[463] Although phototherapy does affect cardiac output and blood flow to other organs (e.g., increased cerebral blood flow) and may be associated with opening of the ductus arteriosus, these effects are not generally problematic.[464,465] In extremely premature infants (<800-g birth weight), prolonged phototherapy and low peak serum bilirubin levels (<9.4 mg/dL) were shown in one study to be independently associated with blindness.[466] This could possibly be related to the direct effects of light on the unshielded immature eye or decreased antioxidant protection by low serum bilirubin levels. Phototherapy should not be used without previous diagnostic evaluation of the cause of the jaundice. The shielding of phototherapy units should never be removed because of the ultraviolet radiation hazards that can result.[467] Although it has been recommended that infant position be changed every 6 hours during phototherapy,[468] data from one study showed that position change

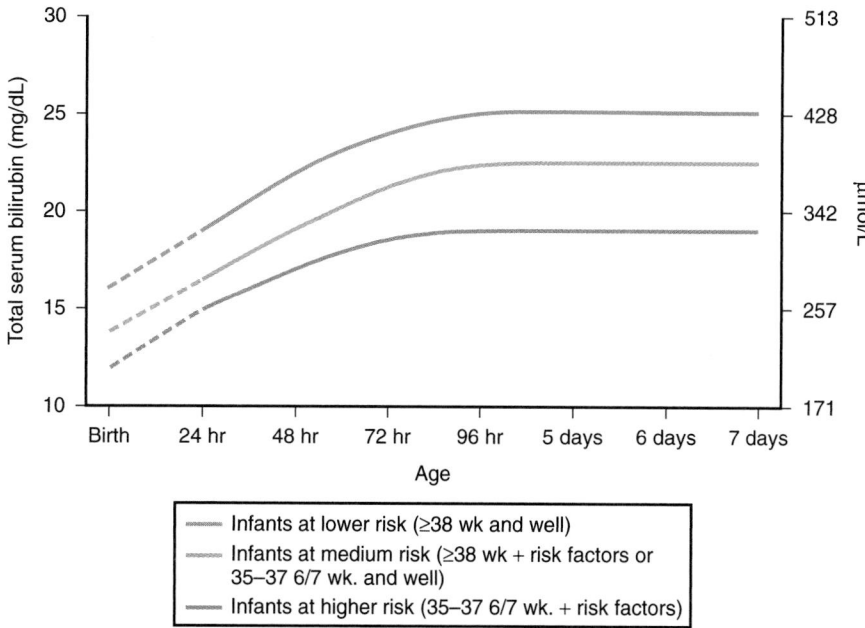

FIGURE 4-12. Guidelines for exchange transfusion in infants 35 or more weeks' gestation. These suggested levels are based on limited evidence, and the levels shown are approximations. During birth hospitalization, exchange transfusion is recommended if total serum bilirubin (TSB) rises to these levels despite intensive phototherapy. For readmitted infants, if the TSB level is above the exchange level, TSB measurement should be repeated every 2 to 3 hours and exchange transfusion considered if TSB remains above the levels indicated after intensive phototherapy for 6 hours. The *dashed lines* for the first 24 hours indicate uncertainty because of a wide range of clinical circumstances and a range of responses to phototherapy. Immediate exchange transfusion is recommended if the infant shows signs of acute bilirubin encephalopathy (hypertonia, arching, retrocollis, opisthotonos, fever, high-pitched cry) or if TSB is 5 mg/dL (85 μmol/L) or greater above these lines. Risk factors include isoimmune hemolytic disease, glucose-6-phosphate dehydrogenase deficiency, asphyxia, significant lethargy, temperature instability, sepsis, and acidosis. Total bilirubin should be used without subtracting direct-reacting or conjugated bilirubin. If the infant is well and 35 to 37⁶/₇ weeks (median risk), TSB levels can be individualized for exchange based on actual gestational age. *(Reproduced with permission from Pediatrics 2004;114:297-316; Copyright © 2004 by the American Academy of Pediatrics.)*

made no difference in serum bilirubin levels.[469] One study of 264 neonates (some with hemolytic jaundice) who completed an average of 121 hours of phototherapy indicated that significant rebound hyperbilirubinemia did not occur.[470] Similarly, no significant rebound hyperbilirubinemia occurred in 163 healthy full-term infants with nonhemolytic jaundice (including breast-feeding and formula and mixed feeding) who underwent an average of 54 to 65 hours of phototherapy.[471] In term, healthy newborns, phototherapy may be stopped when the serum bilirubin level falls below 14 to 15 mg/dL, and hospital discharge need not be delayed to observe for rebound.[432]

Exchange Transfusion

Exchange transfusion is the most rapid method to acutely lower the serum bilirubin concentration. Indications for exchange transfusion vary, have been published elsewhere,[125,456,460,472,473] and can be related to either anemia or elevated serum bilirubin levels. The American Academy of Pediatrics has published guidelines that represent the most widely accepted indications for initiation of exchange transfusion based on risk factors, including the hour-specific total bilirubin level, response to intensive phototherapy, serum bilirubin-to-albumin ratio, and the presence of hemolytic disease, sepsis, acidosis, or other acute conditions (see Fig. 4-12). Additionally, exchange transfusion should be initiated if the infant displays signs of acute bilirubin encephalopathy (see the section "Kernicterus"). In neonatal hemolytic disease, suggested indications for transfusion include (1) anemia (hematocrit <45%), positive direct Coombs test, and bilirubin greater than 4 mg/dL in cord blood; (2) postnatal rise in serum bilirubin concentration that exceeds 1 mg/dL/hr for more than 6 hours; (3) progressive anemia and rate of increase in serum bilirubin greater than 0.5 mg/dL/hr; and (4) continuing progression of anemia despite control of hyperbilirubinemia. Sometimes, exchange transfusion for hemolytic disease can be avoided through the use of high-dose intravenous immunoglobulin therapy.[474] Suggested indications for exchange transfusion because of hyperbilirubinemia alone include (1) bilirubin concentration higher than 15 mg/dL for more than 48 hours, (2) salicylate saturation index higher than 8.0 or 2(4'-hydroxyazobenzene) benzoic acid (HABA) binding less than 50% on two successive determinations 4 hours apart, (3) ratio of total serum bilirubin (mg/dL) to total serum protein (g/dL) greater than 3.7, and (4) molar concentration ratio of serum bilirubin to serum albumin of greater than 0.7.[460]

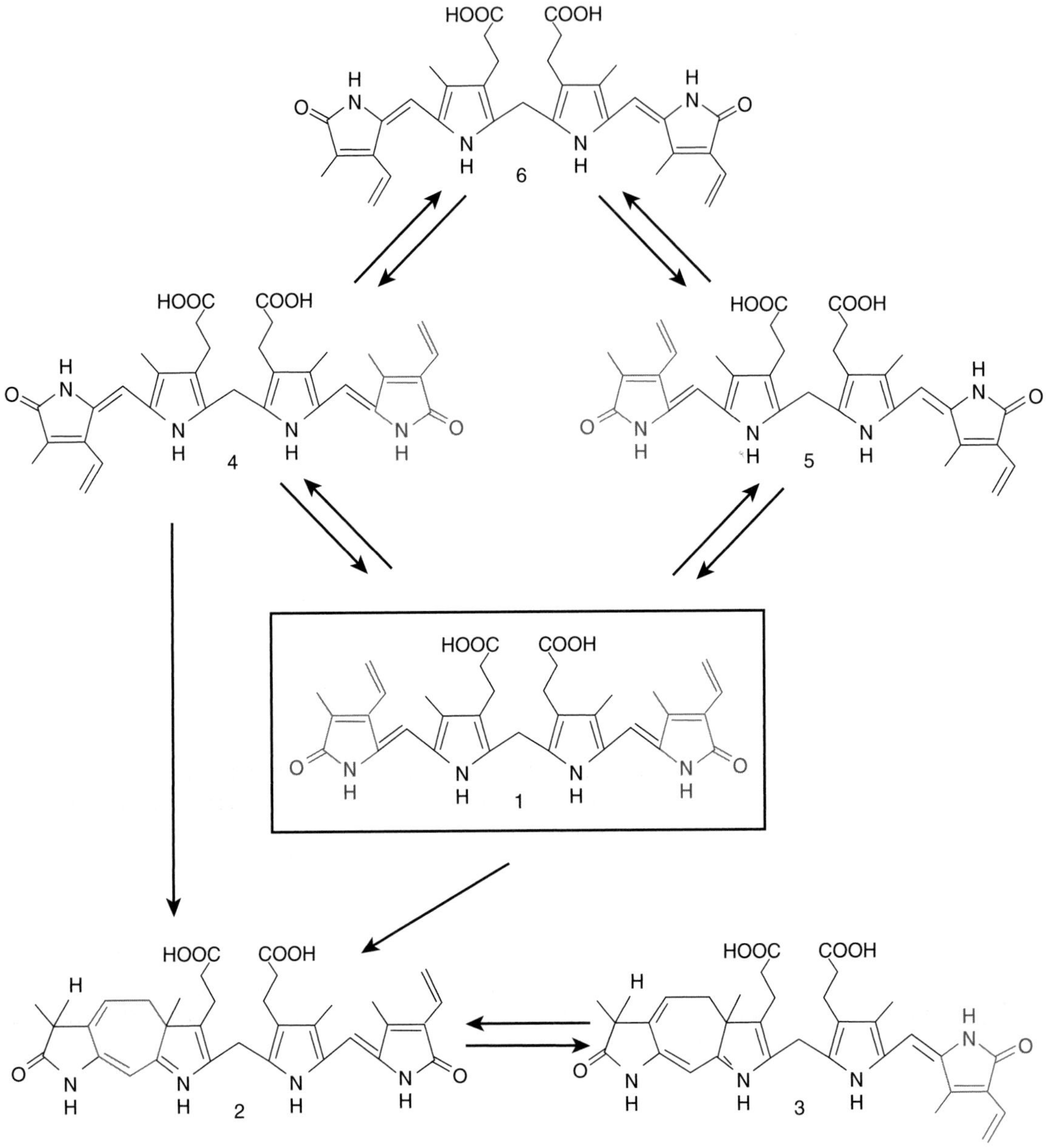

FIGURE 4-13. Products of phototherapy. Light induces isomerization of 4Z,15Z-bilirubin (1) to produce the configurational isomers 4E,15Z-bilirubin (4), 4Z,15E-bilirubin (5), and 4E,15E-bilirubin (6) and the structural isomers Z-lumirubin (2) and E-lumirubin (3) as shown. Isomerization exposes one or both of the propionic acid side chains, which increases the polarities of the isomers with respect to biosynthetic bilirubin (1) and allows excretion in bile without hepatic glucuronidation. The formation of 4E,15Z-bilirubin, 4Z,15E-bilirubin, and 4E,15E-bilirubin is reversible, and these isomers spontaneously revert to the parent 4Z,15Z-bilirubin (1) isomer after excretion in bile. The predominant isomer present in the circulation of infants exposed to light or phototherapy is 4Z,15E-bilirubin (5). Although the structural isomers (2 and 3) are formed more slowly than the configurational isomers, they may contribute more to the overall effect of the treatment because of their relatively faster excretion. *(Redrawn from McDonagh A. Phototherapy: From ancient Egypt to the new millennium. J Perinatol 2001;21:S7-S12. Modified with the author's assistance and permission and reprinted by permission from Macmillan Publishers Ltd: J Perinatol 2001;21:S7-S12, copyright 2001.)*

Although there are many well-described risks with exchange transfusion, mortality should be low (<0.6%) if it is performed properly.[413,475,476]

Pharmacotherapy

A number of pharmacologic approaches to the prevention and treatment of neonatal hyperbilirubinemia have been reviewed.[477] The enterohepatic circulation can be interrupted by the enteral administration of agents that bind bilirubin in the intestine and prevent reabsorption. Such agents include agar,[89,359,364] cholestyramine,[360] activated charcoal,[399] and calcium phosphate.[362,478,479] Increased intestinal peristalsis would be expected to allow less time for bilirubin absorption. Frequent feedings[480] and rectal stimulation[397] are associated with lower serum bilirubin levels. Enteral feeding of bilirubin oxidase, an enzyme that degrades bilirubin to biliverdin, dipyrrols, and other unidentified products,[481] is an additional method to block the enterohepatic circulation but remains experimental at present.[482] Another experimental approach involves the use of intravenous bilirubin oxidase.[483,484]

Because neonatal hepatic BUGT activity has been shown to be low in neonates,[410] it is not surprising that induction of hepatic BUGT results in lower serum bilirubin levels. Such induction in neonates can be accomplished with the prenatal maternal use of phenobarbital or diphenylhydantoin.[485,486] Even very low–birth weight infants (<2000 g) have been shown to respond to in utero phenobarbital therapy with significantly increased serum levels of conjugated bilirubin and decreased need for phototherapy.[487] In the postnatal period, use of phenobarbital by the neonate has the same bilirubin-lowering effect.[488] Clofibrate is advocated by French workers as a simple, nontoxic pharmacologic treatment that induces BUGT and is being used increasingly in France to prevent and treat neonatal jaundice.[489] An alternative approach to treat neonatal hyperbilirubinemia is to block the first enzyme responsible for the production of bilirubin, HO. This can be accomplished by several different metalloporphyrins.[490,491] Sn-protoporphyrin has been used successfully in the experimental management of jaundice in neonates with ABO incompatibility.[492] Treatment of neonatal jaundice by inhibition of HO remains experimental at this time, although clinical trials appear promising. Two studies showed that phototherapy could be abolished by using tin-mesoporphyrin.[493,494] In addition to inhibiting bilirubin production, metalloporphyrins are photosensitizers that can accelerate the destruction of bilirubin by light but also cause other unwanted side effects.[495] Because CO is now suggested to be a significant neurotransmitter, blocking HO activity early in life may not be a completely benign process. Thus, a major concern about metalloporphyrins is the lack of detailed long-term follow-up studies addressing safety issues.[496] At the present time, phototherapy and exchange transfusion remain the primary modalities to control neonatal unconjugated hyperbilirubinemia, and pharmacologic interventions remain largely adjunctive or experimental.

Feeding Strategies

Optimization of breast-feeding in the perinatal period is important.[497] If the bilirubin level is rising, published recommendations support encouraging mothers to breast-feed more frequently,[432,498,499] with an average suggested interval between feeding of 2 hours and no feeding supplements[500] or at least 8 to 10 feedings per 24 hours.[432] A strong dose-response relationship has been shown between feeding frequency and decreased incidence of hyperbilirubinemia.[501] More frequent nursing may not increase intake but has been suggested to increase peristalsis and stool frequency, thus promoting excretion of bilirubin.[456] The frequency of breast-feeding during the first 24 hours of life has been shown to be significantly correlated with the frequency of meconium passage.[501] The serum bilirubin level at which breast-feeding should be discontinued is controversial, and recommendations

include 14,[502] 15,[179] 16 to 17,[499] and 18 to 20 mg/dL.[500] When breast-feeding is interrupted, formula feeding may be initiated for 24 to 48 hours, or breast-feeding and formula feeding can be alternated with each feeding.[432] No studies have addressed the cost-effectiveness of various formulas in their jaundice-lowering effects, although two independent studies have shown that infants exclusively fed Nutramigen (a casein hydrolysate formula, Mead Johnson) have lower jaundice levels than do infants fed routine formula.[503,504] Supplementing breast-fed infants with small volumes of specific nutritional ingredients has been shown to result in increased fecal bilirubin excretion and lower transcutaneous bilirubin levels,[100] but no commercial preparations of these ingredients are currently available. Feeding heated expressed breast milk is also said to reduce serum bilirubin levels.[500] A fall in the serum bilirubin level of 2 to 5 mg/dL[456] is consistent with a diagnosis of breast milk jaundice. Breast-feeding may then be resumed with the acknowledgment that serum bilirubin levels may rise for several days but will gradually level off and decline.[179,498] If breast-feeding is to be resumed after the interruption, it is important to preserve lactation with the use of a breast pump. In one study, interruption of breast-feeding for approximately 50 hours (during which time formula was given) was shown to have the same bilirubin-lowering effect as a similar duration of phototherapy.[505] Interruption of breast-feeding for 24 to 48 hours has been shown to be successful in lowering serum bilirubin levels and avoiding the need for phototherapy in 81 of 87 jaundiced infants.[502] Formula feedings in Asian neonates undergoing phototherapy resulted in a greater decrease in serum bilirubin levels than in infants who were exclusively breast-fed.[471] Careful counseling and support can prevent the interruption in breast-feeding from becoming a permanent discontinuance of nursing.[502]

DISORDERS OF CONJUGATED HYPERBILIRUBINEMIA

Rotor's Syndrome

Rotor's syndrome (RS, OMIM 237450), first described in 1948, is a familial disorder that involves chronic elevation of both the conjugated and unconjugated serum bilirubin fractions.[506,507] Half or more of the total serum bilirubin is conjugated, and total bilirubin levels usually range from 2 to 7 mg/dL but may occasionally reach 20 mg/dL.[508] Liver functions test results are otherwise normal, and there is no evidence of hemolysis. Liver histology is normal when examined with both light and electron microscopy. Oral cholecystograms reveal normal gallbladder opacification. This disorder can occur in early childhood[509] or possibly the first months of life if coinherited with G6PD deficiency or heterozygous β-thalassemia[510] and has no gender predisposition. Family studies suggest an autosomal recessive mode of inheritance.[506,507,511]

Pathophysiology

The primary abnormality in RS is listed in the OMIM as unknown but appears to be a deficiency in the intracellular storage capacity of the liver for binding anions,[512,513] which can be demonstrated by constant infusion of BSP and ICG.[514] Patients with RS demonstrate delayed plasma clearance of both BSP and ICG, and heterozygotes show delayed BSP clearance with values intermediate between normal individuals and those with homozygous RS.[512] GST serves as an intracellular carrier protein for certain organic molecules and acts as an intracellular equivalent to albumin in blood plasma.[515] A patient with RS has been shown to have a deficiency of hepatic GST,[516] and this would be consistent with observations regarding the pathogenesis of this disorder. Deficiency of GST would result in impaired uptake of bilirubin within the cytosol. In addition, because bilirubin conjugates are bound to GST while awaiting excretion from the hepatocyte via the canalicular membrane,[517] deficient intracellular storage would result in leakage of bilirubin conjugates back into the circulation. Serum elevations of both conjugated and nonconjugated bilirubin result.

Another important observation in RS relates to the urinary excretion of coproporphyrin. In normal healthy individuals, only the I and III isomers of coproporphyrin are excreted in urine. In RS there is a marked increase in urinary coproporphyrin excretion, and usually, less than 80% of the total (I + III) is isomer I. Heterozygotes demonstrate urinary coproporphyrin values that are intermediate between those of normal individuals and homozygotes.[518] Urinary excretion of coproporphyrin is believed to be increased because biliary excretion is impaired, similar to findings in other liver diseases.[519]

Diagnosis and Treatment

A diagnosis of RS should be considered in all individuals with elevation of both conjugated and nonconjugated serum bilirubin fractions, along with otherwise normal liver function test results. The diagnosis can be confirmed by the presence of urinary coproporphyrin levels that are 2.5 to 5 times higher than normal.[518] Of the total urinary coproporphyrin isomers I plus III, isomer I constitutes less than 80% of the total in RS.[520] ^{99m}Tc-labeled hepatobiliary iminodiacetic acid (HIDA) cholescintigraphy has also been shown to be useful in diagnosing RS but provides poor to no visualization of the liver.[521,522] Patients with RS require no specific therapy and are asymptomatic. Although jaundice is a lifelong finding, it is associated with no morbidity or mortality.

Dubin-Johnson Syndrome

Dubin-Johnson syndrome (DJS, OMIM 237500), first described in 1954,[523] involves elevation of both the conjugated and unconjugated serum bilirubin fractions.[524] More than half of the total serum bilirubin is conjugated

and total bilirubin levels usually range from 1.5 to 6 mg/dL, although levels as high as 25 mg/dL have been reported during intercurrent illness.[525] It is not unusual for patients with DJS to report vague abdominal complaints, but this is not believed to reflect serious pathology. Even though hepatomegaly is sometime seen, liver functions test results are otherwise normal, including bile acids,[526] and there is no evidence of hemolysis.[523,524,527] Although this syndrome occurs in both sexes, males predominate and are affected at an earlier age. DJS occurs in all races, but Iranian Jews have an increased incidence.[528,529] It is usually diagnosed after puberty, although cases have also been reported in neonates,[530] at which time cholestasis can be significant.[531-535] DJS is inherited as an autosomal recessive trait with heterozygotes manifesting normal serum bilirubin levels.[528,536,537] This syndrome is far more common than RS, and the jaundice can be worsened by pregnancy and oral contraceptives.[538] Frequently, the gallbladder is not visualized in patients with DJS when undergoing oral cholecystography.[524]

A striking characteristic of DJS is brown to black discoloration of the liver. There is still debate about the identity of this pigment, which is located in lysosomes.[539] Though originally thought to be lipofuscin, more recent data provide conflicting evidence for a relationship to melanin,[540-542] polymerized epinephrine, or other metabolites[543,544] that accumulate in lysosomes. It is hypothesized that these pigments accumulate in the liver because of impaired secretion of various metabolites from the hepatocyte into bile.[544] This pigment disappears from the liver during acute viral hepatitis, with subsequent reappearance.[545] Other than this striking pigmentation, the liver is histologically normal. Recently, a black liver was reported in an individual who did not have DJS.[546]

Pathophysiology

The primary defect in DJS is deficient hepatic excretion of non–bile salt organic anions at the apical canalicular membrane by the ABC transport system known variously as cMOAT, MRP2, or ABCC2 (OMIM 601107).[547,548] cMOAT is encoded by a single-copy gene located on chromosome 10q24.[549] Mutations in this gene have been shown to produce a highly defective cMOAT that is associated with DJS.[62,547,548,550-553] Similar findings made in the homologous cMOAT gene of two rat models of hyperbilirubinemia (TR$^-$ and Eisai) have been very helpful in understanding DJS in humans.[62]

Although hepatic BSP clearance tests are no longer performed, they nicely demonstrate the effect of deficient transport via the canalicular membrane, characteristic of DJS.[554] Initially, the clearance rate of intravenously administered BSP from the circulation is rapid and results in BSP retention that is often normal at 45 minutes. However, a subsequent rise in serum BSP concentration occurs at 90 and 120 minutes because the conjugated BSP cannot be excreted and thus refluxes out of the hepatocyte back into the circulation.[554-557] Data suggest that BSP hepatic storage is normal, but there is a 90%

decrease in the BSP excretory transport maximum.[538,556] Other substances (e.g., ICG, rose bengal, and dibromo-sulfophthalein) have also been shown to have a decreased excretory transport maximum, although these substances do not require hepatic biotransformation and do not show the late rise in plasma levels during clearance tests.[558] Hence, in DJS, deficient excretion of bilirubin glucuronides at the canalicular membrane in the presence of otherwise normal intrahepatic metabolism results in reflux of conjugated bilirubin back into the circulation.

An important observation in DJS patients relates to the urinary excretion of coproporphyrins.[559,560] Patients with this disorder have an increase in the urinary excretion of coproporphyrin I with a concomitant decrease in the excretion of coproporphyrin III. This results in total coproporphyrin excretion (I + III) that is normal or only slightly increased but consists of greater than 80% coproporphyrin I (normal, 25%).[560-563] In heterozygotes, the coproporphyrin I/III ratio is intermediate between that of normal individuals and homozygotes,[560,562,563] although there is some overlap between heterozygotes and normal individuals. The explanation for these findings regarding urinary coproporphyrin excretion is unclear. Several pathogenetic mechanisms have been suggested.[560] Fecal coproporphyrin levels are normal.[560] Healthy neonates have been shown to have impressive elevations in urinary coproporphyrin levels, with more than 80% isomer I on the first 2 days of life.[564] By day 10, levels fell to overlap normal adult values.

Diagnosis and Treatment

A diagnosis of DJS should be considered in all individuals with elevated serum conjugated bilirubin levels along with otherwise normal liver function test results. The diagnosis can be confirmed by measuring urinary coproporphyrin levels of isomers I and III. Although the total coproporphyrin level will be approximately normal, more than 80% will be isomer I. This finding is pathognomonic for DJS when congenital erythropoietic porphyria[565] or arsenic poisoning[566] have been excluded. Even though oral cholecystography may fail to visualize the gallbladder, ultrasound examination will show a normal biliary tree. Cholescintigraphy demonstrates prolonged intense visualization of the liver with delayed appearance of the gallbladder and only faint visualization or nonvisualization of the biliary ducts.[522,567,568] Computed tomography of the liver has shown increased attenuation in one report.[569] Because cMOAT transport of leukotrienes into bile is defective in DJS, there is increased excretion of leukotriene metabolites into urine, and this has been suggested to be a new approach to the noninvasive diagnosis of this disease.[570] Another proposed diagnostic tool for DJS involves micro–positron emission tomography (micro-PET) of a copper complex studied in normal and cMOAT-deficient (TR⁻) rats.[571] In normal rats, the radioactive copper complex was cleared quickly from the liver into the intestine, whereas radioactivity accumulated continuously in the liver of TR⁻ rats and was not excreted into the small intestine.

Patients with DJS require no specific therapy. Although jaundice is a lifelong finding, it is associated with no morbidity or mortality, as demonstrated in a 30-year follow-up of 10 Japanese individuals.[553] Avoidance of oral contraceptives has been recommended[572] because they can increase jaundice. Anticipatory guidance regarding pregnancy[538] is appropriate. Increased fetal wastage has been reported in one study.[573] In one case report of neonatal DJS with severe cholestasis, phenobarbital significantly decreased serum levels of bilirubin and bile acids,[531] although chronic phenobarbital therapy is not recommended.[574] Drugs such as rifampin and ursodeoxycholic acid should be used with caution if cMOAT expression is decreased, as in DJS.[575]

REFERENCES

1. Gourley GR. Bilirubin metabolism and kernicterus. Adv Pediatr. 1997;44:173-229.
2. Bhutani VK, Johnson LH, Keren R. Diagnosis and management of hyperbilirubinemia in the term neonate: for a safer first week. Pediatr Clin North Am. 2004;51:843-861, vii.
3. Maisels MJ. Jaundice. In MacDonald MG, Seshia MMK, Mullett MD (eds). Avery's Neonatology: Pathophysiology & Management of the Newborn. Philadelphia, JB Lippincott, 2005, pp 768-846.
4. Städeler G. Ueber die Farbstoffe der Galle. Justus Liebigs Ann Chem. 1864;132:323-354.
5. Schmid R, McDonagh AF. The enzymatic formation of bilirubin. Ann N Y Acad Sci. 1975;244:533-552.
6. Ryter SW, Alam J, Choi AM. Heme oxygenase-1/carbon monoxide: from basic science to therapeutic applications. Physiol Rev. 2006;86:583-650.
7. O'Carra P, Colleran E. Methine bridge selectivity in haem-cleavage reactions: relevance to the mechanism of haem catabolism. Biochem Soc Trans. 1976;4:209-214.
8. Fischer H, Orth H. Die Chemie des Pyrrols. Leipzig, Germany Akademische Verlagsgesellschaft MBH, 1937, p 626.
9. Blumenthal SG, Stucker T, Rassmussen RD, et al. Changes in bilirubins in human prenatal development. Biochem J. 1980;186:693-700.
10. Blumenthal SG, Taggart DB, Ikeda R, et al. Conjugated and unconjugated bilirubins in bile of human and rhesus monkeys—structure of adult human and rhesus monkey bilirubins compared with dog bilirubins. Biochem J. 1977;167:535-548.
11. Colleran E, O'Carra P. Enzymology and comparative physiology of biliverdin reduction. In Berk PD, Berlin NE (eds). International Symposium on Chemistry and Physiology of Bile Pigments. Washington, DC, US Government Printing Office, 1977, p 69.
12. Bartoletti AL, Stevenson DK, Ostrander CR, Johnson JD. Pulmonary excretion of carbon monoxide in the human infant as an index of bilirubin production. I. Effects of gestational age and postnatal age and some common neonatal abnormalities. J Pediatr. 1979;94:952-955.

13. Maisels MJ, Pathak A, Nelson NM, et al. Endogenous production of carbon monoxide in normal and erythroblastotic infants. J Clin Invest. 1971;50:1-8.

14. Bloomer JR, Berk PD, Howe RB, et al. Comparison of fecal urobilinogen excretion with bilirubin production in normal volunteers and patients with increased bilirubin production. Clin Chim Acta. 1970;29:463.

15. Ostrow JD, Jandle JG, Schmid R. The formation of bilirubin from hemoglobin in vivo. J Clin Invest. 1962; 41:1628-1637.

16. Daly JS, Little JM, Troxler RF, Lester R. Metabolism of ³H-myoglobin. Nature. 1967;216:1030-1031.

17. London IM, West R. The formation of bile pigment in pernicious anemia. J Biol Chem. 1950;184:359-364.

18. Gray CH, Scott JJ. The effect of haemorrhage on the incorporation [a-C14] glycine into stercobilin. J Biochem. 1959;71:38-42.

19. Robinson SH, Tsong M, Brown BW, et al. The sources of bile pigment in the rat: studies of early labeled fraction. J Clin Invest. 1966;45:1569-1586.

20. Sedlak TW, Snyder SH. Bilirubin benefits: cellular protection by a biliverdin reductase antioxidant cycle. Pediatrics. 2004;113:1776-1782.

21. McDonagh AF, Palma LA, Schmid R. Reduction of biliverdin and placental transfer of bilirubin and biliverdin in the pregnant guinea pig. Biochem J. 1981;194: 273-282.

22. Bonnett R, Davies JE, Hursthouse MB. Structure of bilirubin. Nature. 1976;262:327-328.

23. Bennhold H. Uber die Vehikelfunktion der Serumeiweisskorper. Ergeb Inn Med Kinderheilkd. 1932;42:273-375.

24. Jacobsen J. Binding of bilirubin to human serum albumin—determination of the dissociation constants. FEBS Lett. 1969;5:112-114.

25. Robertson A, Karp W, Brodersen R. Comparison of the binding characteristics of serum albumins from various animal species. Dev Pharmacol Ther. 1990;15:106-111.

26. Schaffner F, Popper H. Capillarization of hepatic sinusoids in man. Gastroenterology. 1963;44:239-242.

27. Bloomer JR, Berk PD, Vergalla J, Berlin NI. Influence of albumin on the hepatic uptake of unconjugated bilirubin. Clin Sci Mol Med. 1973;45:505-516.

28. Scharschmidt BF, Waggoner JG, Berk PD. Hepatic organic anion uptake in the rat. J Clin Invest. 1975;56: 1280-1292.

29. Zucker SD, Goessling W, Hoppin AG. Unconjugated bilirubin exhibits spontaneous diffusion through model lipid bilayers and native hepatocyte membranes. J Biol Chem. 1999;274:10852-10862.

30. Wolkoff AW, Chung CT. Identification, purification and partial characterization of an organic anion binding protein from rat liver plasma membrane. J Clin Invest. 1980;65:1152-1161.

31. Wolkoff AW, Sosiak A, Greenblutt HC, et al. Immunologic studies on an organic anion-binding protein isolated from rat liver cell plasma membrane. J Clin Invest. 1985;76:454-459.

32. Stremmel W, Gerber M, Glezerov V, et al. Physiochemical and immunohistological studies of a sulfobromophthalein- and bilirubin-binding protein from rat liver plasma membranes. J Clin Invest. 1983;71:1796-1805.

33. Hagenbuch B, Meier PJ. Organic anion transporting polypeptides of the OATP/ SLC21 family: phylogenetic classification as OATP/ SLCO superfamily, new nomenclature and molecular/functional properties. Pflugers Arch. 2004; 447:653-665.

34. Wolkoff AW, Weisiger RA, Jakoby WB. The multiple roles of the glutathione transferases (ligandin). Prog Liver Dis. 1979;6:213-224.

35. Wolkoff AW, Goresky CA, Sellin J, et al. Role of ligandin in transfer of bilirubin from plasma into liver. Am J Physiol. 1979;236:E638-E648.

36. Boyer TD. The glutathione S-transferases: an update. Hepatology. 1989;9:486-496.

37. Dutton GJ. The biosynthesis of glucuronides. In Dutton GJ (ed). Glucuronic Acid, Free and Combined: Chemistry, Biochemistry, Pharmacology and Medicine. London, Academic Press, 1966, pp 186-299.

38. Kiang TK, Ensom MH, Chang TK. UDP-glucuronosyltransferases and clinical drug-drug interactions. Pharmacol Ther. 2005;106:97-132.

39. Senafi SB, Clarke DJ, Burchell B. Investigation of the substrate specificity of a cloned expressed human bilirubin UDP-glucuronosyltransferase: UDP-sugar specificity and involvement in steroid and xenobiotic glucuronidation. Biochem J. 1994;303:233-240.

40. Pogell BM, LeLoir LF. Nucleotide activation of liver microsomal glucuronidation. J Biol Chem. 1961;236: 293-298.

41. Berry C, Hallinan T. Summary of a novel, three-component regulatory model for uridine diphosphate glucuronyltransferase. Biochem Soc Trans. 1976;4:650-652.

42. Kuriyama T. Studies on microsomal nucleoside diphosphatase of rat hepatocytes. Its purification, intramembranous location and turnover. J Biol Chem. 1972;247: 2979-2988.

43. Clarke DJ, Moghrabi N, Monaghan G, et al. Genetic defects of the UDP-glucuronosyltransferase-1 (UGT1) gene that cause familial non-haemolytic unconjugated hyperbilirubinaemias. Clin Chim Acta. 1997;266:63-74.

44. Gong QH, Cho JW, Huang T, et al. Thirteen UDPglucuronosyltransferase genes are encoded at the human UGT1 gene complex locus. Pharmacogenetics. 2001;11: 357-368.

45. Mackenzie PI, Owens IS, Burchell B, et al. The UDP glycosyltransferase gene superfamily: recommended nomenclature update based on evolutionary divergence. Pharmacogenetics. 1997;7:255-269.

46. Burchell B, Blanckaert N. Bilirubin mono- and diglucuronide formation by purified rat liver microsomal bilirubin UDP-glucuronyltransferase. Biochem J. 1984;223:461-465.

47. Maruo Y, Iwai M, Mori A, et al. Polymorphism of UDP-glucuronosyltransferase and drug metabolism. Curr Drug Metab. 2005;6:91-99.

48. Fevery J, Van Damme B, Mechiel R, et al. Bilirubin conjugates in bile of man and rat in the normal state and in liver disease. J Clin Invest. 1972;51:2482-2492.

49. Gordon ER, Goresky CA, Chan TH, Perlin AS. The isolation and characterization of bilirubin diglucuronide, the major bilirubin conjugate in dog and human bile. Biochem J. 1976;155:477-486.

50. Sinaasappel M, Jansen PL. The differential diagnosis of Crigler-Najjar disease, types 1 and 2, by bile pigment analysis. Gastroenterology. 1991;100:783-789.

51. Fevery J, Blanckaert N, Heirwegh KPM, et al. Unconjugated bilirubin and an increased proportion of bilirubin monoconjugates in the bile of patients with Gilbert's syndrome and Crigler-Najjar disease. J Clin Invest. 1977;60:970-979.

52. Fevery J, Blanckaert N, Leroy P, et al. Analysis of bilirubins in biological fluids by extraction and thin-layer chromatography of the intact tetrapyrrole: application to bile of patients with Gilbert's syndrome, hemolysis, or cholelithiasis. Hepatology. 1983;3:177-183.

53. Goresky CA, Gordon ER, Shaffer EA, et al. Definition of a conjugation dysfunction in Gilbert's syndrome: studies of the handling of bilirubin loads and of the pattern of bilirubin conjugates secreted in bile. Clin Sci. 1978; 55:63-71.

54. Adachi Y, Kobayashi H, Kurumi Y, et al. Bilirubin diglucuronide transport by rat liver canalicular membrane vesicles: stimulation by biocarbonate ion. Hepatology. 1991;14:1251-1258.

55. Nishida T, Gatmaitan Z, Roy-Chowdhry J, Arias IM. Two distinct mechanisms for bilirubin glucuronide transport by rat bile canalicular membrane vesicles. Demonstration of defective ATP-dependent transport in rats (TR-) with inherited conjugated hyperbilirubinemia. J Clin Invest. 1992;90:2130-2135.

56. Paulusma CC, Oude ER. The canalicular multispecific organic anion transporter and conjugated hyperbilirubinemia in rat and man. J Mol Med. 1997;75:420-428.

57. Keppler D, Konig J. Hepatic canalicular membrane 5: expression and localization of the conjugate export pump encoded by the MRP2 (cMRP/cMOAT) gene in liver. FASEB J. 1997;11:509-516.

58. Chandra P, Brouwer KL. The complexities of hepatic drug transport: current knowledge and emerging concepts. Pharm Res. 2004;21:719-735.

59. Paulusma CC, Bosma PJ, Zaman GJ, et al. Congenital jaundice in rats with a mutation in a multidrug resistance–associated protein gene. Science. 1996;271: 1126-1128.

60. Kamisako T, Leier I, Cui Y, et al. Transport of monoglucuronosyl and bisglucuronosyl bilirubin by recombinant human and rat multidrug resistance protein 2. Hepatology. 1999;30:485-490.

61. Keppler D, Leier I, Jedlitschky G, et al. The function of the multidrug resistance proteins (MRP and cMRP) in drug conjugate transport and hepatobiliary excretion. Adv Enzyme Regul. 1996;36:17-29.

62. Wada M, Toh S, Taniguchi K, et al. Mutations in the canalicular multispecific organic anion transporter (cMOAT) gene, a novel ABC transporter, in patients with hyperbilirubinemia II/Dubin-Johnson syndrome. Hum Mol Genet. 1998;7:203-207.

63. Erlinger S. Physiology of bile flow. Prog Liver Dis. 1975;4:63-82.

64. Weinbren K, Billing BH. Hepatic clearance of bilirubin as an index of cellular function in the regenerating rat liver. Br J Exp Pathol. 1956;37:199-204.

65. Natzschka JC, Odell GB. The influence of albumin on the distribution and excretion of bilirubin in jaundiced rats. Pediatrics. 1966;37:51-61.

66. Albert S, Mosher M, Shanske A, Arias IM. Multiplicity of hepatic excretory mechanisms for organic anions. J Gen Physiol. 1969;53:238-247.

67. Hargreaves T, Lathe GH. Inhibitory aspects of bile secretion. Nature. 1963;200:1172-1176.

68. Clarenburg R, Kao CC. Shared and separate pathways for biliary excretion of bilirubin and BSP in rats for biliary excretion of bilirubin and BSP in rats. Am J Physiol. 1973;225:192-200.

69. Schoenfield LJ, McGill DB, Hunton DB, et al. Studies of chronic idiopathic jaundice (Dubin-Johnson syndrome). I. Demonstration of hepatic excretory defect. Gastroenterology. 1963;44:101-111.

70. Goresky CA, Haddad HH, Kluger WS, et al. The enhancement of maximal bilirubin excretion with taurocholate-induced increments in bile flow. Can J Physiol Pharmacol. 1974;52:389-403.

71. Roberts RJ, Plaa GS. Effect of phenobarbital on the excretion of an exogenous bilirubin load. Biochem Pharmacol. 1967;16:827-835.

72. Gallagher TF, Mueller MN, Kappas A. Estrogen pharmacology. IV. Studies on the structural basis for estrogen-induced impairment of liver function. Medicine (Baltimore). 1966;45:471-479.

73. Zimmerman HJ. Hepatotoxicity. The Adverse Effects of Drug and Other Chemicals on the Liver. New York, Appleton-Century-Crofts, 1978, pp 436-467.

74. Fevery J, Blanckaert N. Review. What can we learn from analysis of serum bilirubin? J Hepatol. 1986;2:113-121.

75. Muraca M, Fevery J, Blanckaert N. Relationships between serum bilirubins and production and conjugation of bilirubin—studies in Gilbert's syndrome, Crigler-Najjar disease, hemolytic disorders, and rat models. Gastroenterology. 1987;92:309-317.

76. Van Steenbergen W, Fevery J. Effects of uridine diphosphate glucuronosyltransferase activity on the maximal secretion rate of bilirubin conjugates in the rat. Gastroenterology. 1990;99:488-499.

77. Sieg A, Stiehl A, Raedsch R, et al. Gilbert's syndrome: diagnosis by typical serum bilirubin pattern. Clin Chim Acta. 1986;154:41-47.

78. Ullrich D, Fevery J, Sieg A, et al. The influence of gestational age on bilirubin conjugation in newborns. Eur J Clin Invest. 1991;21:83-89.

79. Weiss JS, Guatam A, Lauff JJ, et al. The clinical importance of a protein-bound fraction of serum bilirubin in patients with hyperbilirubinemia. N Engl J Med. 1983; 309:147-150.

80. Brett EM, Hicks JM, Powers DM, Rand RN. Delta bilirubin in serum of pediatric patients: correlations with age and disease. Clin Chem. 1984;30:1561-1564.

81. Van Breemen RB, Fenselau C. Acylation of albumin by 1-*O*-acyl glucuronides. Drug Metab Dispos. 1985;13: 318-320.

82. Stogniew M, Fenselau C. Electrophilic reactions of acyl-linked glucuronides—formation of clofibrate mercapturate in humans. Drug Metab Dispos. 1982;10:609-613.

83. Van Breemen RB. Electrophilic reactions of 1-*O*-acyl Glucuronides [dissertation]. Baltimore, Johns Hopkins University, 1985.

84. Berson SA, Yalow RS, Schreiber SS. Tracer experiments with I131 labeled human serum albumin: distribution

and degradation studies. J Clin Invest. 1953;32: 746-768.

85. Billing BH. Intestinal and renal metabolism of bilirubin including enterohepatic circulation. In Ostrow JD (ed). Bile Pigments and Jaundice. New York, Marcel Dekker, 1986, pp 255-269.

86. Midtvedt T, Gustafsson BE. Microbial conversion of bilirubin to urobilins in vitro and in vivo. Acta Pathol Microbiol Immunol Scand [B]. 1981;89:57-60.

87. Fahmy K, Gray CH, Nicholson DC. The reduction of bile pigments by faecal and intestinal bacteria. Biochim Biophys Acta. 1972;264:85-97.

88. Vitek L, Kotal P, Jirsa M, et al. Intestinal colonization leading to fecal urobilinoid excretion may play a role in the pathogenesis of neonatal jaundice. J Pediatr Gastroenterol Nutr. 2000;30:294-298.

89. Poland RL, Odell GB. Physiologic jaundice: the enterohepatic circulation of bilirubin. N Engl J Med. 1971; 284:1-6.

90. Vitek L, Zelenka J, Zadinova M, Malina J. The impact of intestinal microflora on serum bilirubin levels. J Hepatol. 2005;42:238-243.

91. Hawksworth G, Drasar BS, Hill MJ. Intestinal bacteria and the hydrolysis of glycosidic bonds. J Med Microbiol. 1971;4:451-459.

92. Kent TH, Fischer LJ, Marr R. Glucuronidase activity in intestinal contents of rat and man and relationship to bacterial flora. Proc Soc Exp Biol Med. 1972;140:590-594.

93. Nanno M, Morotomi M, Takayama H, et al. Mutagenic activation of biliary metabolites of benzo(a)pyrene by beta-glucuronidase–positive bacteria in human faeces. J Med Microbiol. 1986;22:351-355.

94. Musa BU, Doe RP, Seal US. Purification and properties of human liver β-glucuronidase. J Biol Chem. 1965;240:2811-2816.

95. Lester R, Schmid R. Intestinal absorption of bile pigments. I. The enterohepatic circulation of bilirubin in the cat. J Clin Invest. 1963;42:736-746.

96. Gourley GR, Arend RA. β-Glucuronidase and hyperbilirubinemia in breast-fed and formula-fed babies. Lancet. 1986;1:644-646.

97. Saxerholt H, Skar V, Midtvedt T. HPLC separation and quantification of bilirubin and its glucuronide conjugates in faeces and intestinal contents of germ-free rats. Scand J Clin Lab Invest. 1990;50:487-495.

98. Gourley GR. Pathophysiology of breast-milk jaundice. In Polin RA, Fox WW (eds). Fetal and Neonatal Physiology. Philadelphia, WB Saunders, 1998, pp 1499-1505.

99. Kreamer BL, Siegel FL, Gourley GR. A novel inhibitor of β-glucuronidase: L-aspartic acid. Pediatr Res. 2001;50:460-466.

100. Gourley GR, Li Z, Kreamer BL, Kosorok MR. A controlled, randomized, double-blind trial of prophylaxis against jaundice among breastfed newborns. Pediatrics. 2005;116:385-391.

101. Newman TB, Easterling MJ, Goldman ES, Stevenson DK. Laboratory evaluation of jaundice in newborns—frequency, cost and yield. Am J Dis Child. 1990;144:364-368.

102. Rutledge JC, Ou CN. Bilirubin and the laboratory. Advances in the 1980's, considerations for the 1990's. Pediatr Clin North Am. 1989;36:189-197.

103. Schreiner RL, Glick MR. Interlaboratory bilirubin variability. Pediatrics. 1982;69:277-281.

104. Lo SF, Doumas BT, Ashwood ER. Performance of bilirubin determinations in US laboratories—revisited. Clin Chem. 2004;50:190-194.

105. Lo SF, Doumas BT, Ashwood ER. Bilirubin proficiency testing using specimens containing unconjugated bilirubin and human serum: results of a College of American Pathologists study. Arch Pathol Lab Med. 2004;128: 1219-1223.

106. Rosenthal P, Keefe MT, Henton D, et al. Total and direct-reacting bilirubin values by automated methods compared with liquid chromatography and with manual methods for determining delta bilirubin. Clin Chem. 1990;36:788-791.

107. Westwood A. The analysis of bilirubin in serum. Ann Clin Biochem. 1991;28:119-130.

108. Vreman HJ, Verter J, Oh W, et al. Interlaboratory variability of bilirubin measurements. Clin Chem. 1996;42: 869-873.

109. Schlebusch H, Axer K, Schneider C, et al. Comparison of five routine methods with the candidate reference method for the determination of bilirubin in neonatal serum. J Clin Chem Clin Biochem. 1990;28:203-210.

110. Mair B, Klempner LB. Abnormally high values for direct bilirubin in the serum of newborns as measured with the DuPont aca. Am J Clin Pathol. 1987;87:642-644.

111. Blanckaert N, Kabra PM, Farina FA. Measurement of bilirubin and its monoconjugates and diconjugates in human serum by alkaline methanolysis and high-performance liquid chromatography. J Lab Clin Med. 1980;96:198-212.

112. Wu TW, Dappen GM, Powers DM. The Kodak EKTACHEM Clinical Chemistry slide for measurement of bilirubin in newborns: principles and performance. Clin Chem. 1982;28:2366-2372.

113. Wu TW, Dappen GM, Spayd RW. The EKTACHEM Clinical Chemistry slide for simultaneous determination of unconjugated and sugar-conjugated bilirubin. Clin Chem. 1984;30:1304-1309.

114. Mullon C, Langer R. Determination of conjugated and total bilirubin in serum of neonates with use of bilirubin oxidase. Clin Chem. 1987;33:1822-1825.

115. Bhutani VK, Gourley GR, Adler S, et al. Noninvasive measurement of total serum bilirubin in a multiracial predischarge newborn population to assess the risk of severe hyperbilirubinemia. Pediatrics. 2000;106:e17.

116. Rubaltelli FF, Gourley GR, Loskamp N, et al. Transcutaneous bilirubin measurement: a multi-centre evaluation of a new device. Pediatrics. 2001;107:1264-1271.

117. Muraca M, Rubaltelli FF, Blanckaert N, Fevery J. Unconjugated and conjugated bilirubin pigments during perinatal development. II. Studies on serum of healthy newborns and of neonates with erythroblastosis fetalis. Biol Neonate. 1990;57:1-9.

118. Arvan D, Shirey TL. Conjugated bilirubin: a better indicator of impaired hepatobiliary excretion than direct bilirubin. Ann Clin Lab Sci. 1985;15:252-259.

119. Schlebusch H, Schneider C. Enzymatic determination of bilirubin in serum of newborns—any advantage over previous methods? Ann Clin Biochem. 1991;28:290-296.

120. Grohmann K, Roser M, Rolinski B, et al. Bilirubin measurement for neonates: comparison of 9 frequently used methods. Pediatrics. 2006;117:1174-1183.

121. Leslie GI, Phillips JB, Cassady G. Capillary and venous bilirubin values: are they really different? Am J Dis Child. 1987;141:1199-1200.

122. Eidelman AI, Schimmel MS. Capillary and venous bilirubin values: they are different—and how! Am J Dis Child. 1989;143:642.

123. Maisels MJ. Capillary vs venous bilirubin values [letter]. Am J Dis Child. 1990;144:521-522.

124. Maisels MJ, Ostrea EM Jr, Touch S, et al. Evaluation of a new transcutaneous bilirubinometer. Pediatrics. 2004; 113:1628-1635.

125. American Academy of Pediatrics Subcommittee on Hyperbilirubinemia. Management of hyperbilirubinemia in the newborn infant 35 or more weeks of gestation. Pediatrics. 2004;114:297-316.

126. Knudsen A, Brodersen R. Skin color and bilirubin in neonates. Arch Dis Child. 1989;64:605-609.

127. Bilgen H, Ince Z, Ozek E, et al. Transcutaneous measurement of hyperbilirubinaemia: comparison of the Minolta jaundice meter and the Ingram icterometer. Ann Trop Paediatr. 1998;18:325-328.

128. Schumacher RE, Thornbery JM, Gutcher GR. Transcutaneous bilirubinometry: a comparison of old and new methods. Pediatrics. 1985;76:10-14.

129. Gossett IH, Oxon BM. A Perspex icterometer for neonates. Lancet. 1960;1:87-88.

130. Odell GB, Schutta HS. Bilirubin encephalopathy. In McCandless DW (ed). Cerebral Energy Metabolism and Metabolic Encephalopathy. New York, Plenum, 1985, pp 229-261.

131. Shapiro SM, Bhutani VK, Johnson L. Hyperbilirubinemia and kernicterus. Clin Perinatol. 2006;33:387-410.

132. Claireaux AE. Pathology of human kernicterus. In Sass-Kortsak A (ed). Kernicterus: A Report Based on a Symposium Held at the IX International Congress of Paediatrics. Toronto, University of Toronto Press, 1961, p 140.

133. Odell GB, Storey GNB, Rosenberg LA. Studies in kernicterus. III. The saturation of serum proteins with bilirubin during neonatal life and its relationship to brain damage at five years. J Pediatr. 1970;76:12-21.

134. Johnson L, Boggs TR Jr. Bilirubin-dependent brain damage: incidence and indication for treatment. In Odell GB, Schaffer R, Simopoulous AP (eds). Phototherapy in the Newborn: An Overview. Washington, DC, National Academy of Sciences,1974, pp 122-149.

135. Seidman DS, Paz I, Stevenson DK, et al. Neonatal hyperbilirubinemia and physical and cognitive performance at 17 years of age. Pediatrics. 1991;88:828-833.

136. Walker PC. Neonatal bilirubin toxicity—a review of kernicterus and the implications of drug-induced bilirubin displacement. Clin Pharmacokinet. 1987;13:26-50.

137. Brodersen R, Stern L. Deposition of bilirubin acid in the central nervous system—a hypothesis for the development of kernicterus. Acta Paediatr Scand. 1990;79:12-19.

138. Brito MA, Brites D, Butterfield DA. A link between hyperbilirubinemia, oxidative stress and injury to neocortical synaptosomes. Brain Res. 2004;1026:33-43.

139. Gardner WA Jr, Konigsmark BW. Familial nonhemolytic jaundice: bilirubinosis and encephalopathy. Pediatrics. 1969;43:365-376.

140. Rubboli G, Ronchi F, Cecchi P, et al. A neurophysiological study in children and adolescents with Crigler-Najjar syndrome type I. Neuropediatrics. 1997;28:281-286.

141. Hsia DYY, Allen FH Jr, Gellis SS, Diamond LK. Erythroblastosis fetalis. VIII. Studies of serum bilirubin in relation to kernicterus. N Engl J Med. 1952;247:668-671.

142. Newman TB, Maisels MJ. Does hyperbilirubinemia damage the brain of healthy full-term infants? Clin Perinatol. 1990;17:331-358.

143. Ose T, Tsuruhara T, Araki M, et al. Follow-up study of exchange transfusion for hyperbilirubinemia in infants in Japan. Pediatrics. 1967;40:196-201.

144. Odell GB. The dissociation of bilirubin from albumin and its clinical implications. J Pediatr. 1959;55:268-279.

145. Wadsworth SJ, Suh B. In vitro displacement of bilirubin by antibiotics and 2-hydroxybenzoylglycine in newborns. Antimicrob Agents Chemother. 1988;32:1571-1575.

146. Harris RC, Lucey JF, MacLean JR. Kernicterus in premature infants associated with low concentrations of bilirubin in the plasma. Pediatrics. 1958;21:875-884.

147. Ahlfors CE, Wennberg RP. Bilirubin-albumin binding and neonatal jaundice. Semin Perinatol. 2004;28:334-339.

148. Ahlfors CE, Marshall GD, Wolcott DK, et al. Measurement of unbound bilirubin by the peroxidase test using Zone Fluidics. Clin Chim Acta. 2006;365:78-85.

149. Wennberg RP, Ahlfors CE, Bhutani VK, et al. Toward understanding kernicterus: a challenge to improve the management of jaundiced newborns. Pediatrics. 2006; 117:474-485.

150. Nakamura H, Takada S, Shimabuku R, et al. Auditory nerve and brainstem responses in newborn infants with hyperbilirubinemia. Pediatrics. 1985;75:703-708.

151. Hung K. Auditory brainstem responses in patients with neonatal hyperbilirubinemia and bilirubin encephalopathy. Brain Dev. 1989;11:297-301.

152. Wennberg RP, Ahlfors CE, Bickers R. Abnormal auditory brainstem response in a newborn infant with hyperbilirubinemia: improvement with exchange transfusion. J Pediatr. 1982;100:624-626.

153. Deliac P, Demarquez JL, Barberot JP, et al. Brainstem auditory evoked potentials in icteric fullterm newborns: alterations after exchange transfusion. Neuropediatrics. 1990;21:115-118.

154. Vohr BR, Karp D, O'Dea C, et al. Behavioral changes correlated with brain-stem auditory evoked responses in term infants with moderate hyperbilirubinemia. J Pediatr. 1990;117:288-291.

155. Vohr BR, Lester B, Rapisardi G, et al. Abnormal brainstem function (brain-stem auditory evoked response) correlates with acoustic cry features in term infants with hyperbilirubinemia. J Pediatr. 1989;115:303-308.

156. Kemper K, Forsyth B, McCarthy P. Jaundice, terminating breast-feeding, and the vulnerable child. Pediatrics. 1989;84:773-778.

157. Kemper KJ, Forsyth BW, McCarthy PL. Persistent perceptions of vulnerability following neonatal jaundice. Am J Dis Child. 1990;144:238-241.

158. Schedle A, Fricker HS. Impact of hyperbilirubinaemia and transient mother-child separation in the neonatal period on mother-child attachment in the 1st year of life. Eur J Pediatr. 1990;149:587-591.

159. Moyer V, Freese DK, Whitington PF, et al. Guideline for the evaluation of cholestatic jaundice in infants: recommendations of the North American Society for Pediatric Gastroenterology, Hepatology and Nutrition. J Pediatr Gastroenterol Nutr. 2004;39:115-128.

160. Ackerman BD, Dyer GY, Leydorf MM. Hyperbilirubinemia and kernicterus in small premature infants. Pediatrics. 1970;45:918-925.

161. Knudsen A. The cephalocaudal progression of jaundice in newborns in relation to the transfer of bilirubin from plasma to skin. Early Hum Dev. 1990;22:23-28.

162. Kramer LI. Advancement of dermal icterus in the jaundiced newborn. Am J Dis Child. 1969;118:454-458.

163. Schneider AP. Breast milk jaundice in the newborn—a real entity. JAMA. 1986;255:3270-3274.

164. Linn S, Schoenbaum SC, Monson RR, et al. Epidemiology of neonatal hyperbilirubinemia. Pediatrics. 1985;75:770-774.

165. Bracci R, Buonocore G, Garosi G, et al. Epidemiologic study of neonatal jaundice—a survey of contributing factors. Acta Paediatr Scand Suppl. 1989;360:87-92.

166. Johnson CA, Liese BS, Hassanein RE. Factors predictive of heightened third-day bilirubin levels: a multiple stepwise regression analysis. Fam Med. 1989;21:283-287.

167. Meyer L, Mailloux J, Blanchet P, et al. Maternal and neonatal morbidity in instrumental deliveries with the Kobayashi vacuum extractor and low forceps. Acta Obstet Gynecol Scand. 1987;66:643-647.

168. Freeman J, Lesko SM, Mitchell AA, et al. Hyperbilirubinemia following exposure to pancuronium bromide in newborns. Dev Pharmacol Ther. 1990;14:209-215.

169. Knudsen A. Prediction of the development of neonatal jaundice by increased umbilical cord blood bilirubin. Acta Paediatr Scand. 1989;78:217-221.

170. Knudsen A, Lebech M. Maternal bilirubin, cord bilirubin, and placenta function at delivery and the development of jaundice in mature newborns. Acta Obstet Gynecol Scand. 1989;68:719-724.

171. Diwan VK, Vaughan TL, Yang CY. Maternal smoking in relation to the incidence of early neonatal jaundice. Gynecol Obstet Invest. 1989;27:22-25.

172. Gourley GR. The pathophysiology of breast milk jaundice. In Polin RA, Fox WW (eds). Fetal and Neonatal Physiology. Philadelphia, WB Saunders, 1992, pp 1173-1179.

173. Gourley GR. Breast-feeding, neonatal jaundice and kernicterus. Semin Neonatol. 2002;7:135-141.

174. Saigal S, Lunyk O, Bennett KJ, Patterson MC. Serum bilirubin levels in breast- and formula-fed infants in the first 5 days of life. Can Med Assoc J. 1982;127:985-989.

175. Kivlahan C, James EJP. The natural history of neonatal jaundice. Pediatrics. 1984;74:364-370.

176. Gartner LM, Arias IM. Studies of prolonged neonatal jaundice in the breast-fed infant. J Pediatr. 1966;68:54-66.

177. Grunebaum E, Amir J, Merlob P, et al. Breast milk jaundice: natural history, familial incidence and late neurodevelopmental outcome of the infant. Eur J Pediatr. 1991;150:267-270.

178. Behrman RE, Kliegman JM. Jaundice and hyperbilirubinemia in the newborn. In Behrman RE, Vaughan VCI, Nelson WE (eds). Nelson Textbook of Pediatrics. Philadelphia, WB Saunders, 1983, pp 378-381.

179. Lascari AD. "Early" breast-feeding jaundice: clinical significance. J Pediatr. 1986;108:156-158.

180. Orlowski JP. Breast milk jaundice—early and late. Cleve Clin Q. 1983;50:339.

181. Arias IM, Gartner LM, Seifter S, Furman M. Prolonged neonatal unconjugated hyperbilirubinemia associated with breast feeding and a steroid, pregnane-3(alpha), 20(beta)-diol in maternal milk that inhibits glucuronide formation in vitro. J Clin Invest. 1964;43:2037-2047.

182. Murphy JF, Hughs I, Verrier Jones ER, et al. Pregnanediols and breast-milk jaundice. Arch Dis Child. 1981;56:474-476.

183. Forsyth JS, Donnet L, Ross PE. A study of the relationship between bile salts, bile salt–stimulated lipase, and free fatty acids in breast milk: normal infants and those with breast milk jaundice. J Pediatr Gastroenterol Nutr. 1990;11:205-210.

184. Gaffney PT, Buttenshaw RL, Ward M, Diplock RD. Breast milk β-glucuronidase and neonatal jaundice. Lancet. 1986;1:1161-1162.

185. Alonso EM, Whitington PM, Whitington SH, et al. Enterohepatic circulation of nonconjugated bilirubin in rats fed with human milk. J Pediatr. 1991;118:425-430.

186. Tazawa Y, Abukawa D, Watabe M, et al. Abnormal results of biochemical liver function tests in breast-fed infants with prolonged indirect hyperbilirubinaemia. Eur J Pediatr. 1991;150:310-313.

187. Zipursky A. Mechanisms of hemolysis. Mead Johnson Symp Perinat Dev Med. 1982;17-24.

188. Wenk RE, Goldstein P, Felix JK. Kell alloimmunization, hemolytic disease of the newborn, and perinatal management. Obstet Gynecol. 1985;66:473-476.

189. Sieg A, Konig R, Ullrich D, Fevery J. Subfractionation of serum bilirubins by alkaline methanolysis and thin-layer chromatography. An aid in the differential diagnosis of icteric diseases. J Hepatol. 1990;11:159-164.

190. Bevis DCA. The antenatal prediction of hemolytic disease of the newborn. Lancet. 1952;1:395-398.

191. Odell GB. Evaluation of fetal hemolysis. N Engl J Med. 1970;282:1204-1205.

192. Frigoletto FD, Greene MF, Benacerraf BR, et al. Ultrasonographic fetal surveillance in the management of the isoimmunized pregnancy. N Engl J Med. 1986;315:430-432.

193. Vintzileos AM, Campbell WA, Storlazzi E, et al. Fetal liver ultrasound measurements in isoimmunized pregnancies. Obstet Gynecol. 1986;62:162-167.

194. Grannum PA, Copel JA, Plaxe SC, et al. In utero exchange transfusion by direct intravascular injection in severe erythroblastosis fetalis. N Engl J Med. 1986;314:1431-1434.

195. Queenan JT. Erythroblastosis fetalis: closing the circle. N Engl J Med. 1986;314:1448-1449.

196. Clarke CA. Prevention of Rh-hemolytic disease. BMJ. 1967;4:484-485.

197. Barss VA, Doubilet PM, John-Sutton M, et al. Cardiac output in a fetus with erythroblastosis fetalis: assessment

using pulsed Doppler. Obstet Gynecol. 1987;70:442-444.

198. Grannum PA, Copel JA. Prevention of Rh isoimmunization and treatment of the compromised fetus. Semin Perinatol. 1988;12:324-335.

199. Feng CS, Wan CP, Lau J, et al. Incidence of ABO haemolytic disease of the newborn in a group of Hong Kong babies with severe neonatal jaundice. J Paediatr Child Health. 1990;26:155-157.

200. Wong WY, Powars DR, Abdalla C, Wu PY. Phototherapy failure in jaundiced newborns with hereditary spherocytosis. Acta Paediatr Scand. 1990;79:368-369.

201. Kaplan M, Hammerman C. Severe neonatal hyperbilirubinemia. A potential complication of glucose-6-phosphate dehydrogenase deficiency. Clin Perinatol. 1998;25:575-590.

202. Beutler E. G6PD deficiency. Blood. 1994;84:3613-3636.

203. Kaplan M, Herschel M, Hammerman C, et al. Studies in hemolysis in glucose-6-phosphate dehydrogenase–deficient African American neonates. Clin Chim Acta. 2006;365:177-182.

204. Kaplan M, Herschel M, Hammerman C, et al. Neonatal hyperbilirubinemia in African American males: the importance of glucose-6-phosphate dehydrogenase deficiency. J Pediatr. 2006;149:83-88.

205. Kaplan M, Renbaum P, Levy-Lahad E, et al. Gilbert syndrome and glucose-6-phosphate dehydrogenase deficiency: a dose-dependent genetic interaction crucial to neonatal hyperbilirubinemia. Proc Natl Acad Sci U S A. 1997;94:12128-12132.

206. Chui DH. Alpha-thalassemia: Hb H disease and Hb Barts hydrops fetalis. Ann N Y Acad Sci. 2005;1054:25-32.

207. Beris P, Darbellay R, Extermann P. Prevention of beta-thalassemia major and Hb Bart's hydrops fetalis syndrome. Semin Hematol. 1995;32:244-261.

208. Laosombat V, Dissaneevate S, Wongchanchailert M, Satayasevanaa B. Neonatal anemia associated with Southeast Asian ovalocytosis. Int J Hematol. 2005;82:201-205.

209. Singhi S, Chookang E, Hall JSE. Intrapartum infusion of aqueous glucose solution, transplacental hyponatraemia, and risk of neonatal jaundice. Br J Obstet Gynaecol. 1984;99:1014-1018.

210. D'Souza SW, Lieberman B, Cadman J, Richards B. Oxytocin induction of labour: hyponatraemia and neonatal jaundice. Eur J Obstet Gynecol Reprod Biol. 1986;22:309-317.

211. Leylek OA, Ergur A, Senocak F, et al. Prophylaxis of the occurrence of hyperbilirubinemia in relation to maternal oxytocin infusion with steroid treatment. Gynecol Obstet Invest. 1998;46:164-168.

212. Maisels MJ, Kring E. Risk of sepsis in newborns with severe hyperbilirubinemia. Pediatrics. 1992;90:741-743.

213. Benaron DA, Bowen FW. Variation of initial serum bilirubin rise in newborn infants with type of illness. Lancet. 1991;338:78-81.

214. Apt L, Downey WS. Melena neonatorum: the "swallowed blood syndrome." J Pediatr. 1955;47:6-12.

215. Jacobs DS, Kasten BL, Demott WR, Wolfson WL. APT Test. Laboratory Test Handbook with DRG Index. St Louis, Mosby/Lexi-Comp, 1984, p 277.

216. Chen D, Wilhite TR, Smith CH, et al. HPLC detection of fetal blood in meconium: improved sensitivity compared with qualitative methods. Clin Chem. 1998;44:2277-2280.

217. Werner EJ. Neonatal polycythemia and hyperviscosity. Clin Perinatol. 1995;22:693-710.

218. Schimmel MS, Bromiker R, Soll RF. Neonatal polycythemia: is partial exchange transfusion justified? Clin Perinatol. 2004;31:545-553.

219. Bosma PJ. Inherited disorders of bilirubin metabolism. J Hepatol. 2003;38:107-117.

220. Gilbert A, Lereboullet P. La cholemie simple familiale. Semaine Medicale. 1901;21:241-243.

221. Odell GB, Gourley GR. Hereditary hyperbilirubinemia. In Lebenthal E (ed). The Textbook of Gastroenterology and Nutrition in Infancy. New York, Raven, 1989, pp 949-967.

222. Watson KJ, Gollan JL. Gilbert's syndrome. Baillieres Clin Gastroenterol. 1989;3:337-355.

223. Berk PD, Noyer C. The familial unconjugated hyperbilirubinemias. Semin Liver Dis. 1994;14:356-385.

224. Ashraf W, van Someren N, Quigley EM, et al. Gilbert's syndrome and Ramadan: exacerbation of unconjugated hyperbilirubinemia by religious fasting. J Clin Gastroenterol. 1994;19:122-124.

225. Naiman JL, Sugasawara EJ, Benkosky SL, Mailhot EA. Icteric plasma suggests Gilbert's syndrome in the blood donor. Transfusion. 1996;36:974-978.

226. Lachaux A, Aboufadel A, Chambon M, et al. Gilbert's syndrome: a possible cause of hyperbilirubinemia after orthotopic liver transplantation. Transplant Proc. 1996;28:2846.

227. Jansen PL, Bosma PJ, Bakker C, et al. Persistent unconjugated hyperbilirubinemia after liver transplantation due to an abnormal bilirubin UDP-glucuronosyltransferase gene promoter sequence in the donor. J Hepatol. 1997;27:1-5.

228. Gates LKJ, Wiesner RH, Krom RA, et al. Etiology and incidence of unconjugated hyperbilirubinemia after orthotopic liver transplantation. Amer J Gastroenterol. 1994;89:1541-1543.

229. Arnold JC, Otto G, Kraus T, et al. Gilbert's syndrome—a possible cause of hyperbilirubinemia after orthotopic liver transplantations. J Hepatol. 1992;14:404.

230. Wilding P, Rollason JG, Robinson D. Patterns of change for various biochemical constituents detected in well population screening. Clin Chim Acta. 1972;41:375-387.

231. Sieg A, Schlierf G, Stiehl A, Kommerell B. Die prävalenz des Gilbert-Syndroms in Deutschland. Dtsch Med Wochenschr. 1987;112:1206-1208.

232. Olsson R, Bliding Å, Jagenburg R, et al. Gilbert's syndrome—does it exist? Acta Med Scand. 1988;244:485-490.

233. Cleary KJ, White PD. Gilbert's and chronic fatigue syndromes in men. Lancet. 1993;341:842.

234. Valesini G, Conti F, Priori R, Balsano F. Gilbert's syndrome and chronic fatigue syndrome. Lancet. 1993;341:1162-1163.

235. Owens D, Evans J. Population studies on Gilbert's syndrome. J Med Genet. 1975;12:152-156.

236. Bailey A, Robinson D, Dawson AM. Does Gilbert's disease exist? Lancet. 1977;1:931-933.

237. Berk PD, Howe RB, Bloomer JR, Berlin NI. Studies of bilirubin kinetics in normal adults. J Clin Invest. 1969;48:2176-2190.

238. Alwall N, Laurell CB, Nilsby I. Studies on hereditary in cases of "nonhemolytic bilirubinemia without direct van den Bergh reaction" (hereditary, nonhemolytic bilirubinemia). Acta Med Scand. 1946;124:114-125.

239. Foulk WT, Butt HR, Owen CA, et al. Constitutional hepatic dysfunction (Gilbert's disease): its natural history and related syndromes. Medicine (Baltimore). 1959;38:25-46.

240. Powell LW, Hemingway E, Billing BH, Sherlock S. Idiopathic unconjugated hyperbilirubinemia (Gilbert's syndrome). A study of 42 families. N Engl J Med. 1967;277:1108-1112.

241. Aono S, Adachi Y, Uyama E, et al. Analysis of genes for bilirubin UDP-glucuronosyltransferase in Gilbert's syndrome. Lancet. 1995;345:958-959.

242. Bosma P, Chowdhury JR, Jansen PH. Genetic inheritance of Gilbert's syndrome. Lancet. 1995;346:314-315.

243. Soffer LJ. Bilirubin excretion as a test for liver function during normal pregnancy. Bull Johns Hopkins Hosp. 1933;52:365-375.

244. Muraca M, Fevery J. Influence of sex and sex steroids on bilirubin uridine diphosphate-glucuronsyltransferase activity of rat liver. Gastroenterology. 1984;87:308-313.

245. Odell GB. Neonatal Hyperbilirubinemia. New York, Grune & Stratton,1980, pp 39-41.

246. Bancroft JD, Kreamer B, Gourley GR. Gilbert syndrome accelerates development of neonatal jaundice. J Pediatr. 1998;132:656-660.

247. Monaghan G, McLellan A, McGeehan A, et al. Gilbert's syndrome is a contributory factor in prolonged unconjugated hyperbilirubinemia of the newborn. J Pediatr. 1999;134:441-446.

248. Akaba K, Kimura T, Sasaki A, et al. Neonatal hyperbilirubinemia and a common mutation of the bilirubin uridine diphosphate-glucuronosyltransferase gene in Japanese. J Hum Genet. 1999;44:22-25.

249. Laforgia N, Faienza MF, Rinaldi A, et al. Neonatal hyperbilirubinemia and Gilbert's syndrome. J Perinat Med. 2002;30:166-169.

250. Trioche P, Chalas J, Francoual J, et al. Jaundice with hypertrophic pyloric stenosis as an early manifestation of Gilbert syndrome. Arch Dis Child. 1999;81:301-303.

251. Hua L, Shi D, Bishop PR, et al. The role of UGT1A1*28 mutation in jaundiced infants with hypertrophic pyloric stenosis. Pediatr Res. 2005;58:881-884.

252. Sampietro M, Lupica L, Perrero L, et al. The expression of uridine diphosphate glucuronosyltransferase gene is a major determinant of bilirubin level in heterozygous beta-thalassaemia and in glucose-6-phosphate dehydrogenase deficiency. Br J Haematol. 1997;99:437-439.

253. Galanello R, Cipollina MD, Dessi C, et al. Co-inherited Gilbert's syndrome: a factor determining hyperbilirubinemia in homozygous beta-thalassemia. Haematologica. 1999;84:103-105.

254. Galanello R, Perseu L, Melis MA, et al. Hyperbilirubinaemia in heterozygous beta-thalassaemia is related to co-inherited Gilbert's syndrome. Br J Haematol. 1997;99:433-436.

255. Tzetis M, Kanavakis E, Tsezou A, et al. Gilbert syndrome associated with beta-thalassemia. Pediatr Hematol Oncol. 2001;18:477-484.

256. Sharma S, Vukelja SJ, Kadakia S. Gilbert's syndrome co-existing with and masking hereditary spherocytosis. Ann Hematol. 1997;74:287-289.

257. Black M, Billing BH. Hepatic bilirubin UDP-glucuronyl transferase activity in liver disease. N Engl J Med. 1969;280:1266-1271.

258. Felsher BF, Craig JR, Carpio N. Hepatic bilirubin glucuronidation in Gilbert's syndrome. J Lab Clin Med. 1973;81:829-837.

259. Auclair C, Hakim J, Boivin H, et al. Bilirubin and para-nitrophenol glucuronyl transferase activities of the liver in patients with Gilbert's syndrome. An attempt at a biochemical breakdown of the Gilbert's syndrome. Enzyme. 1976;21:97-107.

260. Adachi Y, Yamashita M, Nanno T, Yamamoto T. Proportion of conjugated bilirubin in bile in relation to hepatic bilirubin UDP-glucuronyltransferase activity. Clin Biochem. 1990;23:131-134.

261. Martin JF, Vierling JM, Wolkoff AW, et al. Abnormal hepatic transport of indocyanine green in Gilbert's syndrome. Gastroenterology. 1976;70:385-391.

262. Ohkubo H, Okuda K, Jida S. A constitutional unconjugated hyperbilirubinemia combined with indocyanine green intolerance: a new functional disorder. Hepatology. 1981;1:319-324.

263. Berk PD, Blaschke TF, Waggoner JG. Defective bromosulfophthalein clearance in patients with constitutional hepatic dysfunction (Gilbert's syndrome). Gastroenterology. 1972;63:472-481.

264. Billing BH, Williams R, Richards TG. Defects in hepatic transport of bilirubin in congenital hyperbilirubinemia: an analysis of plasma bilirubin disappearance curves. Clin Sci. 1964;27:245-257.

265. Berk PD, Bloomer JR, Hower RB, Berlin NI. Constitutional hepatic dysfunction (Gilbert's syndrome): a new definition based on kinetic studies with unconjugated radiobilirubin. Am J Med. 1970;49:296-305.

266. Okoliesanyi L, Ghidini O, Orlando R, et al. An evaluation of bilirubin kinetics with respect to the diagnosis of Gilbert's syndrome. Clin Sci Mol Med. 1978;54:539-547.

267. Debinski HS, Lee CS, Dhillon AP, et al. UDP-glucuronosyltransferase in Gilbert's syndrome. Pathology. 1996;28:238-241.

268. Ritter JK, Chen F, Sheen Y, et al. A novel complex locus UGT1 encodes human bilirubin, phenol, and other UDP-glucuronosyltransferase isozymes with identical carboxyl termini. J Biol Chem. 1992;267:3257-3261.

269. Jansen PL, Bosma PJ, Chowdhury JR. Molecular biology of bilirubin metabolism. Prog Liver Dis. 1995;13:125-150.

270. Bosma PJ, Chowdhury JR, Bakker C, et al. The genetic basis of the reduced expression of bilirubin UDP-glucuronosyltransferase 1 in Gilbert's syndrome. N Engl J Med. 1995;333:1171-1175.

271. Sampietro M, Lupica L, Perrero L, et al. TATA-box mutant in the promoter of the uridine diphosphate glucuronosyltransferase gene in Italian patients with Gilbert's syndrome. Ital J Gastroenterol Hepatol. 1998;30:194-198.

272. Monaghan G, Ryan M, Seddon R, et al. Genetic variation in bilirubin UPD-glucuronosyltransferase gene promoter and Gilbert's syndrome. Lancet. 1996;347:578-581.

273. Ando Y, Chida M, Nakayama K, et al. The UGT1A1*28 allele is relatively rare in a Japanese population. Pharmacogenetics. 1998;8:357-360.

274. Koiwai O, Nishizawa M, Hasada K, et al. Gilbert's syndrome is caused by a heterozygous missense mutation in the gene for bilirubin UDP-glucuronosyltransferase. Hum Mol Genet. 1995;4:1183-1186.

275. Maruo Y, Sato H, Yamano T, et al. Gilbert syndrome caused by a homozygous missense mutation (Tyr486Asp) of bilirubin UDP-glucuronosyltransferase gene. J Pediatr. 1998;132:1045-1047.

276. Beutler E, Gelbart T, Demina A. Racial variability in the UDP-glucuronosyltransferase 1 (UGT1A1) promoter: a balanced polymorphism for regulation of bilirubin metabolism? Proc Natl Acad Sci U S A. 1998;95:8170-8174.

277. Coelho H, Costa E, Vieira E, et al. A new case of (TA)$_8$ allele in the UGT1A1 gene promoter in a Caucasian girl with Gilbert syndrome. Pediatr Hematol Oncol. 2004;21:371-374.

278. Metreau JM, Yvart J, Dhumeaux D, Berthelot P. Role of bilirubin overproduction in revealing Gilbert's syndrome: is dyserythropoiesis an important factor? Gut. 1978;19:838-843.

279. Sugatani J, Kojima H, Ueda A, et al. The phenobarbital response enhancer module in the human bilirubin UDP-glucuronosyltransferase UGT1A1 gene and regulation by the nuclear receptor CAR. Hepatology. 2001;33:1232-1238.

280. Costa E. Hematologically important mutations: bilirubin UDP-glucuronosyltransferase gene mutations in Gilbert and Crigler-Najjar syndromes. Blood Cells Mol Dis. 2006;36:77-80.

281. Gourley GR, Siegel FL, Odell GB. A rapid method for collection and analysis of bile pigments in humans. Gastroenterology. 1984;86:1322A.

282. Onishi S, Itoh S, Kawade N, et al. An accurate and sensitive analysis by high-pressure liquid chromatography of conjugated and unconjugated bilirubin IX-α in various biological fluids. Biochem J. 1980;185:281-284.

283. Blaschke TF, Berk PD, Rodkey FL, et al. Drugs and the liver. I. Effects of glutethimide and phenobarbital on hepatic bilirubin clearance, plasma bilirubin turnover and carbon monoxide production in man. Biochem Pharmacol. 1974;23:2795-2806.

284. Black M, Fevery J, Parker D, et al. Effect of phenobarbitone on plasma [^{14}C] bilirubin clearance in patients with unconjugated hyperbilirubinemia. Clin Sci Mol Med. 1974;46:1-17.

285. Kutz K, Kandler H, Gugler R, Fevery J. Effect of clofibrate on metabolism of bilirubin, bromosulphophthalein and indocyanine green and on the biliary lipid composition in Gilbert's syndrome. Clin Sci. 1984;66:389-397.

286. Foliot A, Drocourt JL, Etienne JP, et al. Increase in the hepatic glucuronidation of bilirubin in clofibrate-treated rats. Biochem Pharmacol. 1977;26:547-549.

287. Felsher BF, Richard D, Redeker AG. The reciprocal relation between caloric intake and the degree of hyperbilirubinemia in Gilbert's syndrome. N Engl J Med. 1970;283:170-172.

288. Bloomer JR, Barrett PV, Rodkey FL, Berlin NI. Studies of the mechanisms of fasting hyperbilirubinemia. Gastroenterology. 1971;61:479-487.

289. Whitmer DI, Gollan JL. Mechanisms and significance of fasting and dietary hyperbilirubinemia. Semin Liver Dis. 1983;3:42-51.

290. Owens D, Sherlock S. Diagnosis of Gilbert's syndrome: role of reduced caloric intake test. BMJ. 1973;3:559-563.

291. Bakken AF, Thaler MM, Schmid R. Metabolic regulation of heme catabolism and bilirubin production. I. Hormonal control of hepatic heme oxygenase activity. J Clin Invest. 1972;51:530-536.

292. Kirshenbaum G, Shames DM, Schmid R. An expanded model of bilirubin kinetics; effect of feeding, fasting and phenobarbital in Gilbert's syndrome. J Pharmacokinet Biopharm. 1976;4:115-155.

293. Gartner U, Goeser T, Wolkoff AW. Effect of fasting on the uptake of bilirubin and sulfobromophthalein by the isolated perfused liver. Gastroenterology. 1997;113:1707-1713.

294. Ricci GL, Ricci RR. Effect of an intraluminal food-bulk on low calorie induced hyperbilirubinemia. Clin Sci. 1984;66:493-496.

295. Fromke VL, Miller D. Constitutional hepatic dysfunction (CHD; Gilbert's syndrome): a review with special reference to a characteristic increase and prolongation of the hyperbilirubinemic response to nicotinic acid. Medicine (Baltimore). 1972;51:451-464.

296. Rollinghoff W, Paumgartner G, Preisig R. Nicotinic acid test in the diagnosis of Gilbert's syndrome: correlation with the bilirubin clearance. Gut. 1981;22:663-668.

297. Gentile S, Orzes N, Persico M, et al. Comparison of nicotinic acid and caloric restriction induced hyperbilirubinemia in the diagnosis of Gilbert's syndrome. J Hepatol. 1985;1:537-545.

298. Gentile S, Rubba P, Persico M, et al. Improvement of the nicotinic acid test in the diagnosis of Gilbert's syndrome by pretreatment with indomethacin. Hepatogastroenterology. 1985;32:267-269.

299. Gentile S, Marmo R, Persico M, et al. Dissociation between vascular and metabolic effects of nicotinic acid in Gilbert's syndrome. Clin Physiol. 1990;10:171-178.

300. Davidson AR, Rojas Bueno A, Thompson RPH, Williams R. Reduced caloric intake test and nicotinic acid provocation test in the diagnosis of Gilbert's syndrome. BMJ. 1975;2:480.

301. Ohkubo H, Musha H, Okuda K. Studies on nicotinic acid interaction with bilirubin metabolism. Dig Dis Sci. 1979;24:700-704.

302. Gentile S, Tiribelli C, Persico M, et al. Dose dependence of nicotinic acid–induced hyperbilirubinemia and its dissociation from hemolysis in Gilbert's syndrome. J Lab Clin Med. 1986;107:166-171.

303. Dickey W, McAleer JJ, Callender ME. The nicotinic acid provocation test and unconjugated hyperbilirubinaemia. Ulster Med J. 1991;60:49-52.

304. Murthy GD, Byron D, Shoemaker D, et al. The utility of rifampin in diagnosing Gilbert's syndrome. Am J Gastroenterol. 2001;96:1150-1154.

305. Ullrich D, Sieg A, Blume R, et al. Normal pathways for glucuronidation, sulphation and oxidation of paracetamol

in Gilbert's syndrome. Eur J Clin Invest. 1987;17: 237-240.

306. Adachi Y, Katoh H, Fuchi I, Yamamoto T. Serum bilirubin fractions in healthy subjects and patients with unconjugated hyperbilirubinemia. Clin Biochem. 1990;23:247-251.

307. Rudenski AS, Halsall DJ. Genetic testing for Gilbert's syndrome: how useful is it in determining the cause of jaundice? Clin Chem. 1998;44:1604-1609.

308. Berk PB, Isola LM. Specific defects in hepatic storage and clearance of bilirubin. In Ostrow JD (ed). Bile Pigments and Jaundice: Molecular, Metabolic and Medical Aspects. New York, Marcel Dekker, 1986, pp 279-316.

309. Evans DA. Survey of the human acetylator polymorphism in spontaneous disorders. J Med Genet. 1984;21: 243-253.

310. Siegmund W, Fengler JD, Franke G, et al. N-acetylation and debrisoquine hydroxylation polymorphisms in patients with Gilbert's syndrome. Br J Clin Pharmacol. 1991;32:467-472.

311. Herman RJ, Chaudhary A, Szakacs CB. Disposition of lorazepam in Gilbert's syndrome: effects of fasting, feeding, and enterohepatic circulation. J Clin Pharmacol. 1994;34:978-984.

312. de Morais SM, Uetrecht JP, Wells PG. Decreased glucuronidation and increased bioactivation of acetaminophen in Gilbert's syndrome. Gastroenterology. 1992;102: 577-586.

313. Esteban A, Perez-Mateo M. Gilbert's disease: a risk factor for paracetamol overdosage? J Hepatol. 1993;18: 257-258.

314. Wasserman E, Myara A, Lokiec F, et al. Severe CPT-11 toxicity in patients with Gilbert's syndrome: two case reports. Ann Oncol. 1997;8:1049-1051.

315. Ewesuedo RB, Iyer L, Das S, et al. Phase I clinical and pharmacogenetic study of weekly TAS-103 in patients with advanced cancer. J Clin Oncol. 2001;19:2084-2090.

316. Zucker SD, Qin X, Rouster SD, et al. Mechanism of indinavir-induced hyperbilirubinemia. Proc Natl Acad Sci U S A. 2001;98:12671-12676.

317. Black M, Sherlock S. Treatment of Gilbert's syndrome with phenobarbitone. Lancet. 1970;1:1359-1361.

318. Stocker R, McDonagh AF, Glazer AN, Ames BN. Antioxidant activities of bile pigments: biliverdin and bilirubin. Methods Enzymol. 1990;186:301-309.

319. McDonagh AF. Is bilirubin good for you? Clin Perinatol. 1990;17:359-369.

320. Breimer LH, Wannamethee G, Ebrahim S, Shaper AG. Serum bilirubin and risk of ischemic heart disease in middle-aged British men. Clin Chem. 1995;41: 1504-1508.

321. Schwertner HA, Jackson WG, Tolan G. Association of low serum concentration of bilirubin with increased risk of coronary artery disease. Clin Chem. 1994;40:18-23.

322. Crigler JF, Najjar VA. Congenital familial nonhemolytic jaundice with kernicterus. Pediatrics. 1952;10:169-180.

323. Shevell MI, Majnemer A, Schiff D. Neurologic perspectives of Crigler-Najjar syndrome type I. J Child Neurol. 1998;13:265-269.

324. Childs B, Najjar VA. Familial nonhemolytic jaundice with kernicterus. A report of two cases without neurologic damage. Pediatrics. 1956;18:369-377.

325. Blumenschein SD, Kallen RJ, Storey B, et al. Familial nonhemolytic jaundice with late onset of neurologic damage. Pediatrics. 1968;42:786-792.

326. Blaschke TF, Berke PD, Scharschmidt BF, et al. Crigler-Najjar syndrome: an unusual course with development of neurological damage at age eighteen. Pediatr Res. 1974; 8:573-590.

327. Labrune PH, Myara A, Francoual J, et al. Cerebellar symptoms as the presenting manifestations of bilirubin encephalopathy in children with Crigler-Najjar type I disease. Pediatrics. 1992;89:768-770.

328. Chalasani N, Chowdhury NR, Chowdhury JR, Boyer TD. Kernicterus in an adult who is heterozygous for Crigler-Najjar syndrome and homozygous for Gilbert-type genetic defect. Gastroenterology. 1997;112:2099-2103.

329. Arias IM, Gartner LM, Cohen M, et al. Chronic nonhemolytic unconjugated hyperbilirubinemia with glucuronyl transferase deficiency. Am J Med. 1969;47:395-409.

330. Gollan JL, Huang SM, Billing B, Sherlock S. Prolonged survival in 3 brothers with severe type II Crigler-Najjar syndrome: ultrastructural and metabolic studies. Gastroenterology. 1975;68:1543-1555.

331. Gordon ER, Shaffer EA, Sass-Kortsak A. Bilirubin secretion and conjugation in the Crigler-Najjar syndrome type II. Gastroenterology. 1976;70:761-765.

332. Koiwai O, Aono S, Adachi Y, et al. Crigler-Najjar syndrome type II is inherited both as a dominant and as a recessive trait. Hum Mol Genet. 1996;5:645-647.

333. Burchell B, Coughtrie MW, Jansen PL. Function and regulation of UDP-glucuronosyltransferase genes in health and liver disease: report of the Seventh International Workshop on Glucuronidation, September 1993, Pitlochry, Scotland. Hepatology. 1994;20:1622-1630.

334. Seppen J, Bosma PJ, Goldhoorn BG, et al. Discrimination between Crigler-Najjar type I and II by expression of mutant bilirubin uridine diphosphate-glucuronosyltransferase. J Clin Invest. 1994;94:2385-2391.

335. Labrune P, Myara A, Hadchouel M, et al. Genetic heterogeneity of Crigler-Najjar syndrome type I: a study of 14 cases. Hum Genet. 1994;94:693-697.

336. Gantla S, Bakker CT, Deocharan B, et al. Splice-site mutations: a novel genetic mechanism of Crigler-Najjar syndrome type 1. Am J Hum Genet. 1998;62:585-592.

337. Kadakol A, Ghosh SS, Sappal BS, et al. Genetic lesions of bilirubin uridine-diphosphoglucuronate glucuronosyltransferase (UGT1A1) causing Crigler-Najjar and Gilbert Syndromes: correlation of genotype to phenotype. Hum Mutat. 2000;16:297-306.

338. Szabo L, Kovács Z, Ebrey PB. Crigler-Najjar syndrome. Acta Paediatr Hung. 1962;3:49-70.

339. Duhamel G, Blanckaert N, Metreau JM, et al. An unusual case of Crigler-Najjar disease in the adult. Classification into types I and II revisited. J Hepatol. 1985;1: 47-53.

340. van Es HHG, Goldhoorn BG, Paul-Abrahamse M, et al. Immunochemical analysis of uridine diphosphate-glucuronosyltransferase in four patients with Crigler-Najjar syndrome type I. J Clin Invest. 1990;85: 1199-1205.

341. Childs B, Sidbury JB, Migeon CJ. Glucuronic acid conjugation by patients with familial nonhemolytic jaundice and their relatives. Pediatrics. 1959;23:903-913.

342. Szabo L, Ebrey P. Studies on the inheritance of Crigler-Najjar's syndrome by the menthol test. Acta Paediatr Hung. 1963;4:153-159.

343. Hunter JO, Thompson PH, Dunn PM, Williams R. Inheritance of type 2 Crigler-Najjar hyperbilirubinemia. Gut. 1973;14:46-49.

344. Labrune P, Myara A, Hennion C, et al. Crigler-Najjar type II disease inheritance: a family study. J Inherit Metab Dis. 1989;12:302-306.

345. Ertel IJ, Newton WA Jr. Therapy in congenital hyperbilirubinemia: phenobarbital and diethylnicotinamide. Pediatrics. 1969;44:43-48.

346. Crigler JF, Gold NI. Effect of phenobarbital on bilirubin metabolism in an infant with congenital, nonhemolytic, unconjugated hyperbilirubinemia, and kernicterus. J Clin Invest. 1969;48:42-55.

347. Yaffe SJ, Levy G, Matsuzawa T, Baliah T. Enhancement of glucuronide-conjugating capacity in a hyperbilirubinemic infant due to apparent enzyme induction by phenobarbital. N Engl J Med. 1966;275:1461-1466.

348. Kreek MJ, Sleisenger MH. Reduction of serum-unconjugated bilirubin with phenobarbitone in adult nonhaemolytic unconjugated hyperbilirubinaemia. Lancet. 1968;2:73-78.

349. Rubaltelli FF, Novello A, Zancan L, et al. Serum and bile bilirubin pigments in the differential diagnosis of Crigler-Najjar Disease. Pediatrics. 1994;94:553-556.

350. Odell GB, Whitington PF. Crigler-Najjar syndrome, type III: a new variant of hereditary non-hemolytic, nonconjugated hyperbilirubinemia. Hepatology. 1990;12:871.

351. Francoual J, Trioche P, Mokrani C, et al. Prenatal diagnosis of Crigler-Najjar syndrome type I by single-strand conformation polymorphism (SSCP). Prenat Diagn. 2002;22:914-916.

352. Ciotti M, Obaray R, Martin MG, Owens IS. Genetic defects at the UGT1 locus associated with Crigler-Najjar type I disease, including a prenatal diagnosis. Am J Med Genet. 1997;68:173-178.

353. Moghrabi N, Clarke DJ, Burchell B, Boxer M. Cosegregation of intragenic markers with a novel mutation that causes Crigler-Najjar syndrome type I: implication in carrier detection and prenatal diagnosis. Am J Hum Genet. 1993;53:722-729.

354. van der Veere CN, Sinaasappel M, McDonagh AF, et al. Current therapy for Crigler-Najjar syndrome type 1: report of a world registry. Hepatology. 1996;24:311-315.

355. Gorodischer R, Levy G, Krasner J, Jaffe SJ. Congenital nonobstructive, nonhemolytic jaundice. Effect of phototherapy. N Engl J Med. 1970;282:375-380.

356. Agati G, Fusi F, Pratesi S, et al. Bilirubin photoisomerization products in serum and urine from a Crigler-Najjar type I patient treated by phototherapy. J Photochem Photobiol B. 1998;47:181-189.

357. Job H, Hart G, Lealman G. Improvements in long term phototherapy for patients with Crigler-Najjar syndrome type I. Phys Med Biol. 1996;41:2549-2556.

358. Nydegger A, Bednarz A, Hardikar W. Use of daytime phototherapy for Crigler-Najjar disease. J Paediatr Child Health. 2005;41:387-389.

359. Odell GB, Gutcher GR, Whitington PF, Yang G. Enteral administration of agar as an effective adjunct to phototherapy of neonatal hyperbilirubinemia. Pediatr Res. 1983;17:810-814.

360. Arrowsmith WA, Payne RB, Littlewood JM. Comparison of treatments for congenital nonobstructive nonhaemolytic hyperbilirubinemia. Arch Dis Child. 1975;50:197-201.

361. Suresh G, Lucey JF. Lack of deafness in Crigler-Najjar syndrome type 1: a patient survey. Pediatrics. 1997;100:E9.

362. van der Veere CN, Jansen PL, Sinaasappel M, et al. Oral calcium phosphate: a new therapy for Crigler-Najjar disease? Gastroenterology. 1997;112:455-462.

363. Kotal P, van der Veere CN, Sinaasappel M, et al. Intestinal excretion of unconjugated bilirubin in man and rats with inherited unconjugated hyperbilirubinemia. Pediatr Res. 1997;42:195-200.

364. Kemper K, Horwitz RI, McCarthy P. Decreased neonatal serum bilirubin with plain agar: a meta-analysis. Pediatrics. 1988;82:631-638.

365. Sherker AH, Heathcote J. Acute hepatitis in Crigler-Najjar syndrome. Am J Gastroenterol. 1987;82:883-885.

366. Rubaltelli FF, Guerrini P, Reddi E, Jori G. Tin-protoporphyrin in the management of children with Crigler-Najjar disease. Pediatrics. 1989;84:728-731.

367. Galbraith RA, Drummond GS, Kappas A. Suppression of bilirubin production in the Crigler-Najjar type I syndrome: studies with the heme oxygenase inhibitor tin-mesoporphyrin. Pediatrics. 1992;89:175-182.

368. Kappas A, Drummond GS, Galbraith RA. Prolonged clinical use of a heme oxygenase inhibitor: hematological evidence for an inducible but reversible iron-deficiency state. Pediatrics. 1993;91:537-539.

369. Rubaltelli FF. Current drug treatment options in neonatal hyperbilirubinaemia and the prevention of kernicterus. Drugs. 1998;56:23-30.

370. Drummond GS, Kappas A. Chemoprevention of severe neonatal hyperbilirubinemia. Semin Perinatol. 2004;28:365-368.

371. Prager MC, Johnson KL, Ascher NL, Roberts JP. Anesthetic care of patients with Crigler-Najjar syndrome. Anesth Analg. 1992;74:162-164.

372. Whitington PF, Emond JC, Heffron T, Thistlethwaite JR. Orthotopic auxiliary liver transplantation for Crigler-Najjar syndrome type 1. Lancet. 1993;342:779-780.

373. Rela M, Muiesan P, Andreani P, et al. Auxiliary liver transplantation for metabolic diseases. Transplant Proc. 1997;29:444-445.

374. Rela M, Muiesan P, Vilca-Melendez H, et al. Auxiliary partial orthotopic liver transplantation for Crigler-Najjar syndrome type I. Ann Surg. 1999;229:565-569.

375. Kaufman SS, Wood RP, Shaw BW Jr, et al. Orthotopic liver transplantation for type 1 Crigler-Najjar syndrome. Hepatology. 1986;6:1259-1262.

376. Shevell MI, Bernard B, Adelson JW, et al. Crigler-Najjar syndrome type I: treatment by home phototherapy followed by orthotopic hepatic transplantation. J Pediatr. 1987;110:429-431.

377. Sokal EM, Silva ES, Hermans D, et al. Orthotopic liver transplantation for Crigler-Najjar type I disease in six children. Transplantation. 1995;60:1095-1098.

378. McDiarmid SV, Millis MJ, Olthoff KM, So SK. Indications for pediatric liver transplantation. Pediatr Transpl. 1998;2:106-116.

379. Rela M, Muiesan P, Heaton ND, et al. Orthotopic liver transplantation for hepatic-based metabolic disorders. Transpl Int. 1995;8:41-44.

380. Mowat AP. Orthotopic liver transplantation in liver-based metabolic disorders. Eur J Pediatr. 1992;151(Suppl 1): S32-S38.

381. Gridelli B, Lucianetti A, Gatti S, et al. Orthotopic liver transplantation for Crigler-Najjar type I syndrome. Transplant Proc. 1997;29:440-441.

382. Pratschke J, Steinmuller T, Bechstein WO, et al. Orthotopic liver transplantation for hepatic associated metabolic disorders. Clin Transplant. 1998;12:228-232.

383. Toietta G, Mane VP, Norona WS, et al. Lifelong elimination of hyperbilirubinemia in the Gunn rat with a single injection of helper-dependent adenoviral vector. Proc Natl Acad Sci U S A. 2005;102:3930-3935.

384. Schauer R, Stangl M, Lang T, et al. Treatment of Crigler-Najjar type 1 disease: relevance of early liver transplantation. J Pediatr Surg. 2003;38:1227-1231.

385. Jaffe BM, Burgos AA, Martinez-Noack M. The use of jejunal transplants to treat a genetic enzyme deficiency. Ann Surg. 1996;223:649-656.

386. Medley MM, Hooker RL, Rabinowitz S, et al. Correction of congenital indirect hyperbilirubinemia by small intestinal transplantation. Am J Surg. 1995;169:20-27.

387. Kokudo N, Takahashi S, Sugitani K, et al. Supplement of liver enzyme by intestinal and kidney transplants in congenitally enzyme-deficient rat. Microsurgery. 1999;19: 103-107.

388. Ambrosino G, Varotto S, Strom SC, et al. Isolated hepatocyte transplantation for Crigler-Najjar syndrome type 1. Cell Transplant. 2005;14:151-157.

389. Bellodi-Privato M, Aubert D, Pichard V, et al. Successful gene therapy of the Gunn rat by in vivo neonatal hepatic gene transfer using murine oncoretroviral vectors. Hepatology. 2005;42:431-438.

390. Jia Z, Danko I. Single hepatic venous injection of liver-specific naked plasmid vector expressing human UGT1A1 leads to long-term correction of hyperbilirubinemia and prevention of chronic bilirubin toxicity in Gunn rats. Hum Gene Ther. 2005;16:985-995.

391. Thummala NR, Ghosh SS, Lee SW, et al. A non-immunogenic adenoviral vector, coexpressing CTLA4Ig and bilirubin-uridine-diphosphoglucuronateglucuronosyltransferase permits long-term, repeatable transgene expression in the Gunn rat model of Crigler-Najjar syndrome. Gene Ther. 2002;9:981-990.

392. Odell GB. Neonatal Hyperbilirubinemia. New York, Grune & Stratton, 1980, pp 35-49.

393. Boggs TR Jr, Bishop H. Neonatal hyperbilirubinemia associated with high obstruction of the small bowel. J Pediatr. 1965;66:349-356.

394. Porto SO. Jaundice in congenital malrotation of the intestine. Am J Dis Child. 1969;117:684-688.

395. Clarkson JE, Cowan JO, Herbison GP. Jaundice in full-term healthy neonates—a population study. Aust Paediatr J. 1984;20:303-308.

396. Rosta J, Makoi Z, Kertesz A. Delayed meconium passage and hyperbilirubinemia. Lancet. 1986;2:1138.

397. Cottrell BH, Anderson GC. Rectal or axillary temperature measurement: effect on plasma bilirubin and intestinal transit of meconium. J Pediatr Gastroenterol Nutr. 1984; 3:734-739.

398. Poland RL, Odell GB. The binding of bilirubin to agar. Proc Soc Exp Biol Med. 1974;146:1114-1118.

399. Ulstrom RA, Eisenklam E. The enterohepatic shunting of bilirubin in the newborn infant: I. Use of oral activated charcoal to reduce normal serum bilirubin values. J Pediatr. 1964;65:27-37.

400. Thompson GN, McCrossin RB, Penfold JL, et al. Management and outcome of children with congenital hypothyroidism detected on neonatal screening in South Australia. Med J Aust. 1986;145:18-22.

401. Lafranchi S. Diagnosis and treatment of hypothyroidism in children. Compr Ther. 1987;13:20-30.

402. Odell GB. Studies in kernicterus. I. Protein binding of bilirubin. J Clin Invest. 1959;38:823.

403. Stutman HR, Parker KM, Marks MI. Potential of moxalactam and other new antimicrobial agents for bilirubin-albumin displacement in neonates. Pediatrics. 1985;75: 294-298.

404. Brodersen R, Robertson A. Ceftriaxone binding to human serum albumin: competition with bilirubin. Mol Pharmacol. 1989;36:478-483.

405. Park HZ, Lee SP, Schy AL. Ceftriaxone-associated gallbladder sludge. Identification of calcium-ceftriaxone salt as a major component of gallbladder precipitates. Gastroenterology. 1991;100:1665-1670.

406. Yeung CY, Lee FT, Wong HN. Effect of a popular Chinese herb on neonatal bilirubin protein binding. Biol Neonate. 1990;58:98-103.

407. Lambert GH, Muraskas J, Anderson CL, Myers TF. Direct hyperbilirubinemia associated with chloral hydrate administration in the newborn. Pediatrics. 1990;86: 277-281.

408. Jahrig D, Jahrig K, Stiete S, et al. Neonatal jaundice in infants of diabetic mothers. Acta Paediatr Scand Suppl. 1989;360:101-107.

409. Arias IM, Wolfson S, Lucey JF, McKay RJ Jr. Transient familial neonatal hyperbilirubinemia. J Clin Invest. 1965;44:1442-1450.

410. Kawade N, Onishi S. The prenatal and postnatal development of UDP-glucuronyltransferase activity towards bilirubin and the effect of premature birth on this activity in the human liver. Biochem J. 1981;196: 257-260.

411. Obrinsky W, Denley ML, Brauer RW. Sulfobromophthalein sodium excretion test as a measure of liver function in premature infants. Pediatrics. 1952;9:421-438.

412. Vest M, Rossier R. Detoxification in the newborn: the ability of the newborn infant to form conjugates with glucuronic acid, glycine, acetate and glutathione. Ann N Y Acad Sci. 1963;111:183-198.

413. Boggs TR Jr, Westphal MD Jr. Mortality of exchange transfusions. Pediatrics. 1960;26:745-755.

414. Murayama K, Nagasaka H, Tate K, et al. Significant correlations between the flow volume of patent ductus venosus and early neonatal liver function: possible involvement of patent ductus venosus in postnatal liver function. Arch Dis Child Fetal Neonatal Ed. 2006;91:F175-F179.

415. Johnson L, Brown AK. A pilot registry for acute and chronic kernicterus in term and near-term infants. Pediatrics. 1999;104:736.

416. Brown AK, Johnson L. Loss of concern about jaundice and the re-emergence of kernicterus in full term infants

in the era of managed care. In Fanaroff A, Klaus M (eds). St Louis, Mosby–Year Book, 1996, pp xvii-xxviii.

417. Ebbesen F. Recurrence of kernicterus in term and near-term infants in Denmark. Acta Paediatr. 2000;89: 1213-1217.

418. Bhutani VK, Johnson LH. Newborn jaundice and kernicterus—health and societal perspectives. Indian J Pediatr. 2003;70:407-416.

419. Liu LL, Clemens CJ, Shay DK, et al. The safety of newborn early discharge. The Washington State experience. JAMA. 1997;278:293-298.

420. Salem-Schatz S, Peterson LE, Palmer RH, et al. Barriers to first-week follow-up of newborns: findings from parent and clinician focus groups. Jt Comm J Qual Saf. 2004; 30:593-601.

421. Szabo P, Wolf M, Bucher HU, et al. Detection of hyperbilirubinaemia in jaundiced full-term neonates by eye or by bilirubinometer? Eur J Pediatr. 2004;163:722-727.

422. Shell ER. The hospital hustle. Parenting. 1990;4: 57-61.

423. Johnson L. Hyperbilirubinemia in the term infant: when to worry, when to treat. N Y State J Med. 1991;91: 483-487.

424. Joint Commission on Accreditation of Healthcare Organizations. Sentinel event alert issue 18: kernicterus threatens healthy newborns. Sentinel Event Alert. 2001.

425. Kernicterus in full-term infants—United States, 1994-1998. MMWR Morb Mortal Wkly Rep. 2001;50(23): 491-494.

426. Maisels MJ, Newman TB. Kernicterus in otherwise healthy, breast-fed term newborns. Pediatrics. 1995;96: 730-733.

427. American Academy of Pediatrics Subcommittee on Neonatal Hyperbilirubinemia. Neonatal jaundice. Pediatrics. 2001;108:763-765.

428. Johnson LH, Bhutani VK, Brown AK. System-based approach to management of neonatal jaundice and prevention of kernicterus. J Pediatr. 2002;140:396-403.

429. Committee on Fetus and Newborn. Hospital stay for healthy newborns. Pediatrics. 1995;96:788-790.

430. Madlon-Kay DJ. Evaluation and management of newborn jaundice by Midwest family physicians. J Fam Pract. 1998;47:461-464.

431. Maisels MJ, Newman TB. Jaundice in full-term and near-term babies who leave the hospital within 36 hours. The pediatrician's nemesis. Clin Perinatol. 1998;25:295-302.

432. American Academy of Pediatrics. Practice parameter: management of hyperbilirubinemia in the healthy term newborn. Pediatrics. 1994;94:558-565.

433. Newman TB, Hope S, Stevenson DK. Direct bilirubin measurements in jaundiced term newborns. A reevaluation. Am J Dis Child. 1991;145:1305-1309.

434. Keffler S, Kelly DA, Powell JE, Green A. Population screening for neonatal liver disease: a feasibility study. J Pediatr Gastroenterol Nutr. 1998;27:306-311.

435. Bhutani VK, Johnson L, Sivieri EM. Predictive ability of a predischarge hour-specific serum bilirubin for subsequent significant hyperbilirubinemia in healthy term and near-term newborns. Pediatrics. 1999;103:6-14.

436. Johnson L, Bhutani VK. Guidelines for management of the jaundiced term and near-term infant. Clin Perinatol. 1998;25:555-574.

437. Eggert LD, Wiedmeier SE, Wilson J, Christensen RD. The effect of instituting a prehospital-discharge newborn bilirubin screening program in an 18-hospital health system. Pediatrics. 2006;117:e855-e862.

438. Britton JR, Britton HL, Beebe SA. Early discharge of the term newborn: a continued dilemma. Pediatrics. 1994;94: 291-295.

439. Soskolne EL, Schumacher R, Fyock C, et al. The effect of early discharge and other factors on readmission rates of newborns. Arch Pediatr Adolesc Med. 1996;150: 373-379.

440. Ahlfors CE. Effect of ibuprofen on bilirubin-albumin binding. J Pediatr. 2004;144:386-388.

441. Cockington RA, Drew JH, Eberhard A. Outcomes following the use of rational guidelines in the management of jaundiced newborn infants. Aust Paediatr J. 1989;25: 346-350.

442. Ennever JF. Blue light, green light, white light, more light: treatment of neonatal jaundice. Clin Perinatol. 1990;17: 467-481.

443. Pratesi R, Agati G, Fusi F. Phototherapy for neonatal hyperbilirubinemia. Photodermatology. 1989;6:244-257.

444. McDonagh AF, Lightner DA. "Like a shrivelled blood orange"—bilirubin, jaundice and phototherapy. Pediatrics. 1985;75:443-445.

445. McDonagh AF, Palma LA, Lightner DA. Phototherapy for neonatal jaundice: stereospecific and regioselective photoisomerization of bilirubin bound to human serum albumin and NMR characterization of intramolecular cyclized photoproducts. J Am Chem Soc. 1982;104: 6867-6869.

446. Itoh S, Onishi S, Manabe M, Yamakawa T. Wavelength dependence of the geometric and structural photoisomerization of bilirubin bound to human serum albumin. Biol Neonate. 1987;51:10-17.

447. Ennever JF, Dresing TJ. Quantum yields for the cyclization and configurational isomerization of 4E,15Z-bilirubin. Photochem Photobiol. 1991;53:25-32.

448. Onishi S, Isobe K, Itoh S, et al. Metabolism of bilirubin and its photoisomers in newborn infants during phototherapy. J Biochem (Toyko). 1986;100:789-795.

449. Ennever JF, Costarino AT, Polin RA, et al. Rapid clearance of a structural isomer of bilirubin during phototherapy. J Clin Invest. 1987;79:1674-1678.

450. Tan KL. Efficacy of fluorescent daylight, blue, and green lamps in the management of nonhemolytic hyperbilirubinemia. J Pediatr. 1989;114:132-137.

451. Rosenfeld W, Twist P, Concepcion L. A new device for phototherapy. Pediatr Res. 1989;25:227A.

452. Rosenfeld W, Twist P, Concepcion L. A new device for phototherapy treatment of jaundiced infants. J Perinatol. 1990;10:243-248.

453. Gale R, Dranitzki Z, Dollberg S, Stevenson DK. A randomized, controlled application of the Wallaby phototherapy system compared with standard phototherapy. J Perinatol. 1990;10:239-242.

454. van Kaam AH, van Beek RH, Vergunst-van Keulen JG, et al. Fibre optic versus conventional phototherapy for hyperbilirubinaemia in preterm infants. Eur J Pediatr. 1998;157:132-137.

455. Fetus and Newborn Committee, Canadian Paediatric Society. Use of phototherapy for neonatal hyperbilirubinemia. Can Med Assoc J. 1986;134:1237-1245.

456. Cashore WJ, Stern L. The management of hyperbilirubinemia. Clin Perinatol. 1984;11:339-357.

457. Polin RA. Management of neonatal hyperbilirubinemia: rational use of phototherapy. Biol Neonate. 1990;58(Suppl 1):32-43.

458. Grabert BE, Wardwell C, Harburg SK. Home phototherapy. An alternative to prolonged hospitalization of the full-term, well newborn. Clin Pediatr (Phila). 1986;25: 291-294.

459. Ludwig MA. Phototherapy in the home setting. J Pediatr Health Care. 1990;4:304-308.

460. Gourley GR, Odell GB. Bilirubin metabolism in the fetus and neonate. In Lebenthal E (ed). Human Gastrointestinal Development. New York, Raven, 1989, pp 581-621.

461. De Curtis M, Guandalini S, Fasano A, et al. Diarrhea in jaundiced neonates treated with phototherapy: a role of intestinal secretion. Arch Dis Child. 1989;64:1161-1164.

462. Drew JH, Marriage KJ, Bayle V. Phototherapy. Short and long-term complications. Arch Dis Child. 1976;51: 454-458.

463. Scheidt PC, Bryla DA, Nelson KB, et al. Phototherapy for neonatal hyperbilirubinemia: six-year follow-up of the National Institute of Child Health and Human Development Clinical Trial. Pediatrics. 1990;85:455-463.

464. Benders MJ, van Bel F, Van de Bor M. The effect of phototherapy on cerebral blood flow velocity in preterm infants. Acta Paediatr. 1998;87:786-791.

465. Benders MJ, van Bel F, Van de Bor M. Haemodynamic consequences of phototherapy in term infants. Eur J Pediatr. 1999;158:323-328.

466. Yeo KL, Perlman M, Hao Y, Mullaney P. Outcomes of extremely premature infants related to their peak serum bilirubin concentrations and exposure to phototherapy. Pediatrics. 1998;102:1426-1431.

467. Gies HP, Roy CR. Bilirubin phototherapy and potential UVR hazards. Health Phys. 1990;58:313-320.

468. Poland RL, Ostrea EM. Care of the high risk neonate. In Klaus MH, Fanaroff AA (eds). Neonatal Hyperbilirubinemia. Philadelphia, Ardmore Medical, 1986, pp 238-261.

469. Yamauchi Y, Kasa N, Yamanouchi I. Is it necessary to change the babies' position during phototherapy. Early Hum Dev. 1989;20:221-227.

470. Yetman RJ, Parks DK, Huseby V, et al. Rebound bilirubin levels in infants receiving phototherapy. J Pediatr. 1998;133:705-707.

471. Tan KL. Decreased response to phototherapy for neonatal jaundice in breast-fed infants. Arch Pediatr Adolesc Med. 1998;152:1187-1190.

472. Odell GB. Neonatal Hyperbilirubinemia. New York, Grune & Stratton, 1980, p 117.

473. Gartner LM, Lee K-S. Jaundice and liver disease. Part I. Unconjugated hyperbilirubinemia. In Fanaroff AA, Martin RJ (eds). Behrman's Neonatal-Perinatal Medicine. St Louis, CV Mosby, 1983, pp 754-770.

474. Alpay F, Sarici SU, Okutan V, et al. High-dose intravenous immunoglobulin therapy in neonatal immune haemolytic jaundice. Acta Paediatr. 1999;88:216-219.

475. Shapiro M. Safer exchange transfusions with ACD blood. Bibl Haematol. 1965;23:883-886.

476. Weldon VV, Odell GB. Mortality risk of exchange transfusion. Pediatrics. 1968;41:797-801.

477. Valaes TN, Harvey-Wilkes K. Pharmacologic approaches to the prevention and treatment of neonatal hyperbilirubinemia. Clin Perinatol. 1990;17:245-273.

478. van der Veere CN, Schoemaker B, van der Meer R, et al. Rapid association of unconjugated bilirubin with amorphous calcium phosphate. J Lipid Res. 1995;36:1697-1707.

479. van der Veere CN, Schoemaker B, Bakker C, et al. Influence of dietary calcium phosphate on the disposition of bilirubin in rats with unconjugated hyperbilirubinemia. Hepatology. 1996;24:620-626.

480. De Carvalho M, Klaus MH, Merkatz RB. Frequency of breast-feeding and serum bilirubin concentration. Am J Dis Child. 1982;136:737-738.

481. Wu T-W, Li GS. A new bilirubin-degrading enzyme from orange peels. Biochem Cell Biol. 1988;66:1248.

482. Johnson L, Dworanczyk R, Jenkins D. Bilirubin oxidase (BOX) feedings at varying time intervals and enzyme concentrations in infant Gunn rats. Pediatr Res. 1989;25:116A.

483. Kimura M, Matsumura Y, Miyauchi Y, Maeda H. A new tactic for the treatment of jaundice: an injectable polymer-conjugated bilirubin oxidase. Proc Soc Exp Biol Med. 1988;188:364-369.

484. Kimura M, Matsumura Y, Konno T, et al. Enzymatic removal of bilirubin toxicity by bilirubin oxidase in vitro and excretion of degradation products in vivo. Proc Soc Exp Biol Med. 1990;195:64-69.

485. Gartner LM, Lee KS, Vaisman L, et al. Development of bilirubin transport and metabolism in the newborn rhesus monkey. J Pediatr. 1977;90:513-531.

486. Waltman R, Nigrin G, Bonura F, et al. Ethanol in prevention of hyperbilirubinaemia in the newborn. Lancet. 1969;2:1265-1267.

487. Rayburn W, Donn S, Piehl E, Compton A. Antenatal phenobarbital and bilirubin metabolism in the very low birth weight infant. Am J Obstet Gynecol. 1988;159: 1491-1493.

488. Stern L, Khanna NN, Levy G, et al. Effect of phenobarbital on hyperbilirubinemia and glucuronide formation in newborns. Am J Dis Child. 1970;120:26-31.

489. Gabilan JC, Benattar C, Lindenbaum A. Clofibrate treatment of neonatal jaundice. Pediatrics. 1990;86:647-648.

490. Stevenson DK, Rodgers PA, Vreman HJ. The use of metalloporphyrins for the chemoprevention of neonatal jaundice. Am J Dis Child. 1989;143:353-356.

491. Rodgers PA, Stevenson DK. Developmental biology of heme oxygenase. Clin Perinatol. 1990;17:275-291.

492. Kappas A, Drummond GS, Manola T, et al. Sn-protoporphyrin use in the management of hyperbilirubinemia in term newborns with direct Coombs-positive ABO-incompatibility. Pediatrics. 1988;81:485-497.

493. Martinez JC, Garcia HO, Otheguy LE, et al. Control of severe hyperbilirubinemia in full-term newborns with the inhibitor of bilirubin production Sn-mesoporphyrin. Pediatrics. 1999;103:1-5.

494. Valaes T, Drummond GS, Kappas A. Control of hyperbilirubinemia in glucose-6-phosphate dehydrogenase–deficient newborns using an inhibitor of bilirubin production, Sn-mesoporphyrin. Pediatrics. 1998;101:E1.

495. Vreman HJ, Stevenson DK. Metalloporphyrin-enhanced photodegradation of bilirubin in vitro. Am J Dis Child. 1990;144:590-594.

496. Cooke RW. New approach to prevention of kernicterus. Lancet. 1999;353:1814-1815.

497. Neifert MR. The optimization of breast-feeding in the perinatal period. Clin Perinatol. 1998;25:303-326.

498. Gartner LM, Auerbach KG. Breast milk and breastfeeding jaundice. Adv Pediatr 1987;34:249-274.

499. Maisels MJ. Neonatal jaundice. In Avery GB (ed). Neonatalogy—Pathophysiology and Management of the Newborn. Philadelphia, JB Lippincott, 1987, pp 534-629.

500. Gartner LM. Breast milk jaundice. In Levine RL, Maisels MJ (eds). Hyperbilirubinemia in the Newborn. Report of the 85th Ross Conference on Pediatric Research. Columbus, OH, Ross Laboratories, 1983, pp 75-86.

501. Yamauchi Y, Yamanouchi I. Breast-feeding frequency during the first 24 hours after birth in full-term neonates. Pediatrics. 1990;86:171-175.

502. Osborn LM, Bolus R. Breast feeding and jaundice in the first week of life. J Fam Pract. 1985;20:475.

503. Gourley GR, Kreamer B, Arend R. The effect of diet on feces and jaundice during the first 3 weeks of life. Gastroenterology. 1992;103:660-667.

504. Gourley GR, Kreamer B, Cohnen M, Kosorok MR. Neonatal jaundice and diet. Arch Pediatr Adolesc Med. 1999;153:184-188.

505. Amato M, Howald H, von Muralt G. Interruption of breast-feeding versus phototherapy as treatment of hyperbilirubinemia in full-term infants. Helv Paediatr Acta. 1985;40:127-131.

506. Rotor AB, Manahan L, Florentin A. Familial nonhemolytic jaundice with direct van den Bergh reaction. Acta Med Phil. 1948;5:37-49.

507. Namihisa T, Yamaguchi K. The constitutional hyperbilirubinemia in Japan: studies on 139 cases reported during the period 1963-1969. Gastroenterol Jpn. 1973;8:311-321.

508. Wolkoff AW. Inheritable disorders manifested by conjugated hyperbilirubinemia. Semin Liver Dis. 1983;3:65-72.

509. Vest MF, Kaufmann JH, Fritz E. Chronic nonhaemolytic jaundice with conjugated bilirubin in the serum and normal histology: a case study. Arch Dis Child. 1960;36:600-604.

510. Fretzayas A, Koukoutsakis P, Moustaki M, et al. Coinheritance of Rotor syndrome, G-6-PD deficiency, and heterozygous beta thalassemia: a possible genetic interaction. J Pediatr Gastroenterol Nutr. 2001;33:211-213.

511. Pascasio FM, de la Fuenta D. Rotor-Manahan-Florentin syndrome: clinical and genetic studies. Phil J Int Med. 1969;7:151-157.

512. Wolpert E, Pascasio FM, Wolkoff AW. Abnormal sulfobromophthalein metabolism in Rotor's syndrome and obligate heterozygotes. N Engl J Med. 1977;296:1099-1101.

513. Dhumeaux D, Berthelot P. Chronic hyperbilirubinemia associated with hepatic uptake and storage impairment. Gastroenterology. 1975;69:988-993.

514. Wheeler HO, Meltzer JI, Bradley SE. Biliary transport and hepatic storage of sulfobromophthalein sodium in the unanesthetized dog, in normal man, and in patients with hepatic disease. J Clin Invest. 1960;39:1131-1144.

515. Tipping E, Ketterer B. The role of intracellular proteins in the transport and metabolism of lipophilic compounds. In Blaver G, Sund H (eds). Transport by Proteins. Berlin, Walter de Gruyter, 1978, p 369.

516. Adachi Y, Yamamoto T. Partial defect in hepatic glutathione S-transferase activity in a case of Rotor's syndrome. Gastroenterology. 1987;22:34-38.

517. Wolkoff AW, Ketley JN, Waggoner JG, et al. Hepatic accumulation and intracellular binding of conjugated bilirubin. J Clin Invest. 1978;61:142-149.

518. Wolkoff AW, Wolpert E, Pascasio FN, Arias IM. Rotor's syndrome. A distinct inheritable pathophysiologic entity. Am J Med. 1976;60:173-179.

519. Aziz MA, Schwartz S, Watson CJ. Studies on coproporphyrin VIII. Reinvestigation of the isomer distribution in jaundice and liver diseases. J Lab Clin Med. 1964;63:596-604.

520. Shimizu Y, Naruto H, Ida S, Kohakura M. Urinary coproporphyrin isomers in Rotor's syndrome: a study in eight families. Hepatology. 1981;1:173-178.

521. Fretzayas AM, Garoufi AI, Moutsouris CX, Karpathios TE. Cholescintigraphy in the diagnosis of Rotor syndrome. J Nucl Med. 1994;35:1048-1050.

522. Bar-Meir S, Baron J, Seligson U, et al. 99mTc-HIDA cholescintigraphy in Dubin-Johnson and Rotor syndromes. Radiology. 1982;142:743-746.

523. Dubin IN, Johnson FB. Chronic idiopathic jaundice with unidentified pigment in liver cells: a new clincopathologic entity with a report of 12 cases. Medicine (Baltimore). 1954;33:155-197.

524. Dubin IN. Chronic idiopathic jaundice. A review of fifty cases. Am J Med. 1958;24:268-292.

525. Gustein SL, Alpert L, Arias IM. Studies of hepatic excretory function. IV. Biliary excretion of sulfobromophthalein sodium in a patient with Dubin-Johnson syndrome and a biliary fistula. Isr J Med Sci. 1968;4:36-40.

526. Javitt NB, Kondo T, Kuchiba K. Bile acid excretion in Dubin-Johnson syndrome. Gastroenterology. 1978;75:931-932.

527. Sprinz H, Nelson RS. Persistent nonhemolytic hyperbilirubinemia associated with lipochrome-like pigment in liver cells: report of four cases. Ann Intern Med. 1954;41:952-962.

528. Shani M, Seligsohn V, Gilon E, et al. Dubin-Johnson syndrome in Israel. I. Clinical, laboratory and genetic aspects of 101 cases. Q J Med. 1970;39:549-567.

529. Zlotogora J. Hereditary disorders among Iranian Jews. Am J Med Genet. 1995;58:32-37.

530. Lee JH, Chen HL, Chen HL, et al. Neonatal Dubin-Johnson syndrome: long-term follow-up and MRP2 mutations study. Pediatr Res. 2006;59:584-589.

531. Kimura A, Ushijima K, Kage M, et al. Neonatal Dubin-Johnson syndrome with severe cholestasis: effective phenobarbital therapy. Acta Paediatr Scand. 1991;80:381-385.

532. Shieh CC, Chang MH, Chen CL. Dubin-Johnson syndrome presenting with neonatal cholestasis. Arch Dis Child. 1990;65:898-899.

533. Haimi-Cohen Y, Amir J, Merlob P. Neonatal and infantile Dubin-Johnson syndrome. Pediatr Rediol. 1998;28:900.

534. Haimi-Cohen Y, Merlob P, Marcus-Eidlits T, Amir J. Dubin-Johnson syndrome as a cause of neonatal jaundice: the importance of coproporphyrins investigation. Clin Pediatr (Phila). 1998;37:511-513.

535. Kimura A, Yuge K, Kosai KI, et al. Neonatal cholestasis in two siblings: a variant of Dubin-Johnson syndrome? J Paediatr Child Health. 1995;31:557-560.

536. Kondo T, Kuchiba K, Ohtsuka Y, et al. Clinical and genetic studies on Dubin-Johnson syndrome in a cluster area in Japan. Jpn J Hum Genet. 1974;18:378-392.

537. Edwards RH. Inheritance of the Dubin-Johnson-Sprinz syndrome. Gastroenterology. 1975;63:734-749.

538. Cohen L, Lewis C, Arias IM. Pregnancy, oral contraceptives and chronic familial jaundice with predominantly conjugated hyperbilirubinemia (Dubin-Johnson syndrome). Gastroenterology. 1972;62:1182-1190.

539. Muscatello U, Mussini I, Agnolucci MT. Dubin-Johnson syndrome: an electron microscopic study of the liver cell. Acta Hepatosplenol. 1967;14:162-170.

540. Ehrlich JC, Novikoff AB, Platt R, et al. Hepatocellular lipofuscin and the pigment of chronic idiopathic jaundice. Bull N Y Acad Med. 1960;36:488-491.

541. Swartz HM, Sarna, Varma RR. On the nature and excretion of the hepatic pigment in the Dubin-Johnson syndrome. Gastroenterology. 1979;76:958-964.

542. Swartz HM, Chen K, Roth JA. Further evidence that the pigment in the Dubin-Johnson syndrome is not melanin. Pigment Cell Res. 1987;1:69-75.

543. Arias IM, Blumberg W. The pigment in Dubin-Johnson syndrome. Gastroenterology. 1979;77:820-821.

544. Kitamura T, Alroy J, Gatmaitan Z, et al. Defective biliary excretion of epinephrine metabolites in mutant (TR-) rats: relation to the pathogenesis of black liver in the Dubin-Johnson syndrome and Corriedale sheep with an analogous excretory defect. Hepatology. 1992;15:1154-1159.

545. Hunter FM, Sparks RD, Flinner RL. Hepatitis with resulting mobilization of hepatic pigment in a patient with Dubin-Johnson syndrome. Gastroenterology. 1964;47:631-635.

546. Kobayashi Y, Ishihara T, Wada M, et al. Dubin-Johnson–like black liver with normal bilirubin level. J Gastroenterol. 2004;39:892-895.

547. Paulusma CC, Kool M, Bosma PJ, et al. A mutation in the human canalicular multispecific organic anion transporter gene causes the Dubin-Johnson syndrome. Hepatology. 1997;25:1539-1542.

548. Toh S, Wada M, Uchiumi T, et al. Genomic structure of the canalicular multispecific organic anion-transporter gene (MRP2/cMOAT) and mutations in the ATP-binding-cassette region in Dubin-Johnson syndrome. Am J Hum Genet. 1999;64:739-746.

549. van Kuijck MA, Kool M, Merkx GF, et al. Assignment of the canalicular multispecific organic anion transporter gene (CMOAT) to human chromosome 10q24 and mouse chromosome 19D2 by fluorescent in situ hybridization. Cytogenet Cell Genet. 1997;77:285-287.

550. Kajihara S, Hisatomi A, Mizuta T, et al. A splice mutation in the human canalicular multispecific organic anion transporter gene causes Dubin-Johnson syndrome. Biochem Biophys Res Commun. 1998;253:454-457.

551. Tsujii H, König J, Rost D, et al. Exon-intron organization of the human multidrug-resistance protein 2 (MRP2) gene mutated in Dubin-Johnson syndrome. Gastroenterology. 1999;117:653-660.

552. Materna V, Lage H. Homozygous mutation Arg768Trp in the ABC-transporter encoding gene MRP2/cMOAT/ABCC2 causes Dubin-Johnson syndrome in a Caucasian patient. J Hum Genet. 2003;48:484-486.

553. Machida I, Wakusawa S, Sanae F, et al. Mutational analysis of the MRP2 gene and long-term follow-up of Dubin-Johnson syndrome in Japan. J Gastroenterol. 2005;40:366-370.

554. Mendema E, DeFraiure WH, Nieweg HO, et al. Familial chronic idiopathic jaundice. Am J Med. 1960;28:42-50.

555. Charbonnier A, Brisbois P. Etude chromatographique de la BSP au cours de l'epreuve clinique d'epuration plasmatique de ce colorant. Rev Int Hepatol. 1960;10:1163-1213.

556. Shani M, Gilon E, Ben-Ezzer J, Sheba C. Sulfobromophthalein tolerance test in patients with Dubin-Johnson syndrome and their relatives. Gastroenterology. 1970;59:842-847.

557. Abe H, Okuda K. Biliary excretion of conjugated sulfobromophthalein (BSP) in constitutional conjugated hyperbilirubinemias. Digestion. 1975;13:272-283.

558. Erlinger S, Dhumeaux D, Desjeux JF, Benhamou JP. Hepatic handling of unconjugated dyes in the Dubin-Johnson syndrome. Gastroenterology. 1973;64:106-110.

559. Koskelo P, Toivonen I, Aldercreutz H. Urinary coproporphyrin isomer distribution in Dubin-Johnson syndrome. Clin Chem. 1967;13:1006-1009.

560. Frank M, Doss M, de Carvalho DG. Diagnostic and pathogenetic implications of urinary coproporphyrin excretion in the Dubin-Johnson syndrome. Hepatogastroenterology. 1990;37:147-151.

561. Ben-Ezzer J, Seligson U, Shani M, et al. Abnormal excretion of the isomers of urinary coproporphyrin by patients with Dubin-Johnson syndrome in Israel. Clin Sci. 1971;40:17-30.

562. Wolkoff AW, Cohen LE, Arias IM. Inheritance of the Dubin-Johnson syndrome. N Engl J Med. 1973;288:113-117.

563. Kondo T, Kuchiba K, Shimizu Y. Coproporphyrin isomers in Dubin-Johnson syndrome. Gastroenterology. 1976;70:1117-1120.

564. Rocchi E, Balli F, Gibertini P, et al. Coproporphyrin excretion in healthy newborn babies. J Pediatr Gastroenterol Nutr. 1984;3:402-407.

565. Kappas A, Sassa S, Anderson KE. Disorders of porphyrin and heme metabolism. In Standbury JB, Wyngaarden JB, Fredrickson DS, et al (eds). The Metabolic Basis of Inherited Disease. New York, McGraw-Hill, 1983, pp 1299-384.

566. Garcia-Vargas GG, Del Razo LM, Cebrian ME, et al. Altered urinary porphyrin excretion in a human population chronically exposed to arsenic in Mexico. Hum Exp Toxicol. 1994;13:839-847.

567. Kladchareon N, Suwannakul P, Bauchum V. Dubin-Johnson syndrome: report of two siblings with Tc-99m IODIDA cholescintigraphic findings. J Med Assoc Thai. 1988;71:640-642.

568. Pinós T, Constansa JM, Palacin A, Figueras C. A new diagnostic approach to the Dubin-Johnson syndrome. Am J Gastroenterol. 1990;85:91-93.

569. Shimizu T, Tawa T, Maruyama T, et al. A case of infantile Dubin-Johnson syndrome with high CT attenuation in the liver. Pediatr Rediol. 1997;27:345-347.

570. Mayatepek E, Lehmann WD. Defective hepatobiliary leukotriene elimination in patients with the Dubin-Johnson syndrome. Clin Chim Acta. 1996;249:37-46.

571. Yoo J, Reichert DE, Kim J, et al. A potential Dubin-Johnson syndrome imaging agent: synthesis, biodistribution, and microPET imaging. Mol Imaging. 2005;4:18-29.

572. Lindberg MC. Hepatobiliary complications of oral contraceptives. J Gen Intern Med. 1992;7:199-209.

573. Di Zoglio JD, Cardillo E. Dubin-Johnson syndrome and pregnancy. Obstet Gynecol. 1973;42:560-563.

574. Berk PD, Noyer C. The familial conjugated hyperbilirubinemias. Semin Liver Dis. 1994;14:386-394.

575. Corpechot C, Ping C, Wendum D, et al. Identification of a novel 974C→G nonsense mutation of the MRP2/ABCC2 gene in a patient with Dubin-Johnson syndrome and analysis of the effects of rifampicin and ursodeoxycholic acid on serum bilirubin and bile acids. Am J Gastroenterol. 2006;101:2427-2432.

5

Developmental Hemostasis: Relevance to Newborns and Infants

Alan B. Cantor

Development of the human hemostatic system begins in utero and continues until well after birth. As a result, functional levels of many of the procoagulants, coagulation inhibitors, fibrinolytic components, and platelet-associated factors differ from those of older children and adults, with "adult" values often not reached until about 6 months of age. These unique aspects of fetal and neonatal coagulation were first fully documented in the pioneering work of Dr. Maureen Andrew in the 1980s and have been termed "developmental hemostasis." A firm understanding of these differences, as well as access to tables listing the "normal" ranges of various hemostatic factors in infants at different gestational and postnatal ages, is critical to proper interpretation of laboratory tests performed on newborns and infants. Despite broad differences from adults in functional levels of hemostatic factors, healthy newborns rarely have difficulties with hemorrhage or thrombosis. Thus, these differences in prothrombotic and antithrombotic factors are uniquely balanced in the neonate and fetus and represent a normal physiologic state. However, this system provides little reserve, which often contributes to significant morbidity in sick and preterm infants. In addition to these developmental aspects of hemostasis, many inherited bleeding and clotting disorders can present in the newborn period. This chapter reviews the normal development of the hemostatic system, presents data tables for normal ranges at different developmental ages, and briefly reviews inherited disorders of hemostasis and thrombosis that can occur in the newborn period. For additional discussion of the investigation and management of neonatal hemostasis and thrombosis, see recent evidence-based guidelines published by the British Haemostasis and Thrombosis Task Force.[1]

ONTOGENY OF THE HUMAN HEMOSTATIC SYSTEM

Coagulation Factors

The biochemistry and function of the individual coagulation factors are reviewed in detail in Chapter 26. Coagulation proteins do not effectively cross the placental barrier and are independently synthesized by the fetus.[2-14] mRNA transcripts for coagulation factors VII, VIII, IX, and X and fibrinogen are detectable at about 5 weeks of gestation in hepatocytes of the embryo (Fig. 5-1).[15] By 10 weeks of gestation, plasma protein levels of most factors are measurable but range from 10% of the normal adult level for factor IX to about 30% for most of the other coagulation factors.[16] In general, these levels continue to increase gradually in parallel with gestational age (Table 5-1). However, with the exception of fibrinogen and factors V, VIII, and XIII, these levels remain considerably below the normal adult range, even at the time of birth for full-term infants.[16-18] They then continue to gradually increase and near the normal adult range by about 6 months of age (Tables 5-2 and 5-3). Premature infants have an accelerated increase in levels after birth

TABLE 5-1	Coagulation Screening Tests and Coagulation Factor Levels in Fetuses, Full-Term Infants, and Adults				
	FETUSES (WEEKS' GESTATION)			**Newborn**	
Parameter	**19-23 (n = 20)**	**24-29 (n = 22)**	**30-38 (n = 22)**	**(n = 60)**	**Adult (n = 40)**
PT (sec)	32.5 (19-45)	32.2 (19-44)*	22.6 (16-30)*	16.7 (12.0-23.5)†	13.5 (11.4-14.0)
PT (INR)	6.4 (1.7-11.1)	6.2 (2.1-10.6)*	3.0 (1.5-5.0)†	1.7 (0.9-2.7)†	1.1 (0.8-1.2)
APTT (sec)	168.8 (83-250)	154.0 (87-210)*	104.8 (76-128)*	44.3 (35-52)†	33.0 (25-39)
TCT (sec)	34.2 (24-44)†	26.2 (24-28)	21.4 (17.0-23.3)	20.4 (15.2-25.0)*	14.0 (12-16)
Factor I von Clauss (g/L)	0.85 (0.57-1.50)	1.12 (0.65-1.65)	1.35 (1.25-1.65)	1.68 (0.95-2.45)*	3.0 (1.78-4.50)
Factor I Ag (g/L)	1.08 (0.75-1.50)	1.93 (1.56-2.40)	1.94 (1.30-2.40)	2.65 (1.68-3.60)*	3.5 (2.50-5.20)
Factor IIc (%)	16.9 (10-24)	19.9 (11-30)†	27.9 (15-50)*	43.5 (27-64)*	98.7 (70-125)
Factor VIIc (%)	27.4 (17-37)	33.8 (18-48)†	45.9 (31-62)	52.5 (28-78)*	101.3 (68-130)
Factor IXc (%)	10.1 (6-14)	9.9 (5-15)	12.3 (5-24)*	31.8 (15-50)*	104.8 (70-142)
Factor Xc (%)	20.5 (14-29)	24.9 (16-35)	28.0 (16-36)*	39.6 (21-65)*	99.2 (75-125)
Factor Vc (%)	32.1 (21-44)	36.8 (25-50)	48.9 (23-70)*	89.9 (50-140)	99.8 (65-140)
Factor VIIIc (%)	34.5 (18-50)	35.5 (20-52)	50.1 (27-78)*	94.3 (38-150)	101.8 (55-170)
Factor XIc (%)	13.2 (8-19)	12.1 (6-22)	14.8 (6-26)*	37.2 (13-62)*	100.2 (70-135)
Factor XIIc (%)	14.9 (6-25)	22.7 (6-40)	25.8 (11-50)*	69.8 (25-105)*	101.4 (65-144)
PK (%)	12.8 (8-19)	15.4 (8-26)	18.1 (8-28)*	35.4 (21-53)*	99.8 (65-135)
HMWK (%)	15.4 (10-22)	19.3 (10-26)	23.6 (12-34)*	38.9 (28-53)*	98.8 (68-135)

All values are given as means followed in parentheses by the lower and upper boundaries including 95% of the population.
*$P < .01$.
†$P < .05$.

Ag, antigen; APTT, activated partial thromboplastin time; HMWK, high-molecular-weight kininogen; INR, international normalized ratio; PK, prekallikrein; PT, prothrombin time; TCT, thrombin clotting time.

From Reverdiau-Moalic P, Delahousse B, Body G, et al: Evolution of blood coagulation activators and inhibitors in the healthy human fetus. Blood. 1996;88:900-906.

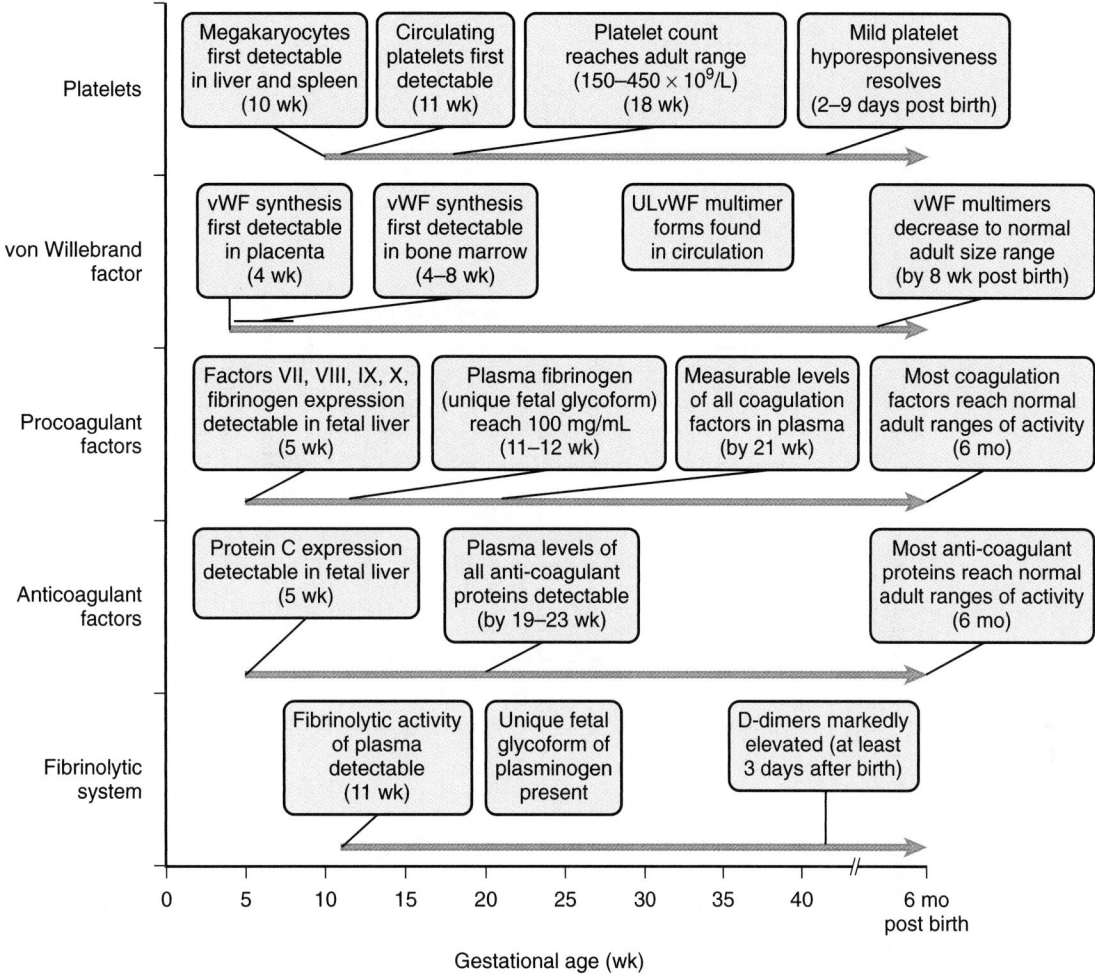

FIGURE 5-1. Development of the hemostasis system in human embryos and newborns. Reported detection or other key developmental changes that occur in the different components of the hemostatic system during gestation and the first 6 months of postnatal life are presented in this schematic timeline. ULVWF, ultralarge von Willebrand factor multimers. *(Adapted from Manco-Johnson MJ. Development of hemostasis in the fetus. Thromb Res. 2005;115[Suppl 1]:55-63.)*

and, in general, "catch up" to the full-term infant range by 3 months' postnatal age (Table 5-4).[19] True reference ranges for extremely premature infants (<30 weeks' gestation) are not available because the majority of these infants have postnatal complications. Table 5-5 provides reference ranges for older children.[20] The nearly normal "adult" levels of fibrinogen and factors V and VIII in neonates make them useful markers for the investigation of possible consumptive coagulopathy or hemophilia A.

Regulation of fetal coagulation protein levels occurs by both transcriptional and translational mechanisms.[15,21] In addition, ratios of hepatocyte to plasma levels of many factors are relatively high in comparison to adults, thus suggesting that delayed hepatocyte release may also contribute to the relatively low coagulation factor levels in fetuses and newborns.[22]

Natural Inhibitors of Coagulation

Like many of the procoagulant factors, functional levels of most coagulation inhibitors in fetuses and neonates are

significantly lower than those in adults (Tables 5-6 and 5-7; also see Table 5-3).[16,18,23] Awareness of these differences is critical to proper interpretation of laboratory studies obtained during evaluation of neonatal thrombosis. Most coagulation inhibitors reach the adult range of activity by 6 months of age.

As reviewed in Chapter 26, at least three mechanisms/pathways exist for inhibition of procoagulant activity: (1) cleavage of factors V and VIII by the protein C/S system; (2) direct inhibition of thrombin by antithrombin III (ATIII), heparin cofactor, and α_2-macroglobulin; and (3) inhibition of factor VIIa by the tissue factor pathway inhibitor (TFPI)/factor Xa complex. When thrombin binds to thrombomodulin on endothelial surfaces, it no longer cleaves fibrinogen but activates protein C. Activated protein C, in complex with protein S, proteolytically inactivates factors V and VIII. At birth, plasma concentrations of protein C are quite low and remain decreased during the first 6 months of life.[17,19,23] Neonates also have about a twofold higher amount of the single-chain form of protein C than adults do and may

Text continues on p. 155.

TABLE 5-2   Reference Values for Coagulation Tests in Healthy Full-Term Infants during the First 6 Months of Life with the ACL Analyzer

Coagulation Tests	Day 1	Day 5	Day 30	Day 90	Day 180	Adult
PT (sec)	13.0 (10.1-15.9)*	12.4 (10.0-15.3)*	11.8 (10.0-14.3)*	11.9 (10.0-14.2)*	12.3 (10.7-13.9)*	12.4 (10.8-13.9)
INR	1.00 (0.53-1.62)	0.89 (0.53-1.48)	0.79 (0.53-1.26)	0.81 (0.53-1.26)	0.88 (0.61-1.17)	0.89 (0.64-1.17)
APTT (sec)	42.9 (31.3-54.5)	42.6 (25.4-59.8)	40.4 (32.0-55.2)	37.1 (29.0-50.1)*	35.5 (28.1-42.9)	33.5 (26.6-40.3)*
TCT (sec)	23.5 (19.0-28.3)*	23.1 (18.0-29.2)	24.3 (19.4-29.2)*	25.1 (20.5-29.7)*	25.5 (19.8-31.2)	25.0 (19.7-30.3)*
Fibrinogen (g/L)	2.83 (1.67-3.99)*	3.12 (1.62-4.62)*	2.70 (1.62-3.78)*	2.43 (1.50-3.79)*	2.51 (1.50-3.87)	2.78 (1.56-4.00)*
Factor II (U/mL)	0.48 (0.26-0.70)	0.63 (0.33-0.93)	0.68 (0.34-1.02)	0.75 (0.45-1.05)	0.88 (0.60-1.16)	1.08 (0.70-1.46)
Factor V (U/mL)	0.72 (0.34-1.08)	0.95 (0.45-1.45)	0.98 (0.62-1.34)	0.90 (0.48-1.32)	0.91 (0.55-1.27)	1.06 (0.62-1.50)
Factor VII (U/mL)	0.66 (0.28-1.04)	0.89 (0.35-1.43)	0.90 (0.42-1.38)	0.91 (0.39-1.43)	0.87 (0.47-1.27)	1.05 (0.67-1.43)
Factor VIII (U/mL)	1.00 (0.50-1.78)*	0.88 (0.50-1.54)*	0.91 (0.50-1.57)*	0.79 (0.50-1.25)*	0.73 (0.50-1.09)	0.99 (0.50-1.49)
VWF (U/mL)	1.53 (0.50-2.87)	1.40 (0.50-2.54)	1.28 (0.50-2.46)	1.18 (0.50-2.06)	1.07 (0.50-1.97)	0.92 (0.50-1.58)
Factor IX (U/mL)	0.53 (0.15-0.91)	0.53 (0.15-0.91)	0.51 (0.21-0.81)	0.67 (0.21-1.13)	0.86 (0.36-1.36)	1.09 (0.55-1.63)
Factor X (U/mL)	0.40 (0.12-0.68)	0.49 (0.19-0.79)	0.59 (0.31-0.87)	0.71 (0.35-1.07)	0.78 (0.38-1.18)	1.06 (0.70-1.52)
Factor XI (U/mL)	0.38 (0.10-0.66)	0.55 (0.23-0.87)	0.53 (0.27-0.79)	0.69 (0.41-0.97)	0.86 (0.49-1.34)	0.97 (0.67-1.27)
Factor XII (U/mL)	0.53 (0.13-0.93)	0.47 (0.11-0.83)	0.49 (0.17-0.81)	0.67 (0.25-1.09)	0.77 (0.39-1.15)	1.08 (0.52-1.64)
PK (U/mL)	0.37 (0.18-0.69)	0.48 (0.20-0.76)	0.57 (0.23-0.91)	0.73 (0.41-1.05)	0.86 (0.56-1.16)	1.12 (0.62-1.62)
HMWK (U/mL)	0.54 (0.06-1.02)	0.74 (0.16-1.32)	0.77 (0.33-1.21)	0.82 (0.30-1.46)*	0.82 (0.36-1.28)*	0.92 (0.50-1.36)
Factor XIIIa (U/mL)	0.79 (0.27-1.31)	0.94 (0.44-1.44)*	0.93 (0.39-1.47)*	1.04 (0.36-1.72)*	1.04 (0.46-1.62)*	1.05 (0.55-1.55)
Factor XIIIb (U/mL)	0.76 (0.30-1.22)	1.06 (0.32-1.80)	1.11 (0.39-1.73)*	1.16 (0.48-1.84)*	1.10 (0.50-1.70)*	0.97 (0.57-1.37)

All factors except fibrinogen are expressed as units per milliliter, with pooled plasma containing 1.0 U/mL. All values are expressed as means followed by the lower and upper boundary encompassing 95% of the population. Between 40 and 77 samples were assayed for each value in newborns. Some measurements were skewed because of a disproportionate number of high values. All infants received 1 mg vitamin K intramuscularly at birth. The following reagents were used for coagulation screening tests: prothrombin time (Dade C rabbit thromboplastin), activated partial thromboplastin time (Dade FS). Measurements were made with an ACL analyzer.

*Values indistinguishable from those of adults.

APTT, activated partial thromboplastin time; HMWK, high-molecular-weight kininogen; INR, international normalized ratio; PK, prekallikrein; PT, prothrombin time; TCT, thrombin clotting time; VWF, von Willebrand factor.

From Andrew M, Paes B, Milner R, et al: Development of the human coagulation system in the full-term infant. Blood. 1987;70:165-172.

TABLE 5-3   Reference Values for Coagulation Tests in Healthy Full-Term Infants and Children with the STA Analyzer

	Day 1	Day 3	1 Month-1 Year	1-5 Years	6-10 Years	11-16 Years	Adults
COAGULATION TESTS							
APTT (sec)*	38.7 (34.3-44.8)†	36.3 (29.5-42.2)†	39.3 (35.1-46.3)†	37.7 (33.6-43.8)†	37.3 (31.8-43.7)†	39.5 (33.9-46.1)†	33.2 (28.6-38.2)
PT (sec)‡	15.6 (14.4-16.4)†	14.9 (13.5-16.4)†	13.1 (11.5-15.3)	13.3 (12.1-14.5)	13.4 (11.7-15.1)†	13.8 (12.7-16.1)†	13.0 (11.5-14.5)
INR	1.26 (1.15-1.35)†	1.20 (1.05-1.35)†	1.00 (0.86-1.22)	1.03 (0.92-1.14)†	1.04 (0.87-1.20)†	1.08 (0.97-1.30)†	1.00 (0.80-1.20)
Fibrinogen (g/L)	2.80 (1.92-3.74)	3.30 (2.83-4.01)	2.42 (0.82-3.83)†	2.82 (1.62-4.01)†	3.04 (1.99-4.09)	3.15 (2.12-4.33)	3.10 (1.9-4.3)
COAGULATION FACTORS							
Factor II (%)	54 (41-69)†	62 (50-73)†	90 (62-103)†	89 (70-109)†	89 (67-110)†	90 (61-107)†	110 (78-138)
Factor V (%)	81 (64-103)†	122 (92-154)	113 (94-141)	97 (67-127)†	99 (56-141)†	89 (67-141)†	118 (78-152)
Factor VII (%)	70 (52-88)†	86 (67-107)†	128 (83-160)	111 (72-150)†	113 (70-156)†	118 (69-200)	129 (61-199)
Factor VIII (%)	182 (105-329)	159 (83-274)	94 (54-145)†	110 (36-185)†	117 (52-182)†	120 (59-200)†	160 (52-290)
Factor IX (%)	48 (35-56)†	72 (44-97)†	71 (43-121)†	85 (44-127)†	96 (48-145)†	111 (64-216)†	130 (59-254)
Factor X (%)	55 (46-67)†	60 (46-75)†	95 (77-122)†	98 (72-125)†	97 (68-125)†	91 (53-122)†	124 (96-171)
Factor XI (%)	30 (7-41)†	57 (24-79)†	89 (62-125)†	113 (65-162)	113 (65-162)	111 (65-139)	112 (67-196)
Factor XII (%)	58 (43-80)†	53 (14-80)†	79 (20-135)†	85 (36-135)†	81 (26-137)†	75 (14-117)†	115 (35-207)
COAGULATION INHIBITORS							
ATIII (%)	76 (58-90)†	74 (60-89)†	109 (72-134)†	116 (101-131)†	114 (95-134)†	111 (96-126)†	96 (66-124)
Protein C, chromogenic (%)	36 (24-44)†	44 (28-54)†	71 (31-112)†	96 (65-127)†	100 (71-129)	94 (66-118)†	104 (74-164)
Protein C, clotting (%)	32 (24-40)†	33 (24-51)†	77 (28-124)†	94 (50-134)†	94 (64-125)†	88 (59-112)†	103 (54-166)
Protein S, clotting (%)	36 (28-47)†	49 (33-67)†	102 (29-162)†	101 (67-136)†	109 (64-154)†	103 (65-140)†	75 (54-103)

Values represent means. Boundaries including 95% of the population are shown in parentheses. All infants received 1 mg vitamin K intramuscularly at the time of birth.
*STA-PTT-A reagent used.
†Denotes values that are significantly different from adult values (*P* < .05).
‡Neoplastine CI reagent used.
APTT, activated partial thromboplastin time; ATIII, antithrombin III; INR, international normalized ratio; PT, prothrombin time.
Reproduced with permission from Monagle P, Barnes C, Ignjatovic V, et al. Developmental haemostasis. Impact for clinical haemostasis laboratories. Thromb Haemost. 2006;95:362-372.

TABLE 5-4   Reference Values for Coagulation Tests in Healthy Premature Infants (30 to 36 Weeks' Gestation) during the First 6 Months of Life

Coagulation Tests	Day 1	Day 5	Day 30	Day 90	Day 180	Adult
PT (sec)	13.0 (10.6-16.2)*	12.5 (10.0-15.3)*	11.8 (10.0-13.6)*	12.3 (10.0-14.6)	12.5 (10.0-15.0)*	12.4 (10.8-13.9)
INR	1.0 (0.61-1.70)	0.91 (0.53-1.48)	0.79 (0.53-1.32)	0.88 (0.53-1.48)	0.91 (0.53-1.48)	0.89 (0.64-1.17)
APTT (sec)	53.6 (27.5-79.4)†	50.5 (26.9-74.1)	44.7 (26.9-62.5)	39.5 (28.3-50.7)	37.5 (27.2-53.3)	33.5 (26.6-40.3)
TCT (sec)	24.8 (19.2-30.4)	24.1 (18.8-29.4)*	24.4 (18.8-29.9)	25.1 (19.4-30.8)	25.2 (18.9-31.5)	25.0 (19.7-30.3)
Fibrinogen (g/L)	2.43 (1.50-3.73)*†	2.80 (1.60-4.18)*†	2.54 (1.50-4.14)	2.46 (1.50-3.52)	2.28 (1.50-3.60)	2.78 (1.56-4.00)
Factor II (U/mL)	0.45 (0.20-0.77)	0.57 (0.29-0.85)†	0.57 (0.36-0.95)	0.68 (0.30-1.06)	0.87 (0.51-1.23)	1.08 (0.70-1.46)
Factor V (U/mL)	0.88 (0.41-1.44)*†	1.00 (0.46-1.54)*	1.02 (0.48-1.56)*	0.99 (0.59-1.39)	1.02 (0.58-1.46)*	1.06 (0.62-1.50)
Factor VII (U/mL)	0.67 (0.21-1.13)	0.84 (0.30-1.38)	0.83 (0.21-1.45)	0.87 (0.31-1.43)	0.99 (0.47-1.51)*	1.05 (0.67-1.43)
Factor VIII (U/mL)	1.11 (0.50-2.13)	1.15 (0.53-2.05)*†	1.11 (0.50-1.99)	1.06 (0.58-1.88)*†	0.99 (0.50-1.87)*†	0.99 (0.50-1.49)
VWF (U/mL)	1.36 (0.78-2.10)	1.33 (0.72-2.19)	1.36 (0.66-2.16)	1.12 (0.75-1.84)*†	0.98 (0.54-1.58)*	0.92 (0.50-1.58)
Factor IX (U/mL)	0.35 (0.19-0.65)†	0.42 (0.14-0.74)†	0.44 (0.13-0.80)	0.59 (0.25-0.93)	0.81 (0.50-1.20)	1.09 (0.55-1.63)
Factor X (U/mL)	0.41 (0.11-0.71)	0.51 (0.19-0.83)	0.56 (0.20-0.92)	0.67 (0.35-0.99)	0.77 (0.35-1.19)	1.06 (0.70-1.52)
Factor XI (U/mL)	0.30 (0.08-0.52)†	0.41 (0.13-0.69)†	0.43 (0.15-0.71)*	0.59 (0.25-0.93)*	0.78 (0.46-1.10)	0.97 (0.67-1.27)
Factor XII (U/mL)	0.38 (0.10-0.66)†	0.39 (0.09-0.69)†	0.43 (0.11-0.75)	0.61 (0.15-1.07)	0.82 (0.22-1.42)	1.08 (0.52-1.64)
PK (U/mL)	0.33 (0.09-0.57)	0.45 (0.25-0.75)	0.59 (0.31-0.87)	0.79 (0.37-1.21)	0.78 (0.40-1.16)	1.12 (0.62-1.62)
HMWK (U/mL)	0.49 (0.09-0.89)	0.62 (0.24-1.00)†	0.64 (0.16-1.12)†	0.78 (0.32-1.24)	0.83 (0.41-1.25)*	0.92 (0.50-1.36)
Factor XIIIa (U/mL)	0.70 (0.32-1.08)	1.01 (0.57-1.45)*	0.99 (0.51-1.47)*	1.13 (0.71-1.55)*	1.13 (0.65-1.61)*	1.05 (0.55-1.55)
Factor XIIIb (U/mL)	0.81 (0.35-1.27)	1.10 (0.68-1.58)*	1.07 (0.57-1.57)*	1.21 (0.75-1.67)	1.15 (0.67-1.63)	0.97 (0.57-1.37)

All factors except fibrinogen are expressed as units per milliliter, with pooled plasma containing 1.0 U/mL. All values are given as means followed by the lower and upper boundary encompassing 95% of the population. Between 40 and 96 samples were assayed for each value in newborns. Some measurements were skewed because of a disproportionate number of high values. All infants received 1 mg vitamin K intramuscularly at birth. The following reagents were used for coagulation screening tests: prothrombin time (Dade C rabbit thromboplastin), activated partial thromboplastin time (Dade FS). Measurements were made with an ACL analyzer.

*Values indistinguishable from those of adults.

†Measurements are skewed because of a disproportionate number of high values.

APTT, activated partial thromboplastin time; Factor VIII, factor VIII procoagulant; HMWK, high-molecular-weight kininogen; INR, international normalized ratio; PK, prekallikrein; PT, prothrombin time; TCT, thrombin clotting time; VWF, von Willebrand factor.

From Andrew M, Paes B, Milner R, et al: Development of the human coagulation system in the healthy premature infant. Blood. 1988;72:1651-1657.

TABLE 5-5 Reference Values for Coagulation Tests in Healthy Children (Aged 1 to 16 Years) and Adults

Coagulation Tests	1-5 Years	6-10 Years	11-16 Years	Adult
PT (sec)	11 (10.6-11.4)	11.1 (10.1-12.1)	11.2 (10.2-12.0)	12 (11.0-14.0)
PT (INR)	1.0 (0.96-1.04)	1.01 (0.91-1.11)	1.02 (0.93-1.10)	1.10 (1.0-1.3)
APTT (sec)	30 (24-36)	31 (26-36)	32 (26-37)	33 (27-40)
Fibrinogen (g/L)	2.76 (1.70-4.05)	2.79 (1.57-4.0)	3.0 (1.54-4.48)	2.78 (1.56-4.0)
Bleeding time (min)	6 (2.5-10)*	7 (2.5-13)*	5 (3-8)*	4 (1-7)
Factor II (U/mL)	0.94 (0.71-1.16)*	0.88 (0.67-1.07)	0.83 (0.61-1.04)*	1.08 (0.70-1.46)
Factor V (U/mL)	1.03 (0.79-1.27)	0.90 (0.63-1.16)*	0.77 (0.55-0.99)*	1.06 (0.62-1.50)
Factor VII (U/mL)	0.82 (0.55-1.16)	0.85 (0.52-1.20)	0.83 (0.58-1.15)*	1.05 (0.67-1.43)
Factor VIII (U/mL)	0.90 (0.59-1.42)	0.95 (0.58-1.32)	0.92 (0.53-1.31)	0.99 (0.50-1.49)
VWF (U/mL)	0.82 (0.60-1.20)	0.95 (0.44-1.44)	1.00 (0.46-1.53)	0.92 (0.50-1.58)
Factor IX (U/mL)	0.73 (0.47-1.04)	0.75 (0.63-0.89)*	0.82 (0.59-1.22)*	1.09 (0.55-1.63)
Factor X (U/mL)	0.88 (0.58-1.16)	0.75 (0.55-1.01)*	0.79 (0.50-1.17)*	1.06 (0.70-1.52)
Factor XI (U/mL)	0.97 (0.56-1.50)	0.86 (0.52-1.20)	0.74 (0.50-0.97)	0.97 (0.67-1.27)
Factor XII (U/mL)	0.93 (0.64-1.29)	0.92 (0.60-1.40)	0.81 (0.34-1.37)*	1.08 (0.52-1.64)
PK (U/mL)	0.95 (0.65-1.30)	0.99 (0.66-1.31)	0.99 (0.53-1.45)	1.12 (0.62-1.62)
HMWK (U/mL)	0.98 (0.64-1.32)	0.93 (0.60-1.30)	0.91 (0.63-1.19)	0.92 (0.50-1.36)
Factor XIIIa (U/mL)	1.08 (0.72-1.43)	1.09 (0.65-1.51)*	0.99 (0.57-1.40)	1.05 (0.55-1.55)
Factor XIIIb (U/mL)	1.13 (0.69-1.56)	1.16 (0.77-1.54)*	1.02 (0.60-1.43)	0.97 (0.57-1.37)

All factors except fibrinogen are expressed as units per milliliter, with pooled plasma containing 1.0 U/mL. All data are expressed as means followed by the upper and lower boundary encompassing 95% of the population. Between 20 and 50 samples were assayed for each value in each age group. Some measurements were skewed because of a disproportionate number of high values. The lower limit, which excludes the lower 2.5 percent of the population, has been given. The following reagents were used for coagulation screening tests: prothrombin time (Dade C rabbit thromboplastin), activated partial thromboplastin time (Dade FS). Measurements were made with an ACL analyzer.

*Values significantly different from those of adults.

APTT, activated partial thromboplastin time; HMWK, high-molecular-weight kininogen; INR, international normalized ratio; PK, prekallikrein; PT, prothrombin time; TCT, thrombin clotting time; VWF, von Willebrand factor.

From Andrew M, Vegh P, Johnston M, et al: Maturation of the hemostatic system during childhood. Blood. 1992;80:1998-2005.

TABLE 5-6 Blood Coagulation Inhibitor Levels in Fetuses, Full-Term Infants, and Adults

Parameter	FETUSES (WEEKS' GESTATION) 19-23 (n = 20)	24-29 (n = 22)	30-38 (n = 22)	Newborns (n = 60)	Adults (n = 40)
AT (%)	20.2 (12-31)*	30.0 (20-39)	37.1 (24-55)†	59.4 (42-80)†	99.8 (65-130)
HCII (%)	10.3 (6-16)	12.9 (5.5-20)	21.1 (11-33)†	52.1 (19-99)†	101.4 (70-128)
TFPI (%)‡	21.0 (16.0-29.2)	20.6 (13.4-33.2)	20.7 (10.4-31.5)†	38.1 (22.7-55.8)†	73.0 (50.9-90.1)
PC Ag (%)	9.5 (6-14)	12.1 (8-16)	15.9 (8-30)†	32.5 (21-47)†	100.8 (68-125)
PC Act (%)	9.6 (7-13)	10.4 (8-13)	14.1 (8-18)*	28.2 (14-42)†	98.8 (68-125)
Total PS (%)	15.1 (11-21)	17.4 (14-25)	21.0 (15-30)†	38.5 (22-55)†	99.6 (72-118)
Free PS (%)	21.7 (13-32)	27.9 (19-40)	27.0 (18-40)†	49.3 (33-67)†	98.7 (72-128)
Free PS/total PS	0.82 (0.75-0.92)	0.83 (0.76-0.95)	0.79 (0.70-0.89)†	0.64 (0.59-0.98)†	0.41 (0.38-0.43)
C4b-BP (%)	1.8 (0-6)	6.1 (0-12.5)	9.3 (5-14)	18.6 (3-40)†	100.3 (70-124)

All values are given as means followed in parentheses by the lower and upper boundaries including 95% of the population.

ACT, activity; AT, antithrombin; BP, binding protein; HCII, heparin cofactor II; PC, protein C; PS, protein S; TFPI, tissue factor pathway inhibitor.

*P < .05.

†P < .01.

‡Twenty samples were assayed for each group, but only 10 for 19- to 23-week-old fetuses.

From Reverdiau-Moalic P, Delahousse B, Body G, et al: Evolution of blood coagulation activators and inhibitors in the healthy human fetus. Blood. 1996;88:900-906.

TABLE 5-7 Reference Values for Inhibitors of Coagulation in Infants during the First 6 Months of Life

Inhibitor Levels	Day 1	Day 5	Day 30	Day 90	Day 180	Adult
HEALTHY FULL-TERM INFANTS						
AT (U/mL)	0.63 (0.39-0.87)	0.67 (0.41-0.93)	0.78 (0.48-1.08)	0.97 (0.73-1.21)*	1.04 (0.84-1.24)*	1.05 (0.79-1.31)
α_2M (U/mL)	1.39 (0.95-1.83)	1.48 (0.98-1.98)	1.50 (1.06-1.94)	1.76 (1.26-2.26)	1.91 (1.49-2.33)	0.86 (0.52-1.20)
C1E-INH (U/mL)	0.72 (0.36-1.08)	0.90 (0.60-1.20)*	0.89 (0.47-1.31)	1.15 (0.71-1.59)	1.41 (0.89-1.93)	1.01 (0.71-1.31)
α_1AT (U/mL)	0.93 (0.49-1.37)*	0.89 (0.49-1.29)*	0.62 (0.36-0.88)	0.72 (0.42-1.02)	0.77 (0.47-1.07)	0.93 (0.55-1.31)
HCII (U/mL)	0.43 (0.10-0.93)	0.48 (0.00-0.96)	0.47 (0.10-0.87)	0.72 (0.10-1.46)	1.20 (0.50-1.90)	0.96 (0.66-1.26)
Protein C (U/mL)	0.35 (0.17-0.53)	0.42 (0.20-0.64)	0.43 (0.21-0.65)	0.54 (0.28-0.80)	0.59 (0.37-0.81)	0.96 (0.64-1.28)
Protein S (U/mL)	0.36 (0.12-0.60)	0.50 (0.22-0.78)	0.63 (0.33-0.93)	0.86 (0.54-1.18)*	0.87 (0.55-1.19)*	0.92 (0.60-1.24)
HEALTHY PREMATURE INFANTS (30-36 WEEKS' GESTATION)						
AT (U/mL)	0.38 (0.14-0.62)†	0.56 (0.30-0.82)	0.59 (0.37-0.81)†	0.83 (0.45-1.21)†	0.90 (0.52-1.28)†	1.05 (0.79-1.31)
α_2M (U/mL)	1.10 (0.56-1.82)†	1.25 (0.71-1.77)	1.38 (0.72-2.04)	1.80 (1.20-2.66)	2.09 (1.10-3.21)	0.86 (0.52-1.20)
C1E-NH (U/mL)	0.65 (0.31-0.99)	0.83 (0.45-1.21)	0.74 (0.40-1.24)†	1.14 (0.60-1.68)*	1.40 (0.96-2.04)	1.01 (0.71-1.31)
α_1AT (U/mL)	0.90 (0.36-1.44)*	0.94 (0.42-1.46)*	0.76 (0.38-1.12)†	0.81 (0.49-1.13)*†	0.82 (0.48-1.16)*	0.93 (0.55-1.31)
HCII (U/mL)	0.32 (0.10-0.60)†	0.34 (0.10-0.69)	0.43 (0.15-0.71)	0.61 (0.20-1.11)	0.89 (0.45-1.40)*†	0.96 (0.66-1.26)
Protein C (U/mL)	0.28 (0.12-0.44)†	0.31 (0.11-0.51)	0.37 (0.15-0.59)†	0.45 (0.23-0.67)†	0.57 (0.31-0.83)	0.96 (0.64-1.28)
Protein S (U/mL)	0.26 (0.14-0.38)†	0.37 (0.13-0.61)	0.56 (0.22-0.90)	0.76 (0.40-1.12)†	0.82 (0.44-1.20)	0.92 (0.60-1.24)

All values are expressed in units per milliliter, with pooled plasma containing 1.0 U/mL. All values are given as means followed by the lower and upper boundary encompassing 95% of the population. Between 40 and 75 samples were assayed for each value in newborns. Some measurements were skewed because of a disproportionate number of high values. The lower limits exclude the lower 2.5% of the population.

α_1AT, α_1-antitrypsin; α_2M, α_2-macroglobulin; AT, antithrombin; C1E-INH, C1 esterase inhibitor; HCII, heparin cofactor II.

*Values indistinguishable from those of adults.

†Values different from those of full-term infants.

From Andrew M, Paes B, Johnston M: Development of the hemostatic system in the neonate and young infant. Am J Pediatr Hematol Oncol. 1990;12:95-104.

exhibit increased protein C glycosylation. Despite these alterations, there is no evidence that protein C from neonates differs functionally from that of adults when compared at equivalent concentrations.[24,25]

In adults, protein S circulates in either a free form or bound to the carrier protein C4b binding protein. In fetuses and neonates, circulating protein S is almost entirely of the free type because levels of C4b binding protein are extremely low.[26,27] Thus, the protein S activity-to-antigen ratio is greater for fetuses and neonates than for adults. Nonetheless, both total and free protein S levels are lower in fetuses and neonates. They rise gradually after birth, with the adult range of free protein S reached by 4 months and total protein S by about 10 months.[1] The interaction of protein S with activated protein C in the plasma of newborns may be modulated by increased levels of α_2-macroglobulin.[28]

Healthy full-term newborns have lower functional ATIII levels than adults do, with an average of 0.55 U/mL based on several studies.[12,13,18,29-32] This is most likely due to a reduced amount of absolute ATIII protein inasmuch as most studies have found no significant difference in the antigen-to–functional activity ratio, immunoelectrophoresis, or chromatographic properties of purified ATIII from neonates and adults.[12,29,32,33] The reduced ATIII levels in neonates probably account, at least in part, for the relative heparin resistance seen in this age group. ATIII levels typically reach the adult range by 3 months of age in full-term healthy infants. Preterm infants with respiratory distress syndrome (RDS) have significantly lower levels of ATIII, typically less than 0.2 U/mL, and the ATIII present often has additional dysfunctional properties.[29,34-37] Lower ATIII levels correlate with increased catheter-related thrombosis, intracranial hemorrhage (ICH), and mortality.

Like ATIII, levels of heparin cofactor II are also substantially lower in infants than adults.[38] A circulating fetal dermatan sulfate proteoglycan has been described that has natural anticoagulant properties mediated through heparin cofactor II.[39] This fetal anticoagulant is also present in the plasma of pregnant women and is produced by the placenta. The length of time that it circulates in newborns is not known; however, it is still present during the first week of life in sick premature infants with RDS.

α_2-Macroglobulin is a more important inhibitor of thrombin in plasma from newborns than in adults.[40] It compensates, in part, for the low levels of ATIII and heparin cofactor in newborns, even in the presence of endothelial cell surfaces.[40,41] However, the overall rate of thrombin inhibition is still lower in newborns than adults.[40]

TFPI binds to factor VIIa/tissue factor complexes in a factor Xa calcium-dependent reaction that results in the inhibition of factor VIIa. After generation of small amounts of thrombin, TFPI prevents further generation of thrombin via tissue factor/factor VIIa. TFPI levels in cord plasma have been reported to be approximately 50% of adult values.[42]

Vitamin K–Dependent Factors

Factors II, VII, IX, and X and proteins C, S, and Z undergo vitamin K (VK)-dependent post-translational γ-carboxylation of certain glutamic acid residues (see Chapter 26). Typically, 9 to 12 glutamic acid residues, often clustered within a 45–amino acid region referred to as a "Gla" domain, are modified.[22,43] γ-Carboxylation of glutamic acids enhances calcium-dependent phospholipid interactions of the coagulation factors and helps catalyze the coagulation cascade. Because of the association of relative VK deficiency and hemorrhagic disease of the newborn (HDN; see detailed description later), development of these VK-dependent factors in utero has been the focus of considerable research. During gestation, a steep gradient of VK concentration is maintained across the placenta, with fetal levels being 10% or less of maternal levels.[22,44-49] This gradient is even further enhanced during the third trimester.[45] Consequently, VK stores in newborns are low, as shown by low levels of VK in the cord blood and liver of aborted fetuses.[44,47,50] The teleologic explanation for maintenance of low fetal VK levels is not known. However, VK has been shown to promote DNA mutagenesis in vivo. For this reason, several investigators have suggested that maintenance of low fetal VK levels might be a mechanism to prevent chromosomal damage during the rapid cellular proliferation of embryogenesis.[51-53] In addition to these low VK levels, deficiency of VK reductase activity (a rate-limiting step in the reaction) as a result of immaturity of the hepatocyte may contribute to inefficient γ-carboxylation of coagulation factors.[22] In fact, undercarboxylated prothrombin and protein C have been detected in up to 7% and 27% of the cord and peripheral blood of healthy term infants, respectively, and these levels correlate with gestational age.[54,55] Even when corrected for this relative VK deficiency, levels of VK-dependent factors are still considerably lower than the normal adult range because the values presented in Tables 5-1 to 5-4, 5-6, and 5-7 were measured in infants who received VK prophylaxis at birth.

VK-dependent glutamic acid carboxylation also occurs on proteins outside the coagulation system, many of which play roles in development. Such proteins include Gas-6, the ligand for the receptor kinases Sky and Axl; the bone growth– and calcification-related factors osteocalcin and matrix Gla protein; the urine calcium binding protein nephrocalcin; and PRPG1 and PRPG2, two proline-rich predicted signaling proteins expressed in the central nervous system (CNS) and endocrine tissues.[43,55,56,57] Thus, VK is predicted to have pleiotropic effects on development.

Although VK is maintained at low levels in the fetus, further deficiency of VK during gestation can reduce functional levels of the VK-dependent coagulation factors to an even greater extent. Maternal use of certain anticonvulsant medications, including phenytoin, phenobarbital, valproic acid, and carbamazepine, is associated with an increased risk of VK deficiency in the fetus and neonate.[22,58] Fetal or neonatal bleeding has been linked to maternal use of these medications on rare occasion. Fetal VK deficiency can be prevented in such cases by antenatal oral administration of 10 mg of VK$_1$ daily to the mother beginning at 36 weeks' gestation.[59]

Warfarin is a potent VK antagonist commonly used for long-term anticoagulation. It crosses the placenta and inhibits VK-dependent carboxylation in the fetus. Its use during pregnancy at 6 to 12 weeks of gestation is associated with an embryopathy syndrome consisting of limb deformities, nasal hypoplasia, ophthalmologic malformations, mental retardation, hypotonia, and ear abnormalities.[60] Warfarin exposure during the second or third trimester is associated with fetal wastage and CNS anomalies. The developmental defects related to warfarin use during pregnancy are thought to be due to bleeding into the developing limb buds or effects on bone and cartilage growth from inhibition of bone-associated Gla proteins, or both.

The Fetal and Neonatal Fibrinolytic System

The enzyme plasmin degrades polymerized fibrin and is responsible for clot dissolution. It is generated from its precursor plasminogen by two known activators, tissue plasminogen activator (tPA) and urokinase plasminogen activator (uPA). These activators, in turn, are inhibited by the plasminogen activator inhibitors PAI-1 and PAI-2. In addition, plasmin itself is inhibited by the circulating blood protein α_2-antiplasmin. See Chapter 27 for more detailed description of the fibrinolytic system. In newborns, plasminogen levels are only 50% of adult values, α_2-antiplasmin levels are 80% of adult values, and plasma concentrations of PAI-1 and tPA are significantly greater than adult values (Table 5-8).[17,19,23,61-64] The increased levels of tPA and PAI-1 found on day 1 of life contrast markedly with values obtained from cord blood, which are significantly lower than adult levels. The discrepancy between newborn and cord plasma concentrations of tPA and PAI-1 may be explained by the enhanced release of both proteins from the endothelium shortly after birth. PAI-2 levels are detectable in cord blood but are significantly lower than they are in pregnant women.[65] Unique glycoforms of plasminogen with an increased content of mannose and sialic acid exist in the fetus.[66-68] This fetal form of plasminogen is less efficiently converted to plasmin by tPA than adult plasminogen is.[66] No significant differences exist in activation kinetics by uPA.[66]

D-Dimers

D-dimers are the breakdown product of fibrin mesh cross-linked by factor XIII. Neonates have markedly elevated D-dimer levels in comparison to older children and adults that persist for at least 3 days after birth (Table 5-9).[18] These high levels suggest activation of the coagulation system at birth, decreased clearance of D-dimers in neonates, or both.

TABLE 5-8   **Reference Values for Components of the Fibrinolytic System during the First 6 Months of Life**

Fibrinolytic System	Day 1	Day 5	Day 30	Day 90	Day 180	Adult
HEALTHY FULL-TERM INFANTS						
Plasminogen (U/mL)	1.95 (1.25-2.65)	2.17 (1.41-2.93)	1.98 (1.26-2.70)	2.48 (1.74-3.22)	3.01 (2.21-3.81)	3.36 (2.48-4.24)
tPA (ng/mL)	9.6 (5.0-18.9)	5.6 (4.0-10.0)*	4.1 (1.0-6.0)*	2.1 (1.0-5.0)*	2.8 (1.0-6.0)*	4.9 (1.4-8.4)
α_2AP (U/mL)	0.85 (0.55-1.15)	1.00 (0.70-1.30)*	1.00 (0.76-1.24)*	1.08 (0.76-1.40)*	1.11 (0.83-1.39)*	1.02 (0.68-1.36)
PAI-1 (U/mL)	6.4 (2.0-15.1)	2.3 (0.0-8.1)*	3.4 (0.0-8.8)*	7.2 (1.0-15.3)	8.1 (6.0-13.0)	3.6 (0.0-11.0)
HEALTHY PREMATURE INFANTS (30-36 WEEKS' GESTATION)						
Plasminogen (U/mL)	1.70 (1.12-2.48)†	1.91 (1.21-2.61)†	1.81 (1.09-2.53)	2.38 (1.58-3.18)	2.75 (1.91-3.59)†	3.36 (2.48-4.24)
tPA (ng/mL)	8.48 (3.00-16.70)	3.97 (2.00-6.93)*	4.13 (2.00-7.79)*	3.31 (2.00-5.07)*	3.48 (2.00-5.85)*	4.96 (1.46-8.46)
α_2AP (U/mL)	0.78 (0.40-1.16)	0.81 (0.49-1.13)†	0.89 (0.55-1.23)†	1.06 (0.64-1.48)*	1.15 (0.77-1.53)	1.02 (0.68-1.36)
PAI-1 (U/mL)	5.4 (0.0-12.2)*†	2.5 (0.0-7.1)*	4.3 (0.0-10.9)*	4.8 (1.0-11.8)*†	4.9 (1.0-10.2)*†	3.6 (0.0-11.0)

Plasminogen units are those recommended by the Committee on Thrombolytic Agents. Values for tPA are given as nanograms per milliliter. For α_2AP, values are expressed as units per milliliter, with pooled plasma containing 1.0 U/mL. Values for PAI-1 are given as units per milliliter, with 1 unit of PAI-1 activity being defined as the amount of PAI-1 that inhibits the 1 IU of human single-chain tPA. All values are given as means followed by the lower and upper boundaries encompassing 95% of the population.
*Values indistinguishable from those of adults.
†Values different from those of full-term infants.
α_2AP, α_2-antiplasmin; PAI-1, plasminogen activator inhibitor 1; tPA, tissue plasminogen activator.
From Andrew M, Paes B, Johnston M: Development of the hemostatic system in the neonate and young infant. Am J Pediatr Hematol Oncol. 1990;12:95-104.

TABLE 5-9	D-Dimer Reference Values for Neonates and Children						
	AGE						
	Day 1	Day 3	1 Month-1 Year	1-5 Years	6-10 Years	11-16 Years	Adults
D-dimers (µg/mL)	1.47 (0.41-2.47)*	1.34 (0.58-2.74)*	0.22 (0.11-0.42)	0.25 (0.09-0.53)*	0.26 (0.10-0.56)*	0.27 (0.16-0.39)*	0.18 (0.05-0.42)
	n = 20 (10F/10M)	*n* = 23 (12F/11M)	*n* = 20 (7F/13M)	*n* = 40 (19F/21M)	*n* = 39 (12F/27M)	*n* = 21 (6F/15M)	*n* = 32 (19F/13M)

Mean and boundaries including 95% of the population of D-dimer (mg/mL) concentrations are shown. Measurements were made with the Liatest D-Di test kit (Diagnostica Stago, France).
*Denotes values that are significantly different from adult values (*P* < .05).
Reproduced with permission from Monagle P, Barnes C, Ignjatovic V, et al. Developmental haemostasis. Impact for clinical haemostasis laboratories. Thromb Haemost. 2006;95:362-372.

von Willebrand Factor

von Willebrand factor (VWF) is a large protein that mediates adhesion of platelets to exposed subendothelium and is involved in platelet aggregation (see Chapter 30). Its synthesis can first be detected as early as 4 weeks of gestation in placental endothelial cells and by 4 to 8 weeks in bone marrow.[22,69,70] In contrast to other coagulation factors, VWF functional levels are considerably elevated in neonates in comparison to the normal adult range (see Tables 5-2 and 5-5). They gradually decline to the normal adult range by about 3 to 6 months. It is important to keep these physiologically elevated levels in mind when using VWF as a marker of inflammation in infants.

VWF is released from endothelial cells and megakaryocytes as large multimers with molecular weights in the millions-of-dalton range. They are then cleaved into smaller multimers by the metalloproteinase ADAMTS-13. Unusually large VWF (ULVWF) multimers are VWF multimer forms larger than those found in normal plasma. These ULVWF multimers are 10 to 20 times more active in shear stress–induced platelet aggregation and bind more avidly to the extracellular matrix of fibroblasts than do the VWF multimer forms found in normal plasma.[71,72] In older children and adults, the presence of ULVWF plasma forms is the hallmark of thrombotic thrombocytopenic purpura, a microangiopathic disorder. It is due to deficiency, acquired or congenital, of ADAMTS-13. ULVWF forms are consistently found in platelet-poor plasma (PPP) from fetuses less than 35 weeks' estimated gestational age (EGA) and most fetuses older than 35 weeks' EGA, as well as in umbilical cord blood.[73,74] These forms are not seen in simultaneously sampled maternal PPP, thus indicating that the ULVWF forms are fetal specific. The ULVWF in fetal PPP is similar to the VWF directly released from endothelial cells. This similarity may be explained by the recent finding of low VWF cleaving protease (ADAMTS-13) activity in many neonates.[75,76] Serial monitoring of PPP from neonates shows a gradual reduction in ULVWF to the normal size range within 8 weeks after birth.[74] The presence of ULVWF during fetal development is probably physiologically relevant because plasma derived from umbilical cord blood shows increased shear stress– and ristocetin-induced

VWF platelet-binding activity in comparison to plasma derived from adults, even when adult platelets are used in the assay.[77] The enhanced hemostatic efficacy of ULVWF may therefore balance the low functional levels of other coagulation factors to achieve reliable hemostasis in the fetus and newborn.

Platelets

Megakaryocytes during Fetal Development

In humans, megakaryocytes are first detectable in the liver and spleen by 10 weeks of gestation.[78] By 30 weeks, megakaryocytes are present in bone marrow and actively contributing to thrombopoiesis. Circulating megakaryocyte progenitors are detectable in the blood of neonates, and their number decreases as a function of postconceptional age (gestational age + days of life).[79]

Several pieces of evidence suggest that fetal liver megakaryocytes have unique features when compared with adult bone marrow–derived megakaryocytes. Megakaryocytes that develop from murine neonatal liver progenitors after transplantation into myeloablated mouse recipients are smaller and have lower ploidy levels than do those derived from transplanted adult bone marrow.[80] These differences disappear by 1 month after transplantation. In addition, several congenital disorders of megakaryopoiesis in humans, such as Down syndrome–transient myeloproliferative disorder (DS-TMD) and thrombocytopenia with absent radii (TAR), resolve spontaneously after the newborn period, thus suggesting specific effects on fetal megakaryopoiesis. In support of this hypothesis, experiments in mice show stage-specific effects of a mutation in the transcription factor GATA-1 associated with DS-TMD and Down syndrome–acute megakaryoblastic leukemia (DS-AMKL) that affect fetal liver megakaryopoiesis but not adult bone marrow megakaryopoiesis.[81] It has been proposed that stage-specific differences in megakaryopoiesis may account for the delayed platelet engraftment in humans often observed when umbilical cord blood is used as a source of hematopoietic stem cells rather than bone marrow or peripheral blood mobilized stem cells.[80] The potential differences between fetal liver and adult bone marrow megakaryocytes could be due to intrinsic differences in the progenitors themselves or their interactions with different microenvironments, or both.

Platelet Number, Size, and Survival during Development

In humans, circulating platelets are first detected by 11 weeks' gestational age.[78] Thereafter, the plasma platelet concentration rises rapidly and reaches the adult range of 150 to 450 × 10⁹/L by about 18 weeks of gestation.[22,23,62,78,82-88] During the earliest phase of platelet production, mean platelet volume (MPV) is larger than the adult range.[22] However, platelet volume "normalizes" soon thereafter and reaches the adult range of 7 to 9 fL.[89,90] It is possible that the larger platelets arise from a unique wave of "primitive" megakaryopoiesis that occurs early in gestation, as demonstrated in several mouse studies,[91,92] but this mechanism remains to be determined in humans. Platelet survival has not been measured in healthy infants. In rabbits, survival of ¹¹¹In oxine–labeled platelets is similar in adult and newborn rabbits.[93] However, in humans, levels of reticulated platelets, which represent those recently released from megakaryocytes, are elevated about 20-fold in comparison to adults.[94] Concentrations of thrombopoietin (TPO), the major cytokine for megakaryocyte progenitor proliferation and development, are increased about twofold in fetal versus adult plasma.[95] These findings suggest possible increased platelet turnover in human fetuses versus adults.

Platelet Structure

Peripheral blood platelets from newborns contain similar numbers of platelet-specific granules as platelets from older children and adults; however, serotonin and adenosine diphosphate (ADP), which are stored in dense granules, are present at concentrations less than 50% of adult values.[96] Newborn platelets contain normal levels of the receptors glycoprotein Ib (GPIb) (part of the VWF binding complex), GPIa/IIa, P-selectin, and Pl^A1. Variable levels of GPIIb/IIIa have been reported, with some studies indicating significantly reduced expression.[97-99] Functional epinephrine receptors are significantly diminished in newborn platelets.[100]

Platelet Function

Platelet aggregometry studies of neonatal and cord blood platelets have shown variable results, but most demonstrate a modest hyporesponsiveness to ADP, epinephrine, collagen, and thrombin when compared with platelets from older children and adults (Fig. 5-2).[101-104] The hyporesponsiveness spontaneously resolves by 2 to 9 days after birth in full-term infants.[105] Several explanations have been proposed to account for this hyporesponsiveness, including impaired calcium channel transport and signal

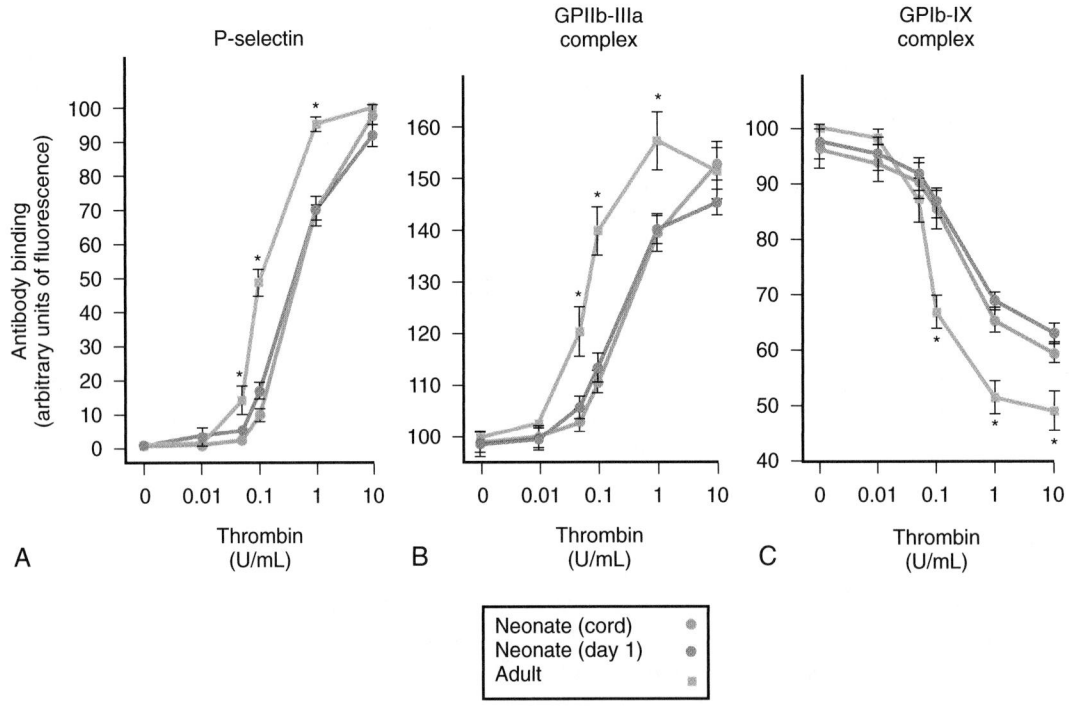

FIGURE 5-2. Effect of thrombin on the surface expression of P-selectin, the glycoprotein (GP) IIb/IIIa complex, and the GPIb/IX complex on neonatal and adult platelets in whole blood. Results were similar for cord and neonatal day 1 values. Expression of P-selectin and GPIIb/IIIa complexes was decreased in newborns, whereas GPIb/IX expression was relatively preserved in newborns in comparison to adults after stimulation with thrombin. Data are expressed as means ± SEM; N = 20. *Asterisks* indicate *P* > .05 for both cord blood and day 1 neonatal platelets in comparison to adult platelets. *(Redrawn from Rajasekhar D, Kestin AS, Bednarek FJ, et al: Neonatal platelets are less reactive than adult platelets to physiological agonists in whole blood. Thromb Haemost 1994;72:957-963.)*

transduction,[22,106-108] decreased availability of α-adrenergic receptors because of either delayed receptor maturation or occupation by catecholamines released during birth,[96,101,102,104,106,109-112] and the presence of inhibitory placenta-derived prostaglandins.[113]

In contrast to the agonists just described, agglutination in response to low concentrations of ristocetin is significantly enhanced in fetal and newborn platelet-rich plasma in comparison to that of adults,[96] probably partly because of high VWF levels and the presence of ULVWF forms in newborn plasma.[73,74,106,114-116] In the end, the hyporesponsiveness to certain platelet agonists and the hyperresponsiveness to VWF appear to balance each other out inasmuch as most healthy term infants do not experience bleeding or thrombotic complications in the newborn period.

Platelet Activation during the Birth Process

There is strong evidence that platelets are activated during the birth process. Cord plasma levels of thromboxane B_2, β-thromboglobulin, and platelet factor 4 are increased; the granular content of cord platelets is decreased; and epinephrine receptor availability is reduced, perhaps as a result of occupation.[117-120] The mechanisms of activation are probably multifactorial and include thermal changes, hypoxia, acidosis, adrenergic stimulation, and the thrombogenic effects of amniotic fluid.

Blood Vessel Wall: Age and Anticoagulant Properties

The endothelium fulfills a complex role in hemostasis in that it prevents thrombotic complications under physiologic conditions and promotes fibrin formation when injured. One of the anticoagulant properties of endothelial cell surfaces is mediated by lipoxygenase and cyclooxygenase metabolites of unsaturated fatty acids. Prostacyclin (prostaglandin I_2 [PGI_2]) production by cord vessels exceeds that by blood vessels in adults.[121] A second endothelial cell–mediated antithrombotic property is promotion of antithrombin (AT) neutralization of thrombin by cell surface proteoglycans. Structurally, there is evidence that the vessel wall glycosaminoglycans of the young differ from those of adults.[122,123] In a rabbit venous model, increased amounts of glycosaminoglycans are seen in the inferior venae cavae of rabbit pups as compared with adults. Similarly, in the rabbit arterial model, greater glycosaminoglycan-mediated AT activity is seen in rabbit pups than in adult rabbits.[124,125]

Maternal Preeclampsia and Fetal Hemostasis

Preeclampsia is a pregnancy-associated syndrome consisting of maternal hypertension and proteinuria. Alterations in maternal coagulation and fibrinolysis, including reduced ATIII and PAI-2 levels and increased tPA antigen, PAI-1 antigen, and fibrin degradation product levels, have been described in women with preterm preeclampsia.[126-130] This suggests a state of enhanced thrombin generation and fibrinolysis in the maternal circulation. Analysis of cord blood from infants born to mothers with preeclampsia shows no statistical difference in the levels of these factors versus those of age-matched controls born to mothers without preeclampsia, thus indicating a probable protective effect of the placenta on the fetal circulation.[126,131]

Summary of Hemostatic Differences between Neonates and Older Children and Adults

In summary, the salient differences in the hemostatic system of neonates and older children or adults are (1) decreased plasma concentrations of many of the procoagulant proteins, including factors II, VII, IX, X, XI, and XII, prekallikrein, and high-molecular weight kininogens; (2) a unique fetal glycoform of fibrinogen; (3) decreased plasma concentrations of the coagulation inhibitors ATIII, heparin cofactor II, TFPI, protein C, and protein S, with a concomitant slower rate of thrombin inhibition; (4) a unique glycoform of plasminogen that is less efficiently converted to plasmin by tPA; (5) markedly elevated D-dimer levels until at least 3 days after birth; (6) increased plasma VWF concentration and elevated levels of circulating ULVWF multimers; and (7) modest, transient hyporesponsiveness of platelets to certain agonists such as collagen and epinephrine, but increased agglutination with low-dose ristocetin. In general, most of these differences resolve within the first 6 months of life.

CLINICAL ASPECTS OF DEVELOPMENTAL HEMOSTASIS

Hemorrhagic Disorders

Although acquired disorders are more commonly seen, severe forms of congenital factor deficiencies or platelet disorders can present in early infancy and should be seriously considered in otherwise healthy infants who are bleeding.[22,34,62,132-136] Recent studies estimate that about 15% to 30% of children with inherited bleeding disorders have hemorrhage in the neonatal period.[137,138] In addition, a third of new cases of severe hemophilia represent new mutations and are therefore not accompanied by any antecedent family history.[138]

Clinical Findings

The clinical manifestations of bleeding disorders are different in newborns than in older children and adults. Bleeding may appear as oozing from the umbilicus, bleeding into the scalp, large cephalohematomas, bleeding after circumcision, bleeding from peripheral phlebotomy sites, and bleeding into the skin. A small but important proportion of infants are seen with ICH as the first manifestation of their bleeding tendency.[136,139-145] Sick infants can bleed from mucous membranes, the bladder, and sites of invasive procedures. Joint bleeding is rare. The most common causes of bleeding in healthy infants are thrombocytopenia secondary to transplacental passage of a maternal antiplatelet antibody, sepsis, VK deficiency, and congenital coagulation factor deficiencies.

Laboratory Evaluation

In addition to a workup for sepsis, laboratory evaluation of infants with bleeding complications should include determination of the prothrombin time (PT), activated partial thromboplastin time (APTT), thrombin clotting time (TCT), fibrinogen level, and platelet count. As discussed earlier, results need to be compared with the expected range of values for neonates because some may not reflect the normal adult range (see later). Abnormalities in test results usually prompt additional tests, such as specific factor assays. For a male child in whom hemophilia A or B is suspected, specific factor assays should be performed regardless of the APTT value. The PT, APTT, and TCT are not prolonged in those with factor XIII and α_2-antiplasmin deficiency. Therefore, levels of these factors must be measured directly if deficiencies are suspected.

Sample Collection

Collection of samples for laboratory investigation of hemostatic defects in neonates, especially premature infants, presents particular challenges because of the patient's small size and increased hematocrit. Specialized microcollection tubes (1 mL) should be available in the neonatal unit. Blood sampling techniques should avoid contamination with intravenous fluids and heparin and should also avoid activating the coagulation system. Slow transit time and contact with plastic tubing are most likely to cause activation. All neonatal samples should be inspected for the presence of fibrin clumps before processing, and those containing clumps should not be used for analysis. Ideally, the volume of anticoagulant in the sample should be based on the volume of plasma, not the total volume of blood, because the increased hematocrit of neonates causes accentuated dilution of the coagulation factors if not taken into account.[1] This is particularly important for neonates with very high hematocrit values, such as those with cyanotic congenital cardiac disease. Overfilled or underfilled samples should not be analyzed.

Screening Coagulation Tests in Neonates

Screening tests of plasma clotting activity, including the PT, APTT, and TCT, are all prolonged during fetal development and in neonates when compared with the normal adult range (see Tables 5-1 to 5-3), probably because of physiologic "deficiencies" of the VK-dependent factors, contact factors, and the presence of fetal glycoforms of fibrinogen.[1] The absolute values for these tests, as well as specific coagulation factor tests, depend on the reagents and analyzer used. Table 5-3 provides reference ranges recently generated by Monagle and co-workers using the STA Compact analyzer and Diagnostica Stago reagents, a system currently used in many clinical laboratories.[18] In contrast to some earlier systems, such as the ACL system, the STA Compact analyzer is not affected by plasma bilirubin levels. The differences observed underscore the need for each clinical laboratory to establish its own normal age-related reference ranges.[18]

Bleeding Time

The bleeding time has traditionally been used as an in vivo test of platelet function, particularly for testing adhesion to injured vasculature.[114] However, it is subject to considerable operator-dependent variability and is not routinely used in newborns. Automated devices modified for newborns and children are available and have been standardized.[146] In contrast to the prolonged coagulation screening tests, multiple studies have shown that bleeding times in infants during the first week of life are significantly shorter than those in adults.[106,114-116,146] This somewhat paradoxical finding can be explained by several mechanisms, including higher plasma concentrations of VWF,[17,19,23] enhanced function of VWF because of a disproportional increase in ULVWF multimers,[73,74] large red cells,[147] and high hematocrits.[148]

Platelet Functional Analyzer

The Platelet Functional Analyzer 100 (PFA-100) system provides an in vitro method of assessing primary platelet-related hemostasis by measuring the time (closure time) required for a platelet plug to occlude a microscopic aperture cut into a membrane coated with collagen and either epinephrine or ADP. It uses the patient's own platelets and plasma. The PFA-100 system is attractive for use in neonates because of the small volume required, rapidity of testing, and standardization of testing cartridges. Like the bleeding time, most studies of neonates' peripheral or cord blood report PFA-100 closure times, for both epinephrine and ADP, that are shorter than those for older children and adults (Table 5-10).[1,149-152] This is probably due to similar mechanisms as described earlier for the shortened bleeding time.[150] Normal ranges for premature infants of different postconceptional ages have not been reported. Although the PFA-100 system may eventually become a standard screening test for platelet function in neonates, older children, and adults, its clinical utility has not yet been clearly established.[153] Thus, further studies will be required to determine the optimal method of assessing primary hemostasis in newborns and children, particularly premature infants.

TABLE 5-10	PFA-100 Closure Time Values from Healthy Cord Blood Samples and Adults			
Study	**CT-Epi (sec): Neonate**	**CT-Epi (sec): Adult**	**CT-ADP (sec): Neonate**	**CT-ADP (sec): Adult**
Boudewijns et al.[149]	108 ± 30 (49-168) (*n* = 80)	85-65 (*n* = 20)	66 ± 13 (40-92) (*n* = 80)	72-120 (*n* = 20)
Roschitz et al.[150]	75 (50-112) (*n* = 70)	106 (84-150) (*n* = 25)	58 (43-98) (*n* = 70)	83 (64-98) (*n* = 25)
Carcao et al.[151]	81 ± 17 (61-108) (*n* = 17)	106 ± 21 (82-142) (*n* = 31)	56 ± 6 (48-65) (*n* = 17)	85 ± 16 (67-111) (*n* = 31)
Israels et al.[152]	82 ± 27 (*n* = 31)	111 ± 22 (*n* = 21)	60 ± 16 (*n* = 31)	91 ± 17 (*n* = 21)

ADP, adenosine triphosphate; CT, closure time; Epi, epinephrine.
Adapted from Saxonhouse MA, Sola MC. Platelet function in term and preterm neonates. Clin Perinatol. 2004;31:15-28.

Hereditary Coagulation Factor Deficiencies

For most hemostatic components, both severe and mild forms of deficiency can occur, with severe deficiencies often characterized by significant bleeding in newborns. Chapter 30 and 31 discuss hereditary factor deficiencies in detail.

Inheritance

Deficiencies of factors II, V, VII, XI, and XII, prekallikrein, and high-molecular-weight kininogen are rare autosomally inherited disorders, with consanguinity present in many families. Deficiencies of factor XII, prekallikrein, and high-molecular-weight kininogen do not result in hemorrhagic complications and thus are not considered further here. Deficiencies of factors VIII and IX are sex linked and the most common congenital bleeding disorders in newborns. Rarely, combined deficiencies of factors II, VII, and IX and/or factors V and VIII occur in the neonatal period.[154,155] The latter is due to mutations in LMAN1 (also called ERGIC-53), a mannose-binding type I transmembrane protein, or its binding partner MCFD2, which together form a specific cargo receptor complex in the endoplasmic reticulum.[155,156] It is typically inherited in an autosomal recessive manner. Tests are available to diagnose most congenital factor deficiencies prenatally so that either termination of pregnancy or management of affected infants can be planned (see Chapters 30 and 31).

Clinical Findings

In the majority of newborns with congenital coagulation factor deficiencies, bleeding does not occur in the perinatal period unless a hemostatic challenge is present. On the other hand, unexplained bleeding in an otherwise healthy newborn should be carefully investigated because it may be due to a congenital coagulation factor deficiency.

ICH is rare in full-term newborns and usually occurs either spontaneously or after insults such as birth asphyxia or trauma, VK deficiency, or severe congenital factor deficiencies. Other risk factors include small birth weight, young gestational age, and ethnic background.[157-165] The

risk for ICH in children with severe hemophilia A or B ranges from 2% to 8%. The location of the ICH is most commonly the subarachnoid area, but subdural and parenchymal bleeding also occurs. Head ultrasound may not detect small parafalcine bleeding, so computed tomography (CT) is the preferred modality when deficiency of a coagulation factor is suspected. Some infants require surgical intervention, and many have long-term neurologic deficits.

Full-term infants with unexplained ICH should be carefully evaluated for congenital or acquired hemostatic defects.[139,157-165] Unfortunately, the diagnosis of ICH may be delayed because of the nonspecific nature of the early clinical findings, including poor feeding, lethargy, apnea, vomiting, and irritability. Further delays can result when secondary coagulopathies such as disseminated intravascular coagulation (DIC) occur or because of confusion related to the physiologically low levels of some coagulation factors in newborns.[166,167] The more extreme clinical manifestations of ICH are usually recognized early and include seizures, meningismus, and a tense fontanelle.

Although severe deficiency of factor VIII is the most common cause of ICH from a coagulation factor deficiency, severe congenital deficiencies of fibrinogen and factors II, V, VII, VIII, IX, X, XI, and XIII can also cause ICH at birth.[168] The incidence of ICH in newborns is unknown and is probably changing because of improvements in perinatal care. The widespread use of ultrasound, a safe modality for monitoring fetuses at risk, has resulted in the detection of ICH in utero. In utero factor replacement has also been accomplished in several infants.[10] Though less common than ICH, subgaleal bleeding with concurrent shock and DIC may be the initial manifestation of a congenital factor deficiency.[169]

Diagnosis

In newborns, the diagnosis of many congenital factor deficiencies based on plasma concentrations can be difficult because of neonates' physiologically low levels at birth (see Tables 5-2 and 5-3). Mild to moderate hereditary deficiencies of factors II, VII, IX, X, and XI result in plasma concentrations that may overlap with the normal neonatal range. In contrast, plasma concentrations resulting from either mild to moderate factor VIII deficiency or severe deficiency of factors V, VII, VIII, IX, X, and XIII can easily be distinguished from physiologic values. Prenatal diagnosis of most hereditary factor deficiencies is performed by amniocentesis or chorionic villus biopsy and is largely confined to severe hemophilia A and B, although deficiencies of factors V, VII, and XIII and VWF have also been diagnosed prenatally.[9,10,170-172]

Treatment

In the presence of active bleeding or a planned hemostatic challenge, the fundamental principle of management is to increase the plasma concentration of the deficient coagulation protein to a minimal hemostatic level. This target level varies, depending on the protein and nature of the hemostatic challenge (see Chapters 30 and 31). When possible, recombinant protein products or detergent-treated pooled donor preparations should be used to reduce the risk of infectious complications. Most products available for the treatment of older children and adults can be used in neonates. Although it has not been well studied, the half-lives and volumes of distribution of recombinant factor VIII (rFVIII) and rFIX appear to be similar in full-term newborns and older children, so standard initial dosing regimens can be used. However, it is critical to monitor trough levels closely and make appropriate dose modifications to ensure achievement of the proper target level. There are a few case reports of extremely premature infants (<1500 g or <30 weeks' EGA) having a slightly shortened half-life of factor VIII (about 6 hours versus 8 to 12 hours in full-term infants and older children).[173,174]

Fresh frozen plasma (FFP) should be given for bleeding emergencies in neonates in whom a coagulation defect is suspected but a specific factor deficiency has not yet been documented. There are case reports of a small number of infants (<4 months) treated successfully with rFVIIa for catastrophic bleeding of varying causes.[175] However, rFVIIa treatment of patients without congenital factor VII deficiency or hemophilia with high-titer inhibitors should be considered investigational at this time. Infants with known or suspected deficiencies in coagulation factors should receive vaccinations by subcutaneous rather than intramuscular route, and arterial puncture should be avoided when possible.

Mode of Delivery

The optimal mode of delivery for infants of hemophilia carrier mothers has yet to be determined.[138] However, normal vaginal delivery appears to be generally safe for many babies with hemophilia.[176] Use of vacuum assistance is associated with an increased risk for significant cranial hematomas in newborns with hemophilia and should be avoided if possible.[138,176]

Specific Coagulation Factor Deficiencies

Fibrinogen Deficiency. Deficiency of fibrinogen is rare. Bleeding secondary to afibrinogenemia has been reported in newborns after circumcision or as umbilical stump bleeding and soft tissue hemorrhage, with some cases being fatal. Reported replacement therapies have included whole blood, cryoprecipitate, FFP, and fibrinogen concentrates.[177-180] One fibrinogen concentrate (Haemocomplettan HS, Centeon/Aventis Behring) is available in Europe and North America.

Factor II Deficiency. Deficiency of prothrombin is very rare. Reported bleeding complications in newborns include gastrointestinal bleeding and ICH.[181,182] Reviews of adult patients have reported bleeding after invasive events such as circumcision and venipuncture or as soft tissue hematomas.[178] Although FFP can be used as initial therapy, factor II concentrate or prothrombin complex concentrate (PCC) is the preferred replacement product.

Factor V Deficiency. Bleeding as a result of severe factor V deficiency has been reported in newborns. Clinical manifestation include ICH, subdural hematoma, bleeding from the umbilical stump, gastric hemorrhage, and soft tissue hemorrhage.[183,184] Antenatal intraventricular hemorrhage was reported in two newborns.[185] Replacement therapy included whole blood, FFP, and the local application of pressure on sites of bleeding. Although thrombotic complications occur in some patients with factor V deficiency, they have not been reported in newborns.[183-187]

Factor VII Deficiency. Severe factor VII deficiency (factor VII level <1%) usually causes significant bleeding equivalent to that seen in patients with severe hemophilia. Patients with factor VII levels greater than 5% generally have mild hemorrhagic episodes. The most commonly reported bleeding complication in newborns with congenital factor VII deficiency is ICH.[188-190] In a review of 75 patients with factor VII deficiency, ICH was observed in 12 (16%). In 5 (42%) of these 12 patients, ICH occurred in the first week of life with a fatal outcome. Congenital factor VII deficiency may occur in infants with Dubin-Johnson syndrome[189,191] or Gilbert's syndrome[192] in certain populations. Bleeding episodes secondary to factor VII deficiency can be treated with FFP, PCC, purified factor VIIa concentrates, or preferably, rFVIIa.[175,188-190,193,194] Lower doses of rFVIIa (15 to 20 µg/kg) than those used for patients with severe hemophilia A or B and high-titer inhibitors (90 µg/kg) are often sufficient to control bleeding in patients with factor VII deficiency.[195,196] However, this has not been carefully defined in prospective clinical trials, and the Food and Drug Administration (FDA) has not yet approved rFVIIa for the treatment of congenital factor VII deficiency. Moreover, dosing has not been optimized for neonates and infants. Caution should be used in combining treatment with rFVIIa and PPC because thrombotic complications have been reported.

Factor VIII Deficiency. The severity of factor VIII deficiency is determined by the plasma concentration of factor VIII, with a level of less than 1% being severe, 1% to 5% being moderate, and 5% to 50% being mild. Severe factor VIII deficiency is the most common inherited bleeding disorder of the neonatal period. In addition, a small number of neonates with moderate and mild hemophilia are seen after a hemostatic challenge.[141,143,197-199] Large cohort studies have revealed that approximately 10% of children with hemophilia have clinical symptoms in the neonatal period.[168] In approximately 50% of factor VIII–deficient children with bleeding in the neonatal period, it occurred after circumcision. Almost 20% had intracranial bleeding. Death may occur from neonatal bleeding. In contrast to older infants and children, bleeding into joints is extremely rare in neonates.[200] Severe factor VIII deficiency can, on rare occasion, occur in female infants as a result of skewed lyonization and be clinically manifested in the neonatal period.[201,202] Management of bleeding secondary to factor VIII deficiency is discussed in detail in Chapter 30.

Factor IX Deficiency. Classification of the severity of factor IX deficiency is identical to that used for factor VIII deficiency. Diagnosis of milder forms of factor IX deficiency is complicated by physiologic levels of factor IX that can be as low as 0.15 U/mL and, in rare infants, by the potential for concurrent VK deficiency. Bleeding after circumcision and ICH can occur in neonates with factor IX deficiency.[141,143,197,203,204] Management of bleeding secondary to factor IX deficiency is discussed in detail in Chapter 30.

Factor X Deficiency. Severe factor X deficiency can be manifested as bleeding in the newborn period.[205-209] ICH was present in a high proportion of reported cases, several of which were fatal. Additional sites of bleeding that have been noted include umbilical, gastrointestinal, and intra-abdominal. Whole blood, FFP, factor X concentrate, and PCC have been used as replacement therapy.

Factor XI Deficiency. Severe deficiency of factor XI is rare. It is different from other coagulation protein deficiencies in that bleeding symptoms are not necessarily tightly correlated with factor plasma concentrations. Bleeding complications as a result of severe factor XI deficiency were reported in two newborns. One bled after circumcision at the age of 3 days and had a factor XI level of 0.07 U/mL. In another newborn, factor XI deficiency with bilateral subdural hemorrhage was diagnosed prenatally.[210-212] Either FFP or cryoprecipitate can be used for the treatment of factor XI–deficient patients if factor XI concentrate is not available.

Factor XIII Deficiency. Severe factor XIII deficiency is typically manifested at birth as bleeding from the umbilical stump or ICH.[142,213-222] Other clinical manifestations of homozygous factor XIII deficiency include delayed wound healing, abnormal scar formation, and recurrent soft tissue hemorrhage with a tendency to form hemorrhagic cysts. ICH occurs even in the absence of trauma in approximately a third of all affected patients.[138] Newborns with heterozygous factor XIII deficiency are not clinically affected.

FFP, cryoprecipitate, or factor XIII concentrates can be used for the treatment of factor XIII–deficient patients. Newborns with known factor XIII deficiency should receive a prophylactic regimen of factor XIII because of the high incidence of ICH. Plasma concentrations of factor XIII greater than 1% are effective, and the very long half-life of factor XIII permits once-per-month therapy. Therefore, prophylactic replacement therapy consists of either small doses of FFP (2 to 3 mL/kg) administered every 4 to 6 weeks, cryoprecipitate at a dose of 1 bag/10 to 20 kg of weight every 3 to 6 weeks, or preferably, factor XIII concentrate at a dose of 10 to 20 U/kg every 4 to 6 weeks, depending on the clinical situation and the preinfusion plasma concentration of factor XIII.[142,213-224]

Hereditary Deficiencies of Multiple Coagulation Factors. Hereditary deficiencies of two or more coagulation proteins have been reported for 16 different combinations of coagulation factors.[225] Combined deficiency of factors V and VIII has been described in patients with mutations in the genes encoding LMAN1 (also called ERGIC-53) and MCFD2.[154,156,226,227] Administration of FFP is usually the initial therapy. Subsequent treatment varies, depending on the specific factors affected.

Hemorrhagic Disease of the Newborn

Historical Background

HDN, as first described by Townsend in 1894, consists of hemorrhage on days 1 through 5 of life from multiple sites in otherwise healthy infants.[228] Subsequently, a causal link between HDN and abnormal blood coagulation was established.[62,229,230] Initial treatment of infants with HDN consisted of intravenous, intramuscular, or subcutaneous injection of blood or serum. Even at this very early time, the difficulty of separating treatment response from spontaneous improvement was recognized. Later, a randomized, controlled trial showed that intramuscular injection of blood was not helpful in preventing the abnormalities in blood coagulation that occurred during the first week of life.[229] The link between VK deficiency and spontaneous hemorrhage was first recognized in chicks in 1929.[231] The association between VK deficiency and HDN quickly followed, as subsequently did treatment of infants with HDN.[62,232-234]

The next historical step was recognition of the link between decreased prothrombin activity and increased

PT on days 2 to 4 of life in the absence of prophylactic VK. Prothrombin activity was observed to return to normal by days 5 to 7 of life.[62,235-238] These observations led to the hypothesis that VK administered prophylactically could prevent HDN.[235,236,239-241] There was uniform agreement that the prophylactic administration of VK to mothers or infants prevented the decrease in prothrombin activity during the first 3 to 4 days of life.[62,234,235,239] On the basis of these studies, VK prophylaxis was widely recommended. Subsequently, the scientific basis for this policy became less clear for several reasons. First, plasma concentrations of other coagulation proteins in addition to prothrombin were shown to be low in newborns. Second, there was increasing recognition that bleeding in neonates was often not due to VK deficiency.[62,230,242-244] Third, administration of high amounts (50 to 70 mg) of a water-soluble form of VK resulted in hemolytic anemia with kernicterus in some infants.[62,245,246] Fourth, many clinicians suggested that VK prophylaxis was not needed for all healthy full-term infants.[244,247-249] Consequently, VK prophylaxis was suspended in some countries, and recurrence of HDN ensued.[62,236,250-261] Most of the controversy concerning prophylactic use of VK can be explained by the design of the trials and subsequent interpretation of their results. The best evidence comes from large randomized, placebo-controlled trials. Such trials have consistently shown a statistically significant benefit from VK prophylaxis in terms of clinical bleeding.[262-264] No randomized, controlled trials with large enough sample size have shown that prophylactic VK does not prevent bleeding.

Prophylactic Vitamin K Administration

VK exists in three forms: VK_1 (phytonadione), which is present in leafy green vegetables; VK_2 (menaquinone), which is synthesized by intestinal bacterial flora; and VK_3 (menadione), which is a synthetic, water-soluble form. VK_3 is rarely used in newborns because at high doses it causes hemolytic anemia, which results in jaundice and potential morbidity.[62,245,246] The recommendations for VK prophylaxis in many countries are reasonably similar.[46] Daily requirements of VK are approximately 1 to 5 μg/kg of body weight for newborns.[46] Most groups recommend a single dose of 0.5 to 1 mg intramuscularly or an oral dose of 2 to 4 mg at birth, with subsequent dosing for breast-fed infants. Oral VK prophylaxis is preferable to parenteral prophylaxis; studies have shown that oral administration of VK is as effective, less expensive, and less traumatic than intramuscular administration in preventing the classic signs and symptoms of VK deficiency.[46] However, orally administered VK_1 or VK_3 is not as effective as intramuscularly injected VK in the prevention of late VK deficiency. In a 1991 randomized, controlled trial in Thailand, infants were given a single 2-mg dose of VK orally, 5 mg orally, or 1 mg intramuscularly.[265] Although mean levels of VK_1 were not significantly different in the treated infants given the various dosage forms, a trend toward higher levels was observed in intramuscularly

treated infants. Strategies for preventing late VK deficiency include repeat administration of oral VK[260,266] or continuous low-dose VK supplementation.[260] A mixed micelle oral VK_1 preparation that is readily absorbed has been tested in children.[46] However, optimal dosing of this preparation to prevent late VK deficiency bleeding remains to be determined.[267]

In addition to general prophylaxis at birth, patients in certain risk groups require additional VK prophylaxis (e.g., infants with α_1-antitrypsin deficiency, chronic diarrhea, cystic fibrosis, or celiac disease). Pregnant women receiving oral anticonvulsant therapy should take 10 mg of oral VK_1 daily beginning at 36 weeks' gestation for the prevention of overt VK deficiency in their infants at birth.[59]

In 1990, a cohort study aimed at determining perinatal risk factors for childhood cancer reported an association between drugs administered in the peripartum period (maternal pethidine or neonatal VK) and childhood cancer (odds ratio, 2.6).[268] A subsequent case-control study by the same group found no association between maternal pethidine and childhood cancer; however, they again reported an increased risk of childhood cancer after neonatal intramuscular VK administration (odds ratio, 1.97).[269] In contrast, a later large case-control study of 2530 children with cancer, one ecologic study, and one meta-analysis have shown no association between VK administration and childhood cancer.[270,271] The current consensus of the American Academy of Pediatrics Committee on Fetus and Newborn is that the risk for increased childhood cancer is probably minimal, if any, and the benefits of VK prophylaxis in terms of reduced bleeding are substantial.[272]

Bleeding Caused by Vitamin K Deficiency in the Newborn

In the absence of prophylactic VK, the incidence of vitamin K–dependent bleeding (VKDB) ranges from 0.25% to 1.7%.[62,262] Infants are at greater risk for hemorrhagic complications from VK deficiency than similarly affected adults are because their plasma concentrations of VK-dependent factors are physiologically decreased.[17,19,23,62,261,273] The clinical manifestation of VKDB can be classified as classic, early, or late on the basis of the timing and type of complications (Table 5-11). Classic VKDB initially occurs on days 2 to 7 of life in breast-fed, healthy full-term infants.[54,62,256,273-276] Causes include poor placental transfer of VK,[45,47-49] marginal VK content in breast milk (<20 μg/L), inadequate milk intake, and a sterile gut.[62] VKDB rarely occurs in formula-fed infants because commercially available formulas are supplemented with VK.[277,278] How often classic VKDB occurs in the absence of VK prophylaxis depends on the population studied, the supplemental formula, and the number of mothers breast-feeding. Early VKDB develops in the first 24 hours of life and is linked to maternal use of specific medications that interfere with VK stores or func-

TABLE 5-11   Forms of Vitamin K Deficiency Bleeding in Infancy

Parameter	Early Form	Classic Form	Late Form
Age	<24 hr	2-7 days	0.5-6 mo
Causes and risk factors	Medications during pregnancy	Breast-feeding	Marginal VK content in breast milk resulting from low VK intake and absorption
	Anticonvulsants	Inadequate VK intake	Cystic fibrosis
	Oral anticoagulants (rifampin, isoniazid)		Diarrhea
			α_1AT deficiency
	Antibiotics (rarely, idiopathic or hereditary)		Hepatitis
			Celiac disease
Localization in order of occurrence	ICH	ICH	ICH (>50%)
	GI	GI	GI
	Umbilicus	Umbilicus	Skin
	Intra-abdominal	ENT region	ENT region
	Cephalhematoma	Injection sites	Injection sites
		Circumcision	Urogenital tract
			Intrathoracic
Occurrence without VK prophylaxis	Very rare	1.5% (1/10,000 births)	4-10/10,000 births*
Prophylaxis	Discontinue or replace offending medications	Adequate VK supply	Adequate VK supply
	Maternal VK prophylaxis	Early and adequate breast-feeding	Adequate breast-feeding
		Formula	Formula
		VK prophylaxis	VK prophylaxis†

α_1AT, α_1-antitrypsin; ENT, ear, nose, and throat region; GI, gastrointestinal bleeding; VK, vitamin K.
*More common in Southeast Asia.
†A single intramuscular injection is better than a single oral dose; repeated small doses are closer to physiologic conditions.

tion, such as some anticonvulsants.[279-281] Late VKDB occurs between weeks 2 and 8 of life and is linked to disorders that compromise ongoing VK supply.[282,283]

Laboratory Diagnosis of Vitamin K Deficiency in the Newborn

Laboratory tests used to detect VK deficiency include screening coagulation tests, specific factor assays, measurement of decarboxylated forms of VK-dependent factors, PIVKA (protein induced by VK antagonists) assays, and direct measurements of VK levels. The results of these tests must always be compared with values for age-matched, healthy, non–VK-deficient infants to distinguish physiologic and pathologic deficiencies.[55,284]

Treatment

An infant suspected of having VK deficiency should be treated immediately with VK while laboratory confirmation is awaited. All infants with VKDB should be given VK either subcutaneously or intravenously, depending on the clinical problem. VK should not be given intramuscularly to infants with VKDB because large hematomas may form at the site of the injection. Absorption of subcutaneously administered VK is rapid, and its effect occurs only slightly slower than that of systemically administered VK. Intravenous VK should be given slowly and with a test dose because it may induce an anaphylactoid reaction. Infants with major bleeding because of

VK deficiency should also be treated with plasma products to rapidly increase levels of VK-dependent proteins. Plasma is the product of choice for treatment of a non–life-threatening hemorrhagic event, whereas PCCs should be considered for the management of life-threatening bleeding.

Liver Disease

The coagulopathies associated with liver disease in newborns are similar to those of adults and reflect the failure of hepatic synthetic function. However, in newborns this problem may be superimposed on the already "physiologic" immaturity of the coagulation system, activation of the coagulation and fibrinolytic systems, poor clearance of activated coagulation factors, and loss of hemostatic proteins into ascitic fluid.[285] Secondary effects of liver disease on platelet number and function also occur in newborns.[286,287] Common causes of hepatic dysfunction in newborns include viral hepatitis, hypoxia, total parenteral nutrition, shock, and fetal hydrops. Rare causes include genetic diseases such as α_1-antitrypsin deficiency,[288] galactosemia,[289] and tyrosinemia.[290]

Laboratory abnormalities induced by acute liver disease include prolongation of the PT and low plasma concentrations of several coagulation proteins, including fibrinogen.[291,292] However, it is important to compare these levels with those of normal age-matched controls (see Tables 5-1 to 5-3) because some of these factors are considerably lower than the adult range. Fibrinogen is present at adult levels in newborns and may be a useful marker. Chronic liver failure with cirrhosis is also characterized by a coagulopathy and mild thrombocytopenia.[288-290,293] Secondary VK deficiency may occur as a result of impaired absorption from the small intestine, particularly in those with intrahepatic and extrahepatic biliary atresia.[294] Patients with clinical bleeding may benefit temporarily from replacement of coagulation proteins with FFP, cryoprecipitate, or exchange transfusion. However, without recovery of hepatic function, replacement therapy is futile. VK should be administered to infants in whom cholestatic liver disease is suspected.

von Willebrand Disease

Although von Willebrand disease (VWD) is the most common inherited bleeding disorder, patients with the disease are rarely seen in the neonatal period. Plasma concentrations of VWF are increased in neonates, as is the proportion of ULVWF multimers.[73,74] Nonetheless, severe deficiency (type 3) and some qualitative VWF disorders (type 2) have been reported in the newborn period.[295-298] Management of VWD is discussed in detail in Chapter 30. Use of arginine vasopressin (DDAVP) in the newborn period is contraindicated because of associated excess free water retention.

Platelet Disorders

Quantitative Platelet Disorders

Healthy full-term infants have platelet counts within the normal adult range (150 to $450 \times 10^9/L$).[62,86] Healthy premature infants typically have platelet counts in the low end of the normal adult range.[62,83,84] The definition of thrombocytopenia in newborns is the same as that in adults: a platelet count less than $150 \times 10^9/L$. Studies of fetuses between 18 and 30 weeks' gestation show a stable platelet count of approximately $250 \times 10^9/L$.[2] Consequently, platelet counts less than $150 \times 10^9/L$ are abnormal and indicate the need for investigation and, sometimes, treatment. Mean volumes of platelets in newborns are similar to those of adults (range, 7 to 9 fL).[86-88] Postnatally, MPV increases slightly over the first 2 weeks of life, concomitantly with an increase in platelet count.[89,90]

Epidemiology. Thrombocytopenia is the most common hemostatic abnormality in newborns admitted to neonatal intensive care units (NICUs).[83,85,87,88,299] A single prospective cohort study[87] and six retrospective reviews[88,300-304] have provided the most reliable information on the occurrence, natural history, mechanisms, and clinical impact of thrombocytopenia in newborns. There is general agreement that thrombocytopenia indicates the presence of an underlying pathologic process; however, the clinical relevance of mild thrombocytopenia is unknown. Thrombocytopenia develops in approximately 22% of infants admitted to the NICUs of tertiary hospi-

tals.[87] In some infants the thrombocytopenia is trivial, with platelet counts between 100 and $150 \times 10^9/L$. However, in 50% of affected infants, platelet counts decrease to less than $100 \times 10^9/L$, and in 20% of infants, platelet counts are lower than $50 \times 10^9/L$.[87] What constitutes a safe platelet count in a neonate remains to be rigorously determined, but many neonatal units attempt to keep the platelet count higher than $50 \times 10^9/L$, although this figure may vary, depending on the postconceptional age of the infant and comorbid conditions.

Pathogenesis. Causes of thrombocytopenia in neonates, like those in older children and adults, can be divided into disorders involving increased platelet destruction, decreased platelet production, or sequestration (Box 5-1). Although many of these causes overlap with those seen in older children and adults, several entities are unique to neonates or may occur in the newborn period and are considered in more detail later. Increased platelet destruction is the mechanism responsible for thrombocytopenia in most infants.[87,305] Characterization of mechanisms responsible for thrombocytopenia is important because they have practical implications in assessing the risk for bleeding and in guiding management.

Increased Platelet Destruction. Thrombocytopenia secondary to increased platelet destruction can be divided into immune and nonimmune causes.

IMMUNE THROMBOCYTOPENIA. Immune thrombocytopenia is defined as an increased rate of platelet clearance caused by platelet-associated immunoglobulin G (IgG) or complement. It is the most common form of increased platelet destruction in newborns and should always be suspected in otherwise healthy infants with isolated severe thrombocytopenia. Neonatal immune thrombocytopenia can be further broken down into one of three processes: transplacental passage of a maternal antibody directed against a nonshared platelet antigen (termed "alloimmune thrombocytopenia" or sometimes "isoimmune thrombocytopenia"), transplacental passage of a cross-reactive maternal autoimmune-derived antiplatelet antibody, or generation of an autoreactive antiplatelet antibody by the newborn itself (termed "autoimmune thrombocytopenia"). The second can be distinguished from the other two by examining the mother for a low platelet count. Differentiation of autoimmune thrombocytopenia from alloimmune thrombocytopenia in neonates is critical because the management and severity of these disorders are quite different. Chapter 33 discusses these two forms of immune thrombocytopenia and their management in detail.

Neonatal Alloimmune Thrombocytopenia. Neonatal alloimmune thrombocytopenia (NAIT) is the most common cause of immune-mediated thrombocytopenia in the newborn period, with an estimated incidence of about 1 in 1000 to 5000 live births in white popula-

Box 5-1	Causes of Thrombocytopenia in Newborns

INCREASED DESTRUCTION OF PLATELETS

Immune Mediated

Neonatal alloimmune thrombocytopenia
Maternal idiopathic thrombocytopenic purpura
Drug-dependent antibody (could be from maternal
  medication use)
Autoimmune thrombocytopenic purpura

Non–Immune Mediated

Pseudothrombocytopenia (platelet clumping) in vitro
Disseminated intravascular coagulation
Asphyxia
Perinatal aspiration
Necrotizing enterocolitis
Hemangiomas (Kasabach-Merritt syndrome)
Neonatal thrombosis
Respiratory distress syndrome
Maternal preeclampsia
Cardiopulmonary bypass (including ECMO)
Familial thrombotic thrombocytopenic purpura

Other

Hyperbilirubinemia
Phototherapy
Polycythemia
Rh hemolytic disease
Total parenteral nutrition

DECREASED PRODUCTION OF PLATELETS

Acquired

Viral infection (e.g., HIV, CMV, Rubella, HHV-6)
Congenital leukemia
Down syndrome–transient myeloproliferative disorder
  (DS-TMD)
Neuroblastoma

Histiocytosis
Osteopetrosis

Inherited

Disorders associated with small platelets
  Wiskott-Aldrich syndrome (WAS)
  X-linked thrombocytopenia (associated with WASP)
Disorders associated with normal-sized platelets
  Thrombocyopenia with absent radii (TAR)
  Amegakaryocytic thrombocytopenia with radioulnar
    synostosis
  Congenital amegakaryocytic thrombocytopenia
    (CAMT)
  Familial platelet disorder with a propensity for the
    development of AML (FPD/AML)
Disorders associated with large platelets
  X-linked macrothrombocytopenia with or without
    anemia (GATA-1 mutations)
  MYH9-related disorders (May-Hegglin anomaly;
    Sebastian's, Fechtner's, and Epstein's syndromes)
  Bernard-Soulier syndrome
  Paris-Trousseau/Jacobsen syndrome
  Velocardiofacial syndrome
  Montreal platelet syndrome
  Gray platelet syndrome
  Platelet-type or pseudo–von Willebrand disease
Other
  Fanconi's anemia
  Metabolic disorders (methylmalonic academia, ketotic
    glycinemia, isovaleric academia, etc.)
  Drug-mediated suppression

SEQUESTRATION

Hypersplenism

AML, acute myelogenous leukemia; CMV, cytomegalovirus; ECMO, extracorporeal membrane oxygenation; HHV-6, human herpesvirus 6; HIV, human immunodeficiency virus; WASP, Wiskott-Aldrich syndrome protein.

---

tions.[306-309] It arises when the mother, who lacks a common platelet antigen, is exposed to the antigen (inherited from the father) on neonatal platelets and generates a neutralizing IgG. This crosses the placenta and mediates premature clearance of fetal and newborn platelets. First-born infants can be affected. Frequently, the thrombocytopenia is severe. It is critical to make the diagnosis because the risk of life-threatening bleeding and CNS morbidity is high, estimated at up to 10% to 15% of cases. A useful diagnostic test is to assay the reactivity of the mother's serum with the father's platelets. If such samples are not available, it is possible to look for reaction of the mother's serum with the newborn's platelets or the presence of antiplatelet antibodies in the newborn's serum. The most common antigen is Pl[A1], although other antigens, such as Bak[a], Pen[a] (more common in Asian populations), Br[b],

and Br[a], have been described.[310] However, not all cases in which the pregnant mother generates allosensitive antiplatelet antibodies result in neonatal thrombocytopenia.

Treatment of NAIT includes transfusion with washed platelets donated by the mother. Because the mother's platelets lack the offending antigen, they should have a normal life span. Many blood banks also maintain registries of Pl[A1]-negative donors who can be contacted for platelet donation in cases involving antibodies against Pl[A1]. If antigen-negative platelets are not available, treatment with intravenous immunoglobulin (IVIG), 1 g/kg as a single daily bolus for 1 or 2 consecutive days, along with random donor platelets if the patient is bleeding, is effective in reducing the rate of platelet destruction. Endogenous platelet counts typically rise by 36 to 48 hours. There is no role for corticosteroids because all of the antibody production occurs in the mother. All infants with NAIT should undergo head ultrasonography or CT to rule out ICH. The natural history of NAIT is gradual resolution of the thrombocytopenia over the first few months of life as the offending antibody is cleared. Close monitoring of the platelet count is indicated for at least the first month of life until the platelet count normalizes. The safety of breast-feeding in the setting of NAIT has not been rigorously studied. One case report suggested that breast-feeding did not significantly worsen the clinical course, even though the breast milk contained anti-platelet IgG.[311]

Immune Thrombocytopenia Caused by Maternal Antiplatelet Autoantibodies. Maternal autoimmune anti-platelet IgG can cross the placenta and result in increased platelet destruction in the fetus. A common cause is maternal systemic lupus erythematosus. Like NAIT, the thrombocytopenia gradually resolves over the first few months of life as the maternal antibodies are cleared. In severe cases, use of IVIG in the neonate may help reduce the rate of platelet destruction. Corticosteroids are of no utility. Drug-dependent antibodies can result in both maternal and neonatal thrombocytopenia.[109]

Autoimmune Thrombocytopenia. True autoimmune thrombocytopenia, in which neonates generate an antibody against their own platelets, is very rare in the newborn period. If present, it typically signals an underlying immune dysregulatory disorder. If heparin-induced thrombocytopenia is suspected, heparin therapy should be discontinued immediately and alternative forms of anticoagulation considered if necessary (see Chapter 33).

NONIMMUNE THROMBOCYTOPENIA

Sepsis and Disseminated Intravascular Coagulation. A common nonimmune cause of thrombocytopenia in the newborn period is sepsis, with or without DIC. Viral (rubella, herpesvirus, echovirus, cytomegalovirus, human herpesvirus 6 [HHV-6], and human immunodeficiency virus [HIV]), protozoal (Toxoplasma), and bacterial infections cause severe thrombocytopenia.[312] Mechanisms responsible for bacterial sepsis–induced thrombocytopenia are multifactorial and include consumption resulting from DIC, endothelial damage, platelet aggregation caused by binding of bacterial products to platelet membranes, and decreased production as a result of marrow infection.[313] Mechanisms responsible for virus-induced thrombocytopenia include loss of sialic acid from platelet membranes because of viral neuraminidase, intravascular platelet aggregation, and impaired megakaryopoiesis (see later). Congenital rubella causes thrombocytopenia in three quarters of infants, with platelet counts ranging from 20 to 60×10^9/L for the first 4 to 8 weeks of life.

In premature infants, thrombocytopenia often complicates other disorders such as RDS, persistent pulmo-nary hypertension, necrotizing enterocolitis, and hyperbilirubinemia treated by phototherapy. Activation of coagulation with platelet consumption occurs in RDS, and mechanical ventilation may be an independent factor contributing to thrombocytopenia.[314] It has been suggested that persistent pulmonary hypertension in new-borns may be due in part to intrapulmonary platelet aggregation and the release of platelet-derived vasoactive substances such as thromboxane A_2.[315] Approximately half of infants with necrotizing enterocolitis are thrombocytopenic, with about 20% having laboratory evidence of DIC.

Exchange Transfusion, Hyperbilirubinemia, and Phototherapy. Intrauterine and exchange transfusions cause thrombocytopenia by a dilutional effect that depends on the amount of blood transfused.[301] After exchange transfusion, platelet counts increase within 3 days and reach pre-exchange levels by about 7 days.[34] Both hyperbilirubinemia and phototherapy are associated with mild thrombocytopenia in newborn humans and shortened platelet survival in rabbits.[305]

Hypoxia and Placental Insufficiency. Acute asphyxia is a consistent cause of DIC and thrombocytopenia.[93] Chronic hypoxia is associated with placental dysfunction, intrauterine growth retardation, and significant thrombocytopenia.

Vascular Malformations. Certain types of large vascular malformations are associated with Kasabach-Merritt syndrome, in which a local consumptive coagulopathy occurs as a result of abnormal endothelium. This causes hypofibrinogenemia, elevated levels of fibrinogen-fibrin degradation products, microangiopathic fragmentation of red cells, and thrombocytopenia (see Chapter 33).[316-320] The thrombocytopenia can be severe, with platelet counts lower than 50×10^9/L. Approximately 50% of affected infants experience systemic bleeding during the first month of life. Sometimes the vascular malformations are not apparent on physical examination and may require imaging studies to detect.

Thrombosis and Familial Thrombotic Thrombocytopenic Purpura. Thrombocytopenia is loosely associated with thromboembolic complications and polycythemia in infants with hematocrit values greater than 70%. However, thrombocytopenia may also indicate the presence of other concurrent disease processes. Infants with a familial form of hemolytic-uremic syndrome or thrombotic thrombocytopenic purpura have a microangiopathic hemolytic anemia in association with transient neurologic or renal abnormalities.

Decreased Platelet Production. Thrombocytopenia secondary to decreased platelet production is rare and accounts for less than 5% of thrombocytopenic infants.[34,83-85] Causes include viral infections, drug-induced thrombocytopenia, congenital leukemia, DS-TMD, neuroblastoma, histiocytosis, osteopetrosis, congenital amegakaryocytic thrombocytopenia (CAMT), TAR, other inherited genetic platelet disorders, and bone marrow failure syndromes.

CONGENITAL VIRAL INFECTION. Congenital viral infections with rubella, herpesvirus, echovirus, cytomegalovirus, HHV-6, and HIV have been associated with thrombocytopenia in the newborn period, in part through deleterious effects on megakaryopoiesis and thrombopoiesis. It may occur via direct infection of megakaryocytes in the case of HIV because the HIV coreceptor CXCR4 is expressed on the surface of human megakaryocytes and their precursor cells.[321]

DRUG-INDUCED THROMBOCYTOPENIA. Transplacental passage of drugs or the use of drugs in neonates can cause thrombocytopenia via bone marrow suppression or the development of drug-dependent antibodies, or both.[109] However, these causes are rare, and evidence for them is weak.[322-325] Agents implicated are salicylates, quinine, hydralazine, tolbutamide, and thiazide diuretics.

CONGENITAL LEUKEMIA AND OTHER MALIGNANCIES. Infantile leukemia, as well as other neonatal malignancies characterized by bone marrow infiltration such as neuroblastoma, can be accompanied by thrombocytopenia in the newborn period. Typically, other hematopoietic lineages are affected and other clinical signs are apparent. An infantile form of myelofibrosis has been described is several families in Saudi Arabia.[326,327]

DOWN SYNDROME–TRANSIENT MYELOPROLIFERATIVE DISORDER. Some children with Down syndrome (trisomy 21) are born with a transient myeloproliferative disorder (DS-TMD) characterized by leukocytosis, predominance of circulating early erythromegakaryocytic precursor cells, pancytopenia, and in some cases, severe liver fibrosis. Remarkably, this myeloproliferation resolves spontaneously over the first few months of life. In about 20% of symptomatic cases, acute megakaryocytic leukemia (DS-AMKL) develops within a few years, sometimes preceded by a myelodysplastic phase.[328] The DS-TMD and DS-AMKL cells harbor acquired mutations in the gene encoding GATA-1, a zinc finger transcription factor essential for normal megakaryocyte and erythroid development.[329-335] Although a wide spectrum of mutations have been identified, including missense, deletion, insertion, and splice site mutations, they essentially all result in the same outcome: exclusive production of a short isoform of GATA-1 that lacks the amino-terminal 83 amino acids of the full-length protein (Fig. 5-3). These mutations are highly specific for DS-TMD and DS-AMKL. There has been only one reported case of such a mutation in AMKL without trisomy 21.[336] Why these mutations are so highly selected for in a Down syndrome genetic background and how they may participate in the pathogenesis of DS-TMD and DS-AMKL are not known.

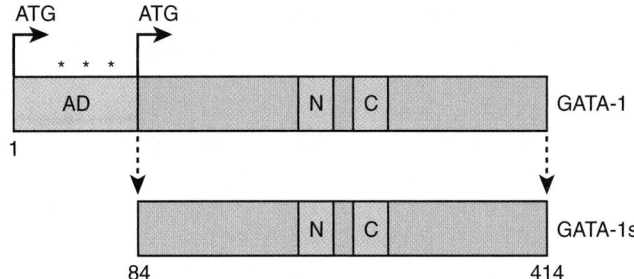

FIGURE 5-3. Acquired mutations of GATA-1 in Down syndrome–transient myeloproliferative disorder and acute megakaryoblastic leukemia. In this schematic diagram of full-length GATA-1, mutations are represented by *asterisks*. Introduction of premature stop codons, or splicing around exon 2, results in exclusive generation of a shorter isoform of GATA-1 (GATA-1s) because of initiation of translation from a downstream in-frame ATG at codon 84. AD, classic transcriptional activation domain; C, C-terminal zinc finger; N, N-terminal zinc finger.

Knock-in mice that recapitulate the truncating GATA-1 mutation show unexpected stage-specific effects on megakaryopoiesis.[81] During fetal liver hematopoiesis, the mutant megakaryocytes markedly hyperproliferate, similar to what is observed for GATA-1–deficient megakaryocytes. However, during adult-stage bone marrow hematopoiesis, megakaryopoiesis and thrombopoiesis appear to be normal. This suggests that the fetal liver and bone marrow cellular contexts interact differentially with the GATA-1–truncated molecule, which may explain restriction of TMD to the neonatal period and infers that additional genetic events occur and lead to clonal evolution of a rare TMD cell to full DS-AMKL.[337]

INHERITED PLATELET DISORDERS

Though considerably less common than consumptive processes or viral suppression, inherited platelet disorders can occur in the newborn period and should be considered in the differential diagnosis of thrombocytopenia in a neonate. They are discussed in more detail in Chapter 29. Several classifications, diagnostic algorithms, and management recommendations have recently been published.[338,339] Brief descriptions, with particular focus on neonatal manifestations, are given here. Infants with aplastic disorders have the greatest risk of serious bleeding in the form of ICH in the first months of life.

DISORDERS WITH SMALL PLATELETS. Wiskott-Aldrich Syndrome. Wiskott-Aldrich syndrome (WAS; OMIM 301000) is an X-linked disorder caused by deficiency of the Wiskott-Aldrich syndrome protein (WASP), which functions in actin dynamics in megakaryocytes and T lymphocytes. It is one of the few disorders characterized by small platelets. The small size of the platelets is not always apparent by standard automated blood cell MPV measurements. Therefore, if the diagnosis is being considered, it is imperative to evaluate platelet size by examination of the peripheral smear and to confirm small platelet volume with cytometer devices calibrated for platelets. The other clinical hallmarks of WAS are immunodeficiency (usually severe) and eczema. Bloody diarrhea is often seen and can be an initial sign. The immunodeficiency is frequently the most significant clinical problem associated with this disease. It is important to recognize the syndrome early so that appropriate interventions can be instituted, including prophylactic treatment against opportunistic infections such as *Pneumocystis carinii*. A destructive component of the thrombocytopenia in WAS is also likely because splenectomy increases platelet counts in a large number of patients. In addition, the thrombocytopenia can be exacerbated by development of immune thrombocytopenic purpura secondary to the immune dysregulation. Bone marrow transplantation is curative for WAS, and early diagnosis is helpful in initiating listing for transplantation before significant complications arise.

X-Linked Thrombocytopenia. X-linked thrombocytopenia (OMIM 313900) is a less severe form of WAS that is manifested predominantly as thrombocytopenia. Typically, there is no or minimal immunologic dysfunction. However, more severe immunologic disturbances may develop in some patients over time. This clinical entity is distinct from X-linked macrothrombocytopenia, which is associated with mutations in GATA-1 (see later).

DISORDERS WITH NORMAL-SIZE PLATELETS. Congenital Amegakaryocytic Thrombocytopenia. CAMT (OMIM 604498) is characterized by severe thrombocytopenia with a markedly reduced number or absence of megakaryocytes. Patients are typically seen shortly after birth with petechiae, bruising, or bleeding. Biallelic inactivating mutations in the gene for c-mpl, the receptor for the major megakaryocyte cytokine TPO, have been identified in a large number of patients. Interestingly, no patients have been reported to date with mutations in the TPO gene itself. Patients with severe CAMT are at high risk for the development of complete bone marrow failure, usually within the first few years of life.[340] Such failure is most likely due to a role of TPO signaling in hematopoietic stem cell function.[341,342] Bone marrow transplantation has been used successfully to treat patients with severe CAMT.

Thrombocytopenia with Absent Radii. TAR syndrome (OMIM 274000) is characterized by hypomegakaryocytic thrombocytopenia and bilateral radial hypoplasia with the presence of thumbs.[343] Other hematopoietic lineages are not affected. Additional skeletal features may include shortening or, rarely, aplasia of the humerus and ulna. The lower limbs are frequently affected, but to a lesser extent. Congenital cardiac disease and cow's milk intolerance have also been associated in some cases. The genetic basis of TAR is unknown. The inheritance pattern is unclear, but some have suggested an autosomal recessive pattern. Recently, Klopocki and colleagues

identified a common interstitial microdeletion of 200 kilobases (kb) on chromosome 1q21.1 in several families with TAR.[344] However, the incomplete penetrance of the phenotype suggests that additional genetic loci may be involved. Patients with TAR have elevated circulating TPO levels, and their platelets exhibit defective TPO receptor (c-mpl) signaling, which suggests a possible role for downstream cytokine signaling in this disorder.[345]

Neither splenectomy nor steroids are beneficial for infants with TAR.[346,347] Platelet transfusions are highly effective but should be reserved for symptomatic infants because prophylactic platelet transfusions could result in refractoriness as a result of allosensitization.[347] By several months of age, increased numbers of megakaryocytes usually appear in the bone marrow, and platelet counts increase.[346,347] A functional platelet defect may be present in some children with TAR.[348]

Amegakaryocytic Thrombocytopenia with Radioulnar Synostosis. Amegakaryocytic thrombocytopenia with radioulnar synostosis (ATRUS, OMIM 605432) is a rare disorder characterized by reduced or absent megakaryocytes, severe thrombocytopenia, possible aplastic anemia, and proximal radioulnar synostosis leading to difficulty with forearm pronation. Sensorineural hearing loss may also be present. Mutations in the gene encoding the homeobox containing transcription factor HOXA11 have been found in some familial cases of ATRUS.[349,350]

Familial Platelet Disorder with a Propensity for the Development of Acute Myelogenous Leukemia. Familial platelet disorder with a propensity for the development of acute myelogenous leukemia (AML) (OMIM 601399) is a rare autosomal dominant disorder characterized by thrombocytopenia, an aspirin-like functional platelet defect, and increased risk for the development of myelodysplastic syndrome (MDS) and AML.[351-353] It is caused by constitutional haploinsufficieny of RUNX-1, a transcription factor involved in multiple stages of hematopoiesis, including megakaryopoiesis, and a frequent target of chromosomal translocations in human leukemias.[351,354] Bone marrow or peripheral blood from these patients has reduced ability to form megakaryocyte colonies, thus indicating a role for RUNX-1 dosage in megakaryopoiesis. A family history of MDS or AML should raise suspicion for this disorder in a newborn with thrombocytopenia and bleeding out of proportion to the platelet count.

DISORDERS WITH LARGE PLATELETS. Paris-Trousseau or Jacobsen's Syndrome. Paris-Trousseau syndrome (OMIM 188925) (also called Jacobsen's syndrome; OMIM 147791) is a constitutional contiguous gene deletion disorder involving the long arm of chromosome 11 (11q23).[355,356] The constellation of findings in these syndromes includes severe congenital cardiac abnormalities, trigonocephaly, mental retardation, dysmorphogenesis of the hands and face, and macrothrombocytopenia.[357] The cause of the thrombocytopenia appears to be related to impaired platelet production because platelet survival time is normal.[358] These patients can also exhibit a predisposition to thrombosis, thus suggesting possible qualitative defects in platelet production. Examination of bone marrow reveals significant dysmegakaryopoiesis with an abundance of micromegakaryocytes and death of large numbers of megakaryocytes during the late stages of maturation.[359] Peripheral blood platelets contain giant alpha granules, which are thought to arise from aberrant alpha granule fusion during prolonged residence in bone marrow.[360] The minimal chromosome regions deleted in Paris-Trousseau and Jacobsen's syndromes associated with thrombocytopenia include genes for the Ets family transcription factors FLI-1 and ETS-1, both of which play roles in megakaryocyte development.[361] Lentiviral expression of FLI-1 in CD34+ cells from patients with Paris-Trousseau thrombocytopenia rescues megakaryocyte differentiation in vitro, thereby providing strong evidence that deficiency of FLI-1 is the cause of impaired thrombopoiesis in these patients.

X-linked Macrothromboctyopenia with and without Anemia. Germline missense mutations in the gene encoding GATA-1 have recently been identified in several families with X-linked macrothrombocytopenia.[362] Some of the mutations impair binding of GATA-1 to its essential cofactor Friend of GATA-1.[362-366] Although all the mutations described produce thrombocytopenia to varying degrees, the more severe mutations also result in dyserythropoietic anemia. In the most severe cases, infants have required in utero red blood cell transfusions and bone marrow transplantation after birth.[362] Mutations in the N-terminal zinc finger of GATA-1 that impair binding to double GATA consensus DNA sites are associated with X-linked thrombocytopenia with β-thalassemia,[367-369] congenital erythropoietic prophyria,[370] X-linked gray platelet syndrome, or any combination of these conditions.[371]

Bernard-Soulier Disorder. Bernard-Soulier disorder (OMIM 231200) is caused by deficiency of the GPIb/IX/V complex on platelets, which binds VWF. Most reported mutations have been in the gene encoding the GPIb subunit, but mutations have also been found in GPIX.[372,373] Homozygous deficiency is associated with severe thrombocytopenia, giant platelets, defective ristocetin-induced platelet aggregation, and clinical bleeding. Heterozygous deficiency typically leads to mild thrombocytopenia with normal ristocetin-induced platelet aggregation in vitro and is now thought to be the underlying cause of benign Mediterranean macrothrombocytopenia.[374]

Velocardiofacial Syndrome. Velocardiofacial syndrome (OMIM 192430) is a contiguous gene deletion disorder involving chromosome 22q11.2. Clinical manifestations include cleft palate, cardiac anomalies, typical facies, learning disabilities, and defective GPIb/IX/V function. The platelet effects are due to heterozygous loss of the GPIbα gene, which resides in this region, and the condition should be considered a mild form of Bernard-Soulier disorder.[375]

MYH9-Related Disorders. MYH9-related disorders include May-Hegglin anomaly (OMIM 155100),

Sebastian's syndrome (OMIM 605249), Fechtner's syndrome (OMIM 153640), and Epstein's syndrome (OMIM 153650). All four disorders involve mutations in the gene encoding nonmuscle myosin heavy-chain type IIA (MYH9) and are inherited in an autosomal dominant fashion.[376] They are all associated with giant platelets but differ in the presence of neutrophil inclusions (Döhle bodies), sensorineural hearing loss, cataracts, and renal defects.[338]

Hypersplenism. As in adults, thrombocytopenia resulting from hypersplenism is usually mild to moderate, with platelet counts ranging from 50 to 100×10^9/L in newborns.

Clinical Impact of Neonatal Thrombocytopenia. Clinically important bleeding is less likely to occur in patients with consumptive platelet disorders than in those with production defects. The bleeding risk is increased in patients who have both thrombocytopenia and a defect in platelet function. Selection of a platelet count at which one should intervene, though a simplistic response, provides a guideline for therapy. A platelet count less than 50×10^9/L places some otherwise healthy full-term newborns at risk for serious ICH.[377] The importance of "moderate" thrombocytopenia (platelet counts between 50 and 100×10^9/L) in sick premature infants has been a subject of controversy. A randomized, controlled trial assessed the potential benefits of platelet concentrate transfusions in 154 premature thrombocytopenic infants during the first 72 hours of life.[378] Treated infants received platelet concentrates to maintain platelet counts higher than 150×10^9/L. No beneficial effect on the incidence or extension of ICH was shown in this study, which was designed to detect an effect of 25% or greater. However, infants who received transfusions had shortened bleeding times and required significantly less blood product support. A more recent retrospective study of 53 neonates with severe thrombocytopenia treated at a single NICU showed no significant difference in major hemorrhage in those transfused to maintain a platelet count greater than 30×10^9/L versus greater than 50×10^9/L.[304]

Treatment. Management of thrombocytopenic infants depends in part on the underlying disorder. If an infant is bleeding, a trial of platelet concentrates (10 to 20 mL/kg) is indicated. The increased platelet count usually shortens the bleeding time and is frequently clinically effective.[116] Autoimmune and alloimmune thrombocytopenia typically does not respond to random donor platelet concentrates and requires specific forms of therapy.

Thrombocytosis in the Newborn. Elevated platelet counts are frequently observed in premature infants at approximately 4 to 6 weeks after birth.[379] There are no clinical manifestations of neonatal thrombocytosis, and therapeutic intervention is not indicated.

Qualitative Platelet Disorders

Despite the physiologic hyporeactivity of neonatal platelets in response to exposure to some agents, healthy infants do not have an increased risk of bleeding. Pathologic impairment of platelet function may occur, to a variable extent, as a result of the use of certain drugs or the presence of pathologic states in either mothers or infants. In mothers, causative factors include the use of some drugs, diabetes,[380-383] dietary abnormalities,[384-389] smoking,[390-392] and ethanol abuse[393]; in infants, they include the use of some drugs, perinatal aspiration syndrome,[301,394-397] hyperbilirubinemia,[398,399] phototherapy,[399,400] renal failure,[401] and hepatic failure.

Phototherapy. When platelets are exposed to a broad-spectrum blue fluorescent light in vitro, aggregation is decreased and microscopic alterations in granules and external membranes occur.[402]

Medications

Aspirin. Salicylate crosses the placenta and can be detected in fetuses after maternal ingestion.[322-325,403-407] Clearance of salicylate is slower in newborns than in adults, and thus infants have a potential risk of bleeding for a prolonged time.[323] However, in vitro studies have not demonstrated increased sensitivity of newborn platelets to salicylates as compared with adult platelets,[118,405] and the evidence linking maternal aspirin ingestion to clinically important bleeding in newborns is weak.[325] There is little reason to have serious concerns about maternal ingestion of aspirin, but it is reasonable to advise mothers to not ingest aspirin unless specifically indicated by their physician.

Indomethacin. Indomethacin is used for nonsurgical closure of a patent ductus arteriosus in premature infants, but it also has antiplatelet activities. Indomethacin, like salicylate, has a longer half-life in newborns than in adults (21 to 24 hours in newborns versus 2 to 3 hours in adults).[408] This extended half-life is probably due to underdevelopment of hepatic drug metabolism or renal excretory function or to altered protein binding.[409,410] Indomethacin inhibits platelet function in newborns, as shown by prolongation of bleeding times.[411,412] Randomized, controlled trials have provided conflicting conclusions on the effect of indomethacin on intraventricular hemorrhage in premature infants.[413]

Maternal Diabetes. The reactivity of platelets from diabetic mothers and their infants is increased, as demonstrated by enhanced thromboxane B_2 production, enhanced platelet aggregation,[382,414] and a lower threshold to many aggregating agents.[414] The enhanced platelet function in diabetes is associated with increased synthesis of a prostaglandin E–like substance that crosses the placenta and affects the fetus.[415] Despite these in vitro findings, the evidence linking enhanced platelet reactivity to clinically significant thromboembolism in newborns of diabetic mothers is weak.[416,417]

Diet. Alterations in the diet of mothers or infants during the postnatal period can affect newborn platelet function. Increases in the ratio of polyunsaturated fatty acids to saturated fatty acids in the diet of mothers who breast-feed their infants result in increases in the concentration of linoleic acid and enhanced thromboxane B_2 production.[384] Infants receiving a diet deficient in essential fatty acids may exhibit arachidonic acid depletion and platelet dysfunction.[385,387] Vitamin E functions as an antioxidant and as an inhibitor of platelet aggregation/release in humans.[388,389,418,419] Instances of vitamin E–deficient infants with increased platelet aggregation that reversed after vitamin E supplementation have been reported.[389,420]

Amniotic Fluid. Amniotic fluid contains procoagulant activity that enhances the generation of thromboxane A_2 by platelets.[394-397] Infants in whom perinatal aspiration syndrome develops have pulmonary hypertension with platelet thrombi in the pulmonary microcirculation. The exact mechanism or mechanisms leading to persistent pulmonary hypertension in these infants is unknown.

Nitric Oxide. Nitric oxide prevents adhesion of platelets to endothelial cells and inhibits ADP-induced aggregation of cord platelets in a manner similar to that in adults.[421-424]

Extracorporeal Membrane Oxygenation. Extracorporeal membrane oxygenation (ECMO) permits transfer of oxygen into blood across a semipermeable membrane and is currently used for infants with life-threatening severe respiratory insufficiency. Underlying respiratory disorders include meconium aspiration syndrome, severe RDS, congenital diaphragmatic hernia, persistent pulmonary hypertension, and sepsis. Hemorrhage, particularly ICH, is one of the most serious complications of this technique. Hardart and Fackler reported an overall incidence of new ICH of about 10% in infants included in the Extracorporeal Life Support Organization Registry ($N = 4550$) from 1992 through 1995.[425] Of 1398 evaluable premature infants (born at <37 weeks' EGA) reported to the registry between 1992 and 2000, ICH developed in 13%.[426] Similar to that found with cardiopulmonary bypass, the increased risk of bleeding during ECMO is due mostly to the use of heparin in combination with other hemostatic defects, including significantly decreased plasma concentrations of coagulation factors and platelet dysfunction secondary to chronic activation.[427-429] Other recognized contributing factors include prolonged hypoxia, ischemia, general anesthesia, acidosis, sepsis, and treatment with epinephrine.[425,427,430-435] In premature infants, the risk for ICH with ECMO correlates inversely with postconceptional age.[426] Although anticoagulation is required for ECMO, the optimal use of heparin has never been tested in clinical trials. Whether lower doses of heparin or the use of low-molecular-weight heparin (LMWH) has a role in ECMO remains to be determined.

Thrombotic Disorders in the Neonate

Congenital Prothrombotic Disorders

Patients with heterozygous defects for recognized inherited prothrombotic disorders are rarely seen with their first thromboembolic complication during childhood unless another pathologic event unmasks the problem. In contrast, patients who are homozygotes or double heterozygotes for a congenital prothrombotic disorder are often initially encountered in the newborn period or during early childhood. The following discussion is limited to the unique aspects of these inherited deficiencies in newborns. Chapter 32 discusses congenital prothrombotic disorders in detail.

Homozygous Prothrombotic Disorders

Though rare, the most commonly reported homozygous prothrombotic disorder encountered during the newborn period is protein C deficiency. Homozygous protein S deficiency is even less common.[436-458] All patients seen in the newborn period had undetectable levels of protein C (or protein S), whereas children with a delayed manifestation had detectable levels ranging between 0.05 and 0.20 U/mL.

Clinical Findings. The classic clinical manifestation of homozygous protein C/protein S deficiency consists of cerebral or ophthalmic damage (or both) in utero, purpura fulminans within hours or days of birth, and on rare occasion, large vessel thrombosis. Purpura fulminans is an acute, lethal syndrome of DIC characterized by rapidly progressive hemorrhagic necrosis of the skin secondary to dermal vascular thrombosis.[459-461] The skin lesions start as small, ecchymotic sites that increase in radial fashion, become purplish black with bullae, and then turn necrotic and gangrenous.[459,461] The lesions develop mainly on the extremities but can occur on the buttocks, abdomen, scrotum, and scalp. They also occur at pressure points, at sites of previous puncture, and at previously affected sites. Moreover, affected infants have severe DIC with hemorrhagic complications.

Diagnosis. The diagnosis of homozygous protein C/protein S deficiency in infants is based on the appropriate clinical picture, a protein C/protein S level that is usually undetectable, a heterozygous state in the parents, and ideally, identification of the molecular defect. The presence of very low levels of protein C/protein S in the absence of clinical manifestations and a family history cannot be considered diagnostic because physiologic plasma levels can be as low as 0.12 U/mL. Homozygous forms of ATIII (or heparin cofactor II) deficiency have

not been confirmed in newborns, but one would anticipate that affected infants might have life-threatening thromboembolic complications. Molecular diagnosis is available for identified families (see Chapter 32).

Initial Treatment. The diagnosis of homozygous protein C/protein S deficiency is usually unanticipated and made at the time of clinical evaluation. Although numerous forms of initial therapy have been used, 10 to 20 mL/kg of FFP every 6 to 12 hours is usually the form of therapy that is most readily available.[462] Plasma levels of protein C achieved with these doses of FFP vary from 15% to 32% 30 minutes after the infusion and from 4% to 10% at 12 hours.[447] Plasma levels of protein S (which was entirely bound to C4b) were 23% at 2 hours and 14% at 24 hours, with an approximate half-life of 36 hours.[463]

A protein C concentrate (Ceprotin) has recently received FDA approval for use in treating congenital protein C deficiency. Recommended initial doses for acute thrombotic episodes and short-term prophylaxis in patients with severe protein C deficiency are 100 to 120 IU/kg in neonates, with subsequent doses of 60 to 80 IU/kg every 6 hours and maintenance doses of 45 to 60 IU/kg thereafter every 6 to 12 hours. However, dosing should be adjusted to maintain peak protein C activity of 100%. After resolution of the acute event, the patient should continue on a dose to maintain the trough protein C activity level above 25% for the duration of treatment. Replacement therapy should be continued until all the clinical lesions resolve, which usually takes place at 6 to 8 weeks. In addition to the clinical course, plasma D-dimer concentrations may be useful for monitoring the effectiveness of protein C replacement.[26]

Long-Term Therapy. Modalities used for the long-term management of infants with homozygous protein C/protein S deficiency include oral anticoagulation therapy, replacement therapy with either FFP or protein C concentrate, or liver transplantation.[455] When oral anticoagulation therapy is initiated, replacement therapy should be continued until the international normalized ratio (INR) is at a therapeutic value so that skin necrosis can be avoided. The therapeutic range for the INR can be individualized to some extent but is usually between 2.5 and 4.5. Risks associated with oral anticoagulation therapy include bleeding with high INR values and recurrent purpuric lesions with low INR values. Frequent monitoring of INR values is required if these complications are to be avoided. Bone development should also be monitored because the long-term effect of warfarin use on the bones of young infants is unknown. Long-term use of LMWH could be considered, but it also has the potential for osteopenia. Moreover, it is expensive and requires twice-daily subcutaneous injections.

Heterozygous Prothrombotic Disorders

Thromboembolic events related to heterozygous genetic prothrombotic disorders rarely occur in infants. When they do, a secondary, acquired insult is usually present. The few case reports in the literature describe a diversity of clinical manifestations that usually reflect the site of the thrombus. Purpura fulminans did not occur in any case.[464-470]

Treatment. Treatment consists of supportive therapy alone, anticoagulation with heparin, thrombolytic therapy, and replacement with specific factor concentrates.[471-473] Removal or treatment of the secondary acquired insult is important. For ATIII deficiency, ATIII concentrates were administered to four infants as either boluses or continuous infusions. Boluses of 52 and 104 U/kg of ATIII concentrate increased ATIII levels from 0.10 U/mL to 0.75 and 1.48 U/mL, respectively, at 1 hour.[473] At 24 hours, levels of ATIII had decreased to approximately 0.20 U/mL. A continuous infusion of ATIII concentrate at a rate of 2.1 U/kg/hr maintained a plasma level of 0.40 to 0.50 U/mL.

Acquired Prothrombotic Disorders

Symptomatic secondary thromboembolic complications occur more frequently in sick newborns than in children of any other age, with an incidence of approximately 2.4 per 1000 hospital admissions to the NICU.[474] Intravascular catheters are responsible for more than 80% of venous and 90% of arterial thrombotic complications.[474] Their contribution to thrombosis is probably multifactorial, including the presence of a foreign surface, endothelial cell damage, impairment of flow, and infusion of noxious substances. Renal vein thrombosis (RVT) is the most common form of non–catheter-related thrombosis. Other risk factors include increased blood viscosity because of a high hematocrit, poor deformability of physiologically large red cells, dehydration, and activation of the coagulation and fibrinolytic systems secondary to a variety of medical problems. Very low ATIII levels have been observed in preterm infants with RDS, which probably contributed to their increased risk for thromboembolic complications.[29]

Venous Catheter–Related Thrombosis

The use of umbilical venous catheters and other forms of central venous catheters is associated with a significant risk for thrombosis.[474-476] According to autopsy studies, 20% to 65% of infants who die with an umbilical venous catheter in place have an associated thrombus. Appropriate placement of umbilical venous catheters is critical to prevention of serious organ impairment, such as portal vein thrombosis and hepatic necrosis. Long-term sequelae of umbilical venous catheters have not been rigorously studied but include portal vein thrombosis with portal hypertension, splenomegaly, gastric and esophageal varices, and hypertension. Until recently, pulmonary embolism was rarely diagnosed in sick newborns because its clinical signs were easily confused with those of RDS. The use of ventilation lung scintigraphy in newborns has facilitated the diagnosis of pulmonary embolism.[477]

Arterial Catheter–Related Thrombosis

Seriously ill infants require indwelling arterial catheters, which are associated with a risk of thrombosis regardless of the vessel or catheter type chosen.[478-482] Catheter-related thrombosis not only occludes catheters but may also obstruct major arterial vessels. In a retrospective examination of approximately 4000 infants who underwent umbilical artery catheterization, 1% had severe symptomatic vessel obstruction. Asymptomatic catheter-related thrombi occur more frequently, as evidenced by postmortem (3% to 59% of cases) and angiographic (10% to 90% of cases) studies.

Diagnosis. Contrast-enhanced angiography is considered the reference test for the diagnosis of arterial thrombosis. Noninvasive techniques such as Doppler ultrasound offer advantages, but their sensitivity and specificity are unknown. A review of 20 neonates with aortic thrombosis treated in one institution revealed that ultrasound failed to identify thrombi in 4 patients, 3 of whom had complete aortic obstruction.[483]

Sequelae. The sequelae of catheter-related thrombosis can be immediate or long term. Acute symptoms reflect the location of the catheter and include renal hypertension, intestinal necrosis, and peripheral gangrene.[484] The long-term side effects of symptomatic and asymptomatic thrombosis of major vessels have not been studied but are probably significant.

Prophylaxis with Heparin. A low-dose continuous heparin infusion (3 to 5 U/hr) is commonly used to maintain catheter patency. The effectiveness of heparin was assessed in seven studies focusing on three outcomes: patency, local thrombus, and ICH.[479-482,485,486] Patency, which is probably linked to the presence of local thrombus, is prolonged with the use of low-dose heparin. Local thrombosis was assessed by ultrasound in two randomized studies. The evidence linking low-dose heparin prophylaxis to ICH in newborns is weak.[482,487] One study had a sample size of only 15 per arm,[482] and another case-control study had a broad odds ratio that ranged from 1.4 to 11.0.[487] Thus, the magnitude of risk for ICH is uncertain. Heparin is used in at least three quarters of American nurseries.[484]

Renal Vein Thrombosis

RVT occurs primarily in newborns and young infants. Approximately 80% of cases occur within the first month and usually within the first week of life. In some infants RVT develops in utero. The incidence in male and female infants is similar, and the left and right sides are affected equally. Bilateral RVT occurs in 24% of pediatric patients.

Clinical Findings and Etiology

The initial symptoms and clinical findings are different in neonates and older patients and are influenced by the extent and rapidity of thrombus formation. Neonates generally have a flank mass, hematuria, proteinuria, thrombocytopenia, and impaired function of the involved kidney. Clinical findings suggesting acute inferior vena cava thrombosis include cold, cyanotic, and edematous lower extremities. RVT results from pathologic states characterized by reduced renal blood flow, increased blood viscosity, hyperosmolality, or hypercoagulability.

Coagulation Abnormalities

The most common coagulation abnormality in RVT is thrombocytopenia, which is usually mild, with average values of 100×10^9/L. Thus, RVT should be considered in the differential diagnosis of thrombocytopenia in neonates. Coagulation may be prolonged and levels of fibrinogen-fibrin degradation products increased. Children with RVT are often evaluated for a congenital prothrombotic disorder, although the significance of thrombophilic markers in this disease is unknown.[466]

Diagnosis and Treatment

Ultrasound is the radiographic test of choice for the diagnosis of RVT because of ease of testing and sensitivity to an enlarged kidney. Treatment options include supportive care, anticoagulation, and thrombolytic therapy. In the 1990s, there has been uniform agreement that aggressive supportive care is indicated. However, the use of anticoagulants and thrombolytic agents is controversial. One approach is to use supportive care for unilateral RVT in the absence of uremia and extension into the inferior vena cava. Heparin therapy should be considered for unilateral RVT that extends into the inferior vena cava or for bilateral RVT because of the risk of pulmonary embolism and complete renal failure. Thrombolytic therapy should be considered in the presence of bilateral RVT and renal failure. Thrombectomy, though a common therapeutic choice in the past, is rarely indicated.

Outcome

RVT has changed from a frequently lethal complication to one that more than 85% of children survive. Unfortunately, no recent studies have assessed long-term morbidity, such as hypertension and renal atrophy.

Spontaneous Venous and Arterial Thrombosis

Spontaneous venous thrombosis occurs in the adrenal veins, inferior vena cava, portal vein, hepatic veins, and venous system of the brain.[484,488] Spontaneous occlusion of arterial vessels in the absence of a catheter is unusual, but it can occur in ill infants. As in catheter-related thrombosis, the clinical findings reflect the vessel that is occluded. Complete occlusion of a vessel can lead to gangrene and loss of the affected limb or to ischemic organ damage. The presence of systemic hypertension in newborns is frequently related to renal artery thrombosis, even in the absence of a catheter.

Anticoagulation Therapy in Newborns

Heparin Therapy in Newborns

The lack of consensus for prophylaxis and treatment of thromboembolic complications in newborns reflects the lack of controlled trials in this area. Recommendations for adult patients provide useful guidelines but probably do not reflect the optimal therapy for newborns. Current therapeutic options include supportive care alone, anticoagulant therapy, thrombolytic therapy, and thrombectomy. For most infants in whom thrombotic complications develop, the cause of thrombosis is a catheter-related thrombus that does not produce clinical symptoms. In most nurseries, catheters are not routinely checked for associated thrombosis; thus, by exclusion, most infants with clinically silent thrombi receive supportive care alone.

Age-Dependent Features. Indications for heparin therapy in newborns remain unclear. Although the benefits of heparin therapy in newborns are probably similar to those in adults, the relative risk that major bleeding will occur with its use may be increased. Infants with thromboses that are extending or infants whose organ or limb viability is threatened by thrombosis may benefit from heparin therapy.

Heparin's anticoagulant activities are mediated primarily through acceleration of inhibition of thrombin and factor Xa by ATIII. Although dosing for heparin therapy in newborns differs from that in adults, optimal dosing cannot be predicted. Several observations suggest that the heparin requirements of neonates are decreased in comparison to those of adults. First, the capacity of plasma from healthy newborns to generate thrombin is both delayed and decreased in comparison to that of adult plasma, but similar to that of plasma from adults receiving therapeutic amounts of heparin.[489,490] Second, at heparin concentrations in the therapeutic range, the capacity of plasma from healthy newborns to generate thrombin is barely measurable.[491] Third, the amount of clot-bound thrombin is decreased in newborns because low plasma concentrations of prothrombin probably reduce heparin requirements.[492] Observations suggesting higher heparin requirements include the following: (1) clearance of heparin is accelerated in newborns,[29,493,494] and (2) plasma concentrations of ATIII are decreased to levels frequently less than 0.40 in premature infants, which may limit heparin's antithrombotic activities[17,19,23473,495]

Therapeutic Range and Dose. Therapeutic ranges reflect the optimal risk-benefit ratio of anticoagulant therapy with regard to recurrent thrombotic events and bleeding complications. In the absence of clinical trials in newborns, one approach is to use heparin in doses that achieve the lower therapeutic range for adults (see Chapter 32).

General guidelines for initial dosing and subsequent dose adjustment of unfractionated heparin in full-term and premature neonates have been published.[496] Average doses of heparin required in newborns are bolus doses of 50 or 100 U/kg, depending on gestational age, and average maintenance doses of 20 to 25 U/kg/hr, again depending on gestational age. Adjustments are made most reliably with heparin assays, with a target-level range of 0.30 to 0.70 U/mL. Because of the short half-life of unfractionated heparin, simple discontinuation of the infusion is typically sufficient to reverse anticoagulation in the event of hemorrhage. For more rapid reversal, protamine sulfate can be used to neutralize heparin in vivo. However, anaphylactoid reactions with hypotension and bradycardia have been associated with protamine use in children and adults, and it should therefore be used with caution.[497]

The use of LMWH offers significant therapeutic advantages over unfractionated heparin, and there is now considerable experience using these preparations in newborns.[484,496,498,499] Potential advantages include more predictable pharmacokinetics, the need for less frequent monitoring than with unfractionated heparin, ease of administration, decreased bleeding, and possibly a lower incidence of heparin-induced thrombocytopenia. Full-term and moderately preterm (28 to 36 week' EGA) infants metabolize heparin at considerably faster rates than older children and adults do and typically require higher doses to maintain the same levels. Very premature infants (<28 weeks) have similar pharmacokinetics for heparin as older children and adults do. General guidelines for initial therapeutic dosing and subsequent sliding-scale dose adjustments of LMWH in neonates of different gestational age have been published.[496] Levels should be monitored with anti-Xa heparin assays on samples drawn via fresh venipuncture 4 hours after the subcutaneous dose is given to achieve levels of 0.5 to 1.0 U/mL for full therapeutic dosing. Levels should be checked every two to four doses for the first week of therapy, then once a week for a month, and then monthly if stable.[496] Infants who do not respond appropriately to heparin therapy, despite adequate levels, may benefit from infusions of ATIII concentrate, even if the levels are close to the normal physiologic range for their age.[496] Intramuscular and arterial puncture and the use of antiplatelet medications should be avoided in newborns receiving heparin therapy, and platelet counts should be monitored periodically.

Like unfractionated heparin, LMWH can be reversed with the use of protamine, with dosing dependent on the last dose of LMWH given.[500] As discussed earlier, protamine must be given slowly, and caution must be exercised to avoid potential hypersensitivity reactions. Repeat doses of protamine may be required to reverse the effects of LMWH because of the relatively shorter half-life of protamine than LMWH. Protocols for reversal of LMWH with protamine in adolescents and adults have been published, and case reports exist for its use in neonates.[501,502]

Close monitoring of the thrombus with objective means such as ultrasound is recommended. The duration of heparin therapy required for the treatment of thromboembolic complications is uncertain. One approach is to treat the infant for 10 to 14 days with heparin alone. If there is subsequent extension of the thrombus in the absence of anticoagulation therapy, treatment with oral anticoagulants may be considered.

Adverse Effects. There are two clinically important adverse effects of heparin therapy: hemorrhage, including ICH, and heparin-induced thrombocytopenia.[503,504] In the absence of an alternative cause, thrombocytopenic patients should be evaluated for heparin-induced thrombocytopenia and treated with alternative therapies.

Oral Anticoagulant Therapy in Newborns

Age-Dependent Features. Oral anticoagulation therapy in children is discussed in Chapter 32, and only specific issues related to newborns are discussed in this section. The oral anticoagulant warfarin works by reducing functional plasma levels of the VK-dependent proteins. At birth, levels of the VK-dependent proteins are similar to those found in adults receiving therapeutic amounts of warfarin for deep venous thrombosis/pulmonary embolism.[17,19,23,82,491,505,506] In addition, stores of VK are low, and a small number of newborns have evidence of functional VK deficiency.[55] These features significantly increase the sensitivity of newborns to warfarin and potentially their risk for bleeding. Oral anticoagulant therapy should be avoided when possible during the first month of life.[55,507] Unfortunately, a small number of infants require extended anticoagulation therapy, and heparin cannot be used for extended periods because of the risk for osteopenia.

Indications, Therapeutic Range, and Dose. The optimal therapeutic INR range is unknown for newborns and almost certainly differs from that for adults. Recommendations for oral anticoagulation therapy in adults can be used as a guideline for determining the lowest effective dose, which to some extent can be individualized. Maintenance doses for warfarin are age dependent, with infants requiring the highest doses (0.32 mg/kg).

Adverse Effects. Close monitoring of oral anticoagulation in newborns is required if both hemorrhagic and recurrent thrombotic complications are to be prevented. Unfortunately, these infants often have poor venous access, as well as complicated medical problems. Weekly or biweekly INR measurements and frequent dose adjustments are required.[508] Doses are affected by diet, medications, and intercurrent illnesses. Breast-fed infants are very sensitive to oral anticoagulants because of low concentrations of VK in breast milk.[62,44,50,277,509] Daily supplementation of breast-fed infants with small amounts of commercial formulas reduces their sensitivity to oral anticoagulants and the risk of sudden increases in INR values. In contrast to breast-fed infants, infants receiving commercial formulas or total parenteral nutrition are resistant to oral anticoagulants because of VK supplementation.[277,510] Reducing or removing VK supplementation in infants receiving total parenteral nutrition significantly decreases the dose requirements. Most infants requiring oral anticoagulants also require other medications on an intermittent and long-term basis. The effects of dosage changes and the introduction of new medications must be closely supervised.

Antiplatelet Agents in Newborns

Antiplatelet agents are rarely used in newborns for antithrombotic therapy. The hyporeactivity of neonatal platelets and the paradoxically short bleeding time suggest that optimal use of antiplatelet agents differs in newborns and adults. Aspirin is the most commonly used antiplatelet agent. The empirical use of low doses of 1 to 5 mg/kg/day has been proposed as adjuvant therapy for patients with Blalock-Taussig shunts, some endovascular stents, and some thrombotic cerebrovascular events.[511] Use of the antiplatelet agent clopidogrel (Plavix) in infants as young as 6 weeks of age has been reported in a small retrospective series.[512] The agent appears to be well tolerated at doses of 1 mg/kg/day.

Thrombolytic Therapy in Newborns

Age-Dependent Features. The activity of thrombolytic agents depends on endogenous concentrations of plasminogen, which are physiologically decreased at birth.[513] Low plasminogen levels result in impairment of the capacity to generate plasmin[63] and a decrease in the capacity to thrombolyse fibrin clots.[513] In addition, fetal glycoforms of plasminogen are less efficiently converted to plasmin by tPA than adult plasminogen is.[66] Thus, neonates have an overall reduced capacity to respond to tPA in comparison to adults. If an infant's condition does not respond to thrombolytic therapy, replacement of plasminogen should be considered.

Indications, Therapeutic Range, and Dose. Infants in whom serious thrombotic complications develop, as defined by organ or limb impairment, may benefit from thrombolytic therapy. The clinical objective is removal of the clot as quickly and safely as possible. Surgical removal of a clot in a major vessel can be curative; however, it is technically difficult and poses a considerable life-threatening risk to infants, who are often premature. In the absence of contraindications, the use of thrombolytic agents in these infants is a preferred approach (see Chapter 32).

CONCLUSIONS

Over the past several decades, the developmental timing and functional maturation of the human hemostatic system have been examined in great detail. These studies show critically important differences in many components of the hemostatic system in premature and full-term newborns versus older children and adults. The reason for this unique physiologic state in the fetus and neonate is not clear but appears to be appropriately balanced for healthy full-term infants. Of clinical importance has been the determination of gestational and postnatal age-specific activity ranges of factors involved in hemostasis, which has allowed appropriate interpretation of clinical data. As newer diagnostic tests and treatments are introduced for older children and adults, it will be critical to carefully evaluate them separately in the context of neonates, both premature and full-term, given their unique physiologic state.

Acknowledgment

The author would like to acknowledge Dr. Paul Monagle and the late Dr. Maureen Andrew for their chapter on developmental hemostasis contained in previous editions of this textbook. Their work formed the basis for the current chapter. The author would also like to thank Dr. Ellis Neufeld and Dr. Marilyn Manco-Johnson for helpful advice.

REFERENCES

1. Williams MD, Chalmers EA, Gibson BE. The investigation and management of neonatal haemostasis and thrombosis. Br J Haematol. 2002;119:295-309.
2. Forestier F, Daffos F, Galacteros F, et al. Hematological values of 163 normal fetuses between 18 and 30 weeks of gestation. Pediatr Res. 1986;20:342-346.
3. Cade JF, Hirsh J, Martin M. Placental barrier to coagulation factors: its relevance to the coagulation defect at birth and to haemorrhage in the newborn. BMJ. 1969;2:281-283.
4. Andrew M, O'Brodovich H, Mitchell L. Fetal lamb coagulation system during normal birth. Am J Hematol. 1988;28:116-118.
5. Kisker CT, Robillard JE, Clarke WR. Development of blood coagulation—a fetal lamb model. Pediatr Res. 1981;15:1045-1050.
6. Holmberg L, Henriksson P, Ekelund H, Astedt B. Coagulation in the human fetus. Comparison with term newborn infants. J Pediatr. 1974;85:860-864.
7. Jensen AH, Josso F, Zamet P, et al. Evolution of blood clotting factor levels in premature infants during the first 10 days of life: a study of 96 cases with comparison between clinical status and blood clotting factor levels. Pediatr Res. 1973;7:638-644.
8. Mibashan RS, Rodeck CH, Thumpston JK, et al. Plasma assay of fetal factors VIIIC and IX for prenatal diagnosis of haemophilia. Lancet. 1979;1:1309-1311.

9. Forestier F, Cox WL, Daffos F, Rainaut M. The assessment of fetal blood samples. Am J Obstet Gynecol. 1988;158:1184-1188.

10. Forestier F, Daffos F, Sole Y, Rainaut M. Prenatal diagnosis of hemophilia by fetal blood sampling under ultrasound guidance. Haemostasis. 1986;16:346-351.

11. Forestier F, Daffos F, Rainaut M, et al. Vitamin K dependent proteins in fetal hemostasis at mid trimester of pregnancy. Thromb Haemost. 1985;53:401-403.

12. Barnard DR, Simmons MA, Hathaway WE. Coagulation studies in extremely premature infants. Pediatr Res. 1979;13:1330-1335.

13. Toulon P, Rainaut M, Aiach M, et al. Antithrombin III (ATIII) and heparin cofactor II (HCII) in normal human fetuses (21st-27th week). Thromb Haemost. 1986; 56:237.

14. Nossel HL, Lanzkowsky P, Levy S, et al. A study of coagulation factor levels in women during labour and in their newborn infants. Thromb Diath Haemorrh. 1966;16:185-197.

15. Hassan HJ, Leonardi A, Chelucci C, et al. Blood coagulation factors in human embryonic-fetal development: preferential expression of the FVII/tissue factor pathway. Blood. 1990;76:1158-1164.

16. Reverdiau-Moalic P, Delahousse B, Body G, et al. Evolution of blood coagulation activators and inhibitors in the healthy human fetus. Blood. 1996;88:900-906.

17. Andrew M, Paes B, Milner R, et al. Development of the human coagulation system in the full-term infant. Blood. 1987;70:165-172.

18. Monagle P, Barnes C, Ignjatovic V, et al. Developmental haemostasis. Impact for clinical haemostasis laboratories. Thromb Haemost. 2006;95:362-372.

19. Andrew M, Paes B, Milner R, et al. Development of the human coagulation system in the healthy premature infant. Blood. 1988;72:1651-1657.

20. Andrew M, Vegh P, Johnston M, et al. Maturation of the hemostatic system during childhood. Blood. 1992;80:1998-2005.

21. Kisker CT, Bohlken D, Perlman S. Regulatory mechanisms controlling prothrombin and the development of blood coagulation factors during gestation. In Suzuki S, Hathaway WE, Bonnar J, Sutor AH (eds). Perinatal Thrombosis-Hemostasis. Tokyo, Pringer Verlag, 1991, p 125.

22. Manco-Johnson MJ. Development of hemostasis in the fetus. Thromb Res. 2005;115(Suppl 1):55-63.

23. Andrew M, Paes B, Johnston M. Development of the hemostatic system in the neonate and young infant. Am J Pediatr Hematol Oncol. 1990;12:95-104.

24. Greffe BS, Marlar RA, Manco-Johnson MJ. Neonatal protein C: molecular composition and distribution in normal term infants. Thromb Res. 1989;56:91-98.

25. Manco-Johnson MJ, Spedale S, Peters M, et al. Identification of a unique form of protein C in the ovine fetus: developmentally linked transition to the adult form. Pediatr Res. 1995;37:365-372.

26. Reverdiau-Moalic P, Gruel Y, Delahousse B, et al. Comparative study of the fibrinolytic system in human fetuses and in pregnant women. Thromb Res. 1991;61:489-499.

27. Schwarz HP, Muntean W, Watzke H, et al. Low total protein S antigen but high protein S activity due to decreased C4b-binding protein in neonates. Blood. 1988; 71:562-565.

28. Cvirn G, Gallistl S, Koestenberger M, et al. Alpha 2-macroglobulin enhances prothrombin activation and thrombin potential by inhibiting the anticoagulant protein C/protein S system in cord and adult plasma. Thromb Res. 2002;105:433-439.

29. Manco-Johnson MJ. Neonatal antithrombin III deficiency. Am J Med. 1989;87:49S-52S.

30. Peters M, Jansen E, ten Cate JW, et al. Neonatal antithrombin III. Br J Haematol. 1984;58:579-587.

31. De Stefano V, Leone G, De Carolis MP, et al. Antithrombin III in full-term and pre-term newborn infants: three cases of neonatal diagnosis of AT III congenital defect. Thromb Haemost. 1987;57:329-331.

32. Andrew M, Massicotte-Nolan PM, Karpatkin M. Plasma protease inhibitors in premature infants: influence of gestational age, postnatal age, and health status. Proc Soc Exp Biol Med. 1983;173:495-500.

33. Hathaway WE, Neumann LL, Borden CA, Jacobson LJ. Immunologic studies of antithrombin III heparin cofactor in the newborn. Thromb Haemost. 1978;39:624-630.

34. Hathaway W, Bonnar J. Bleeding disorders in the newborn infant. In Oliver T (ed). Perinatal Coagulation Monographs in Neonatology. New York, Grune & Stratton, 1978, pp 115-169.

35. Andrew M, Massicotte-Nolan P, Mitchell L, Cassidy K. Dysfunctional antithrombin III in sick premature infants. Pediatr Res. 1985;19:237-239.

36. McDonald MM, Johnson ML, Rumack CM, et al. Role of coagulopathy in newborn intracranial hemorrhage. Pediatrics. 1984;74:26-31.

37. Peters M, Ten Cate JW, Breederveld C, et al. Low antithrombin III levels in neonates with idiopathic respiratory distress syndrome: poor prognosis. Pediatr Res. 1984; 18:273-276.

38. Andersson TR, Bangstad H, Larsen ML. Heparin cofactor II, antithrombin and protein C in plasma from term and preterm infants. Acta Paediatr Scand. 1988;77:485-488.

39. Delorme MA, Xu L, Berry L, et al. Anticoagulant dermatan sulfate proteoglycan (decorin) in the term human placenta. Thromb Res. 1998;90:147-153.

40. Schmidt B, Mitchell L, Ofosu FA, Andrew M. Alpha-2-macroglobulin is an important progressive inhibitor of thrombin in neonatal and infant plasma. Thromb Haemost. 1989;62:1074-1077.

41. Levine JJ, Udall JN Jr, Evernden BA, et al. Elevated levels of alpha 2-macroglobulin–protease complexes in infants. Biol Neonate. 1987;51:149-155.

42. Cvirn G, Gallistl S, Leschnik B, Muntean W. Low tissue factor pathway inhibitor (TFPI) together with low antithrombin allows sufficient thrombin generation in neonates. J Thromb Haemost. 2003;1:263-268.

43. Furie B, Bouchard BA, Furie BC. Vitamin K–dependent biosynthesis of gamma-carboxyglutamic acid. Blood. 1999;93:1798-1808.

44. Shearer MJ, Rahim S, Barkhan P, Stimmler L. Plasma vitamin K_1 in mothers and their newborn babies. Lancet. 1982;2:460-463.

45. Mandelbrot L, Guillaumont M, Leclercq M, et al. Placental transfer of vitamin K_1 and its implications in fetal hemostasis. Thromb Haemost. 1988;60:39-43.

46. von Kries R, Hanawa Y. Neonatal vitamin K prophylaxis. Report of Scientific and Standardization Subcommittee on Perinatal Haemostasis. Thromb Haemost. 1993; 69:293-295.

47. Hiraike H, Kimura M, Itokawa Y. Determination of K vitamins (phylloquinone and menaquinones) in umbilical cord plasma by a platinum-reduction column. J Chromatogr. 1988;430:143-148.

48. Hamulyak K, de Boer-van den Berg MA, Thijssen HH, et al. The placental transport of [^{3}H]vitamin K_1 in rats. Br J Haematol. 1987;65:335-338.

49. Hiraike H, Kimura M, Itokawa Y. Distribution of K vitamins (phylloquinone and menaquinones) in human placenta and maternal and umbilical cord plasma. Am J Obstet Gynecol. 1988;158:564-569.

50. Greer FR, Mummah-Schendel LL, Marshall S, Suttie JW. Vitamin K_1 (phylloquinone) and vitamin K_2 (menaquinone) status in newborns during the first week of life. Pediatrics. 1988;81:137-140.

51. Israels LG, Israels ED. Observations on vitamin K deficiency in the fetus and newborn: has nature made a mistake? Semin Thromb Hemost. 1995;21:357-363.

52. Israels LG, Friesen E, Jansen AH, Israels ED. Vitamin K_1 increases sister chromatid exchange in vitro in human leukocytes and in vivo in fetal sheep cells: a possible role for "vitamin K deficiency" in the fetus. Pediatr Res. 1987;22:405-408.

53. Webster WS, Vaghef H, Ryan B, et al. Measurement of DNA damage by the comet assay in rat embryos grown in media containing high concentrations of vitamin K_1. Toxicol In Vitro. 2000;14:95-99.

54. Shapiro AD, Jacobson LJ, Armon ME, et al. Vitamin K deficiency in the newborn infant: prevalence and perinatal risk factors. J Pediatr. 1986;109:675-680.

55. Bovill EG, Soll RF, Lynch M, et al. Vitamin K_1 metabolism and the production of des-carboxy prothrombin and protein C in the term and premature neonate. Blood. 1993;81:77-83.

56. Ohashi K, Nagata K, Toshima J, et al. Stimulation of sky receptor tyrosine kinase by the product of growth arrest–specific gene 6. J Biol Chem. 1995;270:22681-22684.

57. Price PA, Poser JW, Raman N. Primary structure of the gamma-carboxyglutamic acid–containing protein from bovine bone. Proc Natl Acad Sci U S A. 1976; 73:3374-3375.

58. Cornelissen M, Steegers-Theunissen R, Kollee L, et al. Increased incidence of neonatal vitamin K deficiency resulting from maternal anticonvulsant therapy. Am J Obstet Gynecol. 1993;168:923-928.

59. Cornelissen M, Steegers-Theunissen R, Kollee L, et al. Supplementation of vitamin K in pregnant women receiving anticonvulsant therapy prevents neonatal vitamin K deficiency. Am J Obstet Gynecol. 1993;168: 884-888.

60. Wong V, Cheng CH, Chan KC. Fetal and neonatal outcome of exposure to anticoagulants during pregnancy. Am J Med Genet. 1993;45:17-21.

61. Corrigan JJ Jr. Neonatal thrombosis and the thrombolytic system: pathophysiology and therapy. Am J Pediatr Hematol Oncol. 1988;10:83-91.

62. Aballi AJ, De Lamerens S. Coagulation changes in the neonatal period and in early infancy. Pediatr Clin North Am. 1962;9:785-817.

63. Corrigan JJ Jr, Sleeth JJ, Jeter M, Lox CD. Newborn's fibrinolytic mechanism: components and plasmin generation. Am J Hematol. 1989;32:273-278.

64. Kolindewala JK, Das BK, Dube RK, et al. Blood fibrinolytic activity in neonates: effect of period of gestation, birth weight, anoxia and sepsis. Indian Pediatr. 1987;24: 1029-1033.

65. Lecander I, Astedt B. Specific plasminogen activator inhibitor of placental type PAI 2 occurring in amniotic fluid and cord blood. J Lab Clin Med. 1987;110: 602-605.

66. Edelberg JM, Enghild JJ, Pizzo SV, Gonzalez-Gronow M. Neonatal plasminogen displays altered cell surface binding and activation kinetics. Correlation with increased glycosylation of the protein. J Clin Invest. 1990;86:107-112.

67. Ries M. Molecular and functional properties of fetal plasminogen and its possible influence on clot lysis in the neonatal period. Semin Thromb Hemost. 1997;23: 247-252.

68. Ries M, Easton RL, Longstaff C, et al. Differences between neonates and adults in carbohydrate sequences and reaction kinetics of plasmin and alpha$_2$-antiplasmin. Thromb Res. 2002;105:247-256.

69. Travis PA, Bovill EG, Hamill B, Tindle BH. Detection of factor VIII von Willebrand factor in endothelial cells in first-trimester fetuses. Arch Pathol Lab Med. 1988;112: 40-42.

70. Tuddenham EG, Shearn AM, Peake IR, et al. Tissue localization and synthesis of factor-VIII–related antigen in the human foetus. Br J Haematol. 1974;26:669-677.

71. Moake JL, Turner NA, Stathopoulos NA, et al. Involvement of large plasma von Willebrand factor (vWF) multimers and unusually large vWF forms derived from endothelial cells in shear stress–induced platelet aggregation. J Clin Invest. 1986;78:1456-1461.

72. Sporn LA, Marder VJ, Wagner DD. von Willebrand factor released from Weibel-Palade bodies binds more avidly to extracellular matrix than that secreted constitutively. Blood. 1987;69:1531-1534.

73. Weinstein MJ, Blanchard R, Moake JL, et al. Fetal and neonatal von Willebrand factor (vWF) is unusually large and similar to the vWF in patients with thrombotic thrombocytopenic purpura. Br J Haematol. 1989;72:68-72.

74. Katz JA, Moake JL, McPherson PD, et al. Relationship between human development and disappearance of unusually large von Willebrand factor multimers from plasma. Blood. 1989;73:1851-1858.

75. Takahashi Y, Kawaguchi C, Hanesaka Y, et al. Plasma von Willebrand factor–cleaving protease is low in newborns [abstract]. Thromb Haemost. 2001;86(Suppl):P285.

76. Schmugge M, Dunn MS, Amankwah KS, et al. The activity of the von Willebrand factor cleaving protease ADAMTS-13 in newborn infants. J Thromb Haemost. 2004;2:228-233.

77. Rehak T, Cvirn G, Gallistl S, et al. Increased shear stress– and ristocetin-induced binding of von Willebrand factor to platelets in cord compared with adult plasma. Thromb Haemost. 2004;92:682-687.

78. Bleyer WA, Hakami N, Shepard TH. The development of hemostasis in the human fetus and newborn infant. J Pediatr. 1971;79:838-853.

79. Saxonhouse MA, Christensen RD, Walker DM, et al. The concentration of circulating megakaryocyte progenitors in

preterm neonates is a function of post-conceptional age. Early Hum Dev. 2004;78:119-124.

80. Slayton WB, Wainman DA, Li XM, et al. Developmental differences in megakaryocyte maturation are determined by the microenvironment. Stem Cells. 2005;23: 1400-1408.

81. Li Z, Godinho FJ, Klusmann JH, et al. Developmental stage-selective effect of somatically mutated leukemogenic transcription factor GATA1. Nat Genet. 2005;37:613-619.

82. Hathaway W, Bonnar J. Hemostatic Disorders of the Pregnant Woman and Newborn Infant. New York, Elsevier, 1987.

83. Andrew M, Kelton J. Neonatal thrombocytopenia. Clin Perinatol. 1984;11:359-391.

84. Pearson HA, McIntosh S. Neonatal thrombocytopenia. Clin Haematol. 1978;7:111-122.

85. Gill FM. Thrombocytopenia in the newborn. Semin Perinatol. 1983;7:201-212.

86. Beverley DW, Inwood MJ, Chance GW, et al. 'Normal' haemostasis parameters: a study in a well-defined inborn population of preterm infants. Early Hum Dev. 1984;9: 249-257.

87. Castle V, Andrew M, Kelton J, et al. Frequency and mechanism of neonatal thrombocytopenia. J Pediatr. 1986;108: 749-755.

88. Mehta P, Vasa R, Neumann L, Karpatkin M. Thrombocytopenia in the high-risk infant. J Pediatr. 1980;97: 791-794.

89. Kipper SL, Sieger L. Whole blood platelet volumes in newborn infants. J Pediatr. 1982;101:763-766.

90. Arad ID, Alpan G, Sznajderman SD, Eldor A. The mean platelet volume (MPV) in the neonatal period. Am J Perinatol. 1986;3:1-3.

91. Xu MJ, Matsuoka S, Yang FC, et al. Evidence for the presence of murine primitive megakaryocytopoiesis in the early yolk sac. Blood. 2001;97:2016-2022.

92. Tober J, Koniski A, McGrath KE, et al. The megakaryocyte lineage originates from hemangioblast precursors and is an integral component both of primitive and of definitive hematopoiesis. Blood. 2007;109:1433-1441.

93. Castle V, Coates G, Mitchell LG, et al. The effect of hypoxia on platelet survival and site of sequestration in the newborn rabbit. Thromb Haemost. 1988;59: 45-48.

94. Jilma-Stohlawetz P, Homoncik M, Jilma B, et al. High levels of reticulated platelets and thrombopoietin characterize fetal thrombopoiesis. Br J Haematol. 2001;112: 466-468.

95. Murray NA, Watts TL, Roberts IA. Endogenous thrombopoietin levels and effect of recombinant human thrombopoietin on megakaryocyte precursors in term and preterm babies. Pediatr Res. 1998;43:148-151.

96. Ts'ao CH, Green D, Schultz K. Function and ultrastructure of platelets of neonates: enhanced ristocetin aggregation of neonatal platelets. Br J Haematol. 1976;32: 225-233.

97. Rajasekhar D, Kestin AS, Bednarek FJ, et al. Neonatal platelets are less reactive than adult platelets to physiological agonists in whole blood. Thromb Haemost. 1994; 72:957-963.

98. Hurtaud-Roux M, Hezard N, Lefranc V, et al. Quantification of the major integrins and P-selectin in neonatal

platelets by flow cytometry [abstract]. Thromb Haemost. 2001;86(Suppl):P284.

99. Gruel Y, Boizard B, Daffos F, et al. Determination of platelet antigens and glycoproteins in the human fetus. Blood. 1986;68:488-492.

100. Jones CR, McCabe R, Hamilton CA, Reid JL. Maternal and fetal platelet responses and adrenoceptor binding characteristics. Thromb Haemost. 1985;53:95-98.

101. Stuart MJ, Dusse J, Clark DA, Walenga RW. Differences in thromboxane production between neonatal and adult platelets in response to arachidonic acid and epinephrine. Pediatr Res. 1984;18:823-826.

102. Barradas MA, Mikhailidis DP, Imoedemhe DA, et al. An investigation of maternal and neonatal platelet function. Biol Res Pregnancy Perinatol. 1986;7:60-65.

103. Israels SJ, Daniels M, McMillan EM. Deficient collagen-induced activation in the newborn platelet. Pediatr Res. 1990;27:337-343.

104. Gader AM, Bahakim H, Jabbar FA, et al. Dose-response aggregometry in maternal/neonatal platelets. Thromb Haemost. 1988;60:314-318.

105. Ucar T, Gurman C, Arsan S, Kemahli S. Platelet aggregation in term and preterm newborns. Pediatr Hematol Oncol. 2005;22:139-145.

106. Mull MM, Hathaway WE. Altered platelet function in newborns. Pediatr Res. 1970;4:229-237.

107. Nicolini U, Guarneri D, Gianotti GA, et al. Maternal and fetal platelet activation in normal pregnancy. Obstet Gynecol. 1994;83:65-69.

108. Israels SJ, Cheang T, Roberston C, et al. Impaired signal transduction in neonatal platelets. Pediatr Res. 1999;45:687-691.

109. Whaun JM, Smith GR, Sochor VA. Effect of prenatal drug administration on maternal and neonatal platelet aggregation and PF4 release. Haemostasis. 1980;9:226-237.

110. Corby DG, O'Barr TP. Decreased alpha-adrenergic receptors in newborn platelets: cause of abnormal response to epinephrine. Dev Pharmacol Ther. 1981;2:215-225.

111. Hicsonmez G, Prozorova-Zamani V. Platelet aggregation in neonates with hyperbilirubinaemia. Scand J Haematol. 1980;24:67-70.

112. Alebouyeh M, Lusher JM, Ameri MR, et al. The effect of 5-hydroxytryptamine and epinephrine on newborn platelets. Eur J Pediatr. 1978;128:163-168.

113. Landolfi R, De Cristofaro R, Ciabattoni G, et al. Placental-derived PGI$_2$ inhibits cord blood platelet function. Haematologica. 1988;73:207-210.

114. Harker LA, Slichter SJ. The bleeding time as a screening test for evaluation of platelet function. N Engl J Med. 1972;287:155-159.

115. Feusner JH. Normal and abnormal bleeding times in neonates and young children utilizing a fully standardized template technic. Am J Clin Pathol. 1980;74:73-77.

116. Andrew M, Castle V, Saigal S, et al. Clinical impact of neonatal thrombocytopenia. J Pediatr. 1987;110: 457-464.

117. Suarez CR, Menendez CE, Walenga JM, Fareed J. Neonatal and maternal hemostasis: value of molecular markers in the assessment of hemostatic status. Semin Thromb Hemost. 1984;10:280-284.

118. Stuart MJ, Dusse J. In vitro comparison of the efficacy of cyclooxygenase inhibitors on the adult versus neonatal platelet. Biol Neonate. 1985;47:265-269.

119. Kaplan KL, Owen J. Plasma levels of beta-thromboglobulin and platelet factor 4 as indices of platelet activation in vivo. Blood. 1981;57:199-202.

120. Suarez CR, Gonzalez J, Menendez C, et al. Neonatal and maternal platelets: activation at time of birth. Am J Hematol. 1988;29:18-21.

121. Jacqz EM, Barrow SE, Dollery CT. Prostacyclin concentrations in cord blood and in the newborn. Pediatrics. 1985;76:954-957.

122. Kumar V, Berenson GS, Ruiz H, et al. Acid mucopolysaccharides of human aorta. 1. Variations with maturation. J Atheroscler Res. 1967;7:573-581.

123. Andrew M, Mitchell L, Berry L, et al. An anticoagulant dermatan sulfate proteoglycan circulates in the pregnant woman and her fetus. J Clin Invest. 1992;89:321-326.

124. Nitschmann E, Berry L, Bridge S, et al. Morphologic and biochemical features affecting the antithrombotic properties of the inferior vena cava of rabbit pups and adult rabbits. Pediatr Res. 1998;43:62-67.

125. Nitschmann E, Berry L, Bridge S, et al. Morphological and biochemical features affecting the antithrombotic properties of the aorta in adult rabbits and rabbit pups. Thromb Haemost. 1998;79:1034-1040.

126. Tanjung MT, Siddik HD, Hariman H, Koh SC. Coagulation and fibrinolysis in preeclampsia and neonates. Clin Appl Thromb Hemost. 2005;11:467-473.

127. Saleh AA, Bottoms SF, Welch RA, et al. Preeclampsia, delivery, and the hemostatic system. Am J Obstet Gynecol. 1987;157:331-336.

128. de Boer K, ten Cate JW, et al. Enhanced thrombin generation in normal and hypertensive pregnancy. Am J Obstet Gynecol. 1989;160:95-100.

129. Koh SC, Anandakumar C, Montan S, Ratnam SS. Plasminogen activators, plasminogen activator inhibitors and markers of intravascular coagulation in pre-eclampsia. Gynecol Obstet Invest. 1993;35:214-221.

130. Higgins JR, Walshe JJ, Darling MR, et al. Hemostasis in the uteroplacental and peripheral circulations in normotensive and pre-eclamptic pregnancies. Am J Obstet Gynecol. 1998;179:520-526.

131. Higgins JR, Bonnar J, Norris LA, et al. The effect of pre-eclampsia on coagulation and fibrinolytic activation in the neonate. Thromb Res. 2000;99:567-570.

132. Buchanan GR. Coagulation disorders in the neonate. Pediatr Clin North Am. 1986;33:203-220.

133. Montgomery RR, Marlar RA, Gill JC. Newborn haemostasis. Clin Haematol. 1985;14:443-460.

134. Gobel U, von Voss H, Petrich C, Jurgens H, Oliven A. Etiopathology and classification of acquired coagulation disorders in the newborn infant. Klin Wochenschr. 1979;57:81-86.

135. Gibson B. Neonatal haemostasis. Arch Dis Child. 1989;64:503-506.

136. Gray OP, Ackerman A, Fraser AJ. Intracranial haemorrhage and clotting defects in low-birth-weight infants. Lancet. 1968;1:545-548.

137. Chalmers EA. Neonatal coagulation problems. Arch Dis Child Fetal Neonatal Ed. 2004;89:F475-478.

138. Kulkarni R, Ponder KP, James AH, et al. Unresolved issues in diagnosis and management of inherited bleeding disorders in the perinatal period: a White Paper of the Perinatal Task Force of the Medical and Scientific Advisory Council of the National Hemophilia Foundation, USA. Haemophilia. 2006;12:205-211.

139. Girolami A, De Marco L, Dal Bo Zanon R, et al. Rarer quantitative and qualitative abnormalities of coagulation. Clin Haematol. 1985;14:385-411.

140. Silverstein A. Intracranial bleeding in hemophilia. Arch Neurol. 1960;3:141-157.

141. Yoffe G, Buchanan GR. Intracranial hemorrhage in newborn and young infants with hemophilia. J Pediatr. 1988;113:333-336.

142. Abbondanzo SL, Gootenberg JE, Lofts RS, McPherson RA. Intracranial hemorrhage in congenital deficiency of factor XIII. Am J Pediatr Hematol Oncol. 1988;10: 65-68.

143. Baehner RL, Strauss HS. Hemophilia in the first year of life. N Engl J Med. 1966;275:524-528.

144. Mariani G, Mazzucconi MG. Factor VII congenital deficiency. Clinical picture and classification of the variants. Haemostasis. 1983;13:169-177.

145. Struwe FE. Intracranial haemorrhage and occlusive hydrocephalus in hereditary bleeding disorders. Dev Med Child Neurol Suppl 1970;22(Suppl 22):165+.

146. Widdershoven J, Kollee L, van Munster P, et al. Biochemical vitamin K deficiency in early infancy: diagnostic limitation of conventional coagulation tests. Helv Paediatr Acta. 1986;41:195-201.

147. Aarts PA, Bolhuis PA, Sakariassen KS, et al. Red blood cell size is important for adherence of blood platelets to artery subendothelium. Blood. 1983;62:214-217.

148. Fernandez F, Goudable C, Sie P, et al. Low haematocrit and prolonged bleeding time in uraemic patients: effect of red cell transfusions. Br J Haematol. 1985;59:139-148.

149. Boudewijns M, Raes M, Peeters V, et al. Evaluation of platelet function on cord blood in 80 healthy term neonates using the Platelet Function Analyser (PFA-100); shorter in vitro bleeding times in neonates than adults. Eur J Pediatr. 2003;162:212-213.

150. Roschitz B, Sudi K, Kostenberger M, Muntean W. Shorter PFA-100 closure times in neonates than in adults: role of red cells, white cells, platelets and von Willebrand factor. Acta Paediatr. 2001;90:664-670.

151. Carcao MD, Blanchette VS, Dean JA, et al. The Platelet Function Analyzer (PFA-100): a novel in-vitro system for evaluation of primary haemostasis in children. Br J Haematol. 1998;101:70-73.

152. Israels SJ, Cheang T, McMillan-Ward EM, Cheang M. Evaluation of primary hemostasis in neonates with a new in vitro platelet function analyzer. J Pediatr. 2001;138: 116-119.

153. Podda GM, Bucciarelli P, Lussana F, et al. Usefulness of PFA-100 testing in the diagnostic screening of patients with suspected abnormalities of hemostasis: comparison with the bleeding time. J Thromb Haemost. 2007;5: 2393-2398.

154. Rost S, Fregin A, Ivaskevicius V, et al. Mutations in VKORC1 cause warfarin resistance and multiple coagulation factor deficiency type 2. Nature. 2004;427:537-541.

155. Zhang B, Ginsburg D. Familial multiple coagulation factor deficiencies: new biologic insight from rare genetic bleeding disorders. J Thromb Haemost. 2004;2:1564-1572.

156. Zhang B, Cunningham MA, Nichols WC, et al. Bleeding due to disruption of a cargo-specific ER-to-Golgi transport complex. Nat Genet. 2003;34:220-225.

157. Scher MS, Wright FS, Lockman LA, Thompson TR. Intraventricular hemorrhage in the full-term neonate. Arch Neurol. 1982;39:769-772.

158. Serfontein GL, Rom S, Stein S. Posterior fossa subdural hemorrhage in the newborn. Pediatrics. 1980;65:40-43.

159. Jackson JC, Blumhagen JD. Congenital hydrocephalus due to prenatal intracranial hemorrhage. Pediatrics. 1983;72:344-346.

160. Gunn TR, Mok PM, Becroft DM. Subdural hemorrhage in utero. Pediatrics. 1985;76:605-610.

161. Cartwright GW, Culbertson K, Schreiner RL, Garg BP. Changes in clinical presentation of term infants with intracranial hemorrhage. Dev Med Child Neurol. 1979; 21:730-737.

162. Chaplin ER Jr, Goldstein GW, Norman D. Neonatal seizures, intracerebral hematoma, and subarachnoid hemorrhage in full-term infants. Pediatrics. 1979;63: 812-815.

163. Palma PA, Miner ME, Morriss FH Jr, et al. Intraventricular hemorrhage in the neonate born at term. Am J Dis Child. 1979;133:941-944.

164. Guekos-Thoeni U, Boltshauser E, Willi UV. Intraventricular haemorrhage in full-term neonates. Dev Med Child Neurol. 1982;24:704-705.

165. Mackay RJ, de Crespigny LC, Murton LJ, Roy RN. Intraventricular haemorrhage in term neonates: diagnosis by ultrasound. Aust Paediatr J. 1982;18:205-207.

166. Schmidt B, Zipursky A. Disseminated intravascular coagulation masking neonatal hemophilia. J Pediatr. 1986; 109:886-888.

167. Bray GL, Luban NL. Hemophilia presenting with intracranial hemorrhage. An approach to the infant with intracranial bleeding and coagulopathy. Am J Dis Child. 1987; 141:1215-1217.

168. Smith PS. Congenital coagulation protein deficiencies in the perinatal period. Semin Perinatol. 1990;14:384-392.

169. Rohyans JA, Miser AW, Miser JS. Subgaleal hemorrhage in infants with hemophilia: report of two cases and review of the literature. Pediatrics. 1982;70:306-307.

170. Killick CJ, Barton CJ, Aslam S, Standen G. Prenatal diagnosis in factor XIII-A deficiency. Arch Dis Child Fetal Neonatal Ed. 1999;80:F238-F239.

171. Antonarakis SE, Copeland KL, Carpenter RJ Jr, et al. Prenatal diagnosis of haemophilia A by factor VIII gene analysis. Lancet. 1985;1:1407-1409.

172. Peake IR, Bowen D, Bignell P, et al. Family studies and prenatal diagnosis in severe von Willebrand disease by polymerase chain reaction amplification of a variable number tandem repeat region of the von Willebrand factor gene. Blood. 1990;76:555-561.

173. Gale RF, Hird MF, Colvin BT. Management of a premature infant with moderate haemophilia A using recombinant factor VIII. Haemophilia. 1998;4:850-853.

174. Bidlingmaier C, Bergmann F, Kurnik K. Haemophilia A in two premature infants. Eur J Pediatr. 2005;164: 70-72.

175. Brady KM, Easley RB, Tobias JD. Recombinant activated factor VII (rFVIIa) treatment in infants with hemorrhage. Paediatr Anaesth. 2006;16:1042-1046.

176. Ljung R, Lindgren AC, Petrini P, Tengborn L. Normal vaginal delivery is to be recommended for haemophilia carrier gravidae. Acta Paediatr. 1994;83:609-611.

177. Zenny JC, Chevrot A, Sultan Y, et al. [Intra-osseus hemorrhagic lesions in congenital afibrinogenemia. A new case (author's transl).] J Radiol. 1981;62:263-266.

178. Lewis JH, Spero JA, Ragni MV, Bontempo FA. Transfusion support for congenital clotting deficiencies other than haemophilia. Clin Haematol. 1984;13:119-135.

179. Manios SG, Schenck W, Kunzer W. Congenital fibrinogen deficiency. Acta Paediatr Scand. 1968;57:145-150.

180. Fried K, Kaufman S. Congenital afibrinogenemia in 10 offspring of uncle-niece marriages. Clin Genet. 1980;17: 223-227.

181. Gill FM, Shapiro SS, Schwartz E. Severe congenital hypoprothrombinemia. J Pediatr. 1978;93:264-266.

182. Viola L, Chiaretti A, Lazzareschi I, et al. [Intracranial hemorrhage in congenital factor II deficiency.] Pediatr Med Chir. 1995;17:593-594.

183. Ehrenforth S, Klarmann D, Zabel B, et al. Severe factor V deficiency presenting as subdural haematoma in the newborn. Eur J Pediatr. 1998;157:1032.

184. Kashyap R, Saxena R, Choudhry VP. Rare inherited coagulation disorders in India. Haematologia (Budap). 1996; 28:13-19.

185. Seeler RA. Parahemophilia. Factor V deficiency. Med Clin North Am. 1972;56:119-125.

186. Roberts H, Lefkowitz J. Inherited disorders of prothrombin conversion. In Colman R, Hirsh J, Marder V, et al (eds). Hemostasis and Thrombosis: Basic Principles and Clinical Practice, 5th ed. Philadelphia, JB Lippincott, 1994, pp 200-218.

187. Salooja N, Martin P, Khair K, et al. Severe factor V deficiency and neonatal intracranial haemorrhage: a case report. Haemophilia. 2000;6:44-46.

188. Matthay KK, Koerper MA, Ablin AR. Intracranial hemorrhage in congenital factor VII deficiency. J Pediatr. 1979;94:413-415.

189. Levanon M, Rimon S, Shani M, et al. Active and inactive factor VII in Dubin-Johnson syndrome with factor-VII deficiency, hereditary factor-VII deficiency and on coumadin administration. Br J Haematol. 1972;23:669-677.

190. Schubert B, Schindera, F. Congenital factor VII deficiency in a newborn [abstract]. Paper presented at the Hamophilie-Symposion, Hamburg, Germany, 1988.

191. Seligsohn U, Shani M, Ramot B, et al. Dubin-Johnson syndrome in Israel. II. Association with factor-VII deficiency. Q J Med. 1970;39:569-584.

192. Seligsohn U, Shani M, Ramot B. Gilbert syndrome and factor-VII deficiency. Lancet. 1970;1:1398.

193. Rabiner SF, Winick M, Smith CH. Congenital deficiency of factor VII associated with hemorrhagic disease of the newborn: report of a case. Pediatrics. 1960;25:101-105.

194. Ragni MV, Lewis JH, Spero JA, Hasiba U. Factor VII deficiency. Am J Hematol. 1981;10:79-88.

195. Goodnough LT, Hewitt PE, Silliman CC. Joint ASH and AABB educational session. Hematology Am Soc Hematol Educ Program. 2004, pp 457-472.

196. Wong WY, Huang WC, Miller R, et al. Clinical efficacy and recovery levels of recombinant FVIIa (NovoSeven) in the treatment of intracranial haemorrhage in severe neonatal FVII deficiency. Haemophilia. 2000;6:50-54.

197. Schulman I. Pediatric aspects of the mild hemophilias. Med Clin North Am. 1962;46:93-105.

198. Kozinn PJ, Ritz ND, Horowitz AW. Scalp hemorrhage as an emergency in the newborn. JAMA. 1965;194:567-568.

199. Kozinn PJ, Ritz ND, Moss AH, Kaufman A. Massive hemorrhage—scalps of newborn infants. Am J Dis Child. 1964;108:413-417.

200. Rosendaal FR, Smit C, Briet E. Hemophilia treatment in historical perspective: a review of medical and social developments. Ann Hematol. 1991;62:5-15.

201. Stormorken H, Hessel B, Lunde J, Holmsen IB. Severe factor VIII deficiency in a chromosomally normal female. Thromb Res. 1986;44:113-117.

202. Mannucci PM, Coppola R, Lombardi R, et al. Direct proof of extreme lyonization as a cause of low factor VIII levels in females. Thromb Haemost. 1978;39:544-545.

203. Ljung R, Petrini P, Nilsson IM. Diagnostic symptoms of severe and moderate haemophilia A and B. A survey of 140 cases. Acta Paediatr Scand. 1990;79:196-200.

204. Trotter CW, Hasegawa DK. Hemophilia B. Case study and intervention plan. J Obstet Gynecol Neonatal Nurs. 1983;12:82-85.

205. Girolami A, Molaro G, Calligaris A, De Luca G. Severe congenital factor X deficiency in 5-month-old child. Thromb Diath Haemorrh. 1970;24:175-184.

206. Machin SJ, Winter MR, Davies SC, Mackie IJ. Factor X deficiency in the neonatal period. Arch Dis Child. 1980;55:406-408.

207. de Sousa C, Clark T, Bradshaw A. Antenatally diagnosed subdural haemorrhage in congenital factor X deficiency. Arch Dis Child. 1988;63:1168-1170.

208. Sandler E, Gross S. Prevention of recurrent intracranial hemorrhage in a factor X–deficient infant. Am J Pediatr Hematol Oncol. 1992;14:163-165.

209. Ruane BJ, McCord FB. Factor X deficiency—a rare cause of scrotal haemorrhage. Ir Med J. 1990;83:163.

210. Edson JR, White JG, Krivit W. The enigma of severe factor XI deficiency without hemmorrhagic symptoms. Distinction from Hageman factor and "Fletcher factor" deficiency; family study; and problems of diagnosis. Thromb Diath Haemorrh. 1967;18:342-348.

211. Kitchens CS. Factor XI: a review of its biochemistry and deficiency. Semin Thromb Hemost. 1991;17:55-72.

212. Barozzino T, Sgro M, Toi A, et al. Fetal bilateral subdural haemorrhages. Prenatal diagnosis and spontaneous resolution by time of delivery. Prenat Diagn. 1998;18:496-503.

213. Barry A, Delage JM. Congenital deficiency of fibrin-stabilizing factor. Observation of a new case. N Engl J Med. 1965;272:943-947.

214. Fisher S, Rikover M, Naor S. Factor 13 deficiency with severe hemorrhagic diathesis. Blood. 1966;28:34-39.

215. Britten AF. Congenital deficiency of factor 13 (fibrin-stabilizing factor): Report of a case and review of the literature. Am J Med. 1967;43:751-761.

216. Ozsoylu S, Altay C, Hicsonmez G. Congenital factor 13 deficiency. Observation of two new cases in the newborn period. Am J Dis Child. 1971;122:541-543.

217. Francis J, Todd P. Congenital factor XIII deficiency in a neonate. BMJ. 1978;2:1532.

218. Merchant RH, Agarwal BR, Currimbhoy Z, et al. Congenital factor XIII deficiency. Indian Pediatr. 1992;29:831-836.

219. Seitz R, Duckert F, Lopaciuk S, et al. ETRO Working Party on Factor XIII questionnaire on congenital factor XIII deficiency in Europe: status and perspectives. Study Group. Semin Thromb Hemost. 1996;22:415-418.

220. Blanckaert D, Oueidat I, Chelala J, et al. [Congenital deficiency of fibrin stabilizing factor (factor XIII).] Pediatrie. 1993;48:451-453.

221. Daly HM, Haddon ME. Clinical experience with a pasteurised human plasma concentrate in factor XIII deficiency. Thromb Haemost. 1988;59:171-174.

222. Landman J, Creter D, Homburg R, et al. Neonatal factor XIII deficiency. Clin Pediatr (Phila). 1985;24:352-353.

223. Duckert F, Jung E, Shmerling DH. A hitherto undescribed congenital haemorrhagic diathesis probably due to fibrin stabilizing factor deficiency. Thromb Diath Haemorrh. 1960;5:179-186.

224. Solves P, Altes A, Ginovart G et al. Late hemorrhagic disease of the newborn as a cause of intracerebral bleeding. Ann Hematol. 1997;75:65-66.

225. Mammen EF. Seminars in Thrombosis and Hemostasis. Semin Thromb Hemost. 1983;9:1-72.

226. Zhang B, Ginsburg D. Familial multiple coagulation factor deficiencies. In Colman RW, Hirsh J, Marder VJ, et al. (eds). Hemostasis and Thrombosis: Basic Principles and Clinical Practice. Philadelphia, Lippincott Williams & Wilkins, 2006, pp 953-959.

227. Nichols WC, Seligsohn U, Zivelin A, et al. Mutations in the ER-Golgi intermediate compartment protein ERGIC-53 cause combined deficiency of coagulation factors V and VIII. Cell. 1998;93:61-70.

228. Townsend C. The haemorrhagic disease of the newborn. Arch Pediatr. 1894;11:559.

229. Sanford H, Gasteyer TH, Wyat L. The substances involved in the coagulation of the blood of a newborn [abstract]. Am J Dis Child. 1932;43:58.

230. Clifford S. Hemorrhagic disease of the newborn. A critical consideration. J Pediatr. 1941;18:333.

231. Dam C. Cholesterinstoffwechsel in Huhnereierin und Huhnchen. Biochemischeschr Z. 1929;215:475-492.

232. Dam H, Tage-Hansen E, Plum P. K-avitaminose hos spaeade born som aarag til hemorrhagisk diathese. Ugesk Laeger. 1939;101:896.

233. Brinkhous K, Smith HP, Warner ED. Plasma prothrombin level in normal infancy and in hemorrhagic disease of the newborn. Am J Med Sci. 1937;193:475.

234. Bruchsaler F. Vitamin K and the prenatal and postnatal prevention of hemorrhagic disease in newborn infants. J Pediatr. 1941;18:317.

235. Nygaard K. Prophylactic and curative effect of vitamin K in hemorrhagic disease of the newborn (hypothrombinemia hemorrhagica neonatorum). A preliminary report. Acta Obstet Gynecol Scand. 1939;19:361.

236. Waddell W, Guerry D. The role of vitamin K in the etiology, prevention, and treatment of hemorrhage in the newborn infant. Part II. J Pediatr. 1939;15:802.

237. Dam H, Glavind J, Larsen EH, et al. Investigations into the cause of the physiological hypoprothrombinemia in new-born children. IV. The vitamin K content of woman's milk and cow's milk. Acta Med Scand. 1942;112:211.

238. Quick A, Grossman AM. Prothrombin concentration in newborns. Proc Soc Exp Biol Med. 1939;41:227.

239. Fitzgerald J, Webster A. Effect of vitamin K administered to patients in labor. Am J Obstet Gynecol. 1940;40: 413.

240. Mull J, Bill AH, Skowronska H. Effect on the newborn of vitamin K administered to mothers in labor. J Lab Clin Med. 1941;26:1305.

241. Hellman L, Shettles LB. The prophylactic use of vitamin K in obstetrics. South Med J. 1942;35:289.

242. Kugelmass I. The management of hemorrhagic problems in infancy and childhood. JAMA. 1932;99:895.

243. Aballi A, Lopez Banus V, De Lamerens S, et al. The coagulation defect of fullterm infants. Pediatr Int. 1959;9:315.

244. Potter E. The effect on infant mortality of vitamin K administered during labor. Am J Obstet Gynecol. 1945;50:235.

245. Committee on Nutrition, American Academy of Pediatrics. Vitamin K compounds and water-soluble analogues: use in therapy and prophylaxis in pediatrics. Pediatrics. 1961;28:501-507.

246. Lucey JF, Dolan RG. Hyperbilirubinemia of newborn infants associated with the parenteral administration of a vitamin K analogue to the mothers. Pediatrics. 1959;23: 553-560.

247. Parks J, Sweet LK. Does the antenatal use of vitamin K prevent hemorrhage in the newborn infant? Am J Obstet Gynecol. 1942;44:432.

248. Waddell W, Whitehead BW. Neonatal mortality rates in infants receiving prophylactic doses of vitamin K. South Med J. 1945;38:349.

249. Malia RG, Preston FE, Mitchell VE. Evidence against vitamin K deficiency in normal neonates. Thromb Haemost. 1980;44:159-160.

250. Dyggve H. The prophylactic use of vitamin K in obstetrics. South Med J. 1942;35:289.

251. MacElfresh M. Coagulation during the neonatal period. Am J Med Sci. 1961;242:77.

252. Lawson R. Treatment of hypoprothrombinemia (hemorrhagic disease) of the newborn infant. J Pediatr. 1941;18:224.

253. Motohara K, Endo F, Matsuda I. Effect of vitamin K administration on acarboxy prothrombin (PIVKA-II) levels in newborns. Lancet. 1985;2:242-244.

254. Lane PA, Hathaway WE. Vitamin K in infancy. J Pediatr. 1985;106:351-359.

255. O'Connor ME, Livingstone DS, Hannah J, Wilkins D. Vitamin K deficiency and breast-feeding. Am J Dis Child. 1983;137:601-602.

256. Rose SJ. Neonatal haemorrhage and vitamin K. Acta Haematol. 1985;74:121.

257. Behrmann BA, Chan WK, Finer NN. Resurgence of hemorrhagic disease of the newborn: a report of three cases. CMAJ. 1985;133:884-885.

258. Tulchinsky TH, Patton MM, Randolph LA, et al. Mandating vitamin K prophylaxis for newborns in New York State. Am J Public Health. 1993;83:1166-1168.

259. Binder L. Hemorrhagic disease of the newborn: an unusual etiology of neonatal bleeding. Ann Emerg Med. 1986;15:935-938.

260. McNinch AW, Tripp JH. Haemorrhagic disease of the newborn in the British Isles: two year prospective study. BMJ. 1991;303:1105-1109.

261. von Kries R, Shearer MJ, Gobel U. Vitamin K in infancy. Eur J Pediatr. 1988;147:106-112.

262. Sutherland JM, Glueck HI, Gleser G. Hemorrhagic disease of the newborn. Breast feeding as a necessary factor in the pathogenesis. Am J Dis Child. 1967;113: 524-533.

263. Vietti TJ, Stephens JC, Bennett KR. Vitamin K-1 prophylaxis in the newborn. JAMA. 1961;176:791-793.

264. Vietti TJ, Murphy TP, James JA, Pritchard JA. Observations on the prophylactic use of vitamin K in the newborn infant. J Pediatr. 1960;56:343-346.

265. Hathaway WE, Isarangkura PB, Mahasandana C, et al. Comparison of oral and parenteral vitamin K prophylaxis for prevention of late hemorrhagic disease of the newborn. J Pediatr. 1991;119:461-464.

266. von Kries R, Gobel U. Vitamin K prophylaxis and vitamin K deficiency bleeding (VKDB) in early infancy. Acta Paediatr. 1992;81:655-657.

267. Schubiger G, Berger TM, Weber R, et al. Prevention of vitamin K deficiency bleeding with oral mixed micellar phylloquinone: results of a 6-year surveillance in Switzerland. Eur J Pediatr. 2003;162:885-888.

268. Golding J, Paterson M, Kinlen LJ. Factors associated with childhood cancer in a national cohort study. Br J Cancer. 1990;62:304-308.

269. Golding J, Greenwood R, Birmingham K, Mott M. Childhood cancer, intramuscular vitamin K, and pethidine given during labour. BMJ. 1992;305:341-346.

270. Fear NT, Roman E, Ansell P, et al. Vitamin K and childhood cancer: a report from the United Kingdom Childhood Cancer Study. Br J Cancer. 2003;89:1228-1231.

271. Brousson MA, Klein MC. Controversies surrounding the administration of vitamin K to newborns: a review. CMAJ. 1996;154:307-315.

272. Controversies concerning vitamin K and the newborn. American Academy of Pediatrics Committee on Fetus and Newborn. Pediatrics. 2003;112:191-192.

273. Lehmann J. Vitamin K as a prophylactic in 13,000 infants [abstract]. Lancet. 1944;1:493.

274. Hathaway WE. New insights on vitamin K. Hematol Oncol Clin North Am. 1987;1:367-379.

275. Hall MA, Pairaudeau P. The routine use of vitamin K in the newborn. Midwifery. 1987;3:170-177.

276. Hanawa Y, Maki M, Murata B, et al. The second nationwide survey in Japan of vitamin K deficiency in infancy. Eur J Pediatr. 1988;147:472-477.

277. Haroon Y, Shearer MJ, Rahim S, et al. The content of phylloquinone (vitamin K_1) in human milk, cows' milk and infant formula foods determined by high-performance liquid chromatography. J Nutr. 1982;112: 1105-1117.

278. von Kries R, Becker A, Gobel U. Vitamin K in the newborn: influence of nutritional factors on acarboxyprothrombin detectability and factor II and VII clotting activity. Eur J Pediatr. 1987;146:123-127.

279. Srinivasan G, Seeler RA, Tiruvury A, Pildes RS. Maternal anticonvulsant therapy and hemorrhagic disease of the newborn. Obstet Gynecol. 1982;59:250-252.

280. Mountain KR, Hirsh J, Gallus AS. Neonatal coagulation defect due to anticonvulsant drug treatment in pregnancy. Lancet. 1970;1:265-268.

281. Laosombat V. Hemorrhagic disease of the newborn after maternal anticonvulsant therapy: a case report and literature review. J Med Assoc Thai. 1988;71:643-648.

282. Martin-Bouyer G, Khanh NB, Linh PD, et al. Epidemic of haemorrhagic disease in Vietnamese infants caused by warfarin-contaminated talcs. Lancet. 1983;1:230-232.

283. Sutor AH, Dagres N, Niederhoff H. Late form of vitamin K deficiency bleeding in Germany. Klin Padiatr. 1995;207:89-97.

284. Pietersma-de Bruyn AL, van Haard PM, Beunis MH, et al. Vitamin K_1 levels and coagulation factors in healthy term newborns till 4 weeks after birth. Haemostasis. 1990;20:8-14.

285. Kelly DA, Summerfield JA. Hemostasis in liver disease. Semin Liver Dis. 1987;7:182-191.

286. Rubin MH, Weston MJ, Bullock G, et al. Abnormal platelet function and ultrastructure in fulminant hepatic failure. Q J Med. 1977;46:339-352.

287. Weston MJ, Langley PG, Rubin MH, et al. Platelet function in fulminant hepatic failure and effect of charcoal haemoperfusion. Gut. 1977;18:897-902.

288. Hope PL, Hall MA, Millward-Sadler GH, Normand IC. Alpha-1-antitrypsin deficiency presenting as a bleeding diathesis in the newborn. Arch Dis Child. 1982;57:68-70.

289. Olivera JE, Elcarte R, Erice B, et al. [Galactosemia of early diagnosis with psychomotor retardation.] An Esp Pediatr. 1986;25:267-270.

290. Di Battista C, Rossi L, Marcelli P, et al. [Hereditary tyrosinemia in an acute form: a case report (author's transl).] Pediatr Med Chir. 1981;3:101-104.

291. Dupuy JM, Frommel D, Alagille D. Severe viral hepatitis type B in infancy. Lancet. 1975;1:191-194.

292. Mindrum G, Glueck HI. Plasma prothrombin in liver disease: its clinical and prognostic significance. Ann Intern Med. 1959;50:1370-1384.

293. Aster RH. Pooling of platelets in the spleen: role in the pathogenesis of "hypersplenic" thrombocytopenia. J Clin Invest. 1966;45:645-657.

294. Blanchard RA, Furie BC, Jorgensen M, et al. Acquired vitamin K–dependent carboxylation deficiency in liver disease. N Engl J Med. 1981;305:242-248.

295. Donner M, Holmberg L, Nilsson IM. Type IIB von Willebrand's disease with probable autosomal recessive inheritance and presenting as thrombocytopenia in infancy. Br J Haematol. 1987;66:349-354.

296. Bignell P, Standen GR, Bowen DJ, et al. Rapid neonatal diagnosis of von Willebrand's disease by use of the polymerase chain reaction. Lancet. 1990;336:638-639.

297. Gazengel C, Fischer AM, Schlegel N, et al. Treatment of type III von Willebrand's disease with solvent/detergent-treated factor VIII concentrates. Nouv Rev Fr Hematol. 1988;30:225-227.

298. Pasi KJ, Williams MD, Enayat MS, Hill FG. Clinical and laboratory evaluation of the treatment of von Willebrand's disease patients with heat-treated factor VIII concentrate (BPL 8Y). Br J Haematol. 1990;75:228-233.

299. Pearson HA, Shulman NR, Marder VJ, Cone TE Jr. Isoimmune neonatal thrombocytopenic purpura. Clinical and therapeutic considerations. Blood. 1964;23:154-177.

300. Gajl-Peczalska K. Plasma protein composition of hyaline membrane in the newborn as studies by immunofluorescence. Arch Dis Child. 1964;39:226-231.

301. Austin N, Darlow BA. Transfusion-associated fall in platelet count in very low birthweight infants. Aust Paediatr J. 1988;24:354-356.

302. Lupton BA, Hill A, Whitfield MF, et al. Reduced platelet count as a risk factor for intraventricular hemorrhage. Am J Dis Child. 1988;142:1222-1224.

303. Samuels P, Main EK, Tomaski A, et al. Abnormalities in platelet antiglobulin tests in preeclamptic mothers and their neonates. Am J Obstet Gynecol. 1987;157:109-113.

304. Murray NA, Howarth LJ, McCloy MP, et al. Platelet transfusion in the management of severe thrombocytopenia in neonatal intensive care unit patients. Transfus Med. 2002;12:35-41.

305. Castle V, Coates G, Kelton JG, Andrew M. ^{111}In-oxine platelet survivals in thrombocytopenic infants. Blood. 1987;70:652-656.

306. Blanchette VS, Chen L, de Friedberg ZS, et al. Alloimmunization to the Pl[A1] platelet antigen: results of a prospective study. Br J Haematol. 1990;74:209-215.

307. Dreyfus M, Kaplan C, Verdy E, et al. Frequency of immune thrombocytopenia in newborns: a prospective study. Immune Thrombocytopenia Working Group. Blood. 1997;89:4402-4406.

308. Williamson LM, Hackett G, Rennie J, et al. The natural history of fetomaternal alloimmunization to the platelet-specific antigen HPA-1a (Pl[A1], Zw[a]) as determined by antenatal screening. Blood. 1998;92:2280-2287.

309. Mueller-Eckhardt C, Kiefel V, Grubert A, et al. 348 cases of suspected neonatal alloimmune thrombocytopenia. Lancet. 1989;1:363-366.

310. Manno CS. Management of bleeding disorders in children. Hematology Am Soc Hematol Educ Program. 2005, pp 416-422.

311. Reese J, Raghuveer TS, Dennington PM, Barfield CP. Breast feeding in neonatal alloimmune thrombocytopenia. J Paediatr Child Health. 1994;30:447-449.

312. Patrick CH, Lazarchick J. The effect of bacteremia on automated platelet measurements in neonates. Am J Clin Pathol. 1990;93:391-394.

313. Weinblatt ME, Scimeca PG, James-Herry AG, Pahwa S. Thrombocytopenia in an infant with AIDS. Am J Dis Child. 1987;141:15.

314. Ballin A, Koren G, Kohelet D, et al. Reduction of platelet counts induced by mechanical ventilation in newborn infants. J Pediatr. 1987;111:445-449.

315. Horgan MJ, Carrasco NJ, Risemberg H. The relationship of thrombocytopenia to the onset of persistent pulmonary hypertension of the newborn in the meconium aspiration syndrome. N Y State J Med. 1985;85:245-247.

316. Shim WK. Hemangiomas of infancy complicated by thrombocytopenia. Am J Surg. 1968;116:896-906.

317. Fost NC, Esterly NB. Successful treatment of juvenile hemangiomas with prednisone. J Pediatr. 1968;72:351-357.

318. Johnson DH, Vinson AM, Wirth FH, et al. Management of hepatic hemangioendotheliomas of infancy by transarterial embolization: a report of two cases. Pediatrics. 1984;73:546-549.

319. Orchard PJ, Smith CM 3rd, Woods WG, et al. Treatment of haemangioendotheliomas with alpha interferon. Lancet. 1989;2:565-567.

320. Larsen EC, Zinkham WH, Eggleston JC, Zitelli BJ. Kasabach-Merritt syndrome: therapeutic considerations. Pediatrics. 1987;79:971-980.

321. Kowalska MA, Ratajczak J, Hoxie J, et al. Megakaryocyte precursors, megakaryocytes and platelets express the HIV co-receptor CXCR4 on their surface: determination of response to stromal-derived factor-1 by megakaryocytes and platelets. Br J Haematol. 1999;104:220-229.

322. Corby DG, Schulman I. The effects of antenatal drug administration on aggregation of platelets of newborn infants. J Pediatr. 1971;79:307-313.

323. Levy G, Garrettson LK. Kinetics of salicylate elimination by newborn infants of mothers who ingested aspirin before delivery. Pediatrics. 1974;53:201-210.

324. Ylikorkala O, Makila UM, Kaapa P, Viinikka L. Maternal ingestion of acetylsalicylic acid inhibits fetal and neonatal prostacyclin and thromboxane in humans. Am J Obstet Gynecol. 1986;155:345-349.

325. Haslam RR, Ekert H, Gillam GL. Hemorrhage in a neonate possibly due to maternal ingestion of salicylate. J Pediatr. 1974;84:556-557.

326. Rossbach HC. Familial infantile myelofibrosis as an autosomal recessive disorder: preponderance among children from Saudi Arabia. Pediatr Hematol Oncol. 2006;23:453-454.

327. Sheikha A. Fatal familial infantile myelofibrosis. J Pediatr Hematol Oncol. 2004;26:164-168.

328. Massey GV, Zipursky A, Chang MN, et al. A prospective study of the natural history of transient leukemia (TL) in neonates with Down syndrome (DS): Children's Oncology Group (COG) study POG-9481. Blood. 2006;107:4606-4613.

329. Wechsler J, Greene M, McDevitt MA, et al. Acquired mutations in GATA1 in the megakaryoblastic leukemia of Down syndrome. Nat Genet. 2002;32:148-152.

330. Rainis L, Bercovich D, Strehl S, et al. Mutations in exon 2 of GATA1 are early events in megakaryocytic malignancies associated with trisomy 21. Blood. 2003;102:981-986.

331. Mundschau G, Gurbuxani S, Gamis AS, et al. Mutagenesis of GATA1 is an initiating event in Down syndrome leukemogenesis. Blood. 2003;101:4298-4300.

332. Hitzler JK, Cheung J, Li Y, et al. GATA1 mutations in transient leukemia and acute megakaryoblastic leukemia of Down syndrome. Blood. 2003;101:4301-4304.

333. Greene ME, Mundschau G, Wechsler J, et al. Mutations in GATA1 in both transient myeloproliferative disorder and acute megakaryoblastic leukemia of Down syndrome. Blood Cells Mol Dis. 2003;31:351-356.

334. Xu G, Nagano M, Kanezaki R, et al. Frequent mutations in the GATA-1 gene in the transient myeloproliferative disorder of Down syndrome. Blood. 2003;102:2960-2968.

335. Groet J, McElwaine S, Spinelli M, et al. Acquired mutations in GATA1 in neonates with Down's syndrome with transient myeloid disorder. Lancet. 2003;361:1617-1620.

336. Harigae H, Xu G, Sugawara T, et al. The GATA1 mutation in an adult patient with acute megakaryoblastic leukemia not accompanying Down syndrome. Blood. 2004;103:3242-3243.

337. Cantor AB. GATA transcription factors in hematologic disease. Int J Hematol. 2005;81:378-384.

338. Balduini CL, Cattaneo M, Fabris F, et al. Inherited thrombocytopenias: a proposed diagnostic algorithm from the Italian Gruppo di Studio delle Piastrine. Haematologica. 2003;88:582-592.

339. Bolton-Maggs PH, Chalmers EA, Collins PW, et al. A review of inherited platelet disorders with guidelines for their management on behalf of the UKHCDO. Br J Haematol. 2006;135:603-633.

340. King S, Germeshausen M, Strauss G, et al. Congenital amegakaryocytic thrombocytopenia: a retrospective clinical analysis of 20 patients. Br J Haematol. 2005;131:636-644.

341. Kimura S, Roberts AW, Metcalf D, Alexander WS. Hematopoietic stem cell deficiencies in mice lacking c-Mpl, the receptor for thrombopoietin. Proc Natl Acad Sci U S A. 1998;95:1195-1200.

342. Kaushansky K. Thrombopoietin and the hematopoietic stem cell. Ann N Y Acad Sci. 2005;1044:139-141.

343. Greenhalgh KL, Howell RT, Bottani A, et al. Thrombocytopenia–absent radius syndrome: a clinical genetic study. J Med Genet. 2002;39:876-881.

344. Klopocki E, Schulze H, Strauss G, et al. Complex inheritance pattern resembling autosomal recessive inheritance involving a microdeletion in thrombocytopenia–absent radius syndrome. Am J Hum Genet. 2007;80:232-240.

345. Ballmaier M, Schulze H, Cremer M, et al. Defective c-Mpl signaling in the syndrome of thrombocytopenia with absent radii. Stem Cells. 1998;16(Suppl 2):177-184.

346. Hall JG, Levin J, Kuhn JP, et al. Thrombocytopenia with absent radius (TAR). Medicine (Baltimore). 1969;48:411-439.

347. Hedberg VA, Lipton JM. Thrombocytopenia with absent radii. A review of 100 cases. Am J Pediatr Hematol Oncol. 1988;10:51-64.

348. Homans AC, Cohen JL, Mazur EM. Defective megakaryocytopoiesis in the syndrome of thrombocytopenia with absent radii. Br J Haematol. 1988;70:205-210.

349. Thompson AA, Nguyen LT. Amegakaryocytic thrombocytopenia and radio-ulnar synostosis are associated with HOXA11 mutation. Nat Genet. 2000;26:397-398.

350. Thompson AA, Woodruff K, Feig SA, et al. Congenital thrombocytopenia and radio-ulnar synostosis: a new familial syndrome. Br J Haematol. 2001;113:866-870.

351. Song WJ, Sullivan MG, Legare RD, et al. Haploinsufficiency of CBFA2 causes familial thrombocytopenia with propensity to develop acute myelogenous leukaemia. Nat Genet. 1999;23:166-175.

352. Ho CY, Otterud B, Legare RD, et al. Linkage of a familial platelet disorder with a propensity to develop myeloid malignancies to human chromosome 21q22.1-22.2. Blood. 1996;87:5218-5224.

353. Arepally G, Rebbeck TR, Song W, et al. Evidence for genetic homogeneity in a familial platelet disorder with predisposition to acute myelogenous leukemia (FPD/AML). Blood. 1998;92:2600-2602.

354. Speck NA, Gilliland DG. Core-binding factors in haematopoiesis and leukaemia. Nat Rev Cancer. 2002;2:502-513.

355. Penny LA, Dell'Aquila M, Jones MC, et al. Clinical and molecular characterization of patients with distal 11q deletions. Am J Hum Genet. 1995;56:676-683.

356. Tunnacliffe A, Jones C, Le Paslier D, et al. Localization of Jacobsen syndrome breakpoints on a 40-Mb physical map of distal chromosome 11q. Genome Res. 1999;9: 44-52.

357. Favier R, Jondeau K, Boutard P, et al. Paris-Trousseau syndrome: clinical, hematological, molecular data of ten new cases. Thromb Haemost. 2003;90:893-897.

358. Favier R, Douay L, Esteva B, et al. A novel genetic thrombocytopenia (Paris-Trousseau) associated with platelet inclusions, dysmegakaryopoiesis and chromosome deletion AT 11q23. C R Acad Sci III. 1993;316:698-701.

359. Breton-Gorius J, Favier R, Guichard J, et al. A new congenital dysmegakaryopoietic thrombocytopenia (Paris-Trousseau) associated with giant platelet alpha-granules and chromosome 11 deletion at 11q23. Blood. 1995;85: 1805-1814.

360. Krishnamurti L, Neglia JP, Nagarajan R, et al. Paris-Trousseau syndrome platelets in a child with Jacobsen's syndrome. Am J Hematol. 2001;66:295-299.

361. Hart A, Melet F, Grossfeld P, et al. Fli-1 is required for murine vascular and megakaryocytic development and is hemizygously deleted in patients with thrombocytopenia. Immunity. 2000;13:167-177.

362. Nichols KE, Crispino JD, Poncz M, et al. Familial dyserythropoietic anaemia and thrombocytopenia due to an inherited mutation in GATA1. Nat Genet. 2000;24: 266-270.

363. Freson K, Devriendt K, Matthijs G, et al. Platelet characteristics in patients with X-linked macrothrombocytopenia because of a novel GATA1 mutation. Blood. 2001; 98:85-92.

364. Freson K, Matthijs G, Thys C, et al. Different substitutions at residue D218 of the X-linked transcription factor GATA1 lead to altered clinical severity of macrothrombocytopenia and anemia and are associated with variable skewed X inactivation. Hum Mol Genet. 2002;11: 147-152.

365. Mehaffey MG, Newton AL, Gandhi MJ, et al. X-linked thrombocytopenia caused by a novel mutation of GATA-1. Blood. 2001;98:2681-2688.

366. Del Vecchio GC, Giordani L, De Santis A, De Mattia D. Dyserythropoietic anemia and thrombocytopenia due to a novel mutation in GATA-1. Acta Haematol. 2005;114: 113-116.

367. Raskind WH, Niakan KK, Wolff J, et al. Mapping of a syndrome of X-linked thrombocytopenia with thalassemia to band Xp11-12: further evidence of genetic heterogeneity of X-linked thrombocytopenia. Blood. 2000;95: 2262-2268.

368. Yu C, Niakan KK, Matsushita M, et al. X-linked thrombocytopenia with thalassemia from a mutation in the amino finger of GATA-1 affecting DNA binding rather than FOG-1 interaction. Blood. 2002;100:2040-2045.

369. Balduini CL, Pecci A, Loffredo G, et al. Effects of the R216Q mutation of GATA-1 on erythropoiesis and megakaryocytopoiesis. Thromb Haemost. 2004;91:129-140.

370. Phillips JD, Steensma DP, Pulsipher MA, et al. Congenital erythropoietic porphyria due to a mutation in GATA1: the first trans-acting mutation causative for a human porphyria. Blood. 2007;109:2618-2621.

371. Tubman VN, Levine JE, Campagna DR, et al. X-linked gray platelet syndrome due to a GATA1 Arg216Gln mutation. Blood. 2007;109:3297-3299.

372. Clemetson JM, Kyrle PA, Brenner B, Clemetson KJ. Variant Bernard-Soulier syndrome associated with a homozygous mutation in the leucine-rich domain of glycoprotein IX. Blood. 1994;84:1124-1131.

373. Lanza F, De La Salle C, Baas MJ, et al. A Leu7Pro mutation in the signal peptide of platelet glycoprotein (GP)IX in a case of Bernard-Soulier syndrome abolishes surface expression of the GPIb-V-IX complex. Br J Haematol. 2002;118:260-266.

374. Savoia A, Balduini CL, Savino M, et al. Autosomal dominant macrothrombocytopenia in Italy is most frequently a type of heterozygous Bernard-Soulier syndrome. Blood. 2001;97:1330-1335.

375. Budarf ML, Konkle BA, Ludlow LB, et al. Identification of a patient with Bernard-Soulier syndrome and a deletion in the DiGeorge/velo-cardio-facial chromosomal region in 22q11.2. Hum Mol Genet. 1995;4:763-766.

376. Dong F, Li S, Pujol-Moix N, et al. Genotype-phenotype correlation in MYH9-related thrombocytopenia. Br J Haematol. 2005;130:620-627.

377. Hegde UM. Immune thrombocytopenia in pregnancy and the newborn. Br J Obstet Gynaecol. 1985;92: 657-659.

378. Andrew M, Vegh P, Caco C, et al. A randomized, controlled trial of platelet transfusions in thrombocytopenic premature infants. J Pediatr. 1993;123:285-291.

379. Chan KW, Kaikov Y, Wadsworth LD. Thrombocytosis in childhood: a survey of 94 patients. Pediatrics. 1989;84: 1064-1067.

380. Ostermann H, van de Loo J. Factors of the hemostatic system in diabetic patients. A survey of controlled studies. Haemostasis. 1986;16:386-416.

381. Stuart MJ, Elrad H, Graeber JE, et al. Increased synthesis of prostaglandin endoperoxides and platelet hyperfunction in infants of mothers with diabetes mellitus. J Lab Clin Med. 1979;94:12-26.

382. Kaapa P, Knip M, Viinikka L, Ylikorkala O. Increased platelet thromboxane B_2 production in newborn infants of diabetic mothers. Prostaglandins Leukot Med. 1986;21: 299-304.

383. Stuart MJ, Sunderji SG, Allen JB. Decreased prostacyclin production in the infant of the diabetic mother. J Lab Clin Med. 1981;98:412-416.

384. Kaapa P, Uhari M, Nikkari T, et al. Dietary fatty acids and platelet thromboxane production in puerperal women and their offspring. Am J Obstet Gynecol. 1986;155: 146-149.

385. Friedman Z, Lamberth EL Jr, Stahlman MT, Oates JA. Platelet dysfunction in the neonate with essential fatty acid deficiency. J Pediatr. 1977;90:439-443.

386. Friedman Z, Danon A, Stahlman MT, Oates JA. Rapid onset of essential fatty acid deficiency in the newborn. Pediatrics. 1976;58:640-649.

387. Friedman Z, Seyberth H, Lamberth EL, Oates J. Decreased prostaglandin E turnover in infants with essential fatty acid deficiency. Pediatr Res. 1978;12: 711-714.

388. Machlin LJ, Filipski R, Willis AL, et al. Influence of vitamin E on platelet aggregation and thrombocythemia in the rat. Proc Soc Exp Biol Med. 1975;149:275-277.

389. Lake AM, Stuart MJ, Oski FA. Vitamin E deficiency and enhanced platelet function: reversal following E supplementation. J Pediatr. 1977;90:722-725.

390. Ahlsten G, Ewald U, Kindahl H, Tuvemo T. Aggregation of and thromboxane B_2 synthesis in platelets from newborn infants of smoking and non-smoking mothers. Prostaglandins Leukot Med. 1985;19:167-176.

391. Ahlsten G, Ewald U, Tuvemo T. Maternal smoking reduces prostacyclin formation in human umbilical arteries. A study on strictly selected pregnancies. Acta Obstet Gynecol Scand. 1986;65:645-649.

392. Davis RB, Leuschen MP, Boyd D, Goodlin RC. Evaluation of platelet function in pregnancy. Comparative studies in non-smokers and smokers. Thromb Res. 1987;46:175-186.

393. Ylikorkala O, Halmesmaki E, Viinikka L. Effect of ethanol on thromboxane and prostacyclin synthesis by fetal platelets and umbilical artery. Life Sci. 1987;41:371-376.

394. Stuart M, Wu J, Sunderji S, Ganley C. Effect of amniotic fluid on platelet thromboxane production. J Pediatr. 1987;110:289-292.

395. Segall ML, Goetzman BW, Schick JB. Thrombocytopenia and pulmonary hypertension in the perinatal aspiration syndromes. J Pediatr. 1980;96:727-730.

396. Levin DL, Weinberg AG, Perkin RM. Pulmonary microthrombi syndrome in newborn infants with unresponsive persistent pulmonary hypertension. J Pediatr. 1983;102:299-303.

397. Suzuki S, Wake N, Yoshiaki K. New neonatal problems of blood coagulation and fibrinolysis. II. Thromboplastic effect of amniotic fluid and its relation to lung maturity. J Perinat Med. 1976;4:221-226.

398. Kaapa P. Immunoreactive thromboxane B_2 and 6-keto-prostaglandin F_1 alpha in neonatal hyperbilirubinemia. Prostaglandins Leukot Med. 1985;17:97-105.

399. Maurer HM, Haggins JC, Still WJ. Platelet injury during phototherapy. Am J Hematol. 1976;1:89-96.

400. Karim MA, Clelland IA, Chapman IV, Walker CH. β-Thromboglobulin levels in plasma of jaundiced neonates exposed to phototherapy. J Perinat Med. 1981;9:141-144.

401. Remuzzi G. Bleeding in renal failure. Lancet. 1988;1:1205-1208.

402. Vella Briffa D, Greaves MW. Inhibition of human blood platelet aggregation by photochemotherapy in vitro and in vivo. Br J Dermatol. 1979;101:679-683.

403. Bleyer WA, Breckenridge RT. Studies on the detection of adverse drug reactions in the newborn. II. The effects of prenatal aspirin on newborn hemostasis. JAMA. 1970;213:2049-2053.

404. Rumack CM, Guggenheim MA, Rumack BH, et al. Neonatal intracranial hemorrhage and maternal use of aspirin. Obstet Gynecol. 1981;58:52S-56S.

405. Ts'ao CH. Comparable inhibition of aggregation of PRP of neonates and adults by aspirin. Haemostasis. 1977;6:118-126.

406. Palmisano PA, Cassady G. Salicylate exposure in the perinate. JAMA. 1969;209:556-558.

407. Casteels-van Daele M, Jaeken J, Eggermont E, et al. More on the effects of antenatally administered aspirin on aggregation of platelets of neonates. J Pediatr. 1972;80:685-686.

408. Friedman Z, Whitman V, Maisels MJ, et al. Indomethacin disposition and indomethacin-induced platelet dysfunction in premature infants. J Clin Pharmacol. 1978;18:272-279.

409. Guignard JP, Torrado A, Da Cunha O, Gautier E. Glomerular filtration rate in the first three weeks of life. J Pediatr. 1975;87:268-272.

410. Brown AK, Zuelzer WW. Studies on the neonatal development of the glucuronide conjugating system. J Clin Invest. 1958;37:332-340.

411. Corazza MS, Davis RF, Merritt TA, et al. Prolonged bleeding time in preterm infants receiving indomethacin for patent ductus arteriosus. J Pediatr. 1984;105:292-296.

412. Setzer ES, Webb IB, Wassenaar JW, et al. Platelet dysfunction and coagulopathy in intraventricular hemorrhage in the premature infant. J Pediatr. 1982;100:599-605.

413. Ment LR, Ehrenkranz RA, Duncan CC. Intraventricular hemorrhage of the preterm neonate: prevention studies. Semin Perinatol. 1988;12:359-372.

414. Sagel J, Colwell JA, Crook L, Laimins M. Increased platelet aggregation in early diabetes mellitus. Ann Intern Med. 1975;82:733-738.

415. Halushka PV, Lurie D, Colwell JA. Increased synthesis of prostaglandin-E–like material by platelets from patients with diabetes mellitus. N Engl J Med. 1977;297:1306-1310.

416. Oppenheimer EH, Esterly JR. Thrombosis in the newborn: comparison between infants of diabetic and nondiabetic mothers. J Pediatr. 1965;67:549-556.

417. Cowett RM, Schwartz R. The infant of the diabetic mother. Pediatr Clin North Am. 1982;29:1213-1231.

418. Steiner M, Anastasi J. Vitamin E. An inhibitor of the platelet release reaction. J Clin Invest. 1976;57:732-737.

419. Cox AC, Rao GH, Gerrard JM, White JG. The influence of vitamin E quinone on platelet structure, function, and biochemistry. Blood. 1980;55:907-914.

420. Khurshid M, Lee TJ, Peake IR, Bloom AL. Vitamin E deficiency and platelet functional defect in a jaundiced infant. BMJ. 1975;4:19-21.

421. Varela AF, Runge A, Ignarro LJ, Chaudhuri G. Nitric oxide and prostacyclin inhibit fetal platelet aggregation: a response similar to that observed in adults. Am J Obstet Gynecol. 1992;167:1599-1604.

422. Radomski MW, Palmer RM, Moncada S. Endogenous nitric oxide inhibits human platelet adhesion to vascular endothelium. Lancet. 1987;2:1057-1058.

423. Golino P, Cappelli-Bigazzi M, Ambrosio G, et al. Endothelium-derived relaxing factor modulates platelet aggregation in an in vivo model of recurrent platelet activation. Circ Res. 1992;71:1447-1456.

424. Bodzenta-Lukaszyk A, Gabryelewicz A, Lukaszyk A, et al. Nitric oxide synthase inhibition and platelet function. Thromb Res. 1994;75:667-672.

425. Hardart GE, Fackler JC. Predictors of intracranial hemorrhage during neonatal extracorporeal membrane oxygenation. J Pediatr. 1999;134:156-159.

426. Hardart GE, Hardart MK, Arnold JH. Intracranial hemorrhage in premature neonates treated with extracorporeal membrane oxygenation correlates with conceptional age. J Pediatr. 2004;145:184-189.

427. Cheung PY, Sawicki G, Salas E, et al. The mechanisms of platelet dysfunction during extracorporeal membrane

oxygenation in critically ill neonates. Crit Care Med. 2000;28:2584-2590.

428. Robinson TM, Kickler TS, Walker LK, et al. Effect of extracorporeal membrane oxygenation on platelets in newborns. Crit Care Med. 1993;21:1029-1034.

429. Plotz FB, van Oeveren W, Bartlett RH, Wildevuur CR. Blood activation during neonatal extracorporeal life support. J Thorac Cardiovasc Surg. 1993;105:823-832.

430. Canady AI, Fessler RD, Klein MD. Ultrasound abnormalities in term infants on ECMO. Pediatr Neurosurg. 1993;19:202-205.

431. Chan AK, Leaker M, Burrows FA, et al. Coagulation and fibrinolytic profile of paediatric patients undergoing cardiopulmonary bypass. Thromb Haemost. 1997;77: 270-277.

432. Watson JW, Brown DM, Lally KP, et al. Complications of extracorporeal membrane oxygenation in neonates. South Med J. 1990;83:1262-1265.

433. Zavadil DP, Stammers AH, Willett LD, et al. Hematological abnormalities in neonatal patients treated with extracorporeal membrane oxygenation (ECMO). J Extracorpor Technol. 1998;30:83-90.

434. Jarjour IT, Ahdab-Barmada M. Cerebrovascular lesions in infants and children dying after extracorporeal membrane oxygenation. Pediatr Neurol. 1994;10:13-19.

435. McManus ML, Kevy SV, Bower LK, Hickey PR. Coagulation factor deficiencies during initiation of extracorporeal membrane oxygenation. J Pediatr. 1995;126: 900-904.

436. Andrews NP, Broughton Pipkin F, Heptinstall S. Blood platelet behaviour in mothers and neonates. Thromb Haemost. 1985;53:428-432.

437. Ozkutlu S, Saraclar M, Atalay S, et al. Two-dimensional echocardiographic diagnosis of tricuspid valve noninfective endocarditis due to protein C deficiency (lesion mimicking tricuspid valve myxoma). Jpn Heart J. 1991;32: 139-145.

438. Marlar RA, Sills RH, Groncy PK, et al. Protein C survival during replacement therapy in homozygous protein C deficiency. Am J Hematol. 1992;41:24-31.

439. Pescatore P, Horellou HM, Conard J, et al. Problems of oral anticoagulation in an adult with homozygous protein C deficiency and late onset of thrombosis. Thromb Haemost. 1993;69:311-315.

440. Deguchi K, Tsukada T, Iwasaki E, et al. Late-onset homozygous protein C deficiency manifesting cerebral infarction as the first symptom at age 27. Intern Med. 1992;31: 922-925.

441. Yamamoto K, Matsushita T, Sugiura I, et al. Homozygous protein C deficiency: identification of a novel missense mutation that causes impaired secretion of the mutant protein C. J Lab Clin Med. 1992;119:682-689.

442. Auberger K. Evaluation of a new protein-C concentrate and comparison of protein-C assays in a child with congenital protein-C deficiency. Ann Hematol. 1992;64: 146-151.

443. Grundy CB, Melissari E, Lindo V, et al. Late-onset homozygous protein C deficiency. Lancet. 1991;338: 575-576.

444. Marlar RA, Neumann A. Neonatal purpura fulminans due to homozygous protein C or protein S deficiencies. Semin Thromb Hemost. 1990;16:299-309.

445. Tripodi A, Franchi F, Krachmalnicoff A, Mannucci PM. Asymptomatic homozygous protein C deficiency. Acta Haematol. 1990;83:152-155.

446. Petrini P, Segnestam K, Ekelund H, Egberg N. Homozygous protein C deficiency in two siblings. Pediatr Hematol Oncol. 1990;7:165-175.

447. Marlar RA, Montgomery RR, Broekmans AW. Report on the diagnosis and treatment of homozygous protein C deficiency. Report of the Working Party on Homozygous Protein C Deficiency of the ICTH-Subcommittee on Protein C and Protein S. Thromb Haemost. 1989;61: 529-531.

448. Marlar RA, Adcock DM, Madden RM. Hereditary dysfunctional protein C molecules (type II): assay characterization and proposed classification. Thromb Haemost. 1990;63:375-379.

449. Ben-Tal O, Zivelin A, Seligsohn U. The relative frequency of hereditary thrombotic disorders among 107 patients with thrombophilia in Israel. Thromb Haemost. 1989; 61:50-54.

450. Burrows RF, Kelton JG. Low fetal risks in pregnancies associated with idiopathic thrombocytopenic purpura. Am J Obstet Gynecol. 1990;163:1147-1150.

451. Manco-Johnson MJ, Marlar RA, Jacobson LJ, et al. Severe protein C deficiency in newborn infants. J Pediatr. 1988;113:359-363.

452. Vukovich T, Auberger K, Weil J, et al. Replacement therapy for a homozygous protein C deficiency-state using a concentrate of human protein C and S. Br J Haematol. 1988;70:435-440.

453. Gladson CL, Groncy P, Griffin JH. Coumarin necrosis, neonatal purpura fulminans, and protein C deficiency. Arch Dermatol. 1987;123:1701a-1706a.

454. Casella JF, Lewis JH, Bontempo FA, et al. Successful treatment of homozygous protein C deficiency by hepatic transplantation. Lancet. 1988;1: 435-438.

455. Marlar RA, Montgomery RR, Broekmans AW. Diagnosis and treatment of homozygous protein C deficiency. Report of the Working Party on Homozygous Protein C Deficiency of the Subcommittee on Protein C and Protein S, International Committee on Thrombosis and Haemostasis. J Pediatr. 1989;114:528-534.

456. Rappaport ES, Speights VO, Helbert B, et al. Protein C deficiency. South Med J. 1987;80:240-242.

457. Miletich J, Sherman L, Broze G Jr. Absence of thrombosis in subjects with heterozygous protein C deficiency. N Engl J Med. 1987;317:991-996.

458. Peters C, Casella JF, Marlar RA, et al. Homozygous protein C deficiency: observations on the nature of the molecular abnormality and the effectiveness of warfarin therapy. Pediatrics. 1988;81:272-276.

459. Adcock DM, Brozna J, Marlar RA. Proposed classification and pathologic mechanisms of purpura fulminans and skin necrosis. Semin Thromb Hemost. 1990;16: 333-340.

460. Auletta MJ, Headington JT. Purpura fulminans. A cutaneous manifestation of severe protein C deficiency. Arch Dermatol. 1988;124:1387-1391.

461. Adcock DM, Hicks MJ. Dermatopathology of skin necrosis associated with purpura fulminans. Semin Thromb Hemost. 1990;16:283-292.

462. Estelles A, Garcia-Plaza I, Dasi A, et al. Severe inherited "homozygous" protein C deficiency in a newborn infant. Thromb Haemost. 1984;52:53-56.

463. Mahasandana C, Suvatte V, Chuansumrit A, et al. Homozygous protein S deficiency in an infant with purpura fulminans. J Pediatr. 1990;117:750-753.

464. Dahlback B, Hildebrand B. Inherited resistance to activated protein C is corrected by anticoagulant cofactor activity found to be a property of factor V. Proc Natl Acad Sci U S A. 1994;91:1396-1400.

465. Svensson PJ, Dahlback B. Resistance to activated protein C as a basis for venous thrombosis. N Engl J Med. 1994;330:517-522.

466. Rogers PC, Silva MP, Carter JE, Wadsworth LD. Renal vein thrombosis and response to therapy in a newborn due to protein C deficiency. Eur J Pediatr. 1989;149:124-125.

467. Lobato-Mendizabal E, Ruiz-Arguelles GJ, Toquero-Franco O. [Effect of danazol on heterozygous protein C coagulation deficiency exacerbated by *Salmonella typhi* sepsis.] Bol Med Hosp Infant Mex. 1989;46:343-345.

468. Simioni P, de Ronde H, Prandoni P, et al. Ischemic stroke in young patients with activated protein C resistance. A report of three cases belonging to three different kindreds. Stroke. 1995;26:885-890.

469. Cucuianu M, Blaga S, Pop S, et al. Homozygous or compound heterozygous qualitative antithrombin III deficiency. Nouv Rev Fr Hematol. 1994;36:335-337.

470. Glueck CJ, Glueck HI, Greenfield D, et al. Protein C and S deficiency, thrombophilia, and hypofibrinolysis: pathophysiologic causes of Legg-Perthes disease. Pediatr Res. 1994;35:383-388.

471. Schander K, Niessen M, Rehm A, et al. Diagnose und Therapie eines kongenitalen Antithrombin III Manglels in der neonatalen Periode. Blut. 1980;40:68.

472. Soutar R, Marzinotto V, Andrew M. Overtight nappy precipitating thrombosis in antithrombin III deficiency. Arch Dis Child. 1993;69:599.

473. Shiozaki A, Arai T, Izumi R, et al. Congenital antithrombin III deficient neonate treated with antithrombin III concentrates. Thromb Res. 1993;70:211-216.

474. Schmidt B, Andrew M. Neonatal thrombosis: report of a prospective Canadian and international registry. Pediatrics. 1995;96:939-943.

475. David M, Andrew M. Venous thromboembolic complications in children. J Pediatr. 1993;123:337-346.

476. Andrew M, David M, Adams M, et al. Venous thromboembolic complications (VTE) in children: first analyses of the Canadian Registry of VTE. Blood. 1994;83:1251-1257.

477. O'Brodovich HM, Coates G. Quantitative ventilation-perfusion lung scans in infants and children: utility of a submicronic radiolabeled aerosol to assess ventilation. J Pediatr. 1984;105:377-383.

478. Bejar R, Curbelo V, Coen RW, et al. Diagnosis and follow-up of intraventricular and intracerebral hemorrhages by ultrasound studies of infant's brain through the fontanelles and sutures. Pediatrics. 1980;66:661-673.

479. Jackson JC, Truog WE, Watchko JF, et al. Efficacy of thromboresistant umbilical artery catheters in reducing aortic thrombosis and related complications. J Pediatr. 1987;110:102-105.

480. Horgan MJ, Bartoletti A, Polansky S, et al. Effect of heparin infusates in umbilical arterial catheters on frequency of thrombotic complications. J Pediatr. 1987;111:774-778.

481. Rajani K, Goetzman BW, Wennberg RP, et al. Effect of heparinization of fluids infused through an umbilical artery catheter on catheter patency and frequency of complications. Pediatrics. 1979;63:552-556.

482. Ankola PA, Atakent YS. Effect of adding heparin in very low concentration to the infusate to prolong the patency of umbilical artery catheters. Am J Perinatol. 1993;10:229-232.

483. Vailas GN, Brouillette RT, Scott JP, et al. Neonatal aortic thrombosis: recent experience. J Pediatr. 1986;109:101-108.

484. Schmidt B, Andrew M. Neonatal thrombotic disease: prevention, diagnosis, and treatment. J Pediatr. 1988;113:407-410.

485. Bosque E, Weaver L. Continuous versus intermittent heparin infusion of umbilical artery catheters in the newborn infant. J Pediatr. 1986;108:141-143.

486. David RJ, Merten DF, Anderson JC, Gross S. Prevention of umbilical artery catheter clots with heparinized infusates. Dev Pharmacol Ther. 1981;2:117-126.

487. Lesko SM, Mitchell AA, Epstein MF, et al. Heparin use as a risk factor for intraventricular hemorrhage in low-birth-weight infants. N Engl J Med. 1986;314:1156-1160.

488. Schmidt B, Zipursky A. Thrombotic disease in newborn infants. Clin Perinatol. 1984;11:461-488.

489. Andrew M, Schmidt B, Mitchell L, et al. Thrombin generation in newborn plasma is critically dependent on the concentration of prothrombin. Thromb Haemost. 1990;63:27-30.

490. Schmidt B, Ofosu FA, Mitchell L, et al. Anticoagulant effects of heparin in neonatal plasma. Pediatr Res. 1989;25:405-408.

491. Andrew M, Mitchell L, Vegh P, Ofosu F. Thrombin regulation in children differs from adults in the absence and presence of heparin. Thromb Haemost. 1994;72:836-842.

492. Patel P, Weitz J, Brooker LA, et al. Decreased thrombin activity of fibrin clots prepared in cord plasma compared with adult plasma. Pediatr Res. 1996;39:826-830.

493. Andrew M, Ofosu F, Schmidt B, et al. Heparin clearance and ex vivo recovery in newborn piglets and adult pigs. Thromb Res. 1988;52:517-527.

494. McDonald MM, Jacobson LJ, Hay WW Jr, Hathaway WE. Heparin clearance in the newborn. Pediatr Res. 1981;15:1015-1018.

495. Schmidt B, Buchanan MR, Ofosu F, et al. Antithrombotic properties of heparin in a neonatal piglet model of thrombin-induced thrombosis. Thromb Haemost. 1988;60:289-292.

496. Manco-Johnson MJ, Nuss R. Neonatal thrombotic disorders. NeoReviews. 2000;1:e201-e205.

497. Seifert HA, Jobes DR, Ten Have T, et al. Adverse events after protamine administration following cardiopulmonary bypass in infants and children. Anesth Analg. 2003;97:383-389.

498. Hirsh J, Levine MN. Low molecular weight heparin. Blood. 1992;79:1-17.

499. Michaels LA, Gurian M, Hegyi T, Drachtman RA. Low molecular weight heparin in the treatment of venous and arterial thromboses in the premature infant. Pediatrics. 2004;114:703-707.

500. Monagle P, Chan A, Massicotte P, et al. Antithrombotic therapy in children: the Seventh ACCP Conference on Antithrombotic and Thrombolytic Therapy. Chest. 2004;126:645S-687S.

501. Massonnet-Castel S, Pelissier E, Bara L, et al. Partial reversal of low molecular weight heparin (PK 10169) anti-Xa activity by protamine sulfate: in vitro and in vivo study during cardiac surgery with extracorporeal circulation. Haemostasis. 1986;16:139-146.

502. Wiernikowski JT, Chan A, Lo G. Reversal of antithrombin activity using protamine sulfate. Experience in a neonate with a 10-fold overdose of enoxaparin. Thromb Res. 2007;120:303-305.

503. Murdoch IA, Beattie RM, Silver DM. Heparin-induced thrombocytopenia in children. Acta Paediatr. 1993;82:495-497.

504. Spadone D, Clark F, James E, et al. Heparin-induced thrombocytopenia in the newborn. J Vasc Surg. 1992;15:306-311; discussion 311-302.

505. Hathaway W, Corrigan J. Report of Scientific and Standardization Subcommittee on Neonatal Hemostasis. Normal coagulation data for fetuses and newborn infants. Thromb Haemost. 1991;65:323-325.

506. Corrigan J. Normal hemostasis in fetus and newborn. In Polin R, Fox W (eds). Fetal and Neonatal Physiology. Philadelphia, WB Saunders, 1992, pp 1368-1371.

507. Schmidt B, Andrew M. Report of Scientific and Standardization Subcommittee on Neonatal Hemostasis Diagnosis and Treatment of Neonatal Thrombosis. Thromb Haemost. 1992;67:381-382.

508. Andrew M, Marzinotto V, Brooker LA, et al. Oral anticoagulation therapy in pediatric patients: a prospective study. Thromb Haemost. 1994;71:265-269.

509. von Kries R, Shearer M, McCarthy PT, et al. Vitamin K_1 content of maternal milk: influence of the stage of lactation, lipid composition, and vitamin K_1 supplements given to the mother. Pediatr Res. 1987;22:513-517.

510. von Kries R, Stannigel H, Gobel U. Anticoagulant therapy by continuous heparin-antithrombin III infusion in newborns with disseminated intravascular coagulation. Eur J Pediatr. 1985;144:191-194.

511. Hathaway WE. Use of antiplatelet agents in pediatric hypercoagulable states. Am J Dis Child. 1984;138:301-304.

512. Finkelstein Y, Nurmohamed L, Avner M, et al. Clopidogrel use in children. J Pediatr. 2005;147:657-661.

513. Andrew M, Brooker L, Leaker M, et al. Fibrin clot lysis by thrombolytic agents is impaired in newborns due to a low plasminogen concentration. Thromb Haemost. 1992;68:325-330.

III | Bone Marrow Failure

6

Anatomy and Physiology of Hematopoiesis

Colin A. Sieff and Leonard I. Zon

This chapter offers a review of the anatomy and physiology of normal hematopoiesis that is intended to provide a basis of understanding of the marrow failure syndromes described at length in the following chapter. In this chapter we briefly discuss the phylogeny of hematopoiesis and describe marrow anatomy and the egress of recognizable hematopoietic cells from the marrow into peripheral blood. Then follows a more detailed analysis of the cellular bases of erythrocyte, granulocyte-macrophage, and megakaryocyte development, including discussion of the pluripotent stem cell, the more committed but still undifferentiated progenitor cell, and differentiated precursors of the mature formed elements of blood. Much of this chapter is devoted to the interactions of growth factors and the cells that produce them in the upregulation of hematopoiesis. The mechanisms of downregulation of hematopoiesis by cell interactions and cytokines are touched on here, but they are less well understood despite the fact that they are likely to influence the pathophysiology of aplastic anemia and other marrow failure syndromes.

HISTORY*

That "blood is life" was appreciated by Empedocles in the fifth century BC. The theory that the vasculature contains blood, phlegm, black bile, and yellow bile, all revealed when freshly let blood is permitted to separate, is attributed to Polibus, the son-in-law of Hippocrates.

Servetus recognized the systemic and lesser circulations in the 16th century. He was burned at the stake, in part because he did not accept the dogma that blood must pass through the intraventricular cardiac septum. (Grant disapproval and, more recently, approval without funding have been substituted for immolation. The effects are not entirely dissimilar.)

In view of the present growth of knowledge of hematology, it is remarkable to realize that the concept of the circulation of blood was finally established by Harvey only a little more than 300 years ago. This began the clinical application of blood transfusion, of which Pepys wrote, "It gave rise to many pretty wishes as of the blood of a Quaker to be let into an Archbishop and such like."

In the mid-17th century, Swammerdam observed red blood corpuscles in the microscope and Malpighi discovered the capillary circulation in the lung and omentum. However, it was not until the 19th century that the source of blood cell production began to be suc-cessfully explored. Houston suggested that red cells were derived from leukocytes in the lymphoid system. Zimmerman believed that erythrocytes were derived from platelets, an opinion shared by Hayem. Addison, perhaps not surprisingly, attributed red cell production to the adrenals, and Reikert finally suggested that red cells might be produced in the embryonic liver. In fact, not until 1868 did Neumann demonstrate that red cells arise from precursors in the marrow. The modern understanding of the physiology of hematopoiesis then began.

PHYLOGENY

Much can be learned about the physiology of hematopoiesis from study of the evolution of oxygen transport, a subject reviewed by Lehman and Huntsman.[1]

One of the major advantages of mammalian life over that of invertebrates is the capacity to package large amounts of hemoglobin within cells. This permits the delivery of oxygen to tissues without the enormous increase in oncotic pressure that would be induced by a similar concentration of high-molecular-weight hemoglobin free in plasma. The renewal rate of red cells is a function of the metabolic rate or basal heat production. This is illustrated dramatically in studies of the animal kingdom, ranging from the turtle to the pygmy shrew, and by comparisons of red cell renewal in marmots during periods at ambient and cold temperature,[2] in rats,[3] and in frogs.[4]

Production of blood cells in bone marrow is a late development in phylogeny. Red cells are found in the coelomic cavity of the worm and are produced in the kidneys of the goldfish. The influence of oxygen demand on the production of red cells[5] is illustrated by the effects of hyperoxia on bled rats[6] and the behavior of the European eel, one of the few vertebrate forms that ordinarily lacks erythrocytes in its juvenile state. When the adult eel struggles against the current up the rivers of Europe, hemoglobin-containing nucleated cells appear in its plasma. This influence of oxygen demand on respiratory pigment production is also illustrated in non–red cell–producing organisms such as *Daphnia*, the English water flea, a creature that produces high-molecular-weight hemoglobin in its ovaries when exposed to the low oxygen tension in stagnant ponds. The recent discovery of transcription factors that function as oxygen sensors provides a potential molecular explanation for these regulatory mechanisms.[7-10]

MARROW ANATOMY

The relative red (active) marrow space of a child is much greater than that of an adult, presumably because the high requirements for red cell production during neonatal life demand the resources of the entire production potential of the marrow. During postnatal life the

---

*For an entertaining review from which this precis was in part drawn, see The Growth of Knowledge of Functions of the Blood by A.H.T. Robb-Smith in *Functions of the Blood*, edited by R.G. MacFarlane and A.H.T. Robb-Smith, Oxford, Blackwell Scientific Publications, 1961. For more details, see also *Blood Pure and Simple* by the late Maxwell M. Wintrobe, New York, McGraw-Hill Book Company.

Total marrow space—adult (10 kg)
2600–4000 mL
Active red marrow—1200–1500 g

Total marrow space—child (15 kg)
1600 mL
Active red marrow—1000–1400 g

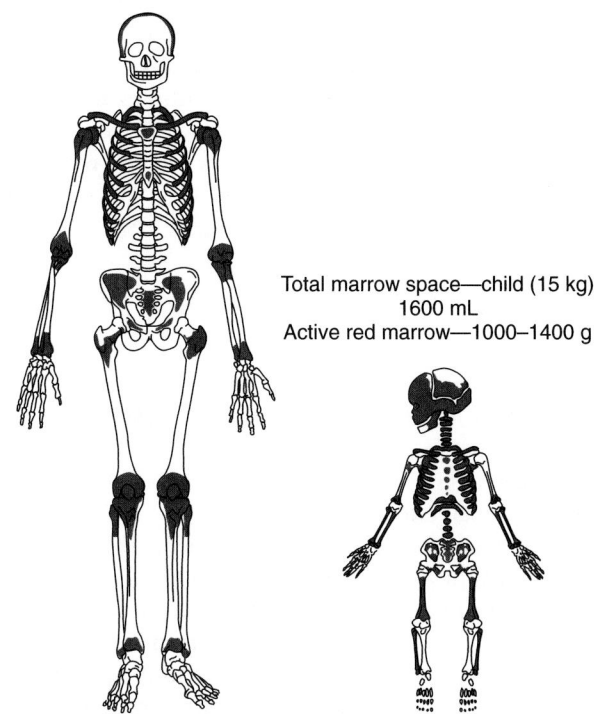

FIGURE 6-1. Comparison of active red marrow–bearing areas in a child and adult. Note the almost identical amount of active red marrow in the child and adult despite a fivefold discrepancy in body weight. *(Redrawn from MacFarlane RC, Robb-Smith AHT [eds]. Functions of the Blood. Oxford, Blackwell Scientific, 1961, p 357.)*

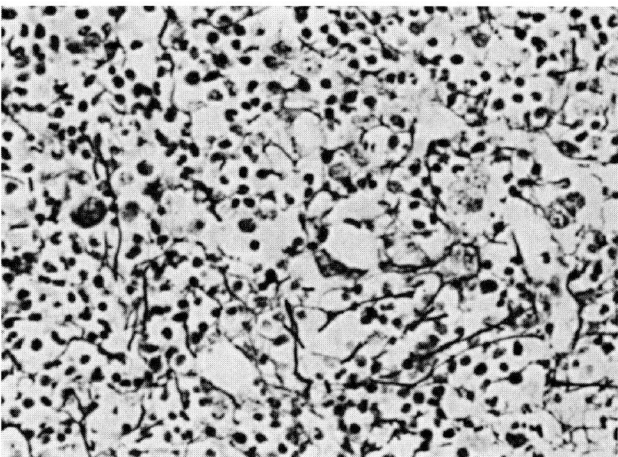

FIGURE 6-2. Bone marrow biopsy of a patient with mild myelofibrosis showing a slight increase in the number of reticulin fibers in a delicate discontinuous fiber network (Gomori stain ×350). *(From Lennert K, Nagai K, Schwarze EW. Patho-anatomical features of the bone marrow. Clin Haematol. 1975;4:331-351.)*

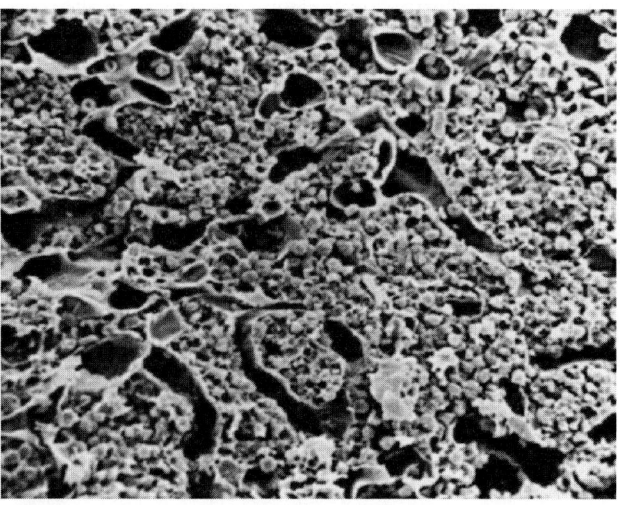

FIGURE 6-3. Scanning electron micrograph of rat femoral marrow. The hematopoietic cells are grouped between the interlacing network of the vascular sinuses. Many cells are dislodged when the marrow is transected, and separate spaces are present where cells had been. *(From Lichtman MA, Chamberlain JK, Santillo PA. Factors thought to contribute to the regulation of egress of cells from marrow. In Silber K, LoBue L, Gordon AS [eds]. The Year in Hematology, 1978. New York, Plenum, 1978, pp 243-279.)*

demands for red cell production ebb, and much of the marrow space is slowly and progressively filled with fat (Fig. 6-1). In certain disease states that are usually associated with anemia, such as myeloid metaplasia, hematopoiesis may return to its former sites in the liver, spleen, and lymph nodes and may also be found in the adrenals, cartilage, adipose tissue, thoracic paravertebral gutters, and even the kidneys.

The microenvironment of the marrow cavity is a vast network of vascular channels or sinusoids in which float fronds of hematopoietic cells, including fat cells. This complex area of cell biology and anatomy has been the subject of several reviews.[11-15] The cells are found in the intrasinusoidal fronds. The vascular and hematopoietic compartments are joined by reticular fibroblastoid cells that form the adventitial surfaces of the vascular sinuses and extend cytoplasmic processes to create a lattice on which blood cells are found. The lattice itself is illustrated by reticulin stains of marrow sections (Fig. 6-2). The comformation of the meshwork of reticulin and the location of hematopoietic cells in the network of vascular sinuses are best illustrated by scanning electron microscopy (Fig. 6-3). The fibroblastoid network provides two major functions—an adhesive framework onto which the developing cells are bound and production by these cells

of essential hematopoietic colony-stimulating factors (CSFs),[16] to be discussed later. Cell-cell adhesion may be mediated by binding of the hematopoietic very late antigen 4 (VLA-4) integrin to stromal fibronectin or vascular cell adhesion molecule 1 (VCAM-1).[17-20] In addition, cytokine receptors such as c-kit can bind to the membrane-bound form of stem cell factor or Steel factor (SCF),[21] and the extracellular matrix proteins secreted by stromal cells may actually provide a binding site for some growth factors or for hematopoietic cells.[22-24] In addition, chemokines, a family of small molecules, may have a role in stromal function. Specifically, stromal cell–

derived factor 1 (SDF-1) is a potent attractant for hematopoietic cells, both mature leukocytes and progenitor cells that express its receptor CXCR4.[25] Gene disruption of both ligand and receptor in mice is embryonically lethal, with defects in B lymphopoiesis and myelopoiesis.[26,27] These defects may relate to a critical role for CXCR4 in bone marrow engraftment in nonobese diabetic (NOD)/severe combined immunodeficiency (SCID) mice[28]; SDF-1 has been shown to activate the integrins VLA-4, VLA-5, and lymphocyte function antigen 1 (LFA-1) on CD34+ cells.[29] Last, there is evidence that SDF-1 may also play a role in the egress of progenitor cells from bone marrow to blood during stem cell mobilization.[30,31]

A schema of the marrow circulation is shown in Figure 6-4. The central and radial arteries ramify in the cortical capillaries, which in turn join the marrow sinusoids and drain into the central sinus. Cells that egress from the marrow sinusoids then join the venous circulation through comitant veins. The inner, or luminal, surface of the vascular sinusoids is lined with endothelial cells, the cytoplasmic extensions of which overlap, or interdigitate with, one another. Escape of developing hematopoietic cells into the sinus for transport to the general circulation occurs through gaps that develop in this endothelial lining and even through endothelial cell cytoplasmic pores.

The location of the different hematopoietic cells is not random. Clumps of megakaryocytes are found adjacent to marrow sinuses. They shed platelets, or fragments of their cytoplasm, directly into the lumen. This reduces

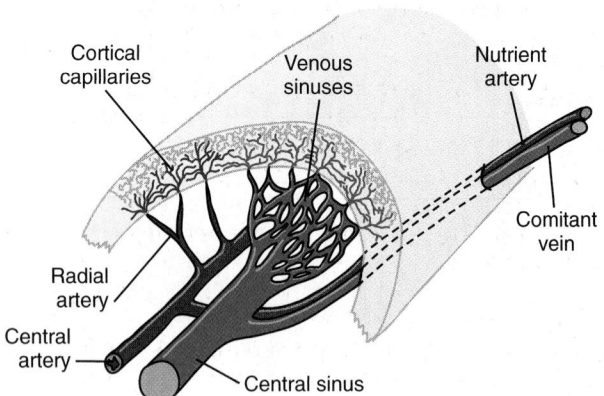

FIGURE 6-4. Schematic representation of the circulation of the marrow. The nutrient artery, central arteries, and radial arteries feed the cortical capillaries. The cortical capillaries anastomose with the marrow sinuses, which drain into the large central sinus. The central sinus enters the comitant vein, through which the marrow effluent enters the systemic venous circulation. An interesting feature of the circulation of marrow is the transit of nearly all arterial blood through cortical capillaries before entering the marrow sinuses. Not shown are the arterial communications from muscular arteries that feed the periosteum and penetrate the cortex to anastomose with intracortical vessels. *(Redrawn from Lichtman MA, Chamberlain JK, Santillo PA. Factors thought to contribute to the regulation of egress of cells from marrow. In Silber K, LoBue L, Gordon AS [eds]. The Year in Hematology, 1978. New York, Plenum, 1978, pp 243-279.)*

the requirement for movement of bulky mature megakaryocytes, a mobility characteristic of the granuloid- and erythroid-differentiated precursors as they approach the point at which they egress from the marrow. A schema that illustrates the transfer of hematopoietic cells into the sinus is shown in Figure 6-5. Disruption of the function of microenvironmental cells inhibits long-term murine marrow cultures.[32] Such disruptions may be responsible for certain cases of aplastic anemia.

HEMATOPOIETIC CELLS

Stem Cells

The concept that sustained hematopoiesis derives from pluripotent stem cells was first suggested by Jacobson and colleagues,[33] who showed that mice can be protected from the lethal effects of whole-body irradiation by exteriorization and shielding of the spleen. This protective effect was shown to be cell mediated by the observation that the injection of spleen cells could initiate recovery and re-establish hematopoiesis in irradiated animals.[34] The clonal nature of hematopoiesis and the concept that a single pluripotent stem cell exhibits the capacity to repopulate the entire hematopoietic system was first demonstrated experimentally by Till and McCulloch,[35] who also used the mouse as an experimental system. They demonstrated that colonies of hematopoietic cells could be observed in the spleen of transplanted, irradiated recipients within 10 days after the transplant. These colonies contained precursors to erythrocytes, granulocytes, macrophages, and megakaryocytes. Subsequent experiments using karyotypically marked donor cells confirmed the clonal origin of the differentiated cells in the colony, thus proving that a single pluripotent stem cell had given rise to these differentiated cells.[36] It was also shown that each colony contained a number of stem cells that could again form a colony of differentiated progeny in a second irradiated recipient, thus demonstrating their self-renewal capacity. This is true only of spleen colony-forming units that are present on day 12 to 14 (CFU-S$_{12}$). Colonies observed on days 7 to 8 after marrow infusion are transient, disappear by day 12, and are neither multipotential nor self-maintaining.[37] Under steady-state conditions, no more than 10% of the CFU-S become committed to differentiation during any given 3-hour period. The demonstration of a stem cell that can differentiate to form progenitor cells for erythropoiesis, granulopoiesis, and megakaryopoiesis is completely consistent with subsequent observations in disease states such as chronic myelogenous leukemia[38,39] and polycythemia vera (PCV),[40,41] in which a clonal origin of abnormal erythroid, granulocytic, and megakaryocytic precursor cells and lymphocytes can be demonstrated (see the Myeloid Leukemia, Myelodysplasia and Myeloproliferative Disease in Children in the companion volume *Oncology of Infancy and Childhood*).

FIGURE 6-5. Schematic diagram of the factors that may be involved in controlling the release of marrow cells. The central relationship between the hematopoietic compartment and the marrow sinus is depicted. The drawing highlights the similarity of the egress process for the three major hematopoietic cells: reticulocytes in the *top* pathway, granulocytes and monocytes in the *central* pathway, and platelets in the *lower* pathway. Immature cells undergo biophysical changes under the influence of cytopoietins that favor egress. In the case of the reticulocyte, enucleation precedes egress. This is shown by the *solid black* inclusion in the perisinal macrophage, which represents nucleophagocytosis before digestion of the erythroblast nucleus. The cytoplasmic protrusion of the megakaryocyte presumably detaches itself from the cell and will further fragment into platelets in the circulation. (*Redrawn from Lichtman MA, Chamberlain JK, Santillo PA. Factors thought to contribute to the regulation of egress of cells from marrow. In Silber K, LoBue L, Gordon AS [eds]. The Year in Hematology, 1978. New York, Plenum, 1978, pp 243-279.*)

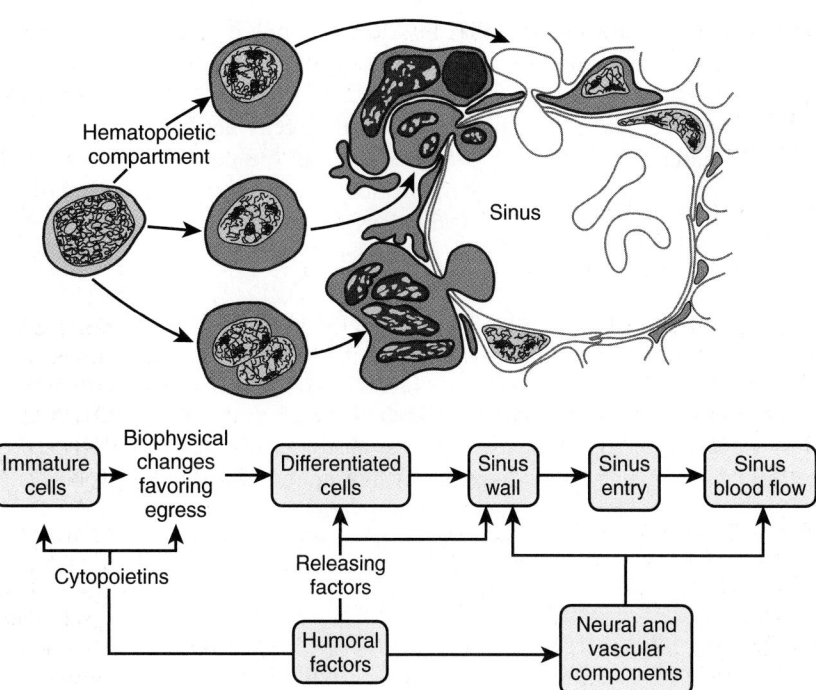

Demonstration of a pluripotent stem cell in adult bone marrow led to a systematic search for the ontogenic origins of hematopoietic stem cells (HSCs). Experiments performed by Metcalf and Moore[42] clearly demonstrated the presence of cells capable of repopulating adult marrow in the yolk sac and the murine fetal liver. Subsequent work has confirmed and extended these observations,[43] although data show that HSCs may arise simultaneously in the yolk sac and the intraembryonic aorta/gonad/mesonephros (AGM) region.[44] A difficulty here is that primordial germ cells also arise or migrate through this region and have been shown to have the potential to generate HSCs.[45] A point of interest that arises is whether the stem cells observed in the yolk sac, fetal liver, and adult marrow and spleen are functionally equivalent in every respect. One experimental finding that suggests functional differences between CFU-S at different stages of development of the mouse was made by Micklem and Ross.[46] Their experimental approach was to transfer spleen cells sequentially from a repopulated recipient to an irradiated recipient. Experiments of this type had previously shown that the capacity for transfer of CFU-S from adult marrow or spleen was finite, and in fact only three serial transfers could be accomplished.[47] Micklem and Ross showed that cells transplanted from the yolk sac to the spleen of an irradiated recipient could be serially transplanted as many as seven times before further proliferative capacity was lost. CFU-S derived from fetal liver was capable of five to six serial transfers.

The placenta has recently been found to be a source of HSCs during development.[48,49] The origin of stem cells within the placenta remains controversial inasmuch as it is possible that the stem cells arrive from intraembryonic sources such as the AGM region or the placenta may be a de novo producer of blood stem cells. It is interesting that the stem cells produced within the aorta appear to be on the arterial surfaces during embryogenesis, and the placenta is rich in this particular process. The placenta is quantitatively a large source of HSCs during development.

Studies of Hellman and co-workers[50] have provided a model of the stem cell compartment in which there is a continuum of cells with decreasing capacity for self-renewal, increasing likelihood for differentiation, and increasing proliferative activity. Cells progress in a unidirectional fashion in this continuum. It is the most primitive cells with the greatest self-renewal capacity that reconstitute long-term hematopoiesis after transfer into irradiated recipient mice. These cells, termed long-term–reconstituting hematopoietic stem cells (LTR-HSCs), were shown to be separable from $CFU-S_{12}$ in a limiting-dilution assay designed to detect and enumerate "cobblestone areas."[51] This assay is derived from the original "Dexter" technique for long-term culture of murine marrow in which CFU-S, colony-forming unit–granulocyte-macrophage (CFU-GM), and burst-forming unit–erythrocyte (BFU-E) flourish for many months on and within an adherent stromal monolayer.[52] The areas of active hematopoiesis have a "cobblestone" appearance. In the limiting-dilution assay, different concentrations of bone marrow cells are plated onto a series of microwells that contain a pre-established stromal monolayer, and at 5 weeks the cobblestone areas that comprise proliferating blast cells within the stromal cell layer are counted.[51] In cell separation experiments, their numbers correlate with a cell fraction that is characterized by low mitochondrial mass per cell (minimal retention of the supravital fluorochrome rhodamine 123); this cell fraction is enriched with marrow-repopulating cells but depleted of CFU-S$_{12}$.[51,53] Even more impressive separation of pre–CFU-S from CFU-S$_{12}$ was obtained by countercurrent elutriation.[54] Intermediate and rapidly sedimenting cells contained greater than 99% CFU-S$_{12}$, as well as the cells responsible for short-term reconstitution. In contrast, long-term–reconstituting cells (>60 days) came from a slowly sedimenting fraction that contained only 0.25% CFU-S$_{12}$.

In summary, LTR-HSCs are cells capable of long-term reconstitution of myelopoiesis and lymphopoiesis. More mature progenitor cells, represented by CFU-S$_{12}$, give rise to spleen colonies 12 to 14 days after injection into irradiated recipients, exhibit less self-renewal and proliferative capacity, and are generally limited to myeloid differentiation. The most mature compartment, represented by cells that give rise to spleen colonies 6 to 8 days after transplantation (CFU-S$_8$), have limited self-renewal and proliferative capacity. The relationship between the in vivo LTR-HSC assay and in vitro assays that measure blast cell colonies capable of forming additional colonies after replating,[55] high–proliferative potential colony-forming cells (HPP-CFCs) that form large monocyte colonies (up to 5×10^4 cells),[56] or cells that survive in long-term cultures[57] is at this point unresolved.

The stem cell model of hematopoiesis has parallels in other organ systems. That rapidly self-renewing epithelial tissues such as skin and intestine have stem cells that continually replenish the cells lost by differentiation is well described. However, demonstration of the existence of neural stem cells[58,59] has raised the possibility that many organ systems might retain a population of self-renewing stem cells. Muscle satellite cells also appear to fulfill this role. These organ- or tissue-specific stem cells arise during early fetal development from embryonic stem (ES) cells of the inner cell mass of the blastocyst that are totipotent and give rise to all body cell types.

Many assays have been proposed as "surrogate" stem cell assays, but until homogeneous populations can be evaluated in both in vitro and in vivo assays it will be impossible to determine the precise cell type measured by these methods. Fauser, Messner, and others[39,60-62] demonstrated colonies in semisolid media that contain granulocytes, erythrocytes, monocytes, and megakaryocytes (CFU-GEMM) in methylcellulose cultures of human bone marrow. A unique type of in vitro blast cell colony that contains small numbers of blast cells with higher self-renewal capacity (secondary colonies on replating) than CFU-GEMM possesses has been described.[55] Evidence for the presence of pluripotent HSCs is also derived from the human "Dexter" technique for liquid culture of marrow in which myeloid progenitors (mostly CFU-GM) are sustained for about 2 months on and within an adherent stromal monolayer.[63,64] The progenitors can be detected by replating into methylcellulose with several growth factors at 5 to 8 weeks, thereby demonstrating that unipotent and multipotent cells are gener-

ated in this culture system. Eaves and colleagues have adapted this long-term culture technique to a limiting-dilution assay in which long-term culture–initiating cells (LTC-ICs) can be quantitated after culture at different concentrations on a stromal layer for 5 weeks, followed by replating in methylcellulose and counting the number of wells that do not contain colonies.[65] The analogous cobblestone area–forming cell (CAFC) assay has also been adapted to human cells.[66] Another method that measures the enormous proliferative capacity of primitive progenitor cells is the HPP-CFC assay, which gives rise to macroscopically (>5 mm) visible in vitro colonies.[56,67] In an effort to establish a more direct measure of the ability of human stem cells to reconstitute hematopoiesis, Kamel-Reid and Dick developed an in vivo assay.[68] In this method human cells are injected into immunodeficient NOD/SCID mice, and 5 to 8 weeks later the animals are sacrificed and tested for the presence of human cells in blood and progenitors in bone marrow. By limiting dilution these SCID-reconstituting cells (SRCs) can be quantitated. Cell fractionation and gene-marking studies provide some evidence that SRCs are more primitive than LTC-ICs.[69,70] Although SRCs may still be a heterogeneous population of cells that includes LTR-HSCs, this assay provides a better measure of stem cell properties than the LTC-IC assay does, especially with regard to the multipotent (i.e., myeloid and lymphoid) and self-renewal properties of HSCs. A tentative relationship of the cells measured in these different assays to the stem cell is shown in Figure 6-6.

Application of these assays plus analysis of HSCs has in general been hindered by the low frequency of the cell in the hematopoietic population and the lack of reagents to identify stem cells. However, it is now possible to purify murine stem cells by several methods. Murine HSCs can be highly purified by density gradient centrifugation combined with labeling with antibodies, lectins, or intracellular dyes (alone or in combination), followed by separation via fluorescence-activated cell sorting (FACS), immunopanning, or immunomagnetic beads. Immunologic reagents that define murine stem cell populations include antibodies to Thy-1, c-kit, and stem cell antigen (Sca-1). Spangrude and co-workers[71] used FACS in combination with negative expression of T-cell, B-cell, granulocyte, and monocyte lineage–specific markers, low expression of Thy-1, and expression of Sca-1 to isolate HSCs. Transplantation of single c-kit$^+$, Thy-1^{lo}, lin$^-$, Sca-1$^+$ (KTLS) cells can ensure long-term survival of lethally irradiated syngeneic recipients,[72] and approximately 20% of such cells are LTR-HSCs. Murine HSCs can be even further enriched by using cell surface receptors of the signaling lymphocyte activation molecule (SLAM) family. HSCs are CD150$^+$, CD244$^-$, CD48$^-$, whereas multipotent progenitors lose CD150 expression and begin to express the other family members CD244 and CD48. Purification of CD150$^+$, CD48$^-$, D41$^-$ cells (CD41 is also expressed on megakaryocyte lineage cells) provides a population of cells in which 45% are LTR-HSCs.[73]

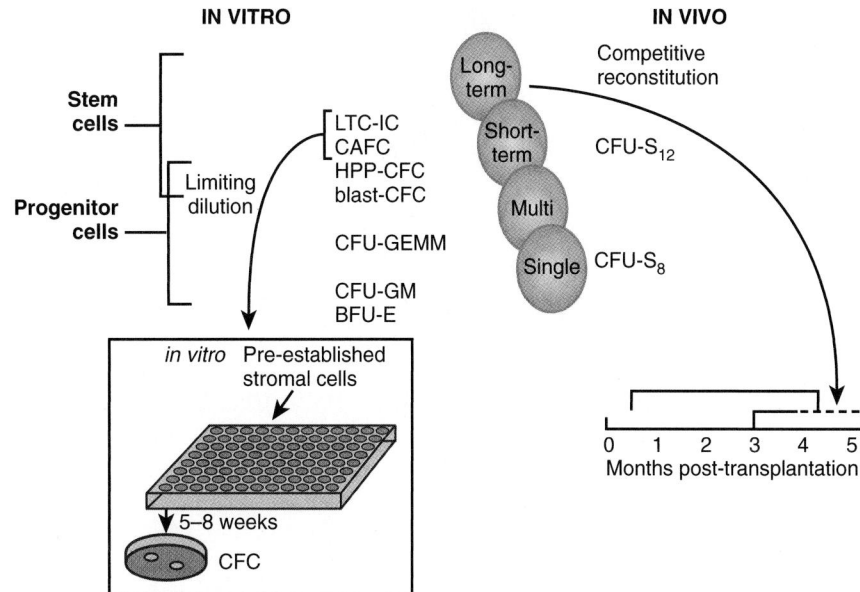

FIGURE 6-6. Schematic view of some general properties and assays for the heterogeneous cells that constitute the stem cell and progenitor cell compartments. As indicated on the diagram, cells capable of permanently reconstituting in vivo hematopoiesis are separable from cells that give rise to day 12 CFU-S, but the precise developmental stage of in vitro long-term culture–initiating cells (LTC-IC), cobblestone area–forming cells (CAFC), high–proliferative potential colony-forming cells (HPP-CFC), and blast CFC is not established. In the progenitor compartment, mixed colonies of almost all lineage combinations have been described. BFU-E, burst-forming unit–erythroid; CFU-GEMM, colony-forming unit–granulocyte-erythrocyte-macrophage-megakaryocyte; CFU-GM, colony-forming unit–granulocyte-macrophage.

Expression of the CD34 antigen has been used to enrich for human stem cells. Although most colony-forming cells (CFCs) express both the CD34 and CD33 antigens, cells that give rise to CFCs in long-term bone marrow culture (i.e., pre-CFCs) can be separated by their expression of CD34, lack of expression of CD33, and intermediate forward light–scattering property.[74] A G_0 CD34$^+$ cell population has been isolated by exploiting the resistance of these cells to 5-fluorouracil (5-FU) in the presence of SCF and interleukin-3 (IL-3).[75] G_0 cells are also c-kit, interleukin-6 receptor (IL-6R), and IL-1R positive; do not form progenitor-derived colonies on direct culture in methylcellulose; but after 5 weeks in culture on stromal cells, do form primary colonies in methylcellulose, 40% of which are replatable. The importance of CD34$^+$ marrow cells is emphasized by in vivo simian studies. Similar to human bone marrow, the CD34 antigen is expressed by a minority of baboon cells, and infusion of these cells after isolation by immunoabsorption chromatography and FACS can reconstitute lymphohematopoiesis in lethally irradiated baboons.[76] Cloning of murine CD34 cDNA has cast some doubt on expression of CD34 by LTR-HSCs, at least in the mouse. A monoclonal antibody raised to a murine CD34-GST fusion protein was used to separate purified Sca-1$^+$, c-kit$^+$, lin$^-$ bone marrow cells into CD34$^{lo/-}$, CD34^{lo}, and CD34$^+$ fractions. Interestingly, long-term multilineage reconstitution was observed after transplantation of the CD34$^{lo/-}$ cells, whereas the CD34$^+$ fraction provided early but unsustained multilineage reconstitution.[72] It is possible that murine and primate LTR-HSCs differ in their expression of CD34; however, the human and primate transplants did not use very highly purified cells, and thus it is also possible that CD34$^{lo/-}$ cells could account for the long-term engraftment. These data are supported by experiments demonstrating that a tiny subset of murine bone marrow cells that exclude the Hoechst 33342 dye (called the side pop-

ulation) contains all the LTR-HSC activity but is CD34$^-$.[77] Primate and human studies have also raised the possibility that HSCs do not express CD34.[78] When primitive human lin$^-$ cells are separated into CD34$^+$ and CD34$^-$ fractions, the capacity to reconstitute hematopoiesis in immunodeficient mice (called SRCs) is found in both cell fractions.[79] Resolution to this controversy may come from the demonstration that resting murine HSCs are CD34$^-$ whereas HSCs activated with 5-FU or cytokines such as granulocyte colony-forming factor (G-CSF) express the CD34 antigen.[80,81] Most interesting, transplantation of activated CD34$^+$ HSCs showed that these HSCs can lose CD34 expression after return of the recipients to the resting steady state and still retain the capacity to reconstitute secondary recipients, thus demonstrating that CD34 expression is reversible.[81]

Progenitor Cells

The pluripotent stem cells of the marrow slowly self-replicate while occasionally (and stochastically) differentiating into cells that are multipotent but have reduced self-renewal capacity (short-term–reconstituting HSCs [STR-HSCs]) and then into either common lymphoid (CLP) or common myeloid progenitors (CMP). These cells can be prospectively isolated according to their expression of unique combinations of cell surface markers (Fig. 6-7).[82-84] Lymphoid differentiation will not be further considered here. The CMP differentiates into all of the progenitors of blood cells other than lymphoid cells. These include more committed progenitors of the granulocyte, monocyte (GMP), and eosinophil lineages or progenitors of the megakaryocyte, erythroid, and basophil (MEP) lineages. These cells can be isolated prospectively, and transplantation into lethally irradiated mice can confer transient but not long-term hematopoiesis.[85]

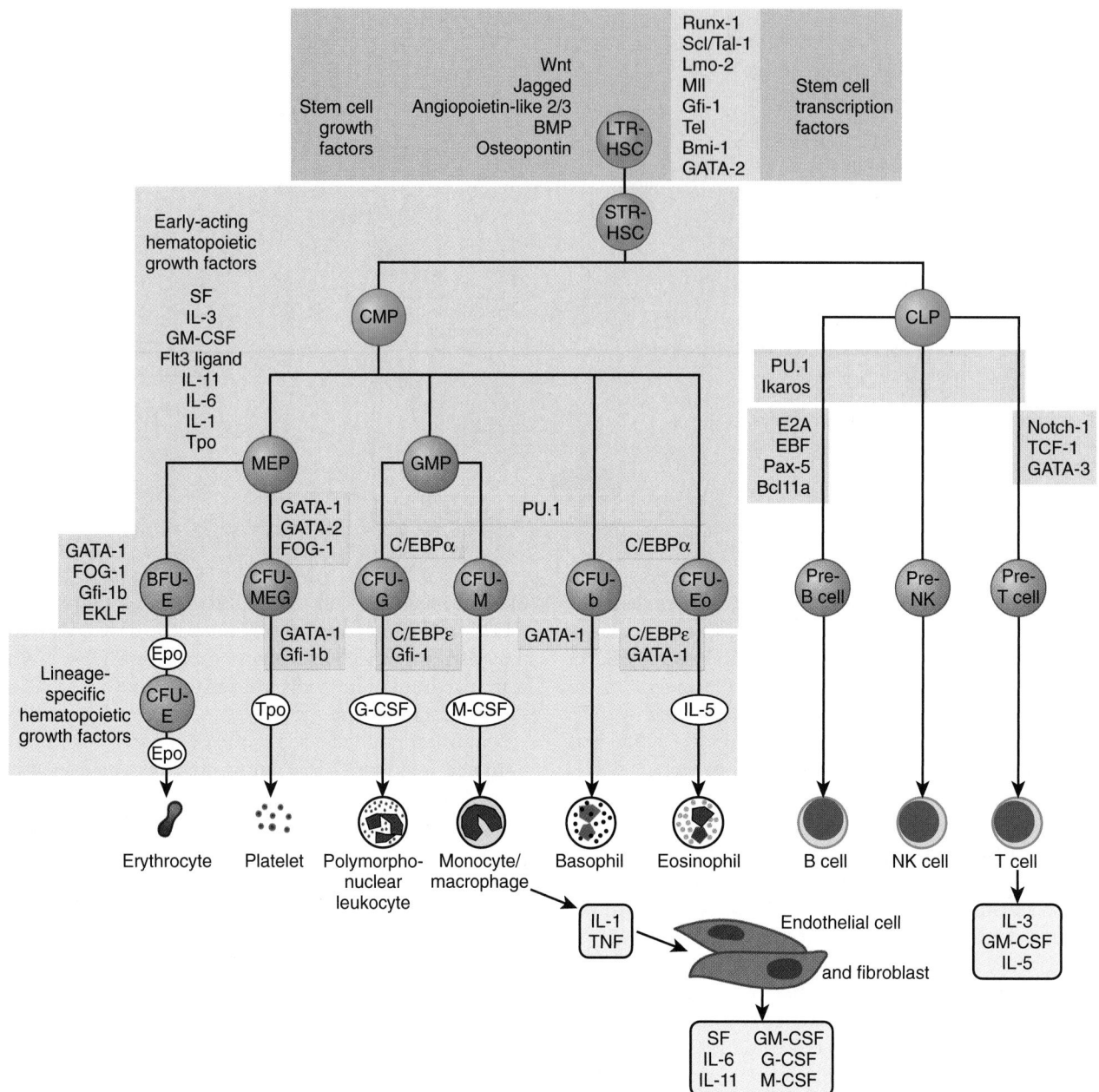

FIGURE 6-7. Major cytokine sources and actions and transcription factor requirements for hematopoietic cells. Cells of the bone marrow microenvironment such as macrophages, endothelial cells, and reticular fibroblastoid cells produce M-CSF, GM-CSF, G-CSF, IL-6, and probably SCF after induction with endotoxin (macrophage) or IL-1/TNF (endothelial cells and fibroblasts). T cells produce IL-3, GM-CSF, and IL-5 in response to antigenic and IL-1 stimulation. These cytokines have overlapping actions during hematopoietic differentiation, as indicated, and for all lineages optimal development requires a combination of early- and late-acting factors. Transcription factors important for survival or self-renewal of stem cells are shown at the top (*light green panel*), and stages of hematopoiesis blocked after the depletion of indicated transcription factors for multipotent and committed progenitors are shown in *light green boxes* throughout. Abbreviations are spelled out in the text.

Erythroid Colony-Forming Cells

The erythroid progenitor compartment is invisible to the light microscope. These committed progenitors of a single lineage are derived from stochastic differentiation of bipotential or multipotential progenitors,[86] which in turn are derived from a tiny population of pluripotential stem cells (see Fig. 6-7). In humans, the most primitive single-lineage–committed erythroid progenitor is the

BFU-E. BFU-E progenitors are so named because in response to the combination of erythropoietin (EPO) and either SCF, IL-3, or granulocyte-macrophage colony-stimulating factor (GM-CSF) in vitro in semisolid (methylcellulose) culture, the progenitor divides several times while still motile, thereby forming subpopulations of erythroid colony-forming units (CFU-E).[87] Each of the latter then form a large colony of proerythroblasts that eventually form more mature erythroblasts and even reticulocytes. The burst-like morphology of the colony is responsible for the name of the progenitor. The entire process requires about 2 weeks in vitro. Bone marrow also contains more mature CFU-E progenitors, which under the influence of EPO, form small colonies of erythroblasts in 7 days.

Granulocyte and Macrophage Colony-Forming Cells

The first colony assays relevant to the study of the production of granulocytes and monocytes in the mouse were described in 1965 by Pluznik and Sachs[88] and in 1966 by Bradley and Metcalf.[89] Analogous assays have been developed in the human system.[90] These groups demonstrated that individual cells derived from mouse spleen or bone marrow could give rise to colonies of up to several thousand differentiated granulocytes, macrophages, or both in soft agar medium. A period of 7 to 8 days was required for full maturation of these colonies (12 to 14 days is required in humans). Appropriate studies were performed to demonstrate the single-cell origin of the colonies. These studies also demonstrated that a single progenitor cell, which was termed the colony-forming unit in culture (CFU-C), was capable of differentiation into both granulocytes and macrophages, thus the designation CFU-GM. Unit gravity sedimentation and other separation methods have been used to demonstrate that CFU-GM represents a cell population distinguishable from pluripotent stem cells.[91] Long-term liquid bone marrow cultures have been particularly helpful in defining the humoral and cell-cell interactions that induce myeloid differentiation.[92] CFU-GM give rise to the more mature granulocyte and macrophage colony-forming units, CFU-G and CFU-M respectively.[89,90] In addition, CFU-GM can be distinguished from the eosinophil progenitor, CFU-Eo, each arising independently from the myeloid stem cell. A progenitor more mature than CFU-GM that differentiates to smaller clusters of mature myeloid cells earlier in culture than CFU-GM does has been described.[56,90,93,94] This is analogous to the erythroid system, in which BFU-E differentiates to the more mature progenitor CFU-E. A pre–CFU-GM similar to the most immature BFU-E but with a slower sedimentation rate and lower cycling index than CFU-GM has been described in humans.[95-97] Thus, the myeloid progenitor population, like the erythroid one, represents a continuum with respect to proliferative potential.

Megakaryocyte Colony-Forming Cells

Figure 6-7 provides an accepted if idealized schema of lineage-restricted megakaryocyte progenitor development. Evidence strongly suggests that the initial phase of differentiation into erythrocyte and megakaryocyte commitment involves a single progenitor capable of giving rise to colonies of differentiated cells, all of which express a nuclear transcription factor known as GATA-1.[98,99] Of great interest is the fact that another transcription factor, NF-E2, has been shown to regulate platelet production.[100] Mice rendered NF-E2 deficient die of bleeding from the absence of platelets. The thrombocytopenia is due to a block late in megakaryocyte maturation. Interestingly, these animals do not show an increase in thrombopoietin (TPO) levels, thus suggesting that the megakaryocyte mass rather than the platelet count regulates TPO production.

Precursors and Mature Cells

The erythroid precursor, or erythroblast, pool represents about a third of the marrow cell population in normal children older than 3 years and adults. Proerythroblasts are the earliest recognizable forms. These cells divide and mature through various stages that involve nuclear condensation and extrusion and hemoglobin accumulation. On average, each erythroblast can form about eight reticulocytes. Measurement of the total marrow proerythroblast content[101] and daily reticulocyte production shows that under normal conditions, replicating proerythroblasts largely maintain the reticulocyte pool by renewal from the progenitor compartment at a rate of about 10% per day.[102]

Erythroid Development

Up to this point we have discussed the nondescript progenitors of erythropoiesis without reference to their physical appearance or to the appearance of their differentiated daughter cells. The best evidence to date suggests that hematopoietic progenitors or stem cells look like lymphoblasts,[103-105] and studies of peripheral blood have shown BFU-E to reside in the nonadherent "null" lymphocyte population.[106]

The pathway of erythroid *precursor* differentiation between the development of proerythroblasts and the mature red cell is known as the erythron and includes the functioning differentiated precursor cells observed in bone marrow aspirates and biopsy sections. The morphology of erythroid precursor maturation is well described in several texts and will not be repeated here. The salient features of the morphologic changes during cell development are related to biochemical and kinetic alterations, as reviewed by Granick and Levere[107] and shown in Figure 6-8. Times spent in each morphologic compartment are shown at the bottom of the figure, but the average transit time from proerythroblast to emergence of the reticulocyte into the circulation is approximately 5 days.[108] In acute anemia, the transit time may decrease to as little as 1 or 2 days by means of skipped divisions.[109] The red cells that emerge are macrocytic and may bear surface i antigen and other fetal characteristics because the abbreviated time in the marrow compartment does not permit complete conversion of i antigen to I antigen or acquisition of certain other adult characteristics.[110] The cells also contain excessive burdens of the rubbish that normally

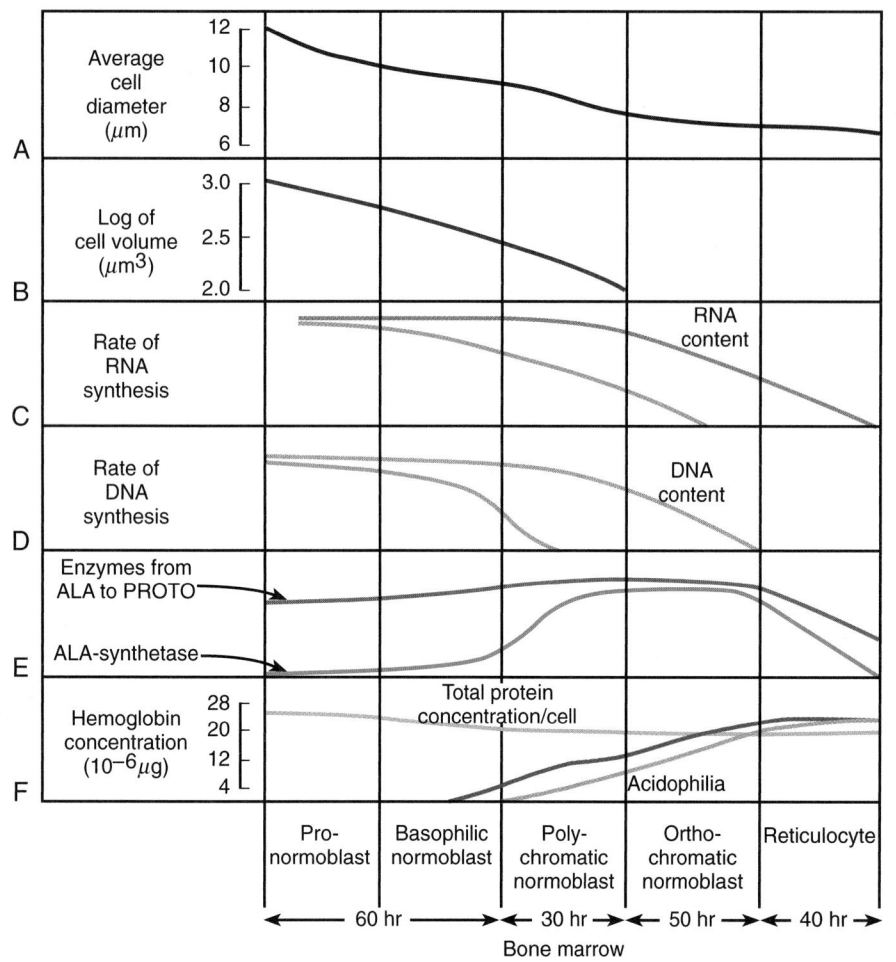

FIGURE 6-8. Erythroid maturation: alterations in cell size, rates of DNA and RNA synthesis, enzymes involved in heme synthesis, and hemoglobin concentration. Substances listed in the *left* column are represented by corresponding *solid black lines*. Unless specified, graphs represent relative values. ALA refers to δ-aminolevulinic acid and PROTO to protoporphyrin. It will be noted that considerable protein synthesis takes place during the earliest phase, after which the nucleolus disappears but mitochondria remain. As the concentration of DNA decreases and that of RNA starts to fall, hemoglobin begins to appear and increases rapidly in amount. *(Redrawn from Granick S, Levere RD. Heme synthesis in erythroid cells. In Moore CV, Brown EB [eds]. Progress in Hematology, vol. 4. New York, Grune & Stratton, 1964, p 1.)*

accumulates during cell assembly[111] because less time is available for the cleansing action of cell proteases and nucleases.[112] Thus, stress erythropoiesis is associated with circulating Pappenheimer bodies (iron granules), basophilic stippling (ribosomes), Heinz bodies (hemoglobin inclusions), and Howell-Jolly bodies (nuclear remnants).

The kinetics of erythropoiesis can be monitored with the use of radioactive iron and surface scanning. The various ferrokinetic patterns in human diseases are shown in Figure 6-9. The total distribution of erythroid marrow can be determined by scintigraphy with ^{111}InCl bound to transferrin, as shown in Figure 6-10. Both ^{59}Fe kinetics and ^{111}InCl scintigraphy can be useful in the diagnosis of marrow failure, but these techniques are rarely necessary. Initial uptake of ^{59}Fe in marrow primarily occurs in pro-erythroblasts and early basophilic erythroblasts.[113]

Neutrophil Production

A model that describes the production and kinetics of neutrophils in human is shown in Figure 6-11. It is highly compartmentalized. The relatively tiny peripheral blood pool is divided into two components in equilibrium: the circulatory granulocyte pool (CGP) and the marginating granulocyte pool (MGP). These pools provide entrance into tissues. The level of circulating cells is buffered by an immense narrow reserve of identifiable precursors, some of which are located in the mitotic compartment and others in a maturing storage compartment. Transit times within each compartment are relatively long, so a huge reserve remains available. The responses of these compartments to various diseases are detailed in Chapter 21. The kinetics of proliferation of recognizable cell precursors has been studied with labeled precursors of DNA. The so-called labeling indices from which measurements of cell cycle times can be made have served as important approaches to study of the pharmacology and toxicity of chemotherapy (see the chapter Chemotherapy in the Pediatric Patient in the companion volume *Oncology of Infancy and Childhood*).

The final stages of granulocyte production, their release from marrow, is also multifaceted.[114] At least four factors may influence granulocyte egress: organization and localization of the cells in relation to vascular channels, development of nuclear and cytoplasmic changes that increase cell deformability, factors that cause cell release, and finally, regulation of blood flow through vascular channels in the marrow.

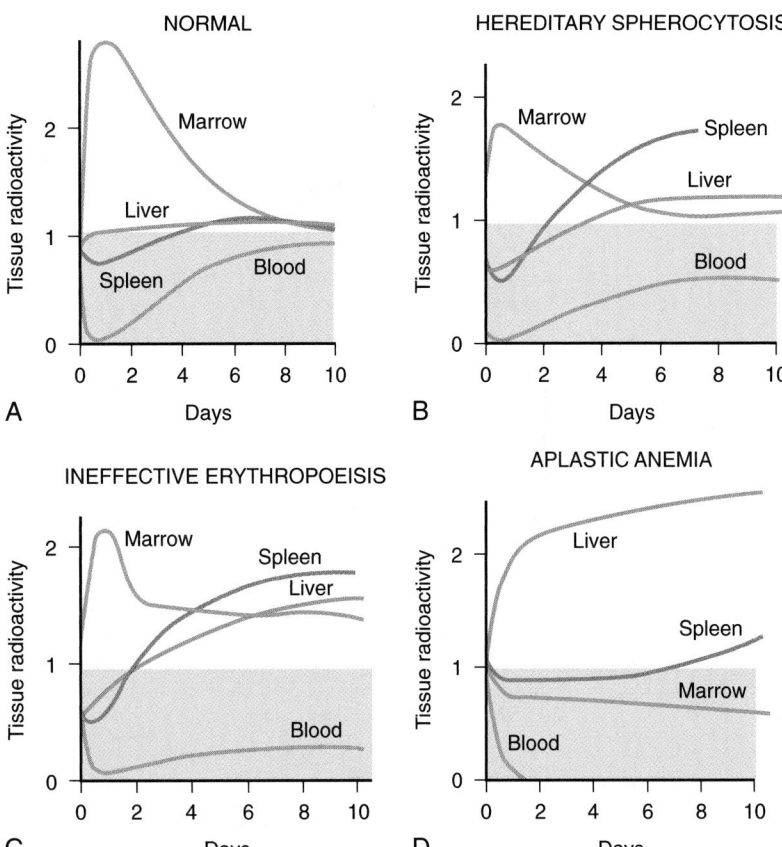

FIGURE 6-9. Pattern of radioactivity in blood and over the sacrum (marrow), liver, and spleen during a ferrokinetic study. Representative data from patients with three different disorders and one normal individual are presented. *(Redrawn from Finch CA, Deubelbeiss K, Cook JD, et al. Ferrokinetics in man. Medicine [Baltimore]. 1970;49:17-53. Copyright 1970 The Williams & Wilkins Company, Baltimore.)*

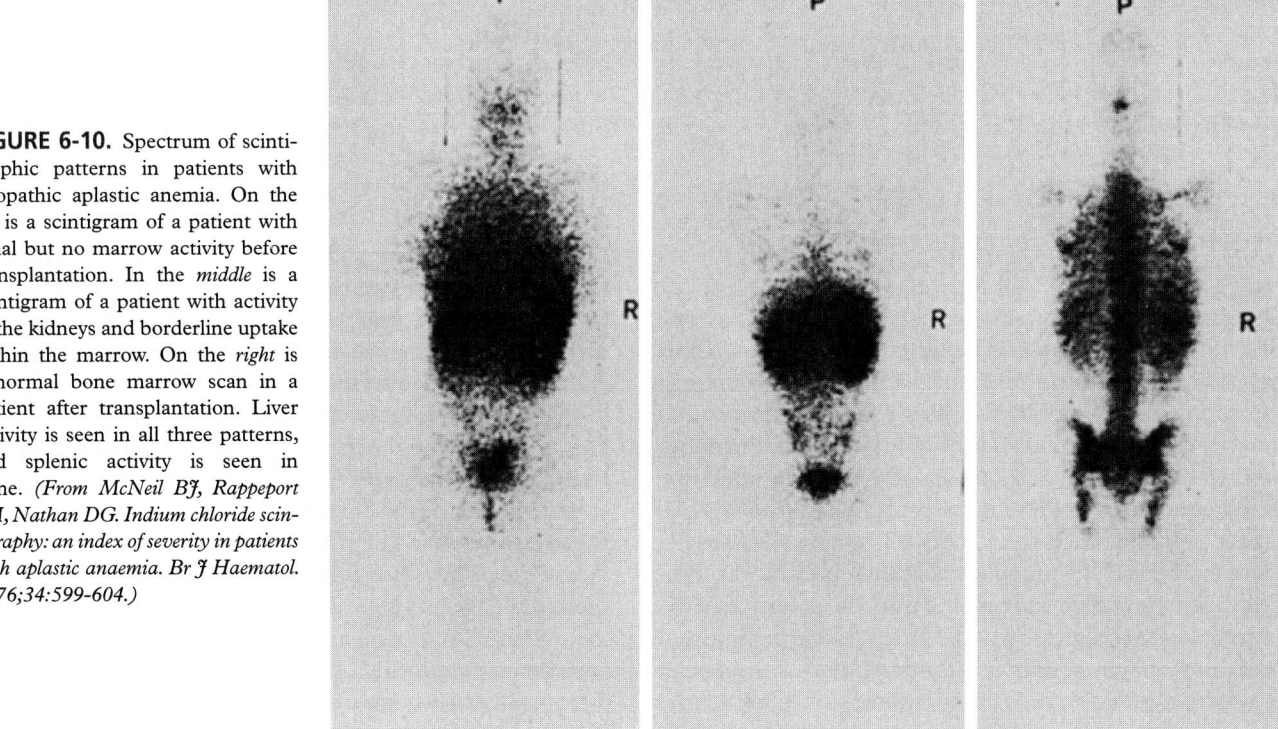

FIGURE 6-10. Spectrum of scintigraphic patterns in patients with idiopathic aplastic anemia. On the *left* is a scintigram of a patient with renal but no marrow activity before transplantation. In the *middle* is a scintigram of a patient with activity in the kidneys and borderline uptake within the marrow. On the *right* is a normal bone marrow scan in a patient after transplantation. Liver activity is seen in all three patterns, and splenic activity is seen in none. *(From McNeil BJ, Rappeport JM, Nathan DG. Indium chloride scintigraphy: an index of severity in patients with aplastic anaemia. Br J Haematol. 1976;34:599-604.)*

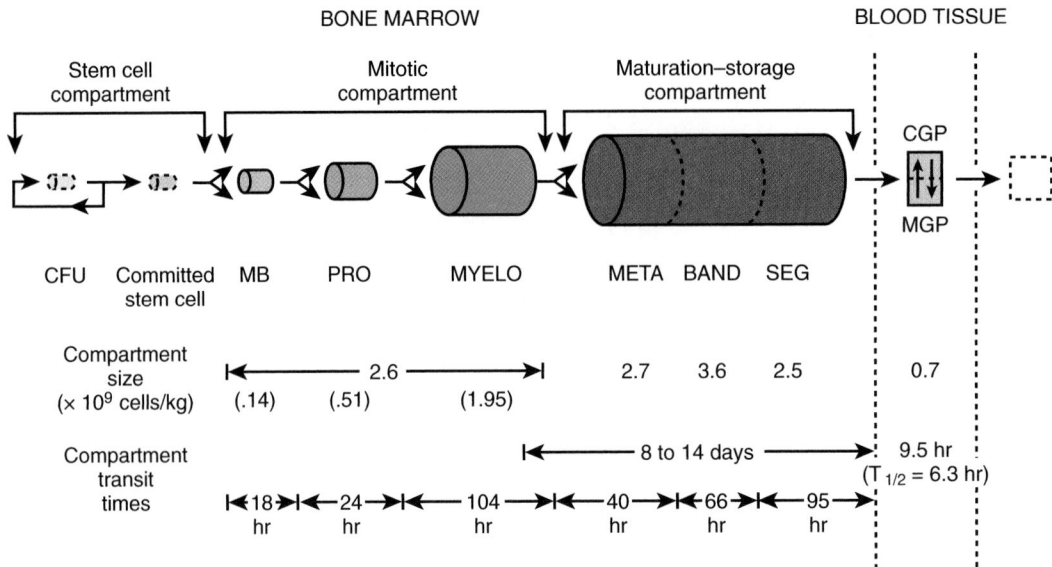

FIGURE 6-11. Model of the production and kinetics of neutrophils in humans. Marrow and blood compartments have been drawn to show their relative sizes. Compartment transit times, as derived from DF ^{32}P studies, are shown on the next to the last line. Values derived from titrated thymidine studies are shown on the last line. CFU, colony-forming unit; CGP, circulatory granulocyte pool; MGP, marginating granulocyte pool; MB, myeloblast; PRO, promyelocyte; MYELO, myelocyte; META, metamyelocyte; BAND, band form; SEG, segmented neutrophil. *(Redrawn from Wintrobe MM, Lee RG, Boggs DR, et al [eds]. Clinical Hematology, 7th ed. Philadelphia, Lea & Febiger, 1975, p 244.)*

TABLE 6-1	**Cytologic Characteristics of Megakaryocyte Maturation Stages**					
Stage	**Nuclear Morphology**	**Cytoplasmic Staining (Wright-Giemsa)**	**Approximate Size Range**	**Demarcation Membranes**	**Granules**	**Suggested Name**
I	Compact (lobed)	Basophilic	6-24 µm	Present by electron microscopy	Few present by electron microscopy	Megakaryoblast
II	Horseshoe	Pink center	14-30 µm	Proliferating to center of cell	Starting to increase	Promegakaryocyte
III	Multilobed	Increasingly more pink than blue	15-56 µm	Extensive but asymmetric	Great numbers	Granular megakaryocyte
IV	Compact but highly lobulated	Wholly eosinophilic	20-50 µm	Evenly distributed	Organized into "platelet field"	Mature megakaryocyte

Bone Marrow Examination and Megakaryocytopoiesis

Despite the fact that the morphology of megakaryocyte development is fairly well established (Fig. 6-12 and Table 6-1), bone marrow examination can be of limited value in the various platelet disorders. Bone marrow smears and biopsy sections provide insufficient data about thrombopoiesis because the final stage of platelet production, extrusion of cytoplasm into the sinusoid and shedding of platelets (to be described later), is not appreciated by these techniques; just the relative numbers of megakaryocytes and their size and ploidy can be determined by routine morphologic methods. It is not surprising that such information is only loosely correlated with platelet production (Fig. 6-13). Furthermore, sampling errors can be responsible for serious misinterpretations. This is a particular hazard with aspirates of neonatal marrow, in which megakaryocytes may be hard to detect regardless of whether platelet production is normal. Furthermore,

megakaryocytes are not evenly distributed in marrow smears. They are more readily found around the edges of the particles and may be mistaken for broken cells by an untrained observer. Megakaryocyte nuclei are often found lying free in marrow smears, where they may be erroneously scored as tumor cells. Biopsy sections provide more accurate assessment of megakaryocyte number and distribution than smears do, although the latter are usually sufficient (except in neonates) if examined carefully. Biopsy should not be attempted in neonates merely to define megakaryocytes; clinical judgment is a safer tool in these patients.

Examination of routine marrow smears and biopsy samples, though instructive, is limited by the two-dimensional views and thickness of the sections. Megakaryocytes have a peculiar predilection to lie next to the endothelial cell lining of the fronds of developing marrow cells, perhaps because TPO is produced by these cells. In general, megakaryocytes are too large to squeeze through

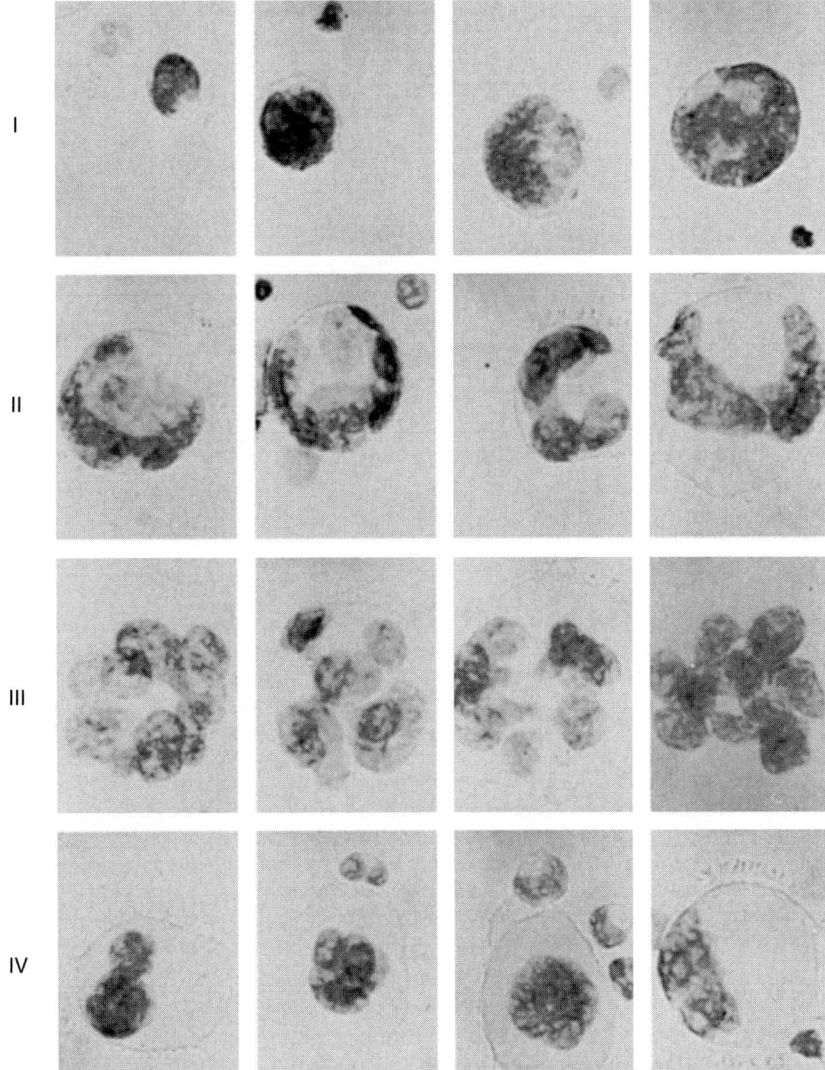

FIGURE 6-12. Photomicrographs of maturation stages of Feulgen-stained guinea pig megakaryocytes (all ×760). Each row illustrates representative nuclear configurations of maturation stages I, II, III, and IV. *(From Levine RF, Hazzard KC, Lamberg JD. The significance of megakaryocyte size. Blood. 1982;60:1122-1131.)*

the sinusoidal meshwork, so they merely push their cytoplasm through the fenestrations. These cytoplasmic structures, called proplatelets, serve as microtubule conduits for platelet packaging and release at sinusoids.[115] The protruding cytoplasm forms demarcation lines and then shatters into platelets, which are swept into blood, regulated in part by fibrinogen interacting with platelet $\alpha_{IIb}\beta_3$ integrin.[116] Megakaryocyte nuclei rarely make the transfenestration journey into the sinusoids and thence blood. If they do, they may be mistakenly interpreted by an unwary microscopist as tumor cells in the blood. Intact or partial megakaryocytes are regularly observed in the blood of patients with marrow-invasive diseases such as certain leukemias, metastatic cancers, granulomatous disorders, and fibrosis.

HEMATOPOIETIC GROWTH FACTORS

Since the pioneering work of Metcalf,[89] Sachs,[88] and their co-workers in the early 1960s, it has been recognized that

normal and leukemic blood progenitor cells can be propagated in culture in the presence of soluble protein growth factors. These factors were originally termed *colony-stimulating factors* based on their ability to support the formation of colonies of blood cells by bone marrow cells plated in semisolid medium.[117] During the 1970s and 1980s it was recognized that there are multiple types of CSFs based on the different types of blood cells found in the colonies that grew in the presence of the different factors, thus leading to the hypothesis that the growth and differentiation of different lineages of blood cells are controlled, at least in part, by exposure of progenitor cells to CSFs with different lineage specificities.[117-119] With molecular cloning of the genes for many of these factors and their receptors during the 1980s and 1990s it became possible to study in detail the structure, function, and biology of the recombinant CSFs, as well as the molecular biology of their respective genes.[117-122] This analysis, along with similar work on regulation of cells in the immune system, led to the realization that there exists a large number of interacting regulatory molecules now

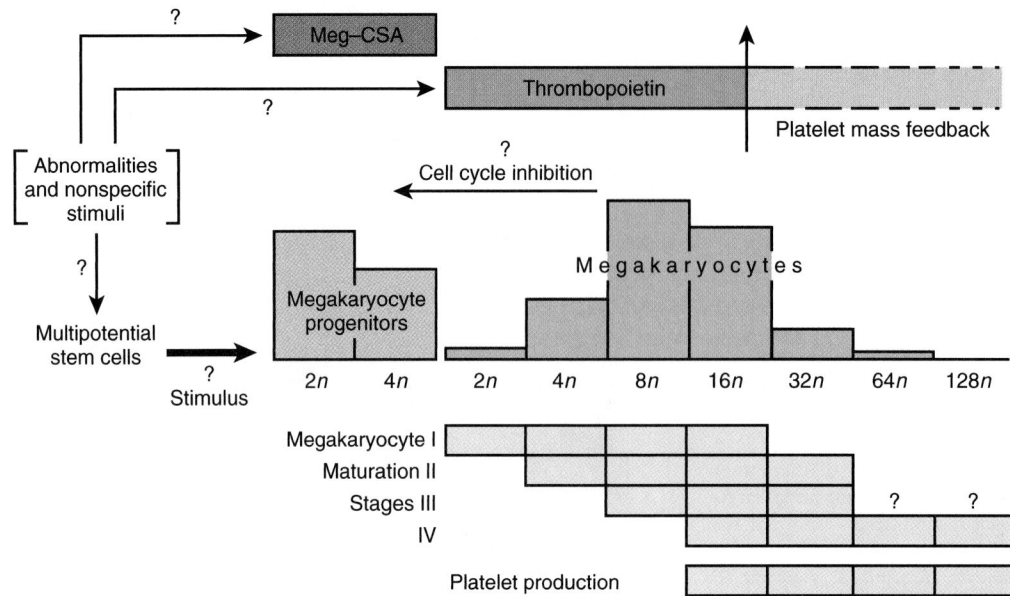

FIGURE 6-13. Thrombopoiesis. Shown *horizontally* in the center is the progression from uncommitted multipotential stem cells, through the proliferating progenitors detected in the in vitro clonogenic assays, to the spectrum of maturing megakaryocytes. The relative DNA levels of megakaryocytes and their precursors are given as ploidy values (*n*), where 2*n* is a diploid cell. The megakaryocytes are also presented *vertically* in terms of their maturation stages, with platelet shedding being the end stage; a detailed classification of these stages in given in Table 6-1 and Figure 6-16. The columns show the maturation stages at particular ploidy ranges. Thus, 4*n* megakaryocytes are found at maturation stages I and II. The *top* row shows a postulated two-level regulatory process with megakaryocyte colony-stimulating activity (Meg-CSA) primarily influencing the proliferation of progenitors and thrombopoietin required for megakaryocyte ploidy amplification and possibly for maturation. It is not certain that these regulators are completely exclusive in their target cell specificities as shown. Furthermore, no clear distinction is currently possible between the specific or nonspecific control of the two factors. Thrombopoietin production is sensitive to variations in platelet mass, as indicated in the figure; it is assumed that this feedback mechanism operates on the source of thrombopoietin. The progenitors might be controlled by cell cycle inhibition, perhaps as a consequence of normal numbers of megakaryocytes. *(Redrawn from Williams N, Levine RF. The origin, development and regulation of megakaryocytes. Br J Haematol. 1982;52:173-180.)*

generally known as cytokines or lymphohematopoietic cytokines that together serve to control the hematopoietic and immune systems and integrate the responses of these systems with those of many other physiologic systems.[120,123-126] These control molecules serve to regulate the growth, development, differentiation, activation, and trafficking of cells within the hematopoietic and immune systems. With elucidation of the sequence of most of the human genome in the final years of the 1990s, even more cytokine and growth factor genes have been discovered and have provided both new insight into how all these systems have evolved with common themes and further challenges to cell biologists in their attempt to understand the functions and interactions of all of the different molecules.

Cytokine gene families that contain at least one member that functions within the hematopoietic or immune system include the lymphohematopoietic cytokines (including many interleukins and CSFs)[117,122]; the receptor tyrosine kinase ligands CSF-1,[127] stem cell factor (SCF; also known as SF),[128] and the ligand for the Flks/Flt3 receptor (FL)[129]; the IL-1 gene family[130]; the chemokines[131]; the tumor necrosis factors (TNFs)[132]; the interferons[133]; the IL-10 gene family[134]; transforming growth factor β (TGF-β)[135]; and the IL-17 gene family.[136] We will briefly describe these families and molecules

among the family members selected as hematopoietic growth factors (HGFs) for further discussion.

Lymphohematopoietic Cytokines

For our purposes, the lymphohematopoietic cytokines are defined as protein ligands for members of the hematopoietin receptor gene family, also known as the cytokine receptor class I gene family.[137] This gene family is characterized by an extracellular domain with pairs of conserved cysteine residues and the distinctive amino acid sequence element Trp-Ser-Xaa-Trp-Ser (WSXWS).[138] These receptors all signal at least partly through the JAK-STAT (Janus kinase–signal transducer and activator of transcription) pathway.[139,140] This rather large family of hematopoietins now includes many interleukins[1] (IL-2, IL-3, IL-4, IL-5, IL-6, IL-7, IL-9, IL-11, IL-12, IL-13, IL-15, IL-21, and IL-23),[122,141-143] GM-CSF,[117,144] G-CSF,[145] EPO,[146] TPO,[147] thymic stromal thymopoietin (TSLP),[148-150] leukemia inhibitory factor (LIF),[151] oncostatin M (OSM), cardiotropin-1 (CT-1), and ciliary neurotrophic factor (CNTF).[152] The hematopoietin receptors on the cell surface signal as multimers, either homomeric or heteromeric, and the family can be further divided into subfamilies based on the molecular composition of their receptor complexes. The lymphohematopoietic cytokines with homodimeric receptors include EPO, TPO, and G-CSF.[122] A second subgroup consisting of GM-CSF, IL-3, and IL-5 in the human system has receptor complexes that share a common subunit known as the β_c chain that forms heterodimers with unique cytokine α subunits to provide selectivity for the respective cytokines.[122] A third group that includes IL-6, IL-11, LIF, OSM,[153] CNTF, and CT-1 all share a common receptor signaling chain known as gp130, but with unique chains that provide ligand specificity.[152] A fourth group of cytokines largely involved in lymphocyte development and activation, including IL-2, IL-4, IL-7, IL-9, IL-15, and IL-21,[154] share a hematopoietin receptor component known as the γ_c chain, originally identified as a component of IL-2R.[126] A fifth group, comprising IL-7 and TSLP, share the IL-7Rα chain,[155] and finally, IL-12 and IL-23, heterodimeric cytokines with a common subunit (p40) shared by each cytokine, also share the IL-12Rβ1 component.[143] Cytokines from the first two groups (EPO, TPO, G-CSF, GM-CSF, IL-3, and IL-5) all have predominant activities on the growth and differentiation of various myeloid cell populations and are traditionally included among the HGFs. Among the gp130 family of cytokines, IL-6 and IL-11 have multiple activities in different biologic systems but in addition, at least in vitro, play important roles in regulating myeloid cell growth and development, and therefore we will also consider them HGFs.[156] Although IL-4, IL-9, IL-12, and LIF display some activity as growth factors for myeloid cells, they all have prominent activity in other system as well and will not be considered further here.[122] The other interleukins, CNTF,[157] and CT-1 (the latter two of which act primarily outside the hematopoietic and immune systems) act predominantly on the growth, development, and activation of various lymphocyte populations, and although these activities are extremely important in controlling the immune system and possibly in indirectly controlling the hematopoietic system, we will leave them aside for simplicity and concentrate on the activity of the previously mentioned lymphohematopoietic HGFs.

Receptor Tyrosine Kinase Ligands

Three HGFs—macrophage CSF (M-CSF, also known as CSF-1[127]), SCF,[129,158] and FL[159]—have been identified that signal through related receptors, which themselves have tyrosine kinase activity.[129] The receptors for these HGFs are all evolutionarily related, as are the ligands themselves, and each plays an important role in controlling blood cell production.[160,161]

Interleukin-1 Gene Family

The IL-1[162,163] gene family has grown substantially and now includes at least IL-1α through IL-1χ, the IL-1 receptor antagonist (IL-1RA), and IL-18.[130,164] IL-1α, IL-1β, and IL-18 all have potent ability to induce cytokine production. IL-18, particularly in combination with

IL-12, induces interferon-γ [IFN-γ],[165] but IL-1α and IL-1β have also been shown to synergize with other HGFs in support of early blood cell proliferation and therefore will be considered further here.[166] The functions of the other novel members of the IL-1 gene family are still unknown.

Chemokines

The chemokines represent a large family of generally small proteins (usually 8 to 12 kd) that are readily identifiable by sequence homology, including characteristic twin cysteine residues near the amino-terminals, which separates the family into CC chemokines if the cysteines are adjacent or into CXC cytokines if they are separated by one residue.[131] Currently, more than 50 members of the gene family have been demonstrated to have important roles in cell trafficking in many systems. The receptor gene family for this cytokine family comprises about 20 members of the G protein–coupled receptor (GPCR) family. However, their biologic function is not limited to chemotaxis inasmuch as several have been shown to effect gene transcription, apoptosis, and cell proliferation. IL-8 is a prominent CXC chemokine that regulates neutrophil trafficking and is therefore a prominent player in inflammatory responses.[131] However, two chemokines, SDF-1 and macrophage inflammatory protein 1α (MIP-1α),[167] have been reported to inhibit the cycling of very early stem cells and hence may be important molecules in halting cycling stem cells and returning them to their normal, quiescent state. SDF-1 is clearly very interesting and important in the hematopoietic system as a chemotactic factor for very primitive stem cells; it provides a possible mechanism for homing of cells both as hematopoiesis moves from the fetal liver to the bone marrow and during transplantation of cells in adults.[168]

Tumor Necrosis Factors

The TNF gene family[137] now includes TNF-α, lymphotoxin α and β, CD27 ligand, CD30 ligand, CD40 ligand, Fas ligand, TRAIL, and Trance.[126] Many of these molecules are involved in regulating the activation and death of various cells, including T lymphocytes. TNF-α itself has many biologic activities, particularly in inflammation. However, it is mentioned here because of its potent and important role in promotion of dendritic cell differentiation and activation.[169,170]

Interferons

Type I interferons (13 species of IFN-α, IFN-β, and IFN-ω) are closely linked on human chromosome 9. The type II IFN-γ demonstrates little if any sequence homology with the type I interferons, but the receptors for all of these cytokines are members of cytokine receptor class 2, which is related to but distinct from cytokine receptor class 1 (hematopoeitin receptors) because they lack the distinctive WSXWS sequence.[171] In addition to their antiviral activities, both type I and type II interferons have multiple other regulatory activities with many cell types, including T cells. In the human system, type I interferons play a prominent role in polarizing helper T cells toward the type 1 (T_H1) phenotype.[126] However, none of these molecules appear to have prominent roles in directly controlling blood cell production and will not be considered further here.[133]

Transforming Growth Factor-β Gene Family

The TGF-β gene family is a large family of genes that includes TGF-β1, TGF-β2, and TGF-β3; bone morphogenetic proteins (BMPs) 2 through 16; growth and differentiation factor (GDF) genes 1 to 10; activin; and inhibin. Like many of the other cytokines, receptors for the TGF-β family members are multimers composed of two different members of the serine/threonine kinase receptor gene family.[135] Receptors with different ligand specificities are generated by combining these gene products in different groupings. TGF-β1 itself is a very important regulator of cell cycling in many cell systems, including the hematopoietic system, and will be considered here further as a negative regulator of hematopoiesis.[172,173] Mutations in its receptor cause the Loeys-Dietz syndrome.[174] The BMPs and GDFs have been implicated in many developmental systems, but interestingly, BMP-4 has been shown to be essential in *Xenopus* for embryonic development of HSCs, and it seems at least possible that this molecule might play a role in mammals as well in blood cell development during embryogenesis, if not in adult hematopoiesis, an area worth following. However, for our purposes, we will include only TGF-β1 itself as an HGF for simplicity's sake.

Action of Hematopoietic Growth Factors

Predominantly Lineage-Specific Hematopoietic Growth Factors: GM-CSF, M-CSF, IL-5, TPO, and EPO

Early on it was recognized that different CSFs could selectively support the growth of specific types of hematopoietic colonies.[117] Thus, when human bone marrow cells are cultured in semisolid medium in the presence of G-CSF, 7 to 8 days later colonies emerge that consist largely of mature neutrophilic granulocytes and their precursors.[145] This led to the model that G-CSF to a large degree interacts with relatively late hematopoietic progenitors that have already committed to the neutrophil lineage (CFU-G) and serves to support their growth and final maturation into functional neutrophils.[145] Similar analysis has revealed that the other major hematopoietic cell lineages have analogous lineage-specific late-acting factors and that these molecules frequently serve as important, if not primary regulators of the respective pathways. Thus, M-CSF supports monocyte/macrophage

colony growth and is important in supporting the growth and maturation of monocyte progenitors (CFU-M)[127]; IL-5 supports eosinophilic granulocyte colony formation and therefore supports the growth and maturation of eosinophil progenitors (CFU-Eo), as well as activating eosinophils[175,176]; EPO is necessary for the growth and maturation of both earlier (BFU-E) and later (CFU-E) progenitors of the erythroid lineage[146]; and TPO directly supports the growth and maturation of megakaryocyte progenitors (CFU-Meg) and the subsequent production of functional platelets.[147,177]

Although regulation of the respective blood cell pathways by the lineage-specific HGFs is likely to be their major function, in no case is this lineage specificity absolutely maintained. G-CSF has been found to influence the migration and proliferation of endothelial cells, cells that express high-affinity receptors for this cytokine.[178] IL-5 serves as a growth factor for activated B cells, particularly in the mouse, and affects the type of immunoglobulin secreted by mature B cells.[179] EPO[180] and TPO[181] have been noted to interact with megakaryocyte and erythroid progenitors, respectively. M-CSF appears to be important in trophoblast development.[127] Finally, populations of early HSCs have been found to express receptors for many cytokines; typically, these cells do not respond to single factors but require combinations of factors to trigger them into cycle.[182,183] "Lineage-specific" factors that have been reported to act in various combinations to trigger cycling of early "stem" cells include G-CSF,[184] M-CSF,[185] and TPO,[186] thus demonstrating that the molecules are not strictly "lineage specific," even within the hematopoietic system. Mice deficient in either the TPO receptor (mpl) or G-CSF are deficient in levels of all progenitor cells, consistent with the idea that these factors are indeed involved in expansion of early-lineage cells.[121] However, when administered in vivo, each of these molecules largely influences the growth and development of the expected lineage, and the designation of lineage specificity therefore seems warranted.

Multilineage Hematopoietic Growth Factors: IL-3 and GM-CSF

Initial analysis of human bone marrow cell cultures grown in the presence of GM-CSF revealed that a variety of different colony types develop over a period of 10 to 14 days.[187] Mature blood cells that could be readily identified included neutrophils, monocytes/macrophages, and eosinophils. This led to designation of the molecule as a "granulocyte-macrophage" colony-stimulating factor, or GM-CSF. When compared with G-CSF, it was found that GM-CSF took longer to produce colonies with identifiable neutrophils, but the ultimate variety of cell types was greater. This led to a model in which GM-CSF acts on progenitors committed to produce either neutrophils or monocytes (CFU-GM), which is a precursor to the G-CSF–responsive CFU-G and the M-CSF–responsive CFU-M.[117,187] These later progenitors apparently retain responsiveness to GM-CSF as well because mature monocytes and neutrophils can be observed in cultures supported by GM-CSF alone. That this model is not strictly correct was shown when recombinant GM-CSF was introduced into human bone marrow cultures in the presence of EPO and it was found that this combination of factors was very effective in supporting the development of erythroid colonies (murine GM-CSF is somewhat less effective in this regard).[188,189] Thus, despite its name, GM-CSF generally interacts with intermediate multilineage progenitors that yield neutrophils, eosinophils, monocytes, erythroid cells, and megakaryocytes (CFU-GEMM). At the time, these activities were similar to those ascribed to IL-3 in the murine system.[190] When human IL-3 was identified, it proved to be able to support multilineage colony formation similar to human GM-CSF, thus indicating that it interacts with slightly different but strongly overlapping subsets of progenitors.[191,192] When compared with GM-CSF, IL-3 is somewhat more effective in supporting multilineage, erythroid, and megakaryocyte colony formation, and GM-CSF is slightly more effective in mediating granulocyte and monocyte/macrophage colony formation.[191,192] In serum-free conditions, the ability of IL-3 to support final neutrophil and monocyte maturation is significantly depressed, thus indicating that later-acting factors, G-CSF or GM-CSF in the case of neutrophils or M-CSF or GM-CSF in the case of monocytes, are necessary for final end cell production.[193]

In addition to acting slightly earlier than GM-CSF, IL-3 is clearly distinguished in its activity by its ability to support the growth and maturation of mast cells and basophils.[194,195] In the mouse, this was one of the first recognized activities of IL-3,[190] and when first administered to primates, basophilia was one of the most prominent findings.[195,196] Hence, IL-3 appears to be capable of supporting the growth and development of basophil and mast cell progenitors. In the human system, both IL-3 and GM-CSF can support the development and differentiation of dendritic cells of either myeloid or lymphoid origin, especially in combination with SCF, FL, and TNF.[197-199]

IL-4 in mice and humans has also been reported to support multilineage colony formation, including colonies that contain cells from the erythroid, megakaryocytic, neutrophilic, and monocytic lineages.[200-202] IL-4 in the mouse supports mast cell growth and therefore shares many activities with IL-3.[179] However, IL-4 plays very important roles in the development and maturation of T and B cells,[179,202,203] particularly in the polarization of cytokine production by helper T cells toward the type 2 (T_H2) response.[204] Therefore, on balance IL-4 is likely to be more important in controlling immune cell development and function and will not be discussed further here. IL-9 in both the murine and human systems has been shown to enhance erythroid colony formation in the presence of EPO[205] and appears to play a role in T- and B-cell development as well.[206] More recently, IL-9 has been shown to have some effects on the growth and activation

of mast cells and may play some role in the pathology of asthma.[207]

Early-Acting Hematopoietic Growth Factors: SCF and FL

SCF[128,129,158] and FL,[159,208,209] both receptor tyrosine kinase ligands, interact with a variety of hematopoietic progenitor cells, perhaps most importantly with very early stem cell populations. SCF also plays an important role in melanocyte growth and development, which is reflected in the coat color effects of mutations in SCF or its receptor c-kit.[128] Genetic analysis of mice clearly shows that mice defective in either SCF (*Sl* mice) or c-kit (*W* mice) have serious hematopoietic (and many other) defects, including macrocytic anemia, mast cell deficiencies, and deficiencies in the stem cell compartment (reviewed by Galli and colleagues[128]). These early studies had already indicated the critical importance of SCF in the survival and development of stem cells. Mutations in the human c-kit gene lead to a similar phenotype in melanocyte development in humans known as the piebald mutation; however, these patients do not have any hematologic problems, probably because severe mutations in this locus are likely to be lethal.[210] In vitro, the activities of SCF are generally most evident when combined with other HGFs; its proliferative activity when used with hematopoietic cells in culture as a single factor is minimal.[128] In fact, culture of murine bone marrow cells with SF alone ultimately yields largely mast cells.[211] However, SF acts synergistically to enhance the activities of most of the other HGFs in culture and is particularly effective when combined with HGFs such as IL-3, IL-1, or IL-11 in promoting the expansion of "blast"-like cells that retain considerable potential for yielding multilineage colonies in secondary culture.[212-214] These colonies, when replated under conditions that support B-lymphocyte development or when transplanted into animals, also yield B and T lymphocytes, thus indicating that SCF-responsive cells include primitive stem cells with both lymphoid and myeloid potential.[215,216] SCF has also been implicated in combination with IL-2 or IL-7 in early stages of T-cell development in the thymus,[217] with IL-7 in pre-B-cell growth,[218] and with IL-7 in enhancing natural killer (NK) cell responsiveness to IL-2.[128] However, that none of these lineages are dramatically affected in *W* or *Sl* mice indicates that SCF-independent mechanisms can compensate in these systems.

SCF,[219] M-CSF,[220] and FL[161] are all expressed as both membrane-bound and soluble forms. In the case of SCF, expression of membrane-bound forms of the molecule in the marrow microenvironment provides a nice model for how this growth factor might act locally. Indeed, cell lines that express exclusively membrane-associated SCF are much more effective in supporting long-term hematopoiesis in vitro than are cell lines that exclusively produce soluble forms of the molecule.[219] This interaction of membrane-associated SCF with c-kit provides one mechanism for the adherence of hematopoietic cells to stroma in that binding of human megakaryocytes to fibroblasts can be blocked by antibodies to c-kit.[221] Finally, membrane-associated forms of SCF in which the cytoplasmic domain is essentially missing results in male but not female sterility, thus suggesting that the cytoplasmic domain may have an as yet undetermined important biologic function.[128,222]

As shown by early genetic studies and confirmed through analysis of the recombinant protein, SCF is not specific for the hematopoietic system. It is also an important growth factor for melanocytes and primordial germ cells, and it appears to play a role in development of the nervous system, perhaps as a neuronal guidance factor, although it has been difficult to demonstrate neurologic defects in *W* or *Sl* mice.[128]

The Flt3 receptor tyrosine kinase was originally identified as a novel receptor present in HSCs; in human marrow, expression is largely limited to the CD34$^+$ cell population.[223-225] FL alone yields low numbers of CFU-GM from human bone marrow but acts synergistically with other cytokines, including IL-3, GM-CSF, EPO, and SCF, to yield enhanced colony formation in terms of both size and number of colonies.[208,226,227] The synergy observed between FL and the other HGFs is comparable to that observed with SCF in similar systems, with the exception that FL has little effect on BFU-E.[209] Multifactor combinations with SCF have been used for expansion of CFCs in long-term cultures; FL has effects comparable to those of SCF when combined with IL-1, IL-3, IL-6, and EPO in 4-week cultures.[228,229] Like SCF, FL in combination with other cytokines such as GM-CSF supports dendritic cell development from CD34$^+$ bone marrow cells.[197] In contrast to SCF, FL does not support the growth and development of mast cells.[208,226] Despite this overlap in bioactivities, mice in which the Flt3 receptor tyrosine kinase has been disrupted appear to have normal hematopoiesis, with the only detectable defects being observed within the B-lymphocyte lineage.[230] However, mice with disruption of both the c-kit and Flt3 receptor tyrosine kinase genes display more severe hematologic complications than do mice with either single mutation, thus suggesting that the two pathways can to some degree compensate for one another.[230] The importance of Flt3 ligand in B-cell growth has also been shown with cultures of primitive B-cell progenitors (CD43$^+$B220^{low}) in combination with either IL-7 or SF.[231] Altogether, these findings argue for an important role for Flt3 ligand in hematopoiesis.

Other Stem Cell Factors: Wnt, Jagged, BMP, and Angiopoietin-like Growth Factors

Several new growth factors have been shown to regulate HSC production during embryogenesis, as well as adulthood. The Wnt family of factors regulates stem cell homeostasis.[232-238] Overexpression of Wnt 3a led to a threefold expansion of HSCs. This is the first time that stem cell number was actually increased in a competitive repopulation assay. In separate experiments, overexpression of β-catenin led to an expansion of HSCs, and sorting by activated β-catenin in HSCs based on a Wnt reporter line that turned cells green when Wnt is activated demonstrated HSC activity. Further studies in chronic myelocytic leukemia demonstrated that Wnt activation was present in leukemia.[239] These studies showed that Wnt activity could drive HSC production; however, other experiments have demonstrated that knockout of β-catenin within HSCs is not required for stem cell homeostasis.[240] Two recent papers demonstrated that constitutively activated β-catenin in HSCs leads to aplastic anemia.[241,242] Activation of the Wnt pathway may not be necessary for stem cell homeostasis, but it may be sufficient to drive HSCs to produce more self-renewal cell divisions.

The Wnt pathway clearly interfaces with HSC production. It is possible that pulses of Wnt will have different activity than a constitutively active Wnt signal. In addition, redundancy within the marrow space among other signaling pathways, including the Notch and BMP pathways, have left the stem cell compartment with significant chances of survival. Wnt acts through canonical and noncanonical pathways. In the former case this leads to activation of β-catenin to the nucleus through the complex involving adenomatous polyposis coli and β-catenin. In the latter, there is stem cell activation by the Rho guanosine triphosphatases (GTPases). Wnt activation acts at multiple places during hematopoiesis, both at the stem cell level and at the pre-B level, as well as at multiple places in T-cell development. Wnt factors bind to canonical Frizzled receptors and activate a signaling pathway. An antagonist Wnt signal, Wnt 5a, suppresses B-cell proliferation and may act to suppress stem cell homeostasis. Other Wnt factors have been found to regulate hematopoiesis, including Wnt 2b and Wnt 10b for human bone marrow CD34$^+$ cells.

The Notch pathway has been shown to regulate HSC production based on retroviral transduction of hematopoietic cells.[243,244] This expands the population of HSCs significantly. Notch works through a ligand-receptor interaction in which Deltas and Jaggeds are presented on the stem cell niche. In general, Jagged2 is thought to be the predominant Notch ligand in marrow and is presented by the osteoblast. Modulation of Jagged2 leads to expansion of HSC production. The Notch pathway has been put into a genetic pathway with Runx1 based on the zebra fish mutant mindbomb.[245] Mindbomb mutants have no Notch signaling because of a defect in an E3 ubiquitin ligase that promotes ligand recycling. This mutant lacks HSCs during development, and overexpression of Runx1 rescues hematopoiesis. A pulse of Notch signaling has been shown to expand HSCs in the zebra fish system. Furthermore, Runx1 rescue of Notch1 mutants was demonstrated in the mouse system, and it was also shown that GATA-2 was a target of the Notch pathway.[246,247] Modulation of Wnt and Notch demonstrates synergy of Wnt 3a and activation of the Notch pathway. It is possible to activate Wnt pathways with the chemical called BIO drug, which is an inhibitor of glycogen synthase kinase 3β (GSK3β). Thus modulation of the Wnt and Notch pathways plays a significant role in stem cell homeostasis.

The BMP family has been demonstrated to induce HSC production in the *Xenopus* and zebra fish systems.[248-255] This leads to expansion of erythroid blood islands during early development. Interestingly, a dominant-negative version of BMP activated later in development leads to enhanced erythropoiesis, thus demonstrating two independent effects of BMP regulation of HSC differentiation and proliferation. Furthermore, BMP has recently been shown to expand HSC production in the AGM region. BMP was shown to expand or maintain HSC production in human ES cells and functions as a key regulator of stress-induced erythropoiesis.[256] BMP also regulates the stem cell niche. It is unclear how BMP and the Notch and Wnt pathways interact.

Angiopoietin-related proteins are potent activators of HSC production.[257] For example, angiopoietin-like 2 and angiopoietin-like 3 were shown to lead to a 20- or 30-fold expansion of long-term HSCs when cultured for 10 days in the presence of the ligands. This was demonstrated by a limiting-dilution competitive repopulation assay. Thus, angiopoietin-like genes must also participate in the stem cell niche. Another growth factor glycoprotein called osteopontin is also involved in stem cell homeostasis and negatively regulates the stem cell pools.[258,259] A number of factors, including TGF-β1, also demonstrate negative regulation. Ligands produced by the stem cells themselves may also regulate stem cell homeostasis.

Synergistic Factors: IL-1, IL-6, and IL-11

Early in the 1980s, factors were identified that had the ability to enhance hematopoietic colony formation supported by other HGFs, particularly early progenitor cells. One factor, designated hematopoietin 1, was subsequently purified and discovered to be IL-1.[185] In this fashion, IL-1 was recognized as having little ability on its own to stimulate hematopoietic colony formation but can act in synergy with other HGFs, notably IL-3, to increase both the frequency of colony formation and the number of cells per colony.[166] Subsequent to discovery of the synergistic activity of IL-1, numerous other cytokines have emerged with similar activity, including IL-6,[260] IL-11,[261] LIF,[262] and IL-12.[263] Of these, IL-6, IL-11, and LIF all signal through a common signal-transducing molecule, the gp130 component of IL-6R.[264] Because these molecules are likely to behave similarly in most systems and because IL-6 and IL-11 have been the most thoroughly studied, we will limit our discussion to these two members of this family. IL-12, which signals through a distinct but perhaps similar pathway to gp130,[265] has interesting effects in combinations with other cytokines[263] but appears to be more important in regulating the development and activities of T and NK cells[266,267] and will therefore not be discussed further here.

The effects of IL-1 on hematopoiesis have been highly complicated by the fact that this cytokine is a potent inducer of secondary cytokine production, frequently by accessory cells in the culture.[268] The induction of other growth factors, notably IL-6, G-CSF, GM-CSF, and IL-11, is likely to contribute to the activity of IL-1 as a synergistic factor in hematopoietic colony formation. Nevertheless, combinations of IL-1 with other factors in cultures of highly purified hematopoietic cells typically yield synergistic effects, thus suggesting that at least some of the effects are direct.[269,270] However, even with highly purified hematopoietic progenitor cell populations, the effects of IL-1 can be indirect. For example, Rodriguez and co-authors reported that IL-1 can prevent the apoptotic death of CD34+lin− human bone marrow cells but that the effect is largely abrogated by antibodies to GM-CSF, which suggests that some progenitor cells in the population can produce their own GM-CSF.[271] Consequently, the survival effect of IL-1 in some systems may also be indirectly mediated by induction of GM-CSF expression in CD34+lin− bone marrow cells themselves.

IL-6 is an extremely pleiotropic cytokine with important effects on the growth and differentiation of T and B cells, on induction of the hepatic acute phase response, and on enhancement of the proliferation of hematopoietic progenitor cells.[223] IL-6 signaling, mediated by two members of the hematopoietin receptor gene family, IL-6R[272] and gp130,[273] was the first example of signaling through a commonly shared receptor subunit, gp130, which is now known to be involved in the signaling of LIF, IL-11, OSM, CNTF, and CT-1.[264,274] Because most cells express gp130, expression of other receptor components such as IL-6R or IL-11R generally determines whether a cell will respond to one of these family members; cells that express receptors for multiple members of this cytokine subgroup generally exhibit identical or nearly identical responses to each member whose receptor component is expressed by the cell.[152,264,275]

The HGF activity of IL-6 was recognized when the cDNA for this cytokine was cloned by functional expression cloning from a human T-cell line that produced weak colony-stimulating activity that supported modest CFU-GM colony formation with murine bone marrow target cells.[276] More detailed analysis of the murine system and subsequently the human system led to the realization that IL-6 has little if any ability to support colony formation on its own but can enhance colony formation when supported by other HGFs, particularly IL-3 and SCF.[212,260] This effect was most prominent with bone marrow cells from mice isolated 2 days after treatment with 5-FU, a drug that enriches for primitive progenitors by selectively killing later, actively cycling cells in the bone marrow.[182] Bone marrow cells treated in this fashion generally yield significant numbers of colonies only when plated in the presence of multiple HGFs. In this system, IL-6 was found to enhance colony formation when supported by IL-3 or SCF. These early cells are typically quiescent in the G_0 phase of the growth cycle, and combined effects of cytokines, such as IL-3 and IL-6, are required to push them into active cycling.[182] Similar effects have been observed in cultures of purified early human hematopoietic progenitor cells.[277]

IL-11 was originally identified as a stimulatory factor for a murine hybridoma cell line,[278] but characterization in various hematopoietic cell culture systems soon revealed a much broader spectrum of biologic effects.[279,280] Evaluation of the various properties of IL-11 led to the realization that the IL-11R complex uses the IL-6 gp130 signal-transducing system. These two HGFs appear to have somewhat overlapping biologic activities.[281] In general, IL-6 has proved to have more effects on T and B cells than IL-11 does[223,280] and similar effects on the hepatic acute phase response[282] and on osteoclast formation,[283] but IL-11 is somewhat more potent in megakaryocytopoiesis.[284] Like IL-6, the effects of IL-11 in hematopoietic cultures are largely observed only when combined with other factors. IL-11 in combination with SCF or FL has proved to be very effective in supporting the growth of primitive hematopoietic progenitors.[227] Early after its discovery, IL-11 was shown to have important effects on the growth and development of megakaryocyte progenitors.[280,284,285] Again, in this system IL-11 had little effect on colony formation on its own but was found to act in synergy with IL-3, with SCF, or more recently, with TPO in supporting CFU-Meg colony formation.[286]

Negative Regulator of Hematopoiesis: TGF-β

A variety of cytokines have been reported to reversibly inhibit cycling of early hematopoietic cells, including the chemokines SDF-1[208] and MIP-1α,[167] as well as TGF-β, perhaps the most potently of all.[287-289] Very interestingly, when individual early cells were plated in wells, either antibody to TGF-β1 or an antisense oligonucleotide to the mRNA for this factor could trigger the release of cells from quiescence in the presence of appropriate combinations of early-acting cytokines, which by themselves failed to trigger cycling of the cells.[288,289]

MOLECULAR BIOLOGY OF THE HEMATOPOIETIC GROWTH FACTORS

Genomic Analysis of Cytokine and Cytokine Receptor Genes

From analysis of the human genome, several common themes and relationships have emerged from the different types of cytokine/growth factor and receptor genes. First, as already noted, most of the cytokines and their receptors exist as members of distinct evolutionarily related gene families; examples of single cytokine or growth factor genes with no relatives are rare. Similarly, the receptors also fall into gene families. Thus, a relatively

small number of primordial growth factor/cytokine genes were duplicated many times to form families of genes that evolved into serving regulatory functions for many different systems. As already discussed, members of the cytokines that signal through the gp130 receptor component are important regulators in many different systems, including embryonic development, the central nervous system, the myocardium, and the hematopoietic and the immune systems.[193] That different physiologic systems share cytokines and receptor components from common gene families gives us more assurance that lessons learned from the relatively accessible hematopoietic system will at least provide guidance as we begin to dissect other systems. Interestingly, in most cases each of the individual cytokines of a particular gene family use members of a single receptor gene family. For example, all of the chemokines use G protein–coupled receptors as their signaling/recognition molecules,[131] whereas all members of the TGF-β gene family use different combinations of serine/threonine kinase receptors as their recognition and signaling molecules.[135] All these receptor-ligand pairs must have evolved in concert as they were selected to control different cellular processes.

Despite the obvious gene duplications that have occurred in all these gene families, there is no absolute rule regarding how the genes are arranged today. In some cases, the related genes are still closely linked in tandem in the genome, as is the case for the IL-3 and GM-CSF genes on chromosome 5 at 5q31.1 (Fig. 6-14). In this case, another duo of related genes, IL-4 and IL-13, are very closely linked to one another but slightly more separated from the IL-3/GM-CSF cluster. Similarly, in the case of the IL-10 gene family, several of the members are closely linked at 1q32 (IL-10, IL-19, IL-20, MDA-7), whereas IL-22 and AK155 are linked at 12q15 (MDA, AK195),[290] another example in which genes have either been split out of a tandem array on one chromosome during recombination or have migrated from the original site of the primordial gene and subsequently undergo further gene duplication and separate evolution events.

Structures of the Hematopoietic Growth Factor Proteins

The availability of cDNA for the individual cytokines allowed rapid determination of their primary amino acid sequence, expression in quantities large enough for direct x-ray determination of their crystal structure, and more broadly, prediction of structures based on those of proteins related even distantly by sequence. One of the clear results of analysis of the structures of the different cytokines was the realization that despite generally low conservation of amino acid sequence, many of the lymphohematopoietic cytokines are distantly related in evolution. Most of the lymphohematopoietic cytokines are believed to assume a tightly packed, antiparallel, four–α-helix bundled structure with either short or long

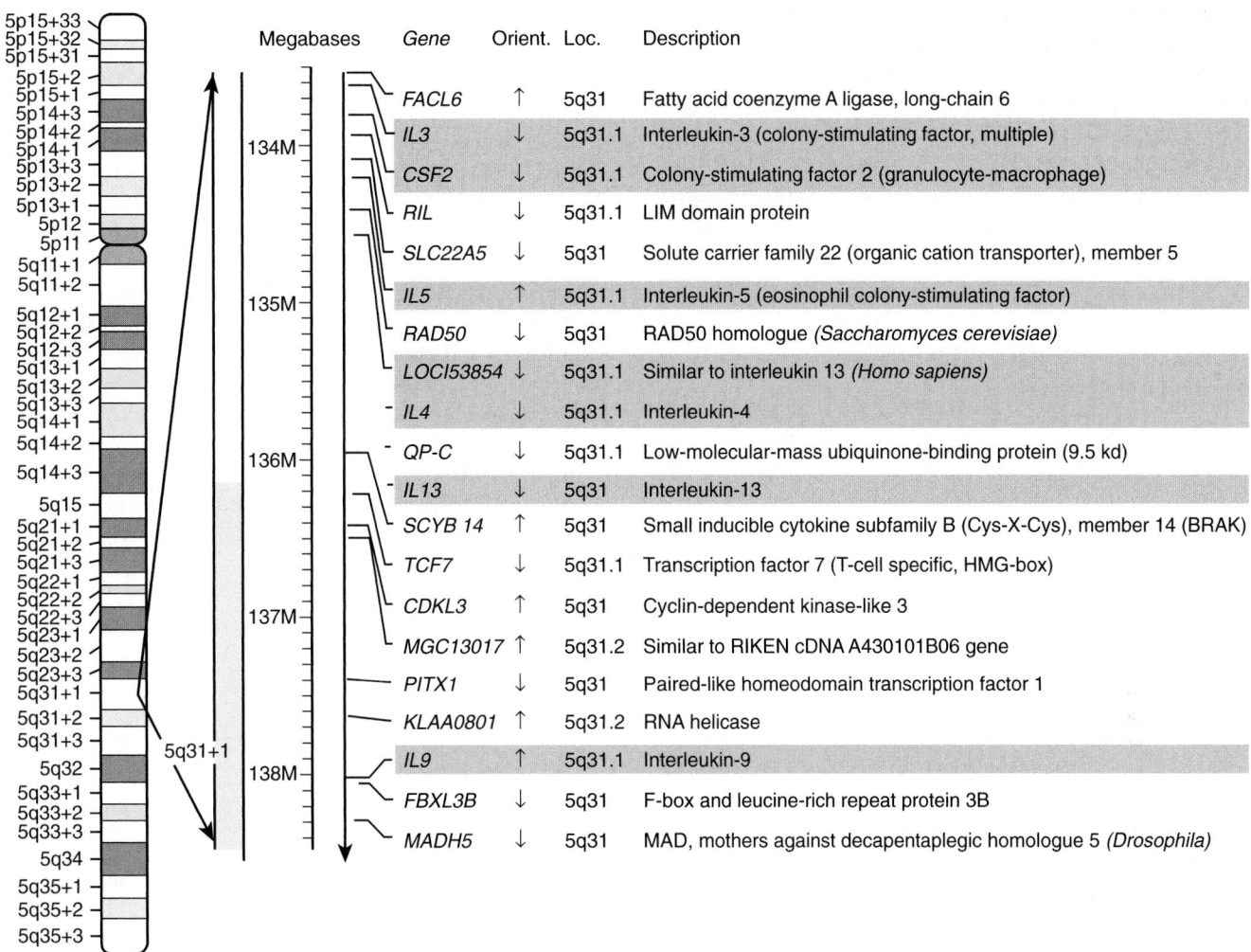

FIGURE 6-14. Cytokine gene cluster at 5q31.1. The region from chromosome 5, which consists of 5 megabases of DNA sequence, is expanded as shown, with the structures of the individual genes, GenBank notations, descriptions, and gene orientations indicated. The region contains approximaley 115 genes, 21 of which are illustrated. The data were collected and assembled from the National Center for Biotechnology Information database.

helical bundles.[122,126] Lymphohematopoietins with the short helical bundle structure include IL-2, IL-3, IL-4, IL-5, IL-7, IL-9, IL-13, IL-15, and GM-CSF. Cytokines with long helical structures include the gp130 signaling proteins IL-6, IL-11, LIF, and OSM; IL-12p35; and the homodimeric receptor signaling proteins EPO, TPO, and G-CSF.[122,177,291] With the exception of IL-12, which is a covalently linked heterodimer of two chains, designated p40 and p35,[267] all these cytokines are believed to act as monomers.

Sequence and structural information suggests that the long helical bundle–structured cytokines are all distantly related in evolution. Members of the IL-6 subfamily, including IL-6, IL-11, and G-CSF, show rather modest sequence similarity but display common gene organization and certain structural features that suggest evolutionary relatedness.[125,291,292] Sequence alignment of IL-6 and G-CSF shows conservation of cysteine residues.[293] Interestingly, a cytokine identified in the chicken, myelomonocytic growth factor (MGF),[294] displays

sequence similarities with G-CSF and IL-6, which suggests that all three are derived from a common ancestral gene. EPO shows some structural features similar to growth hormone and to G-CSF, but at a very low level.[291] In contrast, the amino-terminal half of TPO shows strong sequence similarity with EPO, whereas the carboxy-terminal half is unrelated to any known protein.[295-297] The four–helical bundle structure of EPO is clearly related to the amino-terminal helically structured portion of TPO, whereas the additional domain of TPO, which is heavily glycosylated, may serve to increase the serum half-life of the molecule. Both these family members are believed to act as monomers.

Ligands for the receptor tyrosine kinase gene family members SCF, FL, and M-CSF share many common structural similarities.[128,161,298] All three contain transmembrane domains and are initially synthesized as homodimeric integral membrane proteins. Although the membrane-bound forms are functional, dimeric soluble forms released from the cell by proteolysis also display biologic activity. The extracellular domains have low but significant sequence similarity, including conservation of the position of the cysteine residues involved in disulfide bridge formation.[161] Modeling of these extracellular domains indicates that they, too, are likely to form four–α-helix bundle structures tethered to the membrane through variable spacer domains with dimerization through a cysteine located in the spacer domain.[122,160,161]

Hematopoietic Growth Factor Gene Disruptions

Hematopoietin Receptor Ligands

G-CSF

The combination of technology for regenerating mice from cultured ES cells and the ability to selectively disrupt genes in cultured mammalian cells has led to methodology for studying gene function in vivo (mutants related to HGFs are summarized in Table 6-2).[318] Using this approach, Lieschke and co-workers[313] were able to generate mice with both copies of the G-CSF gene disrupted. These animals develop normally but as adults display a 70% to 80% reduction in levels of circulating neutrophils, a 50% reduction in the number of progenitors in all lineages, and impaired resistance to challenge by infection with *Listeria monocytogenes*. These findings, which are in agreement with earlier observations by Hammond and colleagues[319] in dogs that had developed cross-reacting antibodies to canine G-CSF, demonstrate a central role for G-CSF in controlling neutrophil levels. However, the decline in all populations of progenitors is consistent with a role for G-CSF before commitment to the neutrophil lineage, perhaps at the early stem cell stage as suggested by the synergy of G-CSF and SCF in generating blast cell colonies.[156,320]

TABLE 6-2   Genetic Defects in Receptors or Signaling Proteins

HUMAN MUTATIONS

Gene	Mutation	Phenotype	Reference
IL-2Rγ$_c$	Deletion	SCID	299
JAK3	Deletion	SCID	300
G-CSFR	C-terminal deletion	Kostmann's disease	301
EPOR	C-terminal deletion	Benign erythrocytosis	302

NONHUMAN MUTATIONS

Species	Gene	Name	Phenotype	Reference
Mouse	c-kit	White-spotting	Macrocytic anemia, mast cell deficiency, lack of pigmentation, sterile	303-305
	Steel factor	Steel	Macrocytic anemia, mast cell deficiency, lack of pigmentation, sterile	303-305
	CSF-1	Microphthalmia	Osteopetrosis secondary to decreased osteoclast function	306
	HCP	Motheaten	Immunodeficiency, autoimmune disease, increased sensitivity to erythropoietin	307
Drosophila	JAK homologue	Hopscotch	TumL allele is a gain-of-function mutation that causes leukemia	308, 309

TARGETED DISRUPTION IN MURINE EMBRYONIC STEM CELLS

Gene	Phenotype	Reference
IL-6	Decreased CFU-S and stem cell function	310
GM-CSF	Hematopoiesis normal; progressive accumulation of pulmonary surfactant	311, 312
G-CSF	Neutrophils 25% normal; impaired response to *Listeria monocytogenes* infection	313
EPO	Embryonic lethal—failure of definitive erythropoiesis	314
EPOR	Embryonic lethal—failure of definitive erythropoiesis	314
TPOR (c-mpl)	Platelets 15-20% normal	315
IL-3Rβ	Normal hematopoiesis	316
IL-3/IL-5/GMRβ$_c$	Similar to GM-CSF$^{-/-}$ mice; also low eosinophils and impaired eosinophil response to *Nippostrongylus brasiliensis*	316
Vav	Not required for hematopoiesis	317

CFU-S, colony-forming unit–spleen; CSF-1, colony-stimulating factor 1; EPO, erythropoietin; EPOR, erythropoietin receptor; G-CSFR, granulocyte colony-stimulating factor receptor; GM-CSFR, granulocyte-macrophage colony-stimulating factor receptor; HCP, hematopoietic cell phosphatase; IL, interleukin; JAK, Janus kinase; SCID, X-linked severe combined immunodeficiency; TPOR, thrombopoietin receptor.

EPO and TPO

The TPO and EPO genes have clearly evolved from a common ancestor, and at some point the extra protein-coding region found in the final coding exon of the TPO gene was either removed (in the case of the EPO gene) or added (in the case of the TPO gene) after the early duplication event.

Mice with deletion of either the TPO or the c-mpl gene have been described.[315,321] Although these animals develop normally and do not display significant abnormalities in bleeding times, they have only 15% to 20% of normal levels of circulating platelets. This result implies that TPO is very important for maintaining circulating levels of platelets but that other cytokines might have some capacity to generate platelets at low levels. Interestingly, through an elegant study of various combinations of receptor gene disruptions, Gainsford and associates[322,323] have shown that cytokines with megakaryocyte-stimulating activity in culture, including IL-3, IL-6, IL-11, and LIF, play no role in basal platelet production in mice with the *mpl* gene disruption.

In the case of EPO, gene disruption results in embryonic lethality because of failure of fetal liver erythropoiesis.[314]

IL-6–gp130 Complex Ligands: IL-6 and IL-11

Animals that have been engineered to lack the IL-6 gene develop normally but display significant deficiencies in various immune and inflammatory responses.[324] Interestingly, the hepatic acute phase response in these animals is severely compromised after tissue damage, but only moderately in response to lipopolysaccharide (LPS). The effects of disruption of the IL-6 gene on normal hematopoiesis are relatively minor: a slight decrease in peripheral blood leukocyte counts, a 10% reduction in bone marrow cellularity, a 50% reduction in CFU-S$_{12}$, and fourfold to fivefold reduction in pre-CFU-S.[310] This relatively minor effect of disruption of the IL-6 gene on hematopoiesis points out the difficulty in evaluating the relative importance of cytokines in vivo through in vitro culture systems; IL-6 in cultures of mouse bone marrow cells is one of the most potent synergistic factors for all lineages, yet gene disruption experiments suggest that either it is highly redundant with other cytokines or its role in regulating normal hematopoiesis is relatively minor.[121]

GM-CSFR Complex Ligands: IL-3, GM-CSF, IL-5

The genes for each of these proteins consist of approximately 3000 base pairs divided among four (GM-CSF,[325,326] IL-5,[179,327]) or five (IL-3[326,328]) exons with somewhat similar structure. All these genes have been localized to the long arm of chromosome 5 at 5q31.1,[329] a region commonly disrupted or deleted in patients with various malignant myeloid neoplasms.[330] This region also contains the genes for other important cytokines, including IL-4, IL-9, IL-12p40, and IL-13.[329-331] Detailed

mapping of the region has demonstrated that several of these genes are very closely linked: the GM-CSF and IL-3 genes are tandemly arrayed within 9 kilobases (kb) of one another,[332] whereas IL-4 and IL-13 are separated by only 12.5 kb.[329] This clustering of molecules with similar structure and function, including sharing of receptor components in the case of GM-CSF, IL-3, and IL-5,[333,334] provides further strong support for the evolutionary relatedness of their respective genes.

Mice with homozygous disruption of the GM-CSF gene develop normally and do not display any numerical defects in levels of circulating granulocytes or monocytes or in levels of CFU-GM progenitors in the marrow or spleen.[311,312] However, these animals exhibit alveolar proteinosis with accumulation of surfactant in the lungs as a result of defective aveolar macrophage function. Thus, GM-CSF plays an irreplaceable role in the function/development of certain macrophage populations, but any function played by this cytokine in controlling basal or stimulated production of granulocytes or monocytes can be replaced by other factors.

To evaluate the role of the entire IL-3/GM-CSF/IL-5 complex, Nishinakamura and co-workers[335] engineered a mouse without the β$_c$ receptor component shared by all three cytokines, as well as with a disruption in the IL-3 gene. Mice lacking β$_c$ have a pulmonary alveolar proteinosis–like disease and reduced numbers of peripheral eosinophils, which is explained by the lack of GM-CSF and IL-5 function, respectively. Combined disruption of the IL-3 gene showed no further abnormalities in hematopoiesis, thus demonstrating that the entire IL-3/GM-CSF/IL-5 axis is dispensable for hematopoiesis in both normal and stressed mice.

Receptor Tyrosine Kinase Ligands: M-CSF, SCF, Flt3 Receptor Ligand

With the isolation of the genes encoding SCF and FL, it has become clear that like their receptor genes, the M-CSF, SCF, and FL genes are all evolutionarily related.[160,161] The first of these to be identified was the gene for M-CSF. The more recently cloned gene for FL also shows similar gene structure, with locations of introns reasonably well preserved with those of M-CSF and SCF.

The gene for M-CSF proved to be defective in the spontaneous mutant Osteopetrosis (op/op).[306] Female op/op mice are infertile, thus confirming the role of M-CSF in the biology of the pregnant uterus.[336] Such mice also have a severe deficiency in the ability to produce osteoclasts derived from the monocytic lineage that results in the development of osteopetrosis and failure to form teeth.[337] However, that fact that some macrophage populations do develop in the animals indicates that M-CSF is important in many but not all macrophage-related lineages. The observation that some of the defects in the op/op mouse are corrected as the animals mature has led to speculation that alternative splicing of the mutant M-CSF transcript can lead to the production of some functional M-CSF.[338] This raises the necessity of genetically engineering mice with substantial deletions in this gene to see whether there is some redundancy in HGF function or whether *op* is not a true null mutation.

Naturally occuring mutations in the SCF locus (*Sl*) or in c-kit (*W*), the receptor for SCF, result in profound effects on many stages of hematopoiesis, most notably in the stem cell, erythroid, and mast cell compartments (reviewed by Galli and colleagues[128]). These studies have clearly demonstrated the central role of SCF in controlling hematopoietic cell function. Interestingly, disruption of the flt3 receptor gene has relatively minor effects on hematopoiesis, the most notable being somewhat depressed levels of B-lymphocyte precursors.[230] However, mice with disruption of both the c-kit and Flt3 receptor tyrosine kinase genes display more severe hematologic complications than do mice with either single mutation,[230] thus suggesting that the two factors do, at some level, complement one another in vivo.

Hematopoietic Growth Factor Genes: Regulation of Expression

Expression of Hematopoietic Growth Factor by Monocytes/Macrophages and Dendritic Cells: G-CSF, M-CSF, GM-CSF, IL-6, and Steel Factor

Monocytes/macrophages and related cells, including dendritic cells, Kupfer cells in the liver, and Langerhans cells in the skin, are key cells that serve many important functions in regulating the immune system.[339] Among the functions performed by these cells is the production of many cytokines, including TNF,[340] IL-1,[165] G-CSF,[145] M-CSF,[340] GM-CSF,[118] IL-6,[223] and IL-12,[339] in response to various stimuli, including LPS,[339,340] IL-1, IL-3,[341] GM-CSF,[342] and M-CSF.[343] Other cytokines, such as IL-4,[344] IL-10,[345] and IL-11,[346] downregulate monocyte production of many of these cytokines. Several of the newer cytokines, including IL-18,[165] various members of the IL-17 gene family,[347] and IL-23,[143] are likely to play important roles in controlling cytokine production by monocytes and macrophages.

All these interactions are key components of the interactions between T cells and monocytes in determining the nature and direction of the immune response. Different regulators have been found to induce different subsets of these cytokines. For example, LPS has been shown to induce the expression of IL-1, IL-6, TNF, IL-1RA, GM-CSF and G-CSF.[341] In contrast, IL-3 and GM-CSF failed to induce the expression of either GM-CSF or G-CSF but were found to induce M-CSF expression. M-CSF has been shown to induce peritoneal macrophages to activate expression of GM-CSF and IL-6 at the transcriptional level, but additional signals are necessary to induce the release of functional cytokine proteins from the cells.[348] Murine bone marrow–derived macrophages have been reported to constitutively express the mRNA for M-CSF and SCF, and the level of expression can be enhanced by treating the cultures with pokeweed mitogen.[349]

The different HGF genes in monocytes can be upregulated by a variety of different mechanisms. In the case of IL-6, LPS and *Mycobacterium tuberculosis* activate gene expression at the transcriptional level through activation of the transcription factors NF–IL-6 and NF–κB.[350] In contrast, activation of IL-1 and IL-6 expression by *Salmonella typhimurium* porins is largely mediated by mRNA stabilization.[351] Cytokine activation of monocyte IL-6 expression also occurs by various mechanisms, often involving interactions between NF-κB and NF–IL-6.[352] IL-2, IL-3, and GM-CSF have all been shown to induce monocyte expression of IL-6, and such expression is inhibited, post-transcriptionally, by treatment with IL-4.[341,344] LPS-activated expression of IL-6 is potently inhibited at the transcriptional level by IL-10.[353] Activation of IL-6 expression by the combination of TNF and IFN-γ in the human THP-1 monocytic cell line requires activation of NF-κB. Perhaps surprisingly, treatment of monocytes with the anti-inflammatory cytokine TGF-β also activates IL-6 expression.[354] In the case of G-CSF, expression can be activated by treating monocytes with either IL-1 or LPS (IFN-γ potentiates the LPS response[355]), and IL-4 given simultaneously can block this induction, an effect that is not mediated by mRNA stability but rather at the transcriptional level.[356] However, the IFN-γ enhancement effect appears to be largely at the level of mRNA stability; the half-life of mRNA with LPS treatment alone is roughly 20 minutes, but after exposure to IFN-γ, the half-life increases to 120 minutes.[356] M-CSF gene expression can be activated in HL-60 cells, an event mediated by NF-κB.[357] These interactions between monocytes and T cells and the cytokines that they produce, though complicated, are clearly important in determining the direction and extent of the resulting immune responses and are likely to play a key role in controlling the cytokine network.

Dendritic cells, which have been characterized as potent antigen-presenting cells, are also an important source of HGFs and other cytokines.[358] With the availability of cytokines such as FL, GM-CSF, IL-3, and IL-4, it has become much easier to generate dendritic cells from both myeloid and lymphoid sources in signficant numbers for further studies.[198,359] Originally believed to be largely of myeloid cell origin, it is now recognized that some are probably derived from myeloid cells whereas others have their origins in the lymphoid lineages.[360] Interestingly, different types of dendritic cells, matured under different conditions, can serve to polarize cytokine production by maturing helper T cells[361] and are therefore likely to play key roles in determining the outcomes of immune responses. Murine bone marrow–derived immature dendritic cells (CD86$^-$) produce high levels of IL-1α, IL-1β, TNF-α, and TGF-β1, but upon maturation (CD86$^+$) in the presence of CD40 ligand, levels of TGF-β dropped whereas levels of IL-6, IL-12p40, IL-15, IL-18, and TNF-α increased, as did the ability of the cells to prime naïve T cells.[361] With the newly available cytokines for expanding both myeloid and dendritic cells in culture it will be very interesting to further elaborate how these important cells interact with T cells through the cytokine network in upregulating and downregulating immune responses.

Different populations of fibroblasts, endothelial cells, and epithelial cells can be stimulated to produce cytokines by treatment with LPS,[362] phorbol esters,[326] or other cytokines, including IL-1,[162] TNF,[363] and platelet-derived growth factor (PDGF).[364] In many tissues this is likely to be an integral part of the host response to infection—cytokine production at the site of infection should result in local activation of host defense effector cells and systemic recruitment of more effector cells until the infection is cleared.[365] In the bone marrow, thymus, and spleen, these cell populations are likely to be critical components of the local microenvironment that are involved in the normal proliferation, development, and differentiation of cells of the hematopoietic and lymphopoietic systems. Control of production of the various HGFs in the steady state, however, is still poorly understood.[365]

Fibroblasts and endothelial cells are important sources of many of the HGFs, including G-CSF,[145] M-CSF,[127] GM-CSF,[326] IL-6,[366] IL-11,[280] SCF,[128] and FL.[208,226] Such expression is regulated both transcriptionally and post-transcriptionally by exposure to LPS, phorbol esters, or cytokines such as IL-1, TNF, and IFN-γ.[145,367,368] SCF expression has been reported to be constitutive in human stromal bone marrow cultures, in endothelial cells, and in bone marrow–derived fibroblasts and is not responsive to IL-1.[369]

Although it is not clear that stromal fibroblasts from bone marrow are any more or less capable of cytokine production than fibroblasts from other tissues, because of their proximity to stem and progenitor cells, they have long been studied for their ability to express HGFs. Many of these cells constitutively express the tyrosine kinase receptor ligands M-CSF and SCF.[369,370]

After myeloablation, circulating levels of many HGFs increase dramatically. In some cases this might result from mechanisms that sense low levels of the various blood cells. However, Hachiya and colleagues[371] have found that in culture, TNF and IL-1 synergize with irradiation to upregulate expression of GM-CSF through both mRNA stabilization and activation of gene transcription. These observations raise the possibility that the myeloablative agents themselves may directly induce or enhance HGF production in vivo after various cancer therapy regimens.

Endothelial cells are another important source of HGFs. Human endothelial cells produce G-CSF, GM-CSF, and M-CSF in response to inflammatory cytokines such as IL-1 and TNF.[372,373] In contrast to G-CSF and GM-CSF, SCF mRNA is expressed constitutively by human umbilical vein endothelial cells (HUVECs).[374] Levels of SCF mRNA are further increased in response

to inflammatory mediators, including IL-1 and LPS. Such induction results predominantly from mRNA stabilization by approximately threefold. Increased expression of GM-CSF mRNA in HUVECs is also mediated at least in part by mRNA stabilization.[375] Possibly, induction of SF mRNA in endothelial cells contributes to the elevated plasma levels of this factor in sepsis patients and those with inflammatory diseases.[374] Finally, vascular endothelial cells express M-CSF in response to minimally modified low-density lipoprotein though transcriptional activation mediated by NF-κB; however it is not clear how this might contribute to the biology of macrophage-derived foam cells in the atherosclerotic lesion.[376]

Regulation of Erythropoietin Expression by Hypoxia

EPO has long been recognized as the physiologic regulator of red cell production (reviewed elsewhere[377-379]). It is produced in the kidney and in the fetal liver in response to hypoxia or exposure to cobalt (II) chloride; the mechanism of the switch of production from predominantly fetal liver to predominantly kidney in adults is largely unknown.[380] Beck,[381] Semenza,[382] and their colleagues showed that the EPO gene contains a hypoxia response element (HRE) in the 3′ flanking sequence.

Nuclear factors present in hypoxic but not normoxic cells were identified as a heterodimeric basic helix-loop-helix (bHLH) transcription factor complex designated hypoxia-inducible factor 1 (HIF-1); the complex consists of inducible HIF-1α and constitutively expressed HIF-1β[8,383] (reviewed by Semenza[9]). HIF-1 is induced in a variety of cell types in response to hypoxia or cobalt, which indicates that although it is important in activation of EPO expression, it is also important in the activation of many other hypoxia-inducible genes.[8,384] HIF-1 has been shown to bind to an enhancer sequence located approximately 130 bp downstream from the poly(A) addition signal of the EPO gene. This enhancer segment has been shown to render other promoter-reporter gene constructs hypoxia responsive, with typical inductions in the range of 4- to 15-fold, significantly less than the 50- to 100-fold induction observed with the chromosomal EPO gene in Hep3B cells.[382] In addition to HIF-1 and its role on the 3′ EPO gene enhancer, other studies have identified a 53-bp sequence from the EPO promoter that confers oxygen sensitivity (6- to 10-fold inducibility) to a luciferase reporter gene.[385] The combination of the enhancer and promoter sequences together results in cooperative (50-fold) inducibility of transcription in response to hypoxia that approaches that observed in vivo.

HIF-1α protein levels are regulated by binding to the von Hippel-Lindau (VHL) tumor suppressor, followed by ubiquitin-mediated proteosomal degradation (Fig. 6-15).[386,387] Under normoxic conditions, a prolyl hydroxylase uses molecular O_2, iron (Fe[II]), and α-ketoglutarate to hydroxylate Pro402 and Pro564 in human HIF-1α, which leads to VHL binding and proteosome-mediated

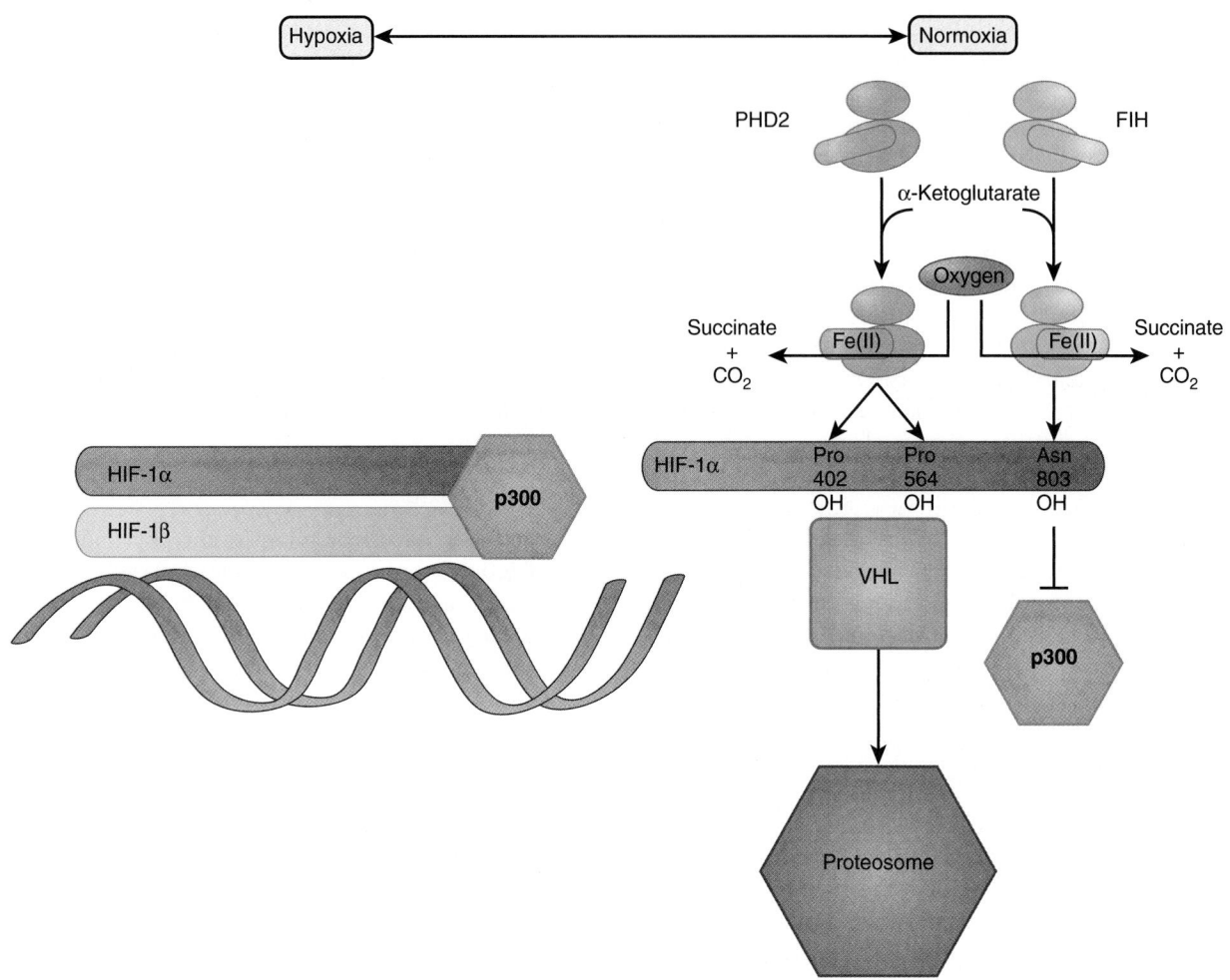

FIGURE 6-15. Hypoxia-inducible regulation of erythropoietin production. Under normoxic conditions, hypoxia-inducible factor 1α (HIF-1α) undergoes prolyl hydroxylation at Pro402 and Pro564, which leads to binding of HIF-1α to von Hippel-Lindau (VHL) protein and subsequent ubiquitin-mediated destruction. This dioxygenase enzymatic reaction is catalyzed by a prolyl hydroxylase termed prolyl hydroxylase domain 2 (PHD2). A second hydroxylation at asparagine 803 prevents binding of HIF-1α to its transcriptional coactivator p300 and is catalyzed by an HIF asparaginyl hydroxylase called factor inhibiting HIF (FIH). Both these reactions are dependent on oxygen, Fe(II), and α-ketoglutarate, which is oxidized to succinate with the release of CO_2. Under hypoxic conditions, both hydroxylases are inhibited, thereby leading to an increase in HIF-1α and recruitment of the p300 coactivator, which together with the ubiquitously expressed HIF-1β, activates transcription.

proteolysis. A second hydroxylation of Asn803 by an asparaginyl hydroxylase (similarly dependent on O_2, Fe[II], and α-ketoglutarate) blocks the C-terminal interaction of HIF-1α with the transcriptional coactivators p300/CREB-binding protein (CBP) (reviewed by Ratcliffe[10]). Under hypoxic conditions, both hydroxylases are inhibited, thereby leading to escape from ubiquitin-mediated proteolysis and an increase in HIF-1α protein, as well as recruitment of p300/CBP and transcriptional activation.[388-391]

Regulation of Thrombopoietin Gene Expression

Cloning and expression of the gene for TPO[392] have provided new insight into the regulation of levels of platelets.[129] Gene disruption studies of c-mpl, the receptor for TPO, in mice have shown that in the absence of function of this pathway, mice have only 15% of the normal levels of circulating platelets.[315] Thus, although redundancy among the growth factors, perhaps including SCF, IL-3,

IL-6, and IL-11, can partially compensate for dysfunctional c-mpl signaling, TPO, like EPO in the erythrocyte lineage, appears to be the major regulator of circulating platelet levels.[177] However, in contrast to the control of EPO production, TPO gene expression does not seem to be transcriptionally regulated or significantly influenced by platelet levels.[393] It may be regulated by megakaryocyte/platelet mass.[394] In adult mice, the major sources of TPO mRNA are the liver and kidney; in both organs the gene is constitutively expressed and is not significantly upregulated during thrombocytopenia. However, circulating levels of TPO increase rapidly during thrombocytopenia and decline as platelet counts return to normal.[395,396] The observation that platelets themselves can remove TPO from thrombocytopenic plasma in vitro has led to the model that TPO is constantly produced and released into circulation but, in normal circumstances, is rapidly removed by circulating platelets and possibly megakaryocytes as well.[394-396] During thrombocytopenia, the platelet shortage fails to remove TPO as fast as it is made, which results in elevated levels and stimulation of platelet production. This mechanism is similar to one proposed some years ago by Stanley and co-workers for the regulation of circulating M-CSF levels directly through consumption by the monocytes themselves.[397]

HEMATOPOIETIC GROWTH FACTOR RECEPTORS

Types of Hematopoietic Growth Factor Receptors

Analysis of the actions of HGFs on purified murine or human stem and progenitor cells (see later) has shown that there is considerable overlap in the action of HGFs. Some insight into the apparent overlap in biologic activities of many cytokines has come from analysis of their structural homologies and from cloning of many of their receptors. These receptors are all type 1 membrane glycoproteins with extracellular N-terminals and single transmembrane domains, and they fall into two major classes. Receptors such as c-kit, c-fms (the M-CSFR), and Flt3 are characterized by a cytoplasmic tyrosine kinase domain (receptor tyrosine kinase), whereas most of the other receptors lack cytoplasmic tyrosine kinase activity and can be divided into four subclasses (Table 6-3). Most of the HGR receptors (HGFRs, class 1) fall into a superfamily with structural features based on two linked fibronectin (FBN) type III domains (Fig. 6-16). Analogous FBN domains are found in the interferon (class 2) receptors, and the class 1 and 2 structures probably evolved from a common primitive adhesion molecule.[398] Whereas the TNF family of receptors (class 3) are characterized by an extracellular fourfold repeat of approximately 40 amino acids that contains six conserved cysteine residues (Cys repeat),[125] the IL-1Rs (class 4) feature extracellular immunoglobulin-like repeats. Although the discussion later is focused mainly on the HGFRs, the receptor tyrosine kinases activate many of the same signaling cascades (see elsewhere[399,400] for reviews).

Structure and Binding Properties

Prototypes for the class 1 structure are the (nonhematopoietic) prolactin and growth hormone receptors.[401-403] These polypeptides share a number of features (Fig. 6-17). The major homology lies in the extracellular domain, which is characterized by four conserved cysteine residues in the N-terminal FBN III repeat and a WSXWS motif in the linked C-terminal FBN III repeat that forms a hydrophobic hinge between the two domains. In addition, the IL-6 family of receptors is composed of members that each have an N-terminal immunoglobulin-like domain, as well as extra FBN III repeats. The cytoplasmic regions of the receptor family show much less homology, although membrane proximal domains rich in prolines (box1, within 20 amino acids of the membrane) and acidic residues (box2), separated by a positionally conserved tryptophan, have been defined. Mutations within the box1/2 domains have inactivated the mitogenic function of the receptors that have been examined,[404] whereas mutations of the conserved tryptophan inactivate some but not other receptors.[405] An additional interesting feature of many of the HGFRs is that receptor subunits are shared. GM-CSF, IL-3, and IL-5 all have receptors with unique α chains that bind their respective ligands with low affinity. They share a common β chain (β_c) that converts ligand binding from low to high affinity in each case and is thought to be critical for signal transduction (reviewed by Miyajima and associates[406]). A similar arrangement is evident with the IL-6, LIF, OSM, IL-11, and CNTF receptors, all of which share a common β chain, namely, gp130. An additional subunit, the low-affinity leukemia inhibitory factor receptor (LIFR), is shared by LIF, OSM, and CNTF. IL-6 and CNTF also use ligand-specific α receptor components, and gp130 is thought to form homodimers when IL-6 binds IL-6Rα and heterodimers with LIFR in the presence of LIF, OSM or CNTF. The finding of shared subunits explains to a

---

TABLE 6-3   Hematopoietic Growth Factor Receptor Classes

Type	Receptor	Cytokine
Tyrosine kinase (Ig repeats)	c-kit, M-CSFR (c-fms)	Four–α-helix bundle
Non–tyrosine kinase		
Class 1: HGFRs (FBN III domains)		Four–α-helix bundle
Shared β_c	IL-3R, GM-CSFR, IL-5R	
Shared gp130	IL-6R, LIFR, IL-11R, IL-12R, OSMR	
Shared γ_c	IL-2R, IL-4R, IL-7R, IL-9R, IL-15R	
Single chain	G-CSFR, EPOR, TPOR (c-mpl)	
Class 2 (FBN III domains)	IFNRα/β, IFNRγ	
Class 3 (Cys repeats)	TNFR I, TNFR II, FAS, CD40	β-Jellyroll wedge
Class 4 (Ig repeats)	IL-1R I and II	β-Trefoil fold

EPOR, erythropoietin receptor; FBN, fibronectin; GM-CSFR, granulocyte-macrophage colony-stimulating factor receptor; G-CSFR, granulocyte colony-stimulating factor receptor; HGFR, hematopoietic growth factor receptor; IFNR, interferon receptor; Ig, immunoglobulin; IL, interleukin; LIFR, leukemia inhibitory factor receptor; M-CSFR, macrophage colony-stimulating factor receptor; OSMR, oncostatin M receptor; TNFR, tumor necrosis factor receptor; TPOR, thrombopoietin receptor.

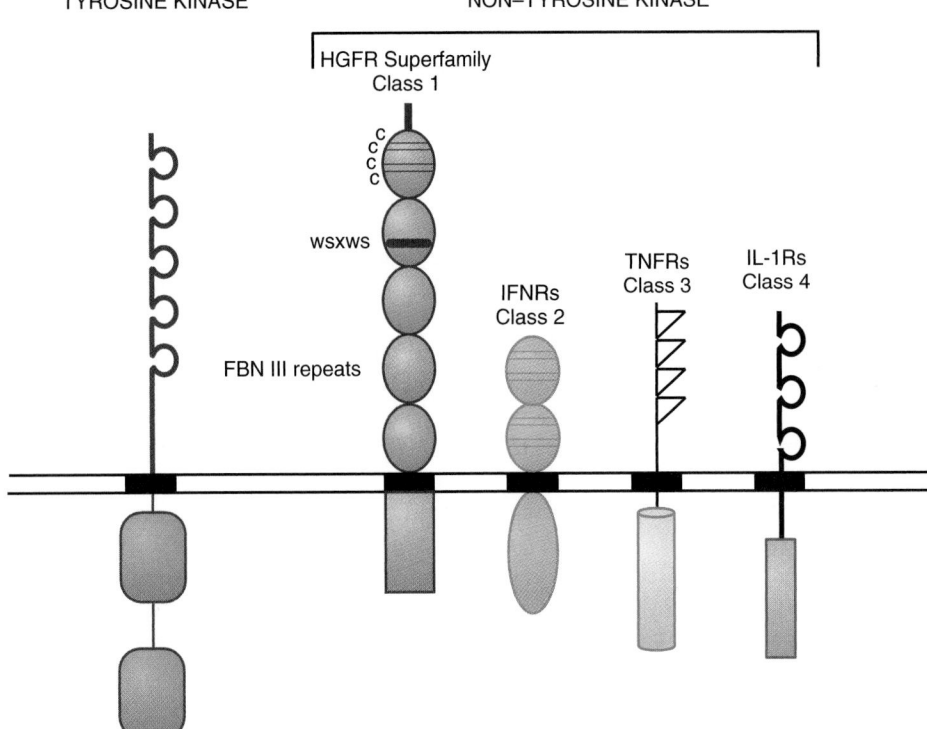

TYROSINE KINASE   NON–TYROSINE KINASE

FIGURE 6-16. Receptors such as c-kit, c-fms (macrophage colony-stimulating factor receptor [M-CSFR]), and Flt3 are characterized by a cytoplasmic tyrosine kinase domain, whereas most of the other receptors lack cytoplasmic tyrosine kinase activity and can be divided into four subclasses. Most of the hematopoietic growth factor receptors (HGFRs) (class 1) fall into a super-family with structural features based on two linked fibronectin (FBN) type III domains; analogous FBN domains are found in the interferon (class 2) receptors (IFNRs); the tumor necrosis factor family of receptors (TNFR, class 3) are characterized by an extracellular four-fold repeat of approximately 40 amino acids that contains six conserved cysteine residues (Cys repeat), and the interleukin-1 receptors (IL-1Rs, class 4) feature extracellular immunoglobulin-like repeats.

certain extent why the actions of GM-CSF and IL-3 overlap on many cells and why IL-6, LIF, and IL-11 all share pleiotropic actions on HSCs and hepatic cells. The fact that IL-12 is a heterodimer of two polypeptides that are similar to IL-6 and IL-6Rα provides an explanation for its biologic activities falling into the IL-6 group, at least on stem cells.[293] The γ chain of IL-2R is now known to be shared by the IL-4,[407,408] IL-7,[409] IL-9,[410] and IL-15[411] receptors. Other members of the HGFR superfamily that act on lineage-restricted cells such as the EPO, G-CSF, and TPO receptors appear to not require an additional subunit for ligand binding or signal transduction.

The number of IL-3, GM-CSF, G-CSF, and EPO receptors per cell is strikingly low (≈1000 sites per cell), whereas those for M-CSF are about 1 log higher. In all cases, affinity of a receptor for its ligand is high, with dissociation constants usually in the picomolar range. Stimulation of target cells can occur at factor concentrations orders of magnitude lower than the equilibrium constant at which 50% of receptors are occupied, and therefore it is apparent that low receptor occupancy is sufficient to produce biologic effects.

Receptor Function

Lineage-Specific Factors and Induction of Differentiation

Do lineage-specific receptors direct differentiation or do intracellular proteins specific for lineage-restricted cells have that function? With respect to receptor-driven events,

a proximal cytoplasmic domain of the G-CSFR is essential for proliferation, whereas a more distal domain is important for induction of acute phase plasma protein expression when the receptor is transfected into hepatoma cell lines[412] or for induction of granulocyte-specific proteins when it is introduced into murine IL-3–dependent FDC-P1 cells.[413] Support for a role of G-CSFR in granulocyte differentiation comes from sequence analysis of the receptor in two patients with severe congenital neutropenia (Kostmann's disease) in whom acute myeloid leukemia eventually developed.[301] Two different point mutations in the G-CSFR gene resulted in truncations of the C-terminal cytoplasmic region of the receptor and coexpression of both mutant and wild-type genes. The mutation was present in the neutropenic phase in one of the patients, thus suggesting that the mutation was not acquired along with the leukemia. Functional analysis by transfection of mutant or wild-type genes into murine 32D.C10 cells showed that the mutation acted as a "dominant negative" and prevented differentiation in response to G-CSF. Other evidence for an inductive role of receptors comes from murine long-term bone marrow cultures infected with a retroviral c-fms vector that yielded a pre-B line with an immunoglobulin heavy-chain gene rearrangment. This line grew in IL-7 or M-CSF; interestingly, the switch to M-CSF led to macrophage maturation, which suggests that signals from this receptor can determine differentiation in these bipotent cells.[414] Last, transduction and stable expression of the EPO receptor (EPOR) in IL-3–dependent Ba/F3 cells result in cells that produce globin mRNA on EPO but not IL-3 stimu-

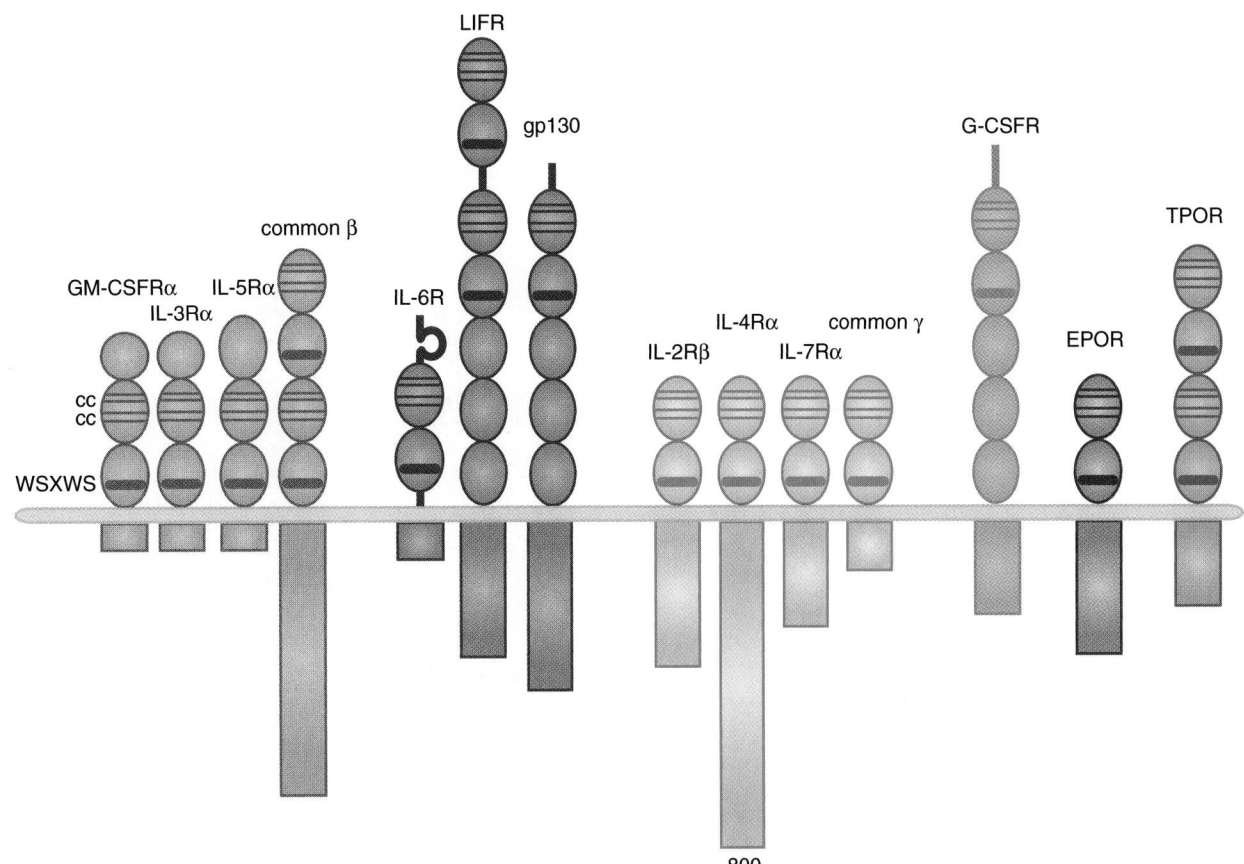

FIGURE 6-17. Diagram of some of the hematopoietic growth factor receptors (HGFRs) that have been cloned. The extracellular domains are all characterized by one or two regions that contain four conserved cysteines and a tryptophan-serine-x-tryptophan-serine (WSXWS) motif, such as the prolactin receptor. Unique features consist of interleukin-6 (IL-6) containing an immunoglobulin-like domain (*open circle*) and granulocyte colony-stimulating factor (G-CSF) containing a fibronectin type III–like region (*cross-hatched*). The intracellular domains show less homology. An additional interesting feature of many of the HGFRs is that receptor subunits are shared, in particular the IL-3R, IL-6R, and IL-2R groups. In contrast, lineage-restricted receptors such as the erythropoietin receptor (EPOR), G-CSF receptor (G-CSFR), and thrombopoietin receptor (TPOR) appear to not require an additional subunit for ligand binding or signal transduction.

lation,[415] and a chimeric receptor that comprises the extracellular domain of GM-Rα and the cytoplasmic domain of EPOR can induce increased glycophorin A expression in Ba/F3 cells, in contrast to the GM-Rα/β$_c$ control.[416] Although these experiments suggest that elements of the cytoplasmic domains of these receptors can direct both proliferation and differentiation, experiments with cell lines must be interpreted with caution. Definitive proof that EPOR is not specifically required for erythroid differentiation comes from retroviral expression of the prolactin receptor in wild-type and EPOR$^{-/-}$ progenitors; these cells differentiate efficiently in prolactin, thus indicating that there is no unique instructive role for EPO in erythropoiesis.[417] However, the prolactin receptor activates similar signaling pathways to EPOR such as STAT5 and therefore could perhaps readily substitute for EPOR function. In contrast, GM-CSF cannot rescue lymphopoiesis in GM-CSFR transgenic mice crossed with IL-7–deficient animals; furthermore, common lymphoid progenitors (CLPs) that express ectopic GM-CSFR differentiate into myelomonocytic cells, thus indicating plasticity in CLPs and an instructive role for GM-CSFR in this context.[418]

Taken together, it is reasonable to conclude that the major role of HGFRs is survival, amplification, and particularly in the case of lineage-specific receptors, completion of an intrinsic differentiation program of committed progenitor cells. However, there is overlap of expression, such as EPOR expression on megakaryocyte progenitors.[419]

Signal Transduction

HGF-Induced Tyrosine Phosphorylation

Several signaling proteins and pathways are common to many different receptor types. A paradigm common to receptors both with and without endogenous tyrosine kinase activity is that ligand binding induces homodimerization or heterodimerization of receptor subunits, followed rapidly by transient tyrosine phosphorylation of the cytoplasmic domain of the receptor itself, cytoplasmic tyrosine kinases, and other cytoplasmic proteins involved in generating different signaling cascades (Fig. 6-18). In the case of receptors with intrinsic tyrosine kinases, ligand-induced activation of their catalytic func-

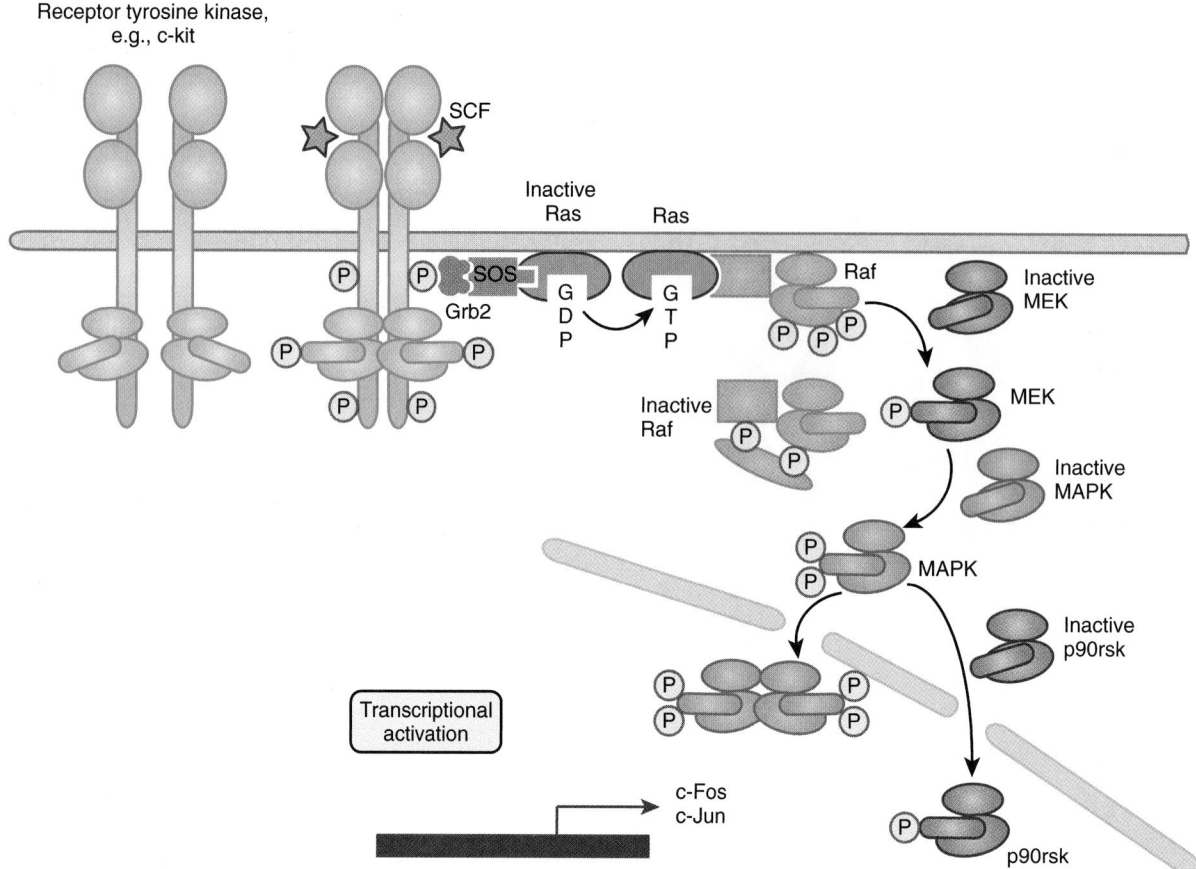

FIGURE 6-18. Signal transduction through a receptor tyrosine kinase such as c-kit. The figure illustrates that the cytosolic domains contain a protein tyrosine kinase catalytic site that forms a functional dimer after ligand binding. The kinases phosphorylate each other, which causes the activation lip to move out of the catalytic site and allows binding of adenosine triphosphate or a protein substrate. The kinase phosphorylates other tyrosines in the receptor cytosolic domain that function as docking sites for other signaling proteins. One of the major pathways is Ras activation and phosphorylation of c-raf, mitogen-activated protein kinase (MAPK) kinase (MEK), MAPK, p90S6k (or p90rsk), and induction of c-fos/c-jun and probably bcl-2, important for cell proliferation and survival. GDP, guanosine diphosphate; GTP, guanosine triphosphate; SCF, stem cell factor.

tion leads to transphosphorylation or autophosphorylation of dimerized receptor subunits and activation of three major signaling cascades: Ras/mitogen-activated protein kinase (MAPK), phosphatidylinositol 3′-kinase (PI3K)/protein kinase B (PKB, also known as Akt), and phospholipase C (PLC)/inositol triphosphate (IP$_3$)/diacylglycerol (DAG)/protein kinase C (PKC). Receptors that lack a tyrosine kinase domain must recruit cytoplasmic tyrosine kinases. For class 1 cytokine receptors, the JAK family fulfills this role, but other nonreceptor kinases have been identified and may also be important. Tyrosine phosphorylation within the receptor cytoplasmic domain creates docking sites for substrates characterized by the presence of Src homology 2 (SH2) domains. These SH2 domains recognize phosphotyrosine in the context of specific short sequences of amino acids.[420] This leads to activation of the three signaling cascades just mentioned (Ras, PI3K, and PLC), as well as activation by JAK of a critical family of signal transducers and activators of transcription (STAT proteins).

There are four known members of the JAK family, JAK1, JAK2, JAK3, and Tyk2 (for reviews see elsewhere[421-423]). All are 130- to 134-kd related proteins that

have an amino-terminal receptor-binding domain, a carboxy-terminal kinase domain, and a middle domain that regulates kinase activity (Fig. 6-19). Although it first appeared that HGFs activate JAK proteins in a rather promiscuous manner, some patterns have emerged (Table 6-4).[465] Thus, receptors that consist of single chains, such as EPOR, G-CSFR, and TPOR, associate with JAK2 (or to a lesser extent with JAK1) in either a constitutive or ligand-dependent manner. Ligand binding and consequent clustering of receptor molecules lead to JAK2 aggregation and transphosphorylation at the lysine–glutamic acid–tyrosine-tyrosine (KEYY) site in the kinase activation loop (see Fig. 6-19). For example, the inactive EPOR exists as a homodimer, and each cytoplasmic domain is irreversibly bound to a molecule of JAK2. Binding of EPO to the extracellular domain of the receptor induces a conformational change that brings the JAK kinase domains together and results in rapid tyrosine transphosphorylation.[456] In vitro experiments show that JAK2 phosphorylation leads to activation of its kinase function, which taken together with evidence of association of JAK2 with EPOR, suggests that JAK2 may act as the "master" protein tyrosine kinase that mediates the

TABLE 6-4 JAK/STAT and Nonreceptor Protein Tyrosine Kinases Activated by Hematopoietic Growth Factor Receptors

Receptor	JAK Family	JAK-Activated STATs	Other Nonreceptor PTKs
c-kit	JAK2[424]		PI3K[425,426]
IFNRα/β	JAK1,[427-429] Tyk2[430]	STAT1,[431] STAT2,[431] STAT3[432]	
IFNRγ	JAK1,[427-429] JAK2[427-429]	STAT1[433]	
IL-3Rα (→βc)	**JAK1,[434] JAK2[434]**	STAT5,[435,436] STAT6[437]	Lyn,[438,439] Fyn,[439] Fes,[440] Tec[441]
GM-CSFRα (→βc)	JAK1,[442,443] **JAK2[442,443]**	STAT5[435,436]	**Fes[440]**
IL-6Rα (→gp130)	**JAK1,[444] JAK2,[444] Tyk2[444]**	STAT1,[445,446] STAT3[444]	**Hck,[447] Btk,[448] Tec[448]**
IL-2Rα (→βc, γc)	**JAK1[449,450]**	STAT3,[451] STAT5[451,452]	**Lck,[453] Fyn,[439] Lyn,[439,454]**
IL-4, -7, -9, -15Rαs (→γc)	**JAK3[449,450]**	STAT6 (IL-4[437])	**Syk[455]**
EPOR	**JAK2[456]**	STAT5[436,457,458]	**Fes[459]**
G-CSFR	**JAK1,[460] JAK2[461,462]**	STAT3[461]	**Lyn,[463] Syk,[463] c-rel[464]**

Nonreceptor tyrosine kinases that associate with receptors are indicated in bold, and references are in superscript.

EPOR, erythropoietin receptor; G-CSFR, granulocyte colony-stimulating factor receptor; GM-CSFR, granulocyte-macrophage colony-stimulating receptor; IFNR, interferon receptor; IL, interleukin; JAK, Janus kinase; PI3K, phosphatidylinositol 3′-kinase; PTK, protein tyrosine kinase; STAT, signal transducer and activator of transcription.

Adapted from a detailed review by Taniguchi T. Cytokine signaling through non-receptor protein tyrosine kinases. Science. 1995;268:251-255.

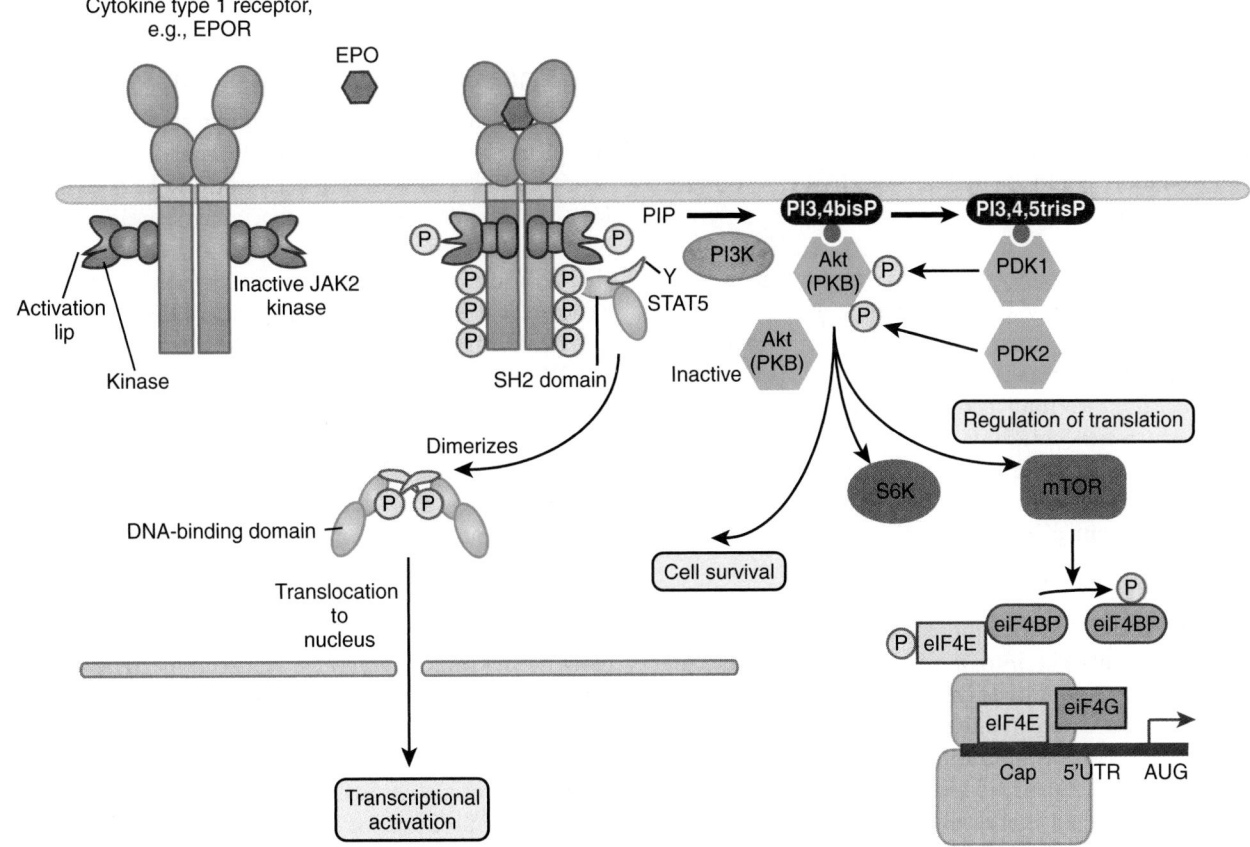

FIGURE 6-19. Signal transduction through a cytokine receptor such as the erythropoietin receptor, with JAK2 being tightly bound to the receptor. The JAKs contain a C-terminal tyrosine kinase domain and an N-terminal receptor-binding domain separated by a regulatory domain. The homodimeric receptor undergoes a conformational change after ligand binding that brings together associated JAK2 molecules, which then phosphorylate each other on a tyrosine in the activation lip and result in tyrosine phosphorylation of the receptor. These tyrosines act as docking sites for STAT5 and other Src homology 2 (SH2) and phosphotyrosine-binding domains containing signal transduction proteins. The STAT proteins have an SH2 domain that contains the completely conserved GTFLLRFSS sequence; mutation of the arginine residue eliminates function. The SH2 domain is critical for recruitment to the receptor and for STAT dimerization. The N-terminal DNA-binding domain is highly conserved and, after STAT dimerization, binds similar symmetrical dyad sequences (e.g., STAT5: TTCC[A→T]GGAA). DNA binding is totally dependent on phosphorylation of a critical tyrosine at the C-terminal. For an excellent review see *Molecular Cell Biology*, 6th ed., 2007. PI3K, phosphatidylinositol 3′-kinase; PI3,4bisP, phosphatidylinositol 3,4-bisphosphate; PI3,4,5trisP, phosphatidylinositol 3,4,5-trisphosphate; PIP, phosphatidylinositol 4-phosphate; PKB, protein kinase B; UTR, untranslated region.

biologic response to EPO. Support comes from observations that a kinase-negative JAK2 acts as a dominant-negative suppressor of the proliferative response to EPO[466] and that the box1/box2 proximal cytoplasmic domain of the EPOR is the region that both binds JAK2 and is essential for receptor function.[456] Furthermore, an acquired JAK2V617F mutation, found in almost all patients with PCV and about half with essential thrombocytosis and myelofibrosis, confers constitutive tyrosine kinase activity on JAK2; it transforms hematopoietic cells when coexpressed with homodimeric cytokine type 1 receptors and is sufficient for the development of PCV in murine recipients of transplanted JAK2V617F stem cells.[467] A number of other substrates are phosphorylated in response to EPO,[468-470] including nonreceptor kinases such the p85 subunit of PI3K, substrates such as PLCγ1 and the adaptor molecule Shc, and the tyrosine phosphatases hematopoietic cell phosphatase (HCP or PTP-1C) and Syp (also known as PTP-1D or SH-PTP2), which downregulate signal transduction; other kinases such as c-fes[459] and Vav are also activated.

The other heterodimeric receptors appear to associate with and activate several JAKs (see Table 6-4 and reviewed by Ihle and associates[421]). The β_c component of the IL-3/GM-CSF receptor is tyrosine-phosphorylated after IL-3 or GM-CSF stimulation.[471,472] The tyrosine kinase that is responsible for ligand-induced receptor phosphorylation could be JAK2[422] or JAK1,[442] but the role of other recruited nonreceptor kinases such as lyn,[438] fyn,[439] or c-fes[440] has not been clearly defined. Truncation mutants of β_c show that the proximal cytoplasmic domain (amino acids 449 to 517) can induce JAK2 tyrosine phosphorylation and kinase activation,[443] and this truncated receptor also retains the capacity to induce myc and pim-1 and promote proliferation in serum-replete but not serum-free conditions.[471,473-475] Both gp130 and LIFR can associate with and activate JAK1, JAK2, and Tyk2, but the pattern of such JAK family activation is distinct in different cell types.[476]

HGF-Induced Activation of STAT Proteins

The paradigm of the response to IFN has provided another major insight into a subsequent step in JAK family signal transduction. The kinase activities of Tyk2 and JAK1 that are activated after IFN-α binding lead to phosphorylation of STAT1α/STAT1β and STAT2. STAT proteins are characterized by an amino-terminal DNA-binding domain, a conserved carboxy-terminal SH2 domain, and a critical tyrosine at the carboxy-terminal (see Fig. 6-19). Tyrosine-phosphorylated STAT1α/β and STAT2 form heterodimers through their SH2 domains, bind to a 48-kd protein, translocate to the nucleus, and activate gene expression by binding to an interferon-stimulated response element (ISRE).[433,477,478] STAT1α is also tyrosine-phosphorylated (at Y701) after IFN-γ binds to the IFN-γR, and this event is associated with tyrosine phosphorylation of JAK1 and JAK2.[428,479] STAT1α homodimerizes, translocates to the nucleus, and binds to

the IFN-γ–activated sequence (GAS), thereby transcriptionally activating genes that contain this sequence in their promoters.

Activation of JAK proteins by HGFRs also leads to phosphorylation and DNA binding of STAT proteins, and four additional members of the STAT family have been cloned, STAT3, STAT4, STAT5, and STAT6 (see Table 6-4). Thus, ligand-induced activation of gp130, the signal-transducing component of the IL-6, LIF, IL-11, OSM, and CNTF family of receptors, leads to tyrosine phosphorylation of the JAK-Tyk family and activation of STAT3.[444,445,476] STAT4 expression is restricted to spermatogonia, as well as thymic and myeloid cells. STAT4 mRNA levels appear to decline when 32Dcl1 cells differentiate in culture with either G-CSF or EPO.[480] An ovine DNA-binding activity induced by prolactin, called mammary gland factor, was cloned and is named STAT5.[481] STAT5 is activated by EPO and growth hormone,[435] as well as by IL-3, GM-CSF, and IL-5.[436] This 92-kd protein exists as two highly related proteins, STAT5A and STAT5B (96% identical), that are encoded by different genes. STAT6 is most closely related to STAT5 and is induced by IL-4.[482]

HGF Signaling through the Ras Pathway

Ras is a "turnstile" through which signals from many receptors are routed.[483] Ras guanosine triphosphate (GTP) associates with and activates Raf-1 and MAPK.[484] Ras is a 21-kd membrane-associated protein that cycles between the active GTP-bound and the inactive guanosine diphosphate (GDP)-bound forms in response to extracellular signals from various HGFRs, including c-kit, IL-3R and GM-CSFR, T-cell receptor, IL-2R, and EPOR.[485-488] Activation of Ras is mediated by guanine nucleotide–releasing factors (GRFs) that catalyze the release of bound GDP and its exchange for GTP, whereas deactivation occurs by GTPase-activating proteins (GAPs) such as p120^GAP and neurofibromin, which accelerate the intrinsic activity of Ras and thereby lead to hydrolysis of GTP to GDP. The mammalian prototype for GRF-mediated Ras activation is the epidermal growth factor receptor (EGFR), the cytoplasmic domain of which bears intrinsic tyrosine kinase activity. After ligand-mediated dimerization, the EGFR is activated through autophosphorylation or transphosphorylation of tyrosine 1068. An adaptor protein, Grb2, binds to this phosphotyrosine through its SH2 domain. This in turn leads to the formation of a ternary complex of EGFR, Grb2, and a GRF called SOS, which is analogous to the *Drosophila* son of sevenless (SOS) protein.[489] SOS contains a proline-rich region that recognizes two SH3 domains of Grb2, and the complex then activates membrane-bound Ras GDP to Ras GTP. The protooncogene *vav* also has Ras GDP/GTP nucleotide exchange activity[490] and is activated through tyrosine phosphorylation after cross-linking of the T-cell antigen receptor–CD3 complex. With respect to the HGFRs, IL-2–mediated activation of IL-2R leads to IL-2Rβ chain tyrosine phosphorylation and association of the receptor with Shc, another adaptor protein that is characterized by both an SH2 domain and a second phosphotyrosine-binding (PTB) domain.[491,492] Shc itself becomes phosphorylated on tyrosine, and this in turn leads to the recruitment of Grb2 and SOS.[493] The IL-3/GM-CSF–mediated signaling cascade involves phosphorylation of the β subunit itself as well as Shc, with subsequent increased levels of Ras GTP and activation of Raf-1, MEK (also called MAPK kinase), and MAPK, followed by induction of c-fos and c-jun (see Fig. 6-18). This activity was mapped to the cytoplasmic domain of β_c between amino acids 626 and 763, whereas a more proximal domain (amino acids 449 to 517) retains the capacity to induce myc and pim-1.[474] The PTB domain of Shc binds to tyrosine 577 of β_c after JAK2-mediated phosphorylation of β_c.[494] Ras activation is important for both proliferative and survival (prevention of apoptosis) functions.[475,495] In the case of EPOR, ligand-induced phosphorylation of Shc and association of Shc with EPOR have also been demonstrated; phosphorylated Shc associates with Grb2, and the Ras and MAPK pathway is activated.[496-500] In summary, these three examples show that Ras is activated by a number of HGFRs and that the Ras-Raf-MEK-MAPK pathway is important for the proliferation and survival of hematopoietic cells.

The Ras pathway may also be important in certain leukemias. Neurofibromin, encoded by the NF-1 gene, is mutated in patients with autosomal dominant neurofibromatosis type 1 (NF-1). NF-1 shows sequence homology with yeast and mammalian GAP genes. Children with neurofibromatosis have an increased risk for juvenile myelomonocytic leukemia (JMML), monosomy 7 syndrome, and acute myeloblastic leukemia (AML).[501,502] Importantly, leukemic cells from children with NF-1 and myelodysplastic syndrome (MDS) show loss of the normal NF-1 allele, thus implicating NF-1 as a tumor suppressor gene.[502] NF-1^{GAP} activity is significantly lower in cell lysates prepared from NF-1–associated leukemias than in normal bone marrow or non–NF-1 leukemic lysates.[503] Bone marrow mononuclear cells from patients with JMML show an increase in CFU-GM in response to GM-CSF, but not IL-3. Interestingly, fetal liver cells from mice that are rendered null for the NF-1 gene show similar hypersensitivity to GM-CSF, thus indicating that NF-1^{GAP} may play a crucial and specific role in the response of myeloid cells to GM-CSF.[503,504] NF-1$^{-/-}$ mice die in utero around day 13.5 to 14.5 as a result of complex cardiac defects, but transplantation of day 11.5 to 13.5 fetal liver cells into lethally irradiated recipients produces a myeloproliferative syndrome similar to the human disease.[504] BCR-ABL is a chimeric oncogenic protein that shows dysregulated tyrosine kinase activity and is implicated in the pathogenesis of Philadelphia chromosome–positive chronic myeloid leukemia. A phosphorylated tyrosine (Y177) in the first exon of BCR binds to the SH2 domain of Grb2 and activates Ras.[505] Mutation of the Y177 BCR-ABL to phenylalanine abolishes Grb2 binding and abrogates both BCR-ABL–induced Ras acti-

vation and transformation of primary bone marrow cultures.[505] In summary, Ras dysregulation may contribute to the increased proliferation that characterizes these two chronic leukemias.

Phosphatases and Receptor Signaling

The C-terminal domain of the EPOR has a negative regulatory role.[506] It is likely that this effect is mediated by a phosphatase that dephosphorylates kinase-associated tyrosines in this region, as has been shown for IL-3R.[507] There is a fascinating report of a Finnish family with dominantly inherited benign erythrocytosis.[508] The proband, an Olympic cross-country skier, has a mutation in EPOR that introduces a premature stop codon and generates a receptor lacking the C-terminal 70 amino acids. This mutation cosegregates with the disease phenotype in this large family. Recent data show that the nontransmembrane protein tyrosine phosphatase SH-PTP1 (also called SHP-1, HCP, and PTP-1C) associates via its SH2 domain with the tyrosine-phosphorylated EPOR.[509] Mutational analysis mapped the binding site most probably to Y429, and this tyrosine is deleted with the C-terminal truncation of the EPOR in the Finnish family with benign erythrocytosis. Factor-dependent cells that express a Y429,431F mutant EPOR show increased sensitivity to EPO, as do cultured erythroid progenitors from patients with benign erythrocytosis.[509] CFU-E progenitors from mice that lack or have impaired SH-PTP1 activity (Motheaten or Motheaten viable) show similar increased sensitivity to EPO.[307,510] Therefore, EPO-induced activation and subsequent tyrosine phosphorylation of EPOR leads to recruitment of SH-PTP1, which then plays a major role in terminating the EPO signal, possibly through dephosphorylation of JAK2[509] or other tyrosine kinases.

Another nonreceptor protein tyrosine phosphatase called SH-PTP2 or SHP2, encoded by the *PTPN11* gene, has 50% to 60% identity with SH-PTP1 in both the SH2 and catalytic domains. Despite this similarity, SH-PTP2 appears to be a positive regulator of some growth factor pathways (for review see Sun and Tonks[511]), in particular, Ras. Approximately 50% of patients with Noonan's syndrome (NS), a developmental disorder characterized by short stature, dysmorphic features, and cardiac defects, have germline mutations in SH-PTP2, and 35% of non-NS JMML patients have somatic mutations in this gene. JMML develops in some patients with NS, and it appears that the mutations in NS/JMML differ from those found in de novo nonsyndromic JMML[512] and differ in the degree to which they activate the phosphatase.[513]

Other Inhibitors of HGF Signaling

Another family of negative regulators is the suppressor of cytokine signaling (SOCS) proteins. SOCS-1 was discovered by three groups, contains an SH2 domain, and has sequence and structural similarities to an immediate early gene called CIS (cytokine-inducible SH2-containing protein).[400,514-516] It is one of an eight-member gene family (SOCS-1 to SOCS-7 and CIS) characterized by a central SH2 domain and a C-terminal conserved motif called a SOCS box. Unlike the constitutively expressed phosphatases, SOCS expression is induced by many cytokines, including IL-3, EPO, TPO, IL-6, and LIF, and the proteins are expressed in hematopoietic and other tissues (for a detailed review see Greenhalgh and Hilton[517]). SOCS-1, expressed predominantly in the thymus, interacts directly with the phosphorylated activation loop of (activated) JAKs, and its N-terminal is thought to inhibit binding of adenosine triphosphate (ATP) to the activation cleft.[400,514,518] Subsequently, the SOCS box was hypothesized to target the SOCS/signaling complex to the proteosome for degradation by recruiting components of the proteasome machinery, including elongins B and C and Cullin 2.[519,520] SOCS-3 has been shown to inhibit signaling by a different mechanism— binding directly to activated receptors and to JAKs without inhibiting JAK activity,[521] whereas CIS can bind to phosphorylated tyrosines on the EPOR and thereby inhibit STAT5 signaling.[522]

SOCS knockouts have provided insight into the important physiologic roles of some of these proteins. SOCS-1$^{-/-}$ mice die before weaning with fatty degeneration of the liver, reduced thymic size, lack of T and B cells, and monocytic infiltration of organs.[523,524] This phenotype is similar to that of mice with elevated IFN-γ, and indeed, SOCS-1$^{-/-}$ mice have increased IFN-γ levels; rescue of the animals can be achieved with antibodies to IFN-γ or by crossing them with IFN-γ$^{-/-}$ mice.[525,526] SOCS-2$^{-/-}$ mice are normal at birth but then become significantly larger than wild-type mice, with thickening of the dermis caused by excess collagen deposition.[527] Therefore, SOCS-2 appears to play an important role in postnatal growth, possibly through the growth hormone/ insulin-like growth factor I (IGF-I) axis. SOCS-3$^{-/-}$ mice are hematopoietically most interesting in that they die at embryonic day 12 to 14 of massive erythrocytosis.[528] Progenitor cells appear to be hyperresponsive to IL-3 and EPO. Thus, SOCS-3 plays a crucial role in inhibiting fetal erythropoiesis. Although CIS-deleted mice show no abnormalities, overexpression of CIS induces a phenotype similar to STAT5a$^{-/-}$ or STAT5b$^{-/-}$ animals.[529-532]

BIOLOGY OF HEMATOPOIESIS

Stem Cells

The formed elements of the blood in vertebrates, including humans, continuously undergo replacement to maintain a constant number of red cells, white cells, and platelets. The number of cells of each type is maintained in a very narrow range in physiologically normal adults— approximately 5000 granulocytes, 5×10^6 red blood cells, and 150,000 to 300,000 platelets per microliter of whole blood (see Appendix for normal values in infancy and childhood). In this section we examine the normal regulatory mechanisms that maintain balanced production of new blood cells. These regulatory systems are far from completely understood, but present evidence strongly supports the following basic principles, schematically depicted in Figure 6-7:

1. A single pluripotent stem cell is capable of giving rise to many committed progenitor cells. These committed progenitors are destined to form differentiated recognizable precursors of the specific types of blood cells.

2. Pluripotent stem cells are capable of self-renewal. Committed progenitor cells are limited in proliferative potential and are not capable of indefinite self-renewal. In addition to their limited proliferative potential, committed progenitors also "die by differentiation,"[533] and their numbers depend on influx from the pluripotent stem cell pool.

3. The proliferative potential and differentiation of stem cells and committed progenitors may be influenced by niche cells or factors derived from them. Thymus-derived lymphocytes appear to contribute to the induction of spleen colony formation in irradiated recipients.[534-537] The hematopoietic role of thymus-derived cells is further supported by experiments demonstrating defective restorative capacity of bone marrow from congenitally athymic[538] or neonatally thymectomized[539] mice or from rigorously T-depleted human bone marrow.[540]

4. Committed progenitor cells are capable of response to humoral or marrow stroma–derived regulators, some produced in reaction to circulating levels of a particular differentiated cell type. In this response, they proliferate and differentiate to form the recognizable blood cells. Under this type of control, amplification of production occurs at the committed progenitor cell level. Most of the regulatory molecules are produced by hematopoietic accessory cells in close proximity to progenitor cells. These molecules are produced as part of an incompletely understood complex regulatory network operating at close range and may involve accessory cell–progenitor cell interactions. For most hematopoietic lineages studied, there appear to be at least two humoral regulators that work sequentially. The immature progenitor of a particular lineage has a greater requirement for a regulator that acts on all or many immature progenitors than its more mature counterparts do. As differentiation proceeds, sensitivity to the late-acting factor increases. This variable degree of response to the late-acting regulators that are present at high concentration during hematopoietic stress (e.g., EPO in anemia) may serve to protect the highly proliferative, but numerically limited immature progenitor compartment from exhaustion or death by differentiation under these stress conditions.

5. Hematopoietic differentiation requires an appropriate microenvironment. In normal humans, this environ-

ment is confined to the bone marrow, whereas in the mouse the microenvironment includes both the spleen and bone marrow. The existence of Steel (*Sl*) strains of mutant mice,[303,541] which exhibit a deficiency in the hematopoietic microenvironment (see later), suggests that interactions between hematopoietic progenitors and the bone marrow microenvironment involve very specific molecular mechanisms.[304] A number of early hematopoietic cells, including pluripotent stem cells and certain committed progenitor cells, have been demonstrated in the circulation of normal individuals and experimental animals.[60,542-544] The capacity of HSCs to negotiate nonhematopoietic tissues via the circulation is especially significant with regard to bone marrow transplantation, which is carried out by infusion of bone marrow or blood cells from the donor into the circulation of the recipient.[545] For example, blockade of hepatic asialoglycoprotein receptors enhances stem cell engraftment in murine spleen and marrow.[546] There is also convincing evidence that murine stem cells (CFU-S) and progenitors (CFU-GM) express "homing" or adhesive lectin receptors that bind to the mannose or galactose (or both) presented on stromal cells. For example, homing of transplanted mouse progenitors can be blocked by synthetic neoglycoproteins with these specificities, thus suggesting that stromal cells are likely to express these sugars.[547] SDF-1/chemokine (CXCR4) signaling and adhesion molecules, including VLA-4/VCAM-1 and CD44/hyaluronic acid interactions, are also important in the regulation of homing.[548]

If only 10% to 20% of stem cells are in cycle in the resting state, what is their role with regard to self-renewal versus differentiation, and what is the role of the noncycling stem cells? The hypothesis that a series of stem cells may contribute clones successively to maintain hematopoiesis throughout the life span of an individual was first advanced by Kay.[549] Support for this hypothesis comes from transplant studies of recipients of small numbers of bone marrow cells[550,551] and from experiments in which mixtures of fetal liver cells from different inbred mouse strains were introduced into *W*-mutant fetuses. *W* mutants exhibit a genetically determined deficiency of HPCs (as well as germ and follicle cells; see later). Long-term monitoring showed clonal dominance followed by the decline of cells of particular genotypes.[551]

The use of retrovirally mediated gene transfer to mark HSCs at first lent support to this hypothesis. Analysis of the viral integration patterns at intervals after transplantation documented concurrent contributions of small numbers of stem cells to hematopoiesis, with changing patterns over time.[552,553] These conclusions are not supported by the work of Harrison and associates, who measured variances at successive intervals in recipients of marrow mixtures from two congenic donors. The high correlations observed in this study suggest that the trans-

planted stem cells continuously produce descendants.[554] However, if 10 to 20 (or more) clones are contributing to hematopoiesis simultaneously, even with clonal succession one might expect variances between two alloenzymes at sequential samplings to be minimized. Furthermore, longer-term analysis of viral integration patterns in multiple-lineage progeny of stem cells transplanted into mice shows that integration patterns are unstable initially but then stabilize and maintain a consistent pattern for many months.[555] Although this consistency does not appear to support the clonal succession hypothesis, the contributory role of unmarked stem cells in these experiments cannot be assessed. Furthermore, it is not possible to determine whether the immediate progeny of the transplanted (and retrovirally marked) stem cells might not all still have self-renewal capacity and subsequently contribute to hematopoiesis successively. Such clones would carry the same integration marker. Long-term analysis of female Safari cats (heterozygous for two glucose-6-phosphate dehydrogenase [G6PD] isoforms) that received transplants of small numbers (1 to 2×10^7/kg) of autologous marrow cells showed extensive variation in G6PD phenotype over a $4\frac{1}{2}$-year period.[556] Computer modeling of the data was consistent with a stochastic model in which stem cells did not replicate more frequently than once every 3 weeks, which challenges many of the current strategies for inserting foreign genes into HSCs. A problem with the transplant approach discussed earlier is that the preparation required for successful transplantation may perturb hematopoiesis and complicate interpretation of the results. Resolution of the problem came from studies in which a nontoxic dose of bromodeoxyuridine (BrdU) was fed to mice in drinking water.[557,558] BrdU is incorporated into DNA by proliferating cells, and measurement of incorporation rates into primitive stem cell populations over time can be used as a monitor of proliferative history. Under steady-state conditions, approximately 5% of LTR-HSCs were in cycle and another 20% in the G_1 phase, with approximately 8% entering the cell cycle per day. By 6 days, 1 month, and 6 months, 50%, 90%, and 99%, respectively, of the stem cell pool had incorporated the label.[558] Because the size of the stem cell pool remains constant, these data indicate that 50% of dividing LTR-HSCs must self-renew; this could be accomplished by asymmetric division or by symmetrical division in which half the cells give rise to LTR-HSCs and the other half to differentiating cells.

Transcription Factors and Stem Cells

Although the factors that control the decision of stem cells to undergo either self-renewal or commitment to differentiate down one of the alternative lineage pathways are poorly understood, in recent years nuclear transcription factors have been characterized that play a role in stem or early progenitor cell proliferation and lineage commitment (reviewed by Orkin and colleagues[559,560]). The tal-1/SCL, Rbtn2/LMO2, and GATA families of transcription factors are important in this regard. In particular, tal-1/SCL, a bHLH transcription factor, is expressed in biphenotypic (lymphoid/myeloid) and T-cell leukemias,[561,562] as well as in both early hematopoietic progenitors and more mature erythroid, mast, megakaryocyte, and endothelial cells.[563,564] Targeted disruption of the tal-1/SCL gene leads to death in utero from absence of blood formation, and lack of in vitro myeloid colony formation suggests a role for this factor very early during hematopoiesis at the pluripotent or myeloid-erythroid stem cell level.[565,566] Another transcription factor implicated in T-cell acute lymphoblastic leukemia (ALL) is the LIM domain nuclear protein rhombotin 2 (rbtn2/LMO2).[567,568] Mice that lack this factor die in utero and have the same bloodless phenotype as the tal-1/SCL$^{-/-}$ animals.[569] Interestingly, although rbtn2/LMO2 does not show sequence-specific DNA binding, immunoprecipitates in erythroid cells show that rbtn2/LMO2 exists in a complex with tal-1/SCL,[570,571] thus suggesting physiologic interaction in vivo. GATA-2 is expressed in the regions of *Xenopus* and zebra fish embryos that are fated to become hematopoietic and is highly expressed in progenitor cells.[564,572-574] Overexpression of GATA-2 in chicken erythroid progenitors leads to proliferation at the expense of differentiation.[575] Targeted disruption of the GATA-2 gene by homologous recombination in ES cells results in reduced primitive hematopoiesis in the yolk sac and embryonic death by day 10 to 11.[576] Definitive hematopoiesis in the liver and bone marrow is profoundly reduced with loss of virtually all lineages, and in vitro differentiation data show a marked deficiency in SCF-responsive definitive erythroid and mast cell colonies and reduced macrophage colonies, which suggests that GATA-2 serves as a regulator of genes that control HGF responsiveness or proliferation of stem or early progenitor cells (or both).

These data contrast with the later time of embryonic death (day 15) from anemia during the mid–fetal liver stage in mice with targeted disruption of c-myb[577] and Rb[578-580] and severe forms of *W* and *Sl* mutations (see later).[305] C-myb has been shown to be absolutely required for normal hematopoietic production during embryogenesis.[581] Embryonic erythropoiesis in c-myb knockout mice is normal, but there is complete failure of erythropoiesis in fetal liver. Progenitors of other lineages, but not megakaryocytes, were also decreased, which indicates that c-myb is required for early definitive cellular expansion.[577] Furthermore, a knockdown allele of c-myb shows that suboptimal levels of c-myb favor macrophage and megakaryocyte differentiation whereas higher levels are particularly important for erythropoiesis and lymphopoiesis.[582] An N-ethyl-N-nitrosourea (ENU)-induced allele of c-myb (M303V) affects the transactivation domain of the protein that interacts with the transcriptional coactivator p300; recessive mice (c-myb$^{M303V/M303V}$) demonstrate increased platelet production, anemia, absence of eosinophils, and defects in B- and T-cell lymphopoiesis.[583] Interestingly, these animals were found to have an increase in transplantable HSCs, thus indicating that c-myb has a negative role in HSC self-renewal. Hence, c-myb appears to have a negative role in HSC and megakaryocyte progenitor proliferation and positive effects on erythropoiesis, eosinophil production, and lymphopoiesis.

Loss of function of the AML-1 gene, which encodes one of the α subunits of the heterodimeric core-binding factor (CBF), results in fetal death by day 12.5 because of failure of production of all definitive hematopoietic lineages.[584] CBF recognition sequences are present in the IL-3R, GM-CSFR, M-CSFR, and T-cell antigen receptor promoters. The AML-1 gene is frequently rearranged in AML and childhood ALL and is expressed in myeloid and lymphoid cells.[568] AML-1 has been shown to interact with a number of repressors, including GROUCHO domain factors. AML-1 is also a regulator of HSC production in the AGM region, as well as in adult stem cell homeostasis. Rescue of AML-1 by a tie2 promoter salvages hematopoiesis during development.

Interestingly, the order of expression of transcription factors is thought to regulate a stem cell hierarchy.[585] This can be demonstrated in purified progenitor cells by looking at a variety of transcription factors, including GATA-1, GATA-2, CCAAT/enhancer-binding protein α (C/EBPα), PU.1, and others. It is clear that competition of hematopoietic transcription factors is a prominent theme. There are GATA-1–PU.1 interactions that regulate an erythroid/myeloid decision, and there are many other decisions, including PAX5, C/EBPα, and PU.1 interactions, for lymphoid and myeloid systems. Such competition for transcription factors and regulation of stem cell differentiation appears to be a mechanism in the hematopoietic system. Manipulation of the process actually leads to altered hematopoiesis that can favor a single lineage. This involves a cell fate change rather than a proliferative event.

Homeobox (HOX) genes encode transcription factors involved in the establishment of body pattern and tissue identity during development.[586] The human genes occur in four clusters, *HOXA* to *HOXD*, on chromosomes 7, 17, 12, and 2, respectively. *HOXA* and *HOXB* genes are expressed in CD34$^+$ cells and downregulated as these cells mature. Intriguingly, murine bone marrow cells engineered to overexpress HOXB4 by retrovirus-mediated gene transfer show a dramatic upregulation in stem cell activity both in vitro and in vivo, although it may not be required for normal hematopoiesis.[587,588] Serial transplantation studies showed a greatly enhanced ability of HOXB4-transduced bone marrow cells to regenerate the most primitive HSC compartment; such regeneration resulted in a 50-fold higher number of transplantable totipotent HSCs in primary and secondary recipients than in serially passaged control cells. This in vivo expansion of HOXB4-transduced HSCs was not accompanied by identifiable anomalies in the blood of these mice, thus suggesting that HOXB4 is an important regulator of very early but not late hematopoietic cell proliferation. Recent data show that ectopic expression of HOXB4 in yolk sac and ES cells confers long-term engraftment capacity in primary and secondary recipients.[589] Daley, Jaenisch, and colleagues reported that nuclei from Rag2 knockout (Rag2$^{-/-}$) tail cells could be transferred into enucleated oocytes and embryonic stem (ntES) cell lines derived from the resulting blastocysts. The Rag2 mutation was then corrected by homologous recombination. Insertion of HOXB4 into the corrected ES cells allowed their expansion into transplantable HSCs. These cells were able to partially correct the defect in immunoglobulin production in Rag2$^{-/-}$ recipients after bone marrow transplantation.[590] The HOX pathway has been expanded to include HOXA7 and HOXA9 as major regulators of hematopoiesis and leukemia formation.[591] The posterior HOX genes therefore drive HSC production; this was highlighted by the finding that mutations in CDX4, a controller of HOX gene expression, leads to absence of HSCs in the zebra fish and lack of control of HOX gene expression for the formation of HSCs.[587]

The Gfi 1 locus was originally identified as an oncogene causing lymphoma based on retroviral insertion.[592] Gfi 1 contains an internal SNAG domain and a six–zinc finger DNA-binding domain. There are two nearly identical genes called Gfi 1 and Gfi 1b. Gfi 1 is restricted to the lymphoid system, whereas Gfi 1b seems to be distributed throughout the entire hematopoietic system. Gfi 1 is also expressed in neutrophils. Gfi 1 knockout animals have a severe reduction in lymphoid progenitors. This leads to an early lack of both CD4$^+$ and CD8$^+$ cells. In addition, IL-7R signaling is suppressed. Gfi 1 is a major regulator of neutrophil maturation. Normal neutrophils are absent in the knockout animals, and yet eosinophils are present in the normal number. The response to G-CSF by neutrophils is preserved, but differentiation does not take place. There is a significant interaction of Gfi 1 with other transcription factors, including PU.1, C/EBPβ, and C/EBPε, which regulate neutrophil maturation.

Gfi 1 has also been shown to be involved in HSC self-renewal. In Gfi 1 knockout animals, HSCs actually increase and outcompete other cells. This leads to stem cell exhaustion. Gfi 1b may also regulate stem cell homeostasis. The HSCs appear to be more active in terms of their cell cycle and have increased proliferation rates. It is clear that p21 is probably one of the mediators of Gfi 1 in HSC production.[593] There is also modulation of STAT3 activity as a consequence of the interaction of Gfi 1 with PIAS3, a factor that simulates transcription factors. This is interesting because other genes such as SCL, Runx1, Notch1, Notch2, RBPJ, integrin1, HOXB4, and β-catenin are dispensable for most HSC activities whereas p21, Bmi 1, tel1, C/EBP, PU.1, and Gfi are actually required.

Growth Factors and Stem Cells

HGFs also appear to influence at least some classes of stem cells. Analysis of the actions of HGFs on "purified" murine or human stem and progenitor cells has led to several major conclusions that should be interpreted in the light that to date, even the most highly purified "stem cell" fractions are still heterogeneous with respect to the content of LTR-HSCs, HSCs with short-term–reconstituting potential, and lineage-committed progenitors. HGFs such as SF and perhaps IL-3, GM-CSF, and G-CSF can independently support the survival of murine or human stem cell populations (or both).[277,5948-596] However, of all these HGFs, only SF has been shown to enhance the survival of murine LTR-HSCs, and no single HGF or combination of HGFs has unequivocally shown the capacity to induce significant self-renewal of LTR-HSCs.[597,598] IL-6–deficient mice show a reduction in CFU-S and failure of IL-6$^{-/-}$ bone marrow cells to contribute to long-term hematopoiesis after serial transfer.[310] In addition to its effect on megakaryocyte and platelet formation, TPO is also vital for stem cell production. Mice that lack the receptor for TPO (c-mpl) show reduced numbers of blast colonies and CFU-S and fail to compete effectively with normal stem cells for reconstitution of hematopoiesis in irradiated recipients, even when transplanted in 10-fold excess.[599] Furthermore, both murine and human repopulating activity segregates with primitive cells that express c-mpl.[600] In the human system, information on HSC self-renewal is not available because no human assay measures this property.

Analysis of mutations that affect the function of stem cells and the hematopoietic microenvironment through HGF interactions have provided important insight. Two murine mutations have been characterized in some detail, the Steel (*Sl*) and dominant White-spotting (*W*) mutations.[303,305,541] Genetically affected mice that are defective at these loci have severe macrocytic anemia associated with increased radiation sensitivity, lack of pigmentation, poor gastrointestinal motility, and sterility. Though phenotypically similar, these mutations map to different chromosomes (*W*, chromosome 5; *Sl*, chromosome 10) and have distinct hematologic characteristics. Best characterized at the molecular level, the *W* mutation results in a functional deficiency of HSCs, particularly erythroid progenitors. Transplantation of normal bone marrow into homozygous *W* recipients completely corrects the hematopoietic abnormalities, whereas transplantation of *W* bone marrow into normal mice fails to reconstitute hematopoiesis.[541,601] The *W* gene is allelic with the c-kit proto-oncogene,[602,603] which as discussed earlier, is known to be a member of a tyrosine kinase receptor family,[604] as is c-fms, the receptor for M-CSF. Several variants of the *W* mutation have been shown to be phenotypic expressions of specific mutations of the c-kit gene, and the severity of the phenotypic changes associated with specific alleles correlates with the degree of functional impairment in kinase activity.[605]

In contrast, the Steel mutation affects the function of cells of the microenvironment. *Sl/Sl^d* bone marrow cells are capable of reconstituting hematopoiesis in irradiated normal mice, whereas transplantation of normal bone marrow into *Sl/Sl^d* animals fails to cure the defect.[606] Deeper insight into the molecular nature of this defect was provided by purification of a factor that is active on mast cells and on post–5-FU mouse bone marrow (enriched for primitive stem cells but depleted of mature progenitors).[607,608] This "stem cell factor" or "mast cell growth factor" was purified and its cDNA cloned. Labeling studies with the purified recombinant protein demonstrate that it is the ligand for c-kit.[609-612] Furthermore, administration of the factor to Sl/Sl^d mice corrects their macrocytic anemia and repairs their mast cell deficiency. Less severe mutations at the Sl locus such as Sl^d are associated with smaller deletions at the Sl locus. The gene encodes a protein that exists in both transmembrane and secreted forms.[609,613,614]

Recently, other growth factor pathways that are important during embryogenesis and have been subverted in certain cancers have also been implicated in stem cell self-renewal. Notch receptors (four members, Notch1 to Notch4) are expressed on the surface of a variety of hematopoietic cells as proteolytically cleaved dimers consisting of an EGF repeat-rich extracellular domain and a transmembrane/intracellular domain that contains two motifs (RAM and ANK) that can bind to a transcriptional repressor, CBF1/RBPJκ (see Kojika and Griffin[615] for a detailed review). After ligand binding (three ligands, Delta, Jagged1, and Jagged2), the transmembrane/intracellular domain is cleaved to release the active intracellular domain of Notch (ICN), which translocates to the nucleus, binds to CBF1/RPBJκ, and transactivates genes such as Hairy and Enhancer of Split 1 (HES-1), a bHLH protein that suppresses transcription of N-box (CACNAG) target genes. Human Notch1 was first identified as a gene called TAN-1 that is involved in some T-cell leukemias by generating an intracellular activated form of Notch1 (ICN1).[616] Remarkably, overexpression of ICN1 in murine stem cells leads to immortalization of cytokine-dependent cell lines that can generate lymphoid or myeloid progeny in vitro and in vivo, thus suggesting a role for Notch1 in stem cell self-renewal.[617] Activating mutations in Notch have been found in many T-cell leukemias.[618] Addition of soluble Jagged1 to cultures of human purified stem and progenitor cells also increased NOD/SCID repopulating activity.[619] A second signaling pathway that may be involved in stem cell self-renewal involves the Sonic hedgehog protein.[620] Shh activates the Smoothened receptor (Smo) by binding to its inhibitor Patched. Smo initiates signaling that regulates transcription factors of the Gli family, which modify expression of genes that encode BMP-4 and its inhibitor Noggin. Shh has recently been shown to induce expansion of human NOD/SCID repopulating cells, possibly through regulation of BMP-4. Last, Wnt signaling may also be involved in stem cell self-renewal. Wnt signals through the receptors Frizzled and lipoprotein receptor–related protein (LRP) to activate a cytoplasmic protein called Disheveled, which in turn stabilizes β-catenin, a transcriptional coactivator that associates with the Tcf/LEF family of transcription factors (reviewed by Taipale and Beachy[621]). Without Wnt signaling, β-catenin is normally destabilized by a cytoplasmic complex that comprises Axin, adenomatous polyposis coli (APC), and GSK3β. Overexpression of activated β-catenin in highly purified murine HSCs appears to be capable of expanding the pool of transplantable cells.[622]

Two models have been proposed to explain the mechanisms that influence the choice of stem cells between self-renewal and commitment. A *stochastic model* was proposed by Till, McCullough, and Siminovitch.[533] In this model, self-renewal or differentiation is considered to occur in a random or stochastic manner, only dictated by a certain probability. Because no extrinsic source of stem cells exists, under steady-state conditions the overall probability of stem cell division resulting in self-renewal must be 0.5; probabilities less or greater than this value would lead to progressive stem cell depletion (aplasia) or expansion (leukemia), respectively. The commitment of stem cells could occur symmetrically, where half the stem cells overall divide to produce progeny that enter a differentiation pathway and half generate progeny in which all remain undifferentiated stem cells. Alternatively, asymmetric division would give rise to one stem cell and one cell committed to differentiation. Analysis of single cells from blast cell colonies has shown that hematopoietic cells can divide asymmetrically; these micromanipulated single cells give rise to colonies that comprise almost all possible lineage combinations.[86] Single-cell analysis of purified human CD34+CD45RA^lo CD71^lo provides evidence for quiescent survival, self-renewal, and asymmetric division.[623] These data provide strong support for a stochastic mechanism to explain both commitment and restriction of differentiation potential. Differentiation of single blast cells into mature cells occurs in these methylcellulose cultures in the absence of an intact microenvironment. A source of HGFs is obligatory, however, as is the case for all colonies grown in semisolid media. It is important to recognize that although these random events occur with a given probability, it must be possible to favor self-renewal versus differentiation as circumstances demand. For example, during the regeneration of hematopoietic tissue after injury by irradiation or cytotoxic drugs, the probability of generating stem cells must increase. How this probability is altered is one of the outstanding unanswered questions in hematopoiesis.

A contrasting model proposed by Curry and Trentin[624] in which it was postulated that the *hematopoietic microenvironment is inductive* (HIM) was based on the observation that domains of a given lineage exist within single spleen colonies. Although this model is no longer tenable in its original formulation, the observation that the osteoblastic niche in bone marrow plays a role in stem cell self-renewal whereas the sinusoidal endothelial niche regulates proliferation, differentiation, and mobilization suggests a mechanism for the external control of stem cell expression. This plus other observations related to the morphology of the focal development of hematopoietic islands attached to adherent cells has led to the postulate that HSCs reside within stromal cell "niches" that play a vital role in supporting stem cell survival, perhaps by intimate cell contact.[15]

Whether a stochastic mechanism or one influenced by environmental cues dictates the outcome of the stem cell's decision to commit to one or another hematopoietic lineage is also uncertain. Recent experiments suggest that cross-antagonism among lineage-specific transcription factors may provide a mechanistic explanation for lineage specification. Forced expression of the erythroid-specific factor GATA-1 in myelomonocytic cells perturbs their ability to differentiate,[625] and evidence is accumulating that this is due to direct physical interaction and cross-antagonism of PU.1, the myeloid transcription factor, and GATA-1; GATA-1 inhibits PU.1 by preventing it from interacting with its cofactor c-jun, whereas PU.1 prevents GATA-1 from binding to DNA.[626-629] Down syndrome patients have mutations in GATA-1 that lead to a truncated protein missing its N-terminus.[630] This appears to give competitive advantage to a yolk sac/fetal liver progenitor in the genesis of leukemia and transient myeloproliferative disorder. Another example is the antagonism between friend of GATA-1 (FOG-1) and C/EBPβ in an eosinophilic cell line in that enforced expression of FOG-1 blocks C/EBPβ-mediated eosinophil differentiation.[631] It is therefore possible that lineage-specific transcription factors not only have potent inductive effects but also exert blocking effects on alternative lineage choices. The observation that forced expression of C/EBPβ in pancreatic cells promotes their differentiation into a hepatic phenotype raises the intriguing possibility that this mechanism underlies stem cell plasticity as well (reviewed by Cantor and Orkin[560]).[632]

Erythropoiesis

It is well established that the level of oxyhemoglobin and the rate of delivery of oxygen to tissues is the fundamental stimulus of erythropoiesis.[5] In species that package hemoglobin in erythrocytes, EPO mediates the response to oxygen demand and does so by interacting with specific receptors[633] found on the surface of committed erythroid progenitor cells[634-636] and erythroblasts.[637] As discussed earlier, insight into the mechanism by which hypoxia induces a transcriptional increase in expression of the EPO gene has come from the identification of HIF-1α.[383,638]

It is believed that BFU-E progenitors do not directly give rise to erythroblasts in vivo except under conditions of extreme anemic stress. Instead, they mature to single erythroid colony-forming units, or CFU-E, that divide in vivo and, under the influence of lower concentrations of EPO, form single, relatively small colonies of proerythroblasts at about 1 week in vitro. Many (at least half) of the CFU-E progenitors will form erythroid colonies in vitro in response to EPO alone. They do not require the additional presence of either GM-CSF or IL-3 because they have differentiated beyond this requirement.[639] All

proerythroblasts can differentiate in the presence of EPO alone. In the steady state, the number of human CFU-E progenitors exceeds the number of BFU-E progenitors by a factor of 10. CFU-E progenitors are larger than BFU-E progenitors, and because a higher fraction of CFU-E than BFU-E progenitors are in the S-phase of DNA synthesis, the former exhibit a higher rate of "suicide" in response to exposure to tritiated thymidine. The membranes of mature BFU-E and CFU-E are CD34+ and HLA-DR+, and various negative and positive selection methods may be used to purify them from sources such as bone marrow and human fetal liver.[103,640] They have the appearance of lymphoblasts.

The bone marrow of an adult mouse contains about 500 CFU-E per 10^5 nucleated cells. In response to anemic stress, such as hemorrhage or hemolysis, nearly the entire burden of accelerated reticulocyte production is born by rapid EPO-dependent influx into the proerythroblast pool from the progenitor compartment.[102,113] This produces an expanded proerythroblast pool. Little or no increase in the mitotic rate of recognizable erythroid precursors occurs.[102] Instead, the late BFU-E and CFU-E proliferate in response to engagement of their EPO receptors by the hormone and, in addition, differentiate to proerythroblasts and beyond. In normal murine marrow, the CFU-E frequency of about 500 per 10^5 nucleated cells increases to 1000 to 2000 CFU-E per 10^5 nucleated cells after experimental hemorrhage or hemolysis. In contrast, hypertransfused mice exhibit a reduced number of CFU-E per 10^5 nucleated marrow cells (values between 10% to 20% of normal have been reported).

During stress erythropoiesis induced by anemia, the orderly progression from immature BFU-E through CFU-E to proerythroblast is interrupted inasmuch as high EPO levels appear to permit or induce differentiation of immature progenitors to proerythroblasts. In the rhesus monkey this premature terminal differentiation may account for the marked increase in fetal hemoglobin content and F cells seen in simian stress erythropoiesis.[641] The ability of human progenitors to generate erythroblasts capable of synthesizing large quantities of fetal hemoglobin is less pronounced.[642] Thus, the accumulation of F cells in peripheral blood in response to anemia is relatively limited.[643] Such red cells are usually macrocytic and carry the i antigen as well, but these two characteristics may relate to a short transit time through the marrow in response to EPO rather than an intrinsic characteristic of the fetal hemoglobin–containing cells themselves (see later). F cells are also present in very small numbers in the blood of normal individuals, but these cells are not macrocytic and do not bear i antigen. F-cell progenitors can easily be detected in the bone marrow of patients with various hemoglobinopathies[644,645] and even in normal marrow.[646]

Transcription Factors and Erythropoiesis

As discussed earlier, targeted disruption of the tal-1/SCL, rbtn2/LMO-2, and GATA-2 genes leads to embryonic lethality secondary to failure of blood production, probably at the HSC level. GATA-1 expression is limited to multipotent progenitors and the erythroid, megakaryocyte, mast, and eosinophil lineages.[98,647,648] Injection of chimeric mice at the blastocyst stage with GATA-1[-/-] ES cells leads to failure of contribution of the GATA-1[-/-] cells to erythrocytes but development into other hematopoietic lineages, as well as other tissues.[649,650] Differentiation assays in vitro show proerythroblast arrest and apoptosis of these cells.[651-653] FOG-1, a transcriptional cofactor of GATA-1, was discovered and found to be essential for erythropoiesis and megakaryopoiesis.[654,655] Evidence that this interaction is essential in vivo comes from studies of a family with severe dyserythropoietic anemia and thrombocytopenia. Affected family members have a mutation in GATA-1 that disrupts its interaction with FOG-1 without affecting DNA-binding affinity.[656] The EKLF transcription factor was found as an activity bound to the CACCC site of the β-globin promoter.[657] It controls globin expression and some aspects of erythroid development. The NF-E2 protein complex binds to the locus control region to regulate globin gene transcription; it is a dimer of a tissue-restricted (erythroid/megakaryocyte/mast cell) subunit of 45 kd and a smaller widely expressed subunit of 18 kd that is essential for platelet but not erythrocyte production.[658,659]

Growth Factors and Erythropoiesis

Regulation of the proliferation and maturation of erythroid progenitors depends on interaction with a number of growth factors. The availability of pure recombinant growth factors, the enrichment of target progenitor cells, and the use of defined "serum-free" culture conditions have provided insight into the role of these factors during hematopoiesis.

EPO is essential for the terminal maturation of erythroid cells. Its major effect appears to be at the level of the CFU-E during adult erythropoiesis, and recombinant preparations[639] are as effective as the natural hormone.[660,661] These progenitors do not require "burst-promoting activity"[662,663] in the form of IL-3 or GM-CSF, and their dependence on EPO is emphasized by the observation that they will not survive in vitro in the absence of EPO. Because most CFU-E progenitors are in cycle, their survival in the presence of EPO is probably tightly linked to their proliferation and differentiation to mature erythrocytes. EPO also acts on a subset of presumptive mature BFU-E, which also require EPO for survival and terminal maturation. A second subset of BFU-E, presumably less mature, survive EPO deprivation if IL-3 or GM-CSF (IL-3 > GM-CSF) is present. When EPO is added to these cultures on day 3, these BFU-E progenitors form typical colonies. Under serum-deprived culture conditions, the combination of IL-3 and GM-CSF results in more BFU-E than either factor alone when EPO is added on day 3.[664] Although EPO is crucial for the terminal differentiation of erythroid progenitors, mice with homozygous null mutations of the EPO or EPOR genes form BFU-E and CFU-E normally, but they fail to differentiate into mature erythrocytes.[314] Both the EPO[-/-] and EPOR[-/-] mutations are embryonically lethal because of failure of definitive (fetal liver) erythropoiesis. However, yolk sac erythropoiesis is only partially impaired, thus indicating the existence of a population of EPO-independent primary erythropoietic precursors. SF has marked synergistic effects on BFU-E cultured in the presence of EPO,[128] although alone it has no colony-forming ability. SF is crucial for the normal development of CFU-E because mice that lack SF (Sl mutants) or its receptor c-kit (W mutants) are severely anemic and have a reduction in fetal liver CFU-E.[665] Further studies showed that SF induces tyrosine phosphorylation of EPOR and that c-kit associates with the cytoplasmic domain of the tyrosine-phosphorylated EPOR. Further insight into the molecular mechanism by which EPO prevents apoptosis in erythroid cells comes from studies of STAT5A[-/-]5B[-/-] mice. During fetal development the embryos are severely anemic; the erythroid progenitors in fetal liver are reduced in number and show increased apoptosis.[666] This result was explained by the finding that STAT5 mediates early induction of the antiapoptotic gene Bcl-X$_L$ through direct binding to its promoter. Interestingly, although adult animals were thought to be hematologically normal, about half have chronic anemia with splenomegaly as a result of an increase in early erythroid precursors; erythropoiesis is ineffective because of an increase in apoptosis in these early normoblasts that have reduced levels of Bcl-X$_L$.[667]

Factors distinct from the classic CSFs may positively regulate erythropoiesis, either directly or indirectly. Limiting-dilution studies of highly purified CFU-E in serum-free culture show that insulin and IGF-I act directly on these cells.[668] The presence of EPO is essential in these studies, in contrast to earlier murine studies of unfractionated cells in which CFU-E respond to IGF-I or insulin in the absence of EPO.[669] Another factor that enhances both BFU-E and CFU-E colony formation is activin. This protein dimer, also known as follicle-stimulating hormone–releasing protein, appears to have a lineage-specific effect on erythropoiesis that is indirect because removal of monocytes or T lymphocytes (or both) abrogates its effect.[670] It is interesting that activin has been identified as the factor produced by vegetal cells during blastogenesis that induces animal ectodermal cells to form primary mesoderm.[671] Hepatocyte growth factor has also been shown to have synergistic effects on CFU-GEMM and BFU-E in EPO-containing cultures.[672]

Negative Regulation of Erythropoiesis

Observations that subsets of lymphocytes with an immunologic suppressor phenotype isolated from normal subjects can inhibit erythroid activity in vitro[673-675] correlate with reports of patients with a variety of disorders in whom anemia or granulocytopenia is associated with expansion of certain T-lymphocyte populations (see also

Chapter 7).[676-678] In the rare disorder T lymphocytosis with cytopenia,[679] in vitro suppression of erythropoiesis has been correlated with the expansion of a T-lymphocyte population that may be the counterpart of the hematopoietic suppressor cells isolated from normal blood. The phenotype of these cells has been described in detail.[679,680] The cell is a large granular lymphocyte that is both E rosette positive and CD8 (classic suppressor phenotype) positive. Suppressor T cells may also be involved in some cases of aplastic anemia[681,682] or neutropenia[683] without an underlying immunologic disorder or overt T-cell proliferation. Exactly how such suppressor T cells interact with hematopoietic progenitors and what surface antigens are "seen" by the suppressors are uncertain. There is evidence to support the concept that suppression of erythroid colony expression in vitro is regulated by T cells and may be genetically restricted.[680,684] Cell-cell interactions in immunologic systems have been well characterized with regard to surface determinants that allow cellular recognition. That certain phenotypes of T cells "recognize" distinct classes of histocompatibility antigens on immunologic cell surfaces has been well described.[685] Thus, the observation that hematopoietic progenitors have a unique distribution of class II hiscompatibility antigens on their cell surface[686-689] suggests a role for these antigens in the cell-cell interactions that regulate hematopoietic differentiation.

TNF also suppresses erythropoiesis in vitro.[690,691] Injection of peritoneal macrophages into Friend murine leukemia virus–infected animal results in rapid, but transient resolution of the massive erythroid hyperplasia associated with this disease. This may be due to elaboration by macrophages of IL-1α, which does not suppress erythropoiesis itself but acts by induction of TNF. This effect is reversed by EPO.[692]

Myelopoiesis

Phagocyte Development

Although a clonogenic assay of granulocyte progenitors was developed almost a decade before the erythroid clonogenic assay, the various factors responsible for granulocyte/macrophage development remain incompletely understood. Excellent reviews of early work in this field have been provided by Metcalf[94] and Moore.[90]

It is now accepted that CFU-GM is derived from the pluripotent progenitor and, under the influence of SCF, IL-3, GM-CSF, G-CSF, or M-CSF (or any combination of these factors), ultimately gives rise to mature granulocytes and monocytes. Monocytes irreversibly leave the circulation[693,694] and differentiate further into fixed-tissue macrophages, a category comprising alveolar macrophages,[695] hepatic Kupffer cells,[696] dermal Langerhans cells,[697] osteoclasts,[698] peritoneal and pleural macrophages, and perhaps brain microglial cells.[699] The enormous diversity of this system and the high turnover rate of granulocytes, as well as the necessity to maintain splenic, marginated, and bone marrow granulocyte pools to meet sudden demands caused by infection, have led to the evolution of an extremely complex regulatory network. Indeed, although many of the factors that allow release of granulocytes from storage pools are distinct from CSF,[13] GM-CSF can inhibit granulocyte motility,[700] as well as serve as an activator of granulocyte superoxide anion generation.[701] This complexity in vivo does not permit studies analogous to those in which erythropoiesis is influenced by hypertransfusion or hemorrhage[702,703] and megakaryocytopoiesis is stimulated by induced thrombocytopenia.[704] Thus, investigators have relied heavily on in vitro progenitor assays to study the regulation of myelopoiesis.

Transcription Factors and Myelopoiesis

A family of transcription factors important for commitment to the myeloid and lymphoid lineages, as well as regulation of myeloid-specific promoters such as those of the myeloperoxidase (MPO) and neutrophil elastase (NE) genes, are factors that were first identified on the basis of their ability to bind to the polyomavirus enhancer–binding protein 2 (PEBP2)/CBF. Two α subunits (CBFα1 and CBFα2 [the human homologue is known as AML-1 or Runx1]) bind DNA with low affinity, and affinity is strengthened in the presence of the non–DNA-binding β subunit (CBFβ). As noted earlier, AML-1[-/-] mice die in utero by day 12.5 because of failure production of all definitive hematopoietic lineages.[584] The C/EBP family of transcription factors bind to DNA through a basic region–leucine zipper domain (bZIP). There are several family members (C/EBPα, C/EBPβ [NF–IL-6], C/EBPγ, C/EBPδ, C/EBPζ, and C/EBPε) that are differentially expressed during myelopoiesis, with increased (C/EBPβ) or increased followed by either partial (C/EBPδ) or marked (C/EBPα) decreased levels of expression during maturation of 32D cl3 cells to terminally differentiated granulocytes.[705] C/EBPα has been implicated in the regulation of hepatocyte and adipocyte differentiation (levels are low in undifferentiated dividing cells but high in quiescent terminally differentiated cells), as well as in myeloid CSF receptor promoter function; AML-1 can act synergistically with C/EBPα to activate the M-CSFR promoter.[706] C/EBPα[-/-] mice show arrested myelopoiesis at the myeloblast stage as a result of failure of expression of G-CSFR and IL-6R.[707,708] Mice that lack C/EBPβ produce monocytes that are defective in bactericidal and tumoricidal function, and their macrophages and fibroblasts, but interestingly not their endothelial cells, fail to produce G-CSF in response to LPS.[709] C/EBPε is produced primarily in myeloid lineages. Knockout mice are viable and fertile but die at 50 to 75 days as a result of opportunistic infections with *Pseudomonas aeruginosa*.[710] Nullizygous animals fail to produce normal neutrophils and eosinophils. Functional abnormalities include diminished release of hydrogen peroxide in response to phytohemagglutinin stimulation because of failure to produce secondary and tertiary granules, which are important reservoirs of membrane-bound components of the reduced nicotinamide adenine dinucleotide phosphate (NADPH) oxidase apparatus. Additional components of secondary and tertiary granules, lactoferrin and gelatinase B, are absent because of failure of transcriptional activation of C/EBPε.[710,711] Interestingly, similar abnormalities characterize the rare neutrophil-specific granule deficiency,[712] and indeed, mutations in C/EBPε have recently been found in these patients.[713-715] The PU.1 (Spi-1) transcription factor is a member of the Ets family and is expressed principally in monocytes/macrophages and B lymphocytes, as well as in erythroid cells and granulocytes.[716,717] Potential target genes include the integrin CD11b, M-CSFR, GM-CSFRα, G-CSFR, and the immunoglobulin λ light chain.[718-722] Mice that lack PU.1 die in utero with absence of monocytes, granulocytes, and T and B lymphocytes; the presence of anemia is variable and thus does not explain the prenatal mortality.[723]

Growth Factors and Myelopoiesis

Murine IL-3 stimulates a broad spectrum of myeloid progenitor cells, including pluripotent stem cells, CFU-GM, CFU-G, CFU-M, BFU-E, CFU-Eo, CFU-Meg, and mast cells. As its name implies, GM-CSF was initially shown to be more restricted as a stimulus of the proliferation and development of CFU-GM. However, murine studies with purified or recombinant factor have shown that it also stimulates the initial proliferation of other progenitors such as BFU-E (see earlier).[189,724] The other murine factors, G-CSF and M-CSF, are more restricted and predominantly stimulate CFU-G and CFU-M, respectively.[725,726]

With the possible exception of GM-CSF, the activities of human CSFs are similar to those of the corresponding murine factors. Both IL-3 and GM-CSF affect a similar broad spectrum of human progenitor cells, including CFU-GEMM, CFU-GM, CFU-G, CFU-M, CFU-Eo, and CFU-Meg. In full serum cultures, IL-3 and GM-CSF alone stimulate the formation of colonies derived from CFU-GM, CFU-G, CFU-M, CFU-Eo, and CFU-Meg. Data from serum-free cultures suggest that in the presence of IL-3 or GM-CSF alone, myeloid colony formation is much reduced and optimal CFU-G or CFU-M proliferation requires the addition of G-CSF or M-CSF, respectively, to the cultures.[193,664] Even in serum-replete conditions, IL-3 acts additively or synergistically with G-CSF to induce more granulocyte colony formation than observed with either factor alone.[192]

Insight into the in vivo role of GM-CSF comes from studies in which the GM-CSF gene was disrupted by homologous recombination in ES cells.[321] GM-CSF knockout mice showed normal basal hematopoiesis, but surfactant lipids and proteins progressively accumulated in the alveolar space, the defining characteristic of idiopathic human pulmonary alveolar proteinosis. Extensive lymphoid hyperplasia associated with lung airways and blood vessels was also found. Surfactant proteins and lipids are synthesized by type II pneumocytes and cleared from the alveolar space by type II cells and alveolar macrophages. Lungs from the null animals showed normal surfactant synthetic capacity and no accumulation in type II pneumocytes. In contrast, alveolar macrophages showed a marked increase in surfactant protein and lipid, which strongly suggests that these cells cannot process surfactant as a result of the lack of GM-CSF. Mice generated with null mutations of the common chain of the GM-CSF/IL-3/IL-5 receptor (β_c) have similar pulmonary pathology and also show low basal numbers of eosinophils and absence of blood and lung eosinophilia in response to infection with the parasite *Nippostrongylous brasiliensis*.[316] The G-CSF gene has also been disrupted by homologous recombination in ES cells.[313] G-CSF[-/-] mice have a chronic neutropenia (20% to 30% of normal levels) and reduced bone marrow myeloid precursors and progenitors. The animals also exhibited a markedly impaired capacity to increase neutrophil and monocyte counts after infection with *Listeria monocytogenes*.

In addition to their effects on progenitor differentiation, the CSFs also induce a variety of functional changes in mature cells. GM-CSF inhibits polymorphonuclear neutrophil migration under agarose,[700] induces antibody-dependent cytotoxicity (ADCC) in human target cells,[701] and increases neutrophil phagocytic activity.[187] Some of these functional changes may be related to the GM-CSF–induced increase in cell surface expression of a family of antigens that function as cell adhesion molecules.[727] The increase in antigen expression is rapid and associated with increased aggregation of neutrophils; both are maximal at the migration inhibitory concentration of 500 pM, and granulocyte-granulocyte adhesion can be inhibited by an antigen-specific monoclonal antibody. GM-CSF also acts as a potent stimulus of eosinophil ADCC, superoxide production, and phagocytosis.[728] G-CSF acts as a potent stimulus of neutrophil superoxide production, ADCC, and phagocytosis,[729] whereas M-CSF activates mature macrophages[730] and enhances macrophage cytotoxicity.

Megakaryocytopoiesis

The cloning of TPO has greatly clarified our understanding of the regulation of megakaryocytopoiesis.[177] Before the discovery of TPO, several factors,[731] including IL-3,[732] IL-6,[733] IL-11,[734] kit ligand,[735,736] and even EPO,[737,738] were shown to stimulate megakaryocytopoiesis and thrombopoiesis in vitro and in vivo. IL-3, IL-6, and IL-11 engage heterodimeric receptors of the β_c (IL-3R) and gp130 families (IL-6R and IL-11R). Kit ligand engages a receptor whose intracellular domain expresses tyrosine kinase activity upon ligand binding. As already emphasized in this chapter, ligand engagement of these receptor families is known to induce early multipotent progenitors to proliferate and even differentiate toward lineage-specific progenitors, and kit ligand, IL-3, and IL-11 participate in the induction of proliferation and differentiation of lineage-specific progenitors. Single-cell analysis of prospectively isolated murine megakaryocyte progenitors shows that a large proportion (≈60%) express EPOR,[419] which is consistent with the potent effect of EPO on megakaryocyte colony formation.[739]

The discovery of TPO provided a major step in understanding megakaryocytopoiesis because this factor induces lineage-restricted megakaryocyte progenitor proliferation, differentiation of these committed progenitors to megakaryoblasts, and finally, differentiation of megakaryoblasts to megakaryocytes, which in turn produce platelets (see Fig. 6-13).

Thrombopoietin

TPO is produced at the site of hematopoiesis. Therefore, although its activity is increased in blood during episodes of thrombopenia, it does not necessarily function as a hormone because it is produced directly at the site of thrombopoiesis. In this sense it differs from EPO, which is not produced at all in marrow stroma. Blood levels may increase in thrombocytopenic states merely because circulating platelets or tissue megakaryocytes, or both, sop up the growth factor and carry it out of the circulation.[395,740] This theory has received support from observations in mice with disruption of the murine transcription factor gene NF-E2[100]; although these animals are thrombocytopenic, they have an increase in megakaryocyte mass and no increase in serum TPO levels.[741]

As reviewed by Kaushansky,[177] the TPO molecule is considerably longer than the other HGF polypeptides. Its 5′ half bears 23% sequence homology to EPO, whereas the 3′ half bears no structural homology to any cytokine and may be removed by a proteolytic mechanism. Indeed, removal of this half does not ablate its physiologic function. The resemblance of the 5′ domain of the molecule to EPO may explain the synergy of TPO and EPO in megakaryocyte colony formation and platelet production.[177,730] It is well recognized that splenectomized individuals with persistent anemia usually have significant thrombocytosis and that many individuals with red cell aplasia and high EPO levels also have thrombocytosis and megakaryocytosis.

The function of TPO has been studied carefully in vivo and in vitro. Lineage-specific CD34+ megakaryocyte progenitors bear receptors for SF, IL-3, IL-11, and TPO, the four major classes of hematopoietic cytokine receptors. Maximal megakaryocyte colony formation probably requires signaling by all four receptors, but TPO is absolutely required for the final stages of megakaryocyte maturation, including maximal ploidy, cytoplasmic volume, and therefore platelet production.

Therapeutic trials of TPO in mice have shown that TPO is species specific. Treatment of mice with murine TPO induces massive thrombocytosis, whereas human TPO is much less active in these animals. More importantly, TPO is active in reducing the platelet nadir in mice and primates rendered thrombcytopenic by chemotherapy or radiation.

Circulating Platelets

The differential diagnosis of thrombocytopenia rests first on evaluation of platelet morphology. In conditions in which megakaryocytopoiesis is accelerated, circulating platelet volume (and usually diameter) is increased. The reasons for this shift in volume are disputed. Some claim that young platelets are larger than old platelets.[742] Others suggest that large megakaryocytes give rise to large platelets.[743] Neither explanation satisfies all experimental and clinical conditions, but in general, thrombocytopenia secondary to increased destruction of platelets is associated with platelets with large volume, and thrombocytopenia related to decreased production of platelets is associated with platelets of normal size. There are major exceptions to this rule. Patients with hyposplenism tend to have large platelets in their blood, regardless of whether thrombopoiesis is increased, and patients with primary abnormalities in platelet function, such as Wiskott-Aldrich or Bernard-Soulier syndrome, have platelet sizes that bear no relationship to platelet production. TPO increases platelet production by increasing both the number and size of individual megakaryocytes. Although TPO is probably solely responsible for the later stages of recognizable megakaryocyte differentiation and proliferation of megakaryocyte progenitors, its function depends, at least in part, on additional stimulation of megakaryocyte progenitors (and probably early megakaryocytes as well) with other growth factors, including IL-3, IL-11, SCF, and EPO.

CLINICAL USE OF HEMATOPOIETIC GROWTH FACTORS

Correction or amelioration of marrow failure syndromes by the administration of HGFs has been and continues to be a major practical goal of research in hematopoiesis. The goal could not be achieved, however, until recombinant DNA technology provided sufficient amounts of the hormones to permit interpretable investigations.

Human Clinical Studies

Several recombinant HGFs are currently under evaluation in a variety of clinical settings. G-CSF and EPO are widely used clinically. G-CSF shortens the hypoplasia that follows chemotherapy and makes more intensive myeloablative chemotherapy regimens possible.

Malignant Disease

G-CSF

In the first phase I/II clinical studies in patients with malignant disease, administration of G-CSF by bolus or continuous intravenous infusion for 5 to 6 days before chemotherapy led to a dose-related increase in polymorphonuclear neutrophils.[744,745] Rapid increases in neutrophil counts were observed, with maximal counts of 80 to 100×10^9/L at doses of 10 to 30 mg/kg/day. A transient depression in neutrophil counts was noted to precede this increase in one study.[746] In another study, recombinant human GM-CSF (rhGM-CSF) was given for 14 days after alternate cycles of intensive chemotherapy.[747] The period of neutropenia was reduced by a median of 80% (52% to 100%) in the chemotherapy/G-CSF cycles, with a return to normal neutrophil counts within 2 weeks after chemotherapy. Infective episodes were observed during the cycles of chemotherapy that did not include G-CSF, whereas no infective episode occurred in those that did. G-CSF treatment after chemotherapy results in a significant reduction in the number of days per patient in which the neutrophil count is less than 1.0×10^9/L.[744] Antibiotic use to treat fever and neutropenia is also reduced, and all the patients could receive their next course of chemotherapy on schedule (versus 29% of patients who did not receive G-CSF). The mature neutrophils produced in response to G-CSF have normal mobility and bactericidal capacity.[748] A double-blind, randomized, placebo-controlled U.S. multicenter trial was conducted in which patients with lung carcinoma who received up to six cycles of cyclophosphamide, doxorubicin, and etoposide were given G-CSF or placebo from days 4 to 17 of each cycle. The results showed a reduction in the median duration of severe neutropenia ($<0.5 \times 10^9$/L) from 6 to 3 days in the G-CSF arm and a 50% reduction in febrile neutropenia, hospitalizations, confirmed infections, and antibiotic use with G-CSF (see Fig. 6-2).[749] This study and other reports[750,751] have led the American Society of Clinical Oncology and the European Organization for Research and Treatment of Cancer to recommend primary use of G-CSF in patients with an expected rate of neutropenia that exceeds 20%.[752,753] The use of G-CSF is recommended to support dose-dense or dose-intense chemotherapy regimens in adult carcinoma patients, but most studies do not show a significant effect on progression-free survival.[753] Patients in the placebo arm of the U.S. multicenter trial[749] in whom fever developed in the first treatment cycle were subsequently treated with G-CSF, which reduced the duration of severe neutropenia from 6 to 3 days and neutropenic fever from 100% in cycle 1 to 1% to 23% in cycle 2. Thus, the prophylactic use of G-CSF in chemotherapy-induced neutropenia is supported. However, the literature does not support the use of G-CSF or GM-CSF once afebrile[754] or febrile neutropenia has developed,[755,756] with the exception of one study.[757] Although days of neutropenia may be shortened, it has been difficult to show an effect on clinically significant end points such as shortened duration of hospitalization, which was seen in only one of the studies.[756]

GM-CSF

rhGM-CSF has been administered in phase I/II studies to several adult groups of patients with advanced malignancy, both before and after chemotherapy.[758-760] Glyco-sylated GM-CSF produced in either mammalian (Chinese hamster ovary) cells or yeast and *Escherichia coli*–derived nonglycosylated GM-CSF have been evaluated with comparable results. A rapid, dose-related increase in polymorphonuclear neutrophils, monocytes, and eosinophils is observed in patients treated before chemotherapy. Neutrophils peak at around 20 to 30×10^9/L with doses of 4 to 32 mg/kg/day, and GM-CSF is well tolerated at doses up to this level. Capillary leak syndrome and venous thrombi are observed at higher doses (64 mg/kg/day).[758] Phase III randomized trials in patients with lymphoma or breast cancer have confirmed that GM-CSF given after chemotherapy is associated with shorter periods of neutropenia and higher leukocyte nadirs.[761-763] However, one of these studies included only patients able to tolerate treatment and was not significant on an intention-to-treat basis. Furthermore, another study of GM-CSF after chemotherapy showed decreased neutropenia after the first treatment cycle only,[764] whereas another two studies showed no improvement in neutrophil counts.[765,766] In one of these studies,[765] patients with small cell lung cancer were given chemotherapy and radiation therapy; when compared with the placebo control, patients in the GM-CSF arm suffered more infections, toxic deaths, and longer hospital stays, and therefore the American Society of Clinical Oncology panel has cautioned against the use of CSFs in combined chemotherapy/radiotherapy regimens.[767,768]

Similar encouraging results have been obtained in children with solid tumors undergoing intensive chemotherapy.[769-771] Significantly shorter durations of severe neutropenia and thrombocytopenia were observed in a study of 25 children in whom yeast-derived GM-CSF was administered at 60 to 1500 µg/m^2/day for 14 days after chemotherapy.[769]

Like G-CSF, GM-CSF also produced an increase in blood progenitor cells of both the erythroid and myeloid lineage. Before chemotherapy, an 18-fold increase in blood CFU-GM and an 8-fold increase in BFU-E was noted; after chemotherapy, GM-CSF produced a much greater increase in progenitors (60-fold) when given during the recovery period.[769]

Erythropoietin

Anemia is frequent in cancer patients and correlates with poor performance status and decreased quality of life (reviewed by Beutel and Ganser[772]). There is good evidence that recombinant human EPO (rhEPO) can increase the hemoglobin level in adults[773,774] and children[775] with anemia associated with cancer or its treatment. Three different EPO preparations are available, epoetin alfa (Epogen [Amgen], Procrit [Ortho Biotech], and Eprex [Ortho Biologicals, not sold in the United States]), epoetin beta (NeoRecormon [Roche], sold in Europe), and darbopoetin alfa (Aranesp [Amgen], sold in the United States, Europe, Canada, and Australia). Differences in the sialic acid carbohydrate composition of epoetin alfa and beta account for an increase in half-life from 8.5 hours (natural EPO) to 20 to 24 hours, whereas hyperglycosylation of darbopoetin results in a half-life of 49 hours.

Two 2003 randomized studies of patients with anemia and either head and neck cancer or breast cancer showed shorter survival in the groups receiving EPO, thus raising concern that EPO can lead to progression of disease.[776,777] Another study of advanced non–small cell lung cancer designed to compare EPO with placebo was stopped early when a safety analysis of 70 patients showed a significant survival advantage in the placebo group. Whether carcinoma cells express EPOR and respond to EPO is controversial. Antibodies to EPOR lack specificity and do not distinguish cell surface from intracellular expression, and functional in vitro effects are frequently limited and found at supraphysiologic doses. However, EPO could still have adverse consequences through indirect effects on endothelial cells or on angiogenesis.[778]

Thrombopoietin

Because of TPO's potent in vitro activity and its role as the factor essential for terminal megakaryocytic differentiation, analogous to EPO for the erythroid lineage, clinical studies designed to assess its effect on platelet production have been reported. Both recombinant human TPO (rhTPO) and pegylated megakaryocyte growth and development factor (PEG-MGDF) are safe and show no organ toxicity, and in normal volunteers, a single bolus of 3 µg/kg/day of PEG-MGDF doubles the blood platelet concentration by day 12 with a return to baseline by day 28 (reviewed by Harker[779]). A stimulatory effect on platelet production was observed when TPO or PEG-MGDF was administered after chemotherapy to more than 100 cancer patients, with a decrease in the time for platelet counts to return to normal and elevated platelet nadirs.[780-782] Further studies showed that TPO and PEG-MGDF were effective in malignancies treated with nonmyeloablative chemotherapy but were less effective in myeloablative regimens followed by stem cell transplantation for the treatment of leukemia (reviewed by Kuter and Begley[783]). Moreover, PEG-MGDF has caused the development of antibodies to TPO that resulted in severe thrombocytopenia (see later), and these cytokines have been withdrawn from clinical use. Small molecules, peptides, and a peptide–Fc antibody combination (AMG 531 "peptibody") that have no sequence homology with TPO but activate the receptor are under investigation (reviewed by Szilvassy[784]).

Bone Marrow Transplantation

GM-CSF, G-CSF, and M-CSF have been evaluated in clinical autotransplantation trials.

GM-CSF

Patients with nonhematopoietic malignancies were treated with high-dose combination chemotherapy, autologous bone marrow transplantation, and rhGM-CSF given by continuous intravenous infusion for 14 days beginning 3 hours after bone marrow infusion. There was a dose-related increase in neutrophil count at day 14 (1411/µL at 2 to 8 mg/kg/day, 2575/µL at 16 mg/kg/day, and 3120/µL at 32 mg/kg/day as compared with 863/µL in 24 historical controls).[785] Though not statistically significant, there was an improved neutrophil response in patients who had not received previous chemotherapy versus those who had (1832 versus 833/µL). Lower morbidity and mortality were also noted in patients who received GM-CSF; bacteremia occurred in 16% of treated patients as compared with 35% of evaluable controls. Comparable results were reported in a study of patients with lymphoid malignancies who received rhGM-CSF as a 2-hour infusion daily for 14 days after chemotherapy, radiotherapy, and autologous bone marrow transplantation.[786] Neutrophil and platelet counts recovered more rapidly, there were fewer days of fever, and the extent of hospitalization was reduced in comparison to a historical control group. In a pediatric study, nine patients received 5 to 10 µg/kg/day GM-CSF after bone marrow transplantation. Neutrophil recovery was accelerated, although there was no difference in fever, infection, or length of hospitalization when compared with historical controls.[787] Similar results were obtained in a larger prospective double-blind randomized study of 40 patients.[788]

The response to GM-CSF after myelosuppression may be dependent on the infusion of sufficient progenitor cells. In an autotransplantation study of patients with ALL, bone marrow was purged with 4-hydroperoxycyclophosphamide and anti–T- or anti–B-cell lineage-specific antibodies before transplantation.[789] Thirty percent of the patients who received more than 64 µg/m²/day GM-CSF achieved an absolute neutrophil count (ANC) of greater than 1000/µL by day 21, whereas none of the nonresponders reached this level by day 27 after transplantation. The responders required only a third as many platelet transfusions, and there was a trend toward fewer red cell transfusions, higher myeloid-erythroid ratio, and earlier day of discharge in the responder group as well. Although the bone marrow cell dose did not differ between the two groups, the number of CFU-GM progenitors infused per kilogram was significantly higher in the responders than in the nonresponders (17.5 [12 to 27] × 10³/kg versus 2 [0 to 7.2] × 10³/kg). Although it is possible that this accounts for the more rapid recovery rather than the rhGM-CSF infusion, the responder group all showed a rapid decrease in ANC within 48 to 72 hours of discontinuing GM-CSF; this is consistent with a stimulatory effect on bone marrow. One can conclude that GM-CSF is effective in this context, provided that sufficient progenitor cells are present.

G-CSF

Recombinant human G-CSF (rhG-CSF) was evaluated in patients with hematopoietic and nonhematopoietic malignancies after intensive chemotherapy and reinfusion of cryopreserved autologous bone marrow.[790] rhG-CSF was given by continuous intravenous infusion starting 24 hours after marrow infusion for a maximum of 28 days; the initial dose of 20 µg/kg/day was reduced after the neutrophil count persistently exceeded $1 \times 10^9/$L. The mean time to neutrophil recovery ($>0.5 \times 10^9$/L) was 11 days, 9 days earlier than in historical controls. This led to significantly fewer days of parental antibiotic therapy, but there was no effect on red cell or platelet recovery. Although the rate of recovery from neutropenia was faster than that reported for rhGM-CSF, the latter studies were phase I dose escalation evaluations, and many patients did not receive an optimal dose of GM-CSF. A prospective randomized study of 221 children receiving allogeneic or autologous bone marrow or peripheral blood stem cells showed more rapid neutrophil recovery in the G-CSF–treated patients, and this translated to clinical benefit in the bone marrow group (platelet transfusion independence and time to discharge).[791] A study compared G-CSF with GM-CSF in exactly the same analogous bone marrow transplant protocol. The G-CSF group contained more patients with breast carcinoma who had previously received chemotherapy, and this group did not show a dose-related increase in neutrophil count after a 14-day continuous intravenous infusion at doses of 16, 32, and 64 µg/kg/day. Overall, however, total leukocyte recovery was slightly more rapid in the G-CSF group than in the GM-CSF group. Administration of G-CSF resulted in two leukocyte peaks. The first at day 10 involved lymphocytes, whereas the second at day 14 consisted of mostly granulocytes; in contrast, GM-CSF produced a single peak at the end of the period of infusion. A major difference was observed with respect to neutrophil migration to an inflammatory site during CSF infusion after hematopoietic reconstitution.[792] Neutrophils did not migrate to skin chambers filled with autologous serum during GM-CSF treatment, a defect not encountered during the administration of G-CSF. There was, however, a similar reduction in the incidence of bacteremia with both GM-CSF and G-CSF (18% and 19%, respectively) in comparison to historical controls (35%).

In conclusion, if neutrophil recovery is the goal after bone marrow transplantation, G-CSF appears to be the factor of choice. It preserves neutrophil function and is well tolerated. The inability to hasten platelet recovery is still the major challenge.

Thrombopoietin

PEG-MGDF was evaluated in a controlled trial of 50 breast cancer patients who received chemotherapy along with autologous bone marrow; the time during which the platelet count remained lower than 20,000/µL was reduced ($P \leq 0.6$), and the time to recovery of normal platelets was significantly shortened. However, when mobilized blood progenitors were given rather than bone marrow, the more rapid recovery made it difficult to demonstrate an effect of PEG-MGDF on duration of thrombocytopenia or platelet transfusion requirements. Furthermore, a phase III randomized placebo-controlled double-blind study of 64 patients failed to show a consistent reduction in the duration of severe thrombocytopenia.[793]

Myelodysplasia

GM-CSF

Despite the theoretical risks of administering CSFs to patients with myeloid stem cell clonal diseases, the factors have been evaluated in patients with refractory anemia (RA), RA with an excess of blasts (RAEB), RAEB in transformation (RAEBIT), and chronic myelomonocytic leukemia.[794-796] In an early study, GM-CSF was given by continuous infusion for 14 days and repeated after a 2-week rest period.[794] Five of the eight patients had received chemotherapy up to 4 weeks before the study. Doses of 30 to 500 µg/m² were used. Blood leukocytes rose 5- to 70-fold and neutrophils 5- to 373-fold, and an absolute increase in monocytes, eosinophils, and lymphocytes was also observed. Three of the eight patients also had a 2- to 10-fold increase in platelet count and improvement in erythropoiesis, and two of the three became transfusion independent. Marrow cellularity increased and the proportion of blasts decreased, although there was a transient and dose-related increase in the absolute number of circulating blasts. In no patient did overt leukemia develop during the period of follow-up (up to 32 weeks). There was no cytogenetic evidence of a reduction in abnormal clones, and it is likely that the stimulatory effect on hematopoiesis affects both normal and abnormal cells. A dose-related increase in neutrophils, monocytes, eosinophils, and lymphocytes was also noted in a study of 11 patients with myelodysplasia. However, four patients with greater than 14% blasts in bone marrow showed an increase in blasts after therapy, and an additional three patients showed an increase in blasts in blood; five patients progressed to acute leukemia either during or within 4 weeks after treatment.[796] Unlike the earlier report, none of these patients had previously received chemotherapy.

G-CSF

A number of patients have also been treated with G-CSF.[797,798] Neutrophil responses were seen in five patients with myelodysplasia who received 50 to 1600 µg/m²/day by 30-minute infusion daily for 6 days. At higher doses (400 µg/m²/day), the increase was sustained and associated with an increase in bone marrow cellularity. No reticulocyte or platelet increases were observed, and no patient progressed to an acute phase. Similar results were reported in a study of 12 patients given G-CSF by daily subcutaneous injection, with dose escalation from 0.1 to 3 µg/kg/day over an 8-week period.[798] Although 10 of the 12 patients showed elevations in neutrophils (5- to 40-fold), an increase in reticulocytes occurred in 5 patients with a reduction in transfusion requirements in 2. There was no response in other cell lineages and no conversion to acute leukemia.

Other HGFs and HGF Combinations

Approximately 20% of patients have an increase in platelet count during treatment with IL-3,[799,800] and a similar proportion have an increase in hematocrit or reduced transfusion requirement with EPO.[7801] This erythroid response can be increased to about 40% if EPO is combined with either G-CSF or GM-CSF.[802,803]

In a review of this subject, Marsh and colleagues concluded that although EPO can increase hemoglobin levels and reduce the need for transfusion, the cost-effectiveness of the approach is uncertain, as is safety with regard to the risk of progression. There is no compelling evidence for a survival benefit with the use of EPO or G-CSF in MDS.[804]

Aplastic Anemia

GM-CSF

Establishing a role for the CSFs in aplastic anemia has challenged investigators. Severe aplastic anemia is a heterogeneous disease that may result either from absent or defective stem cells, from microenvironmental defects, or from immunologically mediated suppression. Mortality is high and therapeutic options are limited to bone marrow transplantation if an appropriate donor is available or to immunosuppression (see Chapters 7 and 8). Although bone marrow transplantation can be curative, treatment with antithymocyte globulin (ATG) and cyclosporine is sometimes effective but not generally curative. For these reasons, rhGM-CSF has been evaluated in a number of phase I/II studies. Administration of rhGM-CSF by bolus or continuous intravenous infusion for 7 or 14 days resulted in increased granulocytes, monocytes, and reticulocytes in six of eight patients.[795] In another small study, rhGM-CSF was given to cohorts of patients in escalating doses of 4 to 64 μg/kg/day by continuous intravenous infusion for 14 days. Although a dose-related effect was not observed, 10 of 11 evaluable patients had partial or complete responses in neutrophil, monocyte, and eosinophil counts, along with increases in bone marrow cellularity. Importantly, the greatest increments occurred in patients with higher pretreatment neutrophil counts and more cellular marrow. Only 10% to 20% of patients show an increase in hemoglobin concentration and platelet count, and in all cases counts return to baseline after cessation of treatment.[794,805] In the first report of rhGM-CSF treatment in childhood, three quarters of the evaluable patients responded with a significant rise in neutrophil count during the 28-day induction period.[806] Although neutrophil counts returned to baseline after cessation of treatment in all the responders with severe aplastic anemia, one patient with moderate aplasia maintained a trilineage response off therapy for longer than 1 year. One cannot extrapolate from such a small experience, but the data underscore the point that responses are more likely in less severely affected cases.

Thus, in summary, it appears as though rhGM-CSF is palliative in aplastic anemia, with greater neutrophil responses evident in less severely affected patients. The most severely affected patients respond poorly.[807] No infections were observed during the study period in several reports, whereas infections were reported in others. Longer-term prospective comparative studies will be necessary to investigate morbidity.

G-CSF

Neutrophil responses have also been reported in a study of 20 children given 400 μg/m²/day G-CSF for 14 days.[808] Twelve patients responded by doubling their neutrophil counts, but other lineages were unaffected. In another pediatric study, high doses of G-CSF (400 to 2000 μg/m²/day) induced neutrophil responses in 6 of 10 patients with very severe aplastic anemia.[809] Long-term treatment may be associated with multilineage responses when given alone[810] or in combination with cyclosporine.[811]

IL-3, IL-6, and EPO

Hematopoietic responses have been reported in a small phase I study of nine aplastic anemia patients given IL-3, 250 to 500 μg/m² (five of nine doubled their neutrophil counts, four of nine showed an increase in reticulocyte counts but no reduction in transfusion requirement, and in one platelet counts increased from 1 to 31×10^9/L).[812] An increase in platelet count was reported in one of six patients entered in a phase I study of IL-6, although a dose-related decrease in neutrophils, monocytes, and lymphocytes was observed; a proportion (approximately a third) of patients given EPO had reduced transfusion requirements or an increase in hemoblobin, or both (reviewed by Kojima[813]). Trilineage responses have been reported in a small number of refractory aplastic anemia patients treated with low-dose GM-CSF plus EPO[814] or G-CSF plus EPO.[815] The effects of EPO are unexpected because endrogenous levels are very high in patients with aplastic anemia.

Human Immunodeficiency Virus Infection

GM-CSF

Human immunodeficiency virus (HIV) infection is associated with several hematologic abnormalities, including neutropenia, anemia, and thrombocytopenia. Anemia and neutropenia can be exacerbated by treatment with azidothymidine, and rhGM-CSF has been evaluated in an effort to enhance immunologic and hematopoietic function and improve tolerance to therapeutic agents. In the first report of the use of rhGM-CSF in humans, cohorts of patients with acquired immunodeficiency syndrome (AIDS) were treated with increasing doses of factor given by 14-day continuous intravenous infusion.[816] Such treatment resulted in a rapid, dose-related increase in neutrophils, bands, and eosinophils, with a slight increase in monocytes. A follow-up study with subcutaneous administration showed that these effects could be sustained for up to 6 months without evidence of tachyphylaxis.[816]

A concern with the use of GM-CSF in AIDS is possible enhancement of HIV replication. In one study of azidothymidine given on an alternate-week schedule with GM-CSF, some patients showed increased viral p24 levels during therapy with GM-CSF. There is evidence, however, that GM-CSF may in fact augment azidothymidine levels in monocytes, which suggests that the combination of azidothymidine and GM-CSF might be advantageous.[817] Such is not the case, however, with newer nucleoside analogues such as dideoxycytidine and dideoxyinosine (reviewed by Mueller).[818] Two clinical studies have documented an increase in HIV p24 antigen in patients undergoing GM-CSF therapy,[819,761] and therefore GM-CSF has been replaced by G-CSF for the treatment of neutropenia.

G-CSF

In a pilot study at the National Institutes of Health, G-CSF was evaluated in 19 pediatric AIDS patients in whom neutropenia developed during treatment with azidothymidine. The neutrophil count increased from a median of 1 to 2.9×10^9/L at doses of 1 to 20 μg/kg/day, and in 17 of the 19 patients continued azidothymidine was well tolerated.[820] Of note was the development of thrombocytopenia in some patients; G-CSF–dependent disseminated intravascular coagulation developed in 2 patients, and an increase in myeloblasts that disappeared after stopping G-CSF treatment was observed in 1 patient.[818]

Erythropoietin

EPO has been used in 12 anemic pediatric patients to determine whether tolerance to azidothymidine could be improved.[818] EPO was well tolerated, and at doses of 150 to 400 U/kg subcutaneously or intravenously three times per week, all patients could be maintained on azidothymidine with a marked (four patients) or moderate (four patients) reduction in transfusion requirements.

Thrombopoietin

PEG-MGDF has been evaluated in six HIV-infected thrombocytopenic patients in a randomized placebo-controlled study.[821] Platelet counts increased 10-fold within 14 days and were sustained for the 16 weeks of the study, with return to previous levels within 2 weeks of cessation of treatment. There was no evidence of increased viral load or anti–PEG-MGDF antibodies. Megakaryocytic apoptosis, which was abnormal before treatment, shifted into the normal range by TPO treatment, thus suggesting that the mechanism of action involves increased effectiveness of the platelets that are produced.

Inherited Bone Marrow Failure Syndromes

The use of HGFs in the treatment of inherited bone marrow failure syndromes has been reviewed in detail.[822,823]

Fanconi's Anemia

GM-CSF has been studied in seven patients with Fanconi's anemia,[824] and trials of IL-3 and G-CSF[822] show that all three HGFs can improve the neutrophil count in most pancytopenic patients, but platelet and hemoglobin levels are unaffected.

Diamond-Blackfan Anemia

Although there is no evidence that Diamond-Blackfan anemia (DBA) is due to deficiency of EPO,[825] IL-3, or GM-CSF[826] or an abnormality of c-kit or its ligand SF,[827,828] it is possible that pharmacologic doses of these factors might stimulate erythropoiesis. Niemeyer and co-workers[829] observed no reticulocyte or hemoglobin responses in nine patients treated with rhEPO doses as high as 2000 U/kg/day. In contrast, three of six patients treated with IL-3 (60 to 125 μg/m^2/day subcutaneously for 4 to 6 weeks) had increases in reticulocytes, and two of the responders remained transfusion independent for 1.5 to 2 years off therapy.[830] Another IL-3 study[831] reported 4 responders out of 18 patients treated with 0.5 to 10 μg/kg subcutaneously. In two responders deep venous thrombosis developed and necessitated discontinuation of treatment, whereas the other two patients sustained their responses, one receiving maintenance IL-3 for 31 months and one off treatment for 12 months after 30 months of therapy. In another study of 13 patients no responses were observed.[832] Thus, 6 patients have had significant erythroid responses to IL-3 out of a total of 37 (16%), a rate similar to that reported by the European working group for DBA (3/25).[833]

Amegakaryocytic Thrombocytopenia

Amegakaryocytic thrombocytopenia (AMT) is a rare disease manifested in infancy or early childhood with thrombocytopenia, frequent anemia, and progression to pancytopenia. Bone marrow megakaryocytes are absent or extremely scarce, and the disease results from mutations in the TPO receptor c-mpl. A phase I/II IL-3 dose escalation study without or with sequential GM-CSF in five children with AMT showed that IL-3 (but not IL-3/GM-CSF) induced platelet responses in two patients and improvement in bruising, bleeding, and transfusion requirements in the other three.[732] The two platelet responders became unresponsive after several months of IL-3 maintenance (125 to 250 μg/m^2/day), whereas another patient became platelet transfusion independent after 4 months of IL-3 and had a trilineage response sustained for almost 2 years.

Severe Congenital Neutropenia (SCN)

Severe congenital neutropenia, or Kostmann disease (see also Chapter 8), is a disorder of myelopoiesis characterized by impaired neutrophil differentiation and ANCs greater than 200/μL. In contrast, monocyte and eosinophil counts are normal or increased. The bone marrow shows maturation arrest at the promyelocyte stage, and these cells are often atypical, with abnormal nuclei and vacuolated cytoplasm. The pathophysiology is uncertain despite the identification of mutations in NE (ELA2) and more recently HAX-1 in recessively inherited disease, including patients from the original Kostmann pedigree.[834] Serum from these patients contains normal or elevated levels of G-CSF, as determined by Western blot[783] and bioassay.[835] Other investigations showed mutations in the C-terminal "differentiation" domain of the G-CSFR in two patients.[301]

The responses of these patients to exogenous G-CSF and GM-CSF are therefore of great interest. One study has compared the effects of GM-CSF and G-CSF in a small number of patients, and G-CSF alone was evaluated in other studies.[836-838] In these investigations G-CSF produced a remarkable increase in neutrophils in all patients. The dose necessary to maintain a neutrophil count greater than 1000/μL varied, with ranges of 3 to 15 μg/kg/day. The monocyte count was also increased. In contrast, rhGM-CSF produced an increase in neutrophils in only one patient, whereas the others showed an increase in eosinophils and monocytes. Although the period on study was short, no new episodes of severe bacterial infection occurred during either GM-CSF or G-CSF treatment, in contrast to the recurrent bacterial and fungal infections that occurred before treatment. A multicenter phase III study of G-CSF in 120 patients with severe chronic neutropenic disorders, including SCN, Shwachman-Diamond syndrome, and myelokathexis, showed complete responses in 108 patients (ANC $> 1.5 \times 10^9$/L), partial responses in 4 patients, and failure to respond in 8 patients.[839] Although the majority of patients respond with an ANC of 1.0×10^9/L or higher at doses ranging from 3 to 20 μg/kg/day, about 25% patients need 20 to 100 μg/kg/day or more.[823]

Somatic mutations of a single allele of the G-CSFR that result in loss of the C-terminal "differentiation" domain of the receptor were described in several SCN patients and shown to act as a dominant negative in transduced cells.[840,841] MDS or AML may eventually develop in these patients.[401] Data from the Severe Congenital Neutropenia International Registry[842] on 506 patients with severe congenital neutropenia, cyclic neutropenia, or idiopathic neutropenia who were treated in phase I to phase III clinical G-CSF trials showed that MDS/AML developed in 23 of 249 patients with SCN/ Schwachman-Diamond syndrome (neutropenia and pancreatic insufficiency), as compared with none of the 97 cyclic or 160 idiopathic neutropenia patients. The observation that MDS/AML develops in SCN but not cyclic or idiopathic neutropenia patients receiving G-CSF is consistent with reports of AML in SCN before the introduction of G-CSF treatment[843,844] and shows that SCN is a preleukemic disease. Additional cytogenetic changes (translocations and monosomy 7) and oncogene (*ras*) mutations are common in the patients in whom MDS/AML eventually develops.[845] The G-CSFR mutation occurs in myeloid cells only and was not present

in first-degree relatives of affected patients, including a sibling with SCN,[846] thus demonstrating that the mutation is acquired. Interestingly, detailed study to identify the risks for leukemic transformation shows increased risk over time (2.9%/yr after 6 years and 8%/yr after 12 years, with a cumulative incidence of 21% after 10 years). Importantly, the risk of MDS/AML developing correlates with the dose of G-CSF; MDS/AML developed in 40% of the poor responders (G-CSF dose greater than the median of 8 μg/kg/day and ANC less than the median of 2188 cells/μL at 6 to 8 months) versus only 11% of the good responders.[847] Similar results were reported by the French Severe Chronic Neutropenia study group.[848]

In summary, treatment with recombinant G-CSF has had a major positive impact on the lives of the majority of these patients. Continued treatment has increased the risk for emergence of leukemic clones in this preleukemic disease, and patients need to be monitored regularly for the acquisition of such clones. Patients who respond poorly to G-CSF should be considered earlier for stem cell transplantation.

Cyclic Neutropenia

Cyclic neutropenia (see also Chapter 8) is a rare HSC disease caused by mutations in NE (ELA2). It is characterized by regular 21-day cyclic fluctuations in numbers of neutrophils, monocytes, eosinophils, lymphocytes, platelets, and reticulocytes. Patients typically have recurrent episodes of fever, malaise, mucosal ulceration, and occasionally life-threatening infection during periods of neutropenia. Six patients were treated with intravenous or subcutaneous rhG-CSF for 3 to 15 months at doses ranging from 3 to 10 μg/kg/day.[849] The median neutrophil count increased from 0.7 to 9.8×10^9/L. In five of the patients, cycling of blood counts continued, but the length of cycles decreased from 21 to 14 days. The number of days of severe neutropenia (<200/μL) was reduced from a mean of 12.7/mo to less than 1/mo, and importantly, the nadir counts increased, neutrophil turnover increased almost fourfold, and migration to a skin window was normal. Average counts of other cells did not increase. One patient with disease of adult onset had a qualitatively different response consisting of an increase in neutrophils and disappearance of the cyclic fluctuations in count. Therapy reduced the frequency of oropharyngeal inflammation, fever, and infections, thus demonstrating that treatment with rhG-CSF is effective management in such patients. These results have been confirmed in other studies and the treatment is well tolerated.[850-852] GM-CSF has not been effective in two patients but eliminated severe neutropenia when given in low dose (0.3 μg/kg/day).[853-855]

Chronic Idiopathic Neutropenia

This disorder of myelopoiesis is characterized by maturation arrest of neutrophil precursors in the bone marrow, neutrophil counts lower than 1.5×10^9/L, and normal other cell lineages. Patients have mucosal ulcers, periodontal disease, and recurrent infections. The pathophysiology is uncertain; in vitro bone marrow culture shows normal numbers of myeloid progenitors, and antineutrophil antibodies are absent. A single patient who received 1 to 3 µg/kg/day rhG-CSF by subcutaneous injection showed normalization of the ANC with healing of chronic oral ulceration, reduction of episodes of recurrent infection, and minimal side effects.[856] Cycling of neutrophils, monocytes, and platelets was induced with a 40-day periodicity; this contrasts with the normal 21-day cycle and out-of-phase fluctuation of neutrophils and monocytes seen in cyclic neutropenia.

Anemia of Chronic Renal Failure

Erythropoietin

Anemia is a major complication of end-stage renal failure and is due primarily to a reduction in EPO production. Other mechanisms that may be involved are shortened red cell survival, iron deficiency, hypersplenism, possible circulating inhibitors of erythropoiesis, and aluminum-induced microcytosis. Several phase I, II, and III studies have documented that rhEPO can induce a dose-dependent increase in effective erythropoiesis.[857-859]

In a phase III study patients received 150 or 300 units of rhEPO three times per week after hemodialysis and reached a target hematocrit of 35% by 8 to 12 weeks.[858,859] The majority of patients required 50 to 125 U/kg intravenously three times per week after dialysis to maintain a hematocrit of approximately 35%. The increase in erythropoiesis needed to normalize hemoglobin requires mobilization of a considerable amount of iron; in patients who improve, rapidly in particular, absolute or relative iron deficiency can develop. If iron is not given, the response to rhEPO becomes blunted; the standard corrective measure is intravenous administration of iron dextran or oral iron supplementation. Regular measurements of ferritin and transferrin saturation are necessary to ensure that iron stores are adequate.

EPO has been well tolerated and has resulted in elimination of transfusion dependency. Hypertension, occasionally with encephalopathy, has been observed, particularly with rapid rises in hematocrit that lead to an increase in peripheral vascular resistance; induction with doses not greater than 150 U/kg is recommended to produce a gradual increase in hemoglobin levels. Some patients require either the initiation of antihypertensive medication or dose adjustment A marked increase in pure red cell aplasia occurred from 1998 to 2004 because of the development of anti-EPO antibodies,[860-8627] with reports of approximately 250 suspected or proven cases. The complication, characterized by reticulocytopenia, absence of erythroid precursors, and severe anemia, has occurred mostly in adults (a few children are included) with renal disease treated with Eprex outside the United States, but cases have been reported in the United States as well. Differences in EPO glycosylation status and drug formulation, processing, storage, and route of administration appear to affect the immunogenicity of EPO. The estimated exposure-adjusted incidence per 100,000 patient years was 18 cases for Eprex without serum albumin (epoetin alfa, Ortho Biotech), 6 for Eprex with serum albumin, 1 for NeoRecormon (epoetin beta), and 0.2 for Epogen (epoetin alfa).[862] Changes in drug formulation and drug monitoring programs have led to an 80% reduction in the incidence of pure red cell aplasia, and EPO should not be withheld for this reason.

The effect of rhEPO in most studies appears to be restricted to the erythroid lineage. However, data from a phase III study of 303 patients showed a significant increase in mean platelet count (224 to 241×10^9/L at 6 months), which is not biologically meaningful. There is also a slight increase in blood urea nitrogen, creatinine, and serum potassium levels. Bone marrow progenitors from patients with end-stage renal failure were studied before and 2 weeks after rhEPO treatment. The concentration of BFU-E, CFU-E, and CFU-Meg increased after therapy. Surprisingly, an increment in CFU-GM also occurred, and the number of progenitors of all classes in cell cycle almost doubled.[863]

Subjective improvement in appetite, energy, sleep pattern, and libido are also noted. A Canadian double-blind placebo-controlled study of rhEPO treatment has provided objective evidence of benefit.

Extending this treatment to patients who do not yet require dialysis has met with similar success.[864] An issue that has yet to be resolved is financial; rhEPO is not inexpensive, and the National Kidney Foundation in the United States has issued guidelines for the use of rhEPO in which all patients with a hematocrit of less than 30% will be eligible. rhEPO is more effective when administered by the subcutaneous route, and this is more convenient for patients and also allows dose reduction.[865,866] In predialysis patients, 100 U/kg subcutaneously provided a response similar to 150 U/kg given intravenously.[865] There is evidence that the bioavailability of subcutaneous EPO is seven times greater than that of the intravenously administered drug, and a large controlled study showed that the mean EPO dose to maintain a stable hematocrit was 32% lower with the subcutaneous than with the intravenous route.[867]

Similar results have been obtained in several rhEPO studies in children (reviewed by Müller-Wiefel and Amon[868]). Anemia was corrected by 3 to 4 months in 24 children with preterminal chronic renal failure (CRF) treated with rhEPO and iron, which was adjusted by careful monitoring of iron status. Hypertension is the most common side effect.[869-872] Interestingly, although the growth failure of children with terminal CRF is unaffected by rhEPO treatment, mean growth velocity in 22 children with preterminal CRF increased from −2.29 to −0.56 within the first 6 months of treatment.[868] Other possible benefits include reports of delay in progression of renal dysfunction in children with preterminal CRF and improvement in cognitive function.

Other Indications for Recombinant Erythropoietin Therapy

Several small clinical trials have evaluated the use of rhEPO for the anemia of prematurity.[873-879] These studies have been reviewed by Mentzer and Shannon,[880] and although differences in patient populations, transfusion criteria, rhEPO dose, and iron therapy make comparisons difficult, rhEPO treatment is safe and stimulates a reticulocyte response. An effect on hematocrit was observed only in the studies in which doses greater than 500 U/kg/wk were used,[873,875,877 878] and there appears to be a modest effect on transfusion requirement. Increasing the dose from 750 to 1500 U/kg/wk was not supported by a large European study of 184 very-low-birth-weight infants.[881]

Preliminary data suggest that rhEPO may be useful in the treatment of patients with the anemia of chronic disease associated with rheumatoid arthritis[882] and the anemia that complicates azidothymidine treatment in patients with AIDS (see earlier).

In simian studies, hemoglobin F levels can be increased by administration of EPO.[883] If similar changes occur in humans, EPO may have a role in the management of sickle cell disease and thalassemia. Several small studies in sickle cell disease have shown that hemoglobin F reticulocytosis can occur in some patients whereas others show an increase in hemoglobin without a sustained F reticulocyte response, a finding that is of some concern because blood viscosity might be increased.[884] There are also data suggesting that hydroxyurea in combination with EPO can augment the F reticulocyte response, although the contribution of EPO is still uncertain.[885,886] In patients with transfusion-dependent or untransfused thalassemia, variable responses to EPO alone have also been reported,[887-890] with some patients showing an increase in hemoglobin and F cells. The only report to show a consistent increase in fetal hemoglobin was a study of 10 untransfused thalassemic patients who received rhEPO (400 to 800 U/kg three times per week), as well as iron and hydroxyurea (4 days/wk). Hemoglobin increased significantly in 8 of the 10 patients with concomitant increases in fetal hemoglobin 5% to 20% above baseline.[890]

Finally, EPO can be used to increase the number of units of blood that can be obtained preoperatively in the context of autologous blood donation.[891]

Stem and Progenitor Cell Mobilization

The effect of G-CSF on progenitor cells is interesting. After melphalan and G-CSF, the absolute number of *circulating* progenitor cells of the granulocyte-macrophage, erythroid, mixed, and megakaryocyte lineages show a dose-related increase of up to 100-fold after 4 days of treatment with rhG-CSF,[892] thereby confirming earlier animal studies.[893,894] The relative proportion of early and late granulocyte progenitors and early progenitors of different lineages remains unchanged; however, CFU-E, normally undetectable in blood, is markedly increased. The mechanism for the increase in all progenitors in blood is unclear; G-CSF has been shown to affect immature blast CFCs, and it is possible that stem cells are stimulated in vivo to produce increased progenitors of all classes; alternatively, G-CSF may indirectly stimulate progenitors by induction of HGF production or by release of bone marrow progenitor cells into the circulation.

These early studies set the stage for attempts at high-dose chemotherapy followed by mobilized blood progenitor cell rescue in a number of chemosensitive tumors such as lymphoma, breast cancer, and multiple myeloma. Time to engraftment is critically related to the number of CD34[+] cells infused, and a number of studies indicate that a dose of 5×10^6 CD34[+] cells/kg or greater results in prompt neutrophil and platelet engraftment.[895-898] G-CSF is the usual HGF used to mobilize progenitors, and multiple apheresis procedures (four or more) are commonly required to achieve this dose of CD34[+] cells. Strategies to increase the yield and thereby reduce the number of apheresis procedures include the combination of G-CSF with chemotherapy, SCF,[898-901] TPO,[902,903] high-affinity IL-3RA,[904] or FL in animal studies.[905-909] Two studies suggest that SCF in combination with G-CSF can decrease the number of apheresis procedures required,[887,910] which might be expected to have several advantages, including reduction of apheresis-associated morbidity, less delay in administration of chemotherapy, and decreased cost.

Toxicity of Colony-Stimulating Factor Treatment

The CSFs tested in all these clinical trials have in general been well tolerated. Both GM-CSF and G-CSF induce *transient leukopenia* in the first 30 minutes after intravenous bolus injection. GM-CSF rapidly induces surface expression of the leukocyte adhesion protein CD11b (MO1) in vitro, and this is accompanied by an increase in neutrophil aggregation.[727] CD11a (LFA-1) and CD11c (gp150, gp95), two other members of this family of cell surface adhesion glycoproteins that have distinct α chains but share a common β chain (CD18) with CD11b, are unaffected by GM-CSF. These results have been corroborated by in vivo studies of sarcoma patients who received 32 or 64 µg/kg/day GM-CSF. A marked increase in CD11b was noted that was evident by 30 minutes and persisted for 12 to 24 hours after treatment.[911] Radionuclide-labeled leukocytes are sequestered in the lungs after GM-CSF treatment,[746] probably because of the aggregability and adhesiveness induced by increased CD11b expression. Breathlessness and hypoxia have been observed in some patients, particularly after short-duration intravenous administration. CD11b is not modulated by G-CSF, and the reason for the transient leukopenia after treatment with G-CSF is at present unclear.

Both GM-CSF and G-CSF have been associated with bone pain coincident with or shortly after administration. Occasional increases in leukocyte alkaline phosphatase or lactate dehydrogenase (or both) have been noted. In contrast, GM-CSF has also induced flu-like symptoms, including fever, flushing, malaise, myalgia, arthralgia, anorexia, and headache. Mild elevations in transaminase levels and rash are also reported. These effects are usually mild, are alleviated by antipyretics, and disappear with continued administration. More serious GM-CSF toxicity has been observed at higher dose levels (>32 μg/kg/day intravenously or >15 μg/kg/day subcutaneously), including capillary leak syndrome with weight gain as a result of fluid retention manifested as pericardial or pleural effusions, ascites, or edema.[758,785] Phlebitis was noted in initial studies when GM-CSF was infused into small veins; large vessel thrombosis has occurred with infusion of high doses into central veins.[758]

Antibodies to Recombinant Factors

The rhGM-CSF that is produced in mammalian cells (Chinese hamster ovary cells) is variably glycosylated on both O-linked and N-linked sites. Production in *E. coli* results in nonglycosylated GM-CSF, and the yeast product is glycosylated at N-linked sites. All three products appear to be equally efficacious, but antibodies have been reported in 4 of 13 patients given the yeast-derived product in phase I/II studies.[912] The IgG antibodies developed by 7 days after the start of the infusion in all four patients, three of whom had received a bolus test dose; the antibodies were non-neutralizing as judged by bone marrow colony-forming assay, and they were directed at sites on the protein backbone of the GM-CSF molecule that are normally protected by O-linked glycosylation but are exposed in the yeast and *E. coli*–derived products. Transient antibodies to TPO have been reported in one cancer patient.[913] However, the development of antibodies in both patients and volunteers given PEG-MGDF led to termination of further clinical development of this TPO formulation because transient decreases in platelet count were noted.[779,914-916] Antibodies to EPO can also develop in patients with the anemia of CRF during treatment with EPO.[917] Some formulations of EPO were associated with an antibody to EPO that resulted in pure red cell aplasia, and this complication is discussed more fully earlier in the section on the use of EPO in renal failure.

No dose-limiting toxicity has been observed with G-CSF. However, one case of pathogenic neutrophil infiltration (acute febrile neutrophilic dermatosis, or Sweet's syndrome) has been reported.[918] In one patient with SCN, cutaneous necrotizing vasculitis (leukoclastic vasculitis) developed during G-CSF treatment.[835,837] As noted earlier, there is also concern that G-CSF will induce or accelerate the development of AML or MDS with monosomy 7 in aplastic anemia and SCN, perhaps more likely in patients with G-CSF receptor mutations that can transduce a proliferative but not a differentiation signal.

As noted earlier, EPO treatment has been associated with increased risk for thromboembolic complications in adults, particularly when target hemoglobin concentrations were in the normal range, and it has a possible adverse effect on progression of breast cancer.[777,919] Two randomized studies in which the targeted hemoglobin level was either in the normal (>13.5 g/dL) or subnormal (10.5 to 11.5 g/dL) range showed an increased risk for adverse cardiovascular effects in the normal hemoglobin groups.[920,921] A 2006 update of a Cochrane review of 57 trials that included more than 9000 patients showed strong evidence that epoetin and darbepoetin increase the risk for thromboembolic complications (relative risk of 1.67, 95% confidence interval of 1.35 to 2.06).[922] There are no comparable large studies in children. As a result of these and other studies, the Food and Drug Administration has recommended the lowest dose possible to increase hemoglobin to a level that avoids transfusion, not to exceed 12 g/dL or a rise of greater than 1 g in any 2 weeks (http://www.fda.gov/cder/drug/InfoSheets/HCP/RHE2007HCP.htm).

CONCLUSION

Advances in molecular and cellular biology have led to an unraveling of some of the most challenging and confusing aspects of the study of hematopoiesis. Therapeutic benefits have emerged from these discoveries. The field of hematopoiesis, once a jumble of unknown factors and activities, has come of age and is providing direct benefits to countless patients.

REFERENCES

1. Lehmann H, Huntsman RG. Why are red cells the shape they are? The evolution of the human red cell. In MacFarlane RG, Robb-Smith AHT (eds). Function of the Blood. Oxford, Blackwell Scientific, 1961, pp 73-148.
2. Brace KC. Life span of the marmot erythrocyte. Blood. 1953;8:648-650.
3. Everett NB, Caffrey RW. Rate of red cell formation in rats at 24 degrees C and 5 degrees C. Anat Rec. 1962;143:339-344.
4. Cline MJ, Waldmann TA. Effect of temperature on erythropoiesis. Am J Physiol. 1962;203:401-403.
5. Grant WC, Root WS. Fundamental stimulus for erythropoiesis. Physiol Rev. 1952;32:449-498.
6. Necas E, Neuwirt J. Response of erythropoiesis to blood loss in hyperbaric air. Am J Physiol. 1969;216:800-803.
7. Goldberg MA, Dunning SP, Bunn HF. Regulation of the erythropoietin gene: evidence that the oxygen sensor is a heme protein. Science. 1988;242:1412-1415.
8. Wang GL, Jiang BH, Rue EA, Semenza GL. Hypoxia-inducible factor 1 is a basic-helix-loop-helix–PAS heterodimer regulated by cellular O_2 tension. Proc Natl Acad Sci U S A. 1995;92:5510-5514.
9. Semenza GL. Regulation of physiological responses to continuous and intermittent hypoxia by hypoxia-inducible factor 1. Exp Physiol. 2006;91:803-806.

10. Ratcliffe PJ. Understanding hypoxia signalling in cells—a new therapeutic opportunity? Clin Med. 2006;6: 573-578.

11. Wolf NS. The haemopoietic microenvironment. Clin Haematol. 1979;8:469-500.

12. Muller-Sieburg CE, Deryugina E. The stromal cells' guide to the stem cell universe. Stem Cells. 1995;13:477-486.

13. Lichtman MA, Chamberlain JK, Santillo PA. Factors thought to contribute to the regulation of egress of cells from marrow. In Silber R, LoBue J, Gordon AS (eds). The Year in Hematology. New York, Plenum, 1978, pp 243-279.

14. Adams GB, Scadden DT. The hematopoietic stem cell in its place. Nat Immunol. 2006;7:333-337.

15. Yin T, Li L. The stem cell niches in bone. J Clin Invest. 2006;116:1195-1201.

16. Bagby GC. Production of multilineage growth factors by hematopoietic stromal cells: an intracellular regulatory network involving mononuclear phagocytes and interleukin-1. Blood Cells. 1987;13:147-159.

17. Miyake K, Weissman IL, Greenberger JS, Kincade PW. Evidence for the role of the integrin VLA-4 in lympho-hemopoiesis. J Exp Med. 1991;173:599-607.

18. Simmons PJ, Masinovsky B, Longenecker BM, et al. Vascular cell adhesion molecule-1 expressed by bone marrow stromal cells mediates the binding of hematopoietic progenitor cells. Blood. 1992;80:388-395.

19. Teixido J, Hemler ME, Greenberger JS, Anklesaria P. Role of beta 1 and beta 2 integrins in the adhesion of CD34[hi] stem cells to bone marrow stroma. J Clin Invest. 1996;90:358-367.

20. Williams DA, Rios M, Stephens C, Patel VP. Fibronectin and VLA-4 in hematopoietic stem cell–microenvironment interactions. Nature. 1991;352:438-441.

21. Kodama H, Nose M, Niida S, et al. Involvement of the c-kit receptor in the adhesion of hematopoietic stem cells to stromal cells. Exp Hematol. 1994;22:979-984.

22. Gordon MY, Riley GP, Watt SM, Greaves MF. Compartmentalization of a haematopoietic growth factor. Nature. 1987;326:403-405.

23. Dexter TM, Coutinho LH, Spooncer E, et al. Stromal cells in haemopoiesis. Ciba Foundation Symp. 1990;148: 76-86; discussion 86-95.

24. Baumheter S, Singer MS, Henzel W, et al. Binding of L-selectin to the vascular sialomucin CD34. Science. 1993; 262:436-438.

25. Aiuti A, Webb IJ, Bleul C, et al. The chemokine SDF-1 is a chemoattractant for human CD34+ hematopoietic progenitor cells and provides a new mechanism to explain the mobilization of CD34+ progenitors to peripheral blood. J Exp Med. 1997;185:111-120.

26. Ma Q, Jones D, Borghesani PR, et al. Impaired B-lymphopoiesis, myelopoiesis, and derailed cerebellar neuron migration in CXCR4- and SDF-1–deficient mice. Proc Natl Acad Sci U S A. 1998;95:9448-9453.

27. Nagasawa T, Hirota S, Tachibana K, et al. Defects of B-cell lymphopoiesis and bone-marrow myelopoiesis in mice lacking the CXC chemokine PBSF/SDF-1. Nature. 1996;382:635-638.

28. Peled A, Petit I, Kollet O, et al. Dependence of human stem cell engraftment and repopulation of NOD/SCID mice on CXCR4. Science. 1999;283:845-848.

29. Peled A, Kollet O, Ponomaryov T, et al. The chemokine SDF-1 activates the integrins LFA-1, VLA-4, and VLA-5 on immature human CD34(+) cells: role in transendothelial/stromal migration and engraftment of NOD/SCID mice. Blood. 2000;95:3289-3296.

30. Hattori K, Heissig B, Tashiro K, et al. Plasma elevation of stromal cell–derived factor-1 induces mobilization of mature and immature hematopoietic progenitor and stem cells. Blood. 2001;97:3354-3360.

31. Sweeney EA, Lortat-Jacob H, Priestley GV, et al. Sulfated polysaccharides increase plasma levels of SDF-1 in monkeys and mice: involvement in mobilization of stem/progenitor cells. Blood. 2002;99:44-51.

32. Zuckerman KS, Rhodes RK, Goodrum DD, et al. Inhibition of collagen deposition in the extracellular matrix prevents the establishment of a stroma supportive of hematopoiesis in long-term murine bone marrow cultures. J Clin Invest. 1985;75:970-975.

33. Jacobson LO, Marks EK, Gaston EO, et al. Role of the spleen in radiation injury. Proc Soc Exp Biol Med. 1949;70:7440-7442.

34. Ford CE, Hamerton JL, Barnes DWH, Loutit JF. Cytological identification of radiation-chimaeras. Nature. 1956;177:452-454.

35. Till JE, McCulloch EA. A direct measurement of the radiation sensitivity of normal mouse bone marrow cells. Radiat Res. 1961;14:213-222.

36. Becker AJ, McCulloch EA, Till JE. Cytological demonstration of the clonal nature of spleen colonies derived from transplanted mouse cells. J Cell Physiol. 1967; 69:65-72.

37. Magli MC, Iscove NN, Odartchenko N. Transient nature of early haematopoietic spleen colonies. Nature. 1982;295: 527-529.

38. Whang J, Frei E 3rd, Tjio JH, et al. The distribution of the Philadelphia chromosome in patients with chronic myelogenous leukemia. Blood. 1963;22:644-673.

39. Fauser AA, Kanz L, Bross KJ, Löhr GW. T cells and probably B cells arise from the malignant clone in chronic mylogenous leukemia. J Clin Invest. 1985;75:1080-1082.

40. Raskind WH, Jacobson R, Murphy S, et al. Evidence for involvement of B lymphoid cells in polycythemia vera and essential thrombocythemia. J Clin Invest. 1985;75:1388-1390.

41. Adamson JW, Fialkow PJ, Murphy S, et al. Polycythemia vera: stem cell and probably clonal origin of the disease. N Engl J Med. 1975;295:913-916.

42. Metcalf D, Moore MAS. Senescence of haematopoietic tissues. In Neuberger A, Tatum EL (eds). Frontiers of Biology, 24th ed. Amsterdam, North-Holland Publishing, 1971, pp 448-465.

43. Huang H, Auerbach R. Identification and characterization of hematopoietic stem cells from the yolk sac of the early mouse embryo. Proc Natl Acad Sci U S A. 1993;90: 10110-10114.

44. Godin I, Dieterlen-lievre F, Cumano A. Emergence of multipotent hemopoietic cells in the yolk sac and para-aortic splanchnopleura in mouse embryos, beginning at 8.5 days postcoitus. Proc Natl Acad Sci U S A. 1995;92: 773-777.

45. Rich IN. Primordial germ cells are capable of producing cells of the hematopoietic system in vitro. Blood. 1995;86:463-472.

46. Micklem HS, Ross E. Heterogeneity and aging of hematopoietic stem cells. Ann Immunol. 1978;129:367-376.

47. Siminovitch L, Till JE, McCulloch EA. Decline in colony-forming ability of marrow cells subjected to serial transplantation into irradiated mice. J Cell Comp Physiol. 1964;64:23-31.

48. Mikkola HK, Gekas C, Orkin SH, Dieterlen-Lievre F. Placenta as a site for hematopoietic stem cell development. Exp Hematol. 2005;33:1048-1054.

49. Ottersbach K, Dzierzak E. The murine placenta contains hematopoietic stem cells within the vascular labyrinth region. Dev Cell. 2005;8:377-387.

50. Hellman S, Botnick LE, Hannon EC, Vignuelle RM. Proliferative capacity of murine hematopoietic stem cells. Proc Natl Acad Sci U S A. 1978;75:490-494.

51. Ploemacher RE, van der Sluijs JP, Voerman SA, Brons NHC. An in vitro limiting-dilution assay of long-term repopulating hematopoietic stem cells in the mouse. Blood. 1989;74:2755-2763.

52. Dexter TM. Cell interactions in vivo. Clin Haematol. 1979;8:453-468.

53. Ploemacher RE, Brons RHC. Separation of CFU-S from primitive cells responsible for reconstitution of the bone marrow hemopoietic stem cell compartment following irradiation: evidence for a pre–CFU-S cell. Exp Hematol. 1989;17:263-266.

54. Jones RJ, Wagner JE, Celano P, et al. Separation of pluripotent haematopoietic stem cells from spleen colony-forming cells. Nature. 1990;347:188-189.

55. Nakahata T, Ogawa M. Identification in culture of a new class of hematopoietic colony forming units with extreme capability to self-renew and generate multipotential colonies. Proc Natl Acad Sci U S A. 1982;79:3943-3947.

56. Bradley TR, Hodgson GS. Detection of primitive macrophage progenitor cells in mouse bone marrow. Blood. 1979;54:1446-1450.

57. Harrison DE, Lerner CP, Spooncer E. Erythropoietic repopulating ability of stem cells from long-term marrow cultures. Blood. 1987;69:1021-1025.

58. Morrison SJ, White PM, Zock C, Anderson DJ. Prospective identification, isolation by flow cytometry, and in vivo self-renewal of multipotent mammalian neural crest stem cells. Cell. 1999;96:737-749.

59. Uchida N, Buck DW, He D, et al. Direct isolation of human central nervous system stem cells. Proc Natl Acad Sci U S A. 2000;97:14720-14725.

60. Fauser AA, Messner HA. Granuloerythropoietic colonies in human bone marrow, peripherial blood, and cord blood. Blood. 1978;52:1243-1248.

61. Fauser AA, Messner HA. Identification of megakaryocytes, macrophages and eosinophils in colonies of human bone marrow containing neutrophilic granulocytes and erythroblasts. Blood. 1979;53:1023-1028.

62. Leary AG, Ogawa M, Strauss LC, Civin CI. Single cell origin of multilineage colonies in culture. J Clin Invest. 1984;74:2193-2197.

63. Coulombel L, Kalousek DK, Eaves CJ, et al. Long-term marrow culture reveals chromosomally normal hematopoietic progenitor cells in patients with Philadelphia chromosome positive chronic myelogenous leukemia. N Engl J Med. 1983;308:1493-1498.

64. Greenberg HM, Newberger PE, Parker LM, et al. Generation of physiologically normal human peripheral blood granulocytes in continuous bone marrow cultures. Blood. 1981;58:724-732.

65. Sutherland HJ, Lansdorp PM, Henkelman DH, et al. Functional characterization of individual human hematopoietic stem cells cultured at limiting dilution on supportive marrow stromal layers. Proc Natl Acad Sci U S A. 1990;87:3584-3588.

66. Breems DA, Blokland EAW, Neben S, Ploemacher RE. Frequency analysis of human primitive haematopoietic stem cell subsets using a cobblestone area forming cell assay. Leukemia. 1994;8:1095-1104.

67. McNiece IK, Stewart FM, Deacon DM, et al. Detection of human CFC with a high proliferative potential. Blood. 1989;74:609-612.

68. Kamel-Reid S, Dick JE. Engraftment of immune-deficient mice with human hematopoietic stem cells. Science. 1988;242:1706-1709.

69. Larochelle A, Vormoor J, Hanenberg H, et al. Identification of primitive human hematopoietic cells capable of repopulating NOD/SCID mouse bone marrow: implications for gene therapy. Nat Med. 1996;2:1329-1337.

70. de Wynter EA, Heyworth CM, Mukaida N, et al. NOD/SCID repopulating cells but not LTC-IC are enriched in human CD34$^+$ cells expressing the CCR1 chemokine receptor. Leukemia. 2001;15:1092-1101.

71. Spangrude GJ, Heimfeld S, Weissman IL. Purification and characterization of mouse hematopoietic stem cells. Science. 1988;241:58-62.

72. Osawa M, Hanada K, Hamada H, Nakauchi H. Long-term lymphohematopoietic reconstitution by a single CD34-low/negative hematopoietic stem cell. Science. 1996;273:242-245.

73. Kiel MJ, Yilmaz OH, Iwashita T, et al. SLAM family receptors distinguish hematopoietic stem and progenitor cells and reveal endothelial niches for stem cells. Cell. 2005;121:1109-1121.

74. Andrews RG, Singer JW, Bernstein ID. Precursors of colony-forming cells in humans can be distinguished from colony-forming cells by expression of the CD33 and CD34 antigens and light scatter properties. J Exp Med. 1989;169:1721-1731.

75. Berardi AC, Wang A, Levine JD, et al. Functional isolation and characterization of human hematopoietic stem cells. Science. 1995;267:104-108.

76. Berenson RJ, Andrews RG, Bensinger WI, et al. Antigen CD34$^+$ marrow cells engraft lethally irradiated baboons. J Clin Invest. 1988;81:951-955.

77. Goodell MA, Brose K, Paradis G, et al. Isolation and functional properties of murine hematopoietic stem cells that are replicating in vivo. J Exp Med. 1996;183:1797-1806.

78. Goodell MA, Rosenzweig M, Kim H, et al. Dye efflux studies suggest that hematopoietic stem cells expressing low or undetectable levels of CD34 antigen exist in multiple species. Nat Med. 1997;3:1337-1345.

79. Bhatia M, Bonnet D, Murdoch B, et al. A newly discovered class of human hematopoietic cells with SCID-repopulating activity. Nat Med. 1998;4:1038-1045.

80. Tajima F, Sato T, Laver JH, Ogawa M. CD34 expression by murine hematopoietic stem cells mobilized by granulocyte colony-stimulating factor. Blood. 2000;96:1989-1993.

81. Sato T, Laver JH, Ogawa M. Reversible expression of CD34 by murine hematopoietic stem cells. Blood. 1999;94:2548-2554.

82. Kondo M, Weissman IL, Akashi K. Identification of clonogenic common lymphoid progenitors in mouse bone marrow. Cell. 1997;91:661-672.

83. Akashi K, Traver D, Miyamoto T, Weissman IL. A clonogenic common myeloid progenitor that gives rise to all myeloid lineages. Nature. 2000;404:193-197.

84. Traver D, Miyamoto T, Christensen J, et al. Fetal liver myelopoiesis occurs through distinct, prospectively isolatable progenitor subsets. Blood. 2001;98:627-635.

85. Na Nakorn T, Traver D, Weissman IL, Akashi K. Myelo-erythroid-restricted progenitors are sufficient to confer radioprotection and provide the majority of day 8 CFU-S. J Clin Invest. 2002;109:1579-1585.

86. Suda T, Suda J, Ogawa M. Disparate differentiation in mouse hemopoietic colonies derived from paired progenitors. Proc Natl Acad Sci U S A. 1984;81:2520-2524.

87. Axelrad AA, McLeod DL, Steeves RA, Heath DS. Properties of cells that produce erythocytic colonies in vitro. In Robinson WA (ed). Hemopoiesis in Culture, DHEW Publication NIH-74-205. Washington, DC, Department of Health, Education, and Welfare, 1974, pp 226-234.

88. Pluznik DH, Sachs L. The cloning of normal "mast" cells in tissues cultures. J Cell Comp Physiol. 1965;66:319-324.

89. Bradley TR, Metcalf D. The growth of mouse bone marrow cells in vitro. Aust J Exp Biol Med Sci. 1966;44:287-293.

90. Moore MAS. Humoral regulation of granulopoiesis. Clin Haematol. 1979;8:263-309.

91. Haskill JS, Moore MAS. Two-dimensional cell separation: a comparison of embryonic and adult haematopoietic stem cells. Nature. 1970;266:853-854.

92. Dexter TM, Allen TD, Lajtha LG. Conditions controlling the proliferation of haemopoietic stem cells in vitro. J Cell Physiol. 1977;91:335-344.

93. Haskill JS, McNeil TA, Moore MA. Density distribution analysis of in vivo and in vitro colony-forming cells in bone marrow. J Cell Physiol. 1970;75:167-179.

94. Metcalf D. Detection and analysis of human granulocyte-monocyte precursors using semi-solid cultures. Clin Haematol. 1979;8:263-285.

95. Jacobsen N, Broxmeyer HE, Grosshard E, Moore MA. Colony-forming units in diffusion chambers (CFU-d) and colony-forming unts in agar culture (CFU-c) obtained from normal human bone marrow: a possible parent-progeny relationship. Cell Tissue Kinet. 1979;12:213-216.

96. Jacobsen N, Broxmeyer HE, Grosshard E, Moore MA. Diversity of human granulopoetic percursor cells: separation of cells that form colonies in diffusion chambers (CFU-d) from populations of colony-forming cells in vitro (CFU-c) by velocity sedimentation. Blood. 1978;52:221-232.

97. Moore MAS, Broxmeyer HE, Sheridan AP, et al. Continuous human bone marrow culture: Ia antigen characterization of probable pluripotental stem cells. Blood. 1980;55:682-690.

98. Martin DIK, Zon LI, Mutter G, Orkin SH. Expression of an erythroid transcription factor in megakaryocytic and mast cell lineages. Nature. 1990;344:444-447.

99. Orkin SH. GATA-binding transcription factors in hematopoietic cells. Blood. 1992;80:575-581.

100. Shivdasani RA, Rosenblatt MF, Zucker-Franklin D, et al. Transcription factor NF-E2 is required for platelet formation independent of the actions of thrombopoietin/MGDF in megakaryocyte development. Cell. 1995;81:695-704.

101. Duebelbeiss KA, Dancey JT, Harker LA, Finch CA. Marrow erythroid and neutrophil cellularity in the dog. J Clin Invest. 1975;55:825.

102. Alpen EL, Cranmore D. Cellular kinetics and iron utilization in bone marrow as observed by Fe-59 radioautography. Ann N Y Acad Sci. 1959;77:753-765.

103. Emerson SG, Sieff CA, Wang EA, et al. Purification of fetal hematopoietic progenitors and demonstration of recombinant multipotential colony-stimulating activity. J Clin Invest. 1985;76:1286-1290.

104. Dicke KA, van Noord MJ, Maat B, et al. Identification of cells in primate bone marrow resembling the hematopoietic stem cell in the mouse. Blood. 1973;42:195-205.

105. Rosse C. Small lymphocyte and transitional cell populations of the bone marrow: their role in the mediation of immune and hemopoietic progenitor cell functions. Int Rev Cytol. 1976;45:155-290.

106. Nathan DG, Chess L, Hillman DG, et al. Human erythroid burst-forming unit: T-cell requirement for proliferation in vitro. J Exp Med. 1978;147:324-339.

107. Granick S, Levere RD. Heme synthesis in erythroid cells. Progr Hematol. 1964;4:1-47.

108. Finch CA, Deubelbeiss K, Cook JD, et al. Ferrokinetics in man. Medicine (Baltimore). 1970;49:17-53.

109. Lord BI. Kinetics of the recognizable erythrocyte precursor cells. Clin Haematol. 1979;9:335-350.

110. Hillman RS, Giblett ER. Red cell membrane alteration associated with "marrow stress." J Clin Invest. 1965;44:1730-1736.

111. Nathan DG. Rubbish in the red cell [editorial]. N Engl J Med. 1969;281:558-559.

112. Etlinger JD, Goldberg AL. Control of protein degradation in reticulocyte extracts by hemin. J Biol Chem. 1980;255:4563-4568.

113. Alpen EL, Cranmore D. Observations on the regulation of erythropoiesis and on cellular dynamics by Fe-59 autoradiography. In Stohlman F Jr (ed). The Kinetics of Cellular Proliferation. New York, Grune & Stratton, 1959, pp 290-300.

114. Lichtman MA, Chamberlain JK, Weed RI, et al. The regulation of the release of granulocytes from normal marrow. In Greenwalt TJ, Jamieson GA (eds). The Granulocyte: Function and Clinical Utilization, 13th ed. New York, Alan R Liss, 1977, pp 53-75.

115. Italiano JE Jr, Patel-Hett S, Hartwig JH. Mechanics of proplatelet elaboration. J Thromb Haemost. 2007;5(Suppl 1):18-23.

116. Larson MK, Watson SP. Regulation of proplatelet formation and platelet release by integrin alpha IIb beta3. Blood. 2006;108:1509-1514.

117. Metcalf D. Hemopoietic regulators and leukemia development: a personal retrospective. Adv Cancer Res. 1994;63:41-91.

118. Clark SC, Kamen R. The human hematopoietic colony-stimulating factors. Science. 1987;236:1229-1237.

119. Metcalf D. The colony stimulating factors. Cancer. 1990;65:2185-2195.

120. Moore MAS. Haemopoietic growth factor interactions: in vitro and in vivo preclinical evaluation. Cancer Surv. 1990;9:7-80.

121. Metcalf D. Cell-cell signalling in the regulation of blood cell formation and function. Immunol Cell Biol. 1998;76:441-447.

122. Alexander WS. Cytokines in hematopoiesis. Int Rev Immunol. 1998;16:651-682.

123. Wong GG, Clark SC. Multiple actions of interleukin-6 within a cytokine network. Immunol Today. 1988;9:137-139.

124. Bazan JF. Neuropoietic cytokines in the hematopoietic fold. Neuron. 1991;7:197-208.

125. Bazan JF. Emerging families of cytokines and receptors. Current Biol. 1993;3:603-606.

126. Kelso A. Cytokines: principles and prospects. Immunol Cell Biol. 1998;76:300-317.

127. Roth P, Stanley ER. The biology of csf-1 and its receptor. Curr Top Microbiol Immunol. 1992;181:141-167.

128. Galli SJ, Zsebo KM, Geissler EN. The kit ligand, stem cell factor. Adv Immunol. 1994;55:1-95.

129. Lyman SD, Jacobsen SE. C-kit ligand and flt3 ligand: stem/progenitor cell factors with overlapping yet distinct activities. Blood. 1998;91:1101-1134.

130. Sims JE, Nicklin MJ, Bazan JF, et al. A new nomenclature for IL-1-family genes. Trends Immunol. 2001;22:536-537.

131. Rollins BJ. Chemokines. Blood. 1997;90:909-928.

132. Shalaby MR, Pennica D, Palladino MA Jr. An overview of the history and biologic properties of tumor necrosis factors. Springer Semin Immunopathol. 1986;9:33-37.

133. Pestka S, Langer JA, Zoon KC, Samuel CE. Interferons and their actions. Annu Rev Biochem. 1987;56:727-777.

134. Blumberg H, Conklin D, Xu WF, et al. Interleukin 20: discovery, receptor identification, and role in epidermal function. Cell. 2001;104:9-19.

135. Massagué J. TGF-beta signal transduction. Annu Rev Biochem. 1998;67:753-791.

136. Fossiez F, Banchereau J, Murray R, et al. Interleukin-17. Int Rev Immunol. 1998;16:541-551.

137. Miyazaki T, Maruyama M, Yamada G, et al. The integrity of the conserved "WS motif" common to IL-2 and other cytokine receptors is essential for ligand binding and signal transduction. EMBO J. 1991;10:3191-3197.

138. Nicola NA. Guidebood to Cytokines and Their Receptors. Oxford, Oxford University Press, 1994.

139. Darnell JE. STATS and gene regulation. Science. 1997;277:1630-1635.

140. Ihle JN. Cytokine receptor signaling. Nature. 1995;377:591-594.

141. Strober W, James SP. The interleukins. Pediatr Res. 1988;24:549-557.

142. Vosshenrich CA, Di Santo JP. Cytokines: Il-21 joins the gamma(c)-dependent network? Curr Biol. 2001;11:R175-R177.

143. Oppmann B, Lesley R, Blom B, et al. Novel p19 protein engages Il-12p40 to form a cytokine, Il-23, with biological activities similar as well as distinct from IL-12. Immunity. 2000;13:715-725.

144. Clark SC. Biological activities of human granulocyte-macrophage colony-stimulating factor. Int J Cell Cloning. 1988;6:365-377.

145. Demetri GD, Griffin JD. Granulocyte colony-stimulating factor and its receptor. Blood. 1991;78:2791-2808.

146. Goldwasser E, Beru N, Smith D. Erythropoietin. Immunol Ser. 1990;49:257-276.

147. Alexander WS. Thrombopoietin. Growth Factors. 1999;17:13-24.

148. Quentmeier H, Drexler HG, Fleckenstein D, et al. Cloning of human thymic stromal lymphopoietin (tslp) and signaling mechanisms leading to proliferation. Leukemia. 2001;15:1286-1292.

149. Reche PA, Soumelis V, Gorman DM, et al. Human thymic stromal lymphopoietin preferentially stimulates myeloid cells. J Immunol. 2001;167:336-343.

150. Sims JE, Williams DE, Morrissey PJ, et al. Molecular cloning and biological characterization of a novel murine lymphoid growth factor. J Exp Med. 2000;192:671-680.

151. Metcalf D. Murine hematopoietic stem cells committed to macrophage/dendritic cell formation: stimulation by flk2-ligand with enhancement by regulators using the gp130 receptor chain. Proc Natl Acad Sci U S A. 1997;94:11552-11556.

152. Taga T, Kishimoto T. Gp130 and the interleukin-6 family of cytokines. Annu Rev Immunol. 1997;15:797-819.

153. Loy JK, Davidson TJ, Berry KK, et al. Oncostatin M: development of a pleiotropic cytokine. Toxicol Pathol. 1999;27:151-155.

154. Asao H, Okuyama C, Kumaki S, et al. Cutting edge: the common gamma-chain is an indispensable subunit of the IL-21 receptor complex. J Immunol. 2001;167:1-5.

155. Pandey A, Ozaki K, Baumann H, et al. Cloning of a receptor subunit required for signaling by thymic stromal lymphopoietin. Nat Immunol. 2000;1:59-64.

156. Ogawa M, Matsunaga T. Humoral regulation of hematopoietic stem cells. Ann N Y Acad Sci. 1999;872:17-23.

157. Marz P, Otten U, Rose-John S. Neural activities of IL-6–type cytokines often depend on soluble cytokine receptors. Eur J Neurosci. 1999;11:2995-3004.

158. Ashman LK. The biology of stem cell factor and its receptor c-kit. Int J Biochem Cell Biol. 1999;31:1037-1051.

159. Lyman SD. Biologic effects and potential clinical applications of flt3 ligand. Curr Opin Hematol. 1998;5:192-196.

160. Bazan J. Genetic and structural homology of stem cell factor and macrophage colony-stimulating factor [letter]. Cell. 1991;65:9-10.

161. Lyman SD, Stocking K, Davison B, et al. Structural analysis of human and murine flt3 ligand genomic loci. Oncogene. 1995;11:1165-1172.

162. Dinarello CA. The interleukin-1 family: 10 years of discovery. FASEB J. 1994;8:1314-1325.

163. Dinarello CA. The biological properties of interleukin-1. Eur Cytokine Netw. 1994;5:517-531.

164. Nakanishi K, Yoshimoto T, Tsutsui H, Okamura H. Interleukin-18 is a unique cytokine that stimulates both th1 and th2 responses depending on its cytokine milieu. Cytokine Growth Factor Rev. 2001;12:53-72.

165. Dinarello CA. IL-18: a TH1-inducing, proinflammatory cytokine and new member of the IL-1 family. J Allergy Clin Immunol. 1999;103:11-24.

166. Zhou YQ, Stanley ER, Clark SC, et al. Interleukin-3 and interleukin-1 alpha allow earlier bone marrow progenitors to respond to human colony-stimulating factor 1. Blood. 1988;72:1870-1874.

167. Mayani H, Little MT, Dragowska W, et al. Differential effects of the hematopoietic inhibitors MIP-1 alpha, TGF-beta, and TNF-alpha on cytokine-induced proliferation of subpopulations of CD34$^+$ cells purified from cord blood and fetal liver. Exp Hematol. 1995;23:422-427.

168. Jo D-Y, Rafii S, Hamada T, Moore MAS. Chemotaxis of primitive hematopoietic cells in response to stromal cell–derived factor-1. J Clin Invest. 2000;105:101-111.

169. Palucka KA, Taquet N, Sanchez-Chapuis F, Gluckman JC. Dendritic cells as the terminal stage of monocyte differentiation. J Immunol. 1998;160:4587-4595.

170. Pasparakis M, Alexopoulou L, Episkopou V, Kollias G. Immune and inflammatory responses in TNF alpha–deficient mice: a critical requirement for TNF alpha in the formation of primary B cell follicles, follicular dendritic cell networks and germinal centers, and in the maturation of the humoral immune response. J Exp Med. 1996;184:1397-1411.

171. Pestka S. The interferon receptors. Semin Oncol. 1997;24:S9-S40.

172. Fortunel NO, Hatzfeld A, Hatzfeld J. Transforming growth factor beta: pleiotropic role in the regulation of hematopoiesis. Blood. 2000;96:3722-3729.

173. Cashman JD, Clark-Lewis I, Eaves AC, Eaves CJ. Differentiation stage–specific regulation of primitive human hematopoietic progenitor cycling by exogenous and endogenous inhibitors in an in vivo model. Blood. 1999;94:3722-3729.

174. Loeys BL, Schwarze U, Holm T, et al. Aneurysm syndromes caused by mutations in the TGF-beta receptor. N Engl J Med. 2006;355:788-798.

175. Sanderson CJ. Interleukin-5, eosinophils, and disease. Blood. 1992;79:3101-3109.

176. Lopez AF, Sanderson CJ, Gamble JR, et al. Recombinant human interleukin-5 (IL-5) is a selective activator of human eosinophil function. J Exp Med. 1988;167:219-224.

177. Kaushansky K. Thrombopoietin: the primary regulator of platelet production. Blood. 1995;86:419-431.

178. Bussolino F, Wang JM, Defilippi P, et al. Granulocyte- and granulocyte-macrophage-colony stimulating factors induce human endothelial cells to migrate and proliferate. Nature. 1989;337:471-473.

179. Yokota T, Arai N, de Vries J, et al. Molecular biology of interleukin 4 and interleukin 5 genes and biology of their products that stimulate B cells, T cells and hemopoietic cells. Immunol Rev. 1988;102:137-187.

180. Berridge MV, Fraser JK, Carter JM, Lin F-K. Effects of recombinant human erythropoietin on megakaryocytes and on platelet production in the rat. Blood. 1988;72:970-977.

181. Kobayashi M, Laver JH, Kato T, et al. Recombinant human thrombopoietin (Mpl ligand) enhances proliferation of erythroid progenitors. Blood. 1995;86:2494-2499.

182. Ogawa M. Differentiation and proliferation of hematopoietic stem cells. Blood. 1993;81:2844-2853.

183. McKinstry WJ, Li CL, Rasko JE, et al. Cytokine receptor expression on hematopoietic stem and progenitor cells. Blood. 1997;89:65-71.

184. Ikebuchi K, Clark SC, Ihle JN, et al. Granulocyte colony-stimulating factor enhances interleukin 3–dependent proliferation of multipotential hemopoietic progenitors. Proc Natl Acad Sci U S A. 1988;85:3455-3449.

185. Stanley ER, Bartocci A, Patinkin D, et al. Regulation of very primitive, multipotent, hemopoietic cells by hemopoietin-1. Cell. 1986;45:667-674.

186. Zeigler FC, de Sauvage F, Widmer HR, et al. In vitro megakaryocytopoietic and thrombopoietic activity of c-mpl ligand (TPO) on purified murine hematopoietic stem cells. Blood. 1994;84:4045-4052.

187. Metcalf D, Begley CG, Johnson GR, et al. Biologic properties in vitro of a recombinant human granulocyte-macrophage colony-stimulating factor. Blood. 1986;67:37-45.

188. Metcalf D. Lineage commitment in the progeny of murine hematopoietic preprogenitor cells: influence of thrombopoietin and interleukin 5. Proc Natl Acad Sci U S A. 1998;95:6408-6412.

189. Sieff CA, Emerson SG, Donahue RE, et al. Human recombinant granulocyte-macrophage colony-stimulating factor: a multilineage hematopoietin. Science. 1985;230:1171-1173.

190. Ihle JN, Keller J, Oroszalan S, et al. Biologic properties of homogeneous interleukin 3. I. Demonstration of WEHI-3 growth factor activity, mast cell growth factor activity, P cell–stimulating activity, and histamine-producing cell-stimulating activity. J Immunol. 1983;131:282-287.

191. Leary AG, Yang Y-C, Clark SC, et al. Recombinant gibbon interleukin 3 supports formation of human multilineage colonies and blast cell colonies in culture: comparison with recombinant human granulocyte-macrophage colony-stimulating factor. Blood. 1987;70:1343-1348.

192. Sieff CA, Niemeyer CM, Nathan DG, et al. Stimulation of human hematopoietic colony formation by recombinant gibbon multi-colony–stimulating factor or interleukin 3. J Clin Invest. 1987;80:818-823.

193. Sonoda Y, Yang Y-C, Wong GG, et al. Analysis in serum-free culture of the targets of recombinant human hemopoietic growth factors: interleukin-3 and granulocyte/macrophage-colony-stimulating factor are specific for early developmental stages. Proc Natl Acad Sci U S A. 1988;85:4360-4364.

194. Ottmann OG, Abboud M, Welte K, et al. Stimulation of human hematopoietic progenitor cell proliferation and differentiation by recombinant human interleukin 3. Comparison and interactions with recombinant human granulocyte-macrophage and granulocyte colony-stimulating factors. Exp Hematol. 1989;17:191-197.

195. Mayer P, Valent P, Schmidt G, et al. The in vivo effects of recombinant human interleukin-3: demonstration of basophil differentiation factor, histamine-producing activity, and priming of GM-CSF–responsive progenitors in nonhuman primates. Blood. 1989;74:613-621.

196. Donahue RE, Seehra J, Metzger M, et al. Human interleukin-3 and GM-SCF act synergistically in stimulating hematopoiesis in primates. Science. 1988;241:1820-1823.

197. Szabolcs P, Moore MA, Young JW. Expansion of immunostimulatory dendritic cells among the myeloid progeny of human CD34$^+$ bone marrow precursors cultured with c-kit ligand, granulocyte-macrophage colony-stimulating factor, and TNF-alpha. J Immunol. 1995;154:5851-5861.

198. Kelly KA, Lucas K, Hochrein H, et al. Development of dendritic cells in culture from human and murine thymic precursor cells. Cell Mol Biol. 2001;47:43-54.

199. McKenna HJ. Role of hematopoietic growth factors/flt3 ligand in expansion and regulation of dendritic cells. Curr Opin Hematol. 2001;8:149-154.

200. Keller U, Aman MJ, Derigs G, et al. Human interleukin-4 enhances stromal cell–dependent hematopoiesis: costimulation with stem cell factor. Blood. 1994;84:2189-2196.

201. Sonoda Y, Okuda T, Yokota S, et al. Actions of human interleukin-4/B-cell stimulatory factor-1 on proliferation and differentiation of enriched hematopoietic progenitor cells in culture. Blood. 1990;75:1615-1621.

202. Kishi K, Ihle JN, Urdal DL, Ogawa M. Murine B-cell stimulatory factor-1 (BSF-1/interleukin-4 (IL-4) is a multilineage colony-stimulating factor that acts directly on primitive hemopoietic progenitors. J Cell Physiol. 1989; 139:463-468.

203. Paul WE. Interleukin-4: a prototypic immunoregulatory lymphokine. Blood. 1991;77:1859-1870.

204. Mosmann TR, Coffman RL. TH1 and TH2 cells: different patterns of lymphokine secretion lead to different functional properties. Annu Rev Immunol. 1989;7: 145-173.

205. Donahue RE, Yang Y-C, Clark SC. Human P40 T-cell growth factor (interleukin-9) supports erythroid colony formation. Blood. 1993;75:2271-2275.

206. Renauld JC, Houssiau F, Louahed J, et al. Interleukin-9. Adv Immunol. 1993;54:79-97.

207. Demoulin JB, Renauld JC. Interleukin 9 and its receptor: an overview of structure and function. Int Rev Immunol. 1998;16:345-364.

208. Hannum C, Culpepper J, Campbell D, et al. Ligand for FLT3/FLK2 receptor tyrosine kinase regulates growth of haematopoietic stem cells and is encoded by variant RNAs. Nature. 1994;368:643-648.

209. Lyman SD, James L, Johnson L, et al. Cloning of the human homologue of the murine flt3 ligand: a growth factor for early hematopoietic progenitor cells. Blood. 1994;83:2795-2801.

210. Spritz RA, Giebel LB, Holmes SA. Dominant negative and loss of function mutations of the c-kit (mast/stem cell growth factor receptor) proto-oncogene in human piebaldism. Am J Hum Genet. 1992;50:261-269.

211. Alexander WS, Lyman SD, Wagner EF. Expression of functional c-kit receptors rescues the genetic defect of W mutant mast cells. EMBO J. 1991;10:3683-3691.

212. Tsuji K, Lyman SD, Sudo T, et al. Enhancement of murine hematopoiesis by synergistic interactions between Steel factor (ligand for c-kit), interleukin-11, and other early acting factors in culture. Blood. 1992;79:2855-2860.

213. Tsuji K, Zsebo KM, Ogawa M. Enhancement of murine blast cell colony formation in culture by recombinant rat stem cell factor, ligand for c-kit. Blood. 1991;78: 1223-1229.

214. Metcalf D, Nicola NA. Direct proliferative actions of stem cell factor on murine bone marrow cells in vitro: effects of combination with colony-stimulating factors. Proc Natl Acad Sci U S A. 1991;88:6239-6243.

215. Hirayama F, Ogawa M. Negative regulation of early T lymphopoiesis by interleukin-3 and interleukin-1 alpha. Blood. 1995;86:4527-4531.

216. Hirayama F, Shih JP, Awgulewitsch A, et al. Clonal proliferation of murine lymphohemopoietic progenitors in culture. Proc Natl Acad Sci U S A. 1992;89:5907-5911.

217. Williams DE, de Vries P, Namen AE, et al. The steel factor. Dev Biol. 1992;151:368-376.

218. McNiece IK, Langley KE, Zsebo KM. The role of recombinant stem cell factor in early B cell development. Synergistic interaction with IL-7. J Immunol. 1991;146: 3785-3790.

219. Toksoz D, Zsebo KM, Smith KA, et al. Support of human hematopoiesis in long-term bone marrow cultures by murine stromal cells selectively expressing the membrane-bound and secreted forms of the human homolog of the steel gene product, stem cell factor. Proc Natl Acad Sci U S A. 1992;89:7350-7354.

220. Cerretti DP, Wignall J, Anderson D, et al. Human macrophage-colony stimulating factor: alternative RNA and protein processing from a single gene. Mol Immunol. 1988;25:761-770.

221. Avraham H, Scadden D, Chi S, et al. Interaction of human bone marrow fibroblasts with megakaryocytes: role of the c-kit ligand. Blood. 1992;80:1679-1684.

222. Brannan CI, Lyman SD, Williams DE, et al. Steel-Dickie mutation encodes a c-Kit ligand lacking transmembrane and cytoplasmic domains. Proc Natl Acad Sci U S A. 1991;88:4671-4674.

223. Akira S, Taga T, Kishimoto T. Interleukin-6 in biology and medicine. Adv Immunol. 1993;54:1-78.

224. Matthews W, Jordan C, Wiegand G, et al. A receptor tyrosine kinase specific to hematopoietic stem and progenitor cell–enriched populations. Cell. 1991;65:1143-1152.

225. Small D, Levenstein M, Kim E, et al. STK-1, the human homolog of Flk-2/Flt-3, is selectively expressed in CD34+ human bone marrow cells and is involved in the proliferation of early progenitor/stem cells. Proc Natl Acad Sci U S A. 1994;91:459-463.

226. Lyman SD, James L, Vanden Bos T, et al. Molecular cloning of a ligand for the flt3/flk-2 tyrosine kinase receptor: a proliferative factor for primitive hematopoietic cells. Cell. 1993;75:1157-1167.

227. Hirayama F, Lyman SD, Clark SC, Ogawa M. The flt3 ligand supports proliferation of lymphohematopoietic progenitors and early B-lymphoid progenitors. Blood. 1995;85:1762-1768.

228. McKenna HJ, de Vries P, Brasel K, et al. Effect of flt3 ligand on the ex vivo expansion of human CD34+ hematopoietic progenitor cells. Blood. 1995;86:3413-3420.

229. Hudak S, Hunte B, Culpepper J, et al. FLT3/FLK2 ligand promotes the growth of murine stem cells and the expansion of colony-forming cells and spleen colony-forming units. Blood. 1995;85:2747-2755.

230. Mackarehtschian K, Hardin JD, Moore KA, et al. Targeted disruption of the flk2/flt3 gene leads to deficiencies in primitive hematopoietic progenitors. Immunity. 1995;3:147-161.

231. Hunte BE, Hudak S, Campbell D, et al. Flk2/flt3 ligand is a potent cofactor for the growth of primitive B cell progenitors. J Immunol. 1996;156:489-496.

232. Staal FJ, Clevers HC. Regulation of lineage commitment during lymphocyte development. Int Rev Immunol. 2001;20:45-64.

233. Austin TW, Solar GP, Ziegler FC, et al. A role for the Wnt gene family in hematopoiesis: expansion of multilineage progenitor cells. Blood. 1997;89:3624-3635.

234. Yamane T, Kunisada T, Tsukamoto H, et al. Wnt signaling regulates hemopoiesis through stromal cells. J Immunol. 2001;167:765-772.

235. Brandon C, Eisenberg LM, Eisenberg CA. WNT signaling modulates the diversification of hematopoietic cells. Blood. 2000;96:4132-4141.

236. Van Den Berg DJ, Sharma AK, Bruno E, Hoffman R. Role of members of the Wnt gene family in human hematopoiesis. Blood. 1998;92:3189-3202.

237. Naito AT, Shiojima I, Akazawa H, et al. Developmental stage–specific biphasic roles of Wnt/beta-catenin signaling in cardiomyogenesis and hematopoiesis. Proc Natl Acad Sci U S A. 2006;103:19812-19817.

238. Wang J, Shackleford GM. Murine Wnt10a and Wnt10b: cloning and expression in developing limbs, face and skin of embryos and in adults. Oncogene. 1996;13:1537-1544.

239. Jamieson CH, Ailles LE, Dylla SJ, et al. Granulocyte-macrophage progenitors as candidate leukemic stem cells in blast-crisis CML. N Engl J Med. 2004;351:657-667.

240. Cobas M, Wilson A, Ernst B, et al. Beta-catenin is dispensable for hematopoiesis and lymphopoiesis. J Exp Med. 2004;199:221-229.

241. Kirstetter P, Anderson K, Porse BT, et al. Activation of the canonical Wnt pathway leads to loss of hematopoietic stem cell repopulation and multilineage differentiation block. Nat Immunol. 2006;7:1048-1056.

242. Scheller M, Huelsken J, Rosenbauer F, et al. Hematopoietic stem cell and multilineage defects generated by constitutive beta-catenin activation. Nat Immunol. 2006;7:1037-1047.

243. Carlesso N, Aster JC, Sklar J, Scadden DT. Notch1-induced delay of human hematopoietic progenitor cell differentiation is associated with altered cell cycle kinetics. Blood. 1999;93:838-848.

244. Ohishi K, Katayama N, Shiku H, et al. Notch signalling in hematopoiesis. Semin Cell Dev Biol. 2003;14:143-150.

245. Burns CE, Traver D, Mayhall E, et al. Hematopoietic stem cell fate is established by the Notch-Runx pathway. Genes Dev. 2005;19:2331-2342.

246. Nakagawa M, Ichikawa M, Kumano K, et al. AML1/Runx1 rescues Notch1-null mutation–induced deficiency of para-aortic splanchnopleural hematopoiesis. Blood. 2006;108:3329-3334.

247. de Pooter RF, Schmitt TM, de la Pompa JL, et al. Notch signaling requires GATA-2 to inhibit myelopoiesis from embryonic stem cells and primary hemopoietic progenitors. J Immunol. 2006;176:5267-5275.

248. Chadwick K, Wang L, Li L, et al. Cytokines and BMP-4 promote hematopoietic differentiation of human embryonic stem cells. Blood. 2003;102:906-915.

249. Li F, Lu S, Vida L, et al. Bone morphogenetic protein 4 induces efficient hematopoietic differentiation of rhesus monkey embryonic stem cells in vitro. Blood. 2001;98:335-342.

250. Xu RH, Ault KT, Kim J, et al. Opposite effects of FGF and BMP-4 on embryonic blood formation: roles of PV.1 and GATA-2. Dev Biol. 1999;208:352-361.

251. Bhatia M, Bonnet D, Wu D, et al. Bone morphogenetic proteins regulate the developmental program of human hematopoietic stem cells. J Exp Med. 1999;189:1139-1148.

252. Lenox LE, Perry JM, Paulson RF. BMP4 and Madh5 regulate the erythroid response to acute anemia. Blood. 2005;105:2741-2748.

253. Kiel MJ, Morrison SJ. Maintaining hematopoietic stem cells in the vascular niche. Immunity. 2006;25:862-864.

254. Kishimoto Y, Lee KH, Zon L, Hammerschmidt M, Schulte-Merker S. The molecular nature of zebrafish swirl: BMP2 function is essential during early dorsoventral patterning. Development. 1997;124:4457-4466.

255. Sadlon TJ, Lewis ID, D'Andrea RJ. BMP4: its role in development of the hematopoietic system and potential as a hematopoietic growth factor. Stem Cells. 2004;22:457-474.

256. Perry JM, Harandi OF, Paulson RF. BMP4, SCF and hypoxia cooperatively regulate the expansion of murine stress erythroid progenitors. Blood. 2007;109:4494-4502.

257. Zhang CC, Kaba M, Ge G, et al. Angiopoietin-like proteins stimulate ex vivo expansion of hematopoietic stem cells. Nat Med. 2006;12:240-245.

258. Stier S, Ko Y, Forkert R, et al. Osteopontin is a hematopoietic stem cell niche component that negatively regulates stem cell pool size. J Exp Med. 2005;201:1781-1791.

259. Haylock DN, Nilsson SK. Osteopontin: a bridge between bone and blood. Br J Haematol. 2006;134:467-474.

260. Ikebuchi K, Wong GG, Clark SC, et al. Interleukin-6 enhancement of interleukin-3–dependent proliferation of multipotential hemopoietic progenitors. Proc Natl Acad Sci U S A. 1987;84:9035-9039.

261. Musashi M, Yang Y-C, Paul SR, et al. Direct and synergistic effects of interleukin 11 on murine hemopoiesis in culture. Proc Natl Acad Sci U S A. 1991;88:765-769.

262. Leary AG, Wong GG, Clark SC, et al. Leukemia inhibitory factor/differentiation-inhibiting activity/human interleukin for DA cells augments proliferation of human hemopoietic stem cells. Blood. 1990;75:1960-1964.

263. Hirayama F, Katayama N, Neben S, et al. Synergistic interaction between interleukin-12 and steel factor in support of proliferation of murine lymphohematopoietic progenitors in culture. Blood. 1994;83:92-98.

264. Zhang XG, Gu JJ, Lu ZY, et al. Ciliary neurotropic factor, interleukin 11, leukemia inhibitory factor, and oncostatin M are growth factors for human myeloma cell lines using the interleukin 6 signal transducer gp130. J Exp Med. 1994;179:1337-1342.

265. Chua AO, Chizzonite R, Desai BB, et al. Expression cloning of a human IL-12 receptor component. A new member of the cytokine receptor superfamily with strong homology to gp130. J Immunol. 1994;153:128-136.

266. Trinchieri G. Interleukin-12: a proinflammatory cytokine with immunoregulatory functions that bridge innate resistance and antigen-specific adaptive immunity. Annu Rev Immunol. 1995;13:251-276.

267. Trinchieri G. Interleukin-12: a cytokine at the interface of inflammation and immunity. Adv Immunol. 1998;70:63-243.

268. Leary AG, Ikebuchi K, Hirai Y, et al. Synergism between interleukin-6 and interleukin-3 in supporting proliferation

of human hematopoietic stem cells: comparison with interleukin-1α. Blood. 1988;71:1759-1763.

269. Srour EF, Brandt JE, Leemhuis T, et al. Relationship between cytokine-dependent cell cycle progression and MHC class II antigen expression by human CD34⁺HLA-DR⁻ bone marrow cells. J Immunol. 1992;148:815-820.

270. Jacobsen SE, Ruscetti FW, Okkenhaug C, et al. Distinct and direct synergistic effects of IL-1 and IL-6 on proliferation and differentiation of primitive murine hematopoietic progenitor cells in vitro. Exp Hematol. 1994;22:1064-1069.

271. Rodriguez C, Lacasse C, Hoang T. Interleukin-1 beta suppresses apoptosis in CD34 positive bone marrow cells through activation of the type I IL-1 receptor. J Cell Physiol. 1996;166:387-396.

272. Yamasaki K, Taga T, Hirata Y, et al. Cloning and expression of the human interleukin-6 (BSF-2/IFN beta 2) receptor. Science. 1988;241:825-828.

273. Hibi M, Murakami M, Saito M, et al. Molecular cloning and expression of an IL-6 signal transducer, gp130. Cell. 1990;63:1149-1157.

274. Pennica D, Shaw KJ, Swanson TA, et al. Cardiotrophin-1. Biological activities and binding to the leukemia inhibitory factor receptor/gp130 signaling complex. J Biol Chem. 1995;270:10915-10922.

275. Nishimoto N, Ogata A, Shima Y, et al. Oncostatin M, leukemia inhibitory factor, and interleukin 6 induce the proliferation of human plasmacytoma cells via the common signal transducer, gp130. J Exp Med. 1994;179:1343-1347.

276. Wong GG, Witek-Giannotti JS, Temple PA, et al. Stimulation of murine hemopoietic colony formation by human IL-6. J Immunol. 1988;140:3040-3044.

277. Leary AG, Zeng HQ, Clark SC, Ogawa M. Growth factor requirements for survival in G₀ and entry into the cell cycle of primitive human hematopoietic progenitors. Proc Natl Acad Sci U S A. 1992;89:4013-4017.

278. Paul SR, Bennett F, Calvetti JA, et al. Molecular cloning of a cDNA encoding interleukin 11, a novel stromal cell–derived lymphopoietic and hematopoietic cytokine. Proc Natl Acad Sci U S A. 1990;87:7512-7516.

279. Du XX, Williams DA. Interleukin-11: a multifunctional growth factor derived from the hematopoietic microenvironment. Blood. 1994;83:2023-2030.

280. Turner KJ, Clark SC. Interleukin-11: biological and clinical perspectives. In Mertelsmann R, Herrmann F (eds). Hematopoietic Growth Factors in Clinical Applications, 2nd ed. New York, Marcel Dekker, 1995, pp 315-336.

281. Yin T, Taga T, Tsang ML-S, et al. Interleukin (IL)-6 signal transducer, gp130, is involved in IL-11 mediated signal transduction [abstract]. Blood. 1992;80:151a.

282. Baumann H, Schendel P. Interleukin-11 regulates the hepatic expression of the same plasma protein genes as interleukin-6. J Biol Chem. 1991;266:20424-20427.

283. Suda T, Udagawa N, Nakamura I, et al. Modulation of osteoclast differentiation by local factors. Bone. 1995;17:87S-91S.

284. Burstein SA, Mei R-L, Henthorn J, et al. Leukemia inhibitory factor and interleukin-11 promote the maturation of murine and human megakaryocytes in vitro. J Cell Physiol. 1992;153:305-312.

285. Paul SR, Bennett F, Calvetti JA, et al. Molecular cloning of a cDNA encoding interleukin-11, a stromal cell–derived

286. Broudy V, Lin N, Kaushansky K. Thrombopoietin (c-mpl ligand) acts synergistically with erythropoietin, stem cell factor, and interleukin-11 to enhance murine megakaryocyte colony growth and increases megakaryocyte ploidy in vitro. Blood. 1995;85:1719-1726.

287. Eaves AC, Eaves CJ. Maintenance and proliferation control of primitive hemopoietic progenitors in long-term cultures of human marrow cells. Blood Cells. 1988;14:355-368.

288. Cardoso AA, Li ML, Batard P, et al. Release from quiescence of CD34⁺ CD38⁻ human umbilical cord blood cells reveals their potentiality to engraft adults. Proc Natl Acad Sci U S A. 1993;90:8707-8711.

289. Li ML, Cardoso AA, Sansilvestri P, et al. Additive effects of steel factor and antisense TGF-beta 1 oligodeoxynucleotide on CD34⁺ hematopoietic progenitor cells. Leukemia. 1994;8:441-445.

290. Dumoutier L, Van Roost E, Ameye G, et al. IL-TIF/IL-22: genomic organization and mapping of the human and mouse genes. Genes Immun. 2000;1:488-494.

291. Boulay JL, Paul WE. Hematopoietin sub-family classification based on size, gene organization and sequence homology. Curr Biol. 1993;3:573-581.

292. Bazan JF. Haemopoietic receptors and helical cytokines. Immunol Today. 1990;11:350-354.

293. Merberg DM, Wolf SF, Clark SC. Sequence similarity between NKSF and the IL-6/G-CSF family. Immunol Today. 1992;13:77-78.

294. Leutz A, Damm K, Sterneck E, et al. Molecular cloning of the chicken myelomonocytic growth factor (CMGF) reveals relationship to interleukin 6 and granulocyte colony stimulating factor. EMBO J. 1989;8:175-181.

295. Sohma Y, Akahori H, Seki N, et al. Molecular cloning and chromosomal localization of the human thrombopoietin gene. FEBS Lett. 1994;353:57-61.

296. Foster DC, Sprecher CA, Grant FJ, et al. Human thrombopoietin: gene structure, cDNA sequence, expression, and chromosomal localization. Proc Natl Acad Sci U S A. 1994;91:13023-13027.

297. Gurney A, Kuang W, Xie M, et al. Genomic structure, chromosomal localization, and conserved alternative splice forms of thrombopoietin. Blood. 1995;85:981-988.

298. Anderson DM, Williams DE, Tushinski R, et al. Alternate splicing of mRNAs encoding human mast cell growth factor and localization of the gene to chromosome 12q22-q24. Cell Growth Differ. 1991;2:373-378.

299. Leonard WJ, Noguchi M, Russell SM, McBride OW. The molecular basis of X-linked severe combined immunodeficiency: the role of the interleukin-2 receptor gamma chain as a common gamma chain, gamma c. Immunol Rev. 1994;138:61-86.

300. Macchi P, Villa A, Gilliani S, et al. Mutations of Jak-3 gene in patients with autosomal severe combined immune deficiency (SCID). Nature. 1995;377:65-68.

301. Dong F, Brynes RK, Tidow N, et al. Mutations in the gene for the granulocyte colony-stimulating-factor receptor in patients with acute myeloid leukemia preceded by severe congenital neutropenia. N Engl J Med. 1995;333:487-493.

302. Jubinsky PT, Nathan DG, Wilson DJ, Sieff CA. A low-affinity human granulocyte-macrophage colony-stimulating factor/murine erythropoietin hybrid receptor functions in murine cell lines. Blood. 1993;81:587-591.

303. Pinkerton PH, Bannerman RM. The hereditary anemias of mice. Hematol Rev. 1968;1:119-192.

304. Witte ON. Steel locus defines new multipotent growth factor. Cell. 1990;63:5-6.

305. Russell ES. Hereditary anemias of the mouse: a review for geneticists. Adv Genet. 1979;20:357-459.

306. Yoshida H, Hayashi S-I, Kunisada T, et al. The murine mutation osteopetrosis is in the coding region of the macrophage colony stimulating factor gene. Nature. 1990;345:442-444.

307. Van Zant G, Shultz L. Hematologic abnormalities of the immunodeficient mouse mutant, viable motheaten (mev). Exp Hematol. 1989;17:81-87.

308. Luo H, Hanratty WP, Dearolf CR. An amino acid substitution in the *Drosophilia* hopTum-l Jak kinase causes leukemia-like hematopoietic defects. EMBO J. 1995;14:1412-1420.

309. Harrison DA, Binari R, Nahreini TS, et al. Activation of a *Drosophila* Janus kinase (JAK) causes hematopoietic neoplasia and developmental defects. EMBO J. 1995;14:2857-2865.

310. Bernad A, Kopf M, Kulbacki R, et al. Interleukin-6 is required in vivo for the regulation of stem cells and committed progenitors of the hematopoietic system. Immunity. 1994;1:725-731.

311. Stanley E, Lieschke GJ, Grail D, et al. Granulocyte/macrophage colony-stimulating factor–deficient mice show no major perturbation of hematopoiesis but develop a characteristic pulmonary pathology. Proc Natl Acad Sci U S A. 1994;91:5592-5596.

312. Dranoff G, Crawford AD, Sadelain M, et al. Involvement of granulocyte-macrophage colony-stimulating factor in pulmonary homeostasis. Science. 1994;264:713-716.

313. Lieschke GJ, Grail D, Hodgson G, et al. Mice lacking granulocyte colony-stimulating factor have chronic neutropenia, granulocyte and macrophage progenitor cell deficiency, and impaired neutrophil mobilization. Blood. 1994;84:1737-1746.

314. Wu H, Liu X, Jaenisch R, Lodish HF. Generation of committed erythroid BFU-E and CFU-E progenitors does not require erythropoietin or the erythropoietin receptor. Cell. 1995;83:59-67.

315. Gurney AL, Carver-Moore K, de Sauvage FJ, Moore MW. Thrombocytopenia in c-mpl–deficient mice. Science. 1994;265:1445-1447.

316. Nishinakamura R, Nakayama N, Hirabayashi Y, et al. Mice deficient for the IL-3/GM-CSF/IL-5 βc receptor exhibit lung pathology and impaired immune response while βIL3 receptor–deficient mice are normal. Immunity. 1995;2:211-222.

317. Zmuidzinas A, Fischer KD, Lira SA, et al. The vav proto-oncogene is required early in embryogenesis but not for hematopoietic development in vitro. EMBO J. 1995;14:1-11.

318. Thomas KR, Capecchi MR. Site-directed mutagenesis by gene targeting in mouse embryo–derived stem cells. Cell. 1987;51:503-512.

319. Hammond WP, Csiba E, Canin A, et al. Chronic neutropenia. A new canine model induced by human granulocyte colony-stimulating factor. J Clin Invest. 1991;87:704-710.

320. Metcalf D. The molecular control of hematopoiesis: progress and problems with gene manipulation. Stem Cells. 1998;16:314-321.

321. de Sauvage FJ, Carver-Moore K, Luoh SM, et al. Physiological regulation of early and late stages of megakaryocytopoiesis by thrombopoietin. J Exp Med. 1996;183:651-656.

322. Gainsford T, Roberts AW, Kimura S, et al. Cytokine production and function in c-mpl–deficient mice: no physiologic role for interleukin-3 in residual megakaryocyte and platelet production. Blood. 1998;91:2745-2752.

323. Gainsford T, Nandurkar H, Metcalf D, et al. The residual megakaryocyte and platelet production in c-mpl–deficient mice is not dependent on the actions of interleukin-6, interleukin-11, or leukemia inhibitory factor. Blood. 2000;95:528-534.

324. Kopf M, Baumann H, Freer G, et al. Impaired immune and acute-phase responses in interleukin-6–deficient mice. Nature. 1994;368:339-342.

325. Miyatake S, Otsuka T, Yokota T, et al. Structure of the chromosomal gene for granulocyte-macrophage colony stimulating factor: comparison of the mouse and human genes. EMBO J. 1985;4:2561-2568.

326. Nimer SD, Uchida H. Regulation of granulocyte-macrophage colony-stimulating factor and interleukin 3 expression. Stem Cells. 1995;13:324-335.

327. Campbell HD, Tucker WQJ, Hort Y, et al. Molecular cloning, nucleotide sequence, and expression of the gene encoding human eosinophil differentiation factor (interleukin 5). Proc Natl Acad Sci U S A. 1987;84:6629-6633.

328. Yang Y-C, Clark SC. Molecular cloning of a primate cDNA and the human gene for IL-3. Lymphokines. 1988;15:375-391.

329. Dolganov G, Bort S, Lovett M, et al. Coexpression of the interleukin-13 and interleukin-4 genes correlates with their physical linkage in the cytokine gene cluster on human chromosome 5q23-31. Blood. 1996;87:3316-3326.

330. Le Beau MM, Espinosa R III, Neuman WL, et al. Cytogenetic and molecular delineation of the smallest commonly deleted region of chromosome 5 in malignant myeloid diseases. Proc Natl Acad Sci U S A. 1993;90:5484-5488.

331. Sieburth D, Jabs EW, Warrington JA, et al. Assignment of genes encoding a unique cytokine (IL12) composed of two unrelated subunits to chromosomes 3 and 5. Genomics. 1992;14:59-62.

332. Yang Y-C, Kovacic S, Kriz R, et al. The human genes for GM-CSF and IL 3 are closely linked in tandem on chromosome 5. Blood. 1988;71:958-961.

333. Tavernier J, Devos R, Cornelis S, et al. A human high affinity interleukin-5 receptor (IL5R) is composed of an IL5-specific α chain and a β chain shared with the receptor for GM-CSF. Cell. 1991;66:1175-1184.

334. Kitamura T, Sato N, Arai K, Miyajima A. Expression cloning of the human IL-3 receptor cDNA reveals a shared beta subunit for the human IL-3 and GM-CSF receptors. Cell. 1991;66:1165-1174.

335. Nishinakamyura R, Miyajima A, Mee PJ, et al. Hematopoiesis in mice lacking the entire granulocyte-macrophage

colony-stimulating factor/interleukin-3/interleukin-5 functions. Blood. 1996;88:2458-2464.

336. Pollard JW, Hunt JS, Wiktor-Jedrzejczak W, Stanley ER. A pregnancy defect in the osteopetrotic (op/op) mouse demonstrates the requirement for Csf-1 in female fertility. Dev Biol. 1991;148:273-283.

337. Wiktor-Jedrzejczak W, Ratajczak MZ, Ptasznik A, et al. Csf-1 deficiency in the op/op mouse has differential effects on macrophage populations and differentiation stages. Exp Hematol. 1992;20:1004-1010.

338. Hume DA, Favot P. Is the osteopetrotic (op/op mutant) mouse completely deficient in expression of macrophage colony-stimulating factor? J Interferon Cytokine Res. 1995;15:279-284.

339. Trinchieri G. Interleukin-12: a cytokine produced by antigen-presenting cells with immunoregulatory functions in the generation of T-helper cells type 1 and cytotoxic lymphocytes. Blood. 1994;84:4008-4027.

340. Dinarello CA. Interleukin-1 and its biologically related cytokines. Adv Immunol. 1989;44:153-205.

341. Cluitmans FH, Esendam BH, Landegent JE, et al. Regulatory effects of T cell lymphokines on cytokine gene expression in monocytes. Lymphokine Cytokine Res. 1993;12:457-464.

342. Horiguchi J, Warren MK, Kufe D. Expression of the macrophage-specific colony-stimulating factor in human monocytes treated with granulocyte-macrophage colony-stimulating factor. Blood. 1987;69:1259-1261.

343. Warren MK, Ralph P. Macrophage growth factor CSF-1 stimulates human monocyte production of interferon, tumor necrosis factor, and colony stimulating activity. J Immunol. 1986;137:2281-2285.

344. Cluitmans FH, Esendam BH, Landegent JE, et al. IL-4 down-regulates IL-2-, IL-3-, and GM-CSF–induced cytokine gene expression in peripheral blood monocytes. Ann Hematol. 1994;68:293-298.

345. Fiorentino DF, Zlotnik A, Mosmann TR, et al. IL-10 inhibits cytokine production by activated macrophages. J Immunol. 1991;147:3815-3822.

346. Trepicchio WL, Bozza M, Pednault G, Dorner AJ. Recombinant human interleukin-11 attenuation of the inflammatory response through down-regulation of pro-inflammatory cytokine release and nitric oxide production. J Immunol. 1996;157:3627-3634.

347. Chabaud M, Durand JM, Buchs N, et al. Human interleukin-17: a T cell–derived proinflammatory cytokine produced by the rheumatoid synovium. Arthritis Rheum. 1999;42:963-970.

348. Evans R, Kamdar SJ, Fuller JA, Krupke DM. The potential role of the macrophage colony-stimulating factor, CSF-1, in inflammatory responses: characterization of macrophage cytokine gene expression. J Leukoc Biol. 1995;58:99-107.

349. Temeles DS, McGrath HE, Kittler EL, et al. Cytokine expression from bone marrow derived macrophages. Exp Hematol. 1993;21:388-393.

350. Zhang Y, Broser M, Rom W. Activation of the interleukin 6 gene by *Mycobacterium tuberculosis* or lipopolysaccharide is mediated by nuclear factors NF IL 6 and NF-kappa B. Proc Natl Acad Sci U S A. 1995;92:3632-3630.

351. Galdiero M, Cipollaro de L, Donnarumma G, et al. Interleukin-1 and interleukin-6 gene expression in human monocytes stimulated with *Salmonella typhimurium* porins. Immunology. 1995;86:612-619.

352. Matsusaka T, Fujikawa K, Nishio Y, et al. Transcription factors NF-IL6 and NF-kappa B synergistically activate transcription of the inflammatory cytokines, interleukin 6 and interleukin 8. Proc Natl Acad Sci U S A. 1993;90:10193-10197.

353. Wang P, Wu P, Siegel MI, et al. IL-10 inhibits transcription of cytokine genes in human peripheral blood mononuclear cells. J Immunol. 1994;153:811-816.

354. Moller A, Schwarz A, Neuner P, et al. Regulation of monocyte and keratinocyte interleukin 6 production by transforming growth factor beta. Exp Dermatol. 1994;3:314-320.

355. de Wit H, Dokter WH, Esselink MT, et al. Interferon-gamma enhances the LPS-induced G-CSF gene expression in human adherent monocytes, which is regulated at transcriptional and posttranscriptional levels. Exp Hematol. 1993;21:785-790.

356. Vellenga E, Dokter W, de Wolf JT, et al. Interleukin-4 prevents the induction of G-CSF mRNA in human adherent monocytes in response to endotoxin and IL-1 stimulation. Br J Haematol. 1991;79:22-26.

357. Yamada H, Iwase S, Mohri M, Kufe D. Involvement of a nuclear factor-kappa B–like protein in induction of the macrophage colony-stimulating factor gene by tumor necrosis factor. Blood. 1991;78:1988-1995.

358. Steinman RM. The dendritic cell system and its role in immunogenicity. Annu Rev Immunol. 1991;9:271-296.

359. Zhou LJ, Tedder TF. A distinct pattern of cytokine gene expression by human CD83+ blood dendritic cells. Blood. 1995;86:3295-3301.

360. Galy A, Travis M, Cen D, Chen B. Human T, B, natural killer, and dendritic cells arise from a common bone marrow progenitor cell subset. Immunity. 1995;3:459-473.

361. Morelli AE, Zahorchak AF, Larregina AT, et al. Cytokine production by mouse myeloid dendritic cells in relation to differentiation and terminal maturation induced by lipopolysaccharide or CD40 ligation. Blood. 2001;98:1512-1523.

362. Watari K, Ozawa K, Tajika K, et al. Production of human granulocyte colony stimulating factor by various kinds of stromal cells in vitro detected by enzyme immunoassay and in situ hybridization. Stem Cells. 1994;12:416-423.

363. Mantovani L, Henschler R, Brach MA, et al. Regulation of gene expression of macrophage-colony stimulating factor in human fibroblasts by the acute phase response mediators interleukin (IL)-1beta, tumor necrosis factor-alpha, and IL-6. FEBS Lett. 1991;280:97-102.

364. Walther Z, May LT, Sehgal PB. Transcriptional regulation of the interferon-beta 2/B cell differentiation factor BSF-2/hepatocyte-stimulating factor gene in human fibroblasts by other cytokines. J Immunol. 1988;140:974-977.

365. Metcalf D, Willson TA, Hilton DJ, et al. Production of hematopoietic regulatory factors in cultures of adult and fetal mouse organs: measurement by specific bioassays. Leukemia. 1995;9:1556-1564.

366. Sironi M, Sciacca FL, Matteucci C, et al. Regulation of endothelial and mesothelial cell function by interleukin-13: selective induction of vascular cell adhesion molecule-1 and amplification of interleukin-6 production. Blood. 1994;84:1913-1921.

367. Hirano T, Akira S, Taga T, Kishimoto T. Biological and clinical aspects of interleukin 6. Immunol Today. 1990;11: 443-449.

368. Van Snick J. Interleukin-6: an overview. Annu Rev Immunol. 1990;8:253-278.

369. Heinrich MC, Dooley DC, Freed AC, et al. Constitutive expression of Steel factor gene by human stromal cells. Blood. 1993;82:771-783.

370. Cerretti DP, Wignall J, Anderson D, et al. Membrane bound forms of human macrophage colony stimulating factor (M-CSF, CSF-1). Prog Clin Biol Res. 1990;352: 63-70.

371. Hachiya M, Koeffler HP, Suzuki G, Akashi M. Tumor necrosis factor and interleukin-1 synergize with irradiation in expression of GM-CSF gene in human fibroblasts. Leukemia. 1995;9:1276-1281.

372. Seelentag WK, Mermod J-J, Montesano R, Vassalli P. Additive effects of interleukin 1 and tumor necrosis factor α on the accumulation of the three granulocyte and macrophage colony-stimulating factor mRNAs in human endothelial cells. EMBO J. 1987;6:2261-2265.

373. Zsebo KM, Yuschenkoff VN, Schiffer S, et al. Vascular endothelial cells and granulopoiesis: interleukin-1 stimulates release of G-CSF and GM-CSF. Blood. 1988;71: 99-103.

374. Koenig A, Yakisan E, Reuter M, et al. Differential regulation of stem cell factor mRNA expression in human endothelial cells by bacterial pathogens: an in vitro model of inflammation. Blood. 1994;83:2836-2843.

375. Bagby GC, Shaw G, Heinrich MC, et al. Interleukin-1 stimulation stabilizes GM-CSF mRNA in human vascular endothelial cells: preliminary studies on the role of the 3′ au rich motif. Prog Clin Biol Res. 1990;352:233-239.

376. Rajavashisth TB, Yamada H, Mishra NK. Transcriptional activation of the macrophage-colony stimulating factor gene by minimally modified LDL. Involvement of nuclear factor-kappa B. Arterioscler Thromb Vasc Biol. 1995;15: 1591-1598.

377. Blanchard KL, Fandrey J, Goldberg MA, Bunn HF. Regulation of the erythropoietin gene. Stem Cells (Dayt). 1993;11(Suppl 1):1-7.

378. Porter DL, Goldberg MA. Regulation of erythropoietin production. Exp Hematol. 1993;21:399-404.

379. Jelkmann W. Erythropoietin: structure, control of production, and function. Physiol Rev. 1992;72:449-489.

380. Eckardt KU, Ratcliffe PJ, Tan CC, et al. Age-dependent expression of the erythropoietin gene in rat liver and kidneys. J Clin Invest. 1992;89:753-760.

381. Beck I, Ramirez S, Weinmann R, Caro J. Enhancer element at the 3′-flanking region controls transcriptional response to hypoxia in the human erythropoietin gene. J Biol Chem. 1991;266:15563-15566.

382. Semenza GL, Koury ST, Nejfelt MK, et al. Cell-type–specific and hypoxia-inducible expression of the human erythropoietin gene in transgenic mice. Proc Natl Acad Sci U S A. 1991;88:8725-8729.

383. Wang GL, Semenza GL. Purification and characterization of hypoxia-inducible factor 1. J Biol Chem. 1995;270: 1230-1237.

384. Semenza GL. HIF-1: mediator of physiological and pathophysiological responses to hypoxia. J Appl Physiol. 2000;88:1474-1480.

385. Blanchard KL, Acquaviva AM, Galson DL, Bunn HF. Hypoxic induction of the human erythropoietin gene: cooperation between the promoter and enhancer, each of which contains steroid receptor response elements. Mol Cell Biol. 1992;12:5373-5385.

386. Maxwell PH, Wiesener MS, Chang GW, et al. The tumour suppressor protein VHL targets hypoxia-inducible factors for oxygen-dependent proteolysis. Nature. 1999;399: 271-275.

387. Jaakkola P, Mole DR, Tian YM, et al. Targeting of HIF-alpha to the von Hippel-Lindau ubiquitylation complex by O2-regulated prolyl hydroxylation. Science. 2001;292: 468-472.

388. Brunelle JK, Bell EL, Quesada NM, et al. Oxygen sensing requires mitochondrial ROS but not oxidative phosphorylation. Cell Metab. 2005;1:409-414.

389. Guzy RD, Hoyos B, Robin E, et al. Mitochondrial complex III is required for hypoxia-induced ROS production and cellular oxygen sensing. Cell Metab. 2005;1:401-408.

390. Lando D, Peet DJ, Whelan DA, et al. Asparagine hydroxylation of the HIF transactivation domain α hypoxic switch. Science. 2002;295:858-861.

391. Lando D, Peet DJ, Gorman JJ, et al. FIH-1 is an asparaginyl hydroxylase enzyme that regulates the transcriptional activity of hypoxia-inducible factor. Genes Dev. 2002;16:1466-1471.

392. Kaushansky K. Thrombopoietin: the primary regulator of megakaryocyte and platelet production. Thromb Haemost. 1995;74:521-525.

393. Stoffel R, Wiestner A, Skoda RC. Thrombopoietin in thrombocytopenic mice: evidence against regulation at the mRNA level and for a direct regulatory role of platelets. Blood. 1996;87:567-573.

394. Nagata Y, Shozaki Y, Nagahisa H, et al. Serum thrombopoietin level is not regulated by transcription but by the total counts of both megakaryocytes and platelets during thrombocytopenia and thrombocytosis. Thromb Haemost. 1997;77:808-814.

395. Kuter DJ, Rosenberg RD. The reciprocal relationship of thrombopoietin (c-Mpl ligand) to changes in the platelet mass during busulfan-induced thrombocytopenia in the rabbit. Blood. 1995;85:2720-2730.

396. Chang M, Suen Y, Meng G, et al. Differential mechanisms in the regulation of endogenous levels of thrombopoietin and interleukin-11 during thrombocytopenia: insight into the regulation of platelet production. Blood. 1996;88: 3354-3362.

397. Bartocci A, Mastrogiannis DS, Migliorati G, et al. Macrophages specifically regulate the concentration of their own growth factor in the circulation. Proc Natl Acad Sci U S A. 1987;84:6179-6183.

398. Bazan JF. Structural design and molecular evolution of a cytokine receptor superfamily. Proc Natl Acad Sci U S A. 1990;87:6934-6938.

399. Endo TA, Masuhara M, Yokouchi M, et al. A new protein containing an SH2 domain that inhibits JAK kinases. Nature. 1997;387:921-924.

400. Naka T, Narazaki M, Hirata M, et al. Structure and function of a new STAT-induced STAT inhibitor. Nature. 1997;387:924-929.

401. Boutin J-M, Jolicoeur C, Okamura H, et al. Cloning and expression of the rat prolactin receptor, a member of the

growth hormone/prolactin receptor gene family. Cell. 1988;53:69-77.

402. Edery M, Jolicoeur C, Levi-Meyrueis C, et al. Identification and sequence analysis of a second form of prolactin receptor by molecular cloning of complementary DNA from rabbit mammary gland. Proc Natl Acad Sci U S A. 1989;86:2112-2116.

403. Leung DW, Spencer SA, Cachianes G, et al. Growth hormone receptor and serum binding protein: purification, cloning and expression. Nature. 1987;330:537-543.

404. Hatakeyama M, Mori H, Doi T, Taniguchi T. A restricted cytoplasmic region of IL-2 receptor beta chain is essential for growth signal transduction but not for ligand binding and internalization. Cell. 1989;59:837-845.

405. Miura O, Cleveland JL, Ihle JN. Inactivation of erythropoietin receptor function by point mutations in a region having homology with other cytokine receptors. Mol Cell Biol. 1993;13:1788-1795.

406. Miyajima A, Mui AL-F, Ogorochi T, Sakamaki K. Receptors for granuylocyte-macrophage colony-stimulating factor, interleukin-3, and interleukin-5. Blood. 1993;82:1960-1974.

407. Kondo M, Takeshita T, Ishii N, et al. Sharing of the interleukin-2 (IL-2) receptor γ chain between receptors for IL-2 and IL-4. Science. 1993;262:1874-1877.

408. Russell S, Keegan AD, Harada N, et al. Interleukin-2 receptor γ chain: a functional component of the interleukin-4 receptor. Science. 1993;262:1880-1883.

409. Noguchi M, Nakamura Y, Russell SM, et al. Interleukin-2 receptor γ chain: a functional component of the interleukin-7 receptor. Science. 1993;262:1877-1880.

410. Kimura Y, Takeshita T, Kondo M, et al. Sharing of the IL-2 receptor gamma chain with the functional IL-9 receptor complex. Int Immunol. 1995;7:115-120.

411. Giri JG, Ahdieh M, Eisenman J, et al. Utilization of the beta and gamma chains of the IL-2 receptor by the novel cytokine IL-15. EMBO J. 1994;13:2822-2830.

412. Ziegler SF, Bird TA, Morella KK, et al. Distinct regions of the human granulocyte-colony-stimulating factor receptor cytoplasmic domain are required for proliferation and gene induction. Mol Cell Biol. 1993;13:2384-2390.

413. Fukunaga R, Ishizaka-Ikeda E, Nagata S. Growth and differentiation signals mediated by different regions in the cytoplasmic domain of granulocyte colony-stimulating factor receptor. Cell. 1993;74:1079-1087.

414. Borzillo GV, Ashmun RA, Sherr CJ. Macrophage lineage switching of murine early pre-B lymphoid cells expressing transduced fms genes. Mol Cell Biol. 1990;10:2703-2714.

415. Liboi E, Carroll M, D'Andrea AD, Mathey-Prevot B. Erythropoietin receptor signals both proliferation and erythroid-specific differentiation. Proc Natl Acad Sci U S A. 1993;90:11351-11355.

416. Jubinsky PT, Nathan DG, Sieff CA. A low-affinity GM-CSF/erythropoietin chimeric receptor functions in murine cell lines [abstract 1037]. Blood. 1991;78:262a.

417. Socolovsky M, Fallon AE, Lodish HF. The prolactin receptor rescues EpoR−/− erythroid progenitors and replaces EpoR in a synergistic interaction with c-kit. Blood. 1998;92:1491-1496.

418. Iwasaki-Arai J, Iwasaki H, Miyamoto T, et al. Enforced granulocyte/macrophage colony-stimulating factor signals do not support lymphopoiesis, but instruct lymphoid to myelomonocytic lineage conversion. J Exp Med. 2003;197:1311-1322.

419. Pronk CJH, Rossi DJ, Mansson R, et al. Elucidation of the phenotypic, functional, and molecular topography of a myeloerythroid progenitor cell hierarchy. Cell Stem Cell. 2007;1:428-442.

420. Songyang Z, Shoelson SE, Chaudhuri M, et al. SH2 domains recognize specific phosphopeptide sequences. Cell. 1993;72:767-778.

421. Ihle JN, Witthuhn BA, Quelle FW, et al. Signaling through the hematopoietic cytokine receptors. Annu Rev Immunol. 1995;13:369-398.

422. Schindler CW. Series introduction. JAK-STAT signaling in human disease. J Clin Invest. 2002;109:1133-1137.

423. Aaronson DS, Horvath CM. A road map for those who know JAK-STAT. Science. 2002;296:1653-1655.

424. Brizzi MF, Zini MG, Aronica MG, et al. Convergence of signaling by interleukin-3, granulocyte-macrophage colony-stimulating factor, and mast cell growth factor on JAK2 tyrosine kinase. J Biol Chem. 1994;269:31680-31684.

425. Lev S, Givol D, Yarden Y. A specific combination of substrates is involved in signal transduction by the kit-encoded receptor. EMBO J. 1991;10:647-654.

426. Herbst R, Lammers R, Schlessinger J, Ullrich A. Substrate phosphorylation specificity of the human c-kit receptor tyrosine kinase. J Biol Chem. 1991;266:19908-19916.

427. Müller M, Briscoe J, Laxton C, et al. The protein tyrosine kinase JAK1 complements defects in interferon-α/β and -γ signal transduction. Nature. 1993;366:129-135.

428. Watling D, Guschin D, Müller M, et al. Complementation by the protein tyrosine kinase JAK2 of a mutant cell line defective in the interferon-γ signal transduction pathway. Nature. 1993;366:166-170.

429. Hunter T. Cytokine connections. Nature. 1993;366:114-116.

430. Velazquez L, Fellous M, Stark GR, Pellegrini S. A protein tyrosine kinase in the interferon α/β signaling pathway. Cell. 1992;70:313-322.

431. Leung S, Qureshi SA, Kerr IM, et al. Role of STAT2 in the alpha interferon signaling pathway. Mol Cell Biol. 1995;15:1312-1317.

432. Darnell JE Jr, Kerr IM, Stark GR. Jak-STAT pathways and transcriptional activation in response to IFNs and other extracellular signaling proteins. Science. 1994;264:1415-1421.

433. Greenlund AC, Farrar MA, Viviano BL, Schreiber RD. Ligand-induced IFN gamma receptor tyrosine phosphorylation couples the receptor to its signal transduction system (p91). EMBO J. 1995;13:1591-1600.

434. Silvennoinen O, Witthuhn BA, Quelle FW, et al. Structure of the murine JAK2 protein tyrosine kinase and its role in IL-3 signal transduction. Proc Natl Acad Sci U S A. 1993;90:8429-8433.

435. Gouilleux F, Pallard C, Dusanter-Fourt I, et al. Prolactin, growth hormone, erythropoietin and granulocyte-macrophage colony stimulating factor induce MGF-Stat5 DNA binding activity. EMBO J. 1995;14:2005-2013.

436. Mui AL-F, Wakao H, O'Farrell A-M, et al. Interleukin-3, granulocyte-macrophage colony stimulating factor and

interleukin-5 transduce signals through two STAT5 homologs. EMBO J. 1995;14:1166-1175.

437. Quelle FW, Shimoda K, Thierfelder W, et al. Cloning of murine Stat6 and human Stat6, Stat proteins that are tyrosine phosphorylated in responses to IL-4 and IL-3 but are not required for mitogenesis. Mol Cell Biol. 1995;15:3336-3343.

438. Torigoe T, O'Connor R, Santoli D, Reed JC. Interleukin-3 regulates the activity of the LYN protein-tyrosine kinase in myeloid-committed leukemic cell lines. Blood. 1992; 80:617-624.

439. Kobayashi N, Kono T, Hatakeyama M, et al. Functional coupling of the src-family protein tyrosine kinases p59fyn and p53/56lyn with the interleukin 2 receptor: implications for redundancy and pleiotropism in cytokine signal transduction. Proc Natl Acad Sci U S A. 1993;90: 4201-4205.

440. Hanazono Y, Chiba S, Sasaki K, et al. c-fps/fes protein-tyrosine is implicated in a signaling pathway triggered by granulocyte-macrophage colony-stimulating factor and interleukin-3. EMBO J. 1993;12:1641-1646.

441. Mano H, Yamashita Y, Sato K, et al. Tec protein-tyrosine kinase is involved in interleukin-3 signaling pathway. Blood. 1995;85:343-350.

442. Shikama Y, Barber DL, D'Andrea A, Sieff CA. A constitutively activated chimeric cytokine receptor confers factor-dependent growth in hematopoietic cell lines. Blood. 1996;88:455-464.

443. Quelle FW, Sato N, Witthuhn BA, et al. JAK2 associates with the β_c chain of the receptor for granulocyte-macrophage colony-stimulating factor, and its activation requires the membrane-proximal region. Mol Cell Biol. 1994;14: 4335-4341.

444. Lütticken C, Wegenka UM, Yuan J, et al. Association of transcription factor APRF and protein kinase Jak1 with the interleukin-6 signal transducer gp130. Science. 1994;263:89-92.

445. Zhong Z, Wen Z, Darnell JE Jr. Stat3: a STAT family member activated by tyrosine phosphorylation in response to epidermal growth factor and interleukin-6. Science. 1994;264:95-98.

446. Akira S, Nishio Y, Inoue M, et al. Molecular cloning of APRF, a novel IFN-stimulated gene factor 3 p91-related transcription factor involved in the gp130-mediated signaling pathway. Cell. 1994;77:63-71.

447. Ernst M, Gearing DP, Dunn AR. Functional and biochemical association of Hck with the LIF/IL-6 receptor signal transducing subunit gp130 in embryonic stem cells. EMBO J. 1994;13:1574-1584.

448. Matsuda T, Takahashi-Tezuka M, Fukada T, et al. Association and activation of Btk and Tec tyrosine kinases by gp130, a signal transducer of the interleukin-6 family of cytokines. Blood. 1995;85:627-633.

449. Miyazaki T, Kawahara A, Fujii H, et al. Functional activation of Jak1 and Jak3 by selective association with IL-2 receptor subunits. Science. 1994;266:1045-1047.

450. Johnston JA, Kawamura M, Kirken RA, et al. Phosphorylation and activation of the Jak-3 Janus kinase in response to interleukin-2. Nature. 1994;370:151-153.

451. Nielsen M, Svejgaard A, Skov S, Odum N. Interleukin-2 induces tyrosine phosphorylation and nuclear translocation of stat3 in human T lymphocytes. Eur J Immunol. 1994;24:3082-3086.

452. Beadling C, Guschin D, Witthuhn BA, et al. Activation of JAK kinases and STAT proteins by interleukin-2 and interferon alpha, but not the T cell antigen receptor, in human T lymphocytes. EMBO J. 1994;13:5605-5615.

453. Hatakeyama M, Kono T, Kobayashi N, et al. Interaction of the IL-2 receptor with the src-family kinase p56lck: identification of novel intermolecular association. Science. 1991;252:1523-1528.

454. Torigoe T, Saragovi HU, Reed JC. Interleukin 2 regulates the activity of the lyn protein-tyrosine kinase in a B-cell line. Proc Natl Acad Sci U S A. 1992;89:2674-2678.

455. Minami Y, Nakagawa Y, Kawahara A, et al. Protein tyrosine kinase Syk is associated with and activated by the IL-2 receptor: possible link with the c-myc induction pathway. Immunity. 1995;2:89-100.

456. Witthuhn BA, Quelle FW, Silvennoinen O, et al. JAK2 associates with the erythropoietin receptor and is tyrosine phosphorylated and activated following stimulation with erythropoietin. Cell. 1993;74:227-236.

457. Gouilleux F, Wakao H, Mundt M, Groner B. Prolactin induces phosphorylation of Tyr694 of Stat5 (MGF), a prerequisite for DNA binding and induction of transcription. EMBO J. 1994;13:4361-4369.

458. Wakao H, Harada N, Kitamura T, et al. Interleukin 2 and erythropoietin activate STAT5/MGF via distinct pathways. EMBO J. 1995;14:2527-2535.

459. Hanazono Y, Chib S, Sasaki K, et al. Erythropoietin induces tyrosine phosphorylation and kinase activity of the c-fps/fes proto-oncogene product in human erythropoietin-responsive cells. Blood. 1993;81:3193-3196.

460. Nicholson SE, Oates AC, Harpur AG, et al. Tyrosine kinase KAK1 is associated with the granulocyte-colony-stimulating factor receptor and both become tyrosine-phosphorylated after receptor activation. Proc Natl Acad Sci U S A. 1994;91:2985-2988.

461. Tian SS, Lamb P, Seidel HM, et al. Rapid activation of the STAT3 transcription factor by granulocyte colony-stimulating factor. Blood. 1994;84:1760-1764.

462. Dong F, van Paassen M, van Buitenen C, et al. A point mutation in the granulocyte colony-stimulating factor receptor (G-CSF-R) gene in a case of acute myeloid leukemia results in the overexpression of a novel G-CSF-R isoform. Blood. 1995;85:902-911.

463. Corey SJ, Burkhardt AL, Bolen JB, et al. Granulocyte colony-stimulating factor receptor signaling involves the formation of a three-component complex with Lyn and Syk protein-tyrosine kinases. Proc Natl Acad Sci U S A. 1994;91:4683-4687.

464. Avalos BR, Hunter MG, Parker JM, et al. Point mutations in the conserved box 1 region inactivate the human granulocyte colony-stimulating factor receptor for growth signal transduction and tyrosine phosphorylation of p75c-rel. Blood. 1995;85:3117-3126.

465. Taniguchi T. Cytokine signaling through nonreceptor protein tyrosine kinases. Science. 1995;268:251-255.

466. Zhuang H, Patel SV, He T-c, et al. Inhibition of erythropoietin-induced mitogenesis by a kinase-deficient form of Jak2. J Biol Chem. 1994;269:21411-21414.

467. Levine RL, Gilliland DG. JAK-2 mutations and their relevance to myeloproliferative disease. Curr Opin Hematol. 2007;14:43-47.

468. Miura O, D'Andrea A, Kabat D, Ihle JN. Induction of tyrosine phosphorylation by the erythropoietin receptor

correlates with mitogenesis. Mol Cell Biol. 1991;11: 4895-4902.

469. Linnekin D, Evans GA, D'Andrea A, Farrar WL. Association of the erythropoietin receptor with protein tyrosine kinase activity. Proc Natl Acad Sci U S A. 1992;89: 6237-6241.

470. Yoshimura A, Lodish HF. In vitro phosphorylation of the erythropoietin receptor and an associated protein, pp130. Mol Cell Biol. 1992;12:706-715.

471. Sakamaki K, Miyajima I, Kitamura T, Miyajima A. Critical cytoplasmic domains of the common beta subunit of the human GM-CSF, IL-3 and IL-5 receptors for growth signal transduction and tyrosine phosphorylation. EMBO J. 1992;11:3541-3549.

472. Duronio V, Clark-Lewis I, Federsppiel B, et al. Tyrosine phosphorylation of receptor beta subunits and common substrates in response to interleukin-3 and granulocyte-macrophage colony-stimulating factor. J Biol Chem. 1992;267:21856-21863.

473. Weiss M, Yokoyama C, Shikama Y, et al. Human granulocyte-macrophage colony-stimulating factor receptor signal transduction requires the proximal cytoplasmic domains of the α and β subunits. Blood. 1993;82:3298-3306.

474. Sato N, Sakamaki K, Terada N, et al. Signal transduction by the high-affinity GM-CSF receptor: two distinct cytoplasmic regions of the common β subunit responsible for different signaling. EMBO J. 1993;12:4181-4189.

475. Kinoshita T, Yokota T, Arai K-I, Miyajima A. Suppression of apoptotic death in hematopoietic cells by signalling through the IL-3/GM-CSF receptors. EMBO J. 1995;14: 266-275.

476. Stahl N, Boulton TG, Farruggella T, et al. Association and activation of Jak-Tyk kinases by CNTF-LIF-OSM–IL-6β receptor components. Science. 1994;263:92-95.

477. Fu X-Y. A transcription factor with SH2 and SH3 domains is directly activated by an interferon α–induced cytoplasmic protein tyrosine kinase(s). Cell. 1992;70:323-335.

478. Fu X-Y, Schindler C, Improta T, et al. The proteins of ISGF-3, the interferon α–induced transcriptional activator, define a gene family involved in signal transduction. Proc Natl Acad Sci U S A. 1992;89:7840-7843.

479. Shuai K, Stark GR, Kerr IM, Darnell JE Jr. A single phosphotyrosine residue of stat91 required for gene activation by interferon γ. Science. 1993;261:1744-1746.

480. Yamamoto K, Quelle FW, Thierfelder WE, et al. Stat4, a novel gamma interferon activation site–binding protein expressed in early myeloid differentiation. Mol Cell Biol. 1994;14:4342-4349.

481. Wakao H, Gouilleux F, Groner B. Mammary gland factor (MGF) is a novel member of the cytokine regulated transcription factor gene family and confers the prolactin response. EMBO J. 1994;13:2182-2191.

482. Hou J, Schindler U, Henzel WJ, et al. An interleukin-4–induced transcription factor: IL-4 Stat. Science. 1994;265: 1701-1706.

483. Feig L. The many roads that lead to Ras. Science. 1993;260:767-768.

484. Moodie SA, Willumsen BM, Weber MJ, Wolfman A. Complexes of Ras-GTP with Raf-1 and mitogen-activated protein kinase kinase. Science. 1993;260: 1658-1660.

485. Satoh T, Nakafuku M, Miyajima A, Kaziro Y. Involvement of ras p21 protein in signal-transduction pathways from interleukin 2, interleukin 3, and granulocyte/macrophage colony-stimulating factor, but not from interleukin 4. Proc Natl Acad Sci U S A. 1991;88:3314-3318.

486. Duronio V, Welham MJ, Abraham S, et al. p21ras activation via hemopoietin receptors and c-kit requires tyrosine kinase activity but not phosphorylation of p21ras GTPase-activating protein. Proc Natl Acad Sci U S A. 1993;89: 1587-1591.

487. Torti M, Marti KB, Altschuler D, et al. Erythropoietin induces p21ras activation and p120GAP tyrosine phosphorylation in human erythroleukemia cells. J Biol Chem. 1992;267:8293-8298.

488. Downward J, Graves JD, Warne PH, et al. Stimulation of p21ras upon T-cell activation. Nature. 1990;346: 719-723.

489. McCormick F. How receptors turn Ras on. Nature. 1993;363:15-16.

490. Gulbins E, Coggeshall KM, Baier G, et al. Tyrosine kinase–stimulated guanine nucleotide exchange activity of vav in T cell activation. Science. 1993;260:822-825.

491. Kavanaugh WM, Williams LT. An alternative to SH2 domains for binding tyrosine-phosphorylated proteins. Science. 1994;266:1862-1865.

492. van der Geer P, Pawson T. The PTB domain: a new protein module implicated in signal transduction. Trends Biochem Sci. 1996;20:277-280.

493. Ravichandran KS, Burakoff SJ. The adapter protein Shc interacts with the interleukin-2 (IL-2) receptor upon upon IL-2 stimulation. J Biol Chem. 1994;269: 1599-1602.

494. Pratt JC, Weiss M, Sieff CA, et al. Evidence for a physical association between the Shc-PTB domain and the β_c chain of the granulocyte-macrophage colony stimulating receptor. J Biol Chem. 1996;271:12137-12140.

495. Inhorn RC, Carlesso N, Durstin M, et al. Identification of a viability domain in the granulocyte/macrophage colony-stimulating factor receptor β-chain involving tyrosine-750. Med Sci. 1995;92:8665-8669.

496. Damen JE, Liu L, Cutler RL, Krystal G. Erythropoietin stimulates the tyrosine phosphorylation of Shc and its association with Grb2 and a 145-Kd tyrosine phosphorylated protein. Blood. 1993;82:2296-2303.

497. Cutler RL, Liu L, Damen JE, Krystal G. Multiple cytokines induce the tyrosine phosphorylation of Shc and its association with Grb2 in hemopoietic cells. J Biol Chem. 1993;268:21463-21465.

498. Komatsu N, Adamson JW, Yamamoto K, et al. Erythropoietin rapidly induces tyrosine phosphorylation in the human erythropoietin-dependent cell line, UT-7. Blood. 1992;80:53-59.

499. Carroll MP, Spivak JL, McMahon M, et al. Erythropoietin induces Raf-1 activation and Raf-1 is required for erythropoietin-mediated proliferation. J Biol Chem. 1991;266:14964-14969.

500. Miura Y, Miura O, Ihle JN, Aoki N. Activation of the mitogen-activated protein kinase pathway by the erythropoietin receptor. J Biol Chem. 1994;269:29962-29969.

501. Bader JL. Neurofibromatosis and cancer. Ann N Y Acad Sci. 1986;486:57-65.

502. Shannon KM, O'Connell P, Martin GA, et al. Loss of the normal NF1 allele from the bone marrow of children with type 1 neurofibromatosis and malignant myeloid disorders. N Engl J Med. 1994;330:597-601.

503. Bollag G, Clapp DW, Shih S, et al. Loss of NF1 results in activation of the Ras signaling pathway and leads to aberrant growth in haematopoietic cells. Nat Genet. 1996;12:144-148.

504. Largaespada DA, Brannan CI, Jenkins NA, Copeland NG. Nf1 deficiency causes Ras-mediated granulocyte/macrophage colony stimulating factor hypersensitivity and chronic myeloid leukaemia. Nat Genet. 1996;12:137-143.

505. Pendergast AM, Quilliam LA, Cripe LD, et al. BCR-ABL–induced oncogenesis is mediated by direct interaction with the SH2 domain of the GRB-2 adaptor protein. Cell. 1993;75:175-185.

506. D'Andrea AD, Yoshimura A, Youssoufian H, et al. The cytoplasmic region of the erythropoietin receptor contains nonoverlapping positive and negative growth-regulatory domains. Mol Cell Biol. 1991;11:1980-1987.

507. Yi T, Mui AL-F, Krystal G, Ihle JN. Hematopoietic cell phosphatase associates with the interleukin-3 (IL-3) receptor β chain and down-regulates IL-3–induced tyrosine phosphorylation and mitogenesis. Mol Cell Biol. 1993;13:7577-7586.

508. de la Chapelle A, Traskelin A-L, Juvonen E. Truncated erythropoietin receptor causes dominantly inherited benign human erythrocytosis. Proc Natl Acad Sci U S A. 1993;90:4495-4499.

509. Klingmüller U, Lorenz U, Cantley LC, et al. Specific recruitment of SH-PTP1 to the erythropoietin receptor causes inactivation of JAK2 and termination of proliferative signals. Cell. 1995;80:729-738.

510. Schultz LD, Schweitzer PA, Rajan TV, et al. Mutations at the murine motheaten locus are within the hematopoietic cell protein-tyrosine phosphatase (Hcph) gene. Cell. 1993;73:1445-1454.

511. Sun H, Tonks NK. The coordinated action of protein tyrosine phophatases and kinases in cell signaling. Trends Biochem Sci. 1994;19:480-485.

512. Kratz CP, Niemeyer CM, Castleberry RP, et al. The mutational spectrum of PTPN11 in juvenile myelomonocytic leukemia and Noonan syndrome/myeloproliferative disease. Blood. 2005;106:2183-2185.

513. Niihori T, Aoki Y, Ohashi H, et al. Functional analysis of PTPN11/SHP-2 mutants identified in Noonan syndrome and childhood leukemia. J Hum Genet. 2005;50:192-202.

514. Endo TA, Masuhara M, Yokouchi M, et al. A new protein containing an SH2 domain that inhibits JAK kinases. Nature. 1997;387:921-924.

515. Yoshimura A, Ohkubo T, Kiguchi T, et al. A novel cytokine-inducible gene CIS encodes an SH2-containing protein that binds to tyrosine-phosphorylated interleukin 3 and erythropoietin receptors. EMBO J. 1995;14:2816-2826.

516. Starr R, Willson TA, Viney EM, et al. A family of cytokine-inducible inhibitors of signalling. Nature. 1997;387:917-921.

517. Greenhalgh CJ, Hilton DJ. Negative regulation of cytokine signaling. J Leukoc Biol. 2001;70:348-356.

518. Nicholson SE, Willson TA, Farley A, et al. Mutational analyses of the SOCS proteins suggest a dual domain requirement but distinct mechanisms for inhibition of LIF and IL-6 signal transduction. EMBO J. 1999;18:375-385.

519. Kamura T, Sato S, Haque D, et al. The Elongin BC complex interacts with the conserved SOCS-box motif present in members of the SOCS, ras, WD-40 repeat, and ankyrin repeat families. Genes Dev. 1998;12:3872-3881.

520. Zhang JG, Farley A, Nicholson SE, et al. The conserved SOCS box motif in suppressors of cytokine signaling binds to elongins B and C and may couple bound proteins to proteasomal degradation. Proc Natl Acad Sci U S A. 1999;96:2071-2076.

521. Sasaki A, Yasukawa H, Shouda T, et al. CIS3/SOCS-3 suppresses erythropoietin (EPO) signaling by binding the EPO receptor and JAK2. J Biol Chem. 2000;275:29338-29347.

522. Yoshimura A, Ohkubo T, Kiguchi T, et al. A novel cytokine-inducible gene CIS encodes an SH2-containing protein that binds to tyrosine-phosphorylated interleukin 3 and erythropoietin receptors. EMBO J. 1995;14:2816-2826.

523. Starr R, Metcalf D, Elefanty AG, et al. Liver degeneration and lymphoid deficiencies in mice lacking suppressor of cytokine signaling-1. Proc Natl Acad Sci U S A. 1998;95:14395-14399.

524. Naka T, Matsumoto T, Narazaki M, et al. Accelerated apoptosis of lymphocytes by augmented induction of Bax in SSI-1 (STAT-induced STAT inhibitor-1) deficient mice. Proc Natl Acad Sci U S A. 1998;95:15577-15582.

525. Alexander WS, Starr R, Fenner JE, et al. SOCS1 is a critical inhibitor of interferon gamma signaling and prevents the potentially fatal neonatal actions of this cytokine. Cell. 1999;98:597-608.

526. Marine JC, Topham DJ, McKay C, et al. SOCS1 deficiency causes a lymphocyte-dependent perinatal lethality. Cell. 1999;98:609-616.

527. Metcalf D, Greenhalgh CJ, Viney E, et al. Gigantism in mice lacking suppressor of cytokine signalling-2. Nature. 2000;405:1069-1073.

528. Marine JC, McKay C, Wang D, et al. SOCS3 is essential in the regulation of fetal liver erythropoiesis. Cell. 1999;98:617-627.

529. Liu X, Robinson GW, Wagner KU, et al. Stat5a is mandatory for adult mammary gland development and lactogenesis. Genes Dev. 1997;11:179-186.

530. Teglund S, McKay C, Schuetz E, et al. Stat5a and Stat5b proteins have essential and nonessential, or redundant, roles in cytokine responses. Cell. 1998;93:841-850.

531. Matsumoto A, Seki Y, Kubo M, et al. Suppression of STAT5 functions in liver, mammary glands, and T cells in cytokine-inducible SH2-containing protein 1 transgenic mice. Mol Cell Biol. 1999;19:6396-6407.

532. Udy GB, Towers RP, Snell RG, et al. Requirement of STAT5b for sexual dimorphism of body growth rates and liver gene expression. Proc Natl Acad Sci U S A. 1997;94:7239-7244.

533. Till JE, McCulloch EA, Siminovich L. A stochastic model of stem cell proliferation based on growth of spleen colony-forming cells. Proc Natl Acad Sci U S A. 1964;51:29-36.

534. Petrov RV, Khaitov RM, Aleinikova NV, Gulak LV. Factors controlling stem cell recirculation. III. Effect of thymus on the migration and differentiation of hemopoietic stem cells. Blood. 1977;49:865-872.

535. Lord BI, Schofield R. The influence of thymus cells in hemopoiesis: stimulation of hemopoietic stem cells in a syngeneic, in vivo situation. Blood. 1973;42:395-404.

536. Trainin N, Resnitzky P. Influence of neonatal thymectomy on cloning capacity of bone marrow cells in mice. Nature. 1969;221:1154-1155.

537. Pritchard LL, Shinpock SG, Goodman JW. Augmentation of marrow growth by thymocytes separated by discontinuous albumin density-gradient centrifugation. Exp Hematol. 1975;3:94-100.

538. Zipori D, Trainin N. Defective capacity of bone marrow from nude mice to restore lethally irradiated recipients. Blood. 1973;42:671-678.

539. Zipori D, Trainin N. Impaired radioprotective capacity and reduced proliferative rate of bone marrow from neonatally thymectomized mice. Exp Hematol. 1975;3:1-11.

540. Martin PJ, Hansen JA, Buckner CD, et al. Effects of in vitro depletion of T cells in HLA-identical allogeneic marrow grafts. Blood. 1985;66:664-672.

541. Bernstein SE, Russell ES, Keighley G. Two hereditary mouse anemias (Sl/Sld and W/Wv) deficient in response to erythropoietin. Ann N Y Acad Sci. 1968;149:475-485.

542. Calvo W, Fleidner TM, et al. Regeneration of blood-forming organs after autologous leukocyte transfusion in lethally irradiated dogs. II. Distribution and cellularity of bone marrow in irradiated and transfused animals. Blood. 1976;47:593.

543. Barr RD, Wang-Peng J, Perry S. Hematopoietic stem cells in human peripheral blood. Science. 1975;109:284-285-289.

544. Clarke BJ, Housman D. Characterization of an erythroid precursor cell of high proliferative capacity in normal human peripheral blood. Proc Natl Acad Sci U S A. 1977;74:1105.

545. Thomas ED, Storb R, Clift RA, et al. Bone marrow transplantation (first of two parts). N Engl J Med. 1975;292:832-843.

546. Samlowski WE, Daynes RA. Bone marrow engraftment is enhanced by competitive inhibition of the hepatic asialoglycoprotein. Proc Natl Acad Sci U S A. 1985;82:2508-2512.

547. Tavassoli M, Hardy CL. Molecular basis of homing of intravenously transplanted stem cells to the marrow. Blood. 1990;76:1059-1070.

548. Lapidot T, Dar A, Kollet O. How do stem cells find their way home? Blood. 2005;106:1901-1910.

549. Kay HEM. Hypothesis: How many cell-generations? Lancet. 1965;2:418-419.

550. Micklem HS, Ansell JD, Wayman JER, Forrester L. The clonal organization of hematopoiesis in the mouse. Prog Immunol. 1983;5:633-640.

551. Mintz B, Anthony K, Litwin S. Monoclonal derivation of mouse myeloid and lymphoid lineages from totipotent hematopoietic stem cells experimentally transplanted in fetal hosts. Proc Natl Acad Sci U S A. 1984;81:7835-7839.

552. Lemischka IR, Raulet DH, Mulligan RC. Developmental potential and dynamic behavior of hematopoietic stem cells. Cell. 1986;45:917-927.

553. Capel B, Hawley R, Covarrusias L, et al. Clonal contributions of small numbers of retrovirally marked hematopoietic stem cells engrafted in unirradiated neonatal W/Wv mice. Proc Natl Acad Sci U S A. 1989;86:4564-4569.

554. Harrison DE, Astle CM, Lerner C. Number and continuous proliferative pattern of transplanted primitive immunohematopoietic stem cells. Proc Natl Acad Sci U S A. 1988;85:822-826.

555. Jordan CT, Lemischka IR. Clonal and systemic analysis of long-term hematopoiesis in the mouse. Genes Dev. 1990;4:220-232.

556. Abkowitz JL, Catlin SN, Guttorp P. Evidence that hematopoiesis may be a stochastic process in vivo. Nat Med. 1996;2:190-197.

557. Bradford GB, Williams B, Rossi R, Bertoncello I. Quiescence, cycling, and turnover in the primitive hematopoietic stem cell compartment. Exp Hematol. 1997;25:445-453.

558. Cheshier SH, Morrison SJ, Liao X, Weissman IL. In vivo proliferation and cell cycle kinetics of long-term self-renewing hematopoietic stem cells. Proc Natl Acad Sci U S A. 1999;96:3120-3125.

559. Shivdasani RA, Orkin SH. The transcriptional control of hematopoiesis. Blood. 1996;87:4025-4039.

560. Cantor AB, Orkin SH. Hematopoietic development: a balancing act. Curr Opin Genet Dev. 2001;11:513-519.

561. Begley CG, Aplan PD, Davey MP, et al. Chromosomal translocation in a human leukemic stem-cell line disrupts the T-cell antigen receptor γ-chain diversity region and results in a previously unreported fusion transcript. Proc Natl Acad Sci U S A. 1989;86:2031-2035.

562. Finger LR, Kagan J, Christopher G, et al. Involvement of the TCL5 gene on human chromosome 1 in T-cell leukemia and melanoma. Proc Natl Acad Sci U S A. 1989;86:5039-5043.

563. Begley CG, Aplan PD, Denning SM, et al. The gene SCL is expressed during early hematopoiesis and encodes a differentiation-related DNA-binding motif. Proc Natl Acad Sci U S A. 1989;86:10128-10132.

564. Mouthon MA, Bernard O, Mitjavila MT, et al. Expression of tal-1 and GATA-binding proteins during human hematopoiesis. Blood. 1993;81:647-655.

565. Robb L, Lyons I, Li R, et al. Absence of yolk sac hematopoiesis from mice with a targeted disruption of the scl gene. Proc Natl Acad Sci U S A. 1995;92:7075-7079.

566. Shivdasani RA, Mayer EL, Orkin SH. Absence of blood formation in mice lacking the T-cell leukaemia oncoprotein tal-1/SCL. Nature. 1995;373:432-434.

567. Boehm T, Foroni L, Kaneko Y, et al. The rhombotin family of cysteine-rich LIM-domain oncogenes: distinct members are involved in T-cell translocations to human chromosomes 11p15 and 11p13. Proc Natl Acad Sci U S A. 1991;88:4367-4371.

568. Rabbitts TH. Chromosomal translocations in human cancer. Nature. 1994;372:143-149.

569. Warren AJ, Colledge WH, Carlton MBL, et al. The oncogenic cysteine-rich LIM domain protein Rbtn2 is essential for erythroid development. Cell. 1994;78:45-57.

570. Wadman I, Li J, Bash RO, et al. Specific in vivo association between the bHLH and LIM proteins implicated in human T cell leukemia. EMBO J. 1994;13:4831-4839.

571. Valge-Archer VE, Osada H, Warren AJ, et al. The LIM protein RBTN2 and the basic helix-loop-helix protein TAL1 are present in a complex in erythroid cells. Proc Natl Acad Sci U S A. 1994;91:8617-8621.

572. Dorfman DM, Wilson DB, Bruns GA, Orkin SH. Human transcription factor GATA-2. Evidence for regulation of preproendothelin-1 gene expression in endothelial cells. J Biol Chem. 1992;267:1279-1285.

573. Leonard M, Brice M, Engel JD, Papayannopoulou T. Dynamics of GATA transcription factor expression during erythroid differentiation. Blood. 1993;82:1071-1079.

574. Visvader J, Adams JM. Megakaryocytic differentiation induced in 416B myeloid cells by GATA-2 and GATA-3 transgenes or 5-azacytidine is tightly coupled to GATA-1 expression. Blood. 1993;82:1493-1501.

575. Briegel K, Lim KC, Plank C, et al. Ectopic expression of a conditional GATA-2/estrogen receptor chimera arrests erythroid differentiation in a hormone-dependent manner. Genes Dev. 1993;7:1097-1109.

576. Tsai FY, Keller G, Kuo FC, et al. An early haematopoietic defect in mice lacking the transcription factor GATA-2. Nature. 1994;371:221-226.

577. Mucenski ML, McLain K, Kier AB, et al. A functional c-myb gene is required for normal murine fetal hepatic hematopoiesis. Cell. 1991;65:677-689.

578. Lee EY-HP, Chang C-Y, Hu N, et al. Mice deficient for Rb are nonviable and show defects in neurogenesis and haematopoiesis. Nature. 1992;359:288-294.

579. Clarke AR, Maandag ER, van Roon M, et al. Requirement for a functional Rb-1 gene in murine development. Nature. 1992;359:328-330.

580. Jacks T, Fazeli A, Schmitt EM, et al. Effects of an RB mutation in the mouse. Nature. 1992;359:295-300.

581. Ramsay RG. c-Myb a stem-progenitor cell regulator in multiple tissue compartments. Growth Factors. 2005;23: 253-261.

582. Emambokus N, Vegiopoulos A, Harman B, et al. Progression through key stages of haemopoiesis is dependent on distinct threshold levels of c-Myb. EMBO J. 2003;22: 4478-4488.

583. Sandberg ML, Sutton SE, Pletcher MT, et al. c-Myb and p300 regulate hematopoietic stem cell proliferation and differentiation. Dev Cell. 2005;8:153-166.

584. Okuda T, van Deursen J, Hiebert SW, et al. AML1, the target of multiple chromosomal translocations in human leukemia, is essential for normal fetal liver hematopoiesis. Cell. 1996;84:321-330.

585. Gery S, Koeffler HP. Transcription factors in hematopoietic malignancies. Curr Opin Genet Dev. 2007;17: 78-83.

586. Boncinelli E, Simeone A, Acampora D, Mavilio F. HOX gene activation by retinoic acid. Trends Genet. 1991;7: 329-334.

587. Davidson AJ, Ernst P, Wang Y, et al. cdx4 mutants fail to specify blood progenitors and can be rescued by multiple hox genes. Nature. 2003;425:300-306.

588. Sauvageau G, Thorsteinsdottir U, Eaves CJ, et al. Overexpression of HOXB4 in hematopoietic cells causes the selective expansion of more primitive populations in vitro and in vivo. Genes Dev. 1995;9:1753-1765.

589. Kyba M, Perlingeiro RC, Daley GQ. HoxB4 confers definitive lymphoid-myeloid engraftment potential on embryonic stem cell and yolk sac hematopoietic progenitors. Cell. 2002;109:29-37.

590. Rideout WM, Hochedlinger K, Kyba M, et al. Correction of a genetic defect by nuclear transplantation and combined cell and gene therapy. Cell. 2002;109:17-27.

591. Eklund EA. The role of HOX genes in malignant myeloid disease. Curr Opin Hematol. 2007;14:85-89.

592. Hock H, Orkin SH. Zinc-finger transcription factor Gfi-1: versatile regulator of lymphocytes, neutrophils and hematopoietic stem cells. Curr Opin Hematol. 2006;13:1-6.

593. Duan Z, Horwitz M. Gfi-1 takes center stage in hematopoietic stem cells. Trends Mol Med. 2005;11:49-52.

594. Bodine DM, Crosier PS, Clark SC. Effects of hematopoietic growth factors on the survival of primitive stem cells in liquid suspension culture. Blood. 1991;78:914.

595. Itoh Y, Ikebuchi K, Hirashima K. Interleukin-3 and granulocyte colony-stimulating factor as survival factors in murine hemopoietic stem cells in vitro. Int J Hematol. 1992;55:139-145.

596. Katayama N, Clark SC, Ogawa M. Growth factor requirement for survival in cell-cycle dormancy of primitive murine lymphohematopoietic progenitors. Blood. 1993;81:610-616.

597. Neben S, Donaldson D, Sieff C, et al. Synergistic effects of interleukin-11 with other growth factors on the expansion of murine hematopoietic progenitors and maintenance of stem cells in liquid culture. Exp Hematol. 1994;22:353-359.

598. Li CL, Johnson GR. Stem cell factor enhances the survival but not the self-renewal of murine hematopoietic long-term repopulating cells. Blood. 1994;84:408-414.

599. Kimura S, Roberts AW, Metcalf D, Alexander WS. Hematopoietic stem cell deficiencies in mice lacking c-Mpl, the receptor for thrombopoietin. Proc Natl Acad Sci U S A. 1998;95:1195-1200.

600. Solar GP, Kerr WG, Zeigler FC, et al. Role of c-mpl in early hematopoiesis. Blood. 1998;92:4-10.

601. McCulloch EA, Siminovich L, Till JE. Spleen colony formation of anemic mice of genotype WWv. Science. 1964;144:844-846.

602. Chabot B, Stephenson DA, Chapman VM, et al. The proto-oncogenic c-kit encoding a transmembrane tyrosine kinase receptor maps to the mouse W locus. Nature. 1988;335:88-89.

603. Geissler EN, Ryan MA, Housman DE. The dominant-white spotting (W) locus of the mouse encodes the c-kit proto-oncogene. Cell. 1988;55:185-192.

604. Yarden Y, Kuang W-J, Yang-Feng T, et al. Human proto-oncogene c-kit: a new cell surface receptor tyrosine kinase for an unidentified ligand. EMBO J. 1987;6:3341-3351.

605. Reith AD, Rottapel R, Giddens E, et al. W mutant mice with mild or severe developmental defects contain distinct point mutations in the kinase domain of the c-kit receptor. Genes Dev. 1990;4:390-400.

606. McCulloch EA, Siminovitch L, Till JE, et al. The cellular basis of the genetically determined hemopoietic defect in anemic mice of genotype Sl/Sld. Blood. 1965;26: 399-410.

607. Williams DE, Eisenman J, Baird A, et al. Identification of a ligand for the c-kit proto-oncogene. Cell. 1990;63: 167-174.

608. Zsebo KM, Wypych J, McNiece IK, et al. Identification, purification, and biological characterization of hematopoietic stem cell factor from buffalo rat liver–conditioned medium. Cell. 1990;63:195-201.

609. Anderson DM, Lyman SD, Baird A, et al. Molecular cloning of mast cell growth factor, a hematopoietin that

is active in both membrane bound and soluble forms. Cell. 1990;63:235-243.

610. Huang E, Nocka K, Beier DR, et al. The hematopoietic growth factor KL is encoded at the Sl locus and is the ligand of the c-kit receptor, the gene product of the W locus. Cell. 1990;63:225-233.

611. Martin FH, Suggs SV, Langley KE, et al. Primary structure and functional expression of rat and human stem cell factor DNAs. Cell. 1990;63:203-211.

612. Nocka K, Buck J, Levi E, Besmer P. Candidate ligand for the c-kit transmembrane kinase receptor: KL, a fibroblast-derived growth factor stimulates mast cells and erythroid progenitors. EMBO J. 1990;9:3287-3294.

613. Flanagan JG, Leder P. The kit ligand: A cell surface molecule altered in steel mutant fibroblasts. Cell. 1990;63: 185-194.

614. Flanagan JG, Chan DC, Leder P. Transmembrane form of the kit ligand growth factor is determined by alternative splicing and is missing in the Sld mutant. Cell. 1991;64: 1025-1035.

615. Kojika S, Griffin JD. Notch receptors and hematopoiesis. Exp Hematol. 2001;29:1041-1052.

616. Ellisen LW, Bird J, West DC, et al. TAN-1, the human homolog of the *Drosophila* notch gene, is broken by chromosomal translocations in T lymphoblastic neoplasms. Cell. 1991;66:649-661.

617. Varnum-Finney B, Xu L, Brashem-Stein C, et al. Pluripotent, cytokine-dependent, hematopoietic stem cells are immortalized by constitutive Notch1 signaling. Nat Med. 2000;6:1278-1281.

618. Weng AP, Ferrando AA, Lee W, et al. Activating mutations of NOTCH1 in human T cell acute lymphoblastic leukemia. Science. 2004;306:269-271.

619. Karanu FN, Murdoch B, Gallacher L, et al. The notch ligand jagged-1 represents a novel growth factor of human hematopoietic stem cells. J Exp Med. 2000;192:1365-1372.

620. Bhardwaj G, Murdoch B, Wu D, et al. Sonic hedgehog induces the proliferation of primitive human hematopoietic cells via BMP regulation. Nat Immunol. 2001;2: 172-180.

621. Taipale J, Beachy PA. The Hedgehog and Wnt signalling pathways in cancer. Nature. 2001;411:349-354.

622. Reya T, Morrison SJ, Clarke MF, Weissman IL. Stem cells, cancer, and cancer stem cells. Nature. 2001;414: 105-111.

623. Lansdorp PM, Dragowska W. Maintenance of hematopoiesis in serum-free bone marrow cultures involves sequential recruitment of quiescent progenitors. Exp Hematol. 1993;21:1321-1327.

624. Curry JL, Trentin JJ. Hemopoietic spleen colony studies. I. Growth and differentiation. Dev Biol. 1967;15: 395-413.

625. Kulessa H, Frampton J, Graf T. GATA-1 reprograms avian myelomonocytic cell lines into eosinophils, thromboblasts, and erythroblasts. Genes Dev. 1995;9:1250-1262.

626. Nerlov C, Querfurth E, Kulessa H, Graf T. GATA-1 interacts with the myeloid PU.1 transcription factor and represses PU.1-dependent transcription. Blood. 2000;95: 2543-2551.

627. Rekhtman N, Radparvar F, Evans T, Skoultchi AI. Direct interaction of hematopoietic transcription factors PU.1 and GATA- 1: functional antagonism in erythroid cells. Genes Dev. 1999;13:1398-1411.

628. Zhang P, Behre G, Pan J, et al. Negative cross-talk between hematopoietic regulators: GATA proteins repress PU.1. Proc Natl Acad Sci U S A. 1999;96:8705-8710.

629. Zhang P, Zhang X, Iwama A, et al. PU.1 inhibits GATA-1 function and erythroid differentiation by blocking GATA-1 DNA binding. Blood. 2000;96:2641-2648.

630. Li Z, Godinho FJ, Klusmann JH, et al. Developmental stage–selective effect of somatically mutated leukemogenic transcription factor GATA1. Nat Genet. 2005;37: 613-619.

631. Querfurth E, Schuster M, Kulessa H, et al. Antagonism between C/EBPbeta and FOG in eosinophil lineage commitment of multipotent hematopoietic progenitors. Genes Dev. 2000;14:2515-2525.

632. Shen CN, Slack JM, Tosh D. Molecular basis of transdifferentiation of pancreas to liver. Nat Cell Biol. 2000;2:879-887.

633. D'Andrea AD, Lodish HF, Wong GG. Expression cloning of the murine erythropoietin receptor. Cell. 1989; 57:277-285.

634. Krantz SB, Goldwasser E. Specific binding of erythropoietin in spleen cells infected with the anemia strain of Friend virus. Proc Natl Acad Sci U S A. 1984;81:7574.

635. Sawada K, Krantz SB, Sawyer ST, Civin CI. Quantitation of specific binding of erythropoietin to human erythroid colony-forming cells. J Cell Physiol. 1988;137:337-345.

636. Sawyer ST, Krantz SB, Sawada K. Receptors for erythropoietin in mouse and human erythroid cells and placenta. Blood. 1989;74:103-109.

637. Akahane K, Tojo A, Fukamachi H, et al. Binding of iodinated erythropoietin to rat bone marrow cells under normal and anemic conditions. Exp Hematol. 1989;17:177-182.

638. Wang GL, Jiang B, Rue EA, Semenza GL. Hypoxia-inducible factor 1 is a basic-helix-loop-basic–PAS heterodimer regulated by cellular O_2 tension. Proc Natl Acad Sci U S A. 1995;92:5510-5514.

639. Sieff CA, Emerson SG, Mufson A, et al. Dependence of highly enriched human bone marrow progenitors on hemopoietic growth factors and their response to recombinant erythropoietin. J Clin Invest. 1986;77:74-81.

640. Lansdorp PM, Dragowska W. Long-term erythropoiesis from constant numbers of CD34$^+$ cells in serum-free cultures initiated with highly purified progenitor cells from human bone marrow. J Exp Med. 1992;175: 1501-1509.

641. Macklis RM, Javid J, Lipton JM, et al. Synthesis of hemoglobin F in adult simian erythroid progenitor–derived colonies. J Clin Invest. 1982;70:752-761.

642. Friedman AD, Linch DC, Miller B, et al. Determination of the hemoglobin F program in human progenitor-derived erythroid cells. J Clin Invest. 1985;75: 1359-1368.

643. Dover GJ, Boyer SH, Zinkham WH. Production of erythrocytes that contains fetal hemoglobin in anemia: transient in vivo changes. J Clin Invest. 1979;63:173-176.

644. Kidoguchi K, Ogawa M, Karam JD, Martin AG. Augmentation of fetal hemoglobin (HbF) synthesis in culture by human erythropoietic precursors in the marrow and peripheral blood: studies in sickle cell anemia and non-hemoglobinopathic adults. Blood. 1978;52:1115-1124.

645. Clarke BJ, Nathan DG, Alter BP, et al. Hemoglobin synthesis in human BFU-E and CFU-E–derived erythroid colonies. Blood. 1979;54:805-817.

646. Papayannopoulou T, Brice M, Stamatoyannopoulos G. Hemoglobin F synthesis in vitro: evidence for control at the level of primitive erythroid stem cells. Proc Natl Acad Sci U S A. 1977;74:2923-2927.

647. Romeo P-H, Prandini M-H, Joulin V, et al. Megakaryocytic and erythrocytic lineages share specific transcription factors. Nature. 1990;344:447-449.

648. Zon LI, Yamaguchi Y, Yee K, et al. Expression of mRNA for the GATA-binding proteins in human eosinophils and basophils: Potential role in gene transcription. Blood. 1993;81:3234-3241.

649. Pevny L, Simon MC, Robertson E, et al. Erythroid differentiation in chimaeric mice blocked by a targeted mutation in the gene for transcription factor GATA-1. Nature. 1991;349:257-260.

650. Simon MC, Pevny L, Wiles MV, et al. Rescue of erythroid development in gene targeted GATA-1 mouse embryonic stem cells. Nat Genet. 1992;1:92-98.

651. Weiss MJ, Keller G, Orkin SH. Novel insights into erythroid development revealed through in vitro differentiation of GATA-1⁻ embryonic stem cells. Genes Dev. 1994;8:1184-1197.

652. Pevny L, Lin C-S, D-Agati V, et al. Development of hematopoietic cells lacking transcription factor GATA-1. Development. 1995;121:163-172.

653. Weiss MJ, Orkin SH. Transcription factor GATA-1 permits survival and maturation of erythroid precursors by preventing apoptosis. Proc Natl Acad Sci U S A. 1995; 92:9623-9627.

654. Tsang AP, Visvader JE, Turner CA, et al. FOG, a multitype zinc finger protein, acts as a cofactor for transcription factor GATA-1 in erythroid and megakaryocytic differentiation. Cell. 1997;90:109-119.

655. Tsang AP, Fujiwara Y, Hom DB, Orkin SH. Failure of megakaryopoiesis and arrested erythropoiesis in mice lacking the GATA-1 transcriptional cofactor FOG. Genes Dev. 1998;12:1176-1188.

656. Nichols KE, Crispino JD, Poncz M, et al. Familial dyserythropoietic anaemia and thrombocytopenia due to an inherited mutation in GATA1. Nat Genet. 2000;24: 266-270.

657. Miller IJ, Bieker JJ. A novel, erythroid cell–specific murine transcription factor that binds to the CACCC element and is related to the Kruppel family of nuclear proteins. Mol Cell Biol. 1993;13:2776-2786.

658. Andrews NC, Erdjument-Bromage H, Davidson MB, et al. Erythroid transcription factor NF-E2 is a haematopoietic-specific basic-leucine zipper protein. Nature. 1993;362:722-728.

659. Andrews NC. The NF-E2 transcription factor. Int J Biochem Cell Biol. 1998;30:429-432.

660. Eaves CJ, Eaves AC. Erythropoietin (Ep) dose-response curves for three classes of erythroid progenitors in normal human marrow and in patients with polycythemia vera. Blood. 1978;52:1196-1210.

661. Eaves AC, Eaves CJ. Erythropoiesis in culture. Clin Haematol. 1984;13:371-391.

662. Iscove NN. Erythropoietin-independent stimulation of early erythropoiesis in adult bone marrow cultures by conditioned media from lectin stimulated mouse spleen cells. In Golde DW, Cline MJ, Metcalf D, Fox CF (eds). Hematopoietic Cell Differentiation. New York, Academic Press, 1978, pp 37-52.

663. Li CL, Johnson GR. Stimulation of multipotential erythroid and other murine haematopoietic progenitor cells by adherent cell lines in the absence of detectable multi-CSF (IL3). Nature. 1985;316:633-636.

664. Sieff CA, Ekern SC, Nathan DG, Anderson JW. Combinations of recombinant colony stimulating factors are required for optimal hematopoietic differentiation in serum-deprived culture. Blood. 1989;73: 688-693.

665. Nocka K, Majumder S, Chabot B, et al. Expression of c-kit gene products in known cellular targets of W mutations in normal and W mutant mice—evidence for an impaired c-kit kinase in mutant mice. Genes Dev. 1989;3: 816-826.

666. Socolovsky M, Fallon AE, Wang S, et al. Fetal anemia and apoptosis of red cell progenitors in Stat5a–/–5b–/– mice: a direct role for Stat5 in Bcl-X(L) induction. Cell. 1999;98:181-191.

667. Socolovsky M, Nam H, Fleming MD, et al. Ineffective erythropoiesis in Stat5a(–/–)5b(–/–) mice due to decreased survival of early erythroblasts. Blood. 2001;98:3261-3273.

668. Sawada K, Krantz SB, Dessypris EN, et al. Human colony-forming units-erythroid do not require accessory cells, but do require direct interaction with insulin-like growth factor I and/or insulin for erythroid development. J Clin Invest. 1989;83:1701-1709.

669. Kurtz A, Jelkmann W. Insulin stimulates erythroid colony formation independently of erythropoietin. Br J Haematol. 1983;53:311-316.

670. Yu J, Shao L, Vaughan J, et al. Characterization of the potentiation effect of activin on human erythroid colony formation in vitro. Blood. 1989;73:952-960.

671. Smith JC, Price BM, van Nimmen K, Huylebroeck D. Identification of a potent *Xenopus* mesoderm–inducing factor as a homologue of activin A. Nature. 1990;345: 729-731.

672. Galimi F, Bagnara GP, Bonsi L, et al. Hepatocyte growth factor induces proliferation and differentiation of multipotent and erythroid hemopoietic progenitors. J Cell Biol. 1994;127:1743-1754.

673. Mangan KF, Chikkappa G, Sieler LZ, et al. Regulation of human blood erythroid burst-forming unit (BFU-E) proliferation by T lymphocyte subpopulations defined by Fc receptors and monoclonal antibodies. Blood. 1982;59:990-996.

674. Torok-Storb BJ, Martin PJ, Hansen JA. Regulation of in vitro erythropoiesis by normal T cells: evidence for two T cell subsets with opposing functions. Blood. 1981;58: 171-174.

675. Lipton JM, Smith BR, et al. Suppression of in vitro erythropoiesis by a subset of large granular lymphocytes. Blood. 1984;64:337a.

676. Hoffman R, Kopel SD, Hsu SD. T cell chronic lymphocytic leukemia: presence in bone marrow and peripheral blood of cells that suppress erythropoiesis in vitro. Blood. 1978;52:255-260.

677. Abdou JI, NaPombejara C, Balentine L, Abdou NL. Suppressor cell–mediated neutropenia in Felty's syndrome. J Clin Invest. 1978;61:738-743.

678. Bagby GC Jr. T lymphocytes involved in inhibition of granulopoiesis in two neutropenic patients are of the cytotoxic/suppressor (T3+T8+) subset. J Clin Invest. 1981;68:1597-1600.

679. Linch DC, Cawley JC, MacDonald SM, et al. Acquired pure red cell aplasia associated with an increase of T cells bearing receptors for the Fc of IgG. Acta Haematol. 1981;65:270-274.

680. Lipton JM, Nadler LM, Canellos GP, et al. Evidence for genetic restriction in the suppression of erythropoiesis by a unique subset of T lymphocytes in man. J Clin Invest. 1983;72:694-706.

681. Torok-Storb BJ, Sieff C, Storb R, et al. In vitro tests for distinguishing possible immune-mediated aplastic anemia from transfusion-induced sensitization. Blood. 1980;55:211-217.

682. Bacigalupo A, Podesta M, Mingari MC, et al. Immunosuppression of hematopoiesis in aplastic anemia: activity of T lymphocytes. J Immunol. 1980;125:1449-1453.

683. Smith BR, Lipton JM, et al. Multiparameter flow cytometric characterization of a unique T-lymphocyte subclass associated with granulocytopenia and pure red cell aplasia. Blood. 1984;64:343a.

684. Torok-Storb BJ, Hansen JA. Modulation of in vitro BFU-E growth by normal Ia-positive T cells is restricted by HLA-DR. Nature. 1982;298:473-474.

685. Krensky AM, Reiss CS, Mier JW, et al. Long-term human cytolytic T-cell lines allospecific for HLA-DR6 antigen are OKT4+. Proc Natl Acad Sci U S A. 1982;79:2365-2369.

686. Falkenburg JHF, Jansen J, van der Vaart-Duinkerken N, et al. Polymorphic and monomorphic HLA-DR determinants on human hematopoietic progenitor cells. Blood. 1984;63:1125-1132.

687. Sieff C, Bicknell D, Caine G, et al. Changes in cell surface antigen expression during hemopoietic differentiation. Blood. 1982;60:703-713.

688. Greaves MF, Katz FE, Myers CD, et al. Selective expression of cell surface antigens on human haemopoietic progenitor cells. In Palek J (ed). Hematopoietic Stem Cell Physiology. New York, Alan R Liss, 1985, pp 301-315.

689. Sparrow RL, Williams N. The pattern of HLA-DR and HLA-DQ antigen expression on clonable subpopulations of human myeloid progenitor cells. Blood. 1986;67:379-384.

690. Roodman DC, Bird A, Hutzler D, Montgomery W. Tumor necrosis factor α and hematopoietic progenitors: effects of tumor necrosis factor on the growth of erythroid progenitors CFU-E and BFU-E and the hematopoietic cell lines K562, HL60, and HEL cells. Exp Hematol. 1987;15:928-935.

691. Broxmeyer HE, Williams DE, Lu L, et al. The suppressive influences of human tumor necrosis factor on bone marrow hematopoietic progenitor cells from normal donors and patients with leukemia: synergism of tumor necrosis factor and interferon-gamma. J Immunol. 1986;136:4487.

692. Furmanski P, Johnson CS. Macrophage control of normal and leukemic erythropoiesis: identification of the macrophage-derived erythroid suppressing activity as interleukin-1 and the mediator of its in vivo action as tumor necrosis factor. Blood. 1990;75:2328-2334.

693. van Furth R, Raeburn JA, van Zwet TL. Characteristics of human mononuclear phagocytes. Blood. 1979;54:485-500.

694. Meuret G. Human monocytopoiesis. Exp Hematol. 1974;2:238-249.

695. Thomas ED, Ramberg RE, Sale GE, et al. Direct evidence for a bone marrow origin of the alveolar macrophage in man. Science. 1976;192:1016-1068.

696. Gale RP, Sparkes RS, Golde DW. Bone marrow origin of hepatic macrophages (Kupffer cells) in humans. Science. 1978;201:937-938.

697. Katz SI, Tamaki K, Sach DS. Epidermal Langerhans cells are derived from cells originating in bone marrow. Nature. 1979;282:324-326.

698. Ash P, Loutit JF, Townsend KM. Osteoclasts derived from haematopoietic stem cells. Nature. 1980;283:669-670.

699. Carr I. The biology of macrophages. Clin Invest Med. 1978;1:59-69.

700. Gasson JC, Weisbart RH, Kaufman SE, et al. Purified human granulocyte-macrophage colony-stimulating factor: direct action on neutrophils. Science. 1984;226:1339-1342.

701. Weisbart RH, Golde DW, Clark SC, et al. Human granulocyte-macrophage colony-stimulating factor is a neutrophil activator. Nature. 1985;314:361-363.

702. Iscove NN. The role of erythropoietin in regulation of population size and cell cycling of early and late erythroid precursors in mouse bone marrow. Cell Tissue Kinet. 1977;10:323-334.

703. Udupa KB, Reissman KR. In vivo erythropoietin requirements of regenerating erythroid progenitors (BFU-e), CFU-e in bone marrow of mice. Blood. 1979;53:1164-1171.

704. Odell TT Jr, McDonald TP, Detwiler TC. Stimulation of platelet production by serum of platelet-depleted rats. Proc Soc Exp Biol Med. 1961;108:428-431.

705. Scott LM, Civin CI, Rorth P, Friedman AD. A novel temporal expression pattern of three C/EBP family members in differentiating myelomonocytic cells. Blood. 1992;80:1725-1735.

706. Zhang DE, Hetherington CJ, Meyers S, et al. CCAAT enhancer-binding protein (C/EBP) and AML1 (CBF alpha2) synergistically activate the macrophage colony-stimulating factor receptor promoter. Mol Cell Biol. 1996;16:1231-1240.

707. Zhang DE, Zhang P, Wang ND, et al. Absence of granulocyte colony-stimulating factor signaling and neutrophil development in CCAAT enhancer binding protein alpha–deficient mice. Proc Natl Acad Sci U S A. 1997;94:569-574.

708. Zhang P, Iwama A, Datta MW, et al. Upregulation of interleukin 6 and granulocyte colony-stimulating factor receptors by transcription factor CCAAT enhancer binding protein alpha (C/EBP alpha) is critical for granulopoiesis. J Exp Med. 1998;188:1173-1184.

709. Tanaka T, Akira S, Yoshida K, et al. Targeted disruption of the NF-IL6 gene discloses its essential role in bacteria killing and tumor cytotoxicity by macrophages. Cell. 1995;80:353-361.

710. Yamanaka R, Barlow C, Lekstrom-Himes J, et al. Impaired granulopoiesis, myelodysplasia, and early lethality in CCAAT/enhancer binding protein epsilon–deficient mice. Proc Natl Acad Sci U S A. 1997;94:13187-13192.

711. Lekstrom-Himes J, Xanthopoulos KG. CCAAT/enhancer binding protein epsilon is critical for effective neutrophil-mediated response to inflammatory challenge. Blood. 1999;93:3096-3105.

712. Gallin JI. Neutrophil specific granule deficiency. Annu Rev Med. 1985;36:263-274.

713. Lekstrom-Himes JA, Dorman SE, Kopar P, et al. Neutrophil-specific granule deficiency results from a novel mutation with loss of function of the transcription factor CCAAT/enhancer binding protein epsilon. J Exp Med. 1999;189:1847-1852.

714. Gombart AF, Shiohara M, Kwok SH, et al. Neutrophil-specific granule deficiency: homozygous recessive inheritance of a frameshift mutation in the gene encoding transcription factor CCAAT/enhancer binding protein-epsilon. Blood. 2001;97:2561-2567.

715. Lekstrom-Himes JA. The role of C/EBP(epsilon) in the terminal stages of granulocyte differentiation. Stem Cells. 2001;19:125-133.

716. Moreau-Gachelin F, Ray D, Tambourin P, et al. The PU.1 transcription factor is the product of the putative oncogene Spi-1. Cell. 1990;61:1165-1166.

717. Klemsz MJ, McKercher SR, Celada A, et al. The macrophage and B cell–specific factor PU.1 is related to the ets oncogene. Cell. 1990;61:113-124.

718. Pongubala JMR, Van Beveren C, Nagulapalli S, et al. Effect of PU.1 phosphorylation on interaction with NF-EM5 and transcriptional activation. Science. 1993;259:1622-1625.

719. Shin MK, Koshland ME. Ets-related protein PU.1 regulates expression of the immunoglobulin J-chain gene through a novel Ets-binding element. Genes Dev. 1993;7:2006-2015.

720. Pahl HL, Scheibe RJ, Zhang D-E, et al. The proto-oncogene PU.1 regulates expression of the myeloid-specific CD11b promotor. J Biol Chem. 1993;268:5014-5020.

721. Zhang DE, Fujioka K, Hetherington CJ, et al. Identification of a region which directs the monocytic activity of the colony-stimulating factor 1 (macrophage colony-stimulating factor) receptor promoter and binds PEBP2/CBF (AML1). Mol Cell Biol. 1994;14:8085-8095.

722. Hohaus S, Petrovick MS, Voso MT, et al. PU.1 (Spi-1) and C/EBP alpha regulate expression of the granulocyte-macrophage colony-stimulating factor receptor alpha gene. Mol Cell Biol. 1995;15:5830-5845.

723. Scott EW, Simon MC, Anastasi J, Singh H. Requirement of transcription factor PU.1 in the development of multiple hematopoietic lineages. Science. 1994;265:1573-1577.

724. Metcalf D, Johnson GR, Burgess AW. Direct stimulation by purified GM-CSF of the proliferation of multipotential and erythroid precursor cells. Blood. 1980;55:138-147.

725. Metcalf D, Nicola NA. Proliferative effects of purified granulocyte colony-stimulating factor (G-CSF) on normal mouse hemopoietic cells. J Cell Physiol. 1983;116:198-206.

726. Metcalf D, Stanley ER. Haematological effects in mice of partially purified colony stimulating factor (CSF) prepared from human urine. Br J Haematol. 1971;21:481-492.

727. Arnaout MA, Wang EA, Clark SC, Sieff CA. Human recombinant granulocyte macrophage colony-stimulating factor increases cell to cell adhesion and surface expression of adhesion promoting surface glycoproteins on mature granulocytes. J Clin Invest. 1986;78:597-601.

728. Lopez AF, To LB, Yang Y-C, et al. Stimulation of proliferation, differentiation, and function of human cells by primate interleukin 3. Proc Natl Acad Sci U S A. 1987;84:2761-2765.

729. Lopez AF, Nicola NA, Burgess AW, et al. Activation of granulocyte cytotoxic function by purified mouse colony stimulating factors. J Immunol. 1983;131:2983-2988.

730. Hamilton JA, Stanley ER, Burgess AW, Shadduck RK. Stimulation of macrophage plasminogen activator activity by colony-stimulating factors. J Cell Physiol. 1980;103:435-445.

731. Debili N, Masse JM, Katz A, et al. Effects of the recombinant hematopoietic growth factors interleukin-3, interleukin-6, stem cell factor, and leukemia inhibitory factor on the megakaryocytic differentiation of CD34+ cells. Blood. 1993;82:84-95.

732. Guinan EC, Lee YS, Lopez KD, et al. Effects of interleukin-3 and granulocyte-macrophage colony-stimulating factor on thrombopoiesis in congenital amegakaryocytic thrombocytopenia. Blood. 1993;81:1691-1698.

733. Hill RJ, Warren MK, Stenberg P, et al. Stimulation of megakaryocytopoiesis in mice by human recombinant interleukin-6. Blood. 1991;77:42-48.

734. Neben S, Turner K. The biology of interleukin 11. Stem Cells. 1993;11(Suppl 2):156-162.

735. Broudy VC, Lin NL, Kaushansky K. Thrombopoietin (c-mpl ligand) acts synergistically with erythropoietin, stem cell factor, and interleukin-11 to enhance murine megakaryocyte colony growth and increases megakaryocyte ploidy in vitro. Blood. 1995;85:1719-1726.

736. Briddell RA, Bruno E, Cooper RJ, et al. Effect of c-kit ligand on in vitro human megakaryocytopoiesis. Blood. 1991;78:2854-2859.

737. Ishibashi T, Koziol JA, Burstein SA. Human recombinant erythropoietin promotes differentiation of murine megakaryocytes in vitro. J Clin Invest. 1987;79:286-289.

738. Longmore GD, Pharr P, Neumann D, Lodish HF. Both megakaryocytopoiesis and erythropoiesis are induced in mice infected with a retrovirus expressing an oncogenic erythropoietin receptor. Blood. 1993;82:2386-2395.

739. Metcalf D, Di Rago L, Mifsud S. Synergistic and inhibitory interactions in the in vitro control of murine megakaryocyte colony formation. Stem Cells. 2002;20:552-560.

740. Emmons RV, Reid DM, Cohen RL, et al. Human thrombopoietin levels are high when thrombocytopenia is due to megakaryocyte deficiency and low when due to increased platelet destruction. Blood. 1996;87:4068-4071.

741. Shivdasani RA, Fielder P, Keller GA, et al. Regulation of the serum concentration of thrombopoietin in thrombocytopenic NF-E2 knockout mice. Blood. 1997;90:1821-1827.

742. Karpatkin S. Heterogeneity of human platelets. I. Metabolic and kinetic evidence suggestive of young and old platelets. J Clin Invest. 1969;48:1073-1082.

743. Paulus JM, Breton-Gorius J, et al. Megakaryocyte ultrastructure and ploidy in human macrothrombocytosis. In Baldini MG, Ebbe S (eds). Platelets, Production, Function, Transfusion and Storage. New York, Grune & Stratton, 1974, pp 131-141.

744. Gabrilove J, Jakubowski A, Scher H, et al. Effect of granulocyte colony-stimulating factor on neutropenia and associated morbidity due to chemotherapy for transitional-cell carcinoma of the urothelium. N Engl J Med. 1988; 318:1414-1422.

745. Morstyn G, Campbell L, Souza LM, et al. Effect of granulocyte colony stimulating factor on neutropenia induced by cytotoxic chemotherapy. Lancet. 1988;1:667-672.

746. Devereaux S, Linch DC, Campos-Costa D, et al. Transient leucopenia induced by granulocyte-macrophage colony-stimulating factor. Lancet. 1987;2:1523-1524.

747. Bronchud MH, Scarffe JH, Thatcher N, et al. Phase I/II study of recombinant human granulocyte colony-stimulating factor in patients receiving intensive chemotherapy for small cell lung cancer. Br J Cancer. 1987;56: 809-813.

748. Kodo H, Tajika K, Takahashi S, et al. Acceleration of neutrophilic granulocyte recovery after bone-marrow transplantation by the administration of recombinant human granulocyte colony-stimulating factor. Lancet. 1988;2:38-39.

749. Crawford J, Ozer H, Stoller R, et al. Reduction by granulocyte colony-stimulating factor of fever and neutropenia induced by chemotherapy in patients with small-cell lung cancer. N Engl J Med. 1991;325:164-170.

750. Pettengell R, Gurney H, Radford JA, et al. Granulocyte colony-stimulating factor to prevent dose-limiting neutropenia in non-Hodgkin's lymphoma: a randomized controlled trial. Blood. 1992;80:1430-1436.

751. Zinzani PL, Pavone E, Storti S, et al. Randomized trial with or without granulocyte colony-stimulating factor as adjunct to induction VNCOP-B treatment of elderly high-grade non-Hodgkin's lymphoma. Blood. 1997;89: 3974-3979.

752. Smith TJ, Khatcheressian J, Lyman GH, et al. 2006 update of recommendations for the use of white blood cell growth factors: an evidence-based clinical practice guideline. J Clin Oncol. 2006;24:3187-3205.

753. Aapro MS, Cameron DA, Pettengell R, et al. EORTC guidelines for the use of granulocyte-colony stimulating factor to reduce the incidence of chemotherapy-induced febrile neutropenia in adult patients with lymphomas and solid tumours. Eur J Cancer. 2006;42:2433-2453.

754. Hartmann LC, Tschetter LK, Habermann TM, et al. Granulocyte colony-stimulating factor in severe chemotherapy-induced afebrile neutropenia. N Engl J Med. 1997;336:1776-1780.

755. Maher DW, Lieschke GJ, Green M, et al. Filgrastim in patients with chemotherapy-induced febrile neutropenia. A double-blind, placebo-controlled trial. Ann Intern Med. 1994;121:492-501.

756. Mayordomo JI, Rivera F, Diaz-Puente MT, et al. Improving treatment of chemotherapy-induced neutropenic fever by administration of colony-stimulating factors. J Natl Cancer Inst. 1995;87:803-808.

757. Aviles A, Guzman R, Garcia EL, et al. Results of a randomized trial of granulocyte colony-stimulating factor in patients with infection and severe granulocytopenia. Anticancer Drugs. 1996;7:392-397.

758. Antman KS, Griffin JD, Elias A, et al. Effect of recombinant human granulocyte-macrophage colony-stimulating factor on chemotherapy-induced myelosuppression. N Engl J Med. 1988;319:593-598.

759. Steward WP, Scarffe JH, Austin R, et al. Recombinant human granulocyte macrophage colony stimulating factor (rhGM-CSF) given as daily short infusions—a phase I dose-toxicity study. Br J Cancer. 1989;59:142-145.

760. Herrmann F, Schulz G, Lindemann A, et al. Hematopoietic responses in patients with advanced malignancy treated with recombinant human granulocyte-macrophage colony-stimulating factor. J Clin Oncol. 1989;7:159-167.

761. Kaplan LD, Kahn JO, Crowe S, et al. Clinical and virologic effects of recombinant human granulocyte-macrophage colony-stimulating factor in patients receiving chemotherapy for human immunodeficiency virus–associated non-Hodgkin's lymphoma: results of a randomized trial. J Clin Oncol. 1991;9:929-940.

762. Jones SE, Schottstaedt MW, Duncan LA, et al. Randomized double-blind prospective trial to evaluate the effects of sargramostim versus placebo in a moderate-dose fluorouracil, doxorubicin, and cyclophosphamide adjuvant chemotherapy program for stage II and III breast cancer. J Clin Oncol. 1996;14:2976-2983.

763. Gerhartz HH, Engelhard M, Meusers P, et al. Randomized, double-blind, placebo-controlled, phase III study of recombinant human granulocyte-macrophage colony-stimulating factor as adjunct to induction treatment of high-grade malignant non-Hodgkin's lymphomas. Blood. 1993;82:2329-2339.

764. Yau JC, Neidhart JA, Triozzi P, et al. Randomized placebo-controlled trial of granulocyte-macrophage colony-stimulating-factor support for dose-intensive cyclophosphamide, etoposide, and cisplatin. Am J Hematol. 1996;51: 289-295.

765. Bunn PAJ, Crowley J, Kelly K, et al. Chemoradiotherapy with or without granulocyte-macrophage colony-stimulating factor in the treatment of limited-stage small-cell lung cancer: a prospective phase III randomized study of the Southwest Oncology Group [published erratum appears in J Clin Oncol 1995;13(11):2860]. J Clin Oncol. 1995;13:1632-1641.

766. Bajorin DF, Nichols CR, Schmoll HJ, et al. Recombinant human granulocyte-macrophage colony-stimulating factor as an adjunct to conventional-dose ifosfamide-based chemotherapy for patients with advanced or relapsed germ cell tumors: a randomized trial. J Clin Oncol. 1995;13: 79-86.

767. American Society of Clinical Oncology. Recommendations for the use of hematopoietic colony-stimulating factors: evidence-based, clinical practice guidelines. J Clin Oncol. 1994;12:2471-2508.

768. Update of recommendations for the use of hematopoietic colony-stimulating factors: evidence-based clinical practice guidelines. American Society of Clinical Oncology. J Clin Oncol. 1996;14:1957-1960.

769. Furman WL. Cytokine support following cytotoxic chemotherapy in children. Int J Pediatr Hematol Oncol. 1995;2:163-171.

770. Burdach S. Molecular regulation of hematopoietic cytokines: implications and indications for clinical use in pediatric oncology. Med Pediatr Oncol Suppl. 1992;2:10-17.

771. Saarinen UM, Hovi L, Riikonen P, et al. Recombinant human granulocyte-macrophage colony-stimulating factor in children with chemotherapy-induced neutropenia. Med Pediatr Oncol. 1992;20:489-496.

772. Beutel G, Ganser A. Risks and benefits of erythropoiesis-stimulating agents in cancer management. Semin Hematol. 2007;44:157-165.

773. Seidenfeld J, Piper M, Flamm C, et al. Epoetin treatment of anemia associated with cancer therapy: a systematic review and meta-analysis of controlled clinical trials. J Natl Cancer Inst. 2001;93:1204-1214.

774. Bohlius J, Langensiepen S, Schwarzer G, et al. Recombinant human erythropoietin and overall survival in cancer patients: results of a comprehensive meta-analysis. J Natl Cancer Inst. 2005;97:489-498.

775. Razzouk BI, Hord JD, Hockenberry M, et al. Double-blind, placebo-controlled study of quality of life, hematologic end points, and safety of weekly epoetin alfa in children with cancer receiving myelosuppressive chemotherapy. J Clin Oncol. 2006;24:3583-3589.

776. Henke M, Laszig R, Rube C, et al. Erythropoietin to treat head and neck cancer patients with anaemia undergoing radiotherapy: randomised, double-blind, placebo-controlled trial. Lancet. 2003;362:1255-1260.

777. Leyland-Jones B. Breast cancer trial with erythropoietin terminated unexpectedly. Lancet Oncol. 2003;4:459-460.

778. Longmore GD. Do cancer cells express functional erythropoietin receptors? N Engl J Med. 2007;356:2447.

779. Harker LA. Physiology and clinical applications of platelet growth factors. Curr Opin Hematol. 1999;6:127-134.

780. O'Malley CJ, Rasko JE, Basser RL, et al. Administration of pegylated recombinant human megakaryocyte growth and development factor to humans stimulates the production of functional platelets that show no evidence of in vivo activation. Blood. 1996;88:3288-3298.

781. Vadhan-Raj S, Murray LJ, Bueso-Ramos C, et al. Stimulation of megakaryocyte and platelet production by a single dose of recombinant human thrombopoietin in patients with cancer. Ann Intern Med. 1997;126:673-681.

782. Fanucchi M, Glaspy J, Crawford J, et al. Effects of polyethylene glycol–conjugated recombinant human megakaryocyte growth and development factor on platelet counts after chemotherapy for lung cancer. N Engl J Med. 1997;336:404-409.

783. Kuter DJ, Begley CG. Recombinant human thrombopoietin: basic biology and evaluation of clinical studies. Blood. 2002;100:3457-3469.

784. Szilvassy SJ. Haematopoietic stem and progenitor cell–targeted therapies for thrombocytopenia. Exp Opin Biol Ther. 2006;6:983-992.

785. Brandt SJ, Peters WP, Atwater SK, et al. Effect of recombinant human granulocyte-macrophage colony-stimulating factor of hematopoietic reconstitution after high-dose chemotherapy and autologous bone marrow transplantation. N Engl J Med. 1988;318:869-876.

786. Nemunaitis J, Singer JW, Buckner CD, et al. Use of recombinant human granulocyte-macrophage colony-stimulating factor in graft failure after bone marrow transplantation. Blood. 1990;76:345-253.

787. Tapp H, Vowels M. Prophylactic use of GM-CSF in pediatric marrow transplantation. Transplant Proc. 1992;24:2267-2268.

788. Trigg ME, Peters C, Zimmerman MB. Administration of recombinant human granulocyte-macrophage colony-stimulating factor to children undergoing allogeneic marrow transplantation: a prospective, randomized, double-masked, placebo-controlled trial. Pediatr Transplant. 2000;4:123-131.

789. Blazar BR, Kersey JH, McGlave PB, et al. In vivo administration of recombinant human granulocyte/macrophage colony-stimulating factor in acute lymphoblastic leukemia patients receiving purged autografts. Blood. 1989;73:849-857.

790. Sheridan WP, Morstyn G, Wolf M, et al. Granulocyte colony-stimulating factor and neutrophil recovery after high-dose chemotherapy and autologous bone marrow transplantation. Lancet. 1989;2:891-895.

791. Dallorso S, Rondelli R, Messina C, et al. Clinical benefits of granulocyte colony-stimulating factor therapy after hematopoietic stem cell transplant in children: results of a prospective randomized trial. Haematologica. 2002;87:1274-1280.

792. Peters WP, Stuart A, Affronti ML, et al. Neutrophil migration is defective during recombinant human granulocyte-macrophage colony-stimulating factor infusion after autologous bone marrow transplantation in humans. Blood. 1988;72:1310-1315.

793. Schuster MW, Beveridge R, Frei-Lahr D, et al. The effects of pegylated recombinant human megakaryocyte growth and development factor (PEG-rHuMGDF) on platelet recovery in breast cancer patients undergoing autologous bone marrow transplantation. Exp Hematol. 2002;30:1044-1050.

794. Vadhan-Raj S, Buescher S, Broxmeyer HE, et al. Stimulation of myelopoiesis in patients with aplastic anemia by recombinant human granulocyte-macrophage colony-stimulating factor. N Engl J Med. 1988;319:1628-1634.

795. Antin JH, Smith BR, Holmes W, Rosenthal DS. Phase I/II study of recombinant human granulocyte-macrophage colony-stimulating factor in aplastic anemia and myelodysplastic syndrome. Blood. 1988;72:705-713.

796. Ganser A, Volkers B, Greher J, et al. Recombinant human granulocyte-macrophage colony-stimulating factor in patients with myelodysplastic syndromes—a phase I/II trial. Blood. 1989;73:31-37.

797. Kobayashi Y, Okabe T, Ozawa K, et al. Treatment of myelodysplastic syndromes with recombinant human granulocyte colony-stimulating factor: a preliminary report. Am J Med. 1989;86:178-182.

798. Negrin RS, Haeuber D, Nagler A, et al. Treatment of myelodysplastic syndromes with recombinant human granulocyte colony-stimulating factor: a phase I/II trial. Ann Intern Med. 1989;110:976-984.

799. Ganser A, Ottmann OG, Seipelt G, et al. Effect of long-term treatment with recombinant human interleukin-3 in patients with myelodysplastic syndromes. Leukemia. 1993;7:696-701.

800. Nimer SD, Paquette RL, Ireland P, et al. A phase I/II study of interleukin-3 in patients with aplastic anemia and myelodysplasia. Exp Hematol. 1994;22:875-880.

801. Hellstrom-Lindberg E. Efficacy of erythropoietin in the myelodysplastic syndromes: a meta-analysis of 205 patients from 17 studies. Br J Haematol. 1995;89:67-71.

802. Hellstrom-Lindberg E, Ahlgren T, Beguin Y, et al. Treatment of anemia in myelodysplastic syndromes with granulocyte colony-stimulating factor plus erythropoietin: results from a randomized phase II study and long-term follow-up of 71 patients. Blood. 1998;92:68-75.

803. Economopoulos T, Mellou S, Papageorgiou E, et al. Treatment of anemia in low risk myelodysplastic syndromes with granulocyte-macrophage colony-stimulating factor plus recombinant human erythropoietin. Leukemia. 1999;13:1009-1012.

804. Marsh JC, Ganser A, Stadler M. Hematopoietic growth factors in the treatment of acquired bone marrow failure states. Semin Hematol. 2007;44:138-147.

805. Champlin RE, Nimer SD, Ireland P, et al. Treatment of refractory aplastic anemia with recombinant human granulocyte-macrophage-colony-stimulating factor. Blood. 1989;73:694-699.

806. Guinan EC, Sieff CA, Oette DH, Nathan DG. A phase I/II trial of recombinant granulocyte-macrophage colony-stimulating factor for children with aplastic anemia. Blood. 1990;76:1077-1082.

807. Nissen C, Tichelli A, Gratwohl A, et al. Failure of recombinant human granulocyte-macrophage colony-stimulating factor therapy in aplastic anemia patients with very severe neutropenia. Blood. 1988;72:2045-2047.

808. Kojima S, Fukuda M, Miyajima Y, Horibe K. Treatment of aplastic anemia in children with recombinant human granulocyte colony-stimulating factor. Blood. 1991;77:937-941.

809. Kojima S, Matsuyama T. Stimulation of granulopoiesis by high-dose recombinant human granulocyte colony-stimulating factor in children with aplastic anemia and very severe neutropenia. Blood. 1994;83:1474-1478.

810. Sonoda Y, Yashige H, Fujii H, et al. Bilineage response in refractory aplastic anemia patients following long-term administration of recombinant human granulocyte colony-stimulating factor. Eur J Haematol. 1992;48:41-48.

811. Gluckman E, Esperou-Bourdeau H. Recent treatments of aplastic anemia. The international group on SAA. Nouv Rev Fr Hematol. 1991;33:507-510.

812. Ganser A, Lindemann A, Seipelt G, et al. Effects of recombinant human interleukin-3 in patients with normal hematopoiesis and in patients with bone marrow failure. Blood. 1990;76:666-676.

813. Kojima S. Cytokine treatment of aplastic anemia. Int J Pediatr Hematol Oncol. 1995;2:135-141.

814. Kurzrock R, Talpaz M, Gutterman JU. Very low doses of GM-CSF administered alone with erythropoietin in aplastic anemia. Am J Med. 1992;93:41-48.

815. Hirashima K, Bessho M, Jinnai I, Murohashi I. Successful treatment of aplastic anemia and refractory anemia by combination therapy with recombinant human granulocyte colony-stimulating factor and erythropoietin. Exp Hematol. 1993;21:1080a.

816. Groopman JE, Mitsuyasu RT, DeLeo MJ, et al. Effects of recombinant human granulocyte-macrophage colony-stimulating factor on myelopoiesis in the acquired immunodeficiency syndrome. N Engl J Med. 1987;317:593-598.

817. Perno CF, Yarchoan R, Conney DA, et al. Replication of human immunodeficiency virus in monocytes: granulocyte/macrophage colony-stimulating factor (GM-CSF) potentiates viral production yet enhances the antiviral effect mediated by 3′-azido-2′3′-dideoxythymidine (AZT) and other dideoxynucleoside congeners of thymidine. J Exp Med. 1989;169:933-951.

818. Mueller BU. Role of cytokines in children with HIV infection. Int J Pediatr Hematol Oncol. 1995;2:151-161.

819. Pluda JM, Yarchoan R, Smith PD, et al. Subcutaneous recombinant granulocyte-macrophage colony-stimulating factor used as a single agent and in an alternating regimen with azidothymidine in leukopenic patients with severe human immunodeficiency virus infection. Blood. 1990;76:463-472.

820. Mueller BU, Jacobsen F, Butler KM, et al. Combination treatment with azidothymidine and granulocyte colony-stimulating factor in children with human immunodeficiency virus infection. J Pediatr. 1992;121:797-802.

821. Cole JL, Marzec UM, Gunthel CJ, et al. Ineffective platelet production in thrombocytopenic human immunodeficiency virus–infected patients. Blood. 1998;91:3239-3246.

822. Gillio AP, Guinan EC. Cytokine treatment of inherited bone marrow failure syndromes. Int J Pediatr Hematol Oncol. 1992;2:123-133.

823. Zeidler C, Welte K. Hematopoietic growth factors for the treatment of inherited cytopenias. Semin Hematol. 2007;44:133-137.

824. Guinan EC, Lopez KD, Huhn RD, et al. Evaluation of granulocyte-macrophage colony-stimulating factor for treatment of pancytopenia in children with fanconi anemia. J Pediatr. 1994;124:144-150.

825. Hammond D, Keighley G. The erythrocyte-stimulating factor in serum and urine in congenital hypoplastic anemia. Am J Dis Child. 1960;100:466-468.

826. Bagnara GP, Zauli G, Vitale L, et al. In vitro growth and regulation of bone marrow enriched CD34+ hematopoietic progenitors in Diamond-Blackfan anemia. Blood. 1991;78:2203-2210.

827. Abkowitz JL, Broudy VC, Bennett LG, et al. Absence of abnormalities of c-kit or its ligand in two patients with Diamond-Blackfan anemia. Blood. 1992;79:25-28.

828. Sieff CA, Yokoyama CT, Zsebo KM, et al. The production of Steel factor mRNA in Diamond-Blackfan anaemia long-term cultures and interactions of Steel factor with erythropoietin and interleukin-3. Br J Haematol. 1992;82:640-647.

829. Niemeyer CM, Baumgarten E, Holldack J, et al. Treatment trial with recombinant human erythropoietin in children with congenital hypoplastic anemia. Contrib Nephrol. 1991;88:276-280.

830. Dunbar CE, Smith DA, Kimball J, et al. Treatment of Diamond-Blackfan anaemia with haematopoietic growth factors, granulocyte-macrophage colony stimulating factor and interleukin 3: sustained remissions following IL-3. Br J Haematol. 1991;79:316-321.

831. Gillio AP, Faulkner LB, Alter BP, et al. Treatment of Diamond-Blackfan anemia with recombinant human interleukin-3 Blood. 1993;82:744-751.

832. Olivieri NF, Feig SA, Valentino L, et al. Failure of recombinant human interleukin-3 therapy to induce erythropoiesis in patients with refractory Diamond-Blackfan anemia. Blood. 1994;83:2444-2450.

833. Bastion Y, Bordigoni P, Debre M, et al. Sustained response after recombinant interleukin-3 in Diamond Blackfan anemia [letter]. Blood. 1994;83:617-618.

834. Klein C, Grudzien M, Appaswamy G, et al. HAX1 deficiency causes autosomal recessive severe congenital neutropenia (Kostmann disease). Nat Genet. 2007;39:86-92.

835. Pietsch T, Buhrer C, Mempel K, et al. Blood mononuclear cells from patients with severe congenital neutropenia are

capable of producing granulocyte colony-stimulating factor. Blood. 1991;77:1234-1237.

836. Bonilla MA, Gillio AP, Ruggeiro M, et al. Effects of recombinant human granulocyte colony-stimulating factor on neutropenia in patients with congenital agranulocytosis. N Engl J Med. 1989;320:1574-1580.

837. Welte K, Zeidler C, Reiter A, et al. Differential effects of granulocyte-macrophage colony-stimulating factor and granulocyte-stimulating factor in children with severe congenital neutropenia. Blood. 1990;75:1056-1063.

838. Boxer LA, Hutchinson R, Emerson S. Recombinant human granulocyte-colony-stimulating factor in the treatment of patients with neutropenia. Clin Immunol Immunopathol. 1992;62:S39-S46.

839. Dale DC, Bonilla MA, Davis MW, et al. A randomized controlled phase III trial of recombinant human granulocyte colony-stimulating factor (filgrastim) for treatment of severe chronic neutropenia. Blood. 1993;81:2496-2502.

840. Dong F, van Buitenen C, Pouwels K, et al. Distinct cytoplasmic regions of the human G-CSF receptor involved in induction of proliferation and maturation. Mol Cell Biol. 1993;13:7774-7781.

841. Dong F, Hoefsloot LH, Schelen AM, et al. Identification of a nonsense mutation in the granulocyte-colony-stimulating factor receptor in severe congenital neutropenia. Proc Natl Acad Sci U S A. 1994;91:4480-4484.

842. Welte K, Boxer LA. Severe chronic neutropenia: pathophysiology and therapy. Semin Hematol. 1997;34:267-278.

843. Gilman PA, Jackson DP, Guild HG. Congenital agranulocytosis: prolonged survival and terminal acute leukemia. Blood. 1970;36:576-585.

844. Rosen RB, Kang SJ. Congenital agranulocytosis terminating in acute myelomonocytic leukemia. J Pediatr. 1979;94:406-408.

845. Kalra R, Dale D, Freedman M, et al. Monosomy 7 and activating RAS mutations accompany malignant transformation in patients with congenital neutropenia. Blood. 1995;86:4579-4586.

846. Tidow N, Pilz C, Teichmann B, et al. Clinical relevance of point mutations in the cytoplasmic domain of the granulocyte colony-stimulating factor receptor gene in patients with severe congenital neutropenia. Blood. 1997;89:2369-2375.

847. Rosenberg PS, Alter BP, Bolyard AA, et al. The incidence of leukemia and mortality from sepsis in patients with severe congenital neutropenia receiving long-term G-CSF therapy. Blood. 2006;107:4628-4635.

848. Donadieu J, Leblanc T, Bader Meunier B, et al. Analysis of risk factors for myelodysplasias, leukemias and death from infection among patients with congenital neutropenia. Experience of the French Severe Chronic Neutropenia Study Group. Haematologica. 2005;90:45-53.

849. Hammond WP IV, Price TH, Souza LM, Dale DC. Treatment of cyclic neutropenia with granulocyte colony-stimulating factor. N Engl J Med. 1989;320:1306-1311.

850. Sugimoto K, Togawal A, Miyazono K. Treatment of childhood-onset cyclic neutropenia with recombinant human granulocyte colony stimulating factor. Eur J Haematol. 1990;45:110-111.

851. Hanada T, Ono I, Nagasawa T. Childhood cyclic neutropenia treated with granulocyte colony-stimulating factor. Br J Haematol. 1990;75:135-137.

852. Dale D, Bolyard A, Hammond W. Cyclic neutropenia: natural history and effects of long-term treatment with recombinant human granulocyte colony-stimulating factor. Cancer Invest. 1993;11:219-223.

853. Wright D, Oette D, Malech H. Treatment of cyclic neutropenia with recombinant human granulocyte-macrophage colony-stimulating factor (rhGM-CSF). Blood. 1989;74:231a.

854. Freund M, Luft S, Schüber C, et al. Differential effect of GM-CSF and G-CSF in cyclic neutropenia. Lancet. 1990;336:313.

855. Kurzrock R, Talpaz M, Gutterman J. Treatment of cyclic neutropenia with very low-doses of GM-CSF. Am J Med. 1991;91:317-318.

856. Jakubowski AA, Souza L, Kelly F, et al. Effects of human granulocyte colony-stimulating factor in a patient with idiopathic neutropenia. N Engl J Med. 1989;320:38-42.

857. Winearls CG, Oliver DO, Pippard MJ, et al. Effect of human erythropoietin derived from recombinant DNA on the anemia of patients maintained by chronic haemodialysis. Lancet. 1986;11:1175-1178.

858. Eschbach JW, Abdulhadi MH, Browne JK, et al. Recombinant human erythropoietin in anemic patients with end-stage renal disease. Ann Intern Med. 1989;111:992-1000.

859. Adamson JW. The promise of recombinant human erythropoietin. Semin Hematol. 1989;26(Suppl 2):5-8.

860. Casadevall N, Nataf J, Viron B, et al. Pure red-cell aplasia and antierythropoietin antibodies in patients treated with recombinant erythropoietin. N Engl J Med. 2002;346:469-475.

861. Peces R, de la Torre M, Alcazar R, Urra JM. Antibodies against recombinant human erythropoietin in a patient with erythropoietin-resistant anemia. N Engl J Med. 1996;335:523-524.

862. Bennett CL, Luminari S, Nissenson AR, et al. Pure red-cell aplasia and epoetin therapy. N Engl J Med. 2004;351:1403-1408.

863. Dessypris EN, Graber SE, Krantz SB, Stone WJ. Effects of recombinant erythropoietin on the concentration and cycling status of human marrow hematopoietic progenitor cells in vivo. Blood. 1988;72:2060-2062.

864. Laupacis A. Changes in quality of life and functional capacity in hemodialysis patients treated with recombinant human erythropoietin. Semin Nephrol. 1990;10(Suppl 1):11-19.

865. Eschbach JW, Kelly MR, Haley NR, et al. Treatment of the anemia of progressive renal failure with recombinant human erythropoietin. N Engl J Med. 1989;321:158-163.

866. Bommer J, Ritz E, Weinrich T, et al. Subcutaneous erythropoietin. Lancet. 1988;2:406.

867. Kaufman JS, Reda DJ, Fye CL, et al. Subcutaneous compared with intravenous epoetin in patients receiving hemodialysis. Department of Veterans Affairs Cooperative Study Group on Erythropoietin in Hemodialysis Patients. N Engl J Med. 1998;339:578-583.

868. Müller-Wiefel DE, Amon O. Erythropoietin treatment of anemia associated with chronic renal failure in children. Int J Pediatr Hematol Oncol. 1995;2:87-95.

869. Offner G, Hoyer PF, Latta K, et al. One year's experience with recombinant erythropoietin in children undergoing continuous ambulatory or cycling peritoneal dialysis. Pediatr Nephrol. 1990;4:498-500.

870. Scigalla P, Bonzel KE, Bulla M, et al. Therapy of renal anemia with recombinant human erythropoietin in children with end-stage renal disease. Contrib Nephrol. 1989;76:227-240.

871. Scharer K, Klare B, Braun A, et al. Treatment of renal anemia by subcutaneous erythropoietin in children with preterminal chronic renal failure. Acta Pediatr. 1993;82:953-958.

872. Onkingco JRC, Ruley EJ, Turner ME. Use of low-dose subcutaneous recombinant human erythropoietin in end-stage renal disease: experience with children receiving continuous cycling peritoneal dialysis. Am J Kidney Dis. 1991;18:446-450.

873. Ohls R, Christensen R. Recombinant erythropoietin compared with erythrocyte transfusion in the treatment of anemia of prematurity. J Pediatr. 1991;119:781-788.

874. Soubasi V, Kremenopoulos G, Diamandi E, et al. In which neonates does early recombinant human erythropoietin treatment prevent anemia of prematurity? Results of a randomized, controlled study. Pediatr Res. 1993;34:675-679.

875. Messer J, Haddad J, Donato L, et al. Early treatment of premature infants with recombinant human erythropoietin. Pediatrics. 1993;92:519-523.

876. Bechensteen AG, Haga P, Halvorsen S, et al. Erythropoietin, protein, and iron supplementation and the prevention of anaemia of prematurity. Arch Dis Child. 1993;69:19-23.

877. Shannon KM, Mentzer WC, Abels RI, et al. Enhancement of erythropoiesis by recombinant human erythropoietin in low birth weight infants: a pilot study. J Pediatr. 1992;120:586-592.

878. Carnielli V, Montini G, Da Riol R, et al. Effect of high doses of human recombinant erythropoietin on the need for blood transfusions in preterm infants. J Pediatr. 1992;121:98-102.

879. Halperin D, Felix M, Wacker P, et al. Recombinant human erythropoietin in the treatment of infants with anemia of prematurity. Eur J Pediatr. 1992;151:661-667.

880. Mentzer WC, Shannon KM. The use of recombinant human erythropoietin in preterm infants. Int J Pediatr Hematol Oncol. 1995;2:97-103.

881. Maier RF, Obladen M, Kattner E, et al. High-versus low-dose erythropoietin in extremely low birth weight infants. The European Multicenter rhEPO Study Group. J Pediatr. 1998;132:866-870.

882. Means RT, Olsen NJ, Krantz SB, et al. Treatment of the anemia of rheumatoid arthritis with recombinant human erythropoietin: clinical and in vitro studies. Arthritis Rheum. 1989;32:638-642.

883. Umemura T, al-Khatti A, Donahue RE, et al. Effects of Interleukin-3 and erythropoietin on in vitro erythropoiesis and F cell formation in primates. Blood. 1989;74:1561-1576.

884. al-Khatti A, Umemura T, Clow J, et al. Erythropoietin stimulates F-reticulocyte formation in sickle cell anemia. Trans Assoc Am Physicians. 1988;101:54-61.

885. Goldberg MA, Brugnara C, Dover GJ, et al. Treatment of sickle cell anemia with hydroxyurea and erythropoietin. N Engl J Med. 1990;323:366-372.

886. Rodgers GP, Dover GJ, Uyesaka N, et al. Augmentation by erythropoietin of the fetal-hemoglobin response to hydroxyurea in sickle cell disease. N Engl J Med. 1993;328:73-80.

887. Rachmilewitz EA, Goldfarb A, Dover G. Administration of erythropoietin to patients with β-thalassemia intermedia: a preliminary trial. Blood. 1991;78:1145-1147.

888. Olivieri NF, Freedman MH, Perrine SP, et al. Trial of recombinant human erythropoietin: three patients with thalassemia intermedia [letter]. Blood. 1992;80:3258-3260.

889. Aker M, Dover G, Schrier S, et al. Sustained increase in the hemoglobin, hematocrit and RBC following long term administration of recombinant human erythropoietin to patients with beta thalassemia intermedia [abstract]. Blood. 1993;82:358a.

890. Loukopoulos D, Voskaridou E, Cozma C, et al. Effective stimulation of erythropoiesis in thalassemia intermedia with recombinant human erythropoietin and hydroxyurea [abstract]. Blood. 1993;82:357a.

891. Goodnough LT, Rudnick S, Price TH, et al. Increased preoperative collection of autologous blood with recombinant human erythropoietin therapy. N Engl J Med. 1989;321:1163-1168.

892. Duhrsen U, Villeval J-L, Boyd J, et al. Effects of recombinant human granulocyte colony-stimulating factor on hematopoietic progenitor cells in cancer patients. Blood. 1988;72:2074-2081.

893. Tamura M, Hattori K, Nomura H, et al. Induction of neutrophilic granulocytes in mice by administration of purified human native granulocyte colony-stimulating factor (G-CSF). Biochem Biophys Res Commun. 1987;142:454-460.

894. Shimamura M, Kobayashi Y, Yuo A, et al. Effect of human recombinant granulocyte colony-stimulating factor on hematopoietic injury in mice induced by 5-fluorouracil. Blood. 1987;69:353-355.

895. Bensinger W, Appelbaum F, Rowley S, et al. Factors that influence collection and engraftment of autologous peripheral-blood stem cells. J Clin Oncol. 1995;13:2547-2555.

896. Weaver CH, Hazelton B, Birch R, et al. An analysis of engraftment kinetics as a function of the CD34 content of peripheral blood progenitor cell collections in 692 patients after the administration of myeloablative chemotherapy. Blood. 1995;86:3961-3969.

897. Pecora AL, Preti RA, Gleim GW, et al. CD34$^+$CD33$^-$ cells influence days to engraftment and transfusion requirements in autologous blood stem-cell recipients. J Clin Oncol. 1998;16:2093-2104.

898. Glaspy JA, Shpall EJ, LeMaistre CF, et al. Peripheral blood progenitor cell mobilization using stem cell factor in combination with filgrastim in breast cancer patients. Blood. 1997;90:2939-2951.

899. Moskowitz CH, Stiff P, Gordon MS, et al. Recombinant methionyl human stem cell factor and filgrastim for peripheral blood progenitor cell mobilization and transplantation in non-Hodgkin's lymphoma patients—results of a phase I/II trial. Blood. 1997;89:3136-3147.

900. Weaver A, Ryder D, Crowther D, et al. Increased numbers of long-term culture–initiating cells in the apheresis product of patients randomized to receive increasing doses of stem cell factor administered in combination with chemotherapy and a standard dose of granulocyte colony-stimulating factor. Blood. 1996;88:3323-3328.

901. Begley CG, Basser R, Mansfield R, et al. Enhanced levels and enhanced clonogenic capacity of blood progenitor cells following administration of stem cell factor plus granulocyte colony-stimulating factor to humans. Blood. 1997;90:3378-3389.

902. Basser RL, Rasko JE, Clarke K, et al. Randomized, blinded, placebo-controlled phase I trial of pegylated recombinant human megakaryocyte growth and development factor with filgrastim after dose-intensive chemotherapy in patients with advanced cancer [published erratum appears in Blood 1997;90(6):2513]. Blood. 1997;89:3118-3128.

903. Rasko JE, Basser RL, Boyd J, et al. Multilineage mobilization of peripheral blood progenitor cells in humans following administration of PEG-rHuMGDF. Br J Haematol. 1997;97:871-880.

904. Fleming WH, Lankford-Turner P, Turner CW, et al. Administration of daniplestim and granulocyte colony-stimulating factor for the mobilization of hematopoietic progenitor cells in nonhuman primates. Biol Blood Marrow Transplant. 1999;5:8-14.

905. Pless M, Wodnar-Filipowicz A, John L, et al. Synergy of growth factors during mobilization of peripheral blood precursor cells with recombinant human Flt3-ligand and granulocyte colony-stimulating factor in rabbits. Exp Hematol. 1999;27:155-161.

906. Brasel K, McKenna HJ, Charrier K, et al. Flt3 ligand synergizes with granulocyte-macrophage colony-stimulating factor or granulocyte colony-stimulating factor to mobilize hematopoietic progenitor cells into the peripheral blood of mice. Blood. 1997;90:3781-3788.

907. Papayannopoulou T, Nakamoto B, Andrews RG, et al. In vivo effects of Flt3/Flk2 ligand on mobilization of hematopoietic progenitors in primates and potent synergistic enhancement with granulocyte colony-stimulating factor. Blood. 1997;90:620-629.

908. Molineux G, McCrea C, Yan XQ, et al. Flt-3 ligand synergizes with granulocyte colony-stimulating factor to increase neutrophil numbers and to mobilize peripheral blood stem cells with long-term repopulating potential. Blood. 1997;89:3998-4004.

909. Sudo Y, Shimazaki C, Ashihara E, et al. Synergistic effect of FLT-3 ligand on the granulocyte colony-stimulating factor–induced mobilization of hematopoietic stem cells and progenitor cells into blood in mice. Blood. 1997;89:3186-3191.

910. Shpall EJ. The utilization of cytokines in stem cell mobilization strategies. Bone Marrow Transplant. 1999;23(Suppl 2):S13-S19.

911. Socinski MA, Cannistra SA, Elias A, et al. Granulocyte-macrophage colony stimulating factor expands the circulating haemopoietic progenitor cell compartment in man. Lancet. 1988;1:1194-1198.

912. Gribben JG, Devereux S, Thomas NSB, et al. Development of antibodies to unprotected glycosylation sites on recombinant human GM-CSF. Lancet. 1990;335:434-437.

913. Vadhan-Raj S, Verschraegen CF, Bueso-Ramos C, et al. Recombinant human thrombopoietin attenuates carboplatin-induced severe thrombocytopenia and the need for platelet transfusions in patients with gynecologic cancer. Ann Intern Med. 2000;132:364-368.

914. Crawford J, Glaspy J, Belani C, et al. A randomized, placebo-controlled, blinded, dose-scheduling trial of pegylated recombinant human megakaryocyte growth and development factor (PEG-rHuMGDF) with filgastrim support in small non-lung cancer (NSCLC) patients treated with paclitaxel and carboplatin during multiple cycles of chemotherapy. Proc Am Soc Clin Oncol. 1998;17:73a.

915. Li J, Yang C, Xia Y, et al. Thrombocytopenia caused by the development of antibodies to thrombopoietin. Blood. 2001;98:3241-3248.

916. Yang C, Xia Y, Li J, Kuter DJ. The appearance of anti-thrombopoietin antibody and circulating thrombopoietin-IgG complexes in a patient developing thrombocytopenia after the injection of PEG-rHuMGDF. Blood. 1999;94:681a.

917. Casadevall N, Nataf J, Viron B, et al. Pure red-cell aplasia and antierythropoietin antibodies in patients treated with recombinant erythropoietin. N Engl J Med. 2002;346:469-475.

918. Glaspy JA, Baldwin GC, Robertson PA, et al. Therapy for neutropenia in hairy cell leukemia with recombinant human granulocyte colony-stimulating factor. Ann Intern Med. 1988;109:789-795.

919. Besarab A, Bolton WK, Browne JK, et al. The effects of normal as compared with low hematocrit values in patients with cardiac disease who are receiving hemodialysis and epoetin. N Engl J Med. 1998;339:584-590.

920. Singh AK, Szczech L, Tang KL, et al. Correction of anemia with epoetin alfa in chronic kidney disease. N Engl J Med. 2006;355:2085-2098.

921. Drueke TB, Locatelli F, Clyne N, et al. Normalization of hemoglobin level in patients with chronic kidney disease and anemia. N Engl J Med. 2006;355:2071-2084.

922. Bohlius J, Wilson J, Seidenfeld J, et al. Erythropoietin or darbepoetin for patients with cancer. Cochrane Database Syst Rev. 2006;3:CD003407.

7 Acquired Aplastic Anemia and Pure Red Cell Aplasia

Akiko Shimamura and David G. Nathan

Acquired and congenital bone marrow failure syndromes are characterized by a reduction in the effective production of mature erythrocytes, granulocytes, and platelets by bone marrow. Bone marrow failure leads to various peripheral blood cytopenias. In some conditions, only one or two cell lines may be affected. In others, such as aplastic anemia, the result is pancytopenia. In this chapter we deal only with the acquired bone marrow failure syndromes, although we use the term rather loosely because seemingly acquired marrow failure syndromes may have a genetic basis. The known inherited/congenital bone marrow failure syndromes are described in detail in Chapter 8. Acquired marrow failure syndromes that affect only granulocytes or platelets are described in Chapters 21 and 33, respectively. Acquired single-lineage deficiency syndromes that involve red cell production (pure red cell aplasia) are also described in this chapter, except that the 5q– syndrome is discussed in Chapter 8 and in more detail in *Oncology of Infancy and Childhood.*

APLASTIC ANEMIA

Decreased production of *mature blood cells* may result from a reduction in the number or function of their *progenitors*. Aplastic anemia is a descriptive term referring to a clinical state in which peripheral blood pancytopenia results from reduced or absent production of blood cells in bone marrow. Aplastic anemia may arise in the setting of inherited/congenital syndromes associated with a predisposition to marrow failure (discussed in Chapter 8), may develop secondary to marrow-toxic stressors in an otherwise seemingly normal host, or may lack any apparent underlying cause. Classification of the aplastic anemias is presented in Box 7-1. A careful medical history, physical examination, and laboratory evaluation are critical to discern inherited versus acquired causes of aplastic anemia. The distinction between inherited and acquired causes of aplastic anemia carries profound implications for medical management and treatment, so a careful search for possible underlying inherited syndromes should be undertaken before initiation of therapy.

Camitta and co-workers classified the severity of aplastic anemia in an effort to make possible the comparison of diverse groups of patients and different therapeutic approaches.[1] Diagnosis of *severe aplastic anemia* requires that the patient have at least two of the following anomalies: a granulocyte count below 500/μL, a platelet count below 20,000/μL, and an absolute reticulocyte count of 40×10^9/L or less. In addition, the bone marrow biopsy specimen must contain less than 25% of the normal cellularity or less than 30% hematopoietic elements. Very severe aplastic anemia is further defined by a granulocyte count lower than 200/μL.[2] *Mild* or *moderate aplastic anemia*, sometimes called "hypoplastic anemia," is distinguished from the severe form by the presence of

| Box 7-1 | Classification of the Aplastic Anemias |

ACQUIRED

Secondary
Radiation
Drugs and chemicals
    Direct toxicity: chemotherapy, benzene
    Idiosyncratic: chloramphenicol, anti-inflammatory
        drugs, antiepileptics, carbonic anhydrase inhibitors
Viruses
    Epstein-Barr virus
    Hepatitis (non-A, -B, -C, -E, or -G)
    Human immunodeficiency virus
Immune diseases
    Eosinophilic fasciitis
    Hypoimmunoglobulinemia
    Systemic lupus erythematosus (uncommon)
Thymoma
Graft-versus-host disease in immunodeficiency
Pregnancy
Paroxysmal nocturnal hemoglobinuria
Myelodysplasia

Idiopathic

INHERITED

Fanconi's anemia
Dyskeratosis congenita
Shwachman-Diamond syndrome
Amegakaryocytic thrombocytopenia
Diamond-Blackfan anemia
Reticular dysgenesis
Familial aplastic anemias
Nonhematologic syndromes (e.g., Down, Dubowitz', and
    Seckel's syndromes)

Modified from Alter BP, Potter NU, Li FP. Classification and aetiology of the aplastic anaemias. Clin Haematol. 1978;7:431-465.

mild or moderate cytopenia and more variable, but still deficient bone marrow cellularity. These distinctions are more than semantic; they are critical for prediction of outcome and selection of therapy.

Epidemiology

Epidemiologic studies performed in Europe estimate that the annual incidence of aplastic anemia is 2 per million per year[3]; by comparison, the incidence of acute leukemia is about 50 per million per year. Higher figures for the incidence of aplastic anemia have been obtained from smaller studies in the United States and earlier surveys in Europe, but these figures may have been inflated by the inclusion of cases of the more common syndrome myelodysplasia. Aplastic anemia is more common in Asia (4 to 7 per million per year[4]) than in the West. Chloramphenicol has been widely used in much of Asia because of its efficacy and low cost, but reductions in its use have not been accompanied by reductions in the incidence of aplastic anemia in Japan[5,6] or elsewhere,[7,8] and no association was observed in case-control studies in Thailand.[9] A recent case-control study[10] in Thailand spanning 1989 to 2002 described an association between aplastic anemia and exposure to benzene or pesticides. Although an increased risk for aplastic anemia was also associated with animal exposure and ingestion of nonbottled or nondistilled water, no significant associations with known infections or hepatitis were observed.

The peak age for the development of aplastic anemia is 15 to 25 years or older than 60 years, with a male-to-female ratio of approximately 1:1.

Causal Factors

When no causative factors are ascertained, the cases are classified as "idiopathic." A search for possible causative agents is warranted because some patients may improve after removal of the offending agent. Many patients have been exposed to several potentially myelosuppressive agents, and the number of possible associations depends in part on the intensity of the investigation. A drug or toxin is often implicated if the exposure is to a previously implicated agent and is appropriately extensive or temporally proximate; sometimes, a drug history is given significance only because all other factors are excluded. Therefore, the course, management, and outcome are related more to the severity of the hematopoietic depression than the cause, and they are generally similar for cases with apparent cause and those that are idiopathic.

Drugs

The incidence of drug- and chemical-related aplastic anemia[11] varies over time and from place to place. Many drugs and toxins have been implicated by inferential and circumstantial evidence; the magnitude of the risk is usually unknown (Box 7-2). The presence of an agent on this list suggests caution regarding its use, but no drug on the list should be proscribed if there are strong clinical indications for its use. From a public health perspective, even drugs associated with an increased risk for marrow failure do not cause large numbers of cases of aplastic anemia.[3]

Note that even confirmed associations do not substantiate causality. Antibiotics thought to be causative may have been administered for the viral infection that led to the aplastic anemia or for symptoms from already established neutropenia in an undiagnosed case of aplastic anemia. Bleeding may be precipitated in undiagnosed thrombocytopenic patients who receive nonsteroidal anti-inflammatory drugs. As an example of known errors in association, among six patients reported to have sniffed glue and become aplastic, five had sickle cell anemia and aplastic crises now known to be due to parvovirus infection.[12]

The incidence of drug-related aplasia in pediatric cases is low, mainly because many of the drugs consid-

---

| Box 7-2 | **Classification of Drugs and Chemicals Associated with Aplastic Anemia*** |

AGENTS THAT REGULARLY PRODUCE MARROW DEPRESSION

Antibiotics: daunorubicin, doxorubicin hydrochloride (Adriamycin), chloramphenicol
Antimetabolites: antifolic compounds, nucleotide analogues
Antimitotics: vinblastine, colchicine
Benzene and chemicals containing benzene: carbon tetrachloride, chlorophenols, kerosene, Stoddard's solvent
Cytotoxic cancer chemotherapy with alkylating drugs: busulfan, melphalan, cyclophosphamide

AGENTS POSSIBLY ASSOCIATED BUT WITH A LOW PROBABILITY RELATIVE TO USE

Chloramphenicol
Insecticides: chlordane, chlorophenothane (DDT), γ-benzene hexachloride (lindane), parathion
Anticonvulsants: carbamazepine, hydantoins, phenacemide
Nonsteroidal anti-inflammatory agents: indomethacin, ibuprofen, oxyphenylbutazone, phenylbutazone, sulindac
Antihistamines: cimetidine, chlorpheniramine, ranitidine
Antiprotozoal drugs: quinacrine, chloroquine
Sulfonamides: some antibiotics, antidiabetics (chlorpropamide, tolbutamide), antithyroid drugs (methimazole, methylthiouracil, propylthiouracil), carbonic anhydrase inhibitors (acetazolamide, methazolamide)
Penicillamine
Metals: gold, arsenic, bismuth, mercury

AGENTS MORE RARELY ASSOCIATED

Allopurinol (may potentiate marrow suppression by cytotoxic drugs)
Antibiotics: flucytosine, mebendazole, methicillin, sulfonamides, streptomycin, tetracycline, trimethoprim/sulfamethoxazole
Carbimazole
Guanidine
Lithium
Methyldopa
Potassium perchlorate
Quinidine
Sedatives and tranquilizers: chlordiazepoxide, chlorpromazine, meprobamate, methyprylon, piperacetazine, prochlorperazine
Thiocyanate

---

*Agents are listed because they have been cited in the literature; inclusion in this list does not imply acceptance by the author of a causal relationship.
Modified from Young NS, Alter BP. Aplastic Anemia: Acquired and Inherited. Philadelphia, WB Saunders, 1994, p 104.

ered to be related to aplasia are not used in childhood, with the exception of antiepileptic drugs, carbonic anhydrase inhibitors, nonsteroidal anti-inflammatory medications, and some antibiotics.

Drug-related aplasia may occur in several ways. Drugs may exert direct cytotoxic or suppressive effects on bone marrow. Myelosuppressive drugs, such as those used in cancer chemotherapy, lead to predictable and dose-related marrow suppression. Benzene, too, can be regularly demonstrated to suppress bone marrow in animals in a dose-linked manner, and most individuals exposed to sufficient amounts of benzene would probably suffer some type of marrow damage. In practice, most drug-related aplastic anemia is "idiosyncratic" and occurs unpredictably in only rare individuals who are prescribed the medication, sometimes weeks to months after its administration is discontinued. This last category of patients may possess a genetic propensity for this phenomenon.

Chloramphenicol

Chloramphenicol was considered to be the most common cause of aplastic anemia at the peak of its use, which began in 1949.[13] A genetic predisposition may exist. The mechanism of the idiosyncratic aplasia remains unknown despite extensive investigation.

Chloramphenicol contains a nitrobenzene ring and thus resembles amidopyrine, a drug known to cause agranulocytosis.[14,15] Chloramphenicol is the prime example of a drug that causes dose-related marrow suppression through mechanisms that include mitochondrial inhibition,[16] as well as idiosyncratic aplastic anemia.[17]

The signs of dose-related toxicity appear more rapidly in patients with hepatic or renal disease because the drug must be inactivated by conjugation with glucuronide in the liver and excreted in urine. High doses and high plasma levels correlate with the characteristic reversible erythroid depression. In vitro, chloramphenicol inhibits the growth of both colony-forming unit, granulocyte macrophage (CFU-GM), and colony-forming unit, erythroid (CFU-E),[18-22] and may also inhibit the hematopoietic microenvironment.[20,23]

Other Drugs

Nonsteroidal anti-inflammatory drugs, which are used more extensively in adults than in children, are associated with aplasia.[3] Nonsteroidal anti-inflammatory drugs associated by occasional case reports with aplastic anemia include aspirin,[24] indomethacin,[25-28] and ibuprofen.[29] Several large studies reported an increased risk for aplastic anemia with phenylbutazone[30,31] and identified even higher probability with some of the other nonsteroidal anti-inflammatory drugs.[3] Another drug associated with a risk for cytopenia in 2 per 100,000 patients is cimetidine.[32,33] Sulfa-containing compounds, which appear as risk factors in most case-control studies of drugs and aplastic anemia, are used in a wide variety of clinical circumstances.[34-43] Other drugs implicated in aplastic

anemia that are commonly used in the pediatric population include anticonvulsants (hydantoins,[44-46] carbamazepine[47-51]) and carbonic anhydrase inhibitors[52] (acetazolamide[53,54] and methazolamide[55,56]). Many of the drugs listed in Box 7-2 have also been associated with agranulocytosis. In general, only a minority of cases of aplastic anemia can be assigned a drug association. The distinction between aplasia secondary to the medication and aplasia arising from the underlying disorder (or occult viral infection) requiring treatment can be difficult.

Chemicals and Toxins

Benzene

Benzene is a particularly dangerous environmental contaminant.[57,58] It is found in organic solvents, coal tar derivatives, and petroleum products.[59-62] Fatal aplastic anemia, leukemia, or both have been reported years later in factory workers exposed to benzene. Benzene concentrates in bone marrow fat,[63] forms water-soluble intermediates,[64-66] and damages DNA.[67-69] It decreases numbers of progenitors and damages stroma. The risk for cytopenia is probably related to cumulative exposure.

Other Aromatic Hydrocarbons

Toxicity thought to be due to other organic solvents may in some instances be caused by benzene contaminants. Neither pure toluene nor xylene is a marrow toxin. Aplastic anemia has been linked by many case reports to insecticides, particularly γ-hexachlorobenzene (lindane) in children.[70] Aromatic hydrocarbons are present in insecticides and herbicides and may be the solvents for these agents. Some organophosphate insecticides have been shown to inhibit in vitro hematopoietic colony formation, as has lindane.[71]

Ionizing Radiation

Marrow aplasia may occur as an acute toxic sequela of irradiation from a nuclear bomb explosion, radioactive fallout, reactor accidents, and accidental exposure in medicine and industry. Bone marrow cells may be affected by high-energy gamma rays, as well as by ingested or absorbed lower-energy alpha particles. The radiation injury is inflicted on the actively replicating pool of precursor and progenitor cells and also on stem cells, in which DNA damage may have a more severe effect. Nonetheless, radiation-related marrow aplasia is infrequent. Even in a restricted episode, such as the Chernobyl reactor accident in 1986, most immediate deaths were due to skin burns and damage to the gastrointestinal and pulmonary systems.

Chronic radiation-induced aplasia is dose related. Patients who underwent irradiation for ankylosing spondylitis had an increased risk for aplastic anemia, and American radiologists have been reported to have an increased death rate from aplasia (for both groups, pathologic distinction between aplasia and myelodysplasia was not made). The incidence of late aplasia in atomic bomb victims was not increased, nor was it increased in patients undergoing radiation therapy for malignancies. Knospe and co-workers suggested that irradiation with an exposure greater than 4.4 Gy was required for the development of aplasia; they also postulated that low doses might damage only stem cells whereas high doses would also damage the supportive hematopoietic stromal microenvironment.[72]

Infectious Agents

Mild pancytopenia frequently develops in patients with bacterial or viral illnesses during or after the infection (see Chapter 36). Patients with bacterial or viral infections often receive antibiotics and other medications, and it is frequently not clear whether an ensuing aplastic anemia was caused by the infection, by the drug, or by the combination of the two or even whether the infectious illness was the result and not the cause of the pancytopenia.

Hepatitis

Although hepatitis is frequently associated with mild depression of blood cell counts, aplasia is a rare sequela, estimated to occur in less than 0.07% of the total number of pediatric hepatitis cases[73] and in less than 2% of those with non-A, non-B hepatitis.[74] Nonetheless, as an identifiable clinical event, a previous episode of hepatitis was recognized in 2% to 5% of aplastic anemia patients in a Western series.[75] The prevalence of previous hepatitis is about twofold this proportion in the Far East.[76] Among children with aplastic anemia in Taiwan, 24% had a history of recent acute hepatitis.[77] The antecedent hepatitis may be subclinical inasmuch as about 50% of patients with aplastic anemia may have elevated hepatic transaminases before their first transfusion. In a report of 32 patients who underwent liver transplantation for hepatic failure after non-A, non-B hepatitis, aplastic anemia developed in 28%.[78] Although aplasia has been reported after both hepatitis A and B virus infection,[79,80] the majority of cases of hepatitis/aplasia syndrome are not associated with serotypable hepatitis virus.[81,82]

Aplastic anemia associated with hepatitis is particularly severe. More than 200 cases of aplastic anemia and hepatitis have been reported, with two thirds of those affected being male and three quarters being younger than 20 years. In one early series, more than 90% died within a year, and the mean survival was only 11 weeks.[83] More recently, successful treatment with bone marrow transplantation (BMT) or with antithymocyte globulin (ATG) and cyclosporin A has been reported.[87]

Flaviviruses

Flaviviruses cause arbovirus hemorrhagic fever, dengue, and other hematodepressive syndromes. Dengue can propagate in bone marrow cultures without direct cytotoxicity, and dengue antigens induce lymphocyte activation and the release of marrow-suppressive cytokines.[88]

Epstein-Barr Virus

Herpesviruses such as Epstein-Barr virus (EBV) are large, complex DNA viruses.[89] EBV causes infectious mononucleosis, which is associated with pancytopenic complications in less than 1% of cases. More than 12 such cases have been reported, and half of these cases had a fatal outcome. In one study, EBV was demonstrated by immunologic and molecular methods in the bone marrow of six patients with aplastic anemia.[90] Only two had a history of typical mononucleosis, although all six had serologic evidence of such, thus suggesting that EBV may be an unrecognized cause of aplastic anemia. EBV's target is B cells, although T cells may also be infected. Because EBV is a common infection, issues of ascertainment can render the causative determination of aplasia difficult.

Cytomegalovirus and Human Herpesvirus 6

Infection with cytomegalovirus (CMV) may lead to graft failure in immunosuppressed bone marrow transplant recipients.[91] CMV can infect marrow stromal cells in vitro and can inhibit their ability to produce growth factors[92]; direct progenitor cell infection by some CMV strains has also been documented.[92,93] Herpesvirus 6 is the cause of erythema subitum[94] and, like CMV, may be found in the marrow of patients with graft failure after transplantation,[95] as well as in hematopoietic progenitors infected in vitro.[96] As with other viruses, both of these are ubiquitous infections, which makes causality difficult to ascertain.

Human Immunodeficiency Virus

Patients with acquired immunodeficiency syndrome (AIDS) often have cytopenias,[97] but their marrow is much more commonly cellular and dysplastic than empty. Colony formation by marrow from patients may be diminished.[98-101] The action of human immunodeficiency virus type 1 (HIV-1), a lentivirus, on hematopoietic cells remains a subject of controversy. HIV-1 infection of CD34+ cells has been difficult to detect in vivo from patient material[100,102] or after tissue culture infection of normal cells.[100,103] The virus apparently directly infects megakaryocytes that bear the CD4 receptor present on T cells.[104] The virus may also affect stroma function, at least in vitro.[105,106] HIV-1 can act indirectly on hematopoiesis through inhibitory lymphokine production; the envelope glycoprotein can stimulate macrophages to produce tumor necrosis factor, which in turn inhibits hematopoietic colony formation.[107] Hematologic suppression can also be due to opportunistic infections, neoplasms, or marrow suppression from the drugs used to treat AIDS and its complications.

Other Viruses

Blood count abnormalities, which are rarely severe, may be observed in the course of rubella, measles, mumps, varicella, and influenza A.[108]

Paroxysmal Nocturnal Hemoglobinuria

Paroxysmal nocturnal hemoglobinuria (PNH) is a disease characterized by variable combinations of mild to severe intravascular hemolysis, thromboses, and aplastic anemia.[109] It is uncommon in adults and even rarer in children. There is a clear association of PNH with aplastic anemia in that pancytopenia and marrow hypoplasia develop in many patients with PNH and PNH clones are detectable in up to 50% to 70% of patients with acquired aplastic anemia.[110-113]

PNH is characterized by an inability to inactivate complement on the erythrocyte cell surface, thereby resulting in increased sensitivity to complement. Deficits were subsequently identified in a family of membrane proteins, all of which were anchored to the cell membrane via glycosylphosphatidylinositol (GPI). GPI binds covalently to specific carboxyl-terminal protein sequences and attaches them to cell membrane phosphatidylinositol residues. The genetic defect in PNH was localized to the X-linked *PIG-A* (phosphatidylinositol glycan class A) gene, whose product functions in the transfer of *N*-acetyl-glucosamine to phosphatidylinositol as an early step in GPI anchor formation. Early tests for PNH, such as the Ham or sucrose hemolysis test, relied on the demonstration of increased sensitivity to complement-mediated red cell lysis. Increased sensitivity and specificity are achieved with flow cytometry assays for the absence of GPI-anchored proteins such as CD59 and CD55.[114] More sensitive tests use aerolysin, a channel-forming toxin that binds GPI-anchored proteins and results in cell lysis but leaves GPI-deficient PNH cells intact.[115] The use of a fluorescently labeled aerolysin variant that binds to GPI but fails to lyse the cells offers increased sensitivity and specificity for detection of the PNH clone.[116]

The clinical significance of small populations of PNH clones is unclear. Small numbers of PNH cells are detectable in healthy controls,[117] although the PNH cells in this context are typically polyclonal. Despite the frequent finding of PNH clones in the bone marrow of patients with aplastic anemia, the clinical syndrome of PNH subsequently develops in only 10% to 15% of patients (reviewed by Parker[118]). In the majority of patients, such clones may persist or disappear. Patients with small asymptomatic PNH clones may respond to the same treatments as other patients with aplastic anemia.

The etiology of marrow aplasia in PNH remains an area of active investigation. Although severe combined immunodeficiency (SCID) mice infused with bone marrow from PNH patients show preferential engraftment with the PNH clones,[115] studies of hematopoiesis in PNH patients have not detected any selective proliferative advantage of the *PIG-A(−)* hematopoietic clones.[120] A subsequent study comparing in vitro proliferation of *PIG-A(−)* and *PIG-A(+)* CD34 cells from PNH patients found a selective growth deficiency in the *PIG-A(+)* cell population rather than an advantage for the *PIG-A* mutant cells; Fas expression was elevated on the

wild-type versus the GPI-deficient cells, thus suggesting increased resistance to apoptosis as one potential mechanism to explain their findings.[121] No proliferative advantage of PNH hematopoietic clones was observed in mice mosaic for the *pig-a* gene.[122,123] To evaluate the hypothesis that autoreactive T cells might preferentially eliminate *PIG-A(+)* hematopoietic stem cells while sparing the PNH clones, the sensitivity of normal versus PNH EBV-transformed B-cell lines to autologous EBV-specific T-cell lines was examined.[124] The PNH cells were no less sensitive to T-cell–mediated cytotoxicity than the non-PNH cells were; thus, the GPI-linked cell surface molecules are not required for killing by T cells. An abnormal distribution of expanded T-cell clones detected by size analysis of the complementarity-determining region 3 (CDR3) in the β variable region (V_{β}) mRNA of the T-cell receptor (TCR) has been noted in PNH patients,[125] although the targets of such T-cell populations remain to be ascertained. The mechanisms underlying clonal expansion of the GPI-negative cells in PNH or aplastic anemia are currently unclear. Despite the presence of clonal populations of PNH cells, patients with PNH do not exhibit an increased incidence of leukemia, and the GPI-negative clones do not behave in a malignant fashion. A recent study suggests that additional genetic or epigenetic events, such as elevation of HMGA2 expression, may contribute to clonal expansion.[126]

Immunologic Diseases

Ten percent of patients with the rare collagen vascular syndrome *eosinophilic fasciitis* have associated aplastic anemia.[127] This condition is usually limited to adults. Thymoma associated with hematopoietic failure is generally, but not exclusively manifested as pure red cell aplasia (PRCA).[128] Some of the adults had also received drugs such as chloramphenicol or sulfonamides, and the aplasia could have been due to the drugs alone or to the combination. An iatrogenic aplasia can be induced by the transfusion of competent lymphocytes into immunodeficient hosts. In these cases, marrow failure arises from the transfusional graft-versus-host disease (GVHD).[129]

Pathophysiology

The purported mechanisms for failure of hematopoiesis are predicated on our current knowledge of normal hematopoiesis (see Chapter 6). Disease could result from decreased numbers or defective function of the cellular or soluble components required for blood cell production or from exogenous factors that result in damage or elimination of hematopoietic cells. Figure 7-1 depicts different mechanisms for the loss of hematopoietic cells in aplastic anemia. In model I, marrow toxins such as irradiation, drugs, or chemicals or direct invasion by viruses might cause hematopoietic stem or progenitor cell death (or both). In model II, an underlying abnormality of the hematopoietic cells may result in a predisposition to hematopoietic stem cell damage, premature stem cell

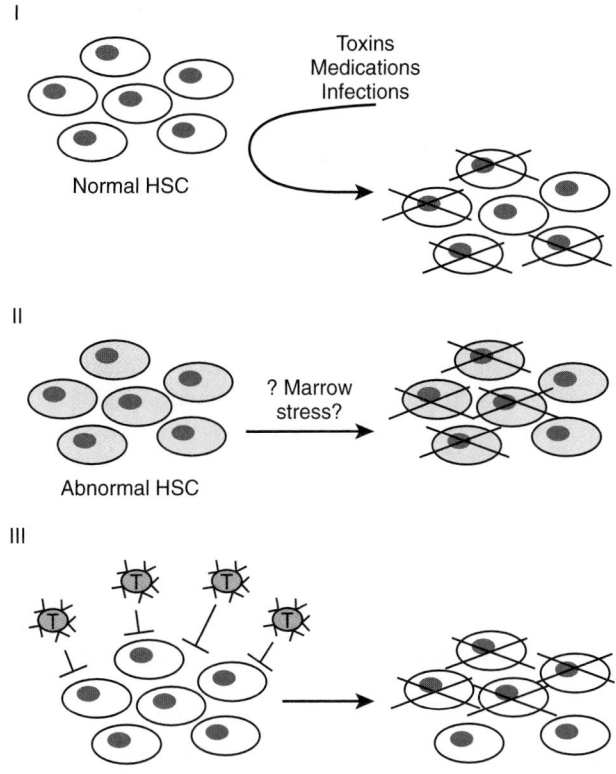

FIGURE 7-1. Models for the pathogenesis of aplastic anemia. **I,** Healthy hematopoietic stem cells and progenitors are damaged by an exogenous agent such as a toxin, medication, or infectious pathogen, with resultant marrow aplasia. **II,** Abnormal marrow cells (e.g., inherited marrow failure syndromes) undergo premature attrition. Marrow aplasia might be exacerbated by external factors. **III,** Immune-mediated attack (cellular or humeral) eliminates hematopoietic stem cells and progenitors. HSC, hematopoietic stem cell.

loss, or insufficient stem cell production (see Chapter 6). In model III, viruses, drugs, toxins, or immune dysregulation may incite a cellular or humoral immunologic reaction against a normal hematopoietic compartment. These possibilities are not mutually exclusive, and supportive data for each model have been described. Current data suggest that aplastic anemia may represent the final seemingly common outcome of different pathogenic mechanisms, with different underlying causes entailing different medical management considerations.

Hematopoietic Stem Cells and Clonality

Patients with aplastic anemia have decreased numbers of blood- and marrow-committed progenitor cells, assayed as myeloid colony-forming cells (CFU-GMs), erythroid colony-forming cells (CFU-Es and burst-forming units, erythrocytes [BFU-Es]), megakaryocytic progenitors (CFU-megas), multipotent colony-forming cells (CFU-GEMMs), and long-term culture-initiating cell (LTC-ICs).[130,131] Hematopoietic cells can also be assessed phenotypically for the presence of the CD34 antigen, which defines a compartment of about 1% of marrow cells that includes progenitors and possibly activated

stem cells.[132-135] CD34+ cells are reduced in aplastic anemia, and almost all patients show not only a severe reduction in numbers of these cells but also poor plating efficiency for colony formation from purified CD34+ cells.[136,137]

Several lines of evidence point to primary abnormalities in the hematopoietic stem cell as a potential cause of aplastic anemia. Multiple studies have noted that simple infusion of stem cells from an identical twin donor without previous conditioning was sufficient to treat the aplasia in many cases.[138-141] These results strongly support a pathogenic stem cell defect and argue against permanent disorders of the bone marrow environment, including immunologic mechanisms, as the cause of stem cell destruction. Low stem cell numbers persist even with hematologic recovery after medical therapy with antithymocyte globulin (ATG) and cyclosporine (see later), and blood cell parameters such as macrocytosis do not return to normal in many cases, again suggestive of an underlying stem cell abnormality. A primary stem cell defect probably also contributes to the observation of clonal hematopoiesis in aplastic anemia,[142] as well as the late development of other hematologic diseases such as myelodysplasia and acute leukemia (see later).

A subset of (and perhaps most) patients with seemingly idiopathic aplastic anemia may actually carry an inherited/congenital predisposition to marrow failure (see Chapter 8). Although the inherited/congenital marrow failure syndromes are often associated with characteristic physical findings, patients may have isolated aplastic anemia as the sole manifestation of their underlying inherited syndrome.[143] In some patients lacking significant physical findings or cytopenia at the time of evaluation, an elevated mean corpuscular volume may be the only clue to an underlying inherited marrow failure syndrome. A careful family history for hematologic abnormalities, predisposition to malignancy, or other characteristic clinical stigmata may be helpful in distinguishing an inherited marrow failure syndrome.[144] For example, a subset of patients with aplastic anemia but without other clinical stigmata of an inherited marrow failure syndrome were found to harbor mutations in the dyskeratosis congenita genes *hTERC*,[145,146] which encodes the RNA component of telomerase, or *hTERT*,[147-149] which encodes the catalytic subunit of the telomerase complex. Telomeres are specialized structures that stabilize the ends of each chromosome to prevent excessive shortening with replication, to distinguish chromosome ends from internal DNA breaks, and to prevent end-to-end fusion. Telomeres consist of 6–base pair (bp) repeated sequences (TTAGGG) associated with a specific protein complex. Telomerase is a ribonucleoprotein enzyme consisting of an H/ACA RNA component (TERC) complexed with a reverse transcriptase (TERT) and additional H/ACA binding proteins, including dyskerin, GAR1, NHP2, and NOP10. When telomerase levels are diminished or absent, telomeres progressively shorten with each cell division. At a critically short telomere length, a checkpoint is triggered for cells to stop dividing and undergo senescence to prevent chromosomal rearrangements.

Shortened telomeres have been observed in the leukocytes of patients with aplastic anemia.[150] Of five patients noted to have mean telomere lengths less than 5 kb, three had acquired cytogenetic abnormalities, thus suggesting that compromise in the telomere's probable role in stabilizing chromosome ends may contribute to the increased incidence of myelodysplasia and acute leukemia. A study by Brummendorf and colleagues reported relatively normal telomere lengths in patients who responded to immunosuppression, whereas untreated or unresponsive patients showed significant telomere shortening.[151] Telomere shortening is a common feature associated with marrow failure, although telomere lengths are particularly short in patients with dyskeratosis congenita, a disorder of telomerase function, even in comparison to other marrow failure patients.[152] Whether telomere shortening in marrow failure patients lacking telomerase mutations represents a primary defect in telomere maintenance or a secondary effect of increased cycling of the few remaining hematopoietic stem cells remains to be clarified.

Immune Destruction

Several lines of data suggest that immune phenomena may result in aplastic anemia (reviewed elsewhere[153,154]). In some syngeneic (identical twin) bone marrow transplants, simple infusion of stem cells is not sufficient to reconstitute hematopoiesis. The requirement for previous conditioning of the host may reflect some operational immunologic process, although it is also consistent with the presence of an underlying clonal abnormality that requires ablation.[155] Histocompatibility studies conducted in Europe, Asia, and the United States have indicated an increased representation of HLA-DR2 among aplastic anemia patients, consistent with a genetically determined immune susceptibility to disease.[155-157] Evidence for specific immune mechanisms is reviewed in the following sections.

Lymphocytes

Autologous recovery has been reported after either mismatched or matched transplants in patients prepared with antilymphocyte sera or cyclophosphamide.[158-160] An immune mechanism for aplastic anemia is suggested by the observation that aplasia often responds to treatment with antilymphocyte globulin (ALG)/ATG, cyclosporine, or both without transplantation. The antilymphocyte preparations contain heterogeneous mixtures of antibodies to many cells, including lymphocytes, and are clearly immunosuppressive, as well as generally cytotoxic. They lead to rapid lymphopenia during and immediately after treatment, and the reduced levels of activated lymphocytes persist for months. Cyclosporine exerts inhibitory T-cell effects and inhibits the transcription of genes for cytokines, including interleukin-2 (IL-2) and interferon-γ.[161] It has many other toxic effects on several tissues,

including the brain and kidney. The attribution of immune dysregulation as causal in aplastic anemia based on therapy must be tempered with caution because ATG and cyclosporine exert multiple effects in addition to immunosuppression. The diverse antibodies in ATG react with a wide range of antigens, including signal transduction and adhesion molecules.[162] The component or components of ATG active in aplastic anemia have not been isolated. Of note, therapies with mixtures of monoclonal antibodies specific for human T cells have not been effective in clinical trials to date (reviewed by Tisdale and colleagues[163]). Furthermore, ATG can increase colony growth in normal, myelodysplastic syndrome (MDS), and aplastic anemia CD34$^+$ bone marrow cells in culture.[164,165] ATG treatment also reduces the expression of Fas antigen on aplastic anemia bone marrow CD34$^+$ cells.[166] Cyclosporine is thought to be more specifically immunosuppressive than ATG, and thus its efficacy further implicates T-cell participation in the pathophysiology of aplastic anemia. Nonetheless, cyclosporine therapy also has a broad range of additional effects. Effective treatment of myelodysplasia with cyclosporine has recently been reported and may suggest that cyclosporine may exert additional effects on bone marrow,[167] although a possible immune mechanism underlying myelodysplasia is also under investigation.[168]

A role for immune dysregulation in aplastic anemia in some patients is further supported by several studies of T-cell characteristics in aplastic anemia. Activated cytotoxic lymphocyte clones have been isolated from patients with aplastic anemia, and in vitro they overproduce inhibitory cytokines and inhibit hematopoiesis.[169-171] Altered helper and cytotoxic T-cell profiles have been reported in patients with aplastic anemia.[172-174] Identification of a T-cell clone with HLA-DRB10405–restricted cytotoxicity for hematopoietic cells has been reported in one patient with aplastic anemia.[175] Analysis of the CDR3 region of CD4 cells derived from patients with aplastic anemia and an HLA-DR2 haplotype showed a high frequency of clones bearing identical CDR3 DNA sequences that were not found in normal controls.[176] A recent flow cytometry study[177] in which antibodies against different TCR V$_\beta$ subfamilies were used and the CDR3 region of the TCR β chain was sequenced described dominant T-cell clones in aplastic anemia patients. The size of these clones and the total number of T cells decreased after successful treatment with ATG and increased with relapse. The V$_\beta$3 CD8$^+$ cell fraction of one patient with aplastic anemia induced increased levels of apoptosis of autologous bone marrow cells, whereas the V$_\beta$3-depleted CD8$^+$ T-cell fraction did not induce autologous apoptosis but continued to be cytotoxic for allogeneic bone marrow mononuclear cells. All of these findings, though suggestive, could also represent secondary manifestations of whatever inciting damage caused the aplastic anemia in the first place. Direct demonstration of genetically restricted suppression of hematopoiesis by a unique subset of T lymphocytes, as has been shown for PRCA,[178] remains a critical area of future active investigation for acquired aplastic anemia.

Lymphokines

Whether overproduction or dysregulated production of inhibitory cytokines represents a primary cause versus a secondary effect of an underlying bone marrow abnormality remains unclear. Interferon-γ, a soluble inhibitor produced by T cells, was found to be produced at high levels in culture from aplastic anemia patients.[179-181] Interferon-γ is expressed in the marrow of most patients with aplastic anemia but not in normal persons or those with other hematologic diseases who have undergone frequent transfusions.[182,183] High pretreatment intracellular interferon-γ levels correlated with response to immunosuppressive therapy (IST).[184a] Other inhibitory cytokines, such as *tumor necrosis factor*[185] and *macrophage inflammatory protein-1*,[186,187] are also overexpressed in patients with aplastic marrow. Both interferon and tumor necrosis factor directly and synergistically inhibit hematopoiesis in vitro.[188] In long-term bone marrow culture, constitutive low-level expression of interferon-γ is sufficient to markedly reduce the output of both committed progenitor cells and LTC-ICs, the stem cell surrogate.[189] Both interferon and tumor necrosis factor enhance the potential for programmed cell death within the CD34+ compartment by increasing Fas antigen expression on target cells.[190] Fas antigen is a cell surface molecule in the tumor necrosis factor receptor family; its activation signals apoptosis.

Microenvironment

In theory, aplastic anemia could be due to a microenvironment that fails to support hematopoiesis—a lesion of "soil" rather than "seed."[72] The anemia of the Sl/Sl[d] murine strain, which is missing stem cell factor (SCF), the ligand for the c-kit receptor, is an example of such a defect.[191] Although defects in some stromal cell function have occasionally been measured in patients, these defects do not appear to be causative in most cases. After marrow transplantation, most stromal cell elements remain of host origin,[192] yet these cells adequately support the donor's stem cells. In the laboratory, aplastic marrow usually provides normal adherent cell function in long-term or Dexter flask-type cultures; however, a patient's marrow is a poor source of clonogenic cells when grown on normal stroma, consistent with the defect in stem and progenitor cell numbers described earlier.[193] Some investigators have reported low fibroblast colony formation in aplastic anemia,[194] but this assay may not reflect stromal cell function.

Hematopoietic growth factor production and plasma levels are usually increased rather than decreased in patients with aplastic anemia (reviewed by Koijima[195]). Circulating levels of erythropoietin, granulocyte colony-stimulating factor (G-CSF) and granulocyte-macrophage colony-stimulating factor (GM-CSF), thrombopoietin, and flt-3 ligand are elevated in patients with aplastic

anemia. SCF levels have been reported to be low to normal. Levels of IL-1, produced by monocytes, may be low in aplastic anemia. Therapeutic trials with these factors have yielded divergent and incomplete responses (reviewed by Marsh[196]), thus casting doubt on the pathophysiologic significance of deficiency of these factors.

Clinical Evaluation

The differential diagnosis of pancytopenia is broad (Box 7-3). The evaluation and diagnostic workup of a patient with presumed acquired aplastic anemia should be directed at eliminating alternative diagnoses for which curative therapies are available or for which therapies for aplastic anemia would be inappropriate (Table 7-1). Because the inherited marrow failure syndromes entail different medical management issues, a careful medical history, family history, physical examination, and appropriate laboratory evaluation to assess for underlying inherited bone marrow failure syndromes should be pursued. The diagnosis of an inherited marrow failure syndrome also carries profound implications for selection of hematopoietic stem cell donors from family members and may be important for family planning. Given the

Box 7-3	Causes of Pancytopenia

HYPOCELLULAR BONE MARROW

Acquired aplastic anemia
Inherited bone marrow failure syndrome (Fanconi's anemia, amegakaryocytic thrombocytopenia, dyskeratosis congenita, Shwachman-Diamond syndrome)
Paroxysmal nocturnal hemoglobinuria
Hypoplastic myelodysplastic syndrome
Virus-associated aplastic anemia

CELLULAR BONE MARROW

Primary Bone Marrow Disease

Myelodysplasia
Paroxysmal nocturnal hemoglobinuria

Secondary to Systemic Disease

Systemic lupus erythematosus, Sjögren's syndrome
Hypersplenism
Vitamin B_{12}, folate deficiency
Infection
Storage disease (Gaucher, Niemann-Pick)
Alcoholism
Sarcoidosis

INFILTRATIVE BONE MARROW DISORDERS

Acute myelogenous leukemia
Acute lymphoblastic leukemia
Hemophagocytic lymphohistiocytosis
Metastatic solid tumors
Osteopetrosis
Myelofibrosis

TABLE 7-1 Clinical Evaluation	
Evaluation	**Rationale**
CLINICAL HISTORY	
Recent illnesses	Infectious cause
Medications	Marrow suppression
Exposure to toxins	Marrow suppression
Family history of blood disorders, malignancy, congenital anomalies	Assess for inherited marrow failure
PHYSICAL EXAMINATION	
Vital signs	Clinical sequelae of cytopenia
Height and weight	Assess for inherited marrow failure
Congenital anomalies, stigmata	Assess for inherited marrow failure
	Assess for other systemic diseases
LABORATORY TESTS	
Complete blood count and differential	Defines severity
Morphology	Malignant versus benign
	Vitamin B_{12} deficiency
	Storage disease
Reticulocyte count	Defines severity
	Differentiate production versus destruction
Bone marrow biopsy	Assess cellularity
	Assess architecture (granuloma, fibrosis, hemophagocytosis, infiltrative or metastatic disease)
Bone marrow aspirate	
Morphology	Malignant versus benign
	Storage disease
	Hemophagocytosis
	Congenital disorder
Cytogenetics	Myelodysplasia
Culture	Infectious agent (e.g., tuberculosis, virus)
Other	DNA/antigen-based viral tests
PERIPHERAL BLOOD CHEMISTRY	
AST, ALT, GGT, bilirubin, LDH	Hepatitis
Coombs' test	Autoimmune cytopenia
BUN, creatinine, electrolytes	Chronic renal failure
Serologic testing/PCR	Hepatitis, EBV, HIV, other virus
Flow cytometry for CD55/CD59	Paroxysmal nocturnal hemoglobinuria
Diepoxybutane or mitomycin C chromosomal breakage	Fanconi's anemia
Autoimmune disease evaluation	Evidence of collagen vascular disease
Histocompatibility testing of patient and family	Establish potential donor pool

ALT, alanine aminotransferase; AST, aspartate aminotransferase; BUN, blood urea nitrogen; EBV, Epstein-Barr virus; GGT, γ-glutamyltransferase; HIV, human immunodeficiency virus; LDH, lactate dehydrogenase; PCR, polymerase chain reaction.

Modified from Guinan E. Clinical aspects of aplastic anemia. Hematol Oncol Clin North Am. 1997;11:1028.

wide clinical variability of the inherited marrow failure syndromes, even among members of a given family, all siblings of a patient with an inherited marrow failure disorder should be tested regardless of whether they appear to carry clinical stigmata of the disease.

History

The chief initial symptoms relate to low blood counts. Bleeding, such as gum oozing, nosebleeds, easy bruising with minimal trauma, or heavy menses, may be seen. Chronic anemia may be manifested as fatigue, decreased activity, or exercise intolerance, although the gradual onset of severe anemia can be surprisingly well compensated in young children. Serious infection is not a frequent initial symptom early in the course of aplastic anemia. Many patients feel well with few symptoms at initial evaluation. A history of steatorrhea or fatty food intolerance may be a manifestation of Shwachman-Diamond syndrome. Gastrointestinal disorders may also be associated with other inherited marrow failures syndromes such as dyskeratosis congenita or Fanconi's anemia. A careful family history for blood disorders, malignancies, or congenital anomalies that might suggest an inherited bone marrow syndrome should be sought. A developmental history can provide helpful screening for potential congenital, metabolic, or storage diseases. A detailed medication, environmental, and infectious history should be obtained, especially for the preceding 1- to 12-month period.

Physical Examination

Clinical appearance is related to the severity and duration of the underlying pancytopenia. Hemorrhagic manifestations from thrombocytopenia occur early and include petechiae (particularly on the border of the hard and soft palate), ecchymoses, epistaxis, and bleeding from mucous membranes. Neutropenia may be associated with oral ulcerations, bacterial infections, and fever; these signs are rarely present early. Evidence of erythropoietic failure, such as pallor, fatigue, and tachycardia, often appears late because the life span of erythrocytes (120 days) far exceeds that of platelets (10 days) or white cells (variable, but measured in hours for granulocytes). Mucous membranes and nail beds may be pale. Lymphadenopathy, splenomegaly, and severe weight loss are uncommon and may suggest other underlying disorders. Short stature, congenital anomalies (especially of the thumbs and forearms), areas of hyperpigmentation or hypopigmentation, or dystrophic nails should alert the examiner to possible inherited bone marrow failure disorders.

Laboratory Studies

Evaluation should include a complete blood count, reticulocyte count, Coombs test to rule out autoimmune destruction, and biochemical profile, including renal and hepatic evaluation. Laboratory tests for possible infectious causes should be performed as indicated clinically.

Careful evaluation of the peripheral blood smear may suggest infection or dietary deficiency. Blood counts are most often uniformly depressed. The blood smear shows a paucity of platelets and leukocytes. The anemia is often macrocytic, although if erythropoiesis is arrested entirely, it may be normocytic. The red cell distribution width, a numeric measure of anisocytosis, is most often normal. Platelet size is not increased, as it is in most cases of immune thrombocytopenia. The absolute reticulocyte count is decreased. Granulocyte numbers are clearly diminished, as may be those of monocytes and lymphocytes.[197,198] Increases in fetal hemoglobin (HbF) and red cell i antigen are manifestations of the fetal-like erythropoiesis seen in "stress" hematopoiesis[199] but occur irregularly in patients with aplastic anemia, have no prognostic value, and can persist in recovered patients.

Blood chemistry panels should be used to evaluate hepatic and renal function. Blood tests to rule out Fanconi's anemia and PNH are important because these diagnoses would entail alternative treatments. A growing array of genetic testing is available to assist in the diagnosis of many of the inherited marrow failure syndromes (see Chapter 8). Patients with stigmata of collagen vascular disease should be appropriately evaluated. Early HLA typing of the patient and family members is helpful in guiding future therapies.

Bone marrow examination must be done by both aspiration and biopsy so that cellularity can be evaluated both qualitatively and quantitatively. The bone marrow in patients with aplastic anemia is hypocellular with empty spicules and increased fat, reticulum cells, plasma cells, and mast cells (Fig. 7-2). Some dyserythropoiesis with megaloblastosis and nuclear-cytoplasmic asynchrony may be seen. Aspirates alone may appear hypocellular because of dilution with peripheral blood, or they may look hypercellular because of areas of focal residual hematopoiesis. Biopsies provide more reliable specimens for assessment of cellularity, as well as critical information regarding bone marrow architecture, such as fibrosis or granulomas. Bone marrow aspirates should also be sent for cytogenetics and possibly fluorescent in situ hybridization (FISH) to assess for abnormalities associated with myelodysplasia or malignancy. In addition, bone marrow may be sent for culture or DNA-based antigen detection of infectious agents such as viruses.

Management and Outcome

Prognosis

Outcome depends on the types of treatments offered, the causes of the aplasia, and the eras and countries being analyzed. In a large series conducted before 1957, Wolff found a survival rate of only 3%.[200] In other series ending no later than 1965, complete recovery was reported in 10% to 35% of patients. In a series of 40 pediatric patients seen before 1958, Diamond and Shahidi found that only 2 patients recovered, 1 of whom suffered recurrence,[201] although these studies may have included patients with moderate disease, for whom spontaneous recovery is more common.[202,203] The long-term prognosis is adversely affected by delayed complications such as clonal disease. A recent study[204] described the natural history of 24 pediatric patients with moderate aplastic anemia monitored at St. Jude Children's Research Hospital for a median of 66 months (range, 10 to 293 months). Moderate aplastic anemia was defined as marrow hypoplasia of less than 50% and at least two cytopenias, such as an absolute neutrophil count less than 1500/mm³, a platelet count less than 100,000/mm³, or reticulocytopenic anemia lasting at least 6 weeks. Sixteen patients (67%) progressed to severe aplastic anemia, 5 (21%) remained in the moderate range, and in 3 patients (12%) the aplastic anemia resolved. It is currently unclear whether early institution of therapy for moderate aplastic anemia confers an improved outcome. Because current therapies are associated with significant side effects, their use in children with moderate aplastic anemia, for whom the marrow aplasia may resolve spontaneously, warrants careful consideration.

Spontaneous Recovery

Spontaneous recovery from aplastic anemia has been reported anecdotally, although most cases were probably moderate rather than severe. Good supportive care (see later) may contribute to such recovery; in one series 14 of 33 children recovered,[205] and children with moderate aplastic anemia have been found to have an excellent prognosis, even without specific treatment.[206] A study of IST in which 21 patients were randomized (some to receive only supportive care) found no improvement in the control group after 3 months.[207] Spontaneous recovery is sufficiently rare in patients with severe aplastic anemia that all modalities of current therapy should be initiated.

Supportive Care

Blood product support should be used judiciously to avoid sensitization, and blood product donors should never be from the patient's family for the same reason. Complete red cell phenotyping is recommended when feasible to minimize the potential risk of erythrocyte antibodies in patients who may receive long-term blood product support. All blood products should be filtered and irradiated. Exposure to potentially hazardous drugs or toxins should be eliminated.

Bleeding

Platelet (and red cell) support has probably had the greatest impact on survival in patients with aplastic anemia and has changed the cause of death from bleeding to infection. Platelets can be provided from several individual units of blood or, preferably, by plateletpheresis from a single donor to reduce antigenic exposure (see Chapter 35).

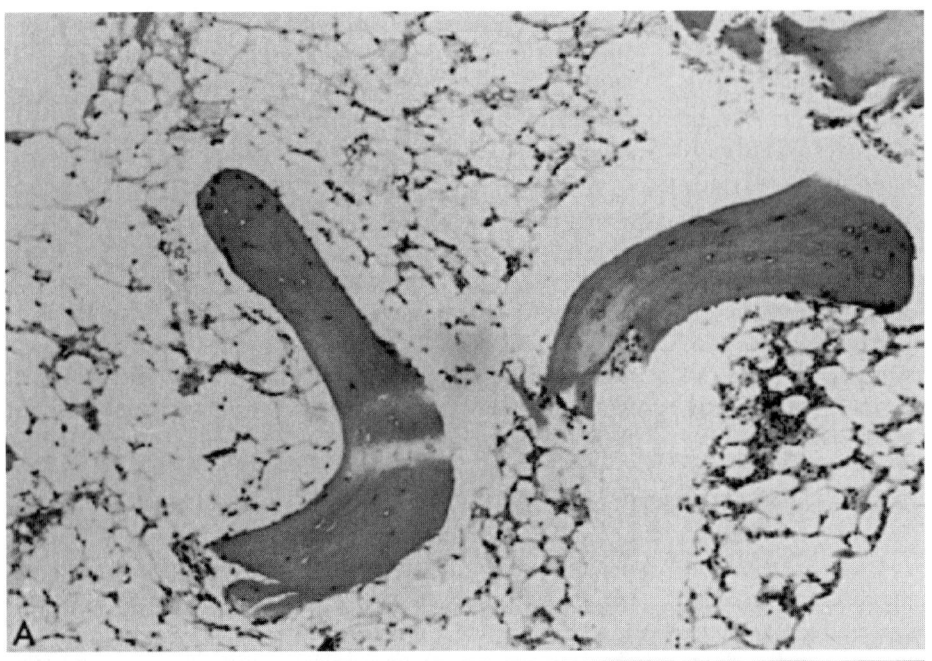

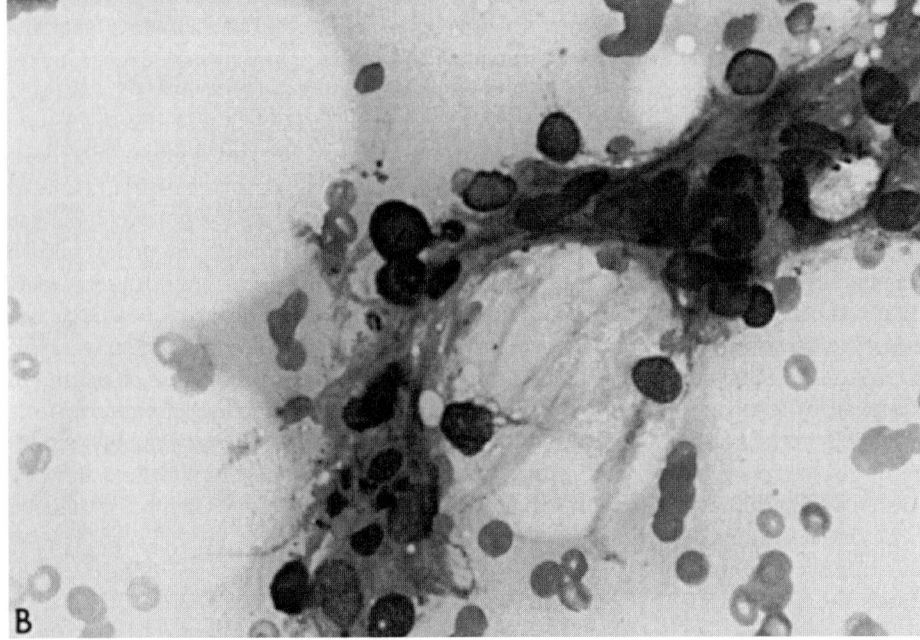

FIGURE 7-2. Bone marrow examination in severe aplastic anemia. **A,** Note the hypocellularity in a biopsy specimen. **B,** Residual cells seen in the aspirate are lymphocytes, stromal cells, plasma cells, and mast cells. *(Courtesy of Dr. Gail Wolfe, Boston.)*

The main role of prophylactic platelet support is reduction of the risk for intracranial hemorrhage, which is a rare but potentially devastating event. The general threshold platelet count has traditionally been 20,000 cells/μL; however, this figure and the entire practice of prophylactic administration of platelet transfusions have been questioned.[208-210] Platelet transfusions at platelet counts below 10,000/μL in stable outpatients with chronic severe aplastic anemia was shown to be feasible and safe in a recent study.[211] Chronic platelet transfusions for aplastic anemia are generally given when the patient has symptoms of bleeding or is at increased risk for bleeding (e.g., toddlers learning to walk, patients with hypertension while taking cyclosporine, patients with fever and infection, recent treatment with ATG).

Other measures to reduce bleeding include maintenance of good dental hygiene, use of a soft toothbrush, stool softeners, and avoidance of trauma. Drugs that may interfere with platelet function, such as aspirin or nonsteroidal anti-inflammatory medications, should be avoided in patients with thrombocytopenia. Antifibrinolytic agents such as aminocaproic acid and tranexamic acid may decrease bleeding, particularly from the gums and nasal mucosa.

Infections

There are few reported studies of infection in patients with aplastic anemia.[212-214] Severe granulocytopenia may last for years. However, the immune systems of granulocytopenic patients remain intact, in contrast to the situation in patients with malignancies who undergo chemotherapy and experience simultaneous neutropenia and immunosuppression. Neutropenia (and perhaps monocytopenia) increases the risk for bacterial infection in patients with aplastic anemia.[197] Because neutropenia precludes the development of an inflammatory response, identification of an infected locus is often difficult. The bacterial organisms may be gram-negative bacilli such as *Escherichia coli*, *Klebsiella pneumoniae*, or *Pseudomonas aeruginosa*, as well as gram-positive cocci, including *Staphylococcus aureus*, *Streptococcus epidermidis*, and other streptococci. Immunosuppression as a result of preparation for BMT or as primary therapy for aplastic anemia may lead to unusual bacterial, fungal, viral, and protozoal infections. Recommendations for specific antibiotics and other anti-infection agents are beyond the scope of this chapter, and regimens are changing rapidly as new generations of treatment are developed.

The use of prophylactic antibiotics has no role in a "well" patient with aplastic anemia. Patients undergoing IST should receive prophylaxis for *Pneumocystis carinii*. In the context of fever and neutropenia, complete evaluation and culture of all possible sites should be followed by the administration of broad-spectrum parenteral antibiotics. Fungal infections occur frequently in neutropenic patients who have received repeated or extended courses of antibiotics; candidiasis and especially aspergillosis, which lead to sinusitis, lung disease, or disseminated infection, are distressingly frequent causes of death in those with aplastic anemia.[212] Antecedent or concurrent administration of steroids increases this risk. Aggressive introduction of antifungal treatment is indicated in a persistently febrile patient who is unresponsive to antibiotics or in the appropriate clinical setting.

Anemia

Red cells should be provided as clinically indicated. Hemoglobin should be maintained at a level consistent with normal activities if routine transfusions are to be used. Chronic anemia can be well tolerated once adaptation has occurred, and some children who can sustain a hemoglobin level greater than 6 to 7 g/dL without transfusions (i.e., a child who is not bleeding) may be carefully observed. Long-term transfusions lead to iron overload with accumulation in critical organs. Permanent damage to the heart, liver, and endocrine glands from iron overload may be prevented by iron chelation therapy.[215]

Treatment

Bone Marrow Transplantation

The general topic of BMT is described in Chapter 9. The discussion that follows is limited to the role of BMT in the treatment of aplastic anemia.

The earliest transplants for aplastic anemia involved identical twins. Subsequent definition of the human histocompatibility gene complex, the development of immunosuppressive regimens, and improved support of severely

pancytopenic patients led to more general application of this form of therapy. Stem cell transplantation between identical twins in the absence of any conditioning regimen was curative in around 50% of cases.[138-141] A recent study showed that the highest long-term survival with identical twin transplants was achieved by using an algorithm of initial transplantation without conditioning followed by a subsequent transplant with conditioning for any patients demonstrating engraftment failure with the first transplant. None of the patients in whom the first transplant failed died before receiving a second transplant, and mortality was similar to that in patients who received conditioning up-front.[141] The European Group for Blood and Marrow Transplantation (EBMT) recently reported actuarial 5-year survival rates among syngeneic twin transplants performed between 1976 and 1998 to be 91%.

Initial outcomes with cyclophosphamide regimens were associated with a high risk of graft rejection.[216] The combination of cyclophosphamide and radiation therapy improved engraftment rates but was limited by increased toxicity and increased rates of GVHD associated with radiation therapy.[217,218] The combination of ATG and cyclophosphamide together with the use of cyclosporine to prevent GVHD and increased stem cell infusion doses have resulted in lower rates of graft rejection (3.7% in one recent series of 81 patients).[219] Exposure to blood products before transplantation was associated with an increased risk for allosensitization and subsequent graft rejection. The detrimental role of transfusions may have decreased with the routine use of leukocyte-free products, as well as with strict avoidance of the use of family members as donors.[220] The addition of fludarabine, a highly immunosuppressive nucleoside analogue, has yielded high rates of engraftment, even in heavily pretransfused patients with aplastic anemia.[221] Outcomes of HLA-matched allogeneic BMT have been reported by large registries, which combine the results of many contributing centers, or in single-center studies by the largest referral centers.[222,223] Recent studies of transplants from HLA-matched family donors report survival rates of up to 88% to 97% with 4 to 10 years of follow-up in children (Table 7-2).[218,219,224,225] Transplantation in patients of advanced age is associated with lower survival and increased rates of GVHD.

GVHD remains another factor limiting outcomes after matched sibling transplants.[226] The reader is referred to Chapter 9 for a full discussion of GVHD. Secondary solid tumors may arise after BMT, with a cumulative incidence of 10% 15 years after transplantation noted in a recent report.[218] Nine of the 11 tumors reported in that study arose in patients who underwent a radiation-containing conditioning regimen. The cyclophosphamide-based conditioning regimens currently reported for matched sibling transplants for aplastic anemia are generally associated with few long-term effects. Growth and development, endocrine function (thyroid and adrenal), and long-term gonadal function (ovarian and testicular)

TABLE 7-2   **Representative Recent Allogeneic Transplantation Studies That Include Pediatric Patients**

Study	Years	Patients	Age (yr)	Years of Follow-up (Median and Range)	Conditioning Regimen (n)	Graft Rejection/ Failure	Graft-versus-Host Disease	Survival	Malignancy
Kojima et al. (Japan)[224]	1984-1998	37	Median, 10 (range, 0-16)	7.4 (0.5-13.8)	Cy, TLI (22) Cy, ATG (9) Cy, ATG, TLI (2)	0	6% acute 3% chronic	97%	0
Gupta et al. (UK)[225]	1989- 2003	33	Median, 17 (range, 4-46)	4.9	Cy, anti-CD52	24%	14% acute, 4% chronic	81%	1 EBV LPS
Ades et al. (France)[218]	1978- 2001	143	73 < 20 yr 60 > 20 yr	15.9 ± 0.7 (Cy-TAI) 4.4 ± 0.8 (Cy-ATG)	Cy-TAI (100) Cy-ATG (33)	3%	79% chronic	58.7% ± 5.2% at 15 years; >90% with Cy-ATG	10.9% (9/100 Cy-TAI, 2/33 Cy-ATG)
Kahl et al. (Seattle)[219]	1988- 2004	81	25.1 (range, 2-63)	9.2 (0.5-16.4)	Cy-ATG	3.70%	24% acute, 26% chronic	88%	1 EBV LPS. 5 solid tumors

ATG, antithymocyte globulin; Cy, cyclophosphamide; EBV LPS, Epstein-Barr virus lymphoproliferative syndrome; TAI, total abdominal irradiation; TLI, total lymphoid irradiation.

are typically preserved. The use of myeloablative radiation-containing regimens may be associated with growth compromise, endocrine dysfunction, and irreversible gonadal failure.[227,228]

The preceding discussion refers to transplants from HLA-matched sibling donors; however, 75% to 80% of transplant patients do not have such a donor. Alternative donors include HLA-matched but unrelated volunteers, phenotypically but not genotypically matched relatives, and partially matched (mismatched) donors. Umbilical cord blood provides an alternative source of stem cells for hematopoietic stem cell transplantation and is discussed in Chapter 9. Ongoing advances in high-resolution HLA typing techniques continue to improve selection of HLA-matched donors. The reader is referred to Chapter 9 for a general discussion of alternative donor bone marrow transplants. Currently, long-term survival after alternative donor stem cell transplantation for aplastic anemia has generally been lower (<50% long-term survival rate) than that after matched sibling donor transplantation.[229] The risk of graft rejection is greater, the higher-intensity conditioning regimens required to promote engraftment entail greater treatment-related toxicity, and the risk for GVHD is higher. The longer delay from diagnosis to transplantation for unrelated donor transplants might also contribute to the higher risk.

Studies to reduce regimen-related toxicity while preserving engraftment are ongoing. Replacement of radiation therapy with fludarabine together with cyclophosphamide and ATG in 38 patients with aplastic anemia undergoing transplantation with an unrelated or family mismatched donor yielded low rates of acute (11%) and chronic (24%) GVHD, but graft failure or rejection rates (18%) remained relatively high. The actuarial 2-year survival rate was 73%.[230] A prospective multi-center study of 87 unrelated donor transplant patients (median age of 18.6 years) who had previously failed therapy for aplastic anemia investigated the effects of de-escalating the dose of radiation from 600-cGy total body irradiation (TBI) down to 200-cGy TBI given together with cyclophosphamide (200 mg/kg) with or without ATG. Engraftment was preserved at the lowest TBI dose, with a graft failure rate of only 2% for HLA-matched unrelated donor transplants. The survival rate was 61% (38/62) for HLA-matched and 40% (10/25) for HLA-mismatched transplant recipients at a median follow-up of 7 years. Outcomes were better for younger patients (<20 years of age), who had a 5-year survival rate of 73%. Rates of GVHD, however, were comparable across all radiation doses (69% to 77% with grade II to IV acute GVHD; 52% to 57% with chronic GVHD). Additional trials are ongoing to investigate whether replacement of cyclophosphamide with fludarabine might reduce toxicity while preserving engraftment.[231] Additional strategies include T-cell depletion[232] (with its attendant high risk of rejection), anti-CD52 antibody,[233] or haploidentical CD34 selection,[234] and research in this field is actively ongoing.

Immunosuppression

Antithymocyte Globulin. ALG and ATG (the sera produced by immunization of horses or rabbits with human thoracic duct lymphocytes or thymocytes) are highly cytotoxic reagents with activity against all blood and marrow cells, including progenitors. These reagents were initially used to decrease the rate of rejection of HLA-matched bone marrow. ALG, cyclophosphamide, or both were also used to permit at least temporary engraftment with mismatched marrow in aplastic patients without a matched donor.[158,159,160,2354,236] Autologous recovery occurred in some of these patients, which encouraged several groups to examine the use of ATG or ALG with and without haploidentical BMT. Treatment with ALG was superior to controls in both response rate and 3-year survival.[207] The use of other agents in addition to ALG therapy can further enhance the therapeutic effect.

ATG or ALG/antilymphocyte serum is often given up to a total cumulative dose of 100 to 160 mg/kg, typically divided over 4 days. Immediate allergic reactions to ALG are rare and can be predicted by skin testing, followed by desensitization in those who are allergic.[237] The patient begins to make antibodies to horse protein about 1 week after the first exposure, at which point equine antibodies are rapidly cleared from the circulation. This reduces the effective dose and enhances immune complex formation. *Serum sickness* as a result of immune complex deposition may be manifested around 11 days after initiation of treatment as fever, a serpiginous rash at the volar-dorsal border of the hands and feet, arthralgia, myalgia, lassitude, and changes in urine sediment. Bronchospasm or liver chemistry abnormalities may also occur. A short course of corticosteroids is usually given (prednisone, 1 mg/kg) to reduce ATG-related side effects. ATG binds to determinants on all cell types in blood and marrow, reduces platelet and granulocyte counts in addition to the lymphocyte counts, and may lead to a positive Coombs test. Thrombocytopenia may require intensive blood product support during this time.[238]

Responses to ATG given as a single agent usually occur within the first 3 months, if at all, and blood count improvement by 3 months correlates with survival.[239] The earliest response to therapy may be heralded by the appearance of a few granulocytes and nucleated red cells in the circulation. Red cell size distribution histograms typically show a macrocytic shoulder.[240] Reticulocytes appear, transfusions decline, and the hemoglobin level increases slowly. The white cell count rises next. The last cell line to return to normal is often the platelets, whose numbers may remain low for months or even years. The recovering red cells are not normal; in addition to macrocytosis, HbF levels are increased and fetal membrane antigens may remain present.[241] Long-term survivors (except those with successful transplants) often have residual abnormalities such as thrombocytopenia, red cell macrocytosis, and elevated HbF levels.[242] Clearly, we do not understand either the mechanism of action of this poorly characterized drug, the ultimate course of patients with ATG-induced remission, or the basis of their partial recovery.

Cyclosporine. Cyclosporine (formerly cyclosporin A) is a fungal cyclic undecapeptide and an effective immunosuppressive agent.[243] Among its many effects, cyclosporine can inhibit T cells and thereby prevent production of IL-2 and interferon-γ.[161] About half of the patients who had failed ATG or ALG treatment subsequently experienced remission with cyclosporine.[244,245] Treatment with cyclosporine alone yielded significantly lower response rates and higher rates of disease progression than did treatment with combined therapy.[246,247]

Oral cyclosporine should be administered twice daily to maintain blood trough levels between 100 and 250 ng/mL as measured by radioimmunoassay, although target levels may vary depending on the laboratory methods used to determine cyclosporine levels. Hematologic responses can take weeks to months, and an initial trial period of 3 to 6 months is generally recommended.

Toxic effects from the use of cyclosporine are not insignificant and include hypertension, hypertensive encephalopathy, azotemia, hirsutism, gingival hypertrophy, coarsening of facial features, tremor, immunodeficiency, increase in serum creatinine levels, transient or irreversible nephrotoxicity, hepatotoxicity, seizures, and *P. carinii* pneumonia.[243] As with ATG, in vitro tests of the effect of cyclosporine on progenitor cells do not predict responses.[248]

Combination Immunosuppressive Therapy. The combination of ATG with cyclosporine has resulted in higher rates of hematologic recovery than with either drug alone.[246,247,249] Importantly, intensive IST has greatly improved the results of therapy in two groups commonly refractory to ALG or ATG alone: patients with very severe disease and children.[250,251] In the National Institutes of Health (NIH) Clinical Center trial,[252] survival curves of those older and younger than 35 years were similar. A large study including both children and adults at the NIH reported a response rate of 67% at 43 months and a 5-year actuarial survival rate of 70% (86% for responders and 16% for nonresponders).[253] The EBMT Working Party on Severe Aplastic Anemia and the Gruppo Italiano Trapianto di Midollo Osseo (GITMO) study of 100 patients, including children (median age, 16 years), with severe aplastic anemia treated with ALG, cyclosporine, prednisolone, and G-CSF found a trilineage hematopoietic response in 77% after one or more courses of ALG.[254] Several trials in children have reported the efficacy of combined ATG and cyclosporine in the pediatric population with an overall response rate of close to 80%.[250,251,255-257]

ATG is typically given over a period of 4 days in combination with a 6- to 12-month course of cyclosporine. The lack of a unified definition for response complicates comparison of different studies, but in general, a complete response refers to normal or functionally normal blood counts, a partial response denotes hemoglobin and platelet counts adequate to avoid the need for transfusion and neutrophil counts typically greater than 500/μL, and no response commonly refers to continued severe aplastic anemia. Improvements in blood counts are delayed and may not be evident for many weeks. In a study including both children and adults, response rates, defined as at least a partial response in two blood cell lineages, were 67% at 3 months and 71% at 6 months after initiation of combined ATG and cyclosporine therapy.[252] Cyclosporine should be tapered gradually with close monitoring of blood counts before each decrease in dosage. A persistent drop in blood counts can often be treated by either an increase in cyclosporine dosage or reinitiation of the full dose. Some patients require continuous cyclosporine, and these patients should be maintained on the lowest effective dose. In a review of ongoing trials by the German multicenter group and the NIH, 29% and 14% of initial responders, respectively, were found to require continuous treatment.[252] Reoccurrence of frank pancytopenia generally requires a second course of ATG followed by full-dose cyclosporine. Patients treated with IST often continue to have subnormal counts and may remain macrocytic. Although the majority of patients respond within 6 months, delayed responses beyond that time may be seen in some patients.

About 20% to 40% of patients in pediatric studies fail to respond to ATG and cyclosporine therapy (Table 7-3), and a recent study of mostly adult patients reported failure to achieve response in around 40% of patients.[259] In most studies, failure of response is typically defined as persistence of severe aplastic anemia. In adult patients failing the first treatment with horse ATG, 63% of those receiving a second course of horse ATG responded,[260] and 77% (23/30) of those initially treated with horse ATG and cyclosporine responded to a second course of rabbit ATG and cyclosporine.[261] Less acute reactions were noted when the source of ATG was varied between the first and second treatments. The time frame to response after a second course of IST was similar to that observed after initial treatment. Patients failing to response to two courses of IST are unlikely to respond to a third treatment course.[262]

Because androgens are effective in treating some patients with aplastic anemia (see later), the effect of combining androgen treatment with ATG was examined in several trials. Champlin and associates reported no difference in response rate or survival in patients with moderate to severe aplastic anemia.[263] Studies by Kaltwasser and colleagues[264] and the EBMT[265] found significantly higher response rates after ALG plus androgens (73% and 56%) than after ALG alone (31% and 40%). A recent retrospective study in adults reported an overall response rate of 77% and overall survival rate of 78% 5 years after treatment with ATG plus androgens.[266] Because some patients with inherited causes of aplastic

---

TABLE 7-3   Pediatric Studies of Immunosuppressive Therapy for Aplastic Anemia

Study	Years	Patient Number	Treatment	Follow-up (yr)	Response	Survival	Relapse	Clonal Abnormality
Fuher et al.[255]	1993-1997	86 (49 vSAA, 30 SAA, 7 MAA)	ALG, Cy, G-CSF	4	80% (OR)	87%	15%	3% clonal abnormalities, 4.7% AML
Kojima et al.[250]	1992-1997	119 (50 vSAA, 36 SAA, 33 MAA)	ATG, Cy, DAN, ± G-CSF	4	71% (OR) vSAA, 61% (OR) SAA + G-CSF, 83% (OR) SAA − G-CSF	83% vSAA, 91-93% MAA + SAA	13% vSAA, 29% MAA/SAA + G-CSF, 64% MAA/SAA − G-CSF	3%
Kojima et al.[258]	1992-1997	113 (39 vSAA, 47 SAA, 27 MAA)	ATG, Cy, DAN, ± G-CSF	Median, 5.3; range, 3.75-8.9	30% CR, 31% PR, 42% NR at 6 months	87%	NR	13.7% cumulative incidence of MDS at 8 years, 21.9% cumulative incidence of clonal cytogenetic abnormalities at 8 years
Goldenberg et al.[257]	1990-2003	14	ATG, Cy ± G-CSF	Median, 4.4; range, 0.8-13.3	93% (OR)	93%	0	0
Fuher et al.[251]	1993-2001	97 vSAA / 49 SAA	ATG, Cy, G-CSF	Median, 4.1	69% (CR) vSAA / 44% (CR) SAA	93% vSAA / 81% SAA	13% vSAA / 14% SAA	NR / NR

ALG, antilymphocyte globulin; ATG, antithymocyte globulin; CR, complete response; Cy, cyclosporine; DAN, danazol; G-CSF, granulocyte colony-stimulating factor; MAA, moderate aplastic anemia; MDS, myelodysplastic syndrome; NR, not reported; OR, overall response; PR, partial response; SAA, severe aplastic anemia; vSAA, very severe aplastic anemia.

anemia may experience hematologic improvement after androgen therapy,[267] it is important to rule out an underlying inherited marrow failure syndrome. The side effects of androgen may be unacceptable to some patients, and their use for acquired aplastic anemia in children is generally limited.

Relapse. Relapse after IST has been reported in around a third of patients in studies that include both children and adults,[258,268] although lower rates of relapse may be attained with slow tapering of cyclosporine and continued maintenance doses at the lowest required cyclosporine dose for some patients. Lack of standardized definitions of relapse hamper comparison between studies. An EBMT study including both children and adults reported an actuarial risk for relapse of 35% at 14 years.[269] Relapses were observed up to 10 years after treatment. Disease severity, age, sex, and cause were not predictive of relapse. Large studies of relapse risk after IST in the pediatric population are scarce. The results of these studies are summarized in Table 7-3.

Tichelli and co-workers studied the efficacy of repeated treatment with ALG in patients with severe aplastic anemia who either failed to respond to an initial course of ALG or experienced hematologic relapse.[260] Independence from transfusion was achieved in 63% and the probability of survival was 52% ± 8% at 10 years. No differences were noted between patients retreated for nonresponse versus relapse. No increases in acute toxicity were noted with additional courses of ALG, although the timing of serum sickness tended to be earlier after repeat ALG administration. Relapse had little effect on survival in patients responding to reinstitution of immunosuppression. A study of 22 patients refractory to combined ATG/cyclosporine reported an overall response rate of only 30% at 6 months. This study included two refractory patients younger than 18 years, neither of whom responded to a second course of IST. Of 21 patients relapsing after ATG/cyclosporine treatment, an overall response rate of 65% was observed.[270] A retrospective study of 18 relapsed or refractory patients reported responses to a third course of an ATG-containing regimen only in those who had previously responded to a prior course of treatment.[262]

Complications of Immunosuppressive Therapy. Patients treated for aplastic anemia with IST have an increased risk for the development of clonal hematopoietic disorders (reviewed elsewhere[271,2720]). Because ATG and cyclosporine are not associated with an increased risk for MDS or leukemia in patients treated for other disorders, these complications are believed to result from the underlying dyspoiesis of aplastic anemia. In an analysis of 860 aplastic anemia patients treated with immunosuppression, 42 malignant conditions were reported, including 19 cases of PNH, 11 cases of myelodysplasia, 15 cases of acute leukemia, 7 solid tumors, and 1 non-Hodgkin's lymphoma.[273] Of 748 aplastic anemia patients

treated by transplantation, nine malignancies were reported: two acute leukemias and seven solid tumors. The cumulative incidence of a malignant tumor developing at 10 years was 18.8% after immunosuppression and 3.1% after transplantation. A recent NIH study of 122 patients treated with immunosuppression showed a 33% actuarial risk of a clonal hematopoietic disorder developing at 10 years.[4] An increased risk for clonal abnormalities as high as 21.9%[258] has been reported in some studies of pediatric patients with aplastic anemia. An increased risk for MDS or acute myelogenous leukemia has also been observed in pediatric patients (Table 7-3). Although an association between the use of G-CSF and risk of clonal disease has been observed,[258] in the absence of randomized studies, the question of causality remains unanswered. These data suggest that a clonal transformation of stem cells may underlie aplastic anemia, at least in a subset of patients. Prolonged survival with ATG/ALG/cyclosporine may permit the expected clonal evolution.

Transplantation versus Immunosuppression

The decision to treat with immunosuppression versus an HLA-identical sibling stem cell transplant for the 25% of patients for whom a suitable donor is available is based on consideration of the risks and benefits, which vary according to patient age and neutrophil count. Up-front toxicities associated with the conditioning regimens, GVHD, and graft rejection are the major problems related to stem cell transplantation, but this treatment offers the potential for long-term cure. Immunosuppressive and cytotoxic therapy is associated with lower acute toxicity but often yields incomplete hematologic recovery and is accompanied by late mortality from long-term complications such as relapse and clonal hematologic disorders. Comparison of outcomes after BMT and IST in children supports the benefit of HLA-matched sibling stem cell transplantation. Kojima and co-authors[224] reported a study of 100 children younger than 17 years with aplastic anemia between 1984 and 1998. Thirty-seven patients received allogeneic bone marrow transplants and 63 received IST with either ATG plus danazol or ATG and cyclosporine with or without danazol. Some patients also received G-CSF. Eleven patients initially treated with IST received subsequent salvage treatment with an unrelated donor transplant. The projected 10-year survival rate was 55% ± 8% with IST and 97% ± 35% with transplantation. The failure-free survival rate at 10 years was 40% ± 8% for the IST group and 97% ± 3% for the transplant group. MDS with monosomy 7 developed in seven patients in the IST group, and the estimated 10-year cumulative incidence of MDS was 20% ± 7%.

A recent report from the EBMT analyzed 1765 patients with aplastic anemia who underwent initial treatment with either an HLA-identical sibling transplant or IST.[222] Analysis was performed on an "intent-to-treat" basis. Patients were 1 to 50 years of age and treated between 1974 and 1996. Five hundred eighty-three patients received HLA-identical sibling transplants and 1182 underwent IST. A comparison of IST versus BMT in patients stratified by age and neutrophil count showed superior failure-free survival with transplantation for children regardless of their neutrophil count. The advantage of transplantation increased with increasing follow-up time, most likely because of the ongoing risks of late relapse and evolution to myelodysplasia and leukemia in the group receiving IST. Children have lower mortality with stem cell transplantation and a longer post-treatment life expectancy, which places them at higher risk than older adults for late complications. Thus, the current recommendation is to treat young patients ($\leq$10 years) with HLA-identical sibling stem cell transplants when a suitable donor is available. Patients with severe disease also do better with BMT. It is important to note that many patients in these studies of long-term outcomes were treated before the development of current combined immunosuppressive regimens containing both ATG and cyclosporine.

For patients lacking a suitable HLA-matched sibling donor, treatment with ATG and cyclosporine is generally the preferred line of therapy given the higher risk of toxicity and morbidity associated with current alternative donor transplant regimens. For patients who fail to respond to an initial course of ATG and cyclosporine, either a second course of ATG/cyclosporine or an alternative donor hematopoietic stem cell transplant may be considered. The risks and benefits of each approach will vary for each patient, but the risks associated with prolonged delay to potential transplantation[274] should be weighed against the most current data on alternative donor regimens.

Hematopoietic Growth Factors

Although patients with aplastic anemia do not have a deficiency of most hematopoietic growth factors (see earlier), it was hypothesized that pharmacologic levels might stimulate hematopoiesis of one or more cell lines.[196] Small trials of GM-CSF, G-CSF, IL-3, IL-1, IL-6, and SCF in mostly adult patients with aplastic anemia do not support the use of growth factors as primary treatment of aplastic anemia, and serious side effects were noted with some agents. To date, no consistent benefit in terms of response rate or survival after the adjunctive use of growth factors such as G-CSF in immunosuppressive regimens has been observed.[250,275] No improvement in overall response rates were noted in a retrospective study of 18 pediatric patients receiving GM-CSF in addition to ATG and cyclosporine.[276] Responses to single or combined growth factors have been reported in a few refractory patients.

G-CSF is associated with flu-like symptoms, bone pain, and splenomegaly. Symptoms of "cytokine flu"—fever, rash, hives, headache, and myalgia—are common but do respond to acetaminophen or resolve with the passage of time. Bone pain may be a symptom of increased marrow activity, although this is more commonly seen with G-CSF. At higher doses, the severity of symptoms increases, and there may be evidence of visceral engorgement and fluid retention.

The potential risk of promoting or stimulating the development of abnormal hematopoietic clones leading to a further increased risk for myelodysplasia or leukemia after prolonged treatment with growth factors remains a concern in patients with aplastic anemia. Although associations between G-CSF treatment and the subsequent development of MDS and leukemia have been reported,[277] in the absence of randomized prospective trials, it is not clear whether this represents an effect of growth factor treatment or merely an association reflecting the natural history of aplastic anemia of sufficient severity to warrant the addition of G-CSF.

Androgens

Androgens no longer have a primary role in the management of aplastic anemia, unless the first-line therapies discussed earlier are unavailable or unsuccessful. As described previously, androgens have been used as adjuncts to immunosuppression.

The mechanism of action has been reviewed extensively by Gardner and Besa.[278] Androgens increase erythropoietin production[279] and stimulate erythroid stem cells.[280] Hemoglobin levels increase in normal males at puberty and in patients treated with androgens for arthritis or breast cancer or in old age. Shahidi and Diamond were the first to report success with testosterone,[281] and large confirmatory series were published in France[282] and Mexico.[283] However, later critical evaluations revealed no evidence supporting the use of androgens. Despite the use of androgens, greater than 75% mortality has been reported in children[204] and adults.[284] Androgen-treated patients often did not do as well as those who were not treated with these hormones.[203,285] The older publications often failed to distinguish patients with moderate and severe aplastic anemia. Camitta and co-workers performed a prospective, multicenter analysis beginning in 1974 and concluded that androgens (whether oral or intramuscular) were no more effective than supportive care alone for severe aplastic anemia.[286,287]

Improvement, if it occurs, is usually greatest in hematocrit, although increases in granulocyte and platelet counts may also be seen. Response may take weeks to months, and trials of at least 3 months are recommended before declaring a patient unresponsive. The major side effect of androgens is liver toxicity. Cholestatic jaundice and hepatomegaly are usually reversible. Peliosis hepatis (blood lakes) has been reported.[288] Hepatic tumors are a serious risk, although the pathologic picture is usually that of a benign adenoma; such tumors may be reversible when use of the androgen is discontinued. Other side effects include masculinization with hirsutism, baldness, deepening of the voice, and enlargement of the genitalia. Acne, flushing of the skin, nausea, and sodium and fluid retention also occur. The appetite is stimulated, and there is weight gain with increased muscular development. The rate of skeletal maturation may be increased, with eventual premature fusion and ultimate short stature.[289] All patients who receive androgens should be monitored with frequent liver function testing, annual liver ultrasound examination, and annual bone age determination.

Corticosteroids

Modest doses of methylprednisolone are generally given during ATG or ALG treatment to lessen the side effects of serum sickness. As a single agent, very high doses of corticosteroids have been reported to lead to responses in a few patients.[290,291] Treatment with high-dose steroids is associated with substantial toxicity, including hypertension, hyperglycemia, fluid retention, potassium wasting, psychosis, aseptic necrosis of the femoral and humeral heads, and increased susceptibility to fungal infections. Given the higher response rate and lower toxicity profile of ATG, high-dose steroids are not recommended as first-line therapy for aplastic anemia.

Splenectomy

Splenectomies were performed until recently, perhaps for want of something better to offer to patients. A review in 1957 indicated improvement in 20 of 35 patients.[292] More recently, the operation has been performed to facilitate supportive care.[293] Unless there are clear indications of hypersplenism significantly impeding platelet and red cell transfusion support, the operation does not seem warranted.

Other Therapies

New therapeutic regimens are aimed at improving rates of hematologic response and minimizing acute and long-term complications of therapy.[163] The current status of a few investigational regimens is summarized in the following sections.

Cyclophosphamide

Administration of high doses of cyclophosphamide is effective IST and is not myeloablative in normal hosts. Historically, a few patients who received high-dose cyclophosphamide as preparation for BMT rejected their grafts and underwent autologous recovery. An early study of treatment with this drug without transplantation indicated a complete response in 7 of 10 patients treated with 45 mg/kg/day for 4 days.[294] A study of 19 previously untreated patients with aplastic anemia reported a 73% overall response rate at 24 months with a 65% probability of achieving a complete response at 50 months and an 85% survival rate at 24 months.[295] No relapses or clonal disorders were observed in the responding patients. A phase III prospective randomized trial compared high-dose cyclophosphamide plus cyclosporine with ATG plus cyclosporine as first-line therapy.[296] The trial was terminated prematurely because of invasive fungal infections and three early deaths in the group treated with cyclophosphamide plus cyclosporine (none were noted in the ATG/cyclosporine group). Responses at 6-month follow-up were seen in 6 of 13 (46%) patients treated with cyclophosphamide plus cyclosporine versus 9 of 12 (75%) treated with ATG plus cyclosporine. Trials of high-dose cyclophosphamide as a single agent in patients refractory to previous IST reported a 53% response rate and 59% survival rate at a median follow-up of 29 months.[297] The generally prolonged time to response and associated toxicity are potentially limiting factors, and additional studies are required to determine whether the development of long-term complications such as relapse or clonal disease will be less frequent than with ATG and cyclosporine.

Recombinant Humanized Anti–Interleukin-2 Receptor Antibody

The IL-2 receptor is found on activated T cells and is required for T-cell expansion.[298] A pilot study of 17 patients with moderate aplastic anemia treated for 3 months with a humanized monoclonal antibody against the IL-2 receptor (daclizumab) reported improved blood counts in 38% of patients.[299] Daclizumab was well tolerated with minimal side effects. Further studies on the use of daclizumab in patients with aplastic anemia are warranted.

Mycophenolate Mofetil

Mycophenolate mofetil (MMF, CellCept) is the prodrug of mycophenolic acid, which inhibits B- and T-cell proliferation through inhibition of inosine monophosphate dehydrogenase, which is involved in guanine nucleotide synthesis.[300] MMF has been in clinical use for prevention of solid organ transplant rejection and treatment of autoimmune diseases. Though generally well tolerated, side effects of MMF include leukopenia and marrow suppression. A study of 104 patients with severe aplastic anemia treated with ATG, cyclosporine, and MMF reported an overall response rate of 62% at 6 months.[301] Relapses were seen in 37% of responders, with more than half of relapses occurring while the patients were still receiving MMF. Clonal abnormalities were noted in 8.7% of patients after a median follow-up of 42 months. No difference in overall survival was noted between children and adults. The addition of MMF did not result in improved rates of response, relapse, or clonal abnormalities in comparison to those reported after treatment with ATG and cyclosporine.

ACQUIRED PURE RED CELL APLASIA

Acquired pure red cell aplasia (APRCA) is a term that embraces a range of incompletely understood aregenerative anemias (sometimes associated with neutropenia and thrombocytopenia) that must be considered in the differential diagnosis of congenital Diamond-Blackfan anemia (see Chapter 8). Unifying characteristics of this broad range of disorders are anemia and a paucity of

TABLE 7-4   Classification of Acquired Pure Red Cell Aplasia

Condition	Type	Mechanism		References
Parvovirus B19 infection	Acute TAC in hemolytic anemia Chronic in immunosuppressed Congenital	Direct infection of erythroid progenitors	P antigen	302-306
Immune	TEC Chronic (usually adults)—SLE, RA, HD, thymoma	Antibody	Red cell progenitors	307-309
	Thymoma			307
	ABO incompatibility after BMT		Blood group antigen A or B	
	EPO		Antibody to EPO	
	T-CLL	Cell mediated MHC restricted or MHC unrestricted	T cell	310
	LGL		T-LGL (CD3⁺/αβ or γδ TCR) or NK-LGL (CD3⁻TCR⁻)	178, 311, 312
Preleukemia and myelodysplasia	5q–	RPS14 haploinsufficiency + other genetic change		313
Drugs and toxins	Phenytoin, azathioprine, isoniazid	Unknown—direct or immune		314

BMT, bone marrow transplantation; EPO, erythropoietin; HD, hemodialysis; LGL, large granular lymphocyte; NK, natural killer; RA, rheumatoid arthritis; RPS, ribosomal protein of the small ribosomal subunit; SLE, systemic lupus erythematosus; TAC, transient aplastic crisis; T-CLL, T-cell chronic lymphatic leukemia; TCR, T-cell receptor; TEC, transient erythroblastopenia of childhood.

recognizable erythroid precursors in bone marrow. The anemia may be macrocytic if some residual "stress" erythropoiesis is present. If there is complete arrest of erythropoiesis, the anemia will be normocytic or even slightly microcytic and hyperchromic if the arrest of erythropoiesis has existed for 2 months or more because red cell volume shrinks as red cells age in the circulation. In some cases, particularly those associated with parvovirus infection, mild neutropenia and even thrombocytopenia may coexist with the anemia. Thus, the term "pure red cell aplasia" may be honored in the breech. APRCA may be classified as outlined in Table 7-4.

Parvovirus B19 Infection

Parvovirus B19 was identified as the cause of outbreaks of aplastic crises in sickle cell anemia patients in 1981.[302,303] This virus is most likely to have caused a similar disease in several earlier descriptions of anemia, fever, and malaise in patients with hereditary spherocytosis or elliptocytosis, immune hemolytic anemia, and thalassemia, to name a few of the conditions whose common feature is shortening of red cell life span.[315-318] Gasser[319] coined the term "transient aplastic crisis" and also noted the presence of gigantic proerythroblasts in bone marrow. Subsequent studies in volunteers established that the virus does not cause significant anemia in individuals with a normal red cell life span.[320] The main target of this small nonenveloped single-stranded DNA virus is the erythroid progenitor, which it enters through binding to the blood group P antigen. Antibodies

(IgM and IgG) to the viral capsid antigen VP1 are neutralizing and confer long-term immunity. Persistent B19 infection can occur in immunodeficient or immunosuppressed patients as a result of either congenital immunodeficiency, lymphoproliferative disorders, organ transplantation, or HIV infection.[304,305] Neutralizing antibodies to VP1 are absent or low and diagnosis requires demonstration of viral DNA in serum by hybridization assay. Fetal infection with parvovirus can lead to miscarriage, hydrops fetalis, or infants born with chronic anemia.[306]

Immune-Mediated Pure Red Cell Aplasia

Much of our understanding of APRCA seen in adults has been derived from the clinical research of Sanford Krantz and Emmanuel Dessypris and their colleagues at Vanderbilt University.[1] The reader is referred to Dr. Dessypris' excellent monograph for a history and reasonable classification and description of these arcane disorders.[321] A more recent set of reviews has been edited by Stephen A. Feig and Melvin H. Freedman[322] and an independent review has been presented by Fisch and associates.[323]

Acute Pure Red Cell Aplasia: Transient Erythroblastopenia of Childhood

Though probably described in the 1960s by Schmid and by DiGiacomo and their colleagues[324,325] who each reported a potpourri of cases of APRCA, transient erythroblastopenia of childhood (TEC) was first clearly enunciated by Wranne in 1970.[326] This frequent disease is well described by Glader in the book edited by Feig and Freedman.[322]

TEC is certainly the most common aregenerative anemia in childhood and is likely to be a very frequent complication of a host of relatively trivial viral infections. It is well established that erythropoiesis is briefly interrupted during such infections in most individuals. but anemia is not documented because the red cell life span is 120 days and the suppression usually lasts for only a week. In many patients the suppression is protracted, and anemia ensues. Spontaneous recovery without any treatment is virtually the rule, but confusion may result if the pediatrician sees the patient at the time of recovery when reticulocytosis is in full spate.[327] This may lead to a false diagnosis of hemolytic anemia and a gigantic, expensive, and totally unnecessary workup that simply produces more anemia in the blood as well as in the pocketbook. It is important to suspect TEC in an otherwise healthy child whose blood smear does not suggest a red cell disorder or leukemia. Bone marrow examination is not indicated in the vast majority of cases.[328] Because neutropenia and mild thrombocytopenia are frequent concomitants of many viral infections, TEC is often not a "pure" red cell disease; however, the anemia is usually the more striking anomaly.

Much effort has been expended in implicating parvovirus serotype 19 as an offender in TEC. Although rare cases have been noted, parvovirus is not usually detected.[329-331] In many cases it appears to be a result of antibodies to erythroid progenitors.[307] It is, however, a serious risk in patients with immune deficiency, such as those undergoing organ or marrow transplantation[332-334] and in patients with foreshortened red cell life span such as those with sickle cell anemia or hemolytic anemia (see Chapter 19).

Chronic Pure Red Cell Aplasia: Circulating Antibodies and Suppressing T Cells

Thymoma is very rare in children. Freedman and Feig[322] reviewed the pediatric literature in 1993 and little has emerged since. Thymoma, when associated with PRCA, may be successfully treated with surgery coupled with immunosuppression or intravenous immunoglobulin.[334-337]

Dessypris and Krantz have carefully described the course of patients in whom antibodies reactive with erythroid precursors suddenly develop that presumably suppress erythroid progenitors (BFU-E and CFU-E), recognizable precursors, or both. Dessypris' monograph[321] and Krantz's more recent review in the volume edited by Feig and Freedman[322] exhaustively document the evidence for such antibodies and their suppressing activities. In brief, the antibodies may arise de novo and hence are considered primary, or in the setting of immune deficiency, neoplastic disease, collagen vascular disease, or infection they are considered secondary. In either case, the antibodies cause severe aregenerative anemia and, though often responsive to immunosuppressive therapy,

commonly return to the circulation and cause relapse unless therapy is continued for protracted periods. Fortunately, antibody-mediated APRCA is quite rare in children. The pathophysiology, course, and treatment of the disease are better understood in adults.

Autoantibodies that bind and inhibit erythropoietin and are responsible for erythroid aplasia were first inferred from the work of Jepson and Lowenstein in 1966.[339] Although similar reports emerged later, three of which were associated with recombinant erythropoietin therapy, the pathophysiologic evidence for such antibodies was marginal until 2002, when French investigators[340] reported a high incidence of antierythropoietin antibodies in patients (largely with renal failure) who had been treated with a particular brand of recombinant erythropoietin that had been altered by a variation in glycosylation and by improper storage and thereby rendered antigenic. The findings have been confirmed worldwide. The offending brand of erythropoietin has since been modified, and the incidence of such autoantibodies has been markedly reduced. Immunosuppressive therapy induces these antibodies to disappear in most cases.[341-347]

A case of primary APRCA associated with T-cell suppression of erythropoiesis by large granular lymphocytes that carried both T-cell and monocyte surface markers was described in 1983 by Lipton and associates.[178] In this case, the T cells recognized erythroid but not myeloid progenitors in the context of HLA and suppressed in vitro erythropoiesis in the patient and in HLA-identical normal individuals. Before and since that report there have been several papers that describe such T cells in cases of APRCA,[311,322,338,348-350] but the Lipton study provides the best evidence for HLA-specific erythroid inhibition by an offending clone of T cells. Interestingly, this patient was rapidly cured by treatment with cyclophosphamide. The cell expanded in many of these cases and, though originally described as a Tγ cell, has been renamed a large granular lymphocyte, and these cells can be of either T cell ($CD3^+$, T cell receptor [TCR] $\alpha\beta$ or $\gamma\delta$), or natural killer cell ($CD3^-$, TCR^-) origin.[312]

Preleukemia (the 5q– Syndrome)

The 5q– syndrome is an acquired clonal defect in which a segment of chromosome 5q bearing at least 40 genes is deleted. Severe aregenerative anemia, absent marrow erythroblasts, abnormal megakaryocytes, and a high incidence of acute myelogenous leukemia are the results. The recent discovery by Ebert and co-workers that the deletion responsible is the gene encoding a ribosomal protein[313] classifies the 5q– syndrome as an acquired and clonal form of Diamond-Blackfan anemia, although one might expect that additional genetic defects must be present to explain the growth advantage of the malignant cells. (It is discussed extensively in *Oncology of Infancy and Childhood*).

Other Causes of Acquired Pure Red Cell Aplasia

Very rarely, children with B-cell proliferative diseases may have concomitant PRCA, but almost all of the therapeutic experience is recorded in adults. Of the few cases of PRCA reported in children, most are in the setting of immunodeficiency. Drug-induced PRCA is by far the most common cause of secondary PRCA in childhood, and azathioprine treatment of renal transplant rejection is by far the most frequent offender.[351] The latter drug usually causes megaloblastic anemia, but it may result in nearly total aplasia. Severe renal failure may also cause PRCA in childhood.

REFERENCES

1. Camitta BM, Thomas ED, Nathan DG, et al. Severe aplastic anemia: a prospective study of the effect of early marrow transplantation on acute mortality. Blood. 1976; 48:63-70.
2. Bacigalupo A, Hows J, Gluckman E, et al. Bone marrow transplantation (BMT) versus immunosuppression for the treatment of severe aplastic anaemia (SAA): a report of the EBMT SAA working party. Br J Haematol. 1988; 70:177-182.
3. Kaufman DW, Kelly JP, Levy M, Shapiro S. The Drug Etiology of Agranulocytosis and Aplastic Anemia. New York, Oxford University Press, 1991.
4. Young NS. Acquired aplastic anemia. In Young NS (ed). Bone Marrow Failure Syndromes. Philadelphia, WB Saunders, 2000, pp 1-46.
5. Shimizu H, Kuroishi T, Tominaga S, et al. Production amount of chloramphenicol and mortality rate of aplastic anemia in Japan. Nippon Ketsueki Gakkai Zasshi. 1979; 42:689-696.
6. Mizuno S, Aoki K, Ohno Y, et al. Time series analysis of age-sex specific death rates from aplastic anemia and the trend in production amount of chloramphenicol. Nagoya J Med Sci. 1982;44:103-115.
7. Szklo M, Sensenbrenner L, Markowitz J, et al. Incidence of aplastic anemia in metropolitan Baltimore: a population-based study. Blood. 1985;66:115-119.
8. Bottiger LE, Furhoff AK, Holmberg L. Drug-induced blood dyscrasias. A ten-year material from the Swedish Adverse Drug Reaction Committee. Acta Med Scand. 1979;205:457-461.
9. Issaragrisil S, Kaufman DW, Anderson T, et al. Low drug attributability of aplastic anemia in Thailand. The Aplastic Anemia Study Group. Blood. 1997;89:4034-4039.
10. Issaragrisil S, Kaufman DW, Anderson T, et al. The epidemiology of aplastic anemia in Thailand. Blood. 2006;107:1299-1307.
11. De Gruchy GC. Drug Induced Blood Disorders. Philadelphia, JB Lippincott, 1975.
12. Powars D. Aplastic anemia secondary to glue sniffing. N Engl J Med. 1965;273:700.
13. Scott J, Cartwright G, Wintrobe M. Acquired aplastic anemia: an analysis of thirty-nine cases and review of the pertinent literature. Medicine (Baltimore). 1958;36:119.
14. Smadel J, Jackson E. Chloromycetin, an antibiotic with chemotherapeutic activity in experimental and viral infections. Science. 1944;106:41B.
15. Smadel J. Chloramphenicol (Chloromycetin) in the treatment of infectious diseases. Am J Med. 1949;7:671.
16. Firkin FC. Mitochondrial lesions in reversible erythropoietic depression due to chloramphenicol. J Clin Invest. 1972;51:2085-2092.
17. Yunis A. Mechanisms underlying marrow toxicity from chloramphenicol and thiamphenicol. In Silber R, LoBue J, Gordon A (eds). The Year in Hematology. New York, Plenum, 1978, p 143.
18. Ratzan RJ, Moore MA, Yunis AA. Effect of chloramphenicol and thiamphenicol on the in vitro colony-forming cell. Blood. 1974;43:363-369.
19. Bostrom B, Smith K, Ramsay NK. Stimulation of human committed bone marrow stem cells (CFU-GM) by chloramphenicol. Exp Hematol. 1986;14:156-161.
20. Sawada H, Tezuka H, Kamamoto T. Effects of chloramphenicol on hemopoietic cells and their microenvironment in vitro. Nippon Ketsueki Gakkai Zasshi. 1985;48: 1323-1331.
21. Hara H, Kohsaki M, Noguchi K, Nagai K. Effect of chloramphenicol on colony formation from erythrocytic precursors. Am J Hematol. 1978;5:123-130.
22. Firkin FC, Sumner MA, Bradley TR. The influence of chloramphenicol on the bone marrow haemopoietic stem cell compartment. Exp Hematol. 1974;2:264-268.
23. Nara N, Bessho M, Hirashima K, Momo H. Effects of chloramphenicol on hematopoietic inductive microenvironment. Exp Hematol. 1982;10:20-25.
24. Wijnja L, Snijder JA, Nieweg HO. Acetylsalicylic acid as a cause of pancytopenia from bone-marrow damage. Lancet. 1966;2:768-770.
25. Menkes E, Kutas GJ. Fatal aplastic anemia following indomethacin ingestion. Can Med Assoc J. 1977; 117:118.
26. Shearer CA. Indomethacin and aplastic anemia. Can Med Assoc J. 1978;118:18.
27. Canada AT Jr, Burka ER. Aplastic anemia after indomethacin. N Engl J Med. 1968;278:743-744.
28. TK Fredrick GR. Indomethacin and aplastic anemia [letter]. N Engl J Med. 1968;279:1290.
29. Gryfe CI. Agranulocytosis and aplastic anemia possibly due to ibuprofen [letter]. Can Med Assoc J. 1976;114: 877.
30. McCarthy D, Chalmers T. Hematological complications of phenylbutazone therapy: review of the literature and report of two cases. Can Med Assoc J. 1964;90:1061.
31. Gaisfort W. Fatality after oxyphenbutazone in Still's disease. BMJ. 1962;2:1517.
32. Chang HK, Morrison SL. Bone-marrow suppression associated with cimetidine. Ann Intern Med. 1979;91: 580.
33. Tonkonow B, Hoffman R. Aplastic anemia and cimetidine. Arch Intern Med. 1980;140:1123-1124.
34. Kutscher AH, Lane SL, Segall R. The clinical toxicity of antibiotics and sulfonamides: a comparative review of the literature based on 104,672 cases treated systemically. J Allergy. 1954;25:135-150.
35. Holsinger DR, Hanlon DG, Welch JS. Fatal aplastic anemia following sulfamethoxypyridazine therapy. Proc Staff Meet Mayo Clin. 1958;33:679-681.

36. Tulloch AL. Pancytopenia in an infant associated with sulfamethoxazole-trimethoprim therapy. J Pediatr. 1976; 88:499-500.

37. Levine B, Rosenberg DV. Aplastic anemia during the treatment of hyperthyroidism with tapazole. Ann Intern Med. 1954;41:844-848.

38. Edell SL, Bartuska DG. Aplastic anemia secondary to methimazole—case report and review of hematologic side effects. J Am Med Womens Assoc. 1975;30:412-413.

39. Aksoy M, Erdem S. Aplastic anaemia after propylthiouracil. Lancet. 1968;1(7556):1379.

40. Jost F. Blood dyscrasias associated with tolbutamide therapy. BMJ. 1959;169:1468.

41. Chapman I, Cheung WH. Pancytopenia associated with tolbutamide therapy. JAMA. 1963;186:595-596.

42. White LL. Fatal marrow aplasia during chlorpropamide therapy [letter]. BMJ. 1962;1:691.

43. Recker RR, Hynes HE. Pure red blood cell aplasia associated with chlorpropamide therapy. Patient summary and review of the literature. Arch Intern Med. 1969;123:445-447.

44. Sparbert M. Diagnostically confusing complications of diphenylhydantoin therapy. Ann Intern Med. 1963;59:914.

45. Witkind E, Waid ME. Aplasia of the bone marrow during Mesantoin therapy. Report of a fatal case. JAMA. 1951;147:757-759.

46. Isaacson S, Gold JA, Ginsberg V. Fatal aplastic anemia after therapy with nuvarone (3-methyl-5-phenylhydantoin). JAMA. 1956;160:1311-1312.

47. Donaldson GW, Graham JG. Aplastic anaemia following the administration of Tegretol. Br J Clin Pract. 1965;19:699-702.

48. Dyer NH, Hughes DT, Jenkins GC. Aplastic anaemia after carbamazepine. BMJ. 1966;5479:108.

49. Pisciotta AV. Hematologic toxicity of carbamazepine. In Penry JK (ed). Advances in Neurology. New York, Raven Press, 1975, p 355.

50. Gayford JJ, Redpath TH. The side-effects of carbamazepine. Proc R Soc Med. 1969;62:615-616.

51. Pellock JM. Carbamazepine side effects in children and adults. Epilepsia. 1987;28(Suppl 3):S64-S70.

52. Wisch N, Fischbein FI, Siegel R, et al. Aplastic anemia resulting from the use of carbonic anhydrase inhibitors. Am J Ophthalmol. 1973;75:130-132.

53. Underwood LC. Fatal bone marrow depression after the treatment with acetazolamide (Diamox). JAMA. 1956;161:1477.

54. Lubeck MJ. Aplastic anemia following acetazolamide therapy. Am J Ophthalmol. 1970;69:684-685.

55. Gangitano JL, Foster SH, Contro RM. Nonfatal methazolamide-induced aplastic anemia. Am J Ophthalmol. 1978;86:138-139.

56. Werblin TP, Pollack IP, Liss RA. Aplastic anemia and agranulocytosis in patients using methazolamide for glaucoma. JAMA. 1979;241:2817-2818.

57. Smith M. Overview of benzene-induced aplastic anaemia. Eur J Haematol. 1996;57(Suppl):107-110.

58. Ross D. Metabolic basis of benzene toxicity. Eur J Haematol. 1996;57(Suppl):111-118.

59. Young Y. Drugs and chemicals as agents of bone marrow failure. In Testa N, Gale RC (eds). Hematopoiesis: Long-Term Effects of Chemotherapy and Radiation. New York, Marcel Dekker, 1988.

60. Snyder R, Kocsis JJ. Current concepts of chronic benzene toxicity. CRC Crit Rev Toxicol. 1975;3:265-288.

61. Fishbein L. An overview of environmental and toxicological aspects of aromatic hydrocarbons. I. Benzene. Sci Total Environ. 1984;40:189-218.

62. Brief RS, Lynch J, Bernath T, Scala RA. Benzene in the workplace. Am Ind Hyg Assoc J. 1980;41:616-623.

63. Sato A, Nakajima T, Fujiwara Y, Hirosawa K. Pharmacokinetics of benzene and toluene. Int Arch Arbeitsmed. 1974;33:169-182.

64. Kalf G, Post G, Snyder R. Solvent toxicology: recent advances in the toxicology of benzene, the glycol ethers, and carbon tetrachloride. Annu Rev Pharmacol Toxicol. 1987;27:399.

65. Sawahata T, Rickert D, Greenlee W. Metabolism of benzene and its metabolites in bone marrow. In Irons RD (ed). Toxicology of the Blood and Bone Marrow. New York, Raven, 1985.

66. Greenlee WF, Sun JD, Bus JS. A proposed mechanism of benzene toxicity: formation of reactive intermediates from polyphenol metabolites. Toxicol Appl Pharmacol. 1981;59:187-195.

67. Lee E, Garner C, Johnson J. A proposed role played by benzene itself in the induction of acute cytopenia: inhibition of DNA synthesis. Res Comm Chem Pathol Pharmacol. 1988;60:27.

68. Kissling M, Speck B. Further studies on experimental benzene induced aplastic anemia. Blut. 1972;25:97-103.

69. Pellack-Walker P, Blumer JL. DNA damage in L5178YS cells following exposure to benzene metabolites. Mol Pharmacol. 1986;30:42-47.

70. Brahams D. Lindane exposure and aplastic anaemia. Lancet. 1994;343:1092.

71. Parent-Massin D, Thouvenot D, Rio B, Riche C. Lindane haematotoxicity confirmed by in vitro tests on human and rat progenitors. Hum Exp Toxicol 1994;13:103-106.

72. Knospe WH, Crosby WH. Aplastic anaemia: a disorder of the bone-marrow sinusoidal microcirculation rather than stem-cell failure? Lancet. 1971;1:20-22.

73. Pikis A, Kavaliotis J, Manios S. Incidence of aplastic anemia in viral hepatitis in children. Scand J Infect Dis. 1988;20:109-110.

74. Perrillo RP, Pohl DA, Roodman ST, Tsai CC. Acute non-A, non-B hepatitis with serum sickness–like syndrome and aplastic anemia. JAMA. 1981;245:494-496.

75. Bottiger LE, Westerholm B. Aplastic anaemia. 3. Aplastic anaemia and infectious hepatitis. Acta Med Scand. 1972;192:323-326.

76. Young NS, Issaragrasil S, Chieh CW, Takaku F. Aplastic anaemia in the Orient. Br J Haematol. 1986;62:1-6.

77. Liang DC, Lin KH, Lin DT, et al. Post-hepatitic aplastic anaemia in children in Taiwan, a hepatitis prevalent area. Br J Haematol. 1990;74:487-491.

78. Tzakis AG, Arditi M, Whitington PF, et al. Aplastic anemia complicating orthotopic liver transplantation for non-A, non-B hepatitis. N Engl J Med. 1988;319:393-396.

79. Smith D, Gribble TJ, Yeager AS, et al. Spontaneous resolution of severe aplastic anemia associated with viral hepatitis A in a 6-year-old child. Am J Hematol. 1978;5:247-252.

80. Kindmark CO, Sjolin J, Nordlinder H, et al. Aplastic anaemia in a case of hepatitis B with a high titer of hepatitis B antigen. Acta Med Scand. 1984;215:89-92.

81. Hibbs JR, Frickhofen N, Rosenfeld SJ, et al. Aplastic anemia and viral hepatitis. Non-A, Non-B, Non-C? JAMA. 1992;267:2051-2054.

82. Brown KE, Tisdale J, Barrett AJ, et al. Hepatitis-associated aplastic anemia. N Engl J Med. 1997;336:1059-1064.

83. Hagler L, Pastore RA, Bergin JJ, Wrensch MR. Aplastic anemia following viral hepatitis: report of two fatal cases and literature review. Medicine (Baltimore). 1975;54:139-164.

84. Savage WJ, Derusso PA, Resar LM, et al. Treatment of hepatitis-associated aplastic anemia with high-dose cyclophosphamide. Pediatr Blood Cancer. 2007;49:947-951.

85. Sanchez R, Rosenthal P, Goldsby R. Immunotherapy for severe aplastic anemia following orthotopic liver transplantation in children. Pediatr Blood Cancer. 2007;49:93-98.

86. Gupta A, Bansal D, Marwaha RK, Trehan A. Hepatitis-associated aplastic anemia: successful outcome following immunosuppressive therapy. Indian J Gastroenterol. 2005;24:175-176.

87. Goldenberg NA, Graham DK, Liang X, Hays T. Successful treatment of severe aplastic anemia in children using standardized immunosuppressive therapy with antithymocyte globulin and cyclosporine A. Pediatr Blood Cancer. 2004;43:711-712.

88. Nakao S, Lai CJ, Young NS. Dengue virus, a flavivirus, propagates in human bone marrow progenitors and hematopoietic cell lines. Blood. 1989;74:1235-1240.

89. Tosato G, Taga K, Angiolillo AL, Sgadari C. Epstein-Barr virus as an agent of haematological disease. Baillieres Clin Haematol. 1995;8:165-199.

90. Baranski B, Armstrong G, Truman JT, et al. Epstein-Barr virus in the bone marrow of patients with aplastic anemia. Ann Intern Med. 1988;109:695-704.

91. Sing GK, Ruscetti FW. The role of human cytomegalovirus in haematological diseases. Baillieres Clin Haematol. 1995;8:149-163.

92. Simmons P, Kaushansky K, Torok-Storb B. Mechanisms of cytomegalovirus-mediated myelosuppression: perturbation of stromal cell function versus direct infection of myeloid cells. Proc Natl Acad Sci U S A. 1990;87:1386-1390.

93. Maciejewski JP, Bruening EE, Donahue RE, et al. Infection of hematopoietic progenitor cells by human cytomegalovirus. Blood. 1992;80:170-178.

94. Carrigan DR, Knox KK. Human herpesvirus 6 (HHV-6) isolation from bone marrow: HHV-6–associated bone marrow suppression in bone marrow transplant patients. Blood. 1994;84:3307-3310.

95. Lusso P, Gallo RC. Human herpesvirus 6. Baillieres Clin Haematol. 1995;8:201-223.

96. Knox KK, Carrigan DR. In vitro suppression of bone marrow progenitor cell differentiation by human herpesvirus 6 infection. J Infect Dis. 1992;165:925-929.

97. Davis BR, Zauli G. Effect of human immunodeficiency virus infection on haematopoiesis. Baillieres Clin Haematol. 1995;8:113-130.

98. Stella CC, Ganser A, Hoelzer D. Defective in vitro growth of the hemopoietic progenitor cells in the acquired immunodeficiency syndrome. J Clin Invest. 1987;80:286-293.

99. Bagnara GP, Zauli G, Giovannini M, et al. Early loss of circulating hemopoietic progenitors in HIV-1–infected subjects. Exp Hematol. 1990;18:426-430.

100. De Luca A, Teofili L, Antinori A, et al. Haemopoietic CD34+ progenitor cells are not infected by HIV-1 in vivo but show impaired clonogenesis. Br J Haematol. 1993;85:20-24.

101. Zauli G, Re MC, Davis B, et al. Impaired in vitro growth of purified (CD34+) hematopoietic progenitors in human immunodeficiency virus-1 seropositive thrombocytopenic individuals. Blood. 1992;79:2680-2687.

102. von Laer D, Hufert FT, Fenner TE, et al. CD34+ hematopoietic progenitor cells are not a major reservoir of the human immunodeficiency virus. Blood. 1990;76:1281-1286.

103. Molina JM, Scadden DT, Sakaguchi M, et al. Lack of evidence for infection of or effect on growth of hematopoietic progenitor cells after in vivo or in vitro exposure to human immunodeficiency virus. Blood. 1990;76:2476-2482.

104. Zucker-Franklin D, Seremetis S, Zheng ZY. Internalization of human immunodeficiency virus type I and other retroviruses by megakaryocytes and platelets. Blood. 1990;75:1920-1923.

105. Cen D, Zauli G, Szarnicki R, Davis BR. Effect of different human immunodeficiency virus type-1 (HIV-1) isolates on long-term bone marrow haemopoiesis. Br J Haematol. 1993;85:596-602.

106. Schwartz GN, Kessler SW, Rothwell SW, et al. Inhibitory effects of HIV-1–infected stromal cell layers on the production of myeloid progenitor cells in human long-term bone marrow cultures. Exp Hematol. 1994;22:1288-1296.

107. Maciejewski JP, Weichold FF, Young NS. HIV-1 suppression of hematopoiesis in vitro mediated by envelope glycoprotein and TNF-alpha. J Immunol. 1994;153:4303-4310.

108. Young Y, Alter B. Aplastic Anemia: Acquired and Inherited. Philadelphia, WB Saunders, 1994.

109. Yeh ET, Rosse WF. Paroxysmal nocturnal hemoglobinuria and the glycosylphosphatidylinositol anchor. J Clin Invest. 1994;93:2305-2310.

110. Schubert J, Vogt HG, Zielinska-Skowronek M, et al. Development of the glycosylphosphatitylinositol-anchoring defect characteristic for paroxysmal nocturnal hemoglobinuria in patients with aplastic anemia. Blood. 1994;83:2323-2328.

111. Schrezenmeier H, Hertenstein B, Wagner B, et al. A pathogenetic link between aplastic anemia and paroxysmal nocturnal hemoglobinuria is suggested by a high frequency of aplastic anemia patients with a deficiency of phosphatidylinositol glycan anchored proteins. Exp Hematol. 1995;23:81-87.

112. Mukhina GL, Buckley JT, Barber JP, et al. Multilineage glycosylphosphatidylinositol anchor–deficient haematopoiesis in untreated aplastic anaemia. Br J Haematol. 2001;115:476-482.

113. Brodsky RA. New insights into paroxysmal nocturnal hemoglobinuria. Hematol Am Soc Hematol Educ Program. 2006;24-28, 516.

114. Hall SE, Rosse WF. The use of monoclonal antibodies and flow cytometry in the diagnosis of paroxysmal nocturnal hemoglobinuria. Blood. 1996;87:5332-5340.

115. Brodsky RA, Mukhina GL, Nelson KL, et al. Resistance of paroxysmal nocturnal hemoglobinuria cells to the glycosylphosphatidylinositol-binding toxin aerolysin. Blood. 1999;93:1749-1756.

116. Brodsky RA, Mukhina GL, Li S, et al. Improved detection and characterization of paroxysmal nocturnal hemoglobinuria using fluorescent aerolysin. Am J Clin Pathol. 2000;114:459-466.

117. Araten DJ, Nafa K, Pakdeesuwan K, Luzzatto L. Clonal populations of hematopoietic cells with paroxysmal nocturnal hemoglobinuria genotype and phenotype are present in normal individuals. Proc Natl Acad Sci U S A. 1999;96:5209-5214.

118. Parker CJ. The pathophysiology of paroxysmal nocturnal hemoglobinuria. Exp Hematol. 2007;35:523-533.

119. Iwamoto N, Kawaguchi T, Horikawa K, et al. Preferential hematopoiesis by paroxysmal nocturnal hemoglobinuria clone engrafted in SCID mice. Blood. 1996;87:4944-4948.

120. Maciejewski J, Sloand E, Sato T, et al. Impaired hematopoiesis in paroxysmal nocturnal hemoglobinuria/aplastic anemia is not associated with a selective proliferative defect in the glycosylphosphatidylinostol-anchored protein-deficient clone. Blood. 1997;89:1173-1181.

121. Chen R, Nagarajan S, Prince GM, et al. Impaired growth and elevated fas receptor expression in PIGA(+) stem cells in primary paroxysmal nocturnal hemoglobinuria. J Clin Invest. 2000;106:689-696.

122. Murakami Y, Kinoshita T, Maeda Y, et al. Different roles of glycosylphosphatidylinositol in various hematopoietic cells as revealed by a mouse model of paroxysmal nocturnal hemoglobinuria. Blood. 1999;94:2963-2970.

123. Tremml G, Dominguez C, Rosti V, et al. Increased sensitivity to complement and a decreased red blood cell life span in mice mosaic for a nonfunctional Piga gene. Blood. 1999;94:2945-2954.

124. Karadimitris A, Notaro R, Koehne G, et al. PNH cells are as sensitive to T-cell–mediated lysis as their normal counterparts: implications for the pathogenesis of paroxysmal nocturnal haemoglobinuria. Br J Haematol. 2000;111:1158-1163.

125. Karadimitris A, Manavalan JS, Thaler HT, et al. Abnormal T-cell repertoire is consistent with immune process underlying the pathogenesis of paroxysmal nocturnal hemoglobinuria. Blood. 2000;96:2613-2620.

126. Inoue N, Izui-Sarumaru T, Murakami Y, et al. Molecular basis of clonal expansion of hematopoiesis in 2 patients with paroxysmal nocturnal hemoglobinuria (PNH). Blood. 2006;108:4232-4236.

127. Hoffman R, Dainiak N, Sibrack L, et al. Antibody-mediated aplastic anemia and diffuse fasciitis. N Engl J Med. 1979;300:718-721.

128. Talerman A, Amigo A. Thymoma associated with aregenerative and aplastic anemia in a five-year-old child. Cancer. 1968;21:1212-1218.

129. Ferrara JL, Deeg HJ. Graft-versus-host disease. N Engl J Med. 1991;324:667-674.

130. Schrezenmeier H, Gerok M, Heimpel H. Assessment of frequency of hematopoietic stem cells in aplastic anemia by limiting dilution type long term marrow culture. Exp Hematol. 1992;20:806.

131. Maciejewski JP, Selleri C, Sato T, et al. A severe and consistent deficit in marrow and circulating primitive hematopoietic cells (long-term culture–initiating cells) in acquired aplastic anemia. Blood. 1996;88:1983-1991.

132. Sutherland HJ, Eaves CJ, Eaves AC, et al. Characterization and partial purification of human marrow cells capable of initiating long-term hematopoiesis in vitro. Blood. 1989;74:1563-1570.

133. Bhatia M, Wang JC, Kapp U, et al. Purification of primitive human hematopoietic cells capable of repopulating immune-deficient mice. Proc Natl Acad Sci U S A. 1997;94:5320-5325.

134. Civin CI, Trischmann T, Kadan NS, et al. Highly purified CD34-positive cells reconstitute hematopoiesis. J Clin Oncol. 1996;14:2224-2233.

135. Berenson RJ, Andrews RG, Bensinger WI, et al. Antigen CD34+ marrow cells engraft lethally irradiated baboons. J Clin Invest. 1988;81:951-955.

136. Maciejewski JP, Anderson S, Katevas P, Young NS. Phenotypic and functional analysis of bone marrow progenitor cell compartment in bone marrow failure. Br J Haematol. 1994;87:227-234.

137. Scopes J, Bagnara M, Gordon-Smith EC, et al. Haemopoietic progenitor cells are reduced in aplastic anaemia. Br J Haematol. 1994;86:427-430.

138. Lu DP. Syngeneic bone marrow transplantation for treatment of aplastic anaemia: report of a case and review of the literature. Exp Hematol. 1981;9:257-263.

139. Champlin RE, Feig SA, Sparkes RS, Galen RP. Bone marrow transplantation from identical twins in the treatment of aplastic anaemia: implication for the pathogenesis of the disease. Br J Haematol. 1984;56:455-463.

140. Storb R. Bone marrow transplantation for aplastic anemia. Cell Transplant. 1993;2:365-379.

141. Hinterberger W, Rowlings PA, Hinterberger-Fischer M, et al. Results of transplanting bone marrow from genetically identical twins into patients with aplastic anemia. Ann Intern Med. 1997;126:116-122.

142. Young NS. The problem of clonality in aplastic anemia: Dr Dameshek's riddle, restated. Blood. 1992;79:1385-1392.

143. Alter BP. Bone marrow failure: a child is not just a small adult (but an adult can have a childhood disease). Hematol Am Soc Hematol Educ Program. 2005:96-103.

144. Fogarty PF, Yamaguchi H, Wiestner A, et al. Late presentation of dyskeratosis congenita as apparently acquired aplastic anaemia due to mutations in telomerase RNA. Lancet. 2003;362:1628-1630.

145. Yamaguchi H, Baerlocher GM, Lansdorp PM, et al. Mutations of the human telomerase RNA gene (TERC) in aplastic anemia and myelodysplastic syndrome. Blood. 2003;102:916-918.

146. Xin ZT, Beauchamp AD, Calado RT, et al. Functional characterization of natural telomerase mutations found in patients with hematologic disorders. Blood. 2007;109:524-532.

147. Yamaguchi H, Calado RT, Ly H, et al. Mutations in TERT, the gene for telomerase reverse transcriptase, in aplastic anemia. N Engl J Med. 2005;352:1413-1424.

148. Vulliamy TJ, Walne A, Baskaradas A, et al. Mutations in the reverse transcriptase component of telomerase

(TERT) in patients with bone marrow failure. Blood Cells Mol Dis. 2005;34:257-263.

149. Armanios M, Chen JL, Chang YP, et al. Haploin-sufficiency of telomerase reverse transcriptase leads to anticipation in autosomal dominant dyskeratosis congenita. Proc Natl Acad Sci U S A. 2005;102:15960-15964.

150. Ball SE, Gibson FM, Rizzo S, et al. Progressive telomere shortening in aplastic anemia. Blood. 1998;91:3582-3592.

151. Brummendorf TH, Maciejewski JP, Mak J, et al. Telomere length in leukocyte subpopulations of patients with aplastic anemia. Blood. 2001;97:895-900.

152. Alter BP, Baerlocher GM, Savage SA, et al. Very short telomere length by flow fluorescent in situ hybridization identifies patients with dyskeratosis congenita. Blood. 2007;110:1439-1447.

153. Brodsky RA, Jones RJ. Aplastic anaemia. Lancet. 2005;365:1647-1656.

154. Young NS, Calado RT, Scheinberg P. Current concepts in the pathophysiology and treatment of aplastic anemia. Blood. 2006;108:2509-2519.

155. Hinterberger W, Raghavachar A, et al. Bone marrow transplantation from genotypically identical twins with aplastic anemia. In Raghavachar A, Schrenzenmeier H, Frickhofen N (eds). Aplastic Anemia: Current Perspectives on the Pathogenesis and Treatment. Vienna, Blackwell-MZV, 1993, p 102.

156. Nakao S, Yamaguchi M, Saito M, et al. HLA-DR2 predicts a favorable response to cyclosporine therapy in patients with bone marrow failure. Am J Hematol. 1992;40:239-240.

157. Nimer SD, Ireland P, Meshkinpour A, Frane M. An increased HLA DR2 frequency is seen in aplastic anemia patients. Blood. 1994;84:923-927.

158. Mathe G, Amiel JL, Schwarzenberg L, et al. Bone marrow graft in man after conditioning by antilymphocytic serum. BMJ. 1970;2:131-136.

159. Thomas ED, Storb R, Giblett ER, et al. Recovery from aplastic anemia following attempted marrow transplantation. Exp Hematol. 1976;4:97-102.

160. Territo MC. Autologous bone marrow repopulation following high dose cyclophosphamide and allogeneic marrow transplantation in aplastic anaemia. Br J Haematol. 1977;36:305-312.

161. Bickel M, Tsuda H, Amstad P, et al. Differential regulation of colony-stimulating factors and interleukin 2 production by cyclosporin A. Proc Natl Acad Sci U S A. 1987;84:3274-3277.

162. Rebellato LM, Gross U, Verbanac KM, Thomas JM. A comprehensive definition of the major antibody specificities in polyclonal rabbit antithymocyte globulin. Transplantation. 1994;57:685-694.

163. Tisdale JF, Dunn DE, Maciejewski J. Cyclophosphamide and other new agents for the treatment of severe aplastic anemia. Semin Hematol. 2000;37:102-109.

164. Killick SB, Marsh JC, Gordon-Smith EC, et al. Effects of antithymocyte globulin on bone marrow CD34+ cells in aplastic anaemia and myelodysplasia. Br J Haematol. 2000;108:582-591.

165. Chen G, Kook H, Zeng W, et al. Is there a direct effect of antithymocyte globulin on hematopoiesis? Hematol J. 2004;5:255-261.

166. Killick SB, Cox CV, Marsh JC, et al. Mechanisms of bone marrow progenitor cell apoptosis in aplastic anaemia and the effect of anti-thymocyte globulin: examination of the role of the Fas-Fas-L interaction. Br J Haematol. 2000;111:1164-1169.

167. Jonasova A, Neuwirtova R, Cermak J, et al. Cyclosporin A therapy in hypoplastic MDS patients and certain refractory anaemias without hypoplastic bone marrow. Br J Haematol. 1998;100:304-309.

168. Young NS, Barrett AJ. Immune modulation of myelodysplasia: rationale and therapy. In Bennett JM (ed). The Myelodysplastic Syndromes: Pathobiology and Clinical Management. New York, Marcel Dekker, 2001.

169. Herrmann F, Griffin JD, Meuer SG, Meyer zum Buschenfelde KH. Establishment of an interleukin 2–dependent T cell line derived from a patient with severe aplastic anemia, which inhibits in vitro hematopoiesis. J Immunol. 1986;136:1629-1634.

170. Tong J, Bacigalupo A, Piaggio G, et al. In vitro response of T cells from aplastic anemia patients to antilymphocyte globulin and phytohemagglutinin: colony-stimulating activity and lymphokine production. Exp Hematol. 1991;19:312-316.

171. Nakao S, Takamatsu H, Yachie A, et al. Establishment of a CD4+ T cell clone recognizing autologous hematopoietic progenitor cells from a patient with immune-mediated aplastic anemia. Exp Hematol. 1995;23:433-438.

172. Zoumbos NC, Ferris WO, Hsu SM, et al. Analysis of lymphocyte subsets in patients with aplastic anaemia. Br J Haematol. 1984;58:95-105.

173. Ruiz-Arguelles GJ, Katzmann JA, Greipp PR, et al. Lymphocyte subsets in patients with aplastic anemia. Am J Hematol. 1984;16:267-275.

174. Tsuda H, Yamasaki H. Type I and type II T-cell profiles in aplastic anemia and refractory anemia. Am J Hematol. 2000;64:271-274.

175. Nakao S, Takami A, Takamatsu H, et al. Isolation of a T-cell clone showing HLA-DRB1*0405–restricted cytotoxicity for hematopoietic cells in a patient with aplastic anemia. Blood. 1997;89:3691-3699.

176. Zeng W, Maciejewski JP, Chen G, Young NS. Limited heterogeneity of T cell receptor BV usage in aplastic anemia. J Clin Invest. 2001;108:765-773.

177. Risitano AM, Maciejewski JP, Green S, et al. In-vivo dominant immune responses in aplastic anaemia: molecular tracking of putatively pathogenetic T-cell clones by TCR beta-CDR3 sequencing. Lancet. 2004;364:355-364.

178. Lipton JM, Nadler LM, Canellos GP, et al. Evidence for genetic restriction in the suppression of erythropoiesis by a unique subset of T lymphocytes in man. J Clin Invest. 1983;72:694-706.

179. Zoumbos NC, Gascon P, Djeu JY, et al. Circulating activated suppressor T lymphocytes in aplastic anemia. N Engl J Med. 1985;312:257-265.

180. Laver J, Castro-Malaspina H, Kernan NA, et al. In vitro interferon-gamma production by cultured T-cells in severe aplastic anaemia: correlation with granulomonopoietic inhibition in patients who respond to anti-thymocyte globulin. Br J Haematol. 1988;69:545-550.

181. Zoumbos NC, Gascon P, Djeu JY, Young NS. Interferon is a mediator of hematopoietic suppression in aplastic

anemia in vitro and possibly in vivo. Proc Natl Acad Sci U S A. 1985;82:188-192.

182. Nakao S, Yamaguchi M, Shiobara S, et al. Interferon-gamma gene expression in unstimulated bone marrow mononuclear cells predicts a good response to cyclosporine therapy in aplastic anemia. Blood. 1992;79:2532-2535.

183. Nistico A, Young NS. γ-Interferon gene expression in the bone marrow of patients with aplastic anemia. Ann Intern Med. 1994;120:463-469.

184. Sloand E, Kim S, Maciejewski JP, et al. Intracellular interferon-gamma in circulating and marrow T cells detected by flow cytometry and the response to immunosuppressive therapy in patients with aplastic anemia. Blood. 2002;100:1185-1191.

185. Schultz JC, Shahidi NT. Detection of tumor necrosis factor-alpha in bone marrow plasma and peripheral blood plasma from patients with aplastic anemia. Am J Hematol. 1994;45:32-38.

186. Holmberg LA, Seidel K, Leisenring W, Torok-Storb B. Aplastic anemia: analysis of stromal cell function in long-term marrow cultures. Blood. 1994;84:3685-3690.

187. Maciejewski JP, Liu JM, Green SW, et al. Expression of stem cell inhibitor (SCI) gene in patients with bone marrow failure. Exp Hematol. 1992;20:1112-1117.

188. Selleri C, Sato T, Anderson S, et al. Interferon-gamma and tumor necrosis factor-alpha suppress both early and late stages of hematopoiesis and induce programmed cell death. J Cell Physiol. 1995;165:538-546.

189. Selleri C, Maciejewski JP, Sato T, Young NS. Interferon-gamma constitutively expressed in the stromal microenvironment of human marrow cultures mediates potent hematopoietic inhibition. Blood. 1996;87:4149-4157.

190. Maciejewski J, Selleri C, Anderson S, Young NS. Fas antigen expression on CD34$^+$ human marrow cells is induced by interferon gamma and tumor necrosis factor alpha and potentiates cytokine-mediated hematopoietic suppression in vitro. Blood. 1995;85:3183-3190.

191. Bussel A, Dumont J, Schenmetzler C, et al. Long-term complete autologous reconstitution following cyclophosphamide and allogeneic marrow infusion in a case of severe aplastic anemia. Nouv Rev Fr Hematol. 1985;27:15-18.

192. Athanasou NA, Quinn J, Brenner MK, et al. Origin of marrow stromal cells and haemopoietic chimaerism following bone marrow transplantation determined by in situ hybridisation. Br J Cancer. 1990;61:385-389.

193. Marsh JC, Chang J, Testa NG, et al. In vitro assessment of marrow 'stem cell' and stromal cell function in aplastic anaemia. Br J Haematol. 1991;78:258-267.

194. Juneja HS, Lee S, Gardner FH. Human long-term bone marrow cultures in aplastic anemia. Int J Cell Cloning. 1989;7:129-135.

195. Koijima S. Hematopoietic growth factors and marrow stroma in aplastic anemia. Int J Hematol. 1998;68:19-28.

196. Marsh JC. Hematopoietic growth factors in the pathogenesis and for the treatment of aplastic anemia. Semin Hematol. 2000;37:81-90.

197. Twomey JJ, Douglass CC, Sharkey O Jr. The monocytopenia of aplastic anemia. Blood. 1973;41:187-195.

198. Elfenbein GJ, Kallman CH, Tutschka PJ, et al. The immune system in 40 aplastic anemia patients receiving conventional therapy. Blood. 1979;53:652-665.

199. Alter BP. Fetal erythropoiesis in stress hematopoiesis. Exp Hematol. 1979;7(Suppl 5):200-209.

200. Wolff J. Anemia caused by infections and toxins, idiopathic aplastic anemia and anemia caused by renal disease. Pediatr Clin North Am. 1957;4:469.

201. Diamond LK, Shahidi NT. Treatment of aplastic anemia in children. Semin Hematol. 1967;4:278-288.

202. Li FP, Alter BP, Nathan DG. The mortality of acquired aplastic anemia in children. Blood. 1972;40:153-162.

203. Lynch RE, Williams DM, Reading JC, Cartwright GE. The prognosis in aplastic anemia. Blood. 1975;45:517-528.

204. Howard SC, Naidu PE, Hu XJ, et al. Natural history of moderate aplastic anemia in children. Pediatr Blood Cancer. 2004;43:545-551.

205. Heyn RM, Ertel IJ, Tubergen DG. Course of acquired aplastic anemia in children treated with supportive care. JAMA. 1969;208:1372-1378.

206. Khatib Z, Wilimas J, Wang W. Outcome of moderate aplastic anemia in children. Am J Pediatr Hematol Oncol. 1994;16:80-85.

207. Champlin R, Ho W, Gale RP. Antithymocyte globulin treatment in patients with aplastic anemia: a prospective randomized trial. N Engl J Med. 1983;308:113-118.

208. Herman JH, Kamel HT. Platelet transfusion. Current techniques, remaining problems, and future prospects. Am J Pediatr Hematol Oncol. 1987;9:272-286.

209. Heyman MR, Schiffer CA. Platelet transfusion therapy for the cancer patient. Semin Oncol. 1990;17:198-209.

210. Patten E. Controversies in transfusion medicine. Prophylactic platelet transfusion revisited after 25 years: con. Transfusion. 1992;32:381-385.

211. Sagmeister M, Oec L, Gmur J. A restrictive platelet transfusion policy allowing long-term support of outpatients with severe aplastic anemia. Blood. 1999;93:3124-3126.

212. Weinberger M, Elattar I, Marshall D, et al. Patterns of infection in patients with aplastic anemia and the emergence of *Aspergillus* as a major cause of death. Medicine (Baltimore). 1992;71:24-43.

213. Keidan AJ, Tsatalas C, Cohen J, et al. Infective complications of aplastic anaemia. Br J Haematol. 1986;63:503-508.

214. Torres HA, Bodey GP, Rolston KV, et al. Infections in patients with aplastic anemia: experience at a tertiary care cancer center. Cancer. 2003;98:86-93.

215. Brittenham GM, Griffith PM, Nienhuis AW, et al. Efficacy of deferoxamine in preventing complications of iron overload in patients with thalassemia major. N Engl J Med. 1994;331:567-573.

216. Champlin RE, Horowitz MM, van Bekkum DW, et al. Graft failure following bone marrow transplantation for severe aplastic anemia: risk factors and treatment results. Blood. 1989;73:606-613.

217. Cohen A, Duell T, Socie G, et al. Nutritional status and growth after bone marrow transplantation (BMT) during childhood: EBMT Late-Effects Working Party retrospective data. European Group for Blood and Marrow Transplantation. Bone Marrow Transplant. 1999;23:1043-1047.

218. Ades L, Mary JY, Robin M, et al. Long-term outcome after bone marrow transplantation for severe aplastic anemia. Blood. 2004;103:2490-2497.

219. Kahl C, Leisenring W, Deeg HJ, et al. Cyclophosphamide and antithymocyte globulin as a conditioning regimen for allogeneic marrow transplantation in patients with aplastic anaemia: a long-term follow-up. Br J Haematol. 2005; 130:747-751.

220. Bordin JO, Heddle NM, Blajchman MA. Biologic effects of leukocytes present in transfused cellular blood products. Blood. 1994;84:1703-1721.

221. Srinivasan R, Takahashi Y, McCoy JP, et al. Overcoming graft rejection in heavily transfused and allo-immunised patients with bone marrow failure syndromes using fludarabine-based haematopoietic cell transplantation. Br J Haematol. 2006;133:305-314.

222. Bacigalupo A, Brand R, Oneto R, et al. Treatment of acquired severe aplastic anemia: bone marrow transplantation compared with immunosuppressive therapy—The European Group for Blood and Marrow Transplantation experience. Semin Hematol. 2000; 37:69-80.

223. Horowitz MM. Current status of allogeneic bone marrow transplantation in acquired aplastic anemia. Semin Hematol. 2000;37:30-42.

224. Kojima S, Horibe K, Inaba J, et al. Long-term outcome of acquired aplastic anaemia in children: comparison between immunosuppressive therapy and bone marrow transplantation. Br J Haematol. 2000;111:321-328.

225. Gupta V, Ball SE, Yi QL, et al. Favorable effect on acute and chronic graft-versus-host disease with cyclophosphamide and in vivo anti-CD52 monoclonal antibodies for marrow transplantation from HLA-identical sibling donors for acquired aplastic anemia. Biol Blood Marrow Transplant. 2004;10:867-876.

226. Bacigalupo A. Bone marrow transplantation for severe aplastic anemia from HLA identical siblings. Haematologica. 1999;84:2-4.

227. Sanders JE. Endocrine complications of high-dose therapy with stem cell transplantation. Pediatr Transplant. 2004;8(Suppl 5):39-50.

228. Eapen M, Ramsay NK, Mertens AC, et al. Late outcomes after bone marrow transplant for aplastic anaemia. Br J Haematol. 2000;111:754-760.

229. Passweg JR, Perez WS, Eapen M, et al. Bone marrow transplants from mismatched related and unrelated donors for severe aplastic anemia. Bone Marrow Transplant. 2006;37:641-649.

230. Bacigalupo A, Locatelli F, Lanino E, et al. Fludarabine, cyclophosphamide and anti-thymocyte globulin for alternative donor transplants in acquired severe aplastic anemia: a report from the EBMT-SAA Working Party. Bone Marrow Transplant. 2005;36:947-950.

231. Deeg HJ, O'Donnell M, Tolar J, et al. Optimization of conditioning for marrow transplantation from unrelated donors for patients with aplastic anemia after failure of immunosuppressive therapy. Blood. 2006;108:1485-1491.

232. Bunin N, Aplenc R, Iannone R, et al. Unrelated donor bone marrow transplantation for children with severe aplastic anemia: minimal GVHD and durable engraftment with partial T cell depletion. Bone Marrow Transplant. 2005;35:369-373.

233. Gupta V, Ball SE, Sage D, et al. Marrow transplants from matched unrelated donors for aplastic anaemia using alemtuzumab, fludarabine and cyclophosphamide based conditioning. Bone Marrow Transplant. 2005;35:467-471.

234. Woodard P, Cunningham JM, Benaim E, et al. Effective donor lymphohematopoietic reconstitution after haplo-identical CD34+-selected hematopoietic stem cell transplantation in children with refractory severe aplastic anemia. Bone Marrow Transplant. 2004;33:411-418.

235. Jeannet M, Speck B, Rubinstein A, et al. Autologous marrow reconstitutions in severe aplastic anemia after ALG pretreatment and HL-A semi-incompatible bone marrow cell transfusion. Acta Haematol. 1976;55:129-139.

236. Silingardi V, Torelli U. Recovery from aplastic anemia after treatment with antilymphocyte globulin. Arch Intern Med. 1979;139:582-583.

237. Bielory L, Wright R, Nienhuis AW, et al. Antithymocyte globulin hypersensitivity in bone marrow failure patients. JAMA. 1988;260:3164-3167.

237. Greco B, Bielory L, Stephany D, et al. Antithymocyte globulin reacts with many normal human cell types. Blood. 1983;62:1047-1054.

238. Young N, Griffith P, Brittain E, et al. A multicenter trial of antithymocyte globulin in aplastic anemia and related diseases. Blood. 1988;72:1861-1869.

240. Bessman JD, Gardner FH. Persistence of abnormal RBC and platelet phenotype during recovery from aplastic anemia. Arch Intern Med. 1985;145:293-296.

241. Alter BP, Rappeport JM, Huisman TH, et al. Fetal erythropoiesis following bone marrow transplantation. Blood. 1976;48:843-853.

242. Freedman MH, Saunders EF, Hilton J, McClure PD. Residual abnormalities in acquired aplastic anemia of childhood. JAMA. 1974;228:201-202.

243. Kahan BD. Cyclosporine. N Engl J Med. 1989;321:1725-1738.

244. Leonard EM, Raefsky E, Griffith P, et al. Cyclosporine therapy of aplastic anaemia, congenital and acquired red cell aplasia. Br J Haematol. 1989;72:278-284.

245. Hinterberger-Fischer M, Hocker P, Lechner K, et al. Oral cyclosporin-A is effective treatment for untreated and also for previously immunosuppressed patients with severe bone marrow failure. Eur J Haematol. 1989;43:136-142.

246. Marsh J, Schrezenmeier H, Marin P, et al. Prospective randomized multicenter study comparing cyclosporin alone versus the combination of antithymocyte globulin and cyclosporin for treatment of patients with nonsevere aplastic anemia: a report from the European Blood and Marrow Transplant (EBMT) Severe Aplastic Anaemia Working Party. Blood. 1999;93:2191-2195.

247. Raghavachar A, Kolbe K, Hoffken K, et al. Standard immunosuppression is superior to cyclosporine/filgrastim in severe aplastic anemia: the German multicenter study. Bone Marrow Transplant. 1999;23:S31.

248. Bacigalupo A, Frassoni F, Podesta M, et al. Cyclosporin A (CyA) does not enhance CFU-c growth in patients with severe aplastic anaemia. Scand J Haematol. 1985;34:133-136.

249. Frickhofen N, Kaltwasser JP, Schrezenmeier H, et al. Treatment of aplastic anemia with antilymphocyte globulin and methylprednisolone with or without cyclosporine.

The German Aplastic Anemia Study Group. N Engl J Med. 1991;324:1297-1304.

250. Kojima S, Hibi S, Kosaka Y, et al. Immunosuppressive therapy using antithymocyte globulin, cyclosporine, and danazol with or without human granulocyte colony-stimulating factor in children with acquired aplastic anemia. Blood. 2000;96:2049-2054.

251. Fuhrer M, Rampf U, Baumann I, et al. Immunosuppressive therapy for aplastic anemia in children: a more severe disease predicts better survival. Blood. 2005;106:2102-2104.

252. Rosenfeld SJ, Kimball J, Vining D, Young NS. Intensive immunosuppression with antithymocyte globulin and cyclosporine as treatment for severe acquired aplastic anemia. Blood. 1995;85:3058-3065.

253. Frickhofen N, Rosenfeld SJ. Immunosuppressive treatment of aplastic anemia with antithymocyte globulin and cyclosporine. Semin Hematol. 2000;37:56-68.

254. Bacigalupo A, Bruno B, Saracco P, et al. Antilymphocyte globulin, cyclosporine, prednisolone, and granulocyte colony-stimulating factor for severe aplastic anemia: an update of the GITMO/EBMT study on 100 patients. European Group for Blood and Marrow Transplantation (EBMT) Working Party on Severe Aplastic Anemia and the Gruppo Italiano Trapianto di Midollo Osseo (GITMO). Blood. 2000;95:1931-1934.

255. Fuhrer M, Burdach S, Ebell W, et al. Relapse and clonal disease in children with aplastic anemia (AA) after immunosuppressive therapy (IST): the SAA 94 experience. German/Austrian Pediatric Aplastic Anemia Working Group. Klin Padiatr. 1998;210:173-179.

256. Matloub YH, Bostrom B, Golembe B, et al. Antithymocyte globulin, cyclosporine, and prednisone for the treatment of severe aplastic anemia in children. A pilot study. Am J Pediatr Hematol Oncol. 1994;16:104-106.

257. Goldenberg NA, Graham DK, Liang X, Hays T. Successful treatment of severe aplastic anemia in children using standardized immunosuppressive therapy with antithymocyte globulin and cyclosporine A. Pediatr Blood Cancer. 2004;43:718-722.

258. Kojima S, Ohara A, Tsuchida M, et al. Risk factors for evolution of acquired aplastic anemia into myelodysplastic syndrome and acute myeloid leukemia after immunosuppressive therapy in children. Blood. 2002;100:786-790.

259. Rosenfeld S, Follmann D, Nunez O, Young NS. Antithymocyte globulin and cyclosporine for severe aplastic anemia: association between hematologic response and long-term outcome. JAMA. 2003;289:1130-1135.

260. Tichelli A, Passweg J, Nissen C, et al. Repeated treatment with horse antilymphocyte globulin for severe aplastic anaemia. Br J Haematol. 1998;100:393-400.

261. Di Bona E, Rodeghiero F, Bruno B, et al. Rabbit antithymocyte globulin (r-ATG) plus cyclosporine and granulocyte colony stimulating factor is an effective treatment for aplastic anaemia patients unresponsive to a first course of intensive immunosuppressive therapy. Gruppo Italiano Trapianto di Midollo Osseo (GITMO). Br J Haematol. 1999;107:330-334.

262. Gupta V, Gordon-Smith EC, Cook G, et al. A third course of anti-thymocyte globulin in aplastic anaemia is only beneficial in previous responders. Br J Haematol. 2005;129:110-117.

263. Champlin RE, Ho WG, Feig SA, et al. Do androgens enhance the response to antithymocyte globulin in patients with aplastic anemia? A prospective randomized trial. Blood. 1985;66:184-188.

264. Kaltwasser JP, Dix U, Schalk KP, Vogt H. Effect of androgens on the response to antithymocyte globulin in patients with aplastic anaemia. Eur J Haematol. 1988;40:111-118.

265. Bacigalupo A, Chaple M, Hows J, et al. Treatment of aplastic anaemia (AA) with antilymphocyte globulin (ALG) and methylprednisolone (MPred) with or without androgens: a randomized trial from the EBMT SAA working party. Br J Haematol. 1993;83:145-151.

266. Leleu X, Terriou L, Duhamel A, et al. Long-term outcome in acquired aplastic anemia treated with an intensified dose schedule of horse antilymphocyte globulin in combination with androgens. Ann Hematol. 2006;85:711-716.

267. Alter BP. Inherited bone marrow failure syndromes. In Nathan DG, Orkin SH, Ginsburg D, Look AT (eds). Nathan and Oski's Hematology of Infancy and Childhood, 6th ed. Philadelphia, WB Saunders, 2003, pp 280-365.

268. Kurre P, Johnson FL, Deeg HJ. Diagnosis and treatment of children with aplastic anemia. Pediatr Blood Cancer. 2005;45:770-780.

269. Schrezenmeier H, Marin P, Raghavachar A, et al. Relapse of aplastic anaemia after immunosuppressive treatment: a report from the European Bone Marrow Transplantation Group SAA Working Party. Br J Haematol. 1993;85:371-377.

270. Scheinberg P, Nunez O, Young NS. Retreatment with rabbit anti-thymocyte globulin and ciclosporin for patients with relapsed or refractory severe aplastic anaemia. Br J Haematol. 2006;133:622-627.

271. Tooze JA, Marsh JC, Gordon-Smith EC. Clonal evolution of aplastic anaemia to myelodysplasia/acute myeloid leukaemia and paroxysmal nocturnal haemoglobinuria. Leuk Lymphoma. 1999;33:231-241.

272. Socie G, Rosenfeld S, Frickhofen N, et al. Late clonal diseases of treated aplastic anemia. Semin Hematol. 2000;37:91-101.

273. Socie G, Henry-Amar M, Bacigalupo A, et al. Malignant tumors occurring after treatment of aplastic anemia. European Bone Marrow Transplantation-Severe Aplastic Anaemia Working Party. N Engl J Med. 1993;329:1152-1157.

274. Deeg HJ, Seidel K, Casper J, et al. Marrow transplantation from unrelated donors for patients with severe aplastic anemia who have failed immunosuppressive therapy. Biol Blood Marrow Transplant. 1999;5:243-252.

275. Locasciulli A, Bruno B, Rambaldi A, et al. Treatment of severe aplastic anemia with antilymphocyte globulin, cyclosporine and two different granulocyte colony-stimulating factor regimens: a GITMO prospective randomized study. Haematologica. 2004;89:1054-1061.

276. Jeng MR, Naidu PE, Rieman MD, et al. Granulocyte-macrophage colony stimulating factor and immunosuppression in the treatment of pediatric acquired severe aplastic anemia. Pediatr Blood Cancer. 2005;45:170-175.

277. Ohara A, Kojima S, Hamajima N, et al. Myelodysplastic syndrome and acute myelogenous leukemia as a late

clonal complication in children with acquired aplastic anemia. Blood. 1997;90:1009-1013.

278. Gardner FH, Besa EC. Physiologic mechanisms and the hematopoietic effects of the androstanes and their derivatives. Curr Top Hematol. 1983;4:123-195.

279. Alexanian R. Erythropoietin and erythropoiesis in anemic man following androgens. Blood. 1969;33:564-572.

280. Singer JW, Adamson JW. Steroids and hematopoiesis. II. The effect of steroids on in vitro erythroid colony growth: evidence for different target cells for different classes of steroids. J Cell Physiol. 1976;88:135-143.

281. Shahidi N, Diamond L. Testosterone-induced remission in aplastic anemia of both acquired and congenital types. Further observations in 24 cases. N Engl J Med. 1961;264:953.

282. Najean Y, Pecking A. Prognostic factors in acquired aplastic anemia. A study of 352 cases. Am J Med. 1979;67:564-571.

283. Sanchez-Medal L, Gomez-Leal A, Duarte L, Guadalupe Rico M. Anabolic androgenic steroids in the treatment of acquired aplastic anemia. Blood. 1969;34:283-300.

284. Davis S, Rubin AD. Treatment and prognosis in aplastic anaemia. Lancet. 1972;1:871-873.

285. Williams DM, Lynch RE, Cartwright GE. Prognostic factors in aplastic anaemia. Clin Haematol. 1978;7:467-474.

286. Camitta BM, Storb R, Thomas ED. Aplastic anemia (first of two parts): pathogenesis, diagnosis, treatment, and prognosis. N Engl J Med. 1982;306:645-652.

287. Camitta BM, Storb R, Thomas ED. Aplastic anemia (second of two parts): pathogenesis, diagnosis, treatment, and prognosis. N Engl J Med. 1982;306:712-718.

288. McGiven AR. Peliosis hepatis: case report and review of pathogenesis. J Pathol. 1970;101:283-285.

289. Bourliere B, Najean Y. Influence of long-term androgen therapy on growth: an analysis of 18 cases of aplastic anemia in children. Am J Dis Child. 1987;141:718-719.

290. Marmont A, Bacigalupo A, VanLint MT, et al. Treatment of severe aplastic anemia with high-dose methylprednisolone and antilyphocyte globulin. In Young NS, Levine AS, Humphries K (eds). Aplastic Anemia: Stem Cell Biology and Advances in Treatment. New York, Alan R Liss, 1984, pp 271-287.

291. Gluckman E, Devergie A, Poros A, Degoulet P. Results of immunosuppression in 170 cases of severe aplastic anaemia. Report of the European Group of Bone Marrow Transplant (EGBMT). Br J Haematol. 1982;51:541-550.

292. Heaton L, Crosby W, Cohen A. Splenectomy in the treatment of hypoplasia of the bone marrow. With a report of twelve cases. Ann Surg. 1957;146:637.

293. Speck B, Gratwohl A, Nissen C, et al. Treatment of severe aplastic anemia. Exp Hematol. 1986;14:126-132.

294. Brodsky RA, Sensenbrenner LL, Jones RJ. Complete remission in severe aplastic anemia after high-dose cyclophosphamide without bone marrow transplantation. Blood. 1996;87:491-494.

295. Brodsky RA, Sensenbrenner LL, Smith BD, et al. Durable treatment-free remission after high-dose cyclophosphamide therapy for previously untreated severe aplastic anemia. Ann Intern Med. 2001;135:477-483.

296. Tisdale JF, Dunn DE, Geller N, et al. High-dose cyclophosphamide in severe aplastic anaemia: a randomised trial. Lancet. 2000;356:1554-1559.

297. Brodsky RA, Chen AR, Brodsky I, Jones RJ. High-dose cyclophosphamide as salvage therapy for severe aplastic anemia. Exp Hematol. 2004;32:435-440.

298. Taniguchi T, Minami Y. The IL-2/IL-2 receptor system: a current overview. Cell. 1993;73:5-8.

299. Maciejewski JP, Sloand EM, Nunez O, et al. Recombinant humanized anti–IL-2 receptor antibody (daclizumab) produces responses in patients with moderate aplastic anemia. Blood. 2003;102:3584-3586.

300. Sievers TM, Rossi SJ, Ghobrial RM, et al. Mycophenolate mofetil. Pharmacotherapy. 1997;17:1178-1197.

301. Scheinberg P, Nunez O, Wu C, Young NS. Treatment of severe aplastic anaemia with combined immunosuppression: anti-thymocyte globulin, ciclosporin and mycophenolate mofetil. Br J Haematol. 2006;133:606-611.

302. Pattison JR, Jones SE, Hodgson J, et al. Parvovirus infections and hypoplastic crisis in sickle-cell anaemia. Lancet. 1981;1:664-665.

303. Serjeant GR, Topley JM, Mason K, et al. Outbreak of aplastic crises in sickle cell anaemia associated with parvovirus-like agent. Lancet. 1981;2:595-597.

304. Kurtzman G, Frickhofen N, Kimball J, et al. Pure red-cell aplasia of 10 years' duration due to persistent parvovirus B19 infection and its cure with immunoglobulin therapy. N Engl J Med. 1989;321:519-523.

305. Frickhofen N, Chen ZJ, Young NS, et al. Parvovirus B19 as a cause of acquired chronic pure red cell aplasia. Br J Haematol. 1994;87:818-824.

306. Brown KE, Green SW, Antunez de Mayolo J, et al. Congenital anaemia after transplacental B19 parvovirus infection. Lancet. 1994;343:895-896.

307. Freedman MH. Pure red cell aplasia in childhood and adolescence: pathogenesis and approaches to diagnosis. Br J Haematol. 1993;85:246-253.

308. Ware RE, Kinney TR. Transient erythroblastopenia in the first year of life. Am J Hematol. 1991;37:156-158.

309. Zaentz SD, Krantz SB. Studies on pure red cell aplasia. VI. Development of two-stage erythroblast cytotoxicity method and role of complement. J Lab Clin Med. 1973;82:31-43.

310. Hoffman R, Kopel S, Hsu SD, et al. T-cell chronic lymphocytic leukemia: presence in bone marrow and peripheral blood of cells that suppress erythropoiesis in vitro. Blood. 1978;52:255-260.

311. Abkowitz JL, Kadin ME, Powell JS, Adamson JW. Pure red cell aplasia: lymphocyte inhibition of erythropoiesis. Br J Haematol. 1986;63:59-67.

312. Loughran TP Jr. Clonal diseases of large granular lymphocytes. Blood. 1993;82:1-14.

313. Ebert BL, Pretz J, Bosco J, et al. Identification of RPS14 as a 5q– syndrome gene by RNA interference screen. Nature. 2008;451:335-339.

314. Thompson DF, Gales MA. Drug-induced pure red cell aplasia. Pharmacotherapy. 1996;16:1002-1008.

315. Horne JL, Kirkpatrick HJR, Lederer H, Leys DG. Familial crises in congenital haemolytic disease. Lancet. 1945;2:33-36.

316. Dameshek W, Bloom ML. The events in the hemolytic crisis of hereditary spherocytosis, with particular refer-

ence to the reticulocytopenia, pancytopenia and an abnormal splenic mechanism. Blood. 1948;3:1381-1410.

317. Owren PA. Congenital hemolytic jaundice. The pathogenesis of the 'hemolytic crisis.' Blood. 1948;3:231-248.

318. Heilmeyer L. Die hamolytischen Anamien. Sang. 1950; 21:105-141.

319. Gasser C. Erythroblastopenie aigue dans les anemies hemolytiques. Sang. 1950;21:237-245.

320. Potter CG, Potter AC, Hatton CSR, et al. Variation of erythroid and myeloid precursors in the marrow and peripheral blood of volunteer subjects infected with human parvovirus (B19). J Clin Invest. 1987;79:1486-1492.

321. Dessypris EN. Pure Red Cell Aplasia. Baltimore, MD, John Hopkins University Press, 1988.

322. Feig SA, Freedman MH. Clinical Disorders and Experimental Models of Erythropoietic Failure. Boca Raton, FL, CRC Press, 1993.

323. Fisch P, Handgretinger R, Schaefer HE. Pure red cell aplasia. Br J Haematol. 2000;111:1010-1022.

324. Schmid JR, Kiely JM, Pease GL, Hargraves MM. Acquired pure red cell agenesis: report of 16 cases and review of the literature. Acta Haematol. 1963;30:255-270.

325. DiGiacomo J, Furst SW, Nixon DD. Primary acquired red cell aplasia in the adult. J Mt Sinai Hosp NY. 1966; 33:382.

336. Wranne J. Transient erythroblastopenia in infancy and childhood. Scand J Haematol. 1970;7:76-81.

327. Cherrick I, Karayalcin G, Lanzkowsky P. Transient erythroblastopenia of childhood. Prospective study of fifty patients. Am J Pediatr Hematol Oncol. 1994;16: 320-324.

328. Hays T, Lane PA Jr, Shafer F. Transient erythroblastopenia of childhood. A review of 26 cases and reassessment of indications for bone marrow aspiration. Am J Dis Child. 1989;143:605-607.

329. Rogers BB, Rogers ZR, Timmons CF. Polymerase chain reaction amplification of archival material for parvovirus B19 in children with transient erythroblastopenia of childhood. Pediatr Pathol Lab Med. 1996;16:471-478.

330. Tugal O, Pallant B, Shebarek N, Jayabose S. Transient erythroblastopenia of the newborn caused by human parvovirus. Am J Pediatr Hematol Oncol. 1994;16:352-355.

331. Bhambhani K, Inoue S, Sarnaik SA. Seasonal clustering of transient erythroblastopenia of childhood. Am J Dis Child. 1988;142:175-177.

332. Heegaard ED, Brown KE. Human parvovirus. Clin Microbiol Rev. 2002;15:485-505.

333. Liang TB, Li DL, Yu J, et al. Pure red cell aplasia due to parvovirus B19 infection after liver transplantation: a case report and review of rhe literature. World J Gastroenterol. 2007;13:2007-2010.

334. Ki CS, Kim JW, Lee NY, et al. Incidence and clinical significance of human parvovirus B19 infection in kidney transplant recipients. Clin Transplant. 2005;19:751-755.

335. Perkins SL. Pediatric red cell disorders and pure red cell aplasia. Am J Clin Pathol. 2004;122(Suppl):S70-S86.

336. Srinivas U, Mahapatra M, Saxena R, Pati HP. Thirty-nine cases of pure red cell aplasia: a single center experience from India. Hematology. 2007;12:245-248.

337. Dhall G, Ginsburg HB, Bodenstein L, et al. Thymoma in children: report of two cases and review of literature. J Pediatr Hematol Oncol. 2004;26:681-685.

338. Larroche C, Mouthon L, Casadevall N, et al. Successful treatment of thymoma-associated pure red cell aplasia with intravenous immunoglobulins. Eur J Haematol. 2000;65:74-76.

339. Jepson JH, Lowenstein L. Inhibition of erythropoiesis by a factor present in the plasma of patients with erythroblastopenia. Blood. 1996;27:425-434.

340. Casadevall N, Nataf J, Viron B, et al. Pure red-cell aplasia and antierythropoietin antibodies in patients treated with recombinant erythropoietin. N Engl J Med. 2002;346: 469-475.

341. Bennett CL, Luminari S, Nissenson AR, et al. Pure red-cell aplasia and epoetin therapy. N Engl J Med. 2004;351: 1403-1408.

342. Lim LC. Acquired red cell aplasia in association with the use of recombinant erythropoietin in chronic renal failure. Hematology. 2005;10:255-259.

343. Locatelli F, Del Vecchio L. Pure red cell aplasia secondary to treatment with erythropoietin. J Nephrol. 2003;16: 461-466.

344. Casadevall N, Eckardt KU, Rossert J. Epoetin-induced autoimmune pure red cell aplasia. J Am Soc Nephrol. 2005;16(Suppl 1):S67-S69.

345. Rossert J. Erythropoietin-induced, antibody-mediated pure red blood cell aplasia. Eur J Clin Invest. 2005;35 (Suppl 3):95-99.

346. Bennett CL, Cournoyer D, Carson KR, et al. Long-term outcome of individuals with pure red cell aplasia and antierythropoietin antibodies in patients treated with recombinant epoetin: a follow-up report from the Research on Adverse Drug Events and Reports (RADAR) Project. Blood. 2005;106(:3343-3347.

347. Summers SA, Matijevic A, Almond MK. Successful reintroduction of recombinant human erythropoietin following antibody induced pure red cell aplasia. Nephrol Dial Transplant. 2004;19:2137-2139.

348. Go RS, Lust JA, Phyliky RL. Aplastic anemia and pure red cell aplasia associated with large granular lymphocyte leukemia. Semin Hematol. 2003;40:196-200.

349. Rose MG, Berliner N. T-cell large granular lymphocyte leukemia and related disorders. Oncologist. 2004;9: 247-258.

350. Linch DC, Cawley JC, MacDonald SM, et al. Acquired pure red cell aplasia associated with an increase of T cells bearing receptors for the Fc of IgG. Acta Haematol. 1980;65:270-274.

351. Narra K, Borghaei H, Al-Saleem T, et al. Pure red cell aplasia in B-cell lymphoproliferative disorder treated with rituximab: report of two cases and review of the literature. Leuk Res. 2006;30:109-114.

8

Inherited Bone Marrow Failure Syndromes

Monica Bessler, Philip J. Mason, Daniel C. Link, and David B. Wilson

Inherited bone marrow failure syndromes (IBMFSs) are genetic disorders characterized by inadequate blood cell production. Bone marrow failure (BMF) may be manifested as an isolated cytopenia (pure red cell aplasia, neutropenia, or thrombocytopenia) or as pancytopenia and the clinical picture of aplastic anemia. Table 8-1 summarizes the more common forms of IBMFSs, the blood cell lineages affected, their association with malignancies, the genes mutated, their mode of inheritance, their chromosomal location, and the pathway involved. Other organ systems are often affected by these genetic abnormalities and result in birth defects or clinical disease in nonhematopoietic organs. Birth defects and extra-hematopoietic manifestations are often characteristic and may be noticed before the onset of BMF. BMF may be present at birth (congenital BMF) or develop later in life. IBMFSs are not always inherited; the genetic mutations responsible may also occur de novo during early embryonic development. Several, but not all of the IBMFSs are characterized by a predisposition for malignant transformation, in particular, malignant transformation of the hematopoietic system, including the development of myelodysplastic syndrome (MDS) and acute leukemia, but also a predisposition for a variety of other forms of cancer.

The prevalence of IBMFSs is difficult to ascertain. Originally, IBMFSs were thought to be mainly diseases of childhood. In children, 25% to 30% of BMF cases were thought to be due to a genetic cause, whereas in adults, an inherited genetic cause was considered only in a minority of patients. However, more recent data suggest that the prevalence of IBMFSs has probably been underestimated, particularly in adults. In addition, improved medical care and long-term survival after bone marrow transplantation (BMT) have extended life expectancy and shifted the management of patients with IBMFSs to adult hematologists.[1]

Timely and correct diagnosis of an IBMFS is of importance because management of an IBMFS differs from that of acquired BMF. Treatment of IBMFSs often requires a complex interdisciplinary approach that includes hematologists, geneticists, endocrinologists, oncologists, orthopedists, neurologists, gastroenterologists, gynecologists, dentists, and other specialists. Furthermore, differentiation between acquired and inherited BMF is of importance not only for affected individuals but also for their family members. Early and correct diagnosis of an IBMFS allows intensified and focused disease surveillance, anticipatory guidance, and avoidance of treatment-related toxicity. Identification of a gene mutation known to be associated with BMF can definitively establish the diagnosis before clinical symptoms advance and help identify an unaffected bone marrow donor in the family. It is therefore important that at the time of initial evaluation maximal effort be made to distinguish acquired from inherited forms of BMF.

Despite the considerable advances that have been made in elucidating the genetic causes of IBMFSs, the mechanisms leading to BMF remain poorly understood. The very nature of the diseases, namely, that the affected bone marrow cells are not dividing, are dying, or are simply absent, confounds laboratory investigations into pathogenesis. Therefore, in the past, investigations of IBMFSs were largely restricted to careful observations and descriptions of clinical manifestations of the patient and family, as well as meticulous study of the clinical course of the disease. However, during the last 10 years a number genes have been identified that when mutated, are responsible for certain forms of IBMFSs (see Table 8-1). Identification of these genes and investigation of their role in hematopoiesis have provided powerful new tools to explore the pathways responsible for BMF. Although IBMFSs have traditionally been classified according to their clinical features, in the future this classification may be supplanted by a definition determined by the affected pathway (see Table 8-1). Interestingly and for many investigators unexpectedly, the pathways affected are often "housekeeping" pathways important for the growth/survival of almost every cell, such as DNA repair, redox-related pathways, telomere maintenance, or ribosome biosynthesis, rather than pathways specific for hematopoiesis. Why hematopoiesis is often preferentially and sometimes even exclusively affected by a derangement in these pathways is intriguing and the focus of current investigations in the field of BMF research.

Accumulating insight into the pathogenetic pathways responsible for IBMFSs and detailed knowledge about the clinical disease continuously reshape our current understanding of IBMFSs and directly impinge on our approach to diagnosis, care, and treatment of patients and their families with IBMFSs. Probably one of the most dramatic emerging insights shared by several IBMFSs is that the severity, onset, and manifestations of disease often vary dramatically and that individuals with the classic clinical features often represent merely the "tip of an iceberg" whose dimensions we are only just beginning to appreciate.[2] IBMFSs or an inherited predisposition to the development of BMF is probably much more common than currently appreciated, not only in the pediatric population but also in adults. With the increased knowledge of how the genetic framework influences the development of BMF, distinguishing between inherited and acquired BMF becomes more difficult. Previously, IBMFSs were restricted mainly to patients with BMF caused by gene mutations with high disease penetrance. Today, it is increasingly being recognized that in addition, a growing number of patients have BMF caused by gene mutations that have lower or very low penetrance, with disease developing only occasionally or just under certain circumstances. Thus, the majority of patients in whom acquired idiopathic aplastic anemia was previously diagnosed in fact have an underlying genetic component responsible for the disease. Gene modifiers and environmental factors are additional factors that influence the penetrance of disease and pathobiology of BMF. Figure 8-1 schematically illustrates the possible interrelationship

TABLE 8-1 Inherited Bone Marrow Failure Syndromes

IBMFS	Inheritance	Peripheral Blood	Malignancies	Gene	Chromosomal Location	Affected Pathway
Fanconi's anemia (FA, MIM 227650)	AR XLR AR AR	Pancytopenia	MDS/AML Squamous cell carcinoma Other tumors	FANCA FANCB FANCC FANCD1	16q24.3 Xp22.31 9q22.3 13q12-13	DNA repair Homologous recombination
	AR		AML Wilms' tumor Medulloblastoma	FANCD2	3q25.3	
	AR AR AR AR AR AR AR		MDS/AML Squamous cell carcinoma Other tumors	FANCE FANCF FANCG FANCI FANCJ FANCL FANCM	6p21.3 11p15 9q13 5q25-q26 17q22-q24 2p16.1 14q21.3	
	AR		Wilms' tumor Medulloblastoma	FANCN	16p12	
Dyskeratosis congenita (DC)	XLR (MIM 305000) AD (MIM 127550)	Pancytopenia	MDS/AML Squamous cell carcinoma Other tumors	DKC1 TERC TERT	Xq28 3q26 5p33	Telomere maintenance Ribosome biogenesis Telomere maintenance Telomere maintenance
			Unknown	TINF2	14q11.2	Telomere maintenance
	AR (MIM 224230)		Unknown	NOP10 NHP2	15q14-q15 5q35.3	Telomere maintenance Ribosome biogenesis
Shwachman-Diamond syndrome (SDS, MIM 260400)	AR	Neutropenia with progression to pancytopenia	MDS/AML	SBDS	7q1.1	Ribosome biogenesis (?) Mitotic spindle maintenance (?)
Cartilage-hair hypoplasia (CHH, MIM 250250)	AR	Neutropenia Lymphopenia Anemia	Lymphoma Basal cell carcinoma	RMRP	9p21-12	Mitochondrial DNA replication Ribosome biogenesis Degradation of *CLB2* mRNA
Pearson's marrow-pancreas syndrome (PS, MIM 557000)	Mitochondrial	Neutropenia with progression to pancytopenia	None	mtDNA del		Mitochondrial function
Diamond-Blackfan anemia (DBA, MIM 105650)	AD	Anemia with rare progression to pancytopenia	MDS/AML Osteosarcoma	RPS19 RPS24 RPS17 RPL35a RPL5 PRL11	19q13.3 10q22-q23 15q25.2 3q29 1p22.1 1p36.12	Ribosome biogenesis
Congenital dyserythropoiesis (CDA) CDA I (MIM 22410) CDA II (MIM 224100†) CDA III (MIM 105600†)	AR AR AD	Anemia	None None None	CDAN1* Unknown Unknown	15q15.1-15.3 20q11.2 15q21-25	Unknown Unknown Unknown

Continues

TABLE 8-1   Inherited Bone Marrow Failure Syndromes—cont'd

	Inheritance	Cytopenia	Malignancy	Gene	Locus	Function
Severe congenital neutropenia caused by *ELA2* mutation (SCN, MIM 202700)	AD	Neutropenia	MDS/AML	*ELA2*	19p13.3	Unfolded protein response (?)
Cyclic neutropenia (CN, MIM 162800)	AD	Neutropenia	None	*ELA2*	19p13.3	Unfolded protein response (?)
Kostmann's syndrome (MIM 610738)	AR	Neutropenia	None	*HAX1*	1q21.3	Regulation of apoptosis (?)
Congenital amegakaryocytic thrombocytopenia (CAMT, MIM 60448)	AR	Thrombocytopenia with progression to pancytopenia	AML	*c-MPL*	1q35	Megakaryopoiesis
Thrombocytopenia with absent radii (TAR, MIM 274000†)	AR? DG?	Thrombocytopenia	AML	Microdeletion + modifier	1q21.1 +?	Unknown
Amegakaryocytic thrombocytopenia with radioulnar synostosis (ARTUS, MIM 605432)	AD	Thrombocytopenia with progression to pancytopenia	AML	*HOXA11*	7p15-p14.2	Morphogenesis
Familial platelet disorder with associated acute myeloid leukemia (FPD/AML, MIM 601399)	AD	Thrombocytopenia	MDS/AML	*AML1*	21q22.3	Hematopoietic cell differentiation
Wiskott-Aldrich syndrome (WAS, MIM 301000)	XLR	Thrombocytopenia Neutropenia	Lymphoma Not reported	*WAS* * *WAS* *	Xp11.22-Xp11.3 Xp11.22-Xp11.3	Signal transduction from cell surface to actin
X-linked thrombocytopenia (XLT, MIM 313900)	XLR	Thrombocytopenia	Lymphoma	*WAS*	Xp11.22-Xp11.3	cytoskeleton
Congenital dyserythropoiesis associated with thrombocytopenia (MIM 300367)	XLR	Thrombocytopenia	None	*GATA1*	Xp11.23	Erythroid and megakaryocytic development
RARE FORMS OF INHERITED BONE MARROW FAILURE						
Nijmegen's breakage syndrome (NBS, MIM 251260)	AR	Pancytopenia	AML Lymphoma	*NSB1* *	8q21	DNA repair
DNA ligase IV (LIG4, MIM 606593)	AR	Pancytopenia	Leukemia	*LIG4*	13q22-q34	DNA repair
Seckel SCKL1, (MIM 210600)	AR	Pancytopenia	Leukemia Lymphoma	*ATR* *PCNT*	3q22-q24 21q22.3	DNA repair Centrosomal function

Disease	Inheritance	Hematologic	Leukemia Lymphoma Neuroblastoma	Gene	Location	Function
Dubowitz (MIM 223370†)	AR	Pancytopenia		Unknown	Unknown	DNA repair (?)
Schminke (SIOD, MIM 242900)	AR	Pancytopenia	Lymphoma (?)	SMARCAL1	2q34-q36	Chromatin remodeling
Ducan/Purtilo (XPL, MIM 308240)	XLR	Pancytopenia	EBV lymphoma	SH2D1A/SAP	Xq25	B- and T-cell function
Nonimmune chronic neutropenia of adults (NI-CINA, MIM 607847)	AD	Neutropenia	None reported, AML (?)	GIF1	1p22	Unknown
Barth (BTHS, MIM 302060)	XLR	Neutropenia	None reported	TAZ1	Xq28	Unknown
Cohen (COH1, MIM 216550)	AR	Neutropenia	None reported	COH1	8q22-q23	Lysosomal protein trafficking
Chédiak-Higashi (CHS1, MIM 606897)	AR	Neutropenia	None reported	LYST	1q42.1-42.2	Lysosomal protein trafficking
Griselli (GS2, MIM 607724)	AR	Neutropenia Thrombocytopenia	None reported	RAB27A	15q14.1	Lysosomal function (?)
Hermansky-Pudlak 2 (HPS2, MIM 608233)	AR	Neutropenia	None reported	AP3B1	5q14.1	Lysosomal protein trafficking Unfolded protein response (?)
Immunodeficiency caused by defect in MAPBP interacting protein P14 (MIM 610798)	AR	Neutropenia	None reported	MAPBPIP	1q21	Lysosome biogenesis
Glycogen storage disease 1b (GSD1B, MIM 23220)	AR	Neutropenia	None reported	G6PT1	11q23	Glycogen storage
Hyper-IgM (XHIM, MIM 308230)	XLR	Neutropenia Pancytopenia	None reported	CD40LG (HIGM1)	Xq26	B-cell activation
WHIM syndrome (MIM 19360)	AD	Neutropenia Lymphopenia	None reported	CXCR4*	2q21	Neutrophil mobilization

*Specific mutations only.
†Responsible gene not identified.
AD, autosomal dominant; AML, acute myeloid leukemia; AR, autosomal recessive; DG, digenic; MDS, myelodysplastic syndrome; MIM, Mendelian Inheritance in Man; WHIM, warts, hypogammaglobulinemia, infections, and myelokathexis; XLR, X-linked recessive; ?, possible.

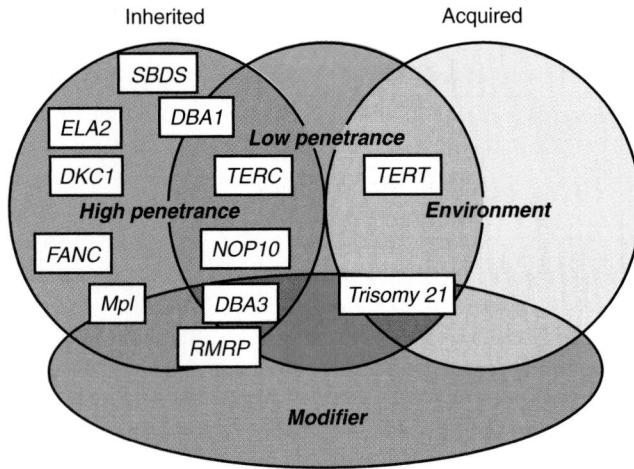

FIGURE 8-1. Interrelationship between disease penetrance of a genetic mutation, the environment, and modifiers in the pathogenesis of bone marrow failure.

between genetic mutation, environment, and modifiers in the pathogenesis of BMF. The increased understanding of the genetic components and their role and importance in the pathogenesis of disease will allow us to improve diagnosis, management, and treatment of patients with BMF.

INHERITED BONE MARROW SYNDROMES ASSOCIATED WITH PANCYTOPENIA

Fanconi's Anemia

Fanconi's anemia (FA) is a genetically and phenotypically heterogeneous disorder. The disease is named after the Swiss pediatrician Guido Fanconi (1892-1979), who first described the syndrome in 1927.[3] Clinically, FA is characterized by a variety of congenital abnormalities, progressive BMF, and a propensity for the development of leukemia and other forms of cancer. Cells from FA patients have a striking hypersensitivity to DNA interstrand cross-links,[4] which has become the basis of a clinical diagnostic test for FA (Box 8-1).[5]

Epidemiology

The incidence of FA is estimated to be approximately 3 per million with a carrier frequency of 1 in 300.[6,7] Males are affected slightly more frequently than females, with a male-to-female ratio of 1.2 : 1.[8,9] FA has been reported in all races and ethnic groups. The world's highest prevalence of FA, caused by a founder effect, is seen in Spanish gypsies, who have a carrier frequency of 1 in 70.[10] A high prevalence of FA is also found in individuals of Ashkenazi Jewish decent, who have an approximate heterozygous frequency of 1 in 89,[11] and in South African Afrikaans, in whom carrier frequency is estimated to be 1 in 83.[12,13]

Clinical Manifestations

The clinical manifestations of FA are heterogeneous (variable penetrance and expressivity; for definitions, see Box 8-2). Affected family members can have a wide variety of abnormalities (variable expressivity).[14-18] Even monozygotic twins have been described to differ in their physical and hematologic manifestations.[16] However, the occurrence of malformations is nonrandom. Siblings are usually concordant for the presence or absence of multiple congenital abnormalities; likewise, the age at onset of hematologic manifestations is similar within an individual family.[19] Thus, the variability in clinical findings appears to be partially linked to the different genotypes (also see later).[20-24] The emergence of revertant cells leading to hematopoietic mosaicism further contributes to disease variability (see later).[25-28] Originally, the diagnosis of FA was based on the presence of both aplastic anemia and a specific, though broad range of physical abnormalities.[29] With the availability of more sensitive and specific tests for the diagnosis of FA, including cytogenetic and molecular diagnostics, it has become increasingly evident that a significant proportion of patients lack congenital abnormalities (25% to 40%)[30,31] or aplastic anemia fails to develop, or both (variable penetrance). Nevertheless, these individuals are still at risk for late complications such as leukemia and cancer.

Congenital Abnormalities

The frequency of congenital abnormalities within the FA population is summarized in Table 8-2. Box 8-3 further details the nature of anomalies found in patients with FA. Figure 8-2A shows a 1-year-old girl with FA, and Figure

TABLE 8-2	Physical Abnormalities in Fanconi's Anemia*	
Abnormality	**Alter,[9] 2003**	**IFAR[16,32]**
Total number of patients	1206	>700
Skin pigment and/or café au lait spots	55%	64%
Short stature	51%	63%
Skeletal abnormality (radial ray, hip, vertebral scoliosis, rib)	71%	—
Upper limbs	43%	49%
Abnormal gonads, male	32%	20%
Abnormal gonads, female	3%	—
Head	26%	—
Central nervous system	—	8%
Eyes	23%	38%
Renal	21%	34%
Birth weight ≤2500 g	11%	—
Developmental disability	11%	16%
Ears, hearing	9%	11%
Legs	8%	—
Cardiopulmonary	6%	13%
Gastrointestinal	5%	14%
No anomalies	25%	30%
Short stature and/or skin only	11%	—

*Data represent percentages of patients with the abnormality. IFAR, International Fanconi Anemia Registry.

8-2C shows a 12-year-old boy with several classic phenotypic features, including short stature, microencephaly, broad nasal bridge, epicanthal folds, micrognathia, café au lait spots and hypopigmentation, and an absent and a triphalangeal thumb. FA patients may have a combination or none of the congenital anomalies listed. The phenotypic variability makes a diagnosis of FA difficult when based only on clinical features.

Endocrinopathies

Data from the International Fanconi Anemia Registry (IFAR) indicate that endocrine abnormalities are present in 81% of FA patients, primarily glucose/insulin abnormalities, growth hormone insufficiency, hypothyroidism, and hypogonadism.[31,33,34]

Short Stature. Although short stature is an integral feature of FA,[17,35] a superimposed endocrinopathy may have an additional impact on growth and is responsive to growth hormone therapy.[36,37] Detection of an anatomic abnormality of the hypothalamic-pituitary region by magnetic resonance imaging is a diagnostic marker of permanent growth hormone deficiency. In patients 18 years or older, osteopenia or osteoporosis is frequent.[34]

Fertility. Female patients with FA usually have a shortened reproductive life because of secondary amenorrhea, irregular menses, anovulatory menstrual cycles, and premature menopause. Congenital abnormalities in the female genitourinary tract further limit fecundity. Though rare, pregnancies have been reported in women with FA. The babies born were normal, and the pregnancies seemed to not have had a significant impact on the mother's hematologic manifestations.[38,39] Pregnancy in women with FA has also been reported after BMT.[40-43] Cryptorchidism, hypogenitalism, hypergonadotropic hypogonadism, and reduced sperm counts are frequent in male patients with FA. Reports of male FA patients fathering children are rare.[44]

Hematologic Abnormalities

Progressive BMF is one of the hallmarks of FA, although the hematologic findings vary. Thrombocytopenia and macrocytosis often precede anemia and neutropenia. Elevated hemoglobin F levels[45] and elevated expression of "i" antigen on red cells usually coincide with macrocytosis and are suggestive of stress hematopoiesis.[46,47] Serum α-fetoprotein levels are consistently elevated in FA patients irrespective of the presence of liver abnormalities.[48] Erythropoietin levels are usually elevated in anemic FA patients. The first hematologic abnormalities in individuals with FA are detected at a median age of 7 years. The majority of FA patients already have pancytopenia at the time of diagnosis (53%). By the age of 40, the cumulative incidence of hematologic abnormalities is 90% to 98%.[21,49]

In rare cases, thrombocytopenia may be present at birth and progress to pancytopenia in the neonatal period or infancy.[19,50,51] Thus, FA also has to be considered in cases of aplastic anemia in neonates and infants. In other patients, hematologic abnormalities never become clinically evident, and the diagnosis of FA is made later in life as a result of late FA-associated complications such as cancer or leukemia. The emergence of revertant cells leading to hematopoietic mosaicism is often associated with a mild or absent hematologic phenotype (also see later). Finally, in a small proportion (2% to 5%) of FA patients, MDS or leukemia is diagnosed but the underlying BMF never becomes clinically apparent.[19,52] Bone marrow examination generally shows reduced cellularity; however, it may also be normocellular or hypercellular, particularly in individuals evolving into MDS or MDS/acute myeloid leukemia (AML). BMF is usually progressive. Fifty percent of individuals who are initially found to have thrombocytopenia progress to pancytopenia within 3 to 4 years. The actuarial risk of progression to pancytopenia is 84% at 20 years after the initial diagnosis of thrombocytopenia.[19]

Bone marrow culture studies show an intrinsic proliferation defect in hematopoietic progenitor cells from FA patients with and without clinical signs of BMF.[53,54] Hematopoietic progenitor cells are exquisitely sensitive to oxidative stress.[53,55,56] Expression of tumor necrosis factor-α (TNF-α) and interferon-γ (IFN-γ) is increased in FA patients.[57-59]

| Box 8-3 | **Specific Types of Anomalies in Fanconi's Anemia** |

SKIN

Generalized hyperpigmentation on the trunk, neck, and intertriginous areas; café au lait spots; hypopigmented areas

BODY

Short stature, delicate features, small size, underweight

UPPER LIMBS

Thumbs: absent or hypoplastic; supernumerary, bifid, or duplicated; rudimentary; short, low-set, attached by a thread; triphalangeal, tubular, stiff, hyperextensible

Radii: absent or hypoplastic (only with abnormal thumbs); absent or weak pulse

Hands: clinodactyly; hypoplastic thenar eminence; six fingers; absent first metacarpal; enlarged, abnormal fingers; short fingers, transverse crease

Ulnae: dysplastic

GONADS

Males: hypogenitalia, undescended testes, hypospadias, abnormal genitalia, absent testis, atrophic testes, azoospermia, phimosis, abnormal urethra, micropenis, delayed development

Females: hypogenitalia; bicornuate uterus; abnormal genitalia; aplasia of the uterus and vagina; atresia of the uterus, vagina, and ovary

OTHER SKELETAL ANOMALIES

Head and face: microcephaly, hydrocephalus, micrognathia, peculiar face, bird-like face, flat head, frontal bossing, scaphocephaly, sloped forehead, choanal atresia, dental abnormalities

Neck: Sprengel's deformity; short, low hairline; webbed

Spine: spina bifida (thoracic, lumbar, cervical, occult sacral), scoliosis, abnormal ribs, sacrococcygeal sinus, Klippel-Feil syndrome, vertebral anomalies, extra vertebrae

EYES

Small eyes, strabismus, epicanthal folds, hypertelorism, ptosis, slanting, cataracts, astigmatism, blindness, epiphora, nystagmus, proptosis, small iris

EARS

Deafness (usually conductive); abnormal shape; atresia; dysplasia; low-set, large or small; infections; abnormal middle ear; absent drum; dimples; rotated; canal stenosis

KIDNEYS

Ectopic or pelvic; abnormal, horseshoe, hypoplastic, or dysplastic; absent; hydronephrosis or hydroureter; infections; duplicated; rotated; reflux; hyperplasia; no function; abnormal artery

GASTROINTESTINAL SYSTEM

High-arched palate, atresia (esophagus, duodenum, jejunum), imperforate anus, tracheoesophageal fistula, Meckel's diverticulum, umbilical hernia, hypoplastic uvula, abnormal biliary ducts, megacolon, abdominal diastasis, Budd-Chiari syndrome

LOWER LIMBS

Feet: toe syndactyly, abnormal toes, flatfeet, short toes, clubfeet, six toes, supernumerary toe

Legs: congenital hip dislocation, Perthes' disease, coxa vara, abnormal femur, thigh osteoma, abnormal legs

CARDIOPULMONARY SYSTEM

Patent ductus arteriosus, ventricular septal defect, abnormal heart, peripheral pulmonic stenosis, aortic stenosis, coarctation, absent lung lobes, vascular malformation, aortic atheromas, atrial septal defect, tetralogy of Fallot, pseudotruncus, hypoplastic aorta, abnormal pulmonary drainage, double aortic arch, cardiac myopathy

OTHER ANOMALIES

Slow development, hyperreflexia, Bell's palsy, central nervous system arterial malformation, stenosis of the internal carotid artery, small pituitary gland, absent corpus callosum

---

*Abnormalities are listed in approximate order of frequency within each category.

Modified from Alter BP. Inherited bone marrow failure syndromes. In Nathan DG, Orkin SH, Ginsburg D, Look AT (eds). Nathan and Oski's Hematology of Infancy and Childhood, vol 1, 6th ed. Philadelphia, WB Saunders, 2003, pp 281-365.

Myelodysplastic Syndrome in Patients with Fanconi's Anemia. The risk of MDS developing in FA patients is estimated to be approximately 6%. In the literature the definition of MDS in FA patients varies, which prevents strict comparison and also suggests that a conventional definition of MDS might not always be appropriate. Nonrandom X-inactivation, suggesting clonal hematopoiesis, may be present at the time of BMF before the onset of MDS.[60,61] Clonal cytogenetic abnormalities are found in 34% to 48% of FA patients.[19,62] The actuarial risk of a chromosomal abnormality developing is 67% by the age of 30 years.[19] Clonal fluctuations are frequent, including the disappearance of clones, the appearance of new clones, and clonal evolution.[62,63] Chromosomal abnormalities in MDS most frequently involve chromosomes 1q, 7 (monosomy, isochromosome, or other structural rearrangement), 6, and 13.[19,64,65] Individuals in whom clonal cytogenetic abnormalities develop have

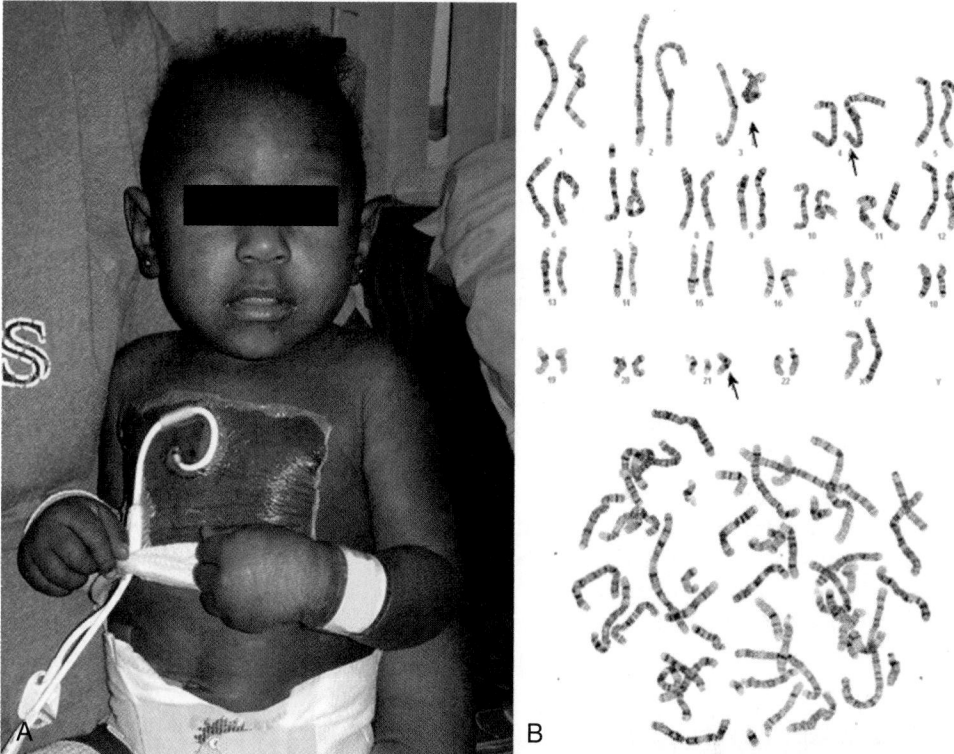

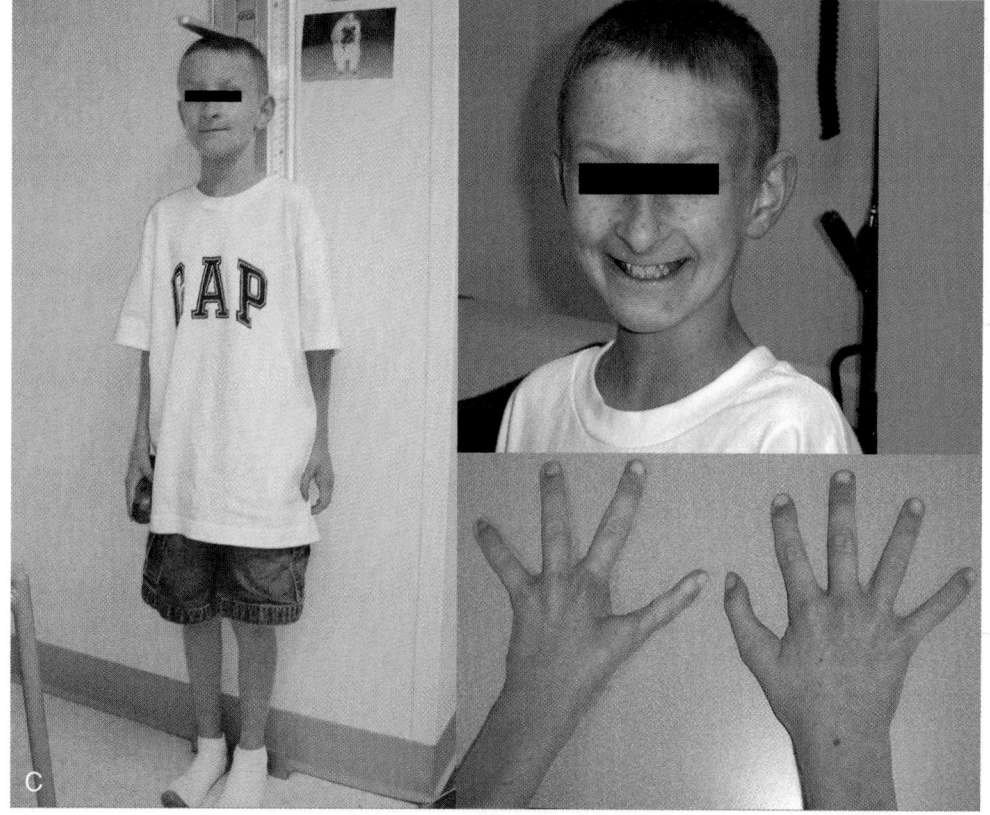

FIGURE 8-2. A, Infant girl with Fanconi's anemia who exhibited several classic phenotypic features, including short stature, microcephaly, broad nasal base, epicanthal folds, micrognathia, and café au lait spots (left side of the forehead). **B,** Cytogenetic findings in peripheral blood lymphocytes in Fanconi's anemia after culture with diepoxybutane. **C,** Twelve-year-old boy with Fanconi's anemia. The classic phenotypic features include short stature, microcephaly, broad nasal base, epicanthal folds, micrognathia, café au lait spots (chin and left temple), absent thumb left (after reconstructive surgery), and triphalangeal thumb left. (**B,** *Courtesy of Shashikanat Kulkarni, Washington University.*)

a reduced survival rate of 35% to 40% as opposed to 92% in FA patients without such abnormities. MDS morphology, as defined by dysplasia in multiple blood cell lineages and found in 32% of patients, has a worse predictive value with a 5-year survival rate of 9%. None of the patients with both morphologic MDS and cytogenetic abnormalities (22%) survived 5 years.[19,62] The yearly risk of progression from MDS to AML is estimated to be about 9%.[66] Gain of the distal portion of chromosome 3q(26-29), frequently present in FA patients even before the onset of MDS, is associated with a poor prognosis, decreased survival, and an increased frequency of MDS and AML.[67-69]

Predisposition to Malignancy. A major phenotype of FA is a predisposition for cancer, including leukemia and solid tumors. The risk of cancer developing is about 800 to 1000 times higher than in the normal population. There are three reports of the occurrence of solid tumors and leukemia in cohorts of patients with FA (see also Table 8-3). One is a retrospective analysis of the literature between 1927 and 2001 that included 1301 patients with FA.[70] The second, from the IFAR at the Rockefeller Institute in New York, included 754 North American patients evaluated between 1982 and 2001.[21] The third is a North American Survey that included 145 patients.[66] The crude risk of leukemia developing is estimated to be between 5% and 10%, and that for MDS is about 5%, with a yearly risk of evolution to leukemia of about 9%. The crude risk of solid tumors developing is estimated to be about 5% to 10%. By the age of 40, the cumulative incidence of leukemia and solid tumors is estimated to be approximately 33% and 26% to 30%, respectively. The median age at development of cancer is 16 years versus 68 years for the same types of cancer in the general population. The risk of solid tumors and leukemia developing increases with age. Thus, patients with mild hematologic and phenotypic abnormalities and the longest survival are at the highest risk for the development of tumors or leukemia.[18] However, with increased survival after hematopoietic stem cell transplantation (HSCT), the frequency of cancer might also increase in patients with more severe disease.[1] The most frequent cancers occur in the neck, head, and upper esophagus, followed by the vulva, anus, and lower esophagus. The role of human papillomavirus in the pathogenesis of squamous cell cancer in patients with FA is controversial.[71,72] The risk for development of squamous cell cancer of the head and neck and particularly the tongue is higher in FA patients after HSCT than in those without HSCT and

TABLE 8-3 Cancer in Patients with Fanconi's Anemia

Type	NO. OF PATIENTS (%)		
	Alter,[70] 2003	Kulter et al.,[21] 2003	Rosenberg et al.,[66] 2003
Reporting period	1927-2001	1982-2001	2001
Patients evaluated	1301	754	145
Hematologic malignancies	214 (16)	128 (17)	32 (22)
Cumulative incidence	—	33 (by age 40)	10 (by age 10)
AML	116 (9)	60 (8)	9 (6)
MDS	89 (7)	53 (7)	23 (16)
ALL	7	5	—
CMML	—	1	—
Lymphoma	2	2	—
Nonhematologic malignancies	89 (7)	73 (10)	18 (12)
Cumulative incidence	—	28 (by age 40)	29 (by age 49)
Squamous cell carcinoma	66 (5)	39 (5)	16 (11)
Oropharynx	26 (2)	19 (3)	6 (4)
Esophagus	9	1	2
Vulva and anus	10	—	—
Vulva	3	8	3
Anus	6	2	2
Cervix	6	6	3
Cutaneous (nonmelanoma)	6	3	—
Hepatic	37(3)	18 (2)	2 (1)
Adenoma	6	11	11
Hepatocellular carcinoma	14	6	22
Renal	0	6 (1)	—
Brain	1	5 (1)	1
Miscellaneous tumors	—	11 (1)	—
Breast	4	3	4
Lung	3	—	2
Gastric	2	—	2
Colon	0	—	1
Osteogenic sarcoma	1	1	1
Retinoblastoma	1	—	1
Other tumors	—	7	1

The three cohorts are not mutually exclusive.
ALL, acute lymphocytic leukemia; AML, acute myeloid leukemia; CMML, chronic myelomonocytic leukemia; MDS, myelodysplastic syndrome.
Modified from Alter BP, Greene MH, Velazquez I, Rosenberg PS. Cancer in Fanconi anemia. Blood. 2003;101:2072.

correlates with the presence and severity of graft-versus-host disease.[49,73] Adenoma of the liver and hepatocarcinoma were found mainly in patients undergoing androgen therapy.[70,74,75] Hepatoadenomas usually regress after cessation of androgen therapy.[76] Multiple neoplasms in patients with FA are not uncommon.[21,70,77]

Leukemia is the most frequent malignancy in patients with FA.[1,21,66,70,78] AML is the most frequent leukemic phenotype, although patients with acute lymphocytic leukemia (ALL) and chronic myelomonocytic leukemia have also been described. The morphologic-histochemical classification developed by the French-American-British (FAB) Cooperative Group[79-82] describes all categories of AML (M0 to M7) in patients with FA, with the exception of M3 (promyelocytic morphology), which has never been reported in patients with FA.[70] The leukemia in FA patients, however, is clinically and molecularly very different from that in the general pediatric and adult population. Chromosomal translocations characteristic of some forms of adult or childhood AML, such as translocation between chromosomes 8 and 21, are not usually found in FA patients with AML.[64] Thus, the conventional FAB classification used to predict a patient's prognosis does not apply to patients with FA and leukemia. However, leukemia in patients with FA shows many molecular and clinical similarities to leukemia occurring in other IBMFSs. Leukemia in FA patients is often difficult to treat, and most patients die within 6 month of diagnosis. Leukemia in patients with FA may arise de novo or develop from MDS. In some FA patients, AML may be the first hematologic manifestation of disease.[52] Leukemic cells often show complex cytogenetic abnormalities, including abnormalities similar to those seen in MDS. Abnormalities of chromosome 7 (monosomy, isochromosome, or other structural rearrangement), followed by abnormalities of 1q (usually duplications), are the most frequent in FA-associated leukemia.[19,64,65,83]

The risk and type of cancer vary for different FA subtypes (also see later). FA patients belonging to complementation group D1 (FA-D1) with biallelic mutations in *FANCD1/BRCA2* have a high risk for the development of malignancies at a very young age, frequently before manifestations of BMF appear, and the cumulative risk for AML or other cancer is 97% by the age of 5.2 years. In addition, the spectrum of cancer is distinct, with medulloblastoma being the predominant malignancy,[24,84,85] possibly because BRCA2 participates in DNA repair outside the FA pathway (see later also). An increased risk for childhood cancer with a very similar spectrum has also been found in families belonging to the FA-N subtype.[86] FANCN/PALB2 binds to BRCA2 and facilitates its binding to chromatin (see later).[87] The interaction between these two proteins explains the similar cancer predisposition in FA individuals belonging to the FA-D1 and FA-N subgroups.

Common to all FA cancer patients is low tolerance for DNA-damaging chemotherapeutic agents. Accordingly, chemotherapeutic regimens often need to be modified, given at low dosage, or avoided in favor of alternative or surgical approaches (also see later).[88]

Diagnosis

The most widely used diagnostic test for FA is hypersensitivity to the clastogenic (chromosome-breaking) effect of diepoxybutane (DEB) or mitomycin C (MMC).[5,89] The increased spontaneous chromosomal instability of FA cells leads to distinctive chromosomal breaks, gaps, and various chromatid interchanges, which were previously used as a cellular marker for FA.[90,91] The frequency of spontaneous chromosomal instability in FA cells is highly variable,[90] and it is thought to be responsible for the increased susceptibility of FA patients to cancer. The sensitivity of FA cells to the clastogenic effect has been studied for numerous cross-linking agents,[4] but DEB and MMC are the agents most widely used for the diagnosis of FA.[5,89] Figure 8-2B shows the increased chromosome breakage after culture in DEB. The diagnosis of FA is made when DEB-treated cultured lymphocytes demonstrate a 3- to 10-fold increase in chromosomal breakage over normal controls.[92] The tests are highly sensitive and fairly specific for FA and are used for the diagnosis of FA before the development of clinical disease and for prenatal diagnosis.[5,93-96] A possible rare exception that can result in a pattern of DEB- or MMC-induced chromosomal breakage similar to that found in FA patients is an individual with specific mutations in the *NBS1* gene in the Nijmegen breakage syndrome.[97-100] However, more frequently, the presence of revertant cells in the specimen may complicate the interpretation of DEB or MMC test results (see later). It is estimated that 10% to 25% of FA patients exhibit two populations of phytohemagglutinin-stimulated lymphocytes, one that is sensitive to the clastogenic effects of DNA cross-linking agents and one that is resistant.[26,101] Thus, the presence of only few metaphases with multiple structural chromosomal changes might indicate FA with somatic mosaicism. In these cases, demonstration of increased chromosomal breakage in patients' DEB- or MMC-treated fibroblasts might help confirm the diagnosis of FA (see later also).

Immunoblotting for FANCD2 Monoubiquitination

Biallelic mutations in 10 of the 13 FA genes (*FANC* genes) lead to failure of FANCD2 monoubiquitination, and failure of FANCD2 monoubiquitination is specific for a defect in the FA pathway (see later). Testing for FANCD2 monoubiquitination by immunoblotting of peripheral blood lymphocytes and fibroblasts has therefore been proposed as an alternative first-line diagnostic tool for the diagnosis of FA.[102,103] Biallelic mutations in *FANCD1/BRCA2*, *FANCJ*, and *FANCN/PALB2*, which have normal FANCD2 monoubiquitination but an abnormal DBE or MMC test (or both), are missed with this diagnostic assay and require additional testing.

Genetic Testing for FANC Gene Mutations

Although only identification of biallelic mutations in a *FANC* gene definitively confirms the diagnosis of FA, genetic testing is not usually recommended as a first-line diagnostic tool for the diagnosis of FA. Possible exceptions are families with a known *FANC* gene mutation and FA in a population with a high frequency of a founder mutation, for example, a case of FA in Spanish gypsies (also see later). The indication, advantages, and difficulties of genetic testing for biallelic mutations in *FANC* genes are discussed later.

Cellular Phenotype of Fanconi's Anemia Cells

In addition to increased spontaneous and induced chromosomal instability, FA cells have several other phenotypic characteristics (Table 8-4). FA cells have increased sensitivity to other DNA-damaging agents, such as ionizing radiation and oxygen radicals.[4,5,109-111,123-125,157-159] FA cells have an abnormality in cell cycle distribution, with an increased number of cells with 4*N* DNA content suggesting a delay in the G$_2$/M or late S phase (or both) of the cell cycle.[145] The increase in cells with 4*N* DNA content is accentuated after treatment with interstrand DNA cross-linking agents. Flow cytometric measurements of the increase in the proportion of cells with 4*N* DNA content after DNA cross-linking agents may be used as an additional criterion for the diagnosis of FA.[112,113] However, similar results have been obtained in patients with ataxia-telangiectasia.[159a] FA cells show accelerated telomere shortening in vitro and an increase in telomere free ends and chromosome end fusions, thus suggesting a defect in maintenance of telomere integrity and increased breakage at telomeric sequences.[115,116]

Differential Diagnosis

Clinically, FA has to be differentiated from other IBMFSs, particularly dyskeratosis congenita (DC), Diamond-Blackfan anemia (DBA), Shwachman-Diamond syndrome (SDS), thrombocytopenia with absent radii (TAR), and other nonclassified forms of BMF. Clinical manifestations, associated physical abnormalities, family history (pattern of inheritance), and increased chromosomal fragility in the DEB or MMC test performed on cultured peripheral lymphocytes or fibroblasts, or both, are helpful in strengthening the diagnosis of FA. However, only identification of pathogenic mutations on both copies of an FA gene (biallelic mutation) may definitely consolidate the diagnosis of FA. Congenital abnormities in FA may have an overlap with malformations seen in other disorders with genetic and nongenetic causes. Thrombocytopenia and radial ray abnormalities are also characteristic of TAR (see later). However, in FA, if the radii are affected, the thumbs are always abnormal; in TAR, in which the radii are absent, thumbs are always present. Other syndromes that have phenotypic overlap with FA include Holt-Oram syndrome (Mendelian

TABLE 8-4	Cellular Abnormalities in Fanconi's Anemia
Feature	**References**
Spontaneous chromosome breaks	90, 101, 104-108
Sensitivity to cross-linking agents	4, 5, 89, 109-111
Prolongation of the G$_2$/M and S phase of the cell cycle	112-114
Accelerated telomere shortening	115-118*
Hypersensitivity to ionizing radiation†	119-122
SENSITIVITY TO OXYGEN	
Poor growth at ambient O$_2$	123-126
Overproduction of O$_2$ radicals	127
Deficient O$_2$ radical defense	128
Deficiency in superoxide dismutase	129, 130
Sensitivity to ionizing radiation during G$_2$	131
Overproduction of TNF-α	132
DIRECT DEFECTS IN DNA REPAIR	
Accumulation of DNA adducts	133
Defective repair of DNA cross-links	134, 135
Hypermutability (by deletion)	136-140
Increased apoptosis	141-143
Abnormal induction of p53	142, 144
Failure to arrest DNA synthesis in response to DNA damage	145, 146
Defective nonhomologous end joining	147-149
Increased homologous recombination	150, 151‡
INTRINSIC STEM CELL DEFECT	
Decreased colony growth in vitro	53, 54, 152-154
Decreased gonadal stem cell survival	155, 156

*Experiments in mice suggest that accelerated telomere shortening is not a direct effect of Fanconi's anemia gene products on telomeres but rather an indirect effect, such as increased sensitivity to oxygen radicals.

†Hypersensitivity to ionizing radiation is controversial. More recent results suggest increased sensitivity in the majority of Fanconi's anemia complementation groups.

‡The defect has been found in only some but not in all Fanconi's anemia complementation groups.

Modified from D'Andrea AD, Grompe M. Molecular biology of Fanconi anemia: implications for diagnosis and therapy. Blood. 1997;90:1725-1736.

Inheritance in Man [MIM] 142900), which is characterized by thumb anomalies and atrial septal defects and caused by mutations in the *TBX5* gene, and the Baller-Gerold (MIM 218600) syndrome and Rothmund-Thomson syndrome (MIM 278400), which are caused by mutations in the *RECQL4* gene and characterized by radial defects, craniosynostosis, and cancer predisposition but no BMF. FA patients may have the VATER (vertebral defects, imperforate anus, tracheoesophageal fistula, and radial and renal dysplasia) or VACTERL (vertebral abnormalities, anal atresia, cardiac abnormalities, tracheoesophageal fistula, and/or esophageal atresia, renal agenesis and dysplasia, and limb defects) association (MIM 192350) or the IVIC syndrome (MIM 147750), which is an acronym for Instituto Venezolano de Investigaciones Científicas, the institution where a family with autosomal dominant radial ray defects, hearing impairment, internal ophthalmoplegia, and thrombocytopenia was first described. Chromosome breakage tests were normal in these families.

The increased chromosomal breakage in FA has to be distinguished from that seen in Bloom's syndrome (MIM 210900), another single-gene disorder with a predisposition for leukemia as a result of mutation in the helicase RecQ protein-like-3 gene (*RECQL3*). Chromosomal aberrations are in general more numerous in FA cells than in Bloom cells. Furthermore, in Bloom's syndrome, most interchanges occur between homologous chromosomes, whereas in FA they are more frequently seen between nonhomologous chromosomes.[91] Interestingly, more recent experimental data suggest that the Bloom and FA pathways may be connected and that protein complexes formed by *RECQL3* are abnormal in cell lines from FA patients.[160,161]

Nijmegen's breakage syndrome (MIM 251260), caused by mutations in the *NBS1* gene and characterized by immunodeficiency and a predisposition to lymphoma, is an additional autosomal recessive chromosomal breakage disease. A small number of patients may have FA-like features, including BMF and the development of myeloid leukemia,[100,162] and certain mutations in the *NSB1* gene cause an increased clastogenic response to MMC and DEB. The similarities between these two disorders suggested an interaction between these proteins. In fact, the NSB1 protein interacts with the FANCD2 protein in two distinct cellular functions, one involved in the DNA cross-link response and other involved in the S-phase checkpoint response (see later).[97,163]

A third disease associated with spontaneous chromosomal breakage and hematopoietic malignancies is ataxia-telangiectasia (MIM 208900), which has autosomal recessive inheritance. Cells from patients with ataxia-telangiectasia are hypersensitive to ionizing radiation but not to cross-linking agents. Furthermore, it is associated with immunodeficiency and progressive cerebellar neuronal degeneration, which clearly distinguish this condition from FA. Interestingly, the product of the gene mutated in ataxia-telangiectasia, ataxia-telangiectasia mutated (ATM), interacts with the pathway affected in FA in response to ionizing radiation by phosphorylating FANCD2 (also see later).

One form of Seckel's syndrome (SCKL1, MIM 210600), caused by mutations in the gene encoding ataxia-telangiectasia and RAD3-related protein (*ATR*), may have some clinical similarities to FA, including anemia and an increased risk for AML. ATR interacts with the FA pathway and is essential for efficient FANCD2 monoubiquitination (also see later).[164]

DNA ligase IV (*LIG4*)-deficient patients are characterized by microcephaly, growth retardation starting in utero, distinctive facial appearance ("bird-like face"), developmental delay, immunodeficiency, pancytopenia, and pronounced clinical and cellular radiosensitivity.

LIG4 deficiency is another rare IBMFS caused by defective DNA repair.[164,165]

Genetics

Inheritance. FA is a genetically heterogeneous recessive disorder. Mutations in at least 13 different genes, all of which have been identified, may be responsible for FA. Inheritance of FA is autosomal or, in rare cases, X-linked.

Complementation Groups. At least 13 genetic subtypes or complementation groups have been identified (FA-A, FA-B, etc.), each with a distinctive disease gene (Fanconi's anemia gene A [*FANCA*], *FANCB*, etc.). The majority of patients belong to complementation group A (approximately 60% to 70%), followed by complementation groups C and G. Table 8-5 shows the complementation groups and the genes responsible for FA and their frequency as estimated from data from the IFAR.[184] Complementation groups were originally defined by somatic cell fusion and the ability of the heterokaryon to correct the MMC hypersensitivity as measured in a growth inhibition assay.[187-190] Correction of the MMC hypersensitivity indicates that the two fusion partners belong to different complementation groups, whereas no correction indicates that they belong to the same complementation group. More recently and as more *FANC* genes are identified, complementation groups are assigned through the correction of MMC hypersensitivity after introduction of the respective wild-type cDNA (complementation by cDNA expression). Retroviruses expressing *FANC* cDNA may be used to correct the phenotype of T cells from FA patients, which determines the complementation group in a rapid, accurate manner.[191]

Fanconi Genes (*FANC* Genes). *FANC* genes have been identified by expression cloning, positional cloning, protein complex purification, or a combination thereof and are summarized in Table 8-5. Figure 8-3 schematically represents the 13 *FANC* genes and their functional domains. Complementation cloning is based on the principle that the wild-type variant of the defective gene will complement or correct the phenotype (the phenotype of FA cells is MMC hypersensitivity; also see earlier). Complementation cloning is a very powerful method that led to the identification of numerous disease genes, including the *FANCC*,[168] *FANCA*,[192] *FANCG*,[173] *FANCF*,[172] and *FANCE*[171] genes. The *FANCA* gene was also identified independently by positional cloning.[193] *FAND2*[170,194] and *FANCJ*[178,179,195] were cloned by using a combination of positional and expression cloning. *FANCD1* and *FANCN* were identified as FA genes by a candidate gene approach. Screening for mutation in the *BRCA2* gene revealed biallelic pathogenic mutations in patients belonging to the FANCD1 complementation group.[169] Similarly, sequencing of *PALB2* revealed biallelic pathogenic mutations very similar to those in *FANCD1* patients, but not *BRCA2*

TABLE 8-5   Thirteen Complementation Groups and Genes Responsible for Fanconi's Anemia

Complementation Group	Responsible Gene	% of FA Patients	Locus	Protein Size (kd)	FANCD2 Monoubiquitination	Main Function of the Protein	Comments	References
FA-A	FANCA	57-65	16q24.30.3	163	+	FA core complex	Phosphorylated after DNA damage	166
FA-B	FANCB	0.3	Xp22.31	95	+	FA core complex		167
FA-C	FANCC	9-15	9q22.3	63	+	FA core complex		168
FA-D1	FANCD1/BRCA2	3-4	13q12-13	380	−	RAD51 recruitment		169
FA-D2	FANCD2	3-6	3p25.3	155, 162	+	Monoubiquitinated protein (part of the FANCI-FAND2 subcomplex) Phosphorylated upon DNA damage	Phosphorylated and monoubiquitinated after DNA damage	170
FA-E	FANCE	1	6p21-22	60	+	FA core complex	Direct binding to FANCD2 Phosphorylated after DNA damage	171
FA-F	FANCF	2	11p15	42	+	FA core complex		172
FA-G	FANCG/XRCC9	8-9	9p13	68	+	FA core complex		173
FA-I	FANCI	Rare	15q25-26	150	+	Monoubiquitinated protein (part of the FANCI-FAND2 subcomplex)	Phosphorylated and monoubiquitinated after DNA damage Binds to FACND2	174-177
FA-J	FANCJ/BACH1/Brip1	1.6-3	17q22-q24	130	−	5′ → 3′ DNA helicase/ATPase	Binding to BRCA1	178, 179
FA-L	FANCL/PHF9/POG/FAAP43	0.1	2p16.1	43	+	FA core complex, ubiquitin ligase		180
FA-M	FANCM/Hef/FAAP250	Rare	14q21.3	250	+	FA core complex, ATPase/translocase ? Sensor for DNA cross-link damage	Helicase/nuclease motif Phosphorylated after DNA damage	181
FA-N	FANCN/PALB2	Rare	16p12	130	−	Binding partner of BRCA2	Binding to BRCA2	87, 182, 183

+, gene required for FANCD2 monoubiquitination; −, gene not required for FANCD2 monoubiquitination; ?, possible; NA, not applicable.
Data from references 184 to 186.

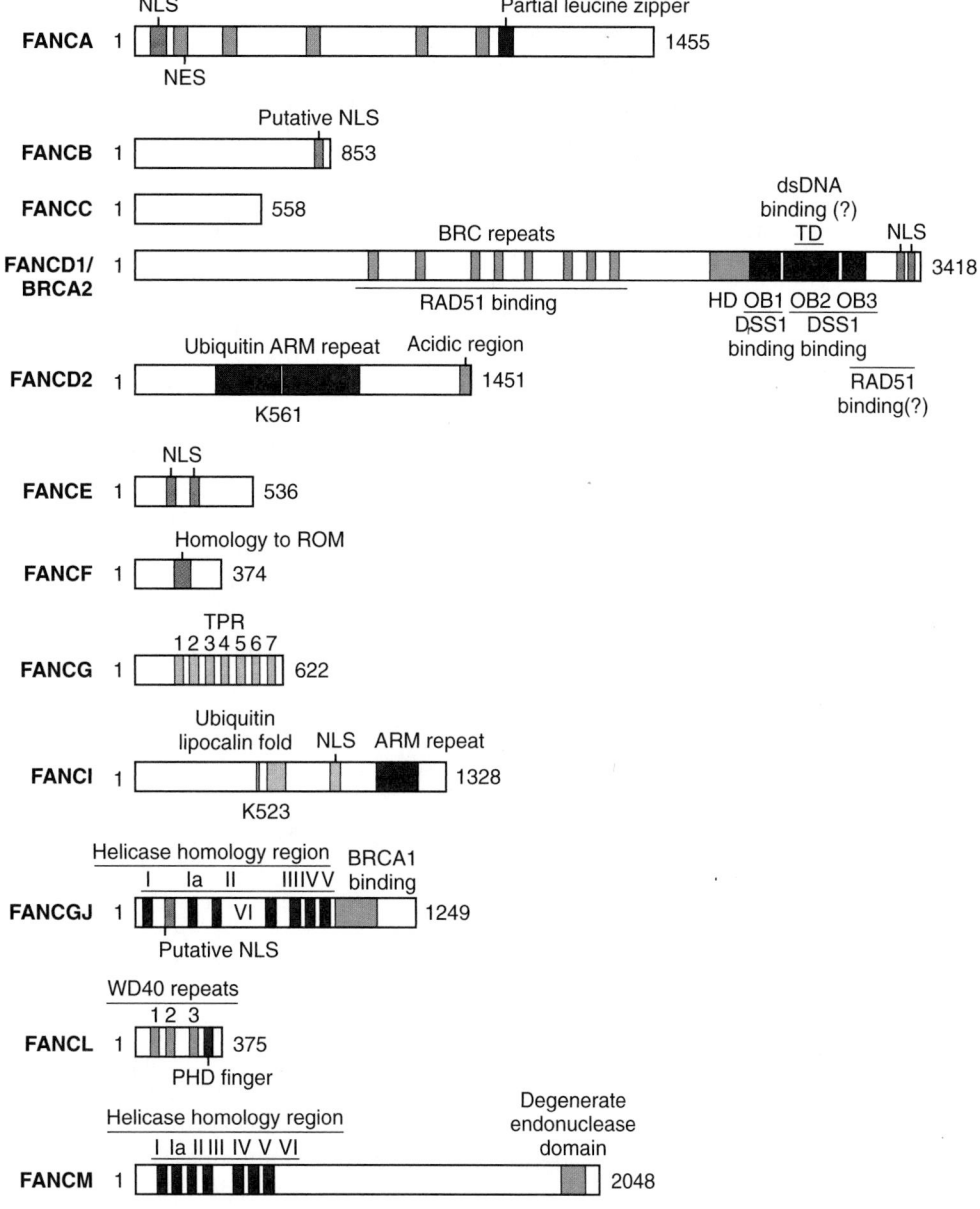

FIGURE 8-3. Schematic representation of the 13 Fanconi's anemia genes and their functional domains. dsDNA, double-stranded DNA; NES, nuclear export sequences; NLS, nuclear localization signals; OB, oligonucleotide/oliosaccharide-binding folds; ssDNA, single-stranded DNA; TD, tower domain; TRP, tetratricopeptide repeat. *(Modified from Taniguchi T, D'Andrea AD. Molecular pathogenesis of Fanconi anemia: recent progress. Blood. 2006;107: 4223-4233.)*

mutations.[86,182] FANCL, FANCB, and FANCM were identified as proteins binding to FANCA. They were initially called Fanconi's anemia–associated proteins (FAAP), followed by a number corresponding to their approximate molecular weight. Mutation screening revealed biallelic mutations in the gene encoding FAAP43 in cells from FA patients belonging to complementation group FANCL[180] and in the gene encoding FAAP250 in cells from patients with FANCM.[181] The gene encoding FAAP95 is on the X chromosome and was found to carry a mutation in the four cell lines from male patients belonging to complementation group FANCB.[167] A fourth protein, FAAP100, has not yet been associated with FA.[160] The most recently identified FA gene is the

FANCI gene, which was identified almost simultaneously by three different groups of investigators.[174-176]

Function of the FANC Proteins. The FANC proteins have been shown to act during the S phase of the cell cycle[97,145,146,161, 196-207] and are thought to participate in DNA repair of lesions encountered during DNA replication.[184,185,208-213] It is generally thought that FANC proteins promote and coordinate three DNA repair pathways: translesion synthesis at replication-blocking lesions and repair of broken replication forks by homologous recombination and possibly through DNA end joining (nonhomologous end joining) in the absence of homologous recombination.[214,215] Thus, it is thought, as schematically summarized in Figure 8-4, that in normal cells the FA pathway serves to minimize the severity of mutational outcomes by favoring error-free DNA repair and error-prone DNA repair that results in base pair substitutions or small deletions over DNA repair that results in larger deletions and chromosomal rearrangements (Box 8-4 summarizes the main DNA repair pathways).[208,218] However, exactly how these proteins function remains elusive.

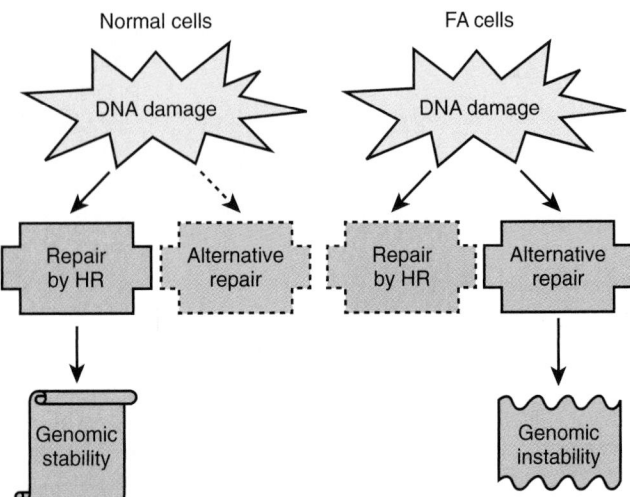

FIGURE 8-4. Presumed function of the Fanconi anemia (FA) DNA repair pathway. In normal cells, the FA pathway ensures correct DNA repair, whereas error-prone alternative pathways are rarely used. In FA cells, error-free DNA repair by homologous recombination (HR) is impaired, so alternative DNA repair pathways are more frequently used and lead to genomic instability and cell death. *(Modified from Levitus M, Joenje H, de Winter JP. The Fanconi anemia pathway of genomic maintenance. Cell Oncol. 2006;28:3-29.)*

Box 8-4	DNA Repair Pathways*

DNA repair pathways are highly regulated pathways that involve detection of DNA lesions, signaling to recruit DNA repair factors, activation of DNA repair enzymes, and disassembly or degradation of DNA repair factors after repair.

EXCISION OF DAMAGED AND MISMATCHED BASES

Nucleotide excision repair, including global genome repair and transcription-coupled repair
Base pair excision repair
Mismatch repair

REPAIR OF DOUBLE-STRANDED BREAKS

Homologous recombination (generally error free)
Nonhomologous end joining (generally error prone)

DNA STRESS REPLICATION PATHWAY; REPLICATION PATHWAY OF DAMAGED TEMPLATES DURING DNA SYNTHESIS

Translesion DNA synthesis (error prone)

*For review, see Kennedy and D'Andrea[216] and Hoeijmakers.[217]

The current model suggests that eight of the proteins responsible for FA—FANCA, FANCB, FANCC, FANCE, FANCF, FANCG, FANCL, and FANCM—are part of a nuclear protein complex (core FA complex) that functions as an ubiquitin ligase, of which FANCL is probably the catalytic subunit.[180] Crystallographic and biologic study demonstrated that FANCE recruits FANCD2 to the FA core complex whereas disease-associated FANCE mutations disrupt the FANCE-FANCD2 interaction.[219] Figure 8-5 schematically summarizes the current view of the FANC protein interconnections in the FA DNA repair pathway. In response to DNA damage or in the S phase of the cell cycle, this complex catalyzes monoubiquitination of the downstream targets, the FANCD2 and FANCI proteins (FANCI-FANCD2 complex). A defect in any of these core proteins results in failure to monoubiquitinate the FANCI-FANCD2 complex, thus underscoring the importance of this modification in the FA pathway. FANCI and FANCD2 are dependent on each other for their respective monoubiquitination. The biochemical mechanism of monoubiquitination of FANCI and FANCD2 is not understood, but the reaction is necessary for association of the FANCI-FANCD2 complex to chromatin and its localization into nuclear foci, where it colocalizes with multiple proteins involved in DNA repair, including BRCA1, RAD51, MRE11-RAD50-NBS1, replication protein A, PCNA, and BRCA2.[97,198,203,221-223] The FANC core complex is also necessary for translocation of the monoubiquitinated FANCI-FANCD2 complex to chromatin. Indeed, FANCA, FANCC, and FANCG also associate with chromatin in response to DNA damage.[220] In addition, FANCD2 is phosphorylated in response to various types of DNA damage,[97,199,200] and it is suspected that FANCI and FANCD2 phosphorylation is part of two separate pathways that are controlled by one of the two checkpoint kinases ATR or ATM.[97,174-176,199,200,224]

The FA gene corresponding to FA-D1 has been identified as the breast cancer susceptibility gene *BRCA2*.[169] In *FANCD1/BRCA2*-defective cells, the core FA complex is intact and FANCD2 is appropriately ubiquitinated, thus suggesting that *FANCD1/BRCA2* acts downstream of the other proteins involved in FA. Recently, biallalic mutations were identified in the gene encoding FANCN/PALB2, a nuclear binding partner of BRCA2.[86,182] FANCN binds to the amino-terminal of BRCA2 and facilitates its binding to chromatin.[87] Similar to *FANCD1/BRCA2*-defective cells, the core FA complex is intact and FANCD2 is appropriately ubiquitinated.

FANCJ has been shown to be mutated in FA and act downstream of FAND2 monoubiquitination. FANCJ is an adenosine triphosphate–dependent helicase that binds and unwinds DNA/DNA and DNA/RNA substrates in a 5′-to-3′ direction.[225] It belongs to the RecQ DEAH helicases, which efficiently unwind DNA structures that occur during homologous recombination and during repair of stalled DNA replication forks. FANCJ contains a C-terminal BRCA1-binding domain, again linking the

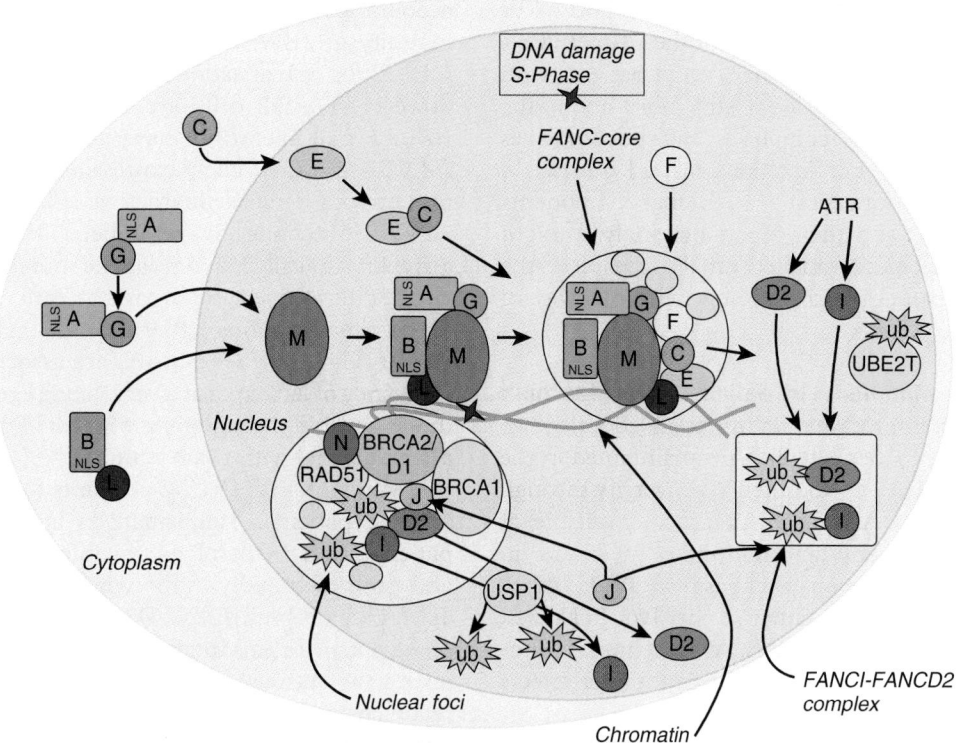

FIGURE 8-5. Schematic summary of the current view of FANC protein interconnections in the Fanconi anemia (FA) DNA repair pathway (also see text). Upon DNA damage and during DNA replication, the FANCI-FANCD2 complex is activated by monoubiquitination. Eight FANC proteins and three additional proteins (FAAP16, FAAP100, and FAAP24, gray cycles) form the FANC core complex necessary for FANCI-FANCD2 monoubiquitination. In addition to the FANC core complex, ATR (ataxia-telangiectasia and RAD3-related protein) is required for efficient FANCI-FAND2 monoubiquitination. FANCI and FAND2 are dependent on each other for their respective monoubiquitination. The activated FANCI-FANCD2 complex migrates to nuclear foci, most likely at the site of DNA damage, where it colocalizes with other DNA repair proteins and to chromatin. The FANC core complex is necessary not only for the monoubiquitination of FANCI and FANCD2 but also for their translocation to chromatin. Indeed, FANCA, FANCC, and FANCG also associate with chromatin in response to DNA damage.[220] The function of the monoubiquitinated FANCI-FANCD2 complex in chromatin remains unknown but may regulate homologous recombination repair or translesion DNA synthesis (or both). *(Modified from Medhurst AL, Laghmani EH, Steltenpool J, et al. Evidence for subcomplexes in the Fanconi anaemia pathway. Blood. 2006;108:2072-2080; Levitus M, Joenje H, de Winter JP. The Fanconi anemia pathway of genomic maintenance. Cell Oncol. 2006;28:3-29; and Taniguchi T, D'Andrea AD. Molecular pathogenesis of Fanconi anemia: recent progress. Blood. 2006;107:4223-4233.)*

FA pathway to the homologous recombination repair pathway.

It has been proposed that the FA core complex is assembled sequentially from subcomplexes (see Fig. 8-5),[226-229] which may have additional functions aside from DNA repair. In fact, the FANCC protein has been reported to interact with a number of other proteins, including STAT1,[230,231] Hsp70,[232,233] cdc2,[227] PKR,[234,235] and p53,[236,237] thus suggesting that FANC proteins/subcomplexes might also have a separate role in cell cycle control, apoptosis, hematopoiesis, and tumorigenesis that is independent of DNA damage recognition/repair (reviewed by Bagby and Alter[238]).

Despite the extensive literature on the function of the FANC proteins, the pathogenesis of BMF in FA remains poorly understood. Although the FA pathway of DNA damage repair and recognition seems to explain the genomic instability and possibly the increased risk for malignancy in patients with FA, its link to the pathogenesis of BMF remains unclear inasmuch as mutations associated with genomic instability outside FA are not

usually associated with BMF. Whether BMF in FA patients is a direct consequence of the FA defect in DNA repair or is caused by impairment of functions apart from DNA repair is the subject of ongoing debate. Naturally, FA DNA repair and non–DNA repair pathways in the pathogenesis of BMF may not be mutually exclusive. For example, the exquisite hypersensitivity of FA hematopoietic progenitor cells to oxidative stress[53,123,239] and the inability of FA hematopoietic progenitors cells to grow unless the culture conditions are optimized to reduce oxidative stress[56] suggest an inability of FA cells to handle oxidative stress. The inability of FA hematopoietic progenitors cells to deal with oxidative stress may occur on several levels, including impairment of the redox-related pathways associated with FANC proteins (function of the FANC proteins outside DNA repair),[55,127,128,240-242] the response to oxidative damage,[199] and impaired repair of oxygen-induced DNA damage (functions of the FANC proteins in DNA damage repair).[53,115,123,124,239,243-249] Thus, it is possible that mutations in FA genes sensitize hematopoietic stem cells to the environmental factors that prevail in BMF, such as increased levels of TNF-α or INF-γ. To find the specific functions of the FA pathways and to link them to the phenotype seen in patients with FA, it will be necessary to learn still more about the individual FANC proteins, complexes, and subcomplexes and their interactions and functions in and outside of DNA repair. The identification of additional components in the FA pathways and their functional analysis might provide additional pieces and eventually complete the jigsaw puzzle surrounding the pathogenetic pathway of BMF in FA.

FANC Gene Mutations in Patients with Fanconi's Anemia.

Detailed information on mutations identified in the *FANC* genes in patients with FA is maintained in the FA Mutation Database at Rockefeller University through the IFAR headed by Arleen D. Auerbach (available at http://www.rockefeller.edu/fanconi/mutate/[21,250]) and in the Leiden Open Variation Database (LOVD; http://chromium.liacs.nl/lovd/) maintained by Ivo Fokkema, John T. den Dunnen, and Peter E. M. Taschner.[251] Frequent FA mutations and mutations with founder effects are presented in Table 8-6.

FANCA is the gene most frequently mutated in FA patients.[21,22,258,259] The mutations are spread throughout the gene and include missense and nonsense mutations, small deletions, insertions, and duplications, as well as splicing mutations.[250] Of note is the substantial number of large genomic, usually intragenic DNA deletions,[13,250,260-264] which account for about 40% of all pathogenic mutations within the *FANCA* gene and are thought to be due to the frequent occurrence of Alu repeats in this genomic region.[250,260] Large gene deletions are not generally detected by routine nucleotide sequence–based mutation detection methods but require more specialized analysis (haplotype analysis) or molecular methods specifically designed for the detection of large gene deletions. Two small deletions (deletion of three nucleotides between positions 3788 and 3790, with c.3788_3790delTCT leading to deletion of phenylalanine at position 1263, 1263delF, and a 4–base pair [bp] deletion at position 1115, c.1115-1118delTTGG, leading to a frameshift and premature stop codon) are the most common pathogenic mutations in the *FANCA* gene, with a frequency of 8.8% and 5.5% in the non-Brazilian and 51.1% and 2.2% in the Brazilian mutated *FANCA* alleles (see Table 8-5).

Mutations in *FANCC* genes account for about 10% to 15% of all FA cases (see Table 8-6).[185,265] The splicing mutation c.711+4A→T (old nomenclature, IVS4+4A→T) in the *FANCC* gene accounts for the majority (80%) of FA cases in Ashkenazi Jewish families (see Table 8-6).[253] Mutations in *FANCG* are responsible for about 8% to 9% of patients with FA. Several mutations with founder effects have been identified in specific populations (see Table 8-6).[254]

Biallelic mutations in *BRCA2* are found in individuals with FA-D1. Biallelic *FANCD1/BRCA2* mutations

account for about 3% to 4% of all FA patients.[184,185] The majority of *FANCD1/BRCA2* mutations in FA lead to frameshifts or truncations (see Table 8-6).[85] Interestingly, however, FA-D1 cells are not biallelic for *FANCD1/BRCA2* null alleles but have at least one hypomorphic *FANCD1/BRCA2* allele expressing a FANCD1/BRCA2 protein with some residual activity. Biallelic null *FANCD1/BRCA2* mutations have never been identified and in mice are embryonically lethal. Biallelic mutations in *FANCD1/BRCA2* have a very high risk of early malignancy. The splice cite mutations c.859+1G→A (IVS7+1G→A) and c.859+1G→A (IVS7+1G→A) are associated with a high frequency of leukemia at a very young age,[85,255,256] whereas the frameshift mutations c.886delGT and c.6174delT are associated with brain tumors.[24,84,85]

Mutation in *FANCD2* accounts for 3% to 6% of FA-affected patients. Malformations are frequent in these patients, and hematologic manifestations appear early and progress rapidly. Although hypomorphic mutations exist, patients with *FANCD2* mutations have a relatively severe form of FA. Mutation analysis revealed 66 mutated alleles, 34 causing aberrant splicing. Many mutations are recurrent and have ethnic associations and shared allelic haplotypes. There were no biallelic null mutations, thus suggesting that in contrast to the *Fancd2* knockout mouse, complete absence of FANCD2 does not exist in patients with *FANCD2* mutations.[266,267]

Mutations in *FANCN/PALB2* were identified in families with the new subtype FA-N and cancer in early childhood. Similar to biallelic *BRCA2* mutations, biallelic *FANCN/PALB2* mutations confer a high risk for childhood cancer.[86,182]

Molecular Diagnosis of Fanconi's Anemia

Currently, molecular diagnostics is not routinely performed for FA because it is expensive, labor intensive, and in some cases, possible only though specialized laboratories using research tests that are currently not approved by the Clinical Laboratory Improvement Amendments (CLIAs). However, only identification of biallelic mutations in a *FANC* gene (or hemizygosity for a mutation in the *FANCB* gene) definitively establishes the diagnosis of FA. Furthermore, molecular diagnostics enables the identification of mutation carriers, facilitates prenatal diagnosis for an existing pregnancy, and allows preimplantation genetic diagnosis (PGD) for partners identified as mutation carriers.[268] For a definition of PGD see Box 8-5. In addition, because the clinical manifestations and severity of disease may vary depending on the affected *FANC* gene and the nature of individual mutations, molecular diagnostics may also influence medical management not only for FA individuals carrying biallelic *FANC* gene mutations but possibly also for heterozygous *FANC* gene mutation carriers (also see later). Currently, an educated candidate gene approach is used to identify the affected the *FANC* gene by taking into account the origin and ethnicity of the affected FA individual.[273] After exclusion of the most frequent mutations,

TABLE 8-6   Frequent FANC Gene Variants and Mutations with a Founder Effect Identified in Patients with Fanconi's Anemia

Gene	Founder Effect	Variation at the DNA level (Old Nomenclature)*	Variation at the Protein Level*	Frequency within the Mutated FA Allele	Population with a Founder Effect (% of All FA Patients)	References
FANCA	Yes	c.3788_3790delTCT†	1263delF	8.8%	51% in Brazilians	250
	No	c.1115-1118delTTGG†	fs	5.5%	2.2% in Brazilians	250
	Yes	Intragenic deletion of exons 12 through 31	del		60% in Afrikaners in South Africa	13
	Yes	c.295C→T	Q55X		Spanish gypsies	10
	Yes	c.65G→A	W22X		Unique to Ashkenazi Jews	252
FANCC	Yes	c.711+4A→T (IVS4+4A→T)	spl?		80% in Ashkenazi Jews	253
	Yes	c.322delG	fs		Dutch	168
FANCG	Yes	c.1087-2A→G	spl?		Portuguese Brazilians	254
	Yes	c.1480+1G→C	spl?		French Acadians	254
	Yes	c.307+1G→C	spl?		Koreans and Japanese	254
	Yes	c.1794_1803del10	fs		Europeans	254
	Yes	313G→T	E105X		44% in Germans	254
FANCD1/BRCA2	Yes	c.6174delT	fs		Unique to Ashkenazi Jews	252
	No	c.859+1G→A (IVS7+1G→A)‡	spl?			85, 255, 256
	No	c.859+1G→A (IVS7+1G→A)‡	spl?			
	No	c.886delGT§	fs			24, 84, 85
	No	c.6174delT§	fs			

*Sequence variations are described according to the Ad-Hoc Committee for Mutation Nomenclature (AHCMN)[257] (for a summary see http://www.hgvs.org/mutnomen/; for the coding DNA reference sequence see http://www.rockefeller.edu/fanconi/mutate/faarefcdna.html), with the first base of the Met codon counted as position 1. Single-letter abbreviations are used for amino acids: E, glutamic acid; F, phenylalanine; Q, glutamine. del, deletion; fs, frameshift, premature stop codon; spl?, splice site mutations with unknown consequences at the protein level; X, stop codon.
†Most frequent FANCA gene mutations.
‡Associated with a high frequency of leukemia at a very young age (acute myelocytic and lymphocytic leukemia).
§Associated with brain tumors.
Data from Fokkema IF, den Dunnen JT, Taschner PE. LOVD: easy creation of a locus-specific sequence variation database using an "LSDB-in-a-box" approach. Hum Mutat. 2005;26:63-68, available at http://chromium.liacs.nl/lovd/; and Levran O, Diotti R, Pujara K, et al. Spectrum of sequence variations in the FANCA gene: an International Fanconi Anemia Registry (IFAR) study. Hum Mutat. 2005;25:142-149.

it might be necessary to determine the complementation group and perform a mutational screen of the entire coding sequence, including methods that will detect large deletions in compound heterozygotes. Protein expression analysis and functional assays are used to test for the pathogenicity of unclassified variants.[274] Although this approach is successful in the majority of FA patients, in some, the responsible gene mutations remain unclear. In addition to the large number of mutations in *FANC* genes associated with FA, a number of nonpathogenic mutations and mutations of unknown pathogenic significance have been identified. The multitude of FA complementation groups, the heterogeneity of the mutation spectrum, and the frequency of large intragenic deletions present a considerable challenge for the molecular diagnosis of FA.

Heterozygous Carriers of FANC Gene Mutations

Heterozygous carriers of *FANC* gene mutations are not at risk for the development of BMF. Similarly, cell lines heterozygous for *FANC* gene mutations do not show the chromosomal instability (either spontaneously or in response to cross-linking agents) characteristic of FA cells with biallelic *FANC* gene mutations. However, an increased frequency of skeletal and genitourinary abnormalities[275] and an increased risk for malignancy have been reported in heterozygous *FANC* gene mutation carriers.[275]

Risk of Malignancy. A strong association exists between heterozygous mutation of *FANC* genes and susceptibility to breast or ovarian cancer,[276] and other forms of malignancy have been identified in heterozygous mutation carriers. Carriers of mutations in *BRCA1* or *BRCA2/ FANCD1* have an 82% risk of breast cancer developing and a 54% (*BRCA1*) and 23% (*BRCA2/FANCD1*) risk for ovarian cancer.[277] Heterozygous *BRCA2/FANCD1* mutations additionally predispose to pancreatic, prostate, and gastric cancer, as well as melanoma.[278,279] Monoallelic truncating *FANCN/PALB2* mutations were also associated with familial breast cancer, although the risk for breast cancer was lower (2.3-fold) than that in *BRCA2* mutation carriers.[183] Heterozygosity for *FANCJ* mutations has been identified in patients with early-onset breast cancer.[225] Heterozygous germline mutations in *FANCC* and *FANCG* and loss of heterozygosity or func-

tional biallelic loss in the tumor sample have been identified in rare patients with pancreatic cancer.[280,281] Furthermore, heterozygous germline mutations of *FANCA* have been identified in a small percentage of patients with AML.[282,283]

Somatic FANC Gene Mutations in Cancer

Cancer cells often accumulate a large number of mutations within an individual cancer cell, many of which promote cell growth and survival. It is therefore thought that a cancer cell with an increased mutation rate, a mutator phenotype, will have a selective advantage in tumor growth and development. Inactivation or mutation of genes involved in maintaining genetic stability is therefore thought to be an early event in cancer development. The FA pathway has been observed to be one of the pathways that maintains genomic stability and is targeted in several forms of sporadic cancer (for review see elsewhere[184,216]); inactivation of *FANCF* by methylation has been observed in ovarian granulosa cell tumors,[284] breast cancer,[285] non–small cell lung cancer,[286] squamous cell head and neck cancer,[286] cervical cancer,[287] testicular germ cell tumors,[288] and possibly ovarian cancer,[289] although the latter was not confirmed.[290] Aberrant or reduced expression of FANCA, FANCC, FANCF, and FANCG was found in AML cells,[282,283,291-293] thus suggesting a role of the FA pathway in leukemogenesis. Inherited and somatic (loss-of-heterozygosity) mutations in *FANCC* and *FANCG* were observed in a subset of early-onset pancreatic cancer.[280,281,294] Loss of BRCA2 expression has been reported in 13% of ovarian adenocarcinomas.[295] FANCD2 expression was found to be absent in 10% to 20% of sporadic and BRCA1-related breast cancers.[296]

Identification of acquired abnormalities in the FA pathway might become clinically important because these tumors are expected to have increased sensitivity to cross-linking agents such as cisplatin, cyclophosphamide, MMC, and other novel agents.[297] Thus, identification of abnormalities in the FA pathway may serve as a biomarker that identifies a subgroup of patients with cancers selectively sensitive to specific chemotherapeutic agents.[233,248] Similarly, inhibition of the FA pathway in cancer may render cancer cells sensitive to chemotherapy.[216,298,299]

Genotype-Phenotype Correlation

Clinical findings in FA are highly variable, although within an individual family the presence or absence of multiple congenital abnormalities or the age at onset of other disease manifestations is usually concordant (see earlier also). More recent studies have demonstrated that disease severity and manifestations, at least in part, are determined by the *FANC* gene affected (FA complementation group) and by the nature of the mutations.[15,21,22] For example, patients with mutations in the *FANCA* gene usually have a milder form of disease and BMF develops at a later age than it does in FA individuals with mutations in the *FANCC* or *FANCG* genes,[22] whereas in FA patients with biallelic *FANCD1* or *FANCN* mutations, cancer develops even before the manifestation of BMF.[24,84-86] Furthermore, splice site mutations in *FACD1* are more frequently associated with the development of leukemia,[85,255,256] whereas frameshift mutations within the same gene more frequently lead to brain tumors (see earlier).[24,84,85] Malformations are frequent in *FANCD2* patients, and hematologic manifestations appear earlier and progress more rapidly than they do in non-*FANCD2* FA patients.[266]

FA-B is X-linked, in contrast to all other forms of FA, which are autosomal. Thus, a single mutation is sufficient to cause a phenotype and disease in males. In females, because of inactivation of one of the two X chromosomes, a phenotype is expressed only in cells with the *FANCB* mutation on the active X chromosome. Because X-chromosome inactivation occurs at random in early embryogenesis and, once determined, persists clonally, one might expect female *FANCB* mutation carriers to have a mild form of FA-B. Interestingly, however, to date no female FA-B patient with clinical manifestations of FA has been reported, and careful clinical examination of females heterozygous for *FANCB* gene mutations showed no manifestations of disease. Molecular studies investigating X-inactivation revealed that only the X chromosome with the normal *FANCB* gene is expressed in blood and bone marrow and also in fibroblasts.[167] This finding indicates a proliferative disadvantage of cells expressing the mutant *FANCB* allele and complete outgrowth by phenotypically normal cells, not only in bone marrow but possibly also in all other tissues. This situation differs from other X-linked IBMFSs such as X-linked DC (see the section "Dyskeratosis Congenita"). For individuals carrying a *FANCB* mutation, however, longer follow-up and examination of additional mutation carriers will be necessary to determine whether some FA-B cells persist in female carriers and whether these persisting FA-B cells are at risk for malignant transformation. Whether somatic *FANCB* inactivation can be found in malignancies (only a single mutation on the active X chromosome is required) remains to be determined.

Somatic Mosaicism and Functional Reversion of Fanconi's Anemia Cells

About 10% to 25% of FA patients have been found to be mosaic in their peripheral blood inasmuch as two populations of lymphocytes can be detected, one with the classic increased sensitivity to cross-linking agents characteristic of FA cells and the other usually a slowly increasing second population that is resistant to treatment with these agents.[26] For definition of genetic mosaicism see Box 8-6. The presence of mosaicism is usually considered if the clinical course of the disease is milder than expected in comparison to individuals with the same genetic abnormality, if the course of the disease improves spontaneously rather than worsens, or in the presence of

Box 8-6	Genetic Mosaicism

Genetic mosaicism is defined as the presence of two or more genetically distinct populations of cells in a single individual that differ from each other at the DNA sequence level but are derived from a single zygote.[300] In Fanconi's anemia (FA), genetic mosaicism results from reversion, which is genetic correction (reversion) of the FA mutation.

classic phenotypic abnormalities but rather mild or absent hematologic disease. The molecular mechanisms of genetic reversion include intragenic recombination (in compound heterozygotes), mitotic gene conversion (nonreciprocal exchange of genetic information as a result of heteroduplex formation between nonsister chromatids),[28] DNA slippage, second-site compensating mutations,[301,302] and site-specific correction by an as yet unknown mechanism.[28] Gene reversion may occur in vivo or in vitro. In FA patients the reverting mutation is thought to occur in progenitor cells with self-renewing capability,[303] possibly stem cells, thereby conferring a proliferative advantage to the revertant cells, which may lead to expansion of the revertant clone and progressive replacement of the FA cells in bone marrow.[26,302,304] Genetic reversion in FA has been documented to date only in hematopoietic cells, not in fibroblasts.[301,302] However, the fact that females heterozygous for *FANCB* mutations have biased X-inactivation in fibroblasts suggests that an intact FA pathway confers a proliferative advantage to nonhematopoietic cells. Thus, the frequency of genetic reversion is largely unknown, and so are its clinical consequences. In many patients genetic reversion is associated with hematologic improvement.[26,302] However, genetic reversion has also been found in leukemic cells from FA patients,[305] thus indicating that genetic reversion may confer a selective growth advantage and resistance of leukemic or preleukemic cells to specific chemotherapy drugs. Furthermore, genetic reversion in hematopoietic cells has no effect on cancer frequency in nonhematopoietic tissue (also see earlier).[306] However, the strong selection for a functional FANC pathway may be used to advantage in gene therapy approaches.[26,302] Genetic mosaicism is responsible at least in part for phenotypic variability, particularly within an individual family, and may create difficulty in interpretation of the chromosomal breakage test (DEB and MMC test, see earlier) or even lead to false-negative testing results.[25,27,28] DEB or MMC testing of fibroblasts should therefore be considered in patients with clinical or genetic suspicion of FA but a negative DEB or MMC test in peripheral blood lymphocytes.

Mouse Models for Fanconi's Anemia

Several mouse models for FA have been generated by introducing mutations into murine *FANC* genes, including *Fancc*,[155,307] *Fanca*,[308] *Fancg*,[309] *Fancd2*,[310] and *Fancd1*.[311] Some models recapitulate the clinical features seen in patients with FA, specifically, microphthalmos, germ cell defects, chromosomal instability, and an increased sensitivity to cross-linking agents. In some models tumors develop at an increased frequency,[310,312,313] and this effect is more pronounced in the absence of p53.[237,314] These models thereby underline the importance of the FA pathway in tumorigenesis. Hematopoietic progenitor cells from mice homozygous for a null mutation in the *Fancc* gene demonstrate a distinct hypersensitivity to IFN-γ that leads to cell death independent of the DNA repair pathway mediated by FAS-induced apoptosis, thus suggesting that IFN-γ hypersensitivity may play a major role in the pathogenesis of BMF in patients with FA.[155,315] Interestingly, however, spontaneous development of aplastic anemia was not observed in these mice.

Clinical Management

Once the diagnosis is confirmed, the family should be referred to a clinical geneticist for counseling and careful examination of family members. Genetic testing or chromosome breakage analysis should be offered to all family members. Early diagnosis is important for correct management of hematologic complications, diagnosis and appropriate treatment of coexisting congenital abnormalities and associated endocrinopathies, and identification of affected but asymptomatic family members and unaffected family members or pregnancies that may serve as potential hematopoietic stem cell donors. In addition, early diagnosis allows targeted cancer surveillance, not only in patients with FA but also in some cases in heterozygous mutation carriers (also see earlier). Management of patients in whom FA is diagnosed depends on the age at diagnosis and the presence or absence of congenital or hematologic abnormalities (see also Fanconi Anemia Standards for Clinical Care, available from the Fanconi Anemia Research Fund at http://www.fanconi.org/[316]). All diagnosed FA patients should have a full hematologic assessment, including examination of bone marrow, and in anticipation of possible HSCT, HLA typing should be performed. Other investigations at diagnosis should include audiometry, ophthalmic examination, renal ultrasound, and an endocrine assessment (see earlier). Referral to specialized surgeons might be necessary for correction of radial ray defects.

Management of Hematologic Disease

Initially, in the absence of hematologic abnormalities or clinical and laboratory signs of mild BMF, monitoring of peripheral blood values and yearly examination of bone marrow might be sufficient (see also elsewhere[317]). Bone marrow examination should include a trephine biopsy and marrow aspirate for examination of marrow cellularity and morphologic changes characteristic of MDS, as well as for cytogenetic examination by G banding and fluorescent in situ hybridization (FISH) analysis, including probes that identify the most frequent cytogenetic abnormalities seen in patients with FA and progression

to MDS or AML (see earlier also). Because of its prognostic value, examination for clonal aberration of 3q should be considered.[68,69] Plans for possible HSCT should be in place because hematologic complications may develop rapidly. With progression of BMF it will become necessary to increase the frequency of hematologic monitoring. HSCT is usually considered in patients with moderate BMF and an available HLA-matched unaffected sibling donor or when BMF becomes severe and an unrelated donor is available. Preventive HSCT in the absence of hematologic disease is highly controversial and currently considered investigational because the risk and time course of disease progression are highly variable and have to be weighed against the morbidity and mortality associated with HSCT.

Management of FA patients with MDS, AML, or both is less standardized. The significance of transient clonal cytogenetic abnormalities is unclear, but if persistent or complex, such abnormalities usually predict a poor prognosis (also see earlier). HSCT with or without induction chemotherapy or enrollment in clinical trials for MDS or MDS/AML is usually considered (see later also).[318] Androgens and hematopoietic growth factors transiently improve BMF in about 50% to 60% of FA patients.[319-322] Side effects of androgen therapy include masculinization, acne, hyperactivity, growth spurt followed by premature closure of the epiphyseal growth plates, liver enzyme abnormalities, hepatic adenomas, and a risk for hepatic adenocarcinomas[75,323] that requires frequent monitoring of liver function and liver ultrasound scans. Hematopoietic growth factors (granulocyte colony-stimulating factor [G-CSF][322] or granulocyte-macrophage colony-stimulating factor [GM-CSF][321]) may transiently improve neutrophil counts and, in rare FA patients, also hemoglobin levels and platelet numbers. The use of hematopoietic growth factors in patients with clonal cytogenetic abnormalities is controversial because of the potential risk of inducing or promoting leukemia. Red cell transfusion therapy and iron chelation (after multiple red cell transfusions) are frequently used in symptomatic FA patients. Platelet transfusions may be indicated in thrombocytopenic patients with bleeding or before surgical procedures.

HSCT from an HLA-matched sibling donor is accepted as the best treatment to cure BMF in FA patients and to prevent progression to MDS and AML. Early experiences with HSCT for the treatment of BMF in FA were disastrous because of excessive regimen-related toxicity.[324-326] Early conditioning regimens consisted of cyclophosphamide alone or in combination with total body irradiation (TBI). Unfortunately, severe toxicities (e.g., gastrointestinal hemorrhage, hemorrhagic cystitis, cardiomyopathy, and skin burns) were common. These poor outcomes prompted in vitro laboratory studies that confirmed the hypersensitivity of FA cells to cyclophosphamide and TBI.[159] Based on these in vitro studies, Gluckman and colleagues[327,328] proposed the use of a less intensive conditioning regimen consisting of low-dose cyclophosphamide and thoracoabdominal irradiation for patients with FA. This approach proved to be a major advance in the treatment of patients with FA who had HLA-matched sibling donors.[329,330] However, it did not afford consistent engraftment in recipients of unrelated donor transplants, with graft rejection rates exceeding 20%,[331] and head and neck cancer was frequent after HSCT. Consequently, irradiation is no longer recommended for the conditioning of patients with FA undergoing HSCT.[332-336] Recent studies suggest that fludarabine-based conditioning regimens are associated with improved survival rates in patients with FA undergoing related or unrelated donor HSCT.[337-342]

PGD may be used in parents with a previously affected child to select embryos that are both unaffected by FA (if a *FANC* gene mutation is known) and HLA matched to the FA-affected sibling. HSCT is performed with the HLA-matched umbilical cord blood of the unaffected newborn.[342,343] The procedure is often successful but is considered ethically controversial.[269-272]

The prognosis for FA patients without HLA-matched siblings after HSCT with unrelated donors is less favorable. Extensive malformations, a positive recipient cytomegalovirus serology, the use of androgens before transplantation, and female donors were associated with a worse outcome.[344] There is also an increased risk for graft rejection in FA cases with somatic mosaicism.[345]

Cancer Surveillance/Treatment

For FA patients who survive the hematologic complications, follow-up surveillance for solid malignancies becomes increasingly important (also see earlier).[1,66,334,345-349] There are no clear guidelines on the treatment of cancer in FA patients, which is complicated because their increased sensitivity to radiation and certain chemotherapeutic agents may result in enhanced toxicity and an increased risk of therapy-induced secondary malignancies.[119,350,351]

Gene Therapy

HSCT may cure hematologic disease in FA patients; unfortunately, however, HLA-matched sibling donor cells are available only for a minority of patients. Gene therapy to correct hematopoietic stem cells, followed by autologous transplantation, therefore offers an attractive alternative for the treatment of hematologic disease in FA patients. Indeed, gene transfer corrects the hypersensitivity of most FA cell lines to DNA cross-linking agents in vitro (with the exception of FANCM, most likely because of insolubility of the protein) and the hypersensitivity of FA knockout mice in vivo. The high incidence of somatic mosaicism and the often ameliorated course of hematologic disease in these patients (frequently referred to as "gene therapy of Nature") suggests that FA cells corrected by gene therapy are likely to have a selective growth/survival advantage. However, gene therapy attempts in FA patients have thus far been rather disappointing,[352-354] mainly because of the lack of permanent

> ### Box 8-7 Dyskeratosis Congenita
>
> Dyskeratosis congenita (DC) is a rare inherited bone marrow failure (BMF) syndrome with X-linked, autosomal dominant, and autosomal recessive inheritance. However, more than half of patients have sporadic disease. Classically, BMF in DC patients is associated with the mucocutaneous triad, including abnormal pigmentation, dystrophic nails, and mucosal leukoplakia. Blood cells from patients with BMF as a result of DC have very short telomeres.[357,358]

gene correction and the difficulty in culturing FA bone marrow cells in vitro. Multiple investigations are currently addressing the major difficulties of gene therapy for FA, including the scarcity of hematopoietic stem cells in FA patients with BMF, the extraordinary fragility of FA hematopoietic progenitor cells, and the increased sensitivity of FA hematopoietic progenitor cells to oxidative stress, which makes it difficult to culture and transduce FA hematopoietic progenitor cells in vitro. There is also a risk that the transduced hematopoietic cells might already have acquired secondary somatic, possibly oncogenic mutations[355] and that correction by gene therapy would promote rather than prevent leukemogenesis in these patients.

Dyskeratosis Congenita

DC, also known as Zinsser-Cole-Engman syndrome, is genetically and phenotypically heterogeneous (Box 8-7). It was first described by Zinsser and recognized as a clinical entity by Cole and Engman.[358-360] DC was originally perceived to be a dermatologic disorder affecting the skin, nails, and mouth.[358-360] Its association with BMF and squamous cell cancer arising from the skin or from leukoplakia in the mouth or anus was recognized later.[361]

Clinical Manifestations

Originally, DC was clinically recognized by the classic diagnostic triad of reticular pigmentation of the skin, nail dystrophy, and mucosal leukoplakia (Fig. 8-6).[358-360] Other symptoms frequently found in patients with classic DC are summarized in Table 8-7[363-367] (for review, see also Docal[368] and Drachtman and Alter[369]). Disease manifestations are highly variable and range from barely detectable to severe forms that cause death in early childhood. Typically, however, affected individuals are normal at birth, mucocutaneous features develop in childhood, BMF develops in adolescence, and they die in the third decade. BMF, immune deficiency, pulmonary complications, and malignancies are the major causes of death in individuals with DC.

The recent identification of five of the genes responsible for DC and the realization that these genes converge into a common pathway have changed our understanding of this disease. It is now thought that individuals in whom

TABLE 8-7   Prevalence of Clinical Features in Patients with Classic Dyskeratosis Congenita

Characteristic	Alter,[9] 2003 (%)	Vulliamy and Dokal,[362] 2006 (%)
Diagnostic mucocutaneous features		
Skin pigmentation	88	89
Nail dystrophy	73	88
Leukoplakia	64	78
Eye abnormalities/epiphora	38	31
Teeth abnormalities/caries/loss	19	17
Learning difficulties/developmental delay/mental retardation	14	25
Pulmonary disease/fibrosis	20	—
Skeletal anomalies		
Osteoporosis/avascular necrosis/scoliosis	14	—
Short stature	14	20
Hyperhidrosis	10	15
Hair loss, early graying	18	16
Urinary tract abnormalities	7	—
Ureteral stricture/phimosis	—	5
Gastrointestinal abnormalities	14	—
Liver fibrosis/ulcer/enteropathy	—	7
Esophageal stricture	—	17
Other conditions	11	—
Gonadal anomalies/hypogonadism/undescended testes	5	6
Intrauterine growth retardation	—	8
Ataxia/cerebellar hypoplasia	—	7
Microencephaly	—	6
Malignancy	12	10

DC is diagnosed on the basis of BMF and the classic cutaneous manifestations represent only a fraction of those who suffer from this condition.[2,370] Whether affected individuals in the absence of cutaneous disease should be labeled with the diagnosis of "dyskeratosis congenita" or whether the disease should be renamed with a term better reflecting the pathogenetic pathway is currently under debate. Here we will use the conventional nomenclature and clinically classify patients as having classic, atypical, or silent DC. Patients who have two or more of the three diagnostic mucocutaneous features or who have one of the mucocutaneous features and hypocellular bone marrow with all three blood cell lineages affected are those with "classic DC." Patients with BMF but lacking mucocutaneous features or patients with clinical manifestations of DC other than hematologic disease or mucocutaneous features, such as pulmonary fibrosis, are those with "atypical DC," and individuals with no clinical manifestations but carrying a pathogenic mutation will be classified as having "silent DC." Much of what we know about DC is biased because early studies focused on patients with the classic clinical manifestations. Little is known about the course of disease, response to treatment, and late complications in patients with atypical or silent DC.

Classic Dyskeratosis Congenita

Mucocutaneous Features. Mucocutaneous abnormalities are the hallmark of classic DC (see Fig. 8-6).[371] The most commonly observed mucocutaneous abnormality (≈90%) is reticulated skin hyperpigmentation on the neck, face, chest, and arms. It may be extensive or localized and tends to increase with age. Other cutaneous manifestations include alopecia, premature hair graying, hyperhidrosis, hyperkeratosis of the palms and soles, and loss of dermal ridges on the fingers and toes.

Nail dystrophy is another frequent finding (≈80%). Progressive nail dystrophy starts with ridging and longitudinal splitting and may proceed via atrophy and thinning to complete nail loss. The severity of nail dystrophy may vary among the digits; fingernails are usually more severely affected than toenails.[372]

Mucosal leukoplakia occurs in the majority of patients (≈70%) and typically involves the tongue, buccal mucosa, and oropharynx, with the tongue being the most frequently affected site.[373,374] Mucosal leukoplakia may be the initial clinical manifestation of disease. Consequently, dentists or oral surgeons may be the first health professionals consulted. Histologic examination reveals hyperkeratosis or a lichenoid reaction. Other sites reported include the urethra, glans penis, vagina, and anorectal region.[371] DC patients have an increased risk of malignancy arising from the preexisting leukoplakia; the incidence of malignant transformation has been estimated to be 35%.[375]

Hematologic Abnormalities. About 85% of patients with classic DC are initially found to have cytopenia of one or more lineages, and pancytopenia develops in more than 95% of patients by 40 years of age. Complications of BMF, such as hemorrhage or opportunistic infection, represent the major cause of death in patients with DC. In patients with atypical DC, BMF may appear before the classic mucocutaneous features and lead to an initial

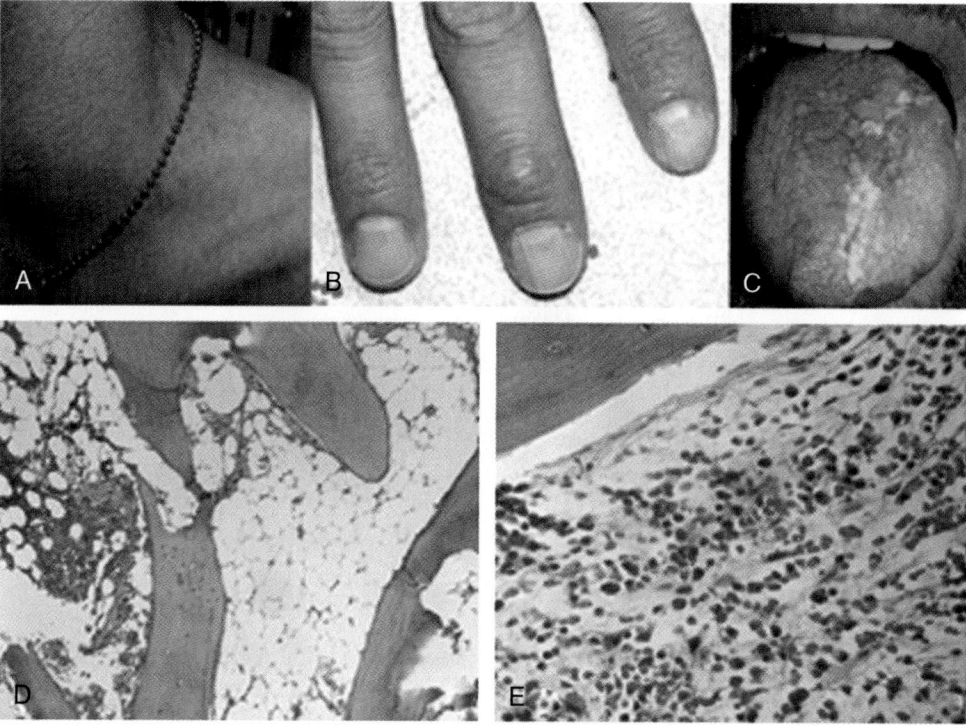

FIGURE 8-6. Physical findings in a 31-year-old patient with classic dyskeratosis congenita (DC). **A,** Reticular skin pigmentation. **B,** Dystrophic fingernails, rather mild in this case. **C,** Leukoplakia of the tongue. **D,** Hypocellular bone marrow. **E,** Hypocellular myelodysplastic syndrome in a different 41-year-old patient with atypical DC caused by a *TERC* gene mutation. *(Courtesy of Susan Bayliss, Washington University.)*

diagnosis of idiopathic aplastic anemia. Hypoplastic MDS and MDS/AML are increasingly diagnosed in patients with DC, especially in those with a milder course or an atypical form of the disease. Indeed, MDS or MDS/AML may be the initial manifestation of patients with atypical DC.

Other Clinical Features. Pulmonary complications are common (≈20%) and include pulmonary fibrosis and vascular abnormalities.[376,377] Pulmonary fibrosis is usually a more prominent finding in older patients or after BMT.[378] In some patients with atypical DC, pulmonary fibrosis may be the only clinical manifestation. Figure 8-7 shows a family with autosomal dominant DC and pulmonary fibrosis. Families with hereditary pulmonary fibrosis of adult onset should be investigated for DC.[379,380]

Ocular findings include epiphora (excessive tearing caused by blocked lacrimal ducts), blepharitis, cataracts, loss of eyelashes, conjunctivitis, ectropion, glaucoma, strabismus, ulcers, ocular albinism, and Coats' retinopathy.[381-384]

Multiple dental caries and early loss of teeth are common.[385-387] Web formation in the upper esophagus, esophageal stricture, and a bifid uvula are other findings in patients with DC.[388-390]

Strictures of the urethra, hypospadias, and phimosis are congenital anomalies found in patients with DC. Underdeveloped testes and azoospermia have been reported in more severe and advanced forms of DC.

Enteropathy and malabsorption associated with chronic diarrhea are underdiagnosed but frequent findings in more advanced forms of DC.[391]

Intellectual disabilities such as learning difficulties are often associated with classic DC. In rare cases an association with schizophrenia has been described.

Osteoporosis and avascular necrosis of the bones frequently complicate the course of the disease. Short statue and an elf-like appearance have been associated with classic DC.

Predisposition to Malignancy

DC is a cancer predisposition syndrome.[9,361,368,369,392] After BMF and pulmonary complications, malignancy is the third leading cause of death. The most frequent malignancies in patients with DC are squamous cell carcinoma of the head and neck (especially the tongue but also the lip, mouth, palate, cheek, nasopharynx, and larynx),[373,375,393,394] the upper and lower gastrointestinal tract (esophagus and anus),[395] and the female genital tract. Other cancers found in patients with DC include skin cancer and adenocarcinoma of the stomach,[396] colon, lung, and pancreas. Malignancies usually develop in the third decade and are therefore more frequently found in individuals with milder and later-onset forms of the disease.

Previously, MDS and MDS/AML were thought to be infrequent in patients with DC; more recently, however, MDS and MDS/AML are increasingly being diagnosed in patients with atypical DC and in patients with late onset of the disease (see also Fig. 8-6E). MDS or MDS/AML may be the first hematologic manifestation of disease. Although DC is rarely a cause of MDS or MDS/AML in children,[397] it should be considered in the differential diagnosis in adults with MDS or MDS/AML. Abnormalities of chromosome 7 (monosomy, isochromosome, or other structural rearrangements) are the

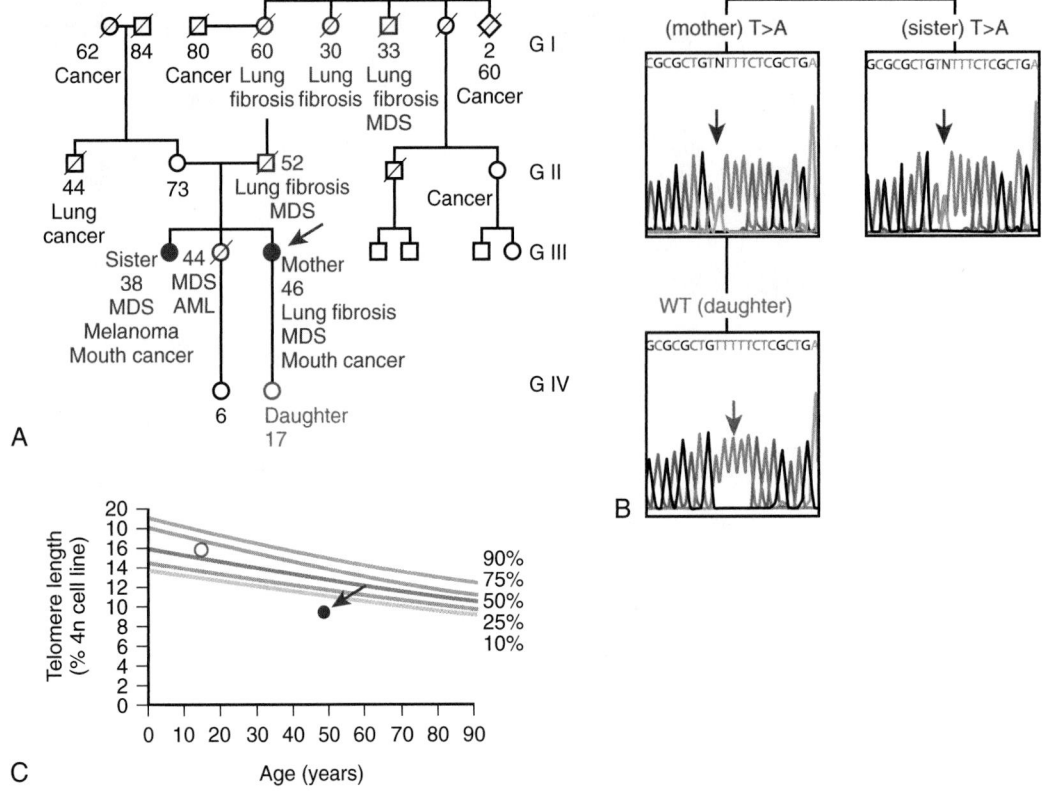

FIGURE 8-7. **A,** Pedigree of a family with dyskeratosis congenita (DC) caused by a *TERC* gene mutation. Note that in addition to myelodysplastic syndrome (MDS), pulmonary fibrosis is a prominent feature in this family with DC. **B,** Chromatogram demonstrating that the mother and her sister are heterozygous for the *TERC* gene mutation whereas the daughter has not inherited the mutation (WT). **C,** Telomere length of the affected mother (below and outside the telomere length distribution of normal controls) and the unaffected daughter (normal telomere length). Colored lines indicate the 10th, 25th, 50th, 75th, and 90th percentiles of telomere length determined in 105 healthy controls between the ages of 1 and 95 years.

most common cytogenetic abnormalities in patients with DC-associated MDS or MDS/AML.

Little is known about the biology of leukemia or other cancers in patients with DC and to what extent these malignancies differ from those seen in patients without DC. The cancer recurrence rate is high in patients with DC.

Laboratory Findings

Common laboratory findings are summarized in Box 8-8. In most patients with DC, the initial hematologic abnormalities are thrombocytopenia or macrocytic anemia followed by pancytopenia. Bone marrow examination often reveals increased cellularity at the outset, thus suggesting an element of hypersplenism. However, hypocellularity then ensues, consistent with the diagnosis of aplastic anemia. Macrocytosis and elevated hemoglobin F levels ("stress erythropoiesis") are common.[383] The number of circulating hematopoietic progenitor cells is decreased, indicative of the impairment in hematopoiesis at the stem cell level.

Bone marrow examination usually shows hypocellular marrow affecting all three blood cell lineages. Hypocellular MDS or MDS/AML is increasingly being found in patients with atypical DC or a late onset of disease. Monosomy 7 is the most frequent clonal

cytogenetic abnormality in DC patients with MDS or MDS/AML.

Long-term culture assays of bone marrow cells from patients with DC show a decreased number of progenitor cells and an impaired capability for colony formation, indicative of a quantitative and qualitative defect.[408]

Immunologic abnormalities may include humoral and cellular defects[366,398] (summarized in Box 8-9). Severe combined immunodeficiency is characteristic of severe forms of DC.

DC cells have increased spontaneous chromosomal instability that leads to distinctive chromosomal breaks, rearrangements,[384,399-401] and sister chromatid exchanges.[384,399,419] Chromosomal instability increases with increasing cell divisions in vitro. However, chromosome breakage does not increase after treatment with alkylating agents such as DEB, MMC, or nitrogen mustard,[399,401-406] which distinguishes DC from FA. Some of the chromosomal abnormalities characteristic of DC include end-to-end fusions, dicentric or tricentric chromosomes, anaphase or telophase bridges, short telomeres, and telomere free ends.

Biased X-inactivation in blood cells, as well as in fibroblasts from buccal mucosa and skin biopsy samples in female mutation carriers, is characteristic of X-linked DC.[417,418]

Box 8-8	Laboratory Findings in Patients with Dyskeratosis Congenita

PERIPHERAL BLOOD

Cytopenia of one or more lineages (80%)
Initial manifestation highly variable
Macrocytosis with or without anemia
Thrombocytopenia
Neutropenia
Pancytopenia
Low number of circulating progenitor cells
Elevated hemoglobin F
Elevated von Willebrand factor

BONE MARROW EXAMINATION

Hypocellular bone marrow affecting all three lineages
Increased number of mast cells
Dyserythropoiesis
Hypocellular myelodysplastic syndrome
Myelodysplastic syndrome/acute myeloid leukemia

IMMUNOLOGIC FINDINGS[368,398]

Humoral abnormalities:
 Hypogammaglobulinemia/hypergammaglobulinemia
Cellular abnormalities:
 Lymphopenia: B cells, T cells, natural killer cells
Functional abnormalities:
 Reduced proliferation upon stimulation
 Increased apoptosis upon stimulation
Anergy
Difficulty in immortalization by Epstein-Barr virus
 transformation (X-linked dyskeratosis congenita)

CYTOGENETICS[384,399-407]

Chromosomal instability: nonclonal complex anomalies in
 cultured cells
Chromosomal breaks, hypodiploidy, micronuclei
Anaphase and telophase bridges*
Short telomeres signal-free ends
End-to-end fusion with no telomeric signal
No increase in chromosomal instability after the
 clastogenic effects of DNA cross-linking agents
Clonal abnormalities in bone marrow cells: monosomy 7
 (myelodysplastic syndrome, myelodysplastic syndrome/
 acute lymphocytic leukemia)

*Laboratory findings in bold are characteristic of dyskeratosis
 congenita.

Box 8-9	Cellular Abnormalities in Dyskeratosis Congenita

Spontaneous chromosome breaks[401,410]
No increased chromosomal breakage after cross-linking
 agents
Hypersensitivity to ionizing radiation (controversial)[413]
Increased sensitivity to certain cytotoxic agents[409,411,412]
Short telomeres*[407,414]
Premature replicative senescence[400,415,416]
Lack of immortalization by TERT (X-linked)[416]
**Biased X-inactivation (female carrier of X-linked
 dyskeratosis congenita)**[417,418]

*Cellular abnormlities in bold are characteristic of dyskeratosis
 congenita.

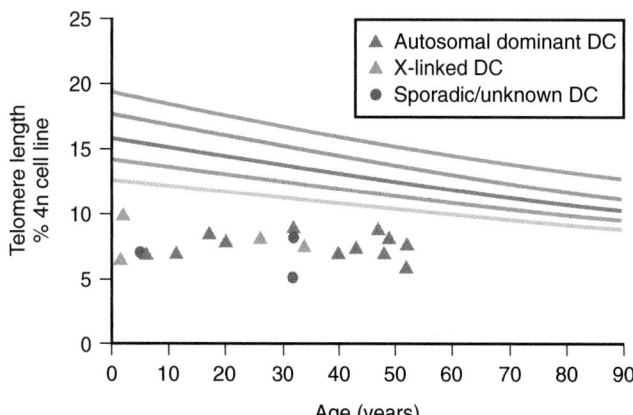

FIGURE 8-8. Telomere length in peripheral blood mononuclear cells in individuals with dyskeratosis congenita (DC) and bone marrow failure (BMF). Note that in all individuals with DC and BMF, telomere lengths are below and outside the telomere length distribution of normal controls. The colored lines indicate the 10th, 25th, 50th, 75th, and 90th percentiles of telomere length determined in 105 healthy controls between the ages of 1 and 95 years.

mere length excludes DC as the cause of BMF.[356,357] However, in some cases with mild clinical manifestations the interpretation of results can be difficult and requires experience with the test method used and should be done in conjunction with the patient's clinical and laboratory data.

Cellular Phenotype of Dyskeratosis Congenita Cells

In addition to increased spontaneous instability, DC cells have several other phenotypic characteristics as summarized in Box 8-9. DC cells have been reported to have increased sensitivity to ionizing radiation and certain chemotherapeutic agents (e.g., bleomycin), although these findings were not consistently found by all investigators.[401,409-412] Decreased proliferation capacity in vitro and premature replicative senescence are also characteristic of DC cells (see Box 8-9).[400,414-416] Cells from some forms of DC (X-linked DC) fail to immortalize after Epstein-Barr virus–induced transformation or after transfection of a plasmid expressing the telomerase catalytic subunit TERT.[416,421]

The presence of short telomeres in circulating peripheral blood cells is the most characteristic finding in patients with BMF and DC.[407,414] Telomere length in individuals with BMF secondary to DC is far below the normal distribution of telomere length in age-matched healthy control individuals (Fig. 8-8).[356,357] In contrast to other IBMFSs, which may have short telomeres in circulating myeloid cells,[117,420] telomeres are exquisitely short in the myeloid and lymphoid cells of patients with DC-associated BMF. Telomere length measurements may be used to screen patients with BMF for DC; normal telo-

Differential Diagnosis

Clinically, DC has to be distinguished from other IBMFSs such FA, DBA, and SDS. Clinical manifestations, associated physical abnormalities, the family history (pattern of inheritance), and the lack of increased chromosomal fragility in the DEB or MMC test performed on cultured peripheral lymphocytes or fibroblasts (or both) are helpful in strengthening the diagnosis of DC. As noted earlier, telomere length outside the normal distribution strongly suggests the diagnosis of DC, whereas normal telomere length excludes DC as a cause of BMF in these patients.[356,357] X-inactivation studies may be helpful in identifying female carriers of the X-linked form of DC.[417,418]

Genetics

Inheritance

There are four distinct forms of inheritance of DC. Historically, before molecular diagnostics was available, inheritance was determined by examining family members for the presence of clinical manifestations. Today, we know that such classification was often mistaken because of the variability of penetrance of gene mutations.

X-linked Dyskeratosis Congenita. The most common form of classic DC is X-linked (MIM 30500), and many families with classic DC and X-linked inheritance have been described. The X-linked form of DC is almost always due to single point mutations in the *DKC1* gene encoding dyskerin (see later).

Autosomal Dominant Dyskeratosis Congenita. Several families have been described with an autosomal dominant form of inheritance of DC (AD DC, MIM 127550). This form of DC exhibits genetic anticipation (see Box 8-11) and may therefore be misclassified as autosomal recessive (AR DC). Several pedigrees in which AD DC is caused by mutations in the *TERC* gene encoding telomerase RNA have been described. In addition, families in whom AD DC appears to be due to mutations in *TERT*, which encodes the telomerase reverse transcriptase, have been reported. AD DC is very often manifested as atypical DC. Because of the often atypical findings, the frequency of AD DC is currently most likely significantly underestimated.[370]

Autosomal Recessive Dyskeratosis Congenita. A number of families have been described with AR DC (MIM 224230). AR DC is usually inferred when neither parent has any signs of DC and two or more children have the disease or when the parents of an affected child are consanguineous. Some families originally thought to have AR DC were found to have AD DC with variable penetrance and expressivity, thus mimicking sporadic or autosomal recessive disease.[422,423] Recently, a homozygous *NOP10* mutation has been associated with AR DC

in a single consanguineous family.[424] However, more likely, the *NOP10* mutations are hypomorphic mutations that are inherited codominantly.

Sporadic Dyskeratosis Congenita. A large proportion of DC cases arise sporadically. Of 123 such male cases from the DC registry in the United Kingdom, 40 were found to have a de novo *DKC1* mutation and 3 were found to have an inherited *TERC* mutation with variable penetrance and expressivity in the affected family. Eighty had neither *TERC* nor *DKC1* mutations. Similarly, all 35 female cases had neither *TERC* nor *DKC1* mutations. These sporadic cases account for more than half of DC patients.[422] Biallelic hypomorphic mutations may mimic sporadic disease, but it is due to codominant expression of the mutant alleles.[423]

The Dyskeratosis Congenita Genes and Their Functions

DKC1 and Dyskerin. X-linked DC is caused by mutations in the *DKC1* gene at Xq28. *DKC1* was identified by positional cloning in families with affected males and biased X-inactivation in female carriers.[367,417,418] The *DKC1*-encoded protein dyskerin is a 58-kd nucleolar protein orthologous to proteins in yeast, flies, and rats (Cbf5p,[425] Nop60B/minifly,[426] and NAP57,[427] respectively).

Dyskerin is associated with box H/ACA RNA molecules in ribonucleoprotein (RNP) complexes (Fig. 8-9). Box H/ACA RNP complexes consist of four different proteins (dyskerin, GAR1, NOP10, and NHP2) and an integral RNA species.[428,429] The box H/ACA RNA determines the function of the RNP complex. The majority of box H/ACA RNAs are small nucleolar RNAs (snoRNA) found in the nucleolus. These snoRNAs guide the protein complex containing dyskerin by complementary base pairing to specific uridine residues of newly synthesized ribosomal RNA (rRNA) molecules, which are then

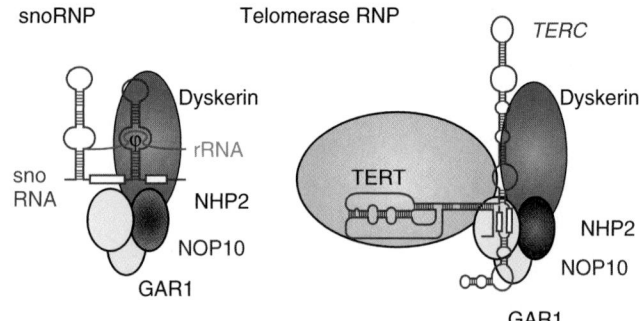

FIGURE 8-9. Dyskerin associates with box H/ACA, small nucleolar RNAs (snoRNA), and telomerase RNA *(TERC)*. Dyskerin is a component of box H/ACA ribonucleoprotein (RNP) particles, where it associates with three other proteins, GAR1, NOP10, and NHP2, and a small noncoding RNA of the class of box H/ACA RNAs. The majority of box H/ACA RNAs are necessary for the modification of uridine residues (pseudouridylation) in ribosomal RNA. The 3' end of the telomerase RNA *TERC* has the structure of box H/ACA RNA and associates with dyskerin and the dyskerin binding partners, as well as with the catalytic component of telomerase, TERT.

modified by pseudouridylation. In snoRNP dyskerin is the enzyme, a pseudouridine synthase, that actually catalyzes the pseudouridylation reaction.[430,431] The role of pseudouridylation is not known, but pseudouridines tend to be found in the conserved sequences of rRNA and transfer RNA (tRNA) in regions of high secondary structure, and it is likely that these modifications stabilize the secondary and tertiary structure of RNA molecules.[432] Other box H/ACA RNAs that associate with dyskerin and the three other proteins of the complex participate in ribosome biogenesis downstream of rRNA modification or messenger RNA (mRNA) splicing or are orphan RNAs, the function of which remains to be determined (for review see Meier[433]).

Telomerase RNA (*TERC*, telomerase RNA component), which along with TERT (telomerase reverse transcriptase) forms the core of the telomerase enzyme, also associates with dyskerin and the other three proteins present in H/ACA-class snoRNP (see Fig. 8-9).[434,435] The conserved secondary structure of the 3′ end of telomerase RNA is very similar to that of H/ACA RNAs.[434] This part of the telomerase RNA and its association with H/ACA RNP components are found only in vertebrates,[436] whereas the H/ACA RNP components themselves are highly conserved among all eukaryotes.[437] The four proteins may be involved in transport, stability, and assembly of the telomerase complex in the nucleolus. At this point there is no evidence that the H/ACA part of telomerase RNA functions as a guide RNA or that dyskerin exhibits any pseudouridylation activity as part of the telomerase complex.

The diverse function of dyskerin in humans raises the interesting question of whether and to what extent the pathogenesis of X-linked DC is caused by defects in telomerase activity or in other functions of RNP, such as rRNA metabolism.

NOP10. Recently, autozygous mutations (homozygous mutations in a consanguineous family) in the *NOP10* gene on chromosome 15q14 have been found to be responsible for disease in a single family.[424] NOP10, like dyskerin, is an essential component of H/ACA RNP complexes and thus participates in the same pathways as dyskerin (see earlier). Whether mutations in *NOP10* cause disease as a result of defects in telomere maintenance or defects in other functions of H/ACA RNP complexes, such as rRNA metabolism, remains to be determined.

TERC, TERT, and Telomerase. AD DC is caused by mutations in the *TERC* gene, also abbreviated as *hTR or TER*, which is found on chromosome 3q26.[438] *TERC* was identified as the gene responsible for AD DC through positional cloning.[438] It encodes the RNA component of the telomerase complex. Telomerase, the enzyme responsible for elongating and maintaining telomeres, synthesizes telomeric DNA repeats by using *TERC* RNA as a template (Box 8-10 and Fig. 8-10A and B).[438] Non-

<table><tr><td>Box 8-10</td><td>Telomeres/Telomerase</td></tr></table>

Telomeres are complex DNA/protein structures at the ends of chromosomes that are needed to protect chromosome ends from degradation and distinguish them from double-stranded breaks.[439] Human telomere DNA consists of thousands of repeats of TTAGGG. In the absence of telomerase in most somatic cells, telomeres do shorten with each cell division.[440] In most tissues, therefore, telomere length decreases with age.[441] When telomeres become critically short, cell cycle arrest or cell death occurs (see Fig. 8-10).[442]

DNA polymerase I cannot copy the extreme end of a DNA strand,[443] so telomeres would tend to get shorter with each cell division. In germ cells,[444] some stem cells,[445,446] and most cancer cells,[442,447] telomeres are maintained by the action of the enzyme *telomerase*,[448] which contains two core components, a reverse transcriptase TERT (telomerase reverse transcriptase) and an RNA molecule, *TERC* (telomerase RNA component), that acts as a template for the synthesis of telomere repeats (see Fig. 8-10).

synonymous mutations have also been identified in the *TERT* gene localized on 5p15.33.[449-452] TERT is the catalytic part of the telomerase complex (see Box 8-10 and Fig. 8-9). *TERT* was identified as a gene responsible for AD DC through a candidate gene approach.[449-451] Telomerase RNA, or the TERC component, which along with TERT forms the core of the telomerase enzyme, also associates with the four proteins present in H/ACA-class RNPs, including dyskerin and NOP10 (telomerase RNP complex, see Fig. 8-9).[434,435]

TINF2. Recently three mutations in exon 6 of *TINF2* encoding TIN2 have been identified in six patients with DC. All mutations were associated with short telomeres. TIN2 associates with the telomere. The mechanism by which the TIN2 mutations cause telomere shortening remains to be determined.[452a]

Other Genes. For about 60% of patients in whom DC and BMF are diagnosed, the mutations or the genes mutated have not been identified. Like patients with DC and BMF caused by mutations in dyskerin, *NOP10*, *TERC*, or *TERT*, these patients also have very short telomeres, thus suggesting that the affected gene or genes participates in the same pathway.

Unraveling of the molecular pathology of DC has greatly advanced our understanding of the disease. The finding that X-linked and AD DC is caused by defects in molecules that are part of the telomerase RNP complex favors the paramount importance of defective telomerase in the pathology of DC. The finding that all patients with DC and BMF have very short telomeres further underscores the importance of telomerase function in this disease. Figure 8-11 summarizes our current model of the pathogenesis of disease in patients with DC.

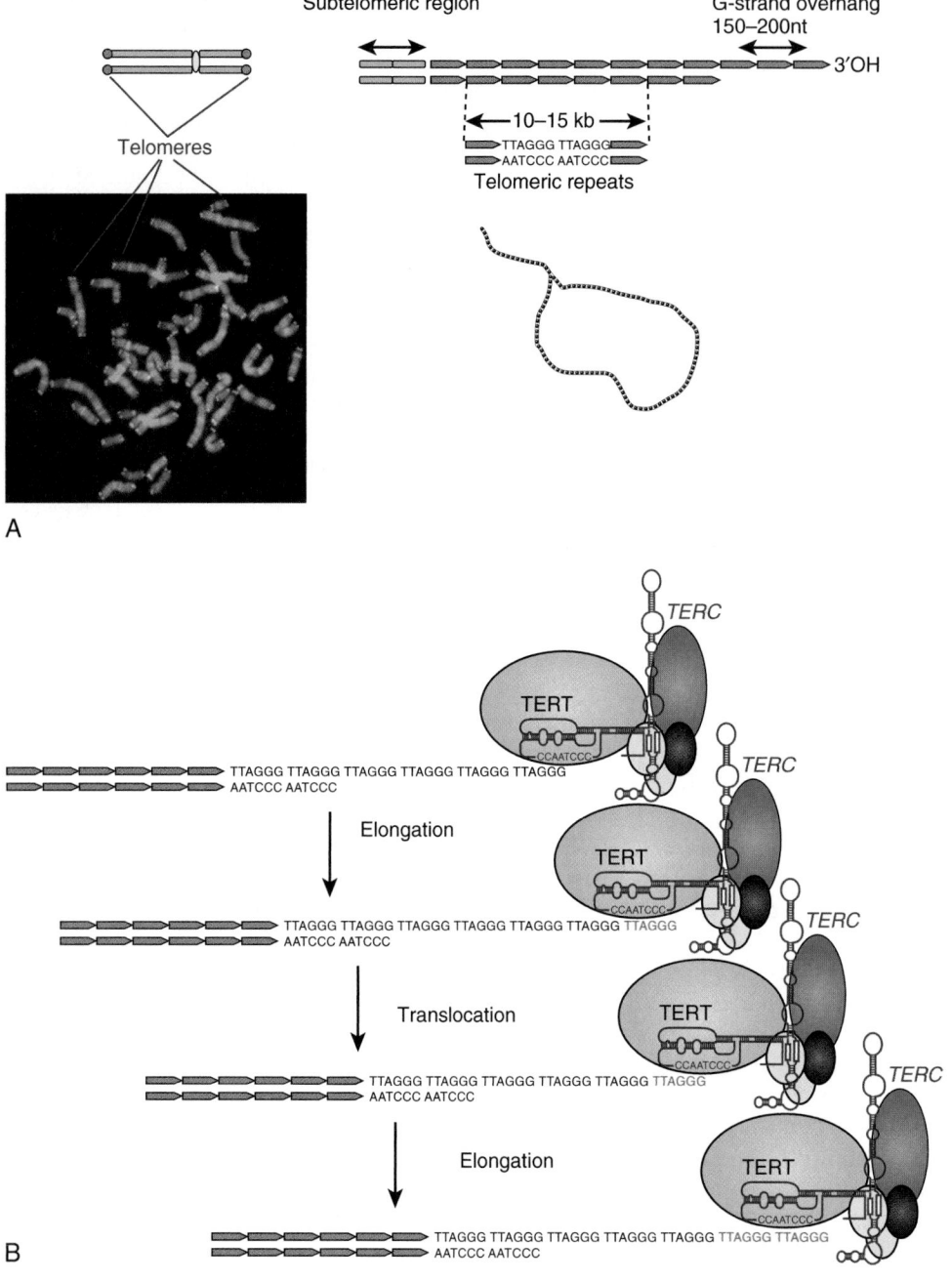

FIGURE 8-10. A, Telomeres and telomere structure. Telomeres are the end of chromosomes. They are complex protein DNA structures that protect telomere ends from degradation and end-to-end fusion (also see Box 8-7). In nondividing cell telomeres often form a loop stucture, which makes the end inaccessible to DNA repair proteins and DNA exonucleases. **B,** Telomerase adds telomeric repeats to the 3' end of telomeres (also see Box 8-10).

Dyskeratosis Congenita Gene Mutations in Patients with Dyskeratosis Congenita

DKC1 Mutations. The mutations in the *DKC1* gene that cause DC are mainly single–amino acid missense mutations[453] (Fig. 8-12A) and can be inherited or occur de novo. The A353G mutation is the most frequent de novo *DKC1* mutation and is found in approximately 40% of patients with DC and *DKC1* mutations.[422] *DKC1* mutations are not randomly distributed but are concentrated in the N-terminal of dyskerin. The crystal structure of the archaeal homologue of the H/ACA RNP complex, the Cbf5-Nop10 complex,[454-456] has enabled modeling of human dyskerin. In this model the majority of residues mutated in cases of DC are tightly clustered in or near the

PUA domain, which is predicted to bind H/ACA RNA, including *TERC* RNA (Fig. 8-13). The mutations would thus be expected to decrease binding of the cognate RNA and lead to instability. Only two mutations have been found in the TruB catalytic domain, one of which, S121G, is located three residues from the essential aspartate required for pseudouridylation and, interestingly, is associated with a severe form of DC also known as Hoyeraal-Hreidarsson syndrome (HHS, MIM 300240) (also see later). The absence of mutations that would predict a "null" allele, such as frameshifts and nonsense mutations, suggests that a dyskerin null mutation is incompatible with life. In support of this notion, a dyskerin null mutation is embryonically lethal in mice.[457]

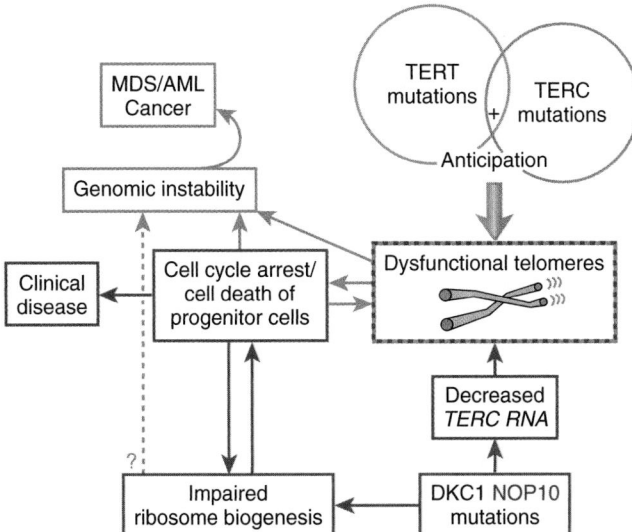

FIGURE 8-11. Model of the pathogenesis of disease in patients with dyskeratosis congenita (DC). Our hypothesis is that excessive telomere shortening and dysfunctional telomeres play a central role in the pathogenesis of DC. Dysfunctional telomeres lead to cell cycle arrest and cell death. In patients with *DKC1* and *NOP10* mutations, *TERC* RNA stability and accumulation are decreased, which leads to decreased telomerase activity and telomere shortening. In addition a possible impairment in ribosome biogenesis also impairs cell survival and proliferation. *TERC* gene mutations and *TERT* mutations cause telomere shortening through haploinsufficiency. The inheritance of shortened telomeres is the molecular mechanism of anticipation in autosomal dominant DC. Dysfunctional telomeres lead to genomic instability, which may contribute to the predisposition to cancer in patients with DC. AMC, acute myeloid leukemia; MDS, myelodyplastic syndrome.

The functional consequences of a subset of pathogenic *DKC1* mutations have been investigated in fibroblasts or mononuclear cells from patients with X-linked DC[458,459] and in XY mouse embryonic stem cells harboring a mutated *Dkc1* allele.[460] Analysis of fibroblasts or mononuclear cells from patients with X-linked DC showed a reduced level of *TERC* RNA and decreased telomerase activity, whereas analysis in mouse cells revealed that not only the level of *Terc* RNA but also the levels of other specific snoRNAs were affected and that overall pseudouridylation activity, in particular, site-specific pseudouridylation involving the affected guide snoRNA, was markedly decreased. Thus, it remains controversial whether X-linked DC is due to defective telomere maintenance, defective ribosome biogenesis, or possibly both.[2,370]

NOP10 Mutation. Recently, autozygous *NOP10* mutations have been identified in one consanguineous family. The mutation leads to replacement of a highly conserved arginine with tryptophan at amino acid position 34 (R34W).[424] The three affected family members were autozygous for the mutation. Heterozygous mutation carriers did not show obvious signs of disease but had shortened telomeres and decreased levels of *TERC* RNA in their peripheral blood cells.[424] The inheritance

of hypomorphic gene mutations may mimic a recessive inheritance pattern. The shortened telomeres and reduced levels of *TERC* RNA in heterozygous mutation carriers, however, suggest that both *NOP10* alleles are expressed codominantly. Whether the mutation affects the function of only telomerase RNP or also other H/ACA RNP complexes remains to be determined.

TERC Gene Mutations. The *TERC* mutations found in patients with DC are shown in Figure 8-12B. Investigation of family members revealed that in all patients with clinical manifestations of DC the *TERC* gene mutations were inherited. Many mutations are found in the pseudoknot domain of the molecule, a domain that mediates binding to the telomerase reverse transcriptase TERT and is essential for telomerase activity. Other mutations are found in the CR7 and H/ACA domains and affect the stability and nuclear accumulation of the *TERC* molecule. In many of these mutations it has been demonstrated that the mutations act by disrupting the secondary structure of the *TERC* molecule rather than by altering nucleotide sequences crucial for function,[461-466] in agreement with the fact that although the secondary structure of *TERC* is highly conserved among different species, the primary sequence is not.[436] Large gene deletions encompassing the *TERC* gene have been identified in two independent families with AD DC. Along with the pathogenic mutations, which have been shown by several groups to severely reduce telomerase activity, there are two polymorphisms that are relatively frequent in people of African descent.[467] These sequence changes, G58A and G228A, do not affect telomerase activity,[461,462,467] and individuals carrying these sequence alterations have normal telomere length independent of the presence of BMF. In addition, the mutation G450A, found in a patient with severe aplastic anemia, apparently had no effect on telomerase or telomere length.[461]

The existence of large deletions and in vitro transfection studies led to the conclusion that haploinsufficiency of *TERC* is the mechanism underlying AD DC.

TERT Gene Mutations. Heterozygosity for nonsynonymous mutations in the *TERT* gene have been identified in individuals with aplastic anemia and short telomeres and more recently also in individuals in whom pulmonary fibrosis was originally diagnosed.[379,380,449-452] The mutations identified are summarized in Figure 8-12C. Mutations located in the N-terminal critical for binding of *TERC* RNA and within the central region of *TERT* defining the catalytic region of the reverse transcriptase impair telomerase activity to a variable degree. Mutations in the C-terminal region affect in vivo telomere synthesis after the assembly of a catalytically active enzyme.[468] The A202T and H412W mutations have been identified more than once in unrelated families. Two small deletions causing a frameshift and a truncated TERT protein and two splicing mutations have been identified in individuals in whom pulmonary fibrosis was originally diagnosed.[379]

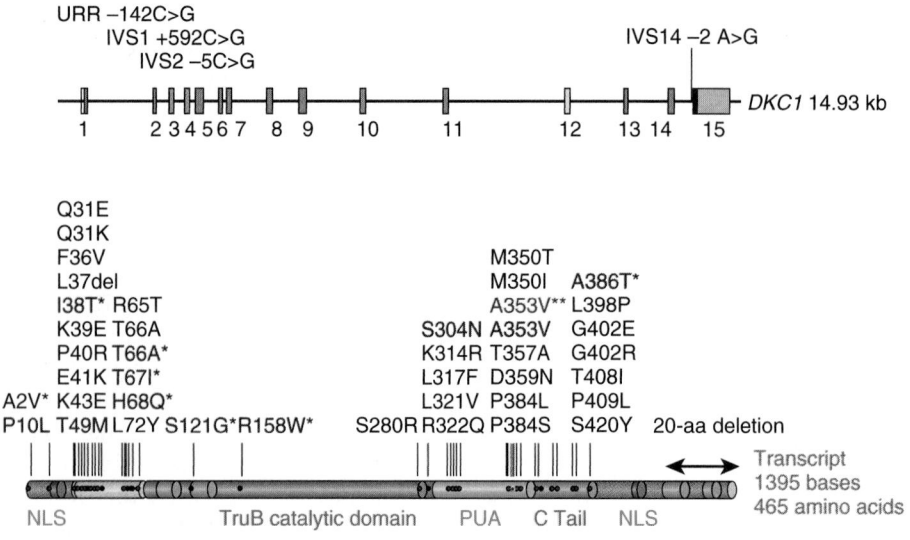

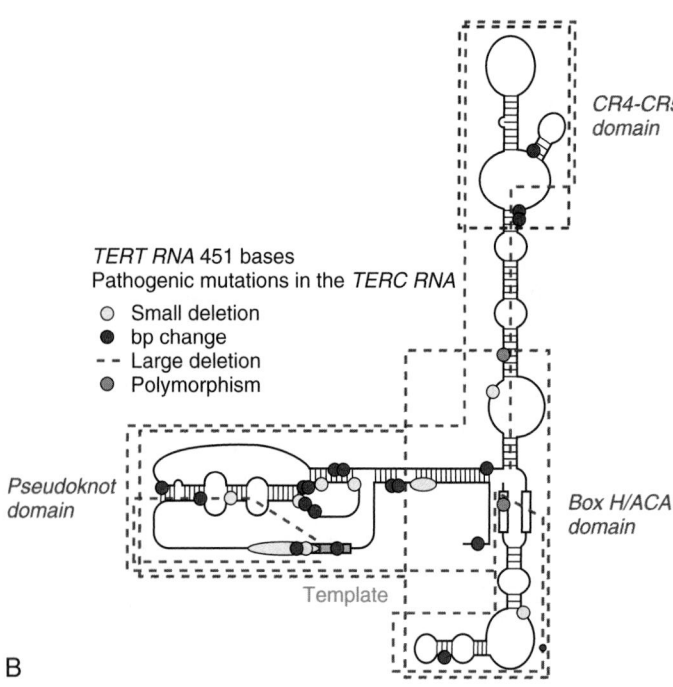

FIGURE 8-12. A, Mutations in the *DKC1* gene. A schematic representation of the *DKC1* gene is presented below the schematic representation of dyskerin protein and its functional domains. Patient-derived mutations are shown. *Asterisks* indicate recurrent mutations. The A353V mutation, shown in red, is a frequent de novo mutation and accounts for about a third of the mutations in *DKC1*. Mutations shown in purple are found in patients with a severe form of dyskeratosis congenita (DC) also known as Hoyeraal-Hreidarsson syndrome. NLS, nuclear localization signal; TruB and PUA, pseudouridine synthase domains. **B,** Mutations in the *TERC* gene as shown in a schematic representation of the tertiary structure of telomerase RNA (*TERC*). The pseudoknot and the CR4-CR5 domain are important for the association of *TERC* with the catalytic subunit TERT and for telomerase activity. Mutations found in families with autosomal dominant DC are shown, including two large deletions, one deleting the 5′ end and the other the 3′ end of *TERC*.

Disease manifestations in families with *TERT* gene mutations are highly variable, and frequently disease does not segregate with the mutation in these families, thus indicating incomplete disease penetrance. Interestingly, individuals with a de novo *TERT* gene deletion secondary to a large chromosomal deletion on chromosome 5p (5p–syndrome, cri du chat syndrome) show accelerated telomere shortening but no clinical features characteristic of DC.[469] In contrast, biallelic *TERT* gene mutations have been identified in patients with classic manifestations of DC and in one individual with HHS, a very severe form of DC (see later also), which suggests that the mutant alleles are expressed codominantly and the residual telomerase activity determines the clinical phenotype.[423,470] Biallelic *TERT* or *TERC* null mutations have never been described, thus suggesting that in contrast to mice, in humans complete lack of telomerase activity is not compatible with life.[410]

***TINF2* Mutations.** Mutation A838G (TIN2 K280E) was found in a large family with aplastic anemia. Mutation G844A (R282H) was identified in three unrelated patients with early onset and severe disease similar to Hoyeraal-Hreidarsson and Ravesz syndrome. The third C845A (R282S) was found in one patient with early onset of severe aplastic anemia and immune deficiency. Both R282H and R282S were de novo mutation and were associated with very short telomeres.[452a]

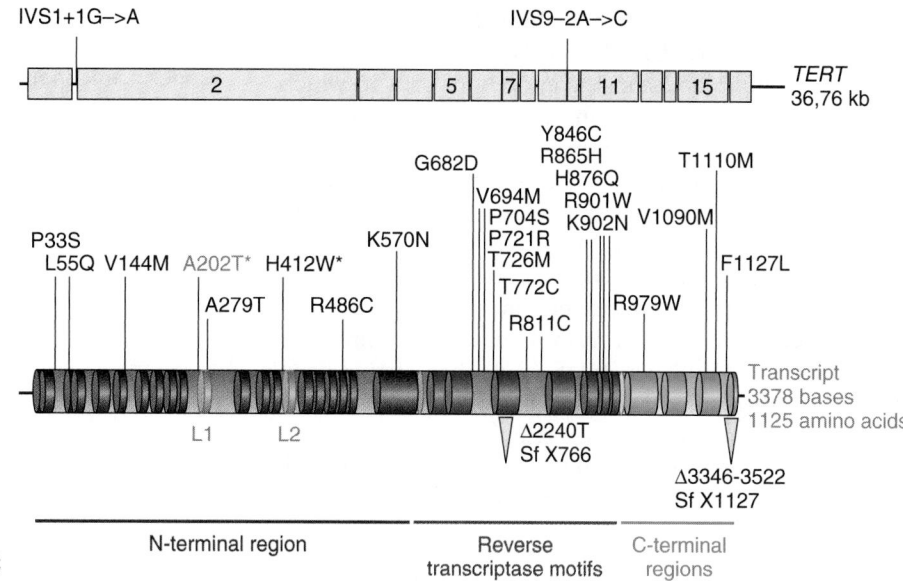

C

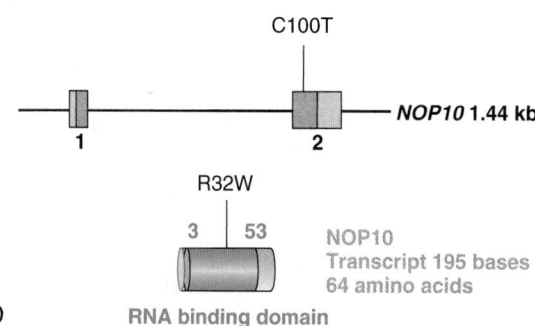

D

FIGURE 8-12—cont'd C, Mutations in the *TERT* gene as shown in a schematic representation of the 16 exons of the *TERT* gene, below the schematic representation of the TERT protein with its functional domains. Patient-derived mutations are shown. Sequence variants of uncertain pathogenicity are shown in gray. Small deletions are indicated below the diagram. L1 and L2 are linker regions; Sf indicates a frameshift, which results in a premature stop codon X. *Asterisks* indicate recurrent mutations. **D,** Mutation in NOP10. A schematic representation of the NOP10 gene is shown, below the NOP10 protein. The mutation identified in one consanguineous family is shown. The patient was homozygous for the mutation.

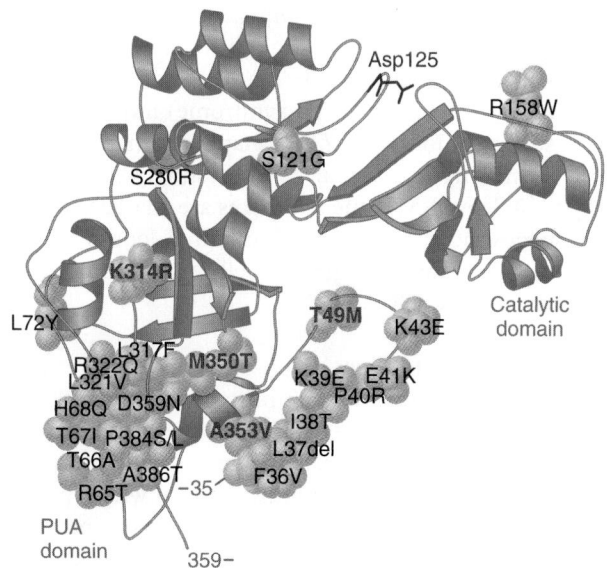

FIGURE 8-13. Clustering of pathogenic mutations in dyskerin. The crystal structure of the archaeal homologue of dyskerin is shown.[454-456] In this model the majority of residues mutated in cases of dyskeratosis congenita are tightly clustered in or near the PUA domain, which is predicted to bind box H/ACA RNA, including *TERC* RNA. *(Modified from Rashid R, Liang B, Baker DL, et al. Crystal structure of a Cbf5-Nop10-Gar1 complex and implications in RNA-guided pseudouridylation and dyskeratosis congenita. Mol Cell. 2006;21:249-260.)*

Genotype-Phenotype Correlation

The disease phenotype of patients with DC is highly variable and largely determined by the gene mutated and the pattern of inheritance (X-linked, autosomal dominant, or autosomal recessive), the nature of the mutation, and the history of inheritance (number of generations that the mutations has been passed on).

***DCK1* Mutations.** The severity of disease in individuals with X-linked DC varies from hardly detectable to a severe form of DC known as HHS (see later), which causes death in early childhood (see Fig. 8-12A). *DKC1* maps to the X chromosome, so the majority of affected individuals are therefore males. The most frequent clinical manifestation is classic DC with mucocutaneous findings in early childhood and progressive BMF in adolescence.

Female carriers of the *DKC1* mutation rarely show signs of hematologic disease. Cutaneous manifestations may be found in female carriers but are usually mild. Female carriers of X-linked DC show a phenomenon known as skewed or *biased X-inactivation*. In females, inactivation of one X chromosome must occur at random early in development to achieve the same dosage of X-linked genes as in male cells. When X-inactivation has been established in a particular cell, it is faithfully passed to all progeny. Thus, in women, tissues are therefore a mosaic in which half the cells have the maternal and half have the paternal X chromosome active. In female carriers of DC, blood consists entirely of cells in which the X chromosome containing the normal dyskerin gene is active,[417,418] which indicates that after random X-inactivation, cells with wild-type dyskerin have a growth or survival advantage (or both) and outgrow mutant cells. Whether this outgrowth takes place in embryogenesis or childhood and whether all tissues are affected are not known. Telomere length in peripheral blood cells in female DC carriers varies from within normal limits to very short.[357] MDS or MDS/AML has never been described in a female *DKC1* mutation carrier. Whether female carriers are at increased risk for the development of cancer in other organs remains to be determined. Biased X-inactivation can be used to determine whether DC in a family is X-linked (see earlier).

TERC Gene Mutations. The clinical phenotype in patients with AD DC caused by *TERC* gene mutations is usually mild. Analysis of family members of individuals with AD DC showed that mutation carriers frequently have only subtle signs of BMF but lack the mucocutaneous features of classic DC (atypical DC, see also Fig. 8-7). Interestingly, the only patient reported to be a compound heterozygote for two different *TERC* gene mutations showed signs of classic DC and early onset of disease, whereas family members with only one of the two mutations did not.[471] *TERC* gene mutations were identified in a subset of adult patients in whom familial or acquired idiopathic aplastic anemia was originally diagnosed and in patients in whom idiopatic pulmonary fibrosis was originally diagnosed.[379,472-474] Investigation of family members revealed that in all patients the *TERC* gene mutations are inherited and that all mutation carriers have short (below the 10th percentile) or very short (below the 1st percentile) telomeres. However, short and very short telomeres were additionally found in individual family members who did not carry the mutation and had no signs of disease.[475] *TERC* gene mutations were likewise identified in some patients with cytopenic MDS or MDS/AML.[474,476] The mutations identified were associated with reduced telomerase activity in vitro and very short telomeres in the mutation carriers with BMF. The presence of *TERC* gene mutations in patients in whom pulmonary fibrosis, aplastic anemia, MDS, or MDS/AML was originally diagnosed indicates that the underlying problem in these patients is the pathology of DC and that the variable expressivity and penetrance of the clinical manifestations in DC lead to a much broader clinical picture than originally anticipated when investigating only individuals with classic DC. Interestingly, *TERC* gene alterations were rarely found in children with aplastic anemia or MDS in the absence of a family history, consistent with the later onset of disease in individuals with AD DC.[397] Pulmonary fibrosis and liver cirrhosis were frequent and sometimes even the first clinical finding in individuals or families with DC and *TERC* gene mutations.

Box 8-11 | Anticipation

Genetic anticipation occurs when an inherited disease develops at increasingly younger ages or with increased severity in each succeeding generation. Thus, if the disease develops in the offspring of patients, it will tend to do so at an earlier age and display more severe clinical manifestations than in their parents. Disease anticipation is found in patients with autosomal dominant dyskeratosis congenita and is caused by the inheritance of increasingly shorter telomeres in subsequent generations.

Anticipation. AD DC is one of a small number of diseases that show genetic anticipation (i.e., the disease becomes more severe and has an earlier age at onset in later generations). Anticipation became apparent when asymptomatic parents of affected individuals were found to also have *TERC* gene mutations (Box 8-11).[438,476] In several cases, examination of these asymptomatic parents revealed that they had signs of mild anemia, such as raised mean corpuscular volume (MCV). In other pedigrees, anemia develops in the parents at an older age than in the children. The mechanism of anticipation appears to be that telomere shortening increases in later generations carrying a defective *TERC* allele.[475,476] Figure 8-14 shows the inheritance of preshortened telomeres in a nuclear family with AD DC caused by a *TERC* gene deletion. Thus, AD DC develops if an individual inherits a defective *TERC* or *TERT* allele and shortened telomeres. It is not known how many generations are needed to produce telomeres short enough to cause the disease. Studies in individuals with a de novo deletion of 5p that includes the *TERT* gene (5p− syndrome) indicate that in the first generation with *TERT* haploinsufficiency, telomere shortening is minimal.[469] Interestingly, in individuals with DC and BMF, the telomeres are all equally short, thus suggesting that there is a minimal length of telomeres required for a progenitor cell to contribute to the peripheral blood cell pool.[469,475]

TERT Gene Mutations. Nonsynonymous mutations, small deletions, and splice site mutations in the telomerase reverse transcriptase *TERT* gene have been identified in individuals in whom aplastic anemia with short telomeres was diagnosed and in individuals in whom pulmonary fibrosis was diagnosed,[379,380,449-452] thus indicating that *TERT* gene mutations may account for cases of atypical DC. Anticipation has also been described in families with AD DC secondary to *TERT* gene mutations.[451] Individuals with heterozygous *TERT* gene mutations rarely have the classic form of DC; the majority have atypical DC. Pulmonary fibrosis is a frequent finding in patients and families with atypical DC caused by *TERT* gene mutations.[379,380,451] Mutation carriers with no signs of disease (silent DC) are often found in families with heterozygous *TERT* gene mutations. Whether telo-

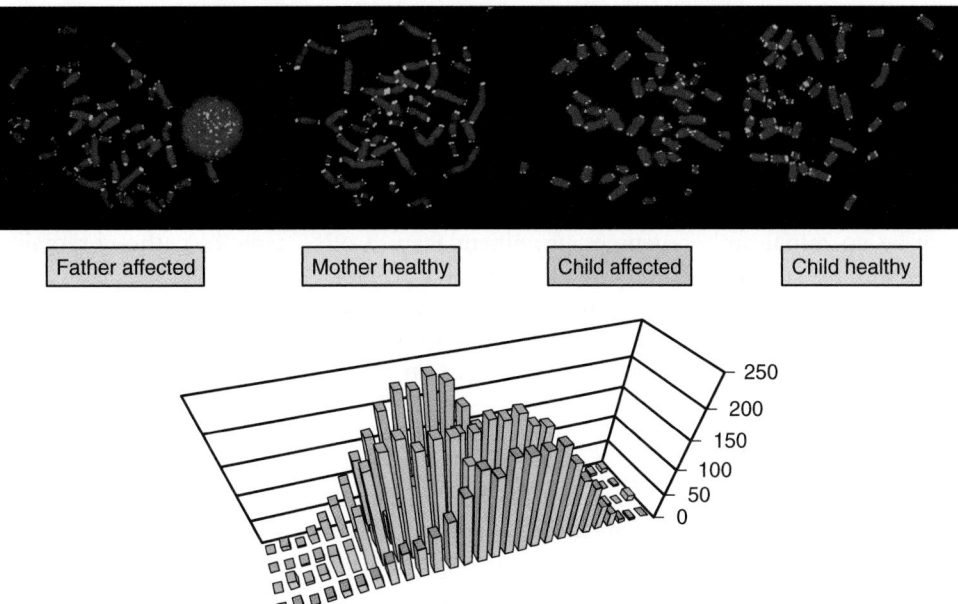

FIGURE 8-14. Inheritance of preshortened telomeres in a family with autosomal dominant dyskeratosis congenita caused by a *TERC* gene deletion. Metaphase spreads of peripheral blood lymphocytes are shown. The green signals at the end of chromosomes show the telomeric repeats hybridized to a fluorescent probe. Below is a graphic representation of the telomere length distribution of each family member. Note that both the affected child and the nonaffected child have inherited preshortened telomeres; in view of their young age, their telomeres should be longer than those of their parents.

Father affected   Mother healthy   Child affected   Child healthy

mere length may identify silent *TERT* gene mutation carriers remains to be determined. Although one would expect that the disease in AD DC secondary to *TERC* or *TERT* mutations would be similar, initial family studies indicate that penetrance and expressivity differ in families heterozygous for *TERC* or *TERT* gene mutations. The most likely explanation is that TERC or TERT is limiting for different tissues and that expression of a functional TERT protein is regulated differently from regulation of *TERC* gene expression. Biallelic *TERT* gene mutations may lead to the classic manifestations of DC and have also been identified in one individual with HHS, a very severe form of DC (also see later), which suggests that the mutant alleles are expressed codominantly and that residual telomerase activity determines the severity of the clinical phenotype.[423,470] Biallelic *TERT* or *TERC* null mutations have never been described, thus suggesting that in contrast to mice, complete lack of telomerase activity is not compatible with life in humans.[423]

Molecular Diagnosis of Dyskeratosis Congenita

Currently, molecular diagnostics is not routinely performed for DC because it is expensive, labor intensive, and limited to specialized laboratories. However, only identification of pathogenic mutations in one of the DC genes definitively establishes the diagnosis of DC. Furthermore, molecular diagnostics enables the identification of mutation carriers, facilitates prenatal diagnosis for an existing pregnancy, and allows PGD for partners identified as mutation carriers. In addition, because the clinical manifestations, severity of disease, prognosis, and response to treatment may vary, depending on the affected gene and the nature of the individual mutation, molecular diagnostics may also influence medical management not only for the DC individual carrying the mutation but also for unaffected family members. Currently, an edu-

cated candidate gene approach in which the gender and family history of the affected DC individual are taken into account is used to identify the affected DC gene. In an affected male after exclusion of the most frequent *DKC1* mutation (A353V), it might be necessary to perform a mutational screen of the entire coding sequence of all three DC genes (usually only *TERC* and *TERT* in an affected female). For *TERC* and *TERT* the screening methods should include techniques that will detect large deletions. Mutation screening is currently successful in only about half of individuals with DC. In addition to the large number of mutations in DC genes associated with DC, a number of nonpathogenic mutations and mutations of unknown pathogenic significance have been identified. Determining the pathogenicity of a particular mutation may be difficult.

Telomere measurement in peripheral blood cells has emerged as a sensitive screening tool for DC in patients with BMF.[356,357] Whether telomere measurements performed on peripheral blood cells may also identify individuals with DC but nonhematopoietic disease manifestations or DC mutation carriers is controversial.[356,357]

Diseases Related to Dyskeratosis Congenita

Idiopathic Aplastic Anemia

A proportion of patients with idiopathic aplastic anemia or hypolastic MDS were found to have mutations in *TERC* or *TERT*.[449,450,472-474] These patients therefore have AD DC. The prevalence of *TERC* mutations among individuals in whom idiopathic aplastic anemia or hypolastic MDS is diagnosed appears to be between 2% and 10%. No *TERC* mutations were found in 284 children with severe aplastic anemia or MDS, in agreement with later onset of the autosomal dominant disease.[397] Because parents are often asymptomatic as a result of the anticipation phenomenon and because of incomplete penetrance of *TERC* and in particular *TERT* gene mutations, a family history is not apparent and a diagnosis of idiopathic aplastic anemia or idiopathic MDS is made.

Hereditary Pulmonary Fibrosis

Pulmonary fibrosis, especially in patients with AD DC, may be an initial and sometimes prominent feature of those with atypical DC. Families with hereditary pulmonary fibrosis of adult onset should be investigated for DC.[379,380] Further investigations are needed to understand the pathogenesis of pulmonary fibrosis in these individuals.

Hoyeraal-Hreidarsson Syndrome

HHS (MIM 300240) is a rare variant of DC that develops in early childhood. It is characterized by intrauterine growth retardation, microcephaly, cerebellar hypoplasia, mental retardation, progressive combined immune deficiency, and aplastic anemia.[477-480] Delayed myelination and hypoplasia of the corpus callosum have been described in patients with HHS.[481] Many but not all patients have a mutation in the *DKC1* gene (see Fig. 8-12A).[482,483] Interestingly, the same mutation (Thr49Met) has been found in four unrelated pedigrees,[422,483,484] and I38T has likewise been found in unrelated HHS patients.[422,485] It is also notable that several cases of HHS are due to the recurrent mutation (A353V) that is responsible for a third of the X-linked *DKC1* cases.[422,453] One of the *DKC1* mutations causing HHS, S121G, is close to the catalytic aspartate residue D125, in the pseudo-uridylation pocket of the protein. In addition, HHS has been found in one individual autozygous (homozygosity in a consanguineous family) for a *TERT* gene mutation and in an individual heterozygous for a *TERT* gene mutation and anticipation, thus indicating that HHS may also be a consequence of a severe telomerase defect alone. In fact, HHS patients have very short telomeres at the time of diagnosis.[356,357,422]

Revesz' Syndrome

The association of progressive bilateral exudative retinopathy (Coats' retinopathy), intrauterine growth retardation, fine sparse hair, fine reticulate skin pigmentation, ataxia secondary to cerebellar hypoplasia, cerebral calcifications, extensor hypertonia, and progressive psychomotor retardation with progressive BMF and death in early childhood, also known as Revesz' syndrome (MIM 268130), might be another severe form of DC.[486-488] Indeed, similar to patients with HHS, individuals with Revesz' syndrome have very short telomeres.[356] Coats' retinopathy has also been described in patients with classic DC.[384] A R282H TIN2 mutation has been identified in one patient with Revesz' syndrome.[452a]

Ataxia-Pancytopenia Syndrome

Ataxia-pancytopenia syndrome is another BMF syndrome with similarities to severe forms of DC. In patients with this syndrome, BMF is associated with severe cerebellar hypoplasia and chromosomal instability without an increase after DEB or MMC testing.[489] MDS and MDS/AML with monosomy 7 are often associated with this syndrome.[489-491] The molecular lesion in patients with ataxia-pancytopenia syndrome and the association with short telomeres suggesting a defect in the telomere maintenance pathway remain to be determined.

Animal Models

Several animal models of dyskerin dysfunction have been described that highlight the importance of rRNA processing in the pathogenesis of DC. Most of what we know about the biochemistry of dyskerin comes from studies of its yeast orthologue Cbf5p (reviewed by Filipowicz and Pogacic[428]; also see earlier). The *cbf5-1* temperature-sensitive mutant was found to have defects in rRNA synthesis and ribosome biogenesis at the restrictive temperature. Null mutations are not viable, whereas hypomorphic point mutations in *Cbf5* are mostly viable at 25° C but show heat- or cold-sensitive growth phenotypes with reduced levels of pseudouridine in rRNA at restrictive temperatures.[492-494] The dyskerin orthologue in *Drosophila* is the protein Nop60B, also known as minifly (*mfl*).[426] Total loss-of-function mutations are lethal, but partial loss-of-function mutations cause pleiotropic defects, including extreme reduction in body size, developmental delay, and reduced female fertility. *mfl* mutants are deficient in pseudouridylation of rRNA and in the production of mature rRNA molecules.[426,495] These results therefore illustrate that decreasing pseudouridylation of rRNA can slow rRNA production and cell growth. Some of the features of these mutants, small size and male sterility, are reminiscent of DC and can be related to the failure of stem cells in tissue renewal.[426,495] In both yeast and *Drosophila*, dyskerin does not associate with telomerase RNA.

In mice the lack of dyskerin is embryonically lethal,[457] whereas hypomorphic *dkc1* mutations in mice and murine ermbryonic stem cells cause defects in both telomere maintenance and ribosome biogenesis.[460,496] Telomere biology in mice differs to some extent from that in humans. Laboratory mice have very long telomeres (50 to 100 kb) in comparison to humans (10 to 15 kb). In mice, telomerase is expressed in almost every tissue, but in humans it is expressed only in germ cells, stem cells, and their immediate progeny and in activated monocytes and lymphocytes. Nevertheless, the study of telomerase-deficient mice (Terc–/–, and Tert–/–) was important for our current understanding of telomere biology and the significance of premature telomere shortening in a living organism.[497] Telomerase null mice, like DC patients, showed genetic anticipation with increasingly shorter telomeres in subsequent generations, as well as a disease phenotype similar to DC, including a shortened life span, early graying, reduced fertility, decreased wound healing, immune deficiency, decreased hematopoietic proliferative capability, and increased chromosomal instability leading to a higher frequency of cancer.[498,499] However, in contrast to mice, homozygosity or compound heterozygosity for telomerase null mutations has never been described in humans, thus suggesting that this would not be compatible with life.

Mechanism of Disease Pathogenesis in Dyskeratosis Congenita

Although some mouse studies support the involvement of rRNA processing defects in the pathogenesis of DC,[460,496,500] the general consensus is that the central component in the pathogenesis of DC is defective telomere maintenance. An interesting question is whether the different clinical manifestations grouped as DC and discussed earlier are due to variations in the extent of telomerase deficiency or whether they relate to secondary effects of the altered gene products. Figure 8-11 summarizes our current model of the pathogenesis of disease in DC.

Clinical Management

Most of what we know regarding therapy and prognosis comes from our experience with patients with classic DC. Care must be taken when extrapolating such experience to patients with atypical DC caused by *TERC* or *TERT* gene mutations. The prognosis for patients with classic DC is usually poor. In males with X-linked and sporadic DC, the median age at death was 20 years.[9] Patients with AD DC have milder disease with a better survival rate. Deaths were usually due to complications from aplastic anemia, BMT, pulmonary fibrosis, or cancer.

Only identification of a pathogenetic mutation can confirm the diagnosis. Once confirmed, the family should be referred to a clinical geneticist familiar with new developments in DC for counseling and careful examination of family members. Genetic testing and possibly telomere measurement should be offered to all family members. Early diagnosis is important for correct management of hematologic complications; appropriate treatment of associated pulmonary, gastrointestinal, ocular, dental, and bone disease; identification of affected presymptomatic family members and unaffected family members or pregnancies that may serve as potential hematopoietic stem cell donors; and targeted cancer surveillance, not only in the patient with DC but also in mutation carriers (also see earlier).

Unfortunately, there is currently no consensus on how to manage patients with DC. Management depends on the age at diagnosis, the presence or absence of clinical signs, the gene affected, the molecular characteristic of the mutation identified, and possibly telomere length. All patients with DC and hematologic manifestations should have a full hematologic assessment, including examination of bone marrow, and in anticipation of possible HSCT, HLA typing should be performed. Other investigations at diagnosis should include pulmonary evaluation and examination of the oropharynx, anal region, and in females, cytologic examination of the vagina and cervical epithelium. The prognosis and life expectancy of family members who have inherited only the short telomeres but not the gene mutation is unknown. Whether these family members should be excluded as potential sibling donors of an affected family member is also unknown.

Management of Hematologic Disease

Treatment of BMF in patients with classic DC is similar to that in patients with FA. Initially, in the absence of hematologic abnormalities or clinical and laboratory signs of mild BMF, monitoring of peripheral blood values might be sufficient. In the presence of hematologic abnormalities, yearly bone marrow examination should include a trephine biopsy and marrow aspirate for the examination of marrow cellularity and morphologic changes characteristic of MDS, as well as for cytogenetic examination by G banding and FISH analysis, including probes that identify the most frequent cytogenetic abnormalities seen in patients with DC and progression to MDS or AML, or both (see earlier also). Plans for possible HSCT should be in place because hematologic complications may develop rapidly. With progression of BMF it will become necessary to increase the frequency of hematologic monitoring, and it may have to be individualized. Androgens and hemopoietic growth factors may improve BMF; however, in many patients the response is only transient.[501] Growth factors usually, if at all, have only a transient effect and should not be used in combination with androgens because of the risk of peliosis and splenic rupture.[502] Unlike idiopathic aplastic anemia, immunosuppressive agents such as antithymocyte globulin and cyclosporine are ineffective in cases of DC and BMF.

The ultimate treatment of BMF is allogenic HSCT. However, historically HSCT for DC has been associated with high morbidity and mortality. Treatment toxicity is a major cause of premature mortality in patients with DC.[378,503-505] Reduced-intensity conditioning regimens without irradiation and bleomycin might improve the outcome of HSCT in patients with DC.[485,506-510]

Management of DC patients with MDS or AML (or both) is even less standardized. The significance of transient clonal cytogenetic abnormalities is unclear, but if persistent or complex, such abnormalities usually predict a poor prognosis. Early hematopoietic stem cell harvest for autologous transplantation at a later time before the development of BMF is investigational and, because of the limited repopulating ability of the affected stem cells, is unlikely to be successful.

Management of Pulmonary Disease

There is currently no treatment of pulmonary disease in DC. Patients with DC should refrain from smoking, avoid drugs with pulmonary toxicity (e.g., bleomycin), and have their lungs shielded from radiation during BMT or cancer treatment.[511] Pulmonary fibrosis in patients with DC does not respond to immunosuppressive therapy. Lung transplantation might be considered in individuals with otherwise mild manifestations of disease.[379,380]

Cancer Surveillance/Treatment

Patients with confirmed DC should avoid excessive exposure to ultraviolet light and use barrier sun creams. Avoidance of smoking and alcohol should be emphasized, particularly in patients with oral leukoplakia.[373,374] DC patients should also undergo regular dental/hygienist review to prevent early tooth loss. It is extremely important to screen for malignancies, especially of the gastrointestinal system. Management of malignancy may be complicated by a number of factors. The diagnosis may be delayed in some cases because of malignant change occurring within an area of persistent leukoplakia, thus resulting in a delay in treatment. There is also a high potential for local recurrence and multiple cancers in these patients. In addition, the presence of BMF makes chemotherapy very difficult and can limit the indications for surgery. The mucosa also has high sensitivity to radiation, which can lead to severe mucosal damage and may thus result in early termination of radiotherapy.

Management of oral malignancy usually includes a regular review and biopsy of the premalignant hyperkeratotic lesion and surgical laser excision of any suspicious areas. Neoadjuvant radiotherapy or surgical resection of confirmed malignancies, along with ipsilateral node clearance with or without adjuvant radiotherapy in accordance with staging of the disease, is the mainstay of treatment.

Gene Therapy

HSCT may cure hematologic disease in DC patients; unfortunately, however, HLA-matched sibling donor cells are available for only a minority of patients. Gene therapy to correct hematopoietic stem cells followed by autologous transplantation might therefore offer an attractive alternative for the treatment of hematologic disease in DC patients. Biased X-inactivation in female *DKC1* mutation carriers suggests that DC cells corrected by gene therapy are likely to have a selective growth/survival advantage. Indeed, gene transfer of *TERT* or *TERC* (or both) corrects the telomere defect in most DC cell lines.[409,512] However, as in many other IBMFSs, there is the problem that the few surviving hematopoietic stem cells might have already acquired secondary somatic and possibly oncogenic mutations and that correction by gene therapy would promote rather then prevent leukemogenesis in these patients.

Shwachman-Diamond Syndrome

SDS (MIM 260400) is a rare recessive multisystem disorder first described in the 1960s that is characterized by exocrine pancreatic insufficiency, bone marrow dysfunction, and skeletal abnormalities (Box 8-12).[513,514]

Box 8-12   Shwachman-Diamond Syndrome

Shwachman-Diamond syndrome (MIM 260400) is a rare recessively inherited bone marrow failure syndrome characterized by exocrine pancreatic insufficiency; bone marrow dysfunction, including increased risk for malignant transformation; and skeletal abnormalities.

Box 8-13   Clinical Diagnostic Criteria for Shwachman-Diamond Syndrome

EXOCRINE PANCREATIC INSUFFICIENCY*

Low serum trypsinogen (in children <3 years old)
Low serum isoamylase (in children >3 years old)
Elevated fecal excretion (72-hour collection) and imaging studies showing fatty infiltration of the pancreas; other causes of steatorrhea should be excluded, including intestinal mucosal disorders and cholestatic liver disease
Abnormal pancreatic stimulation (rarely done today)

HEMATOPOIETIC ABNORMALITIES*

Neutropenia (<1500/μL); can be intermittent or chronic but must be documented at multiple time points (at least three times over a period of more than 3 months)
Anemia: hemoglobin below that for the age-adjusted norm
Thrombocytopenia
Pancytopenia
Myelodysplastic syndrome documented on bone marrow examination
Both exocrine insufficiency and hematopoietic abnormalities must be documented

---

*One of the following

Clinical Manifestations

SDS is an IBMFS with an estimated incidence of 1 per 75,000 live births.[515] It is more commonly diagnosed in boys, with a male-to-female ratio of 1.7:1.[516] The major clinical features associated with SDS have been defined in several large cohort studies and are summarized in Table 8-8.[516-521] It should be noted that with one exception, genetic testing for *SBDS* (Shwachman-Bodian-Diamond syndrome) mutations was not available at the time that these studies were reported. Interestingly, in the study in which the *SBDS* genotype was determined, the phenotype of patients with *SBDS* mutations was similar to that of those who had normal *SBDS* alleles.[521] Nonetheless, it is possible that classifying patients according to *SBDS* mutations may eventually refine the spectrum of clinical features (Box 8-13).

Hematologic Abnormalities

Neutropenia is present in the majority of patients with SDS (range, 77% to 100%); severe neutropenia (as

TABLE 8-8   Major Clinical Features of Shwachman-Diamond Syndrome

Clinical Feature	Aggett et al.,[517] 1980	Mack et al.,[518] 1996*	Smith et al.,[519] 1996	Ginzberg et al.,[516] 1999	Cipolli et al.,[520] 1999	Kuijpers et al.,[521] 2005[†]	Total/ Average
Number of subjects	21	25	21	88	13	23	191
Hematologic[‡]							
Neutropenia	95%	88%	100%	98%	77%	78%	93%
Severe neutropenia (≤500/µL)	67%	60%	33%	—	23%	48%	61%
Anemia	50%	52%	66%	42%	46%	17%	44%
Thrombocytopenia	70%	60%	24%	34%	23%	56%	42%
Pancytopenia	—	44%	10%	19%	23%	13%	21%
Gastrointestinal							
Exocrine pancreatic insufficiency[‡]	100%	100%	100%	100%	100%	100%	100%
Liver (elevated transaminases)	—	56%	—	60%	100%	69%	64%
Skeletal abnormalities	100%	76%	100%	49%	100%	65%	69%
Metaphyseal dysostosis	62%	44%	100%	46%	54%	—	55%
Rib cage abnormalities	52%	32%	—	32%	92%	—	40%
Short stature (<3rd percentile)	95%	67%	—	56%	85%	52%	64%

*Short stature was defined as height below the 5th percentile.
[†]Fifteen of these patients had *SBDS* (Shwachman-Bodian-Diamond syndrome) gene mutations; severe neutropenia is a count less than 600/mL.
[‡]Hematologic abnormalities and exocrine pancreatic insufficiency are defining features of Shwachman-Diamond syndrome, hence the 100% incidence of these findings.

defined by an absolute neutrophil count [ANC] of less than 500/µL) was observed in a mean of 61% of patients (range, 23% to 67%; see Table 8-8). Neutropenia is intermittent in about two thirds of patients and chronic in the remaining third. Although defects in neutrophil chemotaxis are present in most patients with SDS,[522] the clinical significance of this finding is unclear because neutrophils are recruited to sites of infection.[523] Anemia, typically normochromic and normocytic, is present in approximately 50% of cases and is usually associated with a low reticulocyte count.[520] Thrombocytopenia is seen in approximately 50% of cases, sometimes without concomitant neutropenia. Pancytopenia has been reported in 10% to 44% of patients. The presence of or progression to severe aplastic anemia has been reported.[524,525] Defects in B- or T-lymphocyte function (or both) have been described, including impaired specific immunoglobulin response and altered CD4[+] or CD8[+] T-cell subsets.[526] Bone marrow findings are variable and nondiagnostic. Bone marrow cellularity ranges from hypocellular to hypercellular; myelodysplasia and left-shifted granulopoiesis are common.[519] An intrinsic cell defect in hematopoietic progenitors and impaired bone marrow stromal cell function have been reported.[527]

Transformation to Myelodysplastic Syndrome and Acute Myeloid Leukemia

Similar to other congenital BMF syndromes, there is a strong predilection for the development of MDS or MDS/AML in patients with SDS.[528,529] Acquired clonal cytogenetic abnormalities are seen frequently; in a prospective study of 14 patients with SDS monitored for a maximum of 5 years via annual bone marrow evaluation, clonal cytogenetic abnormalities were detected in 29%.[530]

Abnormalities in chromosome 7 are the most common and include monosomy 7, isochromosome 7q, and deletion of 7q. The clinical significance of these cytogenetic abnormalities is uncertain. In particular, isochromosome 7q appears to have a benign course with a low risk of transformation to MDS or MDS/AML[531,532] Transformation to overt MDS or MDS/AML has been reported in 13% to 33% of cases.[519,533] There is a striking male preponderance; in a recent review, 92% of reported cases of MDS or MDS/AML in SDS occurred in males.[529] The malignant clone often displays complex cytogenetic abnormalities frequently involving chromosome 7.

Gastrointestinal Abnormalities

After cystic fibrosis, SDS is the most common cause of congenital exocrine pancreatic insufficiency. Patients are classically seen in early infancy with steatorrhea and failure to thrive. Pathologic analysis shows extensive fatty replacement of pancreatic acini with relative preservation of pancreatic ducts and islets. Exocrine pancreas insufficiency can be assessed by measurement of serum trypsinogen or isoamylase, pancreatic stimulation tests, or fecal fat quantification.[534,535] In addition, imaging of the pancreas may reveal characteristic fatty infiltration (Fig. 8-15).[536-538] For unclear reasons, the pancreatic insufficiency improves with increasing age in most patients. Mild (twofold to threefold) elevation of liver transaminases is often seen in patients younger than 2 years. It is usually of little clinical significance and tends to improve with age.[518]

Skeletal Abnormalities

Most patients with SDS have bony abnormalities, with rib cage abnormalities, metaphyseal dysostosis, and osteopenia being the most common findings (see Table

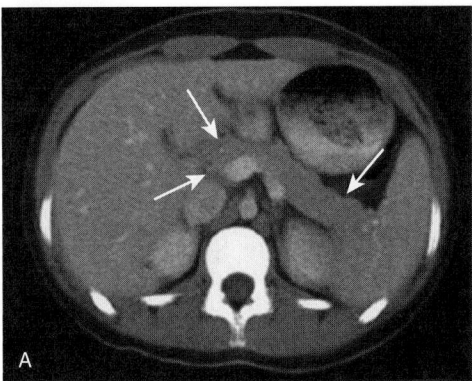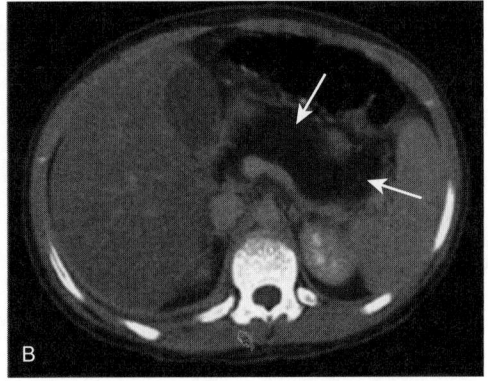

FIGURE 8-15. Fatty infiltration of the pancreas in Shwachman-Diamond syndrome (SDS) shown by transverse computed tomography images of a normal individual (**A**) and patient with SDS (**B**). The density of the normal pancreas (*arrows*) is similar to that of liver. In contrast, the density of the SDS pancreas (*arrows*) is reduced, consistent with fatty infiltration. (*Reproduced with kind permission of Springer Science and Business Media. From Nijs E, Callahan MJ, Taylor GA. Disorders of the pediatric pancreas: imaging features. Pediatr Radiol. 2005;35:358-373.*)

8-8).[539] Growth retardation is also common in SDS patients, but it is not thought to be secondary to malnutrition. More than half of patients with SDS are below the 3rd percentile for height at 1 year. With adequate pancreatic enzyme replacement, most patients show normal growth velocity but remain below or at the 3rd percentile for height.[516]

Miscellaneous Abnormalities

Many patients with SDS suffer from pyschomotor delay[516-518,540] or dental abnormalities.[541,542] There are reports of other endocrine abnormalities such as diabetes mellitus,[517,518] growth hormone deficiency,[543] renal tubular acidosis,[516] cleft palate,[516] and cardiomyopathy.[544]

Differential Diagnosis

Diagnostic criteria for SDS are outlined in Box 8-12[545]; both exocrine pancreatic insufficiency and hematopoietic abnormality must be documented. Other features of SDS, including short stature or skeletal or hepatic abnormalities, though supportive, are not required for the diagnosis. Genetic testing for *SBDS* mutations is merited since their presence confirms the diagnosis of SDS. However, their lack does not exclude the diagnosis because in approximately 10% of cases of clinically defined SDS, no mutations in *SBDS* are present.[546-548] Other causes of exocrine pancreatic insufficiency should be considered, including cystic fibrosis, which can be excluded by performing a sweat test. Pearson's disease is characterized by exocrine pancreatic insufficiency, sideroblastic anemia, vacuolization of hematopoietic cells in bone marrow, and metabolic acidosis.[549,550] It is caused by deletions in mitochondrial DNA (mtDNA).[551] Cartilage-hair hypoplasia (CHH) syndrome is characterized by short stature, metaphyseal dysostosis, cytopenias, and hypoplastic hair.[552] It is secondary to mutations in the RNase mitochondrial RNA processing (*RMRP*) gene encoding the RNA subunit of the RMRP complex.[553]

Genetics

SDS is an autosomal recessive disorder.[554] The gene responsible for SDS was identified by genetic linkage analysis.[547] Boocock and colleagues reported that compound heterozygous mutations of the *SBDS* gene located on chromosome 7 were present in the majority of patients with SDS.[547] Most of these mutations resulted from gene conversion with a neighboring pseudogene (*SBDSP*). Subsequent studies have confirmed that *SBDS* mutations are present in approximately 90% of clinically diagnosed cases of SDS.[547,549,555,556] The majority of mutations occur within exon 2 and are predicted to result in the production of a truncated protein. The remaining mutations are missense and nonsense mutations scattered throughout the protein. Most of the mutations result in a dramatic reduction in SBDS protein production.[547,549] However, patients carrying homozygous null alleles for *SBDS* have not been reported, which suggests that SBDS is essential for life. Consistent with this conclusion, mice lacking the murine orthologue of SBDS are subject to early embryonic lethality.[557] Interestingly, in the subset of patients who do not have *SBDS* mutations, SBDS protein expression in leukocytes is normal, thus indicating that other genetic mutations may be responsible for these cases of SDS.[548,549l]

Recent studies suggest that there may be a spectrum of disease associated with *SBDS* mutations. Nishimura and colleagues reported that two unrelated patients with neonatal spondylometaphyseal dysplasia (SMD) carried compound heterozygous mutations of *SBDS*.[558] Clinical features included severe metaphysial dysplasia, platyspondyly, and neonatal respiratory failure, similar to the Sedaghantian type of SMD.

There is also evidence that halploinsufficiency for *SBDS* may predispose to the development of aplastic anemia. Calado and colleagues reported that 4 of 91 patients with apparently acquired aplastic anemia had heterozygous mutations of *SBDS*.[559] Affected patients had no evidence of exocrine pancreatic insufficiency or bony abnormalities but did have short stature. The significance of this finding is unclear because the number of individuals studied is far too small to predict a statistically significant association between heterozygosity for an *SBDS* mutation and the development of aplastic anemia.

The *SBDS* gene encodes a 250–amino acid protein that is highly conserved throughout evolution but lacks any recognizable functional domain. Although there is evidence that SBDS interacts with the actin cytoskeleton,[560] the primary function of SBDS appears to be regulation of ribosome biogenesis. SBDS protein prominently localizes to the nucleolus of cells in a cell cycle–dependent fashion.[546] SBDS coprecipitates with the 28S ribosomal subunit and associates with nucleophosmin, a protein implicated in ribosome biogenesis and leukemogenesis.[561] In yeast, loss of the *SBDS* orthologue *Sdo1* leads to impaired ribosomal biogenesis.[562] Specifically, Sdo1 appears to facilitate release of Tif6 from the pre-60S ribosomal subunit, which allows final ribosome assembly and activation of translation. Together, these observations place SDS in a growing list of bone marrow disorders caused by impaired ribosome biogenesis.

The mechanism for the increased susceptibility to MDS and MDS/AML in patients with SDS is unclear. Rawls and colleagues showed that inhibition of Sbds expression by RNAi in murine hematopoietic progenitors leads to loss of engraftment potential, thus suggesting that hematopoietic stem cell function in SDS may be impaired.[563] The fact that clonal cytogenetic abnormalities are common in SDS suggests genomic instability within hematopoietic progenitors. There is a single report of short telomeres in the leukocytes of patients with SDS; however, the relevance of this finding to chromosomal instability is unclear.[564] Recent data suggest that SBDS protein localizes to the mitotic spindle and stabilizes microtubules in vitro. Depletion of SBDS leads to mitotic abnormalities and aneuploidy, thus implying that defective spindle stability contributes to the mechanisms of BMF and leukemogenesis in patients with SDS.[565]

Clinical Management

Treatment of SDS includes pancreatic enzyme replacement and administration of fat-soluble vitamins for pancreatic insufficiency. Regular assessment of exocrine pancreatic function is recommended because in approximately 50% of patients, steatorrhea resolves spontaneously with increasing age.[518]

Regular blood counts should be performed every 4 months to monitor for cytopenia. In addition, annual bone marrow examination has been recommended to assess for clonal cytogenetic abnormalities.[545] For patients with severe neutropenia or neutropenia and persistent or recurrent infections, a trial of G-CSF treatment is warranted; response rates are generally high.[534] Similar to severe congenital neutropenia (SCN), current recommendations are that the dose of G-CSF be titrated to

achieve and maintain an ANC of 1000 to 1500/μL.[566] As discussed in the later section on SCN, no clear association of G-CSF with malignant transformation has been demonstrated to date. Nonetheless, patients with SDS should receive the lowest dose of G-CSF required to maintain an acceptable neutrophil count.

Allogeneic HSCT is the only curative therapy for SDS. It is generally reserved for patients with BMF or those who have transformed to AML/MDS. The majority of patients reported received a myeloablative conditioning regimen before HSCT consisting of cyclophosphamide, in combination with either busulfan or TBI, and unrelated bone marrow as a source of stem cells. HSCT in patients with SDS is associated with increased regimen-related toxicity, particularly of the heart and lung. The pathobiology of this increased toxicity is not understood. Data from the French Neutropenia Registry reported a 5-year event-free survival rate of 60% in 10 patients with SDS after HSCT.[567] Similarly, the European Group for Blood and Bone Marrow Transplantation reported a 64.5% overall survival rate with a median follow-up of 1.1 years in 25 patients with SDS after allogeneic HSCT.[568] From these studies it is clear that patients who undergo transplantation for BMF do much better than those receiving a transplant for MDS or AML. Combining these studies, the overall survival rate in patients after HSCT for BMF was 86% (18 of 21) versus 36% (5 of 14) in those after HSCT for MDS/AML. Insufficient follow-up data are available to assess the outcome of nonmyeloablative conditioning regimens in SDS patients with bone marrow aplasia.

Cartilage-Hair Hypoplasia

CHH (MIM 250250), also known as metaphyseal chondroplasia, McKusick type, is an autosomal recessive chondrodysplasia.[569]

Clinical Manifestations

CHH is characterized by metaphyseal dysostosis, short-limbed dwarfism, and fine, sparse hair that lacks the central pigment core. Clinical manifestations are highly heterogeneous and vary between and within families. Other skeletal findings include chest deformity, varus lower limbs, lordosis, and scoliosis. Gastrointestinal problems include aganglionic megacolon (Hirschsprung's disease) and other physical anomalies. The disease is more frequent in the Amish and Finnish populations because of a founder effect, with a carrier frequency of 1 in 19 among the Amish and 1 in 76 among the Finns. Mild to severe macrocytic anemia and lymphopenia are present in the majority of patients, whereas neutropenia is seen in only about a fourth. In the majority of individuals the anemia is mild and resolves spontaneously during early childhood. In more severe cases, the anemia resembles that seen in DBA or may be accompanied by severe immunodeficiency. The severity of the anemia inversely correlates with height. Similar severe immunodeficiency is associated with more severe and persistent anemia. The frequency of lymphoid malignancies and basal cell carcinoma is increased about sevenfold.[570]

Differential Diagnosis

Excluding DBA from the differential diagnosis might be difficult in some cases. Thrombocytosis, increased erythropoietin levels, and increased levels of red cell adenosine deaminase (ADA), characteristic of DBA (see later), may be present in some patients with CHH. Metaphyseal dysplasia has not been reported in patients with DBA. Mutation analysis may be necessary to consolidate the diagnosis.

Genetics

CHH is an autosomal recessive disease. Genetic mapping and DNA sequencing identified the gene encoding the RNA component of *RMRP*, a 265-nucleotide noncoding RNA gene on 9p21-p12.[553] Mutations responsible for CHH are predominantly found in the transcribed and promoter region of the *RMRP* gene (reviewed by Martin and Li[571]). The most frequently found mutation is the A70G transversion, which is the major mutation in Finnish and Amish CHH patients. Other mutations include insertional mutations and duplications between the TATA box and the transcription start site that silence transcription. No patient homozygous or compound heterozygous for the promoter region duplications/insertions have been identified, thus suggesting that these mutations may be lethal. *RMRP* mutations have also been found in a variety of other forms of inherited metaphyseal dysplasia that share features with CHH, including metaphyseal dysplasia without hypotrichosis (MIM 250460), anauxetic dysplasia (MIM 607095), kyphomelic dysplasia (MIM 211350), and Omenn's syndrome (MIM 6035554).[572]

Gene Function

MRPR is the RNA component of the RNP complex RMRP that is involved in several cellular processes, including mtDNA replication,[573] ribosome biogenesis and pre-rRNA processing,[574] and mRNA degradation of cyclin B2 (*CLB2*), thereby regulating cell cycle progression.[575] Which of these pathways is responsible for BMF is unclear; however, differences and similarities to other ribosomal diseases suggest that the defects in ribosome biogenesis might be responsible for the anemia and that degradation of CLB2 contributes to the increased development of lymphoid tumors.[576] Genotype-phenotype correlation studies suggest a strong correlation between the decrease in rRNA cleavage in ribosomal assembly and the degree of bone dysplasia, whereas reduced mRNA cleavage and cell cycle impairment correlate with the presence of hair hypoplasia, immunodeficiency, hematologic abnormalities, and increased cancer risk.[572]

Clinical Management

Severe anemia requiring transfusion is seen rarely in CHH (6%) and often has a poor prognosis. Relapses may occur after recovery. Transfusions and glucocorticoid may improve the anemia. However, possible benefits of the treatment should be carefully weighed against the potential side effects in a condition associated with immune deficiency and short stature. Although many of the patients tended to outgrow their BMF, in some cases the anemia may be severe and persist, as in patients with DBA.[570] In patients with severe combined immunodeficiency, HSCT with or without myeloablation has been shown to provide long-term immune reconstitution.[577]

Pearson's Syndrome

Pearson's marrow-pancreas syndrome (PS, MIM 557000) is a refractory sideroblastic anemia characterized by vacuolization of bone marrow precursors as a result of deletion of mtDNA (Figs. 8-16 and 8-17). Pancreatic dysfunction is frequent but not mandatory for the diagnosis of PS.

Clinical Manifestations

PS is a multisystem disorder that usually becomes evident in early infancy.[549,578,579] Pancytopenia is frequently asso-

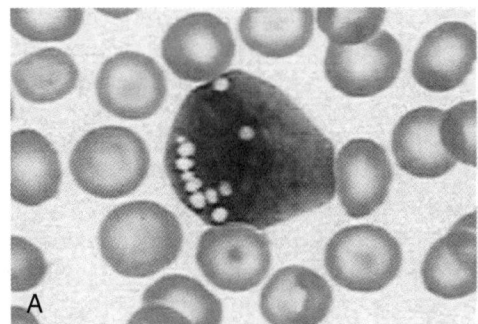
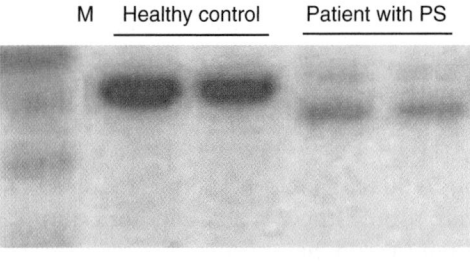

FIGURE 8-16. Characteristics in Pearson's syndrome (PS). **A,** Myeloid bone marrow precursor cell exhibiting prominent cytoplasmatic vacuolization. **B,** Southern blot analysis of the mitochondrial DNA of a patient with PS and a healthy control. The 16.6-kb wild-type mtDNA of the healthy control (lanes 2 and 3) is shown in comparison to the mtDNA of the patient carrying the 4503-bp deletion (lanes 4 and 5) in approximately 70% of the mtDNA molecules as quantified densitometrically. *(From Giese A, Kirschner-Schwabe R, Blumchen K, et al. Prenatal manifestation of pancytopenia in Pearson marrow-pancreas syndrome caused by a mitochondrial DNA deletion. Am J Med Genet A. 2007;143:285-288.)*

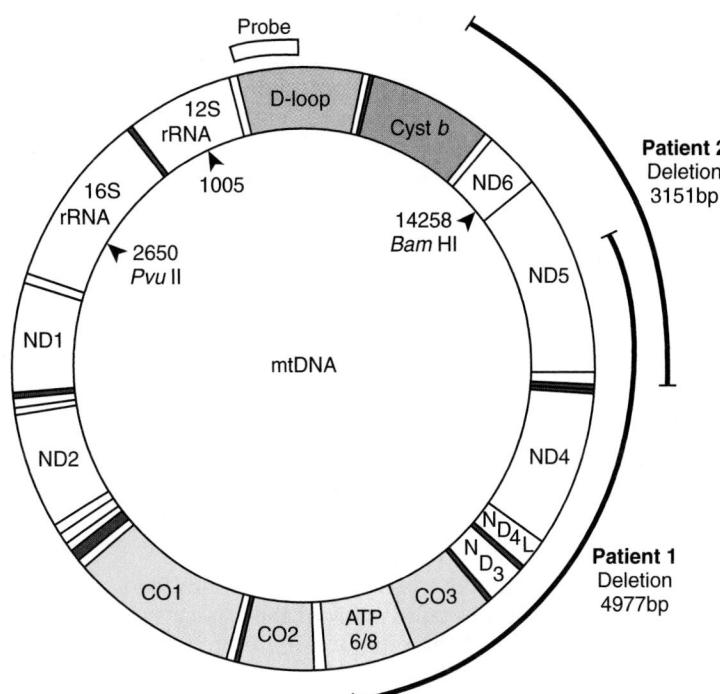

FIGURE 8-17. Example of the type of deletion found in Pearson's syndrome as shown in a schematic diagram of mitochondrial DNA. *(Redrawn from Sano T, Ban K, Ichiki T, et al. Molecular and genetic analyses of two patients with Pearson syndrome. Pediatr Res. 1993;34:105-110.)*

ciated with dysfunction of the exocrine pancreas, hepatic failure, and renal tubulopathy, which may lead to lactic acidosis. Vacuolization of hematopoietic precursor cells is characteristic (see Fig. 8-16). Most PS patients die before the age of 3 years. The major cause of death is metabolic acidosis, followed by liver and renal failure.[580,581] The few surviving children showed hematologic improvement, but typical features of Kearns-Sayre syndrome (MIM 530000) eventually developed.[582,583]

The male-to-female ratio of PS is 0.7:1. Patients from all racial and most ethnic groups have been reported.

Physical anomalies in patients with PS are rare. Approximately a third of patients have exocrine pancreatic insufficiency, and insulin-dependent diabetes develops frequently.

Anemia (usually macrocytic) is present in the majority of patients in whom PS is diagnosed before the age 6 months. Half of the patients have neutropenia and thrombocytopenia. Vacuolated myeloid or erythroid precursors, often with decreased erythroblasts, and ringed sideroblasts are present in almost all patients (see Fig. 8-16).

Differential Diagnosis

Vaculolization of the hematopoietic precursor, fibrosis of the pancreas rather than fatty replacement, and the lack of skeletal anomalies distinguishes PS from SDS. PS has to be differentiated from other refractory anemias in children. Mitochondrial enzyme defects and mtDNA deletions usually establish the diagnosis.

Genetics

PS is maternally inherited and follows a mitochondrial inheritance pattern (Box 8-14). PS is caused by deletions

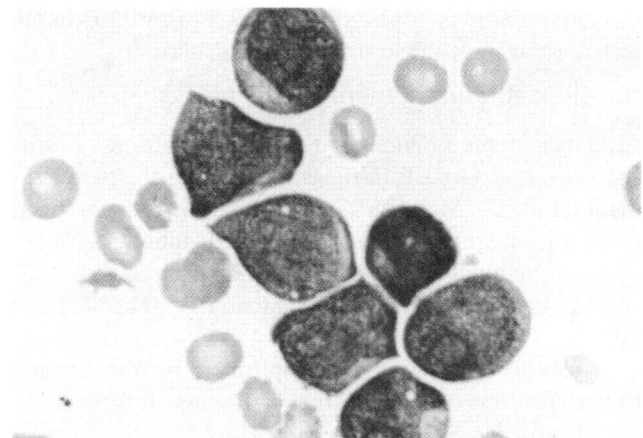

FIGURE 8-18. Blood smear of a child with Down syndrome and transient myeloproliferative disorder. The nucleated cells are megakaryoblasts with small amounts of basophilic cytoplasm, distinct nucleoli, and cytoplasmic blebbing (May-Grünwald-Giemsa stain). *(From Massey GV, Zipursky A, Chang MN, et al. A prospective study of the natural history of transient leukemia [TL] in neonates with Down syndrome [DS]: Children's Oncology Group [COG] study POG-9481. Blood. 2006;107:4606-4613.)*

or duplications of mtDNA (see Fig. 8-17).[550,551] The size of the deletion varies from 2.7 to 7.767 kb[584] (also see Fig. 8-18). The respiratory enzymes involved in the deletions are relevant to oxidative phosphorylation, and alterations include reduced nicotinamide adenine dinucleotide, cytochrome oxidase, adenosine triphosphatase, and tRNA and rRNA.

The severity of the clinical manifestation and the rate of disease progression are variable and correlate with the

Box 8-14	Mitochondrial DNA Disorders

Mitochondria are under genetic control of the mitochondrial and nuclear genomes. Defects in either genome result in mitochondrial disorders. The mitochondrial genome is 16.6 kb in size and encodes 13 enzymes of the respiratory chain, as well as 24 RNA molecules needed for intramitochondrial protein synthesis. Within a cell the mitochondrial genome is present in multiple copies. In healthy individuals, all copies are identical (homoplasmy), whereas in patients with genetic defects of the mitochondrial genome, a mutation can be present in all copies (homoplasmic mutation) or only in some copies (heteroplasmic mutation).

Mitochondrial DNA (mtDNA) is usually maternally inherited. For heteroplasmic disorders such as Pearson's syndrome, the outcome of a specific pregnancy is difficult to predict, mainly because of considerable variation in the mutated DNA inherited by the offspring and because many of the clinical features correlate with the ratio of mutated to wild-type mtDNA.[579,586,587]

Box 8-15	Transient Myeloproliferative Disorder

Transient myeloproliferative disorder (TMD) in newborns with Down syndrome is a clonal proliferation of blast cells with trisomy 21 that have acquired a somatic mutation in the GATA1 gene and are thought to originate from fetal liver hematopoiesis. Both the trisomy 21 and the GATA1 mutation are required for proliferation. Spontaneous remission is common; however, in some cases TMD may be fatal. Acute megakaryoblastic leukemia with leukemic cells carrying the identical GATA1 mutation develops in about 20% of patients with TMD[592] (see also Fig. 7-18).[593]

ratio of mutated to wild-type mtDNA and with the tissue distribution of mutated mtDNA molecules.[585]

Clinical Management

Anemia is treated mainly by red cell transfusions. Erythropoietin and G-CSF have also been used for the treatment of BMF. Malignant transformation has not been reported. The major cause of death is metabolic acidosis, followed by renal and liver failure. The projected median survival time is 4 years, with a plateau rate of 36% at age 10.

Genetic counseling is complicated by the unique genetic features of mtDNA that distinguish it from mendelian disorders, including maternal inheritance, heteroplasmy, the threshold effect, the mitochondrial bottleneck, tissue variation, and selection (Box 8-14).[586-588]

Down Syndrome

Hematologic abnormalities are frequent in Down syndrome (DS). Abnormalities can be seen in any of the three blood cell lineages[589] and in some cases may be associated with other medical conditions frequently found in individuals with DS, such as polycythemia in DS patients with cyanotic heart failure. Neutrophilia, thrombocytopenia, and polycythemia were the most common hematologic abnormalities observed in neonates with DS.[589,590] Increased erythrocyte MCV is frequently present in DS infants, even in the absence of heart disease, and may persist throughout life.[591]

Transient myeloproliferative disorder (TMD) occurs in 10% to 25% of newborns with DS and in phenotypically normal newborns mosaic for trisomy 21 (Fig. 8-18 and Box 8-15).[593-596] TMD is associated with a high inci-

dence of spontaneous remission. Usually, TMD does not cause obvious symptoms and is only an incidental finding of abnormal blood counts and circulating blasts in peripheral blood expressing a megakaryocytic or erythroid phenotype. However, in about 20% of cases the disease may be severe and be manifested as hydrops fetalis or infiltration of the liver or other organs and result in multiorgan failure and death.[597]

TMD is considered a preleukemic condition because in 20% to 30% of patients with TMD, acute megakaryoblastic leukemia (AMKL) will develop within 3 years of TMD. Recently, it has been shown that blast cells in TMD carry unique mutations in the hematopoietic transcription factor GATA-1[598,599] and that the identical mutation can be found in AMKL blasts, thus indicating that AMKL evolves from TMD.[600-603] The mutations occur in exon 2 of the GATA1 gene and lead to the production of a variant GATA-1 protein truncated at its amino-terminal. Experiments in mice showed that expression of the truncated GATA-1 protein leads to hyperproliferation of yolk sac and fetal liver progenitor cells with erythroid/megakaryocytic characteristics, thus indicating that TMD and AMKL originate from a hematopoietic progenitor cell of embryonic/fetal hematopoiesis rather than from mature hematopoiesis in bone marrow, a finding that explains the onset in early childhood and the transient nature of TMD.[604] Interestingly, a similar inherited GATA1 mutation in a family with X-linked anemia and trilineage dysplasia did not show a predisposition to AMKL, which indicates that in humans the GATA1 mutation leads to TMD and AMKL only in those with a genetic background of trisomy 21.[605] The nature of the interaction between the GATA1 mutation and trisomy 21 that leads to clonal expansion of the mutant progenitor remains to be determined (for review see Vyas and Crispino[592] and Kirsammer and colleagues[606]).

AMKL usually has a good prognosis in patients with DS when treated appropriately with regimens that include cytarabine (cytosine arabinoside).[607-611] Increased expression of the chromosome 21–localized genes for cystathionine β-synthase and superoxide dismutase and altered drug metabolism have been implicated in the increased sensitivity of TMD and AMKL blasts to cytarabine.[612] The high frequency of TMD and AMKL in patients with DS and the favorable prognosis of the disease when treated appropriately suggest that all newborns and infants with DS should be routinely screened for signs of TMD and that children with a history of TMD require close surveillance for the development of AMKL.

The insight gained into the pathogenesis of TMD and AMKL in DS patients is thus another notable example of how increased understanding of the pathogenesis of disease development directly influences the care and management of patients.

Familial Marrow Dysfunction

A large group of patients with BMF do not fit any of the classifications described. If more than one family member is affected, in the absence of environmental exposure explaining BMF, these individuals are classified as having familial BMF, not otherwise classified.

Familial BMF or bone marrow dysfunction therefore represents a heterogeneous group of individuals and families. In many, BMF is found in various family members and may include aplastic anemia, MDS, leukemia, and immunodeficiency. The inheritance pattern may suggest dominant, recessive, or X-linked disease. In others, the condition may be manifested as sporadic BMF but with associated physical anomalies suggesting an IBMFS not characteristic of FA or any other known IBMFS.

Pathogenesis of Disease

It is most likely that a significant number of individuals or families in whom familial BMF is diagnosed have disease caused by one of the major IBMFSs discussed earlier. However, because of variable disease penetrance and expressivity, a possible atypical manifestation, failure to identify the pathogenic mutation, and unawareness of the responsible physician, the correct diagnosis has not been made. For example, BMF secondary to *TERC* or *TERT* gene mutations is certainly underdiagnosed because affected individuals often lack the classic mucocutaneous features characteristic of classic DC (see earlier). In others, a syndrome specific for particular clinical findings might have been diagnosed, but association with one of the major forms of BMF has not yet been made. Examples from the past are the VATERL syndrome in individuals with vertebral defects, anal atresia, tracheoesophageal fistula, renal defects, and radial limb defects, some of whom turned out to have FA (see the section on FA); HHS, which turned out to be a severe form of DC (see the section on DC); or the Kearns-Sayre syndrome, which includes patients with PS who outgrew their BMF (see the section on PS). A small proportion of patients might have an IBMFS resulting from causes that are exceedingly rare and therefore have been missed (see also Table 8-1), or the BMF may be due to a mutation in a gene that is not usually associated with BMF.

An example from the past is specific mutations in the *NBS1* gene, usually responsible for the Nijmegen breakage syndrome, that may be manifested as an FA-like phenotype, including pancytopenia and a positive DEB or MMC test (also see the section on FA). Finally, a proportion of individuals with familial BMF have disease caused by mutations in genes that have not yet been identified.

Clinical Management

The overall prognosis in patients with familial BMF is generally less favorable than that in patients with nonfamilial (acquired) BMF. A DEB or MMC test to rule out FA (see the section on FA) and telomere measurements to rule out DC (see the section on DC) are the minimal diagnostic evaluations that should be performed early in the investigation of individuals with familial BMF. Treatment and supportive care, in general, are the same as those described earlier for FA, DC, or acquired aplastic anemia. Antilymphocyte globulin, cyclosporine, androgens, and hematopoietic growth factors have been used with variable success. HSCT from an HLA-matched sibling donor has to be considered carefully because the potential donor may have the same genetic lesion even in the absence of disease. Failure of engraftment or donor cell–derived malignancies (MDS/AML) have been reported in individuals with familial BMF receiving a transplant from an apparently healthy sibling donor.[474,613] In addition, HSCT may be associated with an unexpected toxicity in patients with familial BMF because the underlying genetic defect may render them hypersensitive to radiotherapy or other agents used for HSCT.

INHERITED BONE MARROW FAILURE SYNDROMES ASSOCIATED WITH ISOLATED CYTOPENIAS

Diamond-Blackfan Anemia

DBA (MIM 105650), also known as congenital erythroid hypoplastic anemia, is a rare inherited hypoplastic anemia that usually occurs in early infancy. The disease is named after Louis K. Diamond and Kenneth D. Blackfan, two pediatric hematologists in Boston who first recognized the disease as a distinct clinical entity.[614] DBA is genetically and phenotypically heterogeneous.

Clinical Manifestations

Clinically, DBA is characterized by failure of red cell production, variable congenital anomalies, and a predisposition to malignancy (Box 8-16). DBA is a rare disease with a frequency of 2 to 7 per million live births and has no ethnic or gender predilection.[615,616] Much of our knowledge of the disease has been gained from patient registries in North America,[617] England,[616] Italy,[618] and France.[619] Classically, patients with DBA are seen in early childhood with profound macrocytic or normocytic anemia, reticulocytopenia, and a reduction or absence of erythroid precursors in bone marrow. In more than 90% of patients with DBA the diagnosis is made before the age of 1 year,[617,620,621] but in rare cases severe anemia may develop in utero (nonimmune hydrops fetalis)[622] or later in life.[623] The median age at diagnosis is 8 weeks of age.[620]

Congenital Abnormalities

In about 50% of patients DBA is associated with physical anomalies and growth retardation.[619,620,623,624] In some patients a physical anomaly is the only clinical manifestation of DBA. Table 8-9 summarizes the prevalence

and range of congenital abnormalities found in patients with DBA. Midline craniofacial defects (e.g., cleft palate), renal anomalies, cardiac malformations, and thumb anomalies (e.g., triphalangeal thumbs) are common.[616,620]

Short Stature. Although short stature is an integral feature of DBA and is frequently seen in association with other congenital anomalies,[626] final height is strongly influenced by glucocorticoid therapy, iron overload, and chronic anemia.[616,626] Intrauterine growth retardation has been documented in about 20%,[626] and characteristically there is an absence of catch-up growth after birth.[626]

Hematologic Abnormalities

Anemia, macrocytosis, reticulocytopenia, and absent or decreased numbers of erythroid progenitor cells in bone marrow are the major diagnostic criteria for DBA. In 13% to 20% of individuals, anemia may be present at birth.[616,618] Macrocytosis is evident in the majority of cases; however, it may be masked by iron deficiency or thalassemia trait. Increased hemoglobin F levels and persistent "i" antigen are additional features of stress hematopoiesis frequently seen in patients with DBA.[616] Elevated levels of red cell adenosine deaminase (ADA), a critical enzyme in the purine salvage pathway, are

---

Box 8-16	Diamond-Blackfan Anemia

Diamond-Blackfan anemia (DBA) is a pure red cell aplasia with autosomal dominant inheritance that is usually seen in early infancy. DBA is associated with a reduction or absence of erythroid precursors in bone marrow, variable congenital anomalies, and a predisposition to malignancy. DBA red cells characteristically have increased adenosine deaminase activity. Mutations in ribosomal proteins of the small and large subunit have been associated with DBA.

TABLE 8-9   Congenital Abnormalities in Diamond-Blackfan Anemia

Anomaly	Range of Congenital Anomalies[625]	FREQUENCY (%)			
		Lipton et al.,[620] 2006	Willig et al.,[619] 1999	Ball et al.,[616] 1996	Ramenghi et al.,[618] 1999
No. of patients		420	229	65	88
Head, face, palate	Hypertelorism, cleft palate, high-arched palate, microcephaly, micrognathia, microtia, low-set ears, low hairline, epicanthus, ptosis, flat broad nasal bridge	24	21	36	—
Upper limb	Triphalangeal, duplex or bifid, hypoplastic thumb; flat thenar eminence; syndactyly; absent radial artery	21	9	18	—
Renal, urogenital	Absent kidney, horseshoe kidney, hypospadias	19*	7	NA	—
Cardiopulmonary	Ventricular septal defect, atrial septal defect, coarctation of the aorta, complex cardiac anomalies	15*	7	NA	—
Other					
Eyes	Congenital glaucoma, strabismus, congenital cataract	NA	12	NA	—
Neck	Short neck, webbed neck	NA	4	NA	—
Neuromotor	Learning difficulties	NA	7	NA	—
Short stature		NA	30	33	NA
At least one anomaly†		47	41	37	32
Two or more anomalies		25	24	NA	NA
Short stature alone		NA	NA	11	16

*As found by routine cardial and renal imaging.
†Not including low birth weight or short stature. Many patients had more than one abnormality.

characteristic of DBA erythropoiesis and may be found in 80% to 89% of patients.[619,620,627] Whether macrocytosis, increased fetal hemoglobin, and elevated red cell ADA are integral features of DBA hematopoiesis or rather reflections of stress hematopoiesis is not clear. Macrocytosis, increased fetal hemoglobin, persistent "i" antigen, and elevated red cell ADA may be masked in transfusion-dependent patients. In some individuals, macrocytosis or increased red cell ADA levels are the only manifestations of DBA.[616,628] Parents or siblings of an affected child who have increased red cell ADA levels are likely to be carriers of the pathogenic mutation even in the absence of classic disease (nonclassic DBA).[616,619] In some individuals with DBA the anemia is transient; however, the macrocytosis and elevated red cell ADA levels often persist. Spontaneous remission of anemia in DBA patients has been reported even after years of steroid or transfusion dependence (also see later).[617] Platelet counts are usually normal or mildly increased, although platelet counts greater than $1 \times 10^6/\mu L$ and decreased platelet counts have also been reported.[616] White blood cell counts are generally normal but in some cases decrease with age. In rare cases DBA progresses to the full clinical picture of severe aplastic anemia.[620]

Bone marrow examination reveals normal cellularity, myeloid cells, and megakaryocytes. Lymphocyte counts are often increased. A paucity of erythroid progenitor cells is characteristic. Dyserythropoietic morphology, even ringed sideroblasts, have been reported. Increased iron deposition is seen in patients who have received multiple red cell transfusions. Serum levels of erythropoietin are elevated, and ferrokinetic studies show a delay in plasma iron clearance and low red cell utilization. The slightly shortened autologous red cell survival times and low haptoglobin levels suggest mild hemolysis.[629]

Bone marrow progenitor assays show a severe maturation defect in DBA erythroid progenitor cells, whereas other blood cell lineages are unaffected or only moderately impaired.[6302-633] Erythroid colony size and maturation, as well as colony numbers, are impaired. The defect is intrinsic to the erythroid progenitor cell[631,634,635] and is partially corrected by interleuklin-3 (IL-3) and stem cell factor,[636-639] but not by erythropoietin.[631,632] The rate of apoptosis in erythroid progenitor cell cultures from patients with DBA is increased and accentuated after erythropoietin deprivation.[633] More detailed culture analysis pinpoints the defect to the erythropoietin-dependent phase of expansion and differentiation of erythroid progenitors with no significant defect in the preceding erythropoietin-independent stages.[640] Glucocorticoid treatment increases the erythropoietin sensitivity of both normal and DBA erythroid progenitors, but DBA erythropoietic differentiation and maturation remain suboptimal.[640]

Diagnostic Criteria

Table 8-10 summarizes the diagnostic and major and minor supporting criteria. Patients with "classic DBA" have all of the major diagnostic criteria.[625] Patients with "nonclassic DBA" have at least three diagnostic criteria with one major or two minor supporting criteria, two diagnostic criteria and two major or three minor supporting criteria, or two major supporting criteria.[625]

Predisposition to Malignancy

Patients with DBA have a predisposition to malignancy with a reported frequency of 1.9% to 6.6%.[619,620,646] AML (AML/MDS) is the most frequent reported malignancy, followed by osteosarcoma.[647] Other reported malignancies include hepatocellular carcinoma, gastric carcinoma, fibrous histiocytoma, vaginal melanoma, Hodgkin's and non-Hodgkin's lymphoma, breast cancer, and ALL (reviewed by Alter[9]). The medium age at diagnosis of malignancy was 15 years (range, 1 to 43), as opposed to 68 years in a non-DBA control group.

Differential Diagnosis

Clinically, DBA has to be distinguished from other IBMFSs such FA, DC, SDS, CHH, and PS. Clinical manifestations, associated physical abnormalities, family history, negative chromosome fragility test (DEB or MMC test), and normal telomere length measurements are helpful in strengthening the diagnosis of DBA. Distinguishing DBA from CHH may be difficult. The anemia in CHH is usually less severe but may be similar to that seen in patients with DBA.[570] In the absence of distin-

TABLE 8-10	Diagnostic Criteria for Patients with Diamond-Blackfan Anemia (DBA)		
		SUPPORTING CRITERIA	
Diagnostic Criteria	**Major**	**Minor**	
Age <1 year	Pathogenic mutations*	Elevated red cell ADA	
Macrocytic anemia	Positive family history	Congenital anomalies of DBA	
Reticulocytopenia		Elevated fetal hemoglobin	
Paucity of bone marrow erythroid precursors		No evidence of other IBMFSs	

*Pathogenic mutations have been identified in *RPS19*,[641] *RPS24*,[642] *RPS17*,[643] *RPL35a*,[644] *RPL5*, and *PRL11*.[645] Mutations in additional ribosomal proteins account for additional cases of Diamond-Blackfan anemia.

From Vlachos A, Ball S, Dahl N, et al. Diagnosing and treating Diamond Blackfan anemia: results of an International Clinical Consensus Conference. Br J Haematol 2008 (in press).

ADA, adenosine deaminase.

guishing features, only identification of the responsible mutation may differentiate between the two conditions. Interestingly, either gene product, the RMRP responsible for CHH (see later also) and the ribosomal proteins responsible for DBA, can participate in ribosome biogenesis, which may explain the similarities in hematologic manifestations. In patients with PS, BMF is classically accompanied by characteristic vacuolization of hematopoietic precursors cells.[549]

DBA has to be distinguished from acquired forms of anemia, including transient erythroblastopenia of childhood (TEC, see later and Chapter 7); viral infections, including infection with human immunodeficiency virus and infectious mononucleosis; drug-related anemia; anemia caused by exposure to toxic chemicals; severe renal failure; and anemia after an ABO-incompatible transplant (for a comprehensive list of possible causes of anemia in childhood, see also Lipton[648] and Vlachos and associates[625]).

Genetics

Inheritance

DBA occurs in both familial and sporadic forms. Autosomal dominant inheritance is the most frequently observed pattern of inheritance. Several genes have been identified whose mutations together account for about 45% of DBA patients. All mutations identified affect ribosomal proteins of both the small (RPS) and large (RPL) ribosomal subunit. Mutations in the RPS19 gene on chromosome 19q13.2[641] account for about 25% of patients with DBA; mutations in the RPS24 gene on chromosome 10q22-q23 account for about 3% of DBA patients[642]; a mutation in the RPS17 gene located on chromosome 15q25.2 has been identified in one family[643]; mutations in the RPL35a gene on chromosome 3q29 were found in about 2% of patients with DBA[644]; and

mutations in the RPL5 and PRL11 genes located on chromosome 1p22.1 and 1p36.12, respectively, were found in about 10% and 6.5% of DBA patients.[644] In all families with mutations in ribosomal proteins of the large or small ribosome subunit (RPS or RPL), the disease was either sporadic (caused by de novo mutations) or followed autosomal dominant inheritance. However, an autosomal recessive pattern of inheritance has been reported.[624,649,650] It remains to be determined whether these are indeed due to biallelic mutations or instead are caused by incomplete penetrance of an otherwise dominant mutation mimicking sporadic or autosomal recessive disease.[620,624]

The Diamond-Blackfan Anemia Genes and Their Functions

Following from the observation that a DBA patient had an X;19 chromosomal translocation,[650] the first gene to be identified as being mutated in DBA (DBA1) was the RPS19 gene at 19q13.2.[640] Subsequently, it was established that a fourth of DBA patients harbor a mutation in RPS19,[619,651,652] which encodes the small subunit ribosomal protein 19. The mutations are always heterozygous and include missense, nonsense, frameshift, and splice site mutations, as well as small and large deletions and three translocations (Fig. 8-19). Whereas the nonsense and frameshift mutations are spread evenly throughout the coding region, the missense mutations are clustered. RPS19 haploinsufficiency is thought to be responsible for disease.[653] Analysis of the crystal structure of RPS19 from *Pyrococcus abyssi* suggests that missense mutations in DBA primarily affect the capacity of the protein to be incorporated into preribosomes, thus blocking maturation of pre-40S particles.[654]

Pathogenic mutations have also been found in another gene encoding a protein of the small ribosomal subunit, the RPS24 gene on chromosome 10q22-q23.[645] The locus

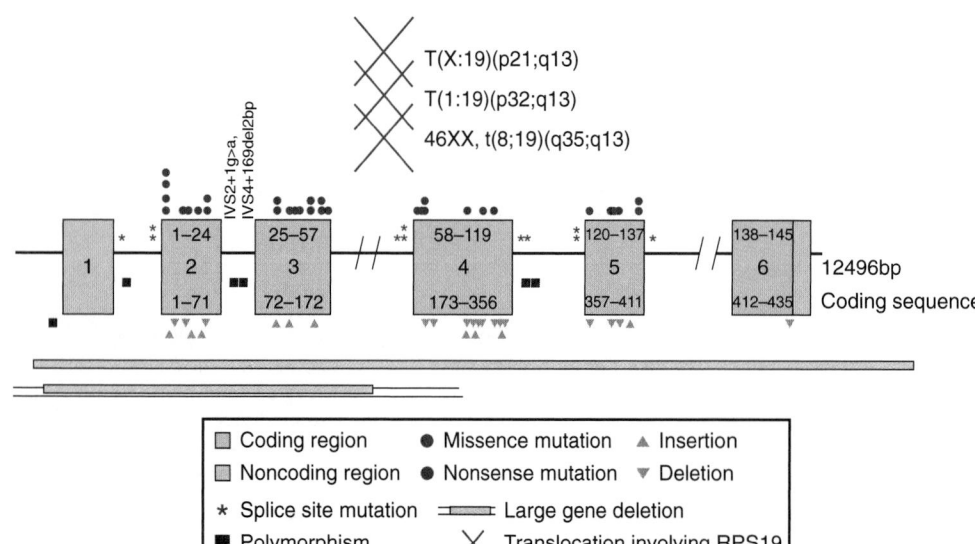

FIGURE 8-19. Mutations in the *RPS19* gene in patients with Diamond-Blackfan anemia as shown in a schematic representation of the six exons with patient-derived mutations. The *red crosses* above the diagram indicate the three translocation that affected the *RPS19* gene. Nonsense and point mutations are shown above the diagram, and small deletions, small insertions, and two large gene deletions are shown below the diagram. (*Kindly provided by Sara Robledo, modified from Lipton JM. Diamond Blackfan anemia: New paradigms for a "not so pure" inherited red cell aplasia. Semin Hematol. 2006;43:167-177.*)

has been designated *DBA3*. Ribosomal proteins are an integral component of ribosomes (Box 8-17). Although ribosomal proteins do not participate in the protein synthesis activity of the ribosome, they are important for maintaining their structure and during ribosome biosynthesis (Box 8-18 and Figs. 8-20 and 8-21). The finding of a second ribosomal protein being affected strongly suggested that DBA is a disorder of ribosome synthesis.[645] *RPS24* mutations are estimated to account for approximately 3% of cases of DBA.[645] Two nonsense mutations and one combined insertion/deletion affecting the intron/exon boundary resulting in a skipped exon 2 were identified in the *RPS24* gene among 215 unrelated probands.

A de novo mutation in a third ribosomal protein of the small subunit, RPS17, has recently been identified in one DBA patient. The mutation affects the translation initiation start codon, with T changing to G. RNA analysis revealed that the mutated allele was expressed.[643]

Box 8-17	**Ribosomes**

Ribosomes are intracellular organelles about 200 Å in diameter that consist of RNA (ribosomal RNA [rRNA]) and protein (ribosomal proteins). In all organisms, ribosomes are the site of protein synthesis and translation of messenger RNA molecules into continuous chains of amino acids (polypeptides or proteins). The ribosome is a ribozyme, which means that it is the rRNA that catalyzes decoding of the message and the formation of peptide bonds. Ribosomal proteins, on the other hand, are important for maturation of rRNA precursors and ensure their correct structure in the ribosome.

Box 8-18	**Ribosome Biogenesis and Pre-rRNA Processing**

Ribosome biogenesis is the new production of ribosomes. In eukaryotes, ribosome biogenesis takes place in the nucleolus, a specialized compartment within the nucleus. Ribosome biogenesis is a complicated, highly regulated process that begins with the synthesis of large preribosomal RNA. Structural rearrangements and cleavage occur as the ribosomal proteins are incorporated to ultimately give rise to mature ribosome subunits. Final maturation of the ribosome subunits takes place in the cytoplasm before they become assembled to form the mature ribosome (see Figs. 7-20 and 7-21). For review see Granneman and Baserga,[655] Fatica and Tollervey,[656] and Fromont-Racine and colleagues.[657]

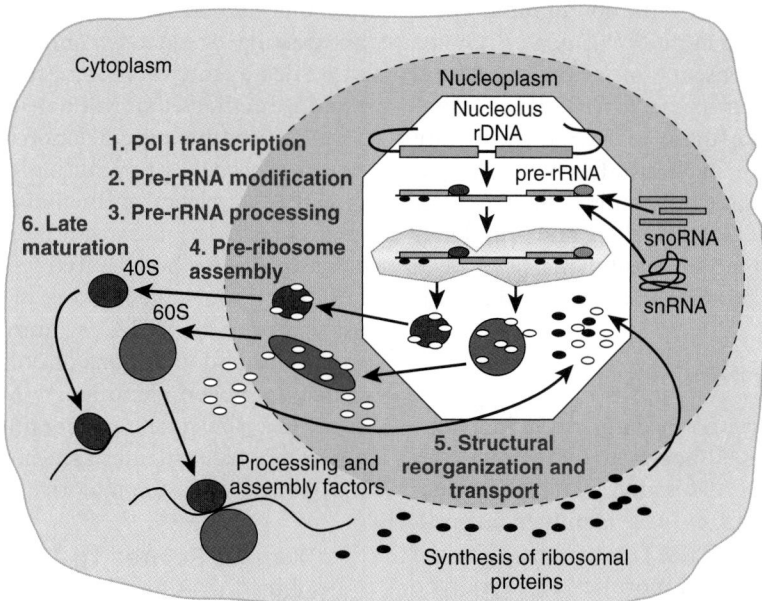

FIGURE 8-20. Diagram of the six major steps in ribosome biogenesis. 1. Pol I transcription. The process starts with transcription of multiple copies of the genes for rRNA (rDNA) to form the large pre-rRNA primary transcript. 2. Pre-rRNA modification. The pre-rRNA is methylated and pseudouridylated under the guidance of small nucleolar RNA (snoRNA). Nonribosomal proteins (*open circles*) and snoRNA (*green rectangles*) associate with the nascent transcript. 3. Pre-rRNA processing. The pre-rRNA undergoes a series of cleavages ultimately resulting in 18S, 5.8S, and 28S rRNA. 5S rRNA, a component of the 60S subunit, is added to the maturing complex. The complex is split into the two precursor particles for the small (40S) and large (60S) ribosomal subunits. 4. Pre-ribosome assembly. Ribosomal proteins (*black circles*) are added to the precursor complexes at various stages of assembly. 5. Structural reorganization and transport. The nearly mature subunits are exported to the cytoplasm through the nuclear pore complexes with the aid of adaptor proteins. 6. Late maturation. The small and large subunits are eventually incorporated into ribosomes in the cytoplasm. Dyskeratosis congenita affects ribosome biogenesis at the step of pre-rRNA modification (step 2); Diamond-Blackfan anemia and cartilage-hair hypoplasia affect ribosome biogenesis at the step of pre-rRNA processing (step 3). snRNA, small nuclear RNA.

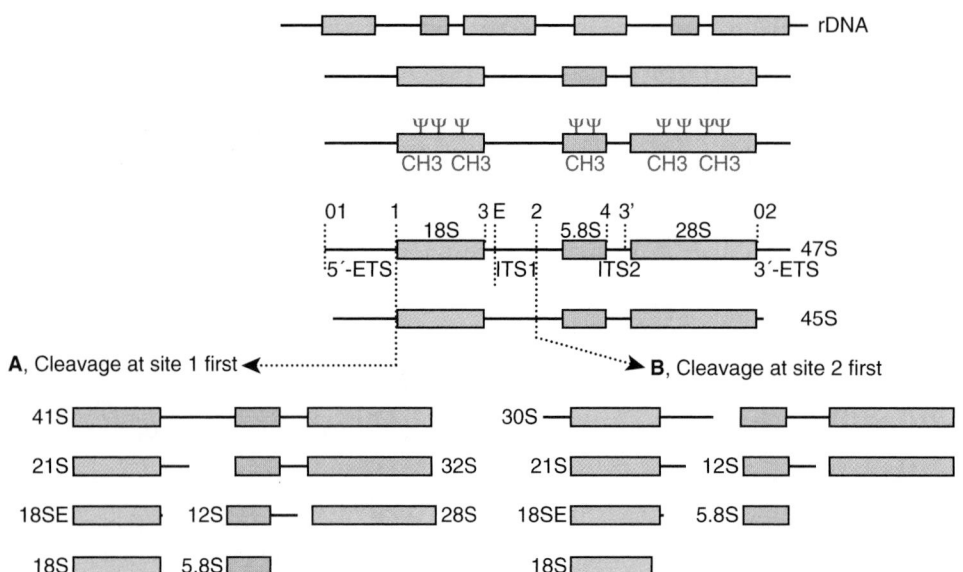

FIGURE 8-21. Pre-rRNA processing in HeLa and lymphoblastoid cell lines (LCL). The 18S, 5.8S, and 28S rRNA is transcribed as a single precursor (45S), which is subsequently processed into mature species by a complex series of cleavage and modification reactions. In addition to the mature rRNA species, the primary precursor (47S) contains two external transcribed spacers at its 5′ and 3′ ends (5′-ETS and 3′-ETS, respectively), as well as two internal transcribed spacers (ITS1 and ITS2). After synthesis of the primary pre-rRNA molecule is completed, the transcribed spacer sequences are removed by a series of endonucleolytic cleavage and exonucleolytic degradation steps. Two alternative pre-rRNA processing pathways, **A** and **B**, have been described in HeLa cells.[658]

Recently, mutations were also identified in three ribosomal proteins of the large subunit, including RPL35a, RPL5, and RPL11.[644,645] Mutations in *RPL35a* include a large genomic deletion, a small deletion, a nonsense mutation, and one missense mutation (G97A, leading to a valine-to-isoleucine substitution of amino acid 33, V33I).[644] Small deletions and insertions causing shift of the reading frame and an early stop codon, nonsense mutations, and one missense mutation (G418A, leading to a glycine-to-serine substitution of amino acid 140, G140S) were identified in the *RPL5* gene.[645] Splice site mutations, small deletions, and insertions accounted for the mutations identified in the *RPL11* gene. Mutations in RPL proteins, like those in RPS proteins, are thought to cause disease by haploinsufficiency.

There was evidence that some families show genetic linkage to chromosome 8p23.2-23.1,[650] and this locus has been designated *DBA2*. No mutations have been identified in ribosomal proteins mapping within this region.[642]

Genotype-Phenotype Correlation

Craniofacial anomalies have not been found in individuals with *RPS19* mutations,[648] nor in the 11 individuals with DBA caused by *RPS24* mutations.[642] No clear genotype-phenotype correlation was identified in individuals with *RPS19*[623,651] or *RPS24*[642] mutations, although null mutations tended to have a more severe phenotype than missense mutations did. The expressivity of individual mutations is highly variable, even within an individual family (Fig. 8-22).[623] The mental retardation noted in individuals with a large deletion of *RPS19* suggested that the concomitant deletion of adjacent genes may account for the additional features in these individuals.[623] Facial anomalies were described in the one patient with DBA secondary to a mutation in *RPS17*.[643] The genotype-phenotype correlation of individuals with RPL mutations remains to be determined.

Molecular Diagnosis of Diamond-Blackfan Anemia

Currently, molecular diagnosis is not routinely performed for DBA because it is expensive and provides a definitive diagnosis in only about 40% of cases. However, only identification of pathogenic mutations in one of the DBA genes definitively establishes the diagnosis of DBA. Furthermore, molecular diagnostics enables the identification of mutation carriers, facilitates prenatal diagnosis for an existing pregnancy, and allows PGD for partners identified as mutation carriers. Mutation analysis should include methods that will detect large deletions. Cases of DBA caused by large deletions are probably underdiagnosed. Anomalies in addition to the ones characteristic for DBA, in particular, mental retardation, are suggestive of a large deletion causing haploinsufficiency for additional genes in the vicinity of the deleted DBA gene. In addition to the large number of mutations in DBA genes associated with DBA, a number of nonpathogenetic mutations and mutations of unknown pathogenic significance have been identified.[659] Determining the pathogenicity of a particular missense mutation may be difficult,[659] whereas nonsense and frameshift mutation are likely to be pathogenic in the majority of cases.

Diseases Related to Diamond-Blackfan Anemia

Aase's Syndrome

Congenital red cell aplasia with a triphalangeal thumb has been described by Aase and Smith as a distinct syndrome.[660] Cleft palate and cardiac anomalies have also been associated with this syndrome.[661] Its clinical manifestations have significant overlap with those characteristic of DBA; thus, Aase's syndrome most likely represents a subset of patients with DBA who have a particular phenotype.[661] Autosomal dominant inheritance and vari-

FIGURE 8-22. *RPS19* mutations in two families with Diamond-Blackfan anemia (DBA). **A,** RPS19 haplotype analysis shown that the *RPS19* mutation in this family most likely occurred as a de novo mutation in the parent and was inherited by all of the four children. The parent had only transient anemia as child, whereas two of the children (6.1. and 6.2) are transfusion dependent and two (6.3 and 6.4) respond to steroids. **B,** Sequence-based mutation analysis of the affected child suggested that in this family DBA was not caused by an *RPS19* mutation. However, haplotype analysis indicates that DBA in this family is caused by a large deletion that includes the first three exons of *RPS19*, thus indicating that gene deletions in the *RPS19* gene might be more common than currently thought.

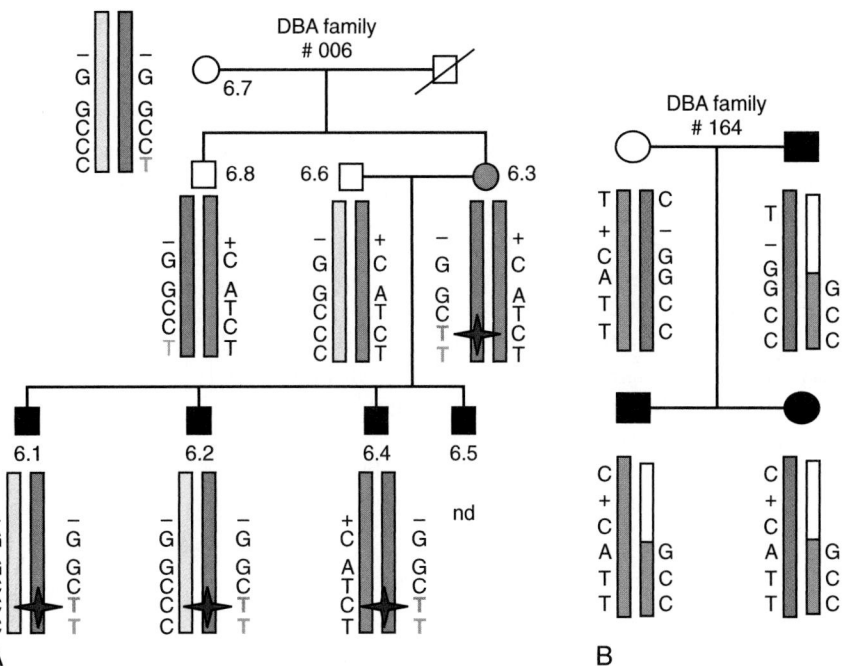

able expressivity have been associated with Aase's syndrome,[662] but no *RPS19* or *RPS24* mutations have been identified in individuals with the classic features of this syndrome.

Myelodysplasia with Deletion of Chromosome 5q (5q– Syndrome)

Patients with a deletion of the long arm of chromosome 5 (5q– syndrome) have severe macrocytic anemia, elevated platelet counts, erythroid hypoplasia in bone marrow, and hypolobulated megakarocytes. Delineation of the critical deletion region on chromosome 5q– includes the *RPS14* gene at position q33.1 and about 40 additional genes.[663] Reducing RPS14 expression in normal CD34[+] cells leads to a gene expression profile similar to that found in bone marrow cells from patients with 5q– MDS and results in selective impairment of erythroid differentiation with only minor effects on megakaryopoiesis or myelopoiesis. Similarly, forced expression of RPS14 restores the erythroid phenotype in bone marrow cells from patients with 5q– MDS, thus suggesting that erythroid hypoplasia is caused by *RPS14* haploinsufficiency.[663] In contrast to patients with DBA, the deletion of *RPS14* in patients with 5q– MDS is not inherited but acquired in early hematopoietic progenitor cells (somatic). Although the mutation explains the erythroid phenotype in patients with MDS and 5q–, the *RPS14* mutation is unlikely to be responsible for the proliferative growth advantage of the mutant progenitor cell. More likely, haploinsufficiency or loss of heterozygosity for one or more additional genes affected by the deletion causes the growth advantage of the mutant cells. Interestingly, MDS with 5q– shows a remarkable response to the thalidomide analogue lenalidomide, the mechanism of which is unknown.

Transient Erythroblastopenia of Childhood

TEC (MIM 227050) is a rare pure red cell aplasia that occurs in children most commonly between 6 months and 4 years of age[664] (see also Chapter 7). Laboratory findings consist of normocytic normochromic anemia and reticulocytopenia, sometimes associated with thrombocytosis and erythroblastopenia of bone marrow.[664] The course is characterized by complete recovery, usually within 1 to 2 months after diagnosis. No therapy is usually necessary, although some children may require red cell transfusion.[664] The absence of macrocytosis, increased fetal hemoglobin, and increased red cell ADA levels in individuals with TEC are used to distinguish TEC from DBA.[664] In addition, congenital abnormalities are not present in patients with TEC.[664] The etiology of TEC is not entirely clear, but is thought to be postinfectious and autoimmune mediated.[665] The majority of TEC cases are sporadic and acquired, but there are a few reports of familial TEC. Linkage analysis suggested allelism for TEC at the *RPS19* gene locus; however, no mutations in the *RPS19* coding region were identified.[666]

Animal Models

Ribosomal mutations have been studied in *Escherichia coli* and *Saccharomyces cerevisiae*.[667] In *Drosophila melanogaster*, mutations in ribosomal proteins are associated with the *Minute* phenotype. Minutes are remarkably similar and share three principal phenotypes—a 2- to 3-day delay in larval development, short thin bristles, and recessive lethality.[668]

In yeast, RPS19 is essential for growth and survival. Decreased expression of RPS19 leads to specific defects in pre-rRNA processing and severely limits the production of small 40S ribosomal subunits.[669,670] Mice homozygous for an *Rps19* null mutation exhibit embryonic lethality, whereas mice with only one active allele, the same genotype that gives rise to DBA in humans, have no detectable abnormality.[671,672] Interestingly, these heterozygous mice appear to express normal levels of RPS19, thus suggesting that mouse cells can compensate for the absence of one functional allele.[671]

The Belly spot and tail (Bst) is a spontaneous semidominant, homozygous lethal mutation in mice that impairs *Rpl24* mRNA splicing and RPL24 production. Mice heterozygous for the mutation have reduced body size, decreased pigmentation, a kinked tail, and retinal abnormalities, but no obvious hematologic abnormalities. Mouse embryonic fibroblasts heterozygous for the Bst mutation have a defect in large subunit assembly and a growth disadvantage in comparison to wild-type fibroblasts.[673]

Mechanism of Disease Pathogenesis in Diamond-Blackfan Anemia

The mechanism whereby mutations in RPS19 or the other ribosomal proteins cause specific defects in red cell maturation is not fully understood and is the focus of current research in the field. RPS19 overexpression improves erythropoiesis in RPS19 mutant CD34+ bone marrow cells from patients with DBA.[674,675] Similarly, a reduction in RPS19 expression in normal CD34+ cells leads to impairment in erythroid differentiation and to some extent also in myeloid differentiation.[676,677]

Reduced RPS19 expression in mammalian cells leads to decreased levels of 18S rRNA production and the accumulation of unprocessed nuclear pre-18S rRNA molecules.[678-680] As in yeast, production of the 40S ribosomal subunit is greatly reduced. Moreover, subtle alterations in rRNA processing could be detected in isolated bone marrow hematopoietic progenitor cells and lymphoblastoid cell lines from patients with DBA secondary to a mutation in *RPS19*,[678-680] but not in cell lines or bone marrow cells from patients with DBA but no *RPS19* mutation, thus suggesting that such alterations affect a different step of pre-rRNA processing. The amount of ribosome subunits and mature ribosomes, however, is normal in steady-state growing cell lines from patients with DBA.[679] Depletion of RPS19 causes a reduction in the steady-state levels of other ribosomal proteins of the small 40S subunit, whereas proteins of the large subunit are unaltered, thus indicating that levels of ribosomal proteins are determined by subunit assembly and that reduction of any ribosomal protein would have the same effect on the small 40S subunit. This suggests that haploinsufficiency for any ribosomal protein of the small subunit may cause DBA.[679]

The fact that ribosomal proteins of the small and large subunit are affected suggests that insufficient functional ribosomes in the maturing erythroid progenitor cell may be the underlying cause of red cell aplasia in patients with DBA. Why the differentiating red cell progenitor in bone marrow is affected by this deficiency whereas other cells are not or are much less affected remains to be determined. A variety of extraribosomal functions have been attributed to several ribosomal proteins of the small and large ribosome subunit. To what extent these extraribosomal functions contribute to the DBA phenotype remains to be determined.

Interestingly, haploinsufficiency for several ribosomal proteins leads to increased tumor formation in zebra fish, a finding suggesting that ribosomal protein genes may act as tumor suppressors.[681] The role of haploinsufficiency of ribosomal proteins in tumorigenesis is the focus of current research in several laboratories.

Clinical Management

The overall actuarial survival rate at 40 years of age is 75%.[620] Survival is significantly better for steroid-responsive patients than for transfusion-dependent patients.[616,619,620,623] The major causes of death are treatment related[618,619,622] and include infection (in particular, *Pneumocystis jiroveci* pneumonia), complications of iron overload, and complications of HSCT. Other causes of death include evolution to severe aplastic anemia and malignancy.

Glucocorticoid Therapy

Steroids and red cell transfusions are the main forms of therapy. Prednisone (or prednisolone) therapy is usually initiated at a dosage of 2 mg/kg/day. For glucocorticoid responders, the prednisone dosage is slowly tapered until the patient is taking an alternate-day dosage that maintains a reasonable hemoglobin level. Many patients remain on small, alternate-day doses of steroids for years. Seventy percent to 80% of patients with DBA are initially steroid responsive, but only 60% to 70% achieve transfusion independence.[616,617,620,623,625] Response to treatment is usually seen within 1 month of treatment. The likelihood of response cannot be predicted.[618,6257] The steroid dose is tapered to the lowest dose necessary to maintain transfusion independence. The maintenance dose of steroids is highly variable, with some requiring only minimal doses.[625,682] The maximum recommended maintenance dose is ≤1 mg/kg/day every other day or ≤0.5 mg/kg/day.[625]

Side effects of steroid therapy include growth retardation, increased risk of infection, diabetes mellitus, hypertension, cushingoid features, pathologic fractures, cataracts, avascular osteonecrosis, osteopenia without fracture, pseudotumor cerebri, and in infants, delay in neuromotor development.[616,625] Steroid therapy is often not recommended in infants younger than 6 months. Individuals taking high doses of steroids require *P. jiroveci* prophylaxis. The steroid maintenance dosage should not exceed 0.5 mg/kg/day and should be continued in the absence of response (for more detailed information, see the consensus document regarding diagnosis and management of DBA[625]).

Transfusion Therapy

Red cell transfusion remains the mainstay of therapy for steroid-resistant disease, as well as for treatment of DBA in early infancy (<6 months of age). Leukocyte-depleted packed red cells should be given every 3 to 6 weeks to maintain a hemoglobin level of about 8 g/dL.[625] The major complication from transfusions is iron overload. Death from complications associated with iron overload is the second most common cause of death in patients with DBA.[619,620,623] Complications of iron overload include endocrinopathy, diabetes, growth failure, and failure to enter puberty, as well as cardiac failure and liver disease. Symptoms of iron overload develop more slowly in patients with DBA than in patients with thalassemia, in whom ineffective erythropoiesis additionally increases iron absorption. Serum ferritin is not a reliable indicator of the body's iron load. Hepatic iron concentration measured from a liver biopsy specimen is the gold standard for estimating hepatic iron concentration. Noninvasive methods of iron measurements include magnetic susceptometry (superconducting quantum interference device [SQUID]) and magnetic resonance imaging (MRI). Iron chelation should begin as soon as patients have increased iron stores (ferritin >1500 mg/dL, hepatic iron >6 to 7 mg/g, which corresponds to a transfusion history of about 170 to 200 mL packed red blood cells/kg). Subcutaneous infusion of deferoxamine has been the standard chelation therapy in patients with DBA. The recently developed oral iron chelators deferiprone, a bidentate (not available in the United States), and deferasirox, a tridentate (available in the United States), may eventually supplant deferoxamine as the standard of iron chelation therapy.[683]

Side effects of deferiprone include neutropenia (6%) and agranulocytosis (0.6%). Fatal agranulocytosis has been described in one patient with DBA taking deferiprone in addition to deferoxamine.[684] The use of deferiprone in patients with DBA should therefore be carefully considered. Iron chelation is contraindicated during pregnancy and should cease when pregnancy is planned or diagnosed.

Hematopoietic Stem Cell Transplantation

HSCT is curative in patients with DBA and may be considered in transfusion-dependent patients who have an HLA-matched sibling donor, patients with DBA progressing to severe aplastic anemia, or patients in whom MDS/AML develops. Five-year post-transplant survival rates are 73% with transplants from sibling donors and 19% with transplants from alternative donors.[620,685] Survival is similar with unrelated marrow and cord blood donors, but a recent report from the Aplastic Anemia Committee of the Japanese Society of Pediatric Hematology suggests that marrow might be superior to cord blood cells.[685] The decision to perform HSCT in patients with DBA is confounded by the possibility of spontaneous remission. HSCT is generally more successful in young patients who have received relatively few transfusions.

Alternative Therapies

Several other therapeutic approaches that have been used over the last 30 years include androgens, erythropoietin, IL-3, stem cell factor, antilymphocyte globulin, cyclosporine, and valproic acid. Although occasional hematologic responses were observed, none of these therapies became a major player in the treatment of DBA. Treatment with metoclopramide, a dopamine antagonist, elicited transfusion independence in a small number of individuals with DBA.[686-688]

Splenectomy was reported in approximately 40 patients, with no beneficial effect noted except in those who had hypersplenism related to transfusions.[643] More than half of the splenectomized patients died, often from infections. Splenectomy is no longer recommended.

More recently, leucine, an amino acid that increases protein synthesis, has been reported to be beneficial in one patient with DBA.[689]

Spontaneous Hematologic Remission

About 20% to 30% of patients experience spontaneous hematologic remission, defined as a stable, physiologically acceptable hemoglobin level maintained for at least 6 months, independent of glucocorticoids, transfusions, or other therapy.[617,620] In the majority of cases hematologic remission occurs within the first decade of life and is stable. However, relapse of hematologic disease has been observed in particular during pregnancy or in women using estrogen-based oral contraception.[620] The molecular basis of the hematologic remission is not understood. In contrast to FA, where hematologic remission is associated with gene reversion, gene mutations persist in patients with DBA who attain hematologic remission.

Pregnancy

Pregnancy in women with DBA is associated with an increased frequency of complications in the mother and child, including preeclampsia, fetal loss, intrauterine death, premature delivery, intrauterine growth retardation, and congenital anomalies.[616,690] It has been suggested that these complications are of vascular-placental origin, and treatment with aspirin has been reported to be beneficial in some cases.[690] Almost half of pregnant patients had transient worsening of anemia during pregnancy. The maternal hemoglobin level should be maintained at greater than 9 to 10 g/dL to avoid maternal anemia, which might lead to intrauterine growth retardation, preterm delivery, or fetal distress. Women planning to become pregnant should be evaluated for conditions that might compromise the outcome of pregnancy, including blood-borne infectious diseases, iron overload and related diabetes mellitus, hypothyroidism, and cardiomyopathy. Iron chelation is contraindicated during pregnancy and should cease when pregnancy is planned or diagnosed. Deferoxamine is teratogenic in rodents but deferasirox is not; however, neither medication is licensed for use in pregnant women.[625]

Cancer Surveillance/Treatment

In addition to an increased risk for AML, there appears to be an association of osteosarcoma and other malignancies with DBA.[647] Bone marrow biopsy plus cytogenetic evaluation is indicated when abnormalities suggestive of MDS or MDS/AML are noted or when the disease progresses to aplastic anemia.[625] Growth hormone therapy is not usually recommended in individuals with DBA and small stature because of the potential increased risk for osteosarcoma.[647] Whether malignancies occurring in patients with DBA differ in their biology and response to treatment from similar malignancies occurring in non-DBA individuals remains to be determined. Similarly, the toxicity of patients with DBA to certain chemotherapy agents used for the treatment of cancer remains to be determined.

Congenital Dyserythropoietic Anemia

Congenital dyserythropoietic anemias (CDAs) are a group of rare genetic disorders characterized by ineffective erythropoiesis and frequent distinctive morphologic abnormalities in bone marrow erythroblasts. The term was used first by Crookston and colleagues,[691] but similar cases had been described previously.[692] Dyserythropoiesis is the major cause of anemia in patients with CDA, although a shortened half-life of the mature cells in circulation may also contribute to anemia (for the definition of dyserythropoiesis see Box 8-19). CDAs are often not considered to belong to the group of IBMFSs. Nevertheless, CDAs are genetic conditions that affect red blood cell production in bone marrow and lead to anemia and reticulocytopenia. Skeletal abnormalities, usually of the limbs, may be associated with some forms of CDA.

Three major forms of CDA[693] and several minor subgroups have been identified.[694] The diagnosis relies on light and electron microscopic examination of erythroblasts in bone marrow and, in the case of CDA type II, also on serologic characteristics.[693] The main characteristics of the three major forms of CDA are summarized in Table 8-11. Shared clinical symptoms include anemia of variable degree, intermittent jaundice, hepatomegaly and splenomegaly, cholelithiasis, and iron overload.

Box 8-19	Ineffective Erythropoiesis/ Dyserythropoiesis

Ineffective erythropoiesis results when in intact, stimulated bone marrow, red blood cell precursors either fail to mature or die in the bone marrow before delivery to the circulation as erythrocytes. Dyserythropoiesis usually defines a qualitative defect in red cells or red cell precursors (or both). Dyserythropoiesis often leads to ineffective erythropoiesis with intramedullary destruction of red cells and their precursors and often a decreased half-life of circulating red blood cells.

Differential Diagnosis

CDA should be considered when the reticulocyte response is suboptimal for the degree of anemia in a patient with erythroid hyperplasia or when there is unexplained hyperbilirubinemia or iron overload. Other congenital anemias and acquired disorders associated with dyserythropoiesis that should be excluded include thalassemia syndromes, hemoglobin C, certain unstable hemoglobins, hereditary sideroblastic anemias, vitamin B_{12} or folate deficiency, iron deficiency, alcohol abuse, liver disease, heavy metal poisoning, and MDS.

Clinical Management

Treatment is essentially symptomatic. Prevention of severe tissue damage secondary to iron overload is important. Splenectomy results in hematologic improvement in some patients with CDA type II,[699] whereas the benefit of splenectomy in other forms of CDA is controversial. Patients with CDA type I show hematologic improvement and a reduction in iron overload in response to recombinant interferon alfa.[655-658,691-694,699-706] Successful treatment with HLA-matched allogeneic HSCT has been reported in severely affected cases of CDA.[698,707-709] In contrast to other IBMFSs, CDA is not associated with a significantly increased risk for leukemia or cancer.

Congenital Dyserythropoietic Anemia Type I

Clinical Characteristics

The incidence of CDA type I is about 1 per 100,000 births per year, and more than 150 patients have been described. Consanguinity may be the cause of an increased incidence in some areas such as the Middle East. In most patients the diagnosis is made during childhood and adolescence. Clinical manifestations in newborns include small stature, hepatosplenomegaly, jaundice, pulmonary hypertension, abnormal liver parameters, and in some cases, transient thrombocytopenia.[710] Red blood transfusions are often required for newborns and infants but are only occasionally necessary later in life. Splenomegaly is evident in 80% to 90% of adult cases. Occasionally, severe erythroid hyperplasia may cause skeletal deformities such as frontal bossing or paravertebral tumors secondary to extramedullary hematopoiesis.

Iron overload with increased ferritin levels is frequent even in untransfused patients. Liver cirrhosis, increased skin pigmentation, and endocrine dysfunction as a result of iron overload have been reported in occasional patients.[711-713] The increased iron loading is due to the enhanced absorption of iron that usually accompanies ineffective erythropoiesis. In fact, hepcidin levels are reduced in CDA type I patients.[714]

Congenital abnormalities are associated with some CDA type I cases and include abnormalities of the fingers, toes, and wrist; short stature; pigeon chest deformity; deformity of the hips, vertebral bodies, and ribs; abnormal skin pigmentation; congenital ptosis; and deafness

TABLE 8-11 Features of Congenital Dyserythropoietic Anemias

Feature	Type I (Fig. 8-23)	Type II (HEMPAS,* Fig. 8-24)	Type III (Fig. 8-25)
Male-to-female ratio	1.1	0.9	0.8
Incidence	<1/100,000/yr	<1/100,000/yr	Very rare
Anemia	Mild to moderate	Moderate	Mild to moderate
Red cell size	Macrocytic	Normocytic or macrocytic	Macrocytic
Bone marrow erythroblasts			
Light microscopy	Megaloblastic, binucleated (2%-5%), chromatin bridges	Normoblastic, binucleated (10%-40%)	Gigantoblasts (10%-40%), often multinucleated
Electron microscopy	Spongy "Swiss cheese" appearance of heterochromatin	Peripheral double membranes (60%)	Nonspecific, intranuclear clefts, karyorrhexis
Altered red cell proteins	Low levels of protein 4.1	Unusual appearance of band 3 protein	
	Impaired globin synthesis	Reticular endoplasmic proteins	
Acid serum hemolysis (Ham test)	Negative	Positive	Negative
Agglutinability			
Anti-i	Normal	Strong	Slight
Anti-I	Slight	Strong	Slight
Glycosylation	Some abnormalities	Markedly abnormal	Some abnormalities
Skeletal abnormalities	± Limb defects[695-697]		
RBC transfusion requirement	In children, rarely in adults		
Iron overload		Frequent, independent of red cell transfusions	
Extramedullary erythropoiesis	Sometimes		
Gallstones			Frequent
Splenomegaly			Mild
Splenectomy	Usually not recommended	96%	100%
Interferon alfa		Effective in the majority of patients	
Hematopoietic stem cell transplantation			Effective (1 case report[698])
Inheritance	Autosomal recessive	Autosomal recessive	Autosomal dominant and sporadic
Gene locus[†]	15q15.1-15.3	20q11.2	15q21-25
Gene mutated	codanin-1 (*CDAN1*)[‡]	*CDAII*	*CDAIII*

*HEMPAS, hereditary erythroblastic multinuclearity with a positive acidified serum lysis test.
[†]Gene locus for some but not all patients in each category.
[‡]Mutated in the majority but not all patients with congenital dyserythropoietic anemia type I.
Data from Alter BP. Inherited bone marrow failure syndromes. In Nathan DG, Orkin SH, Ginsburg D, Look AT (eds). Nathan and Oski's Hematology of Infancy and Childhood, vol 1, 6th ed. Philadelphia, WB Saunders, 2003, pp 281-365; and Wickramasinghe SN, Wood WG. Advances in the understanding of the congenital dyserythropoietic anaemias. Br J Haematol. 2005;131:431-446.

(for review see Tamary and colleagues[715] and Wickramasinghe[716]).

Laboratory Findings

The anemia in CDA type I is moderate with hemoglobin levels between 6.6 and 11.6 g/dL. Red cell morphology includes macrocytosis, severe anisopoikilocytosis, and basophilic stippling. The bone marrow shows erythroid hyperplasia with megaloblastic changes. Diagnostic of CDA type I is the finding of internuclear chromatin bridges between nearly completely separated erythroblasts, which is seen in about 0.6% to 2.8% of the early and late polychromatic erythroblasts (Fig. 8-23).[693,717] Though characteristic of CDA type I, internuclear chromatin bridges may also be found in acquired dyserythropoietic states, such as MDS. The characteristic electron microscopic abnormality in CDA type I is a spongy "Swiss cheese" appearance of heterochromatin in up to 60% of intermediate and late erythroblasts. Additional findings characteristic of CDA type I are summarized in Table 8-11. The acidified serum lysis test is negative, and red cells usually show normal agglutinability with anti-i.[718] The cause of the unbalanced globin chain synthesis in some patients with CDA type I is not known.[713,719]

Patients with CDA type I mount a substantial hematologic response to recombinant interferon alfa-2a or alfa-2b.[700-704] Long-term interferon alfa therapy has been shown to reduce iron overload.[705,706] The basis of the response to interferon is not known.

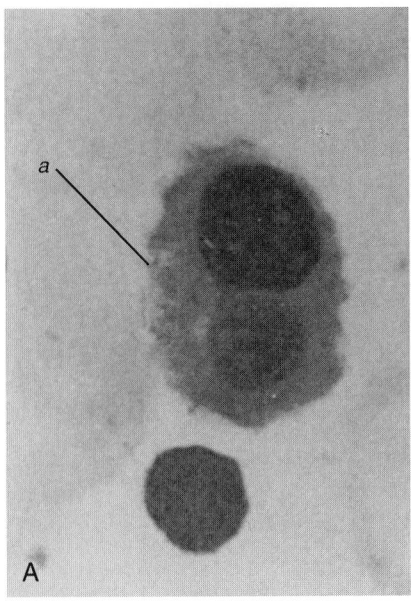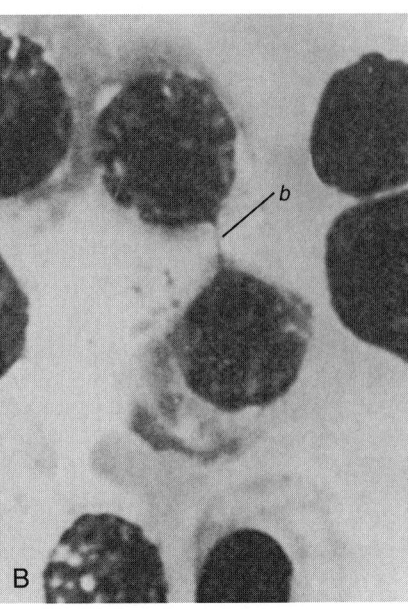

FIGURE 8-23. Bone marrow from a patient with congenital dyserythropoietic anemia type I. **A,** Lowercase *a* indicates a binucleate erythroblast with nuclei of different size and maturity. **B,** Lowercase *b* indicates internuclear chromatin bridges connecting two erythroblasts. *(From Lewis SM, Verwilghen RL [eds]. Dyserythropoiesis. London, Academic Press, 1977.)*

Genetics

CDA type I is inherited as an autosomal recessive disease. Homozygosity mapping of Israeli Bedouin families localized the gene responsible for CDA type I to chromosome 15q15.1-15.3[720] and led to identification of the responsible gene, named *CDAN1*.[721] *CDAN1* has 29 exons and encodes a putative 1226–amino acid protein termed codanin-1. The function of codanin-1 is unknown. There are no identifiable functional domains. CDAN1 mRNA is found at low levels in a wide variety of tissues. The majority of mutations in *CDAN1* are missense mutations causing single–amino acid substitutions in the mutant protein. Nonsense mutations, splice site mutations, and nucleotide insertions or deletions causing a shift in the open reading frame are rare. Homozygosity for 3238 C→T mutation causing an arginine-to-tryptophan substitution at amino acid position 1040 (R1040W) was identified in 45 Bedouin and 11 Israeli Arab families, which suggests a founder effect in these populations. No homozygotes or compound heterozygotes for *CDAN1* null mutations have been identified, thus indicating that residual codanin-1 function is essential during development.[715,721,722] In some families with classic CDA type I, the disease does not segregate with chromosome 15q15.1-15.3 and no mutations were identified in *CDAN1*, which suggests that the disease might be genetically heterogeneous and that mutations in at least one other gene might be responsible for disease expression.[715,721-723]

Congenital Dyserythropoietic Anemia Type II

Clinical Characteristics

The incidence of CDA type II is about 1 in 100,000 births per year, and with more than 300 reported cases, CDA type II is the most frequent form of CDA. CDA type II is also known as hereditary erythroblastic multi-

nuclearity with a positive acidified serum lysis test (HEMPAS, see later).[693] The extent of anemia in patients with CDA type II varies from mild to severe. About 10% of patients require red cell transfusions in infancy and childhood but rarely thereafter.[691,699,724,725] Splenomegaly and the development of gallstones are common. Extramedullary hematopoiesis with the development of paravertebral tumors is rare.[725,726] Progressive iron overload is seen even in untransfused patients, and liver cirrhosis secondary to iron overload develops in about 20%.[744]

Dysmorphic features appear to be less common than in CDA type I. Mental retardation has been reported in some patients with CDA type II.[699,725]

Laboratory Findings

Hemoglobin in patients with CDA type II is generally between 8 and 11 g/dL with a normal MCV.[725] Red cells are usually normocytic with moderate to marked anisocytosis, anisochromasia, and poikilocytosis (including teardrop-shaped poikilocytes); occasional basophil stippling cells; and a few circulating erythroblasts. There is normoblastic erythroid hyperplasia in the bone marrow, with 10% to 35% of binucleate and rarely multinucleate late polychromatic erythroblasts (Fig. 8-24).[699] Electron microscopy shows stretches of double membrane parallel to the inner surface of the erythroblast cell membrane[727,728] that represents excess smooth endoplasmic reticulum containing proteins normally found in this organelle: calreticulin, glucose-regulated protein (GRP78), and protein disulfide isomerase.[729]

The red cells of most patients with CDA type II are lysed in the acidified serum lysis test (Ham test) when mixed with about 30% to 60% of fresh ABO-compatible normal sera but not the patient's own serum.[724,730] The reactive sera contain a naturally occurring IgM antibody that recognizes an antigen present on CDA type II cells

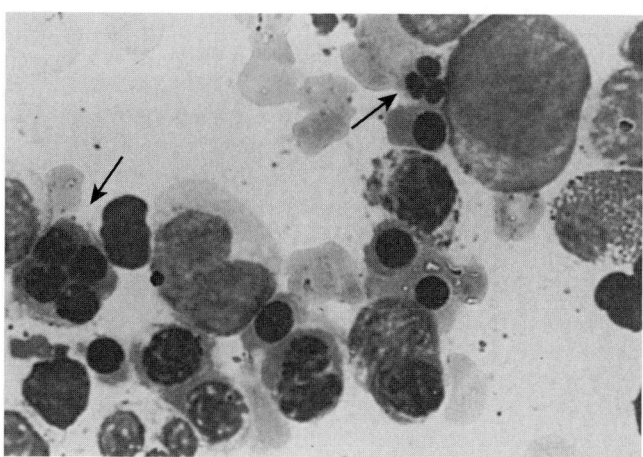

FIGURE 8-24. Bone marrow from a patient with congenital dyserythropoietic anemia type II showing binucleate and multinucleate erythroblasts (arrows). *(Courtesy of Dr. Gail Wolfe, with permission from Alter BP. The bone marrow failure syndromes. In Nathan DG, Oski FA [eds]. Hematology of Infancy and Childhood, 3rd ed. Philadelphia, WB Saunders, 1987, p 159.)*

but not normal cells. CDA type II red cells show increased agglutinability with anti-i antibody. In contrast to red cells from patients with paroxysmal nocturnal hemoglobinuria, which lyse in the acidified serum lysis test even with autologous serum because of complement activation, CDA type II cells lyse because of persistence of "the HEMPAS antigen" on their surface. Thus, CDA type II cells do not lyse in the sucrose lysis test.

Incomplete processing of N-linked oligosaccharides[731,732] leads to defective glycosylation of several usually highly glycosylated membrane proteins such as band 3 (the anion transport protein),[587,733,734] band 4.5 (glucose transporter 1), and glycophorin A.[587,735] It has been speculated that an abnormality in the endoplasmic reticulum may be responsible for the defective glycosylation of red cell membrane constituents in CDA type II.[736] Interestingly, abnormal glycosylation has also been found in other proteins such as serum transferrin (synthesized by hepatocytes). Reduced activity of specific glycosyltransferases has been described in some patients with CDA type II,[731,732] thus suggesting that CDA type II is caused by an abnormality in enzymes involved in N-glycan synthesis.[732,737] However, linkage analysis has not supported this premise.[738] More recently, abnormalities in glycosylation were also found in CDA type I and III red cells,[739] which suggests that abnormal glycosylation is probably a consequence rather than the cause of the dyserythropoiesis.[740]

Genetics

Inheritance of CDA type II is autosomal recessive. Genome-wide linkage analysis has localized the disease gene (*CDAN2*) to a 5-cM region of chromosome 20q11.2.[741] However, thus far sequence analysis of candidate genes has failed to identify the gene responsible gene for CDA type II.[742] In rare families, the disease gene

is not linked to chromosome 20q11.2, a finding indicative of genetic heterogeneity.[743,744]

A zebra fish mutant, *retsina*, shows an erythroid-specific defect very similar to CDA type II. The *retsina* mutation is in the band 3 gene encoding the anion exchanger 1.[745] However, band 3 mutations responsible for CDA type II in humans have not been identified.[746]

CDA Type III

CDA type III is rare. Both familial and sporadic cases have been reported.[747] In familial cases the inheritance pattern is autosomal dominant.[748-750] Splenomegaly was present in some but not others. In contrast to CDA type I and II, iron overload seems to not be clinically significant in patients with familial CDA type III, most likely because of intravascular hemolysis and iron loss by hemosiderinuria. Visual disturbances with macular degeneration and angioid streaks have been described in individual families but are not specific for CDA type III.

In sporadic cases the inheritance is unclear. First- and second-degree relatives are hematologically normal.[752,752] Sporadic cases may occur through a de novo dominant mutation or autosomal recessive inheritance. Alternatively, variability in disease penetrance might cause sporadic disease. Sporadic CDA type III cases are clinically heterogeneous. Hepatosplenomegaly and significant iron overload have been described in some (for review see Wickramasinghe and Wood[694]).

Laboratory Findings

Anisopoikilocytosis, basophilic stippling of red cells, and some very large red cells may be found in the peripheral blood smear. In families with hemosiderinuria, iron deficiency may be found. The bone marrow contains giant multinucleate and mononucleate erythroblasts that may be found throughout erythroid differentiation (Fig. 8-25).[739,748,749,752] Other dysplastic changes include basophilic stippling, nuclear lobulation, and karyorrhexis. Erythroblasts show a variety of nonspecific ultrastructural abnormalities, intranuclear clefts, karyorrhexis, abnormalities in the nuclear membrane, and large autophagic vacuoles.[739] Giant multinucleate and mononucleate erythroblasts may also be seen in MDS and erythroleukemia.

Linkage analysis in one large multiplex family localized the disease gene (*CDAN3*) to chromosome 15q22, distal to the *CDAN1* gene.[747,750]

Additional Variants of Congenital Dyserythropoietic Anemia

A number of forms of CDA cannot be classified as types I, II, or III. In a tentative phenotype-based classification, some of them have been assigned to four groups designated CDA group IV, V, VI, and VII consisting of three or more unrelated families.[694,753] In addition, there are several reports of individual families who have not been further classified.

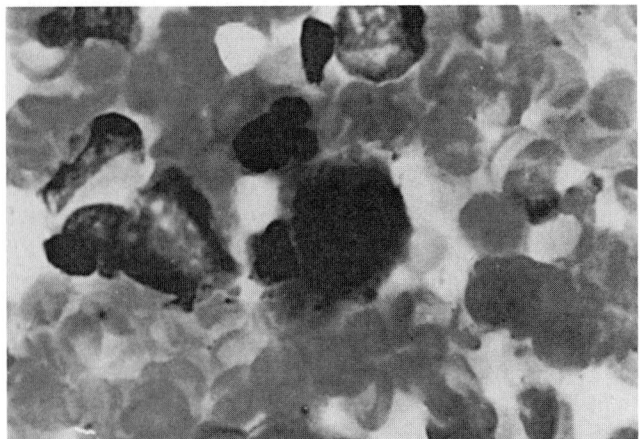

FIGURE 8-25. Bone marrow from a patient with congenital dyseryth-ropoietic anemia type III showing a multinucleate erythroblast. *(Courtesy of Dr. Gail Wolfe, with permission from Alter BP. The bone marrow failure syndromes. In Nathan DG, Oski FA [eds]. Hematology of Infancy and Childhood, 3rd ed. Philadelphia, WB Saunders, 1987, p 159.)*

Congenital Dyserythropoiesis Associated with Thrombocytopenia

X-linked dyserythropoiesis with thrombocytopenia (MIM 305371) is not usually considered a form of CDA; nevertheless, it is associated with mild dyserythropoiesis. X-linked congenital dyserythropoiesis with thrombocyto-penia results from mutations in the transcription factor *GATA1*, which cause either recessive X-linked thrombo-cytopenia and mild dyserythropoiesis or X-linked throm-bocytopenia with the thalassemia minor phenotype and mild dyserythropoiesis.[754-757] Because bleeding secondary to thrombocytopenia and impaired platelet function is the major clinical feature, X-linked dyserythropoiesis with thrombocytopenia is discussed in more detail with the inherited thrombocytopenias (see Chapter 32).

Severe Congenital Neutropenia

SCN (MIM 202700) is a heterogeneous group of disor-ders first described in an extended consanguineous family by the Swedish physician Rolf Kostmann (Box 8-20).[758,759] The disease has thus also been known as Kostmann's syndrome, although this eponym has since been used to define a subset of patients with autosomal recessive inheritance of SCN. The incidence of SCN is estimated to be approximately 1 to 2 cases per million, and both genders are affected equally. SCN has been reported in a broad range of ethnic groups, although there is evi-dence that the incidence of SCN may be lower in Ameri-can blacks than in the general U.S. population.[566]

Clinical Manifestations

SCN is characterized by severe neutropenia at birth with ANCs generally below 200 cells/μL. With infection there may be an increase in neutrophils in blood, but this is always transient and usually modest. Other hematologic parameters are generally normal, although peripheral

| Box 8-20 | **Severe Congenital Neutropenia Associated with *ELA2* Mutations** |

Approximately 60% of cases of severe congenital neutropenia are associated with heterozygous mutations of *ELA2* (MIM 202700). This disorder is characterized by chronic severe neutropenia (absolute neutrophil counts below $0.5 \times 10^9/L$) and is associated with an arrest in myeloid maturation at the promyelocyte/myelocyte stage of granulocytic differentiation. Affected patients have marked susceptibility to infection and a very high risk of progression to acute myeloid leukemia.

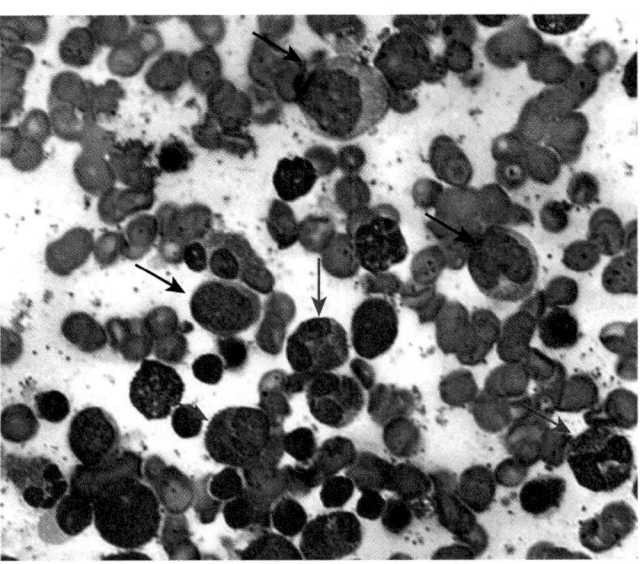

FIGURE 8-26. Bone marrow aspirate from a patient with severe con-genital neutropenia showing a paucity of mature neutrophils, relative accumulation of promyelocytes *(black arrows)*, and marrow eosinophilia *(red arrows)*.

monocytosis and eosinophilia are often observed.[760] Bone marrow cellularity is normal to slightly decreased.[761] Bone marrow in the majority of patients with SCN shows an arrest in myeloid maturation with a relative, but not absolute increase in promyelocytes or myelocytes (Fig. 8-26). The promyelocytes often display vacuolization.[762] Bone marrow eosinophilia and monocytosis are common.[761] The number of progenitors committed to the granulocyte lineage is reduced, and they display decreased responsiveness to G-CSF in vitro.[763-766]

Patients with SCN are prone to infections from birth and may initially have omphalitis.[767] In half of the patients infections develop during the first month of life and in 90% by 6 months. Common types of infection include mouth ulcers, gingivitis, cellulitis, skin abscesses, and otitis media. Pneumonia and deep tissue abscesses occur frequently and are life threatening. The most common causes of infection are *Staphylococci* and *Streptococcus* species. The onset of gingivitis occurs early in childhood, and premature tooth decay and loss result.[768]

There is a high incidence of osteopenia in patients with SCN. In the 422 patients with SCN enrolled in the Severe Chronic Neutropenia International Registry (SCNIR), 28% had bone mineral density measurements or radiographic examinations performed as part of routine care.[566] In this subgroup of patients there was evidence of osteopenia in nearly half. Moreover, pathologic fractures, particularly in vertebrae, have been reported in a substantial minority of patients.[769-771] Although chronic G-CSF treatment has been shown to induce osteopenia in mice,[772] the relationship of long-term G-CSF treatment in humans to osteopenia remains uncertain. A small trial suggested that treatment with bisphosphonates improves the osteopenia in patients with SCN.[771] Given the high incidence of osteopenia and potentially effective therapy, it is reasonable to perform periodic assessment of bone mineral density in all patients with SCN.

Predisposition to Malignancy

Patients with SCN have a markedly increased risk for MDS or AML.[534,773,774] The SCNIR was formed in 1994 to define the natural history of SCN and explore treatment options. As of 2004, 1163 individuals with neutropenia had been enrolled. A recent update of the SCNIR showed that the cumulative incidence of MDS or AML was 21% after 10 years of G-CSF therapy (Fig. 8-27).[774] Even more ominous, the hazard rate for AML/MDS increases with time, reaching 8% per year in patients undergoing G-CSF therapy for 12 years. Approximately

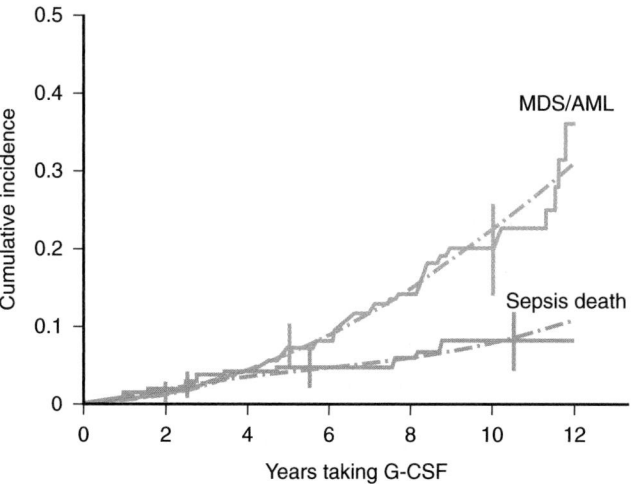

FIGURE 8-27. Cumulative incidence of myelodysplastic syndrome/acute myeloid leukemia (MDS/AML) and death from sepsis in patients with severe congenital neutropenia. The cumulative incidence (cumulative proportion experiencing each event as an initial cause of failure in subjects at risk for each adverse event) is shown by years receiving granulocyte colony-stimulating factor (G-CSF) therapy and 95% confidence intervals at selected years (error bars). The observed cumulative incidence (*stair-step curves*) and smoothed cumulative incidence (*dashed curves*) derived from estimated cause-specific hazard functions are shown. (*Redrawn with permission from Rosenberg PS, Alter BP, Bolyard AA, et al. The incidence of leukemia and mortality from sepsis in patients with severe congenital neutropenia receiving long-term G-CSF therapy. Blood. 2006;107:4628-4635.*)

half of patients in whom myeloid malignancies develop are found to have MDS, typically classified as refractory anemia with excess blasts.[773,775] A consistent feature of myeloid transformation in SCN is the high rate of chromosome 7 abnormalities. In the largest series, nearly 60% of AML/MDS samples displayed complete or partial loss of chromosome 7.[773] Of note, transformation to AML/MDS has been observed in patients with SCN who do or do not have mutations of their *ELA2* gene. Interestingly, malignant transformation is rare (<1%) in individuals with cyclic neutropenia or idiopathic neutropenia.[577]

Differential Diagnosis

A detailed discussion of secondary neutropenia, including immune-mediated, drug-related, and infection-related neutropenia, is provided in the section on the phagocytic system. Inherited causes of congenital neutropenia are shown in Table 8-12. Cyclic neutropenia (MIM 162800), which shares the same gene mutation (*ELA2*) as most cases of SCN, is characterized by 21-day oscillations in the number of circulating neutrophils.[776,777] WHIM syndrome (MIM 193670) (warts, hypogammaglobulinemia, infections, and myelokathexis) can be distinguished from SCN by noting a normal to increased number of mature neutrophils in bone marrow and the presence of *CXCR4* mutations in most cases.[778,779] Both cyclic neutropenia and WHIM syndrome are covered in detail in the phagocytic section. The other disorders can be distinguished by the presence of associated clinical features, including exocrine pancreatic insufficiency (SDS), cardiomyopathy (Barth's syndrome), lactic acidosis (PS), hypoglycemia (glycogen storage disease type Ib), partial albinism (Chediak-Higashi, Griscelli, or p14 deficiency syndromes), and dysgammaglobulinemia (hyper-IgM syndrome); each of these disorders is discussed in detail elsewhere in this text. Genetic testing is becoming an increasingly important tool in the diagnosis of congenital neutropenia.[780] Clinical genetic testing for mutations of most of the genes listed in Table 8-13 is available.[781]

Genetics

SCN demonstrates multiple modes of inheritance, including autosomal recessive, autosomal dominant, X-linked, and sporadic patterns. Accordingly, recent genetic studies have identified multiple gene mutations in SCN, including *ELA2* (MIM 130130), *HAX1* (MIM 605998), *GFI1* (MIM 00871), *CSF3R* (MIM 1389871), and *WAS* (MIM 300392). By far the most common mutations affect the *ELA2* gene encoding neutrophil elastase, which accounts for approximately 60% of all cases (all in autosomal dominant or sporadic SCN).[782-785] To date, more than 50 distinct mutations of the *ELA2* gene have been reported in patients with cyclic neutropenia or SCN (Fig. 8-28). Most of the mutations (≈80%) are missense mutations, although mutations that lead to splicing defects (≈10%) and premature stop codons (≈10%) have also been observed. With a few exceptions, specific *ELA2* muta-

TABLE 8-12   Inherited Disorders Associated with Severe Chronic Neutropenia

Disorder	Inheritance	Genetic Mutation
Severe congenital neutropenia	AD, XL, AR	*ELA2* (sporadic*); *GFI1*, *CSF3R* (AD); *WAS* (XL); *HAX1* (AR)
Cyclic neutropenia	AD	*ELA2*
WHIM syndrome/myelokathexis	AD, AR	*CXCR4* (AD)
Shwachman-Diamond syndrome	AR	*SBDS*
Barth's syndrome	XL	*TAZ*
Pearson's syndrome	Mitochondrial	Variable deletions
Glycogen storage disease type Ib	AR	*G6PT1*
Chédiak-Higashi syndrome	AR	*LYST*
Griscelli's syndrome (type 2)	AR	*RAB27A*
Cartilage-hair hypoplasia	AR	*RMRP*
Dyskeratosis congenita	XL, AD	*DKC1* (XL), *TERC* and *TERT* (AD)
Congenital neutropenia with p14 (MABPIP) deficiency	AR	*P14/MAPBPIP*
Hyper-IgM syndrome	XL; AR	*HIGM1*, *IKBKG* (XL), *AICDA* (AR)

*Sporadic cases are thought to usually represent de novo mutations of *ELA2*.
AD, autosomal dominant; AR, autosomal recessive; WHIM, warts, hypogammaglobulinemia, infections, and myelokathexis; XL, X-linked.

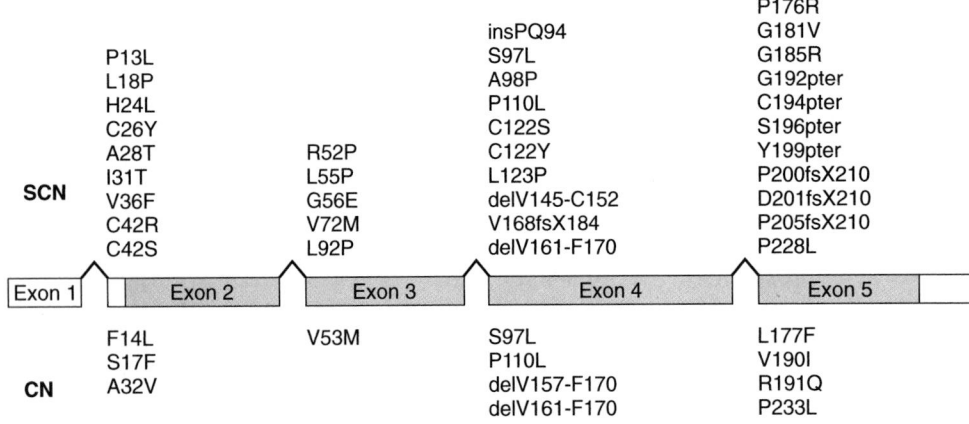

FIGURE 8-28. *ELA2* mutations in severe congenital neutropenia (SCN) and cyclic neutropenia (CN). Mutations associated with SCN (*upper panel*) or CN (*lower panel*) are shown. *Shaded boxes* represent coding exons.

tions are associated with SCN or cyclic neutropenia, but not both, thus suggesting a genotype-phenotype correlation.

The molecular mechanisms by which *ELA2* mutations disrupt granulopoiesis are unclear. Genetic studies provide two important clues. First, in all cases the *ELA2* mutations are heterozygous, which suggests a dominant mechanism of action. Second, a case report of paternal mosaicism for an *ELA2* mutation provides evidence that expression of mutant neutrophil elastase inhibits granulopoiesis in a cell-intrinsic fashion because no toxic paracrine effects of mutant neutrophil elastase on wild-type granulocytic cells in this mosaic individual were observed.[786] Neutrophil elastase is a serine protease stored in the primary (azurophilic) granules of neutrophils and (at a much lower level) monocytes. Although the physiologic substrates have not been fully defined, there are many recognized and potential substrates for neutrophil elastase, including coagulation proteins, growth factors, and extracellular matrix components.[787] However, no consistent effect of *ELA2* mutations on neutrophil elastase proteolytic activity, substrate specificity, or serpin inhibition has been observed.[788] Moreover,

aberrant intracellular trafficking of some, but not all of the neutrophil elastase mutants has been reported.[789,790] There is emerging data suggesting that mutations of *ELA2* may cause disease through induction of the unfolded protein response (UPR).[791,792] In this model, *ELA2* mutations result in the production of misfolded neutrophil elastase protein, activation of the UPR, and ultimately, apoptosis of granulocytic precursors. The propensity of individual neutrophil elastase mutants to misfold may determine the magnitude of UPR-induced apoptosis and ultimately the clinical phenotype. Thus, SCN may represent one of the growing list of disorders caused by protein misfolding.

Homozygous mutations of *HAX1* are associated with autosomal recessively inherited SCN (i.e., Kostmann's syndrome).[793] *HAX1* is a member of the prosurvival bcl2 gene family,[794] thus suggesting that increased susceptibility to apoptosis is the mechanism underlying this form of SCN.

There are three case reports of patients with SCN who have germline mutations in the extracellular domain of their G-CSF receptor (CSFR3) in the absence of *ELA2* mutations.[795-797] These germline G-CSF receptor

TABLE 8-13　Inherited Thrombocytopenia Syndromes

Syndrome	Inheritance	Gene Mutation	Chromosomal Location	Platelet Size, MPV (7-11 fL)	Thrombocytopenia	Associated Findings
MYH9-related thrombocytopenia						Rare progression to MDS/AML
May-Hegglin anomaly (MIM 155100)	AD	*MYH9*	22q11	>11 fL	Mild	Neutrophil inclusion
Fechter's syndrome (MIM 153640)	AD	*MYH9*	22q11	>11 fL	Mild	Neutrophil inclusion Sensorineural hearing loss, nephritis, cataract
Epstein's syndrome (MIM 153650)	AD	*MYH9*	22q11	>11 fL	Mild	Sensorineural hearing loss, nephritis
Sebastian's syndrome (MIM 605294)	AD	*MYH9*	22q11	>11 fL	Mild	Neutrophil inclusion
Mediterranean thrombocytopenia/Bernard-Soulier carrier (MIM 153670)	AD	*GP1BB* Others?	17pter-p12	>11 fL	Mild	None
Bernard-Soulier syndrome (MIM 231200)	AR	*GP1BA*, *GP1BB*	17pter-p12	>11 fL	Moderate to severe	None
Velocardiofacial/DiGeorge's syndrome (MIM 192430)	AD	*GP1BB**	22q11	>11 fL	Mild	Cardiac, facial, parathyroid, and thymus anomalies; cognitive/learning impairment
Familial platelet disorder/AML (MIM 601399)	AD	*AML1*	21q22.2	7-11 fL	Mild to moderate	MDS/AML
Chromosome 10/THC2 (MIM 188000)	AD	*FLJ14813*†		7-11 fL	Mild to moderate	None
Paris-Trousseau thrombocytopenia/Jacobsen's syndrome (MIM 188025)	AD	*FLI1**	11q23	>11 fL Giant alpha granules	Mild to moderate	Psychomotor retardation, facial anomalies
Gray platelet syndrome (MIM 139090)	AD	?	?	>11 fL Absent granules	Mild to moderate	None
Congenital amegakaryocytic thrombocytopenia (MIM 604498)	AR	*MPL*	1p34	7-11 fL	Severe	Aplastic anemia in the 2nd decade, MDS/AML
Thrombocytopenia with absent radii (MIM 274000)	AR? DG?	? micro del +?	? 1q21.1	7-11 fL	Severe	Shortened/absent radii bilaterally
Thrombocytopenia and radial synostosis (MIM 605432)	AD	*HOXA11*	7p15-p14.2	>7-11 fL	Severe	Fused radii, incomplete range of motion
Wiskott-Aldrich syndrome (MIM 301000)	X-linked	*WAS*	Xp11.23-p11.22	<7 fL	Moderate to severe	Immunodeficiency, eczema, lymphoma
X-linked thrombocytopenia (MIM 313900)	X-linked	WAS	Xp11.23-p11.22	<7 fL	Moderate to severe	None
GATA1 mutations (MIM 305371)	X-linked	*GATA1*	Xp11.23	>11 fL	Moderate to severe	Anemia dyserythropoiesis, thalassemia

AD, autosomal dominant; AML, acute myeloid leukemia; AR autosomal recessive; DG, digenic; MDS, myelodysplastic syndrome; micro del, microdeletion; MIM, Mendelian Inheritance in Man; MPV, mean platelet volume.

*Contiguous gene deletion.

†Candidate gene.

Modified from Drachman JG. Inherited thrombocytopenia: when a low platelet count does not mean ITP. Blood. 2004;103:390-398.

mutations are thought to act in a dominant negative fashion by inhibiting receptor trafficking to the cell surface and heterodimerization in response to G-CSF. There are several distinct features of SCN associated with these G-CSF receptor mutations. First, these patients suffer from unusually severe neutropenia that is refractory to suprapharmacologic doses of G-CSF. Second, the bone marrow of these patients displays hypocellularity throughout the myeloid lineage rather than the accumulation of promyelocytes characteristic of most cases of SCN.

Heterozygous germline mutations of *GFI1* have been reported in two families with persistent neutropenia and lymphopenia.[798] *GFI1* encodes a zinc-finger domain transcriptional repressor. The *GFI1* mutations are in the zinc-finger domains and are thought to generate a dominant negative GFI1 mutant protein. Once again, the phenotype of SCN associated with *GFI1* mutations is distinct from that observed in classic SCN in that perturbations in lymphocyte production and function are not typically seen in SCN associated with *ELA2* mutations.

An X-linked form of SCN linked to germline mutations in the *WAS* gene has been identified.[799,800] Unlike classic Wiskott-Aldrich syndrome (WAS), which results from loss-of-function mutations, WAS-associated X-linked neutropenia appears to result from gain-of-function mutations of *WAS* that disrupt an autoinhibitory domain of the WAS protein. Finally, in approximately 25% of cases, the genetic basis of SCN remains obscure.

A recent study suggested that dysregulation of lymphoid enhancer–binding factor 1 (LEF-1) may play a role in the pathogenesis of SCN.[801] LEF-1 is a transcription factor regulated by the canonic Wnt signaling pathway. This study showed that LEF-1 expression is markedly reduced in granulocytic precursors from patients with SCN. Remarkably, restoration of LEF-1 expression in SCN granulocytic precursors partially rescued the block in granulocytic differentiation. These data suggest that loss of LEF-1 may be a key mediator of the block in granulocytic differentiation in SCN. However, no LEF-1 mutations have been detected in SCN, and there is no obvious connection between *ELA2* or *HAX1* mutations and LEF-1 expression.

The genetic factors that contribute to transformation to MDS/AML in patients with SCN are not well defined. Indeed, the spectrum of mutations found in SCN-associated AML is distinct from that seen in de novo AML; whereas mutations in *NPM1*, *FLT3*, *KIT*, and *CEBPA* are relatively common in de novo AML, they are rare in SCN-related AML.[802] Conversely, mutations of the G-CSF receptor are uniquely associated with the development of AML or MDS in patients with SCN.[783,803-805] Of note, these mutations are distinct from the previously discussed germline mutations that affect the extracellular domain of the G-CSF receptor and are thought to inhibit G-CSF signaling in a dominant negative fashion. Instead, these are acquired mutations that introduce a premature stop codon that results in truncation of the distal cytoplasmic portion of the G-CSF receptor and enhanced signaling. In the largest published series, the incidence of G-CSF receptor mutations was 78% (18/23) in individuals with SCN and monosomy 7, MDS, or AML versus 34% (43/125) in individuals without signs of malignant transformation.[783] Because these mutations enhance proliferative signaling by the G-CSF receptor in vivo,[806,807] it has been suggested that G-CSF receptor mutations directly contribute to malignant transformation.

Clinical Management

Historically, patients with SCN had a poor prognosis and often succumbed in the first or second decade of life with recurrent severe bacterial infections. The use of G-CSF has changed the natural history of this disease; the results of a randomized phase III trial comparing G-CSF with no treatment in patients with SCN demonstrated that the majority (>90%) of patients had a significant increase in circulating levels of neutrophils and a reduction in the incidence and severity of bacterial infections.[808] There is substantial patient-to-patient variability in the dose of G-CSF that is required to achieve an acceptable neutrophil count, with some children requiring only 1 to 2 µg/kg on alternate days and others responding only to doses of 50 to 100 µg/kg/day. The SCNIR currently recommends a starting dose of 5 µg/kg/day with upward twofold increases in dose until the ANC in blood is 1000 to 1500/µL[568] Recognized adverse effects of chronic G-CSF therapy include splenomegaly, bone pain, and vasculitis. There are case reports of patients who are refractory to G-CSF treatment alone but respond to combination therapy with G-CSF and glucocorticoids.[795] Of note, GM-CSF treatment is not effective in SCN; it increases circulating eosinophils but not neutrophils.[760] In addition to G-CSF treatment, patients with SCN should receive regular and frequent dental care because the rate of periodontal disease remains high despite G-CSF treatment.[768]

Hematopoietic Stem Cell Transplantation

HSCT from an HLA-identical sibling is curative in patients with SCN who are refractory to G-CSF treatment.[567,809,810] A more difficult question is when to perform transplantation in SCN patients who are doing well with G-CSF and have an HLA-matched sibling donor. The limited published data indicate that transplantation cures a high percentage of patients with neutropenia only but is usually ineffective in children who have progressed to MDS/AML.[809,811] Patients less responsive to G-CSF (defined as an ANC <2188/µL after 6 months of treatment) have the highest risk for AMD/MDS, with a cumulative risk of 40% at 10 years.[774] Moreover, patients who acquire a G-CSF receptor mutation or monosomy 7 appear to have an elevated risk for the development of MDS or AML.[773,783] Though not confirmed in prospective studies, these criteria may help identify patients who should undergo transplantation.

Current recommendations of the SCNIR are to reserve HSCT for patients with SCN who are refractory to G-CSF or who require high doses of G-CSF and have a matched sibling donor.[774] Others, because of the high rate of malignant transformation and the favorable outcome of HSCT when performed before the development of AML or MDS, advocate early HSCT in patients with SCN who have a matched sibling donor.[812] Although there are case reports of successful nonmyeloablative transplantation for SCN,[533,813] there is insufficient data at present to assess its efficacy.

Leukemia Surveillance and the Controversy of Leukemia Promotion by Granulocyte Colony-Stimulating Factor

It should be emphasized that there is no definitive proof that G-CSF directly contributes to leukemic transformation. Indeed, reports of AML/MDS in SCN predate the use of G-CSF. Moreover, myeloid malignancies are rare in children and adults with cyclic neutropenia despite many years of G-CSF treatment.[566] Thus, the contribution of G-CSF to the development of AML/MDS in patients with SCN remains controversial, and therapy with G-CSF should not be withheld from patients with newly diagnosed SCN on this basis. Because of the risk of leukemic transformation in SCN, patients should receive the lowest dose of G-CSF that is required to maintain an acceptable neutrophil count and should undergo yearly bone marrow examination with cytogenetic analysis. For a detailed discussion of congenital neutropenia see Chapter 21.

Inherited Thrombocytopenia

Inherited forms of thrombocytopenia are rare. They are summarized in Table 8-13 (for more detailed discussion see Chapter 32).

Two major forms of inherited thrombocytopenia are discussed in the following sections because of their association with aplastic anemia and because they have to be considered as a possible differential diagnosis in individuals with one of the major forms of IBMFSs discussed in this chapter.

AMEGAKARYOCYTIC THROMBOCYTOPENIA

Congenital amegakaryocytic thrombocytopenia (CAMT, MIM 60448) is a rare IBMFS characterized by isolated thrombocytopenia and a paucity or absence of megakaryocytes in bone marrow (Box 8-21). The isolated thrombocytopenia progresses to severe aplastic anemia in the majority of affected children.

Clinical Manifestations

Thrombocytopenia is usually diagnosed within the first week of life because of petechiae and bleeding. The

---

| **Box 8-21** | **Congenital Amegakaryocytic Thrombocytopenia** |

Congenital amegakaryocytic thrombocytopenia (CAMT, MIM 60448) is a rare inherited bone marrow failure syndrome of infancy characterized by isolated thrombocytopenia, a paucity or absence of megakaryocytes in bone marrow, and no physical anomalies. CAMT exhibits autosomal recessive inheritance and is caused by mutations in the thrombopoietin receptor (TPO-R), more commonly known as the protooncogene *MPL*.

---

thrombocytopenia is usually severe, but platelet size and morphology are normal. The diagnosis is established by bone marrow examination. Thrombopoietin levels are high, consistent with the lack of megakaryocytes and low platelet counts (for review see Geddis[814]). Physical anomalies may be present but are generally nonspecific. An increased incidence of psychomotor retardation has been reported.[815] A less severe form of CAMT is associated with moderate or transient thrombocytopenia. In contrast to thrombocytopenia with absent radii (TAR) (see later), the thrombocytopenia in patients with CAMT worsens over the first 10 years of life and eventually progresses to severe aplastic anemia by the second decade. Transformation to MDS or MDS/AML has been reported.[815]

Differential Diagnosis

Severe CAMT has to be distinguished from other IBMFSs associated with thrombocytopenia, such as TAR and WAS (see Chapter 29). CAMT lacks the forearm abnormalities characteristic of TAR and the microthrombocytes characteristic of WAS. Thrombocytopenia and amegakaryocytosis have been reported in patients with Noonan's syndrome (MIM 163950) caused by mutations of *PTPN11* (see Chapter 29). Patients with CAMT who progress to aplastic anemia may resemble those with other IBMFSs such as FA and DC. The lack of increased chromosomal fragility in the DEB or MMC test performed on cultured peripheral lymphocytes or fibroblasts (or both) is helpful in strengthening the diagnosis of CAMT. Whether telomere length distinguishes CAMT from DC remains to be determined. Severe CAMT has to be distinguished from a long list of acquired thrombocytopenias (see Chapter 29), in particular, intrauterine infections, immune thrombocytopenia of the newborn caused by antiplatelet antibodies (neonatal alloimmune thrombocytopenia), or antiplatelet antibodies secondary to maternal idiopathic thrombocytopenic purpura.

Genetics

CAMT is an autosomal recessive disorder. Mutations in the thrombopoietin receptor gene *c-MPL* on chromosome 1p34 are responsible for disease.[816] Mutations have been identified throughout the *c-MLP* gene, including nonsense, missense, and splicing mutations. Affected individuals are usually compound heterozygous for *c-MLP* mutations, although homozygous mutations have been reported in consanguineous families. Because of consanguinity in affected families, homozygous *c-MPL* mutations in an affected individual are not uncommon.[815] Genetic testing for *c-MPL* mutations is available through approved commercial laboratories.

Genotype-Phenotype Correlation

Patients with CAMT can be divided in two groups: type I patients have complete loss of functional c-Mpl, whereas type II patients have some residual c-Mpl function. Patients with type II CAMT often show transient improvement in the platelet count and have a later onset of pancytopenia than individuals with type I CAMT do.[815,817] Pancytopenia may be the initial clinical manifestation of individuals with type II CAMT. Heterozygous mutation carriers may have impaired megakaryopoiesis despite normal platelet counts.[818]

Clinical Management

The initial treatment of individuals with CAMT is supportive therapy consisting primarily of transfusion of irradiated leukocyte-depleted single-donor platelets to prevent serious bleeding. Platelet increments and platelet survival should be normal. DDAVP is not recommended in small infants because of hyponatremia, but it may be useful in older children. Hematopoietic growth factors and cytokines do not elicit a sustained response in patients with CAMT. HSCT is the only curative treatment of CAMT and should be considered in affected children with a matched sibling donor.[819] Sibling donors heterozygous for a *c-MLP* mutation have been used successfully.[820] HSCT with an unrelated transplant was historically associated with a poor outcome because of regimen-related toxicity and engraftment failure.[815,821,822] Low-intensity conditioning may improve transplant-related mortality and the outcome of HSCT in patients with CAMT.[823] CAMT is likely to be an excellent candidate for future gene therapy because restoration of normal c-MPL in combination with the high levels of endogenous thrombopoietin would provide a selective growth advantage to the corrected hematopoietic stem cell.[824]

THROMBOCYTOPENIA WITH ABSENT RADII

TAR (MIM 274000) is a rare, but well-characterized cause of neonatal thrombocytopenia. The hallmarks of this disorder are shortened forearms as a result of bilateral defects in development of the radii and severe thrombocytopenia at birth.[825]

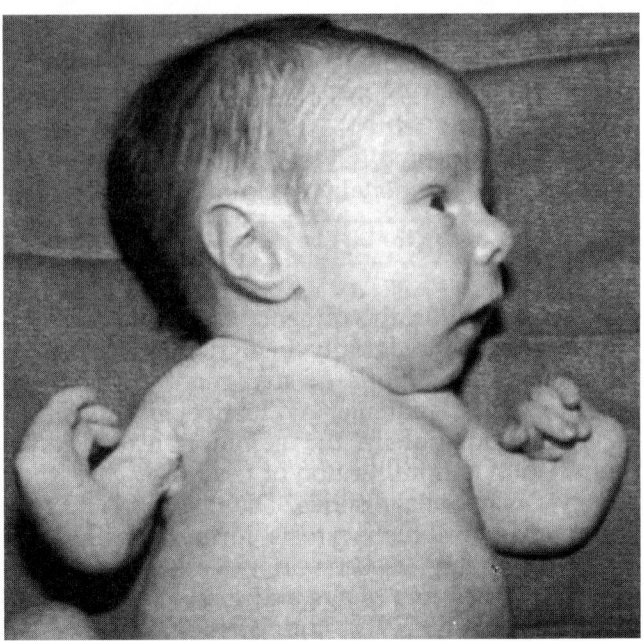

FIGURE 8-29. Patient with thrombocytopenia with absent radii syndrome. *(Reproduced with permission from Luchtman-Jones L, Schwartz AL, Wilson DB. The blood and hematopoietic system: diseases of the fetus and infant. In Fanaroff AA, Martin RJ [eds]. Neonatal-Perinatal Medicine, 7th ed. Philadelphia, Mosby–Year Book, 2000, p 1235.)*

Clinical Manifestations

Patients with TAR have absent radii but may have normal or hypoplastic thumbs (Fig. 8-29). Other skeletal anomalies may accompany the absent radii, including ulnar shortening, thumb hypoplasia, and scapular changes. The hands and fingers, however, are not affected. Lower limb abnormalities are frequent but usually less severe and include hip dislocation, patellar anomalies, absence of tibia/fibula joints, and phocomelia, present in about 50% of individuals.[825-828] Common nonskeletal anomalies observed in individuals with TAR include gastroenteritis and cow's milk allergy,[829] genitourinary malformations, cardiac defects, facial dysmorphisms, short stature, macroencephaly, and capillary hemangiomas.[828,830]

Platelet counts in neonates with this condition are generally below 50,000/μL. Platelet size and morphology are normal. Usually, the degree of thrombocytopenia is greatest at the time of birth. Patients demonstrate mucocutaneous bleeding, and platelet transfusions are frequently required in the first year of life. However, thrombocytopenia becomes less severe during the first year of life, and most affected individuals with TAR will not require platelet transfusions after infancy.[827,831] Levels of thrombopoietin are elevated in patients with TAR, yet such patients fail to respond to recombinant thrombopoietin.[832,833] Bone marrow aspiration reveals a decrease in megakaryocytes, although this is not required to make the diagnosis.[834] Eosinophilia and leukemoid reactions have been reported and are usually transient. The development of aplastic anemia has not been observed, but

AML and ALL have been reported in patients with TAR.[835-837]

Differential Diagnosis

Although the phenotypes of TAR and FA overlap, several features distinguish these conditions. FA patients are rarely thrombocytopenic in the neonatal period; rather, progressive BMF develops in these patients as children or adults. Only about 30% of patients with FA have a radial defect, whereas this skeletal anomaly is the sine qua non of TAR. In a patient with TAR, thumbs may be present in the absence of radii, whereas in FA, absence of the radius is always accompanied by thumb abnormalities. Despite these differences in clinical features, it is prudent to test patients with a clinical picture of TAR for increased chromosome fragility to formally rule out FA.

Amegakaryocytic thrombocytopenia with radioulnar synostosis (ARTUS, MIM 605432), caused by a mutation in the *HOXA11* gene, is usually associated with mild deformity of the forearms, the inheritance pattern is autosomal dominant, and severe thrombocytopenia persists, which distinguishes this condition from TAR syndrome.[838,839] Progression to aplastic anemia has been observed in individuals with ARTUS but not those with TAR.

Trisomy 18 can be manifested as radial hypoplasia and thrombocytopenia but is usually associated with esophageal atresia.

Genetics

The genetic basis of TAR is not fully understood. Autosomal dominant, autosomal recessive, and autosomal dominant with incomplete inheritance have been discussed in the past. In general, the parents of children with TAR syndrome are healthy, and there is no male/female dysequilibrium, which suggests an autosomal recessive inheritance pattern. The very low incidence of siblings with TAR suggests that the syndrome may carry an increased risk for fetal demise. There have been reports of parent-to-child transmission, thus suggesting multiple allelism of TAR.[825]

The molecular etiopathogenesis of TAR remains unknown. c-Mpl is normally expressed on megakaryocytes and platelets in individuals with TAR.[832] However, platelets and megakaryocytes do not respond to thrombopoietin, which suggests a defect in c-Mpl signaling.[840] The homeobox transcription factors (HOX) have been considered as mutated candidate genes in individuals with TAR because of their role in limb development and the identification of mutations in the *HOX11* gene in two families with ARTUS.[838,839] However, sequencing of the *HOXA10*, *HOXA11*, and *HOXD11* coding regions did not reveal mutations in 10 individuals with TAR syndrome.[841]

Recently, high-resolution microarray-based comparative genomic hybridization (array CGH) identified a 200-kb microdeletion on chromosome 1q21.1 in 30 of 30 affected individuals and in 32% of unaffected family members, thus suggesting that a microdeletion on 1q21.1 is necessary but not sufficient and that inheritance of an additional modifier is required to cause a phenotype. In the majority of patients with TAR the deletion was inherited; in 25% the deletion occurred de novo. The deletion was not detected in 700 unrelated normal control individuals, which suggests that the deletion is rare in the normal population and thus the modifier is likely to be more common. Digenic inheritance implies that mutations in each of two unlinked loci have to be present (double heterozygosity) to cause disease and that in an affected family the recurrence rate is about 25%. The nature of the modifier remains to be identified.[842]

Clinical Management

TAR has a much better prognosis than CAMT; the survival curve for TAR plateaus above 70% by 4 years of age. As infants, these patients often require transfusions of single-donor, irradiated platelets to maintain a platelet count above 10,000/μL. After the first year of life, platelet transfusion dependence usually diminishes. DDAVP may be helpful for minor bleeding. Recombinant IL-6 has also been reported to lessen the degree of thrombocytopenia in these patients; however, because of considerable side effects, including fever and chills, IL-6 is no longer used for individuals with TAR.[843] Splenectomy improved persistent thrombocytopenia in an adult patient with TAR. In general, HSCT is not indicated. Treatment of nonhematologic manifestations, in particular, orthopedic interventions, dominate the treatment of TAR later in life. For a detailed discussion of congenital thrombocytopenias, see Chapter 29.

Acknowledgment

M.B., P.M., and D.W. are supported by grant RO-1 CA10532 from the National Institutes of Health (NIH). M.B. has additional support from the Daniella Maria Arturi Foundation and P.M. from NIH grant RO-1 CA1069995. The authors thank Adrianna Vlachos and Jeffrey Lipton for sharing the results of an International Clinical Consensus Conference before publication.

REFERENCES

1. Rosenberg PS, Alter BP, Socie G, Gluckman E. Secular trends in outcomes for Fanconi anemia patients who receive transplants: implications for future studies. Biol Blood Marrow Transplant. 2005;11:672-679.
2. Bessler M, Wilson DB, Mason PJ. Dyskeratosis congenita and telomerase. Curr Opin Pediatr. 2004;16:23-28.
3. Fanconi G. Familiäre, infantile, perniziosaartige Anämie (perniziöses Blutbiod and Konsitution). Jahrb Kinderheilk. 1927:257-280.

4. Auerbach AD, Wolman SR. Susceptibility of Fanconi's anaemia fibroblasts to chromosome damage by carcinogens. Nature. 1976;261:494-496.

5. Auerbach AD. Fanconi anemia diagnosis and the diepoxybutane (DEB) test. Exp Hematol. 1993;21:731-733.

6. Schroeder TM, Tilgen D, Kruger J, Vogel F. Formal genetics of Fanconi's anemia. Hum Genet. 1976;32:257-288.

7. Swift M. Fanconi's anaemia in the genetics of neoplasia. Nature. 1971;230:370-373.

8. Alter BP. Bone marrow failure syndromes. Clin Lab Med. 1999;19:113-133.

9. Alter BP. Inherited bone marrow failure syndromes. In Nathan DG, Orkin SH, Ginsburg D, Look AT (eds). Nathans and Oski's Hematology of Infancy and Childhood, vol 1, 6th ed. Philadelphia, WB Saunders, 2003, pp 281-365.

10. Callen E, Casado JA, Tischkowitz MD, et al. A common founder mutation in FANCA underlies the world's highest prevalence of Fanconi anemia in Gypsy families from Spain. Blood. 2005;105:1946-1949.

11. Verlander PC, Kaporis A, Liu Q, et al. Carrier frequency of the IVS4 + 4 A→T mutation of the Fanconi anemia gene FAC in the Ashkenazi Jewish population. Blood. 1995;86:4034-4038.

12. Rosendorff J, Bernstein R, Macdougall L, Jenkins T. Fanconi anemia: another disease of unusually high prevalence in the Afrikaans population of South Africa. Am J Med Genet. 1987;27:793-797.

13. Tipping AJ, Pearson T, Morgan NV, et al. Molecular and genealogical evidence for a founder effect in Fanconi anemia families of the Afrikaner population of South Africa. Proc Natl Acad Sci U S A. 2001;98:5734-5739.

14. Glanz A, Fraser FC. Spectrum of anomalies in Fanconi anaemia. J Med Genet. 1982;19:412-416.

15. Alter BP. Fanconi's anaemia and its variability. Br J Haematol. 1993;85:9-14.

16. Auerbach A, Buchwald M, Joenje H. Fanconi anaemia. In Vogelstein B, Kinzler KW (eds). The Genetic Basis of Human Cancer. New York, McGraw-Hill, 1999, pp 317-332.

17. De Kerviler E, Guermazi A, Zagdanski AM, et al. The clinical and radiological features of Fanconi's anaemia. Clin Radiol. 2000;55:340-345.

18. Rosenberg PS, Huang Y, Alter BP. Individualized risks of first adverse events in patients with Fanconi anemia. Blood. 2004;104:350-355.

19. Butturini A, Gale RP, Verlander PC, et al. Hematologic abnormalities in Fanconi anemia: an International Fanconi Anemia Registry study. Blood. 1994;84:1650-1655.

20. Gillio AP, Verlander PC, Batish SD, et al. Phenotypic consequences of mutations in the Fanconi anemia FAC gene: an International Fanconi Anemia Registry study. Blood. 1997;90:105-110.

21. Kutler DI, Singh B, Satagopan J, et al. A 20-year perspective on the International Fanconi Anemia Registry (IFAR). Blood. 2003;101:1249-1256.

22. Faivre L, Guardiola P, Lewis C, et al. Association of complementation group and mutation type with clinical outcome in Fanconi anemia. European Fanconi Anemia Research Group. Blood. 2000;96:4064-4070.

23. Wagner JE, Tolar J, Levran O, et al. Germline mutations in BRCA2: shared genetic susceptibility to breast cancer, early onset leukemia, and Fanconi anemia. Blood. 2004;103:3226-3229.

24. Hirsch B, Shimamura A, Moreau L, et al. Association of biallelic BRCA2/FANCD1 mutations with spontaneous chromosomal instability and solid tumors of childhood. Blood. 2004;103:2554-2559.

25. Kwee ML, Poll EH, van de Kamp JJ, et al. Unusual response to bifunctional alkylating agents in a case of Fanconi anaemia. Hum Genet. 1983;64:384-387.

26. Lo Ten Foe JR, Kwee ML, Rooimans MA, et al. Somatic mosaicism in Fanconi anemia: molecular basis and clinical significance. Eur J Hum Genet. 1997;5:137-148.

27. Joenje H, Arwert F, Kwee ML, et al. Confounding factors in the diagnosis of Fanconi anaemia. Am J Med Genet. 1998;79:403-405.

28. Gross M, Hanenberg H, Lobitz S, et al. Reverse mosaicism in Fanconi anemia: natural gene therapy via molecular self-correction. Cytogenet Genome Res. 2002;98:126-135.

29. Fanconi G. Familial constitutional panmyelocytopathy, Fanconi's anemia (F.A.). I. Clinical aspects. Semin Hematol. 1967;4:233-240.

30. Giampietro PF, Adler-Brecher B, Verlander PC, et al. The need for more accurate and timely diagnosis in Fanconi anemia: a report from the International Fanconi Anemia Registry. Pediatrics. 1993;91:1116-1120.

31. Giampietro PF, Verlander PC, Davis JG, Auerbach AD. Diagnosis of Fanconi anemia in patients without congenital malformations: an international Fanconi Anemia Registry Study. Am J Med Genet. 1997;68:58-61.

32. Auerbach A, Buchwald M, Joenje H. Fanconi anemia. In Scriver C, Sly W, Childs B, et al (eds). The Metabolic and Molecular Bases of Inherited Disease. New York, McGraw-Hill, 2001.

33. Wajnrajch MP, Gertner JM, Huma Z, et al. Evaluation of growth and hormonal status in patients referred to the International Fanconi Anemia Registry. Pediatrics. 2001;107:744-754.

34. Giri N, Batista DL, Alter BP, Stratakis CA. Endocrine abnormalities in patients with Fanconi anemia. J Clin Endocrinol Metab. 2007;92:2624-2631.

35. Koubik AC, Franca BH, Ribas Mde O, et al. Comparative study of chronological, bone, and dental age in Fanconi's anemia. J Pediatr Hematol Oncol. 2006;28:260-262.

36. Dupuis-Girod S, Gluckman E, Souberbielle JC, Brauner R. Growth hormone deficiency caused by pituitary stalk interruption in Fanconi's anemia. J Pediatr. 2001;138:129-133.

37. Wajnrajch MP. Physiological and pathological growth hormone secretion. J Pediatr Endocrinol Metab. 2005;18:325-338.

38. Alter BP, Frissora CL, Halperin DS, et al. Fanconi's anaemia and pregnancy. Br J Haematol. 1991;77:410-418.

39. Alter BP. Fanconi's anemia. Current concepts. Am J Pediatr Hematol Oncol. 1992;14:170-176.

40. Dalle JH, Huot C, Duval M, et al. Successful pregnancies after bone marrow transplantation for Fanconi anemia. Bone Marrow Transplant. 2004;34:1099-1100.

41. Morris ES, Darbyshire P, Fairlie F, et al. Two natural pregnancies following allogeneic transplantation for Fanconi anaemia. Br J Haematol. 2008;140:130.

42. Goi K, Sugita K. Pregnancy after bone marrow transplantation in Fanconi anaemia: response to Dalle et al. Br J Haematol. 2007;137:76-77.

43. Veitia RA, Gluckman E, Fellous M, Soulier J. Recovery of female fertility after chemotherapy, irradiation, and bone marrow allograft: further evidence against massive oocyte regeneration by bone marrow–derived germline stem cells. Stem Cells. 2007;25:1334-1335.

44. Liu JM, Auerbach AD, Young NS. Fanconi anemia presenting unexpectedly in an adult kindred with no dysmorphic features. Am J Med. 1991;91:555-557.

45. Jones JH. Foetal haemoglobin in Fanconi type anaemia. Nature. 1961;192:982.

46. Diamond LK, Wang WC, Alter BP. Congenital hypoplastic anemia. Adv Pediatr. 1976;22:349-378.

47. Alter BP. Biology of erythropoiesis. Ann N Y Acad Sci. 1994;731:36-47.

48. Cassinat B, Guardiola P, Chevret S, et al. Constitutive elevation of serum alpha-fetoprotein in Fanconi anemia. Blood. 2000;96:859-863.

49. Rosenberg PS, Socie G, Alter BP, Gluckman E. Risk of head and neck squamous cell cancer and death in patients with Fanconi anemia who did and did not receive transplants. Blood. 2005;105:67-73.

50. Pignatti CB, Bianchi E, Polito E. Fanconi's anemia in infancy. Report of a case diagnosed in the pre-anemic stage. Helv Paediatr Acta. 1977;32:413-418.

51. Landmann E, Bluetters-Sawatzki R, Schindler D, Gortner L. Fanconi anemia in a neonate with pancytopenia. J Pediatr. 2004;145:125-127.

52. Auerbach AD, Weiner MA, Warburton D, et al. Acute myeloid leukemia as the first hematologic manifestation of Fanconi anemia. Am J Hematol. 1982;12:289-300.

53. Alter BP, Knobloch ME, Weinberg RS. Erythropoiesis in Fanconi's anemia. Blood. 1991;78:602-608.

54. Stark R, Thierry D, Richard P, Gluckman E. Long-term bone marrow culture in Fanconi's anaemia. Br J Haematol. 1993;83:554-559.

55. Schindler D, Hoehn H. Fanconi anemia mutation causes cellular susceptibility to ambient oxygen. Am J Hum Genet. 1988;43:429-435.

56. Cohen-Haguenauer O, Peault B, Bauche C, et al. In vivo repopulation ability of genetically corrected bone marrow cells from Fanconi anemia patients. Proc Natl Acad Sci U S A. 2006;103:2340-2345.

57. Schultz JC, Shahidi NT. Tumor necrosis factor-alpha overproduction in Fanconi's anemia. Am J Hematol. 1993;42:196-201.

58. Rosselli F, Sanceau J, Gluckman E, et al. Abnormal lymphokine production: a novel feature of the genetic disease Fanconi anemia. II. In vitro and in vivo spontaneous overproduction of tumor necrosis factor alpha. Blood. 1994;83:1216-1225.

59. Dufour C, Corcione A, Svahn J, et al. TNF-alpha and IFN-gamma are overexpressed in the bone marrow of Fanconi anemia patients and TNF-alpha suppresses erythropoiesis in vitro. Blood. 2003;102:2053-2059.

60. Abkowitz JL, Fialkow PJ, Niebrugge DJ, et al. Pancytopenia as a clonal disorder of a multipotent hematopoietic stem cell. J Clin Invest. 1984;73:258-261.

61. Venkatraj VS, Gaidano G, Auerbach AD. Clonality studies and N-ras and p53 mutation analysis of hematopoietic cells in Fanconi anemia. Leukemia. 1994;8:1354-1358.

62. Alter BP, Caruso JP, Drachtman RA, et al. Fanconi anemia: myelodysplasia as a predictor of outcome. Cancer Genet Cytogenet. 2000;117:125-131.

63. Alter BP, Scalise A, McCombs J, Najfeld V. Clonal chromosomal abnormalities in Fanconi's anaemia: what do they really mean? Br J Haematol. 1993;85:627-630.

64. Auerbach AD, Allen RG. Leukemia and preleukemia in Fanconi anemia patients. A review of the literature and report of the International Fanconi Anemia Registry. Cancer Genet Cytogenet. 1991;51:1-12.

65. Berger R, Le Coniat M, Schaison G. Chromosome abnormalities in bone marrow of Fanconi anemia patients. Cancer Genet Cytogenet. 1993;65:47-50.

66. Rosenberg PS, Greene MH, Alter BP. Cancer incidence in persons with Fanconi anemia. Blood. 2003;101:822-826.

67. Berger R, Bernheim A, Le Coniat M, et al. Chromosomal studies of leukemic and preleukemic Fanconi's anemia patients: examples of acquired "chromosomal amplification." Hum Genet. 1980;56:59-62.

68. Tonnies H, Huber S, Kuhl JS, et al. Clonal chromosomal aberrations in bone marrow cells of Fanconi anemia patients: gains of the chromosomal segment 3q26q29 as an adverse risk factor. Blood. 2003;101:3872-3874.

69. Meyer S, Fergusson WD, Whetton AD, et al. Amplification and translocation of 3q26 with overexpression of EVI1 in Fanconi anemia–derived childhood acute myeloid leukemia with biallelic FANCD1/BRCA2 disruption. Genes Chromosomes Cancer. 2007;46:359-372.

70. Alter BP. Cancer in Fanconi anemia, 1927-2001. Cancer. 2003;97:425-440.

71. Kutler DI, Wreesmann VB, Goberdhan A, et al. Human papillomavirus DNA and p53 polymorphisms in squamous cell carcinomas from Fanconi anemia patients. J Natl Cancer Inst. 2003;95:1718-1721.

72. van Zeeburg HJ, Snijders PJ, Joenje H, Brakenhoff RH. Re: Human papillomavirus DNA and p53 polymorphisms in squamous cell carcinomas from Fanconi anemia patients. J Natl Cancer Inst. 2004;96:968; author reply 968-969.

73. Oksuzoglu B, Yalcin S. Squamous cell carcinoma of the tongue in a patient with Fanconi's anemia: a case report and review of the literature. Ann Hematol. 2002;81:294-298.

74. Johnson FL, Lerner KG, Siegel M, et al. Association of androgenic-anabolic steroid therapy with development of hepatocellular carcinoma. Lancet. 1972;2:1273-1276.

75. Shapiro P, Ikeda RM, Ruebner BH, et al. Multiple hepatic tumors and peliosis hepatis in Fanconi's anemia treated with androgens. Am J Dis Child. 1977;131:1104-1106.

76. Velazquez I, Alter BP. Androgens and liver tumors: Fanconi's anemia and non-Fanconi's conditions. Am J Hematol. 2004;77:257-267.

77. Sarna G, Tomasulo P, Lotz MJ, et al. Multiple neoplasms in two siblings with a variant form of Fanconi's anemia. Cancer. 1975;36:1029-1033.

78. Garriga S, Crosby WH. The incidence of leukemia in families of patients with hypoplasia of the marrow. Blood. 1959;14:1008-1014.

79. Bennett JM, Catovsky D, Daniel MT, et al. Proposals for the classification of the acute leukaemias. French-

American-British (FAB) co-operative group. Br J Haematol. 1976;33:451-458.

80. Bennett JM, Catovsky D, Daniel MT, et al. Criteria for the diagnosis of acute leukemia of megakaryocyte lineage (M7). A report of the French-American-British Cooperative Group. Ann Intern Med. 1985;103:460-462.

81. Bennett JM, Catovsky D, Daniel MT, et al. Proposed revised criteria for the classification of acute myeloid leukemia. A report of the French-American-British Cooperative Group. Ann Intern Med. 1985;103:620-625.

82. Cheson BD, Bennett JM, Kopecky KJ, et al. Revised recommendations of the International Working Group for Diagnosis, Standardization of Response Criteria, Treatment Outcomes, and Reporting Standards for Therapeutic Trials in Acute Myeloid Leukemia. J Clin Oncol. 2003;21:4642-4649.

83. Maarek O, Jonveaux P, Le Coniat M, et al. Fanconi anemia and bone marrow clonal chromosome abnormalities. Leukemia. 1996;10:1700-1704.

84. Offit K, Levran O, Mullaney B, et al. Shared genetic susceptibility to breast cancer, brain tumors, and Fanconi anemia. J Natl Cancer Inst. 2003;95:1548-1551.

85. Alter BP, Rosenberg PS, Brody LC. Clinical and molecular features associated with biallelic mutations in FANCD1/BRCA2. J Med Genet. 2007;44:1-9.

86. Reid S, Schindler D, Hanenberg H, et al. Biallelic mutations in PALB2 cause Fanconi anemia subtype FA-N and predispose to childhood cancer. Nat Genet. 2007;39:162-164.

87. Xia B, Sheng Q, Nakanishi K, et al. Control of BRCA2 cellular and clinical functions by a nuclear partner, PALB2. Mol Cell. 2006;22:719-729.

88. Kutler DI, Auerbach AD, Satagopan J, et al. High incidence of head and neck squamous cell carcinoma in patients with Fanconi anemia. Arch Otolaryngol Head Neck Surg. 2003;129:106-112.

89. Cervenka J, Arthur D, Yasis C. Mitomycin C test for diagnostic differentiation of idiopathic aplastic anemia and Fanconi anemia. Pediatrics. 1981;67:119-127.

90. Schroeder TM, Anschutz F, Knopp A. [Spontaneous chromosome aberrations in familial panmyelopathy.] Humangenetik. 1964;1:194-196.

91. Schroeder TM, German J. Bloom's syndrome and Fanconi's anemia: demonstration of two distinctive patterns of chromosome disruption and rearrangement. Humangenetik. 1974;25:299-306.

92. Auerbach A. Diagnosis of Fanconi anemia by diepoxybutane analysis. In Dracopoli N, Haines J, Korf B, et al (eds). Current Protocols in Human Genetics, supplement 37. Hoboken, NJ, John Wiley & Sons, 2003, pp 8.7.1-8.7.15.

93. Auerbach AD, Adler B, Chaganti RS. Prenatal and postnatal diagnosis and carrier detection of Fanconi anemia by a cytogenetic method. Pediatrics. 1981;67:128-135.

94. Auerbach AD, Sagi M, Adler B. Fanconi anemia: prenatal diagnosis in 30 fetuses at risk. Pediatrics. 1985;76:794-800.

95. Auerbach AD, Min Z, Ghosh R, et al. Clastogen-induced chromosomal breakage as a marker for first trimester prenatal diagnosis of Fanconi anemia. Hum Genet. 1986;73:86-88.

96. Auerbach AD, Liu Q, Ghosh R, et al. Prenatal identification of potential donors for umbilical cord blood transplantation for Fanconi anemia. Transfusion. 1990;30:682-687.

97. Nakanishi K, Taniguchi T, Ranganathan V, et al. Interaction of FANCD2 and NBS1 in the DNA damage response. Nat Cell Biol. 2002;4:913-920.

98. Shimada H, Shimizu K, Mimaki S, et al. First case of aplastic anemia in a Japanese child with a homozygous missense mutation in the NBS1 gene (I171V) associated with genomic instability. Hum Genet. 2004;115:372-376.

99. Gennery AR, Slatter MA, Bhattacharya A, et al. The clinical and biological overlap between Nijmegen breakage syndrome and Fanconi anemia. Clin Immunol. 2004;113:214-219.

100. New HV, Cale CM, Tischkowitz M, et al. Nijmegen breakage syndrome diagnosed as Fanconi anaemia. Pediatr Blood Cancer. 2005;44:494-499.

101. Auerbach AD, Rogatko A, Schroeder-Kurth TM. International Fanconi Anemia Registry: relation of clinical symptoms to diepoxybutane sensitivity. Blood. 1989;73:391-396.

102. Shimamura A, Montes de Oca R, Svenson JL, et al. A novel diagnostic screen for defects in the Fanconi anemia pathway. Blood. 2002;100:4649-4654.

103. Soulier J, Leblanc T, Larghero J, et al. Detection of somatic mosaicism and classification of Fanconi anemia patients by analysis of the FA/BRCA pathway. Blood. 2005;105:1329-1336.

104. Schmid W, Scharer K, Baumann T, Fanconi G. [Chromosomal fragility in familial panmyelopathy (Fanconi type).] Schweiz Med Wochenschr. 1965;95:1461-1464.

105. Swift MR, Hirschhorn K. Fanconi's anemia. Inherited susceptibility to chromosome breakage in various tissues. Ann Intern Med. 1966;65:496-503.

106. Bloom GE, Warner S, Gerald PS, Diamond LK. Chromosome abnormalities in constitutional aplastic anemia. N Engl J Med. 1966;274:8-14.

107. Gmyrek D, Witkowski R, Sylim-Rapport I, Jacobasch G. [Chromosomal aberrations and metabolic disorders of blood cells in Fanconi's anemia before and after transformation into leukosis as exemplified in a patient.] Dtsch Med Wochenschr. 1967;92:1701-1707.

108. German J. Chromosome-breakage syndromes: different genes, different treatments, different cancers. Basic Life Sci. 1980;15:429-439.

109. Sasaki MS, Tonomura A. A high susceptibility of Fanconi's anemia to chromosome breakage by DNA cross-linking agents. Cancer Res. 1973;33:1829-1936.

110. Berger R, Bernheim A, Le Coniat M, et al. [Effect of chlormethin chlorhydrate on the chromosomes in Fanconi's anemia: application to diagnosis and detection of heterozygotes.] C R Seances Acad Sci D. 1980;290:457-459.

111. Carreau M, Alon N, Bosnoyan-Collins L, et al. Drug sensitivity spectra in Fanconi anemia lymphoblastoid cell lines of defined complementation groups. Mutat Res. 1999;435:103-109.

112. Kaiser TN, Lojewski A, Dougherty C, et al. Flow cytometric characterization of the response of Fanconi's anemia cells to mitomycin C treatment. Cytometry. 1982;2:291-297.

113. Kubbies M, Schindler D, Hoehn H, et al. Endogenous blockage and delay of the chromosome cycle despite normal recruitment and growth phase explain poor proliferation and frequent endomitosis in Fanconi anemia cells. Am J Hum Genet. 1985;37:1022-1030.

114. Miglierina R, Le Coniat M, Gendron M, Berger R. Diagnosis of Fanconi's anemia by flow cytometry. Nouv Rev Fr Hematol. 1990;32:391-393.

115. Adelfalk C, Lorenz M, Serra V, et al. Accelerated telomere shortening in Fanconi anemia fibroblasts—a longitudinal study. FEBS Lett. 2001;506:22-26.

116. Callen E, Samper E, Ramirez MJ, et al. Breaks at telomeres and TRF2-independent end fusions in Fanconi anemia. Hum Mol Genet. 2002;11:439-444.

117. Leteurtre F, Li X, Guardiola P, et al. Accelerated telomere shortening and telomerase activation in Fanconi's anaemia. Br J Haematol. 1999;105:883-893.

118. Cabuy E, Newton C, Joksic G, et al. Accelerated telomere shortening and telomere abnormalities in radiosensitive cell lines. Radiat Res. 2005;164:53-62.

119. Alter BP. Radiosensitivity in Fanconi's anemia patients. Radiother Oncol. 2002;62:345-347.

120. Djuzenova CS, Rothfuss A, Oppitz U, et al. Response to X-irradiation of Fanconi anemia homozygous and heterozygous cells assessed by the single-cell gel electrophoresis (comet) assay. Lab Invest. 2001;81:185-192.

121. Gatti RA. The inherited basis of human radiosensitivity. Acta Oncol. 2001;40:702-711.

122. Casado JA, Nunez MI, Segovia JC, et al. Non-homologous end-joining defect in Fanconi anemia hematopoietic cells exposed to ionizing radiation. Radiat Res. 2005;164:635-641.

123. Joenje H, Arwert F, Eriksson AW, et al. Oxygen-dependence of chromosomal aberrations in Fanconi's anaemia. Nature. 1981;290:142-143.

124. Park SJ, Ciccone SL, Beck BD, et al. Oxidative stress/damage induces multimerization and interaction of Fanconi anemia proteins. J Biol Chem. 2004;279:30053-30059.

125. Zhang X, Li J, Sejas DP, Pang Q. Hypoxia-reoxygenation induces premature senescence in FA bone marrow hematopoietic cells. Blood. 2005;106:75-85.

126. Poot M, Gross O, Epe B, et al. Cell cycle defect in connection with oxygen and iron sensitivity in Fanconi anemia lymphoblastoid cells. Exp Cell Res. 1996;222:262-268.

127. Korkina LG, Samochatova EV, Maschan AA, et al. Release of active oxygen radicals by leukocytes of Fanconi anemia patients. J Leukoc Biol. 1992;52:357-362.

128. Gille JJ, Wortelboer HM, Joenje H. Antioxidant status of Fanconi anemia fibroblasts. Hum Genet. 1987;77:28-31.

129. Joenje H, Frants RR, Arwert F, et al. Erythrocyte superoxide dismutase deficiency in Fanconi's anaemia established by two independent methods of assay. Scand J Clin Lab Invest. 1979;39:759-764.

130. Mavelli I, Ciriolo MR, Rotilio G, et al. Superoxide dismutase, glutathione peroxidase and catalase in oxidative hemolysis. A study of Fanconi's anemia erythrocytes. Biochem Biophys Res Commun. 1982;106:286-290.

131. Bigelow SB, Rary JM, Bender MA. G_2 chromosomal radiosensitivity in Fanconi's anemia. Mutat Res. 1979;63:189-199.

132. Rosselli F, Sanceau J, Wietzerbin J, Moustacchi E. Abnormal lymphokine production: a novel feature of the genetic disease Fanconi anemia. I. Involvement of interleukin-6. Hum Genet. 1992;89:42-48.

133. Takeuchi T, Morimoto K. Increased formation of 8-hydroxydeoxyguanosine, an oxidative DNA damage, in lymphoblasts from Fanconi's anemia patients due to possible catalase deficiency. Carcinogenesis. 1993;14:1115-1120.

134. Sasaki MS. Is Fanconi's anaemia defective in a process essential to the repair of DNA cross links? Nature. 1975;257:501-503.

135. Fujiwara Y, Tatsumi M. Cross-link repair in human cells and its possible defect in Fanconi's anemia cells. J Mol Biol. 1977;113:635-649.

136. Papadopoulo D, Guillouf C, Mohrenweiser H, Moustacchi E. Hypomutability in Fanconi anemia cells is associated with increased deletion frequency at the HPRT locus. Proc Natl Acad Sci U S A. 1990;87:8383-8387.

137. Sala-Trepat M, Boyse J, Richard P, et al. Frequencies of HPRT− lymphocytes and glycophorin A variants erythrocytes in Fanconi anemia patients, their parents and control donors. Mutat Res. 1993;289:115-126.

138. Araten DJ, Golde DW, Zhang RH, et al. A quantitative measurement of the human somatic mutation rate. Cancer Res. 2005;65:8111-8117.

139. Laquerbe A, Sala-Trepat M, Vives C, et al. Molecular spectra of HPRT deletion mutations in circulating T-lymphocytes in Fanconi anemia patients. Mutat Res. 1999;431:341-350.

140. Evdokimova VN, McLoughlin RK, Wenger SL, Grant SG. Use of the glycophorin A somatic mutation assay for rapid, unambiguous identification of Fanconi anemia homozygotes regardless of GPA genotype. Am J Med Genet A. 2005;135:59-65.

141. Willingale-Theune J, Schweiger M, Hirsch-Kauffmann M, et al. Ultrastructure of Fanconi anemia fibroblasts. J Cell Sci. 1989;93:651-665.

142. Kupfer GM, D'Andrea AD. The effect of the Fanconi anemia polypeptide, FAC, upon p53 induction and G_2 checkpoint regulation. Blood. 1996;88:1019-1025.

143. Wang J, Otsuki T, Youssoufian H, et al. Overexpression of the Fanconi anemia group C gene (FAC) protects hematopoietic progenitors from death induced by Fas-mediated apoptosis. Cancer Res. 1998;58:3538-3541.

144. Rosselli F, Ridet A, Soussi T, et al. p53-dependent pathway of radio-induced apoptosis is altered in Fanconi anemia. Oncogene. 1995;10:9-17.

145. Akkari YM, Bateman RL, Reifsteck CA, et al. The 4N cell cycle delay in Fanconi anemia reflects growth arrest in late S phase. Mol Genet Metab. 2001;74:403-412.

146. Sala-Trepat M, Rouillard D, Escarceller M, et al. Arrest of S-phase progression is impaired in Fanconi anemia cells. Exp Cell Res. 2000;260:208-215.

147. Escarceller M, Rousset S, Moustacchi E, Papadopoulo D. The fidelity of double strand breaks processing is impaired in complementation groups B and D of Fanconi anemia, a genetic instability syndrome. Somat Cell Mol Genet. 1997;23:401-411.

148. Lundberg R, Mavinakere M, Campbell C. Deficient DNA end joining activity in extracts from Fanconi anemia fibroblasts. J Biol Chem. 2001;276:9543-9549.

149. Escarceller M, Buchwald M, Singleton BK, et al. Fanconi anemia C gene product plays a role in the fidelity of blunt DNA end-joining. J Mol Biol. 1998;279:375-385.

150. Thyagarajan B, Campbell C. Elevated homologous recombination activity in Fanconi anemia fibroblasts. J Biol Chem. 1997;272:23328-23333.

151. Donahue SL, Lundberg R, Saplis R, Campbell C. Deficient regulation of DNA double-strand break repair in Fanconi anemia fibroblasts. J Biol Chem. 2003;278:29487-29495.

152. Saunders EF, Freedman MH. Constitutional aplastic anaemia: defective haematopoietic stem cell growth in vitro. Br J Haematol. 1978;40:277-287.

153. Daneshbod-Skibba G, Martin J, Shahidi NT. Myeloid and erythroid colony growth in non-anaemic patients with Fanconi's anaemia. Br J Haematol. 1980;44:33-38.

154. Lui VK, Ragab AH, Findley HS, Frauen BJ. Bone marrow cultures in children with Fanconi anemia and the TAR syndrome. J Pediatr. 1977;91:952-954.

155. Whitney MA, Royle G, Low MJ, et al. Germ cell defects and hematopoietic hypersensitivity to gamma-interferon in mice with a targeted disruption of the Fanconi anemia C gene. Blood. 1996;88:49-58.

156. Nadler JJ, Braun RE. Fanconi anemia complementation group C is required for proliferation of murine primordial germ cells. Genesis. 2000;27:117-123.

157. D'Andrea AD, Grompe M. Molecular biology of Fanconi anemia: implications for diagnosis and therapy. Blood. 1997;90:1725-1736.

158. Cervenka J, Hirsch BA. Cytogenetic differentiation of Fanconi anemia, "idiopathic" aplastic anemia, and Fanconi anemia heterozygotes. Am J Med Genet. 1983;15:211-223.

159. Auerbach AD, Adler B, O'Reilly RJ, et al. Effect of procarbazine and cyclophosphamide on chromosome breakage in Fanconi anemia cells: relevance to bone marrow transplantation. Cancer Genet Cytogenet. 1983;9:25-36.

159a. Schindler D, Seyschab H, Poot M, et al. Screening test for ataxia telangiectasia. Lancet 1987;2:1389-1399.

160. Meetei AR, Sechi S, Wallisch M, et al. A multiprotein nuclear complex connects Fanconi anemia and Bloom syndrome. Mol Cell Biol. 2003;23:3417-3426.

161. Pichierri P, Franchitto A, Rosselli F. BLM and the FANC proteins collaborate in a common pathway in response to stalled replication forks. EMBO J. 2004;23:3154-3163.

162. Resnick IB, Kondratenko I, Togoev O, et al. Nijmegen breakage syndrome: clinical characteristics and mutation analysis in eight unrelated Russian families. J Pediatr. 2002;140:355-361.

163. Pichierri P, Averbeck D, Rosselli F. DNA cross-link-dependent RAD50/MRE11/NBS1 subnuclear assembly requires the Fanconi anemia C protein. Hum Mol Genet. 2002;11:2531-2546.

164. O'Driscoll M, Gennery AR, Seidel J, et al. An overview of three new disorders associated with genetic instability: LIG4 syndrome, RS-SCID and ATR-Seckel syndrome. DNA Repair (Amst). 2004;3:1227-1235.

165. O'Driscoll M, Cerosaletti KM, Girard PM, et al. DNA ligase IV mutations identified in patients exhibiting developmental delay and immunodeficiency. Mol Cell. 2001;8:1175-1185.

166. Foe JR, Rooimans MA, Bosnoyan-Collins L, et al. Expression cloning of a cDNA for the major Fanconi anaemia gene, FAA. Nat Genet. 1996;14:320-323 (Erratum: Nat Genet. 1996;14:1488.

167. Meetei AR, Levitus M, Xue Y, et al. X-linked inheritance of Fanconi anemia complementation group B. Nat Genet. 2004;36:1219-1224.

168. Strathdee CA, Gavish H, Shannon WR, Buchwald M. Cloning of cDNAs for Fanconi's anaemia by functional complementation. Nature. 1992;356:763-767.

169. Howlett NG, Taniguchi T, Olson S, et al. Biallelic inactivation of BRCA2 in Fanconi anemia. Science. 2002;297:606-609.

170. Timmers C, Taniguchi T, Hejna J, et al. Positional cloning of a novel Fanconi anemia gene, FANCD2. Mol Cell. 2001;7:241-248.

171. de Winter JP, Leveille F, van Berkel CG, et al. Isolation of a cDNA representing the Fanconi anemia complementation group E gene. Am J Hum Genet. 2000;67:1306-1308.

172. de Winter JP, Rooimans MA, van Der Weel L, et al. The Fanconi anaemia gene FANCF encodes a novel protein with homology to ROM. Nat Genet. 2000;24:15-16.

173. de Winter JP, Waisfisz Q, Rooimans MA, et al. The Fanconi anaemia group G gene FANCG is identical with XRCC9. Nat Genet. 1998;20:281-283.

174. Sims AE, Spiteri E, Sims RJ, 3rd, et al. FANCI is a second monoubiquitinated member of the Fanconi anemia pathway. Nat Struct Mol Biol. 2007;14:564-567.

175. Dorsman JC, Levitus M, Rockx D, et al. Identification of the Fanconi anemia complementation group I gene, FANCI. Cell Oncol. 2007;29:211-218.

176. Smogorzewska A, Matsuoka S, Vinciguerra P, et al. Identification of the FANCI protein, a monoubiquitinated FANCD2 paralog required for DNA repair. Cell. 2007;129:289-301.

177. Levitus M, Rooimans MA, Steltenpool J, et al. Heterogeneity in Fanconi anemia: evidence for 2 new genetic subtypes. Blood. 2004;103:2498-2503.

178. Levitus M, Waisfisz Q, Godthelp BC, et al. The DNA helicase BRIP1 is defective in Fanconi anemia complementation group J. Nat Genet. 2005;37:934-935.

179. Levran O, Attwooll C, Henry RT, et al. The BRCA1-interacting helicase BRIP1 is deficient in Fanconi anemia. Nat Genet. 2005;37:931-933.

180. Meetei AR, de Winter JP, Medhurst AL, et al. A novel ubiquitin ligase is deficient in Fanconi anemia. Nat Genet. 2003;35:165-170.

181. Meetei AR, Medhurst AL, Ling C, et al. A human ortholog of archaeal DNA repair protein Hef is defective in Fanconi anemia complementation group M. Nat Genet. 2005;37:958-963.

182. Xia B, Dorsman JC, Ameziane N, et al. Fanconi anemia is associated with a defect in the BRCA2 partner PALB2. Nat Genet. 2007;39:159-161.

183. Rahman N, Seal S, Thompson D, et al. PALB2, which encodes a BRCA2-interacting protein, is a breast cancer susceptibility gene. Nat Genet. 2007;39:165-167.

184. Taniguchi T, D'Andrea AD. Molecular pathogenesis of Fanconi anemia: recent progress. Blood. 2006;107:4223-4233.

185. Levitus M, Joenje H, de Winter JP. The Fanconi anemia pathway of genomic maintenance. Cell Oncol. 2006;28:3-29.

186. Wang W. Emergence of a DNA-damage response network consisting of Fanconi anaemia and BRCA proteins. Nat Rev Genet. 2007;8:735-748.

187. Duckworth-Rysiecki G, Cornish K, Clarke CA, Buchwald M. Identification of two complementation groups in Fanconi anemia. Somat Cell Mol Genet. 1985;11:35-41.

188. Strathdee CA, Duncan AM, Buchwald M. Evidence for at least four Fanconi anaemia genes including FACC on chromosome 9. Nat Genet. 1992;1:196-198.

189. Joenje H, Lo ten Foe JR, Oostra AB, et al. Classification of Fanconi anemia patients by complementation analysis: evidence for a fifth genetic subtype. Blood. 1995;86:2156-2160.

190. Joenje H, Levitus M, Waisfisz Q, et al. Complementation analysis in Fanconi anemia: assignment of the reference FA-H patient to group A. Am J Hum Genet. 2000;67:759-762.

191. Chandra S, Levran O, Jurickova I, et al. A rapid method for retrovirus-mediated identification of complementation groups in Fanconi anemia patients. Mol Ther. 2005;12:976-984.

192. Lo Ten Foe JR, Rooimans MA, Bosnoyan-Collins L, et al. Expression cloning of a cDNA for the major Fanconi anaemia gene, FAA. Nat Genet. 1996;14:320-323.

193. Positional cloning of the Fanconi anaemia group A gene. The Fanconi anaemia/breast cancer consortium. Nat Genet. 1996;14:324-328.

194. Whitney M, Thayer M, Reifsteck C, et al. Microcell mediated chromosome transfer maps the Fanconi anaemia group D gene to chromosome 3p. Nat Genet. 1995;11:341-343.

195. Litman R, Peng M, Jin Z, et al. BACH1 is critical for homologous recombination and appears to be the Fanconi anemia gene product FANCJ. Cancer Cell. 2005;8:255-265.

196. Dean SW, Fox M. Investigation of the cell cycle response of normal and Fanconi's anaemia fibroblasts to nitrogen mustard using flow cytometry. J Cell Sci. 1983;64:265-279.

197. Folias A, Matkovic M, Bruun D, et al. BRCA1 interacts directly with the Fanconi anemia protein FANCA. Hum Mol Genet. 2002;11:2591-2597.

198. Taniguchi T, Garcia-Higuera I, Andreassen PR, et al. S-phase–specific interaction of the Fanconi anemia protein, FANCD2, with BRCA1 and RAD51. Blood. 2002;100:2414-2420.

199. Taniguchi T, Garcia-Higuera I, Xu B, et al. Convergence of the Fanconi anemia and ataxia telangiectasia signaling pathways. Cell. 2002;109:459-472.

200. Pichierri P, Rosselli F. The DNA crosslink-induced S-phase checkpoint depends on ATR-CHK1 and ATR-NBS1-FANCD2 pathways. EMBO J. 2004;23:1178-1187.

201. Rothfuss A, Grompe M. Repair kinetics of genomic interstrand DNA cross-links: evidence for DNA double-strand break-dependent activation of the Fanconi anemia/BRCA pathway. Mol Cell Biol. 2004;24:123-134.

202. Mi J, Kupfer GM. The Fanconi anemia core complex associates with chromatin during S phase. Blood. 2005;105:759-766.

203. Montes de Oca R, Andreassen PR, Margossian SP, et al. Regulated interaction of the Fanconi anemia protein, FANCD2, with chromatin. Blood. 2005;105:1003-1009.

204. Wang X, D'Andrea AD. The interplay of Fanconi anemia proteins in the DNA damage response. DNA Repair (Amst). 2004;3:1063-1069.

205. Wang X, Andreassen PR, D'Andrea AD. Functional interaction of monoubiquitinated FANCD2 and BRCA2/FANCD1 in chromatin. Mol Cell Biol. 2004;24:5850-5862.

206. Park WH, Margossian S, Horwitz AA, et al. Direct DNA binding activity of the Fanconi anemia D2 protein. J Biol Chem. 2005;280:23593-23598.

207. Zhu W, Dutta A. An ATR- and BRCA1-mediated Fanconi anemia pathway is required for activating the G_2/M checkpoint and DNA damage repair upon rereplication. Mol Cell Biol. 2006;26:4601-4611.

208. Hinz JM, Nham PB, Salazar EP, Thompson LH. The Fanconi anemia pathway limits the severity of mutagenesis. DNA Repair (Amst). 2006;5:875-884.

209. Gurtan AM, D'Andrea AD. Dedicated to the core: Understanding the Fanconi anemia complex. DNA Repair (Amst). 2006;5:1119-1125.

210. Sobeck A, Stone S, Costanzo V, et al. Fanconi anemia proteins are required to prevent accumulation of replication-associated DNA double-strand breaks. Mol Cell Biol. 2006;26:425-437.

211. Niedernhofer LJ, Lalai AS, Hoeijmakers JH. Fanconi anemia (cross)linked to DNA repair. Cell. 2005;123:1191-1198.

212. Fei P, Yin J, Wang W. New advances in the DNA damage response network of Fanconi anemia and BRCA proteins. FAAP95 replaces BRCA2 as the true FANCB protein. Cell Cycle. 2005;4:80-86.

213. Collins N, Kupfer GM. Molecular pathogenesis of Fanconi anemia. Int J Hematol. 2005;82:176-183.

214. Niedzwiedz W, Mosedale G, Johnson M, et al. The Fanconi anaemia gene FANCC promotes homologous recombination and error-prone DNA repair. Mol Cell. 2004;15:607-620.

215. Kennedy RD, D'Andrea AD. The Fanconi anemia/BRCA pathway: new faces in the crowd. Genes Dev. 2005;19:2925-2940.

216. Kennedy RD, D'Andrea AD. DNA repair pathways in clinical practice: lessons from pediatric cancer susceptibility syndromes. J Clin Oncol. 2006;24:3799-3808.

217. Hoeijmakers JH. Genome maintenance mechanisms for preventing cancer. Nature. 2001;411:366-374.

218. Thompson LH, Hinz JM, Yamada NA, Jones NJ. How Fanconi anemia proteins promote the four Rs: replication, recombination, repair, and recovery. Environ Mol Mutagen. 2005;45:128-142.

219. Nookala RK, Hussain S, Pellegrini L. Insights into Fanconi anaemia from the structure of human FANCE. Nucleic Acids Res. 2007;35:1638-1648.

220. Qiao F, Moss A, Kupfer GM. Fanconi anemia proteins localize to chromatin and the nuclear matrix in a DNA damage- and cell cycle–regulated manner. J Biol Chem. 2001;276:23391-22396.

221. Grompe M, D'Andrea A. Fanconi anemia and DNA repair. Hum Mol Genet. 2001;10:2253-2259.

222. Howlett NG, Taniguchi T, Durkin SG, et al. The Fanconi anemia pathway is required for the DNA replication stress response and for the regulation of common fragile site stability. Hum Mol Genet. 2005;14:693-701.

223. Hussain S, Wilson JB, Medhurst AL, et al. Direct interaction of FANCD2 with BRCA2 in DNA damage response pathways. Hum Mol Genet. 2004;13:1241-1248.

224. Ho GP, Margossian S, Taniguchi T, D'Andrea AD. Phosphorylation of FANCD2 on two novel sites is required for mitomycin C resistance. Mol Cell Biol. 2006;26: 7005-7015.

225. Cantor S, Drapkin R, Zhang F, et al. The BRCA1-associated protein BACH1 is a DNA helicase targeted by clinically relevant inactivating mutations. Proc Natl Acad Sci U S A. 2004;101:2357-2362.

226. Hoatlin ME, Christianson TA, Keeble WW, et al. The Fanconi anemia group C gene product is located in both the nucleus and cytoplasm of human cells. Blood. 1998;91:1418-1425.

227. Thomashevski A, High AA, Drozd M, et al. The Fanconi anemia core complex forms four complexes of different sizes in different subcellular compartments. J Biol Chem. 2004;279:26201-26209.

228. Medhurst AL, Laghmani EH, Steltenpool J, et al. Evidence for subcomplexes in the Fanconi anaemia pathway. Blood. 2006;108:2072-2080.

229. Leveille F, Ferrer M, Medhurst AL, et al. The nuclear accumulation of the Fanconi anemia protein FANCE depends on FANCC. DNA Repair (Amst). 2006;5: 556-565.

230. Pang Q, Fagerlie S, Christianson TA, et al. The Fanconi anemia protein FANCC binds to and facilitates the activation of STAT1 by gamma interferon and hematopoietic growth factors. Mol Cell Biol. 2000;20:4724-4735.

231. Pang Q, Christianson TA, Keeble W, et al. The Fanconi anemia complementation group C gene product: structural evidence of multifunctionality. Blood. 2001;98: 1392-1401.

232. Pang Q, Keeble W, Christianson TA, et al. FANCC interacts with Hsp70 to protect hematopoietic cells from IFN-gamma/TNF-alpha–mediated cytotoxicity. EMBO J. 2001;20:4478-4489.

233. Pang Q, Christianson TA, Keeble W, et al. The antiapoptotic function of Hsp70 in the interferon-inducible double-stranded RNA–dependent protein kinase–mediated death signaling pathway requires the Fanconi anemia protein, FANCC. J Biol Chem. 2002;277: 49638-49643.

234. Pang Q, Keeble W, Diaz J, et al. Role of double-stranded RNA–dependent protein kinase in mediating hypersensitivity of Fanconi anemia complementation group C cells to interferon gamma, tumor necrosis factor-alpha, and double-stranded RNA. Blood. 2001;97:1644-1652.

235. Zhang X, Li J, Sejas DP, et al. The Fanconi anemia proteins functionally interact with the protein kinase regulated by RNA (PKR). J Biol Chem. 2004;279: 43910-43919.

236. Liebetrau W, Budde A, Savoia A, et al. p53 activates Fanconi anemia group C gene expression. Hum Mol Genet. 1997;6:277-283.

237. Freie B, Li X, Ciccone SL, et al. Fanconi anemia type C and p53 cooperate in apoptosis and tumorigenesis. Blood. 2003;102:4146-4152.

238. Bagby GC, Alter BP. Fanconi anemia. Semin Hematol. 2006;43:147-156.

239. Zhang X, Sejas DP, Qiu Y, et al. Inflammatory ROS promote and cooperate with the Fanconi anemia mutation for hematopoietic senescence. J Cell Sci. 2007;120: 1572-1583.

240. Joenje H, Youssoufian H, Kruyt FA, et al. Expression of the Fanconi anemia gene FAC in human cell lines: lack of effect of oxygen tension. Blood Cells Mol Dis. 1995;21:182-191.

241. Lackinger D, Ruppitsch W, Ramirez MH, et al. Involvement of the Fanconi anemia protein FA-C in repair processes of oxidative DNA damages. FEBS Lett. 1998;440:103-106.

242. Futaki M, Igarashi T, Watanabe S, et al. The FANCG Fanconi anemia protein interacts with CYP2E1: possible role in protection against oxidative DNA damage. Carcinogenesis. 2002;23:67-72.

243. Joenje H, Oostra AB. Effect of oxygen tension on chromosomal aberrations in Fanconi anaemia. Hum Genet. 1983;65:99-101.

244. Joenje H, Oostra AB. Oxygen-induced cytogenetic instability in normal human lymphocytes. Hum Genet. 1986; 74:438-440.

245. Porfirio B, Ambroso G, Giannella G, et al. Partial correction of chromosome instability in Fanconi anemia by desferrioxamine. Hum Genet. 1989;83: 49-51.

246. Rumiantsev AG, Samochatova EV, Afanas'ev IB, et al. [The role of free oxygen radicals in the pathogenesis of Fanconi's anemia.] Ter Arkh. 1989;61:32-36.

247. Liebetrau W, Runger TM, Mehling BE, et al. Mutagenic activity of ambient oxygen and mitomycin C in Fanconi's anaemia cells. Mutagenesis. 1997;12:69-77.

248. Pagano G, Youssoufian H. Fanconi anaemia proteins: major roles in cell protection against oxidative damage. Bioessays. 2003;25:589-595.

249. Sprong D, Janssen HL, Vens C, Begg AC. Resistance of hypoxic cells to ionizing radiation is influenced by homologous recombination status. Int J Radiat Oncol Biol Phys. 2006;64:562-572.

250. Levran O, Diotti R, Pujara K, et al. Spectrum of sequence variations in the FANCA gene: an International Fanconi Anemia Registry (IFAR) study. Hum Mutat. 2005;25: 142-149.

251. Fokkema IF, den Dunnen JT, Taschner PE. LOVD: easy creation of a locus-specific sequence variation database using an "LSDB-in-a-box" approach. Hum Mutat. 2005;26:63-68.

252. Kutler DI, Auerbach AD. Fanconi anemia in Ashkenazi Jews. Fam Cancer. 2004;3:241-248.

253. Whitney MA, Saito H, Jakobs PM, et al. A common mutation in the FACC gene causes Fanconi anaemia in Ashkenazi Jews. Nat Genet. 1993;4:202-205.

254. Auerbach AD, Greenbaum J, Pujara K, et al. Spectrum of sequence variation in the FANCG gene: an International Fanconi Anemia Registry (IFAR) study. Hum Mutat. 2003;21:158-168.

255. Barber LM, Barlow RA, Meyer S, et al. Inherited FANCD1/BRCA2 exon 7 splice mutations associated with acute myeloid leukaemia in Fanconi anaemia D1 are not found in sporadic childhood leukaemia. Br J Haematol. 2005;130:796-797.

256. Alter BP. The association between FANCD1/BRCA2 mutations and leukaemia. Br J Haematol. 2006;133:446-448; author reply 448.

257. den Dunnen JT, Antonarakis SE. Mutation nomenclature extensions and suggestions to describe complex mutations: a discussion. Hum Mutat. 2000;15:7-12.

258. Bouchlaka C, Abdelhak S, Amouri A, et al. Fanconi anemia in Tunisia: high prevalence of group A and identification of new FANCA mutations. J Hum Genet. 2003;48:352-361.

259. Yagasaki H, Hamanoue S, Oda T, et al. Identification and characterization of novel mutations of the major Fanconi anemia gene FANCA in the Japanese population. Hum Mutat. 2004;24:481-490.

260. Levran O, Doggett NA, Auerbach AD. Identification of Alu-mediated deletions in the Fanconi anemia gene FAA. Hum Mutat. 1998;12:145-152.

261. Centra M, Memeo E, d'Apolito M, et al. Fine exon-intron structure of the Fanconi anemia group A (FAA) gene and characterization of two genomic deletions. Genomics. 1998;51:463-467.

262. Morgan NV, Tipping AJ, Joenje H, Mathew CG. High frequency of large intragenic deletions in the Fanconi anemia group A gene. Am J Hum Genet. 1999;65:1330-1341.

263. Wijker M, Morgan NV, Herterich S, et al. Heterogeneous spectrum of mutations in the Fanconi anaemia group A gene. Eur J Hum Genet. 1999;7:52-59.

264. Callen E, Tischkowitz MD, Creus A, et al. Quantitative PCR analysis reveals a high incidence of large intragenic deletions in the FANCA gene in Spanish Fanconi anemia patients. Cytogenet Genome Res. 2004;104:341-345.

265. Gibson RA, Morgan NV, Goldstein LH, et al. Novel mutations and polymorphisms in the Fanconi anemia group C gene. Hum Mutat. 1996;8:140-148.

266. Kalb R, Neveling K, Hoehn H, et al. Hypomorphic mutations in the gene encoding a key Fanconi anemia protein, FANCD2, sustain a significant group of FA-D2 patients with severe phenotype. Am J Hum Genet. 2007;80:895-910.

267. Alter BP, Rosenberg PS, Brody LC. Clinical and molecular features associated with biallelic mutations in FANCD1/BRCA2. J Med Genet. 2007;44:1-9.

268. Kuliev A, Rechitsky S, Tur-Kaspa I, Verlinsky Y. Preimplantation genetics: Improving access to stem cell therapy. Ann N Y Acad Sci. 2005;1054:223-227.

269. Damewood MD. Ethical implications of a new application of preimplantation diagnosis. JAMA. 2001;285:3143-3144.

270. Verlinsky Y, Rechitsky S, Schoolcraft W, et al. Preimplantation diagnosis for Fanconi anemia combined with HLA matching. JAMA. 2001;285:3130-3133.

271. Burgio GR, Gluckman E, Locatelli F. Ethical reappraisal of 15 years of cord-blood transplantation. Lancet. 2003;361:250-252.

272. Wolf SM, Kahn JP, Wagner JE. Using preimplantation genetic diagnosis to create a stem cell donor: issues, guidelines & limits. J Law Med Ethics. 2003;31:327-339.

273. Antonio Casado J, Callen E, Jacome A, et al. A comprehensive strategy for the subtyping of patients with Fanconi anaemia: conclusions from the Spanish Fanconi Anemia Research Network. J Med Genet. 2007;44:241-249.

274. Ameziane N, Errami A, Leveille F, et al. Genetic subtyping of Fanconi anemia by comprehensive mutation screening. Hum Mutat. 2008;29:159-166.

275. Welshimer K, Swift M. Congenital malformations and developmental disabilities in ataxia-telangiectasia, Fanconi anemia, and xeroderma pigmentosum families. Am J Hum Genet. 1982;34:781-793.

276. Berwick M, Satagopan JM, Ben-Porat L, et al. Genetic heterogeneity among Fanconi anemia heterozygotes and risk of cancer. Cancer Res. 2007;67:9591-9596.

277. King MC, Marks JH, Mandell JB. Breast and ovarian cancer risks due to inherited mutations in BRCA1 and BRCA2. Science. 2003;302:643-646.

278. Liede A, Karlan BY, Narod SA. Cancer risks for male carriers of germline mutations in BRCA1 or BRCA2: a review of the literature. J Clin Oncol. 2004;22:735-742.

279. Hahn SA, Greenhalf B, Ellis I, et al. BRCA2 germline mutations in familial pancreatic carcinoma. J Natl Cancer Inst. 2003;95:214-221.

280. Couch FJ, Johnson MR, Rabe K, et al. Germ line Fanconi anemia complementation group C mutations and pancreatic cancer. Cancer Res. 2005;65:383-386.

281. van der Heijden MS, Brody JR, Gallmeier E, et al. Functional defects in the Fanconi anemia pathway in pancreatic cancer cells. Am J Pathol. 2004;165:651-657.

282. Condie A, Powles RL, Hudson CD, et al. Analysis of the Fanconi anaemia complementation group A gene in acute myeloid leukaemia. Leuk Lymphoma. 2002;43:1849-1853.

283. Tischkowitz MD, Morgan NV, Grimwade D, et al. Deletion and reduced expression of the Fanconi anemia FANCA gene in sporadic acute myeloid leukemia. Leukemia. 2004;18:420-425.

284. Dhillon VS, Shahid M, Husain SA. CpG methylation of the FHIT, FANCF, cyclin-D2, BRCA2 and RUNX3 genes in granulosa cell tumors (GCTs) of ovarian origin. Mol Cancer. 2004;3:33.

285. Olopade OI, Wei M. FANCF methylation contributes to chemoselectivity in ovarian cancer. Cancer Cell. 2003;3:417-420.

286. Marsit CJ, Liu M, Nelson HH, et al. Inactivation of the Fanconi anemia/BRCA pathway in lung and oral cancers: implications for treatment and survival. Oncogene. 2004;23:1000-1004.

287. Narayan G, Arias-Pulido H, Nandula SV, et al. Promoter hypermethylation of FANCF: disruption of Fanconi anemia–BRCA pathway in cervical cancer. Cancer Res. 2004;64:2994-2997.

288. Koul S, McKiernan JM, Narayan G, et al. Role of promoter hypermethylation in cisplatin treatment response of male germ cell tumors. Mol Cancer. 2004;3:16.

289. Taniguchi T, Tischkowitz M, Ameziane N, et al. Disruption of the Fanconi anemia–BRCA pathway in cisplatin-sensitive ovarian tumors. Nat Med. 2003;9:568-574.

290. Teodoridis JM, Hall J, Marsh S, et al. CpG island methylation of DNA damage response genes in advanced ovarian cancer. Cancer Res. 2005;65:8961-8967.

291. Xie Y, de Winter JP, Waisfisz Q, et al. Aberrant Fanconi anaemia protein profiles in acute myeloid leukaemia cells. Br J Haematol. 2000;111:1057-1064.

292. Lensch MW, Tischkowitz M, Christianson TA, et al. Acquired FANCA dysfunction and cytogenetic instability in adult acute myelogenous leukemia. Blood. 2003;102:7-16.

293. Tischkowitz M, Ameziane N, Waisfisz Q, et al. Bi-allelic silencing of the Fanconi anaemia gene FANCF in acute myeloid leukaemia. Br J Haematol. 2003;123:469-471.

294. Rogers CD, van der Heijden MS, Brune K, et al. The genetics of FANCC and FANCG in familial pancreatic cancer. Cancer Biol Ther. 2004;3:167-169.

295. Hilton JL, Geisler JP, Rathe JA, et al. Inactivation of BRCA1 and BRCA2 in ovarian cancer. J Natl Cancer Inst. 2002;94:1396-1406.

296. van der Groep P, Hoelzel M, Buerger H, et al. Loss of expression of FANCD2 protein in sporadic and hereditary breast cancer. Breast Cancer Res Treat. 2008;107:41-47.

297. Gallmeier E, Hucl T, Brody JR, et al. High-throughput screening identifies novel agents eliciting hypersensitivity in Fanconi pathway–deficient cancer cells. Cancer Res. 2007;67:2169-2177.

298. Jimeno A, Hidalgo M. Molecular biomarkers: their increasing role in the diagnosis, characterization, and therapy guidance in pancreatic cancer. Mol Cancer Ther. 2006;5:787-796.

299. Mathew CG. Fanconi anaemia genes and susceptibility to cancer. Oncogene. 2006;25:5875-5884.

300. Hirschhorn R. In vivo reversion to normal of inherited mutations in humans. J Med Genet. 2003;40:721-728.

301. Waisfisz Q, Morgan NV, Savino M, et al. Spontaneous functional correction of homozygous Fanconi anaemia alleles reveals novel mechanistic basis for reverse mosaicism. Nat Genet. 1999;22:379-383.

302. Mankad A, Taniguchi T, Cox B, et al. Natural gene therapy in monozygotic twins with Fanconi anemia. Blood. 2006;107:3084-3090.

303. Hamanoue S, Yagasaki H, Tsuruta T, et al. Myeloid lineage–selective growth of revertant cells in Fanconi anaemia. Br J Haematol. 2006;132:630-635.

304. Gregory JJ Jr, Wagner JE, Verlander PC, et al. Somatic mosaicism in Fanconi anemia: evidence of genotypic reversion in lymphohematopoietic stem cells. Proc Natl Acad Sci U S A. 2001;98:2532-2537.

305. Ikeda H, Matsushita M, Waisfisz Q, et al. Genetic reversion in an acute myelogenous leukemia cell line from a Fanconi anemia patient with biallelic mutations in BRCA2. Cancer Res. 2003;63:2688-2694.

306. Alter BP, Joenje H, Oostra AB, Pals G. Fanconi anemia: adult head and neck cancer and hematopoietic mosaicism. Arch Otolaryngol Head Neck Surg. 2005;131:635-639.

307. Chen M, Tomkins DJ, Auerbach W, et al. Inactivation of Fac in mice produces inducible chromosomal instability and reduced fertility reminiscent of Fanconi anaemia. Nat Genet. 1996;12:448-451.

308. Rio P, Segovia JC, Hanenberg H, et al. In vitro phenotypic correction of hematopoietic progenitors from Fanconi anemia group A knockout mice. Blood. 2002;100:2032-2039.

309. Yang Y, Kuang Y, Montes De Oca R, et al. Targeted disruption of the murine Fanconi anemia gene, Fancg/Xrcc9. Blood. 2001;98:3435-3440.

310. Houghtaling S, Timmers C, Noll M, et al. Epithelial cancer in Fanconi anemia complementation group D2 (Fancd2) knockout mice. Genes Dev. 2003;17:2021-2035.

311. Navarro S, Meza NW, Quintana-Bustamante O, et al. Hematopoietic dysfunction in a mouse model for Fanconi anemia group D1. Mol Ther. 2006;14:525-535.

312. Wong JC, Alon N, McKerlie C, et al. Targeted disruption of exons 1 to 6 of the Fanconi anemia group A gene leads to growth retardation, strain-specific microphthalmia, meiotic defects and primordial germ cell hypoplasia. Hum Mol Genet. 2003;12:2063-2076.

313. Carreau M. Not-so-novel phenotypes in the Fanconi anemia group D2 mouse model. Blood. 2004;103:2430.

314. Houghtaling S, Granville L, Akkari Y, et al. Heterozygosity for p53 (Trp53+/−) accelerates epithelial tumor formation in Fanconi anemia complementation group D2 (Fancd2) knockout mice. Cancer Res. 2005;65:85-91.

315. Rathbun RK, Christianson TA, Faulkner GR, et al. Interferon-gamma–induced apoptotic responses of Fanconi anemia group C hematopoietic progenitor cells involve caspase 8–dependent activation of caspase 3 family members. Blood. 2000;96:4204-4211.

316. Nathan DG, Alter BP, Shimamura A, et al. Fanconi anemia; standards for clinical care. In Alter BP, Bagby G (eds). Fanconi Anemia Standards for Clinical Care Conference, 2nd ed. Chicago, Fanconi Anemia Reserach Fund, 2003.

317. Shimamura A. Treatment of hematologic abnormalities in FA. In Nathan DG (ed). Fanconi Anemia Standards for Clinical Care Conference. Chicago, Fanconi Anemia Research Fund, 2003, pp 23-36.

318. Mehta PA, Ileri T, Harris RE, et al. Chemotherapy for myeloid malignancy in children with Fanconi anemia. Pediatr Blood Cancer. 2007;48:668-672.

319. Shahidi NT, Diamond LK. Testosterone-induced remission in aplastic anemia of both acquired and congenital types. Further observations in 24 cases. N Engl J Med. 1961;264:953-967.

320. Diamond LK, Shahidi NT. Treatment of aplastic anemia in children. Semin Hematol. 1967;4:278-288.

321. Guinan EC, Lopez KD, Huhn RD, et al. Evaluation of granulocyte-macrophage colony-stimulating factor for treatment of pancytopenia in children with Fanconi anemia. J Pediatr. 1994;124:144-150.

322. Rackoff WR, Orazi A, Robinson CA, et al. Prolonged administration of granulocyte colony-stimulating factor (filgrastim) to patients with Fanconi anemia: a pilot study. Blood. 1996;88:1588-1593.

323. Shahidi NT, Crigler JF Jr. Evaluation of growth and of endocrine systems in testosterone-corticosteroid–treated patients with aplastic anemia. J Pediatr. 1967;70:233-242.

324. Gluckman E. Radiosensitivity in Fanconi anemia: application to the conditioning for bone marrow transplantation. Radiother Oncol. 1990;18(Suppl 1):88-93.

325. Gluckman E, Auerbach AD, Horowitz MM, et al. Bone marrow transplantation for Fanconi anemia. Blood. 1995;86:2856-2862.

326. Berger R, Bernheim A, Gluckman E, Gisselbrecht C. In vitro effect of cyclophosphamide metabolites on chromosomes of Fanconi anaemia patients. Br J Haematol. 1980;45:565-568.

327. Gluckman E, Devergie A, Dutreix J. Radiosensitivity in Fanconi anaemia: application to the conditioning regimen for bone marrow transplantation. Br J Haematol. 1983;54:431-440.

328. Gluckman E. Bone marrow transplantation in Fanconi's anemia. Stem Cells. 1993;11(Suppl 2):180-183.
329. Guardiola P, Socie G, Pasquini R, et al. Allogeneic stem cell transplantation for Fanconi anaemia. Severe Aplastic Anaemia Working Party of the EBMT and EUFAR. European Group for Blood and Marrow Transplantation. Bone Marrow Transplant. 1998;21(Suppl 2):S24-S27.
330. Ayas M, Al-Jefri A, Al-Mahr M, et al. Allogeneic stem cell transplantation in patients with Fanconi's anemia and myelodysplasia or leukemia utilizing low-dose cyclophosphamide and total body irradiation. Bone Marrow Transplant. 2004;33:15-17.
331. Davies SM, Khan S, Wagner JE, et al. Unrelated donor bone marrow transplantation for Fanconi anemia. Bone Marrow Transplant. 1996;17:43-47.
332. Socie G, Henry-Amar M, Cosset JM, et al. Increased incidence of solid malignant tumors after bone marrow transplantation for severe aplastic anemia. Blood. 1991;78:277-279.
333. Socie G, Devergie A, Girinski T, et al. Transplantation for Fanconi's anaemia: long-term follow-up of fifty patients transplanted from a sibling donor after low-dose cyclophosphamide and thoraco-abdominal irradiation for conditioning. Br J Haematol. 1998;103:249-255.
334. Guardiola P, Socie G, Li X, et al. Acute graft-versus-host disease in patients with Fanconi anemia or acquired aplastic anemia undergoing bone marrow transplantation from HLA-identical sibling donors: risk factors and influence on outcome. Blood. 2004;103:73-77.
335. Ayas M, Al-Jefri A, Al-Mahr M, et al. Stem cell transplantation for patients with Fanconi anemia with low-dose cyclophosphamide and antithymocyte globulins without the use of radiation therapy. Bone Marrow Transplant. 2005;35:463-466.
336. Motwani J, Lawson SE, Darbyshire PJ. Successful HSCT using nonradiotherapy-based conditioning regimens and alternative donors in patients with Fanconi anaemia—experience in a single UK centre. Bone Marrow Transplant. 2005;36:405-410.
337. de la Fuente J, Reiss S, McCloy M, et al. Non-TBI stem cell transplantation protocol for Fanconi anaemia using HLA-compatible sibling and unrelated donors. Bone Marrow Transplant. 2003;32:653-656.
338. Maschan AA, Trakhtman PE, Balashov DN, et al. Fludarabine, low-dose busulfan and antithymocyte globulin as conditioning for Fanconi anemia patients receiving bone marrow transplantation from HLA-compatible related donors. Bone Marrow Transplant. 2004;34:305-307.
339. George B, Mathews V, Shaji RV, et al. Fludarabine-based conditioning for allogeneic stem cell transplantation for multiply transfused patients with Fanconi's anemia. Bone Marrow Transplant. 2005;35:341-343.
340. Bitan M, Or R, Shapira MY, et al. Fludarabine-based reduced intensity conditioning for stem cell transplantation of Fanconi anemia patients from fully matched related and unrelated donors. Biol Blood Marrow Transplant. 2006;12:712-718.
341. Tan PL, Wagner JE, Auerbach AD, et al. Successful engraftment without radiation after fludarabine-based regimen in Fanconi anemia patients undergoing genotypically identical donor hematopoietic cell transplantation. Pediatr Blood Cancer. 2006;46:630-636.
342. Wagner JE, Eapen M, MacMillan ML, et al. Unrelated donor bone marrow transplantation for the treatment of Fanconi anemia. Blood. 2007;109:2256-2262.
343. Grewal SS, Kahn JP, MacMillan ML, et al. Successful hematopoietic stem cell transplantation for Fanconi anemia from an unaffected HLA-genotype–identical sibling selected using preimplantation genetic diagnosis. Blood. 2004;103:1147-1151.
344. Guardiola P, Pasquini R, Dokal I, et al. Outcome of 69 allogeneic stem cell transplantations for Fanconi anemia using HLA-matched unrelated donors: a study on behalf of the European Group for Blood and Marrow Transplantation. Blood. 2000;95:422-429.
345. MacMillan ML, Auerbach AD, Davies SM, et al. Haematopoietic cell transplantation in patients with Fanconi anaemia using alternate donors: results of a total body irradiation dose escalation trial. Br J Haematol. 2000;109:121-129.
346. Deeg HJ, Socie G, Schoch G, et al. Malignancies after marrow transplantation for aplastic anemia and Fanconi anemia: a joint Seattle and Paris analysis of results in 700 patients. Blood. 1996;87:386-392.
347. Alter BP, Greene MH, Velazquez I, Rosenberg PS. Cancer in Fanconi anemia. Blood. 2003;101:2072.
348. Lowy DR, Gillison ML. A new link between Fanconi anemia and human papillomavirus–associated malignancies. J Natl Cancer Inst. 2003;95:1648-1650.
349. Alter BP. Fanconi's anemia, transplantation, and cancer. Pediatr Transplant. 2005;9(Suppl 7):81-86.
350. Huck K, Hanenberg H, Gudowius S, et al. Delayed diagnosis and complications of Fanconi anaemia at advanced age—a paradigm. Br J Haematol. 2006;133:188-197.
351. Williams DA, Croop J, Kelly P. Gene therapy in the treatment of Fanconi anemia, a progressive bone marrow failure syndrome. Curr Opin Mol Ther. 2005;7:461-466.
352. Liu JM, Young NS, Walsh CE, et al. Retroviral mediated gene transfer of the Fanconi anemia complementation group C gene to hematopoietic progenitors of group C patients. Hum Gene Ther. 1997;8:1715-1730.
353. Liu JM, Kim S, Read EJ, et al. Engraftment of hematopoietic progenitor cells transduced with the Fanconi anemia group C gene (FANCC). Hum Gene Ther. 1999;10:2337-2346.
354. Kelly PF, Radtke S, Kalle C, et al. Stem cell collection and gene transfer in Fanconi anemia. Mol Ther. 2007;15:211-219.
355. Galimi F, Noll M, Kanazawa Y, et al. Gene therapy of Fanconi anemia: preclinical efficacy using lentiviral vectors. Blood. 2002;100:2732-2736.
356. Alter BP, Baerlocher GM, Savage SA, et al. Very short telomere length by flow fluorescence in situ hybridization identifies patients with dyskeratosis congenita. Blood. 2007;110:1439-1447.
357. Du H-Y, Pumbo E, Shimamura A, et al. Significance of telomere length measurement in the diagnosis of dyskeratosis congenita. Blood. 2007;110, abstract 836.
358. Zinsser F. Atrophia cutis reticularis cum pigmentatione, dystrophia unguium et leukoplakia oris (poikiloderma atrophicans vascularis Jacobi). Ikonogr Derm (Kyoto) 1906;5:219-223.

359. Cole H, Rauschkolb J, Toomey J. Dyskeratosis congenita with pigmentation, dystrophia unguis and leukokeratosis oris. Arch Derm Syph Suppl. 1930;21:71-95.

360. Engman M. A unique case of reticular pigmentation of the skin with atrophy. Arch Derm Syph Suppl. 1926;13:685-687.

361. Milgrom H, Stoll HL Jr, Crissey JT. Dyskeratosis congenita. A case with new features. Arch Dermatol. 1964;89:345-349.

362. Vulliamy T, Dokal I. Dyskeratosis congenita. Semin Hematol. 2006;43:157-166.

363. Trowbridge AA, Sirinavin C, Linman JW. Dyskeratosis congenita: hematologic evaluation of a sibship and review of the literature. Am J Hematol. 1977;3:143-152.

364. Womer R, Clark JE, Wood P, et al. Dyskeratosis congenita: two examples of this multisystem disorder. Pediatrics. 1983;71:603-609.

365. Wiedemann HP, McGuire J, Dwyer JM, et al. Progressive immune failure in dyskeratosis congenita. Report of an adult in whom *Pneumocystis carinii* and fatal disseminated candidiasis developed. Arch Intern Med. 1984;144:397-399.

366. Solder B, Weiss M, Jager A, Belohradsky BH. Dyskeratosis congenita: multisystemic disorder with special consideration of immunologic aspects. A review of the literature. Clin Pediatr (Phila). 1998;37:521-530.

367. Heiss NS, Knight SW, Vulliamy TJ, et al. X-linked dyskeratosis congenita is caused by mutations in a highly conserved gene with putative nucleolar functions. Nat Genet. 1998;19:32-38.

368. Dokal I. Dyskeratosis congenita in all its forms. Br J Haematol. 2000;110:768-779.

369. Drachtman RA, Alter BP. Dyskeratosis congenita. Dermatol Clin. 1995;13:33-39.

370. Bessler M, Du HY, Gu B, Mason PJ. Dysfunctional telomeres and dyskeratosis congenita. Haematologica. 2007;92:1009-1012.

371. Mallory SB. What syndrome is this characteristic of? Dyskeratosis congenita. Pediatr Dermatol. 1991;8:81-83.

372. Sirinavin C, Trowbridge AA. Dyskeratosis congenita: clinical features and genetic aspects. Report of a family and review of the literature. J Med Genet. 1975;12:339-354.

373. Handley TP, Ogden GR. Dyskeratosis congenita: oral hyperkeratosis in association with lichenoid reaction. J Oral Pathol Med. 2006;35:508-512.

374. Auluck A. Dyskeratosis congenita. Report of a case with literature review. Med Oral Patol Oral Cir Bucal. 2007;12:E369-373.

375. Cannell H. Dyskeratosis congenita. Br J Oral Surg. 1971;9:8-20.

376. Paul SR, Perez-Atayde A, Williams DA. Interstitial pulmonary disease associated with dyskeratosis congenita. Am J Pediatr Hematol Oncol. 1992;14:89-92.

377. Utz JP, Ryu JH, Myers JL, Michels VV. Usual interstitial pneumonia complicating dyskeratosis congenita. Mayo Clin Proc. 2005;80:817-821.

378. Rocha V, Devergie A, Socie G, et al. Unusual complications after bone marrow transplantation for dyskeratosis congenita. Br J Haematol. 1998;103:243-248.

379. Tsakiri KD, Cronkhite JT, Kuan PJ, et al. Adult-onset pulmonary fibrosis caused by mutations in telomerase. Proc Natl Acad Sci U S A. 2007;104:7552-7557.

380. Armanios MY, Chen JJ, Cogan JD, et al. Telomerase mutations in families with idiopathic pulmonary fibrosis. N Engl J Med. 2007;356:1317-1326.

381. Roth K, Lange CE. [Fundus changes in Zinsser-Engman-Cole syndrome (author's transl).] Klin Monatsbl Augenheilkd. 1975;166:695-698.

382. Chambers JK, Salinas CF. Ocular findings in dyskeratosis congenita. Birth Defects Orig Artic Ser. 1982;18:167-174.

383. Reichel M, Grix AC, Isseroff RR. Dyskeratosis congenita associated with elevated fetal hemoglobin, X-linked ocular albinism, and juvenile-onset diabetes mellitus. Pediatr Dermatol. 1992;9:103-106.

384. Kajtar P, Mehes K. Bilateral Coats retinopathy associated with aplastic anaemia and mild dyskeratotic signs. Am J Med Genet. 1994;49:374-377.

385. Wald C, Diner H. Dyskeratosis congenita with associated periodontal disease. Oral Surg Oral Med Oral Pathol. 1974;37:736-744.

386. Yavuzyilmaz E, Yamalik N, Yetgin S, Kansu O. Oral-dental findings in dyskeratosis congenita. J Oral Pathol Med. 1992;21:280-284.

387. Davidovich E, Eimerl D, Aker M, et al. Dyskeratosis congenita: dental management of a medically complex child. Pediatr Dent. 2005;27:244-248.

388. Morrison D, Rose EL, Smith AP, Lesser TH. Dyskeratosis congenita and nasopharyngeal atresia. J Laryngol Otol. 1992;106:996-997.

389. Sawant P, Chopda NM, Desai DC, et al. Dyskeratosis congenita with esophageal stricture and dermatological manifestations. Endoscopy. 1994;26:711-712.

390. Arca E, Tuzun A, Tastan HB, et al. Dyskeratosis congenita with esophageal and anal stricture. Int J Dermatol. 2003;42:555-557.

391. Berezin S, Schwarz SM, Slim MS, et al. Gastrointestinal problems in a child with dyskeratosis congenita. Am J Gastroenterol. 1996;91:1271-1272.

392. Feinberg AP, Coffey DS. Organ site specificity for cancer in chromosomal instability disorders. Cancer Res. 1982;42:3252-3254.

393. Anil S, Beena VT, Raji MA, et al. Oral squamous cell carcinoma in a case of dyskeratosis congenita. Ann Dent. 1994;53:15-18.

394. Handley TP, McCaul JA, Ogden GR. Dyskeratosis congenita. Oral Oncol. 2006;42:331-336.

395. Kawaguchi K, Sakamaki H, Onozawa Y, Koike M. Dyskeratosis congenita (Zinsser-Cole-Engman syndrome). An autopsy case presenting with rectal carcinoma, noncirrhotic portal hypertension, and *Pneumocystis carinii* pneumonia. Virchows Arch A Pathol Anat Histopathol. 1990;417:247-253.

396. Bruna Esteban M, Montalva Oron E, Lopez Delgado A, et al. [Gastric adenocarcinoma in Zinsser-Cole-Engman syndrome.] Cir Esp. 2006;80:176-177.

397. Field JJ, Mason PJ, An P, et al. Low frequency of telomerase RNA mutations among children with aplastic anemia or myelodysplastic syndrome. J Pediatr Hematol Oncol. 2006;28:450-453.

398. Knudson M, Kulkarni S, Ballas ZK, et al. Association of immune abnormalities with telomere shortening in autosomal-dominant dyskeratosis congenita. Blood. 2005;105:682-688.

399. Young NS. Acquired aplastic anemia. Ann Intern Med. 2002;136:534-546.

400. Kehrer H, Krone W. Chromosome abnormalities in cell cultures derived from the leukoplakia of a female patient with dyskeratosis congenita. Am J Med Genet. 1992;42:217-218.

401. Dokal I, Bungey J, Williamson P, et al. Dyskeratosis congenita fibroblasts are abnormal and have unbalanced chromosomal rearrangements. Blood. 1992;80:3090-30906.

402. Phillips RJ, Judge M, Webb D, Harper JI. Dyskeratosis congenita: delay in diagnosis and successful treatment of pancytopenia by bone marrow transplantation. Br J Dermatol. 1992;127:278-280.

403. Putterman C, Safadi R, Zlotogora J, et al. Treatment of the hematological manifestations of dyskeratosis congenita. Ann Hematol. 1993;66:209-212.

404. Forni GL, Melevendi C, Jappelli S, Rasore-Quartino A. Dyskeratosis congenita: unusual presenting features within a kindred. Pediatr Hematol Oncol. 1993;10:145-149.

405. Pritchard SL, Junker AK. Positive response to granulocyte-colony-stimulating factor in dyskeratosis congenita before matched unrelated bone marrow transplantation. Am J Pediatr Hematol Oncol. 1994;16:186-187.

406. Oehler L, Reiter E, Friedl J, et al. Effective stimulation of neutropoiesis with rh G-CSF in dyskeratosis congenita: a case report. Ann Hematol. 1994;69:325-327.

407. Vulliamy TJ, Knight SW, Mason PJ, Dokal I. Very short telomeres in the peripheral blood of patients with X-linked and autosomal dyskeratosis congenita. Blood Cells Mol Dis. 2001;27:353-357.

408. Marsh JC, Will AJ, Hows JM, et al. "Stem cell" origin of the hematopoietic defect in dyskeratosis congenita. Blood. 1992;79:3138-3144.

409. Vernole P, Tullio A, Caporossi D, et al. Bleomycin-induced chromosome aberrations in lymphocytes derived from patients with lamellar ichthyosis. Cancer Genet Cytogenet. 1999;108:154-157.

410. Coulthard S, Chase A, Pickard J, et al. Chromosomal breakage analysis in dyskeratosis congenita peripheral blood lymphocytes. Br J Haematol. 1998;102:1162-1164.

411. Ning Y, Yongshan Y, Pai GS, Gross AJ. Heterozygote detection through bleomycin-induced G_2 chromatid breakage in dyskeratosis congenita families. Cancer Genet Cytogenet. 1992;60:31-34.

412. Pai GS, Yan Y, DeBauche DM, et al. Bleomycin hypersensitivity in dyskeratosis congenita fibroblasts, lymphocytes, and transformed lymphoblasts. Cytogenet Cell Genet. 1989;52:186-189.

413. DeBauche DM, Pai GS, Stanley WS. Enhanced G_2 chromatid radiosensitivity in dyskeratosis congenita fibroblasts. Am J Hum Genet. 1990;46:350-357.

414. Mason PJ, Wilson DB, Bessler M. Dyskeratosis congenita—a disease of dysfunctional telomere maintenance. Curr Mol Med. 2005;5:159-170.

415. Dokal I, Luzzatto L. Dyskeratosis congenita is a chromosomal instability disorder. Leuk Lymphoma. 1994;15:1-7.

416. Wong JM, Collins K. Telomerase RNA level limits telomere maintenance in X-linked dyskeratosis congenita. Genes Dev. 2006;20:2848-2858.

417. Devriendt K, Matthijs G, Legius E, et al. Skewed X-chromosome inactivation in female carriers of dyskeratosis congenita. Am J Hum Genet. 1997;60:581-587.

418. Vulliamy TJ, Knight SW, Dokal I, Mason PJ. Skewed X-inactivation in carriers of X-linked dyskeratosis congenita. Blood. 1997;90:2213-2216.

419. Carter DM, Pan M, Gaynor A, et al. Psoralen-DNA cross-linking photoadducts in dyskeratosis congenita: delay in excision and promotion of sister chromatid exchange. J Invest Dermatol. 1979;73:97-101.

420. Ball SE, Gibson FM, Rizzo S, et al. Progressive telomere shortening in aplastic anemia. Blood. 1998;91:3582-3592.

421. Bodnar AG, Ouellette M, Frolkis M, et al. Extension of life-span by introduction of telomerase into normal human cells. Science. 1998;279:349-352.

422. Vulliamy TJ, Marrone A, Knight SW, et al. Mutations in dyskeratosis congenita: their impact on telomere length and the diversity of clinical presentation. Blood. 2006;107:2680-2685.

423. Du H-Y, Pumbo E, Manly P, et al. Complex inheritance pattern of dyskeratosis congenita in two families with two different mutations in the telomerase reverse transcriptase gene. Blood. Nov 27, 2007 [Epub ahead of print].

424. Walne AJ, Vulliamy T, Marrone A, et al. Genetic heterogeneity in autosomal recessive dyskeratosis congenita with one subtype due to mutations in the telomerase-associated protein NOP10. Hum Mol Genet. 2007;16:1619-1629.

425. Cadwell C, Yoon HJ, Zebarjadian Y, Carbon J. The yeast nucleolar protein Cbf5p is involved in rRNA biosynthesis and interacts genetically with the RNA polymerase I transcription factor RRN3. Mol Cell Biol. 1997;17:6175-6183.

426. Giordano E, Peluso I, Senger S, Furia M. Minifly, a *Drosophila* gene required for ribosome biogenesis. J Cell Biol. 1999;144:1123-1133.

427. Meier UT, Blobel G. NAP57, a mammalian nucleolar protein with a putative homolog in yeast and bacteria. J Cell Biol. 1994;127:1505-1514.

428. Filipowicz W, Pogacic V. Biogenesis of small nucleolar ribonucleoproteins. Curr Opin Cell Biol. 2002;14:319-327.

429. Henras A, Henry Y, Bousquet-Antonelli C, et al. Nhp2p and Nop10p are essential for the function of H/ACA snoRNPs. EMBO J. 1998;17:7078-7090.

430. Ramamurthy V, Swann SL, Paulson JL, et al. Critical aspartic acid residues in pseudouridine synthases. J Biol Chem. 1999;274:22225-22230.

431. Spedaliere CJ, Hamilton CS, Mueller EG. Functional importance of motif I of pseudouridine synthases: mutagenesis of aligned lysine and proline residues. Biochemistry. 2000;39:9459-9465.

432. Charette M, Gray MW. Pseudouridine in RNA: what, where, how, and why. IUBMB Life. 2000;49:341-351.

433. Meier UT. The many facets of H/ACA ribonucleoproteins. Chromosoma. 2005;114:1-14.

434. Mitchell JR, Cheng J, Collins K. A box H/ACA small nucleolar RNA-like domain at the human telomerase RNA 3′ end. Mol Cell Biol. 1999;19:567-576.

435. Pogacic V, Dragon F, Filipowicz W. Human H/ACA small nucleolar RNPs and telomerase share evolutionarily con-

served proteins NHP2 and NOP10. Mol Cell Biol. 2000;20:9028-9040.

436. Chen JL, Blasco MA, Greider CW. Secondary structure of vertebrate telomerase RNA. Cell. 2000;100:503-514.

437. Watanabe Y, Gray MW. Evolutionary appearance of genes encoding proteins associated with box H/ACA snoRNAs: cbf5p in *Euglena gracilis*, an early diverging eukaryote, and candidate Gar1p and Nop10p homologs in archaebacteria. Nucleic Acids Res. 2000;28:2342-2352.

438. Vulliamy T, Marrone A, Goldman F, et al. The RNA component of telomerase is mutated in autosomal dominant dyskeratosis congenita. Nature. 2001;413:432-435.

439. de Lange T. Protection of mammalian telomeres. Oncogene. 2002;21:532-540.

440. Harley CB, Futcher AB, Greider CW. Telomeres shorten during ageing of human fibroblasts. Nature. 1990;345:458-460.

441. Vaziri H, Dragowska W, Allsopp RC, et al. Evidence for a mitotic clock in human hematopoietic stem cells: loss of telomeric DNA with age. Proc Natl Acad Sci U S A. 1994;91:9857-9860.

442. Kim NW, Piatyszek MA, Prowse KR, et al. Specific association of human telomerase activity with immortal cells and cancer. Science. 1994;266:2011-20115.

443. Watson JD. Origin of concatemeric T7 DNA. Nat New Biol. 1972;239:197-201.

444. Wright WE, Piatyszek MA, Rainey WE, et al. Telomerase activity in human germline and embryonic tissues and cells. Dev Genet. 1996;18:173-179.

445. Harle-Bachor C, Boukamp P. Telomerase activity in the regenerative basal layer of the epidermis in human skin and in immortal and carcinoma-derived skin keratinocytes. Proc Natl Acad Sci U S A. 1996;93:6476-6481.

446. Chiu CP, Dragowska W, Kim NW, et al. Differential expression of telomerase activity in hematopoietic progenitors from adult human bone marrow. Stem Cells. 1996;14:239-248.

447. Broccoli D, Young JW, de Lange T. Telomerase activity in normal and malignant hematopoietic cells. Proc Natl Acad Sci U S A. 1995;92:9082-9086.

448. Greider CW, Blackburn EH. Identification of a specific telomere terminal transferase activity in *Tetrahymena* extracts. Cell. 1985;43:405-413.

449. Vulliamy TJ, Walne A, Baskaradas A, et al. Mutations in the reverse transcriptase component of telomerase (TERT) in patients with bone marrow failure. Blood Cells Mol Dis. 2005;34:257-263.

450. Yamaguchi H, Calado RT, Ly H, et al. Mutations in TERT, the gene for telomerase reverse transcriptase, in aplastic anemia. N Engl J Med. 2005;352:1413-1424.

451. Armanios M, Chen JL, Chang YP, et al. Haploinsufficiency of telomerase reverse transcriptase leads to anticipation in autosomal dominant dyskeratosis congenita. Proc Natl Acad Sci U S A. 2005;102:15960-15964.

452. Xin ZT, Beauchamp AD, Calado RT, et al. Functional characterization of natural telomerase mutations found in patients with hematologic disorders. Blood. 2007;109:524-532.

452a. Savage SA, Giri N, Baerlocher GM, et al. TINF2, a component of the shelterin telomere protection complex, is mutated in dyskeratosis congenita. Am J Hum Genet. 2008;82:501-509.

453. Knight SW, Heiss NS, Vulliamy TJ, et al. X-linked dyskeratosis congenita is predominantly caused by missense mutations in the DKC1 gene. Am J Hum Genet. 1999;65:50-58.

454. Rashid R, Liang B, Baker DL, et al. Crystal structure of a Cbf5-Nop10-Gar1 complex and implications in RNA-guided pseudouridylation and dyskeratosis congenita. Mol Cell. 2006;21:249-260.

455. Hamma T, Reichow SL, Varani G, Ferre-D'Amare AR. The Cbf5-Nop10 complex is a molecular bracket that organizes box H/ACA RNPs. Nat Struct Mol Biol. 2005;12:1101-1107.

456. Li L, Ye K. Crystal structure of an H/ACA box ribonucleoprotein particle. Nature. 2006;443:302-307; He J, Navarrete S, Jasinski M, et al. Targeted disruption of Dkc1, the gene mutated in X-linked dyskeratosis congenita, causes embryonic lethality in mice. Oncogene. 2002;21:7740-7744.

457. Mitchell JR, Wood E, Collins K. A telomerase component is defective in the human disease dyskeratosis congenita. Nature. 1999;402:551-555.

459. Wong JM, Kyasa MJ, Hutchins L, Collins K. Telomerase RNA deficiency in peripheral blood mononuclear cells in X-linked dyskeratosis congenita. Hum Genet. 2004;115:448-455.

460. Mochizuki Y, He J, Kulkarni S, et al. Mouse dyskerin mutations affect accumulation of telomerase RNA and small nucleolar RNA, telomerase activity, and ribosomal RNA processing. Proc Natl Acad Sci U S A. 2004;101:10756-10761.

461. Ly H, Calado RT, Allard P, et al. Functional characterization of telomerase RNA variants found in patients with hematologic disorders. Blood. 2005;105:2332-2329.

462. Marrone A, Stevens D, Vulliamy T, et al. Heterozygous telomerase RNA mutations found in dyskeratosis congenita and aplastic anemia reduce telomerase activity via haploinsufficiency. Blood. 2004;104:3936-3942.

463. Theimer CA, Finger LD, Feigon J. YNMG tetraloop formation by a dyskeratosis congenita mutation in human telomerase RNA. RNA. 2003;9:1446-1455.

464. Ly H, Blackburn EH, Parslow TG. Comprehensive structure-function analysis of the core domain of human telomerase RNA. Mol Cell Biol. 2003;23:6849-6856.

465. Comolli LR, Smirnov I, Xu L, et al. A molecular switch underlies a human telomerase disease. Proc Natl Acad Sci U S A. 2002;99:16998-17003.

466. Fu D, Collins K. Distinct biogenesis pathways for human telomerase RNA and H/ACA small nucleolar RNAs. Mol Cell. 2003;11:1361-1372.

467. Wilson DB, Ivanovich J, Whelan A, et al. Human telomerase RNA mutations and bone marrow failure. Lancet. 2003;361:1993-1994.

468. Banik SS, Guo C, Smith AC, et al. C-terminal regions of the human telomerase catalytic subunit essential for in vivo enzyme activity. Mol Cell Biol. 2002;22:6234-6246.

469. Du H-Y, Idol R, Robledo S, et al. Telomerase reverse transcriptase haploinsufficiency and telomere length in individuals with 5p– syndrome. Aging Cell. 2007;6:689-697.

470. Marrone A, Walne A, Tamary H, et al. Telomerase reverse transcriptase homozygous mutations in autosomal recessive dyskeratosis congenita and Hoyeraal-Hreidarsson syndrome. Blood. 2007;110:4198-4205.

471. Ly H, Schertzer M, Jastaniah W, et al. Identification and functional characterization of 2 variant alleles of the telomerase RNA template gene (TERC) in a patient with dyskeratosis congenita. Blood. 2005;106:1246-1252.

472. Vulliamy T, Marrone A, Dokal I, Mason PJ. Association between aplastic anaemia and mutations in telomerase RNA. Lancet. 2002;359:2168-2170.

473. Fogarty PF, Yamaguchi H, Wiestner A, et al. Late presentation of dyskeratosis congenita as apparently acquired aplastic anaemia due to mutations in telomerase RNA. Lancet. 2003;362:1628-1630.

474. Yamaguchi H, Baerlocher GM, Lansdorp PM, et al. Mutations of the human telomerase RNA gene (TERC) in aplastic anemia and myelodysplastic syndrome. Blood. 2003;102:916-918.

475. Goldman F, Bouarich R, Kulkarni S, et al. The effect of TERC haploinsufficiency on the inheritance of telomere length. Proc Natl Acad Sci U S A. 2005;102:17119-17124.

476. Vulliamy T, Marrone A, Szydlo R, et al. Disease anticipation is associated with progressive telomere shortening in families with dyskeratosis congenita due to mutations in TERC. Nat Genet. 2004;36:447-449.

477. Hoyeraal HM, Lamvik J, Moe PJ. Congenital hypoplastic thrombocytopenia and cerebral malformations in two brothers. Acta Paediatr Scand. 1970;59:185-191.

478. Hreidarsson S, Kristjansson K, Johannesson G, Johannsson JH. A syndrome of progressive pancytopenia with microcephaly, cerebellar hypoplasia and growth failure. Acta Paediatr Scand. 1988;77:773-775.

479. Aalfs CM, van den Berg H, Barth PG, Hennekam RC. The Hoyeraal-Hreidarsson syndrome: the fourth case of a separate entity with prenatal growth retardation, progressive pancytopenia and cerebellar hypoplasia. Eur J Pediatr. 1995;154:304-308.

480. Ohga S, Kai T, Honda K, et al. What are the essential symptoms in the Hoyeraal-Hreidarsson syndrome? Eur J Pediatr. 1997;156:80-81.

481. Akaboshi S, Yoshimura M, Hara T, et al. A case of Hoyeraal-Hreidarsson syndrome: delayed myelination and hypoplasia of corpus callosum are other important signs. Neuropediatrics. 2000;31:141-144.

482. Yaghmai R, Kimyai-Asadi A, Rostamiani K, et al. Overlap of dyskeratosis congenita with the Hoyeraal-Hreidarsson syndrome. J Pediatr. 2000;136:390-393.

483. Knight SW, Heiss NS, Vulliamy TJ, et al. Unexplained aplastic anaemia, immunodeficiency, and cerebellar hypoplasia (Hoyeraal-Hreidarsson syndrome) due to mutations in the dyskeratosis congenita gene, DKC1. Br J Haematol. 1999;107:335-339.

484. Sznajer Y, Baumann C, David A, et al. Further delineation of the congenital form of X-linked dyskeratosis congenita (Hoyeraal-Hreidarsson syndrome). Eur J Pediatr. 2003;162:863-867.

485. Cossu F, Vulliamy TJ, Marrone A, et al. A novel DKC1 mutation, severe combined immunodeficiency (T+B– NK– SCID) and bone marrow transplantation in an infant with Hoyeraal-Hreidarsson syndrome. Br J Haematol. 2002;119:765-768.

486. Revesz T, Kardos G, Schuler D. [Rare congenital forms of bone marrow deficiency.] Orv Hetil. 1993;134:1147-1150.

487. Revesz T, Fletcher S, al-Gazali LI, DeBuse P. Bilateral retinopathy, aplastic anaemia, and central nervous system abnormalities: a new syndrome? J Med Genet. 1992;29:673-675.

488. Scheinfeld MH, Lui YW, Kolb EA, et al. The neuroradiological findings in a case of Revesz syndrome. Pediatr Radiol. 2007;37:1166-1170.

489. Gonzalez-del Angel A, Cervera M, Gomez L, et al. Ataxia-pancytopenia syndrome. Am J Med Genet. 2000;90:252-254.

490. Li FP, Hecht F, Kaiser-McCaw B, et al. Ataxia-pancytopenia: syndrome of cerebellar ataxia, hypoplastic anemia, monosomy 7, and acute myelogenous leukemia. Cancer Genet Cytogenet. 1981;4:189-196.

491. Daghistani D, Curless R, Toledano SR, Ayyar DR. Ataxia-pancytopenia and monosomy 7 syndrome. J Pediatr. 1989;115:108-110.

492. Ganot P, Bortolin ML, Kiss T. Site-specific pseudouridine formation in preribosomal RNA is guided by small nucleolar RNAs. Cell. 1997;89:799-809.

493. Ni J, Tien AL, Fournier MJ. Small nucleolar RNAs direct site-specific synthesis of pseudouridine in ribosomal RNA. Cell. 1997;89:565-573.

494. Zebarjadian Y, King T, Fournier MJ, et al. Point mutations in yeast CBF5 can abolish in vivo pseudouridylation of rRNA. Mol Cell Biol. 1999;19:7461-7472.

495. Kauffman T, Tran J, DiNardo S. Mutations in Nop60B, the *Drosophila* homolog of human dyskeratosis congenita 1, affect the maintenance of the germ-line stem cell lineage during spermatogenesis. Dev Biol. 2003;253:189-199.

496. Ruggero D, Grisendi S, Piazza F, et al. Dyskeratosis congenita and cancer in mice deficient in ribosomal RNA modification. Science. 2003;299:259-562.

497. Marciniak RA, Johnson FB, Guarente L. Dyskeratosis congenita, telomeres and human ageing. Trends Genet. 2000;16:193-195.

498. Blasco MA, Lee HW, Hande MP, et al. Telomere shortening and tumor formation by mouse cells lacking telomerase RNA. Cell. 1997;91:25-34.

400. Liu Y, Snow BE, Hande MP, et al. The telomerase reverse transcriptase is limiting and necessary for telomerase function in vivo. Curr Biol. 2000;10:1459-1462.

500. Yoon A, Peng G, Brandenburg Y, et al. Impaired control of IRES-mediated translation in X-linked dyskeratosis congenita. Science. 2006;312:902-906.

501. Dokal I. Inherited aplastic anaemia. Hematol J. 2003;4:3-9.

502. Giri N, Pitel PA, Green D, Alter BP. Splenic peliosis and rupture in patients with dyskeratosis congenita on androgens and granulocyte colony-stimulating factor. Br J Haematol. 2007;138:815-817.

503. Berthou C, Devergie A, D'Agay MF, et al. Late vascular complications after bone marrow transplantation for dyskeratosis congenita. Br J Haematol. 1991;79:335-336.

504. Langston AA, Sanders JE, Deeg HJ, et al. Allogeneic marrow transplantation for aplastic anaemia associated with dyskeratosis congenita. Br J Haematol. 1996;92:758-765.

505. Amarasinghe K, Dalley C, Dokal I, et al. Late death after unrelated-BMT for dyskeratosis congenita following conditioning with alemtuzumab, fludarabine and melphalan. Bone Marrow Transplant. 2007;40:913-914.

506. Gungor T, Corbacioglu S, Storb R, Seger RA. Nonmyeloablative allogeneic hematopoietic stem cell transplantation for treatment of Dyskeratosis congenita. Bone Marrow Transplant. 2003;31:407-410.

507. Dror Y, Freedman MH, Leaker M, et al. Low-intensity hematopoietic stem-cell transplantation across human leucocyte antigen barriers in dyskeratosis congenita. Bone Marrow Transplant. 2003;31:847-850.

508. Ayas M, Al-Musa A, Al-Jefri A, et al. Allogeneic stem cell transplantation in a patient with dyskeratosis congenita after conditioning with low-dose cyclophosphamide and anti-thymocyte globulin. Pediatr Blood Cancer. 2007;49:103-104.

509. de la Fuente J, Dokal I. Dyskeratosis congenita: advances in the understanding of the telomerase defect and the role of stem cell transplantation. Pediatr Transplant. 2007;11:584-594.

510. Ostronoff F, Ostronoff M, Calixto R, et al. Fludarabine, cyclophosphamide, and antithymocyte globulin for a patient with dyskeratosis congenita and severe bone marrow failure. Biol Blood Marrow Transplant. 2007;13:366-368.

511. Yabe M, Yabe H, Hattori K, et al. Fatal interstitial pulmonary disease in a patient with dyskeratosis congenita after allogeneic bone marrow transplantation. Bone Marrow Transplant. 1997;19:389-392.

512. Westin ER, Chavez E, Lee KM, et al. Telomere restoration and extension of proliferative lifespan in dyskeratosis congenita fibroblasts. Aging Cell. 2007;6:383-394.

513. Bodian M, Sheldon W, Lightwood R. Congenital hypoplasia of the exocrine pancreas. Acta Paediatr. 1964;53:282-293.

514. Shwachman H, Diamond LK, Oski FA, Khaw KT. The syndrome of pancreatic insufficiency and bone marrow dysfunction. J Pediatr. 1964;65:645-663.

515. Goobie S, Popovic M, Morrison J, et al. Shwachman-Diamond syndrome with exocrine pancreatic dysfunction and bone marrow failure maps to the centromeric region of chromosome 7. Am J Hum Genet. 2001;68:1048-1054.

516. Ginzberg H, Shin J, Ellis L, et al. Shwachman syndrome: phenotypic manifestations of sibling sets and isolated cases in a large patient cohort are similar. J Pediatr. 1999;135:81-88.

517. Aggett PJ, Cavanagh NP, Matthew DJ, et al. Shwachman's syndrome. A review of 21 cases. Arch Dis Child. 1980;55:331-347.

518. Mack DR, Forstner GG, Wilschanski M, et al. Shwachman syndrome: exocrine pancreatic dysfunction and variable phenotypic expression. Gastroenterology. 1996;111:1593-1602.

519. Smith OP, Hann IM, Chessells JM, et al. Haematological abnormalities in Shwachman-Diamond syndrome. Br J Haematol. 1996;94:279-284.

520. Cipolli M, D'Orazio C, Delmarco A, et al. Shwachman's syndrome: pathomorphosis and long-term outcome. J Pediatr Gastroenterol Nutr. 1999;29:265-272.

521. Kuijpers TW, Alders M, Tool AT, et al. Hematologic abnormalities in Shwachman Diamond syndrome: lack of genotype-phenotype relationship. Blood. 2005;106:356-361.

522. Stepanovic V, Wessels D, Goldman FD, et al. The chemotaxis defect of Shwachman-Diamond syndrome leukocytes. Cell Motil Cytoskeleton. 2004;57:158-174.

523. Grinspan ZM, Pikora CA. Infections in patients with Shwachman-Diamond syndrome. Pediatr Infect Dis J. 2005;24:179-181.

524. Kuijpers TW, Nannenberg E, Alders M, et al. Congenital aplastic anemia caused by mutations in the SBDS gene: a rare presentation of Shwachman-Diamond syndrome. Pediatrics. 2004;114:e387-e391.

525. Woods WG, Krivit W, Lubin BH, Ramsay NK. Aplastic anemia associated with the Shwachman syndrome. In vivo and in vitro observations. Am J Pediatr Hematol Oncol. 1981;3:347-351.

526. Dror Y, Ginzberg H, Dalal I, et al. Immune function in patients with Shwachman-Diamond syndrome. Br J Haematol. 2001;114:712-717.

527. Dror Y, Freedman MH. Shwachman-Diamond syndrome: An inherited preleukemic bone marrow failure disorder with aberrant hematopoietic progenitors and faulty marrow microenvironment. Blood. 1999;94:3048-3054.

528. Dror Y. Shwachman-Diamond syndrome. Pediatr Blood Cancer. 2005;45:892-901.

529. Shimamura A. Shwachman-Diamond syndrome. Semin Hematol. 2006;43:178-188.

530. Dror Y, Durie P, Ginzberg H, et al. Clonal evolution in marrows of patients with Shwachman-Diamond syndrome: a prospective 5-year follow-up study. Exp Hematol. 2002;30:659-669.

531. Cunningham J, Sales M, Pearce A, et al. Does isochromosome 7q mandate bone marrow transplant in children with Shwachman-Diamond syndrome? Br J Haematol. 2002;119:1062-1069.

532. Mellink CH, Alders M, van der Lelie H, et al. SBDS mutations and isochromosome 7q in a patient with Shwachman-Diamond syndrome: no predisposition to malignant transformation? Cancer Genet Cytogenet. 2004;154:144-149.

533. Donadieu J, Leblanc T, Bader Meunier B, et al. Analysis of risk factors for myelodysplasias, leukemias and death from infection among patients with congenital neutropenia. Experience of the French Severe Chronic Neutropenia Study Group. Haematologica. 2005;90:45-53.

534. Ip WF, Dupuis A, Ellis L, et al. Serum pancreatic enzymes define the pancreatic phenotype in patients with Shwachman-Diamond syndrome. J Pediatr. 2002;141:259-265.

535. Schibli S, Corey M, Gaskin KJ, et al. Towards the ideal quantitative pancreatic function test: analysis of test variables that influence validity. Clin Gastroenterol Hepatol. 2006;4:90-97.

536. Adachi M, Tachibana K, Asakura Y, Aida N. Usefulness of pancreatic ultrasonography in the diagnosis of Shwachman-Bodian-Diamond syndrome. Acta Paediatr. 2005;94:1686-1690.

537. Els N, Michael JC, George AT. Disorders of the pediatric pancreas: imaging features. Pediatr Radiol. 2005;V35:358.

538. Nijs E, Callahan MJ, Taylor GA. Disorders of the pediatric pancreas: imaging features. Pediatr Radiol. 2005;35:358-373; quiz 457.

539. Makitie O, Ellis L, Durie PR, et al. Skeletal phenotype in patients with Shwachman-Diamond syndrome and mutations in SBDS. Clin Genet. 2004;65:101-112.

540. Kent A, Murphy GH, Milla P. Psychological characteristics of children with Shwachman syndrome. Arch Dis Child. 1990;65:1349-1352.

541. Hall GW, Dale P, Dodge JA. Shwachman-Diamond syndrome: UK perspective. Arch Dis Child. 2006;91:521-524.

542. Ho W, Cheretakis C, Durie P, Kulkarni G, Glogauer M. Prevalence of oral diseases in Shwachman-Diamond syndrome. Spec Care Dentist. 2007;27:52-58.

543. Kornfeld SJ, Kratz J, Diamond F, et al. Shwachman-Diamond syndrome associated with hypogammaglobulinemia and growth hormone deficiency. J Allergy Clin Immunol. 1995;96:247-250.

544. Savilahti E, Rapola J. Frequent myocardial lesions in Shwachman's syndrome. Eight fatal cases among 16 Finnish patients. Acta Paediatr Scand. 1984;73:642-651.

545. Rothbaum R, Perrault J, Vlachos A, et al. Shwachman-Diamond syndrome: report from an international conference. J Pediatr. 2002;141:266-270.

546. Austin KM, Leary RJ, Shimamura A. The Shwachman-Diamond SBDS protein localizes to the nucleolus. Blood. 2005;106:1253-1258.

547. Boocock GR, Morrison JA, Popovic M, et al. Mutations in SBDS are associated with Shwachman-Diamond syndrome. Nat Genet. 2003;33:97-101.

548. Woloszynek JR, Rothbaum RJ, Rawls AS, et al. Mutations of the SBDS gene are present in most patients with Shwachman-Diamond syndrome. Blood. 2004;104:3588-3590.

549. Pearson HA, Lobel JS, Kocoshis SA, et al. A new syndrome of refractory sideroblastic anemia with vacuolization of marrow precursors and exocrine pancreatic dysfunction. J Pediatr. 1979;95:976-984.

550. Rotig A, Cormier V, Blanche S, et al. Pearson's marrow-pancreas syndrome. A multisystem mitochondrial disorder in infancy. J Clin Invest. 1990;86:1601-1608.

551. Rotig A, Colonna M, Bonnefont JP, et al. Mitochondrial DNA deletion in Pearson's marrow/pancreas syndrome. Lancet. 1989;1:902-903.

552. Makitie O, Kaitila I. Cartilage-hair hypoplasia—clinical manifestations in 108 Finnish patients. Eur J Pediatr. 1993;152:211-217.

553. Ridanpaa M, van Eenennaam H, Pelin K, et al. Mutations in the RNA component of RNase MRP cause a pleiotropic human disease, cartilage-hair hypoplasia. Cell. 2001;104:195-203.

554. Ginzberg H, Shin J, Ellis L, et al. Segregation analysis in Shwachman-Diamond syndrome: evidence for recessive inheritance. Am J Hum Genet. 2000;66:1413-1416.

555. Nicolis E, Bonizzato A, Assael BM, Cipolli M. Identification of novel mutations in patients with Shwachman-Diamond syndrome. Hum Mutat. 2005;25:410.

556. Nakashima E, Mabuchi A, Makita Y, et al. Novel SBDS mutations caused by gene conversion in Japanese patients with Shwachman-Diamond syndrome. Hum Genet. 2004;114:345-348.

557. Zhang S, Shi M, Hui CC, Rommens JM. Loss of the mouse ortholog of the shwachman-diamond syndrome gene (Sbds) results in early embryonic lethality. Mol Cell Biol. 2006;26:6656-6663.

558. Nishimura G, Nakashima E, Hirose Y, et al. The Shwachman-Bodian-Diamond syndrome gene mutations cause a neonatal form of spondylometaphysial dysplasia (SMD) resembling SMD Sedaghatian type. J Med Genet. 2007;44:e73.

559. Calado RT, Graf SA, Wilkerson KL, et al. Mutations in the SBDS gene in acquired aplastic anemia. Blood. 2007;110:1141-1146.

560. Wessels D, Srikantha T, Yi S, et al. The Shwachman-Bodian-Diamond syndrome gene encodes an RNA-binding protein that localizes to the pseudopod of *Dictyostelium* amoebae during chemotaxis. J Cell Sci. 2006;119:370-379.

561. Ganapathi KA, Austin KM, Lee CS, et al. The human Shwachman-Diamond syndrome protein, SBDS, associates with ribosomal RNA. Blood. 2007;110:1458-1465.

562. Menne TF, Goyenechea B, Sanchez-Puig N, et al. The Shwachman-Bodian-Diamond syndrome protein mediates translational activation of ribosomes in yeast. Nat Genet. 2007;39:486-495.

563. Rawls AS, Gregory AD, Woloszynek JR, et al. Lentiviral-mediated RNAi inhibition of Sbds in murine hematopoietic progenitors impairs their hematopoietic potential. Blood. 2007;110:2414-1422.

564. Thornley I, Dror Y, Sung L, et al. Abnormal telomere shortening in leucocytes of children with Shwachman-Diamond syndrome. Br J Haematol. 2002;117:189-192.

565. Austin KM, Gupta ML, Coats SA. Mitotic spindle destabilization and genomic instability in Shwachman-Diamond syndrome. J Clin Invest. 2008;118:1511-1518.

566. Dale DC, Bolyard AA, Schwinzer BG, et al. The severe congenital neutropenia international registry: 10-year follow-up report. Supportive Cancer Therapy (in press).

567. Donadieu J, Michel G, Merlin E, et al. Hematopoietic stem cell transplantation for Shwachman-Diamond syndrome: experience of the French neutropenia registry. Bone Marrow Transplant. 2005;36:787-792.

568. Cesaro S, Oneto R, Messina C, et al. Haematopoietic stem cell transplantation for Shwachman-Diamond disease: a study from the European Group for blood and marrow transplantation. Br J Haematol. 2005;131:231-236.

569. McKusick VA. Metaphyseal dysostosis and thin hair: a "new" recessively inherited syndrome? Lancet. 1964;15:832-833.

570. Williams MS, Ettinger RS, Hermanns P, et al. The natural history of severe anemia in cartilage-hair hypoplasia. Am J Med Genet A. 2005;138:35-40.

571. Martin AN, Li Y. RNase MRP RNA and human genetic diseases. Cell Res. 2007;17:219-226.

572. Thiel CT, Mortier G, Kaitila I, et al. Type and level of RMRP functional impairment predicts phenotype in the cartilage hair hypoplasia–anauxetic dysplasia spectrum. Am J Hum Genet. 2007;81:519-529.

573. Shadel GS, Clayton DA. Mitochondrial DNA maintenance in vertebrates. Annu Rev Biochem. 1997;66:409-435.

574. Lygerou Z, Allmang C, Tollervey D, Seraphin B. Accurate processing of a eukaryotic precursor ribosomal RNA by ribonuclease MRP in vitro. Science. 1996;272:268-270.

575. Gill T, Cai T, Aulds J, et al. RNase MRP cleaves the CLB2 mRNA to promote cell cycle progression: novel method of mRNA degradation. Mol Cell Biol. 2004;24:945-953.

576. Thiel CT, Horn D, Zabel B, et al. Severely incapacitating mutations in patients with extreme short stature identify RNA-processing endoribonuclease RMRP as an essential

cell growth regulator. Am J Hum Genet. 2005;77:795-806.

577. Guggenheim R, Somech R, Grunebaum E, et al. Bone marrow transplantation for cartilage-hair-hypoplasia. Bone Marrow Transplant. 2006;38:751-756.

578. Giese A, Kirschner-Schwabe R, Blumchen K, et al. Prenatal manifestation of pancytopenia in Pearson marrow-pancreas syndrome caused by a mitochondrial DNA deletion. Am J Med Genet A. 2007;143:285-288.

579. Finsterer J. Hematological manifestations of primary mitochondrial disorders. Acta Haematol. 2007;118:88-98.

580. Superti-Furga A, Schoenle E, Tuchschmid P, et al. Pearson bone marrow-pancreas syndrome with insulin-dependent diabetes, progressive renal tubulopathy, organic aciduria and elevated fetal haemoglobin caused by deletion and duplication of mitochondrial DNA. Eur J Pediatr. 1993; 152:44-50.

581. Muraki K, Goto Y, Nishino I, et al. Severe lactic acidosis and neonatal death in Pearson syndrome. J Inherit Metab Dis. 1997;20:43-48.

582. Kleinle S, Wiesmann U, Superti-Furga A, et al. Detection and characterization of mitochondrial DNA rearrangements in Pearson and Kearns-Sayre syndromes by long PCR. Hum Genet. 1997;100:643-650.

583. Lee HF, Lee HJ, Chi CS, et al. The neurological evolution of Pearson syndrome: case report and literature review. Eur J Paediatr Neurol. 2007;11:208-214.

584. Rotig A, Bourgeron T, Chretien D, et al. Spectrum of mitochondrial DNA rearrangements in the Pearson marrow-pancreas syndrome. Hum Mol Genet. 1995;4: 1327-1330.

585. Muraki K, Nishimura S, Goto Y, et al. The association between haematological manifestation and mtDNA deletions in Pearson syndrome. J Inherit Metab Dis. 1997;20: 697-703.

586. Brown DT, Herbert M, Lamb VK, et al. Transmission of mitochondrial DNA disorders: possibilities for the future. Lancet. 2006;368:87-89.

587. Scartezzini P, Forni GL, Baldi M, et al. Decreased glycosylation of band 3 and band 4.5 glycoproteins of erythrocyte membrane in congenital dyserythropoietic anaemia type II. Br J Haematol. 1982;51:569-576.

588. Sano T, Ban K, Ichiki T, et al. Molecular and genetic analyses of two patients with Pearson's marrow-pancreas syndrome. Pediatr Res. 1993;34:105-110.

589. Henry E, Walker D, Wiedmeier SE, Christensen RD. Hematological abnormalities during the first week of life among neonates with Down syndrome: data from a multihospital healthcare system. Am J Med Genet A. 2007; 143:42-50.

590. Webb D, Roberts I, Vyas P. Haematology of Down syndrome. Arch Dis Child Fetal Neonatal Ed. 2007;92: F503-F507.

591. Starc TJ. Erythrocyte macrocytosis in infants and children with Down syndrome. J Pediatr. 1992;121:578-581.

592. Vyas P, Crispino JD. Molecular insights into Down syndrome-associated leukemia. Curr Opin Pediatr. 2007; 19:9-14.

593. Massey GV, Zipursky A, Chang MN, et al. A prospective study of the natural history of transient leukemia (TL) in neonates with Down syndrome (DS): Children's Oncology Group (COG) study POG-9481. Blood. 2006; 107:4606-4613.

594. Schunk GJ, Lehman WL. Mongolism and congenital leukemia. JAMA. 1954;155:250-251.

595. Krivit W, Good RA. Simultaneous occurrence of mongolism and leukemia; report of a nationwide survey. AMA J Dis Child. 1957;94:289-293.

596. Zipursky A, Brown EJ, Christensen H, Doyle J. Transient myeloproliferative disorder (transient leukemia) and hematologic manifestations of Down syndrome. Clin Lab Med. 1999;19:157-167, vii.

597. Al-Kasim F, Doyle JJ, Massey GV, et al. Incidence and treatment of potentially lethal diseases in transient leukemia of Down syndrome: Pediatric Oncology Group Study. J Pediatr Hematol Oncol. 2002;24:9-13.

598. Wechsler J, Greene M, McDevitt MA, et al. Acquired mutations in GATA1 in the megakaryoblastic leukemia of Down syndrome. Nat Genet. 2002;32:148-152.

599. Hitzler JK, Cheung J, Li Y, et al. GATA1 mutations in transient leukemia and acute megakaryoblastic leukemia of Down syndrome. Blood. 2003;101:4301-4304.

600. Mundschau G, Gurbuxani S, Gamis AS, et al. Mutagenesis of GATA1 is an initiating event in Down syndrome leukemogenesis. Blood. 2003;101:4298-4300.

601. Xu G, Nagano M, Kanezaki R, et al. Frequent mutations in the GATA-1 gene in the transient myeloproliferative disorder of Down syndrome. Blood. 2003;102:2960-2968.

602. Ahmed M, Sternberg A, Hall G, et al. Natural history of GATA1 mutations in Down syndrome. Blood. 2004;103: 2480-2489.

603. Pine SR, Guo Q, Yin C, et al. Incidence and clinical implications of GATA1 mutations in newborns with Down syndrome. Blood. 2007;110:2128-2131.

604. Li Z, Godinho FJ, Klusmann JH, et al. Developmental stage-selective effect of somatically mutated leukemogenic transcription factor GATA1. Nat Genet. 2005;37: 613-619.

605. Hollanda LM, Lima CS, Cunha AF, et al. An inherited mutation leading to production of only the short isoform of GATA-1 is associated with impaired erythropoiesis. Nat Genet. 2006;38:807-812.

606. Kirsammer G, Jilani S, Liu H, et al. Highly penetrant myeloproliferative disease in the Ts65Dn mouse model of Down syndrome. Blood. 2008;111:767-775.

607. Ravindranath Y, Abella E, Krischer JP, et al. Acute myeloid leukemia (AML) in Down's syndrome is highly responsive to chemotherapy: experience on Pediatric Oncology Group AML Study 8498. Blood. 1992;80:2210-2214.

608. Creutzig U, Ritter J, Vormoor J, et al. Myelodysplasia and acute myelogenous leukemia in Down's syndrome. A report of 40 children of the AML-BFM Study Group. Leukemia. 1996;10:1677-1686.

609. Lange BJ, Kobrinsky N, Barnard DR, et al. Distinctive demography, biology, and outcome of acute myeloid leukemia and myelodysplastic syndrome in children with Down syndrome: Children's Cancer Group Studies 2861 and 2891. Blood. 1998;91:608-615.

610. Kojima S, Sako M, Kato K, et al. An effective chemotherapeutic regimen for acute myeloid leukemia and myelodysplastic syndrome in children with Down's syndrome. Leukemia. 2000;14:786-791.

611. Webb DK. Optimizing therapy for myeloid disorders of Down syndrome. Br J Haematol. 2005;131:3-7.

612. Taub JW, Ge Y. Down syndrome, drug metabolism and chromosome 21. Pediatr Blood Cancer. 2005;44:33-39.

613. Buijs A, Poddighe P, van Wijk R, et al. A novel CBFA2 single-nucleotide mutation in familial platelet disorder with propensity to develop myeloid malignancies. Blood. 2001;98:2856-2858.

614. Diamond L, Blackfan K. Hypoplastic anemia. Am J Dis Child. 1938;56:464-467.

615. Bresters D, Bruin MC, van Dijken PJ. [Congenital hypoplastic anemia in The Netherlands (1963-1989).] Tijdschr Kindergeneeskd. 1991;59:203-210.

616. Ball SE, McGuckin CP, Jenkins G, Gordon-Smith EC. Diamond-Blackfan anaemia in the U.K.: analysis of 80 cases from a 20-year birth cohort. Br J Haematol. 1996;94:645-653.

617. Vlachos A, Klein GW, Lipton JM. The Diamond Blackfan Anemia Registry: tool for investigating the epidemiology and biology of Diamond-Blackfan anemia. J Pediatr Hematol Oncol. 2001;23:377-382.

618. Ramenghi U, Garelli E, Valtolina S, et al. Diamond-Blackfan anaemia in the Italian population. Br J Haematol. 1999;104:841-848.

619. Willig TN, Niemeyer CM, Leblanc T, et al. Identification of new prognosis factors from the clinical and epidemiologic analysis of a registry of 229 Diamond-Blackfan anemia patients. DBA group of Societe d'Hematologie et d'Immunologie Pediatrique (SHIP), Gesellshaft fur Padiatrische Onkologie und Hamatologie (GPOH), and the European Society for Pediatric Hematology and Immunology (ESPHI). Pediatr Res. 1999;46:553-561.

620. Lipton JM, Atsidaftos E, Zyskind I, Vlachos A. Improving clinical care and elucidating the pathophysiology of Diamond Blackfan anemia: an update from the Diamond Blackfan Anemia Registry. Pediatr Blood Cancer. 2006;46:558-564.

621. Dunbar AE 3rd, Moore SL, Hinson RM. Fetal Diamond-Blackfan anemia associated with hydrops fetalis. Am J Perinatol. 2003;20:391-394.

622. Balaban EP, Buchanan GR, Graham M, Frenkel EP. Diamond-Blackfan syndrome in adult patients. Am J Med. 1985;78:533-538.

623. Campagnoli MF, Garelli E, Quarello P, et al. Molecular basis of Diamond-Blackfan anemia: new findings from the Italian registry and a review of the literature. Haematologica. 2004;89:480-489.

624. Orfali KA, Ohene-Abuakwa Y, Ball SE. Diamond Blackfan anaemia in the UK: clinical and genetic heterogeneity. Br J Haematol. 2004;125:243-252.

625. Vlachos A, Ball S, Dahl N, et al. Diagnosing and treating Diamond Blackfan anemia: results of an International Clinical Consensus Conference. Br J Haematol. 2008 (in press).

626. Chen S, Warszawski J, Bader-Meunier B, et al. Diamond-blackfan anemia and growth status: the French registry. J Pediatr. 2005;147:669-673.

627. Glader BE, Backer K, Diamond LK. Elevated erythrocyte adenosine deaminase activity in congenital hypoplastic anemia. N Engl J Med. 1983;309:1486-1490.

628. Filanovskaya L, Nikitin D, Togo A, et al. The activity of purine nucleotide degradation enzymes and lymphoid cell

629. Feldges D, Schmidt R. [Erythrogenesis imperfecta (Blackfan-Diamond anemia).] Schweiz Med Wochenschr. 1971;101:1813-1814.

630. Freedman MH, Amato D, Saunders EF. Erythroid colony growth in congenital hypoplastic anemia. J Clin Invest. 1976;57:673-677.

631. Nathan DG, Clarke BJ, Hillman DG, et al. Erythroid precursors in congenital hypoplastic (Diamond-Blackfan) anemia. J Clin Invest. 1978;61:489-498.

632. Lipton JM, Kudisch M, Gross R, Nathan DG. Defective erythroid progenitor differentiation system in congenital hypoplastic (Diamond-Blackfan) anemia. Blood. 1986;67:962-968.

633. Perdahl EB, Naprstek BL, Wallace WC, Lipton JM. Erythroid failure in Diamond-Blackfan anemia is characterized by apoptosis. Blood. 1994;83:645-650.

634. Tsai PH, Arkin S, Lipton JM. An intrinsic progenitor defect in Diamond-Blackfan anaemia. Br J Haematol. 1989;73:112-120.

635. Bagnara GP, Zauli G, Vitale L, et al. In vitro growth and regulation of bone marrow enriched CD34+ hematopoietic progenitors in Diamond-Blackfan anemia. Blood. 1991;78:2203-2210.

636. Halperin DS, Estrov Z, Freedman MH. Diamond-Blackfan anemia: promotion of marrow erythropoiesis in vitro by recombinant interleukin-3. Blood. 1989;73:1168-1174.

637. Abkowitz JL, Sabo KM, Nakamoto B, et al. Diamond-blackfan anemia: in vitro response of erythroid progenitors to the ligand for c-kit. Blood. 1991;78:2198-2202.

638. Olivieri NF, Grunberger T, Ben-David Y, et al. Diamond-Blackfan anemia: heterogenous response of hematopoietic progenitor cells in vitro to the protein product of the steel locus. Blood. 1991;78:2211-2115.

639. Sieff C, Guinan E. In vitro enhancement of erythropoiesis by steel factor in Diamond-Blackfan anemia and treatment of other congenital cytopenias with recombinant interleukin 3/granulocyte-macrophage colony stimulating factor. Stem Cells. 1993;11(Suppl 2):113-122.

640. Ohene-Abuakwa Y, Orfali KA, Marius C, Ball SE. Two-phase culture in Diamond Blackfan anemia: localization of erythroid defect. Blood. 2005;105:838-846.

641. Draptchinskaia N, Gustavsson P, Andersson B, et al. The gene encoding ribosomal protein S19 is mutated in Diamond-Blackfan anaemia. Nat Genet. 1999;21:169-175.

642. Gazda HT, Grabowska A, Merida-Long LB, et al. Ribosomal protein S24 gene is mutated in Diamond-Blackfan anemia. Am J Hum Genet. 2006;79:1110-1118.

643. Cmejla R, Cmejlova J, Handrkova H, et al. Ribosomal protein S17 gene (RPS17) is mutated in Diamond-Blackfan anemia. Hum Mutat. 2007;28:1172-1182.

644. Farrar J, Nater M, Caywood E, et al. A large ribosomal subunit protein abnormality in Diamond-Blackfan anemia (DBA) [abstract]. Blood. 2007;110:422.

645. Gazda HT, Sheen MR, Darras N, et al. Mutations of the genes for ribosomal proteins L5 and L11 are a common cause of Diamond-Blackfan anemia [abstract]. Blood. 2007;110:421.

subpopulation in children with Diamond-Blackfan syndrome. Gematologiia i Transfuzinolgiia. 1993;38:19-22.

646. Janov AJ, Leong T, Nathan DG, Guinan EC. Diamond-Blackfan anemia. Natural history and sequelae of treatment. Medicine (Baltimore). 1996;75:77-78.

647. Lipton JM, Federman N, Khabbaze Y, et al. Osteogenic sarcoma associated with Diamond-Blackfan anemia: a report from the Diamond-Blackfan Anemia Registry. J Pediatr Hematol Oncol. 2001;23:39-44.

648. Lipton JM. Diamond Blackfan anemia: New paradigms for a "not so pure" inherited red cell aplasia. Semin Hematol. 2006;43:167-177.

649. Gustavsson P, Willing TN, van Haeringen A, et al. Diamond-Blackfan anaemia: genetic homogeneity for a gene on chromosome 19q13 restricted to 1.8 Mb. Nat Genet. 1997;16:368-371.

650. Gazda H, Lipton JM, Willig TN, et al. Evidence for linkage of familial Diamond-Blackfan anemia to chromosome 8p23.3-p22 and for non-19q non-8p disease. Blood. 2001;97:2145-2150.

651. Willig TN, Draptchinskaia N, Dianzani I, et al. Mutations in ribosomal protein S19 gene and diamond blackfan anemia: wide variations in phenotypic expression. Blood. 1999;94:4294-4306.

652. Cmejla R, Blafkova J, Stopka T, et al. Ribosomal protein S19 gene mutations in patients with Diamond-Blackfan anemia and identification of ribosomal protein S19 pseudogenes. Blood Cells Mol Dis. 2000;26: 124-132.

653. Gazda HT, Zhong R, Long L, et al. RNA and protein evidence for haplo-insufficiency in Diamond-Blackfan anaemia patients with RPS19 mutations. Br J Haematol. 2004;127:105-113.

654. Gregory LA, Aguissa-Toure AH, Pinaud N, et al. Molecular basis of Diamond-Blackfan anemia: structure and function analysis of RPS19. Nucleic Acids Res. 2007;35: 5913-5921.

655. Granneman S, Baserga SJ. Ribosome biogenesis: of knobs and RNA processing. Exp Cell Res. 2004;296:43-50.

656. Fatica A, Tollervey D. Making ribosomes. Curr Opin Cell Biol. 2002;14:313-318.

657. Fromont-Racine M, Senger B, Saveanu C, Fasiolo F. Ribosome assembly in eukaryotes. Gene. 2003;313: 17-42.

658. Hadjiolova KV, Nicoloso M, Mazan S, et al. Alternative pre-rRNA processing pathways in human cells and their alteration by cycloheximide inhibition of protein synthesis. Eur J Biochem. 1993;212:211-215.

659. Huang Q, Robledo S, Wilson DB, et al. A four base pair insertion in exon 1 of the RPS19 gene is a common polymorphism in African-Americans. Br J Haematol. 2006; 135:745-746.

660. Aase JM, Smith DW. Congenital anemia and triphalangeal thumbs: a new syndrome. J Pediatr. 1969;74: 471-474.

661. Alter BP. Thumbs and anemia. Pediatrics. 1978;62: 613-614.

662. Hurst JA, Baraitser M, Wonke B. Autosomal dominant transmission of congenital erythroid hypoplastic anemia with radial abnormalities. Am J Med Genet. 1991;40: 482-484.

663. Ebert BL, Pretz J, Bosco J, et al. Identification of RPS14 as the 5q− syndrome gene by RNA interference screen. Nature. 2008;451:335-339.

664. Glader BE. Diagnosis and management of red cell aplasia in children. Hematol Oncol Clin North Am. 1987;1: 431-447.

665. Dessypris EN, Krantz SB, Roloff JS, Lukens JN. Mode of action of the IgG inhibitor of erythropoiesis in transient erythroblastopenia of children. Blood. 1982;59:114-123.

666. Gustavsson P, Klar J, Matsson H, et al. Familial transient erythroblastopenia of childhood is associated with the chromosome 19q13.2 region but not caused by mutations in coding sequences of the ribosomal protein S19 (RPS19) gene. Br J Haematol. 2002;119:261-264.

667. Warner JR. The economics of ribosome biosynthesis in yeast. Trends Biochem Sci. 1999;24:437-440.

668. Lambertsson A. The minute genes in *Drosophila* and their molecular functions. Adv Genet. 1998;38:69-134.

669. Leger-Silvestre I, Caffrey JM, Dawaliby R, et al. Specific Role for yeast homologs of the Diamond Blackfan anemia–associated Rps19 protein in ribosome synthesis. J Biol Chem. 2005;280:38177-38185.

670. Ferreira-Cerca S, Poll G, Gleizes PE, et al. Roles of eukaryotic ribosomal proteins in maturation and transport of pre-18S rRNA and ribosome function. Mol Cell. 2005;20:263-275.

671. Matsson H, Davey EJ, Draptchinskaia N, et al. Targeted disruption of the ribosomal protein S19 gene is lethal prior to implantation. Mol Cell Biol. 2004;24:4032-4037.

672. Matsson H, Davey EJ, Frojmark AS, et al. Erythropoiesis in the Rps19 disrupted mouse: analysis of erythropoietin response and biochemical markers for Diamond-Blackfan anemia. Blood Cells Mol Dis. 2006;36:259-264.

673. Oliver ER, Saunders TL, Tarle SA, Glaser T. Ribosomal protein L24 defect in belly spot and tail (Bst), a mouse Minute. Development. 2004;131:3907-3920.

674. Hamaguchi I, Flygare J, Nishiura H, et al. Proliferation deficiency of multipotent hematopoietic progenitors in ribosomal protein S19 (RPS19)-deficient Diamond-Blackfan anemia improves following RPS19 gene transfer. Mol Ther. 2003;7:613-622.

675. Hamaguchi I, Ooka A, Brun A, et al. Gene transfer improves erythroid development in ribosomal protein S19–deficient Diamond-Blackfan anemia. Blood. 2002; 100:2724-2731.

676. Ebert BL, Lee MM, Pretz JL, et al. An RNA interference model of RPS19 deficiency in Diamond-Blackfan anemia recapitulates defective hematopoiesis and rescue by dexamethasone: identification of dexamethasone-responsive genes by microarray. Blood. 2005;105:4620-4626.

677. Flygare J, Kiefer T, Miyake K, et al. Deficiency of ribosomal protein S19 in CD34+ cells generated by siRNA blocks erythroid development and mimics defects seen in Diamond-Blackfan anemia. Blood. 2005;105:4627-4634.

678. Choesmel V, Bacqueville D, Rouquette J, et al. Impaired ribosome biogenesis in Diamond-Blackfan anemia. Blood. 2007;109:1275-1283.

679. Idol R, Robledo S, Du H-Y, et al. Cells depleted for RPS19, a protein associated with Diamond Blackfan anemia, show defects in 18S ribosomal RNA synthesis and small ribosomal subunit production. Blood Cells Mol Dis. 2007;39:35-43.

680. Flygare J, Aspesi A, Bailey JC, et al. Human RPS19, the gene mutated in Diamond-Blackfan anemia, encodes a ribosomal protein required for the maturation of 40S ribosomal subunits. Blood. 2007;109:980-986.

681. Amsterdam A, Sadler KC, Lai K, et al. Many ribosomal protein genes are cancer genes in zebrafish. PLoS Biol. 2004;2:E139.

682. Gazda HT, Sieff CA. Recent insights into the pathogenesis of Diamond-Blackfan anaemia. Br J Haematol. 2006;135:149-157.

683. Stumpf JL. Deferasirox. Am J Health Syst Pharm. 2007;64:606-616.

684. Henter JI, Karlén J. Fatal agranulocytosis after deferiprone therapy in a child with Diamond-Blackfan anemia. Blood. 2007;109:5157-5159.

685. Mugishima H, Ohga S, Ohara A, et al. Hematopoietic stem cell transplantation for Diamond-Blackfan anemia: a report from the Aplastic Anemia Committee of the Japanese Society of Pediatric Hematology. Pediatr Transplant. 2007;11:601-607.

686. Abkowitz JL, Schaison G, Boulad F, et al. Response of Diamond-Blackfan anemia to metoclopramide: evidence for a role for prolactin in erythropoiesis. Blood. 2002;100:2687-2691.

687. Nawel G, Fethi M, Kouki R, Mohamed B. Successful treatment of Diamond Blackfan anemia with metoclopramide. J Pediatr Hematol Oncol. 2007;29:728.

688. Leblanc TM, Da Costa L, Marie I, et al. Metoclopramide treatment in DBA patients: no complete response in a French prospective study. Blood. 2007;109:2266-2267.

689. Pospisilova D, Cmejlova J, Hak J, et al. Successful treatment of a Diamond-Blackfan anemia patient with amino acid leucine. Haematologica. 2007;92:e66-e67.

690. Faivre L, Meerpohl J, Da Costa L, et al. High-risk pregnancies in Diamond-Blackfan anemia: a survey of 64 pregnancies from the French and German registries. Haematologica. 2006;91:530-533.

691. Crookston J, Godwin T, Wightmann K, et al. Congenital dyserythropoietic anemia. Paper presented at a meeting of the International Society of Hematology, 1966, Syndey, Australia.

692. Wendt F, Heimpel H. [Congenital dyserythropoietic anemia in a pair of dizygotic twins.] Med Klin. 1967;62:172-177.

693. Heimpel H, Wendt F. Congenital dyserythropoietic anemia with karyorrhexis and multinuclearity of erythroblasts. Helv Med Acta. 1968;34:103-115.

694. Wickramasinghe SN, Wood WG. Advances in the understanding of the congenital dyserythropoietic anaemias. Br J Haematol. 2005;131:431-446.

695. Holmberg L, Jansson L, Rausing A, Henriksson P. Type I congenital dyserythropoietic anaemia with myelopoietic abnormalities and hand malformations. Scand J Haematol. 1978;21:72-79.

696. Brichard B, Vermylen C, Scheiff JM, et al. Two cases of congenital dyserythropoietic anaemia type I associated with unusual skeletal abnormalities of the limbs. Br J Haematol. 1994;86:201-202.

697. Le Merrer M, Girot R, Parent P, et al. Acral dysostosis dyserythropoiesis syndrome. Eur J Pediatr. 1995;154:384-388.

698. Ayas M, al-Jefri A, Baothman A, et al. Transfusion-dependent congenital dyserythropoietic anemia type I successfully treated with allogeneic stem cell transplantation. Bone Marrow Transplant. 2002;29:681-682.

699. Verwilghen RL, Lewis SM, Dacie JV, et al. Hempas: congenital dyserythropoietic anaemia (type II). Q J Med. 1973;42:257-278.

700. Lavabre-Bertrand T, Blanc P, Navarro R, et al. Alpha-interferon therapy for congenital dyserythropoiesis type I. Br J Haematol. 1995;89:929-932.

701. Virjee S, Hatton C. Congenital dyserythropoiesis type I and alpha-interferon therapy. Br J Haematol. 1996;94:581-582.

702. Wickramasinghe SN. Response of CDA type I to alpha-interferon. Eur J Haematol. 1997;58:121-123.

703. Shamseddine A, Taher A, Jaafar H, et al. Interferon alpha is an effective therapy for congenital dyserythropoietic anaemia type I. Eur J Haematol. 2000;65:207-209.

704. Roda L, Pasche J, Fournier A, et al. Congenital dyserythropoietic anemia, type 1, in a Polynesian patient: response to interferon alpha2b. J Pediatr Hematol Oncol. 2002;24:503-506.

705. Lavabre-Bertrand T, Ramos J, Delfour C, et al. Long-term alpha interferon treatment is effective on anaemia and significantly reduces iron overload in congenital dyserythropoiesis type I. Eur J Haematol. 2004;73:380-383.

706. Goede JS, Benz R, Fehr J, et al. Congenital dyserythropoietic anemia type I with bone abnormalities, mutations of the CDAN I gene, and significant responsiveness to alpha-interferon therapy. Ann Hematol. 2006;85:591-595.

707. Iolascon A, Sabato V, de Mattia D, Locatelli F. Bone marrow transplantation in a case of severe, type II congenital dyserythropoietic anaemia (CDA II). Bone Marrow Transplant. 2001;27:213-215.

708. Remacha AF, Badell I, Pujol-Moix N, et al. Hydrops fetalis–associated congenital dyserythropoietic anemia treated with intrauterine transfusions and bone marrow transplantation. Blood. 2002;100:356-358.

709. Ariffin WA, Karnaneedi S, Choo KE, Normah J. Congenital dyserythropoietic anaemia: report of three cases. J Paediatr Child Health. 1996;32:191-193.

710. Shalev H, Kapelushnik J, Moser A, et al. A comprehensive study of the neonatal manifestations of congenital dyserythropoietic anemia type I. J Pediatr Hematol Oncol. 2004;26:746-748.

711. Smithson WA, Perrault J. Use of subcutaneous deferoxamine in a child with hemochromatosis associated with congenital dyserythropoietic anemia, type I. Mayo Clin Proc. 1982;57:322-325.

712. Wickramasinghe SN, Pippard MJ. Studies of erythroblast function in congenital dyserythropoietic anaemia, type I: evidence of impaired DNA, RNA, and protein synthesis and unbalanced globin chain synthesis in ultrastructurally abnormal cells. J Clin Pathol. 1986;39:881-890.

713. Bader-Meunier B, Leverger G, Tchernia G, et al. Clinical and laboratory manifestations of congenital dyserythropoietic anemia type I in a cohort of French children. J Pediatr Hematol Oncol. 2005;27:416-419.

714. Papanikolaou G, Tzilianos M, Christakis JI, et al. Hepcidin in iron overload disorders. Blood. 2005;105:4103-4105.

715. Tamary H, Dgany O, Proust A, et al. Clinical and molecular variability in congenital dyserythropoietic anaemia type I. Br J Haematol. 2005;130:628-634.

716. Wickramasinghe SN. Dyserythropoiesis and congenital dyserythropoietic anaemias. Br J Haematol. 1997;98:785-797.

717. Heimpel H, Forteza-Vila J, Queisser W, Spiertz E. Electron and light microscopic study of the erythroblasts of patients with congenital dyserythropoietic anemia. Blood. 1971;37:299-310.

718. Jean R, Dossa D, Navarro M, et al. [Congenital aplastic anemia, type I.] Arch Fr Pediatr. 1975;32:337-348.

719. Alloisio N, Jaccoud P, Dorleac E, et al. Alterations of globin chain synthesis and of red cell membrane proteins in congenital dyserythropoietic anemia I and II. Pediatr Res. 1982;16:1016-1021.

720. Tamary H, Shalmon L, Shalev H, et al. Localization of the gene for congenital dyserythropoietic anemia type I to a <1-cM interval on chromosome 15q15.1-15.3. Am J Hum Genet. 1998;62:1062-1069.

721. Dgany O, Avidan N, Delaunay J, et al. Congenital dyserythropoietic anemia type I is caused by mutations in codanin-1. Am J Hum Genet. 2002;71:1467-1474.

722. Heimpel H, Schwarz K, Ebnother M, et al. Congenital dyserythropoietic anemia type I (CDA I): molecular genetics, clinical appearance, and prognosis based on long-term observation. Blood. 2006;107:334-340.

723. Ahmed MR, Chehal A, Zahed L, et al. Linkage and mutational analysis of the CDAN1 gene reveals genetic heterogeneity in congenital dyserythropoietic anemia type I. Blood. 2006;107:4968-4969.

724. Crookston JH, Crookston MC, Burnie KL, et al. Hereditary erythroblastic multinuclearity associated with a positive acidified-serum test: a type of congenital dyserythropoietic anaemia. Br J Haematol. 1969;17:11-26.

725. Heimpel H, Anselstetter V, Chrobak L, et al. Congenital dyserythropoietic anemia type II: epidemiology, clinical appearance, and prognosis based on long-term observation. Blood. 2003;102:4576-4581.

726. Imran A, Mawhinney R, Swirsky D, Hall C. Paravertebral extramedullary haemopoiesis occurring in a case of congenital dyserythropoietic anaemia type II. Br J Haematol. 2008;140:1.

727. Verwilghen RL, Tan P, De Wolf-Peeters C, et al. Cell membrane anomaly impeding cell division. Experientia. 1971;27:1467-1468.

728. Wong KY, Hug G, Lampkin BC. Congenital dyserythropoietic anemia type II: ultrastructural and radioautographic studies of blood and bone marrow. Blood. 1972;39:23-30.

729. Alloisio N, Texier P, Denoroy L, et al. The cisternae decorating the red blood cell membrane in congenital dyserythropoietic anemia (type II) originate from the endoplasmic reticulum. Blood. 1996;87:4433-4439.

730. Heimpel H. Congenital dyserythropoietic anemias: epidemiology, clinical significance, and progress in understanding their pathogenesis. Ann Hematol. 2004;83:613-621.

731. Lowenthal RM, Marsden KA, Dewar CL, Thompson GR. Congenital dyserythropoietic anaemia (CDA) with severe gout, rare Kell phenotype and erythrocyte, granulocyte and platelet membrane reduplication: a new variant of CDA type II. Br J Haematol. 1980;44:211-220.

732. Fukuda MN. HEMPAS disease: genetic defect of glycosylation. Glycobiology. 1990;1:9-15.

733. Baines AJ, Banga JP, Gratzer WB, et al. Red cell membrane protein anomalies in congenital dyserythropoietic anaemia, type II (HEMP AS). Br J Haematol. 1982;50:563-574.

734. Mawby WJ, Tanner MJ, Anstee DJ, Clamp JR. Incomplete glycosylation of erythrocyte membrane proteins in congenital dyserythropoietic anaemia type II (CDA II). Br J Haematol. 1983;55:357-368.

735. Tomita A, Parker CJ. Aberrant regulation of complement by the erythrocytes of hereditary erythroblastic multinuclearity with a positive acidified serum lysis test (HEMPAS). Blood. 1994;83:250-259.

736. Delaunay J, Iolascon A. The congenital dyserythropoietic anaemias. Baillieres Best Pract Res Clin Haematol. 1999;12:691-705.

737. Iolascon A, D'Agostaro G, Perrotta S, et al. Congenital dyserythropoietic anemia type II: molecular basis and clinical aspects. Haematologica. 1996;81:543-559.

738. Iolascon A, Miraglia del Giudice E, Perrotta S, et al. Exclusion of three candidate genes as determinants of congenital dyserythropoietic anemia type II (CDA-II). Blood. 1997;90:4197-4200.

739. Wickramasinghe SN, Wahlin A, Anstee D, et al. Observations on two members of the Swedish family with congenital dyserythropoietic anaemia, type III. Eur J Haematol. 1993;50:213-221.

740. Zdebska E, Golaszewska E, Fabijanska-Mitek J, et al. Glycoconjugate abnormalities in patients with congenital dyserythropoietic anaemia type I, II and III. Br J Haematol. 2001;114:907-913.

741. Gasparini P, Miraglia del Giudice E, Delaunay J, et al. Localization of the congenital dyserythropoietic anemia II locus to chromosome 20q11.2 by genomewide search. Am J Hum Genet. 1997;61:1112-1116.

742. Lanzara C, Ficarella R, Totaro A, et al. Congenital dyserythropoietic anemia type II: exclusion of seven candidate genes. Blood Cells Mol Dis. 2003;30:22-29.

743. Iolascon A, De Mattia D, Perrotta S, et al. Genetic heterogeneity of congenital dyserythropoietic anemia type II. Blood. 1998;92:2593-2594.

744. Zdebska E, Iolascon A, Spychalska J, et al. Abnormalities of erythrocyte glycoconjugates are identical in two families with congenital dyserythropoietic anemia type II with different chromosomal localizations of the disease gene. Haematologica. 2007;92:427-428.

745. Paw BH, Davidson AJ, Zhou Y, et al. Cell-specific mitotic defect and dyserythropoiesis associated with erythroid band 3 deficiency. Nat Genet. 2003;34:59-64.

746. Perrotta S, Luzzatto L, Carella M, Iolascon A. Congenital dyserythropoietic anemia type II in human patients is not due to mutations in the erythroid anion exchanger 1. Blood. 2003;102:2704-2705.

747. Sandstrom H, Wahlin A. Congenital dyserythropoietic anemia type III. Haematologica. 2000;85:753-757.

748. Wolff JA, Von Hofe FH. Familial erythroid multinuclearity. Blood. 1951;6:1274-1283.

749. Bergstrom I, Jacobsson L. Hereditary benign erythroreticulosis. Blood. 1962;19:296-303.

750. Lind L, Sandstrom H, Wahlin A, et al. Localization of the gene for congenital dyserythropoietic anemia type III,

CDAN3, to chromosome 15q21-q25. Hum Mol Genet. 1995;4:109-112.

751. Goudsmit R, Beckers D, De Bruijne JI, et al. Congenital dyserythropoietic anaemia, type 3. Br J Haematol. 1972; 23:97-105.

752. Wickramasinghe SN, Parry TE, Williams C, et al. A new case of congenital dyserythropoietic anaemia, type III: studies of the cell cycle distribution and ultrastructure of erythroblasts and of nucleic acid synthesis in marrow cells. J Clin Pathol. 1982;35:1103-1109.

753. Wickramasinghe SN. Congenital dyserythropoietic anemias. Curr Opin Hematol. 2000;7:71-78.

754. Nichols KE, Crispino JD, Poncz M, et al. Familial dyserythropoietic anaemia and thrombocytopenia due to an inherited mutation in GATA1. Nat Genet. 2000;24: 266-270.

755. Mehaffey MG, Newton AL, Gandhi MJ, et al. X-linked thrombocytopenia caused by a novel mutation of GATA-1. Blood. 2001;98:2681-2688.

756. Yu C, Niakan KK, Matsushita M, et al. X-linked thrombocytopenia with thalassemia from a mutation in the amino finger of GATA-1 affecting DNA binding rather than FOG-1 interaction. Blood. 2002;100:2040-2045.

757. Balduini CL, Pecci A, Loffredo G, et al. Effects of the R216Q mutation of GATA-1 on erythropoiesis and megakaryocytopoiesis. Thromb Haemost. 2004;91:129-140.

758. Kostmann R. Infantile genetic agranulocytosis; agranulocytosis infantilis hereditaria. Acta Paediatr Suppl. 1956;45:1-78.

759. Kostmann R. Infantile genetic agranulocytosis. A review with presentation of ten new cases. Acta Paediatr Scand. 1975;64:362-368.

760. Welte K, Zeidler C, Reiter A, et al. Differential effects of granulocyte-macrophage colony-stimulating factor and granulocyte colony-stimulating factor in children with severe congenital neutropenia. Blood. 1990;75:1056-1063.

761. Welte K, Boxer LA. Severe chronic neutropenia: pathophysiology and therapy. Semin Hematol. 1997;34: 267-278.

762. Parmley R, Crist W, Ragab A, et al. Congenital dysgranulopoietic neutropenia: clinical, serologic, ultrastructural, and in vitro proliferative characteristics. Blood. 1980;56: 465-475.

763. Kawaguchi H, Kobayashi M, Nakamura K, et al. Dysregulation of transcriptions in primary granule constituents during myeloid proliferation and differentiation in patients with severe congenital neutropenia. J Leukoc Biol. 2003;73:225-234.

764. Konishi N, Kobayashi M, Miyagawa S, et al. Defective proliferation of primitive myeloid progenitor cells in patients with severe congenital neutropenia. Blood. 1999;94:4077-4083.

765. Hestdal K, Welte K, Lie SO, et al. Severe congenital neutropenia: abnormal growth and differentiation of myeloid progenitors to granulocyte colony-stimulating factor (G-CSF) but normal response to G-CSF plus stem cell factor. Blood. 1993;82:2991-2997.

766. Nakamura K, Kobayashi M, Konishi N, et al. Abnormalities of primitive myeloid progenitor cells expressing granulocyte colony-stimulating factor receptor in patients with severe congenital neutropenia. Blood. 2000;96: 4366-4369.

767. Boxer LA. Neutrophil abnormalities. Pediatr Rev. 2003;24:52-62.

768. Carlsson G, Wahlin YB, Johansson A, et al. Periodontal disease in patients from the original Kostmann family with severe congenital neutropenia. J Periodontol. 2006; 77:744-751.

769. Bishop NJ, Williams DM, Compston JC, et al. Osteoporosis in severe congenital neutropenia treated with granulocyte colony-stimulating factor. Br J Haematol. 1995;89: 927-928.

770. Yakisan E, Schirg E, Zeidler C, et al. High incidence of significant bone loss in patients with severe congenital neutropenia (Kostmann's syndrome). J Pediatr. 1997;131: 592-597.

771. Borzutzky A, Reyes ML, Figueroa V, et al. Osteoporosis in children with severe congenital neutropenia: bone mineral density and treatment with bisphosphonates. J Pediatr Hematol Oncol. 2006;28:205-209.

772. Takahashi T, Wada T, Mori M, et al. Overexpression of the granulocyte colony-stimulating factor gene leads to osteoporosis in mice. Lab Invest. 1996;74:827-834.

773. Freedman MH, Bonilla MA, Fier C, et al. Myelodysplasia syndrome and acute myeloid leukemia in patients with congenital neutropenia receiving G-CSF therapy. Blood. 2000;96:429-436.

774. Rosenberg PS, Alter BP, Bolyard AA, et al. The incidence of leukemia and mortality from sepsis in patients with severe congenital neutropenia receiving long-term G-CSF therapy. Blood. 2006;107:4628-4635.

775. Kalra R, Dale D, Freedman M, et al. Monosomy 7 and activating RAS mutations accompany malignant transformation in patients with congenital neutropenia. Blood. 1995;86:4579-4586.

776. Haurie C, Dale DC, Mackey MC. Cyclical neutropenia and other periodic hematological disorders: a review of mechanisms and mathematical models. Blood. 1998;92: 2629-2640.

777. Horwitz M, Benson KF, Person RE, et al. Mutations in ELA2, encoding neutrophil elastase, define a 21-day biological clock in cyclic haematopoiesis. Nat Genet. 1999;23:433-436.

778. Gorlin RJ, Gelb B, Diaz GA, et al. WHIM syndrome, an autosomal dominant disorder: clinical, hematological, and molecular studies. Am J Med Genet. 2000;91: 368-376.

779. Hernandez PA, Gorlin RJ, Lukens JN, et al. Mutations in the chemokine receptor gene CXCR4 are associated with WHIM syndrome, a combined immunodeficiency disease. Nat Genet. 2003;34:70-74.

780. Boxer LA, Newburger PE. A molecular classification of congenital neutropenia syndromes. Pediatr Blood Cancer. 2007;49:609-614.

781. Drachman JG. Inherited thrombocytopenia: when a low platelet count does not mean ITP. Blood. 2004;103: 390-398.

782. Dale DC, Person RE, Bolyard AA, et al. Mutations in the gene encoding neutrophil elastase in congenital and cyclic neutropenia. Blood. 2000;96:2317-2322.

783. Germeshausen M, Ballmaier M, Welte K. Incidence of CSF3R mutations in severe congenital neutropenia and relevance for leukemogenesis: results of a long-term survey. Blood 2007;109:93-99.

784. Bellanne-Chantelot C, Clauin S, Leblanc T, et al. Mutations in the ELA2 gene correlate with more severe expression of neutropenia: a study of 81 patients from the French Neutropenia Register. Blood. 2004;103:4119-4125.

785. Ancliff PJ, Gale RE, Liesner R, et al. Mutations in the ELA2 gene encoding neutrophil elastase are present in most patients with sporadic severe congenital neutropenia but only in some patients with the familial form of the disease. Blood. 2001;98:2645-2650.

786. Ancliff PJ, Gale RE, Watts MJ, et al. Paternal mosaicism proves the pathogenic nature of mutations in neutrophil elastase in severe congenital neutropenia. Blood. 2002;100:707-709.

787. Bieth J. Leukocyte Elastase. San Diego, CA, Academic Press, 1998.

788. Li FQ, Horwitz M. Characterization of mutant neutrophil elastase in severe congenital neutropenia. J Biol Chem. 2001;276:14230-11441.

789. Benson KF, Li FQ, Person RE, et al. Mutations associated with neutropenia in dogs and humans disrupt intracellular transport of neutrophil elastase. Nat Genet. 2003;35:90-96.

790. Massullo P, Druhan LJ, Bunnell BA, et al. Aberrant subcellular targeting of the G185R neutrophil elastase mutant associated with severe congenital neutropenia induces premature apoptosis of differentiating promyelocytes. Blood. 2005;105:3397-3404.

791. Grenda DS, Murakami M, Ghatak J, et al. Mutations of the ELA2 gene found in patients with severe congenital neutropenia induce the unfolded protein response and cellular apoptosis. Blood. 2007;110:4179-4187.

792. Kollner I, Sodeik B, Schreek S, et al. Mutations in neutrophil elastase causing congenital neutropenia lead to cytoplasmic protein accumulation and induction of the unfolded protein response. Blood. 2006;108:493-500.

793. Klein C, Grudzien M, Appaswamy G, et al. HAX1 deficiency causes autosomal recessive severe congenital neutropenia (Kostmann disease). Nat Genet. 2007;39:86-92.

794. Suzuki Y, Demoliere C, Kitamura D, et al. HAX-1, a novel intracellular protein, localized on mitochondria, directly associates with HS1, a substrate of Src family tyrosine kinases. J Immunol. 1997;158:2736-2744.

795. Dror Y, Ward AC, Touw IP, Freedman MH. Combined corticosteroid/granulocyte colony-stimulating factor (G-CSF) therapy in the treatment of severe congenital neutropenia unresponsive to G-CSF: Activated glucocorticoid receptors synergize with G-CSF signals. Exp Hematol. 2000;28:1381-1389.

796. Druhan LJ, Ai J, Massullo P, et al. Novel mechanism of G-CSF refractoriness in patients with severe congenital neutropenia. Blood. 2005;105:584-591.

797. Sinha S, Zhu QS, Romero G, Corey SJ. Deletional mutation of the external domain of the human granulocyte colony-stimulating factor receptor in a patient with severe chronic neutropenia refractory to granulocyte colony-stimulating factor. J Pediatr Hematol Oncol. 2003;25:791-796.

798. Person RE, Li FQ, Duan Z, et al. Mutations in proto-oncogene GFI1 cause human neutropenia and target ELA2. Nat Genet. 2003;34:308-312.

799. Ancliff PJ, Blundell MP, Cory GO, et al. Two novel activating mutations in the Wiskott-Aldrich syndrome protein result in congenital neutropenia. Blood. 2006;108:2182-2189.

800. Devriendt K, Kim AS, Mathijs G, et al. Constitutively activating mutation in WASP causes X-linked severe congenital neutropenia. Nat Genet. 2001;27:313-317.

801. Skokowa J, Cario G, Uenalan M, et al. LEF-1 is crucial for neutrophil granulocytopoiesis and its expression is severely reduced in congenital neutropenia. Nat Med. 2006;12:1191-1197.

802. Link DC, Kunter G, Kasai Y, et al. Distinct patterns of mutations occurring in de novo AML versus AML arising in the setting of severe congenital neutropenia. Blood. 2007;110:1648-1655.

803. Dong F, Brynes RK, Tidow N, et al. Mutations in the gene for the granulocyte colony-stimulating-factor receptor in patients with acute myeloid leukemia preceded by severe congenital neutropenia. N Engl J Med. 1995;333:487-493.

804. Dong F, Dale DC, Bonilla MA, et al. Mutations in the granulocyte colony-stimulating factor receptor gene in patients with severe congenital neutropenia. Leukemia. 1997;11:120-125.

805. Tidow N, Pilz C, Teichmann B, et al. Clinical relevance of point mutations in the cytoplasmic domain of the granulocyte colony-stimulating factor receptor gene in patients with severe congenital neutropenia. Blood. 1997;89:2369-2375.

806. Hermans MH, Antonissen C, Ward AC, et al. Sustained receptor activation and hyperproliferation in response to granulocyte colony-stimulating factor (G-CSF) in mice with a severe congenital neutropenia/acute myeloid leukemia–derived mutation in the G-CSF receptor gene. J Exp Med. 1999;189:683-692.

807. McLemore ML, Poursine-Laurent J, Link DC. Increased granulocyte colony-stimulating factor responsiveness but normal resting granulopoiesis in mice carrying a targeted granulocyte colony-stimulating factor receptor mutation derived from a patient with severe congenital neutropenia. J Clin Invest. 1998;102:483-492.

808. Dale DC, Bonilla MA, Davis MW, et al. A randomized controlled phase III trial of recombinant human granulocyte colony-stimulating factor (filgrastim) for treatment of severe chronic neutropenia. Blood. 1993;81:2496-2502.

809. Zeidler C, Welte K, Barak Y, et al. Stem cell transplantation in patients with severe congenital neutropenia without evidence of leukemic transformation. Blood. 2000;95:1195-1198.

810. Ferry C, Ouachee M, Leblanc T, et al. Hematopoietic stem cell transplantation in severe congenital neutropenia: experience of the French SCN register. 2004;35:45.

811. Choi SW, Boxer LA, Pulsipher MA, et al. Stem cell transplantation in patients with severe congenital neutropenia with evidence of leukemic transformation. 2005;35:473.

812. Shannon K. Inside blood: Reconsidering how we treat severe congenital neutropenia. Blood. 2006;107:4575-4576.

813. Thachil J, Caswell M, Bolton-Maggs PH, et al. Non-myeloablative transplantation for severe congenital neutropenia. Pediatr Blood Cancer. July 17, 2007 [Epub ahead of print].

814. Geddis AE. Inherited thrombocytopenia: Congenital amegakaryocytic thrombocytopenia and thrombocytopenia with absent radii. Semin Hematol. 2006;43:196-203.

815. King S, Germeshausen M, Strauss G, et al. Congenital amegakaryocytic thrombocytopenia: a retrospective clinical analysis of 20 patients. Br J Haematol. 2005;131:636-644.

816. Ihara K, Ishii E, Eguchi M, et al. Identification of mutations in the c-mpl gene in congenital amegakaryocytic thrombocytopenia. Proc Natl Acad Sci U S A. 1999;96:3132-3136.

817. Ballmaier M, Germeshausen M, Schulze H, et al. c-mpl mutations are the cause of congenital amegakaryocytic thrombocytopenia. Blood. 2001;97:139-146.

818. Tonelli R, Scardovi AL, Pession A, et al. Compound heterozygosity for two different amino-acid substitution mutations in the thrombopoietin receptor (c-mpl gene) in congenital amegakaryocytic thrombocytopenia (CAMT). Hum Genet. 2000;107:225-233.

819. Savoia A, Dufour C, Locatelli F, et al. Congenital amegakaryocytic thrombocytopenia: clinical and biological consequences of five novel mutations. Haematologica. 2007;92:1186-1193.

820. Muraoka K, Ishii E, Ihara K, et al. Successful bone marrow transplantation in a patient with c-mpl–mutated congenital amegakaryocytic thrombocytopenia from a carrier donor. Pediatr Transplant. 2005;9:101-103.

821. MacMillan ML, Davies SM, Wagner JE, Ramsay NK. Engraftment of unrelated donor stem cells in children with familial amegakaryocytic thrombocytopenia. Bone Marrow Transplant. 1998;21:735-737.

822. Lackner A, Basu O, Bierings M, et al. Haematopoietic stem cell transplantation for amegakaryocytic thrombocytopenia. Br J Haematol. 2000;109:773-775.

823. Steele M, Hitzler J, Doyle JJ, et al. Reduced intensity hematopoietic stem-cell transplantation across human leukocyte antigen barriers in a patient with congenital amegakaryocytic thrombocytopenia and monosomy 7. Pediatr Blood Cancer. 2005;45:212-216.

824. Richard RE, Blau CA. Small-molecule–directed mpl signaling can complement growth factors to selectively expand genetically modified cord blood cells. Stem Cells. 2003;21:71-78.

825. Hall JG, Levin J, Kuhn JP, et al. Thrombocytopenia with absent radius (TAR). Medicine (Baltimore). 1969;48:411-439.

826. Ray R, Zorn E, Kelly T, et al. Lower limb anomalies in the thrombocytopenia absent-radius (TAR) syndrome. Am J Med Genet. 1980;7:523-528.

827. Hedberg VA, Lipton JM. Thrombocytopenia with absent radii. A review of 100 cases. Am J Pediatr Hematol Oncol. 1988;10:51-64.

828. Greenhalgh KL, Howell RT, Bottani A, et al. Thrombocytopenia–absent radius syndrome: a clinical genetic study. J Med Genet. 2002;39:876-881.

829. Whitfield MF, Barr DG. Cows' milk allergy in the syndrome of thrombocytopenia with absent radius. Arch Dis Child. 1976;51:337-343.

830. Ahmad R, Pope S. Association of Mayer-Rokitansky-Kuster-Hauser syndrome with thrombocytopenia absent radii syndrome: a rare presentation. Eur J Obstet Gynecol Reprod Biol. May 28, 2007 [Epub ahead of print].

831. Gounder DS, Pullon HW, Ockelford PA, Nicol RO. Clinical manifestations of the thrombocytopenia and absent radii (TAR) syndrome. Aust N Z J Med. 1989;19:479-482.

832. Ballmaier M, Schulze H, Strauss G, et al. Thrombopoietin in patients with congenital thrombocytopenia and absent radii: elevated serum levels, normal receptor expression, but defective reactivity to thrombopoietin. Blood. 1997;90:612-619.

833. Muraoka K, Ishii E, Tsuji K, et al. Defective response to thrombopoietin and impaired expression of c-mpl mRNA of bone marrow cells in congenital amegakaryocytic thrombocytopenia. Br J Haematol. 1997;96:287-292.

834. Letestu R, Vitrat N, Masse A, et al. Existence of a differentiation blockage at the stage of a megakaryocyte precursor in the thrombocytopenia and absent radii (TAR) syndrome. Blood. 2000;95:1633-1641.

835. Camitta BM, Rock A. Acute lymphoidic leukemia in a patient with thrombocytopenia/absent radii (TAR) syndrome. Am J Pediatr Hematol Oncol. 1993;15:335-337.

836. Fadoo Z, Naqvi SM. Acute myeloid leukemia in a patient with thrombocytopenia with absent radii syndrome. J Pediatr Hematol Oncol. 2002;24:134-135.

837. Go RS, Johnston KL. Acute myelogenous leukemia in an adult with thrombocytopenia with absent radii syndrome. Eur J Haematol. 2003;70:246-248.

838. Thompson AA, Nguyen LT. Amegakaryocytic thrombocytopenia and radio-ulnar synostosis are associated with HOXA11 mutation. Nat Genet. 2000;26:397-398.

839. Thompson AA, Woodruff K, Feig SA, et al. Congenital thrombocytopenia and radio-ulnar synostosis: a new familial syndrome. Br J Haematol. 2001;113:866-870.

840. Ballmaier M, Schulze H, Cremer M, et al. Defective c-Mpl signaling in the syndrome of thrombocytopenia with absent radii. Stem Cells. 1998;16(Suppl 2):177-184.

841. Fleischman RA, Letestu R, Mi X, et al. Absence of mutations in the HoxA10, HoxA11 and HoxD11 nucleotide coding sequences in thrombocytopenia with absent radius syndrome. Br J Haematol. 2002;116:367-375.

842. Klopocki E, Schulze H, Strauss G, et al. Complex inheritance pattern resembling autosomal recessive inheritance involving a microdeletion in thrombocytopenia–absent radius syndrome. Am J Hum Genet. 2007;80:232-240.

843. Aquino VM, Mustafa MM, Vaickus L, et al. Recombinant interleukin-6 in the treatment of congenital thrombocytopenia associated with absent radii. J Pediatr Hematol Oncol. 1998;20:474-476.

9 Principles of Bone Marrow and Stem Cell Transplantation

W. Nicholas Haining, Christine Duncan, and Leslie E. Lehmann

Hematopoietic stem cell transplantation (HSCT) has become an accepted treatment of a wide variety of diseases, including hematologic malignancies, bone marrow failure syndromes, immunodeficiency disorders, congenital hematologic defects, and some solid tumors. HSCT generally begins with the administration of high doses of chemotherapy, total body irradiation (TBI), or both to destroy malignant cells and sufficiently immunosuppress the recipient so that the graft will not be rejected. Patients are profoundly immunocompromised as a result and are at risk for opportunistic infections. These infectious risks, together with other complications such as graft rejection, graft-versus-host disease (GVHD), and primary disease recurrence, have been the main barriers to success in HSCT. However, advances in understanding the biology and immunology underlying transplantation, coupled with improvements in supportive care and clinical management of complications, have made HSCT an increasingly efficacious modality for a broadening range of indications.

HISTORY AND OVERVIEW

Infusion of bone marrow in an effort to restore hematopoiesis was first reported in 1939: a patient with aplastic anemia was treated by regular transfusions, as well as the infusion of a small aliquot of fraternal bone marrow.[1] Subsequently, Jacobson and colleagues demonstrated that shielding the spleen from radiation allowed mice receiving lethal doses of radiation to recover normal hematopoiesis.[2,3] Ultimately, such experiments made it clear that hemato-poietic reconstitution of irradiated animals originated from elements in the bone marrow or spleen.[4] These hematopoietic stem cells (HSCs) were also shown to function after cryopreservation and thawing.[5] Investigators subsequently demonstrated that animals did well if histocompatible HSCs were infused but suffered from GVHD if given cells from a histoincompatible donor.[6] Better understanding of the biology of the immune response coupled with the observation that administration of methotrexate was effective for both prophylaxis and treatment of GVHD[7] provided both the theoretical and practical tools necessary for HSCT to be studied in humans.

The first attempt at human bone marrow transplantation (BMT) was carried out in 1957 by E. Donnall Thomas, whose body of work in this area was later recognized by a Nobel Prize. These first experiments were performed in patients with advanced hematologic malignancies and demonstrated that chemotherapy followed by intravenous marrow infusion could result in a transient graft, although all patients subsequently died of progressive disease.[8] In 1959, lethal doses of TBI and bone marrow from an identical twin were used to transplant two patients with advanced acute lymphoblastic leukemia (ALL).[9] Hematopoiesis was established within weeks, although again both patients relapsed and died.

The first successful allogeneic HSCT procedures were performed in 1968 and 1969, with the survival of three patients who underwent transplantation for congenital immunodeficiencies.[10-13]

HSCT is currently used for a variety of malignant and nonmalignant disorders in which replacement of HSC-derived populations of cells provides or restores normal hematopoiesis or other marrow-derived elements. In malignant diseases, infusion of previously collected HSCs abrogates myelosuppression as the dose-limiting toxicity of chemotherapy regimens. Although bone marrow was initially considered the only source of pluripotent HSCs, more recently it has become clear that other sources exist. For example, self-renewing HSCs can be collected from umbilical cord blood (UCB). The low absolute number of HSCs circulating in peripheral blood can be increased after chemotherapy by the administration of hematopoietic growth factors and collected as mobilized peripheral blood stem cells (PBSCs). Exploration of the potential for cell populations derived from tissues such as the liver, nervous system, and muscle to provide HSCs has been initiated.[14-18]

Reinfusion of a patient's own HSCs after the administration of high-dose chemotherapy, radiation therapy, or both is referred to as autologous HSCT. Both tumor contamination and preexisting damage to HSCs from previous therapy limit its application in cases of malignant disease. Moreover, the lack of an allogeneic immunologic response against any residual or recurrent tumor may further have an impact on success. In the case of congenital or acquired benign hematologic conditions, stem cell abnormalities prevent autologous HSCT from being a meaningful option for most patients. Thus, autologous transplants are used mostly for the treatment of lymphomas or solid tumors. Allogeneic HSCT is the infusion of HSCs from a related or unrelated donor. Complications of allogeneic HSCT, such as graft rejection and GVHD, are generally more common or severe with increasing histoincompatibility between the donor and host, and a histocompatible sibling, if available, remains the preferred donor. However, it is estimated that only 15% to 40% of patients will have a matched related donor.[19,20] Available alternatives include HSCT from a related donor that is mismatched[21,22] or from donors in the unrelated donor pool,[23-25] including unrelated UCB collections.[26-28]

Specific conditioning regimens used to prepare patients are reviewed in the next section. In brief, the preparative regimen must reduce or eliminate tumor burden or recipient hematopoietic cells (or both) and provide sufficient immunosuppression to permit engraftment. After conditioning, HSCs are infused intravenously into the host; the day of HSC infusion is termed day 0. Neutrophil engraftment occurs approximately 10 to 24 days after infusion, with red cell and platelet recovery somewhat more delayed. A number of peritransplant and post-transplant complications influence not only survival but also quality of life after transplantation (Box 9-1).

Box 9-1	Complications of Bone Marrow Transplantation

SHORT TERM

Graft rejection
Infection
Bleeding
Acute graft-versus-host disease
Veno-occlusive disease of the liver
Idiopathic pneumonitis
Side effects of radiation therapy, chemotherapy, and
   immunosuppressive therapy (e.g., pancytopenia
   mucositis)

LONG TERM

Late graft failure
Chronic graft-versus-host disease and its sequelae (e.g.,
   bronchiolitis obliterans)
Pulmonary disorders
Infection
Altered intellectual and growth development in children
Endocrine dysfunction
   Hypothyroidism
   Growth retardation (children)
   Pubertal delay, gonadal failure
   Sexual dysfunction (both sexes)
Complications secondary to radiation therapy (e.g.,
   cataracts, radiation nephritis)
Complications secondary to immunosuppressive therapy
   (e.g., aseptic necrosis of bone)
Dental problems
Psychosocial problems
Increased risk for second malignancies

There is a risk of early graft rejection and late graft failure. Early complications of HSCT are due to profound pancytopenia, regimen-related toxicity, immunologic reaction of the graft against host tissues (acute GVHD [aGVHD]) if the transplant is allogeneic, and protracted immune incompetence. Late complications of HSCT are due to chronic end-organ damage from drug and immune insults and ongoing or de novo manifestations of immune dysregulation such as poor immune function or chronic GVHD (cGVHD). Each of these factors and complications is considered in detail later.

Given these obstacles, the evolution of HSCT into a practical and curative therapy has been dependent on a number of important advances, including improved appreciation of the human histocompatibility system and development of more exact methods to establish the degree of histocompatibility between the donor and recipient. The ability to deliver the preparative regimen with greater accuracy, as illustrated both by improvements in TBI dosimetry and strategy and by the ability to monitor busulfan pharmacokinetics, has significantly

decreased regimen-related toxicity. Early and aggressive use of antibiotics, antifungal agents, and antiviral agents has improved survival during the early neutropenic period and during the period of profound and persistent immunosuppression after engraftment. Advances in transfusion support, such as viral screening, irradiation of blood products, and the availability of leukopheresed platelet products, have had enormous impact. Nutritional and other supportive therapies, including the ability to establish long-term vascular access with indwelling lines, has significantly changed the experience and comfort of HSCT recipients. Although HSCT was originally offered only to the rare patient with end-stage disease, improved outcomes because of these and other advances have markedly increased the situations in which the HSCT can provide benefit.

CONDITIONING REGIMENS

The term *conditioning regimen* refers to the preparative drugs or radiation (or both) that are administered to an HSCT recipient before the graft is infused. The purpose of conditioning is threefold: first, to eradicate all malignant cells; second, to be sufficiently immunosuppressive to prevent the immune system of the recipient from rejecting incoming allogeneic cells; and third, to induce enough marrow aplasia that the donor HSCs have a competitive advantage in reconstituting hematopoiesis. Regimens that are capable of achieving all three goals are usually associated with significant toxicity. Therefore, a major goal in HSCT is the development of conditioning regimens that provide an optimal balance between effective myeloablation and manageable toxicity.

The first human BMT by Thomas and colleagues in 1957[9] and a subsequent experience using unrelated donor marrow to treat victims of a radiation accident in Belgrade in 1959[29] established the basic principle of TBI-based conditioning. Work initiated by Santos, Owens, and Sensenbrenner in the 1960s first demonstrated the effectiveness of cyclophosphamide as a conditioning agent.[30] TBI combined with cyclophosphamide has remained the standard conditioning regimen for the last 30 years. More recently, the alkylating agent busulfan has become more widely used as an alternative to TBI, in part because of limited access to costly radiation facilities.[31]

The wide range of indications for HSCT has led to considerable variation in the design of conditioning regimens. For example, high relapse rates after HSCT stimulated attempts to increase the antileukemic efficacy of conditioning regimens by using other high-dose chemotherapy agents in place of or in addition to cyclophosphamide. In contrast, the problem of graft failure/rejection in patients receiving grafts that are T-cell depleted or from genetically disparate donors has led to regimens that increase recipient immunosuppression. Patients with aplastic anemia or severe combined immunodeficiency

(SCID) have preexisting marrow aplasia or immunosuppression, and thus conditioning regimens in these diseases do not require the same degree of myelosuppression as regimens for patients with intact immune function. Similarly, patients with benign hematologic diseases have no need of the antileukemic effect of conditioning, and therefore specialized myeloablative regimens have been developed specifically for these conditions.[32] In addition, as autologous HSC support for high-dose chemotherapy became more common, many new conditioning regimens were developed with an emphasis on potential antitumor effects. Although individual studies demonstrated acceptable or even favorable outcomes related to some of these changes, no consensus on optimal recipient preparation for either autologous or allogeneic stem cell transplantation (SCT) has emerged. More recently, alternative concepts regarding the relative roles of conditioning regimens and the donor immune system in achieving recipient hematopoietic ablation have been applied in preclinical and clinical studies of nonmyeloablative transplantation. Some key issues are highlighted later.

Total Body Irradiation. Several parameters associated with TBI can be adjusted to deliver different amounts of radiation and different degrees of end-organ effect. Total dose, dose rate, fraction size, interfraction interval, and shielding are among the TBI parameters most manipulated in SCT. An ideal schedule would maximize malignant cell killing, hematopoietic ablation, and in the case of allogeneic SCT, immunosuppression while limiting acute and chronic toxicity. In principle, a higher total dose, higher dose rate, and larger fraction size are associated with greater hematopoietic ablative effect (and therefore potentially greater antileukemic efficacy) and with better immunosuppression. Fractionation, or division of the total dose of radiation over time, usually in a twice-daily schedule, theoretically yields improved tolerance of nonhematopoietic tissues and leads to decreased acute toxicity and reduced late effects, but it carries the risk of decreased antileukemic efficacy. However, a series of studies from the 1980s support the use of fractionated radiation, and this remains the standard today.[33,34] Studies from Seattle demonstrated decreased relapse as the total radiation dose increased, but lung, liver, and kidney toxicity was limiting.[35,36] The parameters total dose, fractionation, dose rate, and schedule have largely been extrapolated to pediatric HSCT from adults.[37,38]

Busulfan. Developed in the mid-1970s, busulfan (BU)/cyclophosphamide (CY) rapidly became an established regimen for patients with acute myelocytic leukemia (AML) undergoing either allogeneic[39] or autologous SCT.[40-42] The original regimen, called BU/CY4 (big BU/CY: BU, 4 mg/kg/day for 4 days, followed by CY, 50 mg/kg/day for 4 days) was joined by BU/CY2 (little BU/CY, in which the CY was delivered as 60 mg/kg/day for 2 days),[41-45] and this regimen has been used in patients with acute lymphoblastic leukemia (ALL) or chronic myelog-

enous leukemia (CML).[46,47] The BU/CY regimen has been used extensively in pediatric patients, particularly those with nonmalignant diseases,[48-53] in an attempt to avoid radiation-mediated toxicity.

Total Body Irradiation versus Busulfan. Several randomized studies and meta-analyses have compared BU/CY with TBI-based regimens.[54-62] Overall, the results are similar, although they suggest that both relapse rates and hepatic veno-occlusive disease (VOD) may be less frequent in the TBI-containing regimens. Even though recent data support these observations, variability of the chemotherapy component of TBI-based regimens and potential differences in the antileukemic efficacy of BU/CY4 and BU/CY2 regimens[63] render definitive generalizations difficult. Reports of decreased bioavailability, increased volume of distribution, and increased clearance rate of busulfan in children raise the question of how to interpret studies in which such data are unavailable.[64-67] Alternative busulfan dosing, based on plasma levels, has been suggested,[68,69] and studies comparing "optimal" BU/CY with CY/TBI have not been performed. Busulfan-containing regimens have often been reported to result in greater toxicity than TBI-based regimens; thus, increases in the busulfan dose may further increase regimen-related morbidity.[54,55,57,60,70,71] Monitoring of busulfan pharmacokinetics has generally, but not always demonstrated an association of increased area under the curve with increased VOD.[68,72] Individualizing busulfan dosing may possibly increase the benefit-risk ratio, and the recent availability of an intravenous form of busulfan with more dependable pharmacokinetics now makes such individualization feasible.[73-76]

Alternative Myeloablative Regimens. The addition or substitution of a variety of chemotherapeutic agents to the backbone of CY/TBI—and less commonly BU/CY—has met with mixed success. Etoposide (VP-16), cytarabine, and busulfan have been added to or substituted for cyclophosphamide in TBI-based regimens.[58,77-84] Etoposide and melphalan have also replaced cyclophosphamide in some busulfan-based protocols.[85-88] Fluorouracil, high-dose methotrexate, doxorubicin, cisplatin, carboplatin, thiotepa, melphalan, and many other agents have been used in a variety of high-dose chemotherapeutic regimens supported by autologous SCT. Common conditioning regimens referred to by acronyms are CBV (cyclophosphamide, BCNU [carmustine], VP-16), BACT (BCNU, Ara-C [cytarabine], cyclophosphamide, 6-thioguanine), BEAM (BCNU, etoposide, Ara-C, melphalan), and CBP (cyclophosphamide, BCNU, cisplatin). In the allogeneic setting, alternative regimens have generally shown equivalent benefit in terms of disease control but often at the cost of increased toxicity. No regimen has established unequivocal superiority in terms of disease-free survival (DFS) or overall survival when compared with "standard" regimens. Given the more limited follow-up and the extraordinary diversity of diseases and regimens, establishment of relative efficacy in the realm of autologous SCT is likely to be a complicated and prolonged process.[89-93]

Nonmyeloablative Regimens. One of the target tissues of allogeneic T lymphocytes is the hematopoietic precursors. As a result, the infusion of donor lymphocytes can be sufficient to cause marrow aplasia. Indeed, this is the basis of the marrow aplasia seen in inadvertent cases of transfusional GVHD. Observations made initially in the 1980s by the Seattle group have led to a new approach to conditioning based on the immunologic elimination of normal and malignant hematopoiesis. Because this technique minimizes the doses of conventional conditioning drugs and radiation, it has been termed "nonmyeloablative" or reduced-intensity conditioning.[94-100] Although allogeneic graft-versus–bone marrow can cause the necessary marrow aplasia and antileukemic efficacy, it does not supply the immunosuppression needed to avoid graft rejection. This is usually achieved by preinfusion conditioning with purine analogue chemotherapy, low-dose TBI, or both. A variety of agents, including lower-dose busulfan, melphalan, and cytarabine, have also been used for additional effect and partial HSC depletion.[94-96,98-100] A major advantage of this approach is that the toxicity of conventional myeloablative approaches can be reduced.[101] Comparisons of conventional and nonmyeloablative regimens have shown reduced non–relapse-related mortality, especially in older adults or patients with preexisting illnesses, in whom HSCT is associated with significant toxic death rates.[102,103] The safety and effectiveness of this approach have led to its wider application in recent years. However, the low toxicity of nonmyeloablative regimens is balanced against the increased risk of relapse in acute leukemias and the increased risk of cGVHD.[104] The indications for nonmyeloablative transplantation may therefore remain principally for slower-growing tumors. Because childhood hematologic malignancies rarely fall into this category, the use of nonmyeloablative transplantation in children has been more limited.[96,105,106] Moreover, the increased risk of graft rejection associated with standard HSCT for nonmalignant conditions such as thalassemia and sickle cell anemia have precluded the broad use of nonmyeloablative transplantation for these conditions.

SOURCES OF STEM CELLS

Selection of an appropriate source of HSCs for a patient undergoing HSCT has become a more complex undertaking in recent years. HSCs can be obtained from bone marrow, peripheral blood, or the umbilical vein of newborn infants. The majority of HSCT procedures in the pediatric setting are performed from allogeneic donors, but autologous bone marrow or peripheral blood is used as a source of transplants as well, particularly in patients with solid tumors. For each disease entity, the clinician must consider what sources of stem cells are available and the relative risks and benefits associated with each potential stem cell source. For allogeneic donors, the principal consideration in donor selection is the genetic similarity between donor and recipient.

Typing. Genetic disparity between host and donor can lead to graft rejection or GVHD. The genes encoding the antigens most associated with these complications lie in a group of genes known as the major histocompatibility complex (MHC). In humans, the MHC maps to a region of the short arm of chromosome 6 known as the HLA system. The MHC codes for many genes, and identification and exploration of the functional importance of some of these gene products are still ongoing. Among the best characterized gene products are proteins comprising the class I and class II antigens. In humans, MHC class I molecules include HLA-A, HLA-B, and HLA-C, and MHC class II molecules are called HLA-D. There are at least five subregions, including DR, DQ, and DP, but the number of genes transcribed differs between different HLA class II haplotypes.

MHC class I antigens are present on nearly all human cells (with rare exceptions such as erythrocytes and corneal endothelium). MHC class II antigen expression is more restricted, with expression limited to "professional" antigen-presenting cells, including dendritic cells, B cells, monocytes, macrophages, and Langerhans cells. Class II antigens can also be induced on activated T cells and endothelium. MHC genes are codominantly expressed—that is, each parent contributes half the MHC antigens expressed on each cell of their offspring. MHC class I and II antigens normally function to present partially degraded products of intracellular proteins to T cells. In this way, damaged or virally infected cells can be identified by the immune system. However, in the setting of transplantation, recognition of MHC molecules by T cells is known as *alloimmunity* and is the basis for GVHD and graft rejection.

The genes of the MHC region are highly polymorphic. Matched siblings have inherited the same two copies of chromosome 6 from the parents and thus identical HLA antigens—such a pair of donors are said to be genotypically identical. However, even HLA-identical sibling transplants can be associated with GVHD. Differences in the sequences of intracellular proteins physically associated with MHC molecules are caused by polymorphisms in non-MHC genes, such as blood group antigens and cell adhesion molecules. These polymorphisms are mostly unidentified, and those that are known to elicit alloreactive T-cell responses are termed *minor histocompatibility antigens.*[107] Although these antigens may not be directly responsible for organ and bone marrow rejection, human typing studies suggest that these minor antigens contribute to the generation of GVHD.[108,109]

Historically, HLA typing was performed by using antibodies derived from postpartum sera, from persons who have undergone transplantation or transfusion, or even from persons immunized for the purpose of generating specific serologic reagents. These antibodies were used in a standardized complement-dependent, microcytotoxicity assay with purified T or B lymphocytes as their target cell.[110] The extensive cross-reactivity among products coded by alleles of the HLA-A and HLA-B loci, known as *cross-reactive groups*, made precise delineation of MHC class I antigens by this technique difficult. In contrast, HLA-D specificities were originally defined by their ability to stimulate T-lymphocyte proliferation in a mixed leukocyte culture.[111]

The aforementioned approach, termed *low-resolution typing*, provides sufficient accuracy in the matched sibling setting. However, only approximately 30% of patients have an acceptable sibling donor, and as the infrastructure necessary to identify unrelated donors became available, high-resolution HLA typing techniques that resolve the DNA sequence of specific alleles was essential. The first attempts to use molecular genetic techniques were based on the application of restriction fragment length polymorphism analysis of genomic DNA by Southern blotting with HLA region probes. This technique soon gave way to the current technology in which sequence-specific oligonucleotide probes and, in some cases, direct sequence analysis are performed. This has also led to a great increase in the number of HLA specificities identified. This fine analysis is increasingly being used to determine the haplotypes of patients and potential donors. The implications of more exact typing within families, where the haplotypes are "conserved," are probably confined to the potential identification of differences in minor histocompatibility antigens to allow better selection between possible donors.[108,109,112] In the unrelated donor setting, high-resolution HLA matching has significantly contributed to the lower incidence of GVHD, hence improved outcomes reported in unrelated donor HSCT in the past decade.[113-115] Historically, an allogeneic donor must match the patient at five of the six major loci (A, B, DR) for a transplant to be feasible. Stem cells obtained from UCB are more permissive, and four out of six matches is acceptable. The lower incidence of GVHD when UCB is employed is probably due to the relatively low dose of cells obtained from that source. What degree of mismatching at other loci or which specific loci are most important when mismatch is inevitable has yet to be established.

Allogeneic Stem Cell Transplantation

To date, most allogeneic transplants have used HSCs from a matched sibling donor. However, with improvements in immunosuppression and the ability to prevent or treat GVHD, unrelated donors, umbilical cord blood (UBC), and partially MHC-mismatched donors are now increasingly being used as sources of HSCs. There are presently approximately 10 million unrelated donors listed in more than 72 registries worldwide, including registries of banked unrelated donor UCB collections.

Selection of an allogeneic HSC source is dependent on many variables. In malignant disease, the ease and speed with which a stem cell source can be obtained are important factors. For patients with aggressive malignancies, being able to proceed rapidly to transplantation is particularly desirable. Increasing genetic disparity between donor and host—termed *histoincompatibility*—has historically contributed to both an increased rate of graft rejection and severe aGVHD and cGVHD and is a critical factor in the choice of donor. Even in the setting of HLA-identical siblings, selection can be further refined according to gender, history of donor parity, donor infectious disease status, donor age, and other variables, all of which contribute to the success of transplantation.

For the majority of patients who do not have a matched sibling donor, potential sources include a family member who is phenotypically adequately matched at the HLA loci but is genotypically distinct or a volunteer unrelated donor who shares the majority of HLA alleles with the recipient. The likelihood of locating an appropriate unrelated donor is dependent both on the patient's ethnicity (inasmuch as it determines histocompatibility antigen and haplotype frequency) and on the composition of the donor pool. For example, for whites of middle and northern European descent, the likelihood of finding a six-antigen–matched unrelated donor approaches 50% to 70%.[116] In contrast, the extreme genetic heterogeneity of the African American population coupled with underrepresentation of this population in volunteer registries makes the likelihood of finding a similar matched donor approximately 10% to 15%. Molecular typing techniques demonstrate that the allelic disparities in both whites and nonwhites is much higher than previously expected, thus making the ascertainment of a truly "matched" unrelated donor less likely even as the donor pool expands.[117] Although the implications of specific HLA mismatches are incompletely understood, most studies suggest that high-resolution HLA matching is associated with improved outcome in unrelated donor HSCT.[113-115] Thus, additional strategies to broaden the donor base by using alternative HSCs, such as UCB, that allow greater HLA disparity are being explored.

Sources of Hematopoietic Stem Cells. In the past, most HSCT has used bone marrow mononuclear cells as a source of HSCs. Bone marrow is usually obtained by repeated aspiration of the posterior iliac crests while the donor is under general anesthesia. Multiple aspirations are performed, usually through a limited number of skin holes (one to three per side), to a total volume of 10 to 15 mL/kg recipient body weight. The marrow is filtered through a fine wire mesh to rid the product of aggregates and bony spicules. This is a surprisingly well-tolerated procedure, and serious complications are rare. Risks to the donor are minimized by the fact that the donor is generally a healthy individual undergoing an elective procedure. Potential short- and long-term complications include the risks associated with anesthesia, blood loss and potential transfusion, pain, neurologic deficits, and psychosocial complications. In the most truly altruistic setting, unrelated marrow donor harvest, only 5% to 8% of donors later expressed any ambivalence about their participation. This was most marked if the transplant was subsequently unsuccessful.[118] Once harvested, red cells must be removed from the bone marrow if there is ABO incompatibility before infusion into the recipient.[119] The marrow may be manipulated ex vivo to remove donor T lymphocytes (see later) or tumor cells. It is estimated that only 1% of the donor's pluripotent HSC population is removed in a typical marrow harvest.

HSCs continuously recirculate from the marrow into the peripheral blood; HSCs can therefore be harvested by collection of peripheral blood mononuclear cells, usually by leukapheresis. The frequency of cells that express the surface marker CD34 is widely used as a proxy for actual HSC frequency and allows enumeration of stem cells. HSCs in peripheral blood are rare, and granulocyte colony-stimulating factor (G-CSF) is usually administered to increased the detachment of HSCs from bone marrow niches and promote their egress into the peripheral blood, thereby increasing their frequency.[120-124] Moreover, studies in adults suggest that additional strategies to further mobilize marrow HSCs are possible. AMD3100 is a reversible inhibitor of the CXC chemokine receptor (CXCR4), a receptor on the surface of HSCs that promotes adhesion to the bone marrow milieu. Combining AMD3100 with G-CSF increases HSC yield in adults,[125] but this approach has not been investigated in children. Complications of PBSC harvest have included bone pain as a side effect of G-CSF and inability to collect cells via peripheral access, thus necessitating central line placement.[126,127] Healthy individuals are at risk for splenic rupture from the administration of G-CSF, although this complication is extremely rare.[128] The implications of mobilizing and harvesting PBSCs from pediatric donors have not been fully explored,[129,130] but cytopenia and hemostatic changes of unknown short- and long-term significance have been observed in healthy donors.[131,132]

Since the first description of its use in a child with Fanconi's anemia (FA) in 1989,[133] UCB has become an increasingly investigated HSC source. Placental blood is recovered from the umbilical vein by drainage or catheterization, and techniques to optimize UCB HSC collection are being investigated.[27,134] Cord blood is immediately frozen and stored until needed. If indicated, in the related setting, determination of the HLA type of the fetus can be performed before delivery. Otherwise, typing and analysis are performed on intrapartum or postpartum samples.

Selection of an unrelated donor, whether bone marrow or UCB, is facilitated by the availability of epidemiologic information (e.g., age, sex), as well as HLA typing stored in a database accessible via the Internet. By comparing a patient's HLA type with donors listed and categorized in the registries, one can estimate the likelihood of a successful search, devise search strategies for patients with uncommon HLA types, and sort among potential HSC sources. Although stored UCB can be readily supplied after confirmatory typing, completion of a unrelated bone marrow donor search is more involved. Potential donors must be contacted and give consent to proceed, and the donor center must arrange for appropriate confirmatory studies, donor medical clearance, and scheduling of a harvest date. The time from formal search to BMT averages 4 months.

Engraftment. After allogeneic HSCT, donor stem cells must expand to repopulate hematopoietic niches and differentiate to form mature blood cells. HSCT recipients show accelerated telomere shortening in peripheral blood cells, which is presumably due to the increased replicative demand of donor stem cells.[135] Donor hematopoietic engraftment after allogeneic HSCT can be documented both by analysis of chimerism and by the recovery of peripheral blood cell counts. However, sensitive DNA amplification technologies have demonstrated residual host hematopoiesis for variable periods of time, certainly up to 1 year.[136-138] Mixed lymphoid chimerism is also well documented.[136-139] The implications of mixed chimerism with respect to subsequent relapse remain controversial, probably because the current extremely sensitive assays generate data that are difficult to interpret uniformly and because outcome may well differ by disease type.[140] For example, chimerism after BMT for CML is quite reliably related to subsequent relapse, but this may not be true for other diseases.[139-141]

The rate and probability of engraftment after allogeneic BMT vary with the source of HSCs, the number of HSCs given, the extent of preinfusion cell manipulation, and the GVHD prophylactic regimen used. In general, neutrophil recovery is achieved within 2 to 3 weeks and platelet recovery 1 to 2 weeks thereafter. Peripheral blood stem cell transplantation (PBSCT) is associated with a more rapid rate of engraftment than BMT is, most likely as a result of the higher CD34[+] cell count obtained.[142] Neutrophil engraftment occurs between 1 and 6 days earlier with PBSCT than with BMT and platelet engraftment between 4 and 7 days earlier.[143] Neutrophil and platelet engraftment after UCB transplantation is significantly delayed in comparison to that seen with other stem cell sources[144-148] because of the lower nucleated cell and CD34[+] cell dose in cord blood products. This has limited the application of this modality in adults, and currently, use of two unrelated UCB units for a given patient is being studied.[149]

The use of methotrexate as GVHD prophylaxis is associated with delay in count recovery; conversely, recovery after T-cell–depleted BMT is more rapid. Use of colony-stimulating factors after BMT is associated with more rapid neutrophil recovery after related donor BMT, a finding confirmed in small pediatric series.[139-141,150-155] No change in platelet recovery has been noted. Interestingly, preliminary data do not show any colony-stimulating factor–mediated acceleration of engraftment in patients undergoing unrelated donor BMT.[155]

The number and quality of T cells that are present in grafts from peripheral blood, bone marrow, and UCB confer different rates of GVHD. GVHD, particularly cGVHD, is more frequent in PBSCT than in bone marrow–derived HSCT, although this risk may be offset by an increased graft-versus-leukemia (GVL) effect.[156] In adults, this increased rate of GVHD has not diminished the efficacy of PBCST. However, in children, PBCST has been associated with a worse outcome than when bone marrow is used as a cell source.[157] The precise indications for PBSCs versus bone marrow as a source in pediatric HSCT therefore remain to be defined. Conversely, the lower rate of GVHD with UCB than with either PBSC or bone marrow sources allows less stringent HLA-typing requirements.[158]

Autologous Stem Cell Transplantation

Over the past decade, increasing numbers of cancer patients with either hematologic malignancies or solid tumors have elected to undergo autologous HSCT. In fact, the number now ranges in the tens of thousands worldwide. The fundamental hypothesis supporting this therapeutic approach is the belief that very high doses of cytotoxic agents (dose intensification) increase tumor cell death and that a high-dose treatment regimen can be devised in which the major dose-limiting toxicity is myelosuppression. This toxicity can be ameliorated by infusion of previously collected and cryopreserved autologous stem cells obtained either by bone marrow harvest or by apheresis of peripheral blood. Use of autologous cells to support and reconstitute the host after aggressive ablative or near-ablative therapy has been most thoroughly explored in both Hodgkin's and non-Hodgkin's lymphomas, less well developed in acute and chronic leukemias, and still considered experimental, albeit relatively widely applied, for a growing number of pediatric and adult solid tumors. In addition, the relative merits and disadvantages of autologous cells collected peripherally or from bone marrow are still not firmly established.

Contamination by Tumor Cells. A major limitation of autologous HSCT remains contamination of the stem cell product with residual malignant cells. Although the relative contributions of either residual tumor within the host or tumor reinfused with stem cells to subsequent relapse remain unknown, increasing evidence from gene-marking studies suggests that reinfused cells contribute to relapse.[159] In addition, in vitro assays of tumor cell colony formation and minimal residual disease detection by polymerase chain reaction (PCR) suggest that contamination of the stem cell source by tumor cells is associated with an increased relapse rate after HSCT.[160] No large randomized clinical trial of PBSCs versus bone marrow with respect to DFS has

been reported. However, paired samples of PBSCs and bone marrow have been examined in a variety of settings (e.g., breast cancer, non-Hodgkin's lymphoma), and PBSCs have been found to have lower levels of tumor cell contamination in the steady-state setting.[161] More recent data suggest that the advantage of PBSCs may be abrogated after mobilization,[162-166] although impact on DFS remains unclear.

A variety of methodologies have been developed to eliminate, or purge, tumor cells from stem cell collections. These methods are based on either positive or negative selection. The major clinically applied positive selection strategy is that of stem cell enrichment, most often selection of CD34+ cells. Negative selection is based on technologies that deplete tumor cells to a greater degree than normal stem cells. Strategies include the use of pharmacologic agents (e.g., mafosfamide), immunologic reagents targeting tissue-specific antigens (e.g., neural crest antigens in neuroblastoma), and manipulation of physical or culture properties of cells. Combinations of both negative and positive selection strategies may improve both the yield and purity of stem cell collections.[167,168] Increasing evidence in multiple clinical settings demonstrates an association between minimal residual tumor contamination and relapse[160] and, conversely, suggests that more effective purging strategies may be associated with improved DFS. However, randomized studies comparing purged and unpurged stem cells have yet to be reported.

Engraftment. Trilineage hematologic reconstitution has been achieved after the infusion of autologous bone marrow, bone marrow and PBSCs, and PBSCs alone. The most mature studies consist of patients reconstituting hematopoiesis via autologous marrow, with engraftment after bone marrow infusion being both reliable and durable; the durability of PBSC-reconstituted hematopoiesis, undertaken more recently, is less fully evaluated. The best predictor of engraftment and the rate of hematologic recovery have not been established. Although colony-forming units, burst-forming units–erythroid (BFU-E), nucleated cell count, and other measures have correlated with time to engraftment in some studies, correlations have not been universal and may additionally depend on the patient population, method of cell procurement, and subsequent cell manipulation. CD34+ cell counts have emerged as the most reliable and practical method for predicting engraftment after PBSC infusion, with retrospective analyses demonstrating that the risk of graft failure is substantially higher in patients who received less than 2×10^6 CD34+ cells per kilogram.[169-171]

Reconstitution of hematopoiesis after autologous bone marrow infusion has shown some tendency to be delayed when compared with the allogeneic setting. This delay is presumed to be due to the extent, nature, and duration of previous therapy. In addition, cell manipulation ex vivo (purging) may also contribute to delayed engraftment. Reconstitution after HSCT with autologous bone marrow can be hastened somewhat by the addition of hematopoietic growth factors to the post-SCT supportive care regimen, although the extent and nature of previous therapy may limit response to growth factors. Preliminary information in both the preclinical and clinical arenas suggests that previous aggressive chemotherapy may limit the potential for hematologic recovery.[172-174] Previous intensive chemotherapy supported by the use of growth factors may also contribute to poor engraftment after autologous transplantation. In fact, despite recovery of peripheral blood counts, hematologic marrow reserves as assessed by in vitro measures of hematopoiesis may be blunted for many years after autologous HSCT.[175]

The addition of mobilized PBSCs to bone marrow, with or without subsequent growth factor support, has resulted in a dramatic decrease in days of neutropenia and thrombocytopenia in most series. Furthermore, use of mobilized PBSCs as the sole stem cell source has been almost universally associated with more rapid hematologic recovery. It is still debatable whether the use of hematopoietic growth factors in this setting further enhances the rate of engraftment, but available data suggest that it may. Whether the process of PBSCT will result in durable hematopoiesis over decades is not yet evaluable, but reports of late graft failure are rare. Most studies suggest that the increased rate of engraftment observed with PBSCs results in decreased days in the hospital, use of antibiotics, and need for associated supportive services. The overall impact of PBSCs versus bone marrow as a stem cell source on the outcome or cost of transplantation has yet to be determined.

Myelodysplasia as a Late Complication. It has long been appreciated that intensive chemotherapy, particularly with alkylating agents, may result in an increased risk for subsequent myelodysplastic syndrome (MDS). Many patients who come to autologous transplantation have received treatment with such agents. Over the past several years, increasing numbers of patients have been reported in whom MDS has developed after autologous transplantation, usually 4 to 7 years after HSCT.[176] The actuarial incidence ranges from 5% to 10% in most series,[177-179] although it has been reported to be as high as 18% at 5 to 6 years after HSCT in single-center experiences.[180,181] Risk factors identified have included the use of etoposide for stem cell mobilization,[179] conditioning regimens using TBI,[177,182,183] and the amount of chemotherapy received before HSCT or the interval between diagnosis and HSCT (or both).[183,184] Whether the MDS results from previously damaged reinfused hematopoietic cells or from residual hematopoietic cells sustaining further injury during conditioning is unresolved. Cytogenetic analysis of bone marrow before autologous HSCT can reveal preexisting abnormalities and should be a standard component of the pre-SCT evaluation.[185] However, most patients in whom MDS has developed have been reported to demonstrate normal cytogenetics at the time of transplantation.[178] With more sensitive techniques currently available, such as fluorescence in situ hybridization (FISH), the majority of patients in whom MDS develops after SCT have been shown to harbor the same cytogenetic abnormality in pre-SCT specimens.[186] Similarly, using an X-inactivation–based clonality assay in female patients, clonal hematopoiesis was demonstrated in a small percentage of patients before HSCT; these patients were at significant risk for the development of MDS after HSCT.[176] This suggests that many cases of post-SCT MDS evolve from an abnormal clone already present before HSCT. Appropriate evaluation of hematopoietic status before embarking on autologous stem cell collection and transplantation is an area requiring further study.

Immune Reconstitution

The period after HCST is characterized by profound immunodeficiency, and death as a result of infectious complications remains a major obstacle to the success of transplantation. Myeloablative conditioning leads to wholesale loss of the cells necessary to confer protective immunity, including T and B lymphocytes and natural killer (NK) cells. Whereas neutrophil hematopoiesis can return within weeks of transplantation, recovery of a functional immune system can take much longer, and the risk of opportunistic infection remains high for up to a year, even with uncomplicated transplants.

The degree of immunodeficiency varies with time because of different contributions of donor and recipient immune function at different stages after transplantation. Mature T, B, and NK cells are present in the donor inoculum of bone marrow, peripheral blood, or UCB and contribute to some degree of host immunity in the immediate post-transplant period. The ability of these transferred cells to provide immune protection is dependent on how immunologically "experienced" the donor is. For instance, recipients of grafts from donors who are cytomegalovirus (CMV) immune, that is, who have previously been infected with the virus and have mounted a protective immune response, have a lower rate of CMV disease, presumably because of transferred immunologic memory for that virus.[187] Similarly, recipients whose donors have been vaccinated with a pneumococcal vaccine respond to pneumococcal vaccines more rapidly and with higher antibody titers after transplantation, again suggesting that donor immunity can be transferred to the recipient.[188] However, full immune reconstitution, with the ability to mount a protective immune response to new pathogenic challenges, is dependent on the differentiation of immature immune cells from precursors in the donor graft inoculum.

In most patients, NK cells are the first lymphoid population to recover, and in the first month after transplantation, NK cells can represent the main lymphoid cell in peripheral blood. T cells recover much more slowly, and normal numbers of CD4[+] and CD8[+] T cells are not achieved for 6 to 12 months after HSCT.[189] This delay in T-cell neogenesis is due to the complexity of T-cell development, a process that takes months to complete. It starts with differentiation of stem cells in marrow into early lymphoid progenitors that are capable of migration to the thymus, where further maturation occurs before naïve T cells are released into peripheral blood. During the early period after transplantation, T cells with a naïve phenotype predominate in peripheral blood, thus suggesting repopulation of the T-cell compartment with recent thymic emigrants.[189-191] The relative numbers of recent thymic emigrants can be quantified in the peripheral blood T-cell pool by the quantitative detection of genomic DNA that is present only in thymocytes (T-cell receptor gene excision circle [TREC] DNA). Using these methods, researchers have shown that increased thymic output contributes to the expanding peripheral T-cell pool for 12 to 24 months after HSCT.[192] This thymic output occurs even in adult patients whose thymuses have presumably involuted. The rate of increase in T cells is usually much more rapid in pediatric HSCT patients, however, consistent with the presence of more robust thymic function.[189] The advantage of a functional thymus in immune reconstitution has been demonstrated by the marked decrease in the fraction of naïve peripheral blood T cells in a 15-year-old HSCT patient who had previously undergone thymectomy relative to thymus-bearing HSCT patients.[193] Using quantitative molecular measures of the T-cell repertoire, several studies have shown that it can take as long as 12 to 24 months after HSCT for a full range of T-cell receptor diversity to be present in the T-cell compartment.[190,191,194] This underscores the critical role of naïve thymic emigrants in restoring the full complement of T-cell receptor specificities.

Several factors influence the length of time required for immunologic recovery to occur. Patient age profoundly affects the rate of immune reconstitution, with an inverse correlation between recipient age and the absolute number of T cells 1 year after HSCT.[195] The use of mobilized PBSCs as a source of stem cells appears to be associated with a faster rate of recovery than does the use of HSCs from bone marrow, at least partially because of the infusion of a larger cell dose.[121,196] The intensity of the conditioning regimen also has an impact on the speed of immune reconstitution, and the increasingly intensive preparative regimens used in autologous recipients have delayed recovery to a degree comparable to that seen in patients undergoing allogeneic HSCT.[195] Although hematopoietic engraftment appears to be delayed in UCB recipients, immune reconstitution in children after UCB HSCT is comparable to that in children undergoing unrelated donor BMT.[197] The presence of GVHD can significantly delay immune reconstitution as a result of both disruption of normal T-cell development and the additional immunosuppressive therapy required for man-

agement of the disease.[198] The consequences of delayed immunologic recovery are significant: slow recovery of immune function is associated with an increase in the cumulative incidence of infectious complications and non–relapse-related mortality.[121,199]

PERITRANSPLANT SUPPORTIVE CARE

Transfusion Support

The intensive myeloablative conditioning regimens used in the majority of pediatric HSCT to achieve tumor eradication and successful engraftment result in an extended period of pancytopenia. Virtually all patients undergoing HSCT require red blood cell and platelet transfusions during transplantation, and some patients remain transfusion dependent for months. All blood products should be gamma-irradiated to prevent transfusion-induced GVHD as a result of competent donor T lymphocytes in the cellular product.[200] Multiple processes, including psoralen photochemical treatment and leukocyte filtering, have been investigated for prevention of transfusion-associated GVHD, but gamma irradiation remains the standard of care.[201-204] Additionally, blood products must either be leukofiltered to achieve white blood cell reduction or be CMV seronegative (obtained from a donor previously unexposed to CMV) to prevent the transmission of virus to nonimmune patients. Previous studies indicated that both methods were equally efficacious.[205,206] However, a recent meta-analysis of the available literature suggests that the risk of transfusion-transmitted CMV is lowest when CMV-seronegative products are used for CMV-naïve patients.[207]

The ideal threshold for platelet and red blood cell transfusions in the peritransplant period remains an area of controversy. No studies in the modern era have evaluated the use of prophylactic platelet transfusions versus therapeutic transfusions administered when symptoms of bleeding develop. More recent studies have addressed different therapeutic triggers for prophylactic transfusions, specifically, $10 \times 10^9/L$ versus 30 or $20 \times 10^9/L$.[208,209] A review of studies of prophylactic platelet transfusion triggers found no statistically significant differences between groups with regard to mortality or severe bleeding events.[210] Although no statistical significance was found, these studies were small and no recommendations can supplant the need for clinical judgment in individual situations.

Infection Prophylaxis and Treatment

Even after successful neutrophil engraftment, patients continue to have depressed T-cell function and decreased antibody production and thus remain at risk for a variety of infections. This risk is greatest in the allogeneic and T-cell–depleted transplant settings, where despite phenotypically normal circulating lymphocytes, depressed cellular immunity is present for at least 1 year after HSCT.[211,212] During this time, viral infections continue to present a major risk to patients. Both CMV-seropositive patients and CMV-seronegative patients who have received grafts from seropositive donors are at risk for CMV, with the greatest risk occurring in seropositive recipients of a seronegative donor, in whom reactivation of virus latent in the patient can occur.[213,214] A large multicenter trial found that those undergoing unrelated donor HSCT from CMV-positive donors had an improved overall 5-year survival when compared with patients receiving cells from CMV-negative donors.[215] T-cell depletion abrogated this effect, which suggested that the improved survival was due to transfer of donor immunity. The clinical manifestations of CMV after HSCT include pneumonia/interstitial pneumonitis, colitis, hepatitis, and CMV-related cytopenia. Before the use of ganciclovir for CMV prophylaxis and treatment, CMV infections developed in more than a third of allogeneic SCT patients.[213] Pneumonia developed in almost 20%, with a mortality rate of 85%.[213] With the availability of effective antiviral therapies, almost all patients at risk for CMV disease receive prophylaxis during the first month after transplantation. Randomized studies have found acyclovir, valacyclovir, and ganciclovir prophylaxis initiated at engraftment to be effective in reducing CMV disease before day 100.[216-219] Prophylactic use of acyclovir has been shown to decrease overall mortality for at-risk patients.[220,221] In addition, studies found that prophylactic use of ganciclovir after engraftment was limited by drug-induced cytopenia and other toxicities. There are multiple studies of preemptive CMV treatment based on the results of positive culture, PCR, antigen, or bronchoalveolar lavage (BAL) fluid.[222-225] A review of the published CMV literature since 1995 found no advantage of prophylactic treatment over preemptive treatment in response to screening tests.[225] Moreover, this review found that preemptive therapy based on PCR tests or antigen assay was superior to culture- or BAL-based strategies. Both ganciclovir and foscarnet are considered to be first-line therapy for CMV reactivation or treatment of CMV disease.[226] Ganciclovir and foscarnet are similar in efficacy and primarily differ in terms of side effect profile.[227] CMV-seropositive patients undergoing autologous HSCT have not generally received either screening or prophylaxis,[226] although CMV reactivation and even disease occurs in a small percentage of these patients.

Up to 50% of patients undergoing either autologous or allogeneic HSCT experience reactivation of varicella-zoster virus, usually within the first year after SCT.[228] The vast majority of patients respond to acyclovir treatment. In children, the onset may be earlier, with most disease limited to the skin and few cases of visceral involvement. In general, pediatric patients respond well to antiviral therapy, and fatalities are rare.[229,230] Varicella vaccination is not currently recommended for patients after autologous or allogeneic HSCT. A pilot study of the live attenuated vaccine in autologous patients found the vaccine to be safe, but efficacy data are still pending.[231]

Fungal infection remains a significant problem, especially in those receiving steroids for treatment or prophylaxis of GVHD. A randomized trial demonstrated that prophylactic administration of fluconazole for 75 days after allogeneic HSCT yields ongoing protection against disseminated candidal infections and improved survival.[232] However, prophylactic fluconazole has been associated with the emergence of resistant species such as *Candida krusei*.[233] Low-dose amphotericin B has also been used prophylactically and is as effective as fluconazole, but more toxic.[234] The use of liposomal amphotericin has improved the toxicity profile.[235]

All HSCT patients are at risk for infection with *Pneumocystis carinii* after transplantation. Standard practice is to administer prophylaxis to recipients of autologous HSCT for 6 months after day 0 and for 6 months after discontinuation of immunosuppression for recipients of allogeneic transplants.

Nutrition Support

Provision of nutritional support during HSCT requires an appreciation of the metabolic needs of the individual patient, which are influenced by body composition, underlying nutritional state, and complications of transplantation. Patients who are underweight have been shown to be at higher risk for death than patients of normal weight in the early period after transplantation.[236] The impact of obesity on transplant outcome is debated, with some studies noting no effect and others reporting lower survival in obese patients.[236-238] Both the direct effects of conditioning regimens (mucositis) and complications of HSCT (GVHD, VOD, infection) can induce gastrointestinal damage that compromises the nutritional status of HSCT patients. Enteral feeding has been shown to be effective and safe and to have fewer complications than parenteral nutrition (PN) during HSCT, but it is not always practical for children.[239-241] Several studies have demonstrated the efficacy of PN when enteral nutrition is no longer possible.[242-244] However, in addition to expense, PN has attendant potential complications, including vascular access difficulties, induction of cholestasis, and the potential for hyperglycemia and hyperlipidemia. Thus, the best approach may be to reserve PN for patients unable to tolerate enteral feeding[245]; the occasional patient may be able to maintain nutritional needs orally throughout the transplantation period. Resumption of enteral feeding should be encouraged, and continued monitoring of nutritional intake and weight is necessary not only through engraftment but also after discharge from the hospital. Malnutrition appears to be relatively frequent after HSCT, and even patients with minimal or no GVHD may have significant and prolonged nausea, anorexia, feeding intolerance, and other nutritional problems.

EARLY COMPLICATIONS OF STEM CELL TRANSPLANTATION

Veno-occlusive Disease of the Liver (Sinusoidal Obstruction Syndrome)

VOD, also known as sinusoidal obstruction syndrome, is a clinical syndrome characterized by hepatomegaly, right upper quadrant pain, jaundice, and fluid retention.[246-248] VOD can be a complication of both autologous and allogeneic SCT[247,249-251] and is the result of chemotherapy/radiation-mediated endothelial and hepatocyte damage.[247,250,252,253] Injury to the sinusoidal endothelial cells and hepatocytes in zone 3 of the liver acinus appears to be the initial event and is marked by subendothelial edema and endothelial cell damage with microthromboses, fibrin deposition, and the expression of factor VIII/ von Willebrand factor within venular walls.[254] Later features include deposition of collagen within venular lumens and eventual obliteration and hepatocyte necrosis.[252,255,256] Identified risk factors for VOD include previous chemotherapy regimens that include gemtuzumab, ozogamicin, or busulfan-based conditioning regimens (especially when combined with cyclophosphamide and methotrexate); underlying diseases associated with intensive chemotherapy, including advanced-stage malignancies; total PN for longer than 30 days; higher concentrations of certain chemotherapeutic agents; and unrelated donor transplantation.[249,250,255,257-266]

Hepatomegaly and right upper quadrant pain with fluid retention are the first clinical manifestations of VOD and typically occur 10 to 20 days after chemotherapy.[250] These findings are followed shortly by other clinical indicators of disease, including hyperbilirubinemia, peripheral edema, ascites, sodium avidity, and pulmonary infiltrates/effusion/edema.[247,250] Patients with VOD are at increased risk for renal insufficiency and failure.[250,267] Frank hepatorenal syndrome occurs in approximately half of patients with severe disease,[250] and there are often associated changes in mental status. It is hypothesized that portal hypertension from sinusoidal injury leads to decreased renal perfusion and tubular injury resulting in renal insufficiency.[250,267,268]

Exclusion of other causes of the signs and symptoms of VOD is essential in establishing the diagnosis. Liver biopsy is the gold standard for diagnosis of VOD and, in conjunction with hepatic venous pressure measurements, can provide valuable diagnostic information but unfortunately is associated with considerable morbidity in this population.[269,270] Hepatic venous pressure gradients greater than 10 mm Hg are specific for a diagnosis of VOD but are not highly sensitive.[269] Computed tomography (CT) can be useful in identifying features suggestive of VOD, such as periportal edema, ascites, and a narrow right hepatic vein.[271] The utility of hepatic Doppler ultrasound for the diagnosis of VOD is variable; at times, findings are nonspecific and not always noted early in the disease.[272,273] The presence of ascites, gallbladder wall thickening, hepatomegaly, decreased or reversed flow in the portal vein, and increased mean hepatic artery resistive index is supportive, but not necessarily diagnostic of VOD.[247,272-276] When clinical concern for VOD is high and a liver biopsy is not practical, serial ultrasound can be diagnostically helpful.

Reported overall survival rates for pediatric patients with established VOD range between 50% and 100%.[249,258,264,265,277-280] Reported predictors of mortality for children with VOD include allogeneic transplantation from donors other than matched siblings, concomitant moderate to severe hepatic or cutaneous GVHD, and more severe VOD (higher peak bilirubin, higher maximal weight gain, presence of pleural effusion, requirement for intensive care unit admission).[249,258]

Treatment and prophylactic options for patients with VOD remain limited. The most straightforward preventive technique is to identify patients at highest risk and to consider alternative conditioning regimens when feasible.[246-248] Ursodeoxycholic acid has been used as a preventive agent with inconclusive results.[281-287] Other preventive strategies such as the use of fresh frozen plasma, prostaglandin E_1, N-acetylcysteine, and antithrombin III are potentially effective but need further study.[288-295] Because 70% to 80% of patients recover spontaneously, supportive care with meticulous fluid and blood product management is the mainstay of therapy.[296] Based on histologic observations of microthrombi and fibrin deposition coupled with laboratory evidence of abnormalities of the coagulation cascade, many therapeutic strategies have been directed at promoting thrombolysis or fibrinolysis.[295,297-301] Multiple small studies have investigated the use of thrombolytic agents and anticoagulants (typically tissue plasminogen activator and heparin) for the prevention or treatment of VOD (or both).[295,297-299,302,303] Although these strategies appear to generally be safe, they have not decreased the incidence or improved the outcome of patients with severe disease and have been associated with serious bleeding in some cases.[288,297-299,304-311] Defibrotide, a single-stranded polydeoxyribonucleotide that has antithrombotic and thrombolytic activity, has been demonstrated to be effective for both prevention and treatment of VOD with minimal toxicity.[312-319] Response rates between 35% and 50% have been reported for patients with severe VOD treated with defibrotide.[315,320,321] Surgical intervention is uncommonly used for the treatment of VOD. Liver transplantation has resulted in clinical improvement in about 30% of the small numbers of patients stable enough to undergo the procedure, although the immediate and long-term issues are formidable.[322] Transjugular intrahepatic portosystemic shunting (TIPS) has been performed safely in patients with severe VOD, but it has not been shown to improve overall survival and should be reserved for instances in which fluid retention and ascites are relatively isolated issues.[323-328]

Graft Rejection

Primary graft rejection, defined as failure to recover hematopoietic function of the stem cell graft by day 30, is an uncommon, life-threatening event that occurs after approximately 4% of unrelated donor stem cell transplants and is even less common in related donor transplants.[329] It is an immune-mediated process that occurs because of genetic disparity between the donor and recipient.[22,330,331] Although both donor NK and T cells are considered mediators of graft rejection, it is characterized by the presence of recipient T cells and the absence of donor cells.[332-339] The risk of graft rejection is increased in patients who are mismatched at the HLA-A, HLA-B, or HLA-DRB1 loci; receive a low cell dose; have a positive crossmatch for antidonor lymphocytotoxic antibody; receive T-cell depletion as GVHD prophylaxis; have aplastic anemia, especially if previously multiply transfused; or have storage disorders or osteopetrosis.[329] An altered host microenvironment can also contribute to graft rejection.

Adjustments in both the chemotherapy and radiotherapy components of conditioning regimens, the use of monoclonal antibodies targeting selected populations of recipient T cells, and increases in cell dose (including the use of PBSCs in addition to bone marrow) are among the interventions that have shown some promise in preventing graft rejection. Depletion of host T cells with antithymocyte globulin (ATG) and the use of CD52 monoclonal antibodies are commonly used approaches.[340,341] A number of strategies have been exploited to overcome the increased incidence of graft failure associated with T-cell depletion. First, simply increasing the number of stem cells in the graft has been successful, thus implying that residual host hematopoietic elements are involved in mediating graft rejection. However, such intensification is associated with increased GVHD. Additionally, because the risk of graft failure appears to increase with more exhaustive T-cell depletion, less extensive T-cell removal from the graft with and without T-cell add-back has been attempted.[342-345]

Therapeutic options for patients with graft rejection include a second allogeneic transplantation, infusion of frozen autologous stem cells, use of hematopoietic growth factors, particularly granulocyte-macrophage colony-stimulating factor (GM-CSF), modification of the host's immunologic status, and infusion of donor leukocytes.[231,346-351] Infusion of stem cells with or without additional conditioning can be an effective intervention for the treatment of primary graft failure.[352] It has been studied with bone marrow or PBSCs, although recently the use of unrelated cord blood units[352-355] has been explored. The use of allogeneic PBSCs is appealing in the second transplant setting because PBSCs have been associated with a shorter duration of neutropenia and a higher

neutrophil recovery rate.[346] Graft rejection is a potentially morbid, uncommon complication of HSCT with limited effective therapies. Patients exhibiting signs of graft rejection should be identified as early as possible to maximize potential therapeutic options.

Acute Graft-versus-Host Disease

Grafts from genetically disparate donors, specifically, any donor other than self or an identical twin, can initiate an immune reaction termed *acute graft-versus-host disease*.[356] In general, the greater the degree of genetic difference between the donor and recipient, the higher the risk and severity of aGVHD. The main genetic loci that determine the compatibility of donor and recipient are HLA I and II located on chromosome 6. Each of these loci encode polymorphic glycoproteins—major histocompatibility antigens—that are expressed on the surface of human tissues in a complex with small peptides from degraded intracellular proteins. T-cell receptors on the surface of T cells are finely tuned to recognize the "foreignness" of MHC molecules. Recipient T cells recognize donor antigens and can cause graft rejection. Conversely, donor T cells can recognize recipient antigens and are responsible for the syndrome of aGVHD. The mechanisms by which T cells cause GVHD include both direct effector mechanisms and release of inflammatory mediators that cause tissue damage. The presence of tissue damage either from immunologic events or from direct effects of conditioning can propagate the inflammatory response and trigger further immune responses in a positive feedback loop that has been termed a "cytokine storm."[357-359]

The syndrome of aGVHD was first reported by Barnes and Loutit in 1954.[6] They observed that skin abnormalities and diarrhea developed in lethally irradiated animals given allogeneic spleen cells and that the animals eventually succumbed to a wasting illness. It became clear that for aGVHD to develop, certain criteria had to be in place, and these were summarized by Billingham in 1966[360]: (1) "the graft must contain immunologically competent cells"; (2) "the host must possess important transplantation alloantigens that are lacking in the donor graft, so that the host appears foreign to the graft and is, therefore, capable of stimulating it antigenically;" and (3) "the host itself must be incapable of mounting an effective immunological reaction against the graft, at least for sufficient time for the latter to manifest its immunological capabilities; that is, it must have the security of tenure."

However, the allogeneic immunologic effect also confers potential benefits. Donor graft inocula contain immunologic cells—T cells, NK cells,[361] and possibly others—that are capable of recognizing malignant cells and mediating a GVL and, perhaps, a graft-versus-tumor effect.[362-364] Indeed, patients with hematologic malignancies in whom mild to moderate GVHD develops have a decreased risk for disease relapse.[365-368] Conversely, T-cell depletion from the marrow inocula reduces the risk for

GVHD but can lead to an increased risk for both graft rejection and disease recurrence.[369] The ability to distinguish the populations of T cells that mediate GVHD from those that mount a GVL response remains a central goal in GVHD research.[370] For instance, a well-characterized population within the CD4+ T-cell compartment that constitutively expresses the interleukin-2 (IL-2) receptor α chain (CD25) and the transcription factor FOXP3 has been observed to have marked immunosuppressive activity in vitro and in vivo.[371-373] This cell population, termed regulatory T cells, is able to minimize GVHD in an animal model while retaining the graft-versus-tumor effect of the allogeneic graft. The ability to select and expand[374] human regulatory T cells offers the possibility of a novel approach to mitigating GVHD.

The clinical syndrome of aGVHD develops within 100 (and usually within 60) days of allogeneic SCT. cGVHD is a distinctive clinical syndrome that occurs after day 100 and is discussed later. aGVHD classically involves the skin, liver, and lower gastrointestinal tract, although the degree of involvement of each organ varies. For that reason, the severity of aGVHD is graded by staging the involvement of individual organs and the clinical performance of the patient and then determining an overall grade for the disease. Table 9-1 presents the modified Glucksberg criteria, introduced in 1974,[375] and with several revisions and additions,[376-379] this is the system historically used for assessing aGVHD. As newer methods of both preventing and treating aGVHD were developed, there was concern about the ability of the Glucksberg stage to accurately reflect transplant outcomes. The International Bone Marrow Transplant Registry (IBMTR) constructed a severity index based on organ involvement alone with no need for subjective assessment of performance. This has been shown to correlate well with outcome and is the staging system used in most current studies (Table 9-2).[380]

The first manifestation of GVHD is often a rash, usually a maculopapular eruption commonly involving the palms and soles and the back of the neck and ears at first and later the trunk and extremities. Biopsy specimens from involved areas demonstrate epidermal basal cell vacuolization, followed by epidermal basal cell apoptotic death with lymphoid infiltration.[381] Characteristic eosinophilic bodies may be seen. Unfortunately, the specificity of skin biopsy is not high and it is often unable to

TABLE 9-1	Glucksberg Criteria for Staging and Grading of Acute Graft-versus-Host Disease	
Organ	**Stage**	**Extent of Organ Involvement**
Skin	1	<25%
	2	25%-50%
	3	Generalized erythema
	4	Desquamation, bullous
Liver bilirubin	1	2-3 mg/dL*
	2	3.1-6 mg/dL
	3	6.1-15 mg/dL
	4	>15 mg/dL
Gastrointestinal (children)	1	10-15 mL stool/kg/day
	2	16-20 mL stool/kg/day
	3	21-25 mL stool/kg/day
	4	>25 mL stool/kg/day; severe pain with or without ileus
Gastrointestinal (adult)	1	500-1000 mL stool/day; nausea, anorexia
	2	1000-1500 mL stool/day; histologic diagnosis[†] of upper gastrointestinal graft-versus-host disease
	3	1500-2000 mL stool/day
	4	>2000 mL stool/day; ileus, severe pain
Overall Clinical Grade	**Organ System**	**Clinical Stage**
I (mild)	Skin	1-2
	Liver	1
	Gastrointestinal	0
II (moderate)	Skin	1-3
	Liver	1-2
	Gastrointestinal	1
III (severe)	Skin	2-4
	Liver	2-4
	Gastrointestinal	2-4
IV (life threatening)[‡]	Skin	2-4
	Liver	2-4
	Gastrointestinal	2-4

*Modified Glucksberg scale[216] to prevent overlap in categories.
[†]Data from Weisdorf DJ, Snover DC, Haake R, et al. Acute upper gastrointestinal graft-versus-host disease: clinical significance and response to immunosuppressive therapy. Blood. 1990;76:624-629.
[‡]With severe constitutional symptoms.

TABLE 9-2	International Bone Marrow Transplant Registry Severity Index for Acute Graft-versus-Host Disease			
Severity Index	Maximum Organ Stage	RR of Treatment-Related Mortality (95% CI)	RR Treatment Failure (95% CI)	Glucksberg
0	No GVHD	1.00	1.00	0
A	Skin only stage 1	0.84 (0.6, 1.18)	0.85 (0.68, 1.05)	I
B	Any organ stage 2*	1.90 (1.5, 2.42)	1.21 (1.02-1.43)	I, II, III, IV
C	Any organ stage 3	4.34 (3.33, 5.67)	2.19 (1.78, 2.71)	II, III, IV
D	Any organ stage 4	11.9 (9.12, 15.5)	5.68 (4.57, 7.08)	IV

*Any organ stage 1 other than skin alone (e.g., skin 1, gut 1 = severity index B).
CI, confidence interval; RR, relative risk.

differentiate GVHD from drug allergy or reaction to the conditioning regimen.[382] Bulla formation with epidermal separation and necrosis is seen in advanced stages of skin GVHD.[383] Hepatic GVHD is often manifested as cholestatic jaundice, which must be differentiated from VOD, infection, and drug toxicity.[384,385] Though not without attendant risks of bleeding and pain, liver biopsy may be helpful because characteristic pathologic changes can be observed that aid diagnosis.[386,387] Gastrointestinal involvement is classically seen as watery diarrhea with a "seedy" component and may progress to include crampy abdominal pain, bleeding, and even ileus.[384,385] By convention, stool volume is used to quantitate the severity of gut involvement. Rectal or colonic biopsy may reveal crypt cell necrosis with lymphocytic infiltration and, with increasing severity, crypt abscess or loss and mucosal denudation.[388] These three organs are staged individually for the severity of involvement, after which an overall grade of GVHD is assigned according to criteria developed by Glucksberg and co-workers (see Table 9-1) or the IBMTR (see Table 9-2). However, other clinical findings may be indicative of aGVHD. Involvement of the upper gastrointestinal tract is manifested by symptoms of anorexia, inanition, and vomiting.[378] The differential diagnosis of such symptoms also includes viral or fungal infection, dyspepsia, and gastritis, all common conditions in an immunosuppressed SCT recipient. Endoscopy of the upper gastrointestinal tract with biopsy is minimally invasive and can detect the presence of crypt cell apoptosis with dropout, which is diagnostic of GVHD. Finally, pulmonary involvement with effusions and vascular leak may accompany aGVHD.

Several risk factors for the development aGVHD have been identified. Increasing genetic disparity between the donor and host increases the incidence and severity of GVHD[389-392] and is the most important single predictor of aGVHD. More recently, other genetic risk factors have been evaluated. The existence of polymorphisms in genes between the donor and host offers a plausible mechanism to explain variations in the magnitude of the inflammatory response to tissue injury and hence GVHD. Indeed, specific polymorphisms in the recipient IL-10 promoter region and IL-10 receptor β gene have been found to be associated with a lower rate of GVHD.[393]

Many other candidate genes are currently being examined for similar associations. Moreover, the falling cost and growing scale of genomic sequencing technologies suggest that an increasingly complex and accurate genomic prediction of risk for GVHD is likely to evolve over the coming years.

Other factors increasing the risk for GVHD include older age of the recipient,[390,394,395] use of a female donor for a male recipient, use of parous female donors, and history of previous herpesvirus infection in the recipient.[390,391,394,396] The source of allogeneic stem cells may also affect the risk for subsequent GVHD. For example, the number of T cells collected during pheresis is significantly greater than the number collected during bone marrow harvest. Nonetheless, it appears that the rate of severe aGVHD in patients receiving T-cell–rich PBSCs with standard GVHD prophylaxis may not be greater than that seen after BMT.[124,130,397] Results from large series indicate that there may be a decrease in the severity of aGVHD in UCB transplants.[26,145-147] The reason for this has not been completely elucidated but may be related to the putative relative immunologic "naïveté" of the immune cells contained in the cord graft, or more likely, the lower T-cell dose.

Therapeutic strategies aimed at the prevention (prophylaxis) of aGVHD begin with selection of the best available donor. When a matched sibling donor is not available, HLA matching via molecular techniques is the single most important factor in preventing severe GVHD.[392,398] Considerations of donor sex and parity are advisable if there is a choice of donors. If the patient is seronegative for CMV, use of a CMV-negative donor appears to reduce the risk of GVHD, as well as CMV, after transplantation.[396] Whether the source of HSCs (i.e., bone marrow, PBSCs, UCB) modifies the risk for aGVHD is an area of controversy. Supportive care measures such as the use of protective isolation and gut decontamination also protect against the development of GVHD.[399-401]

Conventional prophylactic approaches have attempted to inhibit T-cell responses by relying on in vivo immunosuppression. Essentially all current pharmacologic regimens use combinations of immunosuppressive agents that target different molecular intermediates of T-cell signaling. Cyclosporine (Sandimmune) and tacrolimus (Prograf) both inhibit calcineurin activity, a serine-threonine phosphatase whose activity is essential for T-cell cytokine transcription.[402] Methotrexate prevents T-cell proliferation,[403] whereas high-dose corticosteroids are lympholytic. Current combinations use cyclosporine or tacrolimus plus methotrexate or prednisone (or both).[404-406] A common prophylactic regimen includes cyclosporine given intravenously at a dose of 1.5 mg/kg every 12 hours until oral administration every 12 hours is tolerated. Doses are adjusted to achieve desired blood levels. Cyclosporine is continued on a tapering schedule through day 180 after transplantation. Methotrexate is given at 15 mg/m^2 on day 1 and at 10 mg/m^2 on days 3, 6, and 11 after marrow infusion. This regimen has been shown to reduce the incidence and severity of aGVHD and improve long-term survival when compared with single-agent therapy in comparable patient cohorts.[407,408] Combinations using newer immunosuppressive agents, such as sirolimus, are also being developed.[409]

As discussed earlier, selective depletion of T lymphocytes from the donor marrow inocula effectively prevents GVHD. T cells can be removed by a variety of techniques, including lectin depletion, anti–T-cell monoclonal antibodies plus complement, coupling with immunotoxin derivatives, or purging with magnetic beads. Each of these techniques may effect up to a 3 log or greater depletion of T cells. Unfortunately, T-cell depletion is associated with an increased risk for graft failure, delayed immune reconstitution, post-SCT lymphoproliferative disease, and in patients with hematologic malignancies, leukemic relapse.[366] Thus, the long-term survival rates of patients who have received T-cell–depleted grafts are similar to those of patients who have received conventional in vivo immunosuppression after transplantation.[410,411] Strategies using "add-back" of donor T cells at various time points after SCT are being explored,[412-415] and the ultimate role of T-cell depletion in SCT has not been completely resolved.

The outcome and long-term survival of patients with aGVHD vary directly with the grade of GVHD and response to treatment. The mainstay of therapy for established aGVHD remains glucocorticoids. Glucocorticoids (generally methylprednisolone) have been used in a variety of schedules and doses.[404,416] The lympholytic effects of very-high-dose corticosteroids must be balanced against the increased risk of infections,[417] and doses higher than 2 mg/kg/day may not increase efficacy.[418] Patients failing to improve or progressing with corticosteroid therapy have been given a variety of other immunosuppressive agents, but secondary treatment of GVHD is often unsuccessful.[419] Generally, cyclosporine is continued at therapeutic levels in patients in whom aGVHD develops, and it may be initiated in patients who have never received the drug. ATG, extracorporeal photochemotherapy,[420] newer immunosuppressive agents such as mycophenolate mofetil,[421] and methods targeting CD5, CD3, IL-2 receptor,[379] and tumor necrosis factor-α

and its receptor have all been attempted with varying, incomplete, or unpredictable responses. Novel and reproducible methods of approaching the treatment of patients with corticosteroid-resistant aGVHD that do not compromise the ability to mount an immune response against infection are needed because the outcome for these patients remains poor.

DELAYED COMPLICATIONS OF TREATMENT

The use of both autologous and allogeneic transplantation for an increasing number of malignant and nonmalignant conditions coupled with marked improvements in supportive care has resulted in a substantial number of long-term survivors. Thus, delayed complications secondary to both the chemoradiotherapy used to prepare patients for SCT and the transplant process itself (e.g., GVHD and propensity for infection) are becoming better defined with regard to incidence, severity, and outcome. It is essential that follow-up occur in conjunction with HSCT specialists so that as consensus statements regarding post-HSCT care are developed, they can be implemented for all patients.

Chronic Graft-versus-Host Disease

GVHD was initially characterized as taking place in two phases: aGVHD generally occurred within the first 100 days after transplantation, whereas cGVHD occurred after day 100 (Table 9-3). It has become evident that certain cases of cGVHD, defined by both clinical and histopathologic criteria, can occur as early as day 50 to 60 after marrow infusion.[422] The pathogenesis of cGVHD is not completely elucidated. It is thought to involve

TABLE 9-3   Comparison of Acute and Chronic Graft-versus-Host Disease

	Acute GVHD	Chronic GVHD
Onset day	7-60 (up to 100)	Day >100 (may be seen from day 60 on)
Manifestations:		
Skin	Erythematous rash	Sclerodermatous changes
Gut	Secretory diarrhea	Dry mouth; sicca syndrome Malabsorption
Liver	Hepatitis/ cholestasis	Cholestasis/ cirrhosis
Other	Fever	Pulmonary dysfunction Alopecia Thrombocytopenia Xerostomia

donor T-cell recognition of minor histocompatibility antigens or loss of peripheral T-cell tolerance leading to symptoms that are very similar to those present in autoimmune disorders. The morbidity and mortality of cGVHD are most severe in patients who have progressive disease after aGVHD and tend to be less severe in those in whom it occurs de novo.[423] Risk factors for the development of cGVHD include HLA disparity between donor and host, previous aGVHD, increasing patient age, and a TBI-based conditioning regimen. A recent review of risk factors in children found that patient age older than 15 years or donor age older than 5 also significantly increases risk.[424] In addition, the use of adult female donors for male recipients increases the likelihood of cGVHD, probably related to donor antibody responses to antigens coded for by genes on the recipient Y chromosome[425]; the impact of pediatric female donors on the incidence of cGVHD has not been evaluated.

cGVHD is a constellation of clinical and pathologic features. The syndrome resembles autoimmune systemic collagen vascular diseases, with protean manifestations potentially involving almost every organ (Table 9-4). Pathologic changes in the skin result from epithelial cell damage characterized by basal cell degeneration and necrosis and, later, epidermal atrophy and dermal fibrosis.[426] Skin involvement may be manifested as lichen planus, areas of local erythema, and areas of hyperpigmentation or hypopigmentation. The skin may be dry, freckled, or ulcerated, and findings are aggravated by exposure to sunlight. Sclerodermatous changes may evolve to flexion contractures that can greatly impair function and may be helped by surgical release procedures. Hair follicles can be involved, with resulting partial or total alopecia. Ocular abnormalities are common and consist of sicca syndrome, including dry eyes and photophobia; decreased tearing is quantitated by the Schirmer test. Dry mouth is a common initial complaint of patients with oral GVHD, and decreased saliva production predisposes to caries. Tongue depapillation or scalloping of the lateral margins of the tongue can be seen. The tongue, buccal mucosa, and gums may have lichen planus–like lesions, which must be differentiated from oral candidiasis. A biopsy specimen typically shows lichenoid changes with epithelial cell necrosis, salivary gland inflammation, lymphocytic infiltrates, and fibrosis. Involvement of the liver with cGVHD is manifested as lymphocytic portal triaditis with resulting obstructive jaundice, which may progress, if untreated, to bridging necrosis and cirrhosis. Gastrointestinal signs include inanition with progressive weight loss, chronic malabsorption, diarrhea, anorexia, nausea, and vomiting. Biopsy demonstrates single-cell apoptosis with crypt destruction and may show fibrosis of the lamina propria. Early cGVHD may be manifested as diffuse myositis and tendonitis. Progressive joint involvement, which may result from the myositis and tendonitis or simply from overlying skin fibrosis, results in decreased range of motion and flexion contractures. Perhaps the most debilitating effect of cGVHD occurs

TABLE 9-4	Clinicopathologic Features of Chronic Graft-versus-Host Disease
System	**Features**
Systemic	Recurrent infections with immunodeficiency
	Weight loss
	Sicca syndrome
	Debility
Skin	Lichen planus, scleroderma, hyperpigmentation or hypopigmentation
	Dry scale, ulceration, erythema, freckling
	Flexion contractures
	Biopsy:
	Epithelial cell damage
	Basal cell degeneration and necrosis
	Epidermal atrophy and dermal fibrosis
Hair	Alopecia
Mouth	Sicca syndrome, depapillation of the tongue with variegations and scalloping of the lateral margins
	Lichen planus and ulcer, angular tightness
	Biopsy:
	Lichenoid changes with mononuclear infiltrates
	Epithelial cell necrosis
	Salivary gland inflammation, lymphocytic infiltrate, fibrosis
Joints	Decreased range of motion, diffuse myositis/tendonitis
Eyes	Decreased tearing; injected sclerae, conjunctivae
Liver	Increase in alkaline phosphatase greater than increase in transaminases and bilirubin
	Cholestasis, cirrhosis
	Biopsy:
	Focal portal inflammation with bile ductule obliteration
	Chronic aggressive hepatitis
	Bridging necrosis
	Cirrhosis
Gastrointestinal	Failure to thrive (children), weight loss (adults)
	Esophageal strictures, malabsorption, chronic diarrhea
	Biopsy:
	Crypt destruction, single-cell dropout
	Fibrosis of the lamina propria
Lung	Cough, dyspnea, wheezing
	Bronchiolitis obliterans or restrictive pulmonary change
	Pneumothorax
Hematology	Refractory thrombocytopenia
	Eosinophilia
	Howell-Jolly bodies

Staging of Chronic Graft-versus-Host Disease

LIMITED CHRONIC GVHD

Localized skin involvement and/or
Hepatic dysfunction secondary to chronic GVHD

EXTENSIVE CHRONIC GVHD

Generalized skin involvement or
Localized skin involvement or hepatic dysfunction (or
    both) as a result of chronic GVHD plus
        Liver histology showing chronic aggressive hepatitis,
            bridging necrosis, cirrhosis, or
        Eye involvement: Schirmer test (<5-mm wetting), or
        Involvement of minor salivary glands or oral mucosa
            demonstrated by buccal biopsy, or
        Involvement of any other target organ

---

with pulmonary involvement, manifested as obstructive lung disease progressing to bronchiolitis obliterans (discussed later). Persistent immunodeficiency with profoundly depressed B- and T-cell responses predisposes to recurrent and severe infections. Patients may have reduced IgG2 and IgG4, decreased mucosal IgA, diminished delayed-type hypersensitivity, and functional asplenia. They remain susceptible to opportunistic infections with encapsulated organisms (primarily pneumococcus), *P. carinii*, varicella-zoster, and herpes simplex and may have a variety of chronic infections, including sinusitis, bronchitis, and conjunctivitis.[427]

Staging of cGVHD is based on the degree of organ involvement (Box 9-2). Limited cGVHD has localized skin involvement with or without hepatic dysfunction. All other manifestations of cGVHD are classified as extensive cGVHD.[426] Limited cGVHD may resolve spontaneously without specific therapy, and these patients have a favorable outcome.[423] Patients with lichenoid skin changes, progressive changes of cGVHD, thrombocytopenia, hyperbilirubinemia, or any combination of these findings have a worse prognosis.[427,428] Recent work has focused on developing a more detailed comprehensive scale to measure symptoms of cGVHD so that response to therapy can be more clearly assessed.[429]

It is essential that patients with cGVHD be managed by a multidisciplinary team with expertise in this complicated and often frustrating condition. Steroids are usually the first approach to therapy, and a regimen of alternating-day cyclosporine and prednisone was shown to be effective in more than half of patients and to have an acceptable toxicity profile.[430] There is no standard approach for patients who are refractory to initial therapy or whose disease flares during taper of immunosuppression.[428] A number of other therapies are being tested, including high-dose pulse steroids,[431] extracorporeal photopheresis,[432] daclizumab (a humanized IL-2 receptor antagonist),[433] mycophenolic acid,[434] rapamycin,[435]

and pentostatin.[436] All of the therapeutic options have a significant impact on immune function, and most fatalities occur from infectious complications as opposed to specific organ toxicity from cGVHD. Meticulous and preemptive management of the complications associated with cGVHD and its therapy is a crucial component of care. Recommendations for patient education, prophylactic interventions, and follow-up are extensively outlined in the Ancillary Therapy and Supportive Care Working Group document of the National Institutes of Health.[437]

Ophthalmologic Problems

A number of different ophthalmologic complications can occur as sequelae of HSCT. Decreased lacrimation secondary to cGVHD may contribute to ocular sicca syndrome and the related complications of photophobia, punctate keratopathy, scar formation, and corneal perforation. Therapy includes artificial tears and lacrimal duct (punctual) plugging, which can be useful even in young children. Patients remain at risk for ocular infections, particularly with herpes simplex viruses. Cyclosporine use is associated with a number of eye complaints, including a well-described syndrome of headache, hypertension, seizures, visual impairment, or any combination of these symptoms, as well as temporary blindness (see "Neurologic Complications" for a detailed description).[438-440] In addition, transplant-related retinopathy can be manifested as optic disc edema, either asymptomatic or accompanied by visual blurring, in patients taking cyclosporine. Ischemic fundal lesions, detected as cotton-wool spots and, in some patients, as optic disc edema, have been reported in patients treated with both TBI and cyclosporine and were not observed in patients who did not have concordance for these risk factors.[441,442] Lesions appeared 3 to 6 months after SCT, with complaints of decreased visual acuity or other visual disturbances. Most patients discontinued cyclosporine, and half were treated with systemic corticosteroids. The majority recovered visual acuity and their ischemic lesions resolved over time, but little further information is available about the course or long-term prognosis of this complication. Occlusive microvascular retinopathy has also been described after autologous SCT in patients receiving high-dose cytarabine and TBI, thus suggesting that particular high-dose chemotherapy regimens may predispose to vascular injury at otherwise safe radiation doses.[443]

Cataracts are a common complication of HSCT. Radiation—TBI, cranial irradiation, or both—is a well-described predisposing factor. Although historically the incidence was as high as 80% in patients receiving single-dose TBI, patients receiving fractionated TBI or chemotherapy-only regimens still have a 20% to 50% incidence of cataracts 5 to 6 years after transplantation.[444,445] The relative risk of cataracts and the need for subsequent cataract surgery may also be related to previous therapy or to glucocorticoid use for prophylaxis or management of GVHD. Overall, reports of large pediatric populations have shown that some type of ophthalmologic abnormality occurs in up to 50% of patients, although visual function remains excellent in virtually all patients.[446-448] Thus, yearly examination by an ophthalmologist is essential, including a Schirmer test to rule out xerophthalmia and a thorough retinal evaluation.

Dental Problems

Disturbances in dental development have been described in children conditioned with TBI, particularly if HSCT took place before 6 years of age.[449,450] Characteristic findings include short dental roots, absence of root development, and microdontia. A review of 52 pediatric patients younger than 10 years at HSCT found that all patients had disturbances in dental root growth, with the most pronounced changes occurring in those 3 to 5 years old at the time of transplantation.[451] Subsequent decreased alveolar bone growth may lead to further compromise of dental development. In addition, oral sicca syndrome (occurring as a complication of either TBI or cGVHD, or both) may result in chronic oral mucosal injury, poor oral hygiene, and subsequent dental decay.[452] The effects of prophylactic interventions are not well reported, but yearly evaluation by a dentist knowledgeable about potential HSCT-related issues is recommended.

Pulmonary Complications

Pulmonary dysfunction of both a restrictive and obstructive nature occurs in approximately 25% of pediatric HSCT patients.[453] Pulmonary complications can be seen after both autologous and allogeneic transplants; however, serious pulmonary dysfunction is more common in the allogeneic setting. Patients with pulmonary complications are known to have higher overall mortality.[453] Obstructive lung disease has been reported in up to 20% of children after allogeneic HSCT, comparable to the incidence in adult patients. Bronchiolitis obliterans (BrOb) is a noninfectious, potentially life-threatening complication of HSCT that has been reported to occur in approximately 8% of allogeneic pediatric HSCT patients.[454] It is a pathologic process that leads to obstruction and eventual obliteration of the small airways.[455] There is characteristic chronic airflow obstruction unresponsive to bronchodilator therapy.[456] The etiology of BrOb is not fully understood. It is thought that immune dysregulation and inflammation are precipitating factors in its development, a theory supported by the association between the syndrome and cGVHD.[457,458] Although BrOb has been most firmly associated with cGVHD, viral infections before day 100 and gastroesophageal reflux have also been identified as risk factors.[456,458-460] Patients typically exhibit dyspnea on exertion and cough, with pulmonary function tests revealing an obstructive pattern. High-resolution CT has been shown to have findings that are both sensitive and specific for BrOb in this population.[461,462] Characteristic findings include air trapping, a mosaic pattern of lung attenuation, and bronchiectasis.[461-463] BrOb is traditionally treated with immunosuppressive agents. Azithromycin has been shown to be a useful adjunct, presumably because of its anti-inflammatory and antibiotic mechanisms of action.[464] Published mortality rates for BrOb after HSCT range between 20% and 100%.[456] The prognosis depends in part on disease tempo and response to first-line therapy.[456,465] Rapid onset and lack of response to steroids define a group of patients with a particularly poor outcome.[465]

Restrictive and diffusion abnormalities have been reported in pediatric patients after SCT.[466,467] These findings may improve over time but do not usually normalize.[466] Risk factors for restrictive lung disease include sclerodermatous-type GVHD, single-fraction TBI, abnormal chest wall growth secondary to radiation, and certain chemotherapeutic agents.[467-472] Treatment depends on the underlying etiology of the pulmonary disease. Because restrictive changes can be asymptomatic, defining the true incidence of this complication depends on the intensity of post-SCT follow-up.

Hematologic Complications

Patients who undergo ABO-incompatible allogeneic HSCT are at risk for immune hemolytic anemias. In the setting of major ABO incompatibility (recipient O and donor A or B, for example), preexisting patient isohemagglutinins can cause lysis of donor red cells. This can potentially cause an acute hemolytic reaction during stem cell infusion, and thus anti-A or anti-B isoagglutinins must be removed from the patient before infusion via pheresis or the stem cell product must undergo red cell depletion. Although the acute issues surrounding transplantation in the setting of major ABO incompatibility are easily managed and not associated with any impact on outcome, pure red cell aplasia may develop in up to a quarter of at-risk patients in the months after HSCT.[473] This occurs when long-lived patient lymphocytes continue to produce antibodies capable of destroying red cell precursors in the graft. Patients who are type O and donors who are type A are at greatest risk, presumably related to the level of isohemagglutinin titers.[474] A relationship of red cell aplasia to post-transplant immunosuppression with cyclosporine alone has been suggested because calcineurin inhibitors permit longer persistence of patient B cells than methotrexate does.[475] Some cases of aplasia will resolve spontaneously over time; plasma exchange with donor-type plasma replacement has also been used, and more recently rituximab, a chimeric anti–B-cell antibody, has been used with success.[476] Minor ABO incompatibility (patient A, donor O, for example) is managed by plasma depletion of the graft before infusion. This situation can also lead to low-level hemolysis in the first months after HSCT as newly formed B lymphocytes produce isohemagglutinins targeting residual patient red cells. Occasionally, in the months to years after transplantation, autoimmune hemolytic anemia, autoimmune thrombocytopenia, or autoimmune neutropenia develops as a result of immune dysregulation after HSCT. Steroids and intravenous immunoglobulin (IVIG) are usually the first therapeutic intervention, but rituximab has been used in this setting as well.[477]

A variety of microangiopathic syndromes have also been described after SCT. The use of cyclosporine for GVHD prophylaxis or treatment has been associated with both thrombotic thrombocytopenic purpura (TTP) and hemolytic-uremic syndrome (HUS), described in the next section.

Renal Complications

HUS may develop at a median of 5 months after HSCT.[478,479] This disorder is generally manifested as moderate hemolysis and renal dysfunction, although some patients have more aggressive findings consisting of severe hypertension and seizures. Factors implicated in the development of this syndrome include exposure to radiation and use of calcineurin inhibitors.[480,481] The majority of reported cases appear to resolve spontaneously over time, although modest persistent anemia and decrements in renal function have been described. TTP is rare in pediatric patients and may result from more pervasive endothelial damage than seen in HUS. It usually occurs in the first months after HSCT and can have associated fever, bloody diarrhea, and neurologic symptoms. Unlike classic TTP, HSCT-associated TTP is not accompanied by deficient von Willebrand multimer proteolysis, and plasma exchange therapy is generally unsuccessful.[482]

The incidence of chronic nephropathy is probably underestimated. Up to 25% of adults undergoing allogeneic HSCT were affected at 10 years; post-transplant hypertension was the most significant predictor of chronic kidney disease.[483] Assessment of renal function by determination of the glomerular filtration rate revealed renal impairment in 41% of pediatric patients 1 year after HSCT and in 11% at 7 years, with exposure to TBI being the most significant risk factor.[484] The long-term impact of transplantation on renal function in pediatric patients is not known,[485] but given the natural decline in renal function with age, monitoring function over time should be part of routine care for survivors of pediatric HSCT.

Neurologic Complications

Patients undergoing HSCT may experience a variety of neurologic complications either directly related to treatment, as a consequence of immunosuppression, or as a result of medications used in supportive care. Acyclovir is used for both prophylaxis and treatment of infection with herpes simplex viruses. Confusion, tremors, delusion, and psychosis have been associated with this drug.[486] Simi-

larly, mental status changes, paresthesias, and uncommonly, seizures have been reported with the antiviral agents ganciclovir and foscarnet.[487,488] Impaired renal function, often seen in HSCT patients, may potentiate the occurrence of these symptoms. Both prednisone and cyclosporine may have neurologic side effects. Mood swings or even frank psychosis accompanying corticosteroid therapy are well described.[489] Cyclosporine administration commonly produces an essential tremor. Seizures, visual disturbances, and encephalopathy are more significant but rarer neurologic complications.[490] It has been postulated that both seizures and acute visual loss arise from the hydrostatic changes accompanying cyclosporine-associated hypertension; as in preeclampsia, hypomagnesemia can be an aggravating factor. These changes affect white matter, most commonly in the occipital area, and are accompanied by characteristic radiologic findings on magnetic resonance imaging (MRI).[440,491] In general, symptoms abate rapidly on discontinuation or decreases in the dose of cyclosporine.[492]

Cerebrovascular accidents, including cerebral hemorrhage, may also be observed after SCT and are usually associated with refractory thrombocytopenia. Large intracranial hemorrhages are generally fatal[493]; patients with isolated subdural hematomas typically do well.[494]

Central nervous system (CNS) infectious complications related to immunosuppression, cGVHD, or both can arise after HSCT. The manifestations of CNS infection can differ from those in an immunocompetent patient in that localizing signs and symptoms may be less dramatic. Autopsy series demonstrate that up to 15% of necropsy patients harbor CNS infections, often clinically unsuspected.[495-497] *Aspergillus* species and *Toxoplasma gondii* are the most common organisms found.[498] Bacterial meningitis or encephalitis/meningoencephalitis caused by a variety of viruses, including CMV, herpes simplex types 1 and 6, adenovirus, and varicella-zoster, can also occur. Opportunistic CNS infections in HSCT recipients are often fatal,[498] and a high level of suspicion is warranted in patients with even minimal neurologic symptoms.

Leukoencephalopathy is a poorly understood sequela of HSCT that is manifested as progressive neurologic deterioration in the months after transplantation. Clinical findings include lethargy, slurred speech, ataxia, seizures, decreased sensorium, dysphagia, spasticity, or even decerebrate posturing. Consistent white matter changes are found on MRI. In a series of 415 patients from Seattle, leukoencephalopathy was observed in 7% of patients, but only in those who had received CNS radiation, intrathecal therapy, or both before HSCT in conjunction with intrathecal methotrexate after HSCT.[499] More recently, a 4% incidence of irreversible leukoencephalopathy was reported in children receiving cyclosporine; a third of the patients died during the period of neurologic decline.[500] Cyclosporine levels were usually therapeutic in the affected patients, and it remains unclear what the risk factors are for this rare but devastating complication.

The effects of different conditioning regimens on neuropsychological functioning have been incompletely investigated. In particular, analysis of very young patients is limited. Nonetheless, it is clear that a significant proportion of young children, including those younger than 2 years, can undergo HSCT with chemotherapy and TBI and subsequently have normal neurologic development,[501] perform well in areas such as sensorimotor and cognitive functioning,[502] and have no decrement in academic achievement.[503] Age at HSCT appears to be the most consistent risk factor predicting subsequent cognitive decline.[503,504]

Endocrine Disorders

Much of the endocrine dysfunction after HSCT results from irradiation and is attenuated in both incidence and severity when radiation is fractionated or when non–radiation-containing conditioning regimens are used. Thyroid dysfunction is one of the most frequent late complications of HSCT. After fractionated TBI, the incidence of compensated hypothyroidism ranges from 13% to 39% and that of overt hypothyroidism is around 15%, with diagnosis occurring at a median of 4 years after HSCT.[505-507] Patients treated with busulfan-based regimens have a lower, but still significant incidence of thyroid complications: 20% compensated and 9% overt hypothyroidism.[508,509] Given that the incidence of thyroid dysfunction increases over time, clinical suspicion and yearly monitoring of thyroid function tests are an important part of long-term care for these patients.

Linear growth after HSCT is hard to predict and is affected by many factors: previous therapy, particularly corticosteroids or cranial or spinal radiotherapy, age at transplantation, conditioning regimen, and development of cGVHD with associated long-term steroid exposure. Growth is most disrupted in children who underwent cranial irradiation before HSCT, followed by a TBI-based conditioning regimen.[510] This group of children is also at greatest risk for growth hormone (GH) deficiency. If deficient, GH replacement can have a positive impact on final height, particularly in children younger than 10 years at the time of HSCT. Therapy is not associated with an increase in relapse; however, a higher incidence of osteochondromas/exostosis was seen in GH-treated patients.[511] Nonetheless, many children do not demonstrate GH deficiency, and the role of exogenous hormone in these children or in children older than 10 at the time of diagnosis of GH deficiency is not clear.[512,513] Overall, the mean loss of height appears to be approximately 6 cm as predicted by both genetic height and height at transplantation.[507] Still, nearly 80% of those undergoing HSCT in childhood will achieve a height that is within 2 SD of adult norms.[514]

Gonadal failure after HSCT is common; predictors include previous gonadotoxic therapy and the preparative regimen used for transplantation. For example, children with aplastic anemia who receive cyclophosphamide as their only cytotoxic agent almost always progress normally through puberty, whereas those receiving a busulfan- or TBI-based ablative regimen are very likely to have delayed development.[513] Thus, these children must be carefully monitored by a pediatric endocrinologist as they approach adolescence so that hormone replacement can be appropriately administered. Females who are postpubertal at the time of HSCT also need to be evaluated for hormone replacement therapy. In addition, they are at risk for gynecologic complications, including reduced uterine size, decreased vaginal and cervical size, atrophic vulvovaginitis, introital stenosis, and loss of pubic hair.[515] No comparable data regarding these complications exist for those prepubertal at the time of HSCT. In postpubertal males, HSCT with or without radiation-based conditioning often results in azoospermia,[516] and sperm banking should be offered to all patients with sufficient spermatogenesis. Significant Leydig cell damage resulting in decreased testosterone and decreased testicular volume is less common.[517] In both sexes, spontaneous recovery of gonadal function has occurred years after HSCT. Fertility resulting in live-born infants has been reported for both male and female SCT patients,[518] particularly after conditioning with cyclophosphamide alone. Successful pregnancies are much less common after busulfan- and TBI-based regimens, and there is an increased risk of spontaneous abortion, preterm labor, and delivery of low- or very-low-birth-weight infants. There does not, however, appear to be an increased incidence of congenital anomalies in the offspring.[517] Concern regarding fertility is one of the major issues for HSCT survivors up to a decade after transplantation.[519]

Bone Problems

The most prominent bony complications after HSCT are decreased bone mineral density (BMD) and osteonecrosis. Patients undergoing transplantation have many potential risk factors for abnormal bone health: exposure to corticosteroids before HSCT or for prophylaxis or treatment of GVHD, calcineurin exposure, gonadal failure, prolonged bed rest, and periods of suboptimal nutrition. Because many patients are asymptomatic, the incidence of osteopenia/osteoporosis in children and the impact on future bone health are not well understood. Small series of pediatric patients indicate that up to 50% of survivors of childhood allogeneic HSCT will have abnormal BMD and thus have an excess risk of fractures and other skeletal complications as they age.[520,521] Osteonecrosis or avascular necrosis, the death of a segment of bone, is a potentially debilitating manifestation of bone disruption and can result in significant pain or fractures. Corticosteroid use and the presence of cGVHD appear to be the major risk factors,[522] and children older than 10 appear to be at more risk than younger children.[523] Joints of the lower limb, particularly the hip, are most often involved, and up to half of patients ultimately require joint replacement.[524] Radiation-induced bone abnormalities, including osteochondromas and metaphyseal growth abnormalities, can occur after TBI-containing transplant regimens; younger patients appear to be at greater risk.[525] Childhood survivors of HSCT should be evaluated regularly to ensure that hormonal and nutritional status is optimized. The role of bisphosphonates in the treatment of these conditions is being investigated. Early data indicate that bisphosphonates can improve BMD, but long-term effects of this intervention in the pediatric population are unknown.[526]

TRANSPLANTATION IN PATIENTS WITH ACQUIRED DISEASES

Aplastic Anemia

Severe aplastic anemia (SAA) is a syndrome characterized by peripheral blood pancytopenia and marrow hypoplasia (see Chapter 7). Historically, the mortality associated with SAA in children can be as high as 50% in the first 6 months.[527] Although a number of immunosuppressive and marrow stimulatory therapies have shown reasonable activity, the only curative treatment remains allogeneic HSCT. The potential efficacy of allogeneic transplantation for patients with SAA was established with the initial publication in 1972 of results achieved in four patients.[528] Randomized studies have since established the superiority of matched allogeneic HSCT over supportive care (androgens in the 1970s, immunosuppressive therapy with ATG in the 1980s and 1990s) in both children and, more recently, adults.[529-532] In the setting of a matched sibling donor, the role of pre-HSCT conditioning is mainly to provide immunosuppression. Cyclophosphamide in combination with ATG is the standard regimen, with cyclosporine and short-course methotrexate given for GVHD prophylaxis. This approach cures almost 90% of patients with none of the sequelae associated with radiation-containing regimens.[533] The stem cell source has traditionally been bone marrow, but many centers have switched to peripheral blood progenitor cell grafts for ease of collection and faster engraftment kinetics. In a retrospective study of European and American registries, patients younger than 20 years had an increased risk for cGVHD and higher overall mortality with peripheral blood versus bone marrow grafts, and bone marrow remains the preferred stem cell source.[534] A course of immunosuppressive therapy before proceeding to matched sibling HSCT also led to an inferior outcome, mostly as a result of increased rates of graft rejection.[535] Young patients with SAA receiving a non–radiation-containing regimen should have preserved fertility after HSCT.[536] In addition, long-term survivors were indistinguishable from healthy controls in terms of reported health, educational achievement, and psychosexual functioning.[537] Given these data and the expected excellent outcomes, patients with SAA who have an available matched sibling donor should be referred expeditiously for BMT to minimize the number of pre-HSCT transfusions and the risk of acquiring serious infections.

Children who lack a matched sibling donor receive immunosuppressive therapy that usually consists of ATG, cyclosporine, and steroids in an attempt to restore normal hematopoiesis. Up to 70% of patients will have a response by 6 months, but only 30% to 50% will have durable responses and remain transfusion independent.[538,539] Additionally, a proportion of patients fail to respond, and responders remain at risk for both relapse of SAA and evolution to MDS/AML.[540,541] The first reports of unrelated donor transplants for SAA used preparative regimens similar to those used with sibling donors. The results were very discouraging, with graft rejection, transplant-related toxicity, and GVHD all being significant problems and survival rates under 40%. Incorporation of TBI into the conditioning regimen decreased the incidence of graft rejection and led to better results in some reports, although the results were also influenced by the time from diagnosis to transplantation and the associated differences in patient condition, number of transfusions, and infectious complications.[542] In the era of improved HLA typing and better transfusion strategies, attempts have been focused on decreasing the intensity of the conditioning regimen, and encouraging results have been reported with cyclophosphamide, ATG, and TBI doses as low as 200 cGy.[543] The long-term results of such approaches, including the durability of donor engraftment, remain to be evaluated. As conditioning regimens become less intense and survival improves, the optimal time to refer SAA patients for unrelated donor HSCT becomes less clear.

Myelodysplasia/Juvenile Myelomonocytic Leukemia

MDS is a heterogeneous group of clonal stem cell disorders that share a propensity to progress to acute leukemia. Though much more common in the adult population, these disorders have been estimated to account for approximately 3% of childhood hematologic malignancies. This figure may be an underestimate inasmuch as a subset of children with de novo AML presumably had antecedent MDS.[53] The French-American-British (FAB) classification system is based on the proportion of leukemic blasts in marrow; most pediatric patients have either refractory anemia (RA), refractory anemia with excess blasts,[492] or RAEB in transformation (RAEB-T). Juvenile myelomonocytic leukemia (JMML), a rare disorder of infants and young children, shares similarities with MDS, and a new classification system has been proposed that allocates pediatric patients with clonal myeloproliferative diseases to three groups: MDS, JMML, and myeloid leukemia of Down syndrome.[544] MDS and JMML are disorders arising from mutated pluripotent stem cells, and thus allogeneic HSCT with a related or unrelated donor remains the only curative approach. Induction chemotherapy before HSCT is not generally recommended for patients with JMML because remission is unlikely to be attained and toxicity is high.[545] A busulfan-versus TBI-based conditioning regimen has been associated with a lower rate of relapse.[546] As transplant-related mortality has decreased, survival has improved, with recent consortium data reporting an approximately 50% 5-year DFS rate; relapse remains the greatest obstacle to cure.[547] *Cis*-retinoic acid appears to decrease the spontaneous proliferation of leukemic progenitor cells in JMML, as well as abrogate their selective hypersensitivity to GM-CSF.[548] It is used after HSCT as therapy for minimal residual disease, although efficacy has not been firmly established.

The role of induction therapy before HSCT for MDS is unclear, but about half the patients can achieve remission after AML-directed therapy,[549] and this approach may improve survival in patients with increased blasts at diagnosis.[545] Conditioning with both TBI- and busulfan-based regimens has been used, with most studies showing no difference in outcome,[550] although some favor busulfan.[551] Overall, the strongest predictor of survival is stage of disease.[552] Children who undergo transplantation for RA/RAEB have event-free survival (EFS) rates of around 70%; patients with RAEB-T were five times more likely to relapse.[553] Currently, approximately half of pediatric patients with MDS can be cured, and thus allogeneic HSCT should be considered early in the disease course.[554]

Acute Lymphoblastic Leukemia

Although more than three quarters of children with newly diagnosed ALL treated with aggressive, multiagent therapy will be cured, management of patients with certain high-risk features or who have relapsed disease remains controversial. There are two situations in which allogeneic SCT is considered to be the standard approach for children in first remission: children with identified high-risk features at diagnosis and children with primary induction failure. The consensus of what constitutes a high-risk patient is greatest for the approximately 2% of children with Philadelphia chromosome–positive (Ph+) ALL, who historically have had a dismal prognosis when treated with conventional ALL-directed chemotherapy.[555,556] Matched sibling HSCT in first remission significantly improved survival; a large European cohort over a 10-year period found a relative risk of 0.3 for relapse or any adverse event with transplantation versus conventional chemotherapy[557] and DFS rates of higher than 60%.[558] As in other transplant scenarios, the decrease in morbidity and mortality associated with unrelated donor transplantation over the past decade has broadened the applicability of this approach. Currently, most patients with Ph+ ALL undergo transplantation in first remission with the best available donor, with a 5-year

EFS rate of 50% after mismatched family or unrelated donor transplantation.[559] The role of transplantation in first remission is less clearly delineated for other high-risk groups, including patients with the 4:11 translocation, T-cell ALL, or hypodiploid ALL. Hypodiploidy is known to be an adverse prognostic factor. Extreme hypodiploidy of less than 44 chromosomes is particularly uncommon and confers an even worse prognosis with an EFS rate of 30%.[560] This has led to the inclusion of such patients in trials of HSCT in first remission for children with a matched family donor and "ultrahigh-risk" features of ALL,[558,561] although the number of hypodiploid cases is too small to make definitive statements about the impact of HSCT on outcome. The historically poor outcome associated with the T-cell phenotype of ALL has been abrogated by the intensive chemotherapy that these children receive on modern protocols.[562] However, there is an ongoing attempt to define high-risk patients within this group, usually those with some combination of a very high white cell count at diagnosis, poor prednisone response, or induction failure, and some reports suggest that outcome for this subgroup may be improved by transplantation in first remison.[563,564] Initial response to therapy is becoming an increasingly important prognostic factor for children with ALL,[565] and those not in remission by the end of induction therapy have an enormous risk of relapse. These children have been included in series of high-risk patients, and although the numbers are small, it appears that undergoing HSCT if remission can be achieved is associated with improved EFS (rate of 56% versus 26%).[563] The 4:11 translocation almost always implies rearrangement of the MLL gene. It is not certain that this abnormality implies a worse outcome in children older than 1 year,[566] but infants who harbor this translocation have an almost fivefold increase in the risk for an adverse event when compared with infants without an MLL rearrangement.[567] Even within this group further distinctions can be made: very young infants with mixed lineage leukemia (MLL)+ ALL and a high white cell count at diagnosis have an EFS rate of less than 5%.[568] A recent international study of infant leukemia found that a poor response to prednisone, in addition to the previously mentioned factors, identified those at the highest risk.[569] It is not definitively known whether HSCT in first remission can improve outcome in this group; however, single-center studies have reported EFS rates of less than 60%,[570,571] and the current version of the international consortium trial is recommending HSCT in first remission for these infants. In summary, it appears that ALL patients with very high-risk features—whatever the specifics of the definition but virtually always including patients who are induction failures or who have the Philadelphia chromosome—have a decreased incidence of relapse and improved survival when they undergo HSCT with stem cells from a matched family donor in first remission and that HSCT confers the greatest advantage in the patients at highest risk.[563] Recent data demonstrating equivalent if not better survival of children with relapsed ALL after unrelated donor versus sibling HSCT[572] make it difficult to know the optimal approach to therapy for those lacking a matched family donor, and a thoughtful discussion of the risks and benefits of unrelated donor HSCT versus chemotherapy is essential.

Once ALL has recurred, the chance of cure drops dramatically. In the late 1980s, the Seattle investigators reported their own experience, as well as reviewed the existing literature, and concluded that HSCT with stem cells from a matched family member cured approximately 40% of children whereas continued chemotherapy resulted in subsequent relapse more than 90% of the time.[573] Over the intervening years it has been discovered that children with relapsed ALL constitute a very heterogeneous group. The two strongest predictors of outcome in patients with recurrent ALL are the duration of the first remission and the site or sites of relapse, and the potential effective therapeutic modalities depend heavily on these factors. Patients experiencing an isolated bone marrow relapse fare more poorly than do those with either an isolated extramedullary relapse (usually involving the CNS or testicles) or those with a combined extramedullary/bone marrow relapse. Consequently, most children with an isolated extramedullary relapse, particularly if occurring while off therapy, are treated with intensive chemotherapy and radiation therapy delivered to the site of relapse rather than allogeneic SCT. This strategy results in very good outcomes, with a recent consortium trial showing that three quarters of children with a first remission of greater than 18 months who experience an isolated CNS relapse can be cured with an approach using systemic and intrathecal chemotherapy and cranial irradiation.[574] Patients who experience an early relapse (defined variably as one occurring during therapy or within 18 to 36 months from diagnosis) present one of the most difficult challenges in ALL therapy. It is clear that chemotherapy alone cannot cure these patients, and most studies show a survival advantage for sibling HSCT.[575] Unfortunately, recurrent disease is a major obstacle to success, and a recent report of children who suffered a bone marrow relapse within 12 months of completing therapy found a 3-year EFS rate of approximately 25% for these patients whether receiving chemotherapy, sibling HSCT, or unrelated donor HSCT.[576] Tellingly, over half of the patients had an adverse event (death, relapse) within 3 months of attaining second remission, and thus achieving sufficient disease control to undergo HSCT complicates evaluation of its efficacy as a modality. Most of the aforementioned studies have involved matched sibling donors; as outcomes with alternative donors have improved, equivalent results with unrelated donor HSCT are now being reported.[572,575] In summary, it has not been determined which patients with ALL in second remission conclusively benefit from allogeneic HSCT. Patients with late isolated extramedullary relapses should not undergo transplantation in most circumstances. For the remaining groups, there are no prospective randomized trials to guide therapy. Some children are unable to tolerate the months of intensive therapy given in relapse protocols and thus should be considered for HSCT.[577] Because most studies reveal a lower incidence of relapse with transplantation that often but not always translates into improved DFS,[578,579] the risks and benefits of transplantation must be carefully considered in each situation by balancing type and match of available donors, medical condition of the patient, and patient and family preference.

Acute Myelocytic Leukemia

Successive clinical trials over the last 25 years have firmly established the role of intensive postremission therapy in the treatment of AML. However, during that time there has been much debate about whether allogeneic HSCT or intensive chemotherapy without stem cell support is the optimum postremission therapy. Allogeneic HSCT offers dose intensity and the possibility of a GVL effect. Alternatively, intensive chemotherapy without stem cell support is feasible for all patients, unlike allogeneic HSCT, and confers less risk of acute and long-term toxicity.

The role of allogeneic HSCT in first clinical remission of AML was initially addressed in a series of prospective trials in the mid-1980s. In 111 consecutive patients, the Seattle group undertook matched sibling allogeneic HSCT for patients who had a donor, whereas the remaining patients received conventional intensification. The probability of 5-year DFS was 49% for HSCT versus 20% for chemotherapy alone.[580] However, since that time, more intensive chemotherapy regimens have been associated with improved disease control in children and adults with AML.[581,582] This has again raised the question of whether allogeneic HSCT is more effective than intensive chemotherapy in the postremission setting. To address this issue, the Children's Cancer Study Group (CCG) conducted a large trial of allogeneic HSCT versus chemotherapy or autologous HSCT in 652 children and adolescents with AML who achieved remission. At the end of induction, patients with five or six HLA antigen–matched relatives were allocated to allogeneic HSCT. All others were randomized between autologous HSCT with 4-hydroperoxycyclophosphamide (4-HC) purging of marrow or four courses of chemotherapy. The results of this trial showed that the outcome with allogeneic HSCT was superior to either chemotherapy or autologous HSCT.[581] For patients treated with an intensive induction regimen, the DFS rate with allogeneic HSCT was 66% versus 53% with chemotherapy and 48% with autologous HSCT.[581] These data underscore the benefit of both intensive induction chemotherapy and first-remission matched sibling donor HSCT in the management of newly diagnosed AML for many patients.

Subsequent studies have attempted to identify patients at increased risk for poor outcomes with chemotherapy alone who would thus derive most benefit from HSCT in first remission. In the pediatric population the consistent prognostic indicators are response to initial induction therapy and cytogenetic markers.[583,584] The Medical Research Council (MRC) AML 10 trial found 5-year survival rates of 67%, 65%, and 23% in patients who respectively achieved complete remission, achieved partial remission (5% to 15% blasts), and had residual disease.[583] Relapse rates in these groups were 34%, 38%, and 87%. This and other studies stratified patients according to favorable, intermediate, and adverse karyotypic abnormalities. Favorable karyotypic abnormalities include t(8;21), inv(16), t(15;17), and in some studies, t(9;11) and t(16;16).[583-586] Adverse abnormalities include −5, −7, del(5q), abn(3q), and complex karyotypes.[586] Patients with neither favorable nor high risk are considered intermediate risk. In the MRC AML 10 trial, patients with favorable and intermediate karyotypic abnormalities had survival rates of 76% and 52%, with relapse rates of 34% and 44%. This was compared with survival and relapse rates of 40% and 61% in patients with adverse karyotypes.[583] The MRC combined cytogenetics and response to initial therapy to delineate good-, standard-, and poor-risk groups in the MRC 10 trial. The good-risk group included patients with favorable karyotypes or FAB type M3, irrespective of response status after one course of chemotherapy or the presence of other karyotypic abnormalities. The standard-risk group included patients in neither the good- nor poor-risk groups. The poor-risk group included patients with adverse karyotypic abnormalities or with resistant disease in the absence of favorable karyotypic abnormalities and not FAB M3.[583] There was no significant difference in the percentage of deaths during first complete remission between any of the groups.[582] There were, however, significant differences between the good-, standard-, and poor-risk groups in regard to relapse-free survival rate (65%, 62%, and 36%), DFS rate (59%, 54%, and 32%), survival from relapse (61%, 17%, and 0%), and 7-year survival rate from complete remission (78%, 60%, and 33%). The 61% salvage rate after relapse in the good-prognosis group suggested that HSCT in the first complete remission may be inappropriate for this group. Though not assessed in the MRC trial, patients with an activating *FLT3* mutation have been shown to have a poor prognosis and benefit from HSCT in first remission.[587] Although specific definitions of risk groups differ between protocols, current AML trials recommend HSCT based on risk group, and ongoing trials from the Children's Oncology Group (COG) and St. Jude Cancer Research Center recommend chemotherapy only for patients in low risk groups and HSCT for intermediate risk only if a family donor is available. HSCT is recommended for high-risk patients even in the absence of a related donor.

Autologous HSCT has been studied for patients who have no allogeneic donor. In many trials, autologous marrow was purged of residual leukemic cells with 4-HC, although no direct benefit of this technique has been proved. Trials in adults and adolescents with AML suggested that autologous HSCT might offer additional therapeutic efficacy over chemotherapy.[549,588] Pediatric trials and a recent meta-analysis did not demonstrate any advantage to this modality in patients in first complete remission, and data are insufficient to assess the influence of AML subclass on outcome.[589-593]

In most studies of patients with relapsed AML, the duration of first remission is strongly predictive of outcome, with 10% to 20% DFS rates in patients relapsing less than 1 year after diagnosis regardless of the treatment modality used.[594,595] Early studies reported DFS rates of up to 30% for those undergoing allogeneic transplantation in untreated first ("early") relapse.[596,597] In contrast, a more recent report of 379 adults with relapsed or refractory AML found the DFS rate of patients who underwent transplantation in untreated first relapse to be no better than 13%.[598] Patients with treatment-refractory disease had an equivalently poor prognosis. However, the DFS rate in patients who were are able to attain a second remission was significantly better at 32%. The outcome of children with relapsed AML was studied by the MRC Childhood Leukemia Working Party.[594] Of the 81 patients in whom curative therapy was attempted, 69% went into a second remission. Approximately two thirds of these patients were consolidated with allogeneic HSCT, with a survival rate of 44% at 3 years. Although this was not a randomized study, patients treated with HSCT had a longer duration of second remission that did those treated with chemotherapy alone.[594] These data support the use of allogeneic HSCT in the treatment of relapsed AML, especially for patients who can achieve a second remission.

Chronic Myelogenous Leukemia

CML is a proliferative stem cell disorder arising from a translocation (9;22) known as the Philadelphia chromosome. The only curative therapy is allogeneic transplantation. However, with the advent of targeted molecular therapies such as imatinib, a tyrosine kinase inhibitor (TKI), daily administration of an oral agent can control the disease for years, if not longer, with minimal side effects. As a result, the role of HSCT with the attendant short- and long-term toxicities is being redefined. The majority of the literature on both HSCT and TKI therapy reflects studies in adults, where current practice is to use TKI as initial therapy in virtually all patients with chronic-phase CML.[599] The risk-benefit profile is different in the pediatric population, and in the largest pediatric series to date, patients receiving either matched sibling ($n = 182$) or unrelated donor ($n = 132$) HSCT had a 63% and 56% DFS rate, respectively. The best outcome was observed in those going to transplantation in the first chronic phase and within 6 months of diagnosis; the DFS rate with a sibling donor for that cohort was 73%.[600] Given these data and newer studies showing outcomes to be virtually identical with sibling or unrelated donors for pediatric leukemia patients, it is still reasonable to offer HSCT as the first therapeutic intervention for pediatric patients with a sibling or fully matched unrelated donor. Alternatively, imatinib could be started at the time of diagnosis with careful monitoring of disease response. Recent data allow response to imatinib at specific time points to be categorized as "failures," and such patients should be offered alternative therapies.[599,601] In young patients, whether this next intervention is allogeneic HSCT or a trial of second-generation TKIs depends on donor availability and physician, family, and patient assessment of the risks and benefits attendant on both strategies. There is some concern that pretreatment with a TKI could have an adverse impact on HSCT outcome, but this does not seem to be a problem, provided that imatinib is discontinued at least 2 weeks before transplantation.[602] Rarely, patients with CML are initially seen in accelerated phase or in myeloid or lymphoid blast crisis. Chemotherapy is administered to try to regain stable phase. Allogeneic HSCT can then offer curative therapy for up to 40% of patients.[59,603] Whether the addition of imatinib before or after HSCT can improve outcome for this group is unknown.

For patients undergoing HSCT, careful monitoring of disease status remains an essential component of post-transplant care. Relapse detected early at the cytogenetic or molecular level responds extraordinarily well to donor lymphocyte infusion (DLI). Currently, most patients receive escalating doses of $CD3^+$ T cells in an attempt to achieve disease control without inducing GVHD.[604] The role of TKI in post-HSCT recurrence—either alone or in combination with DLI—is still being elucidated.[605,606]

Hodgkin's and Non-Hodgkin's Lymphoma

Autologous HSCT has been used in children with Hodgkin's disease (HD) or aggressive non-Hodgkin's lymphoma (NHL) who either relapse or have refractory disease after initial treatment with conventional therapy. Both TBI-based and chemotherapy-only approaches have been used with equal success. There has been increasing consensus about the use of autologous PBSCs versus bone marrow as the stem cell source based on the favorable engraftment characteristics for neutrophils and platelets.[607] The potential of high-dose therapy with autologous rescue to salvage pediatric patients with Burkitt's lymphoma was established in 1986, when a 5-year French experience demonstrated approximately a 50% DFS rate.[608] Similar results in children with Burkitt's and large cell lymphoma (LCL), as well as HD, have been reported more recently from other European centers and in larger combined pediatric and adult series.[609-612] Paralleling the findings in adult patients with lymphoma, DFS is most consistently predicted by the presence of chemotherapy-sensitive disease; long-term survival is unlikely in those with bulky disease at the time of HSCT.[613] The addition of rituximab before or after HSCT (or both) for B-cell lymphomas may further

improve outcome in this group of patients.[614,615] As for T-cell acute lymphoblastic leukemia (T-ALL), allogeneic HSCT is the standard approach for refractory or relapsed T-cell lymphoblastic lymphoma if remission can be attained.[616]

There has also been interest in the role of allogeneic HSCT in the treatment of relapsed/refractory NHL and HD. Retrospective case-controlled studies in adult/pediatric series suggest comparable results. A prospective trial revealed a lower relapse rate in those undergoing allogeneic BMT but no overall survival advantage because of significant transplant-related mortality. As seen in patients undergoing autologous HSCT, chemosensitivity before transplantation was the major prognostic factor for outcome.[617] The advantage conferred by an allogeneic stem cell source may be dependent on the type of lymphoma; a recent study of pediatric patients with anaplastic LCL reported a remarkable 75% DFS rate, with successes even in patients relapsing after autologous HSCT.[618] Whether the decrease in relapse rate seen in these studies reflects a graft-versus-lymphoma effect or merely the infusion of uncontaminated stem cells is not clear.[619] Characterization of patients at particularly high risk for failure should allow better delineation of which patients could benefit from an allogeneic transplant—either alone or as a tandem approach after autologous transplantation[620]—despite the increase in transplant-related mortality and the risk of cGVHD.

Neuroblastoma and Other Solid Tumors

The most extensive HSCT experience with pediatric solid tumors is in patients with advanced-stage neuroblastoma (see Chapter 14 of *Oncology of Infancy and Childhood*). Historically, patients receiving conventional doses of chemotherapy almost always succumbed to disease. In 1999, a landmark trial showed a significant improvement in DFS (34% versus 22%) for patients randomized to consolidation with autologous BMT versus continued intensive nonmyeloablative chemotherapy.[621] Because regimen-related toxicity was acceptable and dose intensification appeared to have an impact on DFS, sequential or "tandem" transplants with the use of two[622] or three[623] cycles of non–cross-resistant agents over a short period of time along with autologous PBSC support have been investigated. It appears that such approaches can further improve outcome, with a reported 3-year DFS rate of 58%[622] and an estimated DFS rate of 45% at 7 years from diagnosis.[624] Relapse remains a significant problem primarily at diffuse osseous sites. Neuroblastoma cells marked in the stem cell product have been identified at sites of relapse,[159] and a variety of positive and negative selection techniques have been used to purge the stem cells before reinfusion, although none have been definitively shown to have an impact on outcome; profound depletion of T cells from the graft has, however, resulted in an increase in life-threatening viral infections.[625] Currently, the role of targeted radionuclides such as metaiodobenzylguanidine (MIBG) is being investigated. MIBG has shown encouraging results in children refractory to conventional approaches, and hepatotoxicity and myelosuppression have been the main toxicities; frequently, autologous stem cell infusion is required after this therapy.[626] Allogeneic transplantation has been evaluated in several small series but does not appear to have a favorable impact on survival.[627] Therapy for minimal residual disease after HSCT is essential, with *cis*-retinoic acid being the most thoroughly evaluated,[621] although potentially more toxic approaches such as antibody therapy are currently under investigation.[628] Most children undergoing autologous HSCT for neuroblastoma are very young, and there has been concern about the quality of life after this intensive therapy. However, the literature suggests that most survivors of this previously almost uniformly fatal disease are neuropsychologically intact.[629,630] Survivors are at risk for a variety of medical complications, the most common being short stature, gonadal failure, and hearing loss (seen in three fourths of patients)[631] and must be closely monitored by appropriate specialists to optimize outcome.

The role of high-dose therapy with autologous PBSC rescue for brain tumors is still being evaluated. The literature is most extensive for tumors with a clear dose-response curve, such as medulloblastoma/primary neuroectodermal tumor (PNET) and germ cell tumors.[632-634] HSCT is most often used in the setting of recurrent disease but is occasionally used at the time of first remission in patients with adverse prognostic features or in very young children in an attempt to avoid radiation therapy.[635] EFS rates range from 30% to 50%, and as is the case for most conditions treated with autologous HSCT, those in remission at the time of transplantation fare best. Ongoing consortium trials hope to standardize therapy and further understand which patients can benefit from this therapeutic approach.

Small single-institution series have been published on the use of either allogeneic or autologous HSCT for other nonhematologic malignancies. Some promise in terms of response rate has been observed for patients with sarcomas who have both minimal residual and chemosensitive disease, but the generalizability and durability of these responses will need to be established before widespread application can be supported.

TRANSPLANTATION IN PATIENTS WITH GENETIC DISEASES

Allogeneic SCT has increasingly been evaluated as a potentially curative approach for children with inherited diseases. The most common inherited diseases that have been treated with SCT are reviewed.

Box 9-3	**Immunodeficiency Disorders Treated by Stem Cell Transplantation**

Classic severe combined immunodeficiency disease (B⁻)
Common severe combined immunodeficiency disease (B⁺)
Adenosine deaminase deficiency
Reticular dysgenesis
Omenn's syndrome
Severe combined immunodeficiency disease associated with short-limbed dwarfism and ectodermal dysplasia
Familial erythrophagocytic lymphohistiocytosis
HLA class II deficiency (bare lymphocyte syndrome)
Purine nucleoside phosphorylase deficiency
X-linked lymphoproliferative disease
Leukocyte adhesion deficiency (CD11/18 deficiency)
Wiskott-Aldrich syndrome

Immunodeficiency Disorders

Severe Combined Immunodeficiency Syndromes

Since the late 1960s, allogeneic BMT has been successfully used to cure children with a number of lethal immunodeficiency diseases (Box 9-3), including SCID and Wiskott-Aldrich syndrome (WAS). SCID is a clinical syndrome arising from a variety of genetic abnormalities that all result in profound deficiencies in T-cell function. Depending on the specific genetic abnormality, B-lymphocyte and NK-cell number and function will be affected as well.[636] In classic X-linked SCID there is profound T-cell lymphopenia and a variable number of nonfunctioning B cells, whereas patients with adenosine deaminase deficiency lack B cells, T cells, and NK cells. Autosomal recessive SCID phenotypes have different combinations of B- and NK-cell presence. Without question, conventional matched sibling allogeneic HSCT for SCID is one of the major success stories of transplantation. Unlike the situation in most transplant settings, because of the underlying immunologic defect, SCID patients with a matched sibling donor do not necessarily require conditioning. After infusion of genotypically matched donor stem cells without cytoreduction, immune reconstitution will take place within several weeks, and evidence of good lymphocyte function will be apparent by 2 to 3 months.[637] Significant aGVHD or cGVHD is uncommon. Dramatically improved long-term survivorship from the range of approximately 50% in the 1970s to greater than 90% currently appears attributable to more rapid and precise diagnosis, followed by transplantation in patients at a younger age and in better condition, and to improved supportive care for the associated infectious complications.[638,639]

The optimal approach for children lacking a matched sibling donor is less clear, and two different strategies have been used: T-cell–depleted haploidentical transplantation generally using a parent as the donor or, more recently, transplantation from a matched unrelated donor.

Early experience with haploidentical HSCT was hampered by graft rejection, frequent severe GVHD, and opportunistic infection, which resulted in poor long-term survival. The development of T-cell depletion protocols improved the outcomes for haploidentical nonconditioned HSCT. The advantage of this approach is that neither cytoreductive therapy nor GVHD prophylaxis is needed, and thus peritransplant mortality is low. T-cell function usually takes several months to appear, patients generally do not have B-cell function mandating lifelong IVIG replacement, and graft rejection necessitating a second or even third transplant occurs in approximately 20% of patients. Buckley reported her 30-year experience using with approach and achieved a 78% survival rate. T-cell function normalized and was most robust in children who were diagnosed early and underwent transplantation within the first 28 days of life.[640] There is some concern about the longevity of T-cell function inasmuch as markers of ongoing thymic-dependent T-cell production diminished markedly when evaluated years after HSCT.[641,642] This has led, particularly in Europe, to the more frequent adoption of complete cytoreduction and the use of matched unrelated donors as a stem cell source for patients lacking a matched sibling donor. This approach allows the development of a fully functional donor immune and hematopoietic system. These advantages must be weighed against the time taken to identify an unrelated donor and the risk of GVHD, the increased risk of acute infectious morbidity and mortality associated with myeloablative therapy, and long-term sequelae, including the likelihood of infertility. Recent reports indicate that use of an unrelated donor confers a survival advantage over mismatched related donors (80% versus 52%), as well as improved reconstitution of a full T-cell repertoire.[639] The role of nonmyeloablative HSCT and the ability of this approach to decrease acute toxicity and mitigate long-term sequelae is being investigated but may be a particularly attractive option in children with severe organ dysfunction at the time of HSCT.[643-645]

Wiskott-Aldrich Syndrome

WAS is an X-linked disorder in which progressive T-cell immunodeficiency is associated with eczema, small platelets, and absolute thrombocytopenia. The pathogenesis of this disorder is associated with aberrant expression of the WAS protein, which is involved in cytoskeletal organization, as well as T- and NK-cell activation.[646] This disorder is reviewed in detail in Chapter 23. As with SCID, matched sibling allogeneic SCT was first undertaken in children with WAS in the late 1960s, and full correction of the hematologic manifestations was reported in 1978.[647] Both TBI- and busulfan-based regimens have been used successfully in conditioning patients with WAS, and the reported survival rate of almost 90% in patients with matched sibling donors is among the best of any patient cohort undergoing allogeneic SCT.[648-651] This approach was thus extended to patients with mismatched family or unrelated donors. Early reports were not encouraging, with survival rates of less than 40% and significant problems related to graft rejection and the development of post-transplant B-cell lymphoproliferative disease.[652-654] Recent data have been more encouraging.[655,656] In a review of the National Marrow Donor Program (NMDP)/IBMTR registry cases, Filipovich and associates found that 85% of boys receiving an unrelated donor transplant before the age of 5 survived, an outcome similar to that seen with sibling donors. In addition, cGVHD was limited in severity and ultimately completely resolved in most affected children.[655] Thus, most children afflicted with WAS are now expeditiously referred for transplantation from the best available donor, with a palliative approach consisting of splenectomy and chronic IVIG administration being used only in rare cases.

Inherited Hematopoietic Disorders

Thalassemia

Thalassemia major (or Cooley's anemia) is the most common transfusion-dependent anemia in the world. Chronic transfusion therapy and chelation to prevent the associated iron overload have modified the natural history of thalassemia and transformed a disease that was uniformly fatal in early childhood into a chronic process with progressive end-organ dysfunction.[657,658] Over time, even medically compliant patients are at risk for complications, including endocrine dysfunction, hepatic cirrhosis, cardiac disease, and transfusion-associated viral infections. In the developed world with sophisticated medical management, life expectancy is 25 to 55 years, depending mostly on compliance with chelation therapy, but in the developing world, the majority of patients still die before their third decade of life.[658,659]

Successful application of HSCT as a curative approach for thalassemia major was first reported in 1982.[660] Subsequently, a very large experience reported by Lucarelli and co-workers[49] unquestionably established the feasibility of SCT for thalassemia, and more than 2000 patients worldwide have received transplants,[661] the overwhelming majority from a matched sibling donor using a busulfan-based conditioning regimen.[662] The Pesaro classification system, based on the presence of hepatic fibrosis as assessed by liver biopsy, the degree of hepatomegaly (an uncertain measurement), and a history of inadequate chelation, allows risk stratification of potential transplant patients younger than 17 years. Class I patients have no risk factors, class 2 patients have one or two risk factors, and class 3 patients have all the risk factors. The probabilities of overall survival, EFS, and graft rejection for patients undergoing HSCT from a matched family donor were 94%, 94%, and 0%, respectively, for class I patients and 80%, 77%, and 9% for class 2 patients. Class 3 patients had only a 53% thalassemia-free survival rate because of increased graft rejection and transplant-related mortality.[49,663] Newer approaches with increased immunosuppression using any combination of hydroxyurea, azathioprine, and fludarabine have yielded improved results for class III patients, with a thalassemia-free survival rate of 80% in patients younger than 17 years.[664] Post-HSCT management of preexisting hepatic and cardiac iron overload and viral infections is essential for optimal outcome and may allow cirrhosis to be reversed.[665,666] Positive effects on bone mineral density in children may also occur.[667] Although matched sibling HSCT is undoubtedly efficacious, the decision to pursue aggressive chelation strategies versus accepting the short- and long-term risks associated with HSCT remains difficult and should occur on an individual basis after consultation with both hematologists and transplant physicians. Historically, HSCT from an unrelated donor had a dismal prognosis in this disease,[661] and HSCT was considered only if a suitable family donor was available. However, improvements in HLA typing and supportive care have had a global impact on transplant outcomes with unrelated donors, and thus HSCT may now be a reasonable option for selected patients with fully matched donors. As with sibling donors, the best results occur in those with less advanced disease, and thalassemia-free survival rates of 80% to 100% for class 1 or 2 patients have been reported in small series.[668,669]

Sickle Cell Disease

Allogeneic HSCT offers a curative approach for patients with sickle cell disease (SCD). Because the clinical course of SCD is highly variable and, particularly with the advent of pneumococcal prophylaxis, childhood morbidity and mortality are low, it is difficult to know which patients should undergo HSCT. Initial studies offered HSCT to the subgroup of patients with the most life-threatening or debilitating symptoms: those with stroke, recurrent acute chest syndrome, or recurrent painful crises. In the seminal report by Walters and colleagues, the DFS rate after busulfan-based myeloablative conditioning was 73%, and the overall survival rate was 91% at 4 years; end-organ damage was stabilized in patients with sustained donor engraftment.[670] Improved management of transplant complications in general and increased attention to SS-specific toxicities (additional immunosuppression to decrease graft rejection, antiseizure prophylaxis, strict management of hypertension) have resulted in consistent gains in cure rates,[671] with EFS rates of greater than 95% in patients who underwent transplantation after January 2000.[672] Newer approaches such as the use of hydroxyurea to decrease the risk of graft rejection by influencing pretransplant bone marrow cellularity[673] or the use of a nonmyeloablative approach to decrease transplant-related morbidity and mortality[674] or even preserve fertility remain to be evaluated.

HSCT has historically been considered only for patients who have an available matched sibling donor. A multi-institutional survey of factors having an impact on the use of HSCT in this population found that less than 15% of affected children had an acceptable sibling donor.[670] The role of unrelated donor HSCT in patients with the most severe manifestations of disease or in those

unable to receive long-term transfusion therapy is unknown, but multi-institutional trials are currently being developed.[675] Unrelated umbilical cord donors are a theoretically attractive option given the decreased incidence of GVHD and the ability to use donors who have greater HLA disparity. Small numbers of transplants have been reported with successful outcomes, although both GVHD and graft rejection remain obstacles to widespread use.[676]

The choice to proceed to matched sibling HSCT remains complicated, particularly if the disease manifestations are moderate or intermittent. No prospective randomized trials are available to inform the decision, and therapy with hydroxyurea, chronic transfusion, and HSCT each have associated risks and benefits. HSCT clearly has the highest upfront risk but also offers the only curative modality. The Belgian experience illustrates that children who undergo transplantation at a young age before significant complications occur do best, with a DFS rate of 93% and overall survival rate of 100%,[677] and serious late complications of SS disease affecting long-term survival, such as pulmonary hypertension, continue to be identified. Unfortunately, even in the reports of HSCT showing the most favorable outcomes, patients are likely to be infertile,[678] and the risk for extensive cGVHD is low but real.[672] Patients (when of an appropriate age) and parents must be aware of the possible therapeutic options so that they can be informed and active participants in the decision-making process.[679]

Fanconi's Anemia

Fanconi's anemia (FA) is an autosomal recessive disorder clinically characterized by a highly variable physical phenotype, progressive marrow failure, and a marked propensity for the development of AML and certain solid tumors (see Chapter 8). HSCT can be curative for the hematologic manifestations of FA, but early experience revealed excessive regimen-associated morbidity and mortality, and in vitro studies confirmed hypersensitivity to alkylating agents and radiation.[680,681] The development of specialized conditioning regimens mostly using low doses of both cyclophosphamide and radiation has spurred the application of HSCT as a treatment option, and results with HLA-identical sibling donors are excellent if performed early in life before the development of MDS or leukemia,[682,683] with 2-year DFS rates as high as 95%.[684] In addition, the first reported transplant using UCB as a stem cell source was successfully undertaken in a child with FA by using cells from an HLA-identical sibling.[133]

In contrast, the outcome with alternative donors has been markedly worse, with survival rates of approximately 30%[685-687]; graft failure and GVHD were the major obstacles. In a recent review of 98 FA patients undergoing unrelated donor HSCT, patients younger than 10 years who had fewer than 20 transfusions and received a fludarabine-containing regimen and T-cell–depleted marrow allografts had better outcomes, with a 3-year survival rate of 52%.[688] Thus, the prognosis for FA patients undergoing alternative donor SCT has greatly improved over time, and early referral for discussion of HSCT is indicated for patients with marrow failure. Data are limited on the use of HSCT in FA patients in whom frank leukemia has developed. Anecdotal reports suggest that there are occasionally long-term survivors, but death from regimen-related toxicity or leukemic relapse is the norm. Recent reports suggesting that these children can tolerate cytoreductive therapy before HSCT may ultimately lead to better outcomes.[689] Although HSCT can restore normal hematopoiesis, meticulous follow-up of these patients is essential because they retain a significant risk for the development of solid tumors, particularly squamous cell carcinomas of the upper gastrointestinal tract and anogenital region. The peak incidence is in the second and third decades of life, and it is unclear whether the preparatory regimen for HSCT increases the underlying risk inherent in the disease.[690,691]

Diamond-Blackfan Anemia

Diamond-Blackfan anemia (DBA) is a rare heritable condition manifested as pure red cell aplasia as a result of an intrinsic erythroid progenitor defect. Approximately a third of patients have associated physical abnormalities, including short stature, cardiac or urogenital abnormalities, cleft palate, and microcephaly.[692] Haploinsufficiency of ribosomal protein S19 (RPS19) is seen in 20% to 25% of patients. DBA is generally diagnosed in the first months of life and is characterized by anemia, macrocytosis, and reticulocytopenia (see Chapter 8). Although approximately two thirds of children initially respond to corticosteroid therapy, significant numbers either fail to respond or lose response over time.[693] The toxicity of this approach, whether sequelae of chronic transfusions or prolonged corticosteroid and cyclosporine use, is significant, in addition to the potential for leukemia developing in early to mid adulthood.[693] Although responses may wax and wane, 15% to 25% of children may obtain a durable spontaneous remission.[694] Allogeneic HSCT can offer a curative option. The first transplant was performed in 1976,[695] and of the 354 patients registered in the DBA registry of North America, 20 have undergone HSCT from family or unrelated donors.[696] Transplants using matched sibling donors were performed with a non–radiation-based regimen and resulted in an 87% DFS rate. Patients undergoing alternative donor transplantation fared poorly, with a 14% survival rate. Sixty-one patients with DBA who underwent HSCT were reported to the IBMTR between 1984 and 2000. The 3-year survival rate was 64%, and having a matched sibling donor and a performance status of at least 90% before HSCT conferred the best prognosis.[697] More recently, the Japanese Aplastic Anemia Registry reported a 100% 5-year survival rate in 13 patients with DBA who received an allogeneic transplant from either sibling or unrelated bone marrow donors; however, 3 of 3 patients receiving unre-

lated cord blood transplants experienced graft failure.[698] Thus, transplantation from a suitable bone marrow donor is a reasonable option, particularly patients who fail to have a sustained response to steroids.

Granulocyte Platelet and Macrophage Disorders

Limited numbers of patients with a variety of qualitative and quantitative disorders of myeloid cell function have achieved successful reconstitution of hematopoietic cells with allogeneic SCT, usually with a busulfan-based regimen (Box 9-4; also see specific diseases in Chapter 21). HSCT has been used successfully for both quantitative granulocyte disorders such as severe congenital neutropenia (SCN or Kostmann's syndrome) and qualitative disorders such as leukocyte adhesion deficiency (LAD), Chédiak-Higashi syndrome (CHS), and chronic granulomatous disease (CGD). Patients with SCN have a 21% cumulative incidence of MDS/AML and an 8% cumulative incidence of mortality from sepsis at 10 years.[699] Those who do not respond to G-CSF and those in whom clonal hematopoiesis develops should proceed expeditiously to HSCT. The SCN registry reported 9 of 11 long-term survivors after related or unrelated HSCT, with 1 survivor having significant cGVHD.[700] Patients with LAD or CD11/CD18 deficiency have impaired neutrophil adhesion, migration, and phagocytosis, and severe infections usually develop early in life. HSCT with related or unrelated donors can be curative.[701,702] Patients with stable-phase CHS may have minimal symptoms but usually progress to an accelerated phase in the first or second decade of life. Acceleration is characterized by pancytopenia, hepatosplenomegaly, and serious infections and is uniformly fatal. HSCT offers a curative option even when patients remain chimeric, and as in other transplant settings, patients with less advanced disease have improved outcomes.[703,704] Medical management of CGD has dramatically improved survival, but HSCT may still be appropriate in patients experiencing recurrent severe infections. After myeloablative conditioning, 22 of 27 patients were cured.[705] Active infection at the time of HSCT was associated with severe GVHD and a worse outcome, so thorough pretransplant evaluation and treatment are essential.

Single-patient reports and small series indicate that HSCT can be curative in patients with congenital platelet disorders, including amegakaryocytic thrombocytopenia

Box 9-4	White Blood Cell Disorders Treated by Stem Cell Transplantation
Chédiak-Higashi syndrome	
Kostmann's syndrome	
Chronic granulomatous disease	
CD11/18 deficiency (leukocyte adhesion deficiency)	
Neutrophil actin defects	
Shwachman-Diamond syndrome	

and severe forms of Glanzmann's thrombasthenia. Most patients had matched sibling donors and received a busulfan-based conditioning regimen. The overall results are encouraging, but regimen-related deaths do occur, and thus the risks associated with HSCT should be balanced against the risks of bleeding episodes and chronic transfusion therapy.[706-708]

Primary hemophagocytic lymphohistiocytosis is the most common congenital macrophage disorder. It is inherited in an autosomal recessive manner and is a disease of infancy or early childhood. Patients have fever, hepatosplenomegaly, and pancytopenia as a result of abnormal proliferation of macrophages and accumulation in the liver, spleen, bone marrow, and CNS. Remission may be attained with immunomodulation consisting of steroids, cyclosporine, and epipodophyllins, but allogeneic HSCT is the only curative modality.[709] As with other diseases, once HSCT from matched related donors was shown to be feasible,[52] the treatment was extended to unrelated donors, usually with a busulfan, etoposide, and cyclophosphamide conditioning regimen, and DFS rates of 45% to 65% were achieved.[710-712] Children who were in remission after pretransplant therapy did best, but cures were still seen in the setting of some degree of disease activity at HSCT. Newer approaches include the use of reduced-intensity conditioning, and a small series reported a 75% DFS rate at a median of 30 months after HSCT; interestingly, three of the nine survivors showed mixed chimerism, albeit with high-level T-cell engraftment, thus suggesting that as with other immunodeficiencies, restoration of T-cell function versus complete myeloablation may suffice for cure.[713]

Osteopetrosis

This rare disorder of osteoclast dysfunction leads to an inability to resorb and remodel bone and the resulting formation of excessive mineralized osteoid and cartilage. Infantile or "malignant" osteopetrosis is inherited in an autosomal recessive manner and causes a severe phenotype. In addition to poor growth and bony encroachment on optic and other cranial nerve foramina causing vision and hearing impairment, eradication of the marrow space ensues with progressive pancytopenia.[714] Murine studies revealed that osteoclasts arise from hematopoietic precursors of the monocytic lineage, and disease reversal was accomplished by engraftment of bone marrow from unaffected animals.[715] Successful HSCT in humans was first reported in 1977, and its applicability has subsequently been shown in many reports,[716-718] mostly using a busulfan-based conditioning regimen. Recently, the European Group for Blood and Marrow Transplantation (EBMT) reported the long-term outcome of 122 children undergoing allogeneic HSCT between 1980 and 2001.[719] The 5-year DFS rate was 73% in those receiving transplants from an HLA-identical sibling versus approximately 40% in those receiving transplants from mismatched family donors or matched unrelated donors. The major causes of failure were lack of engraftment,

attributed in part to disruption of the underlying marrow microenvironment, and pulmonary complications, particularly pulmonary hypertension. Conservation of vision was most likely in those who underwent transplantation before 3 months of age. Patients, especially those older than 2 years at transplantation, are at risk for hypercalcemia as engraftment occurs, and therefore meticulous monitoring of calcium levels is essential in the peritransplant period.[718] At present, HSCT is the only curative option, although calcitriol,[720] interferon gamma,[721] and prednisone[722] have been used to slow progression or ameliorate symptoms, or both. Donor identification and subsequent HSCT should occur expeditiously as soon as the diagnosis is confirmed because neurologic impairment can occur rapidly and may be irreversible, even with successful hematopoietic engraftment.

Storage Disorders

Storage disorders are characterized by accumulation of substrate due to an underlying enzymatic deficiency. This disrupts cellular function and leads to organ impairment. Historically, few treatment options other than palliative and supportive modalities have been available. More recently, the availability of alglucerase (Ceredase) enzyme infusion has dramatically altered the course of patients with Gaucher's disease.[723] Although similar inroads have not yet been made in other diseases, the concepts of gene transfer and somatic cell therapy, as well as infusion of enzymes produced by recombinant techniques, are being investigated in animal models of specific diseases. The rationale for SCT as a therapeutic maneuver is based on the assumption that the most severely affected cell population is hematopoietic in origin or that sufficient transfer of enzyme via enzyme-replete cells can prevent subsequent as well as reverse existing damage. However, the capacity for repair or arrest of damage to affected organ systems, especially the CNS, remains unproven for many storage disorders. Age and neurodevelopmental status before HSCT are consistently the strongest predictors of outcome. Although life expectancy may be prolonged, children severely affected at the time of HSCT are unlikely to experience significant improvement in neurocognitive function. In addition, donor selection is a significant issue inasmuch as siblings may be homozygous or heterozygous for the affected gene. Use of a heterozygous donor does not have an impact on outcome in hematologic disorders such as thalassemia, but whether heterozygosity provides adequate enzyme levels to correct an ongoing process has not been elucidated for this group of disorders.

Several excellent reviews of the results of HSCT for specific storage disorders have been published, with the largest body of literature involving the mucopolysaccharidoses and the leukodystrophies.[724-727] Only for mucopolysaccharidosis IH (Hurler's syndrome), X-linked adrenoleukodystrophy, and infantile globoid cell leukodystrophy (Krabbe's disease) are there sufficient data to suggest that HSCT is indicated in carefully selected cases.[728] Patients with Hurler's disease who undergo HSCT before 2 years of age and achieve donor engraftment can maintain preservation of neurocognitive function and motor development, although the skeletal abnormalities (dysostosis multiplex) do not improve because chondrocytes have difficulty clearing glycosaminoglycan.[729,730] Most transplants for storage disorders have been performed with matched family donors. Graft failure with autologous recovery has also had a negative impact on success; patients receiving unrelated donor[731] T-cell–depleted grafts or reduced-intensity conditioning are at particular risk.[732] Recently, the use of unrelated UCB donors has provided a rapidly available source of stem cells, as well as being a more permissive source in terms of HLA matching and thus increasing the number of acceptable donors. Encouraging outcomes have been reported, although follow-up has been relatively short. After umbilical cord HSCT, 17 of 20 children with Hurler's syndrome are long-term survivors with normal enzyme levels,[733] 11 of 11 asymptomatic newborns with globoid cell leukodystrophy have normal enzyme levels and are making developmental gains,[734] and 3 of 3 young asymptomatic boys with adrenoleukodystrophy have stable MRI findings and normal neurologic examination results.[735] As seen previously with marrow donors, older children with adrenoleukodystrophy and progressive MRI changes had rapid deterioration of neurologic function and poor outcomes. Thus, although a subset of patients with storage disorders can benefit from HSCT, particularly those who are young, have minimal symptoms, or have indolent forms of a disease, patients with aggressive infantile forms or those who have significant neurologic impairment at the time of referral will need alternative therapeutic interventions to improve outcome.

REFERENCES

1. Osgood EE, Riddle MC, Mathews TJ. Aplastic anemia treated with daily transfusions and intravenous marrow; case report. Ann Intern Med. 1939;13:357-367.
2. Jacobson LO, Marks EK, Gaston EO, et al. Effect of spleen protection on mortality following x-irradiation. J Lab Clin Med. 1949;34:1538-1543.
3. Jacobson LO, Simmons EL, Marks EK, et al. Recovery from radiation injury. Science. 1951;113:510-511.
4. Ford CE, Hamerton JL, Barnes DWH, et al. Cytological identification of radiation-chimaeras. Nature. 1956;177:452-454.
5. Barnes DWH, Loutit JF. The radiation recovery factor: preservation by the Polge-Smith-Parkes techniques. J Natl Cancer Inst. 1955;15:901-905.
6. Barnes DWH, Loutit JF. Spleen protection: the cellular hypothesis. In Bacq ZM, Alexander P (eds). Radiobiology Symposium 1954. New York, Academic Press, 1954, pp 134-135.
7. Uphoff DE. Alteration of homograft reaction by A-methopterin in lethally irradiated mice treated with homologous marrow. Proc Soc Exp Biol Med. 1958;99:651-653.
8. Thomas ED, Lochte HL Jr, Lu WC, et al. Intravenous infusion of bone marrow in patients receiving radiation and chemotherapy. N Engl J Med. 1957;257:491-496.
9. Thomas ED, Lochte HL Jr, Cannon JH, et al. Supralethal whole body irradiation and isologous marrow transplantation in man. J Clin Invest. 1959;38:1709-1716.
10. Bach FH, Albertini RJ, Anderson JL, et al. Bone marrow transplantation in a patient with the Wiskott-Aldrich syndrome. Lancet. 1968;2:1364-1366.
11. de Koning J, van Bekkum DW, Dicke KA, et al. Transplantation of bone marrow cells and fetal thymus in an infant with lymphopenic immunological deficiency. Lancet. 1969;1:1223-1227.
12. Good RA, Gatti A, Hong R, et al. Successful marrow transplantation for correction of immunological deficit in lymphopenic agammaglobulinemia and treatment of immunologically induced pancytopenia. Exp Hematol. 1969;19:4.
13. Good RA, Meuwissen HJ, Hong R, et al. Bone marrow transplantation: correction of immune deficit in lymphopenic immunologic deficiency and correction of an immunologically induced pancytopenia. Trans Assoc Am Physicians. 1969;82:278-285.
14. Bjornson CR, Rietze RL, Reynolds BA, et al. Turning brain into blood: a hematopoietic fate adopted by adult neural stem cells in vivo. Science. 1999;283:534-537.
15. Pang W. Role of muscle-derived cells in hematopoietic reconstitution of irradiated mice. Blood. 2000;95:1106-1108.
16. Jackson KA, Mi T, Goodell MA. Hematopoietic potential of stem cells isolated from murine skeletal muscle. Proc Natl Acad Sci U S A. 1999;96:14482-14486.
17. Seale P, Rudnicki MA. A new look at the origin, function, and "stem-cell" status of muscle satellite cells. Dev Biol. 2000;218:115-124.
18. Weissman IL. Translating stem and progenitor cell biology to the clinic: barriers and opportunities. Science. 2000;287:1442-1446.
19. Armitage JO. Bone marrow transplantation. N Engl J Med. 1994;330:827-838.
20. Mentzer WC, Heller S, Pearle PR, et al. Availability of related donors for bone marrow transplantation in sickle cell anemia. Am J Pediatr Hematol Oncol. 1994;16:27-29.
21. Beatty PG, Clift RA, Mickelson EM, et al. Marrow transplantation from related donors other than HLA-identical siblings. N Engl J Med. 1985;313:765-771.
22. Anasetti C, Amos D, Beatty PG, et al. Effect of HLA compatibility on engraftment of bone marrow transplants in patients with leukemia or lymphoma. N Engl J Med. 1989;320:197-204.
23. Champlin R, Coppo P, Howe C. National Marrow Donor Program: progress and challenges. Bone Marrow Transplant. 1993;11(Suppl 1):41-44.
24. Kernan NA, Bartsch G, Ash RC, et al. Analysis of 462 transplantation from unrelated donors facilitated by the National Marrow Donor Program. N Engl J Med. 1993;328:593-601.
25. Anasetti C, Etzioni R, Petersdorf EW, et al. Marrow transplantation from unrelated volunteer donors. Annu Rev Med. 1995;46:169-179.

26. Wagner JE, Kernan NA, Steinbuch M, et al. Allogeneic sibling umbilical-cord-blood transplantation in children with malignant and non-malignant disease. Lancet. 1995;346:214-219.

27. Rubinstein P, Rosenfield RE, Adamson JW, et al. Stored placental blood for unrelated bone marrow reconstitution. Blood. 1993;81:1679-1690.

28. Kurtzberg J, Laughlin M, Graham ML, et al. Placental blood as a source of hematopoietic stem cells for transplantation into unrelated recipients. N Engl J Med. 1996;335:157-166.

29. Mathe G, Jammet H, Pendic B, et al. Transfusions et greffes de moelle osseuse homologue chez des humains irradies a haute dause accidentellement. Rev Fr Etudes Clin Biol. 1959;4:226-238.

30. Santos GW. History of bone marrow transplantation. Clin Haematol. 1983;12:611-639.

31. Tutschka PJ, Santos GW, Elfenbein GJ. Marrow transplantation in acute leukemia following busulfan and cyclophosphamide. Haematol Blood Transfus. 1980;25: 375-380.

32. Storb R, Yu C, Deeg HJ, et al. Current and future preparative regimens for bone marrow transplantation in thalassemia. Ann N Y Acad Sci. 1998;850:276-287.

33. Thomas E, Clift R, Hersman J, et al. Marrow transplantation for acute nonlymphoblastic leukemia in first remission using fractionated or single dose irradiation. Int J Radiat Oncol Biol Phys. 1982;8:817-821.

34. Deeg H, Sullivan K, Buckner C, et al. Marrow transplantation for ANLL in first remission: toxicity and long-term follow-up of patients conditioned with single dose or fractionated total body irradiation. Bone Marrow Transplant. 1986;1:151-157.

35. Buckner C, Clift R, Appelbaum F, et al. A randomized trial of 12 or 15.75 Gy of total body irradiation (TBI) in patients with ANLL and CML followed by marrow transplantation. Exp Hematol. 1989;17:522.

36. Clift R, Buckner C, Appelbaum F, et al. Allogeneic marrow transplantation in patients with chronic myeloid leukemia in the chronic phase: a randomized trial of two irradiation regimens. Blood. 1991;77:1660-1665.

37. Lawton C. Total-body irradiation for bone marrow transplantation. Oncology (Williston Park). 1999;13:5-8, 81-82, 972.

38. Chou RH, Wong GB, Kramer JH, et al. Toxicities of total-body irradiation for pediatric bone marrow transplantation. Int J Radiat Oncol Biol Phys. 1996;34:843-851.

39. Santos GW, Tutschka PJ, Brookmeyer R, et al. Marrow transplantation for acute nonlymphocytic leukemia after treatment with busulfan and cyclophosphamide. N Engl J Med. 1983;309:1347-1353.

40. Santos GW. Antonio Raichs lecture. Autologous bone marrow transplantation. Sangre. 1992;37:471-474.

41. Yeager AM, Kaizer H, Santos GW, et al. Autologous bone marrow transplantation in patients with acute nonlymphocytic leukemia using ex vivo marrow treatment with 4 hydroperoxycyclophosphamide. N Engl J Med. 1986;315: 141-147.

42. Beelen DW, Quabeck K, Graeven U, et al. Acute toxicity and first clinical results of intensive postinduction therapy using a modified busulfan and cyclophosphamide regimen with autologous bone marrow rescue in first remission of acute myeloid leukemia. Blood. 1989;74:1507-1516.

43. Santos GW. Allogeneic and autologous bone marrow transplantation in AML. Leukemia. 1992;6:102-103.

44. Copelan EA, Biggs JC, Thompson JM, et al. Treatment for acute myelocytic leukemia with allogeneic bone marrow transplantation following preparation with BuCy2. Blood. 1991;78:838-843.

45. Tutschka PJ, Copelan EA, Klein JP. Bone marrow transplantation for leukemia following a new busulfan and cyclophosphamide regimen. Blood. 1987;70:1382-1388.

46. Copelan EA, Deeg HJ. Conditioning for allogeneic marrow transplantation in patients with lymphohematopoietic malignancies without the use of total body irradiation. Blood. 1992;80:1648-1658.

47. Copelan EA, Bigges JC, Avalos BR, et al. Radiation-free preparation for allogeneic bone marrow transplantation in adults with acute lymphoblastic leukemia. J Clin Oncol. 1992;10:237-242.

48. Lucarelli G, Clift RA. Bone marrow transplantation in thalassemia. In Forman SJ, Blume KG, Thomas ED (eds). Bone Marrow Transplantation. Boston, Blackwell Scientific, 1994, pp 829-838.

49. Lucarelli G, Galimberti M, Polchi P, et al. Bone marrow transplantation in patients with thalassemia. N Engl J Med. 1990;322:417-421.

50. Rimm IJ, Rappeport JM. Bone marrow transplantation for the Wiskott-Aldrich syndrome. Transplantation. 1990;50:617-620.

51. Hoogerbrugge PM, Brouwer OF, Bordigoni P, et al. Allogeneic bone marrow transplantation for lysosomal storage diseases. Lancet. 1995;345:1398-1402.

52. Blanche S, Caniglia M, Girault D, et al. Treatment of hemophagocytic lymphohistiocytosis with chemotherapy and bone marrow transplantation: a single-center study of 22 cases. Blood. 1991;78:51-54.

53. Hasle H, Arico M, Basso G, et al. Myelodysplastic syndrome, juvenile myelomonocytic leukemia, and acute myeloid leukemia associated with complete or partial monosomy 7. European Working Group on MDS in Childhood (EWOG-MDS). Leukemia. 1999;13:376-385.

54. Davies SM, Ramsay NK, Klein JP, et al. Comparison of preparative regimens in transplants for children with acute lymphoblastic leukemia. J Clin Oncol. 2000;18:340-347.

55. Shank B. Can total body irradiation be supplanted by busulfan in cytoreductive regimens for bone marrow transplantation? Int J Radiat Oncol Biol Phys. 1995;31: 195-196.

56. Hartman AR, Williams SF, Dillon JJ. Survival, disease-free survival and adverse effects of conditioning for allogeneic bone marrow transplantation with busulfan/ cyclophosphamide vs total body irradiation: a meta-analysis. Bone Marrow Transplant. 1998;22:439-443.

57. Ringden O, Remberger M, Ruutu T, et al. Increased risk of chronic graft-versus-host disease, obstructive bronchiolitis, and alopecia with busulfan versus total body irradiation: long-term results of a randomized trial in allogeneic marrow recipients with leukemia. Nordic Bone Marrow Transplantation Group. Blood. 1999;93:2196-2201.

58. Blume KG, Kopecky KJ, Henslee-Downey JP, et al. A prospective randomized comparison of total body irradiation–etoposide versus busulfan-cyclophosphamide as preparatory regimens for bone marrow transplantation in patients with leukemia who were not in first remission: a

Southwest Oncology Group study. Blood. 1993;81:2187-2193.

59. Clift RA, Buckner CD, Thomas ED, et al. Marrow transplantation for chronic myeloid leukemia: a randomized study comparing cyclophosphamide and total body irradiation with busulfan and cyclophosphamide. Blood. 1994;84:2036-2043.

60. Ringden O, Ruutu T, Remberger M, et al. A randomized trial comparing busulfan with total body irradiation as conditioning in allogeneic marrow transplant recipients with leukemia: a report from the Nordic Bone Marrow Transplantation Group. Blood. 1994;83:2723-2730.

61. Devergie A, Blaise D, Attal M, et al. Allogeneic bone marrow transplantation for chronic myeloid leukemia in first chronic phase: a randomized trial of busulfan-Cytoxan versus Cytoxan–total body irradiation as preparative regimen: a report from the French Society of Bone Marrow Graft (SFGM). Blood. 1995;85:2263-2268.

62. Blaise D, Maraninchi D, Archimbaud E, et al. Allogeneic bone marrow transplantation for acute myeloid leukemia in first remission: a randomized trial of a busulfan-cytoxan versus Cytoxan–total body irradiation as preparative regimen: a report from the Groupe d'Etudes de la Greffe de Moelle Osseuse. Blood. 1992;79:2578-2582.

63. Michel G, Gluckman E, Esperou-Bourdeau H, et al. Allogeneic bone marrow transplantation for children with acute myeloblastic leukemia in first complete remission: impact of conditioning regimen without total-body irradiation—a report from the Societe Francaise de Freffe de Moelle. J Clin Oncol. 1994;12:1217-1222.

64. Hassan M, Ljungman P, Bolme P, et al. Busulfan bioavailability. Blood. 1994;84:2144-2150.

65. Grochow LB, Krivit W, Whitley CB, et al. Busulfan disposition in children. Blood. 1990;75:1723-1727.

66. Yeager AM, Wagner JE Jr, Graham ML, et al. Optimization of busulfan dosage in children undergoing bone marrow transplantation: a pharmacokinetic study of dose escalation. Blood. 1992;80:2425-2428.

67. Vassal G, Deroussent A, Chaline D, et al. Is 600 mg/m^2 the appropriate dosage of busulfan in children undergoing bone marrow transplantation. Blood. 1992;79:2475-2479.

68. Schuler U, Schroer S, Kuhnle A, et al. Busulfan pharmacokinetics in bone marrow transplant patients: is drug monitoring warranted? Bone Marrow Transplant. 1994;14:759-765.

69. Shaw PJ, Scharping CE, Brian RJ, et al. Busulfan pharmacokinetics using a single daily high-dose regimen in children with acute leukemia. Blood. 1994;84:2357-2362.

70. Spitzer TR, Peters C, Ortlieb M, et al. Etoposide in combination with cyclophosphamide and total body irradiation or busulfan as conditioning for marrow transplantation in adults and children. Int J Radiat Oncol Biol Phys. 1994;29:39-44.

71. Teinturier C, Hartmann O, Valteau-Couanet D, et al. Ovarian function after autologous bone marrow transplantation in childhood: high-dose busulfan is a major cause of ovarian failure. Bone Marrow Transplant. 1998;22:989-994.

72. Grochow LB, Jones RJ, Brundrett RB, et al. Pharmacokinetics of busulfan: correlation with veno-occlusive disease in patients undergoing bone marrow transplantation. Cancer Chemother Pharmacol. 1989;25:55-61.

73. Cremers S, Schoemaker R, Bredius R, et al. Pharmacokinetics of intravenous busulfan in children prior to stem cell transplantation. Br J Clin Pharmacol. 2002;53:386-389.

74. Kashyap A, Wingard J, Cagnoni P, et al. Intravenous versus oral busulfan as part of a busulfan/cyclophosphamide preparative regimen for allogeneic hematopoietic stem cell transplantation: decreased incidence of hepatic venoocclusive disease (HVOD), HVOD-related mortality, and overall 100-day mortality. Biol Blood Marrow Transplant. 2002;8:493-500.

75. Radich J, Gooley T, Bensinger W, et al. HLA-matched related hematopoietic cell transplantation for chronic-phase CML using a targeted busulfan and cyclophosphamide preparative regimen. Blood. 2003;102:31-35.

76. Tran H, Petropoulos D, Worth L, et al. Pharmacokinetics and individualized dose adjustment of intravenous busulfan in children with advanced hematologic malignancies undergoing allogeneic stem cell transplantation. Biol Blood Marrow Transplant. 2004;10:805-812.

77. Chao NJ, Forman SJ, Schmidt GM, et al. Allogeneic bone marrow transplantation for high-risk acute lymphoblastic leukemia during first complete remission. Blood. 1991;78:1923-1927.

78. Brown RA, Wolff SN, Fay JW, et al. High-dose etoposide, cyclophosphamide, and total body irradiation with allogeneic bone marrow transplantation for patients with acute myeloid leukemia in untreated first relapse: A study by the North American Marrow Transplant Group. Blood. 1995;85:1391-1395.

79. Petersen FB, Lynch MHE, Clift RA, et al. Autologous marrow transplantation for patients with acute myeloid leukemia in untreated first relapse or in second complete remission. J Clin Oncol. 1993;11:1353-1360.

80. Petersen FB, Buckner CD, Appelbaum FR, et al. Etoposide, cyclophosphamide and fractionated total body irradiation as a preparative regimen for marrow transplantation in patients with advanced hematological malignancies: a phase I study. Bone Marrow Transplant. 1992;10:83-88.

81. Krance RA, Forman SJ, Blume KG. Total-body irradiation and high-dose teniposide: a pilot study in bone marrow transplantation for patients with relapsed acute lymphoblastic leukemia. Cancer Treat Rep. 1987;71:645-647.

82. Coccia PF, Strandjord SE, Warkentin PI, et al. High-dose cytosine arabinoside and fractionated total-body irradiation: an improved preparative regimen for bone marrow transplantation of children with acute lymphoblastic leukemia. Blood. 1988;71:888-893.

83. Blume KG, Forman SJ, O'Donnell MR, et al. Total body irradiation and high dose etoposide: a new preparatory regimen for bone marrow transplantation in patients with advanced hematologic malignancies. Blood. 1987;69:1015-1020.

84. Bostrom B, Brunning RD, McGlave P, et al. Bone marrow transplantation for acute nonlymphocytic leukemia in first remission: analysis of prognostic factors. Blood. 1985;65:1191-1196.

85. Chao NJ, Stein AS, Long GD, et al. Busulfan/etoposide—initial experience with a new preparatory regimen for autologous bone marrow transplantation in patients

with acute nonlymphoblastic leukemia. Blood. 1993;81: 319-323.

86. Linker CA, Ries CA, Damon LE, et al. Autologous bone marrow transplantation for acute myeloid leukemia using busulfan plus etoposide as a preparative regimen. Blood. 1993;81:311-318.

87. Matsuyama T, Kojima S, Kato K. Allogeneic bone marrow transplantation for childhood leukemia following a busulfan and melphalan preparative regimen. Bone Marrow Transplant. 1998;22:21-26.

88. Vey N, De Prijck B, Faucher C, et al. A pilot study of busulfan and melphalan as preparatory regimen prior to allogeneic bone marrow transplantation in refractory or relapsed hematological malignancies. Bone Marrow Transplant. 1996;18:495-499.

89. Ayash LJ, Antman K, Cheson BD. A perspective on dose-intensive therapy with autologous bone marrow transplantation for solid tumors. Oncology. 1991;5:25-33.

90. Dicke KA, Spitzer G. Evaluation of the use of high-dose cytoreduction with autologous marrow rescue in various malignancies. Transplantation. 1986;41:4-20.

91. Cheson BD, Lacerna L, Leyland-Jones B, et al. Autologous bone marrow transplantation. Ann Intern Med. 1989;110:51-65.

92. Dallorso S, Manzitti C, Morreale G, et al. High dose therapy and autologous hematopoietic stem cell transplantation in poor risk solid tumors of childhood. Haematologica. 2000;85:66-70.

93. Burnett AK, Kell J, Rowntree C. Role of allogeneic and autologous hematopoietic stem cell transplantation in acute myeloid leukemia. Int J Hematol. 2000;72:280-284.

94. Giralt S, Estey E, Albitar M, et al. Engraftment of allogeneic hematopoietic progenitor cells with purine analog–containing chemotherapy: harnessing graft-versus-leukemia without myeloablative therapy. Blood. 1997;89: 4531-4536.

95. Giralt S, Khouri I, Champlin R. Non myeloablative "mini transplants." Cancer Treat Res. 1999;101:97-108.

96. Slavin S, Nagler A, Naparstek E, et al. Nonmyeloablative stem cell transplantation and cell therapy as an alternative to conventional bone marrow transplantation with lethal cytoreduction for the treatment of malignant and nonmalignant hematologic diseases. Blood. 1998;91:756-763.

97. Storb R, Yu C, Sandmaier B, et al. Mixed hematopoietic chimerism after hematopoietic stem cell allografts. Transplant Proc. 1999;31:677-678.

98. Storb R, Yu C, Barnett T, et al. Stable mixed hematopoietic chimerism in dog leukocyte antigen–identical littermate dogs given lymph node irradiation before and pharmacologic immunosuppression after marrow transplantation. Blood. 1999;94:1131-1136.

99. Sandmaier BM, McSweeney P, Yu C, et al. Nonmyeloablative transplants: preclinical and clinical results. Semin Oncol. 2000;27:78-81.

100. Champlin R, Khouri I, Kornblau S, et al. Reinventing bone marrow transplantation: reducing toxicity using nonmyeloablative, preparative regimens and induction of graft-versus-malignancy. Curr Opin Oncol. 1999;11:87-95.

101. McSweeney P, Niederwieser D, Shizuru J, et al. Hematopoietic cell transplantation in older patients with hematologic malignancies: replacing high-dose cytotoxic therapy

with graft-versus-tumor effects. Blood. 2001;97:3390-3400.

102. Alyea E, Kim H, Ho V, et al. Comparative outcome of nonmyeloablative and myeloablative allogeneic hematopoietic cell transplantation for patients older than 50 years of age. Blood. 2005;105:1810-1814.

103. Baron F, Maris M, Sandmaier B, et al. Graft-versus-tumor effects after allogeneic hematopoietic cell transplantation with nonmyeloablative conditioning. J Clin Oncol. 2005;23:1993-2003.

104. Levine J, Uberti J, Ayash L, et al. Lowered-intensity preparative regimen for allogeneic stem cell transplantation delays acute graft-versus-host disease but does not improve outcome for advanced hematologic malignancy. Biol Blood Marrow Transplant. 2003;9:189-197.

105. Kapelushnik J, Or R, Slavin S, et al. A fludarabine-based protocol for bone marrow transplantation in Fanconi's anemia. Bone Marrow Transplant. 1997;20:1109-1110.

106. Horwitz ME, Barrett AJ, Brown MR, et al. Treatment of chronic granulomatous disease with nonmyeloablative conditioning and a T-cell–depleted hematopoietic allograft. N Engl J Med. 2001;344:881-888.

107. Goulmy E. Minor histocompatibility antigens: from T cell recognition to peptide identification. Hum Immunol. 1997;54:8-14.

108. Goulmy E, Schipper R, Pool J, et al. Mismatches of minor histocompatibility antigens between HLA-identical donors and recipients and the development of graft-versus-host disease after bone marrow transplantation. N Engl J Med. 1996;334:281-285.

109. den Haan JM, Sherman NE, Blokland E, et al. Identification of a graft versus host disease–associated human minor histocompatibility antigen. Science. 1995;268:1476-1480.

110. Terasaki PI, McClelland JD. Microdroplet assay of human serum cytotoxins. Nature. 1964;204:998-1000.

111. Yunis EJ, Amos DB. Three closely linked genetic systems relevant to transplantation. Proc Natl Acad Sci U S A. 1971;68:3031-3035.

112. Petersdorf E, Malkki M, Gooley T, et al. MHC haplotype matching for unrelated hematopoietic cell transplantation. PLoS Med. 2007;4:e8.

113. Petersdorf EW, Gooley TA, Anasetti C, et al. Optimizing outcome after unrelated marrow transplantation by comprehensive matching of HLA class I and II alleles in the donor and recipient. Blood. 1998;92:3515-3520.

114. Speiser DE, Tiercy JM, Rufer N, et al. High resolution HLA matching associated with decreased mortality after unrelated bone marrow transplantation. Blood. 1996;87: 4455-4462.

115. Flomenberg N, Baxter-Lowe L, Confer D, et al. Impact of HLA class I and class II high-resolution matching on outcomes of unrelated donor bone marrow transplantation: HLA-C mismatching is associated with a strong adverse effect on transplantation outcome. Blood. 2004; 104:1923-1930.

116. Beatty PG, Dahlberg S, Mickelson EM, et al. Probability of finding HLA-matched unrelated marrow donors. Transplantation. 1988;45:714-718.

117. Prasad VK, Heller G, Kernan NA, et al. The probability of HLA-C matching between patient and unrelated donor at the molecular level: estimations based on the linkage

disequilibrium between DNA typed HLA-B and HLA-C alleles. Transplantation. 1999;68:1044-1050.

118. Butterworth VA, Simmons RG, Bartsch G, et al. Psychosocial effects of unrelated bone marrow donation: experiences of the National Marrow Donor Program. Blood. 1993;81:1947-1959.

119. Clift RA. Cellular support of the marrow transplant recipient. Prog Clin Biol Res. 1990;337:87-92.

120. Goldman J. Peripheral blood stem cells for allografting. Blood. 1995;85:1413-1415.

121. Storek J, Gooley T, Siadak M, et al. Allogeneic peripheral blood stem cell transplantation may be associated with a high risk of chronic graft-versus-host disease. Blood. 1997;90:4705-4709.

122. Przepiorka D, Anderlini P, Ippoliti C, et al. Allogeneic blood stem cell transplantation in advanced hematologic cancers. Bone Marrow Transplant. 1997;19:455-460.

123. Bensinger WI, Weaver CH, Appelbaum FR, et al. Transplantation of allogeneic peripheral blood stem cells mobilized by recombinant human granulocyte colony-stimulating factor. Blood. 1995;85:1655-1658.

124. Bensinger WI, Martin PJ, Storer B, et al. Transplantation of bone marrow as compared with peripheral-blood cells from HLA-identical relatives in patients with hematologic cancers. N Engl J Med. 2001;344:175-181.

125. Flomenberg N, Devine S, Dipersio J, et al. The use of AMD3100 plus G-CSF for autologous hematopoietic progenitor cell mobilization is superior to G-CSF alone. Blood. 2005;106:1867-1874.

126. Korbling M, Przepiorka D, Huh YO, et al. Allogeneic blood stem cell transplantation for refractory leukemia and lymphoma: potential advantage of blood over marrow allografts. Blood. 1995;85:1659-1665.

127. Schmitz N, Dreger P, Suttorp M, et al. Primary transplantation of allogeneic peripheral blood progenitor cells mobilized by filgrastim (granulocyte colony-stimulating factor). Blood. 1995;85:1666-1672.

128. Tigue CC, McKoy JM, Evens AM, et al. Granulocyte-colony stimulating factor administration to healthy individuals and persons with chronic neutropenia or cancer: an overview of safety considerations from the Research on Adverse Drug Events and Reports Project. Bone Marrow Transplant. 2007;40:185-192.

129. Kanold J, Rapatel C, Berger M, et al. Use of G-CSF alone to mobilize peripheral blood stem cells for collection from children. Br J Haematol. 1994;88:633-635.

130. Korbling M, Chan KW, Anderlini P, et al. Allogeneic peripheral blood stem cell transplantation using normal patient-related pediatric donors. Bone Marrow Transplant. 1996;18:885-890.

131. Falanga A, Marchetti M, Evangelista V, et al. Neutrophil activation and hemostatic changes in healthy donors receiving granulocyte colony-stimulating factor. Blood. 1999;93:2506-2514.

132. Anderlini P, Korbling M, Dale D, et al. Allogeneic blood stem cell transplantation: considerations for donors. Blood. 1997;90:903-908.

133. Gluckman E, Broxmeyer HA, Auerbach AD, et al. Hematopoietic reconstitution in a patient with Fanconi's anemia by means of umbilical-cord blood from an HLA-identical sibling. N Engl J Med. 1989;321:1174-1178.

134. Bertolini F, Lazzari L, Lauri E, et al. Comparative study of different procedures for the collection and banking of umbilical cord blood. J Hematother. 1995;4:29-36.

135. Wynn RF, Cross MA, Hatton C, et al. Accelerated telomere shortening in young recipients of allogeneic bone-marrow transplants. Lancet. 1998;351:178-181.

136. van Leeuwen JEM, van Tol MJD, Joosten AM, et al. Persistence of host-type hematopoiesis after allogeneic bone marrow transplantation for leukemia is significantly related to the recipient's age and/or the conditioning regimen, but it is not associated with an increased risk of relapse. Blood. 1994;83:3059-3067.

137. Hill RS, Petersen FB, Storb R, et al. Mixed hematologic chimerism after allogeneic marrow transplantation for severe aplastic anemia is associated with a higher risk of graft rejection and a lessened incidence of acute graft-versus-host disease. Blood. 1986;67:811-816.

138. Petit T, Raynal B, Socie G, et al. Highly sensitive polymerase chain reaction methods show the frequent survival of residual recipient multipotent progenitors after non–t-cell–depleted bone marrow transplantation. Blood. 1994;84:3575-3583.

139. Mackinnon S, Barnett L, Heller G, et al. Minimal residual disease is more common in patients who have mixed T-cell chimerism after bone marrow transplantation for chronic myelogenous leukemia. Blood. 1994;83:3409-3416.

140. Bertheas MF, Lafage M, Levy P, et al. Influence of mixed chimerism on the results of allogeneic bone marrow transplantation for leukemia. Blood. 1991;78:3103-3106.

141. Roux E, Helg C, Chapuis B, et al. Evolution of mixed chimerism after allogeneic bone marrow transplantation as determined on granulocytes and mononuclear cells by the polymerase chain reaction. Blood. 1992;79:2775-2783.

142. Singhal S, Powles R, Kulkarni S, et al. Comparison of marrow and blood cell yields from the same donors in a double-blind, randomized study of allogeneic marrow vs blood stem cell transplantation. Bone Marrow Transplant. 2000;25:501-505.

143. Cutler C, Antin JH. Peripheral blood stem cells for allogeneic transplantation: a review. Stem Cells. 2001;19:108-117.

144. Gluckman E, Rocha V, Boyer-Chammard A, et al. Outcome of cord-blood transplantation from related and unrelated donors. Eurocord Transplant Group and the European Blood and Marrow Transplantation Group. N Engl J Med. 1997;337:373-381.

145. Thomson BG, Robertson KA, Gowan D, et al. Analysis of engraftment, graft-versus-host disease, and immune recovery following unrelated donor cord blood transplantation. Blood. 2000;96:2703-2711.

146. Rocha V, Wagner J, Sobocinski K, et al. Graft-versus-host disease in children who have received a cord-blood or bone marrow transplant from an HLA-identical sibling. Eurocord and International Bone Marrow Transplant Registry Working Committee on Alternative Donor and Stem Cell Sources. N Engl J Med. 2000;342:1846-1854.

147. Rubinstein P, Carrier C, Scaradavou A, et al. Outcomes among 562 recipients of placental-blood transplants from unrelated donors. N Engl J Med. 1998;339:1565-1577.

148. Barker JN, Davies SM, DeFor T, et al. Survival after transplantation of unrelated donor umbilical cord blood

is comparable to that of human leukocyte antigen–matched unrelated donor bone marrow: results of a matched-pair analysis. Blood. 2001;97:2957-2961.

149. Barker J, Weisdorf D, DeFor T, et al. Transplantation of 2 partially HLA-matched umbilical cord blood units to enhance engraftment in adults with hematologic malignancy. Blood. 2005;105:1343-1347.

150. Locatelli F, Zecca M, Ponchio L, et al. Pilot trial of combined administration of erythropoietin and granulocyte colony-stimulating factor to children undergoing allogeneic bone marrow transplantation. Bone Marrow Transplant. 1994;14:929-935.

151. Tsuchiya S, Minegishi M, Fujie H, et al. Allogeneic bone marrow transplantation for malignant hematologic disorders in children. Tohoku J Exp Med. 1992;168:345-350.

152. Masaoka T, Takaku F, Kato S, et al. Recombinant human granulocyte colony-stimulating factor in allogeneic bone marrow transplantation. Exp Hematol. 1989;17:1047-1050.

153. Powles R, Smith C, Milan S, et al. Human recombinant GM-CSF in allogeneic bone marrow transplant for leukemia: Double blind placebo controlled trial. Lancet. 1990;336:1417-1420.

154. Schriber JR, Chao NJ, Long GD, et al. Granulocyte colony-stimulating factor after allogeneic bone marrow transplantation. Blood. 1994;84:1680-1684.

155. Nemunaitis J, Buckner CD, Appelbaum FR, et al. Phase I/II trial of recombinant granulocyte-macrophage colony stimulating factor following allogeneic bone marrow transplantation. Blood. 1991;77:2065-2071.

156. Cutler C, Giri S, Jeyapalan S, et al. Acute and chronic graft-versus-host disease after allogeneic peripheral-blood stem-cell and bone marrow transplantation: a meta-analysis. J Clin Oncol. 2001;19:3685-3691.

157. Eapen M, Horowitz MM, Klein JP, et al. Higher mortality after allogeneic peripheral-blood transplantation compared with bone marrow in children and adolescents: the Histocompatibility and Alternate Stem Cell Source Working Committee of the International Bone Marrow Transplant Registry. J Clin Oncol. 2004;22:4872-4880.

158. Wagner J, Barker J, DeFor T, et al. Transplantation of unrelated donor umbilical cord blood in 102 patients with malignant and nonmalignant diseases: influence of CD34 cell dose and HLA disparity on treatment-related mortality and survival. Blood. 2002;100:1611-1618.

159. Rill DR, Santana VM, Roberts WM, et al. Direct demonstration that autologous bone marrow transplantation for solid tumors can return a multiplicity of tumorigenic cells. Blood. 1994;84:380-383.

160. Freedman AS, Neuberg D, Mauch P, et al. Long-term follow-up of autologous bone marrow transplantation in patients with relapsed follicular lymphoma. Blood. 1999; 94:3325-3333.

161. Ross AA, Cooper BW, Lazarus HM, et al. Detection and viability of tumor cells in peripheral blood stem cell collections from breast cancer patients using immunocytochemical and clonogenic assay techniques. Blood. 1993;82:2605-2610.

162. Brugger W, Bross KJ, Glatt M, et al. Mobilization of tumor cells and hematopoietic progenitor cells into peripheral blood of patients with solid tumors. Blood. 1994;83:636-640.

163. Lopez M, Lemoine FM, Firat H, et al. Bone marrow versus peripheral blood progenitor cells CD34 selection in patients with non-Hodgkin's lymphomas: different levels of tumor cell reduction. Implications for autografting. Blood. 1997;90:2830-2838.

164. Kanteti R, Miller K, McCann J, et al. Randomized trial of peripheral blood progenitor cell vs bone marrow as hematopoietic support for high-dose chemotherapy in patients with non-Hodgkin's lymphoma and Hodgkin's disease: a clinical and molecular analysis. Bone Marrow Transplant. 1999;24:473-481.

165. Leung W, Chen AR, Klann RC, et al. Frequent detection of tumor cells in hematopoietic grafts in neuroblastoma and Ewing's sarcoma. Bone Marrow Transplant. 1998;22: 971-979.

166. Jacquy C, Soree A, Lambert F, et al. A quantitative study of peripheral blood stem cell contamination in diffuse large-cell non-Hodgkin's lymphoma: one-half of patients significantly mobilize malignant cells. Br J Haematol. 2000;110:631-637.

167. Humpe A, Riggert J, Wolf C, et al. Successful transplantation and engraftment of peripheral blood stem cells after cryopreservation, positive and negative purging procedures, and a second cryopreservation cycle. Ann Hematol. 2001;80:109-112.

168. Tchirkov A, Kanold J, Giollant M, et al. Molecular monitoring of tumor cell contamination in leukapheresis products from stage IV neuroblastoma patients before and after positive CD34 selection. Med Pediatr Oncol. 1998;30:228-232.

169. Urbano-Ispizua A, Brunet S, Solano C, et al. Allogeneic transplantation of CD34⁺-selected cells from peripheral blood in patients with myeloid malignancies in early phase: a case control comparison with unmodified peripheral blood transplantation. Bone Marrow Transplant. 2001;28:349-354.

170. Weaver CH, Hazelton B, Birch R, et al. An analysis of engraftment kinetics as a function of the CD34 content of peripheral blood progenitor cell collections in 692 patients after the administration of myeloablative chemotherapy. Blood. 1995;86:3961-3969.

171. Shpall EJ, Champlin R, Glaspy JA. Effect of CD34⁺ peripheral blood progenitor cell dose on hematopoietic recovery. Biol Blood Marrow Transplant. 1998;4:84-92.

172. Haas R, Mohle R, Fruhauf S, et al. Patient characteristics associated with successful mobilizing and autografting of peripheral blood progenitor cells in malignant lymphoma. Blood. 1994;83:3787-3794.

173. Tricot G, Jagannath S, Vesole D, et al. Peripheral blood stem cell transplants for multiple myeloma: identification of favorable variables for rapid engraftment in 255 patients. Blood. 1995;85:588-596.

174. O'Day SJ, Rabinowe SN, Neuberg D, et al. A phase II study of continuous infusion recombinant human granulocyte-macrophage colony-stimulating factor as an adjunct to autologous bone marrow transplantation for patients with non-Hodgkin's lymphoma in first remission. Blood. 1994;83:2707-2714.

175. Domenech J, Linassier C, Gihana E, et al. Prolonged impairment of hematopoiesis after high-dose therapy followed by autologous bone marrow transplantation. Blood. 1995;85:3320-3327.

176. Mach-Pascual S, Legare RD, Lu D, et al. Predictive value of clonality assays in patients with non-Hodgkin's lymphoma undergoing autologous bone marrow transplant: a single institution study. Blood. 1998;91:4496-4503.

177. Darrington DL, Vose JM, Anderson JR, et al. Incidence and characterization of secondary myelodysplastic syndrome and acute myelogenous leukemia following high-dose chemoradiotherapy and autologous stem-cell transplantation for lymphoid malignancies. J Clin Oncol. 1994;12:2527-2534.

178. Traweek ST, Slovak ML, Nademanee AP, et al. Clonal karyotypic hematopoietic cell abnormalities occurring after autologous bone marrow transplantation for Hodgkin's disease and non-Hodgkin's lymphoma. Blood. 1994;84:957-963.

179. Krishnan A, Bhatia S, Slovak ML, et al. Predictors of therapy-related leukemia and myelodysplasia following autologous transplantation for lymphoma: an assessment of risk factors. Blood. 2000;95:1588-1593.

180. Miller JS, Arthur DC, Litz CE, et al. Myelodysplastic syndrome after autologous bone marrow transplantation: an additional late complication of curative cancer therapy. Blood. 1994;83:3780-3786.

181. Stone RM. Myelodysplastic syndrome after autologous transplantation for lymphoma: the price of progress? Blood. 1994;83:3437-3440.

182. Travis LB, Weeks J, Curtis RE, et al. Leukemia following low-dose total body irradiation and chemotherapy for non-Hodgkin's lymphoma. J Clin Oncol. 1996;14:565-571.

183. Milligan DW, Ruiz De Elvira MC, Kolb HJ, et al. Secondary leukaemia and myelodysplasia after autografting for lymphoma: results from the EBMT. EBMT Lymphoma and Late Effects Working Parties. European Group for Blood and Marrow Transplantation. Br J Haematol. 1999;106:1020-1026.

184. Micallef IN, Lillington DM, Apostolidis J, et al. Therapy-related myelodysplasia and secondary acute myelogenous leukemia after high-dose therapy with autologous hematopoietic progenitor-cell support for lymphoid malignancies. J Clin Oncol. 2000;18:947-955.

185. Chao NJ, Nademanee AP, Long GD, et al. Importance of bone marrow cytogenetic evaluation before autologous bone marrow transplantation for Hodgkin's disease. J Clin Oncol. 1991;9:1575-1579.

186. Abruzzese E, Radford JE, Miller JS, et al. Detection of abnormal pretransplant clones in progenitor cells of patients who developed myelodysplasia after autologous transplantation. Blood. 1999;94:1814-1819.

187. Li C, Greenberg P, Gilbert M, et al. Recovery of HLA-restricted cytomegalovirus (CMV)-specific T-cell responses after allogeneic bone marrow transplant: correlation with CMV disease and effect of ganciclovir prophylaxis. Blood. 1994;83:1971-1979.

188. Molrine D, Antin J, Guinan E, et al. Donor immunization with pneumococcal conjugate vaccine and early protective antibody responses following allogeneic hematopoietic cell transplantation. Blood. 2003;101:831-836.

189. Small TN, Papadopoulos EB, Boulad F, et al. Comparison of immune reconstitution after unrelated and related T-cell–depleted bone marrow transplantation: effect of patient age and donor leukocyte infusions. Blood. 1999;93:467-480.

190. Roux E, Dumont-Girard F, Starobinski M, et al. Recovery of immune reactivity after T-cell–depleted bone marrow transplantation depends on thymic activity. Blood. 2000;96:2299-2303.

191. Dumont-Girard F, Roux E, van Lier RA, et al. Reconstitution of the T-cell compartment after bone marrow transplantation: restoration of the repertoire by thymic emigrants. Blood. 1998;92:4464-4471.

192. Douek DC, Vescio RA, Betts MR, et al. Assessment of thymic output in adults after haematopoietic stem-cell transplantation and prediction of T-cell reconstitution. Lancet. 2000;355:1875-1881.

193. Heitger A, Neu N, Kern H, et al. Essential role of the thymus to reconstitute naive (CD45RA+) T-helper cells after human allogeneic bone marrow transplantation. Blood. 1997;90:850-857.

194. Verfuerth S, Peggs K, Vyas P, et al. Longitudinal monitoring of immune reconstitution by CDR3 size spectra typing after T-cell–depleted allogeneic bone marrow transplant and the effect of donor lymphocyte infusions on T-cell repertoire. Blood. 2000;95:3990-3995.

195. Mackall CL, Stein D, Fleisher TA, et al. Prolonged CD4 depletion after sequential autologous peripheral blood progenitor cell infusions in children and young adults. Blood. 2000;96:754-762.

196. Talmadge JE, Reed E, Ino K, et al. Rapid immunologic reconstitution following transplantation with mobilized peripheral blood stem cells as compared to bone marrow. Bone Marrow Transplant. 1997;19:161-172.

197. Moretta A, Maccario R, Fagioli F, et al. Analysis of immune reconstitution in children undergoing cord blood transplantation. Exp Hematol. 2001;29:371-379.

198. Parkman R, Weinberg KI. Immunological reconstitution following bone marrow transplantation. Immunol Rev. 1997;157:73-78.

199. Small TN, Avigan D, Dupont B, et al. Immune reconstitution following T-cell depleted bone marrow transplantation: effect of age and posttransplant graft rejection prophylaxis. Biol Blood Marrow Transplant. 1997;3:65-75.

200. Brubaker DB. Immunopathogenic mechanisms of post-transfusion graft-vs-host disease. Proc Soc Exp Biol Med. 1993;202:122-147.

201. Corash L, Lin L. Novel processes for inactivation of leukocytes to prevent transfusion-associated graft-versus-host disease. Bone Marrow Transplant. 2004;33:1-7.

202. Grass JA, Hei DJ, Metchette K, et al. Inactivation of leukocytes in platelet concentrates by photochemical treatment with psoralen plus UVA. Blood. 1998;91:2180-2188.

203. Grass JA, Wafa T, Reames A, et al. Prevention of transfusion-associated graft-versus-host disease by photochemical treatment. Blood. 1999;93:3140-3147.

204. Akahoshi M, Takanashi M, Masuda M, et al. A case of transfusion-associated graft-versus-host disease not prevented by white cell–reduction filters. Transfusion. 1992;32:169-172.

205. Bowden RA, Slichter SJ, Sayers M, et al. A comparison of filtered leukocyte-reduced and cytomegalovirus (CMV) seronegative blood products for the prevention of transfusion-associated CMV infection after marrow transplant. Blood. 1995;86:3598-3603.

206. Bowden RA, Slichter SJ, Sayers MH, et al. Use of leukocyte-depleted platelets and cytomegalovirus-seronegative red blood cells for prevention of primary cytomegalovirus infection after marrow transplant. Blood. 1991;78:246-250.

207. Vamvakas EC. Is white blood cell reduction equivalent to antibody screening in preventing transmission of cytomegalovirus by transfusion? A review of the literature and meta-analysis. Transfus Med Rev. 2005;19:181-199.

208. Diedrich B, Remberger M, Shanwell A, et al. A prospective randomized trial of a prophylactic platelet transfusion trigger of 10×10^9 per L versus 30×10^9 per L in allogeneic hematopoietic progenitor cell transplant recipients. Transfusion. 2005;45:1064-1072.

209. Zumberg MS, del Rosario ML, Nejame CF, et al. A prospective randomized trial of prophylactic platelet transfusion and bleeding incidence in hematopoietic stem cell transplant recipients: 10,000/L versus 20,000/ μL trigger. Biol Blood Marrow Transplant. 2002;8:569-576.

210. Stanworth SJ, Hyde C, Heddle N, et al. Prophylactic platelet transfusion for haemorrhage after chemotherapy and stem cell transplantation. Cochrane Database Syst Rev. 2004;4:CD004269.

211. Maury S, Mary JY, Rabian C, et al. Prolonged immune deficiency following allogeneic stem cell transplantation: risk factors and complications in adult patients. Br J Haematol. 2001;115:630-641.

212. Walker CM, van Burik JA, De For TE, et al. Cytomegalovirus infection after allogeneic transplantation: comparison of cord blood with peripheral blood and marrow graft sources. Biol Blood Marrow Transplant. 2007;13:1106-1115.

213. Meyers JD, Flournoy N, Thomas ED. Risk factors for cytomegalovirus infection after human marrow transplantation. J Infect Dis. 1986;153:478-488.

214. Winston DJ, Huang ES, Miller MJ, et al. Molecular epidemiology of cytomegalovirus infections associated with bone marrow transplantation. Ann Intern Med. 1985;102:16-20.

215. Ljungman P, Brand R, Einsele H, et al. Donor CMV serologic status and outcome of CMV-seropositive recipients after unrelated donor stem cell transplantation: an EBMT megafile analysis. Blood. 2003;102:4255-4260.

216. Goodrich JM, Boeckh M, Bowden R. Strategies for the prevention of cytomegalovirus disease after marrow transplantation. Clin Infect Dis. 1994;19:287-298.

217. Winston DJ, Ho WG, Bartoni K, et al. Ganciclovir prophylaxis of cytomegalovirus infection and disease in allogeneic bone marrow transplant recipients. Results of a placebo-controlled, double-blind trial. Ann Intern Med. 1993;118:179-184.

218. Ljungman P, de La Camara R, Milpied N, et al. Randomized study of valacyclovir as prophylaxis against cytomegalovirus reactivation in recipients of allogeneic bone marrow transplants. Blood. 2002;99:3050-3056.

219. Meyers JD. Prevention and treatment of cytomegalovirus infection after marrow transplantation. Bone Marrow Transplant. 1988;3:95-104.

220. Prentice HG, Gluckman E, Powles RL, et al. Long-term survival in allogeneic bone marrow transplant recipients following acyclovir prophylaxis for CMV infection. The European Acyclovir for CMV Prophylaxis Study Group. Bone Marrow Transplant. 1997;19:129-133.

221. Prentice HG, Gluckman E, Powles RL, et al. Impact of long-term acyclovir on cytomegalovirus infection and survival after allogeneic bone marrow transplantation. European Acyclovir for CMV Prophylaxis Study Group. Lancet. 1994;343:749-753.

222. Einsele H, Ehninger G, Hebart H, et al. Polymerase chain reaction monitoring reduces the incidence of cytomegalovirus disease and the duration and side effects of antiviral therapy after bone marrow transplantation. Blood. 1995;86:2815-2820.

223. Hebart H, Muller C, Loffler J, et al. Monitoring of CMV infection: a comparison of PCR from whole blood, plasma-PCR, pp65-antigenemia and virus culture in patients after bone marrow transplantation. Bone Marrow Transplant. 1996;17:861-868.

224. Hebart H, Schroder A, Loffler J, et al. Cytomegalovirus monitoring by polymerase chain reaction of whole blood samples from patients undergoing autologous bone marrow or peripheral blood progenitor cell transplantation. J Infect Dis. 1997;175:1490-1493.

225. Meijer E, Boland GJ, Verdonck LF. Prevention of cytomegalovirus disease in recipients of allogeneic stem cell transplants. Clin Microbiol Rev. 2003;16:647-657.

226. Boeckh M, Fries B, Nichols WG. Recent advances in the prevention of CMV infection and disease after hematopoietic stem cell transplantation. Pediatr Transplant. 2004;8(Suppl 5):19-27.

227. Reusser P, Einsele H, Lee J, et al. Randomized multicenter trial of foscarnet versus ganciclovir for preemptive therapy of cytomegalovirus infection after allogeneic stem cell transplantation. Blood. 2002;99:1159-1164.

228. Koc Y, Miller KB, Schenkein DP, et al. Varicella zoster virus infections following allogeneic bone marrow transplantation: frequency, risk factors, and clinical outcome. Biol Blood Marrow Transplant. 2000;6:44-49.

229. Kawasaki H, Takayama J, Ohira M. Herpes zoster infection after bone marrow transplantation in children. J Pediatr. 1996;128:353-356.

230. Leung TF, Chik KW, Li CK, et al. Incidence, risk factors and outcome of varicella-zoster virus infection in children after haematopoietic stem cell transplantation. Bone Marrow Transplant. 2000;25:167-172.

231. Ljungman P, Wang FZ, Nilsson C, et al. Vaccination of autologous stem cell transplant recipients with live varicella vaccine: a pilot study. Support Care Cancer. 2003;11:739-741.

232. Marr KA, Seidel K, Slavin MA, et al. Prolonged fluconazole prophylaxis is associated with persistent protection against candidiasis-related death in allogeneic marrow transplant recipients: long-term follow-up of a randomized, placebo-controlled trial. Blood. 2000;96:2055-2061.

233. Marr KA, Seidel K, White TC, et al. Candidemia in allogeneic blood and marrow transplant recipients: evolution of risk factors after the adoption of prophylactic fluconazole. J Infect Dis. 2000;181:309-316.

234. Wolff SN, Fay J, Stevens D, et al. Fluconazole vs low-dose amphotericin B for the prevention of fungal infections in patients undergoing bone marrow transplantation: a study of the North American Marrow Transplant Group. Bone Marrow Transplant. 2000;25:853-859.

235. Sastry PS, Parikh PM, Kulkarni PS, et al. Use of liposomal amphotericin B in bone marrow transplant. J Postgrad Med. 2005;51(Suppl 1):S49-S52.

236. Deeg HJ, Seidel K, Bruemmer B, et al. Impact of patient weight on non-relapse mortality after marrow transplantation. Bone Marrow Transplant. 1995;15:461-468.

237. Deeg HJ, Seidel K, Sullivan KM. Body weight and outcome of hematopoietic stem cell transplantation. Am J Med. 1998;104:607-608.

238. Fleming DR, Rayens MK, Garrison J. Impact of obesity on allogeneic stem cell transplant patients: a matched case-controlled study. Am J Med. 1997;102:265-268.

239. Seguy D, Berthon C, Micol JB, et al. Enteral feeding and early outcomes of patients undergoing allogeneic stem cell transplantation following myeloablative conditioning. Transplantation. 2006;82:835-839.

240. Langdana A, Tully N, Molloy E, et al. Intensive enteral nutrition support in paediatric bone marrow transplantation. Bone Marrow Transplant. 2001;27:741-746.

241. Hopman GD, Pena EG, Le Cessie S, et al. Tube feeding and bone marrow transplantation. Med Pediatr Oncol. 2003;40:375-379.

242. Hwang TL, Chiang CL, Wang PN. Parenteral nutrition support after bone marrow transplantation: comparison of total and partial parenteral nutrition during the early posttransplantation period. Nutrition. 2001;17:773-775.

243. Tartarone A, Wunder J, Romano G, et al. Role of parenteral nutrition in cancer patients undergoing high-dose chemotherapy followed by autologous peripheral blood progenitor cell transplantation. Tumori. 2005;91:237-240.

244. Muscaritoli M, Grieco G, Capria S, et al. Nutritional and metabolic support in patients undergoing bone marrow transplantation. Am J Clin Nutr. 2002;75:183-190.

245. Arfons LM, Lazarus HM. Total parenteral nutrition and hematopoietic stem cell transplantation: an expensive placebo? Bone Marrow Transplant. 2005;36:281-288.

246. McDonald GB, Sharma P, Matthews DE, et al. Venoocclusive disease of the liver after bone marrow transplantation: diagnosis, incidence, and predisposing factors. Hepatology. 1984;4:116-122.

247. Bearman SI. The syndrome of hepatic veno-occlusive disease after marrow transplantation. Blood. 1995;85:3005-3020.

248. Richardson P, Guinan E. The pathology, diagnosis, and treatment of hepatic veno-occlusive disease: current status and novel approaches. Br J Haematol. 1999;107:485-493.

249. Cesaro S, Pillon M, Talenti E, et al. A prospective survey on incidence, risk factors and therapy of hepatic venoocclusive disease in children after hematopoietic stem cell transplantation. Haematologica. 2005;90:1396-1404.

250. McDonald GB, Hinds MS, Fisher LD, et al. Venoocclusive disease of the liver and multiorgan failure after bone marrow transplantation: a cohort study of 355 patients. Ann Intern Med. 1993;118:255-267.

251. Ayash LJ, Hunt M, Antman K, et al. Hepatic venoocclusive disease in autologous bone marrow transplantation of solid tumors and lymphomas. J Clin Oncol. 1990;8:1699-1706.

252. Shulman HM, Fisher LB, Schoch HG, et al. Venoocclusive disease of the liver after marrow transplantation: histological correlates of clinical signs and symptoms. Hepatology. 1994;19:1171-1181.

253. Bearman SI, Anderson GL, Mori M, et al. Venoocclusive disease of the liver: development of a model for predicting fatal outcome after marrow transplantation. J Clin Oncol. 1993;11:1729-1736.

254. Shulman HM, Gown AM, Nugent DJ. Hepatic venoocclusive disease after bone marrow transplantation. Immunohistochemical identification of the material within occluded central venules. Am J Pathol. 1987;127:549-558.

255. Wadleigh M, Richardson PG, Zahrieh D, et al. Prior gemtuzumab ozogamicin exposure significantly increases the risk of veno-occlusive disease in patients who undergo myeloablative allogeneic stem cell transplantation. Blood. 2003;102:1578-1582.

256. Shulman HM, McDonald GB, Matthews D, et al. An analysis of hepatic venoocclusive disease and centrilobular hepatic degeneration following bone marrow transplantation. Gastroenterology. 1980;79:1178-1191.

257. Slattery JT, Kalhorn TF, McDonald GB, et al. Conditioning regimen–dependent disposition of cyclophosphamide and hydroxycyclophosphamide in human marrow transplantation patients. J Clin Oncol. 1996;14:1484-1494.

258. Cheuk DK, Wang P, Lee TL, et al. Risk factors and mortality predictors of hepatic veno-occlusive disease after pediatric hematopoietic stem cell transplantation. Bone Marrow Transplant. 2007;40:935-944.

259. Bastie JN, Suzan F, Garcia I, et al. Veno-occlusive disease after an anti-CD33 therapy (gemtuzumab ozogamicin). Br J Haematol. 2002;116:924.

260. Essell JH, Thompson JM, Harman GS, et al. Marked increase in veno-occlusive disease of the liver associated with methotrexate use for graft-versus-host disease prophylaxis in patients receiving busulfan/cyclophosphamide. Blood. 1992;79:2784-2788.

261. Giles FJ, Kantarjian HM, Kornblau SM, et al. Mylotarg (gemtuzumab ozogamicin) therapy is associated with hepatic venoocclusive disease in patients who have not received stem cell transplantation. Cancer. 2001;92:406-413.

262. McDonald GB, Slattery JT, Bouvier ME, et al. Cyclophosphamide metabolism, liver toxicity, and mortality following hematopoietic stem cell transplantation. Blood. 2003;101:2043-2048.

263. McKoy JM, Angelotta C, Bennett CL, et al. Gemtuzumab ozogamicin–associated sinusoidal obstructive syndrome (SOS): an overview from the Research on Adverse Drug Events and Reports (RADAR) Project. Leuk Res. 2007;31:599-604.

264. Reiss U, Cowan M, McMillan A, et al. Hepatic venoocclusive disease in blood and bone marrow transplantation in children and young adults: incidence, risk factors, and outcome in a cohort of 241 patients. J Pediatr Hematol Oncol. 2002;24:746-750.

265. Barker CC, Butzner JD, Anderson RA, et al. Incidence, survival and risk factors for the development of venoocclusive disease in pediatric hematopoietic stem cell transplant recipients. Bone Marrow Transplant. 2003;32:79-87.

266. Hassan M, Ljungman P, Ringden O, et al. The effect of busulphan on the pharmacokinetics of cyclophosphamide

and its 4-hydroxy metabolite: time interval influence on therapeutic efficacy and therapy-related toxicity. Bone Marrow Transplant. 2000;25:915-924.

267. DeLeve LD, Shulman HM, McDonald GB. Toxic injury to hepatic sinusoids: sinusoidal obstruction syndrome (veno-occlusive disease). Semin Liver Dis. 2002;22:27-42.

268. Hingorani SR, Guthrie K, Batchelder A, et al. Acute renal failure after myeloablative hematopoietic cell transplant: incidence and risk factors. Kidney Int. 2005;67:272-277.

269. Shulman HM, Gooley T, Dudley MD, et al. Utility of transvenous liver biopsies and wedged hepatic venous pressure measurements in sixty marrow transplant recipients. Transplantation. 1995;59:1015-1022.

270. Carreras E, Granena A, Navasa M, et al. Transjugular liver biopsy in BMT. Bone Marrow Transplant. 1993;11:21-26.

271. Erturk SM, Mortele KJ, Binkert CA, et al. CT features of hepatic venoocclusive disease and hepatic graft-versus-host disease in patients after hematopoietic stem cell transplantation. AJR Am J Roentgenol. 2006;186:1497-1501.

272. Ghersin E, Brook OR, Gaitini D, et al. Color Doppler demonstration of segmental portal flow reversal: an early sign of hepatic veno-occlusive disease in an infant. J Ultrasound Med. 2003;22:1103-1106.

273. Yoshimoto K, Yakushiji K, Ijuin H, et al. Colour Doppler ultrasonography of a segmental branch of the portal vein is useful for early diagnosis and monitoring of the therapeutic course of veno-occlusive disease after allogeneic haematopoietic stem cell transplantation. Br J Haematol. 2001;115:945-948.

274. Deeg KH, Glockel U, Richter R, et al. Diagnosis of veno-occlusive disease of the liver by color-coded Doppler sonography. Pediatr Radiol. 1993;23:134-136.

275. Brown BP, Abu-Yousef M, Farner R, et al. Doppler sonography: a noninvasive method for evaluation of hepatic venoocclusive disease. AJR Am J Roentgenol. 1990;154:721-724.

276. McCarville MB, Hoffer FA, Howard SC, et al. Hepatic veno-occlusive disease in children undergoing bone-marrow transplantation: usefulness of sonographic findings. Pediatr Radiol. 2001;31:102-105.

277. Hasegawa S, Horibe K, Kawabe T, et al. Veno-occlusive disease of the liver after allogeneic bone marrow transplantation in children with hematologic malignancies: incidence, onset time and risk factors. Bone Marrow Transplant. 1998;22:1191-1197.

278. Meresse V, Hartmann O, Vassal G, et al. Risk factors for hepatic veno-occlusive disease after high-dose busulfan-containing regimens followed by autologous bone marrow transplantation: a study in 136 children. Bone Marrow Transplant. 1992;10:135-141.

279. Ozkaynak MF, Weinberg K, Kohn D, et al. Hepatic venoocclusive disease post–bone marrow transplantation in children conditioned with busulfan and cyclophosphamide: incidence, risk factors, and clinical outcome. Bone Marrow Transplant. 1991;7:467-474.

280. Srivastava A, Poonkuzhali B, Shaji RV, et al. Glutathione S-transferase M1 polymorphism: a risk factor for hepatic venoocclusive disease in bone marrow transplantation. Blood. 2004;104:1574-1577.

281. Tay J, Tinmouth A, Fergusson D, et al. Systematic review of controlled clinical trials on the use of ursodeoxycholic acid for the prevention of hepatic veno-occlusive disease in hematopoietic stem cell transplantation. Biol Blood Marrow Transplant. 2007;13:206-217.

282. Giles F, Garcia-Manero G, Cortes J, et al. Ursodiol does not prevent hepatic venoocclusive disease associated with Mylotarg therapy. Haematologica. 2002;87:1114-1116.

283. Ruutu T, Eriksson B, Remes K, et al. Ursodeoxycholic acid for the prevention of hepatic complications in allogeneic stem cell transplantation. Blood. 2002;100:1977-1983.

284. Ohashi K, Tanabe J, Watanabe R, et al. The Japanese multicenter open randomized trial of ursodeoxycholic acid prophylaxis for hepatic veno-occlusive disease after stem cell transplantation. Am J Hematol. 2000;64:32-38.

285. Essell JH, Schroeder MT, Harman GS, et al. Ursodiol prophylaxis against hepatic complications of allogeneic bone marrow transplantation. A randomized, double-blind, placebo-controlled trial. Ann Intern Med. 1998;128:975-981.

286. Essell JH, Thompson JM, Harman GS, et al. Pilot trial of prophylactic ursodiol to decrease the incidence of veno-occlusive disease of the liver in allogeneic bone marrow transplant patients. Bone Marrow Transplant. 1992;10:367-372.

287. Comcowich SA, Spitzer TR, Tsunoda SM. Ursodiol to prevent hepatic venoocclusive disease. Ann Pharmacother. 1997;31:1249-1252.

288. Batsis I, Yannaki E, Kaloyannidis P, et al. Veno-occlusive disease prophylaxis with fresh frozen plasma and heparin in bone marrow transplantation. Thromb Res. 2006;118:611-618.

289. Inukai T, Sugita K, Goi K, et al. Prevention of hepatic veno-occlusive disease by a combination of heparin and prostaglandin E_1 in children undergoing hematopoietic stem cell transplantation. Rinsho Ketsueki. 2004;45:297-303.

290. Weiss L, Reich S, Zeira M, et al. N-acetylcysteine mildly inhibits the graft-vs.-leukemia effect but not the lymphokine activated cells (LAK) activity. Transpl Immunol. 2007;17:198-202.

291. Ringden O, Remberger M, Lehmann S, et al. N-acetylcysteine for hepatic veno-occlusive disease after allogeneic stem cell transplantation. Bone Marrow Transplant. 2000;25:993-996.

292. Hassan Z, Hellstrom-Lindberg E, Alsadi S, et al. The effect of modulation of glutathione cellular content on busulphan-induced cytotoxicity on hematopoietic cells in vitro and in vivo. Bone Marrow Transplant. 2002;30:141-147.

293. Haussmann U, Fischer J, Eber S, et al. Hepatic veno-occlusive disease in pediatric stem cell transplantation: impact of pre-emptive antithrombin III replacement and combined antithrombin III/defibrotide therapy. Haematologica. 2006;91:795-800.

294. Ibrahim RB, Peres E, Dansey R, et al. Anti-thrombin III in the management of hematopoietic stem-cell transplantation–associated toxicity. Ann Pharmacother. 2004;38:1053-1059.

295. Morris JD, Harris RE, Hashmi R, et al. Antithrombin-III for the treatment of chemotherapy-induced organ dys-

function following bone marrow transplantation. Bone Marrow Transplant. 1997;20:871-878.

296. Helmy A. Review article: updates in the pathogenesis and therapy of hepatic sinusoidal obstruction syndrome. Aliment Pharmacol Ther. 2006;23:11-25.

297. Leahey AM, Bunin NJ. Recombinant human tissue plasminogen activator for the treatment of severe hepatic veno-occlusive disease in pediatric bone marrow transplant patients. Bone Marrow Transplant. 1996;17:1101-1104.

298. Bearman SI, Shuhart MC, Hinds MS, et al. Recombinant human tissue plasminogen activator for the treatment of established severe venoocclusive disease of the liver after bone marrow transplantation. Blood. 1992;80:2458-2462.

299. Bearman SI, Lee JL, Baron AE, et al. Treatment of hepatic venoocclusive disease with recombinant human tissue plasminogen activator and heparin in 42 marrow transplant patients. Blood. 1997;89:1501-1506.

300. Faioni EM, Krachmalnicoff A, Bearman SI, et al. Naturally occurring anticoagulants and bone marrow transplantation: plasma protein C predicts the development of venoocclusive disease of the liver. Blood. 1993;81:3458-3462.

301. Sartori MT, Spiezia L, Cesaro S, et al. Role of fibrinolytic and clotting parameters in the diagnosis of liver venoocclusive disease after hematopoietic stem cell transplantation in a pediatric population. Thromb Haemost. 2005;93:682-689.

302. Bearman SI, Hinds MS, Wolford JL, et al. A pilot study of continuous infusion heparin for the prevention of hepatic veno-occlusive disease after bone marrow transplantation. Bone Marrow Transplant. 1990;5:407-411.

303. Gherlinzoni F, Vianelli N, Valdre L, et al. Recombinant human tissue plasminogen activator without heparin is effective in the treatment of hepatic veno-occlusive disease. Haematologica. 1999;84:191-192.

304. Attal M, Huguet F, Rubie H, et al. Prevention of hepatic veno-occlusive disease after bone marrow transplantation by continuous infusion of low-dose heparin: a prospective, randomized trial. Blood. 1992;79:2834-2840.

305. Forrest DL, Thompson K, Dorcas VG, et al. Low molecular weight heparin for the prevention of hepatic veno-occlusive disease (VOD) after hematopoietic stem cell transplantation: a prospective phase II study. Bone Marrow Transplant. 2003;31:1143-1149.

306. Or R, Nagler A, Shpilberg O, et al. Low molecular weight heparin for the prevention of veno-occlusive disease of the liver in bone marrow transplantation patients. Transplantation. 1996;61:1067-1071.

307. Simon M, Hahn T, Ford LA, et al. Retrospective multivariate analysis of hepatic veno-occlusive disease after blood or marrow transplantation: possible beneficial use of low molecular weight heparin. Bone Marrow Transplant. 2001;27:627-633.

308. Rosenthal J, Sender L, Secola R, et al. Phase II trial of heparin prophylaxis for veno-occlusive disease of the liver in children undergoing bone marrow transplantation. Bone Marrow Transplant. 1996;18:185-191.

309. Marsa-Vila L, Gorin NC, Laporte JP, et al. Prophylactic heparin does not prevent liver veno-occlusive disease following autologous bone marrow transplantation. Eur J Haematol. 1991;47:346-354.

310. Bajwa RP, Cant AJ, Abinun M, et al. Recombinant tissue plasminogen activator for treatment of hepatic veno-occlusive disease following bone marrow transplantation in children: effectiveness and a scoring system for initiating treatment. Bone Marrow Transplant. 2003;31:591-597.

311. Kulkarni S, Rodriguez M, Lafuente A, et al. Recombinant tissue plasminogen activator (rtPA) for the treatment of hepatic veno-occlusive disease (VOD). Bone Marrow Transplant. 1999;23:803-807.

312. Richardson PG, Elias AD, Krishnan A, et al. Treatment of severe veno-occlusive disease with defibrotide: compassionate use results in response without significant toxicity in a high-risk population. Blood. 1998;92:737-744.

313. Chopra R, Eaton JD, Grassi A, et al. Defibrotide for the treatment of hepatic veno-occlusive disease: results of the European compassionate-use study. Br J Haematol. 2000;111:1122-1129.

314. Abecasis MM, Conceicao Silva JP, Ferreira I, et al. Defibrotide as salvage therapy for refractory veno-occlusive disease of the liver complicating allogeneic bone marrow transplantation. Bone Marrow Transplant. 1999;23:843-846.

315. Richardson PG, Murakami C, Jin Z, et al. Multi-institutional use of defibrotide in 88 patients after stem cell transplantation with severe veno-occlusive disease and multisystem organ failure: response without significant toxicity in a high-risk population and factors predictive of outcome. Blood. 2002;100:4337-4343.

316. Versluys B, Bhattacharaya R, Steward C, et al. Prophylaxis with defibrotide prevents veno-occlusive disease in stem cell transplantation after gemtuzumab ozogamicin exposure. Blood. 2004;103:1968.

317. Dignan F, Gujral D, Ethell M, et al. Prophylactic defibrotide in allogeneic stem cell transplantation: minimal morbidity and zero mortality from veno-occlusive disease. Bone Marrow Transplant. 2007;40:79-82.

318. Bulley SR, Strahm B, Doyle J, et al. Defibrotide for the treatment of hepatic veno-occlusive disease in children. Pediatr Blood Cancer. 2007;48:700-704.

319. Chalandon Y, Roosnek E, Mermillod B, et al. Prevention of veno-occlusive disease with defibrotide after allogeneic stem cell transplantation. Biol Blood Marrow Transplant. 2004;10:347-354.

320. Sucak GT, Aki ZS, Yagci M, et al. Treatment of sinusoidal obstruction syndrome with defibrotide: a single-center experience. Transplant Proc. 2007;39:1558-1563.

321. Corbacioglu S, Greil J, Peters C, et al. Defibrotide in the treatment of children with veno-occlusive disease (VOD): a retrospective multicentre study demonstrates therapeutic efficacy upon early intervention. Bone Marrow Transplant. 2004;33:189-195.

322. Schlitt HJ, Tischler HJ, Ringe B, et al. Allogeneic liver transplantation for hepatic veno-occlusive disease after bone marrow transplantation—clinical and immunological considerations. Bone Marrow Transplant. 1995;16:473-478.

323. Azoulay D, Castaing D, Lemoine A, et al. Transjugular intrahepatic portosystemic shunt (TIPS) for severe veno-occlusive disease of the liver following bone marrow transplantation. Bone Marrow Transplant. 2000;25:987-992.

324. de la Rubia J, Carral A, Montes H, et al. Successful treatment of hepatic veno-occlusive disease in a peripheral

blood progenitor cell transplant patient with a transjugular intrahepatic portosystemic stent-shunt (TIPS). Haematologica. 1996;81:536-539.

325. Smith FO, Johnson MS, Scherer LR, et al. Transjugular intrahepatic portosystemic shunting (TIPS) for treatment of severe hepatic veno-occlusive disease. Bone Marrow Transplant. 1996;18:643-646.

326. Fried MW, Connaghan DG, Sharma S, et al. Transjugular intrahepatic portosystemic shunt for the management of severe venoocclusive disease following bone marrow transplantation. Hepatology. 1996;24:588-591.

327. Levy V, Azoulay D, Rio B, et al. Successful treatment of severe hepatic veno-occlusive disease after allogeneic bone marrow transplantation by transjugular intrahepatic portosystemic stent-shunt (TIPS). Bone Marrow Transplant. 1996;18:443-445.

328. Schoppmeyer K, Lange T, Wittekind C, et al. TIPS for veno-occlusive disease following stem cell transplantation. Z Gastroenterol. 2006;44:483-486.

329. Davies SM, Kollman C, Anasetti C, et al. Engraftment and survival after unrelated-donor bone marrow transplantation: a report from the National Marrow Donor Program. Blood. 2000;96:4096-4102.

330. Szydlo R, Goldman JM, Klein JP, et al. Results of allogeneic bone marrow transplants for leukemia using donors other than HLA-identical siblings. J Clin Oncol. 1997;15:1767-1777.

331. Ash RC, Horowitz MM, Gale RP, et al. Bone marrow transplantation from related donors other than HLA-identical siblings: effect of T cell depletion. Bone Marrow Transplant. 1991;7:443-452.

332. Hamby K, Trexler A, Pearson TC, et al. NK cells rapidly reject allogeneic bone marrow in the spleen through a perforin- and Ly49D-dependent, but NKG2D-independent mechanism. Am J Transplant. 2007;7:1884-1896.

333. Taylor MA, Ward B, Schatzle JD, et al. Perforin- and Fas-dependent mechanisms of natural killer cell–mediated rejection of incompatible bone marrow cell grafts. Eur J Immunol. 2002;32:793-799.

334. Raziuddin A, Longo DL, Mason L, et al. Differential effects of the rejection of bone marrow allografts by the depletion of activating versus inhibiting Ly-49 natural killer cell subsets. J Immunol. 1998;160:87-94.

335. Raziuddin A, Longo DL, Mason L, et al. Ly-49 G2+ NK cells are responsible for mediating the rejection of H-2b bone marrow allografts in mice. Int Immunol. 1996;8:1833-1839.

336. Dennert G, Anderson CG, Warner J. T killer cells play a role in allogeneic bone marrow graft rejection but not in hybrid resistance. J Immunol. 1985;135:3729-3734.

337. Jakubowski AA, Small TN, Young JW, et al. T-cell depleted stem cell transplantation for adults with hematologic malignancies: sustained engraftment of HLA-matched related donor grafts without the use of anti-thymocyte globulin. Blood. 2007;110:4552-4559.

338. Vallera DA, Taylor PA, Sprent J, et al. The role of host T cell subsets in bone marrow rejection directed to isolated major histocompatibility complex class I versus class II differences of bm1 and bm12 mutant mice. Transplantation. 1994;57:249-256.

339. Tomita Y, Mayumi H, Eto M, et al. Tumor allograft rejection is mainly mediated by CD8+ cytotoxic T lymphocytes stimulated with class I alloantigens in cooperation with CD4+ helper T cells recognizing class II alloantigens. J Immunol. 1990;144:2425-2435.

340. Simpson D. T-cell depleting antibodies: new hope for induction of allograft tolerance in bone marrow transplantation? BioDrugs. 2003;17:147-154.

341. Hale G, Jacobs P, Wood L, et al. CD52 antibodies for prevention of graft-versus-host disease and graft rejection following transplantation of allogeneic peripheral blood stem cells. Bone Marrow Transplant. 2000;26:69-76.

342. Bunin N, Aplenc R, Iannone R, et al. Unrelated donor bone marrow transplantation for children with severe aplastic anemia: minimal GVHD and durable engraftment with partial T cell depletion. Bone Marrow Transplant. 2005;35:369-373.

343. Bunin N, Aplenc R, Leahey A, et al. Outcomes of transplantation with partial T-cell depletion of matched or mismatched unrelated or partially matched related donor bone marrow in children and adolescents with leukemias. Bone Marrow Transplant. 2005;35:151-158.

344. Elmaagacli AH, Peceny R, Steckel N, et al. Outcome of transplantation of highly purified peripheral blood CD34+ cells with T-cell add-back compared with unmanipulated bone marrow or peripheral blood stem cells from HLA-identical sibling donors in patients with first chronic phase chronic myeloid leukemia. Blood. 2003;101:446-453.

345. Montero A, Savani BN, Shenoy A, et al. T-cell depleted peripheral blood stem cell allotransplantation with T-cell add-back for patients with hematological malignancies: effect of chronic GVHD on outcome. Biol Blood Marrow Transplant. 2006;12:1318-1325.

346. Guardiola P, Kuentz M, Garban F, et al. Second early allogeneic stem cell transplantations for graft failure in acute leukaemia, chronic myeloid leukaemia and aplastic anaemia. French Society of Bone Marrow Transplantation. Br J Haematol. 2000;111:292-302.

347. Nemunaitis J, Singer JW, Buckner CD, et al. Use of recombinant human granulocyte-macrophage colony-stimulating factor in graft failure after bone marrow transplantation. Blood. 1990;76:245-253.

348. Weisdorf DJ, Verfaillie CM, Davies SM, et al. Hematopoietic growth factors for graft failure after bone marrow transplantation: a randomized trial of granulocyte-macrophage colony-stimulating factor (GM-CSF) versus sequential GM-CSF plus granulocyte-CSF. Blood. 1995;85:3452-3456.

349. Mehta J, Powles R, Singhal S, et al. Outcome of autologous rescue after failed engraftment of allogeneic marrow. Bone Marrow Transplant. 1996;17:213-217.

350. Remberger M, Ringden O, Ljungman P, et al. Booster marrow or blood cells for graft failure after allogeneic bone marrow transplantation. Bone Marrow Transplant. 1998;22:73-78.

351. Godder KT, Abhyankar SH, Lamb LS, et al. Donor leukocyte infusion for treatment of graft rejection post partially mismatched related donor bone marrow transplant. Bone Marrow Transplant. 1998;22:111-113.

352. Davies SM, Weisdorf DJ, Haake RJ, et al. Second infusion of bone marrow for treatment of graft failure after allogeneic bone marrow transplantation. Bone Marrow Transplant. 1994;14:73-77.

353. Grandage VL, Cornish JM, Pamphilon DH, et al. Second allogeneic bone marrow transplants from unrelated donors for graft failure following initial unrelated donor bone

marrow transplantation. Bone Marrow Transplant. 1998;21:687-690.

354. Fernandes J, Rocha V, Robin M, et al. Second transplant with two unrelated cord blood units for early graft failure after haematopoietic stem cell transplantation. Br J Haematol. 2007;137:248-251.

355. Miniero R, Busca A, Vai S, et al. Second bone marrow transplant for children who relapsed or rejected their first graft: experience of the Italian Pediatric Hematology and Oncology Group (AIEOP). Bone Marrow Transplant. 1996;18(Suppl 2):135-138.

356. Ferrara J, Reddy P. Pathophysiology of graft-versus-host disease. Semin Hematol. 2006;43:3-10.

357. Ferrara JLM, Deeg HJ. Graft-versus-host disease. N Engl J Med. 1991;324:667-674.

358. Antin JH, Ferrara JLM. Cytokine dysregulation and acute graft-versus-host disease. Blood. 1992;80:2964-2968.

359. Ferrara JL, Levy R, Chao NJ. Pathophysiologic mechanisms of acute graft-vs.-host disease. Biol Blood Marrow Transplant. 1999;5:347-356.

360. Billingham RE. The biology of graft-versus-host disease. In The Harvey Lectures, Series 60. New York, Academic Press, 1966, pp 21-78.

361. Ruggeri L, Capanni M, Urbani E, et al. Effectiveness of donor natural killer cell alloreactivity in mismatched hematopoietic transplants. Science. 2002;295:2097-2100.

362. Antin JH. Graft-versus leukemia: no longer an epiphenomenon. Blood. 1993;82:2273-2277.

363. Barrett AJ, Malkovska V. Graft-versus-leukaemia: understanding and using the alloimmune response to treat haematological malignancies. Br J Haematol. 1996;93:754-761.

364. Truitt RL, Johnson BD, McCabe CM, et al. Graft versus leukemia. In Ferrara JLM, Deeg HJ, Burakoff SJ (eds). Graft-vs-Host Disease. New York, Marcel Dekker, 1997, pp 385-423.

365. Sullivan KM, Weiden PL, Storb R, et al. Influence of acute and chronic graft-versus-host disease on relapse and survival after bone marrow transplantation from HLA-identical siblings as treatment of acute and chronic leukemia. Blood. 1989;73:1720-1728.

366. Horowitz MM, Gale RP, Sondel PM, et al. Graft-versus-leukemia reactions after bone marrow transplantation. Blood. 1990;75:555-562.

367. Ringden O, Hermans J, Labopin M, et al. The highest leukaemia-free survival after allogeneic bone marrow transplantation is seen in patients with grade I acute graft-versus-host disease. Acute and Chronic Leukaemia Working Parties of the European Group for Blood and Marrow Transplantation (EBMT). Leuk Lymphoma. 1996;24:71-79.

368. Locatelli F, Zecca M, Rondelli R, et al. Graft versus host disease prophylaxis with low-dose cyclosporine-A reduces the risk of relapse in children with acute leukemia given HLA-identical sibling bone marrow transplantation: results of a randomized trial. Blood. 2000;95:1572-1579.

369. Martin PJ, Kernan NA. T-cell depletion for GVHD prevention in humans. In Ferrara JLM, Deeg HJ, Burakoff SJ (eds). Graft-vs-Host Disease. New York, Marcel Dekker, 1997, pp 615-637.

370. Zhang Y, Joe G, Hexner E, et al. Host-reactive CD8$^+$ memory stem cells in graft-versus-host disease. Nat Med. 2005;11:1299-1305.

371. Edinger M, Hoffmann P, Ermann J, et al. CD4$^+$CD25$^+$ regulatory T cells preserve graft-versus-tumor activity while inhibiting graft-versus-host disease after bone marrow transplantation. Nat Med. 2003;9:1144-1150.

372. Hoffmann P, Ermann J, Edinger M, et al. Donor-type CD4$^+$CD25$^+$ regulatory T cells suppress lethal acute graft-versus-host disease after allogeneic bone marrow transplantation. J Exp Med. 2002;196:389-399.

373. Trenado A, Charlotte F, Fisson S, et al. Recipient-type specific CD4$^+$CD25$^+$ regulatory T cells favor immune reconstitution and control graft-versus-host disease while maintaining graft-versus-leukemia. J Clin Invest. 2003;112:1688-1696.

374. June C, Blazar B. Clinical application of expanded CD4$^+$25$^+$ cells. Semin Immunol. 2006;18:78-88.

375. Glucksberg H, Storb R, Fefer A, et al. Clinical manifestations of graft-versus-host disease in human recipients of marrow from HLA-matched sibling donors. Transplantation. 1974;18:295-304.

376. Thomas ED, Storb R, Clift RA, et al. Bone-marrow transplantation (first of two parts). N Engl J Med. 1975;292:832-843.

377. Thomas ED, Storb R, Clift RA, et al. Bone-marrow transplantation (second of two parts). N Engl J Med. 1975;292:895-902.

378. Weisdorf DJ, Snover DC, Haake R, et al. Acute upper gastrointestinal graft-versus-host disease: clinical significance and response to immunosuppressive therapy. Blood. 1990;76:624-629.

379. Przepiorka D, Weisdorf D, Martin P, et al. Consensus conference on acute GVHD grading. Bone Marrow Transplant. 1995;15:825-828.

380. Rowlings P, Przepiorka D, Klein J, et al. IBMTR Severity Index for grading acute graft-versus-host disease: retrospective comparison with Glucksberg grade. Br J Haematol. 1997;97:855-864.

381. Sale GE, Lerner KG, Barker EA, et al. The skin biopsy in the diagnosis of acute graft-versus-host disease in man. Am J Pathol. 1977;89:621-635.

382. Kohler S, Hendrickson MR, Chao NJ, et al. Value of skin biopsies in assessing prognosis and progression of acute graft-versus-host disease. Am J Surg Pathol. 1997;21:988-996.

383. Peck GL, Elias PM, Graw RG. Graft-versus-host reaction and toxic epidermal necrolysis. Lancet. 1972;2:1151-1153.

384. McDonald GB, Shulman HM, Sullivan KM, et al. Intestinal and hepatic complications of human bone marrow transplantation. Part I. Gastroenterology. 1986;90:460-477.

385. McDonald GB, Shulman HM, Sullivan KM, et al. Intestinal and hepatic complications of human bone marrow transplantation. Part II. Gastroenterology. 1986;90:770-784.

386. Snover DC, Weisdorf SA, Ramsay NK, et al. Hepatic graft-versus-host disease: a study of the predictive value of liver biopsy in diagnosis. Hepatology. 1984;4:123-130.

387. Shulman HM, Sharma P, Amos D, et al. A coded histologic study of hepatic graft-versus-host disease after

human bone marrow transplantation. Hepatology. 1988;8: 463-470.

388. Sale GE, McDonald GB, Shulman HM, et al. Gastrointestinal graft-versus-host disease in man: a clinicopathologic study of the rectal biopsy. Am J Surg Pathol. 1979; 3:291-299.

389. Beatty PG, Hansen JA, Longton GM, et al. Marrow transplantation from HLA-matched unrelated donors for treatment of hematologic malignancies. Transplantation. 1991;51:443-447.

390. Weisdorf D, Hakke R, Blazar B. Risk factors for acute graft versus host disease in histocompatible donor bone marrow transplantation. Transplantation. 1991;51:1197-1203.

391. Nash RA, Pepe MS, Storb R, et al. Acute graft-versus-host disease: analysis of risk factors after allogeneic marrow transplantation and prophylaxis with cyclosporine and methotrexate. Blood. 1992;80:1838-1845.

392. Petersdorf EW, Longton GM, Anasetti C, et al. The significance of HLA-DRB1 on clinical outcome after HLA-A,B,DR identical unrelated donor marrow transplantation. Blood. 1995;86:1606-1613.

393. Lin M, Storer B, Martin P, et al. Relation of an interleukin-10 promoter polymorphism to graft-versus-host disease and survival after hematopoietic-cell transplantation. N Engl J Med. 2003;349:2201-2210.

394. Gale RP, Bortin MM, Van Bekkum DW, et al. Risk factors for acute graft-versus-host disease. Br J Haematol. 1987;67:397-406.

395. Hansen JA, Gooley TA, Martin PJ, et al. Bone marrow transplants from unrelated donors for patients with chronic myeloid leukemia. N Engl J Med. 1998;338: 962-968.

396. Hagglund H, Bostrom L, Remberger M, et al. Risk factors for acute graft-versus-host disease in 291 consecutive HLA-identical bone marrow transplant recipients. Bone Marrow Transplant. 1995;16:747-753.

397. Ringden O, Remberger M, Runde V, et al. Peripheral blood stem cell transplantation from unrelated donors: a comparison with marrow transplantation. Blood. 1999;94: 455-464.

398. Nademanee A, Schmidt GM, Parker P, et al. The outcome of matched unrelated donor bone marrow transplantation in patients with hematologic malignancies using molecular typing for donor selection and graft-versus-host disease prophylaxis regimen of cyclosporine, methotrexate, and prednisone. Blood. 1995;86:1228-1234.

399. Storb R, Prentice RL, Buckner CD, et al. Graft-versus-host disease and survival in patients with aplastic anemia treated by marrow grafts from HLA-identical siblings: beneficial effect of a protective environment. N Engl J Med. 1983;308:302-306.

400. Petersen FB, Buckner CD, Clift RA, et al. Laminar air flow isolation and decontamination: a prospective randomized study of the effects of prophylactic systemic antibiotics in bone marrow transplant patients. Infection. 1986;14:115-121.

401. Beelen DW, Elmaagacli A, Muller KD, et al. Influence of intestinal bacterial decontamination using metronidazole and ciprofloxacin or ciprofloxacin alone on the development of acute graft-versus-host disease after marrow transplantation in patients with hematologic malignancies: final results and long-term follow-up of an open-label

prospective randomized trial. Blood. 1999;93:3267-3275.

402. Crum Vander Woude A, Bierer BE. Immunosuppression and immunophilin ligands: cyclosporin A, FK506, and rapamycin. In Ferrara JLM, Deeg HJ, Burakoff SJ (eds). Graft-vs-Host Disease. New York, Marcel Dekker, 1997, pp 111-149.

403. Jolivet J, Cowan KH, Curt GA, et al. The pharmacology and clinical use of methotrexate. N Engl J Med. 1983;309:1094-1104.

404. Chao NJ, Deeg HJ. In vivo prevention and treatment of GVHD. In Ferrara JLM, Deeg HJ, Burakoff SJ (eds). Graft-vs-Host Disease. New York, Marcel Dekker, 1997, pp 639-666.

405. Ruutu T, Niederwieser D, Gratwohl A, et al. A survey of the prophylaxis and treatment of acute GVHD in Europe: a report of the European Group for Blood and Marrow, Transplantation (EBMT). Chronic Leukaemia Working Party of the EBMT. Bone Marrow Transplant. 1997;19: 759-764.

406. Peters C, Minkov M, Gadner H, et al. Statement of current majority practices in graft-versus-host disease prophylaxis and treatment in children. Bone Marrow Transplant. 2000;25:405-411.

407. Storb R, Deeg HJ, Pepe M, et al. Methotrexate and cyclosporine versus cyclosporine alone for prophylaxis of graft-versus-host disease in patients given HLA-identical marrow grafts for leukemia: long-term follow-up of a controlled trial. Blood. 1989;73:1729-1734.

408. Gluckman E, Horowitz MM, Champlin RE, et al. Bone marrow transplantation for severe aplastic anemia: influence of conditioning and graft-versus-host disease prophylaxis regimens on outcome. Blood. 1992;79: 269-275.

409. Cutler C, Antin J. Sirolimus for GVHD prophylaxis in allogeneic stem cell transplantation. Bone Marrow Transplant. 2004;34:471-476.

410. Marmont AM, Horowitz MM, Gale RP, et al. T-cell depletion of HLA-identical transplants in leukemia. Blood. 1991;78:2120-2130.

411. Champlin RE, Passweg JR, Zhang MJ, et al. T-cell depletion of bone marrow transplants for leukemia from donors other than HLA-identical siblings: advantage of T-cell antibodies with narrow specificities. Blood. 2000;95:3996-4003.

412. Hale G, Zhang MJ, Bunjes D, et al. Improving the outcome of bone marrow transplantation by using CD52 monoclonal antibodies to prevent graft-versus-host disease and graft rejection. Blood. 1998;92:4581-4590.

413. Clark RE, Pender N. Transplantation of T-lymphocyte depleted marrow with an addback of T cells. Hematol Oncol. 1995;13:219-224.

414. Sehn LH, Alyea EP, Weller E, et al. Comparative outcomes of T-cell–depleted and non–T-cell–depleted allogeneic bone marrow transplantation for chronic myelogenous leukemia: impact of donor lymphocyte infusion. J Clin Oncol. 1999;17:561-568.

415. Drobyski WR. Evolving strategies to address adverse transplant outcomes associated with T cell depletion. J Hematother Stem Cell Res. 2000;9:327-337.

416. Aschan J. Treatment of moderate to severe acute graft-versus-host disease: a retrospective analysis. Bone Marrow Transplant. 1994;14:601-607.

417. Sayer HG, Longton G, Bowden R, et al. Increased risk of infection in marrow transplant patients receiving methylprednisolone for graft-versus-host disease prevention. Blood. 1994;84:1328-1332.

418. Van Lint MT, Uderzo C, Locasciulli A, et al. Early treatment of acute graft-versus-host disease with high- or low-dose 6-methylprednisolone: a multicenter randomized trial from the Italian Group for Bone Marrow Transplantation. Blood. 1998;92:2288-2293.

419. Martin PJ, Schoch G, Fisher L, et al. A retrospective analysis of therapy for acute graft-versus-host disease: secondary treatment. Blood. 1991;77:1821-1828.

420. Greinix HT, Volc-Platzer B, Kalhs P, et al. Extracorporeal photochemotherapy in the treatment of severe steroid-refractory acute graft-versus-host disease: a pilot study. Blood. 2000;96:2426-2431.

421. Basara N, Blau WI, Romer E, et al. Mycophenolate mofetil for the treatment of acute and chronic GVHD in bone marrow transplant patients. Bone Marrow Transplant. 1998;22:61-65.

422. Atkinson K, Horowitz MM, Gale RP, et al. Consensus among bone marrow transplanters for diagnosis, grading and treatment of chronic graft-versus-host disease. Bone Marrow Transplant. 1989;4:247-254.

423. Sullivan KM, Shulman HM, Storb R, et al. Chronic graft-versus-host disease in 52 patients: adverse natural course and successful treatment with combination immunosuppression. Blood. 1981;57:267-277.

424. Zecca M, Prete A, Rondelli R, et al. Chronic graft-versus-host disease in children: incidence, risk factors, and impact on outcome. Blood. 2002;100:1192-1200.

425. Miklos DB, Kim HT, Miller KH, et al. Antibody responses to H-Y minor histocompatibility antigens correlate with chronic graft-versus-host disease and disease remission. Blood. 2005;105:2973-2978.

426. Shulman HM, Sullivan KM, Weiden P, et al. Chronic graft-versus-host syndrome in man: a long-term clinico-pathologic study of 20 Seattle patients. Am J Med. 1980;69:204-217.

427. Bhushan V, Collins RH Jr. Chronic graft-vs-host disease. JAMA. 2003;290:2599-2603.

428. Wingard JR, Piantadosi S, Vogelsang GB, et al. Predictors of death from chronic graft-versus-host disease after bone marrow transplantation. Blood. 1989;74:1428-1435.

429. Lee S, Cook EF, Soiffer R, et al. Development and validation of a scale to measure symptoms of chronic graft-versus-host disease. Biol Blood Marrow Transplant. 2002;8:444-452.

430. Sullivan KM, Witherspoon RP, Storb R, et al. Alternating-day cyclosporine and prednisone for treatment of high-risk chronic graft-v-host disease. Blood. 1988;72:555-561.

431. Akpek G, Lee SM, Anders V, et al. A high-dose pulse steroid regimen for controlling active chronic graft-versus-host disease. Biol Blood Marrow Transplant. 2001;7:495-502.

432. Chan KW. Extracorporeal photopheresis in children with graft-versus-host disease. J Clin Apheresis. 2006;21:60-64.

433. Teachey DT, Bickert B, Bunin N. Daclizumab for children with corticosteroid refractory graft-versus-host disease. Bone Marrow Transplant. 2006;37:95-99.

434. Baudard M, Vincent A, Moreau P, et al. Mycophenolate mofetil for the treatment of acute and chronic GVHD is effective and well tolerated but induces a high risk of infectious complications: a series of 21 BM or PBSC transplant patients. Bone Marrow Transplant. 2002;30:287-295.

435. Johnston LJ, Brown J, Shizuru JA, et al. Rapamycin (sirolimus) for treatment of chronic graft-versus-host disease. Biol Blood Marrow Transplant. 2005;11:47-55.

436. Jacobsohn DA, Chen AR, Zahurak M, et al. Phase II study of pentostatin in patients with corticosteroid-refractory chronic graft-versus-host disease. J Clin Oncol. 2007;25:4255-4261.

437. Couriel D, Carpenter PA, Cutler C, et al. Ancillary therapy and supportive care of chronic graft-versus-host disease: National Institutes of Health Consensus Development Project on Criteria for Clinical Trials in Chronic Graft-versus-Host Disease: V. Ancillary Therapy and Supportive Care Working Group Report. Biol Blood Marrow Transplant. 2006;12:375-396.

438. Rubin AM, Kang H. Cerebral blindness and encephalopathy with cyclosporine A toxicity. Neurology. 1987;37:1072-1076.

439. Schwartz RB, Bravo SM, Klufas R, et al. Cyclosporine neurotoxicity and its relationship to hypertensive encephalopathy. AJR Am J Roentgenol. 1995;165:627-631.

440. Truwit CL, Denaro CP, Lake JR, et al. MR imaging of reversible cyclosporin A–induced neurotoxicity. AJNR Am J Neuroradiol. 1991;12:651-659.

441. Bernauer W, Gratwohl A, Keller A, et al. Microvasculopathy in the ocular fundus after bone marrow transplantation. Ann Intern Med. 1991;115:925-930.

442. Tichelli A, Duell T, Weiss M, et al. Late-onset keratoconjunctivitis sicca syndrome after bone marrow transplantation: incidence and risk factors. European Group on Blood and Marrow Transplantation (EBMT) Working Party on Late Effects. Bone Marrow Transplant. 1996;17:1105-1111.

443. Lopez PF, Sternberg P, Dabbs CK, et al. Bone marrow transplant retinopathy. Am J Ophthalmol. 1991;112:635-646.

444. Benyunes MC, Sullivan KM, Deeg HJ, et al. Cataracts after bone marrow transplantation: long-term follow-up of adults treated with fractionated total body irradiation. Int J Radiat Oncol Biol Phys. 1995;32:661-670.

445. Deeg HJ, Flournoy N, Sullivan KM, et al. Cataracts after total body irradiation and marrow transplantation: a sparing effect of dose fractionation. Int J Radiat Oncol Biol Phys. 1984;10:957-964.

446. De Marco R, Dassio DA, Vittone P. A retrospective study of ocular side effects in children undergoing bone marrow transplantation. Eur J Ophthalmol. 1996;6:436-439.

447. Ng JS, Lam DS, Li CK, et al. Ocular complications of pediatric bone marrow transplantation. Ophthalmology. 1999;106:160-164.

448. Suh DW, Ruttum MS, Stuckenschneider BJ, et al. Ocular findings after bone marrow transplantation in a pediatric population. Ophthalmology. 1999;106:1564-1570.

449. Dahllof G, Forsberg C-M, Ringden O, et al. Facial growth and morphology in long-term survivors after bone marrow transplantation. Eur J Orthod. 1989;11:332-340.

450. Vaughan MD, Rowland CC, Tong X, et al. Dental abnormalities after pediatric bone marrow transplantation. Bone Marrow Transplant. 2005;36:725-729.

451. Holtta P, Hovi L, Saarinen-Pihkala UM, et al. Disturbed root development of permanent teeth after pediatric stem cell transplantation. Dental root development after SCT. Cancer. 2005;103:1484-1493.

452. Dahllof G, Bagesund M, Ringden O. Impact of conditioning regimens on salivary function, caries-associated microorganisms and dental caries in children after bone marrow transplantation. A 4-year longitudinal study. Bone Marrow Transplant. 1997;20:479-483.

453. Eikenberry M, Bartakova H, Defor T, et al. Natural history of pulmonary complications in children after bone marrow transplantation. Biol Blood Marrow Transplant. 2005;11:56-64.

454. Duncan CN, Buonanno MR, Barry EV, et al. Bronchiolitis obliterans following pediatric allogeneic hematopoietic stem cell transplantation. Bone Marrow Transplant. 2008;Feb 25 [Epub ahead of print].

455. Kurland G, Michelson P. Bronchiolitis obliterans in children. Pediatr Pulmonol. 2005;39:193-208.

456. Clark JG, Crawford SW, Madtes DK, et al. Obstructive lung disease after allogeneic marrow transplantation. Clinical presentation and course. Ann Intern Med. 1989;111:368-376.

457. Reznik SI, Jaramillo A, Zhang L, et al. Anti-HLA antibody binding to HLA class I molecules induces proliferation of airway epithelial cells: a potential mechanism for bronchiolitis obliterans syndrome. J Thorac Cardiovasc Surg. 2000;119:39-45.

458. Freudenberger TD, Madtes DK, Curtis JR, et al. Association between acute and chronic graft-versus-host disease and bronchiolitis obliterans organizing pneumonia in recipients of hematopoietic stem cell transplants. Blood. 2003;102:3822-3828.

459. Dudek AZ, Mahaseth H, DeFor TE, et al. Bronchiolitis obliterans in chronic graft-versus-host disease: analysis of risk factors and treatment outcomes. Biol Blood Marrow Transplant. 2003;9:657-666.

460. Santo Tomas LH, Loberiza FR Jr, Klein JP, et al. Risk factors for bronchiolitis obliterans in allogeneic hematopoietic stem-cell transplantation for leukemia. Chest. 2005;128:153-161.

461. Lee ES, Gotway MB, Reddy GP, et al. Early bronchiolitis obliterans following lung transplantation: accuracy of expiratory thin-section CT for diagnosis. Radiology. 2000;216:472-477.

462. Jung JI, Jung WS, Hahn ST, et al. Bronchiolitis obliterans after allogenic bone marrow transplantation: HRCT findings. Korean J Radiol. 2004;5:107-113.

463. Holland HK, Wingard JR, Beschorner WE, et al. Bronchiolitis obliterans in bone marrow transplantation and its relationship to chronic graft-v-host disease and low serum IgG. Blood. 1988;72:621-627.

464. Khalid M, Al Saghir A, Saleemi S, et al. Azithromycin in bronchiolitis obliterans complicating bone marrow transplantation: a preliminary study. Eur Respir J. 2005;25:490-493.

465. Dudek AZ, Mahaseth H. Hematopoietic stem cell transplant–related airflow obstruction. Curr Opin Oncol. 2006;18:115-119.

466. Wieringa J, van Kralingen KW, Sont JK, et al. Pulmonary function impairment in children following hematopoietic stem cell transplantation. Pediatr Blood Cancer. 2005;45:318-323.

467. Hoffmeister PA, Madtes DK, Storer BE, et al. Pulmonary function in long-term survivors of pediatric hematopoietic cell transplantation. Pediatr Blood Cancer. 2006;47:594-606.

468. Wolff D, Reichenberger F, Steiner B, et al. Progressive interstitial fibrosis of the lung in sclerodermoid chronic graft-versus-host disease. Bone Marrow Transplant. 2002;29:357-360.

469. Attard-Montalto SP, Kingston JE, Eden OB, et al. Late follow-up of lung function after whole lung irradiation for Wilms' tumour. Br J Radiol. 1992;65:1114-1118.

470. Ginsberg SJ, Comis RL. The pulmonary toxicity of antineoplastic agents. Semin Oncol. 1982;9:34-51.

471. Movsas B, Raffin TA, Epstein AH, et al. Pulmonary radiation injury. Chest. 1997;111:1061-1076.

472. Abid SH, Malhotra V, Perry MC. Radiation-induced and chemotherapy-induced pulmonary injury. Curr Opin Oncol. 2001;13:242-248.

473. Gmur JP, Burger J, Schaffner A, et al. Pure red cell aplasia of long duration complicating major ABO-incompatible bone marrow transplantation. Blood. 1990;75:290-295.

474. Zhu KE, Li JP, Zhang T, et al. Clinical features and risk factors of pure red cell aplasia following major ABO-incompatible allogeneic hematopoietic stem cell transplantation. Hematology. 2007;12:117-121.

475. Gajewski JL, Petz LD, Calhoun L, et al. Hemolysis of transfused group O red blood cells in minor ABO-incompatible unrelated-donor bone marrow transplants in patients receiving cyclosporine without posttransplant methotrexate. Blood. 1992;79:3076-3085.

476. Sora F, De Matteis S, Piccirillo N, et al. Rituximab for pure red cell aplasia after ABO-mismatched allogeneic peripheral blood progenitor cell transplantation. Transfusion. 2005;45:643-645.

477. Raj K, Narayanan S, Augustson B, et al. Rituximab is effective in the management of refractory autoimmune cytopenias occurring after allogeneic stem cell transplantation. Bone Marrow Transplant. 2005;35:299-301.

478. Bergstein J, Andreoli SP, Provisor AJ, et al. Radiation nephritis following total-body irradiation and cyclophosphamide in preparation for bone marrow transplantation. Transplantation. 1986;41:63-66.

479. Guinan EC, Tarbell NJ, Niemeyer CM, et al. Intravascular hemolysis and renal insufficiency after bone marrow transplantation. Blood. 1988;72:451-455.

480. Holler E, Kolb HJ, Hiller E, et al. Microangiopathy in patients on cyclosporine prophylaxis who developed acute graft-versus-host disease after HLA-identical bone marrow transplantation. Blood. 1989;73:2018-2024.

481. Oran B, Donato M, Aleman A, et al. Transplant-associated microangiopathy in patients receiving tacrolimus following allogeneic stem cell transplantation: risk factors and response to treatment. Biol Blood Marrow Transplant. 2007;13:469-477.

482. van der Plas RM, Schiphorst ME, Huizinga EG, et al. von Willebrand factor proteolysis is deficient in classic, but not in bone marrow transplantation–associated, thrombotic thrombocytopenic purpura. Blood. 1999;93:3798-802.

483. Kersting S, Hene RJ, Koomans HA, et al. Chronic kidney disease after myeloablative allogeneic hematopoietic stem cell transplantation. Biol Blood Marrow Transplant. 2007; 13:1169-1175.

484. Gronroos MH, Bolme P, Winiarski J, et al. Long-term renal function following bone marrow transplantation. Bone Marrow Transplant. 2007;39:717-723.

485. Patzer L, Kentouche K, Ringelmann F, et al. Renal function following hematological stem cell transplantation in childhood. Pediatr Nephrol. 2003;18:623-635.

486. Wade JC, Meyers JD. Neurologic symptoms associated with parenteral acyclovir treatment after marrow transplantation. Ann Intern Med. 1983;98:921-925.

487. Chrisp P, Clissold SP. Foscarnet. A review of its antiviral activity, pharmacokinetic properties and therapeutic use in immunocompromised patients with cytomegalovirus retinitis. Drugs. 1991;41:104-129.

488. Davis CL, Springmeyer S, Gmerek BJ. Central nervous system side effects of ganciclovir. N Engl J Med. 1990;322: 933-934.

489. Hall RC, Popkin MK, Stickney SK, et al. Presentation of the steroid psychoses. J Nerv Ment Dis. 1979;167:229-236.

490. Kahan BD. Cyclosporine. N Engl J Med. 1989;321:1725-1738.

491. Schwartz RB, Jones KM, Kalina P, et al. Hypertensive encephalopathy: findings on CT, MR imaging, and SPECT imaging in 14 cases. AJR Am J Roentgenol. 1992;159:379-383.

492. Reece DE, Frei-Lahr DA, Shepherd JD, et al. Neurologic complications in allogeneic bone marrow transplant patients receiving cyclosporin. Bone Marrow Transplant. 1991;8:393-401.

493. Bleggi-Torres LF, Werner B, Gasparetto EL, et al. Intracranial hemorrhage following bone marrow transplantation: an autopsy study of 58 patients. Bone Marrow Transplant. 2002;29:29-32.

494. Graus F, Saiz A, Sierra J, et al. Neurologic complications of autologous and allogeneic bone marrow transplantation in patients with leukemia: a comparative study. Neurology. 1996;46:1004-1009.

495. Bleggi-Torres LF, de Medeiros BC, Werner B, et al. Neuropathological findings after bone marrow transplantation: an autopsy study of 180 cases. Bone Marrow Transplant. 2000;25:301-307.

496. de Medeiros BC, de Medeiros CR, Werner B, et al. Central nervous system infections following bone marrow transplantation: an autopsy report of 27 cases. J Hematother Stem Cell Res. 2000;9:535-540.

497. Mohrmann RL, Mah V, Vinters HV. Neuropathologic findings after bone marrow transplantation: an autopsy study. Hum Pathol. 1990;21:630-639.

498. Maschke M, Dietrich U, Prumbaum M, et al. Opportunistic CNS infection after bone marrow transplantation. Bone Marrow Transplant. 1999;23:1167-1176.

499. Thompson CB, Sanders JE, Flournoy N, et al. The risks of central nervous system relapse and leukoencephalopathy in patients receiving marrow transplants for acute leukemia. Blood. 1986;67:195-199.

500. Minn AY, Fisher PG, Barnes PD, et al. A syndrome of irreversible leukoencephalopathy following pediatric allogeneic bone marrow transplantation. Pediatr Blood Cancer. 2007;48:213-217.

501. Woolfrey AE, Gooley TA, Sievers EL, et al. Bone marrow transplantation for children less than 2 years of age with acute myelogenous leukemia or myelodysplastic syndrome. Blood. 1998;92:3546-3556.

502. Kramer JH, Crittenden MR, Halberg FE, et al. A prospective study of cognitive functioning following low-dose cranial radiation for bone marrow transplantation. Pediatrics. 1992;90:447-450.

503. Phipps S, Dunavant M, Srivastava DK, et al. Cognitive and academic functioning in survivors of pediatric bone marrow transplantation. J Clin Oncol. 2000;18:1004-1011.

504. Kramer JH, Crittenden MR, DeSantes K, et al. Cognitive and adaptive behavior 1 and 3 years following bone marrow transplantation. Bone Marrow Transplant. 1997; 19:607-613.

505. Boulad F, Bromley M, Black P, et al. Thyroid dysfunction following bone marrow transplantation using hyperfractionated radiation. Bone Marrow Transplant. 1995;15: 71-76.

506. Sanders JE. Endocrine problems in children after bone marrow transplant for hematologic malignancies. The Long-term Follow-up Team. Bone Marrow Transplant. 1991;8(Suppl 1):2-4.

507. Socie G, Salooja N, Cohen A, et al. Nonmalignant late effects after allogeneic stem cell transplantation. Blood. 2003;101:3373-3385.

508. Bakker B, Oostdijk W, Bresters D, et al. Disturbances of growth and endocrine function after busulphan-based conditioning for haematopoietic stem cell transplantation during infancy and childhood. Bone Marrow Transplant. 2004;33:1049-1056.

509. Michel G, Socie G, Gebhard F, et al. Late effects of allogeneic bone marrow transplantation for children with acute myeloblastic leukemia in first complete remission: the impact of conditioning regimen without total-body irradiation—a report from the Societe Francaise de Greffe de Moelle. J Clin Oncol. 1997;15:2238-2246.

510. Sklar C, Mertens A, Walter A, et al. Final height after treatment for childhood acute lymphoblastic leukemia: comparison of no cranial irradiation with 1800 and 2400 centigrays of cranial irradiation. J Pediatr. 1993;123: 59-64.

511. Sanders JE, Guthrie KA, Hoffmeister PA, et al. Final adult height of patients who received hematopoietic cell transplantation in childhood. Blood. 2005;105:1348-1354.

512. Bakker B, Oostdijk W, Geskus RB, et al. Growth hormone (GH) secretion and response to GH therapy after total body irradiation and haematopoietic stem cell transplantation during childhood. Clin Endocrinol (Oxf). 2007;67: 589-597.

513. Sanders JE. Growth and development after hematopoietic cell transplant in children. Bone Marrow Transplant. 2008;41:223-227.

514. Cohen A, Rovelli A, Bakker B, et al. Final height of patients who underwent bone marrow transplantation for hematological disorders during childhood: a study by the Working Party for Late Effects—EBMT. Blood. 1999;93: 4109-4115.

515. Schubert MA, Sullivan KM, Schubert MM, et al. Gynecological abnormalities following allogeneic bone marrow

transplantation. Bone Marrow Transplant. 1990;5: 425-430.

516. Anserini P, Chiodi S, Spinelli S, et al. Semen analysis following allogeneic bone marrow transplantation. Additional data for evidence-based counselling. Bone Marrow Transplant. 2002;30:447-451.

517. Sanders JE, Pritchard S, Mahoney P, et al. Growth and development following marrow transplantation for leukemia. Blood. 1986;68:1129-1135.

518. Gulati SC, Van Poznak C. Pregnancy after bone marrow transplantation. J Clin Oncol. 1998;16:1978-1985.

519. Hammond C, Abrams JR, Syrjala KL. Fertility and risk factors for elevated infertility concern in 10-year hematopoietic cell transplant survivors and case-matched controls. J Clin Oncol. 2007;25:3511-3517.

520. Bhatia S, Ramsay NK, Weisdorf D, et al. Bone mineral density in patients undergoing bone marrow transplantation for myeloid malignancies. Bone Marrow Transplant. 1998;22:87-90.

521. Kaste SC, Shidler TJ, Tong X, et al. Bone mineral density and osteonecrosis in survivors of childhood allogeneic bone marrow transplantation. Bone Marrow Transplant. 2004;33:435-441.

522. Tauchmanova L, De Rosa G, Serio B, et al. Avascular necrosis in long-term survivors after allogeneic or autologous stem cell transplantation: a single center experience and a review. Cancer. 2003;97:2453-2461.

523. Enright H, Haake R, Weisdorf D. Avascular necrosis of bone: a common serious complication of allogeneic bone marrow transplantation. Am J Med. 1990;89:733-738.

524. Socie G, Cahn JY, Carmelo J, et al. Avascular necrosis of bone after allogeneic bone marrow transplantation: analysis of risk factors for 4388 patients by the Societe Francaise de Greffe de Moelle (SFGM). Br J Haematol. 1997;97:865-870.

525. Fletcher BD, Crom DB, Krance RA, et al. Radiation-induced bone abnormalities after bone marrow transplantation for childhood leukemia. Radiology. 1994;191: 231-235.

526. Carpenter PA, Hoffmeister P, Chesnut CH 3rd, et al. Bisphosphonate therapy for reduced bone mineral density in children with chronic graft-versus-host disease. Biol Blood Marrow Transplant. 2007;13:683-690.

527. Li FP, Alter BP, Nathan DG. The mortality of acquired aplastic anemia in children. Blood. 1972;40:153-161.

528. Thomas ED, Buckner CD, Storb R, et al. Aplastic anaemia treated by marrow transplantation. Lancet. 1972;1:284-289.

529. Bayever E, Champlin R, Ho W, et al. Comparison between bone marrow transplantation and antithymocyte globulin in treatment of young patients with severe aplastic anemia. J Pediatr. 1984;105:920-925.

530. Camitta BM, Thomas ED, Nathan DG, et al. A prospective study of androgens and bone marrow transplantation for treatment of severe aplastic anemia. Blood. 1979;53: 504-514.

531. Paquette RL, Tebyani N, Frane M, et al. Long-term outcome of aplastic anemia in adults treated with antithymocyte globulin: comparison with bone marrow transplantation. Blood. 1995;85:283-290.

532. Werner EJ, Stout RD, Valdez LP, et al. Immunosuppressive therapy versus bone marrow transplantation for children with aplastic anemia. Pediatrics. 1989;83:61-65.

533. Kahl C, Leisenring W, Deeg HJ, et al. Cyclophosphamide and antithymocyte globulin as a conditioning regimen for allogeneic marrow transplantation in patients with aplastic anaemia: a long-term follow-up. Br J Haematol. 2005; 130:747-751.

534. Schrezenmeier H, Passweg JR, Marsh JC, et al. Worse outcome and more chronic GVHD with peripheral blood progenitor cells than bone marrow in HLA-matched sibling donor transplants for young patients with severe acquired aplastic anemia. Blood. 2007;110:1397-1400.

535. Kobayashi R, Yabe H, Hara J, et al. Preceding immunosuppressive therapy with antithymocyte globulin and ciclosporin increases the incidence of graft rejection in children with aplastic anaemia who underwent allogeneic bone marrow transplantation from HLA-identical siblings. Br J Haematol. 2006;135:693-696.

536. Sanders JE, Buckner CD, Amos D, et al. Ovarian function following marrow transplantation for aplastic anemia or leukemia. J Clin Oncol. 1988;6:813-818.

537. Eapen M, Ramsay NK, Mertens AC, et al. Late outcomes after bone marrow transplant for aplastic anaemia. Br J Haematol. 2000;111:754-760.

538. Kurre P, Johnson FL, Deeg HJ. Diagnosis and treatment of children with aplastic anemia. Pediatr Blood Cancer. 2005;45:770-780.

539. Young NS, Calado RT, Scheinberg P. Current concepts in the pathophysiology and treatment of aplastic anemia. Blood. 2006;108:2509-2519.

540. Frickhofen N, Heimpel H, Kaltwasser JP, et al. Antithymocyte globulin with or without cyclosporin A: 11-year follow-up of a randomized trial comparing treatments of aplastic anemia. Blood. 2003;101:1236-1242.

541. Kojima S, Hibi S, Kosaka Y, et al. Immunosuppressive therapy using antithymocyte globulin, cyclosporine, and danazol with or without human granulocyte colony-stimulating factor in children with acquired aplastic anemia. Blood. 2000;96:2049-2054.

542. Maury S, Balere-Appert ML, Chir Z, et al. Unrelated stem cell transplantation for severe acquired aplastic anemia: improved outcome in the era of high-resolution HLA matching between donor and recipient. Haematologica. 2007;92:589-596.

543. Deeg HJ, O'Donnell M, Tolar J, et al. Optimization of conditioning for marrow transplantation from unrelated donors for patients with aplastic anemia after failure of immunosuppressive therapy. Blood. 2006;108:1485-1491.

544. Hasle H. Myelodysplastic and myeloproliferative disorders in children. Curr Opin Pediatr. 2007;19:1-8.

545. Woods WG, Barnard DR, Alonzo TA, et al. Prospective study of 90 children requiring treatment for juvenile myelomonocytic leukemia or myelodysplastic syndrome: a report from the Children's Cancer Group. J Clin Oncol. 2002;20:434-440.

546. Matthes-Martin S, Mann G, Peters C, et al. Allogeneic bone marrow transplantation for juvenile myelomonocytic leukaemia: a single centre experience and review of the literature. Bone Marrow Transplant. 2000;26:377-382.

547. Locatelli F, Nollke P, Zecca M, et al. Hematopoietic stem cell transplantation (HSCT) in children with juvenile myelomonocytic leukemia (JMML): results of the EWOG-MDS/EBMT trial. Blood. 2005;105:410-419.

548. Castleberry RP, Emanuel PD, Zuckerman KS, et al. A pilot study of isotretinoin in the treatment of juvenile chronic myelogenous leukemia. N Engl J Med. 1994;331:1680-1684.

549. de Witte T, Suciu S, Verhoef G, et al. Intensive chemotherapy followed by allogeneic or autologous stem cell transplantation for patients with myelodysplastic syndromes (MDSs) and acute myeloid leukemia following MDS. Blood. 2001;98:2326-2331.

550. Sierra J, Perez WS, Rozman C, et al. Bone marrow transplantation from HLA-identical siblings as treatment for myelodysplasia. Blood. 2002;100:1997-2004.

551. Deeg HJ, Storer B, Slattery JT, et al. Conditioning with targeted busulfan and cyclophosphamide for hemopoietic stem cell transplantation from related and unrelated donors in patients with myelodysplastic syndrome. Blood. 2002;100:1201-1207.

552. Castro-Malaspina H, Harris RE, Gajewski J, et al. Unrelated donor marrow transplantation for myelodysplastic syndromes: outcome analysis in 510 transplants facilitated by the National Marrow Donor Program. Blood. 2002;99:1943-1951.

553. Yusuf U, Frangoul HA, Gooley TA, et al. Allogeneic bone marrow transplantation in children with myelodysplastic syndrome or juvenile myelomonocytic leukemia: the Seattle experience. Bone Marrow Transplant. 2004;33:805-814.

554. Niemeyer CM, Kratz CP, Hasle H. Pediatric myelodysplastic syndromes. Curr Treat Options Oncol. 2005;6:209-214.

555. Fletcher JA, Lynch EA, Kimball VM, et al. Translocation (9;22) is associated with extremely poor prognosis in intensively treated children with acute lymphoblastic leukemia. Blood. 1991;77:435-439.

556. Uckun FM, Nachman JB, Sather HN, et al. Clinical significance of Philadelphia chromosome positive pediatric acute lymphoblastic leukemia in the context of contemporary intensive therapies: a report from the Children's Cancer Group. Cancer. 1998;83:2030-2039.

557. Arico M, Valsecchi MG, Camitta B, et al. Outcome of treatment in children with Philadelphia chromosome–positive acute lymphoblastic leukemia. N Engl J Med. 2000;342:998-1006.

558. Satwani P, Sather H, Ozkaynak F, et al. Allogeneic bone marrow transplantation in first remission for children with ultra-high-risk features of acute lymphoblastic leukemia: a Children's Oncology Group study report. Biol Blood Marrow Transplant. 2007;13:218-227.

559. Talano JM, Casper JT, Camitta BM, et al. Alternative donor bone marrow transplant for children with Philadelphia chromosome ALL. Bone Marrow Transplant. 2006;37:135-141.

560. Nachman JB, Heerema NA, Sather H, et al. Outcome of treatment in children with hypodiploid acute lymphoblastic leukemia. Blood. 2007;110:1112-1115.

561. Wheeler KA, Richards SM, Bailey CC, et al. Bone marrow transplantation versus chemotherapy in the treatment of very high-risk childhood acute lymphoblastic leukemia in first remission: results from Medical Research Council UKALL X and XI. Blood. 2000;96:2412-2418.

562. Goldberg JM, Silverman LB, Levy DE, et al. Childhood T-cell acute lymphoblastic leukemia: the Dana-Farber Cancer Institute Acute Lymphoblastic Leukemia Consortium experience. J Clin Oncol. 2003;21:3616-3622.

563. Balduzzi A, Valsecchi MG, Uderzo C, et al. Chemotherapy versus allogeneic transplantation for very-high-risk childhood acute lymphoblastic leukaemia in first complete remission: comparison by genetic randomisation in an international prospective study. Lancet. 2005;366:635-642.

564. Schrauder A, Reiter A, Gadner H, et al. Superiority of allogeneic hematopoietic stem-cell transplantation compared with chemotherapy alone in high-risk childhood T-cell acute lymphoblastic leukemia: results from ALL-BFM 90 and 95. J Clin Oncol. 2006;24:5742-5749.

565. Schrappe M, Reiter A, Zimmermann M, et al. Long-term results of four consecutive trials in childhood ALL performed by the ALL-BFM study group from 1981 to 1995. Berlin-Frankfurt-Munster. Leukemia. 2000;14:2205-2222.

566. Pui CH, Frankel LS, Carroll AJ, et al. Clinical characteristics and treatment outcome of childhood acute lymphoblastic leukemia with the t(4;11)(q21;q23): a collaborative study of 40 cases. Blood. 1991;77:440-447.

567. Pui CH, Raimondi SC, Hancock ML, et al. Immunologic, cytogenetic, and clinical characterization of childhood acute lymphoblastic leukemia with the t(1;19) (q23; p13) or its derivative. J Clin Oncol. 1994;12:2601-2606.

568. Reaman GH, Sposto R, Sensel MG, et al. Treatment outcome and prognostic factors for infants with acute lymphoblastic leukemia treated on two consecutive trials of the Children's Cancer Group. J Clin Oncol. 1999;17:445-455.

569. Pieters R, Schrappe M, De Lorenzo P, et al. A treatment protocol for infants younger than 1 year with acute lymphoblastic leukaemia (Interfant-99): an observational study and a multicentre randomised trial. Lancet. 2007;370:240-250.

570. Kosaka Y, Koh K, Kinukawa N, et al. Infant acute lymphoblastic leukemia with MLL gene rearrangements: outcome following intensive chemotherapy and hematopoietic stem cell transplantation. Blood. 2004;104:3527-3534.

571. Marco F, Bureo E, Ortega JJ, et al. High survival rate in infant acute leukemia treated with early high-dose chemotherapy and stem-cell support. Groupo Espanol de Trasplante de Medula Osea en Ninos. J Clin Oncol. 2000;18:3256-3261.

572. Saarinen-Pihkala UM, Gustafsson G, Ringden O, et al. No disadvantage in outcome of using matched unrelated donors as compared with matched sibling donors for bone marrow transplantation in children with acute lymphoblastic leukemia in second remission. J Clin Oncol. 2001;19:3406-3414.

573. Sanders JE, Thomas ED, Buckner CD, et al. Marrow transplantation for children with acute lymphoblastic leukemia in second remission. Blood. 1987;70:324-326.

574. Barredo JC, Devidas M, Lauer SJ, et al. Isolated CNS relapse of acute lymphoblastic leukemia treated with intensive systemic chemotherapy and delayed CNS radiation: a Pediatric Oncology Group study. J Clin Oncol. 2006;24:3142-3149.

575. Eapen M, Raetz E, Zhang MJ, et al. Outcomes after HLA-matched sibling transplantation or chemotherapy in children with B-precursor acute lymphoblastic leukemia in a

second remission: a collaborative study of the Children's Oncology Group and the Center for International Blood and Marrow Transplant Research. Blood. 2006;107: 4961-4967.

576. Gaynon PS, Harris RE, Altman AJ, et al. Bone marrow transplantation versus prolonged intensive chemotherapy for children with acute lymphoblastic leukemia and an initial bone marrow relapse within 12 months of the completion of primary therapy: Children's Oncology Group study CCG-1941. J Clin Oncol. 2006;24:3150-3156.

577. Saarinen-Pihkala UM, Heilmann C, Winiarski J, et al. Pathways through relapses and deaths of children with acute lymphoblastic leukemia: role of allogeneic stem-cell transplantation in Nordic data. J Clin Oncol. 2006;24:5750-5762.

578. Uderzo C, Valsecchi MG, Bacigalupo A, et al. Treatment of childhood acute lymphoblastic leukemia in second remission with allogeneic bone marrow transplantation and chemotherapy: ten-year experience of the Italian Bone Marrow Transplantation Group and the Italian Pediatric Hematology Oncology Association. J Clin Oncol. 1995;13:352-358.

579. Wheeler K, Richards S, Bailey C, et al. Comparison of bone marrow transplant and chemotherapy for relapsed childhood acute lymphoblastic leukaemia: the MRC UKALL X experience. Medical Research Council Working Party on Childhood Leukaemia. Br J Haematol. 1998;101:94-103.

580. Appelbaum FR, Dahlberg S, Thomas ED, et al. Bone marrow transplantation or chemotherapy after remission induction for adults with acute nonlymphoblastic leukemia. A prospective comparison. Ann Intern Med. 1984; 101:581-588.

581. Woods WG, Neudorf S, Gold S, et al. A comparison of allogeneic bone marrow transplantation, autologous bone marrow transplantation, and aggressive chemotherapy in children with acute myeloid leukemia in remission. Blood. 2001;97:56-62.

582. Stevens RF, Hann IM, Wheatley K, et al. Marked improvements in outcome with chemotherapy alone in paediatric acute myeloid leukemia: results of the United Kingdom Medical Research Council's 10th AML trial. MRC Childhood Leukaemia Working Party. Br J Haematol. 1998; 101:130-140.

583. Wheatley K, Burnett AK, Goldstone AH, et al. A simple, robust, validated and highly predictive index for the determination of risk-directed therapy in acute myeloid leukaemia derived from the MRC AML 10 trial. United Kingdom Medical Research Council's Adult and Childhood Leukaemia Working Parties. Br J Haematol. 1999; 107:69-79.

584. Ravindranath Y, Chang M, Steuber CP, et al. Pediatric Oncology Group (POG) studies of acute myeloid leukemia (AML): a review of four consecutive childhood AML trials conducted between 1981 and 2000. Leukemia. 2005;19:2101-2116.

585. Raimondi SC, Chang MN, Ravindranath Y, et al. Chromosomal abnormalities in 478 children with acute myeloid leukemia: clinical characteristics and treatment outcome in a cooperative Pediatric Oncology Group study—POG 8821. Blood. 1999;94:3707-3716.

586. Grimwade D, Walker H, Oliver F, et al. The importance of diagnostic cytogenetics on outcome in AML: analysis of 1,612 patients entered into the MRC AML 10 trial. The Medical Research Council Adult and Children's Leukaemia Working Parties. Blood. 1998;92:2322-2333.

587. Meshinchi S, Stirewalt DL, Alonzo TA, et al. Activating mutations of RTK/ras signal transduction pathway in pediatric acute myeloid leukemia. Blood. 2003;102:1474-1479.

588. Zittoun RA, Mandelli F, Willemze R, et al. Autologous or allogeneic bone marrow transplantation compared with intensive chemotherapy in acute myelogenous leukemia. European Organization for Research and Treatment of Cancer (EORTC) and the Gruppo Italiano Malattie Ematologiche Maligne dell'Adulto (GIMEMA) Leukemia Cooperative Groups. N Engl J Med. 1995;332: 217-223.

589. Neudorf S, Sanders J, Kobrinsky N, et al. Autologous bone marrow transplantation for children with AML in first remission. Bone Marrow Transplant. 2007;40: 313-318.

590. Burnett AK, Goldstone AH, Stevens RM, et al. Randomised comparison of addition of autologous bone-marrow transplantation to intensive chemotherapy for acute myeloid leukaemia in first remission: results of MRC AML 10 trial. UK Medical Research Council Adult and Children's Leukaemia Working Parties. Lancet. 1998;351:700-708.

591. Suciu S, Mandelli F, de Witte T, et al. Allogeneic compared with autologous stem cell transplantation in the treatment of patients younger than 46 years with acute myeloid leukemia (AML) in first complete remission (CR1): an intention-to-treat analysis of the EORTC/GIMEMAAML-10 trial. Blood. 2003;102:1232-1240.

592. Nathan PC, Sung L, Crump M, et al. Consolidation therapy with autologous bone marrow transplantation in adults with acute myeloid leukemia: a meta-analysis. J Natl Cancer Inst. 2004;96:38-45.

593. Ravindranath Y, Yeager AM, Chang MN, et al. Autologous bone marrow transplantation versus intensive consolidation chemotherapy for acute myeloid leukemia in childhood. Pediatric Oncology Group. N Engl J Med. 1996;334:1428-1434.

594. Webb DK, Wheatley K, Harrison G, et al. Outcome for children with relapsed acute myeloid leukaemia following initial therapy in the Medical Research Council (MRC) AML 10 trial. MRC Childhood Leukaemia Working Party. Leukemia. 1999;13:25-31.

595. Estey EH. Treatment of relapsed and refractory acute myelogenous leukemia. Leukemia. 2000;14:476-479.

596. Clift RA, Buckner CD, Appelbaum FR, et al. Allogeneic marrow transplantation during untreated first relapse of acute myeloid leukemia. J Clin Oncol. 1992;10:1723-1729.

597. Brown RA, Wolff SN, Fay JW, et al. High-dose etoposide, cyclophosphamide, and total body irradiation with allogeneic bone marrow transplantation for patients with acute myeloid leukemia in untreated first relapse: a study by the North American Marrow Transplant Group. Blood. 1995;85:1391-1395.

598. Michallet M, Thomas X, Vernant JP, et al. Long-term outcome after allogeneic hematopoietic stem cell transplantation for advanced stage acute myeloblastic leukemia: a retrospective study of 379 patients reported to the

Societe Francaise de Greffe de Moelle (SFGM). Bone Marrow Transplant. 2000;26:1157-1163.

599. Goldman JM. How I treat chronic myeloid leukemia in the imatinib era. Blood. 2007;110:2828-2837.

600. Cwynarski K, Roberts IA, Iacobelli S, et al. Stem cell transplantation for chronic myeloid leukemia in children. Blood. 2003;102:1224-1231.

601. Hehlmann R, Hochhaus A, Baccarani M. Chronic myeloid leukaemia. Lancet. 2007;370:342-350.

602. Deininger M, Schleuning M, Greinix H, et al. The effect of prior exposure to imatinib on transplant-related mortality. Haematologica. 2006;91:452-459.

603. Visani G, Rosti G, Bandini G, et al. Second chronic phase before transplantation is crucial for improving survival of blastic phase chronic myeloid leukaemia. Br J Haematol. 2000;109:722-728.

604. Guglielmi C, Arcese W, Dazzi F, et al. Donor lymphocyte infusion for relapsed chronic myelogenous leukemia: prognostic relevance of the initial cell dose. Blood. 2002;100:397-405.

605. Savani BN, Montero A, Kurlander R, et al. Imatinib synergizes with donor lymphocyte infusions to achieve rapid molecular remission of CML relapsing after allogeneic stem cell transplantation. Bone Marrow Transplant. 2005;36:1009-1015.

606. Weisser M, Tischer J, Schnittger S, et al. A comparison of donor lymphocyte infusions or imatinib mesylate for patients with chronic myelogenous leukemia who have relapsed after allogeneic stem cell transplantation. Haematologica. 2006;91:663-666.

607. Vose JM, Sharp G, Chan WC, et al. Autologous transplantation for aggressive non-Hodgkin's lymphoma: results of a randomized trial evaluating graft source and minimal residual disease. J Clin Oncol. 2002;20:2344-2352.

608. Philip T, Pinkerton R, Hartmann O, et al. The role of massive therapy with autologous bone marrow transplantation in Burkitt's lymphoma. Clin Haematol. 1986;15:205-217.

609. Bureo E, Ortega JJ, Munoz A, et al. Bone marrow transplantation in 46 pediatric patients with non-Hodgkin's lymphoma. Bone Marrow Transplant. 1995;15:353-359.

610. Ladenstein R, Pearce R, Hartmann O, et al. High-dose chemotherapy with autologous bone marrow rescue in children with poor-risk Burkitt's lymphoma: a report from the European Lymphoma Bone Marrow Transplantation Registry. Blood. 1997;90:2921-2930.

611. Lavoie JC, Connors JM, Phillips GL, et al. High-dose chemotherapy and autologous stem cell transplantation for primary refractory or relapsed Hodgkin lymphoma: long-term outcome in the first 100 patients treated in Vancouver. Blood. 2005;106:1473-1478.

612. Lieskovsky YE, Donaldson SS, Torres MA, et al. High-dose therapy and autologous hematopoietic stem-cell transplantation for recurrent or refractory pediatric Hodgkin's disease: results and prognostic indices. J Clin Oncol. 2004;22:4532-2540.

613. Rapoport AP, Rowe JM, Kouides PA, et al. One hundred autotransplants for relapsed or refractory Hodgkin's disease and lymphoma: value of pretransplant disease status for predicting outcome. J Clin Oncol. 1993;11:2351-2361.

614. Hoerr AL, Gao F, Hidalgo J, et al. Effects of pretransplantation treatment with rituximab on outcomes of autolo-

gous stem-cell transplantation for non-Hodgkin's lymphoma. J Clin Oncol. 2004;22:4561-4566.

615. Khouri IF, Saliba RM, Hosing C, et al. Concurrent administration of high-dose rituximab before and after autologous stem-cell transplantation for relapsed aggressive B-cell non-Hodgkin's lymphomas. J Clin Oncol. 2005;23:2240-2247.

616. Levine JE, Harris RE, Loberiza FR Jr, et al. A comparison of allogeneic and autologous bone marrow transplantation for lymphoblastic lymphoma. Blood. 2003;101:2476-2482.

617. Dhedin N, Giraudier S, Gaulard P, et al. Allogeneic bone marrow transplantation in aggressive non-Hodgkin's lymphoma (excluding Burkitt and lymphoblastic lymphoma): a series of 73 patients from the SFGM database. Societe Francaise de Greffe de Moelle. Br J Haematol. 1999;107:154-161.

618. Woessmann W, Peters C, Lenhard M, et al. Allogeneic haematopoietic stem cell transplantation in relapsed or refractory anaplastic large cell lymphoma of children and adolescents—a Berlin-Frankfurt-Munster group report. Br J Haematol. 2006;133:176-182.

619. Jones RJ, Ambinder RF, Piantadosi S, et al. Evidence of a graft-versus-lymphoma effect associated with allogeneic bone marrow transplantation. Blood. 1991;77:649-653.

620. Carella AM, Cavaliere M, Lerma E, et al. Autografting followed by nonmyeloablative immunosuppressive chemotherapy and allogeneic peripheral-blood hematopoietic stem-cell transplantation as treatment of resistant Hodgkin's disease and non-Hodgkin's lymphoma. J Clin Oncol. 2000;18:3918-3924.

621. Matthay KK, Villablanca JG, Seeger RC, et al. Treatment of high-risk neuroblastoma with intensive chemotherapy, radiotherapy, autologous bone marrow transplantation, and 13-*cis*-retinoic acid. Children's Cancer Group. N Engl J Med. 1999;341:1165-1173.

622. Grupp SA, Stern JW, Bunin N, et al. Tandem high-dose therapy in rapid sequence for children with high-risk neuroblastoma. J Clin Oncol. 2000;18:2567-2575.

623. Kletzel M, Katzenstein HM, Haut PR, et al. Treatment of high-risk neuroblastoma with triple-tandem high-dose therapy and stem-cell rescue: results of the Chicago Pilot II Study. J Clin Oncol. 2002;20:2284-2292.

624. George RE, Li S, Medeiros-Nancarrow C, et al. High-risk neuroblastoma treated with tandem autologous peripheral-blood stem cell–supported transplantation: long-term survival update. J Clin Oncol. 2006;24:2891-2896.

625. Powell JL, Bunin NJ, Callahan C, et al. An unexpectedly high incidence of Epstein-Barr virus lymphoproliferative disease after CD34+ selected autologous peripheral blood stem cell transplant in neuroblastoma. Bone Marrow Transplant. 2004;33:651-657.

626. Matthay KK, Tan JC, Villablanca JG, et al. Phase I dose escalation of iodine-131-metaiodobenzylguanidine with myeloablative chemotherapy and autologous stem-cell transplantation in refractory neuroblastoma: new approaches to Neuroblastoma Therapy Consortium Study. J Clin Oncol. 2006;24:500-506.

627. Matthay KK, Seeger RC, Reynolds CP, et al. Allogeneic versus autologous purged bone marrow transplantation for neuroblastoma: a report from the Children's Cancer Group. J Clin Oncol. 1994;12:2382-2389.

628. Simon T, Hero B, Faldum A, et al. Consolidation treatment with chimeric anti-GD2-antibody ch14.18 in children older than 1 year with metastatic neuroblastoma. J Clin Oncol. 2004;22:3549-3557.

629. Carpentieri SC, Diller LR. Neuropsychological resiliency after treatment for advanced stage neuroblastoma. Bone Marrow Transplant. 2005;35:1117-1122.

630. Notteghem P, Soler C, Dellatolas G, et al. Neuropsychological outcome in long-term survivors of a childhood extracranial solid tumor who have undergone autologous bone marrow transplantation. Bone Marrow Transplant. 2003;31:599-606.

631. Trahair TN, Vowels MR, Johnston K, et al. Long-term outcomes in children with high-risk neuroblastoma treated with autologous stem cell transplantation. Bone Marrow Transplant. 2007;40:741-746.

632. Fagioli F, Biasin E, Mastrodicasa L, et al. High-dose thiotepa and etoposide in children with poor-prognosis brain tumors. Cancer. 2004;100:2215-2221.

633. Guruangan S, Dunkel IJ, Goldman S, et al. Myeloablative chemotherapy with autologous bone marrow rescue in young children with recurrent malignant brain tumors. J Clin Oncol. 1998;16:2486-2493.

634. Modak S, Gardner S, Dunkel IJ, et al. Thiotepa-based high-dose chemotherapy with autologous stem-cell rescue in patients with recurrent or progressive CNS germ cell tumors. J Clin Oncol. 2004;22:1934-1943.

635. Dupuis-Girod S, Hartmann O, Benhamou E, et al. Will high dose chemotherapy followed by autologous bone marrow transplantation supplant cranio-spinal irradiation in young children treated for medulloblastoma? J Neurooncol. 1996;27:87-98.

636. Buckley RH. Primary immunodeficiency diseases due to defects in lymphocytes. N Engl J Med. 2000;343:1313-1324.

637. Wijnaendts L, Le Deist F, Griscelli C, et al. Development of immunologic functions after bone marrow transplantation in 33 patients with severe combined immunodeficiency. Blood. 1989;74:2212-2219.

638. Fischer A, Landais P, Friedrich W, et al. Bone marrow transplantation (BMT) in Europe for primary immunodeficiencies other than severe combined immunodeficiency: a report from the European Group for BMT and the European Group for Immunodeficiency. Blood. 1994;83:1149-1154.

639. Grunebaum E, Mazzolari E, Porta F, et al. Bone marrow transplantation for severe combined immune deficiency. JAMA. 2006;295:508-518.

640. Buckley RH, Schiff SE, Schiff RI, et al. Hematopoietic stem-cell transplantation for the treatment of severe combined immunodeficiency. N Engl J Med. 1999;340:508-516.

641. Myers LA, Patel DD, Puck JM, et al. Hematopoietic stem cell transplantation for severe combined immunodeficiency in the neonatal period leads to superior thymic output and improved survival. Blood. 2002;99:872-878.

642. Patel DD, Gooding ME, Parrott RE, et al. Thymic function after hematopoietic stem-cell transplantation for the treatment of severe combined immunodeficiency. N Engl J Med. 2000;342:1325-1332.

643. Amrolia P, Gaspar HB, Hassan A, et al. Nonmyeloablative stem cell transplantation for congenital immunodeficiencies. Blood. 2000;96:1239-1246.

644. Kikuta A, Ito M, Mochizuki K, et al. Nonmyeloablative stem cell transplantation for nonmalignant diseases in children with severe organ dysfunction. Bone Marrow Transplant. 2006;38:665-669.

645. Woolfrey A, Pulsipher MA, Storb R. Nonmyeloablative hematopoietic cell transplant for treatment of immune deficiency. Curr Opin Pediatr. 2001;13:539-545.

646. Derry JM, Ochs HD, Francke U. Isolation of a novel gene mutated in Wiskott-Aldrich syndrome. Cell. 1994;78:635-644.

647. Parkman R, Rappeport J, Geha R, et al. Complete correction of the Wiskott-Aldrich syndrome by allogeneic bone-marrow transplantation. N Engl J Med. 1978;298:921-927.

648. Brochstein JA, Gillio AP, Ruggiero M, et al. Marrow transplantation from human leukocyte antigen–identical or haploidentical donors for correction of Wiskott-Aldrich syndrome. J Pediatr. 1991;119:907-912.

649. Kapoor N, Kirkpatrick D, Blaese RM, et al. Reconstitution of normal megakaryocytopoiesis and immunologic functions in Wiskott-Aldrich syndrome by marrow transplantation following myeloablation and immunosuppression with busulfan and cyclophosphamide. Blood. 1981;57:692-696.

650. Mullen CA, Anderson KD, Blaese RM. Splenectomy and/or bone marrow transplantation in the management of the Wiskott-Aldrich syndrome: long-term follow-up of 62 cases. Blood. 1993;82:2961-2966.

651. Rimm IJ, Rappeport JM. Bone marrow transplantation for the Wiskott-Aldrich syndrome. Long-term follow-up. Transplantation. 1990;50:617-620.

652. Brochstein JA, Gillio AP, Ruggiero M, et al. Marrow transplantation from human leukocyte antigen–identical or haploidentical donors for correction of Wiskott-Aldrich syndrome. J Pediatr. 1991;119:907-912.

653. Ozsahin H, Le Deist F, Benkerrou M, et al. Bone marrow transplantation in 26 patients with Wiskott-Aldrich syndrome from a single center. J Pediatr. 1996;129:238-244.

654. Sullivan KE, Mullen CA, Blaese RM, et al. A multiinstitutional survey of the Wiskott-Aldrich syndrome. J Pediatr. 1994;125:876-885.

655. Filipovich AH, Stone JV, Tomany SC, et al. Impact of donor type on outcome of bone marrow transplantation for Wiskott-Aldrich syndrome: collaborative study of the International Bone Marrow Transplant Registry and the National Marrow Donor Program. Blood. 2001;97:1598-1603.

656. Pai SY, DeMartiis D, Forino C, et al. Stem cell transplantation for the Wiskott-Aldrich syndrome: a single-center experience confirms efficacy of matched unrelated donor transplantation. Bone Marrow Transplant. 2006;38:671-679.

657. Cunningham MJ, Macklin EA, Neufeld EJ, et al. Complications of beta-thalassemia major in North America. Blood. 2004;104:34-39.

658. Lawson SE, Roberts IA, Amrolia P, et al. Bone marrow transplantation for beta-thalassaemia major: the UK experience in two paediatric centres. Br J Haematol. 2003;120:289-295.

659. Modell B, Khan M, Darlison M. Survival in beta-thalassaemia major in the UK: data from the UK Thalassaemia Register. Lancet. 2000;355:2051-2052.

660. Thomas ED, Buckner CD, Sanders JE, et al. Marrow transplantation for thalassaemia. Lancet. 1982;2:227-229.

661. Gaziev J, Lucarelli G. Stem cell transplantation for thalassaemia. Reprod Biomed Online. 2005;10:111-115.

662. Roberts I. Current status of allogeneic transplantation for haemoglobinopathies. Br J Haematol. 1997;98:1-7.

663. Giardini C, Lucarelli G. Bone marrow transplantation for beta-thalassemia. Hematol Oncol Clin North Am. 1999;13:1059-1064, viii.

664. Sodani P, Gaziev D, Polchi P, et al. New approach for bone marrow transplantation in patients with class 3 thalassemia aged younger than 17 years. Blood. 2004;104:1201-1203.

665. Angelucci E, Muretto P, Nicolucci A, et al. Effects of iron overload and hepatitis C virus positivity in determining progression of liver fibrosis in thalassemia following bone marrow transplantation. Blood. 2002;100:17-21.

666. Muretto P, Angelucci E, Lucarelli G. Reversibility of cirrhosis in patients cured of thalassemia by bone marrow transplantation. Ann Intern Med. 2002;136:667-672.

667. Leung TF, Hung EC, Lam CW, et al. Bone mineral density in children with thalassaemia major: determining factors and effects of bone marrow transplantation. Bone Marrow Transplant. 2005;36:331-336.

668. Hongeng S, Pakakasama S, Chaisiripoomkere W, et al. Outcome of transplantation with unrelated donor bone marrow in children with severe thalassaemia. Bone Marrow Transplant. 2004;33:377-379.

669. La Nasa G, Giardini C, Argiolu F, et al. Unrelated donor bone marrow transplantation for thalassemia: the effect of extended haplotypes. Blood. 2002;99:4350-4356.

670. Walters MC, Patience M, Leisenring W, et al. Bone marrow transplantation for sickle cell disease. N Engl J Med. 1996;335:369-376.

671. Walters MC, Storb R, Patience M, et al. Impact of bone marrow transplantation for symptomatic sickle cell disease: an interim report. Multicenter investigation of bone marrow transplantation for sickle cell disease. Blood. 2000;95:1918-1924.

672. Bernaudin F, Socie G, Kuentz M, et al. Long-term results of related myeloablative stem-cell transplantation to cure sickle cell disease. Blood. 2007;110:2749-2756.

673. Brachet C, Azzi N, Demulder A, et al. Hydroxyurea treatment for sickle cell disease: impact on haematopoietic stem cell transplantation's outcome. Bone Marrow Transplant. 2004;33:799-803.

674. Iannone R, Casella JF, Fuchs EJ, et al. Results of minimally toxic nonmyeloablative transplantation in patients with sickle cell anemia and beta-thalassemia. Biol Blood Marrow Transplant. 2003;9:519-528.

675. Shenoy S. Has stem cell transplantation come of age in the treatment of sickle cell disease? Bone Marrow Transplant. 2007;40:813-821.

676. Adamkiewicz TV, Mehta PS, Boyer MW, et al. Transplantation of unrelated placental blood cells in children with high-risk sickle cell disease. Bone Marrow Transplant. 2004;34:405-411.

677. Vermylen C. Hematopoietic stem cell transplantation in sickle cell disease. Blood Rev. 2003;17:163-166.

678. Brachet C, Heinrichs C, Tenoutasse S, et al. Children with sickle cell disease: growth and gonadal function after hematopoietic stem cell transplantation. J Pediatr Hematol Oncol. 2007;29:445-450.

679. Hankins J, Hinds P, Day S, et al. Therapy preference and decision-making among patients with severe sickle cell anemia and their families. Pediatr Blood Cancer. 2007;48:705-710.

680. Berger R, Bernheim A, Gluckman E, et al. In vitro effect of cyclophosphamide metabolites on chromosomes of Fanconi anaemia patients. Br J Haematol. 1980;45:565-568.

681. Gluckman E, Devergie A, Dutreix J. Radiosensitivity in Fanconi anaemia: application to the conditioning regimen for bone marrow transplantation. Br J Haematol. 1983;54:431-440.

682. Ayas M, Solh H, Mustafa MM, et al. Bone marrow transplantation from matched siblings in patients with Fanconi anemia utilizing low-dose cyclophosphamide, thoracoabdominal radiation and antithymocyte globulin. Bone Marrow Transplant. 2001;27:139-143.

683. Dufour C, Rondelli R, Locatelli F, et al. Stem cell transplantation from HLA-matched related donor for Fanconi's anaemia: a retrospective review of the multicentric Italian experience on behalf of AIEOP-GITMO. Br J Haematol. 2001;112:796-805.

684. Kohli-Kumar M, Morris C, DeLaat C, et al. Bone marrow transplantation in Fanconi anemia using matched sibling donors. Blood. 1994;84:2050-2054.

685. Davies SM, Khan S, Wagner JE, et al. Unrelated donor bone marrow transplantation for Fanconi anemia. Bone Marrow Transplant. 1996;17:43-47.

686. Gluckman E, Auerbach AD, Horowitz MM, et al. Bone marrow transplantation for Fanconi anemia. Blood. 1995;86:2856-2862.

687. Guardiola P, Pasquini R, Dokal I, et al. Outcome of 69 allogeneic stem cell transplantations for Fanconi anemia using HLA-matched unrelated donors: a study on behalf of the European Group for Blood and Marrow Transplantation. Blood. 2000;95:422-429.

688. Wagner JE, Eapen M, MacMillan ML, et al. Unrelated donor bone marrow transplantation for the treatment of Fanconi anemia. Blood. 2007;109:2256-2262.

689. Mehta PA, Ileri T, Harris RE, et al. Chemotherapy for myeloid malignancy in children with Fanconi anemia. Pediatr Blood Cancer. 2007;48:668-672.

690. Kutler DI, Wreesmann VB, Goberdhan A, et al. Human papillomavirus DNA and p53 polymorphisms in squamous cell carcinomas from Fanconi anemia patients. J Natl Cancer Inst. 2003;95:1718-1721.

691. Rosenberg PS, Greene MH, Alter BP. Cancer incidence in persons with Fanconi anemia. Blood. 2003;101:822-826.

692. Fisch P, Handgretinger R, Schaefer HE. Pure red cell aplasia. Br J Haematol. 2000;111:1010-1022.

693. van Dijken PJ, Verwijs W. Diamond-Blackfan anemia and malignancy. A case report and a review of the literature. Cancer. 1995;76:517-520.

694. Janov A, Leong T, Nathan DG, et al. Diamond-Blackfan anemia. Natural history and sequelae of treatment. Medicine (Baltimore). 1996;76:1-11.

695. August CS, King E, Githens JH, et al. Establishment of erythropoiesis following bone marrow transplantation in a patient with congenital hypoplastic anemia (Diamond-Blackfan syndrome). Blood. 1976;48:491-498.

696. Vlachos A, Federman N, Reyes-Haley C, et al. Hematopoietic stem cell transplantation for Diamond Blackfan anemia: a report from the Diamond Blackfan Anemia Registry. Bone Marrow Transplant. 2001;27:381-386.

697. Roy V, Perez WS, Eapen M, et al. Bone marrow transplantation for Diamond-Blackfan anemia. Biol Blood Marrow Transplant. 2005;11:600-608.

698. Mugishima H, Ohga S, Ohara A, et al. Hematopoietic stem cell transplantation for Diamond-Blackfan anemia: a report from the Aplastic Anemia Committee of the Japanese Society of Pediatric Hematology. Pediatr Transplant. 2007;11:601-607.

699. Rosenberg PS, Alter BP, Bolyard AA, et al. The incidence of leukemia and mortality from sepsis in patients with severe congenital neutropenia receiving long-term G-CSF therapy. Blood. 2006;107:4628-4635.

700. Zeidler C, Welte K, Barak Y, et al. Stem cell transplantation in patients with severe congenital neutropenia without evidence of leukemic transformation. Blood. 2000;95:1195-1198.

701. Le Deist F, Blanche S, Keable H, et al. Successful HLA nonidentical bone marrow transplantation in three patients with the leukocyte adhesion deficiency. Blood. 1989;74:512-516.

702. Mancias C, Infante AJ, Kamani NR. Matched unrelated donor bone marrow transplantation in leukocyte adhesion deficiency. Bone Marrow Transplant. 1999;24:1261-1263.

703. Haddad E, Le Deist F, Blanche S, et al. Treatment of Chédiak-Higashi syndrome by allogenic bone marrow transplantation: report of 10 cases. Blood. 1995;85:3328-3333.

704. Yamazaki S, Takahashi H, Fujii H, et al. Split chimerism after allogeneic bone marrow transplantation in Chédiak-Higashi syndrome. Bone Marrow Transplant. 2003;31:137-140.

705. Seger RA, Gungor T, Belohradsky BH, et al. Treatment of chronic granulomatous disease with myeloablative conditioning and an unmodified hemopoietic allograft: a survey of the European experience, 1985-2000. Blood. 2002;100:4344-4350.

706. Al-Ahmari A, Ayas M, Al-Jefri A, et al. Allogeneic stem cell transplantation for patients with congenital amegakaryocytic thrombocytopenia (CAT). Bone Marrow Transplant. 2004;33:829-831.

707. Bellucci S, Damaj G, Boval B, et al. Bone marrow transplantation in severe Glanzmann's thrombasthenia with antiplatelet alloimmunization. Bone Marrow Transplant. 2000;25:327-330.

708. Johnson A, Goodall AH, Downie CJ, et al. Bone marrow transplantation for Glanzmann's thrombasthenia. Bone Marrow Transplant. 1994;14:147-150.

709. Arico M, Danesino C, Pende D, et al. Pathogenesis of haemophagocytic lymphohistiocytosis. Br J Haematol. 2001;114:761-769.

710. Baker KS, DeLaat CA, Steinbuch M, et al. Successful correction of hemophagocytic lymphohistiocytosis with related or unrelated bone marrow transplantation. Blood. 1997;89:3857-3863.

711. Henter JI, Samuelsson-Horne A, Arico M, et al. Treatment of hemophagocytic lymphohistiocytosis with HLH-94 immunochemotherapy and bone marrow transplantation. Blood. 2002;100:2367-2373.

712. Horne A, Janka G, Maarten Egeler R, et al. Haematopoietic stem cell transplantation in haemophagocytic lymphohistiocytosis. Br J Haematol. 2005;129:622-630.

713. Cooper N, Rao K, Gilmour K, et al. Stem cell transplantation with reduced-intensity conditioning for hemophagocytic lymphohistiocytosis. Blood. 2006;107:1233-1236.

714. Tolar J, Teitelbaum SL, Orchard PJ. Osteopetrosis. N Engl J Med. 2004;351:2839-2849.

715. Walker DG. Bone resorption restored in osteopetrotic mice by transplants of normal bone marrow and spleen cells. Science. 1975;190:784-786.

716. Ballet JJ, Griscelli C, Coutris C, et al. Bone-marrow transplantation in osteopetrosis. Lancet. 1977;2:1137.

717. Coccia P. Bone marrow transplantation for osteopetrosis. In Forman SJ, Blume KG, Thomas ED (eds). Bone Marrow Transplantation. Boston, Blackwell Scientific, 1994, pp 874-882.

718. Gerritsen EJ, Vossen JM, Fasth A, et al. Bone marrow transplantation for autosomal recessive osteopetrosis. A report from the Working Party on Inborn Errors of the European Bone Marrow Transplantation Group. J Pediatr. 1994;125:896-902.

719. Driessen GJ, Gerritsen EJ, Fischer A, et al. Long-term outcome of haematopoietic stem cell transplantation in autosomal recessive osteopetrosis: an EBMT report. Bone Marrow Transplant. 2003;32:657-663.

720. Key L, Carnes D, Cole S, et al. Treatment of congenital osteopetrosis with high-dose calcitriol. N Engl J Med. 1984;310:409-415.

721. Key LL Jr, Rodriguiz RM, Willi SM, et al. Long-term treatment of osteopetrosis with recombinant human interferon gamma. N Engl J Med. 1995;332:1594-1599.

722. Reeves JD, Huffer WE, August CS, et al. The hematopoietic effects of prednisone therapy in four infants with osteopetrosis. J Pediatr. 1979;94:210-214.

723. Barton NW, Brady RO, Dambrosia JM, et al. Replacement therapy for inherited enzyme deficiency: macrophage-targeted glucocerebrosidase for Gaucher's disease. N Engl J Med. 1991;324:1464-1470.

724. Guffon N, Souillet G, Maire I, et al. Follow-up of nine patients with Hurler syndrome after bone marrow transplantation. J Pediatr. 1998;133:119-125.

725. Krivit W, Shapiro EG, Peters C, et al. Hematopoietic stem-cell transplantation in globoid-cell leukodystrophy. N Engl J Med. 1998;338:1119-1126.

726. Peters C, Shapiro EG, Anderson J, et al. Hurler syndrome: II. Outcome of HLA-genotypically identical sibling and HLA-haploidentical related donor bone marrow transplantation in fifty-four children. The Storage Disease Collaborative Study Group. Blood. 1998;91:2601-2608.

727. Shapiro E, Krivit W, Lockman L, et al. Long-term effect of bone-marrow transplantation for childhood-onset cerebral X-linked adrenoleukodystrophy. Lancet. 2000;356:713-718.

728. Boelens JJ. Trends in haematopoietic cell transplantation for inborn errors of metabolism. J Inherit Metab Dis. 2006;29:413-420.

729. Hite SH, Peters C, Krivit W. Correction of odontoid dysplasia following bone-marrow transplantation and engraftment (in Hurler syndrome MPS 1H). Pediatr Radiol. 2000;30:464-470.

730. Souillet G, Guffon N, Maire I, et al. Outcome of 27 patients with Hurler's syndrome transplanted from either

related or unrelated haematopoietic stem cell sources. Bone Marrow Transplant. 2003;31:1105-1117.

731. Peters C, Balthazor M, Shapiro EG, et al. Outcome of unrelated donor bone marrow transplantation in 40 children with Hurler syndrome. Blood. 1996;87:4894-4902.

732. Boelens JJ, Wynn RF, O'Meara A, et al. Outcomes of hematopoietic stem cell transplantation for Hurler's syndrome in Europe: a risk factor analysis for graft failure. Bone Marrow Transplant. 2007;40:225-233.

733. Staba SL, Escolar ML, Poe M, et al. Cord-blood transplants from unrelated donors in patients with Hurler's syndrome. N Engl J Med. 2004;350:1960-1969.

734. Escolar ML, Poe MD, Provenzale JM, et al. Transplantation of umbilical-cord blood in babies with infantile Krabbe's disease. N Engl J Med. 2005;352:2069-2081.

735. Beam D, Poe MD, Provenzale JM, et al. Outcomes of unrelated umbilical cord blood transplantation for X-linked adrenoleukodystrophy. Biol Blood Marrow Transplant. 2007;13:665-674.

IV Disorders of Erythrocyte Production

10 | Diagnostic Approach to the Anemic Patient

Carlo Brugnara, Frank A. Oski,* and David G. Nathan

*Deceased.

Most of the chapters thus far have been devoted to descriptions of specific disorders that result in anemia. The purpose of this chapter is to provide both a more general classification of the anemias and an initial diagnostic approach to patients with this laboratory finding. Details of the diagnostic procedures used for ultimate diagnosis of the various anemias are omitted because they are presented in their respective chapters.

DEFINITION OF ANEMIA

Anemia is generally defined as a reduction in red cell mass or blood hemoglobin concentration. The limit for differentiating anemic from normal states is generally set at 2 standard deviations (SD) below the mean for the normal population. This definition will result in 2.5% of the normal population being classified as anemic. Conversely, values for hemoglobin-deficient individuals are distributed in such a fashion that some are placed within the normal range. These individuals, who have the potential for a hemoglobin concentration in the upper part of the normal range, may be recognized only after a response to treatment. Definition of the lower limit of normal for both pediatric and adult patients is critically dependent on the population used to establish the normal range of values.[1] Hematocrit, hemoglobin, and mean corpuscular volume (MCV) are significantly lower in African American than in whites. A third of this difference can be accounted for by the α-globin -3.7-kilobase (kb) deletion.[2] In the absence of a race-specific normal range, the fact that African Americans generally have lower hemoglobin levels than whites do (approximately 0.5 g/dL) could result in 10% of normal African American children being consider anemic just because the proper normal range is not used.[3] Figure 10-1 presents pediatric reference ranges for hemoglobin in non-Hispanic whites, African Americans, and Mexican Americans that were obtained from the National Health and Nutrition Examination Survey (NHANES) III database.

Because the primary function of the red cell is to deliver and release adequate quantities of oxygen to tissues to meet their metabolic demands, it is apparent that some measures of both body oxygen metabolism and accompanying cardiovascular compensation are required to complement the current laboratory definition of anemia. The fact that hemoglobin concentration alone is insufficient to judge whether a patient is "functionally anemic" is best illustrated in a patient with cyanotic congenital heart disease or chronic respiratory insufficiency or in one with mutant hemoglobins that alter hemoglobin's affinity for oxygen (see Chapter 18).

With these caveats in mind, a useful statistical definition of anemia that recognizes the effect of age and sex on the designation of anemia is provided in Table 10-1.[4]

CLASSIFICATION OF ANEMIAS

Anemias may be classified on the basis of physiology or morphology. A combination of both approaches is often used in the initial differential diagnosis.

The best approach for providing an understanding of the multiple disorders capable of producing anemia is to separate the causes of anemia into two categories of functional disturbances:

1. Disorders of effective red cell production, in which the net rate of red cell production is depressed. This can be due to disorders of erythrocyte maturation, in which erythropoiesis is largely ineffectual, or to an

TABLE 10-1	Normal Mean and Lower Limits of Normal for Hemoglobin, Hematocrit, and Mean Corpuscular Volume					
	HEMOGLOBIN (g/dL)		**HEMATOCRIT (%)**		**MEAN CORPUSCULAR VOLUME (μm^3)**	
Age (yr)	Mean	Lower Limit	Mean	Lower Limit	Mean	Lower Limit
0.5-1.9	12.5	11.0	37	33	77	70
2-4	12.5	11.0	38	34	79	73
5-7	13.0	11.5	39	35	81	75
8-11	13.5	12.0	40	36	83	76
12-14						
Female	13.5	12.0	41	36	85	78
Male	14.0	12.5	43	37	84	77
15-17						
Female	14.0	12.0	41	36	87	79
Male	15.0	13.0	46	38	86	78
18-49						
Female	14.0	12.0	42	37	90	80
Male	16.0	14.0	47	40	90	80

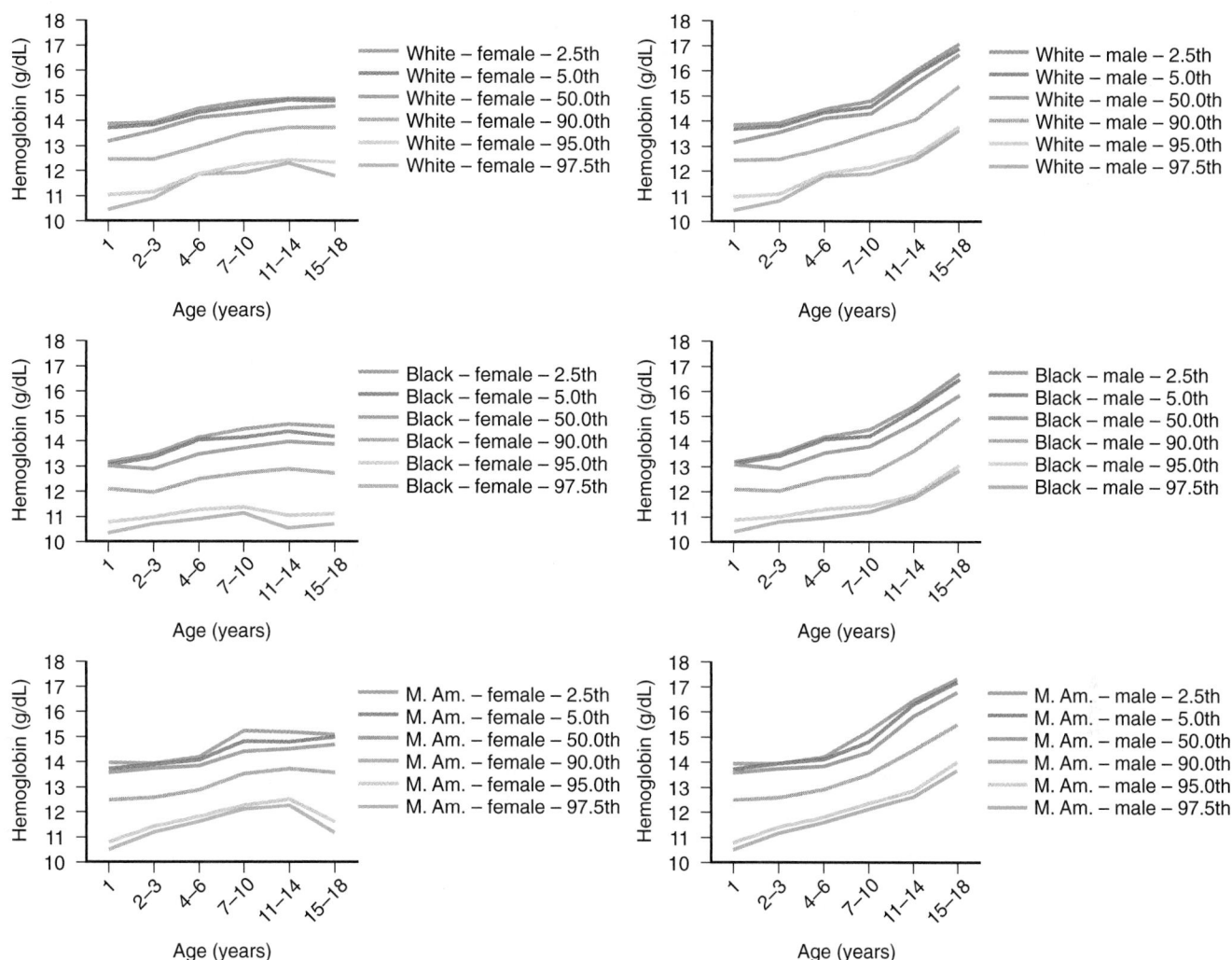

FIGURE 10-1. Pediatric reference ranges for hemoglobin in non-Hispanic whites (*top row*), non-Hispanic blacks (*middle row*), and Mexican Americans (*bottom row*). (*Data were kindly provided by Dr. George Cembrowski and obtained from the National Health and Examination Survey (NHANES) III. Presented at the 2004 meeting of the International Society for Laboratory Hematology [Cembrowski GS, Chan J, Cheng C, Bamforth FJ. NHANES 1999-2000 data used to create comprehensive health-associated race-, sex- and age-stratified pediatric reference intervals for the Coulter MAXM. Lab Hematol. 2004;10:245-246]. Data can also be accessed at http://www.mylaboratoryquality.com. See Reference Intervals.*)

absolute failure of erythropoiesis. In the former, bone marrow contains many erythroblasts that die in situ before reaching the reticulocyte stage. In the latter, there is absolute erythroblastopenia.

2. Disorders in which rapid erythrocyte destruction or red cell loss is primarily responsible for the anemia.

These two categories are not mutually exclusive. More than one mechanism may be present in some anemias, but one functional disorder is generally the major reason for the patient's anemia. Box 10-1 lists the anemias most commonly encountered in infancy and childhood and classifies them into three categories of functional disturbance.

Anemias may also be classified on the basis of red cell size and then further subdivided according to red cell

morphology. In this type of classification, anemias are subdivided into microcytic, normocytic, and macrocytic anemias. This classification is also arbitrary, and categories are not mutually exclusive. For example, macrocytic reticulocytes abound in the hemolytic anemias. Therefore, although mature erythrocytes in the various hemolytic anemias may be normocytic, the MCV of all the cells may be larger than normal because of the contribution of reticulocytes to the volume measurement.[5] Volume distribution curves may reveal the contribution of a subset of large cells to the MCV. Furthermore, during the course of a disease, classification of the patient's anemia may change from one category to another as a result of other clinical or pathologic variables. In Box 10-2 the more common anemias of infancy and childhood are classified on the basis of their characteristic cell size.

Box 10-1 **Physiologic Classification of Anemia**

A. DISORDERS OF RED CELL PRODUCTION IN WHICH THE RATE OF RED CELL PRODUCTION IS LESS THAN EXPECTED FOR THE DEGREE OF ANEMIA
  1. Marrow failure
     a. Aplastic anemia
        Congenital
        Acquired
     b. Pure red cell aplasia
        Congenital
        Diamond-Blackfan syndrome
        Aase's syndrome
        Acquired
        Transient erythroblastopenia of childhood
        Other
     c. Marrow replacement
        Malignancies
        Osteopetrosis
        Myelofibrosis
        Chronic renal disease
        Vitamin D deficiency
     d. Pancreatic insufficiency–marrow hypoplasia syndrome
  2. Impaired erythropoietin production
     a. Chronic renal disease
     b. Hypothyroidism, hypopituitarism
     c. Chronic inflammation
     d. Protein malnutrition
     e. Hemoglobin mutants with decreased affinity for oxygen
B. DISORDERS OF ERYTHROID MATURATION AND INEFFECTIVE ERYTHROPOIESIS
  1. Abnormalities in cytoplasmic maturation
     a. Iron deficiency
     b. Thalassemia syndromes
     c. Sideroblastic anemias
     d. Lead poisoning
  2. Abnormalities in nuclear maturation
     a. Vitamin B_{12} deficiency
     b. Folic acid deficiency
     c. Thiamine-responsive megaloblastic anemia
     d. Hereditary abnormalities in folate metabolism
     e. Orotic aciduria
  3. Primary dyserythropoietic anemias (types I, II, III, IV)
  4. Erythropoietic protoporphyria
  5. Refractory sideroblastic anemia with vacuolization of marrow precursors and pancreatic dysfunction/ deficiency
C. HEMOLYTIC ANEMIAS
  1. Defects in hemoglobin
     a. Structural mutants
     b. Synthetic mutants (thalassemia syndromes)
  2. Defects in the red cell membrane
  3. Defects in red cell metabolism
  4. Antibody mediated
  5. Mechanical injury to the erythrocyte
  6. Thermal injury to the erythrocyte
  7. Oxidant-induced red cell injury
  8. Infectious agent–induced red cell injury
  9. Paroxysmal nocturnal hemoglobinuria
  10. Plasma lipid–induced abnormalities in the red cell membrane

EVALUATION OF THE ANEMIC PATIENT

The initial diagnostic approach to an anemic patient includes a detailed history and physical examination and a minimum of essential laboratory tests. Tables 10-2 and 10-3 list the features of the history and physical examination that are most helpful in providing clues to the cause of the anemia. The initial laboratory tests should include a determination of hemoglobin and hematocrit; measurement of red cell indices, platelet count, white blood cell count and differential, and reticulocyte count; and examination of a peripheral blood smear. After this initial assessment, other useful and simple laboratory procedures may be used, including, when indicated, measurement of erythrocyte porphyrin and serum ferritin concentration, supravital staining of erythrocytes, hemoglobin electrophoresis, a screening test for the presence of unstable hemoglobins, a direct and indirect Coombs test, a screening test for glucose-6-phosphate dehydrogenase deficiency, and examination of bone marrow.

Automated Cell Counting

The most widely used methods for determination of hemoglobin, hematocrit, and red cell indices are now fully automated. When compared with manual techniques, automated methods have the advantages of greater precision and reproducibility and the capacity for completing a large number of measurements quickly.

One of two general principles is used in most of the more popular automated hematology analyzers. They may simply be classified as the electrical impedance principle and the laser light scatter principle.

In automated cell counters using the electrical impedance principle (Abbott, Abbott Park, IL; ABX, Kyoto, Japan; Beckman-Coulter, Miami, FL; Sysmex, Kobe, Japan), cells passing through an aperture cause changes in electrical resistance that are counted as voltage pulses, which are proportional to cell volume. The electrical pulses are amplified and counted during the time that an

Box 10-2	Classification of Anemias Based on Red Cell Size

A. MICROCYTIC ANEMIAS
1. Iron deficiency (nutritional, chronic blood loss)
2. Chronic lead poisoning
3. Thalassemia syndromes
4. Sideroblastic anemias
5. Chronic inflammation
6. Some congenital hemolytic anemias with unstable hemoglobin

B. MACROCYTIC ANEMIAS
1. With megaloblastic bone marrow
   a. Vitamin B_{12} deficiency
   b. Folic acid deficiency
   c. Hereditary orotic aciduria
   d. Thiamine-responsive anemia
2. Without megaloblastic bone marrow
   a. Aplastic anemia
   b. Diamond-Blackfan syndrome
   c. Hypothyroidism
   d. Liver disease
   e. Bone marrow infiltration
   f. Dyserythropoietic anemias

C. NORMOCYTIC ANEMIAS
1. Congenital hemolytic anemias
   a. Hemoglobin mutants
   b. Red cell enzyme defects
   c. Disorders of the red cell membrane
2. Acquired hemolytic anemias
   a. Antibody mediated
   b. Microangiopathic hemolytic anemias
   c. Secondary to acute infections
3. Acute blood loss
4. Splenic pooling
5. Chronic renal disease (usually)

accurately metered volume of the suspension is drawn through the aperture. These devices can directly measure MCV and compute the hematocrit from the MCV and red blood cell count.

In automated cell counters using the laser light scatter principle (Abbott, Abbott Park, IL; Siemens Medical Solutions Diagnostics, Tarrytown, NY), single cells passing through a laser beam induce scattering of laser light, which can be detected and translated into measurements of cell size. In the instruments produced by Siemens, red cells first undergo isovolumetric sphering, and then MCV and the mean corpuscular hemoglobin concentration (MCHC) are measured from the low-angle forward light scattering and the high-angle (refractive index) light scattering, respectively.[6-9]

Some of the potential errors that can be generated by automated cell counters for hemoglobin, hematocrit, and red cell indices are listed in Table 10-4.[10] Cold agglutinins in high titer tend to cause spurious macrocytosis with low red cell counts and very high MCHCs. Warming either the blood or the diluent may eliminate this problem.

Electronic cell counting provides a useful means of categorizing anemias based on the MCV and MCHC. The red cell volume distribution width (RDW) is derived from the red blood cell histogram that accompanies each analysis. The RDW is an index of the variation in red cell size and thus can be used to detect anisocytosis. In a normal patient, the histogram is virtually symmetrical. RDW is calculated as a standard statistical value, the coefficient of variation in distribution of red cell volume. The formula can be expressed as

$$RDW = SD/MCV \times 100$$

TABLE 10-2	Historical Factors of Importance in Evaluating Patients with Anemia
Age	Nutritional iron deficiency is never responsible for anemia in term infants before 6 months of age; rarely seen in premature infants before the time that they have doubled their birth weight. Anemia occurring in the neonatal period is generally the result of recent blood loss, isoimmunization, or initial manifestation of a congenital hemolytic anemia or congenital infection
	Anemia first detected at 3 to 6 months of age suggests a congenital disorder of hemoglobin synthesis or hemoglobin structure
Gender	Consider X-linked disorders in males (G6PD deficiency, pyruvate kinase deficiency)
Race	Hemoglobins S and C more common in blacks; β-thalassemia more common in whites; α-thalassemia trait most common among black and yellow races
Ethnicity	Thalassemia syndromes most common among patients of Mediterranean origin. G6PD deficiency observed more often among Sephardic Jews, Filipinos, Greeks, Sardinians, and Kurds
Neonatal	A history of hyperbilirubinemia in the newborn period suggests the presence of congenital hemolytic anemia, such as the hereditary spherocytosis of G6PD deficiency. Prematurity predisposes to the early development of iron deficiency
Diet	Document sources of iron, vitamin B_{12}, folic acid, or vitamin E in the diet. A history of pica, geophagia, or pagophagia suggests the presence of iron deficiency
Drugs	Oxidant-induced hemolytic anemia, phenytoin (Dilantin)-induced megaloblastic anemia, drug-induced aplastic anemia
Infection	Hepatitis-induced aplastic anemia, infection-induced red cell aplasia, hemolytic anemia
Inheritance	Family history of anemia, jaundice, gallstones, or splenomegaly
Diarrhea	Suspect small bowel disease with malabsorption of folate or vitamin B_{12}. Suspect inflammatory bowel disease with blood loss. Suspect exudative enteropathy with blood loss

G6PD, glucose-6-phosphate dehydrogenase.

TABLE 10-3   Physical Findings as Clues to the Cause of Anemia

Skin	Hyperpigmentation	Fanconi's Aplastic Anemia
	Petechiae, purpura	Autoimmune hemolytic anemia with thrombocytopenia, hemolytic-uremic syndrome, bone marrow aplasia, bone marrow infiltration
	Carotenemia	Suspect iron deficiency in infants
	Jaundice	Hemolytic anemia, hepatitis, aplastic anemia
	Cavernous hemangioma	Microangiopathic hemolytic anemia
	Ulcers on lower extremities	S and C hemoglobinopathies, thalassemia
Facies	Frontal bossing, prominence of the malar and maxillary bones	Congenital hemolytic anemias, thalassemia major, severe iron deficiency
Eyes	Microcornea	Fanconi's aplastic anemia
	Tortuosity of the conjunctival and retinal vessels	S and C hemoglobinopathies
	Microaneurysms of the retinal vessels	S and C hemoglobinopathies
	Cataracts	Glucose-6-phosphate dehydrogenase deficiency, galactosemia with hemolytic anemia in the newborn period
	Vitreous hemorrhages	S hemoglobinopathy
	Retinal hemorrhages	Chronic, severe anemia
	Edema of the eyelids	Infectious mononucleosis, exudative enteropathy with iron deficiency, renal failure
	Blindness	Osteopetrosis
Mouth	Glossitis	Vitamin B_{12} deficiency, iron deficiency
	Angular stomatitis	Iron deficiency
Chest	Unilateral absence of the pectoral muscles	Poland's syndrome (increased incidence of leukemia)
	Shield chest	Diamond-Blackfan syndrome
Hands	Triphalangeal thumbs	Red cell aplasia
	Hypoplasia of the thenar eminence	Fanconi's aplastic anemia
	Spoon nails	Iron deficiency
Spleen	Enlargement	Congenital hemolytic anemia, leukemia, lymphoma, acute infection, portal hypertension

TABLE 10-4   Sources of Spurious Results in Hemoglobin and Red Cell Count Parameters

Erroneous increase in Hb	Lipemia (hypertriglyceridemia, fat emulsion, type I and IV hyperlipoproteinemias)
	Elevated WBC counts (threshold varies from 50 to 250×10^9/L)
	Immunoglobulins (monoclonal IgG, IgM, IgA in Waldenström's or multiple myeloma)
	Hemolysis (when free plasma Hb is markedly elevated because of intravascular hemolysis)
Erroneous increase in RBC counts	High WBC count (especially if greater than 100×10^9/L)
Erroneous increase in MCV	Hyperglycemia (secondary to dilution of a severe hyperglycemic sample)
	Hypernatremia
	Sample storage at room temperature
Erroneous decrease in RBC counts	Cold agglutinin (in association with high MCV and high MCHC)
	Clotting (abnormal mixing, overfilling of sample)

Hb, hemoglobin; MCHC, mean corpuscular hemoglobin concentration; MCV, mean corpuscular volume; RBC, red blood cell; WBC, white blood cell.
From Zandecki M, Genevieve F, Gerard J, Godon A. Spurious counts and spurious results on haematology analysers: a review. Part II: white blood cells, red blood cells, haemoglobin, red cell indices and reticulocytes. Int J Lab Hematol. 2007;29:21-41.

Because RDW reflects the ratio of SD and MCV, a wide red cell distribution curve in a patient with markedly increased MCV may still generate a normal RDW value. RDW in normal individuals ranges from 11.5% to 14.5%, but it may vary as a function of the model of the electronic cell counter used. Normal values for infants and children appear to range from 1.5% to 15.0%. The hemoglobin distribution width (HDW) is calculated in a similar manner from the histogram for MCHC. Coulter instruments do not directly measure the red cell hemoglobin concentration. The MCHC and HDW values provided by these instruments are sensitive to variations in MCV and should be used with caution in the differential diagnosis of anemias.

Bessman and associates have provided a classification of anemias based on MCV and RDW. An updated version that includes MCHC and HDW appears in Table 10-5.[11]

TABLE 10-5 **Relationship of Mean Corpuscular Volume (MCV) and Red Cell Volume Distribution Width (RDW) in a Variety of Disease States**

RDW	MCV		
	Low	Normal	High
Normal	Heterozygous α- and β-thalassemia	Normal Lead poisoning	Aplastic anemia
High	Iron deficiency Hemoglobin H disease S β-thalassemia	Early iron deficiency Liver disease Mixed nutritional deficiencies	Newborns, prematurity Vitamin B$_{12}$ or folate deficiency
		HIGH MCHC/HDW Immune hemolytic anemia SS and SC disease Hereditary spherocytosis/xerocytosis	**HIGH MCHC/HDW** Immune hemolytic anemia

HDW, hemoglobin distribution width; MCHC, mean corpuscular hemoglobin concentration.

Visual analysis of the red cell histograms generated by automated cell counters provides essential clues for the diagnosis of anemias. The presence of either microcytes or macrocytes and increased RDW can readily be appreciated. Histograms for MCHC are particularly useful because they allow prompt identification of dehydrated hyperchromic cells in sickle cell disease, hereditary spherocytosis, hereditary xerocytosis, and immune hemolytic anemias. Moreover, a careful study of volume and hemoglobin concentration histograms allows rapid differentiation of iron deficiency and β-thalassemia trait and differentiation of hemoglobin H and hemoglobin H/CS disease. Figure 10-2 provides the histograms for MCV and MCHC in a normal control and in patients with β-thalassemia trait, iron deficiency, and sickle cell disease.

Automated reticulocyte counting is also available in several hematology analyzers. Automated counting is more precise and accurate than manual counting.[12,13] Absolute reticulocyte counts are easily obtained with these instruments, thereby obviating the limitations of counting reticulocytes only as a percentage or correcting for changes in hematocrit (corrected reticulocyte count). An additional useful feature of automated reticulocyte counters is that stress reticulocytes can easily be identified by their increased volume and RNA content.[13-15] Cellular indices for reticulocytes such as volume, hemoglobin concentration, and hemoglobin content are also available in the Siemens and Sysmex instruments. The reticulocyte hemoglobin content[16] has been shown to be a valuable parameter in identifying iron deficient states in young children and toddlers.[17,18]

The Blood Film

Although automatic blood film machines are now the vogue in clinical laboratories, films made on coverslips are preferable to those made on glass slides because a greater proportion of blood on the coverslip film is technically suitable for microscopic examination. Proper processing of blood films on coverslips is fast becoming a lost art. The details of preparation and examination can be found in a variety of manuals of laboratory hematology, but the lucid and succinct instructions of Wintrobe deserve reproduction here[19]:

1. Use a small drop of blood, only 2 to 3 mm in diameter, taken either from a stylet wound, as described earlier, or from a syringe or needle tip used in venipuncture immediately after the venipuncture has been performed (anticoagulants are not to be used because they will alter the morphologic appearance).
2. Hold the coverslips only by their edges, placing one crosswise over the other, and allow the blood to spread between them for about 2 seconds.
3. Quickly but gently separate the coverslips by pulling them laterally, in opposite directions to one another but in the plane of the spreading film, just before the film reaches the edges (do not squeeze or lift the coverslips from one another).
4. Quickly air-dry the films, either by placing them face up on a clean surface if the humidity is low or by moving them through the air while holding them by their edges with your fingertips.

If the procedure has been carried out successfully, the blood will be spread evenly, and there will be no holes or thick areas in the preparation. A multicolored sheen will be seen on the surface of the dried, unstained film if light glances off it at the proper angle because the thin layer of closely fitting cells acts like a diffraction grating. Later, under the microscope after staining, the red cells will be seen next to each other, but neither overlapping nor in rouleau formation, and central pallor will be visible; lymphocytes will have a readily distinguished cytoplasm rather than a minimal zone bearing closely on the nucleus as occurs with thick films or those that dry too slowly.

Examination of a peripheral blood film is the single most useful procedure in the initial evaluation of a patient

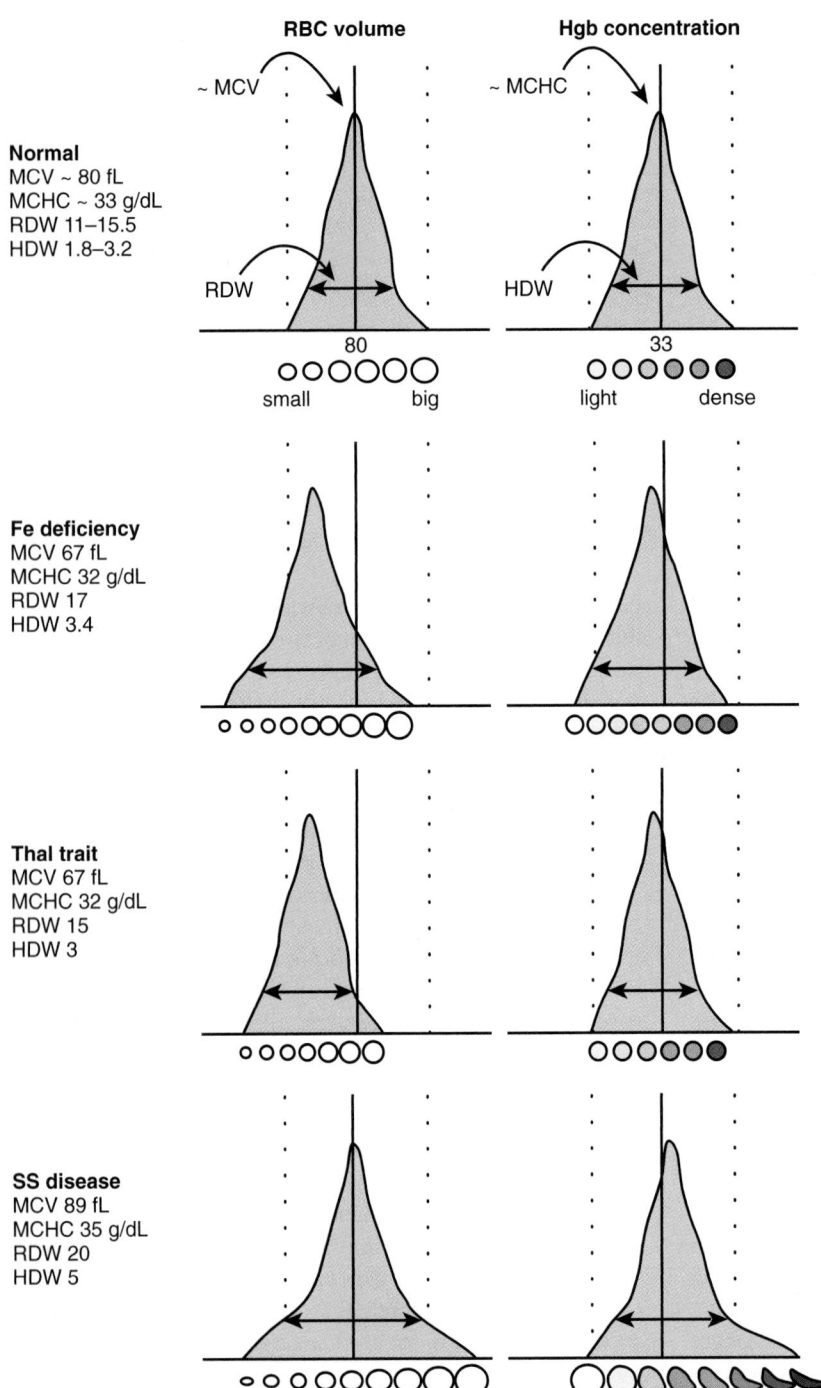

FIGURE 10-2. Histograms for mean corpuscular volume (MCV, *left column*) and mean corpuscular hemoglobin concentration (MCHC, *right column*) in a normal control subject (*first row*), a patient with iron deficiency (*second row*), a subject with heterozygous β-thalassemia (*third row*), and a patient with homozygous hemoglobin S disease (*bottom row*). Goal posts are placed at 60 and 120 fL for MCV and at 28 and 41 g/dL for MCHC. HDW, hemoglobin distribution width; RBC, red blood cell; RDW, red cell volume distribution width.

with anemia. The blood film should first be examined under low power to determine the adequacy of cell distribution and staining. Signs of poor blood film preparation include loss of central pallor in red blood cells, polygonal shapes, and artifactual spherocytes. Artifactual spherocytes, in contrast to true spherocytes, show no variation in central pallor and are larger than normal red cells. One should never attempt to interpret a poorly prepared blood film.

After the adequacy of the blood film is determined by low-power examination, the blood film should be examined first under 50× magnification and then under 1000× magnification. Cells should be graded for size, staining intensity, variation in color, and abnormalities in shape. Red cell hemolytic disorders can be classified according to their predominant morphology. An approach to such a classification is presented in Box 10-3 and is discussed in detail in Chapters 14 through 17.

The blood film should also be examined for the presence of basophilic stippling and red cell inclusions. The significance of some of these findings is described in Table 10-6.

Box 10-3	Classification of Red Cell Hemolytic Disorders by Predominant Morphology*

SPHEROCYTES

Hereditary spherocytosis
ABO incompatibility in neonates
Immunohemolytic anemias with IgG- or C3-coated red cells[†]
Acute oxidant injury (hexose monophosphate shunt defects during hemolytic crisis, oxidant drugs, and chemicals)
Hemolytic transfusion reactions[†]
Clostridium welchii septicemia
Severe burns, other red cell thermal injury
Spider, bee, and snake venom
Severe hypophosphatemia
Hypersplenism[‡]

BIZARRE POIKILOCYTES

Red cell fragmentation syndromes (microangiopathic and macroangiopathic hemolytic anemias)
Acute oxidant injury[‡]
Hereditary elliptocytosis in neonates
Hereditary pyropoikilocytosis

ELLIPTOCYTES

Hereditary elliptocytosis
Thalassemias
(Other hypochromic-microcytic anemias)
(Megaloblastic anemias)

STOMATOCYTES

Hereditary stomatocytosis
Rh$_{null}$ blood group
Stomatocytosis with cold hemolysis
(Liver disease, especially acute alcoholism)
(Mediterranean stomatocytosis)

IRREVERSIBLY SICKLED CELLS

Sickle cell anemia
Symptomatic sickle syndromes

INFRAERYTHROCYTIC PARASITES

Malaria
Babesiasis
Bartonellosis

SPICULATED OR CRENATED RED CELLS

Acute hepatic necrosis (spur cell anemia)
Uremia
Red cell fragmentation syndromes[‡]
Infantile pyknocytosis
Embden-Meyerhof pathway defects[‡]
Vitamin E deficiency[‡]
Abetalipoproteinemia
Heat stroke[‡]
McLeod blood group
(After splenectomy)
(Transiently after massive transfusion of stored blood)
(Anorexia nervosa)[‡]

TARGET CELLS

Hemoglobins S, C, D, and E
Hereditary xerocytosis
Thalassemias
(Other hypochromic-microcytic anemias)
(Obstructive liver disease)
(After splenectomy)
(Lecithin–cholesterol acyltransferase deficiency)

PROMINENT BASOPHILIC STIPPLING

Thalassemias
Unstable hemoglobins
Lead poisoning[‡]
Pyrimidine 5'-nucleotidase deficiency

NONSPECIFIC OR NORMAL MORPHOLOGY

Embden-Meyerhof pathway defects
Hexose monophosphate shunt defects
Unstable hemoglobins
Paroxysmal nocturnal hemoglobinuria
Dyserythropoietic anemias
Copper toxicity (Wilson's disease)
Cation permeability defects
Erythropoietic porphyria
Vitamin E deficiency
Hemolysis with infections[‡]
Rh hemolytic disease in neonates[†]
Paroxysmal cold hemoglobinuria*[‡]
Cold hemagglutinin disease[†]
Hypersplenism
Immunohemolytic anemia[†‡]

*Nonhemolytic disorders of similar morphology are enclosed in parentheses for reference.
[†]Usually associated with a positive Coombs test.
[‡]Disease sometimes associated with this morphology.

DIAGNOSTIC APPROACH

After the laboratory tests have been performed, the results may be used in an initial attempt to diagnostically characterize the patient's anemia, as illustrated by the simple algorithm in Figure 10-3. This algorithm provides two additional diagnostic steps after the initial characterization of anemia based on the complete blood cell count, reticulocyte count, and cellular indices.

If the diagnosis of hemolytic anemia is considered, it is useful to consider the potential pathophysiology before ordering useless and expensive screening tests. The authors have used a simple and reliable approach to

TABLE 10-6   Diagnostic Significance of Red Cell Inclusions

Inclusion	Staining Agent	Diagnostic Significance
Basophilic stippling	Wright stain	Represents aggregated ribosomes. May be observed in thalassemia syndromes, iron deficiency, syndromes accompanied by ineffective erythropoiesis and pyrimidine 5′-nucleotidase deficiency; particularly prominent in unstable hemoglobinopathies and lead poisoning
Howell-Jolly bodies	Wright stain	Represent nuclear remnants. Observed in asplenic and hyposplenic states, pernicious anemia, dyserythropoietic anemias, and severe iron deficiency anemia
Cabot's rings	Wright stain	Appear as basophilic rings, circular, or twisted figures-of-eight. Considered to be nuclear remnants or artifacts. Observed in lead poisoning, pernicious anemia, and hemolytic anemias
Heinz' bodies	Brilliant cresyl blue, methyl violet	Represent denatured or aggregated hemoglobin. Observed in patients with thalassemia syndromes or unstable hemoglobins, after oxidant stress in patients with enzyme deficiencies of the pentose phosphate pathway, and in patients with asplenia or chronic liver disease
Siderocytes	Prussian blue counterstained with safranin O	Represent nonhemoglobin iron within erythrocytes. Seen in increased numbers in the peripheral circulation after splenectomy. Observed in increased numbers in patients with chronic infection, aplastic anemias, or hemolytic anemias

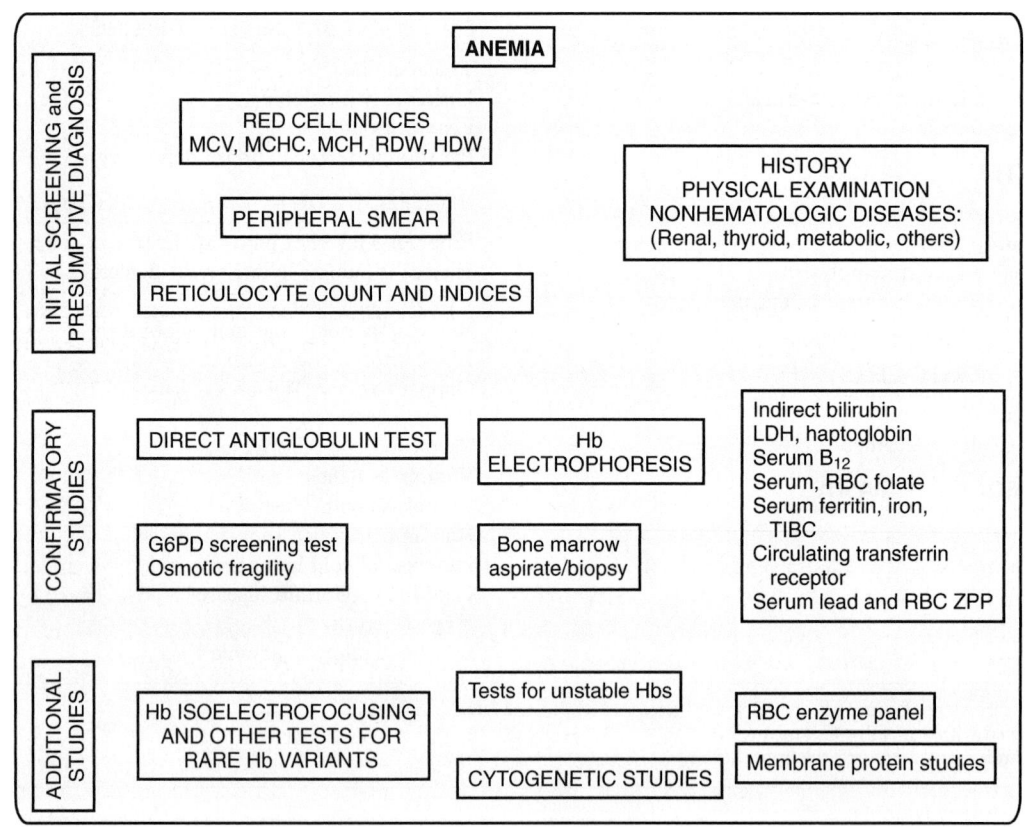

FIGURE 10-3. Algorithm for the differential diagnosis of anemia. Initial characterization of the anemia is based on the complete blood cell count, reticulocyte count, cellular indices, erythrocyte morphology, and history. This step is followed by two additional diagnostic steps: either to confirm a relatively common type of anemia or to diagnose one of the uncommon types of anemia. G6PD, glucose-6-phosphate dehydrogenase; Hb, hemoglobin; HDW, hemoglobin distribution width; LDH, lactate dehydrogenase; MCH, mean corpuscular hemoglobin; MCHC, mean corpuscular hemoglobin concentration; MCV, mean corpuscular volume; RBC, red blood cell; RDW, red cell volume distribution width; TIBC, total iron-binding capacity; ZPP, zinc protoporphyrin.

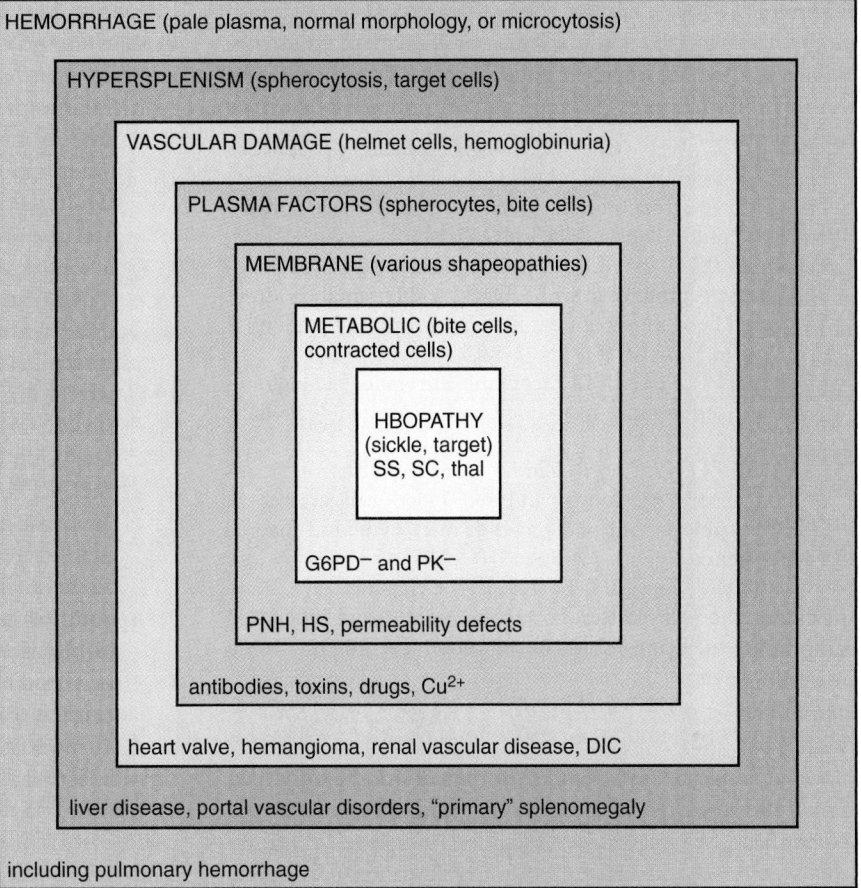

FIGURE 10-4. Assaults on the red cell from the vasculature to the "center" of the cell. The site of damage is in capital letters, the laboratory findings in parentheses, and the common causes in the lower part of the square. Cu^{2+}, copper; DIC, disseminated intravascular coagulation; HBOPATHY, hemoglobinopathy; HS, hereditary spherocytosis; PK, pyruvate kinase; PNH, paroxysmal nocturnal hemoglobinuria; SC, hemoglobin SC; SS, hemoglobin SS; thal, thalassemia.

pathophysiologic analysis that involves consideration of the potential assaults on the red cell from the farthest point to the inner core of the erythrocyte (Fig. 10-4).

The most common cause of rapid red cell loss with reticulocytosis is hemorrhage. In infants and children, unusual causes include hemorrhage beneath the scalp and intraabdominal, urinary tract, and pulmonary hemorrhage. In the latter two situations, hyperbilirubinemia is not present. Indeed, if the hemorrhage is chronic and leads to iron deficiency, the plasma will be pale.

Sequestration in an abnormal spleen will usually cause spherocytosis, but if the hypersplenism is associated with liver disease, target cells will also be present. In this condition, the osmotic fragility test will reveal a sensitive and a resistant population of erythrocytes.

Vascular damage to erythrocytes may be associated with thrombocytopenia and can be caused by hemangiomas (Kasabach-Merritt syndrome); intravascular coagulation, usually secondary to sepsis; damaged artificial heart valves; and renal vascular disease and severe hypertension. Schistocytes, which resemble military helmets of various nationalities, are usually present, and siderinuria and hemoglobinuria are often detected.

Abnormalities in plasma are frequent causes of hemolysis. Antibodies usually induce spherocytosis by causing splenic sequestration, but sometimes they merely fix complement and cause hemoglobinuria without mor-

phologic change. Many drugs and toxins can damage red cells either by oxidant injury with resultant schistocytosis or by direct lysis, as illustrated by bacterial lipases in septic shock. Acute hemolysis may also be caused by excessive release of hepatic copper in Wilson's disease. No morphologic change is noted.

Primary membrane abnormalities that cause hemolysis are usually congenital and are associated with specific morphologic changes. An exception is paroxysmal nocturnal hemoglobinuria, which is an acquired membrane defect associated with no morphologic change. The congenital membrane defects are usually due to abnormalities in structural membrane proteins, such as in hereditary spherocytosis, but they may involve cation channels (hydrocytosis and xerocytosis) and, rarely, membrane lipids (abetalipoproteinemia).

The red cell itself may contribute to its own quietus, as exemplified by glucose-6-phosphate dehydrogenase deficiency, pyruvate kinase deficiency, and deficiencies of the other enzymes involved in erythrocyte metabolic pathways. Morphologic alterations are not predictable.

Finally, the red cell may be sabotaged by its own hemoglobin, such as in sickle cell anemia, the thalassemias, and the unstable hemoglobinopathies.

If the clinician considers these options in an inclusive but systematic fashion, direct screening tests can be ordered and expert consultation avoided.

REFERENCES

1. Beutler E, Waalen J. The definition of anemia: what is the lower limit of normal of the blood hemoglobin concentration? Blood. 2006;107:1747-1750.
2. Beutler E, West C. Hematologic differences between African-Americans and whites: the roles of iron deficiency and α-thalassemia on hemoglobin levels and mean corpuscular volume. Blood. 2005;106:740-745.
3. Dallman PR, Barr GD, Allen CM, Shinefield HR. Hemoglobin concentration in white, black, and Oriental children: is there a need for separate criteria in screening for anemia? Am J Clin Nutr. 1978;31:377-380.
4. Dallman PR, Sijmes MA. Percentile curves for hemoglobin and red cell volume in infancy and childhhod. J Pediatr. 1979;94:26-31.
5. d'Onofrio G, Chirillo R, Zini G, et al. Simultaneous measurement of reticulocyte and red blood cell indices in healthy subjects and patients with microcytic and macrocytic anemia. Blood. 1995;85:818-823.
6. Tycko DH, Metz MH, Epstein EA, Grinbaum A. A flow-cytometric light scattering measurement of red blood cell volume and hemoglobin concentration. J Appl Opt. 1985;24:1355-1365.
7. Fossat G, David M, Harle JR, et al. New parameters in erythrocyte counting. Arch Pathol Lab Med. 1987;111:1150-1154.
8. Mohandas N, Kim YR, Tycko DH, et al. Accurate and independent measurement of volume and hemoglobin concentration of individual red cells by laser light scattering. Blood. 1986;68:506-513.
9. Mohandas N, Johnson A, Wyatt J, et al. Automated quantitation of cell density distribution and hyperdense cell fraction in RBC disorders. Blood. 1989;74:442-447.
10. Zandecki M, Genevieve F, Gerard J, Godon A. Spurious counts and spurious results on haematology analysers: a review. Part II: white blood cells, red blood cells, haemoglobin, red cell indices and reticulocytes. Int J Lab Hematol. 2007;29:21-41.
11. Bessman JD, Gilmer PR Jr, Gardner FH. Improved classification of anemias by MCV and RDW. Am J Clin Pathol. 1983;80:322-326.
12. Savage RA, Skoog DP, Rabinovitch A. Analytic inaccuracy and imprecision in reticulocyte counting: a preliminary report from the College of American Pathologists reticulocyte project. Blood Cells. 1985;11:97-112.
13. Schimenti KJ, Lacerna K, Wamble A, et al. Reticulocyte quantification by flow cytometry, image analysis and manual counting. Cytometry. 1992;13:853-862.
14. Turowski D, Wysocka J, Butkiewicz AM. Peripheral blood reticulocytes and their reference range values for percentage, absolute count, and immature fraction in children, measured with flow cytometry. Folia Histochem Cytobiol. 2000;38:31-36.
15. Lacombe F, Lacoste L, Vial JP, et al. Automated reticulocyte counting and immature reticulocyte fraction measurement. Comparison of ABX Pentra 120 Retic, Sysmex R-2000, flow cytometry and manual counts. Am J Clin Pathol. 1999;112:677-686.
16. Brugnara C, Shiller B, Moran J. Reticulocyte hemoglobin equivalent (Ret He) and assessment of iron-deficient states. Clin Lab Haematol. 2006;28:303-308.
17. Brugnara C, Zurakowski D, DiCanzio J, et al. Reticulocyte hemoglobin content to diagnose iron deficiency in children. JAMA. 1999;281:2225-2230.
18. Ullrich C, Wu A, Armsby C, et al. Screening healthy infants for iron deficiency using reticulocyte hemoglobin content. JAMA. 2005;294:924-930.
19. Wintrobe MM. Clinical Hematology, 7th ed. Philadelphia, Lea & Febiger, 1974.

11

Megaloblastic Anemia

David Watkins, V. Michael Whitehead, and David S. Rosenblatt

Before the mid-1920s, pernicious anemia was a disease dreaded as much as drug-resistant leukemia is today. With its characteristic megaloblastic bone marrow, pernicious anemia was a fatal illness until it was successfully treated with dietary liver in 1926.[1] It is now known that megaloblastic anemia is most often caused by a nutritional deficiency of folates or by a specific malabsorption of cobalamin (vitamin B_{12}) known as pernicious anemia (Box 11-1). Precise means for diagnosing and treating these deficiencies are available. Over the past 80 years, hematologists have gained detailed knowledge of the synthesis, biology, biochemistry, and molecular biology of both cobalamin and folate. It is extraordinary that this knowledge base continues to grow as new discoveries are made.

This chapter reviews aspects of this knowledge as it pertains to pediatric patients in particular. Emphasis is placed on clinical and laboratory diagnosis and on the treatment of overt deficiencies of cobalamin and folate. In addition, attention is focused on subclinical deficiency states as they relate to populations at increased risk, including premature newborns, the elderly, those infected with human immunodeficiency virus (HIV), and those with elevated plasma total homocysteine levels. Consideration is given to the role of these vitamins in the prevention of neural tube defects (NTDs) and cardiovascular disease and in the pathogenesis of cancer. Finally, current knowledge of inborn errors of cobalamin and folate metabolism is presented.

Box 11-1	Causes of Megaloblastic Anemia

COBALAMIN (VITAMIN B_{12})

Defects in Absorption

Inadequate gastric intrinsic factor as a result of
    Pernicious anemia
    Gastritis
    Total gastrectomy
    Mutations in *GIF* (intrinsic factor gene)
Achlorhydria and pepsin deficiency
Disease of the small intestine
    Surgical resection or bypass of the terminal ileum
    Regional enteritis (Crohn's disease)
    Tropical and nontropical sprue
    Infiltrative disease (Whipple's syndrome, lymphoma)
    Competition by parasites (fish tapeworm, blind loop syndrome)
    Imerslund-Gräsbeck syndrome
    Drugs (colchicines, *p*-aminosalicylic acid, neomycin)
    Transcobalamin deficiency

Inadequate Nutrition

Strict vegetarians (vegans)
Maternal deficiency affecting the fetus or infant

Defects in Transport

Transcobalamin deficiency

Defects in Metabolism

Nitrous oxide intoxication
Inherited (cblC, cblD, cblE, cblF, and cblG disease)

FOLATES

Defects in Absorption

Hereditary folate malabsorption
Tropical and nontropical sprue
Infiltrative diseases of the small bowel (Whipple's syndrome, lymphoma)

Inadequate Nutrition

Insufficient or poorly selected diet
Maternal deficiency affecting the fetus or infant

Increased Requirement

Alcoholism
Pregnancy
Lactation
Hemolytic anemia
Hyperthyroidism
Anticonvulsant therapy
Lesch-Nyhan syndrome
Prematurity
Homocystinuria
First trimester during neural tube closure

Folate Inhibitors

Antifolates (methotrexate, pyrimethamine, trimethpoprim)
Sulfones

Inherited Defects

Methylenetetrahydrofolate reductase deficiency
Methionine synthase deficiency (cblE and cblG disease)
Others

OTHER CAUSES

Defects in Purine and Pyrimidine Synthesis

Inherited
    Orotic aciduria
Acquired
    Myelodysplasia and leukemia
    Drug induced
    Human immunodeficiency virus infection

Other

3-Phosphoglycerate dehydrogenase deficiency
Thiamine-responsive anemia
Scurvy
Pyridoxine-responsive anemia

DEFINITIONS

Megaloblastic anemia is a macrocytic anemia that is usually accompanied by leukopenia and thrombocytopenia. It is characterized by a specific megaloblastic bone marrow morphology that affects erythroid, myeloid, and platelet precursors. In this chapter the terms *cobalamin* and *vitamin B$_{12}$* are used interchangeably to refer to corrins that have coenzyme activity or that can be converted to coenzymes in cells (see later). The term *folates* refers to synthetic folic acid and to the various natural folate coenzymes, including reduced dihydrofolates (DHFs) and tetrahydrofolates (THFs) and their single-carbon substituted forms. Natural folate coenzymes are substrates for the enzyme folate polyglutamate synthetase and are converted by it to *folate polyglutamates* containing predominantly six or seven γ-linked glutamate residues. Most folates are present in nature as reduced and substituted folate polyglutamates. These, too, are included under the general term *folates*.

HISTORY

Anemia associated with morphologically abnormal erythrocytes had been observed in patients with pernicious anemia from 1876 to 1877.[2-4] By 1883, macrocytosis had been described. In 1891, Ehrlich stained and described megaloblastic erythroid precursors.[5] Giant myeloid band forms were observed in megaloblastic bone marrow in 1920, and the presence of increased numbers of nuclear segments in circulating neutrophils ("hypersegmentation") was described in 1923. Megaloblastic changes in bone marrow during relapse, with return of normal morphology during remission, were reported in 1921, 5 to 6 years before therapy for the disease was developed. In 1926, Minot and Murphy[1] described conversion of megaloblastic bone marrow to normoblastic bone marrow along with reticulocytosis and correction of the anemia after treatment with dietary liver. The sequence of these events has been summarized in several reviews.[2-4]

Among many subsequent observations, the following are among the most important:

1. Similar clinical syndromes (pernicious anemia of pregnancy and tropical anemia) were described by Wills in 1931 and subsequently demonstrated to be due to deficiency in folates.[6]
2. It was shown that in pernicious anemia, because of atrophy (destruction) of the gastric mucosa,[7] the stomach does not secrete enough of the intrinsic factor needed for absorption of cobalamin from the gut.[8] The disease is caused by failure to absorb adequate quantities of cobalamin.[4,9]
3. Cobalamin injections were found to correct pernicious anemia,[10] and administration of folate to resolve the anemia that was described by Wills. Each vitamin, when given in large doses, could produce some effect

on the hematologic abnormalities caused by deficiency of the other.[11,12]

4. The cobalamin-binding protein transcobalamin was shown to play a role in endocytosis-mediated uptake of cobalamin by cells.[13,14]
5. Assays for cobalamin and folates in serum and tissues permitted chemical definition of the deficiencies in patients with megaloblastic anemia.[15-17]
6. It was recognized that subacute combined degeneration of the spinal cord (SCDSC), a neurologic syndrome, often accompanied classic pernicious anemia but not the megaloblastic anemia caused by folate deficiency.[1,18]
7. It was shown that pernicious anemia is an autoimmune disease[19] caused by lymphocyte-mediated destruction of gastric parietal cells, with the possible immunologic target being H$^+$,K$^+$-adenosine triphosphate (ATPase) on the parietal cell membrane.[20-22]
8. Inherited defects in the metabolism of cobalamin and folates that may cause abnormal development in addition to megaloblastic anemia were identified.[23-26] Identification of the genes affected in these inherited defects has provided insight into cobalamin and folate metabolism in human cells.
9. Purification and subsequent cloning of the genes for intrinsic factor, transcobalamin, and haptocorrin, accumulation of information about their structure, and study of their receptors defined the function of these proteins.[27-32]
10. The pathways for cobalamin biosynthesis by bacteria, including aerobic and anaerobic pathways, were elucidated.[33]
11. Elevated plasma methylmalonic acid and total homocysteine were found to reflect functional deficiency of cobalamin and either folates or cobalamin, respectively, even in patients with vitamin levels within the normal range.[34]
12. It was demonstrated that NTDs, including spina bifida, can be prevented by maternal folate supplementation during the periconceptional interval.[35,36]
13. It was shown that the plasma total homocysteine level, recognized to be a risk factor for arteriosclerotic vascular disease,[37] could be decreased by folate supplementation and that polymorphisms in genes involved in folate metabolism could modulate the total homocysteine level.[38] The total plasma homocysteine level may also influence the incidence of bowel and other cancers.[39]

HEMATOLOGIC DESCRIPTION

Bone Marrow and Blood

The causes of megaloblastic anemia are classified in Box 11-1.

Megaloblastic bone marrow is hyperplastic, with erythropoiesis stimulated by increased levels of erythro-

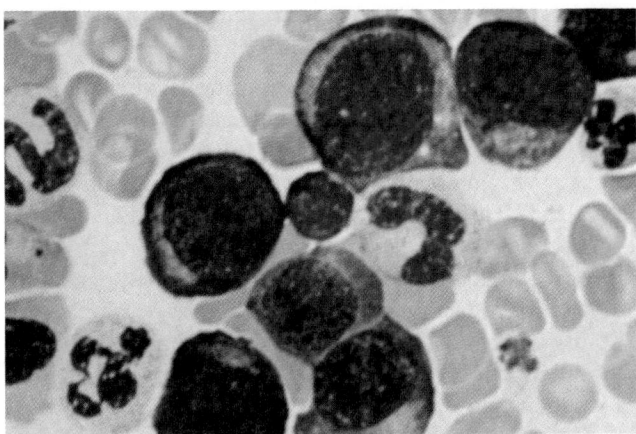

FIGURE 11-1. Bone marrow with megaloblasts. *(Courtesy of Dr. A. V. Hoffbrand, Royal Free Hospital, London.)*

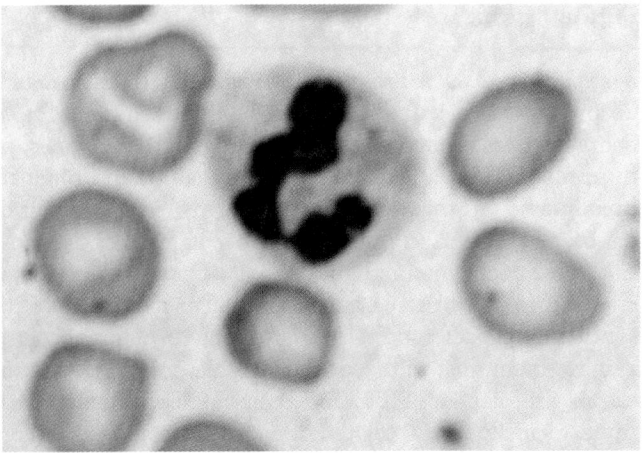

FIGURE 11-2. Multilobar neutrophil. *(Courtesy of Dr. A. V. Hoffbrand, Royal Free Hospital, London.)*

poietin acting on erythroid progenitor cells. Megaloblastic erythroid cells are prone to undergo programmed cell death, or apoptosis,[40,41] thereby leading to a left shift with young erythroid precursors predominating in the bone marrow. This "ineffective erythropoiesis" results in elevated serum levels of lactate dehydrogenase, bile pigments, and iron derived from dying erythroid precursors. Mature erythrocytes have abnormal shapes and are of various sizes, and their mean cell volume (MCV) is much greater than normal. Macrocytic and misshapen erythrocytes survive for a shorter time in blood than normal erythrocytes do.

Erythroid precursors have a normal DNA content together with an elevated RNA content. They have increased RNA per unit of DNA and are thus larger than normal cells at the same level of maturation.[42] Their nuclear chromatin appears looser than normal on stained smears (Fig. 11-1), which gives the characteristic appearance of the megaloblast. Maturation of the nucleus and cytoplasm is asynchronous, with the nucleus appearing less mature than the cytoplasm. For example, polychromatophilic erythroblasts with considerable accumulation of hemoglobin in the cytoplasm may have vesicular, open, or immature nuclei, and more mature orthochromic erythroblasts may contain nuclei that are not the dense, small, purple-staining pyknotic nuclei of normal orthochromes. Experienced observers usually recognize megaloblastic erythropoiesis by noting the vesicular and open nuclear pattern in the earliest erythroblasts (proerythroblasts and basophilic erythroblasts) (see Fig. 11-1).

Myeloid precursors are larger than normal, with giant metamyelocytes and band neutrophils being the most striking features. These cells may persist in bone marrow for 10 to 14 days after the start of treatment.[43] Giant metamyelocytes and band neutrophils are not seen in the megaloblastoid bone marrow of patients with leukemia or myelodysplasia. Similar abnormalities probably affect megakaryocyte precursors but have not been well described. Neutropenia and thrombocytopenia occur

more often with severe megaloblastic anemia, although both may occur in the absence of anemia.

Neutrophil hypersegmentation (Fig. 11-2) is defined as the presence of one or more six-lobed neutrophils or five or more neutrophils with five well-separated lobes among 100 segmented neutrophils. Multilobed neutrophils are a characteristic feature of the peripheral blood of cobalamin- and folate-deficient patients.

Other Tissues

Macrocytosis of buccal cells has been reported in patients with megaloblastic anemia. Similar abnormalities have been described in cells of the tongue, vaginal epithelium, urinary tract, and nasal epithelium. Decreased height of gastric cells and enterocytes has also been described. These changes reverse after treatment of the megaloblastic anemia.[44,45]

COBALAMIN (VITAMIN B₁₂)

Chemistry of Cobalamins

Cobalamins, members of the class of molecules called corrins, have the chemical structure shown in Figure 11-3. They consist of a planar corrin ring, similar to but distinct from that of porphyrins such as heme, with a central cobalt atom that coordinates with four nitrogen atoms of the corrin ring. A nucleotide, 5,6-dimethylbenzimidazole, coordinates with the cobalt atom below the plane of the corrin ring and attaches covalently as well to the corrin ring. The central cobalt atom may exist in three different oxidation states: the oxidized trivalent state (cob[III]alamin), the divalent state (cob[II]alamin), and the fully reduced monovalent state (cob[I]alamin). A number of different groups may be attached to the cobalt atom in the upper axial position (position "X" in Fig. 11-3) when it is in the cob(III)alamin state. Corrins that have coenzyme activity or can be converted to coen-

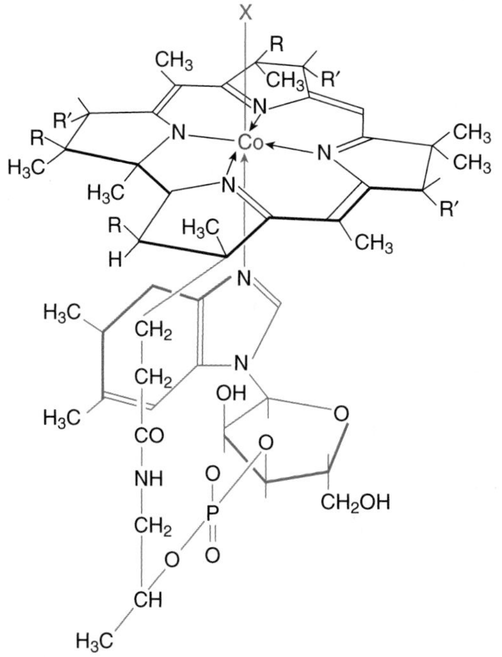

FIGURE 11-3. Cobalamin (vitamin B_{12}, Cbl) consists of a planar corrin ring (black) that coordinates with a central cobalt atom (red), with a 5,6-dimethylbenzimidazole base (blue) covalently attached to the corrin ring and coordinating with the cobalt atom. X (green) represents the upper axial ligand, which varies in different biologic and pharmacologic cobalamins. When X is methyl, the compound is methylcobalamin (MeCbl); when it is adenosyl, the compound is 5-deoxyadenosylcobalamin (AdoCbl); when it is CN, the compound is cyanocobalamin (CNCbl); and when it is OH, the compound is hydroxycobalamin (OHCbl).

zyme forms within the cell include cobalamins with CN (cyanocobalamin, CNCbl), OH (hydroxycobalamin, OHCbl), H_2O (aquocobalamin, H_2OCbl), SH (sulfitocobalamin, SOCbl), glutathionyl (glutathionylcobalamin, GSCbl), methyl (methylcobalamin, MeCbl), or 5'-deoxyadenosyl (adenosylcobalamin, AdoCbl) bound in the upper axial position, as well as cob(II)alamin and cob(I)alamin.[46,47]

Nutritional Sources and Requirements

Although cobalamin is required for metabolism by prokaryotes, animals, and many algae, it is synthesized only by prokaryotes. Two distinct pathways for de novo cobalamin synthesis have been identified, one anaerobic and the other requiring molecular oxygen.[48,49] Eukaryotes lack a biochemical pathway for de novo cobalamin synthesis and are dependent on diet for their cobalamin requirement. Some algae contain large amounts of cobalamin, which they apparently acquire through a symbiotic relationship with cobalamin-synthesizing bacteria.[50] Cobalamin is not required as a vitamin by higher plants, which neither synthesize nor accumulate cobalamin and thus do not contribute it to the diet.

The recommended dietary allowance of cobalamin for adults has been set at 2.4 μg/day, with the aim of ensuring absorption of 1 μg/day, assuming absorption of about 50% from food.[51] The World Health Organization has recommended a daily cobalamin intake of 1 μg for normal adults; 1.3 and 1.4 μg daily for lactating and pregnant women, respectively; and 0.1 μg/day for infants. Studies of chromosomal damage and uracil misincorporation into DNA in different populations suggest that this level may need to be higher, 7 to 10 μg/day, to ensure genomic stability.[52-54]

Because all of the cobalamin needs of humans are met through the diet, inadequate intake causes deficiency. Typical diets in developed countries contain more than adequate amounts of cobalamin, although cobalamin deficiency may occur in vegans, who consume no animal products whatever. Elsewhere, cobalamin deficiency may occur frequently in populations whose diet contains little meat.[51] On the Indian subcontinent, the concentration of vitamin B_{12} in serum and tissues is low in vegans, in lactovegetarians, and in nonvegetarians whose diets nevertheless contain little meat.[55-57] Low cobalamin levels have also been reported in populations in the Middle East, elsewhere in Asia, Africa, Mexico, and Central and South America.

SCDSC secondary to cobalamin deficiency has been described in vegans, but its frequency appears to be very low.[58,59] The reason for this is unknown and merits further study.

Cobalamin-Binding Proteins

Effective transmembrane transport of cobalamins into mammalian cells at the low cobalamin levels found in nature requires mediation of cobalamin-binding proteins interacting with receptors on the cell surface that recognize the cobalamin-protein complex. Three cobalamin-binding proteins play roles in the uptake and transport of cobalamin: intrinsic factor, transcobalamin (previously called transcobalamin II), and haptocorrin (also called transcobalamin I, transcobalamin III, cobalaphilin, and R binder). These proteins have similar primary sequences and intron/exon structure, thus suggesting that they have arisen by duplications of an ancestral gene.[60,61] They show 33% overall homology with each other, and specific regions demonstrate as much as 60% to 80% identity.[62]

Intrinsic Factor

Intrinsic factor, a 45-kd glycoprotein, is synthesized in gastric parietal cells in humans and is required for efficient uptake of dietary cobalamin in the intestine. It is readily digested by pepsin, but not by trypsin.[63] Intrinsic factor binds cobalamins less tightly (K_d = 0.1 to 1.0 nmol/L) than transcobalamin or haptocorrin does.[64] However, its binding affinity for cobalamins is far greater than that for nonfunctional corrin analogues such that the latter are not absorbed from the intestine. Intrinsic factor is encoded by the *GIF* (gastric intrinsic factor) gene on chromosome 11q13.[65]

Transcobalamin

Transcobalamin mediates the entry of cobalamin into a variety of cell types. It is found in plasma, cerebrospinal fluid (CSF), seminal fluid, and transudates and is synthesized in a variety of cells, including fibroblasts, macrophages, enterocytes, renal cells, hepatocytes, spleen, heart, gastric mucosa, and endothelium.[66] Transcobalamin is a nonglycosylated protein with a molecular weight of 43 kd.[67] Plasma turnover is rapid.[68] It binds cobalamin tightly (K_d = 5 to 18 pmol/L) to form holotranscobalamin (holo-TC) but has low affinity for corrins without vitamin B_{12} activity. The *TCN2* gene is localized to chromosome 22q12-13.[61]

Haptocorrin

The *TCN1* gene on chromosome 11q11-q12[69] encodes the haptocorrins, a family of proteins of approximately 46 kd that contain the same protein backbone but differ in their degree of glycosylation. They are synthesized by myeloid and probably other cells. Haptocorrins are present in many secretions, including plasma, bile, saliva, tears, breast milk, amniotic fluid, and seminal fluid, as well as in extracts of granulocytes, salivary gland, platelets, hepatoma cells, and breast tumors.[66,70,71] The fully glycosylated haptocorrin found in plasma has a low isoelectric point and a half-life of 9 days; haptocorrins with higher isoelectric points are cleared more rapidly from plasma into bile. Seventy percent to 90% of the cobalamin in plasma is bound to haptocorrin (holohaptocorrin, holo-HC), with the remainder being associated with transcobalamin; however, only transcobalamin-bound cobalamin is available for uptake by cells other than hepatocytes. Haptocorrins have the greatest affinity for cobalamins of all of the cobalamin-binding proteins (K_d = 3 to 7 pmol/L). In addition, they have considerable binding affinity for other corrins that lack vitamin B_{12} activity. An important function of haptocorrins in vivo may be the binding and excretion of such cobalamin analogues into bile.[72]

Cobalamin Binding

The three-dimensional structure of human transcobalamin has recently been determined. The protein has a two-domain structure with an N-terminal α_6-α_6 barrel and a smaller C-terminal domain. One molecule of cobalamin is bound between the two domains in the base-on conformation.[73] Similar studies with intrinsic factor or haptocorrin are complicated by their carbohydrate content, but studies of isolated domains from intrinsic factor and modeling of the three-dimensional structures of intrinsic factor and haptocorrin are consistent with a similar binding mechanism for cobalamin.[74,75]

Absorption of Dietary Cobalamins

Cobalamin in food is almost entirely protein bound. It is released from protein by the action of acid and pepsin in the stomach, where it binds to the haptocorrin present in saliva and gastric secretions. In the duodenum, the haptocorrin-cobalamin complex is broken down by pancreatic proteases with release of cobalamin, which then binds the intrinsic factor secreted by gastric parietal cells.[76] The intrinsic factor–cobalamin complex binds to receptors in the apical brush border of enterocytes in the distal ileum. Free cobalamin is not recognized by these receptors. The maximum quantity of intrinsic factor–cobalamin that can be bound to receptors in the human intestine is about 1.5 µg.[44]

The ileal receptor is made up of two proteins, cubilin (the product of the *CUBN* gene on chromosome 10p12.1) and amnionless (the product of the *AMN* gene on chromosome 14q32), and has been named "cubam." Cubilin is a 460-kd protein that consists of a 113-residue N-terminal region, followed by 8 epidermal growth factor–like repeats and 27 110–amino acid CUB domains.[77] It binds a variety of ligands in addition to intrinsic factor–cobalamin, including receptor-associated protein, albumin, apolipoprotein A-I/high-density lipoprotein, transferrin, immunoglobulin light chains, and vitamin D–binding protein.[62] It is present in the renal proximal tubule and yolk sac, as well as the ileum.[77] Amnionless is an approximately 48-kd protein that is expressed in the same tissues as cubilin.[78] In a dog model it binds tightly to cubilin and appears to be essential for the production of mature cubilin and its transport to the apical brush border surface.[79] Expression of both cubilin and amnionless is required for uptake of intrinsic factor–cobalamin.[79-81] Another multiligand endocytic receptor, megalin, is coexpressed with cubilin, but it may not play any role in intestinal cobalamin uptake.[77]

Intrinsic factor–cobalamin is rapidly internalized by endocytosis after binding to its receptor.[82] Attachment of cobalamin to transcobalamin appears to occur within enterocytes after its release from intrinsic factor, which is subsequently degraded.[83-85] Holo-TC appears in the portal circulation after about 4 hours. Involvement of the lysosomal compartment in uptake of intrinsic factor–cobalamin is suggested both by impairment of cobalamin uptake by agents that interfere in lysosome function[86] and by the finding of impaired uptake of cobalamin in patients with the cblF disorder, in whom release of free cobalamin from the lysosome into the cytoplasm is impaired.[87]

Cobalamin is excreted in bile, binds to intrinsic factor in the small intestine, and is reabsorbed. This enterohepatic circulation is interrupted in pernicious anemia such that depletion of cobalamin stores occurs more rapidly. Normal body losses have been estimated to be in the range of 2 to 4 µg cobalamin per day.

Cobalamin deficiency may develop in patients with heavy infestations of the fish tapeworm *Diphyllobothrium latum*, which has been shown to be capable of releasing cobalamin from intrinsic factor and accumulating it.[88] Removal of massive quantities of fish tapeworm from patients has corrected megaloblastic anemia. However, it is likely that cobalamin deficiency caused by the worm is restricted to patients with marginal secretion of intrinsic factor or malabsorption of dietary cobalamin. The recent increase in ingestion of raw fish may provide new cases for study and treatment.

Cobalamin malabsorption has been observed in some patients with intestinal blind loops or stenotic areas of the small bowel.[76] Malabsorption decreased after treatment with antibiotics (e.g., tetracyclines), thus suggesting that bacteria proliferating in stagnant intestinal areas compete with the host for cobalamin in the intestinal lumen, but the exact nature of the process remains unclear. The increased serum folate level observed in many of these patients is attributed to the synthesis of large amounts of folates by intestinal bacteria.

Entry of Cobalamin into Cells

Transcobalamin carries just a fraction of the cobalamin present in blood, but only cobalamin bound to transcobalamin is available for uptake by cells other than hepatocytes. Uptake is mediated by a specific membrane receptor present in many types of cells.[13,64,89] Several groups have purified holo-TC receptors from mammalian cell membranes that have differing properties.[90-93] The primary sequence of the physiologic receptor is not known, and no gene has been identified. There is rapid binding of holo-TC to the receptor at the cell surface, followed by slower internalization with degradation of transcobalamin and release of free cobalamin.[94,95] Internalization involves endocytosis, with holo-TC entering the lysosomal compartment; the process is disrupted by treatment with lysosomotropic agents such as chloroquine or ammonium chloride, which prevent acidification of the lysosome.[14,96] Transfer of free cobalamin from the lysosome to the cytoplasm appears to require a specific transport system, but it has not been characterized. This system is defective in patients with cblF disease and results in accumulation of free cobalamin within the lysosome.[97,98]

Cellular Cobalamin Metabolism

Cobalamin functions as a coenzyme in two reactions in humans (Fig. 11-4). MeCbl is required in the synthesis of methionine from homocysteine and 5-methyltetrahydrofolate (5-methyl-THF). This reaction is mediated by the cytoplasmic enzyme methionine synthase (5-methyl-THF:homocysteine *S*-methyltransferase, International Union of Biochemistry Enzyme Commission [EC] 2.1.1.13)[99,100]:

Reaction 1

Homocysteine + 5-methyl-THF → Methionine + THF

AdoCbl (Ado-B$_{12}$) is required for the conversion of methylmalonyl-coenzyme A (CoA) to succinyl-CoA, which is mediated by the mitochondrial enzyme methylmalonyl-CoA mutase (EC 5.4.99.2)[101]:

Reaction 2

Methylmalonyl-CoA → Succinyl-CoA

In prokaryotes, a variety of other enzymes use cobalamin for reactions that do not appear to occur in mammalian cells.

Once inside the cell, cobalamin is partitioned between the cytoplasm, where it is required for the activity of methionine synthase, and the mitochondria, where it is required by methylmalonyl-CoA mutase. Synthesis of the cobalamin coenzyme derivatives MeCbl and AdoCbl requires reduction of exogenous cobalamin, which is typically in the cob(III)alamin state, to cob(I)alamin before addition of the upper axial ligand. The early steps in this process remain poorly understood. GSCbl may play a role.[102] In bacteria, reduction of cob(III)alamin to cob(I)alamin requires the activity of two separate reductases catalyzing the sequential reduction of cob(III)alamin to cob(II)alamin and cob(II)alamin to cob(I)alamin.[103] A number of enzymes that catalyze these reactions in vitro have been identified in mammalian mitochondrial and microsomal extracts,[104-107] but their physiologic relevance has not been established. Two classes of inborn error of cobalamin metabolism, cblC and cblD, affect early steps in cellular cobalamin metabolism. The cblC disorder results in decreased synthesis of both AdoCbl and MeCbl; the cblD disorder may result in decreased synthesis of AdoCbl, MeCbl, or both. The genes underlying these disorders, *MMACHC* (cblC)[108] and *MMADHC* (cblD),[109] have been identified, but their functions have not been established.

Methionine Synthase

Methionine synthase is the major pathway for remethylation of homocysteine in humans. The reaction catalyzed by methionine synthase involves transfer of a methyl group from 5-methyl-THF to an enzyme-bound cob(I)alamin prosthetic group to generate MeCbl; the methyl group is subsequently transferred from MeCbl to homocysteine to form methionine and regenerate cob(I)alamin.[99,100] Maintenance of the enzyme-bound cobalamin in its active, fully reduced state requires the activity of a second protein, methionine synthase reductase. Once every 100 to 200 turnovers, the enzyme-bound cobalamin spontaneously oxidizes to cob(II)alamin; methionine synthase reductase catalyzes reductive remethylation to regenerate MeCbl by using *S*-adenosylmethionine (AdoMet) as methyl group donor[110,111]:

Reaction 3

Homocysteine + AdoMet → Methionine + AdoHcy

The gene encoding human methionine synthase, *MTR*, has been localized to chromosome 1q43.[112-114] It consists of 33 exons spanning over 60 kilobases (kb) of genomic DNA[115] and encodes a gene product of 1265 amino acids. The protein is 55% identical with cobalamin-dependent methionine synthase (MetH) from

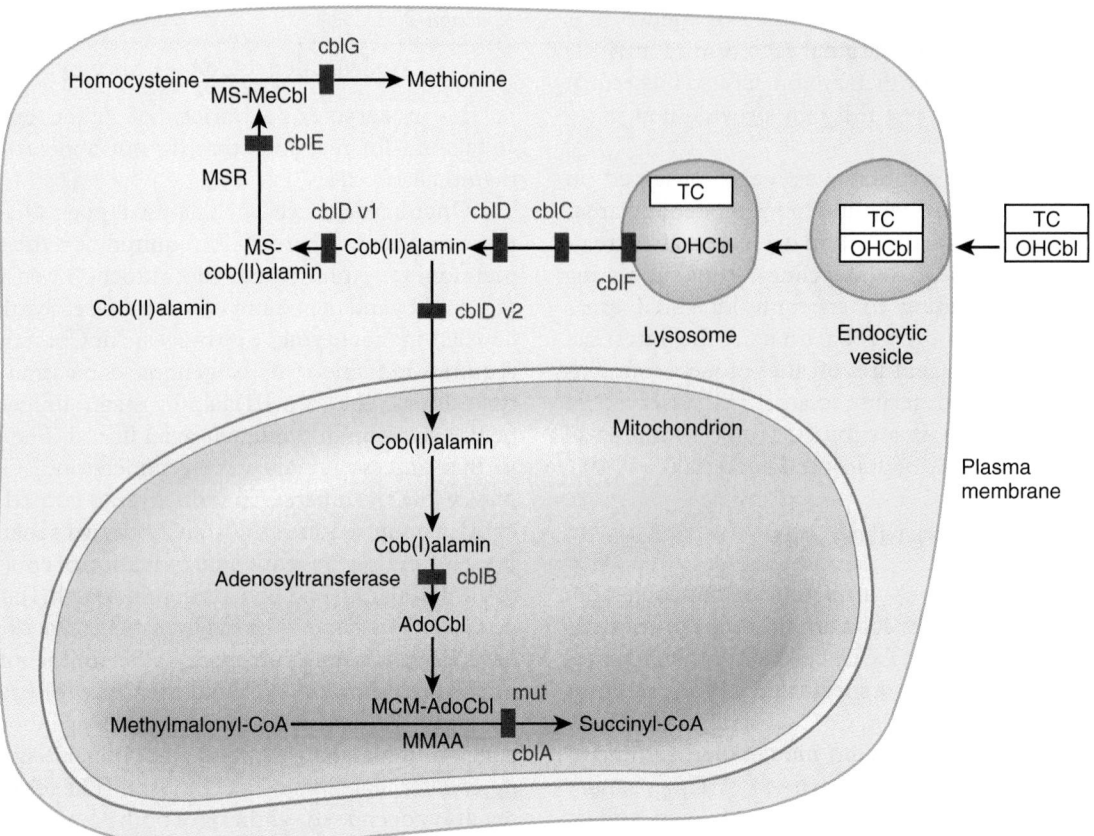

FIGURE 11-4. Scheme of cobalamin metabolism. The sites affected by methylmalonyl-CoA mutase deficiency (*mut*) and inborn errors of cobalamin metabolism (*cblA* to *cblG*) are shown in red. The cblA disorder is caused by defects in the MMAA protein; cblB is caused by defects in the cob(I)alamin adenosyltransferase (MMAB) protein; cblC is caused by defects in the MMACHC protein; cblD, cblD variant 1 (*cblDv1*), and cblD variant 2 (*cblDv2*) are caused by defects in the MMADHC protein; cblE is caused by defects in the methionine synthase reductase (MSR) protein; cblG is caused by defects in the methionine synthase (MS) protein; and the mut disorder is caused by defects in methylmalonyl-CoA mutase (MCM). The protein affected in the cblF disorder is unknown. MCM-AdoCbl, holomethylmalonyl-CoA mutase (mutase with bound adenosylcobalamin); MS-cob(II)alamin, methionine synthase with bound cob(II)alamin; MS-MeCbl, holo methionine synthase (synthase with bound methylcobalamin); TC, transcobalamin.

Escherichia coli,[113] in which enzyme function has been extensively studied. The *E. coli* enzyme is modular, with an amino-terminal homocysteine-binding domain,[116] a methyl-THF–binding domain,[116] a cobalamin-binding domain,[117] and a C-terminal activation domain that contains the AdoMet binding site required for methionine synthase reductase–catalyzed reductive methylation.[118] X-ray crystallography studies have demonstrated the importance of a triad of amino acids (equivalent to Asp783, His785, and Ser836 of the human synthase) in binding cobalamin to the enzyme. This is a component of an extended cobalamin-binding motif common to several cobalamin-utilizing enzymes, including methylmalonyl-CoA mutase.[119] The human enzyme has a similar arrangement of domains. Crystallography studies have shown structural differences in the activation domain, which interacts with the flavin mononucleotide–binding domain of methionine synthase reductase rather than the flavodoxin/flavodoxin reductase system used by the *E. coli* enzyme.[120]

When MeCbl is bound to methionine synthase, its dimethylbenzimidazole base is displaced from the cobalt

and its place is taken by the histidine residue (the "base-off" conformation), which facilitates the methyl transfer reactions of the catalytic cycle.[119] The histidine residue does not appear to be essential for the reductive methylation reaction.[121] Conformational changes in the protein result in apposition of the 5-methyl-THF–binding and the homocysteine-binding domains to the upper surface of the bound cobalamin at appropriate times during the catalytic cycle, as well as apposition of the activation domain to the upper surface of the bound cobalamin during reductive methylation.[122]

Methionine Synthase Reductase

The human methionine synthase reductase gene (*MTRR*) on chromosome 5p15.2-15.3 was identified and cloned on the basis of homology to the flavodoxin/flavodoxin reductase system that plays a similar role in the *E. coli* cobalamin-dependent methionine synthase.[110] *MTRR* encodes a 698–amino acid protein that is a member of the FNR family of electron transferases. Methionine synthase reductase has been shown to support the reduced nicotinamide adenine dinucleotide phosphate (NADPH)-

dependent activation of methionine synthase in vitro.[111] It may also act as an H$_2$OCbl reductase, as well as a stabilizing methionine synthase.[123]

Methionine Metabolism

Methionine is an essential amino acid in humans. The role of methionine synthase is to remethylate the homocysteine generated during cellular metabolism, thereby helping maintain adequate methionine levels, as well as preventing the accumulation of potentially toxic homocysteine. It also represents the only means of converting methyl-THF to THF because the reaction catalyzing the synthesis of methyl-THF from methylene-THF is irreversible under physiologic conditions. A cobalamin-independent enzyme, betaine–homocysteine methyltransferase (EC 2.1.1.5), catalyzes homocysteine remethylation in the liver[124]; however, in situations in which methionine synthase is decreased, as in inborn errors of metabolism or cobalamin deficiency, the betaine-utilizing enzyme is insufficient to prevent accumulation of homocysteine and its sequelae.

Cellular methionine may be used in protein synthesis or adenosylated to form AdoMet by the enzyme adenosine triphosphate (ATP)–L-methionine *S*-adenosyltransferase (EC 2.5.1.6):

Reaction 4

$$\text{Methionine} + \text{adenosine} \rightarrow \text{AdoMet} + 2P_i$$

AdoMet acts as a methyl group donor in at least 39 different AdoMet-dependent transmethylation reactions, including DNA methyltransferase 1, which catalyzes the methylation of cytosine residues at CpG sites of DNA, as well as enzymes catalyzing the methylation of RNA, lipids, proteins (including histones), neurotransmitters, and thiols.[125] These reactions generate *S*-adenosylhomocysteine (AdoHcy), which in turn can be hydrolyzed to homocysteine and adenosine by the enzyme *S*-adenosylhomocysteine hydrolase (EC 3.3.1.1):

Reaction 5

$$\text{AdoMet} + \text{R} \rightarrow \text{AdoHcy} + \text{CH}_3\text{-R}$$

Reaction 6

$$\text{AdoHcy} \rightarrow \text{Homocysteine} + \text{adenosine}$$

Intracellular homocysteine is generated from methionine by this cycle. Homocysteine may be remethylated by methionine synthase or betaine–homocysteine methyltransferase, or it may react with serine to form cystathionine in a reaction catalyzed by cystathionine β-synthase (EC 4.2.1.22). Accumulation of intracellular homocysteine results in increased levels of AdoHcy by mass action because the equilibrium of the reaction catalyzed by AdoHcy hydrolase favors synthesis rather than hydrolysis of AdoHcy.[126] AdoHcy in turn inhibits various AdoMet-dependent methyltransferases,[125] with potential adverse effects on numerous systems.

Synthesis of Adenosylcobalamin

The system responsible for transport of cobalamin from the cytoplasm to the mitochondria is not well understood, nor is the reduction state of the cobalamin that traverses the mitochondrial membrane known. Cobalamin uptake by isolated mitochondria was observed only in swollen mitochondria; under these conditions, OHCbl, AdoCbl, and MeCbl were taken up more effectively than CNCbl was.[127] Uptake was apparently achieved by diffusion, followed by binding of cobalamin to a mitochondrial protein, presumably methylmalonyl-CoA mutase, thereby resulting in unidirectional uptake. It is not clear how well cobalamin uptake under these conditions reflects physiologic processes.

Synthesis of AdoCbl occurs before the coenzyme becomes bound to methylmalonyl-CoA mutase. The terminal step in this process, adenosylation of cob(I)alamin by ATP–cob(I)alamin adenosyltransferase (Reaction 7), occurs in mitochondria:

Reaction 7

$$\text{Cob(I)alamin} + \text{ATP} \rightarrow \text{AdoCbl} + \text{triphosphate}$$

The gene encoding this enzyme, *MMAB*, has been identified and cloned. It is localized to chromosome 12q24 and encodes a 250–amino acid protein that is a member of the PduO family of ATP–cob(I)alamin adenosyltransferases,[128,129] one of three classes of cob(I)alamin adenosyltransferase that have been identified in bacteria. In addition to catalyzing the adenosylation of cob(I)alamin, adenosyltransferase may also act as a chaperone and deliver cobalamin in an activated (base-off) state to methylmalonyl-CoA mutase.[130-132]

Another protein, the product of the *MMAA* gene on chromosome 4q31.1-2, is also required for the function of methylmalonyl-CoA mutase.[133] *MMAA* encodes a protein of 418 amino acids that is a member of a family of auxiliary P-loop guanosine triphosphatases (GTPases), which includes proteins that function as chaperones in the assembly of metal cofactors. Studies of MeaB, an orthologue of MMAA from *Methylobacterium extorquens*, have shown that it interacts physically with methylmalonyl-CoA mutase.[134,135] MeaB (and by extension MMAA) may act in the GTP-dependent assembly of holomethylmalonyl-CoA mutase from apoenzyme and AdoCbl and in the protection of radical intermediates during enzyme activity.[136]

The majority of intracellular cobalamin exists bound to proteins; it appears that cobalamin is not retained in cells unless it is protein bound. Cytoplasmic cobalamin seems to consist exclusively of MeCbl bound to methionine synthase, whereas most cobalamin in the mitochondria is AdoCbl bound to methylmalonyl-CoA mutase.[138]

Methylmalonyl-CoA Mutase

The mitochondrial enzyme methylmalonyl-CoA mutase catalyzes the final step in the pathway that converts propionyl-CoA, generated during the catabolism of branched-chain amino acids, odd-chain fatty acids, and cholesterol, to succinyl-CoA. Mutase is encoded by the *MUT* gene on chromosome 6p12-21.2.[139,140] The human enzyme is a homodimer consisting of 77-kd subunits, with two molecules of AdoCbl bound per dimer.[141,142] The protein is synthesized in the cytoplasm as a precursor containing a leader sequence and is processed to a mature protein in mitochondria.[143] The structure and function of bacterial methylmalonyl-CoA mutase (from *Propionibacterium shermanii*) have been studied extensively. This enzyme is a heterodimer composed of an α and a β subunit. The human enzyme shows 60% sequence identity to the α subunit, the only subunit of the bacterial enzyme that binds AdoCbl,[144] and the results of studies of *P. shermanii* methylmalonyl-CoA mutase seem to be relevant to the human enzyme.

Methylmalonyl-CoA mutase contains the same extended cobalamin-binding motif present in methionine synthase. As with methionine synthase, the enzyme-bound cobalamin cofactor is in the base-off conformation, with a histidine residue from the enzyme replacing the dimethylbenzimidazole base at the central cobalt.[145] Binding of substrate to holoenzyme results in change from an "open" enzyme conformation to a "closed" conformation in which the active site is completely buried, coupled with displacement of the adenosyl group from the cobalt. Subsequent exchange of a carbonyl-CoA radical and a hydrogen atom located on vicinal carbons of the substrate results in conversion of methylmalonyl-CoA to succinyl-CoA.[101]

Biochemical Effects of Cobalamin Deficiency

The biochemical consequences of cobalamin deficiency result from decreased activity of the cobalamin-dependent enzymes methionine synthase and methylmalonyl-CoA mutase. Decreased activity of methionine synthase results in elevated levels of its substrate homocysteine in blood and excretion of homocystine in urine. Methionine levels in blood may be decreased or in the low-normal range. Decreased activity of methylmalonyl-CoA mutase results in accumulation of methylmalonic acid in blood and urine.

Diagnosis of Cobalamin Deficiency

Commonly, macrocytic anemia occurs and is accompanied by neutropenia and thrombocytopenia. The MCV is 120 fL or greater unless coexisting iron deficiency or a chronic inflammatory process is present.[146-149] The blood smear contains oval macrocytes and multilobed neutrophils. However, changing technology, including the use of automated cell counters, and the varying competence of technologists reporting blood smears may mean that oval macrocytes and multilobed neutrophils are not always reported. The bone marrow is usually megaloblastic.

Abnormal biochemical findings include increased levels of lactate dehydrogenase, bilirubin, and iron in serum, as well as increased transferrin saturation, which reflects "ineffective erythropoiesis." Serum cholesterol, lipid, and immunoglobulin levels may be decreased. These changes are not specific to cobalamin deficiency but are corrected with cobalamin therapy.[150,151] Increased serum gastrin and pepsinogen levels and antibody to gastric parietal cells, which signals the presence of atrophic gastritis, are equally nonspecific[152,153] because they do not distinguish those who lack intrinsic factor. The presence of antibody to intrinsic factor in serum is highly specific and indicates that the patient has cobalamin deficiency or that it will develop. However, it is present in 70% or less of patients.[19,152,154]

Serum Cobalamin Levels

The most direct evidence of cobalamin deficiency is an abnormally low serum cobalamin level. Although early studies using microbiologic assays showed that the serum cobalamin level was almost always less than 100 pg/mL (78 pmol/L) in patients with megaloblastic anemia secondary to cobalamin deficiency,[155] megaloblastic bone marrow is found in only 20% to 30% of patients with serum cobalamin levels less than 100 pg/mL. Therefore, significant cobalamin deficiency can occur without hematologic manifestations. Neurologic manifestations of cobalamin deficiency may appear before macrocytosis and classic megaloblastic anemia develop.[156]

The serum cobalamin level has been shown to reflect hepatic cobalamin in small numbers of subjects,[44] but the significance of low serum cobalamin levels without clinical evidence of cobalamin deficiency, abnormal metabolism of methylmalonate or homocysteine, or an abnormal deoxyuridine suppression test has not been determined. In many cases these patients are treated with cobalamin, with variable clinical benefit.[157,158]

In contrast, significant cobalamin deficiency may occur in the absence of low serum cobalamin levels in patients who do not have megaloblastic anemia. In one study the serum cobalamin level was greater than 100 pg/mL in 30% to 40% of patients demonstrated to have significant cobalamin deficiency; in 3% to 5%, the serum cobalamin level was in the normal range.[156,159] This failure of the assay to provide a near-perfect clinical correlation[160] is due in part to technical defects, including the specificity of the cobalamin binder used in some commercial ligand-binding assays. It also reflects the limits of the sensitivity and specificity of newer assays[161,162] when used as the sole measure of cobalamin deficiency, particularly when the assay is applied to populations lacking clinical features of cobalamin deficiency. In patients with megaloblastic anemia, the finding of a normal to increased level of serum folate, together with a reduced ratio of erythrocyte to serum folate, provides strong but indirect evidence of cobalamin deficiency.[163]

These studies suggest that evidence of functional cobalamin deficiency in addition to serum cobalamin levels (e.g., macrocytosis, multilobed neutrophils, and elevated levels of plasma methylmalonic acid and total homocysteine) should be sought when cobalamin sufficiency is evaluated in such populations, as well as in individuals in whom deficiency is suspected. The finding of increased serum levels of methylmalonic acid and total homocysteine provides evidence of functional cobalamin deficiency at the cellular level.

In patients who cannot absorb cobalamin, there is evidence that the amount of cobalamin bound to transcobalamin (holo-TC) decreases before the reduction in total serum cobalamin (mostly holo-HC) occurs.[164] Attempts to improve the clinical accuracy of serum cobalamin determination have focused on measurement of holo-TC, the physiologic component. Recent improvements have been made in the assay,[165,166] but the benefit of this measure over serum cobalamin is the subject of continued study.[158,167-169]

Tests of Cobalamin Absorption

In cases of deficient intestinal cobalamin transport, the diagnosis of cobalamin deficiency used to be confirmed by the demonstration of correction of cobalamin malabsorption by the administration of cobalamin with a source of intrinsic factor (urinary excretion tests, or Schilling tests I and II). Indeed, correction of the cobalamin malabsorption by feeding intrinsic factor and radiolabeled cobalamin together confirmed that a lack of intrinsic factor is the cause of the malabsorption and established that the patient has pernicious anemia.[170] Unfortunately, this "gold standard" for investigating cobalamin absorption is no longer readily available because of the increasing difficulty of obtaining both radiolabeled cobalamin and intrinsic factor. Native human intrinsic factor is no longer available, and hog intrinsic factor is rarely used because of health concerns.[171] Under development is a new test for cobalamin absorption in which changes in serum holo-TC are measured after a physiologic divided dose of cobalamin with plant-derived recombinant human intrinsic factor.[172-174]

Dietary Cobalamin Malabsorption

Malabsorption of dietary cobalamin is a disorder characterized by the inability to release cobalamin from food or its binding proteins.[175-177] It is measured by feeding subjects eggs, meat, or liver from birds or animals fed radiolabeled cobalamin. It is basically restricted to research laboratories and needs to be standardized in each. Patients have reduced serum cobalamin levels with normal free cobalamin absorption (Schilling test). Many have atrophic gastritis and reduced gastric peptic activity. Dietary cobalamin malabsorption affects about 40% of subjects with low serum cobalamin levels and is thus the most common cause of cobalamin deficiency. Proton pump inhibitors, which inhibit gastric acid secretion, can also induce dietary cobalamin malabsorption.[178]

Single-Sample Fecal Excretion Test

The single-sample fecal excretion test of cobalamin absorption avoided the pitfalls of tests that relied on urinary excretion. Labeled cobalamin (free or bound to food) was fed with a nonabsorbable dye (carmine red) together with nonabsorbable [^{51}Cr]chromic chloride. A sample of carmine red–stained stool was counted for ^{51}Cr and ^{57}Co and the ratio of counts compared with that in the sample that was fed. In normal subjects, 36% to 88% of a 1- to 2-μg dose of ^{57}Co-labeled cobalamin was absorbed.[179] This test is not readily available.

Measurement of Plasma Methylmalonic Acid and Total Homocysteine

The presence of methylmalonic acid in the urine of patients with pernicious anemia and its disappearance days or weeks after treatment with cobalamin was described in 1962.[180] Almost all subjects who are cobalamin deficient, both children and adults,[181] accumulate methylmalonic acid in plasma.[34,182-185] Indeed, elevated plasma levels of methylmalonic acid may be found before the appearance of macrocytosis, anemia, or other clinical features of cobalamin deficiency.

Homocysteine accumulates in the plasma of patients deficient in cobalamin, folate, or both.[34,156,159,181,186-188] Plasma homocysteine binds to free SH groups on proteins, and low concentrations may not be detected unless released from proteins by reducing agents, which yields the total plasma homocysteine concentration. Elevated total plasma homocysteine levels are found in more than 80% of patients who are deficient in cobalamin or folates.

An increased neutrophil lobe count and elevated total plasma homocysteine and methylmalonic acid levels indicate functional cobalamin deficiency and add to the interpretation of serum cobalamin and holo-TC measurements.[189] Although elevated plasma methylmalonic acid is more specific than total homocysteine for cobalamin deficiency, this test is more difficult to perform and is less widely available. Methylmalonic acid and total homocysteine levels, as well as holo-TC levels, are increased in patients with renal impairment. The relationship of elevated levels of total plasma homocysteine to NTDs, cerebral and cardiovascular disease, and the incidence of cancer is discussed later in this chapter.

Positive Therapeutic Test

Correction of hematologic, biochemical, and neurologic abnormalities after treatment with cobalamin represents a positive therapeutic test (Fig. 11-5). A single injection of 10 μg CNCbl is given. The test is positive if megaloblastic changes in the erythroid series in bone marrow disappear within 48 hours and at least two of the following occur:

1. Fifty percent decrease in serum iron or lactate dehydrogenase within 48 hours
2. Increase in the reticulocyte count 5 to 10 days after treatment
3. Correction of thrombocytopenia over a 2-week period

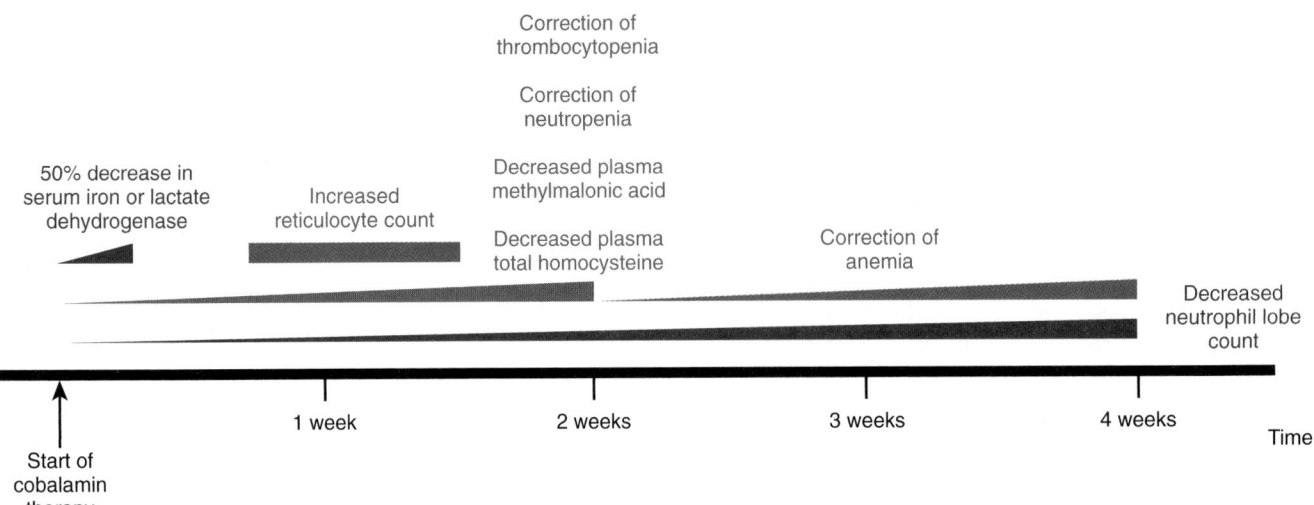

FIGURE 11-5. Timeline of clinical response of cobalamin deficiency after the administration of 10 μg of cyanocobalamin.

4. Correction of neutropenia over a 2-week period
5. Decrease in MCV by 5 fL or more after the reticulocytosis has subsided
6. Correction of anemia over a period of 2 to 4 weeks
7. Decrease in the neutrophil lobe count from the elevated to the normal range over a 4-week period
8. Decrease in elevated plasma methylmalonic acid and total homocysteine levels over a 2-week period

A diagnosis of folate deficiency can be established by treating the patient with a low dose of folic acid (in the range of 0.5 mg/day by mouth for 2 to 3 days) and monitoring for metabolic normalization and reticulocytosis in the succeeding 2 weeks. It should be noted that a dose of 2 to 5 mg of folic acid can induce reticulocytosis in most patients with cobalamin deficiency and 100 to 1000 μg of cobalamin can induce reticulocytosis in patients with folate deficiency.

Serum Cobalamin in Folate Deficiency

The serum cobalamin level may be decreased, even into the deficient range, in patients with megaloblastic anemia secondary to folate deficiency. The level increases over a period of 7 days with folate treatment unless the patient is deficient in cobalamin as well.[190] These changes may reflect alterations in the distribution of cobalamin between cells and plasma.

Deoxyuridine Suppression Test

The deoxyuridine suppression test[191,192] is based on the hypothesis that the activity of thymidylate synthase is decreased in cells deficient in cobalamin or folates because of lack of the folate coenzyme 5,10-methylene-THF polyglutamate. Such deficient cells have increased intracellular deoxyuridylate as a result of this decreased activity, and incubation of these cells with deoxyuridine would further expand the deoxyuridylate pool. In the test, bone marrow cells are incubated first with deoxyuridine and then with ³H-labeled thymidine, each for 1 hour, and

the quantity of ³H incorporated into cell DNA is determined.

In normal cells, thymidylate synthase converts deoxyuridine to thymidine during the initial incubation, with the amount of ³H-thymidine subsequently incorporated reduced to less than 10% of that observed when deoxyuridine preincubation is omitted. In bone marrow cells from a patient who is deficient in cobalamin or folates, preincubation with deoxyuridine reduces incorporation of ³H-thymidine into DNA to only 30% to 40%.

This defect in suppression of ³H-thymidine incorporation into DNA in cobalamin-deficient cells can be corrected by the addition of either MeCbl or 5-formyl-THF (folinic acid) during preincubation with deoxyuridine. Addition of 5-methyl-THF to deoxyuridine corrects the defect in folate-deficient but not in cobalamin-deficient cells. There is uncertainty regarding the biochemical processes actually being modulated during this test, but the deoxyuridine suppression test reliably discriminates between cobalamin and folate deficiency, except in patients with concomitant iron deficiency.

Treatment of Cobalamin Deficiency

Severe Deficiency

Patients with severe anemia may have accompanying heart failure because of the anemia itself, sodium retention, and myocardial hypoxia. Initial treatment includes the administration of oxygen and diuretics and slow red blood cell (RBC) transfusion to avoid circulatory overload. Clinical disasters have occurred during initial therapy. Treatment of severely anemic adults with pernicious anemia was associated with immediate death in 14% in one study[193]; however, more recent studies have not confirmed this result.[152] Disasters include life-threatening hypokalemia and cerebral and cardiovascular accidents (usually strokes secondary to thrombosis or embolism). To minimize the risk for severe metabolic disturbances such as hypokalemia in these patients, an initial dose of 10 µg CNCbl may be given subcutaneously for 2 days. This therapy is sufficient to normalize serum lactate dehydrogenase and iron levels and induce reticulocytosis in 5 to 7 days, but insufficient to normalize plasma methylmalonic acid and total homocysteine levels and replete body stores. For severely affected children, the dose of CNCbl is 0.2 µg/kg/day subcutaneously for 2 days.

The hypokalemia appears to be due to a shift of potassium from the extracellular to the intracellular compartment, accompanied by a delay in renal potassium retention. The clinician should anticipate this complication and provide a potassium supplement if needed. The role of potentially thrombogenic hyperhomocysteinemia in causing thrombosis and stroke during recovery is not known. These complications of initial therapy may affect children with severe cobalamin deficiency as well.

Conventional Therapy

Bone marrow aspiration should be performed before a transfusion is given to establish the presence of megaloblastic anemia and avoid the decrease in erythroid hyperplasia and changes in cell morphology induced by it. The RBC folate blood sample must be obtained before transfusion. Serum cobalamin and folate values are not altered much by transfusion but should be obtained beforehand as well.

Complete correction of megaloblastosis and associated metabolic changes requires anywhere from 15 to 150 µg of CNCbl. Conventional therapy has been 1000 µg of CNCbl or OHCbl by injection daily for 1 week, followed by 100 µg of CNCbl weekly for 1 month and then monthly thereafter. This therapy is believed to replete and sustain body cobalamin stores. Recently, oral and parenteral therapy with CNCbl or OHCbl has been compared and found to yield comparable benefits, particularly in regard to correction of the megaloblastic anemia.[194-196] Indeed, oral therapy with 1 to 2 mg cobalamin daily is cheaper and better tolerated and has become standard treatment in many countries. Whether oral therapy arrests the neurologic toxicity as quickly as parenteral dosing does is not yet known.[197] The answer would depend on the rapidity of delivery of the initial oral dose to the central nervous system (CNS) and on patient-to-patient variability. Another potential problem relates to "timed-release" cobalamin tablets with dissolution times of 3 to 6 hours, which are available in some countries and have been provided to patients by pharmacists.[198] "Timed-release" tablets have not been the subject of study. For these reasons it would be prudent to give an initial injection of cobalamin to patients with neurologic involvement.

Dementia and depression often respond rapidly to therapy, whereas other neurologic abnormalities improve gradually over a period of 6 months and may not return to normal. However, complete recovery from SCDSC in a bedridden patient with positive Babinski reflexes has been observed within 1 to 2 weeks after the start of cobalamin treatment (B. A. Cooper, personal communication).

Patients with pernicious anemia require indefinite replacement therapy. A prudent monthly dose is 100 µg CNCbl subcutaneously, although some patients require higher doses. Similar repletion plus maintenance of stores is achieved with injections of 1000 µg of OHCbl every 3 months[199] or 1000 µg OHCbl for 14 days every 6 to 12 months. The strong tissue binding of OHCbl permits such infrequent injections. Oral therapy consisting of 1 to 2 mg of cobalamin at intervals, with lower dosing in children and monitoring of plasma cobalamin levels periodically, is also an option. In some patients with pernicious anemia, cobalamin levels in serum or plasma can be maintained in the normal range with the daily ingestion of 50 to 200 µg CNCbl taken remote from meals.

In a few patients antibodies develop against the transcobalamin-cobalamin complex.[200,201] These antibodies do not appear to affect health but can result in very high levels of cobalamin in plasma. It is unclear whether this rare cobalamin allergy is more common after OHCbl, MeCbl, or CNCbl injections.

Cobalamin resistance is defined as correction of abnormal metabolite levels and clinical features in subjects with normal serum cobalamin values by treatment with pharmacologic doses of cobalamin. The cobalamin resistance encountered in subjects with diabetes, renal insufficiency, and advanced age may be attributable to kidney failure.[202-206]

In patients with apparent dietary cobalamin malabsorption, normal serum cobalamin levels and tissue stores can be maintained by feeding 10 to 25 µg CNCbl daily. Such treatment should be monitored periodically by measuring serum cobalamin, methylmalonic acid, total homocysteine levels, or any combination of the three. In children with inherited defects of cobalamin metabolism, injection of 1000 µg OHCbl two to three times per week is recommended. The effectiveness of therapy in such cases is monitored by measuring total serum homocysteine, methylmalonic acid, and methionine levels.

Development of Cobalamin Deficiency

Cobalamin deficiency may take years to develop because of the long half-life of cobalamin within the body (about 0.05% to 0.2% is lost per day)[207] and the large hepatic stores of the vitamin. The earliest manifestation in pernicious anemia results from loss of gastric intrinsic factor with reduced absorption of cobalamin from the diet, accompanied by a decrease in holo-TC.[164] Thereafter, levels of cobalamin in the liver and plasma decrease progressively. In most but not all subjects, the plasma cobalamin level falls below the normal range before clinical manifestations of deficiency are detected.[156,159]

The appearance of hypersegmented neutrophils and increased methylmalonic acid and total homocysteine levels in plasma may precede the development of classic megaloblastic anemia. However, bone marrow morphology may show abnormalities, and oval macrocytes may be observed on blood smear. Neurologic and mental disease may develop at this stage and not be recognized as being related to cobalamin deficiency in the absence of anemia, elevated MCV, or decreased concentration of cobalamin in plasma.[156,159] More prolonged deficiency results in anemia with a megaloblastic bone marrow accompanied by neutropenia and thrombocytopenia. These conditions are most commonly (but not exclusively) seen in patients with the most severe anemia.[155]

Patients with deficiency of cobalamin but without symptoms may be identified by laboratory testing, may have unexplained neurologic signs or dementia, or may demonstrate the full picture of megaloblastic anemia. Progression is more rapid in patients with low cobalamin stores and in those with an additional metabolic insult (exposure to nitrous oxide, simultaneous deficiency of folate, or exposure to antifolates).

Pernicious Anemia

Pernicious anemia is the most common cause of severe cobalamin deficiency in adults in developed countries. It results from the lymphocyte-mediated immune destruction of intrinsic factor–producing gastric parietal cells. This acquired lack of intrinsic factor results in malabsorption of cobalamin. Patients who lack intrinsic factor after gastric resection and those few with a genetic mutation yielding defective or undetectable intrinsic factor are not considered to have pernicious anemia.

Pernicious anemia is characterized by autoantibodies directed against the gastric parietal cells (specifically against parietal cell H^+,K^+-ATPase) and against intrinsic factor. Antibodies against gastrin and pepsinogen may be present as well. Progression of this type A chronic atrophic gastritis to gastric atrophy and clinical anemia takes decades. Thus, the frequency of pernicious anemia increases with age, with most new cases being detected in the fifth to seventh decades of life. In the seventh decade and later, the incidence of pernicious anemia reaches 250 to 500 cases per 100,000. However, rare cases have been described in children. Men and women are equally affected. Studies in Sweden, Denmark, and the United Kingdom between 1942 and 1968 reported an incidence of 100 to 130 cases per 100,000. As the population ages, the frequency of pernicious anemia will increase as well.

Pernicious anemia occurs predominantly in whites. It is less common in blacks, in whom it may appear at a younger age,[208] and it has been reported in Asians.[209] Pernicious anemia is more common in northern Europeans than in those of Mediterranean origin. This north-south gradient of case incidence was also detected within the United Kingdom and Holland.[44]

The existence of families with multiple affected individuals[210] and concordance for pernicious anemia in monozygotic twins[211] suggest a genetic component, although the mode of inheritance is not simple. Attempts to link pernicious anemia with HLA phenotypes have been inconclusive. Pernicious anemia may be associated with other autoimmune disorders, including chronic autoimmune thyroiditis, insulin-dependent diabetes mellitus,[212] Addison's disease, Graves' disease, vitiligo, myasthenia gravis,[213] and possibly Sjögren's syndrome.[214] Hypothyroidism is common and should be evaluated clinically and by measurement of hormone levels.[215]

Patients with pernicious anemia are at increased risk for carcinoma of the stomach,[216,217] which may be found before, coincident with, or years after the diagnosis is made. Annual gastroscopy with biopsy of suspicious areas is recommended. Patients showing mucosal dysplasia or chromosomal changes suggesting a premalignant state require more frequent assessment. The current lack of tests to demonstrate cobalamin malabsorption adds extreme complexity to deciding which cobalamin-deficient patients require such monitoring.

Classic Clinical Findings

Cobalamin deficiency, caused by either dietary deficiency or intestinal malabsorption, is manifested clinically through its effects on rapidly proliferating tissues, principally bone marrow and the lining of the intestinal tract, as well as the nervous system. The result is illness in which megaloblastic anemia, gastrointestinal symptoms, or neurologic degeneration (or any combination) may predominate.

Megaloblastic Anemia

Pernicious anemia is often manifested as severe macrocytic anemia accompanied by neutropenia and thrombocytopenia. The gradual onset of the anemia, to which the patient adjusts by gradually curtailing activity, means that the patient may be largely asymptomatic except for some weakness. Impending or actual congestive heart failure may be present, as may postural or activity-induced shortness of breath. Usually, some neurologic or mental symptoms and signs are also present, as are soreness of the tongue (glossitis) and other intestinal symptoms.

Gastrointestinal Features

In some patients the anemia and neurologic deficits are relatively mild and the predominant symptoms are gastrointestinal, including loss of appetite with minor (5% to 10%) weight loss, nausea, constipation, occasional diarrhea, and glossitis aggravated by spicy or "acidic" foods. Failure to notice mild macrocytic anemia or elicit neurologic abnormalities may result in unwarranted intestinal imaging and visualization. Although the gastrointestinal symptoms may be secondary to the "megaloblastic" changes in gut cells, the relationship of morphologic changes in buccal, esophageal, and enteric cells to glossitis, anorexia, constipation, and diarrhea is uncertain.[45]

Neurologic Disease

The neurologic syndrome of cobalamin deficiency is known as *subacute combined degeneration of the spinal cord.*

SCDSC consists of demyelination and degeneration of the posterior and lateral columns of the spinal cord, along with a peripheral neuropathy that is more severe in the lower than the upper extremities.[218,219] Decreased vibration and position sense is usually the first objective manifestations of SCDSC, with pyramidal tract signs being observed later. The latter may be masked by a decrease in tendon reflexes secondary to the peripheral nerve lesions.[220-222] Cerebral symptoms and optic nerve degeneration also occur. Magnetic resonance imaging (MRI) may reveal white matter changes.[203] SCDSC can occur with little evidence of anemia and includes some or all of the following features:

- Degeneration of the posterior spinal columns, which results in decreased vibration sense below the iliac crests in 48%, loss of position sense in the feet in 42%, and ataxia in 64% of patients.
- Degeneration of the pyramidal tracts, which causes spasticity and dorsiflexion of the toes (Babinski reflex) in 56% of patients.
- Peripheral neuropathy with distal paresthesia, anesthesia, and muscular weakness in 90% of patients.
- Dementia mimicking Alzheimer's disease.
- Depression, with or without dementia, in 90% of patients and affecting virtually all symptomatic patients.
- Optic atrophy, which is very rare in pernicious anemia.

Decreased vibration sense, recently described as the "mobile phone sign,"[223] and paresthesias in the legs probably affect most patients with symptomatic pernicious anemia, but SCDSC affects no more than 30%. In one series, paresthesias were noted in 30% of patients, whereas SCDSC was present in only 6% to 9%.

In many patients with SCDSC, MCV is elevated and the serum cobalamin level is in the deficient range. However, patients with neurologic disease but without anemia may have serum cobalamin levels above the range of deficiency. Therefore, the diagnosis of cobalamin deficiency in patients with neurologic problems should not be excluded on the basis of a normal serum cobalamin level.[157] Similarly, in patients with senile dementia or Alzheimer's disease, elevated levels of plasma methylmalonic acid and total homocysteine should be sought.[224]

The pathogenesis of the neurologic lesions in SCDSC is unclear. Similar neurologic lesions can be induced in primates (including humans) and pigs by chronic exposure to nitrous oxide,[225] which also produces megaloblastic anemia in humans. Nitrous oxide reacts with the cob(I)alamin generated during the catalytic cycle of methionine synthase and causes oxidation of the cobalamin prosthetic group and generation of a reactive oxidant, possibly a hydroxyl radical, that can attack and deactivate the enzyme.[226,227] The nitrous oxide–induced neurologic lesion can be prevented in monkeys and pigs with methi-

onine supplements.[225,228] Similarly, SCDSC is observed in patients with inborn errors that affect the function of methionine synthase in the presence of normal methylmalonyl-CoA mutase activity (the cblE and cblG disorders). These data suggest that SCDSC is the result of decreased remethylation of homocysteine, perhaps as a result of changes in the activity of AdoMet-dependent transmethylases.

The frequency of SCDSC as the initial feature of pernicious anemia appears to have increased over the past 40 years. In a study published in 1961,[229] 10% to 15% reported neurologic symptoms. Hall found neurologic signs in 35% of patients with this disease.[230] In 1988, a study in California reported neurologic or mental disorders in 50% of patients with cobalamin deficiency.[231] It is unclear whether the spectrum of the disease has changed or whether more patients without anemia are being recognized through the availability of RBC volume determination (MCV), as well as assays for serum cobalamin.

Subclinical or Preclinical Pernicious Anemia

Erythrocyte macrocytosis, detected by electronic blood cell analysis, identifies patients with pernicious anemia and others with cobalamin deficiency. Still others are identified through screening programs in at-risk populations, such as the institutionalized, the elderly, and those with neurologic or psychiatric impairments. The diagnosis is usually established by finding a low serum cobalamin or plasma holo-TC level together with an elevated plasma methylmalonic acid or total homocysteine level.[188,189,232-237] Current strategies to evaluate suspected cobalamin-deficient patients have been addressed and controversies highlighted.[162,171,238,239] Most disturbing are clinic-based studies in which patients with macrocytic anemia or neurologic deficits, or both, are tested and then treated with cobalamin irrespective of the test results. Some of those with normal metabolite levels clearly respond clinically.[157] Regardless of whether clinical manifestations of cobalamin deficiency are present, many patients showing biochemical evidence of deficiency volunteer that they "feel better" after treatment with pharmacologic doses of cobalamin.

Maternal and Pediatric Cobalamin Deficiency

Maternal Cobalamin Deficiency

Cobalamin deficiency in newborns is most often the result of deficiency in the mother.[240] Mothers following vegan, vegetarian, macrobiotic, and other special diets are at particular risk. Not surprisingly, poverty and malnutrition lead to cobalamin deficiency in mothers and children in many parts of the world.[241-244]

Severely deficient mothers may be sterile,[245] but those with depleted cobalamin stores because of a cobalamin-deficient diet or early pernicious anemia may bear cobalamin-deficient infants. These mothers have low serum and milk cobalamin levels, and their infants are born with low cobalamin stores that are not repleted during breast-feeding. If the mother has circulating anti–intrinsic factor antibodies, they may cross the placenta and impair intestinal cobalamin absorption during the initial weeks of life, particularly if the antibody titer is high.[246] Rare, asymptomatic, nonanemic cases of maternal pernicious anemia have been described.[57,247-249]

Maternal dietary cobalamin deficiency is usually associated with a strict vegetarian (vegan) diet entirely free of animal-derived nutrients,[250] but low serum cobalamin levels are also found in lactovegetarians and lacto-ovovegetarians. This is particularly so in immigrants to the West, where hygienic standards minimize the bacterial content of foods believed to be an important source of dietary cobalamin in Asian countries.[251]

Eating the macrobiotic diet described by Kushi and Jack,[252] which contains little animal protein, can deplete maternal cobalamin stores in as little as 3 years. Elevated urinary methylmalonic acid was found in 15 of 16 breast-fed infants of vegetarian mothers who ate a macrobiotic diet. Methylmalonic acid levels correlated inversely with maternal serum cobalamin levels, half of which were low. Maternal milk cobalamin levels were also low, and levels below 362 pmol/L correlated inversely with infant urinary methylmalonic acid. Functional cobalamin deficiency such as this appears to be much more widespread than hitherto thought.[250,253] Twenty-five of 58 pregnant Canadian adolescents 14.5 to 19 years of age had plasma cobalamin values in the suboptimal range (<148 pmol/L) at 36 weeks' gestation, and 71% of them had hypersegmented neutrophils.[254]

Up to 20% of normal pregnancies are associated with lower than normal serum cobalamin levels in mothers. These levels return to normal after delivery.[255] In a recent study, low maternal cobalamin levels were accompanied by elevated total homocysteine and methylmalonic acid levels and were the principal predictors of low cobalamin and raised total homocysteine and methylmalonic acid levels in the newborn. These abnormalities persisted for 6 weeks in the newborns. The authors concluded that cobalamin status in the neonatal period was strongly associated with maternal cobalamin status and parity.[256] The fact that parity increased the risk of low cobalamin status in mothers suggests that diet alone may be insufficient to replenish maternal cobalamin stores and that cobalamin supplements may be needed during pregnancy and after.

Healthy pregnant Korean women were less likely to have folate deficiency and more likely to have cobalamin deficiency than nonpregnant women were.[257] At the first antenatal visit, 61% of Nepali women had elevated serum methylmalonic acid, and 49% had low serum cobalamin values.[258] These authors recommended cobalamin supplements for this population. Worldwide cobalamin deficiency has been the subject of a detailed review.[51]

Less common causes of maternal cobalamin deficiency are gastric resection with loss of intrinsic factor–producing mucosa, fish tapeworm infestation, intestinal bacterial overgrowth, and sprue affecting the terminal ileum (see Box 11-1). Crohn's disease, ulcerative colitis, and surgical resection involving the terminal ileum may cause cobalamin malabsorption as well. Inhalation of the anesthetic gas nitrous oxide inactivates methionine synthase. Sufficient exposure to nitrous oxide can cause severe functional cobalamin deficiency with megaloblastic anemia and SCDSC in mothers or infants.[259,260] The effect of nitrous oxide exposure on the fetus during maternal nitrous oxide inhalation is unknown.

Cobalamin Deficiency in Newborns and Infants

Detection of cobalamin deficiency in newborns and infants can be challenging for clinicians, but the stakes are high because early treatment can prevent irreversible neurologic damage. The diagnosis is based on a high index of suspicion leading to demonstration of a low serum cobalamin level, an increased plasma total homocysteine level, and an increased plasma methylmalonic acid level, confirmed by response to parenteral cobalamin therapy. Assessment of the mother's diet and cobalamin status is important because maternal cobalamin deficiency is the most common cause of cobalamin deficiency in newborns and infants.

In adults, incipient folate or cobalamin deficiency is often suggested by a raised MCV, indicative of macrocytosis. Unfortunately, this is far less useful in detecting such deficiencies in children. In a study of 146 children 6 months to 12 years of age with an MCV of 90 fL or greater, macrocytosis was related to drug ingestion (anticonvulsants, zidovudine, immunosuppressive agents) in 51 of the cases. Other conditions associated with macrocytosis were congenital heart disease (20 cases), Down syndrome (12 cases), reticulocytosis (11 cases), marrow failure/myelodysplasia (6 cases), and miscellaneous causes (21 cases). No cause was found in 24 cases. No cases of cobalamin or folate deficiency were observed.[261]

In infants born to cobalamin-deficient mothers, severe cobalamin deficiency can develop in the early weeks of life. Indeed, cobalamin deficiency has become equated with severe megaloblastic anemia in children. This restrictive association is based on studies published in the 1960s and 1970s and supported by more recent individual case reports.[262-265] For example, frank megaloblastic anemia developed in a 10-month-old, exclusively breast-fed white boy. His mother had undergone a gastric bypass procedure for morbid obesity 2 years before her pregnancy and was not anemic despite a low serum cobalamin level and an abnormal Schilling test that corrected with intrinsic factor.[266] Cobalamin deficiency has been reported after surgery for necrotizing enterocolitis, particularly when resection has included part of the terminal ileum.[267]

A functional lack of cobalamin can be recognized by an elevated plasma or urinary methylmalonic acid level, an elevated total plasma homocysteine level, or a low plasma cobalamin level in infants born to cobalamin-deficient mothers or mothers consuming vegetarian, macrobiotic, and other diets low in animal protein. Many such infants may not be anemic or may have received transfusions. They can show variable neurologic deficits. Even such subclinical cobalamin deficiency, untreated, can result in long-term neurologic or psychomotor impairment.

Plasma methylmalonic acid and total homocysteine levels were elevated eightfold and twofold above controls in 41 infants receiving a macrobiotic diet. Levels were inversely related to serum cobalamin levels, which were remarkably low. The mothers had been on a macrobiotic diet for 3 or more years, had breast-fed their infants, and had later fed them according to macrobiotic principles. Despite the absence of hematologic or neurologic deficits, these children showed growth retardation and impaired psychomotor development when compared with omnivorous control children.[181,268] In some malnourished or diet-following child populations at risk, even those with the least evidence of deficiency may develop below their full potential. Cobalamin status should be determined in all children suspected of failure to thrive.

In children, perhaps more than adults, functional or quantitative cobalamin deficiency is often clinically obscure. Deficiency of cobalamin is rarely recognized in newborns seen after several months of life with failure to thrive, apathy, anorexia, refusal of solid foods, developmental regression, or any combination of these problems.[265,269,270] Megaloblastic anemia may be present or not. Neurologic deficits may need to be sought with care. The extent to which dietary folates or folate supplements may mask the clinical picture is unknown. Among more recent case reports, several have emphasized the persistence of neurologic deficits despite cobalamin therapy.[248,256,271-277] Cranial MRI studies have shown severe cerebral atrophy and retarded myelination,[263] but the neurologic deficits persisted even after complete resolution of all MRI abnormalities.[278]

Dietary lack of cobalamin in newborns and infants appears to be more common than previously thought, is not restricted to those following specific defined diets, and is not well enough known. For example, a study to assess the efficacy and safety of lowering dietary intake of total fat, saturated fat, and cholesterol to decrease low-density lipoprotein cholesterol in children failed to adequately assess cobalamin nutriture. Self-reported cobalamin intake was significantly reduced, but levels of cobalamin and methylmalonic acid were not measured.[279,280] Cobalamin deficiency should have been of concern with a diet favoring vegetable over animal protein.

The ability of the placenta to accumulate cobalamin results in higher newborn than maternal plasma cobalamin and holo-TC levels[281,282]; as a result, cobalamin deficiency is rarely present at birth, although stores of cobalamin may be reduced. Thus, the increase in meth-

ylmalonic acid level may occur after screening for hereditary organic acidurias, including methylmalonic aciduria, has been performed. However, in premature infants, cobalamin supplements proved more effective than those containing folate in reducing the severity of the anemia of prematurity.[283] Additional therapeutic trials could provide more precision in our knowledge of the cobalamin status of newborns.

The consistency of reports documenting the permanence of neurologic damage induced by cobalamin deficiency in newborns, often despite therapy,[256,272,273,276,278] suggests the need to add cobalamin to folate supplements before and during pregnancy. Added cobalamin would reduce the occurrence of both NTDs[284] and nutritional cobalamin deficiency in newborns, along with its risk of permanent neurologic damage.

The other major causes of inadequate cobalamin availability in newborns, detected within the first year of life or sometimes years later, are inborn errors of cobalamin metabolism (described in a later section).

Treatment of cobalamin deficiency in newborns and infants needs to be aggressive to arrest and reverse the neurologic and psychomotor damage. An initial cobalamin injection is recommended. Parenteral cobalamin at daily and then weekly doses of 100 to 1000 μg CNCbl, OHCbl, or MeCbl provides the best hope of success and replenishes cobalamin stores. However, oral therapy may be effective as well (see earlier). After the initial month, cobalamin injections (or oral dosing) can be spread out further. Once neurologic recovery has occurred, oral cobalamin daily doses of 5 to 10 μg CNCbl or another form can be continued. There are reports of a self-limited "infantile tremor syndrome" arising during cobalamin therapy.[248,271,285]

Cobalamin Deficiency in Older Children and Adolescents

Cobalamin deficiency in older children and adolescents shares many causes seen in adults. It may result from diets lacking cobalamin, prepared by parents or selected by teenagers.[286] Gastric and intestinal diseases may result in malabsorption of cobalamin. Pernicious anemia is extremely rare in children younger than 10 years and rare in teenagers. Obese children, particularly teenagers, are at increased risk of having low cobalamin levels.[287] Low serum cobalamin levels and decreased cobalamin absorption as determined by the Schilling test have been reported in patients infected with HIV but without acquired immunodeficiency syndrome.[243,288-290] Treatment with current highly active antiviral therapy improves cobalamin status. Moreover, treatment with cobalamin and folate reduces total homocysteine levels in such patients.[291]

In a survey on the effects of marginal malnutrition on human function carried out in rural Mexico, a deficient plasma cobalamin level was found in 19% to 41% of individuals. In preschool children, 8% and 33% had deficient and low plasma cobalamin levels, respectively, that persisted for more than a year. Plasma holo-TC was also low. Breast milk cobalamin was low in 31 of 50 lactating women. Deficiency was attributed to dietary lack of cobalamin combined with intestinal malabsorption.[292] In a study of 113 Guatemalan women and their infants, plasma cobalamin was low in 47% of mothers. Most had low holo-TC levels as well. Dietary lack combined with *Giardia lamblia* infection appeared to account for the cobalamin deficiency. Urinary methylmalonic acid was elevated in 12% of infants.[241]

Megaloblastic anemia developed in an 18-year-old woman undergoing diet therapy for phenylketonuria and led to assessment of cobalamin status in 37 adolescent and young adult phenylketonuria patients. Six had low (<150 pmol/L) and six had borderline low (150 to 200 pmol/L) plasma cobalamin levels.[293]

Cobalamin deficiency was identified in a series of infants of families eating a macrobiotic diet, and parents were persuaded to liberalize the family diet. A decade later, adolescents from these families were found to have persisting cobalamin deficiency with low cobalamin and raised methylmalonic acid and total homocysteine levels. These adolescents had impaired cognitive function in comparison to controls.[294,295]

Inborn Errors of Cobalamin Uptake and Transport

Deficiency of Intrinsic Factor

Fewer than 100 children have been identified with megaloblastic anemia and developmental delay as a result of an absence of effective intrinsic factor (intrinsic factor deficiency or congenital pernicious anemia, Mendelian Inheritance in Man [MIM] 261000). Evidence of cobalamin deficiency usually appears after the first year but before the fifth year of life, although clinical deficiency has appeared as late as 12 years of age in patients with partially defective intrinsic factor.[296] Patients have an abnormal Schilling test result that is corrected by exogenous intrinsic factor, but unlike classic pernicious anemia, they have normal gastric acid secretion and normal findings on gastric cytologic examination. In some cases no detectable intrinsic factor is produced[297,298]; in others, there is immunologically reactive but nonfunctional intrinsic factor, including intrinsic factor that has reduced affinity for cubam,[299] reduced affinity for cobalamin,[300] or increased susceptibility to proteolysis.[301] Several mutations have recently been described in the *GIF* gene in patients with intrinsic factor deficiency,[302,303] including some patients in whom Imerslund-Gräsbeck syndrome was clinically diagnosed (see the next section).

Imerslund-Gräsbeck Syndrome

Imerslund-Gräsbeck syndrome, or megaloblastic anemia 1 (MIM 261100), is usually accompanied by clinical manifestations of cobalamin deficiency in children between the ages of 1 and 5 years, although they may appear later.[304-307] At least 300 cases have been described.

Patients typically have failure to thrive, recurrent gastrointestinal or respiratory infections, pallor, and fatigue. Megaloblastic anemia is usually present. Neurologic signs may be relatively mild.[307] In many cases there is proteinuria that is neither of the classic glomerular or tubular type.[308] The disorder was initially recognized among Finns and Norwegians, but it is now more frequently diagnosed in patients from eastern Mediterranean countries. Patients have normal intrinsic factor, no evidence of antibodies to intrinsic factor or H^+,K^+-ATPase, and normal intestinal morphology. There is a selective defect in cobalamin absorption that is not corrected by exogenous intrinsic factor. It is now recognized that Imerslund-Gräsbeck syndrome is a result of deficiency of the intrinsic factor–cobalamin receptor complex, cubam. The proteinuria is a result of disruption of cubam function in the proximal tubule of the kidney.

A number of mutations in the *CUBN* and *AMN* genes have been identified in patients with Imerslund-Gräsbeck syndrome.[80,81,309] All the cases in Finland were due to *CUBN* mutations (three different mutations), whereas all Norwegian cases were due to *AMN* mutations (two mutations). Mutations of both *CUBN* and *AMN* were identified in patients of Middle Eastern origin.[309,310] In some Imerslund-Gräsbeck families, no mutations were identified and linkage to either *CUBN* or *AMN* was excluded, thus suggesting that mutations in at least one additional gene may cause this disorder. Several patients originally thought to have Imerslund-Gräsbeck syndrome on the basis of clinical studies have subsequently been shown to have mutations in the *GIF* gene,[303] thereby leading to the suggestion that sequencing of the *GIF*, *CUB*, and *AMN* genes represents a possible first-line strategy in diagnosing these diseases.

Treatment involves intramuscular injection of cobalamin, initially at 1 mg OHCbl daily for 10 days, followed by monthly injection afterward.[305] Successful treatment has also been reported with oral CNCbl.[172]

Transcobalamin Deficiency

Fewer than 50 patients with transcobalamin deficiency (MIM 275350) are known.[311,312] In these patients severe anemia develops at a much earlier age than in patients with other causes of cobalamin malabsorption, usually in the first months of life. Other symptoms include failure to thrive, weakness, and diarrhea in addition to pallor. The anemia is clearly megaloblastic, but some patients have pancytopenia or even isolated erythroid hypoplasia.[313] The presence of immature white cell precursors in a marrow that is otherwise hypocellular can lead to the misdiagnosis of leukemia. Neurologic disease has appeared from 6 to 30 months after the onset of symptoms.[314-317] Severe immunologic deficiency with defective cellular and humoral immunity has been reported, as has defective granulocyte function. In many patients serum cobalamin levels are normal[315] because most of the serum cobalamin is bound to haptocorrin. Many patients have no detectable transcobalamin, whereas others have immunologically reactive transcobalamin and one patient had transcobalamin capable of binding cobalamin, although the complex did not mediate vitamin uptake into cells.[318,319] Some patients have abnormal intestinal uptake of cobalamin that is not corrected by exogenous intrinsic factor on the Schilling test, thus indicating a role for transcobalamin in cobalamin transport across the enterocyte.

Although all the transcobalamin in fetal and cord blood is of fetal origin, infants with no detectable transcobalamin in their plasma do not demonstrate manifestations of cobalamin deficiency until several days after birth. Homocystinuria was present in two patients and methylmalonic aciduria in three of five patients before they received cobalamin therapy.[311] After discontinuation of therapy, methylmalonic aciduria may return.

Mutations in the *TCN2* gene on chromosome 22q12-13 have now been identified in several patients with transcobalamin deficiency,[312,320,321] including deletions, nonsense mutations, and a mutation resulting in activation of a cryptic intronic splice site. Transcob alamin is synthesized by cultured cells, including fibroblasts and amniocytes, and prenatal diagnosis is possible even when the specific mutation in a family is not known.[322]

Serum cobalamin levels must be kept very high if transcobalamin-deficient patients are to be treated successfully. Levels ranging from 1000 to 10,000 pg/mL have been required and are achieved with doses of oral OHCbl or CNCbl twice weekly (500 to 1000 µg) or with systemic administration of CNCbl or OHCbl (1000 µg) weekly or more often. Folate in the form of folic or folinic acid has been successful in reversing the hematologic findings in most patients, but it should not be given as the sole therapy because of the danger of hematologic relapse and neurologic damage, which was induced in one patient by folate supplementation without cobalamin.[311]

Haptocorrin (R Binder, Transcobalamin I or III) Deficiency

Deficiency or complete absence of haptocorrin in plasma, saliva, and leukocytes has been described in several individuals.[323-327] It is unclear, however, whether haptocorrin deficiency is a cause of disease in any of these patients. Although serum cobalamin levels are low, holo-TC levels are normal and the patients are not clinically deficient in cobalamin. The original report described two brothers, one of whom had optic atrophy, ataxia, long tract signs, and dementia.[323] A later patient had findings resembling SCDSC.[327] Haptocorrin may play a role in the scavenging of cobalamin analogues that may be toxic to the brain.[72]

Inborn Errors of Cobalamin Metabolism

A number of inborn errors of cobalamin metabolism, designated cblA to cblG, have been identified (Table 11-1). These disorders result in homocystinuria, methylmalonic aciduria, or both, depending on whether synthesis of MeCbl, AdoCbl, or both cobalamin cofactors is affected. Only disorders in which synthesis of MeCbl is impaired, either alone (cblE, cblG, cblD variant 1) or in combination with AdoCbl synthesis (cblC, cblD, cblF), are characterized by megaloblastic anemia.

The diagnosis of inborn errors of cobalamin metabolism is usually carried out with the use of cultured fibroblasts from patients because the pathways for cobalamin metabolism are expressed in these cells. Measurement in intact fibroblasts of function of the cobalamin-dependent enzymes methionine synthase and methylmalonyl-CoA mutase and measurement of conversion of labeled CNCbl to its coenzyme derivatives MeCbl and AdoCbl define the biochemical phenotype. Cell complementation analysis is used to accurately identify which complementation class a patient's mutation falls into.[328,329] This is particularly important for groups such as cblE and cblG,

TABLE 11-1 **Diagnostic Studies of Inborn Errors of Cobalamin: Correlation of Genetic Complementation Group with Biochemical Phenotype and Major Clinical Manifestations**

Clinical Manifestations	COMPLEMENTATION GROUP								
	cblA	cblB	cblC	cblD	cblDv1	cblDv2	cblE	CblF	cblG
MAJOR CLINICAL FINDINGS									
Megaloblastic anemia	–	–	+	+	+	–	+	+	+
Methylmalonic aciduria	+	+	+	+	–	+	–	+	–
Homocystinuria	–	–	+	+	+	–	+	+	+
LABORATORY FINDINGS: INTACT CELLS									
[57Co]CNCbl uptake	N	N	D	D	N	N	N	I	N
AdoCbl (%)	D	D	D	D	N	D	N	D	N
MeCbl (%)	N	N	D	D	D	N	D	D	D
Propionate incorporation	D	D	D	D	N	D	N	D	N
Methyl-THF incorporation	N	N	D	D	D	N	D	D	D

AdoCbl (%), adenosylcobalamin as a percentage of total cellular cobalamin; cblDv1, cblD variant 1; cblDv2, cblD variant 2; D, decreased; I, increased; MeCbl (%), methylcobalamin as a percentage of total cellular cobalamin; N, normal; –, finding is absent; +, finding is present.

which are otherwise identical at the clinical and cellular levels.

Inborn errors of cobalamin metabolism are autosomal recessive disorders, with each class being the result of mutations at a different gene. Most of the genes responsible have been identified, and molecular diagnosis is often possible. Common mutations have been identified, as well as mutations that occur frequently in specific ethnic groups, but most mutations are restricted to a single family. Molecular diagnosis of a new patient with no family history therefore requires sequencing of the entire gene. Thus, analysis of patient fibroblasts in culture remains critical for establishing the diagnosis, especially in families in which the responsible mutations are not known.

Prenatal diagnosis by biochemical analysis of cultured amniocytes or chorionic villus cells has been sought for most of the classes of inborn errors of cobalamin metabolism.[330-333] Analysis of amniocytes appears to be more reliable than that of chorionic villus cells. In addition, gas chromatography–mass spectroscopy or liquid chromatography–tandem mass spectroscopy has been used to detect the presence of methylmalonic acid or homocysteine in amniotic fluid. It is now possible to carry out prenatal diagnosis by molecular genetic analysis when the causative mutations segregating in the family have previously been identified. Two independent methods should be used for prenatal diagnosis to minimize the risk of false-negative or false-positive results.[333]

Functional Methionine Synthase Deficiency

Functional methionine synthase deficiency is characterized by elevated plasma homocysteine, homocystinuria, and hypomethioninemia without methylmalonic aciduria. On the basis of complementation analysis, two distinct groups of patients have been identified: cblE and cblG. The clinical and biochemical findings in the two disorders are virtually identical. Patients are usually seen initially in the first 2 years of life, but some have not been symptomatic until adulthood. The most common findings in both cblE and cblG disease include megaloblastic anemia and various neurologic problems, including developmental delay and cerebral atrophy.[334] Other findings include electroencephalographic abnormalities, nystagmus, hypotonia, hypertonia, seizures, blindness, and ataxia. Findings in patients with adult onset of symptoms have typically involved neurologic or psychiatric symptoms. In one patient with onset at 21 years of age, multiple sclerosis was diagnosed.[335] Methylmalonic aciduria is usually absent, thus indicating normal function of the second cobalamin-dependent reaction catalyzed by methylmalonyl-CoA mutase, although one cblE patient had transient methylmalonic aciduria.[336] The significance of this observation is not known.

Fibroblasts from both cblE and cblG patients show decreased synthesis of MeCbl and decreased activity of methionine synthase in the presence of normal AdoCbl

synthesis and methylmalonyl-CoA mutase activity.[334] In fibroblasts from a minority of cblG patients, there is no binding of labeled cobalamin to methionine synthase.[337] The specific activity of methionine synthase is decreased in cblG cell extracts under all assay conditions, whereas in cblE fibroblasts, decreased specific activity is observed only when the assay is conducted under suboptimal reducing conditions, a finding reflecting decreased activity of methionine synthase reductase.[334,338]

The cblG disorder is the result of mutations in the *MTR* gene, which codes for methionine synthase.[112,339,340] Twenty different mutations in the *MTR* gene, including missense and nonsense mutations, deletions, and splice site mutations, have been identified. One mutation, c.3158C→T (p.P1173L), is especially frequent and represented a third of all disease-causing alleles in a panel of cblG patients.[115] This mutation was present only in the heterozygous state, thus suggesting that homozygotes may not be viable. The cblE disorder is the result of mutations at the *MTRR* gene, which encodes methionine synthase reductase. Eighteen different *MTRR* mutations have been identified in cblE patients.[110,341-344] The most frequent are the intronic mutation c.903+469T→C, which leads to the insertion of 140 bp of intronic sequence into mRNA, and c.1361C→T (p.S454L), which is observed in patients of Iberian origin and may be associated with a milder phenotype.

Generally, systemic therapy with OHCbl, at first daily and then once or twice weekly, has been used to treat these disorders. This corrects the anemia and metabolic abnormalities. The neurologic findings have been difficult to reverse, particularly in cblG disease, thus emphasizing the importance of early diagnosis and therapy. A mother carrying a fetus identified by prenatal diagnosis as having the cblE disorder was treated from the second trimester with systemic OHCbl.[330] The baby was treated from birth and has done very well. It is uncertain how much prenatal therapy contributed to this favorable outcome.

Combined Deficiency of Adenosylcobalamin and Methylcobalamin

The cblC, cblD, and cblF disorders are characterized by decreased synthesis of both MeCbl and AdoCbl, with resultant deficient activity of both methionine synthase and methylmalonyl-CoA mutase. Affected individuals have combined homocystinuria and methylmalonic aciduria. The disorders apparently affect early steps in cobalamin metabolism subsequent to hydrolysis of holo-TC in lysosomes. In the cblF disorder, the defect appears to affect the transfer of free cobalamin from lysosomes to the cytoplasm (see Fig. 11-4). The processes affected in the cblC and cblD disorders remain unknown.

The cblC Disorder

The cblC disorder (MIM 277400) is the most common of the inborn errors of cobalamin metabolism, with more than 300 patients identified. Patients have homocystinuria and methylmalonic aciduria; in addition, hypomethioninemia and cystathioninuria are present. The infant is usually seen in the first year of life because of lethargy, poor feeding, failure to thrive, and developmental delay.[345] Most patients have megaloblastic anemia, and some have hypersegmented neutrophils and thrombocytopenia. In others, onset of the disorder occurs later in childhood[346,347] or in adulthood,[348-350] with findings of spasticity, myelopathy, delirium, dementia, or psychosis. A characteristic pigmentary retinopathy with perimacular degeneration has been observed in several patients[347,351-353]; other ocular manifestations have also been reported.[354,355] Some patients have had features of hemolytic-uremic syndrome.[356] Other reported findings in cblC disease include erosive dermatitis, hydrocephalus, and hepatic failure.[357,358]

Fibroblasts from cblC patients show decreased synthesis of both MeCbl and AdoCbl and decreased function of both methionine synthase and methylmalonyl-CoA mutase. Endocytosis of the transcobalamin-cobalamin complex and release of cobalamin from lysosomes into the cytoplasm occur normally,[95] but total intracellular cobalamin levels are markedly decreased in most cases as a result of the inability of cells to retain cobalamin that is not bound to intracellular proteins.

The gene mutated in the cblC disorder, *MMACHC* on chromosome 1p34.1, has recently been identified.[108] The function of its gene product is not yet understood. Mutations have been identified in more than 200 cblC patients. One mutation, c.271dupA, accounted for 40% of the identified mutations and is present primarily in patients of European or western Asian descent. Several additional recurrent mutations showed clustering on the basis of ethnicity. There is some evidence of genotype-phenotype correlation. The common c.271dupA mutation, as well as a c.331C→T (p.R111X) mutation, was associated with early-onset cblC disease, whereas a c.394C→T (p.R132X) mutation was associated with late-onset disease.[108,359]

Therapy for cblC disease can be difficult, particularly in patients with early onset. About a third of patients with onset in the first month of life die.[345] Some patients have improved with OHCbl therapy, 1 mg/day by injection, as assessed by a reduction in methylmalonic acid and homocystine excretion. Studies suggest that OHCbl rather than CNCbl should be used.[360] Therapy with MeCbl or AdoCbl has been used, but it is unclear whether these agents offer a therapeutic advantage. Systemic OHCbl treatment was much more effective than oral therapy, and betaine (250 mg/kg/day) appeared to be helpful when used in combination with OHCbl. Neither folinic acid nor carnitine had any effect.[360] Therapy with daily oral betaine and biweekly injections of OHCbl resulted in a reduction in methylmalonic acid levels, normalization of serum methionine and homocysteine concentrations, and resolution of lethargy, irritability, and failure to thrive. However, complete reversal of the neurologic and retinal findings did not occur, which emphasizes the need for early diagnosis and treatment. Even with good metabolic control, surviving patients generally have moderate to severe developmental delay.[345] The prognosis appears to be better in patients with a later age at onset.

The cblD Disorder

The cblD disorder (MIM 277410) was initially described in a single sibship in 1970. One patient was initially seen at 14 years of age with a history of mild mental retardation, severe behavioral pathology, and a poorly defined neuromuscular problem. There were no hematologic findings in this patient. His younger brother, clinically asymptomatic, was shown to have the same disorder. Cerebrovascular disease secondary to thromboembolism was detected at the age of 18 years in one of the brothers.[361] Both had methylmalonic aciduria and homocystinuria.[362] Fibroblasts from both brothers showed a biochemical phenotype indistinguishable from that of cblC fibroblasts, with decreased synthesis of both AdoCbl and MeCbl and decreased function of both methionine synthase and methylmalonyl-CoA mutase. Differentiation of cblD from cblC was achieved by complementation analysis.[363]

Recently, the cblD disorder has been diagnosed in additional patients with rather different clinical and biochemical findings.[364] Two patients had isolated homocystinuria in the absence of methylmalonic aciduria (cblD variant 1). A third patient had methylmalonic aciduria in the absence of homocystinuria (cblD variant 2). Clinical findings and the results of fibroblast studies for the patients with cblD variant 1 were identical to those of patients with cblE or cblG. Findings in the patient with cblD variant 2 were similar to those of patients with cblA disease. The gene on chromosome 2q23.2 affected in the cblD disorder (*MMADHC*) has recently been identified.[109] The function of the *MMADHC* gene product is not known. Mutations affecting its C-terminal region were associated with isolated homocystinuria, mutations affecting the N-terminal region were associated with isolated methylmalonic aciduria, and truncating mutations were associated with combined homocystinuria and methylmalonic aciduria. It has been suggested that MMADHC is involved in channeling cobalamin to its cytosolic and mitochondrial targets.

The cblF Disorder

At least nine patients with the cblF disorder (MIM 277380) are now known. Clinical findings have been variable, with none shared by all the patients who have been studied. Frequent findings include small size for gestational age, poor feeding, failure to thrive, growth retardation, and persistent stomatitis. Macrocytic anemia, neutropenia, thrombocytopenia, and pancytopenia have been observed. Two patients had minor facial abnormalities, and one had dextrocardia.[97,365-368] Typically, hyperhomocysteinemia and methylmalonic aciduria are present, although elevated homocysteine could not be detected in the blood of the first patient described. Cobalamin absorption and serum cobalamin levels have been decreased in some patients.[87,366,367] One patient died suddenly despite apparent clinical response to therapy with cobalamin.[365]

Fibroblasts from cblF patients show both decreased function of cobalamin-dependent enzymes and decreased synthesis of MeCbl and AdoCbl. Unlike cblC and cblD fibroblasts, large amounts of intracellular cobalamin accumulate, almost all of it unmetabolized free CNCbl present within lysosomes.[97,98,369] The defect in cblF appears to impair transport of the cobalamin that has been released from transcobalamin across the lysosomal membrane into the cytoplasm. The gene affected in this disorder has not been identified. Abnormal intestinal absorption of cobalamin has been observed in two cblF patients, thus suggesting that the same lysosomal transport system plays a role in the transport of cobalamin across ileal cells.[87,366]

The patients with cblF disease appear to respond to systemic therapy with OHCbl, although the first patient responded to oral cobalamin.[97,365-368] A concern in cblF disease is that patients may accumulate cobalamin in lysosomes to such an extent that it impairs other lysosomal functions.

The Methylmalonic Acidurias

Inborn errors affecting activity of the second cobalamin-dependent enzyme, methylmalonyl-CoA mutase, result in accumulation of large amounts of methylmalonic acid in blood, urine, and CSF in the absence of hyperhomocysteinemia. Methylmalonic acid levels are much higher than those seen in adults with cobalamin deficiency, and these patients are prone to life-threatening acidotic crises. Patients with isolated methylmalonic aciduria have been classified on the basis of biochemical studies and somatic cell complementation into three classes: *mut* (mutations in the gene encoding methylmalonyl-CoA mutase) and *cblA* and *cblB* (affecting synthesis of the AdoCbl coenzyme required for methylmalonyl-CoA mutase activity). Methylmalonic aciduria has also been observed in patients with mutations affecting the genes encoding methylmalonyl-CoA epimerase (*MCEE*)[370,371] and succinyl-CoA synthase (*SUCLA2*).[372,373] The incidence of all forms of methylmalonic aciduria in Massachusetts is about 1 in 29,000.

Methylmalonyl-CoA Mutase Deficiency (mut)

Disorders of the mutase apoenzyme result in methylmalonic aciduria that is not responsive to cobalamin therapy. Mutase deficiency has been subdivided into two classes: *mut*[0] cell lines have no residual mutase activity, whereas *mut*[−] cell lines show some residual mutase activity in the presence of added OHCbl, possibly reflecting enzyme with decreased affinity for AdoCbl. Several *mut*[0] cell lines synthesize no detectable protein, whereas others synthesize unstable proteins, and at least one has a mutation

that interferes with translocation of mutase to the mitochondria.[374] Similarly, variable levels of mRNA have been demonstrated in different *mut*[0] lines. There is no complementation between *mut*[0] and *mut*[−] cell lines, but intragenic (interallelic) complementation has been seen among some mut lines.[375,376]

Clinically well at birth, patients with mutase deficiency rapidly become symptomatic with protein feeding. They usually come to medical attention because of lethargy, failure to thrive, muscular hypotonia, respiratory distress, and recurrent vomiting and dehydration. In normal children, the methylmalonic acid level is generally less than 15 to 20 μg/g of creatinine; in contrast, in methylmalonic aciduria, excretion is usually greater than 100 mg and may be as high as several grams per day. In addition to methylmalonic aciduria, these patients may have ketones and glycine in blood and urine and metabolic acidosis with elevated levels of ammonia. Many also have hypoglycemia, leukopenia, and thrombocytopenia. One study[377] demonstrated that methylmalonic acid inhibits the growth of bone marrow stem cells in a concentration-dependent manner. Follow-up of children identified by newborn screening[378] has revealed a number who excrete methylmalonic acid and have mutase deficiency, as demonstrated by complementation analysis, and yet are clinically well and have never been acidotic. It is unclear whether these children are at risk for catastrophic acidosis later in life.

The *MUT* gene on chromosome 6p12-21.2 spans 40 kb and consists of 13 exons.[140,379] Nearly 200 mutations have been identified in the *MUT* gene.[380,381] Many of these mutations are private, but several are common within specific ethnic groups, including c.2150G→T (p.G717V) in mutase-deficient patients of African origin,[382] c.349G→T (p.E117X) in Japanese patients,[383] and c.323C→T (p.R108C) in American Hispanic patients.[381]

Therapy consists of protein restriction, with the goal of limiting the amino acids that are the major source of propionate in humans. Formula deficient in valine, isoleucine, methionine, and threonine is used. Mutase-deficient patients are not responsive to vitamin B[12]. Therapy with carnitine has been advocated in patients who are deficient.[384,385] Lincomycin and metronidazole have been used to reduce enteric propionate production by anaerobic bacteria.[386-388] Even with therapy the prognosis is guarded, and brain infarcts and renal dysfunction have been reported as late complications.[389]

Adenosylcobalamin Deficiency (cblA and cblB Disease)

The cblA and cblB disorders result in cobalamin-responsive methylmalonic aciduria and an intracellular deficiency of AdoCbl. They are distinguished by complementation analysis and by the fact that cblA cell extracts, but not cblB cell extracts, support the synthesis of AdoCbl from exogenous CNCbl. Intact fibroblasts from patients with both disorders do not synthesize AdoCbl from

CNCbl. A similar phenotype is seen in patients with the cblD variant 2 disorder,[364] including the patient previously placed in the cblH complementation class.[390] The cblB disorder results from mutations in the *MMAB* gene, which encodes ATP:cob(I)alamin adenosyltransferase.[128] The cblA disorder results from mutations in the *MMAA* gene, which encodes a protein of as yet unknown function.[133]

Most children with cblA or cblB disease become ill within the first year of life. Symptoms are similar to those seen in mutase deficiency but are less severe. Most cblA patients (90%) respond to cobalamin, with almost 70% being well at the age of 14 years. Less than half of cblB patients (40%) respond to therapy, and only 30% survive long-term.[391] Therapy involves the systemic use of either OHCbl or CNCbl. It is not clear whether AdoCbl offers any therapeutic advantage. Prenatal treatment of a fetus with deficient AdoCbl synthesis, ascertained via amniocentesis, by giving oral vitamin B_{12} to the mother[392] yielded a good therapeutic result. It is uncertain whether therapy starting at birth would have been equally effective.

The cblA and cblB disorders are inherited as autosomal recessive traits. Thirty mutations in the *MMAA* gene have been identified in cblA patients.[133,393-395] One mutation, c.433C→T (p.R145X), accounted for 43% of mutant alleles in a study of primarily North American patients.[393] This mutation was observed much less frequently in Japanese cblA patients; in this population, a c.503delC mutation, not detected in other patient populations, was frequent (8 of 14 mutant alleles).[394] Twenty-three mutations in the *MMAB* gene have been identified in cblB patients.[128,395,396] Many are predicted to affect the active site of the enzyme, identified from the crystal structure of its bacterial orthologue.[397,398] A c.556C→T (p.R186W) mutation represented 33% of affected alleles in the largest of these studies.[396]

FOLATE

Chemistry of Folates

Folates are heterocyclic compounds consisting of a pteroyl group conjugated with one or more glutamic acid units (Fig. 11-6). Folic acid, or pteroylglutamic acid, is an oxidized folate consisting of pteroic acid conjugated with a single glutamate residue. Biologically active folates are derived from folic acid by reduction of its pterin ring to form DHF and THF, by the addition of single carbon units at different redox states to nitrogens 5 or 10 of the pterin, and by conjugation of up to seven total glutamate residues by γ-carboxyl bonding. Intracellular folates exist primarily as one carbon group–substituted tetrahydrofolate polyglutamates. Folate derivatives that play an important role in cellular metabolism include 5-methyl-THF; 5,10-methylene-THF; 5,10-methenyl-THF; 10-formyl-THF; 5-formyl-THF; and 5-formimino-THF. Folic acid

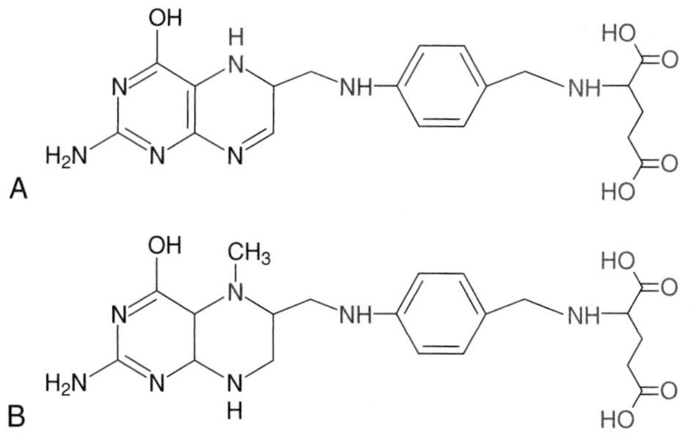

FIGURE 11-6. Structure of folic acid (**A**) and 5-methyltetrahydrofolic acid (**B**). Folic acid consists of pteroic acid (black) conjugated to glutamic acid (blue). Cellular folates are derived from this molecule by reduction to 7,8-dihydrofolate (DHF) and further reduction to 5,6,7,8-tetrahydrofolate (THF); by the addition of one carbon group to THF at nitrogens 5 or 10 (shown in red); and by the addition of up to six additional glutamic acid residues via γ-carboxyl bonding. Forms active in cellular metabolism include 5-methyl-THF (shown); 5-formimino-THF; 5-formyl-THF (folinic acid); 5,10-methylene-THF; 5,10-methenyl-THF; and 10-formyl-THF.

itself is available commercially as a stable yellow powder. It has low solubility in aqueous solutions and at acidic pH. 5-Formyl-THF (folinic acid, leucovorin) is a stable reduced folate that is available commercially. Other reduced folates are photolabile and susceptible to destruction by oxidation; they readily break at the carbon 9–nitrogen 10 bond to produce inactive catabolites.[399]

Nutritional Sources and Requirements

Folate is widely available in vegetables, fruit, and meat.[44,400,401] Foods with very high folate content include liver, kidney, orange juice, and spinach[402-404]; however, the reduced folates in food are labile to light and oxidation and are partly destroyed during processing and cooking. Inadequate folate intake is the most common etiology of folate deficiency causing megaloblastic anemia. The dietary folate requirement is a matter of dispute. The daily intake recommended by the World Health Organization is listed in Table 11-2. It should be noted that techniques for measurement of folate in diets can vary widely and give different results. The mean dietary folate intake in populations in which folate deficiency is unusual is about 3 µg of total folates per kilogram of body weight per day. This is about 150 µg/day for women and 200 µg/day for men. Folate levels measured in 500 liver specimens from such a population, most obtained from victims of trauma, appeared to be adequate.[405] In volunteers ingesting diets of known folate content, plasma and erythrocyte folate levels remained within the normal range when intake was 150 to 200 µg/day.[406,407] Intake of this magnitude was calculated for normal subjects by measurement of a catabolite of folate (*p*-acetamidobenzoyl glutamate) that is excreted in urine.[408,409] The recognition that the elevated total plasma homocysteine levels

TABLE 11-2	Recommended Intake of Folate and Cobalamin (Food and Agriculture Organization of the United Nations, 1988)	
Age	**Folate (µg/kg/day)**	**Cobalamin (µg/day)**
Infants	3.6	0.1
Ages 1-6	3.3	
Adults	3.1*	1.0

*For pregnant or lactating women, supplement with 300 to 1000 µg/day of folate and 0.3 to 0.4 µg/day of cobalamin.

in many patients with cerebral and cardiovascular disease are reduced with folate supplements, plus the reduction in NTDs as a result of giving mothers a folate supplement in the periconceptional period (even those with normal folate levels), suggests that effective folate deficiency can exist in individuals with apparently normal folate concentrations and no megaloblastic anemia.

Efforts to promote folate sufficiency through consumption of a healthy balanced diet have not been successful, and since January 1998, folic acid fortification of all enriched cereal grain products has been mandated in the United States,[410] Canada, and parts of South America. Current levels of folate fortification are 140, 150, and 220 µg/100 g of flour in the United States, Canada, and Chile, respectively.[411] As a result, the incidence of NTD-affected pregnancies has decreased by 26% in the United States and by 48% in Canada.[412,413] Serum and RBC folate levels are higher as well. However, less than 10% of women of childbearing age have reached the recommended RBC folate level of greater than 906 nmol/L,[414,415] which has been shown to reduce the risk for NTDs substantially.[416] There have been repeated pleas to increase the level of folic acid fortification.[417] To date, adding folate to food seems to have not "masked" the anemia of pernicious anemia.[411] Concerns about folate fortification delaying the diagnosis of cobalamin deficiency and promoting cancer growth and issues of choice have delayed mandating the addition of folate to the diet in Europe and elsewhere.[418]

Because 50% of pregnancies are unplanned, it is recommended that a 0.4-mg folic acid daily supplement be taken by women during the childbearing years to ensure adequate folate during the initial 30 days after conception.[414]

Human milk provides enough folate for the infant, but heat-sterilized bovine milk may not. Goat's milk contains little folate, and severe folate deficiency develops in children maintained on it alone.[419]

Subjects with Increased Folate Requirements

Maternal folate intake beyond that recommended to maintain normal RBC and serum folate levels may be necessary for maximum gain in birth weight and prevention of NTDs. Although folate deficiency can be recognized through its hematologic effects, with the lack of

such defects combined with normal total plasma homocysteine levels being interpreted as folate sufficiency, studies linking folate status with NTDs and with arteriosclerotic vascular disease (see later) suggest the need to re-examine what is meant by "folate sufficiency." Increased folate intake may be required for reduction of the risk of cardiovascular and cerebrovascular disease in at least some adults. Whether this reflects a greater need for folate in the general population or in one or more subpopulations with altered folate metabolism remains to be determined.

Folate requirements appear to be greatest in newborn infants and young children[420]; in pregnant women, in whom folate is shunted to the developing fetus and urinary folate loss is increased; and in lactating women, who secrete 50 µg of folate or more per liter of milk. Folate in milk is concentrated above and does not correlate with the level of plasma folate.[421] Other groups with greater than normal folate requirements include patients with tropical and nontropical sprue and other malabsorptive states; those taking antiepileptic medications[422]; women taking high-dose oral contraceptives[423]; and patients with hemolytic anemia, especially those with sickle cell anemia and thalassemia.

Physiology of Folates

Absorption of Folates from the Gut

Dietary folates are principally folate polyglutamates. They are hydrolyzed within the gut lumen or brush border or in the lysosomes of enterocytes to folate monoglutamates by γ-glutamylhydrolase. Transport of monoglutamates occurs primarily in the proximal small intestine and is promoted by a specific carrier-mediated system that is most active at acidic pH and shows similar affinity for reduced and oxidized folates.[424-428] Folate appears in portal venous blood within 15 minutes of entering the stomach and reaches a maximum level in portal venous plasma about 1 hour later. Reduced folates, such as 5-formyl-THF, are rapidly converted to 5-methyl-THF during absorption.[429] A second potential source of folate is that synthesized by bacteria in the colon, some of which exists as monoglutamates. There is evidence for a folate transport system in the colon with the same properties as in the small intestine system.[430-432] It may contribute to whole body folate homeostasis or at least support the folate requirements of colon cells.

Intestinal folate uptake has been attributed to the reduced folate carrier (RFC), which is expressed in human enterocytes, primarily at the brush border membrane but also to some extent at the basolateral membrane.[433-435] However, RFC-mediated folate uptake in vitro is optimal at neutral pH and shows a preference for reduced folates over folic acid, and no mutations have been detected in the *SLC19A1* gene, which encodes the RFC, in patients with hereditary folate malabsorption. This suggested that folate uptake under physiologic conditions is mediated by another carrier system.[436,437]

Recently, a proton-coupled folate transport protein with an acidic optimal pH and similar affinity for reduced folates and folic acid has been identified in the intestine and choroid plexus[438]; identification of mutations in the gene encoding this protein in patients with hereditary folate malabsorption has demonstrated that this is the physiologic intestinal folate transporter.

Some folates presented to the liver and some hepatic folates are excreted into bile and reabsorbed.[439,440] This enterohepatic circulation mediates slower and more even absorption than would occur in its absence. There is evidence that the enterohepatic circulation of folates is impaired with alcohol ingestion,[440,441] thereby contributing to folate deficiency.[442,443] The efficiency of absorption of folic acid, folate polyglutamates, and dietary folate varies in different subjects. In general, absorption of synthetic folic acid is about twice as efficient as that of folate in food, whereas folate from folate-fortified cereal grain food is absorbed about 1.7 times as efficiently as dietary folate.[444]

Transport of Folates in Plasma

Plasma folate consists almost entirely of 5-methyl-THF.[445] Most of it is unbound; some may be bound to albumin, and a small proportion is bound to a folate-binding protein[446-448] derived from the cell surface protein folate receptor α by cleavage of its membrane-anchoring domain.[449,450] Plasma folate-binding protein levels are increased in pregnancy, in folate deficiency, in renal failure, with breast and ovarian cancers, and with some types of inflammation. Its function in plasma is unclear.[451-453] It is present in milk, where it may function to improve absorption of folate by the newborn.[454,455]

Entry of Folates into Cells

Three distinct systems for cellular uptake of folates have been identified in mammals. The RFC supports a low-affinity, high-capacity system for uptake of reduced folates and methotrexate (an antifolate cancer drug) at high concentrations (in the micromolar range); it is less effective in the uptake of folic acid. The RFC appears to be an important folate transporter in many types of cells, including hemopoietic cells, and has been extensively studied in tumor cells. It is encoded by the *SLC19A1* gene on chromosome 21q22.3.[456-460] There is considerable heterogeneity among transcripts produced from this gene.[461-463] Although silencing of *SLC19A1* results in decreased folate uptake in rat intestinal cells in vitro,[464] the RFC does not appear to be the major specific intestinal folate transporter in humans under physiologic conditions. Inactivation of *SLC19A1* in mice results in neonatal lethality because of failure of erythropoiesis.[465]

A second high-affinity, low-capacity system for folate uptake, active at nanomolar folate concentrations, is mediated by members of the folate receptor family, which bind 5-methyl-THF (the predominant circulating form of folate) and folic acid. Three isoforms of the folate receptor are known. Two of these, designated folate receptor α and folate receptor β, are encoded by separate genes, designated *FOLR1* and *FOLR2*, on chromosome 11q13.3-11q13.5.[466] The genes are similar structurally but differ in their 5′ untranslated regions and in their transcriptional regulatory elements. The folate receptors are attached to the cell surface by a glycosylphosphatidylinositol anchor.[450] The circulating folate-binding protein referred to in the previous section is derived from folate receptor α by cleavage from this anchor. It has been suggested that folate receptors, as well as other glycosylphosphatidylinositol-anchored proteins, are sequestered in cell surface structures called caveolae, where folate is taken up by a process called potocytosis.[467] However, it is also possible that folate uptake occurs by endocytosis.[468] Uptake of folate bound to circulating folate-binding protein may be mediated by the large multiligand receptor megalin, which is expressed in intestinal, renal, and other epithelia.[469]

The contribution of these folate receptors to total folate uptake by cells is not known. The level of cell surface folate receptors increases greatly in cultured mouse cells grown in very low folate concentrations, thus suggesting that they play an important role in cellular folate uptake under these conditions.[470] In addition, homozygosity for an inactivated *FOLR1* gene in transgenic mice results in embryonic lethality in the absence of high-dose folate supplementation.[471] Treatment of pregnant rats with antibodies to folate receptors results in embryonic defects that are preventable with folate supplementation.[472] The presence of autoantibodies to folate receptors in mothers has been associated with the occurrence of NTDs in humans.[473]

A third folate transport protein, the proton-coupled folate transporter (PCFT), has recently been described. It is expressed in enterocytes and choroid plexus cells, has an acidic optimal pH, and transports reduced and oxidized folates with similar efficiency.[438] Identification of mutations in its gene in individuals with hereditary folate malabsorption suggests that this carrier is responsible for both intestinal folate uptake and transport of folates across the blood-brain barrier at the choroid plexus.[438]

Biochemistry of Folates

Intracellular folate metabolism involves the transfer of one-carbon groups at various oxidation states from glycine, serine, histidine, and formate to THF; interconversion of different THF derivatives; and transfer of one-carbon units to other molecules in the synthesis of purines, thymidine, and methionine. A scheme of folate metabolism is illustrated in Figure 11-7.

Reduction of folic acid to DHF and reduction of DHF to THF are catalyzed by the enzyme DHF reductase (EC 1.5.1.3.):

Reaction 8

$$Folic\ acid + NADPH + H^+ \rightarrow DHF + NADP$$

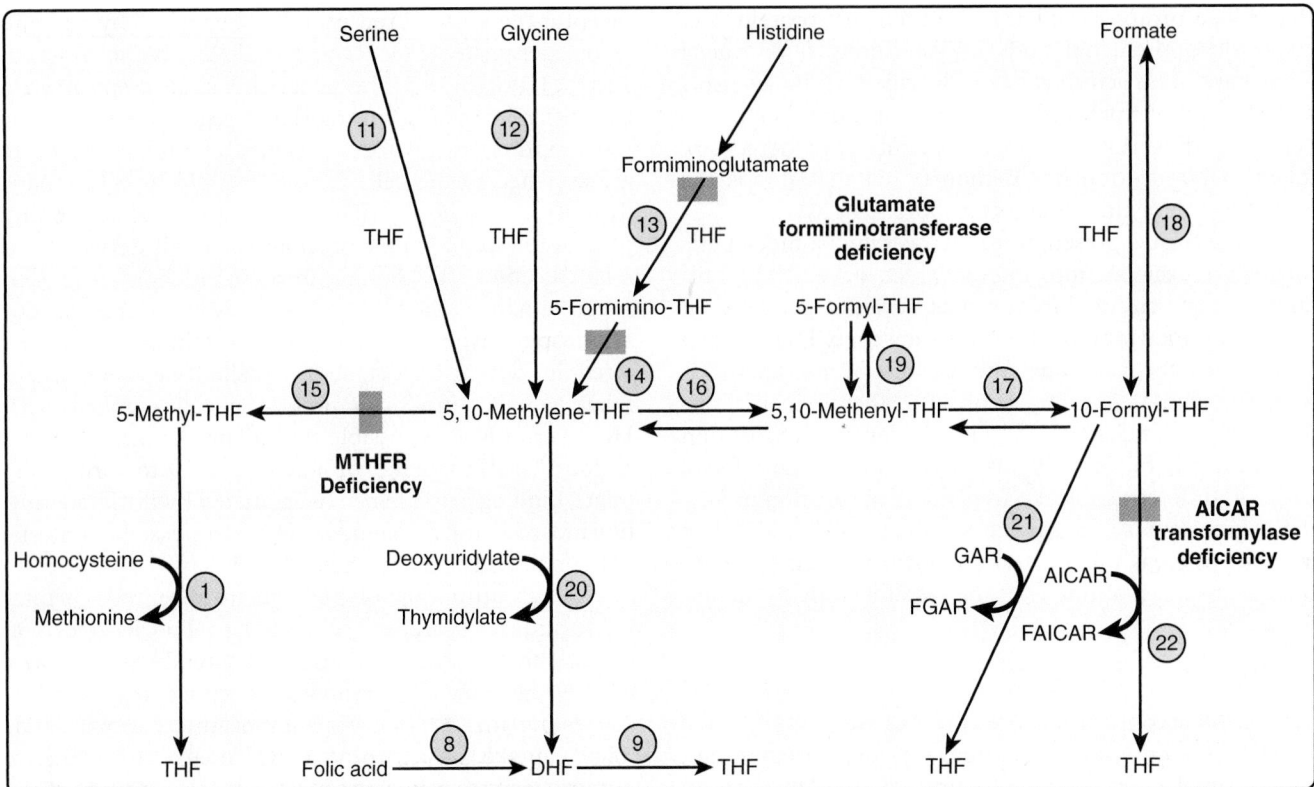

FIGURE 11-7. Cellular folate metabolism. Sources of one-carbon units are shown in the upper part of the figure and reactions that consume one-carbon units are shown in the bottom. Steps blocked in the three confirmed disorders of cobalamin metabolism are shown in orange; note that glutamate formiminotransferase deficiency affects both glutamate formiminotransferase (Reaction 13) and formiminotetrahydrofolate cyclodeaminase (Reaction 14) activities, which are carried on a single protein. Reactions are numbered as in the text. 1, methionine synthase; 8, 9, dihydrofolate reductase; 11, serine hydroxymethyltransferase; 12, glycine cleavage system; 13, glutamate formiminotransferase; 14, formimino-THF cyclodeaminase; 15, methylene-THF reductase; 16, methylene-THF dehydrogenase; 17, methenyl-THF cyclohydrolase; 18, formyl-THF synthetase; 19, methenyl-THF synthetase; 20, thymidylate synthase; 21, glycinamide ribonucleotide (GAR) transformylase; 22, amino-4-imidazolecarboxamide ribonucleotide (AICAR) transformylase.

Reaction 9

$$DHF + NADPH + H^+ \rightarrow THF + NADP$$

This enzyme shows higher affinity and a higher reaction rate for DHF than for folic acid. DHF reductase is required for reduction of any exogenous folic acid or DHF present in the diet, as well as for reduction of DHF generated from methylene-THF in the reaction catalyzed by thymidylate synthase.

A majority of intracellular folates exist as polyglutamylated derivatives, which usually contain a total of six or seven glutamate residues.[474] Synthesis of these folate polyglutamates depends on activity of the enzyme folylpoly-γ-glutamate synthetase (EC 6.3.2.17), which adds glutamate residues one at a time to reduced folates by using ATP as an energy source.

Reaction 10

Folate Glu_n + glutamate + ATP →
$$Folate\ Glu_{n+1} + ADP + P_i$$

DHF and THF are the preferred substrates for human folylpoly-γ-glutamate synthetase, whereas 5-sub-stituted derivatives (5-methyl-THF and 5-formyl-THF) are poor substrates.[475] The affinity of folate polyglutamates for most folate-dependent enzymes is much greater than that of the corresponding monoglutamates. This is critical for cellular folate metabolism because intracellular folate concentrations are far lower than the affinity constants determined in vitro for most folate-dependent enzymes when folate monoglutamate substrates are used. Moreover, folate polyglutamates are channeled between active sites in multifunctional enzymes such as C_1-THF synthase and glutamate formiminotransferase-cyclodeaminase (FTCD), whereas monoglutamates must diffuse between the active sites.[476] Folate polyglutamates do not readily cross the cell or mitochondrial membranes. Polyglutamylation of folates within cells thus contributes to the ability of cells to retain reduced folates in the presence of low extracellular concentrations.

Folate polyglutamates are converted to monoglutamates by the enzyme γ-glutamylhydrolase (EC 3.4.22.12), located in lysosomes and in the intestinal brush border.[477,478] Folate monoglutamates cross cell membranes much better than polyglutamates do, and adequate cellular nutrition is impossible without this hydrolysis.

Sources of One-Carbon Units

Intracellular folates exist predominantly as polyglutamate derivatives, and these are the forms that the various cobalamin-dependent enzymes interact with. In the biochemical schemes described in the following sections, the length of the polyglutamate chains of the folate coenzymes is not indicated.

The majority of one-carbon units for folate metabolism in mammalian cells are derived from catabolism of the amino acids serine and glycine. Interconversion of serine and glycine is catalyzed by the enzyme serine hydroxymethyltransferase (EC 2.1.2.1):

Reaction 11

THF + serine → 5,10-Methylene-THF + glycine

Breakdown of glycine is catalyzed by the glycine cleavage system (EC 2.1.1.10), a four-protein complex composed of P protein, H protein, L protein, and T protein:

Reaction 12

Glycine + THF + NAD$^+$ →
$$5,10\text{-Methylene-THF} + CO_2 + NH_4^+$$

T protein catalyzes the transfer of a one-carbon group from H protein to THF to form methylene-THF.[479,480]

Both these reactions are reversible, although there is no evidence that the glycine cleavage system catalyzes the fixation of NH_3 and CO_2 to form glycine in vivo. Serine hydroxymethyltransferase can catalyze the conversion of glycine to serine when cells are exposed to high levels of glycine.[481] The enzyme is present in both cytoplasm and mitochondria; the two forms are products of separate genes.[482] The glycine cleavage system is present only in mitochondria.

Another source of one-carbon units for folate metabolism is through the degradation of histidine, which generates formiminoglutamate. This compound reacts with THF to form 5-formimino-THF in a reaction catalyzed by glutamate formiminotransferase (EC 2.1.2.5). Formimino-THF is subsequently deaminated to form 5,10-methenyl-THF in a reaction catalyzed by formimino-THF cyclodeaminase (EC 4.3.1.4):

Reaction 13

Formiminoglutamate + THF →
$$5\text{-Formimino-THF} + glutamate$$

Reaction 14

5-Formimino-THF + H$^+$ →
$$5,10\text{-Methenyl-THF} + NH_3$$

Both these reactions are catalyzed by a single bifunctional enzyme, FTCD, which is an octomeric protein arranged as a tetramer of dimers in a planar ring[483,484] and present only in the liver and kidney. Although increased urinary excretion of formiminoglutamic acid (FIGlu) is a biochemical feature of folate deficiency, it is not measured frequently because of technical difficulties and lack of specificity.

Interconversion of Folate Coenzyme Derivatives

Methylene-THF is converted to 5-methyl-THF by the enzyme methylene-THF reductase (MTHFR, EC 1.5.1.20).

Reaction 15

5,10-Methylene-THF + NADH →
$$5\text{-Methyl-THF} + NAD^+$$

Methyl-THF is the predominant form of folate in plasma and intracellular fluids. It is required for activity of the cobalamin-dependent enzyme methionine synthase, as discussed in the section on cobalamin metabolism (Reaction 1). The reaction catalyzed by methionine synthase is the only means of regenerating THF from 5-methyl-THF in humans. Because the reaction catalyzed by MTHFR is irreversible under physiologic conditions and is inhibited by AdoMet, when activity of methionine synthase is impaired as a result of cobalamin deficiency or mutations affecting its activity, folate becomes trapped as methyl-THF and is unavailable for other folate-dependent reactions (the methyl trap hypothesis).[485] Methyl trapping is the reason that both folate and cobalamin deficiencies result in megaloblastic anemia.

5,10-Methylene-THF can also be oxidized by methylene-THF dehydrogenase (EC 1.5.1.5, Reaction 16) to form 5,10-methenyl-THF, which is then converted to 10-formyl-THF by the enzyme methenyl-THF cyclohydrolase (EC 3.5.4.9, Reaction 17). These two activities, together with formyl-THF synthetase (EC6.3.4.4, Reaction 18), are carried out in the cytoplasm of vertebrates by a trifunctional enzyme [486,487] that has been designated C_1-tetrahydrofolate synthase.

Reaction 16

5,10-Methylene-THF + NADP$^+$ →
$$5,10\text{-Methenyl-THF} + NADPH + H^+$$

Reaction 17

5,10-Methenyl-THF + H$_2$O → 10-Formyl-THF + H$^+$

Reaction 18

THF + ATP + formate → 10-Formyl-THF + ADP + P$_i$

A second mitochondrial 5,10-methylene-THF dehydrogenase that preferentially uses NAD rather than NADP has been identified.[488] It is part of a bifunctional enzyme that also includes cyclohydrolase activity and appears to have arisen by duplication of the gene encoding C_1-THF synthase, followed by loss of its formyl-THF synthetase domain and change in its cofactor dependence.[489] The mitochondrial bifunctional enzyme is expressed in embryonic and transformed cells, but not in normal adult tissues.[488] Mitochondrial formyl-THF synthetase activity has also been identified. This activity is catalyzed by an enzyme that was originally described as a mitochondrial C_1-THF synthase[490] but was subsequently shown to lack dehydrogenase and cyclohydrolase activity.[491] This enzyme also appears to have originated by duplication of the C_1-THF synthase gene with subsequent loss of 5,10-methylene-THF dehydrogenase and methenyl-THF cyclohydrolase activity because of mutations.

Conversion of 5,10-methenyl-THF to 5-formyl-THF is catalyzed by the enzyme methenyl-THF synthetase (EC 6.3.3.2).

Reaction 19

5-Formyl-THF + ATP →
$$\text{5,10-Methenyl-THF} + \text{ADP} + P_i$$

5-Formyl-THF does not serve as a cofactor for any reaction in cellular metabolism. Methenyl-THF synthetase is inhibited by 10-formyl-THF, which exists in equilibrium with 5,10-methenyl-THF.[492] This supports the suggestion that 5-formyl-THF acts as a storage form of folate[493,494] that can be converted to metabolically active forms when intracellular levels of 10-formyl-THF fall.

Utilization of Folate One-Carbon Units

Reactions that involve the use of one-carbon units attached to reduced folates include synthesis of methionine, with 5-methyl-THF used as methyl donor (see Reaction 1). Synthesis of thymidylate from deoxyuridylate, the final step in de novo thymidine synthesis, is catalyzed by thymidylate synthase (dTMP synthase, EC 2.1.1.45). In the course of this reaction, folate serves as both a one-carbon donor and a reductant, with the 6-hydrogen of 5,10-methylene-THF being transferred to the methyl group of dTMP. The DHF generated in this reaction is reduced to THF by DHF reductase (see Reaction 9).

Reaction 20

$$\text{5,10-Methylene-THF} + \text{dUMP} \rightarrow \text{DHF} + \text{dTMP}$$

Two steps during de novo purine biosynthesis use 10-formyl-THF as a one-carbon donor to generate carbons 2 and 8 of the purine ring. Conversion of glycinamide ribonucleotide (GAR) to formylglycinamide ribonucleotide (FGAR) is catalyzed by GAR transformylase (EC 2.1.2.2).

Reaction 21

$$\text{GAR} + \text{10-formyl-THF} \rightarrow \text{FGAR} + \text{THF}$$

Conversion of amino-4-imidazolecarboxamide ribonucleotide (AICAR) to formamido-4-imidazolecarboxamide ribonucleotide (FAICAR) is catalyzed by AICAR transformylase (EC 2.1.2.3). AICAR transformylase exists as a bifunctional enzyme with the enzyme that catalyzes the final reaction in purine biosynthesis, inosine 5′-monophosphate (IMP) cyclohydrolase.[495]

Reaction 22

$$\text{AICAR} + \text{10-formyl-THF} \rightarrow \text{FAICAR} + \text{THF}$$

Compartmentalization of Cellular Folate Metabolism

Because folate polyglutamates are unable to cross the mitochondrial membrane, cytosolic and mitochondrial folates form separate compartments. Folate-metabolizing enzymes in mitochondria differ from those present in the cytosol and represent products of alternative splicing (as folylpoly-γ-glutamate synthetase) or separate genes. It has been suggested that the mitochondrial NAD-dependent methylene-THF dehydrogenase favors the synthesis of formyl-THF whereas the cytosolic NADPH-dependent enzyme favors methylene-THF synthesis. Expression of the mitochondrial enzyme, which occurs only in rapidly proliferating tissues, would result in the synthesis of formate, which after crossing the mitochondrial membrane could be used for synthesis of the 10-formyl-THF needed for purine biosynthesis in the cytoplasm.[496]

Folate Deficiency

Next to iron deficiency, folate deficiency is the most common micronutrient deficiency. It is prevalent worldwide and coexists with poverty, malnutrition, and chronic parasitic, bacterial, and viral infections. Women are more frequently affected than men. Inadequate diet, overcooking of vegetables with loss of folates, and malabsorption secondary to tropical sprue are important contributors. Interestingly, vegetarian diets low in animal protein can provide more folate than omnivorous diets such as those eaten in the West.[181] Also at increased risk are the elderly, the very young, and pregnant and lactating mothers. In addition, many Europeans and North Americans fail to consume 200 μg of folates daily. Megaloblastic anemia secondary to folate deficiency is common worldwide, as is anemia with megaloblastosis in patients with multifactorial malnutrition and ill health. The finding of elevated total plasma homocysteine levels in patients with cerebrovascular and cardiovascular disease and their reduction with folate supplements, plus the reduction in NTDs as a result of giving mothers a folate supplement in the periconceptional period (even those with normal folate levels), raise questions about the definition of dietary folate sufficiency (see later).

Diagnosis of Folate Deficiency

The hematologic diagnosis of folate deficiency is similar to that for cobalamin deficiency. The bone marrow is indistinguishable from that in deficiency of cobalamin, and the same abnormalities may be noted in clinical chemistry data. In most patients who are deficient in folate, serum and erythrocyte folate levels are low. The level of serum folate (normal range, 4 to 20 ng/mL [8.8 to 44.0 nmol/L]) decreases rapidly during folate deprivation and falls into the range of deficiency (<3 ng/mL or 6.6 nmol/L) within 2 weeks of cessation of folate intake.[497] The erythrocyte folate level decreases slowly (normal, 200 to 800 ng/mL [440 to 1800 nmol/L]) because deficient erythrocytes replace sufficient ones during the 3- to 4-month turnover of RBCs. Most deficient subjects have erythrocyte folate values that are less than 150 ng/mL (330 nmol/L). With chronic low folate intake or malabsorption, both values fall into the deficient range, whereas patients in whom deficiency develops rapidly from alcohol abuse, from receiving unsupplemented intravenous amino acids, or from some antibiotics may have low serum folate levels only. The level of FIGlu in a 24-hour urine sample with or without a histidine load is often elevated in patients with folate deficiency but is infrequently measured.

Total plasma homocysteine, but not methylmalonic acid, is increased in the majority of patients with folate deficiency.[498] The result of the deoxyuridine suppression test with bone marrow cells is abnormal and is corrected by the addition of 5-formyl-THF, 5-methyl-THF, or other folates during preincubation with deoxyuridine (see earlier).

Erythrocyte Folate Levels in Cobalamin Deficiency

Erythroid precursors in the bone marrow accumulate 5-methyl-THF from plasma and convert it to THF by means of the cobalamin-dependent enzyme methionine synthase. THF is converted to THF polyglutamates and retained in mature RBCs as 5-methyl-THF polygluta-mates. The reaction catalyzed by methionine synthase is impaired in cobalamin-deficient cells, and 5-methyl-THF is a poor substrate for polyglutamylation, such that patients deficient in cobalamin have lower erythrocyte folate levels together with normal or raised serum folate levels.[163,499] This interpretation of the cause of erythrocyte folate changes in cobalamin deficiency is known as the "methylfolate trap hypothesis."

Treatment of Folate Deficiency

Five mg of folic acid daily by mouth (100 µg/kg body weight for children) is sufficient to correct folate deficiency, whether dietary or secondary to malabsorption. The megaloblastic anemia responds to very small doses of folic acid (200 to 500 µg/day), and the response provides verification of the diagnosis because that caused by cobalamin deficiency does not respond to such low doses of folate. Daily treatment with 1 mg is more than adequate. Larger doses are usually given because folic acid is available in 5-mg tablets. There is concern that folate can exacerbate the neurologic damage in patients with cobalamin deficiency by delaying diagnosis and treatment. In patients with inborn errors of cobalamin metabolism mistreated with folate, neurologic degeneration has occurred.[361]

Above oral doses of 200 µg of folic acid, unmetabolized folic acid appears in the circulation.[500] However, such unmetabolized folic acid has never been associated with toxicity in patients such as those with sickle cell disease or other hemolytic anemias who are receiving long-term folic acid supplements. Likewise, the unnatural isomer *dl*-5-formyl-THF has never been associated with toxicity.

Reduction in plasma zinc in newborns was attributed to a dose of 1 mg oral folic acid daily, but not to doses of 0.05 to 0.2 mg/day.[501] Although such lower doses are both effective and prudent, there are no firm data attributing toxicity to folic acid.

Nutritional folate deficiency requires an improved diet or a folate supplement, or both. For patients with folate malabsorption, 5 to 15 mg/day of folate should yield normal or high serum and erythrocyte folate levels.

Clinical responses have been reported in a small number of patients with dementia, restless leg syndrome, and other neurologic ailments treated with large doses of folic or folinic acid.[502-504]

Maternal and Pediatric Folate Deficiency

Maternal Folate Deficiency

The major problem with folate insufficiency in children occurs before rather than after birth. It has been well established that maternal folate deficiency in the periconceptional period is the cause of more than 50% of cases of NTDs, including spina bifida, meningomyelocele, and anencephaly.[35,36,505] Intrauterine growth retardation has also been linked to reduced maternal folate levels and increased total homocysteine levels.[506]

Folate deficiency is common in mothers, particularly where poverty and malnutrition are common, intestinal malabsorption is prevalent, and dietary supplements are not provided.[507] It is usually accompanied by iron deficiency. The growing fetus imposes an increased demand for folate, which is further increased in mothers with thalassemia minor or sickle cell disease.

Several researchers have reported lower serum or RBC folate levels in users of oral contraceptive agents (OCAs) in the past. However, these results preceded the development of lower-dose OCA preparations. This question was re-evaluated in adolescent Canadian females aged 14 to 19 years. Twenty-one percent were using current OCAs, most frequently Triphasil (Wyeth-Ayerst Canada), Marvelon (Organon Canada), Ortho 7/7/7 (Ortho Pharmaceutical), and Cyclen (Ortho Pharmaceutical). Smoking and OCA or alcohol use were not linked to low serum or RBC folate levels.[508] However, OCA use was associated with an unexplained 33% lower serum cobalamin level. Thus, current OCA use seems to not predispose women to future maternal folate insufficiency.

Levels of plasma folate are higher in cord than maternal blood. Perfusion of the human placental cotyledon revealed a two-step maternal-to-fetal transfer of methyl-THF consisting first of a concentrative component. Folate is bound to placental folate-binding proteins/folate receptors on the maternally facing chorionic surface. Gradual release of methyl-THF from this bound pool added to incoming folates generated an intervillous blood folate level three times that in the maternal circulation. In the second step, folates were passively transferred to the fetal circulation along a downhill concentration gradient.[509]

Except in extreme cases, this mechanism was believed to protect the fetus in utero from maternal folate deficiency. Nevertheless, three early abortions and two stillbirths were associated with hyperhomocysteinemia and the homozygous thermolabile 677C→T allele of MTHFR in a woman with low plasma folate. Because treatment with folate and pyridoxine normalized the homocysteine level and favored a subsequent successful pregnancy, it may be that some recurrent miscarriages are associated with hyperhomocysteinemia.[510] Maternal folate deficiency is also related to fetal hypotrophy. In a small well-nourished population, there was a significant correlation between birth weight and both folate status of the mother at 32 weeks of pregnancy and the decrease in her RBC folate levels before delivery.[511] Maternal serum folate concentrations at 18 and 30 weeks correlated negatively with the extent of fetal growth retardation in a study of 289 pregnant women.[512] In 832 women, a low mean daily folate intake was linked to a doubling of the risk for preterm delivery and low infant birth weight.[513] These findings suggest that maternal folate status may affect other birth outcomes beyond causing NTDs. Thus, preferential transfer of folate to the fetus from the placenta may provide limited protection against the deleterious effects of maternal folate insufficiency.

A survey conducted in the United States after food fortification has found modest, yet statistically significant reductions in transposition of the great arteries (12%), cleft palate only (12%), pyloric stenosis (5%), upper limb reduction defects (11%), and omphalocele (21%). More substantial subgroup decreases were observed for renal agenesis in programs that conduct prenatal surveillance (28%), for common truncus among Hispanics (45%), and for upper limb reduction defects among Hispanics (44%).[514]

Deficiency in Newborns and Infants

Levels of plasma and RBC folate fell and total plasma homocysteine levels increased during pregnancy in 404 healthy Danish mothers.[515] Despite this finding, folate deficiency in the infant as a result of folate deficiency in the mother is unusual. Clinical folate deficiency is seldom present at birth. However, the rapid growth in the first few weeks of life demands increased folate. There is a need for folate supplements at this time, particularly for premature infants.[283] Maternal milk folate levels remain elevated during the development of maternal folate deficiency but decrease once deficiency is present.

Folate must be added to hyperalimentation solutions given to newborns in intensive care units. Infections or other illnesses may increase folate needs. Hemolysis secondary to vitamin E deficiency, glucose-6-phosphate dehydrogenase deficiency, or rarer RBC enzyme deficiencies increases demand for folates. Folate absorption is reduced with chronic diarrhea. As mentioned earlier, folate deficiency develops in infants fed goat's milk.[419]

Folate deficiency in infants may not be manifested as classic megaloblastic anemia. After transfusion, neutropenia and thrombocytopenia may be the only hematologic features. Where general malnutrition exists, features of folate deficiency may be overshadowed by the clinical picture of marasmus or protein-calorie malnutrition. The increased requirement for growth and the lack of long-term folate stores make folate deficiency a regular component of starvation. Because folate is stored mainly in the liver, hepatitis and other diseases of the liver may disturb stores and precipitate folate deficiency. Inborn errors of folate metabolism are rare but of considerable interest (discussed later).

Deficiency in Older Children and Adolescents

Malnutrition is the most common cause of folate deficiency in older children. Subgroups at particular risk include those with sickle cell disease, thalassemia major, hepatitis, HIV infection, and malabsorption. Certain drugs and medications predispose to folate deficiency. Folate deficiency has been reported in patients taking chronic antiepileptic medications and older, high-dose oral contraceptives.[422,423] Antifolate drugs such as triamterene and sulfisoxazole-trimethoprim inhibit human DHF reductase to some degree and may induce folate deficiency. Alcohol abuse is associated with folate deficiency and affects a proportion of children and adolescents.

Folates and Neural Tube Defects

Folate insufficiency in the first trimester of pregnancy has been implicated in the occurrence of NTDs in infants.[516,517] Studies have demonstrated that folate supplementation during the periconceptional period (from initiation of pregnancy to closure of the neural tube at about 1 month of gestation) reduces the occurrence[36] and recurrence[35] of NTDs by 50% to 70%. Pregnancies at particular risk may be identified by the maternal total plasma homocysteine level or by MTHFR polymorphism status.[518-520] The most effective way to ensure that pregnant women receive sufficient folate during this period is to fortify foods with folate.[521] Fortification of flour and other enriched grain products with synthetic folic acid has been compulsory in the United States and other countries since 1998.[522] This fortification has been associated with a decrease in the prevalence of NTDs.[514,523,524]

Periconceptional folate supplementation may also be associated with a decreased risk of having a child with nonsyndromic cleft lip with or without cleft palate,[525-527] although not all studies support such an association.[528,529] No consistent effect of the c.677C→T MTHFR polymorphism on orofacial clefting has been observed.[530]

Folates and Down Syndrome

Folate insufficiency or gene polymorphisms (or both) have been linked with other birth defects, in particular Down syndrome.[531,532] A raised total plasma homocysteine concentration is a risk factor for Down syndrome.[533-536] In some studies, the *MTRR* 66A→G, *MTR* 2756A→G, *MTHFR* 677C→T, *MTHFR* 1298A→C, and *RFC1* 80A→G polymorphisms in association with elevated total homocysteine or decreased folate or cobalamin increased the maternal risk of having a child with Down syndrome,[533,537-540] although other studies do not support this finding.[539,541,542] There is a significant increase in the frequency of Down syndrome in mothers who have had a child with spina bifida and vice versa.[543] Fortification of food with folate has not decreased the incidence of Down syndrome as yet, perhaps because a much higher level of folate is needed to prevent the genomic instability associated with marginal folate deficiency.[531]

Folates and Arteriosclerotic Vascular Disease

The premature occurrence of arteriosclerosis in patients with severe homocystinuria first implicated homocysteine as an atherogenic factor.[544] It was subsequently demonstrated that a thermolabile variant of MTHFR was associated with moderate elevation of the total plasma homocysteine concentration and the development of atherosclerotic disease.[545] Thermolability was shown to be due to homozygosity for the T allele of a 677C→T polymorphism in MTHFR that causes conversion of alanine to valine at position 222 of the protein; such conversion results in an approximately 50% decrease in enzyme activity when present in the homozygous state.[38] Epidemiologic studies have shown a significant association between elevated total plasma homocysteine levels and cardiovascular disease and a modest, but statistically significant increased risk of cardiovascular disease in patients with the 677T allele of MTHFR.[546] Heterozygosity for cystathionine β-synthase deficiency may account for a small number of cases of elevated plasma homocysteine as well.[37] Patients participating in the Framingham Heart Study showed a strong correlation between homocysteine levels, carotid stenosis, and low folate levels.[547]

Treatment of subjects who have elevated total plasma homocysteine levels with vitamin B$_6$, folic acid, or betaine normalizes the homocysteine level[548]; such therapy may prevent recurrent or occurrent arteriosclerotic disease.[549] However, three large studies of cobalamin, pyridoxine, and folate treatment to lower total plasma homocysteine failed to reduce the risk for major cardiovascular events in patients with vascular disease.[550-553] Nevertheless, the power of these individual studies may be insufficient to detect the current assessment of an 11% and 19% expected reduction in the incidence of heart attacks and strokes, respectively, for a 25% reduction in the total homocysteine level, and conclusions may need to await a meta-analysis of data from up to a dozen of such studies.[554]

Folates and Cancer

Epidemiologic studies have found an association between folate deficiency and premalignant changes in several epithelial tissues, including the cervix,[555] bronchus,[556] and colon.[39] Some studies demonstrated an apparent reversal of the pathologic lesions with folate supplementation. Difficulty differentiating between megaloblastic and dysplastic changes may have confounded these results. The relationship between folate levels and carcinogenesis has been studied in colorectal cancer. Dietary folate correlates inversely with risk for colorectal adenoma and cancer, and serum homocysteine levels are higher in subjects with colorectal neoplasia.[557] Results from studies of other types of cancer are less clear. A quandary exists that although folate may assist in stabilizing the genome and thus reducing the rate of mutations and the incidence of certain cancers, it may also promote the growth of some malignancies already present.

Folate Antimetabolites

Antifolates are analogues of folic acid that block folate metabolism, thereby interrupting DNA synthesis and causing cell death. They inhibit the enzyme DHF reductase as the primary target.

Methotrexate is an anticancer agent effective in combination chemotherapy for carcinoma of the breast, lung, bone, ovary, head, neck, and elsewhere. It contributes to cure of choriocarcinoma and childhood acute lymphoblastic leukemia. Methotrexate is also used for its immunosuppressive and antiproliferative properties in the treatment of psoriasis, rheumatoid arthritis, and graft-versus-host disease after bone marrow transplantation. Cancer and leukemia cells develop resistance to methotrexate in a variety of ways, including diminished transport of methotrexate (and reduced folates) into the cell; amplification of the *DHFR* gene, with overproduction of DHF reductase; mutations in the *DHFR* gene resulting in a DHF reductase with decreased binding affinity for methotrexate; decreased folate polyglutamate synthetase activity, with resultant diminished polyglutamylation of methotrexate; or increased γ-glutamylhydrolase activity, with decreased retention of methotrexate polyglutamates.[558]

Newer antifolates have been synthesized and tested over the past 40 years.

Pyrimethamine is an antimalarial drug with greater affinity for parasitic than human DHF reductase. Trimethoprim is an antifolate with antibacterial activity and higher affinity for bacterial than human DHF reductase. In combination with sulfisoxazole, which interferes with bacterial synthesis of folic acid, there is a double synergistic antifolate attack on bacteria. Bactrim and Septra are such combinations widely used to treat urinary tract and other infections. They are effective in preventing *Pneumocystis carinii* pneumonia in immunocompromised patients undergoing chemotherapy or in persons infected with HIV.

Inborn Errors of Folate Transport and Metabolism

Hereditary Folate Malabsorption

Hereditary folate malabsorption (MIM 229050) has been reported in fewer than 20 patients.[559-564] It is characterized by megaloblastic anemia, diarrhea, mouth ulcers, failure to thrive, and usually, progressive neurologic deterioration. A majority of the patients documented have been girls. Megaloblastic anemia and low serum folate levels appear in the first few months of life, with excretion of FIGlu and orotic acid in urine. Patients with hereditary folate malabsorption fail to absorb folic acid or reduced folates across the intestinal membrane and the choroid plexus, thereby resulting in decreased folate levels in both blood and CSF. Uptake of folate into cultured and uncultured cells is normal.

Mutations in the *SLC46A1* gene on chromosome 17q11.2, which encodes the PCFT, have now been identified in six patients with hereditary folate malabsorption.[438,565] Identification of mutations in patients with hereditary folate malabsorption and segregation studies in one family make it clear that this is an autosomal recessive disorder.[438,565] The reason for the preponderance of females among patients remains unknown.

Hematologic changes respond to relatively low levels of folate, but levels in CSF may remain low.[566] The clinical response to therapy with folates has varied. Both oral and parenteral administration of folate in pharmacologic doses has corrected the hematologic abnormalities in some patients, with less effect in correcting the low folate levels in CSF. Folinic acid and methyltetrahydrofolic acid may be more effective in entering CSF. In some cases, seizures were reduced in number, and in others, seizures worsened with folate therapy.[361] It is essential to maintain levels of folate in both blood and CSF in the range associated with folate sufficiency. Oral doses of folates in excess of 100 mg daily or systemic therapy may be needed. Intrathecal folate may be needed if CSF levels remain low.

Cellular Folate Uptake Defects

A series of patients with well-characterized abnormalities in folate uptake into cells have been described. It remains unclear whether any of these abnormalities represent primary defects.

In one large family, the prevalence of severe hematologic disease was very high, with anemia, pancytopenia, and leukemia in 34 individuals resulting in the death of 18.[567,568] The proband had severe aplastic anemia that responded to folate therapy. Uptake of methyl-THF was markedly reduced in stimulated lymphocytes from the proband and four family members despite normal uptake of folic acid. The proband and his son also had a lesser reduction in methyl-THF uptake in bone marrow cells. In one son the transport defect developed only after he became neutropenic, thus suggesting that the abnormality may not be the primary defect. In another family, the proband and three daughters had dyserythropoiesis without anemia.[569] An abnormality in methyl-THF uptake was detected in RBCs and bone marrow cells but not in lymphocytes. There was little correlation in the family between clinical findings and cellular folate uptake.

Methylenetetrahydrofolate Reductase Deficiency

MTHFR deficiency is the most common inborn error of folate metabolism (Table 11-3), and at least 85 cases are known.[25,26,570] The clinical manifestations are variable, with many patients initially seen during infancy with severe neurologic disease leading to death, others initially seen as adults, and some remaining clinically asymptomatic.[571] Most come to medical attention as infants because of developmental delay, breathing disorders, gait abnormalities, seizures, and macrocephaly. Patients have been described with schizophrenia and severe MTHFR deficiency, which has focused attention on the role of MTHFR deficiency in psychiatric disease.[572-574]

Homocystinuria is always present in patients with MTHFR deficiency, with the homocystine level ranging from 15 to 667 μmol/24 hr (mean, 130),[25] lower than levels in patients with homocystinuria secondary to cystathionine β-synthase deficiency. More than one determination of homocystine excretion may be needed because false-negative values occur. Serum methionine is in the low-normal range or decreased, whereas in cystathionine β-synthase deficiency, methionine is elevated. Values range from 0 to 18 μmol/L (mean, 12 μmol/L; normal range, 23 to 35 μmol/L).[25] Neurotransmitter levels in the CSF of a few patients have been low. Megaloblastic anemia is rarely present, in contrast to other disorders in which synthesis of methionine from homocysteine is impaired (cobalamin deficiency, cblC, cblD, cblE, cblF, and cblG). This reflects the lack of trapping of folate as methyl-THF in MTHFR deficiency and its availability for purine and pyrimidine biosynthesis.

Findings at autopsy in patients with MTHFR deficiency[575-580] include dilation of cerebral vessels, internal hydrocephalus, and microgyria. Perivascular changes, demyelination, macrophage infiltration, gliosis, and astrocytosis have been reported. A major cause of death was arterial and cerebral venous thrombosis.[575] The neurovascular findings in severe MTHFR deficiency resemble those seen in classic homocystinuria secondary to cystathionine β-synthase deficiency. Patients with the classic findings of SCDSC, similar to that seen in cobalamin deficiency, have been reported.[579,580] Because methyl-THF is the only form of folate that can cross the blood-brain barrier, MTHFR deficiency may result in

TABLE 11-3   **Inherited Defects of Folate Metabolism**

	Hereditary Folate Malabsorption	MTHFR Deficiency	FTCD Deficiency
CLINICAL FINDINGS			
Prevalence	≈20 cases	> 85 cases	13 cases
Megaloblastic anemia	A	N*	N*
Developmental delay	A	A	N*
Seizures	A	A	N*
Speech abnormalities	N	N	A*
Gait abnormalities	N	A	N*
Peripheral neuropathy	N	A	N*
Apnea	N	A	N*
BIOCHEMICAL FINDINGS			
Homocystinuria, homocystinemia	N	A	N
Hypomethioninemia	N	A	N
FIGlu-uria	A*	N	A
Folate absorption	A	N	N
Serum folate	A	A	N*
Red cell folate	A	A*	N*
DEFECTS DETECTABLE IN CULTURED FIBROBLASTS			
Whole Cells			
Methyl-THF uptake	N	N	N
Methyl-THF content	N	A	N
Extracts			
FTCD activity	Activity undetectable in cultured fibroblasts		
MTHFR activity	N	A	N

*Exceptions described in some cases.

A, abnormal (i.e., clinical or laboratory findings present); FIGlu, formiminoglutamic acid; FTCD, formiminotransferase-cyclodeaminase; MTHFR, methylene-THF reductase; N, normal; THF, 5,6,7,8-tetrahydrofolate.

functionally low levels of folate in the brain. Neurologic findings in MTHFR deficiency may be the result of low methionine levels and decreased function of AdoMet-dependent methyltransferase reactions. Alternatively, decreased CNS folate levels may result in impaired purine and pyrimidine synthesis. Because MTHFR has dihydropteridine reductase activity,[581] it may also have a direct role in neurotransmitter synthesis.

The diagnosis of severe MTHFR deficiency is established by measurement of enzyme activity in the liver, leukocytes, or cultured fibroblasts or lymphocytes. The specific activity of MTHFR in cultured fibroblasts is dependent on the stage of the culture cycle, with activity being severalfold greater at confluence than during logarithmic growth[582]; it is thus important to compare activities of patient samples and control cell lines at confluence. MTHFR activity, the proportion of total intracellular folate that is methyl-THF, and the extent of labeled formate incorporation into methionine are inversely correlated with clinical severity.[583,584] When compared with normal enzyme, enzyme from many individuals, including several patients with severe MTHFR deficiency, is unstable when incubated at 55° C, especially in the presence of the cofactor flavin adenine dinucleotide.[545,585]

The human *MTHFR* gene on chromosome 1p36.3 is 2.2 kb in length and consists of 11 exons; it encodes an active protein of about 70 kd.[586,587] MTHFR deficiency shows autosomal recessive inheritance. To date, 41 mutations of the *MTHFR* gene have been identified.[588-595] None occurs frequently in patients from different families. Prenatal diagnosis has been reported with amniocytes and chorionic villus cells.[26,594,596-598] In most cases, MTHFR activity in cell extracts was measured. Because the known *MTHFR* mutations are private, mutation analysis has been limited to families in which the mutations have been sequenced. The existence of common intragenic polymorphisms has allowed the use of linkage analysis to establish the diagnosis.[599]

In addition to mutations that result in severe MTHFR deficiency, several common polymorphisms have been identified. One of them, a 677C→T (cDNA)/A222V (protein) sequence change, results in reduction of MTHFR activity by approximately 50% of control values when the T allele is present in the homozygous state.[38] The T allele represents 30% to 50% of MTHFR alleles in many European, North American, and Japanese populations[600]; its frequency is much lower in Africans and African Americans. This polymorphism is the cause of MTHFR thermolability in both patients with severe MTHFR deficiency and normal individuals. A second polymorphism, 1298A→C (cDNA)/E429A (protein), reduces MTHFR activity to 68% of the wild-type value.[601] Several additional polymorphisms have been identified whose effects on enzyme activity are not known.[602,603]

MTHFR deficiency is difficult to treat, with a poor prognosis once neurologic involvement is evident.

Therefore, it is important to diagnose MTHFR deficiency as early as possible. The following agents have been used for therapy:

1. Folates, to maximize any residual enzyme activity
2. Methyl-THF, to specifically replace the missing product of MTHFR
3. Methionine, to correct deficiency of this amino acid, which requires methyl-THF for synthesis
4. Pyridoxine, because it is a cofactor for cystathionine synthase and thus may lower homocysteine levels
5. Cobalamin, because MeCbl is a cofactor for methionine synthase
6. Carnitine, because of its requirement for adenosylmethionine
7. Betaine, because with homocysteine, it is a substrate for betaine methyltransferase, an enzyme that also converts homocysteine to methionine and is primarily active in the liver.

Betaine has the double advantage of raising methionine and decreasing homocysteine levels. However, because betaine methyltransferase is a liver enzyme, the effects of betaine on the brain are thought to be mediated through changes in circulating levels of metabolites. A summary of the treatment protocols for individual patients with MTHFR deficiency has been published.[25] Such protocols have been highly variable and, for the most part, unsuccessful until the introduction of betaine. Therapy with methionine alone or combined with methyl-THF has not been effective. A regimen consisting of oral betaine, folinic acid, cobalamin, and vitamin B_6 has been suggested.[604] Therapy with betaine after prenatal diagnosis has resulted in the best outcome reported to date.[605]

Glutamate Formiminotransferase Deficiency

Glutamate formiminotransferase deficiency results from mutations in the bifunctional (glutamate formiminotransferase plus cyclodeaminase) enzyme encoded by the *FTCD* gene. It is not clear whether this disorder is associated with any consistent clinical findings. Fewer than 20 patients have been described. FIGlu excretion, either constitutively or in response to a histidine load, is the one constant feature of formiminotransferase deficiency. Patients have ranged in age from 3 months to 42 years at diagnosis. Two distinct phenotypes have been described. The severe form is characterized by mental and physical retardation, abnormal electroencephalographic activity, and dilation of the cerebral ventricles with cortical atrophy. No mental retardation occurs in the mild form, but excretion of FIGlu is greater. Analysis of mutations in the *FTCD* gene has not supported the hypothesis[606] that the mild form is due to a defect in formiminotransferase activity whereas the severe form results from a block in cyclodeaminase.[607]

Several patients had macrocytosis and hypersegmentation of neutrophils, three had delayed speech, two had seizures, and two had mental retardation as their initial signs. Two were identified because they were siblings of known patients. Mental retardation was described in the majority of the original patients from Japan,[608-610] but in only three of the remaining eight patients.[25,611-613] Elevated FIGlu excretion and increased FIGlu levels in blood after a histidine load, as well as high to normal serum folate levels, have been reported. Plasma amino acid levels, including histidine, are usually normal; however, hyperhistidinemia and hyperhistidinuria have been found on occasion, as have low plasma methionine levels. Excretion of hydantoin-5-propionate, the stable oxidation product of the FIGlu precursor 4-imidazolone-5-propionate, and excretion of 4-amino-5-imidazolecarboxamide, an intermediate in purine synthesis, have also been reported.

Hepatic enzyme activity was measured in five patients and was higher (14% to 54% of control values) than would be expected if its deficiency caused the disease. Because FTCD enzyme activity is expressed in the liver and kidney only, cultured cells cannot be used to confirm the diagnosis of formiminotransferase deficiency. There have been reports of measurement of formiminotransferase activity in erythrocytes, but these have not been confirmed.[25]

The human *FTCD* gene on chromosome 21q22.3 consists of 15 exons and generates multiple transcripts.[614] Three *FTCD* mutations have been identified in patients; one patient also had a deletion that eliminated one copy of the *FTCD* gene.[607] Expression of the mutations in vitro demonstrated that they reduced enzyme activity to 30% to 50% of control values, in line with the results of liver assays of affected individuals.[606] These studies confirmed that mutations in the *FTCD* gene underlie cases of formiminotransferase deficiency and demonstrated autosomal recessive inheritance of the disorder.

Two patients in one family[611] responded to folate therapy with decreased FIGlu excretion, whereas six other patients did not.[25] One of two patients responded to methionine supplementation.[612,613] Because the relationship between clinical expression and FIGlu excretion is uncertain, the value of reducing FIGlu excretion is unknown.

Amino-4-Imidazolecarboxamide Ribonucleotide Transformylase Deficiency

A single patient has been reported with deficiency of AICAR transformylase (MIM 60868), one of the 10-formyl-THF–dependent reactions in de novo purine biosynthesis. The patient had profound mental retardation, epilepsy, dysmorphic features, and congenital blindness. Megaloblastic anemia was not observed. Very high levels of AICAR, as well as its diphosphate and triphosphate derivatives, were observed in patient erythrocytes. Two mutations were identified in the *ATIC* gene on chromosome 2q35, which encodes the bifunctional AICAR transformylase–IMP cyclohydrolase enzyme. Enzyme assay demonstrated a profound deficiency in AICAR transformylase activity, with IMP cyclohydrolase activity being 40% of control values.[615]

Other Possible Inborn Errors of Folate Metabolism

Three patients have been reported to have DHF reductase deficiency,[616] but alternative genetic lesions affecting other enzymes involved in folate or cobalamin metabolism have subsequently been identified in two of the patients.[361,617] Three patients were reported to have methenyl-THF cyclohydrolase deficiency, but the diagnosis was retracted in a later publication from the same group.[610]

3-PHOSPHOGLYCERATE DEHYDROGENASE DEFICIENCY

Megaloblastic anemia has been reported in two brothers with 3-phosphoglycerate dehydrogenase (EC 1.1.1.95) deficiency (MIM 601815),[618] a rare disorder (six patients in four families have been reported) that results in impaired ability to synthesize serine from 3-phosphoglycerate. Although serine is a nonessential amino acid, impairment of this pathway results in severely decreased levels of serine in serum and CSF,[619] thus demonstrating that diet alone does not provide sufficient serine to support normal metabolism. Patients with this disorder are characterized by macrocephaly beginning before birth, with severe psychomotor delay and intractable seizures developing during the first year of life. Cataracts, hypogonadism, adduction of the thumbs, and thrombocytopenia were present in some patients.

The disorder is characterized biochemically by markedly decreased levels of serine in CSF and by decreased plasma serine after an overnight fast. The low levels of serine in CSF may reflect relatively low affinity of the neutral amino acid transporter for serine, which leaves the CNS particularly dependent on de novo serine synthesis to meet its metabolic needs.[619] The level of methyl-THF in CSF is also reduced.[618] Under normal conditions, serine is the major source of one-carbon units for cellular folate metabolism, and serine deficiency may therefore result in decreased levels of folate coenzyme forms. Patients have been treated with high doses of serine and in some cases with glycine as well. Treatment has resulted in correction of the biochemical deficits and decreased frequency of seizures, but no progress in psychomotor development has been observed in patients when treatment was started after 1 year of age.[620] One affected individual who was identified by prenatal diagnosis and was treated with serine beginning in the prenatal period has shown normal development.[621]

Two mutations in the *PHGDH* gene on chromosome 1q12 have been identified in patients with 3-phosphoglycerate dehydrogenase deficiency. Five patients, including the brothers with megaloblastic anemia, were homozygous for a c.1468G→A (p.V490M) mutation; the sixth patient was homozygous for a c.1273G→A (p.V425M) mutation. Both mutations resulted in decreased dehydrogenase activity in vitro.[622]

THIAMINE-RESPONSIVE MEGALOBLASTIC ANEMIA

Thiamine-responsive megaloblastic anemia (TRMA; MIM 249270) is a rare autosomal recessive disorder characterized by megaloblastic anemia, diabetes mellitus, and sensorineural deafness that responds to pharmacologic doses of thiamine.[623-625] Additional clinical findings have included optic atrophy, cardiomyopathy, and stroke-like episodes. The bone marrow is characterized by megaloblastic changes and ringed sideroblasts. The disorder has been reported in fewer than 30 families.

Dietary thiamine is taken up by cells and converted to its active coenzyme derivative thiamine pyrophosphate by the enzyme thiamine pyrophosphokinase (EC 2.7.6.2). Thiamine pyrophosphate is required for the activity of four known mammalian enzymes: transketolase, pyruvate dehydrogenase, α-ketoglutarate dehydrogenase, and branched-chain ketoacid dehydrogenase.

TRMA has been shown to be caused by mutations affecting the *SLC19A2* gene on chromosome 1q23.3.[626-629] This gene encodes a thiamine transporter protein that has homology to the RFC (which is encoded by the gene *SLC19A1*). TRMA fibroblasts have decreased thiamine uptake relative to control fibroblasts and, unlike control cells, undergo apoptosis when incubated in medium lacking thiamine.[630] At least 14 mutations in the *SLC19A2* gene have been reported in patients with TRMA.[626]

REFERENCES

1. Minot GR, Murphy WP. Treatment of pernicious anemia by a special diet. JAMA. 1926;87:470-476.
2. Castle WB. The conquest of pernicious anemia. In Wintrobe MM (ed). Blood, Pure and Eloquent. New York, McGraw-Hill, 1979, pp 283-318.
3. Wintrobe MM. Hematology, the Blossoming of a Science: A Story of Inspiration and Effort. Philadelphia, Lea & Febiger, 1985.
4. Chanarin I. A history of pernicious anemia. Br J Haematol. 2000;111:407-415.
5. Ehrlich P. Untersuchungen zur Histologie und Klinik des Blutes. Berlin, Hirschwald, 1891.
6. Wills L. Treatment of "pernicious anaemia of pregnancy" and "tropical anaemia" with special reference to yeast extract as curative agent. BMJ. 1931;1:1059-1064.
7. Fenwick S. On atrophy of the stomach. Lancet. 1870;96: 78-80.
8. Castle WB. Observations on the etiological relationship of achylia gastrica to pernicious anemia. I. The effect of administration to patients with pernicious anemia of the contents of the normal human stomach recovered after ingestion of beef muscle. Am J Med Sci. 1929;178: 748-764.

9. Cooper BA, Castle WB. Sequential mechanisms in the enhanced absorption of vitamin B$_{12}$ by intrinsic factor in the rat. J Clin Invest. 1960;39:199-214.

10. Ungley CC. Vitamin B$_{12}$ in pernicious anaemia. Parenteral administration. BMJ. 1949;2:1370-1377.

11. Hall BE, Watkins CH. Experience with pteroylglutamate synthetic folic acid in treatment of pernicious anemia. J Lab Clin Med. 1947;32:622.

12. Zalusky R, Herbert V, Castle WB. Cyanocobalamin therapy effect in folic acid deficiency. Arch Intern Med. 1962;109:545-554.

13. Cooper BA, Paranchych W. Selective uptake of specifically bound cobalt-58 vitamin B$_{12}$ by human and mouse tumour cells. Nature. 1961;191:393-395.

14. Youngdahl-Turner P, Rosenberg LE, Allen RH. Binding and uptake of transcobalamin II by human fibroblasts. J Clin Invest. 1978;61:133-141.

15. Mollin DL, Ross GIM. The vitamin B$_{12}$ concentrations of serum and urine of normals and of patients with megaloblastic anaemias and other diseases. J Clin Pathol. 1952;5:129.

16. Gottlieb C, Lau KS, Wasserman LR, Herbert V. Rapid charcoal assay for intrinsic factor (IF), gastric juice unsaturated B$_{12}$ binding capacity, antibody to IF, and serum unsaturated B$_{12}$ binding capacity. Blood. 1965;25:875-884.

17. Adams JF, Tankel HI, MacEwan F. Estimation of the total body vitamin B$_{12}$ in the live subject. Clin Sci. 1970;39:107-113.

18. Russell JSR, Batten FE, Collier J. Subacute combined degeneration of the spinal cord. Brain. 1900;23:39-110.

19. Jeffries GH, Hoskins DW, Sleisinger MH. Antibody to intrinsic factor in serum from patients with pernicious anemia. J Clin Invest. 1962;41:1106-1115.

20. Dow CA, De Aizpurua HJ, Pedersen JS, et al. 65-70 kD protein identified by immunoblotting as the presumptive gastric microsomal autoantigen in pernicious anaemia. Clin Exp Immunol. 1985;62:732-737.

21. De Aizpurua HJ, Ungar B, Toh BH. Autoantibody to the gastrin receptor in pernicious anemia. N Engl J Med. 1985;313:479-483.

22. Burman P, Mardh S, Norberg L, Karlsson FA. Parietal cell antibodies in pernicious anemia inhibit H$^+$,K$^+$-adenosine triphosphatase, the proton pump of the stomach. Gastroenterology. 1989;96:1434-1438.

23. Hakami N, Neiman PE, Canellos GP, Lazerson J. Neonatal megaloblastic anemia due to inherited transcobalamin II deficiency in two siblings. N Engl J Med. 1971;285:1163-1170.

24. Levy HL, Mudd SH, Schulman JD, et al. A derangement in B$_{12}$ metabolism associated with homocystinemia, cystathioninemia, hypomethioninemia and methylmalonic aciduria. Am J Med. 1970;48:390-397.

25. Erbe RW. Inborn errors of folate metabolism. In Blakley RL (ed). Folates and Pterins, vol 3, Nutritional, Pharmacological and Physiological Aspects. New York, John Wiley & Sons, 1986, pp 413-465.

26. Marquet J, Chadefaux B, Bonnefont JP, et al. Methylenetetrahydrofolate reductase deficiency: prenatal diagnosis and family studies. Perinat Diagn. 1994;14:29-33.

27. Platica O, Geneczko R, Regec A, et al. Isolation of complementary DNA for human transcobalamin II. Proc Soc Exp Biol Med. 1989;192:95-97.

28. Johnston J, Bollekens J, Allen RH, Berliner N. Structure of the cDNA encoding transcobalamin I, a neutrophil granule protein. J Biol Chem. 1989;264:15754-15757.

29. Hansen MR, Nexo E, Svendsen I, et al. Human intrinsic factor. Its primary structure compared to the primary structure of rat intrinsic factor. Scand J Clin Lab Invest. 1989;49:19-22.

30. Guéant JL, Jokinen O, Schohn H, et al. Purification of intrinsic factor receptor from pig ileum using as affinity medium human intrinsic factor covalently bound to Sepharose. Biochim Biophys Acta. 1989;92:281-288.

31. Dieckgraefe BK, Seetharam B, Banaszak L, et al. Isolation and structural characterization of a cDNA clone encoding rat gastric intrinsic factor. Proc Natl Acad Sci U S A. 1988;5:46-50.

32. Gräsbeck R, Stenman UH, Puutula L, Visuri K. Procedure for detaching bound vitamin B$_{12}$ from its transport proteins. Biochim Biophys Acta. 1968;58:292-295.

33. Warren MJ. Finding the final pieces of the vitamin B$_{12}$ biosynthetic jigsaw. Proc Natl Acad Sci U S A. 2006;103:4799-4800.

34. Savage DG, Lindenbaum J, Stabler SP, Allen RH. Sensitivity of serum methylmalonic acid and total homocysteine determinations for diagnosing cobalamin and folate deficiencies. Am J Med. 1994;96:239-246.

35. MRC Vitamin Study Research Group. Prevention of neural tube defects: results of the Medical Research Council Vitamin Study. Lancet. 1991;338:131-137.

36. Czeizel AE, Dudas I. Prevention of the first occurrence of neural-tube defects by periconceptional vitamin supplementation. N Engl J Med. 1992;327:1832-1835.

37. Dudman NPB, Wilcken DEL, Wang J, et al. Disordered methionine/homocysteine metabolism in premature vascular disease: its occurrence, cofactor therapy, and enzymology. Arterioscler Thromb. 1993;13:1253-1260.

38. Frosst P, Blom HJ, Milos R, et al. A candidate genetic risk factor for vascular disease: a common mutation in methylenetetrahydrofolate reductase. Nat Genet. 1995;10:111-113.

39. Lashner BA, Heidenreich PA, Su GL, et al. Effect of folate supplementation on the incidence of dysplasia and cancer in chronic ulcerative colitis. A case-control study. Gastroenterology. 1989;97:255-259.

40. Finch CA, Coleman DH, Motulsky AG, et al. Erythrokinetics in pernicious anemia. Blood. 1956;11:807-820.

41. London IM, West R. The formation of bile pigment in pernicious anemia. J Biol Chem. 1950;184:359-364.

42. Glazer HS, Mueller JF, Jarrold T, et al. The effect of vitamin B$_{12}$ and folic acid on nucleic acid composition of the bone marrow of patients with megaloblastic anemia. J Lab Clin Med. 1954;43:905-913.

43. Nath BJ, Lindenbaum J. Persistence of neutrophil hypersegmentation during recovery from megaloblastic granulopoiesis. Ann Intern Med. 1979;90:757-760.

44. Chanarin I. The Megaloblastic Anaemias. London, Blackwell Scientific, 1979.

45. Mitchell K, Ferguson MM, Lucie NP, MacDonald DG. Epithelial dysplasia in the oral mucosa associated with pernicious anaemia. Br Dent J. 1986;161:259-260.

46. Pratt JM. Inorganic Chemistry of Vitamin B$_{12}$. New York, Academic Press, 1972.

47. Hogenkamp HPC. The chemistry of cobalamin and related compounds. In Babior BM (ed). Cobalamin:

Biochemistry and Pathophysiology. New York, Wiley-Interscience, 1975, pp 21-74.

48. Battersby AR, Leeper FJ. Biosynthesis of B_{12} in the aerobic organism *Pseudomonas denitrificans*. In Banerjee R (ed). Chemistry and Biochemistry of B_{12}. New York, John Wiley & Sons; 1999, pp 507-536.

49. Scott AI, Roessner CA, Santander PJ. B_{12} biosynthesis: the anaerobic pathway. In Banerjee R (ed). Chemistry and Biochemistry of B_{12}. New York, John Wiley & Sons; 1999, pp 537-556.

50. Croft MT, Lawrence AD, Raux-Deery E, et al. Algae acquire vitamin B_{12} through a symbiotic relationship with bacteria. Nature. 2006;438:90-93.

51. Stabler SP, Allen RH. Vitamin B_{12} deficiency as a worldwide problem. Ann Rev Nutr. 2004;24:299-326.

52. Fenech M, Dreosti IE, Rinaldi JR. Folate, vitamin B_{12}, homocysteine status and chromosome damage rate in lymphocytes of older men. Carcinogenesis. 1997;18:1329-1336.

53. Fenech M, Aitken C, Rinaldi J. Folate, vitamin B_{12}, homocysteine status and DNA damage in young Australian adults. Carcinogenesis. 1998;19:1163-1171.

54. Kapiszewska M, Kalemba M, Wojciech U, Milewicz T. Uracil misincorporation into DNA of leukocytes of young women with positive folate balance depends on plasma vitamin B_{12} concentrations and methylenetetrahydrofolate reductase polymorphisms. a pilot study. J Nutr Biochem. 2005;16:467-478.

55. Banerjee DK, Chatterjea JB. Vitamin B_{12} content of some articles of Indian diets and the effect of cooking on it. Br J Nutr. 1953;17:385-389.

56. Roberts RD, James H, Petrie A, et al. Vitamin B_{12} status in pregnancy among immigrants to Britain. BMJ. 1973;3:67-72.

57. Chanarin I, Stephenson E. Vegetarian diet and cobalamin deficiency: their association with tuberculosis. J Clin Pathol. 1988;41:759-762.

58. Armstrong BK, Davis RE, Nicol DJ, et al. Hematological, vitamin B_{12} and folate studies on Seventh-Day Adventist vegetarians. Am J Clin Nutr. 1974;27:712-718.

59. Abdulla M, Andersson I, Asp NG, et al. Nutrient intake and health status of vegans. Chemical analyses of diets using the duplicate portion sampling technique. Am J Clin Nutr. 1981;34:2464-2477.

60. Platica O, Janeczko R, Quadros EV, et al. The cDNA sequence and the deduced amino acid sequence of human transcobalamin II show homology with rat intrinsic factor and human transcobalamin I. J Biol Chem. 1991;266:7860-7863.

61. Li N, Seetharam S, Seetharam B. Genomic structure of human transcobalamin II: comparison to human intrinsic factor and transcobalamin I. Biochem Biophys Res Commun. 1995;208:756-764.

62. Seetharam B, Yammani RR. Cobalamin transport proteins and their cell-surface receptors. Exp Rev Mol Med. 2003;5:1-18.

63. Allen NC, Seetharam B, Podell ER, Alpers DH. Effect of proteolytic enzymes on the binding of cobalamin to R protein and intrinsic factor. In vitro evidence that a failure to partially degrade protein is responsible for cobalamin malabsorption in pancreatic insufficiency. J Clin Invest. 1978;61:47-54.

64. Sennett C, Rosenberg LE, Mellman IS. Transmembrane transport of cobalamin in prokaryotic and eukaryotic cells. Annu Rev Biochem. 1981;50:1053-1086.

65. Hewitt JE, Gordon MM, Taggart RT, et al. Human intrinsic factor: characterization of cDNA and genomic clones and localization to human chromosome 11. Genomics. 1991;10:432-440.

66. Fernandes-Costa F, Metz J. Vitamin B_{12} binders (transcobalamins) in serum. Crit Rev Clin Lab Sci. 1982;18:1-30.

67. Quadros EV, Rothenberg SP, Pan Y-CE, Stein S. Purification and molecular characterization of human transcobalamin II. J Biol Chem. 1986;261:15455-15460.

68. Pletsch QA, Coffey JW. Intracellular distribution of radioactive vitamin B_{12} in rat liver. J Biol Chem. 1971;246:4619-4629.

69. Yang-Feng TL, Berliner N, Deverajan P, Johnston J. Assignment of two human neutrophil secondary protein granule protein genes, transcobalamin I and neutrophil collagenase, to chromosome 11. Cytogenet Cell Genet. 1991;58:1974.

70. Ogawa K, Kudo H, Kim YC, et al. Expression of vitamin B_{12} R-binder in breast tumors. An immunohistochemical study. Arch Pathol Lab Med. 1988;112:1117-1120.

71. Lee EY, Seetharam B, Alpers DH, DeSchryver-Kecskemeti K. Immunohistochemical survey of cobalamin-binding proteins. Gastroenterology. 1989;97:1171-1180.

72. Kolhouse JF, Kondo H, Allen NC, et al. Cobalamin analogues are present in human plasma and can mask cobalamin deficiency because current isotope dilution assays are not specific for true cobalamin. N Engl J Med. 1978;299:785-792.

73. Wuerges J, Garau G, Geremia S, et al. Structural basis for mammalian vitamin B_{12} transport by transcobalamin. Proc Natl Acad Sci U S A. 2006;103:4386-4391.

74. Fedosov SN, Fedosova NU, Berglund L, et al. Composite organization of the cobalamin binding and cubilin recognition sites of intrinsic factor. Biochemistry. 2005;44:3604-3614.

75. Wuerges J, Geremia S, Randaccio L. Structural study on ligand specificity of human B_{12} transporters. Biochem J. 2007;403:431-440.

76. Seetharam B. Gastrointestinal absorption and transport of cobalamin (vitamin B_{12}). In Johnson LR (ed). Physiology of the Gastrointestinal Tract. New York, Raven Press, 1994, pp 1997-2026.

77. Moestrup SK, Kozyraki R, Kristiansen M, et al. The intrinsic factor–vitamin B_{12} receptor and target of teratogenic antibodies is a megalin-binding peripheral protein with homology to developmental proteins. J Biol Chem. 1998;273:5235-5242.

78. Kalantry S, Manning S, Haub O, et al. The amnionless gene, essential for mouse gastrulation, encodes a visceral-endoderm–specific protein with an extracellular cysteine-rich domain. Nat Genet. 2001;27:412-416.

79. He Q, Madsen H, Kilkenney A, et al. Amnionless function is required for cubilin brush-border expression and intrinsic factor–cobalamin (vitamin B_{12}) absorption in vivo. Blood. 2005;106:1447-1453.

80. Aminoff M, Carter JE, Chadwick RB, et al. Mutations in CUBN, encoding the intrinsic factor–vitamin B_{12} receptor, cubilin, cause hereditary megaloblastic anaemia 1. Nat Genet. 1999;21:309-313.

81. Tanner SM, Aminoff M, Wright FA, et al. Amnionless, essential for mouse gastrulation, is mutated in recessive hereditary megaloblastic anemia. Nate Genet 2003;33: 426-429.

82. Robertson JA, Gallagher ND. In vivo evidence that cobalamin is absorbed by receptor-mediated endocytosis in the mouse. Gastroenterology. 1985;88:908-912.

83. Rothenberg SP, Weiss JP, Cotter R. Formation of transcobalamin II–vitamin B_{12} complex by guinea-pig ileal mucosa in organ culture after in vitro incubation with intrinsic factor–vitamin B_{12}. Br J Haematol. 1978;40: 401-414.

84. Chanarin I, Muir M, Hughes A, Hoffbrand AV. Evidence for intestinal origin of transcobalamin-II during vitamin-B_{12} absorption. BMJ. 1978;1:1453-1455.

85. Kapadia CR, Schafer DE, Donaldson RM, Ebersole ER. Evidence for involvement of cyclic nucleotides in intrinsic factor secretion by isolated rabbit gastric mucosa. J Clin Invest. 1979;64:1044-1049.

86. Robertson JA, Gallagher ND. Intrinsic factor–cobalamin accumulates in the ilea of mice treated with chloroquine. Gastroenterology. 1985;89:1353-1359.

87. Laframboise R, Cooper BA, Rosenblatt DS. Malabsorption of vitamin B_{12} from the intestine in a child with cblF disease: evidence for lysosomal-mediated absorption. Blood. 1992;80:291-292.

88. Nyberg W, Gräsbeck R, Saarni M, von Bonsdorff B. Serum vitamin B_{12} levels and incidence of tapeworm anemia in a population heavily infected with *Diphyllobothrium latum*. Am J Clin Nutr. 1961;9:606-612.

89. Kishimoto T, Tavassoli M, Green R, Jacobsen DW. Receptors for transferrin and transcobalamin II display segregated distribution on microvilli of leukemia L1210 cells. Biochem Biophys Res Commun. 1987;146:1102-1108.

90. Seligman PA, Allen RH. Characterization of the receptor for transcobalamin II isolated from human placenta. J Biol Chem. 1978;253:1766-1772.

91. Quadros EV, Sai P, Rothenberg SP. Characterization of the human placental membrane receptor for transcobalamin II–cobalamin. Arch Biochem Biophys. 1994;308: 192-199.

92. Bose S, Seetharam S, Seetharam B. Membrane expression and interactions of human transcobalamin II receptor. J Biol Chem. 1995;270:8152-8157.

93. Quadros EV, Nakayama Y, Seqeira JM. The binding properties of the human receptor for the cellular uptake of vitamin B_{12}. Biochem Biophys Res Commun. 2005;327: 1006-1010.

94. DiGirolamo PM, Huennekens FM. Transport of vitamin B_{12} into mouse leukemia cells. Arch Biochem Biophys. 1975;168:386-393.

95. Youngdahl-Turner P, Mellman IS, Allen RH, Rosenberg LE. Protein mediated vitamin uptake. Adsorptive endocytosis of the transcobalamin II–cobalamin complex by cultured human fibroblasts. Exp Cell Res. 1979;118: 127-134.

96. Rosenblatt D, Hosack A, Matiaszuk N. Expression of transcobalamin II by amniocytes. Prenat Diag. 1987;7:35-39.

97. Rosenblatt DS, Laframboise R, Pichette J, et al. New disorder of vitamin B_{12} metabolism (cobalamin F) presenting as methylmalonic aciduria. Pediatrics. 1986;78: 51-54.

98. Vassiliadis A, Rosenblatt DS, Cooper BA, Bergeron JJM. Lysosomal cobalamin accumulation in fibroblasts from a patient with an inborn error of cobalamin metabolism (*cblF* complementation group): visualization by electron microscope radioautography. Exp Cell Res. 1991;195: 295-302.

99. Matthews RG. Cobalamin-dependent methionine synthase. In Banerjee R (ed). Chemistry and Biochemistry of B_{12}. New York, Wiley-Interscience, 1999, pp 681-706.

100. Olteanu H, Banerjee R. Cobalamin-dependent remethylation. In Carmel R, Jacobsen DW (eds). Homocysteine in Health and Disease. New York, Cambridge University Press, 2001, pp 135-144.

101. Banerjee R, Chowdhury S. Methylmalonyl-CoA mutase. In Banerjee R (ed). Chemistry and Biochemistry of B_{12}. New York, Wiley-Interscience, 1999, pp 707-730.

102. Pezacka E, Green R, Jacobsen DW. Glutathionylcobalamin as an intermediate in the formation of cobalamin coenzymes. Biochem Biophys Res Commun. 1990;169: 443-450.

103. Walker GA, Murphy S, Huennekens FM. Enzymatic conversion of vitamin B_{12a} to adenosyl-B_{12}: evidence for the existence of two separate reducing systems. Arch Biochem Biophys. 1969;134:95-102.

104. Pezacka EH, Rosenblatt DS. Intracellular metabolism of cobalamin. Altered activities of β-axial-ligand transferase and microsomal cob(III)alamin reductase in *cblC* and *cblD* fibroblasts. J Endocrinol 1994;1:315-323.

105. Watanabe F, Nakano Y, Saido H, et al. Cytochrome b_5/cytochrome b_5 reductase complex in rat liver microsomes has NADH-linked aquacobalamin reductase activity. J Nutr. 1992;122:940-944.

106. Watanabe F, Nakano Y, Saido H, et al. NADPH-cytochrome c (P-450) reductase has the activity of NADPH-linked aquacobalamin reductase in rat liver microsomes. Biochim Biophys Acta. 1992;1119:175-177.

107. Saido H, Watanabe F, Tamura Y, et al. Cytochrome b_5–like hemoprotein/cytochrome b_5 reductase complex in rat liver mitochondria has NADH-linked aquacobalamin reductase activity. J Nutr. 1994;124:1037-1040.

108. Lerner-Ellis JP, Tirone JC, Pawelek PD, et al. Identification of the gene responsible for methylmalonic aciduria and homocystinuria, *cblC* type. Nat Genet. 2006;38: 93-100.

109. Coelho D, Suormala T, Stucki M, et al. Gene identification for the cblD defect of vitamin B_{12} metabolism. N Engl J Med. 2008;358:1454-1464.

110. Leclerc D, Wilson A, Dumas R, et al. Cloning and mapping of a cDNA for methionine synthase reductase, a flavoprotein defective in patients with homocystinuria. Proc Natl Acad Sci U S A. 1998;95:3059-3064.

111. Olteanu H, Banerjee R. Human methionine synthase reductase, a soluble P-450 reductase–like dual flavoprotein, is sufficient for NADPH-dependent methionine synthase activation. J Biol Chem. 2001;276:35558-35563.

112. Leclerc D, Campeau E, Goyette P, et al. Human methionine synthase: cDNA cloning and identification of mutations in patients of the *cblG* complementation group of folate/cobalamin disorders. Hum Mol Genet. 1996;5: 1867-1874.

113. Li YN, Gulati S, Baker PJ, et al. Cloning, mapping and RNA analysis of the human methionine synthase gene. Hum Mol Genet. 1996;5:1851-1858.

114. Chen LH, Liu M-L, Hwang H-Y, et al. Human methionine synthase: cDNA cloning, gene localization, and expression. J Biol Chem. 1997;272:3628-3634.

115. Watkins D, Ru M, Hwang H-Y, et al. Hyperhomocysteinemia due to methionine synthase deficiency, *cblG*: structure of the MTR gene, genotype diversity, and recognition of a common mutation, P1173L. Am J Hum Genet. 2002;71:143-153.

116. Goulding CW, Postigo D, Matthews RG. Cobalamin-dependent methionine synthase is a modular protein with distinct regions for binding homocysteine, methyltetrahydrofolate, cobalamin, and adenosylmethionine. Biochemistry. 1997;36:8082-8091.

117. Banerjee RV, Johnston NL, Sobeski JK, et al. Cloning and sequence analysis of the *Escherichia coli* metH gene encoding cobalamin-dependent methionine synthase and isolation of a tryptic fragment containing the cobalamin-binding domain. J Biol Chem. 1989;264:13888-13895.

118. Dixon MM, Huang S, Matthews RG, Ludwig ML. The structure of the C-terminal domain of methionine synthase: presenting *S*-adenosylmethionine for reductive methylation of B_{12}. Structure. 1996;4:1263-1275.

119. Drennan CL, Matthews RG, Ludwig ML. Cobalamin-dependent methionine synthase: the structure of a methylcobalamin-binding fragment and implications for other B_{12}-dependent enzymes. Curr Opin Struct Biol. 1994;4: 919-929.

120. Wolthers KR, Toogood HS, Jowitt TA, et al. Crystal structure and solution characterization of the activation domain of human methionine synthase. FEBS J. 2007;274: 738-750.

121. Jarrett JT, Amaratunga M, Drennan CL, et al. Mutations in the B_{12}-binding region of methionine synthase: how the protein controls methylcobalamin reactivity. Biochemistry. 1996;35:2464-2475.

122. Bandarian V, Pattridge KA, Lennon BW, et al. Domain alternation switches B_{12}-dependent methionine synthase to the activation conformation. Nat Struct Biol. 2002;9:53-56.

123. Yamada K, Gravel RA, Toraya T, Matthews RG. Human methionine synthase reductase is a molecular chaperone for human methionine synthase. Proc Natl Acad Sci U S A. 2006;103:9476-9481.

124. Garrow TA. Betaine-dependent remethylation. In Carmel R, Jacobsen DW (eds). Homocysteine in Health and Disease. Cambridge, England, Cambridge University Press, 2001, pp 145-152.

125. Clarke S, Banfield K. *S*-adenosylmethionine–dependent methyltransferases. In Carmel R, Jacobsen DW (eds). Homocysteine in Health and Disease. New York, Cambridge University Press, 2001, pp 63-78.

126. de la Haba G, Cantoni GL. The enzymatic synthesis of *S*-adenosyl-L-homocysteine from adenosine and homocysteine. J Biol Chem. 1959;234:603-608.

127. Fenton WA, Ambani LM, Rosenberg LE. Uptake of hydroxocobalamin by rat liver mitochondria. Binding to a mitochondrial protein. J Biol Chem. 1976;251: 6616-6623.

128. Dobson CM, Wai T, Leclerc D, et al. Identification of the gene responsible for the cblB complementation group of vitamin B_{12}–dependent methylmalonic aciduria. Hum Mol Genet. 2002;26:3361-3369.

129. Leal NA, Park SD, Kima PE, Bobik TA. Identification of the human and bovine ATP:Cob(I)alamin adenosyltransferase cDNAs based on complementation of a bacterial mutant. J Biol Chem. 2003;278:9227-9234.

130. Stich TA, Yamanishi M, Banerjee R, Brunold TC. Spectroscopic evidence for the formation of a four-coordinate Co^{2+} cobalamin species upon binding to the human ATP: cobalamin adenosyltransferase. J Am Chem Soc. 2005;127: 7660-7661.

131. Yamanishi M, Labunska T, Banerjee R. Mirror "Base-off" conformation of coenzyme B_{12} in human adenosyltransferase and its downstream target, methylmalonyl-CoA mutase. J Am Chem Soc. 2005;127:526-527.

132. Yamanishi M, Vlasie M, Banerjee R. Adenosyltransferase: an enzyme and an escort for coenzyme B_{12}? Trends Biochem Sci. 2005;30:304-308.

133. Dobson CM, Wai T, Leclerc D, et al. Identification of the gene responsible for the cblA complementation group of vitamin B_{12}–responsive methylmalonic acidemia based on analysis of prokaryotic gene arrangements. Proc Nat Acad Sci U S A. 2002;99:15554-15559.

134. Padovani D, Labunska T, Banerjee R. Energetics of interaction between the G-protein chaperone, MeaB, and B_{12}-dependent methylmalonyl-CoA mutase. J Biol Chem. 2006;81:17838-17844.

135. Korotkova N, Lidstrom ME. MeaB is a component of the methylmalonyl-CoA mutase complex required for protection of the enzyme from inactivation. J Biol Chem. 2004;279:13652-13658.

136. Padovani D, Banerjee R. Assembly and protection of the radical enzyme, methylmalonyl-CoA mutase, by its chaperone. Biochemistry. 2006;45:9300-9306.

137. Moras E, Hosack A, Watkins D, Rosenblatt DS. Mitochondrial vitamin B_{12}–binding proteins in patients with inborn errors of cobalamin metabolism. Mol Genet Metab. 2007;90:140-147.

138. Mellman I, Willard HF, Youngdahl-Turner P, Rosenberg LE. Cobalamin coenzyme synthesis in normal and mutant fibroblasts. Evidence for a processing enzyme activity deficient in *cblC* cells. J Biol Chem. 1979;254: 11847-11853.

139. Ledley FD, Lumetta MR, Zoghbi HY, et al. Mapping of human methylmalonyl CoA mutase (*MUT*) locus on chromosome 6. Am J Hum Genet. 1988;42:839-846.

140. Ledley FD, Lumetta M, Nguyen PN, et al. Molecular cloning of L-methylmalonyl-CoA mutase: gene transfer and analysis of *mut* cell lines. Proc Natl Acad Sci U S A. 1988;85:3518-3521.

141. Kolhouse JF, Utley C, Allen RH. Isolation and characterization of methylmalonyl-CoA mutase from human placenta. J Biol Chem. 1980;255:2708-2712.

142. Fenton WA, Hack AM, Willard HF, et al. Purification and properties of methylmalonyl coenzyme A mutase from human liver. Arch Biochem Biophys. 1982;214:815-823.

143. Fenton WA, Hack AM, Helfgott D, Rosenberg LE. Biogenesis of the mitochondrial enzyme methylmalonyl-CoA mutase. Synthesis and processing of a precursor in a cell-free system and in cultured cells. J Biol Chem. 1984;259:6616-6621.

144. Leadlay PF, Ledley FD. Primary sequence homology between methylmalonyl CoA mutase from *Propionibacte-*

rium shermanii and *Homo sapiens*. In Linnell JC, Bhatt HR (eds). Biomedicine and Physiology of Vitamin B$_{12}$. London, Children's Medical Charity, 1990, pp 341-352.

145. Mancia F, Keep NH, Nakagawa A, et al. How coenzyme B$_{12}$ radicals are generated: the crystal structure of methylmalonyl-coenzyme A mutase at 2 Å resolution. Structure. 1996;4:339-350.

146. Pierce HI, Hillman RS. The value of the serum vitamin B$_{12}$ level in diagnosing B$_{12}$ deficiency. Blood. 1974;43: 915-921.

147. Thong KL, Hanley SA, McBride JA. Clinical significance of a high mean corpuscular volume in nonanemic patients. Can Med Soc J. 1977;117:909-910.

148. Saxena S, Weiner JM, Carmel R. Red blood cell distribution width in untreated pernicious anemia. Am J Clin Pathol. 1988;89:660-663.

149. Carmel R, Karnaze DS. Physician response to low serum cobalamin values. Arch Intern Med. 1986;146: 1161-1165.

150. Kafetz K. Immunoglobulin deficiency responding to vitamin B$_{12}$ in two elderly patients with megaloblastic anaemia. Postgrad Med J. 1985;61:1065-1066.

151. Wright PE, Sears DA. Hypogammaglobulinemia and pernicious anemia. South Med J. 1987;80:243-246.

152. Carmel R. Treatment of severe pernicious anemia: no association with sudden death. Am J Clin Nutr. 1988;48:1443-1444.

153. Lindgren A, Lindstedt G, Kilander AF. Advantages of serum pepsinogen A combined with gastrin or pepsinogen C as first-line analytes in the evaluation of suspected cobalamin deficiency: a study in patients previously not subjected to gastrointestinal surgery. J Intern Med. 1998;244:341-349.

154. Nimo RE, Carmel R. Increased sensitivity of detection of the blocking (type I) anti-intrinsic factor antibody. Am J Clin Pathol. 1987;88:729-733.

155. Mollin DL, Anderson BB, Burman JF. The serum vitamin B$_{12}$ level: its assay and significance. Clin Haematol. 1976;5:521-546.

156. Lindenbaum J, Savage DG, Stabler SP, Allen RH. Diagnosis of cobalamin deficiency: II. Relative sensitivities of serum cobalamin, methylmalonic acid, and total homocysteine concentrations. Am J Hematol. 1990;34: 99-107.

157. Solomon LR. Cobalamin-responsive disorders in the ambulatory care setting: unreliability of cobalamin, methylmalonic acid, and homocysteine testing. Blood. 2005;105:978-985.

158. Goringe A, Ellis R, McDowell I, et al. The limited value of methylmalonic acid, homocysteine and holotranscobalamin in the diagnosis of early B$_{12}$ deficiency. Haematologica. 2006;91:231-234.

159. Lindenbaum J, Healton EB, Savage DG, et al. Neuropsychiatric disorders caused by cobalamin deficiency in the absence of anemia or macrocytosis. N Engl J Med. 1988;318:1720-1728.

160. Cooper BA, Whitehead VM. Evidence that some patients with pernicious anemia are not recognized by radiodilution assay for cobalamin in serum. N Engl J Med. 1978;299:816-818.

161. Carmel R, Brar S, Agrawal A, Penha DP. Failure of assay to identify low cobalamin concentrations. Clin Chem. 2000;46:2017-2018.

162. Carmel R, Serrai M. Diagnosis and management of clinical and subclinical cobalamin deficiency: advances and controversies. Curr Hematol Rep. 2006;5:23-33.

163. Cooper BA, Lowenstein L. Relative folate deficiency of erythrocytes in pernicious anemia and its correction with cyanocobalamin. Blood. 1964;24:502-521.

164. Herzlich B, Herbert V, Drivas G. Depletion of serum holotranscobalamin II. An early sign of negative vitamin B$_{12}$ balance. Lab Invest. 1988;58:332-337.

165. Ulleland M, Eilertsen I, Quadros EV, et al. Direct assay for cobalamin bound to transcobalamin (holotranscobalamin) in serum. Clin Chem. 2002;48: 526-532.

166. Nexo E, Christensen AL, Hvas AM, et al. Quantification of holo-transcobalamin, a marker of vitamin B$_{12}$ deficiency. Clin Chem. 2002;48:561-562.

167. Miller JW, Garrod MG, Rockwood AL, et al. Measurement of total vitamin B$_{12}$ and holotranscobalamin, singly and in combination, in screening for metabolic vitamin B$_{12}$ deficiency. Clin Chem. 2006;52:278-285.

168. Herrmann W, Obeid R, Schorr H, Geisel J. Functional vitamin B$_{12}$ deficiency and determination of holotranscobalamin in populations at risk. Clin Chem Lab Med. 2003;41:1478-1488.

169. Hvas AM, Nexo E. Holotranscobalamin—a first choice assay for diagnosing early vitamin B$_{12}$ deficiency? J Intern Med. 2005;257:289-298.

170. Schilling RF. Intrinsic factor studies. II. The effect of gastric juice on the urinary excretion of radioactivity after the oral administration of radioactive vitamin B$_{12}$. J Lab Clin Med. 1953;42:860-866.

171. Hvas AM, Nexo E. Diagnosis and treatment of vitamin B$_{12}$ deficiency—an update. Haematologica. 2006;91: 1508-1514.

172. Bor M, Çetin M, Aytaç S, et al. Nonradioactive vitamin B$_{12}$ absorption test evaluated in controls and in patients with inherited malabsorption of vitamin B$_{12}$. Clin Chem. 2005;51:2151-2155.

173. Fedosov SN, Laursen NB, Nexo E, et al. Human intrinsic factor expressed in the plant *Arabidopsis thaliana*. Eur J Biochem. 2003;270:3362-3367.

174. Hvas AM, Morkbak AL, Nexo E. Plasma holotranscobalamin compared with plasma cobalamins for assessment of vitamin B$_{12}$ absorption; optimisation of a non-radioactive vitamin B$_{12}$ absorption test (CobaSorb). Clin Chim Acta. 2007;376:150-154.

175. Andrès E, Affenberger S, Vinzio S, et al. Food-cobalamin malabsorption in elderly patients: clinical manifestations and treatment. Am J Med. 2005;118:1154-1159.

176. Carmel R. Malabsorption of food cobalamin. Baillieres Clin Haematol. 1995;8:639-6355.

177. Carmel R. Current concepts in cobalamin deficiency. Annu Rev Med. 2000;51:357-375.

178. Steinberg WM, King CE, Toskes PP. Malabsorption of protein-bound cobalamin but not unbound cobalamin during cimetidine administration. Dig Dis Sci. 1980;25:188-192.

179. Hippe E, Gimsing P, Holländer NH. A simplified method for quantitative determination of vitamin B$_{12}$ absorption. In Zagalak B, Friedrich W (eds). Vitamin B$_{12}$. Proceedings of the Third European Symposium on Vitamin B$_{12}$ and Intrinsic Factor. Berlin, Walter de Gruyter, 1979, pp 939-944.

180. Cox EV, White AM. Methylmalonic acid excretion: an index of vitamin-B_{12} deficiency. Lancet. 1962;2:853-856.

181. Schneede J, Dagnelie PC, van Staveren WA, et al. Methylmalonic acid and homocysteine in plasma as indicators of functional cobalamin deficiency in infants on macrobiotic diets. Pediatr Res. 1994;36:194-201.

182. Stabler SP, Marcell PD, Podell ER, et al. Assay of methylmalonic acid in the serum of patients with cobalamin deficiency using capillary gas chromatography–mass spectrometry. J Clin Invest. 1986;77:1606-1612.

183. Norman EJ. New urinary methylmalonic acid test is a sensitive indicator of cobalamin (vitamin B_{12}) deficiency: a solution for a major unrecognized medical problem. J Lab Clin Med. 1987;110:369-370.

184. Ho CH, Chang HC, Yeh SF. Quantitation of urinary methylmalonic acid by gas chromatography mass spectroscopy and its clinical applications. Eur J Haematol. 1987;38:80-84.

185. Matchar DB, Feussner JR, Millington DS, et al. Isotope-dilution assay for urinary methylmalonic acid in the diagnosis of vitamin B_{12} deficiency. A prospective clinical evaluation. Ann Intern Med. 1987;106:707-710.

186. Kang S-S, Wong PWK, Norusis M. Homocysteinemia due to folate deficiency. Metabolism. 1987;36:458-462.

187. Refsum H, Ueland PM, Svardal AM. Fully automated fluorescence assay for determining total homocysteine in plasma. Clin Chem. 1989;35:1921-1927.

188. Joosten E, Pelemans W, Devos P, et al. Cobalamin absorption and serum homocysteine and methylmalonic acid in elderly subjects with low serum cobalamin. Eur J Haematol. 1993;51:25-30.

189. Clarke R, Refsum H, Birks J, et al. Screening for vitamin B-12 and folate deficiency in older persons. Am J Clin Nutr. 2003;77:1241-1247.

190. Cooper BA, Lowenstein L. Vitamin B_{12}–folate interrelationships in megaloblastic anaemia. Br J Haematol. 1966;12:283-296.

191. Waxman S, Metz J, Herbert V. Defective DNA synthesis in human megaloblastic bone marrow: effects of homocysteine and methionine. J Clin Invest. 1969;48:284-289.

192. Wickramasinghe SN. The deoxyuridine suppression test. In Hall CA (ed). The Cobalamins. Edinburgh, Churchill Livingstone, 1983, pp 196-208.

193. Lawson DH, Parker JL. Deaths from severe megaloblastic anemia in hospitalised patients. Scand J Haematol. 1976;17:347-352.

194. Kuzminski AM, Del Giacco EJ, Allen RH, et al. Effective treatment of cobalamin deficiency with oral cobalamin. Blood. 1998;92:1191-1198.

195. Bolaman Z, Kadikoylu G, Yukselen V, et al. Oral versus intramuscular cobalamin treatment in megaloblastic anemia: a single-center, prospective, randomized, open-label study. Clin Ther. 2003;25:3124-3134.

196. Vidal-Alaball J, Butler CC, Cannings-John R, et al. Oral vitamin B_{12} versus intramuscular vitamin B_{12} for vitamin B_{12} deficiency. Cochrane Database Syst Rev. 2005;3: CD004655.

197. Solomon LR. Oral pharmacological doses of cobalamin may not be as effective as parenteral cobalamin therapy in reversing hyperhomocystinemia and methylmalonic

aciduria in apparently normal subjects. Clin Lab Haematol. 2006;28:275-278.

198. Solomon LR. Oral vitamin B_{12} therapy: a cautionary tale. Blood. 2004;103:2863.

199. Skouby AP. Hydroxocobalamin for initial and long-term therapy for vitamin B_{12} deficiency. Acta Med Scan. 1987;221:339-402.

200. Olesen H, Hom B, Schwartz M. Antibody to transcobalamin II in patients treated with long acting vitamin B_{12} preparations. Scand J Haematol. 1968;5:5.

201. Bowen RAR, Drake SK, Vanjani R, et al. Markedly increased vitamin B_{12} concentrations attributable to IgG-IgM-vitamin B_{12} immune complexes. Clin Chem. 2006;52: 2107-2114.

202. Kuwabara S, Nakazawa R, Azuma N, et al. Intravenous methylcobalamin treatment for uremic and diabetic neuropathy in chronic hemodialysis patients. Intern Med. 1999;38:472-475.

203. Duning T, Nabavi DG, Dziewas R, Kugel H. Chronic renal failure promotes severe variant of vitamin B_{12} deficiency. Eur Nephrol. 2006;56:62-65.

204. Naurath HJ, Joosten E, Riezler R, et al. Effects of vitamin B_{12}, folate, and vitamin B_6 supplements in elderly people with normal serum vitamin concentrations. Lancet. 1995;346:85-89.

205. Lewerin C, Nillson-Ehle H, Matousek M, et al. Reduction of plasma homocysteine and serum methylmalonate concentrations in apparently healthy elderly subjects after treatment with folic acid, vitamin B_{12} and vitamin B_6: a randomised trial. Eur J Clin Nutr. 2003;57: 1426-1436.

206. Birn H, Nexo E, Christensen EI, Nielsen R. Diversity in rat tissue accumulation of vitamin B_{12} supports a distinct role for the kidney in vitamin B_{12} homeostasis. Nephrol Dial Transplant. 2003;18:1095-1100.

207. Reizenstein P, Matthews CME. Vitamin B_{12} kinetics in man. Implications on total-body-B_{12}-determinations, human requirements, and normal and pathological cellular B_{12} uptake. Phys Med Biol. 1966;11:295-306.

208. Carmel R, Johnson CS. Racial patterns in pernicious anemia. Early age at onset and increased frequency of intrinsic-factor antibody in black women. N Engl J Med. 1978;298:647-650.

209. Chan JCW, Liu HSY, Kho BCS, et al. Megaloblastic anaemia in Chinese patients: a review of 52 cases. Hong Kong Med J. 1998;4:269-274.

210. McIntyre PA. Genetic and auto-immune features of pernicious anemia. I. Unreliability of the Schilling test in detecting genetic predisposition to the disease. Johns Hopkins Med J. 1968;122:181-183.

211. Delva PL, MacDonnell JE, MacIntosh OC. Megaloblastic anemia occurring simultaneously in white female monozygotic twins. Can Med Assoc J. 1965;92:1129-1131.

212. Davis RE, McCann VJ, Stanton KG. Type I diabetes and latent pernicious anemia. Med J Aust. 1992;156: 160-162.

213. Toh BH, Van Driel IR, Gleeson PA. Pernicious anemia. N Engl J Med. 1997;337:1441-1448.

214. Andrès E, Blicklé F, Sordet C, et al. Primary Sjögren's syndrome and vitamin B_{12} deficiency: preliminary results in 80 patients. Am J Med. 2006;119:e9-e10.

215. Ottesen M, Feldt-Rasmussen U, Andersen J, et al. Thyroid function and autoimmunity in pernicious anemia before

and during cyanocobalamin treatment. J Endocrinol Invest. 1995;18:91-97.

216. Berendt RC, Jewell LD, Shnitka TK, et al. Multicentric gastric carcinoids complicating pernicious anemia. Origin from the metaplastic endocrine cell population. Arch Pathol Lab Med. 1989;113:399-403.

217. Hsing AW, Hansson LE, McLaughlin JK, et al. Pernicious anemia and subsequent cancer. A population-based cohort study. Cancer. 1993;71:745-750.

218. Botez MI. Neuropsychiatric illness and deficiency of vitamin B_{12} and folate. In Zittoun JA, Cooper BA (eds). Folates and Cobalamins. Berlin, Springer-Verlag, 1989, pp 145-159.

219. Di Trapani G, Barone C, La Cara A, Laurienzo P. Dementia–peripheral neuropathy during combined deficiency of vitamin B_{12} and folate. Light microscopy and ultrastructural study of sural nerve. Ital J Neurol Sci. 1986;7: 545-552.

220. Steiner I, Kidron D, Soffer D, et al. Sensory peripheral neuropathy of vitamin B_{12} deficiency: a primary demyelinating disease? J Neurol. 1988;235:163-164.

221. Zegers de Beyl D, Delecluse F, Verbanck P, et al. Somatosensory conduction in vitamin B_{12} deficiency. Electroencephalogr Clin Neurophysiol. 1988;69:313-318.

222. Perkin GD, Roche SW, Abraham R. Delayed somatosensory evoked potentials in pernicious anaemia with intact peripheral nerves. J Neurosurg Psychiatry. 1989;52: 1017-1018.

223. Kozak N, Schattner A. 'Mobile phone sign' in early vitamin B_{12} deficiency. Q J Med. 2006;99:273-274.

224. Refsum H, Smith AD. Low vitamin B-12 status in confirmed Alzheimer's disease as revealed by serum holo-transcobalamin. J Neurol Neurosurg Psychiatry. 2003;74: 959-961.

225. Weir DG, Keating S, Molloy AM, et al. Methylation deficiency causes vitamin B_{12}–associated neuropathy in the pig. J Neurochem. 1988;51:1949-1952.

226. Drummond JT, Matthews RG. Nitrous oxide degradation by cobalamin-dependent methionine synthase; characterization of the reactants and products in the inactivation reaction. Biochemistry. 1994;33:3732-3741.

227. Drummond JT, Matthews RG. Nitrous oxide inactivation of cobalamin-dependent methionine synthase from *Escherichia coli*: characterization of the damage to the enzyme and prosthetic group. Biochemistry. 1994;33:3742-3750.

228. Scott JM, Dinn JJ, Wilson P, Weir DG. Pathogenesis of subacute combined degeneration: a result of methyl group deficiency. Lancet. 1981;318:334-337.

229. Unglaub WG, Prevatt AL, Goldsmith GA. Recent experiences in diagnosing and treating pernicious anemia. Postgrad Med. 1961;29:399-407.

230. Hall CA. The nondiagnosis of pernicious anemia. Ann Intern Med. 1965;63:951-954.

231. Carmel R, Karnaze DS, Weiner JM. Neurologic abnormalities in cobalamin deficiency are associated with higher cobalamin "analogue" values than are hematologic abnormalities. J Lab Clin Med. 1988;111: 57-62.

232. Nilsson K, Gustafson L, Faldt R, et al. Plasma homocysteine in relation to serum cobalamin and blood folate in a psychogeriatric population. Eur J Clin Invest. 1994;24: 600-606.

233. Lindenbaum J, Rosenberg IH, Wilson PWF, et al. Prevalence of cobalamin deficiency in the Framingham elderly population. Am J Clin Nutr. 1994;60:2-11.

234. Herbert V. Staging vitamin B-12 (cobalamin) status in vegetarians. Am J Clin Nutr. 1994;59:1213S-1222S.

235. Norman EJ, Morrison JA. Screening elderly populations for cobalamin (vitamin B_{12}) deficiency using the urinary methylmalonic acid assay by gas chromatography mass spectrometry. Am J Med. 1993;94:589-594.

236. Pennypacker LC, Allen RH, Kelly JP, et al. High prevalence of cobalamin deficiency in elderly outpatients. J Am Geriatr Soc. 1992;40:1197-1204.

237. Clarke R, Grimley Evans J, Schneede J, et al. Vitamin B_{12} and folate deficiency in later life. Age Ageing. 2004;33: 34-41.

238. Snow CF. Laboratory diagnosis of vitamin B_{12} and folate deficiency. Arch Intern Med. 1999;159:1289-1298.

239. Wickramasinghe SN. Diagnosis of megaloblastic anaemias. Blood Rev. 2006;20:299-318.

240. Rosenblatt DS, Whitehead VM. Cobalamin and folate deficiency: acquired and hereditary disorders in children. Semin Hematol. 1999;36:19-34.

241. Casterline JE, Allen LH, Ruel MT. Vitamin B-12 deficiency is very prevalent in lactating Guatemalan women and their infants at three months postpartum. J Nutr. 1997;127:1966-1972.

242. Rogers LM, Boy E, Miller JW, et al. High prevalence of cobalamin deficiency in Guatemalan schoolchildren: associations with low plasma holotranscobalamin II and elevated serum methylmalonic acid and plasma homocysteine concentrations. Am J Clin Nutr. 2003;77:433-440.

243. Guerra-Shinohara EM, Morita OE, Peres S, et al. Low ratio of *S*-adenosylmethionine to *S*-adenosylhomocysteine is associated with vitamin deficiency in Brazilian pregnant women and newborns. Am J Clin Nutr. 2004;80:1312-1321.

244. Garcia-Casal MN, Osorio C, Landaeta M, et al. High prevalence of folic acid and cobalamin deficiencies in infants, children, adolescents and pregnant women in Venezuela. Eur J Clin Nutr. 2005;59:1064-1070.

245. Sanfillipo JS, Liu YK. Vitamin B_{12} deficiency and infertility: report of a case. Int J Fertil. 1991;36:36-38.

246. Bar-Shany S, Herbert V. Transplacentally acquired antibody to intrinsic factor with vitamin B_{12} deficiency. Blood. 1967;30:777-784.

247. Danielsson L, Enocksson E, Hagenfeldt L, et al. Failure to thrive due to subclinical maternal pernicious anemia. Acta Paediatr Scand. 1988;77:310-311.

248. Emery ES, Homans AC, Colletti RB. Vitamin B_{12} deficiency: a cause of abnormal movements in infants. Pediatrics. 1997;99:255-256.

249. Korenke GC, Hunneman DH, Eber S, Hanefeld F. Severe encephalopathy with epilepsy in an infant caused by subclinical maternal pernicious anaemia: case report and review of the literature. Eur J Pediatr. 2004;163: 196-201.

250. Specker BL, Miller D, Norman EJ, et al. Increased urinary methylmalonic acid excretion in breast-fed infants of vegetarian mothers and identification of an acceptable dietary source of vitamin B-12. Am J Clin Nutr. 1988;47:89-92.

251. Herbert V. Vitamin B-12: plant sources, requirements, and assay. Am J Clin Nutr. 1988;48:852-858.

252. Kushi M, Jack A. The Book of Macrobiotics. The Universal Way of Health, Happiness, and Peace. New York, Japan Publications, 1987.

253. Specker BL, Black A, Allen L, Morrow F. Vitamin B-12: low milk concentrations are related to low serum concentrations in vegetarian women and to methylmalonic aciduria in their infants. Am J Clin Nutr. 1990;52: 1073-1076.

254. Gadowsky SL, Gale K, Wolfe SA, et al. Biochemical folate, B₁₂, and iron status of a group of pregnant adolescents accessed through the public health system in southern Ontario. J Adolesc Health. 1995;16:465-474.

255. Lowenstein L, Lalonde M, Deschenes EB, Shapiro L. Vitamin B₁₂ in pregnancy and the puerperium. Am J Clin Nutr. 1960;8:265-275.

256. Monsen ALB, Ueland PM, Vollset SE, et al. Determinants of cobalamin status in newborns. Pediatrics. 2001;108: 624-630.

257. Park H, Kim YJ, Ha EH, et al. The risk of folate and vitamin B₁₂ deficiencies associated with hyperhomocysteinemia among pregnant women. Am J Perinatol. 2004;21: 469-476.

258. Bondevik GT, Schneede J, Refsum H, et al. Homocysteine and methylmalonic acid levels in pregnant Nepali women. Should cobalamin supplementation be considered? Eur J Clin Nutr. 2001;55:856-864.

259. Layzer RB, Fishman RA, Schafer JA. Neuropathy following abuse of nitrous oxide. Neurology. 1978;28:504-506.

260. Skacel PO, Hewlett AM, Lewis JD, et al. Studies on the haemopoietic toxicity of nitrous oxide in man. Br J Haematol. 1983;53:189-200.

261. Pappo AS, Fields BW, Buchanan GR. Etiology of red blood cell macrocytosis during childhood: impact of new diseases and therapies. Pediatrics. 1992;89:1063-1067.

262. Kühne T, Bubl R, Baumgartner R. Maternal vegan diet causing a serious infantile neurological disorder due to vitamin B₁₂ deficiency. Eur J Pediatr. 1991;150:205-208.

263. Lövblad KO, Ramelli G, Remonda L, et al. Retardation of myelination due to dietary vitamin B₁₂ deficiency: cranial MRI findings. Pediatr Radiol. 1997;27:155-158.

264. Monagle PT, Tauro GP. Infantile megaloblastosis secondary to maternal vitamin B₁₂ deficiency. Clin Lab Haematol. 1997;19:23-25.

265. Sklar R. Nutritional vitamin B₁₂ deficiency in a breast-fed infant of a vegan-diet mother. Clin Pediatr (Phila). 1986;25:219-221.

266. Grange DK, Finlay JL. Nutritional vitamin B₁₂ deficiency in a breastfed infant following maternal gastric bypass. Pediatr Hematol Oncol. 1994;11:311-318.

267. Skidmore MD, Shenker N, Kliegman RM, et al. Biochemical evidence of asymptomatic vitamin B₁₂ deficiency in children after ileal resection for necrotizing enterocolitis. J Pediatr. 1989;115:102-105.

268. Dagnelie PC, van Staveren WA, Hautvast JG. Stunting and nutrient deficiencies in children on alternative diets. Acta Paediatr Scand. 1991;374:111-118.

269. Higginbottom MC, Sweetman L, Nyhan WL. A syndrome of methylmalonic aciduria, homocystinuria, megaloblastic anemia and neurological abnormalities in a vitamin B₁₂–deficient breast-fed infant of a strict vegetarian. N Engl J Med. 1978;299:317-323.

270. Silberstein EP, Wilson RG, Scurlock JM. Methylmalonic aciduria in an infant of a mother with undiagnosed pernicious anaemia. Med J Aust. 1987;146:329-330.

271. Goraya J. Persistence of neurological damage induced by dietary vitamin B-12 deficiency. Arch Dis Child. 1998; 78:395.

272. Centers for Disease Control and Prevention (CDC). Neurologic impairment in children associated with maternal dietary deficiency of cobalamin—Georgia, 2001. MMWR Morb Mortal Wkly Rep. 2003;52(4):61-64.

273. Weiss R, Fogelman Y, Bennett M. Severe vitamin B₁₂ deficiency in an infant associated with a maternal deficiency and a strict vegetarian diet. J Pediatr Hematol Oncol. 2004;26:270-271.

274. Simsek OP, Gönç N, Gümrük F, Çetin M. A child with vitamin B₁₂ deficiency presenting with pancytopenia and hyperpigmentation. J Pediatr Hematol Oncol. 2004;26: 834-836.

275. Roschitz B, Plecko B, Huemer M, et al. Nutritional infantile vitamin B₁₂ deficiency: pathobiochemical considerations in seven patients. Arch Dis Child Fetal Neonat Ed. 2005;90:F281-F282.

276. Codazzi D, Sala F, Parini R, Langer M. Coma and respiratory failure in a child with severe vitamin B₁₂ deficiency. Pediatr Crit Care Med. 2005;6:483-485.

277. Reghu A, Hosdurga S, Sandhu B, Spray C. Vitamin B₁₂ deficiency presenting as oedema in infants of vegetarian mothers. Eur J Pediatr. 2005;164:257-258.

278. von Schenck U, Bender-Götze C, Koletzko B. Persistence of neurological damage induced by dietary vitamin B-12 deficiency in infancy. Arch Dis Child. 1997;77: 137-139.

279. The Writing Group for the DISC Collaborative Research Group. Efficacy and safety of lowering dietary intake of fat and cholesterol in children with elevated low-density lipoprotein cholesterol. The Dietary Intervention Study in Children (DISC). JAMA. 1995;273:1429-1435.

280. Obarzanek E, Hunsberger SA, Van Horn L, et al. Safety of a fat-reduced diet: the Dietary Intervention Study in Children (DISC). Pediatrics. 1997;100:51-59.

281. Fréry N, Huel G, Leroy M, et al. Vitamin B₁₂ among parturients and their newborns and its relationship with birthweight. Eur J Obstet Gynecol Reprod Biol. 1992;45:155-163.

282. Obeid R, Morkbak AL, Munz W, et al. The cobalamin-binding proteins transcobalamin and haptocorrin in maternal and cord blood sera at birth. Clin Chem. 2006;52:263-269.

283. Worthington-White DA, Behnke M, Gross S. Premature infants require additional folate and vitamin B-12 to reduce the severity of the anemia of prematurity. Am J Clin Nutr. 1994;60:930-935.

284. Kirke PN, Molloy AM, Daly LE, et al. Maternal plasma folate and vitamin B₁₂ are independent risk factors for neural tube defects. Q J Med. 1993;86:703-708.

285. Chandra J, Jain V, Narayan S, et al. Tremors and thrombocytosis during treatment of megaloblastic anaemia. Ann Trop Paediatr. 2006;26:101-105.

286. Ashkenazi S, Weitz R, Varsano I, Mimouni M. Vitamin B₁₂ deficiency due to a strictly vegetarian diet in adolescence. Clin Pediatr (Phila). 1987;26:662-663.

287. Pinhas-Hamiel O, Doron-Panush N, Reichman B, et al. Obese children and adolescents. A risk group for low

vitamin B_{12} concentration. Arch Pediatr Adolesc Med. 2006;160:933-936.

288. Burkes RL, Cohen H, Krailo M, et al. Low serum cobalamin levels occur frequently in the acquired immune deficiency syndrome and related disorders. Eur J Haematol. 1987;38:141-147.

289. Harriman GR, Smith PD, Horne MK, et al. Vitamin B_{12} malabsorption in patients with acquired immunodeficiency syndrome. Arch Intern Med. 1989;149: 2039-2041.

290. Kieburtz KD, Giang DW, Schiffer RB, Vakil N. Abnormal vitamin B_{12} metabolism in human immunodeficiency virus infection. Arch Neurol. 1991;48:312-314.

291. Remacha AF, Cadafalch J, Sardà P, et al. Vitamin B-12 metabolism in HIV-infected patients in the age of highly active antiretroviral therapy: role of homocysteine in assessing vitamin B-12 status. Am J Clin Nutr. 2003;77: 420-424.

292. Allen LH, Rosado JL, Casterline JE, et al. Vitamin B-12 deficiency and malabsorption are highly prevalent in Mexican Communities. Am J Clin Nutr. 1995;62: 1013-1019.

293. Hanley WB, Feigenbaum AS, Clarke JT, et al. Vitamin B_{12} deficiency in adolescents and young adults with phenylketonuria. Eur J Pediatr. 1996;155:145-147.

294. van Dusseldorp M, Schneede J, Refsum H, et al. Risk of persistent cobalamin deficiency in adolescents fed a macrobiotic diet in early life. Am J Clin Nutr. 1999;69: 664-671.

295. Louwman MWJ, van Dusseldorp M, van de Vijver FJR, et al. Signs of impaired cognitive function in adolescents with marginal cobalamin status. Am J Clin Nutr. 2000;72:762-769.

296. Katz M, Lee SK, Cooper BA. Vitamin B_{12} malabsorption due to a biologically inert intrinsic factor. N Engl J Med. 1972;287:425-429.

297. Spurling CL, Sacks MS, Jiji RM. Juvenile pernicious anemia. N Engl J Med. 1964;271:995-1003.

298. McIntyre OR, Sullivan LW, Jeffries GH, Silver RH. Pernicious anemia in childhood. N Engl J Med. 1965;272: 981-986.

299. Katz M, Mehlman CS, Allen RH. Isolation and characterization of an abnormal human intrinsic factor. J Clin Invest. 1974;53:1274-1283.

300. Yang Y-M, Ducos R, Rosenberg AJ, et al. Cobalamin malabsorption in three siblings due to an abnormal intrinsic factor that is markedly susceptible to acid and proteolysis. J Clin Invest. 1985;76:2057-2065.

301. Levine JS, Allen RH. Intrinsic factor within parietal cells of patients with juvenile pernicious anemia. A retrospective immunohistochemical study. Gastroenterology. 1985; 88:1132-1136.

302. Yassin F, Rothenberg SP, Rao S, et al. Identification of a 4-base deletion in the gene in inherited intrinsic factor deficiency. Blood. 2004;103:1515-1517.

303. Tanner SM, Li Z, Perko JD, et al. Hereditary juvenile cobalamin deficiency caused by mutations in the intrinsic factor gene. Proc Natl Acad Sci U S A. 2005;102: 4130-4133.

304. Gräsbeck R. Familial selective vitamin B_{12} malabsorption. N Engl J Med. 1972;287:358.

305. Mackenzie IL, Donaldson RM, Trier JS, Mathan VI. Ileal mucosa in familial selective vitamin B_{12} malabsorption. N Engl J Med. 1972;286:1021-1025.

306. Wulffraat NM, de Schryver J, Bruin M, et al. Failure to thrive is an early symptom of the Imerslund Gräsbeck syndrome. Am J Pediatr Hematol Oncol. 1994;16: 177-180.

307. Gräsbeck R. Imerslund-Gräsbeck syndrome (selective vitamin B_{12} malabsorption with proteinuria). Orphanet J Rare Dis. 2006;1:17.

308. Wahlstedt-Fröberg V, Pettersson T, Aminoff M, et al. Proteinuria in cubilin-deficient patients with selective vitamin B_{12} malabsorption. Pediatr Nephrol. 2003;18:417-421.

309. Tanner SM, Li Z, Bisson R, et al. Genetically heterogeneous selective intestinal malabsorption of vitamin B_{12} founder effects, consanguinity, and high clinical awareness explains the aggregations in Scandinavia and the Middle East. Hum Mutat. 2004;23:327-333.

310. Bouchlaka C, Maktouf C, Mahjoub B, et al. Genetic heterogeneity of megaloblastic anaemia type 1 in Tunisian patients. J Hum Genet. 2007;52:262-270.

311. Cooper BA, Rosenblatt DS. Inherited defects of vitamin B_{12} metabolism. Annu Rev Nutr. 1987;7:291-320.

312. Li N, Rosenblatt DS, Kamen B, et al. Identification of two mutant alleles of transcobalamin II in an affected family. Hum Mol Genet. 1994;3:1835-1840.

313. Niebrugge DJ, Benjamin DR, Christie D, Scott CR. Hereditary transcobalamin II deficiency presenting as red cell hypoplasia. J Pediatr. 1982;101:732-735.

314. Burman JF, Mollin DL, Sourial NA, Sladden RA. Inherited lack of transcobalamin II in serum and megaloblastic anaemia: a further patient. Br J Haematol. 1979;43: 27-38.

315. Meyers PA, Carmel R. Hereditary transcobalamin II deficiency with subnormal serum cobalamin levels. Pediatrics. 1984;74:866-871.

316. Thomas PK, Hoffbrand AV, Smith IS. Neurological involvement in hereditary transcobalamin II deficiency. J Neurol Neurosurg Psychiatry. 1982;45:74-77.

317. Zeitlin HC, Sheppard K, Baum JD, et al. Homozygous transcobalamin II deficiency maintained on oral hydroxocobalamin. Blood. 1985;66:1022-1027.

318. Haurani FI, Hall CA, Rubin R. Megaloblastic anemia as a result of an abnormal transcobalamin II (Cardeza). J Clin Invest. 1979;64:1253-1259.

319. Seligman PA, Steiner LL, Allen RH. Studies of a patient with megaloblastic anemia and an abnormal transcobalamin II. N Engl J Med. 1980;303:1209-1212.

320. Li N, Rosenblatt DS, Seetharam B. Nonsense mutations in human transcobalamin II deficiency. Biochem Biophys Res Commun. 1994;204:1111-1118.

321. Namour F, Helfer AC, Quadros EV, et al. Transcobalamin deficiency due to activation of an intra exonic cryptic splice set. Br J Haematol. 2003;123:915-920.

322. Rosenblatt DS, Hosack A, Matiaszuk N. Expression of transcobalamin 2 by amniocytes. Prenat Diagn. 1987;6:195-205.

323. Carmel R, Herbert V. Deficiency of vitamin B_{12}–binding alpha globulin in two brothers. Blood. 1969;33:1-12.

324. Carmel R. A new case of deficiency of the R binder for cobalamin, with observations on minor cobalamin-binding proteins in serum and saliva. Blood. 1982;59:152-156.

325. Jenks J, Begley JA, Howard L. Cobalamin R binder deficiency in a woman with thalassemia. Nutr Rev. 1983;41:277-280.

326. Carmel R. R-binder deficiency. A clinically benign cause of cobalamin pseudodeficiency. JAMA. 1983;250:1886-1890.

327. Sigal SH, Hall CA, Antel JP. Plasma R binder and neurologic disease. N Engl J Med. 1987;317:1330-1332.

328. Fowler B, Whitehouse C, Wenzel F, Wraith JE. Methionine and serine formation in control and mutant human cultured fibroblasts: evidence for methyl trapping and characterization of remethylation defects. Pediatr Res. 1997;41:145-151.

329. Watkins D. Cobalamin metabolism in methionine-dependent human tumour and leukemia cell lines. Clin Invest Med. 1998;21:151-158.

330. Rosenblatt DS, Cooper BA, Schmutz SM, et al. Prenatal vitamin B$_{12}$ therapy of a fetus with methylcobalamin deficiency (cobalamin E disease). Lancet. 1985;325:1127-1129.

331. Zammarchi E, Lippi A, Falorni S, et al. cblC disease: case report and monitoring of a pregnancy at risk by chorionic villus sampling. Clin Invest Med. 1990;13:139-142.

332. Evans MI, Duquette DA, Rinaldo P, et al. Modulation of B$_{12}$ dosage and response in fetal treatment of methylmalonic aciduria (MMA): titration of treatment dose to serum and urine MMA. Fetal Diagn Ther. 1997;12:21-23.

333. Morel CF, Watkins D, Scott P, et al. Prenatal diagnosis for methylmalonic acidemia and inborn errors of vitamin B$_{12}$ metabolism and transport. Mol Genet Metab. 2005;86:160-171.

334. Watkins D, Rosenblatt DS. Functional methionine synthase deficiency (*cblE* and *cblG*): clinical and biochemical heterogeneity. Am J Med Genet. 1989;34:427-434.

335. Carmel R, Watkins D, Goodman SI, Rosenblatt DS. Hereditary defect of cobalamin metabolism (*cblG* mutation) presenting as a neurologic disorder in adulthood. N Engl J Med. 1988;318:1738-1741.

336. Tuchman M, Kelly P, Watkins D, Rosenblatt DS. Vitamin B$_{12}$–responsive megaloblastic anemia, homocystinuria, and transient methylmalonic aciduria in *cblE* disease. J Pediatr. 1988;113:1052-1056.

337. Sillaots SL, Hall CA, Hurteloup V, Rosenblatt DS. Heterogeneity in *cblG*: differential retention of cobalamin on methionine synthase. Biochem Med Metab Biol. 1992;47:242-249.

338. Schuh S, Rosenblatt DS, Cooper BA, et al. Homocystinuria and megaloblastic anemia responsive to vitamin B$_{12}$ therapy. An inborn error of metabolism due to a defect in cobalamin metabolism. N Engl J Med. 1984;310:686-690.

339. Gulati S, Baker P, Li YN, et al. Defects in human methionine synthase in *cblG* patients. Hum Mol Genet. 1996;5:1859-1865.

340. Wilson A, Leclerc D, Saberi F, et al. Functionally null mutations in patients with the *cblG*-variant form of methionine synthase deficiency. Am J Hum Genet. 1998;63:409-414.

341. Wilson A, Leclerc D, Rosenblatt DS, Gravel RA. Molecular basis for methionine synthase reductase deficiency in patients belonging to the *cblE* complementation group of disorders in folate/cobalamin metabolism. Hum Mol Genet. 1999;8:2009-2016.

342. Zavadakova P, Fowler B, Zeman J, et al. CblE type of homocystinuria due to methionine synthase reductase deficiency: clinical and molecular studies and prenatal diagnosis. J Inherit Metab Dis. 2002;25:461-476.

343. Vilaseca MA, Vilarinho L, Zavafakova P, et al. CblE type of homocystinuria: mild clinical phenotype in two patients homozygous for a novel mutation in the *MTRR* gene. J Inherit Metab Dis. 2003;26:361-369.

344. Zavadakova P, Fowler B, Suormala T, et al. *cblE* type of homocystinuria due to methionine synthase reductase deficiency: functional correction by minigene expression. Hum Mutat. 2005;25:239-247.

345. Rosenblatt DS, Aspler AL, Shevell MI, et al. Clinical heterogeneity and prognosis in combined methylmalonic aciduria and homocystinuria (*cblC*). J Inherit Metab Dis. 1997;20:528-538.

346. Shinnar S, Singer HS. Cobalamin C mutation (methylmalonic aciduria and homocystinuria) in adolescence. N Engl J Med. 1984;311:451-454.

347. Mitchell GA, Watkins D, Melançon SB, et al. Clinical heterogeneity in cobalamin C variant of combined homocystinuria and methylmalonic aciduria. J Pediatr. 1986;108:410-415.

348. Augoustides-Savvopoulou P, Mylonas I, Sewell AC, Rosenblatt DS. Reversible dementia in an adolescent with *cblC* disease: clinical heterogeneity within the same family. J Inherit Metab Dis. 1999;22:756-758.

349. Powers JM, Rosenblatt DS, Schmidt RE, et al. Neurological and neuropathologic heterogeneity in two brothers with cobalamin C deficiency. Ann Neurol. 2001;49:396-400.

350. Bodamer OAF, Rosenblatt DS, Appel SH, Beaudet AL. Adult-onset combined methylmalonic aciduria and homocystinuria (*cblC*). Neurology. 2001;56:1113.

351. Robb RM, Dowton SB, Fulton AB, Levy HL. Retinal degeneration in vitamin B$_{12}$ disorder associated with methylmalonic aciduria and sulfur amino acid abnormalities. Am J Ophthalmol. 1984;97:691-696.

352. Traboulsi EI, Silva JC, Geraghty MT, et al. Ocular histopathologic characteristics of cobalamin C type vitamin B$_{12}$ defect with methylmalonic aciduria and homocystinuria. Am J Ophthalmol. 1992;113:269-280.

353. Schimel AM, Mets MB. The natural history of retinal degeneration in association with cobalamin C (cblC) disease. Ophthalmic Genet. 2006;27:9-14.

354. Francis PJ, Calver DM, Barnfield P, et al. An infant with methylmalonic aciduria and homocystinuria (cblC) presenting with retinal haemorrhages and subdural haematoma mimicking non-accidental injury. Eur J Pediatr. 2004;163:420-421.

355. Tsina EK, Marsden DL, Hansen RM, Fulton AB. Maculopathy and retinal degeneration in cobalamin C methylmalonic aciduria and homocystinuria. Arch Ophthalmol. 2005;123:1143-1145.

356. Geraghty MT, Perlman EJ, Martin LS, et al. Cobalamin C defect associated with hemolytic-uremic syndrome. J Pediatr. 1992;120:934-937.

357. Howard R, Frieden IJ, Crawford D, et al. Methylmalonic acidemia, cobalamin C type, presenting with cutaneous manifestations. Arch Dermatol. 1997;133:1563-1566.

358. Andersson HC, Marble M, Shapira E. Long-term outcome in treated combined methylmalonic acidemia and homocystinemia. Genet Med. 1999;1:146-150.

359. Morel CF, Lerner-Ellis JP, Rosenblatt DS. Combined methylmalonic aciduria and homocystinuria (*cblC*): phenotype-genotype correlations and ethnic-specific observations. Mol Genet Metab. 2006;88:315-321.

360. Bartholomew DW, Batshaw ML, Allen RH, et al. Therapeutic approaches to cobalamin-C methylmalonic acidemia and homocystinuria. J Pediatr. 1988;112:32-39.

361. Rosenblatt DS, Fenton WA. Inherited disorders of folate and cobalamin transport and metabolism. In Scriver CR, Beaudet AL, Sly WS, et al. (eds). The Metabolic and Molecular Bases of Inherited Disease. New York, McGraw-Hill, 2001, pp 3897-3933.

362. Goodman SI, Moe PG, Hammond KB. Homocystinuria with methylmalonic aciduria: two cases in a sibship. Biochem Med. 1970;4:500-515.

363. Willard HF, Mellman IS, Rosenberg LE. Genetic complementation among inherited deficiencies of methylmalonyl-CoA mutase activity: evidence for a new class of human cobalamin mutant. Am J Hum Genet. 1978;30:1-13.

364. Suormala T, Baumgartner MR, Coelho D, et al. The cblD defect causes either isolated or combined deficiency of methylcobalamin and adenosylcobalamin synthesis. J Biol Chem. 2004;279:42742-42749.

365. Shih V, Axel SM, Tewksbury JC, et al. Defective lysosomal release of vitamin B_{12} (*cblF*): a hereditary cobalamin metabolic disorder associated with sudden death. Am J Med Genet. 1989;33:555-563.

366. MacDonald, MR, Wiltse HE, Bever JL, Rosenblatt DS. Clinical heterogeneity in two patients with cblF disease. Am J Hum Genet. 1992;51:A353.

367. Wong LTK, Rosenblatt DS, Applegarth DA, Davidson AGF. Diagnosis and treatment of a child with cblF disease. J Clin Invest. 1992;15:A111.

368. Waggoner DJ, Ueda K, Mantia C, Dowton SB. Methylmalonic aciduria (cblF): case report and response to therapy. Am J Med Genet. 1998;79:373-375.

369. Rosenblatt DS, Hosack A, Matiaszuk NV, et al. Defect in vitamin B_{12} release from lysosomes: newly described inborn error of vitamin B_{12} metabolism. Science. 1985;228:1319-1321.

370. Dobson CM, Gradinger A, Longo N, et al. Homozygous nonsense mutation in the *MCEE* gene and siRNA suppression of methylmalonyl-CoA epimerase expression: a novel cause of mild methylmalonic aciduria. Mol Genet Metab. 2006;88:327-333.

371. Bikker H, Bakker HD, Abeling NGGM, et al. A homozygous nonsense mutation in the methylmalonyl-CoA epimerase gene (*MCEE*) results in mild methylmalonic aciduria. Hum Mutat. 2006;27:640-643.

372. Carrozzo R, Dionisi-Vici C, Steuerwald U, et al. *SUCLA2* mutations are associated with mild methylmalonic aciduria, Leigh-like encephalomyopathy, dystonia and deafness. Brain. 2007;130:862-874.

373. Ostergaard E, Hansen FJ, Sorensen N, et al. Mitochondrial encephalomyopathy with elevated methylmalonic acid is caused by *SUCLA2* mutations. Brain. 2007;130:853-861.

374. Fenton WA, Hack AM, Kraus JP, Rosenberg LE. Immunochemical studies of fibroblasts from patients with methylmalonyl-CoA mutase apoenzyme deficiency: detection of a mutation interfering with mitochondrial import. Proc Natl Acad Sci U S A. 1987;84:1421-1424.

375. Raff ML, Crane AM, Jansen R, et al. Genetic characterization of a *MUT* locus mutation discriminating heterogeneity in mut^0 and mut^- methylmalonic aciduria by interallelic complementation. J Clin Invest. 1991;87:203-207.

376. Qureshi AA, Crane AM, Matiaszuk NV, et al. Cloning and expression of mutations demonstrating intragenic complementation in mut^0 methylmalonic aciduria. J Clin Invest. 1994;93:1812-1819.

377. Inoue S, Krieger I, Sarnaik A, et al. Inhibition of bone marrow stem cell growth in vitro by methylmalonic acid: a mechanism for pancytopenia in a patient with methylmalonic aciduria. Pediatr Res. 1981;15:95-98.

378. Ledley FD, Levy HL, Shih V, et al. Benign methylmalonic aciduria. N Engl J Med. 1984;311:1015-1018.

379. Jansen R, Kalousek F, Fenton WA, et al. Cloning of full-length methylmalonyl-CoA mutase from a cDNA library using the polymerase chain reaction. Genomics. 1989;4:198-205.

380. Ledley FD, Rosenblatt DS. Mutations in mut methylmalonic acidemia: clinical and enzymatic correlations. Hum Mutat. 1997;9:1-6.

381. Worgan LC, Niles K, Tirone JC, et al. Spectrum of mutations in *mut* methylmalonic acidemia and identification of a common Hispanic mutation and haplotype. Hum Mutat. 2006;27:31-43.

382. Adjalla CE, Hosack A, Matiaszuk N, Rosenblatt DS. A common mutation among blacks with mut^- methylmalonic aciduria. Hum Mutat. 1998;S248-S250.

383. Ogasawara M, Matsubara Y, Mikami H, Narisawa K. Identification of two novel mutations in the methylmalonyl-CoA mutase gene with decreased levels of mutant mRNA in methylmalonic acidemia. Hum Mol Genet. 1994;3:867-872.

384. Chalmers RA, Stacey TE, Tracey BM, et al. L-Carnitine insufficiency in disorders of organic acid metabolism: response to L-carnitine by patients with methylmalonic aciduria and 3-hydroxy-3-methylglutaric aciduria. J Inherit Metab Dis. 1984;7:109-110.

385. Wolff JA, Thuy L, Haas R, et al. Carnitine reduces fasting ketogenesis in patients with disorders of propionate metabolism. Lancet. 1986;327:289-291.

386. Snyderman SE, Sansaricq C, Norton P, Phansalkar SV. The use of neomycin in the treatment of methylmalonic aciduria. Pediatrics. 1972;50:925-927.

387. Bain MD, Borriello SP, Tracey BM, et al. Contribution of gut bacterial metabolism to human metabolic disease. Lancet. 1988;331:1078-1079.

388. Koletzko B, Bachman C, Wendel U. Antibiotic therapy for improvement of metabolic control in methylmalonic aciduria. J Pediatr. 1990;117:99-101.

389. Mahoney MJ, Bick D. Recent advances in the inherited methylmalonic acidemias. Acta Paediatr Scand. 1987;76:689-696.

390. Watkins D, Matiaszuk N, Rosenblatt DS. Complementation studies in the *cblA* class of inborn error of cobalamin metabolism: evidence for interallelic complementation and for a new complementation class (*cblH*). J Med Genet. 2000;37:510-513.

391. Matsui SM, Mahoney MJ, Rosenberg LE. The natural history of the inherited methylmalonic acidemias. N Engl J Med. 1983;308:857-861.

392. Ampola MG, Mahoney MJ, Nakamura E, Tanaka K. Prenatal therapy of a patient with vitamin B$_{12}$–responsive methylmalonic acidemia. N Engl J Med. 1975;293: 313-317.

393. Lerner-Ellis JP, Dobson CM, Wai T, et al. Mutations in the *MMAA* gene in patients with the *cblA* disorder of vitamin B$_{12}$ metabolism. Hum Mutat. 2004;24:509-516.

394. Yang X, Sakamoto O, Matsubara Y, et al. Mutation analysis of the *MMAA* and *MMAB* genes in Japanese patients with vitamin B$_{12}$–responsive methylmalonic acidemia: identification of a prevalent *MMAA* mutation. Mol Genet Metab. 2004;82:329-333.

395. Martinez MA, Rincon A, Desviat LR, et al. Genetic analysis of three genes causing isolated methylmalonic acidemia: identification of 21 novel allelic variants. Mol Genet Metab. 2005;84:317-325.

396. Lerner-Ellis JP, Gradinger AB, Watkins D, et al. Mutation and biochemical analysis of patients belonging to the *cblB* complementation class of vitamin B$_{12}$–dependent methylmalonic aciduria. Mol Genet Metab. 2006;87:219-225.

397. Saridakis V, Yakunin A, Xu X, et al. The structural basis for methylmalonic aciduria. The crystal structure of archaeal ATP:cobalamin adenosyltransferase. J Biol Chem. 2004;279:23646-23653.

398. St. Maurice M, Mera PE, Taranto MP, et al. Structural characterization of the active site of the PduO-type ATP:co(I)rrinoid adenosyltransferase from *Lactobacillus reuteri*. J Biol Chem. 2007;282:2596-2605.

399. Suh JR, Herbig K, Stover PJ. New perspectives on folate catabolism. Annu Rev Nutr. 2001;21:255-282.

400. Chung ASM, Pearson WN, Darby WJ, et al. Folic acid, vitamin B$_6$, pantothenic acid and vitamin B$_{12}$ in human dietaries. Am J Clin Nutr. 1961;9:573-582.

401. Moscovitch LF, Cooper BA. Folate content of diets in pregnancy: comparison of diets collected at home and diets prepared from dietary records. Am J Clin Nutr. 1973;26:707-714.

402. Zittoun J. Folate and nutrition. Chemioterapia. 1985;4: 388-392.

403. Senti FR, Pilch SM. Analysis of folate data from the second National Health and Nutrition Examination Survey (NHANES II). J Nutr. 1985;115:1398-1402.

404. Herbert V. Making sense of laboratory tests of folate status: folate requirements to sustain normality. In Zittoun JA, Cooper BA (eds). Folates and Cobalamins. Berlin, Springer-Verlag, 1989, pp 119-127.

405. Hoppner K, Lampi B. Folate levels in human liver from autopsies in Canada. Am J Clin Nutr. 1980;33:862-864.

406. Milne DB, Johnson LK, Mahalko JR, Sandstead HH. Folate status of adult males living in a metabolic unit: possible relationships with iron nutriture. Am J Clin Nutr. 1983;37:768-773.

407. Banerjee DK, Maitra A, Basu AK, Chatterjea JB. Minimal daily requirement of folic acid in normal Indian subjects. Indian J Med Res. 1975;63:45-53.

408. McNulty H, McPartlin JM, Weir DG, Scott JM. Folate catabolism in normal subjects. Hum Nutr Appl Nutr. 1987;41:338-341.

409. Scott JM. Catabolism of folates. In Blakley RL, Benkovic SJ (eds). Folates and Pterins, vol 1, Chemistry and Bio-chemistry of Folates. New York, John Wiley & Sons, 1984, pp 307-344.

410. Food and Drug Administration. Food standards: amendment of standards of identity for enriched grain products to require addition of folic acid. Fed Reg. 1998;61: 8781-8797.

411. Oakley GP, Bell KN, Weber MB. Recommendations for accelerating global action to prevent folic acid–preventable birth defects and other folate-deficiency diseases: meeting of experts on preventing folic acid–preventable neural tube defects. Birth Defects Res A Clin Mol Teratol. 2004;70:835-837.

412. Ray JG, Meier C, Vermeulen MJ, et al. Association of neural tube defects and folic acid food fortification in Canada. Lancet. 2002;360:2047-2048.

413. Centers for Disease Control and Prevention (CDC). Spina bifida and anencephaly before and after folic acid mandate—United States, 1995-1996 and 1999-2000. MMWR Morb Mortal Wkly Rep. 2004;53(17):362-365.

414. Dietrich M, Brown CJP, Block G. The effect of folate fortification of cereal-grain products on blood folate status, dietary folate intake, and dietary folate sources among adult non-supplement users in the United States. J Am Coll Nutr. 2005;24:266-274.

415. Pfeiffer CM, Caudill SP, Gunter EW, et al. Biochemical indicators of B vitamin status in the US population after folic acid fortification: results from the National Health and Nutrition Examination Survey 1999-2000. Am J Clin Nutr. 2005;82:442-450.

416. Brown JE, Jacobs DR, Hartman TJ, et al. Predictors of red cell folate level in women attempting pregnancy. JAMA. 1997;277:548-552.

417. Brent RL, Oakley GP. The folate debate. Pediatrics. 2006;117:1418-1419.

418. Botto LD, Lisi A, Robert-Gnansia E, et al. International retrospective cohort study of neural tube defects in relation to folic acid recommendations: are the recommendations working? BMJ. 2005;330:571-576.

419. Taitz LS, Armitage BL. Goats' milk for infants and children. BMJ. 1984;288:428-429.

420. Beaton G. Requirements of Vitamin A, Iron, Folate and Vitamin B$_{12}$: Report of a Joint FAO/WHO Expert Consultation. Rome, Food and Agriculture Organization of the United Nations, 1988.

421. Ek J. Plasma, red cell, and breast milk folacin concentrations in lactating women. Am J Clin Nutr. 1983;38: 929-935.

422. Dansky LV, Rosenblatt DS, Andermann E. Mechanisms of teratogenesis: folic acid and antiepilectic therapy. Neurology. 1992;42:32-42.

423. Shojania AM. Oral contraceptives: effect of folate and vitamin B$_{12}$ metabolism. Can Med Assoc J. 1982;126: 244-247.

424. Selhub J, Rosenberg IH. Folate transport in isolated brush border membrane vesicles from rat intestine. J Biol Chem. 1981;256:4489-4493.

425. Schron CM, Washington C, Blitzer BL. The transmembrane pH gradient drives uphill folate transport in rabbit jejunum. Direct evidence for folate/hydroxyl exchange in brush border membrane vesicles. J Clin Invest. 1985;76:2030-2033.

426. Said HM, Ghishan FK, Redha R. Folate transport by human intestinal brush-border membrane vesicles.

Am J Physiol Gastrointest Liver Physiol. 1987;252: G229-G236.

427. Blakeborough P, Salter DN. Folate transport in entero-cytes and brush-border-membrane vesicles isolated from small intestine of the neonatal goat. Br J Nutr. 1988;59:485-495.

428. Schron CM, Washington C, Blitzer BL. Anion specificity of the jejunal folate carrier: effects of reduced folate analogues on folate uptake and efflux. J Membr Biol. 1988;102:175-183.

429. Whitehead VM, Pratt R, Viallet A, Cooper BA. Intestinal conversion of folinic acid to 5-methyltetrahydrofolate in man. Br J Haematol. 1972;22:63-72.

430. Rong N, Selhub J, Goldin BR, Rosenberg IH. Bacterially synthesized folate in rat large intestine is incorporated into host tissue folate polyglutamates. J Nutr. 1991;121: 1955-1959.

431. Duffy TH, Beckman SB, Huennekens FM. Multiple forms of L1210 dihydrofolate reductase differing in affinity for methotrexate. Biochem Biophys Res Commun. 1984;119:352-358.

432. Kumar CK, Moyers MP, Dudeja PK, Said HM. A protein-tyrosine kinase–regulated, pH dependent, carrier-mediated uptake system for folate in human normal colonic epithelial cell line NCM460. J Biol Chem. 1987;272:6226-6231.

433. Nguyen TT, Dyer DL, Dunning DD, et al. Human intestinal folate transport: cloning, expression, and distribution of complementary RNA. Gastroenterology. 1997;112: 783-791.

434. Chiao JH, Roy K, Tolner B, et al. RFC-1 gene expression regulates folate absorption in mouse small intestine. J Biol Chem. 1997;272:11165-11170.

435. Said HM, Mohammed ZM. Intestinal absorption of water-soluble vitamins: an update. Curr Opin Gastroenterol. 2006;22:140-146.

436. Wang Y, Rajgopal A, Goldman ID, Zhao R. Preservation of folate transport activity with a low-pH optimum in rat IEC-6 intestinal epithelial cell lines that lack reduced folate carrier function. Am J Physiol Cell Physiol. 2004; 288:65-71.

437. Zhao R, Hanscom M, Goldman ID. The relationship between folate transport activity at low pH and reduced folate carrier function in human Huh7 hepatoma cells. Biochim Biophys Acta. 2005;1715: 57-64.

438. Qiu A, Jansen M, Sakaris A, et al. Identification of an intestinal folate transporter and the molecular basis for hereditary folate malabsorption. Cell. 2006;127:917-928.

439. Herbert V. Excretion of folic acid in bile. Lancet. 1965;285:913.

440. Hillman RS, McGuffin R, Campbell C. Alcohol interference with folate enterohepatic cycle. Trans Assoc Am Physicians. 1977;90:145-156.

441. Eisenga BH, Collins TD, McMartin KE. Differential effects of acute ethanol on urinary excretion of folate derivatives in the rat. J Pharmacol Exp Ther. 1989;248: 916-922.

442. Blocker DE, Thenen SW. Intestinal absorption, liver uptake, and excretion of ^{3}H-folic acid in folic acid–deficient, alcohol-consuming nonhuman primates. Am J Clin Nutr. 1987;46:503-510.

443. Lane F, Goff P, McGuffin R, et al. Folic acid metabolism in normal, folate deficient and alcoholic man. Br J Haematol. 1976;34:489-500.

444. Pfeiffer CM, Rogers LM, Bailey LB, Gregory JF. Absorption of folate from fortified cereal-grain products and of supplemental folate consumed with or without food determined by using a dual-label stable-isotope protocol. Am J Clin Nutr. 1997;66:1388-1397.

445. Herbert V, Larrabee AR, Buchanan JM. Studies on the identification of a folate compound of human serum. J Clin Invest. 1962;41:1134-1138.

446. Eichner ER, McDonald CR, Dickson VL. Elevated serum levels of unsaturated folate binding protein: clinical correlates in a general hospital. Am J Clin Nutr. 1978;31: 1988-1992.

447. Waxman S, Schreiber C. Characteristics of folic acid–binding protein in folate-deficient serum. Blood. 1973;42:291-301.

448. Wagner C. Folate-binding proteins. Nutr Rev. 1985;43: 293-299.

449. Sadasivan E, Rothenberg SP. The complete amino acid sequence of a human folate binding protein from KB cells determined from the cDNA. J Biol Chem. 1989; 264:5806-5811.

450. Lacey SW, Sanders JM, Rothberg KG, et al. Complementary DNA for the folate binding protein correctly predicts anchoring to the membrane by glycosyl-phosphatidylinisotol. J Clin Invest. 1989;84: 715-720.

451. Deutsch JC, Elwood PC, Portillo RM, et al. Role of the membrane-associated folate binding protein (folate receptor)* in methotrexate transport by human KB cells. Arch Biochem Biophys. 1989;274:327-337.

452. Ratnam M, Marquardt H, Duhring JL, Freisheim JH. Homologous membrane folate binding proteins in human placenta: cloning and sequencing of a cDNA. Biochemistry. 1989;28:8249-8254.

453. Hansen SI, Holm J, Hoier-Madsen M. A high-affinity folate binding protein in human urine. Radioligand binding characteristics, immunological properties and molecular size. Biosci Rep. 1989;9:93-97.

454. Lonnerdal B. Biochemistry and physiological function of human milk proteins. Am J Clin Nutr. 1985;42: 1299-1317.

455. Said HM, Horne DW, Wagner C. Effect of human milk folate binding protein on folate intestinal transport. Arch Biochem Biophys. 1986;251:114-120.

456. Wong SC, Proefke SA, Bhushan A, Matherly LH. Isolation of human cDNAs that restore methotrexate sensitivity and reduced folate carrier activity in methotrexate transport–defective Chinese hamster ovary cells. J Biol Chem. 1995;270:17468-17475.

457. Williams FM, Flintoff WF. Isolation of a human cDNA that complements a mutant hamster cell defective in methotrexate uptake. J Biol Chem. 1995;270:2987-2992.

458. Prasad PD, Ramamoorthy S, Leibach FH, Ganapathy V. Molecular cloning of the human placental folate transporter. Biochem Biophys Res Commun. 1995;206: 681-687.

459. Moscow JA, Gong M, He R, et al. Isolation of a gene encoding a human reduced folate carrier (RFC1) and analysis of its expression in transport-deficient, metho-

trexate-resistant human breast cancer cells. Cancer Res. 1995;55:3790-3794.

460. Yang-Feng TL, Ma YY, Liang R, et al. Assignment of the human folate transporter gene to chromosome 21q22.3 by somatic cell hybrid analysis and in situ hybridization. Biochem Biophys Res Commun. 1995;210: 874-879.

461. Williams FM, Flintoff WF. Structural organization of the human reduced folate carrier gene: evidence for 5′ heterogeneity in lymphoblast mRNA. Somat Cell Mol Genet. 1998;24:142-156.

462. Tolner B, Roy K, Sirotnak FM. Structural analysis of the human RFC-1 gene encoding a folate transporter reveals multiple promoters and alternatively spliced transcripts with 5′ end heterogeneity. Gene. 1998;211:331-334.

463. Zhang L, Wong SC, Matherly LH. Transcript heterogeneity of the human reduced folate carrier results from the use of multiple promoters and variable splicing of alternative upstream exons. Biochem J. 1998;332:773-780.

464. Balamurugan K, Said HM. Role of reduced folate carrier in intestinal folate uptake. Am J Physiol Cell Physiol. 2006;291:C189-C193.

465. Zhao R, Russell RG, Wang Y, et al. Rescue of embryonic lethality in reduced folate carrier–deficient mice by maternal folic acid supplementation reveals early neonatal failure of hematopoietic organs. J Biol Chem. 2001;276: 10224-10228.

466. Ragoussis J, Senger G, Trowsdale J, Campbell IG. Genomic organization of the human folate receptor genes on chromosome 11q13. Genomics. 1992;14:423-430.

467. Anderson RG, Kamen BA, Rothberg KG, Lacey SW. Potocytosis: sequestration and transport of small molecules by caveolae. Science. 1992;255:410-411.

468. Sabharanjak S, Mayor S. Folate receptor endocytosis and trafficking. Adv Drug Deliv Rev. 2004;56:1099-1109.

469. Birn H, Zhai X, Holm J, et al. Megalin binds and mediates cellular internalization of folate binding protein. FEBS J. 2005;272:4423-4430.

470. Matsue H, Rothberg KG, Takashima A, et al. Folate receptor allows cells to grow in low concentrations of 5-methyltetrahydrofolate. Proc Natl Acad Sci U S A. 1992;89:606-609.

471. Piedrahita JA, Oetama B, Bennett GD, et al. Mice lacking the folic acid–binding protein Folbp1 are defective in early embryonic development. Nat Genet. 1999;23:228-232.

472. Da Costa M, Sequeira JM, Rothenberg SP, Weedon J. Antibodies to folate receptors impair embryogenesis and fetal development in the rat. Birth Defect Res. 2003; 67:837-847.

473. Rothenberg SP, Da Costa M, Sequeira JM, et al. Autoantibodies against folate receptors in women with pregnancy complicated by a neural-tube defect. N Engl J Med. 2004;350:134-142.

474. Foo SK, Shane B. Regulation of folylpoly-γ-glutamate synthesis in mammalian cells. In vivo and in vitro synthesis of pteroylpoly-γ-glutamates by Chinese hamster ovary cells. J Biol Chem. 1982;257:13587-13592.

475. Chen L, Qi H, Korenberg J, et al. Purification and properties of human cytosolic folyl-γ-glutamate synthetase and organization, localization, and differential splicing of its gene. J Biol Chem. 1996;271:13077-13087.

476. MacKenzie RE, Baugh CM. Tetrahydropteroylglutamate derivatives as substrates of two multifunctional proteins

with folate-dependent enzyme activities. Biochim Biophys Acta. 1980;611:187-195.

477. Chandler CJ, Wang TT, Halsted CH. Pteroylglutamate hydrolase from human jejunal brush borders. Purification and characterization. J Biol Chem. 1986;261:928-933.

478. McGuire JJ, Coward JK. Pteroylpolyglutamates: biosynthesis, degradation, and function. In Blakley RL, Benkovic SJ (eds). Folates and Pterins, vol 1, Chemistry and Biochemistry of Folates. New York, John Wiley & Sons, 1984, pp 135-190.

479. Fujiwara K, Okamura-Ikeda K, Motokawa Y. Mechanism of the glycine cleavage reaction. Further characterization of the intermediate attached to H-protein and of the reaction catalyzed by T-protein. J Biol Chem. 1984;259: 10664-10668.

480. Okamura-Ikeda K, Fujiwara K, Motokawa Y. Mechanism of the glycine cleavage reaction. Properties of the reverse reaction catalyzed by T-protein. J Biol Chem. 1987;262: 6746-6749.

481. Schirch L. Folates in serine and glycine metabolism. In Blakley RL, Benkovic SJ (eds). Folates and Pterins, vol 1, Chemistry and Biochemistry of Folates. New York, John Wiley & Sons, 1984, pp 399-432.

482. Garrow TA, Brenner AA, Whitehead VM, et al. Cloning of human cDNAs encoding mitochondrial and cytosolic serine hydroxymethyltransferases and chromosomal localization. J Biol Chem. 1993;268: 11910-11916.

483. Beaudet R, MacKenzie RE. Formiminotransferase cyclodeaminase from porcine liver. An octomeric enzyme containing bifunctional polypeptides. Biochim Biophys Acta. 1976;453:151-161.

484. Murley LL, MacKenzie RE. The two monofunctional domains of octameric formiminotransferase-cyclodeaminase exist as dimers. Biochemistry. 1995;34:10358-10364.

485. Herbert V, Zalusky R. Interrelations of vitamin B_{12} and folic acid metabolism: folic acid clearance studies. J Clin Invest. 1962;41:1263-1276.

486. Paukert JL, Straus LD, Rabinowitz JC. Formyl-methenyl-methylenetetrahydrofolate synthetase-(combined). An ovine protein with multiple catalytic activities. J Biol Chem. 1976;251:5104-5111.

487. Tan LUL, Drury EJ, MacKenzie RE. Methylenetetrahydrofolate dehydrogenase–methenyltetrahydrofolate cyclohydrolase–formyltetrahydrofolate synthetase. A multifunctional enzyme from porcine liver. J Biol Chem. 1977;252:1117-1122.

488. Mejia NR, MacKenzie RE. NAD-dependent methylenetetrahydrofolate dehydrogenase is expressed by immortal cells. J Biol Chem. 1985;260:14616-14620.

489. Christensen KE, Mirza IA, Berghuis AM, Mackenzie IL. Magnesium and phosphate ions enable NAD binding to methylenetetrahydrofolate dehydrogenase–methenyltetrahydrofolate cyclohydrolase. J Biol Chem. 2005;280: 34316-34323.

490. Prasannan P, Pike S, Peng K, et al. Human mitochondrial C1-tetrahydrofolate synthase. Gene structure, tissue distribution of the mRNA, and immunolocalization in Chinese hamster ovary cells. J Biol Chem. 2003;278: 43178-43187.

491. Christensen KE, Patel H, Kuzmanov U, et al. Disruption of the *Mthfd1* gene reveals a monofunctional 10-for-

myltetrahydrofolate synthetase in mammalian mitochondria. J Biol Chem. 2005;280:7597-7602.

492. Field MS, Szebenyi DME, Stover PJ. Regulation of de novo purine biosynthesis by methenyltetrahydrofolate synthetase in neuroblastoma. J Biol Chem. 2006;281: 4215-4221.

493. Dayan A, Bertrand R, Beauchemin M, et al. Cloning and characterization of the human 5,10-methenyltetrahydrofolate synthetase–encoding DNA. Gene 1995;165: 307-311.

494. MacKenzie RE. Biogenesis and interconversion of substituted tetrahydrofolates. In Blakley RL, Benkovic SJ (eds). Folates and Pterins, vol 1, Chemistry and Biochemistry of Folates. New York, John Wiley & Sons, 1984, pp 255-306.

495. Mueller WT, Benkovic SJ. On the purification and mechanism of action of 5-aminoimidazole-4-carboxamide-ribonucleotide transformylase from chicken liver. Biochemistry. 1981;20:337-344.

496. Christensen KE, MacKenzie RE. Mitochondrial one-carbon metabolism is adapted to the specific needs of yeast, plants and mammals. Bioessays. 2006;28:595-605.

497. Herbert V. Experimental nutritional folate deficiency in man. Trans Assoc Am Physicians. 1962;75:307-320.

498. Stabler SP, Marcell PD, Podell ER, et al. Elevation of total homocysteine in the serum of patients with cobalamin or folate deficiency detected by capillary gas chromatography–mass spectrometry. J Clin Invest. 1988;81:466-474.

499. Smulders YM, Smith DEC, Kok RM, et al. Cellular folate vitamer distribution during and after correction for vitamin B$_{12}$ deficiency: a case for the methylfolate trap. Br J Haematol. 2005;132:623-629.

500. Kelly P, McPartlin J, Goggins M, et al. Unmetabolized folic acid in serum: acute studies in subjects consuming fortified food and supplements. Am J Clin Nutr. 1997;65:1790-1795.

501. Fuller NJ, Bates CJ, Evans PH, Lucas A. High folate intakes related to zinc status in preterm infants. Eur J Pediatr. 1992;151:51-53.

502. Reynolds EH. Neurological aspects of folate and vitamin B$_{12}$ metabolism. Clin Haematol. 1976;5:661-696.

503. Lever EG, Elwes RD, Williams A, Reynolds EH. Subacute combined degeneration of the cord due to folate deficiency: response to methyl folate treatment. J Neurol Neurosurg Psychiatry. 1986;49:1203-1207.

504. Brockner P, Lods JC. Folate deficiency in geriatric patients. In Zittoun JA, Cooper BA (eds). Folates and Cobalamins. Berlin, Springer-Verlag, 1989, pp 179-189.

505. Botto LD, Moore CA, Khoury MJ, Erickson DJ. Neural-tube defects. N Engl J Med. 1999;341:1509-1519.

506. Lindblad B, Zaman S, Malik A, et al. Folate, vitamin B$_{12}$, and homocysteine levels in South Asian women with growth-retarded fetuses. Acta Obstet Gynecol Scand. 2005;84:1055-1061.

507. Subar AF, Block G, James LD. Folate intake and food sources in the US population. Am J Clin Nutr. 1989;50:508-516.

508. Green TJ, Houghton LA, Donovan U, et al. Oral contraceptives did not affect biochemical folate indexes and homocysteine concentrations in adolescent females. J Am Diet Assoc. 1998;98:49-55.

509. Henderson GI, Perez T, Schenker S, et al. Maternal-to-fetal transfer of 5-methyltetrahydrofolate by the perfused human placental cotylodon: evidence for a concentrative role by placental folate receptors in fetal folate delivery. J Lab Clin Med. 1995;126:184-203.

510. Quere I, Bellet H, Hoffet M, et al. A woman with five consecutive fetal deaths: case report and retrospective analysis of hyperhomocysteinemia prevalence in 100 consecutive women with recurrent miscarriages. Fertil Steril. 1998;69:152-154.

511. Frelut ML, de Courcy GP, Christades JP, et al. Relationship between maternal folate status and fetal hypotrophy in a population with good socio-economic level. Int J Vitam Nutr Res. 1995;65:267-271.

512. Tamura T, Goldenberg RL, Johnston KE, et al. Serum concentrations of zinc, folate, vitamins A and E, and proteins, and their relationships to pregnancy. Acta Obstet Gynecol Scand. 1997;165:63-70.

513. Scholl TO, Hediger ML, Schall JI, et al. Dietary and serum folate: their influence on the outcome of pregnancy. Am J Clin Nutr. 1996;63:520-525.

514. Canfield MA, Collins JS, Botto LD, et al. Changes in the birth prevalence of selected birth defects after grain fortification with folic acid in the United States: findings from a multi-state population-based study. Birth Defect Res A Clin Mol Teratol. 2005;73:679-689.

515. Milman N, Byg KE, Hvas AM, et al. Erythrocyte folate, plasma folate and plasma homocysteine during normal pregnancy and postpartum: a longitudinal study comprising 404 Danish women. Eur J Haematol. 2006;76: 200-205.

516. Smithells RW, Sheppard S, Schorah CJ. Vitamin deficiencies and neural tube defects. Arch Dis Child. 1976;51: 944-950.

517. Christensen B, Rosenblatt DS. Effects of folate deficiency on embryonic development. Ballieres Clin Haematol. 1995;8:617-637.

518. Steegers-Theunissen RPM, Boers GH, Trijbels FJ, et al. Maternal hyperhomocysteinemia: a risk factor for neural tube defects? Metabolism. 1994;43:1475-1480.

519. Mills JL, McPartlin J, Kirke PN, et al. Homocysteine metabolism in pregnancies complicated by neural-tube defects. Lancet. 1995;345:149-151.

520. van der Put NMJ, Steegers-Theunissen RPM, Frosst P, et al. Mutated methylenetetrahydrofolate reductase as a risk factor for spina bifida. Lancet. 1995;346: 1070-1071.

521. Cuskelly GJ, McNulty H, Scott JM. Effect of increasing dietary folate on red-cell folate: implications for prevention of neural tube defects. Lancet. 1996;347:657-659.

522. Eichholzer M, Tonz O, Zimmermann R. Folic acid: public health challenge. Lancet. 2006;367:1352-1361.

523. Williams LJ, Mai CT, Edmonds LD, et al. Prevalence of spina bifida and anencephaly during the transition to mandatory folic acid fortification in the United States. Teratology. 2002;66:33-39.

524. Honein MA, Paulozzi LJ, Mathews TJ, et al. Impact of folic acid fortification of the US food supply on the occurrence of neural tube defects. JAMA. 2001;285: 2981-2986.

525. Wong WY, Eskes TKAB, Kuijpers-Jagtman A-M, et al. Nonsyndromic orofacial clefts: association with maternal hyperhomocysteinemia. Teratology. 1999;60:253-257.

526. van Rooij IALM, Ocké MC, Straatman H, et al. Periconceptional folate intake by supplement and food reduces

the risk of nonsyndromic cleft lip with or without cleft palate. Prev Med. 2004;39:689-694.

527. Wilcox AJ, Lie RT, Solvoll K, et al. Folic acid supplements and risk of facial clefts: national population based case-control study. BMJ. 2007;334:464-467.

528. Shaw GM, Carmichael SL, Laurent C, Rasmussen SA. Maternal nutrient intakes and risk of orofacial clefts. Epidemiology. 2006;17:285-291.

529. Badovinac RL, Werler MM, Williams PL, et al. Folic acid–containing supplement consumption during pregnancy and risk for oral clefts: a meta-analysis. Birth Defect Res A Clin Mol Teratol. 2007;79:8-15.

530. Vollset SE, Botto LD. Neural tube defects, other congenital malformations and single nucleotide polymorphisms in the 5,10-methylenetetrahydrofolate reductase (*MTHFR*) gene: a meta-analysis. In Ueland PM, Rozen R (eds). *MTHFR* Polymorphisms and Disease. Georgetown, TX, Landes Bioscience, 2005, pp 125-143.

531. James SJ. Maternal metabolic phenotype and risk of Down syndrome: beyond genetics. Am J Med Genet A. 2004;127:1-4.

532. Eskes TKAB. Abnormal folate metabolism in mothers with Down syndrome offspring: review of the literature. Eur J Obstet Gynecol Reprod Biol. 2006;124:130-133.

533. Bosco P, Guéant-Rodriguez RM, Anello G, et al. Methionine synthase (MTR) 2756 (A→G) polymorphism, double heterozygosity methionine synthase 2756 AG/methionine synthase reductase (MTRR) 66 AG, and elevated homocysteinemia are three risk factors for having a child with Down syndrome. Am J Med Genet A. 2003;121:219-224.

534. Sheth JJ, Sheth FJ. Gene polymorphism and folate metabolism: a maternal risk factor for Down syndrome. Indian Pediatr. 2003;40:115-123.

535. Takamura N, Kondoh T, Ohgi S, et al. Abnormal folic acid–homocysteine metabolism as maternal risk factors for Down syndrome in Japan. Eur J Nutr. 2004;43:285-287.

536. da Silva LRJ, Vergani N, Galdieri LDC, et al. Relationship between polymorphisms in genes involved in homocysteine metabolism and maternal risk for Down syndrome in Brazil. Am J Med Genet. 2005;135A:263-267.

537. James SJ, Pogribna M, Pogribny IP, et al. Abnormal folate metabolism and mutation in the methylenetetrahydrofolate reductase gene may be maternal risk factors for Down syndrome. Am J Clin Nutr. 1999;70:495-501.

538. Hobbs CA, Sherman SL, Yi P, et al. Polymorphisms in genes involved in folate metabolism as maternal risk factors for Down syndrome. Am J Hum Genet. 2000;67:623-630.

539. O'Leary VB, Parle-McDermott A, Molloy AM, et al. MTRR and MTHFR polymorphism: link to Down syndrome? Am J Med Genet. 2002;107:151-155.

540. Scala I, Granese B, Sellitto M, et al. Analysis of seven maternal polymorphisms of genes involved in homocysteine/folate metabolism and risk of Down syndrome offspring. Genet Med. 2006;8:409-416.

541. Chadefaux-Vekemans B, Coudé M, Muller F, et al. Methylenetetrahydrofolate reductase polymorphism in the etiology of Down syndrome. Pediatr Res. 2002;51:766-767.

542. Coppedè F, Marini G, Bargagna S, et al. Folate gene polymorphisms and the risk of Down syndrome pregnancies in young Italian women. Am J Med Genet A. 2006;140A:1083-1091.

543. Barkai G, Arbuzova S, Berkenstadt M, et al. Frequency of Down syndrome and neural-tube defects in the same family. Lancet. 2003;361:1331-1335.

544. McCully KS. Vascular pathology of homocysteinemia: implications for the pathogenesis of arteriosclerosis. Am J Pathol. 1969;56:111-128.

545. Kang S-S, Wong PWK, Susmano A, et al. Thermolabile methylenetetrahydrofolate reductase: an inherited risk factor for coronary artery disease. Am J Hum Genet. 1991;48:536-545.

546. Castro R, Rivera I, Blom HJ, et al. Homocysteine metabolism, hyperhomocysteinaemia and vascular disease: an overview. J Inherit Metab Dis. 2006;29:3-20.

547. Selhub J, Jacques PF, Bostom AG, et al. Relationship between plasma homocysteine and vitamin status in the Framingham study population. Impact of folic acid fortification. Public Health Rev. 2000;28:117-145.

548. Franken DG, Boers GH, Blom HJ, et al. Treatment of mild hyperhomocysteinemia in vascular disease patients. Arterioscler Thromb. 1994;14:465-470.

549. Boushey CJ, Beresford SAA, Omenn GS, Motulsky AG. A quantitative assessment of plasma homocysteine as a risk factor for vascular disease. Probable benefits of increasing folic acid intakes. JAMA. 1995;274:1049-1057.

550. Toole JF, Malinow MR, Chambless LE, et al. Lowering homocysteine in patients with ischemic stroke to prevent recurrent stroke, myocardial infarction, and death: the Vitamin Intervention for Stroke Prevention (VISP) randomized controlled trial. JAMA. 2004;291:565-575.

551. Heart Outcomes Prevention 2 Investigators. Homocysteine lowering with folic acid and B vitamins in vascular disease. N Engl J Med. 2006;354:1578-1588.

552. Bonaa KH, Njolstad I, Ueland PM, et al. Homocysteine lowering and cardiovascular events after acute myocardial infarction. N Engl J Med. 2006;354:1578-1588.

553. Loscalzo J. Homocysteine trials—clear outcomes for complex reasons. N Engl J Med. 2006;354:1629-1632.

554. B-Vitamin Treatment Trialists' Collaboration. Homocysteine-lowering trials for prevention of cardiovascular events: a review of the design and power of the large randomized trials. Am Heart J. 2006;151:282-287.

555. Butterworth CE, Hatch KD, Gore H, et al. Improvement in cervical dysplasia associated with folic acid therapy in users of oral contraceptives. Am J Clin Nutr. 1982;35:73-82.

556. Heimberger DC, Alexander CB, Birch R, et al. Improvement in bronchial squamous metaplasia in smokers treated with folate and vitamin B_{12}. Report of a preliminary randomized, double-blind intervention trial. JAMA. 1988;259:1525-1530.

557. Kim YI. Folate and carcinogenesis: evidence, mechanisms, and implications. J Nutr Biochem. 1999;10:66-88.

558. Jolivet J. Methotrexate and 5-fluorouracil: cellular interactions with folates. In Zittoun JA, Cooper BA (eds). Folates and Cobalamins. Berlin, Springer-Verlag, 1989, pp 247-254.

559. Lanzkowsky P, Erlandson ME, Bezan AI. Isolated defect of folic acid absorption associated with mental retardation and cerebral calcification. Blood. 1969;34:452-465.

560. Lanzkowsky P. Congenital malabsorption of folate. Am J Med. 1970;48:580-583.

561. Corbeel L, Van den Berghe G, Jaeken J, et al. Congenital folate malabsorption. Eur J Pediatr. 1985;143:284-290.

562. Urbach J, Abrahamov A, Grossowicz N. Congenital isolated folic acid malabsorption. Arch Dis Child. 1987;62:78-80.

563. Santiago-Borrero PJ, Santini R, Pérez-Santiago E, et al. Congenital isolated defect of folic acid absorption. J Pediatr. 1973;82:450-455.

564. Geller J, Kronn D, Jayabose S, Sandoval C. Hereditary folate malabsorption. Family report and review of the literature. Medicine (Baltimore). 2002;81:51-68.

565. Zhao R, Min SH, Qiu A, et al. The spectrum of mutations in the PCFT gene, coding for an intestinal folate transporter, that are the basis for hereditary folate malabsorption. Blood. 2007;110:1147-1152.

566. Steinschneider M, Sherbany A, Pavlakis S, et al. Congenital folate malabsorption: reversible clinical and neurophysiologic abnormalities. Neurology. 1990;40:1315.

567. Branda RF, Moldow CF, MacArthur JR, et al. Folate-induced remission of aplastic anemia with familial defect of cellular folate uptake. N Engl J Med. 1978;298:469-475.

568. Arthur DC, Danzyl TJ, Branda RF. Cytogenetic studies of a family with a hereditary defect of cellular folate uptake and high incidence of hematologic disease. In Butterworth CE, Hutchinson M (eds). Nutritional Factors in the Induction and Maintenance of Malignancy. New York, Academic Press, 1983, pp 101-111.

569. Howe RB, Branda RF, Douglas SD, Brunning RD. Hereditary dyserythropoiesis with abnormal membrane folate transport. Blood. 1979;54:1080-1090.

570. Thomas MA, Rosenblatt DS. Severe methylenetetrahydrofolate reductase deficiency. In Ueland PM, Rozen R (eds). *MTHFR* Polymorphisms and Disease. Georgetown, TX, Landes Bioscience, 2005, pp 41-53.

571. Haworth JC, Dilling LA, Surtees RAH, et al. Symptomatic and asymptomatic methylenetetrahydrofolate reductase deficiency in two adult brothers. Am J Med Genet. 1993;45:572-576.

572. Freeman JM, Finkelstein JD, Mudd SH. Folate-responsive homocystinuria and "schizophrenia." A defect in methylation due to deficient 5,10-methylenetetrahydrofolate reductase activity. N Engl J Med. 1975;292:491-496.

573. Pasquier F, Lebert F, Petit H, et al. Methylenetetrahydrofolate reductase deficiency revealed by a neuropathy in a psychotic adult. J Neurol Neurosurg Psychiatry. 1994;57:765-766.

574. Regland B, Johansson BV, Gottfries CG. Homocysteinemia and schizophrenia as a case of methylation deficiency. J Neural Transm. 1994;98:143-152.

575. Kanwar YS, Manaligod JR, Wong PWK. Morphologic studies in a patient with homocystinuria due to 5,10-methylenetetrahydrofolate reductase deficiency. Pediatr Res. 1976;10:598-609.

576. Wong PWK, Justice P, Hruby M, et al. Folic acid nonresponsive homocystinuria due to methylenetetrahydrofolate reductase deficiency. Pediatrics. 1977;59:749-756.

577. Haan EA, Rogers JG, Lewis GP, Rowe PB. 5,10-Methylenetetrahydrofolate reductase deficiency. Clinical and biochemical features of a further case. J Inherit Metab Dis. 1985;8:53-57.

578. Baumgartner ER, Stokstad ELR, Wick H, et al. Comparison of folic acid coenzyme distribution patterns in patients with methylenetetrahydrofolate reductase and methionine synthase deficiencies. Pediatr Res. 1985;19:1288-1292.

579. Clayton PT, Smith I, Harding B, et al. Subacute combined degeneration of the cord, dementia and parkinsonism due to an inborn error of folate metabolism. J Neurol Neurosurg Psychiatry. 1986;49:920-927.

580. Beckman DR, Hoganson G, Berlow S, Gilbert EF. Pathological findings in 5,10-methylene-tetrahydrofolate reductase deficiency. Birth Defects. 1987;23:47-64.

581. Matthews RG, Kaufman S. Characterization of the dihydropterin reductase activity of pig liver methylenetetrahydrofolate reductase. J Biol Chem. 1980;255:6014-6017.

582. Rosenblatt DS, Erbe RW. Methylenetetrahydrofolate reductase in cultured human cells. I. Growth and metabolic studies. Pediatr Res. 1977;11:1137-1141.

583. Rosenblatt DS, Cooper BA, Lue-Shing S, et al. Folate distribution in cultured human cells. Studies on 5,10-CH$_2$-H$_4$PteGlu reductase deficiency. J Clin Invest. 1979;63:1019-1025.

584. Boss GR, Erbe RW. Decreased rates of methionine synthesis by methylene tetrahydrofolate reductase–deficient fibroblasts and lymphoblasts. J Clin Invest. 1981;67:1659-1664.

585. Kang S-S, Zhou J, Wong PWK, et al. Intermediate homocysteinemia: a thermolabile variant of methylenetetrahydrofolate reductase. Am J Hum Genet. 1988;43:414-421.

586. Goyette P, Pai A, Milos R, et al. Gene structure of human and mouse methylenetetrahydrofolate reductase (*MTHFR*). Mamm Genome. 1998;9:652-656.

587. Goyette P, Sumner JS, Milos R, et al. Human methylenetetrahydrofolate reductase: isolation of cDNA, mapping and mutation identification. Nat Genet 1994;7:195-200.

588. Goyette P, Frosst P, Rosenblatt DS, Rozen R. Seven novel mutations in the methylenetetrahydrofolate reductase gene and genotype/phenotype correlations in severe methylenetetrahydrofolate reductase deficiency. Am J Hum Genet. 1995;56:1052-1059.

589. Goyette P, Christensen B, Rosenblatt DS, Rozen R. Severe and mild mutations in cis for the methylenetetrahydrofolate reductase (*MTHFR*) gene, and description of five novel mutations in MTHFR. Am J Hum Genet. 1996;59:1268-1275.

590. Sibani S, Christensen B, O'Ferrall E, et al. Characterization of six novel mutations in the methylenetetrahydrofolate reductase (*MTHFR*) gene in patients with homocystinuria. Hum Mutat. 2000;15:280-287.

591. Sibani S, Leclerc D, Weisberg I, et al. Characterization of mutations in severe methylenetetrahydrofolate reductase deficiency reveals an FAD-responsive mutation. Hum Mutat. 2003;21:509-520.

592. Kluijtmans LAJ, Wendel U, Stevens EMB, et al. Identification of four novel mutations in severe methylenetetrahydrofolate reductase deficiency. Eur J Hum Genet. 1998;6:257-265.

593. Tonetti C, Amiel J, Munnich A, Zittoun J. Impact of new mutations in the methylenetetrahydrofolate reductase

gene assessed on biochemical phenotypes: a familial study. J Inherit Metab Dis. 2001;24:833-842.

594. Tonetti C, Burtscher A, Bories D, et al. Methylenetetrahydrofolate reductase deficiency in four siblings: a clinical, biochemical, and molecular study of the family. Am J Hum Med Genet. 2000;91:363-367.

595. Tonetti C, Saudubray JM, Echenne B, et al. Relations between molecular and biological abnormalities in 11 families from siblings affected with methylenetetrahydrofolate reductase deficiency. Eur J Pediatr. 2003;162: 466-475.

596. Wendel U, Claussen U, Diekmann E. Prenatal diagnosis for methylenetetrahydrofolate reductase deficiency. J Pediatr. 1983;102:938-940.

597. Shin YS, Pilz G, Endres W. Methylenetetrahydrofolate reductase and methyltetrahydrofolate methyltransferase in human fetal tissues and chorionic villli. J Inherit Metab Dis. 1986;9(Suppl 2):275-276.

598. Christensen E, Brandt NJ. Prenatal diagnosis for 5,10-methylenetetrahydrofolate reductase deficiency. N Engl J Med. 1985;13:50-51.

599. Morel CF, Scott P, Christensen E, et al. Prenatal diagnosis for severe methylenetetrahydrofolate reductase deficiency by linkage analysis and enzymatic assay. Mol Genet Metab. 2005;85:115-120.

600. Botto LD, Yang Q. 5,10-Methylenetetrahydrofolate reductase gene variants and congenital anomalies: a HuGE review. Am J Epidemiol. 2000;151:862-877.

601. Weisberg I, Tran P, Christensen B, et al. A second genetic polymorphism in methylenetetrahydrofolate reductase (MTHFR) associated with decreased enzyme activity. Mol Genet Metab. 1998;64:169-172.

602. Leclerc D, Sibani S, Rozen R. Molecular biology of methylenetetrahydrofolate reductase (*MTHFR*) and overview of mutations/polymorphisms. In Ueland PM, Rozen R (eds). *MTHFR* Polymorphisms and Disease. Georgetown, TX, Landes Bioscience, 2005, pp 1-20.

603. Leclerc D, Rozen R. Génétique moléculaire de *MTHFR*. Les polymorphismes ne sont pas tous bénins. Med Sci. 2007;23:297-302.

604. Cooper BA. Anomalies congénitales du métabolisme des folates. In Zittoun JA, Cooper BA (eds). Folates et Cobalamines. Paris, Doin, 1987, pp 193-208.

605. Brandt NJ, Christensen E. Treatment of methylenetetrahydrofolate reductase deficiency from the neonatal period. The Society for the Study of Inborn Errors of Metabolism. The Netherlands, Amersfoort, 1986, p 23. Abstract.

606. Hilton JF, Christensen KE, Watkins D, et al. The molecular basis of glutamate formiminotransferase deficiency. Hum Mutat. 2003;22:57-73.

607. Rowe PB. Inherited disorders of folate metabolism. In Stanbury JB, Wyngaarden JB, Fredrickson DS, et al. (eds). The Metabolic Basis of Inherited Disease. New York, McGraw-Hill, 1983, pp 498.

608. Arakawa T, Ohara K, Takahashi Y, et al. Formiminotransferase-deficiency syndrome: a new inborn error of folic acid metabolism. Ann Pediatr. 1965;206:1-11.

609. Arakawa T, Fujii M, Ohara K. Erythrocyte formiminotransferase activity in forminotransferase deficiency syndrome. Tohoku J Exp Med. 1966;88:195-202.

610. Arakawa T. Congenital defects in folate utilization. Am J Med. 1970;48:594-598.

611. Perry TL, Applegarth DA, Evans ME, et al. Metabolic studies of a family with massive forminiminoglutamic aciduria. Pediatr Res. 1975;9:117-122.

612. Duran M, Ketting D, de Bree PK, et al. A case of formiminoglutamic aciduria. Clinical and biochemical studies. Eur J Pediatr. 1981;136:319-323.

613. Russell A, Statter M, Abzug-Horowitz S. Methionine dependent glutamic acid formiminotransferase deficiency: human and experimental studies in its therapy. Monogr Hum Genet. 1978;9:65-74.

614. Solans A, Estivill X, de la Luna S. Cloning and characterization of human FTCD on 21q22.3, a candidate gene for glutamate formiminotransferase deficiency. Cytogenet Cell Genet. 2000;88:43-49.

615. Marie S, Heron B, Bitoun P, et al. AICA-ribosiduria: a novel, neurologically devastating inborn error of purine biosynthesis caused by mutation of ATIC. Am J Hum Genet. 2004;74:1276-1281.

616. Tauro GP, Danks DM, Rowe PB, et al. Dihydrofolate reductase deficiency causing megaloblastic anemia in two families. N Engl J Med. 1976;294:466-470.

617. Hoffbrand AV, Tripp E, Jackson BFA, et al. Hereditary abnormal transcobalamin II previously diagnosed as congenital dihydrofolate reductase deficiency. N Engl J Med. 1984;310:789-790.

618. de Koning TJ, Duran M, Dorland L, et al. Beneficial effects of L-serine and glycine in the management of seizures in 3-phosphoglycerate dehydrogenase deficiency. Ann Neurol. 1998;44:261-265.

619. de Koning TJ, Klomp LWJ. Serine deficiency syndromes. Curr Opin Neurol. 2004;17:197-204.

620. de Koning TJ. Treatment with amino acids in serine deficiency disorders. J Inherit Metab Dis. 2006;29:347-351.

621. de Koning TJ, Klomp LWJ, van Oppen ACC, et al. Prenatal and early postnatal treatment in 3-phosphoglycerate dehydrogenase deficiency. Lancet. 2004;364:2221-2222.

622. Klomp LWJ, de Koning TJ, Malingré HEM, et al. Molecular characterization of 3-phosphoglcerate dehydrogenase deficiency—a neurometabolic disorder associated with reduced L-serine biosynthesis. Am J Hum Genet. 2000;67:1389-1399.

623. Rogers LE, Porter FS, Sidbury JB. Thiamine-responsive megaloblastic anemia. J Pediatr. 1969;74:494-504.

624. Viana MB, Carvalho RI. Thiamine-responsive megaloblastic anemia, sensorineural deafness, and diabetes mellitus: a new syndrome? J Pediatr. 1978;93:235-238.

625. Neufeld EJ, Fleming JC, Tartaglini E, Steinkamp MP. Thiamine-responsive megaloblastic anemia syndrome: a disorder of high-affinity thiamine transport. Blood Cells Mol Dis. 2001;27:135-138.

626. Labay V, Raz T, Baron D, et al. Mutations in SLC19A2 cause thiamine-responsive megaloblastic anemia associated with diabetes mellitus and deafness. Nat Genet. 1999;22:300-304.

627. Fleming JC, Tartaglini E, Steinkamp MP, et al. The gene mutated in thiamine-responsive anaemia with diabetes and deafness (TRMA) encodes a functional thiamine transporter. Nat Genet. 1999;22:305-308.

628. Diaz GA, Banikazemi M, Oishi K, et al. Mutations in a new gene encoding a thiamine transporter cause a thiamine-responsive megaloblastic anaemia syndrome. Nat Genet. 1999;22:309-312.

629. Alzahrani AS, Baitei E, Zou M, Shi Y. Thiamine transporter mutation: an example of monogenic diabetes mellitus. Eur J Endocrinol. 2006;155:787-792.

630. Stagg AR, Fleming JC, Baker MA, et al. Defective high-affinity thiamine transporter leads to cell death in thiamine-responsive megaloblastic anemia syndrome fibroblasts. J Clin Invest. 1999;103:723-729.

Disorders of Iron Metabolism and Sideroblastic Anemia

Nancy C. Andrews, Christina K. Ullrich, and Mark D. Fleming

Box 12-1	Iron-Containing Proteins*

HEME PROTEINS

Hemoglobin
Myoglobin
Cytochrome *a, b, c*
Cytochrome P-450
Tryptophan-1,2-dioxygenase
Catalase
Myeloperoxidase

IRON-DEPENDENT ENZYMES

Aldehyde oxidase
Reduced nicotinamide adenine dinucleotide
 dehydrogenase
Tyrosine hydroxylase
Succinate dehydrogenase
Prolyl hydroxylase
Tryptophan hydrolase
Xanthine oxidase
Ribonucleotide reductase
Aconitase
Phosphoenolpyruvate carboxykinase

*Partial list.
Adapted from Griffin IJ, Abrams SA. Iron and breastfeeding.
 Pediatr Clin North Am. 2001;48:401-413.

Iron lacks the glitter of gold and the sparkle of silver but outshines both in biologic importance. This plebeian metal is vital to the function of a wide variety of critical enzymes, including catalases, aconitases, ribonucleotide reductase, peroxidases, and cytochromes, that exploit the flexible redox chemistry of iron to execute a number of chemical reactions essential for our survival (Box 12-1). In addition, we depend on hemoglobin, another iron-containing protein, to transport inhaled oxygen from the lungs to peripheral tissues. Human existence is inextricably linked to iron, and disturbances in its metabolism may have dire consequences.

PHYSIOLOGIC CHEMISTRY OF IRON

Iron and Oxidation

The key to the biologic utility of iron is its ability to exist in either of two stable oxidation states: Fe^{2+} (ferrous) or Fe^{3+} (ferric). This property permits iron to act as a redox catalyst by reversibly donating or accepting electrons. An excellent example is the electron transport chain of oxidative phosphorylation, in which adenosine triphosphate (ATP) is generated from glucose by the orderly transfer of electrons through a network of iron-containing mitochondrial cytochromes.

When dissolved in aqueous solution, ferrous iron rapidly oxidizes to its ferric form, which is insoluble at physiologic pH. The resulting ferric hydroxide salts (rust)

are of no metabolic utility. To achieve stable solubility under physiologic conditions, iron must be complexed to iron-binding agents termed chelators. Chelators are synthesized by all organisms ranging from microbes (e.g., deferoxamine produced by *Streptomyces pilosis*) to humans (e.g., transferrin in human plasma). These molecules are crucial to the acquisition of iron from the environment and to its transport and storage within the body.

Iron-Protein Complexes

Iron-protein complexes capitalize on the properties of the metal to perform metabolic functions. Stable coordination complexes form between iron and electron-donating amino acids in proteins. Iron acts as the chemical workhorse, and protein structure dictates biologic specificity.

Individual iron atoms can interact directly with amino acid side groups in proteins, as in ribonucleotide reductase. Alternatively, iron may form coordination complexes with other small molecules. Protoporphyrin IX donates four of the six electrons needed to form a stable coordination complex with iron. Heme, the iron–protoporphyrin IX complex, is so stable that removal of the iron moiety requires the enzyme heme oxygenase. The functional properties of heme are determined by the nature of the associated protein or small molecule ligands supplying the remaining two electrons. The best-characterized heme protein is hemoglobin, in which a globin histidine residue donates the fifth electron and the sixth comes from molecular oxygen.[1] This configuration enables hemoglobin to transport oxygen safely throughout the body.

Iron and sulfur atoms can form stable complexes ("clusters") that catalyze enzymatic reactions. The Krebs cycle enzyme aconitase, for example, contains an iron-sulfur (Fe/S) cluster. As discussed later in this chapter, the iron content of the Fe/S cluster of a related aconitase-like molecule allows it to "sense" iron concentrations within the cell and to act as an iron regulatory protein (IRP) to modulate the translation of genes of iron metabolism.

Iron Toxicity

The ability of iron to catalyze redox reactions also accounts for its toxicity. As an enzymatic cofactor, the metal is involved in the restructuring of cellular components, including proteins, carbohydrates, and nucleic acids. Unbound iron has unbridled redox activity, however, and may wreak havoc. We live in an oxygen-rich atmosphere and our bodies require oxygen for many metabolic processes. However, oxygen is highly reactive and thus is toxic. The reactive oxygen intermediates superoxide (O_2^-) and hydrogen peroxide (H_2O_2) are generated by normal cellular reactions. Oxidative stress develops when production of reactive oxygen species exceeds the body's processing capacity. Under these circumstances, reactive oxygen intermediates may be converted to injurious free radicals by the iron-catalyzed Fenton reaction[2]:

$$O_2^- + Fe^{3+} \rightarrow O_2 + Fe^{2+}$$

$$Fe^{2+} + H_2O_2 \rightarrow Fe^{3+} + HO\cdot + OH^-$$

$$O_2^- + H_2O_2 \rightarrow O_2 + HO\cdot + OH^-$$

Hydroxyl radicals (HO•) attack many biologic macromolecules, including proteins and DNA. They also promote peroxidation of membrane lipids, a problem exacerbated by iron overload and pathologic membrane binding of iron. Intracellular structures are particularly susceptible to iron-dependent peroxidation. In iron-overloaded cells, injured lysosomes become fragile and leaky.[3] Release of lysosomal proteases causes further cell injury and may ultimately lead to cell death. This process contributes to the severe tissue damage seen in the liver, heart, joints, and pancreas of patients with iron overload disorders (see later).

Iron is not normally present in cell membranes. However, in both sickle cell disease and thalassemia, iron, heme, ferritin, and denatured hemoglobin adhere to the inner surface of the red cell plasma membrane and thereby contribute to the pathogenesis of these congenital anemias.[4,5] The membrane complex containing denatured hemoglobin has been termed *hemichrome*.[6] The red cell anion transport protein band 3 appears to nucleate the formation of these iron aggregates.[7,8] Injured cells decorated with membrane iron deposits are removed by a functioning spleen in patients with thalassemia and hemoglobin SC disease, but they circulate in functionally asplenic patients with homozygous hemoglobin SS disease. Membrane-associated iron promotes free radical formation and further membrane damage, marked by generation of the lipid peroxidation product malonyldialdehyde and by cross-linking of membrane proteins.[4,5] Membranes become rigid and thus contribute to the formation of irreversibly sickled cells that occlude the microcirculation.

Sometimes reactive oxygen intermediates can be beneficial. Neutrophils contain a membrane-associated reduced nicotinamide adenine dinucleotide phosphate (NADPH) oxidase that produces superoxide to kill ingested microorganisms (reviewed by Clark[9]). Superoxide and secondary reactive oxygen intermediates are potent antimicrobial agents. Congenital defects in this NADPH oxidase, collectively termed *chronic granulomatous disease* (see Chapter 21), are characterized by a serious defect in defense against bacterial pathogens.

Neutrophils and iron also injure tissues in inflammatory diseases such as rheumatoid arthritis.[10] Synovial macrophages ingest red cell hemoglobin introduced by intermittent joint hemorrhage. Iron is deposited in the synovial membrane, proximate to superoxide and hydrogen peroxide generated by neutrophils and macrophages participating in the inflammatory reaction. Iron catalyzes the conversion of these compounds to free radical species, which promote lipid peroxidation. Iron therapy exacer-

bates this process. In contrast, antioxidants and iron chelators retard free radical generation, thereby affording some theoretical protection against injury in rheumatoid arthritis.[11,12]

These deleterious properties of iron are threatening only when the element is in a "free" state or in an abnormal compartment within the cell. Protection of cell structures from iron-dependent free radical damage is crucial to survival. When iron is bound to protein either directly or in the form of heme, the generation of free radicals is largely abrogated. Thus, tight chelation of iron is a means of controlling its reactivity. As discussed later, cytoplasmic ferritin allows iron to be stored safely within cells by sequestering it in an innocuous form. Expression of ferritin is induced by oxidative stress.[13] Both prokaryotic and eukaryotic cells contain ferritins, and mice lacking one of the two ferritin genes do not develop past the early embryonic stages.[14] Thus, ferritin appears to be necessary for most, if not all living cells.

ACQUISITION AND DISTRIBUTION OF IRON

Although the average adult has 4 to 5 g of iron, a meticulous balance exists between dietary uptake and loss. About 0.5 to 1 mg of iron is lost each day through sloughing of cells from skin and mucosal surfaces (Fig. 12-1).[15] Because menstruating females lose an average of an additional 1 mg of iron daily, their dietary iron requirement is increased.[16] Neither the liver nor the kidney has a significant capability to excrete iron in humans. Consequently, absorption appears to be the primary means of regulating body iron stores.[17] During neonatal and childhood growth spurts, iron requirements increase in response to augmentation of body mass.

Iron Absorption

Iron absorption occurs predominantly in the proximal duodenum.[18,19] The physical state of iron entering the duodenum greatly influences its absorption. At physiologic pH, ferrous iron is rapidly converted to the insoluble ferric form. Acid produced by the stomach serves to lower the pH in the duodenum and thereby enhance the solubility and uptake of iron (see later). Heme is absorbed separately from and more efficiently than inorganic iron,[18] independent of duodenal pH. Consequently, meat is an excellent nutritive source of iron. Heme iron absorption is poorly understood, but a heme oxygenase inhibitor has been shown to block heme catabolism in the intestine and result in an iron-deficient state.[20]

A number of dietary factors influence iron absorption.[21] Ascorbate and citrate increase iron uptake, in part by acting as weak chelators to help solubilize the metal in the duodenum. Iron is readily transferred from these compounds to the absorptive epithelium. Conversely, plant phytates, bran, and tannins inhibit iron absorp-

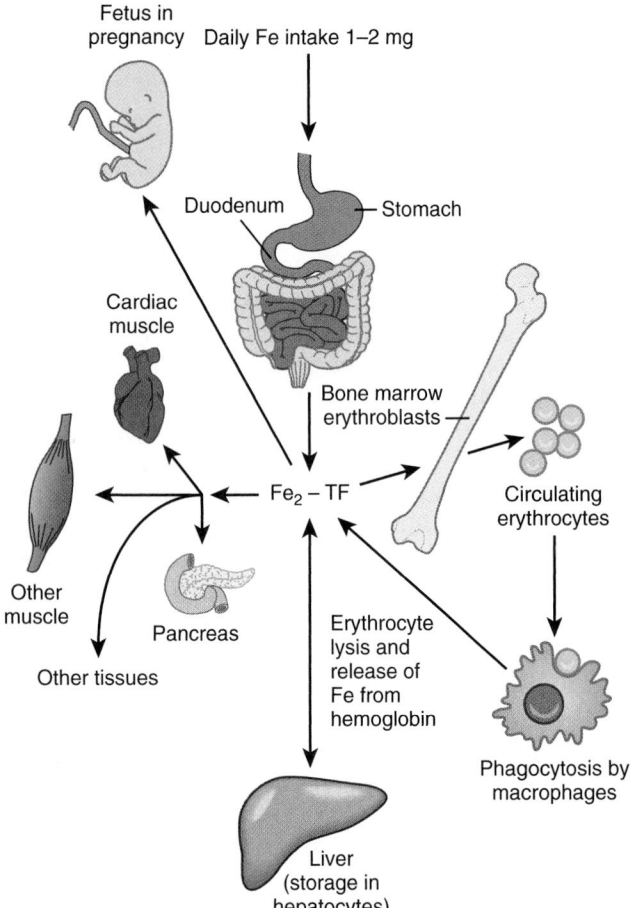

FIGURE 12-1. The body's iron economy. Although the average adult has 4 to 5 g of body iron, only 1 mg of dietary iron enters and leaves the iron economy on an average day. Dietary iron enters through the duodenum and becomes bound to plasma transferrin for delivery to tissues. The erythron is the largest site of iron utilization, but all cells require the metal. Storage iron is found primarily in the liver. Reticuloendothelial macrophages carry out iron recycling. Iron is lost from the body with bleeding and with exfoliation of skin and mucosal cells. Fe_2 – TF, diferric transferrin. *(Adapted with permission from Andrews NC. Iron homeostasis: insights from genetics and animal models. Nat Rev Genet. 2000;1:208-217.)*

tion.[21-23] These compounds also chelate iron but prevent its uptake by the absorption machinery (see later).

Through a combination of genetic and biochemical approaches, much has been learned about the absorption of nonheme iron over the past decade. Nonheme iron arrives at the apical surface of the absorptive duodenal enterocyte in its ferric (Fe^{3+}) form. It is reduced through the action of a brush border ferric reductase. This enzyme may be duodenal cytochrome b, a heme protein that is homologous to b_{561} cytochromes.[24] Expression of duodenal cytochrome b is significantly greater in the proximal duodenum than elsewhere and increases in iron deficiency.

Ferrous (Fe^{2+}) iron is then taken up by the enterocyte through the action of divalent metal transporter 1 (DMT1, formerly known as Nramp2, DCT1).[25-27] Transport requires movement of protons along with metal ions in the same direction (symport) to generate an electrical

gradient. DMT1 functions only at low pH; it has little or no activity at neutral pH. DMT1 is widely expressed, but duodenal levels increase dramatically in iron-deficient animals.[27,28]

DMT1 can also transport other divalent metal ions, including Cd^{2+}, Co^{2+}, Cu^{2+}, Mn^{2+}, Pb^{2+}, and Zn^{2+}.[27] Competition studies have shown that lead, manganese, cobalt, and zinc can share the intestinal absorption pathway used by iron. Increased iron absorption induced by iron deficiency also enhances the uptake of these elements. Because iron deficiency often coexists with lead intoxication, this interaction has vast public health significance and can produce particularly serious medical complications in children.[29] Interestingly, as discussed later, copper absorption and metabolism appear to be handled by an entirely different mechanism.

After iron enters the absorptive enterocyte through the action of DMT1, it has at least two possible fates. It can be retained by the cell and subsequently be lost when the enterocyte dies and is sloughed into the intestinal lumen, or it can be transported across the basolateral membrane to enter the body. Iron retained by the enterocyte is used for cellular metabolism or incorporated into ferritin. Exported iron leaves the cell through the action of a unique basolateral transmembrane iron transporter, ferroportin (FPN1, also known as SLC40A1, MTP1, IREG1).[30-33]

Basolateral iron transfer also requires a change in the oxidation state of the metal, probably mediated by the multicopper ferroxidase hephaestin,[34,35] which bears strong homology to the plasma protein ceruloplasmin. A comprehensive model of intestinal iron absorption, primarily derived from studies in mice, is shown in Figure 12-2. This model pertains only to nonheme iron transport; details of heme iron uptake have not yet been worked out. A candidate intestinal heme transporter was reported but subsequently proven to be a folate transporter instead.[36] Although this is a good representation of what takes place in mice, it is possible that human iron absorption is significantly different.

Normally, only about 10% of dietary nonheme iron entering the duodenum is absorbed. However, this value increases significantly with iron deficiency.[37] In contrast, iron overload reduces, but does not completely eliminate absorption, thus reaffirming the fact that body iron stores regulate absorption. Finch[37] and subsequent investigators have designated this modulation the "stores regulator." In addition, both iron deficiency anemia and the anemia associated with ineffective erythropoiesis induce a marked increase in iron absorption. This effect is greater than that seen with variations in iron stores, and it has been designated the "erythroid regulator."[37] Additionally, hypoxia increases iron absorption, independent of anemia.

The peptide hormone hepcidin links the actions of all these regulators through a unifying molecular mechanism. Hepcidin is a 25–amino acid peptide produced in the liver from a larger precursor (reviewed by Nemeth and Ganz[38]). It circulates in serum and binds to the iron

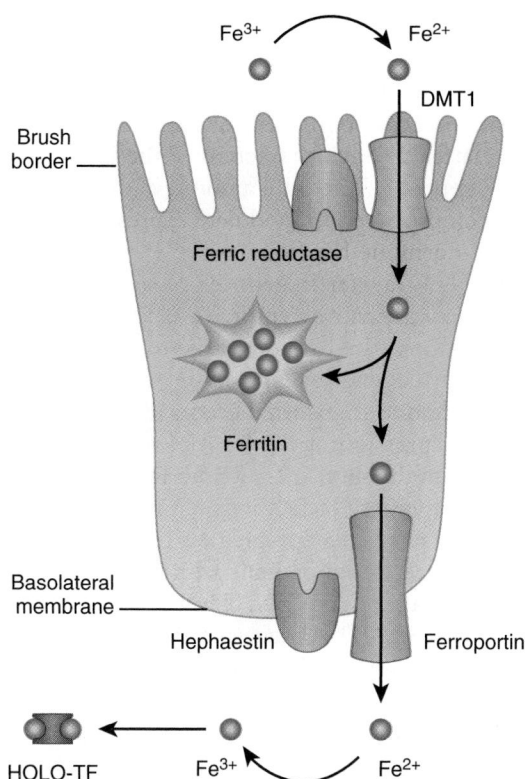

Fe³⁺ → Fe²⁺
DMT1
Brush border
Ferric reductase
Ferritin
Basolateral membrane
Hephaestin   Ferroportin
HOLO-TF   Fe³⁺ ← Fe²⁺

FIGURE 12-2. Duodenal iron transfer. The microstructure of the iron absorption apparatus is depicted in this cartoon. Iron is taken up by enterocytes lining the duodenal villi. These absorptive cells start out as undifferentiated precursors in the intestinal crypts. Crypt cells appear to be programmed for an iron absorption "set-point" that is determined in response to iron needs. As the cells differentiate, they migrate up the villi and begin to express iron transporter proteins. According to current models, nonheme iron uptake occurs in mature enterocytes through the enzymatic reduction of iron, transmembrane import into the cell by DMT1, transmembrane export from the cell by ferroportin, and enzymatic oxidation by hephaestin before loading onto apotransferrin to produce diferric transferrin (HOLO-TF). *(Adapted with permission from Andrews NC. Iron homeostasis: insights from genetics and animal models. Nat Rev Genet. 2000;1:208-217.)*

exporter ferroportin on the basolateral surface of absorptive enterocytes, which causes ferroportin to be internalized and degraded.[39] In this way, hepcidin controls cellular iron egress. Hepcidin thus regulates iron absorption at the level of the intestinal epithelium in that any iron unable to leave the enterocytes is lost when these cells senesce and are sloughed into the gut lumen.

Expression of hepcidin is induced in response to iron overload[40,41] and inflammation[42,43] and repressed in response to increased erythropoietic activity[43,44] and hypoxia.[43] Regulation appears to be at the level of hepcidin gene transcription. However, the signals that govern hepcidin transcription in response to these stimuli are incompletely understood. Only the inflammatory cytokine interleukin-6 has been definitely shown to be involved in regulation of hepcidin expression by physiologic changes outside the liver.[45-47]

Most of the total body iron is ultimately incorporated into hemoglobin in erythroid precursors. An average

adult produces 200 billion red cells daily to achieve a red cell renewal rate of 0.8% per day. Each red cell contains more than 1 billion atoms of iron, and each milliliter of packed red blood cells contains 1 mg of iron. To meet this daily need for 2×10^{20} atoms (or 20 mg) of elemental iron, iron is recycled from senescent red cells and returned to the circulation. Plasma iron turnover (PIT) represents the mass turnover of transferrin-bound iron in the circulation (expressed as milligrams per kilogram per day).[48] Accelerated erythropoiesis increases PIT and enhances iron uptake from the gastrointestinal tract.[49] Although hepcidin appears to be the effector molecule that alters intestinal absorption, an upstream, circulating factor that communicates the iron needs of the erythron must exist.[37,50] Several candidate factors have been considered unlikely, including transferrin[51] and erythropoietin.[52]

This erythroid control of hepcidin expression is particularly apparent in patients with thalassemia intermedia, in whom marked iron overload develops even without transfusions. The accelerated (but ineffective) erythropoiesis taking place in thalassemia substantially boosts iron absorption. Hepcidin expression is markedly decreased.[53-56] Increased PIT also leads to increased gastrointestinal iron absorption in pregnancy, in which PIT is accelerated by placental removal of iron. This increases the availability of the element to meet the needs of the growing and developing fetus. Decreased expression of hepcidin is probably involved in this situation as well, but definitive studies have not yet been reported.

Intercellular Iron Transport

As illustrated in Figure 12-1, only a small proportion of total body iron enters and leaves the body each day. Consequently, intercellular iron transport is quantitatively more important than intestinal absorption. The greatest mass of iron is found in erythroid cells, which make up about 60% to 80% of the total body endowment in normal individuals. The reticuloendothelial system recycles a substantial amount of iron from effete red cells that approximates the amount used by the erythron for production of new hemoglobin.

Approximately 0.1% (4 mg) of total body iron circulates in plasma as an exchangeable pool. In normal individuals, nearly all circulating plasma iron is bound to transferrin. Transferrin serves three purposes: (1) it renders iron soluble under physiologic conditions, (2) it prevents iron-mediated free radical toxicity, and (3) it facilitates transport into cells. Transferrin is by far the most important physiologic supplier of iron to red cells.[57] In fact, plasma transferrin serves to deliver iron to most tissues of the body. It is an 80-kd glycoprotein that has homologous N-terminal and C-terminal iron binding domains.[58] The molecule is related to several other proteins, including ovotransferrin in bird and reptile eggs,[59] lactoferrin in extracellular secretions and neutrophil granules,[60,61] and melanotransferrin (p97), a protein produced by melanoma cells.[62] The functions of these related proteins are incompletely understood.

The liver is the major site of synthesis and secretion of transferrin.[63] Other tissues, including Sertoli cells of the testis, oligodendrocytes of the central nervous system (CNS), lymphocytes, muscle cells, and mammary cells, can, however, also produce the protein.[64-69] Local synthesis within the brain and testis apparently provides transferrin for these tissues because serum transferrin does not penetrate their unique capillary barriers. The blood-testis barrier prevents free flow of proteins from the circulation into the lumen of the seminiferous tubules. The Sertoli cells of the testis synthesize a significant quantity of transferrin that bathes developing germ cells.[68,69] These rapidly dividing cells require substantial amounts of iron for normal growth and differentiation. The transferrin supplied by Sertoli cells is believed to be vital to spermatocyte development. However, forced overexpression of transferrin in the testes appears to be deleterious for spermatogenesis.[70]

Transferrin mRNA and protein have also been detected in oligodendrocytes.[65] Like the testis, the CNS has limited access to serum molecules because of the blood-brain barrier. Unlike the testis, however, the CNS has no cohort of rapidly proliferating cells. Iron may be needed instead to support a vast array of redox reactions that produce specialized neurotransmitter compounds such as γ-aminobutyric acid. The question of whether synthesis of transferrin by oligodendrocytes is absolutely required for distribution of iron to neural tissues remains unanswered. Interestingly, however, mice with an inactivating mutation in the transferrin gene[71] have been reported to have subtle abnormalities in CNS architecture.[72]

Activated T lymphocytes also synthesize and secrete transferrin.[67] At rest, mature T cells do not generate transferrin and do not express surface transferrin receptors. After mitogenic stimulation, however, both proteins are produced.[67,73] Synthesis of transferrin is restricted to CD4+ helper lymphocytes. Transferrin mRNA production and transferrin receptor synthesis by these cells precede cell division and have been postulated to be part of an autocrine regulatory loop.[67]

Transferrin genes have been cloned from many different species. A basic similarity exists both in the protein structure of the transferrin molecule and in its genomic organization. Human transferrin mRNA is 2.3 kilobases (kb) in length and encodes 679 amino acids, including a 19–amino acid leader sequence.[74] It is located on chromosome 3q, near genes for the transferrin receptor and melanotransferrin (p97).

Transferrin production is regulated at multiple levels. Several *cis*-acting control regions exist upstream of the gene. The transferrin promoter contains binding sites for tissue-specific nuclear factors that activate transcription differentially in the liver and other tissues (e.g., Sertoli cells).[75] Transferrin gene expression is also modulated by iron, hormones, and inflammatory stimuli.[76-80] In the setting of iron deficiency, serum transferrin levels rise substantially as a result of enhanced synthesis of transferrin mRNA by the liver.[78] In contrast, inflammation depresses levels of both serum transferrin and serum iron, the latter through the action of the iron regulatory hormone hepcidin. The total amount of diferric transferrin has been proposed to modulate expression of the iron regulatory hormone hepcidin.[81]

Control of transferrin gene expression contrasts with that of the transferrin receptor. Transferrin is abundant and serves as a buffer to prevent the toxicity of free iron. Consequently, its expression does not have to be altered acutely to respond to external events. Primary control of transferrin expression at the level of message transcription allows modulation of systemic iron metabolism in response to a variety of factors such as inflammation or the hormonal changes of pregnancy. Liver-derived serum transferrin levels fall in patients with genetic or acquired iron overload, although mRNA levels have been reported to be unchanged.[82] This suggests that hepatic transferrin is also controlled at the level of translation or secretion. Interestingly, the quantity of transferrin mRNA in nonhepatic tissues (including the testis, kidney, and spleen) is not affected by iron deficiency. The liver-derived transferrin, therefore, appears to have the unique responsibility of responding to iron status.

X-ray crystal structures have been determined for transferrin and related proteins (reviewed elsewhere[83-85]). All members of the transferrin protein superfamily exhibit similar polypeptide folding. The N-terminal and C-terminal domains are globular moieties of about 330 amino acids; each of these domains is divided into two subdomains, with the iron and anion binding sites located in the intersubdomain cleft on either side of a central plane of symmetry, thus suggesting an origin by gene duplication from a primordial protein containing a single iron binding site. The binding cleft opens with iron release and closes with iron binding.[86] The N-terminal and C-terminal binding sites are very similar. No cooperativity exists in binding of iron by the two sites, and the protein can be proteolytically cleaved into two halves, each of which retains iron-binding capability.[87,88] Transferrin binds ferric iron much more avidly than ferrous iron.[89]

The precise mechanism by which iron is loaded onto transferrin as it leaves intestinal epithelial cells or reticuloendothelial cells is unknown. Ferroportin has been postulated to mediate iron export from these cells. The copper-dependent ferroxidase ceruloplasmin and its homologue hephaestin probably also play a role. Compelling evidence indicates that ceruloplasmin is involved in mobilizing tissue iron stores to produce diferric transferrin.[90-92] Transferrin binds iron avidly with a dissociation constant of approximately 10^{-22} mol/L.[89] Ferric iron binds only in the company of an anion (usually carbonate), which serves as a bridging ligand between the metal and protein and excludes water from two coordination sites.[89,93,94] Without the anion cofactor, iron binding is negligible; with it, ferric transferrin is resistant to all but the most potent chelators. The remaining four coordination sites provided by the transferrin protein are a histidine nitrogen, an aspartic acid carboxylate oxygen, and two tyrosine phenolate oxygens.[83,95,96] The available evidence suggests that anion binding takes place before iron binding. Release of iron from transferrin involves protonation of the carbonate anion to loosen the metal-protein bond.

The sum of all iron binding sites on transferrin constitutes the total iron-binding capacity (TIBC) of plasma. Thus, on a molar basis, TIBC is twice the concentration of transferrin protein because each transferrin molecule can bind two iron atoms. Under normal circumstances, about a third of transferrin's iron binding pockets are filled. Consequently, except for the situation of iron overload, in which all transferrin binding sites are occupied, non–transferrin-bound iron in the circulation is present at very low concentrations.[97] The distribution of plasma and tissue iron can be traced with the use of ^{59}Fe as a radioactive tag by reinfusing a subject with autologous transferrin loaded with radiolabeled iron. Blood samples can be analyzed at timed intervals to determine the rate of loss of the radioactive label. Such ferrokinetic studies indicate that the normal half-life of iron in the circulation is about 75 minutes.[48] The absolute amount of iron released from transferrin per unit time is the PIT (see earlier).

Such radioactive tracer studies indicate that at least 80% of the iron bound to circulating transferrin is delivered to the bone marrow and incorporated into newly formed reticulocytes.[98,99] Other major sites of iron delivery include the liver, which is a primary depot for stored iron, and the spleen. Hepatic iron is found in both reticuloendothelial cells and hepatocytes. Reticuloendothelial cells acquire iron primarily by phagocytosis and breakdown of aging red cells; they extract the iron from heme and return it to the circulation bound to transferrin. Hepatocytes take up iron by at least two different pathways. The relative amounts of iron in each of these cell types depend on clinical circumstances, as discussed in detail later.

Given the preeminent role of bone marrow in the clearance of labeled iron from the circulation, ferrokinetic studies provide a window on erythropoietic activity. Conditions that augment erythrocyte production increase PIT. For example, hemolytic anemias such as hereditary spherocytosis and sickle cell disease induce rapid delivery of transferrin-bound iron to the marrow. In contrast, disorders that reduce red cell production, such as Diamond-Blackfan anemia and aplastic anemia, prolong PIT.

When erythrocytes are produced and released into the circulation in a normal fashion, the process of erythropoiesis is termed *effective*. In patients with certain anemias, however, the abnormal, nascent red cells are destroyed before they leave the marrow cavity. In this situation, erythropoiesis is *ineffective*, which means simply that the erythropoietic precursors have failed to accomplish their primary task: delivery of intact erythrocytes to the circulation. The ferrokinetic profile in this case shows rapid removal of iron from transferrin with delayed entry of label into the pool of circulating red cell hemoglobin. β^+-Thalassemia is an important example of this pattern. In β^+-thalassemia, ineffective erythropoiesis is coupled with markedly enhanced PIT.

Intracellular Iron Metabolism

Transferrin and the Transferrin Cycle

Although transferrin was first characterized more than 60 years ago,[100] its receptor eluded investigators until the early 1980s, when monoclonal antibodies prepared against tumor cells were found to recognize the transferrin receptor glycoprotein.[101] Subsequently, receptor-mediated endocytosis of iron bound to transferrin has been characterized in detail. A diagram showing key features of the transferrin receptor is presented in Figure 12-3. Each subunit of the disulfide-linked homodimer contains 760 amino acids.[102-104] Oligosaccharides account for about 5% of the 90-kd subunit's molecular mass.[105] Four glycosylation sites (three *N* linked and one *O* linked)

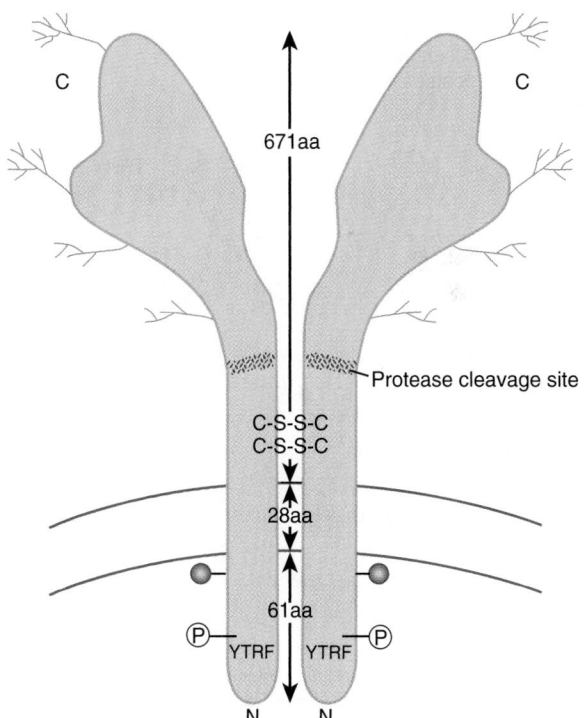

FIGURE 12-3. Structure of the dimeric transferrin receptor. The N-terminals of both subunits are inside the cell, and the C-terminals are outside. The 61–amino acid (aa) intracellular domain has three structural features that appear to play a role in endocytosis: a tyrosine-threonine-arginine-phenylalanine (YTRF) amino acid motif, a phosphorylated serine residue (*encircled* "P"), and a covalently linked molecule of palmitic acid (*solid circle*). The transmembrane domain is 28 amino acids long. The extracellular domain has 671 amino acids, including disulfide linkages (C-S-S-C), as well as four glycosylation sites (*branched lines*). A potential protease cleavage site is located between amino acids 100 and 101.

are found in the protein.[106,107] Glycosylation-defective mutants have fewer disulfide bridges, less transferrin binding, and less cell surface expression. The transmembrane domain, located between amino acids 62 and 89, functions as an internal signal peptide because there is none at the N-terminal end.[108] A molecule of fatty acid (usually palmitate) is also covalently linked to each subunit at the internal edge of the transmembrane domain and may play a role in membrane localization. Interestingly, nonacylated mutants mediate faster iron uptake.[109,110] The transferrin binding regions of the protein have not been definitively identified. However, the crystal structure of the ectodomain of the transferrin receptor has been reported.[111] Although no one has yet succeeded in cocrystallizing the receptor with transferrin, binding studies of mutant transferrin receptor proteins have yielded important insights.[112]

Iron is taken into cells by receptor-mediated endocytosis of diferric transferrin (Fig. 12-4).[113-116] Receptors on the outer face of the plasma membrane bind iron-loaded transferrin with very high affinity. The C-terminal domain of transferrin appears to mediate receptor binding.[117] Diferric transferrin binds with much higher affinity than monoferric transferrin or apotransferrin does.[118-120] The dissociation constant (K_d) for bound diferric transferrin ranges from 10^{-7} to 10^{-9} mol/L at physiologic pH, depending on the species and tissue. The K_d of monoferric transferrin is approximately 10^{-6} mol/L. The concentration of circulating transferrin is about 25 μmol/L. Therefore, cellular transferrin receptors are ordinarily fully saturated.

After binding to its receptor on the cell surface, transferrin is internalized through a constitutive mechanism that begins with invagination of clathrin-coated pits and the formation of endocytic vesicles. This process requires the short, 61–amino acid intracellular tail of the transferrin receptor molecule.[121-124] Receptors with truncated N-terminal cytoplasmic domains do not recycle properly. This portion of the molecule contains a conserved tyrosine-threonine-arginine-phenylalanine (YTRF) sequence that functions as a signal for endocytosis. Genetically engineered addition of a second YTRF sequence enhances receptor endocytosis.[125]

An ATP-dependent proton pump lowers the pH of the internalized endosome to about 5.5.[126-128] Acidification of the endosome weakens the association between iron and transferrin and promotes a conformational change in the transferrin receptor to enhance binding of apotransferrin and facilitate release of iron.[129] An endosomal ferrireductase must reduce iron from the Fe^{3+} state to Fe^{2+}, either at the same time that it is released from transferrin or soon afterward. This reductase was recently shown to be STEAP3, a membrane protein localized to transferrin cycle endosomes in erythroid precursors.[130] Related proteins may serve similar functions at other sites.[131]

The iron released from transferrin must leave the endosome and enter the cytoplasm and mitochondria for use in heme biosynthesis, Fe/S cluster formation, storage, and other purposes. This transmembrane transport step is also mediated by DMT1.[132,133] DMT1 is unusual in that it is expressed on two very different types of membranes—the apical membrane of intestinal enterocytes and the endosomal membrane of transferrin uptake vesicles in nonpolarized cells. Once transported out of the endosome or across the plasma membrane, iron must be delivered to sites of use or stored in the form of ferritin. Unlike copper (see later), however, there are no known cytosolic protein chaperones for iron, and how iron traverses the cell is unknown. In erythroid cells, iron is delivered across the mitochondrial inner membrane by mitoferrin 1 (SLC25A37),[134] where it is incorporated into heme by the enzyme ferrochelatase.

The fate of transferrin and the transferrin receptor is distinct from that of iron. Rather than entering lysosomes for degradation, as do ligands in other receptor-mediated endocytosis pathways, intact receptor-bound apotransferrin recycles to the cell surface, where neutral pH promotes detachment into the circulation. Thus, preservation and reuse of transferrin are accomplished

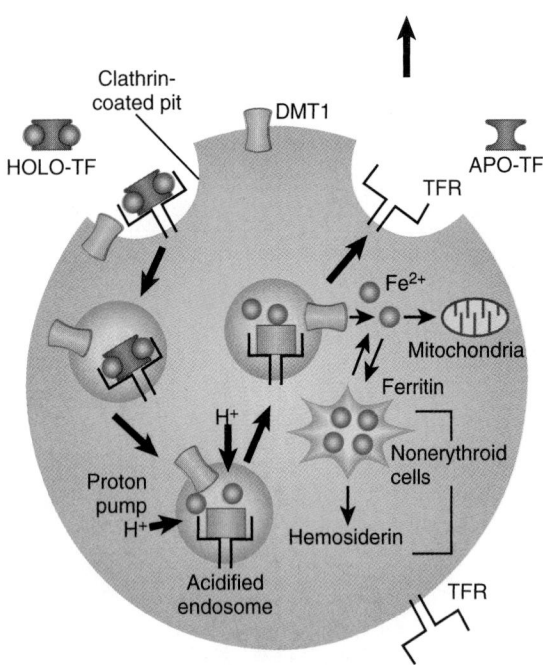

FIGURE 12-4. The endocytotic transferrin cycle. Apotransferrin (APO-TF) binds two atoms of iron per molecule to form diferric transferrin (HOLO-TF). Diferric transferrin binds to the transferrin receptor (TFR) on the cell surface. The complex is internalized by invagination of clathrin-coated pits to form specific endosomes. The endosomes import protons, thus lowering the pH within the organelle and decreasing the affinity of transferrin for iron. Liberated iron is translocated through the endosome membrane to the cytoplasm by DMT1. The iron released is shuttled to mitochondria for synthesis of heme and to ferritin for storage. The apotransferrin-transferrin receptor complex recycles to the cell surface, where neutral pH promotes release of apotransferrin into serum for reuse. Details are given in the text. *(Adapted with permission from Andrews NC. Iron homeostasis: insights from genetics and animal models. Nat Rev Genet. 2000;1:208-217.)*

by pH-dependent changes in the affinity of transferrin for its receptor.[126,128,135] Exported apotransferrin binds additional iron atoms and undergoes further rounds of iron delivery to cells. The average transferrin molecule, with a half-life of 8 days, may be used hundreds of times for delivery of iron.

Topologically, the cell exterior and the endosome interior are equivalent compartments. The primary role of the transferrin–transferrin receptor interaction is to sequester iron near the cell membrane, thereby increasing the likelihood of iron uptake. DMT1 may reside on the plasma membrane of the cell before endocytosis. If so, it should be oriented to transport iron directly into the cell, without the assistance of transferrin (as diagrammed in Fig. 12-4). Such non–transferrin-bound iron uptake activities have been characterized in tissue culture cells (see later). This uptake system could function constitutively but inefficiently in tissues in which pH is low enough to provide protons for DMT1 function.

It was once a widely accepted belief that the transferrin cycle was important, if not necessary for uptake of iron by all mammalian cells. However, two lines of evidence indicate that such is not the case. First, mice and human patients with severe deficiencies of plasma transferrin have iron deficiency anemia but excess iron in nonhematopoietic tissues.[57,71,136-141] This finding indicates that uptake of iron bound to transferrin is important for red blood cell hemoglobinization and maturation but transferrin is not essential for delivery of iron to most other tissues. Second, mouse embryos lacking transferrin receptor die midway through gestation as a result of severe anemia, but nonhematopoietic tissues appear to generally be intact.[142] Aside from the erythron, only the developing CNS shows an apparent requirement for transferrin receptor. In its absence, primitive neuroepithelial cells undergo apoptosis at a greatly increased rate. Taken together, these observations indicate that the transferrin cycle is of primary importance in erythropoiesis and neurogenesis but of lesser importance in other mammalian tissues, at least early in embryonic development.

Non–Transferrin-Bound Iron Uptake

Both hypotransferrinemia and iron overload lead to complete saturation of available plasma transferrin, and non–transferrin-bound iron circulates in a chelatable, low-molecular-weight form (reviewed by Cabantchik and colleagues[143]). This iron is weakly complexed to albumin, citrate, amino acids, sugars, and other small molecules, and it behaves differently from iron associated with transferrin. Nonhematopoietic tissues (particularly the liver, endocrine organs, kidneys, and heart) preferentially take up non–transferrin-bound iron. Radiolabeled iron administered to mice with and without available transferrin-binding capacity is distributed in markedly different patterns.[57] In normal animals with excess plasma iron-binding capacity, hematopoietic tissues are the primary sites of uptake. When free transferrin iron binding sites

are absent, however, most iron is deposited in the liver and pancreas, thus indicating that these organs serve as the initial iron reservoirs in the situation of iron overload. Notably, this pattern of distribution is similar to that seen in idiopathic hemochromatosis.

Kaplan and co-workers have studied cellular assimilation of iron from $FeNH_4$ citrate in HeLa cells.[144,145] Intriguingly, they found that its transferrin-independent uptake increases in direct proportion to the concentration of this compound, similar to hepatic uptake of non–transferrin-bound iron in patients with saturated transferrin. They speculated that this is a protective alternative pathway that removes the toxic metal from the circulation. Other investigators have described similar uptake in a hepatic cell line and have shown that it is interrupted by the addition of chelating compounds.[146]

A nontransferrin iron uptake mechanism with different properties has been described in K562 erythroleukemia cells.[147,148] In the absence of ferric transferrin, uptake of iron into K562 cells is sensitive to treatment with trypsin, thus suggesting that it requires a protein carrier. Higher ambient iron concentrations do not increase cellular iron uptake. As discussed earlier, this transport may be accomplished by the same machinery responsible for passage of iron out of transferrin cycle endosomes into the cytoplasm. These two processes accomplish essentially the same task. However, the fact that DMT1 functions only at acidic pH suggests that it probably does not, by itself, account for all non–transferrin-bound iron transport.

Non–transferrin-bound iron is highly toxic to cells.[149] Plasma non–transferrin-bound iron can potentiate the formation of free radicals through the Fenton reaction (see earlier) and thereby induce cell membrane damage. Cardiac cells are particularly susceptible to this damage. Hence, therapeutic chelation must effectively remove plasma non–transferrin-bound iron.

Role of Iron in Cell Proliferation and Differentiation

Iron is indispensable for DNA synthesis and a host of metabolic processes. Iron starvation arrests cell proliferation, presumably because ribonucleotide reductase and other enzymes require the metal.[150] Although transferrin receptors are expressed on all dividing cells in numbers that roughly reflect their growth rate,[151] the erythron is the tissue that relies most heavily on delivery of iron by transferrin, as discussed in detail earlier. However, the transferrin cycle also appears to play a significant, if expendable role in other cell types.

Studies of mature T lymphocytes exemplify the general relationship between expression of transferrin receptor and cell proliferation. Transferrin receptors, absent from resting T cells, have long been recognized as a marker of T-cell activation. Initiation of cell division by a mitogen such as phytohemagglutinin dramatically increases both surface expression of transferrin receptor and iron uptake.[152] Along the same lines, tumor cells upregulate transferrin receptor expression to optimize acquisition of iron for proliferation.

Blockade of transferrin receptor function can halt cell division. For instance, certain monoclonal antibodies against the transferrin receptor curb proliferation of tumor cells in vitro and in vivo.[153-158] Some 159 of these antibodies actually prevent binding of transferrin to its receptor, whereas others suppress receptor recycling but do not abrogate ligand binding.[154] Interestingly, some reports have suggested that the transferrin receptor may have an additional role in activated T cells, apart from its iron uptake function. Anti–transferrin receptor monoclonal antibodies have been described that can trigger T-cell activation and secretion of interleukin-2. These antibodies presumably activate a signal transduction pathway beginning with the transferrin receptor but independent of iron trafficking. The transferrin receptor also appears to have a role in early lymphocyte development. Embryonic stem cells in which both transferrin receptor genes have been inactivated fail to differentiate into circulating lymphocytes in vivo in chimeric mice.[159] It is not yet clear whether this is due to defective iron delivery or perturbation of some other, as yet unknown function of the transferrin receptor.

Chelators that deplete intracellular iron and limit its bioavailability in extracellular fluids further demonstrate the central role of iron in cell proliferation. Agents such as deferoxamine, desferrithiocin, and pyridoxal isonicotinoyl hydrazone inhibit the growth of a variety of tumor cells in culture[160,161] and greatly reduce T-cell proliferation.[162-165] A likely inhibitory mechanism is iron deprivation, with reduced ribonucleotide reductase activity and lower levels of deoxyribonucleotides. This, in turn, leads to mitotic arrest in the S phase of the cell cycle.[166] The addition of iron to the medium reverses the growth inhibition. Chelators may also induce apoptosis, or programmed cell death, through other mechanisms that are not yet understood.

Erythroid precursors need an extraordinary amount of iron to support hemoglobin synthesis and differentiation into mature red cells. The density of transferrin receptors on the cell surface is modulated during erythroid development. Transferrin receptors first appear in measurable numbers on colony-forming unit–erythroid (CFU-E) cells and increase to 300,000 per cell on proerythroblasts and as many as 800,000 per cell on basophilic erythroblasts at the time of maximal iron uptake. Numbers then fall to 100,000 per cell on circulating reticulocytes and to negligible levels on mature red cells.[167] A precise correlation exists between iron requirement and transferrin receptor number, thus indicating that the abundance of transferrin receptors on the cell surface is a major determinant of erythroid iron uptake. In culture, a monoclonal antibody to the transferrin receptor that permits ligand binding but subsequently slows receptor recycling partially blocks erythroid iron uptake. The level of iron uptake is sufficient for cell division but not hemoglobin synthesis.[168]

Beug's group[169] demonstrated that an anti–transferrin receptor monoclonal antibody blocks differentiation of chick erythroid cells at the erythroblast or early reticulocyte stage and promotes premature, pyknotic cell death. The antibody apparently prevents normal cycling of transferrin receptors and inhibits efficient iron uptake. Its effects were specific for erythroid differentiation because it did not inhibit proliferation of a variety of other cell lines. Ferric salicylaldehyde-isonicotinyl-hydrazone (Fe-SIH) was added to antibody-treated cells to determine whether direct delivery of iron by this compound could rescue the normal erythroid program. Interestingly, Fe-SIH only partially restored maturation of antibody-treated avian cells. The investigators postulated that insufficient levels of heme or hemoglobin might shut off production of the proteins required for differentiation. These data are in accord with those of Ponka and Schulman,[170] who have shown that the rate of heme synthesis is influenced by the efficiency of iron uptake. A wealth of literature demonstrates that oxidized heme (hemin) promotes differentiation of erythroleukemia cell lines in tissue culture.[171-174] Conversely, deficient heme biosynthesis abrogates chemical induction of differentiation in an erythroleukemia cell line subclone.[175]

Other reports indicate that heme biosynthesis indirectly regulates the transcription of globin, transferrin receptor, and ferritin genes.[176-178] Heme also regulates globin mRNA translation by an elegant mechanism involving a kinase that binds heme to modulate translation factor activity (reviewed by Chen[179]). Although some of the precise mechanisms remain to be elucidated, it is clear that iron uptake, heme biosynthesis, and globin protein production are coordinately regulated. Interrelated regulatory networks apparently allow red cell precursors to maximize hemoglobin formation without accumulating excess globin proteins, unbound iron, or toxic protoporphyrin intermediates.

REGULATION OF PROTEINS OF IRON METABOLISM

Ferritin

Once inside the cytoplasm, iron is probably bound by unidentified carrier molecules that may assist in delivery to various intracellular locations, including mitochondria (for heme biosynthesis) and ferritin (for storage). The identities of the intracellular iron carrier molecules remain unknown. The amount of iron in transit within the cell at any given time is small and difficult to measure. This minute pool of transit iron, which is believed to be in the Fe^{2+} oxidation state, is the biologically active and potentially toxic form of the element. Metabolically inactive iron, stored in ferritin and hemosiderin, is nontoxic and in equilibrium with this exchangeable transit iron.

Both prokaryotes and eukaryotes produce ferritin molecules for iron storage. Mammalian ferritin molecules are complex 24-subunit heteropolymers of H (for heavy or heart) and L (for light or liver) protein subunits. L subunits are 19.7 kd in mass, with isoelectric points of 4.5 to 5.0; H subunits are 21 kd in mass, with isoelectric points of 5.0 to 5.7. The subunits of the ferritin molecule probably arose by gene duplication, although the degree of nucleotide sequence homology between the two is only about 50%. They assemble to form a sphere with a central cavity in which up to several thousand atoms of crystalline iron can be stored in the form of poly-iron-phosphate oxide.[180] Eight channels through the sphere are lined by hydrophilic amino acid residues (along the threefold axes of symmetry), and six more are lined by hydrophobic residues (along the fourfold axes).[181] Strong interspecies amino acid conservation is seen in the residues that line the hydrophilic channels, whereas marked variation is seen in those along the hydrophobic passages. The hydrophilic channels terminate with aspartic acid and glutamic acid residues and are lined by serine, histidine, and cysteine residues (all of which potentially bind metal ligands).

Although the two ferritin chains are homologous, only H ferritin has ferroxidase activity. A mechanism involving dioxygen converts ferrous to ferric iron, thereby promoting incorporation into ferritin.[182,183] The composition of ferritin shells varies from H-subunit homopolymers to L-subunit homopolymers and includes all possible combinations between the two. Isoelectric focusing of ferritin from a particular tissue reveals multiple bands representing shells with different subunit compositions. These isoferritins, as they are called, show tissue-specific variation. Ferritin from liver, for instance, is rich in L subunits, as is that from the spleen. In contrast, the heart has ferritin rich in H subunits. Increased H-subunit content correlates with increased iron utilization, whereas increased L-subunit content correlates with increased iron storage.[184] The H-to-L ratio increases with increased cell proliferation.[185] Thus, ferritin provides a flexible reserve of iron.

Despite the fact that it does not, itself, have enzymatic activity, a mutation in L ferritin has been shown to cause a distinctive iron deposition disease in humans. In patients carrying a nucleotide insertion altering the carboxy-terminus of L ferritin, iron overload develops in the basal ganglia and leads to a neurodegenerative disease with variable extrapyramidal features.[186]

Ferritin molecules aggregate into clusters that are engulfed by lysosomes and degraded. The end product of this process, hemosiderin, is an amorphous agglomerate of denatured protein and lipid interspersed with iron oxide molecules.[187] In cells overloaded with iron, lysosomes accumulate large amounts of hemosiderin, which can be visualized by Prussian blue (Perls) staining. Although the iron enmeshed in this insoluble compound constitutes an end-stage product of cellular iron storage, it remains in equilibrium with soluble ferritin. Ferritin iron, in turn, is in equilibrium with iron complexed to low-molecular-weight carrier molecules. Therefore, introduction of an effective chelator into the cell captures iron from the low-molecular-weight "toxic" iron pool, draws iron out of ferritin, and eventually depletes iron from hemosiderin as well, though only very slowly. As might be expected, the bioavailability of hemosiderin iron is much lower than that of iron stored in ferritin.

The large number of processed pseudogenes that exist for each subunit initially confounded pinpointing the chromosomal location of ferritin genes. Functional ferritin genes for the H and L subunits are located on human chromosomes 11 and 19, respectively.[188] In addition, there is an intronless gene encoding a mitochondrion-specific, H-like ferritin molecule located on human chromosome 5q.[189] The function of mitochondrial ferritin remains uncertain, although the fact that its expression is increased in erythroid precursors from patients with sideroblastic anemia suggests that it is involved in mitochondrial iron management.[189,190]

Ferritin formation is controlled at multiple levels—transcription, message stabilization, translation, and subunit assembly. In the liver and in HeLa cells, iron rapidly induces the synthesis of L-subunit mRNA, with no effect on H-subunit transcription.[191,192] In contrast, induced differentiation of HL-60 promyelocytic leukemia cells and mouse erythroleukemia cells increases production of H-subunit mRNA.[193,194] Tumor necrosis factor induces H-chain transcription in human myoblasts.[195] Iron, heme, reactive oxygen species, and oxidative stress all enhance transcription and translation of the ferritin heavy chain (reviewed by Rouault[196]).

Cytoplasmic ferritin mRNA forms a stable complex with several proteins. Both iron and interleukin-1β enhance translation of ferritin messenger ribonucleoprotein.[197] Influx of iron into cells shifts the message onto the ribosomes, thereby enhancing the synthesis of ferritin subunits.[198] This translational control mechanism involves an RNA-protein interaction that links the expression of genes encoding ferritin, the transferrin receptor, enzymes of heme biosynthesis, DMT1, ferroportin, and other proteins. Munro and colleagues[198] initially showed that ferritin synthesis was regulated at the level of message translation. Comparison of the 5' untranslated regions of ferritin mRNA encoding both heavy and light chains showed striking conservation of a 28-bp sequence motif that was predicted to form a stable RNA stem-loop structure and was necessary for translational control of ferritin (Fig. 12-5, inset).[199,200]

Subsequently designated the iron response element (IRE), this RNA stem-loop is recognized by at least two specific RNA-binding proteins called IRP1 and IRP2 for iron regulatory proteins 1 and 2. IRP1 is a 98-kd soluble polypeptide with striking homology to the mitochondrial tricarboxylic acid cycle enzyme aconitase.[201] The crystal structure of IRP1 bound to an IRE was recently reported.[202]

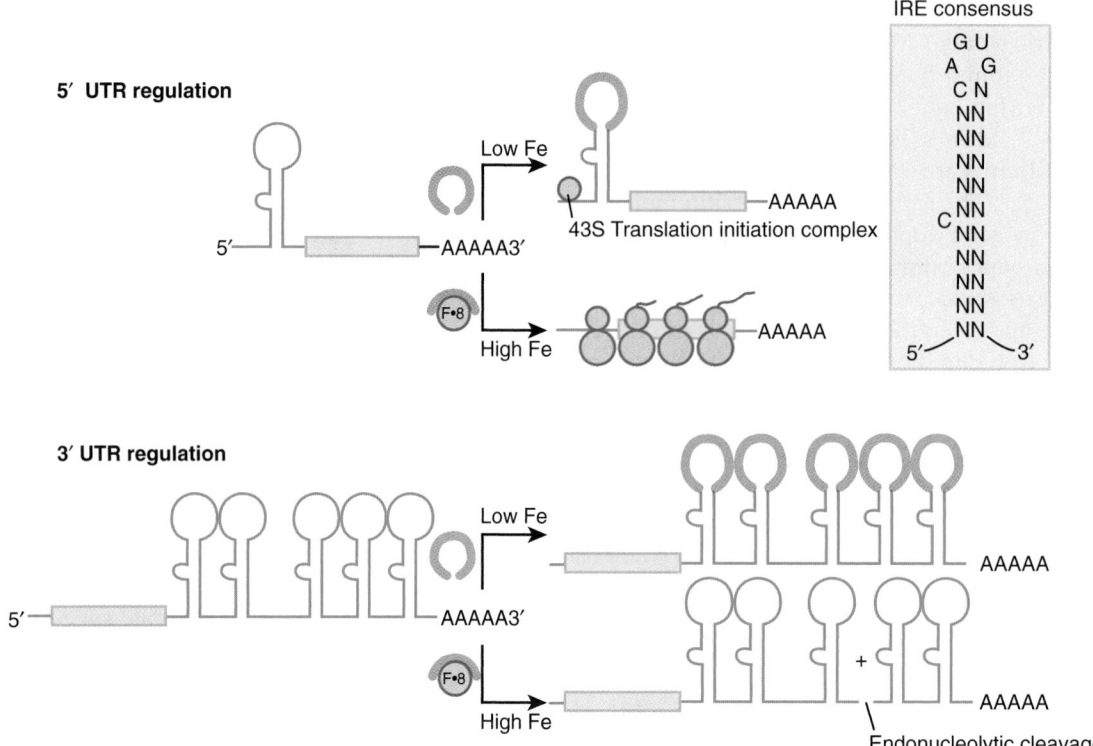

FIGURE 12-5. IRE/IRP regulation. Two mechanisms of action of iron regulatory proteins (IRPs) are shown. An IRP molecule binds to an iron response element (IRE) stem-loop structure located in noncoding mRNA sequences. A consensus IRE structure is shown in the *inset*. Under low-iron conditions, IRP binds avidly to RNA. With abundant iron, no binding occurs. Binding of IRP to IRE elements in the 5′ untranslated region (UTR) (e.g., in ferritin mRNA) blocks translation. In contrast, binding of IRP to 3′ UTR IRE elements (e.g., in transferrin receptor mRNA) prevents site-specific nucleolytic cleavage, thereby stabilizing the message. In this way, a single regulatory element plays two different roles in the translational regulation of proteins involved in cellular iron metabolism.

IRP1 and mitochondrial aconitase have identical amino acid residues in the region corresponding to the aconitase active site, and IRP1 probably serves as the major cytosolic aconitase. The enzymatic active site of IRP1 contains a 4Fe/4S cluster. When the iron concentration in the cytosol is high, the cluster is complete, and this form of IRP1 has aconitase activity but cannot bind mRNA. Under these circumstances, the ferritin message is translated efficiently. Conversely, when the iron concentration is low, aconitase activity is absent, RNA binding is avid, and ferritin message translation is blocked because translation initiation complexes cannot form properly.[203-208] Thus, IRP1 is a dual-function protein, with ambient iron controlling the switch by its participation in the 4Fe/4S cluster. Other molecules that modulate the switch include ascorbic acid, nitric oxide, and heme.[209-211] This mechanism allows ferritin protein expression to be rapidly downregulated without degradation of mRNA. The importance of IRP-mediated translational control is underscored by the fact that hyperferritinemia and ferritin-containing cataracts develop in patients with mutations in the L-ferritin IRE but these patients do not have abnormalities in iron homeostasis.[212,213] Furthermore, it appears that an iron overload disorder resembling hereditary hemochromatosis develops in rare patients with mutations in the H-ferritin IRE, presumably because increased H-ferritin expression leads to increased cellular iron assimilation, retention, or both.[214]

A second IRE-binding protein, IRP2, also modulates post-transcriptional expression of mRNA by binding to IREs in much the same way. Initially isolated in the liver, IRP2 has been found in all tissues examined and is more abundant than IRP1 in some.[215,216] Although the two proteins differ in molecular mass (90 kd for IRP1 and 118 kd for IRP2), the key difference is that IRP2 lacks aconitase activity[217] and does not contain an Fe/S cluster to function as a "ferrostat." Rather, IRP2 protein levels are modulated directly by iron or by heme and the molecule is actively degraded when iron or heme (or both) are abundant.[215,218-220] IRP1 and IRP2 function differently when oxygen tension changes, and IRP2 appears to be more important in vivo, in settings in which tissue oxygen tension is relatively low.[221]

The Transferrin Receptor

IRPs also modulate expression of the transferrin receptor gene. The gene encoding the transferrin receptor is located on human chromosome 3q26.2-qter, near the gene encoding transferrin at 3q21.[222] It consists of 19 exons spread over 31 kb.[223] The transferrin receptor mRNA is approximately twice the length needed to encode the receptor protein. Its lengthy 3′ untranslated region contains five potential RNA stem-loop structures that are structurally similar to those of the ferritin IREs.[224-226] These conserved regions of the mRNA bind the same proteins as the IREs of the ferritin mRNA do.[226] The attached protein increases the stability of the transferrin receptor message by obscuring an endonucleolytic cleavage site.[227] The result is a larger amount of transferrin receptor mRNA in the cell. A deficit of cellular iron, then, raises transferrin receptor mRNA levels at least in part through enhanced message stability. However, IRE regulation is probably not responsible for the primary increases in transferrin receptor number in erythroid cells because this occurs at the transcriptional level and is unaffected by iron status. Relatively little is understood about the tissue-specific transcriptional regulation of the transferrin receptor.[228]

The versatile regulatory functions of IREs may also confer iron-dependent regulation on other proteins. IREs are present in the 5′ untranslated regions of the mRNA encoding the erythroid form of the heme biosynthetic enzyme δ-aminolevulinic acid synthase, mitochondrial aconitase, and ferroportin.[30,31,33,229-231] A single 3′ IRE is found in one splicing isoform of DMT1 mRNA.[232] As the rate-limiting enzyme in heme biosynthesis, the IRE in the erythroid form of δ-aminolevulinic acid synthase produces a conceptually satisfying link between iron and heme production. However, the functions of the IREs in the other mRNAs are not yet understood. It is postulated that all IREs serve the common purpose of coupling changes in the iron status of the cell with its ability to utilize and store the element (see Fig. 12-5). When the intracellular iron concentration is low, the IRE of ferritin mRNA binds IRP and reduces ferritin synthesis because additional iron storage capacity is not needed in this circumstance. Simultaneously, the level of transferrin receptor mRNA increases as the IRP stabilizes the message, thereby increasing expression of the transferrin receptor. Together, these events increase the flow of iron into cells while protecting against iron toxicity. When iron levels in the cell are high, the opposite scenario is operative. Although the IRPs accomplish these regulatory feats under extremes of iron status, the importance of IREs and IRPs in modulating gene expression in normal humans and animals is not fully understood. Recently, novel IRE-containing genes have been identified, with roles less directly related to iron homeostasis.[233-235]

In an attempt to sort out the unique functions of IRP1 and IRP2 and to evaluate their roles in vivo, targeted mutagenesis was used to generate mutant mice lacking each of the proteins.[236-241] Surprisingly, IRP1 knockout mice had no identifiable defects, but IRP2 knockout mice had abnormalities in several tissues. Initially, the most striking aspect of the IRP2 knockout phenotype was a late-onset neurologic disorder associated with abnormal deposition of iron in white matter tracts and nuclei throughout the brain.[239] The mice dem-

onstrated ataxia, bradykinesia, and tremors. However, these findings could not readily be explained by known activities of IRP2, and a second group reported that an independently targeted line of mice did not have obvious neurodegeneration.[238] It is possible that the discrepancy may be explained by differential severity of a neurologic phenotype on different genetic backgrounds. More recently, both groups have reported that IRP2-deficient mice have mild microcytosis because of functional erythroid iron deficiency, as well as other subtle perturbations in systemic iron homeostasis.[236,242]

Serum Ferritin and Transferrin Receptors

Although most ferritin is located within cells, a measurable amount of the protein exists in serum. Intracellular concentrations, particularly in the liver, are several orders of magnitude higher than serum concentrations. Therefore, a small amount of cellular lysis could liberate a relatively large amount of ferritin. However, the vast majority of serum ferritin appears to be secreted. There are probably several cell types that are sources of secreted extracellular ferritin, including iron-recycling macrophages and hepatocytes. Circulating ferritin consists almost exclusively of L-chain subunits.[243] In contrast, intracellular ferritin contains a mixture of H and L subunits. In addition, unlike intracellular ferritin, circulating ferritin is glycosylated, thus suggesting that it passes through the endoplasmic reticulum and Golgi apparatus as do other secreted proteins.

Serum ferritin levels decline with iron deficiency and rise with iron loading.[244] In the absence of liver disease, infection, or chronic inflammation, serum ferritin is roughly proportional to total body iron stores. The correlation between serum ferritin levels and body iron stores is useful in the evaluation of patients with possible iron deficiency or iron overload. A low serum ferritin level (less than 12 µg/L) invariably represents iron deficiency, and high serum ferritin levels are found in patients with iron overload. Extreme serum ferritin levels should be interpreted cautiously, however, because the correlation between ferritin levels and body iron stores is approximately linear only for storage reserves of iron ranging between 1 and 3 g. In addition, normal circulating ferritin values vary with sex and age. These considerations must be factored into any evaluation of iron stores based on ferritin values, particularly in children.

Various conditions modify serum ferritin levels. Inflammation increases the serum ferritin concentration severalfold.[245] Infections, particularly chronic conditions such as tuberculosis or osteomyelitis, may also increase levels substantially, presumably because of the associated inflammatory response. Chronic renal disease and chronic liver disease are likewise associated with elevated levels. A number of tumors are variably associated with an increased level of circulating ferritin. For example, ferritin is an important prognostic factor in childhood neuroblastoma, in which serum ferritin levels correlate with disease severity.[246]

The mechanisms by which inflammation and tumors increase the quantity of plasma ferritin are not fully understood. Treatment with interleukin-1β, a prime mediator of the inflammatory response, increases synthesis of ferritin in human hepatoma cells,[197] whereas tumor necrosis factor has been shown to increase ferritin mRNA levels in murine cells in culture.[195] These cytokines may also increase ferritin synthesis in cells secreting the protein. In addition, the inflammatory cytokine interleukin-6 induces hepcidin expression,[45] which results in increased macrophage iron storage and probably contributes to increased serum ferritin. Furthermore, serum ferritin elevated out of proportion to iron stores is a hallmark feature of ferroportin disease (see later).[247]

Soluble transferrin receptors are also found in serum. Small vesicles containing transferrin receptors are shed from reticulocytes during their maturation to erythrocytes.[248] In addition to these vesicle-associated receptors, the extracellular portion of the transferrin receptor lacking its transmembrane anchor can be found in the circulation.[249-251] One mechanism by which soluble transferrin receptors are generated is a membrane-associated protease activity that clips the molecule between amino acids 100 and 101, at the base of its extracellular stem.[252,253] This cleavage is potentiated by mutation of an O-linked glycosylation site at amino acid 104, thus suggesting that differential glycosylation may play a regulatory role.[254] The transferrin binding domain is intact in these soluble receptors, and they are likely to be complexed with transferrin in serum.

Because maturing red cells shed their transferrin receptors, the amount of soluble transferrin receptor in plasma reasonably reflects the degree of erythropoiesis. Measurement of serum levels of soluble transferrin receptor provides a means of estimating erythropoietic activity that is simpler than the relatively cumbersome PIT determination.[255] Serum transferrin receptor (sTfR) is present in substantially lower amounts in patients with aplastic anemia relative to normal individuals. In contrast, values in patients with anemia caused by ineffective erythropoiesis are markedly increased. Patients with iron deficiency also have increased levels of circulating soluble transferrin receptors. This may result in part from the increase in cellular transferrin receptor expression produced by iron starvation and in part from the increased erythroid turnover associated with the ineffective erythropoiesis of iron deficiency. sTfR and serum ferritin values can be considered together as the ratio of sTfR to the log of ferritin (sTfR-F index). Values greater than 1.5 suggest iron deficiency alone or in combination with an inflammatory condition; values less than 1.5 are characteristic of the anemia of chronic inflammation.[256] The sTfR-F index also appears to be sensitive enough to detect iron deficiency before iron-restricted erythropoiesis is clinically apparent.[257] sTfR and the sTfR-F index are both decreased in patients with iron overload.[258,259]

EXTREMES OF IRON BALANCE

Iron disorders are invariably abnormalities in iron balance, distribution, or both. Iron deficiency is primarily due to acquired causes. In contrast, primary iron overload usually results from genetic abnormalities that perturb the regulation of intestinal iron absorption. Disorders affecting other steps in transport may be manifested as inappropriate iron accumulation in some tissues and iron deficiency in other tissues.

Iron Deficiency

Epidemiology of Iron Deficiency

Iron deficiency is the most frequent and widespread nutritional deficiency in the world[260] because it is common in developing and developed countries alike. In fact, iron deficiency is the only micronutrient deficiency that is also prevalent in virtually all developed countries.[260] To this end, one of the U.S. national health objectives for 2010 is to reduce iron deficiency in vulnerable populations such as toddlers and women of childbearing age by 3% to 4%.[261]

Increasing rates of breast-feeding and the availability of iron-fortified formula (see later), in conjunction with initiatives such as the U.S. Special Supplemental Food Program for Women, Infants and Children and the American Academy of Pediatrics' promotion of formula in place of cow's milk, have greatly reduced the prevalence of iron deficiency *anemia* in infants in developed countries. Nonetheless, iron deficiency, both with and without anemia, remains relatively common. According to the Fourth National Health and Nutrition Examination Survey (NHANES IV), iron deficiency without anemia exists in 7% of toddlers aged 1 to 2 years, 9% of adolescent girls, and 16% of women of childbearing age.[262] Adolescents participating in strenuous training are another pediatric subpopulation at risk for iron deficiency. For example, young military recruits and elite adolescent athletes have an increased risk of nonanemic iron deficiency.[263-265]

Socioeconomic factors are associated with iron deficiency anemia in children. For example, infants and children of low-income and minority backgrounds have higher documented rates of iron deficiency anemia.[266-268] Although food insecurity is known to be associated with iron deficiency anemia,[269] other factors such as bottle-feeding patterns may also play a role in the prevalence of iron deficiency.[270] The iron status of young children correlates closely with the iron status of their mothers, thus indicating that a constellation of factors in the child's environment influence iron intake and therefore iron status.[271]

Phases of Development of Iron Deficiency

Because most of the body's iron is directed toward synthesis of hemoglobin, erythrocyte production is among the first casualties of iron deficiency to become clinically apparent in usual laboratory evaluations. However, it actually represents a late stage of iron depletion. Iron deficiency progresses through three discernible phases:

1. *Prelatent iron deficiency* occurs when tissue stores are depleted, without a change in hematocrit or serum iron levels. This stage of iron deficiency may be detected by low serum ferritin measurements.
2. *Latent iron deficiency* occurs when reticuloendothelial macrophage iron stores are depleted. The serum iron level drops and TIBC increases without a change in hematocrit. This stage may be detected by a routine check of fasting, early morning transferrin saturation. Erythropoiesis begins to be limited by a lack of available iron, and sTfR levels increase. The reticulocyte hemoglobin content (CHr) decreases because newly produced erythrocytes are iron deficient.[272] The bulk of the erythrocyte population appears normal. For this reason, sole reliance on indicators derived from the entire erythrocyte population frequently fails to detect this stage of iron deficiency.[272,273]
3. *Frank iron deficiency* anemia is associated with erythrocyte microcytosis and hypochromia. It is detected when iron deficiency has persisted long enough that a large proportion of the circulating erythrocytes were produced after iron became limiting.

Etiology of Iron Deficiency

The development of iron deficiency is a result of the interaction between iron intake, physiologic iron requirements, and the potential for blood loss.

Inadequate Iron Intake

Dietary Sources. Heme, derived from animal tissues, is the most readily absorbed form of iron. Uptake occurs independently of gastric pH and, like the uptake of nonheme iron, is increased in patients with high marrow erythroid activity. Much of the world's population eats little or no meat, with their nutrition derived from cultivated grasses such as rice. These plants are relatively poor sources of iron,[22] which contributes to the fact that iron deficiency anemia is the most common nutritional anemia worldwide.

In developing countries, nutritional iron deficiency is often compounded by chronic blood loss from parasitic infections and malaria (see later). In industrialized countries, however, iron deficiency is usually due to insufficient dietary intake to meet physiologic needs. Because of their rapid growth and increased need for iron, infants, toddlers, female adolescents, and childbearing women are especially vulnerable.

Consumption of cow's milk may contribute to iron deficiency through several mechanisms. Cow's milk and human milk both have low iron content, but the bioavailability of iron in human milk is greater.[274] Therefore, the transition from human milk to cow's milk may place toddlers at risk for iron deficiency. Indeed, the prevalence of iron deficiency increases with the duration of bottle-feeding of cow's milk.[270] Cow's milk also compounds iron deficiency by replacing iron-rich foods in the diet. In addition, components of cow's milk, such as calcium and caseinophosphopeptide, can directly interfere with iron absorption.[275,276] Furthermore, whole cow's milk contains proteins that may irritate the lining of the gastrointestinal tract in infants, and even low-grade but chronic hemorrhage may produce significant iron deficiency.[277] The neonatal growth spurt requires a tremendous quantity of iron, thus compounding the disadvantages of cow's milk. For these reasons, current recommendations exclude cow's milk from the infant's diet in the first year of life, limit subsequent consumption of cow's milk to 24 ounces per day, suggest that non–breast-fed infants should receive iron-fortified formulas, and advise an additional source of iron for infants who are breast-fed after 4 to 6 months of age, when they have depleted the excess iron that was present in newborn stores and erythrocytes.[278,279]

Poor Bioavailability. Although iron is abundant in the environment, it is nearly insoluble in aqueous solution, which makes acquisition of the common element a major challenge. Most environmental iron exists as insoluble salts. Gastric acidity assists in conversion to absorbable forms, but the efficiency of this process is limited.[280] Many plant products contain iron, but absorption frequently is limited both by low solubility and by powerful natural chelators that bind ambient iron. Phytates (organic polyphosphates) found in wheat products, for example, bind iron with tremendous avidity. The challenge of acquiring sufficient iron from the environment may have been an important factor in the spread of genes for hemochromatosis disorders.

High gastric pH reduces the solubility of inorganic iron and thereby impedes absorption. Surgical interventions, such as vagotomy or hemigastrectomy for peptic ulcer disease, formerly were the major causes of impaired gastric acidification with secondary iron deficiency, particularly in adults. The histamine H_2 blockers and the more recently introduced acid pump blockers, used to treat peptic ulcer disease and acid reflux, may cause defective iron absorption.[281,282] There is, however, little evidence that they substantially alter iron status in those without preexisting iron deficiency.[283-285]

The impaired function of gastric parietal cells associated with pernicious anemia not only reduces the production of intrinsic factor but also lessens gastric acidity and hence compromises absorption of iron. In addition, megaloblastic enterocytes absorb iron poorly. Frank iron deficiency can accompany the anemia produced by cobalamin deficiency.[286-288] However, the rarity of pernicious anemia in children makes this complication uncommon in pediatric populations.

A number of environmental factors can produce dietary iron deficiency by interfering with iron absorption, including metals such as cobalt, which share the iron absorption machinery. Lead may fall into this category, although it remains to be definitively established whether DMT1 is the primary intestinal lead transporter in vivo.[27] Regardless of the mechanism, it is clear that iron deficiency increases the rate of uptake of both iron and lead from the gastrointestinal tract. Iron deficiency and lead intoxication frequently coexist.

Malabsorption. Some disorders disrupt the integrity or surface area of the enteric mucosa and thereby hamper iron absorption (Box 12-2). Inflammatory bowel disease,

---

Box 12-2	Causes of Iron Deficiency Anemia

INADEQUATE ABSORPTION

Poor bioavailability (absorption of heme Fe > Fe^{2+} > Fe^{3+})
Antacid therapy/high gastric pH
Bran, tannins, phytates, starch
Other metals (Co, Pb)
Loss/dysfunction of absorptive enterocytes

INSUFFICIENT/INACCESSIBLE IRON STORES

Gastrointestinal Blood Loss

Epistaxis
Gastritis
Ulcer
Meckel's diverticulum
Milk-induced enteropathy
Parasitosis
Varices
Tumor or polyps
Inflammatory bowel disease
Arteriovenous malformation
Colonic diverticula
Hemorrhoids

Vaginal Blood Loss

Increased menstrual flow
Tumor

Urinary Blood Loss

Chronic infection
Tumor

Pulmonary Blood Loss

Pulmonary hemosiderosis
Tuberculosis
Bronchiectasis

Inflammation/infection

Defects in intestinal iron uptake (e.g., TMPRSS6 mutations)

INADEQUATE PRESENTATION TO ERYTHROID PRECURSORS

Atransferrinemia
Anti–transferrin receptor antibodies

ABNORMAL INTRACELLULAR TRANSPORT/UTILIZATION

Erythroid iron trafficking defects (e.g., DMT1 mutations)
Defects in heme biosynthesis

---

particularly Crohn's disease, may injure extensive segments of the small intestine, including the jejunum and duodenum. Invasion of the submucosa by inflammatory cells and disruption of the tissue architecture impair iron absorption and uptake of dietary nutrients.[289] Occult gastrointestinal bleeding exacerbates the problem. The result is iron deficiency anemia complicated by the anemia of chronic inflammation. Furthermore, Crohn's disease frequently involves the terminal ileum, with the concurrent development of cobalamin deficiency. These disorders are not diagnostic enigmas. Patients with extensive bowel involvement are very ill. Diminishing the underlying inflammatory process best treats the iron deficiency.

Tropical sprue and celiac disease can also interfere with iron absorption.[289] Degeneration of the intestinal lining cells along with chronic inflammation causes profound malabsorption, although some patients with deranged iron absorption lack gross or even histologic changes in the structure of the bowel mucosa. The anemia in these patients is often complicated by a superimposed, generalized nutritional deficiency.[290] Celiac disease frequently improves with ingestion of a gluten-free diet, with secondary correction of the anemia.

Iron absorption may be disrupted when substantial segments of bowel, particularly the proximal duodenum, are removed surgically. Intractable inflammatory bowel disease, traumatic abdominal injury, and structural complications such as intestinal volvulus or intussusception all may necessitate intestinal resection. Iron deficiency develops slowly afterward and may not become evident for several years after the surgical procedure.

Malabsorption of iron is rare in the absence of gross or microscopic structural defects of the intestine or the anemia of chronic inflammation (see later). However, several families with an autosomal recessively inherited predisposition to iron deficiency and systemic iron malutilization have been described.[291-294] These individuals exhibit iron deficiency anemia at early age that is characterized by a nearly complete lack of response to oral iron supplementation and a slow, incomplete response to parenteral iron therapy—so-called iron-refractory, iron deficiency anemia (IRIDA). Recently, it has been shown that individuals with IRIDA have biallelic inactivating mutations in the TMPRSS6 protein, a transmembrane serine protease expressed in the liver, that leads to inappropriate hepcidin overexpression and eventuates in impaired iron absorption and iron recycling.[294,295] Although mutations in DMT1 might also be expected to lead to a somewhat similar congenital iron deficiency anemia phenotype, in fact, reported patients with DMT1 mutations have iron-restricted erythropoiesis in the setting of systemic iron overload.[296-300]

Systemic Iron Loss

Gastrointestinal Blood Loss. Blood loss is the leading cause of iron deficiency worldwide. The gastrointestinal tract is both the site of iron uptake and the most common site of blood loss, particularly when bleeding is not readily apparent. However, bleeding from other sites should also be considered if iron deficiency has not otherwise been explained.

Anatomic defects of the gastrointestinal tract commonly cause blood loss and consequent iron deficiency. The most frequent congenital defect is Meckel's diverticulum, which results from a persistent omphalomesenteric duct. This abnormality can produce abdominal pain and, occasionally, intestinal obstruction in young children. Adolescents with Meckel's diverticulum may have occult blood loss and secondary iron deficiency.[301] Peptic ulcer disease is extremely uncommon in children but should be considered as a cause of gastrointestinal blood loss when the clinical setting suggests it.

Other structural defects of the gastrointestinal tract may cause bleeding as well. Arteriovenous malformations involving the superficial blood vessels occur in patients with hereditary hemorrhagic telangiectasia (Osler-Weber-Rendu syndrome). These defective vessels frequently bleed to a degree that engenders iron deficiency. Although the disorder is transmitted as an autosomal dominant trait, the characteristic vascular lesions rarely attain clinical significance before young adulthood. The condition is easily recognized because the mucosal lining of the oropharynx and nasal cavity exhibits characteristic telangiectases.

The leading cause of gastrointestinal blood loss worldwide is parasitic infestation. Hookworm infection, caused primarily by *Necator americanus* or *Ancylostoma duodenale*, is endemic to much of the world and is often asymptomatic. Microscopic blood loss leads to significant iron deficiency, particularly in children.[302] More than 1 billion people, most in tropical or subtropical areas, are infested with parasites. Combined, their total daily blood loss exceeds 11 million L. The larvae spawn in moist soil and penetrate the skin of unprotected feet. Hookworm infection, once prevalent in the southeastern United States, declined precipitously with better sanitation and routine use of footwear when outside.

Trichuris trichiura, the culprit in trichuriasis or whipworm infection, is believed to infest the colon of 600 to 700 million people. Only 10% to 15% of these individuals have worm burdens sufficiently great to produce clinical disease. However, most are children between the ages of 2 and 10 years. Growth retardation, in addition to iron deficiency, occurs with heavy infestation.[303] Trichuriasis is the most common helminthic infection encountered in Americans returning from visits to tropical or subtropical regions of the world.

Urinary Blood Loss. Occasionally, blood loss into the urinary tract outstrips iron absorption. However, urinary blood loss is usually apparent and sufficiently alarming that patients seek medical attention before substantial iron deficiency develops. Iron deficiency resulting from hematuria secondary to renal disease is relatively uncommon.

The best characterized cause of significant renal blood loss is Berger's disease, which produces relapsing episodes of gross or microscopic hematuria. The disorder occurs most commonly in older children and young adults. It is characterized by diffuse mesangial proliferation or focal and segmental glomerulonephritis. Diffuse mesangial deposits of IgA are the hallmark of the disorder. Although the disease spontaneously remits in some children, progression to end-stage renal disease may occur. Occasionally, Goodpasture's syndrome produces substantial urinary blood loss. Immunofluorescent staining of biopsy specimens reveals the characteristic antibodies to basement membrane lining the glomeruli. Blood loss into the urinary bladder can occur in association with infectious cystitis. Hematuria to the point of iron deficiency is extremely uncommon, however.

Pulmonary Blood Loss. Although pulmonary blood loss may be sufficiently severe to produce iron deficiency, it is distinctly rare. Idiopathic pulmonary hemosiderosis primarily affects children and young adolescents (reviewed by Specks[304]). This potentially deadly disorder is characterized by slow but intractable hemorrhage into the bronchioles and alveoli. Iron deficiency anemia is a major part of the clinical picture of pulmonary hemosiderosis inasmuch as pulmonary macrophages are distinct from the normal iron-recycling circuit and iron trapped within these cells is effectively lost from the functional systemic pool. Consequently, a paradoxical situation evolves in which iron deficiency anemia develops in the presence of a surfeit of total body iron. Bronchoalveolar lavage reveals hemosiderin-laden macrophages that are characteristic of the disorder. Chronic pulmonary infection with bronchiectasis, once considered to be a frequent cause of pulmonary hemorrhage, is now rare. Formation of toxic products is induced by the iron that accumulates in these cells, which leads to the activation of macrophages. These cells begin to damage the delicate lining of the bronchoalveolar tree and produce severe fibrosis. Oxygen exchanges poorly across the damaged alveolar surfaces, thereby lowering the efficiency of oxygen/carbon dioxide exchange. Late in the course of pulmonary hemosiderosis, the radiographic picture of the lungs is striking and frequently shows marked retraction and scarring.[305] The restrictive lung disease and substantial pulmonary arterial shunting across the lung may eventually be fatal.

Most often the cause of pulmonary hemosiderosis evades elucidation. In a number of patients, it occurs in conjunction with disorders of immune dysfunction, including celiac disease[306] and Goodpasture's syndrome.[307,308] Treatment of the associated disorder can lead to remission of the pulmonary process, consistent with an immunologic mechanism of the lung injury.[309] Chloroquine treatment has been used with modest success in some patients.[310] Cyclophosphamide has produced responses in a number of patients.[311] A combination of prednisone and azathioprine has also been used.[312] Other immunosuppressive agents may prove to be even more effective as immunologic suppressers in the treatment of this condition, but the infrequency of the disorder means that a large, multicenter trial is needed to collect definitive treatment information. Although the prognosis was once believed to be very poor for all patients with idiopathic pulmonary hemosiderosis, more recent data suggest that such may not be the case.[309]

Menstrual Blood Loss. Blood loss associated with menstruation predisposes women to iron deficiency. In a sample of healthy, menstruating, nonpregnant Danish women 18 to 30 years of age not receiving iron supplementation, serum ferritin levels correlated inversely with the duration and intensity of menstrual bleeding.[313] Menorrhagia or dysfunctional uterine bleeding may lead to frank iron deficiency anemia. In many cases, dysfunctional uterine bleeding is due to anovulation, a common phenomenon in pubertal females. Progestational agents or oral contraceptives may ameliorate the dysfunctional uterine bleeding or menorrhagia. If this approach does not resolve the abnormal bleeding, other causes such as pelvic abnormalities or disorders of hemostasis, particularly von Willebrand's disease, should be considered. Women with menorrhagia, especially menorrhagia present since menarche, have a high incidence of von Willebrand's disease (13%), which in the general population is 1% to 2%.[314,315]

Consequences of Iron Deficiency

Although anemia is the most prominent manifestation of iron deficiency, there may be other clinically significant sequelae of iron deficiency, even in the absence of anemia. Organ and tissue dysfunction, including impaired immunity, decreased muscle performance and neurocognitive function, and poor weight gain, may occur with iron deficiency. Significant inroads in understanding some of these effects, particularly cognitive dysfunction in young children, have been made in the past few years.

Neurocognitive Effects

The association between iron deficiency anemia and impaired neurocognitive function is well established, and this association holds even when potential confounders such as psychosocial and environmental factors are taken into account. Infants and toddlers, who are undergoing critical neurocognitive development, may be at particular risk for such effects.[316]

Iron deficiency that has not yet progressed to anemia is also associated with impaired mental and motor functioning.[317,318] For example, when tested with the Bayley Scale of Infant Development, nonanemic, iron-deficient infants had lower developmental scores than iron-sufficient infants did, and these abnormalities were detected in children as young as 9 to 12 months.[317] In addition, the degree of developmental deficits in infants may correlate with the level of iron deficiency.[319] Older populations of children, such as nonanemic iron-deficient preschoolers, have lower mental development scores,[320] and school-age children and adolescents have lower math and verbal scores than their iron-sufficient peers do.[320-323]

In some investigations, dietary iron supplementation has reversed the cognitive dysfunction.[317,318,323] For example, in the study of 9- to 12-month-old infants cited earlier, iron replacement increased Mental Development Index scores substantially in only 7 days.[317] Numerous other studies, however, failed to show improvement in depressed performance.[319,324-326] Lozoff and colleagues have also demonstrated that these effects remain evident as long as 19 years later and that children of low socioeconomic status may be disproportionately affected.[327]

Iron deficiency may increase the risk for lead exposure through either pica or increased absorption. Concomitant lead toxicity can further hamper the psychological development of these children.[328] Information on the long-term effects of iron deficiency during infancy highlights the importance of early detection and intervention. Health care providers must therefore work actively to prevent and detect iron deficiency during infancy.

The mechanism by which iron deficiency impairs neurologic function is unknown. Iron deficiency could impair neurotransmitter mechanisms. It has been shown to decrease expression of dopamine receptors in the rat brain.[329] Iron deficiency may also interfere with myelination and alters myelin proteins and lipids in oligodendrocytes.[330] In addition, several enzymes in neural tissue require iron for normal function.[331] The cytochromes involved in energy production, for example, are predominantly heme proteins.

Pica. Pica, the compulsive consumption of nonnutritive substances, is a recurrent symptom in patients with iron deficiency. The precise pathophysiology of pica is unknown, but it is probably attributable to CNS iron deficiency. Patients often consume laundry starch, ice, soil, or clay. Both clay and starch can bind iron in the gastrointestinal tract and exacerbate the deficiency.[332,333] A dramatic example of the problems produced with clay consumption occurred in the 1950s in iron-deficient children along the border between Iran and Turkey.[334,335] These youngsters had other peculiar abnormalities, including massive hepatosplenomegaly, poor wound healing, and a bleeding diathesis. Presumably, the children initially had simple iron deficiency associated with pica, including geophagia. The soil contained compounds that bound both iron and zinc.[335] Secondary zinc deficiency was thought to cause the hepatomegaly and other unusual features.[334]

Epithelial Changes

Iron deficiency produces significant gastrointestinal tract abnormalities, reflecting the enormous proliferative capacity of this tissue. Angular stomatitis and glossitis with painful swelling of the tongue may develop. The flattened, atrophic, lingual papillae make the tongue smooth and shiny. A rare complication of iron deficiency is the Plummer-Vinson syndrome with the formation of a postcricoid esophageal web. Long-standing, severe iron deficiency affects the cells that generate the fingernails and produces koilonychia, or spooning. The nail substance is soft, so ordinary pressure on the fingertips, as occurs with writing, for instance, produces a concave deformity. Most of these abnormalities are now uncommon in industrialized nations.

Iron Deficiency Anemia

On physical examination, pallor, tachycardia, splenomegaly and a systolic murmur may be appreciated. The microcytic, hypochromic anemia of iron deficiency impairs tissue oxygenation and produces the symptoms of pallor, weakness, fatigue, and lightheadedness. Thalassemia trait (see Chapter 20) also produces microcytic cells and is sometimes confused with iron deficiency. Iron deficiency alters red cell size unevenly. Electronic blood analyzers determine the mean red cell volume (MCV), as well as the range of variation in red cell size (expressed as the red cell distribution width [RDW]). RDW and the cell hemoglobin distribution width (both determined as part of electronically processed complete blood cell counts) are normal in patients with thalassemia trait but high in those with iron deficiency.[336] Other common features of thalassemia trait are basophilic stippling and target cells. These characteristics are not sufficiently distinctive to be diagnostically useful, however. A simple, reliable approach is to examine the color of plasma. It is watery in iron deficiency and straw colored in thalassemia trait.

The plasma membranes of iron-deficient red cells are abnormally stiff, and such cells are more prone to hemolysis.[337] This rigidity could contribute to poikilocytic changes, seen particularly with severe iron deficiency. Small, stiff, misshapen cells are cleared by the reticuloendothelial system, thereby further contributing to low-grade hemolysis. The cause of this alteration in membrane fluidity is unknown.

Thrombocytosis with platelet counts in the range of 500,000 to 700,000 cells/fL occurs frequently in iron-deficient patients. Megakaryocytes and normoblasts are derived from a common committed progenitor cell, the colony-forming unit–granulocyte, erythrocyte, macrophage, megakaryocyte (CFU-GEMM). Thrombopoietin, the molecule that stimulates the growth of megakaryocytes and the production of platelets, is homologous to erythropoietin (see Chapter 6). The high levels of erythropoietin produced by iron deficiency anemia conceivably could cross-react with megakaryocyte thrombopoietin receptors and modestly raise the platelet count. However, this hypothesis has not been proved experimentally.

Diagnosis of Iron Deficiency

Because they are inexpensive and widely available, hematologic markers are frequently used to assess iron status. A hemoglobin content less than the 5th percentile in a reference population is often used to define anemia.

Changes in erythrocyte parameters accompanying iron deficiency anemia include a decrease in MCV, reflecting microcytosis, and an increase in RDW, reflecting anisocytosis, as described earlier. Because these parameters represent averages of the entire red blood cell population, iron deficiency must be present for some time before it deviates from these measures.

The American Academy of Pediatrics and the U.S. Centers for Disease Control and Prevention recommend the use of hemoglobin to screen children at risk for iron deficiency. Because only the later stages of iron deficiency result in anemia, relying on hemoglobin (or hematocrit) to screen for iron deficiency misses many children who are, in fact, iron deficient and in whom adverse consequences, such as potentially irreversible neurocognitive impairment, may have already begun to occur. For example, based on NHANES data, a hemoglobin concentration of less than 11 g/dL has a sensitivity of 30% for detecting iron deficiency, as defined by ferritin, erythrocyte protoporphyrin, and transferrin saturation.[338] That adverse consequences of iron deficiency may occur in the absence of anemia highlights the importance of diagnostic approaches that detect iron deficiency early, without relying on hematologic indicators that are altered only after iron deficiency has progressed.

Biochemical parameters based on iron metabolism are often used to diagnose and in fact define iron deficiency. A low serum ferritin level is a very specific and early indicator of iron deficiency. Plasma iron concentrations fall as iron is depleted, but they are also affected by diurnal variation and dietary intake. The availability of plasma iron binding sites, or TIBC, increases as iron stores fall. Serum iron concentration divided by TIBC may be calculated to yield transferrin saturation, a measure of occupied binding sites on transferrin. These biochemical tests may be altered by physiologic states unrelated to iron stores. For example, ferritin, serum iron, and TIBC are acute phase reactants. In the setting of inflammation, ferritin, a positive acute phase reactant, may overestimate iron stores. Ferritin has in fact been shown to be a poor indicator of iron deficiency in the pediatric population.[272]

Because of the limitations of both hematologic and biochemical tests, novel methods of diagnosing iron deficiency have been sought. sTfR is a truncated form of the receptor that is cleaved from reticulocytes and erythroid cells and circulates in plasma largely attached to transferrin. sTfR is upregulated in iron deficiency. Though not uniformly available in all clinical laboratories, it may be an important adjunct in diagnosing iron deficiency,[339,340] particularly insofar as it may help distinguish iron deficiency anemia from the anemia of inflammation.[341]

CHr is another test available only in selected laboratories because it is unique to instruments manufactured by Bayer (Tarrytown, NY). CHr was recently evaluated prospectively as a means of routinely screening infants and toddlers.[273] In this setting a CHr cutoff of 27.5 pg had 83% sensitivity and 72% specificity, whereas a hemoglobin concentration of less than 11 g/dL was a poor predictor of iron deficiency, with only 26% sensitivity. CHr has also been used to accurately assess the iron status of potential adult blood donors.[342]

Treatment of Iron Deficiency

The most important steps in the evaluation and treatment of iron deficiency are determining the cause and correcting the abnormality. Malignancy of the gastrointestinal tract, the most worrisome etiology in adults with iron deficiency, is vanishingly rare in children. Growth spurts, poor dietary patterns, menstrual losses, and benign gastrointestinal bleeding are much more common. After initial diagnostic investigations, oral iron supplementation usually replaces stores most efficiently.

Oral Supplementation

Iron salts offer inexpensive, effective therapy for iron deficiency. Although ferrous sulfate is most often recommended, patients frequently complain of gastrointestinal discomfort, constipation, and bloating, as well as stool discoloration, thus making its use unacceptable to many. Interestingly, in a randomized, controlled trial comparing 3 mg/kg/day of ferrous sulfate drops with placebo in 278, 12-month-old infants, there was no difference in the frequency of vomiting, diarrhea, or fussiness, and infants in the placebo group had a higher incidence of constipation (95% versus 1%).[343] Iron is frequently provided to children at a dose of 3 mg/kg/day divided into three-times-a-day dosing. Single-dose daily regimens, however, are tolerated as well as three-times-a-day regimens.[344] Administration of iron on an empty stomach at night will lessen the gastrointestinal difficulties. The decreased gastrointestinal motility of sleep will also enhance absorption.

The absorptive capacity of the normal duodenum for iron is essentially saturated with about 25 mg of elemental iron in ionic form. Ferrous gluconate, which is roughly equivalent in cost, contains about 50 mg of elemental iron per tablet. This form of replacement may produce fewer problems than ferrous sulfate and is excellent as the initial treatment of iron deficiency. Ascorbic acid supplementation enhances iron absorption, although it has a relatively minor effect in individuals ingesting normal, balanced diets.[345] Combination tablets containing iron salts and ascorbic acid are significantly more expensive than separate tablets for each. Even with faithful use of oral iron, adequate replacement of body stores in patients with moderate iron deficiency anemia requires several months. With ongoing blood loss, replacement of stores with oral iron becomes very difficult.

Polysaccharide/iron complexes differ from iron salts. Polar oxygen groups in the sugars form coordination complexes with iron atoms. The well-hydrated microspheres of polysaccharide iron remain in solution over a wide range of pH values. Most patients tolerate this form of iron better than the iron salts, even though the 150 mg

Box 12-3	**Reasons for Poor Response to Oral Iron**

Noncompliance
Ongoing blood loss
Insufficient duration of therapy
High gastric pH
   Antacids
   Histamine H_2 blockers
   Gastric proton pump inhibitors
Inhibitors of iron absorption/utilization
   Lead
   Aluminum intoxication (hemodialysis patients)
   Chronic inflammation
   Neoplasia
Incorrect diagnosis
   Thalassemia disorder
   Sideroblastic anemia
   Anemia of chronic inflammation

of elemental iron per tablet is substantially greater than that provided by iron salts.

Iron supplements must be stored in a childproof manner. Unintentional iron poisoning from iron supplements is a leading cause of poisoning-related injury in young children and frequently occurs when children obtain improperly stored iron.[346]

Box 12-3 lists potential causes of a poor response to oral iron supplementation. A variety of barriers, including treatment-associated factors and system-wide barriers, contribute to the shortcomings in iron deficiency screening and correction that have been documented.[347]

Parenteral Iron Replacement

Parenteral iron is now available in the United States in three intravenous forms: iron dextran, iron gluconate, and iron sucrose.[348-351] This medication is indicated when (1) oral iron is poorly tolerated; (2) rapid replacement of iron stores is needed; (3) gastrointestinal iron absorption is compromised; or (4) erythropoietin therapy is necessary, particularly in renal dialysis patients. Iron dextran can also be administered by intramuscular injection, but this route is discouraged because it can be painful and leakage into subcutaneous tissue produces long-standing skin discoloration. A "Z-track" injection into the muscle minimizes the chance of subcutaneous leakage. The suboptimal muscle mass frequently associated with nutritional deficiency further complicates this mode of replacement. Intravenous infusion circumvents these problems altogether. With either route of administration, a small test dose should be given and the patient observed by a physician for 30 minutes to rule out an anaphylactic reaction to the medication. Such reactions do occur but are infrequent. The newer iron sucrose and iron gluconate preparations are believed to be less likely to cause complications, but there is less accumulated experience with these preparations, and many practitioners still use iron dextran routinely.

Ten percent to 15% of patients experience transient mild to moderate arthralgias the day after intramuscular or intravenous administration of iron dextran. Acetaminophen usually relieves the discomfort effectively. Iron dextran is generally avoided in patients with rheumatoid arthritis because it may provoke painful flares of their disease.[12] The symptoms may result from release of inflammatory cytokines such as interleukin-1 and tumor necrosis factor. Iron dextran is cleared from the circulation by macrophages, which are probably activated to release proinflammatory peptides.

In uncomplicated cases of iron deficiency, intravenous replacement may produce subjective improvement in symptoms within a few days. Peak reticulocytosis occurs after about 10 days, and complete correction of the anemia takes 4 to 6 weeks, although the hematocrit rises sufficiently in 1 or 2 weeks to provide symptomatic relief for most patients.[345] CHr is a very sensitive measure of response.[352] Brugnara and colleagues have demonstrated that a rise in CHr is appreciated within 2 to 4 days of the administration of intravenous iron.[352]

Refractory bleeding that cannot be prevented, as occurs, for example, with hereditary hemorrhagic telangiectasia, presents a management problem. Oral iron supplementation often fails to keep pace with losses. Blood transfusions replace red cells in the short term and iron in the long term, but infection and alloimmunization make such therapy unacceptable for many patients. Intermittent iron replacement with infusions of intravenous iron is the most reasonable alternative. Replacements should occur over short intervals two or three times a year, with the aim of repleting body stores. A simple formula can be used to determine the replacement dose of iron dextran:

$$\text{Dose (mL)} = 0.0442 \times (\text{Desired Hb} - \text{Observed Hb}) \times \\ \text{Lean body weight} + (0.26 \times \text{Lean body weight})$$

Alternatively, there is a calculator provided on the Internet at http://www.infed.com/calcltor.htm. The maximum adult dose of iron dextran is 14 mL.

Over many years this treatment can produce massive deposition of hemosiderin (from iron dextran) in macrophages, the liver, and the pancreas despite the fact that plasma transferrin is iron deficient because of increased iron delivery to erythroid precursors. This supports the concept that tissue iron content is unimportant for erythropoiesis and that erythropoiesis relies exclusively on iron from transferrin.[99,142]

Iron Replacement in Infants

Because the fetus accumulates iron at the mother's expense in the third trimester of pregnancy, full-term infants are born with adequate iron stores to last approximately 6 months. Preterm infants are at greater risk for iron deficiency, with their stores depleted by 3 to 4 months of age.

Human breast milk initially contains relatively high amounts of iron, but the level decreases, independent of maternal iron status, to approximately 0.3 mg/L after 5 months of lactation (reviewed by Griffin and Abrams[353]). The iron is present in several forms: in casein, in whey, in fat, and to a small extent, in the abundant protein lactoferrin. The rate of absorption of iron from human milk has been estimated to be 20% to 50%, which is adequate early in life when iron stores are still high but inadequate to meet an older infant's needs. Based on all available information, the Committee on Nutrition of the American Academy of Pediatrics has recommended the following[278]:

1. Breast milk should be provided for at least 5 to 6 months when feasible. During that period, young infants can mobilize iron from their large stores. Iron supplementation of 1 mg/kg/day should be provided to infants who are exclusively fed breast milk beyond 6 months of age.
2. Infants who are not breast-fed should be nourished with an iron-supplemented formula (at least 12 mg/L) until the end of the first year of life.
3. Iron-enriched cereals should be among the first foods introduced with a solid diet.
4. Cow's milk should be avoided during the first year because it contains substances that chelate iron and it sometimes induces occult gastrointestinal hemorrhage in young infants.

Maternal Iron Stores and Effects on the Fetus

When the mother is iron deficient, the placenta is concerned only with the welfare of the fetus and will continue to remove iron from the mother to support fetal development, even at the cost of negative maternal iron balance. For years, investigators debated the effect of maternal iron deficiency on the fetus. Early findings by Cook and colleagues indicated that the iron storage status of the mother does not affect the infant's iron status as measured by ferritin.[354] The controversy was fueled by the indirect and imprecise assays of neonatal iron status, such as the cord blood ferritin level or transferrin saturation. These parameters in cord blood are subject to all the vicissitudes that affect their values in later life. Accurate determination of neonatal iron status was difficult, if not impossible. The one point on which nearly universal agreement existed was that neonatal anemia secondary to maternal iron deficiency is rare.

It is likely that in fact maternal iron status over a wide range of values does affect the iron stores of the neonate. The most compelling data have come from a study of women who underwent elective abortions.[355,356] The iron status of the mothers was determined from transferrin saturation, plasma ferritin levels, and hemoglobin values. This information was correlated with the iron status of the fetuses, which was determined by atomic absorption spectroscopy of the complete abortus. This procedure determined the absolute fetal iron content. Fetal iron stores varied linearly with maternal hemoglobin, which ranged between 6 g/dL (severe iron deficiency) and 13 g/dL (adequate, though possibly low iron stores).

Fetal iron stores, in turn, may influence neonatal outcomes. Maternal iron deficiency before midpregnancy is associated with an increased risk for preterm delivery. Maternal anemia detected during the last trimester of pregnancy is not associated with an increase risk for preterm birth. This anemia probably reflects the expansion of maternal plasma volume rather than actual maternal iron stores.

Neonatal iron stores are also influenced by other maternal factors apart from iron stores. Maternal diabetes is associated with decreased fetal stores, as evidenced by lower cord blood ferritin and an increased demand for iron reflected by higher soluble transferrin receptor levels.[357] This may be due to neonatal polycythemia and increased erythropoietic drive associated with maternal diabetes. Similarly, maternal smoking is also associated with increased cord hemoglobin and decreased iron stores.[358]

The infant's gestational age is related to the development of adequate iron stores, as described earlier. The timing of umbilical cord clamping at birth may also affect neonatal iron stores. A randomized, controlled trial of delayed clamping (2 minutes after delivery) versus usual clamping found that infants in the delayed umbilical cord clamping group had higher ferritin and total body iron stores at 6 months of age.[359] The effect of delayed clamping was particularly pronounced in infants otherwise at risk for iron deficiency, such as those not receiving iron-fortified milk or formula, mothers with low ferritin levels at birth, and lower-birth-weight infants.

Iron supplementation of gravidas during the first 28 weeks is associated with higher mean birth weight and a lower incidence of low-birth-weight infants, but not maternal anemia or higher preterm delivery rates.[360] Consequently, at this time there is insufficient evidence to support or reject the routine practice of prophylactic iron supplementation during pregnancy as opposed to supplementing iron-deficient gravidas or pregnant women at risk for iron deficiency.

Iron Overload

The Evolutionary Advantage of Iron Overload

The fact that multiple mutations in diverse populations all lead to iron overload (see later) raises the possibility that these conditions once conferred a selective advantage. As previously noted, iron deficiency is the most common nutritional cause of anemia in the world. Anemia was probably a selective disadvantage earlier in human history. A genetic change that increased the efficiency of iron absorption may therefore have been an advantage. A person who survived into the third decade would have reproduced and passed genes to the next generation, including those that increase iron absorption. Survival into the fifth decade, when severe iron overload begins

to produce problems, was uncommon until recently. However, a problem develops with this tidy theory when the inhabitants of Asia are considered. The incidence of iron overload is reportedly quite low in this region of the world, the home of most of the Earth's population.

Hereditary Hemochromatosis

Hereditary hemochromatosis is a condition that originates from a genetic predisposition to iron overload as a result of mutations in one of several genes involved in iron metabolism (see later). It is caused by an alteration in the iron absorption mechanism that fractionally increases the uptake of dietary iron.[361,362] Although the rate and extent of iron loading vary widely among patients, dangerous levels of tissue iron develop in many people by middle age. Iron deposits in cells of the liver, heart, endocrine tissues, and skin. It promotes oxidative cell damage, which leads to fibrosis and, when unrecognized, to the classic manifestations of "bronze diabetes," including liver dysfunction, increased melanization of the epidermis, and pancreatic insufficiency.[363] Because erythropoiesis is normal, iron can be removed through phlebotomies performed regularly. If untreated, hemochromatosis may be a lethal disease and result in death from cirrhotic liver failure or, less often, from cardiomyopathy.

Pediatricians are often asked to evaluate children who have close relatives with hemochromatosis. This is a complicated task because iron loading occurs gradually over a period of many years and may not be apparent before adulthood. Although the genes responsible for most forms of hemochromatosis have been identified, at this time commercial laboratories test for only one form of the disease. However, this situation is likely to change over the next few years and simplify presymptomatic diagnosis. Until then, assessment should take into account the family history, serum transferrin saturation, serum ferritin levels, and if indicated, quantitative liver iron determined by analysis of a biopsy sample (Fig. 12-6).

In the United States, Canada, Australia, and the northwestern part of Europe, most patients with hemochromatosis are homozygous for a unique missense mutation designated C282Y (for cysteine 282 to tyrosine) in the gene encoding HFE, a protein that resembles class I major histocompatibility (MHC) molecules.[364] The HFE gene lies on chromosome 6p, near the HLA-A locus. It was discovered through a positional cloning approach that took advantage of the fact that patients with the C282Y mutation are descended from a common ancestor who probably lived in a Celtic population in the British Isles 60 to 70 generations ago.[365]

Like class I MHC proteins, HFE forms a heterodimer with β_2-microglobulin and is expressed on the cell surface. However, unlike other family members, HFE cannot bind a small peptide. Its structure, as determined by x-ray crystallography, does not allow enough space within the groove that is involved in peptide binding by MHC class I molecules.[366] Some insight into the function of HFE was gained from observations that it forms a

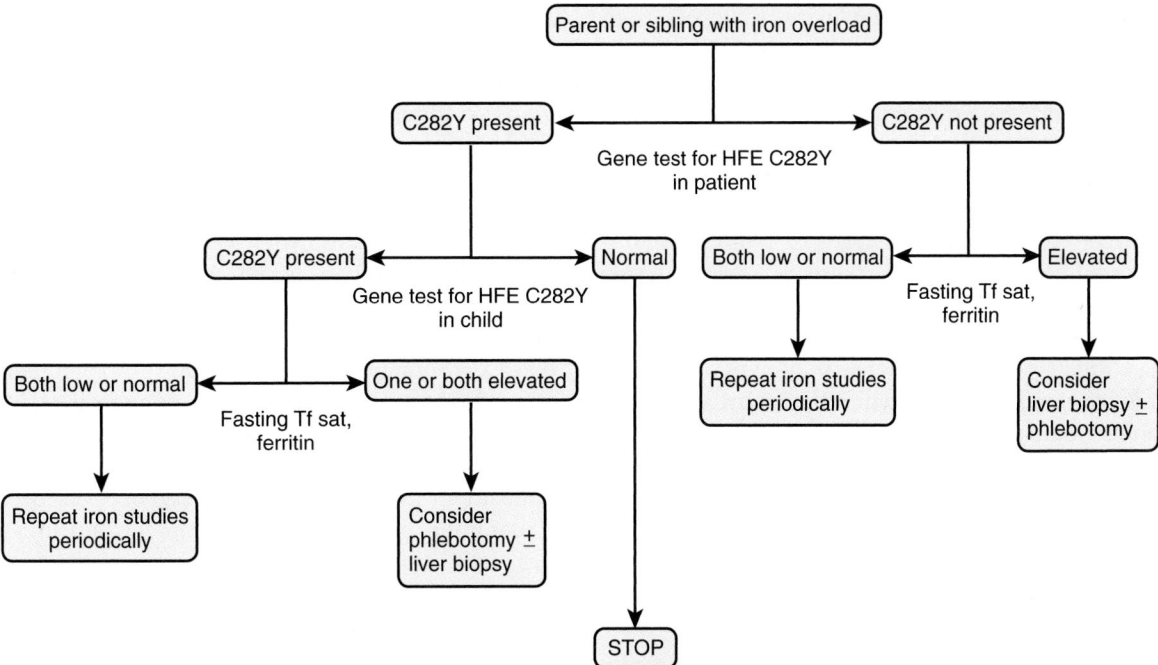

FIGURE 12-6. Algorithm for the workup of children at risk for iron overload. *(Adapted with permission from Andrews NC. Inherited iron overload disorders. Curr Opin Pediatr. 2000;12:596-602.)*

high-affinity complex with the transferrin receptor.[366] HFE binds to a site that overlaps the binding site for ferric transferrin, which results in competition between HFE and transferrin for occupancy of the transferrin receptor.[367] Studies in transfected cells overexpressing HFE indicate that the HFE-transferrin receptor association alters cellular iron uptake. However, the effect of HFE on iron homeostasis is not directly attributable to its effect on cellular iron uptake. As discussed later, we now know that HFE and several other forms of hemochromatosis result from aberrant expression of the iron regulatory hormone hepcidin.

In patients with HFE hemochromatosis, serum transferrin becomes saturated with iron before clinical signs appear. The increased serum iron is deposited in parenchymal cells of the liver, heart, pancreas, and other tissues. In knockout mice lacking murine Hfe, an iron overload disorder develops that closely resembles human hemochromatosis.[368,369] The mutant allele for HLA-linked hemochromatosis is prevalent in the United States. Studying a cross section of the American population, Steinberg and colleagues found that 9.5% of non-Hispanic whites, 2% of non-Hispanic blacks, and approximately 5% of the population overall were C282Y carriers.[370] Testing for the HFE C282Y mutation allows identification of patients in whom clinical hemochromatosis may develop. Heterozygotes rarely have clinically significant iron overload, but homozygotes are at risk. Published data give conflicting estimates of the proportion of patients homozygous for C282Y in whom complications of the disease will develop; such estimates range from less than 1% to greater than 20%. It is clear, however, that some individuals have severe iron loading as young adults whereas others may never manifest signs or symptoms of hemochromatosis. There must be both environmental and genetic modifiers that affect the extent of iron loading. Current efforts are aimed at defining these modifiers to aid in predicting in which genetically at-risk individuals clinically significant iron overload will develop.

Other polymorphisms and potential mutations have been described in the HFE coding sequence. One of these polymorphisms, H63D (histidine 63 to aspartic acid) is prevalent throughout the world and found in as many as a quarter of asymptomatic patients. Although clinical laboratories currently test for and report the H63D polymorphism, most patients with one or two copies of the H63D allele are probably not at risk for iron loading. Other polymorphisms associated with altered amino acids or altered mRNA splicing have also been reported (reviewed by Camaschella and co-workers[371]). Some of these polymorphisms do appear to be associated with iron overload, but most clinical laboratories do not look exhaustively for them.

Since the identification of HFE, it has become clear that there are at least four other types of hemochromatosis. A disorder that may be clinically indistinguishable from HFE-associated hemochromatosis results from homozygosity for mutations in the gene encoding transferrin receptor 2 (TFR2).[372] TFR2 is highly homologous to the transferrin receptor, particularly in its extracellular domain, but it binds transferrin with much lower affinity.[373,374] It is primarily expressed in the liver and in erythroid cells. Its function remains incompletely understood, as does the reason why loss of the protein results in iron overload. Similar to the transferrin receptor, TFR2 forms a protein complex with HFE, which is believed to be involved in regulation of hepcidin expression.[375]

Two other types of hemochromatosis are easier to distinguish from HFE-associated hemochromatosis. Juvenile hemochromatosis, also called type 2 hemochromatosis, is a more severe disorder with accelerated iron loading that typically leads to death by the third decade.[376] Patients have iron deposition in the same pattern as that seen in those with HFE-associated hemochromatosis, but the rapid accumulation of metal leads to a different clinical picture dominated by cardiac disease and endocrine dysfunction. Patients are often identified when they fail to enter puberty. If these patients are recognized before end-stage organ disease develops, they can be treated by aggressive phlebotomy. Juvenile hemochromatosis is inherited in an autosomal recessive pattern and is caused by mutations in *HAMP*, the gene encoding hepcidin,[377] or in an unrelated gene encoding hemojuvelin (*HJV*, also called *HFE2, RGMC*).[378] Hemojuvelin is a cell surface protein that acts as a bone morphogenetic protein (BMP) coreceptor to stimulate hepcidin expression, presumably in response to as yet unidentified BMP signals.[379] Targeted disruption of the murine hemojuvelin gene results in a phenotype very similar to human juvenile hemochromatosis, with a near absence of hepcidin mRNA expression.[380,381]

Although all of the forms of hemochromatosis discussed thus far (caused by mutations in *HFE, TFR2, HAMP*, and *HJV*) are associated with inappropriately low hepcidin production, there is one hemochromatosis disorder that is not. A subset of patients carrying mutations in *SLC40A1*, the gene encoding ferroportin, have autosomal dominant hemochromatosis that is similar to other forms of the disease.[382-384] Apparently, these mutations render ferroportin resistant to hepcidin regulation. A second class of ferroportin mutations cause a distinct autosomal recessive disorder characterized by macrophage iron loading, an early rise in serum ferritin levels, comparatively less saturation of transferrin with iron, and no major increase in total body iron stores.[247,385,386] Both forms of "ferroportin disease" are autosomal dominant because functional ferroportin exists in cells as a multimer and mutation of one subunit is deleterious for transport function.[387]

African Iron Overload Syndrome

During the 1960s, several groups of investigators reported that iron overload occurred at a very high rate among sub-Saharan Africans.[388-391] Many patients had massive iron stores approaching or exceeding those seen in individuals with hemochromatosis. Some indigenous inhabitants of the region prepared alcoholic beverages in nongalvanized steel drums, thus raising the possibility that iron overload resulted from the high iron content of these beverages. Iron loading was thought to be exacerbated by an increase in gastrointestinal iron absorption induced by alcohol. The term *Bantu siderosis* was coined to describe the condition.[391]

Later reports suggested that African iron overload was not simply the result of increased intake.[392-394] In only a fraction of the group who drank the beverage did iron overload develop. In fact, a more extensive study showed that similar degrees of iron overload occurred in people who consumed little, if any of this brew. Although the pattern of inheritance has not been definitively worked out, the disorder may be autosomal codominant, with obligate heterozygotes expressing an intermediate level of iron loading. African iron overload is not associated with HFE mutations.[395]

Intriguingly, African iron overload syndrome most closely resembles nonhemochromatosis ferroportin disease in the cellular distribution of iron. In contrast to other forms of hereditary hemochromatosis, in which the iron is almost entirely confined to parenchymal cells, reticuloendothelial macrophages display massive iron deposition in the African variety of iron overload.[388] A common missense mutation in ferroportin, Q248H, has been implicated as a possible genetic factor.[396,397] However, the ultimate clinical consequences of iron overload are similar to those seen in all other forms of hemochromatosis, irrespective of the cause of the accumulation. African iron overload syndrome is not confined to any ethnic group, although it appears to be restricted to the inhabitants of sub-Saharan Africa. In some areas, the incidence may be as high as 10%, which makes it one of the most common, clinically significant iron disorders in any population.

An important, unanswered question is whether mutated genes causing this syndrome are found in people of African descent elsewhere in the world. No comprehensive study of iron overload has been performed in African Americans, but preliminary data suggest that a substantial portion of this population may be at risk.[398,399] There has not yet been an exhaustive examination of hemochromatosis disease genes in this group.

Neonatal Hemochromatosis

Neonatal hemochromatosis (NH) is a rare condition characterized by neonatal liver failure associated with systemic iron overload, parenchymal iron deposition, thrombocytopenia, and coagulopathy in the absence of evidence of any known causative agent or condition, including Down syndrome, metabolic liver disease (e.g., tyrosinemia, galactosemia), congenital infection (e.g., herpesviruses), or congenital anemia (e.g., α-thalassemia, hydrops fetalis secondary to ABO/Rh incompatibility) (reviewed elsewhere[400-403]). In addition to fetal diseases, NH has been associated with maternal autoimmune disorders, including lupus erythematosus and Sjögren's syndrome. Although iron chelation and antioxidant cocktails have been studied and occasionally have led to some clinical improvement, the outcome in NH is nearly always fatal in the absence of prompt hepatic transplantation.[404-406] The rare individuals who have survived without transplantation have recovered full organ function,[407,408] and the disease usually does not recur in those who have undergone transplantation successfully, thus suggesting that the hepatic insult is developmental or transient in nature.

Mutations in several of the "adult" hemochromatosis genes have not been identified in NH patients, and there is substantial evidence of a nonmendelian or otherwise unconventional hereditary predisposition to NH.[401,402,409] Specifically, the possibility of mitochondrial inheritance or inheritance of a maternally imprinted gene has been raised by the discovery of several kindreds in which women have borne affected children fathered by different men. However, neither of these types of inheritance can account for the tendency for a mother's first pregnancy to be spared of or mildly affected by the disorder whereas subsequent pregnancies have a greater than 50% risk for the development of clinically overt NH. These latter observations, in particular, have spawned the current leading hypothesis that NH is the consequence of prenatal alloimmune liver injury.[410,411] In this model, which parallels the paradigm of neonatal alloimmune thrombocytopenia (see Chapter 33), the mother is sensitized to a fetal antigen during a first pregnancy and subsequent pregnancies provoke an amnestic immune response that results in a severe clinical phenotype. What the antigen might be or how it perturbs iron metabolism is unknown. Nonetheless, a recent clinical trial demonstrated that clinically significant liver disease can be avoided in the vast majority of at-risk fetuses by treating the expectant mother with intravenous immunoglobulin beginning in the early second trimester of gestation, thus further substantiating the alloimmune hypothesis.[412]

Iron Overload Caused by Erythroid Hyperplasia and Ineffective Erythropoiesis

The connection between hematopoiesis and iron absorption is most strikingly apparent in patients with ineffective erythropoiesis. With disorders such as β^+-thalassemia (thalassemia intermedia) and X-linked sideroblastic anemia, the fractional absorption of ingested iron is increased. Patients with these disorders can manifest iron overload without transfusion.[413]

The mechanism by which bone marrow activity modulates gastrointestinal iron absorption is only partially understood. A soluble factor appears to be released that depresses hepcidin production.[414] Recently, it was reported that GDF15, a member of the transforming growth factor β superfamily, is induced in patients with thalassemia and that GDF15 suppresses expression of hepcidin by human hepatocytes.[415] It is not yet clear, however, whether this is the major or the only factor contributing to the "erythroid regulator."

In humans, depressed hepcidin levels and, consequently, robust absorption of iron from the gastrointestinal tract are associated most often with ineffective erythropoiesis.[56] Some patients with pyruvate kinase deficiency, a condition frequently associated with reticulocyte counts as high as 70%, manifest iron overload without transfusion. Hemolytic anemias with effective erythropoiesis rarely lead to iron loading. Without some

compounding variable, such as hereditary hemochromatosis trait, iron loading without transfusion is not generally seen with conditions such as sickle cell anemia or hereditary spherocytosis, in which the erythroid cells mature and leave the bone marrow before they are destroyed.

Consequences of Iron Overload

The effects of iron overload on some organs, such as the skin, are trivial, whereas hemosiderotic harm to other organs, such as the liver, can be fatal. Few notable symptoms precede advanced injury. Abdominal discomfort, lethargy, depression, arthralgias, erectile dysfunction, and fatigue are common but nonspecific complaints. Dyspnea with exertion and peripheral edema indicate significant cardiac compromise and reflect advanced iron loading.

As the major site of iron storage, the liver is a conspicuous target for excessive iron deposition. Mild to moderate hepatomegaly develops early, followed by shrinkage produced by fibrosis and micronodular cirrhosis. Hepatic tenderness may be present, but hemosiderotic liver damage produces little inflammation. Consequently, significant hepatic iron deposition and even fibrosis can occur with very little increase in serum transaminase levels. Disturbances in liver synthetic function indicate advanced disease. Liver biopsy is still the "gold standard" for determining the extent of hepatic iron deposition, although noninvasive imaging techniques do have a role. Hematoxylin-eosin staining reveals a brownish pigment in the hepatocytes that staining with Perls Prussian blue unmasks as iron. Large amounts of iron are also deposited in Kupffer cells in patients with ferroportin disease, African iron overload syndrome, or transfusional iron overload. Electron microscopy reveals substantial hemosiderin aggregates in addition to large quantities of ferritin.

Congestive cardiomyopathy is the most common heart problem that occurs with iron overload, but other abnormalities have been described, including pericarditis, restrictive cardiomyopathy, and angina without coronary artery disease.[416-419] There is strong correlation between the cumulative number of blood transfusions and functional cardiac derangements in children with thalassemia.[420] Findings on physical examination are surprisingly benign, even in patients with heavy cardiac iron deposition. Once evidence of cardiac failure appears, however, heart function deteriorates rapidly, and medical intervention is frequently ineffective. Biventricular failure produces pulmonary congestion, peripheral edema, and hepatic engorgement. These potentially lethal cardiac complications have, in some cases, been reversed by vigorous iron extrication.[421]

Iron deposition in the bundle of His and the Purkinje system can lead to conduction defects.[422,423] Sudden death is common in these patients, presumably as a result of arrhythmias. At one time, patients treated with the chelator deferoxamine for transfusional iron overload received supplements of ascorbic acid in the range of 15 to 30 mg/kg/day to promote iron mobilization. Reports of sudden death prompted cessation of this practice.[424] Given carefully at lower doses (2 to 4 mg/kg) by an experienced practitioner, ascorbic acid is a safe adjunct to chelation therapy in patients with transfusional iron overload.

Cardiac dysfunction can also occur with very little tissue iron deposition. The total quantity of iron is less important than the unbound, or "toxic," iron fraction in the circulation. The concentration of unbound iron in tissues is extremely low and virtually impossible to measure. This toxic iron is precisely the component that is bound and neutralized by iron chelators. Therefore, cardiac damage is best prevented in patients with transfusional iron overload by maintaining a constant, low level of chelator in the circulation (and consequently in the tissues where the protection is rendered).

Dysfunction of the endocrine pancreas is common in patients with iron overload.[425,426] Overt diabetes mellitus requiring insulin therapy develops in some patients. The disturbances in carbohydrate metabolism may be more subtle, however. An oral glucose tolerance test often unmasks abnormal insulin production. Vigorous removal of excess iron may reverse the islet cell dysfunction.[427] Exocrine pancreatic function, in contrast, is usually well preserved.

Pituitary dysfunction may produce several endocrine disturbances.[428] Reduced gonadotropin levels are common. When coupled with primary reductions in gonadal synthesis of sex steroids, sexual maturation is delayed in children with transfusional iron overload.[429] Secondary infertility is common. Although Addison's syndrome is uncommon with iron overload, production of adrenocorticotropic hormone is occasionally deficient. A metapyrone stimulation test shows delayed or diminished pituitary secretion of this hormone.[430] Thyroid function is usually well preserved in patients with iron overload. In contrast, parathyroid activity is frequently compromised. Functional hypoparathyroidism can be demonstrated in many patients by inducing hypocalcemia with an intravenous bolus of ethylenediaminetetraacetic acid (EDTA) while monitoring the production of parathyroid hormone.[431]

Hyperpigmentation is a nonspecific skin response to a variety of insults, including excessive exposure to ultraviolet light, thermal injury, and drug eruptions. Cutaneous iron deposition damages the skin and enhances melanin production by melanocytes. Ultraviolet light exposure and iron are often synergistic in the induction of skin pigmentation, and consequently, many patients with siderosis tan very readily. Fair-skinned people who tan poorly may never exhibit hyperpigmentation despite very large body iron burdens. In contrast, a striking, almond-colored hue frequently develops in patients with moderate baseline pigmentation. With a particularly heavy iron overload, visible iron deposits sometimes appear in the skin as a grayish discoloration.

Arthropathy is a common problem in patients with hereditary hemochromatosis but rare in patients with secondary iron overload.[432,433] Patients with hemochromatosis typically exhibit involvement of small joints, particularly in the hands, but large joints, such as the hip, may also be involved. Chondrocalcinosis is a late but characteristic feature of the arthropathy seen in hereditary hemochromatosis. Other troubling musculoskeletal problems include severe, recurrent cramps and disabling myalgias. Muscle biopsy shows iron deposits in myocytes, but the pathophysiologic connection to the pain and cramps is unclear.

Iron Overload and Opportunistic Infections

Withholding iron from potential pathogens is believed to be a natural part of the host defense repertoire.[434] Because transferrin binds iron with extremely high affinity and two thirds of the iron binding sites of the protein are normally unoccupied, there is very little free iron available in plasma and extracellular fluids. Not surprisingly, both transferrin and its homologue lactoferrin are bacteriostatic in vitro for many bacteria.[435-437] However, the very high transferrin saturations attained in patients with iron overload compromise the bacteriostatic properties of the proteins, and transferrin can serve as a source of iron for some microorganisms.[438] Various infections with unusual organisms have been reported in patients with iron overload (Box 12-4).[439-442] Host defense is compromised even further in patients with sideroblastic anemia and secondary iron overload because of abnormal neutrophil function. Although aggressive antimicrobial therapy is often successful, some infections, such as the mucormycosis produced by *Rhizopus oryzae*, are usually fatal.

Acute Iron Poisoning

Acute iron poisoning from the accidental ingestion of large doses of medicinal iron is a medical emergency. Significant gastrointestinal symptoms occur with doses as low as 20 mg/kg of elemental iron, and systemic toxicity becomes evident with ingestions of 60 mg/kg (reviewed by McGuigan[443]). Treatment consists of removing as

Box 12-4	Infectious Agents Associated with Iron Overload

BACTERIAL

Listeria monocytogenes
Yersinia enterocolitica
Salmonella typhimurium
Klebsiella pneumoniae
Vibrio vulnificus
Escherichia coli

FUNGAL

Cunninghamella bertholeatiae
Rhizopus oryzae

much residual iron as possible from the gastrointestinal tract and administering intravenous deferoxamine, which chelates the toxic non–transferrin-bound iron.[443,444] It is appropriate to consult a toxicologist or poison center for assistance.

DISORDERS OF IRON UTILIZATION

Anemia of Chronic Inflammation

The anemia of chronic inflammation, also called the anemia of chronic disease, is a well-recognized condition associated with a broad spectrum of maladies. It was elegantly described in a classic review by Cartwright almost half a century ago.[445] Typically a mild to moderate, normochromic and normocytic anemia, the RDW is slightly elevated as a result of a mild anisocytosis. This is often the only hint on the blood smear that the anemia is due to insufficient iron available for erythropoiesis. Serum iron and serum transferrin levels are usually low. Serum ferritin levels are generally increased but may not be when coexistent with iron deficiency. Similarly, sTfR levels are normal unless iron deficiency accompanies the disorder. Not surprisingly, the diagnosis of anemia of chronic inflammation may be challenging to make. Inflammation is the key to the condition.

Bone marrow examination with Perls Prussian blue stain usually reveals deposits of iron in the reticuloendothelial cells. This characteristic feature of the anemia of chronic inflammation reflects ineffective iron recycling. Normoblasts that fail to mature properly and effete erythrocytes are engulfed by reticuloendothelial macrophages in the marrow, liver, and spleen. The phagocytes degrade the protein and lipid and recycle the iron from hemoglobin onto transferrin for reuse. The anemia of chronic inflammation disturbs this cycle, with iron left trapped in the reticuloendothelial cells.

Much has been learned about the pathogenesis of the anemia of chronic inflammation over the past few years. Initially, studies of patients with an unusual metabolic disorder complicated by anemia and hepatic adenomas provided a clue that increased hepcidin expression might account for both the reticuloendothelial block and the decreased intestinal iron absorption characteristic of the anemia of inflammation.[44] Subsequent investigations confirmed that hepcidin expression was elevated in patients with inflammation associated with a variety of infectious and noninfectious conditions.[42,446] Hepcidin production is induced by the inflammatory cytokine interleukin-6 through a direct effect on the hepcidin promoter.[45-47,447]

Patients with the anemia of chronic inflammation may have unusually low plasma erythropoietin levels for their degree of anemia.[448] This finding was previously attributed to proinflammatory cytokines, which were shown to suppress production of erythropoietin by cells in culture.[449] However, erythropoietin responsiveness is also suppressed in an animal model of anemia of inflammation developed by transgenic expression of hepcidin in noninflamed animals.[450] In addition, hepcidin has been reported to have a direct effect on erythroid colony formation in vitro.[451] Taken together, these findings suggest that induction of hepcidin in response to inflammation results in most, if not all of the characteristic features of the anemia of inflammation.

Control of the inflammation (e.g., by colectomy in patients with ulcerative colitis) usually eliminates the anemia and corrects the disturbances in iron metabolism. In general, the anemia is recalcitrant when the inflammation is uncontrolled. However, it is likely that new treatment strategies will be developed that take advantage of our current understanding of the pathogenesis of the anemia of inflammation and regulation of hepcidin production.

SIDEROBLASTIC ANEMIAS

The sideroblastic anemias are a heterogeneous group of congenital and acquired bone marrow disorders defined by the presence of pathologic iron deposits within the mitochondria of erythroid precursors. On Prussian blue or Perls iron-stained bone marrow aspirate smears or biopsies, these iron-encrusted mitochondria appear as coarse granules that typically form a halo or "ring" around the nucleus, thus giving rise to the term "ringed sideroblast," which is, by definition, an abnormal cell[452] (Fig. 12-7). Mitochondrial localization of the iron deposits can be confirmed by electron microscopy, but it is not used routinely for diagnostic purposes. A recent report suggests that the iron deposits may contain a mitochondrial ferritin molecule encoded by a nuclear gene that is distinct from those encoding H- and L-ferritin polypeptides.[189,190]

Up to 30% to 40% of the erythroid precursors in normal, iron-replete bone marrow contain several fine, more peripherally placed iron deposits that represent iron

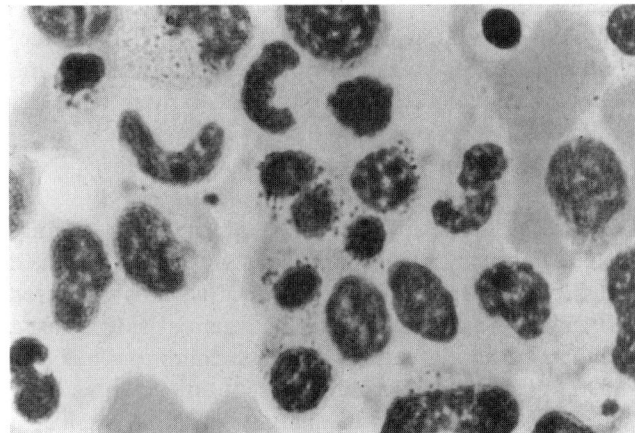

FIGURE 12-7. Prussian blue stain of a bone marrow aspirate from a patient with sideroblastic anemia. The granules that circle the nucleus of the normoblasts are iron-laden mitochondria.

TABLE 12-1 Clinical and Genetic Features of the Molecularly Defined Congenital Sideroblastic Anemias

	XLSA	XLSA/A	TRMA	MLASA	PMPS
Inheritance	X-linked	X-linked	Autosomal	Autosomal	Sporadic/maternal*
Gene	*ALAS2*	*ABCB7*	*SLC19A2*	*PUS1*	Variable
Sex	M >> F	M	M = F	M = F	M ≈ F
Carrier	+	+	−/+	ND	NA
MCV	↓↓	↓	↑	N/↑	↓
Erythrocyte PPIX	↓	↑	N/↑	ND	↑
Vitamin response	Pyridoxine	—	Thiamine	—	—
Other affected tissues/ cell lines	—	Nv	My, Meg, Nv, P, H	M	My, Meg, P, L, K, Nv, M

*Nearly all cases of PMPS are sporadic, but rare maternally inherited cases are reported.
↓, Decreased; ↑, increased; H, heart; K, kidney; L, liver; M, muscle; MCV, mean corpuscular volume; Meg, megakaryocytic; MLASA, mitochondrial myopathy with lactic acidosis and sideroblastic anemia; My, myeloid; N, within normal limits; NA, not applicable; ND, not determined; Nv, nervous system; P, pancreas; PMPS, Pearson's marrow-pancreas syndrome; PPIX, protoporphyrin IX; TRMA, thiamine-responsive megaloblastic anemia; XLSA, X-linked sideroblastic anemia; XLSA/A, X-linked sideroblastic anemia with ataxia.
Modified from Fleming MD. The genetics of inherited sideroblastic anemias. Semin Hematol. 2002;39:270-281; and Bottomley SS. Congenital sideroblastic anemias. Curr Hematol Rep. 2006;5:41-49.

in cytosolic ferritin. Such cells are termed "sideroblasts" and are absent or decreased in iron deficiency or the anemia of inflammation. "Siderocytes" are mature, enucleated peripheral blood erythrocytes that contain stainable iron, which may be the consequence of residual mitochondria from ringed sideroblasts or cellular ferritin, organelle, and nucleic acid concretions left over from terminal erythroid maturation.[452] Both are recognized as "Pappenheimer bodies" on conventional Wright-Giemsa–stained peripheral blood smears and are abundant in patients with sideroblastic anemia and a number of other anemias, including thalassemia syndromes and hemoglobinopathies.

In addition to the obligatory ringed sideroblasts, the bone marrow in patients with sideroblastic anemia is typically hypercellular with erythroid hyperplasia. Ineffective erythropoiesis frequently eventuates in elevated body iron stores and may be so severe that it results in clinically significant iron overload with secondary organ dysfunction. All patients are anemic, and thrombocytopenia and neutropenia develop in some, particularly acquired, neoplastic forms. The anemia may be normocytic, microcytic, or macrocytic and is typically characterized by a relative reticulocytopenia (Table 12-1 and Box 12-5; reviewed by Fleming[453] and Bottomley[454]).

Congenital Sideroblastic Anemias

Genetically defined, congenital sideroblastic anemias may be inherited in an autosomal recessive, an X-linked recessive, or infrequently, a maternal fashion (reviewed elsewhere[453,454]). Most cases of congenital sideroblastic anemia are considered to be inherited conditions but defy genetic characterization at the present time. In classifying the known causes of congenital sideroblastic anemia, it is helpful to consider the MCV of the anemia, whether other hematopoietic cell lineages are affected, and whether syndromic associations or other distinctive clinical findings are present (see Table 12-1).

Box 12-5 | **Acquired Sideroblastic Anemias**

TOXIC

Ethanol
Lead

DRUG

Chloramphenicol
Isoniazid and other antituberculous drugs
Penicillamine
Lincomycin

NUTRITIONAL

Copper deficiency

NEOPLASTIC

Myelodysplastic syndromes
    Refractory anemia with ringed sideroblasts
    Refractory anemia with ringed sideroblasts and marked thrombocytosis

Adapted from Ammus S, Yunis AA. Drug-induced red cell dyscrasias. Blood Rev. 1989;3:71-82.

X-Linked Sideroblastic Anemia

X-linked sideroblastic anemia (XLSA) is the prototype of all congenital sideroblastic anemias. As the name implies, the disorder is linked to the X chromosome and disproportionately affects men and boys, although females may be affected because of skewed X-chromosome inactivation or Turner's syndrome.[455-457] The cardinal features of XLSA include (1) a congenital microcytic, hypochromic anemia with a large RDW and erythrocyte dimorphism (particularly in carrier females) and Pappenheimer bodies apparent on the peripheral blood smear; (2) an abundance of ringed sideroblasts, especially in late erythroid precursors; and (3) a variable clinical response to pharmacologic doses of pyridoxine (vitamin B$_6$).[454] Systemic iron overload may also develop as a result of chronic, severe, ineffective erythropoiesis.[458,459] Nearly all patients with XLSA have missense mutations in the protein-coding regions of the erythroid-specific isoform of the heme biosynthesis enzyme δ-aminolevulinic acid synthase (ALAS2) (reviewed elsewhere[453,454]); rare patients have promoter mutations,[460] and unusual affected females carriers harbor nonsense or frameshift mutations.[461] The missense mutations tend to cluster in amino acids surrounding the catalytic site or the subunit interface of the homodimer, thereby leading to enzymes with decreased stability or decreased affinity for the cofactor pyridoxal phosphate, which can account for the clinical response to large doses of pyridoxine.[462] Because ALAS2 is the rate-limiting step in heme biosynthesis in the erythron, mutations inevitably impair the production of heme in developing erythroblasts. How heme deficiency leads to the hallmark ringed sideroblast is uncertain; however, the characteristic hypochromia and microcytosis are almost certainly the result of the protean effects of heme on erythroid transcription, mRNA stability, and translation.

The age at clinical onset of XLSA varies greatly. Anemia develops in some individuals within a few months of birth, whereas in others it occurs later in childhood and often even in adulthood. Generally, the anemia is progressive, with transfusions often required to maintain an adequate hemoglobin level. Frequent transfusions can hasten the development of iron overload. Oral pyridoxine therapy is useful in many patients with XLSA. Often, however, correction of the anemia is incomplete. Some patients become more pyridoxine responsive after their excess body iron stores are depleted.[463] A few children who failed pyridoxine therapy have responded to the parenteral administration of pyridoxal-5-phosphate.[464] Unfortunately, many children with XLSA improve little, if at all with either of these interventions. Because pyridoxine is inexpensive and lacks deleterious side effects, all children with sideroblastic anemia should receive a trial of vitamin therapy. Splenectomy is ill advised because of thrombotic risks.[454] There is one case report of successful allogeneic peripheral stem cell transplantation for refractory sideroblastic anemia.[465]

X-Linked Sideroblastic Anemia with Ataxia

X-linked sideroblastic anemia with ataxia (XLSA/A) is a very rare, distinct X-linked form of sideroblastic anemia caused by missense mutations in the mitochondrial ATP-binding cassette transporter ABCB7.[466-468] Patients with XLSA/A typically have static or slowly progressive cerebellar ataxia and only later are found to have a mild sideroblastic anemia with morphologic features similar to those of classic XLSA.[469,470] However, they do not require transfusion therapy, systemic iron overload does not develop, and they do not respond to pyridoxine therapy. ABCB7 and its yeast orthologue Atm1p are essential genes involved in the biogenesis of cytosolic Fe/S clusters.[471-477] Interestingly, another protein implicated in Fe/S cluster biogenesis in yeast and zebra fish, GRX5, has

been shown to be mutated in a single patient with severe sideroblastic anemia and iron overload.[478-480] In all cases, these Fe/S cluster biogenesis mutants appear to disrupt regulation of IRP1 RNA binding activity,[477,479] thus raising the possibility that this is a common mechanism for the development of sideroblasts.

Thiamine-Responsive Megaloblastic Anemia

Children with thiamine-responsive megaloblastic anemia (TRMA), also known as Rogers' syndrome, exhibit a characteristic triad of megaloblastic anemia with ringed sideroblasts, diabetes mellitus, and deafness.[481,482] The clinical manifestations of TRMA are progressive and may also include optic atrophy and nonthrombotic, nonembolic strokes. The anemia is characteristically macrocytic, and erythroid maturation in bone marrow, as the name implies, is megaloblastic and associated with variable numbers of ringed sideroblasts. Patients may also have leukopenia. The gene responsible for TRMA encodes a transmembrane thiamine transporter designated SLC19A2.[483-486] TRMA patients are not thiamine deficient but rather have a defect in high-affinity thiamine uptake in a number of cell types.[487] The megaloblastic marrow maturation is probably related to defective thiamine-dependent steps in nucleic acid synthesis[488]; however, the pathogenesis of sideroblasts remains obscure. Therapy with pharmacologic doses of thiamine ameliorates the anemia and may abrogate progression of the neurologic and pancreatic phenotypes.[481,489,490]

Pearson's Marrow-Pancreas Syndrome

Pearson's marrow-pancreas syndrome (PMPS) is a fatal, multisystemic disorder of infancy with marked disturbances in bone marrow and pancreatic function.[491] The initial manifestation is often a severe, transfusion-dependent macrocytic anemia associated with a variable degree of neutropenia and thrombocytopenia. Marrow examination characteristically shows vacuolization in the erythroid and myeloid precursors and ringed sideroblasts.[492] Exocrine pancreatic dysfunction as a result of pancreatic fibrosis is characteristic, and hepatic, renal, and neurologic dysfunction develops in some patients as well. The variability and pleiotropy of the disorder can be accounted for by the fact that PMPS is a mitochondrial cytopathy; nearly half of the patients share heteroplasmy for a common, nearly 5-kb deletion of mitochondrial DNA that is associated with other mitochondrial disorders, particularly Kearns-Sayre syndrome, and the distribution of defective mitochondrial genomes will necessarily influence expression of the disorder.[493,494] Defective energy production appears to be the central disturbance, and no treatment other than supportive care currently exists.

Mitochondrial Myopathy with Lactic Acidosis and Sideroblastic Anemia

Mitochondrial myopathy with lactic acidosis and sideroblastic anemia (MLASA) is a recently recognized autosomal recessive disorder of mitochondrial dysfunction caused by mutations in the gene for pseudouridine synthase 1 (PUS1).[495-500] Most cases are associated with a unique founder mutation present in the Persian-Jewish population. Individuals with MLASA have highly variable neurologic abnormalities that most characteristically consist of exercise intolerance and lactic acidosis but may include severe hypotonia, muscle wasting, developmental delay, and mental retardation. The anemia, which is typically slightly macrocytic, is equally variable despite a common genotype, with some patients having asymptomatic anemia and others requiring transfusional support. PUS1, which localizes to mitochondria, the cytosol, and nuclei, is one of several enzymes that modify uridine residues in long-lived RNA (e.g., tRNA) to the alternate base pseudouridine. This modification is thought to enhance the stability of these molecules and enhance protein translation.

Acquired Sideroblastic Anemias

A number of drugs and toxins that impair heme biosynthesis or perturb mitochondrial iron metabolism can produce sideroblastic anemia (Box 12-5) (reviewed by Ammus and Yunis[501]). The most important of these agents is lead. This element inhibits several enzymes in the heme biosynthetic pathway, including δ-aminolevulinic acid dehydratase, coproporphyrinogen oxidase, and ferrochelatase.[502] Lead screening, therefore, is mandatory in any child suspected of having sideroblastic anemia because lead poisoning can be treated. Isoniazid also produces sideroblastic anemia by causing functional depletion of pyridoxine, which inhibits heme biosynthesis.[503,504] Prophylactic treatment with pyridoxine is now part of the standard therapeutic regimen with this drug.

Acquired, clonal neoplastic sideroblastic anemias such as refractory anemia with ringed sideroblasts (RARS) and other myelodysplastic syndromes (MDSs) are exceptionally uncommon in the pediatric age group, except perhaps in children who have previously received chemotherapy for cancer.[505] The extent to which the considerable experience with these disorders in adults might be applicable to children is uncertain; however, when compared with other categories of MDS, RARS has a lesser propensity to evolve to acute leukemia and may often be associated with iron overload in the absence of significant transfusional support.[506] Intriguingly, some patients have been shown to have mutations within the mitochondrial genome that alter the coding sequence for cytochrome *c* oxidase.[507]

COPPER METABOLISM

Copper Physiology and Transport

A total of 100 to 150 mg of copper is present in an adult human. As with iron, the fetus accumulates large amounts of copper near the end of gestation, particularly in the liver, where concentrations are 5 to 10 times greater at birth than in adulthood. These stores do not decrease to adult levels until 5 to 15 years of age. The liver has the highest copper content, which together with muscle and bone, accounts for 50% to 75% of total body copper. The normal net copper intake is 2 to 5 mg in an adult and 0.04 to 0.15 mg/kg in a growing child. After about 6 months of age, normal plasma copper levels range between 70 and 140 mg/dL. Values are lower in early infancy.[508] Depressed plasma copper levels are a good indicator of early copper deficiency; however, functional tests of enzymatic activity (e.g., ceruloplasmin) may be better.

Like iron, copper is essential for normal cell growth and metabolism but toxic in excess. Unlike iron, however, copper balance is regulated by excretion, as well as by absorption.[509,510] The gastrointestinal tract absorbs about 30% of the copper present in an average diet. The liver promptly disposes of much of that copper in bile, whereas a lesser amount is lost through the intestinal mucosa.[511]

Plasma copper, which is held much more constant than plasma iron, exists in two forms. Albumin and amino acids loosely bind 10% to 15% of circulating copper. Ceruloplasmin, a multicopper ferroxidase, tightly binds the remaining copper in plasma. Ceruloplasmin was once thought to be a copper transport protein; however, it is now clear that it functions primarily to change the oxidation state of iron, thereby aiding in release of iron from storage cells, including hepatocytes and macrophages (as discussed earlier). In human patients[512-515] and mice[92] lacking ceruloplasmin, a distinct clinical syndrome characterized by neurodegeneration, hepatic iron overload, diabetes, impaired iron recycling by reticuloendothelial cells, and mild iron deficiency anemia develops.

Copper is an essential component of cytochrome oxidase, the terminal oxidase of the electron transport chain required for combining hydrogen with oxygen to form water. As such, the element is essential for the oxidative generation of ATP. The enzyme tyrosinase is a copper-containing protein required for the synthesis of melanin. Thus, copper-deficient animals have depressed levels of cytochrome oxidase in most tissues, along with loss of hair pigment. Another copper metalloenzyme, lysyl oxidase, plays a role in the cross-linking of collagen and elastin. Lysyl oxidase deficiency may cause the vascular defects, including aortic aneurysm, seen in copper-deficient animals and patients with Menkes' disease (see later).[509]

Copper trafficking is relatively well understood (reviewed by Kim and colleagues[516]). A multitransmembrane domain protein, CTR1, appears to be the major transporter that brings copper into mammalian cells.[517-519] Knockout mice lacking CTR1 die early in gestation with findings that may be attributable to severe copper deficiency. Once copper is inside cells, it moves to its sites of utilization escorted by specific chaperone proteins (reviewed elsewhere[520,521]). These proteins appear to be conserved from yeast to mammals. Targeted disruption of one of these proteins, Atox1, in mice leads a poorly viable, copper-deficient phenotype, thus indicating that its copper chaperone function is important but not essential.[522]

Two inherited defects of human copper metabolism have given insight into copper transport within cells. Menkes' disease, or Menkes' kinky hair syndrome, is a congenital disorder characterized by a low serum copper concentration, reduced activity of copper metalloenzymes, slow growth, hypopigmented kinky hair, cerebral degeneration, and an X-linked pattern of inheritance.[523] Parenteral copper administration, like all other attempts to treat the disease, is ineffective, and death before 3 years of age is typical. By contrast, in the autosomal recessive disorder Wilson's disease, the predominant clinical phenotypes—liver disease and neurodegeneration—are due to copper cytotoxicity.

Positional cloning led to identification of the genes mutated in Menkes' and Wilson's diseases.[524-529] Each is a P-type adenosine triphosphatase transmembrane copper transporter (Cu-ATPase) containing Gly-Met-Thr-Cys-X-X-Cys copper-binding motifs at their N-termini. The Menkes protein is involved in transport of copper in intestinal enterocytes, as well as a number of other cell types. Deficiency of the Menkes proteins leads to paradoxical systemic copper deficiency as a result of impaired intracellular intestinal copper transport accompanied by intracellular copper accumulation in certain cell types, particularly the kidney. By contrast, deficiency of the Wilson disease Cu-ATPase leads to cellular copper accumulation in the liver, basal ganglia, and kidney, along with impaired production of ceruloplasmin and hepatobiliary copper excretion. Interestingly, although Menkes' disease patients are copper deficient, anemia is not a prominent feature of the syndrome (see later). Wilson's disease may be manifested in children as fulminant hepatic failure associated with severe acute intravascular hemolysis.[530,531]

Hematologic Aspects of Copper Deficiency

Copper deficiency commonly causes hypochromic, microcytic anemia among farm animals in areas of the world where the soil is poor in copper.[532-535] In humans, the predominant clinical feature of copper deficiency is most commonly peripheral neuropathy. Because of milk's low copper content (about 0.12 mg/L), infants who consume a diet consisting largely of milk may be at risk for marginal copper nutrition or deficiency.[536] Nutritional copper deficiency can be due to extraordinary dietary circumstances, such as inadvertent omission of copper from intravenous alimentation formulations for an extended time or treatment of severely malnourished patients with a copper-deficient milk diet.[509,510,537] Impaired copper absorption may be a consequence of a variety of renal and gastrointestinal disturbances, including nephrotic syndrome, inflammatory bowel disease and other forms of malabsorption, or bariatric or other intestinal surgery.[538,539] Excessive zinc supplementation may

also lead to copper deficiency because zinc readily induces intestinal epithelial metallothionein, which preferentially chelates intestinal copper and prevents absorption.[509,540] Coexisting iron deficiency or severe malnutrition can obscure the manifestations of copper deficiency.

In humans, the anemia of copper deficiency is most typically normocytic, but it may be microcytic or macrocytic. Leukopenia with very marked neutropenia is particularly prevalent; thrombocytopenia is unusual. Bone marrow aspirates from copper-deficient individuals are often hypocellular and show a relative erythroid hyperplasia with prominent vacuolization of erythroid precursors and variable degrees of dyserythropoiesis or megaloblastoid changes (or both), with or without the presence of ringed sideroblasts. As many recent reports indicate, resistance to treatment with typical hematemics combined with the morphology may suggest the errant diagnosis of MDS (reviewed by Haddad and associates[541]). The coexistence of peripheral neuropathy, also typical of copper deficiency, may suggest the correct diagnosis. Osteoporosis may occur with severe copper deficiency.

Oral treatment with 0.1 to 0.3 mg/kg of copper per day (two or three times the estimated daily requirement) as 0.5% copper sulfate (containing about 2 mg of copper per milliliter) produces prompt reticulocytosis and correction of the anemia and neutropenia. Intravenous copper may also be given in severe deficiency states. Generally, the dietary imbalance that produced the deficiency can be corrected when the problem is recognized.

LEAD POISONING

Sources of Lead

Lead is a toxic metal without any function in the human body. Because of its useful properties, lead has been mined for several centuries. As a result, progressively larger amounts have been removed from the depths of the earth and introduced into the biosphere. Enough lead has found its way into humans that at least in the industrialized parts of the world, all people have some lead in the body and hence in the blood. It has thus become customary to refer to the blood lead values found in apparently healthy populations as "normal" blood lead levels. This term is an obvious misnomer because it implies some kind of minimum physiologic requirement for lead.

Airborne lead enters the human body through inhalation; about 35% is absorbed and 15% to 18% is retained.[542] Intake of airborne lead is greater in children because they breathe at a lower height, where the lead concentration is greater, and have a greater respiratory rate per unit of body weight.[543] Sources of inhaled lead include combustion engines that burn leaded fuel and primary and secondary (recycling) lead smelters. Lead can also be ingested through the intake of contaminated food, water, and beverages. Lead absorption is increased by deficiencies of essential minerals, such as iron and calcium.[544] High maternal lead levels can result in fetal lead toxicity.[545]

Children living in older houses are exposed to the additional risk of lead in paint. Although lead in air, food, and beverages can be considered "*low-dose*" sources, lead in paint is by far the most concentrated source. As much as 40% lead by weight is present in dried paint used before World War II. Since then, lead levels in paint have been progressively reduced. For many years it was believed that lead poisoning in children occurs primarily as a result of pica (the urge to ingest nonfood material), with consequent ingestion of paint chips.[546] Although this is not an uncommon occurrence, it is neither the only nor even the prevailing mechanism of ingestion of lead paint. Small children, through their ordinary hand-to-mouth activities (such as thumb sucking) directly ingest dust and thus take in large amounts of lead. Despite legislative efforts and scientific advances in the United States, millions of dwellings still contain leaded paint. These dwellings present an obvious risk, particularly to children of the poor, who tend to live in the oldest houses. The state of repair of the dwelling is almost as important as the lead content of the paint; peeling or flaking paint is obviously more accessible to small children. Because iron deficiency often induces pica, lead poisoning is more common in iron-deficient children.

Less common sources of lead include fumes from old battery casings; illegally distilled whiskey; printed paper, particularly colored magazines; and lead-painted toys. An uncommon source of lead that may result in severe poisoning is improperly glazed earthenware vessels used to store acidic beverages (such as fruit juices or cider).

Biochemical and Hematologic Effects of Lead

Lead has strong affinity for the sulfhydryl groups of cysteine, the amino group of lysine, the carboxyl groups of glutamic and aspartic acids, and the hydroxyl group of tyrosine. Lead binds to proteins, modifies their tertiary structure, and inactivates their enzymatic properties. Enzymes that are rich in sulfhydryl groups appear to be most sensitive. Mitochondria are particularly sensitive to lead. Many prominent effects of lead on heme synthesis are mediated through alterations of the mitochondrial membrane. Heme synthesis starts and ends inside the mitochondria; intermediate steps take place in the cytoplasm. In all cells, heme is an essential component of molecules of the cytochrome system, also located inside the mitochondria. Additionally, in erythropoietic precursors, very large amounts of heme are formed to make hemoglobin. Lead interferes at several points in the heme synthetic pathway in all cells. The two most important steps affected are those catalyzed by δ-aminolevulinic

acid dehydratase (a cytoplasmic enzyme) and ferrochelatase (an intramitochondrial enzyme). Both these enzymes depend on critical sulfhydryl groups for their activities. The inhibition by lead of ferrochelatase, which catalyzes the ultimate insertion of iron into protoporphyrin, results in the accumulation of protoporphyrins in maturing erythrocytes. Ultimately, despite the presence of a normal or increased intracellular content of iron, the mitochondria are starved for iron. Metalloporphyrins inhibit several mitochondrial enzymes, and the increased concentration of zinc protoporphyrin resulting from lead toxicity further impairs mitochondrial function.[547] There is a relationship between the concentration of lead that inhibits ferrochelatase in mitochondria and the ambient concentration of iron in the medium. At any concentration of lead, inhibition of ferrochelatase is most marked when the iron concentration is the lowest.[548] This biochemical mechanism explains the greater elevation of erythrocyte protoporphyrin observed, at equal lead exposure, in children with concomitant iron deficiency.[549] A progressive, exponential increase in erythrocyte protoporphyrin concentration is observed at blood lead levels of 5 to 90 μg/dL.[550] The erythrocyte protoporphyrin level is an indicator of adverse metabolic effects. It is very effective as a screening test for severe lead poisoning, but it cannot be used to screen for blood lead levels below 40 to 50 μg/dL.

The bulk of lead in blood (>90%) is contained in erythrocytes, but blood lead content is independent of the hematocrit. Basophilic stippling results from deposition of ribosomal DNA and mitochondrial fragments.[551] Moderate basophilic stippling may be seen in iron deficiency and thalassemia trait, but stippling is particularly prominent in the polychromatophilic erythrocytes in lead poisoning, unstable hemoglobinopathies, including severe β-thalassemia, and pyrimidine-5′-nucleotidase deficiency. Anemia is observed in children with lead poisoning, primarily in severe cases or in those with concomitant iron deficiency.[548] This is not an unexpected finding because the defect in heme synthesis affects only a very small fraction of the total protoporphyrin production and clinically significant anemia usually develops in the late stages. It is not uncommon to observe severe neurologic toxicity in the absence of anemia in children. On the other hand, lead intoxication and iron deficiency anemia tend to occur in the same lower socioeconomic population and are aggravated by each other. Iron-deficient children are more severely affected because iron deficiency increases lead ingestion through pica, increases lead absorption, enhances the defect in heme synthesis, and increases the toxicity of lead.

Other enzymes of heme biosynthesis are also affected by lead, but less severely. Uroporphyrinogen synthetase activity is inhibited only by a rather high (10^{-4} mol/L) lead concentration.[547] Coproporphyrinogen decarboxylase, another mitochondrial enzyme, also is inhibited by lead.[547] There is a marked increase in urinary coproporphyrin levels in lead intoxication. Measurement of urinary coproporphyrin has been widely used for the diagnosis of childhood lead poisoning, particularly in emergency departments. Although this test has been superseded by the easier measurement of erythrocyte protoporphyrin, it is important to recognize its usefulness in discriminating between recent and past lead exposure. Because of the protracted persistence of protoporphyrin within erythrocytes, significant elevations may be observed as long as 2 to 3 months after exposure to lead.[552] In contrast, increased coproporphyrin production, as a result of its high solubility, is immediately reflected in excess urinary excretion. Hence, when exposure to lead is current, both the erythrocyte protoporphyrin level and the urinary coproporphyrin level are increased; when exposure to lead is no longer present, there is a discrepancy between the elevated erythrocyte protoporphyrin level and normal urinary coproporphyrin excretion.

The process of heme synthesis is not exclusive to the erythron. All cells contain essential heme proteins, particularly in the respiratory cytochrome system, also located in the mitochondria. The most visible effects of lead on heme synthesis are those detectable in peripheral blood because this is the easiest tissue to sample. However, the ubiquitous presence of active heme synthesis in the mitochondria of all body cells and the affinity of lead for mitochondria result in widespread impairment of cellular function. Lead intoxication inhibits the synthesis of cytochrome P-450, the key enzyme in the mixed oxidase system. It appears likely that the toxic effects of lead, particularly in the nervous system, reflect the derangement in heme synthesis.[553]

In adults, peripheral neuropathy, abdominal colic, and anemia are the most common initial signs of lead poisoning. In children, the clinical effects of excessive exposure to lead are apparent primarily in the CNS; alterations in renal function and anemia occur only in the most severe cases. Acute encephalopathy can be the first manifestation of severe childhood lead poisoning. The onset is usually marked by seizures, often intractable, followed by coma and cardiorespiratory arrest. The syndrome may be fatal within 24 to 48 hours. Survivors often suffer permanent neurologic damage.[554] Acute encephalopathy may be accompanied by Fanconi's syndrome with aminoaciduria, glycosuria, and hyperphosphaturia.[555]

Chronic symptoms of lead toxicity are vague and include abdominal pain, vomiting, general malaise, and behavioral changes. These symptoms are nonspecific and of little diagnostic help, particularly in the youngest children, aged 1 to 3 years, who are the most frequently affected. The threshold blood lead level at which encephalopathy occurs in children is difficult to define. *Acute lead poisoning* with clinical signs other than encephalopathy has been observed at blood lead levels ranging between 60 and 450 µg/dL. On the other hand, it is possible to observe blood lead levels as high as 200 µg/dL in children without overt neurologic symptoms. The probability of overt neurologic problems increases with the blood lead level and becomes significant when the blood lead level rises above 70 µg/dL. For these reasons and because of the impending risk of an unpredictable clinical deterioration, children found to have blood lead levels of 70 µg/dL or greater should be treated as medical emergencies, even in the absence of symptoms.[556]

As a result of the greater awareness of childhood lead poisoning by physicians, extensive screening programs in large cities, and the reduction of lead in the air subsequent to the wider use of lead-free gasoline, severe lead poisoning is extremely rare. Additionally, there is a greater awareness of the subclinical effects of lead and the fact that there is no threshold below which body lead levels can be considered safe. In view of the evidence of adverse effects of exposure to lead, even at low levels, there has been progressive lowering of the "acceptable" blood lead level. Therefore, it is important to not confuse "intervention level" (decided on pragmatic considerations) with "safe" levels.

The insidious nature of lead toxicity mandates the detection of excessive exposure in apparently asymptomatic children before irreparable damage occurs. Screening for lead poisoning is made particularly difficult by the fact that the most commonly affected children are those of preschool age, who are also the least accessible, as a group, to mass testing. Screening in this age group is most often performed by pediatricians at routine office visits. It would be desirable, instead, for screening programs to reach out to the community and focus on the most economically deprived children, who have the least access to medical care, as well as the highest risk.

Nationwide programs for screening children must be directed primarily at identifying those in need of medical attention. The definition of *lead poisoning* now includes the category of children with blood lead levels of 10 to 19 µg/dL. Yet it has been shown that at this level the potential loss of IQ is so low that most people would agree that it is trivial.[557,558] Although medical intervention is not necessary for this group, educational and dietary advice is recommended. Children in need of medical attention are those with blood lead levels of 20 µg/dL or higher. Above this level, cognitive issues become significant.[557,558] Severe lead poisoning is defined as levels above 45 µg/dL.

Treatment of Lead Poisoning

The first and most essential step in treating childhood lead poisoning is identification and removal of the source of lead. Without elimination of the exposure, any treatment is futile. Environmental analysis, including home visits, is recommended to ascertain and remove the source of lead. Although complete removal of lead from the environment remains a formidable task for modern society, it offers the only viable solution to prevent lead toxicity in children. Multiple studies have shown that neurotoxicity is unlikely to be reversible, regardless of treatment, once lead intoxication is discovered. Because lead exposure is additive, removal of automobile-generated lead from the air has already had a profound impact on the problem of urban lead poisoning. However, residual lead-based paint continues to be a major problem.

Children who are symptomatic require urgent treatment. However, because the symptoms of lead poisoning may be elusive, treatment is indicated even in their absence if there is clear evidence of excessive body burden of lead. The goal of treatment is prevention of subclinical damage without producing complications of the therapy itself; it is necessary to exercise judicious compromise. Two parenteral treatments are used in severe lead poisoning: dimercaprol (formerly called BAL for British antilewisite) and CaNaEDTA. Both these agents chelate lead and induce its excretion. Dimercaprol is an oily, malodorous compound that is unpleasant to patients. It forms an emetic compound with iron, so iron therapy should not be given to a patient receiving dimercaprol.[559] It is dissolved in peanut oil and thus is contraindicated in children allergic to peanuts. Approximately half of patients treated with dimercaprol have side effects, many of which can be ameliorated by the concurrent use of antihistamines.[556]

CaNaEDTA is water soluble and best administered by continuous intravenous infusion. When administered intramuscularly (a less preferable and much more painful option), 2% procaine should be added to avoid severe local pain. CaNaEDTA may itself be toxic, particularly to the kidneys. Overdosage may induce tubular necrosis directly or renal toxicity as a result of hypercalcemia. CaNaEDTA is also able to chelate zinc, thus presenting another risk. Because δ-aminolevulinic acid dehydratase, a zinc-dependent enzyme, is already damaged by lead, the additional removal of zinc leads to its complete paralysis. This results in a burst of neurotoxic δ-aminolevulinic acid into plasma, which may aggravate (and even induce) convulsions. For these reasons, CaNaEDTA should never be given alone to symptomatic children or to asymptomatic children with blood lead levels of 70 μg/dL or greater; instead, it should be given after administration of dimercaprol to prevent these acute effects.[559] An additional note of caution is necessary with regard to the use of EDTA. Besides CaNaEDTA, a commercial preparation of disodium EDTA is also available and occasionally used for hyperparathyroidism. Disodium EDTA should never be used for the treatment of lead poisoning because it may induce acute hypocalcemia, which may be fatal. Only CaNaEDTA should be used for the treatment of lead poisoning. Hospital pharmacies should exercise maximum caution in dispensing disodium EDTA, which could be fatal if erroneously given to a child with lead poisoning but without hypercalcemia.

Because of their different pharmacologic properties, dimercaprol and CaNaEDTA are advantageously used in combination to treat children with symptomatic lead poisoning, with or without concomitant encephalopathy, as well as asymptomatic children with blood lead levels greater than 70 μg/dL.[556] The combined use of dimer-caprol and CaNaEDTA is both safer and more effective than the use of CaNaEDTA alone. Treatment should always start first with dimercaprol to avoid precipitating encephalopathy.[559] Involvement of an experienced toxicologist is strongly advised for safe, effective management of these patients.

Succimer is a derivative of dimercaprol in which the methyl groups are replaced by carboxylic groups. This results in excellent water solubility, thus allowing it to be used orally. Although the advantages of an oral chelator are obvious, it is crucial to be cautious in the use of succimer because with its great water solubility and affinity for lead, it may result in increased absorption if used in a lead-laden environment. For this reason, succimer should be used only when it is absolutely certain that the child has been removed from the lead-containing environment and is in a safe home. In a recent trial, succimer was shown to be effective in reducing blood lead levels in patients with levels of 20 to 45 μg/dL.[560] Importantly, however, it did not reverse neurologic and cognitive deficits. For this reason, the authors concluded that it is not indicated in children with moderate lead levels (20 to 45 μg/dL). Experience with this drug in treating children with blood lead levels of 70 μg/dL or higher is very limited. In these cases, as well as in symptomatic children, it may still be prudent to treat with a combination of dimercaprol and CaNaEDTA.

Regardless of the treatment, it is important to remember that improvement in blood lead levels does not mean that all lead has been removed. Blood levels are likely to rebound 1 to 2 weeks after therapy as tissue lead (particularly from bone) enters the circulation. Children with a large body burden of lead, such as those with clinical symptomatology or blood lead levels in excess of 70 μg/dL, invariably require several cycles of chelation therapy before a substantial reduction in the body burden of lead is obtained.[559] The need for additional cycles of therapy can be established by measurement of urinary lead excretion during the first days of treatment. The lead excreted should be related to the amount of EDTA given. Children who excrete lead in larger proportions are in greater need of additional cycles of therapy. It is not uncommon for a child to require several months of chelation therapy, initially with both dimercaprol and CaNaEDTA and later with CaNaEDTA alone, before urinary lead excretion declines and the blood lead level stabilizes below 30 μg/dL. Only at that point can chelation therapy be stopped.[559]

REFERENCES

1. Karlin KD. Metalloenzymes, structural motifs, and inorganic models. Science. 1993;261:701-708.
2. Gutteridge JMC, Rowley DA, Halliwell B. Superoxide-dependent formation of hydroxyl radicals in the presence of iron salts. Biochem J. 1981;199:263-265.
3. Frigerio R, Mela Q, Passiu G, et al. Iron overload and lysosomal stability in β⁰-thalassaemia intermedia and trait: correlation between serum ferritin and serum N-

acetyl-β-D-glucosaminidase levels. Scand J Haematol. 1984;33:252-255.

4. Hebbel RP. The sickle erythrocyte in double jeopardy: autoxidation and iron decompartmentalization. Semin Hematol. 1990;27:51-69.

5. Repka T, Shalev O, Reddy R, et al. Nonrandom association of free iron with membranes of sickle and beta-thalassemic erythrocytes. Blood. 1993;82:3204-3210.

6. Kuross SA, Rank BH, Hebbel RP. Iron compartments associated with sickle cell RBC membranes: a mechanism for targeting of oxidative damage. Prog Clin Biol Res. 1989;319:601-610.

7. Schluter K, Drenckhan D. Co-clustering of denatured hemoglobin with band 3: its role in binding of autoantibodies against band 3 to abnormal and aged erythrocytes. Proc Natl Acad Sci U S A. 1986;83:6137-6141.

8. Waugh SM, Willardson BM, Kannan R, et al. Heinz bodies induce clustering of band 3, glycophorin and ankyrin in sickle cell erythrocytes. J Clin Invest. 1986;78:1155-1160.

9. Clark RA. Activation of the neutrophil respiratory burst oxidase. J Infect Dis. 1999;179(Suppl 2):S309-S317.

10. Dabbagh AJ, Trenam CW, Morris CJ, Blake DR. Iron in joint inflammation. Ann Rheum Dis. 1993;52:67-73.

11. Blake DR, Hall ND, Treby DA, et al. Protection against superoxide and hydrogen peroxide in synovial fluid from rheumatoid patients. Clin Sci (Lond). 1981;61:483-486.

12. Winyard PG, Blake DR, Chirico S, et al. Mechanism of exacerbation of rheumatoid synovitis by total dose iron dextran infusion. In vivo demonstration of iron promoted oxidant stress. Lancet. 1987;1:69-72.

13. Cairo G, Tacchini L, Pogliaghi G, et al. Induction of ferritin synthesis by oxidative stress. J Biol Chem. 1995;270:700-703.

14. Ferreira C, Bucchini D, Martin ME, et al. Early embryonic lethality of H ferritin gene deletion in mice. J Biol Chem. 2000;275:3021-3024.

15. Cook JD, Skikne BS, Lynch SR, Reusser ME. Estimates of iron sufficiency in the US population. Blood. 1986;68:726-731.

16. Bothwell TH, Charlton RW. A general approach of the problems of iron deficiency and iron overload in the population at large. Semin Hematol. 1982;19:54-67.

17. McCance RA, Widdowson EM. The absorption and excretion of iron following oral and intravenous administration. J Physiol. 1938;94:148-154.

18. Gitlin D, Cruchaud A. On the kinetics of iron absorption in mice. J Clin Invest. 1962;41:344-350.

19. Muir A, Hopfer U. Regional specificity of iron uptake by small intestinal brush-border membranes from normal and iron-deficient mice. Am J Physiol. 1985;248:G376-G379.

20. Kappas A, Drummond GS, Galbraith RA. Prolonged clinical use of a heme oxygenase inhibitor: hematological evidence for an inducible but reversible iron-deficiency state. Pediatrics. 1993;91:537-539.

21. Zijp IM, Korver O, Tijburg LB. Effect of tea and other dietary factors on iron absorption. Crit Rev Food Sci Nutr. 2000;40:371-398.

22. Gillooly M, Bothwell TH, Charlton RW, et al. Factors affecting the absorption of iron from cereals. Br J Nutr. 1984;51:37-46.

23. Gillooly M, Bothwell TH, Torrance JD, et al. The effects of organic acids, phytates and polyphenols on the absorption of iron from vegetables. Br J Nutr. 1983;49:331-342.

24. McKie AT, Barrow D, Latunde-Dada GO, et al. An iron-regulated ferric reductase associated with the absorption of dietary iron. Science. 2001;291:1755-1759.

25. Fleming MD, Trenor CC 3rd, Su MA, et al. Microcytic anaemia mice have a mutation in Nramp2, a candidate iron transporter gene. Nat Genet. 1997;16:383-386.

26. Gunshin H, Fujiwara Y, Custodio AO, et al. Slc11a2 is required for intestinal iron absorption and erythropoiesis but dispensable in placenta and liver. J Clin Invest. 2005;115:1258-1266.

27. Gunshin H, Mackenzie B, Berger UV, et al. Cloning and characterization of a mammalian proton-coupled metal-ion transporter. Nature. 1997;388:482-488.

28. Canonne-Hergaux F, Gruenheid S, Ponka P, Gros P. Cellular and subcellular localization of the Nramp2 iron transporter in the intestinal brush border and regulation by dietary iron. Blood. 1999;93:4406-4417.

29. Piomelli S. Childhood lead poisoning in the '90s. Pediatrics. 1994;93:508-510.

30. Abboud S, Haile DJ. A novel mammalian iron-regulated protein involved in intracellular iron metabolism. J Biol Chem. 2000;275:19906-19912.

31. Donovan A, Brownlie A, Zhou Y, et al. Positional cloning of zebrafish ferroportin1 identifies a conserved vertebrate iron exporter. Nature. 2000;403:776-781.

32. Donovan A, Lima CA, Pinkus JL, et al. The iron exporter ferroportin/Slc40a1 is essential for iron homeostasis. Cell Metab. 2005;1:191-200.

33. McKie AT, Marciani P, Rolfs A, et al. A novel duodenal iron-regulated transporter, IREG1, implicated in the basolateral transfer of iron to the circulation. Mol Cell. 2000;5:299-309.

34. Vulpe CD, Kuo YM, Murphy TL, et al. Hephaestin, a ceruloplasmin homologue implicated in intestinal iron transport, is defective in the sla mouse. Nat Genet. 1999;21:195-199.

35. Li L, Vulpe CD, Kaplan J. Functional studies of hephaestin in yeast: evidence for multicopper oxidase activity in the endocytic pathway. Biochem J. 2003;375:793-798.

36. Qiu A, Jansen M, Sakaris A, et al. Identification of an intestinal folate transporter and the molecular basis for hereditary folate malabsorption. Cell. 2006;127:917-928.

37. Finch C. Regulators of iron balance in humans. Blood. 1994;84:1697-1702.

38. Nemeth E, Ganz T. Regulation of iron metabolism by hepcidin. Annu Rev Nutr. 2006;26:323-342.

39. Nemeth E, Tuttle MS, Powelson J, et al. Hepcidin regulates cellular iron efflux by binding to ferroportin and inducing its internalization. Science. 2004;306:2090-2093.

40. Muckenthaler M, Roy CN, Custodio AO, et al. Regulatory defects in liver and intestine implicate abnormal hepcidin and Cybrd1 expression in mouse hemochromatosis. Nat Genet. 2003;34:102-107.

41. Pigeon C, Ilyin G, Courselaud B, et al. A new mouse liver-specific gene, encoding a protein homologous to human antimicrobial peptide hepcidin, is overexpressed

during iron overload. J Biol Chem. 2001;276:7811-7819.

42. Nemeth E, Valore EV, Territo M, et al. Hepcidin, a putative mediator of anemia of inflammation, is a type II acute-phase protein. Blood. 2003;101:2461-2463.

43. Nicolas G, Chauvet C, Viatte L, et al. The gene encoding the iron regulatory peptide hepcidin is regulated by anemia, hypoxia, and inflammation. J Clin Invest. 2002; 110:1037-1044.

44. Weinstein DA, Roy CN, Fleming MD, et al. Inappropriate expression of hepcidin is associated with iron refractory anemia: implications for the anemia of chronic disease. Blood. 2002;100:3776-3781.

45. Nemeth E, Rivera S, Gabayan V, et al. IL-6 mediates hypoferremia of inflammation by inducing the synthesis of the iron regulatory hormone hepcidin. J Clin Invest. 2004;113:1271-1276.

46. Verga Falzacappa MV, Vujic Spasic M, Kessler R, et al. STAT3 mediates hepatic hepcidin expression and its inflammatory stimulation. Blood. 2007;109:353-358.

47. Wrighting DM, Andrews NC. Interleukin-6 induces hepcidin expression through STAT3. Blood. 2006;108:3204-3209.

48. Huff RL, Hennessey TG, Austin RE, et al. Plasma and red cell iron turnover in normal subjects and in patients having various hematopoietic disorders. J Clin Invest. 1950;29:1041-1052.

49. Weintraub LR, Conrad ME, Crosby WH. Regulation of the intestinal absorption of iron by the rate of erythropoiesis. Br J Haematol. 1965;2:432-438.

50. Beutler E, Buttenwieser E. The regulation of iron absorption. I. A search for humoral factors. J Lab Clin Med. 1960;55:274-280.

51. Aron J, Baynes R, Bothwell TH, et al. Does plasma transferrin regulate iron absorption? Scand J Haematol. 1985; 35:451-454.

52. Raja KB, Pippard MJ, Simpson RJ, Peters TJ. Relationship between erythropoiesis and the enhanced intestinal uptake of ferric iron in hypoxia in the mouse. Br J Haematol. 1986;64:587-593.

53. Adamsky K, Weizer O, Amariglio N, et al. Decreased hepcidin mRNA expression in thalassemic mice. Br J Haematol. 2004;124:123-124.

54. Weizer-Stern O, Adamsky K, Amariglio N, et al. mRNA expression of iron regulatory genes in beta-thalassemia intermedia and beta-thalassemia major mouse models. Am J Hematol. 2006;81:479-483.

55. Gardenghi S, Marongiu MF, Ramos P, et al. Ineffective erythropoiesis in β-thalassemia is characterized by increased iron absorption mediated by down-regulation of hepcidin and up-regulation of ferroportin. Blood. 2007;109:5027-5035.

56. Kearney SL, Nemeth E, Neufeld EJ, et al. Urinary hepcidin in congenital chronic anemias. Pediatr Blood Cancer. 2007;48:57-63.

57. Craven CM, Alexander J, Eldridge M, et al. Tissue distribution and clearance kinetics of non–transferrin-bound iron in the hypotransferrinemic mouse: a rodent model for hemochromatosis. Proc Natl Acad Sci U S A. 1987;84: 3457-3461.

58. Huebers HA, Finch CA. The physiology of transferrin and transferrin receptors. Physiol Rev. 1987;67:520-582.

59. Williams J, Elleman TC, Kingston IB, et al. The primary structure of hen ovotransferrin. Eur J Biochem. 1982;122: 297-303.

60. Mazurier J, Metz-Boutigue MH, Jollès J, et al. Human lactotransferrin: molecular, functional and evolutionary comparisons with human serum transferrin and hen ovotransferrin. Experientia. 1983;39:135-141.

61. Metz-Boutigue MH, Jolies J, Mazurier J, et al. Human lactotransferrin: Amino acid sequence and structural comparison with other transferrins. Eur J Biochem. 1984; 145:659-676.

62. Brown JP, Hewick RM, Hellström I, et al. Human melanoma-associated antigen p97 is structurally and functionally related to transferrin. Nature. 1982;296:171-173.

63. Aisen P, Leibman A, Zweier J. Stoichiometric and site characteristics of the binding of iron to human transferrin. J Biol Chem. 1978;253:1930-1937.

64. Chen LH, Bissell MJ. Transferrin mRNA level in the mouse mammary gland is regulated by pregnancy and extracellular matrix. J Biol Chem. 1987;262:17247-17250.

65. Gerber MR, Connor JR. Do oligodendrocytes mediate iron regulation in the human brain? Ann Neurol. 1989; 26:95-98.

66. Levin MJ, Tuil D, Uzan G, et al. Expression of transferrin gene during development of non-hepatic tissues: high level of transferrin mRNA in fetal muscle and adult brain. Biochem Biophys Res Commun. 1984;122:212-217.

67. Lum JB, Infante AJ, Makker DM, et al. Transferrin synthesis by inducer T-lymphocytes. J Clin Invest. 1986;77: 841-849.

68. Skinner MK, Cosand WL, Griswold MD. Purification and characterization of testicular transferrin secreted by rat Sertoli cells. Biochem J. 1984;218:313-320.

69. Sylvester SR, Griswold MD. Localization of transferrin and transferrin receptors in rat testes. Biol Reprod. 1984; 31:195-203.

70. Lecureuil C, Staub C, Fouchecourt S, et al. Transferrin overexpression alters testicular function in aged mice. Mol Reprod Dev. 2007;74:197-206.

71. Trenor CC 3rd, Campagna DR, Sellers VM, et al. The molecular defect in hypotransferrinemic mice. Blood. 2000;96:1113-1118.

72. Dickinson T, Connor JR. Histological analysis of selected brain regions of hypotransferrinemic mice. Brain Res. 1994;635:169-178.

73. Pattanapanyasat K, Hoy TG. Expression of cell surface transferrin receptor and intracellular ferritin after in vitro stimulation of peripheral blood T lymphocytes. Eur J Haematol. 1991;47:140-145.

74. Schaeffer E, Lucero MA, Jeltsch JM, et al. Complete structure of the human transferrin gene. Comparison with analogous chicken gene and human pseudogene. Gene. 1987;56:109-116.

75. Chaudhary J, Skinner MK. Comparative sequence analysis of the mouse and human transferrin promoters: hormonal regulation of the transferrin promoter in Sertoli cells. Mol Reprod Dev. 1998;50:273-283.

76. Adrian GS, Korinek BW, Bowman BH, Yang F. The human transferrin gene: 5′ region contains conserved sequences which match the control elements regulated by

heavy metals, glucocorticoids and acute phase reaction. Gene. 1986;490:167-175.

77. Huggenvik JI, Idzerda RL, Haywood L, et al. Transferrin messenger ribonucleic acid: molecular cloning and hormonal regulation in rat Sertoli cells. Endocrinology. 1987;120:332-340.

78. Idzerda RL, Huebers H, Finch CA, McKnight GS. Rat transferrin gene expression: tissue-specific regulation by iron deficiency. Proc Natl Acad Sci U S A. 1986;83:3723-3727.

79. Lucero MA, Schaeffer E, Cohen GN, Zakin MM. The 5' region of the human transferrin gene: structure and potential regulatory sites. Nucleic Acids Res. 1986;14:8692.

80. Tsutsumi M, Skinner MK, Sanders-Bush E. Transferrin gene expression and synthesis by cultured choroid plexus epithelial cells. Regulation by serotonin and cyclic adenosine 3', 5'-monophosphate. J Biol Chem. 1989;264:9626-9631.

81. Frazer DM, Anderson GJ. The orchestration of body iron intake: how and where do enterocytes receive their cues? Blood Cells Mol Dis. 2003;30:288-297.

82. Pietrangelo A, Rocchi E, Ferrari A, et al. Regulation of hepatic transferrin, transferrin receptor and ferritin genes in human siderosis. Hepatology. 1991;14:1083-1089.

83. Baker EN, Lindley PF. New perspectives on the structure and function of transferrins. J Inorganic Biochem. 1992;47:147-160.

84. Hirose M. The structural mechanism for iron uptake and release by transferrins. Biosci Biotechnol Biochem. 2000;64:1328-1336.

85. Mizutani K, Mikami B, Hirose M. Domain closure mechanism in transferrins: new viewpoints about the hinge structure and motion as deduced from high resolution crystal structures of ovotransferrin N-lobe. J Mol Biol. 2001;309:937-947.

86. MacGillivray RT, Moore SA, Chen J, et al. Two high-resolution crystal structures of the recombinant N-lobe of human transferrin reveal a structural change implicated in iron release. Biochemistry. 1998;37:7919-7928.

87. Williams J. The formation of iron-binding fragments of hen ovotransferrin by limited proteolysis. Biochem J. 1974;141:745-752.

88. Zak O, Aisen P. Preparation and properties of a single-sited fragment from the C-terminal domain of human transferrin. Biochim Biophys Acta. 1985;829:348-353.

89. Aisen P, Listowsky I. Iron transport and storage proteins. Annu Rev Biochem. 1980;49:357-393.

90. Osaki S, Johnson DA. Mobilization of liver iron by ferroxidase (ceruloplasmin). J Biol Chem. 1969;244:5757-5758.

91. Osaki S, Johnson DA, Frieden E. The possible significance of the ferrous oxidase activity of ceruloplasmin in normal human serum. J Biol Chem. 1966;241:2746-2751.

92. Harris ZL, Durley AP, Man TK, Gitlin JD. Targeted gene disruption reveals an essential role for ceruloplasmin in cellular iron efflux. Proc Natl Acad Sci U S A. 1999;96:10812-10817.

93. Harris DC, Aisen P. Physical biochemistry of the transferrins. In Loehr TM, Gray HB, Lever ABP (eds). Iron Carriers and Iron Proteins. Weinheim, Germany, VCH Publishers, 1989, pp 139-351.

94. Shongwe MS, Smith CA, Ainscough EW, et al. Anion binding by human lactoferrin: Results from crystallographic and physicochemical studies. Biochemistry. 1992;31:4451-4458.

95. Anderson BF, Baker HM, Norris GE, et al. Structure of human lactoferrin: Crystallographic structure analysis and refinement at 2.8 Å resolution. J Mol Biol. 1989;209:711-734.

96. Bailey S, Evans RW, Garatt RC, et al. Molecular structure of serum transferrin at 3.3-Å resolution. Biochemistry. 1988;27:5804-5812.

97. Breuer W, Hershko C, Cabantchik ZI. The importance of non–transferrin bound iron in disorders of iron metabolism. Transfus Sci. 2000;23:185-192.

98. Finch CA, Huebers H, Eng M, Miller L. Effect of transfused reticulocytes on iron exchange. Blood. 1982;59:364-369.

99. Jandl JH, Katz JH. The plasma-to-cell cycle of transferrin. J Clin Invest. 1963;42:314-326.

100. Laurell C, Ingelman B. The iron-binding protein of swine serum. Acta Chem Scand. 1947;1:770.

101. Sutherland R, Delia D, Schneider C, et al. Ubiquitous cell-surface glycoprotein on tumor cells is proliferation-associated receptor for transferrin. Proc Natl Acad Sci U S A. 1981;78:4515-4519.

102. Jing SQ, Trowbridge IS. Identification of the intermolecular disulfide bonds of the human transferrin receptor and its lipid-attachment site. EMBO J. 1987;6:327-331.

103. Kuhn LC, McClelland A, Ruddle FH. Gene transfer, expression and molecular cloning of the human transferrin receptor gene. Cell. 1984;37:95-103.

104. Schneider C, Kurkinen M, Greaves M. Isolation of cDNA clones for the human transferrin receptor. EMBO J. 1983;2:2259-2263.

105. Reckhow CL, Enns CA. Characterization of the transferrin receptor in tunicamycin-treated A431 cells. J Biol Chem. 1988;263:7297-7301.

106. Hayes GR, Enns CA, Lucas JJ. Identification of the O-linked glycosylation site of the human transferrin receptor. Glycobiology. 1992;2:355-359.

107. Williams AM, Enns CA. A region of the C-terminal portion of the human transferrin receptor contains an asparagine-linked glycosylation site critical for receptor structure and function. J Biol Chem. 1993;268:12780-12786.

108. Zerial M, Melancon P, Schneider C, Garoff H. The transmembrane segment of the human transferrin receptor functions as a signal peptide. EMBO J. 1986;5:1543-1550.

109. Alvarez E, Girones N, Davis RJ. Inhibition of receptor-mediated endocytosis of diferric transferrin is associated with covalent modification of the transferrin receptor with palmitic acid. J Biol Chem. 1990;265:16644-16655.

110. Jing SQ, Trowbridge IS. Nonacylated human transferrin receptors are rapidly internalized and mediate iron uptake. J Biol Chem. 1990;265:11555-11559.

111. Lawrence CM, Ray S, Babyonyshev M, et al. Crystal structure of the ectodomain of human transferrin receptor. Science. 1999;286:779-782.

112. West AP Jr, Giannetti AM, Herr AB, et al. Mutational analysis of the transferrin receptor reveals overlapping HFE and transferrin binding sites. J Mol Biol. 2001;313:385-397.

113. Iacopetta BJ, Morgan EH. The kinetics of transferrin endocytosis and iron uptake from transferrin in rabbit reticulocytes. J Biol Chem. 1983;258:9108-9115.

114. Iacopetta BJ, Rothenberger S, Kuhn LC. A role for the cytoplasmic domain in transferrin receptor sorting and coated pit formation during endocytosis. Cell. 1988;54:485-489.

115. Klausner RD, Ashwell G, van Renswoude J, et al. Binding of apotransferrin to K562 cells: explanation of the transferrin cycle. Proc Natl Acad Sci U S A. 1983;80:2263-2266.

116. Klausner RD, Van Renswoude J, Ashwell G, et al. Receptor-mediated endocytosis of transferrin in K562 cells. J Biol Chem. 1983;258:4715-4724.

117. Zak O, Trinder D, Aisen P. Primary receptor-recognition site of human transferrin is in the C-terminal lobe. J Biol Chem. 1994;269:7110-7114.

118. Huebers H, Csiba E, Huebers E, Finch CA. Molecular advantage of diferric transferrin in delivering iron to reticulocytes: a comparative study. Proc Soc Exp Biol Med. 1985;179:222-226.

119. Huebers HA, Huebers E, Csiba E, Finch CA. Heterogeneity of the plasma iron pool: explanation of the Fletcher-Huehns phenomenon. Am J Physiol. 1984;247:R280-R283.

120. Young SP, Bomford A, Williams R. The effect of the iron saturation of transferrin on its binding and uptake by rabbit reticulocytes. Biochem J. 1984;219:505-510.

121. Girones N, Alvarez E, Seth A, et al. Mutational analysis of the cytoplasmic tail of the human transferrin receptor. Identification of a sub-domain that is required for rapid endocytosis. J Biol Chem. 1991;266:19006-19012.

122. McGraw TE, Maxfield FR. Human transferrin receptor internalization is partly dependent upon an aromatic amino acid in the cytoplasmic domain. Cell Regul. 1990;1: 369-377.

123. Miller K, Shipman M, Trowbridge IS, Hopkins CR. Transferrin receptors promote the formation of clathrin lattices. Cell. 1991;65:621.

124. Rothenberger S, Iacopetta BJ, Kuhn LC. Endocytosis of the transferrin receptor requires the cytoplasmic domain but not its phosphorylation site. Cell. 1987;49:423-431.

125. Collawn JF, Lai A, Domingo D, et al. YTRF is the conserved internalization signal of the transferrin receptor, and a second YTRF signal at position 30-34 enhances endocytosis. J Biol Chem. 1993;268:21686-21692.

126. Dautry-Varsat A, Ciechanover A, Lodish HF. pH and the recycling of transferrin during receptor-mediated endocytosis. Proc Natl Acad Sci U S A. 1983;80:2258-2262.

127. Paterson S, Armstrong NJ, Iacopetta BJ, et al. Intravesicular pH and iron uptake by immature erythroid cells. J Cell Physiol. 1984;120:225-232.

128. Van Renswoude J, Bridges KR, Harford JB, Klausner RD. Receptor-mediated endocytosis and the uptake of iron in K562 cells: Identification of a non-lysosomal acidic compartment. Proc Natl Acad Sci U S A. 1982;79:6186-6190.

129. Giannetti AM, Halbrooks PJ, Mason AB, et al. The molecular mechanism for receptor-stimulated iron release from the plasma iron transport protein transferrin. Structure. 2005;13:1613-1623.

130. Ohgami RS, Campagna DR, Greer EL, et al. Identification of a ferrireductase required for efficient transferrin-dependent iron uptake in erythroid cells. Nat Genet. 2005;37:1264-1269.

131. Ohgami RS, Campagna DR, McDonald A, Fleming MD. The Steap proteins are metalloreductases. Blood. 2006; 108:1388-1394.

132. Canonne-Hergaux F, Zhang AS, Ponka P, Gros P. Characterization of the iron transporter DMT1 (NRAMP2/DCT1) in red blood cells of normal and anemic mk/mk mice. Blood. 2001;98:3823-3830.

133. Fleming MD, Romano MA, Su MA, et al. Nramp2 is mutated in the anemic Belgrade (b) rat: evidence of a role for Nramp2 in endosomal iron transport. Proc Natl Acad Sci U S A. 1998;95:1148-1153.

134. Shaw GC, Cope JJ, Li L, et al. Mitoferrin is essential for erythroid iron assimilation. Nature. 2006;440:96-100.

135. Klausner RD, van Renswoude J, Ashwell G, et al. Receptor-mediated endocytosis of transferrin in K562 cells. J Biol Chem. 1983;258:4715-4724.

136. Bernstein SE. Hereditary hypotransferrinemia with hemosiderosis, a murine disorder resembling human atransferrinemia. J Lab Clin Med. 1987;110:690-705.

137. Goya N, Miyazaki S, Kodate S, Ushio B. A family of congenital atransferrinemia. Blood. 1972;40:239-245.

138. Hamill RL, Woods JC, Cook BA. Congenital atransferrinemia: a case report and review of the literature. Am J Clin Pathol. 1991;96:215-218.

139. Heilmeyer L, Keller W, Vivell O, et al. Congenital transferrin deficiency in a seven-year old girl. German Medical Monthly. 1961;86:1745-1751.

140. Kaplan J, Craven C, Alexander J, et al. Regulation of the distribution of tissue iron. Lessons learned from the hypotransferrinemic mouse. Ann N Y Acad Sci. 1988;526: 124-135.

141. Simpson RJ, Konijn AM, Lombard M, et al. Tissue iron loading and histopathological changes in hypotransferrinaemic mice. J Pathol. 1993;171:237-244.

142. Levy JE, Jin O, Fujiwara Y, et al. Transferrin receptor is necessary for development of erythrocytes and the nervous system. Nat Genet. 1999;21:396-399.

143. Cabantchik ZI, Breuer W, Zanninelli G, Cianciulli P. LPI-labile plasma iron in iron overload. Best Pract Res Clin Haematol. 2005;18:277-287.

144. Kaplan J, Jordan I, Sturrock A. Regulation of the transferrin-independent iron transport system in cultured cells. J Biol Chem. 1991;266:2997-3004.

145. Sturrock A, Alexander J, Lamb J, et al. Characterization of a transferrin-independent uptake system for iron in HeLa cells. J Biol Chem. 1990;265:3139-3145.

146. Randell EW, Parkes JG, Olivieri NF, Templeton DM. Uptake of non–transferrin bound iron by both reductive and non-reductive processes is modulated by intracellular iron. J Biol Chem. 1994;269:16046-16053.

147. Inman RS, Coughlan MM, Wessling-Resnick M. Extracellular ferrireductase activity of K562 cells is coupled to transferrin-independent iron transport. Biochemistry. 1994;33:11850-11857.

148. Inman RS, Wessling-Resnick M. Characterization of transferrin-independent iron transport in K562 cells. Unique properties provide evidence for multiple pathways of iron uptake. J Biol Chem. 1993;268:8521-8528.

149. Hershko C, Graham G, Bates GW, Rachmilewitz EA. Non-specific serum iron in thalassemia: an abnormal

serum iron fraction of potential toxicity. Br J Haematol. 1978;40:255-263.

150. Hoffbrand AV, Ganeshaguru K, Hooton JW, Tattersall MH. Effect of iron deficiency and desferrioxamine on DNA synthesis in human cells. Br J Haematol. 1976;33:517-526.

151. Frazier JL, Caskey JH, Yoffe M, Seligman PA. Studies of the transferrin receptor on both human reticulocytes and nucleated human cells in culture. J Clin Invest. 1982;69:853-865.

152. Larrick JW, Cresswell P. Modulation of cell surface iron transferrin receptors by cellular density and state of activation. J Supramol Struct. 1979;11:579-586.

153. Lesley JF, Schulte RJ. Inhibition of cell growth by monoclonal anti–transferrin receptor antibodies. Mol Cell Biol. 1985;5:1814-1821.

154. Trowbridge IS, Lesley JF, Domingo D, et al. Monoclonal antibodies to transferrin receptor and assay of their biological effects. Methods Enzymol. 1987;147:265-279.

155. White S, Taetle R, Seligman PA, et al. Combinations of anti–transferrin receptor monoclonal antibodies inhibit human tumor cell growth in vitro and in vivo: evidence for synergistic anti-proliferative effects. Cancer Res. 1990;50:6295-6301.

156. Daniels TR, Delgado T, Rodriguez JA, et al. The transferrin receptor part I: Biology and targeting with cytotoxic antibodies for the treatment of cancer. Clin Immunol. 2006;121:144-158.

157. Jones DT, Trowbridge IS, Harris AL. Effects of transferrin receptor blockade on cancer cell proliferation and hypoxia-inducible factor function and their differential regulation by ascorbate. Cancer Res. 2006;66:2749-2756.

158. Qing Y, Shuo W, Zhihua W, et al. The in vitro antitumor effect and in vivo tumor-specificity distribution of human-mouse chimeric antibody against transferrin receptor. Cancer Immunol Immunother. 2006;55:1111-1121.

159. Ned RM, Swat W, Andrews NC. Transferrin receptor 1 is differentially required in lymphocyte development. Blood. 2003;102:3711-3718.

160. Gao J, Richardson DR. The potential of iron chelators of the pyridoxal isonicotinoyl hydrazone class as effective antiproliferative agents, IV: the mechanisms involved in inhibiting cell-cycle progression. Blood. 2001;98:842-850.

161. Reddel RR, Hedley DW, Sutherland RL. Cell cycle effects of iron depletion on T-47D human breast cancer cells. Exp Cell Res. 1985;161:277-284.

162. Bierer BE, Nathan DG. The effect of desferrithiocin, an oral iron chelator, on T cell function. Blood. 1990;76:2052-2059.

163. Chaudhri G, Clark IA. Reactive oxygen species facilitate the in vitro and in vivo lipopolysaccharide-induced release of tumor necrosis factor. J Immunol. 1989;143:1290-1294.

164. Pattanapanyasat K, Webster HK, Tongtawe P, et al. Effect of orally active hydroxypyridinone iron chelators on human lymphocyte function. Br J Haematol. 1992;82:13-19.

165. Polson RJ, Jenkins R, Lombard M, et al. Mechanisms of inhibition of mononuclear cell activation by the iron-chelating agent desferrioxamine. Immunology. 1990;71:176-181.

166. Lederman HM, Cohen A, Lee JW, et al. Deferoxamine: a reversible S-phase inhibitor of human lymphocyte proliferation. Blood. 1984;64:748-753.

167. Brittenham GM. The red cell cycle. In Brock JH, Halliday JW, Pippard MJ, Powell LW (eds). Iron Metabolism in Health and Disease. London, WB Saunders, 1994, pp 31-62.

168. Shannon KM, Larrick JW, Fulcher SA, et al. Selective inhibition of the growth of human erythroid bursts by monoclonal antibodies against transferrin or transferrin receptor. Blood. 1986;67:1631-1638.

169. Schmidt JA, Marshall J, Hayman MJ, et al. Control of erythroid differentiation. Cell. 1986;46:41-51.

170. Ponka P, Schulman HM. Regulation of heme biosynthesis: distinct regulatory features in erythroid cells. Stem Cells (Dayt). 1993;11(Suppl 1):24-35.

171. Bonanou-Tzedaki SA, Sohi M, Arnstein HR. Regulation of erythroid cell differentiation by haemin. Cell Differentiation. 1981;10:267-279.

172. Mager D, Bernstein A. The role of heme in the regulation of the late program of Friend cell erythroid differentiation. J Cell Physiol. 1979;100:467-479.

173. Ross J, Sautner D. Induction of globin mRNA accumulation by hemin in cultured erythroleukemic cells. Cell. 1976;8:513-520.

174. Rutherford TR, Clegg JB, Weatherall DJ. K562 human leukaemic cells synthesise embryonic haemoglobin in response to haemin. Nature. 1979;280:164-165.

175. Rutherford TR, Weatherall DJ. Deficient heme synthesis as the cause of noninducibility of hemoglobin synthesis in a Friend erythroleukemia cell line. Cell. 1979;16:415-423.

176. Battistini A, Coccia EM, Marziali G, et al. Intracellular heme coordinately modulates globin chain synthesis, transferrin receptor number, and ferritin content in differentiating Friend erythroleukemia cells. Blood. 1991;78:2098-2103.

177. Battistini A, Marziali G, Albertini R, et al. Positive modulation of hemoglobin, heme and transferrin receptor synthesis by murine interferon-alpha and -beta in differentiating Friend cells. Pivotal role of heme synthesis. J Biol Chem. 1991;266:528-535.

178. Coccia EM, Profita V, Fiorucci G, et al. Modulation of ferritin H-chain expression in Friend erythroleukemia cells: transcriptional and translational regulation by hemin. Mol Cell Biol. 1992;12:3015-3022.

179. Chen JJ. Regulation of protein synthesis by the heme-regulated eIF2alpha kinase: relevance to anemias. Blood. 2007;109:2693-2699.

180. Harrison PM, Fischbach FA, Hoy TG, Haggis GH. Ferric oxyhydroxide core of ferritin. Nature. 1967;216:1188-1190.

181. Harrison PM, Arosio P. The ferritins: molecular properties, iron storage function and cellular regulation. Biochim Biophys Acta. 1996;1275:161-203.

182. Levi S, Luzzago A, Cesareni G, et al. Mechanism of ferritin iron uptake: activity of the H-chain and deletion mapping of the ferro-oxidase site. A study of iron uptake and ferro-oxidase activity of human liver, recombinant H-chain ferritins, and two H-chain deletion mutants. J Biol Chem. 1988;263:18086-18092.

183. Theil EC, Takagi H, Small GW, et al. The ferritin iron entry and exit problem. Inorganica Clin Acta. 1999;297:242-251.

184. Drysdale J, Jain SK, Boyd D. Human ferritins: genes and proteins. In Spik G, Montreuil J, Crichton RR, Mazurier J (eds). Proteins of Iron Storage and Transport. New York, Elsevier, 1985, p 343.

185. McClarty G, Chan AK, Choy BK, Wright JA. Increased ferritin gene expression is associated with increased ribonucleotide reductase gene expression and the establishment of hydroxyurea resistance in mammalian cells. J Biol Chem. 1990;265:7539-7547.

186. Curtis AR, Fey C, Morris CM, et al. Mutation in the gene encoding ferritin light polypeptide causes dominant adult-onset basal ganglia disease. Nat Genet. 2001;28:350-354.

187. Wixom RL, Prutkin L, Munro HN. Hemosiderin: nature, formation and significance. Int Rev Exp Pathol. 1980;22:193-225.

188. Worwood M, Brook JD, Cragg SJ, et al. Assignment of human ferritin genes to chromsomes 11 and 19q13.3-19 qter. Hum Genet. 1985;69:371-374.

189. Levi S, Corsi B, Bosisio M, et al. A human mitochondrial ferritin encoded by an intronless gene. J Biol Chem. 2001;276:24437-24440.

190. Cazzola M, Invernizzi R, Bergamaschi G, et al. Mitochondrial ferritin expression in erythroid cells from patients with sideroblastic anemia. Blood. 2003;101:1996-2000.

191. Cairo G, Bardella L, Schiaffonati L, et al. Multiple mechanisms of iron-induced ferritin synthesis in HeLa cells. Biochem Biophys Res Comm. 1985;133:314-321.

192. White K, Munro HN. Induction of ferritin synthesis by iron is regulated at both transcriptional and translational levels. J Biol Chem. 1988;263:8938-8942.

193. Beaumont C, Jain SK, Bogard M, et al. Ferritin synthesis in differentiating Friend erythroleukemia cells. J Biol Chem. 1987;262:10619-10623.

194. Chou CC, Gatti RA, Fuller ML, et al. Structure and expression of ferritin genes in a human promyelocytic cell line that differentiates in vitro. Mol Cell Biol. 1986;6:566-573.

195. Torti SV, Kwak EL, Miller SC, et al. The molecular cloning and characterization of murine ferritin heavy chain, a tumor necrosis factor–inducible gene. J Biol Chem. 1988;263:12638-12644.

196. Rouault TA. The role of iron regulatory proteins in mammalian iron homeostasis and disease. Nat Chem Biol. 2006;2:406-414.

197. Rogers JT, Bridges KR, Durmowicz GP, et al. Translational control during the acute phase response: ferritin synthesis in response to interleukin-1. J Biol Chem. 1990;265:14572-14578.

198. Zahringer J, Baliga BS, Munro HN. Novel mechanism for translation control in regulation of ferritin synthesis by iron. Proc Natl Acad Sci U S A. 1976;73:857-861.

199. Aziz N, Munro HN. Iron regulates ferritin mRNA translation through a segment of its 5′-untranslated region. Proc Natl Acad Sci U S A. 1987;84:8478-8482.

200. Hentze MW, Rouault TA, Caughman SW, et al. A cis-acting element is necessary and sufficient for translational regulation of human ferritin expression in response to iron. Proc Natl Acad Sci U S A. 1987;84:6730-6734.

201. Rouault TA, Tang CK, Kaptain S, et al. Cloning of the cDNA encoding an RNA regulatory protein—the human iron-responsive element–binding protein. Proc Natl Acad Sci U S A. 1990;87:7958-7962.

202. Walden WE, Selezneva AI, Dupuy J, et al. Structure of dual function iron regulatory protein 1 complexed with ferritin IRE-RNA. Science. 2006;314:1903-1908.

203. Constable A, Quick S, Gray NK, Hentze MW. Modulation of the RNA-binding activity of a regulatory protein by iron in vitro: switching between enzymatic and genetic function? Proc Natl Acad Sci U S A. 1992;89:4554-4558.

204. Emory-Goodman A, Hirling H, Scarpellino L, et al. Iron regulatory factor expressed from recombinant baculovirus: conversion between the RNA-binding apoprotein and Fe-S cluster containing aconitase. Nucleic Acids Res. 1993;21:1457.

205. Gray NK, Hentze MW. Iron regulatory protein prevents binding of the 43S translation pre-initiation complex to ferritin and eALAS mRNAs. EMBO J. 1994;13:3882-3891.

206. Haile DJ, Rouault TA, Tang CK, et al. Reciprocal control of RNA-binding and aconitase activity in the regulation of the iron-responsive element binding protein: role of the iron-sulfur cluster. Proc Natl Acad Sci U S A. 1992;89:7536-7540.

207. Kaptain S, Downey WE, Tang C, et al. A regulated RNA binding protein also possesses aconitase activity. Proc Natl Acad Sci U S A. 1991;88:10109-10113.

208. Muckenthaler M, Gray NK, Hentze MW. IRP-1 binding to ferritin mRNA prevents the recruitment of the small ribosomal subunit by the cap-binding complex eIF4F. Mol Cell. 1998;2:383-388.

209. Hentze MW, Kuhn LC. Molecular control of vertebrate iron metabolism: mRNA-based regulatory circuits operated by iron, nitric oxide, and oxidative stress. Proc Natl Acad Sci U S A. 1996;93:8175-8182.

210. Lin J-J, Daniels-McQueen S, Patino MM, et al. Derepression of ferritin messenger RNA translation by hemin in vitro. Science. 1990;247:74.

211. Toth I, Bridges KR. Ascorbic acid enhances ferritin mRNA translation by an IRP/aconitase switch. J Biol Chem. 1995;270:19540-19544.

212. Beaumont C, Leneuve P, Devaux I, et al. Mutation in the iron responsive element of the L ferritin mRNA in a family with dominant hyperferritinemia and cataract. Nat Genet. 1995;11:444-446.

213. Girelli D, Olivieri O, Gasparini P, Corrocher R. Molecular basis for the hereditary hyperferritinemia-cataract syndrome [letter]. Blood. 1996;87:4912-4913.

214. Kato J, Fujikawa K, Kanda M, et al. A mutation, in the iron-responsive element of H ferritin mRNA, causing autosomal dominant iron overload. Am J Hum Genet. 2001;69:191-197.

215. Guo B, Phillips JD, Yu Y, Leibold EA. Iron regulates the intracellular degradation of iron regulatory protein 2 by the proteasome. J Biol Chem. 1995;270:21645-21651.

216. Samaniego F, Chin J, Iwai K, et al. Molecular characterization of a second iron-responsive element binding protein, iron regulatory protein 2. Structure, function, and post-translational regulation. J Biol Chem. 1994;269:30904-30910.

217. Guo B, Yu Y, Leibold EA. Iron regulates cytoplasmic levels of a novel iron-responsive element–binding protein without aconitase activity. J Biol Chem. 1994;269:24252.

218. Wang J, Chen G, Muckenthaler M, et al. Iron-mediated degradation of IRP2, an unexpected pathway involving a 2-oxoglutarate–dependent oxygenase activity. Mol Cell Biol. 2004;24:954-965.

219. Iwai K, Drake SK, Wehr NB, et al. Iron-dependent oxidation, ubiquitination, and degradation of iron regulatory protein 2: implications for degradation of oxidized proteins. Proc Natl Acad Sci U S A. 1998;95:4924-4928.

220. Yamanaka K, Ishikawa H, Megumi Y, et al. Identification of the ubiquitin-protein ligase that recognizes oxidized IRP2. Nat Cell Biol. 2003;5:336-340.

221. Meyron-Holtz EG, Ghosh MC, Rouault TA. Mammalian tissue oxygen levels modulate iron-regulatory protein activities in vivo. Science. 2004;306:2087-2090.

222. Rabin M, McClelland A, Kühn L, Ruddle FH. Regional localization of the human transferrin receptor gene to 3q26mqter. Am J Hum Genet. 1985;37:1112-1116.

223. McClelland A, Kuhn LC, Ruddle FH. The human transferrin receptor gene: Genomic organization, and the complete primary structure of the receptor deduced for a cDNA sequence. Cell. 1984;39:267-274.

224. Koeller DM, Casey JL, Hentze MW, et al. A cytosolic protein binds to structural elements within the iron-responsive regulatory region of the transferrin receptor mRNA. Proc Natl Acad Sci U S A. 1989;86:3574-3578.

225. Mullner EW, Kuhn LC. A stem-loop in the 3'-untranslated region mediates iron-dependent regulation of transferrin receptor mRNA stability in the cytoplasm. Cell. 1988;53:815.

226. Mullner EW, Neupert B, Kuhn LC. A specific mRNA binding factor regulates the iron-dependent stability of cytoplasmic transferrin receptor mRNA. Cell. 1989; 58:373.

227. Binder R, Horowitz JA, Basilion JP, et al. Evidence that the pathway of transferrin receptor mRNA degradation involves an endonucleolytic cleavage within the 3' UTR and does not involve poly(A) tail shortening. EMBO J. 1994;13:1969-1980.

228. Lok CN, Ponka P. Identification of an erythroid active element in the transferrin receptor gene. J Biol Chem. 2000;275:24185-24190.

229. Cox TC, Bawden MJ, Martin A, May BK. Human erythroid 5'-aminolevulinate synthase: promoter analysis and identification of an iron-responsive element in the mRNA. EMBO J. 1991;10:1891.

230. Dandekar T, Stripecke R, Gray NK, et al. Identification of a novel iron-responsive element in murine and human erythroid delta-aminolevulinic acid synthase mRNA. EMBO J. 1991;10:1903-1909.

231. Zheng L, Kennedy MC, Blondin GA, et al. Binding of cytosolic aconitase to the iron responsive element of porcine mitochondrial aconitase mRNA. Arch Biochem Biophys. 1992;299:356.

232. Hubert N, Hentze MW. Previously uncharacterized isoforms of divalent metal transporter (DMT)-1: implications for regulation and cellular function. Proc Natl Acad Sci U S A. 2002;99:12345-12350.

233. Sanchez M, Galy B, Dandekar T, et al. Iron regulation and the cell cycle: identification of an iron-responsive element in the 3'-untranslated region of human cell division cycle 14A mRNA by a refined microarray-based screening strategy. J Biol Chem. 2006;281:22865-22874.

234. Sanchez M, Galy B, Hentze MW, Muckenthaler MU. Identification of target mRNAs of regulatory RNA-binding proteins using mRNP immunopurification and microarrays. Nat Protoc. 2007;2:2033-2042.

235. Sanchez M, Galy B, Muckenthaler MU, Hentze MW. Iron-regulatory proteins limit hypoxia-inducible factor-2alpha expression in iron deficiency. Nat Struct Mol Biol. 2007;14:420-426.

236. Cooperman SS, Meyron-Holtz EG, Olivierre-Wilson H, et al. Microcytic anemia, erythropoietic protoporphyria and neurodegeneration in mice with targeted deletion of iron regulatory protein 2. Blood. 2005;106:1084-1091.

237. Galy B, Ferring D, Hentze MW. Generation of conditional alleles of the murine iron regulatory protein (IRP)-1 and -2 genes. Genesis. 2005;43:181-188.

238. Galy B, Holter SM, Klopstock T, et al. Iron homeostasis in the brain: complete iron regulatory protein 2 deficiency without symptomatic neurodegeneration in the mouse. Nat Genet. 2006;38:967-969; discussion 969-970.

239. LaVaute T, Smith S, Cooperman S, et al. Targeted deletion of the gene encoding iron regulatory protein-2 causes misregulation of iron metabolism and neurodegenerative disease in mice. Nat Genet. 2001;27:209-214.

240. Meyron-Holtz EG, Ghosh MC, Iwai K, et al. Genetic ablations of iron regulatory proteins 1 and 2 reveal why iron regulatory protein 2 dominates iron homeostasis. EMBO J. 2004;23:386-395.

241. Smith SR, Cooperman S, Lavaute T, et al. Severity of neurodegeneration correlates with compromise of iron metabolism in mice with iron regulatory protein deficiencies. Ann N Y Acad Sci. 2004;1012:65-83.

242. Galy B, Ferring D, Minana B, et al. Altered body iron distribution and microcytosis in mice deficient in iron regulatory protein 2 (IRP2). Blood. 2005;106:2580-2589.

243. Worwood M. Serum ferritin. Clin Sci. 1986;70:215.

244. Lipschitz DA, Cook JD, Finch CA. A clinical evaluation of serum ferritin as an index of iron stores. N Engl J Med. 1974;290:1213.

245. Elin RJ, Wolff SM, Finch CA. Effect of induced fever on serum iron and ferritin concentrations in man. Blood. 1977;49:147.

246. Riley RD, Heney D, Jones DR, et al. A systematic review of molecular and biological tumor markers in neuroblastoma. Clin Cancer Res. 2004;10:4-12.

247. Pietrangelo A. The ferroportin disease. Blood Cells Mol Dis. 2004;32:131-138.

248. Pan BT, Blostein R, Johnstone RM. Loss of the transferrin receptor during the maturation of sheep reticulocytes in vitro. An immunological approach. Biochem J. 1983; 210:37-47.

249. Beghe C, Wilson A, Ershler WB. Prevalence and outcomes of anemia in geriatrics: a systematic review of the literature. Am J Med. 2004;116(Suppl 7A):3S-10S.

250. Beguin Y, Huebers HA, Josephson B, Finch CA. Transferrin receptors in rat plasma. Proc Natl Acad Sci U S A. 1988;85:637-640.

251. Kohgo Y, Nishisato T, Kondo H, et al. Circulating transferrin receptors in human serum. Br J Haematol. 1986;64: 277-281.

252. Baynes RD, Shih YJ, Hudson BG, Cook JD. Production of the serum form of the transferrin receptor by a cell membrane–associated serine protease. Proc Soc Exp Biol Med. 1993;204:65-69.

253. Shih YJ, Baynes RD, Hudson BG, et al. Serum transferrin receptor is a truncated form of tissue receptor. J Biol Chem. 1990;265:19077-19081.

254. Rutledge EH, Root BJ, Lucas JJ, Enns CA. Elimination of the O-linked glycosylation site at Thr 104 results in the generation of a soluble human transferrin receptor. Blood. 1994;83:580.

255. Cook JD. The measurement of serum transferrin receptor. Am J Med Sci. 1999;318:269-276.

256. Punnonen K, Irjala K, Rajamaki A. Serum transferrin receptor and its ratio to ferritin in the diagnosis of iron deficiency. Blood. 1997;89:1052-1057.

257. Suominen P, Punnonen K, Rajamaki A, Irjala K. Serum transferrin receptor and transferrin receptor–ferritin index identify healthy subjects with subclinical iron deficits. Blood. 1998;92:2934-2939.

258. Baynes RD, Cook JD, Bothwell TH, et al. Serum transferrin receptor in hereditary hemochromatosis and African siderosis. Am J Hematol. 1994;45:288-292.

259. Looker AC, Loyevsky M, Gordeuk VR. Increased serum transferrin saturation is associated with lower serum transferrin receptor concentration. Clin Chem. 1999;45:2191-2199.

260. Iron Deficiency Anaemia: Assessment, Prevention and Control. A Guide for Programme Managers. Geneva, World Health Organization. 2001.

261. Healthy people 2010. Washington, DC, US Department of Health and Human Services, 2000.

262. Looker A. Iron deficiency—United States, 1999-2000. MMWR Morb Mortal Wkly Rep. 2002;51:897-899.

263. Merkel D, Huerta M, Grotto I, et al. Prevalence of iron deficiency and anemia among strenuously trained adolescents. J Adolesc Health. 2005;37:220-223.

264. Dubnov G, Constantini NW. Prevalence of iron depletion and anemia in top-level basketball players. Int J Sport Nutr Exerc Metab. 2004;14:30-37.

265. Risser WL, Lee EJ, Poindexter HB, et al. Iron deficiency in female athletes: its prevalence and impact on performance. Med Sci Sports Exerc. 1988;20:116-121.

266. Schneider JM, Fujii ML, Lamp CL, et al. The use of multiple logistic regression to identify risk factors associated with anemia and iron deficiency in a convenience sample of 12-36-mo-old children from low-income families. Am J Clin Nutr 2008;87:614-620.

267. Brotanek JM, Gosz J, Weitzman M, Flores G. Iron deficiency in early childhood in the United States: risk factors and racial/ethnic disparities. Pediatrics. 2007;120:568-575.

268. Bogen DL, Duggan AK, Dover GJ, Wilson MH. Screening for iron deficiency anemia by dietary history in a high-risk population. Pediatrics 2000;105:1254-1259.

269. Skalicky A, Meyers AF, Adams WG, et al. Child food insecurity and iron-deficiency anemia in low-income infants and toddlers in the United States. Matern Child Health J. 2006;10:177-186.

270. Brotanek JM, Halterman JS, Auinger P, et al. Iron deficiency, prolonged bottle-feeding, and racial/ethnic disparities in young children. Arch Pediatr Adolesc Med. 2005;159:1038-1042.

271. Cook JD, Boy E, Flowers C, Daroca Mdel C. The influence of high-altitude living on body iron. Blood 2005;106:1441-1446.

272. Brugnara C, Zurakowski D, DiCanzio J, et al. Reticulocyte hemoglobin content to diagnose iron deficiency in children. JAMA. 1999;281:2225-2230.

273. Ullrich C, Wu A, Armsby C, et al. Screening healthy infants for iron deficiency using reticulocyte hemoglobin content. JAMA. 2005;294:924-930.

274. Picciano MF, Deering RH. The influence of feeding regimens on iron status during infancy. Am J Clin Nutr. 1980;33:746-753.

275. Hallberg L, Rossander-Hulten L, Brune M, Gleerup A. Bioavailability in man of iron in human milk and cow's milk in relation to their calcium contents. Pediatr Res. 1992;31:524-527.

276. Ani-Kibangou B, Bouhallab S, Molle D, et al. Improved absorption of caseinophosphopeptide-bound iron: role of alkaline phosphatase. J Nutr Biochem. 2005;16:398-401.

277. Tunnessen WW Jr, Oski FA. Consequences of starting whole cow milk at 6 months of age. J Pediatr. 1987;111:813-816.

278. American Academy of Pediatrics Committee on Nutrition: The use of whole cow's milk in infancy. Pediatrics. 1992;89:1105-1109.

279. American Academy of Pediatrics Committee on Nutrition: Iron fortification of infant formulas. Pediatrics. 1999;104:119.

280. Conrad ME, Barton JC. Factors affecting iron balance. Am J Hematol. 1981;10:199.

281. Golubov J, Flanagan P, Adams P. Inhibition of iron absorption by omeprazole in rat model. Dig Dis Sci. 1991;36:405-408.

282. Hutchinson C, Geissler CA, Powell JJ, Bomford A. Proton pump inhibitors suppress absorption of dietary non-haem iron in hereditary haemochromatosis. Gut. 2007;56:1291-1295.

283. Koop H. Review article: metabolic consequences of long-term inhibition of acid secretion by omeprazole. Aliment Pharmacol Ther. 1992;6:399-406.

284. Koop H, Bachem MG. Serum iron, ferritin, and vitamin B_{12} during prolonged omeprazole therapy. J Clin Gastroenterol. 1992;14:288-292.

285. Sharma VR, Brannon MA, Carloss EA. Effect of omeprazole on oral iron replacement in patients with iron deficiency anemia. South Med J. 2004;97:887-889.

286. Lagarde S, Jovenin N, Diebold MD, et al. Is there any relationship between pernicious anemia and iron deficiency? Gastroenterol Clin Biol. 2006;30:1245-1249.

287. Marignani M, Delle Fave G, Mecarocci S, et al. High prevalence of atrophic body gastritis in patients with unexplained microcytic and macrocytic anemia: a prospective screening study. Am J Gastroenterol. 1999;94:766-772.

288. Demiroglu H, Dundar S. Pernicious anaemia patients should be screened for iron deficiency during follow up. N Z Med J. 1997;110:147-148.

289. Beeken WL. Absorptive defects in young people with regional enteritis. Pediatrics. 1973;52:69-74.

290. Sutton DR, Stewart JS, Baird IM, Coghill NF. "Free" iron loss in atrophic gastritis, post-gastrectomy states, and adult coeliac disease. Lancet. 1970;2:387-389.

291. Buchanan GR, Sheehan RG. Malabsorption and defective utilization of iron in three siblings. J Pediatr. 1981;98: 723-728.

292. Hartman KR, Barker JA. Microcytic anemia with iron malabsorption: An inherited disorder of iron metabolism. Am J Hematol. 1996;51:269-275.

293. Pearson HA, Lukens JN. Ferrokinetics in the syndrome of familial hypoferremic microcytic anemia with iron malabsorption. J Pediatr Hematol Oncol. 1999;21:412-417.

294. Finberg KE, Heeney MM, Campagna DR, et al. Mutations in TMPRSS6 cause iron-refractory, iron deficiency anemia (IRIDA). Nat Genet. 2008;45:569-571.

295. Du X, She E, Gelbart T, et al. The serine protease TMPRSS6 is required to sense iron deficiency. Science. 2008;320:1088-1092.

296. Iolascon A, Camaschella C, Pospisilova D, et al. Natural history of recessive inheritance of DMT1 mutations. J Pediatr 2008;152:136-139.

297. Lam-Yuk-Tseung S, Camaschella C, Iolascon A, Gros P. A novel R416C mutation in human DMT1 (SLC11A2) displays pleiotropic effects on function and causes microcytic anemia and hepatic iron overload. Blood Cells Mol Dis. 2006;36:347-354.

298. Beaumont C, Delaunay J, Hetet G, et al. Two new human DMT1 gene mutations in a patient with microcytic anemia, low ferritinemia, and liver iron overload. Blood. 2006;107:4168-4170.

299. Iolascon A, d'Apolito M, Servedio V, et al. Microcytic anemia and hepatic iron overload in a child with compound heterozygous mutations in DMT1 (SCL11A2). Blood. 2006;107:349-354.

300. Mims MP, Guan Y, Pospisilova D, et al. Identification of a human mutation of DMT1 in a patient with microcytic anemia and iron overload. Blood. 2005;105:1337-1342.

301. Firor HV. The many faces of Meckel's diverticulum. South Med J. 1980;73:1507-1511.

302. Crompton DW. The public health importance of hookworm disease. Parasitology. 2000;121:S39-S50.

303. Ramdath DD, Simeon DT, Wong MS, Grantham-McGregor SM. Iron status of schoolchildren with varying intensities of *Trichuris trichiura* infection. Parasitology. 1995;110:347-351.

304. Specks U. Diffuse alveolar hemorrhage syndromes. Curr Opin Rheumatol. 2001;13:12-17.

305. Buschman DL, Ballard R. Progressive massive fibrosis associated with idiopathic pulmonary hemosiderosis. Chest. 1993;104:293-295.

306. Bouros D, Panagou P, Rokkas T, Siafakas NM. Bronchoalveolar lavage findings in a young adult with idiopathic pulmonary haemosiderosis and coeliac disease. Eur Respir J. 1994;7:1009-1012.

307. van der Ent CK, Walenkamp MJ, Donckerwolcke RA, et al. Pulmonary hemosiderosis and immune complex glomerulonephritis. Clin Nephrol. 1995;43:339-341.

308. Le Clainche L, Le Bourgeois M, Fauroux B, et al. Long-term outcome of idiopathic pulmonary hemosiderosis in children. Medicine (Baltimore). 2000;79:318-326.

309. Saeed MM, Woo MS, MacLaughlin EF, et al. Prognosis in pediatric idiopathic pulmonary hemosiderosis. Chest. 1999;116:721-725.

310. Bush A, Sheppard MN, Warner JO. Chloroquine in idiopathic pulmonary haemosiderosis. Arch Dis Child. 1992; 67:625-627.

311. Colombo JL, Stolz SM. Treatment of life-threatening primary pulmonary hemosiderosis with cyclophosphamide. Chest. 1992;102:959-960.

312. Rossi GA, Balzano E, Battistini E, et al. Long-term prednisone and azathioprine treatment of a patient with idiopathic pulmonary hemosiderosis. Pediatr Pulmonol. 1992;13:176-180.

313. Milman N, Clausen J, Byg KE. Iron status in 268 Danish women aged 18-30 years: influence of menstruation, contraceptive method, and iron supplementation. Ann Hematol 1998;77:13-19.

314. Kadir RA, Economides DL, Sabin CA, et al. Frequency of inherited bleeding disorders in women with menorrhagia. Lancet. 1998;351:485-489.

315. Lukes AS, KKadir RA, Peyvandi F, Kouides PA. Disorders of hemostasis and excessive menstrual bleeding: prevalence and clinical impact. Fertil Steril. 2005;84:1338-1344.

316. Oski FA. The nonhematologic manifestations of iron deficiency. Am J Dis Child. 1979;133:315-322.

317. Oski FA, Honig AS, Helu B, Howanitz P. Effect of iron therapy on behavior performance in nonanemic, iron-deficient infants. Pediatrics. 1983;71:877-880.

318. Akman M, Cebeci D, Okur V, et al. The effects of iron deficiency on infants' developmental test performance. Acta Paediatr. 2004;93:1391-1396.

319. Lozoff B, Brittenham GM, Viteri FE, et al. Developmental deficits in iron-deficient infants: effects of age and severity of iron lack. J Pediatr. 1982;101:948-952.

320. Pollitt E. The developmental and probabilistic nature of the functional consequences of iron-deficiency anemia in children. J Nutr. 2001;131:669S-675S.

321. Halterman JS, Kaczorowski JM, Aligne CA, et al. Iron deficiency and cognitive achievement among school-aged children and adolescents in the United States. Pediatrics. 2001;107:1381-1386.

322. Bruner AB, Joffe A, Duggan AK, et al. Randomised study of cognitive effects of iron supplementation in non-anaemic iron-deficient adolescent girls. Lancet. 1996;348: 992-996.

323. Pollitt E, Saco-Pollitt C, Leibel RL, Viteri FE. Iron deficiency and behavioral development in infants and preschool children. Am J Clin Nutr. 1986;43:555-565.

324. Lozoff B, Wolf AW, Jimenez E. Iron-deficiency anemia and infant development: effects of extended oral iron therapy. J Pediatr. 1996;129:382-389.

325. Lozoff B, Jimenez E, Hagen J, et al. Poorer behavioral and developmental outcome more than 10 years after treatment for iron deficiency in infancy. Pediatrics. 2000;105: E51.

326. Walter T, De Andraca I, Chadud P, Perales CG. Iron deficiency anemia: adverse effects on infant psychomotor development. Pediatrics. 1989;84:7-17.

327. Lozoff B, Jimenez E, Smith JB. Double burden of iron deficiency in infancy and low socioeconomic status: a longitudinal analysis of cognitive test scores to age 19 years. Arch Pediatr Adolesc Med. 2006;160:1108-1113.

328. Wasserman G, Graziano JH, Factor-Litvak P, et al. Independent effects of lead exposure and iron deficiency anemia on developmental outcome at age 2 years. J Pediatr. 1992;121:695-703.

329. Erikson KM, Jones BC, Hess EJ, et al. Iron deficiency decreases dopamine D(1) and D(2) receptors in rat brain. Pharmacol Biochem Behav. 2001;69:409-418.

330. Ortiz E, Pasquini JM, Thompson K, et al. Effect of manipulation of iron storage, transport, or availability on myelin composition and brain iron content in three different animal models. J Neurosci Res. 2004;77:681-689.

331. Beard JL. Iron biology in immune function, muscle metabolism and neuronal functioning. J Nutr. 2001;131: 568S-579S; discussion 580S.

332. Thomas FB, Falko JM, Zuckerman K. Inhibition of intestinal iron absorption by laundry starch. Gastroenterology. 1976;71:1028-1032.

333. Crosby WH. Clay ingestion and iron deficiency anemia. Ann Intern Med. 1982;97:456.

334. Prasad AS. Recognition of zinc-deficiency syndrome. Nutrition. 2001;17:67-69.

335. Cavdar AO, Arcasoy A, Cin S, et al. Geophagia in Turkey: iron and zinc deficiency, iron and zinc absorption studies and response to treatment with zinc in geophagia cases. Prog Clin Biol Res. 1983;129:71-97.

336. Liu TC, Seong PS, Lin TK. The erythrocyte cell hemoglobin distribution width segregates thalassemia traits from other nonthalassemic conditions with microcytosis. Am J Clin Pathol. 1997;107:601-607.

337. Anderson C, Aronson I, Jacobs P. Erythropoiesis: erythrocyte deformability is reduced and fragility increased by iron deficiency. Hematology. 2000;4:457-460.

338. White KC. Anemia is a poor predictor of iron deficiency among toddlers in the United States: for heme the bell tolls. Pediatrics. 2005;115:315-320.

339. Olivares M, Walter T, Cook JD, et al. Usefulness of serum transferrin receptor and serum ferritin in diagnosis of iron deficiency in infancy. Am J Clin Nutr. 2000;72: 1191-1195.

340. Skikne BS. Circulating transferrin receptor assay—coming of age. Clin Chem. 1998;44:7-9.

341. Vazquez Lopez MA, Carracedo A, Lendinez F, et al. The usefulness of serum transferrin receptor for discriminating iron deficiency without anemia in children. Haematologica. 2006;91:264-265.

342. Radtke H, Meyer T, Kalus U, et al. Rapid identification of iron deficiency in blood donors with red cell indexes provided by Advia 120. Transfusion. 2005;45:5-10.

343. Reeves JD, Yip R. Lack of adverse side effects of oral ferrous sulfate therapy in 1-year-old infants. Pediatrics. 1985;75:352-355.

344. Zlotkin S, Arthur P, Antwi KY, Yeung G. Randomized, controlled trial of single versus 3-times-daily ferrous sulfate drops for treatment of anemia. Pediatrics 2001;108: 613-616.

345. Cook JD, Reddy MB. Effect of ascorbic acid intake on nonheme-iron absorption from a complete diet. Am J Clin Nutr. 2001;73:93-98.

346. Morris CC. Recent trends in pediatric iron poisonings. South Med J. 2000;93:1229.

347. Biondich PG, Downs SM, Carroll AE, et al. Shortcomings in infant iron deficiency screening methods. Pediatrics. 2006;117:290-294.

348. Charytan C, Levin N, Al-Saloum M, et al. Efficacy and safety of iron sucrose for iron deficiency in patients with dialysis-associated anemia: North American clinical trial. Am J Kidney Dis. 2001;37:300-307.

349. Fishbane S, Kowalski EA. The comparative safety of intravenous iron dextran, iron saccharate, and sodium ferric gluconate. Semin Dial. 2000;13:381-384.

350. Kosch M, Bahner U, Bettger H, et al. A randomized, controlled parallel-group trial on efficacy and safety of iron sucrose (Venofer) vs iron gluconate (Ferrlecit) in haemodialysis patients treated with rHuEpo. Nephrol Dial Transplant. 2001;16:1239-1244.

351. Yorgin PD, Belson A, Sarwal M, Alexander SR. Sodium ferric gluconate therapy in renal transplant and renal failure patients. Pediatr Nephrol. 2000;15:171-175.

352. Brugnara C, Laufer MR, Friedman AJ, et al. Reticulocyte hemoglobin content (CHr): early indicator of iron deficiency and response to therapy. Blood. 1994;83: 3100-3101.

353. Griffin IJ, Abrams SA. Iron and breastfeeding. Pediatr Clin North Am. 2001;48:401-413.

354. Rios E, Lipschitz DA, Cook JD, Smith NJ. Relationship of maternal and infant iron stores as assessed by determination of plasma ferritin. Pediatrics. 1975;55:694-699.

355. Ahmad SH, Amir M, Ansari Z, Ahmed KN. Influence of maternal iron deficiency anemia on the fetal total body iron. Indian Pediatr. 1983;20:643-646.

356. Ahmad SH, Ansari Z, Matto GM, et al. Serum iron in babies of anemic mothers—II. Indian Pediatr. 1984;21: 759-763.

357. Verner AM, Manderson J, Lappin TR, et al. Influence of maternal diabetes mellitus on fetal iron status. Arch Dis Child Fetal Neonatal Ed. 2007;92:F399-F401.

358. Sweet DG, Savage G, Tubman TR, et al. Study of maternal influences on fetal iron status at term using cord blood transferrin receptors. Arch Dis Child Fetal Neonatal Ed. 2001;84:F40-F43.

359. Chaparro CM, Neufeld LM, Tena Alavez G, et al. Effect of timing of umbilical cord clamping on iron status in Mexican infants: a randomised controlled trial. Lancet. 2006;367:1997-2004.

360. Cogswell ME, Parvanta I, Ickes L, et al. Iron supplementation during pregnancy, anemia, and birth weight: a randomized controlled trial. Am J Clin Nutr. 2003;78: 773-781.

361. Cox TM, Peters TJ. Uptake of iron by duodenal biopsy specimens from patients with iron-deficiency anaemia and primary haemochromatosis. Lancet. 1978;1:123-124.

362. Lynch SR, Skikne BS, Cook JD. Food iron absorption in idiopathic hemochromatosis. Blood. 1989;74:2187-2193.

363. von Recklinghausen FD. Uber haemochromatose. Tageblatt der versammlung Deutsch Naturforscher und Artze in Herdelbert. 1889;62:324-325.

364. Feder JN, Gnirke A, Thomas W, et al. A novel MHC class I–like gene is mutated in patients with hereditary haemochromatosis. Nat Genet. 1996;13:399-408.

365. Jazwinska EC, Pyper WR, Burt MJ, et al. Haplotype analysis in Australian hemochromatosis patients: evidence for a predominant ancestral haplotype exclusively associated with hemochromatosis. Am J Hum Genet. 1995;56: 428-433.

366. Lebron JA, Bennett MJ, Vaughn DE, et al. Crystal structure of the hemochromatosis protein HFE and characterization of its interaction with transferrin receptor. Cell. 1998;93:111-123.

367. Lebron JA, West AP Jr, Bjorkman PJ. The hemochromatosis protein HFE competes with transferrin for binding to the transferrin receptor. J Mol Biol. 1999;294:239-245.

368. Levy JE, Montross LK, Cohen DE, et al. The C282Y mutation causing hereditary hemochromatosis does not produce a null allele. Blood. 1999;94:9-11.

369. Zhou XY, Tomatsu S, Fleming RE, et al. HFE gene knockout produces mouse model of hereditary hemochromatosis. Proc Natl Acad Sci U S A. 1998;95:2492-2497.

370. Steinberg KK, Cogswell ME, Chang JC, et al. Prevalence of C282Y and H63D mutations in the hemochromatosis (HFE) gene in the United States. JAMA. 2001;285:2216-2222.

371. Camaschella C, Roetto A, De Gobbi M. Genetic haemochromatosis: genes and mutations associated with iron loading. Best Pract Res Clin Haematol. 2002;15:261-276.

372. Camaschella C, Roetto A, Cali A, et al. The gene TFR2 is mutated in a new type of haemochromatosis mapping to 7q22. Nat Genet. 2000;25:14-15.

373. Kawabata H, Germain RS, Vuong PT, et al. Transferrin receptor 2-α supports cell growth both in iron-chelated cultured cells and in vivo. J Biol Chem. 2000;275:16618-16625.

374. Kawabata H, Yang R, Hirama T, et al. Molecular cloning of transferrin receptor 2. A new member of the transferrin receptor–like family. J Biol Chem. 1999;274:20826-20832.

375. Goswami T, Andrews NC. Hereditary hemochromatosis protein, HFE, interaction with transferrin receptor 2 suggests a molecular mechanism for mammalian iron sensing. J Biol Chem. 2006;281:28494-28498.

376. Brissot P, de Bels F. Current approaches to the management of hemochromatosis. Hematology Am Soc Hematol Educ Program. 2006:36-41.

377. Roetto A, Papanikolaou G, Politou M, et al. Mutant antimicrobial peptide hepcidin is associated with severe juvenile hemochromatosis. Nat Genet. 2003;33:21-22.

378. Papanikolaou G, Samuels ME, Ludwig EH, et al. Mutations in HFE2 cause iron overload in chromosome 1q-linked juvenile hemochromatosis. Nat Genet. 2004;36:77-82.

379. Babitt JL, Huang FW, Wrighting DM, et al. Bone morphogenetic protein signaling by hemojuvelin regulates hepcidin expression. Nat Genet. 2006;38:531-539.

380. Huang FW, Pinkus JL, Pinkus GS, et al. A mouse model of juvenile hemochromatosis. J Clin Invest. 2005;115:2187-2191.

381. Niederkofler V, Salie R, Arber S. Hemojuvelin is essential for dietary iron sensing, and its mutation leads to severe iron overload. J Clin Invest. 2005;115:2180-2186.

382. De Domenico I, Ward DM, Musci G, Kaplan J. Iron overload due to mutations in ferroportin. Haematologica. 2006;91:92-95.

383. Njajou OT, Vaessen N, Joosse M, et al. A mutation in SLC11A3 is associated with autosomal dominant hemochromatosis. Nat Genet. 2001;28:213-214.

384. Zoller H, McFarlane I, Theurl I, et al. Primary iron overload with inappropriate hepcidin expression in V162del ferroportin disease. Hepatology. 2005;42:466-472.

385. Montosi G, Donovan A, Totaro A, et al. Autosomal-dominant hemochromatosis is associated with a mutation in the ferroportin (SLC11A3) gene. J Clin Invest. 2001;108:619-623.

386. Schimanski LM, Drakesmith H, Merryweather-Clarke AT, et al. In vitro functional analysis of human ferroportin (FPN) and hemochromatosis-associated FPN mutations. Blood. 2005;105:4096-4102.

387. De Domenico I, Ward DM, Langelier C, et al. The molecular mechanism of hepcidin-mediated ferroportin down-regulation. Mol Biol Cell. 2007;18:2569-2578.

388. Bothwell TH, Bradlow BA. Siderosis in the Bantu: a combined histopathological and chemical study. Arch Pathol. 1960;70:279-292.

389. Bothwell TH, Charlton RW, Seftel HC. Oral iron overload. S Afr Med J. 1965;39:892-900.

390. Gordeuk VR, Boyd RD, Brittenham GM. Dietary iron overload persists in rural sub-Saharan Africa. Lancet. 1986;1:1310-1313.

391. Seftel HC, Malkin C, Schmaman A, et al. Osteoporosis, scurvy, and siderosis in Johannesburg bantu. BMJ. 1966;5488:642-646.

392. Gordeuk V, Mukiibi J, Hasstedt SJ, et al. Iron overload in Africa. Interaction between a gene and dietary iron content. N Engl J Med. 1992;326:95-100.

393. Moyo VM, Gangaidzo IT, Gomo ZA, et al. Traditional beer consumption and the iron status of spouse pairs from a rural community in Zimbabwe. Blood. 1997;89:2159-2166.

394. Moyo VM, Mandishona E, Hasstedt SJ, et al. Evidence of genetic transmission in African iron overload. Blood. 1998;91:1076-1082.

395. McNamara L, MacPhail AP, Gordeuk VR, et al. Is there a link between African iron overload and the described mutations of the hereditary haemochromatosis gene? Br J Haematol. 1998;102:1176-1178.

396. Beutler E, Barton JC, Felitti VJ, et al. Ferroportin 1 (SCL40A1) variant associated with iron overload in African-Americans. Blood Cells Mol Dis. 2003;31:305-309.

397. Gordeuk VR, Caleffi A, Corradini E, et al. Iron overload in Africans and African-Americans and a common mutation in the SCL40A1 (ferroportin 1) gene. Blood Cells Mol Dis. 2003;31:299-304.

398. Barton JC, Acton RT, Rivers CA, et al. Genotypic and phenotypic heterogeneity of African Americans with primary iron overload. Blood Cells Mol Dis. 2003;31:310-319.

399. Brown KE, Khan CM, Zimmerman MB, Brunt EM. Hepatic iron overload in blacks and whites: a comparative autopsy study. Am J Gastroenterol. 2003;98:1594-1598.

400. Shneider BL. Neonatal liver failure. Curr Opin Pediatr. 1996;8:495-501.

401. Knisely AS, Mieli-Vergani G, Whitington PF. Neonatal hemochromatosis. Gastroenterol Clin North Am. 2003;32:877-889, vi-vii.

402. Cox TM, Halsall DJ. Hemochromatosis—neonatal and young subjects. Blood Cells Mol Dis. 2002;29:411-417.

403. Whitington PF. Fetal and infantile hemochromatosis. Hepatology. 2006;43:654-660.

404. Sigurdsson L, Reyes J, Kocoshis SA, et al. Neonatal hemochromatosis: outcomes of pharmacologic and surgi-

cal therapies. J Pediatr Gastroenterol Nutr. 1998;26: 85-89.

405. Grabhorn E, Richter A, Burdelski M, et al. Neonatal hemochromatosis: long-term experience with favorable outcome. Pediatrics. 2006;118:2060-2065.

406. Rodrigues F, Kallas M, Nash R, et al. Neonatal hemo-chromatosis—medical treatment vs. transplantation: the king's experience. Liver Transpl. 2005;11:1417-1424.

407. Bellini C, Mazzella M, Scopesi F, Serra G. Spontaneous recovery in neonatal hemochromatosis. J Hepatol. 2004; 41:882-883.

408. Ekong UD, Melin-Aldana H, Whitington PF. Regression of severe fibrotic liver disease in 2 children with neonatal hemochromatosis. J Pediatr Gastroenterol Nutr. 2008;46: 329-333.

409. Shneider BL. Genetic counseling in neonatal hemochro-matosis. J Pediatr Gastroenterol Nutr. 2002;34:328.

410. Whitington PF. Neonatal hemochromatosis: a congenital alloimmune hepatitis. Semin Liver Dis. 2007;27:243-250.

411. Whitington PF, Malladi P. Neonatal hemochromatosis: is it an alloimmune disease? J Pediatr Gastroenterol Nutr. 2005;40:544-549.

412. Whitington PF, Hibbard JU. High-dose immunoglobulin during pregnancy for recurrent neonatal haemochroma-tosis. Lancet. 2004;364:1690-1698.

413. Pippard MJ, Callender ST, Warner GT, Weatherall DJ. Iron absorption and loading in beta-thalassaemia inter-media. Lancet. 1979;2:819-821.

414. Weizer-Stern O, Adamsky K, Amariglio N, et al. Down-regulation of hepcidin and haemojuvelin expression in the hepatocyte cell-line HepG2 induced by thalassaemic sera. Br J Haematol. 2006;135:129-138.

415. Tanno T, Bhanu NV, Oneal PA, et al. High levels of GDF15 in thalassemia suppress expression of the iron regulatory protein hepcidin. Nat Med. 2007;13: 1096-1101.

416. Fitchett DH, Coltart DJ, Littler WA, et al. Cardiac involve-ment in secondary haemochromatosis: a catheter biopsy study and analysis of myocardium. Cardiovasc Res. 1980;14:719-724.

417. Liu P, Olivieri N. Iron overload cardiomyopathies: new insights into an old disease. Cardiovasc Drugs Ther. 1994;8:101-110.

418. Sanyal SK, Johnson W, Jayalakshmamma B, Green AA. Fatal "iron heart" in an adolescent: biochemical and ultra-structural aspects of the heart. Pediatrics. 1975;55: 336-341.

419. Schellhammer PF, Engle MA, Hagstrom JW. Histochemi-cal studies of the myocardium and conduction system in acquired iron-storage disease. Circulation. 1967;35:631-637.

420. Wolfe L, Olivieri N, Sallan D, et al. Prevention of cardiac disease by subcutaneous deferoxamine in patients with thalassemia major. N Engl J Med. 1985;312:1600-1603.

421. Rahko PS, Salerni R, Uretsky BF. Successful reversal by chelation therapy of congestive cardiomyopathy due to iron overload. J Am Coll Cardiol. 1986;8:436-440.

422. Buja LM, Roberts WC. Iron in the heart. Etiology and clinical significance. Am J Med. 1971;51:209-221.

423. Olson LJ, Edwards WD, McCall JT, et al. Cardiac iron deposition in idiopathic hemochromatosis: histologic and analytic assessment of 14 hearts from autopsy. J Am Coll Cardiol. 1987;10:1239-1243.

424. Nienhuis AW. Vitamin C and iron. N Engl J Med. 1981; 304:170-171.

425. Flynn DM, Fairney A, Jackson D, Clayton BE. Hormonal changes in thalassaemia major. Arch Dis Child. 1976;51: 828-836.

426. Oerter KE, Kamp GA, Munson PJ, et al. Multiple hormone deficiencies in children with hemochromatosis. J Clin Endocrinol Metab. 1993;76:357-361.

427. Bomford A, Williams R. Long term results of venesection therapy in idiopathic haemochromatosis. Q J Med. 1976;45:611-623.

428. Costin G, Kogut MD, Hyman CB, Ortega JA. Endocrine abnormalities in thalassemia major. Am J Dis Child. 1979;133:497-502.

429. Schafer AI, Cheron RG, Dluhy R, et al. Clinical conse-quences of acquired transfusional iron overload in adults. N Engl J Med. 1981;304:319-324.

430. Schafer AI, Rabinowe S, Le Boff MS, et al. Long-term efficacy of deferoxamine iron chelation therapy in adults with acquired transfusional iron overload. Arch Intern Med. 1985;145:1217-1221.

431. Gertner JM, Broadus AE, Anast CS, et al. Impaired para-thyroid response to induced hypocalcemia in thalassemia major. J Pediatr. 1979;95:210-213.

432. Ines LS, da Silva JA, Malcata AB, Porto AL. Arthropathy of genetic hemochromatosis: a major and distinctive man-ifestation of the disease. Clin Exp Rheumatol. 2001;19: 98-102.

433. von Kempis J. Arthropathy in hereditary hemochromato-sis. Curr Opin Rheumatol. 2001;13:80-83.

434. Weinberg ED. The iron-withholding defense system. ASM News. 1993;59:559-562.

435. Bullen JJ, Rogers HJ, Lewin JE. The bacteriostatic effect of serum on *Pasteurella septica* and its abolition by iron compounds. Immunology. 1971;20:391-406.

436. Lawrence TH 3rd, Biggers CJ, Simonton PR. Bacterio-static inhibition of *Klebsiella pneumoniae* by three human transferrins. Ann Hum Biol. 1977;4:281-284.

437. Reiter B, Brock JH, Steel ED. Inhibition of *Escherichia coli* by bovine colostrum and post-colostral milk. II. The bac-teriostatic effect of lactoferrin on a serum susceptible and serum resistant strain of *E. coli*. Immunology. 1975; 28:83-95.

438. Otto BR, Verweij-van Vught AM, MacLaren DM. Transferrins and heme-compounds as iron sources for pathogenic bacteria. Crit Rev Microbiol. 1992;18:217-233.

439. Abbott M, Galloway A, Cunningham JL. Haemochroma-tosis presenting with a double *Yersinia* infection. J Infect. 1986;13:143-145.

440. Brennan RO, Crain BJ, Proctor AM, Durack DT. *Cun-ninghamella*: a newly recognized cause of rhinocerebral mucormycosis. Am J Clin Pathol. 1983;80:98-102.

441. Bullen JJ, Spalding PB, Ward CG, Gutteridge JM. Hemo-chromatosis, iron and septicemia caused by *Vibrio vulni-ficus*. Arch Intern Med. 1991;151:1606-1609.

442. Capron JP, Capron-Chivrac D, Tossou H, et al. Spontane-ous *Yersinia enterocolitica* peritonitis in idiopathic hemo-chromatosis. Gastroenterology. 1984;87:1372-1375.

443. McGuigan MA. Acute iron poisoning. Pediatr Ann. 1996;25:33-38.

444. Mills KC, Curry SC. Acute iron poisoning. Emerg Med Clin North Am. 1994;12:397-413.

445. Cartwright GE. The anemia of chronic disorders. Semin Hematol. 1966;3:351-375.

446. Kemna E, Pickkers P, Nemeth E, et al. Time-course analysis of hepcidin, serum iron, and plasma cytokine levels in humans injected with LPS. Blood. 2005;106: 1864-1866.

447. Lee P, Peng H, Gelbart T, et al. Regulation of hepcidin transcription by interleukin-1 and interleukin-6. Proc Natl Acad Sci U S A. 2005;102:1906-1910.

448. Means RT. Pathogenesis of the anemia of chronic disease: a cytokine-mediated anemia. Stem Cells. 1995;13:32-37.

449. Faquin WC, Schneider TJ, Goldberg MA. Effect of inflammatory cytokines on hypoxia-induced erythropoietin production. Blood. 1992;79:1987-1994.

450. Roy CN, Mak HH, Akpan I, et al. Hepcidin antimicrobial peptide transgenic mice exhibit features of the anemia of inflammation. Blood. 2007;109:4038-4044.

451. Dallalio G, Law E, Means RT Jr. Hepcidin inhibits in vitro erythroid colony formation at reduced erythropoietin concentrations. Blood. 2006;107:2702-2704.

452. Cartwright GE, Deiss A. Sideroblasts, siderocytes, and sideroblastic anemia. N Engl J Med. 1975;292:185-193.

453. Fleming MD. The genetics of inherited sideroblastic anemias. Semin Hematol. 2002;39:270-281.

454. Bottomley SS. Congenital sideroblastic anemias. Curr Hematol Rep. 2006;5:41-49.

455. Bottomley SS, Wise PD, Wasson EG, Carpenter NJ. X-linked sideroblastic anemia in ten female probands due to ALAS2 mutations and skewed X chromosome inactivation. Am J Hum Genet. 1998;63:A352.

456. Cazzola M, May A, Bergamaschi G, et al. Familial-skewed X-chromosome inactivation as a predisposing factor for late-onset X-linked sideroblastic anemia in carrier females. Blood. 2000;96:4363-4365.

457. Aivado M, Gattermann N, Rong A, et al. X-linked sideroblastic anemia associated with a novel ALAS2 mutation and unfortunate skewed X-chromosome inactivation patterns. Blood Cells Mol Dis. 2006;37:40-45.

458. Lee PL, Barton JC, Rao SV, et al. Three kinships with ALAS2 P520L (c. 1559 C → T) mutation, two in association with severe iron overload, and one with sideroblastic anemia and severe iron overload. Blood Cells Mol Dis. 2006;36:292-297.

459. Collins TS, Arcasoy MO. Iron overload due to X-linked sideroblastic anemia in an African American man. Am J Med. 2004;116:501-502.

460. Bekri S, May A, Cotter PD, et al. A promoter mutation in the erythroid-specific 5-aminolevulinate synthase (ALAS2) gene causes X-linked sideroblastic anemia. Blood. 2003;102:698-704.

461. Cortesao E, Vidan J, Pereira J, et al. Onset of X-linked sideroblastic anemia in the fourth decade. Haematologica. 2004;89:1261-1263.

462. Astner I, Schulze JO, van den Heuvel J, et al. Crystal structure of 5-aminolevulinate synthase, the first enzyme of heme biosynthesis, and its link to XLSA in humans. EMBO J. 2005;24:3166-3177.

463. Cotter PD, May A, Li L, et al. Four new mutations in the erythroid-specific 5-aminolevulinate synthase (ALAS2) gene causing X-linked sideroblastic anemia: increased pyridoxine responsiveness after removal of iron overload by phlebotomy and coinheritance of hereditary hemochromatosis. Blood. 1999;93:1757-1769.

464. Mason DY, Emerson PM. Primary acquired sideroblastic anaemia: response to treatment with pyridoxal-5-phosphate. BMJ. 1973;1:389-390.

465. Gonzalez MI, Caballero D, Vazquez L, et al. Allogeneic peripheral stem cell transplantation in a case of hereditary sideroblastic anaemia. Br J Haematol. 2000;109:658-660.

466. Allikmets R, Raskind WH, Hutchinson A, et al. Mutation of a putative mitochondrial iron transporter gene (ABC7) in X-linked sideroblastic anemia and ataxia (XLSA/A). Hum Mol Genet. 1999;8:743-749.

467. Maguire A, Hellier K, Hammans S, May A. X-linked cerebellar ataxia and sideroblastic anaemia associated with a missense mutation in the ABC7 gene predicting V411L. Br J Haematol. 2001;115:910-917.

468. Pondarré C, Campagna DR, Antiochos B, et al. Abcb7, the gene responsible for X-linked sideroblastic anemia with ataxia, is essential for hematopoiesis. Blood. 2007; 109:3567-3569.

469. Pagon RA, Bird TD, Detter JC, Pierce I. Hereditary sideroblastic anaemia and ataxia: an X linked recessive disorder. J Med Genet. 1985;22:267-273.

470. Hellier KD, Hatchwell E, Duncombe AS, et al. X-linked sideroblastic anaemia with ataxia: another mitochondrial disease? J Neurol Neurosurg Psychiatry. 2001;70:65-69.

471. Bekri S, Kispal G, Lange H, et al. Human ABC7 transporter: gene structure and mutation causing X-linked sideroblastic anemia with ataxia with disruption of cytosolic iron-sulfur protein maturation. Blood. 2000;96:3256-3264.

472. Leighton J. ATP-binding cassette transporter in *Saccharomyces cerevisiae* mitochondria. Methods Enzymol. 1995; 260:389-396.

473. Leighton J, Schatz G. An ABC transporter in the mitochondrial inner membrane is required for normal growth of yeast. EMBO J. 1995;14:188-195.

474. Kispal G, Csere P, Guiard B, Lill R. The ABC transporter Atm1p is required for mitochondrial iron homeostasis. FEBS Lett. 1997;418:346-350.

475. Csere P, Lill R, Kispal G. Identification of a human mitochondrial ABC transporter, the functional orthologue of yeast Atm1p. FEBS Lett. 1998;441:266-270.

476. Kispal G, Csere P, Prohl C, Lill R. The mitochondrial proteins Atm1p and Nfs1p are essential for biogenesis of cytosolic Fe/S proteins. EMBO J. 1999;18:3981-3989.

477. Pondarré C, Antiochos BB, Campagna DR, et al. The mitochondrial ATP-binding cassette transporter Abcb7 is essential in mice and participates in cytosolic iron-sulfur cluster biogenesis. Hum Mol Genet. 2006;15:953-964.

478. Rodriguez-Manzaneque MT, Tamarit J, Belli G, et al. Grx5 is a mitochondrial glutaredoxin required for the activity of iron/sulfur enzymes. Mol Biol Cell. 2002; 13:1109-1121.

479. Wingert RA, Galloway JL, Barut B, et al. Deficiency of glutaredoxin 5 reveals Fe-S clusters are required for vertebrate haem synthesis. Nature. 2005;436:1035-1039.

480. Camaschella C, Campanella A, De Falco L, et al. The human counterpart of zebrafish shiraz shows sideroblastic-like microcytic anemia and iron overload. Blood. 2007;110:1353-1358.

481. Porter FS, Rogers LE, Sidbury JB Jr. Thiamine-responsive megaloblastic anemia. J Pediatr. 1969;74:494-504.

482. Neufeld EJ, Fleming JC, Tartaglini E, Steinkamp MP. Thiamine-responsive megaloblastic anemia syndrome: a disorder of high-affinity thiamine transport. Blood Cells Mol Dis. 2001;27:135-138.

483. Fleming JC, Tartaglini E, Steinkamp MP, et al. The gene mutated in thiamine-responsive anaemia with diabetes and deafness (TRMA) encodes a functional thiamine transporter. Nat Genet. 1999;22:305-308.

484. Labay V, Raz T, Baron D, et al. Mutations in SLC19A2 cause thiamine-responsive megaloblastic anaemia associated with diabetes mellitus and deafness. Nat Genet. 1999;22:300-304.

485. Diaz GA, Banikazemi M, Oishi K, et al. Mutations in a new gene encoding a thiamine transporter cause thiamine-responsive megaloblastic anaemia syndrome. Nat Genet. 1999;22:309-312.

486. Dutta B, Huang W, Molero M, et al. Cloning of the human thiamine transporter, a member of the folate transporter family. J Biol Chem. 1999;274:31925-31929.

487. Stagg AR, Fleming JC, Baker MA, et al. Defective high-affinity thiamine transporter leads to cell death in thiamine-responsive megaloblastic anemia syndrome fibroblasts. J Clin Invest. 1999;103:723-729.

488. Boros LG, Steinkamp MP, Fleming JC, et al. Defective RNA ribose synthesis in fibroblasts from patients with thiamine-responsive megaloblastic anemia (TRMA). Blood. 2003;102:3556-3561.

489. Abboud MR, Alexander D, Najjar SS. Diabetes mellitus, thiamine-dependent megaloblastic anemia, and sensorineural deafness associated with deficient alpha-ketoglutarate dehydrogenase activity. J Pediatr. 1985;107:537-541.

490. Borgna-Pignatti C, Marradi P, Pinelli L, et al. Thiamine-responsive anemia in DIDMOAD syndrome. J Pediatr. 1989;114:405-410.

491. Pearson HA, Lobel JS, Kocoshis SA, et al. A new syndrome of refractory sideroblastic anemia with vacuolization of marrow precursors and exocrine pancreatic dysfunction. J Pediatr. 1979;95:976-984.

492. Stoddard RA, McCurnin DC, Shultenover SJ, et al. Syndrome of refractory sideroblastic anemia with vacuolization of marrow precursors and exocrine pancreatic dysfunction presenting in the neonate. J Pediatr. 1981;99:259-261.

493. McShane MA, Hammans SR, Sweeney M, et al. Pearson syndrome and mitochondrial encephalomyopathy in a patient with a deletion of mtDNA. Am J Hum Genet. 1991;48:39-42.

494. Rotig A, Cormier V, Blanche S, et al. Pearson's marrow-pancreas syndrome. A multisystem mitochondrial disorder in infancy. J Clin Invest. 1990;86:1601-1608.

495. Bykhovskaya Y, Casas K, Mengesha E, et al. Missense mutation in pseudouridine synthase 1 (PUS1) causes mitochondrial myopathy and sideroblastic anemia (MLASA). Am J Hum Genet. 2004;74:1303-1308.

496. Bykhovskaya Y, Mengesha E, Fischel-Ghodsian N. Pleiotropic effects and compensation mechanisms determine tissue specificity in mitochondrial myopathy and sideroblastic anemia (MLASA). Mol Genet Metab. 2007;91:148-156.

497. Casas KA, Fischel-Ghodsian N. Mitochondrial myopathy and sideroblastic anemia. Am J Med Genet A. 2004;125:201-204.

498. Fernandez-Vizarra E, Berardinelli A, Valente L, et al. Nonsense mutation in pseudouridylate synthase 1 (PUS1) in two brothers affected by myopathy, lactic acidosis and sideroblastic anaemia (MLASA). J Med Genet. 2007;44:173-180.

499. Patton JR, Bykhovskaya Y, Mengesha E, et al. Mitochondrial myopathy and sideroblastic anemia (MLASA): missense mutation in the pseudouridine synthase 1 (PUS1) gene is associated with the loss of tRNA pseudouridylation. J Biol Chem. 2005;280:19823-19828.

500. Zeharia A, Fischel-Ghodsian N, Casas K, et al. Mitochondrial myopathy, sideroblastic anemia, and lactic acidosis: an autosomal recessive syndrome in Persian Jews caused by a mutation in the PUS1 gene. J Child Neurol. 2005;20:449-452.

501. Ammus S, Yunis AA. Drug-induced red cell dyscrasias. Blood Rev. 1989;3:71-82.

502. Lubran MM. Lead toxicity and heme biosynthesis. Ann Clin Lab Sci. 1980;10:402-413.

503. Haden HT. Pyridoxine-responsive sideroblastic anemia due to antituberculous drugs. Arch Intern Med. 1967;120:602-606.

504. Tomkin GH. Isoniazid as a cause of neuropathy and sideroblastic anaemia. Practitioner. 1973;211:773-777.

505. Niemeyer CM, Baumann I. Myelodysplastic syndrome in children and adolescents. Semin Hematol. 2008;45:60-70.

506. Nearman ZP, Szpurka H, Serio B, et al. Hemochromatosis-associated gene mutations in patients with myelodysplastic syndromes with refractory anemia with ringed sideroblasts. Am J Hematol. 2007;82:1076-1079.

507. Gatterman N, Retzlaff S, Wang Y-L, et al. Heteroplasmic point mutations of mitochondrial DNA affecting subunit I of cytochrome c oxidase in two patients with acquired idiopathic sideroblastic anemia. Blood. 1997;90:4961-4972.

508. Salmenperä L, Perheentupa J, Pakarinen P, Siimes MA. Cu nutrition in infants during prolonged exclusive breast-feeding: low intake by rising serum concentrations of Cu and ceruloplasmin. Am J Clin Nutr. 1986;43:251.

509. Danks DM. Copper deficiency in humans. Annu Rev Nutr. 1988;8:235.

510. Williams DM. Copper deficiency in humans. Semin Hematol. 1983;20:118.

511. Wijmenga C, Klomp LW. Molecular regulation of copper excretion in the liver. Proc Nutr Soc. 2004;63:31-39.

512. Yoshida K, Furihata K, Takeda S, et al. A mutation in the ceruloplasmin gene is associated with systemic hemosiderosis in humans. Nat Genet. 1995;9:267-272.

513. Harris ZL, Takahashi Y, Miyajima H, et al. Aceruloplasminemia: molecular characterization of this disorder of iron metabolism. Proc Natl Acad Sci U S A. 1995;92:2539-2543.

514. Okamoto N, Wada S, Oga T, et al. Hereditary ceruloplasmin deficiency with hemosiderosis. Hum Genet. 1996;97:755-758.

515. Takahashi Y, Miyajima H, Shirabe S, et al. Characterization of a nonsense mutation in the ceruloplasmin gene

resulting in diabetes and neurodegenerative disease. Hum Mol Genet. 1996;5:81-84.

516. Kim BE, Nevitt T, Thiele DJ. Mechanisms for copper acquisition, distribution and regulation. Nat Chem Biol. 2008;4:176-185.

517. Kuo Y-M, Zhou B, Cosco D, Gitschier J. The copper transporter CTR1 provides an essential function in mammalian embryonic development. Proc Natl Acad Sci U S A. 2001;98:6836-6841.

518. Lee J, Prohaska JR, Thiele DJ. Essential role for mammalian copper transporter Ctr1 in copper homeostasis and embryonic development. Proc Natl Acad Sci U S A. 2001;98:6842-6847.

519. Andrews NC. Mining copper transport genes. Proc Natl Acad Sci U S A. 2001;98:6543-6545.

520. Culotta VC, Lin SJ, Schmidt P, et al. Intracellular pathways of copper trafficking in yeast and humans. Adv Exp Med Biol. 1999;448:247-254.

521. Rosenzweig AC, O'Halloran TV. Structure and chemistry of the copper chaperone proteins. Curr Opin Chem Biol. 2000;4:140-147.

522. Hamza I, Faisst A, Prohaska J, et al. The metallochaperone Atox1 plays a critical role in perinatal copper homeostasis. Proc Natl Acad Sci U S A. 2001;98:6848-6852.

523. Menkes JH, Alter M, Steigleder GK, et al. A sex-linked recessive disorder with retardation of growth, peculiar hair and focal cerebral and cerebellar degeneration. Pediatrics. 1962;29:764-779.

524. Bull PC, Thomas GR, Rommens JM, et al. The Wilson's disease gene is a putative copper transporting P-type ATPase similar to the Menkes gene. Nat Genet. 1993; 5:327-337.

525. Chelly J, Tumer S, Tonnesen T, et al. Isolation of a candidate gene for Menkes disease that encodes a potential heavy metal binding protein. Nat Genet. 1993;3:14-19.

526. Mercer JF, Livingston J, Hall B, et al. Isolation of a partial candidate gene for Menkes disease by positional cloning. Nat Genet. 1993;3:20-25.

527. Vulpe C, Levinson B, Whitney S, et al. Isolation of a candidate gene for Menkes disease and evidence that it encodes a copper-transporting ATPase. Nat Genet. 1993; 3:7-13.

528. Yamaguchi Y, Heiny ME, Gitlin JD. Isolation and characterization of a human liver cDNA as a candidate gene for Wilson's disease. Biochem Biophys Res Commun. 1993;197:271-277.

529. Tanzi RE, Petrukhin K, Chernov I, et al. The Wilson's disease gene is a copper transporting ATPase with homology to the Menkes disease gene. Nat Genet. 1993;5:344-350.

530. Walia BN, Singh S, Marwaha RK, et al. Fulminant hepatic failure and acute intravascular haemolysis as presenting manifestations of Wilson's disease in young children. J Gastroenterol Hepatol. 1992;7:370-373.

531. Kraut JR, Yogev R. Fatal fulminant hepatitis with hemolysis in Wilson's disease. Criteria for diagnosis. Clin Pediatr (Phila). 1984;23:637-640.

532. Gubler CJ, Lahey ME, Chase MS, et al. Studies on copper metabolism. III. The metabolism of iron in copper deficient swine. Blood. 1952;7:1075.

533. Lahey ME, Gubler CJ, Chase MS, et al. Studies on copper metabolism. II. Hematologic manifestations of copper deficiency in swine. Blood. 1952;7:1053.

534. Cartwright GE, Gubler CJ, Bush JA, Wintrobe MM. Studies on copper metabolism. XVII. Further observations on the anemia of copper deficiency in swine. Blood. 1956;11:143.

535. Lee GR, Nacht S, Lukens JN, Cartwright GE. Iron metabolism in copper-deficient swine. J Clin Invest. 1968;47:2058-2069.

536. Levy Y, Zeharia A, Grunebaum M, et al. Copper deficiency in infants fed cow milk. J Pediatr. 1985;106:786-788.

537. Castillo-Duran C, Uauy R. Copper deficiency impairs growth of infants recovering from malnutrition. Am J Clin Nutr. 1988;47:710.

538. Celsing F, Blomstrand E, Werner B, et al. Effects of iron deficiency on endurance and muscle enzyme activity in man. Med Sci Sports Exerc. 1986;18:156-161.

539. Goyens P, Brasseur D, Cadranel S, et al. Copper deficiency in infants with active celiac disease. J Pediatr Gastroenterol Nutr. 1985;4:677-680.

540. Yuzbasiyan-Gurkan V, Grider A, Nostrant T, et al. Treatment of Wilson's disease with zinc: X. Intestinal metallothionein induction. Lab Clin Med 1992;120:380-386.

541. Haddad AS, Subbiah V, Lichtin AE, et al. Hypocupremia and bone marrow failure. Haematologica. 2008;93:e1-e5.

542. Lin-Fu JS. Vulnerability of children to lead exposure and toxicity (first of two parts). N Engl J Med. 1973;289:1229-1233.

543. Knelson JH. Problem of estimating respiratory lead dose in children. Environ Health Perspect. 1974;7:53-57.

544. Mahaffey KR. Exposure to lead in childhood. The importance of prevention. N Engl J Med. 1992;327:1308-1309.

545. Hamilton S, Rothenberg SJ, Khan FA, et al. Neonatal lead poisoning from maternal pica behavior during pregnancy. J Natl Med Assoc. 2001;93:317-319.

546. Chisolm JJ, Harrison HE. The exposure of children to lead. Pediatrics. 1956;18:943.

547. Sassa S. Toxic effects of lead, with particular reference to porphyrin and heme metabolism. In DeMatteis F, Aldridge W (eds). Handbook of Experimental Pharmacology, New Series, vol 44. Berlin, Springer-Verlag, 1973, p 333.

548. Piomelli S, Seaman C, Kapoor S. Lead-induced abnormalities of porphyrin metabolism. The relationship with iron deficiency. Ann N Y Acad Sci. 1987;514:278.

549. Piomelli S. The diagnostic utility of measurements of erythrocyte porphyrins. Hematol Oncol Clin North Am. 1987;1:419-430.

550. Piomelli S. A micromethod for free erythrocyte porphyrins: the FEP test. J Lab Clin Med. 1973;81:932-940.

551. Bessis MC, Breton-Gorius J. Ferritin and ferruginous micelles in normal erythroblsts and hypochromic hypersideremic anemias. Blood. 1959;14:423.

552. Piomelli S, Lamola AA, Poh-Fitzpatrick MF, et al. Erythropoietic protoporphyria and lead intoxication: the molecular basis for difference in cutaneous photosensitivity. I. Different rates of disappearance of protoporphyrin from the erythrocytes, both in vivo and in vitro. J Clin Invest. 1975;56:1519-1527.

553. Silbergeld EK. Mechanisms of lead neurotoxicity, or looking beyond the lamppost. FASEB J. 1992;6:3201-3206.

554. Byers RK, Lord EE. Late effects of lead poisoning on mental development. Am J Dis Child. 1943;6:471.

555. Chisolm JJ. Aminoaciduria as a manifestation of renal tubular injury in lead intoxication and a comparison with patterns of aminoaciduria sen in other disease. J Pediatr. 1962;60:1.

556. Treatment guidelines for lead exposure in children. American Academy of Pediatrics Committee on Drugs. Pediatrics. 1995;96:155-160.

557. Schwartz J. Low-level lead exposure and children's IQ: a meta-analysis and search for a threshold. Environ Res. 1994;65:42-55.

558. Pocock SJ, Smith M, Baghurst P. Environmental lead and children's intelligence: a systematic review of the epidemiological evidence. BMJ. 1994;309:1189-1197.

559. Piomelli S, Rosen JF, Chisolm JJ Jr, Graef JW. Management of childhood lead poisoning. J Pediatr. 1984; 105:523-532.

560. Rogan WJ, Dietrich KN, Ware JH, et al. The effect of chelation therapy with succimer on neuropsychological development in children exposed to lead. N Engl J Med. 2001;344:1421-1426.

13 The Porphyrias

John D. Phillips and James P. Kushner

The porphyrias are disorders caused by reduced activity of enzymes that constitute the heme biosynthetic pathway. Almost all are inherited. The porphyric disorders, with the exception of porphyria cutanea tarda (PCT), are uncommon, and clinical manifestations in children are quite rare. Porphyrins are planar molecules composed of four pyrrole rings connected by four methene groups and are also referred to as tetrapyrroles (Fig. 13-1A). Porphyrins are intensely colored compounds (the word porphyria is derived from the Greek *porphuros*, meaning red-purple). All porphyrins, because of the alternating single- and double-bond structure of the porphyrin macrocycle, avidly absorb light in a region near 400 nm of the spectrum (the Soret band). Porphyrins also have four minor absorption bands at higher wavelengths. Once excited by light, porphyrins emit photons in the red region of the spectrum, a phenomenon responsible for their fluorescent properties. The emitted photons mediate the skin damage, which occurs in sun-exposed skin in some of the porphyric disorders.

The porphyrin precursors δ-aminolevulinic acid (ALA) and porphobilinogen (PBG) (a monopyrrole) are colorless compounds that do not fluoresce. Recent evidence suggests that these compounds are responsible for the neurovisceral manifestations of several of the porphyric disorders. A convenient classification scheme divides the porphyric disorders into three groups according to their clinical manifestations (Box 13-1). Alternative schemes have been proposed by which the porphyrias are classified according to the organ in which the enzymatic defect is most apparent (hepatic porphyrias versus erythropoietic porphyrias), but these schemes are less useful to the clinician. Most heme synthesis takes place in erythroid precursors and is used for the generation of hemoglobin, but approximately 15% of the daily production takes place in the liver,[1] mainly for the formation of cytochrome P-450 enzymes. Heme is also a component of numerous other cellular proteins, including cytochromes, myoglobin, catalase, peroxidase, guanylate cyclase, and others; the heme biosynthetic pathway is present in all cells.

With the exception of ferrochelatase (FECH), the terminal enzyme in the pathway that catalyzes the insertion of iron into protoporphyrin IX, all enzymes in the pathway that use cyclic tetrapyrroles require fully reduced porphyrinogens as substrates. Porphyrinogens are flexible, colorless, reduced compounds with hydrogen atoms added to each of the bridge carbons and to nitrogens of the pyrrole rings (see Fig. 13-1B). Porphyrinogens are very sensitive to oxidation. When the heme biosynthetic intermediates uroporphyrinogen and coproporphyrinogen are oxidized to the corresponding porphyrins, they can no longer serve as substrates (Fig. 13-2) and are excreted in urine and stool. Protoporphyrinogen oxidase (PPO) also requires the reduced compound protoporphyrinogen as substrate. Nonenzymatic oxidation of the substrate to protoporphyrin results in excretion of protoporphyrin in stool.

Hans Fischer[2] originally developed the porphyrin nomenclature currently used. Protoporphyrin IX was the ninth isomer of protoporphyrin synthesized by Fischer and corresponded to the only isomer of protoporphyrin

| Box 13-1 | **Clinical Classification of the Porphyrias** |

PHOTOSENSITIVITY SYMPTOMS

Congenital erythropoietic porphyria (4)★
Porphyria cutanea tarda (5)†
Hepatoerythropoietic porphyria (5)★
Erythropoietic protoporphyria (8)★

NEUROVISCERAL SYMPTOMS

Aminolevulinate dehydratase porphyria (2)★
Acute intermittent porphyria (3)‡

PHOTOSENSITIVITY AND NEUROVISCERAL SYMPTOMS

Hereditary coproporphyria (6)‡
Variegate porphyria (7)‡

Numbers in parentheses designate the enzymatic defect responsible for the disorder (see Fig. 13-2).

★Clinical manifestations usually recognized in childhood.
†Clinical manifestations rarely recognized in childhood.
‡Clinical manifestations rarely occur before puberty except in children with homozygous or compound heterozygous genotypes.

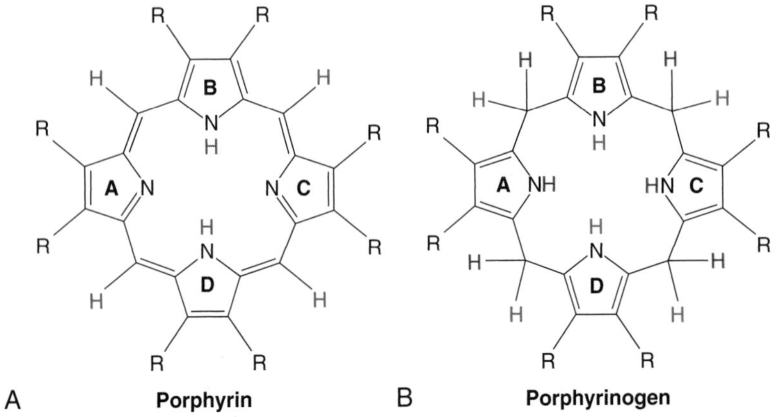

FIGURE 13-1. Porphyrin and porphyrinogens. Porphyrins are tetrapyrroles. **A,** Porphyrins are the oxidized form of porphyrinogens. The alternating single- and double-bond sequence at the periphery of the molecule imparts the color and fluorescent properties of porphyrins and produces a rigid planar shape. **B,** Porphyrinogens, the reduced form, are colorless, do not fluoresce, and are highly flexible.

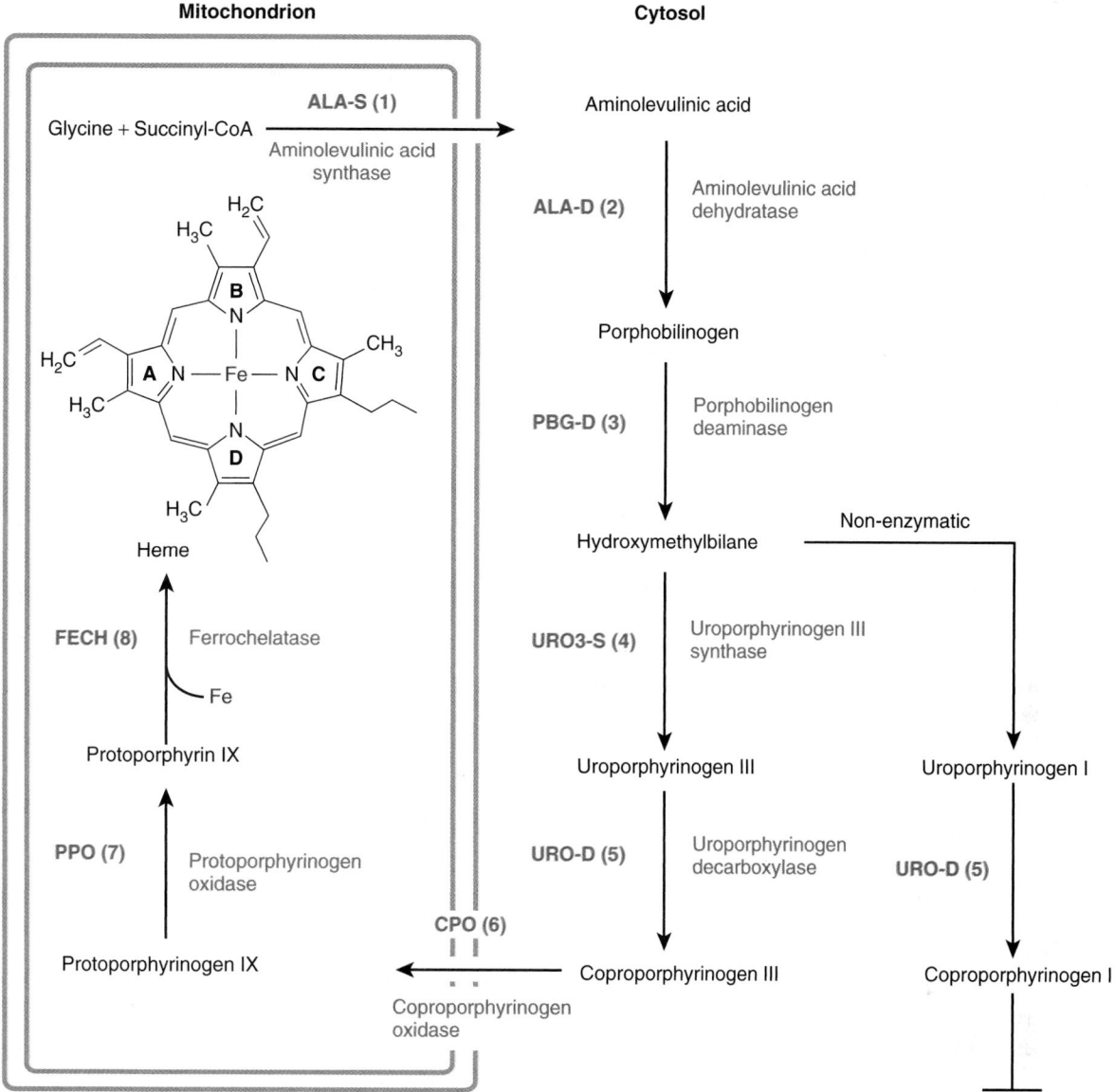

FIGURE 13-2. Heme biosynthetic pathway. The eight enzymes required to synthesize heme are named (*green*). Abbreviations used throughout this chapter are in *blue*. Synthesis starts in mitochondria, depicted by the *double orange line*, continues in the cytosol, and terminates in mitochondria. Enzyme 6, coproporphyrinogen oxidase, is located in the mitochondrial intermembrane space. Enzyme 7, protoporphyrinogen oxidase, is an integral membrane protein located on the outer surface of the inner membrane. Enzyme 8, ferrochelatase, an integral membrane protein, is located on the matrix side of the inner mitochondrial membrane.

found in nature. Uroporphyrinogen and coproporphyrinogen can occur in four isomeric forms, but only the I and III forms occur in nature. The I and III isomers of uroporphyrinogen differ solely in the position of the acetate and propionate side chains on the D ring (see Fig. 13-1), but only the III isomer can ultimately be converted to protoporphyrin IX and heme.

In eukaryotic cells, the heme biosynthetic pathway is divided between three compartments: the mitochondrial matrix, the mitochondrial intermembrane space, and the cytosol (Fig. 13-2). The pathway enzymes have been intensively studied in recent years. All of the genes have been cloned, and mutations responsible for the porphyrias have been identified. The crystal struc-

tures of all the enzymes have been determined, and these structures have provided models for the mechanisms of catalysis and the effects of specific mutations (Table 13-1).

Here, we will dissect the complex heme biosynthetic pathway into four basic processes, and each porphyric disorder will be described in the context of the process that is defective:

1. Formation of the pyrrole
2. Assembly of the tetrapyrrole
3. Modification of the tetrapyrrole side chains
4. Enzymatic oxidation of protoporphyrinogen IX to protoporphyrin IX and insertion of iron

TABLE 13-1	Porphyrias, Causative Genes, Chromosomal Locations and Protein Codes					
Disease	**Gene**	**Location**	**OMIM**	**EC**	**PDB**
None	ALA-S1	3p21.1	125290	2.3.1.37	2BWN*
X-linked sideroblastic anemia	ALA-S2	Xp11.21	301300	2.3.1.37	
Aminolevulinate dehydratase deficiency porphyria	ALA-D	9q34	125270	4.2.1.24	1PV8
Acute intermittent porphyria	PBG-D	11q23.3	609806	4.3.1.8	1PDA*
Congenital erythropoietic porphyria	URO3-S	10q25.2	263700	4.2.1.75	1JR2
Porphyria cutanea tarda	URO-D	1p34	176100	4.1.1.37	1URO
Hereditary coproporphyria	CPO	3q12	121300	1.3.3.3	1R3Q
Variegate porphyria	PPO	1q22	600923	1.3.3.4	1SEZ*
Erythropoietic protoporphyria	FECH	18q21.3	177000	4.99.1.1	2HRC

*Structure of bacterial homologue.
EC, Enzyme Commission number; OMIM, Online Mendelian Inheritance in Man; PDB, Protein Data Base.

FORMATION OF THE PYRROLE

The δ-Aminolevulinate Synthases

Regulatory mechanisms controlling heme synthesis in erythroid precursors and in the liver differ. In the liver, heme biosynthesis must respond rapidly to changing metabolic requirements. In erythroid cells, the pathway is regulated to permit a high steady-state level of heme synthesis, and regulation is tied to the availability of iron. The first and rate-limiting enzyme in the pathway in all cells condenses glycine and succinyl coenzyme A to yield ALA (Fig. 13-3). This highly exergonic reaction occurs in the mitochondrial matrix and involves cleavage of the thioester bond of succinyl coenzyme A. Two ALA synthase (ALA-S) enzymes have evolved to accommodate the requirements of the liver (and other tissues) and the unique demands of the erythron. The first, ALA-S1, is expressed ubiquitously but at very low levels in erythroid precursors. The dominant form of ALA-S in erythroid cells is ALA-S2. The gene encoding ALA-S1 maps to the short arm of chromosome 3,[3] whereas ALA-S2 is encoded on the X-chromosome.[4] The two forms of ALA-S are 62% identical at the amino acid level.[5] Although these two forms of ALA-S are regulated differently, both forms require pyridoxal 5-phosphate (PLP) as a cofactor, and both are expressed as homodimers. Pyridoxine deficiency is therefore associated with hypochromic anemia.

ALA synthases are highly conserved between species, and the crystal structure of a bacterial ALA-S (from *Rhodobacter capsulatus*) has been determined[6] (Fig. 13-4). The crystal structure supports the enzyme mechanism that had been suggested by biochemical studies.[7]

In eukaryotes, both forms of ALA-S are synthesized in the cytosol and then translocated to the mitochondrial matrix, the site of generation of succinyl coenzyme A by the tricarboxylic acid cycle. Both forms contain an amino-terminal mitochondrial targeting sequence that also contains heme binding domains designated as heme regulatory motifs (HRMs).[8] Binding of heme to the HRM inhibits mitochondrial import of both forms of ALA-S, which represents a post-translational point of

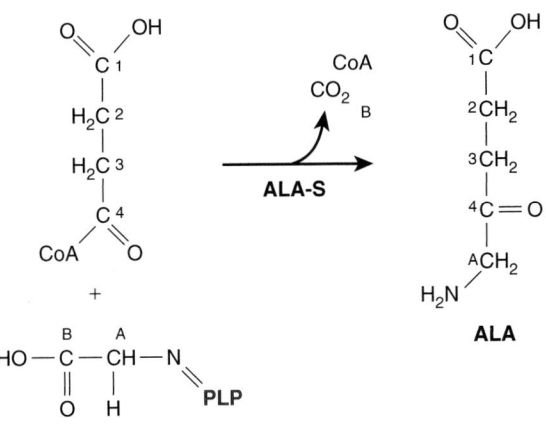

FIGURE 13-3. Synthesis of δ-aminolevulinic acid (ALA). In mitochondria, glycine is decarboxylated after forming a Schiff base with the cofactor pyridoxal phosphate (PLP). The reaction continues by condensation with succinyl coenzyme A (succinyl-CoA), followed by release and recycling of CoA. The origin of the carbon atoms in ALA and CO_2 is indicated with either numbers or letters.

end-product feedback inhibition of the pathway.[9] The effect is greater for ALA-S1 than for ALA-S2. In addition, developing erythroid cells express a heme transporter that prevents the accumulation of unbound heme in the cytosol (FLVCR).[10]

The genes for both ALA-S1 and ALA-S2 are transcriptionally regulated, but by quite different mechanisms. Extensive studies in avian embryonic liver cells indicated that hemin, a chloride salt of heme, represses transcription of ALA-S1,[11] but the precise mechanism responsible for this effect has not been defined. Transcription of ALA-S1 is upregulated by the peroxisomal proliferator–activated receptor γ coactivator 1α (PGC-1α),[12] a coactivator of nuclear receptors and transcription factors.[13] Transcriptional regulation of ALA-S1 by PGC-1α is mediated by the interaction of Nrf-1 (nuclear regulatory factor 1) and FOXO-1 (a forkhead family member) with the ALA-S1 promoter.[14] When cellular glucose levels are low, transcription of PGC-1α is upregulated,[15,16] thereby leading to increased levels of ALA-S1 and creat-

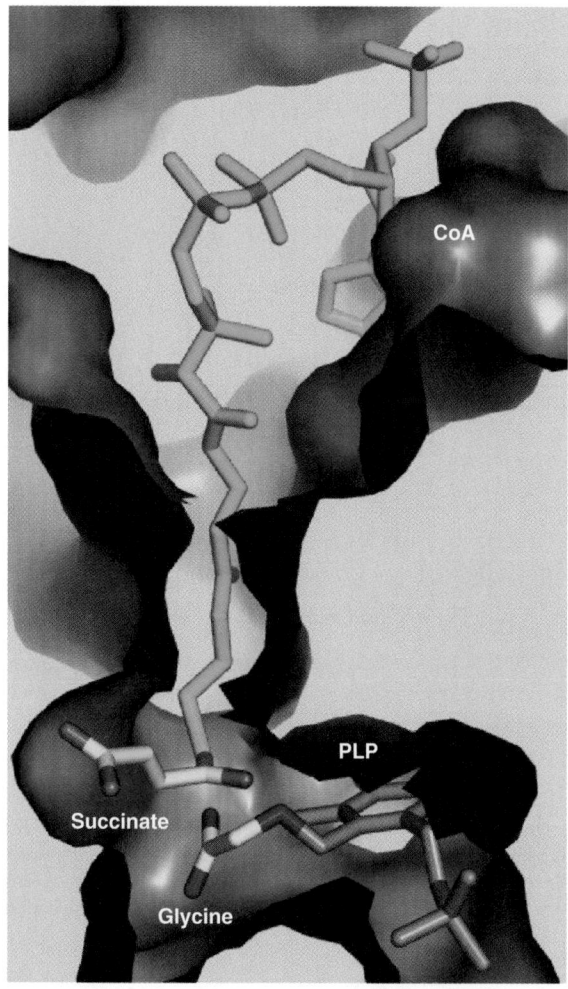

FIGURE 13-4. The active site of aminolevulinate synthase (ALA-S) from *Rhodobacter capsulatus*. Pyridoxal phosphate (PLP, *orange*) forms a covalent linkage with a lysine residue. Glycine is bound through a transient Schiff base with PLP. Condensation with the succinate moiety of succinyl CoA (CoA in *green*) allows the release of CoA, ALA, and PLP. The PLP cofactor is then bound again for subsequent rounds of catalysis. *(Figure based on the coordinates 2BWN, available from the Protein Data Bank.)*

ing conditions capable of precipitating acute attacks of the neurovisceral porphyrias. Upregulation of PGC-1α probably explains the clinical observation that fasting may precipitate attacks whereas glucose infusions are useful therapeutically.[17,18]

There are two alternate splice forms of ALA-S1 in humans. The major form lacks exon 1B (Fig. 13-5) and is destabilized by heme.[19,20] The minor form includes exon 1B and is resistant to heme-mediated destabilization.[21] It is apparent that heme regulates ALA-S1 by multiple mechanisms, including transcription, translation, and translocation of the protein from the cytosol to the mitochondria. The regulatory effects of heme are mediated by the concentration of heme in small "pools" of heme not bound to hemoproteins.[22,23] Factors depleting unbound heme pools result in induction of ALA-S1, an effect that is the prime factor in precipitating acute attacks of the neurovisceral porphyrias. No disease-causing mutations of ALA-S1 have been identified in humans, but downregulation of ALA-S1 by infusion of glucose or hemin (or both) forms the basis of therapy for acute porphyric attacks.[17]

In contrast to ALA-S1, ALA-S2 is transcriptionally regulated by erythroid-specific factors (including GATA1) that interact with promoter sequences found in many genes differentially regulated in red cells.[24] Translational regulation also plays a major role in regulating expression of ALA-S2. The ALA-S2 transcript contains a 5′ iron responsive element (IRE) that interacts with an IRE-binding protein (IRP).[25] The IRE-IRP complex prevents translation of ALA-S2 mRNA. Addition of an iron-sulfur cluster (Fe/S) to IRP1 changes the conformation of the protein and reduces its affinity for IRE. Fe/S clusters are generated and exported by mitochondria, thus linking regulation of heme biosynthesis in the red cell to the availability of iron and mitochondrial function.[26-28] Mutations in ALA-S2 cause X-linked sideroblastic anemia. This disorder and the spectrum of causative ALA-S2 mutations are described in detail in Chapter 12.

δ-Aminolevulinate Dehydratase

Once synthesized, ALA exits mitochondria by an unknown mechanism probably involving a transporter. In the cytosol, two molecules of ALA undergo a condensation reaction catalyzed by aminolevulinate dehydratase (ALA-D, also known porphobilinogen synthase) to form the monopyrrole porphobilinogen (Fig. 13-6). The crystal structure of human ALA-D and ALA-D from many other species indicates that the enzyme functions as a tetramer of homodimers formed from eight identical subunits.[29,30] Each of the homodimers contains one active site.[31] Each of the eight subunits binds a zinc atom, and the enzyme is inactivated by replacement of the zinc with lead, hence the hypochromia of lead poisoning. Four zinc molecules are essential for catalysis. The remaining four zincs serve to stabilize the tertiary structure of the enzyme.[32-34] Each active site binds two molecules of ALA through the formation of Schiff base linkages with active-site lysine residues, one for each of the two substrate molecules. One molecule of ALA contributes the acetate side chain and the aminomethyl groups of PBG. The other contributes the propionate side chain and the pyrrole nitrogen (Fig. 13-6).

In contrast to ALA-S, there is a single ALA-D gene located on chromosome 9q34[34a] (see Table 13-1). The gene consists of two alternatively spliced noncoding exons (1A and 1B) and 11 coding exons[34b] (see Fig. 13-5). The translational start site is located in exon 2. A housekeeping promoter is located upstream of exon 1A, and a second erythroid-specific promoter is located between exons 1A and 1B. The erythroid promoter contains binding sites for erythroid-specific transcription factors, including GATA1.[34b] Although the housekeeping and erythroid transcripts differ, they both encode identical proteins because they share the same translational start site in exon 2.

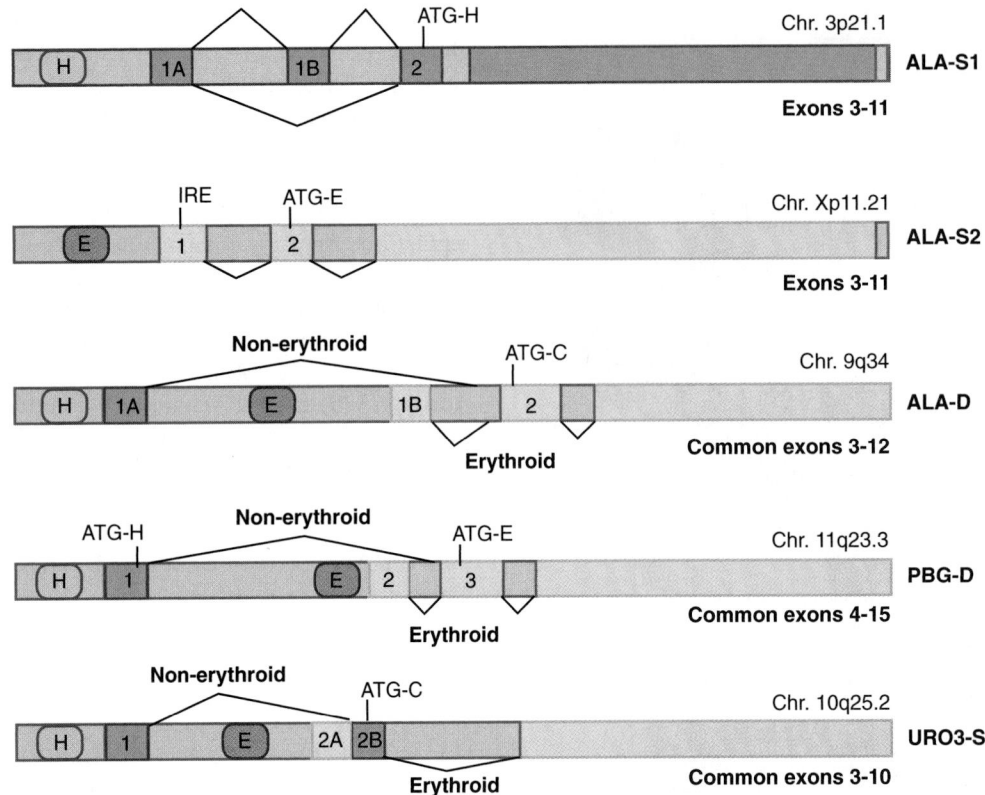

FIGURE 13-5. Genomic organization of the promoters for early steps in heme synthesis. Chr., chromosomal location for the gene. Two distinct genes encode aminolevulinate synthase (ALA-S), a housekeeping form (ALA-S1) and an erythroid-specific form (ALA-S2). An iron regulatory element (IRE) in exon 1 of ALA-S2 controls post-transcriptional gene expression. The next three genes use specific promoters for erythroid (E) or nonerythroid tissues (H). The ATG start sites are designated: C, common; E, erythroid; H, housekeeping. ALA-D, aminolevulinate dehydratase; PBG-D, porphobilinogen deaminase; URO3-S, uroporphyrinogen III synthase.

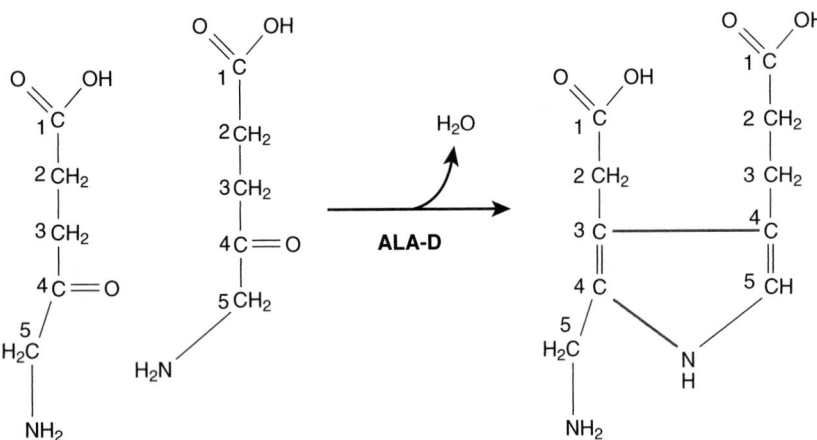

FIGURE 13-6. Reaction catalyzed by aminolevulinate dehydratase (ALA-D). In the cytosol, two molecules of δ-aminolevulinic acid (ALA) condense to form porphobilinogen. The carbon atoms of each molecule of ALA are numbered for reference.

A common polymorphism of ALA-D, K59N,[35] has been detected in approximately 10% of white individuals,[36,37] 3% of African Americans,[36] and 6% to 11% of Asians.[37] This polymorphism has been designated the ALA-D2 allele. The ALA-D2 allele retains normal enzyme activity and appears to have higher affinity for both zinc and lead than the ALA-D1 allele does.[38] Lead entering plasma is rapidly taken up by red cells and binds to ALA-D by displacing zinc and inactivating the enzyme.[39] Multiple studies have shown an association between the ALA-D2 allele and high blood lead levels,[36,38] but it

remains unclear whether this allele is associated with increased susceptibility or increased resistance to lead toxicity.[39]

Although the quaternary structure of human ALA-D is that of a homo-octamer, recent studies have also detected a homohexamer form of ALA-D composed of three homodimers. The homohexamer has low enzyme activity. The octameric and hexameric forms of ALA-D are described as morpheeins, which indicates that dissociation of the high-activity octamer is followed by a conformational change and then reassembly as the structurally different low-activity hexamer. Conformational changes in the component dimers may result from substrate binding, but the most dramatic effects result from ALA-D mutations causing ALA-D porphyria.

In all tissues the enzymatic activity of ALA-D greatly exceeds the activity of ALA-S. The abundance of ALA-D in comparison to all of the heme biosynthetic enzymes has been ascribed to the finding that ALA-D plays several roles: it serves as a proteasome inhibitor affecting the adenosine triphosphate (ATP)/ubiquitin-dependent degradation of proteins, plays a role in chaperone-assisted protein folding, and is an enzyme in the heme biosynthetic pathway.[40]

Aminolevulinate Dehydratase Deficiency Porphyria

ALA-D deficiency porphyria (ADP) is caused by homozygosity or compound heterozygosity for mutations of the ALA-D gene.

Frequency. ADP is an autosomal recessive disorder resulting from loss-of-function mutations of ALA-D. The disorder is exceedingly rare, and fewer than 10 cases have been reported, 2 in one family.[41] Most of the cases have represented compound heterozygotes. Eleven disease-causing ALA-D mutations have been described, 10 of which are point mutations leading to amino acid substitutions.[42,43] The sole exception is the deletion of two sequential bases resulting in a frameshift yielding a premature stop codon.[44] Estimates of the frequency of heterozygosity for loss-of-function alleles of ALA-D, based on half-normal or less enzyme activity in the erythrocytes of asymptomatic northern Europeans, range from 1% to 2%.[45,46] The extreme rarity of homozygosity or compound heterozygosity for ALA-D mutations suggests a high incidence of embryonic lethality when two mutant alleles of ALA-D are present.

Clinical Manifestations. The clinical manifestations of ADP resemble those of the neurovisceral porphyrias but vary greatly in severity. The first two cases reported by Doss and colleagues[47,48] in Germany involved unrelated 15-year-old boys. Both suffered recurrent attacks of abdominal pain, nausea, vomiting, constipation, tachycardia, and a motor neuropathy causing paralysis. In a third German patient reported by Doss and associates,[49] symptoms also developed at age 15, including abdominal pain and a severe polyneuropathy. All three German patients were compound heterozygotes for ALA-D mutations.

The youngest reported patient with ADP was a Swedish boy in whom muscle hypotonia was recognized at birth. At the age of 3 years, recurrent attacks of abdominal pain, vomiting, and motor polyneuropathy developed. This child also proved to be a compound heterozygote for ALA-D mutations.[50] A liver transplant was performed at the age of 6 under the assumption that the metabolic defect was most profound in the liver. No

change in excretion of ALA was observed after the transplant, thus strongly suggesting that red cells were the major source of this porphyrin precursor. The child died at the age of 9 of pneumonia and respiratory deficiency.[51]

The oldest reported patient with ADP was a Belgian man in whom a motor neuropathy and markedly increased urinary excretion of ALA developed at the age of 63.[52] ALA-D activity in his erythrocytes was dramatically reduced to 1% of normal controls. The syndrome developed together with a clonal myeloproliferative disorder, namely, polycythemia vera. Molecular studies revealed heterozygosity for a loss-of-function mutation (G133R) present in the polycythemia clone that became clinically manifested with clonal expansion.[53] This represents the only case in which a fully penetrant phenotype occurred in a heterozygote.

In two other cases, partial biochemical evidence of ALA-D deficiency was detected in heterozygotes, but by a completely different mechanism. The first was a healthy Swedish newborn undergoing neonatal screening for hereditary tyrosinemia.[54] Erythrocyte ALA-D activity was 12% of normal, and there were slight elevations in urinary ALA and coproporphyrin, as well as an increase in erythrocyte protoporphyrin. The child proved to be heterozygous for an F12L mutation, a catalytically inactive mutant that also affects the secondary structure of the protein and favors the formation of (with wild-type protein) the low-activity hexameric form of ALA-D.[43,55] Despite the ALA-D defect, the child remained healthy and developed normally.

The second case of partial biochemical expression in a heterozygous ALA-D mutant occurred in a 23-year-old American man and was also due to the F12L mutation.[56] This patient had an acute porphyric attack that was clinically and biochemically compatible with hereditary coproporphyria (HCP). Indeed, a mutation of coproporphyrinogen oxidase (CPO) was identified. Because of a greater than usual increase in urinary ALA excretion and an increase in erythrocyte zinc protoporphyrin, an additional defect in ALA-D was suspected. Subnormal erythrocyte ALA-D activity was detected, and molecular studies revealed heterozygosity for the F12L mutation.

Pathogenesis. The pathogenesis of the symptom complex associated with ADP is poorly understood. It has been suggested that ALA may act as a neurotoxin based on structural similarities between ALA and glutamate and ALA and γ-aminobutyric acid (GABA).[57] High concentrations of ALA may interact with GABA receptors or inhibit uptake of glutamate. ALA has been demonstrated to bind to GABA receptors in vitro, and GABA receptors are highly expressed by oligodendrocytes.[58] In addition, oligodendrocytes are highly sensitive to glutamate-dependent metabolic pathways, which could be impaired by the effect of ALA on glutamate uptake.[59] A possible role for ALA as a neurotoxin is supported in patients with hereditary tyrosinemia, who exhibit neurovisceral symptoms associated with marked inhibition of ALA-D by succinylacetone[60] (see later).

Laboratory Diagnosis. Although ADP is rare, it should be suspected when an acute attack of abdominal pain suggests the possibility of a porphyric attack, especially when a prominent distal motor neuropathy is present. The dramatic reduction in ALA-D activity (to levels of 5% or less) results in the urinary excretion of large amounts of ALA and normal or minimally increased levels of PBG, a finding that distinguishes ADP from other neurovisceral porphyrias. Urinary excretion of coproporphyrin is markedly increased. The mechanism responsible for the increase in urinary excretion of coproporphyrin is not known, but similar findings occur when ALA-D is inhibited in lead poisoning and when ALA is administered orally to normal individuals.[61] Zinc protoporphyrin accumulates in erythrocytes in patients with ADP, again by a poorly understood mechanism.

Heterozygous parents and siblings of probands with ADP have approximately half-normal ALA-D activity as measured in red cell lysates. Erythrocyte ALA-D assays are available in reference laboratories in the United States and Europe. Gene sequencing is available for mutation analysis of ALA-D through the Department of Human Genetics at the Mount Sinai School of Medicine in New York.

It is important to emphasize that ALA-D activity can be subnormal in disorders other than ADP. Patients with lead poisoning often exhibit clinical signs and symptoms similar to those found in patients with ADP and other neurovisceral porphyrias. Lead in plasma is taken up by red cells and inhibits ALA-D activity by displacing zinc atoms from the enzyme.[39] The result is excess ALA in blood and urine, excess urinary excretion of coproporphyrin, and accumulation of zinc protoporphyrin in erythrocytes, findings also associated with ADP. The abnormal accumulation and excretion of porphyrins may be due, in part, to inhibitory effects of lead on CPO and FECH[62] but are more likely due to disposition of the excess ALA, as occurs in ADP. Lead poisoning can be distinguished from ADP by measuring the blood lead level.

Patients with hepatorenal tyrosinemia type I, an autosomal recessive disorder caused by deficiency of fumarylacetoacetate hydrolase (FAH), manifest acute episodes of porphyric-like neurologic crises and secrete large amounts of ALA in urine.[63] The FAH defect results in the generation of succinylacetone, a structural analogue of ALA and a potent inhibitor of ALA-D.[64]

A single patient with an acquired reversible, unidentified inhibitor of ALA-D, high urinary ALA levels, and a porphyria-like acute attack has been reported.[65] In addition, both styrene and bromobenzene have been shown to inhibit ALA-D in rats.[66,67] Humans exposed to these compounds have moderately decreased erythrocyte ALA-D activity but do not suffer clinical consequences.

ADP is a rare disorder that must be differentiated from other causes of ALA-D deficiency. Biochemical and molecular evidence is essential to establish the diagnosis of ADP.

Treatment. Clear recommendations for the treatment of ADP are difficult because the number of reported cases is small and the results of therapy have been variable. Suppression of ALA-S1 by the infusion of heme (heme arginate) proved effective in three German patients (all adolescent boys),[48,49] and infusions of glucose, narcotic analgesics, and hemin were effective in a 14-year-old American boy.[42] Hemin infusion proved ineffective in a Swedish infant.[50] The Swedish child underwent liver transplantation at the age of 7,[68] but there were few biochemical or clinical changes. The findings in the Swedish infant suggest that the main source of excess ALA was the erythron.

Avoidance of drugs known to induce acute attacks in other neurovisceral porphyrias, generally by depleting hepatic heme pools and inducing ALA-S1, is suggested but has not been proved to be useful.

ASSEMBLY OF THE TETRAPYRROLE

Porphobilinogen Deaminase

A polymer of four molecules of PBG is generated by porphobilinogen deaminase (PBG-D, a.k.a. hydroxymethylbilane synthase), a cytosolic enzyme. The polymer, an unstable tetrapyrrole, is designated hydroxymethylbilane (HMB) (Fig. 13-7). PBG-D functions as a monomer, and the crystal structure of the enzyme from several sources has been determined.[69] Purification of PBG-D from both mammals and bacteria has yielded an enzyme with a dipyrrole (dipyromethane) in the active site. The dipyrrole serves as a cofactor and is required for enzyme activity. A novel mechanism has been proposed to explain how PBG-D acquires the dipyrrole.[70] PBG-D first binds HMB and then deaminates and polymerizes two additional molecules of PBG to form a hexapyrrole. The distal tetrapyrrole is cleaved and released as HMB. The proximal dipyrrole remains covalently bound through a thioester linkage and serves as the cofactor for subsequent rounds of catalysis[71] (Fig. 13-8). The source of the first HMB molecule to bind to PBG-D remains unexplained. Polymers of PBG can be formed nonenzymatically,[72] but incubation of apo–PBG-D with PBG yields very little holoenzyme with the dipyrrole cofactor bound.[73] It seems likely that the sequence of events involves nonenzymatic condensation of four molecules of PBG to form the aminomethylbilane, which interact with PBG-D. Though a poor substrate, aminomethylbilane is deaminated to form HMB, which is capable of forming a covalent thioester bond with PBG-D leading to assembly of the initial hexapyrrole.[70]

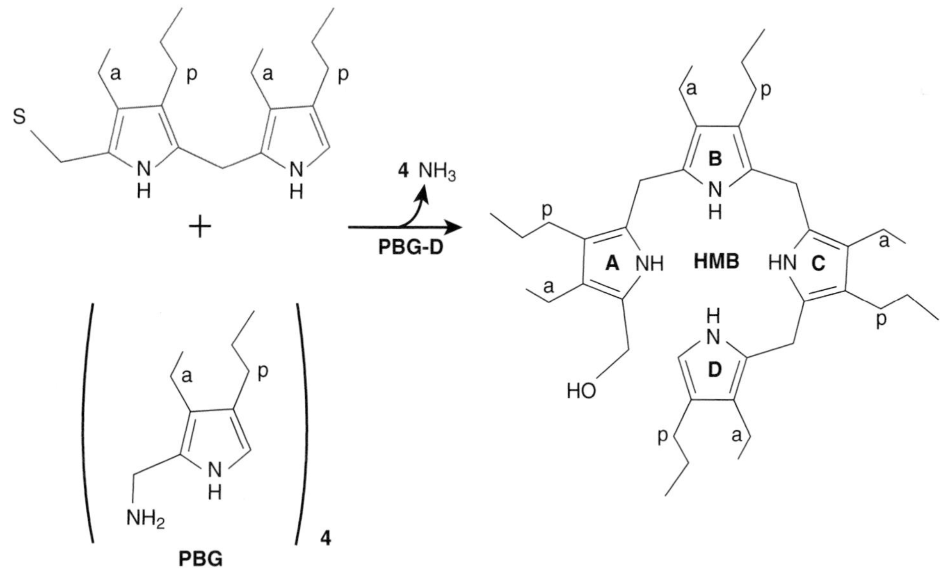

FIGURE 13-7. Reaction catalyzed by porphobilinogen deaminase (PBG-D). A dipyrrole cofactor, dipyromethane (*red*), is covalently linked to the enzyme via a thioester bond. Four molecules of PBG are added, each releasing an amino group. Once a hexapyrrole has been formed, the terminal tetrapyrrole is cleaved and released as hydroxymethyl-bilane (HMB). The acetate (a) and propionate (p) side chains of the mono-pyrroles are labeled.

The human PBG-D gene has been cloned and mapped to chromosome 11q23-11qter.[74,75] The gene spans 10 kilobases (kb) and contains 15 exons.[76] Two separate promoters control transcription and allow tissue-specific regulation of gene expression, a mechanism also used by ALA-D and uroporphyrinogen III synthase (URO3-S) (see Fig. 13-5). The housekeeping promoter lies upstream of exon 1 and is active in all tissues. The erythroid-specific promoter lies upstream of exon 2 and resembles other erythroid-specific promoters.[77] Processing of the transcript initiated by the housekeeping promoter results in splicing of exon 1 to exon 3 and loss of exon 2. Transcription initiated by the erythroid promoter results in a transcript containing exons 2 through 15. Translation of erythroid mRNA is initiated at an AUG located in exon 3 because exon 2 lacks an AUG codon.[76] The AUG translational start codon in exon 1 of the housekeeping transcript is spliced in frame with the AUG in exon 3, thereby resulting in a protein 17 amino acids longer at the amino-terminus than the erythroid protein.[78]

Acute Intermittent Porphyria

Acute intermittent porphyria (AIP) is caused by mutations of the PBG-D gene. More than 300 PBG-D mutations have been described.[79] The spectrum of mutations includes point mutations, deletions, duplications, and insertions, and they have been found in the housekeeping promoter, in exons 1 and 3 through 15, and in each of the 14 introns. Exon 12 appears to be a mutational hot spot with 46 identified mutations.[79]

Frequency. AIP is transmitted as an autosomal dominant trait, although occasional homozygotes or compound heterozygotes have been reported.[57,80-83] AIP is the most common of the acute neurovisceral porphyrias, but estimates of prevalence vary according to the screening method used (clinical manifestations, erythrocyte PBG-

D assays, molecular methods). Prevalence estimates based on clinical diagnoses range from 3 to 5 per 100,000 in Finland, Australia, and the United States.[84,85] Estimates of prevalence in Sweden are higher at 1 in 10,000, mainly because of a founder effect in northern Sweden.[86] When subnormal erythrocyte PBG-D activity is used for screening, the incidence of AIP in European populations is as high as 20 to 200 per 100,000.[87,88] Estimates based on erythrocyte PBG-D activity must be interpreted with caution because the normal range is wide, with considerable overlap between low-normal and high-activity carrier values. Additionally, improper sample processing, storage, and shipping lead to decreased enzymatic activity.[17] Molecular screening for PBG-D mutations on a large scale in a general population has not been done. It is likely that the prevalence of undetected gene carriers in the population may be high because most gene carriers remain free of symptoms throughout their lives and only 10% to 20% experience acute attacks.[89] In all series, clinical symptoms occur more commonly in women than men.

Clinical Manifestations. Clinical manifestations of AIP may occur before puberty in homozygotes or compound heterozygotes for PBG-D mutations, but most cases occur after puberty.[80,82,83,90] Pediatricians are likely to encounter adolescent patients with symptomatic AIP, particularly adolescent girls after menarche. Virtually all of the clinical signs and symptoms that characterize attacks of AIP are due to neurovisceral dysfunction (Table 13-2). Diffuse abdominal pain, often accompanied by nausea, vomiting, abdominal distention, and constipation, is the most common symptom of an acute attack.[85,91-95] The abdominal pain is usually unremitting and severe but may occasionally be cramping. Decreased bowel sounds and even signs of ileus are generally present, although some attacks may be associated with enhanced gut motility and diarrhea. Tachycardia is present in up to

TABLE 13-2   Signs and Symptoms of an Acute Porphyric Attack

Signs and Symptoms	Frequency*	Comments
GASTROINTESTINAL		
Abdominal pain	Common	Generally constant and not localized
Nausea and vomiting	Common	Accompanies abdominal pain
Constipation	Common	Urinary retention may occur also
Diarrhea	Uncommon	
NEUROLOGIC		
Pain in the back, chest, neck, head, extremities	Occasional	Pain may migrate to the abdomen. May be accompanied by a sensory neuropathy
Paresis	Common	More proximal than distal. Arms involved more often than the legs
Respiratory paralysis	Uncommon	Occurs with progressive motor neuropathy and paresis
Mental symptoms	Occasional	Ranges from agitation to psychosis
Convulsions	Uncommon	Mainly occurs with hyponatremia
CARDIOVASCULAR		
Tachycardia	Common	Rate control with β-blockers may be needed
Systemic arterial hypertension	Occasional	May become chronic and affect renal function

*Common, greater than 61%; occasional, 21% to 60%; uncommon, less than 20%.

80% of attacks,[94] but in some series the frequency is as low as 37%.[91] Other symptoms secondary to sympathetic overactivity or autonomic neuropathy include hypertension, tremors, sweating, and restlessness. Anxiety is a particularly common symptom, both during acute attacks and between attacks.[96] A variety of other neuropsychiatric symptoms associated with AIP ranging from hypomania to overt psychotic behavior have been described,[97-99] and psychiatric symptoms may be the only manifestation of biochemically evident AIP.[100,101]

Peripheral neuropathy may occur with or without an acute attack of abdominal pain. The neuropathy, caused by axonal degeneration, is manifested mainly as muscle weakness in the extremities.[102] Nerve conduction abnormalities may be minor, even with symptomatic weakness, but sophisticated studies of slow motor fiber conduction have been abnormal, even in the absence of symptoms.[103,104] Cranial neuropathies are uncommon, although blindness secondary to optic nerve involvement or occipital lobe involvement has been reported.[105,106]

Seizures may occur during an acute attack and are often associated with hyponatremia.[107] When serum sodium levels are normal, it is difficult to determine whether the seizure is due to porphyria or to coexistent idiopathic epilepsy. In a large study including 268 patients, the lifetime prevalence of seizures was 5.1% in those who had suffered at least one acute attack and 2.2% in known carriers.[107] Seizures occurring during latent periods are likely to be related to AIP. It is essential to establish a firm diagnosis of idiopathic epilepsy in patients with AIP who experience seizures because many antiseizure medications may precipitate acute attacks (see later). If seizures are associated with the hyponatremia of an acute attack, prolonged antiseizure therapy is not necessary.

Hyponatremia is a common finding during acute attacks.[91,108] Hyponatremia may be due to inappropriate secretion of antidiuretic hormone,[109] but renal salt wasting has been implicated in patients with the lowest serum sodium levels.[91] Serum sodium values below 120 nmol/L are generally found only in severe attacks.[110]

The likelihood of full recovery after an acute attack has increased dramatically over the last 25 years, undoubtedly because of the introduction of effective therapy with hemin or heme arginate (see later). The risk of death, however, has not been eliminated. A review of 136 patients hospitalized with acute attacks at the University of Minnesota between 1940 and 1998 (i.e., both before and after the introduction of hemin therapy) found that 29 (21%) had died during an acute attack.[111] In a study from Finland and Russia, 7 of 55 patients (13%) died as the result of an acute attack between 1966 and 2002 (hematin therapy was first used in 1971[112] but was not widely used until 1978[113,114]). In another study of 47 Finnish patients ascertained between 1967 and 1989, six deaths (12.8%) occurred as the result of an acute attack.[89]

Pathogenesis. Heterozygotes for PBG-D mutations have approximately half-normal enzyme activity in all tissues, which is usually sufficient for heme homeostasis. The enzymatic defect becomes manifested when demand for hepatic heme is increased and ALA-S1 is induced. The result is increased production of ALA and PBG, which creates a situation in which the half-normal activity of PBG-D becomes rate limiting and PBG (and ALA) accumulate in hepatocytes, circulate in plasma, and are excreted in urine. Drugs are the most commonly recognized factors that increase the demand for hepatic heme, especially those metabolized by hemoprotein enzymes of the cytochrome P-450 family. Barbiturates, anticonvulsants, and steroid hormones are well-recognized precipitating factors in patients with AIP, but other factors not

Box 13-2	Selected Drugs Unsafe for Patients with Neurovisceral Porphyrias*

Angiotensin-converting enzyme inhibitors
Barbiturates
Carbamazepine
Chlorpropamide
Danazol
Diphenylhydantoin
Ergots
Estrogens
Glutethimide
Griseofulvin
Mephenytoin
Metoclopramide
Primidone
Progesterone
Rifampin
Succinimides
Sulfasalazine
Sulfonamides
Sulfonylureas
Valproic acid

*A complete list of unsafe and safe drugs is available at two websites: http://www.porphyriafoundation.com and http://www.porphyria-europe.com.

directly connected with P-450 metabolism have also been incriminated, including fasting, dieting, and the stress of an acute illness.[115-117] Most drugs taken by patients with AIP and other neurovisceral porphyrias have been classified as unsafe, potentially unsafe, probably safe, or safe. Isolated case reports have resulted in many drugs being classified as unsafe or potentially unsafe, so caution needs to be exercised when drawing conclusions. Some drugs, however, have repeatedly been associated with acute porphyric attacks and must be avoided. A selection of such drugs is presented in Box 13-2.

The current prevailing view is that symptoms of the porphyric attack result from the toxic effects of ALA or PBG (or both) rather than from a deficiency of heme in neurons.[57,118] The most striking evidence in support of this view is a report of a young woman with AIP who suffered repeated, life-threatening attacks. An allogeneic liver transplant normalized urinary excretion of ALA and PBG within a day and eliminated her recurrent neurovisceral attacks.[118] In a second case, liver transplantation corrected the biochemical findings in a patient with variegate porphyria (VP).[119] These impressive case reports support the causative role of hepatic overproduction of ALA and PBG in acute neurovisceral attacks, but it is premature to consider liver transplantation as a broadly applicable treatment, especially with the efficiency of hemin or heme arginate infusions (see later).

Laboratory Diagnosis. The signs and symptoms of an acute porphyric attack are quite nonspecific, and correct diagnosis requires both consideration of a neurovisceral

porphyria and performance of a highly specific laboratory test. An acute porphyria is frequently not considered until fruitless, expensive imaging studies (and often unnecessary surgical exploration) are complete.

Increased urinary excretion of PBG is the key diagnostic finding in patients suffering an acute attack of AIP, HCP, or VP. Most methods used to quantify urinary PBG excretion rely on formation of a violet pigment when the sample is reacted with *p*-dimethylaminobenzaldehyde (Ehrlich's aldehyde). Because Ehrlich's aldehyde reacts with other compounds secreted in urine, mainly urobilinogen, PBG must be partially purified. Ion exchange chromatography effectively separates PBG and ALA from interfering substances.[120] PBG can then be reacted with Ehrlich's aldehyde. ALA is condensed with ethyl acetoacetate to form a pyrrole, which will react with Ehrlich's aldehyde. Ion exchange chromatography is a rapid, specific assay when performed in an experienced laboratory and measures both ALA and PBG. Typical reference ranges for excretion of PBG are 0 to 18 μmol/day (0 to 4 mg/day); values for ALA range from 0 to 60 μmol/day (0 to 8 mg/day). In contrast, during an acute attack, urinary PBG excretion generally ranges from 220 to 880 μmol/day and ALA excretion ranges from 100 to 450 μmol/day.[17]

A simplified method for measuring PBG at the bedside or in the emergency department uses a small anion exchange column packed in a kit that includes all the required reagents and a color chart. The trace PBG kit (Thermo Trace/DMA, Arlington, TX) can detect PBG at concentrations greater than 6 mg/L.[121] The kit does not measure ALA.

Urinary porphyrin excretion (mainly uroporphyrin) is increased during acute attacks of AIP, but this finding is much less specific than increased excretion of PBG and ALA. Fecal and plasma porphyrin levels are generally normal. In contrast, increased urinary porphyrin excretion during an acute attack of HCP or VP consists mainly of coproporphyrin, and stool porphyrin excretion is also increased. Markedly increased stool coproporphyrin and protoporphyrin are found in VP. Fluorescence scanning of diluted plasma at neutral pH readily distinguishes VP from the other neurovisceral porphyrias, even during asymptomatic periods.[122,123]

A word of caution is required when interpreting urinary porphyrin values. Minimal elevations of urinary coproporphyrin may be found in patients with liver disease, marrow disorders, and a host of other illnesses. An incorrect diagnosis of porphyria is commonly made by overinterpreting minimal elevations in urinary coproporphyrin, which can lead to a delay in establishing the true cause of the abdominal pain and other neurovisceral symptoms.

Assays of PBG-D activity in erythrocyte lysates have been widely used to confirm the diagnosis of AIP and to detect asymptomatic family members once an index case has been identified. Erythrocyte PBG-D activity is approximately half-normal in most patient with PCT.

Normal PBG-D activity, however, does not exclude a diagnosis of AIP because of differential splicing of the PBG-D transcript in the liver and the red cell. Mutations in exon 1 of the PBG-D gene affect activity of the enzyme in the liver, but the erythrocyte enzyme is encoded only by exons 2 through 15.[76] Furthermore, the normal range for erythrocyte PBG-D activity is wide, and low-normal values overlap with high mutation carrier values. Falsely low values can be obtained when samples are processed, stored, or shipped improperly. It is important to emphasize that a valid half-normal measurement of erythrocyte PBG-D activity does not distinguish between asymptomatic (latent) and clinically manifested cases of AIP. Only urinary PBG levels can make this distinction.

Detection of PBG-D mutations by DNA analysis has proved to be more reliable than PBG-D enzyme assays and is now the preferred method for confirming a diagnosis of AIP and for identifying asymptomatic carriers. DNA studies have demonstrated that enzymatic assays may misclassify up to 15% of individuals tested.[124,125] Detection of mutations for AIP patients and their relatives is now readily available through the Department of Human Genetics at the Mount Sinai School of Medicine in New York.

Treatment. Treatment of an acute attack of AIP (and the other neurovisceral porphyrias) is designed to repress the activity of hepatic ALA-S1 and to offer supportive care and relief of symptoms. Intravenous infusions of heme result in a rapid reduction in levels of ALA and PBG in plasma and urine.[112,114,126] Heme binds to plasma hemopexin and albumin and is then taken up by hepatocytes, where it expands the heme pool and represses ALA-S1. Many small, uncontrolled trials have demonstrated both biochemical and clinical responses to infusion of heme.[112,114,126-130] In one study involving 22 patients suffering 57 acute attacks, all patients responded favorably; however, therapy was most beneficial when administered early in the attack,[128] a finding confirmed by others.[129,131] A single placebo-controlled trial found dramatic biochemical benefits of heme infusion, although clinical benefits were more difficult to confirm.[132]

Heme is not soluble at neutral pH, but solubilized hemin (heme chloride) and heme arginate have been administered to many patients. In the United States, a lyophilized preparation of hemin (Panhematin, Ovation Pharmaceuticals, Deerfield, IL) has been approved by the Food and Drug Administration for the treatment of acute porphyric attacks. Hemin is unstable when reconstituted with sterile water, and degradation may cause an anticoagulant effect and phlebitis at the site of infusion.[133,134] Phlebitis can be avoided by the use of intravenous catheters that extend to larger veins (e.g., the superior vena cava). Instability and the locally irritating effects of lyophilized hemin can be attenuated by solubilizing it in 25% albumin,[127] a method now recommended.[17] The recommended regimen for heme therapy is 3 to 4 mg/kg infused once daily on 4 consecutive days.

Clinical improvement generally occurs within 1 or 2 days, but when neuronal damage is severe because of a delay in initiating therapy, complete recovery may take months. The key to success is initiation of therapy as soon as an attack is recognized and completion of a 4-day course. Rare side effects of therapy include constitutional symptoms such as fever, myalgia, and malaise, but one case of marked hypotension[135] and another of transient renal failure[136] have been reported. The latter case was associated with an excessive dose (1000 mg) of hemin.

Heme arginate (Normosang, Orphan Pharmaceuticals, Paris) is more stable than hemin in solution, is equally effective, and is widely available in Europe and South Africa but remains an experimental drug in the United States. Phlebitis is a rare complication with heme arginate,[137] and the shelf life is considerably longer than that of hemin. Adenoviral-mediated expression of PBG-D corrects the metabolic defect in a mouse model of AIP,[138] but no studies have been performed in humans. Intravenous infusions of recombinant human PBG-D have been administered to normal subjects and asymptomatic PBG-D mutation carriers.[139] Transient decreases in plasma concentrations of PBG were noted, and no serious side effects occurred. No trials of recombinant PBG-D for the treatment of symptomatic AIP have been reported.

Intravenous infusions of glucose (300 to 500 g/day, administered as 10% glucose) may be effective when an attack is mild or until hemin is obtained[17]; however, glucose is far less effective than hemin. The mechanism of the glucose effect relates to the finding that transcription of ALA-S1 is upregulated by PGC-1α[12] and transcription of PGC-1α is controlled by the availability of glucose. Under conditions of low glucose, PGC-1α production is increased, thereby leading to increased levels of ALA-S1 and heme, conditions promoting a porphyric attack. Just the opposite would occur under conditions of high glucose. Regulation of ALA-S1 by PGC-1α ties together the observation that caloric deprivation can precipitate an acute porphyric attack with the benefits of high-dose glucose.[140] Insulin may also downregulate PGC-1α,[12] and it has been suggested that the combination of glucose and insulin may be more effective than glucose alone.[18]

Acute attacks require treatment of symptoms in addition to therapy directed at ALA-S1. Pain is often severe, and full doses of morphine or other opioids are both safe and effective. Phenothiazines in modest doses are safe and useful for control of nausea and anxiety.[17] Hypertension and tachycardia may respond to β-adrenergic blocking agents,[141,142] but these drugs should be used with caution when patients are hypovolemic because increased catecholamine secretion is often an important compensatory mechanism. Seizures during an acute attack can be a particularly vexing problem inasmuch as most antiseizure drugs have the potential to worsen the intensity of the attack. Clonazepam and gabapentin may be safe,[143-145] and benzodiazepines are probably safe.[17]

Hyponatremia and hypomagnesemia should be corrected because these abnormalities are common and may induce seizures.

Long-term management of patients with acute neurovisceral porphyrias is focused on the prevention of future attacks. Avoidance of unsafe drugs is critical, as is maintenance of a balanced, calorically adequate diet. In some women, acute attacks occur only in the luteal phase of the menstrual cycle. In such cases, gonadotropin-releasing hormone (GnRH) analogues can be highly effective.[146,147] Prolonged use of GnRH analogues in young women may cause irreversible bone loss, but low-dose transdermal estradiol may safely prevent this complication.[148,149] Both cyclic and noncyclic attacks may be prevented by frequent infusions of hemin[113]; however, the expense and the potential for iron overload (8 mg of iron per 100 mg of hemin) makes this option unattractive.

Levels of progesterone, an inducer of hepatic heme synthesis, are elevated in pregnancy, but pregnancy is well tolerated by most women with acute porphyrias. In a large series reported from Finland of 176 pregnancies in women with AIP or VP, porphyric symptoms occurred in less than 10%.[89] Worsening symptoms during pregnancy may be due to harmful drugs,[150,151] inadequate nutrition, or both.[17]

An unexplained finding in patients with AIP and VP is a 35- to 70-fold increased risk for the development of hepatocellular carcinoma.[152-156] It has been suggested that DNA damage induced by ALA may be responsible for these observations.[157,158]

Uroporphyrinogen III Synthase

The product of the PBG-D reaction, HMB (see Fig. 13-8), serves as the substrate for URO3-S. URO3-S catalyzes the asymmetric cyclization of HMB to the III isomer of uroporphyrinogen. The reaction involves "flipping" of the D ring to yield the asymmetric product (Fig. 13-9). Rearrangement of the D ring occurs by a complex mechanism involving cleavage and formation of carbon-carbon bonds.[159,160] Spontaneous cyclization of HMB can also occur (Fig. 13-10), but the product, uroporphyrinogen I, cannot ultimately be converted to heme. URO3-S functions as a monomer. Although the primary sequence is highly divergent, the crystal structure of human URO3-S and a bacterial URO3-S is nearly identical.[161,162] The structure of URO3-S from the bacterium *Thermus thermophilus* has been determined with the uroporphyrinogen III product bound.[162] The structure suggests that the enzyme prevents the formation of uroporphyrinogen I by positioning the A and D rings to favor the formation of uroporphyrinogen III (see Fig. 13-10).

The human URO3-S gene is localized to chromosome 10q25.2-26.3[163] (see Table 13-1) and contains 10

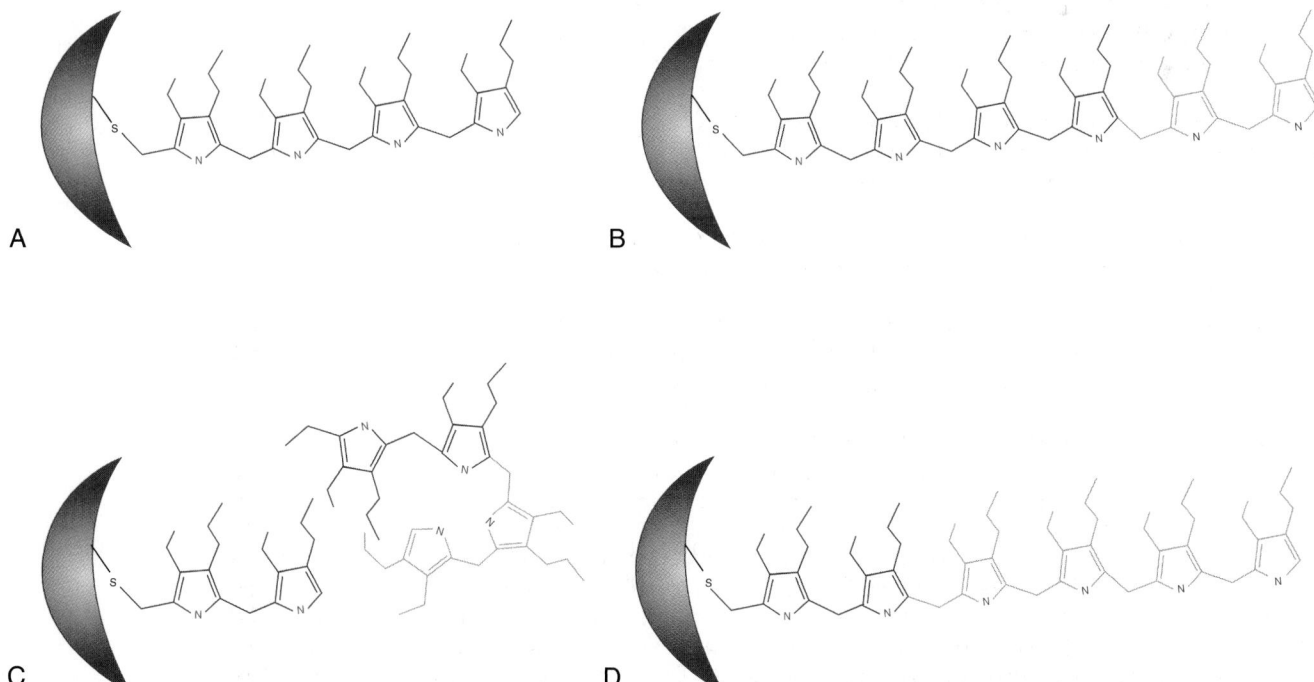

FIGURE 13-8. Initial reaction cycle of porphobilinogen deaminase (PBG-D). **A,** Post-translationally, a molecule of hydroxymethylbilane (*red*) is added to the apoprotein. **B,** Two additional molecules of porphobilinogen (*green*) are added. **C,** The distal tetrapyrrole is cleaved to form the product hydroxymethylbilane (*red* and *green*). **D,** In subsequent rounds of catalysis, the dipyrrole cofactor (*red*) remains bound in the active site, and four molecules of porphobilinogen (*green*) are added sequentially and then cleaved and released as hydroxymethylbilane.

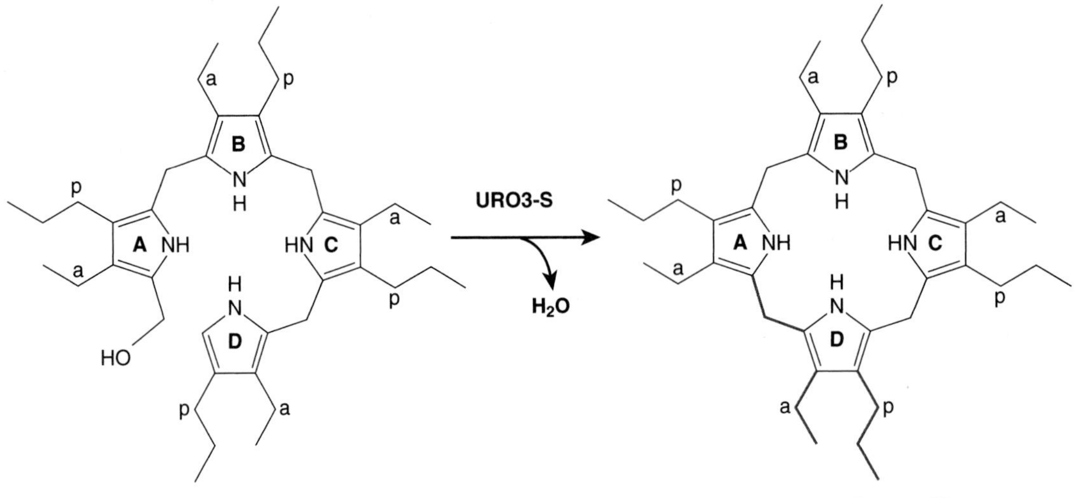

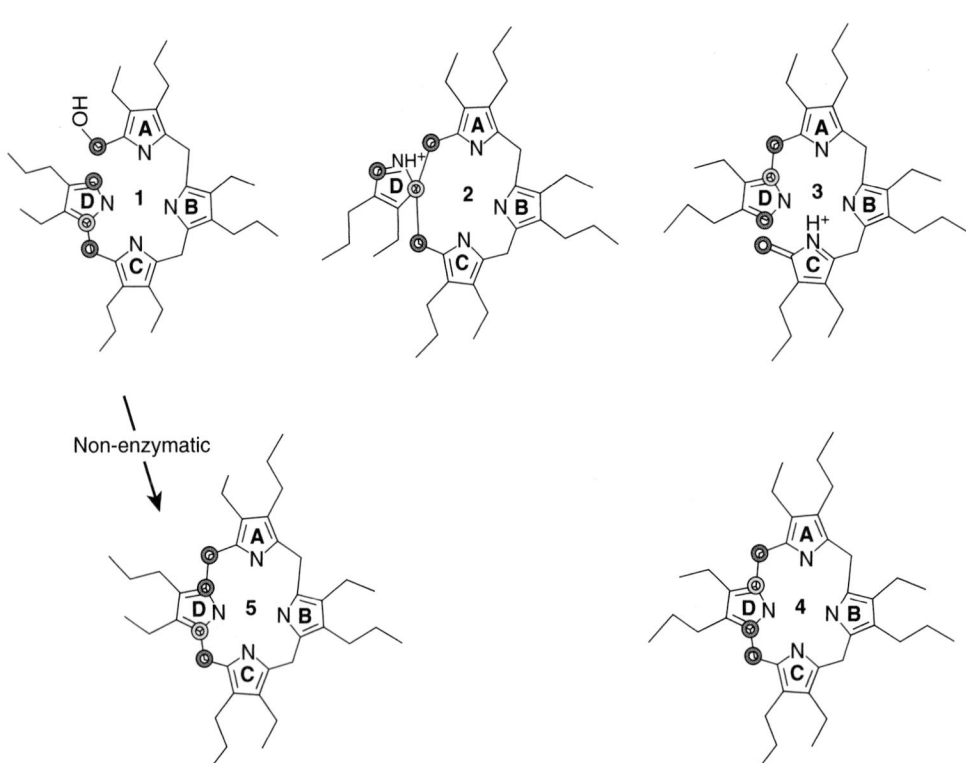

FIGURE 13-9. Reaction catalyzed by uroporphyrinogen III synthase. Uroporphyrinogen III synthase (URO3-S) enzymatically closes the tetrapyr-role ring with concomitant "flipping" of the D ring. The acetate (a) and propionate (p) side chains are labeled. In the uroporphyrinogen III product, the acetate and propionate groups of the D ring are reversed.

Non-enzymatic

Uroporphyrinogen I

Uroporphyrinogen III

FIGURE 13-10. Proposed mechanism for formation of uroporphyrinogen III. Hydroxymethylbilane (HMB), structure 1, forms a spirolactam intermediate, structure 2. The intermediate is resolved by cleaving the carbon bond between pyrrole rings C and D on the opposite side, structure 3. The final step is closure of the macrocycle, structure 4, to form the III isomer of uroporphyrinogen. HMB can also cycle nonenzymatically to form uroporphyrinogen I, structure 5.

coding exons.[164] The translational start site is located in exon 2B (see Fig. 13-5). Both housekeeping and erythroid-specific transcripts are produced. The housekeeping promoter lies upstream of exon 1.[165] The housekeeping transcript results from a splicing event that joins exons 1 and 2B. The erythroid-specific promoter lies within intron 1 and contains eight GATA1 binding sites. The erythroid-specific transcript contains all of exon 2. Although the housekeeping and erythroid transcripts are expressed from different promoters, they produce identical proteins.

Congenital Erythropoietic Porphyria (Günther's Disease)

Congenital erythropoietic porphyria (CEP) is a rare form of porphyria in humans caused by mutations in URO3-S. Fewer than 200 cases have been reported. The disorder is of historical interest in that it was the first porphyria to be recognized as an inherited trait and the first to be characterized biochemically.[166-168] CEP also occurs in squirrels,[169] cows,[170] and other species.[171] More than 30 URO3-S mutations have been reported, including exonic and promoter point mutations, deletions, insertions, and splice site mutations.[172-176]

Frequency. The rarity of CEP makes estimating its frequency difficult, but the disorder has been described in multiple ethnic groups.[177] The frequency of heterozygosity for URO3-S mutations is not known because heterozygotes have no phenotype and population-based sequencing screens have not been done. Though rare, CEP is recognized more frequently than ALA-D porphyria, perhaps because of the dramatic cutaneous phenotype.

Clinical Manifestations. Cutaneous photosensitivity is the most dramatic feature of CEP and is usually recognized in early infancy. The diagnosis may be suspected because of the dark brown color of urine-soaked diapers that demonstrate a distinctive, intense red-pink fluorescence when illuminated with long-range ultraviolet light (e.g., Wood's light)[178] (Fig. 13-11). The severity of the skin lesions varies widely and is related to the amount of residual URO3-S activity,[179] which in turn determines the magnitude of porphyrin accumulation and excretion. In most cases the photosensitivity is severe and characterized by skin fragility, bullous lesions, ulcerations, and secondary infections.[177] If exposure to sunlight is not rigorously avoided, mutilation of the face and hands is the ultimate outcome (Fig. 13-12). A common finding in CEP and the other porphyric disorders associated with photosensitivity is the presumably protective response of extensive hypertrichosis.[177] Photo-induced damage to nails and ocular structures may also occur.[177,180,181] A unique finding in children with CEP is red-brown discoloration of the teeth as a result of deposition of por-

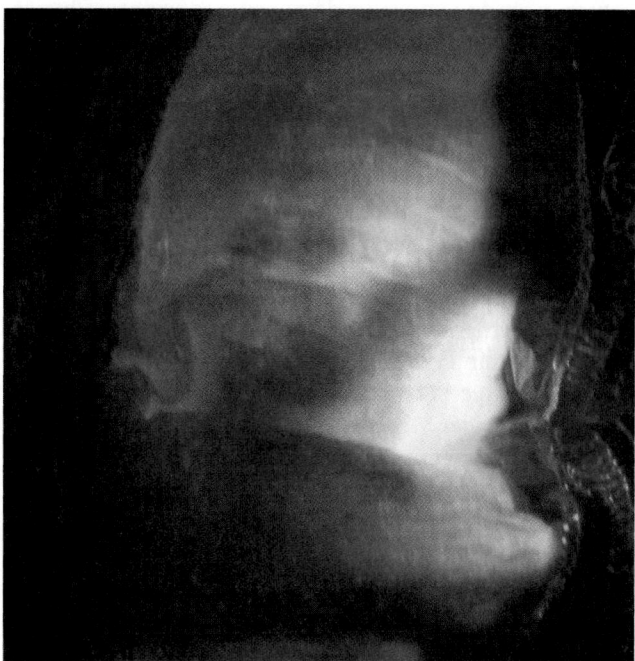

FIGURE 13-11. The diaper from a child with congenital erythropoietic porphyria. Urine porphyrins, primarily uroporphyrin I, fluoresce with a brilliant pink color when illuminated with a Wood's light.

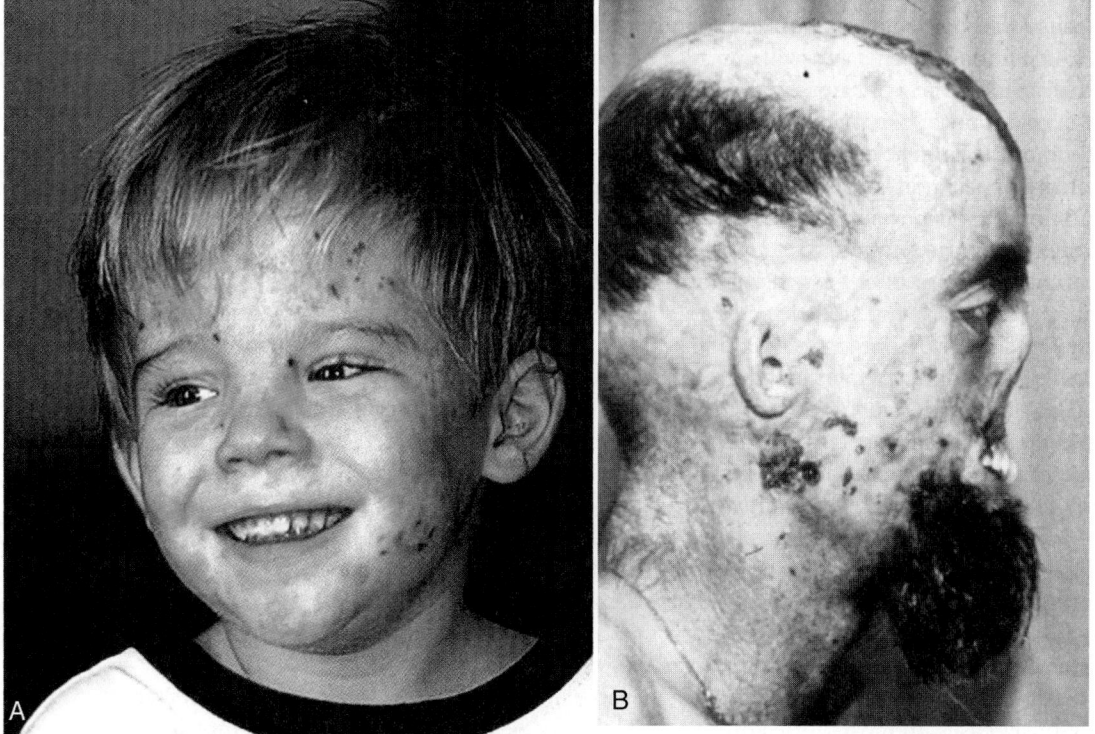

FIGURE 13-12. Skin changes in congenital erythropoietic porphyria (CEP). **A,** A 3-year-old boy with early facial photodermatitis. **B,** Severe case of CEP in an adult. Sun exposure has led to blistering, erosions, secondary infections, and subsequent photomutilation.

phyrins in dentine and enamel during tooth development.[182] The teeth fluoresce when illuminated with Wood's light.

Hemolytic anemia of varying severity is found in nearly all cases, but detailed morphologic findings in blood and bone marrow have been reported infrequently. Ineffective erythropoiesis may also be present. Poikilocytosis, nucleated red cells, and basophilic stippling are common, and the marrow demonstrates erythroid hyperplasia and may manifest marked dyserythropoiesis.[183-186] Fluorescence microscopy may demonstrate fluorocytes in peripheral blood, but this is more dramatic in bone marrow.[171,183,186,187] Splenomegaly generally accompanies the hemolytic anemia, and the magnitude of splenic enlargement reflects the severity of hemolysis. Leukopenia and symptomatic thrombocytopenia may occur as a result of splenic sequestration.[188]

A variety of osteolytic skeletal lesions have been described when the disease reaches the stage of mutilation.[177] Vitamin D deficiency secondary to sun avoidance may play a role in the development of osteolysis.[189] The role of porphyrins deposited in bone is uncertain, but at postmortem examination the skeleton is fluorescent under long-range ultraviolet light.[190]

Pathogenesis. Loss-of-function mutations in URO3-S lead to accumulation of the HMB substrate in erythrocyte precursors, which is readily converted nonenzymatically to uroporphyrinogen I (see Fig. 13-10). Residual URO3-S activity is generally less than 10% of normal. Uroporphyrinogen I may be auto-oxidized to uroporphyrin I or may serve as a substrate for uroporphyrinogen decarboxylase (URO-D) (see Fig. 13-2) and ultimately generate coproporphyrinogen I. This results in a metabolic "dead end" inasmuch as the next enzyme in the pathway, CPO, is stereospecific and will accept only coproporphyrinogen III as a substrate. Uroporphyrin I and, to a lesser extent, coproporphyrin I accumulate in erythroid precursors. Erythrocyte fragility and hemolysis result by an undefined mechanism and liberate porphyrins into plasma. Uroporphyrin I mediates the cutaneous photosensitivity[191] and is excreted in urine. Coproporphyrin I is excreted in stool and, to a lesser extent, in urine.

Two phenotypic forms of CEP have been reported. In one, a partial defect in URO-D combined with a congenital dyserythropoietic anemia produced mutilating photosensitivity and massive uroporphyrinuria.[192] The pattern of urinary porphyrin excretion differed from CEP in that large amounts of heptacarboxyl porphyrin were found in addition to even larger amounts of uroporphyrin. In the other, a mutation in the erythroid-specific transcription factor GATA1 resulted in subnormal URO3-S in red cells and a phenotype of CEP, thalassemia intermedia, and thrombocytopenia.[193]

CEP may become evident in adult life, and clinical symptoms are generally less severe than in the more typical early-onset cases. In most of the adult-onset cases, moderate URO3-S defects became evident only when an acquired marrow disorder developed.[194-199]

Laboratory Diagnosis. Urinary porphyrin excretion is massively increased in CEP, in some cases up to 1000 times normal. The pattern of porphyrin excretion, determined by high-performance liquid chromatography (HPLC), is characteristic. The dominant urine porphyrin is uroporphyrin I, with smaller amounts of coproporphyrin I.[200,201] Assays of URO3-S have been performed on erythrocytes and cultured cells, but the assays are available in just a few research laboratories.[202,203] The most practical way to confirm the diagnosis of CEP is through direct sequencing of the gene, a procedure available through the Department of Human Genetics at the Mount Sinai School of Medicine in New York. URO3-S mutations can be detected in chorionic villi or cultured amniotic cells.[204] This may be useful in subsequent pregnancies when parents have had a child with CEP.

Treatment. The only curative therapy for CEP is an allogeneic marrow transplant. Eleven patients with CEP who have undergone allogeneic transplantation have been reported.[193,205-209] The published experience suggests that early transplantation is preferred, but this approach is not universally applicable because of potential donor availability, treatment-related morbidity, and financial constraints. Allogeneic transplants should probably be restricted to the more severe cases of CEP because conservative management can yield longevity of 40 to 60 years.

The morbidity associated with marrow allografts could be avoided by autologous hematopoietic stem cell transplantation if stem cells could be stably transfected with normal URO3-S cDNA. This has been accomplished in a murine model of CEP with a lentivirus vector.[210] Complete correction of the phenotype was achieved. No studies of this type have yet been reported in humans with CEP.

Avoidance of sunlight is at the core of conservative management and can be achieved with protective clothing and effective sunscreens. Conventional sunscreens containing para-aminobenzoic acid are ineffective, and opaque "pancake" makeup is preferred. Splenectomy may reduce the severity of hemolysis and correct the leukopenia and thrombocytopenia, but beneficial effects on photosensitivity are often transient.[211] Erythropoiesis and endogenous porphyrin production can be suppressed with aggressive transfusion regimens,[212] although transfusion-induced iron overload results.[213]

MODIFICATION OF THE TETRAPYRROLE SIDE CHAINS

Uroporphyrinogen Decarboxylase

Uroporphyrinogen III is converted to coproporphyrinogen III by sequential removal of the carboxyl groups of the four acetate side chains to yield four methyl groups. This reaction is catalyzed by cytosolic URO-D

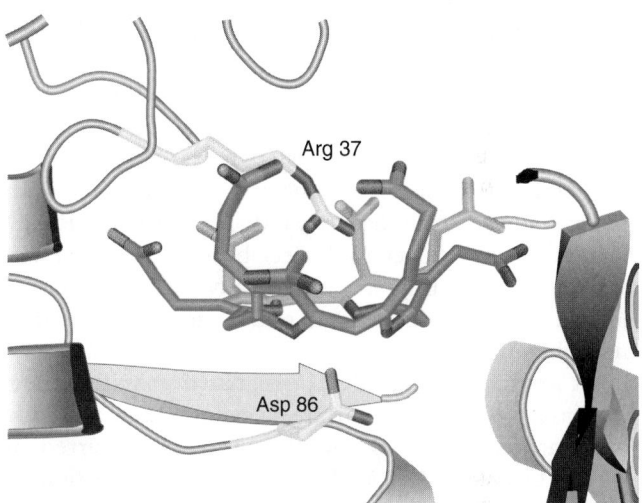

FIGURE 13-13. Reaction catalyzed by uroporphyrinogen decarboxylase (URO-D). Uroporphyrinogen undergoes four successive decarboxylations, starting at the asymmetric D ring. The acetate side chains (a) are decarboxylated to form methyl groups. URO-D will decarboxylate both the I and III isomers of uroporphyrinogen, but coproporphyrinogen I is not a substrate for coproporphyrinogen oxidase.

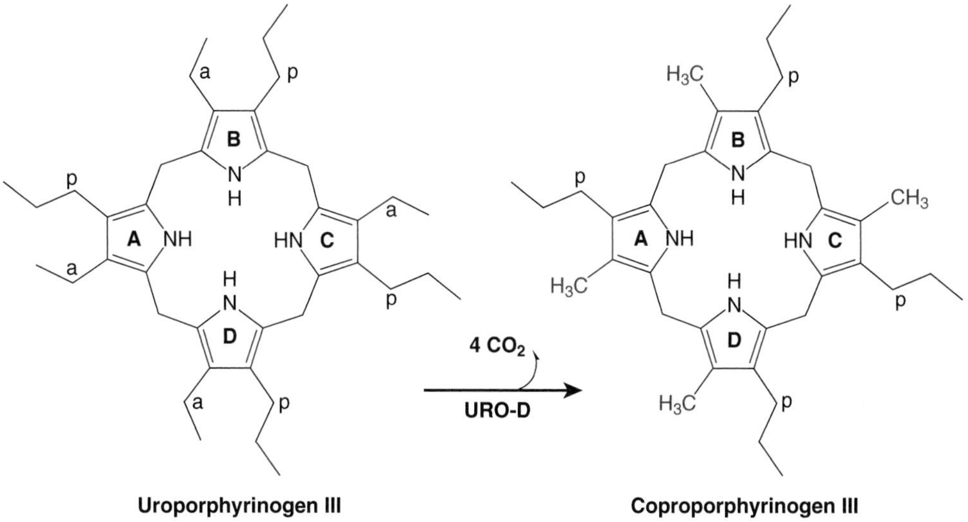

Uroporphyrinogen III

4 CO₂

URO-D

Coproporphyrinogen III

(Fig. 13-13). Decarboxylation of uroporphyrinogen III begins at the asymmetric D ring and proceeds in a clockwise manner.[214] Uroporphyrinogen III is the preferred substrate. The enzyme will accept uroporphyrinogen I as a substrate, but the product, coproporphyrinogen I, cannot be converted to heme.

Human URO-D is encoded by a single gene located on chromosome 1p34[215,216] (see Table 13-1). Unlike ALA-D, PBG-D, and URO3-S, there is no erythroid-specific promoter in the URO-D gene.[217] URO-D mRNA is highly expressed in developing erythrocytes, but the mechanism responsible for erythroid-specific upregulation is not known.[218]

URO-D has been purified from human erythrocytes,[219,220] from bovine liver,[221] and from yeast and bacteria.[222] Unlike most decarboxylases, URO-D does not require cofactors or prosthetic groups for activity. Determination of the crystal structure of human URO-D has revealed that URO-D functions as a homodimer.[223,224] Each monomer contains an active-site cleft. The active site can accommodate only the flexible porphyrinogen macrocycle[225] (Fig. 13-14). Oxidation of the bridge carbons connecting the pyrrole rings renders the molecule rigid and planar and may explain why uroporphyrin is not a substrate for URO-D.

Porphyria Cutanea Tarda

PCT is due to subnormal activity of URO-D in the liver. The disorder is characterized clinically by a photosensitive dermatosis that is usually less severe than in CEP. Expression of the clinical phenotype is associated with one or more risk factors, including homozygosity for the C282Y mutation of the hemochromatosis gene (*HFE*), hepatitis C, alcohol abuse, and the use of medicinal estrogens.[226-233] The frequency of these risk factors is far higher than the observed incidence of PCT, thus suggesting that susceptibility factors, either genetic or environmental and yet to be identified, are important determinants of disease expression.[234]

FIGURE 13-14. Crystal structure of uroporphyrinogen decarboxylase with uroporphyrinogen III bound in the active site. Uroporphyrinogen III (*green*) is shown in the active site. The fully reduced bridge carbons permit uroporphyrinogen to adopt the domed configuration positioning the 4-pyrrole nitrogens for hydrogen bonding with aspartic acid 86 (Asp86). The positive charge of arginine 37 (Arg37) interacts with the negatively charged propionate groups of uroporphyrinogen to correctly position the substrate in the active site. *(Figure based on the coordinates 1R3Y, available from the Protein Data Bank.)*

Two major variants have been identified. The first, designated familial PCT (F-PCT), is associated with heterozygosity for mutations at the URO-D locus.[235-237] F-PCT is transmitted as an autosomal dominant trait. Affected individuals display approximately half-normal URO-D activity and half-normal URO-D protein in all tissues.[236,238] There is considerable variation in URO-D activity inasmuch as different mutations have varied effects on enzyme activity.[239] F-PCT accounts for approximately 25% of clinically observed cases.[234,240,241] Most carriers of a mutant URO-D allele do not express a porphyric phenotype unless one or more of the risk factors mentioned earlier are also present.[234] Clinical expression of F-PCT in childhood is rare.[242-247] The authors have evaluated three children with F-PCT, two of whom were brothers who were also homozygous for the C282Y *HFE* mutation.

The second major variant—and the most prevalent form of PCT—is designated sporadic PCT (S-PCT) and accounts for approximately 70% of cases.[234] In S-PCT, reduced activity of URO-D is restricted to the liver. No URO-D mutations have been identified in patients with S-PCT, and there is no evidence of a liver-specific URO-D transcript.[248] Nevertheless, S-PCT may cluster in families and thus suggests the presence of predisposing genetic factors.[249] The concentration of URO-D protein is normal in all cells, including hepatocytes, yet when the disease phenotype is expressed, enzyme activity is markedly reduced in the liver. A normal URO-D protein concentration coupled with subnormal URO-D enzymatic activity strongly suggests the presence of an enzyme inhibitor.[250-252] Risk factors identified when S-PCT is clinically evident are identical to those associated with F-PCT.[226,234]

A third rare variant of PCT occurs in children who have inherited two mutant alleles of URO-D.[226,253-256] This variant has been designated hepatoerythropoietic porphyria (HEP) because porphyrins accumulate in both the liver and red cells. Severely reduced levels of URO-D resulting from the genetic defect become rate limiting. Activity in red cell lysates is generally less than 10% of normal[257] but may be as high as 20% in patients with a mild phenotype.[255]

A fourth variant of PCT, designated toxic PCT, has been associated with exposure to halogenated aromatic hydrocarbons. An epidemic of toxic PCT occurred in Turkey between 1956 and 1961 after the ingestion of wheat treated with the fungicide hexachlorobenzene.[187,258] Many of the Turkish cases were children. Later studies in animals established that halogenated aromatic hydrocarbons diminish hepatic URO-D activity.[259-265] PCT in humans has also been reported after exposure to 2,3,7,8-tetrachlorodibenzo-*p*-dioxin (TCDD)[266,267] and to dichlorophenols and trichlorophenols.[268]

Frequency. PCT is the most common of the porphyric disorders, but the incidence varies in different populations. In white populations of northern European origin, the incidence may be as high as 2 to 5 per 20,000, probably because of the high incidence of hemochromatosis gene mutations in this group.[268] In contrast, PCT is uncommon in African Americans but does occur in the Bantus of South Africa, in whom iron overload develops from drinking beer brewed in iron pots.[269] PCT has occurred commonly in patients undergoing chronic hemodialysis[270-272]; however, substitution of erythropoietin for red cell transfusions has reduced the incidence.

The high frequency of PCT, with a quarter of cases associated with URO-D mutations, would predict that HEP should not be rare. Instead, fewer than 40 cases have been reported.[255] This is best explained by embryonic lethality of the extremely low residual activity of mutant URO-D enzymes or the lethal effect of null alleles.

Clinical Manifestations. Skin fragility on the dorsal aspect of the hands is often the initial finding, but blistering lesions (bullae) then appear on all sun-exposed areas. The fluid-filled bullae rupture and the denuded area heals slowly, often forming thick eschars and eventually hyperpigmented patches (Fig. 13-15). Facial hypertrichosis is common, particularly in children and women. Facial hypertrichosis may be localized to periorbital regions (Fig. 13-16A) or can be manifested in a lanugo-like diffuse facial pattern with or without pigmentation (see Fig. 13-16B). In some patients, scleroderma-like skin changes develop, mainly in light-exposed areas.[273,274] When PCT becomes chronic, milia (small, cyst-like collections of keratin) are common on the hands.[275] Similar photocutaneous findings have been seen in patients with pseudoporphyria, a disorder in which plasma and urine porphyrins are normal. The skin findings are probably due to other photosensitizing compounds. Nonsteroidal anti-inflammatory drugs have been implicated in most cases.[276]

The cutaneous manifestations of HEP can be very dramatic and may resemble those seen in CEP.[277] Recurrent blisters and erosions complicated by infection can lead to severe scarring, scleroderma-like changes, and photomutilation.[80,257] In other cases, the skin is less severely damaged and appears more like mild PCT.[278,279] Hemolytic anemia and splenomegaly may be present, findings not associated with PCT.[257]

Evidence of abnormal liver function is nearly always present in patients with PCT, even in those without hepatitis C. In some reports, approximately 80% of males with PCT have been infected with hepatitis C,[230,280] but the association of hepatitis C with PCT is lower in northern

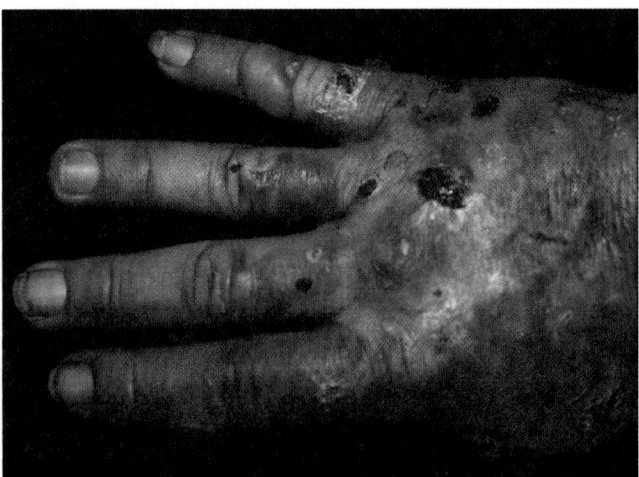

FIGURE 13-15. Hand of a patient with porphyria cutanea tarda. Bullous lesions form (note the large blister on the fifth digit), rupture, and leave ulcerations that heal slowly. The resultant scars are both hypopigmented and hyperpigmented.

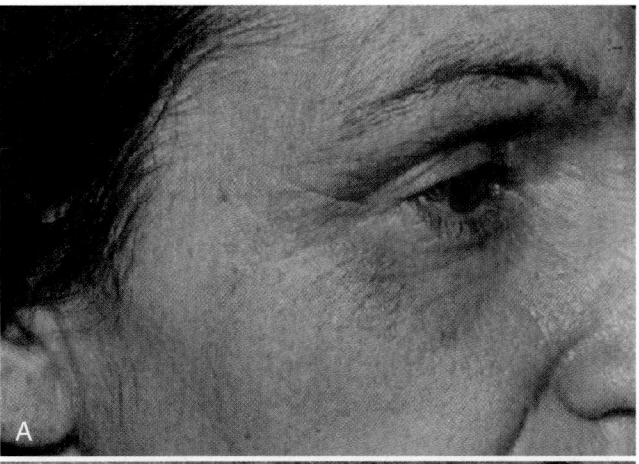

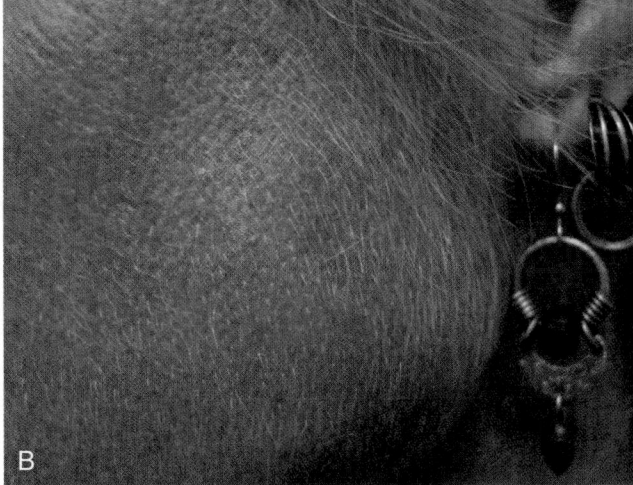

FIGURE 13-16. Facial hypertrichosis with porphyria cutanea tarda (PCT). **A,** Characteristic periorbital facial hair in a 60-year-old woman in whom PCT developed while receiving postmenopausal oral estrogen replacement. **B,** Diffuse lanugo-like facial hair in a 26-year-old woman in whom PCT developed while taking an oral contraceptive.

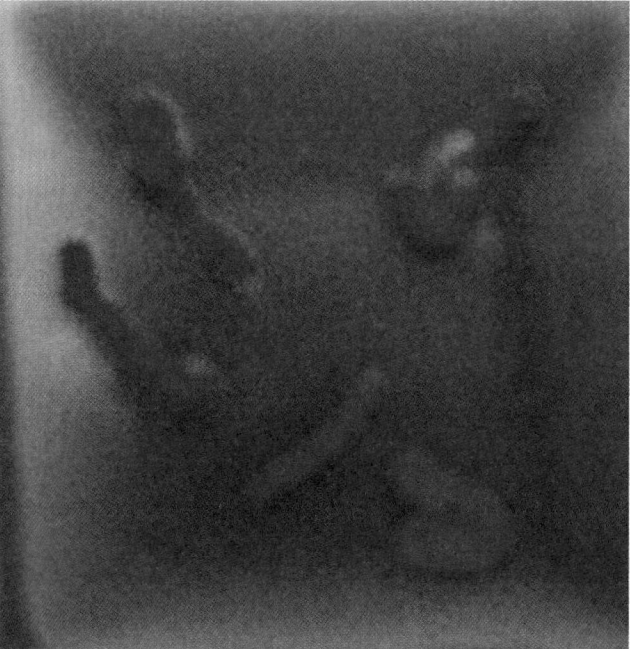

FIGURE 13-17. Percutaneous liver biopsy specimens from five patients with porphyria cutanea tarda. The massive amount of porphyrins in hepatocytes results in striking fluorescence under illumination with a Wood's light.

Europe.[280,281] The high concentration of porphyrins in the liver results in brilliant fluorescence of liver biopsy samples illuminated with Wood's light (Fig. 13-17). Microscopic examination reveals needle-shaped, fluorescent porphyrin crystals in hepatocytes.[282] Other histologic findings are not specific,[283] but increased hepatocellular iron stores are a nearly constant finding.[284-286]

Pathogenesis. More than 50 URO-D mutations have been identified in patients with PCT.[287,288] The functional consequences of many of these mutations have been studied,[288] but heterozygosity for mutant URO-D alleles alone cannot explain the phenotype because half-normal URO-D activity is not rate limiting. Immunoreactive URO-D in the liver of patients with clinically evident F-PCT is half-normal, yet enzyme activity is 25% of normal or less.[289] No URO-D mutations are found in patients with S-PCT, and immunoreactive URO-D in all tissues is normal. When S-PCT becomes clinically evident, immunoreactive URO-D in the liver remains normal, but

enzyme activity is reduced to approximately 25% of normal, the same level of activity found in F-PCT.[290,291] These findings indicate that the specific activity of hepatic URO-D is affected. Furthermore, the catalytic activity of URO-D returns to normal after phlebotomy-induced iron depletion,[289] thus suggesting that an iron-dependent process is responsible for the reduction in specific activity of hepatic URO-D. Similar findings, a reduction in URO-D activity without a change in URO-D protein, have been noted in several animal models of PCT.[292-296] Collectively, these data suggest a common mechanism in the pathogenesis of PCT, namely, generation of an inhibitor of URO-D by an iron-dependent mechanism.

The inhibitor of URO-D in humans with PCT and in animal models of PCT has been identified as uroporphomethene. Uroporphomethene differs from uroporphyrinogen by oxidation of a single bridge carbon between adjacent pyrrole rings[297] (Fig. 13-18). Uroporphomethene is sufficiently flexible to adapt to the spatial requirements of the active site of URO-D, but variance from the structure of uroporphyrinogen prevents the inhibitor from serving as a substrate.[297]

Generation of the uroporphomethene inhibitor probably requires liver-specific isozymes of cytochrome P-450[298]; however, the mechanism of the iron effect remains unidentified. Iron clearly plays a central role inasmuch as iron depletion through phlebotomy therapy reverses the clinical and biochemical phenotype. Replacement of iron removed by phlebotomy produces a prompt relapse.[299] Iron depletion prevents or dramatically attenuates the porphyric phenotype in animal models of PCT, and iron

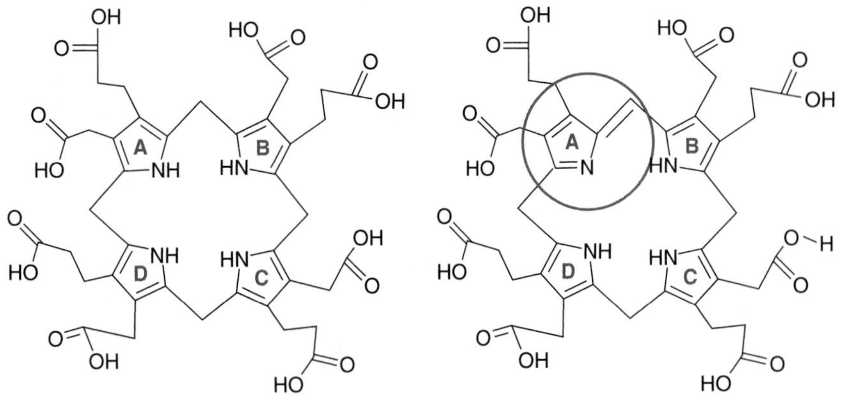

$C_{40}H_{44}N_4O_{16}$
Exact mass: 836.28
Mol. wt.: 836.79

Uroporphyrinogen I

$C_{40}H_{42}N_4O_{16}$
Exact mass: 834.26
Mol. wt.: 834.78

Uroporphomethene I

FIGURE 13-18. Structures of uroporphyrinogen and the uroporphomethene inhibitor of uroporphyrinogen decarboxylase. Oxidation of a single bridge carbon leads to rearrangement of the double bonds of the pyrrole and loss of an additional proton from a pyrrole nitrogen (seen in the *green circle*). The chemical composition and molecular mass are given below each compound.

supplementation accelerates development of the phenotype.[231,264] Despite these data, PCT develops in very few patients with hemochromatosis or other disorders associated with iron overload. Hepatic iron loading, therefore, is not sufficient to produce the PCT phenotype. Other factors, both genetic and environmental, appear to be required to create susceptibility to PCT.

The cutaneous findings in PCT, as in other porphyrias associated with photosensitivity, result from the interaction of light at a wavelength of approximately 400 nm (the Soret band) with porphyrins that accumulate in the skin.[300] The photo-excited porphyrin returns to a stable state by emitting energy as a photon that disrupts membranes and intracellular organelles.[301] The photodynamic reaction activates inflammatory mediators, which damage the epidermal basement membrane and cause fragility of the skin and blistering.[302] Another prominent site of photodamage is at the vascular level of the skin, where thickening of superficial dermal vessel walls is a constant finding.[303,304]

Laboratory Diagnosis. Laboratory testing is essential for confirmation of the clinical diagnosis of PCT and HEP. The appearance of the skin and skin biopsy findings resemble those of other photosensitizing porphyrias and pseudoporphyria. A useful initial approach to establishing that a porphyric disorder is present is to measure the total porphyrin content of plasma.[305] A normal value excludes the diagnosis of PCT and HEP. If the plasma porphyrin level is high, additional testing is required to distinguish PCT and HEP from HCP and VP. Chromatographic separation and quantification of urinary and stool porphyrins serve this purpose. In PCT and HEP, greatly increased amounts of uroporphyrin and heptacarboxyl porphyrin are excreted in urine (Fig. 13-19). Urinary excretion of coproporphyrin may be slightly increased.[285,306] Daily urine porphyrin excretion averages 3000 µg (normal, <50 µg) and may be considerably higher. Cutaneous symptoms are usually mild or absent

when uroporphyrin excretion is less than 1000 µg/day. A distinctive tetracarboxylic porphyrin, isocoproporphyrin, is excreted in feces, but total fecal porphyrin excretion is normal or minimally increased.[307] HEP can be distinguished from PCT by the presence of anemia and an increase in erythrocyte zinc protoporphyrin.[308]

Erythrocyte URO-D assays can be useful but are not widely available. Furthermore, distinguishing between F-PCT and S-PCT is not critical for patient management. Very low activity of URO-D in erythrocyte lysates can distinguish HEP from F-PCT and would affect therapeutic choices, but directly determining URO-D mutation status is more precise and facilitates genetic counseling.

In patients with PCT, additional laboratory testing is indicated to determine body iron burden (serum iron, total iron-binding capacity, and serum ferritin), liver function status, hemochromatosis genotype, and the presence or absence of antibodies to hepatitis C and human immunodeficiency virus.

Treatment. Two effective forms of therapy have been widely used in patients with PCT, phlebotomy and low-dose chloroquine. Phlebotomy is preferred in patients with marked increases in hepatic iron stores, as determined by liver biopsy and serum ferritin values. Removal of 500 mL of blood every 2 weeks for 3 to 4 months will usually surfice,[285,309] but additional treatment is required for patients with hemochromatosis. The objective is to produce iron depletion, not iron deficiency. A useful target is a serum ferritin value of approximately 50 µg/L. Skin lesions clear when urine porphyrin excretion falls below 1000 µg/day, but it may take a year or more for the urine to become completely normal. Relapses are infrequent, especially if risk factors (alcohol and oral estrogens) are avoided. Transdermal estrogen administration after phlebotomy-induced remission of PCT in women, however, appears to be safe.[227]

Low-dose chloroquine therapy is an effective alternative treatment and at some centers is preferred for patients

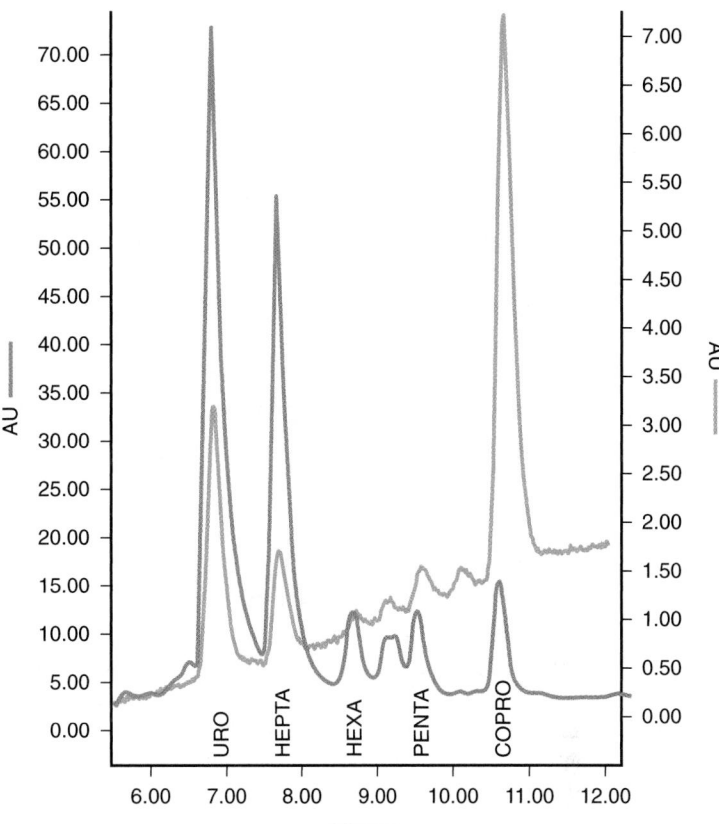

FIGURE 13-19. Urine porphyrin profile in porphyria cutanea tarda (PCT). Urine porphyrins were separated by high-performance liquid chromatography and quantified fluorometrically. The tracing from a normal person is shown in *blue* with the scale on the right (0 to 7 absorbance units). The profile of urine porphyrins from a patient with PCT is shown in *red*, with the scale on the left (0 to 70 absorbance units). Uroporphyrin (URO) and 7-carboxyl porphyrin (HEPTA) predominate in the PCT sample, whereas coproporphyrin (COPRO) is the main porphyrin present in normal urine. The intermediate porphyrins with 6- and 5-carboxyl groups (HEXA and PENTA) are also increased in the PCT sample.

with modest iron overload.[310] The time required to produce clinical remission is longer than with phlebotomy, but ultimately, the results are equivalent. Chloroquine at a dose of 125 mg by mouth twice weekly (or hydroxychloroquine at a dose of 100 mg by mouth twice weekly) will gradually reduce plasma and urinary porphyrins.[311-313] Chloroquine concentrates in the liver, where a water-soluble complex with uroporphyrin is formed and promotes urinary excretion.[314] Higher doses of chloroquine should be avoided because marked hepatotoxicity may occur, an effect that is unique to patients with PCT.[315,316] There is some risk of retinopathy with low-dose regimens,[317] and transient, modest elevations in transaminase values may occur.[285] Because of these potential reactions to low-dose chloroquine regimens, many centers prefer phlebotomy unless comorbid conditions render it unsuitable.

In contrast to PCT, phlebotomy is not effective therapy for HEP,[257] and responses to chloroquine are infrequent and suboptimal.[318] Treatment of HEP, as with CEP, is focused on symptomatic relief by avoidance of sunlight, use of protective clothing, and topical application of opaque sun screens.

Coproporphyrinogen Oxidase

Coproporphyrinogen III, the product of the URO-D reaction, is transported across the outer mitochondrial membrane by an ATP-binding cassette transporter des-

ignated ABCB6.[319] CPO, located in the mitochondrial intermembrane space, catalyzes sequential oxidative decarboxylation of the propionate groups of pyrrole rings A and B of coproporphyrinogen III to form protoporphyrinogen IX (Fig. 13-20). CPO uses two molecules of O_2 and releases 2 molecules of CO_2 and H_2O_2.[320] It has been suggested that the mechanism of the oxidative decarboxylation requires molecular oxygen to act as the intermediate electron acceptor,[321] but recent data suggest that oxygen reacts directly with the targeted pyrrole ring to yield a hydroperoxide that acts as the electron acceptor.[322] The nuclear-encoded CPO protein possesses an unusually long leader sequence that is required for mitochondrial localization.[9]

CPO in humans, all eukaryotes, and some prokaryotes is an oxygen-dependent enzyme.[323] The crystal structure of both human and yeast oxygen-dependent CPO has been determined.[321,324] The enzyme functions as a homodimer.[323] The structure of CPO allows the enzyme to maintain the substrate as the reduced porphyrinogen, yet permits access of oxygen to the active site for the oxidative decarboxylation reaction and release of H_2O_2.[321,324] The human CPO gene has been cloned and is located on chromosome 3q12.[325] The CPO promoter region encodes an Sp-1–like element, a GATA site, and a novel regulatory element that interacts in a synergistic manner in erythroid cells.[326] The GATA site is not required for transcription in nonerythroid tissues, but the novel regulatory element is necessary. There is increased

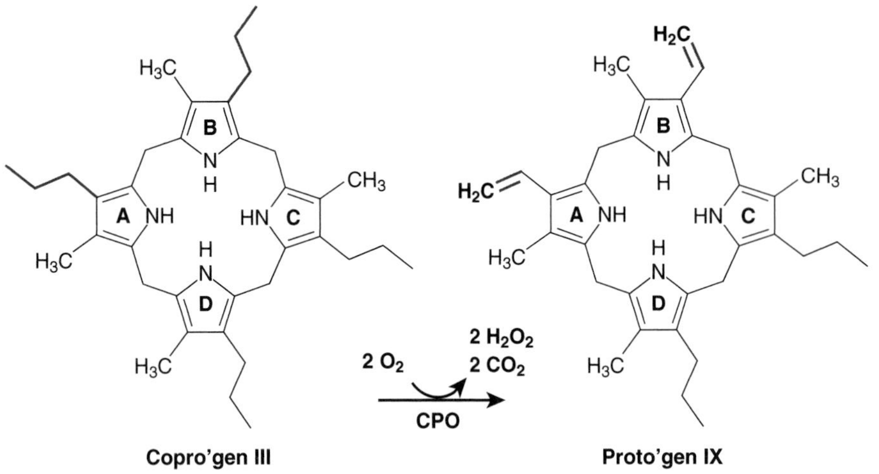

FIGURE 13-20. Reaction catalyzed by coproporphyrinogen oxidase (CPO). The propionate groups on rings A and B of the tetrapyrrole are sequentially oxidatively decarboxylated with the formation of vinyl groups. The reaction consumes 2 molecules of molecular oxygen and produces protoporphyrinogen IX (proto'gen IX), plus 2 molecules of carbon dioxide and hydrogen peroxide. Copro'gen, coproporphyrinogen.

expression of CPO in erythroid cells, a finding consistent with erythroid upregulation mediated by the GATA site.[327]

Hereditary Coproporphyria

Mutations in CPO are the cause of HCP. The disorder is transmitted as an autosomal dominant trait with low penetrance. Affected individuals and nonpenetrant mutation carriers have half-normal CPO activity.[328] Acute neurovisceral attacks are identical to those that occur in patients with AIP, but photo-induced skin lesions are occasionally present. Onset before puberty is extremely rare, although several early-onset cases attributable to homozygosity or compound heterozygosity for CPO mutations have been reported.[329,330] Homozygosity for a specific CPO mutation is responsible for a rare form of homozygous HCP, designated harderoporphyria, with onset in infancy and with a prominent erythroid phenotype.[331] Harderoporphyrin is a tricarboxylic porphyrin in which the propionate on the A ring is oxidized to a vinyl group but the propionate on the B ring is not. Harderoporphyrin was named for an unusual porphyrin found in the rat harderian gland. It was later learned that the porphyrin found in the rat was a glycoconjugate of protoporphyrin and not a tricarboxylic porphyrin, thus rendering the term harderoporphyrin a misnomer.[332]

Frequency. The prevalence of HCP is not known, but it is clearly lower than the prevalence of AIP. Homozygous HCP is very uncommon; however, important clinical manifestations occur in children. Harderoporphyria is even more rare, with only six cases reported.

Clinical Manifestations. Acute neurovisceral attacks in patients with HCP are clinically indistinguishable from the acute attacks in patients with AIP. In a series of 53 German patients,[333] abdominal pain was the most common symptom (89%). Neurologic, psychiatric, and cardiovascular symptoms occurred in 25% to 33% of cases. Cutaneous symptoms occurred in only 14%. Similar findings were reported in an earlier series from the United Kingdom, but the incidence of cutaneous findings was slightly higher.[334] The cutaneous findings are the sole feature of HCP that distinguishes an attack from AIP. Most acute attacks of HCP are precipitated by drugs (see Box 13-2)[335]; however, attacks may also occur in association with menstrual cycles. The cutaneous photosensitivity is manifested mainly as bullous lesions and is generally present only in acute attacks. The bullae resemble those seen in PCT, but chronic scarring reactions are uncommon because the photosensitivity is intermittent. Rarely, intermittent photosensitivity may be the only clinical sign of HCP.[334] In children who are homozygotes or compound heterozygotes for CPO mutations, the disorder is an early-onset phenocopy of clinically affected adults who are simple heterozygotes. Growth retardation, hypertrichosis, and skin pigmentation are additional findings in early-onset cases.[329,330]

The clinical manifestations of harderoporphyria are quite different. Hemolytic anemia, intense jaundice, and hepatosplenomegaly are present at or shortly after birth.[331,336] Bullous skin lesions develop if therapy for neonatal jaundice is undertaken. The urine appears red. Nucleated erythrocytes are present on the peripheral blood smear. Exchange transfusions have been helpful. With time, the hepatomegaly resolves but the splenomegaly remains. The hemolytic anemia becomes partially compensated, and additional transfusions are not necessary. The cutaneous photosensitivity persists, and by the teenage years, the skin resembles that seen in PCT. Acute neurovisceral attacks do not occur.

Five of the six reported cases of harderoporphyria occurred in three families, and in all cases homozygosity for a mutation present in exon 6 (K404E) was detected.[337] The sixth patient, a Japanese newborn with jaundice, hemolytic anemia, hepatomegaly, and photosensitivity, proved not to be homozygous for a CPO mutation. This infant was heterozygous for the K404E mutation, inherited from the father, but enzyme activity was not measured in the child or the parents. A promoter mutation in one maternal allele was suspected as the cause of the harderoporphyria phenotype in the child.[338]

Pathogenesis. Accumulation and excretion of coproporphyrin are best explained by loss-of-function mutations in CPO, but acute neurovisceral attacks, as in AIP, require induction of hepatic ALA-S. More than 30 CPO mutations have been described in patients with HCP and homozygous HCP.[339] The mutation responsible for harderoporphyria, K404E, is of special interest because it affects mainly the second decarboxylation reaction in the conversion of coproporphyrinogen III to protoporphyrinogen IX. One other mutation, R401W, that was found in a patient with HCP was expressed in vitro, and a defect in the second decarboxylation reaction was also found.[339] These findings suggest that a region around residues 401 and 404 is important for retaining the tricarboxylic intermediate (harderoporphyrin) in the active site and permitting the second oxidative decarboxylation. The distinctive erythroid phenotype of harderoporphyria is difficult to explain but must be related to a peculiar toxic effect of harderoporphyrin. The accompanying photosensitivity is probably due to the photodynamic properties of coproporphyrin. The roles of ALA and PBG in the pathogenesis of the acute neurovisceral attacks are as described for AIP.

Laboratory Diagnosis. Increased levels of fecal coproporphyrin III are the most prominent findings and are always present in clinically affected cases.[333] The ratio of coproporphyrin III to coproporphyrin I in feces is markedly increased, even in asymptomatic heterozygotes.[333] Urinary excretion of coproporphyrin is strikingly increased during acute attacks but generally returns to normal during remission. Similarly, urinary excretion of ALA and PBG is increased during attacks but then returns to normal. The laboratory findings in homozygous HCP are the same; however, the abnormalities are more dramatic.

Laboratory findings in harderoporphyria are characterized by the presence of harderoporphyrin in feces along with increased amounts of coproporphyrin III. Urinary excretion of coproporphyrin is also increased, and trace amounts harderoporphyrin may be found. There is no increase in the urinary excretion of ALA or PBG. Modest increases in erythrocyte protoporphyrin are detected, but harderoporphyrin is not present in red cells.[336,337] Iron overload as a consequence of chronic hemolysis and ineffective erythropoiesis has also been reported.[337]

Assays for CPO activity have been used but are difficult to perform and are not widely available. Red cells are not a ready source of the enzyme because CPO is localized in mitochondria. Lymphocytes or cultured cells are required.[72] DNA sequencing is the most direct approach, but the biochemical phenotype is so distinctive that a secure diagnosis can be made by simply analyzing fecal and urine porphyrins. Misdiagnosis of HCP is a common problem because urinary coproporphyrin excretion may be minimally increased in many nonporphyric conditions.

Treatment. Acute neurovisceral attacks are treated as in AIP. Hemin therapy is useful.[340] Although the skin lesions resemble those of PCT, phlebotomy and chloroquine are not effective. The chronic photosensitivity associated with homozygous HCP and harderoporphyria is best managed by avoidance of sunlight, protective clothing, and opaque sunscreens. The extreme jaundice and hemolytic anemia in newborns with harderoporphyria responds to exchange transfusions. Phototherapy should be avoided. The chronic compensated hemolytic anemia requires supplementation with folic acid and may require orally administered iron chelators.

ENZYMATIC OXIDATION OF PROTOPORPHYRINOGEN IX TO PROTOPORPHYRIN IX AND INSERTION OF IRON

Protoporphyrinogen Oxidase

Protoporphyrinogen IX is oxidized to protoporphyrin IX by PPO (Fig. 13-21). PPO is functionally conserved in eukaryotes despite low sequence identity. PPO is an intrinsic protein of the inner mitochondrial membrane and requires molecular oxygen and the cofactor flavin adenine dinucleotide (FAD). Three molecules of oxygen serve as terminal acceptors in the six-electron oxidation reaction, and hydrogen peroxide is generated rather than water.[341-343] The reaction proceeds via three two-electron oxidations rather than one six-electron oxidation.[344]

The crystal structure of tobacco PPO revealed that the enzyme functions as a homodimer.[345] Each monomer contains one noncovalently bound FAD molecule. PPO is synthesized in the cytosol and locates to the outer surface of the inner mitochondrial membrane. The human PPO protein does not contain a cleavable leader sequence but contains a mitochondrial targeting sequence within the first 175 residues. The 28 N-terminal residues have some features of a presequence that functions as an independent mitochondrial targeting sequence.[346] Deletion of these residues, however, does not prevent translocation to mitochondria, thus indicating that more distal regions are required for efficient import and insertion into the inner mitochondrial membrane.[347] There is a single 1.8-kb transcript of PPO in all tissues.[343] The human PPO gene is located on chromosome 1q22-q23.[348,349] The 5′ flanking region of human PPO contains a GATA1 binding site, which suggests the potential for erythroid-specific regulation. Induction of erythroid differentiation in mouse erythroleukemia cells with dimethyl sulfoxide leads to increased expression of PPO.[349]

Variegate Porphyria

VP is transmitted as an autosomal dominant trait resulting from subnormal activity of PPO.[350] The clinical and biochemical features of the disease were first described

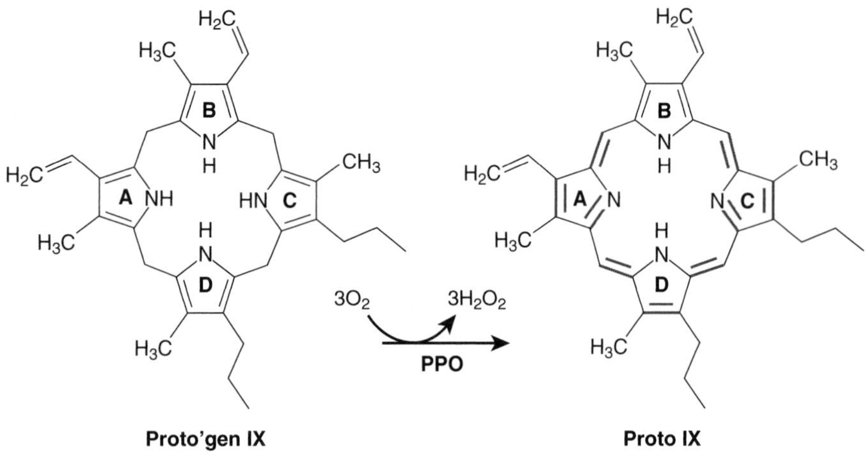

FIGURE 13-21. Reaction catalyzed by protoporphyrinogen oxidase (PPO). Protoporphyrinogen IX (Proto'gen IX) is oxidized to protoporphyrin IX (Proto IX) with the loss of six protons. Three molecules of molecular oxygen are consumed, and three molecules of hydrogen peroxide are formed in the reaction.

in 1937,[351] but VP was not recognized as a distinct porphyric disorder until the description by Dean and Barnes in 1955.[352] The term VP was applied when it was recognized that patients had either cutaneous photosensitivity, a predisposition to acute neurovisceral attacks, or both. Onset before puberty is extremely rare, but early onset with marked photosensitivity has been reported in children homozygous for PPO mutations or with compound heterozygous genotypes.[80]

Frequency. The prevalence of VP in Europe is established at 0.5 per 100,000.[81] The prevalence is higher in Finland at 1.3 per 100,000,[353] but the disease is extraordinarily common in South Africa, where its prevalence is estimated at 3 per 1000 in the white population.[91] The high prevalence in South Africa is due to a founder mutation introduced from the Netherlands in 1688.[354] The connection with the Netherlands has been confirmed by haplotype association studies in South African and Dutch families with VP.[355] Clinical penetrance in earlier reports was estimated at approximately 90%,[356] but the advent of molecular genotyping and sensitive biochemical markers has reduced the estimate to approximately 40% of PPO mutation carriers.[355,357]

Clinical Manifestations. The acute attacks in patients with VP are identical to those seen in AIP but occur at a lower frequency and a later age.[91] Skin manifestations in VP are similar to those in PCT[358] and are of long duration. In a heterozygous western European population of 103 clinically affected patients with VP, 59% had skin lesions only, 20% had acute neurovisceral attacks only, and 21% had both.[359] This distribution is similar to that observed in a 1980 report from South Africa.[356] In contrast, recent reports from South Africa and Finland indicate a marked reduction in acute attacks and a less dramatic decrease in photosensitivity, changes thought to be due to systematic detection of mutant PPO alleles in families and avoidance of potentially harmful drugs.[91,357]

Homozygous VP in two young siblings was first described by Korda and colleagues in 1984.[360] The clini-

cal phenotype differed dramatically from adult-onset VP. Marked photosensitivity from birth, mental retardation, and seizures were described, although no acute neurovisceral attacks occurred. Since then, more than a dozen additional cases have been described.[361-366] Severe cutaneous manifestations beginning in infancy have been a constant finding. Short stature is common, but mental retardation and seizures are not. A peripheral sensory neuropathy and deformities of the hands were noted in some patients, but in no cases were neurovisceral attacks described.

Pathogenesis. A wide variety of PPO mutations in families with VP have been reported in different ethnic groups.[357,359,367,368] A single mutation, R59N, is found in almost all cases in South Africa.[369,370] There appears to be no correlation between specific mutations and the severity of the clinical syndrome. In all cases, the activity of PPO is approximately half-normal.[371,372] The cutaneous manifestations of VP are due to the photodynamic properties of protoporphyrin and coproporphyrin. The acute neurovisceral attacks are due to episodic overproduction of ALA and PBG. The extreme photosensitivity seen in early-onset VP is mediated by very elevated plasma porphyrins.[373] Most of the early-onset cases have been heteroallelic for PPO mutations (i.e., compound heterozygotes) with markedly reduced PPO activity.[365]

Laboratory Diagnosis. When acute attacks of VP occur, fecal protoporphyrin and coproporphyrin and urinary coproporphyrin are markedly elevated.[357] VP can be distinguished from HCP and AIP by detection in plasma of a characteristic fluorescence emission spectrum with a maximum at 626 nm.[122] This emission spectrum results from a dicarboxyl porphyrin bound to plasma proteins.[374] Detection of the 626-nm peak in plasma is a useful method of identifying asymptomatic gene carriers and is more sensitive than fecal porphyrin analysis.[355,375] Urinary ALA and PBG are increased during acute attacks but may be normal during remissions.

Homozygous VP is characterized by markedly increased erythrocyte zinc protoporphyrin levels and elevated stool protoporphyrin and coproporphyrin levels. PPO activity can be measured in cells that contain mitochondria,[376] but enzyme assays are not widely available. Direct fluorometric measurement of plasma porphyrins is probably the most rapid method of establishing the diagnosis of VP. Sequencing of the PPO gene is being applied more widely and is available through the Department of Human Genetics at the Mount Sinai School of Medicine in New York.

Treatment. Treatment of acute attacks is as described for AIP and HCP. Protection from sunlight is the only practical way to manage the photosensitivity. Phlebotomy therapy, chloroquine, and hemin are not effective.[350,377,378] A single patient with symptomatic VP has been treated with a liver transplant.[119] The indication for transplantation was advanced alcohol-induced cirrhosis. After transplantation, fecal porphyrin values returned to normal and no further cutaneous or neurovisceral symptoms occurred. Improved treatment, detection of latent family members, and avoidance of potentially harmful drugs have improved the outcome and reduced disease-related morbidity.[91,355]

Ferrochelatase

The final step in the heme biosynthetic pathway, insertion of iron into protoporphyrin IX, occurs on the matrix side of the inner mitochondrial membrane, a reaction catalyzed by FECH (Fig. 13-22). Human FECH has been crystallized and the enzyme functions as a homodimer.[379] Each monomer of FECH contains a nitric oxide–sensitive 2Fe-2S iron-sulfur cluster bound to a cysteine-rich site at the C-terminal.[380] It has been suggested that a direct interaction occurs between PPO on the outer surface of the inner mitochondrial membrane and FECH on the inner surface.[345] This arrangement would permit direct transfer of protoporphyrin IX from PPO to the active site of FECH. This mechanism has been questioned, however, inasmuch as experiments using isolated mitochondria indicate that a complex between enzymes is not required for synthesis of heme.[381]

The human FECH gene has been cloned and mapped to chromosome 18q21.3.[382] The same transcriptional start site is used in erythroid and nonerythroid tissues and contains binding sites for both housekeeping and erythroid-specific promoter elements.[383] FECH is synthesized in the cytosol and targeted to mitochondria by sequences in the leader peptide,[384] followed by cleavage to produce the active, mature protein. The first 62 amino acids in the leader sequence are sufficient for mitochondrial targeting, but an additional 11 residues are required for efficient proteolytic processing.[385] Expression of FECH is regulated by intracellular iron levels, probably related to the enzyme's requirement for iron-sulfur clusters.[327] Additional regulatory effects occur through interactions with hypoxia-inducible factor.[386]

Erythropoietic Protoporphyria

Erythropoietic protoporphyria (EPP) is an inherited disorder of heme biosynthesis characterized clinically by the onset in childhood or infancy of acute photosensitivity of sun-exposed skin. The disorder was first recognized in 1953 by Kosenow and Treibs[387] but was clinically characterized and named EPP by Magnus and associates in 1961.[388] The inherited nature of the disease was first reported by Haeger-Aronsen in 1963.[389] In most cases, EPP is due to deficient activity of FECH associated with loss-of-function mutations of the FECH gene, but in some cases, EPP results from mutant alleles of the mitochondrial iron importer mitoferrin.[390,391] In a minority of patients with EPP, the excess protoporphyrin IX generated in erythrocytes causes severe cholestatic liver disease requiring liver transplantation.[392]

Frequency. The prevalence of clinically manifested EPP has been difficult to estimate but is probably close to that of AIP. In the European immigrant population of South Africa, clinically evident EPP is estimated to occur in 6.6 individuals per million.[393] The prevalence in the United Kingdom is approximately 7.7 per million.[394]

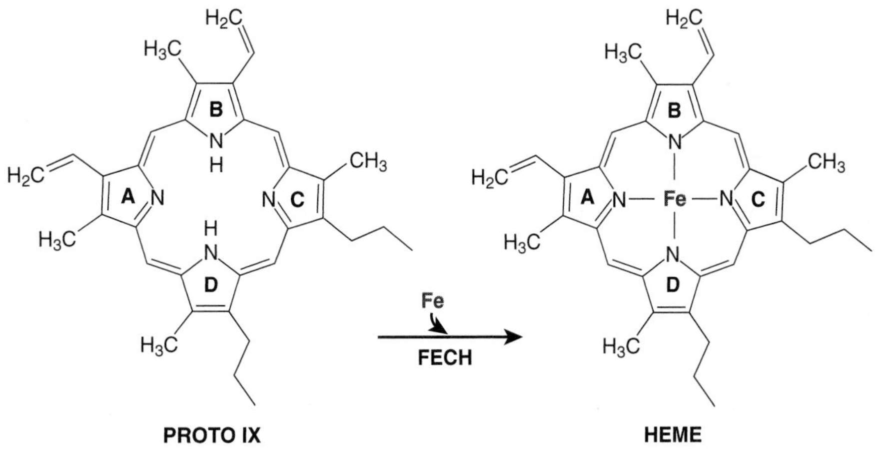

FIGURE 13-22. Reaction catalyzed by ferrochelatase (FECH). The final step in the synthesis of heme is insertion of ferrous iron into the protoporphyrin IX (Proto IX) macrocycle with the release of two protons.

PROTO IX

HEME

Prevalence estimates for Northern Ireland and the Netherlands have approached 13 per million,[395,396] a finding attributed to a founder effect.[397] A report from Slovenia estimated an even higher prevalence at 17.5 per million.[398] EPP is pan-ethnic but is extremely rare in individuals of African descent.[393]

Clinical Manifestations. The dominant clinical feature of EPP is cutaneous photosensitivity in response to sun exposure with onset in infancy or childhood.[399,400] The clinical picture is very different from that of the other photosensitizing porphyrias. A characteristic burning pain, erythema, and edema develop as an acute response to sun exposure.[394] Early in the course of EPP, the burning discomfort may occur in the absence of objective cutaneous findings.[401,402] Bullous lesions, pigment changes, and scarring are very uncommon. Instead, the skin develops a leathery characteristic that mimics premature aging. The symptoms and objective skin findings change little over time, but increased sun tolerance has been reported during pregnancy.[403,404]

A mild, microcytic anemia is common,[400,405-407] presumably caused by impaired heme synthesis. Iron may accumulate in the cytosol and mitochondria of erythroblasts, but such findings are uncommon.[408] A similar microcytic anemia develops in a mouse model of EPP because of homozygosity for mutant FECH alleles.[409] Serum ferritin values in humans with EPP are reduced, but erythropoiesis does not appear to be limited by iron.[406]

Gallstones develop in approximately 10% of patients with EPP and tend to occur early in life.[400,410] The gallstones contain protoporphyrin IX, which becomes insoluble in bile and alters the solubility of other components of bile.[411,412] When gallstones develop in children, a diagnosis of EPP should be considered.[413] Minor abnormalities in liver function tests, mainly elevations in transaminases, are common,[399] and liver biopsy may demonstrate deposition of protoporphyrin and periportal fibrosis.[400,414-417]

Severe cholestatic liver disease progressing to portal hypertension and fatal decompensated cirrhosis will develop in between 1% and 5% of patients with EPP.[392,418,419] Rarely, acute liver failure may be the initial feature of EPP.[420,421] Approximately 50 fatal cases of EPP-related liver disease have been reported,[392,395,422-424] including two teenagers and an 11-year-old child.[395]

Pathogenesis. More than 85 mutations in the FECH gene have been detected.[393,425,426] The mode of mendelian transmission had been described as autosomal dominant with incomplete penetrance, but heterozygotes expressing the clinical phenotype have consistently shown FECH activity between 15% and 20% of normal.[427] This was explained by a proposed dominant negative effect in which both mutant-mutant homodimers and mutant–wild type homodimers are catalytically inactive, with only wild type–wild type homodimers being responsible for

the measured enzyme activity. This theory was discarded with the discovery of a hypomorphic FECH allele that is common in the population.[428-430] An intragenic polymorphism (IVS 3-48C) in intron 3 is responsible for low expression of the hypomorphic allele. This polymorphism favors the use of a cryptic acceptor splice site 63 bases upstream of the normal splice site. The aberrantly spliced mRNA contains a premature stop codon and is degraded by a nonsense-mediated decay mechanism.[430] The result is a lower steady-state level of wild-type FECH mRNA. Virtually all clinically evident cases of EPP are due to coinheritance of the hypomorphic allele in *trans* to a loss-of-function mutant allele. This genetic combination was found in 98% of French patients with EPP[431] and at a similar frequency in South African patients.[393] The frequency of the IVS 3-48C hypomorphic allele varies widely in different populations and is related to the observed differences in the prevalence of EPP.[431,432]

The rare exception to the compound heterozygous mutant/hypomorph genotype is inheritance of two loss-of-function FECH alleles. The autosomal recessive form of EPP was found in 3% of patients with EPP in the United Kingdom[426] and in occasional cases from other countries.[393,427,433-435] The autosomal recessive form of EPP may carry a higher risk for severe liver disease.

The genetics of EPP is complicated further by the discovery of a phenocopy caused by a mutation in the gene encoding mitoferrin, the principal mitochondrial iron importer.[390,391] Eight patients from six families referred to a liver center because of advanced liver disease were found to be heterozygous for a 477-base insertion in intron 2 of the mitoferrin gene that generates a stop codon at codon 156 in exon 3. None of the patients had FECH-coding mutations or the IVS 3-48C polymorphism.[390] One South African family with a highly penetrant EPP phenotype, yet no mutant FECH alleles, has also been described.[393] Affected members of this family had high levels of erythrocyte zinc protoporphyrin rather than the usual free erythrocyte protoporphyrin, thus suggesting that impaired iron delivery to mitochondria was the underlying defect.

Laboratory Diagnosis. The free erythrocyte protoporphyrin concentration is markedly increased in symptomatic EPP.[400,436] Values ranging from 6- to 100-fold greater than normal have been reported. Elevated erythrocyte protoporphyrin levels are also found in patients with iron deficiency and lead poisoning, but in these conditions the elevation is less dramatic and it is zinc protoporphyrin that is present.[437] Zinc protoporphyrin can easily be distinguished spectrally from the free protoporphyrin found in EPP.[438] Zinc protoporphyrin can also be distinguished from free protoporphyrin by chromatographic techniques.[72] An elevated plasma porphyrin level confirms the presence of a porphyric disorder, but false-negative results may be obtained in patients with EPP because protoporphyrin is particularly susceptible to photodegradation.[439] Care must be taken to shield the plasma sample from sunlight or fluorescent lighting.

Fecal protoporphyrin excretion may be increased up to 15-fold, although values vary widely from patient to patient.[440] Urinary excretion of ALA and PBG is normal. Protoporphyrin, a highly hydrophobic compound, is not excreted in urine.

Assays for FECH activity are not widely available. Detection of FECH mutations is the most direct approach to confirm the diagnosis of EPP. Molecular studies are also the only reliable method for identifying asymptomatic cases in families with an affected proband.

Treatment. Treatment of EPP has two objectives. First, an attempt should be made to minimize the harmful effects of exposure to sunlight. Protective clothing and opaque sunscreens can be helpful, as with other photosensitizing porphyrias. Tolerance to sunlight can be improved in most patients with EPP by inducing carotenemia. This can best be accomplished by administering β-carotene beadlets (Lumitene, Tishcon Corp., Westbery, NY) in doses ranging from 120 to 300 mg/day.[441,442] The only side effect is a dose-related, yellow-orange discoloration of the skin.[443,444] The mechanism of action of β-carotene probably involves quenching of singlet oxygen species or free radicals.[445]

The second objective of therapy is to minimize the hepatotoxic effects of protoporphyrin. Cholestyramine can interrupt the enterohepatic circulation of protoporphyrin excreted in bile and promote fecal excretion. This has been moderately effective in some patients.[411] Oral administration of bile salts (ursodeoxycholic acid or chenodeoxycholic acid) can increase excretion of protoporphyrin into bile.[446,447] A variety of other measures have been used when liver function deteriorates, including plasmapheresis, hemodialysis, exchange transfusions, and suppression of erythropoiesis.[392] In the small proportion of patients with EPP in whom liver failure develops, liver transplantation is the only effective therapy.[392,448,449] Liver transplantation, however, does not address the underlying overproduction of protoporphyrin in the native marrow, and recurrent disease can develop in the transplanted liver.[449-451] This complication was successfully managed in a 15-year-old boy with a bone marrow allograft from an HLA-matched sibling who did not have EPP.[452]

REFERENCES

1. Garnick S, Sassa S. δ-Aminolevulinic acid synthase and the control of heme and chlorophyll synthesis. In Vogel H (ed). Metabolic Regulation. New York, Academic Press, 1971, p 77.

2. Moore MR. Historical introduction to porphyrins and porphyrias. In Dailey HA (ed). Biosynthesis of Heme and Chlorophylls, vol 1. New York, McGraw-Hill, 1990, pp 1-54.

3. Cotter PD, Drabkin HA, Varkony T, et al. Assignment of the human housekeeping delta-aminolevulinate synthase gene (ALAS1) to chromosome band 3p21.1 by PCR analysis of somatic cell hybrids. Cytogenet Cell Genet. 1995;69:207-208.

4. Cox TC, Bawden MJ, Abraham NG, et al. Erythroid 5-aminolevulinate synthase is located on the X chromosome. Am J Hum Genet. 1990;46:107-111.

5. Larkin MA, Blackshields G, Brown NP, et al. Clustal W and Clustal X version 2.0. Bioinformatics. 2007;23: 2947-2948.

6. Astner I, Schulze JO, van den Heuvel J, et al. Crystal structure of 5-aminolevulinate synthase, the first enzyme of heme biosynthesis, and its link to XLSA in humans. EMBO J. 2005;24:3166-3177.

7. Hunter GA, Zhang J, Ferreira GC. Transient kinetic studies support refinements to the chemical and kinetic mechanisms of aminolevulinate synthase. J Biol Chem. 2007;282:23025-23035.

8. Lathrop JT, Timko MP. Regulation by heme of mitochondrial protein transport through a conserved amino acid motif. Science. 1993;259:522-525.

9. Dailey TA, Woodruff JH, Dailey HA. Examination of mitochondrial protein targeting of haem synthetic enzymes: in vivo identification of three functional haemresponsive motifs in 5-aminolaevulinate synthase. Biochem J. 2005;386:381-386.

10. Quigley JG, Yang Z, Worthington MT, et al. Identification of a human heme exporter that is essential for erythropoiesis. Cell. 2004;118:757-766.

11. Whiting MJ. Synthesis of delta-aminolaevulinate synthase by isolated liver polyribosomes. Biochem J. 1976;158:391-400.

12. Handschin C, Lin J, Rhee J, et al. Nutritional regulation of hepatic heme biosynthesis and porphyria through PGC-1alpha. Cell. 2005;122:505-515.

13. Wu Z, Puigserver P, Andersson U, et al. Mechanisms controlling mitochondrial biogenesis and respiration through the thermogenic coactivator PGC-1. Cell. 1999; 98:115-124.

14. Virbasius JV, Scarpulla RC. Activation of the human mitochondrial transcription factor A gene by nuclear respiratory factors: a potential regulatory link between nuclear and mitochondrial gene expression in organelle biogenesis. Proc Natl Acad Sci U S A. 1994;91:1309-1313.

15. Scassa ME, Guberman AS, Ceruti JM, Canepa ET. Hepatic nuclear factor 3 and nuclear factor 1 regulate 5-aminolevulinate synthase gene expression and are involved in insulin repression. J Biol Chem. 2004;279:28082-28092.

16. Scassa ME, Guberman AS, Varone CL, Canepa ET. Phosphatidylinositol 3-kinase and Ras/mitogen-activated protein kinase signaling pathways are required for the regulation of 5-aminolevulinate synthase gene expression by insulin. Exp Cell Res. 2001;271:201-213.

17. Anderson KE, Bloomer JR, Bonkovsky HL, et al. Recommendations for the diagnosis and treatment of the acute porphyrias. Ann Intern Med. 2005;142:439-450.

18. Phillips JD, Kushner JP. Fast track to the porphyrias. Nat Med. 2005;11:1049-1050.

19. Cable EE, Miller TG, Isom HC. Regulation of heme metabolism in rat hepatocytes and hepatocyte cell lines: delta-aminolevulinic acid synthase and heme oxygenase

are regulated by different heme-dependent mechanisms. Arch Biochem Biophys. 2000;384:280-295.

20. Roberts AG, Elder GH. Alternative splicing and tissue-specific transcription of human and rodent ubiquitous 5-aminolevulinate synthase (ALAS1) genes. Biochim Biophys Acta. 2001;1518:95-105.

21. Roberts AG, Redding SJ, Llewellyn DH. An alternatively-spliced exon in the 5′-UTR of human ALAS1 mRNA inhibits translation and renders it resistant to haem-mediated decay. FEBS Lett. 2005;579:1061-1066.

22. Grandchamp B, Bissell DM, Licko V, Schmid R. Formation and disposition of newly synthesized heme in adult rat hepatocytes in primary culture. J Biol Chem. 1981; 256:11677-11683.

23. Yannoni CZ, Robinson SH. Early-labelled haem in erythroid and hepatic cells. Nature. 1975;258:330-331.

24. Srivastava G, Borthwick IA, Maguire DJ, et al. Regulation of 5-aminolevulinate synthase mRNA in different rat tissues. J Biol Chem. 1988;263:5202-5209.

25. Cox TC, Bawden MJ, Martin A, May BK. Human erythroid 5-aminolevulinate synthase: promoter analysis and identification of an iron-responsive element in the mRNA. EMBO J. 1991;10:1891-1902.

26. Napier I, Ponka P, Richardson DR. Iron trafficking in the mitochondrion: novel pathways revealed by disease. Blood. 2005;105:1867-1874.

27. Rouault TA, Tong W-H. Iron-sulphur cluster biogenesis and mitochondrial iron homeostasis. Nat Rev Mol Cell Biol. 2005;6:345-351.

28. Wingert RA, Galloway JL, Barut B, et al. Deficiency of glutaredoxin 5 reveals Fe-S clusters are required for vertebrate haem synthesis. Nature. 2005;436:1035-1039.

29. Erskine PT, Norton E, Cooper JB, et al. X-ray structure of 5-aminolevulinic acid dehydratase from *Escherichia coli* complexed with the inhibitor levulinic acid at 2.0 Å resolution. Biochemistry. 1999;38:4266-4276.

30. Frankenberg N, Erskine PT, Cooper JB, et al. High resolution crystal structure of a Mg^{2+}-dependent porphobilinogen synthase. J Mol Biol. 1999;289:591-602.

31. Anderson PM, Desnick RJ. Purification and properties of delta-aminolevulinate dehydrase from human erythrocytes. J Biol Chem. 1979;254:6924-6930.

32. Bevan DR, Bodlaender P, Shemin D. Mechanism of porphobilinogen synthase. Requirement of Zn^{2+} for enzyme activity. J Biol Chem. 1980;255:2030-2035.

33. Dent AJ, Beyersmann D, Block C, Hasnain SS. Two different zinc sites in bovine 5-aminolevulinate dehydratase distinguished by extended x-ray absorption fine structure. Biochemistry. 1990;29:7822-7828.

34. Jaffe EK, Abrams WR, Kaempfen HX, Harris KA Jr. 5-Chlorolevulinate modification of porphobilinogen synthase identifies a potential role for the catalytic zinc. Biochemistry. 1992;31:2113-2123.

34a. Kaya AH, Plewinska M, Wong DM, Desnick RJ, Wetmur JG. Human delta-aminolevulinate dehydratase (ALAD) gene: structure and alternative splicing of the erythroid and housekeeping mRNAs. Genomics. 1994;19: 242-248.

34b. Potluri VR, Astrin KH, Wetmur JG, Bishop DF, Desnick RJ. Human delta-aminolevulinate dehydratase: chromosomal localization to 9q34 by in situ hybridization. Hum Genet. 1987;76:236-239.

35. Battistuzzi G, Petrucci R, Silvagni L, et al. δ-Aminolevulinate dehydrase: a new genetic polymorphism in man. Ann Hum Genet. 1981;45:223-229.

36. Astrin KH, Bishop DF, Wetmur JG, et al. δ-Aminolevulinic acid dehydratase isozymes and lead toxicity. Ann N Y Acad Sci. 1987;514:23-29.

37. Benkmann HG, Bogdanski P, Goedde HW. Polymorphism of delta-aminolevulinic acid dehydratase in various populations. Hum Hered. 1983;33:62-64.

38. Sithisarankul P, Schwartz BS, Lee BK, et al. Aminolevulinic acid dehydratase genotype mediates plasma levels of the neurotoxin, 5-aminolevulinic acid, in lead-exposed workers. Am J Ind Med. 1997;32:15-20.

39. Jaffe EK, Martins J, Li J, et al. The molecular mechanism of lead inhibition of human porphobilinogen synthase. J Biol Chem. 2001;276:1531-1537.

40. Guo GG, Gu M, Etlinger JD. 240-kDa proteasome inhibitor (CF-2) is identical to delta-aminolevulinic acid dehydratase. J Biol Chem. 1994;269:12399-12402.

41. Wolff C, Piderit F, Armas-Merino R. Deficiency of porphobilinogen synthase associated with acute crisis. Diagnosis of the first two cases in Chile by laboratory methods. Eur J Clin Chem Clin Biochem. 1991;29:313-315.

42. Akagi R, Kato N, Inoue R, et al. δ-Aminolevulinate dehydratase (ALAD) porphyria: the first case in North America with two novel ALAD mutations. Mol Genet Metab. 2006;87:329-336.

43. Jaffe EK, Stith L. ALAD porphyria is a conformational disease. Am J Hum Genet. 2007;80:329-337.

44. Akagi R, Shimizu R, Furuyama K, et al. Novel molecular defects of the delta-aminolevulinate dehydratase gene in a patient with inherited acute hepatic porphyria. Hepatology. 2000;31:704-708.

45. Doss M, Laubenthal F, Stoeppler M. Lead poisoning in inherited delta-aminolevulinic acid dehydratase deficiency. Int Arch Occup Environ Health. 1984;54:55-63.

46. Thunell S, Holmberg L, Lundgren J. Aminolaevulinate dehydratase porphyria in infancy. A clinical and biochemical study. J Clin Chem Clin Biochem. 1987;25:5-14.

47. Doss M, von Tiepermann R, Schneider J, Schmid H. New type of hepatic porphyria with porphobilinogen synthase defect and intermittent acute clinical manifestation. Klin Wochenschr. 1979;57:1123-1127.

48. Gross U, Sassa S, Jacob K, et al. 5-Aminolevulinic acid dehydratase deficiency porphyria: a twenty-year clinical and biochemical follow-up. Clin Chem. 1998;44:1892-1896.

49. Doss MO, Stauch T, Gross U, et al. The third case of Doss porphyria (delta-amino-levulinic acid dehydratase deficiency) in Germany. J Inherit Metab Dis. 2004;27:529-536.

50. Plewinska M, Thunell S, Holmberg L, et al. δ-Aminolevulinate dehydratase deficient porphyria: identification of the molecular lesions in a severely affected homozygote. Am J Hum Genet. 1991;49:167-174.

51. Maruno M, Furuyama K, Akagi R, et al. Highly heterogeneous nature of delta-aminolevulinate dehydratase (ALAD) deficiencies in ALAD porphyria. Blood. 2001;97: 2972-2978.

52. Hassoun A, Verstraeten L, Mercelis R, Martin JJ. Biochemical diagnosis of an hereditary aminolaevulinate dehydratase deficiency in a 63-year-old man. J Clin Chem Clin Biochem. 1989;27:781-786.

53. Akagi R, Nishitani C, Harigae H, et al. Molecular analysis of delta-aminolevulinate dehydratase deficiency in a patient with an unusual late-onset porphyria. Blood. 2000; 96:3618-3623.

54. Akagi R, Yasui Y, Harper P, Sassa S. A novel mutation of delta-aminolaevulinate dehydratase in a healthy child with 12% erythrocyte enzyme activity. Br J Haematol. 1999;106:931-937.

55. Breinig S, Kervinen J, Stith L, et al. Control of tetrapyrrole biosynthesis by alternate quaternary forms of porphobilinogen synthase. Nat Struct Biol. 2003;10: 757-763.

56. Akagi R, Inoue R, Muranaka S, et al. Dual gene defects involving delta-aminolaevulinate dehydratase and coproporphyrinogen oxidase in a porphyria patient. Br J Haematol. 2006;132:237-243.

57. Solis C, Martinez-Bermejo A, Naidich TP, et al. Acute intermittent porphyria: studies of the severe homozygous dominant disease provides insights into the neurologic attacks in acute porphyrias. Arch Neurol. 2004;61:1764-1770.

58. Von Blankenfeld G, Trotter J, Kettenmann H. Expression and developmental regulation of a GABA$_A$ receptor in cultured murine cells of the oligodendrocyte lineage. Eur J Neurosci. 1991;3:310-316.

59. Alberdi E, Sanchez-Gomez MV, Marino A, Matute C. Ca^{2+} influx through AMPA or kainate receptors alone is sufficient to initiate excitotoxicity in cultured oligodendrocytes. Neurobiol Dis. 2002;9:234-243.

60. Tschudy DP, Hess RA, Frykholm BC. Inhibition of delta-aminolevulinic acid dehydrase by 4,6-dioxoheptanoic acid. J Biol Chem. 1981;256:9915-9923.

61. Jacob K, Egeler E, Gross U, Doss MO. Investigations on the formation of urinary coproporphyrin isomers I-IV in 5-aminolevulinic acid dehydratase deficiency porphyria, acute lead intoxication and after oral 5-aminolevulinic acid loading. Clin Biochem. 1999;32:119-123.

62. Warren MJ, Cooper JB, Wood SP, Shoolingin-Jordan PM. Lead poisoning, haem synthesis and 5-aminolaevulinic acid dehydratase. Trends Biochem Sci. 1998;23:217-221.

63. Mitchell G, Larochelle J, Lambert M, et al. Neurologic crises in hereditary tyrosinemia. N Engl J Med. 1990;322: 432-437.

64. Sassa S, Kappas A. Hereditary tyrosinemia and the heme biosynthetic pathway. Profound inhibition of delta-aminolevulinic acid dehydratase activity by succinylacetone. J Clin Invest. 1983;71:625-634.

65. Akagi R, Prchal JT, Eberhart CE, Sassa S. An acquired acute hepatic porphyria: a novel type of delta-aminolevulinate dehydratase inhibition. Clin Chim Acta. 1992;212: 79-84.

66. Fujita H, Ishihara N. Reduction of delta-aminolevulinate dehydratase concentration by bromobenzene in rats. Br J Ind Med. 1988;45:640-644.

67. Fujita H, Koizumi A, Furusawa T, Ikeda M. Decreased erythrocyte delta-aminolevulinate dehydratase activity after styrene exposure. Biochem Pharmacol. 1987;36:711-716.

68. Thunell S, Henrichson A, Floderus Y, et al. Liver transplantation in a boy with acute porphyria due to aminolaevulinate dehydratase deficiency. Eur J Clin Chem Clin Biochem. 1992;30:599-606.

69. Helliwell JR, Nieh YP, Habash J, et al. Time-resolved and static-ensemble structural chemistry of hydroxymethylbilane synthase. Faraday Discuss. 2003;122:131-144; discussion 171-190.

70. Shoolingin-Jordan PM, Al-Dbass A, McNeill LA, et al. Human porphobilinogen deaminase mutations in the investigation of the mechanism of dipyrromethane cofactor assembly and tetrapyrrole formation. Biochem Soc Trans. 2003;31:731-735.

71. Brownlie PD, Lambert R, Louie GV, et al. The three-dimensional structures of mutants of porphobilinogen deaminase: toward an understanding of the structural basis of acute intermittent porphyria. Protein Sci. 1994;3: 1644-1650.

72. Elder GH, Smith SG, Smyth SJ. Laboratory investigation of the porphyrias. Ann Clin Biochem. 1990;27:395-412.

73. Shoolingin-Jordan PM, Warren MJ, Awan SJ. Discovery that the assembly of the dipyrromethane cofactor of porphobilinogen deaminase holoenzyme proceeds initially by the reaction of preuroporphyrinogen with the apoenzyme. Biochem J. 1996;316:373-376.

74. Raich N, Romeo PH, Dubart A, et al. Molecular cloning and complete primary sequence of human erythrocyte porphobilinogen deaminase. Nucleic Acids Res. 1986;14: 5955-5968.

75. Wang AL, Arredondo-Vega FX, Giampietro PF, et al. Regional gene assignment of human porphobilinogen deaminase and esterase A4 to chromosome 11q23 leads to 11qter. Proc Natl Acad Sci U S A. 1981;78:5734-5738.

76. Chretien S, Dubart A, Beaupain D, et al. Alternative transcription and splicing of the human porphobilinogen deaminase gene result either in tissue-specific or in housekeeping expression. Proc Natl Acad Sci U S A. 1988;85: 6-10.

77. Mignotte V, Eleouet JF, Raich N, Romeo PH. Cis- and trans-acting elements involved in the regulation of the erythroid promoter of the human porphobilinogen deaminase gene. Proc Natl Acad Sci U S A. 1989;86:6548-6552.

78. Grandchamp B, De Verneuil H, Beaumont C, et al. Tissue-specific expression of porphobilinogen deaminase. Two isoenzymes from a single gene. Eur J Biochem. 1987; 162:105-110.

79. Hrdinka M, Puy H, Martasek P. May 2006 update in porphobilinogen deaminase gene polymorphisms and mutations causing acute intermittent porphyria: comparison with the situation in Slavic population. Physiol Res. 2006;55(Suppl 2):S119-S136.

80. Elder GH. Hepatic porphyrias in children. J Inherit Metab Dis. 1997;20:237-246.

81. Elder GH, Hift RJ, Meissner PN. The acute porphyrias. Lancet. 1997;349:1613-1617.

82. Hessels J, Voortman G, van der Wagen A, et al. Homozygous acute intermittent porphyria in a 7-year-old boy with massive excretions of porphyrins and porphyrin precursors. J Inherit Metab Dis. 2004;27:19-27.

83. Llewellyn DH, Smyth SJ, Elder GH, et al. Homozygous acute intermittent porphyria: compound heterozygosity for adjacent base transitions in the same codon of the porphobilinogen deaminase gene. Hum Genet. 1992;89:97-98.

84. Grandchamp B. Acute intermittent porphyria. Semin Liver Dis. 1998;18:17-24.

85. Mustajoki P, Koskelo P. Hereditary hepatic porphyrias in Finland. Acta Med Scand. 1976;200:171-178.

86. Kauppinen R, von und zu Fraunberg M. Molecular and biochemical studies of acute intermittent porphyria in 196 patients and their families. Clin Chem. 2002;48:1891-1900.

87. Mustajoki P, Kauppinen R, Lannfelt L, et al. Frequency of low erythrocyte porphobilinogen deaminase activity in Finland. J Intern Med. 1992;231:389-395.

88. Nordmann Y, Puy H, Da Silva V, et al. Acute intermittent porphyria: prevalence of mutations in the porphobilinogen deaminase gene in blood donors in France. J Intern Med. 1997;242:213-217.

89. Kauppinen R, Mustajoki P. Prognosis of acute porphyria: occurrence of acute attacks, precipitating factors, and associated diseases. Medicine (Baltimore). 1992;71:1-13.

90. Hultdin J, Schmauch A, Wikberg A, et al. Acute intermittent porphyria in childhood: a population-based study. Acta Paediatr. 2003;92:562-568.

91. Hift RJ, Meissner PN. An analysis of 112 acute porphyric attacks in Cape Town, South Africa: evidence that acute intermittent porphyria and variegate porphyria differ in susceptibility and severity. Medicine (Baltimore). 2005;84:48-60.

92. Nordmann Y, Puy H. Human hereditary hepatic porphyrias. Clin Chim Acta. 2002;325:17-37.

93. Goldberg A. Acute intermittent porphyria: a study of 50 cases. Q J Med. 1959;28:183-209.

94. Stein JA, Tschudy DP. Acute intermittent porphyria. A clinical and biochemical study of 46 patients. Medicine (Baltimore). 1970;49:1-16.

95. Waldenstrom J. The porphyrias as inborn errors of metabolism. Am J Med. 1957;22:758-773.

96. Millward LM, Kelly P, King A, Peters TJ. Anxiety and depression in the acute porphyrias. J Inherit Metab Dis. 2005;28:1099-1107.

97. Cashman MD. Psychiatric aspects of acute porphyria. Lancet. 1961;1:115-116.

98. Patience DA, Blackwood DH, McColl KE, Moore MR. Acute intermittent porphyria and mental illness—a family study. Acta Psychiatr Scand. 1994;89:262-267.

99. Santosh PJ, Malhotra S. Varied psychiatric manifestations of acute intermittent porphyria. Biol Psychiatry. 1994;36:744-747.

100. Boon FF, Ellis C. Acute intermittent porphyria in a children's psychiatric hospital. J Am Acad Child Adolesc Psychiatry. 1989;28:606-609.

101. Ellencweig N, Schoenfeld N, Zemishlany Z. Acute intermittent porphyria: psychosis as the only clinical manifestation. Isr J Psychiatry Relat Sci. 2006;43:52-56.

102. Albers JW, Fink JK. Porphyric neuropathy. Muscle Nerve. 2004;30:410-422.

103. Meyer UA, Schuurmans MM, Lindberg RL. Acute porphyrias: pathogenesis of neurological manifestations. Semin Liver Dis. 1998;18:43-52.

104. Mustajoki P, Seppalainen AM. Neuropathy in latent hereditary hepatic porphyria. BMJ. 1975;2:310-312.

105. Kupferschmidt H, Bont A, Schnorf H, et al. Transient cortical blindness and biooccipital brain lesions in two patients with acute intermittent porphyria. Ann Intern Med. 1995;123:598-600.

106. Sze G. Cortical brain lesions in acute intermittent porphyria. Ann Intern Med. 1996;125:422-423.

107. Bylesjo I, Forsgren L, Lithner F, Boman K. Epidemiology and clinical characteristics of seizures in patients with acute intermittent porphyria. Epilepsia. 1996;37:230-235.

108. Morales Ortega X, Wolff Fernandez C, Leal Ibarra T, et al. [Porphyric crisis: experience of 30 episodes.] Medicina (B Aires). 1999;59:23-27.

109. Usalan C, Erdem Y, Altun B, et al. Severe hyponatremia due to SIADH provoked by acute intermittent porphyria. Clin Nephrol. 1996;45:418.

110. Pischik E, Bulyanitsa A, Kazakov V, Kauppinen R. Clinical features predictive of a poor prognosis in acute porphyria. J Neurol. 2004;251:1538-1541.

111. Jeans JB, Savik K, Gross CR, et al. Mortality in patients with acute intermittent porphyria requiring hospitalization: a United States case series. Am J Med Genet. 1996;65:269-273.

112. Bonkowsky HL, Tschudy DP, Collins A, et al. Repression of the overproduction of porphyrin precursors in acute intermittent porphyria by intravenous infusions of hematin. Proc Natl Acad Sci U S A. 1971;68:2725-2729.

113. Lamon JM, Frykholm BC, Bennett M, Tschudy DP. Prevention of acute porphyric attacks by intravenous haematin. Lancet. 1978;2:492-494.

114. Lamon JM, Frykholm BC, Hess RA, Tschudy DP. Hematin therapy for acute porphyria. Medicine (Baltimore). 1979;58:252-269.

115. Felsher BF, Redeker AG. Acute intermittent porphyria: effect of diet and griseofulvin. Medicine (Baltimore). 1967;46:217-223.

116. Paxton JW, Moore MR, Deattie AD, Goldberg A. 17-Oxosteroid conjugates in plasma and urine of patients with acute intermittent porphyria. Clin Sci Mol Med. 1974;46:207-222.

117. Welland FH, Hellman ES, Gaddis EM, et al. Factors affecting the excretion of porphyrin precursors by patients with acute intermittent porphyria. I. The effect of diet. Metabolism. 1964;13:232-250.

118. Soonawalla ZF, Orug T, Badminton MN, et al. Liver transplantation as a cure for acute intermittent porphyria. Lancet. 2004;363:705-706.

119. Stojeba N, Meyer C, Jeanpierre C, et al. Recovery from a variegate porphyria by a liver transplantation. Liver Transpl. 2004;10:935-938.

120. Mauzerall D, Granick S. The occurrence and determination of delta-amino-levulinic acid and porphobilinogen in urine. J Biol Chem. 1956;219:435-446.

121. Deacon AC, Peters TJ. Identification of acute porphyria: evaluation of a commercial screening test for urinary porphobilinogen. Ann Clin Biochem. 1998;35:726-732.

122. Poh-Fitzpatrick MB. A plasma porphyrin fluorescence marker for variegate porphyria. Arch Dermatol. 1980;116:543-547.

123. Hift RJ, Davidson BP, van der Hooft C, et al. Plasma fluorescence scanning and fecal porphyrin analysis for the diagnosis of variegate porphyria: precise determination of sensitivity and specificity with detection of protoporphy-

rinogen oxidase mutations as a reference standard. Clin Chem. 2004;50:915-923.

124. Kauppinen R, Mustajoki S, Pihlaja H, et al. Acute intermittent porphyria in Finland: 19 mutations in the porphobilinogen deaminase gene. Hum Mol Genet. 1995;4: 215-222.

125. Puy H, Deybach JC, Lamoril J, et al. Molecular epidemiology and diagnosis of PBG deaminase gene defects in acute intermittent porphyria. Am J Hum Genet. 1997;60: 1373-1383.

126. Watson CJ, Pierach CA, Bossenmaier I, Cardinal R. Use of hematin in the acute attack of the "inducible" hepatic prophyrias. Adv Intern Med. 1978;23:265-286.

127. Bonkovsky HL, Healey JF, Lourie AN, Gerron GG. Intravenous heme-albumin in acute intermittent porphyria: evidence for repletion of hepatic hemoproteins and regulatory heme pools. Am J Gastroenterol. 1991;86:1050-1056.

128. Mustajoki P, Nordmann Y. Early administration of heme arginate for acute porphyric attacks. Arch Intern Med. 1993;153:2004-2008.

129. Mustajoki P, Tenhunen R, Tokola O, Gothoni G. Haem arginate in the treatment of acute hepatic porphyrias. Br Med J (Clin Res Ed). 1986;293:538-539.

130. Nordmann Y, Deybach JC. [Acute attacks of hepatic porphyria: specific treatment with heme arginate.] Ann Med Interne (Paris). 1993;144:165-167.

131. Goetsch CA, Bissell DM. Instability of hematin used in the treatment of acute hepatic porphyria. N Engl J Med. 1986;315:235-238.

132. Herrick AL, McColl KE, Moore MR, et al. Controlled trial of haem arginate in acute hepatic porphyria. Lancet. 1989;1:1295-1297.

133. Green D, Furby FH, Berndt MC. The interaction of the factor VIII/von Willebrand factor complex with hematin. Thromb Haemost. 1986;56:277-282.

134. Green D, Ts'ao CH. Hematin: effects on hemostasis. J Lab Clin Med. 1990;115:144-147.

135. Khanderia U. Circulatory collapse associated with hemin therapy for acute intermittent porphyria. Clin Pharm. 1986;5:690-692.

136. Dhar GJ, Bossenmaier I, Cardinal R, et al. Transitory renal failure following rapid administration of a relatively large amount of hematin in a patient with acute intermittent porphyria in clinical remission. Acta Med Scand. 1978;203:437-443.

137. Tenhunen R, Mustajoki P. Acute porphyria: treatment with heme. Semin Liver Dis. 1998;18:53-55.

138. Johansson A, Nowak G, Moller C, et al. Adenoviral-mediated expression of porphobilinogen deaminase in liver restores the metabolic defect in a mouse model of acute intermittent porphyria. Mol Ther. 2004;10: 337-343.

139. Sardh E, Rejkjaer L, Andersson DE, Harper P. Safety, pharmacokinetics and pharmacodynamics of recombinant human porphobilinogen deaminase in healthy subjects and asymptomatic carriers of the acute intermittent porphyria gene who have increased porphyrin precursor excretion. Clin Pharmacokinet. 2007;46:335-349.

140. Tschudy DP, Welland FH, Collins A, Hunter G Jr. The effect of carbohydrate feeding on the induction of delta-aminolevulinic acid synthetase. Metabolism. 1964;13: 396-406.

141. Beattie AD, Moore MR, Goldberg A, Ward RL. Acute intermittent porphyria: response of tachycardia and hypertension to propranolol. BMJ. 1973;3:257-260.

142. Schoenfeld N, Epstein O, Atsmon A. The effect of beta-adrenergic blocking agents on experimental porphyria induced by 3,5-diethoxycarbonyl-1,4-dihydrocollidine (DDC) in vivo and in vitro. Biochim Biophys Acta. 1976; 444:286-293.

143. Bonkowsky HL, Sinclair PR, Emery S, Sinclair JF. Seizure management in acute hepatic porphyria: risks of valproate and clonazepam. Neurology. 1980;30:588-592.

144. Hahn M, Gildemeister OS, Krauss GL, et al. Effects of new anticonvulsant medications on porphyrin synthesis in cultured liver cells: potential implications for patients with acute porphyria. Neurology. 1997;49:97-106.

145. Chaix Y, Gencourt C, Grouteau E, Carriere JP. [Acute intermittent porphyria associated with epilepsy in a child: diagnostic and therapeutic difficulties.] Arch Pediatr. 1997;4:971-974.

146. Anderson KE, Spitz IM, Bardin CW, Kappas A. A gonadotropin releasing hormone analogue prevents cyclical attacks of porphyria. Arch Intern Med. 1990;150:1469-1474.

147. Anderson KE, Spitz IM, Sassa S, et al. Prevention of cyclical attacks of acute intermittent porphyria with a long-acting agonist of luteinizing hormone–releasing hormone. N Engl J Med. 1984;311:643-645.

148. De Block CE, Leeuw IH, Gaal LF. Premenstrual attacks of acute intermittent porphyria: hormonal and metabolic aspects—a case report. Eur J Endocrinol. 1999;141:50-54.

149. Andersson C, Innala E, Backstrom T. Acute intermittent porphyria in women: clinical expression, use and experience of exogenous sex hormones. A population-based study in northern Sweden. J Intern Med. 2003;254:176-183.

150. Milo R, Neuman M, Klein C, et al. Acute intermittent porphyria in pregnancy. Obstet Gynecol. 1989;73:450-452.

151. Shenhav S, Gemer O, Sassoon E, Segal S. Acute intermittent porphyria precipitated by hyperemesis and metoclopramide treatment in pregnancy. Acta Obstet Gynecol Scand. 1997;76:484-485.

152. Andersson C, Bjersing L, Lithner F. The epidemiology of hepatocellular carcinoma in patients with acute intermittent porphyria. J Intern Med. 1996;240:195-201.

153. Linet MS, Gridley G, Nyren O, et al. Primary liver cancer, other malignancies, and mortality risks following porphyria: a cohort study in Denmark and Sweden. Am J Epidemiol. 1999;149:1010-1015.

154. Andant C, Puy H, Bogard C, et al. Hepatocellular carcinoma in patients with acute hepatic porphyria: frequency of occurrence and related factors. J Hepatol. 2000;32: 933-939.

155. Kauppinen R. Porphyrias. Lancet. 2005;365:241-252.

156. von und zu Fraunberg M, Pischik E, Udd L, Kauppinen R. Clinical and biochemical characteristics and genotype-phenotype correlation in 143 Finnish and Russian patients with acute intermittent porphyria. Medicine (Baltimore). 2005;84:35-47.

157. Onuki J, Chen Y, Teixeira PC, et al. Mitochondrial and nuclear DNA damage induced by 5-aminolevulinic acid. Arch Biochem Biophys. 2004;432:178-187.

158. Onuki J, Teixeira PC, Medeiros MH, et al. Is 5-aminolevulinic acid involved in the hepatocellular carcinogenesis of acute intermittent porphyria? Cell Mol Biol (Noisy-le-grand). 2002;48:17-26.

159. Battersby AR, Fookes CJ, Matcham GW, McDonald E. Biosynthesis of the pigments of life: formation of the macrocycle. Nature. 1980;285:17-21.

160. Battersby AR, McDonald E. Biosynthesis of porphyrins and corrins. Philos Trans R Soc Lond B Biol Sci. 1976; 273:161-180.

161. Mathews MA, Schubert HL, Whitby FG, et al. Crystal structure of human uroporphyrinogen III synthase. EMBO J. 2001;20:5832-5839.

162. Schubert H, Phillips JD, Heurox A, Hill CP. Structure and mechanistic implications of a uroporphyrinogen III synthase–product complex. Biochemistry 2008;47:8648-8655.

163. Astrin KH, Warner CA, Yoo HW, et al. Regional assignment of the human uroporphyrinogen III synthase (UROS) gene to chromosome 10q25.2-q26.3. Hum Genet. 1991;87:18-22.

164. Aizencang G, Solis C, Bishop DF, et al. Human uroporphyrinogen-III synthase: genomic organization, alternative promoters, and erythroid-specific expression. Genomics. 2000;70:223-231.

165. Aizencang GI, Bishop DF, Forrest D, et al. Uroporphyrinogen III synthase. An alternative promoter controls erythroid-specific expression in the murine gene. J Biol Chem. 2000;275:2295-2304.

166. Goldberg A, Rimington C. History, classification, geographical distribution and incidence of the porphyrias. In Goldberg A, Rimington C (eds). Diseases of Porphyrin Metabolism. Springfield, IL, Charles C Thomas, 1962, pp 3-20.

167. Goldberg A, Rimington C. Porphyria in animals. In Goldberg A, Rimington C (eds). Diseases of Porphyrin Metabolism. Springfield, IL, Charles C Thomas, 1962, pp 155-174.

168. Günther H. Die haematoporphyrie. Dtsch Arch Klin Med. 1911;105:89-146.

169. Levin EY, Flyger V. Uroporphyrinogen 3 cosynthetase activity in the fox squirrel (*Sciurus niger*). Science. 1971; 174:59-60.

170. Pence ME, Liggett AD. Congenital erythropoietic protoporphyria in a Limousin calf. J Am Vet Med Assoc. 2002;221:277-279.

171. Levin EY. Comparative aspects of porphyria in man and animals. Ann N Y Acad Sci. 1975;244:481-495.

172. Desnick RJ, Astrin KH. Congenital erythropoietic porphyria: advances in pathogenesis and treatment. Br J Haematol. 2002;117:779-795.

173. Shady AA, Colby BR, Cunha LF, et al. Congenital erythropoietic porphyria: identification and expression of eight novel mutations in the uroporphyrinogen III synthase gene. Br J Haematol. 2002;117:980-987.

174. Solis C, Aizencang GI, Astrin KH, et al. Uroporphyrinogen III synthase erythroid promoter mutations in adjacent GATA1 and CP2 elements cause congenital erythropoietic porphyria. J Clin Invest. 2001;107:753-762.

175. Wiederholt T, Poblete-Gutierrez P, Gardlo K, et al. Identification of mutations in the uroporphyrinogen III cosynthase gene in German patients with congenital erythropoietic porphyria. Physiol Res. 2006;55(Suppl 2): S85-S92.

176. Xu W, Kozak CA, Desnick RJ. Uroporphyrinogen-III synthase: molecular cloning, nucleotide sequence, expression of a mouse full-length cDNA, and its localization on mouse chromosome 7. Genomics. 1995;26:556-562.

177. Fritsch C, Bolsen K, Ruzicka T, Goerz G. Congenital erythropoietic porphyria. J Am Acad Dermatol. 1997;36: 594-610.

178. Pollack SS, Rosenthal MS. Images in clinical medicine. Diaper diagnosis of porphyria. N Engl J Med. 1994; 330:114.

179. Warner CA, Poh-Fitzpatrick MB, Zaider EF, et al. Congenital erythropoietic porphyria. A mild variant with low uroporphyrin I levels due to a missense mutation (A66V) encoding residual uroporphyrinogen III synthase activity. Arch Dermatol. 1992;128:1243-1248.

180. Chumbley LC. Scleral involvement in symptomatic porphyria. Am J Ophthalmol. 1977;84:729-733.

181. Douglas WH. Congenital porphyria: general and ocular manifestations. Trans Ophthalmol Soc U K. 1972;92:541-553.

182. Trodahl JN, Schwartz S, Gorlin RJ. The pigmentation of dental tissues in erythropoietic (congenital) porphyria. J Oral Pathol. 1972;1:159-171.

183. Gross S. Hematologic studies on erythropoietic porphyria: a new case with severe hemolysis, chronic thrombocytopenia, and folic acid deficiency. Blood. 1964;23:762-775.

184. Gross S, Schoenberg MD, Mumaw VR. Electron microscopy of the red cells in erythropoietic porphyria. Blood. 1965;25:49-55.

185. Haining RG, Cowger ML, Shurtleff DB, Labbe RF. Congenital erythropoietic porphyria. I. Case report, special studies and therapy. Am J Med. 1968;45:624-637.

186. Varadi S. [Haematological aspects in a case of erythropoietic porphyria.] Br J Haematol. 1958;4:270-280.

187. Schmid R, Schwartz S, Watson CJ. Porphyrin content of bone marrow and liver in the various forms of porphyria. AMA Arch Intern Med. 1954;93:167-190.

188. Aldrich RA, Hawkinson V, Grinstein M, Watson CJ. Photosensitive or congenital porphyria with hemolytic anemia. I. Clinical and fundamental studies before and after splenectomy. Blood. 1951;6:685-698.

189. Pullon HW, Bellingham AJ, Humphreys S, Cundy TF. The osteodystrophy of congenital erythropoietic porphyria. Bone. 1991;12:89-92.

190. Bhutani LK, Sood SK, Das PK, et al. Congenital erythropoietic porphyria. An autopsy report. Arch Dermatol. 1974;110:427-431.

191. Bickers DR, Keogh L, Rifkind AB, et al. Studies in porphyria. VI. Biosynthesis of porphyrins in mammalian skin and in the skin of porphyric patients. J Invest Dermatol. 1977;68:5-9.

192. Kushner JP, Pimstone NR, Kjeldsberg CR, et al. Congenital erythropoietic porphyria, diminished activity of uroporphyrinogen decarboxylase and dyserythropoiesis. Blood. 1982;59:725-737.

193. Phillips JD, Steensma DP, Spangrude GJ, Kushner JP. Congenital erythropoietic porphyria, β-thalassemia intermedia and thrombocytopenia due to a GATA1 mutation. Blood. 2005;106:154a.

194. Deybach JC, de Verneuil H, Phung N, et al. Congenital erythropoietic porphyria (Günther's disease): enzymatic studies on two cases of late onset. J Lab Clin Med. 1981;97:551-558.

195. Kramer S, Viljoen E, Meyer AM, Metz J. The anemia of erythropoietic porphyria with the first description of the disease in an elderly patient. Br J Haematol. 1965;11: 666.

196. Murphy A, Gibson G, Elder GH, et al. Adult-onset congenital erythropoietic porphyria (Günther's disease) presenting with thrombocytopenia. J R Soc Med. 1995;88: 357P-358P.

197. Pain RW, Welch FW, Woodroffe AJ, Handley DA, Lockwood WH. Erythropoietic uroporphyria of Günther first presenting at 58 years with positive family studies. BMJ. 1975;3:621-623.

198. Weston MJ, Nicholson DC, Lim CK, et al. Congenital erythropoietic uroporphyria (Günther's disease) presenting in a middle aged man. Int J Biochem. 1978;9:921-926.

199. Yamauchi K, Kushibiki Y. Pyridoxal 5-phosphate therapy in a patient with myelodysplastic syndrome and adult onset congenital erythropoietic porphyria. Br J Haematol. 1992;81:614-615.

200. Murphy GM. Diagnosis and management of the erythropoietic porphyrias. Dermatol Ther. 2003;16:57-64.

201. Sassa S. Modern diagnosis and management of the porphyrias. Br J Haematol. 2006;135:281-292.

202. Shoolingin-Jordan PM, Leadbeater R. Coupled assay for uroporphyrinogen III synthase. Methods Enzymol. 1997;281:327-336.

203. Tsai SF, Bishop DF, Desnick RJ. Coupled-enzyme and direct assays for uroporphyrinogen III synthase activity in human erythrocytes and cultured lymphoblasts. Enzymatic diagnosis of heterozygotes and homozygotes with congenital erythropoietic porphyria. Anal Biochem. 1987;166:120-133.

204. Ged C, Moreau-Gaudry F, Taine L, et al. Prenatal diagnosis in congenital erythropoietic porphyria by metabolic measurement and DNA mutation analysis. Prenat Diagn. 1996;16:83-86.

205. Dupuis-Girod S, Akkari V, Ged C, et al. Successful match-unrelated donor bone marrow transplantation for congenital erythropoietic porphyria (Günther disease). Eur J Pediatr. 2005;164:104-107.

206. Faraci M, Morreale G, Boeri E, et al. Unrelated HSCT in an adolescent affected by congenital erythropoietic porphyria. Pediatr Transplant. 2008;12:117-120.

207. Shaw PH, Mancini AJ, McConnell JP, et al. Treatment of congenital erythropoietic porphyria in children by allogeneic stem cell transplantation: a case report and review of the literature. Bone Marrow Transplant. 2001;27:101-105.

208. Taibjee SM, Stevenson OE, Abdullah A, et al. Allogeneic bone marrow transplantation in a 7-year-old girl with congenital erythropoietic porphyria: a treatment dilemma. Br J Dermatol. 2007;156:567-571.

209. Tezcan I, Xu W, Gurgey A, et al. Congenital erythropoietic porphyria successfully treated by allogeneic bone marrow transplantation. Blood. 1998;92:4053-4058.

210. Robert-Richard E, Moreau-Gaudry F, Lalanne M, et al. Effective gene therapy of mice with congenital erythropoietic porphyria is facilitated by a survival advantage of corrected erythroid cells. Am J Hum Genet. 2008;82:113-124.

211. Rosenthal IM, Lipton EL, Asrow G. Effect of splenectomy on porphyria erythropoietica. Pediatrics. 1955;15:663-675.

212. Piomelli S, Poh-Fitzpatrick MB, Seaman C, et al. Complete suppression of the symptoms of congenital erythropoietic porphyria by long-term treatment with high-level transfusions. N Engl J Med. 1986;314:1029-1031.

213. Haining RG, Cowger ML, Labbe RF, Finch CA. Congenital erythropoietic porphyria. II. The effects of induced polycythemia. Blood. 1970;36:297-309.

214. Jackson AH, Sancovich HA, Ferrmola AM, et al. Macrocyclic intermediates in the biosynthesis of porphyrins. Philos Trans R Soc Lond. 1976;273:191-206.

215. de Verneuil H, Grandchamp B, Foubert C, et al. Assignment of the gene for uroporphyrinogen decarboxylase to human chromosome 1 by somatic cell hybridization and specific enzyme immunoassay. Hum Genet. 1984;66:202-205.

216. Dubart A, Mattei MG, Raich N, et al. Assignment of human uroporphyrinogen decarboxylase (URO-D) to the p34 band of chromosome 1. Hum Genet. 1986;73: 277-279.

217. Romana M, Dubart A, Beaupain D, et al. Structure of the gene for human uroporphyrinogen decarboxylase. Nucleic Acids Res. 1987;15:7343-7356.

218. Romeo PH, Raich, N, Dubart A, et al. Molecular cloning and nucleotide sequence of a complete human uroporphyrinogen decarboxylase cDNA. J Biol Chem. 1986; 261:9825-9831.

219. de Verneuil H, Sassa S, Kappas A. Purification and properties of uroporphyrinogen decarboxylase from human erythrocytes. A single enzyme catalyzing the four sequential decarboxylations of uroporphyrinogens I and III. J Biol Chem. 1983;258:2454-2460.

220. Elder GH, Tovey JA, Sheppard DM. Purification of uroporphyrinogen decarboxylase from human erythrocytes. Immunochemical evidence for a single protein with decarboxylase activity in human erythrocytes and liver. Biochem J. 1983;215:45-55.

221. Straka JG, Kushner JP. Purification and characterization of bovine hepatic uroporphyrinogen decarboxylase. Biochemistry. 1983;22:4664-4672.

222. Elder GH, Roberts AG. Uroporphyrinogen decarboxylase. J Bioenerg Biomembr. 1995;27:207-214.

223. Phillips JD, Whitby FG, Kushner JP, Hill CP. Characterization and crystallization of human uroporphyrinogen decarboxylase. Protein Sci. 1997;6:1343-1346.

224. Whitby FG, Phillips JD, Kushner JP, Hill CP. Crystal structure of human uroporphyrinogen decarboxylase. EMBO J. 1998;17:2463-2471.

225. Phillips JD, Whitby FG, Kushner JP, Hill CP. Structural basis for tetrapyrrole coordination by uroporphyrinogen decarboxylase. EMBO J. 2003;22:6225-6233.

226. Bonkovsky HL, Poh-Fitzpatrick M, Pimstone N, et al. Porphyria cutanea tarda, hepatitis C, and HFE gene mutations in North America. Hepatology. 1998;27:1661-1669.

227. Bulaj ZJ, Franklin MR, Phillips JD, et al. Transdermal estrogen replacement therapy in postmenopausal women previously treated for porphyria cutanea tarda. J Lab Clin Med. 2000;136:482-488.

228. Egger NG, Carlson GL, Shaffer JL. Nutritional status and assessment of patients on home parenteral nutrition: anthropometry, bioelectrical impedance, or clinical judgment? Nutrition. 1999;15:1-6.

229. Enriquez de Salamanca R, Morales P, Castro MJ, et al. The most frequent HFE allele linked to porphyria cutanea tarda in Mediterraneans is His63Asp. Hepatology. 1999;30:819-820.

230. Fargion S, Piperno A, Cappellini MD, et al. Hepatitis C virus and porphyria cutanea tarda: evidence of a strong association. Hepatology. 1992;16:1322-1326.

231. Sampietro M, Fracanzani AL, Corbetta N, et al. High prevalence of hepatitis C virus type 1b in Italian patients with porphyria cutanea tarda. Ital J Gastroenterol Hepatol. 1997;29:543-547.

232. Sampietro M, Piperno A, Lupica L, et al. High prevalence of the His63Asp HFE mutation in Italian patients with porphyria cutanea tarda. Hepatology. 1998;27:181-184.

233. Stuart KA, Busfield F, Jazwinska EC, et al. The C282Y mutation in the haemochromatosis gene (HFE) and hepatitis C virus infection are independent cofactors for porphyria cutanea tarda in Australian patients. J Hepatol. 1998;28:404-409.

234. Bulaj ZJ, Phillips JD, Ajioka RS, et al. Hemochromatosis genes and other factors contributing to the pathogenesis of porphyria cutanea tarda. Blood. 2000;95:1565-1571.

235. Anderson KE, Sassa S, Bishop DF, Desnick RJ. Disorders of heme biosynthesis: X-linked sideroblastic anemia and the porphyrias. In Scriver CR, Sly WS, Childs B, et al. (eds). The Metabolic and Molecular Bases of Inherited Disease, 8th ed. New York, McGraw-Hill, 2001, pp 2991-3062.

236. Benedetto AV, Kushner JP, Taylor JS. Porphyria cutanea tarda in three generations of a single family. N Engl J Med. 1978;298:358-362.

237. Wyckoff EE, Kushner JP. Heme biosynthesis, the porphyrias, and the liver. In Arias IM, Boyer JL, Fausto N, et al. (eds). The Liver: Biology and Pathobiology, 3rd ed. New York, Raven Press, 1994, pp 505-527.

238. Hansen JL, Pryor MA, Kennedy JB, Kushner JP. Steady-state levels of uroporphyrinogen decarboxylase mRNA in lymphoblastoid cell lines from patients with familial porphyria cutanea tarda and their relatives. Am J Hum Genet. 1988;42:847-853.

239. Garey JR, Hansen JL, Harrison LM, et al. A point mutation in the coding region of uroporphyrinogen decarboxylase associated with familial porphyria cutanea tarda. Blood. 1989;73:892-895.

240. Magness ST, Tugores A, Diala ES, Brenner DA. Analysis of the human ferrochelatase promoter in transgenic mice. Blood. 1998;92:320-328.

241. Mendez M, Poblete-Gutierrez P, Garcia-Bravo M, et al. Molecular heterogeneity of familial porphyria cutanea tarda in Spain: characterization of 10 novel mutations in the UROD gene. Br J Dermatol. 2007;157:501-507.

242. Battle AM, Stella AM, De Kaminsky AR, et al. Two cases of infantile porphyria cutanea tarda: successful treatment with oral S-adenosyl-L-methionine and low-dose oral chloroquine. Br J Dermatol. 1987;116:407-415.

243. Cotton JB, Abeille A, Jeune R, et al. [Porphyria cutanea tarda in a 4-year-old child with uroporphyrinogen decarboxylase deficiency.] Pediatrie. 1986;41:617-627.

244. Doutre MS, Beylot C, Bioulac P, Nordmann Y. [Hereditary porphyria cutanea in children. Enzymatic studies (author's transl).] Ann Dermatol Venereol. 1981;108: 751-757.

245. Lambert DG, Beer F, Dalac S, Hourdain MJ. Familial porphyria cutanea tarda in a 7-year-old girl. Dermatologica. 1988;176:202-204.

246. Rogers M, Kamath KR, Poulos V. Porphyria cutanea tarda in a seven year old child. Australas J Dermatol. 1984;25: 107-112.

247. Welland FH, Carlsen RA. Porphyria cutanea tarda in an 8-year-old boy. Arch Dermatol. 1969;99:451-454.

248. Garey JR, Franklin KF, Brown DA, et al. Analysis of uroporphyrinogen decarboxylase complementary DNAs in sporadic porphyria cutanea tarda. Gastroenterology. 1993;105:165-169.

249. Roberts AG, Elder GH, Newcomb RG, et al. Heterogeneity of familial porphyria cutanea tarda. J Med Genet. 1988;25:669-676.

250. Billi de Catabbi S, Sterin-Speziale N, Fernandez MC, Minutolo C, et al. Time course of hexachlorobenzene-induced alterations of lipid metabolism and their relation to porphyria. Int J Biochem Cell Biol. 1997;29:335-344.

251. Cantoni L, dal Fiume D, Ferraroli A, et al. Different susceptibility of mouse tissues to porphyrogenic effect of 2,3,7,8-tetrachlorodibenzo-p-dioxin. Toxicol Lett. 1984; 20:201-210.

252. Francis JE, Smith AG. Oxidation of uroporphyrinogens by hydroxyl radicals. Evidence for nonporphyrin products as potential inhibitors of uroporphyrinogen decarboxylase. FEBS Lett. 1988;233:311-314.

253. Edwards C, Griffen L, Bulaj Z, et al. Estimates of the frequency of morbid complications of hemochromatosis. In Barton J, Edwards C (eds). Hemochromatosis: Genetics, Pathophysiology, Diagnosis and Treatment. Cambridge, England, Cambridge University Press, 2000, pp 312-317.

254. Meguro K, Fujita H, Ishida N, et al. Molecular defects of uroporphyrinogen decarboxylase in a patient with mild hepatoerythropoietic porphyria. J Invest Dermatol. 1994;102:681-685.

255. Phillips JD, Whitby FG, Stadtmueller BM, et al. Two novel uroporphyrinogen decarboxylase (URO-D) mutations causing hepatoerythropoietic porphyria (HEP). Transpl Res. 2007;149:85-91.

256. Romana M, Grandchamp B, Dubart A, et al. Identification of a new mutation responsible for hepatoerythropoietic porphyria. Eur J Clin Invest. 1991;21:225-229.

257. Koszo F, Elder GH, Roberts A, Simon N. Uroporphyrinogen decarboxylase deficiency in hepatoerythropoietic porphyria: further evidence for genetic heterogeneity. Br J Dermatol. 1990;122:365-370.

258. Cam C, Nigogosyan G. Acquired toxic porphyria cutanea tarda due to hexachlorobenzene. JAMA. 1963;183:90-93.

259. Francis JE, Smith AG. Polycyclic aromatic hydrocarbons cause hepatic porphyria in iron-loaded C57BL/10 mice: comparison of uroporphyrinogen decarboxylase inhibition with induction of alkoxyphenoxazone dealkylations. Biochem Biophys Res Commun. 1987;146:13-20.

260. Franklin MR, Phillips JD, Kushner JP. Cytochrome P450 induction, uroporphyrinogen decarboxylase depression, porphyrin accumulation and excretion, and gender influence in a 3-week rat model of porphyria cutanea tarda. Toxicol Appl Pharmacol. 1997;147:289-299.

261. Smith AG, Carthew P, Clothier B, et al. Synergy of iron in the toxicity and carcinogenicity of polychlorinated

biphenyls (PCBs) and related chemicals. Toxicol Lett. 1995;82-83:945-950.

262. Smith AG, Clothier B, Robinson S, et al. Interaction between iron metabolism and 2,3,7,8-tetrachlorodibenzo-*p*-dioxin in mice with variants of the Ahr gene: a hepatic oxidative mechanism. Mol Pharmacol. 1998;53:52-61.

263. Smith AG, Francis JE, Green JA, et al. Sex-linked hepatic uroporphyria and the induction of cytochromes P450IA in rats caused by hexachlorobenzene and polyhalogenated biphenyls. Biochem Pharmacol. 1990;40:2059-2068.

264. Sweeny GD, Jones KG, Cole FM, et al. Iron deficiency prevents liver toxicity of 2,3,7,8-tetrachlorodibenzo-*p*-dioxin. Science. 1979;204:332-335.

265. Urquhart AJ, Elder GH, Roberts AG, et al. Uroporphyria produced in mice by 20-methylcholanthrene and 5-aminolaevulinic acid. Biochem J. 1988;253:357-362.

266. Doss M, Sauer H, von Tiepermann R, Colombi AM. Development of chronic hepatic porphyria (porphyria cutanea tarda) with inherited uroporphyrinogen decarboxylase deficiency under exposure to dioxin. Int J Biochem. 1984;16:369-373.

267. McConnell R, Anderson K, Russell W, et al. Angiosarcoma, porphyria cutanea tarda, and probable chloracne in a worker exposed to waste oil contaminated with 2,3,7,8-tetrachlorodibenzo-*p*-dioxin. Br J Ind Med. 1993;50:699-703.

268. Lynch RE, Lee GR, Kushner JP. Porphyria cutanea tarda associated with disinfectant misuse. Arch Intern Med. 1975;135:549-552.

269. Barnes HD. Porphyria in the Bantu races on the Witwatersrand. S Afr Med J. 1955;29:781-784.

270. Poh-Fitzpatrick MB, Masullo AS, Grossman ME. Porphyria cutanea tarda associated with chronic renal disease and hemodialysis. Arch Dermatol. 1980;116:191-195.

271. Garcia Parrilla J, Ortega R, Pena ML, et al. Porphyria cutanea tarda during maintenance haemodialysis. BMJ. 1980;280:1358.

272. Goldsman CI, Taylor JS. Porphyria cutanea tarda and bullous dermatoses associated with chronic renal failure: a review. Cleve Clin Q. 1983;50:151-161.

273. Castanet J, Lacour JP, Perrin C, et al. Sclerodermatous changes revealing porphyria cutanea tarda. Acta Derm Venereol. 1994;74:310-311.

274. Francoeur CJ Jr, Epinette WW. Sclerodermoid plaques in a middle-aged man. Sclerodermoid porphyria cutanea tarda (PCT). Arch Dermatol. 1991;127:1571-1572, 1574-1575.

275. Fritsch C, Lang K, von Schmiedeberg S, et al. Porphyria cutanea tarda. Skin Pharmacol Appl Skin Physiol. 1998;11:321-335.

276. Harber LC, Bickers DR. Porphyria and pseudoporphyria. J Invest Dermatol. 1984;82:207-209.

277. Elder GH, Smith SG, Herrero C, et al. Hepatoerythropoietic porphyria: a new uroporphyrinogen decarboxylase defect or homozygous porphyria cutanea tarda? Lancet. 1981;1:916-919.

278. de Verneuil H, Beaumont C, Deybach JC, et al. Enzymatic and immunological studies of uroporphyrinogen decarboxylase in familial porphyria cutanea tarda and hepatoerythropoietic porphyria. Am J Hum Genet. 1984;36:613-622.

279. Fujita H, Sassa S, Toback AC, Kappas A. Immunochemical study of uroporphyrinogen decarboxylase in a patient with mild hepatoerythropoietic porphyria. J Clin Invest. 1987;79:1533-1537.

280. Chuang TY, Brashear R, Lewis C. Porphyria cutanea tarda and hepatitis C virus: a case-control study and meta-analysis of the literature. J Am Acad Dermatol. 1999;41:31-36.

281. Stolzel U, Kostler E, Koszka C, et al. Low prevalence of hepatitis C virus infection in porphyria cutanea tarda in Germany. Hepatology. 1995;21:1500-1503.

282. James KR, Cortes JM, Paradinas FJ. Demonstration of intracytoplasmic needle-like inclusions in hepatocytes of patients with porphyria cutanea tarda. J Clin Pathol. 1980;33:899-900.

283. Cortes JM, Oliva H, Paradinas FJ, Hernandez-Guio C. The pathology of the liver in porphyria cutanea tarda. Histopathology. 1980;4:471-485.

284. Edwards CQ, Griffen LM, Goldgar DE, et al. HLA-linked hemochromatosis alleles in sporadic porphyria cutanea tarda. Gastroenterology. 1989;97:972-981.

285. Grossman ME, Bickers DR, Poh-Fitzpatrick MB, et al. Porphyria cutanea tarda. Clinical features and laboratory findings in 40 patients. Am J Med. 1979;67:277-286.

286. Lundvall O, Weinfeld A, Lundin P. Iron storage in porphyria cutanea tarda. Acta Med Scand. 1970;1-2:37-53.

287. Elder G. Porphyria cutanea tarda and related disorders. In Kadish KM, Smith KM, Guilard R (eds). The Porphyrin Handbook, vol 14. New York, Academic Press, 2003.

288. Phillips JD, Parker TL, Schubert HL, et al. Functional consequences of naturally occurring mutations in human uroporphyrinogen decarboxylase. Blood. 2001;98:3179-3185.

289. Elder GH, Urquhart AJ, De Salamanca RE, et al. Immunoreactive uroporphyrinogen decarboxylase in the liver in porphyria cutanea tarda. Lancet. 1985;2:229-232.

290. Elder GH, Lee GB, Tovey JA. Decreased activity of hepatic uroporphyrinogen decarboxylase in sporadic porphyria cutanea tarda. N Engl J Med. 1978;299:274-278.

291. Kushner JP, Barbuto AJ, Lee GR. An inherited enzymatic defect in porphyria cutanea tarda: decreased uroporphyrinogen decarboxylase activity. J Clin Invest. 1976;58:1089-1097.

292. Franklin MR, Phillips JD, Kushner JP. Uroporphyria in the uroporphyrinogen decarboxylase-deficient mouse: interplay with siderosis and polychlorinated biphenyl exposure. Hepatology. 2002;36:805-811.

293. Phillips JD, Jackson LK, Bunting M, et al. A mouse model of familial porphyria cutanea tarda. Proc Natl Acad Sci U S A. 2001;98:259-264.

294. Billi de Catabbi S, Rios de Molina MC, San Martin de Viale LC. Studies on the active centre of rat liver porphyrinogen carboxylase: in vivo effect of hexachlorobenzene. Int J Biochem. 1991;23:675-679.

295. Cantoni L, Graziani A, Rizzardini M, Saletti MC. Porphyrinogenic effect of hexachlorobenzene and 2,3,7,8-tetrachlorodibenzo-para-dioxin: is an inhibitor involved in uroporphyrinogen decarboxylase inactivation? IARC Sci Publ. 1986;77:449-456.

296. Smith AG, Francis JE. Chemically-induced formation of an inhibitor of hepatic uroporphyrinogen decarboxylase in inbred mice with iron overload. Biochem J. 1987;246:221-226.

297. Phillips JD, Bergonia HA, Reilly CA, et al. A porphomethene inhibitor of uroporphyrinogen decarboxylase causes

porphyria cutanea tarda. Proc Natl Acad Sci U S A. 2007; 104:5079-5084.

298. Sinclair PR, Gorman N, Dalton T, et al. Uroporphyria produced in mice by iron and 5-aminolaevulinic acid does not occur in Cyp1a2(−/−) null mutant mice. Biochem J. 1998;330:149-153.

299. Felsher BF, Jones ML, Redeker AG. Iron and hepatic uroporphyrin synthesis. Relation in porphyria cutanea tarda. JAMA. 1973;226:663-665.

300. Poh-Fitzpatrick MB. Molecular and cellular mechanisms of porphyrin photosensitization. Photodermatology. 1986;3:148-157.

301. Poh-Fitzpatrick MB. Porphyrias: photosensitivity and phototherapy. Methods Enzymol. 2000;319:485-493.

302. Herrmann G, Wlaschek M, Bolsen K, et al. Photosensitization of uroporphyrin augments the ultraviolet A–induced synthesis of matrix metalloproteinases in human dermal fibroblasts. J Invest Dermatol. 1996;107:398-403.

303. Maynard B, Peters MS. Histologic and immunofluorescence study of cutaneous porphyrias. J Cutan Pathol. 1992;19:40-47.

304. Timonen K, Niemi KM, Mustajoki P, Tenhunen R. Skin changes in variegate porphyria. Clinical, histopathological, and ultrastructural study. Arch Dermatol Res. 1990; 282:108-114.

305. Poh-Fitzpatrick MB, Lamola AA. Direct spectrofluorometry of diluted erythrocytes and plasma: a rapid diagnostic method in primary and secondary porphyrinemias. J Lab Clin Med. 1976;87:362-370.

306. Pimstone NR. Porphyria cutanea tarda. Semin Liver Dis. 1982;2:132-142.

307. Elder GH. Differentiation of porphyria cutanea tarda symptomatica from other types of porphyria by measurement of isocoproporphyrin in faeces. J Clin Pathol. 1975;28:601-607.

308. Lim HW, Poh-Fitzpatrick MB. Hepatoerythropoietic porphyria: a variant of childhood-onset porphyria cutanea tarda. Porphyrin profiles and enzymatic studies of two cases in a family. J Am Acad Dermatol. 1984;11: 1103-1111.

309. Di Padova C, Marchesi L, Cainelli T, et al. Effects of phlebotomy on urinary porphyrin pattern and liver histology in patients with porphyria cutanea tarda. Am J Med Sci. 1983;285:2-12.

310. Valls V, Ena J, Enriquez-De-Salamanca R. Low-dose oral chloroquine in patients with porphyria cutanea tarda and low-moderate iron overload. J Dermatol Sci. 1994;7: 169-175.

311. Ashton RE, Hawk JL, Magnus IA. Low-dose oral chloroquine in the treatment of porphyria cutanea tarda. Br J Dermatol. 1984;111:609-613.

312. Kordac V, Semradova M. Treatment of porphyria cutanea tarda with chloroquine. Br J Dermatol. 1974;90:95-100.

313. Taljaard JJ, Shanley BC, Stewart-Wynne EG, et al. Studies on low dose chloroquine therapy and the action of chloroquine in symptomatic porphyria. Br J Dermatol. 1972; 87:261-269.

314. Scholnick PL, Epstein J, Marver HS. The molecular basis of the action of chloroquine in porphyria cutanea tarda. J Invest Dermatol. 1973;61:226-232.

315. Felsher BF, Redeker AG. Effect of chloroquine on hepatic uroporphyrin metabolism in patients with porphyria cutanea tarda. Medicine (Baltimore). 1966;45:575-583.

316. Vogler WR, Galambos JT, Olansky S. Biochemical effects of chloroquine therapy in porphyria cutanea tarda. Am J Med. 1970;49:316-321.

317. Malkinson FD, Levitt L. Hydroxychloroquine treatment of porphyria cutanea tarda. Arch Dermatol. 1980;116: 1147-1150.

318. Moran-Jimenez MJ, Ged C, Romana M, et al. Uroporphyrinogen decarboxylase: complete human gene sequence and molecular study of three families with hepatoerythropoietic porphyria. Am J Hum Genet. 1996;58:712-721.

319. Krishnamurthy PC, Du G, Fukuda Y, et al. Identification of a mammalian mitochondrial porphyrin transporter. Nature. 2006;443:586-589.

320. Yoshinaga T, Sano S. Coproporphyrinogen oxidase. II. Reaction mechanism and role of tyrosine residues on the activity. J Biol Chem. 1980;255:4727-4731.

321. Lee DS, Flachsova E, Bodnarova M, et al. Structural basis of hereditary coproporphyria. Proc Natl Acad Sci U S A. 2005;102:14232-14237.

322. Silva PJ, Ramos MJ. A comparative density-functional study of the reaction mechanism of the O₂-dependent coproporphyrinogen III oxidase. Bioorg Med Chem. 2008;16:2726-2733.

323. Martasek P, Camadro JM, Raman CS, et al. Human coproporphyrinogen oxidase. Biochemical characterization of recombinant normal and R231W mutated enzymes expressed in E. coli as soluble, catalytically active homodimers. Cell Mol Biol (Noisy-le-grand). 1997;43:47-58.

324. Phillips JD, Whitby FG, Warby CA, et al. Crystal structure of the oxygen-dependant coproporphyrinogen oxidase (Hem13p) of Saccharomyces cerevisiae. J Biol Chem. 2004;279:38960-38968.

325. Cacheux V, Martasek P, Fougerousse F, et al. Localization of the human coproporphyrinogen oxidase gene to chromosome band 3q12. Hum Genet. 1994;94:557-559.

326. Takahashi S, Taketani S, Akasaka JE, et al. Differential regulation of coproporphyrinogen oxidase gene between erythroid and nonerythroid cells. Blood. 1998;92:3436-3444.

327. Taketani S, Adachi Y, Nakahashi Y. Regulation of the expression of human ferrochelatase by intracellular iron levels. Eur J Biochem. 2000;267:4685-4692.

328. Elder GH, Evans JO, Thomas N. The primary enzyme defect in hereditary coproporphyria. Lancet. 1976;2:1217-1219.

329. Grandchamp B, Phung N, Nordmann Y. Homozygous case of hereditary coproporphyria. Lancet. 1977;2:1348-1349.

330. Martasek P, Nordmann Y, Grandchamp B. Homozygous hereditary coproporphyria caused by an arginine to tryptophane substitution in coproporphyrinogen oxidase and common intragenic polymorphisms. Hum Mol Genet. 1994;3:477-480.

331. Lamoril J, Puy H, Gouya L, et al. Neonatal hemolytic anemia due to inherited harderoporphyria: clinical characteristics and molecular basis. Blood. 1998;91:1453-1457.

332. Gorchein A, Danton M, Lim CK. Harderoporphyrin: a misnomer. Biomed Chromatogr. 2005;19:565-569.

333. Kuhnel A, Gross U, Doss MO. Hereditary coproporphyria in Germany: clinical-biochemical studies in 53 patients. Clin Biochem. 2000;33:465-473.

334. Brodie MJ, Thompson GG, Moore MR, et al. Hereditary coproporphyria. Demonstration of the abnormalities in haem biosynthesis in peripheral blood. Q J Med. 1977;46:229-241.

335. Goldberg A, Rimington C, Lochhead AC. Hereditary coproporphyria. Lancet. 1967;1:632-636.

336. Nordmann Y, Grandchamp B, de Verneuil H, et al. Harderoporphyria: a variant hereditary coproporphyria. J Clin Invest. 1983;72:1139-1149.

337. Schmitt C, Gouya L, Malonova E, et al. Mutations in human CPO gene predict clinical expression of either hepatic hereditary coproporphyria or erythropoietic harderoporphyria. Hum Mol Genet. 2005;14:3089-3098.

338. Takeuchi H, Kondo M, Daimon M, et al. Neonatal-onset hereditary coproporphyria with male pseudohermaphrodism. Blood. 2001;98:3871-3873.

339. Lamoril J, Puy H, Whatley SD, et al. Characterization of mutations in the CPO gene in British patients demonstrates absence of genotype-phenotype correlation and identifies relationship between hereditary coproporphyria and harderoporphyria. Am J Hum Genet. 2001;68:1130-1138.

340. Manning DJ, Gray TA. Haem arginate in acute hereditary coproporphyria. Arch Dis Child. 1991;66:730-731.

341. Ferreira GC, Andrew TL, Karr SW, Dailey HA. Organization of the terminal two enzymes of the heme biosynthetic pathway. Orientation of protoporphyrinogen oxidase and evidence for a membrane complex. J Biol Chem. 1988;263:3835-3839.

342. Ferreira GC, Dailey HA. Mouse protoporphyrinogen oxidase. Kinetic parameters and demonstration of inhibition by bilirubin. Biochem J. 1988;250:597-603.

343. Dailey HA, Dailey TA. Protoporphyrinogen oxidase of *Myxococcus xanthus*. Expression, purification, and characterization of the cloned enzyme. J Biol Chem. 1996;271:8714-8718.

344. Akhtar M. Mechanism and stereochemistry of the enzymes involved in the conversion of uroporphyrinogen III into haem. In Shoolingin-Jordan PM (ed). Biosynthesis of Tetrapyrroles. Amsterdam, Elsevier, 1991, pp67-99.

345. Koch M, Breithaupt C, Kiefersauer R, et al. Crystal structure of protoporphyrinogen IX oxidase: a key enzyme in haem and chlorophyll biosynthesis. EMBO J. 2004;23:1720-1728.

346. von und zu Fraunberg M, Nyroen T, Kauppinen R. Mitochondrial targeting of normal and mutant protoporphyrinogen oxidase. J Biol Chem. 2003;278:13376-13381.

347. Morgan RR, Errington R, Elder GH. Identification of sequences required for the import of human protoporphyrinogen oxidase to mitochondria. Biochem J. 2004;377:281-287.

348. Roberts AG, Whatley SD, Daniels J, et al. Partial characterization and assignment of the gene for protoporphyrinogen oxidase and variegate porphyria to human chromosome 1q23. Hum Mol Genet. 1995;4:2387-2390.

349. Taketani S, Inazawa J, Abe T, et al. The human protoporphyrinogen oxidase gene (PPOX): organization and location to chromosome 1. Genomics. 1995;29:698-703.

350. Kirsch RE, Meissner PN, Hift RJ. Variegate porphyria. Semin Liver Dis. 1998;18:33-41.

351. van den Bergh AAH, Grotepass W. Ein bemerkenswerter Fall von Porphyrie. Wein Klin Wochenschr. 1937;50:830-831.

352. Dean G, Barnes HD. The inheritance of porphyria. BMJ. 1955;2:89-94.

353. Mustajoki P. Variegate porphyria. Twelve years' experience in Finland. Q J Med. 1980;49:191-203.

354. Dean G. The Porphyrias: A Study of Inheritance and Environment, 2nd ed. London, Pitman Medical, 1971.

355. Hift RJ, Meissner D, Meissner PN. A systematic study of the clinical and biochemical expression of variegate porphyria in a large South African family. Br J Dermatol. 2004;151:465-471.

356. Eales L, Day RS, Blekkenhorst GH. The clinical and biochemical features of variegate porphyria: an analysis of 300 cases studied at Groote Schuur Hospital, Cape Town. Int J Biochem. 1980;12:837-853.

357. von und zu Fraunberg M, Timonen K, Mustajoki P, Kauppinen R. Clinical and biochemical characteristics and genotype-phenotype correlation in Finnish variegate porphyria patients. Eur J Hum Genet. 2002;10:649-657.

358. Day RS. Variegate porphyria. Seminar Dermatol. 1986;5:138-154.

359. Whatley SD, Puy H, Morgan RR, et al. Variegate porphyria in Western Europe: identification of PPOX gene mutations in 104 families, extent of allelic heterogeneity, and absence of correlation between phenotype and type of mutation. Am J Hum Genet. 1999;65:984-994.

360. Korda V, Deybach JC, Martasek P, et al. Homozygous variegate porphyria. Lancet. 1984;1:851.

361. Hift RJ, Meissner PN, Todd G, et al. Homozygous variegate porphyria: an evolving clinical syndrome. Postgrad Med J. 1993;69:781-786.

362. Kauppinen R, Timonen K, von und zu Fraunberg M, et al. Homozygous variegate porphyria: 20 y follow-up and characterization of molecular defect. J Invest Dermatol. 2001;116:610-613.

363. Palmer RA, Elder GH, Barrett DF, Keohane SG. Homozygous variegate porphyria: a compound heterozygote with novel mutations in the protoporphyrinogen oxidase gene. Br J Dermatol. 2001;144:866-869.

364. Poblete-Gutierrez P, Wolff C, Farias R, Frank J. A Chilean boy with severe photosensitivity and finger shortening: the first case of homozygous variegate porphyria in South America. Br J Dermatol. 2006;154:368-371.

365. Roberts AG, Puy H, Dailey TA, et al. Molecular characterization of homozygous variegate porphyria. Hum Mol Genet. 1998;7:1921-1925.

366. Meissner P. Medical aspects of porphyrins. In Kadish KM, Smith KM, Guilard R (eds). The Porphyrin Handbook, vol 14. New York, Academic Press, 2003.

367. Frank J, Aita VM, Ahmad W, et al. Identification of a founder mutation in the protoporphyrinogen oxidase gene in variegate porphyria patients from Chile. Hum Hered. 2001;51:160-168.

368. Schneider-Yin X, Gouya L, Meier-Weinand A, et al. New insights into the pathogenesis of erythropoietic protoporphyria and their impact on patient care. Eur J Pediatr. 2000;159:719-725.

369. Meissner PN, Dailey TA, Hift RJ, et al. A R59W mutation in human protoporphyrinogen oxidase results in decreased enzyme activity and is prevalent in South Africans with variegate porphyria. Nat Genet. 1996;13:95-97.

370. Warnich L, Kotze MJ, Groenewald IM, et al. Identification of three mutations and associated haplotypes in the protoporphyrinogen oxidase gene in South African families with variegate porphyria. Hum Mol Genet. 1996;5:981-984.

371. Brenner DA, Bloomer JR. The enzymatic defect in variegate prophyria. Studies with human cultured skin fibroblasts. N Engl J Med. 1980;302:765-769.

372. Deybach JC, de Verneuil H, Nordmann Y. The inherited enzymatic defect in porphyria variegata. Hum Genet. 1981;58:425-428.

373. Mustajoki P, Tenhunen R, Niemi KM, et al. Homozygous variegate porphyria. A severe skin disease of infancy. Clin Genet. 1987;32:300-305.

374. Longas MO, Poh-Fitzpatrick MB. A tightly bound protein-porphyrin complex isolated from the plasma of a patient with variegate porphyria. Clin Chim Acta. 1982;118:219-228.

375. Long C, Smyth SJ, Woolf J, et al. Detection of latent variegate porphyria by fluorescence emission spectroscopy of plasma. Br J Dermatol. 1993;129:9-13.

376. Meissner P, Adams P, Kirsch R. Allosteric inhibition of human lymphoblast and purified porphobilinogen deaminase by protoporphyrinogen and coproporphyrinogen. A possible mechanism for the acute attack of variegate porphyria. J Clin Invest. 1993;91:1436-1444.

377. Cramers M, Jepsen LV. Porphyria variegata: failure of chloroquin treatment. Acta Derm Venereol. 1980;60:89-91.

378. Timonen K, Mustajoki P, Tenhunen R, Lauharanta J. Effects of haem arginate on variegate porphyria. Br J Dermatol. 1990;123:381-387.

379. Wu CK, Dailey HA, Rose JP, et al. The 2.0 A structure of human ferrochelatase, the terminal enzyme of heme biosynthesis. Nat Struct Biol. 2001;8:156-160.

380. Burden AE, Wu C, Dailey TA, et al. Human ferrochelatase: crystallization, characterization of the [2Fe-2S] cluster and determination that the enzyme is a homodimer. Biochim Biophys Acta. 1999;1435:191-197.

381. Proulx KL, Woodard SI, Dailey HA. In situ conversion of coproporphyrinogen to heme by murine mitochondria: terminal steps of the heme biosynthetic pathway. Protein Sci. 1993;2:1092-1098.

382. Whitcombe DM, Carter NP, Albertson DG, et al. Assignment of the human ferrochelatase gene (FECH) and a locus for protoporphyria to chromosome 18q22. Genomics. 1991;11:1152-1154.

383. Taketani S, Inazawa J, Nakahashi Y, et al. Structure of the human ferrochelatase gene. Exon/intron gene organization and location of the gene to chromosome 18. Eur J Biochem. 1992;205:217-222.

384. Karr SR, Dailey HA. The synthesis of murine ferrochelatase in vitro and in vivo. Biochem J. 1988;254:799-803.

385. Cobbold C, Roberts A, Badminton M. Erythropoietic protoporphyria: a functional analysis of the leader sequence of human ferrochelatase. Mol Genet Metab. 2006;89:227-232.

386. Liu YL, Ang SO, Weigent DA, et al. Regulation of ferrochelatase gene expression by hypoxia. Life Sci. 2004;75:2035-2043.

387. Kosenow W, Treibs A. Lichtübererempfind Lichtveit und Porphyrinämie. Z Kinderheilk. 1953;73:82-92.

388. Magnus IA, Jarrett A, Prankerd TA, Rimington C. Erythropoietic protoporphyria. A new porphyria syndrome with solar urticaria due to protoporphyrinaemia. Lancet. 1961;2:448-451.

389. Haeger-Aronsen B. Erythropoietic protoporphyria. A New type of inborn error of metabolism. Am J Med. 1963;35:450-454.

390. Bloomer JR, Wang Y, Shaw GC, et al. Variant erythropoietic protoporphyria (EPP): a disorder with severe EPP phenotype, no mutations in ferrochelatase DNA, and abnormal mitoferrin expression. Hepatology. 2007;46:881A.

391. Shaw GC, Cope JJ, Li L, et al. Mitoferrin is essential for erythroid iron assimilation. Nature. 2006;440:96-100.

392. Anstey AV, Hift RJ. Liver disease in erythropoietic protoporphyria: insights and implications for management. Postgrad Med J. 2007;83:739-748.

393. Parker M, Corrigall AV, Hift RJ, Meissner PN. Molecular characterization of erythropoietic protoporphyria in South Africa. Br J Dermatol. 2008;May 2. [Epub ahead of print].

394. Holme SA, Anstey AV, Finlay AY, et al. Erythropoietic protoporphyria in the U.K.: clinical features and effect on quality of life. Br J Dermatol. 2006;155:574-581.

395. Todd DJ. Erythropoietic protoporphyria. Br J Dermatol. 1994;131:751-766.

396. Baart de la Faille H, Bijlmer-Iest JC, van Hattum J, et al. Erythropoietic protoporphyria: clinical aspects with emphasis on the skin. Curr Probl Dermatol. 1991;20:123-134.

397. Went LN, Klasen EC. Genetic aspects of erythropoietic protoporphyria. Ann Hum Genet. 1984;48:105-117.

398. Marko PB, Miljkovic J, Gorenjak M, et al. Erythropoietic protoporphyria patients in Slovenia. Acta Dermatovenerol Alp Panonica Adriat. 2007;16:99-102, 104.

399. Cox TM, Alexander GJ, Sarkany RP. Protoporphyria. Semin Liver Dis. 1998;18:85-93.

400. DeLeo VA, Poh-Fitzpatrick M, Mathews-Roth M, Harber LC. Erythropoietic protoporphyria. 10 years experience. Am J Med. 1976;60:8-22.

401. Labrousse AL, Salmon-Ehr V, Eschard C, et al. Recurrent painful hand crisis in a four-year-old girl, revealing an erythropoietic protoporphyria. Eur J Dermatol. 1998;8:515-516.

402. Lecluse AL, Kuck-Koot VC, van Weelden H, et al. Erythropoietic protoporphyria without skin symptoms—you do not always see what they feel. Eur J Pediatr. 2008;167:703-706.

403. Bewley AP, Keefe M, White JE. Erythropoietic protoporphyria improving during pregnancy. Br J Dermatol. 1998;139:145-147.

404. Poh-Fitzpatrick MB. Human protoporphyria: reduced cutaneous photosensitivity and lower erythrocyte porphyrin levels during pregnancy. J Am Acad Dermatol. 1997;36:40-43.

405. Bottomley SS, Tanaka M, Everett MA. Diminished erythroid ferrochelatase activity in protoporphyria. J Lab Clin Med. 1975;86:126-131.

406. Holme SA, Worwood M, Anstey AV, et al. Erythropoiesis and iron metabolism in dominant erythropoietic protoporphyria. Blood. 2007;110:4108-4110.

407. Mathews-Roth MM. Anemia in erythropoietic protoporphyria [letter]. JAMA. 1974;230:824.

408. Rademakers LH, Koningsberger JC, Sorber CW, et al. Accumulation of iron in erythroblasts of patients with

erythropoietic protoporphyria. Eur J Clin Invest. 1993;23: 130-138.

409. Lyoumi S, Abitbol M, Andrieu V, et al. Increased plasma transferrin, altered body iron distribution, and microcytic hypochromic anemia in ferrochelatase-deficient mice. Blood. 2007;109:811-818.

410. Schmidt H, Snitker G, Thomsen K, Lintrup J. Erythropoietic protoporphyria. A clinical study based on 29 cases in 14 families. Arch Dermatol. 1974;110:58-64.

411. Bloomer JR. The liver in protoporphyria. Hepatology. 1988;8:402-407.

412. Lee RG, Avner DL, Berenson MM. Structure-function relationships of protoporphyrin-induced liver injury. Arch Pathol Lab Med. 1984;108:744-746.

413. Todd DJ. Gallstones in children. Am J Dis Child. 1991;145:971-972.

414. Cripps DJ, Scheuer PJ. Hepatobiliary changes in erythropoietic protoporphyria. Arch Pathol. 1965;80:500-508.

415. MacDonald DM, Germain D, Perrot H. The histopathology and ultrastructure of liver disease in erythropoietic protoporphyria. Br J Dermatol. 1981;104:7-17.

416. Mooyaart BR, de Jong GM, van der Veen S, et al. Hepatic disease in erythropoietic protoporphyria. Dermatologica. 1986;173:120-130.

417. Rademakers LH, Cleton MI, Kooijman C, et al. Early involvement of hepatic parenchymal cells in erythrohepatic protoporphyria? An ultrastructural study of patients with and without overt liver disease and the effect of chenodeoxycholic acid treatment. Hepatology. 1990;11: 449-457.

418. Mathews-Roth MM. The consequences of not diagnosing erythropoietic protoporphyria. Arch Dermatol. 1980;116: 407.

419. Nordmann Y. Erythropoietic protoporphyria and hepatic complications. J Hepatol. 1992;16:4-6.

420. Reisenauer AK, Soon SL, Lee KK, Hanifin JM. Erythropoietic protoporphyria presenting with liver failure in adulthood. Dermatology. 2005;210:72-73.

421. Singer JA, Plaut AG, Kaplan MM. Hepatic failure and death from erythropoietic protoporphyria. Gastroenterology. 1978;74:588-591.

422. Bonkovsky HL, Schned AR. Fatal liver failure in protoporphyria. Synergism between ethanol excess and the genetic defect. Gastroenterology. 1986;90:191-201.

423. Ishibashi A, Ogata R, Sakisaka S, et al. Erythropoietic protoporphyria with fatal liver failure. J Gastroenterol. 1999;34:405-409.

424. Meerman L. Erythropoietic protoporphyria. An overview with emphasis on the liver. Scand J Gastroenterol Suppl. 2000;232:79-85.

425. Rufenacht UB, Gouya L, Schneider-Yin X, et al. Systematic analysis of molecular defects in the ferrochelatase gene from patients with erythropoietic protoporphyria. Am J Hum Genet. 1998;62:1341-1352.

426. Whatley SD, Mason NG, Khan M, et al. Autosomal recessive erythropoietic protoporphyria in the United Kingdom: prevalence and relationship to liver disease. J Med Genet. 2004;41:e105.

427. Goerz G, Bunselmeyer S, Bolsen K, Schurer NY. Ferrochelatase activities in patients with erythropoietic protoporphyria and their families. Br J Dermatol. 1996;134: 880-885.

428. Gouya L, Deybach JC, Lamoril J, et al. Modulation of the phenotype in dominant erythropoietic protoporphyria by a low expression of the normal ferrochelatase allele. Am J Hum Genet. 1996;58:292-299.

429. Gouya L, Puy H, Lamoril J, et al. Inheritance in erythropoietic protoporphyria: a common wild-type ferrochelatase allelic variant with low expression accounts for clinical manifestation. Blood. 1999;93:2105-2110.

430. Gouya L, Puy H, Robreau AM, et al. The penetrance of dominant erythropoietic protoporphyria is modulated by expression of wildtype FECH. Nat Genet. 2002;30:27-28.

431. Gouya L, Martin-Schmitt C, Robreau AM, et al. Contribution of a common single-nucleotide polymorphism to the genetic predisposition for erythropoietic protoporphyria. Am J Hum Genet. 2006;78:2-14.

432. Saruwatari H, Ueki Y, Yotsumoto S, et al. Genetic analysis of the ferrochelatase gene in eight Japanese patients from seven families with erythropoietic protoporphyria. J Dermatol. 2006;33:603-608.

433. Herrero C, To-Figueras J, Badenas C, et al. Clinical, biochemical, and genetic study of 11 patients with erythropoietic protoporphyria including one with homozygous disease. Arch Dermatol. 2007;143:1125-1129.

434. Lamoril J, Boulechfar S, de Verneuil H, et al. Human erythropoietic protoporphyria: two point mutations in the ferrochelatase gene. Biochem Biophys Res Commun. 1991;181:594-599.

435. Poh-Fitzpatrick MB, Wang X, Anderson KE, et al. Erythropoietic protoporphyria: altered phenotype after bone marrow transplantation for myelogenous leukemia in a patient heteroallelic for ferrochelatase gene mutations. J Am Acad Dermatol. 2002;46:861-866.

436. Reed WB, Wuepper KD, Epstein JH, et al. Erythropoietic protoporphyria. A clinical and genetic study. JAMA. 1970; 214:1060-1066.

437. Lamola AA, Yamane T. Zinc protoporphyrin in the erythrocytes of patients with lead intoxication and iron deficiency anemia. Science. 1974;186:936-938.

438. Lamola AA, Piomelli S, Poh-Fitzpatrick MG, et al. Erythropoietic protoporphyria and lead intoxication: the molecular basis for difference in cutaneous photosensitivity. II. Different binding of erythrocyte protoporphyrin to hemoglobin. J Clin Invest. 1975;56:1528-1535.

439. Poh-Fitzpatrick MB, DeLeo VA. Rates of plasma porphyrin disappearance in fluorescent vs. red incandescent light exposure. J Invest Dermatol. 1977;69:510-512.

440. Poh-Fitzpatrick MB. Protoporphyrin metabolic balance in human protoporphyria. Gastroenterology. 1985;88: 1239-1242.

441. Mathews-Roth MM, Pathak UA, Fitzpatrick TB, et al. Beta-carotene as an oral photoprotective agent in erythropoietic protoporphyria. JAMA. 1974;228:1004-1008.

442. Thomsen K, Schmidt H, Fischer A. Beta-carotene in erythropoietic protoporphyria: 5 years' experience. Dermatologica. 1979;159:82-86.

443. Mathews-Roth MM. Erythropoietic protoporphyria—diagnosis and treatment. N Engl J Med. 1977;297:98-100.

444. Mathews-Roth MM, Pathak MA, Fitzpatrick TB, et al. Beta carotene therapy for erythropoietic protoporphyria and other photosensitivity diseases. Arch Dermatol. 1977; 113:1229-1232.

445. Moshell AN, Bjornson L. Photoprotection in erythropoietic protoporphyria: mechanism of photoprotection by beta carotene. J Invest Dermatol. 1977;68:157-160.

446. Gross U, Frank M, Doss MO. Hepatic complications of erythropoietic protoporphyria. Photodermatol Photoimmunol Photomed. 1998;14:52-57.

447. Van Hattum J, Baart de la Faille H, Van den Berg JW, et al. Chenodeoxycholic acid therapy in erythrohepatic protoporphyria. J Hepatol. 1986;3:407-412.

448. Seth AK, Badminton MN, Mirza D, et al. Liver transplantation for porphyria: who, when, and how? Liver Transpl. 2007;13:1219-1227.

449. McGuire BM, Bonkovsky HL, Carithers RL Jr, et al. Liver transplantation for erythropoietic protoporphyria liver disease. Liver Transpl. 2005;11:1590-1596.

450. de Torres I, Demetris AJ, Randhawa PS. Recurrent hepatic allograft injury in erythropoietic protoporphyria. Transplantation. 1996;61:1412-1413.

451. Rollwagen FM. Hepatic allograft injury in erythropoietic protoporphyria. Transplantation. 1997;63:485-486.

452. Rand EB, Bunin N, Cochran W, et al. Sequential liver and bone marrow transplantation for treatment of erythropoietic protoporphyria. Pediatrics. 2006;118:e1896-e1899.

V Hemolytic Anemias

14 Autoimmune Hemolytic Anemia

Russell E. Ware

The vast majority of erythrocyte disorders that occur in the pediatric age group result from abnormalities within the red blood cell (RBC); that is, they are intracorpuscular defects. These intrinsic RBC defects include a wide variety of inherited genetic mutations, as well as acquired nutritional deficiencies, and lead to defects in globin chain and heme synthesis, abnormal membrane structural proteins, or defective intracellular enzymes. Particularly in the congenital conditions, intracorpuscular defects often result in a shortened erythrocyte life span, premature destruction of the erythrocytes (hemolysis), and anemia.

A less common category of erythrocyte disorders includes conditions characterized by abnormalities external to the red cells, known as extracorpuscular defects. Examples include environmental stress (oxidation, toxins, heat, or mechanical injury), microangiopathic erythrocyte damage (hemolytic-uremic syndrome [HUS] or thrombotic thrombocytopenic purpura [TTP]), or immune-mediated RBC destruction. Like many of the intrinsic conditions, extrinsic erythrocyte disorders are typically associated with hemolysis and anemia.

Disorders that result from abnormal interactions between erythrocytes and the immune system are collectively referred to as immune-mediated hemolytic anemia. The most common type is autoimmune hemolytic anemia (AIHA), characterized by the presence of autoantibodies that bind to the erythrocyte surface membrane and lead to premature red cell destruction. Specific characteristics of the autoantibodies, particularly the isotype, thermal reactivity, and ability to fix complement, help shape the resulting clinical picture. In all patients with AIHA, however, the autoantibody leads to shortened RBC survival, hemolysis, and anemia. Additional types of immune-mediate hemolytic anemia reflect abnormal interactions between erythrocytes and varied components of the complement and hemostasis systems, as well as the vessel wall. The reticuloendothelial system, primarily the spleen, plays a critical role in premature destruction of erythrocytes in all forms of immune-mediated hemolytic anemia.

This chapter begins with a description of the spleen, whose anatomy and physiology provide a unique environment for the clearance of normal and abnormal erythrocytes. Three important clinical forms of primary AIHA are then described: (1) warm-reactive AIHA, characterized by an autoantibody (usually immunoglobulin G [IgG]) that binds preferentially to erythrocyte antigens at 37° C, fixes complement in some cases, and leads primarily to extravascular hemolysis; (2) paroxysmal cold hemoglobinuria (PCH), in which an IgG erythrocyte autoantibody binds optimally at 4° C, fixes complement efficiently, and causes mainly intravascular hemolysis; and (3) cold agglutinin disease, characterized by an autoantibody (typically IgM) that binds optimally to erythrocytes below 37° C, fixes complement efficiently, and also leads primarily to intravascular hemolysis. These three disorders are discussed together because of their

many similarities, although differences in pathophysiology and therapy are emphasized. Secondary forms of AIHA are then described, including Evans syndrome and autoimmune lymphoproliferative syndrome (ALPS). The next section describes paroxysmal nocturnal hemoglobinuria (PNH), a rare and fascinating acquired hematologic disorder that features hemolysis caused by abnormal interactions between erythrocytes and the complement system. Unlike true AIHA, the defect in PNH is intracorpuscular, but the clinical findings may be similar. Advances in the understanding of PNH are described, including its recognition as an acquired clonal stem cell disorder and identification of specific acquired mutations in the phosphatidylinositol glycan class A (*PIGA*) gene in affected patients. Finally, miscellaneous extracorpuscular disorders that lead to schistocytic hemolytic anemia are described, including congenital and acquired microangiopathy, preeclampsia, and environmental stressors such as heat, toxins, or mechanical injury.

THE SPLEEN

Historical Perspective

Since ancient times the spleen has occupied a mysterious niche among organs within the human body. Its proposed functions and necessity for good health were subjects of debate and discussion for centuries, as recently reviewed.[1] Only in the last few decades has this enigmatic organ begun to yield its secrets and reveal its prominent and vital role in providing important hematologic and immunologic functions.

Hippocrates believed that the spleen helped balance the body's "humors," a process necessary to promote harmony and stability. Plato and Aristotle agreed with this notion of the spleen absorbing unhealthy body fluids but further suggested, based on its location, that it assisted or balanced the liver. Galen noted the anatomic connections among the spleen, liver, and stomach and concluded that the spleen had true digestive functions that included the filtering of humoral impurities. Subsequently, the spleen gained a reputation for controlling feelings and emotions, including laughter, ill temper, melancholy, and others. Shakespeare often referred to the spleen as an organ of anger, merriment, or other strong emotion.

During the Renaissance, when the study of anatomy and physiology became popularized, the spleen's microscopic patterns supported a role for filtration; however, only circulatory connections between the spleen and the stomach, liver, and other digestive organs could be identified. Moreover, survival of both animals and humans after surgical splenectomy demonstrated that the spleen was not absolutely required for life. Only in the modern era, with the discovery of individual blood cells, have investigators begun to elucidate the true functions of the

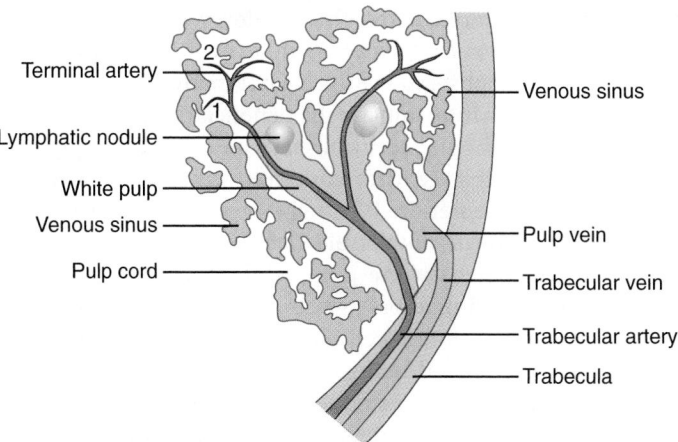

FIGURE 14-1. Blood circulation in the spleen. As blood enters the spleen, the arterial vessels are surrounded by lymphatic sheaths and nodules that constitute the white pulp. The majority of arterial blood terminates in the venous sinuses (red pulp), where filtration and quality control of erythrocytes take place. Erythrocytes return to the venous circulation via the venous sinuses. *(From Fawcett D. A Textbook of Histology, 11th ed. Philadelphia, WB Saunders, 1985, p 474.)*

spleen. We now recognize that the spleen has vital roles in blood filtration and immunologic competence.

Anatomy and Physiology

The spleen can be identified in human embryogenesis during week 5 of gestation, although the development of characteristic splenic architecture with influx of red and white blood cells occurs much later in gestation. At birth the spleen weighs about 10 g and then grows steadily to 30 g at 1 year of age, to 60 g by 5 years, and finally to the adult size of approximately 200 g.[2] The spleen is located under the confines of the left anterior aspect of the rib cage and can have a triangular, crescent, or rhomboidal shape. Though not accurate as a measure of total splenic volume, spleen size is usually estimated clinically by length alone, specifically, how far below the left costal margin the tip of the spleen can be palpated. Frequently, an enlarged spleen is most easily palpated at the midclavicular line, but it can extend prominently toward the midline or even to the midaxillary line in some patients.

The spleen receives 3-5% of the total cardiac output, thus making it a highly perfused organ.[3] Blood enters and leaves the spleen primarily through the splenic artery and vein, respectively, both located at the hilum on the concave (medial) side of the organ. Within the splenic parenchyma, the splenic arterial branches have little overlap, thereby allowing classification of the spleen into lobes and segments separated by relatively avascular planes.

Histologically, the spleen can be separated into two distinct regions, the red pulp and the white pulp, so named because of the blood cells most commonly found in each area. The red pulp represents a large open circulation within the spleen through which erythrocytes pass slowly for filtration and culling functions. In contrast, the white pulp consists primarily of collections of lymphocytes and macrophages that form small white nodules (1 to 2 mm in diameter) distributed throughout the splenic parenchyma. These two regions provide the vital functions of blood filtration and immunologic response, respectively, which are made possible through a unique

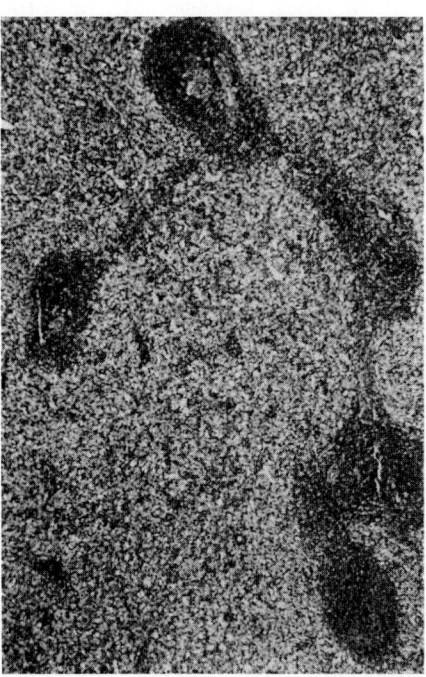

FIGURE 14-2. Lymphoid follicles in the white pulp appearing as budlike outgrowths from the periarteriolar lymphoid sheath. *(From Neiman RS, Orazi A [eds]. Disorders of the Spleen, 2nd ed. Philadelphia, WB Saunders, 1999, p 10.)*

circulation pattern found within the spleen. Figure 14-1 illustrates the arterial and venous circulations of the spleen and the close proximity of the red and white pulp.

As the largest arteries within the spleen branch progressively into the smallest arterioles, the white pulp can be recognized as a circumferential ring of leukocytes that surround the vessel, also known as the periarterial (or periarteriolar) lymphoid sheath (PALS). The PALS consists primarily of T lymphocytes, and this cylindrical cuff of cells becomes thinner as the artery becomes smaller. Spheroidal lymphoid follicles arise at intervals from the PALS, usually where arterial branch points occur, and these follicles contain primarily B lymphocytes (Fig. 14-2). When immunologically stimulated, these primary lymphoid follicles develop into secondary follicles with germinal centers, similar to the processes and architecture observed within lymph nodes. Lymphocytes within the white pulp are the beneficiaries of plasma "skimmed" from the central arterial blood supply. Whereas blood cells tend to continue within the vessel, plasma elements enter the PALS via tiny vessels that arise perpendicular to the flow of blood. Soluble antigens are thus herded into the white pulp, where they encounter dendritic cells and macrophages that function as professional antigen-presenting cells and allow proper immune stimulation of T and B lymphocytes.

After plasma is redirected toward the white pulp, the blood cells that continue through the splenic circulation are mostly erythrocytes, and they form the red pulp as they exit the arteries. Occasionally, erythrocytes pass directly from the arterial to the venous circulation via traditional endothelialized capillaries, a process known as the closed (rapid) splenic circulation, which is primarily nutritive. Much more commonly, however, erythrocytes leave the arterial circulation and empty into large pools called the splenic cords, where they encounter macrophages and other immune effector cells. Erythrocytes must survive these intimate encounters in this hypoxic and acidic environment and then pass from the cords through an endothelialized barrier into the splenic sinuses and finally back to the venous circulation. This open (slow) circulation allows careful filtration of individual erythrocytes, with repair or phagocytosis of cells that cannot successfully negotiate the return trip.

Important Functions of the Spleen

All RBCs pass through the spleen many times each day.[4,5] The spleen serves as an efficient filter for erythrocytes and is able to perform grooming (removal of antibodies or other surface molecules), culling (destruction of cells), and pitting functions (removal of intracellular material). While moving slowly through the hostile environment of the splenic cords, erythrocytes are carefully examined for abnormalities, a process constituting a biologic form of quality control. Macrophages in the red pulp identify abnormal erythrocytes, such as those that have IgG or complement on their surface, and either remove a portion of their membrane or fully engulf them. Newly made reticulocytes spend their first day or two in the spleen,[6] during which the cells appear to be groomed with removal of cytoplasmic organelles and surface adhesion molecules. Normal mature erythrocytes, in contrast, typically endure macrophage scrutiny without difficulty. To leave the red pulp, erythrocytes must then pass back from the splenic cords through potential spaces in the endothelial lining of the splenic sinuses. To negotiate these tiny apertures, known as the cords of Billroth, the erythrocytes must deform themselves substantially (Fig. 14-3). Cordal macrophages phagocytose erythrocytes that cannot deform themselves sufficiently, such as senescent cells; as erythrocytes age, they lose volume, gain density, and

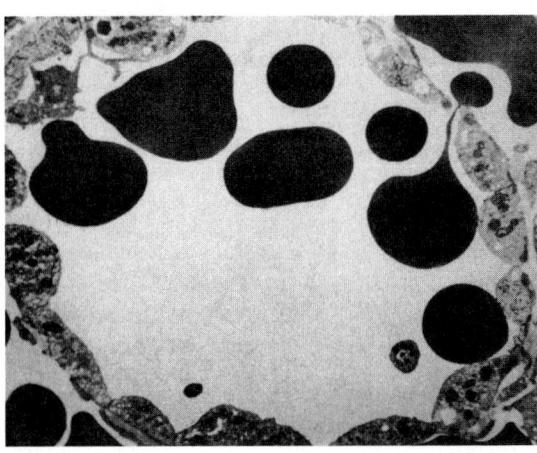

FIGURE 14-3. Deformation of erythrocytes returning from the splenic cords (red pulp) back into the venous sinus. The erythrocytes must pass through very small potential spaces in the sinus wall known as the cords of Billroth. *(From Neiman RS, Orazi A [eds]. Disorders of the Spleen, 2nd ed. Philadelphia, WB Saunders, 1999, p 18.)*

eventually lose the deformability that allows reentry into the splenic sinus. In certain pathologic conditions, such as immune-mediated hemolytic anemia, as well as a variety of erythrocyte membrane, hemoglobin, and enzyme disorders, younger erythrocytes will also be trapped in the splenic cords. Erythrocytes with intracellular inclusions, such as nuclear remnants known as micronuclei (Howell-Jolly bodies), denatured hemoglobin (Heinz bodies), siderotic granules (Pappenheimer bodies), or malarial parasites, have their inclusions "pitted" out before they pass through the endothelial slits and return to the circulation.

The spleen also provides several important immunologic functions. Skimming of plasma into the PALS allows particulate antigens to interact with dendritic cells and other antigen-presenting cells, which initiates the immune response for T- and B-lymphocyte response and proliferation. Polysaccharide antigens in particular require this unique immunologic environment for optimal antibody response.[7,8] Intravenous antigens, such as those found during infection or after immunization, are primarily processed by the spleen.[9] Not surprisingly, normal splenic function is required for optimal early (IgM) response to most intravenous antigens, as well as the secondary (IgG) response.[10] In contrast, antigens administered by the intramuscular or subcutaneous routes do not require normal splenic function for a robust immune response.[11,12] Finally, blood-borne bacteria, particularly encapsulated organisms, are removed by splenic macrophages located in the PALS and in the cords. Without a functioning spleen, patients are susceptible to overwhelming bacterial sepsis and to exaggerated parasitemia from *Plasmodium, Babesia,* or other organisms.[13,14]

To a much lesser extent, the human spleen can also serve as a reservoir for circulating blood cells. About 50 mL of blood is usually contained in a normal spleen, as well as 30% of the platelet mass. In the abnormal state (see later), the spleen can enlarge and trap a larger portion of the circulating blood cells, a condition known as hypersplenism. The spleen may also serve a small role in iron metabolism and homeostasis. Unlike the spleen in other species, however, it has no appreciable role in human hematopoiesis.

Abnormalities of the Spleen

Congenital asplenia is found in children with the rare Ivemark syndrome, in which the body has bilateral "right-sidedness" with trilobed lungs and a centralized liver.[15] Cardiac defects are common, as well as a risk of infection.[16] Even rarer patients have congenital asplenia with no other abnormalities.[16a] This resembles mice with a targeted deletion of Hox 11.[16b] Uptake of radionuclide by functioning splenic tissue can be difficult to document because the anatomic features are distorted and liver tissue can obscure any splenic uptake. Circulating erythrocytes with Howell-Jolly bodies or intracellular vesicles that appear as "pits" or "pocks" allow the diagnosis of asplenia to be established noninvasively.[17] Figure 14-4 illustrates the Howell-Jolly bodies that are found in the peripheral blood smear of an asplenic person. The converse arrangement of bilateral "left-sidedness" leads to congenital polysplenia with several spleens of varying size. In most patients the splenic tissue in polysplenia has normal function. Cardiac defects are common, as well as hepatobiliary abnormalities.[18,19]

Accessory spleens can be identified in 15% of normal persons.[20] In most of these individuals, a single accessory spleen measuring only 1 to 2 cm in diameter is present either in the splenic hilum or in the tail of the pancreas. Multiple accessory spleens can exist, however, as well as ectopic spleens in locations ranging from the abdomen to the pelvis and scrotum. The function of accessory spleens depends on the quality and quantity of blood flow; in most instances their filtration capabilities are minimal, but antibody responses may be present.

Splenoptosis, or wandering spleen, occurs when the spleen is not fixed within the retroperitoneum.[21] The resulting mass can be palpated anywhere in the abdomen and may require reattachment (splenopexy) or even splenectomy if symptoms of sequestration or torsion develop.[22] Splenosis refers to the autotransplantation of splenic tissue into the omentum or peritoneal surfaces of the abdominal cavity. Splenosis typically occurs after fracture or rupture of the spleen as a result of spillage and subsequent implantation of splenocytes. Although some protection against infection may be afforded by splenosis,[23] filtering functions and immunologic responses are limited by the relatively small total amount of splenic tissue and reduced blood supply.

Sequestration refers to enlargement of the spleen that occurs when blood enters the organ but is unable to exit properly. This condition is most often observed in children with sickle cell anemia when venous return of blood is hindered by intrasplenic sickling of erythrocytes within the red pulp. Splenic sequestration also occurs in other settings with abnormal erythrocytes, however, including congenital spherocytosis. Splenic sequestration can develop acutely with sudden pooling of blood within the spleen and result in rapid and painful expansion of the splenic parenchyma and capsule. Children exhibit pallor, fatigue, severe anemia, and occasionally hypovolemic shock.[24] Occasionally, splenic sequestration develops over a period of days or weeks and is then termed subacute or chronic because it is accompanied by relatively asymptomatic splenomegaly.

Hypersplenism refers to the condition of splenomegaly with non–immune-mediated trapping of peripheral blood cells and results in mild to moderate cytopenia.[25] Hypersplenism can develop in patients with abnormal erythrocytes, metabolic storage disorders, or other causes of chronic congestive splenomegaly. In these clinical settings, the spleen first enlarges because of progressive trapping of erythrocytes or storage material and then subsequently becomes a reservoir for all circulating blood cells. Typically, the peripheral platelet count is lower than normal, but the leukocyte count can also be low. If surgery is required, peripheral blood counts normalize after splenectomy.

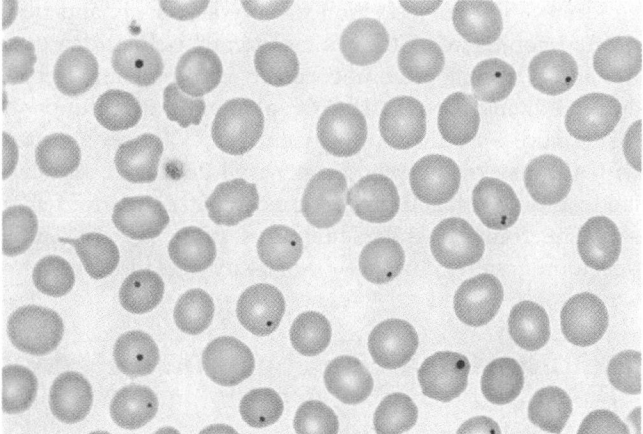

FIGURE 14-4. Howell-Jolly bodies in peripheral blood erythrocytes. These nuclear remnants are identified as small inclusions within circulating erythrocytes and have several characteristic and required features by light microscopy: (1) they are spherical inclusions 0.5 to 2.0 μm in diameter, about the size of a small platelet; (2) they have a smooth contour and no surrounding halo, which distinguishes them from platelets juxtaposed to an erythrocyte; (3) they are always in the same focal plane as the erythrocyte because they are intracellular; (4) they are never refractile, unlike talc or dust particles; and (5) they are homogeneous in appearance, unlike other intracellular inclusions such as Pappenheimer bodies or malarial parasites. Howell-Jolly bodies are normally removed when erythrocytes pass through the cords of Billroth into the venous sinus. Their presence in peripheral blood indicates lack of splenic filtrative function.

Surgery Involving the Spleen

Although the spleen has important hematologic and immunologic functions, in some instances surgical removal is beneficial. A variety of congenital anomalies of the spleen, as well as numerous pathophysiologic processes, are indications for splenectomy.

Benign tumors of the spleen are relatively rare in childhood but primarily include congenital cysts (epidermoid or lymphangiomatous) or pseudocysts that result from liquefaction of splenic parenchyma after infarction or hemorrhage. These tumors may require splenectomy, depending on their size. Malignant splenic tumors are almost always lymphomatous or leukemic in origin, with cancerous cells found diffusely or in a nodular pattern throughout the splenic parenchyma. Perhaps somewhat surprisingly, very few solid tumors metastasize to the spleen. As a general guideline, splenectomy is not usually indicated in the setting of malignancy.

Splenomegaly requiring splenectomy can develop in a variety of clinical settings, including metabolic storage disorders such as Gaucher's disease, transfusion-acquired iron overload from chronic erythrocyte transfusions, or splenic congestion resulting from portal hypertension, among others. Commonly, splenectomy is the recommended therapeutic option for splenic enlargement in patients with primary erythrocyte abnormalities. Congenital hemoglobin, enzyme, and membrane disorders lead to trapping of the abnormal erythrocytes within the splenic cords and gradual expansion of the red pulp. In these settings, splenectomy can relieve the signs and symptoms of splenomegaly, including abdominal discomfort, anemia, hypersplenism, and dependence on transfusions.

Total surgical splenectomy is generally performed by open laparotomy via a left subcostal incision. Laparoscopic splenectomy has become a popular and safe alternative in children[26,27] but requires careful attention and may be technically difficult with very large spleens. With the laparoscopic approach, small amounts of residual splenic tissue may be left or accessory spleens may be missed,[28] which can be a problem for patients with immune-mediated hematologic disorders. When splenectomy is recommended for AIHA or immune thrombocytopenic purpura (ITP), all splenic tissue must be removed to prevent recurrent autoantibody production. Over the past decade, subtotal (partial) splenectomy has become a viable therapeutic alternative to total splenectomy. The partial splenectomy approach is possible because the spleen can be divided into distinct lobes and segments.[29] Removal of 80% to 90% of the enlarged spleen usually provides relief from splenomegaly while retaining sufficient splenic tissue for immune competence. Partial splenectomy has been used successfully in children with nonparasitic splenic cysts,[30] hereditary spherocytosis,[31] homozygous β-thalassemia,[32] and sickle cell disease,[33] although splenic regrowth may limit its long-term efficacy.[34] Even children with massive splenomegaly can successfully undergo partial splenectomy.[35] Based on animal studies, a third of the normal spleen mass is required for normal plasma filtration and antibody formation.[36] When compared to splenic tissue reimplanted either by surgical autotransplantation or splenosis,[37,38] partial splenectomy provides superior retained immune function. Laparoscopic partial splenectomy combines these two new approaches and may represent an ideal option for selected patients who require surgical splenectomy; it is becoming more commonly available for children.[39,40]

The primary danger after total splenectomy is fatal bacterial sepsis, sometimes referred to as overwhelming postsplenectomy infection (OPSI). First recognized more than 50 years ago,[41] bacteremia evolving rapidly into fatal sepsis with or without meningitis can abruptly develop in a patient without splenic function. Pathogens associated with OPSI are primarily encapsulated bacterial organisms and include *Streptococcus pneumoniae*, *Haemophilus influenzae* type b, and *Neisseria meningitidis*. The presumed pathophysiologic origin of OPSI is loss of plasma filtration by the spleen, which allows bacteria to multiply within the bloodstream and evolve from low-grade bacteremia to fulminant sepsis. Risk factors for OPSI include younger age at initial clinical evaluation, younger age at splenectomy, and failure to comply with prophylactic antibiotics or vaccinations. The true risk for the development of OPSI has been estimated in two large studies, although many of the patients were from the prevaccination era. First, in a literature review covering 35 years from 1952 to 1987 (5902 patients), the incidence of infection after splenectomy in children younger than 16 years was 4.4% with a mortality rate of 2.2%; for adults the corresponding values were 0.9% and 0.8%, respectively. Children younger than 5 years and especially infants had a much higher risk for sepsis.[42] In a later survey of 226 splenectomized patients with hereditary spherocytosis that included 5461 years of postoperative follow-up, the estimated mortality rate was 0.73/1000 years for the entire group, but somewhat higher for children.[43] The introduction of polysaccharide and now protein-conjugated vaccines has greatly helped decrease the incidence of pneumococcal bacteremia and sepsis and will help offset the lack of splenic filtration function for children undergoing splenectomy. However, even with the use of presplenectomy immunization, prophylactic antibiotics, and prompt medical attention for fever, a splenectomized child still has a finite risk of OPSI developing with substantial morbidity and mortality.

IMMUNE-MEDIATED HEMOLYTIC ANEMIA

Historical Perspective

Erythrocyte hemolysis characterized by anemia, shortened RBC survival, jaundice, and occasionally hemoglobinuria has been recognized as a clinical entity for more than a century.[44,45] In the early 1900s it was noted that the serum from some patients with hemolytic anemia had the ability to agglutinate or hemolyze erythrocytes in vitro; such sera contained "agglutinins" or "hemolysins," respectively, which suggested an immunologic basis for the hemolysis.[46] The majority of patients with hemolytic anemia did not have these laboratory findings, however, and the mechanism by which their erythrocytes were destroyed was then unknown. In fact, for many years it was quite difficult to distinguish acquired immune hemolytic anemia (an extracorpuscular defect) from the intracorpuscular defect known as congenital hemolytic jaundice (now called hereditary spherocytosis).

A major advance occurred in 1945, when Coombs and co-workers reported the use of rabbit antihuman globulin serum to detect Rh agglutinins.[47] This substance, soon referred to as the Coombs reagent, amplified weak agglutinins present on sensitized red cells and allowed serologic identification of previously undetectable autoantibodies on the erythrocyte surface. The authors presciently noted that their reagent "promises to be of practical use" but probably did not foresee that it would completely revolutionize the field of immunohematology. Their subsequent demonstration that the sensitizing agent on erythrocytes was γ-globulin strengthened the idea of an autoimmune process,[48] and it was later documented that IgG warm-reactive antibodies were the most common form of AIHA.[49] By the late 1950s, it was finally possible to distinguish accurately between intrinsic erythrocyte defects and immune-mediated extrinsic erythrocyte destruction.[50]

Over the next 2 decades, several additional important advances were reported. Complement components, as well as γ-globulin, were found on the red cell surface of patients with immune-mediated hemolytic anemia, and by the late 1960s, the role of complement in immune-mediated destruction of erythrocytes was firmly established.[51-55] Interactions between IgG-sensitized red cells and monocytes were investigated,[56-58] including differences related to IgG subtypes[59,60] or erythrocyte antigens.[61] These studies started to elucidate the complex immune mechanisms of erythrocyte clearance by the human reticuloendothelial system.

The development of an animal model, specifically, guinea pigs deficient in complement components C3 or C4, represented an experimental breakthrough that led to greater understanding of both the pathophysiology[62-64] and treatment[65,66] of immune-mediated hemolytic anemia. With this model, the important contributions of antibody, complement, and the reticuloendothelial system to the pathophysiology of erythrocyte hemolysis could be studied. Taken together, these laboratory investigations led to models of immune-mediated clearance of erythrocytes by the reticuloendothelial system that are still accepted today.

Over the next 15 years there were relatively fewer advances in the field, chiefly ones involving increased precision of serologic diagnosis,[67,68] occasional new therapeutic options,[69-71] or large clinical reviews of patient outcome.[72,73] Over the past 20 years, however, there has been an increase in our knowledge of the immunologic abnormalities and mechanistic pathways that may be important in the generation and expansion of erythrocyte autoantibodies in AIHA. In addition, novel therapies directed at specific targets in the immune system have emerged and expanded the treatment armamentarium

for AIHA. The stage is set for research on individual T and B lymphocytes in patients with AIHA, with the goal of understanding the pathogenesis of AIHA at the molecular level. Specific questions remain unanswered regarding the formation of autoreactive antibodies, loss of self-tolerance, and lack of regulation and suppression of these autoantibodies by the immune system.

Classification

AIHA can be classified in a variety of ways, such as by the thermal sensitivity or isotype of the autoantibodies, but a simple and convenient classification scheme separates the disorders into a primary versus a secondary process (Box 14-1). In primary AIHA, hemolytic anemia is the only clinical finding, and there is no identifiable underlying systemic illness to explain the presence of erythrocyte autoantibodies. Some children with this form of AIHA will, however, have had a recent infectious illness. Warm-reactive AIHA is the most common form of primary AIHA in children and usually involves IgG autoantibodies that sensitize erythrocytes and lead to extravascular immune clearance and hemolysis. A second category of primary AIHA is PCH, which is especially common in children after a viral-like illness. PCH is a particularly interesting form of AIHA characterized by an IgG autoantibody that binds at cold temperatures, fixes complement efficiently, and causes intravascular hemolysis. The third major form of primary AIHA, cold agglutinin disease, is more commonly observed in adults, but in children it typically follows *Mycoplasma* infections. In this disorder, an IgM autoantibody binds to erythrocytes optimally below 37° C and fixes complement; erythrocytes undergo either intravascular hemolysis or immune-mediated extravascular clearance from surface-bound complement components.

Box 14-1	**Classification of Autoimmune Hemolytic Anemia (AIHA) in Children**

PRIMARY AIHA*

Warm-reactive autoantibodies, usually IgG
Paroxysmal cold hemoglobinuria, usually IgG
Cold-agglutinin disease, usually IgM

SECONDARY AIHA†

Systemic autoimmune disease (e.g., lupus, malignancy)
Immunodeficiency
Evans syndrome
Autoimmune lymphoproliferative syndrome
Infection (*Mycoplasma*, viruses)
Drug induced

---

*Occurs in the majority of affected children and often follows a viral-like syndrome, but in the absence of another systemic illness.
†Occurs in association with another systemic process.

Secondary AIHA occurs in the context of another clinical diagnosis, with hemolytic anemia being only one manifestation of a systemic illness. Secondary AIHA can occur in patients with generalized autoimmune disease, such as systemic lupus erythematosus (SLE) or other autoimmune inflammatory disorders. AIHA also occurs in patients with malignancy, immunodeficiency states, exposure to drugs, or specific infections. Because AIHA may be the initial manifestation, however, it is imperative that each patient with AIHA be evaluated for the presence of an underlying illness. Evans' syndrome is a unique entity that features autoimmune pancytopenia, although erythrocytes and platelets are most frequently involved. Evans' syndrome often has a severe and relapsing clinical course, and most patients require aggressive systemic therapy. Finally, ALPS is now increasingly being recognized as an important underlying condition in some children with AIHA.

PRIMARY AUTOIMMUNE HEMOLYTIC ANEMIA

Incidence

Primary AIHA is not a rare disorder. The disease has been estimated to affect 1 in 80,000 persons in the general population per year,[74] thus making it more common than acquired aplastic anemia[75,76] but less common than ITP.[77] In the pediatric age group, AIHA may even occur in infants and toddlers, especially after an infection[72,78,79]; teenagers with AIHA are more likely to have an associated underlying systemic illness and therefore have secondary disease.[80-82] Cold agglutinin disease can occur in the pediatric age group but is particularly common in older persons.[83-86] In summary, AIHA can affect persons of any age, race, ethnicity, or nationality. The issue of gender preference is somewhat more controversial; in children, boys may be affected slightly more often, whereas affected teenagers are more commonly female.[72,79,87]

Natural History

The prognosis for the majority of children with primary AIHA is good.[73,87-90] Overall, young patients with cold-reactive erythrocyte autoantibodies appear to have a better clinical outcome than those with warm-reactive antibodies. The former patients tend to have an acute self-limited illness but may require aggressive short-term supportive care. In contrast, the clinical course in children with warm-reactive AIHA is often chronic and characterized by intermittent remissions and relapses, and these patients generally require long-term therapy.

Older series reported a high mortality rate for patients with AIHA, but these studies included many adults with AIHA secondary to malignancy.[49,91] Later series, including several that focused exclusively on children, have demonstrated a much better prognosis. Buchanan and colleagues[88] reported that 77% of children with AIHA had an acute self-limited disease and that the majority of children responded well to short-term therapy; these results have been confirmed in later reviews. Mortality in children with primary AIHA appears to be no greater than 10%, with death occurring primarily in older children with chronic refractory disease, some of whom possibly had unrecognized Evans syndrome or ALPS.

Heisel and Ortega[80] attempted to define prognostic factors for AIHA in childhood. They concluded that children between 2 and 12 years of age had the best prognosis; these patients tended to have an abrupt onset of symptoms with low numbers of reticulocytes but otherwise normal blood counts. The children who fared worse were either infants younger than 2 years or teenagers; these patients had a more prolonged onset of symptoms, had higher reticulocyte counts with nucleated erythrocyte precursors in their peripheral blood, and often had decreased platelet counts.[80] Other studies have confirmed the observation that younger children with an abrupt onset of symptoms have a better prognosis than older patients do.[72,79]

Clinical Manifestations

Proper evaluation of a pediatric patient with AIHA begins with a careful history and physical examination. Many children with AIHA first come to medical attention because of signs and symptoms referable to anemia, such as pallor and weakness, and less commonly dizziness or exercise intolerance. The anemia is usually well compensated from a cardiovascular standpoint, so symptoms of congestive heart failure or circulatory collapse are rare. Occasionally, a patient has jaundice, typically noted in the sclerae, as a result of accelerated erythrocyte destruction and increased bilirubin turnover. The symptom of dark urine generally reflects intravascular hemolysis rather than bilirubin and has been described by patients in a variety of colorful and flavorful terms, including cola, iced tea, mahogany, or even motor oil. Less commonly, the patient will report abdominal pain or fever.

Children with AIHA often have a benign previous medical history, although questions should be asked regarding previous similar episodes. The review of systems should include a query about recent or concurrent medications and careful questioning regarding the possibility of an underlying illness such as a systemic autoimmune disease, inflammatory disorder, or malignancy. The family history is usually negative in AIHA; rare instances of apparent familial AIHA[72,92,93] probably reflect a tendency toward a generalized autoimmune disorder such as SLE.

On physical examination a child with AIHA is often pale and jaundiced with pallor and icterus, especially apparent in the conjunctivae and palms. The patient should have no physical stigmata of congenital disorders such as Blackfan-Diamond anemia, Fanconi anemia, or constitutional aplastic anemia. Jaundice may be apparent, particularly if the hemolysis is brisk, and is caused by the breakdown and recycling of unconjugated bilirubin from the destroyed erythrocytes. Depending on the skill of the examiner, scleral icterus can be detected at a bilirubin concentration of 2 to 3 mg/dL. Examination of the heart typically reveals tachycardia and an early systolic flow murmur as a result of the high-output anemic state. The liver and spleen may be palpable, in the latter case secondary to an increase in red pulp.[94] However, the presence of massive splenomegaly, hepatomegaly, or enlarged lymph nodes should suggest an underlying infection or malignant process.

Routine Laboratory Evaluation

Similar to that seen with other forms of anemia in young patients, such as aplastic anemia or transient erythroblastopenia of childhood, the degree of anemia in AIHA may be surprisingly marked at initial evaluation. A child with AIHA often has a hemoglobin concentration of 4 to 7 g/dL with no apparent cardiovascular compromise. RBC indices are not generally helpful in establishing the diagnosis because a normal mean corpuscular volume will reflect the weighted average of small microspherocytes and large reticulocytes. Erythrocyte agglutination within the sample tube may give an artificially large mean corpuscular volume on an automated counter.[95] An elevated mean corpuscular hemoglobin concentration (>36 g/dL) is more suggestive of hereditary spherocytosis because a spherocyte has a smaller volume than a normal erythrocyte but contains the normal amount of hemoglobin (see Chapter 15). The leukocyte count and platelet count should be within the normal range. Concurrent thrombocytopenia may indicate a bone marrow failure syndrome (e.g., aplastic anemia) or microangiopathic hemolytic anemia (e.g., HUS or TTP). The combination of AIHA and immune-mediated thrombocytopenia (Evans syndrome) is characterized by broader immune dysregulation.[96] Granulocytopenia may also be present in Evans syndrome as a reflection of the immune-mediated pancytopenia.

Evaluation of the peripheral blood smear is very useful in establishing the diagnosis of AIHA. Numerous small spherocytes are usually present in warm-reactive AIHA; splenic ingestion of a portion of the erythrocyte allows the cell to "sphere," or re-form into a more entropically favored spherical shape.[56] Surface complement may also induce erythrocyte sphering.[97] Occasionally, teardrop shapes or even schistocytes may be observed[98]; the presence of target cells is more consistent with a hemoglobinopathy or primary hepatic disease. Polychromasia is a common finding in AIHA because the bone marrow releases large numbers of reticulocytes and even nucleated RBCs to compensate for the accelerated

erythrocyte destruction. Erythrophagocytosis, first described in 1891,[99] is an unusual finding on the peripheral blood smear but visually illustrates the process of immune-mediated clearance of erythrocytes by monocytes and macrophages of the reticuloendothelial system. Figure 14-5A shows the peripheral blood smear from a patient with warm-reactive AIHA and illustrates numerous small microspherocytes and large reticulocytes. Numerous Howell-Jolly bodies are present because this patient had previously undergone splenectomy. In contrast, Figure 14-5B shows the blood smear of a patient with hereditary spherocytosis and illustrates the morphologic similarities between these two conditions. Spherocytes are seen less commonly in cold-reactive AIHA, but erythrocyte agglutination can be observed on the blood film if the binding affinity of the antibody reaches room temperature. Figure 14-5C illustrates agglutinated red cells in a patient with cold-reactive (IgM-mediated) AIHA; at higher power, nucleated immature erythroid cells released prematurely from the bone marrow can be seen. Figure 14-5D illustrates the phenomenon of erythrophagocytosis by a monocyte on the peripheral blood smear of a child with PCH.

Reticulocytosis is usually present in AIHA because of the bone marrow's compensation for the shortened red cell survival in peripheral blood.[100] Absolute reticulocyte counts are typically 200 to 600×10^9/L, which represents 10% to 30% of the circulating erythrocytes. However, reticulocytopenia is well described in AIHA and probably occurs in 10% of pediatric patients.[101-103] Several explanations have been offered for a low reticulocyte count in the presence of accelerated erythrocyte clearance. The autoantibody may react with antigens on erythroid precursors and lead to immune-mediated clearance within the marrow by resident macrophages. Alternatively, erythrocyte autoantibodies may induce apoptosis of bone marrow erythroblasts.[104] Finally, AIHA may be characterized by a well-compensated anemia that remains subclinical until infection with parvovirus B19 temporarily shuts off erythropoiesis and leads to worse and symptomatic anemia.[105,106] Regardless of its mechanism, however, the presence of reticulocytopenia should not influence therapy or prognosis in AIHA.

Aspiration of bone marrow is not generally necessary for children with AIHA but may be helpful to exclude a malignant process, myelodysplasia, or a bone marrow failure syndrome. In AIHA, the marrow aspirate usually reveals marked erythroid hyperplasia with a myeloid-erythroid ratio below unity. Mild dyserythropoiesis may be observed but should not be a common finding; substantial dyserythropoiesis should suggest an alternative diagnosis such as myelodysplasia.

Results of urine examination may be unremarkable. In patients with AIHA and intravascular hemolysis, however, free plasma hemoglobin is cleared through the renal filtration system, which leads to darkened urine. When hemoglobinuria is present, urine dipstick analysis will indicate the presence of blood, but microscopic

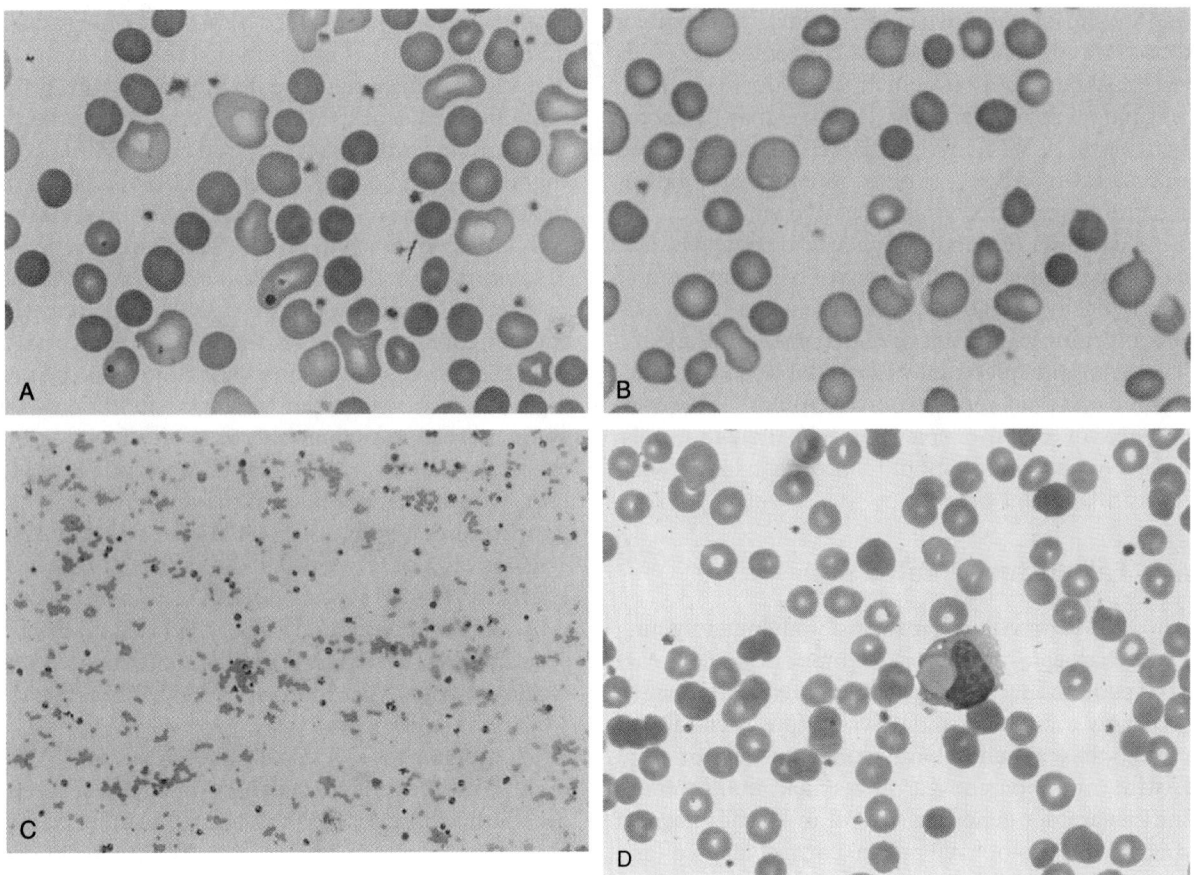

FIGURE 14-5. Examination of peripheral blood in autoimmune hemolytic anemia (AIHA). **A,** Blood from a patient with IgG (warm-reactive) AIHA illustrates many small microspherocytes and larger reticulocytes (×1000). **B,** Blood from a patient with hereditary spherocytosis illustrates the morphologic similarities between these two conditions. **C,** Agglutinated erythrocytes from a patient with IgM (cold-reactive) AIHA are clearly visible at low power (×400). **D,** Erythrophagocytosis by a peripheral blood monocyte (×1000).

examination will reveal few if any RBCs. Chronic hemoglobinuria will lead to accumulation of hemosiderin in uroepithelial cells, which can be detected in the urinary sediment.

The results of a variety of serum chemistry analyses may be abnormal because of erythrocyte hemolysis, but routine measurement should not be essential to establish the diagnosis of AIHA. Elevations in levels of lactate dehydrogenase and aspartate aminotransferase reflect the release of intraerythrocyte enzymes; in contrast, the level of serum alanine aminotransferase or other hepatic enzymes should not be elevated in AIHA. The serum haptoglobin level is almost always low because this protein acts as a scavenger for free plasma hemoglobin. However, haptoglobin is not synthesized well in young infants and is an acute phase reactant[107]; for these reasons, quantitation of serum haptoglobin may not be helpful in the evaluation of a patient with AIHA (or for that matter in any patient). The total serum bilirubin concentration is elevated in most patients with AIHA, although levels greater than 5 mg/dL are unusual and suggest hepatic impairment or the presence of Gilbert syndrome. Because the elevated bilirubin concentration in AIHA reflects accelerated erythrocyte destruction rather than

intrinsic hepatic disease, virtually all of the bilirubin is unconjugated. The direct (conjugated) fraction should not exceed 10% to 20% of the total bilirubin concentration.

Specialized Laboratory Evaluation

The most important and useful laboratory test to establish the diagnosis of AIHA is the direct antiglobulin test (DAT, formerly known as the Coombs test), which identifies antibodies and complement components on the surface of circulating erythrocytes. Therefore, a thorough understanding of the individual laboratory steps that constitute the DAT is essential for accurate interpretation of the test results.

Anticoagulated erythrocytes from the patient are first washed several times to remove all plasma proteins and are then incubated at 37° C with polyclonal rabbit antiserum that binds to human γ-globulin and human complement (usually C3). First described more than 60 years ago,[47] this "Coombs reagent" is clearly the most important diagnostic laboratory tool for a patient with AIHA. IgM autoantibodies are pentameric and can act as a bridge between adjacent erythrocytes (Fig. 14-6A). In

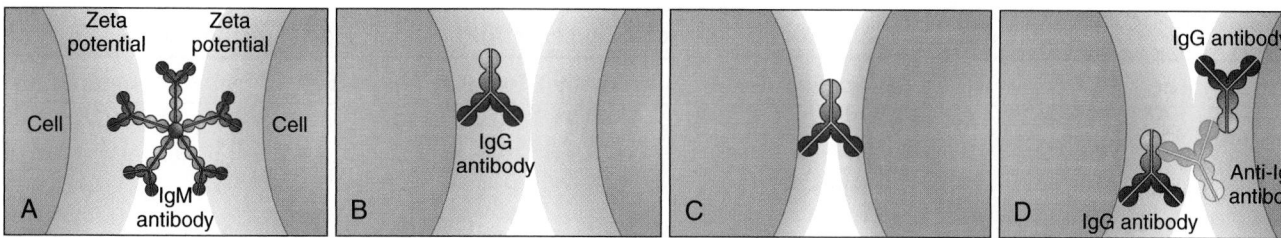

FIGURE 14-6. Interactions between immunoglobulin molecules and the erythrocyte during agglutination tests and the direct antiglobulin test (DAT). **A,** An IgM autoantibody can simultaneously bind two erythrocytes because of its multiple antigen-binding sites. The large size of the IgM molecule allows it to bridge the zeta potential between erythrocytes and cause agglutination. **B,** An IgG autoantibody is too small to bridge the zeta potential. **C,** Hence there is no agglutination of erythrocytes unless the zeta potential is reduced. **D,** On addition of the Coombs reagent, a rabbit antiglobulin that recognizes human IgG, the zeta potential is successfully bridged and red cells agglutinate.

contrast, IgG autoantibodies are smaller and unable to bridge the surface repulsion between adjacent erythrocytes known as the zeta potential (Fig. 14-6B) unless the distance imposed by the zeta potential is reduced (Fig. 14-6C). The broad-spectrum Coombs reagent binds to erythrocyte autoantibodies, bridges the zeta potential, and causes agglutination (Fig. 14-6D).

A positive DAT result with the polyspecific Coombs reagent leads to testing with more specific antisera to discriminate between IgG and complement on the RBC surface. The presence of IgG on the erythrocyte is sufficient evidence for an IgG autoantibody; simultaneous detection of complement indicates that the antibody can fix complement as well. In contrast, the presence of complement alone (with no IgG detected) suggests a cold-reactive autoantibody that fixes complement at lower temperatures but binds poorly to the erythrocyte at 37° C; in this setting, the serum should be analyzed for either the presence of an IgM autoantibody or the unique IgG Donath-Landsteiner autoantibody (described in a later section).

The DAT report for a patient with AIHA should describe the agglutination results of the polyspecific Coombs reagent and, if positive, the results of subsequent testing with the specific IgG and C3 reagents. DAT can be performed at temperatures lower than 37° C, such as 4° C, 10° C, or room temperature (23° C), to assist in the detection of cold-reactive autoantibodies and characterization of their thermal reactivity and amplitude. DAT results are scored on the basis of the amount of agglutination, usually on a scale of 1 to 4.

On occasion, results of the DAT are negative despite good clinical evidence of autoimmune hemolysis.[108] One explanation for this apparent paradox is that the amount of IgG present on the erythrocyte may be below the threshold for detection by standard Coombs reagent testing. In this setting a more sensitive assay for surface-bound IgG, such as enzyme-linked immunosorbent assay,[109] gel card analysis,[110] or flow cytometry,[111] may be helpful in identifying IgG on the cell surface. Alternatively, the lack of surface IgG may indicate the presence of a surface antibody other than an IgG molecule, such as an IgA autoantibody[68,112-114] or even a warm-reactive IgM autoantibody.[115-117]

Also of interest is the observation that DAT results may be positive in an otherwise normal person.[108] This is apparently a biologically false-positive result because no evidence of AIHA develops in these individuals, even with extended follow-up.[118,119] Analysis of the immune system of such persons revealed normal T-cell subsets, although the number of B cells was significantly increased.[120]

Differential Diagnosis

The typical patient with AIHA has clear evidence of hemolytic anemia, including jaundice and splenomegaly on physical examination and spherocytes with reticulocytosis on the peripheral blood smear. In this setting the differential diagnosis includes certain forms of nonimmune hemolytic anemia, including intrinsic RBC membrane or enzyme defects, as well as other rare extrinsic causes of hemolysis. Hereditary spherocytosis, described more fully in Chapter 15, can be confused with AIHA. A positive result in the osmotic fragility test, often erroneously considered to be pathognomonic for the diagnosis of hereditary spherocytosis, is also observed in patients with AIHA or congestive splenomegaly. Patients with other rare disorders such as clostridial sepsis[121] or early stages of Wilson's disease[122] can likewise have numerous spherocytes and hemolytic anemia. Patients with microangiopathic hemolytic anemia, such as HUS or TTP, typically have more schistocytes than spherocytes and usually have severe thrombocytopenia as well. In all clinical settings, the diagnosis of AIHA is most easily and accurately made on the basis of positive DAT results.

If the patient has anemia and reticulocytopenia, the differential diagnosis should include other acquired forms of hypoplastic anemia, such as transient erythroblastopenia of childhood or acquired aplastic anemia. In addition, patients with nonimmune hemolytic anemia in whom transient hypoplastic anemia develops as a result of parvovirus B19 infection may display this clinical picture.[123] In these patients the underlying hemolytic anemia may not be clinically recognizable until the parvovirus infection worsens the anemia and leads to clinical symptoms.

TABLE 14-1	Common Characteristics of Erythrocyte Autoantibodies in Autoimmune Hemolytic Anemia		
Characteristic	Warm-Reactive	Paroxysmal Cold Hemoglobinuria	Cold Agglutinin
Immunoglobulin isotype	IgG	IgG	IgM
Thermal reactivity	37° C	4° C	4° C
Fixes complement	Variable	Yes	Yes
Direct antiglobulin test			
4° C	Not performed	IgG, C3	C3
37° C	IgG ± C3	C3	C3
Plasma titer	Low/absent	Moderate	High
Hemolysin	No	Yes	Variable
Antigenic specificity	Rh and others	P	I/i
Site of red blood cell destruction	Spleen	Intravascular	Liver, intravascular

Characteristics of Erythrocyte Autoantibodies

The sine qua non of both primary and secondary AIHA is the presence of antibodies that bind to erythrocytes. As a direct consequence of the binding of these erythrocyte autoantibodies, circulating erythrocytes have a shortened life span with hemolysis and accelerated clearance by the reticuloendothelial system. The clinical complexity and variability of AIHA depend in large part on the immunologic characteristics of the autoantibody, including its isotype, thermal reactivity, ability to fix complement, binding affinity, and antigenic specificity. Elucidation of each of these characteristics is important in understanding the pathophysiology and clinical course of AIHA in a given patient.[86,124-129] Table 14-1 summarizes the important characteristics of erythrocyte autoantibodies in AIHA, with an emphasis on differences among the three major clinical conditions: warm-reactive AIHA, PCH, and cold agglutinin disease.

Antibody Isotype

One of the most important tasks for the immunohematology laboratory in the evaluation of a new patient with AIHA is to determine the isotype of the erythrocyte autoantibody. In most cases the pathogenic antibody is identified as an IgG molecule.[74,89,130,131] In general, IgG autoantibodies bind to RBC antigens optimally at 37° C, hence the descriptive term warm-reactive autoantibodies. All IgG molecules are heterodimers, with two heavy chains linked noncovalently to two light chains. The heavy and light chains together form two variable antigen-binding sites known as the Fab portions, and the heavy chains also contain a constant structural domain (the Fc portion) that includes the binding site for complement and the binding site for the Fc receptor.

There are four subtypes of IgG antibodies designated IgG1, IgG2, IgG3, and IgG4. These different subtypes have important implications for the fixation of complement, hemolysis, and clearance by the reticuloendothelial

TABLE 14-2	Frequency of IgG Subclasses Identified in Warm-Reactive (IgG Autoantibody) Autoimmune Hemolytic Anemia	
IgG Subclass	% Total Cases
IgG1	74.0
IgG2	0.7
IgG3	2.1
IgG4	0.9
Multiple, including IgG1	20.1
Multiple, not including IgG1	0.3
None detectable	1.9

Adapted from Engelfriet CP, Overbeeke MA, von dem Borne AE: Autoimmune hemolytic anemia. Semin Hematol 1992; 29:3-12.

system. IgG1 and IgG3 antibodies fix complement better than IgG2 and IgG4 antibodies do.[132,133] A patient who had only IgG4 autoantibody on his erythrocytes was reported to have little hemolysis, presumably because of weak interactions with the Fc receptor on macrophages.[134] Adapted from a review of several thousand patients with AIHA by Engelfriet and colleagues,[131] Table 14-2 lists the relative occurrence of each IgG subclass identified in patients with AIHA and warm IgG autoantibody. IgG1 autoantibodies were by far the predominant subclass identified, followed by multiple subclasses that typically included IgG1.

Less commonly, IgG antibodies are cold reactive; these autoantibodies are characteristic of childhood PCH but have also been reported rarely in cold hemagglutinin disease.[135] In the unusual setting of a pregnant woman with AIHA, certain IgG autoantibodies can cross the placenta and cause acquired neonatal AIHA.[136-138]

In other patients with AIHA, IgM autoantibodies are identified, particularly after infection with an organism such as *Mycoplasma pneumoniae*.[139] In one series, IgM autoantibodies characterized a significant proportion of instances of AIHA in early childhood.[140] The IgM molecule is a pentameric structure that contains five covalently linked domains, each of which is structurally similar to a single IgG molecule. Because of their large size, IgM autoantibodies can span the zeta potential between adjacent erythrocytes. Erythrocytes that are connected by a bridging IgM molecule become too dense to remain in suspension and thus agglutinate.

IgG and IgM autoantibodies characterize the vast majority of instances of AIHA, but rarely an IgA autoantibody is identified.[68,113,114,141] IgA antibodies do not react with the standard Coombs reagent, and therefore special research reagents must be used for their identification.[108] Testing for IgA autoantibodies should be considered and specifically requested whenever the DAT fails to detect surface-bound IgG or C3 in a patient who otherwise appears to have AIHA. Finally, a combination of different isotypes, especially simultaneous IgG and IgM autoantibodies, has been reported on several occasions.[142-145]

Thermal Reactivity

The thermal reactivity (sometimes called the thermal amplitude) of an erythrocyte autoantibody is another important parameter to determine. Although the core temperature of humans is 37° C, temperatures in superficial vessels (particularly in the face and digits) may fall below 30° C. Binding of antibody to erythrocytes can be considered a process of dynamic equilibrium, depending on the location of a given erythrocyte within the circulation. The thermal reactivity of most IgG autoantibodies is 37° C, so binding to erythrocytes occurs best at normal body temperature. These antibodies are therefore referred to as warm-reactive autoantibodies. Occasionally, warm-reactive IgM autoantibodies are identified, although they are rare.[115-117,140]

Cold-reactive (Donath-Landsteiner) IgG autoantibodies bind optimally at 4° C and are clinically important as the cause of PCH. Because of their unusual characteristics, results of the DAT are often negative or demonstrate only the presence of complement because cold-reacting antibodies are removed during the washing of erythrocytes. A special procedure must therefore be followed to detect the Donath-Landsteiner antibody characteristic of PCH. Specific testing for this antibody should be performed early in the clinical course, ideally before therapy is initiated.

The Donath-Landsteiner autoantibody is a biphasic hemolysin, which means that it binds to erythrocytes and fixes complement at 4° C, but on warming to 37° C, the complement cascade is amplified and leads to hemolysis. Two samples of blood should be drawn simultaneously from the patient and kept at 37° C to prevent in vitro autoantibody binding and hemolysis. The serum samples are separated from the erythrocytes by centrifugation (preferably at a warm temperature) and then incubated with normal erythrocytes and a source of complement, either in a melting ice bath or at 37° C. Both reactions are then warmed to 37° C and analyzed for the presence

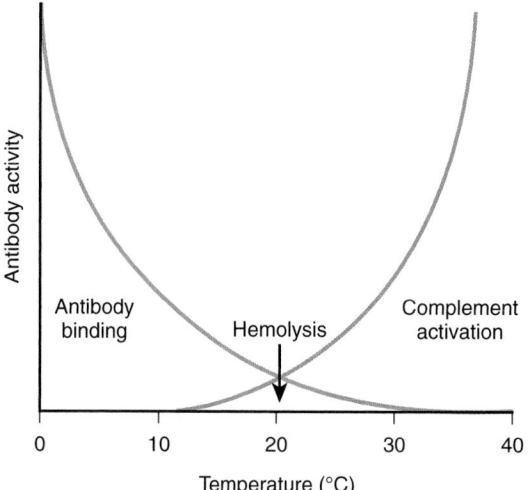

FIGURE 14-7. Thermal reactivity curve of a cold-reactive IgM autoantibody. The antibody is optimally reactive at 0° C to 4° C, whereas complement is fixed most efficiently at 37° C. The overlap area is the so-called zone of hemolysis and determines the amount of hemolysis observed. *(Adapted from Issitt PD, Anstee DJ. Applied Blood Group Serology, 3rd ed. Miami, Montgomery Scientific Publications, 1985, p 545.)*

of hemolysis. In the first sample, cold incubation allows the IgG autoantibody to bind and fix complement, after which the subsequent warming step allows complement amplification to occur with resultant RBC lysis. In contrast, the sample maintained at 37° C shows no lysis because no significant IgG autoantibody binding occurred at the warmer temperature to allow complement fixation.

In contrast to many IgG autoantibodies, IgM autoantibodies typically bind optimally to erythrocytes at 0° C to 4° C and hence are called cold-reactive antibodies. The thermal range over which the autoantibody is active is crucial and determines the amount of hemolysis observed (Fig. 14-7). An IgM autoantibody binds optimally in the cold, but complement activation proceeds optimally at warmer temperatures. The overlap between the range of antibody activity and complement activation is the so-called zone of hemolysis.[146]

Complement Fixation

The ability of an erythrocyte autoantibody to fix complement plays a critical role in the pathophysiology of immune clearance and the clinical manifestations of hemolysis because complement augments the destructive effects of the autoantibody. The process of complement deposition, amplification, and pore formation involves a complex series of intravascular enzymatic events.

In the classical complement activation pathway, the Fc portion of the bound immunoglobulin molecule interacts with C1q, the first component of the complement cascade. Two IgG molecules in close proximity are required to bind C1q to the erythrocyte (Fig. 14-8A), whereas a single IgM molecule is sufficient to bind C1q (Fig. 14-8B). Components C1r and C1s then bind to

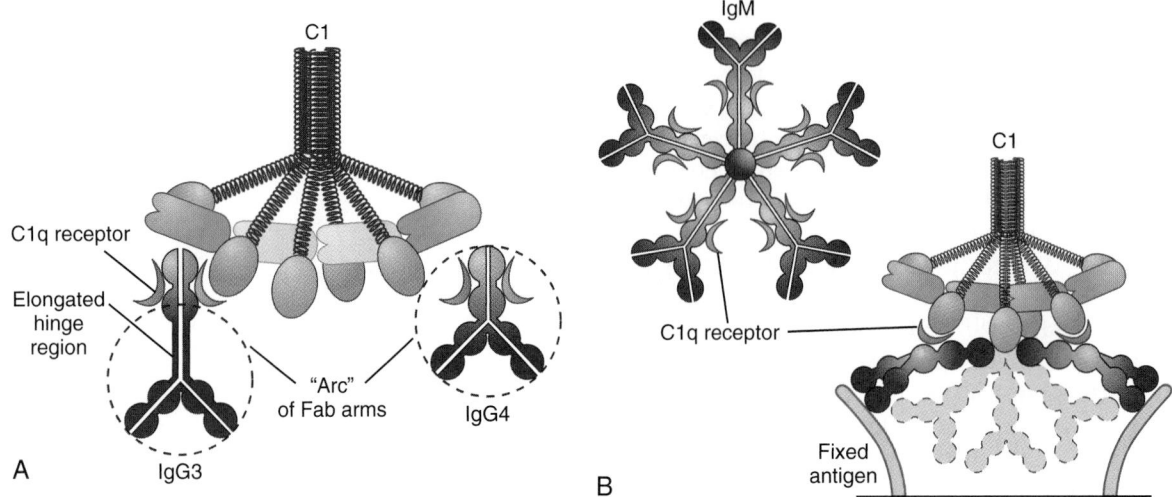

FIGURE 14-8. Binding of C1, the first component of complement, to antibodies. **A,** Binding of C1 to IgG molecules occurs through the Fc portion of the immunoglobulin molecule. Binding is inhibited by interference from the Fab arms, which is minimized when the hinge region is elongated, as in an IgG3 molecule; hence IgG3 fixes complement more efficiently than IgG4 does. **B,** Complement binding sites of IgM molecules are not available when the antibody is in its fluid-phase planar form. When two of the monomers are affixed, however, the IgM molecule assumes an arched form and C1 binding sites become available for reaction.

C1q to form a multiunit protein complex on the red cell surface. This active complex binds and enzymatically cleaves C4, followed by additional enzymatic events that lead to the deposition of component C3b on the surface of the erythrocyte. At this point the erythrocyte may be cleared by the spleen, liver, or other parts of the reticuloendothelial system that recognize C3b via specific surface receptors. Alternatively, amplification of the complement cascade may continue and lead to formation of the C5b-7 membrane attack complex, followed by fixation of C8 and C9 and finally by polymerization of C9 to form pores within the cell membrane (Fig. 14-9). These pores breach the erythrocyte membrane integrity and cause hemolysis of the cell.

IgM autoantibodies fix complement very efficiently because distinct binding sites within the IgM pentamer are close enough to bind C1q (see Fig. 14-8B). In fact, the "hemolysins" that were identified at the turn of the century were actually IgM autoantibodies that fixed complement efficiently and completely, thereby resulting in membrane pore formation and erythrocyte lysis. Rarely, IgM antibodies that do not fix complement have been reported.[140,147] In contrast, IgG autoantibodies do not fix complement as efficiently as their IgM counterparts, in part because of the necessity of two distinct IgG molecules being in close proximity to allow the initial binding of C1q.[51] If the target autoantigens on the erythrocyte membrane are not mobile or are spaced too far apart, complement cannot be fixed. Moreover, all IgG molecules do not have equivalent complement-fixing ability; the IgG1 and IgG3 subclasses are able to fix complement far better than the IgG2 and IgG4 subtypes can.[132,133] Donath-Landsteiner antibodies, even though they are IgG autoantibodies, fix complement very efficiently and thus lead to brisk intravascular lysis.

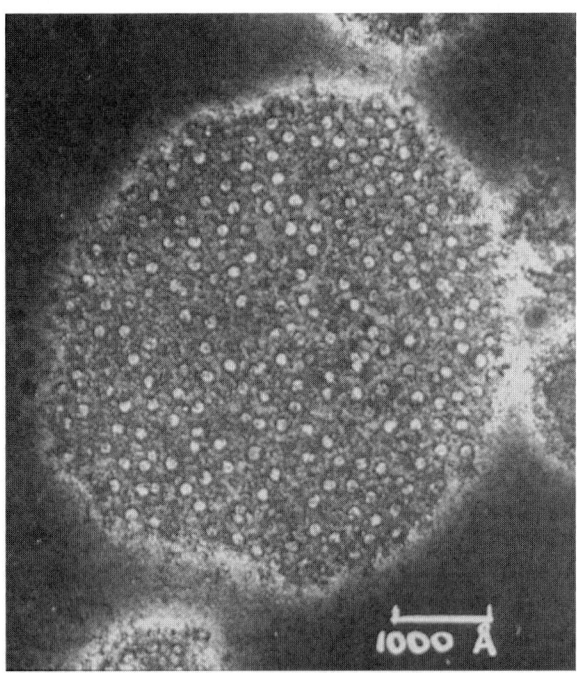

FIGURE 14-9. Electron micrograph of lesions that appear in the cell membrane after completion of the membrane attack complex. The dark lesions are hydrophilic complexes of protein about 10 nm in diameter.

Antibody Binding Affinity

The binding affinity of an erythrocyte autoantibody for its antigen has implications both for the likelihood of in vitro detection and for the pathophysiologic process of erythrocyte clearance.[125,129] An IgG autoantibody typically has high affinity for its antigen on the erythrocyte surface and can therefore be identified readily by the DAT. For this same reason, the indirect antiglobulin test may fail to detect an IgG autoantibody because there is very little unbound antibody circulating in plasma. In contrast, most IgM autoantibodies have little binding affinity at 37° C and are therefore more easily detected as high-titer unbound antibody within plasma.

Antigenic Specificity

When serologic specificity in most patients with warm-reactive AIHA is tested, reactivity with all cells tested is commonly identified. This "panreactive," "nonspecific," or "no specificity defined" pattern of reactivity suggests that the autoantibody is binding to a surface antigenic structure that is common to all human erythrocytes. Interestingly, the autoantibody may not react with cells that lack the entire Rh protein complex; experiments with these rare Rh$_{null}$ erythrocytes provide evidence that the Rh protein cluster is the main antigenic determinant for many warm-reactive autoantibodies.[53,146] Other studies have confirmed that autoantibodies bind to Rh in about 50% of patients with warm-reactive AIHA,[127,128,148] although other candidate autoantigens have been identified.[149]

Occasionally, autoantibody reactivity against a particular Rh antigen such as c or e is identified,[85,150] but this is not common. Warm autoantibodies with defined specificity against unusual protein antigens, including protein 4.1,[151] band 3,[152] Wrb,[67] Kpb,[153] N,[154] and many others, have been described. Reactivity with the ABO blood group antigens[155,156] or with other major systems such as Lewis or Kell is extremely rare in warm-reactive AIHA.[131,146,157] In contrast, IgM autoantibodies often have reactivity against polysaccharides on the red cell rather than surface proteins. The I/i surface structure is a prototypical polysaccharide autoantigen on the red cell surface and is the target of many IgM antibodies that develop in response to infection.[139] In addition to the important I/i surface antigens, other autoantigens have also been reported in cold-reactive AIHA,[85,86,158-160] including the polysaccharide P autoantigen in PCH.[161]

Elucidation of the antigenic specificity of autoreactive erythrocyte antibodies provides information that is useful for several reasons. One is the likelihood of finding compatible blood for transfusion. If an autoantibody is a panreactive antibody that binds to all cells with no apparent specificity, fully compatible blood will probably not be found. Identification of antigenic specificity may also help predict intravascular lysis resulting from activation of complement. If the antigen is within the Rh complex, the antigenic density on erythrocytes makes complement activation remote and complement-mediated intravascular hemolysis less likely. The P antigen system, in contrast, is densely populated on the erythrocyte surface and capable of binding sufficient Donath-Landsteiner IgG antibodies to fix complement efficiently and lead to substantial intravascular lysis.[54]

Immune Clearance of Sensitized Erythrocytes

Much of our understanding about the pathophysiology of immune-mediated erythrocyte clearance derives from experiments performed more than 30 years ago. An elegant series of in vitro and in vivo studies by Jandl and associates[50,56,57,59] and by Rosse[54,55,61] clarified the roles of antibody, complement, and the reticuloendothelial system in the pathophysiology of autoimmune erythrocyte clearance. In the early 1970s, Frank and colleagues developed a guinea pig model for AIHA that permitted dissection of the steps involved in the clearance of erythrocytes coated with antibody or complement. Using ^{51}Cr-labeled RBCs that were sensitized in vitro with rabbit IgG or IgM anti–guinea pig erythrocyte antibodies, these investigators analyzed the rates and patterns of clearance, as well as the sites of sequestration. IgG-coated erythrocytes were removed predominantly by the spleen, regardless of concurrent complement activation, and the amount of surface IgG correlated with the rate of splenic clearance. The liver was the predominant clearance site when very large amounts of IgG were present. Fc receptors on macrophages were responsible for the binding and phagocytosis of IgG-coated erythrocytes.[62,63] In contrast to these findings for IgG-mediated hemolysis, IgM-coated erythrocytes were cleared rapidly within the liver, and the amount of bound IgM correlated with the rate of erythrocyte clearance. However, there was an absolute dependence on complement for the clearance of IgM-coated cells, and macrophage receptors for the C3b molecule were responsible for binding and phagocytosis of erythrocytes.[62,64] Several investigators have attempted to mimic erythrocyte-monocyte interactions and correlate in vitro results with in vivo hemolysis,[162-165] but with limited success.

These and other laboratory experiments, coupled with careful clinical observations, have led to the development of a general understanding about immune-mediated clearance of erythrocytes in AIHA (Fig. 14-10). In warm-reactive AIHA, the IgG autoantibodies coat autologous erythrocytes and may fix complement. The sensitized cells pass through the spleen and other parts of the reticuloendothelial system, where they interact with complement and Fc receptors on macrophages. The human macrophage has three distinct classes of receptor for the Fc portion of the IgG molecule, designated FcγRI, FcγRII, and FcγRIII. Although each form of Fc receptor binds IgG with similar specificity, binding affinity varies for individual subclasses of IgG autoantibodies.[166] The sensitized erythrocytes may be fully ingested by macrophages; however, if only a portion of the surface membrane is removed, the erythrocyte re-forms into a spherocyte that is identifiable on the peripheral blood smear. For IgG-coated erythrocytes, the majority of immune clearance occurs within the cords of the spleen[167]; hence the hemolysis is extravascular. If the IgG antibody fixes complement, the erythrocyte can also be cleared by

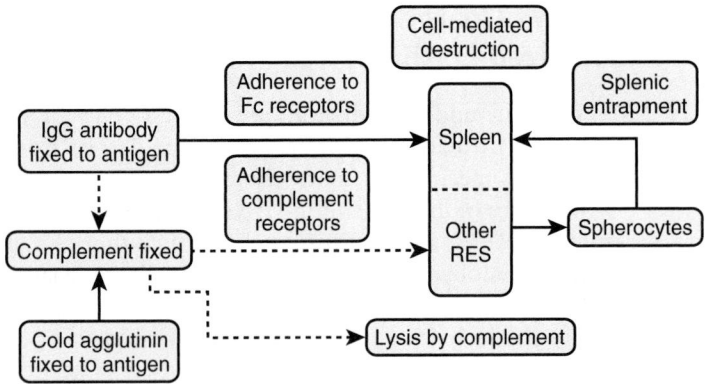

FIGURE 14-10. Immune-mediated clearance of erythrocytes in autoimmune hemolytic anemia. In warm-reactive disease, IgG autoantibodies are bound to erythrocytes but typically do not fix complement efficiently. The coated cells enter the spleen and other parts of the reticuloendothelial system (RES), where they interact with Fc receptors on macrophages. Erythrocytes may be completely engulfed and destroyed by this interaction or may have only a portion of their membrane removed. In this case the red cells will reshape into spherocytes, which are then doomed on their next passage through the spleen. In cold-reactive disease, complement is typically fixed very efficiently, and intravascular lysis by the complement cascade can occur. Alternatively, the presence of surface-bound complement (C3) can lead to extravascular red cell destruction by the spleen and RES.

macrophages bearing receptors for complement receptors.[59,63,168]

In cold agglutinin disease or PCH, the autoreactive antibody binds preferentially at 4° C and fixes complement efficiently. At normal body temperature there is virtually no antibody identifiable on the cell surface, but complement components, particularly C3b, can be identified with the Coombs reagent. If complement is activated to completion on the cell surface in vivo, the erythrocytes will hemolyze intravascularly and cause hemoglobinemia, followed by hemoglobinuria. When C3b is present on the red cell surface without further activation of complement, however, macrophages within the reticuloendothelial system can bind the erythrocytes via specific complement receptors and engulf them in a manner similar to that in warm-reactive AIHA.[169,170] Complement-coated erythrocytes are cleared extravascularly by macrophages located primarily within the liver rather than the spleen.

Therapy

The need to treat a patient with AIHA depends on the severity and rapidity with which the anemia develops. A child with relatively mild anemia (hemoglobin concentration of 9 to 12 g/dL), especially one who has recently had a viral-like illness, may benefit from observation alone. If the patient has a more severe degree of anemia (hemoglobin concentration of 6 to 9 g/dL) or if the hemoglobin concentration is observed to fall precipitously, therapy should be instituted. Optimal therapy depends on the clinical picture, as well as the form of AIHA. If the autoantibodies are cold reactive, for example, the patient should be kept warm with avoidance of all cold stimuli. Strict adherence to this recommendation is difficult, but it is often the best therapy for a patient with cold-reactive autoantibodies. If severe intravascular hemolysis is present, it is imperative that good renal blood flow and urine output be maintained.[90]

Therapy for acute warm-reactive AIHA in children should begin with close observation, judicious use of erythrocyte transfusions, and administration of corticosteroids. Additional therapy includes the administration of intravenous immunoglobulin (IVIG), plasma

(exchange) transfusion in selected settings, and more recently, targeted therapy with rituximab. Other therapeutic modalities such as cyclosporine, vinblastine, danazol, azathioprine, cyclophosphamide, and other agents have not been widely used in the pediatric age group and therefore have a limited therapeutic role for childhood AIHA. Table 14-3 lists these various treatment modalities; clinical responses and mechanisms of action are described in later sections.

When the anemia is severe enough to cause cardiovascular compromise, usually at a hemoglobin level lower than 5 g/dL, the use of erythrocyte transfusions to provide additional oxygen-carrying capacity should be strongly considered. Although the transfusion process is complicated and can be somewhat intimidating, erythrocyte transfusion may be lifesaving for a patient with AIHA, who may die as a result of complications related to anemia.[171] If clinically warranted, erythrocyte transfusions should never be withheld because of fear of a hemolytic transfusion reaction. The fate of transfused cells will probably not be worse than that of the patient's own erythrocytes, and they may provide temporary support until additional therapy slows the rate of hemolysis. In short, no child with AIHA should die of anemia.

The first problem related to the transfusion of a patient with AIHA is identification of compatible erythrocytes. It is important to provide a relatively large amount of serum and cells for testing well in advance of an anticipated erythrocyte transfusion. Particularly if the antigenic specificity is panreactive, the crossmatch will probably identify no units of blood that are fully compatible. In this instance, certain units that are "least incompatible" with the patient's serum will be identified. For patients who have previously received transfusions, it is critical to identify alloantibodies that may be masked by the stronger autoantibody.[172-174] Adsorption techniques are designed to remove autoantibodies and allow the identification of clinically important alloantibodies.[175,176]

The second difficulty associated with transfusion of a patient with AIHA is the actual transfusion itself. Fortunately, acute symptomatic transfusion reactions are not seen frequently, even with transfusion of units of blood that may have strong in vitro reactivity with the patient's serum.[172,177] The transfused cells have an in vivo survival

TABLE 14-3   Treatment Modalities for Autoimmune Hemolytic Anemia

Treatment*	Dose	Comments
Red blood cell transfusions	Sufficient to reach 6-8 g/dL	Incompatibility may cause hemolysis Alloantibodies may be present
Corticosteroids	1-2 mg/kg IV q6h acutely 5-30 mg PO qod chronically	Effective for IgG more than IgM High doses for short-term use only
Intravenous immunoglobulin	1 g/kg/day for 1-5 days	Expensive, inconvenient to administer Effective in only a third of patients

Exchange transfusion or
  plasmapheresis
		Daily until stable; effective for IgM more than IgG
		    Requires large-caliber intravenous access

Splenectomy		Curative in 60-80% of patients Risk of postsplenectomy sepsis
Rituximab	375 mg/m² IV weekly × 4	B cell ablative, immunosuppressive
Danazol	50-800 mg/day PO	Hepatic dysfunction Androgenic side effects
Vincristine	1 mg/m² IV every week	Neurotoxicity
Cyclophosphamide	50-100 mg/day PO	Carcinogenic
Azathioprine	25-200 mg/day PO	Immunosuppressive
Cyclosporine	2-10 mg/kg/day PO	Nephrotoxicity, hypertension Immunosuppression

*See text for further description and discussion of each therapeutic agent.

that is approximately equivalent to that of endogenous erythrocytes, so they often have a beneficial effect even if they circulate only for a short time. On occasion, however, the transfusion results in severe hemolysis with hemoglobinemia, hemoglobinuria, and renal failure. For this reason, it is prudent to begin the transfusion at a slow rate and check both plasma and urine samples periodically for free hemoglobin. For patients with cold-reactive antibodies, it is useful to warm the patient and the entire room; a blood warmer should be used to raise the temperature of the transfused blood.

A recent report described the successful use of polymerized bovine hemoglobin to provide lifesaving oxygen-carrying capacity in a woman dying of AIHA.[178] Though intriguing as an alternative to erythrocyte transfusion, the use of erythrocyte substitutes such as perfluorochemicals or cell-free hemoglobin-based oxygen carriers must be considered highly experimental at this time.[179] Additional research in this area may identify safe alternatives to transfusions that may eventually benefit children with AIHA.

The use of corticosteroids is widely accepted therapy for AIHA, particularly for patients with IgG antibodies. From the initial report more than 50 years ago,[180] glucocorticoids have been used to interfere with the basic pathophysiologic process and immune destruction observed in AIHA. The guinea pig model of AIHA demonstrated that steroids increase the survival of both IgG- and IgM-sensitized erythrocytes by decreasing sequestration within the spleen and liver, respectively.[63,64] Corticosteroids are believed to inhibit Fc receptor–mediated clearance of sensitized erythrocytes,[66,181] which probably accounts for their effect within 24 to 48 hours

of administration. Corticosteroids may also inhibit autoantibody synthesis, although this effect requires several weeks to occur.

In a patient with warm-reactive AIHA or PCH, a typical dosing regimen of corticosteroids is 1 to 2 mg/kg of methylprednisolone given intravenously every 6 to 8 hours for the first 24 to 72 hours, usually while the patient is the sickest. Oral prednisone at 2 mg/kg/day may then be used when the patient's clinical condition is more stable. Typically, these high doses are required for only 2 to 4 weeks, followed by slow tapering of the dose, which may take 3 months or longer. Tapering of the corticosteroid dose should be aimed toward the use of a single morning dose, preferably every other day, but must be based on the patient's hemoglobin concentration, reticulocyte count, and DAT result. In general, tapering should be slower when active disease is evident. An overall response rate of approximately 80% has been reported.[182] On occasion, corticosteroid therapy may be beneficial in cold agglutinin disease.[183]

IVIG became a popular therapy for ITP in the 1980s.[184] Able to induce a potent blockade of the reticuloendothelial system,[185] IVIG was therefore an attractive option for the treatment of AIHA as well. Unfortunately, AIHA in many patients in early trials appeared to be refractory to IVIG therapy.[186,187] Bussel and colleagues[71] then reported that very high doses of IVIG (5 g/kg given over a 5-day period) were necessary to produce a therapeutic benefit, perhaps because the reticuloendothelial system was enlarged in AIHA patients. Even at this high dose, however, only approximately a third of patients with warm-reactive AIHA had a response to IVIG therapy.[71,188] Prognostic factors that predicted response to IVIG included a lower pretreatment hemoglobin concentration and the presence of hepatomegaly.[189] Based on these results, as well as on a variety of safety and cost issues,[190] IVIG should not be considered standard treatment for AIHA in children. However, continued investigation of its potential role in modulation of the immune response may shed light on important mechanisms of autoantibody production and immune-mediated erythrocyte clearance.[191]

Exchange transfusion is a reasonable therapeutic option for AIHA in the acute setting because circulating erythrocyte autoantibodies, soluble activated complement components, and sensitized erythrocytes can all be removed from the patient simultaneously.[192] Alternatively, however, plasmapheresis or plasma exchange has been used to remove pathogenic autoantibodies and paraproteins,[193-196] even in very small children.[197] It is generally accepted that patients with IgM autoantibodies respond better to plasmapheresis than those with IgG autoantibodies do,[198] presumably because of differences in the size and binding characteristics of the two molecules, although plasmapheresis can be effective in IgG-mediated hemolysis as well.[199] The larger size of IgM molecules keeps them within the intravascular space and amenable to removal by plasmapheresis. In contrast, IgG autoantibodies diffuse into the extravascular space; thus, plasmapheresis removes only a fraction of the total IgG autoantibodies. In addition, IgM autoantibodies are less tightly affixed than IgG autoantibodies to erythrocytes at warm temperatures and are more likely to be removed by plasmapheresis. For this reason the extracorporeal circuit should be warmed during exchange transfusion of a patient with cold-reactive autoantibodies.[200] Recently, however, the benefits of plasma exchange to improve survival of transfused blood cells has been questioned.[201]

For a child with chronic or refractory AIHA, more aggressive therapy is often required to alleviate the symptoms of anemia and help the child achieve a more normal lifestyle. Long-term use of corticosteroids or immunoglobulin is generally unacceptable because of side effects, cost, and inconvenience. A variety of additional therapeutic agents are available, however, as well as surgical intervention. No simple treatment algorithm can be proposed that is correct for all children with AIHA. The clinician should individualize therapy for each patient based on the hematologic response and side effects.

Targeted therapy against the source of autoantibody production (antibody-secreting B lymphocytes) has recently become a reality. Rituximab (Rituxan) is a humanized murine monoclonal antibody directed against the human CD20 antigen, which is present only on B lymphocytes. Rituximab induces B-cell apoptosis[202] and is highly effective therapy against B-cell lymphoma.[203] Recently reviewed as a therapeutic option for children with a variety of autoimmune hematologic disorders,[204] rituximab offers a relatively safe and effective treatment of chronic or refractory AIHA. The earliest reports

involved adult patients with AIHA, but excellent response rates have now been reported in case reports and small series of children with AIHA.[205-207] Rituximab quickly eliminates circulating B cells, and their recovery make take several months, yet serum immunoglobulin levels rarely decline and replacement IVIG is not clinically indicated. Reactivated viral infections have been reported rarely in immunosuppressed patients.[204] Rituximab offers an opportunity to eliminate autoreactive B lymphocytes and "reboot" part of the humoral immune system, and in practice it can obviate the need for nonspecific chemotherapy and surgical splenectomy. Prospective trials with rituximab are warranted to determine its efficacy versus more conventional therapy for childhood AIHA.

Splenectomy is the time-honored therapy for a patient with chronic AIHA.[182,208] The rationale for splenectomy is based in part on the animal model of AIHA, which demonstrated that IgG-sensitized erythrocytes were cleared almost exclusively within the spleen, regardless of whether complement was activated.[65] In keeping with this model, patients with IgG autoantibodies respond better to splenectomy than do patients with IgM autoantibodies.[209] However, preoperative prediction of the clinical response to splenectomy, based on splenic uptake of radiolabeled red cells,[210] is variable at best.[72,91] In 12 patients with AIHA, Parker and colleagues[211] found poor correlation between ^{51}Cr-labeled red cell survival and eventual response to splenectomy. Only three of five patients with a highly elevated spleen-to-liver uptake ratio had a clinical remission after splenectomy, whereas three of five with a very low ratio also underwent remission after splenectomy. The authors concluded that radiolabeled red cell survival studies were not reliable indicators of the clinical response to splenectomy in AIHA.[211] Splenectomy may also benefit patients with AIHA by removing a major site of autoantibody production, similar to the pathophysiologic effect of antiplatelet autoantibody production in ITP.[78]

Coon[212] reported 52 patients with AIHA who underwent splenectomy. There was no surgical mortality and low morbidity, and an excellent response was seen in 64% and improved status in another 21% of patients. However, splenectomy should be avoided in young children if possible because of the risk of postsplenectomy sepsis secondary to encapsulated bacterial organisms. Before splenectomy, children should be immunized with polyvalent polysaccharide vaccines against *S. pneumoniae* and *N. meningitidis* to enhance the humoral immune response against these potentially lethal pathogens. The addition of protein-conjugated vaccines against *S. pneumoniae* and *H. influenzae* type b into the routine infant immunization series has helped provide additional effective immunity against these organisms. Children who undergo splenectomy should receive penicillin twice daily for at least 2 years after surgery; some clinicians prefer lifelong penicillin prophylaxis because fatal sepsis occurring years after splenectomy has been described.[213,214]

Erythromycin should be used if the patient is allergic to penicillin. After splenectomy, prompt medical attention should be sought for children with fever (temperature >38.5° C [101.5° F]) because of the possibility of bacterial sepsis.

Additional therapeutic agents have been used less often in children with AIHA. High-dose pulse dexamethasone, which caused initial but fleeting excitement for patients with chronic ITP, had a beneficial effect for some adults with warm-reactive AIHA.[215] Danazol, a semisynthetic androgen, also has efficacy in some patients with AIHA,[70,216,217] although no young children were included in these reports. One report suggested that danazol was more effective when used as first-line therapy in conjunction with corticosteroids,[217] whereas another demonstrated excellent responses even in patients with refractory AIHA who had previously received therapy, including splenectomy.[70] The mechanisms of action of danazol are not known, but decreased titers of cell-bound IgG and complement have been noted in most patients who had a response.[70] Danazol has been shown to decrease IgG production,[218] thus suggesting that this therapy may have multiple mechanisms of action that could be beneficial for a patient with AIHA. The primary side effects of danazol, however, are elevations in hepatic transaminases and mild masculinizing effects, which essentially preclude its routine use in young or female patients.

Cytotoxic agents have been used in the treatment of AIHA, with the presumed intent of reducing autoantibody formation. Vincristine and vinblastine have limited use in the pediatric age group but should be considered for a patient with refractory AIHA.[69,219,220] In vitro incubation of platelets with vinca alkaloids, followed by transfusion of these "loaded" platelets, has been used to poison the reticuloendothelial macrophages directly.[219] Other cytotoxic agents, including cyclophosphamide, 6-mercaptopurine, and 6-thioguanine, have been successful in adults, but no trials involving children with AIHA have been reported to date. A typical daily dose of cyclophosphamide for an adult with AIHA is 50 to 100 mg orally. Because these agents are generally myelosuppressive and potentially mutagenic,[221] they should be used with great caution in children. The use of high-dose cyclophosphamide, designed to provide immunoablation without complete myeloablation, has been reported anecdotally for severe refractory AIHA.[222-224] Of nine patients with chronic refractory AIHA who received high-dose cyclophosphamide, six achieved complete remission and three had a partial remission. An important side effect of this immunoablative therapy is profound myelosuppression, although it was short-lived and not associated with serious infection.[224] The long-term efficacy of this aggressive approach remains unproven at the current time, but the regimen deserves prospective testing in selected children with life-threatening disease.

Azathioprine is an immunosuppressive agent that affects both the humoral and cellular arms of the immune response, but its greatest effects are on T lymphocytes.[182] By affecting helper T-cell function, azathioprine can interfere with autoantibody synthesis. Azathioprine is unlikely to induce clinical remission as a single drug but could be used as a corticosteroid-sparing agent. A treatment dose of azathioprine ranges from 25 to 200 mg/day orally, and side effects include leukopenia, thrombocytopenia, and hepatic injury. Because the goal of azathioprine therapy is a reduction in autoantibody synthesis, responses may not be noted until after 3 months of therapy.[182]

Cyclosporine, another immunosuppressive agent that focuses primarily on T lymphocytes, has been reported to have been successful in a few patients with steroid-resistant AIHA.[225] Because of the significant side effects associated with long-term use of cyclosporine, however, including nephrotoxicity, hypertension, and even a risk of malignancy, it should not be used routinely in children with AIHA. Targeted therapy against T lymphocytes with Campath 1H monoclonal antibodies has shown promising but short-lived responses in refractory disease.[226]

Several additional miscellaneous agents have been reported anecdotally to have beneficial effects in the treatment of AIHA. The response of a patient with cold agglutinin disease to interferon alfa therapy merits additional investigation.[227] The effects of soluble growth factors on erythrocyte phagocytosis by macrophages in AIHA suggests a potential role for cytokine therapy.[228]

Finally, complete lymphoid ablation and myeloablation, followed by reconstitution with compatible healthy hematopoietic stem cells, could theoretically cure systemic autoimmune diseases. The use of stem cell transplantation for autoimmune disorders such as AIHA has been proposed, and suggested guidelines have been published.[229] For children with refractory AIHA, transplantation of autologous stem cells has been attempted, but with limited success.[230,231] Human leukocyte antigen (HLA)-matched allogeneic stem cells may provide an additional graft-versus-autoimmunity effect,[230] although the current morbidity and mortality associated with allogeneic bone marrow transplantation must be carefully weighed against the adverse effects of conventional therapy. Moreover, AIHA can actually develop after bone marrow transplantation for other indications,[232,233] presumably in the setting of a weakened immune system with lymphocyte dysregulation. At this time, stem cell transplantation should not be considered a reasonable therapeutic option for children with primary AIHA unless they have refractory and life-threatening disease.

Pathogenesis of Autoantibody Formation

The erythrocyte autoantibodies produced in AIHA are clearly pathogenic, and the amount of antibody bound to the cell surface is proportional to the rate of erythrocyte removal by the reticuloendothelial system. Less is known about the origin of autoantibody formation, however, and why certain individuals have in vivo expansion of autoreactive lymphocytes that should normally be suppressed or eliminated by the immune system. The pathogenesis of autoantibody formation in AIHA has recently been reviewed,[234,235] with several mechanisms proposed for the loss of self-tolerance, including cytokine imbalance, excessive lymphocyte activation, and molecular mimicry between self and foreign antigens, among others.

Older case reports suggest a genetic predisposition for the development of AIHA, with an association noted between AIHA and certain immune response genes, especially the HLA-B locus.[236] Patients with HLA-B8[237] or HLA-B27[238] may have an increased risk for AIHA,[237] whereas HLA-DQ6 may confer protection against AIHA.[239] Genetic loci in mice associated with the development of AIHA have been reported,[240] and a single nucleotide polymorphism in the human CTLA-4 gene locus may confer increased risk for AIHA.[241] Chromosomal abnormalities have been associated with the development of autoimmune cytopenia.[242,243]

Normal polyclonal antibodies develop after in vivo stimulation of B lymphocytes, especially after vaccination or infection. The erythrocyte autoantibodies that develop in most patients with AIHA also represent a polyclonal B-lymphocyte response; even classic warm-reactive AIHA will usually have multiple IgG isotypes and often detectable IgA autoantibodies.[244] For AIHA to develop, these polyclonal autoreactive B lymphocytes must avoid the normal immune tolerance mechanisms of apoptosis and suppression and then proliferate without proper immune surveillance.[245]

Sequence analysis of the immunoglobulin gene rearrangements used by AIHA autoantibodies has revealed a restricted repertoire of variable gene usage and evidence of somatic mutations,[246-248] which suggests that autoreactive B lymphocytes in AIHA undergo traditional in vivo polyclonal antigen-driven selection and mutation. Self-antigens that lead to the breakdown of normal immunologic tolerance mechanisms could actually be neoantigens that develop during inflammatory processes.[249] Although the autoreactive cells generated during immune responses are typically eliminated by apoptosis or suppressed to prevent their deleterious effects, naturally occurring autoantibodies are easily detectable in most healthy individuals, often without apparent immunization against target antigens.[250] Some of these autoantibodies have specificity against immunoglobulins[251] and presumably play a role in the suppression of other antibodies, thus illustrating a complex immunoregulatory process that can go awry and lead to the formation of pathogenic anti-RBC autoantibodies.[252] Long-lived plasma cells can produce these pathogenic autoantibodies for extended periods.[253] In the case of patients with chronic lymphocytic leukemia and AIHA, typically the leukemic cells have intraclonal diversity[254] and may not directly produce pathogenic antibodies.[255]

Although B lymphocytes have the most critical role in autoantibody formation, the traditional concepts of self/nonself discrimination and antigen-driven somatic mutation that characterize adaptive immunity have recently been modified with the elucidation of a more primitive innate immune system. Cell surface pattern recognition receptors, especially the Toll-like receptor family, allow binding of ligand to specific autoantigens and activation of B lymphocytes and dendritic cells, which can lead to autoantibody production.[256] This "Toll hypothesis" is important for certain B-lymphocyte subsets with a low activation threshold, which leads to their expansion in autoimmune models and autoantibody secretion.[257] Dysregulation of intracellular activation and signaling molecules, especially Lyn kinase, may also lead to enhanced autoantibody formation.[258,259]

In addition to B lymphocytes, it is also possible that other elements of the cellular immune system are involved in the pathophysiology that leads to AIHA. T lymphocytes orchestrate the immune response by interacting with antigen-presenting mononuclear cells and helping B cells produce specific antibody. Experimental results from a murine model of AIHA have implicated T lymphocytes in the pathogenesis of the disorder,[260] and T-lymphocyte reactivity with epitopes on the Rh and band 3 molecules has been described.[261-263] AIHA with substantial morbidity and mortality has been reported in patients after bone marrow transplantation[264,265]; the success of stem cell "add back" as treatment of this complication[266] suggests that T lymphocytes could be part of the pathogenesis of AIHA. AIHA also is a well-recognized clinical manifestation of infection with human immunodeficiency virus (HIV),[267,268] which is known to have profound effects on the T-lymphocyte compartment.

The role of cytokines in the pathophysiology of AIHA is also under investigation. Increased levels of regulatory cytokines, including interleukin-4 (IL-4), IL-6, IL-10, and IL-13, have been reported in AIHA.[269,270] An imbalance of the IL-10/IL-12 ratio, reflecting a prevalence of T_H2 over T_H1 cytokines, has also been observed.[271] Successful treatment of refractory AIHA with an anti-human IL-6 receptor monoclonal antibody indicates the importance of cytokine signaling pathways in the pathophysiology of this disorder.[272] Finally, altered expression of FcγRIII on macrophages appears to influence the clearance of antibody-sensitized erythrocytes,[273] thus illustrating the importance of macrophages in the pathophysiology of AIHA and the potential for targeted therapy. Taken together, these data support the hypothesis that polyclonal autoreactive B lymphocytes are present in the immune repertoire of normal individuals but expand and proliferate only after specific immune stimulation in certain clinical settings, such as genetically susceptible individuals or those with T-lymphocyte dysregulation or cytokine-mediated monocyte/macrophage abnormalities, with subsequent loss of normal tolerance mechanisms.

SECONDARY AUTOIMMUNE HEMOLYTIC ANEMIA

The classification scheme presented in Box 14-1 indicates that AIHA can be a primary disorder or can occur in association with other underlying conditions. The latter cases are known as secondary AIHA because they occur in the setting of much broader immune dysregulation. In one large series composed of mostly adults, patients with secondary AIHA represented more than half of the total patients with warm-reactive AIHA.[131] All patients with AIHA should be evaluated for the presence of another underlying illness.

Systemic Disorders

A common form of secondary AIHA occurs in patients with SLE, another recognized autoimmune disease.[274] Other generalized autoimmune and inflammatory disorders, including Sjögren's syndrome,[275] scleroderma,[276] dermatomyositis,[277] ulcerative colitis,[278] Crohn's disease,[279] and autoimmune thyroiditis,[280] have been associated with AIHA. The belief is that these persons have a genetic susceptibility for immune dysregulation, which leads to the expansion and proliferation of autoreactive B lymphocytes and causes the systemic disorder, including AIHA.

AIHA can occur in the setting of malignancy and is sometimes identified clinically before the diagnosis of cancer. In adults, the erythrocyte autoantibodies may reflect an abnormal B-lymphocyte clone found in chronic lymphocytic leukemia,[281] lymphoma,[282] or multiple myeloma.[283] AIHA may also occur in young patients with lymphoma,[284,285] leukemia,[286] or myelodysplasia.[287] Survival of lymphoma patients in whom AIHA develops is poor.[282] Although the cause of AIHA in patients with cancer is not known, an underlying immune deficiency may be the origin of both the autoimmune phenomenon and the malignancy.

Immunodeficiency

Immune cytopenia, including AIHA, can develop in children with congenital immunodeficiency, probably because of the lack of proper immune regulation.[288] In some cases the underlying immunodeficiency may not yet be clinically recognized, as illustrated by four children with autoimmune cytopenia (two with AIHA, two with ITP) who had unsuspected common variable immunodeficiency (CVID).[289] Autoimmune cytopenia will develop in about 11% of patients with CVID, often during childhood.[290] Treatment of AIHA in patients with CVID is similar to that of primary AIHA; corticosteroids, IVIG, splenectomy, and even rituximab have been used successfully.[289-292] Wiskott-Aldrich syndrome (WAS) is another congenital immunodeficiency that can lead to immune-mediated cytopenia. In one large single-center cohort of 55 patients, AIHA developed in 36% of the patients with WAS before the age of 5 years.[293] Similarly, AIHA can also develop in patients with acquired immunodeficiency. Patients infected with HIV are particularly susceptible to the development of erythrocyte autoantibodies,[267,268] probably because of both the polyclonal B-lymphocyte activation and lack of immune regulation by T lymphocytes. Children with marked immunosuppression, such as after solid organ transplantation, are susceptible to the development of AIHA.[294] A recent report documented the efficacy of rituximab for AIHA that developed in children after cardiac transplantation.[295]

Evans' Syndrome

A special association exists between AIHA and other autoimmune cytopenias, especially thrombocytopenia. First described by Evans and colleagues more than 50 years ago,[96] the combination of autoimmune anemia and thrombocytopenia (and occasionally granulocytopenia) is known as Evans' syndrome. In an older review of childhood Evans' syndrome, the typical clinical course was noted to be chronic and relapsing, and the therapy was generally unsatisfactory.[296] A recent review confirmed this challenging and highly variable clinical course but noted that the advent of potent immunosuppressive drugs, rituximab, and stem cell transplantation now offers improved therapeutic options.[297] A variety of immunoregulatory abnormalities have been suggested in this disorder,[298] although no single underlying specific immune defect has been identified. The autoantibodies are apparently directed against specific antigens on each of the various blood cell types; that is, the antibodies against erythrocytes, platelets, and occasionally granulocytes are not cross-reactive.[299] Because many children with Evans' syndrome have refractory life-threatening disease, aggressive therapy is often warranted. Multiagent therapy including vincristine and cyclosporine has been advocated,[300] and recently, stable remissions have been achieved with rituximab therapy alone.[301] Historically, bone marrow transplantation for children with Evans' syndrome has been associated with a poor clinical outcome, although some successful allogeneic transplants have been reported.[297,302] The diagnosis of Evans' syndrome is essentially one of exclusion because other conditions (described in subsequent sections) such as ALPS, microangiopathic hemolytic anemia, schistocytic anemia, and even PNH can mimic its clinical findings.

Autoimmune Lymphoproliferative Syndrome

In 1967, Canale and Smith[303] described a new condition of significant generalized lymphadenopathy with manifestations of autoimmune disease and a chronic clinical course that occurs before the age of 2 years; the authors presciently postulated a primary immunologic disorder. Decades later, two murine models of autoimmunity (lpr and gld mice) were noted to have similar features.

After these mice were found to have mutations in Fas and Fas ligand, respectively,[304,305] similar mutations were identified in the human condition,[306-308] then named *autoimmune lymphoproliferative syndrome*. Children with ALPS have defective lymphocyte apoptosis as a result of failure of developing lymphocytes to undergo Fas-mediated cell death[309]; an excess number of TCRαβ[+]CD3[+]CD4[-]CD8[-] (double-negative) T lymphocytes are characteristically found in the lymph nodes and peripheral blood.[310,311]

National Institutes of Health criteria for establishing the diagnosis of ALPS have been published and include the following three required findings: (1) chronic non-malignant lymphoproliferation, (2) defective in vitro Fas-mediated lymphocyte apoptosis, and (3) 1% or more double-negative T lymphocytes in the peripheral blood or lymphoid tissues. Supportive diagnostic evidence includes autoimmune antibodies and genetic mutations in the Fas-mediated apoptosis pathway.[312] Most patients with ALPS will have lymphadenopathy, organomegaly, and various autoimmune disorders, including AIHA or ITP. In one series of 34 consecutive patients, 21 (62%) had a positive DAT result, in most cases to IgG alone, although only 10 had a history of hemolytic anemia.[313] An elevated risk of malignancy, especially Hodgkin's and non-Hodgkin's lymphoma, has also been documented.[314]

The majority of ALPS patients have specific genetic mutations in either Fas or Fas ligand, although mutations in other genes within the Fas-mediated signaling pathway, such as caspase-8 or caspase-10, have also been identified.[315] Approximately 25% of patients with ALPS have no genetic mutation that can yet be identified. Perforin mutations in a clinical variant of ALPS has recently been reported,[316] thus suggesting that a variety of genetic mutations leading to immunologic dysfunction may result in lymphoproliferation and autoimmunity. Clinical overlap between Evans syndrome and ALPS is also recognized; 12 children with the diagnosis of Evans syndrome were found to have elevated numbers of circulating double-negative T lymphocytes and defective Fas-mediated apoptosis.[317] Taken together, these data indicate that all children with AIHA, especially those with the diagnosis of Evans syndrome, should be evaluated carefully for an underlying immunologic disorder such as ALPS.

Infections

The majority of young children with PCH have recently had a viral-like illness,[79,87,90] although an infectious pathogen is rarely identified. Historically, PCH developed in patients with syphilis, but this is rarely observed today. On occasion, however, a well-defined infection can trigger AIHA with either warm-reactive or cold-reactive erythrocyte autoantibodies. Numerous infectious agents have been reported, including *M. pneumoniae*,[318] Epstein-Barr virus,[319] varicella,[320] hepatitis C,[321] rubella,[322] parvovirus,[323] mumps, and cytomegalovirus, among others. Most of these autoantibodies are IgM with a specificity for the I/i polysaccharide antigen system on the red cells[139]; reac-

tivity of anti-I antibodies with mycoplasmal antigens suggests that the autoantibodies may result from immunologic cross-reactivity.[324]

Acute bacterial infections can cause immune-mediated hemolytic anemia from a different mechanism. The T antigen on the erythrocyte surface is known as a "cryptic" antigen because it is not normally available for antibody binding. In the presence of bacteria with neuraminidase activity, such as clostridial or pneumococcal species, removal of sialic acid leads to exposure of the RBC T antigen. Because many people have naturally occurring cold-reactive IgM antibodies with anti-T specificity, immune-mediated hemolysis and even microangiopathic schistocytic anemia can result.[325,326] Although the practice is controversial, erythrocytes should probably be washed in this clinical setting to avoid transfusing additional anti-T antibodies.[327]

Drugs

Though not common in childhood, drug-induced auto-antibodies must be included as a cause of secondary AIHA. Classically described after therapy with methyldopa,[328] red cell antibodies have been reported in association with dozens of different pharmaceutical agents.[329] Medications of particular importance in the pediatric age range that can cause AIHA include a variety of antibiotics: penicillins,[330,331] cephalosporins,[332-334] tetracycline,[335] erythromycin,[336] and ribavirin.[337] Common agents such as acetaminophen[338] and ibuprofen[339] have also been implicated in hemolysis. Drug-induced hemolytic anemia typically results from the generation of antidrug antibodies that cross-react with erythrocytes, although the drug may be required to form a hapten or even a ternary complex with the erythrocyte.[329,340,341]

Therapy

Therapy for patients with secondary AIHA must be twofold: the hemolytic anemia must be treated, and for best results the underlying systemic illness must be addressed as well. For example, treatment of a generalized autoimmune or inflammatory disorder or administration of antibiotics for a specific infection can also have a beneficial effect on AIHA. Discontinuation of the offending drug will help ameliorate hemolysis from drug-induced autoantibodies. In most cases of warm-reactive secondary AIHA, administration of corticosteroids is effective in reducing hemolysis. Short bursts or tapering courses of steroids can be used safely in patients with secondary AIHA, even if they are immunodeficient. In contrast, splenectomy is less likely to be successful in adults with secondary AIHA in association with malignancy than in those with primary AIHA.[342] Successful results with rapamycin and arsenic trioxide in murine models of lymphoproliferation and autoimmunity[343,344] suggest that novel therapeutic strategies may soon be available for patients with AIHA secondary to ALPS.

PAROXYSMAL NOCTURNAL HEMOGLOBINURIA

A rare condition, PNH has fascinated hematologists for more than a century. In its classic manifestation, patients with PNH have ongoing intravascular hemolysis with intermittent episodes of dark urine (hemoglobinuria), most commonly on awakening in the morning. The hemolysis of PNH is due to abnormal interactions between erythrocytes and the complement system. However, unlike AIHA, PNH is actually an intracorpuscular defect because the hemolysis results from increased sensitivity of the patient's erythrocytes to physiologic complement-mediated lysis. In addition, PNH is a complex disease with protean clinical manifestations, only one of which is hemolytic anemia. The secrets of this enigmatic disorder have only recently yielded to the efforts of modern molecular biology, culminating with identification of the *PIGA* gene, which is mutated in patients with PNH. Current challenges relate to elucidation of the pathogenetic events that lead to PNH, as well as issues of early diagnosis and optimal clinical management.

Historical Perspective

Clinicians first described PNH in the latter part of the 19th century,[345,346] although it took many years to recognize several important facts: (1) the dark pigment in urine was actually hemoglobin; (2) the serum of patients with PNH did not induce hemolysis of normal erythrocytes, thus distinguishing PNH from PCH; (3) the hemolysis was due to an intrinsic defect in the patient's own erythrocytes; and (4) the hemolysis was due to the lytic action of serum complement. Many of the initial insights into the pathophysiology of the hemolysis were due to the efforts of Dr. Thomas Ham, who first clearly demonstrated that acidified serum enhanced the hemolysis of PNH erythrocytes[347-349]; the test that bears his name was for many years the definitive laboratory method to establish the diagnosis of PNH. It was later recognized that complement lysis sensitivity was not all or none in that patients often had a population of erythrocytes with 15- to 25-fold increased complement sensitivity (type III cells), another population with 3- to 5-fold increased sensitivity (type II cells), and a population of normal type I erythrocytes.[350-352] Flow cytometry has now replaced the time-honored Ham test, as well as the sucrose lysis and complement lysis sensitivity tests, as the preferred diagnostic laboratory method for the diagnosis of PNH.[353]

Clinical Manifestations and Therapy

Passing of dark urine is the classic symptom for which the disorder is named. Patients with PNH have hemoglobinuria rather than hematuria as a result of chronic intravascular hemolysis from complement. Although the original descriptions accurately indicated that dark urine occurs more often on awakening, the cause of this temporal variation is not clear. Possibly, accelerated hemolysis occurs during sleep because of the presence of relative hypercapnia leading to slight acidosis and complement activation, which becomes evident in the morning urine. Many patients with PNH have dark urine throughout the day, whereas this symptom never develops in some. The typical patient reports an episode every few weeks, although some have chronic unrelenting hemolysis. Patients may describe hemoglobinuria with colorful language ranging from iced tea to cola to mahogany to motor oil, or they may describe the urine as various combinations of red, orange, brown, and black (Fig. 14-11A). Stress or infections tend to trigger hemolysis, although there is often no identifiable reason. Therapy with oral corticosteroids (1 to 2 mg/kg/day of prednisone) can ameliorate the hemolysis and is often recommended for 24 to 72 hours around the time of an acute hemolytic episode. Eculizumab, a humanized monoclonal antibody against terminal complement protein C5, has recently been shown to significantly reduce intravascular hemolysis and improve quality of life in adults with PNH.[354] Eculizumab is not currently licensed in the United States for the treatment of children with PNH.

The clinical manifestations of PNH include much more than simply hemolytic anemia.[355] Box 14-2 lists the more common signs and symptoms observed in patients with PNH. In addition to hemolysis, patients with PNH tend to have an increased number of infections, particularly those that are sinopulmonary and blood-borne. A more severe clinical complication is venous thrombosis, which occurs in a third of patients and often in unusual locations such as the hepatic veins, where it leads to Budd-Chiari syndrome (Fig. 14-11B), in the mesenteric veins, or in the sagittal veins (Fig. 14-11C). The complications of venous thrombosis can be fatal because the

Box 14-2	**Signs and Symptoms Commonly Observed in Paroxysmal Nocturnal Hemoglobinuria**

Intravascular hemolysis
  Dark urine
  Iron deficiency
  Acute renal failure
Infections
  Sinopulmonary
  Blood-borne
Venous thrombosis
  Occurs in a third of patients
  Unusual locations
Defective hematopoiesis
  Macrocytosis, pancytopenia
  Association with aplastic anemia
Transition
  Myelodysplasia
  Nonlymphoblastic leukemia

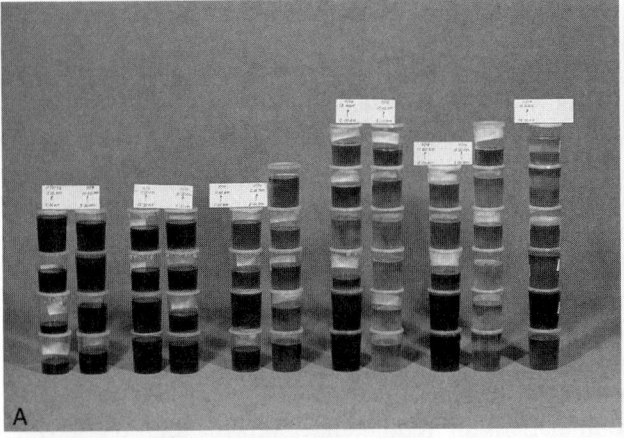

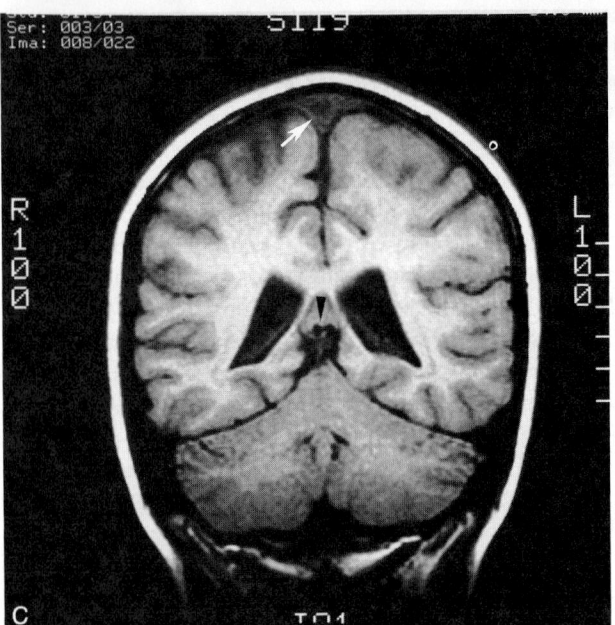

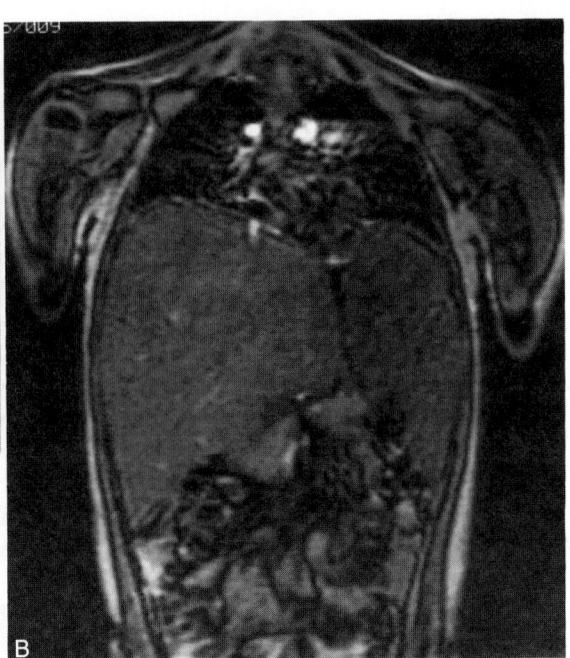

FIGURE 14-11. Clinical manifestations of paroxysmal nocturnal hemoglobinuria (PNH). **A,** Hemoglobinuria produced over a period of several days, with urine samples ranging from normal yellow to black. **B,** Massive hepatosplenomegaly that developed in a 14-year-old child with PNH and Budd-Chiari syndrome. **C,** A fatal superior sagittal sinus thrombosis that developed in a 16-year-old girl with PNH. In this T1-weighted coronal image at the level of the posterior internal cerebral veins, the normally expected black flow signal void in the superior sagittal sinus (*white arrow*) is replaced with an intermediate signal as a result of the thrombus. This appearance contrasts with the normal black venous flow void that is preserved in the internal cerebral veins (*black arrowhead*). (*A, Courtesy of Dr. Wendell Rosse; C, courtesy of Drs. Frank Keller and Jeffrey Hogg.*)

hypercoagulability observed in PNH is very difficult to treat, even with thrombolytic agents. The development of venous thrombosis is a risk factor for poor long-term survival, at least for white patients.[356] In patients of Asian ancestry with PNH, however, venous thrombosis rarely develops, thus suggesting a genetic predisposition for the hypercoagulable state in PNH.[357]

Defective hematopoiesis is present in the majority of patients with PNH, either at initial evaluation or during the course of the disease.[357] Although many patients are aplastic, most have peripheral macrocytic anemia with erythroid hyperplasia in the bone marrow; some evolve into severe aplastic anemia with hypoplastic marrow and suffer the clinical consequences of pancytopenia. Treatment with antithymocyte globulin (ATG) seems to help a portion of patients, particularly those with hypoplastic marrow; the presence of a PNH clone may lead to some increased hemolysis[358] but portends a favorable response to immunosuppressive therapy.[359] Finally, PNH can evolve into myelodysplasia or acute nonlymphoblastic leukemia, which typically occurs within the first 5 years

of disease.[360] The incidence of leukemic transformation is only 1% to 3%, but this rate far exceeds that in the general population.

Though primarily a disease of adults, PNH definitely occurs in children and adolescents, and the diagnosis should be considered in any child with unexplained cytopenia or thrombosis. In a cohort of 26 young patients with PNH, several important differences from the clinical descriptions in adults were noted.[361] In many children, PNH was initially misdiagnosed, with an average of almost 2 years from initial symptoms to the correct diagnosis. Very few children had dark urine as an initial symptom, and in only 65% of children did clinically evident hemoglobinuria ever develop. Thrombosis occurred in approximately a third of patients, and some died of this complication. All patients had laboratory evidence of defective or ineffective hematopoiesis, either at diagnosis or over the course of their disease. The survival curve for these patients indicated that the 10-year survival rate was only 60%, although several deaths were due to complications of pancytopenia in an era before modern antibiotic and transfusion therapy. Because bone marrow transplantation can be curative therapy for PNH,[362] it should be considered in selected patients with this disorder if an HLA-matched sibling donor is available. A recent summary of 11 pediatric patients with PNH from the Netherlands over a 20-year period reported successful transplantation in 4 of 5 patients.[363] Transplants from unrelated stem cell donors are associated with substantial morbidity and mortality, however, and despite anecdotal success[363,364] cannot be recommended routinely for patients with PNH.

Biochemical Basis

Important clues to the etiology of PNH emerged in the 1980s with the identification of two complement regulatory proteins, CD55 (decay accelerating factor [DAF])[365] and CD59 (membrane inhibitor of reactive lysis).[366] The abnormal peripheral blood cells in patients with PNH were noted to be lacking both CD55 and CD59. As a result of these deficiencies, randomly deposited complement factors and C3 convertase complexes cannot be cleared from the erythrocyte membrane, which leads to formation of the membrane attack complex, pores, and cell lysis.[350]

The commonality of these two complement regulatory proteins goes beyond function because both use a novel motif for anchoring into the plasma membrane (Fig. 14-12). Unlike the majority of surface proteins, which contain a highly hydrophobic domain that serves as a transmembrane region between the intracellular domain and the extracellular domain of the polypeptide,

certain proteins use a glycosylphosphatidylinositol (GPI) anchor for membrane attachment.[367,368] GPI-linked proteins are covalently attached at their C-terminal to a variable glycan moiety, which is itself attached to a phosphatidylinositol molecule in the outer leaflet of the cell membrane lipid bilayer. This glycolipid structure is assembled within the endoplasmic reticulum and is coupled to the protein precursor as a preformed unit.[368,369] Initially described for the alkaline phosphatase enzyme,[370] GPI linkage is now known to be used by a diverse set of surface proteins (Box 14-3), including acetylcholinesterase,[371] Thy-1,[372] lymphocyte function–associated antigen,[373] FcγRIII,[374] the complement regulatory proteins CD55 and CD59,[365,366] CD157 involved in neutrophil diapedesis,[375] and others. The functional advantages of GPI linkage for surface proteins remain speculative, but observations suggest increased lateral diffusional mobility,[376,377] second messenger generation,[378] signal transduction,[379,380] and the ability to be cleaved from the cell surface into the extracellular milieu.[381]

The primary defect in PNH resides in the incomplete bioassembly of GPI anchors because all GPI-linked surface proteins have absent or diminished expression on the surface of the abnormal PNH cells.[382-384] Biochemical analysis of GPI-deficient cells has localized the defect in PNH to an early step in GPI anchor biosynthesis.[385] Mammalian mutant cell lines deficient in GPI-linked surface proteins were then established and classified into different complementation classes.[386] Class A, C, and H mutants cannot transfer the initial *N*-acetylglucosamine to the phosphatidylinositol acceptor, which suggests that at least three genes control this step. Fusion experiments

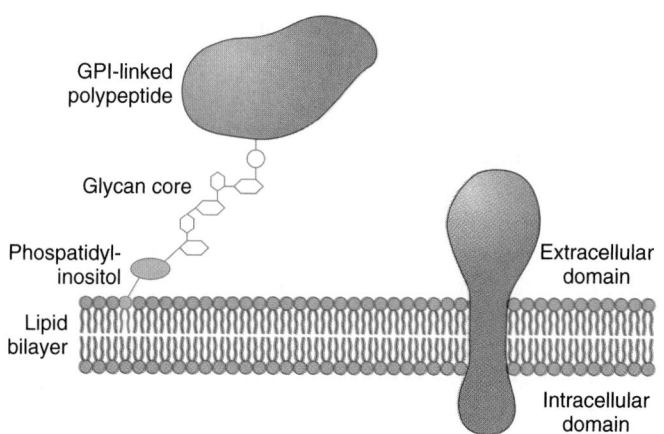

FIGURE 14-12. Glycosylphosphatidylinositol (GPI) anchor for attachment of surface proteins to the cell membrane. The structure of a GPI-linked protein is shown on the *left*. The GPI anchor consists of a phosphatidylinositol molecule in the outer leaflet of the lipid bilayer connected to a glycan core composed of multiple sugars and side chains. The polypeptide is then linked to the anchor at its C-terminal via an amide bond. The result is a surface protein with a fluid and mobile attachment to the cell surface. The entire polypeptide is present in the extracellular milieu. In contrast, a transmembrane protein is shown on the *right* and consists of an extracellular domain, a short transmembrane domain, and an intracellular domain.

Box 14-3	Important Surface Proteins Absent from Affected Hematopoietic Cells in Paroxysmal Nocturnal Hemoglobinuria

Complement regulatory proteins
    Decay-accelerating factor (CD55)
    Membrane inhibitor of reactive lysis (CD59)
Immunologically important proteins
    Lymphocyte function antigen-3 (LFA-3, CD58)
    Fc receptor gamma III (FcγRIII, CD16)
    Endotoxin-binding protein receptor (CD14)
Receptors
    Urokinase receptor (UPAR)
    Folate receptor
Enzymes
    Alkaline phosphatase
    Acetylcholinesterase
    5′-Ectonucleotidase
Proteins with unknown functions
    CD24
    CD48
    CD52 (Campath-1)
    CD66c
    CD67
    JMH-bearing protein

of PNH cells with murine GPI-deficient cell lines further identified the defect as a class A mutation in all patients tested.[385,387] Thus, despite the possibility of various enzymatic defects along the biosynthetic pathway of the GPI anchor, all patients with PNH reported to date have a class A defect.

Altered expression of GPI-linked surface proteins on the abnormal cells in PNH has led to a simpler and more accurate diagnostic test than the older methods of complement-mediated lysis. Peripheral blood erythrocytes and granulocytes can be analyzed by flow cytometry for surface expression of GPI-linked proteins such as CD16, CD48, CD55, or CD59.[353,355] Erythrocytes that are completely deficient in GPI-linked surface proteins are present in almost all patients and correspond to the PNH type III cells. Partially deficient cells can be detected in approximately 50% of patients and correspond to type II cells.[353] Cells with normal GPI-linked surface expression (type I cells) are typically present as well. Identification of these cell populations by flow cytometry analysis is illustrated in Figure 14-13. Surface expression of CD59

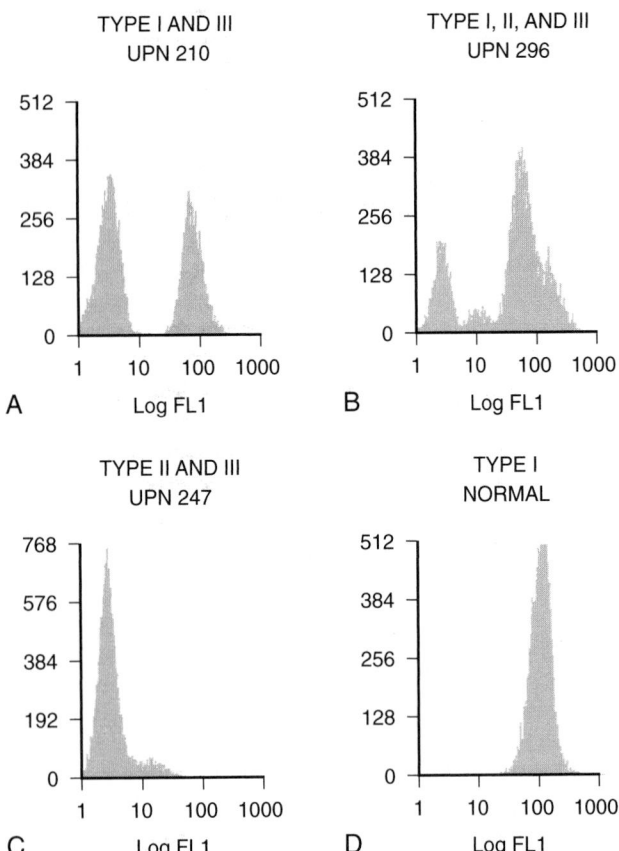

FIGURE 14-13. Immunophenotype analysis of erythrocytes in paroxysmal nocturnal hemoglobinuria by flow cytometry. Examples of surface CD59 expression are shown for three patients and a control subject. **A,** Data for unique patient number (UPN) 210, who had both type I and type III erythrocytes. **B,** Data for UPN 296 with type I, II, and III cells. **C,** Data for UPN 247, who had predominantly type III erythrocytes and a few type II cells. **D,** Normal expression from a control subject. (*Data from Ware RE, Rosse WF, Hall SE. Immunophenotypic analysis of reticulocytes in paroxysmal nocturnal hemoglobinuria. Blood. 1995;86:1586.*)

on circulating erythrocytes from a patient with type I and type III cells is shown in Figure 14-13A, that for a patient with type I, II, and III cells in Figure 14-13B, and that for a patient with predominantly type III cells but a few type II cells in Figure 14-13C. Flow cytometry for a normal control is shown in Figure 14-13D. More recently, flow cytometric analysis of PNH has been improved by the introduction of a fluorescent aerolysin (FLAER) reagent that binds to all GPI-linked surface proteins.[388] Flow cytometry using the FLAER reagent is highly sensitive for PNH and has even led to a new category of disease known as "laboratory" or "subclinical" PNH because of the detection of extremely low numbers of PNH cells, sometimes below 0.01%.[355]

Molecular Basis

Analyses of glucose-6-phosphate dehydrogenase allozymes[389] and a monoclonal pattern of X-chromosome inactivation[390] have documented that PNH is a clonal hematologic disorder. The abnormal clone is believed to originate at the level of a primitive multipotent bone marrow progenitor cell in that all cells of the myeloerythroid lineage are affected, including erythrocytes, granulocytes, platelets, and monocytes. Lymphocytes and natural killer cells are also deficient in GPI to varying degrees, however, thus suggesting that PNH is actually a clonal stem cell disorder. The abnormal PNH clone may be too minimal to be clinically apparent, can be relatively minor and affect 10% to 25% of circulating erythrocytes and granulocytes, or can become dominant with more than 95% GPI-deficient circulating cells.[355]

The recognition that all patients with PNH have a class A complementation defect suggested that a single gene was responsible for this disorder. By using the strategy of a human cDNA expression library, a gene was identified that repaired the defect in a class A GPI-deficient cell line.[391] Designated *PIGA* because it repaired the phosphatidylinositol glycan defect in a class A mutant, this cDNA encoded a novel polypeptide with homology to other known glycosyltransferases. *PIGA* was subsequently considered to be a candidate gene for PNH, and relatively quickly several groups reported that *PIGA* is the gene defective in PNH.[392-396] Interestingly, the majority of mutations are short insertions or deletions (one to two nucleotides) that occur throughout the coding region of the *PIGA* gene.[397] These nucleotide changes cause frameshift mutations because the triplet nucleotide coding sequence is altered; usually a premature termination codon follows the frameshift mutation. Missense mutations that substitute a single amino acid residue account for the minority of *PIGA* abnormalities reported.[398]

Chromosomal assignment of *PIGA* to the X chromosome[392,399] and assignment of other genes involved in GPI anchor biosynthesis (*PIGF* and *PIGH*) to autosomes[399] helped explain the predominant class A defect in PNH. Whereas a single *PIGA* mutation could result in abnormal GPI anchor biosynthesis, mutations in both alleles of other genes involved in GPI anchor biosynthesis would be required to produce clinically overt disease. Recently, an autosomal recessive form of GPI deficiency has been reported[400] to be due to an inherited point mutation in the promoter of *PIGM*, a mannosyltransfer-ase-encoding gene critical in GPI anchor synthesis. In two unrelated consanguineous families, this inherited *PIGM* deficiency led to venous thrombosis and neurologic dysfunction, but not to bone marrow failure or hemolysis. This congenital variant of GPI deficiency without evidence of bone marrow dysfunction suggests that the pathogenesis of PNH involves more than just absence of GPI anchor bioassembly.

Do *PIGA* Mutations Cause Paroxysmal Nocturnal Hemoglobinuria?

The pathophysiology of the various clinical manifestations of PNH presumably reflects the absence or diminished expression of specific GPI-linked surface proteins. Hemoglobinuria is readily explained by the absence of surface CD55 and CD59, which allows chronic complement-mediated intravascular hemolysis. In contrast, the cause of the hypercoagulable state in PNH is not well understood. PNH platelets lack the GPI-linked complement regulatory proteins CD55 and CD59 and respond to the deposition of terminal complement components by vesiculation of portions of their plasma membrane. The resultant platelet microparticles have increased pro-coagulant properties.[401] PNH cells also lack the receptor for the GPI-linked urokinase plasminogen activator, which may result in impaired fibrinolysis.[402] However, patients with PNH have normal plasma levels of natural anticoagulants, including proteins C and S, thrombo-modulin, and antithrombin III, and no known inherited thrombophilic mutations.

The defective hematopoiesis that affects so many patients with PNH is also not well understood. Although GPI-linked surface proteins are likely to be important for normal hematopoiesis, no specific molecule has been identified whose absence leads to marrow hypoplasia. An unusual association is well recognized between PNH and aplastic anemia, however, in that one usually evolves clinically into the other.[403,404] For example, in some patients with severe aplastic anemia, PNH will eventually develop, often after successful immunosuppressive therapy such as ATG or cyclosporine.[405] In contrast, in others with nearly normal blood counts and hypercellular bone marrow, hypoplasia will slowly develop, usually as a terminal event.[357]

Several models have been proposed for the pathogenesis and development of PNH. A one-step model originally proposed more than 40 years ago stated that a single genetic defect leads directly to PNH.[403] Although this model was attractive because of its simplicity, laboratory evidence using embryonic stem cells[406] and murine

models[407] indicated that an acquired *PIGA* mutation did not lead to aplastic anemia or clonal dominance by the abnormal cells. A subsequent two-step model[408,409] suggested that aplastic anemia would occur first and then a *PIGA* mutation would develop within a remaining stem cell. The resulting PNH progeny would then be able to grow preferentially over their normal hematopoietic counterparts. However, the identification of multiple clones with distinct *PIGA* mutations in individual patients with PNH,[396,410,411] coupled with the identification of rare hematopoietic cells with *PIGA* mutations in normal healthy persons,[412-414] indicates that the two-step model is also too simplistic.

As illustrated in Figure 14-14, a newer multistep model proposed that *PIGA* mutations develop initially as randomly acquired events,[415] thus explaining their presence in the bone marrow and peripheral blood of normal adults. These *PIGA* mutant cells do not proliferate, however, unless marrow damage occurs, perhaps by autoimmune attack against primarily normal hematopoietic progenitor cells. In the setting of marrow damage, additional genetic events, perhaps including those that confer resistance to apoptosis,[416-418] then lead to a growth

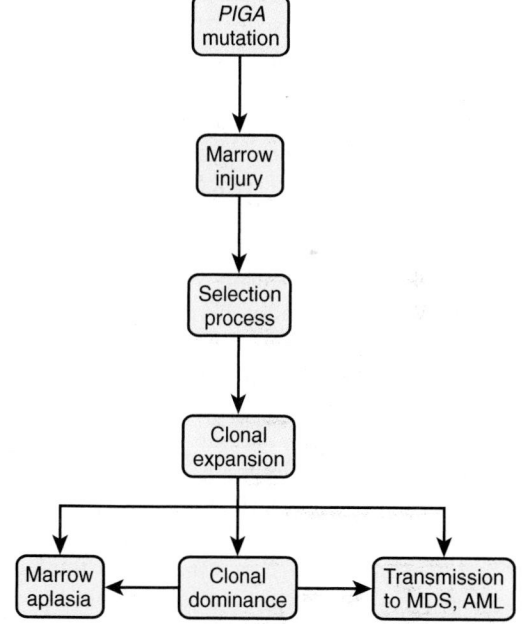

FIGURE 14-14. Multistep model for the pathogenesis and evolution of paroxysmal nocturnal hemoglobinuria (PNH). In contrast to previous models that hypothesized either a one-step or two-step model, a multistep process is proposed. *PIGA* mutations are acquired randomly and are present in most normal healthy persons. In the setting of an aplastogenic event with marrow injury, such as an autoimmune attack on hematopoiesis, surviving cells undergo a selection process. Genetic mechanisms, including those conferring resistance to apoptosis, allow continued clonal expansion and sometimes clonal dominance of the abnormal PNH clone. Additional genetic events occasionally lead to myelodysplasia or aplasia. AML, acute myeloid leukemia; MDS, myelodysplastic syndrome. *(From Ware RE, Heeney MM, Pickens CV, et al. A multistep model for the pathogenesis and evolution of PNH. In Omine M, Kinoshita T [eds]. Paroxysmal Nocturnal Hemoglobinuria and Related Disorders: Molecular Aspects of Pathogenesis. Heidelberg, Germany, Springer-Verlag, 2003.)*

advantage of the *PIGA* mutant cells, clonal expansion, and eventual clonal dominance. Later genetic events can lead to evolution to myelodysplasia or even malignant transformation into leukemia. This multistep model is supported by the recent description of two unrelated patients whose *PIGA* mutant cells also had an acquired rearrangement of the *HMGA2* gene.[419] The recognition that *HMGA2* is a transcriptional factor gene deregulated in many benign lipomas and other mesenchymal tumors led the authors to suggest that PNH might also be considered a "benign tumor of the bone marrow."[419] This intriguing notion is supported by the observations that PNH cell populations are not typically malignant, expand but respect normal tissue boundaries, respond appropriately to physiologic signals, and have no autonomous growth. Mutations in the *HMGA2* gene, which is located on chromosome 12, have also been associated with clonal expansion in polycythemia vera.[420]

SCHISTOCYTIC HEMOLYTIC ANEMIA

Overview

The term *schistocyte* is derived from the Greek word σξιζω (schizo), which translates "to tear" and describes erythrocytes that are broken, torn, or sheared. These bizarre poikilocytes are sometimes referred to as schizocytes, but because this term might be confused with the schizont phase of malarial erythrocyte infection, the term schistocyte is generally preferred. Schistocytic hemolytic anemia is characterized by the development of red cell fragments after exposure of erythrocytes to excessive environmental stress or shearing force within the vasculature. This unusual form of hemolytic anemia arises in various pathophysiologic settings, but each clinical condition features increased external force on the erythrocytes.

RBCs encounter tremendous force as they travel normally through the circulation, including collisions, turbulence, pressure fluctuations, shearing stress, and interactions with a variety of solid surfaces. Erythrocytes are exposed to some of the highest force in the left ventricle as they pass through the aortic valve and flow into the aorta. Among these various forces, experiments have shown that shearing force is the most difficult for erythrocytes to withstand and hemolysis occurs after a threshold is reached. Erythrocytes can withstand shear force of up to 15,000 dynes/cm^2 without hemolysis if this force arises at a fluid-fluid interface,[421] but hemolysis occurs at much lower shear force at a fluid-solid interface. In vitro, hemolysis occurs between 1500 and 3000 dynes/cm^2, especially if the solid surface has irregularities.[422,423] Moreover, the mechanical fragility of erythrocytes is affected by temperature, lipids, viscosity, and plasma proteins.[421]

The clinical features of schistocytic hemolytic anemia reflect primarily intravascular hemolysis because the erythrocytes are damaged and broken within the blood vessels. Anemia with pallor and fatigue is more common than jaundice, and dark urine is often present as the primary manifestation of intravascular hemolysis. Erythrocyte fragmentation leads to hemoglobinemia and hemoglobinuria, as well as elevation of serum lactate dehydrogenase. The serum bilirubin level is usually modestly elevated as a result of extravascular clearance of the damaged erythrocytes. Examination of the peripheral blood smear (Fig. 14-15) reveals schistocytes with characteristic triangular or crescent shapes, which represent erythrocytes that have recently undergone fragmentation. Spherocytes (sometimes called spheroschistocytes) can also be present and represent broken cells that have resealed their membranes and formed into a sphere, analogous to the process that occurs in immune-mediated hemolytic anemia. Teardrop shapes may be seen in response to the anemia, along with polychromasia (reticulocytosis). Depending on the pathophysiologic

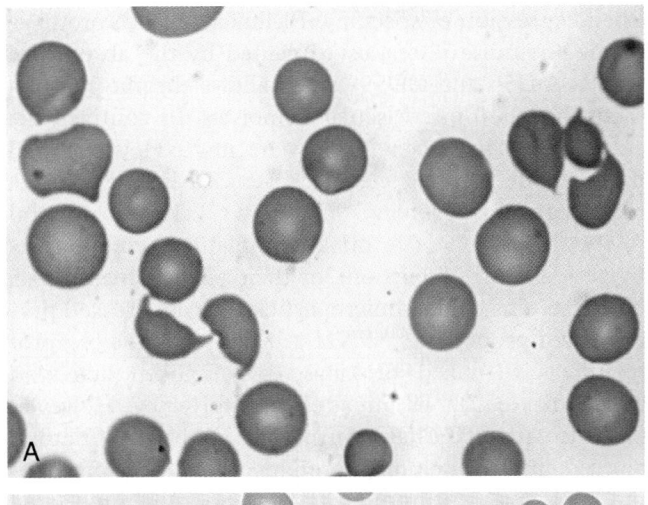

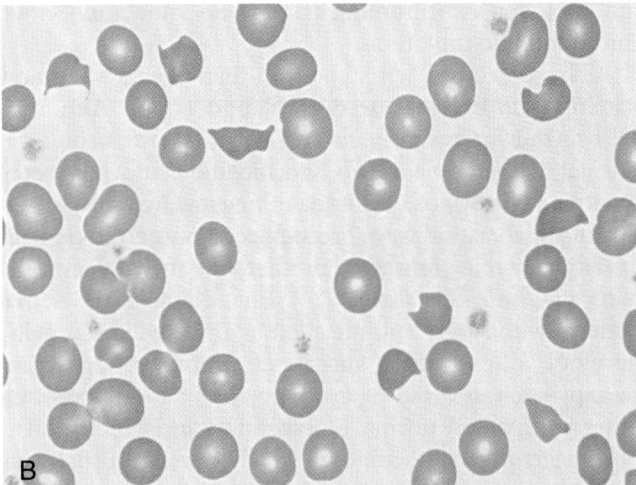

FIGURE 14-15. Schistocytic hemolytic anemia. **A,** Congenital schistocytic anemia. **B,** Acquired schistocytic anemia. The peripheral blood smear (×1000) contains several erythrocytes with characteristic sheared, triangular, or crescent shapes reflecting cells that have recently undergone fragmentation. Spherocytes are also identified and represent broken cells that have resealed their membranes and adopted a spherical shape.

changes, there may also be laboratory evidence of intravascular coagulation and thrombocytopenia from platelet trapping or consumption. Schistocytic hemolytic anemia with renal failure and thrombocytopenia is called HUS; the additional presence of fever and neurologic dysfunction is called TTP.

Microangiopathic Hemolytic Anemia

The term microangiopathic hemolytic anemia was used almost 50 years ago by Brain and co-workers[424] to describe schistocytic hemolysis in conjunction with "disease of small blood vessels." Studying a large cohort of patients with schistocytic hemolytic anemia and acute or chronic renal failure, these authors demonstrated that the amount of erythrocyte fragmentation correlated with the degree of microangiopathic disease, and they postulated that schistocytes develop as a direct consequence of vascular injury. Histologically, microangiopathy was most prominent in the kidney, where arteriolar damage and intraluminal thrombi were noted.[424] An instructive case report of a patient with fatal microangiopathic hemolytic anemia appeared several years later; large numbers of microclots composed of fine fibrin strands were identified within the renal and pulmonary arterioles.[425] With scanning electron microscopy, individual erythrocytes were found to be tangled in the fibrin strands, which caused cellular deformation, breakage, and sphering. Figure 14-16 illustrates a "hanged" red blood cell in this destructive intraluminal milieu.[425] Identification of these fine fibrin strands within the small arteriolar circulation provides a pathophysiologic mechanism for schistocyte formation: the small clots do not fully occlude the vessel; hence blood flows at arterial speed and pressure, and erythrocytes are sheared at this irregular fluid-solid interface. Microangio-

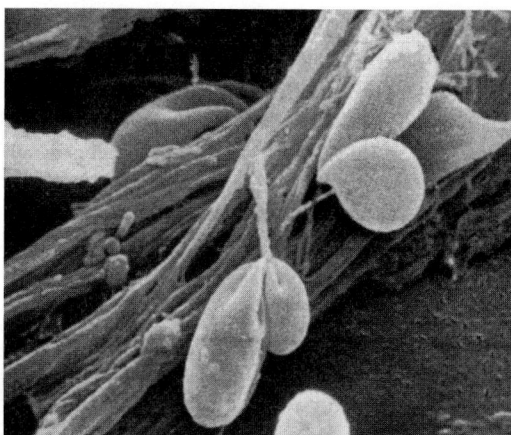

FIGURE 14-16. Hanged red blood cell. A dense fibrin band is seen with several finer strands, over which erythrocytes can be found hanging. With the shearing force available within the arterial circulation, such erythrocytes will be broken across these thin fibrin strands and thereby result in schistocytes. *(From Bull BS, Kuhn IN. The production of schistocytes by fibrin strands [a scanning electron microscope study]. Blood. 1970;35:104.)*

pathic schistocytic hemolytic anemia can therefore occur in any disorder of the small blood vessels that features the intravascular formation of fibrin (or large von Willebrand factor [VWF] multimers, see later).

Genetic Basis

In the vast majority of patients, microangiopathic schistocytic hemolytic anemia appears sporadically, although sometimes a trigger or associated medical condition can be identified. However, the rare occurrence of congenital or familial microangiopathic hemolytic anemia in conjunction with thrombocytopenia and renal dysfunction (HUS/TTP), with a clinical course that tends to be chronic and relapsing,[426-428] suggested a genetic basis in some cases. Mutations in two distinct pathways have now been identified in patients with familial disease, thereby providing insight into the pathophysiologic mechanisms of microangiopathic schistocytic hemolysis.

Abnormally large circulating multimers of VWF have been recognized for many years in patients with HUS/TTP.[428,429] Endothelial cells normally release VWF as very large multimers (sometimes reaching 5 to 20 million daltons) that undergo continuous limited proteolytic degradation by a VWF-cleaving protease. The *ADAMTS13* gene encoding this protease is located on chromosome 9q34 and is a member of the *ADAMTS* (a disintegrin-like and metalloproteinase with thrombospondin motifs) family of zinc metalloproteinase genes. Mutations in *ADAMTS13* that lead to a deficiency of VWF-cleaving protease activity have been identified in families with relapsing TTP,[430-432] thus demonstrating that physiologic degradation of VWF is essential for normal in vivo hemostasis. Acquired deficiency of the ADAMTS13 enzyme also occurs in association with autoantibody formation against the VWF-cleaving protease; ADAMTS13 inhibitors can be detected in most patients with an initial acute episode of TTP, but not in cases of HUS.[433,434] Very large undegraded VWF multimers presumably initiate or participate in intravascular coagulation, which leads to arteriolar fibrin and VWF deposition, platelet trapping, and microangiopathic schistocytic hemolytic anemia.

A seemingly different pathophysiologic process for the development of schistocytic hemolytic anemia involves abnormal complement regulation. Factor H is a 150-kd plasma protein that normally regulates the alternative pathway of complement activation. Without proper binding and inhibition of factor H, the C3b produced by C3 convertase is allowed to activate the alternative pathway unchecked. In a porcine model, factor H deficiency is associated with dysregulated complement activation and the development of fatal glomerulonephritis.[435] In humans, missense mutations in the factor H gene (*HF1*) have been identified in both dominant and recessive familial cases of microangiopathic hemolytic anemia.[436,437] Similarly, mutations in the complement inhibitor factor I[438] and membrane cofactor protein (MCP)[439] have been associated with atypical HUS, defined as disease not associated with exposure to Shiga toxin. Whether all these mutations in complement regulatory proteins lead directly to complement deposition within the kidney, which then leads to microangiopathy, has not been proved, but damage to the endothelium appears to be important.[440] Perhaps complement activation and deposition onto the renal endothelium leads to exaggerated local release of VWF, which then promotes local microangiopathy in a mechanism analogous to that observed in patients with deficiency of VWF-cleaving protease activity. Damage to the renal endothelium could create an irregular fluid-solid interface against which the erythrocytes must pass, thus making schistocyte formation more likely.

Clinical Settings

As noted earlier, when microangiopathic schistocytic hemolytic anemia occurs with acute renal failure and severe thrombocytopenia, the triad is referred to as HUS; the concomitant presence of fever and neurologic deterioration forms a pentad known as TTP. Both these related clinical syndromes typically occur sporadically and are associated with substantial morbidity and mortality. These disorders are discussed more fully elsewhere in the book.

Schistocytic microangiopathy has also been reported in the setting of immune vasculitis. Schistocytic hemolytic anemia can develop in patients with a variety of connective tissue disorders, including SLE,[441] systemic sclerosis,[442] diabetes mellitus,[443] Kawasaki's disease,[444] Wegener's granulomatosis,[445] and antiphospholipid antibody syndrome.[446] The common pathophysiologic process is believed to involve renal involvement by the systemic process, especially small vessel (renal arteriolar) damage. Correlation of autoantibody titers with the degree of microangiopathy,[446] coupled with a case report of neonatal lupus erythematosus with severe microangiopathic hemolytic anemia,[447] suggests that autoantibodies can mediate this process. In the case of microangiopathic hemolytic anemia in association with SLE, the prognosis and outcome appear to be distinct, as opposed to the situation with relapsing TTP.[448]

On some occasions, microangiopathic schistocytic hemolytic anemia occurs in clinical settings that are associated with widespread microangiopathy. Disseminated malignancy, especially adenocarcinoma of the breast or stomach, can lead to schistocytic hemolysis and thrombocytopenia.[449,450] In patients with cancer, laboratory evidence of ongoing intravascular coagulation consistent with a widespread microangiopathic process is observed. Similarly, in patients with systemic infections, schistocytic microangiopathic hemolysis can occasionally develop.[326,451,452] Disseminated intravascular coagulation can lead to schistocytic hemolysis as erythrocytes encounter systemic intravascular fibrin deposition. Schistocytic hemolytic anemia has also been described after allogeneic or autologous stem cell transplantation, usually in conjunction with thrombocytopenia and renal dysfunction. Microangiopathic hemolytic anemia that occurs as a late complication after transplantation is associated with substantial morbidity and mortality; the use of calcineurin inhibitors such as tacrolimus as post-transplant immunosuppressive therapy is an added risk factor.[453]

Microangiopathic disorders associated with pregnancy include preeclampsia, characterized by hypertension and proteinuria, and the more dangerous eclampsia, which can lead to severe hypertension, seizures, and even death. In pregnant women, the development of schistocytic hemolytic anemia, elevated liver enzymes, and a low platelet count is known as the HELLP syndrome. Long recognized but poorly understood, new evidence suggests that HELLP is often a severe manifestation of antiphospholipid syndrome.[454] This triad of abnormalities necessitates aggressive management, including transfusions, plasmapheresis, and especially glucocorticoids.[455] HELLP during a pregnancy may be the first manifestation of antiphospholipid syndrome, but it often recurs and can lead to fetal demise even with aggressive heparin and aspirin therapy.[456] Perhaps the best "therapy" is elective delivery of the infant, which usually leads to complete resolution of the syndrome.[457] Although the etiology and pathophysiologic changes during HELLP have not been fully elucidated, clinical and laboratory observations indicate that schistocytic hemolytic anemia during pregnancy is an ominous development that warrants aggressive intervention during gestation but usually resolves completely after delivery.

Microangiopathic hemolytic anemia can also occur after exposure to a variety of drugs and toxins. Cocaine abuse[458] and the therapeutic use of quinine,[459] immunosuppressants such as cyclosporine[460] and FK506 (tacrolimus),[461] and antineoplastic and other agents[462-465] have all been associated with the development of microangiopathic schistocytic hemolytic anemia. The pathophysiologic process of drug-induced microangiopathy is not known, but it probably follows nephrotoxicity with drug-induced renal endothelial and microvascular damage. Loxoscelism, which refers to the systemic effects after *Loxosceles reclusa* (brown recluse) spider bites, can be associated with a brisk spheroschistocytic immune-mediated hemolytic anemia that includes both intravascular and extravascular hemolysis.[466,467]

Finally, schistocytic hemolysis can occur with hypertension. In patients with pulmonary hypertension, either as a primary disorder[468] or secondary to congenital heart disease,[469] microangiopathic hemolytic anemia can develop from changes within the pulmonary vasculature. Fibrin deposition in the pulmonary arterial and arteriolar circulation can shear erythrocytes efficiently and lead to schistocyte formation. Severe systemic hypertension, sometimes referred to as "malignant" hypertension, can also lead to schistocytic hemolysis; the proposed pathophysiologic process in this setting involves not only intrinsic renal arteriolar changes but also elevated arterial pressure, which increases the shearing force.[470]

Hypertension as a manifestation of antiphospholipid syndrome can be accompanied by thrombotic microangiopathy.[471] Pharmacologic treatment of malignant hypertension can typically reverse the schistocytic hemolytic process, although in rare case reports bilateral nephrectomy was required to control the hypertension and ameliorate the hemolytic anemia.[470]

Therapy

Treatment for patients with microangiopathic schistocytic hemolytic anemia should be individualized according to the degree of anemia and the presence of an associated medical condition. Whenever possible, specific therapy for the underlying process leading to the microangiopathic anemia should be instituted. Transfusion support is warranted if the schistocytic hemolysis is massive or if the anemia is severe enough to be symptomatic. The fate of transfused erythrocytes will probably be the same as that of endogenous RBCs; thus, transfusions should be administered carefully and judiciously. However, erythrocyte transfusions can be lifesaving for patients with schistocytic hemolytic anemia and cardiovascular compromise.

Although a low platelet count can accompany microangiopathic hemolytic anemia, hemorrhagic bleeding is not the norm, even with severe thrombocytopenia. Platelet transfusions are usually unnecessary and can actually lead to worsening of the patient's condition because of in vivo aggregation and consumption.

In patients with congenital schistocytic hemolytic anemia, regular infusions of fresh frozen plasma can help ameliorate the laboratory abnormalities and prevent clinical complications.[472,473] Particularly in patients with documented deficiency of VWF-cleaving protease, prophylactic treatment with fresh frozen plasma can be effective, even with long-term use.[474]

Exchange plasmapheresis has emerged as the most effective acute intervention for patients with severe microangiopathic schistocytic hemolytic anemia due to TTP. The beneficial effects of plasmapheresis derive from both the infusion of fresh frozen plasma and the removal of free hemoglobin, fragments of broken erythrocyte membranes, and any plasma substances promoting intravascular coagulation and platelet aggregation. For patients in whom life-threatening disease develops, plasmapheresis is the therapy of choice[475,476] and is more effective than corticosteroids, aspirin, dipyridamole, or splenectomy.[477] Exchange plasmapheresis is now recommended early in the clinical course, soon after the diagnosis of TTP. However, the patient should be weaned from this therapeutic intervention slowly over a period of several weeks because relapses and periodic exacerbations are often observed when daily plasmapheresis is discontinued. A patient with relapsing refractory microangiopathic hemolytic anemia secondary to autoantibodies to the VWF-cleaving protease may respond to rituximab therapy.[478]

Large Vessel Schistocytic Hemolytic Anemia

In addition to the microangiopathic processes that can lead to schistocyte formation, there are several large vessel or "macrovascular" disorders that also can cause mechanical shearing of erythrocytes. The most common of these large vessel schistocytic disorders occurs in association with hemangiomas, which can lead to hemolytic anemia with intravascular coagulation and severe thrombocytopenia (Kasabach-Merritt syndrome). Most of the cutaneous lesions that lead to Kasabach-Merritt syndrome are not actually hemangiomas at all; they have a kaposiform (spindle cell) hemangioendothelioma pattern on histologic examination, consistent with their aggressive vascular proliferation.[479,480] True capillary hemangiomas, though common in infancy, do not cause erythrocyte fragmentation. In contrast, large cavernous hemangiomas can develop in the liver, spleen, or other organs and cause schistocytic hemolytic anemia at any age.[481-483] However, no single effective therapy has been identified for hemangiomas causing schistocytic hemolysis. Improvement has been reported anecdotally and in small series with the use of steroids and antifibrinolytic agents,[484] embolization,[485] laser therapy,[486] local radiation therapy,[487] and chemotherapy.[488] Initial success with interferon alfa therapy has been dampened by reports of spastic diplegia in association with its use.[489] Newer approaches directed against the angiogenesis process itself, such as the use of angiostatin or related molecules,[490] may eventually prove to be a successful targeted therapy for hemangiomas.

Schistocytic hemolytic anemia is also a well-described complication of valvular heart disease that results from excessive shearing force on the erythrocytes at the interface with the abnormal heart valve. Although mild hemolysis can occur with both congenital and acquired abnormalities of the heart valves, "cardiac" schistocytic hemolysis is most severe after the insertion or failure of a prosthetic heart valve.[491,492] In the immediate postoperative period, erythrocytes can be sheared on valvular surfaces that lack smooth endothelium, thereby leading to schistocyte formation, hemoglobinuria, and anemia. Flow disturbances identified on echocardiography include rapid acceleration, fragmentation, and collision jets that lead to high shear stress and hemolysis.[493] Occasionally, intravascular hemolysis is severe enough to cause massive hemolysis with profound anemia. Transfusions may be required in the short term while the patient awaits endothelialization of the prosthetic valve, although erythropoietin therapy may reduce the transfusion requirement.[494] Surgical correction is often required for patients with chronic or life-threatening transfusion-dependent intravascular hemolysis. The successful use of pentoxifylline for this condition warrants further investigation.[495]

Finally, an infant with fetal schistocytic hemolytic anemia in association with an umbilical vein varix was reported.[496] Turbulent flow through this large vessel was noted by ultrasonographic examination, and severe schistocytic hemolytic anemia was identified at birth. The infant received aggressive supportive care, including erythrocyte transfusions, and survived.

Miscellaneous Forms of Schistocytic Hemolytic Anemia

The term "march hemoglobinuria" refers to the transient intravascular hemolysis that can occur after strenuous exercise.[497] This relatively rare form of schistocytic hemolytic anemia was originally noted in soldiers after prolonged marching drills and has been attributed to physical trauma to erythrocytes within the soles of the feet. The phenomenon seems to occur only in selected individuals, but it can be associated with severe hemoglobinuria and even renal failure.[498] A better name for this form of hemolysis might be "exertional hemoglobinuria" because it can occur after a variety of exercises, including running, swimming, karate, and even playing of conga drums.[499-501] One study reported that transfused erythrocytes also had shortened survival after exercise, thus documenting the extracorpuscular nature of the defect.[502] Avoidance of the offending physical trauma is usually sufficient to resolve the hemolysis. For persons in whom hemoglobinuria develops after running, insertion of protective insoles may protect against the physical pounding of erythrocytes.[503]

Thermal burns are the most common form of burn injury that causes anemia, although chemical burns can also induce hemolysis.[504] Erythrocytes that are directly exposed to the burn become injured, and this damage either leads to their immediate lysis or results in shape changes that shorten their survival in vivo. If the damage is severe, the erythrocytes circulating through the skin at the time of the injury undergo intravascular hemolysis within hours, thereby giving rise to hemoglobinemia, hemoglobinuria, and anemia. Less damaged erythrocytes continue to circulate but undergo sphering and are prematurely removed by the spleen.[505] This extravascular hemolysis may occur several days or weeks after the burn injury and may lead to marked late-onset hemolytic anemia. Despite earlier reports suggesting a high incidence of positive DAT results after burn injury, there is little evidence for immune-mediated hemolytic anemia in this setting.[506]

Although an initial burn injury may be sufficient to cause anemia, concomitant therapies can also contribute to hemolytic anemia.[507] For example, the liberal use of silver sulfadiazine provides an oxidative stress that can induce hemolysis, especially in patients with glucose-6-phosphate dehydrogenase deficiency.[508] Many burn patients require transfusions of fresh frozen plasma, which can induce hemolysis via passively acquired isohemagglutinins. Finally, infections and the antibiotics used to treat these infections can induce hemolysis. Thus, hemolytic anemia associated with burns is often multifactorial. Immediate and delayed hemolytic anemia occurs as a direct consequence of the burn injury, whereas additional therapies can lead to further hemolysis.

REFERENCES

1. McClusky DA III, Skandalakis LJ, Colborn G, Skandalakis JE. Tribute to a triad: history of splenic anatomy, physiology, and surgery—Part 1. World J Surg. 1999;23:311-325.
2. Neiman RS, Orazi A. Embryology and anatomy. In Neiman RS (ed). Disorders of the Spleen, 2nd ed. Philadelphia, WB Saunders, 1999, p 3.
3. Peters AM, Walport MJ, Bell RN, Lavender JP. Methods of measuring splenic blood flow and platelet transit time with In-111-labeled platelets. J Nucl Med. 1984;25:86-90.
4. Hirasawa Y, Tokuhiro H. Electron microscopic studies on the normal spleen: especially on the red pulp and the reticulo-endothelial cells. Blood. 1970;35:201-312.
5. Weiss L, Tavassoli M. Anatomical hazards to the passage of erythrocytes through the spleen. Semin Hematol. 1970;7:372-380.
6. Berendes M. The proportion of reticulocytes in the erythrocytes of the spleen as compared with those of circulating blood, with special reference to hemolytic states. Blood. 1959;14:558-563.
7. Hosea SW, Burch CG, Brown EJ, et al. Impaired immune response of splenectomized patients to polyvalent pneumococcal vaccine. Lancet. 1981;1:804-807.
8. Ruben FL, Hankins WA, Ziegler Z, et al. Antibody responses to meningococcal polysaccharide vaccine in adults without a spleen. Am J Med. 1984;76:115-121.
9. Rowley DA. The formation of circulating antibody in the splenectomized human being following intravenous injection of heterologous erythrocytes. J Immunol. 1950;65:515-521.
10. Sullivan JL, Ochs HD, Schiffman G, et al. Immune response after splenectomy. Lancet. 1978;1:178-181.
11. Saslaw S, Bouroncle BA, Wall RL, Doan CA. Studies on the antibody response in splenectomized persons. N Engl J Med. 1959;261:120-125.
12. Motohashi SJ. The effect of splenectomy on the production of antibodies. J Med Res. 1972;43:473.
13. Schnitzer B, Sodeman TM, Mead ML, Contacos PG. An ultrastructural study of the red pulp of the spleen in malaria. Blood. 1973;41:207-218.
14. Rosner F, Zarrabi MH, Benach JL, Habicht GS. Babesiosis in splenectomized adults. Review of 22 reported cases. Am J Med. 1984;76:696-701.
15. Ivemark BI. Implications of agenesis of the spleen on the pathogenesis of cono-truncus anomalies in childhood: analysis of the heart malformations of the splenic agenesis syndrome, with fourteen new cases. Acta Paediatr Suppl. 1955;44(Suppl 104):7-110.
16. Phoon CK, Neill CA. Asplenia syndrome: insight into embryology through an analysis of cardiac and extra cardiac anomalies. Am J Cardiol. 1994;73:581-587.
16a. Gilbert B, Menetrey C, Belin V, et al. Familial isolated congenital asplenia: a rare, frequently hereditary dominant condition, often detected too late as a cause of over-

whelming pneumococcal sepsis. Report of a new case and review of 31 others. Eur J Pediatr. 2002;161:368-372.

16b. Roberts CW, Shutter JR, Korsmeyer SJ. Hox 11 controls the genesis of the spleen. Nature. 1994;368:747-749.

17. Holroyde CP, Oski FA, Gardner FH. The "pocked" erythrocyte: red cell alterations in the reticuloendothelial immaturity of the neonate. N Engl J Med. 1960; 281:516.

18. Moller JH, Nakih A, Anderson RC, Edwards JE. Congenital cardiac disease associated with polysplenia: a developmental complex of bilateral "left-sidedness." Circulation. 1967;36:789-799.

19. Karrer FM, Hall RJ, Lilly JR. Biliary atresia and the polysplenia syndrome. J Pediatr Surg. 1991;26:524-527.

20. Eraklis AJ, Filler RM. Splenectomy in childhood: a review of 1413 cases. J Pediatr Surg. 1972;7:382-388.

21. Balik E, Yazici M, Taneli C, et al. Splenoptosis (wandering spleen). Eur J Pediatr Surg. 1993;3:174-175.

22. Balm R, Willekens FG. Torsion of a wandering spleen. Eur J Surg. 1993;159:249-251.

23. Schwartz AD, Dadash-Zadeh M, Goldstein R, et al. Antibody response to intravenous immunization following splenic tissue autotransplantation in Sprague-Dawley rats. Blood. 1977;49:779-783.

24. Emond AM, Collis R, Darvill D, et al. Acute splenic sequestration crisis in homozygous sickle cell disease: natural history and management. J Pediatr. 1985;107: 201-206.

25. Jandl JH, Aster RH. Increased splenic pooling and the pathogenesis of hypersplenism. Am J Med. 1967;253: 383-398.

26. Qureshi FG, Ergun O, Sandulache VC, et al. Laparoscopic splenectomy in children. JSLS. 2005;9:389-392.

27. de Lagausie P, Bonnard A, Benkerrou M, et al. Pediatric laparoscopic splenectomy: benefits of the anterior approach. Surg Endosc. 2004;18:80-82.

28. Targarona EM, Espert JJ, Balagué C, et al. Residual splenic function after laparoscopic splenectomy: a clinical concern. Arch Surg. 1998;133:56-60.

29. Liu DL, Xia S, Xu W, et al. Anatomy of vasculature of 850 spleen specimens and its application in partial splenectomy. Surgery. 1996;119:27-33.

30. Cazuderna P, Vajda P, Schaarschmidt K, et al. Nonparasitic splenic cysts in children: a multicentric study. Eur J Pediatr Surg. 2006;16:415-419.

31. Bader-Meunier B, Gauthier F, Archambaud F, et al. Long-term evaluation of the beneficial effect of subtotal splenectomy for management of hereditary spherocytosis. Blood. 2001;97:399-403.

32. de Montalembert M, Girot R, Revillon Y, et al. Partial splenectomy in homozygous beta thalassemia. Arch Dis Child. 1990;65:304-307.

33. Svarch E, Vilorio P, Nordet I, et al. Partial splenectomy in children with sickle cell disease and repeated episodes of splenic sequestration. Hemoglobin. 1996;20:393-400.

34. Rice HE, Oldham KT, Hillery CA, et al. Clinical and hematological benefits of partial splenectomy for congenital hemolytic anemias in children. Ann Surg. 2003;237: 281-288.

35. Diesen DL, Zimmerman SA, Thornburg CD, et al. Partial splenectomy for children with congenital hemolytic anemia and massive splenomegaly. J Pediatr Surg 2008; 43:466-472.

36. Zer M, Freud E. Subtotal splenectomy in Gaucher's disease: towards a definition of critical splenic mass. Br J Surg. 1992;79:742-744.

37. Traub A, Giebink GS, Smith C, et al. Splenic reticuloendothelial function after splenectomy, spleen repair, and spleen autotransplantation. N Engl J Med. 1987;317: 1559-1564.

38. Lüdtke FE, Schuff-Werner P, Lion KA, Speer CP. Immunorestorative effects of reimplanted splenic tissue and splenosis. J Surg Res. 1990;49:413-418.

39. Dutta S, Price VE, Blanchette V, Langer JC. A laparoscopic approach to partial splenectomy for children with hereditary spherocytosis. Surg Endosc. 2006;20:1719-1724.

40. Uranues S, Grossman D, Ludwig L, Bergamaschi R. Laparoscopic partial splenectomy. Surg Endosc. 2007;21: 57-60.

41. King H, Shumacker HB Jr. Susceptibility to infection after splenectomy performed in infancy. Ann Surg. 1951; 136:239-242.

42. Holdsworth RJ, Irving AD, Cuschieri A. Postsplenectomy sepsis and its mortality rate: actual versus perceived risks. Br J Surg. 1991;78:1031-1038.

43. Schilling RF. Estimating the risk for sepsis after splenectomy in hereditary spherocytosis. Ann Intern Med. 1995; 122:187-188.

44. Hayem G. Sur une variété particulière d'ictère chronique. Ictère infectieux chronique splénomégalique. Presse Med. 1898;6:121-125.

45. Donath J, Landsteiner K. Über paroxysmale Hämoglobinurie. Munch Med Wochenschr. 1904;51: 1590-1593.

46. Landsteiner K. Über Beziehungen zwischen dem Blutserum und den Korperzellen. Munch Med Wochenschr. 1903;50:1812-1814.

47. Coombs RRA, Mourant AE, Race RR. A new test for the detection of weak and "incomplete" Rh agglutinins. Br J Exp Pathol. 1945;26:255-266.

48. Coombs RRA, Mourant AE. On certain properties of antisera prepared against human serum and its various protein fractions: their use in the detection of sensitization of human red cells with "incomplete" Rh antibody, and on the nature of this antibody. J Pathol Bacteriol. 1947;59: 105-111.

49. Dausset J, Colombani J. The serology and the prognosis of 128 cases of autoimmune hemolytic anemia. Blood. 1959;14:1280-1301.

50. Jandl JH, Jones AR, Castle WB. The destruction of red cells by antibodies in man. I. Observations on the sequestration and lysis of red cells altered by immune mechanisms. J Clin Invest. 1957;30:1428.

51. Borsos T, Rapp HJ. Complement fixation on cell surfaces by 19S and 7S antibodies. Science. 1965;150:505-506.

52. Eyster ME, Jenkins DE Jr. Erythrocyte coating substances in patients with positive direct antiglobulin reactions. Correlation of gammaG-globulin and complement coating with underlying diseases, overt hemolysis and response to therapy. Am J Med. 1969;46:360-371.

53. Eyster ME, Jenkins DE Jr. Gamma G erythrocyte autoantibodies: comparison of in vivo complement coating and in vitro "Rh" specificity. J Immunol. 1970;105: 221-226.

54. Rosse WF. Fixation of the first component of complement (C'1a) by human antibodies. J Clin Invest. 1968;47: 2430-2445.

55. Rosse WF. Quantitative immunology of immune hemolytic anemia. I. The fixation of C1 by autoimmune antibody and heterologous anti-IgG antibody. J Clin Invest. 1971;50:727-733.

56. LoBuglio AF, Cotran RS, Jandl JH. Red cells coated with immunoglobulin G: binding and sphering by mononuclear cells in man. Science. 1967;158:1582-1585.

57. Abramson N, LoBuglio AF, Jandl JH, Cotran RS. The interaction between human monocytes and red cells. Binding characteristics. J Exp Med. 1970;132:1191-1206.

58. Kay NE, Douglas SD. Monocyte-erythrocyte interaction in vitro in immune hemolytic anemias. Blood. 1977;50: 889-897.

59. Abramson N, Gelfand EW, Jandl JH, Rosen FS. The interaction between human monocytes and red cells. Specificity for IgG subclasses and IgG fragments. J Exp Med. 1970;132:1207-1215.

60. Huber H, Douglas SD, Nusbacher J, et al. IgG subclass specificity of human monocyte receptor sites. Nature. 1971;229:419-420.

61. Kurlander RJ, Rosse WF, Logue GL. Quantitative influence of antibody and complement coating of red cells on monocyte-mediated cell lysis. J Clin Invest. 1978;61: 1309-1319.

62. Schreiber AD, Frank MM. Role of antibody and complement in the immune clearance and destruction of erythrocytes. I. In vivo effects of IgG and IgM complement-fixing sites. J Clin Invest. 1972;51:575-582.

63. Atkinson JP, Frank MM. Complement-independent clearance of IgG-sensitized erythrocytes: inhibition by cortisone. Blood. 1974;44:629-637.

64. Atkinson JP, Frank MM. Studies on the in vivo effects of antibody. Interaction of IgM antibody and complement in the immune clearance and destruction of erythrocytes in man. J Clin Invest. 1974;54:339-348.

65. Atkinson JP, Schreiber AD, Frank MM. Effects of corticosteroids and splenectomy on the immune clearance and destruction of erythrocytes. J Clin Invest. 1973;52: 1509-1517.

66. Schreiber AD, Parsons J, McDermott P, Cooper RH. Effect of corticosteroids on the human monocyte IgG and complement receptors. J Clin Invest. 1975;56:1189-1197.

67. Issitt PD, Pavone BG, Goldfinger D, et al. Anti-Wr[b], and other autoantibodies responsible for positive direct antiglobulin tests in 150 individuals. Br J Haematol. 1976;34: 5-18.

68. Reusser P, Osterwalder B, Burri H, Speck B. Autoimmune hemolytic anemia associated with IgA—diagnostic and therapeutic aspects in a case with long-term follow-up. Acta Haematol. 1987;77:53-56.

69. Ahn YS, Harrington WJ, Byrnes JJ, et al. Treatment of autoimmune hemolytic anemia with Vinca-loaded platelets. JAMA. 1983;249:2189-2194.

70. Ahn YS, Harrington WJ, Mylvaganam R, et al. Danazol therapy for autoimmune hemolytic anemia. Ann Intern Med. 1985;102:298-301.

71. Bussel JB, Cunningham-Rundles C, Abraham C. Intravenous treatment of autoimmune hemolytic anemia with very high dose gammaglobulin. Vox Sang. 1986;51: 264-269.

72. Habibi B, Homberg J-C, Schaison G, Salmon C. Autoimmune hemolytic anemia in children. A review of 80 cases. Am J Med. 1974;56:61-69.

73. Carapella de Luca E, Casadei AM, di Piero G, et al. Auto-immune haemolytic anaemia in childhood. Follow-up in 29 cases. Vox Sang. 1979;36:13-20.

74. Schreiber AD. Autoimmune hemolytic anemia. In Austen KF, Frank MM, Atkinson JP, Cantor H (eds). Samter's Immunologic Diseases, vol 2, 6th ed. Philadelphia, Lippincott Williams & Wilkins, 2001, pp 738-749.

75. Maluf EM, Pasquini R, Eluf JN, et al. Aplastic anemia in Brazil: incidence and risk factors. Am J Hematol. 2002; 71:268-274.

76. Kaufman DW, Kelly JP, Issaragrisil S, et al. Relative incidence of agranulocytosis and aplastic anemia. Am J Hematol. 2006;81:65-67.

77. Segal JB, Powe NR. Prevalence of immune thrombocytopenia: analyses of administrative data. J Thromb Haemost. 2006;4:2377-2383.

78. Oliveira MC, Oliveira BM, Murao M, et al. Clinical course of autoimmune hemolytic anemia: an observational study. J Pediatr (Rio J). 2006;82:58-62.

79. Sokol RJ, Hewitt S, Stamps BK. Autoimmune haemolysis associated with Donath-Landsteiner antibodies. Acta Haematol. 1982;68:268-277.

80. Heisel MA, Ortega JA. Factors influencing prognosis in childhood autoimmune hemolytic anemia. Am J Pediatr Hematol Oncol. 1983;5:147-152.

81. Salawu L, Durosinmi MA. Autoimmune haemolytic anaemia: pattern of presentation and management outcome in a Nigerian population: a ten-year experience. Afr J Med Med Sci. 2002;31:97-100.

82. Wynn RF, Stevens RF, Bolton-Maggs PH, et al. Paroxysmal cold haemoglobinuria of childhood: a review of the management and unusual presenting features of six cases. Clin Lab Haematol. 1998;20:373-375.

83. Rosse WF, Hillmen P, Schreiber AD. Immune-mediated hemolytic anemia. Hematology. 2004;1:48-62.

84. Gertz MA. Cold agglutinin disease and cryoglobulinemia. Clin Lymphoma. 2005;5:290-293.

85. Gehrs BC, Friedberg RC. Autoimmune hemolytic anemia. Am J Hematol. 2002;69:258-271.

86. Nydegger UE, Kazatchkine MD, Miescher PA. Immunopathologic and clinical features of hemolytic anemia due to cold agglutinins. Semin Hematol. 1991;28: 66-77.

87. Vaglio S, Arista MC, Perrone MP, et al. Autoimmune hemolytic anemia in childhood: serologic features in 100 cases. Transfusion. 2007;47:50-54.

88. Buchanan GR, Boxer LA, Nathan DG. The acute and transient nature of idiopathic immune hemolytic anemia in childhood. J Pediatr. 1976;88:780-783.

89. Nordhagen R, Stensvold K, Winsnes A, et al. Paroxysmal cold hemoglobinuria. The most frequent autoimmune hemolytic anemia in children? Acta Paediatr Scand. 1984;73:258-262.

90. Petz LD. Treatment of autoimmune hemolytic anemias. Curr Opin Hematol. 2001;8:411-416.

91. Allgood JW, Chaplin H Jr. Idiopathic acquired autoimmune hemolytic anemia. A review of forty-seven cases treated from 1955 through 1965. Am J Med. 1967;43: 254-273.

92. Dobbs CE. Familial auto-immune hemolytic anemia. Arch Intern Med. 1965;116:273-276.

93. Toolis F, Parker AC, White A, Urbaniak S. Familial autoimmune haemolytic anaemia. Br Med J. 1977;1: 1392.

94. Myhre Jensen O, Kristensen J. Red pulp of the spleen in autoimmune haemolytic anaemia and hereditary spherocytosis: morphometric light and electron microscopy studies. Scand J Haematol. 1986;36:263-266.

95. Weiss GB, Bessman JD. Spurious automated red cell values in warm autoimmune hemolytic anemia. Am J Hematol. 1984;17:433-435.

96. Evans RS, Takahashi K, Duane RT, et al. Primary thrombocytopenic purpura and acquired hemolytic anemia. Evidence for a common etiology. Arch Intern Med. 1951;87:48-65.

97. Brown DL, Nelson DA. Surface microfragmentation of red cells as a mechanism for complement-mediated immune spherocytosis. Br J Haematol. 1973;24:301-305.

98. Farolino DL, Rustagi PK, Currie MS, et al. Teardrop-shaped red cells in autoimmune hemolytic anemia. Am J Hematol. 1986;21:415-418.

99. Ehrlich P. Farbenanalytische Untersuchungen zur Histologie und Klinik des Blutes. Berlin, Hirschwald, 1891, p 104.

100. Stefanelli M, Barosi G, Cazzola M, Orlandi E. Quantitative assessment of erythropoiesis in haemolytic disease. Br J Haematol. 1980;45:297-308.

101. Olcay L, Duzova, A, Gumruk F. A warm antibody mediated acute hemolytic anemia with reticulocytopenia in a four-month-old girl requiring immunosuppressive therapy. Turk J Pediatr. 1999;41:239-244.

102. Jastaniah WA, Pritchard SL, Wu JK, Wadsworth LD. Hyperuricemia and reticulocytopenia in association with autoimmune hemolytic anemia in two children. Am J Clin Pathol. 2004;122:849-854.

103. Liesveld JL, Rowe JM, Lichtman MA. Variability of the erythropoietic response in autoimmune hemolytic anemia: analysis of 109 cases. Blood. 1987;69:820-826.

104. Van De Loosdrecht AA, Hendriks DW, Blom NR, et al. Excessive apoptosis of bone marrow erythroblasts in a patient with autoimmune haemolytic anaemia with reticulocytopenia. Br J Haematol. 2000;108:313-315.

105. Bertrand Y, Lefrere JJ, Leverger G, et al. Autoimmune haemolytic anaemia revealed by human parvovirus linked erythroblastopenia. Lancet. 1985;2:382-383.

106. Smith MA, Shah NS, Lobel JS. Parvovirus B19 infection associated with reticulocytopenia and chronic autoimmune hemolytic anemia. Am J Pediatr Hematol Oncol. 1989;11:167-169.

107. Sadrzadeh SM, Bozorgmehr J. Haptoglobin phenotypes in health and disorders. Am J Clin Pathol. 2004;121: S97-S104.

108. Garratty G. Immune hemolytic anemia associated with negative routine serology. Semin Hematol. 2005;42:156-164.

109. Sokol RJ, Hewitt S, Booker DJ, Stamps R. Small quantities of erythrocyte bound immunoglobulins and autoimmune haemolysis. J Clin Pathol. 1987;40:254-257.

110. Dutta P, Chatterjee T, Tyagi S, et al. Gel card in the diagnosis of autoimmune hemolytic anemia. Indian J Pathol Microbiol. 2005;48:322-324.

111. Chaudhary R, Das SS, Gupta R, Khetan D. Application of flow cytometry in detection of red-cell-bound IgG in Coombs-negative AIHA. Hematology. 2006;11: 295-300.

112. Angevine CD, Anderson BR, Barnett EV. A cold agglutinin of the IgA class. J Immunol. 1966;96:578-586.

113. Suzuki S, Amano T, Mitsunaga M, et al. Autoimmune hemolytic anemia associated with IgA autoantibody. Clin Immunol Immunopathol. 1981;21:247-256.

114. Kowal-Vern A, Jacobson P, Okuno T, Blank J. Negative direct antiglobulin test in autoimmune hemolytic anemia. Am J Pediatr Hematol Oncol. 1986;8:349-351.

115. Freedman J, Wright J, Lim FC, Garvey MB. Hemolytic warm IgM autoagglutinins in autoimmune hemolytic anemia. Transfusion. 1987;27:464-467.

116. Shirey RS, Kickler TS, Bell W, et al. Fatal immune hemolytic anemia and hepatic failure associated with a warm-reacting IgM autoantibody. Vox Sang. 1987;52:219-222.

117. Friedmann AM, King KE, Shirey RS, et al. Fatal autoimmune hemolytic anemia in a child due to warm-reactive immunoglobulin M antibody. J Pediatr Hematol Oncol. 1998;20:502-505.

118. Worlledge SM. The interpretation of a positive direct antiglobulin test. Br J Haematol. 1978;39:157-162.

119. Gorst DW, Rawlinson VI, Merry AH, Stratton F. Positive direct antiglobulin test in normal individuals. Vox Sang. 1980;38:99-105.

120. Bareford D, Longster G, Gilks L, Tovey LA. Follow-up of normal individuals with a positive antiglobulin test. Scand J Haematol. 1985;35:348-353.

121. Poon LM, Kuperan P. Fatal *Clostridium* septicaemia associated with massive intravascular haemolysis in a previously healthy woman. Ann Acad Med Singapore. 2007;36:213-214.

122. Grudeva-Popova JG, Spasova MI, Chepileva KG, Zaprianov ZH. Acute hemolytic anemia as an initial clinical manifestation of Wilson's disease. Folia Med. 2000; 42:42-46.

123. Broliden K, Tolfvenstam T, Norbeck O. Clinical aspects of parvovirus B19 infection. J Int Med. 2006;260:285-304.

124. Garratty G. Mechanisms of immune red cell destruction, and red cell compatibility testing. Hum Pathol. 1983;14: 204-212.

125. Wolf MW, Roelcke D. Incomplete warm hemolysins. I. Case reports, serology, and immunoglobulin classes. Clin Immunol Immunopathol. 1989;51:55-67.

126. Wolf MW, Roelcke D. Incomplete warm hemolysins. II. Corresponding antigens and pathogenetic mechanisms in autoimmune hemolytic anemias induced by incomplete warm hemolysins. Clin Immunol Immunopathol. 1989;51: 68-76.

127. Smith LA. Autoimmune hemolytic anemias: characteristics and classification. Clin Lab Sci. 1999;12:110-114.

128. Wang Z, Shi J, Zhou Y, Ruan C. Detection of red blood cell–bound immunoglobulin G by flow cytometry and its application in the diagnosis of autoimmune hemolytic anemia. Int J Hematol. 2001;73:188-193.

129. Znazen R, Kaabi H, Hmida S, et al. Detection of serum hemolysins in autoimmune hemolytic anemia. Trans Clin Biol. 2006;13:341-345.

130. Zarandona JM, Yazer MH. The role of the Coombs test in evaluating hemolysis in adults. Can Med Assoc J. 2006;174:305-307.

131. Engelfriet CP, Overbeeke MA, von dem Borne AE. Autoimmune hemolytic anemia. Semin Hematol. 1992;29: 3-12.

132. Ishizaka T, Ishizaka K, Salmon S, Fudenberg H. Biologic activities of aggregated γ-globulin. VIII. Aggregated immu-

noglobulins of different classes. J Immunol. 1967;99: 82-91.

133. Augener W, Grey HM, Cooper N, Müller-Eberhard HJ. The reaction of monomeric and aggregated immunoglobulins with C1. Immunochemistry. 1971;8:1011-1020.

134. von dem Borne AE, Beckers D, van der Meulen FW, Engelfriet CP. IgG4 autoantibodies against erythrocytes, without increased haemolysis: a case report. Br J Haematol. 1977;37:137-144.

135. Silberstein LE, Berkman EM, Schreiber AD. Cold hemagglutinin disease associated with IgG cold-reactive antibody. Ann Intern Med. 1987;106:238-242.

136. Durand JM, Salas S, Gauthier C, et al. Danger of anti-erythrocyte antibodies during pregnancy. Rev Med Interne. 1999;20:693-695.

137. Passi GR, Kriplani A, Pati HP, Choudhry VP. Isoimmune hemolysis in an infant due to maternal Evans' syndrome. Indian J Pediatr. 1997;64:893-895.

138. Motta M, Cavazza A, Migliori C, Chirico G. Autoimmune haemolytic anaemia in a newborn infant. Arch Dis Child Fetal Neonatal Ed. 2003;88:F341-F342.

139. Wilson ML, Menjivar E, Kalapatapu V, et al. *Mycoplasma pneumoniae* associated with hemolytic anemia, cold agglutinins, and recurrent arterial thrombosis. South Med J. 2007;100:215-217.

140. Salama A, Mueller-Eckhardt C. Autoimmune haemolytic anaemia in childhood associated with non–complement binding IgM autoantibodies. Br J Haematol. 1987;65: 67-71.

141. Gottsche B, Salama A, Mueller-Eckhardt C. Autoimmune hemolytic anemia associated with an IgA autoanti-Gerbich. Vox Sang. 1990;58:211-214.

142. Sokol RJ, Hewitt S, Stamps BK. Autoimmune hemolysis: mixed warm and cold antibody type. Acta Haematol. 1983;69:266-274.

143. Silberstein LE, Shoenfeld Y, Schwartz RS, Berkman EM. Combination of IgG and IgM autoantibodies in chronic cold agglutinin disease: immunologic studies and response to splenectomy. Vox Sang. 1985;48:105-109.

144. Shulman IA, Branch DR, Nelson JM, et al. Autoimmune hemolytic anemia with both cold and warm autoantibodies. JAMA. 1985;253:1746-1748.

145. Freedman J, Lim FC, Musclow E, et al. Autoimmune hemolytic anemia with concurrence of warm and cold red cell autoantibodies and a warm hemolysin. Transfusion. 1985;25:368-372.

146. Issitt PD, Anstee DJ. Applied Blood Group Serology, 4th ed. Durham, NC, Montgomery Scientific Publications, 1998, p 1004.

147. Szymanski IO, Huff SR, Selbovitz LG, Sherwood GK. Erythrocyte sensitization with monomeric IgM in a patient with hemolytic anemia. Am J Hematol. 1984;17:71-77.

148. Barker RN, Casswell KM, Reid ME, et al. Identification of autoantigens in autoimmune haemolytic anaemia by a non-radioisotope immunoprecipitation method. Br J Haematol. 1992;82:126-132.

149. Leddy JP, Falany JL, Kissel GE, et al. Erythrocyte membrane proteins reactive with human (warm-reacting) anti–red cell autoantibodies. J Clin Invest. 1993;91:1672-1680.

150. Lim YA, Kim MK, Hyun BH. Autoimmune hemolytic anemia predominantly associated with IgA anti-E and anti-c. J Korean Med Sci. 2002;17:708-711.

151. Wakui H, Imai H, Kobayashi R, et al. Autoantibody against erythrocyte protein 4.1 in a patient with auto-immune hemolytic anemia. Blood. 1988;72:408-412.

152. Janvier D, Sellami F, Missud F, et al. Severe autoimmune hemolytic anemia caused by a warm IgA autoantibody directed against the third loop of band 3 (RBC anion-exchange protein 1). Transfusion. 2002;42:1547-1552.

153. Win N, Kaye T, Mir N, et al. Autoimmune haemolytic anaemia in infancy with anti-Kpb specificity. Vox Sang. 1996;71:187-188.

154. Immel CC, McPherson M, Hay SN, et al. Severe hemolytic anemia due to auto anti-N. Immunohematology. 2005;21:63-65.

155. Szymanski IO, Roberts PL, Rosenfield RE. Anti-A auto-antibody with severe intravascular hemolysis. N Engl J Med. 1976;294:995-996.

156. Sokol RJ, Booker DJ, Stamps R, Windle JA. Autoimmune haemolysis and red cell autoantibodies with ABO blood group specificity. Haematologia. 1995;26:121-129.

157. Marsh WL, Oyen R, Alicea E, et al. Autoimmune hemolytic anemia and the Kell blood groups. Am J Hematol. 1979;7:155-162.

158. von dem Borne AE, Mol JJ, Joustra-Maas N, et al. Autoimmune haemolytic anaemia with monoclonal IgM (K) anti-P cold autohaemolysins. Br J Haematol. 1982;50: 345-350.

159. Longster GH, Johnson E. IgM anti-D as auto-antibody in a case of "cold" auto-immune haemolytic anaemia. Vox Sang. 1988;54:174-176.

160. Rousey SR, Smith RE. A fatal case of low titer anti-Pr cold agglutinin disease. Am J Hematol. 1990;35: 286-287.

161. Levine P, Celano MJ, Falkowski F. The specificity of the antibody in paroxysmal cold hemoglobinuria (P.C.H.). Transfusion. 1963;3:278-280.

162. Garratty G, Nance SJ. Correlation between in vivo hemolysis and the amount of red cell–bound IgG measured by flow cytometry. Transfusion. 1990;30:617-621.

163. Zupanska B, Sokol RJ, Booker DJ, Stamps R. Erythrocyte autoantibodies, the monocyte monolayer assay and in vivo haemolysis. Br J Haematol. 1993;84:144-150.

164. Biondi C, Cotorruelo C, Garcia Borras S, et al. Erythrophagocytosis assay in patients with autoimmune hemolytic anemia. Medicine (B Aires). 2001;61:49-52.

165. Biondi CS, Cotorruelo CM, Ensinck A, et al. Use of the erythrophagocytosis assay for predicting the clinical consequences of immune blood cell destruction. Clin Lab. 2004;50:265-270.

166. Ravetch JV, Bolland S. IgG Fc receptors. Annu Rev Immunol. 2001;19:275-290.

167. Ferreira JA, Feliu E, Rozman C, et al. Morphologic and morphometric light and electron microscopic studies of the spleen in patients with hereditary spherocytosis and autoimmune haemolytic anaemia. Br J Haematol. 1989;72:246-253.

168. Fischer JT, Petz LD, Garratty G, Cooper NR. Correlations between quantitative assay of red cell–bound C3, serologic reactions, and hemolytic anemia. Blood. 1974;44: 359-373.

169. Logue GL, Rosse WF, Gockerman JP. Measurement of the third component of complement bound to red blood cells in patients with the cold agglutinin syndrome. J Clin Invest. 1973;52:493-501.

170. Jaffe CH, Atkinson JP, Frank MM. The role of complement in the clearance of cold agglutinin–sensitized erythrocytes in man. J Clin Invest. 1976;58:942-949.

171. Garratty G, Petz LD. Transfusing patients with autoimmune haemolytic anaemia. Lancet. 1993;341:1220.

172. Sokol RJ, Hewitt S, Booker DJ, Morris BM. Patients with red cell autoantibodies: selection of blood for transfusion. Clin Lab Haematol. 1988;10:257-264.

173. James P, Rowe GP, Tozzo GG. Elucidation of alloantibodies in autoimmune haemolytic anaemia. Vox Sang. 1988;54:167-171.

174. Engelfriet CP, Reesink HW, Garratty G, et al. The detection of alloantibodies against red cells in patients with warm-type autoimmune haemolytic anaemia. Vox Sang. 2000;78:200-207.

175. Petz LD. Transfusing the patient with autoimmune hemolytic anemia. Clin Lab Med. 1982;2:193-210.

176. Wallhermfechtel MA, Pohl BA, Chaplin H. Alloimmunization in patients with warm autoantibodies. A retrospective study employing three donor alloabsorptions to aid in antibody detection. Transfusion. 1984;24:482-485.

177. Salama A, Berghofer H, Mueller-Eckhardt C. Red blood cell transfusion in warm-type autoimmune haemolytic anaemia. Lancet. 1992;340:1515-1517.

178. Mullon J, Giacoppe G, Clagett C, et al. Transfusions of polymerized bovine hemoglobin in a patient with severe autoimmune hemolytic anemia. N Engl J Med. 2000;342:1638-1643.

179. Klein HG. The prospects for red-cell substitutes. N Engl J Med. 2000;342:1666-1668.

180. Dameshek W, Rosenthal MC, Schwartz LI. The treatment of acquired hemolytic anemia with adrenocorticotrophic hormone (ACTH). N Engl J Med. 1951;244:117-127.

181. Fries LF, Brickman CM, Frank MM. Monocyte receptors for the Fc portion of IgG increase in number in autoimmune hemolytic anemia and other hemolytic states and are decreased by glucocorticoid therapy. J Immunol. 1983;131:1240-1245.

182. Collins PW, Newland AC. Treatment modalities of autoimmune blood disorders. Semin Hematol. 1992;29:64-74.

183. Meytes D, Adler M, Virag I, et al. High dose methylprednisolone in acute immune cold hemolysis. N Engl J Med. 1985;312:318.

184. Ware R, Kinney TR. Therapeutic considerations in childhood idiopathic thrombocytopenic purpura. Crit Rev Oncol Hematol. 1987;7:169-181.

185. Fehr J, Hofmann V, Kappeler U. Transient reversal of thrombocytopenia in idiopathic thrombocytopenic purpura by high-dose intravenous gamma globulin. N Engl J Med. 1982;306:1254-1258.

186. Salama A, Mueller-Eckhardt C, Kiefel V. Effect of intravenous immunoglobulin in immune thrombocytopenia: competitive inhibition of reticuloendothelial system function by sequestration of autologous red blood cells? Lancet. 1983;2:193-195.

187. Mueller-Eckhardt C, Salama A, Mahn I, et al. Lack of efficacy of high-dose intravenous immunoglobulin in autoimmune hemolytic anemia: a clue to its mechanism. Scand J Hematol. 1985;34:394-400.

188. Hilgartner MW, Bussel J. Use of intravenous gamma globulin for the treatment of autoimmune neutropenia of childhood and autoimmune hemolytic anemia. Am J Med. 1987;83:25-29.

189. Flores G, Cunningham-Rundles C, Newland AC, et al. Efficacy of intravenous immunoglobulin in the treatment of autoimmune hemolytic anemia: results in 73 patients. Am J Hematol. 1993;44:237-242.

190. Mahadevia PJ. The pocketbook: pharmacoeconomic issues related to intravenous immunoglobulin therapy. Pharmacotherapy. 2005;25:94S-100S.

191. Sapir T, Blank M, Shoenfeld Y. Immunomodulatory effects of intravenous immunoglobulins as a treatment for autoimmune diseases, cancer, and recurrent pregnancy loss. Ann N Y Acad Sci. 2005;1051:743-778.

192. Koo AP. Therapeutic apheresis in autoimmune and rheumatic diseases. J Clin Apheresis. 2000;15:18-27.

193. Azuma E, Nishihara H, Hanada M, et al. Recurrent cold hemagglutinin disease following allogeneic bone marrow transplantation successfully treated with plasmapheresis, corticosteroid, and cyclophosphamide. Bone Marrow Transplant. 1996;18:243-246.

194. Olcay L, Koc A. Autoimmune hemolytic anemia preceding T-ALL in a five-year-old girl. Pediatr Hematol Oncol. 2005;22:207-213.

195. Siami GA, Siami FS. Plasmapheresis and paraproteinemia: cryoprotein-induced diseases, monoclonal gammopathy, Waldenström's macroglobulinemia, hyperviscosity syndrome, multiple myeloma, light chain disease, and amyloidosis. Ther Apheresis. 1999;3:8-19.

196. McConnell ME, Atchison JA, Kohaut E, et al. Successful use of plasma exchange in a child with refractory immune hemolytic anemia. Am J Pediatr Hematol Oncol. 1987;9:158-160.

197. McCarthy LJ, Danielson CF, Fernandez C, et al. Intensive plasma exchange for severe autoimmune hemolytic anemia in a four-month-old infant. J Clin Apheresis. 1999;14:190-192.

198. Current status of therapeutic plasmapheresis and related techniques. Report of the AMA panel on therapeutic plasmapheresis. Council on Scientific Affairs. JAMA. 1985;253:819-825.

199. Roy-Burman A, Glader BE. Resolution of severe Donath-Landsteiner autoimmune hemolytic anemia temporally associated with institution of plasmapheresis. Crit Care Med. 2002;30:931-934.

200. Andrzejewski C Jr, Gault E, Briggs M, et al. Benefit of a 37°C extracorporeal circuit in plasma exchange therapy for selected cases with cold agglutinin disease. J Clin Apheresis. 1988;4:13-17.

201. Ruivard M, Tournihac O, Montel S, et al. Plasma exchanges do not increase red blood cell transfusion efficiency in severe autoimmune hemolytic anemia: a retrospective case-control study. J Clin Apheresis. 2006;21:202-206.

202. Shan D, Ledbetter JA, Press OW. Signaling events involved in anti-CD20–induced apoptosis of malignant human B cells. Can Immunol Immunother. 2000;48:673-683.

203. Davis TA, Grillo-Lopez AJ, White CA, et al. Rituximab anti-CD20 monoclonal antibody therapy in non-Hodgkin's lymphoma: safety and efficacy of re-treatment. J Clin Oncol. 2000;18:3135-3143.

204. Giulino LB, Bussel JB, Neufeld EJ, Pediatric and Platelet Immunology Committees of the TMH Clinical Trial Network. Treatment with rituximab in benign and

malignant hematologic disorders in children. J Pediatr. 2007;150:338-344.

205. Quartier P, Brethon B, Philippet P, et al. Treatment of childhood autoimmune haemolytic anemia with rituximab. Lancet. 2001;358:1511-1513.

206. Motto DG, Williams JA, Boxer LA. Rituximab for refractory childhood autoimmune hemolytic anemia. Isr Med Assoc J. 2002;4:1006-1008.

207. Zecca M, Nobili B, Ramenghi U, et al. Rituximab for the treatment of refractory autoimmune hemolytic anemia in children. Blood. 2003;101:3857-3861.

208. Chertkow G, Dacie JV. Results of splenectomy in autoimmune haemolytic anaemia. Br J Haematol. 1956;2: 237-249.

209. Dacie JV. Autoimmune hemolytic anaemia. Arch Intern Med. 1975;135:1293-1300.

210. Mollison PL. Survival curves of incompatible red cells. An analytical review. Transfusion. 1986;26:43-50.

211. Parker AC, Macpherson AIS, Richmond J. Value of radiochromium investigation in autoimmune haemolytic anaemia. BMJ. 1977;1:208-209.

212. Coon WW. Splenectomy in the treatment of hemolytic anemia. Arch Surg. 1985;120:625-628.

213. Grinblat J, Billoa Y. Overwhelming pneumococcal sepsis 25 years after splenectomy. Am J Med Sci. 1975;270: 523-524.

214. McMullin M, Johnston G. Long term management of patients after splenectomy. BMJ. 1993;307:1372-1373.

215. Meyer O, Stahl D, Beckhove P, et al. Pulsed high-dose dexamethasone in chronic autoimmune haemolytic anaemia of warm type. Br J Haematol. 1997;98:860-862.

216. Chan AC, Sack K. Danazol therapy in autoimmune hemolytic anemia associated with systemic lupus erythematosus. J Rheumatol. 1991;18:280-282.

217. Pignon J-M, Poirson E, Rochant H. Danazol in autoimmune haemolytic anaemia. Br J Haematol. 1993;83: 343-345.

218. Agnello V, Pariser K, Gell J, et al. Preliminary observations on danazol therapy of systemic lupus erythematosus: effects on DNA antibodies, thrombocytopenia and complement. J Rheumatol. 1983;10:682-687.

219. Gertz MA, Petitt RM, Pineda AA, et al. Vinblastine-loaded platelets for autoimmune hemolytic anemia. Ann Intern Med. 1981;95:325-326.

220. Medellin PL, Patten E, Weiss GB. Vinblastine for autoimmune hemolytic anemia. Ann Intern Med. 1982;96:123.

221. Seiber SM, Adamson RH. Toxicity of antineoplastic agents in man: chromosomal aberrations, antifertility effects, congenital malformations, and carcinogenic potential. Adv Cancer Res. 1975;22:57-155.

222. Panceri R, Fraschini D, Tornotti G, et al. Successful use of high-dose cyclophosphamide in a child with severe autoimmune hemolytic anemia. Haematologica. 1992;77: 76-78.

223. Brodsky RA, Petri M, Smith BD, et al. Immunoablative high-dose cyclophosphamide without stem-cell rescue for refractory, severe autoimmune disease. Ann Intern Med. 1998;129:1031-1035.

224. Moyo VM, Smith D, Brodsky I, et al. High-dose cyclophosphamide for refractory autoimmune hemolytic anemia. Blood. 2002;100:704-706.

225. Dündar S, Ozdemir O, Ozcebe O. Cyclosporin in steroid-resistant autoimmune haemolytic anaemia. Acta Haematol. 1991;86:200-202.

226. Marsh JC, Gordon-Smith EC. CAMPATH-1H in the treatment of autoimmune cytopenias. Cytotherapy. 2001;3:189-195.

227. O'Connor BM, Clifford JS, Lawrence WD, Logue GL. Alpha-interferon for severe cold agglutinin disease. Ann Intern Med. 1989;111:255-256.

228. Berney T, Shibata T, Merino R, et al. Murine autoimmune hemolytic anemia resulting from Fcγ receptor–mediated erythrophagocytosis: protection by erythropoietin but not by interleukin-3, and aggravation by granulocyte-macrophage colony-stimulating factor. Blood. 1992;79: 2960-2964.

229. Tyndall A, Gratwohl A. Blood and marrow stem cell transplants in auto-immune disease: a consensus report written on behalf of the European League against Rheumatism (EULAR) and the European Group for Blood and Marrow Transplantation (EBMT). Bone Marrow Transplant. 1997;19:643-645.

230. De Stefano P, Zecca M, Giorgiani G, et al. Resolution of immune haemolytic anaemia with allogeneic bone marrow transplantation after an unsuccessful autograft. Br J Haematol. 1999;106:1063-1064.

231. Paillard C, Kanold J, Halle P, et al. Two-step immunoablative treatment with autologous peripheral blood CD34+ cell transplantation in an 8 year old boy with autoimmune haemolytic anaemia. Br J Haematol. 2000;110:900-902.

232. Horn B, Viele M, Mentzer W, et al. Autoimmune hemolytic anemia in patients with SCID after T cell–depleted BM and PBSC transplantation. Bone Marrow Transplant. 1999;24:1009-1013.

233. Azuma E, Nishihara H, Hanada M, et al. Recurrent cold hemagglutinin disease following allogeneic bone marrow transplantation successfully treated with plasmapheresis, corticosteroid and cyclophosphamide. Bone Marrow Transplant. 1996;18:243-246.

234. Toriani-Terenzi C, Fagiolo E. IL-10 and the cytokine network in the pathogenesis of human autoimmune hemolytic anemia. Ann N Y Acad Sci. 2005;1051:29-44.

235. Semple JW, Freedman J. Autoimmune pathogenesis and autoimmune hemolytic anemia. Semin Hematol. 2005;42: 122-130.

236. Abdel-Khalik A, Paton L, White AG, et al. Human leucocyte antigens A, B, C, and DRW in idiopathic "warm" autoimmune haemolytic anaemia. BMJ. 1980;280: 760-761.

237. Kleiner-Baumgarten A, Schlaeffer F, Keynan A. Multiple autoimmune manifestations in a splenectomized subject with HLA-B8. Arch Intern Med. 1983;143:1987-1989.

238. Lortholary O, Valeyre D, Gayraud M, et al. Autoimmune haemolytic anaemia and idiopathic pulmonary fibrosis associated with HLA-B27 antigen. Eur J Haematol. 1990;45:112-113.

239. Wang-Rodriguez J, Rearden A. Reduced frequency of HLA-DQ6 in individuals with a positive direct antiglobulin test. Transfusion. 1996;36:979-984.

240. Kikuchi S, Amano H, Amano E, et al. Identification of 2 major loci linked to autoimmune hemolytic anemia in NZB mice. Blood. 2005;106:1323-1329.

241. Pavkovic M, Georgievski B, Cevreska L, et al. CTLA-4 exon 1 polymorphism in patients with autoimmune blood disorders. Am J Hematol. 2003;72:147-149.

242. Davies JK, Telfer P, Cavenagh JD, et al. Autoimmune cytopenias in the 22q11.2 deletion syndrome. Clin Lab Haematol. 2003;25:195-197.

243. Gordon J, Silberstein L, Moreau L, Nowell PC. Trisomy 3 in cold agglutinin disease. Cancer Genet Cytogenet. 1990;46:89-92.

244. Sokol RJ, Booker DH, Stamps R, et al. IgA red cell auto-antibodies and autoimmune hemolysis. Transfusion. 1997; 37:175-181.

245. Perl A. Pathogenesis and spectrum of autoimmunity. Methods Mol Med. 2004;102:1-8.

246. Sanz I, Casali P, Thomas JW, et al. Nucleotide sequences of eight human natural autoantibody V_H regions reveals apparent restricted use of V_H families. J Immunol. 1989; 142:4054-4061.

247. Potter NK. Molecular characterization of cold agglutinins. Trans Sci. 2000;22:113-119.

248. Silberstein LE, Jefferies LC, Goldman J, et al. Variable region gene analysis of pathologic human autoantibodies to the related i and I red blood cell antigens. Blood. 1991;78:2372-2386.

249. Ohmori H, Kanayama N. Mechanisms leading to autoantibody production: link between inflammation and autoimmunity. Curr Drug Targets Inflamm Allergy. 2003;2: 232-241.

250. Quintana FJ, Cohen IR. The natural autoantibody repertoire and autoimmune disease. Biomed Pharacother. 2004;58:276-281.

251. Terness PI, Navolan D, Dufter C, et al. Immunosuppressive anti-immunoglobulin autoantibodies: specificity, gene structure and function in health and disease. Cell Mol Biol. 2002;48:271-278.

252. Stahl D, Lacroix-Desmazes S, Heudes D, et al. Altered control of self-reactive IgG by autologous IgM in patients with warm autoimmune hemolytic anemia. Blood. 2000;95:328-335.

253. Hoyer BF, Manz RA, Radbruch A, Hiepe F. Long-lived plasma cells and their contribution to autoimmunity. Ann N Y Acad Sci. 2005;1050:124-133.

254. Ruzickova S, Pruss A, Odendahl M, et al. Chronic lymphocytic leukemia preceded by cold agglutinin disease: intraclonal immunoglobulin light-chain diversity in V(H)4-34 expressing single leukemic B cells. Blood. 2002; 100:3419-3422.

255. Efremov DG, Ivanovski M, Burrone OR. The pathologic significance of the immunoglobulins expressed by chronic lymphocytic leukemia B-cells in the development of autoimmune hemolytic anemia. Leuk Lymphoma. 1998;28: 285-293.

256. Martin DA, Elkon KB. Autoantibodies make a U-turn: the toll hypothesis for autoantibody specificity. J Exp Med. 2005;202:1465-1469.

257. Viau M, Zouali M. B-lymphocytes, innate immunity, and autoimmunity. Clin Immunol. 2005;114:17-26.

258. Zouali M. B cell diversity and longevity in systemic autoimmunity. Mol Immunol. 2002;38:895-901.

259. Ochi H, Takeshita H, Suda T, et al. Regulation of B-1 cell activation and its autoantibody production by Lyn kinase–regulated signallings. Immunology. 1999;98:595-603.

260. Young JL, Hooper DC. Characterization of autoreactive helper T cells in a murine model of autoimmune hemolytic disease. Immunology. 1993;80:13-21.

261. Barker RN, Hall AM, Standen GR, et al. Identification of T-cell epitopes on the rhesus polypeptides in autoimmune hemolytic anemia. Blood. 1997;90:2701-2715.

262. Shen CR, Youssef AR, Devine A, et al. Peptides containing a dominant T-cell epitope from red cell band 3 have in vivo immunomodulatory properties in NZB mice with autoimmune hemolytic anemia. Blood. 2003;102:3800-3806.

263. Shen CR, Ward FJ, Devine A. Characterization of the dominant autoreactive T-cell epitope in spontaneous autoimmune haemolytic anaemia of the NZB mouse. J Autoimmun. 2002;18:149-157.

264. O'Brien TA, Eastlund T, Peters C, et al. Autoimmune haemolytic anaemia complicating haematopoietic cell transplantation in paediatric patients: high incidence and significant mortality in unrelated donor transplants for non-malignant diseases. Br J Haematol. 2004;127: 67-75.

265. Sanz J, Arriaga F, Montesinos P, et al. Autoimmune hemolytic anemia following allogeneic hematopoietic stem cell transplantation in adult patients. Bone Marrow Transplant. 2007;39:555-561.

266. Hilgendorf I, Wolff D, Wilhelm S, et al. T-cell–depleted stem cell boost for the treatment of autoimmune haemolytic anaemia after T-cell–depleted allogeneic bone marrow transplantation complicated by adenovirus infection. Bone Marrow Transplant. 2006;37:977-978.

267. Koduri PR, Singa P, Nikolinakos P. Autoimmune hemolytic anemia in patients infected with human immunodeficiency virus-1. Am J Hematol. 2002;70: 174-176.

268. Saif MW. HIV-associated autoimmune hemolytic anemia: an update. AIDS Patient Care STDS. 2001;15:217-224.

269. Fagiolo E, Terenzi CT. Enhanced IL-10 production in vitro by monocytes in autoimmune haemolytic anaemia. Immunol Invest. 1999;28:347-352.

270. Barcellini W, Clerici G, Montesano R, et al. In vitro quantification of anti–red blood cell antibody production in idiopathic autoimmune haemolytic anaemia: effect of mitogen and cytokine stimulation. Br J Haematol. 2000;111:452-460.

271. Fagiolo E, Toriani-Terenzi. Th1 and Th2 cytokine modulation by IL-10/IL-12 imbalance in autoimmune heaemolytic anaemia (AIHA). Autoimmunity. 2002;35: 39-44.

272. Kunitomi A, Konaka Y, Yagita M, et al. Humanized anti–interleukin 6 receptor antibody induced long-term remission in a patient with life-threatening refractory autoimmune hemolytic anemia. Int J Hematol. 2004;80: 246-249.

273. Meyer D, Schiller C, Westermann J, et al. FcγRIII (CD16)-deficient mice show IgG isotype–dependent protection to experimental autoimmune hemolytic anemia. Blood. 1998;92:3997-4002.

274. Fong KY, Loisou S, Boey ML, Walport MJ. Anticardiolipin antibodies, haemolytic anaemia and thrombocytopenia in systemic lupus erythematosus. Br J Rheumatol. 1992;31:453-455.

275. Kondo H, Sakai S, Sakai Y. Autoimmune haemolytic anaemia, Sjögren's syndrome and idiopathic thrombocytopenic purpura in a patient with sarcoidosis. Acta Haematol. 1993;89:209-212.

276. Jones E, Jones JV, Woodbury JFL, et al. Scleroderma and hemolytic anemia in a patient with deficiency of IgA and C4: a hitherto undescribed association. J Rheumatol. 1987;14:609-612.

277. Hay EM, Makris M, Winfield J, Winfield DA. Evans' syndrome associated with dermatomyositis. Ann Rheum Dis. 1990;49:793-794.

278. Veloso T, Fraga J, Carvalho J, et al. Autoimmune hemolytic anemia in ulcerative colitis. A case report with review of the literature. J Clin Gastroenterol. 1991;13: 445-447.

279. Hochman JA. Autoimmune hemolytic anemia associated with Crohn's disease. Inflamm Bowel Dis. 2002;8:98-100.

280. Kang MY, Hahm JR, Jung TS, et al. A 20-year-old woman with Hashimoto's thyroiditis and Evans' syndrome. Yonsei Med J. 2006;47:432-436.

281. Mauro FR, Foa R, Cerretti R, et al. Autoimmune hemolytic anemia in chronic lymphocytic leukemia: clinical, therapeutic, and prognostic features. Blood. 2000;95:2786-2792.

282. Sallah S, Sigounas G, Vos P, et al. Autoimmune hemolytic anemia in patients with non-Hodgkin's lymphoma: characteristics and significance. Ann Oncol. 2000;11:1571-1577.

283. Pereira A, Mazzara R, Escoda L, et al. Anti-Sa cold agglutinin of IgA class requiring plasma-exchange therapy as early manifestation of multiple myeloma. Ann Hematol. 1993;66:315-318.

284. Koksal Y, Calikan U, Ucar C, et al. Autoimmune hemolytic anemia as presenting manifestation of primary splenic anaplastic large cell lymphoma. Turk J Pediatr. 2006;48: 354-356.

285. Xiros N, Binder T, Anger B, et al. Idiopathic thrombocytopenic purpura and autoimmune hemolytic anemia in Hodgkin's disease. Eur J Haematol. 1988;40:437-441.

286. Arbaje YM, Beltran G. Chronic myelogenous leukemia complicated by autoimmune hemolytic anemia. Am J Med. 1990;88:197-199.

287. Sokol RJ, Hewitt S, Booker DJ. Erythrocyte autoantibodies, autoimmune haemolysis, and myelodysplastic syndromes. J Clin Pathol. 1989;42:1088-1091.

288. Blanchette VS, Hallett JJ, Hemphill JM, et al. Abnormalities of the peripheral blood as a presenting feature of immunodeficiency. Am J Hematol. 1978;4:87-92.

289. Heeney MM, Zimmerman SA, Ware RE. Childhood autoimmune cytopenia secondary to unsuspected common variable immunodeficiency. J Pediatr. 2003;143:662-665.

290. Wang J, Cunningham-Rundles C. Treatment and outcome of autoimmune hematologic disease in common variable immunodeficiency (CVID). J Autoimmun. 2005;25: 57-62.

291. Leickly FE, Buckley RH. Successful treatment of autoimmune hemolytic anemia in common variable immunodeficiency with high-dose intravenous gamma globulin. Am J Med. 1987;82:159-162.

292. Wakim M, Shah A, Arndt PA, et al. Successful anti-CD20 monoclonal antibody treatment of severe autoimmune hemolytic anemia due to warm reactive IgM autoantibody in a child with common variable immunodeficiency. Am J Hematol. 2004;76:152-155.

293. Dupuis-Girod S, Medioni J, Haddad E, et al. Autoimmunity in Wiskott-Aldrich syndrome: risk factors, clinical features, and outcome in a single-center cohort of 35 patients. Pediatrics. 2003;111:e622-e627.

294. Bapat AR, Schuster SJ, Dahlke M, Ballas SK. Thrombocytopenia and autoimmune hemolytic anemia following renal transplantation. Transplantation. 1987;44:157-159.

295. Tubman VN, Smoot L, Heeney MM. Acquired immune cytopenias post–cardiac transplantation respond to rituximab. Pediatr Blood Cancer. 2007;48:339-344.

296. Pui C-H, Wilimas J, Wang W. Evans syndrome in childhood. J Pediatr. 1980;97:754-758.

297. Norton A, Roberts I. Management of Evans syndrome. Br J Haematol. 2005;132:125-137.

298. Wang W, Herrod H, Pui C-H, et al. Immunoregulatory abnormalities in Evans syndrome. Am J Hematol. 1983;15: 381-390.

299. Pegels JG, Helmerhorst FM, van Leeuwen EF, et al. The Evans syndrome: characterization of the responsible autoantibodies. Br J Haematol. 1982;51:445-450.

300. Williams JA, Boxer LA. Combination therapy for refractory idiopathic thrombocytopenia in adolescents. J Pediatr Hematol Oncol. 2003;25:232-235.

301. El-Hallak M, Binstadt BA, Leichtner AM, et al. Clinical effects and safety of rituximab for treatment of refractory pediatric autoimmune diseases. J Pediatr. 2007;150: 376-382.

302. Urban C, Lackner H, Sovinz P, et al. Successful unrelated cord blood transplantation in a 7-year-old body with Evans syndrome refractory to immunosuppression and double autologous stem cell transplantation. Eur J Haematol. 2006;76:526-530.

303. Canale VC, Smith CH. Chronic lymphadenopathy simulating malignant lymphoma. J Pediatr. 1967;70:891-899.

304. Takahasi T, Tanaka M, Brannan CI, et al. Generalized lymphoproliferative disease in mice, caused by a point mutation in the Fas ligand. Cell. 1994;76:969-976.

305. Watanabe-Fukunaga R, Brannan CI, Copeland NG, et al. Lymphoproliferation disorder in mice explained by defects in Fas antigen that mediates apoptosis. Nature. 1992;356: 314-317.

306. Fisher GH, Rosenberg FJ, Straus SE, et al. Dominant interfering Fas gene mutations impair apoptosis in a human autoimmune lymphoproliferative syndrome. Cell. 1995;81:935-946.

307. Rieux-Laucat F, Le Deist F, Hivroz C, et al. Mutations in Fas associated with human lymphoproliferative syndrome and autoimmunity. Science. 1995;268:1347-1349.

308. Drappa J, Vaishnaw Ak, Sullivan KE, et al. Fas gene mutations in the Canale-Smith syndrome, an inherited lymphoproliferative disorder associated with autoimmunity. N Engl J Med. 1996;335:1643-1649.

309. Rieux-Laucat F, Fischer A, Deist FL. Cell-death signaling and human disease. Curr Opin Immunol. 2003;15: 325-331.

310. Sneller MC, Wang J, Dale JK, et al. Clinical, immunologic, and genetic features of an autoimmune lymphoproliferative syndrome associated with abnormal lymphocyte apoptosis. Blood. 1997;89:1341-1348.

311. Bleesing JJ, Brown MR, Straus SE, et al. Immunophenotypic profiles in families with autoimmune lymphoproliferative syndrome. Blood. 2001;98:2466-2473.

312. Straus SE, Sneller M, Lenardo MJ, et al. An inherited disorder of lymphocyte apoptosis: the autoimmune lymphoproliferative syndrome. Ann Intern Med. 1999;130: 591-601.

313. Stroncek DF, Carter LB, Procter JL, et al. RBC autoantibodies in autoimmune lymphoproliferative syndrome. Transfusion. 2001;41:18-23.

314. Straus SE, Jaffe ES, Puck JM, et al. The development of lymphomas in families with autoimmune lymphoproliferative syndrome with germline Fas mutations and defective lymphocyte apoptosis. Blood. 2001;98:194-200.

315. Puck JM, Straus SE. Somatic mutations—not just for cancer anymore. N Engl J Med. 2004;351:1388-1390.

316. Clementi R, Chiocchetti A, Cappellano G, et al. Variations of the perforin gene in patients with autoimmunity/lymphoproliferation and defective Fas function. Blood. 2006;108:3079-3084.

317. Teachey DT. Manno CS, Axsom KM, et al. Unmasking Evans syndrome: T-cell phenotype and apoptotic response reveal autoimmune lymphoproliferative syndrome (ALPS). Blood. 2005;105:2443-2448.

318. Murray HW, Masur H, Senterfit LB, Roberts RB. The protean manifestations of *Mycoplasma pneumoniae* infection in adults. Am J Med. 1975;58:229-242.

319. Rollof J, Eklund PO. Infectious mononucleosis complicated by severe immune hemolysis. Eur J Haematol. 1989;43:81-82.

320. Terada K, Tanaka H, Mori R, et al. Hemolytic anemia associated with cold agglutinin during chickenpox and a review of the literature. J Pediatr Hematol Oncol. 1998;20:149-151.

321. Ramos-Casals M, Garcia-Carrasco M, Lopez-Medrano F, et al. Severe autoimmune cytopenias in treatment-naïve hepatitis C virus infection: clinical description of 35 cases. Medicine (Baltimore). 2003;82:87-96.

322. Konig AL, Schabel A, Sugg U, et al. D. Autoimmune hemolytic anemia caused by IgG lambda-monotypic cold agglutinins of anti-Pr specificity after rubella infection. Transfusion. 2001;41:488-492.

323. De la Rubia J, Moscardó F, Arriaga F, et al. Acute parvovirus B19 infection as a cause of autoimmune hemolytic anemia. Haematologica. 2000;85:995-997.

324. Costea N, Yakulis VJ, Heller P. Inhibition of cold agglutinins (anti-I) by *M. pneumoniae* antigens. Proc Soc Exp Biol Med. 1972;139:476-479.

325. Huang DT, Chi H, Lee HC, et al. T-antigen activation for prediction of pneumococcus-induced hemolytic uremic syndrome. Pediatr Infect Dis J. 2006;25:608-610.

326. Waters AM, Kerecuk L, Luk D, et al. Hemolytic uremic syndrome associated with invasive pneumococcal disease: the United Kingdom experience. J Pediatr. 2007;151:140-144.

327. Williams RA, Brown EF, Hurst D, Franklin LC. Transfusion of infants with activation of T antigen. J Pediatr. 1989;115:949-953.

328. Murphy WG, Kelton JG. Methyldopa-induced autoantibodies against red blood cells. Blood Rev. 1988;2:36-42.

329. Arndt PA, Garratty G. The changing spectrum of drug-induced immune hemolytic anemia Semin Hematol. 2005;42:137-144.

330. Petz LD, Fudenberg HH. Coombs-positive hemolytic anemia caused by penicillin administration. N Engl J Med. 1966;274:171-178.

331. Seldon MR, Bain B, Johnson CA, Lennox CS. Ticarcillin-induced immune haemolytic anaemia. Scand J Haematol. 1982;28:459-460.

332. Arndt PA, Leger RM, Garratty G. Serology of antibodies to second- and third-generation cephalosporins associated with immune hemolytic anemia and/or positive direct antiglobulin tests. Transfusion. 1999;39:1239-1246.

333. Viner Y, Hashkes PJ, Yakubova R, et al. Severe hemolysis induced by ceftriaxone in a child with sickle-cell anemia. Pediatr Infect Dis J. 2000;19:83-85.

334. Malloy CA, Kiss JE, Challapalli M. Cefuroxime-induced immune hemolysis. J Pediatr. 2003;143:130-132.

335. Simpson MB, Pryzbylik J, Innis B, Denham MA. Hemolytic anemia after tetracycline therapy. N Engl J Med. 1985;312:840-842.

336. Wong KY, Boose GM, Issitt CH. Erythromycin-induced hemolytic anemia. J Pediatr. 1981;98:647-649.

337. Knowles SR, Phillips EJ, Dresser L, Matukas L. Common adverse events associated with the use of ribavirin for severe acute respiratory syndrome in Canada. Clin Infect Dis. 2003;37:1139-1142.

338. Manor E, Marmor A, Kaufman S, Leiba H. Massive hemolysis caused by acetaminophen. JAMA. 1976;236:2777-2778.

339. Korsager S, Sorensen H, Jensen OH, Falk JV. Antiglobulin-tests for detection of auto-immunohaemolytic anaemia during long-term treatment with ibuprofen. Scand J Rheumatol. 1981;10:174-176.

340. Salama A, Mueller-Eckhardt C. On the mechanisms of sensitization and attachment of antibodies to RBC in drug-induced immune hemolytic anemia. Blood. 1987;69:1006-1010.

341. Kakaiya R, Cseri J, Smith S, et al. A case of acute hemolysis after ceftriaxone: immune complex mechanism demonstrated by flow cytometry. Arch Path Lab Med. 2004;128:905-907.

342. Akpek G, McAneny D, Weintraub L. Comparative response to splenectomy in Coombs-positive autoimmune hemolytic anemia with or without associated disease. Am J Hematol. 1999;61:98-102.

343. Teachey DT, Obzut DA, Axsom K, et al. Rapamycin improves lymphoproliferative disease in murine autoimmune lymphoproliferative syndrome (ALPS). Blood. 2006;108:1965-1971.

344. Bobe P, Bonardelle D, Benihoud K, et al. Arsenic trioxide: a promising novel therapeutic agent for lymphoproliferative and autoimmune syndromes in MRL/lpr mice. Blood. 2006;108:3967-3975.

345. Gull WW. A case of intermittent haematinuria, with remarks. Guys Hosp Rep. 1866;12:381-392.

346. Strübing P. Paroxysmale hämoglobinurie. Dtsch Med Wochenschr. 1882;8:1-3, 17-21.

347. Ham TH. Chronic haemolytic anemia with paroxysmal nocturnal haemoglobinuria. A study of the mechanism of haemolysis in relation to acid-base equilibrium. N Engl J Med. 1937;217:915-917.

348. Ham TH. Studies on the destruction of red blood cells. I. Chronic hemolytic anemia with paroxysmal nocturnal hemoglobinuria: an investigation of the mechanism of hemolysis with observations on five cases. Arch Intern Med. 1939;64:1271-1305.

349. Ham TH, Dingle JH. Studies on destruction of red blood cells. II. Chronic hemolytic anemia with paroxysmal nocturnal hemoglobinuria: certain immunological aspects of the hemolytic mechanism with special reference to serum complement. J Clin Invest. 1939;18:657-672.

350. Rosse WF, Dacie JV. Immune lysis of normal human and paroxysmal nocturnal hemoglobinuria red blood cells. I. The sensitivity of PNH red cells to lysis by complement and specific antibody. J Clin Invest. 1966;45:736-748.

351. Rosse WF. Variations in the red cells in paroxysmal nocturnal hemoglobinuria. Br J Hematol. 1973;24:327.

352. Rosse WF, Adams JP, Thorpe AM. The population of cells in paroxysmal nocturnal hemoglobinuria of intermediate sensitivity to complement lysis—significance and mechanism of increased immune lysis. Br J Haematol. 1974;28:181-190.

353. Hall SE, Rosse WF. The use of monoclonal antibodies and flow cytometry in the diagnosis of paroxysmal nocturnal hemoglobinuria. Blood. 1996;87:5332-5340.

354. Hillmen P, Young NS, Schubert J, et al. The complement inhibitor eculizumab in paroxysmal nocturnal hemoglobinuria. N Engl J Med. 2006;355:1233-1243.

355. Parker C, Omine M, Richards S, et al. Diagnosis and management of paroxysmal nocturnal hemoglobinuria. Blood. 2005;106:3699-3709.

356. Socié G, Mary J-Y, de Gramont A, et al. Paroxysmal nocturnal haemoglobinuria: long-term follow-up and prognostic factors. Lancet. 1996;348:573-577.

357. Nishimura J-I, Kanakura Y, Ware RE, et al. Clinical course and flow cytometric analysis of paroxysmal nocturnal hemoglobinuria in the United States and Japan. Medicine (Baltimore). 2004;83:193-207.

358. Tran MH, Fadeyi E, Scheinberg P, Klein HG. Apparent hemolysis following intravenous antithymocyte globulin treatment in a patient with marrow failure and a paroxysmal nocturnal hemoglobinuria clone. Transfusion. 2006;46:1244-1247.

359. Nakao S, Sugimori C, Yamazaki H. Clinical significance of a small population of paroxysmal nocturnal hemoglobinuria–type cells in the management of bone marrow failure. Int J Hematol. 2006;84:118-122.

360. Devine DV, Gluck WL, Rosse WF, Weinberg JB. Acute myeloblastic leukemia in paroxysmal nocturnal hemoglobinuria: evidence of evolution for the abnormal paroxysmal nocturnal hemoglobinuria clone. J Clin Invest. 1987;79:314-317.

361. Ware RE, Hall SG, Rosse WF. Paroxysmal nocturnal hemoglobinuria with onset in childhood and adolescence. N Engl J Med. 1991;325:991-996.

362. Lee JL, Lee JH, Lee JH, et al. Allogeneic hematopoietic cell transplantation for paroxysmal nocturnal hemoglobinuria. Eur J Hematol. 2003;71:114-118.

363. Van den Heuvel-Eibrink MM, Bredius RG, te Winkel ML, et al. Childhood paroxysmal nocturnal hemoglobinuria (PNH), a report of 11 cases in the Netherlands. Br J Haematol. 2005;128:571-577.

364. Woodard P, Wang W, Pitts N, et al. Successful unrelated donor bone marrow transplantation for paroxysmal nocturnal hemoglobinuria. Bone Marrow Transplant. 2001;27:589-592.

365. Medof ME, Walter EI, Roberts WL, et al. Decay accelerating factor of complement is anchored to cells by a C-terminal glycolipid. Biochemistry. 1986;25:6740-6747.

366. Stefanová I, Hilgert I, Kristofová H, et al. Characterization of a broadly expressed human leucocyte surface antigen MEM-43 anchored in membrane through phosphatidylinositol. Mol Immunol. 1989;26:153-161.

367. Low MG. Biochemistry of the glycosyl-phosphatidylinositol membrane protein anchors. Biochem J. 1987;244:1-13.

368. Low MG, Saltiel AR. Structural and functional roles of glycosyl-phosphatidylinositol in membranes. Science. 1988;239:268-275.

369. Bangs JD, Hereld D, Krakow JL, et al. Rapid processing of the carboxyl terminus of a trypanosome variant surface glycoprotein. Biochemistry. 1985;82:3207-3211.

370. Low MG, Zilversmit DB. Role of phosphatidylinositol in attachment of alkaline phosphatase to membranes. Biochemistry. 1980;19:3913-3918.

371. Haas R, Brandt PT, Knight J Rosenberry TL. Identification of amine components in a glycolipid membrane–binding domain at the C-terminus of human erythrocyte acetylcholinesterase. Biochemistry. 1986;25:3098-3105.

372. Fatemi SH, Haas R, Jentoft N, et al. The glycophospholipid anchor of Thy-1. J Biol Chem. 1987;262:4728-4732.

373. Dustin ML, Selvaraj P, Mattaliano RJ, Springer TA. Anchoring mechanisms for LFA-3 cell adhesion glycoprotein at membrane surface. Nature. 1987;329:846-848.

374. Selvaraj P, Rosse WF, Silber R, Springer TA. The major Fc receptor in blood has a phosphatidylinositol anchor and is deficient in paroxysmal nocturnal haemoglobinuria. Nature. 1988;333:565-567.

375. Ortolan E, Tibaldi EV, Ferranti B, et al. CD157 plays a pivotal role in neutrophil transendothelial migration. Blood. 2006;108:4214-4222.

376. Ishihara A, Hou Y, Jacobson K. The Thy-1 antigen exhibits rapid lateral diffusion in the plasma membrane of rodent lymphoid cells and fibroblasts. Proc Natl Acad Sci U S A. 1987;84:1290-1293.

377. Noda M, Yoon K, Rodan GA, Koppel DE. High lateral mobility of endogenous and transfected alkaline phosphatase: a phosphatidylinositol-anchored membrane protein. J Cell Biol. 1987;105:1671-1677.

378. Romero G, Luttrell L, Rogol A, et al. Phosphatidylinositol-glycan anchors of membrane proteins: potential precursors of insulin mediators. Science. 1988;240:509-511.

379. Yeh ETH, Reiser H, Bamezai A, Rock KL. TAP transcription and phosphatidylinositol linkage mutants are defective in activation through the T cell receptor. Cell. 1988;52:665-674.

380. Presky DH, Low MG, Shevach EM. The role of phosphatidylinositol (PI)-anchored proteins in T cell activation [abstract]. FASEB J. 1989;A1654.

381. Roy-Choudhury S, Mishra VS, Low MG, Das M. A phospholipid is the membrane-anchoring domain of a protein growth factor of molecular mass 34 kDa in placental trophoblasts. Proc Natl Acad Sci U S A. 1988;85:2014-2018.

382. Nicholson-Weller A, March JP, Rosenfeld SI, Austen KF. Affected erythrocytes of patients with paroxysmal nocturnal hemoglobinuria are deficient in the complement regulatory protein, decay accelerating factor. Proc Natl Acad Sci U S A. 1983;80:5066-5070.

383. Selvaraj P, Dustin ML, Silber R, et al. Deficiency of lymphocyte function–associated antigen 3 (LFA-3) in paroxysmal nocturnal hemoglobinuria. J Exp Med. 1987;166:1011-1025.

384. Holguin MH, Fredrick LR, Bernshaw NJ, et al. Isolation and characterization of a membrane protein from normal human erythrocytes that inhibits reactive lysis of the erythrocytes of paroxysmal nocturnal hemoglobinuria. J Clin Invest. 1989;84:7-17.

385. Takahashi M, Takeda J, Hirose S, et al. Deficient biosynthesis of *N*-acetylglucosaminyl-phosphatidylinositol, the first intermediate of glycosyl phosphatidylinositol anchor biosynthesis, in cell lines established from patients with paroxysmal nocturnal hemoglobinuria. J Exp Med. 1993;177:517-521.

386. Sugiyama E, DeGasperi R, Urakaze M, et al. Identification of defects in glycosylphosphatidylinositol anchor biosynthesis in the Thy-1 expression mutants. J Biol Chem. 1991;266:12119-12122.

387. Norris J, Hoffman S, Ware RE, et al. Glycosyl-phosphatidylinositol anchor synthesis in paroxysmal nocturnal hemoglobinuria: partial or complete defect in an early step. Blood. 1994;83:816-821.

388. Brodsky RA, Mukhina GL, Li S, et al. Improved detection and characterization of paroxysmal nocturnal hemoglobinuria using fluorescent aerolysin. Am J Clin Pathol. 2000;114:459-466.

389. Oni SB, Osunkoya BO, Luzzato L. Paroxysmal nocturnal hemoglobinuria: evidence for monoclonal origin of abnormal red cells. Blood. 1970;36:145-152.

390. Ohashi H, Hotta T, Ichikawa A, et al. Peripheral blood cells are predominantly chimeric of affected and normal cells in patients with paroxysmal nocturnal hemoglobinuria: simultaneous investigation on clonality and expression of glycophosphatidylinositol-anchored proteins. Blood. 1994;83:853-859.

391. Miyata T, Takeda J, Iida Y, et al. The cloning of PIG-A, a component in the early step of GPI-anchor biosynthesis. Science. 1993;259:1318-1320.

392. Takeda J, Miyata T, Kawagoe K, et al. Deficiency of the GPI anchor caused by a somatic mutation of the PIG-A gene in paroxysmal nocturnal hemoglobinuria. Cell. 1993;73:703-711.

393. Bessler M, Mason PJ, Hillmen P, et al. Paroxysmal nocturnal haemoglobinuria (PNH) is caused by somatic mutations in the PIG-A gene. EMBO J. 1994;13:110-117.

394. Miyata T, Yamada N, Iida Y, et al. Abnormalities of PIG-A transcripts in granulocytes from patients with paroxysmal nocturnal hemoglobinuria. N Engl J Med. 1994;330:249-255.

395. Ware RE, Rosse WF, Howard TA. Mutations within the Piga gene in patients with paroxysmal nocturnal hemoglobinuria. Blood. 1994;83:2418-2422.

396. Yamada N, Miyata T, Maeda K, et al. Somatic mutations of the PIG-A gene found in Japanese patients with paroxysmal nocturnal hemoglobinuria. Blood. 1995;85:885-892.

397. Rosse WF, Ware RE. The molecular basis of paroxysmal nocturnal hemoglobinuria. Blood. 1995;86:3277-3286.

398. Nishimura J, Murakami Y, Kinoshita T. Paroxysmal nocturnal hemoglobinuria: an acquired genetic disease. Am J Hematol. 1999;62:175-182.

399. Ware RE, Howard TA, Kamitani T, et al. Chromosomal assignment of genes involved in glycosylphosphatidylinositol anchor biosynthesis: implications for the pathogenesis of paroxysmal nocturnal hemoglobinuria. Blood. 1994;83:3753-3757.

400. Almeida AM, Murakami Y, Layton DM, et al. Hypomorphic promoter mutation in *PIGM* causes inherited glycosylphosphatidylinositol deficiency. Nat Med. 2006; 12:846-851.

401. Wiedmer T, Hall SE, Ortel TL, et al. Complement-induced vesiculation and exposure of membrane prothrombinase sites in platelets of paroxysmal nocturnal hemoglobinuria. Blood. 1993;82:1192-1196.

402. Ploug M, Plesner T, Rønne E, et al. The receptor for urokinase-type plasminogen activator is deficient on peripheral blood leukocytes in patients with paroxysmal nocturnal hemoglobinuria. Blood. 1992;79:1447-1455.

403. Lewis SM, Dacie JV. The aplastic anaemia–paroxysmal nocturnal haemoglobinuria syndrome. Br J Haematol. 1967;13:236-251.

404. Rosse WF. Paroxysmal nocturnal hemoglobinuria in aplastic anemia. Clin Haematol. 1985;14:105-125.

405. Schubert J, Vogt HG, Zielinska-Skowronek M, et al. Development of the glycosylphosphatidylinositol-anchoring defect characteristic for paroxysmal nocturnal hemoglobinuria in patients with aplastic anemia. Blood. 1994;83:2323-2328.

406. Rosti V, Tremml G, Soares V, et al. Murine embryonic stem cells without pig-a gene activity are competent for hematopoiesis with the PNH phenotype but not for clonal expansion. J Clin Invest. 1997;100:1028-1036.

407. Murakami Y, Kinoshita T, Maeda Y, et al. Different roles of glycosylphosphatidylinositol in various hematopoietic cells as revealed by a mouse model of paroxysmal nocturnal hemoglobinuria. Blood. 1999;94:2963-2970.

408. Rotoli B, Luzzatto L. Paroxysmal nocturnal haemoglobinuria. Baillieres Clin Haematol. 1989;2:113-138.

409. Young NS. Hematopoietic cell destruction by immune mechanisms in acquired aplastic anemia. Semin Hematol. 2000;37:3-14.

410. Bessler M, Mason P, Hillmen P, Luzzatto L. Somatic mutations and cellular selection in paroxysmal nocturnal haemoglobinuria. Lancet. 1994;343:951-953.

411. Nishimura J, Inoue N, Wada H, et al. A patient with paroxysmal nocturnal hemoglobinuria bearing four independent PIG-A mutant clones. Blood. 1997;89:3470-3476.

412. Araten DJ, Nafa K, Pakdeesuwan K, Luzzatto L. Clonal populations of hematopoietic cells with paroxysmal nocturnal hemoglobinuria genotype and phenotype are present in normal individuals. Proc Natl Acad Sci U S A. 1999;96:5209-5214.

413. Ware RE, Pickens CV, DeCastro DM, Howard TA. Circulating PIG-A mutant T lymphocytes in healthy adults and patients with bone marrow failure syndromes. Exp Hematol. 2001;29:1403-1409.

414. Hu R, Mukhina GL, Piantadosi S, et al. PIG-A mutations in normal hematopoiesis. Blood. 2005;105:3848-3854.

415. Ware RE, Heeney MM, Pickens CV, et al. A multistep model for the pathogenesis and evolution of PNH. In Omine M, Kinoshita T (eds). Paroxysmal Nocturnal Hemoglobinuria and Related Disorders: Molecular Aspects of Pathogenesis. Heidelberg, Germany, Springer-Verlag, 2003.

416. Brodsky RA, Vala MS, Barber JP, et al. Resistance to apoptosis caused by PIG-A gene mutations in paroxysmal

nocturnal hemoglobinuria. Proc Natl Acad Sci U S A. 1997;94:8756-8760.

417. Horikawa K, Nakakuma H, Kawaguchi T, et al. Apoptosis resistance of blood cells from patients with paroxysmal nocturnal hemoglobinuria, aplastic anemia, and myelodysplastic syndrome. Blood. 1997;90:2716-2722.

418. Ware RE, Nishimura J, Moody MA, et al. The PIG-A mutation and absence of glycosylphosphatidylinositol-linked proteins do not confer resistance to apoptosis in paroxysmal nocturnal hemoglobinuria. Blood. 1998;92:2541-2550.

419. Inoue N, Izui-Sarumaru T, Murakami Y, et al. Molecular basis of clonal expansion of hematopoiesis in two patients with paroxysmal nocturnal hemoglobinuria (PNH). Blood. 2006;108:4232-4236.

420. Storlazzi CT, Albano F, Locunsolo C, et al. t(3;12)(q26;q14) in polycythemia vera is associated with upregulation of the HMGA2 gene. Leukemia. 2006;20:2190-2193.

421. Blackshear PL Jr, Dorman FD, Steinbach JH, et al. Shear wall interaction and hemolysis. Trans Am Soc Artif Intern Organs. 1966;12:113-120.

422. Nevaril CG, Lynch EC, Alfrey CP Jr, Hellums JD. Erythrocyte destruction and damage induced by shearing stress. J Lab Clin Med. 1968;71:784-790.

423. Monroe JM, True DE, Williams MC. Surface roughness and edge geometrics in hemolysis with rotating disc flow. J Biomed Mater Res. 1981;15:923-939.

424. Brain MC, Dacie JV, Hourihane DO. Microangiopathic haemolytic anaemia: the possible role of vascular lesions in pathogenesis. Br J Haematol. 1962;8:358-374.

425. Bull BS, Kuhn IN. The production of schistocytes by fibrin strands (a scanning electron microscope study). Blood. 1970;35:104-111.

426. Chintagumpala MM, Hurwitz RL, Moake JL, et al. Chronic relapsing thrombotic thrombocytopenic purpura in infants with large von Willebrand factor multimers during remission. J Pediatr. 1992;120:49-53.

427. Daghistani D, Jimenez JJ, Moake JL, et al. Familial infantile thrombotic thrombocytopenic purpura. J Pediatr Hematol Oncol. 1996;18:171-174.

428. Savasan S, Taub JW, Buck S, et al. Congenital microangiopathic hemolytic anemia and thrombocytopenia with unusually large von Willebrand factor multimers and von Willebrand factor–cleaving protease. J Pediatr Hematol Oncol. 2001;23:364-367.

429. Furlan M, Robles R, Galbusera M, et al. von Willebrand factor–cleaving protease in thrombotic thrombocytopenic purpura and the hemolytic-uraemic syndrome. N Engl J Med. 1998;339:1578-1584.

430. Levy GG, Nichols WC, Lian EC, et al. Mutations in a member of the ADAMTS gene family cause thrombotic thrombocytopenic purpura. Nature. 2001;413:488-494.

431. Matsumoto M, Kokame K, Soejima K, et al. Molecular characterization of ADAMTS13 gene mutations in Japanese patients with Upshaw-Schulman syndrome. Blood. 2004;103:1305-1310.

432. Licht C, Stapenhorst L, Simon T, et al. Two novel ADAMTS13 gene mutations in thrombotic thrombocytopenic purpura/hemolytic-uremic syndrome. Kidney Int. 2004;66:955-958.

433. Hovinga JA, Studt JD, Alberio L, Lammle B. von Willebrand factor–cleaving protease (ADAMTS-13) activity determination in the diagnosis of thrombotic microangiopathies: the Swiss experience. Semin Hematol. 2004;41:75-82.

434. Ferrari S, Scheiflinger F, Rieger M, et al. Prognostic value of anti-ADAMTS 13 antibody features (Ig isotype, titer, and inhibitory effect) in a cohort of 35 adult French patients undergoing a first episode of thrombotic microangiopathy with undetectable ADAMTS 13 activity. Blood. 2007;109:2815-2822.

435. Hogasen K, Jansen JH, Mollnes TE, et al. Hereditary porcine membranoproliferative glomerulonephritis type II is caused by factor H deficiency. J Clin Invest. 1995;95:1054-1061.

436. Warwicker P, Goodship THJ, Donne RL, et al. Genetic studies into inherited and sporadic hemolytic uremic syndrome. Kidney Int. 1998;53:836-844.

437. Ying L, Katz Y, Schlesinger M, et al. Complement factor H gene mutation associated with autosomal recessive atypical hemolytic uremic syndrome. Am J Hum Genet. 2000;65:1538-1546.

438. Nilsson SC, Karpman D, Vaziri-Sani F, et al. A mutation in factor I that is associated with atypical hemolytic uremic syndrome does not affect the function of factor I in complement regulation. Mol Immunol. 2007;44:1835-1844.

439. Fremeaux-Bacchi V, Moulton EA, Kavanagh D, et al. Genetic and functional analyses of membrane cofactor protein (CD46) mutations in atypical hemolytic uremic syndrome. J Am Soc Nephrol. 2006;17:1775-1776.

440. Zipfel PF. Hemolytic uremic syndrome: how do factor H mutants mediate endothelial damage? Trends Immunol. 2001;22:345-348.

441. Jain R, Chartash E, Susin M, Furie R. Systemic lupus erythematosus complicated by thrombotic microangiopathy. Semin Arthritis Rheum. 1994;24:173-182.

442. Steen VD. Renal involvement in systemic sclerosis. Clin Dermatol. 1994;12:253-258.

443. James SH, Meyers AM. Microangiopathic hemolytic anemia as a complication of diabetes mellitus. Am J Med Sci. 1998;315:211-215.

444. Tucker LB. Vasculitis, Kawasaki disease, and hemolytic uremic syndrome. Curr Opin Rheum. 1994;6:530-536.

445. Lim HE, Jo SK, Kim SW, et al. A case of Wegener's granulomatosis complicated by diffuse pulmonary hemorrhage and thrombotic thrombocytopenic purpura. Korean J Intern Med. 1998;13:68-71.

446. Espinosa G, Bucciarelli S, Cervera R, et al. Thrombotic microangiopathic haemolytic anaemia and antiphospholipid antibodies. Ann Rheum Dis. 2004;63:730-736.

447. Hariharan D, Manno CS, Seri I. Neonatal lupus erythematosus with microvascular hemolysis. J Pediatr Hematol Oncol. 2000;22:351-354.

448. Dold S, Singh R, Sarwar H, et al. Frequency of microangiopathic hemolytic anemia in patients with systemic lupus erythematosus exacerbation: distinction from thrombotic thrombocytopenic purpura, prognosis, and outcome. Arthritis Rheum. 2005;53:982-985.

449. Pinckard JK, Wick MR. Tumor-related thrombotic pulmonary microangiopathy: review of pathologic findings and pathophysiologic mechanisms. Ann Diagn Pathol. 2000;4:154-157.

450. Brenner B. Arterial thrombotic syndromes in cancer patients. Haemostasis. 2001;31:43-44.

451. HIV associated thrombotic microangiopathy. Postgrad Med J. 2002;78:520-525.

452. Myers KA, Marrie TJ. Thrombotic microangiopathy associated with *Streptococcus pneumoniae* bacteremia: case report and review. Clin Infect Dis. 1993;17:1037-1040.

453. Oran B, Donato M, Aleman A, et al. Transplant-associated microangiopathy in patients receiving tacrolimus following allogeneic stem cell transplantation: risk factors and response to treatment. Biol Blood Marrow Transplant. 2007;13:469-477.

454. Clark EA, Silver RM, Branch DW. Do antiphospholipid antibodies cause preeclampsia and HELLP syndrome? Curr Rheumatol Rep. 2007;9:219-225.

455. Martin JN Jr, Rose CH, Briery CM. Understanding and managing HELLP syndrome: the integral role of aggressive glucocorticoids for mother and child. Am J Obstet Gynecol. 2006;195:914-934.

456. Le Thi Thuong D, Tieulie N, Costedoat N, et al. The HELLP syndrome in the antiphospholipid syndrome: retrospective study of 16 cases in 15 women. Ann Rheum Dis. 2005;64:273-278.

457. Baxter JK, Weinstein L. HELLP syndrome: the state of the art. Obstet Gynecol Surv. 2004;59:838-845.

458. Volcy J, Nzerue CM, Oderinde A, et al. Cocaine-induced acute renal failure, hemolysis, and thrombocytopenia mimicking thrombotic thrombocytopenic purpura. Am J Kidney Dis. 2000;35:E3.

459. Crum NF, Gable P. Quinine-induced hemolytic-uremic syndrome. South Med J. 2000;93:726-728.

460. Oteo JF, Alonso-Pulpón L, Diez JL. Microangiopathic hemolytic anemia secondary to cyclosporine therapy in a heart and liver transplant recipient. J Heart Lung Transplant. 1996;15:322-324.

461. Trimarchi HM, Truong LD, Brennan S, et al. FK506-associated thrombotic microangiopathy: report of two cases and review of the literature. Transplantation. 1999;67:539-544.

462. Gundappa RK, Sud K, Kohli HS, et al. Mitomycin-C induced hemolytic uremic syndrome: a case report. Ren Fail. 2002;24:373-377.

463. Fung MC, Storniolo AM, Nguyen B, et al. A review of hemolytic uremic syndrome in patients treated with gemcitabine therapy. Cancer. 1999;85:2023-2032.

464. Shahab N, Haidu S, Doll DC. Vascular toxicity of antineoplastic agents. Semin Oncol. 2006;33:121-138.

465. Gordon LI, Kwaan HC. Cancer- and drug-associated thrombotic thrombocytopenic purpura and hemolytic syndrome. Semin Hematol. 1997;34:140-147.

466. Lane DR, Youse JS. Coombs-positive hemolytic anemia secondary to brown recluse spider bite: a review of the literature and discussion of treatment. Cutis. 2004;74:341-347.

467. Elbahlawan LM, Stidham GL, Bugnitz MC, et al. Severe systemic reaction to *Loxosceles reclusa* spider bites in a pediatric population. Pediatr Emerg Care. 2005;21:177-180.

468. Jubelirer SJ. Primary pulmonary hypertension. Its association with microangiopathic hemolytic anemia and thrombocytopenia. Arch Intern Med. 1991;151:1221-1223.

469. Suzuki H, Nakasato M, Sato S, et al. Microangiopathic hemolytic anemia and thrombocytopenia in a child with atrial septal defect and pulmonary hypertension. Tohoku J Exp Med. 1997;181:379-384.

470. Ruggenenti P, Remuzzi G. Malignant vascular disease of the kidney: nature of the lesions, mediators of disease progression, and the case for bilateral nephrectomy. Am J Kidney Dis. 1996;27:459-475.

471. Uthman I, Khamashta M. Antiphospholipid syndrome and the kidneys. Semin Arthritis Rheum. 2006;35:360-367.

472. Chintagumpala MM, Hurwitz RL, Moake JL, et al. Chronic relapsing thrombotic thrombocytopenic purpura in infants with large von Willebrand factor multimers during remission. J Pediatr. 1992;120:49-53.

473. Lowe EJ, Werner EJ. Thrombotic thrombocytopenic purpura and hemolytic uremic syndrome in children and adolescents. Semin Thromb Hemost. 2005;31:717-730.

474. Barbot J, Costa E, Guerra M, et al. Ten years of prophylactic treatment with fresh-frozen plasma in a child with chronic relapsing thrombotic thrombocytopenic purpura as a result of a congenital deficiency of von Willebrand factor–cleaving protease. Br J Haematol. 2001;113:649-651.

475. Moake JL. Thrombotic thrombocytopenic purpura and the hemolytic uremic syndrome. Arch Pathol Lab Med. 2002;126:1430-1433.

476. Murrin RJ, Murray JA. Thrombotic thrombocytopenic purpura: aetiology, pathophysiology and treatment. Blood Rev. 2006;20:51-60.

477. Bell WR, Braine JG, Ness PM, Kickler TS. Improved survival in thrombotic thrombocytopenic purpura-hemolytic uremic syndrome. Clinical experience in 108 patients. N Engl J Med. 1991;325:398-403.

478. Kosugi S, Matsumoto M, Ohtani Y, et al. Rituximab provided long-term remission in a patient with refractory relapsing thrombotic thrombocytopenic purpura. Int J Hematol. 2005;81:433-436.

479. Enjolras O, Wassef M, Mazoyer E, et al. Infants with Kasabach-Merritt syndrome do not have "true" hemangiomas. J Pediatr. 1997;130:631-640.

480. Vin-Christian K, McCalmont TH, Frieden IJ. Kaposiform hemangioendothelioma. An aggressive, locally invasive vascular tumor that can mimic hemangioma of infancy. Arch Dermatol. 1997;133:1573-1578.

481. Pampin C, Devillers A, Treguier C, et al. Intratumoral consumptions of indium-111–labeled platelets in a child with splenic hemangioma and thrombocytopenia. J Pediatr Hematol Oncol. 2000;22:256-258.

482. Billio A, Pescosta N, Rosanelli C, et al. Treatment of Kasabach-Merritt syndrome by embolisation of a giant liver hemangioma. Am J Hematol. 2001;66:140-141.

483. Au WY, Tang SC, Chan KW, et al. Pulmonary renal syndrome and thrombotic thrombocytopenic purpura in a patient with giant cavernous hemangioma of the leg. Arch Intern Med. 2002;162:221-222.

484. Morad AB, McClain KL, Ogden AK. The role of tranexamic acid in the treatment of giant hemangiomas in newborns. J Pediatr Hematol Oncol. 1995;15:383-385.

485. Zeng Q, Li Y, Chen Y, et al. Gigantic cavernous hemangioma of the liver treated by intra-arterial embolization with pingyangmycin-lipiodol emulsion: a multi-center study. Cardiovasc Intervent Radiol. 2004;27:481-485.

486. Burstein FD, Simms C, Cohen SR, et al. Intralesional laser therapy of extensive hemangiomas in 100 consecutive pediatric patients. Ann Plastic Surg. 2000;44:188-194.

487. Cui Y, Zhou LY, Dong MK, et al. Ultrasonography guided percutaneous radiofrequency ablation for hepatic cavernous hemangioma. World J Gastroenterol. 2003;9:2132-2134.

488. Hu B, Lachman R, Phillips J, et al. Kasabach-Merritt syndrome–associated kaposiform hemangioendothelioma successfully treated with cyclophosphamide, vincristine, and actinomycin D. J Pediatr Hematol Oncol. 1998;20:567-569.

489. Powell J. Update on hemangiomas and vascular malformations. Curr Opin Pediatr. 1999;11:457-463.

490. Paller AS. Responses to anti-angiogenic therapies. J Invest Dermatol. 2000;5:83-86.

491. Ismeno G, Renzulli A, Carozza A, et al. Intravascular hemolysis after mitral and aortic valve replacement with different types of mechanical prostheses. Int J Cardiol. 1999;69:179-183.

492. Vesey JM, Otto CM. Complications of prosthetic heart valves. Curr Cardiol Rep. 2004;6:106-111.

493. Yeo TC, Freeman WK, Schaff HV, Orszulak TA. Mechanisms of hemolysis after mitral valve repair: assessment by serial echocardiography. J Am Coll Cardiol. 1998;32:717-723.

494. Hirawat S. Lichtman SM, Allen SL. Recombinant human erythropoietin use in hemolytic anemia due to prosthetic heart valves: a promising treatment. Am J Hematol. 2001;66:224-226.

495. Geller S, Gelber R. Pentoxifylline treatment for microangiopathic hemolytic anemia caused by mechanical heart valves. Md Med J. 1999;48:173.

496. Batton DG, Amanullah A, Comstock C. Fetal schistocytic hemolytic anemia and umbilical vein varix. J Pediatr Hematol Oncol. 2000;22:259-261.

497. Davidson RJL. March or exertional haemoglobinuria. Semin Hematol. 1969;6:150-161.

498. Pollard TD, Weiss IW. Acute tubular necrosis in a patient with march hemoglobinuria. N Engl J Med. 1970;283:803-804.

499. Streeton JA. Traumatic haemoglobinuria caused by karate exercises. Lancet. 1967;2:191-192.

500. Schwartz KA, Flessa HC. March hemoglobinuria. Report of a case after basketball and conga drum playing. Ohio State Med J. 1973;69:448-449.

501. Abarbanel J, Benet AE, Lask D, Kimche D. Sports hematuria. J Urol. 1990;143:887-890.

502. Joshua H, De Vries A. Effect of exercise of red blood cell in march hemoglobinuria. Am J Clin Pathol. 1966;46:341-344.

503. Sagov SE. March hemoglobinuria treated with rubber insoles: two case reports. J Am Coll Health Assoc. 1970;19:146.

504. Sigurdsson J, Björnsson A, Gudmundsson ST. Formic acid burn—local and systemic effects. Report of a case. Burns. 1983;9:358-361.

505. Bhargava M, Agarwal KN, Kumar S. Site of red cell destruction in the anaemia of experimental burns. Br J Haematol. 1969;17:179-185.

506. Vertel RM, Summerlin WT, Pruitt BA Jr, O'Neill JA Jr. Coombs' tests after thermal burns. J Trauma. 1967;7:871-874.

507. Sevitt S, Stone P, Jackson D, et al. Acute Heinz-body anaemia in burned patients. Lancet. 1973;2:471-475.

508. Eldad A, Neuman A, Weinberg A, et al. Silver sulphadiazine–induced haemolytic anaemia in a glucose-6-phosphate dehydrogenase–deficient burn patient. Burns. 1991;17:430-432.

15

Disorders of the Red Cell Membrane

Rachael F. Grace and Samuel E. Lux

The erythrocyte membrane is the most thoroughly studied biologic membrane. It is a small structure, less than 0.1% of the cell's thickness and only about 1% of its weight, but its easy accessibility has enabled researchers to characterize both its primary structure and a number of its important functions. During erythropoiesis it responds to erythropoietin and imports the billion or so iron atoms that each red cell needs to complete the synthesis of hemoglobin. It sequesters the reductants required to protect hemoglobin and other cell proteins from corrosion by oxygen and selectively retains other vital components, such as organic phosphates, manufactured with precious adenosine triphosphate (ATP) energy, but lets metabolic detritus escape. Some evidence hints that it may even help regulate metabolism by reversibly binding and inactivating many glycolytic enzymes.[1] In the circulation it carefully balances cation and water con-

centrations so that red cells do not shrivel or explode. Simultaneously, it exchanges tremendous numbers of bicarbonate and chloride anions ($\approx$10 to 30 billion per second per red cell), which aids transfer of carbon dioxide from tissues to the lungs.[2] It also maintains a slippery exterior so that red cells do not adhere to endothelial cells or aggregate and clog capillaries. Finally, buttressed by the "membrane skeleton," a protein scaffold that lines the inner membrane surface, the membrane achieves the critical combination of strength and flexibility needed to survive 4 months in the circulation. Failure of any of these or numerous other functions shortens red cell survival, a process termed hemolysis. In fact, all hemolysis is ultimately due to membrane failure.

The red cell membrane was originally characterized as an example of the fluid mosaic model proposed by Singer and Nicolson more than 35 years ago.[3] In this model the erythrocyte membrane is composed of mobile, asymmetrically distributed proteins and lipids that interact in a variety of ways. The model has been revised in the intervening $3^{1}/_{2}$ decades because many membrane proteins are not freely mobile but instead diffuse in complicated patterns or are confined to discrete domains.[4-6] In this chapter we first discuss normal membrane structure with an emphasis on aspects that are most involved in the genesis of membrane disease. We then focus on abnormalities of red blood cell membranes, particularly hereditary spherocytosis (HS) and hereditary elliptocytosis (HE), the two most common and best-understood disorders.

MEMBRANE LIPIDS

Lipid Composition

Lipids account for about 50% of the weight of the red cell membrane (Table 15-1) or about 1.6% of the weight of the hemoglobin. Phospholipids and unesterified (free) cholesterol predominate and are present in nearly equal proportions (cholesterol-phospholipid molar ratio of 0.80).[7,16,17] Small amounts of glycolipids, principally globoside (73% of the glycosphingolipids) (Fig. 15-1), are

also present.[14] The average red cell contains about 250 million phospholipid molecules, 195 million cholesterol molecules, 10 million glycolipid molecules, and 6 million protein molecules in a membrane whose total surface area is about 140 μm^2.[18] Phosphatidylcholine (PC), phosphatidylethanolamine (PE), sphingomyelin (SM), and phosphatidylserine (PS) are the predominant phospholipids (see Table 15-1). Their structures are shown in Figure 15-1. Small amounts of phosphatidic acid (PA), phosphatidylinositol (PI), and lysophosphatidylcholine (Lyso-PC) are also present.

At physiologic pH, PS, PA, and PI have a net negative charge, whereas the other phospholipids are electrically neutral. The polar head groups of PC and SM tend to lie parallel to the membrane surface (Fig. 15-2). The head groups of PE and PS are smaller and more cone shaped, which may help them fit in the inner bilayer.

With the exception of SM and Lyso-PC, the phospholipids have two fatty acids attached to a glycerol backbone. They are usually of similar length and attached through an ester linkage, although sometimes, particularly in PE, one of the fatty acids is a vinyl ether (plasmalogen).[13] Typically, the fatty acid attached to glycerol farthest from the polar head group (*sn*-1 position) is saturated and the nearer (*sn*-2) one is unsaturated.[19] PE and

TABLE 15-1	Composition of Normal Human Red Cell Membranes					
Component	Wt%		Grams per Membrane (×10¹³)	Approximate Number of Molecules per Membrane (×10⁶)	% in Outer Half of Bilayer*	% in Inner Half of Bilayer*
Proteins and glycoproteins†	55		5.7‡	6		
Lipids	45		4.7	475		
Phospholipids§		28	3.0	250¶		
Sphingomyelin (SM)		6.8	0.73	60	85	15
Phosphatidylcholine (PC)		7.0	0.75	65	70	30
Phosphatidylethanolamine (PE)		7.4	0.79	65	20	80
Phosphatidylserine (PS)		4.3	0.46	40	0	100
Phosphatidylinositols (PI)		1.0	0.10	8	0	100
PI			0.34	0.036	3	
PIP			0.22	0.024	2	
PIP₂			0.39	0.042	3	
Phosphatidic acid (PA)		1.0	0.10	8	10	90
Lysophosphatidylcholine (Lyso-PC)		0.3	0.03	3	Unknown	Unknown
Lysophosphatidylethanolamine (Lyso-PE)		0.3	0.03	3	Unknown	Unknown
Cholesterol§	13		1.3	195	≈50	~50
Glycolipids¶	3		0.3	10	100	0
Free fatty acids**	1		0.1	20	Unknown	Unknown
	100		10.4	481		

*Based on data from Blau and Bittman,[7] Low and Finean,[8] Verkleij et al.,[9] and Zachowski.[10]
†An average of three reported values by Fairbanks et al.[11]
‡Calculated from data in Table 15-2.
§Based on compiled data from Ferrell and Huestis.[12]
¶Number of phospholipid molecules per membrane based on an average molecular weight of 723 calculated from the average red cell phospholipid polar head group and fatty acid composition.[13]
¶Based on the data from Sweeley and Dawson.[14]
**An average of two reported values compiled by Cooper.[15]
PIP, phosphatidylinositol 4-phosphate; PIP₂, phosphatidylinositol 4,5-bisphosphate.

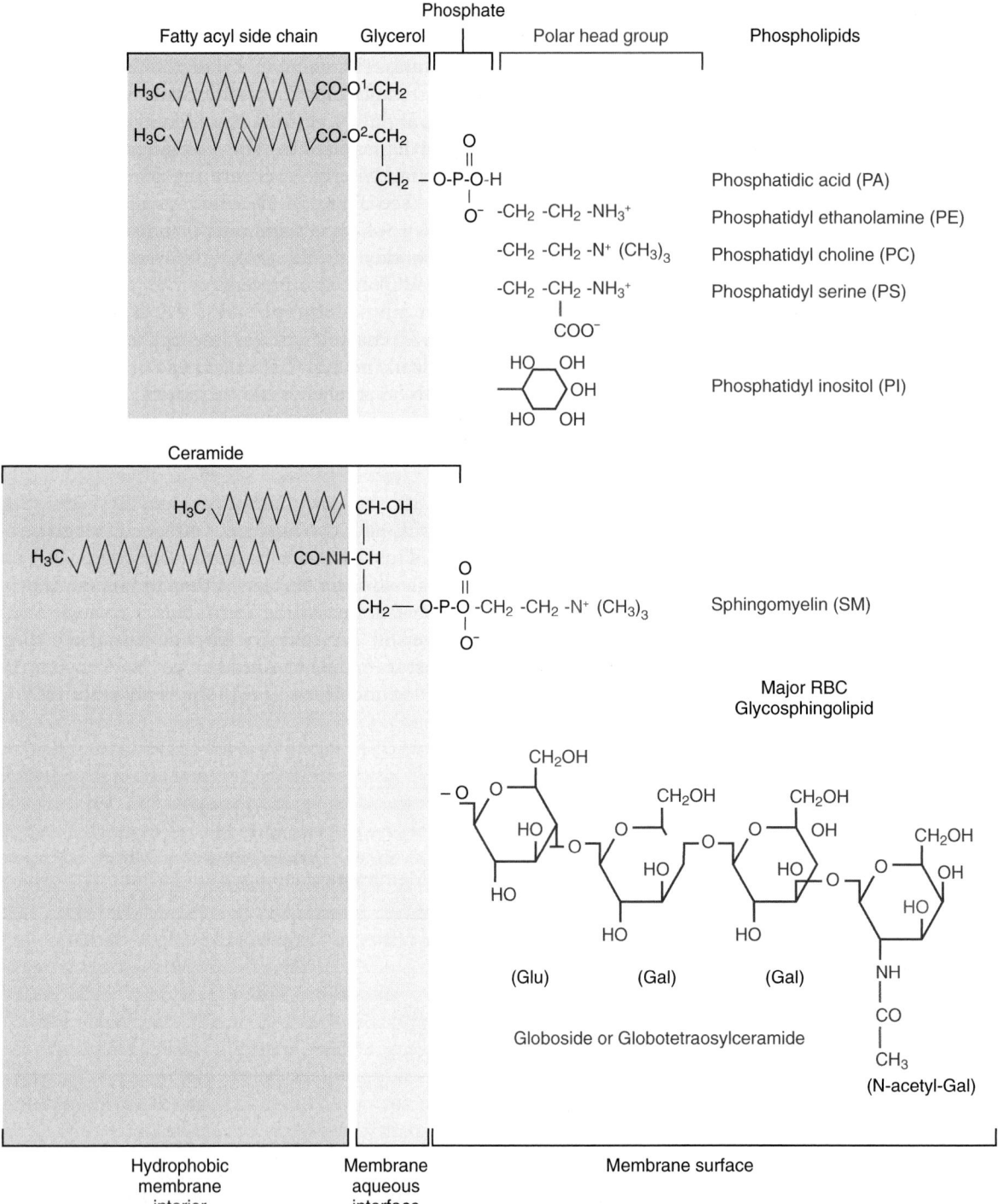

FIGURE 15-1. Chemical structures of the major phospholipids and the major glycosphingolipid (globoside or GL-4) of the red blood cell (RBC) membrane. Note that phosphatidylcholine (PC) and sphingomyelin (SM) share the same polar moiety (choline) and that SM and globoside share the same nonpolar moiety (ceramide).

PS are more unsaturated than PC. In contrast, both acyl side chains are usually saturated in SM, and the amide-linked chain (see Fig. 15-1) is often very long and interdigitates with the hydrocarbon chains of the opposite side of the bilayer. The SM amide linkage also makes its interface region more polar. The *lyso*phospholipids have only one fatty acid and are named for the hemolysis induced because of their detergent-like properties.

Asymmetric Organization of Lipids in the Bilayer

The majority of phospholipids in the red cell membrane are in a planar bilayer with their polar head groups exposed at each surface and their hydrophobic fatty acyl side chains buried in the bilayer core. The phospholipid head groups tend to adopt regular, superlattice-like lateral distributions.[20]

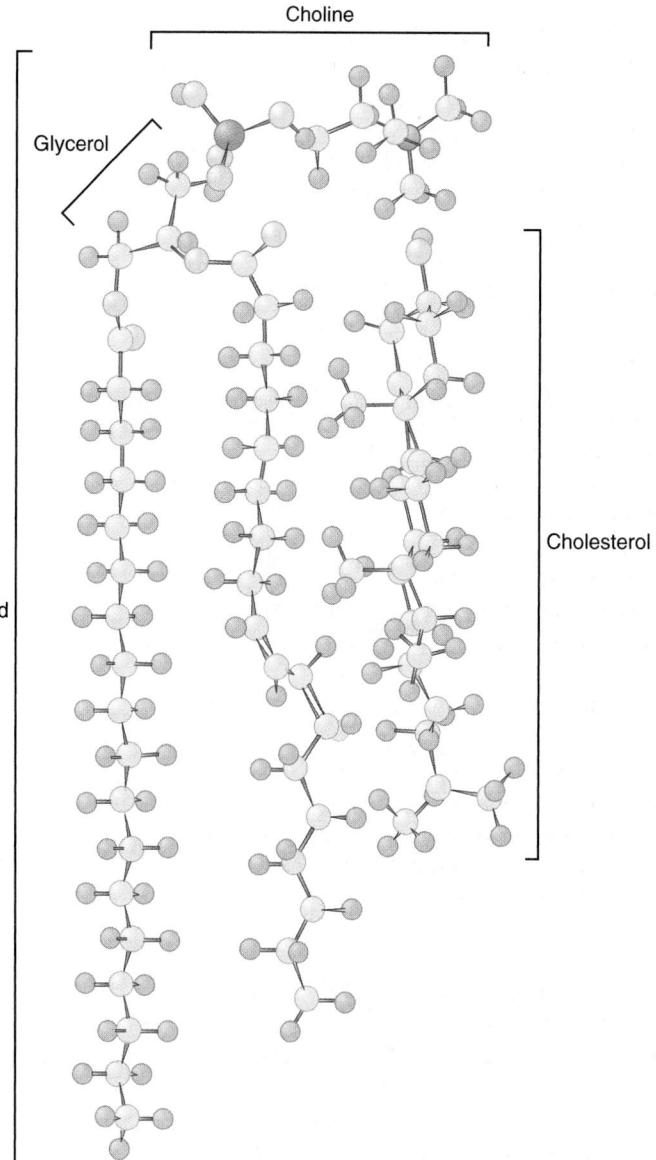

FIGURE 15-2. Approximate orientation of cholesterol and phospholipid (here phosphatidylcholine [PC]) molecules to each other in the membrane bilayer. On average, the cholesterol rings are believed to associate with the first 8 to 10 carbons of the phospholipid acyl chains. Note that the fatty acyl chain attached to the sn-1 position of the glycerol on PC is saturated and straight whereas the sn-2 side chain is unsaturated and kinked (tan, carbon; light blue, hydrogen; yellow, oxygen; orange, phosphorus; green, nitrogen).

Glycolipids and Cholesterol

Glycolipids and cholesterol are intercalated between the phospholipids in the bilayer, with their long axes perpendicular to the bilayer plane (see Fig. 15-2). Red cell glycolipids are located entirely in the external half of the bilayer, and their carbohydrate moieties extend into the aqueous phase. They carry many important red cell antigens, including A, B, H, Le[a], Le[b], and P, and serve other important functions. The P glycolipid, for example, serves as the receptor for parvovirus B19,[21] the agent responsible for most erythroid aplastic crises.

Cholesterol is present on both sides of the bilayer[7,22] and is nearly saturated in the red cell membrane—that is, its concentration is just below the concentration at which major changes in its organization and accessibility to enzymatic modification occur.[23] Its distribution is not known but it is probably slightly more prevalent in the outer half[24,25] because of its high affinity for SM, which is concentrated in the outer bilayer. However, because all of the membrane cholesterol is available for exchange within seconds ($T_{1/2} \approx 1$ second)[26] and has first-order kinetics, inner and outer membrane cholesterol must be exchangeable at an even greater rate. This facilitates membrane bending because movement of cholesterol can offset the difference in surface pressure caused by bending and compression of one of the bilayers relative to the other. Depletion of cholesterol promotes inward curvature of the membrane, whereas enrichment of cholesterol favors outward deflection.[23]

Cholesterol molecules are relatively buried because the 3-OH group, the part of the molecule that is at the aqueous interface, lies approximately at the level of the carbonyl group of the phospholipid fatty acids (see Fig. 15-2).[19,27] Cholesterol has important functions in buffering the fluidity of phospholipid side chains and in forming "lipid rafts," as will be described. In addition, some cholesterol binds directly to some membrane proteins and activates or inactivates them,[28-30] probably through a sterol-sensing domain.[31] Whether this is important in the function of mature red cells is unknown.

Trans Asymmetry

Red cell membrane lipids, like membrane proteins (to be discussed), are asymmetrically distributed across the bilayer plane.[32-34] Choline phospholipids (PC and SM) are concentrated in the outer half of the bilayer, whereas aminophospholipids (PE and PS) and PI are largely confined to the inner half (see Table 15-1). The evidence has been critically reviewed.[10,35-37]

The asymmetric distribution of phospholipids reflects a steady state involving a constant exchange (flip/flop) of phospholipids between the two bilayer hemileaflets.[35,36] In the red cell membrane this transmembrane diffusion is slow, lasting several hours to a day.[38,39] In contrast, the enzymatic translocation of phospholipids in biologic membranes, described in the following paragraphs, is much faster (minutes). At least three distinct activities are involved in regulating membrane phospholipid asymmetry. They are discussed in recent reviews.[40-43]

Flippase. The Mg-ATP–dependent aminophospholipid translocase, or "flippase," is responsible for localization of PS in the inner leaflet by rapidly translocating it from the outer to the inner leaflet against an electrochemical gradient. The stoichiometry between PS translocation and ATP hydrolysis is close to one. PE is translocated to a slight degree. The half-times for translocation of PS and PE are about 5 and 60 minutes, respectively, at 37° C.[44] Similar activity exists in all mammalian red cells[45] and probably in all cells and some cell organelles. Flippase is likely to contain a critical cysteine because it is inhibited by sulfhydryl-modifying reagents.[40] It is also inhibited by the pseudosubstrates of P-type adenosine triphosphatases (ATPases), such as vanadate, and by high concentrations of Ca^{2+}.

Unfortunately, despite almost 2 decades of effort, the aminophospholipid translocase is not fully characterized.[40] Erythrocyte Mg^{2+}-ATPase, purified and reconstituted into proteoliposomes, enhances the movement of PS analogues, but the active fraction contains multiple proteins ranging from 35 to 120 kd. Although it is possible that the translocase contains multiple subunits, definitive proof that Mg^{2+}-ATPase is responsible for flippase activity has not yet been achieved.

One candidate for the aminophospholipid translocase is ATP8A1 (ATPase II), a Mg^{2+}-ATPase first described in bovine chromaffin granules.[46] Close homologues of this protein are found in human red cells.[47,48] The cDNA predicts a unique P-type ATPase in which several amino acids that are involved in ion translocation in other P-ATPases are replaced by hydrophobic groups. Yeasts lacking a homologous protein, Drs2, are defective in aminophospholipid transport.[46] However, the story is complicated because Drs2 is located in the Golgi apparatus, not in the plasma membrane, and is one of a four similar and mostly redundant proteins in yeast.[42] Furthermore, the purified murine ATP8A1 enzyme,

despite having almost all the characteristics of the red cell aminophospholipid transporter when assayed in vitro, is not activated by N-methyl-PS,[47] which is transported by the red cell membrane flippase, as well as native PS, so it is still unclear whether this enzyme is the physiologic aminophospholipid translocase. If not, the true translocase is probably closely related. The ATP8A1 gene has not yet been deleted, which will provide an important test.

Floppase. The Mg-ATP–requiring phospholipid translocase, or "floppase," is responsible for movement of phospholipids from the inner to the outer leaflet of the bilayer,[41] and it is less specific than the flippase.[49,50] The outward lipid movement by the floppase is also much slower than the inward movement of PS by the flippase. Recent evidence suggests that the floppase is one of the family of ATP-binding cassette (ABC) transporters, of which the multidrug resistance transporter (ABCB1, MDR1, or P-glycoprotein) is the best known.

ABCB1 has broad specificity for short-chain lipids and xenobiotics and is unlikely to be the floppase.[41,42,51] Similarly, ABCA1 (ABC1), which exports cholesterol and is deficient in Tangier disease,[52] is an unlikely candidate. This is also true for ABCB4 (MDR1), which is specific for PC[51] and is involved in the secretion of PC into bile[53] but is selectively expressed in the liver, not in red cells. However, there is some evidence in support of ABCC1 (MRP1).[54,55] The efflux of short-chain fluorescent phospholipid analogues of PC, SM, and PS can be measured in erythrocytes and requires ATP and reduced glutathione. This activity is lost in mice lacking the gene equivalent to MRP1,[54] and long-term (48-hour) inhibition of activity leads to loss of PC and SM from the outer bilayer but no change in the distribution of PE or PS.[56] However, it is not yet certain that ABCC1 can transport full-length, native phospholipids, which is a required property of the physiologic floppase.

Scramblase. In conjunction with the two ATP-requiring transporters flippase and floppase, the Mg-ATP–independent, Ca^{2+}-dependent phospholipid "scramblase" facilitates rapid, bidirectional movement of all phospholipids in the bilayer, thereby resulting in the collapse of phospholipid asymmetry,[57] which may occur in less than a minute under some circumstances. Indeed, a high Ca^{2+} concentration can disrupt phospholipid asymmetry by activation of the scramblase and inhibition of the flippase. It is generally accepted that under physiologic conditions (cytosolic Mg-ATP concentration in the millimolar range and Ca^{2+} in the submicromolar range), phospholipid asymmetry is maintained by activation of the flippase and floppase and inactivation of the scramblase. Under these conditions, all phospholipids are slowly but continuously moved to the outer leaflet by the floppase, whereas the aminophospholipids PS and PE are immediately shuttled back to inner leaflet by the flippase.

A single polypeptide of approximately 37 kd with scramblase activity has been purified from red cell membranes. It mediates the Ca^{2+}-dependent redistribution of fluorescently labeled phospholipids between leaflets of reconstituted proteoliposomes,[58] and the cloned protein (PLSCR) has other features suggesting that it binds Ca^{2+} and is attached to membranes.[59,60] However, it does not appear to be the authentic red cell scramblase because blood cells from the knockout mouse are not deficient in activation-induced lipid scrambling![61] Thus, the scramblase, like the flippase and floppase, remains to be conclusively identified.

Loss of Phospholipid Asymmetry

High intracellular Ca^{2+} concentrations in red cells lead to loss of phospholipid asymmetry as a result of activation of the scramblase and inhibition of the flippase. Because normal red cells maintain very low intracellular Ca^{2+} concentrations, their membranes preserve an asymmetric phospholipid distribution through their entire 120-day life span.

Phospholipid Asymmetry Is Lost in Sickle and Thalassemic Red Cells. Changes in the equilibrium distribution of phospholipids could occur under conditions in which flippase is inhibited and either the scramblase is activated or floppase or scramblase activity accelerates to a degree that overwhelms the translocase, or both. A subpopulation of circulating sickle red cells show exposure of PS on their surface.[62] There is large variability in the numbers of sickle red cells that expose PS in sickle cell patients (0.5% to >10%). Phospholipid flip-flop is increased and phospholipid asymmetry is lost in sickle cells,[63-65] in which several forms of skeletal protein damage have been documented,[66-68] including decreased phospholipid translocase activity[63] and uncoupling of the lipid bilayer from the underlying skeleton in the sickle cell spicules.[69] A subpopulation of thalassemic red cells also show exposure of PS on their surface,[70] and phospholipid asymmetry is altered in diabetic red cells,[71] which like sickle cells,[72,73] tend to adhere to endothelial cells.[71]

Externalized Phosphatidylserine Triggers Clotting and Phagocytosis. It is generally believed that red cells, as well as essentially all other cells, sequester aminophospholipids on the cytoplasmic side of the plasma membrane because the exposed lipids trigger the conversion of prothrombin to thrombin and promote intravascular clotting.[74-76] Loss of phospholipid asymmetry may also activate the alternative complement pathway.[77]

In addition, macrophages bind and ingest cells, or even liposomes, that have PS exposed on their outer surfaces.[78-81] Exposure of PS is one of the earliest events in apoptosis, and the PS receptor seems to have evolved to scavenge dead or dying cells that have activated scramblase during apoptosis.

Several adhesive surface receptors on macrophages, including CD14, CD36, CD68, and the class B scavenger protein SR-BI,[82] may participate in recognition and removal of PS-exposing cells during apoptosis. However, these receptors do not discriminate between PS and other anionic phospholipids. The PS-specific receptor is not yet fully defined. A candidate receptor called PSR has been cloned by using a monoclonal antibody that blocks binding of PS,[83] and the phenotype in knockout mice is consistent with a protein that functions to clear dead cells[84]; however, subsequent work suggests that it is not the desired receptor (reviewed by Williamson and Schlegel[85]).

Finally, there is some speculation that the aminophospholipid translocase might foster endocytosis by "pumping" PS and PE into the inner bilayer.[86] Even a small excess of inner bilayer phospholipids would tend to make the membrane invaginate (see later).

Scott's Syndrome: A Defect in the Phospholipid Scramblase?

Scott's syndrome is a very rare autosomal recessive disorder characterized by decreased scramblase activity.[87,88] As a consequence, activated platelets fail to expose sufficient PS on their surface to assemble prothrombinase, and affected individuals have a bleeding tendency.[89] Erythrocytes and other cells also lack scramblase, but without apparent consequence. Whether this is due to mutations in the scramblase itself or is a secondary consequence of some other defect is unknown. The putative red cell scramblase gene (*PLSCR*) has been sequenced and is normal.[90]

Eryptosis

Red Cells May Undergo a Kind of Apoptosis in Response to Oxidative Damage. It is unclear whether the PS receptor participates in the removal of erythrocytes that bear surface PS, such as sickled cells or thalassemic cells, but it seems likely that it does. After an initial report by Bratosin and colleagues in 2001,[91] multiple recent papers by Lang and associates describe a process resembling apoptosis in damaged erythrocytes that they term "eryptosis" (reviewed by Lang and co-workers in 2006[92]). The process seems to be a *forme fruste* of apoptosis because it is not induced by classic apoptotic agents such as staurosporine and because mature red cells lack mitochondria and nuclei.[91] It is characterized by decreased red cell volume, membrane blebbing, activation of the protease calpain, and exposure of PS at the outer membrane leaflet, which leads to phagocytosis by macrophages. Eryptosis is triggered by oxidative stress, influx of Ca^{2+} ions, red cell dehydration, osmotic shock, prostaglandin E_2, and a variety of other stimuli and is inhibited by erythropoietin.[92]

The process resembles that induced by caspases, and recent investigations show that mature red cells contain Fas, Fas ligand, Fas-associated death domain, and caspases 8 and 3 and that oxidatively stressed cells recapitulate apoptotic events, including translocation of Fas into lipid rafts (see later), formation of a Fas-associated complex, and activation of caspases 8 and 3.[93-95] Activation of Fas is also associated with inhibition of the aminophospholipid translocase (flippase) and activation of the scramblase.[96] Thus, exposure of PS on red cells, as on nucleated cells, may often be the consequence of apoptotic events.

If these findings can be confirmed by other groups, they raise the possibility that the hemolysis in many conditions may be mediated by eryptosis, especially conditions associated with increased oxidant damage or cell dehydration (or both), such as sickle cell anemia, thalassemia, Heinz body hemolytic anemias, Hb CC disease, glucose-6-phosphate dehydrogenase (G6PD) deficiency, and hereditary xerocytosis. Moreover, if this is true, interference with the process may be therapeutic.

Recent reports show that Foxos (Forkhead O genes) regulate the cellular response to oxidative stress[97,98] and that the absence of Foxo3, in particular, leads to a marked decrease in expression of antioxidant enzymes in erythroid precursors and marked susceptibility of mature red cells to the reactive oxygen species that red cells generate during their daily oxygen-carrying duties or to exogenous oxidants. It will be interesting to see whether these red cells also die of eryptosis, as would be predicted from the aforementioned studies, and whether manipulation of the Foxo pathway can be used to treat anemias characterized by oxidant damage.

Cis Asymmetry

Macroscopic Domains. Red cell lipids also exist in different domains *within* each of the bilayer planes (*cis* asymmetry). Fluorescent phospholipids partition into doughnut-shaped lipid domains up to several microns in diameter within the membrane of red cells or ghosts.[99] These lipid-rich domains are intrinsic structural features of the membrane, not just "gel-phase" or "fluid-phase" domains.[99] They increase in size when membrane proteins aggregate, and they are lacking in large liposomes made solely of membrane lipids, which suggests that proteins play a role in their formation. How and why this occurs is a mystery.

Microscopic Domains: Protein-Bound Lipids. Lipids also partition on a more microscopic scale within the membrane. Early experiments[100] detected a layer of tightly associated "boundary lipids" attached to membrane proteins that intruded into the bilayer core, but subsequent work[101] suggested that such lipids were bound only transiently ($<10^{-7}$ second) and probably were not distinguishable from other lipids in the bilayer on the time scale of enzyme reactions and other cellular events. However, there are probably exceptions to this generalization because specific lipids are required for the enzymatic functions of some transport proteins, such as the sodium and calcium pumps or the cholesterol-binding proteins described earlier, and because some membrane proteins, such as glycophorin A (GPA; to be discussed), bind anionic (PS, PI) but not choline (PC, SM) phospholipids[102-104] and those lipids are relatively tightly bound.[105] Positively charged amino acids are concentrated on the cytoplasmic side of the bilayer-spanning domains of glycophorins and other membrane proteins,

in part because their position determines the orientation of the protein.[106,107] Although it is not well documented, anionic phospholipids probably cluster near these regions of positive charge. Surface-bound membrane proteins such as spectrin and protein 4.1, which bind preferentially to anionic phospholipids,[108,109] may also contribute to the nonrandom topography of inner membrane phospholipids, and conversely, the lipids appear to contribute to stability of the membrane skeleton.[110]

Membrane Lipid Rafts. Membrane lipid rafts reflect lateral heterogeneity in the lipid bilayer of the plasma membrane and have been implicated in a variety of sorting and signaling processes in cells.[111,112] They appear to be present in all cells and can be functionally isolated as detergent-resistant membranes by virtue of their property of being insoluble in cold, nonionic detergents. Cholesterol and SM are the principal lipids,[111,113] although recent evidence suggests that the rafts also contain large amounts of phosphoinositides.[114] The relatively saturated acyl chains in SM makes SM molecules pack tightly together and interact favorably with the cholesterol ring system. As a consequence, the SM-cholesterol complex is more resistant to solubilization with nonionic detergents. Red cell lipid rafts contain a complex mixture of membrane proteins, including stomatin, flotillin-1 and flotillin-2, the Duffy protein receptor, heterotrimeric Gα_s, and proteins bearing glycosylphosphatidylinositol (GPI) chains, such as CD55, CD58, and CD59.[115-117] Proteins with myristate or palmitate side chains may also tend to partition into the rafts,[118-120] whereas proteins with prenyl side chains are excluded.[119] The large integral membrane proteins that form intramembranous particles (to be discussed) are also excluded.[113] Altogether, raft proteins constitute about 4% of the red cell's membrane proteins. Depletion of cholesterol from the red cell membrane abrogates raft formation and the ability of raft-associated proteins to form membrane microdomains. When red cell cytosolic Ca^{2+} is increased, some of the lipid rafts are shed in large (micro) and small (nano) vesicles. The microvesicles are highly enriched in stomatin, whereas the nanovesicles contain predominantly synexin, a protein involved in vesicle fusion, and sorcin.[117] The flotillins are not found in either vesicle. This means that there are different kinds of lipid rafts in the membrane, with different fates. Although the function of the rafts in normal red cell physiology remains to be determined, it is interesting to note that they appear to play a critical role in the membrane remodeling necessary for invasion of red cells by malarial parasites (reviewed by Murphy and colleagues[121]).

Bilayer Couple Hypothesis

The shape of the lipid bilayer is responsive to very slight variations ($<0.4\%$) in the surface area of its inner and outer halves.[122,123] This is termed the "*bilayer couple effect*."[124] It reflects the tight packing of membrane lipids,

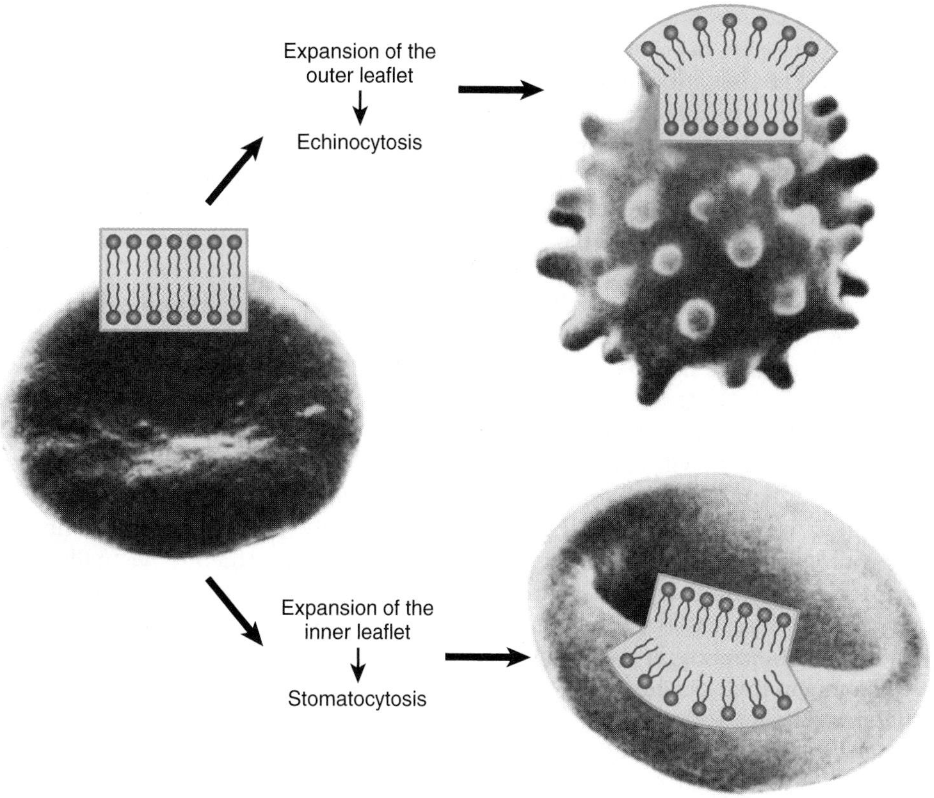

Expansion of the
outer leaflet

Echinocytosis

Expansion of the
inner leaflet

Stomatocytosis

FIGURE 15-3. Bilayer couple hypothesis. Compounds or processes that selectively expand the outer leaflet of the lipid bilayer will produce uniform membrane spiculation (echinocytosis). Selective expansion of the inner leaflet of the bilayer leads to membrane invagination and cup-shaped red cells (stomatocytosis). *(Adapted from Palek J, Jarolim P. Clinical expression and laboratory detection of red cell membrane protein mutations. Semin Hematol. 1993;30:249, with permission.)*

the independent motion of lipids in each half of the bilayer, and the extreme thinness of the membrane (<0.1% of the diameter of the cell). Processes that expand the outer bilayer (or contract the inner) will produce uniform membrane spiculation, called *echinocytosis* (Fig. 15-3). Conversely, relative expansion of the inner bilayer will lead to membrane invagination and cup-shaped red cells (i.e., *stomatocytosis*). Strongly charged amphipathic compounds, such as phospholipids, cause echinocytosis.[123,125] They are trapped in the outer bilayer by their fixed charge. Permeable amphipaths (e.g., weak acids and bases that can cross the membrane in their uncharged form) will cause the membrane to extend toward the side of greater accumulation.[126,127] In general, cationic compounds will accumulate in the negatively charged inner bilayer and anionic compounds will partition to the neutral outer bilayer. Even subtle effects, such as differences in the cross-sectional area of lipid head groups or fatty acyl tails, can lead to changes in membrane curvature.[125]

The bilayer couple hypothesis predicts that shape changes resulting from expansion of one lipid leaflet can be reversed by a commensurate alteration in the other. For example, the intensely spiculated red cells of patients with abetalipoproteinemia can be almost completely converted to biconcave discs by the addition of small amounts (0.1 mM) of chlorpromazine, a cationic amphipath.[128] Unfortunately, this simple test has not been widely applied to pathologic red cells, so it is difficult to estimate how often bilayer couple effects dictate cell shape in vivo.

There is some evidence suggesting that shape is not totally explained by the bilayer couple hypothesis, which

has led some researchers to support a protein scaffold theory, in which complex interactions of the spectrin-actin network, the lipid bilayer, and intracellular water interact to shape the erythrocyte.[129] The plasma lipid bilayer contributes bending rigidity; the membrane skeleton contributes stretch and shear elasticity.[130]

Membrane Phosphoinositides

The polar head group of this interesting class of phospholipids contains PI or its phosphorylated forms phosphatidylinositol 4-phosphate (PIP) and phosphatidylinositol 4,5-bisphosphate (PIP_2). In nucleated cells, phosphoinositides are precursors of important intracellular second messengers such as inositol 1,4,5-triphosphate (IP_3) and diacylglycerol. In mature erythrocytes, phosphoinositides represent 2% to 5% of the total phospholipids. They reside at the inner membrane surface and undergo rapid phosphorylation and dephosphorylation.[131] They help regulate Ca^{2+} transport; interact with membrane proteins such as glycophorin C (GPC), spectrin, and protein 4.1 (see later); and may influence discocyte-echinocyte shape transformation.

Lipid Mobility

Acyl Side Chains

Purified Lipids Exist in Gel or Liquid Crystalline States. Purified phospholipids exhibit discrete transitions from the liquid crystalline to the gel phase that are dependent on the length and degree of unsaturation of their acyl side chains. Above the temperature of this transition, the acyl side chains waggle very rapidly (10^8 to 10^9 times per second) from side to side, with progressively greater excursions as one proceeds from the glycerol ester linkage to the terminal methyl group.[132] The presence of a double bond in the acyl chain increases the disorder and flexibility all along the hydrocarbon chain,[133,134] especially toward the terminal methyl end. Below the temperature needed for transition from the liquid crystalline to the gel phase, acyl chains of purified lipids are extended in stiff, parallel, hexagonally packed arrays that are more nearly solid than liquid.

Cholesterol Creates an Intermediate State between Gel and Liquid Lipids.
Cholesterol buffers the extremes of the gel and liquid crystalline states. At temperatures above the gel-liquid phase transition, cholesterol partially immobilizes the acyl chains of phospholipids, particularly the proximal 8 to 10 carbons that are adjacent to the bulky steroid nucleus.[132] Below this transition, cholesterol disrupts ordering of the acyl chains, in effect preserving membrane fluidity.[135,136] The net result is that cholesterol tends to abolish the gel-to–liquid crystalline transition and creates a condition of intermediate fluidity in which the proximal ends of the hydrocarbon chains are extended and relatively rigid and the distal ends are disordered and fluid.

The red cell membrane contains relatively large amounts of cholesterol (cholesterol-phospholipid ratio, 0.8 mol/mol) and is relatively less fluid than other plasma membranes.[137] The inner bilayer is somewhat more fluid than the outer,[138] probably because it contains more unsaturated fatty acids. The significance of this difference is unknown.

The steady-state polarization of fluorescent probes such as 1,6-diphenyl-1,3,5-hexatriene is widely used to measure lipid "fluidity." However, it is difficult to know whether the polarization changes are due to true alterations in lipid fluidity or to changes in lipid organization that alter the location and spectroscopic properties of the probe or its interactions with membrane proteins.[139]

Lateral Diffusion

Phospholipids move about rapidly within each plane of *model* lipid bilayers.[137,140,141] From the measured lateral diffusion constants (2 to 5×10^{-8} cm^2/sec), one can calculate that phospholipids exchange places with each other about 10^7 times per second. This rate is somewhat dampened in the red cell membrane (estimated diffusion constant of 1.4×10^{-8} cm^2/sec),[142] but the difference is about what would be expected in view of the effects of cholesterol on the lateral mobility of phospholipids.[141]

Lipid Renewal Pathways

Mature Erythrocytes Cannot Synthesize Lipids.
Mature erythrocytes are unable to synthesize fatty acids, phospholipids, or cholesterol de novo and depend on lipid exchange and fatty acid acylation as mechanisms for phospholipid repair and renewal (Fig. 15-4). Outer bilayer phospholipids (PC, SM) exchange slowly (approximate turnover time of 5 days)[143] with the phospholipids of plasma lipoproteins.[144,145] Inner bilayer phospholipids (PS, PE) are unable to participate in this process and are virtually unexchangeable.[143]

Esterification Depletes Red Cell Cholesterol.
Fatty acids and lysophosphatides exchange more rapidly. Red cell membrane cholesterol (unesterified) also exchanges readily with the unesterified cholesterol in plasma lipoproteins ($T_{1/2} = 7$ hours), where it is partially converted to *esterified* cholesterol by the action of *lecithin-cholesterol acyltransferase (LCAT)*. Because the newly formed cholesteryl ester cannot return to the red cell membrane (there is virtually no esterified cholesterol in the membrane), LCAT catalyzes a unidirectional pathway (see Fig. 15-4) that depletes the membrane of cholesterol and decreases its surface area. Conversely, if LCAT is absent or inhibited, excess membrane cholesterol accumulates and expands the membrane surface area.[146]

Fatty Acid Acylation May Repair Phospholipid Side Chains.
The fatty acid acylation pathway is an active metabolic pathway that requires ATP energy. This system combines fatty acids with lysophosphatides (principally Lyso-PC) to remake the native phospholipid (see Fig. 15-4).[147-149] The acylase enzyme and its phospholipid products are located in the inner bilayer.[150] In theory, this enzyme should facilitate the renewal of lost or damaged fatty acid side chains and should prevent the accumulation of deleterious lysophosphatides within the membrane; however, it is not certain that the phospholipases necessary to remove damaged fatty acids operate in the red cell.

These renewal pathways, though limited, permit slow replacement of membrane lipid components. Approximately 30 days is required before erythrocyte lipids reach equilibrium after a change in dietary fatty acids.[151] Theoretically, this could be pathologically significant in persons on unusual diets (e.g., infants receiving a high intake of medium-chain triglycerides); however, no pathologic consequences have been reported to date.

MEMBRANE PROTEIN COMPOSITION

The red cell membrane (or "ghost") contains at least a dozen major proteins[7] and more than 300 minor ones.[152] The major proteins of the red cell membrane (Fig. 15-5; Table 15-2) and their disorders have been intensively studied,[168-170] and in most cases their genes have been cloned. It is important to realize that enumeration and characterization of all the proteins of the red cell membrane may never be achieved because the membrane is not a separate, discontinuous structure but one that

PLASMA LIPOPROTEINS   RED CELL

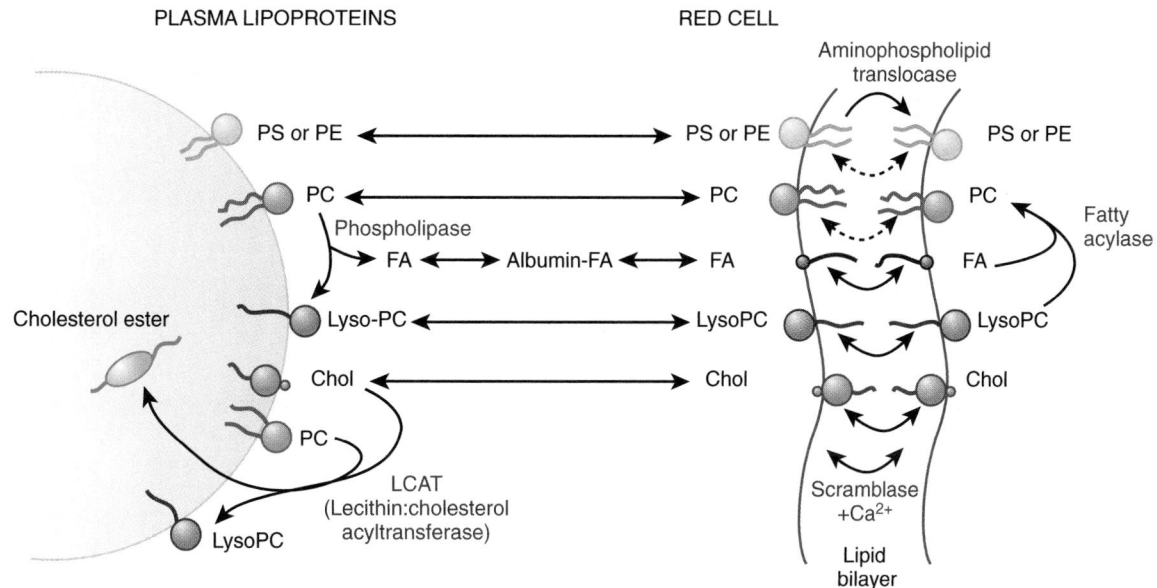

FIGURE 15-4. Pathways for lipid exchange and fatty acid replacement in the red cell membrane. Chol, cholesterol; FA, fatty acid; Lyso-PC, lysophosphatidylcholine; PC, phosphatidylcholine; PE, phosphatidylethanolamine; PS, phosphatidylserine.

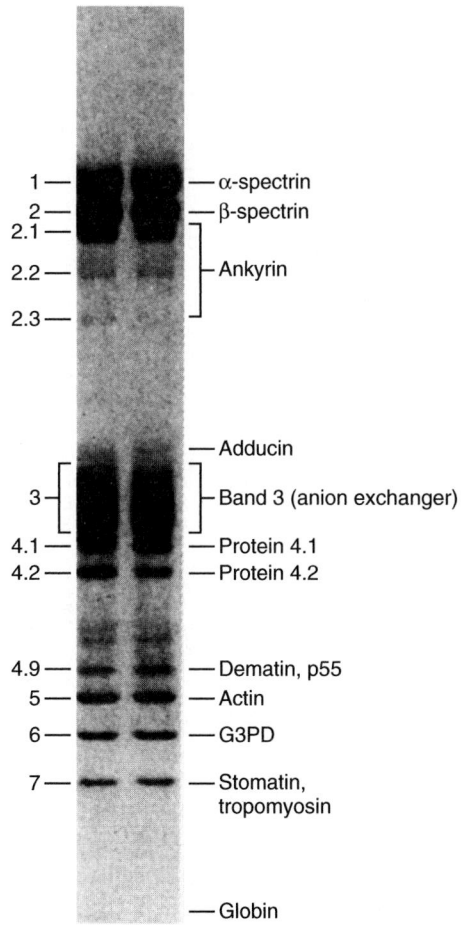

FIGURE 15-5. Major proteins of the red blood cell membrane. The proteins are separated by sodium dodecyl sulfate gel electrophoresis with the Fairbanks-Agre gel system[11,153] and stained with Coomassie blue. The glycophorins and the Rh proteins bind this dye poorly and are not visible. G3PD, glyceraldehyde-3-phosphate dehydrogenase. *(Adapted from Costa FF, Agre P, Watkins PC, et al. Linkage of dominant hereditary spherocytosis to the gene for the erythrocyte membrane-skeleton protein ankyrin. N Engl J Med. 1990;323:1046, with permission.)*

is in equilibrium with both the cytoplasm and the extracellular space. Many of the minor membrane proteins are technically challenging to isolate because of their low concentration, their insolubility, or their sensitivity to even minor variations in isolation conditions.

The protein constituents of the red cell membrane are classically defined by hypotonic hemolysis of red cells,[171] followed by polyacrylamide gel electrophoresis (PAGE) in sodium dodecyl sulfate (SDS).[7] In general, membrane proteins are classified as either *integral* or *peripheral*. Integral membrane proteins penetrate or traverse the lipid bilayer and interact with the hydrophobic lipid core. They include band 3, the anion exchange channel, and the glycophorins, which generate a negative charge at the cell surface, function as receptors, and display surface antigens (Fig. 15-6). Integral membrane proteins form the randomly distributed 8- to 10-nm intramembranous particles seen on freeze-cleave electron microscopy of red cell membranes. Peripheral proteins interact with integral proteins or lipids at the membrane surface but do not penetrate into the bilayer core. In the red cell, the major peripheral membrane proteins are located on the cytoplasmic membrane face and include enzymes such as glyceraldehyde-3-phosphate dehydrogenase (G3PD) and the structural proteins of the membrane skeleton. The red cell membrane skeleton is operationally defined as the insoluble proteinaceous residue that remains after extraction of red cells[172] or their ghosts[173] with the nonionic detergent Triton X-100. The membrane skeleton contains 55% to 60% of the membrane protein mass and includes such proteins as spectrin, actin, protein 4.1, p55, adducin, dematin, tropomyosin (TM), tropomodulin (TMod), ankyrin, and part of band 3 and protein 4.2 (see Fig. 15-6).

TABLE 15-2   Major Erythrocyte Membrane Proteins

SDS Gel Band[a]	Protein	Human Gene Name	MOLECULAR MASS (kd) — Gel	MOLECULAR MASS (kd) — Calc[b]	Monomer Molecules per Cell[c] (×10³)	Oligomeric State	Proportion[d] (%)	Peripheral or Integral	Chromosome Location	Associated Diseases
1	α-Spectrin	SPTA1	240	281	242 ± 20	Heterodimer/	14	P	1q21	HE, HPP, HS
2	β-Spectrin	SPTB	220	246	242 ± 20	tetramer/ oligomer	13	P	14q22-q23.2	HS, HE, HPP
2.1[e]	Ankyrin[e]	ANK1	210	206	124 ± 11[e]	Monomer	5[e]	P	8p11.2	HS
2.9[f]	α-Adducin	ADD1	103	81	≈30	Heterodimer/tetramer	1	P	4p16.3	HS (mice)
	β-Adducin	ADD2	97	80	≈30	tetramer	1	P	2p14-p13	HS (mice)
3[f]	Band 3, AE1	SLC4A1	90-100[g]	102[h]	≈1200	Dimer or tetramer	26	I	17q21-q22	HS, SAO, RTA, HAc, HSt, HC
4.1	Protein 4.1	EPB41	80 + 78[i]	66[j]	≈200	Monomer	3	P	1p36.1	HE
4.2	Protein 4.2	EPB42	72	77	≈250	?Dimer	4	P	15q15	HS[k]
4.9[f]	Dematin[l]	EPB49	48 + 52	43 + 45	≈140	Trimer	1	P	8p21.1	—
	p55	MPP1	55	53	≈80	?Dimer	1	P	Xq28	—
5[f]	β-Actin	ACTB	43	42	≈500	Oligomer (≈14)	5	P	7p15-p12	—
5[f]	Tropomodulin	TMOD	43	41	≈30	Monomer	1	P	9q22.3	—
6	G3PD	GAPDH	35	36	≈500	Tetramer	5[m]	P	12p13.31-p13.1	None
7[f]	Stomatin	EPB72	31	32	≈500	Heterodimer[n]	4	I	9q34.1	—
	Tropomyosin	TPM3	27 + 29	≈30[n]	≈70	?	<1	P	1q22-q23	—
8[f]	Peroxiredoxin-1	PRDX1	23	22	?	Dimer or decamer	1-2	P	1p34.1	OH (mice)
	Peroxiredoxin-2[o]	PRDX2	23	22	≈200[o]	Dimer or decamer	1-2	P	19p13.2 (?13q12)[o]	OH (mice)
PAS-1[p]	Glycophorin A	GYPA	36[q]	14[h]	≈1000	Dimer	3[p]	I	4q28.2-q31.1	None
PAS-2[p]	Glycophorin C[r]	GYPC	32[q]	14[h]	≈150		0.3[p]	I	2q14-q21	HE
PAS-3[p]	Glycophorin B	GYPB	20[q]	8[h]	≈200	?Dimer	0.4[p]	I	4q28.2-q31.1	None
	Glycophorin D[r]	GYPD	23[q]	11[h]	≈50		0.1[p]	I	2q14-q21	HE
	Glycophorin E	GYPE	—[s]	6[h]	—[s]	—[s]	—[s]	I	4q28.2-q31.1	

[a]Numbering system of Fairbanks et al.[11] Bands 1 to 8 refer to gels stained with Coomassie blue. PAS-1 to PAS-3 refers to gels stained with periodic acid–Schiff. The data for spectrin and ankyrin were measured directly by radioimmunoassay,[154] as were the data for glycophorins.[155]

[b]Calculated from amino acid sequences.

[c]Based on an estimate of 5.7×10^{-13} g protein per ghost[7] and on the approximate proportion of each protein, estimated from densitometry of SDS gels.

[d]Proteins 1 to 8 were estimated from published[11,156,157] and unpublished (Lux SE and John KM) data.

[e]Protein 2.1 is full-length ankyrin and is the major isoform. Other isoforms are evident on SDS gels, including band 2.2 (195 kd), band 2.3 (75 kd), and band 2.6 (145 kd). Band 2.2 is produced by alternative splicing. The origin of the other bands is unknown.

[f]The α- and β-adducins lie at the high-molecular-weight end of SDS gel band 3, a region that is sometimes called band 2.9. Band 4.9 contains both dematin and p55. Band 5 contains β-actin and tropomodulin. Band 7 contains stomatin and tropomyosin, and band 8 contains peroxiredoxin-1 and peroxiredoxin-2.

[g]The protein runs as a broad band on SDS gels because of heterogeneous glycosylation.

[h]The calculated molecular weight does not include the contribution of the carbohydrate chains.

[i]Protein 4.1 is a doublet (4.1a and 4.1b) on SDS gels. Protein 4.1a is derived from 4.1b by slow deamidation.[158] Its proportion is a measure of red cell age.

[j]Protein 4.1 homologues are encoded by at least four genes[159] and exist in a very large number of isoforms.[160-163] The major erythroid gene product is listed here.

[k]Deficiency of protein 4.2 is associated with a variety of red cell morphologies, but spherocytes predominate.[164]

[l]The 52-kd isoform of dematin contains a 22–amino acid, N-terminal, adenosine triphosphate binding domain that the 48-kd dematin lacks.[164,165] The two proteins are derived from the same gene. They form a trimer containing two 48-kd subunits and one 52-kd subunit.[164]

[m]The amount of G3PD associated with the membrane varies from person to person (≈3 to 6 wt%).

[n]Red cell tropomyosin is a heterodimer of 27- and 29-kd subunits. There are about 70,000 copies of each chain per red cell. The two major human tropomyosin isoforms found in red cells are hTM5 and hTM5b and derive from the γ- and α-TPM3 genes, respectively.[166] We have not been able to find the exact sequence of these two isoforms.

[o]Peroxiredoxin-2 is also known as calpromotin, thioredoxin peroxidase B, thiol-specific antioxidant protein (TSA), protector protein (PRP), natural killer-enhancing factor B, acidic peroxidoxin, and torin. It translocates between the cytoplasm (dimer) and the membrane (decamer). There are about 14 million protein molecules in the cytoplasm but only about 200,000 on the membrane judging from SDS gels. The gene is located at 13q12 on the cytogenetic map and at 19p13.2 on the human genome sequence map. This dichotomy is currently unexplained.

[p]The glycophorins are visible only on PAS-stained gels.

[q]Molecular weights, including carbohydrate, were estimated from mobility on SDS gels.[156,167]

[r]Glycophorins C and D are synthesized from the same mRNA but with different translational start sites.[167]

[s]Glycophorin E mRNA has been identified, but it is not certain that the mRNA is translated.

G3PD, glyceraldehyde-3-phosphate dehydrogenase; HAc, hereditary acanthocytosis; HC, hereditary cryohydrocytosis; HE, hereditary elliptocytosis; HPP, hereditary pyropoikilocytosis; HS, hereditary spherocytosis; HSt, hereditary stomatocytosis; OH, oxidant hemolysis; RTA, renal tubular acidosis; SAO, Southeast Asian ovalocytosis; SDS, sodium dodecyl sulfate.

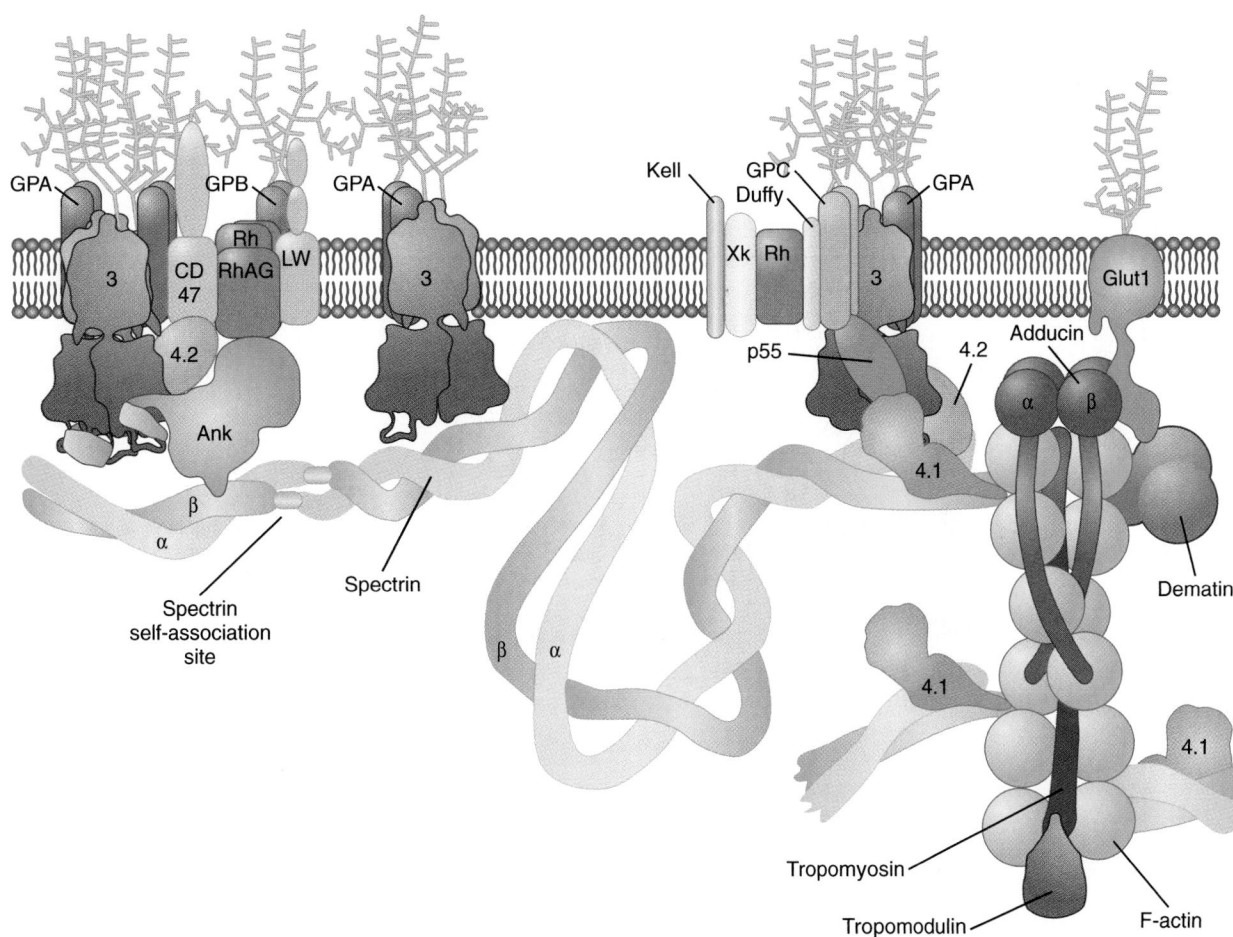

FIGURE 15-6. Schematic model of the red cell membrane. The proteins are drawn roughly to scale, although it is not clear that spectrin ever folds away from the membrane in the manner shown. The relative positions of some of the proteins, particularly within the band 3 tetramer–Rh/RhAG–protein 4.2–CD47 complex and the band 3 dimer–Kell–Xk–Rh–Duffy–GPC–GPA complex, are not known. Recent evidence suggests that band 3 dimers are located near the spectrin-actin junction, where proteins 4.1 and 4.2 bind, as well in untethered positions within the lipid bilayer. In addition, to show its various interactions, the actin protofilament is drawn perpendicular to the membrane plane, jutting out into the cytoplasm, whereas it actually lies parallel to the membrane. The complexes of proteins associated with band 3 are not stoichiometric—that is, some proteins are present in much smaller numbers than others (e.g., Rh, Kell, Xk, Duffy, LW). As a consequence the band 3 complexes shown must vary in their composition. Ank, ankyrin; GPA, glycophorin A; GPB, glycophorin B; GPC, glycophorin C; RhAG, Rh-associated glycoprotein.

INTEGRAL MEMBRANE PROTEINS

Band 3 (AE1, SLC4A1)

Band 3, the major integral membrane protein of the red blood cell, accounts for 25% to 30% of the cell membrane protein (≈1.2 million copies per cell). It is also called anion exchange protein 1 (AE1), but its official title is solute carrier family 4 (anion exchanger), member 1, or SLC4A1. The human band 3 gene is located on chromosome 17q21-q22 and encodes a 911–amino acid polypeptide of 102 kd.[174,175] Band 3 migrates as a diffuse band on SDS gels (see Fig. 15-5) as a result of heterogeneous *N*-glycosylation with a short complex oligosaccharide or an extended polylactosaminyl chain.[176] Residues 1 to 403 generate the 43-kd N-terminal cytoplasmic domain, which functions (1) as an anchor point for the membrane skeleton through interactions with the peripheral membrane proteins ankyrin, protein 4.1, and

protein 4.2 and (2) as a binding reservoir for hemoglobin, denatured hemoglobin, and glycolytic enzymes. Residues 509 to 911 form a 52-kd channel that exchanges HCO_3^- and Cl^-, thereby facilitating the critical function of red cells in the uptake of CO_2 in tissues and subsequent release of CO_2 in the lungs. The carboxy-terminal of band 3, which resides on the cytoplasmic side of the membrane, also binds carbonic anhydrase II.[177]

Cytoplasmic Domain

The N-Terminal Portion of Band 3 Is the Cytoplasmic Binding Domain. The cytoplasmic domain of band 3 is readily released from the red cell membrane as a 43-kd fragment after treatment with chymotrypsin or trypsin.[178] The first 45 amino acids are highly acidic and stretch into the cytoplasm (Fig. 15-7). The remainder of the cytoplasmic domain is remarkably mobile, with expansion at high pH and contraction at low pH,[181] because of a conformational transition that is not fully understood.

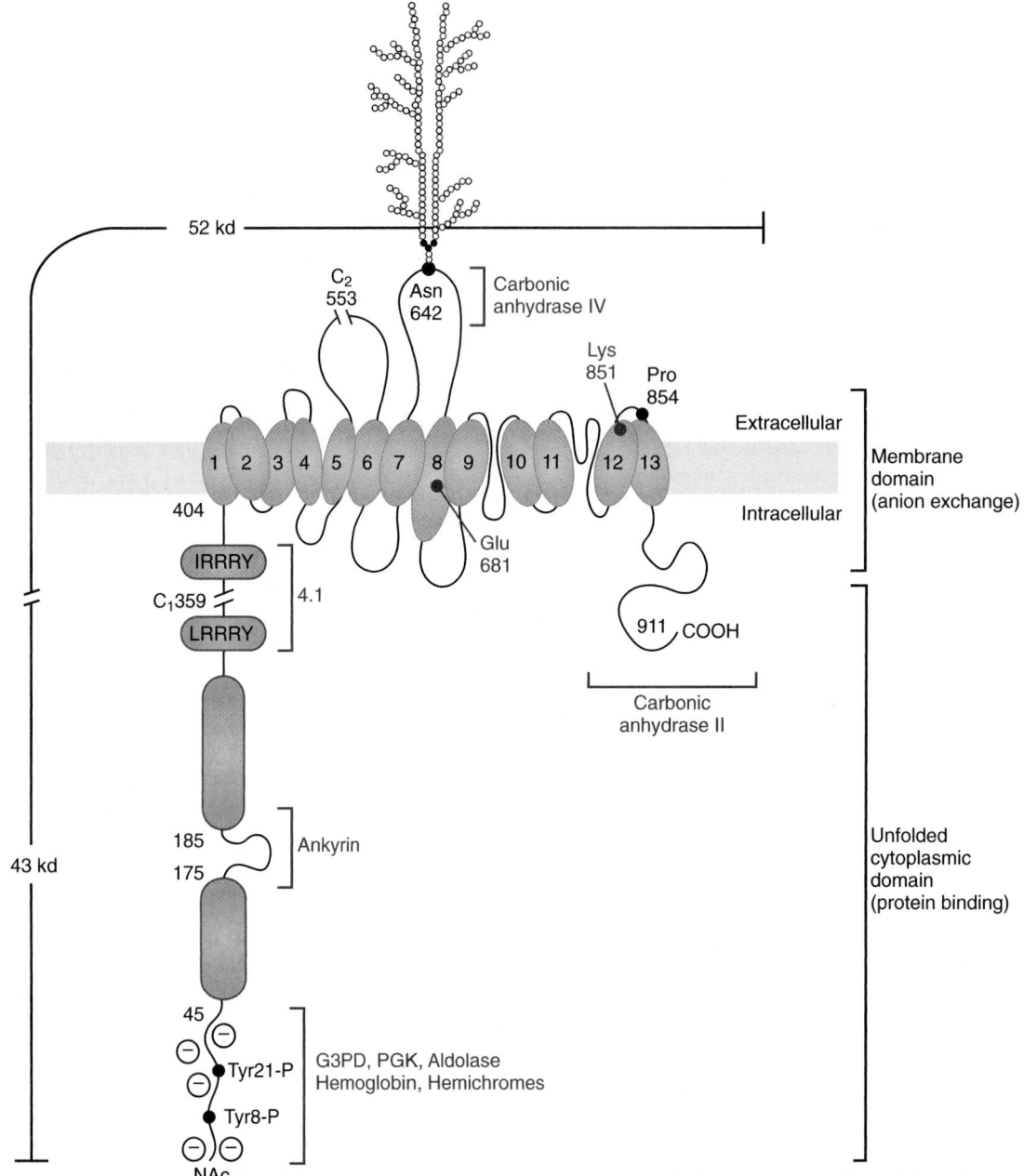

FIGURE 15-7. Organizational model of human erythrocyte band 3 (anion exchange protein, AE1). The protein is divided into two structurally and functionally distinct domains: an approximately 43-kd cytoplasmic domain (amino acids [aa] 1 to 359) that contains binding sites for several cellular proteins and an approximately 52-kd transmembrane domain (aa 360 to 911) that forms the anion exchange channel. The two regions can be separated by cleavage of chymotrypsin at the inner membrane (C_1). A second chymotrypsin site (C_2) is accessible at the external surface. *Cytoplasmic domain:* The highly acidic N-terminal end (aa 1 to 45) binds deoxyhemoglobin, hemichromes, and the glycolytic enzymes phosphoglycerate kinase (PGK), aldolase, and glyceraldehyde-3-phosphate dehydrogenase (G3PD). Enzyme attachment is blocked by phosphorylation of tyrosines 8 and 21. Antibodies to the N-terminal end also interfere with binding of ankyrin, but the main ankyrin site is aa 175 to 185. Protein 4.1 binds to two sites with the (I/L)RRRY motif, near the end of the domain. The binding site for protein 4.2 has not been clearly identified. *Membrane domain:* One current model[179] suggests that band 3 contains 13 α-helical membrane-spanning segments and two additional transmembrane (TM) regions with nonhelical conformations, all of which are connected by hydrophilic loops. Almost nothing is known about how the various TM segments are positioned relative to each other. There is good evidence that Glu681 is required for anion transport and that TM8 and probably TM1+2 and TM13 form part of the channel. Presumably, the unique nonhelical TM segments between TM regions 9-10 and 11-12 are also involved. Pro854 is the site of the Diego[a] blood group antigen[180] and must be extracellular. A complex carbohydrate structure is attached to Asn642. Carbonic anhydrase II (CA-II) binds to the C-terminal of band 3, and CA-IV binds to the extracellular loop between TM7 and TM8. Both are perfectly positioned to shuttle HCO_3^- ions to or from plasma through band 3. *(Adapted with permission from Walensky LD, Narla M, Lux SE. Disorders of the red cell membrane. In Handin RI, Lux SE, Stossel TP [eds]. Blood: Principles and Practice of Hematology, 2nd ed. Philadelphia, JB Lippincott, 2003, pp 1709-1858, with permission.)*

The Acidic N-Terminal Sequence of Band 3 Binds Hemoglobin.
Hemoglobin binds weakly to the acidic N-terminal of band 3 ($K_{d\ [deoxy\ Hb]} = 0.31$ mM), but because the concentration of hemoglobin is so high in red cells, roughly half of the band 3 molecules are bound to hemoglobin under physiologic conditions.[182,183] X-ray crystal structures show that the first 11 amino acids of band 3 penetrate the 2,3-diphosphoglycerate (2,3-DPG) binding cavity in the center of hemoglobin.[182] Because the cavity closes when hemoglobin is oxygenated, only deoxyhemoglobin binds to band 3. Thus, band 3 lowers O_2 affinity, but when hemoglobin is only partially saturated with band 3, its cooperativity is also reduced.[184] This has led to the idea that band 3–bound hemoglobin could preferentially bind O_2 at low pO_2 values and then release it upon saturation with 2,3-DPG in the cytoplasm.[184]

Denatured Hemoglobin Molecules Copolymerize with the Cytoplasmic Domain of Band 3 and Form Aggregates, Which May Play a Role in Red Cell Senescence.
Hemichromes, a partially denatured form of hemoglobin, bind to band 3 more avidly than hemoglobin does, thereby resulting in the formation of hemichrome–band 3 aggregates.[183,185,186] This clustering of band 3 is believed to generate a cell surface epitope identified by autologous IgG antibodies that targets the cell for phagocytosis (see the later section "Red Cell Membrane Alterations of Senescent Red Cells").[187] The formation of such a senescence antigen by band 3 copolymerization with hemichromes may also contribute to the clearance of sickle, β-thalassemic, and hemoglobin Köln red cells, all of which contain unstable hemoglobin that oxidatively degrades into hemichromes. Band 3 clustering can generate multivalent epitopes composed of surface sialylated poly-*N*-acetyllactosaminyl chains, which in turn can be recognized by anti–band 3 IgG autoantibodies and by macrophages directly.[188]

The N-Terminal Sequence Also Binds Glycolytic Enzymes, Which Probably Form a Membrane Metabolon.
The first 23 amino acids of band 3 contain two tandem repeats terminating in the sequences DDY⁸ED and EEY²¹ED. Glyceraldehyde-3-phosphate dehydrogenase (G3PD),[189] phosphoglycerate kinase (PGK),[190] and aldolase[191,192] all bind in this region. Aldolase requires both sites to bind, G3PD binds separately to each, and PGK binds to the more distal site.[193] In confirmation, the red cells from a child with a mutant band 3 that lacks the first 11 amino acids (Bd 3 Neapolis) contain no membrane-bound aldolase.[194]

Approximately 65% of G3PD, 50% of PGK, and 40% of aldolase are membrane bound in the intact red cell,[189,195] and they are inhibited when attached to the membrane.[191,192,196] In addition, lactate dehydrogenase (LDH) and pyruvate kinase (PK) also localize to the membrane, even though they do *not* bind to band 3 (Fig. 15-8).[197] All five enzymes are displaced into cytoplasm by an antibody to the N-terminal of band 3, by phosphorylation of tyrosines 8 and 21, which lie in the middle of the two binding sites, or by deoxygenation, which causes hemoglobin to bind to the N-terminal of band 3 (see later).[197]

The data suggest that at least the distal enzymes in the glycolytic pathway form a complex (a "metabolon") that is bound to band 3 and can be regulated by tyrosine phosphorylation, by the state of oxygenation,[197-199] and perhaps by substrates and cofactors of the enzymes.[189-191] Antibodies show that the enzymes are present in discrete clumps along the membrane, which also supports this idea (see Fig. 15-8). It is not clear whether more proximal glycolytic or pentose phosphate pathway enzymes are also part of this putative metabolon, but there is evidence that diphosphoglyceromutase may be.[200] Interestingly, the existence of a membrane-bound complex of glycolytic enzymes was postulated more than 40 years ago[201] and was indirectly observed more than 25 years ago,[202] but the nuclear magnetic resonance (NMR) methods used in the latter studies were considered suspect at the time and the interpretation was not generally accepted.

The obvious reason for a complex of glycolytic enzymes would be to increase the efficiency of the pathway by channeling glycolytic intermediates from one enzyme to the next (see Fig. 15-8). Furthermore, it would make sense if it were attached to band 3, which transports the phosphate needed to make ATP. However, a glycolytic metabolon might also have other functions. There is relatively recent evidence that human red cells can compartmentalize ATP, thereby allowing its direct use by membrane pumps without release into the cytoplasm.[203] This is another discredited old idea[204] that has been revived. Na^+,K^+-ATPase (the Na, K pump) is metabolically linked to ATP produced by PGK[205] and may be physically associated with PGK or neighboring enzymes.[202] There are only about 290 Na^+,K^+-ATPase molecules per red cell,[206] so perhaps other pumps are also involved.

Some mammalian band 3s lack the acidic N-terminal binding sites on band 3 and do not bind G3PD, which suggests that the interaction of band 3 with glycolytic enzymes either is a late evolutionary adaption[207] or is inconsequential or an artifact. However, deoxygenation of intact human red cells increases glycolysis,[208] and mild oxidants, which stimulate tyrosine phosphorylation in human erythrocytes, also elevate glycolytic rates.[1]

The Cytoplasmic Domain of Band 3 Functions as an Attachment Site for Membrane Skeleton Proteins.
Ankyrin links the major membrane skeletal protein spectrin to the plasma membrane of the red cell by binding to a β-hairpin loop formed by amino acids 175 to 185 in the cytoplasmic domain of band 3[209]; however, this is probably not the only binding site because removal of the β-hairpin does not cause nearly as much hemolysis as loss of ankyrin or band 3 does.[210] Binding blocks access to the N-terminal of band 3, which is nearby (Fig. 15-9; see also Fig. 15-7). Ankyrin's linkage of spectrin to band 3 forms the basis of the skeletal-membrane attachment,

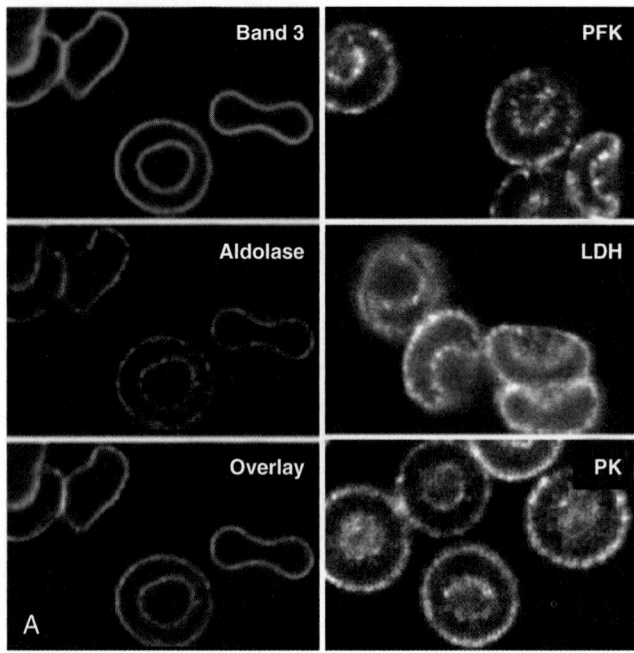

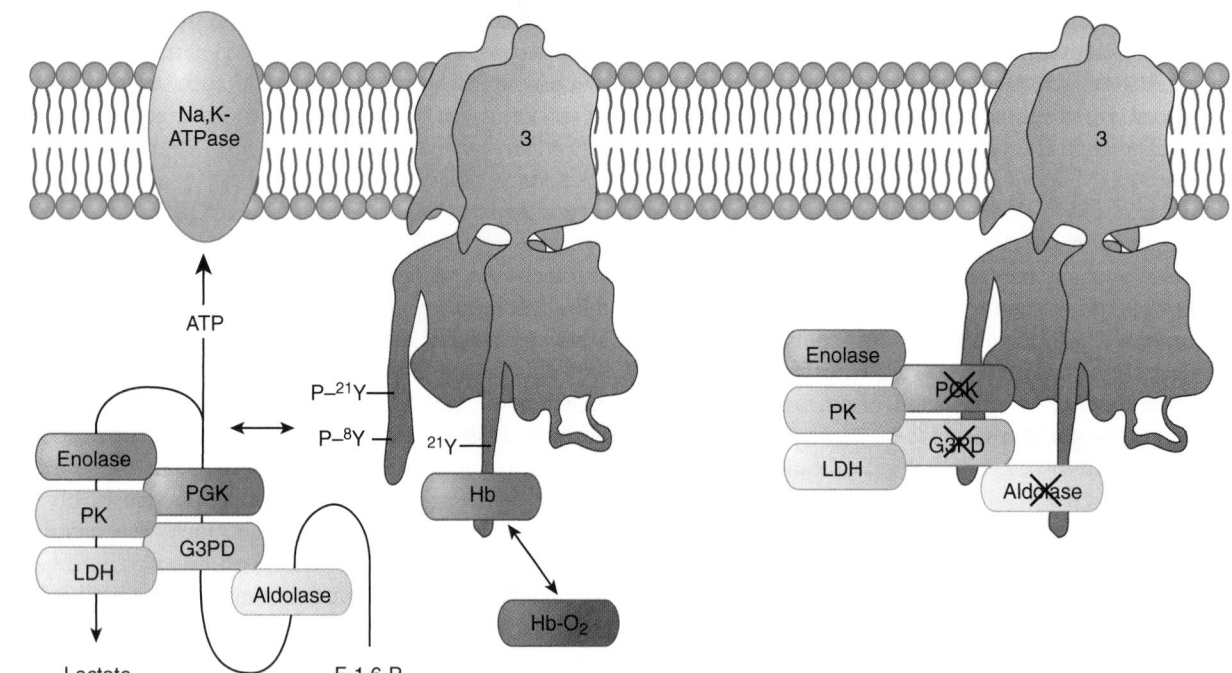

FIGURE 15-8. Postulated glycolytic metabolon. **A,** Fluorescent imaging of band 3 and aldolase on the *left* and phosphofructokinase (PFK), lactate dehydrogenase (LDH), and pyruvate kinase (PK) on the *right*. Note that band 3 is uniformly and exclusively in the membrane whereas the five enzymes are mostly attached to the membrane (some cytoplasmic staining, especially for LDH) and have a punctate appearance as though they are clustered. Glyceraldehyde-3-phosphate dehydrogenase (G3PD) stains similarly but is not shown. Aldolase, PFK, and G3PD bind to band 3; PK and LDH do not. However all are displaced by a fragment of the band 3 binding site, by phosphorylation of the site, or by deoxyhemoglobin, thus suggesting that all are bound in a complex or "metabolon." **B,** Schematic of the postulated glycolytic metabolon. When the enzyme complex is bound to band 3 (*right*), it is inactive. The complex can be displaced and activated (*left*) by phosphorylation of Tyr8 and Tyr21 on band 3 or by binding of deoxyhemoglobin. There is some evidence that part of the adenosine triphosphate (ATP) produced is retained at the membrane and used by the Na⁺,K⁺-ATPase or other membrane pumps. Note that the inorganic phosphate needed for ATP production conveniently enters the cell through band 3. Band 3 also transports phospho*enol*pyruvate, pyruvate, and lactate, all substrates or products of the putative complex. *(Photomicrographs from Campanella ME, Chu H, Low PS. Assembly and regulation of a glycolytic enzyme complex on the human erythrocyte membrane. Proc Natl Acad Sci U S A. 2005;102:2402-2407.)*

which is essential to the mechanical and viscoelastic properties of the red cell. Ankyrin$_R$ preferentially binds to band 3 tetramers and may be required for stabilization of the tetramer.[211,212] It is estimated that 70% of band 3 exists as dimers and 30% as tetramers and higher-order oligomers, with the latter species predominantly associated with the membrane skeleton through interactions with ankyrin.[214]

Protein 4.1, which links the spectrin-actin–based skeleton to the plasma membrane in part via interactions with GPC, has also been shown to bind to the cytoplasmic domain of band 3 at specific (I/L) RRRY sequences near the inner membrane surface (see Fig. 15-7).[215,216]

However, there is controversy regarding whether protein 4.1 binds to band 3 in vivo.[213,217] The different experiments are difficult to reconcile, but recent in vivo experiments suggests that 4.1–band 3 interactions are important.[218] Zebra fish with severe hemolytic anemia because of lack of band 3 can be rescued by expressing normal band 3 in their erythrocytes, but only if the band 3 contains both (I/L)IRRRY sites. Deletion of one site halves the number of fish rescued, and deletion of both sites prevents any rescue from occurring.[218] Because band 3 and ankyrin compete for binding to tetrameric band 3,[213] it may be that protein 4.1 binds preferentially to dimeric band 3 (see Fig. 15-6).

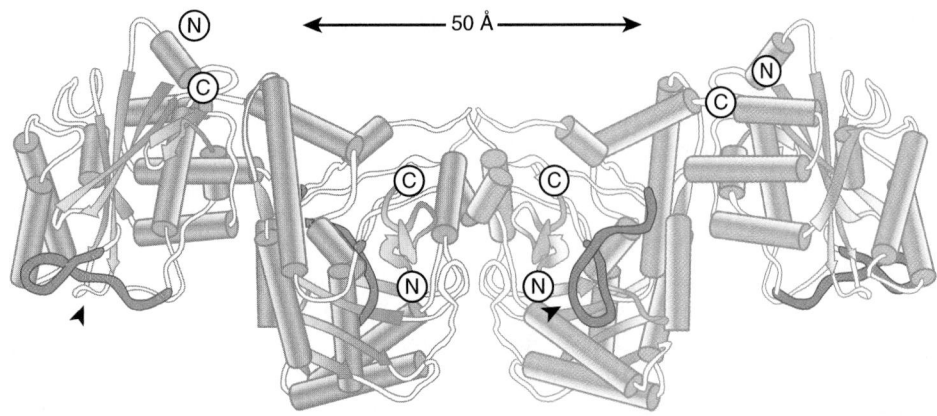

FIGURE 15-9. Crystal structure of the band 3 cytoplasmic domain. The deduced structure of the band 3 tetramer is shown. One dimer is blue, the other green. This is the conformation that binds ankyrin. The ankyrin binding loop[209] is colored a darker blue and the N- and C-terminal ends of the domain are marked by "N" and "C," respectively. Note that the tetramer structure brings two ankyrin sites together on the same side of the molecule (*arrowheads*). Because ankyrin has two band 3 binding sites and would bind with much higher affinity if both were engaged, this may explain why essentially only band 3 tetramers bind ankyrin.[211,212] Note also that the C-terminal ends of the cytoplasmic domain, where protein 4.1 binds, lie close to the ankyrin sites. This may explain why binding of ankyrin and 4.1 is mutually exclusive.[213] (*Redrawn from Walensky LD, Narla M, Lux SE. Disorders of the red cell membrane. In Handin RI, Lux SE, Stossel TP [eds]. Blood: Principles and Practice of Hematology, 2nd ed. Philadelphia, JB Lippincott, 2003, pp 1709-1858, with permission.*)

Protein 4.2, a 77-kd peripheral membrane protein of the red cell, also interacts with the cytoplasmic domain of band 3. The binding site is not well defined. Red cells from patients with the cytoplasmic band 3 mutations Glu40→Lys and Pro327→Arg show some deficiency of protein 4.2, thus suggesting that both proximal and distal cytoplasmic band 3 sequences may be involved. It is not clear whether protein 4.2 binds to the ankyrin-linked band 3 tetramers or the "free" band 3 dimers, but indirect evidence suggests the latter. In red cells from patients with HS who lack protein 4.2, the mobile fraction of band 3 rotates faster and shows greater lateral diffusion, and a greater fraction of band 3 is in the tetramer form, which suggests that band 3 dimers are preferentially lost as the cells become spheroidal.[219,220] Because protein 4.2 binds to the tail end of spectrin,[221] we suspect that it bridges between band 3 dimers and spectrin and that band 3 dimers localize near the spectrin-actin junction (see Fig. 15-6), but additional experiments are needed to test this hypothesis. Whatever the organizational arrangements, it appears that protein 4.2 depends on band 3 to be expressed in the membrane. Membranes from band 3 knockout mice completely lack 4.2,[222] and membranes from 4.2 knockout mice are partially deficient in band 3.[223]

Membrane Domain

The 52-kd Membrane Domain Contains an Anion Exchange Channel. The anatomy of the membrane domain of band 3 has been an active area of interest, with the goal of research efforts focused on understanding how the membrane domain's topology enables the 1.2 million channels in each red cell to exchange 10^{10} to 10^{11} HCO_3^- and Cl^- anions per second.[2] The membrane domain contains 13 α-helical membrane-spanning segments and two additional transmembrane regions with nonhelical conformations, all of which are connected by hydrophilic loops (see Fig. 15-7).[179] A fatty acid is esterified to Cys843. Its function is unknown.

Chemical modification of band 3 at Glu681 (which is found in transmembrane domain 8) by Woodward's reagent K (WRK) abolishes chloride transport, thus implicating this critical glutamic acid in channel function.[224] The key role of Glu681 in chloride translocation by human band 3 was confirmed by mouse band 3 mutagenesis (where Glu699 is the equivalent residue).[225] The membrane domain of band 3 can also accomplish sulfate transport, which requires cotransport with a proton supplied by glutamic acid.[226] Interestingly, WRK modification of band 3 does not interfere with sulfate transport except that proton cotransport is no longer required, thereby implicating Glu681 in the important proton donor step during sulfate transport.[225] Because sulfate-proton cotransport occurs in both inward and outward directions in the native protein and because Glu681 can be modified from both sides of the membrane, Glu681 must have access to both the intracellular and extracellular faces of the membrane.

Identification of Glu681 as a component of the band 3 permeability barrier has prompted thorough investigation of the confusing topology of the latter half of the membrane domain.[179,227-232] The current model, derived from this and other work, is shown in Figure 15-7. (1) Amino acids Met664-Ser690 form transmembrane domain 8 (TM8), which is longer than typical transmembrane domains. It appears to form part of the anion exchange channel. (2) Glu681 is located near the carboxy-terminal of TM8, probably at the portion of the channel that separates the inside and outside of the cell. (3) Amino acids on a polar face of TM12 and TM13 are required for anion exchange, thus suggesting that these domains may line the channel and participate in transport. Lys851, which reacts with an important inhibitor of anion exchange (4,4'-diisothiocyanostilbene-2,2'-disulfonate [DIDS]) is part of the polar face on TM12. The neighboring Ser852-Leu857 amino acids appear to function as a substrate charge filter.[232] (4) Eleven independent patients with hereditary cryohydrocytosis or HS have been identified who have five different mutations in band 3 that astonishingly, cause the anion channel to become a *cation* conductance channel![233,234] The mutations are clustered between the end of TM8 and the beginning of TM10, thus strongly suggesting that this region is also involved in the transport function. (5) There are nonhelical segments between TM9-TM10 and TM11-TM12 that are not externally accessible except for a segment in the middle of the latter loop (Pro815-Arg827), which is sometimes accessible from the extracellular space. (6) Arg656-Met663 (external loop from the carbohydrate side chain to TM8) may form a vestibule-like structure that draws anions toward the transport channel. Carbonic anhydrase IV, a GPI-linked protein, binds to band 3 in this region,[235] probably between Arg656 and Ile661, and forms part of a CO_2/HCO_3^- transport metabolon.

The Transport Channel Exchanges Chloride and Bicarbonate Rapidly ($T_{1/2}$ = 50 msec), Which Facilitates CO_2 Transport from Tissues to the Lungs. In peripheral tissues, CO_2 is rapidly converted to HCO_3^- at the surface of band 3 by carbonic anhydrase IV and is transported into the red cell, or it diffuses into the cell and is then converted to HCO_3^- by carbonic anhydrase II, which binds to the carboxy-terminal of band 3.[177] The H^+ by-product of the carbonic anhydrase reaction binds to hemoglobin and facilitates release of O_2 to tissues (i.e., the Bohr effect); this process is reversed in the lungs (Fig. 15-10). As the red cell circulates, intracellular HCO_3^- is exchanged for extracellular chloride. As a result, HCO_3^- is transported in plasma, as well as within the red cell, which increases transport of CO_2 from tissues to the lungs by approximately 60%.[2] HCO_3^--Cl^- exchange is believed to occur via a "ping-pong" mechanism whereby an intracellular anion enters the transport channel and is translocated outward and released, with the channel remaining in the outward configuration until an extracellular anion enters and activates the reverse cycle.[236] As discussed earlier, the amino acids of a subset of the transmembrane segments form the transport channel. Although monomeric band 3 has been shown to independently transport anions,[237] image analysis of negatively stained, two-dimensional crystals of band 3 dimers has demonstrated an apparent channel at the contact site between two monomers, thus suggesting that anion transport may occur via the dimer.[238] Further data suggest that band 3 dimerization produces allosteric effects that may modify channel function.[239]

Although HCO_3^- and Cl^- are the predominant physiologically relevant anions exchanged by band 3, the specificity of the channel is actually quite broad, and larger anions such as sulfate, phosphate, pyruvate, and superoxide are also transported, albeit at much slower rates.[240] Several potent and experimentally useful inhibitors of band 3 anion transport are also known, with the most commonly used being stilbene disulfonates such as DIDS.[240]

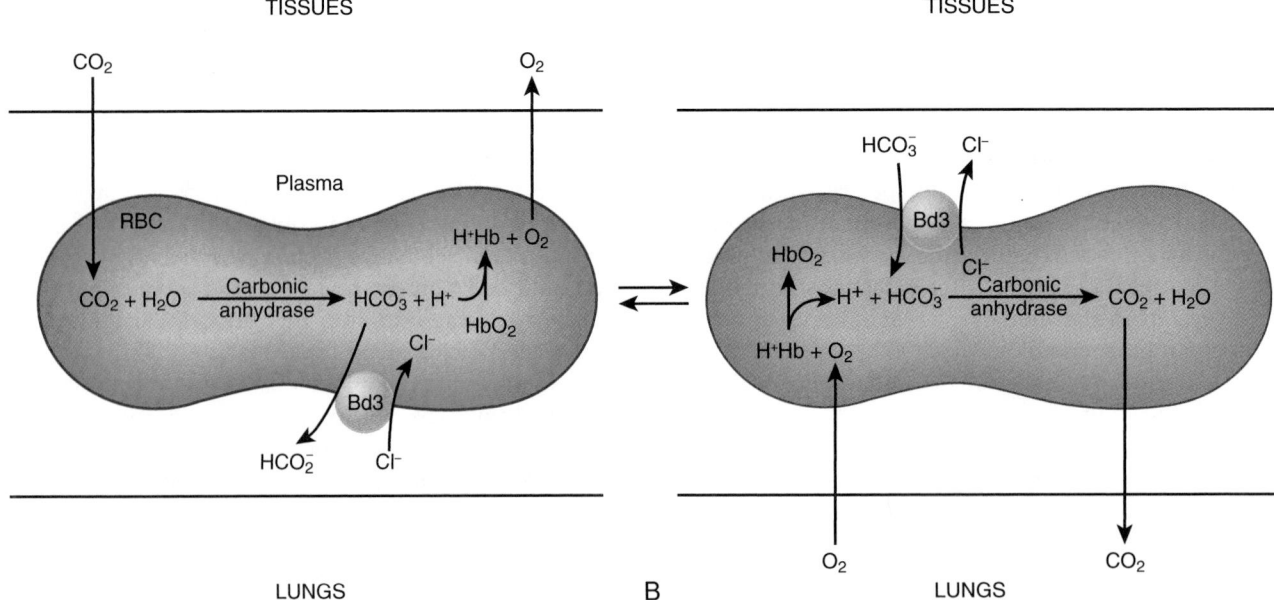

FIGURE 15-10. Function of band 3 in O_2 and CO_2 transport. **A,** Tissue CO_2 is converted into HCO_3^- and H^+ in the red cell by carbonic anhydrase. Band 3–mediated exchange of HCO_3^- for Cl^- (Hamburger shift) allows HCO_3^- to be carried in plasma, as well as in red cells, and increases CO_2 uptake by about 60%. H^+ binds to hemoglobin and facilitates release of O_2 (Bohr effect) and tissue oxygenation. **B,** These processes are reversed in the lungs, with promotion of hemoglobin oxygenation and release of CO_2. *(After Weith JO, Anderson OS, Brahm J, et al. Chloride-bicarbonate exchange in red blood cells: physiology of transport and chemical modification of binding sites. Philos Trans R Soc Lond [Biol]. 1982;299:383.)*

The Extracellular Surface of the Band 3 Membrane Domain Is the Site of Specific Blood Group Antigens.

Asn642, located in the extracellular loop between TM7 and TM8, is derivatized with a complex lactosaminoglycan that is variable in length and contains the I/i blood group antigens (see Fig. 15-7).[241-243] In fetal cells, the carbohydrate chain is unbranched and has i specificity, whereas in adults, there is a branched structure that yields I reactivity. In rare circumstances, the I antigen is absent from adult red cells as a result of a branching enzyme deficiency.[244] The extracellular domains of band 3 also contain antigens of the Diego blood group system[180] and other polymorphisms accounting for many other antigen subtypes.[245-252] The Wr^b blood group antigen is generated by the association of band 3 with GPA in the red cell membrane (see next paraglaph).[252]

The Integral Membrane Protein Glycophorin A and the Membrane Domain of Band 3 Are Functionally Associated.

Although explicit protein binding data have yet to confirm a specific interaction between GPA and band 3, there is mounting evidence that the two red cell membrane proteins have a physiologically relevant association. Expression of the Wright (Wr) blood group antigen (a receptor for the malarial agent *Plasmodium falciparum*) requires interaction between GPA and band 3. Specifically, the presence of Glu658 in band 3 is required for normal expression of this blood group antigen,[253] and an Ala65→Pro mutation in GPA has been shown to cause aberrant Wright antigen expression.[254] Furthermore, a monoclonal antibody directed against the Wr^b antigen immunoprecipitates both proteins.[255] Anti-GPA antibodies have been shown to immobilize GPA *and* band 3 in the red cell membrane as determined by in situ fluorescence recovery after photobleaching (FRAP) assays.[256]

Coexpression of GPA and band 3 in *Xenopus* oocytes facilitates the expression of band 3. A loss-of-function mutation in band 3 at Gly701 leads to impaired protein targeting to the cell surface in *Xenopus* oocytes; the aberrant phenotype is rescued by coexpression of the mutant band 3 with GPA, which suggests a chaperone-like role for GPA in band 3 targeting.[257] GPA also enhances band 3 transport.[258] The effect is significant. For example, SO_4^{2-} transport is diminished 60% in the absence of GPA.[259] This appears to be due to an effect of GPA on band 3 flexibility such that band 3 can adopt a rigid, high-transport structure when GPA is present and a more flexible, lower-transport structure in its absence. Finally, red cells from band 3 knockout mice are completely deficient in GPA, thus showing that band 3 is also important for expression and trafficking of GPA.[260]

Band 3 Mutations

More than 20 different mutations in band 3 are known to cause HS as a result of decreased synthesis, membrane insertion, stability, and protein 4.2 binding of the aberrant band 3 protein. These are discussed in detail in the section "Hereditary Spherocytosis" later in the chapter.

Deletion of amino acids 401 to 408 in band 3 causes Southeast Asian ovalocytosis (SAO),[261,262] an autosomal dominant condition characterized by rounded ellipto-cytic cells, mild or absent hemolysis, and the presence of unusually rigid and heat-tolerant red cells that resist malarial invasion.[263] Multiple mutations in the membrane domain of band 3 and in the C-terminal tail have been independently associated with the autosomal dominant form of distal renal tubular acidosis (dRTA), a condition characterized by impaired distal nephron secretion of hydrogen ions (reviewed by Toye[264]). The phenotype is believed to result from faulty targeting of band 3 to the apical rather than the basolateral membrane of collecting tubule type A intercalated cells, as opposed to a defect in anion transport.[265] Mutation of Gly701 (located in the intracellular loop between TM8 and TM9) is associated with autosomal recessively inherited dRTA, with the phenotype again deriving from faulty band 3 trafficking.[257] Incomplete processing of the band 3 *N*-linked lactosaminoglycan moiety as a result of a deficiency in the relevant glycosyltransferase occurs in congenital dyserythropoietic anemia type II (CDA II or hereditary erythroblastic multinuclearity with a positive acidified serum lysis test [HEMPAS]), although it is probably not the primary molecular defect. A rare Pro868→Leu mutation in TM13 of band 3 causes hereditary acanthocytosis; affected red cells exhibit decreased ankyrin binding and increased anion transport.[266] Moreover, as noted earlier, mutations in band 3 that convert it from an anion to a cation channel are associated with phenotypes of hereditary cryohydrocytosis or HS.[233] Interestingly, band 3 knockout mice can exhibit a fatal hypercoagulable state that is believed to derive from disruption of red cell membrane phospholipid asymmetry, which can produce a cell surface suitable for activating thrombosis.[267] Knockout mice that survive the neonatal period have severe hemolytic anemia, and the band 3–null red cells are spherocytic with increased osmotic fragility (OF) because of membrane surface loss.[222]

Band 3 and Malaria

P. falciparum parasites are believed to invade red cells via two distinct pathways, one that is dependent on the sialic acids on GPA or GPC and a sialic acid–independent pathway that is linked to band 3. Recent work shows that expression of a parasite protein called PfRh4 correlates with switching to the sialic acid–independent pathway.[268] Liposomes containing purified band 3 inhibit invasion,[269] as does a monoclonal antibody against extracellular epitopes of band 3.[270] Peptides corresponding to the two nonhelical regions in Figure 15-7 also partially block invasion,[271] thus suggesting that these regions serve as receptors. MSP1 (*P. falciparum* merozoite surface protein 1) furnishes the ligand.[271]

Nonerythroid Band 3

Band 3 is a member of a highly conserved anion exchanger gene family (also named solute carrier family 4A

[SLC4A]) that is composed of AE1 (SLC4A1),[174,175] AE2 (SLC4A2),[272,273] AE3 (SLC4A3),[274] and their associated spliceoforms. AE1 is expressed in erythrocytes, testes, and kidneys. The kidney isoform of AE1 is found in type A intercalated cells of the collecting tubules and lacks the N-terminal 66 amino acids that interact with glycolytic enzymes and certain membrane skeletal elements in red cells.[275] Another splice variant of AE1 is found in cardiac myocytes.[276] AE2 is widely distributed (e.g., kidney, stomach, lymphocytes, choroid plexus) and probably represents the general tissue anion antiporter. AE3 localizes to excitable tissues such as the heart, brain, and retina. The role of anion exchangers in polarized epithelial cells, such as intercalated cells of the kidney, is to facilitate bicarbonate reabsorption and acid secretion. The CO_2 that diffuses into the cell is converted to H^+ and HCO_3^- by carbonic anhydrase, which is associated with the anion exchanger at the basolateral membrane. Whereas H^+ is ejected from the cell via the apical membrane H^+,K^+-ATPase, HCO_3^- exits at the basolateral membrane in exchange for chloride.

Glycophorins

The glycophorins are a family of integral membrane glycoproteins that account for the majority of the surface charge of the red cell. The extracellular domains of the glycophorins contain an abundance of sialic acid, which generates a layer of negative charge at the cell surface and thereby prevents adherence of red cells to each other and to the vessel walls. Surface epitopes of the glycophorins, including variants generated by protein defects, account for a wide diversity of blood group antigens in the MNSs system. Glycophorins also serve as receptors for infective agents such as *P. falciparum*. Recent data suggest that glycophorins may also function as chaperones by facilitating the targeting of specific integral membrane proteins to the plasma membrane. The glycophorins belong to the broad family of integral membrane proteins that pass through the lipid bilayer as a single α helix. Because other members of the "single-pass" membrane proteins include growth factor receptors and receptor kinases, the glycophorins have been considered potential candidates for mediating transmembrane signaling in red cells.

Glycophorin A

The GPA gene is located on the long arm of chromosome 4 (4q31) and encodes a 36-kd protein that is the major sialoglycoprotein of the red cell (~10^6 copies per cell, see Table 15-2). Of historical note, GPA was the first membrane protein to have its complete amino acid sequence determined. Amino acids 1 to 61 give rise to the extracellular N-terminal domain, which contains a complex oligosaccharide attached to Asn26[277] and 15 serine or threonine O-linked tetrasaccharides with sialic acid moieties (Fig. 15-11A).[278,279] The carbohydrate component

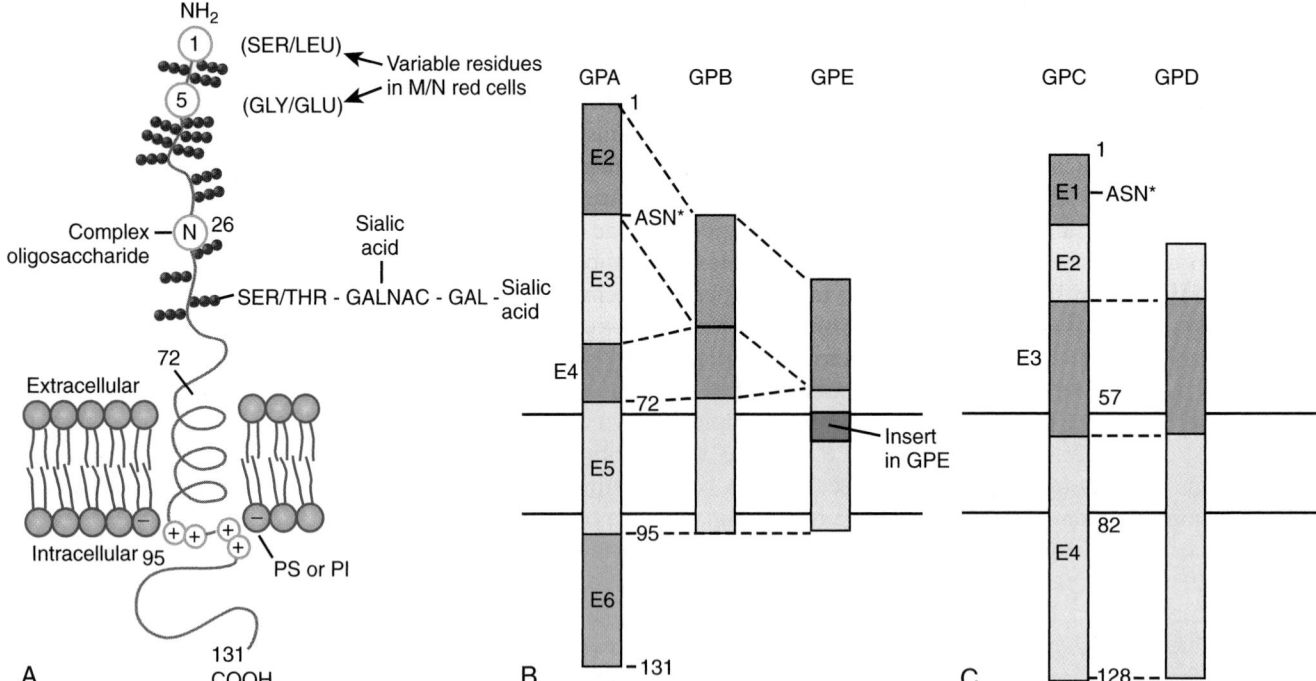

FIGURE 15-11. Structure of red cell glycophorins. **A,** Organization of glycophorin A (GPA), the major red cell sialoglycoprotein. The external domain has 15 tetrasaccharides attached to serine or threonine residues and one complex oligosaccharide attached to asparagine 26. Residues 1 and 5 are Ser and Gly in M red cells and Leu and Glu in N cells. PI, phosphatidylinositol; PS, phosphatidylserine. **B,** Schematic representation of the domain combinations of GPA, GPB, and GPE. Each *box* represents the portion of each protein encoded by a specific exon or insertion sequence. ASN* is the site of attachment of the complex carbohydrate. **C,** Schematic representation of the domains contributing to GPC and GPD. (*After Becker PS, Lux SE. Disorders of the red cell membrane skeleton: hereditary spherocytosis and hereditary elliptocytosis. In Scriver CR, Beaudet AL, Sly WS, Valle D [eds]. The Metabolic Bases of Inherited Disease, 7th ed. New York, McGraw-Hill, 1995; and Fukuda M. Molecular genetics of the glycophorin A gene cluster. Semin Hematol. 1993;30:138.*)

of GPA accounts for 60% of its molecular mass. Experimentally, the glycophorins run anomalously on SDS gels because the abundant carbohydrate interferes with detergent binding. In addition, the carbohydrate interferes with Coomassie blue staining such that special stains (e.g., periodic acid–Schiff) are required to visualize the glycophorins. The amino-terminal of GPA contains the site of the MN blood group antigens; specifically, amino acids 1 and 5 along with the sialic acid residues on adjacent O-linked tetrasaccharides dictate the antigenicity.[280] Whereas amino acids 1 and 5 are serine and glycine in MM red cells, leucine and glutamic acid in the corresponding positions characterize NN cells (Table 15-3). The transmembrane domain of GPA is composed of amino acids 62 to 95 and traverses the lipid bilayer as a single α helix. The membrane domain interacts with negatively charged lipids such as PS and PI.[102,313] Self-association of the Leu75-Ile76-XX-Gly79-Val80-XX-Gly83-Val84-XX-Thr87 motif within the transmembrane domain results in homodimerization into a right-handed pair of α helices.[314,315] NMR spectroscopy has shown that Ile76, Val80, and Val84 on the α helix of one monomer interface with Leu75, Gly79, Gly83, and Thr87 on the second monomer.[316] The extracellular domain also contributes to this dimeric interaction,[317] which is strong enough to resist dissociation by detergents.

Recent evidence shows that the cytoplasmic domain of GPA (amino acids 96 to 131) is important for enhancing the trafficking of band 3 to the membrane[317] and that the GPA–band 3 association increases band 3 anion transport (see the section "Band 3").[259] Conversely, GPA is also dependent on band 3 for trafficking or for stable incorporation in the red cell membrane inasmuch as mice that lack band 3 also lack GPA.[260]

Interestingly, treatment of red cells with antibodies (or monovalent Fab fragments) to GPA induces cellular rigidity as measured by ektacytometry, and the quantity of GPA that becomes associated with the membrane skeleton in experimental systems increases.[318] Both these changes are dependent on the presence of the cytoplasmic tail of GPA, which suggests that the cytoplasmic domain binds to the membrane skeleton in response to a transmembrane signal initiated by antibody treatment.[319] Hypothetically, the cellular rigidity induced by adherence of pathogens to glycophorins may serve the beneficial role of heightening reticuloendothelial clearance of infected cells[319] or may help impede invasion by parasites.

GPA has been used as a specific marker for the erythroid lineage because of its early detection in proerythroblasts.[320] In addition, assays to gauge radiation exposure and consequent somatic mutation based on measuring the frequencies of variant GPA phenotypes in red cells have been developed.[321]

Glycophorin B

The gene for glycophorin B (GPB) lies just downstream of GPA on chromosome 4 and is believed to have arisen by gene duplication.[322,323] The first 26 amino acids of the extracellular N-terminal domain are almost identical to the N blood group form of GPA except that the latter form lacks the N-linked complex oligosaccharide (see Fig. 15-11B).[280] In addition to N blood group reactivity, GPB carries the S, s, and U blood group antigens, with the S and s antigens differing by substitutions at residue 29 (S = Met, s = Thr) (see Table 15-3).[324] Distally, GPB lacks a portion of the extracellular domain corresponding to exon 3 of GPA and almost all of the cytoplasmic domain.

TABLE 15-3	Variants of Glycophorins A, B, and E	
Variant	**Defect**	**References**
AMINO-TERMINAL		
M	Ser-Ser*-Thr*-Thr*-Gly-Val...	280, 281
N	Leu-Ser*-Thr*-Thr*-Glu-Val...	280, 281
M^c	Ser-Ser*-Thr*-Thr*-Glu-Val...	282
M^g	Leu-Ser-Thr-Asn-Glu-Val...	283
H^e (Henshaw)	Trp-Ser*-Thr*-Ser*-Gly-Val...	284
OTHER		
En(a–)	Absence of glycophorin A†	156, 281, 285, 286
S–s–U–	Absence of glycophorin B†	156, 287, 288
M^k	Absence of glycophorins A and B†	156, 289
MiI (Miltenberger I), MiII, MiVII, MiVIII	Variants of glycophorin A that differ by one or two amino acids	290-294
MiIII, MiJ.L., MiV, MiVI, MiIX, MiX, Ph, Pj, Dantu, St^a (types A, B & C),	Variants caused by the formation of Lepore-like and anti-Lepore–like hybrids of glycophorins A, B, and E	156, 290, 295-310
Cad	Carbohydrate variant with an abnormal O-linked oligosaccharide containing an extra β(1→4)-linked galactosamine on the penultimate galactose residue of both glycophorins A and B	311, 312

*O-glycosylation site (see Fig. 15-11).
†Caused by homologous recombination and unequal crossing over as a result of partial gene deletions.

Glycophorins C and D

Glycophorin C (GPC) and glycophorin D (GPD) have a general domain structure similar to that of GPA and GPB (see Figure 15-11C), but they are encoded by a distinct gene located on chromosome 2 (2q14-2q21).[325] GPD is generated from the same mRNA as GPC by means of an alternative initiation codon.[167] GPC is a 32-kd protein bearing one *N*-linked oligosaccharide and approximately 12 *O*-linked oligosaccharides in the N-terminal, extracellular domain. The desialylated form of GPC is exposed on the surface of early erythroid progenitors (burst-forming unit–erythrocyte [BFU-E]) and is a useful marker of early normal or leukemic erythroid differentiation.[326] Normally, glycosylated GPC first appears at the colony-forming unit–erythrocyte (CFU-E) stage.[327] Amino acids 41 to 50 of the extracellular domain contain the Gerbich blood group antigens. Like GPA and GPB, the transmembrane domain passes through the lipid bilayer as a single α helix. The cytoplasmic domain of GPC forms a ternary complex with protein 4.1 and p55 and helps attach the spectrin-actin–based skeleton to the plasma membrane. The 30-kd membrane binding domain (MBD) of protein 4.1 interacts with amino acids 82 to 98 of GPC and the corresponding residues 61 to 77 of GPD.[328] p55 is a member of the membrane-associated guanylate kinase (MAGUK) family of proteins and contains a single PDZ domain that binds to GPC at residues 112 to 128 and to GPD at the corresponding amino acids 91 to 107.[328,329] The ternary complex of GPC/GPD, protein 4.1, and p55 (see Fig. 15-6) aids in maintaining and perhaps regulating red cell membrane deformability and mechanical stability. Unlike GPA and GPB, GPC and GPD are expressed in a variety of tissues (although at lower levels than in erythroid cells and with different glycosylation patterns)[330,331] and may have an analogous functions in the membrane mechanics of nonerythroid cells.

Glycophorin E

The gene for glycophorin E (GPE) lies just downstream of GPB on chromosome 4 and encodes a 78–amino acid protein with structural similarities to GPB (see Fig. 15-11B).[332] The extracellular domain of GPE corresponds to exon 2 of GPB, but the amino acid sequence specifies blood group M rather than N.[332] The transmembrane domain is encoded by exon 5 and contains an eight–amino acid insertion. Like GPB, GPE has a markedly truncated cytoplasmic domain. GPE is believed to have arisen by gene duplication of GPB, which in turn derived from ancestral duplication of GPA.[323] Thus, GPA, GPB, and GPE define an erythroid-specific family of integral membrane sialoglycoproteins. The level of expression of GPE and its specific functional role have not been determined, and we cannot exclude the possibility that it is a pseudogene.

Glycophorin Mutations

Defects in Glycophorins A, B, and E Give Rise to Nearly 40 Variant Phenotypes of the MNS Blood Group System.[333]

Complete loss of GPA, GPB, or both, often by gene deletion from unequal recombination of the neighboring loci, gives rise to En(a–), (S–s–), and M[k]M[k] red cells, respectively (see Table 15-3) (Fig. 15-12). En(a–) red cells, for example, are completely deficient in GPA and have weak MN blood group antigens.[285,286] The affected red cells compensate for a potential 60% loss of surface charge by increasing the glycosylation of band 3

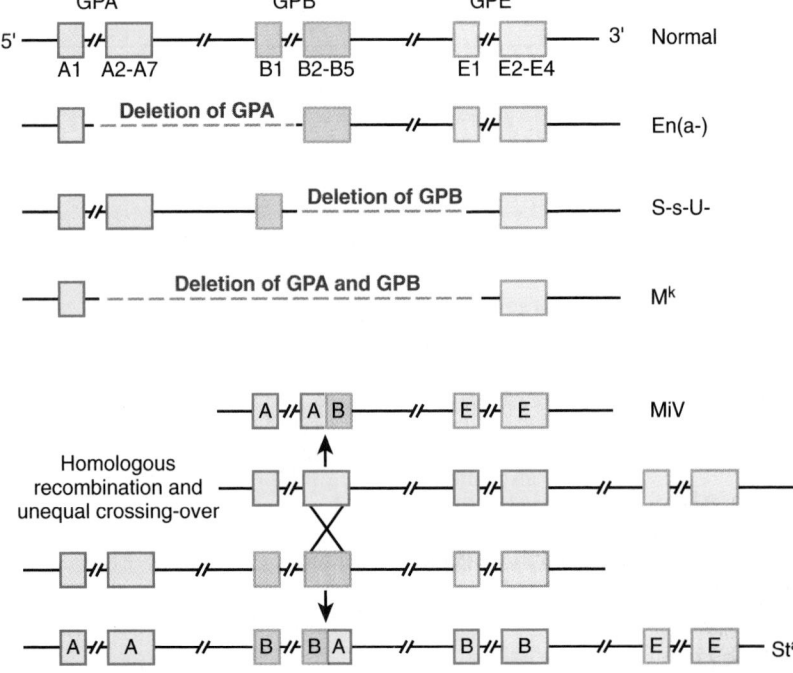

FIGURE 15-12. Organization of the glycophorin A (GPA), B (GPB), and C (GPE) genes on chromosome 4 and probable deletions in the En(a–), S–s–U–, M[k], Miltenburger type V (MiV), and Stones (St[a]) variants. The MiV and St[a] variants arise from unequal crossing over, analogous to the Lepore hemoglobins. In MiV red cells, the normal GPB gene is replaced by a fusion gene (Lepore-type recombination). In St[a] erythrocytes, the product of the reciprocal exchange is inserted between the GPA and GPB loci, but no normal genes are lost (anti-Lepore–type recombination). *(Adapted from Vignal A, London J, Rahuel C, Cartron JP. Promoter sequence and chromosomal organization of the genes encoding glycophorins A, B, and E. Gene. 1990;95:289-293.)*

such that the overall surface charge is reduced by only approximately 20%.[287] Given the proximity and homology of the GPA, GPB, and GPE genes, hybrid glycophorin molecules may be generated by recombination events during meiosis. In the MiV variant, for example, Lepore-like recombination yields a fusion gene containing the N-terminal of GPA and the C-terminal of GPB.[304] In the St[a] variant, anti-Lepore recombination produces the reverse hybrid (N-terminal GPB with C-terminal GPA), which is inserted between the normal GPA and GPB genes, neither of which is lost.[304] Interestingly, none of the GPA and GPB variants produce detectable changes in erythropoiesis or in the shape, function, or life span of the affected red cells. Rare individuals with complete absence of GPA and GPB apparently exhibit no erythrocyte abnormalities.[276] Similarly, GPA knockout mice have a normal phenotype except that they have 60% less O-linked oligosaccharides than normal red cells do.[334] Thus, either GPA, GPB, and GPE do not serve any critical basal functions in red cells or such functions are assumed by other proteins such as GPC or band 3 when GPA/GPB/GPE is deficient. If GPA really has no nonredundant function, it is surprising that deletions and other mutations are not more common because GPA is a major receptor for *P. falciparum* malaria (see later) and must be under intense evolutionary pressure.

Variations in Glycoproteins C and D Affect the Gerbich Antigen System. Mutations in exons 1, 2, and most of 3 modify the N-terminal extracellular domain of GPC and GPD and thus alter the antigenicity of red cells but do not affect cellular mechanical properties.[331,335] Examples include Gerbich-type cells, which lack exon 2; Yus-type cells, which lack exon 3; and Webb-type cells, which have a missense mutation of GPC that converts Asn at position 8 to Ser, thereby precluding N-glycosylation at this site.[336,337] By contrast, in the Leach phenotype there is complete loss of GPC and GPD secondary to deletion of exons 3 and 4[338,339] or a frameshift mutation.[339] Affected individuals do not have significant hemolysis, but their red cells are elliptocytic[340,341] and exhibit decreased membrane deformability and mechanical stability.[335,342,343] GPC-deficient cells also demonstrate partial deficiencies of protein 4.1 and p55,[344] and therefore the disturbance in membrane mechanical properties exhibited by Leach cells probably derives from a deficiency of the GPC/protein 4.1/p55 ternary complex. Individuals with homozygous protein 4.1 deficiency likewise exhibit a deficiency of GPC ($\approx$70%) in their elliptocytic red cells,[345,346] thus underscoring that the cellular content of each component of the ternary complex depends on the expression level of the others. Interestingly, absence of the *Drosophila* protein neurexin IV, which contains a cytoplasmic domain homologous to that of GPC, results in mislocalization of Coracle (the *Drosophila* homologue of protein 4.1) at septate junctions, with attendant defects in the formation of septate-junction septa and intercellular barriers (such as the blood-nerve barrier).[347]

Glycophorins as Receptors for Malarial Invasion

Experiments by Perkins published in 1981 identified GPA as the probable red cell surface attachment site for *P. falciparum* upon merozoite invasion.[348] Subsequently, erythrocytes deficient in GPA were shown to resist malarial invasion, presumably by lacking the requisite attachment site for parasitic invasion.[349] It has since been learned that there are alternative pathways for malarial invasion of red cells that depend on the strain of *P. falciparum* and the ability of the parasite to switch its invasion requirements.[350] For example, sialic acid–dependent invasion results from binding of the merozoite protein EBA175 to the Neu5Ac-(α2,3)-Gal moiety on the O-linked tetrasaccharides of GPA.[351] Another sialic acid–dependent but EBA175-independent pathway is believed to involve merozoite binding to GPB.[352] The structure of EBA175 bound to the relevant glycan has recently been published.[353] Identification of specific *P. falciparum* strains that invade neuraminidase-treated red cells (i.e., desialylated cells)[350,354] and GPA/GPB-deficient M^kM^k cells[355] highlighted the existence of a sialic acid–independent mechanism for malarial invasion. One such mechanism may involve merozoite adhesion to band 3.[269]

Protein 4.1–deficient red cells (which exhibit partial GPC deficiency) and GPC/GPD-deficient Leach-type cells both demonstrate significant resistance to malarial invasion in vitro,[356] thus suggesting that GPC/GPD may also function as an extracellular attachment site for *P. falciparum*. The fact that up to 50% of the Melanesian population in the malarious coastal areas of Papua New Guinea have red blood cells that are Gerbich blood group negative as a result of a deletion in the third exon of the GPC gene also implicates GPC. Recently, GPC has been shown to be the receptor for a second sialic acid–dependent pathway for falciparum malaria.[357-359] The *P. falciparum* erythrocyte binding antigen 140 (EBA140, also called BAEBL) binds with high affinity to the surface of human erythrocytes and facilitates entry of the parasite. EBA140 does not bind to Ge-negative red cells lacking exon 3, nor can the parasite invade such cells via this pathway. It appears that binding depends on the N-linked oligosaccharide of GPC, at least for one variant of EBA140.[359] The existence of so many ways for the parasite to invade erythrocytes, as well as the ability to switch between invasion pathways, obviously complicates efforts to create a malarial vaccine.

Stomatin

Stomatin, or band 7.2b, is of particular interest because it is diminished by 95% to 98% in the classic type of hereditary stomatocytosis, a severe hemolytic anemia characterized by red cell membranes that are extremely leaky to Na[+] and K[+] ions. The disease is discussed in a later section ("Inherited Disorders of Red Cell Cation Permeability and Volume"). Recent data make it clear that hereditary stomatocytosis is not caused by the absence of stomatin, and its role in the pathophysiology of the disease is one of the biggest mysteries in the red cell membrane field.

Stomatin is a Small Integral Membrane Protein That May Regulate an Na+ Channel.

The 31.5-kd stomatin protein (approximately 28 kd on SDS gels) has been isolated[360,361] and cloned.[361-363] It is a positively charged, homo-oligomeric (n = 9 to 12), phosphorylated (cyclic adenosine monophosphate [cAMP]-dependent kinase), palmitoylated integral membrane protein with a single transmembrane helix, a small external segment, and a relatively large cytoplasmic domain.[360,362-365] As noted earlier, it is located, at least in part, in membrane lipid rafts.[115,116] Stomatin is a member of a protein superfamily—the PID superfamily, which stands for *p*roliferation, *i*on, and *d*eath. Red cells contain other members of this family, such as SLP-2[366] and STORP,[367] but nothing is known about their functions or interactions. The stomatin gene (*EPB72*) is located on chromosome 9 at 9q34.1.

Stomatin is expressed in all tissues and in red cells of all tested species, from human to frog,[363] and stomatin-like proteins, of which there are at least 50, are found throughout evolution, even in very primitive organisms such as *Rhizobium*.[368] A homologue of stomatin, MEC-2, has been cloned from *Caenorhabditis elegans*.[369-372] It is involved in touch sensation and is linked to an Na+ channel called the DEG/ENaC channel. The channel is believed to be mechanically gated by linkage to the extracellular matrix and the membrane skeleton or cytoskeleton. Displacement of the membrane (e.g., by touch) pulls the channel open. MEC-2 greatly increases the activity of the Na+ channel. The analogous protein, stomatin-like protein 3 (SLP-3), has recently been found in mice and has a similar function.[373] When expressed in heterologous cells, human stomatin binds to H+-gated Na+ channels and mutes their transport activity.[374] By analogy, stomatin may localize, structurally support, activate, or regulate an Na+ channel in the red cell, perhaps one that is sensitive to shear stress.

Stomatin Interacts with Peroxiredoxin-2 and the Red Cell Glucose Transporter.

Stomatin also interacts with peroxiredoxin-2 (see later)[375] and binds and represses Glut1, the erythrocyte glucose transporter.[376,377] The relationship to peroxiredoxin-2 is interesting because this peroxide-reducing protein binds Ca^{2+} and translocates to the membrane,[375,378] where it seems to be involved in activation of a K+ egress channel (the Gárdos channel).[379] The interaction with the glucose transporter reinforces the emerging concept that stomatin and its paralogues somehow regulate transporters.

Other Integral Membrane Proteins

Although band 3 and the glycophorins are the major integral membrane constituents of the red cell membrane, a large number of other integral membrane proteins with specific functions have also been identified and characterized.

Aquaporin

Aquaporin-1 (AQP1), a 28-kd channel-forming protein (originally called CHIP28), is the major water channel in red cells.[380] The human *AQP1* gene is located on chromosome 7p14 and encodes a 269–amino acid polypeptide with six membrane-spanning domains. Besides red cells, AQP1 is also expressed in the kidney and in endothelial cells in lung. There are approximately 200,000 copies of AQP1 per cell, and the protein carries antigens of the *Colton blood group*. It exists as a tetramer in the red cell membrane, and the crystal structure of the protein has recently been determined.[381] Human red cells lacking AQP1 exhibit markedly reduced osmotic water permeability. Humans with complete deficiency of AQP1 have defective urinary-concentrating ability, as well as decreased pulmonary vascular permeability.[382,383] AQP1 knockout mice appear normal but become severely dehydrated and lethargic after water deprivation for 36 hours when compared with control mice.[384] Interestingly, implanted tumors grow very poorly in AQP1(−/−) mice because of reduced vascularity and very poor cell migration.[385] These studies show that AQP1 also has an unexpected role in cell migration and hence in angiogenesis and wound healing.

Aquaporin-3 is the glycerol permeability channel in human red cells and carries the high-frequency blood group antigen GIL.[386,387] In mice, aquaporin-9 appears to be the glycerol channel.[388]

Rh Proteins (RhD, RhCE, and RhAG)

The Rh blood group system is composed of at least 40 independent antigens carried by two nonglycosylated, palmitoylated proteins encoded by two homologous genes, *RHD* and *RHCE*, located on chromosome 1.[389-391] *RHCE* encodes the CcEe set of antigens and *RHD* encodes the D antigen. Rh antigen expression at the red cell surface requires the presence of Rh-associated glycoprotein (RhAG), which exhibits 36% sequence identity with Rh proteins and is encoded by a gene located on chromosome 6. All three Rh proteins are predicted to have 12 membrane-spanning domains. There are approximately 10,000 to 30,000 copies of RhD and RhCE proteins and 100,000 to 200,000 copies of RhAG per cell. The interaction between RhAG and Rh proteins in the membrane appears to be stabilized by C-terminal and N-terminal domain interactions. In addition to the interaction between the three Rh subunits, the Rh core complex also contains several other proteins[391]—LW glycoprotein (intercellular adhesion molecule 4 [ICAM-4]), integrin-associated protein (IAP, CD47), GPB, protein 4.2, and ankyrin.[392]

Although the function of the Rh protein complex in the normal red cell has yet to be fully defined, RhAG functions as an ammonium transporter in mouse and human red cells[393] and can complement defects in ammonium transport in yeast.[394] It may also be partly responsible (along with aquaporin) for the exceptionally high permeability of CO_2 in the erythrocyte.[395] The importance of the Rh complex in regulating red cell membrane structure is revealed by the altered phenotype of Rh_{null} red cells, which exhibit stomatocytic morphology with loss of membrane surface area, cell dehydration, cation permeability abnormalities, and shortened red cell survival leading to a mild compensated hemolytic anemia.[396]

Kidd Glycoprotein

The Kidd glycoprotein is the urea transporter in the red cell membrane.[397] The human Kidd glycoprotein gene is located on chromosome 18q11-q12 and encodes a 391–amino acid polypeptide with 10 membrane-spanning domains. There are 14,000 copies of Kidd glycoprotein per cell, and the protein carries the antigens of the Kidd blood group system.[398] The urea transporter in red cells functions by rapidly transporting urea into and out of red cells as they pass through the high urea concentration in the renal medulla and thereby prevent red cell dehydration.[399] Urea transport across $Kidd_{null}$ red cell membranes is approximately a thousand times slower than across normal membranes.[400] However, no changes in red cell shape or survival have been noted in persons who lack the Kidd glycoprotein.

Xk Protein

Xk protein (also called Kx), a 37-kd protein (444 amino acids) with 10 membrane-spanning domains, is encoded by a gene on the short arm of the X chromosome,[401] Although the Xk protein has structural but not sequence similarity with a family of proteins involved in transport of neurotransmitters, its transport substrate or substrates have not been defined. The Xk protein carries the Kx blood group antigen. In the red cell membrane the Xk protein is covalently linked to the Kell glycoprotein by a disulfide bond.[402] Lack of the Xk protein in McLeod's syndrome results in acanthocytic red cells, compensated hemolytic anemia, and in later life, muscle wasting and choreiform movements.

Kell Glycoprotein

Kell glycoprotein is a 93-kd (732 amino acids) single-pass type II membrane protein encoded by a gene on chromosome 7q33.[403] It has sequence homology with a family of neutral endopeptidases and has been shown to be an endothelin-3 converting enzyme.[404] In addition to cleaving the precursor of endothelin-3, Kell glycoprotein can also cleave the precursors of endothelin-1 and endothelin-2, but much less effectively. Because endothelins are potent vasoactive peptides, it is thought that the Kell glycoprotein may be involved in the regulation of vascular tone. The Kell glycoprotein carries the antigens in the Kell blood group system. In contrast to the red cell pathology seen in Xk-deficient red cells, Kell glycoprotein deficiency does not result in red cell alterations.[405]

Duffy Glycoprotein

The Duffy glycoprotein is a promiscuous chemokine receptor[406] that binds a variety of proinflammatory cytokines of both the C-X-C class (acute inflammation) and the C-C class (chronic inflammation), including interleukin-8 (IL-8), melanoma growth stimulatory activity (MGSA), monocyte chemotactic protein 1 (MCP-1), and RANTES (regulated on activation, normal T cell expressed and secreted). The Duffy glycoprotein gene is located on chromosome 1q22-23 and encodes a 333–amino acid polypeptide with seven membrane-spanning domains.[407] There are 6000 to 13,000 copies of Duffy glycoprotein per cell, and the protein carries the antigens of the Duffy blood group system. The Duffy glycoprotein is the receptor for the malarial parasite *Plasmodium vivax*, and Duffy glycoprotein–deficient red cells are refractory to invasion by *P. vivax*.[408] The function of Duffy glycoprotein in normal red cell physiology remains to be defined.

Lutheran Glycoprotein

The Lutheran blood group glycoprotein (Lu gp) belongs to the immunoglobulin superfamily and is the receptor on erythroid cells for the extracellular matrix protein laminin[409] (reviewed by Eyler and Telen[410]). It is also highly expressed in endothelial cells. The glycoprotein consists of five disulfide-bonded extracellular, immunoglobulin superfamily domains, a single hydrophobic transmembrane domain, and a cytoplasmic tail. Two isoforms of this membrane protein (85- and 78-kd isoforms) are expressed by alternative splicing of a single gene located on human chromosome 19q13.2. Both isoforms bind laminin. The two isoforms are distinguished by differences in their cytoplasmic domains—the 78-kd isoform has a truncated cytoplasmic tail. There are approximately 1500 to 4000 copies of Lu gp on the mature red cell. Although the function of Lu gp in normal red cells remains to be defined, it has been shown to mediate adhesion of sickle red cells to laminin.[411] Interactions between the $\alpha_4\beta_1$ integrin on sickle cells and the Lu gp on endothelial cells may also be important.[412] Because Lu gp is expressed late during erythroid differentiation, it has been suggested that it may play a functional role in mediating erythroblast–extracellular matrix interactions in the bone marrow that regulate egress of reticulocytes from bone marrow into the circulation.

LW Glycoprotein

The LW glycoprotein (LW gp, also termed ICAM-4) present on the red cell membrane also belongs to the immunoglobulin superfamily.[413] It was recently reviewed.[414] The glycoprotein consists of two extracellular immunoglobulin-like domains that show very strong sequence homology with the protein superfamily known as intracellular adhesion molecules (ICAMs). The 40- to 42-kd LW gp is encoded by a gene on chromosome 19. There are approximately 4000 copies of LW gp on the mature red cell. Preliminary evidence suggests that extracellular domains of LW gp can interact with the integrins LFA1 (CD11/CD18),[415] $\alpha_4\beta_1$, and α_v.[416] LW gp is activated by epinephrine and may also play a role in adhesion of sickle cells.[417] In contrast to Lu gp, which is expressed late during erythroid development, LW gp is expressed early during erythropoiesis. Based on this expression pattern, it has been suggested that LW gp may play a role in the erythroblast-macrophage interactions that are critical for erythropoiesis.

Glucose Transporter (Glut-1)

Glut-1 was the first of 14 members of the glucose transporter family identified.[417a] It is an integral membrane protein with 12 transmembrane segments and is the major glucose transporter in many cells. Glut-1 also transports dehydroascorbic acid (DHA), an oxidized intermediate of vitamin C, and recent evidence suggests that this is its primary function in the red cell, and that Glut-4, a related glucose transporter, may transport most of the glucose.[417b] The switch of Glut-1 from glucose to DHA is associated with an increase in stomatin expression and doesn't occur in patients with hereditary stomatocytosis and stomatin deficiency.[417b] The red cell

has roughly 400,000 copies of Glut-1 per cell, which is the highest number of any human cell. High erythroid expression of Glut-1 is limited to mammals that lack the ability to synthesize vitamin C.[417b]

Glut-1 associates with dematin and adducin in a complex that is presumably located near the spectrin-actin molecular junctions[417c] (see Fig. 15-6). The data suggest that dematin and perhaps adducin bind to a 64-amino acid cytoplasmic loop on Glut-1.

MEMBRANE SKELETON PROTEINS

Spectrin

Erythroid spectrin is the major constituent of the red cell skeleton and accounts for 50% to 75% of the membrane skeletal mass.[172,173] The spectrin-based skeleton is anchored to the plasma membrane by an ankyrin-mediated linkage to band 3[418] and protein 4.1–mediated attachment to glycophorin C.[419] Recent evidence that α-spectrin binds protein 4.2[221] suggests that there may be additional connections. As a result of these vertical attach-

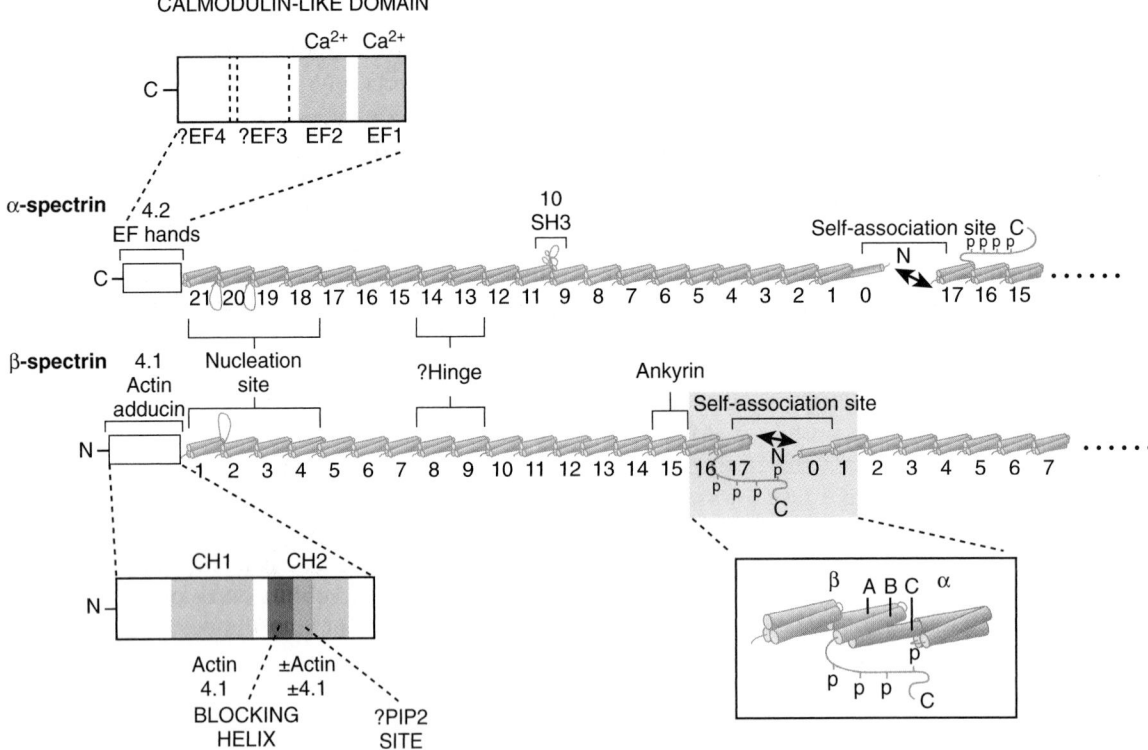

FIGURE 15-13. Spectrin structure. The α and β chains are aligned antiparallel with respect to their N- and C-terminal ends. The approximately 106–amino acid "spectrin repeats"[421] are numbered from the N-terminal of each chain. Each repeat is composed of three α helices (A, B, and C).[422] The SH3 domain, which extrudes from between helix B and helix C of repeat 9, is conventionally numbered as repeat 10, although it is not a spectrin repeat. Similarly, by convention the partial spectrin repeat that begins the α-spectrin chain is called α0, whereas the partial spectrin repeat at the end of the β-spectrin chain is called β17. Note that the spectrin self-association site is formed by joining complementary parts of two partial repeats that are left over at the "head" ends of the two chains (*inset*). The α chain contributes helix C and the β-chain, helices A and B. Some repeats are specialized, such as β15, which forms the ankyrin binding site, and parts of the first four repeats at the "tail" of each chain, which nucleate interchain, heterodimer interactions. Repeats α13-α14 and β8-β9 are more flexible and may form a hinge.[423] *Rectangles* denote peptide segments that differ from the repeats and the SH3 domain. They include the actin/protein 4.1/adducin binding sites and a calmodulin-like Ca[2+] binding region (EF hands) that also binds protein 4.2. The structures of these two domains are shown in more detail in the *insets*. (*Adapted from Walensky LD, Narla M, Lux SE. Disorders of the red cell membrane. In Handin RI, Lux SE, Stossel TP (eds). Blood: Principles and Practice of Hematology, 2nd ed. Philadelphia, JB Lippincott, 2003, pp 1709-1858, with permission.*)

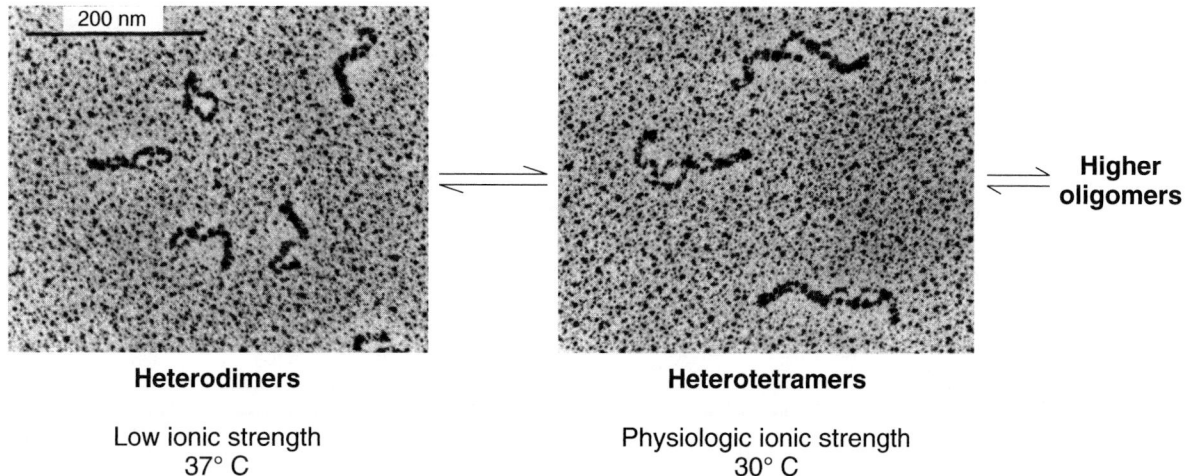

FIGURE 15-14. Electron micrographs (rotary shadowed) of spectrin heterodimers and heterotetramers. Note that the α and β chains of heterodimers are flexible and twisted about each other and that heterotetramers are made by end-to-end association of dimers. The chains are attached at the ends and sometimes separate in the middle. The scale marker indicates 200 nm (2000 Å). Factors that favor the dimer or tetramer-oligomer state are listed under the photographs. The dimer-tetramer-oligomer equilibrium is kinetically frozen at 0° C. Spectrin extracted and maintained at 0° C retains the distribution of dimers and tetramers that exist on the membrane.

ments, spectrin represents approximately 25% of the membrane-associated mass of the red cell. Spectrin is composed of two large polypeptide chains that associate side by side in an antiparallel arrangement[420]; the 280-kd α chain and the 246-kd β chain are structurally similar but functionally distinct (Fig. 15-13). Electron micrographs of spectrin reveal a slender, twisted, worm-like molecule that is 100 nm in length (Fig. 15-14).[424] Spectrin is a highly flexible protein that assumes a variety of conformational and oligomerization states; in concert with its associated membrane skeletal proteins, spectrin generates a deformable juxtamembranous meshwork that provides the circulating red cell with both stability and flexibility.

The Spectrin Family in Humans Is Encoded by at Least Seven Distinct Genes. Two genes encoding α-spectrin and five genes encoding β-spectrin have been characterized.[425] The αI (or $α_R$) spectrin gene (*SPTA*) is located on chromosome 1q22-q23 adjacent to the Duffy blood group and encodes the erythroid-specific α chain.[426] The αII (or $α_G$) spectrin (also called α-fodrin) gene (*SPTAN1*) has been mapped to chromosome 9q34.1 and encodes an α-spectrin homologue found in nearly all cells except mature red cells.[427] The βI (or $β_R$) spectrin gene (*SPTB*) is located on chromosome 14q23-q24.2 and encodes the β subunit of the erythroid-specific spectrin, designated βIΣ1.[428] The βI gene promoter region contains specific GATA-1 and CACCC-related protein binding sites that account for specific, high-level expression in erythroid cells.[429] Differential 3′ processing of βI-spectrin pre-mRNA generates an alternative βI-spectrin subunit that is found in the brain (predominantly cerebellum) and muscle and designated βIΣ2.[430]

The βII (or $β_G$) spectrin (also called β-fodrin) gene (*SPTBN1*) has been mapped to chromosome 2p21 and encodes the generally expressed β subunit of spectrin, which shares 60% amino acid identity with βI-spectrin.[431]

Thus, erythrocyte spectrin (or spectrin$_R$) is composed of αI and βIΣ1 chains, and the widely expressed spectrin (called fodrin, tissue spectrin, brain spectrin, or spectrin$_G$) contains αII and βII subunits. Muscle spectrin is believed to contain predominantly αII and βIΣ2 subunits. Alternative splicing of the spectrin genes, in addition to interchangeability of the α- and β-chain isoforms in heterodimer formation, gives rise to a rich diversity of spectrin proteins that probably exhibit distinct localizations and functions.

The most recently cloned spectrin subunits, designated βIII, βIV, and βV, have been localized to chromosomes 11q13, 19q13.13, and 15q21, respectively.[432-435] βIII-spectrin is predominantly expressed in the central nervous system, especially the cerebellum. Defects in the protein are associated with spinocerebellar ataxia type V.[436] βIV-spectrin associates with the electrogenic Na+ channel in the axon's initial segments and the nodes of Ranvier in neurons by acting through ankyrin$_G$ (see later).[433] Mice lacking this βIV-spectrin have the quivering (qv) mutation, characterized by progressive ataxia with hind limb paralysis, deafness, and tremor.[437] A truncated isoform of βIV-spectrin is associated with a subnuclear structure (promyelocytic leukemia bodies) and may be part of a nuclear scaffold.[434] βV-spectrin is detected prominently in the outer segments of photoreceptor rods and cones and in the basolateral membrane and cytosol of gastric epithelial cells.[435] Presumably, these homologues of β-spectrin perform specialized functions related to their association with the intracellular and nuclear compartments.

Spectrins Consist Mostly of Tandem 106–Amino Acid Repeats. Each spectrin chain is composed of a series of 106–amino acid repeats, and each repeat is formed by three α helices that are folded into a triple-helical bundle.[422,438,439] The α- and β-spectrins contain 20 and 16 full repeats, respectively.[426,428] An SH3 domain within the α chain is conventionally called repeat α10, though it is not a true spectrin repeat (see Fig 15-13A). As will be discussed, the α0 and β17 repeats are complementary partial repeats that join to form a full repeat and link spectrins together (see Fig. 15-13A). The primary sequence of each repeat exhibits extensive heptad (seven-residue) symmetry, with conserved hydrophobic residues situated in the first and fourth positions of each heptad motif (designated as positions a and d in Fig. 15-15A).[422,438] Each spectrin repeat forms a triple-helical

structure that is approximately 5 nm long and 2 nm wide (see Fig. 15-15B) and rotated 60 degrees (right-handed) relative to the neighboring repeats.[438]

The prototypical three-dimensional structure of the spectrin repeats was determined by expression studies and x-ray crystallographic analysis of a spectrin repeat from αII-spectrin.[438,439] The first 28 amino acids of the repeat form a straight α helix designated helix A. The polypeptide chain then reverses itself and forms a second 34–amino acid, long straight α helix designated

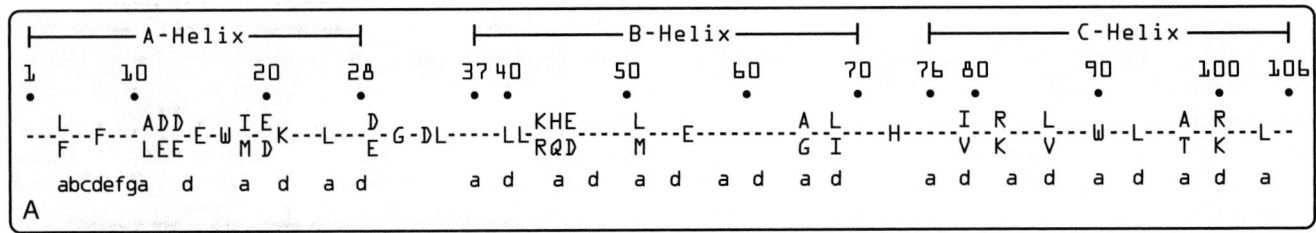

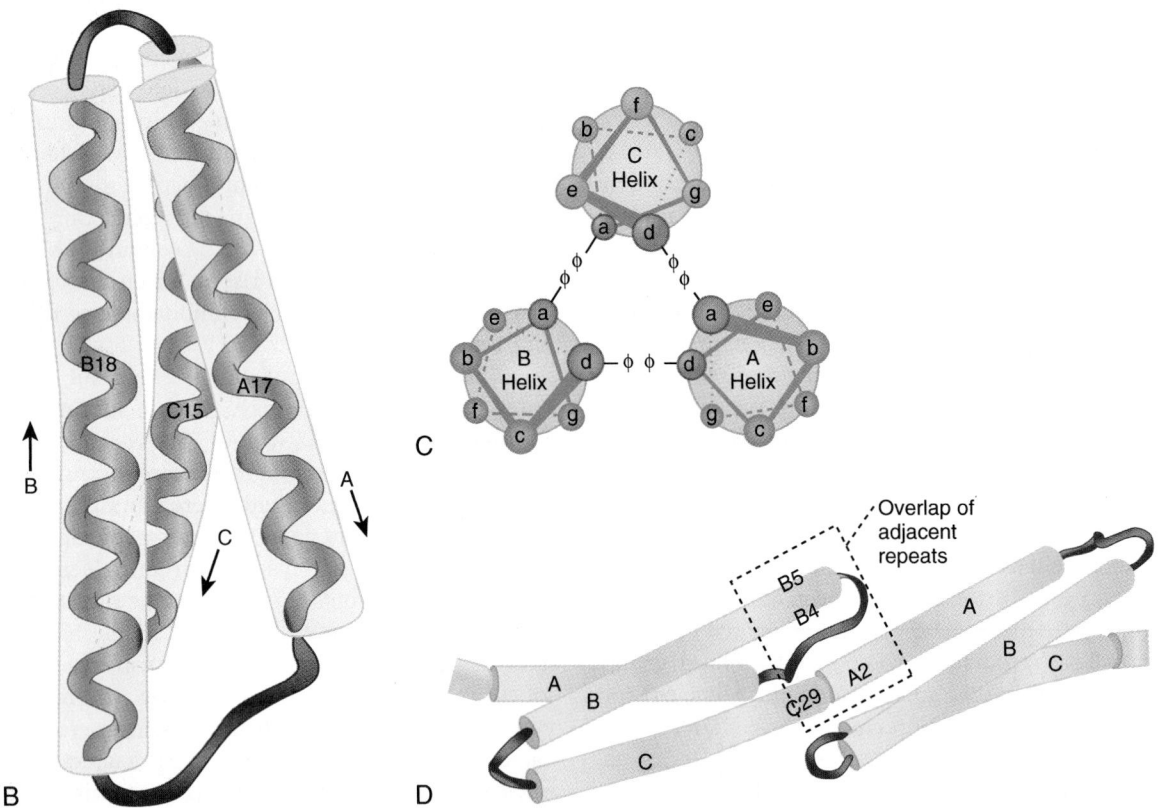

FIGURE 15-15. Structure of spectrin repeats. **A,** Consensus sequence of a typical 106–amino acid, human erythrocyte spectrin repeat phased according to crystallographic data,[438] which identifies three α helices per repeat. Less conserved amino acids are marked with a *dash*. The amino acids in the repeat are designated "a" through "g." The distance from one "a" to the next corresponds to two turns of the α helix. Residues "a" and "d" are the major contact points between helices. They tend to be hydrophobic and are conserved in most spectrins. **B,** Model of a single repeat based on the crystal structure of *Drosophila* αII spectrin.[438] The positions of the nearly invariant tryptophans at A17 (amino acid 17 of the repeat) and C15 (repeat amino acid 90) are shown. They interact with surrounding residues, including B18 (repeat amino acid 54), at the central junction where the A helix crosses over from B to C. **C,** Cross section of a typical repeat. Note that the A, B, and C helices are in a triangular array and that the "a" and "d" residues lie on one face of each helix. The side chains of these amino acids are usually hydrophobic (Φ) and interact with each other to stabilize the triple helical configuration. Salt bonds between the typically polar amino acids at positions "e" and "g" also help attach the B-C and A-C helices to each other. **D,** Interconnection of two adjacent repeats. The A and C helices are colinear and form one long helix. The distal repeat of each pair is rotated 60 degrees (right-handed). Note that the B helix of the proximal repeat overlaps the A helix of the following repeat. Interactions in the overlap region among conserved hydrophobic residues, such as C29, B4, and B5 (repeat amino acids 104, 40, and 41, respectively), and the mostly hydrophobic residues at A2 (repeat amino acid 2) probably stabilize the connection and limit mobility at the repeat junction. *(Redrawn from Walensky LD, Narla M, Lux SE. Disorders of the red cell membrane. In Handin RI, Lux SE, Stossel TP [eds]. Blood: Principles and Practice of Hematology, 2nd ed. Philadelphia, JB Lippincott, 2003, pp 1709-1858, with permission.)*

helix B. After another reverse turn, a third α helix is formed and is composed of 31 amino acids with a bend in the middle of the structure. The three helices are arranged in a triangular array held together by hydrophobic interactions between the hydrophobic faces of the helices and by electrostatic interactions, particularly between helices A-C and B-C, where mostly polar amino acids are found in positions e and g of the helices (see Fig. 15-15C).

Interestingly, the three helices are tilted away from each other by 10 to 20 degrees such that the C-terminal end of each repeat is wider than the N-terminal end (see Fig. 15-15B). This tilted structure enables the subsequent repeat to attach without any adjustment in the architecture of the preceding repeats. Thus, the C helix of one triple-helical bundle connects to the A helix of the subsequent triple-helical bundle to form one long α helix (see Fig. 15-15D). The tight connection between repeats causes the B helix of a proximal repeat to overlap the A helix of the distal repeat; the resultant interaction between the two helices restricts movement at the junction between repeats, thereby limiting the overall range of motion of αII chains. Spectrin-type repeats in other proteins show similar features.[421] However, the crystal structures of two connected repeats of chicken brain α-spectrin suggest that flexibility in the spectrin structure may be preserved by conformational rearrangement within the repeat (causing movement in the position of an interhelical loop, for example) and by various degrees of bending at the linker region.[440] The stability of individual spectrin repeats varies widely, and some repeats are unstable at physiologic temperatures, which would also introduce flexibility.[441] Two of the less stably folded repeats, α13-α14 and β8-β9, are adjacent to each other in the spectrin molecule (see Fig. 15-13) and may form a hinge.[423] Measurements of the force required to unfold a spectrin repeat show that the repeats function as elastic springs.[442] When intact red cells deform, certain spectrin repeats partially unfold, which presumably contributes to the elasticity.[443]

Side-to-Side Interactions between α and β Chains Results in Zipper-like Dimerization. Nucleation sites located at repeats 18 to 21 of the α chain and 1 to 4 of the β-chain are implicated in triggering the zipping up of α and β chains (see Fig. 15-13).[444] The key interactions are between the A and B helices of β1 and the C and A helices of α21 and between the C and A helices of β2 and the A and B helices of α20.[445] These helices form complementary electrostatic surfaces that draw the two chains together.[446] After the initial tight association of the complementary nucleation sites, a conformational change is propagated that causes the remainder of the α and β chains to pair together and form a supercoiled rope-like structure.[444] However, the side-to-side interactions beyond the nucleation site are relatively weak,[447] which may be important in allowing the α and β chains to slide past each other when the spectrin molecule flexes in the plane of the heterodimer. A common polymorphism of the α-spectrin allele α^{LELY} encodes α chains that lack one of the nucleation sites and therefore do not form stable heterodimers.[448,449] This clinically relevant allele is discussed further in the section "Hereditary Elliptocytosis."

Spectrin Tetramerization Occurs in Head-to-Head Fashion by Association of Incomplete Repeats at the Ends of the α and β Chains. The "self-association" sequences required for tetramerization are located at the N-terminal of the α-spectrin chain and the C-terminal of the β-spectrin chain (i.e., at the opposite end of the chain from where the nucleation site is found; see Fig. 15-13).[424,450] For spectrin dimers to associate into tetramers, the dimer bonds located at the opposite end of the chains from the nucleation sites must reversibly open to allow the formation of two new αβ attachments. Thus, opening of the αβ contact, whether present as the internal bond of heterodimers or the αβ attachment site for tetramers, is the rate-limiting step in dimer-tetramer interconversion.[451] The specific structure of the spectrin self-association site has been determined by analysis of mutant spectrins[452] and synthetic spectrin fragments[451,453] and by proteolytic studies.[454] The free C helix at the N-terminal of α-spectrin (α0) associates with the free A and B helices at the C-terminal of β-spectrin (β17) to form a stable triple-helical bundle repeat; in this manner, spectrin heterodimers associate to form tetramers and higher-order oligomers in head-to-head fashion (see Fig. 15-13). The isolated α-chain C helix and the free β-chain A and B helices will associate only if there is at least one adjacent triple-helical repeat present. The formation of spectrin tetramers and higher-order oligomers is critical for maintaining the mechanical strength of the membrane skeleton.[455] Mutations in α- or β-spectrin that interfere with formation of the interchain triple-helical bundle prevent spectrin tetramerization and higher-order oligomerization, thereby weakening the membrane skeleton; such defects in spectrin are the most common causes of hereditary elliptocytosis and hereditary pyropoikilocytosis.

Spectrin Exists Predominantly as Tetramers In Vivo. Whereas physiologic ionic strength and lower temperatures (25° C) favor tetramer formation, low ionic strength and physiologic temperatures favor dissociation to dimers.[456,457] At 0° C, the dimer-tetramer equilibrium is virtually kinetically frozen because of the high activation energy.[450] The oligomerization state of spectrin can be studied directly by extracting spectrin from red cell membranes at various temperatures and by manipulating in vitro conditions to alter the degree of oligomerization.[450,454,455,457] In red cell ghosts, driving the equilibrium toward dimerization produces exceedingly fragile structures, thus underscoring the importance of spectrin tetramerization in membrane skeletal stability.[455] Quantitation of spectrin eluted from normal ghosts at 0° C indicates that approximately 5% of the spectrin is in the dimer form, 50% exists as a tetramer, and the remainder is divided between higher-order oligomers and very-high-molecular-weight complexes of spectrin, actin, protein 4.1, and dematin.[456]

The Quaternary Structure of Spectrin In Vivo Is Unclear. Although electron micrographs show that spectrin has an end-to-end length of 200 nm, simple calculations show that spectrin tetramers must have a length of just about 65 to 75 nm in vivo if the hexameric spectrin array (see later) is only a single layer thick and has an area equal to the area of the red cell, 140 μm². This correlates with the observed length of spectrin filaments in unstretched skeletons.[458] It is not completely clear how spectrin is folded in this physiologic filament. There is some evidence that the molecules condense by twisting the α and β subunits about a common axis. In this model, the degree to which the chains condense is regulated by varying the pitch and diameter of the twisted double strand; native spectrin dimers have approximately 10 turns with a pitch of 7 nm and a diameter of 5.9 nm.[459,460] However, the available pictures do not show this structure very clearly, and it is hard to imagine how spectrin would become so highly wound during its synthesis and assembly into the skeleton in vivo. More studies are needed.

Spectrin Contains Important Functional Domains Involved in Protein-Protein Interactions. In addition to the critical sequences involved in spectrin nucleation and self-association, the α and β chains interface with other proteins via defined structural domains (see Fig. 15-13).

Ankyrin Binding Site. The β subunit of spectrin contains structural domains that interact with multiple membrane skeletal proteins, including ankyrin, protein 4.1, actin, and adducin. The 15th repeat and the first part of the 16th repeat of β-spectrin form the binding site for ankyrin.[461] Spectrin's strongest link to the erythrocyte plasma membrane is achieved by the interaction of β-spectrin with ankyrin, which in turn binds to the integral membrane protein band 3.[209,418,462] In nonerythroid cells, ankyrin homologues mediate the linkage of spectrin to other proteins of the plasma membrane, including Na+,K+-ATPase[463] and voltage-dependent sodium channels.[464]

F-Actin, Protein 4.1, and Adducin Binding Sites. The N-terminal 301 amino acids of β-spectrin bind protein 4.1[465] and actin[466,467] and share sequence homology with several actin-binding proteins, including calponin, α-actinin, dystrophin, filamin, ABP120, adducin, and fimbrin. There are two of these "calponin homology domains" (CH1 and CH2) in tandem in β-spectrin. Recent studies show that protein 4.1 and actin bind to each of these domains.[468] Binding to CH2, the more C-terminal CH domain, is normally inhibited by an α helix at its N-terminal end, which may serve a regulatory role. Binding of protein 4.1 to the region is greatly enhanced by PIP₂ (see Fig. 15-13).[468]

The interaction of spectrin with actin is enhanced by protein 4.1 binding.[469-471] The tail ends of spectrin tetramers and oligomers bind to short, double-helical protofilaments of F-actin with the aid of protein 4.1. Approximately six spectrins can be accommodated on each actin protofilament, and this leads to the characteristic hexagonal network that forms the basic framework of the membrane skeleton (Fig. 15-16). The actin–protein 4.1 complexes, which reside at the nodal junctions of the network, are associated with multiple other proteins, including adducin, dematin, TM, TMod, and p55. Assembly of the spectrin-actin skeleton is further enhanced by adducin, a heteromeric calmodulin-binding phosphoprotein that recruits spectrin to the fast-growing ends of actin filaments in addition to binding, bundling, and barbed-end capping of actin.[472-475] The N-terminal domain and first two spectrin repeats participate in forming the spectrin-adducin-actin complex.[476]

EF Hands: Ca²⁺ and Protein 4.2 Binding Sites and Role in Spectrin-Actin Binding. The C-terminal of α-spectrin, like α-actinin, contains two pairs of EF hands (see Fig. 15-13), which are structures that bind and mediate the regulatory effects of calcium.[477,478] The N-terminal EF hands (EF₁,₂) are structurally similar to calmodulin[479] and bind Ca²⁺ with low affinity ($K_d = 0.48$ mM). Binding of Ca²⁺ to EF₁ triggers a conformational change that allows EF₂ to bind Ca²⁺.[480] The C-terminal EF hands (EF₃,₄) are degenerate.

Recent work has shown that the EF hand domain binds protein 4.2 with high affinity ($K_d = 2.9 \times 10^{-9}$ M).[221] Binding capacity is augmented by micromolar concentrations of Ca²⁺, and the Ca²⁺ effect is blocked by calmodulin, which itself binds to the EF hand domain in the presence of Ca²⁺. Because 4.2 binds to band 3, this suggests that a portion of band 3 may also be located near the spectrin-actin junctions. It also suggests that protein 4.2 may form a secondary site for attaching the membrane skeleton to the lipid bilayer.

The relationships of the EF hand domain, the calponin homology domains, and F-actin are not known in spectrin but are likely to resemble those in α-actinin (Fig. 15-17). That is, the EF hand domains are likely to abut the actin/4.1 binding CH domains and may help regulate actin binding. Previously, the EF domains have been considered impotent in erythroid spectrin, although they are known to bind Ca²⁺ and affect the function of αIIβII-spectrin (fodrin).[477] However, the discovery that deletion of just the C-terminal 13 amino acids in the EF domain of the sph¹ᴶ mouse leads to a severe, spherocytic hemolytic anemia and failure of the mutant spectrin to assemble into the membrane skeleton[484] shows that the EF domain must have an important physiologic function. In addition, PfEMP3, a protein from the malarial parasite *P. falciparum* that appears on the red cell membrane late in the parasite's life cycle, binds to α-spectrin in the EF domain region and disrupts the spectrin-actin-4.1 complex, perhaps as a precursor to release of new parasites into the circulation.[482] These observations suggest that the EF

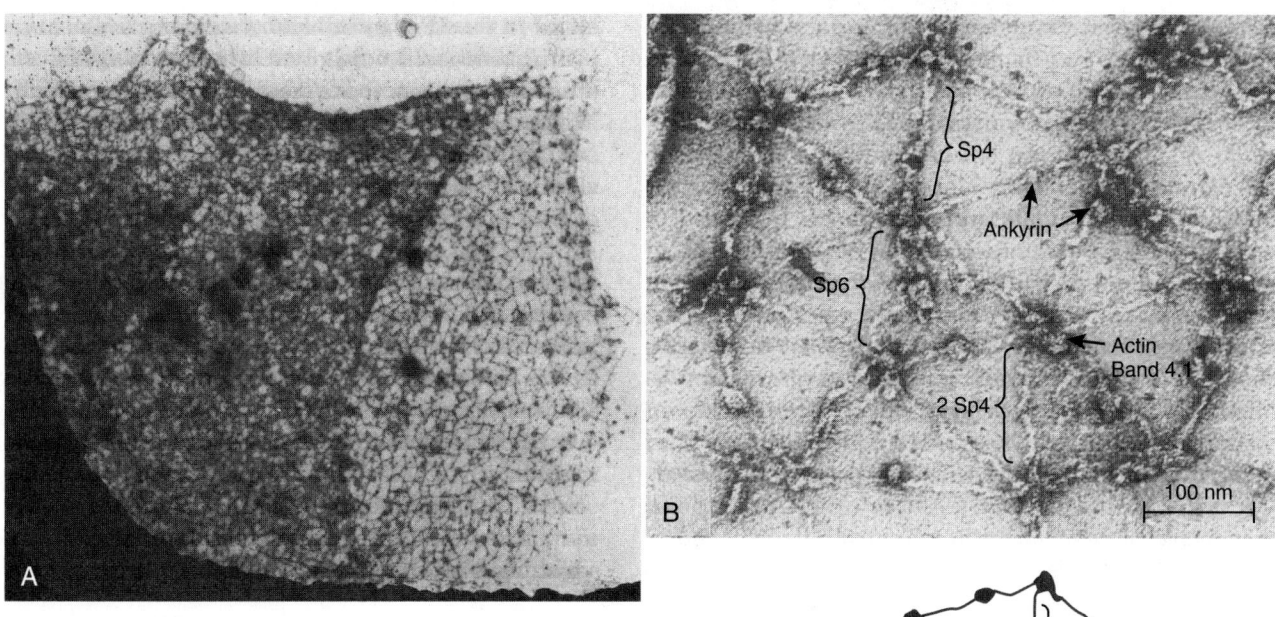

FIGURE 15-16. Electron microscopy of red cell membrane skeletons. The negative-stained skeletons have been stretched during preparation to reveal details of their structure. **A,** Low-power magnification to emphasize the ordered, net-like structure. **B** and **C,** High-power magnification and schematic showing the predominantly hexagonal organization of the skeleton. The location of various skeletal elements is shown in **C.** Sp4, spectrin tetramer; Sp6, spectrin hexamer. *(From Palek J, Sahr KE. Mutations of the red blood cell membrane proteins: from clinical evaluation to detection of the underlying genetic defect. Blood. 1992;80:308.)*

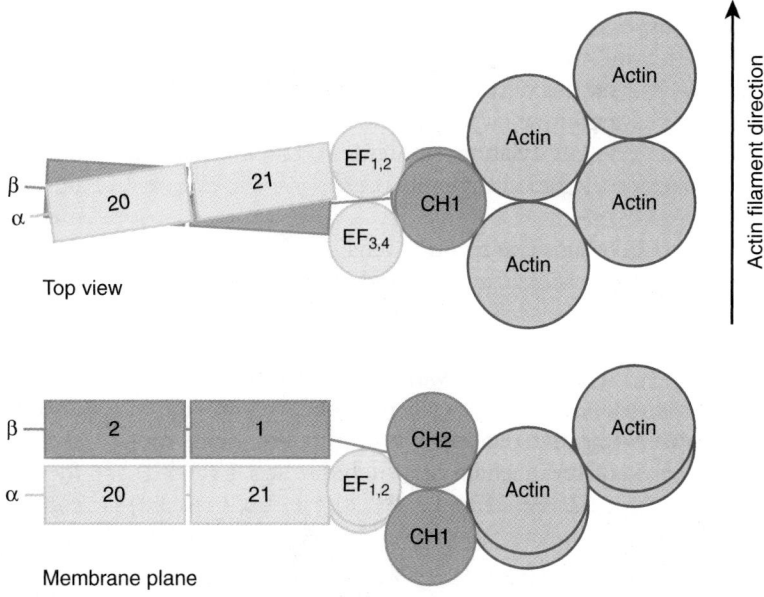

FIGURE 15-17. Structural model, roughly to scale, of the tail end of spectrin deduced from the structure of α-actinin.[481] **Top,** View looking down on the membrane. The *arrow* indicates the direction of the actin filament. **Bottom,** View from within the plane of the membrane skeleton. The top view has been rotated 90 degrees *toward* the viewer (*arrow* pointing up out of the plane). CH1 and CH2 are the actin-4.1 binding sites in the N-terminal, actin binding domain of β-spectrin. $EF_{1,2}$ and $EF_{3,4}$ are the N-terminal and C-terminal pairs of EF hands, respectively, in the EF domain, which lies at the C-terminal end of α-spectrin. The intimate relationship between the EF hands and CH domains suggests that the EF hands may regulate actin binding, and recent evidence supports that hypothesis.[482,483]

domain is important for actin binding, and recent direct evidence supports this speculation. A minispectrin composed of the actin binding and EF domains and the four adjacent spectrin repeats in each chain that form the nucleation site binds to F-actin with the aid of protein 4.1, as expected, but this binding is markedly decreased if the EF hands are missing or even if just the last 13 amino acids of α-spectrin are deleted, as in the sph[1J] mouse.[483]

SH3 Domain. The 10th "repeat" of α-spectrin encodes an Src homology (SH3) domain. SH3 domains generally function as sites of protein-protein attachment at cell membranes. The function of the erythroid α-spectrin SH3 domain and the protein or proteins that bind to it in the red cell are not known. One candidate belongs to a family of tyrosine kinase–binding proteins.[485] Interestingly, plasmepsin II, the aspartic protease of *P. falciparum*, cleaves spectrin mainly within the SH3 domain of α-spectrin, thus suggesting that specific targeting of the SH3 domain by *P. falciparum* may be part of the strategy to dismantle the membrane skeleton.[486]

PH Domain. All β-spectrins *except* the major erythroid isoform (βIΣ1) have a C-terminal extension that contains a pleckstrin homology (PH) domain.[421,487] The specialized 100-residue PH domain has been identified in proteins involved in signal transduction (e.g., protein kinases and their substrates, phospholipase C isoforms, guanosine triphosphatases [GTPases], GTPase-activating proteins, GTPase exchange factors) and in membrane skeletal organization (e.g. dynamin, β-spectrin) and is believed to mediate membrane targeting of proteins.[487,488] The muscle isoform of erythroid spectrin (βIΣ2) also contains a PH domain,[430] and recent studies have shown that mature red cells contain some of this isoform, which is clumped in submicron-size patches within the membrane skeleton.[489] The erythroid spectrin PH domain binds with equal affinity to PIP$_2$ and phosphatidylinositol 3,4,5-triphosphate.[490,491] The function of the PH domain in red cells is untested, but it seems likely that it contributes to the attachment of spectrin to the membrane.

Phosphorylation Sites. Instead of a PH domain, the C-terminal region of βIΣ1-spectrin contains a 52–amino acid extension just beyond the site of self-association that is phosphorylated by a membrane-associated casein kinase I (see Fig. 15-13).[492,493] There are five Ser and one Thr that are phosphorylated in sequential fashion.[494] In vitro phosphorylation of β-spectrin has no effect on spectrin self-association.[450,495,496] However, increased phosphorylation of β-spectrin in vivo has been shown to decrease membrane mechanical stability, whereas decreased phosphorylation strengthens the mechanical properties of the red cell membrane.[497]

Tryptic Domains. The tryptic domains of spectrin have important historical, structural, and clinical significance. Gentle proteolysis of spectrin generates nine structural domains, each composed of several 106–amino acid repeats.[420,498] Thus, spectrin was initially demonstrated to contain a series of proteolytically resistant domains joined by protease-sensitive regions. Five tryptic fragments represent most of the α chain and include the αI (80 kd), αII (46 kd), αIII (52 kd), αIV (52 kd), and αV (41 kd) domains; the β chain is digested into four domains, including βI (17 kd), βII (65 kd), βIII (33 kd), and βIV (74 kd). Many of the molecular defects in HE have been identified as abnormalities in spectrin domain maps after proteolytic digestion (see "Hereditary Elliptocytosis").

Spectrin Is Synthesized Early in Erythroid Development. Spectrin is abundant in pronormoblasts[499] and is detectable in undifferentiated erythroleukemia cells[500] and possibly in immature committed erythroid stem cells, BFU-E and CFU-E.[501] α-Spectrin is synthesized in at least a threefold excess over that of β-spectrin[502-504] and has a distinctly slower degradative pathway.[505] The limited synthesis and more rapid degradation of β-spectrin suggest that its association with the membrane is the rate-limiting step in spectrin assembly.[504,505] The difference in the rate of α- and β-spectrin production is relevant to the molecular pathophysiology that underlies spectrin-related red cell membrane disorders (see "Hereditary Elliptocytosis" and "Hereditary Spherocytosis").

Mutations in Erythroid Spectrin Affect the Integrity of the Red Cell and Lead to Clinical Disease. Spectrin defects are the major cause of HE and are also important in the pathogenesis of HS (see "Hereditary Elliptocytosis" and "Hereditary Spherocytosis").

Actin

The red cell contains β-actin, which is the actin subtype found in a wide variety of nonmuscle cells.[506] Whereas red cell actin shares structural and functional similarities with the β-actin found in nonerythroid cells,[507] the assembly of *protofilaments*, or short, double-helical F-actin filaments composed of 12 to 14 monomers, is a characteristic feature of red cell actin.[508] Actin protofilaments are stabilized by (1) interactions with spectrin, protein 4.1, and tropomyosin; (2) capping of the pointed or slow-growing end by tropomodulin[509]; and (3) capping of the barbed or fast-growing end by adducin.[510] Thus, another unique feature of the membrane-associated actin filaments in red cells is that actin filaments are capped by adducin instead of CapZ, the ubiquitous barbed-end capping protein of nonerythroid cells.[511] Interestingly, this occurs despite the fact that red cells contain CapZ.[511] However, when β-adducin is deleted in red cells, CapZ expression is upregulated ninefold, presumably as a compensatory mechanism.[512]

Actin protofilaments function within the red cell skeleton meshwork as junctional centers intertriangulated by spectrin (see Fig. 15-16). The protofilaments lie parallel to the lipid bilayer within 20 degrees of the membrane plane.[513] This suggests that the protofilaments may also function as attachments between the membrane skeleton and the lipid bilayer. Spectrin dimers bind to the side of actin filaments at a site near the tail of the spectrin molecule (see Figs. 15-13 and 15-17).[466] Spectrin tetramers are bivalent and therefore cross-link actin filaments, although binding is weak ($K_d \approx 10^{-3}$ M) and ineffectual in the absence of protein 4.1.[470] Spectrin-actin interactions are specifically enhanced by protein 4.1 and adducin (see "Protein 4.1" and "Adducin").

Rac1 and Rac2 GTPases regulate actin structures, and mice that lack both GTPases are prone to the development of a microcytic hemolytic anemia with marked anisocytosis and poikilocytosis.[514] Membrane skeletal junctions are aggregated, and there is pronounced irregularity of the hexagonal spectrin meshwork. These changes are accompanied by decreased cellular deformability, an increased actin-to-spectrin ratio, and increased phosphorylation (Ser724) of adducin, an F-actin capping protein. Actin and phosphorylated adducin are more easily extracted by Triton X-100 from Rac1(–/–)/Rac2 (–/–) red cells, indicative of weaker association to the cytoskeleton. Osteopontin phosphorylates or activates multiple proteins in human erythroblasts, including Rac-1 GTPase and adducin. Osteopontin knockout mice are anemic and also show defects in F-actin filaments.[515] The results indicate that Rac GTPases regulate organization of the red cell membrane skeleton. It is unclear whether this occurs dynamically in the mature red cell or just during erythropoiesis.

Protein 4.1

Red cell protein 4.1 (technically the 4.1R homologue) is a major component of the erythrocyte membrane skeleton, with approximately 200,000 copies present in each red cell. Protein 4.1 confers both stability and flexibility to circulating red cells by potentiating the interaction of spectrin tetramers with F-actin[470,516] and by linking this membrane skeletal scaffold to the plasma membrane through vertical interactions with glycophorin C (GPC).[419] In the mature red cell, 4.1 exists as a 588–amino acid protein that is 4.7 nm in diameter and has a molecular weight of 66 kd, although it runs as an 80-kd protein on SDS gels. Two forms of the protein are resolved on high-resolution SDS gels, an 80-kd protein designated 4.1a and a 78-kd protein designated 4.1b. Protein 4.1a derives from 4.1b by progressive deamidation of Asn502 during the life span of the red cell; thus, 4.1a is more prominent in senescent red cells.[517] Proteolysis of 4.1 generates four structural domains: an N-terminal 30-kd membrane binding domain (MBD) (also called the FERM domain[518]), a 16-kd linker domain, a 8- to 10-kd spectrin-actin binding domain (SABD), and a 22- to 24-kd C-terminal domain (CTD) (Fig. 15-18).[519] Two post-translational modifications of the CTD include the previously mentioned deamidation of Asn502 coincident with red cell aging[517] and O-linked glycosidation of cytosolic 4.1 with N-acetylglucosamine.[520] The functional significance of these modifications is unclear. Protein 4.1 is phosphorylated in vitro and in vivo by protein kinase A (PKA), protein kinase C (PKC), and casein kinase II. In each case, 4.1 phosphorylation leads to a marked decrease in its ability to bind spectrin and promote the spectrin-actin interaction.[521,522] PKC phosphorylation of 4.1 inhibits its binding to membranes by blocking its interaction with band 3[523] and GPC.[522]

Spectrin-Actin Binding Domain (SABD)

Protein 4.1 Significantly Enhances the Interaction of Spectrin with Actin. In physiologic solvent conditions, spectrin tetramers bind weakly to F-actin ($K_d \approx 10^{-3}$ M), whereas the addition of protein 4.1 generates a high-affinity ternary complex ($K_d \approx 10^{-12}$ M).[470] The 10-kd domain of 4.1 specifically facilitates spectrin-actin interactions[516] and is encoded by an alternatively spliced exon 16 and a constitutive exon 17.[524,525] The 21–amino acid peptide encoded by exon 16 and amino acids 37 to 43 encoded by the constitutive exon 17 form the spectrin binding site.[524,525] The F-actin binding site[526] is located within the first 26 amino acids of exon 17, particularly a critical 8–amino acid sequence (LKKNFMES),[527] and thus the actin site is straddled by the bipartite spectrin binding site.[527,528] The stoichiometry of 4.1-actin binding is 1:1, and the interaction is highly cooperative such that binding of one 4.1 molecule induces a conformational change in the actin protofilament that promotes further 4.1 binding.[526,528] Thus, the available data suggest that protein 4.1 facilitates spectrin-actin binding by bridging spectrin and actin in a strong ternary complex.

The interactions of spectrin, actin, and 4.1 within the red cell membrane skeleton are dynamic and thus enable red cell membranes to be stable yet deformable as the cells course through the circulation. Phosphorylation of protein 4.1 by PKA, which labels Ser331 in the 16-kd domain and Ser467 in the 10-kd domain, inhibits binding of 4.1 to spectrin-actin.[529] The interaction is also inhibited by tyrosine phosphorylation at Tyr418, which is located in the 10-kd domain.[530] Formation of the ternary complex is further regulated by Ca^{2+} and calmodulin,[531] with attendant consequences on red cell membrane stability.[532] The critical role of protein 4.1 in maintaining red cell membrane stability is underscored by the erythrocyte membrane fragility and resultant hemolysis observed in patients who lack protein 4.1 (see "Hereditary Elliptocytosis"). Interestingly, normal membrane stability is completely restored when patient red cell ghosts are reconstituted with a 64–amino acid fusion protein containing the spectrin-actin binding site (i.e., the 21 amino acids encoded by exon 16 and the first 43 amino acids encoded by exon 17).[528] This finding highlights the critical functional role of the 10-kd domain of 4.1 in red cell function.

The Spectrin-Actin Binding Domain Also Interacts with Myosin. Protein 4.1 binds to heavy meromyosin with 1:1 stoichiometry and partially inhibits the actin-activated Mg^{2+}-ATPase activity of myosin.[533] This interaction may be relevant in modulating Mg^{2+}-ATPase–dependent function in erythroid cells.[533]

Membrane Binding Domain (MBD)

The 30-kd Membrane Binding Domain of Protein 4.1 is Conserved among an Entire Family of Proteins Known as ERM Proteins. The ERM family is composed of a diverse and interesting group of proteins, including ezrin, radixin, moesin, merlin (or schwannomin), talin, coracle, and several tyrosine phosphatases (e.g., PTPH1, PTPMEG).[534,535] Merlin, for example, is a tumor suppressor protein that binds to the C-terminal end of αII (or α_G) spectrin[536] and regulates cell growth and organization of the actin-based cytoskeleton.[537] The merlin gene

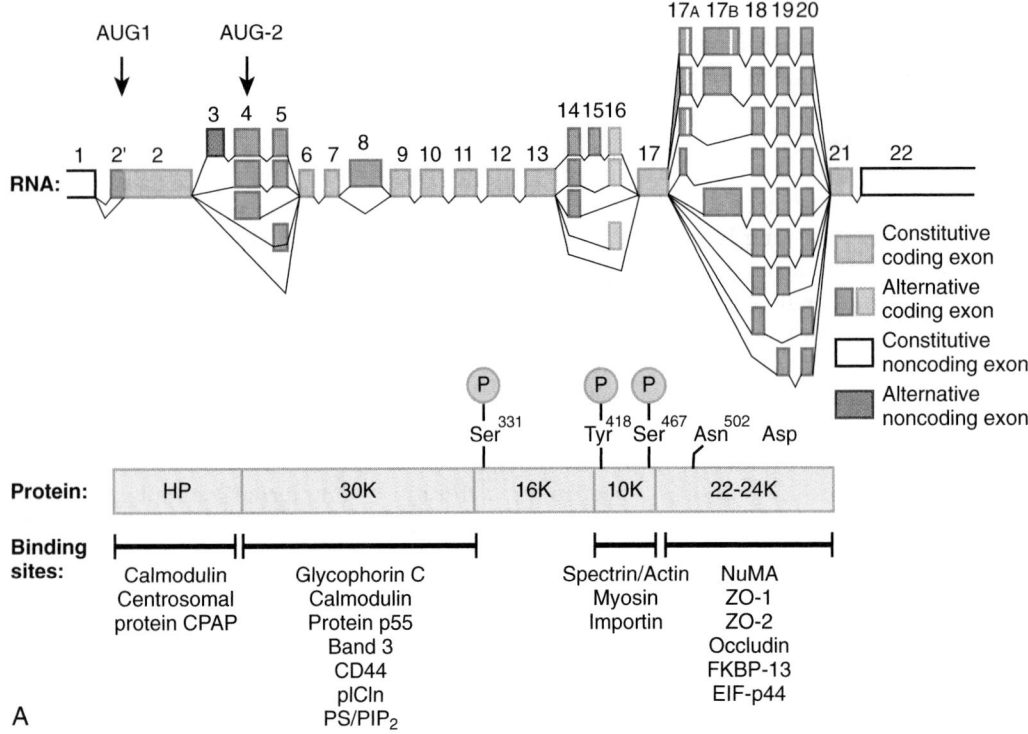

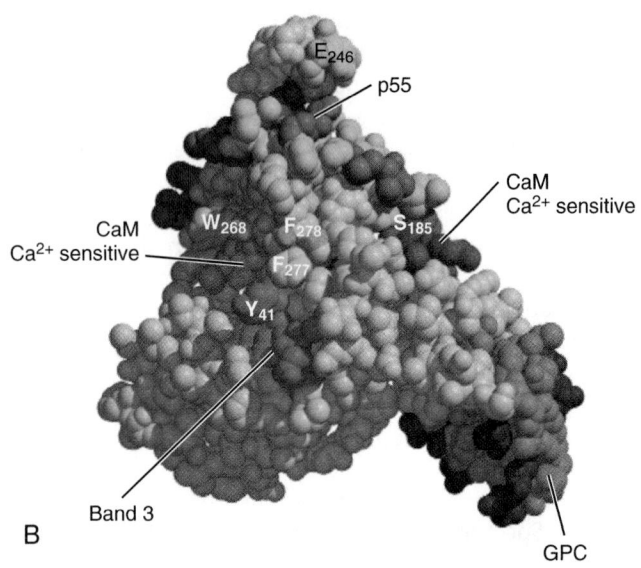

FIGURE 15-18. Protein 4.1. **A,** Alternative splicing map of protein 4.1 mRNA. Erythrocyte 4.1 is translated from AUG-2 and includes a 63–base pair (21–amino acid) erythroid-specific sequence (*orange*) that is critical for spectrin-actin interactions. The nonerythroid protein that begins at AUG-1 contains an additional headpiece (HP) domain. Many combinations of exons are expressed, particularly in the C-terminal domain, although many are observed only in nonerythroid tissues. *Middle,* Domain map of protein 4.1 indicating binding sites, phosphorylation sites, and the location of a C-terminal asparagine that is deamidated in old red cells. The deamidation reaction accounts for the variability in the apparent molecular weight of the C-terminal domain. **B,** Structure of the protein 4.1 membrane binding (30K) domain. Various subdomains are marked where specific proteins bind. Critical amino acids in each region are numbered. *(Adapted from Conboy JG. Structure, function, and molecular genetics of erythroid membrane skeletal protein 4.1 in normal and abnormal red blood cells. Semin Hematol. 1993;30:58; and Han BG, Nunomura W, Takakuwa Y, et al. Protein 4.1R core domain structure and insights into regulation of cytoskeletal organization. Nat Struct Biol. 2000;7:871.)*

is defective in neurofibromatosis type 2 and is absent in virtually all schwannomas and many meningiomas and ependymomas. Despite the diverse functions of ERM proteins, they each use the conserved 30-kd MBD, or the FERM domain, to facilitate interactions with cellular membranes.

Protein 4.1 Links the Membrane Skeleton to the Plasma Membrane through Interactions with the Integral Membrane Protein Glycophorin C/D. The majority of membrane-associated 4.1 is bound to the carboxy-terminal of GPC/GPD via the 30-kd MBD (see Fig. 15-18).[419] Although 4.1 also associates with GPA in vitro, there is considerable evidence indicating that the physiologically relevant interaction is the association of 4.1 with GPC/GPD. For example, (1) 4.1-deficient red cells also lack

GPC/GPD but not GPA[419]; (2) any residual GPC/GPD in 4.1-deficient red cells is only loosely bound to the membrane skeleton and becomes tightly bound if the cells are reconstituted with 4.1[419]; (3) stripped, inside-out membrane vesicles from normal red cells bind five times more 4.1 than do vesicles prepared from red cells lacking GPC/GPD[155]; (4) treatment of membrane vesicles with antibodies that block the 4.1 binding sites on GPC/GPD reduces the ability of 4.1 to promote spectrin-actin binding to the vesicles by 85%[217]; and (5) GPC/GPD-deficient red cells, like 4.1-deficient cells, are elliptocytic and mechanically unstable, whereas GPA-deficient cells are morphologically and structurally normal.[327]

Protein 4.1 and GPC/GPD can occur as a ternary complex with p55, a MAGUK protein. The residues Tyr94 to Arg166 of the 30-kd MBD of protein 4.1 interact with a positively charged peptide in the cytoplasmic domain of GPC localized to residues 82 to 98.[155,538,539] The residues Tyr214 to Glu246 of the 4.1 MBD bind to p55 at a positively charged, 39–amino acid segment found between the SH3 domain and the guanylate kinase domain[538]; p55, in turn, binds via its PDZ domain to the C-terminal amino acids 112 to 128 of GPC.[328,540]

The 4.1 Membrane Binding Domain Also Interacts with Other Integral Membrane Proteins of the Red Cell, Including Band 3 and CD44. Binding sites for the 4.1 MBD include two positively charged motifs, LRRRY and IRRRY, located near the beginning of the band 3 transmembrane domain.[541] Approximately 20% or less of the 4.1 in red cells is believed to associate with band 3,[542] and 4.1–band 3 interactions do not link the spectrin-actin–based skeleton to the plasma membrane.[217] Instead, the protein 4.1–band 3 interaction may function to modulate the association of band 3 with ankyrin. In vitro, protein 4.1 competes with ankyrin for binding to band 3. Displacement of 4.1 from band 3 decreases membrane deformability and increases membrane mechanical stability, presumably because of the resultant increase in band 3–ankyrin interactions.[213] Whether 4.1 regulates band 3–ankyrin binding in vivo remains to be demonstrated. One experiment implies that it may. Zebra fish lacking red cell band 3 have a nearly bloodless phenotype, which can be rescued by injecting normal mouse band 3 cRNA into the early band 3(–/–) fish embryos.[543] Rescue is markedly reduced if mouse band 3 containing a mutation in either the LRRRY or IRRRY site is used and is nearly abolished if both sites are mutated.

The MBD also binds to CD44, a transmembrane glycoprotein present in erythroid and nonerythroid cells. The binding sites on CD44 are the positively charged motifs SRRRC and QKKKL, which are homologous to the interacting peptides found in band 3.[544] Analogous to band 3, protein 4.1 competes with ankyrin for CD44 binding and thus may regulate CD44-ankyrin interactions.[544] Ca^{2+}-dependent and Ca^{2+}-independent calmodulin binding sites have been located within the MBD (see Fig. 15-18),[545] and MBD interactions with transmembrane proteins are subject to regulation by Ca^{2+}-calmodulin. For example, Ca^{2+}-calmodulin specifically reduces the affinity of the 4.1-CD44 interaction,[544] as well as 4.1 interactions with band 3, GPC, and p55. Thus, the intracellular concentration of Ca^{2+} is an important influence on the dynamic nature of protein 4.1's MBD–integral membrane protein associations. The crystal structure of the MBD domain of protein 4.1 (see Fig. 15-18B) provides a mechanistic understanding of the binding of 4.1 to various membrane proteins and the regulation of these interactions by Ca^{2+} and calmodulin.[546]

The discovery that both protein 4.1 and protein 4.2 are located near the tail end of spectrin[221] makes it likely that a subset of band 3 is also located there. The probable subset is band 3 dimers because the tetramers are known to bind ankyrin. The number of band 3 dimers ($\approx$400,000) is sufficient to accommodate both proteins (see Table

15-2). The proximity of the calmodulin-like EF hands on α-spectrin to the calponin homology domains on β-spectrin, where 4.1 binds (see Fig. 15-17), also raises the interesting possibility that the EF hands interact with either the Ca^{2+}-sensitive or the Ca^{2+}-insensitive calmodulin binding sites on 4.1.

Protein 4.1 Also Interacts with the Plasma Membrane through Direct Associations with Phosphatidylserine Moieties and Polyphosphoinositides. The interaction with negatively charged phospholipids may account for some of the low-affinity binding of protein 4.1 to membranes, thus suggesting that the membrane may directly serve as a depot for 4.1 that is temporarily unbound from its protein targets. A recent study showed that binding of protein 4.1 to PS is a two-step process in which 4.1 first interacts with serine head groups through the positively charged amino acids YKRS in the MBD domain and subsequently forms a tight hydrophobic interaction with fatty acid moieties.[547] Importantly, it was shown that acyl chain interactions with 4.1 impair its ability to interact with band 3, GPC, and calmodulin.

PIP_2 enhances binding of protein 4.1 to GPC and spectrin, inhibits its binding to band 3, and does not affect binding to p55.[548] Furthermore, GPC is more readily extracted by Triton X-100 from ATP-depleted red cells, which implies that the 4.1-GPC interaction may be regulated by PIP_2 in situ.

C-Terminal Domain (CTD)

Although the functions of the SABD and MBD of 4.1 have been known for years, the functions of the 16-kd domain and CTD in red cells are poorly understood. Several human mutations in the 4.1 CTD have recently been identified.[549] Rather than affect the primary structure and assembly of 4.1 within the membrane skeleton, the CTD mutations depress the accumulation of 4.1 mRNA and reduce the amount of functional protein in the red cell.[549] The 4.1 CTD also contains a consensus sequence for binding to FKBP13, an immunophilin that is enriched in red cell membranes.[550] The purpose of this interaction is unclear.

4.1 Genes

There are five paralogous genes in the 4.1 family: 4.1R, 4.1G, 4.1N, 4.1B, and 4.1O.

4.1R. The human 4.1R gene, designated *EPB4.1*, maps to human chromosome 1p36.1 and is more than 200 kilobases (kb) in length. 4.1R is the erythroid form of protein 4.1, but it is expressed in some nonerythroid cells in the brain, kidney, heart, and stomach[551,552] and has a number of interesting functions that are relevant only to nucleated cells. For example, the SABD binds to nuclear actin,[553] and the CTD binds to NuMA,[554] a nuclear mitotic apparatus protein involved in organizing the spindle apparatus during mitosis and in reassembling the nucleus at the end of mitosis.[555] Overexpression of either domain interferes with nuclear assembly.[556] Specific spliceoforms of 4.1R contain defined residues that enable importin-mediated nuclear import[557]; these 4.1R spliceoforms are associated with the nuclear matrix and colocalize with several proteins involved in mRNA splicing.[558,559] In resting cells, 4.1R associates with centrosomes,[560] and in dividing cells, 4.1R colocalizes with the mitotic spindle and the midbody at defined time points during the cell cycle.[559] Protein 4.1R is critical for spindle assembly and the formation of centrosome-nucleated and motor-dependent self-organized microtubule asters.[561,562] The 4.1R MBD interacts with pICln, an actin-binding protein thought to play a role in cell volume regulation.[563] It is hypothesized that pICln may join the 4.1R-linked membrane skeleton to a volume-sensitive membrane channel.[563] 4.1R is also located in the tight junctions of epithelial cells, where the CTD specifically interacts with ZO-2, a tight junction MAGUK protein.[564] The exact functions of 4.1R at all these novel sites are unknown, as well as whether the functions are specific to 4.1R rather than the other 4.1 paralogues.

4.1G. 4.1G is the closest homologue to 4.1R and is the general, widely expressed version of protein 4.1.[550,565] The human 4.1G gene (*EPB41L2*) has been mapped to chromosome 6q22-23. Mouse 4.1G is a 988–amino acid protein with a predicted molecular weight of 110 kd that is 53% identical to mouse 4.1R.[550] 4.1G colocalizes with the immunophilin FKBP13, which binds to the 4.1G CTD.[550]

4.1N. 4.1N is a neuronal homologue of 4.1R that is expressed in almost all central and peripheral neurons.[566] The human 4.1N gene (*EPB41L1*) maps to human chromosome 20q11.2-13.1. Like 4.1R (see later), 4.1N has multiple spliceoforms, the predominant 135-kd form being found in the brain and a smaller 100-kd isoform enriched in peripheral tissues.[566] Immunohistochemical studies reveal several patterns of neuronal staining, with localization in the neuronal cell body, dendrites, and axons.[566] A distinct punctate-staining pattern is observed in certain neuronal locations, consistent with a synaptic localization; in neuronal cultures, 4.1N colocalizes with the postsynaptic density protein of 95 kd (PSD95, a postsynaptic marker) and with glutamate receptor type 1 (GluR1, an excitatory postsynaptic marker), thus confirming that 4.1N is a component of the synapse.[566] By analogy to the role of 4.1R in red cells, 4.1N may function to confer stability and plasticity to the neuronal membrane via interactions with multiple binding partners, including the neuronal cytoskeleton, integral membrane channels and receptors, and MAGUK proteins. Like the 4.1R CTD, the 4.1N CTD also interacts with NuMA.[567] PC12 cells stimulated to differentiate with nerve growth factor exhibit translocation of 4.1N into the nucleus concomitant with cell cycle arrest at the G_1 phase.[567] Thus, nuclear 4.1N may mediate the antiproliferative effect of nerve growth factor by antagonizing the role of NuMA in mitosis. Interestingly, 4.1N expression

is detected in embryonal neurons at the earliest stage of postmitotic differentiation.[566]

4.1B. 4.1B is another neuronal paralogue of 4.1R that is focally expressed in brain and selected other tissues.[568] Human 4.1B (*EPB41L3*) maps to human chromosome 18p11.32. Alternative splicing produces a brain isoform that lacks the 21–amino acid peptide important in spectrin-actin binding, as well as a skeletal and heart muscle isoform that incorporates this sequence into the SABD.[568] Interestingly, 4.1B is highly expressed in certain neuronal populations of the brain that do not contain 4.1N, namely Purkinje cells of the cerebellum and thalamic nuclei. This finding demonstrates the selective and complementary nature of 4.1 gene expression. 4.1B is enriched at sites of cell-cell contact.[568]

4.1O. Protein 4.1O is a smaller (553 amino acids) relative of protein 4.1 that contains a FERM domain and is primarily expressed in the ovary.[569] Its gene is located on human chromosome 9q21-9q22. Nothing is known of its function.

Alternative Splicing of the 4.1R Gene

The 4.1R gene undergoes complex alternative pre-mRNA splicing. It contains at least 24 exons, 13 of which are alternatively spliced (see Fig. 15-18).[160-163] The two major isoforms of 4.1R derive from alternate use of two distinct translation initiation codons. The 17-bp motif at the 5′ end of exon 2 encodes an in-frame ATG start site used by early erythroid cells and most nonerythroid cells to produce a 135-kd 4.1R isoform that contains a 209–amino acid N-terminal extension. The upstream translation initiation sequence is spliced out late in erythroid differentiation and a downstream ATG is used instead to produce the prototypical 80-kd isoform of 4.1R found in mature red cells.[570,571] Selective incorporation of exon 16 late in erythroid differentiation inserts a 21–amino acid sequence into the 10-kd domain of 4.1R to generate the domain essential for spectrin-actin binding. In nucleated cells, incorporation of exon 5 and exon 16 into the 4.1R transcript yields a gene product capable of importin-mediated nuclear import.[557] Selective exclusion of exon 17b from the CTD of 4.1R occurs in cultured mammary epithelial cells induced to divide, whereas nondividing cells in suspension uniformly include this exon; thus, incorporation of a specific exon correlates dramatically with changes in cell morphology induced by altering cell culture conditions.[572] Understanding the functional significance of each of the many 4.1R spliceoforms continues to be an active area of research.

4.1R Mutations

Mutations in the human 4.1R gene cause hereditary elliptocytosis, a disease characterized by red cells with (1) elliptical rather than discoid morphology, (2) decreased membrane stability, and (3) decreased circulatory half-life, all of which lead to varying degrees of hemolytic anemia (see "Hereditary Elliptocytosis").[573] Targeted deletion of 4.1R in mice produces an analogous phenotype of moderate hemolytic anemia with a decreased hematocrit and increased reticulocyte count.[551] The erythrocytes of 4.1R knockout mice have an abnormal spherocytic morphology, decreased membrane stability, and reduced expression of 4.1R-interacting proteins, including spectrin, p55, Xk, Kell, Duffy, Rh, band 3, and GPC,[551,551a] suggesting that all these proteins may interact directly or indirectly with 4.1R near the spectrin-actin junctions (see Fig. 15-6).[551a] Interestingly, knockout mice exhibit specific neurobehavioral deficits in movement, coordination, balance, and learning that correspond to selective localization of 4.1R in granule cells of the cerebellum and dentate gyrus.[552] Thus, the data generated by 4.1R knockout mice underscore the relevance of 4.1R to the cellular physiology of both erythroid *and* nonerythroid cells.

Protein p55

Protein p55 is a membrane-associated guanylate kinase (MAGUK) homologue found in the red cell membrane as part of a ternary complex with glycophorin C (GPC) and 4.1R.[574] The p55 gene has been localized to Xq28 and is situated just distal to the factor VIII locus.[575] The protein is heavily palmitoylated, which contributes to its tight association with the plasma membrane.[576] The

structure of p55 is composed of five domains, including an N-terminal PDZ domain, an SH3 domain, a central 4.1R binding region, a tyrosine phosphorylation zone, and a C-terminal guanylate kinase domain (Fig. 15-19).[577] The single PDZ domain of p55 interacts with C-terminal residues 112 to 128 of GPC.[328,329] The binding site lies in a hydrophobic groove on one side of the PDZ domain.[578] The central 39–amino acid, positively charged motif binds to the 30-kd domain of 4.1R. Interestingly, this 4.1 binding domain is conserved in other MAGUK proteins.[579] It is not known whether p55 shares functional characteristics with other MAGUKs, which participate, for example, in ion channel clustering, signal transduction, and regulation of cell proliferation and tumor suppression. It is clear, however, that p55 forms a tight complex with GPC and 4.1R[580] such that red cells lacking either 4.1R or GPC are also deficient in p55.[344] There are 80,000 copies of p55 per red cell,[576] a number less than the available binding sites for p55 on GPC and 4.1R. Thus, it remains to be determined whether there are functional differences between GPC-4.1R complexes that contain p55 and those that do not.

Adducin

Adducin is a heteromeric membrane skeleton protein that functions in regulated assembly of the spectrin-actin network. Adducin is composed of an 81-kd α subunit associated with either an 80-kd β subunit or a 70-kd γ

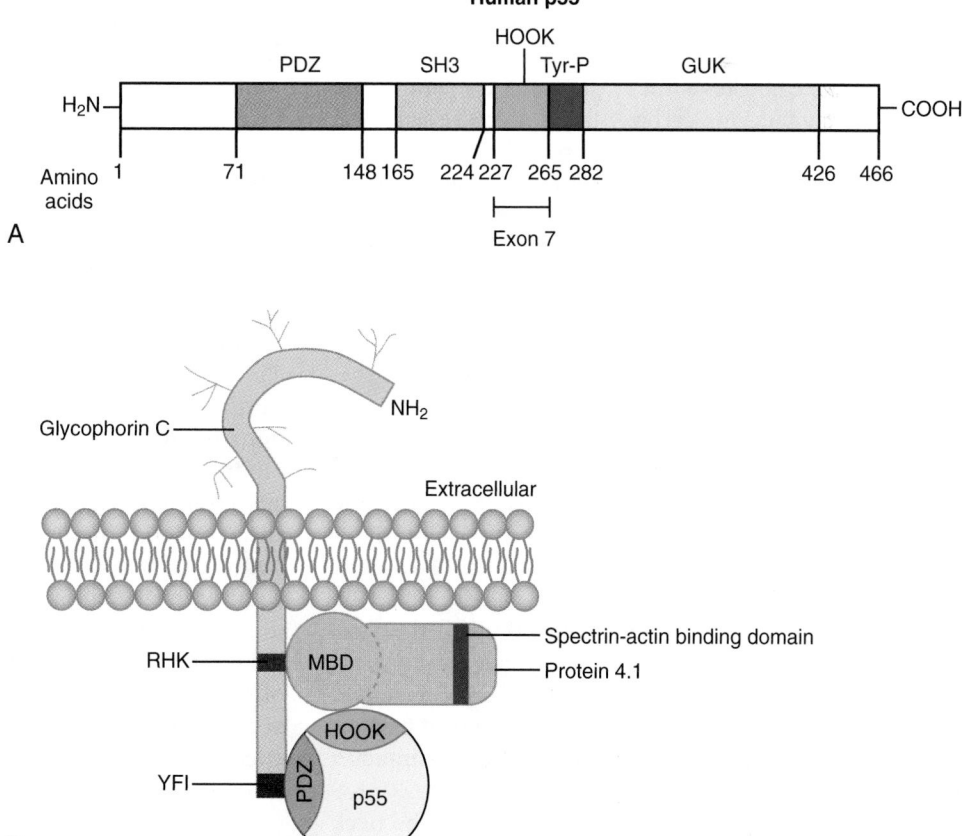

FIGURE 15-19. Model of p55 and its interactions. **A,** Domain structure of p55. 4.1, protein 4.1R binding site (HOOK domain; exon 7); GUK, guanylate kinase domain; PDZ, PSD-95/discs large/ZO-1 domain; SH3, Src homology 3 domain; Tyr-P, site of tyrosine phosphorylation. Protein p55 belongs to the membrane-associated guanylate kinase (MAGUK) protein family. **B,** Ternary interactions between glycophorin C (GPC), protein 4.1, and p55. Note that p55 and GPC bind at two distinct sites on the 30K membrane binding domain (MBD) or FERM domain of protein 4.1R (the p55 site resides in exon 10 of protein 4.1R; the GPC site in exon 8). Although p55 is shown as being distant from the lipid bilayer, it is probably adjacent because it is heavily palmitoylated. (*Adapted from Chishti AH. Function of p55 and its nonerythroid homologues. Curr Opin Hematol. 1998;5:116.*)

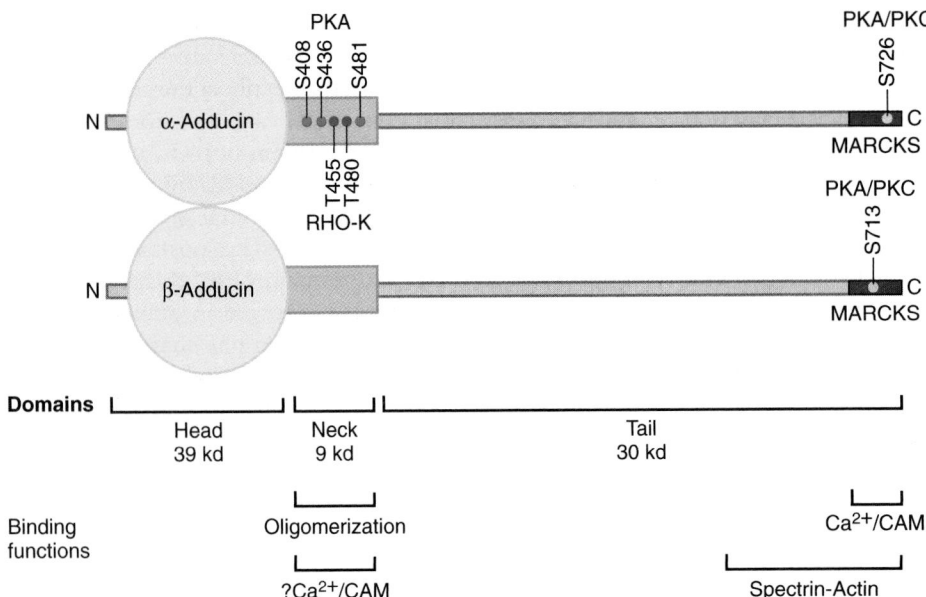

Domains

| Head | Neck | Tail |
| 39 kd | 9 kd | 30 kd |

Binding functions

Oligomerization

?Ca²⁺/CAM

Ca²⁺/CAM

Spectrin-Actin

FIGURE 15-20. Domain organization of adducin. This model of the structure of the αβ-adducin heterodimer shows the three structural domains, the phosphorylation sites, and the identified binding regions. Although the dimer is shown for simplicity, the $\alpha_2\beta_2$ heterotetramer is probably the physiologic form. Binding functions include αβ oligomerization, spectrin-actin binding, and Ca^{2+}-dependent calmodulin (Ca^{2+}/CAM) binding. MARCKS, myristoylated alanine-rich C kinase substrate; PKA, protein kinase A; PKC, protein kinase C; Rho-K, Rho kinase. *(Adapted from Matsuoka Y, Hughes CA, Bennett V. Adducin regulation. Definition of the calmodulin-binding domain and sites of phosphorylation by protein kinases A and C. J Biol Chem. 1996;271:25157.)*

subunit.[472,581,582] The predominant form of adducin in red cells is the $a_2\beta_2$ heterotetramer. The human genes for adducins α (*ADD1*), β (*ADD2*), and γ (*ADD3*) have been mapped to human chromosomes 4p16.3, 2p13-p14, and 10q24.2-q24.3, respectively. Whereas α and γ subunits are widely expressed throughout the body, β-adducin is selectively expressed in brain and hematopoietic tissues.[581-583] The subunits of adducin are approximately 50% identical to each other at the amino acid level[581,582] and are composed of three distinct domains (Fig. 15-20).[581,584] The N-terminal 39-kd domain forms the globular head region, which is protease resistant and generally more basic than the remainder of the protein.[585] A 9-kd neck region links the N-terminal domain to the 30-kd carboxy tail. The carboxy tail is protease sensitive, is composed almost entirely of hydrophilic residues, and contains a highly basic 22-residue C-terminal motif homologous to the myristoylated alanine-rich C kinase substrate (MARCKS) protein (see Fig. 15-20).[581] There are multiple alternative spliceoforms of adducin subunits, many of which generate truncated isoforms that may subserve tissue-specific functions.[586-589]

Adducin Binds, Bundles, and Caps Actin, in Addition to Enhancing the Association of Spectrin with Actin. In solution, adducin exists as a mixture of heterodimers and tetramers, with the 39-kd head domains contacting one another to form a globular core.[584] An important oligomerization site has been localized within the 9-kd neck domain.[474] The adducin tails, which extend from the head and neck domains, interact directly with the fast-growing ends of actin filaments and together recruit spectrin to the membrane skeletal complex.[474] The N-terminal, actin binding domain and the first two repeats of β-spectrin are involved in complex formation.[476] Adducin-actin interactions require both the C-terminal MARCKS domain and the oligomerization site present in the neck domain.[474] In red cells, adducin also functions as the

barbed-end capping protein and stabilizes actin network assemblies by preventing both elongation and depolymerization at the barbed ends of actin filaments.[473] CapZ, the major barbed-end capping protein found in most cells, is also present in red cells but is confined to the cytoplasm and binds to the membrane only if adducin is removed.[511] Of note, the entire adducin protein is required for capping activity, consistent with the presence of stoichiometric amounts of adducin and actin protofilaments in the red cell membrane skeleton.[473]

Adducin Activity Is Regulated by Phosphorylation and Ca²⁺-Calmodulin. The C-terminal MARCKS domain contains a serine phosphorylation site targeted by both PKA and PKC.[590] There are also three additional PKA sites located in the neck domain of α-adducin (see Fig. 15-20).[590] PKA phosphorylation reduces both the affinity of adducin for spectrin-actin complexes and the ability of adducin to enhance spectrin-actin binding.[590] Phosphorylation of the MARCKS domain by PKC inhibits actin capping activity and prevents adducin-mediated recruitment of spectrin to actin protofilaments.[591] The MARCKS domain also contains a Ca²⁺-dependent calmodulin binding site.[590] PKA or PKC phosphorylation of the MARCKS domain inhibits calmodulin binding.[590] Calmodulin binding reduces both adducin-actin binding and adducin-mediated enhancement of spectrin-actin binding.[475] Calmodulin also blocks the binding of a second spectrin molecule to an adducin-actin-spectrin complex.[472] Once bound to the MARCKS domain, calmodulin reduces the rate of PKA phosphorylation of β-adducin and the rate of PKC phosphorylation of α- and β-adducin.[590] Despite these in vitro effects, it appears that PKC phosphorylation of adducin has little effect on red cell membrane mechanical stability.[522] α-Adducin is also subject to Rho kinase phosphorylation (see Fig. 15-20), which enhances the interaction of α-adducin with actin filaments and secondarily with spectrin. Myosin phosphatase dephosphorylates α-adducin, but this activity is inhibited by Rho kinase–mediated phosphorylation of myosin phosphatase.[592] Thus, adducin activity is tightly regulated in vivo by Ca^{2+}-dependent calmodulin binding and a complexity of differential phosphorylation states. In general, Rho kinase phosphorylation tends to foster interaction of adducin with actin and spectrin, and PKA/PKC phosphorylation or calmodulin binding tends to inhibit such interaction.

Adducin and Dematin Bind to Glut-1. Recently, Chishti and his colleagues have discovered that adducin and dematin both bind to Glut-1,[417c] a glucose and dehydroascorbic acid transporter[417a,417b] (see Fig. 15-6). It is not clear whether adducin and dematin also bind to each other. Since Glut-1 is relatively abundant (~400,000 copies per RBC), this complex forms a third major attachment site between the membrane skeleton and the lipid bilayer.

Red Cells Lacking β-Adducin Are Similar to Erythrocytes from Patients with Mild Hereditary Spherocytosis. Mice with a targeted deletion of β-adducin have osmotically fragile, spherocytic, and dehydrated red cells.[583] Incorporation of α-adducin into the membrane skeleton is decreased by 30%, perhaps because of decreased α-subunit stability in the absence of its heteromeric partner.[583] Interestingly, there is a compensatory fivefold increase in the amount of γ-adducin associated with the red cell membrane skeleton.[583] The defective red cell phenotype and resultant hemolytic anemia produced by β-adducin deficiency underscore a role of β-adducin in stabilizing the red cell membrane skeletal network.

Adducin Is Enriched at Sites of Cell-Cell Contact in Nonerythroid Cells. The predominant adducin subunits found in nonerythroid cells are α- and γ-adducin,[581,582] with β-adducin expression mostly being limited to hematopoietic and neural tissues.[583] In cultured epithelial cells, adducin promptly localizes to sites of intercellular contact in response to the addition of calcium (0.3 mM) to the medium. Treatment with nanomolar concentrations of phorbol esters, which stimulate PKC phosphorylation of adducin, redistributes adducin away from the cell-cell contact sites.[593] Transfection of Madin-Darby canine kidney (MDCK) cells with a mutated, unphosphorylatable form of adducin results in a dramatic change in intracellular localization from the usual intercellular contact sites to a diffuse, punctate cytoplasmic distribution. These data indicate that focal cytoskeletal assembly and stability are regulated by calcium and PKC-induced modulation of adducin function. Interestingly, phosphoadducin-specific antibodies localize the phosphorylated form of adducin in hippocampal neurons to postsynaptic sites, the specialized regions of neuronal membranes that undergo dynamic morphologic changes and membrane skeletal rearrangement in response to extracellular signals.[591]

Polymorphisms in the Adducin Genes Have Been Genetically Linked to Certain Forms of Essential Hypertension. In rat models, a single point mutation in the α-adducin gene accounts for 50% of hypertension cases, with the mechanism of action related to changes in actin polymerization and increased Na^+,K^+-ATPase activity, which results in elevated renal tubular salt reabsorption.[594-596] A Gly460Trp polymorphism in α-adducin is associated with a salt-sensitive form of essential hypertension in certain human populations,[597] but not in others.[598-601] Intracellular erythrocyte sodium content and renal fractional excretion of sodium are significantly decreased, and Na^+,K^+-ATPase, Na^+-K^+-Cl^- cotransport, and Li^+-Na^+ countertransport are increased in subjects with the 460Trp polymorphism.[602,603] Homozygosity for the allele is estimated to be responsible for about 10% of cases of low-renin hypertension.

Dematin (Protein 4.9)

Dematin is an actin-binding protein that bundles actin filaments into cables.[604] Because actin bundles are not seen in electron micrographs of red cell skeletons, it probably has other functions in erythrocytes. One of these may be to help attach the membrane skeleton to Glut-1 and the lipid bilayer.[417c] The dematin gene has been mapped to human chromosome 8p21.1 and is widely expressed throughout the body. Red cells contain both a 48-kd gene product and a 52-kd spliceoform that incorporates a 22–amino acid insertion[164,605]; additional alternative spliceoforms have been identified in the brain.[606] The protein is composed of two domains, a rod-shaped N-terminal tail and a C-terminal actin-binding headpiece that shares homology with villin, an actin-bundling protein localized to the epithelial brush border.[605] The 22–amino acid insertion contains an ATP binding site within a conserved 11–amino acid motif that is also found in protein 4.2.[165] The native protein exists as a trimer composed of two 48-kd subunits and one 52-kd subunit held together by disulfide bonds.[164] Dematin is phosphorylated by PKA and PKC,[607] with cAMP-dependent phosphorylation completely abolishing its actin-bundling capability.[608] Phosphorylation at the cAMP-dependent site Ser74 induces a conformational change in the structure of the headpiece that is presumably responsible for this change in function.[609] Dematin interacts with the Ras–guanine nucleotide exchange factor Ras-GRF2 in extracts from brain, blocks transcriptional activation of Jun by Ras-GRF2, and activates ERK1 via a Ras-GRF2–independent pathway.[610] Because Rho GTPases regulate actin organization, dematin may help organize and stabilize actin within the membrane skeletal network.

Knockout of the dematin headpiece leads to a very mild spherocytic hemolytic anemia,[611] thus suggesting that the actin-binding activity of dematin is either redundant or not critical for membrane stability. When dematin and β-adducin knockouts are combined, the effect on membrane shape, stability, and life span is much more severe.[612] This suggests that the adducin–dematin–Glut-1 complex is a physiologically important connection between the membrane skeleton and the lipid bilayer.

Tropomyosin

TM is a heterodimeric protein (reviewed by Gunning and colleagues[613]) that functions in red cells to stabilize F-actin protofilaments in uniform segments measuring 37 nm long.[166,614] The α-helical 27- and 29-kd subunits of TM form a rod-like coiled coil in vivo and migrate in the region of band 7 when subjected to SDS gel electrophoresis (see Fig. 15-5).[615] The two major human TM isoforms found in red cells are designated hTM5 and hTM5b and derive from the γ- and α-TM genes, respectively.[166] hTM5 and hTM5b are each composed of 248–amino acid residues, measure 33 to 35 nm in length, and have high affinity for F-actin and TMod. They are shorter than muscle TM. Each actin protofilament binds two TM molecules such that one TM binds to 1 of the 12 to 14 monomeric actin filaments contained in the protofilament double helix.[615] Thus, all of the actin protofilaments within the red cell membrane skeleton are coated with TM, which strengthens the filamentous network. The corresponding sizes of TM and actin protofilaments have led to the hypothesis that TM functions as a molecular ruler, along with actin-capping proteins, in dictating the length of the actin protofilaments. The amino-terminal of TM binds with high affinity to tropomodulin (TMod), the capping protein for the pointed or slow-growing end of actin. Two molecules of TM bind per TMod in a cooperative manner.[616] This interaction limits the cooperativity of actin-TM associations, thereby restricting the length of actin filaments beyond the length of TM itself.[617] Binding of TM to actin is unaffected by spectrin, but spectrin-actin interactions are inhibited by saturating concentrations of TM,[618] and red cell membranes that lack TM are markedly more fragile than normal.[619] The actin binding domain of β-spectrin is more easily exchanged into the membrane skeleton of TM-depleted red cell membranes, thus indicating that TM strengthens spectrin-actin-4.1 binding.[619] Only endogenous TM and not the longer muscles isoforms can restore mechanical stability to the TM-depleted membranes. These findings suggests that actin-TM interactions may dictate the site specificity, strength, or extent of spectrin binding along the actin filament and that endogenous TM is required for these effects.

Caldesmon

Caldesmon is a 71-kd protein identified in red cells in 1:1 stoichiometry with TM. In conjunction with TM, actin-bound caldesmon has been shown to modify actin-activated myosin ATPase activity.[620] It has been speculated that caldesmon may function as the inhibitory component of an incompletely characterized contractile system that may be present within the red cell.

Tropomodulin

TMod is a 41-kd protein that functions as an actin-capping protein at the pointed or slow-growing end of actin filaments. The C-terminal end of TMod has pointed-end actin-capping activity, whereas the N-terminal portion binds with high affinity to two molecules of TM,[616] which results in further strengthening of actin capping.[621] Among TM homologues, TMod binds with highest affinity to the shorter nonmuscle erythrocyte isoforms (hTM5 and hTM5b) and not as well to the longer muscle TM.[166,617,622] An intact coiled coil at the N-terminal of TM is required for TMod binding.[623] The interaction of TMod with TM inhibits the head-to-tail associations of TM molecules along actin filaments, thereby restricting the lengths of TM-stabilized actin filaments.[624] TMod remains attached to the red cell membrane even after removal of spectrin, actin, and TM. The membrane binding site for TMod and the significance of this membrane interaction are unknown.

Myosin

Red cells contain a nonmuscle myosin composed of two light chains (19 and 25 kd) and one heavy chain (200 kd).[625,626] The protein has two globular heads, a rod-like tail that self-associates to form bipolar filaments, and the characteristic actin-activated Mg^{2+}-ATPase activity.[626] There are approximately 80 actin monomers for every myosin molecule in the red cell, an actin-myosin ratio comparable to that in other nonmuscle cells.[627] Interestingly, neonatal red cells have 2.5 times the myosin of adult cells, perhaps accounting for the enhanced motility of neonatal reticulocytes.[628] The spectrin-actin binding domain of 4.1R binds to myosin and partially inhibits its actin-activated Mg^{2+}-ATPase activity.[533] Thus, 4.1R binding may function as a means of regulating myosin activity in erythroid cells.

Ankyrin

Erythrocyte ankyrin (ankyrin-1 or ankyrin$_R$) is a 206-kd protein[629] that links spectrin to band 3 and thus forms the basis of the skeleton-membrane attachment so critical to the mechanical and viscoelastic properties of the red cell. Ankyrin$_R$ is encoded by the *ANK1* gene, which has been localized to the short arm of chromosome 8 near the centromere (8p11.2).[630] The protein is composed of three domains: an 89-kd membrane domain (amino acids 2 to 827) that interacts with band 3 (and other integral membrane proteins in nonerythroid cells), a 62-kd spectrin binding domain (amino acids 828 to 1382), and a 55-kd C-terminal domain (CTD) (amino acids 1383 to 1881) that modulates ankyrin's interactions with spectrin and band 3 (Fig. 15-21). Alternative

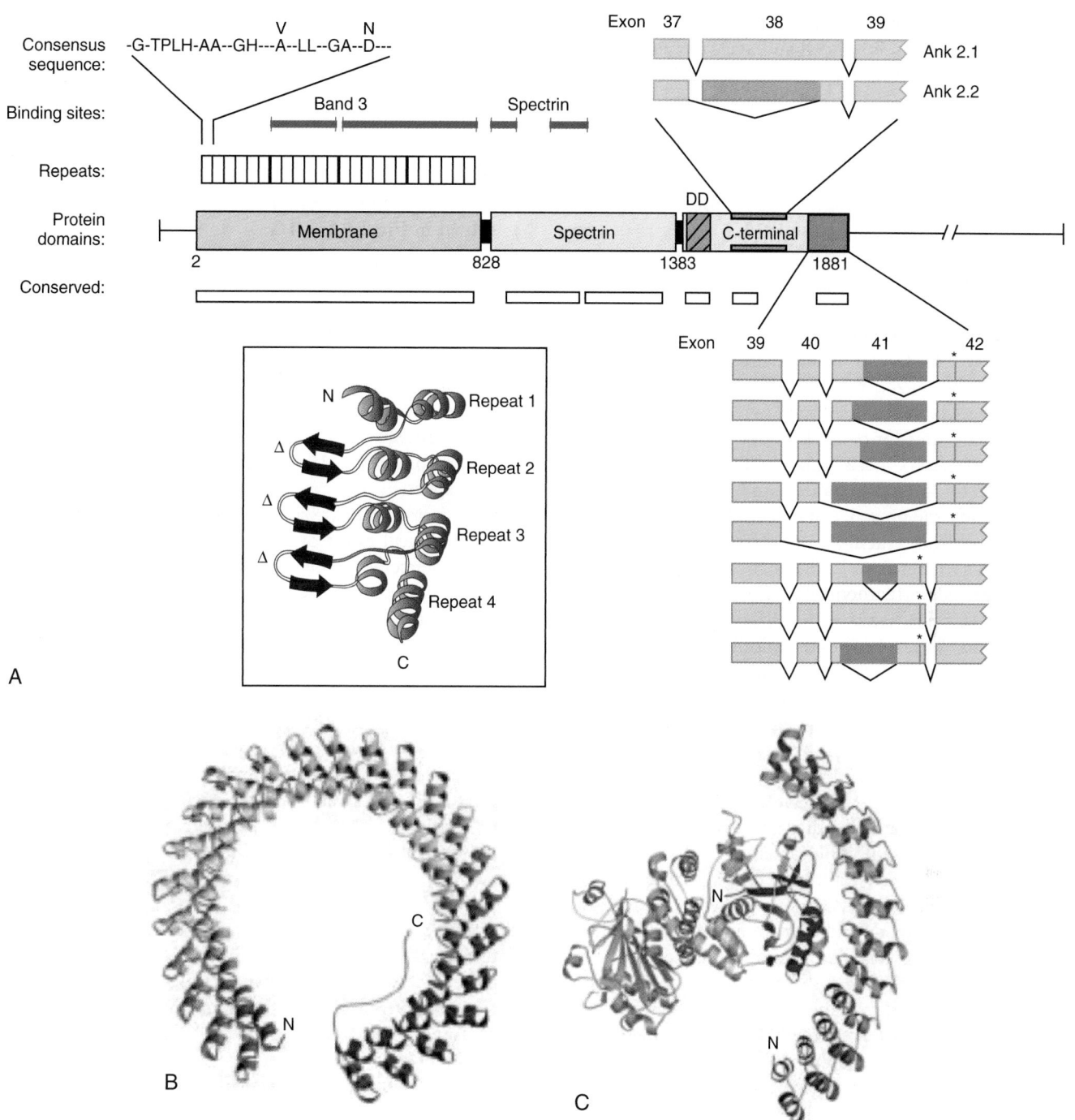

FIGURE 15-21. A, Model of the erythroid ankyrin (Ank1 or AnkR) structure. The *membrane domain* (89 kd) contains 24 "Ank" repeats (33 amino acids each) grouped functionally into subdomains of six repeats. Their consensus sequence is shown at the *top left* in single-letter amino acid code. *Dashes* indicate less conserved residues. There are two binding sites for band 3, one involving repeats 7 to 12 and one involving repeats 13 to 24. The *spectrin domain* (62 kd) contains the binding site or sites for spectrin. These two domains are the most conserved. The *C-terminal (regulatory) domain* (55 kd) is thought to modulate the binding functions of the other two domains. A conserved death domain (DD) resides at the beginning of this domain. It is similar to death domains in proteins involved in apoptosis, but its function in ankyrins is unknown. In the middle of the domain a highly acidic inhibitory region in exon 38 is spliced out of full-length ankyrin (ankyrin 2.1) to make ankyrin 2.2. At least eight isoforms of the last three exons exist. In addition, isoforms lacking exons 38 and 39, 36 through 39, and 36 through 41 have been detected. The *asterisk* and *vertical line* under it indicate the location of the translation terminator codon. The *inset* shows the structure of four consecutive ankyrin repeats.[631] Each repeat forms an L-shaped structure. A β-hairpin loop (*arrows*) makes up the bottom of the L, and two antiparallel α-helical coils form the vertical stem. The hairpin loops of neighboring repeats interact to create an antiparallel β-sheet, and the α helices interact to form helical bundles. The small *triangles* in the *inset* indicate the junction between adjacent repeats. **B,** Model of the membrane domain based on the structure of half the domain[632] and viewed along the spiral axis. **C,** Model of the interaction between a dimer of the cytoplasmic domain of band 3 (*gray* and *purple*) and repeats 13 to 24 of ankyrin (*green*). Residues predicted to bind to ankyrin are shown in *purple*. (**A,** *Redrawn from Walensky LD, Narla M, Lux SE. Disorders of the red cell membrane. In Handin RI, Lux SE, Stossel TP [eds]. Blood: Principles and Practice of Hematology, 2nd ed. Philadelphia, JB Lippincott, 2003, pp 1709-1858, with permission. **B** and **C,** redrawn from Michaely P, Tomchick DR, Machius M, Anderson RG. Crystal structure of a 12 ANK repeat stack from human ankyrin_R. EMBO J. 2002;21:6387.)*

splicing, particularly in the CTD, generates several ankyrin species in the red cell and accounts for the presence of ankyrin bands 2.1, 2.2, 2.3, and 2.6 on SDS gel electrophoresis (see Fig. 15-5).[629] Disruption of the ankyrin–band 3 interaction by exposing intact red cells to alkaline pH causes marked membrane instability, thereby emphasizing the importance of the ankyrin linkage to red cell physiology.[633] Indeed, defects in ankyrin are the most common cause of HS (see the section "Hereditary Spherocytosis").[634]

Membrane Domain

The 89-kd N-Terminal Domain of Ankyrin Contains 24 Consecutive 33–Amino Acid Repeats.[629] The ankyrin repeats are organized functionally into four subdomains of six repeats each[635] and contain two distinct and cooperative binding sites for band 3.[636] One band 3 binding site occurs at repeats 7 to 12 (subdomain 2) and the other at repeats 13 to 24 (subdomains 3 and 4) (see Fig. 15-21A and C). Thus, the presence of two binding sites on ankyrin for dimeric band 3 facilitates the tetramerization of band 3 upon ankyrin binding.[214] The high-affinity binding interface for ankyrin on the cytoplasmic domain of band 3 ($K_d \approx 10^{-7}$ to 10^{-8} M) has been localized to an external loop (amino acids 175 to 185) in the middle of the cytoplasmic domain (see Fig. 15-9).[637,638] Removal of this loop abolishes affinity for ankyrin.[209] Surprisingly, however, red cells containing the loop-deleted ankyrin are only mildly spherocytic and unstable, much less so than red cells that lack ankyrin or band 3.[210] This suggests that either there are additional ankyrin–band 3 interactions or that loss of ankyrin or band 3 affects other interactions attaching the lipid bilayer and membrane skeleton. Both may be true. There is some evidence that ankyrin also interacts with the N-terminal of band 3, both proteins interact with protein 4.2 (see later), and ankyrin and 4.2 both interact with spectrin and with elements of the Rh complex (see Fig. 15-6).[392,639,640] The fact that the ankyrin binding site is mutated in Rh proteins and RhAG from some weak D and Rh(null) variants, respectively, suggests that the Rh-RhAG/ankyrin interaction is crucial for biosynthesis or stability of the Rh complex.[640]

Ankyrin Repeats Are Found in Hundreds of Proteins in All Phyla and Are One of the Most Common Protein Sequence Motifs. The ankyrin repeat motif[641] functions as a site of protein-protein interaction in a broad range of proteins involved in development, cell cycle control, oncogenesis, transport, and many other functions.[642,643] Ankyrin repeats form a novel L-shaped structure consisting of a β hairpin (bottom of the L) followed by two α helices that pack side to side in an antiparallel fashion (stem of the L) (see Fig. 15-21A and B).[631,632,644] In ankyrin, the repeats correspond to individual exons.[645] They start at the tip of the β hairpin and line up side to side like overlapping L's, with the hairpins forming a β sheet that is perpendicular to the plane of the α helices. The concave and convex surfaces of the connected repeats provide an ideal interface for protein-protein interac-

tions, thus making the ankyrin repeat a versatile binding partner. A model of the 24 repeats of ankyrin resembles one twist of a spring (see Fig. 15-21B), and recent mechanical studies show that ankyrin repeats have spring-like properties[646]; some speculate that they may serve as mechanoreceptors to link external mechanical forces to signal transduction or changes in ion transport.[646,647] A model of how red cell band 3 might interact with ankyrin is shown in Figure 15-21C.

Spectrin Domain

The central 62-kd domain of ankyrin binds to β-spectrin and attaches the spectrin-actin–based skeleton to the plasma membrane. Ankyrin-spectrin interactions are cooperative such that ankyrin binding promotes spectrin tetramer and oligomer formation.[648] The spectrin binding interface involves regions at the beginning and middle of the domain (see Fig. 15-21A).[649,650] The site in the middle of the spectrin domain is highly conserved among erythroid and nonerythroid ankyrins and probably represents a critical point of spectrin attachment; the amino acid sequence at the beginning of the domain is less well conserved among ankyrins and may account for selective interactions with distinct β-spectrin homologues.[650] The binding site on spectrin is formed by the last third of β-spectrin repeat 14 and repeat 15 (see Fig. 15-13).[461] β-Spectrin repeat 15 is distinguished by the lack of a conserved tryptophan at position 45 of the repeat (amino acid 1811 of β-spectrin I) and by a nonhomologous 43-residue segment in the terminal third of the repeat; the first 30 residues of repeat 15 are highly conserved among erythroid and nonerythroid β-spectrins and are believed to be critical for ankyrin binding.[461]

C-Terminal (Regulatory) Domain

The 55-kd CTD contains sequences that regulate ankyrin interactions[651,652] and has been dubbed the "regulatory domain."[629] Alternative splicing within the CTD yields at least 15 ankyrin isoforms that differ in size and presumably function (see Fig. 15-21A).[645] For example, one isoform of ankyrin, represented by band 2.2, lacks an acidic 162–amino acid peptide present in full-sized ankyrin (band 2.1). Omission of this sequence generates an activated ankyrin that exhibits enhanced binding to band 3 and spectrin[652] and facilitates binding of ankyrin to additional distinct targets in nonerythroid membranes.[653] The identification of a membrane-associated protease that cleaves ankyrin suggests that cleavage of a repressor region within the CTD may activate ankyrin.[653] The CTD also contains a region homologous to the "death domain" of proteins implicated in apoptosis,[654] thus suggesting that ankyrins may additionally play a role in this signaling pathway. The function of the death domain in red cell ankyrin is unknown, but the death domain of Ank3 interacts with Fas in renal epithelial cells and triggers apoptosis.[655] There is a reasonable possibility that the C-terminal region of ankyrin also contains other functional domains because the most C-terminal amino acids are reasonably well conserved.

Phosphorylation

Phosphorylation of ankyrin regulates its interactions with spectrin and band 3. In vitro, up to seven phosphates are added to ankyrin by casein kinase I[656] and three to four phosphates are contributed by casein kinase II.[657] Unphosphorylated ankyrin preferentially binds to spectrin tetramers and oligomers rather than spectrin dimers.[648,656,658] This preference is abolished by phosphorylation, which also reduces the capacity of ankyrin binding to band 3.[659]

Ankyrin Genes

There Are Three Ankyrin Genes: *ANK1*, *ANK2*, and *ANK3*. The corresponding proteins ankyrin$_R$ (ankyrin-1), ankyrin$_B$ (ankyrin-2), and ankyrin$_G$ (ankyrin-3) exhibit distinct patterns of expression in the body and have multiple spliceoforms. Whereas ankyrin$_B$ and ankyrin$_G$ both contain membrane and spectrin domains highly homologous to those of ankyrin$_R$, distinctions arise from heterogeneous CTDs and domain insertions, differential cellular and intracellular localizations, and an eclectic array of binding partners. Nonerythroid ankyrins link the spectrin-actin–based skeleton to a large number of structurally diverse integral membrane proteins other than band 3. Examples include transporters such as AE2, Na$^+$,K$^+$-ATPase, the electrogenic and amiloride-sensitive Na$^+$ channels, the Na$^+$-Ca^{2+} exchanger, H$^+$,K$^+$-ATPase, the Rh/RhAG ammonium transporter, the voltage-regulated K$^+$ KCNQ2/3 channels, and the hepatic system A amino acid transporter; receptors such as the IP$_3$ receptor and the ryanodine receptor; and adhesive proteins such as CD44, E-cadherin, and the neural cell adhesion molecules neurofascin, L1, NrCAM, NgCAM, and neuroglian. Ankyrins are capable of associating with a wide variety of target proteins as a result of their versatile ANK repeats.[643,660,661] There is no specific motif that specifies an ankyrin binding site in these proteins. They seem to have developed by convergent evolution. The diversity of ankyrin homologues and spliceoforms has been implicated in establishing and maintaining the spatial organization of integral membrane proteins within specialized subcellular compartments.

Ankyrin$_R$ Is Also Expressed in Nonerythroid Cells. In addition to its critical role as a component of the red cell membrane skeleton, ankyrin$_R$ is found in muscle cells, macrophages, endothelium, and specific neuronal populations. In muscle cells, for example, the full-sized ankyrin$_R$ localizes to the sarcolemma and nuclei and functions to stabilize the myocyte membrane skeleton.[662] In addition, muscle cells express small ankyrin$_R$ spliceoforms (20 to 26 kd) that contain homologous C-terminal sequences in addition to a unique, hydrophobic N-terminal extension. The hydrophobic peptide is believed to insert directly into the sarcoplasmic reticulum membrane and functions to stabilize the sarcoplasmic reticulum through an ankyrin-based linkage to the contractile apparatus.[662,663] In the brain, ankyrin$_R$ isoforms are first expressed during the postmitotic phase of neuronal development[664] and ultimately localize to the cell bodies and dendrites of selective neuronal populations, with particularly robust expression in the Purkinje and granule cells of the cerebellum.[665]

Ankyrin$_B$ (*ANK2*) and Ankyrin$_G$ (*ANK3*) Are Both Expressed in Most Cells but Have Distinct Functions. Ankyrin$_B$ and Ankyrin$_G$ are located on chromosomes 4q25-q27 and 10q21, respectively. There are many splice variants of both ankyrins that add or delete various functional domains and that are differentially expressed in different tissues.[666,667] Among the variants are very large ankyrins that contain a large, extended, hydrophilic, filamentous tail domain inserted between the spectrin domain and the CTD.[668]

The 440-kd α-ankyrin$_B$ is specifically associated with the plasma membranes of unmyelinated and premyelinated axons and, accordingly, is the predominant ankyrin found in neonatal brain.[668] The inserted domain targets the protein to unmyelinated and premyelinated sites, and expression is subsequently downregulated upon axonal myelination.[669] Ankyrin$_B$ knockout mice exhibit hypoplasia of the corpus callosum and pyramidal tracts, ventriculomegaly, optic nerve degeneration, and death by postnatal day 21.[670] This phenotype shares similarities to mice and humans with deficiencies of L1, a member of the L1 CAM family of cell adhesion molecules. These data suggest that 440-kd α-ankyrin$_B$, in conjunction with L1, plays an essential role in the maintenance of premyelinated axons during development.

Ankyrin$_B$ also exists in a complex with Na$^+$,K$^+$-ATPase, the Na$^+$-Ca^{2+} exchanger, and the IP$_3$ receptor within the T tubules of cardiomyocytes.[671] It is presumed that the complex shuttles Ca^{2+} from the sarcoplasmic reticulum across the plasma membrane. Loss-of-function mutations of ankyrin B are quite common in white populations (2%)[672] and cause a dominantly inherited cardiac arrhythmia with an increased risk for stress-induced cardiac death ("sick sinus syndrome").[673,674]

The 200-kd isoform of ankyrin$_G$, which has a typical three-domain ankyrin structure, is expressed in the plasma membranes of many cells throughout the body, particularly epithelial and muscle cells.[666] The 480- and 270-kd spliceoforms of ankyrin$_G$ localize to axon initial segments and the nodes of Ranvier, an axonal membrane site where ion fluxes propagate neuronal action potentials.[675] Ankyrin$_G$ cooperates with spectrin βIV[437] to localize voltage-gated Na$^+$ channels, KCNQ2/3 channels, neurofascin, and NrCAM to axon initial segments and the nodes of Ranvier.[675-678] Mice that fail to express ankyrin$_G$ in the cerebellum become ataxic because of loss of Purkinje neurons, cannot localize voltage-gated sodium channels to axon initial segments, and have difficulty initiating action potentials.[679] Similarly, mice lacking spectrin βIV have diminished protein under the membrane and membrane blebbing at the nodes of Ranvier and axon initial segments.[680]

Ankyrin$_G$ and βII-spectrin collaborate to stabilize the lateral domain of bronchial (and perhaps other) epithelial cells and localize Na⁺,K⁺-ATPase and E-cadherin at sites of cell-cell contact.[681-683] The two molecules also seem to be involved in biogenesis of the lateral membrane.[681,682]

Other ankyrin$_G$ isoforms are found in the endoplasmic reticulum, Golgi apparatus, and early endosomes[684]; in late lysosomes[685]; and in coated pits, where the representative isoform binds to clathrin and plays a role in the budding of clathrin-coated pits during endocytosis.[686]

Ankyrin$_R$ Mutations

Mice with Normoblastosis (*nb/nb*) Produce a Defective Ankyrin That Causes Severe Hemolytic Anemia. Red cells from *nb/nb* mice contain a nonsense mutation in ankyrin just between the spectrin binding domain and the CTD that leads to the production of decreased amounts of a shortened (157 kd) ankyrin.[687,688] As a result, *nb/nb* red cells are also moderately spectrin deficient despite normal spectrin synthesis.[503,687] The resultant red cells exhibit severe osmotic fragility and a shortened life span because of a defective membrane skeleton. Interestingly, ataxia also develops in mature *nb/nb* mice secondary to dropout of Purkinje cells in the cerebellum.[689] Ankyrin$_R$ is highly expressed in the cerebellar Purkinje cells of normal mice; the observed reduction of ankyrin$_R$ in the Purkinje cells of *nb/nb* mice may contribute to cell fragility and degeneration.

***ANK1* Mutations Are the Most Common Cause of Hereditary Spherocytosis in Humans.** Ankyrin$_R$ mutations lead to combined deficiencies of ankyrin and spectrin. The defective cells produce a variable clinical manifestation ranging from mild hemolysis to severe transfusion-dependent anemia[634] (see "Hereditary Spherocytosis").

Protein 4.2

Protein 4.2 is an 80-kd peripheral membrane protein that participates in stabilizing the red cell membrane skeleton through interactions with band 3, CD47, spectrin, ankyrin, and the lipid bilayer. Protein 4.2 shares homology with transglutaminases and is part of a transglutaminase gene cluster on chromosome 15q15, but it lacks transglutaminase activity, having an Ala instead of a required Cys at its active site.[690,691] It is first detected in late erythroblasts and is the last of the major erythrocyte membrane proteins to be made.[692] There are eight spliceoforms that arise from alternative splicing of exon 3, exon 5, or 90 bp in exon 1.[692,693] The major form lacks the 90-bp segment. The others are all minor species in the mature red cell. The protein is found mostly in erythroid tissues[694] and the lens.[695] Reports of protein 4.2 detected in other tissues by immunologic methods[696] are not adequately controlled for antibody cross-reactivity with tissue transglutaminases.

Protein 4.2 Structure

Band 3 Binding. Protein 4.2 binds to band 3 with a K_d of 10^{-6} to 10^{-7} M. The band 3 binding site on 4.2 has been mapped to amino acids 187 to 211 (Fig. 15-22).[697] This sequence encompasses a palmitoylation site on Cys203, and palmitoylation enhances band 3 binding.[697] The binding site for protein 4.2 on band 3 has not been clearly identified; however, red cells from patients with the cytoplasmic band 3 mutations Glu40→Lys and Pro327→Arg show some deficiency of protein 4.2, thus suggesting that both proximal and distal cytoplasmic band 3 sequences may be involved (see Fig. 15-7). Red

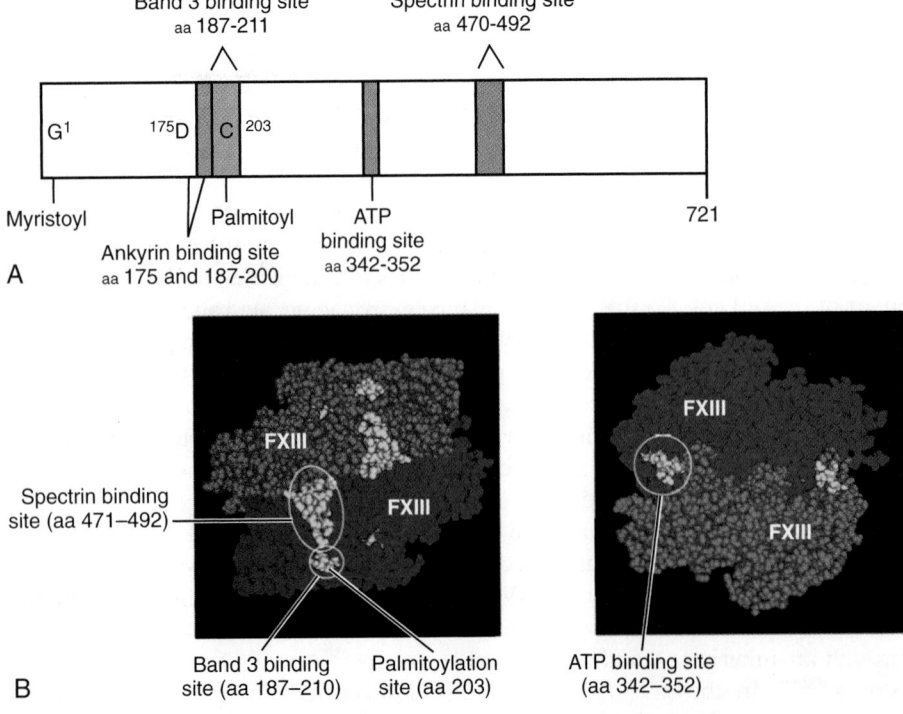

FIGURE 15-22. A, Schematic of protein 4.2 indicating its functional regions and post-translational modifications. aa, amino acid. **B,** Protein 4.2 sequence mapped onto the three-dimensional surface of a related transglutaminase, factor XIII. The dimer of factor XIII is shown, with one molecule in *blue* and one in *magenta*. Note that the spectrin binding site lies near the dimer interface and adjacent to the band 3 binding site on one side of the molecule and that the ATP binding site lies on the opposite side of the molecule.

cells that lack band 3 also lack protein 4.2 despite normal protein 4.2 synthesis.[222] Conversely, band 3 is partially deficient in red cells that lack protein 4.2.[223] As noted earlier, it is not clear whether protein 4.2 binds to the ankyrin-linked band 3 tetramers or the "free" band 3 dimers. Studies of band 3 mobility suggest that 4.2 binds to band 3 dimers, but 4.2 also binds to ankyrin, which attaches to band 3 tetramers.[219,220] Because only a fraction of protein 4.2 remains attached to the membrane skeleton (which retains ankyrin-linked band 3 *tetramers*) after band 3 *dimers* are extracted with Triton X-100,[172] it probably binds to both.

Ankyrin Binding. Protein 4.2 also interacts with ankyrin. The two proteins associate in solution[698] and there is indirect evidence that they interact on the membrane. Red cells containing protein 4.2 Komatsu (Asp175→Tyr) lack 4.2, and the recombinant protein fails to bind ankyrin.[699,700] Mapping studies localize the ankyrin binding site to a neighboring region (amino acids 187 to 200),[701] just next to the band 3 binding site (see Fig. 15-22). It seems likely that ankyrin interacts with 4.2 bound to tetrameric band 3, but this is also unknown.

CD47 Binding. Recent work shows that protein 4.2 interacts with the Rh complex through CD47.[639,702,703] Patients lacking protein 4.2 nearly lack CD47,[639,702] and patients with partial deficiency of 4.2 have less CD47 attached to the membrane skeleton.[138] However, mice lack this association[702] (and, interestingly, protein 4.2 is easier to extract from the membrane in mice). On the other hand, mice and humans with absent CD47 or low expression of the protein do not have reduced protein 4.2.[702] This and other recent work[392] provides convincing evidence for an association of the band 3 complex (band 3, ankyrin, GPA, and 4.2) with the Rh complex (RhAg, Rh polypeptides, GPB, LW, and CD47).

Spectrin Binding. Korsgren and colleagues first showed that protein 4.2 binds spectrin.[219] They identified both high- ($K_d \approx 10^{-9}$ M) and low-affinity ($K_d \approx 10^{-7}$ M) sites. Reconstituting 4.2-stripped membrane vesicles with 4.2 increased spectrin binding capacity from approximately 50% to about 80% of normal.[219] The binding site on 4.2 has been mapped to amino acids 470 to 492 (see Fig. 15-22).[704] This peptide contains a segment homologous to ERM proteins, such as protein 4.1.

Post-translational Modifications. Protein 4.2 has a nucleotide-binding P-loop (residues 342 to 352) and binds ATP with a K_d of around 10^{-6} M.[165] This is well below the concentration of ATP in the red cell (1.5 to 1.9 mM), so 4.2 should be nearly saturated with ATP under physiologic conditions. The consequences of this binding are unknown.

Protein 4.2 is myristoylated on its N-terminal glycine[705] and is palmitoylated on Cys203,[706] which sug-

gests that the protein may interact with lipid bilayers. It is likely that most of the 4.2 molecules are myristylated.[705] The extent of palmitoylation is unknown. The myristoyl group seems to influence cellular localization because nonmyristoylated 4.2 does not go to the plasma membrane.[707] As noted earlier, the palmitoyl group enhances binding of protein 4.2 to band 3 at least threefold.[697]

Topology. When the aforementioned sites are mapped onto the surface of factor XIII, a homologous transglutaminase, the putative spectrin and band 3 sites are predicted to lie quite close to each other on the front face of the molecule (see Fig. 15-22B). The ATP-binding loop, on the other hand, is predicted to lie on the rear face, adjacent to the dimer interface. The predicted spectrin site also lies next to the dimer interface on the front. Such topology suggests that it will be important to investigate the effects of ATP and spectrin binding on 4.2 oligomerization and test whether spectrin and band 3 cooperate or compete for binding to protein 4.2.

Protein 4.2 Deficiency Is a Cause of Hereditary Spherocytosis and Ovalostomatocytosis

Mutations in the human protein 4.2 gene are associated with the production of dysmorphic and osmotically fragile red cells, which results in hemolytic anemia (see "Hereditary Spherocytosis"). Protein 4.2–null mice also exhibit mild HS.[223] The defective red cells demonstrate loss of membrane surface area and defective cation transport, with cell shrinkage being associated with increased Na^+ permeability.[223] Whereas the spectrin and ankyrin content of the 4.2-null red cells is normal, there is decreased band 3 protein and a corresponding decline in anion transport activity.[223]

Peroxiredoxins

There are six known mammalian peroxiredoxins (Prdx1 to Prdx6). Peroxiredoxin-2 is the most common in red blood cells and is the third most abundant protein in the cell. Peroxiredoxin-1 and peroxiredoxin-6 are present in smaller amounts. The peroxiredoxins are widely distributed and conserved in evolution. They protect cells from insult by reactive oxygen species and regulate signal transduction pathways that influence cell growth and apoptosis.[708]

Peroxiredoxin-2

Peroxiredoxin-2, also known as thioredoxin peroxidase B, calpromotin, thiol-specific antioxidant protein, protector protein, natural killer–enhancing factor B, acidic peroxidoxin, torin, and band 8, is 198 resides in length ($\approx$22 kd) and is a soluble cytoplasmic protein that translocates to the membrane in the presence of Ca^{2+}. There are approximately 14 million copies per cell,[379,709] but only about 200,000 molecules appear to be associated with the membrane in normal red cells judging from the intensity of band 8 on SDS gels. Accumulation of peroxiredoxin-2 is maximal in early erythroid development, before the start of hemoglobin synthesis.[710] In common with the glutathione peroxidases, peroxiredoxins are able to reduce hydrogen peroxide (H_2O_2) and lipid hydroperoxides to water or the corresponding alcohol, respectively. The activity of peroxiredoxin-2 depends on a pair of highly conserved cysteine residues that catalyze the peroxide reduction step. Thioredoxin is the hydrogen donor. Peroxiredoxin-2 is especially abundant in the adrenal glands, brain, and lung, as well as in blood.

In the red cell, peroxiredoxin-2 activates the Gárdos channel, a charybdotoxin-sensitive Ca^{2+}-dependent, K^+ channel, which leads to loss of K^+ and water.[379] Such activation is associated with increased Ca^{2+}-dependent binding of dimeric peroxiredoxin-2 to the red cell membrane as a pentamer of the dimers.[375,378] Peroxiredoxin-2 is especially abundant on the red cell membranes of sickle cells, particularly the dense, dehydrated fraction of sickle cells.[711] Interestingly, peroxiredoxin-2 binds stomatin,[375] a protein that is nearly absent in hereditary stomatocytosis, a severe hemolytic anemia associated with markedly increased Na^+ and K^+ permeability (see later discussion).

Recent experiments show that peroxiredoxin-2 is extremely efficient at scavenging H_2O_2.[712] It can rapidly detect and remove even the small amounts generated endogenously by hemoglobin auto-oxidation. In the process the enzyme is oxidized to a disulfide-linked homodimer. Because there is very little thioredoxin reductase activity in red cells, the oxidized enzyme is recycled slowly. However, the concentration of peroxiredoxin-2 is so high that it is still highly effective at protecting the red cell against low concentrations of H_2O_2. This is shown by the fact that mice lacking peroxiredoxin-2 have a Heinz body hemolytic anemia, with Heinz bodies appearing spontaneously at about 2 weeks of age.[713] Smears show burrs, spherocytes, and dense cells.

Peroxiredoxin-1

Despite its low concentration, peroxiredoxin-1 also seems to play an important oxidant-protective role in the red cell. In peroxiredoxin-1 knockout mice, severe oxidant-type hemolytic anemias begin to develop at about 9 months of age, and several types of cancer develop later.[714] The anemias feature an increase in reactive oxygen species, protein oxidation, hemoglobin instability, and Heinz body formation.

ORGANIZATION OF THE MEMBRANE SKELETON

By analogy, the skeleton is sometimes compared to a sweater, which reveals its nodes and individual filaments when stretched, but not when collapsed. Stretched skeletons reveal complexes of F-actin (the nodes) cross-linked by molecular filaments of spectrin in a geodesic dome-like arrangement when viewed by high-resolution, negative-stain electron microscopy (see Fig. 15-16).[508,715,716]

Dematin, adducin, and protein 4.1 colocalize with these complexes on immunoelectron microscopy (Fig. 15-23).[715] Most of the complexes are connected by spectrin tetramers (85%) and three-armed hexamers (10%) (see Fig. 15-16).[716] Ankyrin- and band 3–containing globular complexes attach to spectrin about 80 nm from its distal end or 20 nm from the site of self-association (see Fig. 15-16). The average thickness of the skeletal protein layer has been estimated to be 3 to 6 nm from x-ray diffraction data[717] and 7 to 10 nm from electron micrographs.[718] These dimensions suggest that the skeleton is only one or two molecules thick on average, which means it must cover about 25% to 50% of the inner membrane surface area—and even more if a hydration shell around the proteins is included. This corresponds reasonably to micrographs of unspread skeletons, where the contracted, collapsed spectrin filaments appear to cover most but not all of the inner membrane surface.[458]

A model of the membrane skeleton based on this and other evidence is shown in Figure 15-6. Similar models have existed, with gradual refinement, since 1979.[719] Spectrin dimers are depicted as a twisted, flexible polymers joined head to head to form tetramers and higher-order oligomers. Self-association occurs between the N-terminal end of the spectrin α chain and the C-terminal end of the β chain (see Fig. 15-13), as described in detail in the earlier section on spectrin. Spectrin mole-

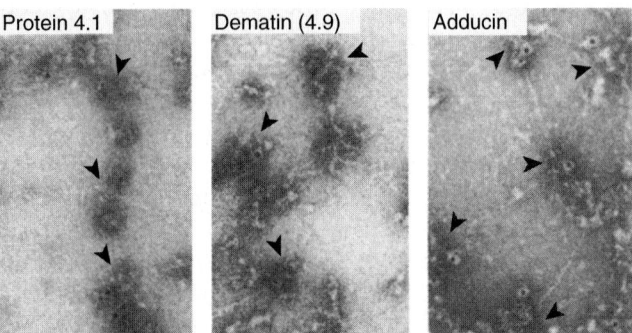

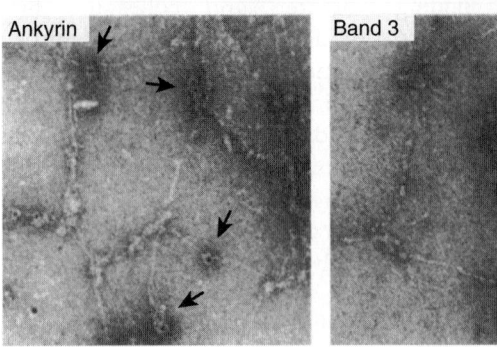
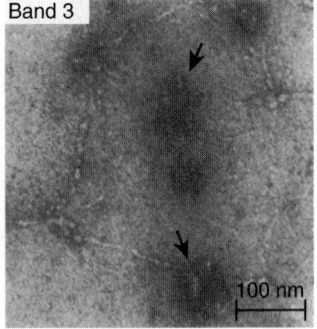

FIGURE 15-23. Immunogold labeling of proteins in red cell membrane skeletons. Expanded membrane skeletons were incubated with affinity-purified antibodies to the membrane skeletal proteins indicated and then washed and stained with 5 nm gold-labeled anti-IgG. Note that protein 4.1, dematin, and adducin are located in junctional complexes (*arrowheads*) whereas band 3 and ankyrin reside in globular structures (*arrows*) on spectrin filaments, midway between junctional complexes. *(From Liu S-C, Derick LH. Molecular anatomy of the red blood cell membrane skeleton: structure-function relationships. Semin Hematol. 1992;29:231.)*

cules are linked into a two-dimensional network by interactions with a complex of actin protofilaments, protein 4.1, dematin, adducin, tropomyosin, and tropomodulin (see Fig. 15-6). These associations occur at the tail ends of the bifunctional spectrin tetramer, where protein 4.2 also binds.[221] The predicted complexes are morphologically similar to isolated spectrin-actin-4.1 complexes and to structures observed in situ in normal ghosts (see Figs. 15-16 and 15-23). They appear to serve as a branch point or "molecular junction" in skeletal construction. On average, six spectrin molecules emanate from each complex, although there is some variation. This is evident in the hexagonal arrangement of spectrin in spread skeletons (see Fig. 15-16). In unperturbed skeletons, most spectrin molecules probably fold up to about a third of their length and do not extensively overlap or intertwine.[458,459]

Individual spectrin tetramers and oligomers are attached to the overlying lipid bilayer through high-affinity interactions with ankyrin and band 3, probably with the assistance of protein 4.2. Current evidence suggests that band 3 is a mixture of dimers and tetramers in the membrane[214] and that the tetramer binds only one molecule of ankyrin.[720,721] If so, about 40% of the band 3 molecules are involved in anchoring the membrane skeleton through ankyrin. Although the spectrin tetramer contains two ankyrin binding sites, there is only enough ankyrin to fill one, and on average, only one is filled in situ. We speculate that the remaining band 3 dimers may be attached to proteins 4.1 and 4.2 near the spectrin-actin junctions and provide another point of attachment in conjunction with interactions between protein 4.1, protein p55, and GPC (see Fig. 15-6). Interactions between ankyrin, protein 4.2, and the Rh/RhAG complex and between dematin, adducin, and Glut-1 also contribute to linkage of the membrane skeleton and lipid bilayer.

Modulation of Membrane Skeletal Structure

Red cell membrane proteins are subject to a large number of post-translational modifications or other regulatory effects: phosphorylation, fatty acid acylation, methylation, glycosylation, deamidation, ubiquitination, calpain cleavage, polyphosphoinositide and calmodulin regulation, oxidation, and modification by polyanions. A detailed discussion of most of these pathways has been published[131] but is beyond the scope of this chapter.

Phosphorylation

Almost all of the membrane skeletal proteins are phosphorylated by one or more protein kinases, including casein kinases (spectrin, ankyrin, band 3, protein 4.1, and dematin), PKA (spectrin, ankyrin, adducin, protein 4.1, and dematin), PKC (adducin, protein 4.1, and dematin), and tyrosine kinases (band 3 and protein 4.1).[131]

In all cases studied so far, phosphorylation inhibits membrane protein interactions: (1) ankyrin phosphorylation (casein kinase) abolishes the preference of ankyrin

for spectrin tetramer[648,656] and (2) decreases binding to band 3.[659] (3) Phosphorylation of protein 4.1 (several kinases) diminishes its binding to spectrin and its ability to promote spectrin-actin binding[522,530,722,723] and decreases its attachment to the membrane.[724] (4) Phosphorylation by PKC also inhibits binding of protein 4.1 to band 3[523] and glycophorin C.[522] (5) Phosphorylation of dematin by PKA prevents actin bundling.[725] (6) Phosphorylation of Tyr8 and Tyr21 at the N-terminal end of band 3 blocks the binding of glycolytic enzymes[198] and presumably hemoglobin and results in increased glycolysis.[1] In contrast, despite extensive study,[450,495,496,726] no functional effect of spectrin phosphorylation on in vitro protein-protein interactions has yet been identified. However, increased phosphorylation of β-spectrin in vivo has been shown to decrease membrane mechanical stability, whereas decreased phosphorylation strengthens the mechanical properties of the red cell membrane.[727]

Polyanions

Physiologic concentrations of organic polyanions such as 2,3-DPG and ATP weaken and dissociate the membrane skeleton[728,729] and increase the lateral mobility of band 3 in ghosts.[730] Although some studies suggest that even supraphysiologic concentrations of 2,3-DPG have little or no effect on intact erythrocytes[731,732] in terms of membrane rigidity, there is convincing evidence that increased 2,3-DPG levels decrease membrane mechanical stability.[729] It has been suggested that the developmental switch from fetal to adult hemoglobin, by diminishing available free 2,3-DPG (which does not bind to fetal hemoglobin), may explain the abatement of cell fragmentation and hemolytic anemia that accompanies maturation of infants with HE and infantile poikilocytosis.[729]

Calcium and Calmodulin

There is good evidence that calmodulin modifies the membrane properties of the red cell.[532] Physiologic concentrations of calmodulin, sealed in red cell ghosts, destabilize membranes in the presence but not the absence of micromolar concentrations of Ca^{2+}. Recent studies suggest that the effect may result from interactions of calmodulin with protein 4.1.[531] Submicromolar concentrations of calmodulin, even lower than those that exist in the red cell (≈ 3 to $6\ \mu M$), block protein 4.1–induced gelation of actin in the presence of spectrin.[531] The effect is Ca^{2+} dependent. It begins at a Ca^{2+} concentration of 10^{-6} to $10^{-7}\ M$, which is relatively low, but still higher than the free Ca^{2+} concentration in the erythrocyte (2 to $4 \times 10^{-8}\ M$). Surprisingly, Ca^{2+}-calmodulin does not block spectrin-actin-4.1 complex formation under these conditions,[531] only the extensive cross-linking needed to cause gelation. The Ca^{2+}-dependent and Ca^{2+}-independent calmodulin binding sites in protein 4.1 are located within the membrane binding domain.[545] Ca^{2+}-calmodulin specifically reduces the affinity of the 4.1-CD44 interaction,[544] as well as 4.1 interactions with band 3, GPC, and p55.

Ca^{2+} augments the binding of protein 4.2 to the EF hand domain at the C-terminal of the spectrin α chain, and the effect is blocked by calmodulin.[221] Calmodulin also binds to the spectrin β chain in a Ca^{2+}-dependent manner[733]; however, the affinity of spectrin for calmodulin is not great, and it is unclear whether this effect occurs at the concentrations of calmodulin that exist in erythrocytes.

β-Adducin is another calmodulin-binding red cell membrane protein ($K_d = 2.3 \times 10^{-7}$ M).[734] The adducin that is bound to spectrin and actin fosters the attachment of a second, neighboring spectrin. In the presence of Ca^{2+} ($>10^{-7}$ M), calmodulin binding reduces both adducin-actin binding and adducin-mediated enhancement of spectrin-actin binding.[475] Calmodulin also blocks the binding of a second spectrin molecule to an adducin-actin-spectrin complex.[472] The physiologic consequences of these effects are unclear.

Several other Ca^{2+}-dependent events do not require the presence of calmodulin. One of them is the so-called Gárdos phenomenon[735] (described later in this chapter), a unidirectional K^+ and water loss that produces cellular dehydration. The Ca^{2+} concentration required to trigger the Gárdos channel is low (in the micromolar range) and thus physiologically significant. As discussed elsewhere in this textbook, this pathway contributes to the dehydration of sickle red cells.

A second calmodulin-independent Ca^{2+} effect involves calpain, one of a family of Ca^{2+}-stimulated neutral proteases that are present in a variety of tissues, including red cells.[131] Susceptible membrane substrates include adducin, ankyrin, protein 4.1, and to a lesser extent, spectrin and band 3.

Finally, Ca^{2+} also induces phospholipid scrambling, as discussed earlier in the chapter.

Thus, increases in intracellular calcium produce a range of deleterious effects. Although these phenomena are well studied in vitro, their role in erythrocyte pathology, particularly in acquired disorders associated with abnormal red cell shape, is not well understood.

Biogenesis of the Membrane Skeleton

Synthesis of Band 3 Initiates Assembly of a Stable Membrane Skeleton. Spectrin and ankyrin synthesis is detectable at very early stages of erythroid development in avian and mammalian erythroid cells (reviewed elsewhere[736-738]). However, these proteins turn over rapidly and they do not assemble into a permanent network. Synthesis of band 3 (the anion exchange protein) and protein 4.1 begins at the proerythroblast stage and increases throughout terminal erythroid maturation, up to the late erythroblast stage. During the same time, mRNA levels and synthesis of spectrin and ankyrin decline. Even so, the proportion (and actual amounts) of newly assembled spectrin and ankyrin on the membrane progressively increase, and these proteins become more stable, as indicated by their slower turnover. This increased recruitment plus stabilization of spectrin and ankyrin, despite declining synthesis, is thought to be related to the progressive increase in the synthesis of band 3 and protein 4.1 because these proteins are the principal sites for attachment of the skeleton to the membrane.[736]

Skeletal Proteins Are Synthesized in Excess. The synthesis of membrane skeletal proteins is wasteful. Only a fraction of newly synthesized spectrin, ankyrin, and protein 4.1 is assembled into the permanent skeletal network. The excess proteins are rapidly catabolized.[737,739,740] Furthermore, skeletal protein synthesis is highly asymmetric. This is most striking in the case of spectrin, where threefold to fourfold more α-spectrin is produced than β-spectrin. Yet the two chains are assembled into the membrane skeleton in equimolar amounts as mixed heterodimers. Because of this high α-spectrin–to–β-spectrin synthetic ratio, heterozygotes for a deleted or synthetically inactive α-spectrin allele are asymptomatic because sufficient α-spectrin is still made to pair with all the β-spectrin.

Rate-Limiting Steps of Membrane Skeletal Assembly. As discussed earlier, the principal rate-limiting step in membrane skeletal assembly is the synthesis of band 3, which contains a high-affinity ankyrin binding site that recruits and stabilizes spectrin and ankyrin on the membrane.[741,742] This view, however, has to be reconciled with observations that some patients with dominantly inherited HS and partial band 3 deficiency do not have a proportional decrease in the amounts of spectrin and ankyrin in their membranes.[634,743] The probable explanation is that band 3 is synthesized in excess. About fivefold more band 3 is made than spectrin or ankyrin, but only the tetrameric fraction of band 3 binds ankyrin with high affinity.[214,721,743] Excess dimeric band 3 is selectively lost in band 3–deficient spherocytes.[743] More convincing evidence that band 3 is not absolutely required for membrane skeletal assembly is the finding that mouse red cells with complete deficiency of band 3 assemble a functional and nearly structurally normal spectrin-based membrane skeleton.[222] This indicated that other membrane sites must bind spectrin and ankyrin in the absence of band 3. The ankyrin/protein 4.2–Rh/RhAG and protein 4.1–p55/GPC complexes are good candidates.

The second rate-limiting step is the availability of ankyrin, which provides the high-affinity binding sites for β-spectrin. This is best illustrated by studies of membrane skeletal synthesis in *nb/nb* spherocytic mice[503] and in a severe form of human HS associated with combined deficiency of spectrin and ankyrin.[502] In both disorders ankyrin synthesis is markedly reduced, which leads to decreased assembly of spectrin and ankyrin on the membrane despite normal spectrin synthesis.

The third rate-limiting step involves the synthesis of β-spectrin. Because α- and β-spectrin polypeptides are assembled on the membrane in equimolar amounts and because β-spectrin binds to ankyrin with high affinity, the availability of β-spectrin seems to regulate the amount of membrane-assembled α/β-spectrin heterodimers. This regulatory role of β-spectrin is illustrated by the effects of erythropoietin on membrane protein assembly. Erythropoietin stimulates the synthesis of β-spectrin and increases the assembly of α/β-spectrin heterodimers on the membrane.[744] In contrast, α-spectrin, which is made in excess, does not seem to have a limiting role in skeletal assembly. α-Spectrin becomes rate limiting only when its synthesis is markedly reduced, as it is in some patients with recessive HS or HPP.

Membrane Remodeling during Enucleation and Reticulocyte Maturation.

At the orthochromatic erythroblast stage, when membrane biogenesis is nearly complete, the cell membrane undergoes a series of critical remodeling steps. The cell nucleus is surrounded by an actin ring, which probably participates in expulsion of the nucleus from the erythroblast. Recent work shows that this process requires the Rac GTPase mDia2, one of the formin proteins that nucleate linear actin filaments.[745] Rac1 and Rac2 bind to mDia2 in a guanosine triphosphate (GTP)-dependent manner, and mDia2 causes the contractile actin ring to form. At the same time, the spectrin skeleton, proteins that attach to it, and selected other proteins segregate into the incipient reticulocyte, and some surface receptors cluster in the membrane surrounding the soon to be extruded nucleus.[499,746] This sorting process is poorly understood.

Further membrane remodeling takes place by exocytosis as the young multilobular reticulocyte attains the biconcave shape (Fig. 15-24).[747,748] This is best studied for transferrin receptors, which enter reticulocytes by endocytosis and are segregated into vesicles called "exosomes" within large membrane-bounded sacs called multivesicular bodies. These bodies fuse with the plasma membrane and discharge the exosomes and their protein cargo (see Fig. 15-24). The transferrin receptor is lost with heat shock protein 70, which binds to the cytoplasmic domain and seems to act as a chaperone.[749] A variety of membrane proteins are lost by this mechanism, including the nucleoside transporter; LFA3; $\alpha_4\beta_1$ integrin, which binds fibronectin; small GTP-binding proteins such as Rab 4p, Rab 5p, and adenosine diphosphate (ADP) ribosylation factor; and GPI-linked proteins such as acetylcholinesterase, CD55, and CD59. Naturally occurring IgM antibodies to lysophosphatidyl choline bind the released exosomes, lead to the deposition of C3, and are probably involved in exosome clearance.[750]

Autophagocytosis also plays an important role in removal of mitochondria, cytoplasmic organelles, and some membrane receptors. Cholesterol-loaded reticulocytes from mice that lack the high-density lipoprotein (HDL) receptor and apoliploprotein E, and that are fed cholesterol, are anemic and contain targeted, macrocytic red cells with large abnormal autophagolysosomes.[751] The cholesterol-loaded reticulocytes also retain ribosomes and transferrin receptor. Removal of cholesterol, incubation in normolipemic serum, or transfusion into

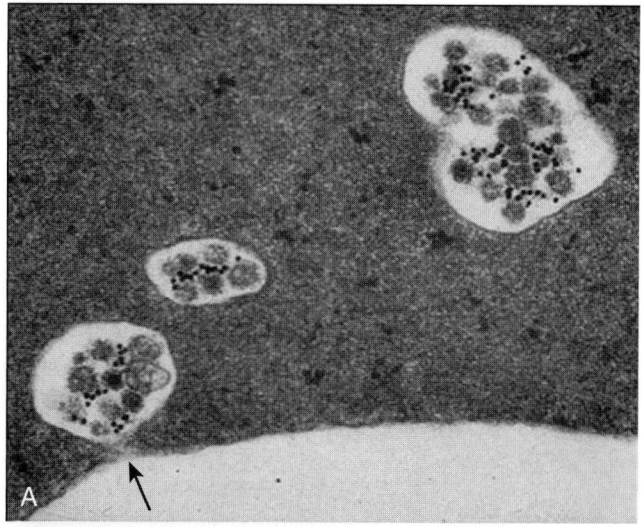

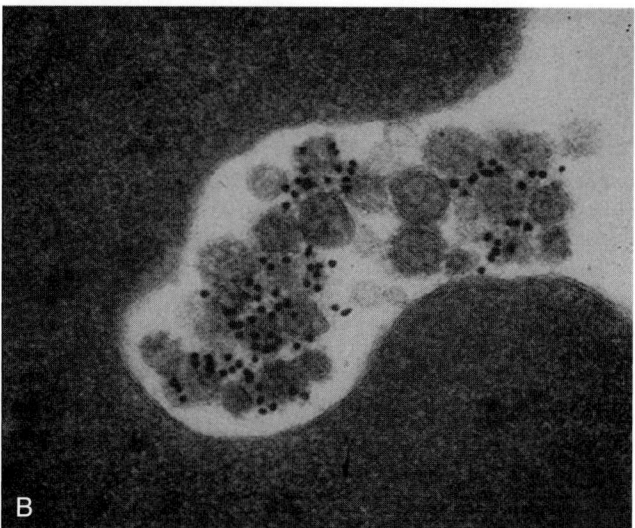

FIGURE 15-24. Maturation of the reticulocyte membrane. **A,** Note that as reticulocytes mature, transferrin receptors, labeled with gold-bound antibodies, collect in small vesicles (exosomes) within intracellular sacs called multivesicular bodies (MVBs). MVBs approach the plasma membrane and begin to fuse (*arrow*), with eventual release (**B**) of exosomes from the cell. A variety of membrane proteins are released by this mechanism. *(From Johnstone RM. Revisiting the road to the discovery of exosomes. Blood Cells Mol Dis. 2005;34:214-219.)*

normal recipients leads to expulsion of the autophagolysosomes and reinitiation of reticulocyte maturation.[751] How cholesterol accumulation inhibits reticulocyte maturation remains to be determined.

RED CELL MEMBRANE DEFORMABILITY AND STABILITY

Material Properties

The material properties of the membrane reflect the properties of both the lipid bilayer and the skeleton. During deformation of the red cell membrane, bending is restricted by the incompressibility of the lipid bilayer

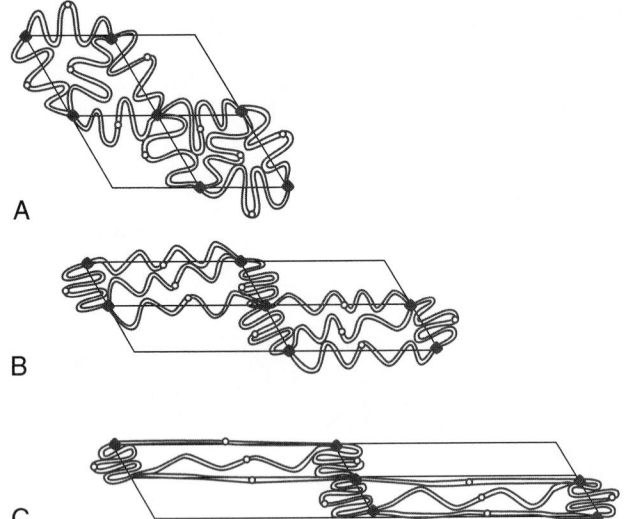

A

B

C

FIGURE 15-25. Model of the effects of deformation on the membrane skeleton. The red cell membrane cannot expand its area. When force applied to a section of nondeformed membrane (**A**) extends the lipid bilayer and its attached spectrin molecules (**B**), the bilayer and spectrin molecules in the nonstressed dimension must shrink to maintain a constant area. Eventually, spectrins reach the limit of their length (**C**). Further extension will disrupt membrane-skeleton inter-connections and lead to membrane fragmentation. *Open circles*, sites of spectrin-spectrin association; *solid diamonds*, spectrin-actin-4.1 junctions. *(Redrawn from Mohandas N, Chasis JA. Red cell deformability, membrane material properties, and shape: regulation by transmembrane, skeletal, and cytosolic proteins and lipids. Semin Hematol. 1993;30:171.)*

and is facilitated by rapid translocation of cholesterol from the inner to the outer half of the bilayer.[752] The lipid bilayer cannot expand its surface area more than 3% to 4%. Consequently, when red cells are suspended in hypotonic solutions, such as during OF testing, they swell to a spherical shape and then rupture and discharge their hemoglobin into the supernatant.[753]

The membrane skeleton determines both the solid and the semisolid properties of the membrane.[754] The solid properties are exemplified by an elastic extension of cells that completely restore their normal shape after the applied force has been removed. An example is a cell that has been deformed when passing through fenestrations of the splenic sinus wall. This elastic recovery of the biconcave shape is facilitated by the unique molecular anatomy of the skeletal lattice. In normal red cells, individual spectrin molecules are arranged in a hexagonal array and are folded in a compact configuration. The junctional complexes are close to each other and are linked by shortened spectrin tetramers, thus allowing large unidirectional extensions without disruption of the lattice (Fig. 15-25). The skeletal connections are unperturbed during such deformations. On the other hand, application of large or prolonged force allows the skeletal elements to reorganize and make new connections. This produces a permanent "plastic" deformation (see later). When the force is excessive, membrane fragmentation ensues. An example is the poikilocytosis produced in microangiopathic blood vessels, where red cells may

adhere to damaged endothelium and be stretched by the vascular torrent or may be clotheslined by fibrin strands.[755] After release, many of the cells are either permanently deformed or fragmented.

Cellular and Molecular Determinants of Red Cell Deformability

The need to undergo large deformations is best exemplified in the wall of the splenic sinus, where red cells have to "squeeze" through narrow slits between the endothelial cells that line the splenic sinus wall (see the later section on splenic structure). Such whole-cell deformability is determined by three factors: (1) cell geometry, specifically, a large cell surface-to-volume ratio, which allows cells to undergo large deformations at a constant volume; (2) viscosity of the cell contents, which is principally determined by the properties and concentration of hemoglobin in the cells; and (3) intrinsic viscoelastic properties of the red cell membrane.[754] Among these factors, the contribution of the surface-to-volume ratio is the most important, as exemplified by the cellular lesion of hereditary spherocytes, discussed later in this chapter. On the other hand, the intrinsic deformability of the red cell membrane has a relatively small effect on red cell survival. This is best illustrated by the red cell membrane properties of Southeast Asian ovalocytes, which carry a mutant band 3 protein. As will be discussed, both the intact Southeast Asian ovalocytosis (SAO) red cells and their membranes are extremely rigid, yet the SAO red cells have normal or nearly normal survival in vivo.

Several molecular alterations increase membrane rigidity. One is accretion of denatured hemoglobin, which may contribute to the membrane rigidity of Heinz body–containing red cells.[756] Another is transamidative or oxidative cross-linking, which rigidifies the membrane in vitro.[757] Oxidative cross-linking may also be important in vivo, as evidenced by aggregates of oxidant–cross-linked proteins in red cells containing unstable hemoglobins.[758] On the other hand, transamidative cross-linking is probably not physiologically significant because the high Ca[2+] concentrations needed for the reaction are unlikely to be attained in vivo.

Integral proteins may also regulate membrane deformability. For example, treatment of red cells by antibodies against GPA, including their Fab fragments, leads to reduced deformability via transmembrane signaling. Red cells that lack the cytoplasmic domain of GPA (e.g., Miltenberger V red cells) are not influenced by such treatment.[256,759] Another important factor is the aggregation state of band 3. Membrane rigidity is increased when band 3 molecules are cross-linked with antibodies or, as in SAO (see later), when mutant band 3s spontaneously stack into linear aggregates.[760,761] This finding presumably also explains the marked restriction of band 3 mobility in SAO red cells. Because aggregates of SAO band 3 contain ankyrin, which attaches the skeleton to the membrane, the decreased mobility of SAO band 3 may impede skeletal deformation when red cells deform and thereby result in a rigid erythrocyte.

Membrane Structural Integrity and Fragmentation. The skeleton is also the principal determinant of membrane stability. As noted earlier, it is possible to manipulate the proportion of spectrin dimers and tetramers in situ by exposing ghosts to temperatures and salt concentrations that favor or discourage spectrin self-association. Ghosts enriched in spectrin dimers are strikingly fragile.[455] Similarly, HE and HPP are often due to α- or β-spectrin mutations that weaken spectrin self-association (see later). In such cells the hexagonal skeletal lattice is dis-

rupted,[762] usually in association with red cell fragmentation and poikilocytosis.

Lipid Bilayer Loss and Microvesiculation. The fluid lipid bilayer is stabilized by both the underlying membrane skeleton and transmembrane proteins. In vitro, the bilayer can be uncoupled from the skeleton at the tips of spiculated red cells by force or by various treatments (Fig. 15-26).[763,764] The lipids are released in the form of microvesicles that contain integral proteins but lack skeletal components.[764] Such loss of membrane material may underlie the surface area deficiency of red cells subjected to prolonged storage[765,766] or ATP-depleted red cells.[767] Aggregation of the band 3–containing intramembrane particles in the membrane also destabilizes the lipid bilayer.[768] The particle-free regions bleb and release lipid microvesicles. As discussed later, all these pathways may contribute to the surface deficiency of hereditary spherocytes.

Plastic Deformation of Red Cells. The role of the membrane skeleton in red cell shape is best illustrated by irreversibly sickled cells or hereditary elliptocytes, in which the abnormal shape is retained in the ghosts and membrane skeletons.[769,770] This process is probably an example of "plastic deformation," the result of prolonged exposure of red cells to deforming forces, with the proteins of the deformed skeleton undergoing active rearrangement that permanently stabilizes the cells in the deformed shape (Fig. 15-27).[754] Existing protein-protein contacts disconnect and new associations form. In HE, shape transformations may be facilitated by the weakened skeletal protein interactions. In vitro, plastic deformation occurs more rapidly in normal red cells with skeletons weakened by exposure to urea.[771]

In addition, both normal and abnormal red cell shapes can be stabilized by intermolecular cross-linking

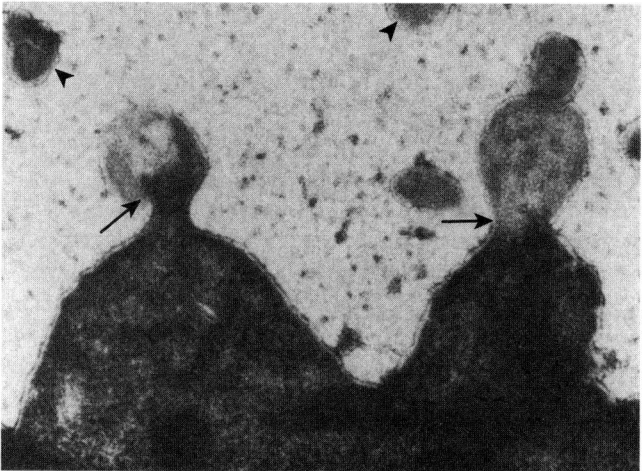

FIGURE 15-26. Microvesiculation. Red cell ghosts treated with hypertonic saline form spicules. At the end of the spicules the lipid bilayer often separates from the underlying membrane skeleton. The *arrows* point to the boundary between the skeleton (dark material below) and the unsupported lipids (light material above), which are unstable and tend to be released as vesicles (*arrowheads*). A similar process is thought to occur in a variety of disorders associated with spiculation, such as spur cell anemia and hereditary spherocytosis.

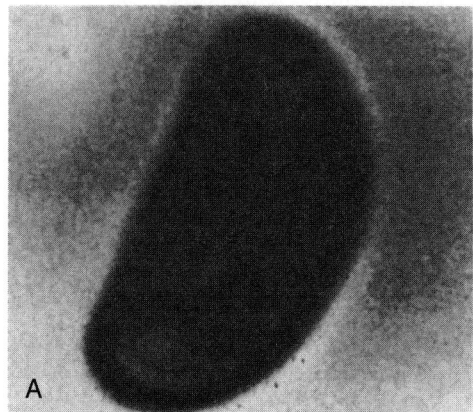
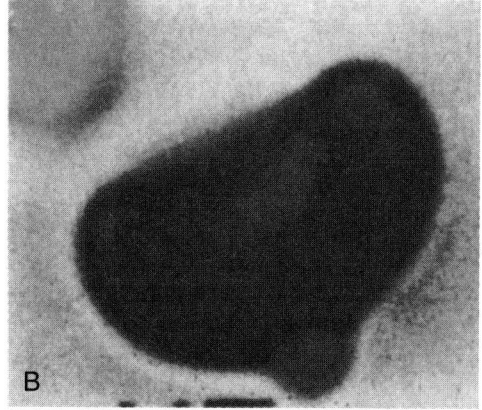

FIGURE 15-27. Plastic deformation. **A,** Discocytic shape of a red cell at rest in solution. If a nipple of membrane from such a cell is aspirated into a micropipette and released immediately, it snaps back to its original position. However, if the aspirated membrane is deformed for some time, a permanent nipple forms (**B**) as a result of reorganization of the membrane skeleton in the stressed portion of the membrane. This semisolid behavior is called "plastic deformation" and is believed to be responsible for the irregular shape of poikilocytes, especially in diseases such as hereditary pyropoikilocytosis, where skeletal reorganization is fostered by genetically weakened skeletal interconnections. *(From Mohandas N, Chasis JA. Red cell deformability, membrane material properties, and shape: regulation by transmembrane, skeletal, and cytosolic proteins and lipids. Semin Hematol. 1993;30:171-192.)*

of membrane proteins, either as a result of the formation of intermolecular disulfide bridges induced by oxidants or as a result of transamidative protein cross-linking catalyzed by a Ca^{2+}-activated cytosolic transglutaminase.[757] These protein modifications are like endogenous fixatives and permanently stabilize cell shape in vitro.

The Red Cell Surface

The red cell surface is rich in sialic acid residues, which accounts for its negative surface charge. Ninety percent of these residues reside on glycophorin A; the remainder are shared by other glycophorins, the anion exchange protein and other integral proteins, and glycolipids. Alterations in surface charge distribution are deleterious. For example, surface charge clustering may contribute to adhesion of sickle red cells to the surface of endothelial cells.[772] Several proteins are removed from the surface of reticulocytes that participate in cell-cell and cell-matrix interactions during erythroid differentiation.[746,773] One example, $\alpha_4\beta_1$ integrin, interacts with vascular cell adhesion molecule 1 (VCAM-1), an endothelial cell adhesion molecule, and may contribute to attachment of sickle cells to the endothelium.[773]

The structure and genetic origins of red cell surface antigens residing either on glycolipids, on externally exposed portions of transmembrane proteins or their carbohydrate side chains, or on the proteins linked via a GPI anchor are discussed in Chapter 35. Furthermore, as discussed earlier, several surface receptors are involved in attachment of malarial parasites to the cells, including glycophorins, band 3 protein, and the Duffy blood group antigen.

Glycosylphosphatidylinositol-Anchored Surface Proteins. To connect externally exposed hydrophilic proteins with the hydrophobic lipid bilayer, Nature has devised a hydrophobic GPI anchor that is embedded in the outer leaflet of the bilayer. Among the large number of GPI-linked surface proteins, a group of complement regulatory proteins are clinically the most important.[774] Defective biosynthesis of the GPI anchor precludes attachment of these proteins to the membrane and causes increased susceptibility to hemolysis by complement, as clinically manifested by paroxysmal nocturnal hemoglobinuria (see Chapter 14). Because this glycolipid anchor is embedded only in the outer leaflet of the bilayer, GPI-anchored surface proteins, such as CD59, are not restricted by the membrane skeleton, in contrast to most transmembrane proteins, and are much more laterally mobile.[774,775] This high mobility may be important in recruiting complement regulatory proteins to sites of complement activation. These regulatory proteins are preferentially enriched in lipid rafts and in the lipid vesicles that are released from abnormal red cells,[776] such as vesicles derived from spicules of deoxygenated sickle cells. Consequently, GPI-linked proteins are diminished in the densest fraction of sickle cells, thus rendering them more susceptible to complement-mediated injury.[776]

Lateral Mobility of Transmembrane and Surface Proteins. The mobility of membrane surface molecules influences the interaction of red cells with the outside environment. For example, cell agglutination requires rapid lateral movement of surface antigens. Their immobilization (e.g., by glutaraldehyde) inhibits agglutination.[777]

The lateral mobility of proteins that are anchored exclusively in the outer leaflet of the bilayer (e.g., GPI-linked proteins) is very fast. Conversely, transmembrane proteins, such as band 3, are much less mobile. In the case of band 3, the limited mobility occurs because of (1) specific binding to ankyrin and the skeleton; (2) steric hindrance by spectrin strands, which entangle the internal portions of band 3; (3) self-association of band 3 into tetramers and higher oligomers; and (4) interaction of band 3 with other transmembrane proteins, such as the glycophorins and Rh/RhAG complex.[778]

MEMBRANE PERMEABILITY

Normally, the red cell membrane is nearly impermeable to monovalent and divalent cations, thereby maintaining a high potassium, low sodium, and very low calcium content. In contrast, the red cell is highly permeable to water and anions, which are readily exchanged by the water channel and the anion transport protein, respectively. Glucose is taken up by the glucose transporter,[779] whereas larger charged molecules, such as ATP and related compounds, do not cross the normal red cell membrane.

The transport pathways for cations and anions in the human red cell membrane can be divided into five categories (Fig. 15-28):

- Exchangers, such as the Na^+-H^+ exchanger and anion exchanger discussed earlier
- Cotransporters, in which the transmembrane movements of more than one solute are coupled in the same direction (e.g., the K^+-Cl^- cotransporter and the Na^+-K^+-$2Cl^-$ cotransporter)
- The Ca^{2+}-activated K^+ channel (Gárdos channel), discussed later
- The cation "leak" pathways, which allow Na^+ and K^+ to move in the direction of their concentration gradients
- Membrane pumps, such as the ouabain-inhibitable Na^+,K^+ pump and the Ca^{2+} pump

A detailed review of these pathways is beyond the scope of this chapter. Interested readers are referred to several excellent recent reviews that discuss them in the pathophysiology of sickle cell disease.[780,781]

An important feature of a normal red cell is its ability to maintain a constant volume. One of the very intriguing, yet unanswered questions is how cells "sense" changes in cell volume and activate appropriate volume regulatory pathways. One possibility is that they sense mechanical events, such as membrane stretching.[782] Such a mecha-

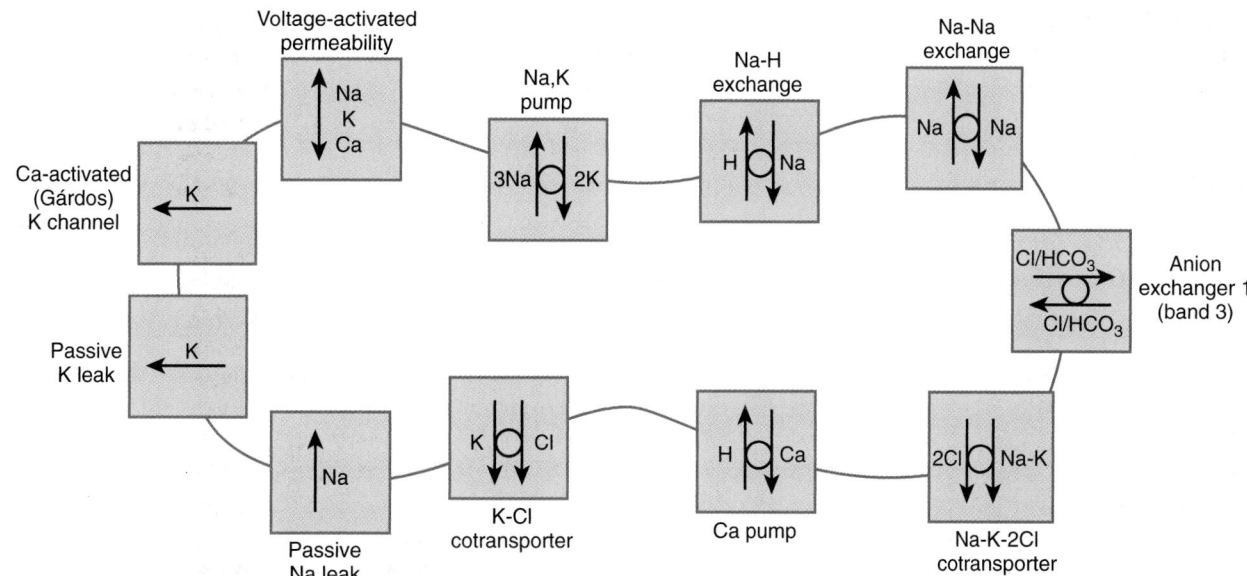

FIGURE 15-28. Red cell membrane ion transport channels, ion exchange channels, and passive permeability pathways. *(Redrawn from Walensky LD, Narla M, Lux SE. Disorders of the red cell membrane. In Handin RI, Lux SE, Stossel TP [eds]. Blood: Principles and Practice of Hematology, 2nd ed. Philadelphia, JB Lippincott, 2003, pp 1709-1858, with permission.)*

nism is unlikely to operate in red cells, which by virtue of their large surface area, can undergo a substantial increase in volume without stretching. Another possibility is that cell volume is controlled by the crowding of cytoplasmic macromolecules.[782]

Water Permeability

The water permeability of many cell types is similar to the permeability of pure lipid bilayer membranes, in which water is postulated to enter through small "cavities" in the bilayer.[783] When phospholipids are in the liquid crystalline state, these cavities are thought to be caused by noncooperative rotation and kinking around the C-C bonds.[783] In addition, water permeability may be facilitated by lipids with large polar head groups, such as gangliosides and lysophospholipids, which when dispersed in water, prefer a micellar rather than a bilayer configuration. Additionally, integral proteins are likely to enhance water diffusion by producing localized discontinuities in the lipid bilayer.[783]

The membranes of red cells and some kidney tubules differ from the membranes of most other cells in that they have high water permeability that is endowed by a molecular water channel called AQP1, which has been cloned[380] and had its structure solved[381] (see the earlier section on aquaporin). AQP1 facilitates rehydration of red cells after their shrinkage in the hypertonic environment of the renal medulla.[784]

Transport Pathways Leading to Cellular Dehydration

Two pathways exert a critical volume regulatory effect that can lead to red cell dehydration and destruction

(Fig. 15-29). One is the K^+-Cl^- cotransporter, a typical carrier-mediated cotransport pathway that is particularly active in reticulocytes. It is activated by cell swelling, acidification, depletion of intracellular Mg^{2+}, and thiol oxidation. It is increased in sickle red cells and hemoglobin C erythrocytes, which accounts, in part, for the cellular dehydration of these cells.[785,786]

The second transporter is the Gárdos channel, which causes selective loss of K^+ in response to an increase in intracellular ionized calcium.[735] This channel appears to be regulated by a cytoplasmic protein called calpromotin or peroxiredoxin-2 and by cAMP. The channel is inhibited by insect toxins such as charybdotoxin and by the Ca^{2+} channel blockers nitrendipine and nifedipine. In sickle cells, the combination of the Gárdos pathway and the K^+-Cl^- cotransporter accounts for the net loss of K^+ and water and the subsequent cellular dehydration.[786]

Disruption of the Permeability Barrier in Abnormal Red Cells

The effects of breaching the red cell permeability barrier are well illustrated by complement hemolysis. Activation of complement on the red cell surface leads to formation of the membrane attack complex, which is composed of the terminal complement components embedded in the lipid bilayer. This multimolecular complex acts as a cation channel and allows passive movement of sodium, potassium, and calcium across the membrane according to their concentration gradients. Attracted by fixed anions such as hemoglobin, ATP, and 2,3-DPG, sodium accumulates in the cells in excess of potassium loss and in excess of the compensatory efforts of the Na^+,K^+ pump (see later). The resulting increase in intracellular monovalent cations and water is followed by cell swelling

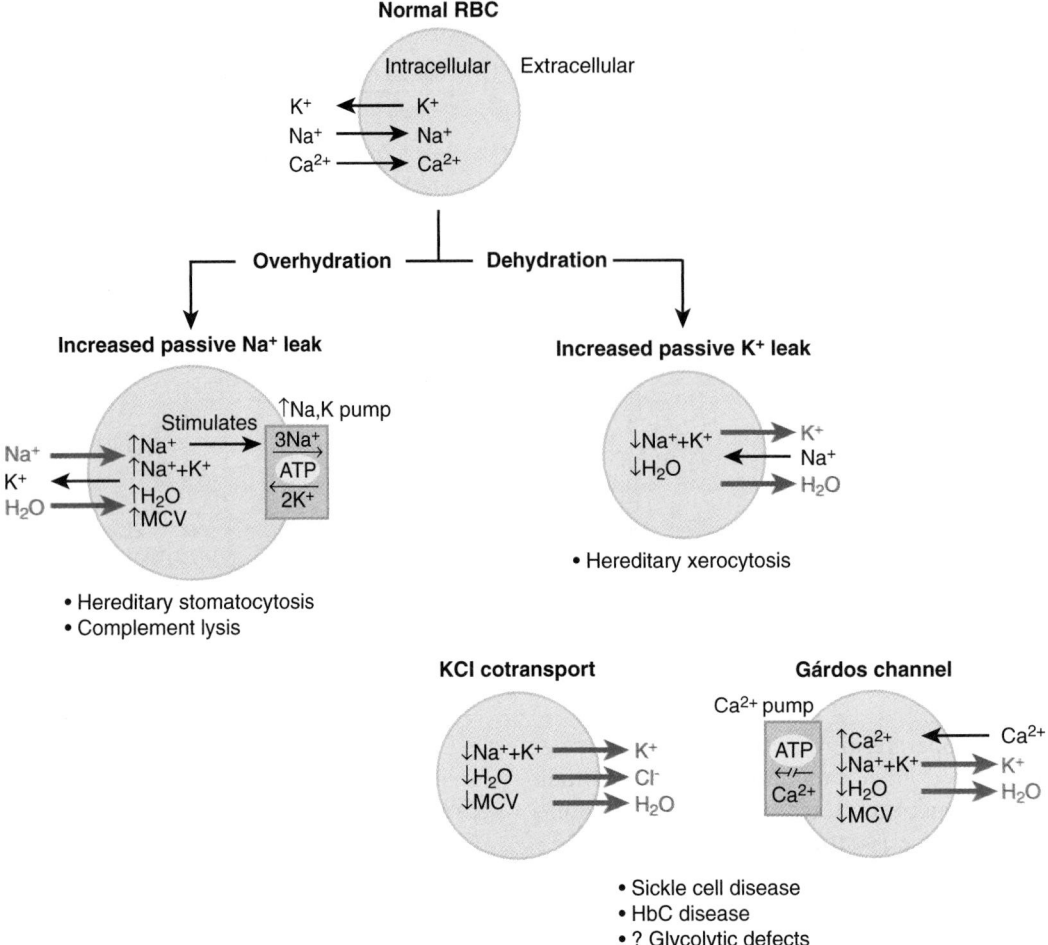

FIGURE 15-29. Cation changes leading to dehydration or overhydration of red cells. *Left*, Overhydration is caused by a massive, unbalanced influx of Na$^+$ that overwhelms the Na$^+$,K$^+$ pump and leads to an increase in total monovalent cations (Na$^+$ + K$^+$) and cell water. *Right*, Dehydration is caused by excess, unbalanced K$^+$ leakage or by activation of K$^+$-losing channels such as the K$^+$-Cl$^-$ cotransport channel or the Ca^{2+}-activated Gárdos pathway. Dehydration is associated with a decline in total monovalent cations (Na$^+$ + K$^+$) and cell water. *(Redrawn from Walensky LD, Narla M, Lux SE. Disorders of the red cell membrane. In Handin RI, Lux SE, Stossel TP [eds]. Blood: Principles and Practice of Hematology, 2nd ed. Philadelphia, JB Lippincott, 2003, pp 1709-1858, with permission.)*

(see Fig. 15-29) and ultimately by colloid osmotic hemolysis.

Another leak pathway has been described in sickle cells. It involves an influx of Na$^+$ and Ca^{2+} and an efflux of K$^+$ during deoxygenation and sickling.[785,786] Although the molecular basis of this diffusional pathway is unknown, the magnitude of the Na$^+$ and K$^+$ leaks correlates with the degree of morphologic sickling and with lipid bilayer–skeleton uncoupling, thus suggesting that it is caused by mechanical events.[786] This conclusion is further supported by the observation that Ca^{2+} permeability is increased by mechanical stress.[787] The mechanism of activation of these channels is unknown, but one of the possibilities involves deformation of the submembrane skeleton.

Membrane Pumps

To maintain low intracellular concentrations of sodium and calcium and a high potassium concentration, the membrane is endowed with two cation pumps, both of which use intracellular ATP as an energy source. The ouabain-inhibitable Na$^+$,K$^+$ pump, extrudes sodium and takes up potassium, with a stoichiometry of 3Na$^+$ pumped outward for 2K$^+$ pumped inward. This exactly balances the normal passive leaks (Na$^+$ influx = 1.0 to 2.0 mEq/L RBCs/hr; K$^+$ efflux = 0.8 to 1.5 mEq/L RBCs/hr). The enzyme is activated by intracellular Na$^+$ (K_m = 25 mM) and extracellular K$^+$ (K_m = 2.5 mM).[788] Because plasma K$^+$ is high enough to saturate the extracellular K$^+$ site, Na$^+$ and K$^+$ transport is primarily regulated by increases in red cell Na$^+$ concentration, and cell K$^+$ losses are rectified only if there is a concomitant Na$^+$ gain to stimulate active transport. Even then the ratio between the inward Na$^+$ leak and the outward K$^+$ leak must not be less than the physiologic ratio of 3:2. At lower ratios, the Na$^+$,K$^+$ pump, driven by the Na$^+$ leak and internal Na$^+$ concentration, will not balance the leaks and will actually exacerbate K$^+$ loss.[789,790] Consequently, conditions in which K$^+$ loss approaches or exceeds Na$^+$ gain lead to irreversible depletion of K$^+$ and cell dehydration.

The calmodulin-activated, Mg^{2+}-dependent Ca^{2+} pump extrudes Ca^{2+} and maintains a very low intracellular free Ca^{2+} concentration (~20 to 40 nM). It protects red cells from the multiple deleterious effects of Ca^{2+} (echinocytosis, membrane vesiculation, calpain activation, membrane proteolysis, and cell dehydration) described earlier in the chapter.

RED CELL MEMBRANE ALTERATIONS OF SENESCENT RED CELLS

Pleiotropic Effects of Red Cell Aging

Removal of senescent red cells from the circulation is a subject of long-standing interest. As discussed in a comprehensive review of the literature published before 1988,[791] the concept of red cell senescence is based on the results of radioactive labeling of a cohort of reticulocytes and bone marrow erythroblasts. In many species, including humans, the fraction of labeled cells remains constant for a defined period, followed by a rapid decline of radioactivity, thus suggesting that the red cells are removed from the circulation in an age-dependent manner. Many techniques have been used to isolate senescent red cells, including methods based on differences in cell density, osmotic fragility, and cell size (reviewed by Clark[791]). Density separation is most widely used, but the results obtained by this technique must be interpreted with caution. Although red cells exhibit a progressive increase in density as they age in vivo, not all dense red cells are senescent.[791-793]

In addition to in vitro separation techniques, various in vivo animal models have been used to study red cell aging.[791] For example, red cells can be labeled with biotin and then removed at defined times with avidin, which complexes tightly to biotin.[794] The senescent cells defined by these techniques exhibit numerous membrane abnormalities.[791,792,794] Of particular note is the loss of potassium and water, which leads to cell dehydration and increased cell density, and the loss of surface area, presumably caused by gradual release of membrane microvesicles.[791,795] The latter phenomenon is probably caused by constant exposure of red cells to the shearing forces of the microcirculation. In addition, membrane proteins and lipids in old red cells are oxidized, as evidenced by high-molecular-weight aggregates containing hemoglobin, spectrin, and band 3[796] and by adducts of proteins and malonylaldehyde, a product of lipid peroxidation.

In addition to red cell membrane abnormalities, red cell aging is associated with a decline in many red cell enzyme activities.[797] However, the red cell ATP concentration is normal.[791] Likewise, no major abnormalities have been detected in Ca^{2+} transport, and there is no compelling evidence that Ca^{2+} accumulates in senescent cells (reviewed by Clark[791]).

An Autologous Autoantibody Targets Senescent Red Cells for Destruction by Macrophages

Although some of the previously discussed alterations may compromise red cell microcirculatory flow, none is likely to destroy old cells. Kay first showed that senescent red cells have small amounts (a few hundred molecules per cell) of autologous IgG on their surface that target the cells for destruction by macrophages.[798] Recent studies suggest that the senescent autoantibody arises from a distinctive subset of B cells, termed B-1, that express CD5.[799] The nature of the "senescent cell antigen" has been a source of some dispute, but it appears to be aggregated and modified band 3 molecules.[794,800-806] There is some evidence that the epitope resides on the band 3 carbohydrate.[807,808] Band 3 clusters have been visualized by immunofluorescence microscopy and detected by biochemical methods in aged red cells.[801,804] Aggregation probably results from cumulative oxidative damage because similar damage, including the binding of autologous IgG, takes place on oxidized red cells or red cells containing Heinz bodies, a product of oxidative denaturation of hemoglobin.[68,801,804,809,810] The senescent cell antigen is also exposed on red cells infected with *P. falciparum*.[811,812]

It should be noted, however, that intramembrane particles, which are mostly band 3, are not reproducibly clustered in cells that bear senescent IgG.[813] This suggests either that the clustered band 3 molecules are rare enough or in small enough clusters that they were missed by electron microscopy or that other band 3 modifications account for increased binding of autologous IgG. For example, band 3 could be structurally modified by proteolysis or oxidation or by other post-translational modification, or band 3 molecules could be vertically displaced, with new antigenic sites exposed or existing sites rendered more accessible to antibodies.

In addition to targeting senescent red cells for macrophage destruction, band 3 antibodies also trigger deposition of complement on senescent cells,[810,814] which would aid cell removal through CR1 receptors on phagocytes. As noted earlier, this process may be facilitated by loss of GPI-linked complement regulatory proteins such as CD55 and CD59 in exosomes and by microvesiculation as red cells age.

Gradual loss of CD47 may also be important. CD47 molecules are recognized by an inhibitory receptor, signal regulation protein-α, on macrophages.[815] This receptor sends a negative signal that can block the phagocytic response. Old red cells have about 30% less CD47 than young red cells do. Depletion of macrophages in mice results in a decrease in the amount of CD47 on red cells and accumulation of senescent red cells.[815]

Although the role of autologous IgG in the destruction of senescent erythrocytes is widely accepted, two observations suggest that other mechanisms must be considered. First, blockade of the Fc portion of autologous "senescent" IgG with protein G fails to inhibit red cell phagocytosis.[816] Second, red cell survival is the same in agammaglobulinemic mice as in controls.[816] However, the latter data may not be applicable to humans because removal of mouse red cells from the circulation is random.[791]

Red cells uniquely express the LW blood group antigen, renamed ICAM-4 (or CD242), which interacts with various β_2 integrins, including CD11c/CD18, on macrophages. Antibodies to either component inhibit erythrophagocytosis and removal of senescent red cells, which suggests that this interaction contributes to the process.[817,818]

Altered phospholipid asymmetry might also contribute to removal of senescent erythrocytes. This could occur from damage to the aminophospholipid translocase by products of lipid peroxidation.[819] Disordered phospholipid asymmetry leads to removal of cells by macrophages as discussed earlier (see "Loss of Phospholipid Asymmetry"). Although there is no convincing evidence that senescent red cells expose PS on their surface, this hypothesis is favored by some,[820] presumably because it is a proven mechanism for removing other types of damaged cells.

Other alterations of possible pathologic significance include postsynthetic modification of red cell proteins by nonenzymatic glycosylation[821] or carboxymethylation.[822,823] Glycosylation of membrane proteins, such as hemoglobin (to form hemoglobin A_{1c}), occurs gradually over the life of the cell and is proportional to the glucose concentration. Methylation of membrane proteins occurs primarily in older red cells. Ankyrin and protein 4.1 are the principal substrates.

Transamidation of membrane proteins may also play a role in aging. Aged red cells from mice lacking transglutaminase-2 are more osmotically resistant than aged normal red cells,[824] thus suggesting that the knockout red cells lose less membrane surface as they age. Transglutaminase-2 catalyzes the formation of peptide bonds between ε-amino groups on lysine side chains and side-chain carboxyls on aspartic and glutamic acids in the presence of Ca^{2+}.

HEREDITARY SPHEROCYTOSIS

HS (Box 15-1) is a common inherited hemolytic anemia in which defects of spectrin or proteins that participate in the attachment of spectrin to the membrane, ankyrin, protein 4.2, or band 3 lead to spheroidal, osmotically fragile cells that are selectively trapped in the spleen, thereby resulting in a shortened red cell life span.

History

HS was first recognized about 140 years ago by two Belgian physicians, Vanlair and Masius,[825] who gave a remarkably thorough account of the disease. They

Box 15-1	Diseases in Which Spherocytosis is the Predominant Morphology

COMMON

Hereditary spherocytosis
Immunohemolytic anemias (warm-antibody type)
ABO incompatibility in neonates

UNCOMMON TO RARE

Clostridial sepsis
Hemolytic transfusion reactions
Severe burns and other red cell thermal injuries
Spider, bee, and snake venom
Severe hypophosphatemia
Acute red cell oxidant injury (glucose-6-phosphate dehydrogenase deficiency during hemolytic crisis)

described a woman who suffered from the clinical symptoms now known as the hallmarks of HS—anemia, jaundice, splenomegaly, and recurrent abdominal pain. The authors noted that most of the woman's red cells were spherical and hypothesized that a combination of splenic enlargement and liver atrophy led to their rapid destruction and the patient's anemia. They also noted that the patient's sister had suffered from an identical illness. In the 1890s, the British physicians Wilson and Stanley recognized the hereditary nature of the disease and were the first to identify the characteristic pathologic appearance of the spleen engorged with red cells.[826,827] Subsequently, a report by Minkowski in 1900 in the German literature[828] received wide attention, and many additional papers soon appeared, including Chauffard's classic description of osmotic fragility[829] and reticulocytosis[830] as hallmark laboratory features of the disease. The first successful splenectomy for HS was unintentionally performed by Wells in England 20 years before splenectomy became widely accepted[831] and 3 years before Wilson's description of HS. While operating on a jaundiced woman for a supposed uterine fibroid, Wells encountered and removed an enormous spleen. The patient recovered and her jaundice disappeared. Forty years after Wells' splenectomy, Dawson[831] found abnormal erythrocyte osmotic fragility (OF) during an examination of the woman and her son. Thus, the major clinical features of HS were defined by the 1920s, although nothing was known about the pathophysiology of the disease. Readers interested in more details about these and other aspects of the history of HS should consult the chapters by Dacie, Crosby, and Wintrobe in *Blood, Pure and Eloquent.*[832]

Prevalence and Genetics

HS occurs in all racial and ethnic groups. It is particularly common in northern Europeans, in whom approximately 1 in 5000 persons is affected.[833] This is probably an underestimate inasmuch as surveys of red cell OF suggest that mild forms of the disease may be four or five times more common than believed.[834-836] There are no good estimates of the prevalence in other populations, but clinical experience suggests that it is less common in African Americans and Southeast Asians.

HS exhibits both dominant and nondominant phenotypes. About 75% of patients have typical autosomal dominant disease,[833,837,838] with the remaining 25% exhibiting nondominant inheritance.[839-845] Homozygotes for dominant HS are rare, occurring at an estimated frequency of once in 100 million births, with only two reported cases in the literature.[838,846] In about half of the patients with nondominant disease, HS is due to de novo autosomal dominant mutations, which tend to occur at CpG dinucleotides and are associated with small insertions or deletions.[839,840] In the remaining patients with nondominant inheritance, both parents are clinically normal but may exhibit subtle laboratory abnormalities that suggest a carrier state.[837,840,845] These patients probably have an autosomal recessive form of the disease, although it is not always possible to exclude dominant HS with reduced penetrance or dominant HS caused by a new mutation.[837]

HS is caused by unique familial mutations in different chromosomes at loci involving the membrane skeletal proteins. The mutations that cause HS are consistent within families but vary between almost every family. The first two genetic loci for HS that were described were a deletion of chromosome 8p11.1-p21.2, which eliminated the gene for ankyrin,[847,848] and a deletion of chromosome 14q23-q24.2, which eliminated the gene for β-spectrin.[849] Other loci have since been described in the genes for α-spectrin, band 3, and protein 4.2. Because most mutations are unique within each family, it is rarely clinically useful to determine the specific molecular defect in patients with HS. Readers who are interested in tables listing each mutation reported to cause HS should consult a related chapter by one of the authors (S.E.L).[850]

Clinical Features

Silent Carrier State

The parents of patients with "nondominant" HS are clinically asymptomatic and do not have anemia, splenomegaly, hyperbilirubinemia, or spherocytosis on peripheral blood smears.[845] However, most do have subtle laboratory signs of HS, including slight reticulocytosis (average, 2.1% ± 0.8%), diminished haptoglobin levels, slightly elevated OF, or slightly shortened times in the acidified glycerol lysis test (AGLT). The incubated OF test is probably the most sensitive measure of this condition, particularly the 100% lysis point, which is significantly elevated in carriers (0.43 ± 0.05 g NaCl/dL) in comparison to normal subjects (0.23 ± 0.07 g NaCl/dL).[837] However, no single test is sufficient. Carriers can be detected reliably only by considering the results of a battery of tests. From the incidence of autosomal recessive HS (1 in 40,000; that is, ≈12.5% of all occurrences of HS, the frequency of which is 1 in 5000 in the United States),[833] one can estimate that roughly 1% of

the population should be silent carriers. Interestingly, screening of normal Norwegian[836] or German[837] blood donors with an OF test or AGLT shows a 0.9% to 1.1% incidence of previously unsuspected "very mild" HS. Presumably, most of these individuals are silent carriers.

Typical Hereditary Spherocytosis

The typical clinical picture of HS combines evidence of hemolysis (anemia, jaundice, reticulocytosis, gallstones,

---

Box 15-2 | Characteristics of Hereditary Spherocytosis

CLINICAL MANIFESTATIONS

Anemia
Splenomegaly
Intermittent jaundice
  From hemolysis
  From biliary obstruction
Aplastic crises
Inheritance
  Dominant ≈75%
  Nondominant ≈25%
Rare manifestations
  Leg ulcers
  Extramedullary hematopoietic tumors
  Spinocerebellar ataxia
  Myocardiopathy
Excellent response to splenectomy

LABORATORY FEATURES

Reticulocytosis
Spherocytosis
Elevated mean corpuscular hemoglobin content
Increased osmotic fragility (especially the incubated osmotic fragility test)
Normal Coombs test
Decreased red cell spectrin, spectrin and ankyrin, band 3, or protein 4.2

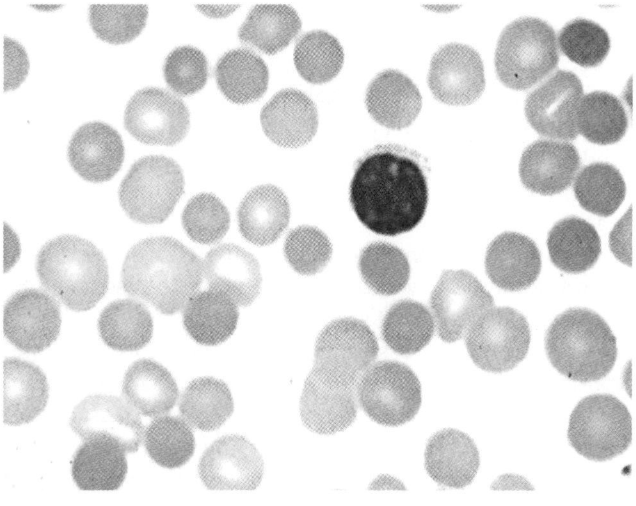

FIGURE 15-30. Peripheral blood smear from a patient with typical hereditary spherocytosis. Small, dense round microspherocytes are scattered throughout the smear.

TABLE 15-4   Clinical Classification of Hereditary Spherocytosis

	Trait	Mild Spherocytosis	Moderate Spherocytosis	Moderately Severe* Spherocytosis	Severe*,† Spherocytosis
Hemoglobin (g/dL)	Normal	11-15	8-12	6-8	<6
Reticulocytes (%)	1-3	3-8	≥8	≥10	≥10
Bilirubin (mg/dL)	0-1	1-2	≥2	2-3	≥3
Spectrin content (% of normal)‡	100	80-100	50-80	40-80	20-50
Peripheral smear	Normal	Mild spherocytosis	Spherocytosis	Spherocytosis	Spherocytosis and poikilocytosis
Osmotic fragility					
Fresh blood	Normal	Normal or slightly increased	Distinctly increased	Distinctly increased	Distinctly increased
Incubated blood	Slightly increased	Distinctly increased	Distinctly increased	Distinctly increased	Markedly increased

*Values in untransfused patients.

†By definition, patients with severe spherocytosis are transfusion dependent.

‡Spectrin content is relevant only for patients with spectrin or ankyrin defects. Patients with hereditary spherocytosis who lack band 3 or protein 4.2 have mild to moderate spherocytosis with normal or nearly normal amounts of spectrin and ankyrin. Normal spectrin content is 245 ± 27 (SD) × 10⁵ spectrin dimers per erythrocyte.

Adapted from Eber SW, Armbrust R, Schröter W. Variable clinical severity of hereditary spherocytosis: relation to erythrocytic spectrin concentration, osmotic fragility and autohemolysis. J Pediatr. 1990;177:409.

and splenomegaly) with spherocytosis (spherocytes on a peripheral blood smear and positive OF test or AGLT results) and a positive family history (Box 15-2; Fig. 15-30). Mild, moderate, and severe forms of HS have been defined according to differences in hemoglobin and bilirubin concentrations and the reticulocyte count (Table 15-4).[837,851]

HS is typically diagnosed in infancy or childhood, but it may occur at any age.[852] In children, anemia is the most common initial finding (50%), followed by splenomegaly, jaundice, or a positive family history.[853] No comparable data exist for adults. The majority of patients with HS have incompletely compensated hemolysis and mild to moderate anemia. The anemia is often asymptomatic except for fatigue and mild pallor or, in children, nonspecific parental complaints such as irritability. Jaundice is seen at some time in about half of the patients, usually in association with viral infections. When jaundice is present, it is acholuric (i.e., unconjugated [indirect] hyperbilirubinemia without detectable direct bilirubinuria). Palpable splenomegaly is detectable in about half of infants and most (75% to 95%) older children and adults.[853-855] Typically, the spleen is modestly enlarged (2 to 6 cm below the costal margin), but it may be massive.[856,857] There is no proven correlation between the size of the spleen and the severity of HS, although given the pathophysiology and response of the disease to splenectomy, such a correlation probably exists.

Typical HS is associated with both dominant and nondominant inheritance. In many patients the nondominant disease is more severe, but there is considerable overlap.[837,839,845] Clinical severity and the response to splenectomy roughly parallel the degree of spectrin (or ankyrin) deficiency in patients with defects in either protein.[837,845,851,858,859] It is not known whether analogous correlations are true for patients with other HS-related mutations.

Mild Hereditary Spherocytosis

Red cell production and destruction are balanced or nearly balanced in 20% to 30% of patients with HS.[854,860] These persons are considered to have "compensated hemolysis" and are usually asymptomatic. In some patients, diagnosis may be difficult because the hemolysis, splenomegaly, and spherocytosis are unusually mild. In this group of patients, reticulocyte counts are generally less than 6%, and only 60% of patients have significant spherocytosis on peripheral blood smears.[837] In addition, red cell spectrin and ankyrin levels are typically greater than 80% of normal.[837]

Hemolysis may become severe with illnesses that cause splenomegaly, such as infectious mononucleosis.[861] Hemolysis may also be exacerbated by pregnancy[862,863] or exercise,[863] to the point where it may impair athletic performance in endurance sports. In many of these patients, HS is diagnosed during family studies or discovered when splenomegaly or gallstones are diagnosed in adult patients. Although mild HS is usually familial, it develops sporadically in families with more severe disease.[864] Presumably, this is due to the coinheritance of modifying genes, such as those affecting spectrin or ankyrin synthesis or splenic function.

It is unclear why patients with HS and compensated hemolysis, with normal hemoglobin levels, continue to have erythroid hyperplasia. It is difficult to reconcile this phenomenon with the generally accepted theory that erythropoiesis is regulated by tissue hypoxia. One possibility is that the erythroid hyperplasia is caused by the concentration of 2,3-DPG, which reportedly is low in hereditary spherocytes before splenectomy (although the

P_{50} of blood from HS patients is normal).[865,866] Another possibility is that the dehydrated HS red cells are rheologically impaired and do not perfuse the juxtaglomerular renal vessels (where erythropoietin is produced) normally, even when the hematocrit is normal. Observations that erythropoietin is inappropriately elevated (up to eight times normal) in HS patients supports this hypothesis.[867,868] However, if this hypothesis is correct, erythropoietin production should correlate inversely with red cell deformability in any disorder (e.g., sickle cell anemia, hereditary xerocytosis) regardless of the hemoglobin level.

Moderate and Severe Hereditary Spherocytosis

A small fraction of patients with HS (5% to 10%) have moderately severe to severe anemia. Patients with "moderately severe" disease typically have a hemoglobin value of 6 to 8 g/dL, a reticulocyte count of about 10%, a bilirubin level of 2 to 3 mg/dL, and 40% to 80% of the normal red cell spectrin content. This category includes patients with both dominant and recessive HS and a variety of molecular defects.

Patients with "severe" disease, by definition, have life-threatening anemia and are transfusion dependent (see Table 15-4). They almost always have recessive HS. Most of these patients probably have isolated, severe spectrin deficiency (<40% of normal), which is thought to be due to a defect in α-spectrin.[869] Some may have ankyrin defects.[870] Patients with severe HS are also distinguished by red cell morphology. They often have some irregularly contoured or budding spherocytes and bizarre poikilocytes, in addition to typical spherocytes.[870,871] Such cells are rare before splenectomy in patients with moderately severe disease, although some may be seen after splenectomy. In addition to the risks associated with recurrent transfusions, patients with "severe" disease frequently experience aplastic crises and may exhibit growth retardation, delayed sexual maturation, or aspects of thalassemic facies.[856,857,871]

Hereditary Spherocytosis in Pregnancy

In general, unsplenectomized patients with HS have no significant complications during pregnancy except for anemia, which worsens as a result of plasma volume expansion[872] and sometimes because of increased hemolysis.[862,863] Hemolytic crises during pregnancy requiring transfusion have been reported.[863] Folic acid deficiency is also a risk.[873,874] One group reported that 20% of patients with HS received transfusions during pregnancy,[863] but in our experience, pregnant patients with HS rarely need transfusions.

Hereditary Spherocytosis in Neonates

HS is often manifested as jaundice in the first few days of life.[875-877] Perhaps as many as half of all patients with HS have a history of neonatal jaundice,[878] and 91% of infants discovered to have HS in the first week of life are jaundiced (bilirubin level > 10 mg/dL).[876] In a French study population of 402 jaundiced neonates requiring phototherapy, 1% were found to have HS.[879] Hyperbilirubinemia usually appears in the first 2 days of life, and bilirubin levels may rise rapidly,[875,877,878] driven by the combination of hemolysis and the reduced capacity of the neonatal liver to conjugate bilirubin. Newborns with both HS and the trait for Gilbert's syndrome, a common polymorphism in the promoter region of the uridine diphosphate–glucuronosyltransferase gene (*UGT1A1*), often have hyperbilirubinemia.[880] Homozygosity for the Gilbert syndrome polymorphism may aggravate neonatal anemia in HS.[881] Kernicterus is a risk[875]; thus, exchange transfusions are sometimes necessary, but in most patients, the jaundice is controlled with phototherapy.

Only 43% of neonates with HS are anemic at birth (hemoglobin level < 15 g/dL), and severe anemia is rare.[876] Most patients have normal hemoglobin levels at birth, which then decrease sharply over the first 3 weeks of life and lead to a transient, severe anemia.[882] In up to three fourths of infants, the anemia is severe enough to warrant transfusion or treatment with erythropoietin (see later). This anemia appears to be aggravated by an inability of the infant's red cells to mount an appropriate erythropoietic response to anemia and to the development of splenic function. Most infants will outgrow the need for transfusion by the end of the first year of life.[882]

Hydrops fetalis has been reported in a few rare patients and is associated with homozygosity or compound heterozygosity for spectrin or band 3 defects.[841,846,883] If hydrops fetalis is detected in utero, these infants may require intrauterine transfusions. No instances of hydrops fetalis have been associated with ankyrin deficiency. It is possible that infants with ankyrin defects, similar to ankyrin-deficient *nb/nb* mice,[884,885] are partially protected in utero by the expression of ankyrin-related proteins in embryonic and fetal erythroblasts.

The diagnosis of HS is sometimes more difficult in the neonatal period than later in life. Splenomegaly is uncommon; at most the spleen tip is palpable, and reticulocytosis is variable and not usually severe.[877,878] Only 35% of affected neonates have a reticulocyte count greater than 10%.[876] In addition, the haptoglobin level is not a reliable indicator of hemolysis during the first few months of life.[886] An even greater problem is that 33% of neonates with HS do not have significant numbers of spherocytes on their peripheral blood smears.[876] Moreover, because fetal red cells are more osmotically resistant than adult cells when fresh, and more osmotically sensitive after incubation at 37° C for 24 hours,[876,887] the OF test occasionally gives false-positive (incubated) or false-negative (unincubated) results unless fetal controls are used. Fortunately, these results have been published,[876] and they appear to reliably differentiate neonates with HS, particularly when the incubated OF test is used.[876-878] However, in our experience it is rarely necessary to use fetal controls. The standard OF test suffices to make the diagnosis in conjunction with the blood smear, Coombs test, and other data. Studying erythrocytes from the parents is also very useful in the diagnosis of HS, particularly if the infant has received a transfusion.[888]

No evidence exists that patients with HS who show symptoms as neonates have a more severe form of the disease. However, some neonates with HS have trouble "getting their bone marrows started" (i.e., generating an appropriate erythropoietic response to their hemolysis) and become progressively more anemic and require transfusion. The reason for this is unknown. In our experience it is more common after an exchange transfusion, but it also occurs in untransfused infants. Fortunately, the problem is transient, except in rare patients with severe HS, and usually remits after one or two transfusions. If the child is otherwise well, we allow the hemoglobin level to fall to 5.5 to 6.5 g/dL before giving transfusions to try to stimulate the marrow and only raise the hemoglobin level to 9 to 11 g/dL after transfusion to avoid suppressing the desired marrow response. After the bone marrow responds, the course of the disease depends on the equilibrium between rates of red cell production and destruction.

Administration of recombinant human erythropoietin (rHuEPO) to infants with HS and relative erythroid hypoplasia was shown to be beneficial in reducing blood transfusions in an uncontrolled, open label study.[889] In this study, 13 of 16 infants given 1000 IU rHuEPO per kilogram by weekly subcutaneous injection had increases in their absolute reticulocyte count and hemoglobin values. The infants were given the same dose of rHuEPO weekly based on their initial weight (at a range of initial ages from 16 to 119 days), a weekly hemoglobin level of less than 8 g/dL, and an absolute reticulocyte count of 200×10^9/L or less. More recent studies have shown similar effectiveness with different doses and different frequencies.[890] Therefore, erythropoietin therapy in infants with HS has become more standard, although weekly erythropoietin injections can be challenging for parents. Nevertheless, further studies of recombinant erythropoietin therapy for neonatal anemia in HS and a poor retic response are needed to determine the optimal time to initiate treatment, the optimal dose, and the duration of therapy.

Close observation of infants with HS is necessary to avoid complications of severe anemia. All infants with HS should have hemoglobin and reticulocyte measurements every 1 to 2 months during the first 6 months of life. In the second 6 months of life, these intervals may be increased to every 2 to 3 months. In the second year of life, blood cell counts can be measured every 4 months. Infants with more severe disease must be observed carefully to avoid unnecessary side effects of severe anemia.

Etiology: Membrane Protein Defects

The primary molecular defects in HS reside in membrane skeleton proteins, particularly the proteins whose vertical interactions connect the membrane skeleton to the lipid bilayer: spectrin, ankyrin, protein 4.2, and band 3 (see Fig. 15-6). Red cells from the majority of European and American patients with HS, both the dominant and nondominant forms, have deficiencies of spectrin and ankyrin.[845,851,871,891] The degree of spectrin deficiency (and by deduction ankyrin deficiency) correlates well with the spheroidicity of HS red cells, the severity of hemolysis, and the response of patients to splenectomy (Fig. 15-31A).[837,845,892] The mechanical properties of the cells, particularly their ability to withstand shear stress, also correlate with their spectrin content (see Fig. 15-31B).[892,893] Microscopically, HS red

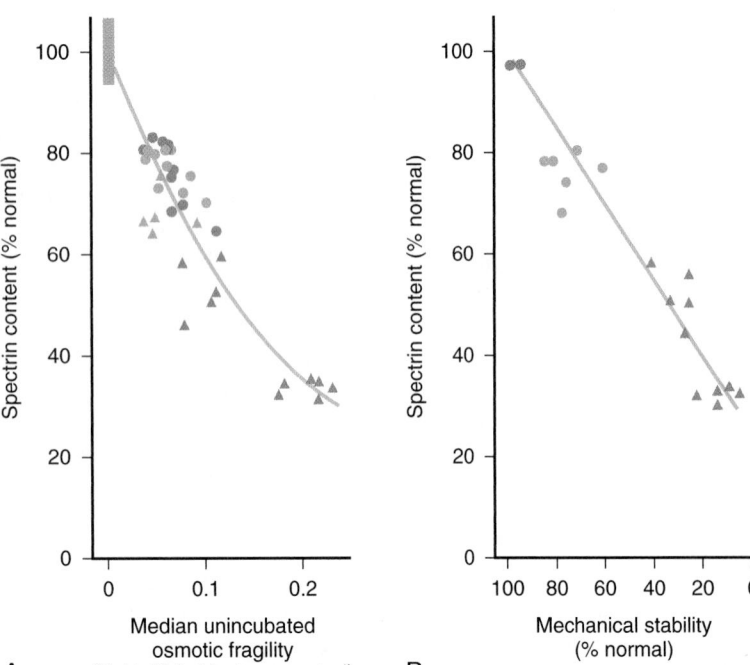

FIGURE 15-31. Correlation of spectrin content with (**A**) unincubated osmotic fragility and (**B**) mechanical stability in hereditary spherocytosis. *Circles* are patients with typical autosomal dominant HS. *Triangles* are patients with nondominant spherocytosis. *Reddish brown* symbols denote patients who have had a splenectomy. The *blue rectangle* in **A** is the normal range. (*A, Adapted from Agre P, Asimos A, Casella JF, et al. Inheritance pattern and clinical response to splenectomy as a reflection of erythrocyte spectrin deficiency in hereditary spherocytosis. N Engl J Med. 1986;315:1579; B, adapted from Chasis JA, Agre PA, Mohandas N. Decreased membrane mechanical stability and in vivo loss of surface area reflect spectrin deficiencies in hereditary spherocytosis. J Clin Invest. 1988;82:617-623.*)

cells show fewer spectrin filaments interconnecting spectrin-actin–protein 4.1 junctional complexes, but overall skeletal architecture is preserved,[894] except in the most severe forms of the disease. A minority of European and American patients with HS have deficiencies of band 3 and protein 4.2 (dominant HS) or protein 4.2 alone (recessive HS).[839,891,895-899] In contrast, these are the most common forms of HS in Japan.[900] In Korean patients, ankyrin and spectrin deficiency is most commonly observed, but protein 4.2 deficiency occurs more commonly than in European or American patients.[901]

α-Spectrin Defects: Recessive Hereditary Spherocytosis

In humans, α-spectrin synthesis exceeds β-spectrin synthesis by 3 or 4 to 1.[902] Heterozygotes for α-spectrin synthetic defects produce enough normal α-spectrin chains to pair with all or nearly all of the β chains that are made. Thus, α-spectrin defects are apparent only in the homozygous or compound heterozygous state and are therefore associated with recessive inheritance. An estimated 5% or less of patients with HS are affected by α-spectrin mutations. In affected patients, the clinical manifestations are often severe, and most patients are transfusion dependent.[845,858,871] The characteristics of HS secondary to α-spectrin deficiency are listed in Box 15-3.

Patients who are homozygotes or compound heterozygotes for α-spectrin defects that produce a 50% to 75% deficiency in spectrin suffer from severe HS. In a report of lethal HS associated with dramatic spectrin deficiency (26% of normal), pulse-labeling studies of BFU-E–derived erythroblasts revealed a marked decrease in α-spectrin synthesis.[841] Although the underlying molecular basis of this defect is unknown, a family history of mild, dominantly inherited HS in the mother and slightly increased OF in the hematologically normal father suggests that the proband inherited at least two genetic defects, which in a simple heterozygote would have minimal adverse consequences. Wichterle and coauthors[903] described a patient with severe HS who was a compound heterozygote for two different α-spectrin gene defects: in one allele there was a splicing defect associated with an upstream intronic mutation, α^{LEPRA}; in the other allele there was another mutation, α^{PRAGUE} (Fig. 15-32).

Box 15-3	Characteristics of Hereditary Spherocytosis Secondary to α-Spectrin Deficiency

<5% of cases of hereditary spherocytosis
Autosomal recessive
α-Spectrin^{LEPRA}, a common, low-expression splicing defect, often paired with a second, presumably null allele
Severe hemolysis and anemia, often transfusion dependent
50% to 75% spectrin deficiency
Red cell morphology not well defined

The α^{LEPRA} allele, a common defect in those with α-spectrin mutations, produces six times less of the correctly spliced α-spectrin transcript than the normal allele does. In many patients with nondominant HS and spectrin deficiency, α^{LEPRA} is in linkage dysequilibrium with α$^{Bug\ Hill}$, which contains an amino acid substitution in the αII domain in the same spectrin molecule.[845,858,869,871] It appears that the combination of the α^{LEPRA} or α^{LEPRA} + α$^{Bug\ Hill}$ alleles with other defects in α-spectrin in *trans* leads to significant spectrin-deficient spherocytic anemia. Interestingly, even in the most severe forms of α-spectrin–linked recessive HS, obligate heterozygotes show little or no spectrin deficiency.[845,858,871]

β-Spectrin Defects: Dominant Hereditary Spherocytosis

Deficiency of the limiting β-spectrin chains restricts the formation of αβ-spectrin heterodimers. Thus, defects in β-spectrin, which affect 15% to 30% of those with HS, are apparent in the heterozygous state and associated with dominant inheritance. The characteristics of HS secondary to β-spectrin deficiency are listed in Box 15-4.

Cloning of the β-spectrin gene, a large gene spanning more than 200 kb, preceded the identification of heterozygous point mutations in a number of unrelated families with dominant HS. Mutations described in β-spectrin have included initiation codon disruptions,[904] frameshift and nonsense mutations, gene deletions, and splicing

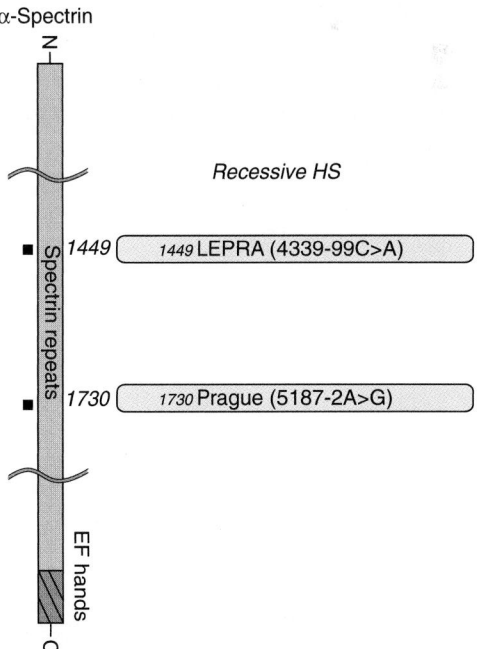

FIGURE 15-32. Two α-spectrin mutations associated with recessive hereditary spherocytosis (HS) are shown next to a schematic representation of the α-spectrin peptide. *(Adapted with permission from Walensky LD, Narla M, Lux SE. Disorders of the red cell membrane. In Handin RI, Lux SE, Stossel TP [eds]. Blood: Principles and Practice of Hematology, 2nd ed. Philadelphia, JB Lippincott, 2003, pp 1709-1858.)*

defects (Fig. 15-33). The following examples of β-spectrin defects are caused by these unique mutations. Spectrin[Kissimmee] is an unstable β-spectrin that lacks the ability to bind protein 4.1 and, as a consequence, binds poorly to actin.[905-907] This variant is due to a point mutation, Trp202→Arg, in a conserved region near the NH$_2$-terminal of β-spectrin, which forms part of the distal (CH2) protein 4.1 binding site.[905] Truncated β-spectrin

mutations caused by a large genomic deletion that leads to skipping of exons 22 and 23, β-spectrin[Durham], or to splicing mutations, β-spectrin[Winston-Salem] and β-spectrin[Guemene-Penfao], have also been described.[908-910] Moreover, screening of the β-spectrin gene in patients with HS and spectrin deficiency has identified a number of nonsense and frameshift mutations.[911-913] One of these, spectrin[Houston], a frameshift mutation caused by a single nucleotide deletion, was found in patients from several unrelated kindreds[911] and may be a relatively common β-spectrin mutation associated with dominant HS.

Patients with HS caused by β-spectrin mutations have mild to moderate hemolysis and anemia. Interestingly, in HS patients in whom peripheral blood morphology has been described, those with β-spectrin mutations have had a small population (5% to 10%) of acanthocytes or spiculated spherocytes, as well as spherocytes.

Ankyrin Defects

Spectrin heterodimers are stable only when bound to the membrane,[914] and ankyrin, the high-affinity binding site, is normally present in limited amounts. As a result,

Box 15-4	Characteristics of Hereditary Spherocytosis Secondary to β-Spectrin Mutations

15% to 30% of cases of hereditary spherocytosis
Almost all individual, dominant null mutations
Spectrin content decreased 15% to 40%
Mild to moderate anemia
Blood smear with spherocytosis plus 5% to 10% spiculated red cells
Spherocytosis plus elliptocytosis in some patients with C-terminal mutations (i.e., spherocytic elliptocytosis)

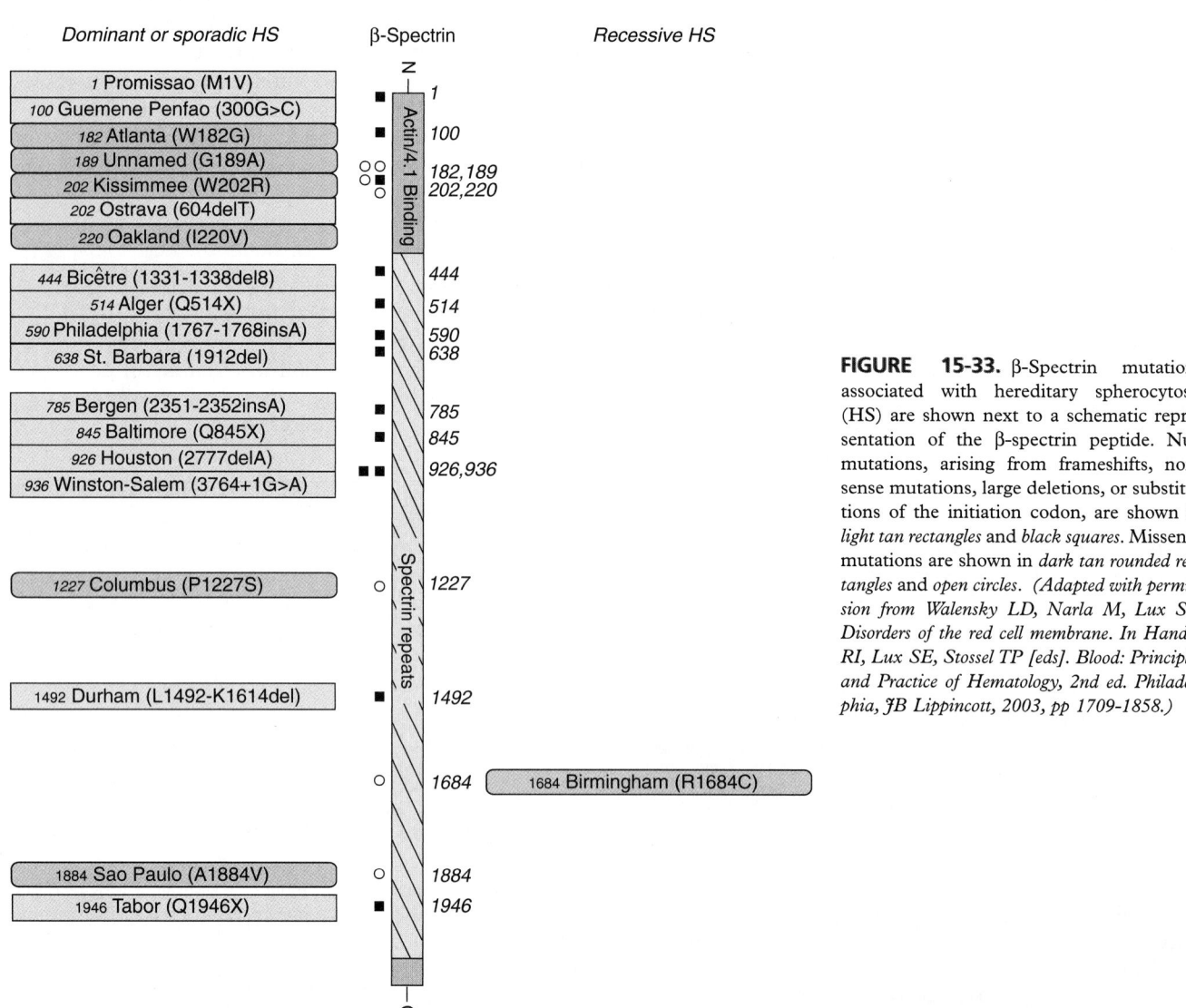

FIGURE 15-33. β-Spectrin mutations associated with hereditary spherocytosis (HS) are shown next to a schematic representation of the β-spectrin peptide. Null mutations, arising from frameshifts, nonsense mutations, large deletions, or substitutions of the initiation codon, are shown in *light tan rectangles* and *black squares.* Missense mutations are shown in *dark tan rounded rectangles* and *open circles.* (Adapted with permission from Walensky LD, Narla M, Lux SE. Disorders of the red cell membrane. In Handin RI, Lux SE, Stossel TP [eds]. Blood: Principles and Practice of Hematology, 2nd ed. Philadelphia, JB Lippincott, 2003, pp 1709-1858.)

Box 15-5	Hereditary Spherocytosis Secondary to Ankyrin Mutations

30% to 60% of cases of hereditary spherocytosis in the United States and Europe; 5% to 10% in Japan

Autosomal dominant and autosomal recessive

Dominant mutations are null mutations and are nearly all unique

Recessive mutations are missense and promoter defects: the $-108T\rightarrow C$ promoter mutation is common

Both spectrin and ankyrin equally deficient: 15% to 50% deficiency

Mild to moderately severe anemia

Blood smear with spherocytosis and no other abnormal morphology

ankyrin defects are typically expressed as a dominant defect, although recessive mutations have been described. The characteristics of HS caused by ankyrin defects are listed in Box 15-5.

Evidence implicating defects of ankyrin in patients with HS comes from a variety of sources, including biochemical analysis, genetic studies, and study of a murine model of HS. The initial biochemical studies suggested an ankyrin defect in two patients with an atypical, unusually severe form of HS characterized by bizarrely shaped microspherocytes and transfusion-dependent anemia.[870] Both red cell spectrin and ankyrin levels were approximately 50% of normal, apparently because of failure of ankyrin synthesis or synthesis of an unstable molecule.[859] Ankyrin mRNA concentrations were also 50% of normal, and pulse-chase studies showed that newly synthesized ankyrin did not accumulate in the cytoplasm and reached only 50% of normal levels on the membrane. In contrast, spectrin mRNA concentrations were normal. However, only 50% of the synthesized spectrin attached to the membrane, presumably because of the lack of ankyrin sites. These results were the initial indication that ankyrin deficiency or dysfunction leads to spectrin deficiency in HS.

Additional studies have provided evidence that ankyrin deficiency is present in the erythrocytes of many patients with typical dominant HS. Savvides and colleagues[891] measured red cell spectrin and ankyrin levels by radioimmunoassay in the erythrocyte membranes of 39 patients from 20 typical kindreds with dominant HS. Values ranged from 40% to 100% of the normal cellular levels of $242,000 \pm 20,500$ spectrin heterodimers and $124,500 \pm 11,000$ ankyrin heterodimers. Both spectrin and ankyrin levels were less than the normal range in 75% to 80% of the kindreds. The degree of spectrin and ankyrin deficiency was very similar in 19 of the 20 kindreds studied. Similar data have been observed in other studies.[851,896-898,901,915,916] The finding of concomitant spectrin and ankyrin deficiency is not unexpected. Decreased ankyrin synthesis could lead to decreased assembly of spectrin on the membrane because ankyrin is the principal spectrin binding site.

Initial genetic studies supported the hypothesis that a defect in the ankyrin gene could be associated with HS. Initially, studies of atypical patients with HS and karyotypic abnormalities, including translocations and interstitial deletions, defined a locus for HS at chromosomal segments 8p11.2-21.1.[847,917-920] After the ankyrin gene was cloned, it was localized to this same region, 8p11.2.[847] Fluorescence-based in situ hybridization of lymphocyte metaphase spreads from a patient with HS, mental retardation, and an interstitial deletion of chromosome 8, band p11.1-p21, with an ankyrin genomic probe provided direct evidence that one copy of the erythrocyte ankyrin gene was deleted.[847] The ankyrin content in the patient's red blood cell membranes was reduced by 50%. A similar phenotype has been reported in another patient with an 8p11.1-p21.3 deletion.[848] These results demonstrated that a deficiency of ankyrin secondary to a gene deletion could be a cause of HS.

Genetic studies have now clearly shown that a defect in the ankyrin gene is the most common cause of dominant HS. The linkage between HS and the ankyrin gene was demonstrated in a large family with typical dominant HS by the use of restriction fragment length polymorphisms.[921] Studies of ankyrin cDNA revealed that a third of patients with dominant HS and spectrin and ankyrin deficiencies expressed only one of their two ankyrin alleles in reticulocyte RNA, thus demonstrating reduced ankyrin expression from one, presumably mutant allele.[922] A series of reports then demonstrated the precise defects in the ankyrin gene that cause HS.[923] Analysis of these mutations revealed the following: (1) ankyrin mutations are common and affect patients with both dominant and nondominant HS, (2) mutations that abolish the normal ankyrin product are common in dominant HS (e.g., frameshift and nonsense mutations), and (3) defects upstream of the coding region in the ankyrin gene erythroid promoter are common in nondominant HS.

The most common ankyrin variant in patients with recessive HS is a $T\rightarrow C$ nucleotide substitution in the ankyrin gene promoter -108 bp from the translation start site. The allele frequency of this variant was found to be 29% in a German HS population and 2% in normal individuals.[923] It has also been associated with nondominant HS with ankyrin deficiency in Italy.[839] The -108 sequence variant is usually in *cis* with a $G\rightarrow A$ nucleotide substitution 153 bp from the start site.[924] These defects are silent in obligate heterozygotes; therefore, patients with nondominant HS must have a second mutation.[924] Functional defects associated with these promoter mutations have been demonstrated in a transgenic animal model.[925]

Variations in the clinical severity and red cell ankyrin content of similar mutations indicate that other factors modify the expression of the primary ankyrin defects. For example, ankyrin[Marburg] and ankyrin[Einbeck] are frameshift mutations that occur in the NH_2-terminal (membrane) domain and do not produce a detectable product in mature red cells. They would be expected to have a similar phenotype, but patients with ankyrin[Marburg] have moderate to severe HS and moderate ankyrin deficiency (64% of normal), whereas patients with ankyrin[Einbeck] have very mild disease and normal ankyrin levels. Understanding this and similar phenotypic variations will be one of the critical problems in HS research in the next few years.

Ankyrin mutations are estimated to account for 30% to 60% of cases of HS in northern European populations and 5% to 10% of cases of HS in Japanese populations. Peripheral blood smears demonstrate only prominent spherocytosis. Hemolysis can be mild to severe, and patients with recessive mutations typically have a more severe clinical course. The majority of ankyrin mutations are private; that is, each individual kindred has a unique mutation (Fig. 15-34). One frameshift mutation associated with severe dominant HS, ankyrin[Florianopolis], has been identified in patients with HS from three different kin-

dreds with different genetic backgrounds.[926] Analysis of an ankyrin gene polymorphism in these individuals demonstrated that this mutation is found on different ankyrin alleles, thus suggesting that the ankyrin[Florianopolis] mutation has occurred more than once.

Band 3 Defects: Dominant Hereditary Spherocytosis

A primary defect in band 3 is present in approximately 20% to 30% of patients with dominant HS.[927] Erythrocyte membranes from these patients are deficient in band 3 with a concomitant deficiency of protein 4.2.[928] The characteristics of HS caused by band 3 deficiency are listed in Box 15-6.

A variety of band 3 mutations have been described, and these mutations are spread out throughout the band 3 gene and occur in both the cytoplasmic and membrane-spanning domains (Fig. 15-35). Band 3 mutations

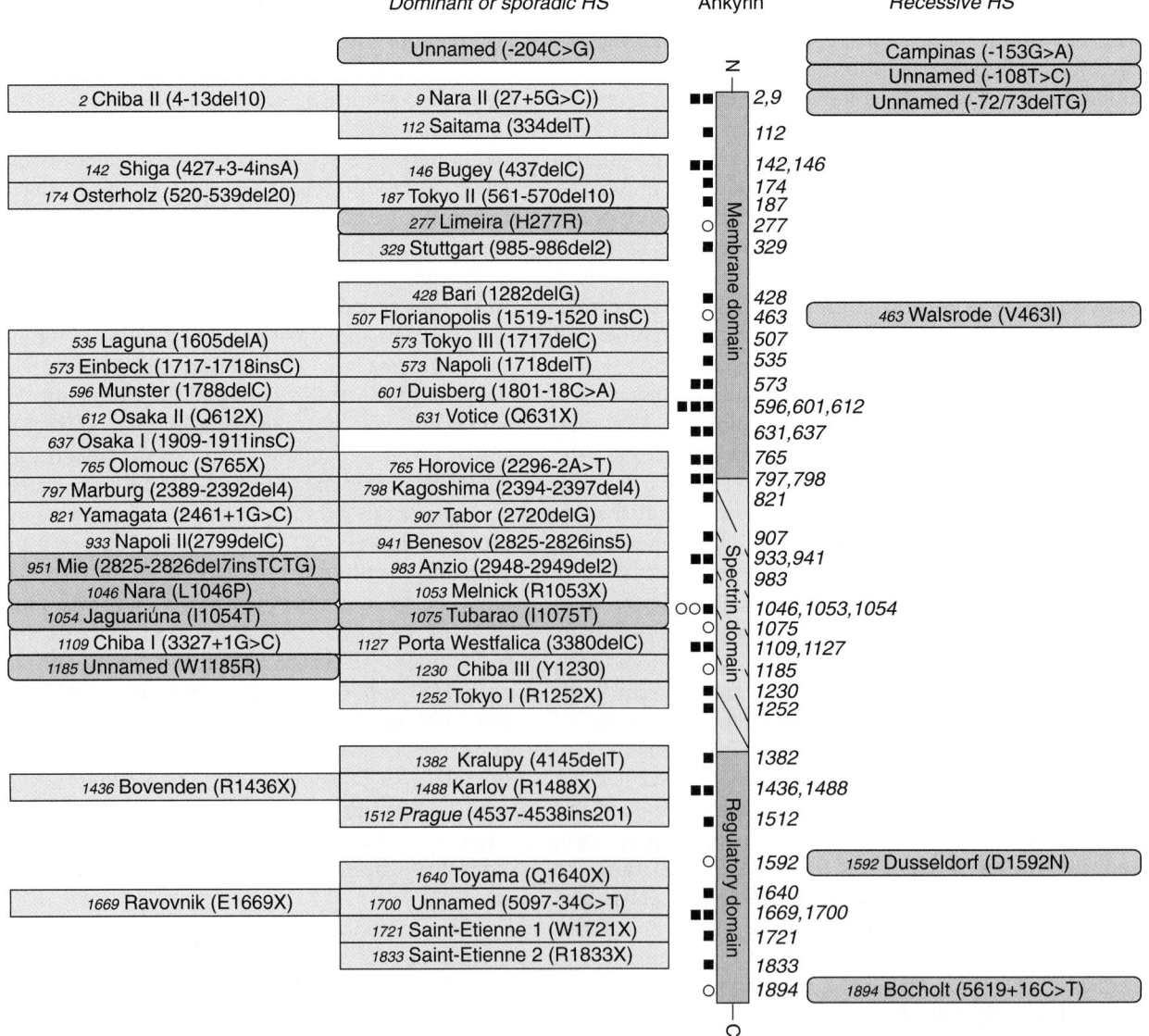

FIGURE 15-34. Ankyrin mutations associated with hereditary spherocytosis (HS). Null mutations, arising from frameshifts or nonsense mutations, are shown in *light tan rectangles* and *black squares*. Missense and putative promoter mutations are shown in *dark tan rounded rectangles* and *open circles*. *(Adapted with permission from Walensky LD, Narla M, Lux SE. Disorders of the red cell membrane. In Handin RI, Lux SE, Stossel TP [eds]. Blood: Principles and Practice of Hematology, 2nd ed. Philadelphia, JB Lippincott, 2003, pp 1709-1858.)*

generally fall into two groups. One group is associated with mild band 3 deficiency and affects protein 4.2 or ankyrin binding. The other group is associated with more severe band 3 deficiency as a result of a mutation that causes mRNA instability or a mutant band 3 protein that is degraded or not otherwise inserted into the membrane.[928] Similar to the other molecular defects that cause HS, band 3 mutations are unique familial defects with no common mutations among affected groups.

One of the first described band 3 mutants associated with HS was band 3[Prague].[929] This mutant is due to a 10-nucleotide duplication in the band 3 gene that leads to a shift in the reading frame and results in premature chain termination by altering the C-terminal after amino acid 821. The mutation affects the last transmembrane helix and probably alters insertion of band 3 into the membrane because the mutant protein is not detectable in mature red cells.

Conserved arginine residues are frequent sites of mutations in the transmembrane domain of the band 3 gene. Arginine 490 appears to be a particular hot spot for HS-related band 3 mutations.[930,931] The affected argi-

Box 15-6	**Hereditary Spherocytosis Secondary to Band 3 Mutations**

20% to 30% of cases of hereditary spherocytosis
Individual, dominant functionally null mutations. No common defects
15% to 40% decrease in band 3 and similar decrease in protein 4.2
Mild to moderate hemolysis and anemia
Spherocytosis with a small number of characteristic mushroom-shaped or "pincered" cells

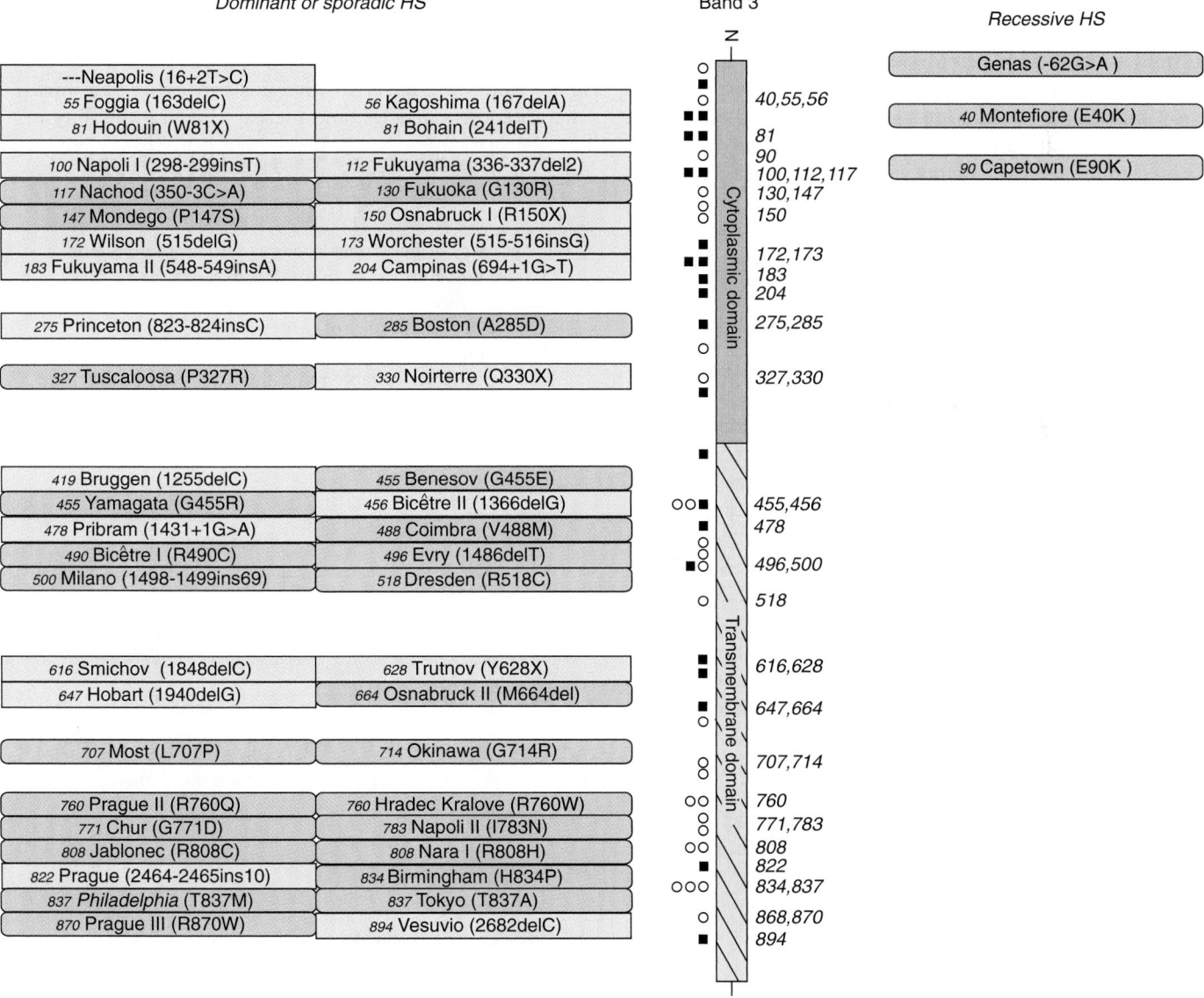

FIGURE 15-35. Band 3 mutations associated with hereditary spherocytosis (HS). Null mutations arising from either frameshift or nonsense mutations are shown in *light tan rectangles* and *black squares*, as is a mutation associated with loss of the translation start site (band 3[Neapolis]). Missense mutations or short in-frame deletions or insertions are shown in *dark tan rounded rectangles* and *open circles*. (*Adapted with permission from Walensky LD, Narla M, Lux SE. Disorders of the red cell membrane. In Handin RI, Lux SE, Stossel TP [eds]. Blood: Principles and Practice of Hematology, 2nd ed. Philadelphia, JB Lippincott, 2003, pp 1709-1858.*)

nine residues are located in the same position on the inside edge of most transmembrane proteins and are believed to help orient the membrane-spanning segments. Thus, as predicted, in vitro studies have demonstrated that these arginine substitutions, as well as several other HS-associated band 3 missense mutations, exhibit defective cellular trafficking from the endoplasmic reticulum to the plasma membrane,[932,933] perhaps as a result of misfolding.

Other band 3 mutations causing HS have been described, including nonsense mutations,[923,934] frameshift mutations,[935] partial gene duplications, other missense mutations, and splicing defects.[846,883,936-938] Determination of the crystal structure of the cytoplasmic domain of band 3 is beginning to provide insight into the biologic significance of the missense mutations.[939,940] A few of the HS mutations have been associated with significant protein 4.2 deficiency or with acanthocytosis alone (see later).

Clinically, most patients with band 3 mutations have mild to moderate hemolysis and anemia. The band 3 protein is reduced by 15% to 40% in HS red cells. On average, band 3 defects are somewhat milder than ankyrin or β-spectrin defects, although there is considerable overlap in severity. Patients with HS and band 3 deficiencies have a small number (≤1%) of button, mushroom-shaped, or "pincered" erythrocytes, in addition to spherocytes, on peripheral blood smears. This morphologic characteristic is not observed in the other membrane protein defects.

Because band 3 functions as an anion exchanger and a shortened form of band 3 is expressed in the intercalated cells of the kidney cortical collecting ducts, patients with HS and band 3 deficiency have been examined for a defect in acid-base homeostasis. Patients who are homozygous for band 3 defects, such as band 3[Coimbra],[883] or patients with defects in band 3 mRNA processing, such as band 3[Pribram] or band 3[Campinas],[941,942] have been found to suffer from hemolytic anemia and renal tubular acidosis (RTA). However, the majority of HS patients with mutations in band 3 do not have RTA.[943-946] The lack of RTA in patients with dominant HS and band 3 mutants supports the hypothesis that dominant RTA results from the association of mutant band 3 with wild-type band 3 into hetero-oligomers in the kidney, but not in erythroid cells, thereby leading to intracellular retention or mistargeting of both proteins.[928] It is poorly understood why some residues are critical in the kidney but not in the red cell, with mutations leading to the phenotype of RTA but not HS, or why some residues are critical in the erythrocyte but not the kidney and lead to the phenotype of HS but not RTA. These are important questions to be addressed in future studies.

Protein 4.2 Defects: Recessive Hereditary Spherocytosis

Investigators have described families with recessive HS in which erythrocytes from affected homozygous patients

lack protein 4.2. HS caused by protein 4.2 deficiency is most common in Japan, although a few patients have been described in other populations.[895,947,948] The characteristics of this form of HS are summarized in Box 15-7.

The molecular defects causing protein 4.2 deficiency have been described in multiple families (Fig. 15-36). The most common mutation is 4.2[Nippon], in which the red cells contain only a small quantity of a 74/72-kd doublet of protein 4.2 instead of the usual abundant 72-kd species because of an Ala142→Thr mutation that affects processing of protein 4.2 mRNA.[949] Protein 4.2[Nippon]-deficient membranes lose 70% of their ankyrin with low–ionic strength extraction, and the ankyrin loss is blocked by preincubation of the membranes with purified 4.2, which suggests that protein 4.2 stabilizes ankyrin on the membrane.[950,951] This hypothesis is supported by the observation that the amount of protein 4.2 is low in the red cell membranes of ankyrin-deficient nb/nb mice and in HS patients who lack one ankyrin gene. In addition, red cells from patients homozygous for 4.2[Nippon] are fragile and have heat-sensitive skeletons, clumped intramembranous particles, and increased lateral mobility of

Box 15-7	Hereditary Spherocytosis Secondary to Protein 4.2 Mutations

<5% of cases of hereditary spherocytosis in the United States and Europe; 45% to 50% in Japan.
Autosomal recessive
95% to 100% deficiency of protein 4.2
4.2[Nippon] common in Japan
Blood smear with variable red cell morphology in different patients: spherocytes, acanthocytes, ovalostomatocytes, normal discocytes

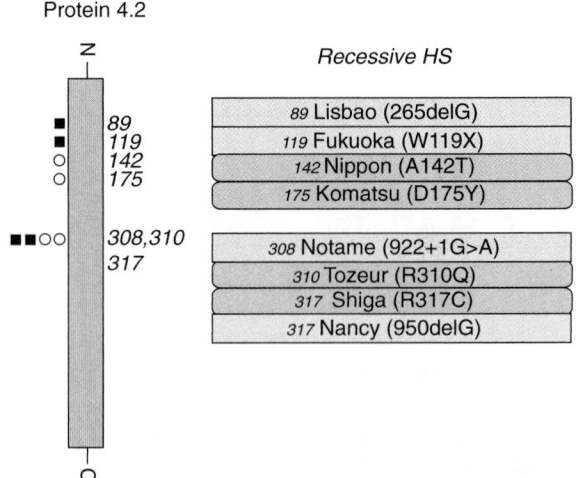

FIGURE 15-36. Protein 4.2 mutations associated with recessive hereditary spherocytosis (HS). Null mutations, arising from frameshifts or nonsense mutations, are shown in *light tan rectangles* and *black squares*. Missense mutations are shown in *dark tan rounded rectangles* and *open circles*. (Adapted with permission from Walensky LD, Narla M, Lux SE. Disorders of the red cell membrane. In Handin RI, Lux SE, Stossel TP [eds]. *Blood: Principles and Practice of Hematology*, 2nd ed. Philadelphia, JB Lippincott, 2003, pp 1709-1858.)

band 3.[951] However, ankyrin lability is not evident in other patients with protein 4.2 deficiency.[952,953] In addition, erythrocyte protein 4.2 deficiency has also been associated with mutations of band 3.[936,950,954,955] However, it is difficult to assess the significance of these reports because all patients with band 3 deficiency have an equivalent loss of protein 4.2.

Clinically, patients with HS secondary to protein 4.2 deficiency have mild anemia. The peripheral smear sometimes demonstrates typical spherocytosis but more often contains ovalocytes or stomatocytes. The mechanism behind this unique and variable red cell morphology is currently unknown.

Secondary Defects

A large number of secondary abnormalities have been identified over the years. They are catalogued and discussed in detail in previous editions of this chapter.[956]

Tight Binding of Spectrin to the Membrane. Inextractable spectrin was first observed some years ago in 2 of 12 patients with HS, in whom spectrin failed to elute from the membrane after exposure to a low–ionic strength buffer for 72 hours.[957] These are conditions that generally produce greater than 90% spectrin extraction. A third patient was subsequently discovered.[958] The molecular basis of this phenomenon has not been investigated, although the possibility that it might be secondary to a defect in ankyrin or β-spectrin is likely. In addition, some tightly bound spectrin is palmitoylated, and this fraction might be increased.[959]

Increased Membrane Hemoglobin. HS membranes contain increased amounts of hemoglobin and catalase.[960] This relatively nonspecific finding is observed in a number of hemolytic anemias, particularly if red cell dehydration occurs. The molecular basis for finding this is not understood.

Enolase Deficiency. Two reports of apparent HS combined with partial enolase deficiency (~50%) have been published.[961,962] In the first patient, the results of red cell OF and autohemolysis tests were typical for HS, although spherocytes were not apparent on the blood smear. Dominant inheritance was suggested by the history but could not be established. However, dominant inheritance of both HS and partial enolase deficiency was clearly evident in the second family when both diseases could be traced through four generations. In this kindred, the enolase-deficient spherocytes resisted lysis in the acidified glycerol lysis test, another characteristic of typical HS (see later). The similarity of these two patients suggests that they may represent a unique subgroup of HS. In particular, the combination of dominant inheritance and half-normal levels of enolase raises the possibility that the primary defect could lie in an enolase-binding membrane protein, assuming that such a protein exists.

Diminished Membrane Phosphorylation. The discovery that red cell membrane proteins are phosphorylated was followed by numerous reports that phosphorylation was defective in HS. These reports are summarized and analyzed in early editions of this book.[956] Overall, the effects were variable and generally were demonstrable only in ghosts incubated in low–ionic strength buffers for relatively long periods. Initial rates of phosphorylation in HS ghosts were normal,[963-965] as was membrane protein phosphorylation of intact spherocytes from splenectomized individuals.[965] It appears that the phosphorylation defects were probably secondary effects.

Membrane Lipids. The principal lipid abnormality of hereditary spherocytes is symmetrical loss of membrane lipids as part of the overall loss of membrane surface, the hallmark of the pathobiology of HS. The relative proportions of cholesterol and the various phospholipids are normal,[966] and the phospholipids show the usual transmembrane asymmetry, even in severe instances.[867,967] It has been reported that very-long-chain fatty acids are missing from certain classes of phospholipids,[968] but this has not been confirmed.[969] It is unclear whether this difference is due to technical factors or to genetic heterogeneity of the disease. Even if real, it seems likely that the changes in fatty acid composition would be secondary to the underlying membrane protein defects.

Cations and Transport. It has been known for many years that HS red cells are intrinsically more leaky to Na^+ and K^+ ions than normal cells are.[970-972] A similar defect exists in the erythrocytes of *sph/sph* mice with HS.[973] The excessive Na^+ influx activates Na^+,K^+-ATPase and the monovalent cation pump, and the accelerated pumping,[974] in turn, increases ATP turnover and glycolysis. Interestingly, protein 4.2–deficient erythrocytes have increased anion transport, whereas erythrocytes deficient in spectrin, ankyrin, or band 3 have normal or decreased anion transport.[975] At one time it was believed that this modest Na^+ leak was responsible for the hemolysis of hereditary spherocytes,[971] particularly cells trapped in the unfavorable metabolic environment of the spleen, but it is now clear that this is incorrect because the magnitude of the Na^+ flux does not correlate with the extent of hemolysis in HS.[976] In addition, patients with hereditary stomatocytosis (see later) have a much greater defect in Na^+ permeability but microspherocytes do not develop and they sometimes have very little hemolysis. The leakage of Na^+ into red cells in hereditary stomatocytosis is accompanied by the entry of water and cell swelling, a finding that contrasts with the well-established dehydration of hereditary spherocytes.

The dehydration of HS red cells is likely to be inflicted, at least in part, by the adverse environment of the spleen because spherocytes from surgically removed spleens are the most dehydrated.[977] The pathways causing HS red cell dehydration have not been clearly defined. One likely candidate is the Gárdos channel, a Ca^{+2}-

activated K^+ channel that is known to mediate erythrocyte dehydration in sickle cell anemia and thalassemia. A recent study examined Gárdos channel activity in mice with erythrocytes devoid of protein 4.1 and showed that the Gárdos channel is functionally upregulated in these erythrocytes and allows more K^+ leakage when in a calcium-rich environment.[978] When mouse erythrocytes devoid of protein 4.1 were exposed to clotrimazole, a known Gárdos channel blocker, hemolysis worsened, thus indicating that the Gárdos channel and red cell dehydration protect HS red cells by compensating for the reduced membrane surface area caused by the defective, 4.1-deficient membrane skeleton. Another possible candidate behind the mechanism of cell dehydration is increased K^+-Cl^- cotransport, which is activated by acid pH.[979] HS red cells, particularly from unsplenectomized subjects, have a low intracellular pH[865] because of the low pH of the splenic environment (see later). The K^+-Cl^- cotransport pathway is also activated by oxidation,[980] which is likely to be inflicted by splenic macrophages. Hyperactivity of the Na^+,K^+ pump, triggered by increased intracellular Na^+, can dehydrate red cells directly because three Na^+ ions are extruded in exchange for only two K^+ ions.[974] The loss of monovalent cations is accompanied by water. Polymorphisms in the cation channels that decrease K^+ loss and red cell dehydration in HS are likely to make the disease worse and are a possible mechanism of clinical variability.

Glycolysis. In general, glycolysis is mildly accelerated in HS red cells,[971,981,982] mostly to support increased cation pumping, and 2,3-DPG concentrations are slightly depressed,[865,866,983] probably because of activation of 2,3-DPG phosphatase by the acidic intracellular pH of the cell. The latter abnormalities are at least partly due to splenic detention because the acidosis and 2,3-DPG deficiency both improve after splenectomy.[865,866]

Phospho*enol*pyruvate Transport. An apparently specific decrease in carrier-mediated transport of phospho*enol*pyruvate has been noted in the red cells of some patients with HS.[984] Unfortunately, only unsplenectomized patients have been studied, so it is possible that the defect is caused by the metabolic derangements that these cells acquire during their detention in the spleen. However, it is more likely caused by diminished anion exchange. Band 3 transports pyruvate and probably phospho*enol*pyruvate. If so, reduced phospho*enol*pyruvate transport would be expected in patients with HS and band 3 deficiency, and indeed, reduced phospho*enol*pyruvate transport has been reported only in the Japanese HS population, in which band 3 deficiency is common.

Pathophysiology

Loss of Membrane Surface by Vesiculation

The primary membrane lesions described earlier, all involving vertical interactions between the skeleton and the bilayer, fit the theory that HS is caused by local disconnection of the skeleton and bilayer, followed by vesiculation of the unsupported surface components. This, in turn, leads to a progressive reduction in membrane surface area and to a shape called a spherocyte, although it usually ranges between a thickened discocyte and a spherostomatocyte.[985] The phospholipid and cholesterol content of isolated spherocytes is decreased by 15% to 20%, consistent with the loss of surface area.[986-989]

Biomechanical measurements show that HS membranes are fragile. The force required to fragment the membrane is diminished and is proportional to the density of spectrin on the membrane.[892,893] Membrane elasticity and bending stiffness are also reduced and are proportional to spectrin density.[990] In addition, HS red cells lose membrane more readily than normal red cells do when metabolically deprived or when their ghosts are subjected to conditions facilitating vesiculation.[989-993] However, this has not been shown to occur in metabolically healthy spherocytes, perhaps because it occurs slowly (1% to 2% per day) under such conditions. Nonetheless, massive vesiculation is evident in mice and zebra fish with severe spherocytic hemolytic anemia (see later).[994-997]

Because budding red cells are rarely observed in typical blood smears from patients with HS, the postulated vesiculation may either involve microscopic vesicles or occur in the reticuloendothelial system. More recent studies suggest that vesiculation may occur in the bone marrow of patients with HS because similar decreases in red cell surface area have been found in reticulocytes in HS as in mature red blood cells.[998] When membrane vesicles are induced in normal red cells, they originate at the tips of spicules, where the lipid bilayer uncouples from the underlying skeleton (see Fig. 15-26).[999] The vesicles are small (about 100 nm) and devoid of hemoglobin and skeletal proteins, so they are invisible during conventional examination of stained blood films. In studies with an atomic force microscope, tiny (50 to 80 nm) bumps have been detected on the surface of red cells obtained from patients with HS whose red cells are actively hemolyzing (Fig. 15-37).[1000] The bumps could be microvesicles, although this needs to be proved with more conventional microscopic techniques. They are less than the length of a spectrin molecule (100 nm) and are not present on red cells from splenectomized patients.

The observation that spectrin or spectrin/ankyrin deficiencies are common in HS has led to the suggestion that they are the primary cause of spherocytosis. According to this hypothesis (Fig. 15-38, hypothesis 1), interactions of spectrin with bilayer lipids or proteins are required to stabilize the membrane. Spectrin-deficient areas would tend to bud off, thereby leading to spherocytosis. However, this conjecture does not explain how spherocytes develop in patients whose red cells are deficient in band 3 or protein 4.2 but have normal amounts of spectrin.[891,950]

An alternative hypothesis argues that the bilayer is stabilized by interactions between lipids and the abun-

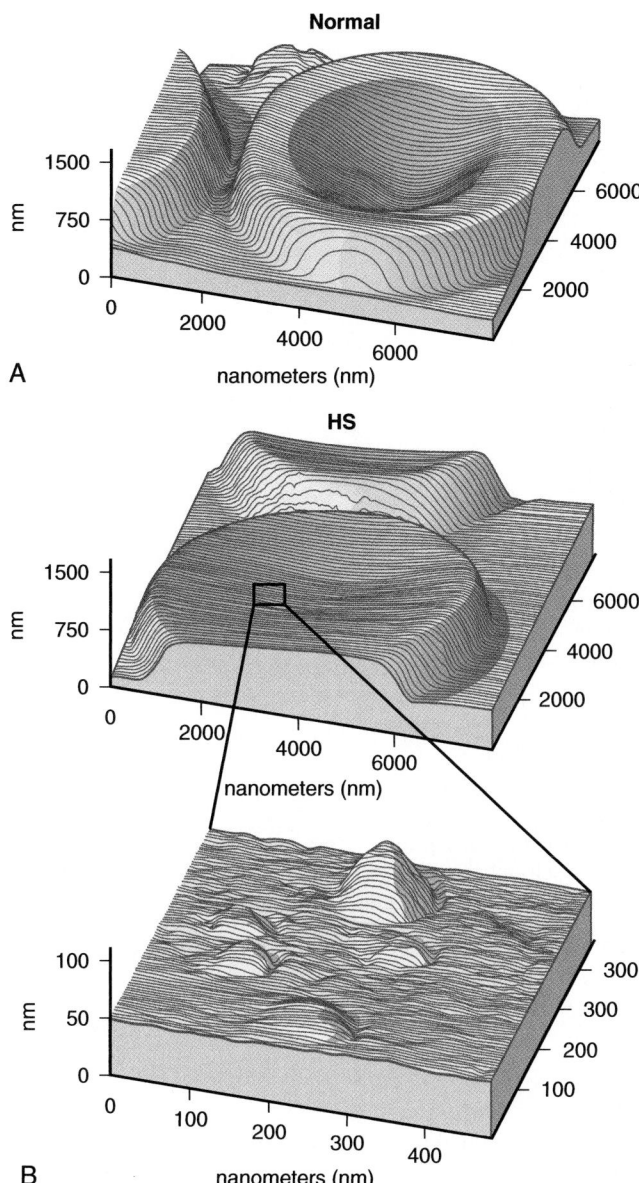

Normal

HS

A

B

FIGURE 15-37. Comparison of the surface of a normal red cell (**A**) and a hereditary spherocyte (HS) (before splenectomy) (**B**) by atomic force microscopy. Note that at high magnification, 50- to 80-nm pseudopodia are evident on the surface of the spherocyte, which may represent membrane microvesicles (bottom of **B**). These structures were not observed after splenectomy. *(Adapted with permission from Walensky LD, Narla M, Lux SE. Disorders of the red cell membrane. In Handin RI, Lux SE, Stossel TP [eds]. Blood: Principles and Practice of Hematology, 2nd ed. Philadelphia, JB Lippincott, 2003, pp 1709-1858.)*

dant band 3 molecules (see Fig. 15-38, hypothesis 2). Each band 3 molecule contains about 13 hydrophobic transmembrane helices, many of which must interact with lipids. These interactions presumably spread beyond the first layer of lipids and influence the mobility of lipids in successive layers. In deficient red cells, the area between band 3 molecules would increase on average, and the stabilizing effect would diminish. Transient fluctuations in the local density of band 3 could aggravate this situation and allow unsupported lipids to be lost and thus result in spherocytosis. This hypothesis is supported by

targeted disruption of the band 3 gene in mice. Erythrocytes from these mice lose massive amounts of membrane surface despite a normal membrane skeleton.[995] This concept is also consistent with early studies of intramembrane particle aggregation, which leads to particle-free domains, as discussed earlier in the chapter. These domains are unstable and give rise to surface blebs that are subsequently released from the cells as vesicles.[1001]

Spectrin-deficient and ankyrin-deficient red cells could become spherocytic by a similar mechanism. Because spectrin filaments corral band 3 molecules and limit their lateral movement, a decrease in spectrin would allow band 3 molecules to diffuse and cluster transiently, thereby fostering vesiculation. However, it is most likely that both of the aforementioned hypotheses operate to a different degree, depending on the membrane skeletal protein that is deficient—hypothesis 1 dominating in spectrin and ankyrin disorders and hypothesis 2 dominating in band 3 and protein 4.2 defects.

Loss of Cellular Deformability

Hereditary spherocytes hemolyze because of the rheologic consequences of their decreased surface-to-volume ratio. The red cell membrane is very flexible, but it can expand its surface area only about 3% before rupturing.[1002] Thus, erythrocytes become less and less deformable as surface area is lost. For HS red cells, poor deformability is a hindrance only in the spleen because the cells have a nearly normal life span after splenectomy.[1003,1004]

Splenic Sequestration and Conditioning

In the spleen most of the arterial blood empties directly into the splenic cords, a tortuous maze of interconnecting narrow passages formed by reticular cells and lined with phagocytes.[1005-1010] Histologically, this is an "open" circulation, but most of the blood that enters the cords normally travels by fairly direct (i.e., functionally closed) pathways. If passage through these channels is impeded, red cells are diverted deeper into the labyrinthine portions of the cords, where blood flow is slow and the cells may be detained for minutes to hours. Whichever route is taken, to reenter the circulation, red cells must squeeze through spaces between the endothelial cells that form the walls of the venous sinuses (Fig. 15-39). Even when maximally distended, these narrow slits are always much smaller than red cells, which are greatly distorted during their passage.[1007,1008] Experiments have shown that spherocytes are selectively sequestered at this cord-sinus juncture.[1011-1013] As a consequence, spleens from patients with HS have massively congested cords and relatively empty sinuses.[1005,1014-1016] On electron micrographs, few spherocytes are seen in transit through the sinus wall,[1005,1015,1017] which is in contrast to the situation in normal spleens, where cells in transit are readily found.[1009]

During detention in the spleen, HS red cells undergo additional damage marked by further loss of surface area and an increase in cell density. Many of these "condi-

Hypothesis 1:

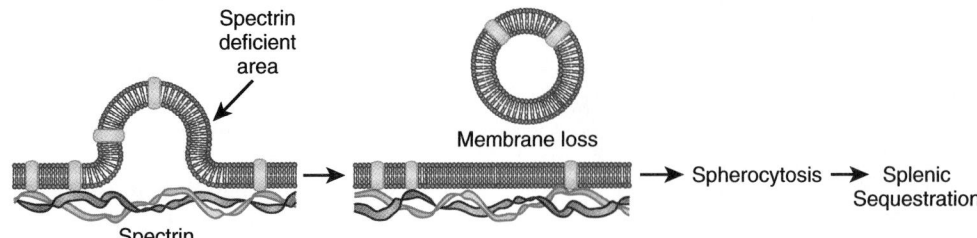

Hypothesis 2:

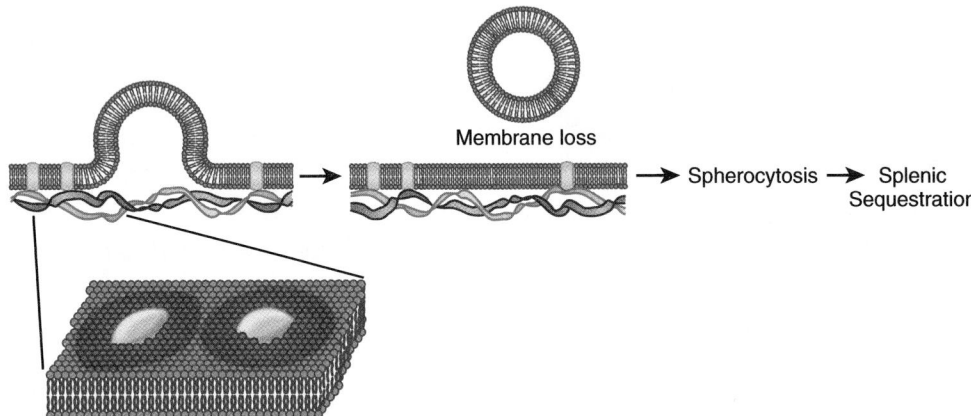

FIGURE 15-38. Two hypotheses concerning the mechanism of membrane loss in hereditary spherocytosis. Hypothesis 1 assumes that the "membrane" (i.e., the lipid bilayer and the integral membrane proteins) is directly stabilized by interactions with spectrin or other elements of the membrane skeleton. Because spectrin-deficient areas lack support, they bud off and thereby lead to spherocytosis. Hypothesis 2 assumes that the membrane is stabilized by interactions of band 3 (tan protein) with neighboring lipids. The influence of band 3 extends into the lipid milieu because the first layer of immobilized lipids slows the lipids in the next layer and so on. The partially immobilized lipids are depicted as a darker blue ring around the protein. In band 3–deficient cells, the area between lipid molecules increases, and unsupported lipids are lost. Spectrin-ankyrin deficiency allows band 3 molecules to diffuse and cluster transiently, with the same consequences. *(Adapted with permission from Walensky LD, Narla M, Lux SE. Disorders of the red cell membrane. In Handin RI, Lux SE, Stossel TP [eds]. Blood: Principles and Practice of Hematology, 2nd ed. Philadelphia, JB Lippincott, 2003, pp 1709-1858.)*

tioned" red cells escape the hostile environment of the spleen and reenter the circulation. In unsplenectomized patients with HS, two populations of spherocytes are detectable: a minor population of hyperchromic "microspherocytes" that form the "tail" of very fragile cells in the unincubated OF test and a major population that may be only slightly more spheroidal than normal.

By 1913 it was known that HS red cells obtained from the splenic vein were more osmotically fragile than those in the peripheral circulation.[1018] In addition, this OF was confirmed by other hematologists of the time.[831,1019] However, its significance was not clear until the classic studies in the 1950s by Emerson, Young, and their colleagues, who showed that osmotically fragile microspherocytes are concentrated in and emanate from the splenic pulp (Fig. 15-40).[1013,1020] After splenectomy, spherocytosis persists, but the tail of hyperfragile red cells is no longer evident on OF testing. These and other data led to the conclusion that the spleen detains and "conditions" circulating HS red cells in a way that increases their spheroidicity and hastens their demise.[1013,1021,1022] The kinetics of this process was illustrated in vivo by Griggs and associates, who found that a cohort of ^{59}Fe-

labeled HS red cells gradually shifted from the major, less fragile population to the more fragile, conditioned population 7 to 11 days after their release into the circulation.[1022] Although most conditioned HS red cells that escape the spleen are probably recaptured and destroyed, the damage incurred is sufficient to permit extrasplenic recognition and removal because conditioned spherocytes, isolated from the spleen and reinfused postoperatively, are eliminated rapidly.[1022,1023]

The mechanism of splenic conditioning is less certain. It is difficult to obtain accurate information about the cordal environment, but existing data suggest that it is metabolically inhospitable,[1012,1021,1024,1025] though perhaps less so than originally believed.[1010] Crowded red cells must compete for limited supplies of glucose[1024] in acidic surroundings (pH $\approx$ 6.6 to 7.2),[1010,1012,1021,1025] where glycolysis is inhibited.[1026,1027] The acidic environment also induces Cl$^-$ and water entry and cell swelling,[1028] but as discussed earlier, it also stimulates the K$^+$-Cl$^-$ cotransporter, which produces a net loss of K$^+$ and water from the cells. The adverse effects of the cordal environment are further compounded by the presence of oxidant-producing macrophages. It has also been suggested that

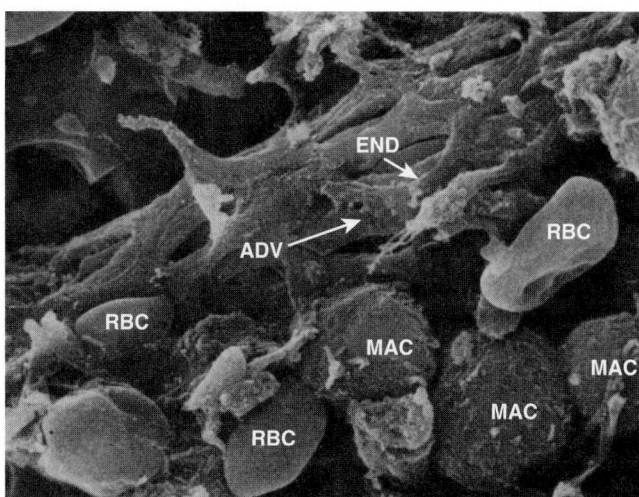

FIGURE 15-39. Scanning electron micrograph of a splenic sinus viewed from within the splenic cords. The narrow transmural slits between the endothelial cells (END) and adventitial cells (ADV) of the sinus are evident. The edges of these slits probably touch each other in a normal spleen, so the openings are potential structures rather than fixed pores. They are revealed here because of a drying artifact. Note that the adjacent erythrocytes (RBC) are considerably larger than the slits and therefore must be flexible to pass into the splenic sinuses and return to the venous circulation. If they are unable to pass into the sinuses, macrophages (MAC) lie in wait. *(From Weiss L. A scanning electron microscopic study of the spleen. Blood. 1974;43:665-691.)*

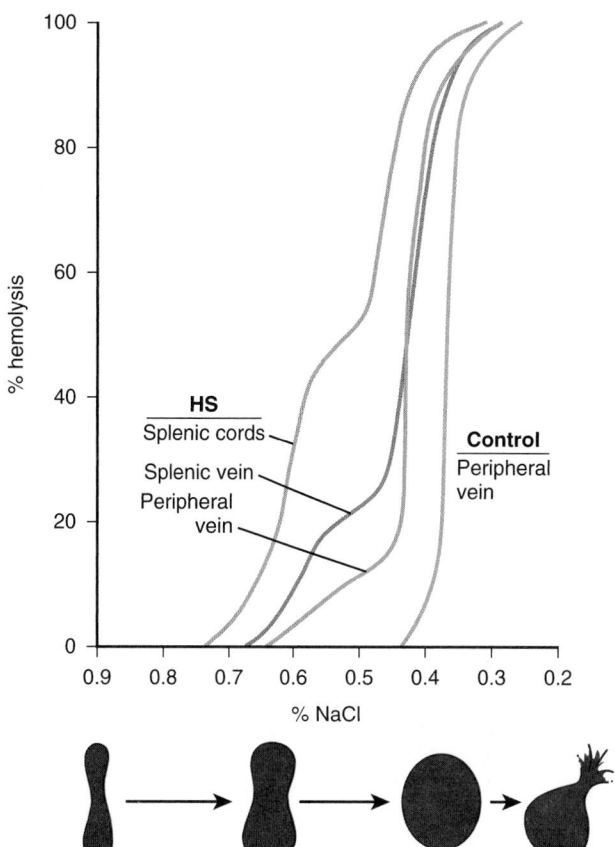

FIGURE 15-40. Osmotic fragility in hereditary spherocytosis (HS). In the osmotic fragility test, red cells are suspended in salt solutions of varying tonicity between isotonic saline (0.9% NaCl) (*left*) and distilled water (*right*). Normal red cells swell in hypotonic media and eventually reach a limiting spheric shape, beyond which they hemolyze (*bottom*). Spherocytes, which begin with a lower than normal surface-to-volume ratio, can swell less before they reach their limiting volume; hence, their osmotic fragility curve is shifted to the left (higher salt concentrations). They are said to be osmotically fragile. Before splenectomy, a small proportion of the red cells are extra fragile and produce a "tail" on the osmotic fragility curve. The cells have been conditioned by the spleen as shown by their higher concentration in the splenic vein and especially the splenic cords. *(Adapted with permission from Walensky LD, Narla M, Lux SE. Disorders of the red cell membrane. In Handin RI, Lux SE, Stossel TP [eds]. Blood: Principles and Practice of Hematology, 2nd ed. Philadelphia, JB Lippincott, 2003, pp 1709-1858.)*

methylation of erythrocyte membrane proteins could contribute to the splenic conditioning of spectrin-deficient HS red cells.[1029] Hence, the spherocyte, detained in the splenic cords because of its surface deficiency, is stressed by erythrostasis in a metabolically threatening environment.

Erythrostasis

The spherocyte is particularly vulnerable to erythrostasis. This is the basis of the well-known autohemolysis test.[1030] During prolonged sterile incubation in the absence of supplemental glucose, red cells undergo a series of changes that culminate in hemolysis. The sequence of the changes is the same for HS and normal red cells; however, because HS cells are abnormally leaky and bear unstable membranes, their degeneration is accelerated. The importance of the autohemolysis test lies in understanding the pathophysiology and history of HS inasmuch as it is no longer used clinically.

HS red cells are initially jeopardized because their membrane permeability to Na^+ is mildly increased.[970,971] Their propensity to accumulate Na^+ and water is normally balanced by increased Na^+ pumping; however, the increased dependence on glycolysis is detrimental in erythrostasis, where substrate is limited.[971] HS red cells exhaust serum glucose and become ATP depleted more rapidly than normal red cells do. As ATP levels fall, ATP-dependent Na^+,K^+ and Ca^{2+} pumps fail, and the cells gain Na^+ and water and swell. Later, when the Ca^{2+}-dependent K^+ (Gárdos) pathway is activated, K^+ loss predominates

and the cells lose water and shrink. The Na^+ gain is accelerated in HS red cells but is insufficient by itself to induce hemolysis. However, HS red cells are doubly jeopardized. As noted earlier, they are inherently unstable and fragment excessively during metabolic depletion.[989-993] Membrane lipids (and probably integral membrane proteins) are lost at more than twice the normal rate.[991] At first this surface loss is balanced by cell dehydration, but eventually (30 to 48 hours), membrane loss predominates, the cells exceed their critical hemolytic volume, and autohemolysis ensues.

Consequences of Splenic Trapping

Calculations indicate that the average normal red cell passes through the splenic cords about 14,000 times during its lifetime and has an average transit time of 30 to 40 seconds, surprisingly close to measured transient times in normal human spleens in vivo.[1031] The calculated residence time of the average HS red cell in the splenic cords is much longer, perhaps as long as 15 to 150 minutes, but still far short of the time required for metabolic depletion to occur. This conclusion is supported by direct analysis of splenic red cells. HS red cells obtained from the splenic pulp and containing 80% to 100% conditioned cells are moderately cation depleted and show changes in ADP and 2,3-DPG concentrations consistent with metabolism in an acidic environment, but their ATP levels are normal.[977] Others have reported similar results.[1032,1033]

The data suggest that splenic conditioning is caused by mechanisms other than ATP depletion. For example, K^+ loss and membrane instability may be exacerbated by the high concentrations of acids and oxidants that must exist in a spleen filled with activated macrophages lunching on trapped HS red cells. In vitro, oxidants from activated phagocytes can diffuse across the membranes of bystander red cells and damage intracellular proteins within minutes. Red cells moving through the rapid transit pathways in the spleen might escape damage, but those caught in cordal traffic would be vulnerable. Oxidants, even in relatively low concentrations, cause selective K^+ loss by a variety of mechanisms[1034-1036] and also damage membrane skeletal proteins.[1037-1043] Finally, there is preliminary evidence that HS red cells may be abnormally sensitive to oxidants.[1044] When exposed to peroxides, they undergo remarkable blebbing and, presumably, vesiculation. If a similar process occurs in the spleen, it could be responsible for the excessive surface loss observed in conditioned cells.

Residence in the spleen may also activate proteolytic enzymes in the red cell membrane. Membrane proteins of red cells from patients with HS and splenomegaly are excessively digested during in vitro incubations, and the degree of proteolysis correlates with splenic size.[1045] Whether this occurs in vivo is uncertain, but if so it could contribute to skeletal weakness and membrane loss.

The possibility that macrophages may directly condition HS red cells should also be considered. It is well known that spherocytosis often results from the interaction of IgG-coated red cells with macrophages, but HS red cells do not have abnormal levels of surface IgG.[1046] Macrophages also bear receptors for oxidized lipids (scavenger receptor) and PS, but there is no evidence at present that HS red cells expose the relevant ligands. The involvement of macrophages is supported by observations that large doses of corticosteroids markedly ameliorate HS in unsplenectomized patients,[1047,1048] similar to the effects produced by splenectomy. Hemoglobin production, reticulocytosis, and the fecal urobilinogen level decline; red cell life span doubles; and hyperspheroidal, conditioned red cells disappear from the circulation. It is well known that similar doses of corticosteroids inhibit splenic processing and destruction of IgG- or C3b-coated red cells in patients with immunohemolytic anemias, probably by suppressing macrophage-induced red cell sphering and phagocytosis.[1049,1050] Electron microscopy shows that splenic erythrophagocytosis is common in HS, particularly in the splenic cords.[1015,1017,1051] In addition, phagocytes expressed from the cords of patients with HS contain bits of ghost-like "debris,"[1052] presumably resulting from membrane fragmentation.

Summary of Pathophysiology

HS red cells are selectively detained by the spleen, which is detrimental and leads to a loss of membrane surface that fosters further splenic trapping and eventual destruction (Fig. 15-41). The primary membrane defects involve deficiencies or defects in spectrin, ankyrin, protein 4.2, or band 3, but much remains to be learned about why these proteins are defective and how this causes surface loss. Obvious membrane budding and fragmentation are

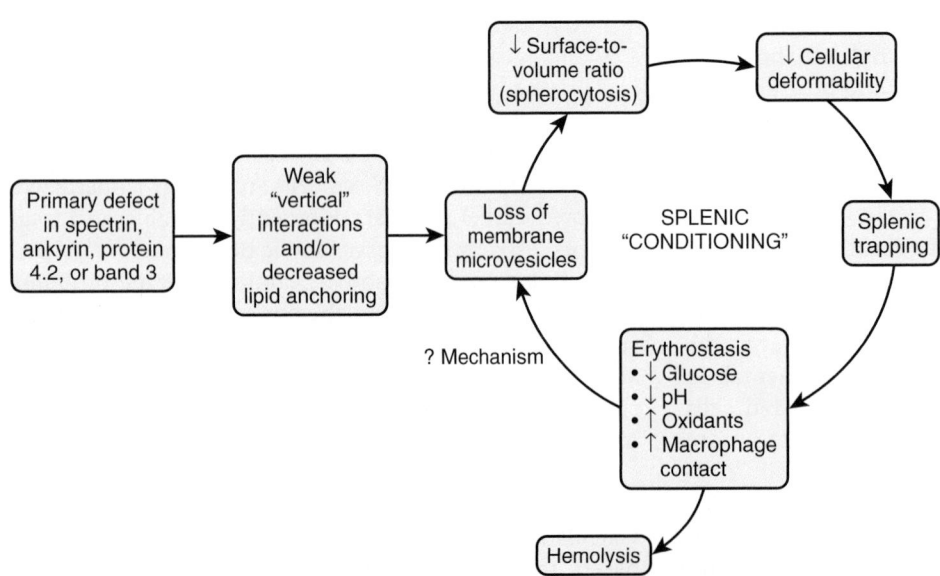

FIGURE 15-41. Pathophysiology of splenic conditioning and destruction of hereditary spherocytosis. *(Redrawn from Walensky LD, Narla M, Lux SE. Disorders of the red cell membrane. In Handin RI, Lux SE, Stossel TP [eds]. Blood: Principles and Practice of Hematology, 2nd ed. Philadelphia, JB Lippincott, 2003, pp 1709-1858, with permission.)*

rare in patients with HS. The HS skeleton (including band 3) may not adequately support all regions of the lipid bilayer, thereby leading to the loss of small areas of untethered lipids and integral membrane proteins. It is not clear whether this is due directly to deficiency of spectrin and ankyrin or whether spectrin/ankyrin deficiency operates indirectly by increasing the lateral mobility of band 3 molecules and decreasing their stabilization of the lipid bilayer.

The mechanisms of splenic conditioning and red cell destruction are also uncertain. Kinetic considerations make it unlikely that HS red cells are continuously trapped in the cords for the long periods required to induce passive sphering and autohemolysis by metabolic depletion; however, repetitious accrual of metabolic damage remains a possibility. A unique susceptibility of the HS red cell to the acidic, oxidant-rich environment of the spleen and active intervention of macrophages in the processing of damaged spherocytes must also be considered.

Laboratory Characteristics

Most of the classic laboratory features of HS are those found in other forms of hemolytic anemia, such as reticulocytosis, erythroid hyperplasia of the bone marrow, indirect hyperbilirubinemia, and increased fecal urobilinogens.[853,854,1053] The plasma hemoglobin level is often normal,[1054] and the haptoglobin value is only variably reduced[1055] because most of the hemoglobin that is released when HS red cells are destroyed is catabolized at the site of destruction, so-called extravascular hemolysis. For the same reasons the LDH level is also often normal. The spherocytic morphology distinguishes HS from other forms of hemolytic anemia, along with laboratory tests that measure biophysical properties of the affected red cells, such as the OF test. Biochemical and molecular testing is performed only in research laboratories because these tests are not as clinically useful.

Red Cell Morphology

Spherocytes (see Fig. 15-30) are the hallmark of HS. They are dense, round, and hyperchromic; lack central pallor; and have a decreased mean cell diameter. They are always present in blood smears from patients with moderate or moderately severe HS but are obvious in only 25% to 35% of patients with mild HS.[837,853,854] Hereditary spherocytes are technically misnamed because they range in shape from thickened discocytes to spherostomatocytes when examined under the scanning electron microscope.[985]

In most patients with HS, spherocytes and microspherocytes are the only abnormal cells on the peripheral smear (other than polychromatophils). Rarely, a few stomatospherocytes may be seen. However, specific morphologic abnormalities have been described in association with certain membrane defects in HS (Fig. 15-42). Patients with ankyrin defects and combined ankyrin/

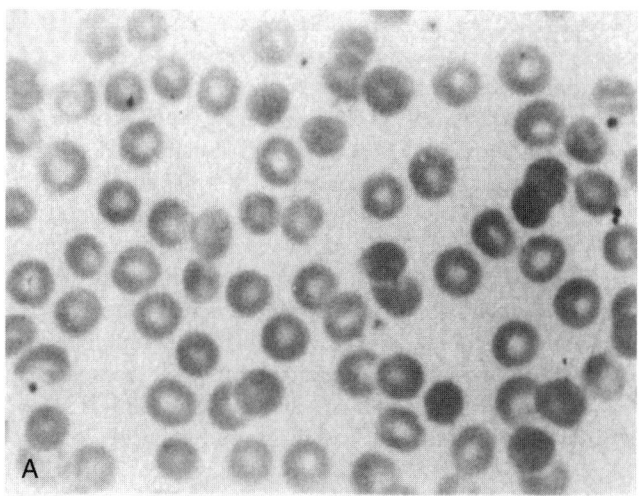

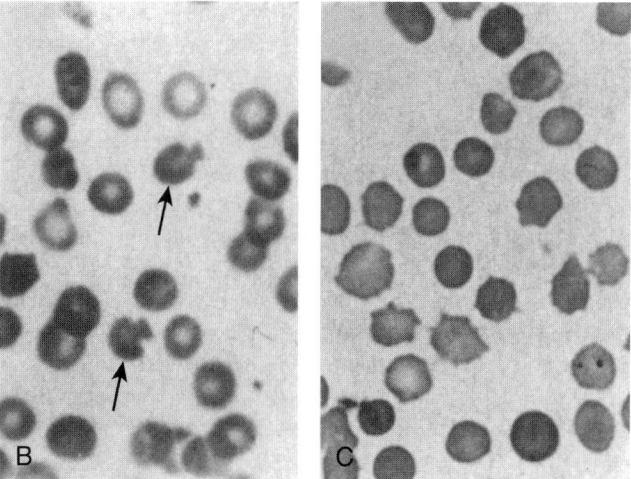

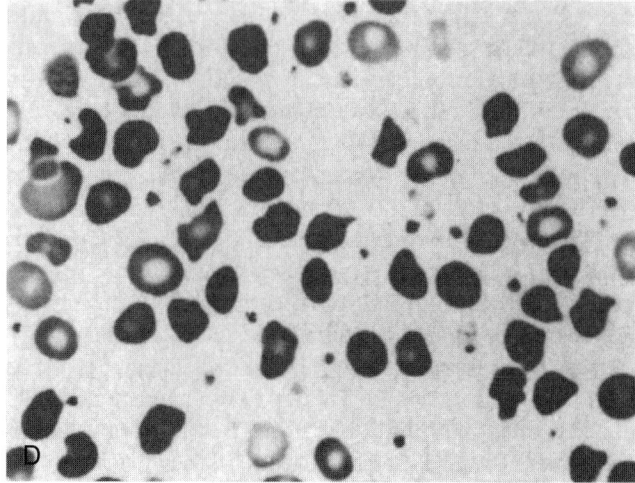

FIGURE 15-42. Red cell morphology in hereditary spherocytosis (HS). **A,** HS caused by an ankyrin defect. Microspherocytes are evident among red cells with some central pallor. **B,** Band 3–deficient HS. Mushroom-shaped ("pincered") red cells (*arrows*) are found in about 80% of patients with this form of HS.[1056] **C,** HS caused by a β-spectrin mutation. Echinocytes and acanthocytes (5% to 15%) are usually observed in addition to typical spherocytes.[906,911] **D,** Severe HS with spherocytes and bizarre poikilocytes. *(From Palek J, Lambert S. Genetics of the red cell membrane. Semin Hematol. 1990;27:290.)*

spectrin deficiency, the most common subgroup, have typical spherocytes and microspherocytes on the peripheral blood smear (see Fig. 15-42A).[923] In addition to spherocytes, acanthocytes or hyperchromic echinocytes are present in many patients with β-spectrin defects (see Fig. 15-42C).[906,911] Other patients with β-spectrin defects, especially truncated β chains, have spherocytic elliptocytosis. In severe HS caused by homozygous α-spectrin mutations, compound heterozygous α-spectrin mutations, or severe ankyrin/spectrin deficiency, misshapen spherocytes, spiculated red cells, and bizarre poikilocytes may be seen and even dominate the blood smear (see Fig. 15-42D). Most patients with band 3–deficient HS have a small number of mushroom-shaped red cells or pincered cells on their peripheral blood smears (see Fig. 15-42B).[1056] Red cell morphology is variable in protein 4.2 deficiency and may even be normal. Acanthopoikilocytes and ovalostomatocytes[1057] have also been observed. Other patients have typical spherocytosis.[950]

In contrast to red cells in autoimmune hemolytic anemia, studies have recently shown that HS red cells lose their surface area in the bone marrow inasmuch as similar decreases in red cell surface area have been found in reticulocytes in HS as in mature red blood cells.[998] HS erythrocytes then gradually lose surface area in the circulation, as is typical with normal erythrocytes. Nucleated red cells are uncommon in blood smears,[853] except in the most severe forms of HS.[871] Howell-Jolly bodies are also uncommon before splenectomy (4% of patients)[853] and suggest reticuloendothelial blockade.

Red Cell Indices

Most patients have mild to moderate HS with mild anemia (hemoglobin level of 9 to 12 g/dL) or no anemia at all (so-called compensated hemolysis). In moderate to severe HS, the hemoglobin concentration ranges from 6 to 9 g/dL. In patients with the most severe disease, the hemoglobin concentration may drop to as low as 4 to 5 g/dL.

The mean corpuscular hemoglobin concentration (MCHC) of HS red cells is increased because of relative cellular dehydration.[854] Spherocyte Na^+ concentrations are normal or slightly increased, but the K^+ concentration and water content are low, particularly in cells harvested from the splenic pulp.[977,1058-1060] The average MCHC exceeds the upper limit of normal (36%) in about half of the patients with HS, but all patients have some dehydrated cells.[854] An MCHC greater than 35 g/dL has a sensitivity of 70% and a specificity of 86%.[1061] Combining the MCHC with the red cell distribution width (RDW) may lead to a specificity approaching 100%.[1061]

Mean corpuscular volume (MCV) falls within the normal range in HS,[854] except in severe HS, in which the MCV may be slightly low.[871] However, MCV is relatively low for the age of the cells (reticulocytes have a high MCV) in all patients with HS as a result of the dehydrated state of HS red cells. Reticulocyte MCV is also low, which contrasts with the spherocytosis in autoim-

mune hemolytic anemia, in which the reticulocyte indices are normal.

Detection of hyperdense red cells by dual-angle laser scattering is now used as a diagnostic tool.[1062] The Technicon H1 blood counter and its successors (Technicon Corp., Tarrytown, NY), which measure MCV by light scattering, provide a histogram of MCHCs that has been claimed to be accurate enough to identify nearly all patients with HS.[1060,1063,1064] In a sample of HS red cells, there is a right shift of the hemoglobin concentration histogram with a population of hyperdense cells (MCHC > 40 g/dL) because of red cell dehydration and broadening of the volume curve because of the mixture of microspherocytes and large reticulocytes (Fig. 15-43). This simple method may be one of the easiest and most accurate ways to diagnose HS, particularly when one member of a family is already known to have HS and an inexpensive method of screening other family members is desired. Some studies have shown that in HS patients with an intact spleen, the percentage of microcytes reflects the severity of disease and the percentage of hyperdense cells discriminates HS patients from normal individuals.[1065] Similar diagnostic information can be obtained through the use of aperture impedance (Coulter) analyzers.[1061] The elevated MCHC and wide RDW suggests the diagnosis of HS.

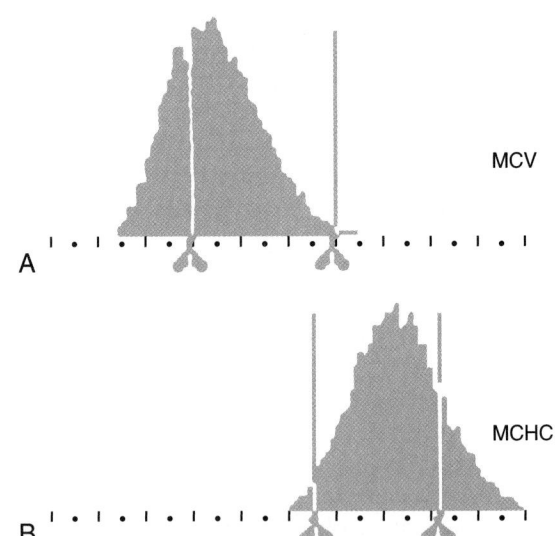

FIGURE 15-43. Histogram of the distribution of mean corpuscular volume (MCV) (**A**) and mean corpuscular hemoglobin concentration (MCHC) (**B**) in the red cells of a patient with hereditary spherocytosis before splenectomy. The *vertical lines* mark the normal limits of distribution. For the volume distribution, they separate microcytic (<60 fL) and macrocytic (>120 fL) cells from normocytic red cells (60 to 120 fL). For the hemoglobin concentration distribution, they separate hypochromic (<28 g/dL) and hyperdense (>41 g/dL) cells from normochromic cells (28 to 41 g/dL). The data were collected with a Technicon H1 laser scattering blood counter. Note that the patient with hereditary spherocytosis has subpopulations of microcytes (low MCV) and dehydrated cells (high MCHC). All patients in this study (N = 21) had similar subpopulations. (*Redrawn from Pati AR, Patton WN, Harris RI. The use of the Technicon H1 in the diagnosis of hereditary spherocytosis. Clin Lab Haematol. 1989;11:27-30.*)

Fragility and Autohemolysis Tests

Osmotic Fragility Test. OF testing (see Fig. 15-40) is performed by suspending red cells in increasingly hypotonic buffered NaCl.[1021,1066,1067] In hypotonic solutions, normal erythrocytes are able to increase their volume by swelling until they become spherical and burst, with release of hemoglobin into the supernatant. Cells that begin with a decreased surface-to-volume ratio, such as spherocytes or stomatocytes, reach the spherical limit at a higher NaCl concentration than normal cells do and are termed osmotically fragile. Freshly drawn red cells from approximately a fourth of individuals with HS will have a normal OF, with the OF curve approximating the number of spherocytes seen on the peripheral smear.[855,1068] When the spleen is present, a subpopulation of very fragile erythrocytes that have been conditioned by the spleen form the "tail" of the OF curve. This tail disappears after splenectomy.

The incubated OF test is thought to be more sensitive than the unincubated OF test, although this is not well proven. The incubated OF test is performed the same way as the unincubated test (as earlier) except that the whole blood sample is first incubated for 24 hours at 37° C. During incubation, the HS erythrocytes become metabolically depleted and lose membrane fragments rapidly, which accentuates their spheroidicity and increases the sensitive of the OF test. OF testing, particularly the incubated OF test, is the most sensitive test routinely available for diagnosing HS.[1068] The sensitivity of OF testing is surprising because OF reflects a combination of secondary properties of HS red cells—loss of surface area relative to the loss of K^+ and water—instead of the primary molecular defect in the membrane skeletons. Although HS patients with a negative incubated OF test have been described,[1069] the incubated OF test is the gold standard for the diagnosis of HS.

Acidified Glycerol Lysis Test and Pink Test. The glycerol lysis test, in which glycerol is used to retard the osmotic swelling of red cells, was developed as an alternative to the OF test. In this test, red cells are incubated in glycerol–sodium phosphate–buffered hypotonic saline solution. Glycerol slows the entry of water into cells so that the time for the cells to lyse is prolonged and can be measured accurately. The glycerol lysis time is shortened for HS red cells because of the reduced surface-to-volume ratio.

The original glycerol lysis test lacked sensitivity and specificity.[1070] An acidified version, the AGLT, was more sensitive for some researchers[1069] but was not completely specific.[1071] For unknown reasons, the accuracy of the standard AGLT is greatly improved if the samples are preincubated at room temperature for 24 hours (incubated AGLT).[1072-1074] Under these conditions, the sensitivity and specificity of the test approach 100%, similar to that for the incubated OF test.

Eber and associates[835] found that changing the concentration of the sodium phosphate buffer from 5.3 to 9.3 mmol/L gives 100% sensitivity and specificity without the need for preincubation. The modified test is easy to perform and requires very little blood. Ethylenediaminetetraacetic acid (EDTA)-anticoagulated blood (20 μL) is diluted into a solution of 9.3 mmol/L sodium phosphate and buffered 2 mol/L glycerol-saline (pH 6.90), and the fall in absorbance at 625 nm (largely turbidity) is measured as the red cells hemolyze. The half-time for lysis in the AGLT is longer than 30 minutes for normal samples and less than 5 minutes for HS samples. The simplicity of this test allows it to be used for rapid screening of a large number of blood samples.

Another adaptation of the original glycerol lysis test, called the *Pink test*, is more reproducible and accurate than the original[1075] but requires a 1-day preincubation.[1076] Modifications of the test have made it adaptable to microsize samples (e.g., fingerstick blood samples).[1076,1077] However, direct comparisons suggest that it is less specific than the OF test or incubated AGLT.[1072] Because the modified AGLT has also been adapted to microsamples,[1076,1077] it would appear to be the test of choice if OF testing is not available.

Hypertonic Cryohemolysis Test. This method is based on the fact that HS red cells are particularly sensitive to cooling at 0° C in hypertonic solutions, which causes the cells to lyse and release hemoglobin.[1078,1079] It has been claimed that this test is 94% to 100% sensitive for HS, but its specificity is only 94% for normal individuals and 86% for patients with autoimmune hemolytic anemia. The advantages of this test are its simplicity, high sensitivity, and the ability to use EDTA-preserved blood specimens. The limitations lie in its inadequate specificity, and therefore it is currently rarely used for clinical diagnosis.

Autohemolysis Test. Autohemolysis of erythrocytes after 48 hours at 37° C is normally less than 5% in the absence of glucose or less than 1% in the presence of glucose. Autohemolysis of spherocytes is increased to 15% to 45% in the absence of glucose.[855,1030,1080] In HS, the degree of autohemolysis is reduced by the addition of glucose,[855,1059,1080] whereas in red cell glycolytic disorders and acquired disorders such as immune-mediated anemias, the degree of autohemolysis is not reduced. Although this differentiation may be helpful occasionally, the autohemolysis test is time consuming and cumbersome, gives variable results, and is rarely performed.

Ektacytometry

The ektacytometer can be used to assess the surface-to-volume ratio and membrane mechanical strength of red cells in patients with hemolytic disorders.[1081-1083] The ektacytometer is described in detail in the sections on HE and HPP. The best method for demonstrating the low surface-to-volume ratio of hereditary spherocytes is osmotic gradient ektacytometry, a modification of the original technique that is useful in the diagnosis of

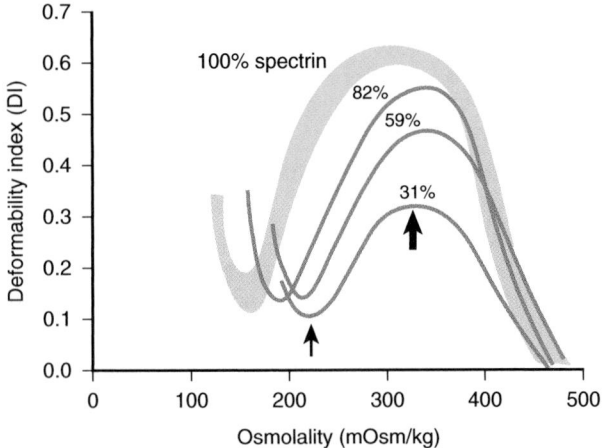

FIGURE 15-44. Osmotic gradient ektacytometry of HS erythrocytes with differing degrees of spectrin deficiency. In HS red cells (*brown lines*), the minimum deformability index observed in the hypotonic region (*thin arrow*) is shifted to the right of the control region (*blue shaded area*), thus indicating a decrease in the cell surface area–to-volume ratio. The maximum deformability index (DI_{max}) associated with spectrin-deficient HS red cells (*thick arrow*) is less than that of control cells because of the reduced surface area of HS cells. The more pronounced the spectrin deficiency, the greater the loss of surface area and the lower the DI_{max}. The osmolality in the hyperosmolar region at which the DI reaches half its maximum value is a measure of the hydration state of the red cells. It is decreased in HS patients with the lowest spectrin content, indicative of cellular dehydration. (*Adapted from Tse WT, Lux SE. Hereditary spherocytosis and hereditary elliptocytosis. In Scriver CR, Beaudet AL, Sly WS, Valle D [eds]. The Metabolic and Molecular Bases of Inherited Disease, 8th ed. New York, McGraw-Hill, 2001. p 4665.*)

HS.[1084,1085] In this method, the "deformability index" (a measure of the average elongation of sheared red cells) is measured as a function of the osmolarity of the suspended medium, which is continuously varied (Fig. 15-44). The osmolarity of the suspending medium at which the red cell deformability index reaches a minimum is the same as the osmolarity at which 50% of the red cells hemolyze in an OF test.[1084] This value is an indirect measure of the surface area–to-volume ratio of the red cells.[1085] The maximum deformability index reflects the surface area of the red cells. In HS, the curve is shifted to the right because of the reduced surface area–to-volume ratio of the cells. The height of the curve is also decreased in HS as a result of the decreased absolute surface area of the erythrocytes. One study demonstrated a 100% rate of detection of HS with osmotic gradient ektacytometry and only a 66% rate of detection of HS with the OF test in the same population.[1085] Although this method provides useful diagnostic information, only a few laboratories are equipped with the instrument for this test.

Membrane Protein, RNA, and DNA Measurements

Specialized tests are occasionally used to study patients with complicated disease or those for whom additional information is desired. Useful tests for these purposes include structural and functional studies of erythrocyte membrane proteins, such as protein quantitation, limited tryptic digestion of spectrin, membrane protein synthesis and assembly, or ion transport studies. Membrane fragility may be examined with an ektacytometer.

Membrane protein concentrations are usually assessed with SDS gels. Individual stained bands are quantified by densitometry or by eluting the dye from an excised band and measuring its concentration spectrophotometrically. This technique is satisfactory for detecting spectrin deficiency (expressed as a spectrin-to–band 3 ratio),[851] although it is not as accurate as radioimmunoassay[891] or enzyme-linked immunoassay.[851] With densitometry, spectrin and ankyrin deficiencies may be underestimated because it normalizes them to band 3, which is partially lost along with membrane lipids as spherocytes circulate. As a result, the spectrin-to–band 3 ratio is lower after splenectomy. This is even more true for ankyrin, which is present in smaller amounts and migrates close to β-spectrin on gels. SDS gels do not routinely give reliable results even with a gel system that optimizes spectrin/ankyrin separation.[871] The popular Laemmli gels are unsatisfactory because ankyrin migrates between the spectrin bands in this system. Immunoassays, on the other hand, work well.[851,859] SDS gels are satisfactory for detecting band 3 deficiency (elevated spectrin-to–band 3 ratio) or protein 4.2 deficiency, and they are useful in combination with antibody staining (Western blots) for detecting mutant proteins of altered size. Band 3 can also be quantified by fluorescence, taking advantage of the fact that eosin maleimide reacts exclusively with band 3 on the surface of intact red cells.

However, SDS gels do not always identify the abnormal protein in HS because missense mutations may cause functional defects rather than quantitative defects and because protein deficiencies may be as small as 10%. Therefore, several other approaches have been described in an attempt to define specific molecular defects. In families with multiple affected members, linkage analysis has been performed to include or exclude the candidate genes. In addition, suspected proteins can be sequenced by direct nucleotide sequence analysis of polymerase chain reaction (PCR)-amplified cDNA or genomic DNA. Currently, no commercial laboratories will identify the molecular defects in HS membrane proteins, and therefore these analyses are performed only by a few research laboratories. Nevertheless, the HS membrane protein mutations are mostly defects restricted to specific families and do not predict the severity of the disease, and thus the ability to detect the exact molecular defect is not often clinically important.

Differential Diagnosis

In general, HS is easily diagnosed in patients with the typical laboratory findings of spherocytosis, such as Coombs-negative hemolysis, increased OF, and a positive family history. However, HS must be differentiated from other causes of spherocytosis, and there are several situations in which diagnosis can be difficult. Other causes of spherocytosis are listed in Box 15-1.

ABO Incompatibility in Neonates. In the neonatal period it may be challenging to differentiate HS from ABO incompatibility.[1086] Anemia, hyperbilirubinemia, circulating microspherocytes, and altered OF are found in both conditions, and results of the direct Coombs test are sometimes negative in ABO incompatibility. However, in most affected infants with ABO incompatibility, anti-A (or anti-B) antibodies can be eluted from the red cells, and free anti-A (or anti-B) IgG antibodies can be detected in the infant's serum.

Immunohemolytic Anemias. Rarely, patients with immunohemolytic anemia and spherocytosis also have so few antibody molecules attached to their red cells that results of the direct Coombs test are negative. In these rare cases, differentiation of the disease from HS is possible only with the use of radioactive antiglobulin reagents, the so-called super-Coombs test.[1087]

Heinz Body Hemolytic Anemias. Spherocytosis is also seen in Heinz body hemolytic anemias during an acute hemolytic crisis and occasionally in the steady state. However, in this situation, bite cells or blister cells (or both) and various dense, irregular cells are always present on the peripheral blood smear, and Heinz bodies can often be detected in red cells supravitally stained with methyl violet.

Aplastic Crises. Diagnostic difficulty may also arise in HS patients who are seen during an aplastic crisis (see later). Early in the crisis, the acute nature of the symptoms may suggest an acquired process, and the absence of reticulocytes may divert the physician from a diagnosis of hemolytic anemia. Later, as marrow function returns, physicians may occasionally be misled by the properties of the emerging young HS red cells, which are less spherocytic and osmotically fragile than usual.

Conditions That Camouflage Hereditary Spherocytosis

HS may be camouflaged by disorders that increase the surface-to-volume ratio of red cells, such as iron deficiency,[1088] vitamin B_{12} or folate deficiency,[1089] obstructive jaundice,[986] β-thalassemia,[1090] or hemoglobin SC disease.[1091] In these types of difficult cases, additional tools, such as immunoassays for red cell membrane proteins and osmotic gradient ektacytometry, may be necessary to confirm the diagnosis of HS.

Iron deficiency corrects the abnormal shape, fragility, and high MCHC of hereditary spherocytes but does not improve their life span.[1088] Megaloblastic anemia can

likewise mask the morphologic characteristics of HS.[1089] OF is also improved. The masking effect is observed in both vitamin B_{12} and folate deficiency and is rapidly reversed after correction of the nutritional deficit.

When obstructive jaundice develops, spherocytosis is transiently improved, and results of the OF test and hemolysis laboratory indices normalize.[986] This improvement is due to the expansion of red cell membrane surface area that follows the increased uptake of cholesterol and phospholipids from the abnormal plasma lipoproteins released by the obstructed liver. In normal cells, this increase in surface area leads to the formation of target cells, but in spherocytes, it leads to the appearance of discocytes. For example, we have seen a 6-year old child in whom jaundice and symptoms of biliary obstruction developed. She had a palpable spleen tip, evidence of mild compensated hemolysis (hemoglobin concentration of 14 g/dL; reticulocyte count of 3.3%), a normal peripheral blood smear, and normal results of an OF test (fresh and incubated cells). Abdominal radiographic studies showed calcified stones in the gallbladder and common bile duct. After cholecystectomy and relief of the partial biliary obstruction, the child's hemolysis worsened (reticulocyte count of 10.8%), and anemia (hemoglobin concentration of 10.2 g/dL), spherocytosis, and abnormal results on an incubated OF test developed. She subsequently underwent splenectomy with clinical improvement.

The coexistence of HS and β-thalassemia trait has been described in a few case reports and has been reported to worsen,[1092,1093] ameliorate,[1090,1094] or have no effect on the clinical status of the patient. In a large French family with independently segregating HS and β-thalassemia trait, patients with both traits had signs of both diseases: small, hemoglobin A_2–rich, osmotically fragile cells and some spherocytes on peripheral blood smears. However, the HS phenotype in these patients was less severe than that of family members with HS but without β-thalassemia trait.[1090]

Coinheritance of HS and hemoglobin SC disease may exacerbate the hemoglobinopathy.[1091] A 15-year-old boy with both diseases was much more anemic than his siblings with SC hemoglobin disease and experienced five splenic sequestration crises. However, the two diseases may also disguise each other morphologically. Only a few spherocytes or target cells were evident on the boy's blood smear, and the surface-to-volume ratio of his red cells (and probably their OF) was normal. This is probably due to the balancing effects of HS (loss of surface area) and hemoglobin SC (loss of cell volume) on red cells.

Sickle trait may also be worsened by HS.[1095,1096] Yang and colleagues[1097] reported two patients with the combination who suffered multiple splenic sequestration crises. On the other hand, spontaneous regression of HS, presumably as a result of the development of a hyposplenic state, has also been observed in two family members who had HS and sickle cell trait.[1098]

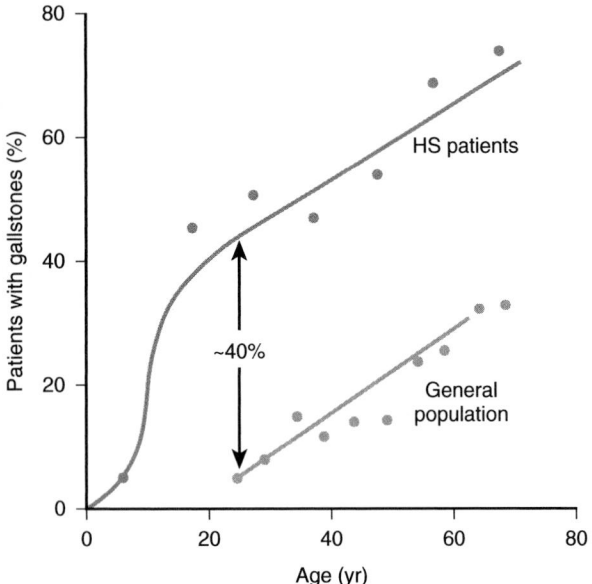

FIGURE 15-45. Proportion of normal and hereditary spherocytosis (HS) patients with gallstones as a function of age. The graph is redrawn from data in a study[1100] of gallbladder disease in 152 consecutive patients seen at The Cleveland Clinic before 1952. Only patients whose gallbladders were examined at surgery or by cholecystography are included. Data for the general population are derived from an autopsy series of patients who did not have hemolytic anemia.[1101] Note that the prevalence of gallstones in HS patients rises sharply between the ages of 10 and 30 years and parallels the general population after 30 years of age. *(Adapted with permission from Walensky LD, Narla M, Lux SE. Disorders of the red cell membrane. In Handin RI, Lux SE, Stossel TP [eds]. Blood: Principles and Practice of Hematology, 2nd ed. Philadelphia, JB Lippincott, 2003, pp 1709-1858.)*

Complications

Most patients with HS have well-compensated hemolysis and are rarely symptomatic. These patients seek medical attention only when complications occur. Complications are generally related to chronic hemolysis and anemia.

Gallstones

The formation of bilirubinate gallstones is one of the most common complications of HS and is a major impetus for splenectomy in many patients. Instances of gallstones occurring in infancy[1099] have been reported, but most appear in adolescents and young adults. In a retrospective study of 152 consecutive patients with HS conducted before the development of ultrasonography, gallstones were detected in only 5% of children younger than 10 years who were adequately examined and in approximately 50% of HS patients between 10 and 30 years of age (Fig. 15-45).[1100] The increase in incidence of gallstones after the age of 30 parallels the incidence in the general population,[1101] which suggests that cholelithiasis secondary to HS is primarily manifested in the second and third decades.

The incidence of gallstones in HS patients is related to the ability of the liver to metabolize increased amounts of bilirubin. A common polymorphism in the promoter of the uridine diphosphate–glucuronyl transferase gene (*UGT1A*) causes decreased enzyme production and, in the homozygous form, Gilbert's syndrome. Recent studies have clearly demonstrated that coinheritance of Gilbert's syndrome and HS increases the risk for cholelithiasis.[1102-1105] One retrospective study of 103 children with HS showed that the rate of gallstone formation was 2.19 times higher in patients with a homozygous mutation in the *UGT1A* gene than in those with a heterozygous mutation and 4.5 times higher than in HS patients lacking the Gilbert polymorphism.[1102] Recent studies also demonstrate that gallstones develop at a younger age in HS patients with a homozygous mutation in the *UGT1A* gene.[1106] Therefore, analysis of this allele is useful in predicting the risk for cholelithiasis in HS.

Because the pigment stones typical of HS are easily detected by ultrasonography, all patients with HS should undergo ultrasound examinations about every 5 years if the spleen is intact and just before splenectomy. Unfortunately, longitudinal studies using modern techniques (i.e., liver and biliary tree ultrasonography) are not available, thus making the true incidence and natural history of gallstones in this population unknown. Indeed, many patients with gallstones are asymptomatic, and it is unclear in how many patients symptomatic gallbladder disease or biliary obstruction will develop. Anecdotal reports in the old HS literature suggested that 40% to 50% of HS patients with cholelithiasis had symptoms and that a high proportion of patients with stone-containing gallbladders had histologic evidence of cholecystitis.[1107] However, studies that include large numbers of patients with mild HS show a much lower incidence of symptomatic gallbladder disease.[1108] Clearly, more accurate data about the long-term complications of pigment stone disease are needed to assess the risk-to-benefit ratio of splenectomy in HS and the need for cholecystectomy in asymptomatic patients with cholelithiasis.

Because of the lack of knowledge about the natural history of cholelithiasis in HS, the treatment of gallbladder disease in HS patients is debatable. Once gallstones are found, an initial observation period is recommended.[1109] Surgery is indicated for recurrent symptoms or signs of biliary obstruction. If a patient is undergoing splenectomy, ultrasound of the gallbladder is indicated before surgery to assess for the necessity of concomitant cholecystectomy.[1110] Prophylactic cholecystectomy or splenectomy solely to prevent the formation of gallstones is not indicated. One analysis[1111] offers the following recommendations for adult patients who have not undergone splenectomy and in whom gallstones develop: for patients younger than 39 years, both splenectomy and cholecystectomy should be performed even if the patient has no symptoms; for patients between 39 and 52 years of age, both operations should only be performed if the patient has biliary colic; if a patient is older than 52 years, cholecystectomy alone should be performed for biliary colic.

TABLE 15-5	**Classification of Crises**				
Type	**Anemia**	**Reticulocytes**	**Jaundice**	**Cause**	**Comment**
Hemolytic	Increased	Increased	Increased	Viral infections leading to splenomegaly	Frequent, usually mild
Aplastic	Increased	Decreased	Decreased	Parvovirus B19	Occurs once Severe. Risk to pregnant contacts
Megaloblastic	Increased	No change or decreased	No change or increased	Relative folic acid deficiency	Rare, preventable

Crises

Patients with HS, like patients with other hemolytic diseases such as sickle cell disease, face a number of potential crises. Table 15-5 summarizes the types of crises that occur in patients with HS.

Hemolytic Crises. Hemolytic crises are probably the most common form of crisis in HS. They usually occur with viral syndromes, particularly in children younger than 6 years.[1112] They are characterized by a mild transient increase in jaundice, splenomegaly, anemia, and reticulocytosis. No medical intervention is usually required. Some of these patients may actually be in the recovery phase of an aplastic crisis. Severe hemolytic crises occur rarely. Characteristic features include jaundice, anemia, vomiting, abdominal pain, and tender splenomegaly. In such cases, hospitalization, red cell transfusion, and careful monitoring may be required.

Aplastic Crises. Aplastic crises are less common than hemolytic crises but are more serious and may lead to severe anemia and result in congestive heart failure or even death.[856] These crises are usually caused by parvovirus B19, the cause of erythema infectiosum (fifth disease).[1113] Parvovirus B19 infection may be accompanied by fever, chills, lethargy, vomiting, diarrhea, myalgia, and a maculopapular rash on the face (slapped cheek appearance), trunk, and extremities.[1114] In addition, an HS patient having an aplastic crisis may experience anemia, jaundice, pallor, and weakness.[1115,1116] Parvovirus B19 selectively infects erythropoietic precursors and inhibits their growth by inducing apoptosis and cell cycle arrest at G_2.[1117-1120] Parvovirus infections are often associated with mild neutropenia ($\approx$20%) or thrombocytopenia ($\approx$40%), and instances of transient pancytopenia have been reported.[1113,1121-1123] Parvovirus may infect several members of a family simultaneously.[1123-1127]

The sequence of events in an aplastic crisis is well described in the classic article of Owren[1115] and is illustrated in Figure 15-46. During the aplastic phase, the hematocrit and reticulocyte count fall, marrow erythroblasts disappear, and unused iron accumulates in serum. As production of new red cells declines, the cells that remain age, and microspherocytosis and OF increase. Bilirubin levels may decrease as the number of abnormal red cells that can be destroyed declines. Return of marrow

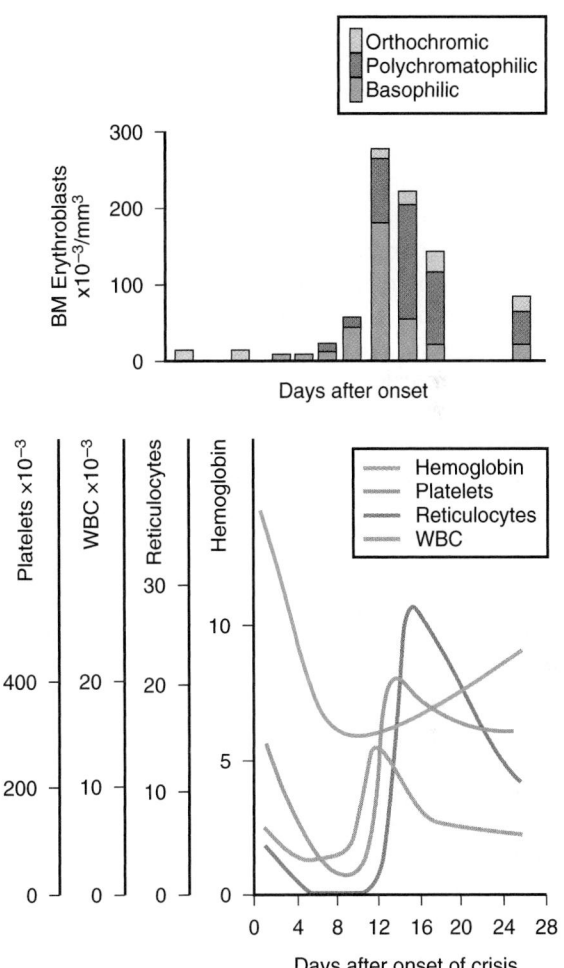

FIGURE 15-46. The temporal sequence of a severe aplastic crisis in a patient with hereditary spherocytosis who previously had well-compensated hemolysis. Note the profound reticulocytopenia and mild leukopenia and thrombocytopenia in the early phases of the reaction. Note also that the re-emergence of reticulocytes is heralded by the sequential return of peripheral blood granulocytes and platelets and bone marrow (BM) normoblasts. As in this patient, jaundice frequently declines during an aplastic crisis because of a decrease in the total number of abnormal red cells that have to be destroyed. WBC, white blood cells. (*Data from Owren PA. Congenital hemolytic jaundice. The pathogenesis of the "hemolytic crisis." Blood. 1948;3:231.*)

function is heralded by a fall in the serum iron concentration and the emergence of granulocytes, platelets, and finally, reticulocytes. During this recovery phase, serum phosphorus can drop to dangerously low levels.[1128] Furthermore, the lack of reticulocytes early in the recovery phase should not eliminate hemolytic anemias from diagnostic consideration.

Infection with parvovirus B19 is a particular danger to susceptible pregnant women because it can infect the fetus and lead to fetal anemia, nonimmune hydrops fetalis, and fetal demise.[1129-1131] The risk of nonimmune hydrops fetalis in the fetus of a woman who becomes infected with B19 during pregnancy is probably low. Nevertheless, because the virus is highly contagious and is easily transmitted to patients and staff[1132,1133] and because only half to two thirds of pregnant women have acquired protective antibodies,[1134] it has been suggested that patients who have or are suspected of having an aplastic crisis be placed on precautions while hospitalized and that IgG-negative contacts who are pregnant be tested for evidence of seroconversion. Nonimmune hydrops fetalis can be detected by ultrasonography and treated with intrauterine transfusions.[1135]

During an aplastic crisis, many asymptomatic patients with HS and compensated hemolysis receive medical attention. As would be expected, aplastic crises develop at the same time in many family members with undiagnosed HS who are infected with parvovirus B19.[1123,1124,1136-1138] Diagnostic confusion may arise during re-emergence of marrow function, when the physician may mistake an aplastic crisis for a hemolytic one. Because aplastic crises generally last 10 to 14 days[1115] (about half the life span of HS red cells),[1031,1139] the hemoglobin value typically falls to about half its usual level before recovery occurs. Thus, aplastic crises are a serious threat to young children with HS, particularly those with more severe forms of the disease. Intensive medical management is required in these cases.

The diagnosis of parvovirus infection can be made with serum PCR or immunologic tests. Pathologic examination of the bone marrow demonstrates giant pronormoblasts, which are a hallmark of the cytopathic effects of parvovirus B19.[1140,1141] Treatment is supportive until the aplastic episode self-resolves. In children with severe anemia, red cell transfusions may be necessary. In immunocompromised patients, intravenous immunoglobulin assists in clearing the virus. Respiratory and contact precautions, from before the onset of symptoms to at least 1 week after symptoms appear, assist in preventing spread of the virus. Immunity after parvovirus infection is lifelong.

Megaloblastic Crises. Rarely, HS patients may have megaloblastic crises as a result of folate deficiency. These crises occur in patients whose dietary intake of folic acid is inadequate for the increased needs of the red cell precursors in the bone marrow. Therefore, megaloblastic crises typically occur in patients with HS who are recovering from an aplastic crisis or who are pregnant.[873,874] In these patients, dietary intake of folic acid is inadequate for the increased needs of the erythroid HS bone marrow. A megaloblastic crisis in pregnancy has been reported as the first manifestation of HS. All patients with hemolytic anemia, including HS before splenectomy, should routinely receive folic acid supplements ($\approx$1 mg/day) to prevent this complication.

Other Complications

Gout and Leg Ulcers. Rarely, gout,[1142,1143] indolent leg ulcers,[1144,1145] or a chronic erythematous dermatitis on the legs develops in adults with HS.[1146,1147] Splenectomy appears to be curative.

Extramedullary Hematopoiesis. Extramedullary masses of hematopoietic tissue, particularly alongside the posterior thoracic or lumbar spine[831,1143,1148-1153] or in the hila of the kidneys, may also develop in adults with HS.[831] These masses may spontaneously bleed and lead to hemothorax.[1151] In one unusual instance, extramedullary hematopoiesis simulated an adrenal mass in a 9-year-old boy with HS.[1154] Surprisingly, these tumors frequently arise in patients with mild HS, perhaps because they often do not undergo splenectomy, and are the first manifestations of HS. The masses gradually enlarge and may be mistaken for neoplasms.[1143] Biopsy may lead to extensive bleeding. If necessary, open biopsy should be performed. These bone marrow tumors can be diagnosed by magnetic resonance imaging (MRI),[1155] which may make biopsies unnecessary. The masses stop growing and undergo fatty metamorphosis after splenectomy, but they do not shrink in size.[1148,1149]

Hematologic Malignancy. Over a dozen occurrences of HS and hematologic malignancy, including myeloproliferative disorders, multiple myeloma, and leukemia, have been reported.[1156-1159] It has been suggested that this association is due to long-standing hematopoietic stress or chronic reticuloendothelial stimulation because splenic clearance of abnormal red cells induces proliferation of lymphocytes and plasma cells, as well as macrophages.[1160] Patients with HS have a mild polyclonal hypergammaglobulinemia,[1156-1158,1160] and there is some evidence favoring the association of myeloma and chronic gallbladder disease.[1156,1161] However, it is not currently clear whether there is a true connection between HS and myeloma or myeloproliferative disease or a chance association.

Hemochromatosis. Untreated HS may exacerbate hemochromatosis in patients who are heterozygous for the hereditary disease.[1162-1165] Several patients with HS subsequently died of liver failure or hepatoma.

Heart Disease. Untreated HS may aggravate underlying heart disease and precipitate heart failure.[1166] Gradually worsening congestive heart failure may rarely be the initial manifestation in an elderly patient with HS in whom progressively worsening anemia has developed as marrow senescence evolves.

Angioid Streaks. These brownish or gray streaks resembling veins in the optic fundus have been described in adult members of several HS kindreds.[1167,1168] The rate of occurrence of this association is unknown. Angioid streaks are relatively common in some other hematologic disorders, notably sickle cell disease and thalassemia,[1167,1169] and may be complicated by retinal vascular proliferation that requires treatment.[1170]

Pseudohyperkalemia. Because HS red cells leak potassium ions more rapidly than normal red cells do, serum samples from HS patients may demonstrate pseudohyperkalemia if allowed to sit for a long time before electrolytes are analyzed.[1171]

Splenic Rupture. Although splenomegaly is a common symptom in HS patients, cases of splenic rupture are rare.[1172] This contrasts significantly with the splenomegaly that accompanies acute viral infections such as Epstein-Barr virus, in which splenic rupture occurs at higher frequency. It is unclear why this difference exists, although it may reflect the unique pathophysiology of splenic enlargement in the different conditions. Children with HS and splenomegaly should not be restricted from normal activities. However, older children and adults with splenic enlargement that extends below the rib cage should avoid activities that may inflict a powerful, direct blow to the abdomen, such as football or ice hockey.

Nonerythroid Manifestations. Kindreds with HS and neurologic manifestations have been described. In the older literature, multiple case reports describe patients with HS and various neurologic abnormalities such as Freidrich-like disease, cerebellar disturbances, muscle atrophy, and a tabes-like syndrome.[1173-1176] More recently, patients with certain ankyrin gene deletions have been reported who have psychomotor retardation, hypogonadism, and various neurologic manifestations.[847,848,870,917-919] Additional reports describe patients with ankyrin-deficient HS and slowly progressive spinocerebellar disease.[1173] The discoveries that erythroid ankyrin[662-665] and β-spectrin[430] are expressed in the cerebellum and spinal cord and that delayed cerebellar ataxia develops in mice with a lack of ankyrin because of slow loss of Purkinje cells[1177] suggest that unique types of ankyrin and β-spectrin mutations may affect the neurologic system, in addition to red blood cells.

Families with HS and hypertrophic cardiomyopathy have also been reported. For example, a three-generation Russian family with cosegregating HS and hypertrophic cardiomyopathy has been described.[1178] Two brothers with HS, a movement disorder, and myopathy have also been reported.[1179] These cases are interesting because spectrin and ankyrin are known to be expressed in muscle.

Splenectomy

Splenectomy cures all patients with typical mild to moderate HS by eliminating anemia and hyperbilirubinemia and reducing the reticulocyte count to nearly normal levels (1% to 3%). In most patients, red cell survival becomes normal or remains only slightly shortened. Spherocytosis and altered OF persist, but the "tail" of the OF curve, created by conditioning of a subpopulation of spherocytes by the spleen, disappears. After splenectomy, patients with the most severe forms of HS still show shortened erythrocyte survival and hemolysis, but their clinical improvement is striking.[845,871] Splenectomy appears to have a more beneficial effect on spectrin/ankyrin-deficient erythrocytes than on band 3–deficient erythrocytes.[1180]

Currently, the major decisions about treatment are who should undergo splenectomy, what kind of operation should be performed, and how patients should be cared for postoperatively. However, the indications for splenectomy should be weighed carefully inasmuch as a small fraction of patients will die of overwhelming postsplenectomy infections.[1181-1185] Because the risk of postsplenectomy sepsis is very high in infancy and early childhood, splenectomy should be delayed until the age of 5 to 9 if possible and until at least 3 years of age in all children, even if transfusions are required chronically in the interim. There is no evidence that further delay is useful, and it may be harmful because the risk of cholelithiasis increases dramatically in children after 10 years of age.[1100]

Risks of Splenectomy

Immediate Postsplenectomy Complications. Early complications of splenectomy include local infection, such as a subphrenic abscess, and bleeding. Pancreatitis has been reported immediately after splenectomy, presumably as a result of injury to the tail of the pancreas incurred during removal of the spleen.[1186]

Postsplenectomy Sepsis. Overwhelming serious bacterial infection with encapsulated bacterial organisms is one of the most significant risks of splenectomy. The risk is highest with encapsulated organisms, such as *Streptococcus pneumoniae*, *Neisseria meningitidis*, and *Haemophilus influenzae*. Postsplenectomy sepsis can be rapidly fatal, and it is unclear how the risk for postsplenectomy infection changes over time. Some studies have suggested that the risk is highest immediately after splenectomy and lessens over time. Other studies conclude that the risk of sepsis is present indefinitely after splenectomy.[1187,1188]

It is difficult to estimate the risk for postsplenectomy infections after infancy.[1189] The surveys of Schwartz and colleagues[1184] and Green and co-workers[1181] are limited to adults and largely predate immunization for *S. pneumoniae* and other bacteria. These surveys show an incidence of fulminant sepsis in adults of 0.2 to 0.5 per 100 person-years of follow-up and a death rate of 0.1 per 100 person-years. In addition, other serious bacterial infections (e.g., pneumonia, meningitis, peritonitis, and bacteremia) in adults were much more common (4.5/100 person-years) than normal, particularly in the first few years after the operation. The incidence of postsplenectomy sepsis appears to be higher in children, particularly younger children.[1189-1192] More recently, in a 30-year follow up of more than 200 splenectomized adult HS patients, Schilling[1185] reported a postsplenectomy mortality rate of 0.073 per 100 person-years, which is substantially lower than the risk reported in the earlier studies.[1181,1184] Three of the four deaths occurred 18 or more years after the operation, and none of the patients who died had received pneumococcal vaccine or prophylactic antibiotics.

The majority of studies of postsplenectomy sepsis in adults and children have serious methodologic problems. Most studies are case reports or retrospective reports subject to recall bias. The patients included in the studies have heterogeneous diseases and are often splenectomized for a variety of indications. Furthermore, in most studies the adults patients are not fully immunized and do not receive antibiotic prophylaxis. Further research is necessary to quantitate the risk over time for postsplenectomy sepsis in HS patients treated according to current practice guidelines.

With development of the *H. influenzae* type b conjugate vaccine, meningococcal conjugate and nonconjugate vaccines, and pneumococcal conjugate and nonconjugate vaccines, the risk of postsplenectomy sepsis should in theory be reduced. However, most members of the older population who were splenectomized before 1990 have not received all of these vaccines (unpublished data). Furthermore, most of these patients do not continue to take their antibiotic prophylaxis in adulthood (unpublished data). Waghorn examined current cases of overwhelming postsplenectomy infection and found that only 31% of 77 patients with overwhelming postsplenectomy infection received the pneumococcal vaccine.[1193] In this study, few patients were found to be adequately educated on antibiotic prophylaxis and fever management. This study indicates the necessity for quality improvement in the care of HS patients after splenectomy.

Babesiosis and Malaria. Splenectomized HS patients are at increased risk for serious parasitic infections, such as babesiosis[1194-1196] and malaria.[1197] Babesiosis is a tick-transmitted zoonotic infection by an intraerythrocytic protozoan that is endemic in Europe and in the northeastern, upper midwestern, and coastal northwestern United States.[1198] In the United States the etiologic agent of babesiosis is *Babesia microti*. The clinical symptoms usually begin with chills, anorexia, and fatigue, followed by intermittent fever and symptoms that include myalgia, arthralgia, headache, and vomiting.[1198] In healthy patients, the infection is often asymptomatic or mild. In patients with asplenia, severe illness with hemolytic anemia can occur, including fulminant illness resulting in death. Diagnosis is made by microscopic identification on Giemsa- or Wright-stained thick or thin blood smears. Serologic tests for *Babesia* antibodies and PCR are also available. Because the primary vector for the parasite is the tick *Ixodes scapularis*, which is shared by the agents

causing Lyme disease and ehrlichiosis, these infections should be considered as well.[1198] Current treatment includes clindamycin and oral quinine for 7 to 10 days.[1198] Exchange blood transfusions should be considered for severely ill patients, especially those with parasitemia of greater than 10%. Splenectomized HS patients, when traveling in endemic areas, should attempt to avoid tick bites by wearing long pants and using tick repellants.

Although animal experiments demonstrate that the spleen is essential in eliminating malaria parasitemia,[1199] only anecdotal reports demonstrate an increased risk for malaria in asplenic individuals.[1197,1200,1201] There are no studies that definitively demonstrate an increased risk for severe malaria in asplenic individuals. Nevertheless, the authors know experienced hematologists practicing in areas endemic for malaria who will not allow their patients to be splenectomized. This "local knowledge" suggests the risk is higher than the limited number of reports suggests. Accordingly, we believe that splenectomized HS patients should strictly adhere to malaria chemoprophylaxis when traveling in endemic areas or avoid such areas altogether.

Thrombosis and Thromboembolic Diseases. Many studies demonstrate an overall increased risk for thrombosis in patients after splenectomy performed for various underlying conditions.[1202-1204] Hirsh and Dacie reviewed 80 patients who were splenectomized because of anemia.[1202] Of these patients, 13% had thromboembolic complications, including two deaths. The time from splenectomy to thrombosis ranged from 4 months to 10 years. A meta-analysis of 12 studies examining the risk for thrombosis after splenectomy found that the risk for postsplenectomy thrombosis was 1.5% to 55%.[1203]

Unlike other pathologic red cell states associated with increased thrombosis, such as thalassemia, erythrocytes from patients with HS and HE do not demonstrate increased exposure of PS on their outer surfaces.[1205] Whether thrombosis after splenectomy for anemia is incited by changes in the membrane surface of pathologic erythrocytes[1206] or in circulating vesicles released from them, or is due to other factors, such as associated diseases, nutritional status, genetic modifiers, infection, environment, or treatment modalities, is unknown.[1207] Furthermore, it is likely that the risk for thrombosis after splenectomy varies according to the underlying disease. Nonetheless, major large vessel and organ thrombosis is a common finding in murine models of HS and may be a risk postsplenectomy in humans with HS.[1207,1208] Further studies specifically examining the risk for thrombosis after splenectomy in HS are needed to test this possibility.

Portal Vein Thrombosis. Many investigators have examined the risk for portal vein thrombosis after splenectomy performed for various underlying conditions. Capellini and co-investigators reviewed the data on coagulation and splenectomy in 2005 and found that the overall incidence of postsplenectomy portal vein thrombosis in the United States was 6.3% to 10%.[1209] A Dutch study reviewed 563 patients with splenectomies and found that 9 patients had portal vein thrombosis (2%), with a higher frequency in patients with hematologic diseases.[1210] Another study of 101 splenectomized patients found an 8% rate of postoperative thrombosis.[1203] In this study, 74% of the patients with portal vein thrombosis were splenectomized for an underlying hematologic disease. In the aforementioned studies, the majority of patients who experienced a postoperative thrombotic event were taking Lovenox at the time of thrombosis. The variability in the reported incidence of postsplenectomy portal vein thrombosis between studies might be due to the high rate of silent disease, in that most patients found to have portal vein thrombosis via ultrasound for study purposes are asymptomatic. It has also been hypothesized that the risk for postsplenectomy portal vein thrombosis is increased after more invasive intraoperative manipulations because of large spleen size or difficulty during surgery for trauma. There have been no reported studies to date examining the risk for portal vein thrombosis specifically in patients with HS, so the exact risk in this population is not known. However, an increased rate of portal vein thrombosis may contribute to an increased risk for pulmonary hypertension (see later).

Ischemic Heart Disease and Stroke. The risk for ischemic heart disease and stroke may increase after splenectomy for HS. In one study, Robinette and Fraumeni[1204] observed that death from ischemic heart disease occurred 1.86 times more often in splenectomized young men than in matched control subjects during a 28-year period of follow-up. These findings have been corroborated by others.[1211] In a retrospective review of 232 patients with HS, Schilling found that splenectomized patients older than 40 years had a 5.9 times increased rate of arteriosclerotic events (stroke, myocardial infarction, and coronary or carotid artery surgery) in comparison to HS patients with intact spleens.[1212]

Pulmonary Hypertension. The prevalence and significance of pulmonary hypertension after splenectomy are not known. Pulmonary hypertension has been reported in splenectomized patients with HS,[1213-1216] as well as in many splenectomized patients with other types of anemia.[1217-1222] Hoeper and associates found an 11.5% incidence of postoperative asplenia in 61 patients with pulmonary hypertension versus a 0% incidence in patients without pulmonary hypertension.[1215] Histopathologic examination of individuals with pulmonary hypertension after splenectomy demonstrated abundant microthrombotic lesions. Of the seven patients who had pulmonary hypertension and splenectomies, three were splectomized because of anemia from HS. Jais and colleagues also examined the rate of splenectomy in patients with pulmonary hypertension and found it to be 8.6%, which was 20 times that expected for the general population.[1223] In

this study, of the patients with HS, the interval between splenectomy and the diagnosis of pulmonary hypertension was as long as 30 to 35 years. A meta-analysis examining the risks associated with splenectomy found an increased risk for pulmonary hypertension regardless of the indication for splenectomy.[1224] The risk seemed to be enhanced by various triggering risk factors and appeared to be present indefinitely, with the greatest risk many years after surgery.

Postulated Mechanisms of Hypercoagulability after Splenectomy in Anemic Patients. The etiology of the association between splenectomy and thrombosis appears to be complex. Chronic postsplenectomy thrombocytosis with platelet aggregation, microthrombosis, stasis, and possible vasoconstrictive effects leading to pulmonary capillary obstruction has been suggested as a cause of pulmonary hypertension after splenectomy.[1225,1226] Loss of the filter function of the spleen, thus allowing abnormal erythrocytes to remain in the circulation, which triggers platelet activation and subsequent trapping of these activated platelets in the pulmonary bed, has been implicated. Furthermore, dysregulation of vascular tone after splenectomy for anemia may contribute to an increased risk for thrombosis. After splenectomy for anemia, increased free hemoglobin is released into serum, which decreases serum nitric oxide, possibly disturbing normal regulation of vascular tone and causing vasocontriction. An animal model supporting this hypothesis has been described.[1227] The investigators divided New Zealand white rabbits into three groups: one group injected with sonicated (damaged) blood, a second group injected with normal blood after ligation of the splenic artery, and a third group injected with sonicated blood after ligation of the splenic artery. The only group found to have pulmonary thromboembolism was the third group, which received damaged red blood cells and underwent ligation of the splenic artery. This study may indicate that both abnormal red blood cell membranes and splenectomy are necessary for the development of pulmonary hypertension in human patients.

The development of postsplenectomy portal hypertension secondary to portal vein thrombosis (see earlier) may contribute to the development of pulmonary hypertension.[1228-1231] In this scenario, portal hypertension leads to intrapulmonary shunting and hypoxic pulmonary vasoconstriction, which is then implicated in the pathogenesis of pulmonary hypertension.[1231]

Many have postulated that the risk for thrombosis increases after splenectomy performed for anemia because as the anemia improves, patients have an increase in cholesterol level, serum hematocrit,[1212] and platelet count, all known risk factors for thrombosis. In the Framingham study, the incidence of stroke was two times higher in patients with high versus low hemoglobin.[1232] Schilling and colleagues examined the risk for arteriosclerotic events (i.e., arterial thrombotic events) in families with HS.[1233] They found the risk for arteriosclerotic events in patients with HS and a spleen to be a fifth the risk in unaffected family members, thus implying that HS with a spleen may be protective against arteriosclerotic disease. However, it is not clear whether this protective effect is due to a lower hematocrit and lower cholesterol level rather than the presence of the spleen.

The risk for thrombosis after splenectomy may also increase because of increasing circulating damaged red blood cells. In patients with thalassemia, red cells are recognized as being more procoagulant than healthy red cells. The prothrombinase assay can use thalassemic red blood cells as a source of phospholipids, which requires them to act as activated platelets. Damaged red blood cells are more procoagulant and become more prevalent after splenectomy because they are no longer filtered through the spleen. "Blood dust" shed from fragmenting erythrocytes with PS exposed on the surface may activate the clotting cascade. In support of this concept, frequent red cell transfusions are protective in splenectomized thalassemia major patients, probably by allowing fewer damaged red blood cells in the circulation.[1203] It is unclear whether this same phenomenon would be true in HS patients.

The risk for thrombosis after splenectomy for HS is not well defined, and further studies are needed to confirm this risk. Nevertheless, a conservative approach to splenectomy is supported by this correlation. Furthermore, once a patient with HS has been splenectomized, a thoughtful approach to clotting risk is recommended, in so far as attempting to limit additional hypercoagulable risk factors.

Indications for Splenectomy

In view of the potential risks, splenectomy should be performed only if there are clear indications. All patients with severe spherocytosis who are transfusion dependent or have growth failure or skeletal changes should undergo splenectomy. Splenectomy is usually recommended for patients with moderate HS if they suffer from reduced vitality or physical stamina as a result of anemia, if later in life anemia compromises vascular perfusion of vital organs, or if leg ulcers or extramedullary hematopoietic tumors develop. Whether patients with moderate HS and asymptomatic anemia should undergo splenectomy remains controversial. Partial (subtotal) splenectomy may be indicated in some of these patients (see later). Splenectomy can be deferred, probably indefinitely, in patients with mild HS and compensated hemolysis. In young symptomatic children with HS, splenectomy should be delayed until at least 3 years of age and, if possible, until 6 to 9 years of age because of the risk for infection. In addition, after the early school years, the number of febrile infections is reduced, which decreases the frequency of postsplenectomy fever evaluations.

Treatment of patients with mild to moderate HS and gallstones is also debatable, particularly because new treatments for gallstones, such as laparoscopic cholecystectomy, endoscopic sphincterotomy, and extracorporal cholelithotripsy, lower the risk of this complication.[1234,1235] If such patients have symptomatic gallstones, the authors and others favor combined cholecystectomy and splenectomy,[1236,1237] especially if acute cholecystitis or biliary obstruction has occurred. Prophylactic cholecystectomy at the time of splenectomy is not indicated in patients who do not have cholelithiasis.[1238]

Surgical Procedures

Laparoscopic Splenectomy. When splenectomy is warranted, laparoscopic splenectomy has become the method of choice in many centers.[1239-1245] The procedure can be combined with laparoscopic cholecystectomy if desired.[1236,1237,1249,1242] The benefits of laparoscopic splenectomy are less postoperative discomfort, quicker return to preoperative diet and activities, shorter hospitalization, decreased cost, and smaller scars.[1241,1242] The drawbacks of a laparoscopic approach are longer operative time,[1239,1242,1243] risk of conversion to standard splenectomy,[1240,1244,1246] chance of missing an accessory spleen,[1243,1247] potential difficulty in controlling bleeding,[1246] and capsular fracture with subsequent splenosis.[1248] Recent studies have compared the laparoscopic approach with the open surgical approach and have demonstrated longer operating times but shorter hospital stay and decreased pain in the laparoscopic group.[1249-1251] The majority of studies to date support the laparoscopic approach to splenectomy as the method of choice in centers in which the surgical staff is experienced.

Partial (Subtotal) Splenectomy. The emergence of antibiotic-resistant pneumococci and increasing evidence suggesting an increased risk for thrombosis after splenectomy have led to re-examination of the role of alternative treatment modalities. Partial splenectomy has been suggested for selected patients with HS, especially those with only moderate disease. The goal of this operation is to decrease hemolysis while maintaining residual splenic phagocytic function. In practice, at least 80% to 90% of the enlarged organ is removed (Fig. 15-47). Partial splenectomy is mostly performed as an open operation, but a laparoscopic approach has been reported.[1252] The procedure is more time consuming than total splenectomy, and the time needed for recovery is longer (4- to 7-day hospitalization), but studies have shown that partial splenectomy is safe and reduces the rate of hemolysis.[1253-1257]

In an initial study by Tchernia and colleagues,[1253] the frequency of complications after partial splenectomy was low, and regrowth of the splenic remnant was not observed during a 4-year follow-up period. Long-term follow-up of 40 patients, monitored for up to 12 years after partial splenectomy, demonstrated that mean hemoglobin increased from 9.2 to 12.7 g/dL and the absolute reticulocyte count decreased from 523 to 267 × 10^9 cells/L (Fig. 15-48).[1254] In children with at least 10 years of follow-up, no differences in hemoglobin and reticulocyte levels were noted between the partial and total splenec-

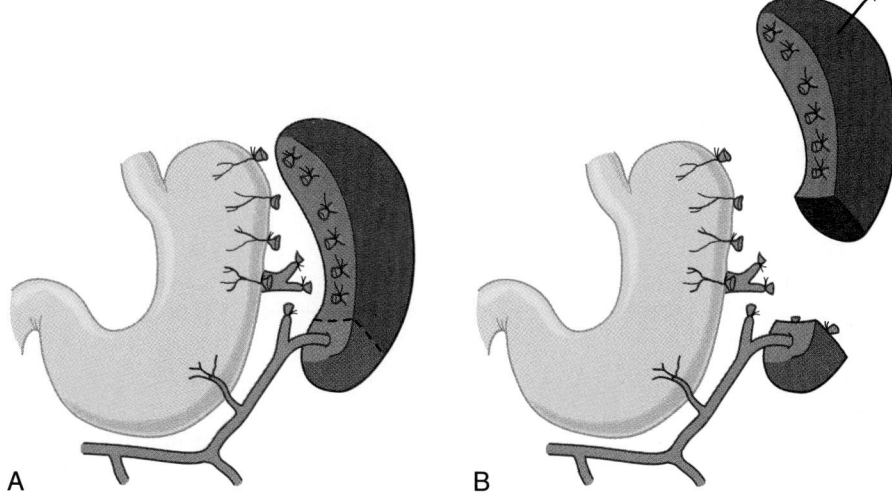

FIGURE 15-47. Surgical technique used for partial (~80%) splenectomy. **A,** All vascular pedicles supplying the spleen are divided except those arising from the left gastroepiploic vessels. **B,** The upper pole of the spleen is removed at the boundary between the well-perfused and poorly perfused tissue. *(Adapted from Tchernia G, Gauthier F, Mielot F, et al. Initial assessment of the beneficial effect of partial splenectomy in hereditary spherocytosis. Blood. 1993;81: 2014.)*

tomy groups.[1254] Significant splenic regrowth was seen in the first year after partial splenectomy, but after the initial growth, the rate of splenic growth in this study was much reduced (see Fig. 15-48). Nevertheless, 8% of patients in this study, particularly those with severe HS, required total splenectomy after partial splenectomy because of splenic regrowth and resumption of hemolysis. Moreover, in 4 of 18 patients in whom the gallbladder was not removed during the initial surgery, subsequent cholecystectomy was necessary.[1254]

Splenic tissue has tremendous regeneration potential, as attested to by reports of previously splenectomized individuals with HS in whom enlarged accessory spleens or ectopic splenic tissue together with recurrent hemolysis developed later in life. Thus, it is not surprising that splenic regrowth has been a problem necessitating reoperation in those with severe HS.[1255-1257] Some authors postulate that the spleen will grow back to its age-equivalent size 2 to 3 years after partial splenectomy. After conventional partial splenectomy, the surgical revision rate for recurrent hemolysis is estimated to be 10% after 5 years and 33% after 10 years.[1256] Moreover, it is important to note that the longest follow-up of partial splenectomy for HS is 10 to 15 years, and therefore the percentage of HS patients with splenic regrowth and recurrent hemolysis many years after partial splenectomy is unknown.

A new procedure called near-total splenectomy, in which a more radical approach to open resection is taken to reduce the risk for continued hemolysis as a result of splenic regrowth, yet maintain splenic function, has recently been performed in Germany. Near-total splenectomy leaves a splenic remnant of 10 cm³ as a residual. One longitudinal cohort study of 42 patients demonstrated that this procedure may be safe and effective, with no patients requiring postprocedure transfusions and no postprocedure hemolysis developing.[1258] More experience and longer follow-up are needed before partial, or near-total, splenectomy can be recom-

mended as a routine procedure for the majority of patients with HS.

Embolization. Several case studies have reported partial splenic arterial embolization as an alternative to splenectomy to treat hemolysis in patients with HS.[1259,1260] The technique has also been used to decrease operative blood loss in patients with very large spleens before laparoscopic splenectomy.[1261] Because experience with this procedure is limited, it cannot be recommended as routine therapy.

Postsplenectomy Changes

After splenectomy, spherocytosis persists but conditioned microspherocytes disappear, and changes typical of the postsplenectomy state, including Howell-Jolly bodies, target cells, siderocytes, and acanthocytes, become evident in the peripheral blood smear. On average, MCV and mean red cell surface area increase and MCHC and OF decrease, but the effects are modest (5% to 10%).[1262] In typical dominant HS, reticulocyte counts fall to normal or nearly normal levels,[845] although red cell life span, if carefully measured, remains slightly shortened (96 ± 13 days).[1004] In all but the most severe occurrences, anemia and jaundice remit and do not recur.

Splenectomy Failure

The rare splenectomy failure (i.e., recurrence of hemolysis) is usually caused by an accessory spleen that was missed during surgery[1255,1263] or by another red cell disorder, such as PK deficiency.[1264,1265] Accessory spleens are present in 15% to 40% of patients and must always be sought.[1107,1186,1266] Recurrence of hemolytic anemia years or even decades[1255] after splenectomy should raise suspicion of an accessory spleen, particularly if Howell-Jolly bodies are no longer evident on peripheral blood smears. The absence of "pitted" red cells with crater-like surface indentations, readily seen by interference contrast microscopy, is also a sensitive measure of recrudescent splenic

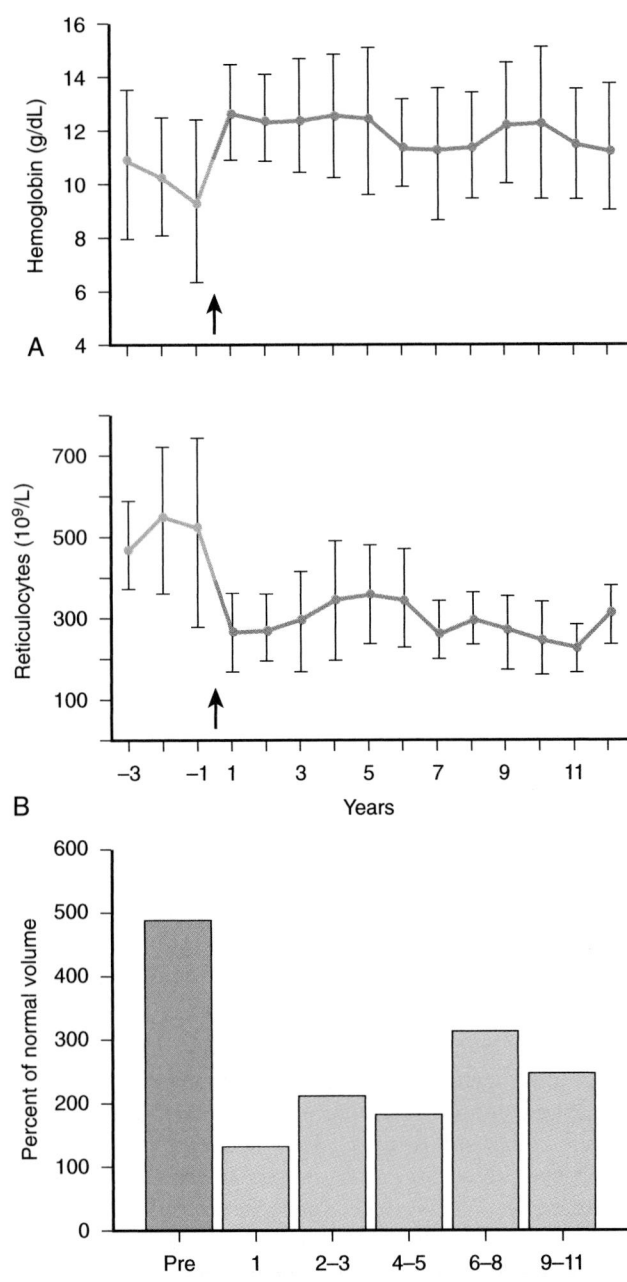

FIGURE 15-48. Long-term follow-up of partial splenectomy in hereditary spherocytosis. Data are the results of 12 years of experience with the procedure in 40 patients (aged 1 to 25 years). **A** and **B,** Change in hemoglobin and reticulocyte count with time before and after subtotal splenectomy (*arrow*). The mean and standard deviations are shown. Both the rise in hemoglobin and the fall in reticulocytes have been sustained for more than a decade. **C,** Size of the spleen during the same period. There is some regrowth of the splenic remnant, especially in the first few years. It remains to be seen whether the remnant reaches a stable size or, as some studies have indicated, continues to grow. (*Adapted with permission from Walensky LD, Narla M, Lux SE. Disorders of the red cell membrane. In Handin RI, Lux SE, Stossel TP [eds]. Blood: Principles and Practice of Hematology, 2nd ed. Philadelphia, JB Lippincott, 2003, pp 1709-1858.*)

function.[1267,1268] The ectopic splenic tissue can be confirmed by a radiocolloid liver/spleen scan or a scan using ^{51}Cr-labeled, heat-damaged red cells.[1263,1269]

Other Therapies

Vaccination and Antibiotic Prophylaxis

All candidates for splenectomy should receive a complete series of vaccinations against encapsulated organisms, including pneumococcus, meningococcus, and *H. influenzae* (Table 15-6). Yearly influenza immunizations are recommended to reduce the chance of secondary bacterial infections. Recent studies (unpublished results) have shown that the majority of adults who were splenectomized as children are not up to date with their vaccinations. In a study examining current cases of overwhelming postsplenectomy infection, only 31% of 77 patients with such infection received the pneumococcal vaccine.[1193] It is important to emphasize the importance of immunizations to the affected parents of children with HS.

Pneumococcal Vaccines. All patients older than 2 years should receive the 23-valent pneumococcal polysaccharide vaccine (PCV23) at least 2 weeks before splenectomy. In addition, all patients should receive two doses, at least 8 weeks apart, of the 7-valent pneumococcal conjugate vaccine (PCV7) before splenectomy.[1270] After both PCV23 and PCV7 have been given, it is not necessary to give booster vaccines of PCV23. However, some physicians continue with this regimen because of the lack of data on the necessity of giving booster vaccines for PCV23 after PCV7 is administered and because of the lack of studies on the safety of PCV7 in populations older than 5 years.

Haemophilus Influenzae Type b Vaccine. The conjugated *H. influenzae* type b vaccine should be given to all patients at least 2 weeks before splenectomy. No studies have been performed on the need for reimmunization, which is not recommended at this time.

Meningococcal Vaccines. All patients undergoing splenectomy after age 2 should be immunized with the meningococcal conjugate vaccine (MCV4). Similar to the *H. influenzae* vaccine, no studies have been performed on reimmunization, which therefore is not recommended at this time.

Antibiotic Prophylaxis

Prophylactic antibiotics are recommended after splenectomy with an emphasis on protection against pneumococcal sepsis (i.e., penicillin V or equivalent, 125 mg orally twice daily in young children [<5 years of age] and 250 mg twice daily in older children and adults). For patients allergic to penicillin, erythromycin is recommended. Antibiotic prophylaxis is recommended at least

TABLE 15-6   Recommended Immunizations at Least 2 Weeks before and after Splenectomy

Vaccination	AGE AT SPLENECTOMY	
	6 to 23 Months	Older than 2 Years
PCV7	As per routine schedule	2 doses, ≥2 mo apart*
PPV23	No	1 dose every 3-5 yr, at least 8 wk after PCV7
MCV4	No	1 dose
MPSV4	No	1 dose if MCV4 is unavailable
Influenza	Yearly	Yearly
Hib	As per routine schedule	1 dose*

*Children or adults who received the primary series as infants do not need to be immunized further.

Hib, *Haemophilus influenzae* type b conjugate vaccine; MCV4, meningococcal conjugate vaccine; MPSV4, meningococcal polysaccharide vaccine; PCV7, pneumococcal conjugate vaccine; PPV23, pneumococcal polysaccharide vaccine.

through childhood and, for teenagers and adults, for at least the first 5 years after surgery.

Some physicians recommend lifelong antibiotic prophylaxis because it is unclear that the risk for overwhelming postsplenectomy infection changes over time. The emergence of penicillin-resistant pneumococci (5% in 1989 to ≥35% in 1997) has led many to reconsider this recommendation, particularly because previous antibiotic use is a risk factor for the development of penicillin resistance in pneumococci.[1271] Patient who do not take prophylactic antibiotics should have a supply of oral antibiotics on hand, which they should take immediately if fever higher than 101.5° C develops. They should then seek medical attention right away.

The risk for infection is decreased in immunized patients because 50% to 70% of postsplenectomy sepsis is due to *S. pneumoniae* and about 80% of pneumococcal disease is due to strains contained in the two vaccines. However, it is likely that strains omitted from the vaccines will rise in frequency as pathogens because of selection. Further risk reduction would be anticipated from the chronic use of prophylactic penicillin. Nevertheless, the risk cannot be reduced to zero. Postsplenectomy infections occur occasionally in successfully immunized patients,[1272-1274] and compliance with prophylactic medication regimens is a problem, particularly in teenagers.[1275]

The occurrence of penicillin-resistant pneumococci is increasing very rapidly all over the world.[1276-1278] In some countries, more than half of all isolates are resistant.[1279] In the United States, the prevalence is approximately 35%, but it is much higher in some localities and is rising.[1276,1278,1280] Although most of the strains show some sensitivity to penicillin, some are highly resistant and others are multiply resistant.[1280-1282] The emergence of these strains will greatly complicate the use of antibiotics for pneumococcal prophylaxis during the next decades.

Folic Acid

Patients with HS should take folic acid (0.5 to 1 mg/day orally) before splenectomy to prevent folate deficiency.

Animal and Fish Models of Hereditary Spherocytosis

Animal models, such as the well characterized mouse and zebra fish models, have assisted in our understanding of the pathophysiology of HS. Four types of spherocytic hemolytic anemia have been identified in the common house mouse *Mus Musculus*[1283]: *ja/ja* (jaundice); *sph/sph* (spherocytosis) and its alleles *sph^{1J}/sph^{1J}* (hemolytic anemia), *sph^{2J}/sph^{2J}* (now lost), *sph^{2BC}/sph^{2BC}*, and *sph^{DEM}/sph^{DEM}*; *nb/nb* (normoblastosis); and *wan/wan*. The nomenclature indicates that anemia is observed only in the homozygous state and that the mutants represent four loci: *ja*, *sph*, *nb*, and *wan*. All defects are autosomal recessive and cause severe hemolysis with spherocytosis, jaundice, bilirubin gallstones, and hepatosplenomegaly,[1284] except in the *sph^{DEM}/sph^{DEM}* mice, which have HE. Another recessive spherocytic hemolytic anemia has been described in the deer mouse *Peromyscus maniculatus*.[1285] This disorder is less severe and closely resembles the autosomal dominant form of human HS. The spectrin content of deer mouse erythrocytes is reduced by about 20% (unpublished data).

Spectrin Mutants

The *ja/ja* mutant has a defect in the spectrin β chain (Arg1160→Stop) and produces no detectable spectrin.[1286] The *sph/sph* variants lack α chains but have small amounts of β-spectrin. These mice do not produce α-spectrin because of either decreased synthesis, function, or stability. The *sph* and *sph^{2BC}* alleles are frameshift mutations and null alleles.[1287,1288] The sph^{1J} allele lacks the last 13 amino acids of α-spectrin and causes marked spherocytosis.[1289] Thus, the amino acids in the C-terminal of the spectrin tail are functionally important in attaching spectrin to actin. The *sph^{DEM}/sph^{DEM}* mouse is missing exon 11 and 46 amino acids near the amino-terminal of repeat 5. These mice have elliptocytes, spherocytes, and poikilocytes and therefore clinically appear to be a cross between HS and HE (see later).[1289]

Cardiac thrombi, fibrotic lesions, and renal hemochromatosis are found in *ja/ja* and *sph/sph* mice who die after the first few days of life.[1290] Transplantation of hematopoietic cells from *sph/sph* mice is sufficient to induce thrombotic events in the transplant recipients.[1291] In mice with α-spectrin mutations, 70% to 100% experience cerebral infarction.[1292,1293] Studies of red cell adhesion in these mice demonstrate 10-fold higher adhesion to thrombospondin than with normal red blood cells and increased adhesion to laminin.[1294] Therefore, it is hypothesized that changes in the red cell adhesive characteristics contribute to the thrombotic events in these mice.

Reisling (*ris*) is an induced mutation in zebra fish that results in a nearly bloodless phenotype that causes severe anemia and congestive heart failure.[997] The *ris* phenotype is caused by a null mutation in β-spectrin. The red blood cells of affected zebra fish are spherocytic rather than elliptocytic, the normal zebra fish red cell shape. Scanning electron micrographs show membrane loss, as is in other forms of severe HS.

Ankyrin Mutants

Mice with the *nb/nb* mutation have a primary defect in ankyrin. This defect is due to a single nucleotide deletion leading to a frameshift and premature chain termination in the regulatory region of ankyrin.[1295,1296] The *nb/nb* red cells have 50% to 70% of normal spectrin levels but only a trace of ankyrin mRNA and protein.[1177,1284] This is in striking contrast to ankyrin defects in human HS, in which ankyrin and spectrin levels are comparably depressed.[891,851] Fetal *nb/nb* mice have no anemia and normal reticulocyte counts at birth,[884] possibly because of expression of ankyrin-related proteins in utero.[885] Humans may also be protected in utero, at least partially, because hydrops fetalis has not been reported in patients with probable ankyrin defects (i.e., combined spectrin/ankyrin deficiency), even in patients who become transfusion dependent after birth.

The *nb/nb* mice also lack ankyrin in their cerebellar Purkinje cells,[886,1177] which leads to an age-related loss of Purkinje cells during the first 5 to 7 months of life and the emergence of cerebellar ataxia.[1177] Spinocerebellar degeneration and related syndromes have also been reported in a few adult humans with HS,[1173-1176] although it is not yet known whether ankyrin is affected.

Band 3 Mutants

Complete deficiency of band 3 was first described in cattle with a recessive form of HS. In cows, homozygosity for a nonsense mutation in the band 3 gene leads to absence of band 3 and protein 4.2.[1297] Red cell membranes are unstable and show loss of surface area, as demonstrated by invagination, vesiculation, and extrusion of microvesicles. Affected cattle have defective anion transport and a mild acidosis but mild hemolysis in comparison to other band 3–deficient species.

In mice, targeted disruption of the band 3 gene causes severe spherocytic hemolytic anemia with exuberant loss of the membrane surface as vesicles, tubules, and myelin form.[995] Red cell membranes also lack protein 4.2 and GPA.[1298] Surprisingly, the content of membrane skeletal proteins and the architecture of negative-stained, spread skeletons is normal or nearly normal.[1299] Therefore, band 3 appears to be required for stabilizing membrane lipids but not for assembly of the membrane skeleton. For unclear reasons, these band 3–deficient mice have a significant propensity for thrombosis and often die in the neonatal period.[1300]

A new mouse model, *wan/wan*, in a C3H/HeJ background with a null defect in the band 3 gene was discovered.[1301] These mice have a severe anemia that is lethal in the neonatal period. However, when *wan/wan* mice are crossed with wild-type mice of a different strain, *Mus castaneous*, the F_2 generation shows variable hematologic severity. The genetic modifier causing this variability in hematologic abnormalities has been localized to a small chromosomal region containing the β-spectrin gene.[1301]

Finally, zebra fish with band 3 mutations associated with the *retsina* (*ret*) phenotype suffer from severe anemia with a complete arrest in erythroid maturation at the late erythroblast stage.[218] The rare *ret/ret* red blood cells are spherocytic rather than elliptical. Many of these arrested erythroblasts have bilobed nuclei reminiscent of those seen in congenital dyserythropoietic anemia, and demonstrate defects in cytokinesis.

Protein 4.2 Mutant

Mice with targeted deletions of the protein 4.2 gene survive normally and have only mildly spherocytic anemia and hemolysis.[1302]

Protein 4.1 Mutants

Mice lacking the protein 4.1 gene because of targeted deletion have moderate hemolysis and decreased red cell membrane stability.[1303] In addition to lacking protein 4.1, these mice are also deficient in protein p55, ankyrin, spectrin, and a complex of integral membrane proteins (band 3, glycophorin C, Xk, Kell, Duffy, and Rh).[551a] Their red cell morphology is remarkable for a spherocytic rather than an elliptocytic shape, probably related to the spectrin deficiency. Two zebra fish models with protein 4.1 deficiency have been established, *merlot* and *chablis*, and these mutants have very severe hemolytic anemia characterized by spherocytosis and increased OF.[994]

β-Adducin Mutant

Mice lacking β-adducin have been produced by gene targeting.[583] They have a mild spherocytic hemolytic anemia[583] and mild defects in learning and memory.[1303a]

HEREDITARY ELLIPTOCYTOSIS AND HEREDITARY PYROPOIKILOCYTOSIS

HE is characterized by the presence of elliptical or oval erythrocytes on peripheral blood smears (Fig. 15-49). Clinically, these disorders range from the asymptomatic

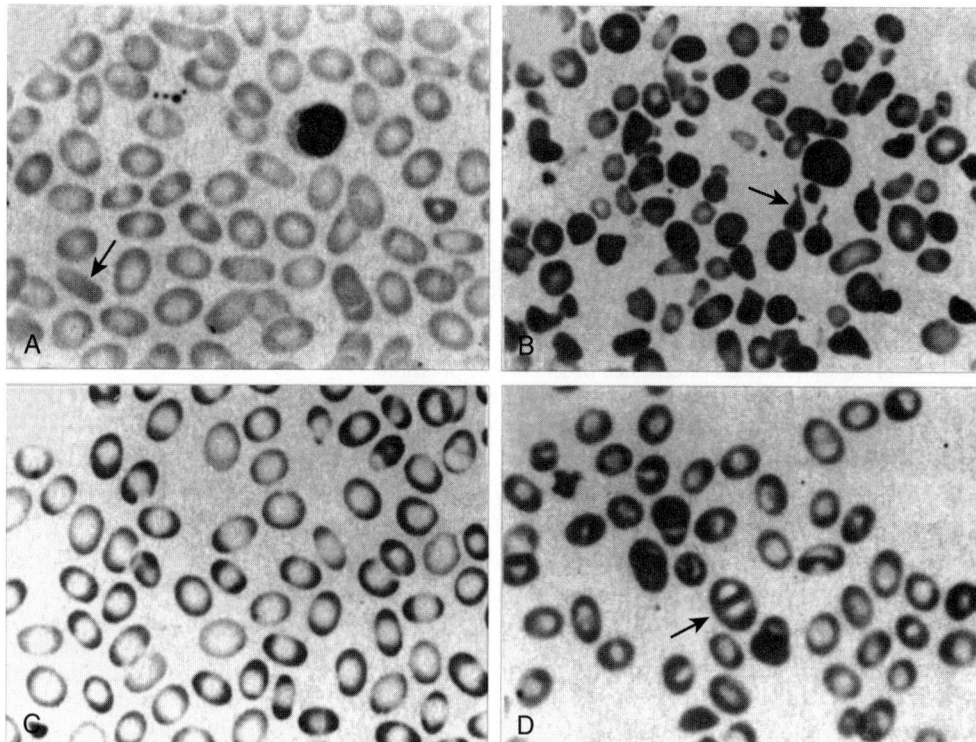

FIGURE 15-49. Peripheral blood smears from subjects with various forms of hereditary elliptocytosis (HE). **A,** Simple heterozygote with mild common HE associated with an elliptogenic spectrin mutation. Note the predominant elliptocytosis with some rod-shaped cells (*arrow*) and virtual absence of poikilocytes. **B,** Hereditary pyropoikilocytosis. Note the prominent microspherocytosis, micropoikilocytosis, and fragmentation. Only a few elliptocytes are present. Some poikilocytes are in the process of budding (*arrow*). **C,** Spherocytic elliptocytosis. Rounded elliptocytes dominate the morphology. In some patients, spherocytes or microelliptocytes are seen. **D,** Southeast Asian ovalocytosis. The majority of cells are oval; some contain either a longitudinal slit or a transverse ridge (*arrow*). The latter are sometimes referred to as theta cells and are characteristic of the disease.

carrier state to severe hemolysis to death in utero as a result of hydrops fetalis. Erythrocyte biochemical defects range from none to severe. In the past, hereditary elliptocytic disorders have been considered to simply be variants of HS and worthy of little further attention. However, the membrane defects and their pathophysiologic consequences in HE differ fundamentally from those of HS and must be regarded separately.

History

HE was first reported in 1904 by Dresbach,[1304] a physiologist at Ohio State University in Columbus, who discovered the condition in one of his histology students during a laboratory exercise in which the students were examining their own blood. This report elicited some controversy because the student died soon thereafter, leading to speculation that the student actually suffered from incipient pernicious anemia.[1305] A number of famous pathologists supported Dresbach's view that the elliptocytosis was a primary disorder,[1306] and this view was substantiated during the next 2 decades by reports of Bishop[1307] and Huck and Bigalow.[1308] Demonstration of the disease in three generations of one family clearly established the hereditary nature of this disorder.[1309,1310]

In the 1930s and 1940s there was some debate about whether HE was a disease or just a morphologic curiosity.[1309-1314] Early on, some confusion also existed in the differentiation of HE from sickle cell anemia, from hypochromic elliptocytosis (probably thalassemia), and later, from HS.[1312] These reports emphasize the morphologically deceptive nature of HE and its hemolytic variants. Additional historical and clinical features of the disease

are found in the reports of Wyandt and associates,[1313] Wolman and Ozge,[1314] and Dacie.[1315]

Prevalence and Genetics

In the United States, HE has been estimated to occur in 1 in 2000 to 4000 of the population.[1313,1316] The true incidence of HE is unknown because its clinical severity is heterogeneous and many patients are asymptomatic. HE is more common in areas of endemic malaria, specifically in people of African and Mediterranean ancestry.[1316-1324] The higher frequency of HE in these populations suggests that this disease may confer some resistance to malaria. In a study of HE in Benin, Western Africa, an incidence of 1.6% was observed.[1317]

HE variants are inherited predominantly in an autosomal dominant manner. Typically, individuals who are heterozygous for an elliptocytic variant have asymptomatic elliptocytosis without anemia. Individuals who are homozygotes or compound heterozygotes for HE variants may suffer mild to severe hemolysis with moderate to marked anemia. Spontaneous elliptocytogenic mutations have been reported. Presumably, they are also inherited in an autosomal dominant fashion. In one kindred with Alport's syndrome, mental retardation, midface hypoplasia, and elliptocytosis, inheritance was X-linked and associated with a submicroscopic deletion on the X chromosome.[1325]

HE is heterogeneous with multiple genetic loci, including reports of mutations in the α-spectrin, protein 4.1, and glycophorin C genes.[1326,1327] The mutations described include deletions, point mutations, insertions, and processing defects. The incidence of one common

---

TABLE 15-7   Clinical Subtypes of Hereditary Elliptocytosis

Clinical Manifestations	Laboratory Features

COMMON HE
Asymptomatic
Dominant inheritance: one parent with HE
No splenomegaly
Variants:
  Some neonates with moderately severe hemolytic anemia and an HPP-like smear. Converts to typical mild HE by ≈1 year
  Some patients with mild to moderate chronic hemolysis caused by either coinheritance of the low-expression α-spectrin variant α^{LELY}, coexistence of chronic disease producing splenomegaly, or unknown factors
	Blood smear: elliptocytes, rod forms, few or no poikilocytes
	No anemia, little or no hemolysis (reticulocytes = 1% to 3%)
	Normal osmotic fragility
	Usually a defect in α- or β-spectrin leading to decreased spectrin self-association, or a defect in protein 4.1 leading to partial deficiency or dysfunction

HOMOZYGOUS COMMON HE AND HPP
Moderate to severe hemolytic anemia
Splenomegaly
Intermittent jaundice
Aplastic crises
Recessive inheritance: typically one parent with HE and one with α^{LELY} or both parents with HE
Good improvement after splenectomy
	Blood smear: bizarre poikilocytes, fragments, ± spherocytes, ± elliptocytes
	Reticulocytosis
	Decreased MCV because of red cell fragmentation
	Increased osmotic fragility
	α-Spectrin defects:
	  Decreased red cell and spectrin heat stability
	  Marked defect in spectrin self-association
	In the more severe variants, partial spectrin deficiency (indicated by more spherocytes on the blood smear)

SPHEROCYTIC HE
Mild to moderate hemolytic anemia
Splenomegaly
Intermittent jaundice
Aplastic crises
Dominant inheritance pattern
Excellent response to splenectomy
	Blood smear: rounded elliptocytes, ± spherocytes. May see variable morphology within a kindred
	Reticulocytosis
	Increased osmotic fragility
	Glucose-responsive autohemolysis
	Variable molecular defects:
	  C-terminal truncations of β-spectrin
	  Protein 4.2 deficiency (some patients) leading to ovalostomatocytosis, which resembles spherocytic HE
	  Glycophorin C deficiency (rare)

SOUTHEAST ASIAN OVALOCYTOSIS Asymptomatic Dominant inheritance (homozygous lethal) Lowland aboriginal tribes, especially in Melanesia and Malaysia Very rigid red cells that resist invasion by some strains of malarial parasites	Blood smear: rounded elliptocytes, some with a transverse bar that divides the central clear space Little or no hemolysis or anemia Normal osmotic fragility Mutant band 3 that lacks anion exchange function and tends to aggregate, leading to a rigid membrane

HE, hereditary elliptocytosis; HPP, hereditary pyropoikilocytosis; MCV, mean corpuscular volume.
From Walensky LD, Narla M, Lux SE. Disorders of the red cell membrane. In Handin RI, Lux SE, Stossel TP (eds). Blood: Principles and Practice of Hematology, 2nd ed. Philadelphia, JB Lippincott, 2003, with permission.

---

elliptocytic mutation of α-spectrin, α$^{I/65-68}$, approaches 1% in Central Africa. It has a worldwide distribution in people of African ancestry. Genetic haplotyping studies suggest that this mutation may have a "founder affect," originating in Central Africa similar to the Benin type of sickle hemoglobin.[1317] This observation further supports the possibility that there has been genetic selection for HE because it imparts some resistance to malaria.[1328]

Clinical Syndromes

Most of the reported patients with HE can be classified into one of four clinical categories: common HE, HPP, spherocytic HE, and SAO (Table 15-7). With the exception of SAO, which is homogeneous in molecular genetic terms (see later), these classifications denote clinical phenotypes and not specific molecular causes, although correlations between the two exist. Numerous molecular defects in the membrane proteins of patients with HE have been identified, and HE can also be classified on the basis of these defects.

Common Hereditary Elliptocytosis

Common HE is, by far, the most prevalent form of HE, particularly in African populations.[1317,1318] The clinical characteristics of the common HE trait vary enormously, with several clinical subtypes defined. It is important to note that different clinical patterns may be seen in members of the same family and that the clinical manifestation in single individuals may exhibit variability over time. Thus, the clinical patterns are probably more useful for illustrating the spectrum of common HE than for classifying the disease.

Silent Carrier State. This condition was identified by analyzing asymptomatic members of kindreds with HE or HPP. Affected persons have red cells with normal morphologic characteristics and no evidence of hemolysis, but detailed investigations show a subtle defect in their membrane skeletons, with decreased red cell thermal stability, decreased mechanical stability of isolated skeletons, an increased fraction of spectrin dimers in 0°C spectrin extracts, abnormal tryptic peptide maps of spectrin, or various combinations of these defects.[1320-1324,1329,1330] It is notable that some patients classified as "silent carriers" have the same molecular defect as patients with mild common HE,[1323,1324,1330,1331] thus emphasizing the variability of clinical expression.

Typical Common Hereditary Elliptocytosis (Mild Hereditary Elliptocytosis or Heterozygous Common Hereditary Elliptocytosis). This is the most common clinical form of HE.[1332-1346] Patients are asymptomatic, and HE is often diagnosed incidentally when individuals are undergoing screening for an unrelated condition. These persons are not anemic and only very rarely exhibit splenomegaly. Red cell survival may be normal,[1345] but more often there is a very mild, compensated hemolysis with a slight reticulocytosis and a decreased haptoglobin level.[1337,1339,1343,1347] In these patients, HE is hardly more than a morphologic curiosity. The peripheral blood smear shows prominent elliptocytosis with little red cell budding or fragmentation and no spherocytosis. Elliptocytes (by definition) usually exceed 30% of the red cells and, in some instances, approach 100% (see Fig. 15-49A).[1313,1330,1331,1343,1347] Very elongated elliptocytes are common (>10%). These patients are easily separated from normal individuals, who have less than 2% to 5% elliptocytes.[1339,1341,1347] Somewhat higher proportions of elliptocytes are seen in patients with anemia, particularly megaloblastic anemias, hypochromic-microcytic anemias, myelodysplastic syndromes, and myelofibrosis,[1348] but even in these individuals elliptocytes do not exceed 35%.[1341] Thus, the diagnosis of common HE is rarely difficult.

Common Hereditary Elliptocytosis with Chronic Hemolysis. More severe variants of common HE occur frequently, sometimes within members of the same kindred.[1336,1349-1352] In general, the marked compensated hemolysis is accompanied by evidence of membrane instability on the peripheral blood smear: budding red cells, fragments, and other bizarre poikilocytes. In patients with α-spectrin mutations, significant hemolysis is often due to coinheritance of a spectrin allele that leads to

decreased α-spectrin expression, such as the α^{LELY} allele, and one of the more deleterious HE alleles affecting α-spectrin (see later).[1337,1353-1358] Of the common mutations, spectrin $\alpha^{I/74}$ is more severe than spectrin $\alpha^{I/46-50a}$ and much more severe than spectrin $\alpha^{I/65-68}$. Patients with α^{LELY} in *trans* to $\alpha^{I/74}$ ($\alpha^{LELY}/\alpha^{I/74}$) have marked hemolysis and elliptopoikilocytosis when compared with their siblings with wild-type α-spectrin and $\alpha^{I/74}$ ($+/\alpha^{I/74}$), whereas patients with $\alpha^{LELY}/\alpha^{I/65-68}$ have more elliptocytes than their siblings with $+/\alpha^{I/65-68}$ but no significant hemolysis.[1356] Less often, hemolysis is caused by inheritance of a mutant spectrin that is grossly dysfunctional.[1349] This is indicated by dominant transmission of the hemolytic syndrome and by an unusually high fraction of spectrin dimers in 0° C spectrin extracts.

Common Hereditary Elliptocytosis with Sporadic Hemolysis. Uncompensated hemolysis may also develop in patients with common HE in response to stimuli that cause hyperplasia of the reticuloendothelial system, particularly if the spleen is involved. Examples include viral hepatitis, cirrhosis, infectious mononucleosis, bacterial infections, and malaria.[1344,1359-1361] Hemolysis has also been observed with thrombotic thrombocytopenic purpura and with disseminated intravascular coagulation, which suggests that elliptocytes may be especially susceptible to microangiopathic damage.[1362] For unknown reasons, pregnancy and cobalamin (vitamin B_{12}) deficiency may also transiently aggravate the disease.[863,1363]

Hereditary Elliptocytosis with Infantile Poikilocytosis. Infants with mild common HE sometimes begin life with moderately severe hemolytic anemia characterized by marked red cell budding, fragmentation, and poikilocytosis and by neonatal jaundice, which may require an exchange transfusion.[1321,1338,1347,1364-1369] Usually enough elliptocytes are present to suggest the diagnosis, but sometimes this is not so and the disorder is mistaken for sepsis, infantile pyknocytosis, or microangiopathic or oxidant-induced hemolytic anemia.[1366,1367] Neonatal HE can easily be distinguished from the latter conditions if the parents' blood smears are examined because one will show common HE. However, it is more difficult to distinguish HE with neonatal poikilocytosis from HPP (see later). Most α-spectrin variants have been associated with the neonatal poikilocytosis syndrome. Factors that determine susceptibility are unknown. With time, fragmentation and hemolysis decline, and the clinical picture of common HE emerges.[1370] This transition requires 4 months to 2 years. Subsequently, the disease is clinically indistinguishable from typical common HE. The prevalence is unknown, but in the authors' experience, it is not rare.

The fragmenting neonatal red cells are very sensitive to heat, like hereditary pyropoikilocytes (see later), but unlike pyropoikilocytes, this sensitivity lessens over time.[1369] During conversion, the poikilocytic red cells are dense and rich in hemoglobin F, whereas the smooth elliptocytes are light and enriched in hemoglobin A. This finding suggests that the change in the disease corresponds to the change from fetal to adult erythropoiesis. No variations in the primary α-spectrin defect or its functional effects on spectrin self-association occur during conversion, so other skeletal interactions must differ in fetal and adult red cells. Mentzer and associates[1371] made the interesting suggestion that 2,3-DPG is the critical agent. Because it is not bound by hemoglobin F, the concentration of 2,3-DPG is elevated in fetal red cells. The free anion is known to weaken spectrin-actin–protein 4.1 interactions[1372-1374] and to increase the fragility of isolated ghosts at physiologic concentrations in vitro.[1363] Whether this occurs in intact red cells is unclear.[1375,1376] If it does, the underlying defect in spectrin self-association would certainly be aggravated.

Homozygous Common Hereditary Elliptocytosis. A number of patients who are homozygotes or compound heterozygotes for typical HE have been reported.[1332,1347,1377-1382] Some have had very severe, even fatal transfusion-dependent hemolytic anemia (hemoglobin levels of 2 to 6 g/dL) with marked fragmentation, poikilocytosis, spherocytosis, and elliptocytosis. Others experience hemolysis to a lesser degree (hemoglobin level of 7 to 11 g/dL). It appears that these differences reflect variations in severity of the many α-spectrin mutations that produce HE.[1347,1383] Clinically, the disease resembles HPP,[1347,1383] except for the mildest forms. Patients have an excellent response to splenectomy.

Hereditary Elliptocytosis with Dyserythropoiesis. In a small number of families with otherwise typical common HE, the sporadic occurrence of hemolysis and anemia is at least partially due to the development of dysplastic and ineffective erythropoiesis. All patients reported with this rare syndrome are from Italy and have somewhat less elongated red cells than is typical for common HE. All reported patients also show the characteristic findings of ineffective erythropoiesis, relatively low reticulocyte counts, indirect hyperbilirubinemia, and high serum iron and ferritin concentrations.[1384,1385] The erythrocytes from some patients are macrocytic. Other patients have a few spherocytes, but these are probably an artifact because OF is normal.[1384] The patient's bone marrow is hyperplastic, with decreased late erythroblasts and dysplastic features (asynchrony of nuclear-cytoplasmic maturation, binuclearity, internuclear bridges, and small numbers of ringed sideroblasts). Anemia and, presumably, erythroid dysplasia usually commence during adolescence or early adult life and advance gradually over years. Splenectomy is not curative for these patients. The data available suggest that dysplasia and elliptocytosis cosegregate because no individuals with dysplasia have been observed who did not also have elliptocytosis.[1384,1385] If so, these families must represent the occurrence of a unique subtype of typical common HE. This suggestion is supported by the fact that none of the typical HE protein defects were observed in one well-studied family.

Hereditary Pyropoikilocytosis

This uncommon disorder is manifested in infancy or early childhood as severe hemolytic anemia (hemoglobin level of 4 to 8 g/dL)[1347] characterized by extreme poikilocytosis with budding red cells, fragments, spherocytes, triangulocytes, and other bizarrely shaped cells, as well as few or no elliptocytes in some patients (see Fig. 15-49B).[1323,1386-1391] The morphology of the blood smear somewhat resembles that seen in patients who have severe thermal burns, which explains the name of the disorder. It is more similar to that observed in homozygous common HE and common HE with neonatal poikilocytosis. Most of the patients are individuals of African origin. Patients typically exhibit hyperbilirubinemia in the neonatal period or marked anemia in the first few months of life.[1390] Red cell fragmentation, erythroblastosis, and splenomegaly are also characteristic.[1390,1392] Complications of severe anemia, including growth retardation, frontal bossing, and early gallbladder disease, have been reported.[1388,1389] The red cells are very osmotically fragile, particularly after incubation.[1377,1387-1389] In the most severely affected patients, there is significant microcytosis with very low MCVs (25 to 75 fL) because of the large number of fragmented red cells.[1324,1325,1331,1347,1387,1388] Another characteristic feature of these cells is their remarkable thermal sensitivity. Hereditary pyropoikilocytes fragment at 45° C to 46° C (normal, 49° C) after short periods of heating (10 to 15 minutes).[1389] After splenectomy, hemolysis is markedly decreased, with the hemoglobin level typically ranging from 10 to 14 g/dL with 3% to 10% reticulocytes.[1347,1388,1389]

Although HPP was initially considered to be a separate disease, there is convincing evidence that it is related to HE. As noted earlier, HPP is clinically and morphologically similar to the more severe forms of hemolytic elliptocytosis. In addition, for many patients, one parent or sibling has typical common HE, and in some of these kindreds, an identical molecular defect is observed in siblings with phenotypically different diseases (i.e., HPP and common HE). In other families, all the first-degree relatives have normal phenotypes. A number of biochemical and molecular defects are shared between HE and HPP. However, only HPP red cells are typically markedly deficient in spectrin.[1347,1392-1394] The genetics of HPP suggest that each patient falls into one of three inheritance patterns.[1395] The first consists of patients who are homozygous for a structural variant of spectrin located in the region of the spectrin αβ heterodimer self-association. The second includes patients who are compound heterozygotes for structural defects of spectrin. In the third pattern, typically one parent has an α-spectrin mutation and another parent has no detectable biochemical abnormality.[1393] Studies of spectrin synthesis and mRNA levels reveal that such asymptomatic parents carry a silent "thalassemia-like" defect of spectrin synthesis. When coinherited with the elliptocytogenic spectrin mutation in the offspring with HPP, this thalassemia-like defect enhances expression of the mutant spectrin in the cells and leads to a superimposed spectrin deficiency. The spectrin deficiency is thought to be responsible for the large number of spherocytes and relative paucity of elliptocytes in some patients.

Spherocytic Hereditary Elliptocytosis

This dominant disorder is a phenotypic hybrid of common HE and HS. It has been reported only in white families of European descent, is not linked to the Rh gene, and appears to be a unique subtype.[1311,1344,1396-1399] The prevalence of spherocytic HE is unknown, but judging from the number of published reports, it is relatively rare and probably accounts for no more than 5% of HE in patients of European ancestry. Unlike common HE, almost all affected patients have some hemolysis. It is usually mild to moderate and is often incompletely compensated. The elliptocytes are fewer and plumper than in common HE (see Fig. 15-49C), and some spherocytes, microspherocytes, and microelliptocytes are often present. Poikilocytes and red cell fragments are uncommon, which distinguishes this disorder from common HE with hemolysis. Red cell morphology may vary, even within the same family. Some family members may have relatively prominent spherocytes and as few as 10% to 20% elliptocytes, whereas in others, elliptocytes predominate and spherocytes are rare.[1311,1396] This may cause diagnostic confusion initially, particularly if the propositus has few elliptocytes. Family studies almost always reveal some members with obvious elliptocytosis.

Spherocytic elliptocytes are osmotically fragile,[1311,1396,1398,1399] particularly after incubation. Excessive mechanical fragility and increased autohemolysis that responds to glucose are also characteristic. Gallbladder disease is common, and aplastic crises are a risk.[1396,1398] The pathologic course of spherocytic HE mimics that of HS.[1400-1402] Splenic sequestration is evident, red cells are conditioned during splenic passage, and hemolysis abates after splenectomy.[1396,1398,1401]

The molecular pathology of classic spherocytic HE is unknown. However, patients with COOH-terminal truncations of α-spectrin (see later) have many of the clinical features of spherocytic HE and probably represent an example of the disorder.[1403-1411] Patients with such truncations typically have moderate hemolysis and anemia, punctuated by recurrent, severe hemolytic crises.[1404,1405,1408] Blood smears show plump and usually smooth elliptocytes, although in a few instances poikilocytosis was prominent.[1404,1405,1407]

Patients who lack glycophorin C (see later) also have positive OF tests and rounded, smooth elliptocytes.[1412,1413] They should probably also be classified as having a recessive (and unusually mild) variant of spherocytic HE. Patients who lack protein 4.2 (another recessive condition) sometimes display features of spherocytic HE, such as ovalostomatocytosis[895,1057]; however, protein 4.2 deficiency more often resembles HS, morphologically and

pathophysiologically, and is better classified as a variant of that disorder.

Rare patients appear to be compound heterozygotes for HS and HE. One Turkish girl is a particularly good candidate.[1414] Her mother had mild HS and her father most likely had very mild common HE, whereas she suffered from moderately severe hemolytic anemia (hemoglobin level, 8.4 g/dL; reticulocyte count, 24%; bilirubin level, 1.6 mg/dL) with frontal bossing, osteoporosis, splenomegaly, and a mixture of microspherocytes and rounded elliptocytes.

Southeast Asian Ovalocytosis

SAO, which has a unique phenotype, molecular defect, and geographic distribution, is discussed later in this chapter.

Treatment

Typical common HE is mild and splenectomy is rarely required. Serial interval ultrasound examinations, beginning at approximately 6 years of age, to detect gallstones should be performed in patients with brisk hemolysis. Splenectomy to decrease hemolysis, ameliorate anemia, and avoid the formation of bilirubinate gallstones has been the cornerstone of therapy for patients with severe hemolytic HE and HPP. Most practitioners believe that the indications for splenectomy in HS should also be applied to patients with symptomatic HE and HPP. Patients with HE and HPP who have been splenectomized have experienced increased hematocrit values, decreased reticulocytosis, and improvement in clinical symptoms. The risk for thrombosis after splenectomy for HE is unclear, although cases have been reported.[1415] If hemolysis is still active after splenectomy, folic acid (1 mg) should be administered daily. Recommendations for antibiotic prophylaxis, immunization, and monitoring during intercurrent illnesses are similar to those noted for HS patients before and after splenectomy.

Neonates should be treated as any patient with hemolytic anemia. Phototherapy and exchange transfusions are warranted in neonates with severe anemia and pathologic hyperbilirubinemia. Splenectomy is never indicated in the neonatal period. Patients with extreme hemolysis should receive tranfusions until they are 2 to 3 years of age, when immunizations are effective and splenectomy can be performed safely.

Laboratory Methods to Define Abnormal Spectrin Structure in Hereditary Elliptocytosis

Thermal Sensitivity of Red Cells and Spectrin

Red cells heated to temperatures approaching 50° C for short periods become unstable and fragment spontaneously,[1416-1418] probably because of denaturation of spectrin.[1419] Normal spectrin denatures at 49° C (10-minute exposure),[1299,1419] and normal red cells fragment at the same temperature.[1389,1420] As noted earlier, almost all patients with HPP and some patients with other forms of HE have thermally sensitive red cells. Hereditary pyropoikilocytes and red cells from infants with common HE and neonatal poikilocytosis fragment after 10 minutes at 44° C to 46° C.[1369,1389] Red cells from some but not all patients with common HE fragment at 47° C to 48° C.[1299,1389] As expected, purified spectrin from these red cells is also heat sensitive.[1299,1419] This test is limited because we do not understand, in molecular terms, why specific mutations are thermally sensitive. However, it remains one of the simplest tests available for assessing HPP in laboratories that do not specialize in membrane protein analysis.

Abnormal Spectrin Oligomerization

In many patients with HE and all patients with HPP, spectrin dimers are not properly converted to tetramers and higher oligomers in vitro or on the membrane. This important functional property is easily assessed in low-temperature spectrin extracts. At 0° C, the equilibrium between spectrin dimer and tetramer is greatly slowed. If spectrin is extracted from the membrane at 0° C and carefully protected from warming during separation of dimers, tetramers, and oligomers (usually on nondenaturing polyacrylamide gels), the proportion of each spectrin species reflects its relative proportion on the membrane.[1421] Patients with defects in spectrin self-association have abnormally high proportions of spectrin dimer in 0° C spectrin extracts (i.e., more than 10% of the total spectrin dimers and tetramers).[1351,1420,1422] The fraction of spectrin dimers is an important functional assessment in patients with α-spectrin defects. It correlates well with clinical severity and accurately predicts unusually severe mutations.[1357] Conversely, discordance between the degree of hemolysis and the fraction of spectrin dimers may alert the physician to an underlying, secondary complication (see the earlier section on common HE with chronic hemolysis).

Ektacytometry

The ektacytometer can be used to assess red cell membrane deformability and stability in patients with hemolytic disorders (see earlier).[1081-1083] Isolated red cell ghosts are subjected to high shear stress in a laser diffraction viscometer, and the "deformability index" (a measure of the average elongation of the sheared ghosts) is recorded as a function of time. Fragile ghosts fragment more quickly than normal, which causes their "deformability" to fall. The technique is a useful screening test because membrane stability is reduced in almost all membrane skeletal diseases, including HE and HPP. In addition, the ektacytometer can be modified to measure cellular deformability at different osmolalities, a technique termed osmotic gradient ektacytometry.[1084] The resulting curves depend on both membrane surface area and cell volume and are a sensitive measure of the surface loss that characterizes many skeletal defects.

Tryptic Maps of Spectrin

Limited tryptic digestion of spectrin extracted from erythrocytes, performed at 0° C, followed by SDS-PAGE or isoelectric focusing combined with SDS-PAGE (two-dimensional gels), separates the resulting trypsin-resistant domains of α- and β-spectrin.[1423,1424] In the past, these gels were used to create characteristic, reproducible maps. Among the peptides on these maps, the 80-kd αI-domain peptide, which contains the self-association site of normal α-spectrin, is the most prominent. Many of the known elliptocytogenic α-spectrin mutations affect the 80-kd domain and yield peptide maps containing one or more fragments of the domain. Historically, tryptic peptide mapping has been a useful tool to map the approximate sites of the underlying spectrin mutations; the mutations have subsequently been defined by PCR and sequencing of the corresponding region of cDNA or genomic DNA.

Genetic Analysis

Genomic DNA isolated from peripheral blood leukocytes or reverse-transcribed reticulocyte or bone marrow mRNA can be amplified by PCR with specific DNA oligonucleotide primers flanking the region suspected to contain a mutation. The amplification product is then subjected to nucleic acid sequencing or other forms of analysis. Screening techniques can be used when there are no biochemical clues to the location of the mutation. These techniques are particularly advantageous when the genes of large proteins, such as spectrin or ankyrin, are analyzed. Genomic DNA is tested in most patients because the mutant mRNA species may not accumulate in significant amounts. The single-strand conformation polymorphism (SSCP) method is a simple, sensitive, and appropriately popular example of such a screening test. Labeled, PCR-amplified DNA fragments (100 to 400 bp) are denatured, and the single strands are refolded before running on a nondenaturing gel.[1425,1426] Even a single nucleotide change usually alters the folding pattern enough to allow mutant and normal fragments to separate on the gel (70% to 90% of mutations). In some regions where common elliptocytogenic mutations have been identified, multiplex PCR techniques or simple restriction endonuclease digestion of amplified DNA can be used to rapidly screen for these mutations. Unfortunately, DNA testing for HS and HE mutations is not available commercially and very few private laboratories will do the analysis. It is hoped that commercial testing will become available as the cost of DNA sequencing comes down in the next few years.

Etiology of Common Hereditary Elliptocytosis and Related Disorders

Spectrin Defects

Abnormalities in either α- or β-spectrin are associated with many occurrences of HE and HPP. The majority

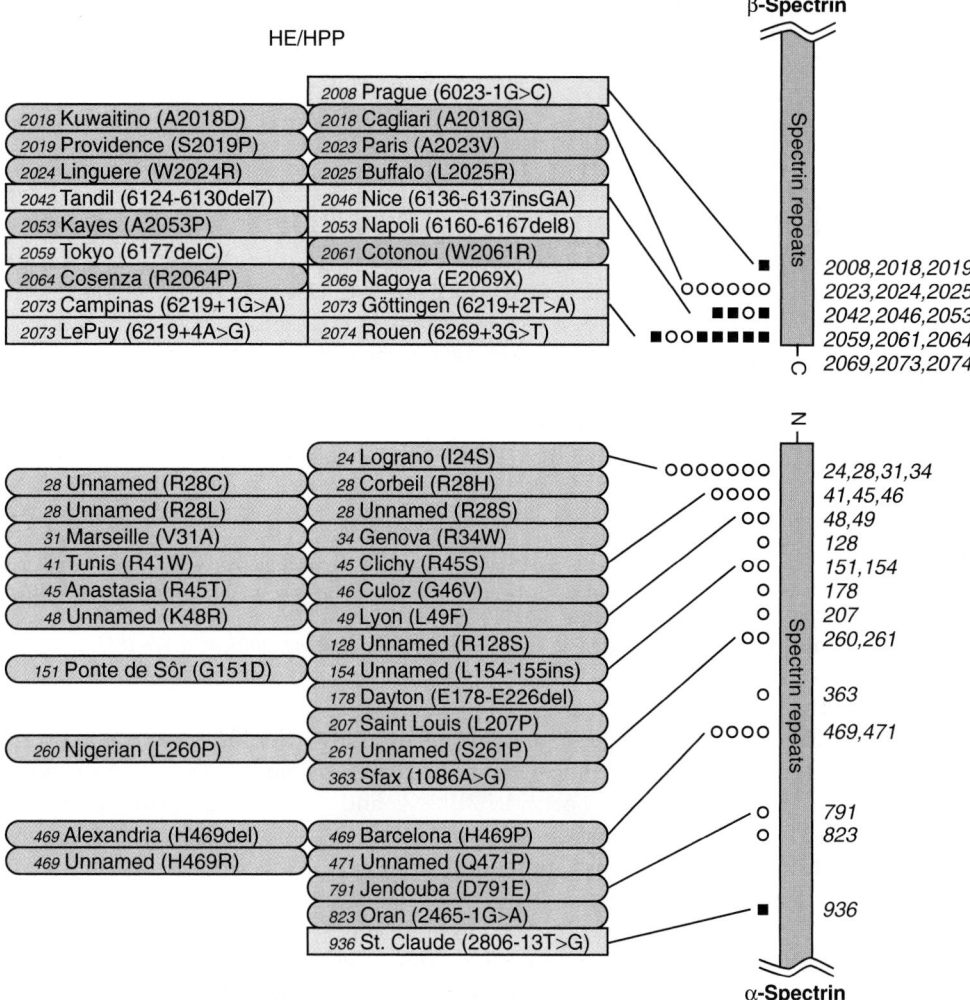

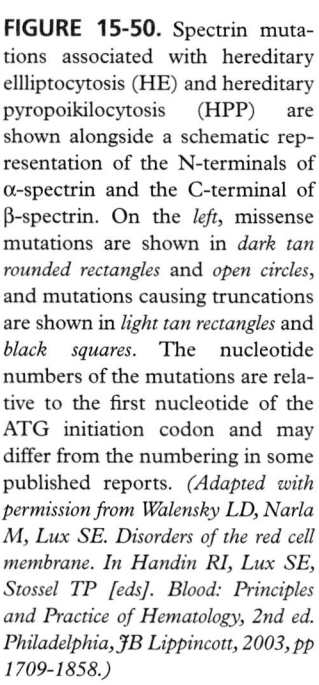

FIGURE 15-50. Spectrin mutations associated with hereditary ellliptocytosis (HE) and hereditary pyropoikilocytosis (HPP) are shown alongside a schematic representation of the N-terminals of α-spectrin and the C-terminal of β-spectrin. On the *left*, missense mutations are shown in *dark tan rounded rectangles* and *open circles*, and mutations causing truncations are shown in *light tan rectangles* and *black squares*. The nucleotide numbers of the mutations are relative to the first nucleotide of the ATG initiation codon and may differ from the numbering in some published reports. (*Adapted with permission from Walensky LD, Narla M, Lux SE. Disorders of the red cell membrane. In Handin RI, Lux SE, Stossel TP [eds]. Blood: Principles and Practice of Hematology, 2nd ed. Philadelphia, JB Lippincott, 2003, pp 1709-1858.*)

are due to mutations in the spectrin heterodimer self-association site (Fig. 15-50), with defective ability of spectrin dimers to form tetramers resulting in destabilization of the erythrocyte membrane skeleton. The decreased spectrin self-association is reflected by an increased proportion of spectrin dimers in 0° C, low–ionic strength extracts of spectrin and decreased conversion of spectrin dimers to tetramers in solution, in ghosts, and on inside-out vesicles. The fragile spectrin-spectrin links weaken the membrane skeleton and diminish resistance of the isolated membrane or skeleton to shear stress.[1082,1323]

The severity of the spectrin mutation in HE correlates with the degree of impairment in spectrin self-association and spectrin structural disruption, as measured by the degree of deviation of the mutant spectrin backbone from the crystal structure of the normal spectrin repeat,[1427] as well as with the amount of mutant spectrin that is produced, which is strongly influenced by the spectrin α[LELY] polymorphism (see later).[1357,1428,1429] Of key clinical importance, mutations within or near the site of self-association produce a more profound defect in spectrin function and a more severe clinical phenotype than do point mutations in more distant spectrin repeats.

α-Spectrin Self-Association Site Defects

Most of the HE defects are in the 80-kd αI domain at the NH$_2$-terminal of the α-spectrin chain. Nine tryptic cleavage defects of the normal 80-kd αI domain peptide have been identified by tryptic mapping and are characterized by loss of the normal 80-kd peptide and appearance of one of the following: a new 78-kd peptide ($\alpha^{I/78}$), a new 74-kd peptide ($\alpha^{I/74}$), a new 65- or 68-kd peptide ($\alpha^{I/65-68}$), a new 61-kd peptide ($\alpha^{I/61}$), a new 46-kd peptide ($\alpha^{I/46}$), a new 50- or 46-kd peptide ($\alpha^{I/46-50a}$), a new 50-kd peptide with a more basic isoelectric point than $\alpha^{I/46-50a}$ ($\alpha^{I/50b}$), two new peptides of 43 and 42 kd ($\alpha^{I/43}$), or two new peptides of 36 and 33 kd ($\alpha^{I/36-33}$). Codon 28, which contains a CpG nucleotide, is a mutation "hot spot." Mutations in this codon are associated with spectrin deficiency and cause mild to severe HE.

The αβ-spectrin heterodimer self-association contact site is a combined triple-helical repeat in which two helices (A and B) are contributed by the COOH-terminal of β-spectrin and the third helix (C) is a portion of the NH$_2$-terminal of α-spectrin (Fig. 15-51; see also Fig. 15-13). These three helices pair up,[1320,1430] as they do all along the spectrin chain, and create the bond responsible for spectrin self-association. The existence and functional

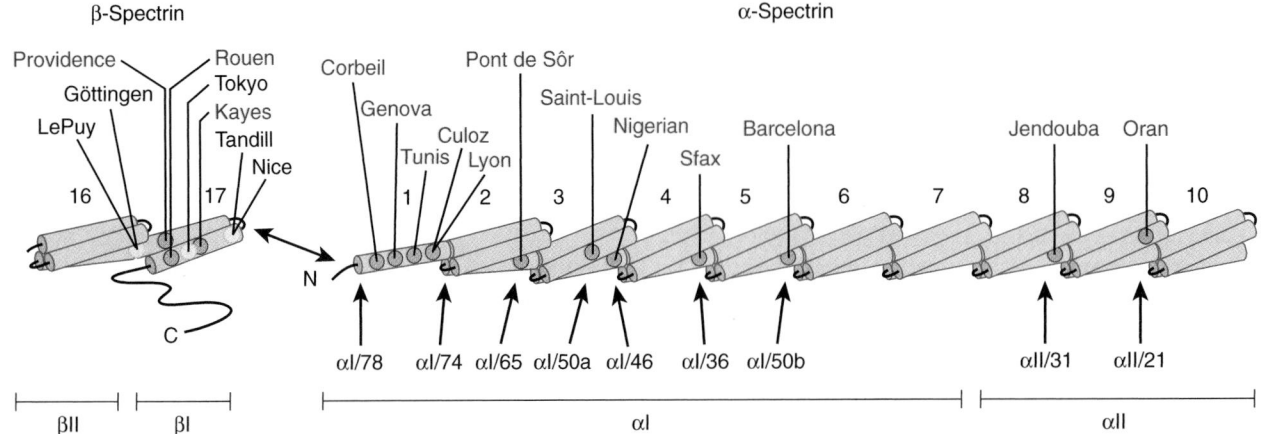

FIGURE 15-51. Triple-helical model of mutations in the αβ-spectrin self-association site associated with hereditary ellliptocytosis and hereditary pyropoikilocytosis. The abnormal tryptic cleavage sites observed in α-spectrin defects are indicated. Nearly all the α-spectrin mutations are missense mutations or in-frame deletions or insertions (*red circles*). Many of the more distal mutations are in helix C near the junction between one spectrin repeat and the next and are thought to interfere with cooperative effects linking spectrin self-association to spectrin-ankyrin and ankyrin–band 3 interactions. Most β-chain defects are C-terminal truncations (*yellow circles*) or missense mutations directly affecting spectrin self-association (*red circles*). The truncations also impair synthesis of the mutant spectrin and often lead to a spherocytic elliptocytosis phenotype. *(Adapted with permission from Walensky LD, Narla M, Lux SE. Disorders of the red cell membrane. In Handin RI, Lux SE, Stossel TP [eds]. Blood: Principles and Practice of Hematology, 2nd ed. Philadelphia, JB Lippincott, 2003, pp 1709-1858.)*

importance of this "atypical repeat" are proved by the study of human mutants, biochemical studies of wild-type and mutant recombinant peptides,[1431-1433] and molecular modeling.[1434-1437] Most α-spectrin defects, commonly attributable to missense mutations, occur in helix C of the triple-helical repeats.

Spectrin $\alpha^{I/74}$ is a heterogeneous collection of defects that result in enhanced tryptic cleavage after Arg45 or Lys48 in an extra helical segment (helix C) that juts out from the NH$_2$-terminal end of the α-spectrin chain. This is the end that participates in formation of the spectrin self-association contact site. The corresponding (COOH-terminal) end of the α chain also contains extra helices (helices A and B) in repeat 17, followed by a phosphorylated segment.

Spectrin $\alpha^{I/74}$ mutations disrupt one of the three interacting terminal helices of the contact site and markedly disrupt spectrin self-association. As a result, they are generally the most severe of the common α-spectrin mutations that cause HE and HPP. Patients who are homozygous for $\alpha^{I/74}$ defects usually have life-threatening hemolysis and an HPP-like syndrome.[1347,1357] Spectrin deficiency and the appearance of spherocytes along with elliptocytes and poikilocytes are common features of the most severe forms of HE and HPP.

In most instances, the primary defect in spectrin $\alpha^{I/74}$ variants is an amino acid substitution near the site of enhanced tryptic cleavage in the α chain.[1438,1439] Examples are Arg28Cys, Arg28Leu, Arg28Ser, Arg34Trp, Gly46Val, Lys48Arg, and Leu49Phe. Codon 28, a CpG dinucleotide, is a "hot spot" for mutation and has been associated with four different sequence variations. In addition, in an increasing number of HE and HPP kindreds with $\alpha^{I/74}$ mutations, the primary defect occurs in helices A or B of repeat 17 of β-spectrin (e.g., Ala2018Gly,

Ser2019Pro, Ala2053Pro, and Trp2016Arg). These two helices are adjacent to the $\alpha^{I/74}$ cleavage site in helix C at the NH$_2$ terminal of the α chain.

Spectrin $\alpha^{I/46-50a}$ is also heterogeneous and variable in severity. Generally, it is less severe than the disorder caused by spectrin $\alpha^{I/74}$ and more severe than that associated with spectrin $\alpha^{I/65-68}$.[1429,1440] Examples include Leu207Pro, Leu260Pro, and Ser261Pro mutations. This disorder is common in black populations, particularly the L260P defect,[1317,1441] which has an incidence of 0.5% in Benin.[1317]

Spectrin $\alpha^{I/65-68}$ is a common α-spectrin mutation (Leu154LeuLeu) that is widely distributed in blacks in West Africa, where the prevalence of HE is 0.67%,[1442] in blacks in Central Africa,[1429] and in their descendants in the West Indies and North America.[1443-1449] It is also seen in Arab populations and is the most common cause of HE in North Africa. The disorder is quite mild. It causes very mild common HE in North Africans, who sometimes have little or no elliptocytosis (i.e., are silent carriers). Even homozygotes have only mild to moderate hemolysis. Studies indicate that with one exception,[1443] all patients have an extra leucine inserted between codons 154 and 155, probably because of duplication of codon 154.[1444,1450] The high rate of occurrence of $\alpha^{I/65-68}$ and its homogeneous expression strongly suggest that it has experienced genetic selection.[1317] This has led to the hypothesis that it may provide some protection from malaria or other tropical diseases caused by blood-borne parasites. This theory has not yet been tested systematically, although there is preliminary evidence that growth of *P. falciparum* is inhibited in $\alpha^{I/65-68}$ erythrocytes.[1451]

Readers interested in descriptions of additional α-spectrin mutations that cause HE can refer to an earlier chapter by one of the authors (S.E.L.).[850]

β-Spectrin Self-Association Site Defects

Almost 20 mutations in the β-spectrin chain have been associated with HE or HPP. These mutations occur at the COOH-terminal region of β-spectrin and tend to be truncations or missense mutations that disrupt formation of the atypical triple-helix repeat, thereby weakening spectrin self-association (see Figs. 15-49 and 15-50). The molecular defects causing the truncated β-spectrin include frameshift mutations,[1405-1407,1452,1453] exon skipping,[1403,1408-1412,1454] and a nonsense mutation.[1455] Several of the missense mutations described result in excess proline residues.[1456] Because proline residues are known to disrupt α helices, this substitution emphasizes the importance of the atypical triple-helix conformation of the spectrin self-association site. Patients with β-spectrin missense mutations have common HE. However, patients with frameshift mutations leading to truncated β-spectrin have spherocytic HE. Patients who are homozygous for a β-spectrin mutation tend to have HPP and a more severe clinical course.

Spectrin Defects outside the Heterodimer Self-Association Site

Mutant spectrins outside the heterodimer self-association site, such as spectrin[St. Claude], spectrin[Oran], spectrin[Jendouba], and spectrin[Detroit], have been described in patients with HE and HPP. These mutations appear to be less severe than those that directly affect spectrin self-association in that the simple heterozygous state is asymptomatic. Patients who are homozygous for these mutations have HE or HPP.

Spectrin[St. Claude], identified in 3% of asymptomatic individuals from Benin, Africa,[1427] and in a white family of Afrikaans origin in South Africa,[1457] is caused by a splice junction mutation that leads to two variant mRNA species.[1379] One species encodes a truncated α-spectrin chain that is not assembled on the membrane. The other species encodes a protein that lacks exon 20 but is attached to the membrane[1427] and exhibits reduced spectrin-ankyrin binding.[1457] Because α-spectrin is produced in excess, heterozygous patients are asymptomatic. Spectrin[Oran] is a variant of the αII domain that is expressed at low levels.[1378] It causes no symptoms in the heterozygous state but causes severe HE in the homozygous state. The abnormal spectrin is caused by abnormal cleavage after Arg890[1378,1381] because of a mutation in the acceptor splice site upstream of exon 18 that causes exon 18 to be skipped. Spectrin[Jendouba] is a variant associated with asymptomatic HE, a mild defect in spectrin self-association,[1458] and abnormal tryptic cleavage after Lys788 as a result of an Asp→Glu mutation at codon 791. A large β-spectrin chain variant, spectrin[Detroit], with an estimated molecular mass of 330 kd has been isolated from two families.[1459,1460] Further study of one of the patients and his family members demonstrated that HE was caused by coinheritance of an α-spectrin chain variant rather than by the elongated β-spectrin chain. Family members with normal α-spectrin and heterozygous for the elongated β-chain variant had normal red cell morphology and no clinical abnormalities, but their erythrocyte membranes were more rigid and fragile than normal. The fragility is probably a consequence of both weaker spectrin dimer association and spectrin deficiency (total spectrin was about 80% of normal).

Low-Expression α-Spectrin Allele: α[LELY] Polymorphism

Some patients with HE and HPP are heterozygous for a structural variant of spectrin involving the self-association site but have a more severe phenotype than expected, including marked hemolysis and anemia that require treatment with blood transfusions or splenectomy. These patients, who also have spectrin deficiency, are usually categorized as having HE with chronic hemolysis or HPP. It has been postulated that the differences in clinical expression are at least partially due to a second defect in α-spectrin or a low-expression allele that affects spectrin production or accumulation. The parents who transmit the postulated defect are clinically and biochemically normal. The best characterized of these low-expression alleles is the α[LELY] allele (low-expression Lyon), which affects approximately 30% of the α-spectrin alleles of white Europeans, 20% of the alleles of the Japanese and Africans, and 22% of the alleles of the Chinese.[1356,1461] Therefore, approximately 42% of white Europeans are heterozygous for this allele and 9% are homozygous. The genetic advantage of the α[LELY] allele has not yet been uncovered.

The α[LELY] allele is caused by a combination of two mutations. One mutation is a C→T substitution at position −12 of intron 45, immediately upstream of exon 46, which causes the six amino acids encoded by exon 46 to be skipped 50% of the time. The second mutation is an amino acid substitution, Leu→Val at codon 1857 in exon 40, caused by a C→G substitution.[1462,1463] This mutation is found in helix B of the α-spectrin repeat and causes more rapid cleavage between the αIV and αV tryptic peptide domains, which creates an increased concentration of the 41-kd αV domain (i.e., the α[V/41] polymorphism).[1356] The effects of these two mutations are shown in Figure 15-52.

The α[LELY] allele is clinically silent by itself, even when in the homozygous state, probably because α-spectrin is normally synthesized in threefold or fourfold excess.[1464] In patients who are heterozygous for α[LELY] and an α-spectrin mutation causing HE, the limited synthesis of α[LELY] protein decreases the amount of spectrin containing α[LELY] that is incorporated into the membrane by approximately 50% and increases the relative incorporation of spectrin containing the mutant HE α chain. α[LELY] is poorly expressed as a result of the mutation in intron 45, described earlier, which causes defective spectrin nucleation because the six deleted amino acids encoded by exon 46 lie within the nucleation site that joins the α- and β-spectrin chains.[1465,1466] α Chains that lack exon

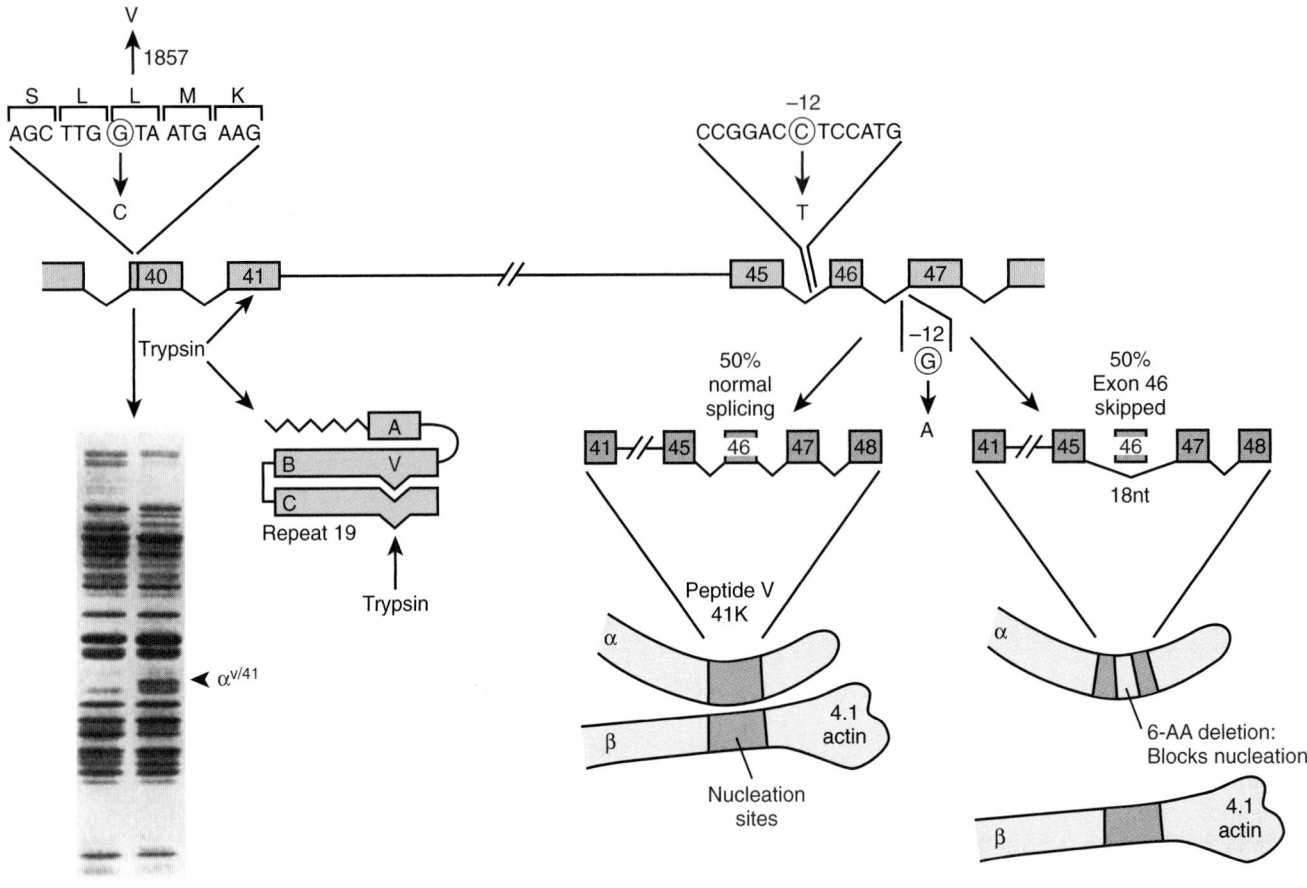

FIGURE 15-52. Nature of the low-expression α^{LELY} allele. The allele contains two linked mutations: a marker mutation, the $\alpha^{V/41}$ defect, and a splicing mutation, the α^{LELY} defect. *Left,* The $\alpha^{V/41}$ defect is caused by a G→C substitution at the beginning of exon 40, which changes a Leu1857→ Val in helix B of spectrin repeat 19. The valine impinges on the neighboring helix C of the repeat and makes it more trypsin sensitive, thereby leading to more rapid release of $\alpha^{V/41}$ peptide from the trypsin-treated spectrin derived from the α^{LELY} allele. Sodium dodecyl sulfate gels of trypsin-treated normal and α^{LELY}-containing spectrin are shown at the *bottom left.* The $\alpha^{V/41}$ peptide is marked. *Right,* The linked splicing mutation is a C→ T substitution at position −12 in the acceptor splice site of intron 45 (a second linked mutation, G→A at position −12 of intron 46, may also contribute). This causes exon 46 to be skipped in 50% of α^{LELY} spectrin molecules *(far right).* Exon 46 is very small, only six amino acids (AA), but it lies in the center of the nucleation site required for side-to-side association of the spectrin α and β chains. The half of α^{LELY} spectrin that lacks exon 46 cannot form spectrin heterodimers and is destroyed. Note that the other 50% of α^{LELY} spectrin contains exon 46 and will be functionally normal (though marked by the $\alpha^{V/41}$ tryptic peptide). *(Adapted with permission from Walensky LD, Narla M, Lux SE. Disorders of the red cell membrane. In Handin RI, Lux SE, Stossel TP [eds]. Blood: Principles and Practice of Hematology, 2nd ed. Philadelphia, JB Lippincott, 2003, pp 1709-1858.)*

46 fail to assemble into stable spectrin dimers and are rapidly degraded.

The effect of the α^{LELY} allele can be quite dramatic. In one family, a patient who was heterozygous for the $\alpha^{I/74}$ mutation (+/$\alpha^{I/74}$) had very mild disease and almost no morphologic abnormality, whereas a relative who had also inherited the α^{LELY} allele ($\alpha^{I/74}/\alpha^{LELY}$) had severe elliptocytosis.[1356] Similarly, in another family the α^{LELY} allele increased the proportion of spectrin $\alpha^{I/65-68}$ in heterozygotes from 45% to 65% of the total spectrin.[1356] This was associated with an increase in the proportion of elliptocytes from none or only a few to nearly 100%. Conversely, when the α^{LELY} allele is on the same chromosome as an α-spectrin mutation, it mutes the elliptocytic phenotype.[1322]

Spectrin α^{LELY} should be distinguished from the thalassemia-like defects of α-spectrin synthesis that when coinherited with some of the α-spectrin mutations, produce a phenotype of HPP. The latter defects are characterized by reduced α-spectrin mRNA levels and diminished α-spectrin synthesis.[1393,1467] In contrast, although the synthesis of α^{LELY} subunits is decreased because of poor incorporation of the peptide lacking exon 46, production of α^{LELY} mRNA is normal.

Protein 4.1 Defects

The link between protein 4.1 deficiency and elliptocytosis was first described in a consanguineous Algerian family (Fig. 15-53).[1332,1380] Partial absence of the protein is found in the 4.1(−) trait, which appears to be a common cause of elliptocytosis and accounts for 30% to 40% of occurrences in some Arab and European populations.[1339,1340,1383,1468] However, this deficiency is not observed in individuals of African ancestry.[1318]

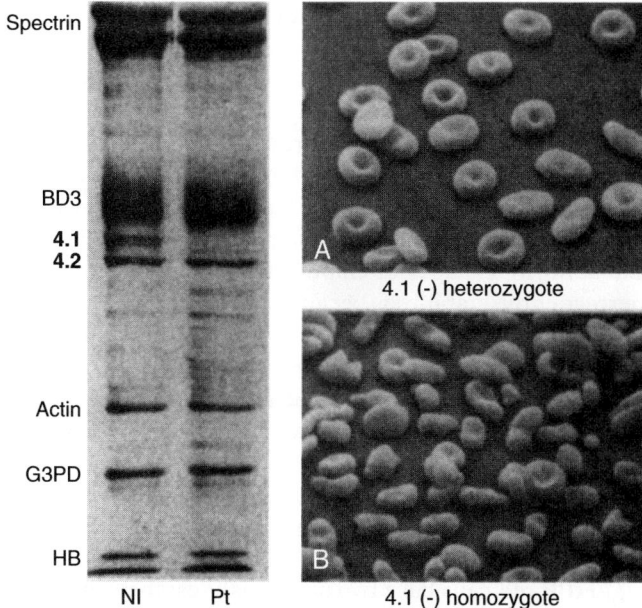

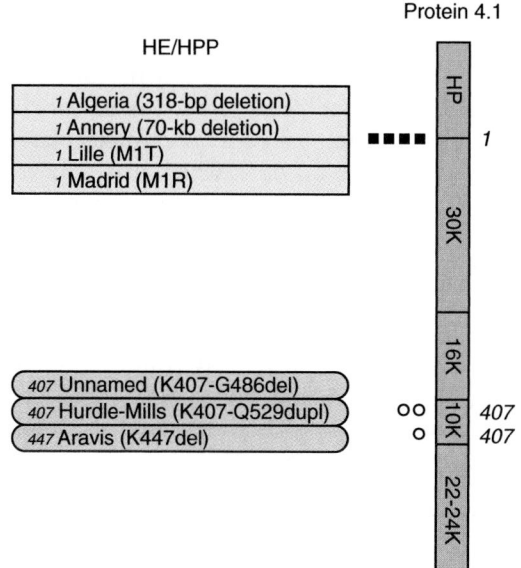

FIGURE 15-53. Deficiency of protein 4.1 in hereditary elliptocytosis. *Left,* Sodium dodecyl sulfate gels of red cell membrane proteins from a normal individual (Nl) and a patient with homozygous hereditary elliptocytosis who lacks protein 4.1 (Pt). *Right,* Scanning electron micrographs of red blood cells in 4.1-deficient patients. **A,** Elliptocytes in a patient with heterozygous hereditary elliptocytosis and 50% protein 4.1. **B,** Elliptocytes, poikilocytes, and fragmented red cells in a patient with homozygous hereditary elliptocytosis and no 4.1. BD, band 3; G3PD, glyceraldehyde-3-phosphate dehydrogenase; HB, hemoglobin. *(Reprinted from Tchernia G, Mohandas N, Shohet SB. Deficiency of cytoskeletal membrane protein band 4.1 in homozygous hereditary elliptocytosis: implications for erythrocyte membrane stability. J Clin Invest. 1981; 68:454.)*

FIGURE 15-54. Protein 4.1 mutations associated with hereditary elliptocytosis are shown alongside a schematic representation of the protein. On the *left,* four mutations abolishing the translation start site are shown in the *light tan rectangles* and *black squares.* A large deletion and a large insertion affecting the spectrin-actin binding domain are shown in the *dark tan rounded rectangles* and *open circles,* as is a missense mutation at codon 447. The nucleotide numbers of the mutations are relative to the first nucleotide of the ATG initiation codon and may differ from the numbering in some published reports. *(Adapted with permission from Walensky LD, Narla M, Lux SE. Disorders of the red cell membrane. In Handin RI, Lux SE, Stossel TP [eds]. Blood: Principles and Practice of Hematology, 2nd ed. Philadelphia, JB Lippincott, 2003, pp 1709-1858.)*

In the original Algerian kindred,[1332] protein 4.1(−) mRNA is not translated[1469] because of a 318-bp deletion that includes the downstream translation initiation site used in reticulocytes (see Fig. 15-18A).[1470] In other patients, point mutations in the downstream initiator codon (AUG→AGG[1380] and AUG→ACG[1471]) have been identified (Fig. 15-54). Interestingly, expression of protein 4.1 is relatively unimpaired in nonerythroid tissues and early erythroblasts[1472-1475] because most of the protein 4.1 isoforms in these tissues initiate translation at the alternatively spliced, upstream translation initiation site.

Protein 4.1(−) heterozygotes have clinically mild common HE with prominent elliptocytosis, often approaching 100%, and little or no hemolysis.[1476] These patients have 50% of the normal amount of protein 4.1.

Erythrocytes from patients homozygous for the protein 4.1(−) trait (i.e., complete protein 4.1 deficiency) are elliptical, fragmented, and poikilocytic (see Fig. 15-53B).[1332,1380,1477] They are very osmotically fragile and possess normal thermal stability. Membranes from homozygous protein 4.1(−) red cells fragment much more rapidly than normal at moderate sheer stress, an indication of their intrinsic instability.[1082] Membrane mechanical stability can be completely restored by reconstituting the deficient red cells with normal protein 4.1 or the spectrin-actin binding site from protein 4.1.[1330,1478]

In addition to complete protein 4.1 deficiency, erythrocytes from protein 4.1(−) homozygotes lack protein p55[1479,1480] and have only 30% of the normal content of GPC and GPD.[1380,1480-1482] This adds evidence to the hypothesis that GPC is one of the membrane attachment sites for protein 4.1.[1483] In addition, protein 4.9 is absent from isolated membrane skeletons but not from intact red cell membranes, and membrane phospholipid asymmetry is perturbed.[1332,1484] Electron microscopic studies of homozygous 4.1(−) erythrocyte membranes have revealed a markedly disrupted skeletal network with disruption of the intramembrane particles, thus suggesting that protein 4.1 plays an important role in maintenance of not only the skeletal network but also the integral proteins of the membrane structure.[1485] Homozygous patients have a severe transfusion-dependent hemolytic anemia but demonstrate a good response to splenectomy.[1332,1380,1477]

Protein 4.1 Structural Defects. Variants of protein 4.1 with abnormal molecular weights have also been described in association with HE.[1340,1486-1489] For example, a shortened protein 4.1 was discovered in an Italian family with very mild common HE and mechanically unstable red cells. The patients are heterozygous for a protein 4.1 variant that has lost the two exons encoding the spectrin/

actin binding domain (see Fig. 15-54). The mutant protein runs as a doublet of 65 and 68 kd on SDS gels and seems to be present in nearly normal amounts. It is presumed but has not been proved to be functionally inept. Another example is a high-molecular-weight variant, protein 4.1[Hurdle-Mills],[1340] which was discovered in a family of Scottish-Irish ancestry with very mild common HE. The patients are heterozygous for a duplication of three exons that include the spectrin-actin binding domain (see Fig. 15-54).[1486,1487] Membrane function appears to be preserved because red cell membranes have normal mechanical stability.[1490] It is not clear how this functionally normal variant causes HE. Other examples of variants of protein 4.1 with abnormal molecular weights have been described.[1488,1489]

Glycophorin C Defects

Elliptocytes are noted on peripheral blood smears of patients whose erythrocytes carry the rare Leach phenotype of Gerbich-negative (Ge–) cells.[1412,1413,1491-1495] These erythrocytes are devoid of GPC and GPD and, presumably secondarily, are also deficient in protein p55 and protein 4.1. It has been speculated that the protein 4.1 deficiency in Leach erythrocytes is the cause of their elliptocytic shape. Interestingly, the relative deficiency of protein 4.1 in Leach erythrocytes is less than the degree of GPC deficiency in homozygous protein 4.1(–) erythrocytes. These findings add supportive evidence to the hypothesis that GPC and protein p55 provide a binding site for protein 4.1 in the red cell.[1479]

The Leach phenotype is usually due to a deletion of 7 kb of genomic DNA that removes exons 3 and 4 from the GPC/GPD locus.[1491,1492] Patients carrying the Leach phenotype suffer from mild spherocytic HE with increased erythrocyte OF.[1412,1493-1495] In some individuals, no elliptocytes are detected on peripheral smear.[1481]

In contrast to GPC and GPD deficiency, individuals whose erythrocytes lack GPA, GPB, or both are asymptomatic and have erythrocytes of normal shape and mechanical stability.

Pathophysiology of Hereditary Elliptocytosis/Hereditary Pyropoikilocytosis

Spectrin Mutations

The principal functional consequence of the elliptocytogenic spectrin mutations is weakening or even disruption of the spectrin dimer-tetramer contact and, consequently, the two-dimensional integrity of the membrane skeleton. These "horizontal" defects are readily detected by ultrastructural examination of membrane skeletons, which reveals disruption of the normally uniform hexagonal lattice. As a result, membrane skeletons, cell membranes, and the red cells are mechanically unstable. In patients who have severely dysfunctional spectrin mutations or in subjects who are homozygous or compound heterozygous for such mutant proteins, this membrane instability

is sufficient to cause hemolytic anemia with red cell fragmentation.

The mechanism for the formation of elliptocytes is less clear. In common HE, red cell precursors are round and become progressively more elliptical as they age in vivo.[1313,1341,1496] Red cells distorted by shear stress in vitro or flowing through the microcirculation in vivo have elliptical or parachute-like shapes, respectively.[1497] Perhaps the abnormal shapes of elliptocytes and poikilocytes are permanently stabilized because the weakened skeletal interactions facilitate skeletal reorganization after prolonged or repetitive cellular deformation. Skeletal reorganization is likely to involve breakage of the unidirectionally stretched protein connections and formation of new contacts that reduce stress on the skeleton and stabilize the deformed shape.[1497] This process, first proposed in 1978, has been shown to account for permanent deformation of irreversibly sickled cells.[1498]

HPP red cells have two abnormalities: they contain a mutant spectrin that disrupts spectrin self-association, and they are partially deficient in spectrin.[1392,1393] This is either due to an elliptocytogenic α-spectrin mutation and a defect involving reduced α-spectrin synthesis or due to two elliptocytogenic spectrin alleles. In the latter situation, the spectrin deficiency might be a consequence of spectrin instability, which would reduce the amount of spectrin available for membrane assembly. In red cells carrying a lot of unassembled spectrin dimers, the fact that one ankyrin is bound per one spectrin tetramer (i.e., two spectrin heterodimers) may also contribute to the spectrin deficiency. At best, only about half of the spectrin dimers could succeed in attaching to the available ankyrin binding sites. Probably, this attachment would be less because unphosphorylated ankyrin binds spectrin dimers about 10 times less avidly than it does spectrin tetramers.[1499] The phenotype of HPP, characterized by the presence of fragments and elliptocytes, together with evidence of red cell surface area deficiency (i.e., microspherocytes), suggests that the membrane dysfunction involves both "vertical" interactions (a consequence of the spectrin deficiency) and "horizontal" interactions (a consequence of the elliptocytogenic spectrin mutations).

Protein 4.1 Variants

Hereditary elliptocytes that are deficient in protein 4.1 are similar in shape and membrane instability to elliptocytes that result from spectrin mutations.[1497] This suggests that protein 4.1 deficiency principally affects spectrin-actin contact (i.e., a horizontal interaction) rather than the skeletal attachment to GPC (a vertical interaction).

Permeability of Hereditary Elliptocytosis Red Cells

Red cells in HE consume more ATP and 2,3-DPG than normal erythrocytes do,[1500] probably because of increased transmembrane Na$^+$ movement.[1501] As a result of the underlying skeletal defect, HE and HPP red cells are abnormally permeable to Na$^+$, K$^+$, and Ca^{2+} ions.[1388,1501] The excessive Ca^{2+} leak was originally thought to be the primary molecular lesion in a patient with severe microcytic hemolytic anemia and red cell thermal instability,[1388] but the patient was subsequently shown to have a spectrin mutation and, probably, HPP.[1440]

Common Hereditary Elliptocytosis and Malaria

Epidemiologic studies of the elliptocytogenic mutations of spectrin in central and western Africa suggest that their prevalence is considerably greater than would be expected for sporadic mutations. The prevalence of the spectrin $\alpha^{I/65-68}$ mutation approaches 1%,[1318] and the mutation is always associated with the same α-spectrin haplotype.[1502] Similar findings were reported for two α-spectrin mutations producing the spectrin $\alpha^{I/46-50a}$ phenotype (Leu207→Pro and Leu260→Pro). These data are of considerable interest in light of recent in vitro studies demonstrating diminished malarial parasite entry or growth in red cells that contain some of the elliptocytogenic spectrin mutants or are deficient in protein 4.1.[1451,1503,1504]

SOUTHEAST ASIAN OVALOCYTOSIS

SAO, also known as Melanesian ovalocytosis or stomatocytic elliptocytosis, is observed in the aboriginal populations of Melanesia and Malaysia and in portions of Indonesia and the Philippines.[1505-1511] The abnormality is very common in Melanesia, particularly in lowland and island tribes, in whom malaria is endemic,[1506,1511-1513] and it affects 1% to 15% of the population.[1514,1515] SAO has been detected rarely in white and African American individuals.[1516-1519] SAO is inherited in an autosomal dominant pattern.[1505-1508,1512,1520] In screening of large populations with SAO, no homozygotes have been identified,[1521,1522] thus suggesting that homozygosity leads to embryonic or fetal lethality.

Resistance to Malaria

In vivo, there is evidence that SAO provides some protection against all forms of malaria, particularly against heavy infections and cerebral malaria.[1506,1507,1512,1513,1523-1526] The prevalence of SAO increases with age in populations challenged by malaria, which suggests that individuals with SAO have a selective advantage.[1523] In vitro, SAO red cells are resistant to invasion by malarial parasites,[1527-1530] apparently because the membrane is 10 to 20 times more rigid than normal.[1531-1534] Other membrane characteristics reflect this property, including unusually high heat resistance, lack of endocytosis in response to drugs that produce dramatic endocytosis in normal cells, and strong resistance to crenation, even after several days of storage in plasma or buffered salt solutions.[1531] However, other population studies show no correlation between the SAO mutation and the prevalence of malaria,[1515,1535] which may be due to the fact that some parasite strains invade SAO red cells efficiently whereas others do not.[1536] This supports the concept that malaria parasites can use different receptors or pathways for invasion (see the earlier section on band 3 and malaria).

Etiology

The finding of tight linkage between an abnormal proteolytic digest of band 3 protein and the SAO phenotype led to detection of the underlying molecular defect.[1520] All carriers of the SAO phenotype are heterozygotes. One band 3 allele is normal and the other contains two mutations in *cis*: a deletion of nine codons encoding amino acids 400 through 408, located at the end of the cytoplasmic domain and the beginning of the first transmembrane segment of band 3, and replacement of Lys56 by Glu.[1533,1534,1537-1540] The Lys56→Glu substitution is an asymptomatic polymorphism known as band 3^{Memphis} that is in linkage disequilibrium with the 9 amino acid deletion. The mutant SAO band 3 exhibits tight binding to ankyrin,[1520] increased tyrosine phosphorylation,[1541,1542] inability to transport anions,[1543,1544] and markedly restricted lateral and rotational mobility in the membrane.[1520,1533]

Clinical Features and Morphology

Most of the cells are rounded elliptocytes, but a few are traversed by one or two transverse bars that divide the central clear space (see Fig. 15-49D).[1505,1509-1511,1520,1545] These "theta cells" or "stomatocytic elliptocytes" are not seen in any other condition. Thus, identification of multiple theta cells on a peripheral blood smear strongly suggests SAO. Some stomatocytes may also be present. The strong resistance of red cells to crenation after several days of storage[1531] provides an additional clue to the diagnosis. However, the most specific diagnostic test for SAO is amplification of the deleted region from the band 3 gene in genomic DNA or reticulocyte cDNA. This produces a single band in control red cells and a doublet in SAO cells, with the second band shorter by 27 bp.[1533,1537,1546]

Hemolysis is apparently mild or absent,[1505,1507,1509,1510] although neonatal hyperbilirubinemia and mild hemolytic anemia have been described.[1547,1548] One patient had compensated hemolysis (no anemia) with mild splenomegaly, an absolute reticulocyte count of 150 to 300 × 10^{-3} (normal, 10 to 100 × 10^{-3}), mild hyperbilirubinemia, and gallstones.[1549] This indicates that membrane rigidity is not a major determinant of red cell survival. In another well-studied patient,[1510] red cell Na$^+$ and K$^+$ permeability was increased, glucose consumption was elevated to compensate for increased cation pumping, and the cells were osmotically resistant. Curiously, many blood group antigens are poorly expressed on the surface of SAO red cells,[1511] possibly because the rigid membrane inhibits their clustering and impedes agglutination.

SAO band 3 also is a recessive mutation for dRTA. The disease develops in patients who are compound heterozygotes for SAO and other band 3 mutations causing dRTA.[1550,1551] The reason is because sufficient heterodimers of normal and SAO band 3 reach the plasma membrane to prevent acidosis, whereas heterodimers of SAO and other dRTA band 3 molecules become trapped in the endoplasmic reticulum and lead to deficient Cl⁻ excretion.[1552]

Molecular Basis of Membrane Rigidity

SAO red cells are unique among elliptocytes in that they are rigid and hyperstable rather than unstable.[1532] The SAO band 3 mutation is the first example of a defect in an integral membrane protein leading to red cell membrane rigidity, a property that had previously been attributed to the membrane skeleton.[1553] The explanation for the rigidity is presently not clear. One hypothesis proposes that conformational changes in the cytoplasmic domain of SAO band 3 preclude lateral movement (extension) of the skeletal network during deformation.[1534,1554] A second possibility is that SAO band 3 binds abnormally tightly to ankyrin and thus to the underlying skeleton.[1513] The increased propensity of SAO band 3 to aggregate into higher oligomers may be important because the oligomers can strengthen attachment of band 3 to ankyrin.[1555] The tendency of SAO band 3 to form linear arrays would also decrease its mobility within the bilayer.[1556] Finally, SAO band 3 may adhere to the skeleton in a nonspecific manner, possibly because of denaturation of the membrane-spanning domain.[1557] Studies of the structure of the first transmembrane span of wild-type and SAO band 3 show that a bend between the cytoplasmic domain and the first transmembrane domain is absent in SAO cells; this leads to the formation of a stable helix in the region,[1558] possibly because of retraction of the polar amino acids that normally lie in the cytoplasm into the first transmembrane segment in SAO band 3.[1559] Other studies using chemical modification and proteolysis show that SAO band 3 is misfolded and affects the structure of its normal band 3 partner or partners.[1560]

The resistance of SAO red cells to malaria is presumably related to the altered properties of SAO band 3. Band 3 serves as one of the *P. falciparum* malaria receptors because invasion by the parasite in vitro is inhibited by band 3–containing liposomes.[1561] In normal red cells, parasite invasion is associated with marked membrane remodeling and redistribution of band 3–containing intramembrane particles.[1562] Intramembrane particles cluster at the site of parasite invasion and form a ring around the orifice through which the parasite enters the cell. The invaginated red cell membrane, which sur-

rounds the invading parasite, is free of intramembrane particles. The reduced lateral mobility of band 3 protein in SAO red cells may preclude band 3 receptor clustering and thus prevent attachment or entry of the parasites.[1520,1533] Resistance to malaria has also been attributed to diminished anion exchange as a result of the inability of SAO band 3 to transport anions.[1544] In addition, SAO red cells consume ATP at a higher rate than normal cells do, and the ensuing partial depletion of ATP levels in ovalocytes has been proposed to account, at least in part, for the resistance of these cells to malaria invasion in vitro.[1531] However, diminished anion transport and ATP depletion do not appear to play a critical role in the resistance of SAO erythrocytes to malaria in vivo. This is evidenced by the fact that band 3–deficient HS red cells are considerably less resistant to malaria invasion than SAO red cells are, although both cell types have a similar decrease in anion transport, and by the fact that resistance of SAO red cells to malaria is detected in vitro even when red cell ATP levels are maintained.

HYDROPS FETALIS SYNDROMES AND DISORDERS OF THE ERYTHROCYTE MEMBRANE

Defects in the erythrocyte membrane have been well characterized in patients with severe neonatal hemolytic anemia secondary to recessive HS, homozygous HE and HPP, and hereditary xerocytosis. Several well-documented kindreds with fatal or nearly fatal anemia and hydrops fetalis associated with erythrocyte membrane defects have been described. In several patients, defects were identified in spectrin, the principal structural protein of the erythrocyte membrane.[841,1435,1442] In the other patients, homozygosity for a band 3 defect was discovered (see earlier). Membrane defects have been suspected, but not proven in numerous other patients with nonimmune hydrops fetalis with severe hemolytic anemia.

STOMATOCYTOSIS AND XEROCYTOSIS

Red cell hydration is largely determined by the intracellular concentration of monovalent cations. A net increase in Na⁺ and K⁺ ions causes water to enter and form "stomatocytes" or "hydrocytes," whereas a net loss of monovalent cations produces dehydrated red cells, or "xerocytes" (see Fig. 15-29). In the past 35 years, numerous descriptions of congenital or familial hemolytic anemias associated with abnormal cation permeability and, in some cases, disturbed red cell hydration have been reported. These cases span the range from severe stomatocytosis to severe xerocytosis. They can be divided into six provisional clinical categories based on differences in severity, morphology, cation content, lipid and protein composition, genetics, and response to splenectomy: severe stomatocytosis,[1563-1579] mild stomatocytosis,[1580-1582] cryohydrocytosis,[1583-1589] stomatocytic xerocytosis,[1590] pseudohyperkalemia,[779,1591-1602] and xerocytosis (Table 15-8).[992,1591-1593,1595,1598,1603-1622] Although these divisions are useful as a method of categorization, it is likely that these categories are not unique entities, and the divisions are not clinically meaningful. Indeed, none of these apparent disorders are precisely defined in either clinical or molecular terms.

Osmotic gradient ektacytometry is a rapid and sensitive measure of red cell membrane hydration.[1084] The ektacytometer measures red cell deformability, osmotic resistance, and cell hydration. However, the equipment required is not readily available in most clinical centers. Therefore, other measures must be used in making the difficult diagnosis of a disorder of red cell membrane permeability.

Hereditary Stomatocytosis (Hydrocytosis, Overhydrated Stomatocytosis)

Hereditary stomatocytosis, the name given by Lock and co-workers[1569] to the first reported instance, is characterized by erythrocytes with a mouth-shaped (stoma) area of central pallor on peripheral blood smears (Fig. 15-55A). The clinical severity of hereditary stomatocytosis, a rare disorder, is variable; some patients experience hemolysis and anemia, whereas others are asymptomatic.

Stomatocyte membranes are remarkably permeable to Na^+ and K^+ ions, particularly Na^+ ions. Intracellular Na^+ is increased and K^+ is decreased, but the total monovalent cation content ($Na^+ + K^+$) is high, which leads to an increase in cell water and cell volume. As a consequence, the "edematous cells" are sometimes called hydrocytes or overhydrated stomatocytes.

Pathophysiology

The major detectable defect in hereditary stomatocytosis is a marked asymmetric increase in passive Na^+ and K^+ permeability (the amount of Na^+ in is greater than the amount of K^+ out). Permeabilities as great as 15 to 40 times normal are observed.[1563,1573,1612] Because the influx of Na^+ exceeds the loss of K^+, stomatocytic red cells progressively gain cations and water and swell. As a result, their average density is less than normal (Fig. 15-56), and the swollen stomatocytes are osmotically fragile. Unlike normal cells, aged stomatocytes are less dense and more stomatocytic than stomatocytic reticulocytes.[1563]

In stomatocytosis, monovalent cation transporters are stimulated by the influx of Na^+, particularly the Na^+,K^+ pump and the K^+-Cl^- cotransporter,[1571] but are unable to keep up with the exaggerated cation leaks. Na^+,K^+ pump kinetics is normal,[1580] and the number of pumps is increased severalfold,[1563,1615] even after corrections for red cell age.[1623]

Bifunctional imidoesters, which cross-link proteins, reverse the abnormal shape and permeability of hereditary stomatocytes and normalize their survival in the circulation.[1563] The critical proteins involved have not been identified with these agents because many red cell membrane proteins are cross-linked at the concentrations required to achieve this effect. Stomatocytes are relatively rigid[1570] and expend extraordinary amounts of ATP in pumping Na^+ and K^+ in an attempt to maintain homeostasis. They are vulnerable to splenic sequestration, and predictably, splenectomy has been beneficial in some patients with severe hemolysis,[1563,1571,1572,1574,1581] but not without risk (see later).[1222]

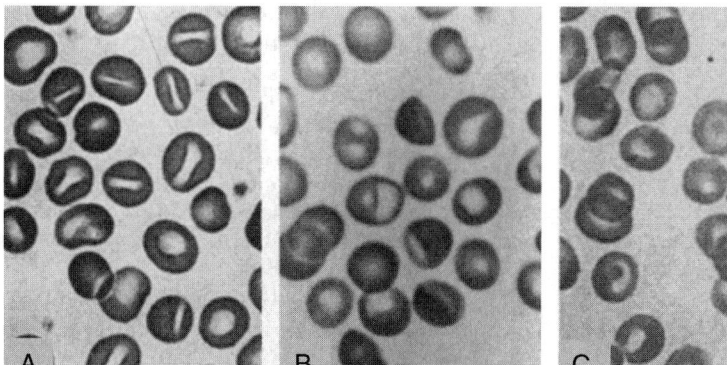
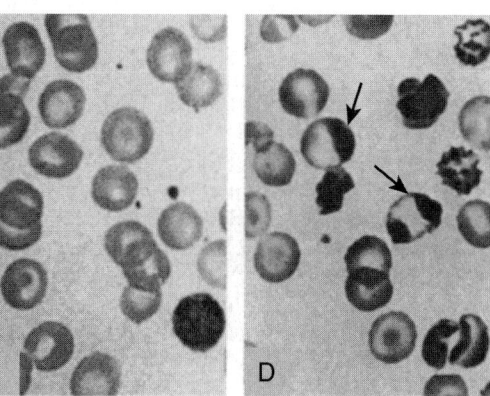

FIGURE 15-55. Peripheral blood morphology in hereditary stomatocytosis and hereditary xerocytosis. **A,** Stomatocytosis. Many stomatocytes and occasional spherocytes are seen. **B,** Cryohydrocytosis. Some of the stomatocytes are bowl shaped, some have curvilinear slits, and some have a transverse bar dividing the central clearing. **C,** Xerocytosis (typical). Some target cells are evident, but most red cells are morphologically unremarkable. **D,** Xerocytosis (severe). Target cells, echinocytes, and dense crenated cells predominate. In occasional cells (*arrow*) the hemoglobin appears to be puddled in one portion of the cell. (*A, From Turpin F, Lortholary P, Lejeune F, Claer R. Un cas d'anémie hémolytique avec stomatocytose. Nouv Rev Fr Hematol. 1971;11:585-594; **B,** from Miller G, Townes PL, MacWhinney JB. A new congenital hemolytic anemia with deformed erythrocytes ("stomatocytes") and remarkable susceptibility of erythrocytes to cold hemolysis in vitro. I. Clinical and hematologic studies. Pediatrics. 1965;35:906; **C,** from Jaffe ER, Gottfried EL. Hereditary nonspherocytic hemolytic disease associated with an altered phospholipid composition of the erythrocytes. J Clin Invest. 1968;47:1375-1388; **D,** from Glader BE, Fortier N, Albala MM, Nathan DG. Congenital hemolytic anemia associated with dehydrated erythrocytes and increased potassium loss. N Engl J Med. 1974;291:491.*)

TABLE 15-8   Features of Hereditary Stomatocytosis-Xerocytosis Syndromes

	STOMATOCYTOSIS (OVERHYDRATED STOMATOCYTOSIS)		INTERMEDIATE SYNDROMES		XEROCYTOSIS (DEHYDRATED STOMATOCYTOSIS)	
	Severe Hemolysis	Mild Hemolysis	Cryohydrocytosis	Stomatocytic Xerocytosis	Pseudohyperkalemia	Xerocytosis*
Hemolysis	Severe	Mild-moderate	Mild-moderate	Mild	Mild or none	Moderate
Anemia	Severe	Mild-moderate	Mild-moderate	None	None	Mild-moderate
Blood smear	Stomatocytes	Stomatocytes	Stomatocytes or normal	Stomatocytes	Targets, few stomatocytes	Some targets; occasional echinocytes, stomatocytes
MCV (80-100 μm³)†	110-150	95-130	90-105	91-98	82-104	84-122
MCHC (32%-36%)	24-30	26-29	34-38	33-39	33-39	34-38
Unincubated osmotic fragility	Very increased	Increased	Normal	Slightly decreased	Slightly decreased	Very decreased
RBC Na^+ (5-12 mEq/L)	60-100	30-60	15-50	10-20	10-25	10-30
RBC K^+ (90-103 mEq/L)	20-55	40-85	55-65	75-85	75-100	60-90
RBC $Na^+ + K^+$ (95-110 mEq/L)	110-140	115-145	75-105	87-109	87-109	75-99
RBC passive membrane leak‡	20-40	≈3-10	1-6	?	1-2	2-4
Cold autohemolysis	No	No	Yes	No	No	No
Pseudohyperkalemia	?Yes	?Yes	Yes	?	Yes	Sometimes
Perinatal ascites	No	?	No	?	No	Sometimes
Stomatin nearly absent	Yes	?	±No	?	?	No
Phosphatidylcholine content	Normal	±Increased	Normal	Normal	Normal	Increased
Effect of splenectomy	Good	Good	Fair-none	?	?	Poor
Thromboembolism post splenectomy	Yes	?	?No	?	?	Yes
Genetics	AD	AD	AD	AD	AD 16q23-q24	AD 16q23-q24

*Hereditary xerocytosis is identical to dehydrated hereditary stomatocytosis and to high-phosphatidylcholine hemolytic anemia.

†Normal values are given in parentheses.

‡Defined as ouabain- and bumetanide-resistant $^{86}Rb^+$ influx at 37° C and expressed as the ratio of patient to normal residual leak (normal = 0.06 to 0.10 mmol/L RBC/hr).

AR, autosomal recessive; AD, autosomal dominant; MCHC, mean corpuscular hemoglobin concentration; MCV, mean corpuscular volume; PC, phosphatidylcholine; RBC, red blood cell.

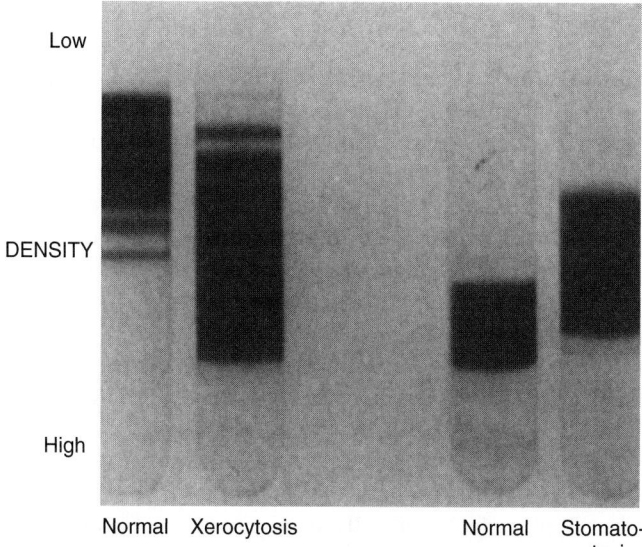

FIGURE 15-56. Separation of stomatocytes and xerocytes by density. *Left,* Normal and hereditary xerocytosis samples. The cells were separated on Stractan density gradients. The xerocytes extend to higher densities than normal red cells do. *Right,* Normal and hereditary stomatocytosis samples. Many of the stomatocytes are lighter than the control red cells. *(From Lande WM, Mentzer WC. Haemolytic anaemia associated with increased cation permeability. Clin Haematol. 1985;14:89.)*

Stomatin

The red cell membranes of all or almost all patients with the classic overhydrated form of stomatocytosis lack a 31-kd protein called stomatin or band 7.2b (Fig. 15-57).[1565,1566,1571,1575,1624,1625] Stomatin, a member of a large family of related proteins, is an integral membrane phosphoprotein whose function is not completely understood.[360,361,1575,1626-1631] The importance of stomatin is underscored by its wide tissue and species distribution. In humans, stomatin mRNA has been detected in every tissue and cell tested. Reactivity to a monoclonal antibody directed against human erythrocyte stomatin has been observed in the erythrocyte membranes of a wide variety of species, including the frog, rat, chicken, rabbit, pig, cow, and sheep.[1626] It has been hypothesized that stomatin may support, activate, or regulate an unidentified ion channel.[1575,1627,1628]

Although hereditary stomatocytosis appears to be a dominantly inherited condition and affected individuals are presumably heterozygotes, stomatin protein is almost absent, even though mRNA levels[1627] and the coding sequence of the gene[1632-1634] are normal. Immunochemistry detects some stomatin in a few red cells, particularly reticulocytes.[1576] Overall, there is about 2% to 5% of the normal amount of stomatin in red cells. Stomatin immunoreactivity in nonerythroid tissues is normal. This suggests that stomatin is made but is lost or destroyed in hereditary stomatocytes as the cells mature in the bone marrow and in the circulation. Mice with targeted disruption of stomatin are clinically and hematologically normal,[1635] which supports the idea that stomatin deficiency is secondary and not directly involved in patho-

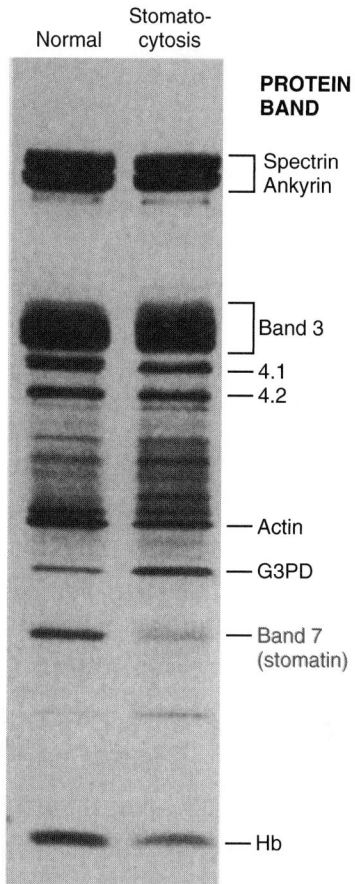

FIGURE 15-57. Stomatin deficiency in hereditary stomatocytosis. Sodium dodecyl sulfate gels of normal and stomatocytosis red cell membranes show that the principal (31-kd) band in the band 7 region (stomatin) is missing. A similar picture is observed in most patients with severe hereditary stomatocytosis. Immunoblots confirm that stomatin is nearly absent in these cells. G3PD, glyceraldehyde-3-phosphate dehydrogenase; Hb, hemoglobin. *(Reprinted from Rix M, Bjerrum PJ, Wieth JO, Frandsen B. Congenital stomatocytosis with hemolytic anemia—with abnormal cation permeability and defective membrane proteins. Ugeskr Laeger. 1991;153:724.)*

genesis of the cation leak and hemolysis. As discussed in the first section of the chapter, stomatin resides in detergent-resistant lipid domains called lipid rafts. Recent studies show that the amount of actin and tropomodulin (TMod) associated with these rafts is markedly reduced in hereditary stomatocytes.[1578] In addition, Ca^{2+}-induced exovesiculation is enhanced in stomatocytes, and the released vesicles contain greatly increased amounts of lipid raft proteins such as annexin VII, sorcin, copine 1, and the flotillins, but decreased amounts of stomatin and annexin V.[1578] In contrast, ATP-dependent endovesiculation is reduced in stomatin-deficient hereditary stomatocytes (but not in other forms of stomatocytosis).[1579] Interestingly, cross-linking imidoesters fix this defect, as well as the monovalent cation leak.[1579] These data suggest that there may be a defect in the interaction of stomatin with the membrane skeleton in stomatocytes, although why that would cause massive monovalent cation leaks is a mystery. Unfortunately, nothing is known about interactions between the membrane skeleton and stomatin or between TMod or actin and the lipid bilayer, so it is difficult to guess which proteins might be involved. It is also hard to guess why stomatin is deficient. Stomatin could be lost with other raft proteins in exocytic vesicles, but the vesicles are stomatin deficient not stomatin replete. In cultured erythroid cells from patients with hereditary stomatocytosis, stomatin immunoreactivity is confined to multivesicular complexes and the nucleus and is not seen on the plasma membrane.[1577] This suggests that stomatin deficiency may result from a trafficking defect, which might also affect other membrane proteins. One can imagine a defect in the trafficking mechanism itself or the loss of a chaperone, or stomatin could be abnormally modified by a post-translational process and preferentially recognized and destroyed by a protease or the proteosome.

Clinical Features

Typical Stomatin-Deficient Stomatocytosis. Diagnostic features of the classic type of hereditary stomatocytosis include the unique red cell morphology (5% to 50% stomatocytes) (see Fig. 15-55A), severe hemolysis, macrocytosis (110 to 150 fL), elevated erythrocyte Na^+ concentration of 60 to 100 mEq/L (normal range, 5 to 12 mEq/L), reduced K^+ concentration of 20 to 55 mEq/L (normal range, 90 to 103 mEq/L), and increased total $Na^+ + K^+$ content of 110 to 140 mEq/L (normal range, 95 to 110 mEq/L). The excess monovalent cations elevate cell water and thereby produce large, osmotically fragile cells with a low MCHC (24% to 30%). In many patients, hereditary stomatocytes are also moderately deficient in 2,3-DPG.[1563,1570,1615] Perhaps a portion of the 1,3-DPG normally used for 2,3-DPG synthesis is diverted through PGK to provide extra ATP for cation transport.[776] The 2,3-DPG deficiency mildly enhances oxygen affinity and causes additional water entry and cell swelling. Some patients[1568,1590] with hereditary stomatocytosis have an unexplained decrease in red cell glutathione; however, it is unlikely that this decrease is pathophysiologically significant. Stomatocytosis, like other hemolytic anemias, is often complicated by iron overload and cholelithiasis.

Hereditary Stomatocytosis Variants. Hereditary stomatocytosis is probably more heterogeneous than suggested earlier. Some patients with severe permeability defects have little or no hemolysis.[1614] In addition, studies of 44 Japanese patients with stomatocytosis show that the proportion of stomatocytes and the degree of Na^+ influx do not correlate with each other and that neither correlates with the amount of hemolysis or anemia.[1624] Furthermore, stomatin deficiency was not observed in Japanese patients with the most severe permeability defects and was present only to a mild degree in five of nine patients with more moderate Na^+ leaks. This suggests that hereditary stomatocytosis is a complex mixture of diseases or that factors other than those that regulate Na^+ leak and stomatin content are critical to demise of the stomatocyte.

Treatment: Splenectomy Is Dangerous

Splenectomy reduces the hemolytic rate in patients with severe hereditary stomatocytosis[1563,1564,1571,1572,1581] and can be beneficial; however, a high proportion of patients have experienced thrombotic complications, at times with disastrous results.[1222] Venous thrombi predominate and sometimes lead to portal hypertension or thromboembolism and pulmonary hypertension.[1222,1636,1637] Thrombotic episodes have not been reported before splenectomy. The cause of the hypercoagulable state after splenectomy in patients with hereditary stomatocytosis is uncertain. There is evidence that stomatocytes have about fourfold more PS on their surfaces than control cells do.[1638] As described earlier (see the section "Asymmetric Organization of Lipids in the Bilayer"), PS exposed on the outer surfaces of cells is highly thrombogenic.[74-76] Such cells are cleared by macrophages, which have PS receptors on their surface.[78-81] This function would presumably be impaired after splenectomy. In vitro, erythrocytes from two splenectomized individuals with hereditary stomatocytosis showed mildly increased adherence to endothelial monolayers.[1638,1639] Conceivably, this might also contribute to a hypercoagulable state.

Hereditary Xerocytosis (High-Phosphatidylcholine Hemolytic Anemia, Dehydrated Hereditary Stomatocytosis)

Hereditary xerocytosis is probably the most common of the membrane cation permeability defects. Several families with this disorder, in which red cells are markedly dehydrated, have been described,[992,1591-1593,1595,1598,1603-1622] and because the disease is often clinically mild, it is likely that many patients go undiagnosed. Physiologically, the major red cell abnormality is a change in the relative membrane permeability to potassium. Efflux of K^+ is increased twofold to fourfold and approximates Na^+ influx. There is no metabolic or hemoglobin abnormality to account for this permeability lesion, and red cell Ca^{2+} content is not increased. The nature of the permeability defect is unknown. Monovalent cation pump activity is increased appropriately for the slightly elevated Na^+ content, but the Na^+,K^+ pump cannot compensate for K^+ losses in excess of Na^+ gain. In fact, the action of the pump significantly exacerbates the rate of K^+ loss because three Na^+ ions are pumped out for every two K^+ ions returned.[1640,1641] As a consequence, xerocytes gradually become cation depleted and lose water in response to decreased intracellular osmolality. This is easily detected by centrifugation on Stractan density gradients (see Fig. 15-56).

Molecular Pathology

The gene for xerocytosis has been mapped to 16q23-q24.[1592,1642,1643] Nevertheless, little is known about the molecular pathology of the disease. When measured, the proportion of red cell membrane PC is increased (12 to 20 fmol/cell; normal range, 10 to 12 fmol/cell).[1613] The combination of hereditary xerocytosis and high PC is sometimes given the name high-PC hemolytic anemia (HPCHA),[1598,1605,1609,1612,1613,1615] but there appears to be little reason to distinguish HPCHA from hereditary xerocytosis.[1613] Early studies suggested that the excess PC was due to diminished transfer of PC fatty acids to PE,[1609] a pathway that is normally stimulated by cellular dehydration.[1644] It is not clear why this pathway is inhibited in hereditary xerocytosis or how it relates to the underlying membrane leakiness and hemolysis.

Xerocytic red cells are also shear sensitive[1608] and are exceptionally prone to membrane fragmentation in response to metabolic stress.[992] This finding suggests a membrane skeletal defect, but none of the well-characterized membrane protein genes reside in the 16q23-q24 interval (see Table 15-2). Results of conventional analyses of red cell membrane proteins have been normal,[992] except for an increase in the proportion of membrane-associated G3PD in one family.[16456] Quantitatively, all membrane components are increased because xerocytes have 15% to 25% more surface area than normal, probably due to the increased amount of phospholipids. Xerocytes are relatively rigid cells[758] and have a dehydration-induced membrane injury.[1608] This poorly defined lesion is also found in irreversibly sickled cells[1646] and presumably is important in the pathophysiology of hemolysis. Hereditary xerocytes are unusually sensitive to oxidants.[1647,1648] Exposure of xerocytes to concentrations of H_2O_2 that do not affect normal cells causes a rapid loss of intracellular K^+, conversion of hemoglobin to methemoglobin, and cross-linking of hemoglobin to spectrin.[1648,1649] Similar sensitivity occurs in dehydrated normal red cells. Conversely, rehydrated xerocytes exhibit a normal reaction to H_2O_2. Native xerocytes have the abnormal spectrin-globin complex, and the amount correlates with the extent of dehydration in various cellular fractions and with membrane rigidity.[1650] Oxidation of normal erythrocytes with peroxide generates the spectrin-globin complex and rigid membranes.[1037] Complex formation is blocked by carbon monoxide, which prevents hemoglobin oxidation, but is not blocked by lipid antioxidants. This implies a direct role for hemoglobin in cross-linking spectrin. However, the relationship of these findings to the pathophysiology of hereditary xerocytosis is unclear.

A constellation of clinical findings, including xerocytosis, pseudohyperkalemia, perinatal ascites, and even hydrops fetalis, have been described in the fetal and newborn period.[1592,1593,1599,1618,1619] Genetic studies of patients with this constellation of disorders also show linkage to 16q23-q24.[1592] The mechanism of ascites in these patients is unclear and appears to be unrelated to anemia or hypoalbuminemia. There is one report of neonatal hepatitis in a patient,[1623] but it seems unlikely that hepatitis would have been missed in others. Although treatments such as fetal transfusion and fetal albumin infusion have been described, the efficacy of these interventions is difficult to assess because of the apparent high rate of self-resolution of symptoms in late gestation and the early neonatal period in these patients.[1619,1651,1652]

Familial Pseudohyperkalemia. Of note, Stewart and co-workers[1596,1597] reported a family with a dominantly inherited disorder characterized by loss of erythrocyte K^+ through passive K^+ leak across the red cell membrane that is exaggerated in the cold. Electrolyte analysis of plasma obtained from blood samples stored for just a few hours at room temperature or below may falsely suggest that affected individuals are hyperkalemic. Familial pseudohyperkalemia is symptomless, and affected patients do not experience hemolysis or anemia. Therefore, the key clinical importance of this disorder is that these patients are not truly hyperkalemic and have a normal electrocardiogram. These patients are at risk of mistakenly receiving hyperkalemic therapy and developing severe hypokalemia. The disorder resembles cryohydrocytosis (see later), except that K^+ loss and dehydration predominate instead of Na^+ gain and cryohemolysis. Studies of patients with hereditary stomatocytosis and particularly those with xerocytosis have shown that many of these variants also cause pseudohyperkalemia.[1591,1592,1594,1595,1653] Further evidence of overlap between these syndromes is that some forms of familial pseudohyperkalemia are linked to the xerocytosis locus at 16q23-q24.[1592,1594,1642]

Clinical and Laboratory Features

In all families with hereditary xerocytosis that have been studied, inheritance is autosomal dominant. Red cell features used for diagnosis include an increased MCHC, increased MCV, and *decreased* OF (i.e., *resistance* to osmotic lysis). The combination of an elevated MCV and MCHC is unique and suggests the diagnosis of hereditary xerocytosis. Hereditary xerocytes appear to be macrocytic despite their dehydration. This, however, is partially an artifact of cellular stiffness. In Coulter-type electronic counters, conversion of pulse height (from the resistance of a cell passing through an electric field) to cellular volume depends on cell shape. Xerocytes do not deform to the same degree as normal cells do, which causes the electronically measured MCV to be about 10% too high.[1654] This behavior also affects the hematocrit value, which is calculated from the MCV. Most patients have compensated hemolysis with little or no anemia.

Most patients also have nearly normal erythrocyte morphology, with only a few target cells and an occasional echinocyte or stomatocyte (see Fig. 15-55C). However, in the most severely affected patients,[1604] particularly after splenectomy, blood smears display contracted and spiculated red cells in which the hemoglobin appears to be aggregated in one portion of the cell (see Fig. 15-55D). The characteristic biochemical abnormalities are a reduced K^+ concentration and total monovalent cation content. In older erythrocytes, K^+ levels approach half-normal.[1613] The clinical course is also remarkable for iron overload in the absence of transfusions,[1655] particularly in patients who are heterozygous for a hemochromatosis gene.[1622] This often requires treatment.

Red cell 2,3-DPG concentrations are moderately decreased in hereditary xerocytosis,[992,1604,1606,1607,1656] as in hereditary stomatocytosis. The reasons are unknown. Because loss of the polyvalent DPG is compensated for by an influx of monovalent chloride ions and water, patients with xerocytosis and unusually low DPG levels have fewer dehydrated red cells than expected for the degree of cation loss, and in rare cases have no dehydrated cells at all.[1657] Patients with low DPG levels also have increased whole-blood oxygen affinity and, consequently, may have little apparent anemia.[1616,1656] However, such patients have relative polycythemia and are more anemic than their hemoglobin level suggests. Autohemolysis is increased and responds to glucose, similar to the pattern seen in HS.[992,1606,1611,1615]

Treatment

Splenectomy is absolutely contraindicated for hereditary xerocytosis. The limited experience available suggests that removing the spleen does not significantly reduce hemolysis.[1604,1605] Presumably, xerocytes are so functionally compromised that they are easily detected and eliminated in other areas of the reticuloendothelial system. Moreover, splenectomy appears to dramatically increase the risk for venous thrombosis and venous thromboembolism in patients with hereditary xerocytosis.[1222,1605,1657] The cause of the hypercoaguable state after splenectomy in these patients is not known. Fortunately, most patients maintain a hemoglobin level of at least 9 g/dL, so surgical intervention is not typically considered.

Intermediate Syndromes

Hydrocytosis and xerocytosis represent the extremes of a spectrum of red cell permeability defects. A number of families with features of both conditions have been reported. The reported patients seem to fall into two groups whose red cells differ principally in morphology, OF, and sensitivity to cold.

Cryohydrocytosis

Patients with this autosomal dominant disorder[1583-1589] have a mild hemolytic anemia characterized by marked autohemolysis that is greater at 4° C than at 37° C.[1583,1585,1586,1653] The cold autohemolysis is sensitive to the method of anticoagulation. It is increased in the cold in heparin- or EDTA-anticoagulated plasma and in defibrinated plasma but not in acid citrate dextrose.[1583,1589] This may reflect unusual pH sensitivity of the abnormal red cells because cold hemolysis is accentuated at pH 8 (the pH of blood in the first three anticoagulants at 4° C) in comparison to pH 7.6 (the pH of acid citrate dextrose–anticoagulated plasma at 4° C).[1583,1589]

Blood smears show stomatocytes, some of which have an eccentric or curvilinear slit or a transverse bar bisecting the area of central pallor (see Fig. 15-55B).[1583,1653] MCV and MCHC are normal or slightly increased; however, measurements are difficult because as blood samples cool for storage, MCV rises rapidly and MCHC falls.[1585,1586] Therefore, red cell measurements in these patients must be completed before a blood sample is allowed to cool. Fresh erythrocytes are Na^+ loaded and K^+ depleted. Although the total concentration of Na^+ and K^+ is normal, measurements are complicated by the ion shifts that occur in storage of the red cells. In the cold, Na^+ and K^+ permeability is markedly increased; however, because Na^+ entry greatly predominates, the red cells rapidly swell and lyse.

The primary molecular lesion of these erythrocytes in a subset of patients was recently elucidated. In an analysis of 11 families with stomatocytic hemolytic anemia defined by marked membrane permeability at 0° C, an associated mutation was found in the intramembrane domain of the band 3 (or AE1) anion exchanger encoded by the *SLC4A1* gene.[1587] The mutations in the band 3 chloride-bicarbonate exchanger convert the anion exchanger into a leaky cation channel.

In two patients with cryohydrocytosis, stomatin was deficient when red cell membrane proteins were analyzed.[1566,1588] The stomatin-deficient red cells were found to be associated with a higher K^+ leak than were the stomatin-containing red cells in patients with cryohydrocytosis.[1588] Both of the stomatin-deficient patients also had an associated neurologic syndrome consisting of seizures, mental retardation, cataracts, and hepatosplenomegaly.[1588] Patients who have this constellation of symptoms and are deficient in stomatin are now identified as having type II hereditary cryohydrocytosis. All other cases of cryohydrocytosis described have had stomatin-containing red cells and have not had a neurologic syndrome.[1585,1586] These patients have type I hereditary cryohydrocytosis. Thrombotic complications, or hematologic improvement, has not been reported after splenectomy in the case series describing these patients, but very few patients with this disorder have been reported.

Stomatocytic Xerocytosis

In 1971, Miller and colleagues[1590] described 54 patients with dominantly inherited stomatocytosis in a large Swiss-German family. Apparent heterozygotes (51 of 54 patients) had mild hemolysis, 1% to 25% stomatocytes on their peripheral blood smears, and no anemia. Intracellular K^+ and total monovalent cation levels were mildly decreased, and fresh red cells were osmotically resistant. Three probable homozygotes from a consanguineous mating had mild anemia, moderately severe hemolysis, marked stomatocytosis (20% to 35%), and greater cation permeability[1583,1623]; however, because net Na^+ and K^+ levels were relatively balanced, cell hydration was not seriously deranged. The molecular defect in this kindred is unknown.

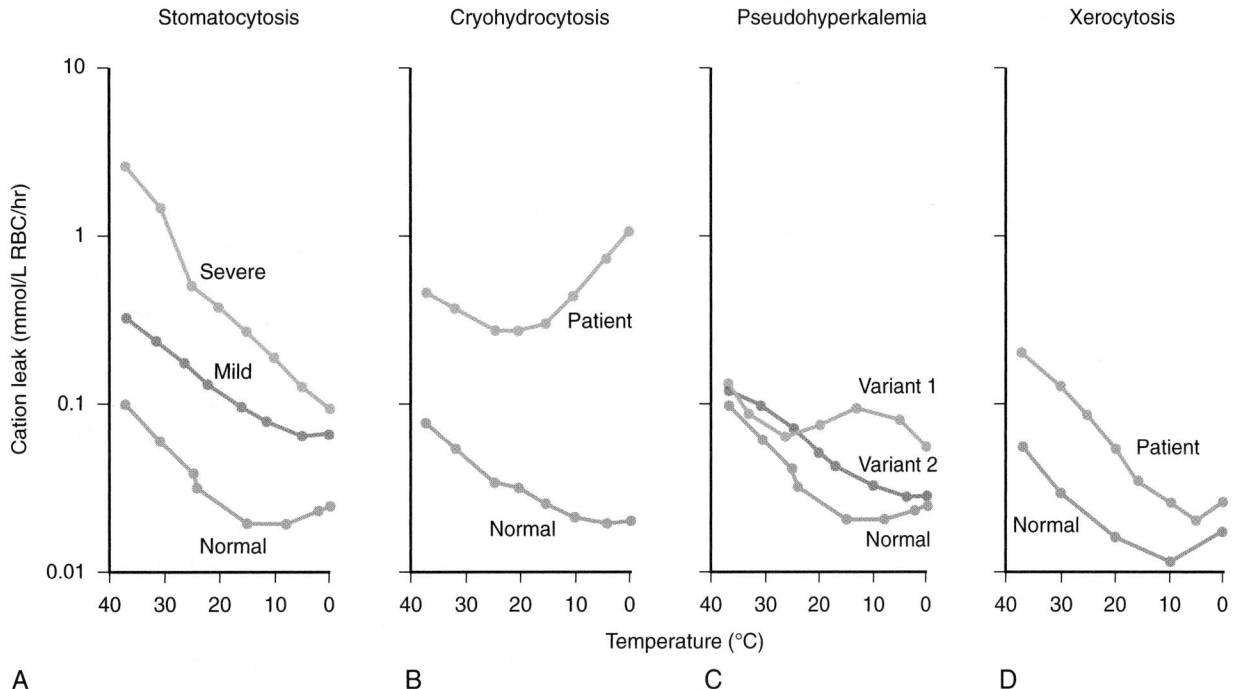

FIGURE 15-58. Passive permeability of monovalent cations as a function of temperature in the hereditary stomatocytosis-xerocytosis disorders (*blue and brown circles*) in comparison to normal individuals (*green circles*). Stomatocytosis[1582,1658] (**A**), cryohydrocytosis[1586] (**B**), pseudohyperkalemia[1591,1659] (**C**), and xerocytosis[1592] (**D**) red cells are shown. Passive permeability is defined as uptake of $^{86}Rb^+$ across the red cell membrane in the presence of oubain (to inhibit the Na^+,K^+-ATPase pump) and bumetanide (to inhibit the Na^+-K^+-$2Cl^-$ cotransporter). RBC, red blood cell. (*Adapted with permission from Walensky LD, Narla M, Lux SE. Disorders of the red cell membrane. In Handin RI, Lux SE, Stossel TP [eds]. Blood: Principles and Practice of Hematology, 2nd ed. Philadelphia, JB Lippincott, 2003, pp 1709-1858.*)

Classification Based on the Temperature Dependence of Cation Leaks

Gordon Stewart and colleagues have classified disorders of red cell membrane cation permability based on the effects of temperature on the cation leak.[1582,1586,1592,1658] The membrane leak is measured by the residual influx of $^{86}Rb^+$ (a radioactive substitute for K^+) across the red cell membrane in the presence of ouabain (to inhibit the Na^+,K^+-ATPase pump) and bumetanide (to inhibit the Na^+-K^+-$2Cl^-$ cotransporter). This is a measure of the passive permeability of monovalent cations, although it does not exclude the contributions of the Gárdos channel and the K^+-Cl^- cotransporter. These transporters do not significantly contribute to cation permeability in normal red cells but may contribute more significantly in pathologic erythrocytes. Nevertheless, the estimate of monovalent cation leak is useful in understanding the pathophysiology of these permeability disorders and is clinically useful in the absence of genetic testing.

Normal red cells have a low leak that falls with temperature, with the minimum reached at approximately 10° C (Figs. 15-58 and 15-59).[1658] The reason for this minimum is unknown. The capacity of the Na^+,K^+ pump far exceeds the normal leak rate at physiologic temperatures, but pump activity falls sharply below room temperature and approximates the normal leak at 0° C (see Fig. 15-59). The temperature profile of the passive leak

varies in each disorder (see Fig. 15-58). In classic, severe stomatin-deficient stomatocytosis, the leak rate, particularly Na^+ leak, is extremely high at body temperatures and exceeds the capacity of the Na^+,K^+ pump, which leads to cell swelling and hemolysis (see Fig. 15-58A). Stomatocytosis patients with milder leaks are better compensated by the Na^+,K^+ pump and experience less hemolysis (see Fig. 15-58A).[1582] Patients with cryohydrocytosis have a similar mild to moderate cation leak at body temperature that causes mild to moderate hemolysis. However, in cryohydrocytosis, the cation leak increases dramatically below ambient temperatures and greatly exceeds the capacity of the Na^+,K^+ pump below 10° C to 15° C, at which point it causes severe hemolysis (see Figs. 15-58B and 15-59).

Individuals with pseudohyperkalemia typically have a nearly normal cation leak at physiologic temperatures and therefore little or no hemolysis. The slope of the leak is flatter than normal and sometimes even rises at temperatures below ambient, so K^+ loss occurs during storage at room temperature (see Fig. 15-58C).

The temperature profile of the cation leak in hereditary xerocytosis parallels the normal temperature profile, but the leak is threefold to fourfold greater (see Fig. 15-58D). Although the leak is relatively small, it favors K^+, which creates a problem because the Na^+,K^+ pump extrudes three Na^+ ions for every two K^+ ions returned. Hence, the red cell cannot compensate for leaks of K^+_{out}

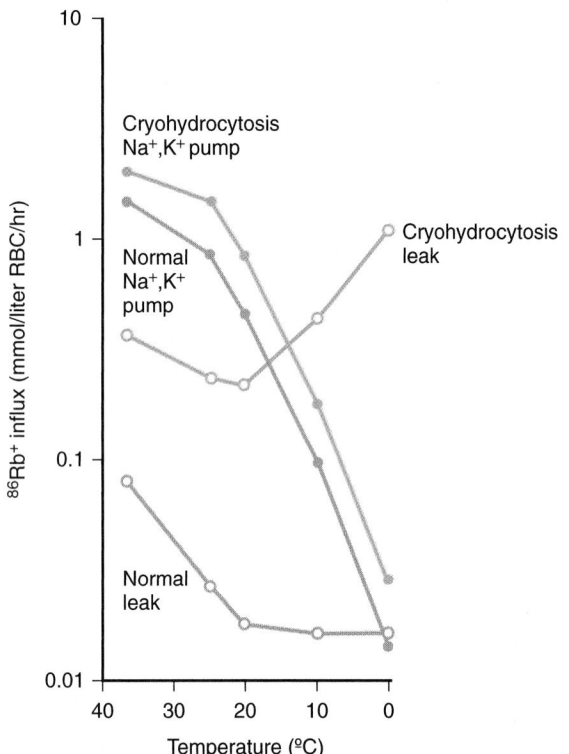

FIGURE 15-59. Comparison of passive monovalent cation permeability (*open circles*) and the capacity of the Na^+,K^+ pump (*solid circles*) in hereditary cryhydrocytosis (*blue circles*) and normal individuals (*green circles*). Note that the rate of cation leak greatly exceeds the pump rate in cryohydrocytosis at low temperatures, which causes the cells to swell and hemolyze. RBC, red blood cell. (*Adapted with permission from Walensky LD, Narla M, Lux SE. Disorders of the red cell membrane. In Handin RI, Lux SE, Stossel TP [eds]. Blood: Principles and Practice of Hematology, 2nd ed. Philadelphia, JB Lippincott, 2003, pp 1709-1858.*)

relative to Na^+_{in} that exceed the normal 2:3 ratio. Therefore, the pump exacerbates the loss of intracellular cations and water and probably contributes to the dehydration of xerocytes.

Other Disorders Characterized by Stomatocytosis

Acquired Stomatocytosis

In normal individuals, 3% or less of the red cells on peripheral blood smears are stomatocytic,[1659,1660] although more stomatocytic forms are evident (up to 10%) if sensitive techniques such as scanning electron microscopy are used.[1661] Because stomatocytes may occasionally occur as a drying artifact in limited areas of the smear, one must take care to examine multiple areas on several smears before diagnosing stomatocytosis. In wet preparations, stomatocytes are bowl shaped (uniconcave). Such preparations are useful in excluding artifactual stomatocytes, but the presence of bowl-shaped cells cannot be used as proof of stomatocytes because target cells are also bowl shaped in solution.[1662]

Drugs. In a prospective study of 4291 peripheral blood smears, Davidson and co-workers[1663] found increased numbers of stomatocytes in 2.3% of the preparations. Fifty-nine percent of these smears had 5% to 20% stomatocytes, 35% had 20% to 50% stomatocytes, and 6% had more than 50% stomatocytes. In this and other studies, a wide variety of drugs and diagnoses were associated with stomatocytosis.[389,1590,1663-1665] Further studies are needed to determine which associations are specific and reproducible. As discussed earlier in the chapter in the section on the bilayer couple hypothesis, amphophilic, lipid-soluble drugs can cause red cells to assume a stomatocytic shape if the drug partitions preferentially into the inner half of the lipid bilayer. The affected red cells are misshapen but are not cation loaded or hydrocytic and do not usually hemolyze. Vinca alkaloids (e.g., vincristine and vinblastine), in doses used for chemotherapy for leukemias and lymphomas, often induce hemolysis, sometimes with increased membrane Na^+ permeability and stomatocytosis.[1666] This is a particular problem in the rare instances in which these drugs must be given to patients with cancer who also have HS. We have seen two such patients, and in both cases very severe hemolysis occurred. Presumably, the explanation is that spherocytes and stomatocytes both have a decreased surface-to-volume ratio. Imposing a stomatocytic stress on HS red cells will make them even more spheroidal and hasten their demise.

Alcoholism. Acquired stomatocytosis is common in alcoholics, particularly in those with acute alcoholism, and may be associated with moderate hemolysis.[1659,1660] Red cell cation measurements have not been reported; however, severe hydrocytosis is unlikely because the results of OF tests have been normal.[1660]

Long-Distance Runners. Some marathon and long-distance runners develop mild stomatocytosis transiently after completing a race[1666,1667] (e.g., 12.8% ± 1.8% stomatocytes immediately after a race versus a baseline of 4.3% ± 1.8%).[1667]

Rh_{null} and Rh_{mod} Disease

The Rh(D) antigen and other antigens of the Rh group (cCeE) are part of two minor red cell membrane proteins encoded by two closely linked genes, one encoding the D polypeptide and the other encoding the Cc/Ee proteins. The antigenic expression of these proteins is a consequence of alternative splicing of their pre-mRNA.[389,1668] Patients who lack all Rh antigens (Rh_{null})[1669] have a moderately severe hemolytic anemia (^{51}Cr-labeled red cell half-life of 10 to 14 days)[396,1670-1672] characterized by stomatocytosis and spherocytosis. OF is only mildly increased,[396,1672] but ektacytometric analysis shows significant loss of membrane surface, particularly in denser (and presumably older) cells.[396] Red cell membrane K^+ permeability is about twice normal, which is compatible with a mild xerocytosis syndrome.[396,1673] Stomatocytosis and hemolysis are also features of Rh_{mod} disease, a related anomaly in which expression of Rh antigens is suppressed but not absent because of the influence of a suppressor gene.[1674,1675]

Tangier Disease

Tangier disease, caused by mutations in the gene encoding ATP-binding cassette 1 (ABCA1), is a rare autosomal recessive condition in which homozygotes have splenomegaly, absent or very low levels of high density lipoproteins (HDL), reduced levels of low-density lipoproteins (LDL) (typically 40% of normal), hypertriglyceridemia, mild corneal clouding, peripheral neuropathy, bone marrow foam cells (70% of patients), and characteristic orange, cholesterol ester–laden tonsils.[1676] ABCA1 is a major determinant of plasma HDL cholesterol and is critically involved in cellular trafficking of cholesterol and choline phospholipids. ABCA1 mediates the first step in reverse cholesterol transport, the transfer of cholesterol and phospholipids to lipid-poor apoproteins.[1677,1678] Cholesterol ester levels are greatly elevated in tissue macrophages in Tangier disease because of the lack of HDL, which normally return cholesterol esters to the liver. The HDL deficiency is caused by hypercatabolism of the lipoprotein. Normally, HDL binds to specific receptors on macrophages, is internalized (presumably to load up on cholesterol esters), and then recycles to the membrane surface. In Tangier disease, HDL is misrouted to macrophage lysosomes and destroyed.

Hematologic examination of one patient with Tangier disease disclosed stomatocytosis, hemolysis (hemoglobin concentration of 8.5 g/dL; reticulocyte count of 6% to 9%), and osmotically sensitive red cells.[1679] The membrane cholesterol level was low, the cholesterol-to-phospholipid ratio was decreased, and phospholipid analysis showed high phosphatidyl choline and low sphingomyelin levels. Red cell cation concentrations and permeabilities were not investigated. Because hematologic data have rarely been reported in patients with Tangier disease, it is difficult to be certain that this patient's data are not exceptional. However, previous reports of unexplained hemolysis in three patients suggest that they are not.[1680-1682]

Mediterranean Stomatocytosis

Multiple independent observations were made more than 30 years ago that stomatocytosis was common among Mediterranean individuals who migrated to Australia.[1683-1686] Clinically, these individuals had mild to moderate hemolytic anemia, normal red cell cations, and normal OF. In addition, they had macrothrombocytopenia (40,000 to 150,000 platelets 3 μm³ to 120 μm³ in size) and splenomegaly. In 1975, a study of healthy Mediterranean immigrants confirmed this finding, with 36% of individuals having more than 5% stomatocytes but no anemia.[1687] The hematologic findings of Mediterranean stomatocytosis have recently been linked to a rare inherited metabolic condition, phytosterolemia, in which

absorption of all sterols, including both cholesterol and phytosterols, is massively increased.[1688] Phytosterolemia is caused by mutations in either *ABCG5* or *ABCG8*, adjacent to chromosome 2p21.[1689,1690] The protein product of these genes normally forms a dimeric ATP-binding cassette protein in the enteric mucosa that aids in rejecting sterols into the gut. A recent study demonstrated that five pedigrees with Mediterranean stomatocytosis also had phytosterolemia with the typical mutations linked to this disease.[1688] Thus, the stomatocytosis and macrothrombocytopenia may be due to toxic effects from circulating sterols. In light of these findings, phytosterolemia should be considered in any patient found to have stomatocytic hemolysis or large platelets, or both.

Other Disorders Characterized by Xerocytosis

Adenosine Triphosphate Depletion

When red cell ATP concentrations decrease to less than 5% to 15% of normal, the cells leak cations and become rigid and echinocytic.[1691] In plasma or other Ca²⁺-containing media, a specific K⁺ permeability lesion (the Gárdos channel) is superimposed on the unchecked normal leak of Na⁺ and K⁺ and leads to cation depletion and dehydration.[1692] Coincidentally, poorly defined changes occur in the membrane skeletal structure.[1693,1694]

Presumably, these phenomena are involved in the hemolysis that occurs in inherited defects of glycolysis such as PK deficiency. Studies by Nathan and coworkers,[1695] Mentzer and Baehner,[1696] and Glader[1697] showed that PK-deficient red cells rapidly lose ATP and K⁺ and become dehydrated, spiculated, and viscous when incubated in vitro, particularly under conditions in which residual mitochondrial production of ATP is curtailed. Contracted, crenated red cells are observed in PK deficiency,[1698,1699] as well as other disorders of red cell glycolysis. These "deflated echinocytes" are more rigid than normal[1700] and are relatively scarce in unsplenectomized patients,[1698,1699] which implies that they are premorbid cells given temporary reprieve by removal of the spleen.

Little is known about the status of membrane proteins in red cells with compromised ATP production.[1692] Small amounts of disulfide-linked spectrin complexes and marked diminution of spectrin extractability were detected in a patient with glucose phosphate isomerase deficiency,[1701] which suggests that membrane protein damage may be pathologically relevant in these disorders.

Irreversibly Sickled Cells

Irreversibly sickled cells are circulating erythrocytes from patients with sickle cell anemia that retain a sickled shape when oxygenated because of an acquired defect in the membrane skeleton.[1702] Biochemically, irreversibly sickled cells are deficient in total monovalent cations and water.[1703] The mechanism of their formation and the nature of the acquired membrane defects responsible for their abnormal shape, cation content, and surface topography are discussed in Chapter 19.

OTHER CAUSES OF DECREASED ERYTHROCYTE MEMBRANE SURFACE AREA

Excluding hereditary spherocytosis, only a few conditions cause decreased membrane surface area leading to spherocytosis on the peripheral blood smear.

Immune Adherence

Immunohemolytic anemias are the most common cause of acquired spherocytosis in infants and children: AB(H)-related hemolysis in neonates and warm antibody–type autoimmune (or drug-related) hemolytic anemias in older children and adults. (For unknown reasons, Rh-related hemolysis in neonates rarely causes spherocytosis, whereas it does so readily later in life.) Patients who suffer from severe transfusion reactions with immunohemolysis may also have spherocytes on their peripheral blood smears. The pathophysiology of these disorders is discussed in Chapter 14.

Thermal Injury

More than 140 years ago, Schultze[1704] observed that membrane budding, fragmentation, and microspherocytosis developed in red cells heated to temperatures approaching 50° C for short periods. This phenomenon was further defined by the careful studies of Ham and co-workers and others[1416-1418] and is now believed to be due to heat denaturation of spectrin or other membrane proteins.[1419] Similar changes are observed acutely in patients with major cutaneous burns, presumably because of exposure of red cells in the skin and subcutaneous tissue to heat. During the first 24 to 48 hours after the burn, intravascular hemolysis develops, which is associated with red cell fragmentation and spherocytosis.[1705,1706] The severity of the reaction is related to the extent and degree of the burn. Generally, hemolysis is evident in patients with third-degree burns involving 15% to 20% or more of body surface area.[1705,1707] In severely burned patients, up to 30% of the red cell mass may be destroyed. This acute hemolytic process is usually complete by the third day after the burn and is followed by a persistent anemia resembling "anemia of chronic disease" seen in various disorders and described in Chapter 12.[1708,1709] An unusual variant of red cell thermal injury has been reported after the infusion of red cells that were inadvertently overheated in a blood warmer.[1710,1711]

Mechanical Injury

Hemolysis can be caused by direct physical trauma to the red cell membrane. This occurs in a variety of disorders, which are grouped under the terms microangiopathic and macroangiopathic hemolytic anemias. Membrane damage leading to intravascular hemolysis is apparently inflicted by the interaction of red cells (flowing at arterial speed) with prosthetic materials, damaged endothelial surfaces, or intravascular fibrin strands.[1712-1714] Dense microspherocytes are almost always produced by this process, but usually bizarre-shaped schizocytes and red cell fragments dominate the morphology. How such cells form is still not completely clear because simple fragmentation of red cells generates spherocytes but not schizocytes. Perhaps red cells draped over fibrin strands or attached to abnormal surfaces not only are distorted by shear but also are held in the distorted position for some time, thereby permitting rearrangement of the stressed membrane skeleton and assumption of a new, irreversibly misshapen form. This concept is strengthened by the observation that fragmentation is worsened by the presence of underlying membrane skeletal weakness.[1362]

Hypophosphatemia

Red cell glucose metabolism is compromised in patients with severe hypophosphatemia (serum phosphorus level < 0.3 mg/dL).[1715,1716] ATP and DPG levels decline and the oxygen affinity of hemoglobin increases.[1717,1718] If the red cell ATP concentration falls to very low levels (10% to 20% of normal), a severe hemolytic anemia characterized by marked microspherocytosis, spheroacanthocytosis, and red cell rigidity results.[1715,1719] The hemolysis is reversible after phosphate repletion and ATP regeneration. Severe hypophosphatemia can occur with gastrointestinal malabsorption, use of phosphate binders, starvation, diabetes mellitus, and increased urinary losses as a result of tubular dysfunction, as well as after nutritional repletion (e.g., refeeding of patients with anorexia nervosa[1720] or severe malnutrition[1721]).

Toxins and Venoms

Clostridial Sepsis

Clostridium welchii and *Clostridium perfringens* septicemias are seen in a variety of clinical situations but must particularly be considered in patients with penetrating wounds, septic abortions, peritonitis after a perforated viscus, or cholecystitis or cholangitis; in immunosuppressed patients with gastrointestinal or hematologic malignancies; and in neonates with necrotizing enterocolitis.[1722-1737] In patients with clostridial sepsis, severe, rapidly progressive intravascular hemolysis and microspherocytosis may occur.[1722,1723,1730,1736,1737] Hemolysis of the entire red cell mass has been reported.[1722,1729,1732,1738-1740] Complications include shock, acute renal failure, and death. Transfusion therapy may be ineffective. Antibiotics and hyperbaric oxygen have occasionally been used successfully to treat clostridial infections.[1726,1731,1732]

The mechanism of red cell damage is uncertain and may vary between patients. The bacteria produce several hemolytic toxins, including α-toxin, a 43-kd protein that contains an NH_2-terminal phospholipase domain and a COOH-terminal domain required for hemolysis,[1731,1741,1742] and θ-toxin, a 54-kd cholesterol-binding protein[1743-1746] that aggregates and forms membrane pores[1744,1747] leading to colloid osmotic hemolysis. α-Toxin appears to induce hemolysis through activation of sphingomyelin metabolism.[1748] *C. perfringens* also contains a neuraminidase that cleaves terminal sialic acids from red cell glycoproteins in some patients.[1749] The underlying galactose residues form the Thomsen-Friedenreich cryptoantigen (or T antigen). This antigen is easily detected because affected erythrocytes are agglutinated by peanut lectin.[1725] Because anti-T antibodies are present in almost all adult plasma, activation of T antigen can lead to significant hemolysis.[1730,1731,1733,1750] In infected infants and children who lack T antibodies, transfusion may lead to massive hemolysis and death. Rarely, T-antigen activation may precede the intravascular hemolysis and lead to early detection of clostridial sepsis and lifesaving therapeutic intervention.[1725]

In one patient with severe hemolysis, red cells showed profound proteolytic damage to membrane proteins, particularly spectrin, and no significant lipid alterations.[1751]

Venoms

The venoms of cobras and certain vipers and rattlesnakes may produce severe hemolysis and spherocytosis.[1752-1756] Spherocytic hemolytic anemia may also be seen in patients bitten by the common brown spiders (*Loxosceles reclusus* and *Loxosceles lata*) of South America and the central and southern sections of the United States[1757,1758] and in individuals with massive numbers of stings by honeybees, wasps, or yellow jackets.[1758-1761] Hemolysis in a child stung by a Portuguese man-of-war jellyfish has also been reported.[1762]

A full description of the numerous toxins in these venoms and their mechanisms of action is beyond the scope of this chapter. In general, the mechanisms of hemolysis after envenomation are not fully understood. The venoms of snakes and insects often contain phospholipases (particularly phospholipase A_2)[1763] and protein toxins that enhance their action. Examples of toxins include the mastoparans of wasp and hornet venoms[1764-1766] and melittin, a polypeptide contained in honeybee (*Apis mellifera*) venom[17678-1770] that immobilizes and clusters erythrocyte band 3 and thereby produces protein-free areas of the lipid bilayer that are susceptible to phospholipase action.[1769]

Hemolysis after brown recluse spider bites is characteristically delayed 1 to 5 days and is caused by a different mechanism.[1771] In affected patients, a transient, spherocytic, hemolytic anemia develops and produces positive Coombs test results[1772-1775] with erythrophagocytosis and deposition of IgG and C3 on the red cell surface. Venom from the brown recluse spider induces activation of an endogenous metalloproteinase that results in cleavage of glycophorin from the erythrocyte membrane, which facilitates the complement-mediated hemolysis.[1776-1778] The hemolysis usually subsides within a week, but it may be fatal.[1771,1779,1780] Complement appears to play a critical role because complement-deficient guinea pigs are resistant to the venom.[1781] The glycoprotein CD59 may play a previously unrecognized role in protection of the membrane from venom-induced injury.[1782] The venom also contains a phospholipase D that may contribute to the hemolysis.[1783]

Except for spider bites, which may be clinically deceptive initially, the potential for a hemolytic catastrophe should be obvious in patients who have been bitten or stung.[1771] An early sign of impending hemolysis may be a rapid rise in the serum K^+ level caused by prelytic leakage of this ion from the red cells. Once hemolysis is established, therapy other than transfusions is usually of little use. In patients with snake bites, localization or drainage of the venom and prompt administration of antivenom can be lifesaving.

Hypersplenism

Occasionally, transient hemolysis associated with spherocytosis and splenic sequestration of red cells develops in patients with infections associated with splenomegaly.[1784-1786] In some instances this may be attributed to latent red cell defects such as HS, but in others, no red cell abnormalities can be identified. Typically, the latter patients have subacute infections with persistent fever, splenomegaly, and numerous cells of lymphocytic or reticuloendothelial derivation (atypical lymphocytes, monocytes, histiocytes, or plasma cells) in their peripheral blood. Only a minor population of the red cells (10% to 50%) are spherical on peripheral blood smears or unincubated OF tests. Conceivably, the combination of delayed splenic passage caused by splenomegaly and pyrogenic stimulation of the reticuloendothelial system is sufficient to permit detention and conditioning of even normal red cells—a form of hypersplenism.

DISORDERS ASSOCIATED WITH INCREASED MEMBRANE SURFACE: TARGET CELLS

Red cells increase their surface area by an increase in membrane lipids. In dried smears the excess surface accumulates and bulges outward in the red cell's central clearing, thereby producing the characteristic target cell morphology. Target cells are also seen when red cell volume is diminished as a result of decreased hemoglobin synthesis (e.g., thalassemia or iron deficiency), abnormal hemoglobin charge or aggregation (e.g., hemoglobins S, C, D, and E), or decreased cell cations and water. In these instances there is a relative increase in the surface-to-volume ratio. With the exception of dehydrated red cells, an increase in membrane surface, whether relative or absolute, has little effect on red cell deformability or life span and hence is usually innocuous.

Obstructive Liver Disease

Target cells are particularly characteristic of biliary obstruction[1662,1787] but also occur in other forms of liver disease. Like spur cells (see later), they form when red cells accumulate excess lipids from abnormal lipoproteins. However, unlike spur cells, target cells are characterized by a balanced increase in both free cholesterol and phospholipids.[1788-1790] The increase in phospholipid is confined to phosphatidyl choline (PC).[1788]

The pathogenesis of the lipid accumulation in target cells is relatively clear. The process is extracorpuscular and reversible and is due to an abnormal serum component. Normal cells acquire target cell surface area, morphologic characteristics, and osmotic resistance when transfused into patients with obstructive jaundice or incubated in the patients' serum, whereas target cells from such patients lose the patients' excess lipids and revert to biconcave discs in normal persons or their sera.[1787] Cooper and co-workers[1788] found a close relationship between the cholesterol-to-phospholipid ratios of target cells and serum lipoproteins, particularly low density lipoproteins (LDL). It is known that in obstructive jaundice a unique, abnormal lipoprotein called LP-X accumulates in the LDL density class,[1791,1792] possibly caused, at least in part, by an acquired deficiency of the hepatic enzyme LCAT. LP-X contains approximately equal amounts of free cholesterol and PC, plus a small amount of protein, cholesterol esters, triglycerides, and lithocholic acid.[1792] Normal red cells rapidly acquire excess cholesterol, PC, and surface area when incubated with LP-X in vitro,[1790] and it seems likely that this may be the source of lipids for membrane expansion and targeting in vivo.

Familial Lecithin-Cholesterol Acyltransferase Deficiency

Familial LCAT deficiency is a rare autosomal recessive disorder characterized by anemia, corneal opacities, hyperlipemia, proteinuria, chronic nephritis, and premature atherosclerosis.[1793] More extensive description of familial LCAT deficiency can be found in a recent review.[1794] LCAT deficiency is relatively asymptomatic during childhood. Proteinuria and corneal opacities are among the earliest manifestations. The latter consist of minute grayish dots that concentrate near the edge of the cornea, similar to arcus senilis. Almost all of the reported patients have had a moderate normochromic anemia (hemoglobin level of 8 to 11 g/dL) characterized by prominent target cell formation and decreased osmotic fragility.[1795-1798] Hematologic studies suggest that the anemia is due to a combination of moderate hemolysis and decreased erythropoietic compensation, but interpretation of the evidence is complicated by the coexisting renal disease. Other studies have shown that the red cells

are abnormally susceptible to peroxidative threat and have mechanically fragile membranes.[1796] There is no obvious explanation for these changes, but it is possible that they contribute to the shortened red cell life span. LCAT deficiency is caused by a variety of mutations in the LCAT gene; affected individuals are either homozygotes or compound heterozygotes for these mutations.[1799,1800] Modeling of the mutations has provided insight into the structure and function of LCAT.[1801] As expected from the absence of LCAT activity, there is a pronounced decrease in cholesteryl esters and an increase in free cholesterol and PC in plasma lipoproteins. Because LCAT is required for normal lipoprotein formation and catabolism, nascent lipoproteins and abnormal lipoprotein remnants accumulate in plasma. One of the latter is LP-X.[1802] As discussed in the previous section, this lipoprotein is believed to be responsible for target cell formation in patients with the acquired LCAT deficiency of obstructive liver disease.[1790] Free cholesterol and PC levels are markedly elevated in the red cell membranes of patients with LCAT deficiency[1793]; however, total red cell phospholipid levels are normal because the increase in PC is balanced by a decrease in PE and SM. As with liver disease, red cell targeting and lipid abnormalities can be induced by incubation of normal red cells in LCAT-deficient lipoproteins and reversed by incubation in normal serum.[1803] Other plasma membranes are also probably affected by the abnormal LCAT-deficient lipoproteins. For example, accumulations of lipid in endothelial membranes may underlie the atherosclerotic and nephritic complications seen in some patients. Phagocytosis of abnormal lipoproteins by reticuloendothelial cells leads to the appearance of foam cells and sea-blue histiocytes in the bone marrow, spleen, and other organs.[1795,1804] Serum and red cell lipids are improved in vivo when LCAT is supplied by infusion of normal plasma; however, the short half-life of this protein, 4 to 5 days, and the large amounts of plasma required make chronic replacement therapy impractical.

Fish Eye Disease

Fish eye disease is caused by partial deficiency of LCAT and is also associated with mutations in the LCAT gene.[1793,1799] It is characterized by corneal opacities (which give the disease its name), hypertriglyceridemia, and very low levels of HDLs. One report noted increased target cells and decreased OF.[1805]

Splenectomy

In the first several weeks after splenectomy, the number of target cells gradually increases,[1662,1806-1808] eventually (in otherwise normal persons) reaching levels of 2% to 10%. This change is associated with increases in osmotic resistance, membrane lipid content, and mean surface area relative to volume, indicative of expansion of the red cell membrane surface. By deduction, the spleen must normally remove surplus membrane from such cells, a process referred to as "surface remodeling."[1809,1810] Experimental studies have clearly documented that the stress reticulocytes induced by acute blood loss or hemolysis undergo extensive surface remodeling and suggest that normal reticulocytes are remodeled to a lesser degree. In addition to membrane lipids, transferrin receptors, fibronectin receptors, and a high-molecular-weight membrane protein complex[1811] are also removed during the remodeling process. Autophagocytosis and expulsion of phagolysosomes are hypothesized to be the major mechanism of the remodeling.[751] Postsplenectomy blood smears also show increased numbers of acanthocytes, poikilocytes, and red cells burdened with useless or potentially harmful inclusions (e.g., Heinz bodies, Howell-Jolly bodies, siderotic granules, and endocytic vesicles).[1267,1268,1812,1813] The presence of these inclusions attests to the "culling" and "pitting" functions of the spleen.[1813]

SPICULATED RED CELLS: ECHINOCYTES AND ACANTHOCYTES

There are two basic types of spiculated red cells—echinocytes and acanthocytes. Echinocytes typically have a serrated outline with small, uniform projections more or less spread evenly over the circumference of the cell, whereas acanthocytes have a few spicules of varying size that project irregularly from the red cell surface. These differences are easily detected on scanning electron micrographs and can usually be discerned in wet preparations, but it is often quite difficult to make the distinction in dried smears. In general, echinocytes appear crenated in smears, that is, as cells with relatively uniform scalloped edges, whereas acanthocytes appear contracted, dense, and irregular (Fig. 15-60).

Echinocytes are readily produced in vitro by washing red cells in saline,[1814] by the interaction of red cells with glass surfaces,[1814] by amphipathic molecules that partition into and expand the outer half of the lipid bilayer,[1815] and by molecules that inhibit band 3 transport.[1815] High pH values, ATP depletion, and accumulation of Ca^{2+} also cause echinocytosis.[1816-1819] In vivo, echinocytes are most often found in patients with advanced uremia[1819] or with defects in glycolytic metabolism,[1698] after splenectomy,[1814] and in some patients with microangiopathic hemolytic anemia. Echinocytes are also commonly seen in neonates, especially those who are premature,[1820] and in divers after decompression from pressures greater than 3 to 4 bar.[1821] They are seen transiently after transfusions with large amounts of stored blood because red cells become echinocytic after a few days of storage. Acanthocytes and echinocytes may be found in patients with neuroacanthocytosis,[1822,1823] severe hepatocellular damage,[1824] infantile pyknocytosis,[1825] anorexia nervosa,[1826,1827] In(Lu) blood groups,[1828] and hypothyroidism.[1829] Occasionally, they are the predominant morphologic feature in patients with myelodysplasia.[1830,1831]

Neuroacanthocytosis

Neuroacanthocytosis refers to a group of diseases in which neurologic changes are found in the setting of acanthocytes in the peripheral blood smear. More information about this group of disorders has recently been described and summarized.[1832] In some cases of neuroacanthocytosis, acanthocytes are not detected in the peripheral smear. However, because routine genetic testing and classic laboratory findings are not available for most of these disorders, detection of acanthocytes is one of the hallmarks of clinical diagnosis. The most sensitive and specific method for measuring acanthocytes is the use of isotonically diluted blood combined with an unfixed wet blood preparation, with the normal range of less than 6.3% acanthocytes in the total erythrocytes.[1833] The mechanism of acanthocyte formation in the neuroacanthocytoses is unknown. However, abnormalities in band 3 have been implicated and are supported by preliminary data.[1834,1835] The subsets of neuroacanthocytoses are abetalipoproteinemia, McLeod's syndrome, choreaacanthocytosis, Huntington's disease–like 2, and pantothenate kinase–associated neurodegeneration.

Abetalipoproteinemia

Abetalipoproteinemia (Bassen-Kornzweig syndrome) is the paradigm of the disorders associated with acantho-

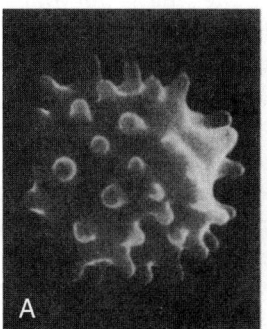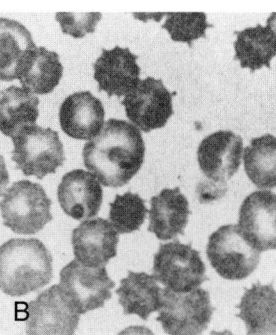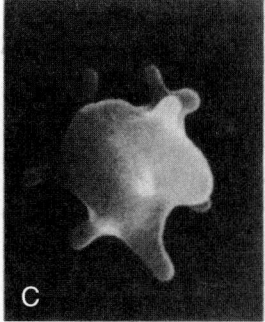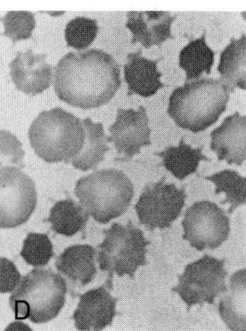

FIGURE 15-60. Morphology of echinocytes and acanthocytes. **A,** Scanning electron micrograph of a spherical echinocyte. **B,** Peripheral blood smear of echinocytes in a splenectomized patient with pyruvate kinase deficiency. **C,** Scanning electron micrograph of an acanthocyte. **D,** Peripheral smear of acanthocytes in a patient with hepatitis and spur cell anemia.

cytosis.[1822,1837] Progressive ataxic neurologic disease, retinitis pigmentosa, fat malabsorption, and acanthocytosis are the primary manifestations of this disorder.[1837] Failure to synthesize or secrete serum apolipoprotein B–containing lipoproteins causes defective intestinal absorption of lipids and extremely low serum cholesterol and triglyceride levels. Because of deficient absorption of fat-soluble vitamin E, severe, but often reversible neurologic problems such as spinocerebellar degenerative ataxic disorder with peripheral neuropathy and retinitis pigmentosa leading to blindness develop in individuals with abetalipoproteinemia.[1838,1839] Some studies have demonstrated delay or prevention of neurologic manifestations with chronic administration of vitamin E.[1838,1839]

This rare disease is caused by various mutations in the gene encoding microsomal triglyceride transfer protein (MTP), which catalyzes the transport of triglyceride, cholesterol ester, and phospholipid from phospholipid surfaces.[1840-1842] MTP forms a heterodimer with a multifunctional protein called disulfide isomerase, which is located in the lumen of hepatic microsomes and intestinal epithelia, the sites of lipoprotein synthesis.[1842-1844] Disulfide isomerase is the only tissue-specific component, other than apolipoprotein B, required for secretion of apolipoprotein B–containing lipoproteins.[1845]

Related entities (hypobetalipoproteinemia, normotriglyceridemic abetalipoproteinemia, and chylomicron retention disease) exist and are associated with partial production of apolipoprotein B–containing lipoproteins or with secretion of lipoproteins containing truncated forms of apolipoprotein B.[1021] Patients with these diseases may also manifest acanthocytosis and neurologic disease, depending on the severity of the lipoprotein defect. The majority of patients with heterozygous hypobetalipoproteinemia do not have acanthocytosis.

Characteristically, 50% to 90% of the red cells are acanthocytes in abetalipoproteinemia.[1846] The shape defect is not evident in nucleated red cells or reticulocytes and worsens as the erythrocytes age. Membrane protein composition is normal, but membrane lipid composition is not. The PC concentration is decreased by about 20%, and the amount of SM is correspondingly increased. The cholesterol-to-phospholipid ratio is normal to mildly elevated.[1847-1849] These changes reflect abnormalities in the distribution of plasma phospholipids and a decrease in LCAT activity.[1850] The relative increases in cholesterol and SM concentration both decrease lipid fluidity,[1848] particularly in the outer half of the bilayer,[1851] and presumably contribute to the acanthocytic shape. They probably do so by expanding the outer bilayer relative to the inner bilayer because drugs that selectively intercalate into the inner bilayer convert acanthocytes to biconcave discs.[1852] However, this is almost impossible to prove because the difference in surface area of the outer bilayers of an acanthocyte and a discocyte is less than 1%.

Because of fat malabsorption and the absence of LDL, which transports vitamin E,[1853] the red cells of these patients are markedly deficient in vitamin E.[1854]

Exposure to lipid-soluble oxidants such as H_2O_2 leads to an increase in lipid peroxides, a decrease in phospholipids rich in unsaturated fatty acids such as PE and PS, damage to membrane proteins, and hemolysis. Oxidant sensitivity can be prevented by treatment with a water-soluble form of vitamin E (e.g., D-α-tocopherol polyethylene glycol succinate).[1854]

Despite increased lipid viscosity and vitamin E deficiency, the hemolysis experienced by these patients is mild.[1847] This is in striking contrast to spur cell anemia (see later), in which hemolysis of similarly shaped cells is often quite severe. It has been suggested that the difference is explained by the fact that the spleen is normal in abetalipoproteinemia whereas it is enlarged and congested by portal hypertension in spur cell anemia. It remains unclear whether this is a sufficient explanation.

Chorea-Acanthocytosis Syndrome

This syndrome was first described by Estes and coworkers.[1855,1856] Since then, this autosomal recessive disorder has been well characterized as a progressive movement disorder consisting of acanthocytosis, myopathy, and cognitive and behavior changes beginning in adolescence or adult life (8 to 62 years).[1835] The movement disorder is most typically characterized by limb chorea, but it can also be manifested as parkinsonism, orofacial dyskinesia, lip and tongue biting, involuntary vocalizations leading to mutism, seizures, and decreased or absent tendon reflexes.[1857,1858] The lingual-buccal-facial dyskinesia and oral self-mutilation are most characteristic of chorea-acanthocytosis. The myopathy causes distal muscle wasting and hypotonia, as well as increased creatine phosphokinase. The extent of mental deterioration varies but often resembles that of frontal lobe syndrome.[1859]

The mutant protein in chorea-acanthocytosis, chorein, encoded by the gene *VPS13A* on chromosome 9q21, has been identified and more than 70 different mutations have been reported to date.[1860-1863] The function of chorein is unknown, but *VPS13A* is a member of a conserved gene family involved in membrane protein trafficking.[1864] Loss of chorein may be diagnostic for this disorder because it is not seen in similar disorders such as Huntington's disease or McLeod's syndrome.[1862,1865] However, routine genetic testing is not available. Therefore, diagnosis of this disorder is made through radiologic and clinical findings, as well as evidence of muscle disease. MRI and pathologic examination show atrophy of the basal ganglia, particularly the caudate and putamen. In some patients, little or no hemolysis occurs; in others, acanthocytosis precedes the onset of neurologic symptoms.[1859] In still others, acanthocytes do not appear until late in the disease course.[1866] Splenomegaly, probably caused by the hemolysis, is noted in some patients.[1867] Elevated levels of creatine phophokinase are found in most patients.

Of note, one family has been described with a defect near the COOH-terminal end of band 3, Pro868Leu.[1868]

Hematologically, affected individuals of this kindred have 20% to 25% acanthocytes and mild anemia with reticulocytosis. However, this family's defect seems to be a distinct disorder separate from the more typically described chorea-acanthocytosis.

McLeod's Syndrome

McLeod's syndrome is a multisystemic disorder with hematologic, muscular, neurologic, and cardiac manifestations.[1869,1870] The McLeod blood group phenotype, first discovered in a dental school student named Hugh McLeod, is an X-linked anomaly of the Kell blood group system in which either red cells, white cells, or both react poorly with Kell antisera but behave normally in other blood group reactions. Affected cells lack Kx, the product of the XK gene, which is a 444–amino acid integral membrane protein precursor of the Kell antigen that has structural features suggesting a transport protein.[1869,1871-1873] As expected, Kx is defective in patients with McLeod's syndrome.[1869,1874-1878] Male hemizygotes who lack Kx on their red cells have variable acanthocytosis (8% to 85%) and mild, compensated hemolysis (3% to 7% reticulocytes).[1823,1879,1880] Some teardrop erythrocytes and bizarre poikilocytes are also present. Female heterozygotes have occasional acanthocytes (as expected by the Lyon hypothesis) and very mild hemolysis,[1823,1879] although some of these women have more severe symptoms.[1874]

Most patients with McLeod's syndrome have a subclinical myopathy associated with an elevated creatine phosphokinase level.[1876,1881,1882] The neuropathy may first be manifested as areflexia and later characterized by basal ganglia atrophy causing dystonic or choreiform movements, psychiatric symptoms, and cognitive changes.[1881-1887] These features, combined with acanthocytosis, can mimic the chorea-acanthocytosis syndrome described in the previous section. However, in contrast to chorea-acanthocytosis, cardiac symptoms such as dilated cardiomyopathy and arrhythmias also develop in most individuals with Mcleod's syndrome.[1876,1887]

The XK gene is located less than 500 kb beyond the chronic granulomatous disease locus on the short arm of the X chromosome (p21.1).[1888] Consequently, males with deletions encompassing both loci have both chronic granulomatous disease and McLeod's syndrome.[1889] It is important to recognize patients with McLeod's syndrome because if they receive transfusions, antibodies may develop that are compatible only with the McLeod syndrome red cells.[1890,1891]

Huntington's Disease–Like 2

In 2001, Margolis and colleagues described a pedigree with an autosomal dominant, Huntington-like disease attributable to CAG/CTG repeats in a novel site.[1892] Huntington's disease–like 2 has since been characterized as a hyperkinetic disorder similar to Huntington's disease that mostly or exclusively affects patients of African ancestry. This neuroacanthocytosis typically is manifested in the third decade by weight loss, dystonia, rigidity, chorea, behavioral changes, and acanthocytosis.[1893,1894] Brain imaging demonstrates marked striatal atrophy and moderate cortical atrophy, similar to Huntington's disease. The CTG/CAG trinucleotide repeat expansion has been found within a variably spliced exon on the junctophilin 3 gene (*JPH3*) on chromosome 16q24.3.[1895]

Pantothenate Kinase–Associated Neurodegeneration

This autosomal recessive progressive movement disorder is caused by a mutation in the pantothenate kinase gene, *PANK2*, on chromosome 20p13.[1896,1897] In the classic form of this neuroacanthocytosis, patients are seen within the first decade of life with a rapidly progressive motor disease leading to loss of ambulation. The atypical and intermediate forms occur later in life and progress more gradually. Pigmented retinopathy typically develops in individuals with an earlier onset of symptoms. In those with a later onset, psychiatric and speech disorders also tend to develop. The motor disease is characterized by rigidity in the lower and, later, the upper extremities. Choreic-type movements often coincide with the rigidity. Because of the effects on voluntary movement and muscular tone, difficulty chewing and swallowing also develops.[1898] Ten percent of patients have acanthocytes on the peripheral smear.[1835]

Diagnosis of this disorder is made clinically and radiologically. Pallidal abnormalities on brain MRI, described as the "'eye of the tiger'" sign, consist of decreased signal intensity on T2-weighted images, compatible with iron deposits, and a small area of hyperintensity in the internal segment.[18990] All patients with this disorder have the "eye of the tiger" sign on brain MRI.[1900,1901] However, this sign is not specific to pantothenate kinase–associated neurodegeneration.[1900,1902] Historically, this disease was called Hallervorden-Spatz disease, named after Julius Hallervorden and Hugo Spatz, who originally described the disorder. In 2001, Zhou and co-authors suggested it be renamed pantothenase kinase–associated neurogeneration to avoid the objection to its eponym because Hallervorden and Spatz actively participated in the euthanasia program in Germany during World War II.[1897]

Vitamin E Deficiency

Premature infants (<36 weeks' gestation or weighing <2000 g) and children or adults with steatorrhea are susceptible to vitamin E deficiency because of decreased absorption of the vitamin.[1903-1905] Discussion of this disorder in preterm infants is now mostly of historical interest.[1906] Infants with this syndrome were fed formulas that were very low in vitamin E and very high in polyunsaturated fatty acids. As the interactions among dietary iron, polyunsaturated fatty acids, and vitamin E were defined, infant formulas were altered so that this condition has virtually disappeared in most nurseries. However, vitamin

E deficiency may cause a hemolytic anemia in infancy in patients with disorders that cause fat malabsorption, such as cystic fibrosis, abetalipoproteinemia, or chronic neonatal cholestasis.[1907-1912] Furthermore, vitamin E deficiency is also seen in individuals with mutations of the tocopherol transport protein gene involved in vitamin E metabolism.[1913,1914]

The features of severe vitamin E deficiency in infants are hemolysis, thrombocytosis, and generalized edema.[1915-1917] Infants with fat malabsorption may also have a rash or other signs of vitamin or protein malnutrition. Peripheral blood smears are often normal but sometimes show variable numbers of irregularly contracted, spiculated cells (acanthocytes or pyknocytes) and small numbers of spherocytes and fragmented red cells.[1908,1916] The mechanism of hemolysis is uncertain. Vitamin E is a lipid-soluble antioxidant, and in its absence, lipid peroxidation occurs with damage to the double bonds of unsaturated fatty acids. Phospholipids rich in unsaturated acyl chains, such as PE, are particularly susceptible.[1849,1854,1918] However, there is some evidence that damage to the sulfhydryl groups of membrane proteins may also contribute to the hemolysis.[1919] In addition, vitamin E has been shown to have a membrane-stabilizing effect against hemolysis induced by hemin.[1920]

Anorexia Nervosa

Acanthocytosis is common in many patients with severe anorexia nervosa.[1826,1827] The cause of the acanthocytosis is unknown. In individuals with anorexia, plasma lipid and low density lipoprotein (LDL) levels are typically normal or slightly decreased. However, even in patients with low levels of LDL,[1921] acanthocytosis may not be due solely to the lipoprotein deficiency because patients with much lower concentrations of LDL (e.g., those with hypobetalipoproteinemia) usually have normal red cell morphology. Severe starvation or malnutrition from causes other than anorexia nervosa can also produce acanthocytosis[1922-1924] or target cells and hypobetalipoproteinemia.[1925]

Despite the acanthocytosis, only approximately 20% to 30% of these patients experience normocytic anemia.[1926-1928] Red cell life span is normal or only slightly shortened. Leukopenia and neutropenia are common, and mild thrombocytopenia is often seen.[1826,1827,1927-1929] Based on morphology, these cytopenias are due to a hypoproliferative bone marrow,[1826] and their severity correlates with weight.[1930] The hypoplastic marrow is also deficient in fat, which is replaced by an amorphous ground substance, perhaps acid mucopolysaccharide.[1927,1931]

Spur Cell Anemia (Hepatocellular Damage)

The anemia seen in patients with liver disease has a complex etiology. Common causes include blood loss, hypersplenism, iron deficiency, folic acid deficiency, and marrow suppression from ingestion of alcohol, hepatitis

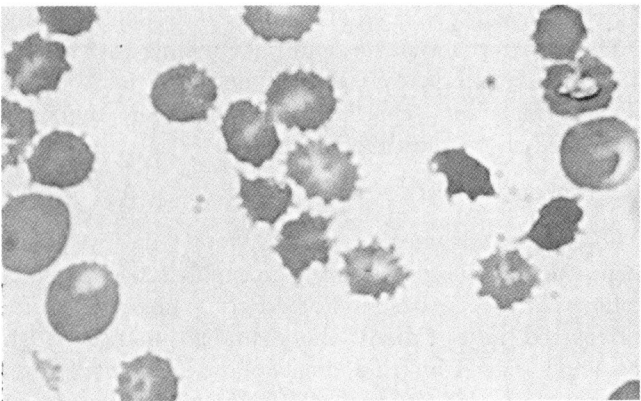

FIGURE 15-61. Peripheral blood smear from a patient with alcoholic cirrhosis and spur cell anemia.

virus infection, and other poorly understood factors.[1932,1933] In addition, in some patients, acquired abnormalities of the red cell membrane may contribute to the anemia. Two morphologic syndromes are recognized. In one, target cells predominate. In the other, a syndrome of brisk hemolysis develops in association with acanthocytes, or "spur" cells, so-called spur cell anemia (Fig. 15-61).[1824,1933-1950]

Typically, target cells are associated with obstructive liver disease, and acanthocytes are associated with hepatocellular disease. In practice, the situation is more complex. It is not uncommon for both cell morphologies to coexist, and some experimental data suggest that they are different stages of the same process. For example, when the bile duct is ligated in a rat, acanthocytes appear within 8 hours, but they convert to target cells if the obstruction persists for 7 days or longer.[1951,1952] Nevertheless, acanthocytes (spur cells) and target cells differ in many important respects, and only spur cells are considered in this section.

Spur cell anemia has most often been described in patients with alcoholic cirrhosis.[1824,1935-1937,1948,1949] However, it is also reported in those with cardiac cirrhosis,[1936] metastatic liver disease,[1940] hemochromatosis,[1939] neonatal hepatitis,[1943] cholestasis,[1933,1934] Wilson's disease, and severe acute hepatitis. The range of diseases in which spur cells are found suggests that it may occur in any disease in which damage to hepatocytes is severe.

Typically, patients have moderately severe hemolysis (hematocrit of 20% to 30%), marked indirect hyperbilirubinemia, splenomegaly, and clinical and laboratory evidence of severe hepatic dysfunction. By definition, more than 20% acanthocytes are evident in multiple areas on several peripheral blood smears. Morphologically, the acanthocytes of spur cell anemia are indistinguishable from those seen in patients with abetalipoproteinemia. In some patients, significant numbers of echinocytes and target cells may be present and spherocytes may develop, presumably as a result of vesiculation. Occasionally, this may cause some

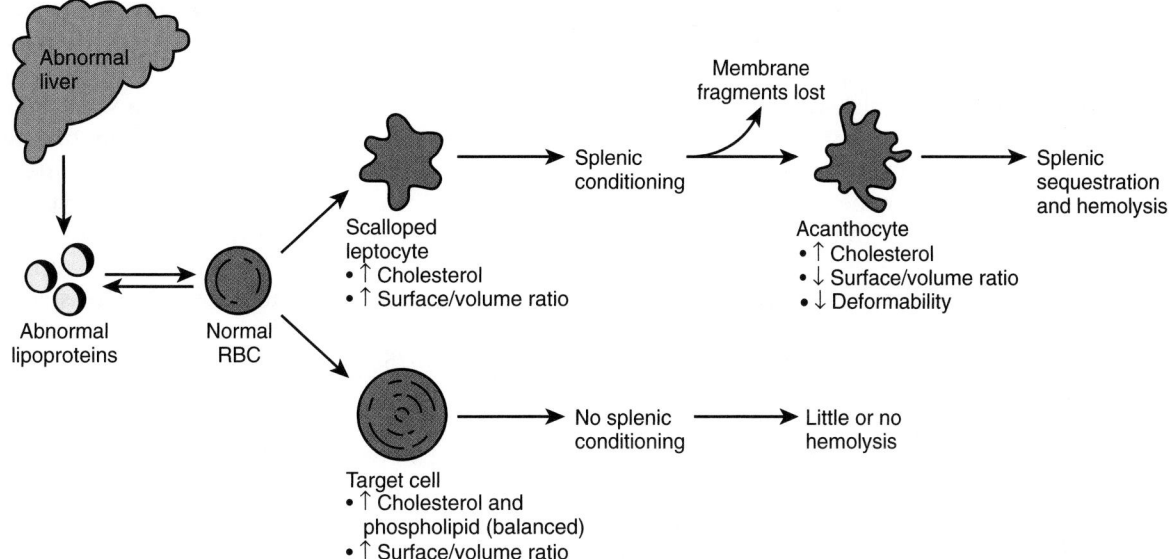

FIGURE 15-62. Schematic illustration of the pathophysiologic course of acanthocyte (spur cell) and target cell formation in liver disease. *(Adapted with permission from Walensky LD, Narla M, Lux SE. Disorders of the red cell membrane. In Handin RI, Lux SE, Stossel TP [eds]. Blood: Principles and Practice of Hematology, 2nd ed. Philadelphia, JB Lippincott, 2003, pp 1709-1858.)*

diagnostic confusion. In our experience, however, many of these "spherocytes" have fine spicules, evident on close examination, which distinguishes them from true microspherocytes.

The red cell life span of spur cells is markedly shortened because of splenic sequestration,[1824,1936,1941,1944] and as expected, the hemolysis abates after splenectomy.[1944] Unfortunately, splenectomy is a dangerous and often fatal procedure in these very sick patients and is not generally recommended.[1944] In addition, spur cell anemia has been reported in a splenectomized patient.[1938] Some success has been reported in treating the anemia of these patients with phospholipid infusions,[1945] flunarizine,[1946] or a combination of flunarizine, pentoxifylline, and cholestyramine[1953]; however, these approaches are still experimental. Cure of the anemia has also been achieved through liver transplantation,[1954] but the disease recurs if the transplant fails.[1955]

The clinical syndrome of spur cell anemia can be produced by at least two different pathogenic mechanisms. In one group, typically consisting of patients with alcoholic cirrhosis,[1824,1937,1942] the disorder is due to an acquired abnormality of red cell lipids. The pathophysiology of spurring in these patients has been defined and reviewed by Cooper and associates[1788,1824,1944,1947,1948] and is illustrated in Figure 15-62. It occurs in two stages: cholesterol loading and splenic remodeling. In the first stage, abnormal, cholesterol-laden, apolipoprotein AII–deficient lipoproteins, produced by the patient's diseased liver, transfer their excess cholesterol to circulating erythrocytes and increase the membrane cholesterol concentration, the cholesterol-to-phospholipid ratio (Fig. 15-63), and membrane surface area.[1788,1949] This is an acquired process and can be mimicked in vitro by incubation of

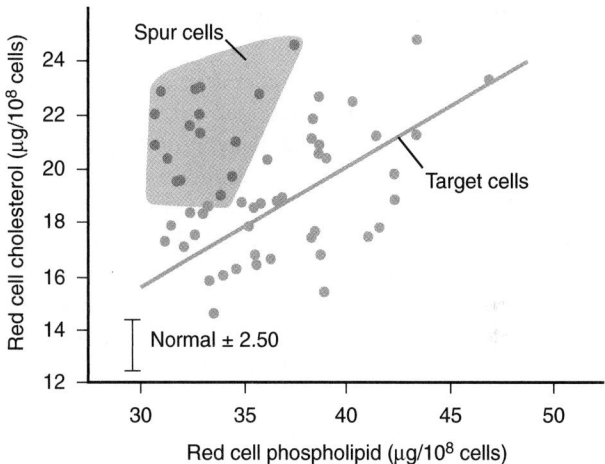

FIGURE 15-63. Cholesterol and phospholipid content of target cells *(blue circles)* and spur cells *(brown circes)*. Note that target cells tend to have a balanced increase in cholesterol and phospholipid whereas spur cells are usually selectively enriched in cholesterol. *(Adapted from Cooper RA, Diloy-Puray M, Lando P, Greenverg MS. An analysis of lipoproteins, bile acids, and red cell membranes associated with target cells and spur cells in patients with liver disease. J Clin Invest. 1972;31:3182.)*

normal red cells in spur cell plasma[1824,1944] or in artificial media containing cholesterol-phospholipid dispersions with a cholesterol-to-phospholipid ratio greater than 1.0. On scanning electron micrographs, these cholesterol-laden cells are flattened and often folded, with an undulating periphery.[1948] They appear scalloped or crenated on dried smears.[1824,1944] In vivo, in the second stage, scalloped cells are converted to spur cells by a process of splenic conditioning (see Fig. 15-62) Over a period of 1 to 7 days, membrane lipids and surface area are lost, cellular rigidity increases, presumably because of the decline in surface-to-volume ratio, and the cell assumes a typical acanthocytic form.[1824,1944] Splenectomy prevents both the formation of spur cells and their premature destruction; however, as noted earlier, it is a high-risk procedure and is seldom indicated.

The cholesterol-laden, incipient spur cell is presumably detained and remodeled by the spleen because it is less deformable than normal. The molecular explanation for this change in deformability is unknown. There is evidence that cholesterol affects the function of band 3.[1950] Cholesterol may also influence band 3 oligomerization or its interaction with other membrane proteins. In addition, it might affect the ratio of band 3 molecules with the anion channel open to the outside versus those with the channel open to the inside. Wong believes that an increase in inward-facing band 3 molecules contracts the membrane skeleton and causes echinocytosis or acanthocytosis whereas an increase in outward-facing band 3 molecules causes stomatocytosis.[1956] A slight increase in the cholesterol-to-phospholipid ratio to above normal markedly alters cholesterol organization in the membrane[1951] and increases the helical content of one or more of the major membrane proteins,[1957] conceivably including band 3. Involvement of band 3 is also suggested by the acanthocytic morphology of rare individuals carrying the band 3 HT variant.[1868]

Other studies have identified a defect in phospholipid repair.[1958] Spur cells and cholesterol-laden normal red cells exhibit decreased fatty acid acylation of phospholipids. Furthermore, red cell membrane lipid "rafts" are cholesterol-rich microdomains that contain unique proteins.[112,116] Changes in intracellular electrolytes causes shedding of these lipid "rafts."[117] It is unclear whether increasing membrane cholesterol would further increase this process. All these processses may play a role in this anemia, but further studies are needed to better understand this process.

A second group of patients with liver disease and spur cell anemia exists in which red cell membrane lipids are normal and incubation of normal red cells in the patients' plasma does not induce spurring.[1936,1940,1941] The pathophysiology of this condition is unknown and largely unstudied. It has been reported in patients with alcoholic cirrhosis[1936,1941] and metastatic liver disease.[1940] This is the form of the disease that the authors have seen in children with spur cells and severe hepatocellular dysfunction.

Infantile Pyknocytosis

In 1959, Tuffy and colleagues[1825] described a syndrome of neonatal jaundice and hemolysis associated with variable numbers of distorted, irregularly contracted, spiculated cells, which they called pyknocytes. Morphologically, these cells are very similar (and possibly identical) to acanthocytes. Normal full-term infants have 0.3% to 1.9% pyknocytes/acanthocytes on peripheral blood smears. In premature infants the normal range is 0.3% to 5.6%. Affected infants typically have jaundice and

slight hepatosplenomegaly in the first few days of life. Pyknocytosis and hemolytic anemia peak at 3 to 4 weeks of age and then decline spontaneously. Clinical severity is variable; however, some infants are severely affected (hemoglobin level of 4 to 6 g/dL, 15% to 20% reticulocytes, 25% to 50% pyknocytes), and some require exchange transfusions. Transfused erythrocytes become pyknocytic and survive poorly,[1825,1959,1960] indicative of an extracorpuscular defect. The syndrome is seen in both premature and term infants. The only consistent chemical abnormality is a mild elevation in serum aspartate transaminase (50 to 250 IU). Parents and siblings are normal.

The cause of this syndrome has not been clearly defined, and for unknown reasons, the diagnosis is seldom made today. Infants with severe G6PD deficiency,[1961] neonatal Heinz body hemolytic anemia,[1825,1962] vitamin E deficiency,[1908,1916] glycolytic enzyme deficiencies,[1698] neonatal hepatitis,[1943] severe HE,[1471] and microangiopathic hemolytic anemia may have hemolysis and pyknocytes, and infantile pyknocytosis is sometimes misdiagnosed in these infants. However, in most of the original case reports, evidence is sufficient to exclude these disorders, which suggests that infantile pyknocytosis may be a valid entity.[1963] The transient nature, mild transaminase elevation, morphologic features, and extracorpuscular etiology suggest a metabolic defect, possibly involving a circulating oxidant; however, other hypotheses are equally tenable.

Uremia

Red cell survival is reduced in patients with advanced renal failure.[1964-1966] An extracorporeal factor is involved because red cells from uremic patients survive normally when infused into normal persons whereas normal red cells survive poorly in uremic patients.[1965] The factor is nondialyzable, and some studies suggest that it is parathyroid hormone (PTH).[1967-1969] PTH levels are elevated in renal failure because of hyperphosphatemia and secondary hyperparathyroidism. PTH levels correlate closely with red cell survival and with the erythropoietin doses necessary to achieve an adequate hematocrit response in patients with chronic renal failure who are undergoing dialysis.[1969,1970] 1,25-Dihydroxycholecalciferol, a vitamin D analogue, improves the anemia in patients with renal failure and increases sensitivity to erythropoietin.[1971] In patients found to be resistent to this therapy, parathyroidectomy for secondary hyperparathyroidism with advanced renal failure often improves the hemolysis and erythropoietin sensitivity.[1971,1972] In vitro, relevant levels of PTH or its bioactive NH_2-terminal peptide augment entry of Ca^{2+} into red cells through a cAMP-independent pathway and cause the cells to develop filamentous extensions and lose membrane surface, presumably by vesiculation.[1968] These effects are largely blocked by the Ca^{2+} channel blocker verapamil. It is possible that they are responsible for the increased numbers of echinocytes observed in some uremic patients because increased intracellular Ca^{2+} is markedly echinocytogenic.[1973] Nevertheless, the reduction in red cell survival and production of echinocytes in uremia may be due to other factors. In a randomized, controlled trial, L-carnitine supplementation in hemodialysis patients was associated with an increase in red cell survival when compared with hemodialysis patients receiving placebo therapy.[1974]

In(Lu) Gene

The major antigens of the Lutheran blood group system are Lu^a and Lu^b. They are located on two low-abundance glycoproteins of 78 kd, on which the basal cell adhesion molecule (BCAM) resides, and 85 kd, on which the Lutheran blood group resides.[1975] In addition to being expressed on the red blood cell membrane, the Lu antigens are expressed by a wide variety of tissues, including the heart, brain, lung, liver, and muscle in the adult, as well as the liver, lung, and kidney in the fetus. Furthermore, Lu glycoproteins are the red cell receptors for laminin and may be involved in the pathogenesis of sickle cell vaso-occlusive crises.[1976,1977] Recent studies have indicated that the Lu glycoproteins may also be involved in the metastasis of certain types of malignancy.[1978]

About 1 person in 5000 inherits a dominantly acting inhibitor called In(Lu)[1828,1979] that partially suppresses expression of Lu^a and Lu^b such that they are undetectable by standard agglutination tests. Such inhibition is the most common cause of the null Lutheran phenotype Lu(a–b–). The In(Lu) gene product inhibits expression of CD44, an adhesive protein; MER2, a common red cell antigen; CR1, the C3b/C4b complement receptor; AnWj, the erythroid *H. influenzae* receptor; and the glycolipid antigens P1 and i, as well as the Lu antigens.[1980] Although several of these proteins are widely expressed, the action of In(Lu) is limited solely to red cells.[1980,1981] Patients with the In(Lu) Lu(a–b–) phenotype have abnormally shaped red cells but no hemolysis.[1828] The morphology varies from normal or mild poikilocytosis to acanthocytosis. The Lu antigens directly interact with spectrin, independently of protein 4.1, which may partially explain the abnormal red cell morphology in some patients with the In(Lu) phenotype.[1982] The OF of fresh In(Lu) Lu(a–b–) red cells is normal, but during in vitro incubation, the cells lose K^+ and become osmotically resistant.

Hypothyroidism

Patients with hypothyroidism often (20% to 65%) have a small number (0.5% to 2%) of acanthocytes on peripheral blood smears.[1829,1983,1984] Given the high incidence of hypothyroidism relative to other disorders that cause acanthocytosis, it has been suggested that the presence of acanthocytes should prompt physicians to consider thyroid testing, especially in adults. This approach has led to the diagnosis of previously unsuspected hypothyroidism.[1985]

OTHER MEMBRANE DISORDERS

Oxidant Hemolysis

Oxidant damage is incurred by the red cell membrane in a variety of inherited disorders involving abnormal hemoglobins that create defects in the cells' endogenous system for detoxification of oxidants. Such disorders include sickle cell disease, thalassemias, unstable hemoglobinopathies, G6PD deficiency, and defects in glutathione metabolism. Membrane oxidant damage may also result from encounters with exogenous oxidants, such as copper. Acute copper-induced hemolysis has been reported in humans after accidental or suicidal ingestion of copper or copper-containing compounds, copper sulfate therapy for burns, copper contamination of hemodialysis units, and Wilson's disease.[1986-1992] In the first three instances, acute intoxication is characterized by flushing, chills, nausea and vomiting, diarrhea, abdominal pain, a metallic taste in the mouth, excessive salivation, headache, weakness, and acute intravascular hemolysis.[1986-1991,1993]

Wilson's Disease (Hepatolenticular Degeneration)

Wilson's disease is an autosomal recessive disorder of copper metabolism that develops between 3 and 52 years of age and is characterized by defective biliary excretion of copper, low plasma levels of ceruloplasmin, and toxic accumulation of copper in the liver, erythrocytes, kidneys, cornea, and brain.[1994,1995] The clinical consequences of toxic copper overload include cirrhosis, hemolysis, corneal Kayser-Fleischer rings, and a progressive neurologic syndrome.[1996-2009] Early diagnosis followed by effective treatment can lead to reversal of the clinical symptoms, including hemolysis.

Hemolysis is an early feature of Wilson's disease; it is seen in about 20% of patients with liver disease[1996] and may be the initial manifestation of the disorder.[1997-2004,2010-2014] Because the disease is treatable and because hemolysis may presage fulminant liver disease by days to years,[2000,2002,2003] the clinician must always consider Wilson's disease in children and young adults with Coombs-negative hemolytic anemia both with and without overt liver disease. Thrombocytopenia may also occur,[2015] and the condition has been misdiagnosed as thrombotic thrombocytopenia purpura or hemolytic-uremic syndrome. Typically, these previously well children have chemical evidence of liver disease, mild hepatosplenomegaly, a low ceruloplasmin concentration, increased erythrocyte and hepatic copper levels, and increased urinary copper excretion. The liver disease has more of a metabolic phenotype (decreased synthesis of albumin and clotting factors compared to the degree of transaminitis), but more acute, fulminant presentations are also observed. Jaundice is often seen and may be severe. The hemolysis observed in Wilson's disease is acute, but the clinical features, though similar to those of acute copper poisoning, are usually more subtle. Hemoglobin may be detected on urinalysis, but gross hemoglobinuria is unusual. Peripheral blood smears do not usually show characteristic changes, although spur cells and target cells have been documented in patients with concurrent severe liver disease.

The Wilson's disease gene, the copper-transporting ATPase *ATP7B*, and the Wilson's disease protein, WNDP, belong to the large family of cation-transporting P-type ATPases.[2016-2020] A wide variety of mutations have been described in this gene in patients with Wilson's disease.[2021-2024] The belief is that in Wilson's disease, copper initially accumulates in hepatocytes because of absence of the copper-transporting protein, which is required for incorporation of copper into ceruloplasmin. Copper eventually reaches a toxic level in the liver and is released into the bloodstream by hepatocellular necrosis.[2002] Plasma copper is rapidly taken up by red cells.[2025] Intravascular hemolysis occurs as a consequence of oxidative damage. The oxidative effects of copper are manifold. In vitro, copper inactivates numerous red cell glycolytic and hexose monophosphate shunt enzymes; directly oxidizes reduced nicotinamide adenine dinucleotide phosphate (NADPH) and glutathione; oxidizes and denatures hemoglobin; damages membrane ATPases, fatty acid acylase, and probably other membrane enzymes; generates lipid peroxides; and cross-links membrane skeletal proteins into disulfide-bonded high-molecular-weight complexes, thereby increasing membrane permeability and rigidity.[2003,2026] However, many of these effects have not been demonstrated at concentrations of copper observed in hemolyzing erythrocytes (150 to 400 mg/dL red cells = 2.4 to 6.3×10^{-5} mol/L).[2004,2008] In vivo studies have indicated marked inhibition of hexokinase and G6PD from red blood cells in patients with untreated Wilson's disease in comparison to patients taking penicillamine and healthy children.[2027] In addition, decreased glutathione levels were found in patients with untreated Wilson's disease, as well as decreased antioxidant enzymes such as superoxide dismutase, catalase, glutathione peroxidase, and glutathione reductase. Although thus far it has not been possible to determine the exact cause of the demise of red cells, initial studies indicate that free copper (non–ceruloplasmin bound) leads to oxidative injury resulting in altered erythrocyte metabolism and antioxidant status in patients with Wilson's disease.

REFERENCES

1. Harrison ML, Rathinavelu P, Arese P, et al. Role of band 3 tyrosine phosphorylation in the regulation of erythrocyte glycolysis. J Biol Chem. 1991;266:4106-4111.
2. Weith JO, Anderson OS, Brahm J, et al. Chloride-bicarbonate exchange in red blood cells: physiology of transport and chemical modification of binding sites. Philos Trans R Soc Lond [Biol]. 1982;299: 383-399.
3. Singer SJ, Nicolson GL. The fluid mosaic model of the structure of cell membranes. Science. 1972;175: 720-731.
4. Jacobson K, Sheets ED, Simson R: Revisiting the fluid mosaic model of membranes. Science. 1995;268:1441-1442.
5. Leitner DM, Brown FL, Wilson KR: Regulation of protein mobility in cell membranes: A dynamic corral model. Biophys J. 2000;78:125-135.
6. White SH, Ladokhin AS, Jayasinghe S, Hristova K. How membranes shape protein structure. J Biol Chem. 2001; 276:32395-32398.
7. Blau L, Bittman R. Cholesterol distribution between the two halves of the lipid bilayer of human erythrocyte ghost membranes. J Biol Chem. 1978;253:8366-8368.
8. Low MG, Finean JB. Modification of erythrocyte membranes by a purified phosphatidylinositol-specific phospholipase C (*Staphylococcus aureus*). Biochem J. 1977;162: 235-240.
9. Verkleij AJ, Zwaal RFA, Roelofsen B, et al. The asymmetric distribution of phospholipids in the human red cell membrane: a combined study using phospholipase and freeze-etch electron microscopy. Biochim Biophys Acta. 1973;323:178-193.
10. Zachowski A. Phospholipids in animal eukaryotic membranes: transverse asymmetry and movement. Biochem J. 1993;294:1-14.
11. Fairbanks G, Steck TL, Wallach DFH. Electrophoretic analysis of the major polypeptides of the human erythrocyte membrane. Biochemistry. 1971;10:2606-2617.
12. Ferrell JE Jr, Huestis WH. Phosphoinositide metabolism and the morphology of human erythrocytes. J Cell Biol. 1984;98:1992-1998.
13. Van Deenen LLM, De Gier J. Lipids of the red blood cell membrane. In Surgenor DM (ed). The Red Blood Cell, 2nd ed. New York, Academic Press, 1974, p 148.
14. Sweeley CC, Dawson G. Lipids of the erythrocyte. In Jamieson GA, Greenwalt TJ (eds). Red Cell Membrane Structure and Function. Philadelphia, JB Lippincott, 1969, p 172.
15. Cooper RA. Lipids of human red cell membranes: normal composition and variability in disease. Semin Hematol. 1970;7:296-332.
16. Turner JD, Rouser G. Precise quantitative determination of human blood lipids by thin layer and triethylaminoethyl cellulose column chromatography. Ann Biochem. 1970;38:437-445.
17. Ways P, Hanahan DJ. Characterization and quantification of red cell lipids in normal man. J Lipid Res. 1964;5:318-328.
18. Weinstein RS. The morphology of adult red cells. In Surgenor DM (ed). The Red Blood Cell, vol 1, 2nd ed. New York, Academic Press, 1974, pp 214-269.
19. Ohvo-Rekila H, Ramstedt B, Leppimaki P, Slotte JP. Cholesterol interactions with phospholipids in membranes. Prog Lipid Res. 2002;41:66-97.
20. Virtanen JA, Cheng KH, Somerharju P. Phospholipid composition of the mammalian red cell membrane can be rationalized by a superlattice model. Proc Natl Acad Sci U S A. 1998;95:4964-4969.
21. Brown K, Anderson SM, Young NS. Erythrocyte P antigen: cellular receptor for B19 parvovirus. Science. 1993;262:114-117.

22. Lange Y, Slayton JM. Interaction of cholesterol and lysophosphatidylcholine in determining red cell shape. J Lipid Res. 1982;23:1121-1127.

23. Lange Y, Cutler HB, Steck TL. The effect of cholesterol and other intercalated amphipaths on the contour and stability of the isolated red cell membrane. J Biol Chem. 1980;255:9331-9337.

24. Hale JE, Schroeder F. Asymmetric transbilayer distribution of sterol across plasma membranes determined by fluorescence quenching of dehydroergosterol. Eur J Biochem. 1982;122:649-661.

25. Fisher KA. Analysis of membrane halves: cholesterol. Proc Natl Acad Sci U S A. 1976;73:173-177.

26. Steck TL, Ye J, Lange Y. Probing red cell membrane cholesterol movement with cyclodextrin. Biophys J. 2002;83:2118-2125.

27. Huang CH. A structural model for the cholesterol-phosphatidylcholine complexes in bilayer membranes. Lipids. 1977;12:348-356.

28. Yeagle PL. Modulation of membrane function by cholesterol. Biochimie. 1991;73:1303-1310.

29. Murata M, Peranen J, Schreiner R, et al. VIP21/caveolin is a cholesterol-binding protein. Proc Natl Acad Sci U S A. 1995;92:10339-10343.

30. Porter JA, Young KE, Beachy PA. Cholesterol modification of hedgehog signaling proteins in animal development. Science. 1996;274:255-259.

31. Osborne TF, Rosenfeld JM. Related membrane domains in proteins of sterol sensing and cell signaling provide a glimpse of treasures still buried within the dynamic realm of intracellular metabolic regulation. Curr Opin Lipidol. 1998;9:137-140.

32. Bergelson LD, Barsukov LI. Topological asymmetry of phospholipids in membranes. Science. 1977;197:224-230.

33. Op den Kamp JAF. Lipid asymmetry in membranes. Annu Rev Biochem. 1979;48:47-71.

34. Fujimoto K, Umeda M, Fujimoto T. Transmembrane phospholipid distribution revealed by freeze-fracture replica labeling. J Cell Sci. 1996;109:2453-2460.

35. Devaux PF. Protein involvement in transmembrane lipid asymmetry. Annu Rev Biophys Biomol Struct. 1992;21:417-439.

36. Devaux PF. Lipid transmembrane asymmetry and flip-flop in biological membranes and in lipid bilayers. Curr Opin Struct Biol. 1993;3:489-494.

37. Bevers EM, Comfurius P, Dekkers DW, Zwaal RF. Lipid translocation across the plasma membrane of mammalian cells. Biochim Biophys Acta. 1999;1439:317-330.

38. van Meer G, Op den Kamp JA. Transbilayer movement of various phosphatidylcholine species in intact human erythrocytes. J Cell Biochem. 1982;19:193-204.

39. Middelkoop E, Lubin BH, Op den Kamp JA, Roelofsen B. Flip-flop rates of individual molecular species of phosphatidylcholine in the human red cell membrane. Biochim Biophys Acta. 1986;855:421-424.

40. Daleke DL, Lyles JV. Identification and purification of aminophospholipid flippases. Biochim Biophys Acta. 2000;1486:108-127

41. Daleke DL. Regulation of transbilayer plasma membrane phospholipid asymmetry. J Lipid Res. 2003;44:233-242

42. Devaux PF, Lopez-Montero I, Bryde S. Proteins involved in lipid translocation in eukaryotic cells. Chem Phys Lipids. 2006;141:119-132.

43. Holthuis JC, Levine TP. Lipid traffic: floppy drives and a superhighway. Nat Rev Mol Cell Biol. 2005;6:209-220.

44. Morrot G, Hervè P, Zachowski A, et al. Aminophospholipid translocase of human erythrocytes: phospholipid substrate specificity and effect of cholesterol. Biochemistry. 1989;28:3456-3462.

45. Connor J, Schroit AJ. Transbilayer movement of phosphatidylserine in nonhuman erythrocytes: evidence that the aminophospholipid transporter is a ubiquitous membrane protein. Biochemistry. 1989;28:9680-9685.

46. Tang X, Halleck MS, Schlegel RA, Williamson P. A novel subfamily of P-type ATPases with aminophospholipid transporting activity. Science. 1996;272:1495-1497.

47. Paterson JK, Renkema K, Burden L, et al. Lipid specific activation of the murine P4-ATPase Atp8a1 (ATPase II). Biochemistry. 2006;45:5367-5376.

48. Soupene E, Kuypers FA. Identification of an erythroid ATP-dependent aminophospholipid transporter. Br J Haematol. 2006;133:436-438.

49. Connor J, Pak CH, Zwaal RFA, Schroit AJ. Bidirectional transbilayer movement of phospholipid analogs in human red blood cells. J Biol Chem. 1992;267:19412-19417.

50. Bitbol M, Devaux PF. Measurement of outward translocation of phospholipids across human erythrocyte membrane. Proc Natl Acad Sci U S A. 1998;85:6783-6787.

51. van Helvoort A, Smith AJ, Sprong H, et al. MDR1 P-glycoprotein is a lipid translocase of broad specificity, while MDR3 P-glycoprotein specifically translocates phosphatidylcholine. Cell. 1996;87:507-517.

52. Rust S, Rosier M, Funke H, et al. Tangier disease is caused by mutations in the gene encoding ATP-binding cassette transporter 1. Nat Genet. 1999;22:352-355.

53. Smit JJ, Schinkel AH, Oude Elferink RP, et al. Homozygous disruption of the murine mdr2 P-glycoprotein gene leads to a complete absence of phospholipid from bile and to liver disease. Cell 1993;75:451-462.

54. Dekkers DWC, Comfurius P, Schroit AJ, et al. Transbilayer movement of NBD-labeled phospholipids in red blood cell membranes: outward-directed transport by the multidrug resistance protein 1 (MRP1). Biochemistry. 1998;37:14833-14837.

55. Kamp D, Haest CWM. Evidence for a role of the multidrug resistance protein (MRP) in the outward translocation of NBD-phospholipids in the erythrocyte membrane. Biochim Biophys Acta. 1998;1372:91-101.

56. Dekkers DW, Comfurius P, van Gool RG, et al. Multidrug resistance protein 1 regulates lipid asymmetry in erythrocyte membranes. Biochem J. 2000;350:531-535.

57. Williamson P, Kulick A, Zachowski A, et al. Ca²⁺ induces transbilayer redistribution of all major phospholipids in human erythrocytes. Biochemistry. 1992;31:6355-6360.

58. Basse F, Stout JG, Sims PJ, Wiedmer T. Isolation of an erythrocyte membrane protein that mediates Ca²⁺-dependent transbilayer movement of phospholipid. J Biol Chem. 1996;271:17205-17210.

59. Zhou QS, Sims PJ, Wiedmer T. Identity of a conserved motif in phospholipid scramblase that is required for Ca^{2+}-accelerated transbilayer movement of membrane phospholipids. Biochemistry. 1998;37:2356-2360.

60. Zhao J, Zhou QS, Wiedmer T, Sims PJ. Palmitoylation of phospholipid scramblase is required for normal function in promoting Ca^{2+}-activated transbilayer movement of membrane phospholipids. Biochemistry. 1998;37:6361-6366.

61. Zhou Q, Zhao J, Wiedmer T, Sims PJ. Normal hemostasis but defective hematopoietic response to growth factors in mice deficient in phospholipid scramblase 1. Blood. 2002;99:4030-4038.

62. de Jong K, Larkin SK, Styles L, et al. Characterization of the phosphatidylserine-exposing subpopulation of sickle cells. Blood. 2001;98:860-867.

63. Blumenfeld N, Zachowski A, Galacteros F, et al. Transmembrane mobility of phospholipids in sickle erythrocytes: effect of deoxygenation on diffusion and asymmetry. Blood. 1991;77:849-854.

64. Franck PFH, Chiu DT, Op den Kamp JA, et al. Accelerated transbilayer movement of phosphatidylcholine in sickled erythrocytes: a reversible process. J Biol Chem. 1983;258:8436-8442.

65. Lubin B, Chiu D, Bastacky J, et al. Abnormalities in membrane phospholipid organization in sickled erythrocytes. J Clin Invest. 1981;67:1643-1649.

66. Platt OS, Falcone JF, Lux SE. Molecular defect in the sickle erythrocyte skeleton. Abnormal spectrin binding to sickle inside-out vesicles. J Clin Invest. 1985;75:266-271.

67. Schwartz RS, Rybicki AC, Heath RH, Lubin BH. Protein 4.1 in sickle erythrocytes. Evidence for oxidative damage. J Biol Chem. 1987;62:15666-15672.

68. Waugh SM, Willardson BM, Kannan R, et al. Heinz bodies induce clustering of band 3, glycophorin, and ankyrin in sickle cell erythrocytes. J Clin Invest. 1986;78:1155-1160.

69. Liu SC, Derick LH, Zhai S, Palek J. Uncoupling of the spectrin based skeleton from the lipid bilayer in sickled red cells. Science. 1991;252:574-576.

70. Kuypers FA, Yuan J, Lewis RA, et al. Membrane phospholipid asymmetry in human thalassemia. Blood. 1998;91:3044-3051.

71. Wautier JL, Paton RC, Wautier MP, et al. Increased adhesion of erythrocytes to endothelial cells in diabetes mellitus and its relationship to vascular complications. N Engl J Med. 1981;305:237-242.

72. Hebbel RP, Yamada O, Moldow CF, et al. Abnormal adherence of sickle erythrocytes to cultured vascular endothelium. Possible mechanism for microvascular occlusion in sickle cell disease. J Clin Invest. 1980;65:154-160.

73. Hebbel RP, Boogaerts MA, Eaton JW, Steinberg MH. Erythrocyte adherence to endothelium in sickle-cell anemia. A possible determinant of disease severity. N Engl J Med. 1980;302:992-995.

74. Bevers EM, Comfurius P, van Rijn JL, et al. Generation of prothrombin-converting activity and the exposure of phosphatidyl serine at the outer surface of platelets. Eur J Biochem. 1982;122:429-436.

75. Chiu D, Lubin B, Roelofsen B, Van Deenen LLM. Sickled erythrocytes accelerate clotting in vitro: An effect of abnormal membrane lipid asymmetry. Blood. 1981;58:398-401.

76. Zwaal RFA, Comfurius P, van Deenen LL. Membrane asymmetry and blood coagulation. Nature. 1977;268:358-360.

77. Test ST, Mitsuyoshi J. Activation of the alternative pathway of complement by calcium-loaded erythrocytes resulting from loss of membrane phospholipid asymmetry. J Lab Clin Med. 1997;130:169-182.

78. Allen TM, Williamson P, Schlegel RA. Phosphatidylserine as a determinant of reticuloendothelial recognition of liposome models of the erythrocyte surface. Proc Natl Acad Sci U S A. 1988;85:8067-8071.

79. McEvoy L, Williamson P, Schlegel RA. Membrane phospholipid asymmetry as a determinant of erythrocyte recognition by macrophages. Proc Natl Acad Sci U S A. 1986;83:3311-3315.

80. Tanaka Y, Schroit AJ. Insertion of fluorescent phosphatidylserine into the plasma membrane of red blood cells: recognition by autologous macrophages. J Biol Chem. 1983;258:11335-11343.

81. Fadok VA, Voelker DR, Campbell PA, et al. Exposure of phosphatidylserine on the surface of apoptotic lymphocytes triggers specific recognition and removal by macrophages. J Immunol. 1992;148:2207-2216.

82. Zwaal RF, Schroit AJ. Pathophysiologic implications of membrane phospholipid asymmetry in blood cells. Blood. 1997;89:1121-1132.

83. Fadok VA, Bratton DL, Rose DM, et al. A receptor for phosphatidylserine-specific clearance of apoptotic cells. Nature. 2000;405:85-90.

84. Li MO, Sarkisian MR, Mehal WZ, et al. Phosphatidylserine receptor is required for clearance of apoptotic cells. Science. 2003;302:1560-1563.

85. Williamson P, Schlegel RA. Hide and seek: the secret identity of the phosphatidylserine receptor. J Biol. 2004;3:14-14.4.

86. Devaux PF. Static and dynamic lipid asymmetry in cell membranes. Biochemistry. 1991;30:1163-1173.

87. Toti F, Satta N, Fressinaud E, et al. Scott syndrome, characterized by impaired transmembrane migration of procoagulant phosphatidylserine and hemorrhagic complications, is an inherited disorder. Blood. 1996;87:1409-1415.

88. Weiss HJ, Lages B. Family studies in Scott syndrome. Blood. 1997;90:475-476.

89. Weiss HJ. Scott syndrome: a disorder of platelet coagulant activity. Semin Hematol. 1994;31:312-319.

90. Zhou Q, Sims PJ, Wiedmer T. Expression of proteins controlling transbilayer movement of plasma membrane phospholipids in the B-lymphocytes from a patient with Scott syndrome. Blood. 1998;92:1707-1712.

91. Bratosin D, Estaquier J, Petit F, et al. Programmed cell death in mature erythrocytes: a model for investigating death effector pathways operating in the absence of mitochondria. Cell Death Differ. 2001;8:1143-1156.

92. Lang F, Lang KS, Lang PA, et al. Mechanisms and significance of eryptosis. Antioxid Redox Signal. 2006;8:1183-1192.

93. Mandal D, Moitra PK, Saha S, Basu J. Caspase 3 regulates phosphatidylserine externalization and phagocytosis of oxidatively stressed erythrocytes. FEBS Lett. 2002;513:184-188.

94. Mandal D, Mazumder A, Das P, et al. Fas-, caspase 8-, and caspase 3–dependent signaling regulates the activity of the aminophospholipid translocase and phosphatidylserine externalization in human erythrocytes. J Biol Chem. 2005;280:39460-39467.

95. Kagan VE, Gleiss B, Tyurina YY, et al. A role for oxidative stress in apoptosis: oxidation and externalization of phosphatidylserine is required for macrophage clearance of cells undergoing Fas-mediated apoptosis. J Immunol. 2002;169:487-499.

96. Gleiss B, Gogvadze V, Orrenius S, Fadeel B. Fas-triggered phosphatidylserine exposure is modulated by intracellular ATP. FEBS Lett. 2002;519:153-158.

97. Tothova Z, Kollipara R, Huntly BJ, et al. FoxOs are critical mediators of hematopoietic stem cell resistance to physiologic oxidative stress. Cell. 2007;128:325-339.

98. Marinkovic D, Zhang X, Yalcin S, et al. Foxo3 is required for the regulation of oxidative stress in erythropoiesis. J Clin Invest. 2007;117:2133-2144.

99. Rodgers W, Glaser M. Characterization of lipid domains in erythrocyte membranes. Proc Natl Acad Sci U S A. 1991;88:1364-1368.

100. Jost PC, Nadakavukaren KK, Griffith OH. Phosphatidylcholine exchange between the boundary lipid and bilayer domains in cytochrome oxidase containing membranes. Biochemistry. 1977;16:3110-3114.

101. Smith RL, Oldfield E. Dynamic structure of membranes by deuterium NMR. Science. 1984;225:280-288.

102. Armitage IM, Shapiro DL, Furthmayr H, Marchesi VT. ^{31}P nuclear magnetic resonance evidence for polyphosphoinositide associated with the hydrophobic segment of glycophorin A. Biochemistry. 1977;16:1317-1320.

103. Mendelsohn R, Dluhy RA, Crawford T, Mantsch HH. Interaction of glycophorin with phosphatidylserine: a Fourier transform infrared investigation. Biochemistry. 1984;23:1498-1504.

104. Ong RL. ^{31}P and ^{19}F NMR studies of glycophorin-reconstituted membranes: preferential interaction of glycophorin with phosphatidylserine. J Membr Biol. 1984;78:1-7.

105. Yeagle PL, Kelsey D. Phosphorus nuclear magnetic resonance studies of lipid-protein interactions: human erythrocyte glycophorin and phospholipids. Biochemistry. 1989;28:2210-2215.

106. Boyd D, Beckwith J. The role of charged amino acids in the localization of secreted and membrane proteins. Cell. 1990;62:1031-1033.

107. Parks GD, Lamb RA. Topology of eukaryotic type II membrane proteins: importance of N-terminal positively charged residues flanking the hydrophobic domain. Cell. 1991;64:777-787.

108. Rybicki AC, Heath R, Lubin B, Schwartz RS. Human erythrocyte protein 4.1 is a phosphatidylserine binding protein. J Clin Invest. 1988;81:255-260.

109. An X, Guo X, Sum H, et al. Phosphatidylserine binding sites in erythroid spectrin: location and implications for membrane stability. Biochemistry. 2004;43:310-315.

110. Manno S, Takakuwa Y, Mohandas N. Identification of a functional role for lipid asymmetry in biological membranes: phosphatidylserine–skeletal protein interactions modulate membrane stability. Proc Natl Acad Sci U S A. 2002;99:1943-1948.

111. Simons K, Ikonen E. Functional rafts in cell membranes. Nature. 1997;387:569-572.

112. Brown DA, London E. Functions of lipid rafts in biological membranes. Annu Rev Cell Dev Biol. 1998;14:111-136.

113. Koumanov KS, Tessier C, Momchilova AB, et al. Comparative lipid analysis and structure of detergent-resistant membrane raft fractions isolated from human and ruminant erythrocytes. Arch Biochem Biophys. 2005;434:150-158.

114. Murphy SC, Fernandez-Pol S, Chung PH, et al. Cytoplasmic remodeling of erythrocyte raft lipids during infection by the human malaria parasite *Plasmodium falciparum*. Blood. 2007;110:2139-2199.

115. Samuel BU, Mohandas N, Harrison T, et al. The role of cholesterol and glycosylphosphatidylinositol-anchored proteins of erythrocyte rafts in regulating raft protein content and malaria infection. J Biol Chem. 2001;276:29319-29329.

116. Salzer U, Prohaska R. Stomatin, flotillin-1, and flotillin-2 are major integral proteins of erythrocyte lipid rafts. Blood. 2001;97:1141-1143.

117. Salzer U, Hinterdorfer P, Hunger U, et al. Ca^{2+}-dependent vesicle release from erythrocytes involves stomatin-specific lipid rafts, synexin (annexin VII) and sorcin. Blood. 2002;99:2569-2577.

118. Arni S, Keilbaugh SA, Ostermeyer AG, Brown DA. Association of GAP-43 with detergent-resistant membranes requires two palmitoylated cysteine residues. J Biol Chem. 1998;273:28478-28485.

119. Melkonian JA, Ostermeyer AG, Chen JZ, et al. Role of lipid modifications in targeting proteins to detergent-resistant membrane rafts. Many raft proteins are acylated, while few are prenylated. J Biol Chem. 1999;274:3910-3917.

120. Moffet S, Brown DA, Linder ME. Lipid-dependent targeting of G proteins into rafts. J Biol Chem. 2000;275:2191-2198.

121. Murphy SC, Hiller NL, Harrison T, et al. Lipid rafts and malaria parasite infection of erythrocytes. Mol Membr Biol. 2006;23:81-88.

122. Beck JS. Relations between membrane monolayers in some red cell shape transformations. J Theor Biol. 1978;75:487-501.

123. Ferrell JE Jr, Lee KJ, Huestis WH. Membrane bilayer balance and erythrocyte shape: a quantitative assessment. Biochemistry. 1985;24:2849-2857.

124. Sheetz MP, Singer SJ. Biological membranes as bilayer couples: a molecular mechanism of drug erythrocyte interactions. Proc Natl Acad Sci U S A. 1974;71:4457-4461.

125. Christiansson A, Kuypers FA, Roelofsen B, et al. Lipid molecular shape effects erythrocyte morphology: a study involving replacement of native phosphatidylcholine with different species followed by treatment of cells with sphingomyelinase C or phospholipase A. J Cell Biol. 1985;101:1455-1462.

126. Isomaa B, Hagerstrand H, Paatero G. Shape transformation induced by amphiphiles in erythrocytes. Biochim Biophys Acta. 1987;899:93-103.

127. Sheetz MP, Painter RG, Singer SJ. Biological membranes as bilayer couples. III. Compensatory shape changes induced in membranes. J Cell Biol. 1976;70:193-203.

128. Lange Y, Steck TL. Mechanism of red blood cell acanthocytosis and echinocytosis in vivo. J Membr Biol. 1984;77:153-159.

129. Nakao M. New insights into regulation of erythrocyte shape. Curr Opin Hematol. 2002;9:127.

130. Lim HWG, Wortis M, Mukhopadhyay R. Stomatocyte-discocyte-echinocyte sequence of the human red blood cell: evidence for the bilayer-couple hypothesis from membrane mechanics. Proc Natl Acad Sci U S A. 2002; 99:16766-16769.

131. Cohen CM, Gascard P. Regulation and post-translational modification of the erythrocyte membrane and membrane-skeletal proteins. Semin Hematol. 1982;29: 244-292.

132. McConnell HM, McFarland BG. The flexibility gradient in biological membranes. Ann N Y Acad Sci. 1972;195: 207-217.

133. Barton PG, Gunstone FD. Hydrocarbon chain packing and molecular motion in phospholipid bilayers formed from unsaturated lecithins. J Biol Chem. 1975;250: 4470-4476.

134. Seelig A, Seelig J. Effect of a single cis double bond on the structure of a phospholipid bilayer. Biochemistry. 1977;16:45-50.

135. Oldfield E, Chapman D. Effects of cholesterol and cholesterol derivatives on hydrocarbon chain mobility in lipids. Biochem Biophys Res Commun. 1971;43:610-616.

136. Demel RA, De Kruijff B. The function of sterols in membranes. Biochim Biophys Acta. 1976;457:109-132.

137. Lee AG, Birdsall NJM, Metcalfe JC. Measurement of fast lateral diffusion of lipids in vesicles and in biological membranes by 1H nuclear magnetic resonance. Biochemistry. 1973;12:1650-1659.

138. Seigneuret M, Devaux PF. ATP dependent asymmetric distribution of spin labeled phospholipids in the erythrocyte membrane: relation to shape changes. Proc Natl Acad Sci U S A. 1984;81:3751-3755.

139. Mely-Goubert B, Freedman MH. Lipid fluidity and membrane protein monitoring using 1,6-diphenyl-1,3,5-hexatriene. Biochim Biophys Acta. 1980;601:315-327.

140. Devaux P, McConnell HM. Lateral diffusion in spin labeled phosphatidyl choline multilayers. J Am Chem Soc. 1992;94:4475-4481.

141. Wu ES, Jacobson K, Papahadjopoulos D. Lateral diffusion in phospholipid multilayers measured by fluorescence recovery after photobleaching. Biochemistry. 1977;16:3936-3941.

142. Koppel DE, Sheetz MP, Schindler M. Matrix control of protein diffusion in biological membranes. Proc Natl Acad Sci U S A. 1981;78:3576-3580.

143. Reed CF. Incorporation of orthophosphate ^{32}P into erythrocyte phospholipids in normal subjects and in patients with hereditary spherocytosis. J Clin Invest. 1968;47:2630-2638.

144. Shohet SB. Release of phospholipid fatty acid from human erythrocytes. J Clin Invest. 1970;49:1668-1678.

145. Renooij W, Van Golde LMG. The transposition of molecular classes of phosphatidyl choline across the rat erythrocyte membrane and their exchange between the red cell membrane and plasma lipoproteins. Biochim Biophys Acta. 1977;470:465-474.

146. Norum KR, Gjone E, Glomset JA. Familial lecithin: cholesterol acyltransferase deficiency, including fish eye disease. In Scriver CS, Beaudet AL, Sly WS, Valle D (eds). The Metabolic Basis of Inherited Disease, 6th ed. New York, McGraw-Hill, 1989, pp 1181-1194.

147. Mulder E, Van Deenen LLM. Metabolism of red cell lipids. I. Incorporation in vitro of fatty acids into phospholipids from mature erythrocytes. Biochim Biophys Acta. 1965;106:106.

148. Oliveria MM, Vaughan M. Incorporation of fatty acids into phospholipids of erythrocyte membranes. J Lipid Res. 1964;5:156.

149. Shohet SB, Nathan DG, Karnovsky ML. Stages in the incorporation of fatty acids into red blood cells. J Clin Invest. 1968;47:1096-1108.

150. Renooij W, Van Golde LMG, Zwaal RF, et al. Preferential incorporation of fatty acids at the inside of human erythrocyte membranes. Biochim Biophys Acta. 1974;363:287-292.

151. Farquhar JW, Ahrens EH Jr. Effects of dietary fats on human erythrocyte fatty acid patterns. J Clin Invest. 1963;42:675-685.

152. Pasini EM, Kirkegaard M, Mortensen P, et al. In-depth analysis of the membrane and cytosolic proteome of red blood cells. Blood. 2006;108:791-801.

153. Agre P, Orringer EP, Bennett V. Deficient red-cell spectrin in severe, recessively inherited spherocytosis. N Engl J Med. 1982;306:1155-1161.

154. Savvides P, Shalev O, John KM, Lux SE. Combined spectrin and ankyrin deficiency is common in autosomal dominant hereditary spherocytosis. Blood. 1993;82:2953-2960.

155. Hemming NJ, Anstee DJ, Mawby WJ, et al. Localization of the protein 4.1-binding site on human erythrocyte glycophorins C and D. Biochem J. 1994;299:191-196.

156. Fukuda M. Molecular genetics of the glycophorin A gene cluster. Semin Hematol. 1993;30:138-151.

157. Pinder JC, Gratzer WB. Structural and dynamic states of actin in the erythrocyte. J Cell Biol. 1983;96:768-775.

158. Inaba M, Guptka KC, Kuwabara M, et al. Deamidation of human erythrocyte membrane protein 4.1: possible role in ageing. Blood. 1992;79:3355-3361.

159. Peters LL, Weier HU, Walensky LD, et al. Four paralogous protein 4.1 genes map to distinct chromosomes in mouse and human. Genomics. 1998;54:348-350.

160. Baklouti F, Huang SC, Vulliamy TJ, et al. Organization of the human protein 4.1 genomic locus: new insights into the tissue-specific alternative splicing of the pre-mRNA. Genomics. 1997;39:289-302.

161. Huang JP, Tang CJ, Kou GH, et al. Genomic structure of the locus encoding protein 4.1. Structural basis for complex combinational patterns of tissue-specific alternative RNA splicing. J Biol Chem. 1993;268:3758-3766.

162. Conboy JG. Structure, function, and molecular genetics of erythroid membrane skeletal protein 4.1 in normal and abnormal red blood cells. Semin Hematol. 1993;30:58-73.

163. Gascard P, Lee G, Coulombel L, et al. Characterization of multiple isoforms of protein 4.1R expressed during erythroid terminal differentiation. Blood. 1998;92: 4404.

164. Azim AC, Knoll JH, Beggs AH, Chishti AH. Isoform cloning, actin binding, and chromosomal localization of human erythroid dematin, a member of the villin super-family. J Biol Chem. 1995;270:17407-17413.

165. Azim AC, Marfatia SM, Korsgren C, et al. Human erythrocyte dematin and protein 4.2 (pallidin) are ATP binding proteins. Biochemistry. 1996;35:3001-3006.

166. Sung LA, Gao KM, Yee LJ, et al. Tropomyosin isoform 5b is expressed in human erythrocytes: implications of tropomodulin-TM5 or tropomodulin-TM5b complexes in the protofilament and hexagonal organization of membrane skeletons. Blood. 2000;95:1473-1480.

167. Cartron JP, Le Van Kim C, Colin Y. Glycophorin C and related glycoproteins: structure, function, and regulation. Semin Hematol. 1993;30:152-168.

168. Tse WT, Lux SE. Red blood cell membrane disorders. Br J Haematol. 1999;104:2.

169. Gallagher PG. Update on the clinical spectrum and genetics of red blood cell membrane disorders. Curr Hematol Rep. 2004;3:85-91.

170. Delaunay J. The molecular basis of hereditary red cell membrane disorders. Blood Rev. 2007;21:1-20.

171. Dodge JT, Mitchell C, Hanahan DJ. The preparation and chemical characteristics of hemoglobin-free ghosts of human erythrocytes. Arch Biochem Biophys. 1963;100:119-130.

172. Sheetz MP. Integral membrane protein interaction with Triton cytoskeletons of erythrocytes. Biochim Biophys Acta. 1979;557:122.

173. Yu J, Fischman DA, Steck TL. Selective solubilization of proteins and phospholipids from red blood cell membranes by nonionic detergents. J Supramol Struct. 1973;1:233.

174. Lux SE, John KM, Kopito RR, Lodish HF. Cloning and characterization of band 3, the human erythrocyte anion-exchange protein (AE1). Proc Natl Acad Sci U S A. 1989;86:9089-9093.

175. Tanner MJ, Martin PG, High S. The complete amino acid sequence of the human erythrocyte membrane anion-transport protein deduced from the cDNA sequence. Biochem J. 1988;256:703-712.

176. Landolt-Marticorena C, Charuk JH, Reithmeier RA. Two glycoprotein populations of band 3 dimers are present in human erythrocytes. Mol Membr Biol. 1998;15:153-158.

177. Vince JW, Reithmeier RA. Carbonic anhydrase II binds to the carboxyl terminus of human band 3, the erythrocyte Cl⁻/HCO₃⁻ exchanger. J Biol Chem. 1998;273:28430-28437.

178. Bennett V, Stenbuck PJ. Association between ankyrin and the cytoplasmic domain of band 3 isolated from the human erythrocyte membrane. J Biol Chem. 1980;255:6424-6432.

179. Zhu Q, Lee DW, Casey JR. Novel topology in C-terminal region of the human plasma membrane anion exchanger, AE1. J Biol Chem. 2003;278:3112-3120.

180. Zelinski T. Erythrocyte band 3 antigens and the Diego blood group system. Transfus Med Rev. 1998;12:36-45.

181. Low PS. Structure and function of the cytoplasmic domain of band 3: center of erythrocyte membrane–peripheral protein interactions. Biochim Biophys Acta. 1986;864:145-167.

182. Walder JA, Chatterjee R, Steck TL, et al. The interaction of hemoglobin with the cytoplasmic domain of band 3 of the human erythrocyte membrane. J Biol Chem. 1984;259:10238-10246.

183. Waugh SM, Low PS. Hemichrome binding to band 3: nucleation of Heinz bodies on the erythrocyte membrane. Biochemistry. 1985;24:34-39.

184. Zhang Y, Manning LR, Falcone J, et al. Human erythrocyte membrane band 3 protein influences hemoglobin cooperativity. Possible effect on oxygen transport. J Biol Chem. 2003;278:39565-39571.

185. Waugh SM, Walder JA, Low PS. Partial characterization of the copolymerization reaction of erythrocyte membrane band 3 with hemichromes. Biochemistry. 1987;26:1777-1783.

186. Kannan R, Labotka R, Low PS. Isolation and characterization of the hemichrome-stabilized membrane protein aggregates from sickle erythrocytes. Major site of autologous antibody binding. J Biol Chem. 1988;263:13766-13773.

187. Rettig MP, Low PS, Gimm JA, et al. Evaluation of biochemical changes during in vivo erythrocyte senescence in the dog. Blood. 1999;93:376-384.

188. Beppu M, Ando K, Kikugawa K. Poly-*N*-acetyllactosaminyl saccharide chains of band 3 as determinants for anti–band 3 autoantibody binding to senescent and oxidized erythrocytes. Cell Mol Biol. 1996;42:1007-1024.

189. Kliman HJ, Steck TL. Association of glyceraldehyde-3-phosphate dehydrogenase with the human red cell membrane. A kinetic analysis. J Biol Chem. 1980;255:6314-6321.

190. De BK, Kirtley ME. Interaction of phosphoglycerate kinase with human erythrocyte membranes. J Biol Chem. 1977;252:6715-6720.

191. Strapazon E, Steck T. Interaction of aldolase and the membrane of human erythrocytes. Biochemistry. 1977;16:2966.

192. Murthy SN, Liu T, Kaul RK, et al. The aldolase-binding site of the human erythrocyte membrane is at the NH₂ terminus of band 3. J Biol Chem. 1981;256:11203-11208.

193. Chu H, Low PS. Mapping of glycolytic enzyme-binding sites on human erythrocyte band 3. Biochem J. 2006;400:143-151.

194. Perrotta S, Borriello A, Scaloni A, et al. The N-terminal 11 amino acids of human erythrocyte band 3 are critical for aldolase binding and protein phosphorylation: implications for band 3 function. Blood. 2005;106:4359-4366.

195. Jenkins J, Madden D, Steck T. Association of phosphofructokinase and aldolase with the membrane of the intact erythrocyte. J Biol Chem. 1984;259:9374.

196. Tsai IH, Murthy SN, Steck TL. Effect of red cell membrane binding on the catalytic activity of glyceraldehyde-3-phosphate dehydrogenase. J Biol Chem. 1982;257:1438-1442.

197. Campanella ME, Chu H, Low PS. Assembly and regulation of a glycolytic enzyme complex on the human erythrocyte membrane. Proc Natl Acad Sci U S A. 2005;102:2402-2407.

198. Low PS, Allen DP, Zioncheck TF, et al. Tyrosine phosphorylation of band 3 inhibits peripheral protein binding. J Biol Chem. 1987;262:4592-4596.

199. Low PS, Rathinavelu P, Harrison ML. Regulation of glycolysis via reversible enzyme binding to the membrane protein, band 3. J Biol Chem. 1993;268:14627-14631.

200. Fossel ET, Solomon AK. Ouabain-sensitive interaction between human red cell membrane and glycolytic enzyme complex in cytosol. Biochim Biophys Acta. 1978;510:99-111.

201. Green DE, Murer E, Hultin HO, et al. Association of integrated metabolic pathways with membranes. I. Glycolytic enzymes of the red blood corpuscle and yeast. Arch Biochem Biophys. 1965;112:635-647.

202. Fossel ET, Solomon AK. Relation between red cell membrane $(Na^+ + K^+)$-ATPase and band 3 protein. Biochim Biophys Acta. 1981;649:557-571

203. Hoffman JF. ATP compartmentation in human erythrocytes. Curr Opin Hematol. 1997;4:112-115.

204. Feig SA, Segel GB, Shohet SB, Nathan DG. Energy metabolism in human erythrocytes. II. Effects of glucose depletion. J Clin Invest. 1972;51:1547-1554.

205. Mercer RW, Dunham PB. Membrane-bound ATP fuels the Na/K pump. Studies on membrane-bound glycolytic enzymes on inside-out vesicles from human red cell membranes. J Gen Physiol. 1981;78:547-568.

206. Erdmann E, Hasse W. Quantitative aspects of ouabain binding to human erythrocyte and cardiac membranes. J Physiol. 1975;251:671-682.

207. Weber RE, Voelter W, Fago A, et al. Modulation of red cell glycolysis: interactions between vertebrate hemoglobins and cytoplasmic domains of band 3 red cell membrane proteins. Am J Physiol Regul Integr Comp Physiol. 2004;287:R454-R464.

208. Messana I, Orlando M, Cassiano L, et al. Human erythrocyte metabolism is modulated by the O_2-linked transition of hemoglobin. FEBS Lett. 1996;390:25-28.

209. Chang SH, Low PS. Identification of a critical ankyrin-binding loop on the cytoplasmic domain of erythrocyte membrane band 3 by crystal structure analysis and site-directed mutagenesis. J Biol Chem. 2003;278:6879-6884.

210. Stefanovic M, Markham NO, Parry EM, et al. An 11–amino acid beta-hairpin loop in the cytoplasmic domain of band 3 is responsible for ankyrin binding in mouse erythrocytes. Proc Natl Acad Sci U S A. 2007;104:13972-13977.

211. Van Dort HM, Moriyama R, Low PS. Effect of band 3 subunit equilibrium on the kinetics and affinity of ankyrin binding to erythrocyte membrane vesicles. J Biol Chem. 1998;273:14819-14826.

212. Yi SJ, Liu SC, Derick LH, et al. Red cell membranes of ankyrin-deficient nb/nb mice lack band 3 tetramers but contain normal membrane skeletons. Biochemistry. 1997;36:9596-9604.

213. An XL, Takakuwa Y, Nunomura W, et al. Modulation of band 3–ankyrin interaction by protein 4.1. Functional implications in regulation of erythrocyte membrane mechanical properties. J Biol Chem. 1996;271:33187-33191.

214. Casey JR, Reithmeier RA. Analysis of the oligomeric state of band 3, the anion transport protein of the human erythrocyte membrane, by size exclusion high performance liquid chromatography. Oligomeric stability and origin of heterogeneity. J Biol Chem. 1991;266:15726-15737.

215. Pasternack GR, Anderson RA, Leto TL, Marchesi VT. Interactions between protein 4.1 and band 3. An alternative binding site for an element of the membrane skeleton. J Biol Chem. 1985;260:3676-3683.

216. Lombardo CR, Willardson BM, Low PS. Localization of the protein 4.1–binding site on the cytoplasmic domain of erythrocyte membrane band 3. J Biol Chem. 1992;267:9540-9546.

217. Workman RF, Low PS. Biochemical analysis of potential sites for protein 4.1–mediated anchoring of the spectrin-actin skeleton to the erythrocyte membrane. J Biol Chem. 1998;11:6171-6176.

218. Paw BH, Davidson AJ, Zhou Y, et al. Cell-specific mitotic defect and dyserythropoiesis associated with erythroid band 3 deficiency. Nat Genet. 2003;34:59-64.

219. Golan DE, Corbett JD, Korsgren C, et al. Control of band 3 lateral and rotational mobility by band 4.2 in intact erythrocytes: release of band 3 oligomers from low-affinity binding sites. Biophys J. 1996;70:1534-1542.

220. Rybicki AC, Schwartz RS, Hustedt EJ, Cobb CE. Increased rotational mobility and extractability of band 3 from protein 4.2–deficient erythrocyte membranes: evidence of a role for protein 4.2 in strengthening the band 3–cytoskeleton linkage. Blood. 1996;88:2745-2753.

221. Korsgren C, Birkenmeier CS, Barker JE, et al. The C-terminus of alpha spectrin binds protein 4.2 and is necessary for optimal spectrin-actin binding [abstract]. Blood. 2005;106(Suppl 1):239a.

222. Peters LL, Shivdasani RA, Liu SC, et al. Anion exchanger 1 (band 3) is required to prevent erythrocyte membrane surface loss but not to form the membrane skeleton. Cell. 1996;86:917-927.

223. Peters LL, Jindel HK, Gwynn B, et al. Mild spherocytosis and altered red cell ion transport in protein 4.2–null mice. J Clin Invest. 1999;103:1527-1537.

224. Jennings ML, Smith JS. Anion-proton cotransport through the human red blood cell band 3 protein. Role of glutamate 681. J Biol Chem. 1992;267:13964-13971.

225. Chernova MN, Jiang L, Crest M, et al. Electrogenic sulfate/chloride exchange in *Xenopus* oocytes mediated by murine AE1 E699Q. J Gen Physiol. 1997;109:345-360.

226. Milanick MA, Gunn RB. Proton-sulfate cotransport: external proton activation of sulfate influx into human red blood cells. Am J Physiol. 1984;247:C247-C259.

227. Tang XB, Fujinaga J, Kopito R, Casey JR. Topology of the region surrounding Glu681 of human AE1 protein, the erythrocyte anion exchanger. J Biol Chem. 1998;273:22545-22553.

228. Tang XB, Kovacs M, Sterling D, Casey JR. Identification of residues lining the translocation pore of human AE1, plasma membrane anion exchange protein. J Biol Chem. 1999;274:3557-3564.

229. Fujinaga J, Tang XB, Casey JR. Topology of the membrane domain of human erythrocyte anion exchange protein, AE1. J Biol Chem. 1999;274:6626-6633.

230. Popov M, Tam LY, Li J, Reithmeier RA. Mapping the ends of transmembrane segments in a polytopic mem-

brane protein. Scanning *N*-glycosylation mutagenesis of extracytosolic loops in the anion exchanger, band 3. J Biol Chem. 1997;272:18325-18332.

231. Popov M, Li J, Reithmeier RA. Transmembrane folding of the human erythrocyte anion exchanger (AE1, band 3) determined by scanning and insertional *N*-glycosylation mutagenesis. Biochem J. 1999;339:269-279.

232. Zhu Q, Casey JR. The substrate anion selectivity filter in the human erythrocyte Cl⁻/HCO₃⁻ exchange protein, AE1. J Biol Chem. 2004;279:23565-23573.

233. Bruce LJ, Robinson HC, Guizouarn H, et al. Monovalent cation leaks in human red cells caused by single amino-acid substitutions in the transport domain of the band 3 chloride-bicarbonate exchanger, AE1. Nat Genet. 2005;37:1258-1263.

234. Guizouarn H, Martial S, Gabillat N, Borgese F. Point mutations involved in red cell stomatocytosis convert the electroneutral anion exchanger 1 to a nonselective cation conductance. Blood. 2007;110:2158-2165.

235. Sterling D, Alvarez BV, Casey JR. The extracellular component of a transport metabolon. Extracellular loop 4 of the human AE1 Cl⁻/HCO₃⁻exchanger binds carbonic anhydrase IV. J Biol Chem. 2002;277:25239-25246.

236. Tanner MJ. Molecular and cellular biology of the erythrocyte anion exchanger (AE1). Semin Hematol. 1993;30:34.

237. Lindenthal S, Schubert D. Monomeric erythrocyte band 3 protein transports anions. Proc Natl Acad Sci U S A. 1991;88:6540-6544.

238. Wang DN, Kuhlbrandt W, Sarabia VE, Reithmeier RA. Two-dimensional structure of the membrane domain of human band 3, the anion transport protein of the erythrocyte membrane. EMBO J. 1993;12:2233-2239.

239. Salhany JM. Allosteric effects in stilbenedisulfonate binding to band 3 protein (AE1). Cell Mol Biol. 1996;42:1065-1096.

240. Jennings ML. Structure and function of the red blood cell anion transport protein. Annu Rev Biophys Chem. 1989;18:397.

241. Fukuda M, Dell A, Fukuda MN. Structure of fetal lactosaminoglycan. The carbohydrate moiety of band 3 isolated from human umbilical cord erythrocytes. J Biol Chem. 1984;259:4782-4791.

242. Fukuda M, Dell A, Oates JE, Fukuda MN. Structure of branched lactosaminoglycan, the carbohydrate moiety of band 3 isolated from adult human erythrocytes. J Biol Chem. 1984;259:8260-8273.

243. Jay DG. Glycosylation site of band 3, the human erythrocyte anion-exchange protein. Biochemistry. 1986;25:554-556.

244. Fukuda M, Fukuda M, Hakomori S. Developmental change and genetic defect in the carbohydrate structure of band 3 glycoprotein of human erythrocyte membrane. J Biol Chem. 1979;254:3700-3703.

245. Bruce LJ, Tanner MJ. Structure-function relationships of band 3 variants. Cell Mol Biol. 1996;42:953-973.

246. Jarolim P, Murray JL, Rubin HL, et al. Blood group antigens Rb(a), Tr(a), and Wd(a) are located in the third ectoplasmic loop of erythroid band 3. Transfusion. 1997;37:607-615.

247. Jarolim P, Murray JL, Rubin HL, et al. A Thr552→Ile substitution in erythroid band 3 gives rise to the Warrior blood group antigen. Transfusion. 1997;37:398-405.

248. Zelinski T, Punter F, McManus K, Coghlan G. The ELO blood group polymorphism is located in the putative first extracellular loop of human erythrocyte band 3. Vox Sang. 1998;75:63-65.

249. Zelinski T, McManus K, Punter F, et al. A Gly565→Ala substitution in human band 3 accounts for the Wu blood group polymorphism. Transfusion 1998;38:745-748.

250. Jarolim P, Rubin HL, Zakova D, et al. Characterization of seven low incidence blood group antigens carried by erythrocyte band 3 protein. Blood. 1998;92:4836-4843.

251. Jarolim P, Kalabova D, Reid ME. Substitution Glu-480Lys in erythroid band 3 corresponds to the Fr(a) blood group antigen and supports existence of the second ectoplasmic loop of band 3. Transfusion. 2004;44:684-689

252. Huang CH, Reid ME, Xie SS, Blumenfeld OO. Human red blood cell Wright antigens: a genetic and evolutionary perspective on glycophorin A–band 3 interaction. Blood. 1996;87:3942-3947

253. Bruce LJ, Ring SM, Anstee DJ, et al. Changes in the blood group Wright antigens are associated with a mutation at amino acid 658 in human erythrocyte band 3: a site of interaction between band 3 and glycophorin A under certain conditions Blood. 1995;85:541-547.

254. Poole J, Banks J, Bruce LJ, et al. Glycophorin A mutation Ala65→Pro gives rise to a novel pair of MNS alleles ENEP (MNS39) and HAG (MNS41) and altered Wrb expression: direct evidence for GPA/band 3 interaction necessary for normal Wrb expression. Transfus Med. 1999;9:167-174.

255. Telen MJ, Chasis JA. Relationship of the human erythrocyte Wrb antigen to an interaction between glycophorin A and band 3. Blood. 1990;76:842-848.

256. Knowles DW, Chasis JA, Evans EA, Mohandas N. Cooperative action between band 3 and glycophorin A in human erythrocytes: immobilization of band 3 induced by antibodies to glycophorin A. Biophys J. 1994;66:1726-1732.

257. Tanphaichitr VS, Sumboonnanonda A, Ideguchi H, et al. Novel AE1 mutations in recessive distal renal tubular acidosis. Loss-of-function is rescued by glycophorin A. J Clin Invest. 1998;102:2173-2179.

258. Groves JD, Tanner MJ. Glycophorin A facilitates the expression of human band 3–mediated anion transport in *Xenopus* oocytes. J Biol Chem. 1992;267:22163-22170.

259. Bruce LJ, Pan RJ, Cope DL, et al. Altered structure and anion transport properties of band 3 (AE1, SLC4A1) in human red cells lacking glycophorin A. J Biol Chem. 2004;279:2414-2420.

260. Hassoun H, Hanada T, Lutchman M, et al. Complete deficiency of glycophorin A in red blood cells from mice with targeted inactivation of the band 3 (AE1) gene. Blood. 1998;91:2146-2151.

261. Liu SC, Zhai S, Palek J, et al. Molecular defect of the band 3 protein in southeast Asian ovalocytosis. N Engl J Med. 1990;323:1530-1538.

262. Jarolim P, Palek J, Amato D, et al. Deletion in erythrocyte band 3 gene in malaria-resistant Southeast Asian ovalocytosis. Proc Natl Acad Sci U S A. 1991;88:11022-11026.

263. Mohandas N, Winardi R, Knowles D, et al. Molecular basis for membrane rigidity of hereditary ovalocytosis. A novel mechanism involving the cytoplasmic domain of band 3. J Clin Invest. 1992;89:686-692.

264. Toye AM. Defective kidney anion-exchanger 1 (AE1, band 3) trafficking in dominant distal renal tubular acidosis (dRTA). Biochem Soc Symp. 2005;72:47-63.

265. Devonald MA, Smith AN, Poon JP, et al. Non-polarized targeting of AE1 causes autosomal dominant distal renal tubular acidosis. Nat Genet. 2003;33:125-127.

266. Bruce LJ, Kay MM, Lawrence C, Tanner MJ. Band 3 HT, a human red-cell variant associated with acanthocytosis and increased anion transport, carries the mutation Pro868→Leu in the membrane domain of band 3. Biochem J. 1993;293:317-320.

267. Hassoun H, Wang Y, Vassiliadis J, et al. Targeted inactivation of murine band 3 (AE1) gene produces a hypercoagulable state causing widespread thrombosis in vivo. Blood. 1998;92:1785-1792.

268. Stubbs J, Simpson KM, Triglia T, et al. Molecular mechanism for switching of P. falciparum invasion pathways into human erythrocytes. Science. 2005;309:1384-1387.

269. Okoye VCN, Bennett V. Plasmodium falciparum malaria. Band 3 as a possible receptor during invasion of human erythrocytes. Science. 1985;227:169-171.

270. Clough B, Paulitschke M, Nash GB, et al. Mechanism of regulation of malarial invasion by extraerythrocytic ligands. Mol Biochem Parasitol. 1995;69:19-27.

271. Goel VK, Li X, Chen H, et al. Band 3 is a host receptor binding merozoite surface protein 1 during the Plasmodium falciparum invasion of erythrocytes. Proc Natl Acad Sci U S A. 2003;100:5164-5169.

272. Demuth DR, Showe LC, Ballantine M, et al. Cloning and structural characterization of a human non-erythroid band 3–like protein. EMBO J. 1986;5:1205-1214.

273. Alper SL, Kopito RR, Libresco SM, Lodish HF. Cloning and characterization of a murine band 3–related cDNA from kidney and from a lymphoid cell line. J Biol Chem. 1988;263:17092-17099.

274. Kopito RR, Lee BS, Simmons DM, et al. Regulation of intracellular pH by a neuronal homolog of the erythrocyte anion exchanger. Cell. 1989;59:927-937.

275. Brosius FC, Alper SL, Garcia AM, Lodish HF. The major kidney band 3 gene transcript predicts an amino-terminal truncated band 3 polypeptide. J Biol Chem. 1989;264:7784-7787.

276. Richards SM, Jaconi ME, Vassort G, Puceat M. A spliced variant of AE1 gene encodes a truncated form of band 3 in heart: the predominant anion exchanger in ventricular myocytes. J Cell Sci. 1999;112:1519-1528.

277. Irimura T, Tsuji T, Tagami S, et al. Structure of a complex-type sugar chain of human glycophorin A. Biochemistry. 1981;20:560-566.

278. Gahmberg CG, Andersson LC. Role of sialic acid in the mobility of membrane proteins containing O-linked oligosaccharides on polyacrylamide gel electrophoresis in sodium dodecyl sulfate. Eur J Biochem. 1982;122:581-586.

279. Morrow B, Rubin CS. Biogenesis of glycophorin A in K562 human erythroleukemia cells. J Biol Chem. 1987;262:13812-13820.

280. Furthmayr H. Structural comparison of glycophorins and immunochemical analysis of genetic variants. Nature. 1978;271:519-524.

281. Dahr W, Gielen W, Beyreuther K, Kruger J. Structure of the Ss blood group antigens. I. Isolation of Ss active glycopeptides and differentiation of the antigens by modification of methionine. Hoppe Seylers Z Physiol Chem. 1980;361:145-152.

282. Dahr W, Kordowicz M, Beyreuther K, Kruger J. The amino acid sequence of the Mc-specific major red cell membrane sialoglycoprotein: an intermediate of the blood group M and N active molecules. Hoppe Seylers Z Physiol Chem. 1981;362:363-366.

283. Dahr W, Beyreuther K, Gallasch E, et al. Amino acid sequence of the blood group Mg-specific major human erythrocyte membrane sialoglycoprotein. Hoppe Seylers Z Physiol Chem. 1981;362:81-85.

284. Dahr W, Kordowicz M, Judd WJH, et al. Structural analysis of the Ss sialoglycoprotein specific for Henshaw blood group from human erythrocyte membranes. Eur J Biochem. 1984;141:51-55.

285. Tanner M, Anstee D. The membrane change in En(a–) human erythrocytes. Biochem J. 1976;153:271-277.

286. Dahr W, Uhlenbruck G, Leikola J, et al. Studies on the membrane glycoprotein defect of En(a–) erythrocytes, I. Biochemical aspects. J Immunogenet. 1976;3:329-346.

287. Tanner MJA, Anstee DJ, Judson PA. A carbohydrate deficient membrane glycoprotein in human erythrocytes of phenotype S–s–. Biochem J. 1977;165:157-161.

288. Huang C-H, Johe K, Moulds JJ, et al. Delta glycophorin (glycophorin B) gene deletion in two individuals homozygous for the S–s–U– blood group phenotype. Blood. 1987;70:1830-1835.

289. Tokunaga E, Sasakawa S, Tamaka K, et al. Two apparently healthy Japanese individuals of type M^kM^k have erythrocytes which lack both blood group MN and Ss-active sialoglycoproteins. J Immunogenet. 1979;6:383-390.

290. Anstee DJ. The blood group MNSs active sialoglycoproteins. Semin Hematol. 1981;15:13-31.

291. Blanchard D, Asseraf A, Prigent MJ, Cartron JP. Miltenberger cClass I and II erythrocytes carry a variant of glycophorin A. Biochem J. 1983;213:399-404.

292. Dahr W, Newman RA, Contreras M, et al. Structures of Miltenberger class I and II specific major human erythrocyte membrane sialoglycoproteins. Eur J Biochem. 1984;138:259-265.

293. Dahr W, Beyreuther K, Moulds JJ. Structural analysis of the major human erythrocyte membrane sialoglycoproteins from Miltenberger class VII cells. Eur J Biochem. 1987;166:27-30.

294. Dahr W, Vengelen-Tyler V, Dybkjaer E, Beyreuther K. Structural analysis of glycophorin A from Miltenberger class VIII erythrocytes. Biol Chem Hoppe Seyler. 1989;370:855-859.

295. Johe KK, Smith AJ, Blumenfeld OO. Amino acid sequence of MiIII glycophorin: demonstration of γ-α and α-γ junction regions and expression of γ pseudoexon by direct protein sequencing. J Biol Chem. 1991;266:7256.

296. Johe KK, Vengelen-Tyler V, Leger R, Blumenfeld OO. Synthetic peptides homologous to human glycophorins

of the Miltenberger complex of variants of MNSs blood group system specify the epitopes for Hil, S JL, Hop, and Mur antisera. Blood. 1991;78:2456-2461.

297. Mawby WJ, Anstee DJ, Tanner MJ. Immunochemical evidence for hybrid sialoglycoproteins of human erythrocytes Nature. 1981;291:161-162.

298. Tanner MJ, Anstee DJ, Mawby WJ. A new human erythrocyte variant (Ph) containing an abnormal membrane sialoglycoprotein. Biochem J. 1980;187:493-500.

299. Johe KK, Smith AJ, Vengelen-Tyler V, Blumenfeld OO. Amino acid sequence of an α-δ glycophorin hybrid: A structure reciprocal to Stᵃ δ-α glycophorin hybrid. J Biol Chem. 1989;264:17486-17492.

300. Anstee DJ, Mawby WJ, Tanner MJ. Abnormal blood-group-Ss–active sialoglycoproteins in the membrane of Miltenberger class III, IV, and V erythrocytes. Biochem J. 1979;183:193-203.

301. Huang C-H, Guizzo ML, Kikuchi M, Blumenfeld OO. Molecular genetic analysis of a hybrid gene encoding Stᵃ glycophorin of the human erythrocyte membrane. Blood. 1989;74:836-843.

302. Blumenfeld OO, Smith AJ, Moulds JJ. Membrane glycophorins of Dantu blood group erythrocytes. J Biol Chem. 1987;262:11864-11870.

303. Blanchard D, Cartron JP, Rouger P, Salmon C. Pʲ variant, a new, hybrid MNSs glycoprotein of the human red-cell membrane. Biochem J. 1982;203:419.

304. Huang C-H, Blumenfeld OO. Identification of recombination events resulting in three hybrid genes encoding human MiV, MiV(J.L.), and Stᵃ glycophorins. Blood. 1991;77:1813-1320.

305. Huang C-H, Blumenfeld OO. Molecular genetics of human erythrocyte MiIII and MiVI glycophorins. Use of a pseudoexon in construction of two δ-α-δ hybrid genes resulting in antigenic diversification. J Biol Chem. 1991;266:7248-7255.

306. Huang C-H, Blumenfeld OO. Multiple origins of the human glycophorin Stᵃ gene. Identification of hot spots for independent unequal homologous recombinations. J Biol Chem. 1991;266:23306-23314.

307. Huang C-H, Kikuchi M, McCreary J, Blumenfeld OO. Gene conversion confined to a direct repeat of the acceptor splice site generates allelic diversity at human glycophorin (GYP) locus. J Biol Chem. 1992;267:3336-3342.

308. Huang C-H, Skov F, Daniels G, et al. Molecular analysis of human glycophorin MiIX gene shows a silent segment transfer and untemplated mutation resulting from gene conversion via sequence repeats. Blood. 1992;80:2379-2387.

309. Huang C-H, Blumenfeld OO. Characterization of a genomic hybrid specifying the human erythrocyte antigen Dantu: Dantu gene is duplicated and linked to a δ glycophorin gene deletion. Proc Natl Acad Sci U S A. 1988;85:9640-9644.

310. Kudo S, Fukuda M. Structural organization of g lycophorin A and B genes: Glycophorin B gene evolved by homologous recombination at Alu repeat sequences. Proc Natl Acad Sci U S A. 1989;86:4619-4623.

311. Cartron JP, Blanchard D. Association of human erythrocyte membrane glycoproteins with blood group Cad specificity. Biochem J. 1982;207:497.

312. Blanchard D, Cartron JP, Fournet B, et al. Primary structure of the oligosaccharide determinant of blood group Cad specificity. J Biol Chem. 1983;258:7691-7695.

313. Mendelsohn R, Dluhy RA, Crawford T, Mantsch HH. Interaction of glycophorin with phosphatidylserine: a Fourier transform infrared investigation. Biochemistry. 1984;23:1498-1504.

314. Smith SO, Bormann BJ. Determination of helix-helix interactions in membranes by rotational resonance NMR. Proc Natl Acad Sci U S A. 1995;92:488-491.

315. Brosig B, Langosch D. The dimerization motif of the glycophorin A transmembrane segment in membranes: importance of glycine residues. Protein Sci. 1998;7:1052-1056.

316. MacKenzie KR, Prestegard JH, Engelman DM. A transmembrane helix dimer: structure and implications. Science. 1997;276:131-133.

317. Young MT, Tanner MJ. Distinct regions of human glycophorin A enhance human red cell anion exchanger (band 3; AE1) transport function and surface trafficking. J Biol Chem. 2003;278:32954-32961.

318. Chasis JA, Mohandas N, Shohet SB. Erythrocyte membrane rigidity induced by glycophorin A–ligand interaction. Evidence for a ligand-induced association between glycophorin A and skeletal proteins. J Clin Invest. 1985;75:1919-1926.

319. Chasis JA, Reid ME, Jensen RH, Mohandas N. Signal transduction by glycophorin A: role of extracellular and cytoplasmic domains in a modulatable process. J Cell Biol. 1988;107:1351-1357.

320. Andersson LC, Gahmberg CG, Teerenhovi L, Vuopio P. Glycophorin A as a cell surface marker of early erythroid differentiation in acute leukemia. Int J Cancer. 1979;24:717-720.

321. Langlois RG, Bigbee WL, Kyoizumi S, et al. Evidence for increased somatic cell mutations at the glycophorin A locus in atomic bomb survivors. Science. 1987;236:445-448.

322. Siebert PD, Fukuda M. Molecular cloning of a human glycophorin B cDNA: nucleotide sequence and genomic relationship to glycophorin A. Proc Natl Acad Sci U S A. 1987;84:6735-6739.

323. Rearden A, Magnet A, Kudo S, Fukuda M. Glycophorin B and glycophorin E genes arose from the glycophorin A ancestral gene via two duplications during primate evolution. J Biol Chem. 1993;268:2260-2267.

324. Dahr W, Beyreuther K, Steinbach H, et al. Structure of the Ss blood group antigens, II: a methionine/threonine polymorphism within the N-terminal sequence of the Ss glycoprotein. Hoppe Seylers Z Physiol Chem. 1980;361:895-906.

325. Colin Y, Rahuel C, London J, et al. Isolation of cDNA clones and complete amino acid sequence of human erythrocyte glycophorin C. J Biol Chem. 1986;261:229-233.

326. Villeval JL, Le Van Kim C, Bettaieb A, et al. Early expression of glycophorin C during normal and leukemic human erythroid differentiation. Cancer Res. 1989;49:2626-2632.

327. Chasis J, Mohandas N. Red blood cell glycophorins. Blood. 1992;8:1869.

328. Hemming NJ, Anstee DJ, Staricoff MA, et al. Identification of the membrane attachment sites for protein 4.1 in the human erythrocyte. J Biol Chem. 1995;270:5360-5366.

329. Marfatia SM, Morais-Cabral JH, Kim AC, et al. The PDZ domain of human erythrocyte p55 mediates its binding to the cytoplasmic carboxyl terminus of glycophorin C. Analysis of the binding interface by in vitro mutagenesis. J Biol Chem. 1997;272:24191-24197.

330. Le Van Kim C, Colin Y, Mitjavila MT, et al. Structure of the promoter region and tissue specificity of the human glycophorin C gene. J Biol Chem. 1989;264:20407-20414.

331. Colin Y. Gerbich blood groups and minor glycophorins of human erythrocytes. Transfus Clin Biol. 1995;2:259-268.

332. Kudo S, Fukuda M. Identification of a novel human glycophorin, glycophorin E, by isolation of genomic clones and complementary DNA clones utilizing polymerase chain reaction. J Biol Chem. 1990;265:1102-1110.

333. Blumenfeld OO, Huang CH. Molecular genetics of glycophorin MNS variants. Transfus Clin Biol. 1997;4:357-365.

334. Arimitsu N, Akimitsu N, Kotani N, T et al. Glycophorin A requirement for expression of O-linked antigens on the erythrocyte membrane. Genes Cells. 2003;8:769-777.

335. Reid M, Anstee D, Jensen RH, Mohandas N. Normal membrane function of abnormal b-related erythrocyte sialoglycoproteins. Br J Haematol. 1987;67:467-472.

336. Chang S, Reid ME, Conboy J, et al. Molecular characterization of erythrocyte glycophorin C variants. Blood. 1991;77:644-648.

337. Telen MJ, Le Van Kim C, Guizzo ML, et al. Erythrocyte Webb-type glycophorin C variant lacks N-glycosylation due to an asparagine to serine substitution. Am J Hematol. 1991;37:51-52.

338. Anstee D, Ridgewell K, Tanner M, et al. Individuals lacking the Gerbich blood-group antigens have alterations in the human erythrocyte membrane sialoglycoproteins β and γ. Biochem J. 1984;221:97.

339. Telen MJ, Le Van Kim C, Chung A, et al. Molecular basis for elliptocytosis associated with glycophorin C and D deficiency in the Leach phenotype. Blood. 1991;78:1603-1606.

340. Anstee D, Parsons S, Ridgewell K, et al. Two individuals with elliptocytic red cells apparently lack three minor sialoglycoproteins. Biochem J. 1984;218:615.

341. Daniels G, Shaw M-A, Judson P, et al. A family demonstrating inheritance of the Leach phenotype, a Gerbich-negative phenotype associated with elliptocytosis. Vox Sang. 1986;50:117.

342. Nash GB, Palmer J, Reid ME. Effects of deficiencies of glycophorins C and D on the physical properties of the red cell. Br J Haematol. 1990;76:282-287.

343. Reid ME, Chasis JA, Mohandas N. Identification of a functional role for human erythrocyte sialoglycoproteins β and γ (C and D). Blood 1987;69:1068-1072.

344. Alloisio N, Dalla Venezia N, Rana A, et al. Evidence that red blood cell protein p55 may participate in the skeleton-membrane linkage that involves protein 4.1 and glycophorin C. Blood. 1993;82:1323-1327.

345. Dhermy D, Garbarz M, Lecomte MC, et al. Hereditary elliptocytosis: clinical, morphological and biochemical studies of 38 cases. Nouv Rev Fr Hematol. 1986;28:129-140.

346. Dalla Venezia N, Gilsanz F, Alloisio N, et al. Homozygous 4.1(−) hereditary elliptocytosis associated with a point mutation in the downstream initiation codon of protein 4.1 gene. J Clin Invest. 1992;90:1713-1717.

347. Baumgartner S, Littleton JT, Broadie K, et al. A Drosophila neurexin is required for septate junction and blood-nerve barrier formation and function. Cell. 1996;87:1059-1068.

348. Perkins M. Inhibitory effects of erythrocyte membrane proteins on the in vitro invasion of the human malarial parasite (Plasmodium falciparum) into its host cell. J Cell Biol. 1981;90:563-567.

349. Pasvol G, Wainscoat JS, Weatherall DJ. Erythrocytes deficiency in glycophorin resist invasion by the malarial parasite Plasmodium falciparum. Nature. 1982;297:64-66.

350. Dolan SA, Miller LH, Wellems TE. Evidence for a switching mechanism in the invasion of erythrocytes by Plasmodium falciparum. J Clin Invest. 1990;86:618-624.

351. Orlandi PA, Klotz FW, Haynes JD. A malaria invasion receptor, the 175-kilodalton erythrocyte binding antigen of Plasmodium falciparum recognizes the terminal Neu5Ac(α2-3)Gal- sequences of glycophorin A. J Cell Biol. 1992;116:901-909.

352. Dolan SA, Proctor JL, Alling DW, et al. Glycophorin B as an EBA-175 independent Plasmodium falciparum receptor of human erythrocytes. Mol Biochem Parasitol. 1994;64:55-63.

353. Tolia NH, Enemark EJ, Sim BK, Joshua-Tor L. Structural basis for the EBA-175 erythrocyte invasion pathway of the malaria parasite Plasmodium falciparum. Cell. 2005;122:183-193.

354. Sharma A, Mishra NC, Biswas S. Receptor heterogeneity and invasion on erythrocytes by Plasmodium falciparum merozoites in Indian isolates. Indian J Exp Biol. 1994;32:486-488.

355. Hadley TJ, Klotz FW, Pasvol G, et al. Falciparum malaria parasites invade erythrocytes that lack glycophorin A and B (M^kM^k). Strain differences indicate receptor heterogeneity and two pathways for invasion. J Clin Invest. 1987;80:1190-1193.

356. Chishti AH, Palek J, Fisher D, et al. Reduced invasion and growth of Plasmodium falciparum into elliptocytic red blood cells with a combined deficiency of protein 4.1, glycophorin C, and p55. Blood. 1996;87:3462-3469.

357. Maier AG, Duraisingh MT, Reeder JC, et al. Plasmodium falciparum erythrocyte invasion through glycophorin C and selection for Gerbich negativity in human populations. Nat Med. 2003;9:87-92.

358. Lobo CA, Rodriguez M, Reid M, Lustigman S. Glycophorin C is the receptor for the Plasmodium falciparum erythrocyte binding ligand PfEBP-2 (baebl). Blood. 2003;101:4628-4631.

359. Mayer DC, Jiang L, Achur RN, et al. The glycophorin C N-linked glycan is a critical component of the ligand for the Plasmodium falciparum erythrocyte receptor BAEBL. Proc Natl Acad Sci U S A. 2006;103:2358-2362.

360. Wang D, Mentzer WC, Cameron T, Johnson RM. Purification of band 7.2b, a 31-kDa integral membrane phosphoprotein absent in hereditary stomatocytosis. J Biol Chem. 1991;266:17826-17831.

361. Hiebl-Dirschmied CM, Adolf GR, Prohaska R. Isolation and partial characterization of the human erythrocyte band 7 integral membrane protein. Biochim Biophys Acta. 1991;1065:195-202.

362. Stewart GW, Hepworth-Jones BE, Keen JN, et al. Isolation of cDNA coding for an ubiquitous membrane protein deficient in high Na+, low K+ stomatocytic erythrocytes. Blood. 1992;79:1593-1601.

363. Hiebl Dirschmied C, Entler B, Glotzman C, et al. Cloning and nucleotide sequence of cDNA encoding human erythrocyte band 7 integral membrane protein. Biochim Biophys Acta. 1991;1090:123-124.

364. Snyers L, Umlauf E, Prohaska R. Oligomeric nature of the integral membrane protein stomatin. J Biol Chem. 1998;273:17221-17226.

365. Snyers L, Umlauf E, Prohaska R. Cysteine 29 is the major palmitoylation site on stomatin. FEBS Lett. 1999;449:101-104.

366. Wang Y, Morrow JS. Identification and characterization of human SLP-2, a novel homologue of stomatin (band 7.2b) present in erythrocytes and other tissues. J Biol Chem. 2000;275:8062-8071.

367. Gilles F, Glenn M, Goy A, et al. A novel gene STORP (STOmatin-Related Protein) is localized 2 kb upstream of the promyelocytic gene on chromosome 15q22. Eur J Haematol. 2000;64:104-113.

368. You Z, Gao X, Ho MM, Borthakur D. A stomatin-like protein encoded by the slp gene of *Rhizobium etli* is required for nodulation competitiveness on the common bean. Microbiology. 1998;144:2619-2627.

369. Huang M, Gu G, Ferguson EL, Chalfie M. A stomatin-like protein necessary for mechanosensation in *C. elegans*. Nature. 1995;378:292-295.

370. Mannsfeldt AG, Carroll P, Stucky CL, Lewin GR. Stomatin, a MEC-2 like protein, is expressed by mammalian sensory neurons. Mol Cell Neurosci. 1999;13:391-404.

371. Sedensky MM, Siefker JM, Morgan PG. Model organisms: new insights into ion channel and transporter function. Stomatin homologues interact in *Caenorhabditis elegans*. Am J Physiol Cell Physiol. 2001;280:C1340-C1348.

372. Goodman MB, Ernstrom GG, Chelur DS, et al. MEC-2 regulates *C. elegans* DEG/ENaC channels needed for mechanosensatiion. Nature. 2002;415:1039-1042.

373. Wetzel C, Hu J, Riethmacher D, et al. A stomatin-domain protein essential for touch sensation in the mouse. Nature. 2007;445:206-209.

374. Price MP, Thompson RJ, Eshcol JO, et al. Stomatin modulates gating of acid-sensing ion channels. J Biol Chem. 2004;279:53886-53891.

375. Moore RB, Shriver SK. Protein 7.2b of human erythrocyte membranes binds to calpromotin. Biochem Biophys Res Commun. 1997;232:294-297.

376. Zhang JZ, Hayashi H, Ebina Y, et al. Association of stomatin (band 7.2b) with Glut1 glucose transporter. Arch Biochem Biophys. 1999;372:173-178.

377. Zhang JZ, Abbud W, Prohaska R, Ismail-Beigi F. Overexpression of stomatin depresses GLUT-1 glucose transporter activity. Am J Physiol Cell Physiol. 2001;280:C1277-C1283.

378. Plishker GA, Chevalier D, Seinsoth L, Moore RB. Calcium-activated potassium transport and high molecular weight forms of calpromotin. J Biol Chem. 1992;267:21839-21843.

379. Moore RB, Mankad MV, Shriver SK, et al. Reconstitution of Ca2+-dependent K+ transport in erythrocyte membrane vesicles requires a cytoplasmic protein. J Biol Chem. 1991;266:18964-18968.

380. Preston GM, Carroll TP, Guggino WB, Agre P. Appearance of water channels in *Xenopus* oocytes expressing red cell CHIP28 protein. Science. 1992;256:385-387.

381. Sui H, Han BG, Lee JK, et al. Structural basis of water specific transport through the AQP1 water channel. Nature. 2001;414:872-878.

382. King LS, Choi M, Fernandez PC, et al. Defective urinary-concentrating ability due to a complete deficiency of aquaporin-1. N Engl J Med. 2001;345:175-179.

383. King LS, Nielsen S, Agre P, Brown RH. Decreased pulmonary vascular permeability in aquaporin-1–null humans. Proc Natl Acad Sci U S A. 2002;99:1059-1063.

384. Ma T, Yang B, Gillespie A, et al. Severely impaired urinary concentrating ability in transgenic mice lacking aquaporin-1 water channels. J Biol Chem. 1998;273:4296-4299.

385. Saadoun S, Papadopoulos MC, Hara-Chikuma M, Verkman AS. Impairment of angiogenesis and cell migration by targeted aquaporin-1 gene disruption. Nature. 2005;434:786-792.

386. Roudier N, Verbavatz JM, Maurel C, et al. Evidence for the presence of aquaporin-3 in human red blood cells. J Biol Chem. 1998;273:8407-8412.

387. Roudier N, Ripoche P, Gane P, et al. AQP3 deficiency in humans and the molecular basis of a novel blood group system, GIL. J Biol Chem. 2002;277:45854-45859.

388. Liu Y, Promeneur D, Rojek A, et al. Aquaporin 9 is the major pathway for glycerol uptake by mouse erythrocytes, with implications for malarial virulence. Proc Natl Acad Sci U S A. 2007;104:12560-12564.

389. Avent ND, Reid ME. The Rh blood group system: a review. Blood. 2000;95:375-387.

390. Haung CH, Liu PZ, Cheng JG. Molecular biology and genetics of Rh blood group system. Semin Hematol. 2000;37:150-165.

391. Van Kim CL, Colin Y, Cartron JP. Rh proteins: key structural and functional components of the red cell membrane. Blood Rev. 2006;20:93-110.

392. Nicolas V, Le Van Kim C, Gane P, et al. Rh-RhAG/ankyrin-R, a new interaction site between the membrane bilayer and the red cell skeleton, is impaired by Rh (null)–associated mutation. J Biol Chem. 2003;278:25526-25533.

393. Ripoche P, Bertrand O, Gane P, et al. Human Rhesus-associated glycoprotein mediates facilitated transport of NH3 into red blood cells. Proc Natl Acad Sci U S A. 2004;101:17222-17227.

394. Marini AM, Matassi G, Raynal V, et al. The human Rhesus-associated RhAG protein and a kidney homo-

logue promote ammonium transport in yeast. Nat Genet. 2000;26:341-344.

395. Endeward V, Cartron JP, Ripoche P, Gros G. Red cell membrane CO_2 permeability in normal human blood and in blood deficient in various blood groups, and effect of DIDS. Transfus Clin Biol. 2006;13:123-127.

396. Ballas SK, Clark MR, Mohandas N, et al. Red cell membrane and cation deficiency in Rh null syndrome. Blood. 1984;63:1046-1055.

397. Olives B, Neau P, Bailly P, et al. Cloning and functional expression of a urea transporter from human bone marrow cells. J Biol Chem. 1994;269:31649-31652.

398. Olives B, Mattei MG, Huet M, et al. Kidd blood group and urea transport function of human erythrocytes are carried by the same protein. J Biol Chem. 1995;270:15607-15610.

399. Macey RI, Yousef LW. Osmotic stability of red cells in renal circulation requires rapid urea transport. Am J Physiol. 1988;254:C669-C674.

400. Frohlich O, Macey RI, Edwards-Moulds J, et al. Urea transport deficiency in Jk (ab–) erythrocytes. Am J Physiol. 1991;260:C778-C783.

401. Ho M, Chelly J, Carter N, et al. Isolation of a gene for McLeod syndrome encodes a novel membrane transport protein. Cell. 1994;77:869-880.

402. Russo D, Redman C, Lee S. Association of Xk and Kell blood group proteins. J Biol Chem. 1998;273:13950-13956.

403. Lee S, Zambas E, Green ED, Redman C. Organization of the gene encoding the human Kell blood group protein. Blood. 1995;85:1364-1370.

404. Lee S, Lin M, Mele A, et al. Proteolytic processing of big endothelin-3 by the Kell blood group protein. Blood. 1999;94:1440-1450.

405. Lee S, Russo D, Redman CM. The Kell blood group system: Kell and XK membrane proteins. Semin Hematol. 2000;37:113-121.

406. Pogo O, Chaudhuri A. The Duffy protein: A malarial and chemokine receptor. Semin Hematol. 2000;37:122-129.

407. Chaudhuri A, Polyakova J, Zbrzezna V, et al. Cloning of glycoprotein D cDNA, which encodes the major subunit of the Duffy blood group system and the receptor for the *Plasmodium vivax* malaria parasite. Proc Natl Acad Sci U S A. 1993;90:10793-10797.

408. Hadley TJ, Peiper SC. From malaria to chemokine receptor: the emerging physiologic role of the Duffy blood group antigen. Blood. 1997;89:3077-3091.

409. Parsons SF, Mallinson G, Holmes CH, et al. The Lutheran blood group glycoprotein, another member of the immunoglobulin superfamily, is widely expressed in human tissues and is developmentally regulated in human liver. Proc Natl Acad Sci U S A. 1995;92:5496-5500.

410. Eyler CE, Telen MJ. The Lutheran glycoprotein: a multifunctional adhesion receptor. Transfusion. 2006;46:668-677.

411. Udani M, Zen Q, Cottman M, et al. Basal cell adhesion molecule/Lutheran protein. The receptor critical for sickle cell adhesion to laminin. J Clin Invest. 1998;101:2550-2558.

412. El Nemer W, Wautier MP, Rahuel C, et al. Endothelial Lu/BCAM glycoproteins are novel ligands for red blood cell alpha4beta1 integrin: role in adhesion of sickle red blood cells to endothelial cells. Blood. 2007;109:3544-3551.

413. Bailly P, Hermand P, Callebault I, et al. The LW blood group glycoprotein is homologous to intracellular adhesion molecules. Proc Natl Acad Sci U S A. 1994;91:5306-5310.

414. Delahunty M, Zennadi R, Telen MJ. LW protein: a promiscuous integrin receptor activated by adrenergic signaling. Transfus Clin Biol. 2006;13:44-49.

415. Bailly P, Tontti E, Hermand P, et al. The red cell LW blood group glycoprotein is an intracellular adhesion molecule (ICAM-4) which binds to CD11/CD18 leukocyte integrin. Eur J Immunol. 1995;25:3316-3320.

416. Spring FA, Parsons SF, Ortlepp S, et al. Intracellular adhesion molecule-4 binds $\alpha_4\beta_1$ and α_V integrins through novel integrin-binding mechanisms. Blood. 2001;98:458-466.

417. Zennadi R, Moeller BJ, Whalen EJ, et al. Epinephrine-induced activation of LW-mediated sickle cell adhesion and vaso-occlusion in vivo. Blood. 2007;110:2708-2717.

417a. Mueckler M, Caruso C, Baldwin SA, et al. Sequence and structure of a human glucose transporter. Science. 1985;229:941-945.

417b. Montel-Hagen A, Kinet S, Manel N, et al. Erythrocyte Glut1 triggers dehydroascorbic acid uptake in mammals unable to synthesize vitamin C. Cell. 2008;132:1039-1048.

417c. Khan AA, Hanada T, Mohseni M, et al. Dematin and adducin provide a novel link between the spectrin cytoskeleton and human erythrocyte membrane by directly interacting with glucose transporter-1. J Biol Chem. 2008;283;14600-14609.

418. Bennett V, Stenbuck PJ. The membrane attachment protein for spectrin is associated with band 3 in human erythrocyte membranes. Nature. 1979;280:468-473.

419. Reid ME, Takakuwa Y, Conboy J, et al. Glycophorin C content of human erythrocyte membrane is regulated by protein 4.1. Blood. 1990;75:2229-2234.

420. Speicher DW, Morrow JS, Knowles WJ, Marchesi VT. A structural model of human erythrocyte spectrin. Alignment of chemical and functional domains. J Biol Chem. 1982;257:9093-9101.

421. *http://pfam.sanger.ac.uk/family?entry = spectrin&type = Family.*

422. Speicher DW, Marchesi VT. Erythrocyte spectrin is comprised of many homologous triple helical segments. Nature. 1984;311:177-180.

423. MacDonald RI, Cummings JA. Stabilities of folding of clustered, two-repeat fragments of spectrin reveal a potential hinge in the human erythroid spectrin tetramer. Proc Natl Acad Sci U S A. 2004;101:1502-1507.

424. Shotton DM, Burke BE, Branton D. The molecular structure of human erythrocyte spectrin. Biophysical and electron microscopic studies. J Mol Biol. 1979;131:303-329.

425. Bennett V, Baines AJ. Spectrin and ankyrin based pathways: Metazoan inventions for integrating cells into tissues. Physiol Rev. 2001;81:1353-1392.

426. Sahr KE, Laurila P, Kotula L, et al. The complete cDNA and polypeptide sequences of human erythroid alpha-spectrin. J Biol Chem. 1990;265:4434-4443.

427. Leto TL, Fortugno-Erikson D, Barton D, et al. Comparison of nonerythroid alpha-spectrin genes reveals

strict homology among diverse species. Mol Cell Biol. 1988;8:1-9.

428. Winkelmann JC, Chang JG, Tse WT, et al. Full-length sequence of the cDNA for human erythroid beta-spectrin. J Biol Chem. 1990;265:11827-11832.

429. Gallagher PG, Sabatino DE, Romana M, et al. A human beta-spectrin gene promoter directs high level expression in erythroid but not muscle or neural cells. J Biol Chem. 1999;274:6062-6073.

430. Winkelmann JC, Costa FF, Linzie BL, Forget BG. Beta spectrin in human skeletal muscle. Tissue-specific differential processing of 3′ beta spectrin pre-mRNA generates a beta spectrin isoform with a unique carboxyl terminus. J Biol Chem. 1990;265:20449-20454.

431. Hu RJ, Watanabe M, Bennett V. Characterization of human brain cDNA encoding the general isoform of beta-spectrin. J Biol Chem. 1992;267:18715-18722.

432. Sakaguchi G, Orita S, Naito A, et al. A novel brain-specific isoform of beta spectrin: isolation and its interaction with Munc13. Biochem Biophys Res Commun. 1998;248:846-851.

433. Berghs S, Aggujaro D, Dirkx R Jr, et al. βIV spectrin, a new spectrin localized at axon initial segments and nodes of Ranvier in the central and peripheral nervous system. J Cell Biol. 2000;151:985-1001.

434. Tse WT, Tang J, Jin O, et al. A new spectrin, βIV, has a major truncated isoform that associates with promyelocytic leukemia protein nuclear bodies and nuclear matrix. J Biol Chem. 2001;276:23974-23985.

435. Stabach PR, Morrow JS. Identification and characterization of βV spectrin, a mammalian ortholog of *Drosophila* βH spectrin. J Biol Chem. 2000;275:21385-21395.

436. Ikeda Y, Dick KA, Weatherspoon MR, et al. Spectrin mutations cause spinocerebellar ataxia type 5. Nat Genet. 2006;38:184-190.

437. Parkinson NJ, Olsson CL, Hallows JL, et al. Mutant β-spectrin 4 causes auditory and motor neuropathies in quivering mice. Nat Genet. 2001;29:61-65.

438. Yan Y, Winograd E, Viel A, et al. Crystal structure of the repetitive segments of spectrin. Science. 1993;262:2027-2030.

439. Winograd E, Hume D, Branton D. Phasing the conformational unit of spectrin. Proc Natl Acad Sci U S A. 1991;88:10788-10791.

440. Grum VL, Li D, MacDonald RI, Mondragon A. Structures of two repeats of spectrin suggest models of flexibility. Cell. 1999;98:523-535.

441. An X, Guo X, Zhang X, et al. Conformational stabilities of the structural repeats of erythroid spectrin and their functional implications. J Biol Chem. 2006;281:10527-10532.

442. Paramore S, Ayton GS, Mirijanian DT, Voth GA. Extending a spectrin repeat unit. I: linear force-extension response. Biophys J. 2006;90:92-100.

443. Johnson CP, Tang HY, Carag C, et al. Forced unfolding of proteins within cells. Science. 2007;317:663-666.

444. Speicher DW, Weglarz L, DeSilva TM. Properties of human red cell spectrin heterodimer (side-to-side) assembly and identification of an essential nucleation site. J Biol Chem. 1992;267:14775-14782.

445. Li D, Tang HY, Speicher DW. A structural model of the erythrocyte spectrin heterodimer initiation site determined using homology modeling and chemical cross-linking. J Biol Chem. 2008;283:1553-1562.

446. Begg GE, Harper SL, Morris MB, Speicher DW. Initiation of spectrin dimerization involves complementary electrostatic interactions between paired triple-helical bundles. J Biol Chem. 2000;275:3279-3287.

447. Li D, Harper S, Speicher DW. Initial propagation of spectrin heterodimer assembly involves distinct energetic processes. Biochemistry. 2007;46:10585-10594.

448. Wilmotte R, Marechal J, Morle L, et al. Low expression allele alpha LELY of red cell spectrin is associated with mutations in exon 40 (alpha V/41 polymorphism) and intron 45 and with partial skipping of exon 46. J Clin Invest. 1993;91:2091-2096.

449. Wilmotte R, Harper SL, Ursitti JA, et al. The exon 46–encoded sequence is essential for stability of human erythroid alpha-spectrin and heterodimer formation. Blood. 1997;90:4188-4196.

450. Ungewickell E, Gratzer W. Self-association of human spectrin. A thermodynamic and kinetic study. Eur J Biochem. 1978;88:379-385.

451. DeSilva TM, Peng KC, Speicher KD, Speicher DW. Analysis of human red cell spectrin tetramer (head-to-head) assembly using complementary univalent peptides. Biochemistry. 1992;31:10872-10878.

452. Tse WT, Lecomte MC, Costa FF, et al. Point mutation in the beta-spectrin gene associated with alpha I/74 hereditary elliptocytosis. Implications for the mechanism of spectrin dimer self-association. J Clin Invest. 1990;86:909-916.

453. Ursitti JA, Kotula L, DeSilva TM, et al. Mapping the human erythrocyte beta-spectrin dimer initiation site using recombinant peptides and correlation of its phasing with the alpha-actinin dimer site. J Biol Chem. 1996;271:6636-6644.

454. Speicher DW, DeSilva TM, Speicher KD, et al. Location of the human red cell spectrin tetramer binding site and detection of a related "closed" hairpin loop dimer using proteolytic footprinting. J Biol Chem. 1993;268:4227-4235.

455. Liu SC, Palek J. Spectrin tetramer-dimer equilibrium and the stability of erythrocyte membrane skeletons. Nature. 1980;285:586-588.

456. Liu SC, Windisch P, Kim S, Palek J. Oligomeric states of spectrin in normal erythrocyte membranes: biochemical and electron microscopic studies. Cell. 1984;37:587-594.

457. Morrow JS, Marchesi VT. Self-assembly of spectrin oligomers in vitro: a basis for a dynamic cytoskeleton. J Cell Biol. 1981;88:463-468.

458. Ursitti JA, Pumplin DW, Wade JB, Bloch RJ. Ultrastructure of the human erythrocyte cytoskeleton and its attachment to the membrane. Cell Motil Cytoskel. 1991;19:227-243.

459. McGough AM, Josephs R. On the structure of erythrocyte spectrin in partially expanded membrane skeletons. Proc Natl Acad Sci U S A. 1990;87:5208-5212.

460. Ursitti JA, Wade JB. Ultrastructure and immunocytochemistry of the isolated human erythrocyte membrane skeleton. Cell Motil Cytoskel. 1993;25:30-42

461. Kennedy SP, Warren SL, Forget BG, Morrow JS. Ankyrin binds to the 15th repetitive unit of erythroid and nonerythroid beta-spectrin. J Cell Biol. 1991;115:267-277.

462. Bennett V, Stenbuck PJ. Identification and partial purification of ankyrin, the high affinity membrane attach-

ment site for human erythrocyte spectrin. J Biol Chem. 1979;254:2533-2541.

463. Devarajan P, Scaramuzzino DA, Morrow JS. Ankyrin binds to two distinct cytoplasmic domains of Na,K-ATPase alpha subunit. Proc Natl Acad Sci U S A. 1994;91:2965-2969.

464. Srinivasan Y, Elmer L, Davis J, et al. Ankyrin and spectrin associate with voltage-dependent sodium channels in brain. Nature. 1988;333:177-180.

465. Becker PS, Tse WT, Lux SE, Forget BG. Beta spectrin Kissimmee: a spectrin variant associated with autosomal dominant hereditary spherocytosis and defective binding to protein 4.1. J Clin Invest. 1993;92:612-616.

466. Cohen CM, Tyler JM, Branton D. Spectrin-actin associations studied by electron microscopy of shadowed preparations. Cell. 1980;21:875-883.

467. Karinch AM, Zimmer WE, Goodman SR. The identification and sequence of the actin-binding domain of human red blood cell beta-spectrin. J Biol Chem. 1990;265:11833-11840.

468. An X, Debnath G, Guo X, et al. Identification and functional characterization of protein 4.1R and actin-binding sites in erythrocyte beta spectrin: regulation of the interactions by phosphatidylinositol-4,5-bisphosphate. Biochemistry. 2005;44:10681-10688.

469. Ungewickell E, Bennett PM, Calvert R, et al. In vitro formation of a complex between cytoskeletal proteins of the human erythrocyte. Nature. 1979;280:811-814.

470. Ohanian V, Wolfe LC, John KM, et al. Analysis of the ternary interaction of the red cell membrane skeletal proteins spectrin, actin, and 4.1. Biochemistry. 1984;23:4416-4420.

471. Cohen CM, Foley SF. Biochemical characterization of complex formation by human erythrocyte spectrin, protein 4.1 and actin. Biochemistry. 1984;23:6091-6098.

472. Gardner K, Bennett V. Modulation of spectrin-actin assembly by erythrocyte adducin. Nature. 1987;328:359-362.

473. Kuhlman PA, Hughes CA, Bennett V, Fowler VM. A new function for adducin. Calcium/calmodulin-regulated capping of the barbed ends of actin filaments. J Biol Chem. 1996;271:7986-7991.

474. Li X, Matsuoka Y, Bennett V. Adducin preferentially recruits spectrin to the fast growing ends of actin filaments in a complex requiring the MARCKS-related domain and a newly defined oligomerization domain. J Biol Chem. 1998;273:19329-19338.

475. Mische SM, Mooseker MS, Morrow JS. Erythrocyte adducin: a calmodulin-regulated actin-bundling protein that stimulates spectrin-actin binding. J Cell Biol. 1987;105:2837-2845.

476. Li X, Bennett V. Identification of the spectrin subunit and domains required for formation of spectrin/adducin/actin complexes. J Biol Chem. 1996;271:15695-15702.

477. Wallis CJ, Wenegieme EF, Babitch JA. Characterization of calcium binding to brain spectrin. J Biol Chem. 1992;267:4333-4337.

478. Dubreuil RR, Brandin E, Reisberg JH, et al. Structure, calmodulin-binding, and calcium-binding properties of recombinant alpha spectrin polypeptides. J Biol Chem. 1991;266:7189-7193.

479. Travé G, Lacombe PJ, Pfuhl M, et al. Molecular mechanism of the calcium-induced conformational change in the spectrin EF-hands. EMBO J. 1995;14:4922-4931.

480. Buevich AV, Lundberg S, Sethson I, et al. NMR studies of calcium-binding to mutant alpha-spectrin EF-hands. Cell Mol Biol Lett. 2004;9:167-186.

481. Tang J, Taylor DW, Taylor KA. The three-dimensional structure of α-actinin obtained by cryoelectron microscopy suggests a model for Ca^{2+}-dependent actin binding. J Mol Biol. 2001;310:845-858.

482. Pei X, Guo X, Coppel R, et al. *Plasmodium falciparum* erythrocyte membrane protein 3 (PfEMP3) destabilizes erythrocyte membrane skeleton. J Biol Chem. 2007;282:26754-26758.

483. Korsgren C, Lux SE. The carboxyterminal EF-hands of erythroid α-spectrin are necessary for optimal spectrin-actin–protein 4.1 binding. Manuscript submitted for publication.

484. Wandersee NJ, Birkenmeier CS, Bodine DM, et al. Mutations in the murine erythroid alpha-spectrin gene alter spectrin mRNA and protein levels and spectrin incorporation into the red blood cell membrane skeleton. Blood. 2003;101:325-330.

485. Ziemnicka-Kotula D, Xu J, Gu H, et al. Identification of a candidate human spectrin Src homology 3 domain–binding protein suggests a general mechanism of association of tyrosine kinases with the spectrin-based membrane skeleton. J Biol Chem. 1998;273:13681-13692.

486. Le Bonniec S, Deregnaucourt C, Redeker V, et al. Plasmepsin II, an acidic hemoglobinase from the *Plasmodium falciparum* food vacuole, is active at neutral pH on the host erythrocyte membrane skeleton. J Biol Chem. 1999;274:14218-14223.

487. Macias MJ, Musacchio A, Ponstingl H, et al. Structure of the pleckstrin homology domain from beta-spectrin. Nature. 1994;369:675-677.

488. Ingley E, Hemmings BA. Pleckstrin homology (PH) domains in signal transduction. J Cell Biochem. 1994;56:436-443.

489. Pradhan D, Tseng K, Cianci CD, Morrow JS. Antibodies to βIΣ2 spectrin identify inhomogeneities in the erythrocyte membrane skeleton. Blood Cells Mol Dis. 2004;32:408-410.

490. Wang DS, Shaw G. The association of the C-terminal region of beta I sigma II spectrin to brain membranes is mediated by a PH domain, does not require membrane proteins, and coincides with a inositol-1,4,5 triphosphate binding site. Biochem Biophys Res Commun. 1995;217:608-615.

491. Rameh LE, Arvidsson A, Carraway KL, et al. A comparative analysis of the phosphoinositide binding specificity of pleckstrin homology domains. J Biol Chem. 1997;272:22059-22066.

492. Tao M, Conway R, Cheta S. Purification and characterization of a membrane-bound protein kinase from human erythrocytes. J Biol Chem. 1980;255:2563.

493. Harris HW Jr, Lux SE. Structural characterization of the phosphorylation sites of human erythrocyte spectrin. J Biol Chem. 1980;255:11512-11520.

494. Tang HY, Speicher DW. In vivo phosphorylation of human erythrocyte spectrin occurs in a sequential manner. Biochemistry. 2004;43:4251-4562.

495. Shahbakhti F, Gratzer WB. Analysis of the self-association of human red cell spectrin. Biochemistry. 1986;25:5969-5975.

496. Anderson JM, Tyler JM. State of spectrin phosphorylation does not affect erythrocyte shape or spectrin binding to erythrocyte membranes. J Biol Chem. 1980;255:1259-1265.

497. Manno S, Takakuwa Y, Nagao K, Mohandas N. Modulation of erythrocyte membrane mechanical function by beta-spectrin phosphorylation and dephosphorylation. J Biol Chem. 1995;270:5659-5665.

498. Speicher DW, Morrow JS, Knowles WJ, Marchesi VT. Identification of proteolytically resistant domains of human erythrocyte spectrin. Proc Natl Acad Sci U S A. 1980;77:5673-5677.

499. Geiduschek JB, Singer SJ. Molecular changes in the membranes of mouse erythroid cells accompanying differentiation. Cell. 1979;16:149-163.

500. Eisen H, Bach R, Emery R. Induction of spectrin in erythroleukemic cells transformed by Friend virus. Proc Natl Acad Sci U S A. 1977;74:3898-3902.

501. Hasthorpe S. Quantification of spectrin-containing erythroid precursor cells in normal and perturbed erythropoiesis. Exp Hematol. 1980;8:1001-1008.

502. Hanspal M, Yoon SH, Yu H, et al. Molecular basis of spectrin and ankyrin deficiencies in severe hereditary spherocytosis: evidence implicating a primary defect of ankyrin. Blood. 1991;77:165-173.

503. Bodine DM, Birkenmeier CS, Barker JE. Spectrin deficient inherited hemolytic anemias in the mouse: characterization by spectrin synthesis and mRNA activity in reticulocytes. Cell. 1984;37:721-729.

504. Moon RT, Lazarides E. Beta-spectrin limits alpha-spectrin assembly on membranes following synthesis in a chicken erythroid cell lysate. Nature. 1983;305:62-65.

505. Woods CM, Lazarides E. Degradation of unassembled alpha- and beta-spectrin by distinct intracellular pathways: regulation of spectrin topogenesis by beta-spectrin degradation. Cell. 1985;40:959-969.

506. Pinder J, Gratzer W. Structural and dynamic states of actin in the erythrocyte. J Cell Biol. 1983;96:768.

507. Tilney LG, Detmers P. Actin in erythrocyte ghosts and its association with spectrin. Evidence for a nonfilamentous form of these two molecules in situ. J Cell Biol. 1975;66:508-520.

508. Byers T, Branton D. Visualization of the protein associations in the erythrocyte membrane skeleton. Proc Natl Acad Sci U S A. 1985;82:6153.

509. Fowler V, Sussmann M, Miller P, et al. Tropomodulin is associated with the free (pointed) ends of the thin filaments in rat skeletal muscle. J Cell Biol. 1993;120:411.

510. Kuhlman P, Hughes C, Bennett V, Fowler V. A new function for adducin: calcium/calmodulin-regulated capping of the barbed ends of actin filaments. J Biol Chem. 1996;271:7986.

511. Kuhlman PA, Fowler VM. Purification and characterization of an alpha 1 beta 2 isoform of CapZ from human erythrocytes: cytosolic location and inability to bind to Mg^{2+} ghosts suggest that erythrocyte actin filaments are capped by adducin. Biochemistry. 1997;36:13461-13472.

512. Porro F, Costessi L, Marro ML, et al. The erythrocyte skeletons of beta-adducin deficient mice have altered levels of tropomyosin, tropomodulin and EcapZ. FEBS Lett. 2004;576:36-40.

513. Picart C, Discher DE. Actin protofilament orientation at the erythrocyte membrane. Biophys J. 1999;77:865-878.

514. Kalfa TA, Pushkaran S, Mohandas N, et al. Rac GTPases regulate the morphology and deformability of the erythrocyte cytoskeleton. Blood. 2006;108:3637-3645.

515. Kang JA, Zhou Y, Weis TL, et al. Osteopontin regulates actin cytoskeleton and contributes to cell proliferation in primary erythroblasts. J Biol Chem. 2008;283:6997-7006.

516. Correas I, Leto TL, Speicher DW, Marchesi VT. Identification of the functional site of erythrocyte protein 4.1 involved in spectrin-actin associations. J Biol Chem. 1986;261:3310-3315.

517. Inaba M, Gupta KC, Kuwabara M, et al. Deamidation of human erythrocyte protein 4.1: possible role in aging. Blood. 1992;79:3355-3361.

518. Chishti A, Kim A, Marfatia S, et al. The FERM domain: a unique module involved in the linkage of cytoplasmic proteins to the membrane. Trends Biochem Sci. 1998;23:281.

519. Leto TL, Marchesi VT. A structural model of human erythrocyte protein 4.1. J Biol Chem. 1984;259:4603-4608.

520. Holt GD, Haltiwanger RS, Torres CR, Hart GW. Erythrocytes contain cytoplasmic glycoproteins: *O*-linked GlcNAc on band 4.1. J Biol Chem. 1987;262:14847.

521. Cohen CM, Gascard P. Regulation and post-translational modification of erythrocyte membrane and membrane-skeletal proteins. Semin Hematol. 1992;29:244-292.

522. Manno S, Takakuwa Y, Mohandas N. Modulation of erythrocyte membrane mechanical function by protein 4.1 phosphorylation. J Biol Chem. 2005;280:7581-7587.

523. Danilov YN, Fennell R, Ling E, Cohen CM. Selective modulation of band 4.1 binding to erythrocyte membranes by protein kinase C. J Biol Chem. 1990;265:2556-2562.

524. Schischmanoff PO, Winardi R, Discher DE, et al. Defining of the minimal domain of protein 4.1 involved in spectrin-actin binding. J Biol Chem. 1995;270:21243-21250.

525. Discher DE, Winardi R, Schischmanoff PO, et al. Mechanochemistry of protein 4.1's spectrin-actin-binding domain: ternary complex interactions, membrane binding, network integration, structural strengthening. J Cell Biol. 1995;130:897-907.

526. Morris MB, Lux SE. Characterization of the binary interaction between human erythrocyte protein 4.1 and actin. Eur J Biochem. 1995;231:644-650.

527. Gimm JA, An X, Nunomura W, Mohandas N. Functional characterization of spectrin-actin–binding domains in 4.1 family of proteins. Biochemistry. 2002;41:7275-7282.

528. Discher DE, Winardi R, Schischmanoff PO, et al. Mechanochemistry of protein 4.1's spectrin-actin–binding domain: ternary complex interactions, membrane

binding, network integration, structural strengthening. J Cell Biol. 1995;130:897-907.

529. Horne WC, Prinz WC, Tang EK. Identification of two cAMP-dependent phosphorylation sites on erythrocyte protein 4.1. Biochim Biophys Acta. 1990;1055:87-92.

530. Subrahmanyam G, Bertics PJ, Anderson RA. Phosphorylation of protein 4.1 on tyrosine-418 modulates its function in vitro. Proc Natl Acad Sci U S A. 1991;88: 5222-5226.

531. Tanaka T, Kadowaki K, Lazarides E, Sobue K. Ca²⁺-dependent regulation of the spectrin/actin interaction by calmodulin and protein 4.1. J Biol Chem. 1991;266: 1134-1140.

532. Takakuwa Y, Mohandas N. Modulation of erythrocyte membrane material properties by Ca²⁺ and calmodulin. Implications for their role in regulation of skeletal protein interactions. J Clin Invest. 1988;82:394-400.

533. Pasternack GR, Racusen RH. Erythrocyte protein 4.1 binds and regulates myosin. Proc Natl Acad Sci U S A. 1989;86:9712-9716.

534. Tsukita S, Yoneumura S. ERM proteins: head-to-tail regulation of actin-plasma membrane interaction. Trends Biochem Sci. 1997;22:53.

535. Chishti AH, Kim AC, Marfatia SM, et al. The FERM domain: a unique module involved in the linkage of cytoplasmic proteins to the membrane. Trends Biochem Sci. 1998;23:281-282.

536. Scoles DR, Huynh DP, Morcos PA, et al. Neurofibromatosis 2 tumour suppressor schwannomin interacts with beta II-spectrin. Nat Genet. 1998;18:354-359.

537. La Jeunesse DR, McCartney BM, Fehon RG. Structural analysis of *Drosophila* merlin reveals functional domains important for growth control and subcellular localization. J Cell Biol. 1998;141:1589.

538. Marfatia SM, Leu RA, Branton D, Chishti AH. Identification of the protein 4.1 binding interface on glycophorin C and p55, a homologue of the *Drosophila* discs–large tumor suppressor protein. J Biol Chem. 1995;270: 715-719.

539. Nunomura W, Takakuwa Y, Parra M, et al. Regulation of protein 4.1R, p55, and glycophorin C ternary complex in human erythrocyte membrane. J Biol Chem. 2000;275: 24540-24546.

540. Marfatia SM, Cabral JHM, Kim AC, et al. The PDZ domain of human erythrocyte p55 mediates its binding to the cytoplasmic carboxyl terminus of glycophorin C: analysis of binding interface by in vitro mutagenesis. J Biol Chem. 1997;272:24191-24197.

541. Jons T, Drenckhahn D. Identification of the binding interface involved in linkage of cytoskeletal protein 4.1 to the erythrocyte anion exchanger. EMBO J. 1992;11: 2863-2867.

542. Hemming NJ, Anstee DJ, Staricoff MA, et al. Identification of the membrane attachment sites for protein 4.1 in the human erythrocyte. J Biol Chem. 1995;270:5360-5366.

543. Paw BH, Davidson AJ, Zhou Y, et al. Cell-specific mitotic defect and dyserythropoiesis associated with erythroid band 3 deficiency. Nat Genet. 2003;34:59-64.

544. Nunomura W, Takakuwa Y, Tokimitsu R, et al. Regulation of CD44–protein 4.1 interaction by Ca²⁺ and calmodulin. Implications for modulation of CD44-ankyrin interaction. J Biol Chem. 1997;272:30322-30328.

545. Nunomura W, Takakuwa Y, Parra M, et al. Ca²⁺-dependent and Ca²⁺-independent calmodulin binding sites in erythrocyte protein 4.1. Implications for regulation of protein 4.1 interaction with transmembrane proteins. J Biol Chem. 2000;275:6360-6367.

546. Han BG, Nunomura W, Takakuwa Y, et al. Protein 4.1R core domain structure and insights into regulation of cytoskeletal organization. Nat Struct Biol. 2000;7:871-875.

547. An XL, Takakuwa Y, Manno S, et al. Structure and functional characterization of protein 4.1R–phosphatidylserine interaction. J Biol Chem. 2001;276:35778-35785.

548. An X, Zhang X, Debnath G, et al. Phosphatidylinositol-4,5-biphosphate (PIP₂) differentially regulates the interaction of human erythrocyte protein 4.1 (4.1R) with membrane proteins. Biochemistry. 2006;45:5725-5732.

549. Moriniere M, Ribeiro L, Dalla Venezia N, et al. Elliptocytosis in patients with C-terminal domain mutations of protein 4.1 correlates with encoded messenger RNA levels rather than with alterations in primary protein structure. Blood. 2000;95:1834-1841.

550. Walensky LD, Gascard P, Fields ME, et al. The 13-kD FK506 binding protein, FKBP13, interacts with a novel homologue of the erythrocyte membrane cytoskeletal protein 4.1. J Cell Biol. 1998;141:143-153.

551. Shi Z-T, Afzal V, Coller B, et al. Protein 4.1R–deficient mice are viable but have erythroid membrane skeleton abnormalities. J Clin Invest. 1999;103:331-340.

551a. Salomao M, Zhang X, Yang Y, et al. Protein 4.1R-dependent multiprotein complex: New insights into the structural organization of the red blood cell membrane. Proc Natl Acad Sci U S A. 2008;105:8026-8031.

552. Walensky LD, Shi Z-T, Blackshaw S, et al. Neurobehavioral deficits in mice lacking the erythrocyte membrane cytoskeletal protein 4.1. Curr Biol. 1998;8:1269-1272.

553. Krauss SW, Chen C, Penman S, Heald R. Nuclear actin and protein 4.1: essential interactions during nuclear assembly in vitro. Proc Natl Acad Sci U S A. 2003;100: 10752-10757.

554. Mattagajasingh SN, Huang SC, Hartenstein JS, et al. A nonerythroid isoform of protein 4.1R interacts with the nuclear mitotic apparatus (NuMA) protein. J Cell Biol. 1999;145:29-43.

555. Compton DA, Cleveland DW. NuMA, a nuclear protein involved in mitosis and nuclear reformation. Curr Opin Cell Biol. 1994;6:343.

556. Krauss SW, Heald R, Lee G, et al. Two distinct domains of protein 4.1 critical for assembly of functional nuclei in vitro. J Biol Chem. 2002;277:44339-44346.

557. Gascard P, Nunomura W, Lee G, et al. Deciphering the nuclear import pathway for the cytoskeletal red cell protein 4.1R. Mol Biol Cell. 1999;10:1783-1798.

558. De Carcer G, Lallena MJ, Correas I. Protein 4.1 is a component of the nuclear matrix of mammalian cells. Biochem J. 1995;312:871-877.

559. Krauss SW, Larabell CA, Lockett S, et al. Structural protein 4.1 in the nucleus of human cells: dynamic rearrangements during cell division. J Cell Biol. 1997;137:275-289.

560. Krauss SW, Chasis JA, Rogers C, et al. Structural protein 4.1 is located in mammalian centrosomes. Proc Natl Acad Sci U S A 1997;94:7297-7302.

561. Krauss SW, Lee G, Chasis JA, et al. Two protein 4.1 domains essential for mitotic spindle and aster microtubule dynamics and organization in vitro. J Biol Chem. 2004;279:27591-25798.

562. Krauss SW, Spence JR, Bahmanyar S, et al. Downregulation of protein 4.1R, a mature centriole protein, disrupts centrosomes, alters cell cycle progression, and perturbs mitotic spindles and anaphase. Mol Cell Biol. 2008;28:2283-2294.

563. Tang CJ, Tang TK. The 30-kD domain of protein 4.1 mediates its binding to the carboxyl terminus of pICln, a protein involved in cellular volume regulation. Blood. 1998;92:1442-1447.

564. Mattagajasingh SN, Huang SC, Hartenstein JS, Benz EJ Jr. Characterization of the interaction between protein 4.1R and ZO-2. A possible link between the tight junction and the actin cytoskeleton. J Biol Chem. 2000;275:30573-30585.

565. Parra M, Gascard P, Walensky LD, et al. Cloning and characterization of 4.1G (EPB41L2), a new member of the skeletal protein 4.1 (EPB41) gene family. Genomics. 1998;49:298-306.

566. Walensky LD, Blackshaw S, Liao D, et al. A novel neuron-enriched homolog of the erythrocyte membrane cytoskeletal protein 4.1. J Neurosci. 1999;19:6457-6467.

567. Ye K, Compton DA, Lai MM, et al. Protein 4.1N binding to nuclear mitotic apparatus protein in PC12 cells mediates the antiproliferative actions of nerve growth factor. J Neurosci. 1999;19:10747.

568. Parra M, Gascard P, Walensky LD, et al. Molecular and functional characterization of protein 4.1B, a novel member of the protein 4.1 family with high level, focal expression in brain. J Biol Chem. 2000;275:3247-3255.

569. Ni X, Ji C, Cao G, et al. Molecular cloning and characterization of the protein 4.1O gene, a novel member of the protein 4.1 family with focal expression in ovary. J Hum Genet. 2003;48:101-106.

570. Baklouti F, Huang SC, Tang TK, et al. Asynchronous regulation of splicing events within protein 4.1 pre-mRNA during erythroid differentiation. Blood. 1996;87:3934-3941.

571. Chasis JA, Coulombel L, Conboy J, et al. Differentiation-associated switches in protein 4.1 expression. Synthesis of multiple structural isoforms during normal human erythropoiesis. J Clin Invest. 1993;91:329-338.

572. Schischmanoff PO, Yaswen P, Parra MK, et al. Cell shape-dependent regulation of protein 4.1 alternative pre-mRNA splicing in mammary epithelial cells. J Biol Chem. 1997;272:10254-10259.

573. Conboy J, Mohandas N, Tchernia G, Kan YW. Molecular basis of hereditary elliptocytosis due to protein 4.1 deficiency. N Engl J Med. 1986;315:680-685.

574. Chishti AH. Function of p55 and its nonerythroid homologues. Curr Opin Hematol. 1998;5:116-121.

575. Metzenberg AB, Gitschier J. The gene encoding the palmitoylated erythrocyte membrane protein, p55, originates at the CpG island 3′ to the factor VIII gene. Hum Mol Genet. 1992;1:97-101.

576. Ruff P, Speicher DW, Husain-Chishti A. Molecular identification of a major palmitoylated erythrocyte membrane protein containing the src homology 3 motif. Proc Natl Acad Sci U S A. 1991;88:6595-6599.

577. Kim AC, Metzenberg AB, Sahr KE, et al. Complete genomic organization of the human erythroid p55 gene (MPP1), a membrane-associated guanylate kinase homologue. Genomics. 1996;31:223-229.

578. Kusunoki H, Kohno T. Solution structure of human erythroid p55 PDZ domain. Proteins. 2006;64:804-807.

579. Marfatia SM, Leu RA, Branton D, Chishti AH. Identification of the protein 4.1 binding interface on glycophorin C and p55, a homologue of the *Drosophila* discs–large tumor suppressor protein. J Biol Chem. 1995;270:715-719.

580. Marfatia SM, Lue RA, Branton D, Chishti AH. In vitro binding studies suggest a membrane-associated complex between erythroid p55, protein 4.1, and glycophorin C. J Biol Chem. 1994;269:8631-8634.

581. Joshi R, Gilligan DM, Otto E, et al. Primary structure and domain organization of human alpha and beta adducin. J Cell Biol. 1991;115:665-675.

582. Katagiri T, Ozaki K, Fujiwara T, et al. Cloning, expression and chromosome mapping of adducin-like 70 (ADDL), a human cDNA highly homologous to human erythrocyte adducin. Cytogenet Cell Genet. 1996;74:90-95.

583. Gilligan DM, Lozovatsky L, Gwynn B, et al. Targeted disruption of the beta adducin gene (Add2) causes red blood cell spherocytosis in mice. Proc Natl Acad Sci U S A. 1999;96:10717-10722.

584. Hughes CA, Bennett V. Adducin: a physical model with implications for function in assembly of spectrin-actin complexes. J Biol Chem. 1995;270:18990-18996.

585. Joshi R, Bennett V. Mapping the domain structure of human erythrocyte adducin. J Biol Chem. 1990;265:13130-13136.

586. Suriyapperuma SP, Lozovatsky L, Ciciotte SL, et al. The mouse adducin gene family: alternative splicing and chromosomal localization. Mamm Genome. 2000;11:16-23.

587. Lin B, Nasir J, McDonald H, et al. Genomic organization of the human alpha-adducin gene and its alternately spliced isoforms. Genomics. 1995;25:93-99.

588. Sinard JH, Stewart GW, Stabach PR, et al. Utilization of an 86 bp exon generates a novel adducin isoform (beta 4) lacking the MARCKS homology domain. Biochim Biophys Acta. 1998;1396:57-66.

589. Gilligan DM, Lozovatsky L, Silberfein A. Organization of the human beta-adducin gene (ADD2). Genomics. 1997;43:141-148.

590. Matsuoka Y, Hughes CA, Bennett V. Adducin regulation. Definition of the calmodulin-binding domain and sites of phosphorylation by protein kinases A and C. J Biol Chem. 1996;271:25157-25166.

591. Matsuoka Y, Li X, Bennett V. Adducin is an in vivo substrate for protein kinase C: phosphorylation in the MARCKS-related domain inhibits activity in promoting spectrin-actin complexes and occurs in many cells, including dendritic spines of neurons. J Cell Biol. 1998;142:485-497.

592. Kimura K, Fukata Y, Matsuoka Y, et al. Regulation of the association of adducin with actin filaments by Rho-associated kinase (Rho-kinase) and myosin phosphatase. J Biol Chem. 1998;273:5542-5548.

593. Kaiser HW, O'Keefe E, Bennett V. Adducin: Ca^{++}-dependent association with sites of cell-cell contact. J Cell Biol. 1989;109:557-569.

594. Bianchi G, Tripodi G, Casari G, et al. Two point mutations within the adducin genes are involved in blood pressure variation. Proc Natl Acad Sci U S A. 1994;91: 3999-4003.

594. Tripodi G, Szpirer C, Reina C, et al. Polymorphism of gamma-adducin gene in genetic hypertension and mapping of the gene to rat chromosome 1q55. Biochem Biophys Res Commun. 1997;237:685-689.

596. Manunta P, Cusi D, Barlassina C, et al. Alpha-adducin polymorphisms and renal sodium handling in essential hypertensive patients. Kidney Int. 1998;53:1471-1478.

597. Cusi D, Barlassina C, Azzani T, et al. Polymorphisms of alpha-adducin and salt sensitivity in patients with essential hypertension. Lancet. 1997;349:1353-1357.

598. Alam S, Liyou N, Davis D, et al. The 460Trp polymorphism of the human alpha-adducin gene is not associated with isolated systolic hypertension in elderly Australian Caucasians. J Hum Hypertens. 2000;14: 199-203.

599. Busch CP, Harris SB, Hanley AJ, et al. The ADD1 G460W polymorphism is not associated with variation in blood pressure in Canadian Oji-Cree. J Hum Genet. 1999;44:225-229.

600. Wang WY, Adams DJ, Glenn CL, Morris BJ. The Gly-460Trp variant of alpha-adducin is not associated with hypertension in white Anglo-Australians. Am J Hypertens. 1999;12:632-636.

601. Ishikawa K, Katsuya T, Sato N, et al. No association between alpha-adducin 460 polymorphism and essential hypertension in a Japanese population. Am J Hypertens. 1998;11:502-506.

602. Grant FD, Romero JR, Jeunemaitre X, et al. Low-renin hypertension, altered sodium homeostasis, and an alpha-adducin polymorphism. Hypertension. 2002;39:191-196.

603. Glorioso N, Filigheddu F, Cusi D, et al. α-Adducin 460Trp allele is associated with erythrocyte Na transport rate in North Sardinian primary hypertensives. Hypertension. 2002;39:357-362.

604. Siegel DL, Branton D. Partial purification and characterization of an actin-bundling protein, band 4.9, from human erythrocytes. J Cell Biol. 1985;100:775.

605. Rana AP, Ruff P, Maalouf GJ, et al. Cloning of human erythroid dematin reveals another member of the villin family. Proc Natl Acad Sci U S A. 1993;90:6651-6655.

606. Kim AC, Azim AC, Chishti AH. Alternative splicing and structure of the human erythroid dematin gene. Biochim Biophys Acta. 1998;1398:382-386.

607. Horne WC, Leto TL, Marchesi VT. Differential phosphorylation of multiple sites in protein 4.1 and protein 4.9 by phorbol ester-activated and cyclic AMP–dependent protein kinases. J Biol Chem. 1985;260:9073-9076.

608. Husain-Chishti A, Levin A, Branton D. Abolition of actin-bundling by phosphorylation of human erythrocyte protein 4.9. Nature. 1988;334:718-721.

609. Jiang ZG, McKnight CJ. A phosphorylation-induced conformation change in dematin headpiece. Structure. 2006;14:379-387.

610. Lutchman M, Kim AC, Cheng L, et al. Dematin interacts with the Ras-guanine nucleotide exchange factor Ras-GRF2 and modulates mitogen-activated protein kinase pathways. Eur J Biochem. 2002;269:638-649.

611. Khanna R, Chang SH, Andrabi S, et al. Headpiece domain of dematin is required for the stability of the erythrocyte membrane. Proc Natl Acad Sci U S A. 2002;99:6637-6642.

612. Chen H, Khan AA, Liu F, et al. Combined deletion of mouse dematin-headpiece and beta-adducin exerts a novel effect on the spectrin-actin junctions leading to erythrocyte fragility and hemolytic anemia. J Biol Chem. 2007;282:4124-4135.

613. Gunning P, O'Neill G, Hardeman E. Tropomyosin-based regulation of the actin cytoskeleton in time and space. Physiol Rev. 2008;88:1-35.

614. Fowler VM. Regulation of actin filament length in erythrocytes and striated muscle. Curr Opin Cell Biol. 1996; 8:86-96.

615. Fowler VM, Bennett V. Erythrocyte membrane tropomyosin. Purification and properties. J Biol Chem. 1984; 259:5978-5989.

616. Kostyukova AS, Choy A, Rapp BA. Tropomodulin binds two tropomyosins: a novel model for actin filament capping. Biochemistry. 2006;45:12068-12075.

617. Sung LA, Lin JJ. Erythrocyte tropomodulin binds to the N-terminus of hTM5, a tropomyosin isoform encoded by the gamma-tropomyosin gene. Biochem Biophys Res Commun. 1994;201:627-634.

618. Mak AS, Roseborough G, Baker H. Tropomyosin from human erythrocyte membrane polymerizes poorly but binds F-actin effectively in the presence and absence of spectrin. Biochim Biophys Acta. 1987;912:157-166.

619. An X, Salomao M, Guo X, et al. Tropomyosin modulates erythrocyte membrane stability. Blood. 2007;109: 1284-1288.

620. der Terrossian E, Deprette C, Lebbar I, Cassoly R. Purification and characterization of erythrocyte caldesmon. Hypothesis for an actin-linked regulation of a contractile activity in the red blood cell membrane. Eur J Biochem. 1994;219:503-511.

621. Fowler VM. Capping actin filament growth: tropomodulin in muscle and nonmuscle cells. Soc Gen Physiol Ser. 1997;52:79-89.

622. Sussman MA, Fowler VM. Tropomodulin binding to tropomyosins. Isoform-specific differences in affinity and stoichiometry. Eur J Biochem. 1992;205:355-362.

623. Greenfield NJ, Fowler VM. Tropomyosin requires an intact N-terminal coiled coil to interact with tropomodulin. Biophys J. 2002;82:2580-2591.

624. Sung LA, Fowler VM, Lambert K, et al. Molecular cloning and characterization of human fetal liver tropomodulin. A tropomyosin-binding protein. J Biol Chem. 1992;267:2616-2621.

625. Wong AJ, Kiehart DP, Pollard TD. Myosin from human erythrocytes. J Biol Chem. 1985;260:46-49.

626. Fowler VM, Davis JQ, Bennett V. Human erythrocyte myosin: identification and purification. J Cell Biol. 1985;100:47-55.

627. Matovcik LM, Groschel-Stewart U, Schrier SL. Myosin in adult and neonatal human erythrocyte membranes. Blood. 1986;67:1668-1674.

628. Colin FC, Schrier SL. Myosin content and distribution in human neonatal erythrocytes are different from adult erythrocytes. Blood. 1991;78:3052.

629. Lux SE, John KM, Bennett V. Analysis of cDNA for human erythrocyte ankyrin indicates a repeated struc-

ture with homology to tissue-differentiation and cell-cycle control proteins. Nature. 1990;344:36-43.

630. Lux SE, Tse WT, Menninger JC, et al. Hereditary spherocytosis associated with deletion of human erythrocyte ankyrin gene on chromosome 8. Nature. 1990;345: 736-739.

631. Gorina S, Pavletich NP. Structure of the p53 tumor suppressor bound to the ankyrin and SH3 domains of 53BP2. Science. 1996;274:1001-1005.

632. Michaely P, Tomchick DR, Machius M, Anderson RG. Crystal structure of a 12 ANK repeat stack from human ankyrin$_R$. EMBO J. 2002;21:6387-6396.

633. Low PS, Willardson BM, Mohandas N, et al. Contribution of the band 3–ankyrin interaction to erythrocyte membrane mechanical stability. Blood. 1991;77:1581-1586.

634. Eber SW, Gonzalez JM, Lux ML, et al. Ankyrin-1 mutations are a major cause of dominant and recessive hereditary spherocytosis. Nat Genet. 1996;13:214-218.

635. Michaely P, Bennett V. The membrane-binding domain of ankyrin contains four independently folded subdomains, each comprised of six ankyrin repeats. J Biol Chem. 1993;268:22703-22709.

636. Michaely P, Bennett V. The ANK repeats of erythrocyte ankyrin form two distinct but cooperative binding sites for the erythrocyte anion exchanger. J Biol Chem. 1995;270:22050-22057.

637. Davis L, Lux SE, Bennett V. Mapping the ankyrin-binding site of the human erythrocyte anion exchanger. J Biol Chem. 1989;264:9665-9672.

638. Ding Y, Kobayashi S, Kopito R. Mapping of ankyrin binding determinants on the erythroid anion exchanger, AE1. J Biol Chem. 1996;271:22494-22498.

639. Bruce LJ, Ghosh S, King MJ, et al. Absence of CD47 in protein 4.2–deficient hereditary spherocytosis in man: an interaction between the Rh complex and the band 3 complex. Blood. 2002;100:1878-1885.

640. Nicolas V, Mouro-Chanteloup I, Lopez C, et al. Functional interaction between Rh proteins and the spectrin-based skeleton in erythroid and epithelial cells. Transfus Clin Biol. 2006;13:23-28.

641. *http://pfam.sanger.ac.uk/family?acc = PF00023.*

642. Mosavi LK, Cammett TJ, Desrosiers DC, Peng ZY. The ankyrin repeat as molecular architecture for protein recognition. Protein Sci. 2004;13:1435-1448.

643. Li J, Mahajan A, Tsai MD. Ankyrin repeat: a unique motif mediating protein-protein interactions. Biochemistry. 2006;45:15168-15178.

644. Jacobs MD, Harrison SC. Structure of an IB/NF-B complex. Cell. 1998;95:749-758.

645. Gallagher PG, Tse WT, Scarpa AL, et al. Structure and organization of the human ankyrin-1 gene. Basis for complexity of pre-mRNA processing. J Biol Chem. 1997;272:19220-19228.

646. Lee G, Abdi K, Jiang Y, et al. Nanospring behaviour of ankyrin repeats. Nature. 2006;440:246-249.

647. Howard J, Bechstedt S. Hypothesis: a helix of ankyrin repeats of the NOMPC-TRP ion channel is the gating spring of mechanoreceptors. Curr Biol. 2004;14: R224-R226.

648. Cianci CD, Giorgi M, Morrow JS. Phosphorylation of ankyrin down-regulates its cooperative interaction with spectrin and protein 3. J Cell Biochem. 1988;37:301-315.

649. Davis LH, Bennett V. Mapping the binding sites of human erythrocyte ankyrin for the anion exchanger and spectrin. J Biol Chem. 1990;265:10589-10596.

650. Platt OS, Lux SE, Falcone JF. A highly conserved region of human erythrocyte ankyrin contains the capacity to bind spectrin. J Biol Chem. 1993;268:24421-24426.

651. Hall TG, Bennett V. Regulatory domains of erythrocyte ankyrin. J Biol Chem. 1987;262:10537-10545.

652. Davis LH, Davis JQ, Bennett V. Ankyrin regulation: an alternatively spliced segment of the regulatory domain functions as an intramolecular modulator. J Biol Chem. 1992;267:18966-18972.

653. Davis J, Davis L, Bennett V. Diversity in membrane binding sites of ankyrins. Brain ankyrin, erythrocyte ankyrin, and processed erythrocyte ankyrin associate with distinct sites in kidney microsomes. J Biol Chem. 1989;264:6417-6426.

654. Cleveland JL, Ihle JN. Contenders in FasL/TNF death signaling. Cell. 1995;81:479.

655. Del Rio M, Imam A, DeLeon M, et al. The death domain of kidney ankyrin interacts with Fas and promotes Fas-mediated cell death in renal epithelia. J Am Soc Nephrol. 2004;15:41-51.

656. Lu PW, Soong CJ, Tao M. Phosphorylation of ankyrin decreases its affinity for spectrin tetramer. J Biol Chem. 1985;260:14958-14964.

657. Wei T, Tao M. Human erythrocyte casein kinase II: characterization and phosphorylation of membrane cytoskeletal proteins. Arch Biochem Biophys. 1993;307: 206-216.

658. Weaver DC, Pasternack GR, Marchesi VT. The structural basis of ankyrin function. II. Identification of two functional domains. J Biol Chem. 1984;259:6170-6175.

659. Soong CJ, Lu PW, Tao M. Analysis of band 3 cytoplasmic domain phosphorylation and association with ankyrin. Arch Biochem Biophys. 1987;254:509-517.

660. Michaely P, Bennett V. Mechanism for binding site diversity on ankyrin. Comparison of binding sites on ankyrin for neurofascin and the Cl^-/HCO_3^- anion exchanger. J Biol Chem. 1995;270:31298-31302.

661. Bennett V. Ankyrins: adaptors between diverse plasma membrane proteins and the cytoplasm. J Biol Chem. 1992;267:8703.

662. Zhou D, Birkenmeier CS, Williams MW, et al. Small, membrane-bound, alternatively spliced forms of ankyrin 1 associated with the sarcoplasmic reticulum of mammalian skeletal muscle. J Cell Biol. 1997;136:621-631.

663. Porter NC, Resneck WG, O'Neill A, et al. Association of small ankyrin 1 with the sarcoplasmic reticulum. Mol Membr Biol. 2005;22:421-432.

664. Lambert S, Bennett V. Postmitotic expression of ankyrin$_R$ and beta R-spectrin in discrete neuronal populations of the rat brain. J Neurosci. 1993;13:3725-3735.

665. Kordeli E, Bennett V. Distinct ankyrin isoforms at neuron cell bodies and nodes of Ranvier resolved using erythrocyte ankyrin-deficient mice. J Cell Biol. 1991;114:1243-1259.

666. Peters LL, John KM, Lu FM, et al. Ank3 (epithelial ankyrin), a widely distributed new member of the ankyrin gene family and the major ankyrin in kidney, is expressed

in alternatively spliced forms, including forms that lack the repeat domain. J Cell Biol. 1995;130:313-330.

667. Bennett V, Baines AJ. Spectrin and ankyrin-based pathways: metazoan inventions for integrating cells into tissues. Physiol Rev. 2001;81:1353-1392.

668. Kunimoto M, Otto E, Bennett V. A new 440-kD isoform is the major ankyrin in neonatal rat brain. J Cell Biol. 1991;115:1319-1331.

669. Chan W, Kordeli E, Bennett V. 440-kD Ankyrin_B: Structure of the major developmentally regulated domain and selective localization in unmyelinated axons. J Cell Biol. 1993;123:1463-1473.

670. Scotland P, Zhou D, Benveniste H, Bennett V. Nervous system defects of ankyrin_B (−/−) mice suggest functional overlap between the cell adhesion molecule L1 and 440-kD ankyrin_B in premyelinated axons. J Cell Biol. 1998;143:1305-1315.

671. Mohler PJ, Davis JQ, Bennett V. Ankyrin-B coordinates the Na/K ATPase, Na/Ca exchanger, and InsP₃ receptor in a cardiac T-tubule/SR microdomain. PLoS Biol. 2005;3:e423.

672. Mohler PJ, Healy JA, Xue H, et al. Ankyrin-B syndrome: enhanced cardiac function balanced by risk of cardiac death and premature senescence. PLoS ONE. 2007;2:e1051.

673. Mohler PJ, Schott JJ, Gramolini AO, et al. Ankyrin-B mutation causes type 4 long-QT cardiac arrhythmia and sudden cardiac death. Nature. 2003;421:634-639.

674. Mohler PJ, Splawski I, Napolitano C, et al. A cardiac arrhythmia syndrome caused by loss of ankyrin-B function. Proc Natl Acad Sci U S A. 2004;101:9137-9142.

675. Kordeli E, Lambert S, Bennett V. Ankyrin_G. A new ankyrin gene with neural-specific isoforms localized at the axonal initial segment and node of Ranvier. J Biol Chem. 1995;270:2352-2359.

676. Davis JQ, Lambert S, Bennett V. Molecular composition of the node of Ranvier: identification of ankyrin-binding cell adhesion molecules neurofascin (mucin_+/third FNIII domain⁻) and NrCAM at nodal axon segments. J Cell Biol. 1996;135:1355-1367.

677. Zhang, X, Bennett, V. Restriction of 480/270-kd ankyrin_G to axon proximal segments requires multiple ankyrin_G-specific domains. J Cell Biol. 1998;142:1571-1581.

678. Pan Z, Kao T, Horvath Z, et al. A common ankyrin-G–based mechanism retains KCNQ and Na_V channels at electrically active domains of the axon. J Neurosci. 2006;26:2599-2613.

679. Zhou D, Lambert S, Malen PL, et al. Ankyrin_G is required for clustering of voltage-gated Na channels at axon initial segments and for normal action potential firing. J Cell Biol. 1998;143:1295-1304.

680. Lacas-Gervais S, Guo J, Strenzke N, et al. BetaIVSigma1 spectrin stabilizes the nodes of Ranvier and axon initial segments. J Cell Biol. 2004;166:983-990.

681. Kizhatil K, Bennett V. Lateral membrane biogenesis in human bronchial epithelial cells requires 190-kDa ankyrin-G. J Biol Chem. 2004;279:16706-16714.

682. Kizhatil K, Yoon W, Mohler PJ, et al. Ankyrin-G and beta2-spectrin collaborate in biogenesis of lateral membrane of human bronchial epithelial cells. J Biol Chem. 2007;282:2029-2037.

683. Kizhatil K, Davis JQ, Davis L, et al. Ankyrin-G is a molecular partner of E-cadherin in epithelial cells and early embryos. J Biol Chem. 2007;282:26552-26561.

684. Devarajan P, Stabach PR, Mann AS, et al. Identification of a small cytoplasmic ankyrin (AnkG119) in the kidney and muscle that binds beta I sigma spectrin and associates with the Golgi apparatus. J Cell Biol. 1996;133:819-830.

685. Hoock TC, Peters LL, Lux SE. Isoforms of ankyrin-3 that lack the NH-2 terminal repeats associate with mouse macrophage lysosomes. J Cell Biol. 1997;136:1059-1070.

686. Michaely P, Kamal A, Anderson RGW, Bennett V. A requirement for ankyrin binding to clathrin during coated pit budding. J Biol Chem. 1999;50:35908-35913.

687. White RA, Birkenmeier CS, Lux SE, Barker JE. Ankyrin and the hemolytic anemia mutation, nb, map to mouse chromosome 8: presence of the nb allele is associated with a truncated erythrocyte ankyrin. Proc Natl Acad Sci U S A. 1990;87:3117-3121.

688. Birkenmeier CS, Gifford EJ, Barker JE. Normoblastosis, a murine model for ankyrin-deficient hemolytic anemia, is caused by a hypomorphic mutation in the erythroid ankyrin gene Ank1. Hematol J. 2003;4:445-449.

689. Peters LL, Birkenmeier CS, Bronson RT, et al. Purkinje cell degeneration associated with erythroid ankyrin deficiency in nb/nb mice. J Cell Biol 1991;114:1233-1241.

690. Korsgren C, Lawler J, Lambert S, et al. Complete amino acid sequence and homologies of human erythrocyte membrane protein band 4.2. Proc Natl Acad Sci U S A. 1990;87:613.

691. Sung LA, Chien S, Chang LS, et al. Molecular cloning of human protein 4.2: a major component of the erythrocyte membrane. Proc Natl Acad Sci U S A. 1990;87:955-959.

692. Wada H, Kanzaki A, Yawata A, et al. Late expression of red cell membrane protein 4.2 in normal human erythroid maturation with seven isoforms of the protein 4.2 gene. Exp Hematol. 1999;27:54-62.

693. Korsgren C, Cohen CM. Organization of the gene for human erythrocyte membrane protein 4.2: structural similarities with the gene for the subunit of factor XIII. Proc Natl Acad Sci U S A. 1991;88:4840-4844.

694. Zhu L, Kahwash SB, Chang LS. Developmental expression of mouse erythrocyte protein 4.2 mRNA: evidence for specific expression in erythroid cells. Blood. 1998;91:695-705.

695. Sung LA, Lo WK. Immunodetection of membrane skeletal protein 4.2 in bovine and chicken eye lenses and erythrocytes. Curr Eye Res. 1997;16:1127-1133.

696. Friedrichs B, Koob R, Kraemer D, Drenckhahn D. Demonstration of immunoreactive forms of erythrocyte protein 4.2 in nonerythroid cells and tissues. Eur J Cell Biol. 1989;48:121-127.

697. Bhattacharyya R, Das AK, Moitra PK, et al. Mapping of a palmitoylatable band 3–binding domain of human erythrocyte membrane protein 4.2. Biochem J. 1999;340:505-512.

698. Korsgren C, Cohen CM. Associations of human erythrocyte protein 4.2. Binding to ankyrin and to the cytoplasmic domain of band 3. J Biol Chem. 1988;263:10212-10218.

699. Toye AM, Ghosh S, Young MT, et al. Protein-4.2 association with band 3 (AE1, SLCA4) in Xenopus oocytes:

effects of three natural protein-4.2 mutations associated with hemolytic anemia. Blood. 2005;105:4088-4095.

700. Su Y, Ding Y, Jiang M, et al. Protein 4.2 Komatsu (D175Y) associated with the lack of interaction with ankyrin in human red blood cells. Blood Cells Mol Dis. 2007;38:221-228.

701. Su Y, Ding Y, Jiang M, et al. Associations of protein 4.2 with band 3 and ankyrin. Mol Cell Biochem. 2006; 289:159-166.

702. Mouro-Chanteloup I, Delaunay J, Gane P, et al. Evidence that the red cell skeleton protein 4.2 interacts with the Rh membrane complex member CD47. Blood. 2003;101:338-344.

703. Dahl KN, Parthasarathy R, Westhoff CM, et al. Protein 4.2 is critical to CD47-membrane skeleton attachment in human red cells. Blood. 2004;103:1131-1136.

704. Mandal D, Moitra PK, Basu J. Mapping of a spectrin-binding domain of human erythrocyte membrane protein 4.2. Biochem J. 2002;364:841-847.

705. Risinger MA, Dotimas EM, Cohen CM. Human erythrocyte protein 4.2, a high copy number membrane protein, is N-myristylated. J Biol Chem. 1992;267:5680-5685.

706. Das AK, Bhattacharya R, Kundu M, et al. Human erythrocyte membrane protein 4.2 is palmitoylated. Eur J Biochem. 1994;224:575-580.

707. Risinger MA, Korsgren C, Cohen CM. Role of N-myristylation in targeting of band 4.2 (pallidin) in nonerythroid cells. Exp Cell Res.h 1996;229:421-431.

708. Butterfield LH, Merino A, Golub SH, Shau H. From cytoprotection to tumor suppression: the multifactorial role of peroxiredoxins. Antioxid Redox Signal. 1999;1:385-402.

709. Shau H, Butterfield LH, Chiu R, Kim A. Cloning and sequence analysis of candidate human natural killer enhancing factor genes. Immunogenetics. 1994;40:129-134.

710. Rabilloud T, Berthier R, Vincon M, et al. Early events in erythroid differentiation: accumulation of the acidic peroxidoxin (PRP/TSA/NKEF-B). Biochem J. 1995;312:699-705.

711. Moore RB, Shriver SK, Jenkins LD, et al. Calpromotin, a cytoplasmic protein, is associated with the formation of dense cells in sickle cell anemia. Am J Hematol. 1997;56:100-106.

712. Low FM, Hampton MB, Peskin AV, Winterbourn CC. Peroxiredoxin 2 functions as a noncatalytic scavenger of low-level hydrogen peroxide in the erythrocyte. Blood. 2007;109:2611-2617.

713. Lee TH, Kim SU, Yu SL, et al. Peroxiredoxin II is essential for sustaining life span of erythrocytes in mice. Blood. 2003;101:5033-5038.

714. Neumann CA, Krause DS, Carman CV, et al. Essential role for the peroxiredoxin Prdx1 in erythrocyte antioxidant defence and tumour suppression. Nature. 2003;424:561-565.

715. Liu S-C, Derick LH. Molecular anatomy of the red blood cell membrane skeleton: Structure-function relationships. Semin Hematol. 1992;29:231-243.

716. Liu S-C, Derick LH, Palek J. Visualization of the hexagonal lattice in the erythrocyte membrane skeleton. J Cell Biol. 1987;104:527-536.

717. McCaughan L, Krimm S. X-ray and neutron scattering density profiles of the intact human red blood cell membrane. Science. 1980;207:1481-1483.

718. Tsukita S, Tsukita S, Ishikawa H. Cytoskeletal network underlying the human erythrocyte membrane. Thin-section electron microscopy. J Cell Biol. 1980;85:567-576.

719. Lux SE. Dissecting the red cell membrane skeleton. Nature 1979;281:426-429.

720. Hargreaves WR, Giedd KN, Verkleij A, Branton D. Reassociation of ankyrin with band 3 in erythrocyte membranes and in lipid vesicles. J Biol Chem. 1980;255:11965-11972.

721. Thevenin BJM, Low PS. Kinetics and regulation of the ankyrin–band 3 interaction of the human red blood cell membrane. J Biol Chem. 1990;265:16166-16172.

722. Ling E, Danilov YN, Cohen CM. Modulation of red cell band 4.1 function by cAMP-dependent kinase and protein kinase C phosphorylation. J Biol Chem. 1988;263:2209-2216.

723. Eder PS, Soong CJ, Tao M. Phosphorylation reduces the affinity of protein 4.1 for spectrin. Biochemistry. 1986;25:1764-1770.

724. Chao T-S, Tao M. Modulation of protein 4.1 binding to inside-out membrane vesicles by phosphorylation. Biochemistry. 1991;30:10529-10535.

725. Husain-Chishti A, Faquin W, Wu C-C, Branton D. Purification of erythrocyte dematin (protein 4.9) reveals an endogenous protein kinase that modulates actin-bundling activity. J Biol Chem. 1989;264:8985-8991.

726. Harris HW Jr, Levin N, Lux SE. Comparison of the phosphorylation of human erythrocyte spectrin in the intact red cell and in various cell-free systems. J Biol Chem. 1980;255:11521-11525.

727. Manno S, Takakuwa Y, Nagoa K, Mohandas N. Modulation of erythrocyte membrane mechanical function by beta-spectrin phosphorylation and dephosphorylation. J Biol Chem. 1995;270:5969-5975.

728. Sheetz MP, Casaly J. 2,3-Diphosphoglycerate and ATP dissociate erythrocyte membrane skeletons. J Biol Chem. 1980;255:9955-9960.

729. Mentzer WC Jr, Iarocci TA, Mohandas N, et al. Modulation of erythrocyte membrane mechanical fragility by 2,3 diphosphoglycerate in the neonatal poikilocytosis/elliptocytosis syndrome. J Clin Invest. 1987;79:943-949.

730. Schindler M, Koppel D, Sheetz MP. Modulation of membrane protein lateral mobility by polyphosphates and polyamines. Proc Natl Acad Sci U S A. 1980;77:1457-1461.

731. Suzuki Y, Nakajima T, Shiga T, et al. Influence of 2,3-diphosphoglycerate on the deformability of human erythrocytes. Biochim Biophys Acta. 1990;1029:85-90.

732. Waugh RE. Effects of 2,3-diphosphoglycerate on the mechanical properties of erythrocyte membrane. Blood. 1986;68:231-238.

733. Anderson JP, Morrow JS. The interaction of calmodulin with erythrocyte spectrin. Inhibition of protein 4.1–stimulated actin binding. J Biol Chem. 1987;262:6365-6372.

734. Gardner K, Bennett V. A new erythrocyte membrane-associated protein with calmodulin binding activity.

Identification and purification. J Biol Chem. 1986;261: 1339-1348.

735. Gárdos G. The role of calcium in the potassium permeability of human erythrocytes. Acta Physiol Acad Sci Hung. 1959;15:121-125.

736. Hanspal M, Palek J. Biogenesis of normal and abnormal red blood cell membrane skeletons. Semin Hematol. 1992;29:305-319.

737. Lazarides E. From genes to structural morphogenesis: The genesis and epigenesis of a red blood cell. Cell 1987;51:345-356.

738. Lazarides E, Woods C. Biogenesis of the red blood cell membrane skeleton and the control of erythroid morphogenesis. Annu Rev Cell Biol. 1989;5:427-452.

739. Hanspal M, Palek J. Synthesis and assembly of membrane skeletal proteins in mammalian red cell precursors. J Cell Biol. 1987;105:1417-1424.

740. Hanspal M, Hanspal J, Kalraiya R. Asynchronous synthesis of membrane skeletal proteins during terminal maturation of murine erythroblasts. Blood. 1992;80: 530-539.

741. Hanspal M, Hanspal JS, Sahr KE, et al. Molecular basis of spectrin deficiency in hereditary pyropoikilocytosis. Blood. 1993;82:1652-1660.

742. Woods CM, Boyer B, Vogt PK, Lazarides E. Control of erythroid differentiation: Asynchronous expression of the anion transporter and the peripheral components of the membrane skeleton in AEV- and S13-transformed cells. J Cell Biol. 1986;103:1789-1798.

743. Jarolim P, Rubin HL, Liu S C, et al. Duplication of 10 nucleotides in the erythroid band 3 (AE1) gene is a kindred with hereditary spherocytosis and band 3 protein deficiency (band 3 PRAGUE). J Clin Invest. 1994;93:121-130.

744. Hanspal M, Kalraiya R, Hanspal J. Erythropoietin enhances the assembly of αβ spectrin heterodimers on the murine erythroblast membranes by increasing β spectrin synthesis. J Biol Chem. 1991;266:15626-15630.

745. Ji P, Jayapal SR, Lodish HF. Enucleation of cultured mouse fetal erythroblasts requires Rac GTPases and mDia2. Nat Cell Biol. 2008;10:314-321.

746. Patel VP, Lodish HF. A fibronectin matrix is required for differentiation of murine erythroleukemia cells into reticulocytes. J Cell Biol. 1987;105:3105-3112.

747. Johnstone RM. Revisiting the road to the discovery of exosomes. Blood Cells Mol Dis. 2005;34:214-219.

748. Blanc L, De Gassart A, Géminard C, et al. Exosome release by reticulocytes—an integral part of the red blood cell differentiation system. Blood Cells Mol Dis. 2005;35:21-26.

749. Géminard C, Nault F, Johnstone RM, Vidal M. Characteristics of the interaction between Hsc70 and the transferrin receptor in exosomes released during reticulocyte maturation. J Biol Chem. 2001;276:9910-9916.

750. Blanc L, Barres C, Bette-Bobillo P, Vidal M. Reticulocyte-secreted exosomes bind natural IgM antibodies: involvement of a ROS-activatable endosomal phospholipase iPLA2. Blood. 2007;110:3407-3016.

751. Holm TM, Braun A, Trigatti BL, et al. Failure of red blood cell maturation in mice with defects in the high-density lipoprotein receptor SR-BI. Blood. 2002;99: 1817-1824.

752. Lange Y, Dolde J, Steck TL. The rate of transmembrane movement of cholesterol in the human erythrocyte. J Biol Chem. 1981;256:5321-5323.

753. Rand RP, Burton AC. Area and volume changes in hemolysis of single erythrocytes. J Cell Comp Physiol. 1963;61:245-253.

754. Mohandas N, Chasis JA. Red cell deformability, membrane material properties, and shape: Regulation by transmembrane, skeletal, and cytosolic proteins and lipids. Semin Hematol. 1993;30:171-192.

755. Bull BS, Kuhn IN. The production of schistocytes by fibrin strands (a scanning electron microscope study). Blood. 1970;35:104.

756. Reinhart WH, Sung LA, Chien S. Quantitative relationship between Heinz body formation and red blood cell deformability. Blood. 1986;68:1376-1383.

757. Smith BD, La Celle PL, Siefring J, et al. Effects of the calcium mediated enzymatic cross linking of membrane proteins on cellular deformability. J Membr Biol. 1981;61:75-80.

758. Flynn TP, Allen DW, Johnson GJ, White JG. Oxidant damage of the lipids and proteins of the erythrocyte membranes in unstable hemoglobin disease. Evidence for the role of lipid peroxidation. J Clin Invest. 1983;71: 1215-1223.

759. Chasis JA, Reid ME, Jensen RH, Mohandas N. Signal transduction by glycophorin A: role of extracellular and cytoplasmic domains in a modulatable process. J Cell Biol. 1988;107:1351-1357.

760. Liu SC, Palek J, Yi SJ, et al. Molecular basis of altered red blood cell membrane properties in Southeast Asian ovalocytosis: role of the mutant band 3 protein in band 3 oligomerization and retention by the membrane skeleton. Blood. 1995;86:349-358.

761. Che A, Cherry RJ, Bannister LH, Dluzewski AR. Aggregation of band 3 in hereditary ovalocytic red blood cell membranes. Electron microscopy and protein rotational diffusion studies. J Cell Sci. 1993;105:655-660.

762. Liu S-C, Derick LH, Agre P, Palek J. Alteration of the erythrocyte membrane skeletal ultrastructure in hereditary spherocytosis, hereditary elliptocytosis, and pyropoikilocytosis. Blood. 1990;76:198-205.

763. Liu S-C, Derick LH, Duquette MA, Palek J. Separation of the lipid bilayer from the membrane skeleton during discocyte-echinocyte transformation of human erythrocyte ghosts. Eur J Cell Biol. 1989;49:358-365.

764. Knowles DW, Tilley L, Mohandas N, Chasis JA. Erythrocyte membrane vesiculation: model for the molecular mechanism of protein sorting. Proc Natl Acad Sci U S A. 1997;94:12969-12974.

765. Wagner GM, Chiu DTY, Qju JH, et al. Spectrin oxidation correlates with membrane vesiculation in stored RBC's. Blood. 1987;69:1777-1781.

766. Wolfe LC. The membrane and the lesions of storage in preserved red cells. Transfusion. 1985;25:185-203.

767. Lutz HU, Liu S C, Palek J. Release of spectrin free vesicles from human erythrocytes during ATP depletion. Characterization of spectrin free vesicles. J Cell Biol. 1977;73:548-560.

768. Elgsaeter A, Shotton DM, Branton D. Intramembrane particle aggregation in erythrocyte ghosts II. The influence of spectrin aggregation. Biochim Biophys Acta. 1976;426:101-122.

769. Lux SE, John KM, Karnovsky MJ. Irreversible deformation of the spectrin actin lattice in irreversibly sickled cells. J Clin Invest. 1976;58:955-963.

770. Tomaselli MB, John KM, Lux SE. Elliptical erythrocyte membrane skeletons and heat-sensitive spectrin in hereditary elliptocytosis. Proc Natl Acad Sci U S A. 1981;78:1911-1915.

771. Khodadad JK, Waugh RE, Podolski JL, et al. Remodeling the shape of the skeleton in the intact red cell. Biophys J. 1996;70:1036-1044.

772. Hebbel RP. Beyond hemoglobin polymerization: The red blood cell membrane and sickle cell disease pathophysiology. Blood. 1991;77:214-237.

773. Swerlick RA, Eckman JR, Kumar A, et al. $\alpha_4\beta_1$-Integrin expression on sickle reticulocytes: Vascular cell adhesion molecule-1–dependent binding to endothelium. Blood. 1993;82:1891-1899.

774. Rosse WF. The glycolipid anchor of membrane surface proteins. Semin Hematol. 1993;30:219-231.

775. Discher DE, Mohandas N, Evans EA. Molecular maps of red cell deformation: hidden elasticity and in situ connectivity. Science. 1994;266:1032-1035.

776. Test ST, Butikofer P, Yee MC, et al. Characterization of the complement sensitivity of calcium-loaded human erythrocytes. Blood. 1991;78:3056-3065.

777. Victoria EJ, Muchmore EA, Sudora EJ, Masouredis SP. The role of antigen mobility in anti Rh(D) induced agglutination. J Clin Invest. 1975;56:292-301.

778. Bruce LJ, Beckmann R, Ribeiro ML, et al. A band 3–based macrocomplex of integral and peripheral proteins in the RBC membrane. Blood. 2003;101:4180-4188.

779. Mueckler MM, Caruso C, Baldwin SA, et al. Sequence and structure of a human glucose transporter. Science. 1985;229:941-945.

780. Brugnara C. Erythrocyte dehydration in pathophysiology and treatment of sickle cell disease. Curr Opin Hematol. 1995;2:132-138.

781. Bookchin RM, Lew VL. Sickle red cell dehydration; mechanisms and interventions. Curr Opin Hematol. 2002;9:107-110.

782. Parker JC. In defense of cell volume? Am J Physiol. 1993;265:1191-1200.

783. De Gier J. Permeability barriers formed by membrane lipids. Bioelectrochem Bioenerg. 1992;27:1-10.

784. Smith BL, Baumgarten R, Nielsen S, et al. Concurrent expression of erythroid and renal aquaporin CHIP and appearance of water channel activity in perinatal rats. J Clin Invest. 1993;92:2035-2041.

785. Brugnara C. Membrane transport of Na and K and cell dehydration in sickle erythrocytes. Experientia. 1993;49:100-109.

786. Joiner CH. Cation transport and volume regulation in sickle red blood cells. Am J Physiol. 1993;264:C251-C270.

787. Johnson RM, Gannon SA. Erythrocyte cation permeability induced by mechanical stress: a model for sickle cell cation loss. Am J Physiol. 1990;259:C746-C751.

788. Garrahan PJ, Glynn IM. Factors affecting the relative magnitude of the sodium:potassium and sodium:sodium exchanges catalyzed by the sodium pump. J Physiol. 1967;192:189.

789. Clark MR, Guatelli JC, White AT, Shohet SB. Study of dehydrating effect of the red cell Na$^+$/K$^+$ pump in nystatin

treated cells with varying Na$^+$ and water content. Biochim Biophys Acta. 1981;646:422-432.

790. Joiner CH, Platt OS, Lux SE. Cation depletion by the sodium pump in red cells with pathologic cation leaks. J Clin Invest. 1986;78:1487-1496.

791. Clark MR. Senescence of red blood cells: Progress and problems. Physiol Rev. 1988;68:503-554.

792. Beutler E. Isolation of the aged. Blood Cells. 1988;14:1-5.

793. Dale GL, Norenberg SL. Density fractionation of erythrocytes by Percoll/Hypaque results in only a slight enrichment for aged cells. Biochim Biophys Acta. 1990;1036:183-187.

794. Rettig MP, Low PS, Gimm JA, et al. Evaluation of biochemical changes during in vivo erythrocyte senescence in the dog. Blood. 1999;93:376-384.

795. Waugh RE, Mohandas N, Jackson CW, et al. Rheologic properties of senescent erythrocytes: loss of surface area and volume with red blood cell age. Blood. 1992;79:1351-1358.

796. Jain SK. Evidence for membrane lipid peroxidation during the in vivo aging of human erythrocytes. Biochim Biophys Acta. 1988;937:205-210.

797. Beutler E. Biphasic loss of red cell enzyme activity during in vivo aging. Prog Clin Biol Res. 1985;95:317-325.

798. Kay MMB. Mechanism of removal of senescent cells by human macrophages in situ. Proc Natl Acad Sci U S A. 1975;72:3521-3525.

799. Hardy RR, Wei CJ, Hayakawa K. Selection during development of VH11$^+$ B cells: a model for natural autoantibody-producing CD5$^+$ B cells. Immunol Rev. 2004;197:60-74.

800. Kay MMB. Localization of senescent cell antigen on band 3. Proc Natl Acad Sci U S A. 1984;81:5753-5757.

801. Schlüter K, Drenckhahn D. Co-clustering of denatured hemoglobin with band 3: Its role in binding of autoantibodies against band 3 to abnormal and aged erythrocytes. Proc Natl Acad Sci U S A. 1986;83:6137-6141.

802. Lutz HU, Stringaro-Wipf G. Senescent red cell bound IgG is attached to band 3 protein. Biomed Biochim Acta. 1983;42:117-121.

803. Kay MMB, Marchalonis JJ, Hughes J, et al. Definition of a physiologic aging autoantigen by using synthetic peptides of membrane protein band 3: Localization of the active antigenic sites. Proc Natl Acad Sci U S A. 1990;87:5734-5738.

804. Kannan R, Labotka R, Low PS. Isolation and characterization of the hemichrome-stabilized membrane protein aggregates from sickle erythrocytes. Major site of autologous antibody binding. J Biol Chem. 1988;263:13766-13773.

805. Turrini F, Mannu F, Arese P, et al. Characterization of the autologous antibodies that opsonize erythrocytes with clustered integral membrane proteins. Blood. 1993;81:3146-3145.

806. Hornig R, Lutz HU. Band 3 protein clustering on human erythrocytes promotes binding of naturally occurring anti–band 3 and anti-spectrin antibodies. Exp Gerontol. 2000;35:1025-1044.

807. Ando K, Kikugawa K, Beppu M. Involvement of sialylated poly-*N*-acetyllactosaminyl sugar chains of band 3 glycoprotein on senescent erythrocytes in anti–

band 3 autoantibody binding. J Biol Chem. 1994;269: 19394-19398.

808. Ando K, Kikugawa K, Beppu M. Induction of band 3 aggregation in erythrocytes results in anti–band 3 autoantibody binding to the carbohydrate epitopes of band 3. Arch Biochem Biophys. 1997;339:250-257.

809. Beppu M, Mizukami A, Nagoya M, Kikugawa K. Binding of anti–band 3 autoantibody to oxidatively damaged erythrocytes. Formation of senescent antigen on erythrocyte surface by an oxidative mechanism. J Biol Chem. 1990;265:3226-3233.

810. Lutz HU, Bussolino F, Flepp R, et al. Naturally occurring anti–band-3 antibodies and complement together mediate phagocytosis of oxidatively stressed human erythrocytes. Proc Natl Acad Sci U S A. 1987;84:7368-7372.

811. Winograd E, Greenan JRT, Sherman IW. Expression of senescent antigen on erythrocytes infected with a knobby variant of the human malaria parasite *Plasmodium falciparum*. Proc Natl Acad Sci U S A. 1987;84:1931-1935.

812. Giribaldi G, Ulliers D, Mannu F, et al. Growth of *Plasmodium falciparum* induces stage-dependent haemichrome formation, oxidative aggregation of band 3, membrane deposition of complement and antibodies, and phagocytosis of parasitized erythrocytes. Br J Haematol. 2001;113:492-499.

813. Lelkes G, Fodor I, Lelkes G, et al. The distribution and aggregatability of intramembrane particles in phenylhydrazine-treated human erythrocytes. Biochim Biophys Acta. 1988;945:105-110.

814. Arese P, Turrini F, Schwarzer E. Band 3/complement-mediated recognition and removal of normally senescent and pathological human erythrocytes. Cell Physiol Biochem. 2005;16:133-146.

815. Khandelwal S, van Rooijen N, Saxena RK. Reduced expression of CD47 during murine red blood cell (RBC) senescence and its role in RBC clearance from the circulation. Transfusion. 2007;47:1725-1732.

816. Gershon H. Is the sequestration of aged erythrocytes mediated by natural autoantibodies? Isr J Med Sci. 1992;28:818-828.

817. Ihanus E, Uotila LM, Toivanen A, et al. Red-cell ICAM-4 is a ligand for the monocyte/macrophage integrin CD11c/CD18: characterization of the binding sites on ICAM-4. Blood. 2007;109:802-810.

818. Toivanen A, Ihanus E, Mattila M, et al. Importance of molecular studies on major blood groups—intercellular adhesion molecule-4, a blood group antigen involved in multiple cellular interactions. Biochim Biophys Acta. 2008;1780:456-466.

819. Herrmann A, Devaux PF. Alteration of the aminophospholipid translocase activity during in vivo and artificial aging of human erythrocytes. Biochim Biophys Acta. 1990;1027:41-46.

820. Kiefer CR, Snyder LM. Oxidation and erythrocyte senescence. Curr Opin Hematol. 2000;7:113-116.

821. Vlassara H, Valinsky J, Brownlee M, et al. Advanced glycosylation end products on erythrocyte cell surface induce receptor mediated phagocytosis by macrophages. A model for turnover of aging cells. J Exp Med. 1987;166:539-549.

822. Barber JR, Clarke S. Membrane protein carboxyl methylation increases with human erythrocyte age. J Biol Chem. 1983;258:1189-1196.

823. Galletti P, Ingrosso D, Nappi A, et al. Increased methyl esterification of membrane proteins in aged red-blood cells. Preferential esterification of ankyrin and band-4.1 cytoskeletal proteins. Eur J Biochem. 1983;135:25-31.

824. Bernassola F, Boumis G, Corazzari M, et al. Osmotic resistance of high-density erythrocytes in transglutaminase 2–deficient mice. Biochem Biophys Res Commun. 2002;291:1123-1127.

825. Vanlair CF, Masius JB: De la microcythemie. Bull R Acad Med Belg. 1871;5:515.

826. Wilson C: Some cases showing hereditary enlargement of the spleen. Trans Clin Soc (London). 1890;23:162.

827. Wilson C, Stanley D: A sequel to some cases showing hereditary enlargement of the spleen. Trans Clin Soc (London). 1893;26:163.

828. Minkowski O: Über eine hereditäre, unter dem Bilde eines chronischen Ikterus mit Urobilinurie, Splenomegalie und Nierensiderosis verlaufende Affektion. Verh Dtsch Kongr Med. 1900;18:316.

829. Chauffard MA: Pathogénie de l'ictère congénital de l'adulte. Semaine Méd (Paris). 1907;27:25.

830. Chauffard MA: Les ictères hémolytiques. Semaine Méd (Paris). 1908;28:49.

831. Dawson of Penn. The Hume Lectures on haemolytic icterus. BMJ. 1931;1:921-928, 963-966.

832. Wintrobe MM: Blood, Pure and Eloquent. New York, McGraw-Hill, 1980.

833. Morton NE, MacKinney AA, Kosower N, et al. Genetics of spherocytosis. Am J Hum Genet. 1962;14:170.

834. Godal HC, Heist H: High prevalence of increased osmotic fragility of red blood cells among Norwegian donors. Scand J Haematol. 1981;27:30.

835. Eber SW, Pekrun A, Neufeldt A, Schroter W. Prevalence of increased osmotic fragility of erythrocytes in German blood donors: Screening using a modified glycerol lysis test. Ann Hematol. 1992;64:88.

836. Kutter D. Hereditary spherocytosis is more frequent than expected: what to tell the patient? Bull Soc Sci Med Grand Duche Luxemb. 2005;1:7-22.

837. Eber SW, Armbrust R, Schröter W: Variable clinical severity of hereditary spherocytosis: Relation to erythrocytic spectrin concentration, osmotic fragility and autohemolysis. J Pediatr. 1990;177:409.

838. Race RR: On the inheritance and linkage relations of acholuric jaundice. Ann Eugenics. 1942;11:365.

839. Miraglia del Giudice E, Lombardi C, Francese M, et al. Frequent de novo monoallelic expression of β-spectrin gene (SPTB) in children with hereditary spherocytosis and isolated spectrin deficiency. Br J Haematol. 1998;101:251.

840. Miraglia del Giudice E, Nobili B, Francese M, et al. Clinical and molecular evaluation of non-dominant hereditary spherocytosis. Br J Haematol. 2001;112:42.

841. Whitfield CF, Follweiler JB, Lopresti-Morrow L, Miller BA. Deficiency of spectrin synthesis in burst-forming units–erythroid in lethal hereditary spherocytosis. Blood. 1991;78:3043.

842. Olim G, Marques S, Saldanha C, et al. Red cell abnormalities in a kindred with an uncommon form of hereditary spherocytosis. Acta Méd Portug. 1984;6:137.

843. Bernard J, Boiron M, Estager J. Une grand famille hémolytique: Trieze cas de maladie de Minkowski-Chauffard observés dans la même fratrie. Semaine Hôp Paris. 1952;28:3741.

844. Duru F, Gurgey, A, Ozturk G, et al. Homozygosity for dominant form of hereditary spherocytosis. Br J Haematol. 1992;82:596.

845. Agre P, Asimos A, Casella JF, McMillan C. Inheritance pattern and clinical response to splenectomy as a reflection of erythrocyte spectrin deficiency in hereditary spherocytosis. N Engl J Med. 1986;315:1579.

846. Perrotta S, Nigro V, Conte ML, et al. Dominant hereditary spherocytosis due to band 3 Neapolis produces a life-threatening anemia at the homozygous state [abstract]. Blood. 1998;92(Suppl):9a.

847. Lux SE, Tse WT, Menninger JC, et al. Hereditary spherocytosis associated with deletion of the human erythrocyte ankyrin gene on chromosome 8. Nature. 1990;345:736.

848. Okamoto N, Wada Y, Nakamura Y, et al. Hereditary spherocytic anemia with deletion of the short arm of chromosome 8. Am J Med Genet. 1995;58:225.

849. Fukushima Y, Byers MG, Watkins PC, et al. Assignment of the gene for β-spectrin (SPTB) to chromosome 14q23-q24.2 by in situ hybridization. Cytogenet Cell Genet. 1990;53:232-233.

850. Walensky LD, Narla M, Lux SE. Disorders of the red cell membrane. In Handin RI, Lux SE, Stossel TP (eds). Blood: Principles and Practice of Hematology, 2nd ed. Philadelphia, JB Lippincott, 2003, pp 1709-1858.

851. Pekrun A, Eber SW, Kuhlmey A, Schroter W. Combined ankyrin and spectrin deficiency in hereditary spherocytosis. Ann Hematol. 1993;67:89.

852. Friedman EW, Williams JC, Van Hook L. Hereditary spherocytosis in the elderly. Am J Med. 1988;84:513.

853. Krueger HC, Burgert EO Jr. Hereditary spherocytosis in 100 children. Mayo Clin Proc. 1966;41:821.

854. MacKinney AA Jr, Morton NE, Kosower NS, Schilling RF. Ascertaining genetic carriers of hereditary spherocytosis by statistical analysis of multiple laboratory tests. J Clin Invest. 1962;41:554.

855. Young LE, Izzo MJ, Platzer RF. Hereditary spherocytosis: I. Clinical, hematologic and genetic features in 28 cases, with particular reference to the osmotic and mechanical fragility of incubated erythrocytes. Blood. 1951;6:1073.

856. Debre R, Lamy M, See G, Schrameck G. Congenital and familial hemolytic disease in children. Am J Dis Child. 1938;56:1189-1192.

857. Diamond LK. Indications for splenectomy in childhood: Results in fifty-two operated cases. Am J Surg. 1938;39:400.

858. Agre P, Casella JF, Zinkham WH, et al. Partial deficiency of erythrocyte spectrin in hereditary spherocytosis. Nature. 1985;314:380.

859. Hanspal M, Yoon SH, Yu H, et al. Molecular basis of spectrin and ankyrin deficiencies in severe hereditary spherocytosis: Evidence implicating a primary defect of ankyrin. Blood. 1991;77:165.

860. Jensson O, Jonasson JL, Magnusson S. Studies on hereditary spherocytosis in Iceland. Acta Med Scand. 1977;201:187.

861. Gehlbach SH, Cooper BA. Haemolytic anaemia in infectious mononucleosis due to inapparent congenital spherocytosis. Scand J Haematol. 1970;7:141.

862. Ho-Yen DO. Hereditary spherocytosis presenting in pregnancy. Acta Haematol (Basel). 1984;72:29-33.

863. Pajor A, Lehoczky D, Szakacs Z. Pregnancy and hereditary spherocytosis: Report of 8 patients and a review. Arch Gynecol Obstet. 1993;253:37.

864. Garwicz S: Atypical spherocytosis, a disease of spleen as well as of red blood cells. Lancet. 1975;1:956.

865. Palek J, Mirevova L, Brabec V. 2,3-Diphosphoglycerate metabolism in hereditary spherocytosis. Br J Haematol. 1969;17:59.

866. Fernandez LA, Erslev AJ. Oxygen affinity and compensated hemolysis in hereditary spherocytosis. J Lab Clin Med. 1972;80:780.

867. Guarnone R, Centenara E, Zappa M, et al. Erythropoietin production and erythropoiesis in compensated and anaemic states of hereditary spherocytosis. Br J Haematol. 1996;92:150.

868. Rocha S, Costa E, Catarino C, et al. Erythropoietin levels in the different clinical forms of hereditary spherocytosis. Br J Haematol. 2005;13:534-542.

869. Tse WT, Gallagher PG, Jenkins PB, et al. Amino-acid substitution in α-spectrin commonly coinherited with nondominant hereditary spherocytosis. Am J Hematol. 1997;54:233.

870. Coetzer TL, Lawler J, Liu S, et al. Partial ankyrin and spectrin deficiency in severe, atypical hereditary spherocytosis. N Engl J Med. 1988;318:230.

871. Agre P, Orringer EP, Bennett V. Deficient red-cell spectrin in severe, recessively inherited spherocytosis. N Engl J Med. 1982;306:1155.

872. Maberry MC, Mason RA, Cunningham FG, Pritchard JA. Pregnancy complicated by hereditary spherocytosis. Obstet Gynecol. 1992;79:735.

873. Delamore IW, Richmond J, Davies SH. Megaloblastic anaemia in congenital spherocytosis. BMJ. 1961;1:543.

874. Kohler HG, Meynell MJ, Cooke WT. Spherocytic anaemia, complicated by megaloblastic anaemia of pregnancy. BMJ. 1960;1:779.

875. Burman D. Congenital spherocytosis in infancy. Arch Dis Child. 1958;33:335.

876. Schröter W, Kahsnitz E. Diagnosis of hereditary spherocytosis in newborn infants. J Pediatr. 1983;103:460.

877. Trucco JI, Brown AK. Neonatal manifestations of hereditary spherocytosis. Am J Dis Child. 1967;113:263.

878. Stamey CC, Diamond LK. Congenital hemolytic anemia in the newborn. Am J Dis Child. 1957;94:616.

879. Saada V, Cynober T, Brossard Y, et al. Incidence of hereditary spherocytosis in a population of jaundiced neonates. Pediatr Hematol Oncol. 2006;23:387-397.

880. Berardi A, Lugli L, Ferrari F, et al. Kernicterus associated with hereditary spherocytosis and UGT1A1 promoter polymorphism. Biol Neonate. 2006;90:243-246.

881. Iolascon A, Faienza MF, Moretti A, et al. UGT1 promoter polymorphism accounts for increased neonatal appearance of hereditary spherocytosis. Blood. 1998;91:1093.

882. Delhommeau F, Cynober T, Schischmanoff PO, et al. Natural history of hereditary spherocytosis during the first year of life. Blood. 2000;95:393.

883. Ribeiro ML, Alloisio N, Almeida H, et al. Severe hereditary spherocytosis and distal renal tubular acidosis associated with the total absence of band 3. Blood. 2000;96:1602.

884. Peters LL, White RA, Birkenmeier CS, et al. Changes in cytoskeletal mRNA expression and protein synthesis during murine erythropoiesis in vivo. Proc Natl Acad Sci U S A. 1992;89:5749-5753.

885. Peters LL, Turtzo C, Birkenmeier CS, Barker JE. Distinct fetal Ank-1 and Ank-2 related proteins and mRNAs in normal and nb/nb mice. Blood 1993;81:2144.

886. Bergstrand CG, Czar B. Serum haptoglobin in infancy. J Clin Lab Invest. 1961;13:576.

887. Erlandson ME, Hilgartner M. Hemolytic disease in the neonatal period and early infancy. J Pediatr. 1959; 54:566.

888. Miraglia del Giudice E, Perrotta S, Lombardi C, Iolascon A. Decision making at the bedside: Diagnosis of hereditary spherocytosis in a transfused infant. Haematologica. 1998;83:347.

889. Tchernia G, Delhommeau F, Perrotta S, et al. Recombinant erythropoietin therapy as an alternative to blood transfusions in infants with hereditary spherocytosis. Hematol J. 2000;1:146.

890. Hosono S, Hosono A, Mugishima H, et al. Successful recombinant erythropoietin therapy for a developing anemic newborn with hereditary spherocytosis. Pediatr Int. 2006;48:178-180.

891. Savvides P, Shalev O, John KM, Lux SE. Combined spectrin and ankyrin deficiency is common in autosomal dominant hereditary spherocytosis. Blood 1993;82: 2953.

892. Chasis JA, Agre PA, Mohandas N. Decreased membrane mechanical stability and in vivo loss of surface area reflect spectrin deficiencies in hereditary spherocytosis. J Clin Invest. 1988;82:617.

893. Waugh RE, Agre P. Reductions of erythrocyte membrane viscoelastic coefficients reflect spectrin deficiencies in hereditary spherocytosis. J Clin Invest. 1988;81: 133.

894. Liu S-C, Derick LH, Agre P, Palek J. Alteration of the erythrocyte membrane skeletal ultrastructure in hereditary spherocytosis, hereditary elliptocytosis, and pyropoikilocytosis. Blood. 1990;76:198.

895. Yawata Y, Kanzaki A, Yawata A. Genotypic and phenotypic expressions of protein 4.2 in human erythroid cells. Gene Funct Dis. 2000;2:61.

896. Premetis E, Stamoulakatou A, Loukopoulos D. Erythropoiesis: hereditary spherocytosis in Greece: collective data on a large number of patients. Hematology. 1999; 4:361.

897. Ricard MP, Gilsanz F, Millan I. Erythroid membrane protein defects in hereditary spherocytosis. A study of 62 Spanish cases. Haematologica. 2000; 85:994.

898. Lanciotti M, Perutelli P, Valetto A, et al. Ankyrin deficiency is the most common defect in dominant and non dominant hereditary spherocytosis. Haematologica. 1997;82:460.

899. Miraglia del Giudice E, Iolascon A, Pinto L, et al. Erythrocyte membrane protein alterations underlying clinical heterogeneity in hereditary spherocytosis. Br J Haematol. 1994;88:52.

900. Yawata Y, Kanzaki A, Yawata A, et al. Characteristic features of the genotype and phenotype of hereditary spherocytosis in the Japanese population. Int J Hematol. 2000;71:118.

901. Lee YK, Cho HI, Park SS, et al. Abnormalities of erythrocyte membrane proteins in Korean patients with hereditary spherocytosis. J Korean Med Sci. 2000;15: 284.

902. Hanspal M, Palek J. Biogenesis of normal and abnormal red blood cell membrane skeletons. Semin Hematol. 1992;29:305.

903. Wichterle H, Hanspal M, Palek J, Jarolim P. Combination of two mutant spectrin alleles underlies a severe spherocytic hemolytic anemia. J Clin Invest. 1996;98: 2300.

904. Basseres DS, Vicentim DL, Costa FF, et al. β-Spectrin Promiss-ao: a translation initiation codon mutation of the β-spectrin gene (ATG→GTG) associated with hereditary spherocytosis and spectrin deficiency in a Brazilian family. Blood. 1998;91:368.

905. Becker PS, Tse WT, Lux SE, Forget BG. Beta spectrin Kissimmee: a spectrin variant associated with autosomal dominant hereditary spherocytosis and defective binding to protein 4.1. J Clin Invest. 1993;92: 612.

906. Wolfe LC, John KM, Falcone JC, et al. A genetic defect in the binding of protein 4.1 to spectrin in a kindred with hereditary spherocytosis. N Engl J Med. 1982;307: 1367.

907. Becker PS, Morrow JS, Lux SE. Abnormal oxidant sensitivity and β-chain structure of spectrin in hereditary spherocytosis associated with defective spectrin–protein 4.1 binding. J Clin Invest. 1987;80:557.

908. Garbarz M, Galand C, Bibas D, et al. A 5 splice region G→C mutation in exon 3 of the human β-spectrin gene leads to decreased levels of α-spectrin mRNA and is responsible for dominant hereditary spherocytosis (spectrin Guemene-Penfao). Br J Haematol. 1998; 100:90.

909. Hassoun H, Vassiliadis JN, Murray J, et al. Hereditary spherocytosis with spectrin deficiency due to an unstable truncated β spectrin. Blood. 1996;87:2538.

910. Hassoun H, Vassiliadis JN, Murray J, et al. Molecular basis of spectrin deficiency in beta-spectrin Durham. A deletion within β spectrin adjacent to the ankyrin-binding site precludes spectrin attachment to the membrane in hereditary spherocytosis. J Clin Invest. 1995;96:2623.

911. Hassoun H, Vassiliadis JN, Murray J, et al. Characterization of the underlying molecular defect in hereditary spherocytosis associated with spectrin deficiency. Blood. 1997;90:398.

912. Dhermy D, Galand C, Bournier O, et al. Hereditary spherocytosis with spectrin deficiency related to null mutations of the β-spectrin gene. Blood Cells Mol Dis. 1998;24:251.

913. Basseres DS, Tavares AC, Acosta FF, et al. Novel β-spectrin variants associated with hereditary spherocytosis. Blood. 1997;90:4b.

914. Woods CM, Lazarides E. Spectrin assembly in avian erythroid development is determined by competing reactions of subunit homo- and hetero-oligomerization. Nature. 1986;321:85.

915. Saad ST, Costa FF, Vicentim DL, Salles TS, Pranke PH. Red cell membrane protein abnormalities in hereditary spherocytosis in Brazil. Br J Haematol. 1994;88:295.

916. Rizk SH, Ibrahim AM, Gafaar TM, et al. Red cell membrane defects and inheritance in 20 Egyptian families with hereditary spherocytosis: Correlation with clinical severity. Cell Vision. 1996;3:137.

917. Chilcote RR, Le Beau MM, Dampier C, et al. Association of red cell spherocytosis with deletion of the short arm of chromosome 8. Blood. 1987;69:156.

918. Cohen H, Walker H, Delhanty JD, et al. Congenital spherocytosis, B19 parvovirus infection and inherited deletion of the short arm of chromosome 8. Br J Haematol. 1991;78:251.

919. Kitatani M, Chiyo H, Ozaki M, et al. Localization of the spherocytosis gene to chromosome segment 8p11.22-8p21.1. Hum Genet. 1988;78:94.

920. Kimberling WJ, Fulbeck T, Dixon L, Lubs HA. Localization of spherocytosis to chromosome 8 or 12 and report of a family with spherocytosis and a reciprocal translocation. Am J Hum Genet. 1975;27:586.

921. Costa FF, Agre P, Watkins PC, et al. Linkage of dominant hereditary spherocytosis to the gene for the erythrocyte membrane-skeleton protein ankyrin. N Engl J Med. 1990;323:1046.

922. Jarolim P, Rubin HL, Brabec V, Palek J. Comparison of the ankyrin (AC)n microsatellites in genomic DNA and mRNA reveals absence of one ankyrin mRNA allele in 20% of patients with hereditary spherocytosis. Blood. 1995;85:3278.

923. Eber SW, Gonzalez JM, Lux ML, et al. Ankyrin-1 mutations are a major cause of dominant and recessive hereditary spherocytosis. Nat Genet. 1996;13:214-218.

924. Leite RC, Basseres DS, Ferreira JS, et al. Low frequency of ankyrin mutations in hereditary spherocytosis: Identification of three novel mutations. Hum Mutat. 2000;16:529.

925. Gallagher PG, Sabatino DE, Basseres DS, et al. Erythrocyte ankyrin promoter mutations associated with recessive hereditary spherocytosis cause significant abnormalities in ankyrin expression. J Biol Chem. 2001;276:41683.

926. Gallagher PG, Ferreira JD, Costa FF, et al. A recurrent frameshift mutation of the ankyrin gene associated with severe hereditary spherocytosis. Br J Haematol. 2000;111:1190.

927. Jarolim P, Rubin HL, Brabec V, et al. Mutations of conserved arginines in the membrane domain of erythroid band 3 lead to a decrease in membrane-associated band 3 and to the phenotype of hereditary spherocytosis. Blood. 1995;85:634.

928. Tanner MJ. Band 3 anion exchanger and its involvement in erythrocyte and kidney disorders. Curr Opin Hematol. 2002;9:133.

929. Jarolim P, Rubin HL, Liu SC, et al. Duplication of 10 nucleotides in the erythroid band 3 (AE1) gene in a kindred with hereditary spherocytosis and band 3 protein deficiency (band 3^PRAGUE). J Clin Invest. 1994;93:121.

930. Dhermy D, Galand C, Bournier O, et al. Heterogenous band 3 deficiency in hereditary spherocytosis related to different band 3 gene defects. Br J Haematol. 1997;98:32.

931. Lima PR, Sales TS, Costa FF, Saad ST. Arginine 490 is a hot spot for mutation in the band 3 gene in hereditary spherocytosis. Eur J Haematol. 1999;63:360.

932. Dhermy D, Burnier O, Bourgeois M, Grandchamp B. The red blood cell band 3 variant (band 3Bicétrel: R490C) associated with dominant hereditary spherocytosis causes defective membrane targeting of the molecule and a dominant negative effect. Mol Membr Biol. 1999;16:305.

933. Quilty JA, Reithmeier RA. Trafficking and folding defects in hereditary spherocytosis mutants of the human red cell anion exchanger. Traffic. 2000;1:987.

934. Jenkins PB, Abou-Alfa GK, Dhermy D, et al. A nonsense mutation in the erythrocyte band 3 gene associated with decreased mRNA accumulation in a kindred with dominant hereditary spherocytosis. J Clin Invest. 1996;97:373.

935. Bianchi P, Zanella A, Alloisio N, et al. A variant of the EPB3 gene of the anti-Lepore type in hereditary spherocytosis. Br J Haematol. 1997;98:283.

936. Bracher NA, Lyons CA, Wessels G, et al. Band 3 Cape Town (E90K) causes severe hereditary spherocytosis in combination with band 3 Prague III. Br J Haematol. 2001;113:689.

937. Alloisio N, Maillet P, Carre G, et al. Hereditary spherocytosis with band 3 deficiency. Association with a nonsense mutation of the band 3 gene (allele Lyon), and aggravation by a low-expression allele occurring in trans (allele Genas). Blood. 1996;88:1062.

938. Alloisio N, Texier P, Vallier A, et al. Modulation of clinical expression and band 3 deficiency in hereditary spherocytosis. Blood. 1997;90:414.

939. Zhang D, Kiyatkin A, Bolin JT, Low PS. Crystallographic structure and functional interpretation of the cytoplasmic domain of erythrocyte membrane band 3. Blood. 2000;96:2925.

940. Low PS, Zhang D, Bolin JT. Localization of mutations leading to altered cell shape and anion transport in the crystal structure of the cytoplasmic domain of band 3. Blood Cells Mol. Dis 2001;27:81.

941. Jarolim P, Murray JL, Rubin HL, et al. Characterization of 13 novel band 3 gene defects in hereditary spherocytosis with band 3 deficiency. Blood. 1996;88:4366.

942. Lima PR, Gontijo JA, Lopes de Faria JB, et al. Band 3 Campinas: A novel splicing mutation in the band 3 gene (AE1) associated with hereditary spherocytosis, hyperactivity of Na^+/Li^+ countertransport and an abnormal renal bicarbonate handling. Blood. 1997;90:2810.

943. Bruce LJ, Cope DL, Jones GK, et al. Familial distal renal tubular acidosis is associated with mutations in the red cell anion exchanger (band 3, AE1) gene. J Clin Invest. 1997;100:1693.

944. Jarolim P, Shayakul C, Prabakaran D, et al. Autosomal dominant distal renal tubular acidosis is associated in three families with heterozygosity for the R589H mutation in the AE1 (band 3) Cl^-/HCO_3^- exchanger. J Biol Chem. 1998;273:6380.

945. Karet FE, Gainza FJ, Györy AZ, et al. Mutations in the chloride-bicarbonate exchanger gene AE1 cause autosomal dominant but not autosomal recessive distal renal tubular acidosis. Proc Natl Acad Sci USA. 1998;95:6337-6342.

946. Toye AM, Bruce LJ, Unwin RJ, et al. Band 3 Walton, a C-terminal deletion associated with distal renal tubular acidosis, is expressed in the red cell membrane but retained internally in kidney cells. Blood. 2002;99:342.

947. Beauchamp-Nicoud A, Morle L, Lutz HU, et al. Heavy transfusions and presence of an anti–protein 4.2 antibody in 4.2(–) hereditary spherocytosis (949delG). Haematologica. 2000;85:19.

948. Perrotta S, Iolascon A, Polito R, et al. 4.2 Nippon mutation in a non-Japanese patient with hereditary spherocytosis. Haematologica. 1999;84:660.

949. Bouhassira EE, Schwartz RS, Yawata Y, et al. An alanine to threonine substitution in protein 4.2 cDNA is associated with a Japanese form of hereditary hemolytic anemia (protein 4.2Nippon). Blood. 1992;79:1846.

950. Rybicki AC, Heath R, Wolf JL, et al. Deficiency of protein 4.2 in erythrocytes from a patient with a Coombs negative hemolytic anemia: Evidence for a role of protein 4.2 in stabilizing ankyrin on the membrane. J Clin Invest. 1988;81:893.

951. Inoue T, Kanzaki A, Yawata A, et al. Electron microscopic and physicochemical studies on disorganization of the cytoskeletal network and integral protein (band 3) in red cells of band 4.2 deficiency with a mutation (codon 142: GCT→ACT). Int J Hematol. 1994;59:157-175.

952. Ideguchi H, Nishimura J, Nawata H, Hamasaki N. A genetic defect of erythrocyte band 4.2 protein associated with hereditary spherocytosis. Br J Haematol. 1990;74:347.

953. Ghanem A, Pothier B, Marechal J, et al. A haemolytic syndrome associated with the complete absence of red cell membrane protein 4.2 in two Tunisian siblings. Br J Haematol. 1990;75:414.

954. Rybicki AC, Qiu JJ, Musto S, et al. Human erythrocyte protein 4.2 deficiency associated with hemolytic anemia and a homozygous ^{40}glutamic acid→lysine substitution in the cytoplasmic domain of band 3 (band 3^{Montefiore}). Blood. 1993;81:2155.

955. Jarolim P, Palek J, Rubin HL, et al. Band 3 Tuscaloosa: Pro^{327}→Arg^{327} substitution in the cytoplasmic domain of erythrocyte band 3 protein associated with spherocytic hemolytic anemia and partial deficiency of protein 4.2. Blood. 1992;80:523.

956. Lux SE. Disorders of the red cell membrane. In Nathan DG, Oski FA (eds). Hematology of Infancy and Childhood, 3rd ed. Philadelphia, WB Saunders, 1987, p 444.

957. Sheehy R, Ralston GB. Abnormal binding of spectrin to the membrane of erythrocytes in some cases of hereditary spherocytosis. Blut. 1978;36:145.

958. Price Evans DA, Mackie MJ, Anand R. Diminished extractable spectrin in the erythrocytes of a patient with "sporadic" hereditary spherocytosis. Acta Haematol. 1986;76:136.

959. Mariani M, Maretzki D, Lutz HU. A tightly membrane-associated subpopulation of spectrin is ^{3}H palmitoylated. J Biol Chem. 1993;268:12996.

960. Allen DW, Cadman S, McCann SR, Finkel B. Increased membrane binding of erythrocyte catalase in hereditary spherocytosis and in metabolically stressed normal cells. Blood. 1977;49:113.

961. Boulard-Heitzmann P, Boulard M, Tallineau C, et al. Decreased red cell enolase activity in a 40-year-old woman with compensated hemolysis. Scand J Haematol. 1984;33:401.

962. Lachant NA, Jennings MA, Tanaka KR. Partial erythrocyte enolase deficiency: A hereditary disorder with variable clinical expression. Blood. 1986;68(Suppl 1):55a.

963. Beutler E, Guinto E, Johnson C. Human red cell protein kinase in normal subjects and patients with hereditary spherocytosis, sickle cell disease, and autoimmune hemolytic anemia. Blood. 1976;48:887.

964. Boivin P, Delaunay J, Galand C. Altered erythrocyte membrane protein phosphorylation in an unusual case of hereditary spherocytosis. Scand J Haematol. 1979;23:251.

965. Wolfe LC, Lux SE. Membrane protein phosphorylation of intact normal and hereditary spherocytic erythrocytes. J Biol Chem. 1978;253:3336.

966. De Gier J, Van Deenen LLM. Phospholipid and fatty acid characteristics of erythrocytes in some cases of anaemia. Br J Haematol. 1964;10:246.

967. Vermeulen WP, Briede JJ, Bunt G, et al. Enhanced Mg^{2+}-ATPase activity in ghosts from HS erythrocytes and in normal ghosts stripped of membrane skeletal proteins may reflect enhanced aminophospholipid translocase activity. Br J Haematol. 1995;90:56.

968. Kuiper PJ, Livne A. Differences in fatty acid composition between normal erythrocytes and hereditary spherocytosis affected cells. Biochim Biophys Acta. 1972;260:755.

969. Zail SS, Pickering A. Fatty acid composition of erythrocytes in hereditary spherocytosis. Br J Haematol. 1979;42:399.

970. Bertles JE. Sodium transport across the surface of red blood cells in hereditary spherocytosis. J Clin Invest. 1957;36:816.

971. Jacob HS, Jandl JH. Cell membrane permeability in the pathogenesis of hereditary spherocytosis (HS). J Clin Invest. 1964;43:1704.

972. Zipursky A, Israels LG. Significance of erythrocyte sodium flux in the pathophysiology and genetic expression of hereditary spherocytosis. Pediatr Res. 1971;5:614.

973. Joiner CH, Franco RS, Jiang M, et al. Increased cation permeability in mutant mouse red cells with defective membrane skeletons. Blood. 1994;86:4307.

974. Wiley JS. Red cell survival in hereditary spherocytosis. J Clin Invest. 1970;49:666.

975. De Franceschi L, Olivieri O, Miraglia del Giudice E, et al. Membrane cation and anion transport activities in erythrocytes of hereditary spherocytosis: Effects of different membrane protein defects. Am J Hematol. 1997;55:121.

976. Vives Corrons JL, Besson I. Red cell membrane Na$^+$ transport systems in hereditary spherocytosis: Relevance to understanding the increased Na$^+$ permeability. Ann Hematol. 2001;80:535.

977. Mayman D, Zipursky A. Hereditary spherocytosis: The metabolism of erythrocytes in the peripheral blood and in the splenic pulp. Br J Haematol. 1974;27:201.

978. De Franceschi L, Rivera A, Fleming MD, et al. Evidence for a protective role of the Gardos channel against hemolysis in murine spherocytosis. Blood. 2005;106:1454-1459.

979. Lauf PK, Adragna NC. K-Cl cotransport: Properties and molecular mechanism. Cell Physiol Biochem. 2000; 10:341.

980. Olivieri O, Bonollo M, Friso S, et al. Activation of K^+/Cl^- cotransport in human erythrocytes exposed to oxidative agents. Biochim Biophys Acta. 1993;1176:37.

981. Loder PB, Babarczy G, de Gruchy GC. Red cell metabolism in hereditary spherocytosis. Br J Haematol. 1967; 13:95.

982. Mohler DN. Adenosine triphosphate metabolism in hereditary spherocytosis. J Clin Invest. 1965;44:1417.

983. Kagimoto T, Hayashi F, Yamasaki M, et al. Phosphorus 31 NMR study on nucleotides and intracellular pH of hereditary spherocytes. Experientia (Basel). 1978;34: 1092.

984. Ideguchi H, Hamasaki N, Ikehara Y. Abnormal phosphoenolpyruvate transport in erythrocytes of hereditary spherocytosis. Blood. 1981;58:426.

985. LeBlond PF, De Boisfleury A, Bessis M. Erythrocytes shape in hereditary spherocytosis. A scanning electron microscopic study and relationship to deformability. Nouv Rev Fr Hematol. 1973;13:873.

986. Cooper RA, Jandl JH. The role of membrane lipids in the survival of red cells in hereditary spherocytosis. J Clin Invest. 1969;48:736.

987. Johnsson R. Red cell membrane proteins and lipids in spherocytosis. Scand J Haematol. 1978;20:341.

988. Langley GR, Feldherhof CH. Atypical autohemolysis in hereditary spherocytosis as a reflection of two cell populations: Relationship of cell lipids to conditioning by the spleen. Blood. 1968;32:569.

989. Reed CF, Swisher SN. Erythrocyte lipid loss in hereditary spherocytosis. J Clin Invest. 1966;45:777.

990. Waugh RE. Effects of inherited membrane abnormalities on the viscoelastic properties of erythrocyte membranes. Biophys J. 1987;51:363.

991. Cooper RA, Jandl JH. The selective and conjoint loss of red cell lipids. J Clin Invest. 1969;48:906.

992. Snyder LM, Lutz HU, Sauberman N, et al. Fragmentation and myelin formation in hereditary xerocytosis and other hemolytic anemias. Blood. 1978;52:750.

993. Weed RI, Bowdler AJ. Metabolic dependence of the critical hemolytic volume of human erythrocytes: Relationship to osmotic fragility and autohemolysis in hereditary spherocytosis and normal red cells. J Clin Invest. 1966;45:1137.

994. Shafizadeh E, Paw BH, Foott H, et al. Characterization of zebrafish merlo/chablis as non-mammalian vertebrate models for severe congenital anemia due to protein 4.1 deficiency. Development. 2002;129:4359-4370.

995. Peters LL, Shivdasani RA, Liu SC, et al. Anion exchanger 1 (band 3) is required to prevent erythrocyte membrane surface loss but not to form the membrane skeleton. Cell. 1996;86:917.

996. Paw BH. Cloning of the zebrafish retsina blood mutation: A genetic model for dyserythropoiesis and erythroid cytokinesis. Blood Cells Mol Dis. 2001; 27:62.

997. Liao EC, Paw PH, Peters LL, et al. Hereditary spherocytosis in zebrafish riesling illustrates evolution of erythroid beta-spectrin structure, and function in red cell morphogenesis and membrane stability. Development. 2000;127:5123-5132.

998. Da Costa L, Mohandas N, Sorette M, et al. Temporal differences in membrane loss lead to distinct reticulocyte features in hereditary spherocytosis and in immune hemolytic anemia. Blood. 2001;98:2894-2899.

999. Liu S-C, Derick LH, Duquette MA, Palek J. Separation of the lipid bilayer from the membrane skeleton during discocyte-echinocyte transformation of human erythrocyte ghosts. Eur J Cell Biol. 1989;49:358.

1000. Zachée P, Boogaerts MA, Hellamans L, Snauwaert J. Adverse role of the spleen in hereditary spherocytosis: Evidence by the use of the atomic force microscope. Br J Haematol. 1992;80:264.

1001. Elgsaeter A, Shotton DM, Branton D. Intramembrane particle aggregation in erythrocyte ghosts: II. The influence of spectrin aggregation. Biochim Biophys Acta. 1976;426:101.

1002. Evans EA, Waugh R, Melnik C. Elastic area compressibility modulus of red cell membranes. Biophys J. 1976;16:585.

1003. Baird R, McPherson AI, Richmond J. Red blood cell survival after splenectomy in congenital spherocytosis. Lancet. 1971;2:1060.

1004. Chapman RG. Red cell life span after splenectomy in hereditary spherocytosis. J Clin Invest. 1968;47:2263.

1005. Barnhart MI, Lusher JM. The human spleen as revealed by scanning electron microscopy. Am J Hematol. 1976; 1:243.

1006. Chen L-T, Weiss L. Electron microscopy of red pulp of human spleen. Am J Anat. 1972;134:425.

1007. Chen L-T, Weiss L. The role of the sinus wall in the passage of erythrocytes through the spleen. Blood. 1973; 41:529.

1008. Weiss L, Tavassoli M. Anatomical hazards to the passage of erythrocytes through the spleen. Semin Hematol. 1970;7:372.

1009. Weiss L. A scanning electron microscopic study of the spleen. Blood. 1974;43:665.

1010. Groom AC. Microcirculation of the spleen: New concepts, new challenges. Microvasc Res. 1987;34:269.

1011. Johnsson R, Vuopio P. Studies on red cell flexibility in spherocytosis using a polycarbonate membrane filtration method. Acta Haematol. 1978;60:329.

1012. Murphy JR. The influence of pH and temperature on some physical properties of normal erythrocytes and erythrocytes from patients with hereditary spherocytosis. J Lab Clin Med. 1967;69:758.

1013. Young LE, Platzer RF, Ervin DM, Izzo MJ. Hereditary spherocytosis: II. Observations on the role of the spleen. Blood. 1951;6:1099.

1014. Ferreira JA, Feliu E, Rozman C, et al. Morphologic and morphometric light and electron microscopic studies of the spleen in patients with hereditary spherocytosis and autoimmune haemolytic anaemia. Br J Haematol. 1989;72:246.

1015. Molnar Z, Rappaport H. Fine structure of the red pulp of the spleen in hereditary spherocytosis. Blood. 1972; 39:81.

1016. Wiland OK, Smith EB. The morphology of the spleen in congenital hemolytic anemia (hereditary spherocytosis). Am J Clin Pathol. 1956;26:619.

1017. Fujita T, Kashimura M, Adachi K. Scanning electron microscopy (SEM) studies of the spleen—normal and pathological. Scan Electron Microsc. 1982;1:435.

1018. Banti G: Splenomegalie hemolytique au hemopoietique: Le role de la rate dans l'hemolyse. Sémaine Med. 1913; 33:313.

1019. MacAdam W, Shiskin C. The cholesterol content of the blood in anaemia and its relation to splenic function. Q J Med. 1922;16:193.

1020. Emerson CP Jr, Shen SC, Ham TH, et al. Studies on the destruction of red blood cells: IX. Quantitative methods for determining the osmotic and mechanical fragility of red cells in the peripheral blood and splenic pulp; the mechanism of increased hemolysis in hereditary spherocytosis (congenital hemolytic jaundice) as related to the function of the spleen. Arch Intern Med. 1956;97:1.

1021. Dacie JV. Familial haemolytic anaemia (acholuric jaundice), with particular reference to changes in fragility produced by splenectomy. Q J Med (New Series) 1943;12:101.

1022. Griggs RC, Weisman R Jr, Harris JW. Alterations in osmotic and mechanical fragility related to in vivo erythrocyte aging and splenic sequestration in hereditary spherocytosis. J Clin Invest. 1960;39:89.

1023. MacPherson AIS, Richmond J, Donaldson GW, Muir AR. The role of the spleen in congenital spherocytosis. Am J Med. 1971;50:35.

1024. Jandl JH, Aster RH. Increased splenic pooling and the pathogenesis of hypersplenism. Am J Med Sci. 1967; 253:383.

1025. LaCelle PL. pH in the mouse spleen and its effect on erythrocyte flow properties. Blood. 1974;44(Suppl 1): 910.

1026. Minakami S, Yoshikawa HL. Studies on erythrocyte glycolysis: III. The effects of active cation transport, pH and inorganic phosphate concentration on erythrocyte glycolysis. J Biochem (Tokyo). 1966;59:145.

1027. Rakitzis ET, Mills GC. Relation of red cell hexokinase activity to extracellular pH. Biochim Biophys Acta. 1967;141:439.

1028. Parker JC. Ouabain-insensitive effects of metabolism on ion and water content in red blood cells. Am J Physiol. 1971;221:338.

1029. Ingrosso D, D'Angelo S, Perrotta S, et al. Cytoskeletal behaviour in spectrin and in band 3 deficient spherocytic red cells: Evidence for differentiated splenic conditioning role. Br J Haematol. 1996;93:38.

1030. Dacie JV. Observations on autohemolysis in familial acholuric jaundice. J Pathol Bacteriol. 1941;52:331.

1031. Ferrant A, Leners N, Michaux JL, et al. The spleen and haemolysis: Evaluation of the intrasplenic transit time. Br J Haematol. 1987;65:331.

1032. Motulsky AG, Casserd F, Giblett R, et al. Anemia and the spleen. N Engl J Med 1958;259:1215-1219.

1033. Prankerd TAJ. Studies on the pathogenesis of haemolysis in hereditary spherocytosis. Q J Med. 1960;24: 199.

1034. Maridonneau I, Braquet P, Garay RP. Na$^+$ and K$^+$ transport damage induced by oxygen free radicals in human red cell membranes. J Biol Chem. 1983;258:3107.

1035. Orringer EP, Parker JC. Selective increase of potassium permeability in red blood cells exposed to acetylphenylhydrazine. Blood. 1977;50:1013.

1036. Orringer EP. A further characterization of the selective K movements observed in human red blood cells following acetylphenylhydrazine exposure. Am J Hematol. 1984;16:355.

1037. Snyder LM, Fortier NL, Trainor J, et al. Effect of hydrogen peroxide exposure on normal human erythrocyte deformability, morphology, surface characteristics and spectrin hemoglobin crosslinking. J Clin Invest. 1985; 76:1971.

1038. Beppu M, Mizukami A, Nagoya M, Kikugawa K. Binding of anti–band 3 autoantibody to oxidatively damaged erythrocytes: Formation of senescent antigen on erythrocyte surface by an oxidative mechanism. J Biol Chem. 1990;265:3226.

1039. Lutz HU, Bussolino F, Flepp R, et al. Naturally occurring anti–band-3 antibodies and complement together mediate phagocytosis of oxidatively stressed human erythrocytes. Proc Natl Acad Sci U S A. 1987;84:7368.

1040. Becker PS, Cohen CM, Lux SE. The effect of mild diamide oxidation on the structure and function of human erythrocyte spectrin. J Biol Chem. 1986;261: 4620.

1041. Caprari P, Bozzi A, Ferroni L, et al. Oxidative erythrocyte membrane damage in hereditary spherocytosis. Biochem Int. 1992;26:265.

1042. Platt OS, Falcone JF. Membrane protein lesions in erythrocytes with Heinz bodies. J Clin Invest. 1988;82: 1051.

1043. Schwartz RS, Rybicki AC, Heath RH, Lubin BH. Protein 4.1 in sickle erythrocytes. Evidence for oxidative damage. J Biol Chem. 1987;62:15666.

1044. Malorni W, Iosi F, Donelli G, et al. A new, striking morphologic feature for the human erythrocyte in hereditary spherocytosis: The blebbing pattern. Blood. 1993;81: 2821.

1045. De Matteis MC, De Angelis V, Sorrentino F, et al. Role of spleen in hereditary spherocytosis: Evidence for increased in vitro proteolysis of red cell membrane. Br J Haematol. 1991;79:108.

1046. Szymanski IO, Odgren PR, Fortier NL, Snyder LM. Red blood cell associated IgG in normal and pathologic states. Blood. 1980;55:48.

1047. Coleman DH, Finch CA. Effect of adrenal steroids in hereditary spherocytic anemia. J Lab Clin Med. 1956;47: 602.

1048. Duru F, Gürgey A. Effect of corticosteroids in hereditary spherocytosis. Acta Paediatr Jpn. 1994;36:666.

1049. Atkinson JP, Schreiber AS, Frank MM. Effects of corticosteroids and splenectomy on the immune clearance and destruction of erythrocytes. J Clin Invest. 1973;52: 1509.

1050. Schreiber AD, Parsons J, McDermott P, Cooper RA. Effect of corticosteroids on the human monocyte IgG and complement receptors. J Clin Invest. 1975;56: 1189.

1051. Matsumoto N, Ishihara T, Shibata M, et al. Electron microscopic studies of the spleen and liver in hereditary spherocytosis. Acta Pathol Jpn. 1973;23:507.

1052. Bowman HS, Oski FA. Splenic macrophage interaction with red cells in pyruvate kinase deficiency and hereditary spherocytosis. Vox Sang. 1970;19:168.

1053. Watson CJ. Studies of urobilinogen. III. The per diem excretion of urobilinogen in the common forms of jaundice and disease of the liver. Arch Intern Med. 1937; 59:206.

1054. Sears DA, Anderson RP, Foy AL, et al. Urinary iron excretion and renal metabolism of hemoglobin in hemolytic disease. Blood. 1966;28:708.

1055. Muller-Eberhard U, Javid J, Liem HH, et al. Plasma concentrations of hemopexin, haptoglobin and heme in patients with various hemolytic diseases. Blood. 1968; 32:811.

1056. Palek J, Sahr KE. Mutations of the red blood cell membrane proteins: from clinical evaluation to detection of the underlying genetic defect. Blood. 1992;80:308.

1057. Hayette S, Morle L, Bozon M, et al. A point mutation in the protein 4.2 gene (allele 4.2 Tozeur) associated with hereditary haemolytic anaemia. Br J Haematol. 1995; 89:762.

1058. Maizels M. The anion and cation content of normal and anaemic bloods. Biochem J. 1936;30:821.

1059. Selwyn JG, Dacie JV. Autohemolysis and other changes resulting from the incubation in vitro of red cells from patients with congenital hemolytic anemia. Blood. 1954; 9:414.

1060. Mohandas N, Kim YR, Tycko DH, et al. Accurate and independent measurement of volume and hemoglobin concentration of individual red cells by laser light scattering. Blood. 1986;68:506.

1061. Michaels LA, Cohen AR, Zhao H, et al. Screening for hereditary spherocytosis by use of automated erythrocyte indexes. J Pediatr. 1997;130:957.

1062. Ricard MP, Gilsanz F. Assessment of the severity of hereditary spherocytosis using routine haematological data obtained with dual angle laser scattering cytometry. Clin Lab Haematol. 1996;18:75.

1063. Gilsanz F, Ricard MP, Millan I. Diagnosis of hereditary spherocytosis with dual-angle differential light scattering. Am J Clin Pathol. 1993;100:119.

1064. Pati AR, Patton WN, Harris RI. The use of the Technicon H1 in the diagnosis of hereditary spherocytosis. Clin Lab Haematol. 1989;11:27.

1065. Cynober T, Mohandas N, Tchernia G. Red cell abnormalities in hereditary spherocytosis: relevance to diagnosis and understanding variable expression of clinical severity. J Lab Clin Med. 1996;128:259.

1066. Parpart AK, Lorenz PB, Parpart ER, et al. The osmotic resistance (fragility) of human red cells. J Clin Invest. 1947;26:636.

1067. Godal HC, Nyvold N, Russtad A. The osmotic fragility of red blood cells: A re-evaluation of technical conditions. Scand J Haematol. 1979;23:55.

1068. Young LE. Observations on inheritance and heterogeneity of chronic spherocytosis. Trans Assoc Am Physicians. 1955;68:141.

1069. Zanella A, Izzo C, Rebulla P, et al. Acidified glycerol lysis test: A screening test for spherocytosis. Br J Haematol. 1980;45:481.

1070. Zanella A, Milani S, Fagnani G, et al. Diagnostic value of the glycerol lysis test. J Lab Clin Med. 1983; 102:743.

1071. Rutherford CJ, Postlewaight BF, Hallowes M. An evaluation of the acidified glycerol lysis test. Br J Haematol. 1986;63:119.

1072. Bucx MJ, Breed WP, Hoffman JJ. Comparison of acidified glycerol lysis test, Pink test and osmotic fragility test in hereditary spherocytosis: Effect of incubation. Eur J Haematol. 1988;40:227.

1073. Hoffmann JJ, Swaak-Lammers N, Breed WP, Strengers JL. Diagnostic utility of the pre-incubated acidified glycerol lysis test in haemolytic and non-haemolytic anaemias. Eur J Haematol. 1991;47: 367.

1074. Marik T, Brabec V. Acidified glycerol lysis test in various haemolytic anaemias. Folia Haematol Int Mag Klin Morphol Blutforsch. 1990;117:259.

1075. Vettore L, Zanella A, Molaro GL, et al. A new test for the laboratory diagnosis of spherocytosis. Acta Haematol (Basel). 1984;72:258.

1076. Sureda-Balari A, Villarrvoia-Espinosa J, Fernandez-Fuertes I. A new modification of the "Pink test" for the diagnosis of hereditary spherocytosis. Acta Haematol. 1989;82:213.

1077. Pinto L, Iolascon A, Miraglia del Giudice E, Nobili B. A modification of the "Pink test" may improve the diagnosis of hereditary spherocytosis. Acta Haematol. 1989; 82:53.

1078. Iglauer A, Reinhardt D, Schröter W, Pekrun A. Cryohemolysis test as a diagnostic tool for hereditary spherocytosis. Ann Hematol. 1999;78:555-557.

1079. Streichman S, Gescheidt Y. Cryohemolysis for the detection of hereditary spherocytosis: Correlation studies with osmotic fragility and autohemolysis. Am J Hematol. 1998;58:206.

1080. Young LE, Izzo MJ, Swisher SN, Young LE. Studies on spontaneous in vitro autohemolysis in hemolytic disorders. Blood. 1956;11:977.

1081. Chasis JA, Mohandas N. Erythrocyte membrane deformability and stability: two distinct membrane properties that are independently regulated by skeletal protein interactions. J Cell Biol. 1986;103:343.

1082. Mohandas N, Clark MR, Health BP, et al. A technique to detect reduced mechanical stability of red cell membranes: Relevance to elliptocytic disorders. Blood. 1982;59:768.

1083. Mohandas N, Clark MR, Jacobs MS, Shohet SB. Analysis of factors regulating erythrocyte deformability. J Clin Invest. 1980;66:563.

1084. Clark MR, Mohandas N, Shohet SB. Osmotic gradient ektacytometry: comprehensive characterization of red cell volume and surface maintenance. Blood. 1983; 61:899.

1085. Johnson RM, Ravindranath Y. Osmotic scan ektacytometry in clinical diagnosis. J Pediatr Hematol Oncol. 1996;18:122.

1086. Zipursky A, Chintu C, Brown E, Brown EJ. The quantitation of spherocytes in ABO hemolytic disease. J Pediatr. 1979;94:965.

1087. Gilliland BC, Baxter E, Evans RS. Red cell antibodies in acquired hemolytic anemia with negative antiglobulin serum tests. N Engl J Med. 1971;85:252.

1088. Crosby WH, Conrad ME. Hereditary spherocytosis: Observations on hemolytic mechanisms and iron metabolism. Blood. 1960;15:662.

1089. Blecher TE. What happens to the microspherocytosis of hereditary spherocytosis in folate deficiency? Clin Lab Haematol. 1988;10:403.

1090. Pautard B, Feo C, Dhermy D, et al. Occurrence of hereditary spherocytosis and beta thalassaemia in the same family: globin chain synthesis and visco diffractometric studies. Br J Haematol. 1988;70:239-245.

1091. Warkentin TE, Barr RD, Ali MA, Mohandas N. Recurrent acute splenic sequestration crisis due to interacting genetic defects: Hemoglobin SC disease and hereditary spherocytosis. Blood. 1990;75:266.

1092. Aksoy M, Erdem S. The combination of hereditary spherocytosis and heterozygous beta-thalassaemia: a family study. Acta Haematol. 1968;39:183-191.

1093. White BP, Farver M. Coexistence of hereditary spherocytosis and beta-thalassemia: Case report of severe hemolytic anemia in an American black. S D J Med. 1991;44:257-261.

1094. Miraglia del Giudice E, Perrotta S, Nobili B, et al. Coexistence of hereditary spherocytosis (HS) due to band 3 deficiency and beta-thalassaemia trait: partial correction of HS phenotype. Br J Haematol. 1993;85:553-557.

1095. Vicari P, Arantes AM, Figueiredo MS. Sickle cell trait associated with hereditary spherocytosis: a potentially life-threatening coexistence. Acta Haematol. 2003; 110:223.

1096. Ustun C, Kutlar F, Holley L, et al. Interaction of sickle cell trait with hereditary spherocytosis: splenic infarcts and sequestration. Acta Haematol. 2003;109:46-49.

1097. Yang YM, Donnell C, Wilborn W, et al. Splenic sequestration associated with sickle cell trait and hereditary spherocytosis. Am J Hematol. 1992;40:110.

1098. Babiker MA, El Seed FA. A family with sickle cell trait and hereditary spherocytosis. Scand J Haematol. 1984;33:54.

1099. Gairdner D. The association of gall-stones with acholuric jaundice in children. Arch Dis Child. 1939;14:109.

1100. Bates GC, Brown CH. Incidence of gallbladder disease in chronic hemolytic anemia (spherocytosis). Gastroenterology. 1952;21:104.

1101. Mentzer SH. Clinical and pathologic study of cholecystitis and cholelithiasis. Surg Gynecol Obstet. 1926; 42:782.

1102. del Giudice EM, Perrotta S, Nobili B, et al. Coinheritance of Gilbert syndrome increases the risk for developing gallstones in patients with hereditary spherocytosis. Blood. 1999;94:2259.

1103. Sharma S, Vukelja SJ, Kadakia S. Gilbert's syndrome co-existing with and masking hereditary spherocytosis. Ann Hematol. 1997;74:287.

1104. Katz ME, Weinstein IM. Extreme hyperbilirubinemia in a patient with hereditary spherocytosis, Gilbert's syndrome, and obstructive jaundice. Am J Med Sci. 1978;275:373.

1105. Economou M, Tsatra I, Athanassiou-Metaxa M. Simultaneous presence of Gilbert syndrome and hereditary spherocytosis: interaction in the pathogenesis of hyperbilirubinemia and gallstone formation. Pediatr Hematol Oncol. 2003;20:493-495.

1106. Tamary H, Aviner S, Freud E, et al. High incidence of early cholelithiasis detected by ultrasonography in children and young adults with hereditary spherocytosis. J Pediatr Hematol Oncol. 2003;25:952-954.

1107. Lawrie GM, Ham JM. The surgical treatment of hereditary spherocytosis. Surg Gynecol Obstet. 1974;139: 208.

1108. MacKinney AA Jr. Hereditary spherocytosis. Clinical family studies. Arch Intern Med. 1965;116:257.

1109. Ransohoff DF, Gracie WA. Treatment of gallstones. Ann Intern Med. 1993;119:606.

1110. Pappis CH, Galanakis S, Moussatos G, et al. Experience of splenectomy and cholecystectomy in children with chronic haemolytic anemia. J Pediatr Surg. 1989;24: 543.

1111. Marchetti M, Quaglini S, Barosi G. Prophylactic splenectomy and cholecystectomy in mild hereditary spherocytosis: analyzing the decision in different clinical scenarios. J Intern Med. 1998;24:217-226.

1112. Tissieres P, Kernen Y, Gervaix A, et al. Varicella zoster virus induced haemolytic crisis in a child with congenital spherocytosis. Eur J Pediatr. 2000;159:788.

1113. Brown KE. Haematological consequences of parvovirus B19 infection. Baillieres Best Pract Res Clin Haematol. 2000;13:245.

1114. Cherry JD. Parvovirus infections in children and adults. Adv Pediatr. 1999;46:245.

1115. Owren PA. Congenital hemolytic jaundice. The pathogenesis of the hemolytic crisis. Blood. 1948;3:231.

1116. Lefrére JJ, Courouce AM, Bertrand Y, et al. Human parvovirus and aplastic crisis in chronic hemolytic anemias: A study of 24 observations. Am J Hematol. 1986;23:271.

1117. Mortimer PP, Humphries RK, Moore JG, et al. A human parvovirus-like virus inhibits haematopoietic colony formation in vitro. Nature. 1983;302:426.

1118. Ozawa K, Kurtzman G, Young N. Replication of the B19 parvovirus in human bone marrow cell cultures. Science. 1986;233:883.

1119. Yaegashi N, Niinuma T, Chisaka H, et al. Parvovirus B19 infection induces apoptosis of erythroid cells in vitro and in vivo. J Infect. 1999;39:68.

1120. Morita E, Tada K, Chisaka H, et al. Human parvovirus B19 induces cell cycle arrest at G_2 phase with accumulation of mitotic cyclins. J Virol. 2001;75:7555.

1121. Hanada T, Koike K, Takeya T, et al. Human parvovirus B19–induced transient pancytopenia in a child with hereditary spherocytosis. Br J Haematol. 1988;70:113.

1122. Saunders PW, Reid MM, Cohen BJ. Human parvovirus induced cytopenias: A report of five cases. Br J Haematol. 1986;53:407.

1123. Goss GA, Szer J. Pancytopenia following infection with human parvovirus B19 as a presenting feature of hereditary spherocytosis in two siblings. Aust N Z J Med. 1997;27:86.

1124. Robins MM. Familial crisis in hereditary spherocytosis: Report of six affected siblings. Clin Pediatr (Phila). 1965;4:210.

1125. Skinnider LF, McSheffrey BJ, Sheridan D, Deneer H. Congenital spherocytic hemolytic anemia in a family presenting with transient red cell aplasia from parvovirus B19 infection. Am J Hematol. 1998;58:341.

1126. Murphy PT, O'Donnell JR. B19 parvovirus infection causing aplastic crisis in 3 out of 5 family members with hereditary spherocytosis. Ir J Med Sci. 1990;159: 182.

1127. Green DH, Bellingham AJ, Anderson MJ. Parvovirus infection in a family associated with aplastic crisis in an affected sibling pair with hereditary spherocytosis. J Clin Pathol. 1984;37:1144.

1128. Sahara N, Tamashima S, Ihara M. Hereditary spherocytosis associated with severe hypophosphatemia in patients recovering from aplastic crisis. Rinsho Ketsueki. 1998;39: 386-391.

1129. von Kaisenberg CS, Jonat W. Fetal parvovirus B19 infection. Ultrasound Obstet Gynecol. 2001;18:280.

1130. Markenson GR, Yancey MK. Parvovirus B19 infections in pregnancy. Semin Perinatol. 1998;22:309.

1131. Rodis JF. Parvovirus infection. Clin Obstet Gynecol. 1999;42:107.

1132. Bell LM, Nasides SJ, Stoffman P, et al. Human parvovirus B19 infection among hospital staff members after contact with infected patients. N Engl J Med 1989;321:485.

1133. Brown KE, Young NS. Epidemiology and pathology of erythroviruses. Contrib Microbiol. 2000;4:107.

1134. Valeur-Jensen AK, Pedersen CB, Westergaard P, et al. Risk factors for parvovirus B19 infection in pregnancy. JAMA. 1999;281:1099.

1135. Rodis JF, Borgida AF, Wilson M, et al. Management of parvovirus infection in pregnancy and outcomes of hydrops: A survey of members of the Society of Perinatal Obstetricians. Am J Obstet Gynecol. 1998;179:985.

1136. Ng JP, Cumming RL, Horn EH, Hogg RB. Hereditary spherocytosis revealed by human parvovirus infection. Br J Haematol. 1987;65:379.

1137. Summerfield GP, Wyatt GP. Human parvovirus infection revealing hereditary spherocytosis. Lancet. 1985;2:1070.

1138. McLellan NJ, Rutter N. Hereditary spherocytosis in sisters unmasked by parvovirus infection. Postgrad Med J. 1987;63:49.

1139. Stefanelli M, Barosi G, Cazzola M, Orlandi E. Quantitative assessment of erythropoiesis in haemolytic disease. Br J Haematol. 1980;45:297.

1140. Ozawa K, Kurtzman G, Young N. Productive infection by B19 parvovirus of human erythroid bone marrow cells in vitro. Blood. 1987;70:384.

1141. Koduri PR. Novel cytomorphology of the giant proerythroblasts of parvovirus B19 infection. Am J Hematol. 1998;58:95.

1142. Tileston W. Hemolytic jaundice. Medicine (Baltimore). 1922;1:355.

1143. Hanford RB, Schneider GF, MacCarthy JD. Massive thoracic extramedullary hemopoiesis. N Engl J Med. 1960;263:120.

1144. Lawrence P, Aronson I, Saxe N, Jacobs P. Leg ulcers in hereditary spherocytosis. Clin Exp Dermatol. 1991;16:28.

1145. Giraldi S, Abbage KT, Marinoni LP, et al. Leg ulcer in hereditary spherocytosis. Pediatr Dermatol. 2003;20:427-428.

1146. Beinhauer LG, Gruhn JG. Dermatologic aspects of congenital spherocytic anemia. Arch Dermatol. 1957;75:642.

1147. Leverkus M, Schwaaf A, Brocker EB, et al. Recurrent hemolysis-associated pseudoerysipelas of the lower legs in a patients with congenital spherocytosis. J Am Acad Dermatol. 2004;51:1019-1023.

1148. Abe T, Yachi A, Ishii Y, et al. Thoracic extramedullary hematopoiesis associated with hereditary spherocytosis. Intern Med. 1992;31:1151.

1149. Martin J, Palacio A, Petit J, Martin C. Fatty transformation of thoracic extramedullary hematopoiesis following splenectomy: CT features. J Comput Assist Tomogr. 1990;14:477.

1150. Pulsoni A, Ferrazza G, Malagnino F, et al. Mediastinal extramedullary hematopoiesis as first manifestation of hereditary spherocytosis. Ann Hematol. 1992;65:196.

1151. Xiros N, Economopoulos T, Papageorgiou E, et al. Massive hemothorax due to intrathoracic extramedullary hematopoiesis in a patient with hereditary spherocytosis. Ann Hematol. 2001;80:38.

1152. Kugler D, Jager D, Barth J. A patient with pancreatitis, anaemia and an intrathoracic tumor. Diagnosis: tumour-simulating asymptomatic intrathoracic extramedullary haematopoiesis (EMH) in a patient with hereditary spherocytosis. Eur Respir J. 2006;27:856-859.

1153. Jalbert F, Chaynes P, Lagarrigue J. Asymptomatic spherocytosis presenting with spinal cord compression: case report. J Neurosurg Spine. 2005;2:491-494.

1154. Calhoun SK, Murphy RC, Shariati N, Jacir N, Bergman K. Extramedullary hematopoiesis in a child with hereditary spherocytosis: An uncommon cause of an adrenal mass. Pediatr Radiol. 2001;31:879.

1155. Pietsch B, Sigmund G, Wurtemberger G. Nuclear spin tomographic findings in compensated chronic hemolysis. A case report of a hereditary spherocytosis. Aktuelle Radiol. 1993;3:266.

1156. Schafer AI, Miller JB, Lester EP, et al. Monoclonal gammopathy in hereditary spherocytosis: A possible pathogenic relation. Ann Intern Med. 1978;88:45.

1157. Fukata S, Tamai H, Nagai K, et al. A patient with hereditary spherocytosis and silicosis who developed an IgA (lambda) monoclonal gammopathy. Jpn J Med. 1987;26:81.

1158. Lempert KD. Gammopathy and spherocytosis. Ann Intern Med. 1978;89:145.

1159. Martinez-Climent JA, Lopez-Andreu JA, Ferris-Tortajada J, et al. Acute lymphoblastic leukaemia in a child with hereditary spherocytosis. Eur J Pediatr. 1995;154:753.

1160. Jandl JH, Files NM, Barnett SB, MacDonald RA. Proliferative response of the spleen and liver to hemolysis. J Exp Med. 1965;122:299.

1161. Isobe T, Osserman EF. Pathologic conditions associated with plasma cell dyscrasias: A study of 806 cases. Ann N Y Acad Sci. 1971;190:507.

1162. Blacklock HA, Meerkin M. Serum ferritin in patients with hereditary spherocytosis. Br J Haematol. 1981;49:117.

1163. Edwards CQ, Skolnick MH, Dadone MM, Kushner JP. Iron overload in hereditary spherocytosis: Association with HLA-linked hemochromatosis. Am J Hematol. 1982;13:101.

1164. Fargion S, Cappellini MD, Piperno A, et al. Association of hereditary spherocytosis and idiopathic hemochromatosis: A synergistic effect in determining iron overload. Am J Clin Pathol. 1986;86:645.

1165. Mohler DN, Wheby MS. Hemochromatosis heterozygotes may have significant iron overload when they also have hereditary spherocytosis. Am J Med Sci. 1986;292:320.

1166. Morita M, Hashizume M, Kanematsu T, et al. Hereditary spherocytosis with congestive heart failure: Report of a case. Surg Today. 1993;23:458.

1167. Clarkson JG, Altman RD. Angioid streaks. Surv Ophthalmol. 1982;26:235.

1168. McLane NJ, Grizzard WS, Kousseff BG, et al. Angioid streaks associated with hereditary spherocytosis. Am J Ophthamol. 1984;97:444.

1169. Gibson JM, Chaudhuri PR, Rosenthal AR. Angioid streaks in a case of beta thalassemia major. Br J Ophthalmol. 1983;67:29.

1170. Deutman AF, Kovacs B. Argon laser treatment in complications of angioid streaks. Am J Ophthalmol. 1979;88:12.

1171. Alani FS, Dyer T, Hindle E, et al. Pseudohyperkalemia associated with hereditary spherocytosis in four members of a family. Postgrad Med J. 1994;70:749-751.

1172. Berne JD, Asensio JA, Falabella A, et al. Traumatic rupture of the spleen in a patient with hereditary spherocytosis. J Trauma. 1997;42:323-326.

1173. d'Eramo N, Levi M. Neurological symptoms in anemia. In Neurological Symptoms in Blood Diseases. Baltimore, University Park Press, 1972, p 1.

1174. Curshmann H. Über funikuläre Myelose bei hämolytischem Ikterus. Dtsch A Nervenheilkd 1931;122:119.

1175. Dumolard C, Sarrovy C, Portier A. Ataxie cerebelleuse associée à un syndrome de splenomegalie chronique avec anemie. Bull Soc Med Hop (Paris). 1938;54:71.

1176. Lemaire A, Dumolard A, Portici A. Deux cas familiaux de maladie de Friedreich avec maladie hemolytique chez des indigenes Algeriens. Bull Soc Med Hop (Paris). 1937;53:1084.

1177. Peters LL, Birkenmeier CS, Bronson RT, et al. Purkinje cell degeneration associated with erythroid ankyrin deficiency in nb/nb mice. J Cell Biol. 1991;114:1233.

1178. Moiseyev VS, Korovina EA, Polotskaya EL, et al. Hypertrophic cardiomyopathy associated with hereditary spherocytosis in three generations of one family. Lancet. 1987;2:853.

1179. Spencer SE, Walker FO, Moore SA. Chorea-amyotrophy with chronic hemolytic anemia: a variant of chorea-amyotrophy with acanthocytosis. Neurology. 1987;37:645.

1180. Reliene R, Mariani M, Zanella A, et al. Splenectomy prolongs in vivo survival of erythrocytes differently in spectrin/ankyrin- and band 3–deficient hereditary spherocytosis. Blood. 2002;100:2208.

1181. Green JB, Shackford SR, Sise MJ, Fridlund P. Late septic complications in adults following splenectomy for trauma: A prospective analysis in 144 patients. J Trauma. 1986;26:999.

1182. Evans DI. Postsplenectomy sepsis 10 years or more after operation. J Clin Pathol. 1985;38:309.

1183. Holdsworth RJ, Irving AD, Cuschieri A. Postsplenectomy sepsis and its mortality rate: actual versus perceived risks. Br J Surg. 1991;78:1031.

1184. Schwartz PE, Serioff S, Mucha P, et al. Postsplenectomy sepsis and mortality in adults. JAMA. 1982;248:2279.

1185. Schilling RF. Estimating the risk for sepsis after splenectomy in hereditary spherocytosis. Ann Intern Med. 1995;122:187.

1186. Eraklis AJ, Filler RM. Splenectomy in childhood: A review of 1413 cases. J Pediatr Surg. 1972;7:382.

1187. Schilling, RJ. Estimating the risk of sepsis after splenectomy in hereditary spherocytosis. Ann Intern Med. 1995;122:187-188.

1188. Waghorn DJ, Mayon-White RT. A study of 42 episodes of overwhelming post-splenectomy infection: is current guidance for asplenic individuals being followed? J Infect. 1997;35:289.

1189. Hansen K, Singer DB. Asplenic-hyposplenic overwhelming sepsis: Postsplenectomy sepsis revisited. Pediatr Dev Pathol. 2001;4:105.

1190. Pederson FK. Postsplenectomy infections in Danish children splenectomized 1969-1978. Acta Paediatr Scand. 1983;72:589.

1191. Posey DL, Marks C. Overwhelming postsplenectomy sepsis in childhood. Am J Surg. 1983;145:318.

1192. Chaikof EL, McCabe CJ. Fatal overwhelming postsplenectomy infection. Am J Surg. 1985;149:534.

1193. Waghorn DJ. Overwhelming infection in asplenic patients: current best practice preventive measures are not being followed. J Clin Pathol. 2001;54:214-218.

1194. Mathewson HO, Anderson AE, Hazard GW. Self-limited babesiosis in a splenectomized child. Pediatr Infect Dis. 1984;3:148-149.

1195. Mylonakis E. When to suspect and how to monitor babesiosis. Am Fam Physician. 2001;63:1969-1974.

1196. White DJ, Talarico J, Chang HG, et al. Human babesiosis in New York State: review of 139 hospitalized cases and analysis of prognostic factors. Arch Intern Med. 1998;158:2149-2154.

1197. Bach O, Baier M, Pullwitt A, et al. Falciparum malaria after splenectomy: a prospective controlled study of 33 previously splenectomized Malawian adults. Trans R Soc Trop Med Hyg. 2005;99:861-867.

1198. Pickering LK, Baker CJ, Long SS, McMillan JA (eds). Red Book: 2006 Report of the Committeee on Infectious Diseases, 27th ed. Elk Grove Villiage, IL, American Academy of Pediatrics, 2006, pp 223-224.

1199. Oster CN, Koontz LC, Wyler DJ. Malaria in asplenic mice: effects of splenectomy, congenital asplenia, and splenic reconstitution on the course of infection. Am J Trop Med Hyg. 1980;29:1138.

1200. Demar M, Legrand E, Hommel D, et al. *Plasmodium falciparum* malaria in splenectomized patients: two case reports in French Guiana and a literature review. Am J Trop Med Hyg. 2004;71:290-293.

1201. Looareesuwan S, Suntharasamai P, Webster HK, Ho M. Malaria in splenectomized patients: report of four cases and review. Clin Infect Dis. 1993;16:361-363.

1202. Hirsh J, Dacie JV. Persistent post-splenectomy thrombocytosis and thrombo-embolism: a consequence of continuing anaemia. Br J Haematol. 1966;12:44-53.

1203. Cappellini, MD, Robbiolo L, Bottasso BM, et al. Venous thromboembolism and hypercoagulability in splenectomized patients with thalassemia intermedia. Br J Haematol. 2000;111:467-473.

1204. Robinette CD, Fraumeni JF Jr. Splenectomy and subsequent mortality in veterans of the 1939-45 war. Lancet. 1977;2:127.

1205. Kuypers FA. Phospholipid asymmetry in health and disease. Curr Opin Hematol. 1998;5:122.

1206. Andrews DA, Low PS. Role of red blood cells in thrombosis. Curr Opin Hematol. 1999;6:76.

1207. Barker JE, Wandersee NJ. Thrombosis in heritable hemolytic disorders. Curr Opin Hematol. 1999;6:71.

1208. Kaysser TM, Wandersee NJ, Bronson RT, Barker JE. Thrombosis and secondary hemochromatosis play major roles in the pathogenesis of jaundiced and spherocytic mice, murine models for hereditary spherocytosis. Blood. 1997;90:4610.

1209. Cappellini MD, Grespi E, Cassinerio E, et al. Coagulation and splenectomy: an overview. Ann N Y Acad Sci. 2005;1054:317-324.

1210. Mohren M, Markmann I, Dworschak U, et al. Thromboembolic complications after splenectomy for hematologic diseases. Am J Hematol 2004;76:143-147.

1211. Schilling RF. Hereditary spherocytosis: A study of splenectomized persons. Semin Hematol. 1976;13:169.

1212. Schilling RF: Spherocytosis, splenectomy, strokes, and heart attacks. Lancet. 1997;350:1677.

1213. Jardine DL, Laing AD. Delayed pulmonary hypertension following splenectomy for HS. Int Med J. 2004;34:214-216.

1214. Verresen D, De Backer W, Van Meerbeeck J, et al. Spherocytosis and pulmonary hypertension coincidental occurrence or causal relationship? Eur Respir J. 1991;4:629.

1215. Hoeper MM, Niedermeyer J, Hoffmeyer F, et al. Pulmonary hypertension after splenectomy? Ann Intern Med. 1999;130:506.

1216. Hayag-Barin JE, Smith RE, Tucker FC Jr. Hereditary spherocytosis, thrombocytosis, and chronic pulmonary emboli: A case report and review of the literature. Am J Hematol. 1998;57:82.

1217. Bonderman D, Jakowitsch J, Adlbrecht C, et al. Medical conditions increasing the risk of chronic thromboembolic pulmonary hypertension. Thromb Haemost. 2005;93:512-516.

1218. Lang I, Kerr K. Risk factors for chronic thromboembolic pulmonary hypertension. Proc Am Thorac Soc. 2003;3:568-570.

1219. Singer ST, Kuypers FA, Styles L, et al. Pulmonary hypertension in thalassemia: association with platelet activation and hypercoagulable state. Am J Hematol. 2006;81:670-675.

1220. Aessopos A, Stamatelos G, Skoumas V, et al. Pulmonary hypertension and right heart failure in patients with beta-thalassemia intermedia. Chest. 1995;107:50.

1221. Sonakul D, Fucharoen S. Pulmonary thromboembolism in thalassemic patients. Southeast Asian J Trop Med Public Health. 1992;23(Suppl 2):25.

1222. Stewart GW, Amess JAL, Eber SW, et al. Thromboembolic disease after splenectomy for hereditary stomatocytosis. Br J Haematol. 1996;93:303.

1223. Jais X, Ioos V, Jardim C, et al. Splenectomy and chronic thromboembolic pulmonary hypertension. Thorax 2005;60:1031-1034.

1224. Piomelli S. Workshop summaries: the splenectomy controversy. Ann N Y Acad Sci. 2005;1054:511-513.

1225. Marvin KS, Spellberg RD. Pulmonary hypertension secondary to thrombocytosis in a patient with myeloid metaplasia. Chest. 1993;103:642.

1226. Rostagno C, Prisco D, Abbate R, Poggesi L. Pulmonary hypertension associated with long-standing thrombocytosis. Chest 1991;99:1303.

1227. Kisanuki A, Kietthubthew S, Asada Y, et al. Intravenous injection of sonicated blood induces pulmonary microthromboembolism in rabbits with ligation of the splenic artery. Thromb Res. 1997;85:95.

1228. McGrew W, Avant GR. Hereditary spherocytosis and portal vein thrombosis. J Clin Gastroenterol. 1984;6:381.

1229. Perel Y, Dhermy D, Carrere A, et al. Portal vein thrombosis after splenectomy for hereditary stomatocytosis in childhood. Eur J Pediatr. 1999;158:628.

1230. Bertolotti M, Loria P, Martella P, et al. Bleeding jejunal varices and portal thrombosis in a splenectomized patient with hereditary spherocytosis. Dig Dis Sci. 2000;45:373.

1231. Teramoto S, Matsuse T, Ouchi Y. Splenectomy-induced portal hypertension and pulmonary hypertension. Ann Intern Med. 1999;131:793.

1232. Kannel WB. Current status of the epidemiology of brain infarction associated with occlusive arterial disease. Stroke. 1971;2:295.

1233. Schilling RE, Gangnon RE, Traver M. Arteriosclerotic events are less frequent in persons with chronic anemia: evidence from families with hereditary spherocytosis. Am J Hematol. 2006;81:315-317.

1234. Rescorla FJ, Breitfeld PP, West KW, et al. A case controlled comparison of open and laparoscopic splenectomy in children. Surgery. 1998;124:670.

1235. Esposito C, Gonzalez Sabin MA, Corcione F, et al. Results and complications of laparoscopic cholecystectomy in childhood. Surg Endosc. 2001;15:890.

1236. Patton ML, Moss BE, Haith LR, et al. Concomitant laparoscopic cholecystectomy and splenectomy for surgical management of hereditary spherocytosis. Am Surg. 1997;63:536.

1237. Yamagishi S, Watanabe T. Concomitant laparoscopic splenectomy and cholecystectomy for management of hereditary spherocytosis associated with gallstones. J Clin Gastroenterol. 2000;30:447.

1238. Sandler A, Winkel G, Kimura K, Soper R. The role of prophylactic cholecystectomy during splenectomy in children with hereditary spherocytosis. J Pediatr Surg. 1999;34:1077.

1239. Lobe TE, Presbury GJ, Smith BM, et al. Laparoscopic splenectomy. Pediatr Ann. 1993;22:671-674.

1240. Smith BM, Schropp KP, Lobe TE, et al. Laparoscopic splenectomy in childhood. J Pediatr Surg. 1994;29:975.

1241. Silvestri F, Russo D, Fanin R, et al. Laparoscopic splenectomy in the management of hematological diseases. Haematologica. 1995;80:47.

1242. Yoshida K, Yamazaki Y, Mizuno R, et al. Laparoscopic splenectomy in children. Preliminary results and comparison with the open technique. Surg Endosc. 1995;9:1279.

1243. Rescorla FJ. Cholelithiasis, cholecystitis, and common bile duct stones. Curr Opin Pediatr. 1997;9:276.

1244. Park A, Heniford BT, Hebra A, Fitzgerald P. Pediatric laparoscopic splenectomy. Surg Endosc. 2000;14:527-531.

1245. Danielson PD, Shaul DB, Phillips JD, et al. Technical advances in pediatric laparoscopy have had a beneficial impact on splenectomy. J Pediatr Surg. 2000;35:1578.

1246. Gigot JF, de Ville de Goyet J, Van Beers BE, et al. Laparoscopic splenectomy in adults and children: Experience with 31 patients. Surgery 1996;119:384.

1247. Esposito C, Schaarschmidt K, Settimi A, Montupet P. Experience with laparoscopic splenectomy. J Pediatr Surg. 2001;36:309-311.

1248. Kumar RJ, Borzi PA. Splenosis in a port site after laparoscopic splenectomy. Surg Endosc. 2001;15:413.

1249. Qureshi FG, Ergun O, Sandulache VC, et al. Laparoscopic splenectomy in children. JSLS. 2005;9:389-392.

1250. Minkes RK, Lagzdins M, Langer JC. Laparoscopic versus open splenectomy in children. J Pediatr Surg. 2000;35:699-701.

1251. Reddy VS, Phan HH, O'Neill JA, et al. Laparoscopic versus open splenectomy in the pediatric population: a contemporary single center experience. Am Surg. 2001; 67:859-863.

1252. Vasilescu C, Stanciulea O, Tudor S, et al. Laparoscopic subtotal splenectomy in hereditary spherocytosis: to preserve the upper or lower pole of the spleen? Surg Endosc. 2006;20:748-752.

1253. Tchernia G, Gauthier F, Mielot F, et al. Initial assessment of the beneficial effect of partial splenectomy in hereditary spherocytosis. Blood. 1993;81:2014.

1254. Bader-Meunier B, Gauthier F, Archambaud F, et al. Long-term evaluation of the beneficial effect of subtotal splenectomy for management of hereditary spherocytosis. Blood. 2001;97:399.

1255. De Buys Roessingh AS, De Lagausie P, Rohrlich P, et al. Follow-up of partial splenectomy in children with hereditary spherocytosis. J Pediatr Surg. 2002;37:1459.

1256. Rice HE, Oldham KT, Hillery CA, et al. Clinical and hematologic benefits of partial splenectomy for congenital hemolytic anemias in children. Ann Surg. 2003; 237:281-288.

1257. Tchernia G, Bader-Meunier B, Berterottiere P, et al. Effectiveness of partial splenectomy in hereditary spherocytosis. Curr Opin Hematol. 1997;4:136-141.

1258. Stoehr GA, Stauffer UG, Eber SW. Near-total splenectomy: a new technique for the management of hereditary spherocytosis. Ann Surg. 2005;241:40-47.

1259. Jimenez M, Azcona C, Castro L, et al. Partial splenic embolization in a child with hereditary spherocytosis. Eur J Pediatr. 1995;154:501.

1260. Kimura F, Ito H, Shimizu A, et al. Partial splenic embolization for the treatment of hereditary spherocytosis. AJR Am J Roentgenol. 2003;181:1021-1024.

1261. Poulin EC, Thibault C. Laparoscopic splenectomy for massive splenomegaly: operative technique and case report. Can J Surg. 1995;38:69.

1262. De Haan LD, Werre JM, Ruben AM, et al. Alterations in size, shape and osmotic behaviour of red cells after splenectomy: A study of their age dependence. Br J Haematol. 1988;69:71.

1263. Bart JB, Appel MF. Recurrent hemolytic anemia secondary to accessory spleens. South Med J. 1978;71:608.

1264. Brook J, Tanaka KR. Combination of pyruvate kinase (PK) deficiency and hereditary spherocytosis (HS). Clin Res. 1970;18:176A.

1265. Valentine WN. Hereditary spherocytosis revisited. West J Med. 1978;128:35.

1266. Rutkow IM. Twenty years of splenectomy for hereditary spherocytosis. Arch Surg. 1981;116:306.

1267. Buchanan GR, Holtkamp CA. Pocked erythrocyte counts in patients with hereditary spherocytosis before and after splenectomy. Am J Hematol. 1987;25: 253.

1268. Kvindesdal BB, Jensen MK. Pitted erythrocytes in splenectomized subjects with congenital spherocytosis and in subjects splenectomized for other reasons. Scand J Haematol. 1986;37:41.

1269. Satou S, Yokota E, Sugihara J, et al. Case report—relapse of hereditary spherocytosis following splenectomy. Nippon Ketsueki Gakkai Zasshi. 1985;48:1337-1340.

1270. Stoehr GA, Rose MA, Eber SW, et al. Immunogenicity of sequential pneumococcal vaccination in subjects splenectomised for hereditary spherocytosis. Br J Haematol. 2006;132:788-790.

1271. Pai VB, Nahata MC. Duration of penicillin prophylaxis in sickle cell anemia: issues and controversies. Pharmacotherapy. 2000;20:110.

1272. Buchanan GR, Smith SJ. Pneumococcal septicemia despite pneumococcal vaccine and prescription of penicillin prophylaxis in patients with sickle cell anemia. Am J Dis Child. 1986;140:428.

1273. Gonzaga RA. Fatal post-splenectomy pneumococcal sepsis despite prophylaxis. Lancet. 1984;2:694.

1274. Wong WY, Overturf GD, Powers DR. Infection caused by *Streptococcus pneumoniae* in children with sickle cell disease: epidemiology, immunologic mechanisms, prophylaxis and vaccination. Clin Infect Dis. 1992;14: 1124.

1275. Buchanan GR, Siegel JD, Smith SJ, DePasse BM. Oral penicillin prophylaxis in children with impaired splenic function: a study of compliance. Pediatrics 1982;70: 926-930.

1276. Caputo GM, Appelbaum PC, Liu HH. Infections due to penicillin-resistant pneumococci. Clinical, epidemiologic, and microbiologic features. Arch Intern Med. 1993;153:1301.

1277. Chesney PJ. The escalating problem of antimicrobial resistance in *Streptococcus pneumoniae*. Am J Dis Child. 1992;146:912.

1278. Tomasz A. Antibiotic resistance in *Streptococcus pneumoniae*. Clin Infect Dis. 1997;24(Suppl 1):S85.

1279. Marton A, Gulyas M, Munoz R, Tomasz A. Extremely high incidence of antibiotic resistance in clinical isolates of *Streptococcus pneumoniae* in Hungary. J Infect Dis. 1991;163:542.

1280. Appelbaum PC. Microbiological and pharmacodynamic considerations in the treatment of infection due to antimicrobial-resistant *Streptococcus pneumoniae*. Clin Infect Dis. 2000;31(Suppl 2):S29.

1281. Friedland IR, McCracken GH Jr. Management of infections caused by antibiotic-resistant *Streptococcus pneumoniae*. N Engl J Med. 1994;331:377.

1282. Wong WY, Powars DR, Hiti AL. Multi-drug resistance to *Streptococcus pneumoniae* in sickle cell anemia. Am J Hematol. 1995;48:278.

1283. Peters LL, Barker JE. Spontaneous and targeted mutations in erythrocyte membrane skeleton genes: mouse models of hereditary spherocytosis. In Zon LI (ed). Hematopoiesis. New York, Oxford University Press, 1999.

1284. Bodine DM, Birkenmeier CS, Barker JE. Spectrin deficient inherited hemolytic anemias in the mouse: Characterization by spectrin synthesis and mRNA activity in reticulocytes. Cell. 1984;37:721.

1285. Anderson R, Huestis RR, Motulsky AG. Hereditary spherocytosis in the deer mouse. Its similarity to the human disease. Blood. 1960;15:491.

1286. Bloom ML, Kaysser TM, Birkenmeier CS, Barker JE. The murine mutation jaundiced is caused by replacement of an arginine with a stop codon in the mRNA encoding the ninth repeat of beta-spectrin. Proc Natl Acad Sci U S A. 1994;91:10099.

1287. Wandersee NJ, Birkenmeier CS, Gifford EJ, et al. Murine recessive hereditary spherocytosis, sph/sph, is caused by a mutation in the erythroid alpha-spectrin gene. Hematol J. 2000;1:235.

1288. Wandersee NJ, Birkenmeier CS, et al. Identification of three mutations in the murine erythroid alpha-spectrin gene causing hereditary spherocytosis in mice. Blood. 1998;92:8a.

1289. Wandersee NJ, Birkenmeier CS, Bodine DM, et al. Mutations in the murine erythroid alpha-spectrin gene alter spectrin mRNA and protein levels and spectrin incorporation into the red cell membrane skeleton. Blood. 2003;101:325-330.

1290. Kaysser TM, Wandersee NJ, Bronson RT, Barker JE. Thrombosis and secondary hemochromatosis play major roles in the pathogenesis of jaundiced and spherocytic mice, murine models for hereditary spherocytosis. Blood. 1997;90:4610.

1291. Wandersee NJ, Lee JC, Kaysser TM, et al. Hematopoietic cells from alpha spectrin–deficient mice are sufficient to induce thrombotic events in hematopoietically ablated recipients. Blood. 1998;92:4856-4863.

1292. Wandersee NJ, Roesch AN, Hamblen NR, et al. Defective spectrin integrity and neonatal thrombosis in the first mouse model for severe hereditary elliptocytosis. Blood. 2001;97:543-550.

1293. Wandersee NJ, Tait JF, Barker JE. Erythroid phosphatidyl serine exposure is not predictive of thrombotic risk in mice with hemolytic anemia. Blood Cells Mol Dis. 2000;26:75-83.

1294. Wandersee NJ, Olson SC, Holzhauer SL, et al. Increased erythrocyte adhesion in mice and humans with hereditary spherocytosis and hereditary elliptocytosis. Blood. 2004;103:710-716.

1295. White RA, Birkenmeier CS, Lux SE, Barker JE. Ankyrin and the hemolytic anemia mutation, nb, map to mouse chromosome 8: Presence of the nb allele is associated with a truncated erythrocyte ankyrin. Proc Natl Acad Sci U S A. 1990;87:3117.

1296. Birkenmeier CS, Gifford EJ, Barker JE. Mutations of the erythroid ankyrin gene: A hypomorph and a null. Blood. 2000;96:594a.

1297. Inaba M, Yawata A, Koshino I, et al. Defective anion transport and marked spherocytosis with membrane instability caused by hereditary total deficiency of red cell band 3 in cattle due to a nonsense mutation. J Clin Invest. 1996;97:1804.

1298. Hassoun H, Hanada T, Lutchman M, et al. Complete deficiency of glycophorin A in red blood cells from mice with targeted inactivation of the band 3 (AE1) gene. Blood. 1998;91:2146.

1299. Tomaselli MB, John KM, Lux SE. Elliptical erythrocyte membrane skeletons and heat-sensitive spectrin in hereditary elliptocytosis. Proc Natl Acad Sci U S A. 1981;78:1911.

1300. Hassoun H, Wang Y, Vassiliadis J, et al. Targeted inactivation of murine band 3 (AE1) gene produces a hypercoagulable state causing widespread thrombosis in vivo. Blood. 1998;92:1785.

1301. Peters LL, Swearingen RA, Anderson SG, et al. Idenitification of quantitative trait loci that modify the severity of hereditary spherocytosis in wan, a new mouse model of band-3 deficiency. Blood 2004;103:3233-3240.

1302. Peters LL, Jindel HK, Gwynn B, et al. Mild spherocytosis and altered red cell ion transport in protein 4.2–null mice. J Clin Invest. 1999;103:1527.

1303. Shi ZT, Afzal V, Coller B, et al. Protein 4.1R–deficient mice are viable but have erythroid membrane skeleton abnormalities. J Clin Invest. 1999;103:331.

1303a. Rabenstein RL, Addy NA, Caldarone BJ, et al. Impaired synaptic plasticity and learning in mice lacking beta-adducin, an actin-regulating protein. J Neurosci. 2005;25:2138-2145.

1304. Dresbach M. Elliptical human red corpuscles. Science. 1904;19:469.

1305. Flint A. Elliptical human erythrocytes. Science. 1904; 19:796.

1306. Dresbach M. Elliptical human erythrocytes. Science. 1905;21:473

1307. Bishop FW. Elliptical human erythrocytes. Arch Intern Med. 1914;14:388.

1308. Huck JG, Bigelow RM. Poikilocytes in otherwise normal blood (elliptical human erythrocytes). Bull Johns Hopkins Hosp. 1923;34:390.

1309. Hunter WC, Adams RB. Hematologic study of three generations of a white family showing elliptical erythrocytes. Ann Intern Med. 1929;2:1162.

1310. Hunter WC. Further study of a white family showing elliptical erythrocytes. Ann Intern Med. 1932;6:775.

1311. Giffin HZ, Watkins CH. Ovalocytosis with features of hemolytic icterus. Trans Assoc Am Physicians. 1939;54:355.

1312. Penfold J, Lipscomb JM. Elliptocytosis in man, associated with hereditary haemorrhagic telangiectasis. Q J Med. 1943;12:157.

1313. Wyandt H, Bancroft PM, Winship TO. Elliptic erythrocytes in man. Arch Intern Med. 1941;68:1043.

1314. Wolman IJ, Ozge A. Studies on elliptocytosis. I. Hereditary elliptocytosis in the pediatric age period: A review of recent literature. Am J Med Sci. 1957;234:702.

1315. Dacie JV. The lifespan of the red blood cell and circumstances of its premature death. In Wintrobe MM (ed). Blood, Pure and Eloquent. New York, McGraw-Hill, 1980, p 210.

1316. McCarty SH. Elliptical red blood cells in man. A report of eleven cases. J Lab Clin Med. 1934;19:612.

1317. Glele-Kakai C, Garbarz M, Lecomte MC, et al. Epidemiological studies of spectrin mutations related to hereditary elliptocytosis and spectrin polymorphisms in Benin. Br J Haematol. 1996;95:57.

1318. Lecomte MC, Dhermy D, Gautero H, et al. Hereditary elliptocytosis in West Africa: frequency and repartition of spectrin variants. C R Acad Sci Paris. 1988;306:43.

1319. Ganesan J, George R, Lie-Injo LE. Abnormal haemoglobins and hereditary ovalocytosis in the Ulu Jempul district of Kuala Pilah, West Malaysia. Southeast Asian J Trop Med Public Health. 1976;7:430.

1320. Tse WT, Lecomte MC, Costa FF, et al. Point mutation in the β-spectrin gene associated with I/74 hereditary elliptocytosis. Implications for the mechanism of spectrin dimer self-association. J Clin Invest. 1990;86:909.

1321. Lawler J, Liu SC, Palek J, Prchal J. Molecular defect of spectrin in hereditary pyropoikilocytosis: Alterations in the trypsin resistant domain involved in spectrin self-association. J Clin Invest. 1982;701019.

1322. Dalla Venezia N, Wilmotte R, Morle L, et al. An α-spectrin mutation responsible for hereditary elliptocytosis associated in cis with the αV/41 polymorphism. Hum Genet. 1993;90:641.

1323. Mentzer WC, Turetsky T, Mohandas N, et al. Identification of the hereditary pyropoikilocytosis carrier state. Blood 1984;63:1439.

1324. Palek J, Lux SE. Red cell membrane skeletal defects in hereditary and acquired hemolytic anemias. Semin Hematol. 1983;20:189.

1325. Jonsson JJ, Renieri A, Gallagher PG, et al. Alport syndrome, mental retardation, midface hypoplasia, and elliptocytosis: A new X linked contiguous gene deletion syndrome? J Med Genet. 1998;35:273.

1326. Tse WT, Lux SE. Red blood cell membrane disorders. Br J Haematol. 1999;104:2.

1327. Gallagher PG, Ferriera JD. Molecular basis of erythrocyte membrane disorders. Curr Opin Hematol. 1997;4:128.

1328. Gallagher, PG. Hereditary elliptocytosis: spectrin and protein 4.1R. Semin Hematol. 2004;41:42-164.

1329. Lambert S, Zail S. Partial deficiency of protein 4.1 in hereditary elliptocytosis. Am J Hematol. 1987;26:263.

1330. Palek J. Hereditary elliptocytosis, spherocytosis and related disorders: Consequences of a deficiency or a mutation of membrane skeletal proteins. Blood Rev. 1987;1:147.

1331. Palek J. Hereditary elliptocytosis and related disorders. Clin Haematol. 1985;14:45.

1332. Tchernia G, Mohandas N, Shohet SB. Deficiency of cytoskeletal membrane protein band 4.1 in homozygous hereditary elliptocytosis: implications for erythrocyte membrane stability. J Clin Invest. 1981;68:454.

1333. Morle L, Alloisio N, Ducluzeau MT, et al. Spectrin Tunis (α^{I/78}): a new alpha I variant that causes asymptomatic hereditary elliptocytosis in the heterozygous state. Blood. 1988;71:508.

1334. Morle L, Morle F, Roux AF, et al. Spectrin Tunis (Sp α^{I/78}), an elliptocytogenic variant, is due to the CGG→TGG codon change (Arg→Trp) at position 35 of the αI domain. Blood. 1989;75:828.

1335. Lecomte MC, Dhermy D, Garbarz M, et al. Hereditary elliptocytosis with spectrin molecular defect in a white patient. Acta Haematol (Basel). 1984;71:235.

1336. Alloisio N, Guetorni D, Morle L, et al. Sp α^{I/65} hereditary elliptocytosis in North Africa. Am J Hematol. 1986;23:113.

1337. Guetarni D, Roux AF, Alloisio N, et al. Evidence that expression of Sp α^{I/65} hereditary elliptocytosis is compounded by a genetic factor that is linked to the homologous α-spectrin allele. Hum Genet. 1990;85:627-630.

1338. Marchesi SL, Knowles WT, Morrow JS, et al. Abnormal spectrin in hereditary elliptocytosis. Blood. 1986;67:141.

1339. Feddal S, Brunet G, Roda L, et al. Molecular analysis of hereditary elliptocytosis with reduced protein 4.1 in the French Northern Alps. Blood. 1991;78:2113.

1340. McGuire M, Smith BL, Agre P. Distinct variants of erythrocyte protein 4.1 inherited in linkage with elliptocytosis and Rh type in three white families. Blood. 1988;72:287.

1341. Florman AL, Wintrobe MM. Human elliptical red corpuscles. Bull Johns Hopkins Hosp. 1938;63:209.

1342. Garrdo-Lacca G, Merino C, Luna G. Hereditary elliptocytosis in a Peruvian family. N Engl J Med. 1957;256:311.

1343. Geerdink RA, Helleman PW, Verloop MC. Hereditary elliptocytosis and hyperhaemolysis: a comparative study of 6 families with 145 patients. Acta Med Scand. 1966;179:715.

1344. Jensson O, Jonasson TH, Olafsson O. Hereditary elliptocytosis in Iceland. Br J Haematol. 1967;13:844.

1345. Motulsky AG, Singer K, Crosby WH, Smith V. The life span of the elliptocyte: hereditary elliptocytosis and its relationship to other familial hemolytic diseases. Blood. 1954;9:57.

1346. Pothier B, Alloisio N, Marechal J, et al. Assignment of spectrin α^{I/74} hereditary elliptocytosis to the α or β-chain of spectrin through in vitro dimer reconstitution. Blood. 1990;75:2061.

1347. Coetzer T, Lawler J, Prchal JT, Palek J. Molecular determinants of clinical expression of hereditary elliptocytosis and pyropoikilocytosis. Blood. 1987;70:766.

1348. Rummens JL, Verfaillie C, Criel A, et al. Elliptocytosis and schistocytosis in myelodysplasia: report of two cases. Acta Haematol. 1986;75:174.

1349. Coetzer T, Sahr K, Prchal J, et al. Four different mutations in codon 28 of alpha spectrin are associated with structurally and functionally abnormal spectrin α^{I/74} in hereditary elliptocytosis. J Clin Invest. 1991;88:743.

1350. Garbarz M, Lecomte MC, Feo C, et al. Hereditary pyropoikilocytosis and elliptocytosis in a white French family with the spectrin α^{I/74} variant related to a CGT to CAT codon change (Arg to His) at position 22 of the spectrin αI domain. Blood. 1990;75:1691.

1351. Lawler J, Liu SC, Palek J, Prchal J. Molecular defect of spectrin in a subgroup of patients with hereditary elliptocytosis. Alteration in the alpha-subunit involved in spectrin self association. J Clin Invest. 1984;73:1688.

1352. Lecomte MC, Feo C, Gautero H, et al. Severe hereditary elliptocytosis in two related Caucasian children with a decreased amount of spectrin (Sp) α chain. J Cell Biochem. 1989;13B:230.

1353. Baklouti F, Marechal J, Morle L, et al. Occurrence of the αI 22Arg→His (CGT→CAT) spectrin mutation in Tunisia: potential association with severe elliptopoikilocytosis. Br J Haematol. 1991;78:108.

1354. Baklouti F, Marechal J, Wilmotte R, et al. Elliptocytogenic α^{I/36} spectrin Sfax lacks nine amino acids in helix 3 of repeat 4. Evidence for the activation of a cryptic 5-splice site in exon 8 of spectrin alpha-gene. Blood. 1992;79:2464.

1355. Dalla Venezia N, Alloisio N, Forissier A, et al. Elliptopoikilocytosis associated with the α 469 His→Pro mutation in spectrin Barcelona (α^{I/50-46b}). Blood. 1993;82:1661.

1356. Alloisio N, Morle L, Marechal J, et al. Sp α^{V/41}: a common spectrin polymorphism at the αIV-αV domain junction. Relevance to the expression level of hereditary elliptocytosis due to α-spectrin variants located in trans. J Clin Invest. 1991;87:2169.

1357. Coetzer T, Palek J, Lawler J, et al. Structural and functional heterogeneity of a spectrin mutations involving the spectrin heterodimer self-association site: relationships to hematologic expression of homozygous hereditary elliptocytosis and hereditary pyropoikilocytosis. Blood. 1990;75:2235.

1358. Randon J, Boulanger L, Marechal J, et al. A variant of spectrin low expression allele α^{LELY} carrying a hereditary elliptocytosis mutation in codon 28. Br J Haematol. 1994;88:534.

1359. Ozer L, Mills GC. Elliptocytosis with haemolytic anaemia. Br J Haematol. 1964;10:468.

1360. Kruetrachuo M, Asawapokee N. Hereditary elliptocytosis and *Plasmodium falciparum* malaria. Ann Trop Med Parasitol. 1972;66:161.

1361. Nkrumah FK. Hereditary elliptocytosis associated with severe haemolytic anaemia and malaria. Afr J Med Sci. 1972;3:131.

1362. Jarolim P, Palek J, Coetzer TL, et al. Severe hemolysis and red cell fragmentation due to a combination of a spectrin mutation with a thrombotic microangiopathy. Am J Hematol. 1989;32:50-56.

1363. Schoomaker EB, Butler WM, Diehl LF. Increased heat sensitivity of red blood cells in hereditary elliptocytosis with acquired cobalamin (vitamin B$_{12}$) deficiency. Blood. 1982;59:1213.

1364. Lecomte MC, Garbarz M, Grandchamp B, et al. Sp α$^{I/78}$: A mutation of the αI spectrin domain in a white kindred with HE and HPP phenotypes. Blood. 1989;74:1126.

1365. Lane PA, Shew RL, Iarocci TA, et al. Unique α-spectrin mutant in a kindred with common hereditary elliptocytosis. J Clin Invest. 1987;79:989.

1366. Austin RF, Desforges JF. Hereditary elliptocytosis: an unusual presentation of hemolysis in the newborn associated with transient morphologic abnormalities. Pediatrics. 1969;44:196.

1367. Carpentieri U, Gustavson LP, Haggard ME. Pyknocytosis in a neonate: an unusual presentation of hereditary elliptocytosis. Clin Pediatr (Phila). 1977;16:76.

1368. Josephs HW, Avery ME. Hereditary elliptocytosis associated with increased hemolysis. Pediatrics. 1965;16:741.

1369. Zarkowsky HS. Heat-induced erythrocyte fragmentation in neonatal elliptocytosis. Br J Haematol. 1979;41:515.

1370. Prchal JT, Castleberry RP, Parmley RT, et al. Hereditary pyropoikilocytosis and elliptocytosis: Clinical, laboratory, and ultrastructural features in infants and children. Pediatr Res. 1982;16:484.

1371. Mentzer WC Jr, Iarocci TA, Mohandas N, et al. Modulation of erythrocyte membrane mechanical stability by 2,3-diphosphoglycerate in the neonatal poikilocytosis/elliptocytosis syndrome. J Clin Invest. 1987;79:943.

1372. Manno S, Takakuwa Y, Nagao K, Mohandas N. Modulation of erythrocyte membrane mechanical function by beta-spectrin phosphorylation and dephosphorylation. J Biol Chem. 1995;270:5659.

1373. Schindler M, Koppel D, Sheetz MP. Modulation of membrane protein lateral mobility by polyphosphates and polyamines. Proc Natl Acad Sci U S A. 1980;77:1457.

1374. Wolfe LC, Lux SE, Ohanian V. Spectrin-actin binding in vitro; effect of protein 4.1 and polyphosphates. J Supramol Struct Cell Biochem. 1981;5(Suppl 5):123.

1375. Suzuki Y, Nakajima T, Shiga T, Maeda N. Influence of 2,3-diphosphoglycerate on the deformability of human erythrocytes. Biochim Biophys Acta. 1990;1029:85.

1376. Waugh RE. Effects of 2,3-diphosphoglycerate on the mechanical properties of erythrocyte membrane. Blood. 1986;68:231.

1377. Garbarz M, Lecomte MC, Dhermy D, et al. Double inheritance of an α$^{I/65}$ spectrin variant in a child with homozygous elliptocytosis. Blood. 1986;67:1661.

1378. Alloisio N, Morle L, Pothier B, et al. Spectrin Oran (α$^{II/21}$), a new spectrin variant concerning the αII domain and causing severe elliptocytosis in the homozygous state. Blood. 1988;71:1039.

1379. Lecomte MC, Feo C, Gautero H, et al. Severe recessive poikilocytic anaemia with a new spectrin α-chain variant. Br J Haematol. 1990;74:497.

1380. Dalla Venezia N, Gilsanz F, Alloisio N, et al. Homozygous 4.1(−) hereditary elliptocytosis associated with a point mutation in the downstream initiation codon of protein 4.1 gene. J Clin Invest. 1992;90:1713-1717.

1381. Alloisio N, Wilmotte R, Marechal J, et al. A splice site mutation of α-spectrin gene causing skipping of exon 18 in hereditary elliptocytosis. Blood. 1993;81:2791.

1382. Haddy TB, Rana SR. Homozygous hereditary elliptocytosis with hemolytic anemia. South Med J. 1984;77:631.

1383. Dhermy D, Garbarz M, Lecomte M, et al. Hereditary elliptocytosis: clinical, morphological, and biochemical studies of 38 cases. Nouv Rev Fr Hematol. 1986;28:129.

1384. Torlontano G, Fioritoni G, Salvati AM. Hereditary haemolytic ovalocytosis with defective erythropoiesis. Br J Haematol. 1979;43:435.

1385. Jankovic M, Sansone G, Conter V, et al. Atypical hereditary ovalocytosis associated with defective dyserythropoietic anemia. Acta Haematol. 1993;89:35.

1386. Floyd PB, Gallagher PG, Valentino LA, et al. Heterogeneity of the molecular basis of hereditary pyropoikilocytosis and hereditary elliptocytosis associated with increased levels of the spectrin α$^{I/74}$-kilodalton tryptic peptide. Blood. 1991;78:1364.

1387. Dacie JV, Mollison PL, Richardson N, et al. Atypical congenital haemolytic anaemia. Q J Med. 1953;22:79.

1388. Wiley JS, Gill FM. Red cell calcium leak in congenital hemolytic anemia with extreme microcytosis. Blood. 1976;47:197.

1389. Zarkowsky HS, Mohandas N, Speaker CB, Shohet SB. A congenital haemolytic anaemia with thermal sensitivity of the erythrocyte membrane. Br J Haematol. 1975;29:537.

1390. DePalma L, Luban NL. Hereditary pyropoikilocytosis: Clinical and laboratory analysis in eight infants and young children. Am J Dis Child. 1993;147:93.

1391. Ramos MC, Schafernak KT, Peterson LC. Hereditary pyropoikilocytosis: a rare but potentially severe form of congenital hemolytic anemia. J Pediatr Hematol Oncol. 2007;29:128-129.

1392. Coetzer T, Palek J. Partial spectrin deficiency in hereditary pyropoikilocytosis. Blood. 1986;59:919.

1393. Hanspal M, Hanspal JS, Sahr KE, et al. Molecular basis of spectrin deficiency in hereditary pyropoikilocytosis. Blood. 1993;82:1652.

1394. Costa DB, Lozovatsky L, Gallagher PG, Forget BG. A novel splicing mutation of the alpha-spectrin gene in the original hereditary poikilocytosis kindred. Blood. 2005; 106:4367-4369.

1395. Gallagher PG. Hereditary elliptocytosis: spectrin and protein 4.1R. Semin Hematol. 2004;41:142-164.

1396. Cutting HO, McHugh WJ, Conrad FG, Marlow AA. Autosomal dominant hemolytic anemia characterized by ovalocytosis: A family study of seven involved members. Am J Med. 1965;39:21.

1397. Dacie JV. Hereditary elliptocytosis (HE). In The Haemolytic Anaemias, vol 1, 3rd ed. Edinburgh, Churchill Livingstone, 1985, p 216.

1398. Greenberg LH, Tanaka KR. Hereditary elliptocytosis with hemolytic anemia—a family study of five affected members. Calif Med. 1969;110:389.

1399. Weiss HJ. Hereditary elliptocytosis with hemolytic anemia. Am J Med. 1963;35:455.

1400. Matsumoto N, Ishihara T, Takahashi M, et al. Fine structure of the spleen in hereditary elliptocytosis. Acta Pathol Jpn. 1976;26:533-542.

1401. Wilson HE, Long MJ. Hereditary ovalocytosis (elliptocytosis) with hypersplenism. Arch Intern Med. 1955; 95:438.

1402. Dhermy D, Lecomte MC, Garbarz M, et al. Spectrin α-chain variant associated with hereditary elliptocytosis. J Clin Invest. 1982;70:707.

1403. Garbarz M, Tse WT, Gallagher PG et al. Spectrin Rouen ($\beta^{220-218}$), a novel shortened beta-chain variant in a kindred with hereditary elliptocytosis. Characterization of the molecular defect as exon skipping due to a splice site mutation. J Clin Invest. 1991;88:76.

1404. Lecomte MC, Gautero H, Bournier O, et al. Elliptocytosis-associated spectrin Rouen ($\beta^{220/218}$) has a truncated but still phosphorylatable beta chain. Br J Haematol. 1992;80:242.

1405. Pothier B, Morle L, Alloisio N, et al. Spectrin Nice ($\beta^{220/216}$): A shortened beta-chain variant associated with an increase of the $\alpha^{I/74}$ fragment in a case of elliptocytosis. Blood. 1987;69:1759.

1406. Tse WT, Gallagher PG, Pothier B, et al. An insertional frameshift mutation of the β-spectrin gene associated with elliptocytosis in spectrin Nice ($\beta^{220/216}$). Blood. 1991;78:517.

1407. Garbarz M, Boulanger L, Pedroni S, et al. Spectrin β Tandil, a novel shortened β-chain variant associated with hereditary elliptocytosis is due to a deletional frameshift mutation in the β-spectrin gene. Blood. 1992;80:1066.

1408. Eber SW, Morris SA, Schroter W, Gratzer WB. Interactions of spectrin in hereditary elliptocytes containing truncated spectrin beta-chains. J Clin Invest. 1988; 81:523.

1409. Yoon SH, Yu H, Eber S, Prchael JT. Molecular defect of truncated β-spectrin associated with hereditary elliptocytosis. Beta-spectrin Gottingen. J Biol Chem. 1991;266: 8490.

1410. Gallagher PG, Tse WT, Costa F, et al. A splice site mutation of the β-spectrin gene causing exon skipping in hereditary elliptocytosis associated with a truncated β-spectrin chain. J Biol Chem. 1991;266:15154.

1411. Jarolim P, Wichterle H, Hanspal M, et al. β spectrin^{PRAGUE}: a truncated spectrin producing spectrin deficiency, defective spectrin heterodimer self-association

and a phenotype of spherocytic elliptocytosis. Br J Haematol. 1995;91:502.

1412. Dahr W, Moulds J, Baumeister G, et al. Altered membrane sialoglycoproteins in human erythrocytes lacking the Gerbich blood group antigen. Biol Chem Hoppe Seyler. 1985;366:201.

1413. Daniels GL, Reid ME, Anstee DJ, et al. Transient reduction in erythrocyte membrane sialoglycoprotein β associated with the presence of elliptocytes. Br J Haematol. 1988;70:477.

1414. Aksoy M, Erdem S, Dincol G, et al. Combination of hereditary elliptocytosis and hereditary spherocytosis. Clin Genet. 1974;6:46.

1415. Skarsgard E, Doski J, Jaksic T, et al. Thrombosis of the portal venous system after appendectomy for pediatric hematologic disease. J Pediatr Surg. 1993;28:1109-1112.

1416. Ham TH, Shen SC, Fleming EM, et al. Studies on the destruction of red blood cells: IV. Thermal injury: Action of heat in causing increased spheroidicity, osmotic and mechanical fragilities and hemolysis of erythrocytes: Observations on the mechanisms of destruction in such erythrocytes in dogs and in a patient with a fatal thermal burn. Blood. 1948;3:373-403.

1417. Ham TH, Sayre RW, Dunn RF, Murphy JR. Physical properties of red cells as related to effects in vivo: II. Effect of thermal treatment on rigidity of red cells, stroma and the sickle cell. Blood. 1968;32:862.

1418. Kimber RJ, Lander H. The effect of heat on human red cell morphology, fragility and subsequent survival in vivo. J Lab Clin Med. 1964;64:922.

1419. Chang K, Williamson JR, Zarkowsky HS. Effect of heat on the circular dichroism of spectrin in hereditary pyropoikilocytosis. J Clin Invest. 1979;64:326.

1420. Liu S-C, Palek J, Prchal J, Castleberry RP. Altered spectrin dimer-dimer association and instability of erythrocyte membrane skeletons in hereditary pyropoikilocytosis. J Clin Invest. 1981;68:597.

1421. Liu SC, Windisch P, Kim S, Palek J. Oligomeric states of spectrin in normal erythrocyte membranes: biochemical and electron microscopic studies. Cell. 1984; 37:587.

1422. Liu S-C, Palek J, Prchal J. Defective spectrin dimer-dimer association in hereditary elliptocytosis. Proc Natl Acad Sci U S A. 1982;79:2072.

1423. Shotton DM, Burke BE, Branton D. The molecular structure of human erythrocyte spectrin. Biophysical and electron microscopic studies. J Mol Biol. 1979;131: 303.

1424. Speicher DW, Morrow JS, Knowles WJ, Marchesi VT. Identification of proteolytically resistant domains of human erythrocyte spectrin. Proc Natl Acad Sci U S A. 1980;77:5673.

1425. Orita M, Iwahana H, Kanazawa H, et al. Detection of polymorphisms of human DNA by gel electrophoresis as single-strand conformation polymorphisms. Proc Natl Acad Sci U S A. 1989;86:2766.

1426. Sarkar G, Yoon H-S, Sommer SS. Screening for mutations by RNA single-strand conformation polymorphism (rSSCP): comparison with DNA-SSCP. Nucleic Acids Res. 1992;20:871.

1427. Fournier CM, Nicolas G, Gallagher PG, et al. Spectrin St. Claude, a splicing mutation of the human α-spectrin gene associated with severe poikilocytic anemia. Blood. 1997;89:4584.

1428. Silveira P, Cynober T, Dhermy D, et al. Red blood cell abnormalities in hereditary elliptocytosis and their relevance to variable clinical expression. Am J Clin Pathol. 1997;108:391.

1429. Palek J, Lambert S. Genetics of the red cell membrane skeleton. Semin Hematol. 1990;27:290.

1430. Speicher DW, Morrow JS, Knowles WJ, Marchesi VT. A structural model of human erythrocyte spectrin: alignment of chemical and functional domains. J Biol Chem. 1982;257:9093.

1431. Kotula L, DeSilva TM, Speicher DW, Curtis PJ. Functional characterization of recombinant human red cell alpha-spectrin polypeptides containing the tetramer binding site. J Biol Chem. 1993;268:14788.

1432. Lecomte MC, Nicolas G, Dhermy D, et al. Properties of normal and mutant polypeptide fragments from the dimer self-association sites of human red cell spectrin. Eur Biophys J. 1999;28:208.

1433. Nicolas G, Pedroni S, Fournier C, et al. Spectrin self-association site: characterization and study of beta-spectrin mutations associated with hereditary elliptocytosis. Biochem J. 1998;332:81.

1434. Park S, Mehboob S, Luo BH, et al. Studies of the erythrocyte spectrin tetramerization region. Cell Mol Biol Lett. 2001;6:571.

1435. Gallagher PG, Petruzzi MJ, Weed SA, et al. Mutation of a highly conserved residue of αI spectrin associated with fatal and near-fatal neonatal hemolytic anemia. J Clin Invest. 1997;99:267.

1436. Zhang Z, Weed SA, Gallagher PG, Morrow JS. Dynamic molecular modeling of pathogenic mutations in the spectrin self-association domain. Blood. 2001;98:1645.

1437. Park S, Johnson ME, Fung LW. Nuclear magnetic resonance studies of mutations at the tetramerization region of human alpha spectrin. Blood. 2002;100:283.

1438. Delaunay J, Dhermy D. Mutations involving the spectrin heterodimer contact site: clinical expression and alterations in specific function. Semin Hematol. 1993;30:21.

1439. Lorenzo F, Miraglia del Giudice E, Alloisio N, et al. Severe poikilocytosis associated with a de novo a 28 Arg→Cys mutation in spectrin. Br J Haematol. 1993;83:152.

1440. Lawler J, Palek J, Liu SC, et al. Molecular heterogeneity of a hereditary pyropoikilocytosis: identification of a second variant of the spectrin α-subunit. Blood. 1983;62:1182.

1441. Gallagher PG, Tse WT, Coetzer T, et al. A common type of the spectrin alpha I 46-50a-kD peptide abnormality in hereditary elliptocytosis and pyropoikilocytosis is associated with a mutation distant from the proteolytic cleavage site. Evidence for the functional importance of the triple helical model of spectrin. J Clin Invest. 1992;89:892-898.

1442. Gallagher PG, Weed SA, Tse WT, et al. Recurrent fatal hydrops fetalis associated with a nucleotide substitution in the erythrocyte beta-spectrin gene. J Clin Invest. 1995;95:1174-1182.

1443. Boulanger L, Dhermy D, et al. A second allele of spectrin α-gene associated with the α$^{I/65}$ phenotype (allele Ponte de Sor). Blood. 1994;84:2056.

1444. Roux AF, Morle F, Guetarni D, et al. Molecular basis of Sp αI/65 hereditary elliptocytosis in North Africa: insertion of a TTG triplet between codons 147 and 149 in the α-spectrin gene from five unrelated families. Blood. 1989;73:2196.

1445. Dhermy D, Garbarz M, Lecomte MC, et al. Abnormal electrophoretic mobility of spectrin tetramers in hereditary elliptocytosis. Hum Genet. 1986;74:363.

1446. Lawler J, Coetzer TL, Palek J, et al N. Sp α I/65: a new variant of the a subunit of spectrin in hereditary elliptocytosis. Blood. 1985;66:706.

1447. Lecomte MC, Dhermy D, Garbarz M, et al. Pathologic and non-pathologic variants of the spectrin molecule in two black families with hereditary elliptocytosis. Hum Genet. 1985;71:351.

1448. Lecomte MC, Dhermy D, Solis C, et al. A new abnormal variant of spectrin in black patients with hereditary elliptocytosis. Blood. 1985;65:1208.

1449. del Giudice EM, Ducluzeau MT, Alloisio N, et al. α I/65 hereditary elliptocytosis in southern Italy: evidence for an African origin. Hum Genet. 1992;89:553.

1450. Sahr KE, Tobe T, Scarpa A, et al. Sequence and exon-intron organization of the DNA encoding the alpha I domain of human spectrin: application to the study of mutations causing hereditary elliptocytosis. J Clin Invest. 1989;84:1243.

1451. Schulman S, Roth EF Jr, Cheng B, et al. Growth of *Plasmodium falciparum* in human erythrocytes containing abnormal membrane proteins. Proc Natl Acad Sci U S A. 1990;87:7339.

1452. Wilmotte R, Miraglia del Giudice E, Marechal J, et al. A deletional frameshift mutation in spectrin beta-gene associated with hereditary elliptocytosis in spectrin Napoli. Br J Haematol. 1994;88:437.

1453. Kanzaki A, Rabodonirina M, Yawata Y, et al. A deletional frameshift mutation of the beta-spectrin gene associated with elliptocytosis in spectrin Tokyo (beta$^{220/216}$). Blood. 1992;80:2115.

1454. Basseres DS, Pranke PH, Sales TS, et al. Beta-spectrin Campinas: a novel shortened β-chain variant associated with skipping of exon 30 and hereditary elliptocytosis. Br J Haematol. 1997;97:579.

1455. Maillet P, Inoue T, Kanzaki A, et al. Stop codon in exon 30 (E2069X) of β-spectrin gene associated with hereditary elliptocytosis in spectrin Nagoya. Hum Mutat. 1996;8:366.

1456. Johnson CP, Massimiliano G, Ortiz V, et al. A pathogenic proline mutation in the linker between spectrin repeats: disease due to spectrin unfolding. Blood. 2006;109:3538-3543.

1457. Burke JP, Van Zyl D, Zail SS, Coetzer TL. Reduced spectrin-ankyrin binding in a South African hereditary elliptocytosis kindred homozygous for spectrin St Claude. Blood. 1998;92:2591.

1458. Alloisio N, Wilmotte R, Morle L, et al. Spectrin Jendouba: An α II/31 spectrin variant that is associated with elliptocytosis and carries a mutation distant from the dimer self-association site. Blood. 1992;80:809.

1459. Johnson RM, Ravindranath Y, Brohn F, Hussain M. A large erythroid spectrin beta-chain variant. Br J Haematol. 1992;80:6.

1460. Pranke PH, Basseres DS, Costa FF, Saad ST. Expression of spectrin α I/65 hereditary elliptocytosis in patients from Brazil. Br J Haematol. 1996;94:470.

1461. Marechal J, Wilmotte R, Kanzaki A, et al. Ethnic distribution of allele α^{LELY}, a low-expression allele of red-cell spectrin α-gene. Br J Haematol. 1995;90:553.

1462. Wilmotte R, Marechal J, Morle L, et al. Low expression allele α^{LELY} of red cell spectrin is associated with mutations in exon 40 (α V/41 polymorphism) and intron 45 and with partial skipping of exon 46. J Clin Invest. 1993;91:2091.

1463. Wilmotte R, Marechal J, Delaunay J. Mutation at position −12 of intron 45 (C→T) plays a prevalent role in the partial skipping of exon 46 from the transcript of allele α^{LELY} in erythroid cells. Br J Haematol. 1999; 104:855.

1464. Hanspal M, Palek J. Synthesis and assembly of membrane skeletal proteins in mammalian red cell precursors. J Cell Biol. 1987;105:1417.

1465. Amin KM, Scarpa AL, Winkelmann JC, et al. The exon-intron organization of the human erythroid beta-spectrin gene. Genomics. 1993;18:118.

1466. Wilmotte R, Harper SL, Ursitti JA, et al. The exon 46-encoded sequence is essential for stability of human erythroid α-spectrin and heterodimer formation. Blood. 1997;90:4188.

1467. Gallagher PG, Tse WT, Marchesi SL, et al. A defect in α-spectrin mRNA accumulation in hereditary pyropoikilocytosis. Trans Assoc Am Physicians. 1991;104:32.

1468. Feo CJ, Fischer S, Piau JP, et al. 1st instance of the absence of an erythrocyte membrane protein (band 4(1)) in a case of familial elliptocytic anemia. Nouv Rev Fr Hematol. 1980;22:315.

1469. Conboy J, Mohandas N, Tchernia G, Kan YW. Molecular basis of hereditary elliptocytosis due to protein 4.1 deficiency. N Engl J Med. 1986;315:680.

1470. Peters B, Kaiser HW, Magin TM. Skin-specific expression of ank-3⁹³, a novel ankyrin-3 splice variant. J Invest Dermatol. 2001;116:216.

1471. Garbarz M, Devaux I, Bournier O, et al. Protein 4.1 Lille, a novel mutation in the downstream initiation codon of protein 4.1 gene associated with heterozygous 4.1(−) hereditary elliptocytosis. Hum Mutat. 1995;5:339.

1472. Conboy JG, Chan JY, Chasis JA, et al. Tissue- and development-specific alternative RNA splicing regulates expression of multiple isoforms of erythroid membrane protein 4.1. J Biol Chem. 1991;266:8273.

1473. Tang TK, Qin Z, Leto T, et al. Heterogeneity of mRNA and protein products arising from the protein 4.1 gene in erythroid and non-erythroid tissues. J Cell Biol. 1990;110:617.

1474. Chasis JA, Coulombel L, Conboy J, et al. Differentiation-associated switches in protein 4.1 expression: synthesis of multiple structural isoforms during normal human erythropoiesis. J Clin Invest. 1993;91:329.

1475. Conboy JG, Chasis JA, Winardi R, et al. An isoform-specific mutation in the protein 4.1 gene results in hereditary elliptocytosis and complete deficiency of protein 4.1 in erythrocytes but not in nonerythroid cells. J Clin Invest. 1993;91:77.

1476. Alloisio N, Morle L, Dorleac E, et al. The heterozygous form of 4.1(−) hereditary elliptocytosis [the 4.1(−) trait]. Blood. 1985;65:46.

1477. Alloisio N, Dorleac E, Girot R, Delaunay J. Analysis of the red cell membrane in a family with hereditary elliptocytosis—total or partial absence of protein 4.1. Hum Genet. 1981;59:68.

1478. Takakuwa Y, Tchernia G, Rossi M, et al. Restoration of normal membrane stability to unstable protein 4.1–deficient erythrocyte membranes by incorporation of purified protein 4.1. J Clin Invest. 1986;78:80.

1479. Alloisio N, Dalla Venezia N, Rana A, et al. Evidence that red blood cell protein p55 may participate in the skeleton-membrane linkage that involves protein 4.1 and glycophorin C. Blood. 1993;82:1323.

1480. Alloisio N, Morle L, Bachir D, et al. Red cell membrane sialoglycoprotein in homozygous and heterozygous 4.1(−) hereditary elliptocytosis. Biochim Biophys Acta. 1985;816:57.

1481. Sondag D, Alloisio N, Blanchard D, et al. Gerbich reactivity in 4.1(−) hereditary elliptocytosis and protein 4.1 level in blood group Gerbich deficiency. Br J Haematol. 1987;65:43.

1482. Lambert S, Conboy J, Zail S. A molecular study of heterozygous protein 4.1 deficiency in hereditary elliptocytosis. Blood. 1988;72:1926.

1483. Reid ME, Takakuwa Y, Conboy J, et al. Glycophorin C content of human erythrocyte membrane is regulated by protein 4.1. Blood. 1990;75:2229.

1484. Rybicki AC, Heath R, Lubin B, Schwartz RS. Human erythrocyte protein 4.1 is a phosphatidylserine binding protein. J Clin Invest. 1988;81:255.

1485. Yawata A, Kanzaki A, Gilsanz F, et al. A markedly disrupted skeletal network with abnormally distributed intramembrane particles in complete protein 4.1–deficient red blood cells (allele 4.1 Madrid): implications regarding a critical role of protein 4.1 in maintenance of the integrity of the red blood cell membrane. Blood. 1997;90:2471.

1486. Conboy J, Marchesi S, Kim R, et al. Molecular analysis of insertion/deletion mutations in protein 4.1 in elliptocytosis: II. Determination of molecular genetic origins of rearrangements. J Clin Invest. 1990;86: 524.

1487. Marchesi S, Conboy J, Agre P, et al. Molecular analysis of insertion/deletion mutations in protein 4.1 in elliptocytosis: I. Biochemical identification of rearrangements in the spectrin/actin binding domain and functional characterizations. J Clin Invest. 1990;86:515.

1488. Moriniere M, Ribeiro L, Dalla Venezia N, et al. Elliptocytosis in patients with C-terminal domain mutations of protein 4.1 correlates with encoded messenger RNA levels rather than with alterations in primary protein structure. Blood. 2000;95:1834.

1489. Venezia ND, Maillet P, Morle L, et al. A large deletion within the protein 4.1 gene associated with a stable truncated mRNA and an unaltered tissue-specific alternative splicing. Blood. 1998;91:4361.

1490. Conboy JG. Structure, function, and molecular genetics of erythroid membrane skeletal protein 4.1 in normal and abnormal red blood cells. Semin Hematol. 1993; 30:58-73.

1491. Tanner MJ, High S, Martin PG, et al. Genetic variants of human red-cell membrane sialoglycoprotein beta. Study of the alterations occurring in the sialoglycoprotein-beta gene. Biochem J. 1988;250:407-414.

1492. Winardi R, Reid M, Conboy J, Mohandas N. Molecular analysis of glycophorin C deficiency in human erythrocytes. Blood. 1993;81:2799.

1493. Anstee DJ, Ridgwell K, Tanner MJ, et al. Individuals lacking the Gerbich blood-group antigen have alterations in the human erythrocyte membrane sialoglycoproteins beta and gamma. Biochem J. 1984;221:97.

1494. Anstee DJ, Parsons SF, Ridgwell K, et al. Two individuals with elliptocytic red cells apparently lack three minor erythrocyte membrane sialoglycoproteins. Biochem J. 1984;218:615.

1495. Daniels GL, Shaw MA, Judson PA, et al. A family demonstrating inheritance of the Leach phenotype: a Gerbich-negative phenotype associated with elliptocytosis. Vox Sang. 1986;50:117.

1496. Rebuck JW, van Slyck EJ. An unsuspected ultrastructural fault in human elliptocytes. Am J Clin Pathol. 1968; 49:19.

1497. Mohandas N, Chasis JA. Red cell deformability, membrane material properties, and shape: regulation by transmembrane, skeletal, and cytosolic proteins and lipids. Semin Hematol. 1993;30:171.

1498. Liu S-C, Derick LH, Palek J. Dependence of the permanent deformation of red blood cell membranes on spectrin dimer-tetramer equilibrium: implication for permanent membrane deformation of irreversibly sickled cells. Blood. 1993;81:522.

1499. Lu P-W, Soong C-J, Tao M. Phosphorylation of ankyrin decreases its affinity for spectrin tetramer. J Biol Chem. 1985;260:14958.

1500. De Gruchy GC, Loder PB, Hennessy IV. Haemolysis and glycolytic metabolism in hereditary elliptocytosis. Br J Haematol. 1962;8:168.

1501. Peters JC, Rowland M, Israels LG, Zipursky A. Erythrocyte sodium transport in hereditary elliptocytosis. Can J Physiol Pharmacol. 1966;44:817.

1502. Gallagher PG, Kotula L, Wang Y, et al. Molecular basis and haplotyping of the α II domain polymorphisms of spectrin: application to the study of hereditary elliptocytosis and pyropoikilocytosis. Am J Hum Genet. 1996;59:351.

1503. Facer CA. Malaria, hereditary elliptocytosis, and pyropoikilocytosis. Lancet. 1989;1:897.

1504. Chishti AH, Palek J, Fisher D, et al. Reduced invasion and growth of *Plasmodium falciparum* into elliptocytic red blood cells with a combined deficiency of protein 4.1, glycophorin C, and p55. Blood. 1996;87:3462.

1505. Amato D, Booth PB. Hereditary ovalocytosis in Melanesians. Papua New Guinea Med J. 1977;20:26.

1506. Castelino D, Saul A, Myler P, et al. Ovalocytosis in Papua New Guinea—dominantly inherited resistance to malaria. Southeast Asian J Trop Med Public Health. 1981;12:549.

1507. Cattani JA, Gibson FD, Alpers MP, Crane GG. Hereditary ovalocytosis and reduced susceptibility to malaria in Papua New Guinea. Trans R Soc Trop Med Hyg. 1987;81:705.

1508. Fix AG, Baer AS, Lie-Injo LE. The mode of inheritance of ovalocytosis/elliptocytosis in Malaysian Orang Asli families. Hum Genet. 1982;61:250.

1509. Harrison KL, Collins KA, McKenna HW. Hereditary elliptical stomatocytosis; a case report. Pathology. 1976; 8:307.

1510. Honig GR, Lacson PS, Maurer HS. A new familial disorder with abnormal erythrocyte morphology and increased permeability of the erythrocytes to sodium and potassium. Pediatr Res. 1971;5:159.

1511. Booth PB, Serjeantson S, Woodfield DG, Amato D. Selective depression of blood group antigens associated with hereditary ovalocytosis among Melanesians. Vox Sang. 1977;32:99.

1512. Baer A, Lie-Injo LE, Welch QB, Lewis AN. Genetic factors and malaria in the Temuan. Am J Hum Genet. 1976;28:179.

1513. Serjeantson S, Bryson K, Amato D, Babona D. Malaria and hereditary ovalocytosis. Hum Genet. 1977;37:161.

1514. Kimura M, Tamam M, Soemantri A, et al. Distribution of a 27-bp deletion in the band 3 gene in South Pacific islanders. J Hum Genet. 2003;48:642-645.

1515. Kimura M, Soemantri A, Ishida T. Malaria species and Southeast Asian ovalocytosis defined by a 27-bp deletion in the erythrocyte band 3 gene. Southeast Asian J Trop Med Public Health. 2002;33:4-6.

1516. Ravindranath Y, Goyette G Jr, Johnson RM. Southeast Asian ovalocytosis in an African-American family. Blood. 1994;84:2823.

1517. Coetzer TL, Beeton L, van Zyl D, et al. Southeast Asian ovalocytosis in a South African kindred with hemolytic anemia. Blood 1996;87:1656.

1518. Schischmanoff PO, Cynober T, Mielot F, et al. Southeast Asian ovalocytosis in white persons. Hemoglobin. 1999; 23:47.

1519. Ramos-Kuri M, Carrillo Farga J, Zúñiga J, et al. Molecular demonstration of SLC4A1 gene deletion in two Mexican patients with Southeast Asian ovalocytosis. Hum Biol. 2005;77:399-405.

1520. Liu S-C, Zhai S, Palek J, et al. Molecular defect of the band 3 protein in Southeast Asian ovalocytosis. N Engl J Med. 1990;323:1530.

1521. Liu SC, Jarolim P, Rubin HL, et al. The homozygous state for the band 3 protein mutation in Southeast Asian ovalocytosis may be lethal. Blood. 1994;84: 3590.

1522. Mgone CS, Koki G, Paniu MM, et al. Occurrence of the erythrocyte band 3 (AE1) gene deletion in relation to malaria endemicity in Papua New Guinea. Trans R Soc Trop Med Hyg. 1996;90:228.

1523. Foo LC, Rekhra J-V, Chiang GL, Mak JW. Ovalocytosis protects against severe malaria parasitemia in the Malayan aborigines. Am J Trop Med Hyg. 1992; 47:271.

1524. Allen SJ, O'Donnell A, Alexander ND, et al. Prevention of cerebral malaria in children in Papua New Guinea by Southeast Asian ovalocytosis band 3. Am J Trop Med Hyg. 1999;60:1056.

1525. Bunyaratvej A, Butthep P, Kaewkettong P, Yuthavong Y. Malaria protection in hereditary ovalocytosis: relation to red cell deformability, red cell parameters and degree of ovalocytosis. Southeast Asian J Trop Med Public Health. 1997;28(Suppl 3):38.

1526. Genton B, al-Yaman F, Mgone CS, et al. Ovalocytosis and cerebral malaria. Nature. 1995;378:564.

1527. Hadley T, Saul A, Lamont G, et al. Resistance of Melanesian elliptocytes (ovalocytes) to invasion by *Plasmodium knowlesi* and *Plasmodium falciparum* malaria parasites in vitro. J Clin Invest. 1983;71:780.

1528. Dluzewski AR, Nash GB, Wilson RJ, et al. Invasion of hereditary ovalocytes by *Plasmodium falciparum* in vitro and its relation to intracellular ATP concentration. Mol Biochem Parasitol. 1992;55:1.

1529. Kidson C, Lamont G, Saul A, Nurse GT. Ovalocytic erythrocytes from Melanesians are resistant to invasion by malaria parasites in culture. Proc Natl Acad Sci U S A. 1981;78:5829.

1530. Cortes A, Benet A, Cooke BM, et al. Ability of *Plasmodium falciparum* to invade Southeast Asian ovalocytes varies between parasite lines. Blood. 2004;104:2961-2966.

1531. Saul A, Lamont G, Sawyer WH, Kidson C. Decreased membrane deformability in Melanesian ovalocytes from Papua New Guinea. J Cell Biol. 1984;98:1348.

1532. Mohandas N, Lie-Injo LE, Friedman M, Mak JW. Rigid membranes of Malayan ovalocytes: a likely genetic barrier against malaria. Blood. 1984;63:1385.

1533. Mohandas N, Winardi R, Knowles D, et al. Molecular basis for membrane rigidity of hereditary ovalocytosis: A novel mechanism involving the cytoplasmic domain of band 3. J Clin Invest. 1992:89:686.

1534. Schofield AE, Tanner MJ, Pinder JC, et al. Basis of unique red cell membrane properties in hereditary ovalocytosis. J Mol Biol. 1992;223:949.

1535. O'Donnell A, Raiko A, Clegg JB, et al. Southeast Asian ovalocytosis and pregnancy in a malaria-endemic region of Papua New Guinea. Am J Trop Med Hyg. 2007;76:631-633.

1536. Cortés A, Benet A, Cooke BM, et al. Ability of *Plasmodium falciparum* to invade Southeast Asian ovalocytes varies between parasite lines. Blood. 2004;104:2961-2966.

1537. Jarolim P, Palek J, Amato D, et al. Deletion in the band 3 gene in malaria resistant Southeast Asian ovalocytosis. Proc Natl Acad Sci U S A. 1991;88:11022-11026.

1538. Mueller TJ, Morrison M. Detection of a variant of protein 3, the major transmembrane protein of the human erythrocyte. J Biol Chem. 1977;252:6573.

1539. Jarolim P, Rubin HL, Zhai S, et al. Band 3 Memphis: a widespread polymorphism with abnormal electrophoretic mobility of erythrocyte band 3 protein caused by substitution AAG→GAG (Lys→Glu) in codon 56. Blood. 1992;80:1592.

1540. Yannoukakos D, Vasseur C, Driancourt C, et al. Human erythrocyte band 3 polymorphism (band 3 Memphis): characterization of the structural modification (Lys 56→ Glu) by protein chemistry methods. Blood. 1991;78:1117.

1541. Jones GL. Red cell membrane proteins in Melanesian ovalocytosis autophosphorylation and proteolysis. Proc Aust Biochem Soc. 1984;16:34.

1542. Jones GL, McLemore-Edmundson H, Wesche D, Saul A. Human erythrocyte band 3 has an altered N-terminus in malaria-resistant Melanesian ovalocytosis. Biochim Biophys Acta. 1991;1096:33.

1543. Schofield AE, Rearden DM, Tanner MJA. Defective anion transport activity of the abnormal band 3 in hereditary ovalocytic red cells. Nature. 1992;335:836.

1544. Tanner MJ, Bruce L, Groves JD, et al. The defective red cell anion transporter (band 3) in hereditary Southeast Asian ovalocytosis and the role of glycophorin A in the expression of band 3 anion transport activity in *Xenopus* oocytes. Biochem Soc Trans. 1992;20:542-546.

1545. O'Donnell A, Allen SJ, Mgone CS, et al. Red cell morphology and malaria anaemia in children with Southeast-Asian ovalocytosis band 3 in Papua New Guinea. Br J Haematol. 1998;101:407.

1546. Tanner MJ, Bruce L, Martin PG, et al. Melanesian hereditary ovalocytes have a deletion in red cell band 3. Blood. 1991;78:2785-2786.

1547. Laosombat V, Dissaneevate S, Peerapittayamongkol C, Matsuo M. Neonatal hyperbilirubinemia associated with Southeast Asian ovalocytosis. Am J Hematol. 1999; 60:136.

1548. Laosombat V, Dissaneevate S, Wongchanchailert M, Satayasevanaa B. Neonatal anemia associated with Southeast Asian ovalocytosis. Int J Hematol. 2005;82:201-205.

1549. Reardon DM, Seymour CA, Cox TM, et al. Hereditary ovalocytosis with compensated haemolysis. Br J Haematol. 1993;85:197.

1550. Wrong O, Bruce LJ, Unwin RJ, et al. Band 3 mutations, distal renal tubular acidosis, and Southeast Asian ovalocytosis. Kidney Int. 2002;62:10-19.

1551. Yenchitsomanus PT. Human anion exchanger1 mutations and distal renal tubular acidosis. Southeast Asian J Trop Med Public Health. 2003;34:651-658.

1552. Sawasdee N, Udomchaiprasertkul W, Noisakran S, et al. Trafficking defect of mutant kidney anion exchanger 1 (kAE1) proteins associated with distal renal tubular acidosis and Southeast Asian ovalocytosis. Biochem Biophys Res Commun. 2006;350:723-730.

1553. Mohandas N, Chasis JA, Shohet SB. The influence of membrane skeleton on red cell deformability, membrane material properties, and shape. Semin Hematol. 1983; 20:225.

1554. Kuma H, Inoue K, Fu G, et al. Secondary structures of synthetic peptides corresponding to the first membrane-contact portion of normal band 3 and its deletion mutant (Southeast Asian ovalocytosis). J Biochem (Tokyo). 1998;124:509.

1555. Liu S-C, Palek J, Yi SJ, et al. Molecular basis of altered red blood cell membrane properties in Southeast Asian ovalocytosis: Role of the mutant band 3 protein in band 3 oligomerization and retention by the membrane skeleton. Blood. 1995;86:349.

1556. Che A, Cherry RJ, Bannister LH, Dluzewski AR. Aggregation of band 3 in hereditary ovalocytic red blood cell membranes. Electron microscopy and protein rotational diffusion studies. J Cell Sci. 1993;105:655.

1557. Moriyama R, Ideguchi H, Lombardo CR, et al. Structural and functional characterization of band 3 from Southeast Asian ovalocytes. J Biol Chem. 1992;267:25792.

1558. Chambers EJ, Bloomberg GB, Ring SM, Tanner MJ. Structural studies on the effects of the deletion in the red cell anion exchanger (band 3, AE1) associated with South East Asian ovalocytosis. J Mol Biol. 1999;285:1289.

1559. Cheung JC, Reithmeier RA. Membrane integration and topology of the first transmembrane segment in normal and Southeast Asian ovalocytosis human erythrocyte anion exchanger 1. Mol Membr Biol. 2005;22:203-214.

1560. Kuma H, Abe Y, Askin D, et al. Molecular basis and functional consequences of the dominant effects of the mutant band 3 on the structure of normal band 3 in Southeast Asian ovalocytosis. Biochemistry. 2002;41:3311-3320.

1561. Okoye VC, Bennett V. *Plasmodium falciparum* malaria. Band 3 as a possible receptor during invasion of human erythrocytes. Science. 1985;227:169.

1562. Dluzewski AR, Fryer PR, Griffiths S, et al. Red cell membrane protein distribution during malarial invasion. J Cell Sci. 1989;92:691.

1563. Zarkowsky HS, Oski FA, Sha'afi R. Congenital hemolytic anemia with high-sodium, low-potassium red cells: I. Studies of membrane permeability. N Engl J Med. 1968;278:573.

1564. Bienzle U, Niethammer D, Kleeberg U, et al. Congenital stomatocytosis and chronic haemolytic anaemia. Scand J Haematol. 1975;15:339.

1565. Eber SW, Lande WM, Iarocci TA, et al. Hereditary stomatocytosis: consistent association with an integral membrane protein deficiency. Br J Haematol. 1989;72:452-455.

1566. Lande WM, Thiemann PV, Mentzer WC Jr. Missing band 7 membrane protein in two patients with high Na, low K erythrocytes. J Clin Invest. 1982;70:1273.

1567. Lo SS, Hitzig WH, Marti HR. Stomatozytose. Schweiz Med Wochenschr. 1970;100:1977.

1568. Lo SS, Marti HR, Hitzig WH. Haemolytic anaemia associated with decreased concentration of reduced glutathione in red cells. Acta Haematol. 1971;46:14.

1569. Lock SP, Smith RS, Hardisty RM. Stomatocytosis: A hereditary red cell anomaly associated with haemolytic anaemia. Br J Haematol. 1961;7:303-314.

1570. Mentzer WC Jr, Smith WB, Goldstone J, Shohet SB. Hereditary stomatocytosis membranes and metabolism studies. Blood 1975;46:659-669.

1571. Morlé L, Pothier B, Alloisio N, et al. Reduction of membrane band 7 and activation of volume stimulated (K$^+$, Cl$^-$)-cotransport in a case of congenital stomatocytosis. Br J Haematol. 1989;71:141-146.

1572. Schroter W, Ungefehr K, Tillmann W. Role of the spleen in congenital stomatocytosis associated with high sodium-low potassium erythrocytes. Klin Wochenschr. 1981;59:173.

1573. Rix M, Bjerrum PJ, Wieth JO, Frandsen B. Medfodt stomatocytose med haemolytisk anaemi-med abnorm kationpermeabilitet og defekte membranproteiner. [Congenital stomatocytosis with hemolytic anemia-with abnormal cation permeability and defective membrane proteins.] Ugeskr Laeger. 1991;153:724-726.

1574. Meadow SR. Stomatocytosis. Proc R Soc Med. 1967;60:13.

1575. Stewart GW, Hepworth-Jones BE, Keen JN, et al. Isolation of cDNA coding for an ubiquitous membrane protein deficient in high Na$^+$, low K$^+$ stomatocytic erythrocytes. Blood. 1992;79:1593-601.

1576. Fricke B, Argent AC, Chetty MC, et al. The "stomatin" gene and protein in overhydrated hereditary stomatocytosis. Blood. 2003;102:2268-2277.

1577. Fricke B, Parsons SF, Knöpfle G, et al. Stomatin is mistrafficked in the erythrocytes of overhydrated hereditary stomatocytosis, and is absent from normal primitive yolk sac–derived erythrocytes. Br J Haematol. 2005;131:265-277.

1578. Wilkinson DK, Turner EJ, Parkin ET, et al. Membrane raft actin deficiency and altered Ca^{2+}-induced vesiculation in stomatin-deficient overhydrated hereditary stomatocytosis. Biochim Biophys Acta. 2008;1778:125-132

1579. Turner EJ, Jarvis HG, Chetty MC, et al. ATP-dependent vesiculation in red cell membranes from different hereditary stomatocytosis variants. Br J Haematol. 2003;120:894-902.

1580. Oski FA, Naiman JL, Blum SF, et al. Congenital hemolytic anemia with high-sodium, low-potassium red cells. Studies of three generations of a family with a new variant. N Engl J Med. 1969;280:909-916.

1581. Mutoh S, Sasaki R, Takaku F, et al. A family of hereditary stomatocytosis associated with normal level of Na-K-ATPase activity of red blood cells. Am J Hematol. 1983;14:113.

1582. Jarvis HG, Chetty MC, Nicolaou A, et al. A novel stomatocytosis variant showing marked abnormalities in intracellular [Na] and [K] with minimal haemolysis. Eur J Haematol. 2001;66:412-414.

1583. Miller G, Townes PL, MacWhinney JB. A new congenital hemolytic anemia with deformed erythrocytes ("stomatocytes") and remarkable susceptibility of erythrocytes to cold hemolysis in vitro. I. Clinical and hematologic studies. Pediatrics. 1965;35:906.

1584. Gore DM, Chetty MC, Fisher J, et al. Familial pseudohyperkalaemia Cardiff: a mild version of cryohydrocytosis. Br J Haematol. 2002;117:212-214.

1585. Haines PG, Jarvis HG, King S, et al. Two further British families with the "cryohydrocytosis" form of hereditary stomatocytosis. Br J Haematol. 2001;113:932-937.

1586. Coles SE, Chetty MC, Ho MM, et al. Two British families with variants of the "cryohydrocytosis" form of hereditary stomatocytosis. Br J Haematol. 1999;105:1055-1065

1587. Bruce LJ, Robinson HC, Guizouarn H, et al. Monovalent cation leaks in human red cells caused by single amino-acid substitutions in the transport domain of the band 3 chloride-bicarbonate exchanger, AE1. Nat Genet. 2005;37:1258-1263.

1588. Fricke B, Jarvis HG, Reid CD, et al. Four new cases of stomatin-deficient hereditary stomatocytosis syndrome: association of the stomatin-deficient cryohydrocytosis variant with neurological dysfunction. Br J Haematol. 2004;125:796-803.

1589. Jarvis HG, Gore DM, Briggs C, et al. Cold storage of "cryohydrocytosis" red cells: the osmotic susceptibility of the cold-stored erythrocyte. Br J Haematol. 2003;122:859-868.

1590. Miller DR, Rickles FR, Lichtman MA, et al. A new variant of hereditary hemolytic anemia with stomatocytosis and erythrocyte cation abnormality. Blood. 1971;38:184.

1591. Haines PG, Crawley C, Chetty MC, et al. Familial pseudohyperkalaemia Chiswick: a novel congenital thermotropic variant of K and Na transport across the human red cell membrane. Br J Haematol. 2001;112:469-474.

1592. Grootenboer S, Schischmanoff PO, Laurendeau I, et al. Pleiotropic syndrome of dehydrated hereditary stomatocytosis, pseudohyperkalemia, and perinatal edema maps to 16q23-q24. Blood. 2000;96:2599-2605.

1593. Grootenboer S, Barro C, Cynober T, et al. Dehydrated hereditary stomatocytosis: A cause of prenatal ascites. Prenat Diagn. 2001;21:1114.

1594. Carella M, Stewart GW, Ajetunmobi JF, et al. Genetic heterogeneity of hereditary stomatocytosis syndromes showing pseudohyperkalemia. Haematologica. 1999;84: 862-863.

1595. Kilpatrick ES, Burton ID. Pseudohyperkalaemia, pseudohyponatraemia and pseudohypoglycaemia in a patient with hereditary stomatocytosis. Ann Clin Biochem. 1997;34:561-563.

1596. Stewart GW, Corrall RJ, Fyffe JA, et al. Familial pseudohyperkalemia. Lancet. 1979;2:175-181.

1597. Stewart GW, Ellory JC. A family with mild hereditary xerocytosis showing high membrane cation permeability at low temperatures. Clin Sci. 1985;69:309-319.

1598. Jaffe ER, Gottfried EL. Hereditary nonspherocytic hemolytic disease associated with an altered phospholipid composition of the erythrocytes. J Clin Invest. 1968;47:1375-1388.

1599. Delaunay J, Stewart G, Iolascon A. Hereditary dehydrated and overhydrated stomatocytosis: recent advances. Curr Opin Hematol. 1999;6:110-114.

1600. Luciani JC, Lavabre-Bertrand T, Fourcade J, et al. Familial pseudohyperkalaemia. Lancet. 1980;1:491.

1601. Meenaghan M, Follett GF, Brophy PJ. Temperature sensitivity of potassium flux into red blood cells in the familial pseudohyperkalaemia syndrome. Biochim Biophys Acta. 1985;821:72-78.

1602. James DR, Stansbie D. Familial pseudohyperkalaemia: inhibition of erythrocyte K^+ efflux at $4°$ C by quinine. Clin Sci (Lond). 1987;73:557-560.

1603. Clark ME, Mohandas N, Caggiano V, Shohet SB. Effects of abnormal cation transport on deformability of desiccytes. J Supramol Struct. 1978;8:521-532.

1604. Glader BE, Fortier N, Albala MM, Nathan DG. Congenital hemolytic anemia associated with dehydrated erythrocytes and increased potassium loss. N Engl J Med. 1974;291:491.

1605. Lane PA, Kuypers FA, Clark MR, et al. Excess of red cell membrane proteins in hereditary high-phosphatidylcholine hemolytic anemia. Am J Hematol. 1990;34: 186.

1606. McGrath KM. Dehydrated hereditary stomatocytosis—a report of two families and a review of the literature. Pathology. 1984;16:146.

1607. Nolan GR. Hereditary xerocytosis: a case history and review of the literature. Pathology. 1984;16:151.

1608. Platt OS, Lux SE, Nathan DG. Exercise-induced hemolysis in xerocytosis: erythrocyte dehydration and shear sensitivity. J Clin Invest. 1981;68:631.

1609. Shohet SB, Livermore BM, Nathan DG, Jaffe ER. Hereditary hemolytic anemia associated with abnormal membrane lipids: mechanism of accumulation of phosphatidyl choline. Blood. 1971;38:445.

1610. Shohet SB, Nathan DG, Livermore BM, et al. Hereditary hemolytic anemia associated with abnormal membrane lipids. II. Ion permeability and transport abnormalities. Blood 1973;42:1-8.

1611. Wiley JS, Ellory JC, Shuman MA, et al. Characteristics of the membrane defect in the hereditary stomatocytosis syndrome. Blood. 1975;46:337.

1612. Yawata Y, Takemoto Y, Yoshimoto M, et al. The Japanese family of congenital hemolytic anemia with high red cell phosphatidyl choline and increased sodium transport. Acta Haematol Jpn. 1982;45:672.

1613. Clark MR, Shohet SB, Gottfried EL. Hereditary hemolytic disease with increased red blood cell phosphatidylcholine and dehydration: one, two, or many disorders? Am J Hematol. 1993;42:25.

1614. Ogburn PL Jr, Ramin KD, Danilenko-Dixon D, et al. In utero erythrocyte transfusion for fetal xerocytosis associated with severe anemia and non-immune hydrops fetalis. Am J Obstet Gynecol. 2001;185:238-239.

1615. Wiley JS, Cooper RA, Adachi K, Asakura T. Hereditary stomatocytosis: association of low 2,3-diphosphoglycerate with increased cation pumping by the red cell. Br J Haematol. 1979;41:133.

1616. Vives-Corrons JL, Besson I, Aymerich M, et al. Hereditary xerocytosis: a report of six unrelated Spanish families with leaky red cell syndrome and increased heat stability of the erythrocyte membrane. Br J Haematol. 1995;90:817.

1617. Entezami M, Becker R, Menssen HD, et al. Xerocytosis with concomitant intrauterine ascites: first description and therapeutic approach. Blood. 1996;87:5392-5393.

1618. Grootenboer S, Schischmanoff PO, Cynober T, et al. A genetic syndrome associating dehydrated hereditary stomatocytosis, pseudohyperkalaemia and perinatal oedema. Br J Haematol. 1998;103:383.

1619. Vicente-Gutiérrez MP, Castelló-Almazán I, Salvía-Roiges MD, et al. Nonimmune hydrops fetalis due to congenital xerocytosis. J Perinatol. 2005;25:63-65.

1620. Gore DM, Layton M, Sinha AK, et al. Four pedigrees of the cation-leaky hereditary stomatocytosis class presenting with pseudohyperkalaemia. Novel profile of temperature dependence of Na^+-K^+ leak in a xerocytic form. Br J Haematol. 2004;125:521-527.

1621. Syfuss PY, Ciupea A, Brahimi S, et al. Mild dehydrated hereditary stomatocytosis revealed by marked hepatosiderosis. Clin Lab Haematol. 2006;28:270-274.

1622. Rees DC, Portmann B, Ball C, et al. Dehydrated hereditary stomatocytosis is associated with neonatal hepatitis. Br J Haematol. 2004;126:272-276.

1623. Wiley JS, Shaller CC. Selective loss of calcium permeability on maturation of reticulocytes. J Clin Invest. 1977;59:1113.

1624. Kanzaki A, Yawata Y. Hereditary stomatocytosis: phenotypical expression of sodium transport and band 7 peptides in 44 cases. Br J Haematol. 1992;82: 133.

1625. Olivieri O, Girelli D, Vettore L, et al. A case of congenital dyserythropoietic anaemia with stomatocytosis, reduced bands 7 and 8 and normal cation content. Br J Haematol. 1992;80:258.

1626. Hiebl-Dirschmied C, Entler B, Glotzmann C, et al. Cloning and nucleotide sequence of cDNA encoding human erythrocyte band 7 integral membrane protein. Biochim Biophys Acta. 1991;1090:123.

1627. Stewart GW, Argent AC, Dash BC. Stomatin: a putative cation transport regulator in the red cell membrane. Biochim Biophys Acta. 1993;1225:15.

1628. Gallagher PG, Forget BG. Structure, organization, and expression of the human band 7.2b gene, a candidate gene for hereditary hydrocytosis. J Biol Chem. 1995;270: 26358.

1629. Seidel G, Prohaska R. Molecular cloning of hSLP-1, a novel human brain-specific member of the band 7/MEC-2 family similar to *Caenorhabditis elegans* UNC-24. Gene. 1998;225:23.

1630. Umlauf E, Mairhofer M, Prohaska R. Characterization of the stomatin domain involved in homo-oligomerization and lipid raft association. J Biol Chem. 2006;281: 23349-23356.

1631. Fricke B, Parsons SF, Knöpfle G, et al. Stomatin is mistrafficked in the erythrocytes of overhydrated hereditary stomatocytosis, and is absent from normal primitive yolk sac–derived erythrocytes. Br J Haematol. 2005;131:265-277.

1632. Stewart GW, Argent AC. Integral band 7 protein of the human erythrocyte membrane. Biochem Soc Trans. 1992;20:785.

1633. Gallagher PG, Segel G, Marchesi SL, Forget BG. The gene for erythrocyte band 7.2b in hereditary stomatocytosis. Blood. 1992;80(Suppl 1):276a.

1634. John KM, Lux SE. Unpublished data.

1635. Zhu Y, Paszty C, Turetsky T, et al. Stomatocytosis is absent in "stomatin"-deficient murine red blood cells. Blood. 1999;93:2404.

1636. Murali B, Drain A, Seller D, et al. Pulmonary thromboendarterectomy in a case of hereditary stomatocytosis. Br J Anaesth. 2003;91:739-741.

1637. Bergheim J, Ernst P, Brinch L, et al. Allogeneic bone marrow transplantation for severe post-splenectomy thrombophilic state in leaky red cell membrane haemolytic anaemia of the stomatocytosis class. Br J Haematol. 2003;121:119-122.

1638. Gallagher PG, Chang SH, Rettig MP, et al. Altered erythrocyte endothelial adherence and membrane phospholipid asymmetry in hereditary hydrocytosis. Blood. 2003;101:4625-4627.

1639. Smith BD, Segel GB. Abnormal erythrocyte endothelial adherence in hereditary stomatocytosis. Blood. 1997;89: 3451.

1640. Ellory JC, Gibson JS, Stewart GW. Pathophysiology of abnormal cell volume in human red cells. Contrib Nephrol. 1998;123:220.

1641. Kaplan JH. Biochemistry of Na,K-ATPase. Annu Rev Biochem. 2002;71:511.

1642. Carella M, Stewart G, Ajetunmobi JF, et al. Genomewide search for dehydrated hereditary stomatocytosis (hereditary xerocytosis): mapping of locus to chromosome 16 (16q23-qter). Am J Hum Genet. 1998;63:810.

1643. Iolascon A, Stewart GW, Ajetunmobi JF, et al. Familial pseudohyperkalemia maps to the same locus as dehydrated hereditary stomatocytosis (hereditary xerocytosis). Blood. 1999;93:3120.

1644. Dise CA, Goodman DBP, Rasmussen H. Selective stimulation of erythrocyte membrane phospholipid fatty acid turnover associated with decreased volume. J Biol Chem. 1980;255:5201.

1645. Fairbanks G, Dino JE, et al. Membrane alterations in hereditary xerocytosis: Elevated binding of glyceraldehyde-3-phosphate dehydrogenase. In Kruckeberg WC, Eaton JW, et al (eds). Erythrocyte Membranes: Recent Clinical and Experimental Advances. New York, Alan R Liss, 1978, p 173.

1646. Platt OS. Exercise-induced hemolysis in sickle cell anemia: shear-sensitivity and erythrocyte dehydration. Blood 1982;59:1055.

1647. Harm W, Fortier NL, Lutz HU, et al. Increased erythrocyte lipid peroxidation in hereditary xerocytosis. Clin Chim Acta. 1979;99:121.

1648. Sauberman N, Fortier NL, Joshi W, et al. Spectrin-hemoglobin crosslinkages associated with in vitro oxidant hypersensitivity in pathologic and artificially dehydrated red cells. Br J Haematol. 1983;54:15.

1649. Snyder LM, Sauberman N, Condara H, et al. Red cell membrane response to hydrogen peroxide–sensitivity in hereditary xerocytosis and in other abnormal red cells. Br J Haematol. 1981;48:435.

1650. Fortier N, Snyder LM, Garver F, et al. The relationship between in vivo generated hemoglobin skeletal protein complex and increased red cell membrane rigidity. Blood. 1988;71:1427.

1651. Sanchez M, Palacio M, Borrell A, et al. Prenatal diagnosis and management of fetal xerocytosis associated with ascites. Fetal Diagn Ther. 2005;20:402-405.

1652. Ogburn PL, Ramin KD, Danilenko-Dixon D, et al. In utero erythrocyte tranfusion for fetal xerocytosis associated with severe anemia and non-immune hydrops fetalis. Am J Obstet Gynecol. 2001;185:238-239.

1653. Chetty MC, Stewart GW. Pseudohyperkalaemia and pseudomacrocytosis caused by inherited red-cell disorders of the "hereditary stomatocytosis" group. Br J Biomed Sci. 2001;58:48.

1654. Sauberman N, Fairbanks G, Lutz HU, et al. Altered red blood cell surface area in hereditary xerocytosis. Clin Chim Med. 1981;114:149.

1655. Delaunay J. The hereditary stomatocytoses: genetic disorders of the red cell membrane permeability to monovalent cations. Semin Hematol. 2004;41:165-172.

1656. Albala MM, Fortier NL, Glader BE. Physiologic features of hemolysis associated with altered cation and 2,3-diphosphoglycerate content. Blood. 1978;52:135.

1657. Jais X, Till SJ, Cynober T, et al. An extreme consequence of splenectomy in dehydrated hereditary stomatocytosis: gradual thrombo-embolic pulmonary hypertension and lung-heart transplantation. Hemoglobin. 2003;27:139-147.

1658. Coles SE, Stewart GW. Temperature effects on cation transport in hereditary stomatocytosis and allied disorders. Int J Exp Pathol. 1999;80:251-258.

1659. Douglass CC, Twomey JJ. Transient stomatocytosis with hemolysis: a previously unrecognized complication of alcoholism. Ann Intern Med. 1970;72:159.

1660. Wislöff F, Boman D. Acquired stomatocytosis in alcoholic liver disease. Scand J Haematol. 1979;23:43.

1661. Simpson LO. Blood from healthy animals and humans contains nondiscocytic erythrocytes. Br J Haematol. 1989;73:561.

1662. Barrett AM. A special form of erythrocyte possessing increased resistance to hypotonic saline. J Pathol Bacteriol. 1938;46:603.

1663. Davidson RJ, How J, Lessels S. Acquired stomatocytosis: its prevalence and significance in routine haematology. Scand J Haematol. 1977;19:47.

1664. Ducrou W, Kimber RJ. Stomatocytes, haemolytic anaemia and abdominal pain in Mediterranean migrants. Some examples of a new syndrome? Med J Aust. 1969;2:1087.

1665. Ohsaka A, Kano Y, Kanzaki A, et al. A transient hemolytic reaction and stomatocytosis following vinca alkaloid administration. Acta Haematol Jpn. 1989;52:7.

1666. Reinhart WH, Chien S. Stomatocytic transformation of red blood cells after marathon running. Am J Hematol. 1985;19:201.

1667. Reinhart WH, Bartsch P, Straub PW. Red cell morphology after a 100-km run. Clin Lab Haematol. 1989;11:105-110.

1668. Huang CH, Liu PZ, Cheng JG. Molecular biology and genetics of the Rh blood group system. Semin Hematol. 2000;37:150.

1669. Vos GH, Vos D, Kirk RL, Sanger R. A sample of blood with no detectable Rh antigens. Lancet. 1961;1:14.

1670. Seidl S, Spielmann W, Martin H. Two siblings with Rh$_{null}$ disease. Vox Sang. 1972;23:182.

1671. Senhauser DA, Mitchell MW, Gault DB, Owens JH. Another example of phenotype Rh$_{null}$. Transfusion. 1970;10:89.

1672. Sturgeon P. Hematological observations on the anemia associated with blood type Rh$_{null}$. Blood 1970;36:310.

1673. Lauf PK, Joiner CH. Increased potassium transport and ouabain binding in human Rh$_{null}$ red blood cells. Blood 1976;48:457.

1674. McGuire DM, Rosenfield RE, Wong KY, et al. Rh$_{mod}$. A second kindred (Craig). Vox Sang. 1976;30:430.

1675. Saji H, Hosoi T. A Japanese Rh$_{mod}$ family: serological and haematological observations. Vox Sang. 1979;37:296.

1676. Oram JF. Tangier disease and ABCA1. Biochim Biophys Acta. 2000;1529:321.

1677. Oram JF, Lawn RM. ABCA1. The gatekeeper for eliminating excess tissue cholesterol. J Lipid Res. 2001;42:1173.

1678. Schmitz G, Langmann T. Structure, function and regulation of the ABC1 gene product. Curr Opin Lipidol. 2001;12:129.

1679. Reinhart WH, Gossi U, Butikofer P, et al. Haemolytic anaemia in an alpha-lipoproteinaemia (Tangier disease): morphological, biochemical, and biophysical properties of the red blood cell. Br J Haematol. 1989;72:272.

1680. Hoffman HN, Fredrickson DS. Tangier disease (familial high density lipoprotein deficiency): clinical and genetic features in two adults. Am J Med. 1965;39:582.

1681. Kummer H, Laissue J, Speiss H, et al. Familiäre Analphalipoproteinämie (Tangier-Krankheit). Schweiz Med Wochenschr. 1968;98:406.

1682. Shaklady MM, Djardjouras EM, Lloyd JK. Red-cell lipids in familial alphalipoprotein deficiency (Tangier disease). Lancet. 1968;2:151.

1683. Ducrou W, Kimber RJ. Stomatocytes, haemolytic anemia and abdominal pain in Mediterranean migrants. Some examples of a new syndrome? Med J Aust. 1969;2:1087-1091.

1684. Norman JG. Stomatocytosis in migrants in Mediterranean origin [letter]. Med J Aust. 1969;1:315.

1685. Jackson, JM, Knight D. Stomatocytosis in migrants of Mediterranean origin [letter]. Med J Aust. 1969;1:939-940.

1686. Lander H. More maladies in Mediterranean migrants: stomatocytosis and macrothrombocytopenia. Med J Aust. 1971;1:438-440.

1687. von Behrens WE. Splenomegaly, macrothrombocytopenia and stomatocytosis in healthy Mediterranean subjects (splenomegaly in Mediterranean macrothrombocytopenia). Scand J Haematol. 1975;14:258-267.

1688. Rees DC, Iolascon A, Carella M, et al. Stomatocytic haemolysis and macrothrombocytopenia (Mediterranean stomatocytosis/macrothrombocytopenia) is the haematological presentation of phytosterolaemia. Br J Haematol. 2005;130:297-309.

1689. Patel SB, Salen G, Hidaka H, et al. Mapping a gene involved in regulating dietary cholesterol absorption: the sitosterolemia locus is found at chromosome 2p21. J Clin Invest. 1998;102:1041-1044.

1690. Berge KE, Tian H, Graf GA, et al. Accumulation of dietary cholesterol in sitosterolemia caused by mutations in adjacent ABC transporters. Science. 2000;290:1771-1775.

1691. Weed RI, LaCelle PL, Merrill EW. Metabolic dependence of red cell deformability. J Clin Invest. 1969;48:795.

1692. Hoffman JF. ATP compartmentation in human erythrocytes. Curr Opin Hematol. 1997;4:112.

1693. Lux SE, John KM, Ukena TE. Diminished spectrin extraction from ATP-depleted human erythrocytes. Evidence relating spectrin to changes in erythrocyte shape and deformability. J Clin Invest. 1978;61:815.

1694. Palek J, Liu SC, Snyder LM. Metabolic dependence of protein arrangement in human erythrocyte membranes. I. Analysis of spectrin-rich complexes in ATP-depleted red cells. Blood 1978;51:385.

1695. Nathan DG, Oski FA, Sidel VW, Diamond LK. Extreme hemolysis and red cell distortion in erythrocyte pyruvate kinase deficiency. II. Measurements of erythrocyte glucose consumption, potassium flux and adenosine triphosphate stability. N Engl J Med. 1965;272:118.

1696. Mentzer WC Jr, Baehner RL, Schmidt-Schonbein H, et al. Selective reticulocyte destruction in erythrocyte pyruvate kinase deficiency. J Clin Invest. 1971;50:688.

1697. Glader BE. Salicylate-induced injury of pyruvate kinase deficient erythrocytes. N Engl J Med. 1976;294:916.

1698. Oski FA, Nathan DG, Sidel VW, Nathan LK. Extreme hemolysis and red cell distortion in erythrocyte pyruvate kinase deficiency. I. Morphology, erythrokinetics and family enzyme studies. N Engl J Med. 1964;270:1023.

1699. Leblond PF, Lyonnais J, Delage JM. Erythrocyte populations in pyruvate kinase deficiency anaemia following splenectomy. I. Cell morphology. Br J Haematol. 1978;39:55.

1700. Leblond PF, Coulombe L, Lyonnais J. Erythrocyte populations in pyruvate kinase deficiency anaemia following splenectomy: II. Cell deformability. Br J Haematol. 1978;31:63.

1701. Coetzer T, Zail SS. Erythrocyte membrane proteins in hereditary glucose phosphate isomerase deficiency. J Clin Invest. 1979;63:552.

1702. Lux SE, John KM, Karnovsky MJ. Irreversible deformation of the spectrin-actin lattice in irreversibly sickled cells. J Clin Invest. 1976;58:955.

1703. McGoron AJ, Joiner CH, Palascak MB, et al. Dehydration of mature and immature sickle red blood cells during fast oxygenation/deoxygenation cycles: role of KCl cotransport and extracellular calcium. Blood. 2000;95:2164.

1704. Schultze M. Ein Heizbarer objectisch und seine Verwendung bei Untersuchungen des Blutes. Arch Mikrok Anat. 1865;1:1.

1705. Shen SC, Ham TH, Fleming AB. Studies on the destruction of red blood cells: III. Mechanism and complication of hemoglobinuria in patients with thermal burns: spherocytosis and increased osmotic fragility of red blood cells. N Engl J Med. 1943;229:701.

1706. Topley E. The usefulness of counting "heat-affected" red cells as a guide to the risk of the later disappearance of red cells after burns. J Clin Pathol. 1961;14:295.

1707. James GW III, Purnell OJ, Evans ET. The anemia of thermal injury: I. Studies of pigment excretion. J Clin Invest. 1951;30:181.

1708. James GW III, Abbott LD, Brooks JW, Evans EI. The anemia of thermal injury: III. Erythropoiesis and hemoglobin metabolism studied with N^{15}-glycine in dog and man. J Clin Invest. 1954;33:150.

1709. Moore FD, Peacock WC, Blakely E, Cope O. The anemia of thermal burns. Ann Surg. 1946;124:811-839.

1710. McCollough J, Polesky HF, Nelson C, Hoff T. Iatrogenic hemolysis: a complication of blood warmed by a microwave device. Anesth Analg. 1972;51:102.

1711. Staples PJ, Griner PF. Extracorporeal hemolysis of blood in a microwave blood warmer. N Engl J Med. 1971;285:317.

1712. Bull BS, Kuhn IN. The production of schistocytes by fibrin strands (a scanning electron microscope study). Blood. 1970;35:104.

1713. Brain MC, Dacie JV. Microangiopathic haemolytic anaemia: the possible role of vascular lesions in pathogenesis. Br J Haematol. 1962;8:358.

1714. Nevaril CG, Lynch EC. Erythrocyte damage and destruction induced by shearing stress. J Lab Clin Med. 1968;71:784.

1715. Jacob HS, Amsden T. Acute hemolytic anemia with rigid red cells in hypophosphatemia. N Engl J Med. 1971;285:1446.

1716. Lichtman MA, Miller DR, Cohen J, Waterhouse C. Reduced red cell glycolysis, 2,3-diphosphoglycerate and adenosine triphosphate concentration, and increased hemoglobin-oxygen affinity caused by hypophosphatemia. Ann Intern Med. 1971;74:562.

1717. Kalan G, Derganc M, Primocic J. Phosphate metabolism in red blood cells of critically ill neonates. Pflugers Arch. 2000;440:R109.

1718. Larsen VH, Waldau T, Gravesen H, Siggaard-Anderson O. Erythrocyte 2,3-diphosphoglycerate depletion associated with hypophosphatemia detected by routine arterial blood gas analysis. Scand J Clin Lab Invest Suppl. 1996;224:83.

1719. Melvin JD, Watts RG. Severe hypophosphatemia: a rare cause of intravascular hemolysis. Am J Hematol. 2002;69:223-224.

1720. Kaiser U, Barth N. Haemolytic anaemia in a patient with anorexia nervosa. Acta Haematol. 2001;106:133-135.

1721. Worley G, Claerhout SJ, Combs SP. Hypophosphatemia in malnourished children during refeeding. Clin Pediatr (Phila). 1998;37:347-352.

1722. Dean HM, Decker CL, Baker LD. Temporary survival in clostridial hemolysis with absence of circulating red cells. N Engl J Med. 1967;277:700.

1723. Myers G, Ngoi SS, Cennerazzo W, et al. Clostridial septicemia in an urban hospital. Surg Gynecol Obstet. 1992;174:291.

1724. Ifthikaruddin JJ, Holmes JA. *Clostridium perfringens* septicaemia and massive intravascular haemolysis as a terminal complication of autologous bone marrow transplant. Clin Lab Haematol. 1992;14:159.

1725. Batge B, Filejski W, Kurowski V, et al. Clostridial sepsis with massive intravascular hemolysis: Rapid diagnosis and successful treatment. Intensive Care Med. 1992;18:488.

1726. Tsai IK, Yen MY, Ho IC, et al. *Clostridium perfringens* septicemia with massive hemolysis. Scand J Infect Dis. 1989;21:467.

1727. Becker RC, Giuliani M, Savage RA, Weick JK. Massive hemolysis in *Clostridium perfringens* infections. J Surg Oncol. 1987;35:13.

1728. Bennett JM, Healey PJM. Spherocytic hemolytic anemia and acute cholecystitis caused by *Clostridium welchii*. N Engl J Med. 1963;268:1070.

1729. Mera CL, Freedman MH. *Clostridium* liver abscess and massive hemolysis: unique demise in Fanconi's aplastic anemia. Clin Pediatr (Phila). 1984;23:126.

1730. Mupanemunda RH, Kenyon CF, Inwood MJ, Leigh K. Bacterial-induced activation of erythrocyte T-antigen complicating necrotizing enterocolitis: a case report. Eur J Pediatr. 1993;152:325.

1731. Placzek MM, Gorst DW. T activation haemolysis and death after blood transfusion. Arch Dis Child. 1987;62:743.

1732. Warren S, Schreiber JR, Epstein MF. Necrotizing enterocolitis and hemolysis associated with *Clostridium perfringens*. Am J Dis Child. 1984;138:686.

1733. Williams RA, Brown EF, Hurst D, Franklin LC. Transfusion of infants with activation of erythrocyte T antigen. J Pediatr. 1989;115:949.

1734. Alvarez A, Rives S, Nomdedeu B, Pereira A. Massive hemolysis in *Clostridium perfringens* infection. Haematologica. 1999;84:571.

1735. Singer AJ, Migdal PM, Oken JP, et al. *Clostridium perfringens* septicemia with massive hemolysis in a patient with Hodgkin's lymphoma. Am J Emerg Med. 1997;15:152.

1736. McArthur HL, Dalal BI, Kollmannsberger C. Intravascular hemolysis as a complication of perfringens sepsis. J Clin Oncol. 2006;24:2387-2388.

1737. Daly JJ, Haeusler MN, Hogan CJ, Wood EM. Massive intravascular haemolysis with T-activation and disseminated intravascular coagulation due to clostridial sepsis. Br J Haematol. 2006;134:533.

1738. Loran MJ, McErlean M, Wilner G. Massive hemolysis associated with *Clostridium perfringens* sepsis. Am J Emerg Med. 2006;24:881-883.

1739. Abdominal pain, total intravascular hemolysis, and death in a 53 year old woman [clinical conference]. Am J Med. 1990;88:667.

1740. Terebelo HR, McCue RL, Lenneville MS. Implication of plasma free hemoglobin in massive clostridial hemolysis. JAMA. 1982;248:2028.

1741. Titball RW, Leslie DL, Harvey S, Kelly D. Hemolytic and sphingomyelinase activities of *Clostridium perfringens* alpha-toxin are dependent on a domain homologous to that of an enzyme from the human arachidonic acid pathway. Infect Immun. 1991;59:1872.

1742. Leslie D, Fairweather N, Pickard D, et al. Phospholipase C and haemolytic activities of *Clostridium perfringens* alpha-toxin cloned in *Escherichia coli*: sequence and homology with a *Bacillus cereus* phospholipase C. Mol Microbiol. 1989;3:383.

1743. Walker N, Holley J, Naylor CE, et al. Identification of residues in the carboxy-terminal domain of *Clostridium perfringens* theta-toxin (phospholipase C) which are required for its biological activities. Arch Biochem Biophys. 2000;384:24-30.

1744. Iwamoto M, Ohno-Iwashita Y, Ando S. Role of the essential thiol group in the thiol-activated cytolysin from *Clostridium perfringens*. Eur J Biochem. 1987;194:25.

1745. Iwamoto M, Ohno-Iwashita Y, Ando S. Effect of isolated C-terminal fragment of theta toxin (perfringolysin O) on toxin assembly and membrane lysis. Eur J Biochem. 1990;194:25.

1746. Tweten RK. Cloning and expression in *Escherichia coli* of the perfringolysin O (theta toxin) from *Clostridium perfringens* and characterization of the gene product. Infect Immun. 1988;56:3228.

1747. Harris RW, Sims PJ, Tweten RK. Kinetic aspects of the aggregation of *Clostridium perfringens* theta-toxin on erythrocyte membranes. A fluorescence energy transfer study. J Biol Chem. 1991;266:6936.

1748. Ochi S, Oda M, Matsuda H, et al. *Clostridium perfringens* alpha-toxin activates the sphingomyelin metabolism system in sheep erythrocytes. J Biol Chem. 2004;279: 12181-12189.

1749. Hubl W, Mostbeck B, Hartleb H, et al. Investigation of the pathogenesis of massive hemolysis in a case of *Clostridium perfringens* septicemia. Ann Hematol. 1993;67: 145.

1750. Ramasethu J, Luban N. T activation. Br J Haematol. 2001;112:259.

1751. Simpkins H, Kahlenberg A. Structural and compositional changes in the red cell membrane during *Clostridium welchii* infection. Br J Haematol. 1971;21:173.

1752. Iyaniwura TT. Snake venom constituents: biochemistry and toxicology (Part 1). Vet Hum Toxicol. 1991;33: 468.

1753. Perkash A, Sarup BM. Red cell abnormalities after snake bite. J Trop Med Hyg. 1972;75:85.

1754. Reid HA. Cobra-bites. BMJ. 1964;2:540.

1755. Gibly RL, Walter FG, Nowlin SW, Berg RA. Intravascular hemolysis associated with North American crotalid envenomation. J Toxicol Clin Toxicol. 1998;36:337.

1756. Flachsenberger W, Leigh CM, Mirtschin PJ. Spheroechinocytosis of human red blood cells caused by snake, red-back spider, bee and blue-ringed octopus venoms and its inhibition by snake sera. Toxicon. 1995;33:791.

1757. Foil LD, Norment BR. Envenomation by *Loxosceles reclusa*. J Med Entomol. 1979;16:18.

1758. Dacie JV. Haemolytic anemias due to drugs, chemicals and venoms: glucose-6-phosphate dehydrogenase deficiency and favism. In The Haemolytic Anaemias, Congenital and Acquired, 2nd ed. New York, Grune & Stratton, 1967, p 993.

1759. Monzon C, Miles J. Hemolytic anemia following a wasp sting. J Pediatr. 1980;96:1039.

1760. Schulte KL, Kochen MM. Haemolytic anemia in an adult after a wasp sting. Lancet. 1981;2:478.

1761. Bousquet J, Huchard G, Michel FB. Toxic reactions induced by Hymenoptera venom. Ann Allergy. 1984; 52:371.

1762. Guess HA, Saviteer PL, Morris CR. Hemolysis and acute renal failure following a Portuguese man-of-war sting. Pediatrics. 1982;70:979.

1763. Diaz C, Leon G, Rucavado A, et al. Modulation of the susceptibility of human erythrocytes to snake venom myotoxic phospholipases A_2: Role of negatively charged phospholipids as potential membrane binding sites. Arch Biochem Biophys. 2001;391:56.

1764. Argiolas A, Pisano JJ. Facilitation of phospholipase A_2 activity by mastoparans, a new class of mast cell degranulation peptides from wasp venom. J Biol Chem. 1983; 25:13697.

1765. Ho CL, Hwang LL. Structure and biological activities of a new mastoparan isolated from the venom of the hornet *Vespa basalis*. Biochem J. 1991;274:453.

1766. Katsu T, Kuroko M, Morikawa T, et al. Interaction of wasp venom mastoparan with biomembranes. Biochim Biophys Acta. 1990;1027:85.

1767. Claque MJ, Cherry RJ. A comparative study of band 3 aggregation in erythrocyte membranes by melittin and other cationic agents. Biochim Biophys Acta. 1989;980: 93.

1768. Dempsey CE. The actions of melittin on membranes. Biochim Biophys Acta. 1990;1031:143.

1769. Dufton MJ, Hider RC, Cherry RJ. The influence of melittin on the rotation of band 3 protein in the human erythrocyte membrane. Eur Biophys J. 1984;11:17.

1770. Hui SW, Stewart CM, Cherry RJ. Electron microscopic observation of the aggregation of membrane proteins in human erythrocyte by melittin. Biochim Biophys Acta. 1990;1023:335.

1771. Nance WE. Hemolytic anemia of necrotic anachnoidism. Am J Med. 1961;31:801.

1772. Eichner ER. Spider bite hemolytic anemia: positive Coombs' test, erythrophagocytosis, and leukoerythroblastic smear. Am J Clin Pathol. 1984;81:683.

1773. Hardman JT, Beck ML, Hardman PK, Stout LC. Incompatibility associated with the bite of a brown recluse spider (*Loxosceles reclusa*). Transfusion. 1983;23: 233.

1774. Madrigal GC, Ercolani RL, Wenzl JE. Toxicity from a bite of the brown spider (*Loxosceles reclusus*): skin necrosis, hemolytic anemia, and hemoglobinuria in a nine-year-old child. Clin Pediatr (Phila). 1972;11:641.

1775. Wright SW, Wrenn KD, Murray L, Seger D. Clinical presentation and outcome of brown recluse spider bite. Ann Emerg Med. 1997;30:28.

1776. Futrell JM, Morgan PN, Su SP, Roth SI. Location of brown recluse venom attachment sites on human erythrocytes by the ferritin-labeled antibody technique. Am J Pathol. 1979;95:675.

1777. Kurpiewski G, Campbell BJ, Forrester LJ, Barrett JT. Alternate complement pathway activation by recluse spider venom. Int J Tissue React. 1981;3:39.

1778. Tambourgi DV, Morgan BP, de Andrade RM, et al. *Loxosceles intermedia* spider envenomation induces activation of an endogenous metalloproteinase, resulting in cleavage of glycophorins from the erythrocyte surface and facilitating complement-mediated lysis. Blood. 2000;95:683.

1779. Taylor EH, Denny WF. Hemolysis, renal failure and death, presumed secondary to bite of brown recluse spider. South Med J. 1966,59:1209.

1780. Vorse H, Seccareccio P, Woodruff K, Humphrey GB. Disseminated intravascular coagulopathy following fatal brown spider bite (necrotic arachnidism). J Pediatr. 1972;80:1035.

1781. Gebel HM, Finke JH, Elgert KD, et al. Inactivation of complement by *Loxosceles reclusa* spider venom. Am J Trop Med Hyg. 1979;28:756.

1782. Holt DS, Botto M, Bygrave AE, et al. Targeted deletion of the CD59 gene causes spontaneous intravascular hemolysis and hemoglobinuria. Blood. 2001;98:442.

1783. Bernheimer AW, Campbell BJ, Forrester LJ. Comparative toxicology of *Loxosceles reclusa* and *Corynebacterium pseudotuberculosis*. Science. 1985;228:590.

1784. Jandl JH, Jacob HS. Hypersplenism due to infection: a study of five cases manifesting hemolytic anemia. N Engl J Med. 1961;264:1063.

1785. Harris IM, McAlister J, Prankerd TA. Splenomegaly and the circulating red cell. Br J Haematol. 1958;4:97.

1786. Crane GG. The anemia of hyperreactive malarious splenomegaly. Rev Soc Bras Med Trop. 1992;25:1.

1787. Cooper RA, Jandl JH. Bile salts and cholesterol in the pathogenesis of target cells in obstructive jaundice. J Clin Invest. 1968;47:809.

1788. Cooper RA, Diloy-Puray M, Lando P, Greenverg MS. An analysis of lipoproteins, bile acids, and red cell membranes associated with target cells and spur cells in patients with liver disease. J Clin Invest. 1972;31:3182.

1789. Neerhout RC. Abnormalities of erythrocyte stromal lipids in hepatic disease: erythrocyte stromal lipids in hyperlipemic states. J Lab Clin Med. 1968;71:438.

1790. Verkleij AJ, Nanta ICD, Werre JM, et al. The fusion of abnormal plasma lipoprotein (LP-X) and the erythrocyte membrane in patients with cholestasis studied by electron microscopy. Biochim Biophys Acta. 1976;436:366.

1791. Narayanan S. Biochemistry and clinical relevance of lipoprotein X. Am Clin Lab Sci. 1984;14:371.

1792. Seidel D, Alaupovic P, Furman RH. A lipoprotein characterizing obstructive jaundice: I. Method for quantitative separation and identification of lipoproteins in jaundice subjects. J Clin Invest. 1969;48:1211.

1793. Glomset JA, Assmann G, et al. Lecithin:choloesterol acyltransferase deficiency and fish eye disease. In Scriver CS, Beuadet AL, Sly WS, et al (eds). The Metabolic and Molecular Bases of Inherited Disease. New York, McGraw-Hill, 1995, p 1933.

1794. Santamarina-Fojo S, Hoeg JM, Assmann G, et al. Lecithin cholesterol acyltransferase deficiency and fish-eye disease. In Scriver CR, Beaudet AL, Sly WS, et al (eds). The Metabolic and Molecular Bases of Inherited Diseases, 8th ed. New York, McGraw-Hill, 2001, pp 2817-2834.

1795. Gjone E, Torsvik H, Norum KR. Familial plasma cholesterol ester deficiency: a study of the erythrocytes. Scand J Clin Lab Invest. 1968;21:327.

1796. Jain SK, Mohandas N, Sensabaugh GF. Hereditary plasma lecithin-cholesterol acyl transferase deficiency: a heterozygous variant with erythrocyte membrane abnormalities. J Lab Clin Med. 1982;99:816.

1797. Murayama N, Asano Y, Hosoda S. Decreased sodium influx and abnormal red cell membrane lipids in a patient with familial plasma lecithin:cholesterol acyltransferase deficiency. Am J Hematol. 1984;16:129.

1798. Suda T, Akamatsu A, Nakaya Y, Desaki J. Alterations in erythrocyte membrane lipid and its fragility in a patient with familial lecithin:cholesterol acyltransferase (LCAT) deficiency. J Med Invest. 2002;49:147.

1799. Kuivenhoven JA, Pritchard H, Hill J, et al. The molecular pathology of lecithin:cholesterol acyltransferase (LCAT) deficiency syndromes. J Lipid Res. 1997;38:191-205.

1800. Miettinen HE, Gylling H, Tenhunen J, et al. Molecular genetic study of Finns with hypoalphalipoproteinemia and hyperalphalipoproteinemia: A novel Gly230 Arg mutation (LCAT^{Fin}) of lecithin:cholesterol acyltransferase (LCAT) accounts for 5 percent of cases with very low serum HDL cholesterol levels. Arterioscler Thromb Vasc Biol. 1998;18:591.

1801. Peelman F, Verschelde JL, Vanloo B, et al. Effects of natural mutations in lecithin:cholesterol acyltransferase on the enzyme structure and activity. J Lipid Res. 1999;40:59-69.

1802. Gjone E, Javitt NB, et al. Studies of lipoprotein-X (LP-X) and bile acids in familial lecithin:cholesterol acyltransferase deficiency. Acta Med Scand. 1973;194:377.

1803. Norum KR, Gjone E. The influence of plasma from patients with familial lecithin:cholesterol acyltransferase deficiency on the lipid pattern of erythrocytes. Scand J Clin Lab Invest. 1968;22:94.

1804. Jacobsen CD, Gjone E, Hovig T. Sea-blue histiocytes in familial lecithin:cholesterol acyltransferase deficiency. Scand J Haematol. 1972;9:106.

1805. Frohlich J, Hoag G, McLeod R, et al. Hypoalphalipoproteinemia resembling fish eye disease. Acta Med Scand. 1987;221:291.

1806. Singer K, Miller EB, Dameshek W. Hematologic changes following splenectomy in man, with particular reference to target cells, hemolytic index and lysolecithin. Am J Med Sci. 1941;202:171-187.

1807. Singer K, Weisz L. The life cycle of the erythrocyte after splenectomy and the problems of splenic hemolysis and target cell formation. Am J Med Sci. 1945;210:301.

1808. DeHaan LD, Werre JM, Ruben AM, et al. Alterations in size, shape and osmotic behaviour of red cells after splenectomy: a study of their age dependence. Br J Haematol. 1988;69:71.

1809. Shattil SJ, Cooper RA. Maturation of macroreticulocyte membranes in vivo. J Lab Clin Med. 1972;79:215.

1810. Come SE, Shohet SB, Robinson SH. Surface remodeling vs whole-cell hemolysis of reticulocytes produced with erythroid stimulation or iron-deficiency anemia. Blood. 1974;44:817.

1811. Lux SE, John KM. Isolation and partial characterization of a high molecular weight red cell membrane protein complex normally removed by the spleen. Blood. 1977;50:625.

1812. Smith CH, Khakoo Y. Burr cells: classification and effect of splenectomy. J Pediatr. 1970;76:99.

1813. Crosby WH. Normal function of the spleen relative to red blood cells: a review. Blood. 1959;14:399.

1814. Brecher G, Haley JE, Wallerstein RO. Spiculed erythrocytes after splenectomy: acanthocytes or non-specific poikilocytes? Nouv Rev Fr Hematol. 1972;12:751-754.

1815. Iglic A, Kralj-Iglic V, Hagerstrand H. Amphiphile induced echinocyte-spheroechinocyte transformation of red blood cell shape. Eur Biophys J. 1998;27:335.

1816. Wong P. A basis of echinocytosis and stomatocytosis in the disc-sphere transformations of the erythrocyte. J Theor Biol. 1999;196:343.

1817. Nakao M, Nakao T, Yamazoe S. Adenosine triphosphate and shape of erythrocytes. J Biochem. 1961;45:487.

1818. Palek J, Stewart G, Lionetti FJ. The dependence of shape of human erythrocyte ghosts on calcium, magnesium, and adenosine triphosphate. Blood. 1974;44:583.

1819. Aherne WA. The "burr" red cell and azotaemia. J Clin Pathol. 1957;10:252.

1820. Feo CJ, Tchernia G, Subtil E, Leblond PF. Observation of echinocytosis in eight patients: a phase contrast and SEM study. Br J Haematol. 1978;40:519.

1821. Carlyle RF, Nichols G, Rowles PM. Abnormal red cells in blood of men subjected to simulated dives. Lancet. 1979;1:1114.

1822. Bassen FA, Kornzweig AL. Malformation of the erythrocytes in a case of atypical retinitis pigmentosa. Blood. 1950;5:381.

1823. Symmans WA, Shepard CS, Marsh WL, et al. Hereditary acanthocytosis associated with the McLeod phenotype of the Kell blood group system. Br J Haematol. 1979;42:575.

1824. Cooper RA. Anemia with spur cells: a red cell defect acquired in serum and modified in the circulation. J Clin Invest. 1969;48:1820.

1825. Tuffy P, Brown AK, Zuelzer WW. Infantile pyknocytosis: a common erythrocyte abnormality of the first trimester. Am J Dis Child. 1959;98:227.

1826. Kay J, Stricker RB. Hematologic and immunologic abnormalities in anorexia nervosa. South Med J. 1983;76:1008.

1827. Mant MJ, Faragher BS. The haematology of anorexia nervosa. Br J Haematol. 1972;23:737.

1828. Udden MM, Umeda M, Hirano Y, Marcus DM. New abnormalities in the morphology, cell surface receptors, and electrolyte metabolism of In(Lu) erythrocytes. Blood. 1987;69:52.

1829. Wardrop C, Hutchison HE. Red-cell shape in hypothyroidism. Lancet. 1969;1:1243.

1830. Doll DC, List AF, Dayhoff DA, et al. Acanthocytosis associated with myelodysplasia. J Clin Oncol. 1989;7:1569.

1831. Ohsaka A, Yawata Y, Enomoto Y, et al. Abnormal calcium transport of acanthocytes in acute myelodysplasia with myelofibrosis. Br J Haematol. 1989;73:568.

1832. Danek A (ed). Neuroacanthocytosis Syndromes. Dordrecht, Netherlands, Springer, 2004.

1833. Storch A, Kornhass M, Schwarz J. Testing for acanthocytosis: A prospective reader-blinded study in movement disorder patients. J Neurol. 2005;252:84.

1834. Bosman G, Walker RH. Acanthocytosis-related changes in erythrocyte band 3: clues for a mechanism and inspiration for future research. Mov Disord. 2005;20:1675.

1835. Walker RH, Danek A, Dobson-Stone C, et al. Developments in neuroacanthocytosis: expanding the spectrum of choreatic syndromes. Mov Disord. 2006;21:11.

1836. Salt HB, Wolff OH, Lloyd JK, et al. On having no beta-lipoprotein. A syndrome comprising α-beta-lipoproteinaemia, acanthocytosis, and steatorrhoea. Lancet. 1960;2:326.

1837. Dieplinger H, Kronenberg F. Genetics and metabolism of lipoprotein(a) and their clinical implications (Part 1). Wien Klin Wochenschr. 1999;111:5.

1838. Muller DPR, Lloyd JK, Bird AC. Long-term management of abetalipoproteinaemia. Arch Dis Child. 1977;52:209.

1839. Chowers I, Banin E, Merin S, et al. Long-term assessment of combined vitamin A and E treatment for the prevention of retinal degeneration in abetalipoproteinaemia and hypobetalipoproteinaemia patients. Eye. 2001;15:525-530.

1840. Wetterau JR, Aggerbeck LP, Bouma ME, et al. Absence of microsomal triglyceride transfer protein in individuals with abetalipoproteinemia. Science. 1992;258:999.

1841. Berriot-Varoqueaux N, Aggerbeck LP, Samson-Bouma M, Wetterau JR. The role of the microsomal triglyceride transfer protein in abetalipoproteinemia. Annu Rev Nutr. 2000;20:663.

1842. Gordon DA, Jamil H. Progress towards understanding the role of microsomal triglyceride transfer protein in apolipoprotein-B lipoprotein assembly. Biochim Biophys Acta. 2000;1486:72.

1843. Black DD, Hay RV, Rohwer-Nutter PL, et al. Intestinal and hepatic apolipoprotein B gene expression in abetalipoproteinemia. Gastroenterology. 1991;101:520.

1844. Glickman RM, Glickman JN, Magun A, Brin M. Apolipoprotein synthesis in normal and abetalipoproteinemic intestinal mucosa. Gastroenterology. 1991;101:749.

1845. Lieper JM, Bayliss JD, Pease RJ, et al. Microsomal triglyceride transfer protein, the abetalipoproteinemia gene product, mediates the secretion of apolipoprotein B–containing lipoproteins from heterologous cells. J Biol Chem. 1994;269:21951.

1846. Gheeraert P, DeBuyzere M, Delanghe J, et al. Plasma and erythrocyte lipids in two families with heterozygous hypobetalipoproteinemia. Clin Biochem. 1988;21:371.

1847. Simon ER, Ways P. Incubation hemolysis and red cell metabolism in acanthocytosis. J Clin Invest. 1964;43:1311.

1848. Barenholz Y, Yechiel E, Cohen R, Deckelbaum RJ. Importance of cholesterol-phospholipid interaction in determining dynamics of normal and abetalipoproteinemia red blood cell membrane. Cell Biophys. 1981;3:115.

1849. Iida H, Takashima Y, Maeda S, et al. Alterations in erythrocyte membrane lipids in abetalipoproteinemia: phospholipid and fatty acyl composition. Biochem Med. 1984;32:79.

1850. Cooper RA, Gulbrandsen CL. The relationship between serum lipoproteins and red cell membranes in abetalipoproteinemia: deficiency of lecithin:cholesterol acyltransferase. J Lab Clin Med. 1971;78:323.

1851. Flamm M, Schachter D. Acanthocytosis and cholesterol enrichment decrease lipid fluidity of only the outer human erythrocyte membrane leaflet. Nature. 1982;298:290.

1852. Lange Y, Steck TL. Mechanism of red blood cell acanthocytosis and echinocytosis in vivo. J Membr Biol. 1984;77:153.

1853. McCormick EC, Cornwell DG, et al. Studies on the distribution of tocopherol in human serum lipoproteins. J Lipid Res. 1969;1:211.

1854. Dodge JT, Cohen G, Kayden HJ, Phillips GB. Peroxidative hemolysis of red blood cells from patients with abetalipoproteinemia (acanthocytosis). J Clin Invest. 1967;46:357.

1855. Estes JW, Morléy JT, Levine IM, Emerson CP. A new hereditary acanthocytosis syndrome. Am J Med. 1967;42:868.

1856. Levine IM, Estes JW, Looney JM. Hereditary neurological disease with acanthocytosis. Arch Neurol. 1968;19:403.

1857. Dobston-Stone C, Rampoldi L, Velayos Baeza A, et al. Choreoacanthocytosis. In GeneReviews at GeneTests: Medical Genetics Information Resource [database online]. Seattle, University of Washington, 2005. Available at *http://www.geneclincs.org/profiles/chac*.

1858. Danek A, Walker RH. Neuroacanthocytosis. Curr Opin Neurol. 2005;18:386-392.

1859. Hardie RJ, Pullon HW, Harding AE, et al. Neuroacanthocytosis: a clinical, haematological and pathological study of 19 cases. Brain. 1991;114:13.

1860. Rampoldi L, Dobson-Stone C, Rubio JP, et al. A conserved sorting-associated protein is mutant in chorea-acanthocytosis. Nat Genet. 2001;28:119.

1861. Ueno S, Maruki Y, Nakamura M, et al. The gene encoding a newly discovered protein, chorein, is mutated in chorea-acanthocytosis. Nat Genet. 2001;28:121.

1862. Dobson-Stone C, Velayos-Baeza A, Filippone LA, et al. Chorein detection for the diagnosis of chorea-acanthocytosis. Ann Neurol. 2004;56:299.

1863. Dobston-Stone C, Danek A, Rampoldi L, et al. Mutational spectrum of the CHAC gene in patients with chorea-acanthocytosis. Eur J Hum Genet. 2002;10:773.

1864. Velayos-Baeza A, Vettori A, Copley RR, et al. Analysis of the human VPS13 gene family. Genomics. 2004;84:536.

1865. Dobson-Stone C, Velayos-Baeza A, Jansen A, et al. Identification of a VPS13A founder mutation in French Canadian families with chorea-acanthocytosis. Neurogenetics. 2005;6:151.

1866. Sorrentino G, De Renzo A, Miniello S, et al. Late appearance of acanthocytes during the course of chorea-acanthocytosis. J Neurol Sci. 1999;163:175.

1867. Clark MR, Aminoff MJ, Chiu DT, et al. Red cell deformability and lipid composition in two forms of acanthocytosis: enrichment of acanthocytic populations by density gradient centrifugation. J Lab Clin Med. 1989;113:469.

1868. Bruce LJ, Kay MM, Lawrence C, Tanner MJ. Band 3 HT, a human red-cell variant associated with acanthocytosis and increased anion transport, carries the mutation Pro868→Leu in the membrane domain of band 3. Biochem J. 1993;293:317.

1869. Redman CM, Russo D, Lee S. Kell, Kx and the McLeod syndrome. Baillieres Best Pract Res Clin Haematol. 1999;12:621.

1870. Jung HH, Danek A, Dobson-Stone C, et al. McLeod neuroacanthocytosis syndrome. In GeneReviews at GeneTests: Medical Genetics Information Resource [database online]. Seattle, University of Washington, 2004. Available at *http://www.geneclinics.org/profiles/mcleod*.

1871. Redman CM, Marsh WL, Scarborough A, et al. Biochemical studies on McLeod phenotype red cells and isolation of Kx antigen. Br J Haematol. 1988;68:131.

1872. Khamlichi S, Bailly P, Blanchard D, et al. Purification and partial characterization of the erythrocyte Kx protein deficient in McLeod patients. Eur J Biochem. 1995;228:931.

1873. Russo D, Redman C, Lee S. Association of XK and Kell blood group proteins. J Biol Chem. 1998;273:13950.

1874. Ho M, Chelly J, Carter N. Isolation of the gene for McLeod syndrome that encodes a novel membrane transport protein. Cell. 1994;77:869.

1875. Ho MF, Chalmers RM, Davis MB, et al. A novel point mutation in the McLeod syndrome gene in neuroacanthocytosis. Ann Neurol. 1996;39:672.

1876. Danek A, Rubio JP, Rampoldi L, et al. McLeod neuroacanthocytosis: genotype and phenotype. Ann Neurol. 2001;50:755.

1877. Lee S, Russo DC, Reiner AP, et al. Molecular defects underlying the Kell null phenotype. J Biol Chem. 2001;276:27281.

1878. Supple SG, Iland HJ, Barnett MH, Pollard JD. A spontaneous novel XK gene mutation in a patient with McLeod syndrome. Br J Haematol. 2001;115:369.

1879. Jung HH, Hergersberg M, Kneifel S, et al. McLeod syndrome: a novel mutation, predominant psychiatric manifestations, and distinct striatal imaging findings. Ann Neurol. 2001;49:384.

1880. Taswell HF, Lewis JC, Marsh WL, et al. Erythrocyte morphology in genetic defects of the Rh and Kell blood group systems. Mayo Clin Proc. 1977;52:157.

1881. Wimmer BM, Marsh WL, Taswell HF, Galey WR. Haematological changes associated with the McLeod phenotype of the Kell blood group system. Br J Haematol. 1977;36:219.

1882. Marsh WL, Marsh NJ, Moore A, et al. Elevated serum creatine phosphokinase in subjects with McLeod syndrome. Vox Sang. 1981;40:403.

1883. Swash M, Schwartz MS, Carter ND, et al. Benign X-linked myopathy with acanthocytosis (McLeod syndrome): its relationship to X-linked muscular dystrophy. Brain. 1983;106:717.

1884. Witt TN, Danek A, Reither M, et al. McLeod syndrome: A distinct form of neuroacanthocytosis: report of two cases and literature review with emphasis on neuromuscular manifestations. J Neurol. 1992;239:302.

1885. Danek A, Uttner I, Vogl T, et al. Cerebral involvement in McLeod syndrome. Neurology. 1994;44:117.

1886. Takashima H, Sakai T, Iwashita H, et al. A family of McLeod syndrome, masquerading as chorea-acanthocytosis. J Neurol Sci. 1994;124:56.

1887. Malandrini A, Fabrizi GM, Truschi F, et al. Atypical McLeod syndrome manifested as X-linked chorea-acanthocytosis, neuromyopathy and dilated cardiomyopathy: report of a family. J Neurol Sci. 1994;124:89.

1888. Bertelson CJ, Pogo AO, Chaudhuri A, et al. Localization of the McLeod locus (XK) within Xp21 by deletion analysis. Am J Hum Genet. 1988;42:703.

1889. Francke U, Ochs HD, de Martinville B, et al. Minor Xp21 chromosome deletion in a male associated with expression of Duchenne muscular dystrophy, chronic granulomatous disease, retinitis pigmentosa, and McLeod syndrome. Am J Hum Genet. 1985;37:250.

1890. Giblett ER, Klebanoff SJ, Pincus SH. Kell phenotypes in chronic granulomatous disease: a potential transfusion hazard. Lancet. 1971;1:1235.

1891. Hart MVD, Szaloky A, van Loghem JJ. A "new" antibody associated with the Kell blood group system. Vox Sang. 1968;15:456.

1892. Margolis RL, O'Hearn E, Rosenblatt A, et al. A disorder similar to Huntington's disease is associated with a novel CAG repeat expansion. Ann. Neurol. 2001;50:373.

1893. Holmes SE, O'Hearn, E, Rosenblatt A, et al. A repeat expansion in the gene encoding junctophilin-3 is associated with Huntington disease–like 2. Nat Genet. 2001;29:377-378. Note: Erratum: Nat Genet. 2002; 30:123.

1894. Margolis RL, Holmes SE, Rosenblatt A, et al. Huntington's disease like–2 (HDL2) in North America and Japan. Ann Neurol. 2004;56:570-674.

1895. Taylor TD, Litt M, Kramer P, et al. Homozygosity mapping of Hallervorden-Spatz syndrome to chromosome 20p12.3-p13. Nat Genet. 1996;14:479.

1896. Walker RH, Rasmussen A, Rudnicki D, et al. Huntington's disease like–2 can present as chorea-acanthocytosis. Neurology. 2003;61:730.

1897. Zhou B, Westaway SK, Levinson B, et al. A novel pantothenate kinase gene (PANK2) is defective in Hallervorden-Spatz syndrome. Nat Genet. 2001;28:345.

1898. Elejalde BR, de Elejalde MMJ, Lopez F. Hallervorden-Spatz disease. Clin Genet. 1979;16:1.

1899. Angelini L, Nardocci N, Rumi V, et al. Hallervorden-Spatz disease: clinical and MRI study of 11 cases diagnosed in life. J Neurol. 1992;239:417.

1900. Hayflick SJ, Westaway SK, Levinson B, et al. Genetic, clinical, and radiographic delineation of Hallervorden-Spatz syndrome. N Engl J Med. 2003;348:33.

1901. Pellecchia MT, Valente EM, Cif L, et al. The diverse phenotype and genotype of pantothenate kinase–associated neurodegeneration. Neurology. 2005;64:1810-1812.

1902. Kumar N, Boes CJ, Babovic-Vuksanovic D, Boeve BF. The "eye-of-the-tiger" sign is not pathognomonic of the PANK2 mutation. Arch. Neurol. 2006;63:292-293.

1903. Melhorn DK, Gross S. Vitamin E–dependent anemia in the premature infant: II. Relationships between gestational age and absorption of vitamin E. J Pediatr. 1971; 79:581.

1904. Ehrenkranz RA. Vitamin E and the neonate. Am J Dis Child. 1980;134:1157.

1905. Zipursky A. Vitamin E deficiency anemia in newborn infants. Clin Perinatol. 1984;11:393.

1906. Gallagher PG, Ehrenkranz RA. Nutritional anemias in infancy. Perinat Hematol. 1995;22:671.

1907. Dolan TF Jr. Hemolytic anemia and edema as the initial signs in infants with cystic fibrosis. Clin Pediatr (Phila). 1976;15:597.

1908. Monzon CM, Woodruff CW. Anemia and edema as presenting signs in cystic fibrosis: a case report. J Med. 1986;17:135.

1909. Elias E, Muller DP, Scott J. Association of spinocerebellar disorders with cystic fibrosis or chronic childhood cholestasis and very low serum vitamin E. Lancet. 1981;2:1319.

1910. Alvarez F, Landrieu P, Feo C, et al. Vitamin E deficiency is responsible for neurologic abnormalities in cholestatic children. J Pediatr. 1985;107:422.

1911. Sokol RJ, Guggenheim MA, Heubi JE, et al. Frequency and clinical progression of the vitamin E deficiency neurologic disorder in children with prolonged neonatal cholestasis. Am J Dis Child. 1985;139:1211.

1912. Harding AE, Matthews S, Jones S, et al. Spinocerebellar degeneration associated with a selective defect of vitamin E absorption. N Engl J Med. 1985;313:32.

1913. Qian J, Atkinson J, Manor D. Biochemical consequences of heritable mutations in the alpha-tocopherol transfer protein. Biochemistry. 2006;45:27.

1914. Stocker A. Molecular mechanisms of vitamin E transport. Ann N Y Acad Sci. 2004;1031:44.

1915. Melhorn DK, Gross S. Vitamin E–dependent anemia in the premature infant: I. Effects of large doses of medicinal iron. J Pediatr. 1971;79:569.

1916. Oski FA, Barness LA. Vitamin E deficiency: a previously unrecognized cause of hemolytic anemia in the premature infant. J Pediatr. 1967;70:211.

1917. Ritchie JH, Fish MB, McMasters V, Grossman M. Edema and hemolytic anemia in premature infants: a vitamin E deficiency syndrome. N Engl J Med. 1968; 279:1185.

1918. Jacob HS, Lux SE. Degradation of membrane phospholipids and thiols in peroxide hemolysis: studies in vitamin E deficiency. Blood. 1968;32:549.

1919. Brownlee NR, Huttner JJ, Panganamala RV, Cornwell DG. Role of vitamin E in glutathione-induced oxidant stress: methemoglobin, lipid peroxidation, and hemolysis. J Lipid Res. 1977;18:635.

1920. Wang F, Wang T, Lai J, et al. Vitamin E inhibits hemolysis induced by hemin as a membrane stabilizer. Biochem Pharmacol. 2006;71:6.

1921. Amrein PC, Friedman R, Kosinski K, Ellman L. Hematologic changes in anorexia nervosa. JAMA. 1979;241: 2190.

1922. Eto Y, Kitagawa T. Wolman's disease with hypobetalipoproteinemia and acanthocytosis: clinical and biochemical observations. J Pediatr. 1970;77:862.

1923. Gracey M, Hilton HB. Acanthocytes and hypobetalipoproteinemia. Lancet. 1973;1:679.

1924. Paramathypathy K, Aw SE. Acanthocytosis with beta-lipoprotein deficiency in an Indian girl. Med J Aust. 1970;2:1081.

1925. Fondu P, Mozes N, Neve P, et al. The erythrocyte membrane disturbances in protein-energy malnutrition: nature and mechanisms. Br J Haematol. 1980;44: 605.

1926. Kaiser U, Barth N. Haemolytic anaemia in a patient with anorexia nervosa. Acta Haematol. 2001;106:133.

1927. Miller KK, Grinspoon SK, Ciampa J, et al. Medical findings in outpatients with anorexia nervosa. Arch Intern Med. 2005;165:5.

1928. Msra M, Aggarwal A, Miller K, et al. Effects of anorexia nervosa on clinical, hematologic, biochemical, and bone density parameters in community-dwelling adolescent girls. Pediatrics. 2004;114:6.

1929. Warren MP, Vande Wiele RL. Clinical and metabolic features of anorexia nervosa. Am J Obstet Gynecol. 1973;117:435.

1930. Herpertz-Dahlmann B, Remschmidt H. Weight-dependent changes in the hematology of anorexia nervosa. Monatsschr Kinderheilkd. 1988;136:739.

1931. Smith RR, Spivak JL. Marrow cell necrosis in anorexia nervosa and involuntary starving. Br J Haematol. 1985; 60:3.

1932. Kimber CD, Deller J, Ibbotson RN, Lander H. The mechanism of anaemia in chronic liver disease. Q J Med. 1965;34:33.

1933. Balistreri WF, Leslie MH, Cooper RA. Increased cholesterol and decreased fluidity of red cell membranes (spur cell anemia) in progressive intrahepatic cholestasis. Pediatrics. 1981;67:461.

1934. Cynamon HA, Isenberg JN, Gustavson LP, Gourley WK. Erythrocyte lipid alterations in pediatric cholestatic liver disease: spur cell anemia of infancy. J Pediatr Gastroenterol Nutr. 1985;4:542.

1935. Doll DC, Doll NJ. Spur cell anemia. South Med J. 1982;75:1205.

1936. Douglass CC, McCall MS, Frenel EP. The acanthocyte in cirrhosis with hemolytic anemia. Ann Intern Med. 1968;68:390.

1937. Grahn EP, Dietz AA, Stefani SS, Donnelly WJ. Burr cells, hemolytic anemia and cirrhosis. Am J Med. 1968;45:78.

1938. Greenberg MS, Choi ES. Post-splenectomy spur cell hemolytic anemia. Am J Med Sci. 1975;269:277.

1939. Hitchins R, Naughton L, Kerlin P, Cobcroft R. Spur cell anemia (acanthocytosis) complicating idiopathic hemochromatosis. Pathology. 1988;20:59.

1940. Keller JW, Majerus PW, Finke EH. An unusual type of spiculated erythrocyte in metastatic liver disease and hemolytic anemia: report of a case. Ann Intern Med. 1971;74:732.

1941. Silber R, Amorosi E, Lhowe J, Kayden HJ. Spur-shaped erythrocytes in Laennec's cirrhosis. N Engl J Med. 1966;275:639.

1942. Smith JA, Lonergan ET, Sterling K. Spur cell anemia: hemolytic anemia with red cells resembling acanthocytes in alcoholic cirrhosis. N Engl J Med. 1964;276:396.

1943. Tchernia G, Navarro J, Becart R, Casasoprana A. Hemolytic anemia with acanthocytosis and dyslipidemia associated with 2 neonatal hepatitis cases. Arch Fr Pediatr. 1968;25:729.

1944. Cooper RA, Kimball DB, Dorocher JR. Role of the spleen in membrane conditioning and hemolysis of spur cells in liver disease. N Engl J Med. 1974;290:1279.

1945. Salvioli G, Rioli G, Lugli R, Salati R. Membrane lipid composition of red blood cells in liver disease: Regression of spur cell anaemia after infusion of polyunsaturated phosphatidylcholine. Gut 1978;19:844.

1946. Fossaluzza V, Rossi P. Flunarizine treatment for spur cell anaemia. Br J Haematol. 1983;55:715.

1947. Cooper RA, Leslie MH, Fischkoff S, et al. Factors influencing the lipid composition and fluidity of red cell membranes in vitro: production of red cells possessing more than two cholesterols per phospholipid. Biochemistry. 1978;17:327.

1948. Cooper RA, Leslie MH, Knight D, Detweiler DK. Red cell cholesterol enrichment and spur cell anemia in dogs fed a cholesterol-enriched atherogenic diet. J Lipid Res. 1980;21:1082.

1949. Duhamel G, Forgez P, Nalpas B, et al. Spur cells in patients with alcoholic liver cirrhosis are associated with reduced plasma levels of apo A-II, HDL, and LDL. J Lipid Res. 1983;24:1612.

1950. Schubert D, Boss K. Band 3 protein–cholesterol interactions in erythrocyte membranes: possible role in anion

transport and dependency on membrane phospholipid. FEBS Lett. 1982;150:4.

1951. Lange Y, Cutler HB, Steck TL. The effect of cholesterol and other interrelated amphipaths on the contour and stability of the isolated red cell membrane. J Biol Chem. 1980;255:9331.

1952. Seigneuret M, Favre E, Morrot G, Devaux PF. Strong interactions between a spin-labeled cholesterol analog and erythrocyte proteins in the human erythrocyte membrane. Biochim Biophys Acta. 1985;813:174.

1953. Aihara K, Azuma H, Ikeda Y, et al. Successful combination therapy—flunarizine, pentoxifylline, and cholestyramine—for spur cell anemia. Int J Hematol. 2001;73:3.

1954. Chitale AA, Sterling RK, Post AB, et al. Resolution of spur cell anemia with liver transplantation: a case report and review of the literature. Transplantation. 1998;65:993-995.

1955. Malik P, Bogetti D, Sileri P, et al. Spur cell anemia in alcoholic cirrhosis: cure by orthotopic liver transplantation and recurrence after liver graft failure. Int Surg. 2002;87:4.

1956. Wong P. A basis of the acanthocytosis in inherited and acquired disorders. Med Hypotheses. 2004;62:966-969.

1957. Rooney MW, Lange Y, Kauffman JW. Acyl chain organization and protein secondary structure in cholesterol-modified erythrocyte membranes. J Biol Chem. 1984;259:8281.

1958. Allen DW, Manning N. Abnormal phospholipid metabolism in spur cell anemia: decreased fatty acid incorporation into phosphatidylethanolamine and increased incorporation into acylcarnitine in spur cell anemia erythrocytes. Blood. 1994;84:1283.

1959. Ackerman BD. Infantile pyknocytosis in Mexican-American infants. Am J Dis Child. 1969;117:417.

1960. Keimowitz R, Desforges JF. Infantile pyknocytosis. N Engl J Med. 1965;273:1152.

1961. Zannos-Mariola L, Kattamis C, Paidoucis M. Infantile pyknocytosis and glucose-6-phosphate dehydrogenase deficiency. Br J Haematol. 1962;8:258.

1962. Allison AC. Acute haemolytic anaemia with distortion and fragmentation of erythrocytes in children. Br J Haematol. 1957;3:1.

1963. Eyssette-Guerreau S, Bader-Meunier B, Garcon L, et al. Infantile pyknocytosis: a cause of haemolytic anaemia of the newborn. Br J Haematol. 2006;133:4.

1964. Joske RA, McAlister JM, Prankerd TA. Isotope investigations of red cell production and destruction in chronic renal disease. Clin Sci (Oxford). 1956;15:511.

1965. Loge JP, Lange RD, Moore CV. Characterization of the anemia associated with chronic renal insufficiency. Am J Med. 1958;24:4.

1966. Nathan DG, Schupak E, Stohlman F Jr, Merrill JP. Erythropoiesis in anephric man. J Clin Invest. 1964;43:2158.

1967. Akmal M, Telfer N, Ansari AN, Massry SG. Erythrocyte survival in chronic renal failure: role of secondary hyperparathyroidism. J Clin Invest. 1985;76:1695.

1968. Bogin E, Massry SG, Levi J, et al. Effect of parathyroid hormone on osmotic fragility of human erythrocytes. J Clin Invest. 1982;69:1017.

1969. Saltissi D, Carter GD. Association of secondary hyperparathyroidism with red cell survival in chronic haemodialysis patients. Clin Sci. 1985;68:29.

1970. Rao DS, Shih MS, Mohini R. Effect of serum parathyroid hormone and bone marrow fibrosis on the response to erythropoietin in uremia. N Eng J Med. 1993; 328:3.

1971. Lin CL, Hung CC, Yang CT, Huang CC. Improved anemia and reduced erythropoietin needs by medical or surgical intervention of secondary hypoparathyroidism in hemodialysis patients. Ren Fail. 2004;26:289-295.

1972. Yasunaga C, Matsuo K, Yanagida T, et al. Early effects of parathyroidectomy on erythropoietin production in secondary hypoparathyroidism. Am J Surg. 2002; 183:2.

1973. White JG. Effects of an ionophore A23187 on the surface morphology of normal erythrocytes. Am J Pathol. 1974;77:507.

1974. Arduini A, Bonomini M, Clutterbuck EJ, et al. Effect of L-carnitine administration on erythrocyte survival in haemodialysis patients. Nephrol Dial Transplant. 2006;21:2671.

1975. Parsons SF, Mallinson G, Judson PA, et al. Evidence that the Lu^b blood group antigen is located on red cell membrane glycoproteins of 85 and 78 kd. Transfusion. 1987;27:61.

1976. El Nemar W, Gane P, Colin Y, et al. The Lutheran blood group glycoproteins, the erythroid receptors for laminin, are adhesion molecules. J Biol Chem. 1998;273:27.

1977. Udani M, Zen Q, Cottman M, et al. Basal cell dhesion molecule/Lutheran protein: the receptor critical for sickle cell adhesion to laminin. J Clin Invest. 1998;101: 11.

1978. Eyler CE, Telen MJ. The Lutheran glycoprotein: a multifunctional adhesion receptor. Transfusion. 2006;46: 668.

1979. Shaw MA, Leak MR, Daniels GL, Tippett P. The rare Lutheran blood group phenotype Lu(a–b–): A genetic study. Ann Hum Genet. 1984;48:229-237.

1980. Telen MJ. The Lutheran antigens and proteins affected by Lutheran regulatory genes. In Agre PC, Cartron JP (eds). Protein Blood Group Antigens of the Human Red Cell: Structure, Function and Clinical Significance. Baltimore, Johns Hopkins University Press, 1992, p 70.

1981. Parsons SE, Mallinson G, Holmes CH, et al. The Lutheran blood group glycoprotein, another member of the immunoglobulin superfamily, is widely expressed in human tissues and is developmentally regulated in human liver. Proc Natl Acad Sci U S A. 1995;92:5496.

1982. Kroviarski Y, El Nemer W, Gane P, et al. Direct interaction between the Lu-B-CAM adhesion glycoproteins and erythroid spectrin. Br J Haematol. 2004;126:255.

1983. Horton L, Coburn RJ, England JM, Himsworth RL. The haematology of hypothyroidism. Q J Med. 1976;45: 101.

1984. Perillie PE, Tembrevilla C. Red-cell changes in hypothyroidism. Lancet. 1975;2:1151.

1985. Betticher DC, Pugin P. Hypothyroidism and acanthocytes: Diagnostic significance of blood smear. Schweiz Med Wochenschr. 1991;121:1127.

1986. Chuttani HK, Gupta PS, Gulati S, Gupta DN. Acute copper sulfate poisoning. Am J Med. 1965;39:849.

1987. Fairbanks VF. Copper sulfate induced hemolytic anemia: inhibition of glucose-6-phosphate dehydrogenase and other possible etiologic mechanisms. Arch Intern Med. 1967;120:428.

1988. Holtzman NA, Elliott DA, Heller RH. Copper intoxication. N Engl J Med. 1966;275:347.

1989. Manzler AD, Schreiner AW. Copper-induced acute hemolytic anemia: a new complication of hemodialysis. Ann Intern Med. 1970;73:409.

1990. Roberts RH. Hemolytic anemia associated with copper sulfate poisoning. Miss Doctor. 1956;33:292.

1991. Clopton DA, Saltman P. Copper-specific damage in human erythrocytes exposed to oxidative stress. Biol Trace Elem Res. 1997;56:231.

1992. Yang CC, Wu ML, Deng JF. Prolonged hemolysis and methemoglobinemia following organic copper fungicide ingestion. Vet Hum Toxicol. 2004;46:6.

1993. Oski FA. Chickee, the copper [editorial]. Ann Intern Med. 1970;73:485.

1994. Loudianos G, Gitlin JD. Wilson's disease. Semin Liver Dis. 2000;20:353.

1995. Sternlieb I. Wilson's disease. Clin Liver Dis. 2000;4: 229.

1996. Walshe JM. Wilson's disease: the presenting symptoms. Arch Dis Child. 1962;37:253.

1997. Buchanan GR. Acute hemolytic anemia as a presenting manifestation of Wilson's disease. J Pediatr. 1975;86: 245.

1998. Forman SJ, Kumar KS, Redeker AG, Hochstein P. Hemolytic anemia in Wilson disease: clinical findings and biochemical mechanisms. Am J Hematol. 1980;9: 269.

1999. Groter W. Hamolytische Krisen als Fruhmanifestation der Wilson'schen Krankheit. Dtsch Z Nervenheilkd. 1959;179:401.

2000. Lehr H, Pauschinger M, Pittke E, et al. Haemolytic anaemia as initial manifestation of Wilson's disease. Blut. 1988;56:45.

2001. Robitaille GA, Piscatelli RL, Majeski EJ, Gelehrter TD. Hemolytic anemia in Wilson's disease. JAMA. 1977;237: 2402.

2002. Roche-Sicot J, Benhamou JP. Acute intravascular hemolysis and acute liver failure associated as a first manifestation of Wilson's disease. Ann Intern Med. 1977;86: 301.

2003. Willms B, Blume KG, Löhr GW. Hemolytic anemia in Wilson's disease (hepato-lenticular degeneration). Klin Wochenschr. 1972;50:995-1002.

2004. Deiss A, Lee GR, Cartwright GE. Hemolytic anemia in Wilson's disease. Ann Intern Med. 1970;73:413.

2005. Dobyns WB, Goldstein NP, Gordon H. Clinical spectrum of Wilson's disease (hepatolenticular degeneration). Mayo Clin Proc. 1979;54:35.

2006. Hoagland HC, Goldstein NP. Hematologic (cytopenic) manifestations of Wilson's disease. Mayo Clin Proc. 1978;53:498.

2007. Iser JH, Stevens BJ, et al. Hemolytic anemia of Wilson's disease. Gastroenterology. 1974;67:290.

2008. McIntyre N, Clink HM, Levi AJ. Hemolytic anemia in Wilson's disease. N Engl J Med. 1967;276:439.

2009. Meyer RJ, Zalusky R. The mechanisms of hemolysis in Wilson's disease: study of a case and review of the literature. Mt Sinai J Med. 1977;44:530.

2010. Michel M, Lafaurie M, Noel V, et al. Hemolytic anemia disclosing Wilson's disease. Report of 2 cases. Rev Med Interne. 2001;22:280.

2011. Pirisi M, Branca B, Avellini C, Solinas A. A 15 year old girl with fever, jaundice, haemolysis, and sudden clinical deterioration. Postgrad Med J. 2002;78:250, 253-254

2012. Dabrowska E, Jablonska-Kaszewska I, Ozieblowski A, Falkiewicz B. Acute haemolytic syndrome and liver failure as the first manifestations of Wilson's disease. Med Sci Monit. 2001;7(Suppl 1):246-251.

2013. Mellacheruvu S, Vergara C. A 32-year-old patient with hemolytic anemia and fulminant hepatic failure. Conn Med. 2006;70:293-295

2014. Asfaha S, Almansori M, Qarni U, Gutfreund KS. Plasmapheresis for hemolytic crisis and impending acute liver failure in Wilson disease. J Clin Apher. 2007;22:295-298.

2015. Prella M, Baccalà R, Horisberger JD, et al. Haemolytic onset of Wilson disease in a patient with homozygous truncation of ATP7B at Arg1319. Br J Haematol. 2001;114:230-232

2016. Petrukhin K, Fischer SG, Pirastu M, et al. Mapping, cloning and genetic characterization of the region containing the Wilson disease gene. Nat Genet. 1993;5:338.

2017. Bull PC, Thomas GR, Rommens JM, et al. The Wilson disease gene is a putative copper transporting P-type ATPase similar to the Menkes gene. Nat Genet. 1993;5:327.

2018. Yamaguchi Y, Heiny ME, Gitlin JD. Isolation and characterization of a human liver cDNA as a candidate gene for Wilson disease. Biochem Biophys Res Commun. 1993;197:271.

2019. Mercer JF. The molecular basis of copper-transport diseases. Trends Mol Med. 2001;7:64.

2020. Camakaris J, Voskoboinik I, Mercer JF. Molecular mechanisms of copper homeostasis. Biochem Biophys Res Commun. 1999;261:225.

2021. Thomas GR, Forbes JR, Roberts EA, et al. The Wilson disease gene: spectrum of mutations and their consequences. Nat Genet. 1995;9:210.

2022. Figus A, Angius A, Loudianos G, et al. Molecular pathology and haplotype analysis of Wilson disease in Mediterranean populations. Am J Hum Genet. 1995;57:1318.

2023. Shah AB, Chernov I, Zhang HT, et al. Identification and analysis of mutations in the Wilson disease gene (ATP7B): population frequencies, genotype-phenotype correlation, and functional analyses. Am J Hum Genet. 1997;61:317.

2024. Grudeva-Popova JG, Spasova MI, Chepileva KG, Zaprianov ZH. Acute hemolytic anemia as an initial clinical manifestation of Wilson's disease. Folia Med (Plovdiv). 2000;42:42.

2025. Gubler CJ, Labey ME, Cartwright GE, Wintrobe MM. Studies on copper metabolism. IX. Transportation of copper in blood. J Clin Invest. 1953;32:405.

2026. Hochstein P, Kumar KS, Forman SJ. Mechanisms of copper toxicity in red cells. In Brewer GJ (ed). The Red Cell. New York, Alan R Liss. 1978.

2027. Attri S, Sharma N, Jahagirdar S, et al. Erythrocyte metabolism and antioxidant status of patients with Wilson disease with hemolytic anemia. Pediatr Res. 2006;59;593.

16 Pyruvate Kinase Deficiency and Disorders of Glycolysis

William C. Mentzer, Jr.

The mature erythrocyte, devoid of nucleus, mitochondria, ribosomes, and other organelles, has no capacity for cell replication, protein synthesis, or oxidative phosphorylation. The glycolytic production of adenosine triphosphate (ATP), the sole known energy source of erythrocytes, is sufficient to meet their limited metabolic requirements. The discovery that hemolytic anemia may result from any of several glycolytic enzymopathies has underscored the dependence of erythrocytes on glycolysis. In this chapter the clinical, biochemical, and genetic features associated with abnormalities in erythrocyte glycolysis are described in detail.

Hereditary hemolytic anemias resulting from altered erythrocyte metabolism are distinguished from hereditary spherocytosis by the absence of spherocytes on the peripheral blood smear, by normal osmotic fragility of fresh erythrocytes, by a partial therapeutic response to splenectomy, and by a recessive mode of inheritance. Hemoglobin structure and synthesis are normal. Because no specific morphologic abnormality is associated with these disorders, they have become known as congenital nonspherocytic hemolytic anemias (CNSHAs).[1] Although CNSHAs are usually transmitted in an autosomal recessive fashion, phosphoglycerate kinase (PGK) deficiency is an X-linked abnormality, and adenosine deaminase (ADA) overproduction is an autosomal dominant disorder. Symptoms and signs may be limited to the manifestations of hemolysis or, if the enzymopathy is present in other tissues, may involve other organ systems. The pattern of involvement of nonerythroid tissues may be of assistance in diagnosis.[2]

Initial attempts to classify these anemias were based on the autohemolysis test, in which saline-washed erythrocytes were incubated without glucose in vitro at 37° C under sterile conditions and the percentage of hemolysis was determined after 48 hours.[3,4] Autohemolysis was greater than normal in almost all patients with CNSHA. If glucose was added before incubation, hemolysis was reduced in control subjects and in some patients with CNSHA (type I) but was unchanged or actually increased in others (type II). Type II erythrocytes did not metabolize glucose well[3] and contained subnormal amounts of ATP but markedly increased amounts of 2,3-diphosphoglycerate (2,3-DPG), thus suggesting a defect in glycolysis below the site of 2,3-DPG synthesis. In 1961, Valentine and associates[5] identified the glycolytic defect to be a deficiency of erythrocyte pyruvate kinase (PK) in three patients with CNSHA. Subsequently, abnormalities of other glycolytic enzymes have also been associated with CNSHA, as indicated in Figure 16-1. Specific alterations in protein structure underlie many of the enzyme deficiency states, and many of the underlying mutations have been identified.[6-8]

The presence of a glycolytic enzymopathy should be suspected when chronic hemolysis occurs in the absence of marked abnormalities in erythrocyte morphology or osmotic fragility. An exception to the usually unremarkable red cell morphology in CNSHA is the pronounced

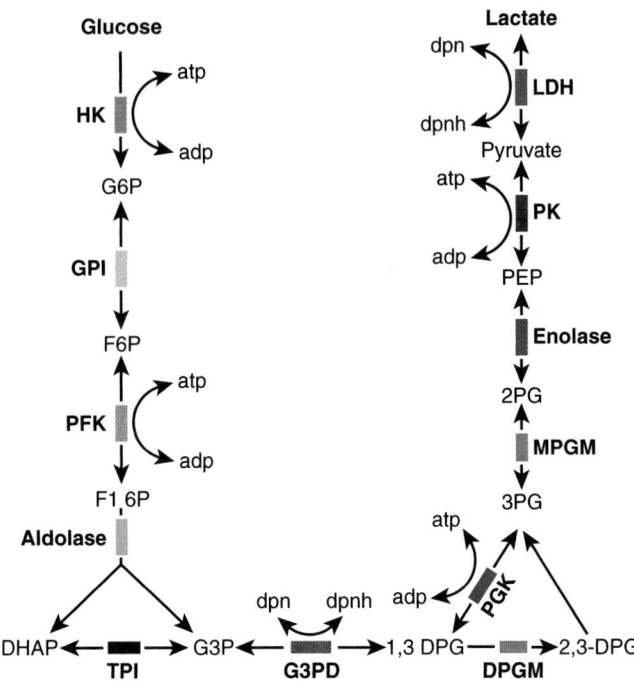

FIGURE 16-1. The Embden-Meyerhof pathway. Recognized enzyme defects are indicated by *solid bars*. adp, adenosine diphosphate; atp, adenosine triphosphate; DHAP, dihydroxyacetone phosphate; DPGM, 2,3-disphosphoglycerate mutase; F1,6P, fructose 1,6-phosphate; F6P, fructose 6-phosphate; G3PD, glucose-3-phosphate dehydrogenase; G6P, glucose 6-phosphate; GPI, glucose phosphate isomerase; HK, hexokinase; LDH, lactate dehydrogenase; MPGM, monophosphoglycerate mutase; PEP, phosphoenolpyruvate; PFK, phosphofructokinase; PG, phosphoglycerate; PK, pyruvate kinase; TPI, triose phosphate isomerase.

basophilic stippling found in pyrimidine-5′-nucleotidase (P-5′-N) deficiency.[9] Hemoglobin electrophoresis, stains for inclusion bodies, hemoglobin heat stability, acid hemolysis, and appropriate studies for immune hemolysis are normal. Despite its initial usefulness in directing the attention of investigators to the glycolytic pathway, further experience with the autohemolysis test has shown that it lacks specificity and has, at best, limited value in the evaluation of CNSHA.[10] Unfortunately, no other simple, convenient laboratory screening test has been developed that will unequivocally reveal the presence of a glycolytic enzymopathy. Therefore, the appropriate diagnostic strategy for the evaluation of a suspected enzymopathy is first to eliminate easily identified causes of hemolysis, such as hemoglobinopathies or spherocytosis, before proceeding to tests for enzyme disorders.[11] Definitive diagnosis depends on quantitative assay of the activity of the suspected enzyme or identification of a specific mutation by DNA analysis. The availability of such assays is limited, but screening tests for deficiencies in PK, triose phosphate isomerase (TPI), and glucose phosphate isomerase (GPI) can be carried out in any well-equipped clinical laboratory.[12] The in vitro properties of mutant enzyme proteins vary (Table 16-1), and characterization of such properties has improved understanding of the genetics

TABLE 16-1	Parameters Commonly Used In Vitro to Characterize Mutant Enzyme Protein
V_{max}	Maximal enzyme velocity obtainable with saturating substrate concentrations
K_m	The substrate concentration yielding half-maximal activity; an index of catalytic efficiency
pH optimum	The pH at which maximal enzyme activity is present
Heat stability	Resistance of enzyme protein to heat denaturation
Electrophoretic mobility	Migration of enzyme protein in an electric field
Specific activity	Enzyme activity per defined amount of enzyme protein (e.g., milligram); enzyme protein is measured immunologically with antienzyme antibodies

and pathogenesis of anemias associated with defective glycolytic enzymes. Measurement of glycolytic intermediates extracted from freshly obtained erythrocytes has provided confirmation of the in vivo significance of in vitro abnormalities in enzyme function. The usual finding is accumulation of proximal intermediates and depletion of distal intermediates, thereby giving rise to a characteristic transition or crossover pattern at the locus of an abnormal enzyme. Secondary crossovers sometimes take place and are due to the influence of altered concentrations of metabolites on key regulatory enzymes such as hexokinase (HK), phosphofructokinase (PFK), and PK. As a result of secondary crossovers, the pattern of glycolytic intermediates may become so complex that it has only limited usefulness in the identification of an enzymopathy. In contrast, measurement of intracellular metabolites is currently the most convenient way to screen for abnormalities in nucleotide metabolism. Red cell ATP levels are below normal with overproduction of ADA, whereas P-5′-N deficiency is associated with increased concentrations of red cell ATP and reduced levels of glutathione. The apparent increase in ATP is, in fact, due to the presence of large amounts of cytidine and uridine nucleotides, which are also measured in the enzymatic assay for ATP. Spectral analysis of a deproteinized extract of red cells provides a straightforward means of identifying such nucleotides, and it is a simple method to screen patients for suspected P-5′-N deficiency.[9]

Caution is needed in interpreting the results of quantitative assays of enzyme activity. First, only surviving cells are available for sampling in circulating blood, and the metabolic circumstances of these favored cells cannot necessarily be extrapolated to indicate the status of cells already hemolyzed. Second, assay in vitro under optimal conditions may not adequately reflect the performance of an enzyme under less favorable circumstances in vivo. Third, the high specific activity of certain enzymes in

leukocytes may result in spurious normal values for erythrocyte enzyme activity unless contaminating leukocytes are removed before assay or their contribution to total activity is compensated for by appropriate calculations. Fourth, transfusion therapy with normal erythrocytes within several months before assay may obscure the presence of an enzyme defect. Fifth, the mean enzyme activity that is determined fails to portray the distribution of activity within individual erythrocytes. The endowment of intracellular enzymes is fixed, and protein synthetic ability disappears at the reticulocyte stage; thereafter, the inevitable denaturation of enzyme protein that accompanies cell aging reduces enzymatic activity at a rate characteristic for each enzyme. Transient accentuation of reticulocytosis, therefore, is often accompanied by rising mean enzyme activity. Certain glycolytic enzymes (notably HK and PK) are strikingly more active in reticulocytes than in postreticulocyte red cells, and the majority of this excess activity is rapidly lost coincident with reticulocyte maturation.[13-15] The true magnitude of an enzyme deficiency may not be apparent unless comparison is made to blood that is equally rich in reticulocytes[14] or corrections are applied that eliminate the contribution of the reticulocyte subfraction to total enzyme activity.[15]

Finally, there is evidence that reversible binding of glyceraldehyde-3-phosphate dehydrogenase (G3PD), HK, and PFK to the band 3 membrane protein is involved in the regulation of glycolysis,[16] and altered binding of mutant forms of these enzymes (and perhaps others) is not assessed in conventional assays performed on hemolysates.

HEXOKINASE DEFICIENCY

Clinical Manifestations

CNSHA has been attributed to deficient erythrocyte HK activity in 22 patients (Table 16-2). Severely affected individuals may exhibit neonatal hyperbilirubinemia and thereafter require transfusion at regular intervals for intractable anemia. In patients with mild disease, the hemolysis is fully compensated for and anemia is absent. However, jaundice, reticulocytosis, and splenomegaly are usually present in such patients. Gallstones may be evident, even in early childhood.[25] Hyperhemolytic episodes are not a feature of the disorder. The results of red cell morphologic examination are usually unremarkable, but occasional burr cells, target cells, stippled cells, and densely stained spiculated cells may be observed after splenectomy. The osmotic fragility of fresh erythrocytes is normal, but a fragile population of cells may appear after incubation at 37° C.

Biochemistry

In human red cells, HK is a monomer (molecular weight, 112,000).[35] It is encoded by a gene (*HK1*) located on

TABLE 16-2 Hexokinase Variants Associated with Hemolytic Anemia

Reference	No. of Cases	CLINICAL FEATURES			PROPERTIES OF RBC HEXOKINASE			
		Inheritance	Hemolytic Anemia	Other	Activity (% of Normal)	Kinetic Abnormalities	Stability In Vitro	Electrophoretic Mobility
17	1	—	+	Congenital malformations	13-24*	0	—	—
18	1	Recessive	++		15-20*	+	Normal	Abnormal
19	1	Recessive	++		16*	0	—	Abnormal
20	1	Recessive	+++	Hydrops fetalis	17			
21	1	Recessive	+		20*	0	Normal	Normal
22, 23	1	Recessive	++	Low platelet and fibroblast hexokinase activity	20*	0	Low	Normal
24	1	Recessive	++	Low platelet hexokinase activity	25*	+	Normal	Abnormal
25	1	Recessive	+		25*	0	Low	Normal
26	2	Dominant	+	Spherocytes, ovalocytes	30*	0	Low	Normal
27	1	Recessive	+	Psychomotor retardation	45†	+	Normal	Normal
28	1	Recessive	+		50*	0	Normal	Normal
29	1	—	+	Congenital malformations	33*	+	—	—
30	2	Recessive	+		40-53*	+	Low	Normal
31	1	—	+		50*	+	—	—
32	1				53			
33	5	Dominant	+	WBC hexokinase activity low	45-91†	+	Normal	Abnormal
34	2	Dominant	++		75*	+	Normal	Abnormal

*Maximal enzyme activity (V_{max}) compared with reticulocytosis controls.
†Maximal enzyme activity (V_{max}) compared with normal red cells.
RBC, red blood cell; WBC, white blood cell.

chromosome 10q22.[20] HK activity declines as red cells age. Loss of activity is particularly striking during reticulocyte maturation. In human reticulocytes, two major isoenzymes of HK have been identified by chromatographic techniques.[36] One (HKR) has an apparent half-life in vivo of only 10 days, whereas the other (HK1) has a longer half-life of 66 days. These two proteins are the products of two closely similar messenger RNAs (mRNAs) that are transcribed from a single gene (*HK1*) by the use of alternate promoters. Exon one is unique to each mRNA species, but the remaining 17 exons are identical.[37] Differential loss of these two isoenzymes appears to explain the biphasic character of the decay in HK activity during erythrocyte aging. An ATP- and ubiquitin-dependent proteolytic system capable of degrading about 80% of HK activity may explain the rapid loss of HK in rabbit reticulocytes,[38] or the loss may be secondary to an intrinsic property of the HK molecule itself.[39] Previous oxidative injury appears to be necessary for recognition and destruction of HK by the ubiquitin-dependent system.[40] Because ATP- and ubiquitin-dependent proteolysis is limited to reticulocytes,[38] it cannot be responsible for the loss of HK in aging human red cells.

HK is the glycolytic enzyme with the lowest activity in normal red cells, and a variety of observations indicate that it plays a rate-limiting role in erythrocyte glycolysis.[41-45] The maximal activity of erythrocyte HK from deficient patients has varied from 13% to 91% of normal (see Table 16-2). In evaluating these findings, comparisons of enzyme activity between red cell populations of equivalent age must be made. In the case described by Valentine and associates,[45] for example (Fig. 16-2), although HK activity was 62% of the normal value for mature erythrocytes, it was only 14% of the activity found in blood with high reticulocyte counts. Separation of young and old red cell populations by centrifugation revealed only the expected moderate diminution (to 0.11 mol/min/10^{10} red blood cells) of HK activity in older cells from this patient.[45] HK activity was even lower (0.075 mol/min/10^{10} red blood cells) in an asymptomatic brother, yet no evidence of undue hemolysis was present. However, Figure 16-2 shows that the brother's cells are actually far less deficient with respect to cell age than the immature cells of the propositus. The impact of HK deficiency is clearly greater in energetic young erythrocytes, whereas cells that survive to an older age can meet their limited metabolic requirements even at very low HK levels.[46] As the erythrocyte ages, in vivo changes in stability or kinetics peculiar to mutant HK may also render older cells liable to undergo premature hemolysis. In rats and rabbits, HK from immature erythrocytes has a higher K_m (Michaelis constant) for glucose than mature cells do, but such is not the case in normal human erythrocytes.[46]

In keeping with their enzymatic defect, HK-deficient erythrocytes have usually demonstrated subnormal glucose consumption and lactate production in vivo. Such cells also metabolize fructose poorly but utilize mannose or galactose normally[45] because these substrates are not metabolized by HK. Some HK-deficient erythrocytes are capable of normal glucose consumption at the glucose concentrations (5 mmol/L) customarily found in

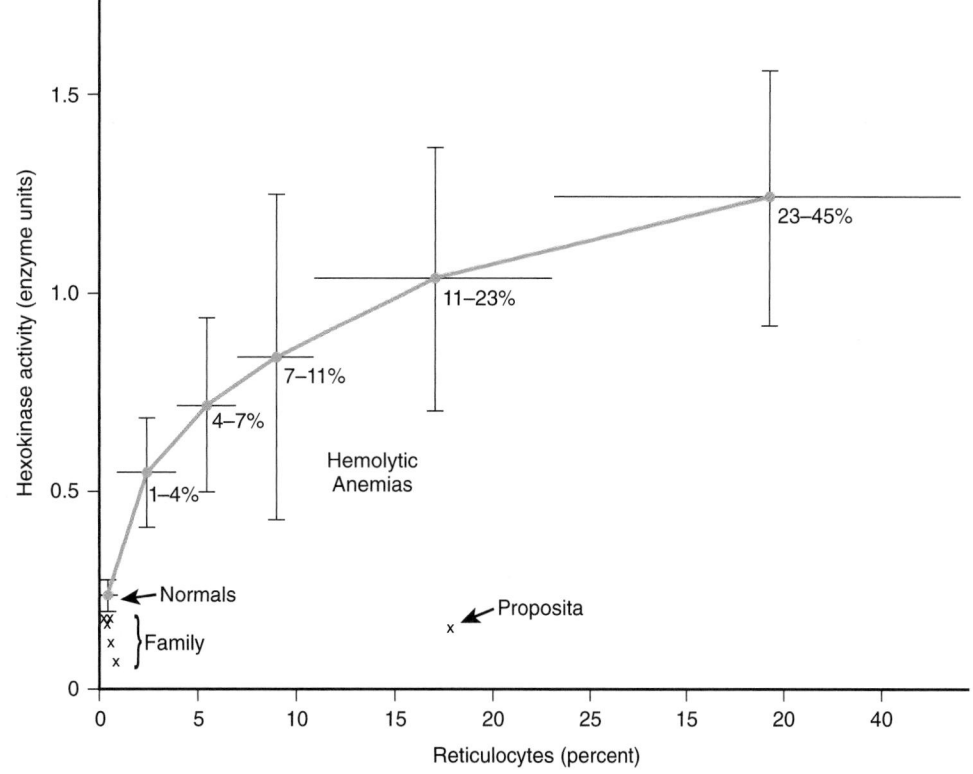

FIGURE 16-2. Hexokinase (HK) activity observed in 54 patients with hemolytic anemia of various causes plotted against percentages of reticulocyte in cells assayed. Patients are grouped according to reticulocyte levels. Mean HK activity for each group is plotted against the mean reticulocyte percentage in cells of that group. Standard deviations are indicated by *vertical bars.* Values for a single HK-deficient patient (proposita) and her family are designated separately. *(From Valentine WN, Oski FA, Paglia DE, et al: Erythrocyte hexokinase and hereditary hemolytic anemia. In Beutler E [ed]: Hereditary Disorders of Erythrocyte Metabolism. New York, Grune & Stratton, 1968, pp 288-300.)*

plasma but utilize glucose poorly or not at all at lower glucose concentrations, either because of an abnormally low affinity for glucose[34] or because of enzyme instability under conditions of low substrate availability.[30] Such erythrocytes may encounter a particularly unfavorable metabolic environment within the spleen. The concentration of glucose in normal splenic homogenates has been found by Necheles and co-workers[34] to be only 5 to 11 μmol/g of tissue, and in a patient with HK deficiency the concentration was even lower (1.1 μmol/g of tissue). Furthermore, because splenic tissue metabolizes glucose rapidly,[47] prolonged vascular pooling in the spleen is probably accompanied by profound local hypoglycemia. Erythrocytes with unfavorable kinetics for glucose metabolism are clearly at a disadvantage in competing with reticuloendothelial cells for such a reduced glucose supply. Another disadvantage of the splenic environment is its relative acidity. The optimal pH of erythrocyte HK is approximately 8; at lower pH values, diminished enzyme activity may be expected. Possibly of greater importance, at low pH values, glucose 6-phosphate, a potent inhibitor of HK, accumulates because of PFK inhibition.[48] An erythrocyte that has diminished HK activity under optimal pH conditions will be further compromised in the acidic environment of the spleen. The clinical improvement that follows splenectomy attests to the importance of this organ in the pathogenesis of hemolysis. Detailed isotopic studies to define red cell kinetics and sites of hemolysis have yet to be reported. Although no splenic sequestration of chromated autologous erythrocytes was noted in two patients,[25,31] in another sequestration was present. Thus, in this disorder the red cells may be damaged by the spleen and die elsewhere.

Significant alterations in intracellular metabolites are associated with defective HK function. The erythrocyte ATP concentration is sometimes,[31,35] but not always[21,24,29,33] subnormal. The glucose-6-phosphate concentration is reduced to approximately half normal, and the concentrations of other more distal intermediates, most notably 2,3-DPG, are also usually reduced. These metabolites may exert a significant regulatory influence on glycolysis. For example, Brewer[49] has shown that concentrations of 2,3-DPG in the physiologic range inhibit HK, so the low 2,3-DPG levels in HK-deficient red cells may facilitate the performance of available HK. The increased affinity of hemoglobin for oxygen expected to be associated with subnormal 2,3-DPG levels has been documented in one anemic patient with HK deficiency by Delivoria-Papadopoulos and co-workers[50] and by Oski and associates.[51] This patient, whose hemoglobin-oxygen affinity (P-50) was 19 mm Hg (normal, 27 ± 1.2), was capable of just minimal exercise despite only moderate anemia (hemoglobin, 9.8 g/dL). On exercise, her central venous partial pressure of oxygen (PO_2) promptly fell to minimal levels as oxygen consumption rose. Increased oxygen delivery was achieved primarily by an increase in cardiac output because the unfavorable oxygen affinity curve precluded any substantial further desaturation of hemoglobin.[51]

Thus, the altered concentration of intracellular metabolites induced by HK deficiency may, as in this patient, accentuate symptoms associated with anemia.

Because of its reactive sulfhydryl group, HK is susceptible to oxidant inactivation in the absence of sufficient glutathione.[52] Both normal and low glutathione levels have been reported in HK deficiency, but Heinz bodies have not been observed. Resting hexose monophosphate (HMP) shunt activity, measured with ^{14}C-glucose-1, was quantitatively normal in one patient despite subnormal glucose consumption, but stimulation with methylene blue was suboptimal.[45] Failure of the shunt at low glucose concentrations has also been noted in an HK mutant with a high K_m for glucose.[32] Methylene blue–stimulated methemoglobin reduction was subnormal in the single instance that it was evaluated.[17] When HK-inactivating antibodies are incorporated into normal red cells by the process of hypotonic lysis and isotonic reannealing, enzyme-deficient cells exhibit a greatly impaired response to HMP shunt stimulation by methylene blue.[42] These studies, though not indicating a central role for defective shunt activity in the pathogenesis of hemolysis, do suggest that under unusual circumstances, HK-deficient cells might be compromised by a limited shunt. Such circumstances might arise on exposure to a potent oxidant in the low glucose environment of the spleen.

Genetics

Inheritance of HK deficiency is autosomal recessive. Biochemical identification of asymptomatic carriers is not always possible because enzyme activity often falls within the low-normal range. In a few pedigrees (see Table 16-2), the heterozygous state appears to be severe enough to result in hemolytic anemia. One such heterozygote appeared to be doubly heterozygous for HK and glucose-6-phosphate dehydrogenase (G6PD) deficiency.[53]

The qualitative abnormalities characteristic of mutant HK (see Table 16-2) may reflect either a structural or a regulatory gene mutation. On electrophoresis, mutant HK lacks one or more of the normal bands of activity, but no bands migrating in an abnormal position have been observed. The various bands represent the presence of several isozymes of HK. Diminished synthesis of one or more isozymes with predominance of the remaining isozymes accounts for the electrophoretic differences observed (see Table 16-2). DNA analysis has defined two separate HK mutations in a compound heterozygote who exhibited nonspherocytic hemolytic anemia.[20,54,55] One was a missense mutation (T1667→C) and the other was a deletion of exon 5 (96 base pairs [bp]). Expression of each HK mutation in a bacterial system allowed recovery of sufficient purified enzyme to determine that the missense mutation completely abolished HK activity whereas the deletion reduced activity to about 10% of normal.[55] In another individual,[24] a homozygous missense mutation in the active site of HK1 (2039 C→G in exon 15) was discovered.[56] In a Japanese family, a stillborn fetus with HK deficiency was found to be homozygous for a large deletion that removed exons 5 through 8 in HK mRNA and led to premature termination of translation.[20] The kinetic abnormalities noted in many other mutant forms of HK undoubtedly also reflect as yet undefined structural abnormalities in enzyme protein.[17,18,22,27,28,32]

Studies of the tissue distribution of HK deficiency have been performed in blood cells and cultured fibroblasts. Electrophoresis of leukocyte or platelet HK reveals an anodal isozyme (Hk3) distinct from those of the erythrocyte (Hk1 and Hk2), as well as a shared isozyme (Hk1).[57,58] Leukocyte HK activity has been normal in some patients,[30,45] but the qualitative abnormality in leukocyte HK described by Necheles and colleagues,[34] as well as the case of generalized HK deficiency in all blood cells reported by Rijksen and co-workers,[24] indicates that to some extent the enzyme is under common genetic control in different tissues. When platelet HK activity has been low, platelet function has been normal despite subtle defects in in vitro energy metabolism.[59] Cultured fibroblasts from two individuals with different HK mutants contained HK with properties and activity like those found in red cells,[23] thus suggesting that this source of fetal tissue could be used for prenatal diagnosis.

A murine model of HK deficiency, termed Downeast anemia, is due to homozygous inheritance of a mutation that markedly decreases the expression of HK1 in erythroid tissues, spleen, and kidney. The mutation is the result of insertion of a transposon into intron 4 of the *HK1* gene. Mice exhibit nonspherocytic hemolytic anemia, marked reticulocytosis, splenomegaly, and striking accumulation of iron in the liver and kidney. Echinocytes and red cells split into two poles of hemoglobin connected only by thin strands of membrane are features of erythrocyte morphology in affected homozygous mice that are of interest because they have not been reported in human HK deficiency.[60]

Therapy

Treatment consists of red cell transfusion as indicated, supplemental folic acid, and close observation for cholelithiasis. Splenectomy may alleviate but does not eliminate the anemia.[18,22,24,30,34,45]

GLUCOSE PHOSPHATE ISOMERASE DEFICIENCY

Clinical Manifestations

A deficiency of erythrocyte GPI has been reported in more than 60 patients with congenital hemolytic anemia.[61] Hemolytic anemia usually appears in infancy and often requires red cell transfusion therapy. Hyperbilirubinemia,[62] hydrops fetalis,[63,64] or death[65] may occur during the neonatal period. Several patients have experienced hyperhemolytic crises after infections or drug exposure.[62,66] In some of these individuals, G6PD, as well as GPI, has been deficient.[66,67] Hemolytic anemia is usually the sole clinical manifestation of GPI deficiency. A subset of patients also exhibit neurologic dysfunction.[68-73] In one patient, neuromuscular abnormalities were correlated with a severe reduction in muscle and cerebrospinal fluid GPI activity.[71] Blockade of glycolysis at the GPI step may divert the flow of glucose metabolism in the direction of glycogen synthesis. Several patients with GPI deficiency have been reported to have increased hepatic glycogen stores,[74,75] and in one, muscular fatigue was severe enough to suggest a diagnosis of glycogen storage disease.[75] An animal model of GPI deficiency and chronic hemolytic anemia has been developed in the mouse. The clinical and biochemical features of the disease in mice closely resemble those found in humans.[76]

Red cell morphologic characteristics are generally similar to those seen in other types of CNSHA. In severely anemic patients, dense, spiculated, or "whiskered" microspherocytes have been noted after splenectomy. In one instance, sufficient numbers of such cells were present before splenectomy to suggest the diagnosis of hereditary spherocytosis.[77] In another, the predominant morphologic abnormality was stomatocytosis.[78] The reticulocytosis may be profound. Mean corpuscular volume is elevated (97 to 139 fL). With incubation at 37° C, a variable fraction of erythrocytes may exhibit abnormally increased osmotic fragility, whereas fresh cells are usually normal. Survival of chromated autologous red cells is reduced, often[79-81] but not invariably,[65,79,82] with evidence of splenic sequestration.

Biochemistry

GPI is a dimer[83] composed of two identical subunits, each with a molecular weight of approximately 60,000.[81,83] Subunit synthesis is directed by a single genetic locus on chromosome 19.[84] The crystal structure of human GPI has been defined.[85] GPI is a multifunctional protein. The dimeric form exhibits glycolytic enzyme activity, whereas the monomeric form functions as a cytokine. Monomeric GPI is 100% homologous to neuroleukin, a neurotrophic growth factor secreted by lectin-stimulated T cells[61,86,87]; to autocrine motility factor, which stimulates cell motility and the growth of metastases[88]; and to a differentiation and maturation mediator for human myeloid leukemia cells in tissue culture.[89] Altered neuroleukin function may explain the neurologic disorder associated with several GPI mutations.[61,73]

The metabolic events that precede hemolysis of GPI-deficient erythrocytes are poorly understood. Erythrocyte glycolysis is impaired in vivo, as reflected by an increased ratio of substrate to product (i.e., glucose 6-phosphate to fructose 6-phosphate) in freshly obtained GPI-deficient cells.[67,77,90-95] Paradoxically, with only occasional exceptions,[77,96] such cells are fully capable of glycolysis in vitro.[67,82,97-00] In contrast to HK deficiency, in which 2,3-DPG levels are low, sufficient glycolysis generally occurs in GPI deficiency to maintain the 2,3-DPG concentration at or above the normal level.[88,90,92,96,100] Except for three patients with diminished ATP concentrations, two of whom also exhibited reduced in vitro glycolysis for cell age,[68,78,83] the erythrocyte ATP concentration has been normal.

A profound defect in recycling of fructose-6-phosphate through the pentose phosphate pathway has been observed repeatedly in GPI-deficient red cells.[77,99,100] The increased formation of Heinz bodies[65,78] and glutathione instability[69,94] after exposure to acetylphenylhydrazine, an abnormal ascorbate cyanide test, and diminished concentrations of red cell glutathione[78,82,91,92,94] in fresh erythrocytes all suggest that diminished shunt activity in vivo may contribute to hemolysis.

With rare exceptions,[71] mutant forms of red cell GPI exhibit considerable thermal lability in vitro, thus making it likely that enzyme lability in vivo as red cells age will lead to premature metabolic collapse and hemolysis. Separation of red cells by centrifugation into young and old subpopulations has usually demonstrated accelerated decay of enzyme activity in the older cells.[82,101] Arnold and co-workers[101] simulated the in vivo process of aging by incubating red cells in vitro at 37° C for 8 days and changing the incubation medium often to ensure that glucose availability and pH remained constant. GPI activity declined by 66% in GPI-deficient red cells during incubation, with a level of only 6% of normal being reached, and lactate production, normal at the onset, was reduced to 11% of normal. In contrast, normal reticulocyte-rich blood lost only 6% of the original GPI activity after 8 days, and lactate production fell only 7%. If mannose rather than glucose was used, GPI-deficient and normal red cells made equivalent amounts of lactate, and there was little or no loss in lactate production after 8 days. The normal glycolytic rate noted with mannose, which is isomerized by mannose phosphate isomerase and thus bypasses the GPI reaction, clearly pinpoints defective GPI activity as the cause of glycolytic failure in GPI-deficient cells. ATP depletion with consequent erythrocyte rigidity and reticuloendothelial entrapment would be anticipated to follow failure of glycolysis. GPI-deficient red cells are, indeed, less deformable than normal cells, particularly when comparison is made to young, reticulocyte-rich populations of cells.[89,90,102,103] Goulding studied a 9-year-old patient with GPI deficiency and priapism and concluded that the priapism was the consequence of abnormal erythrocyte deformability.[104] Studies by Coetzer and Zail revealed aggregation of membrane spectrin in GPI-deficient erythrocytes.[105] The extent of the aggregation is a function of cell age.

Even reticulocytes may be severely GPI deficient.[74] Deficient reticulocytes with limited anaerobic glycolytic capability may also be incapable of effective oxidative phosphorylation in the acidic, hypoglycemic splenic environment (see the section "Pyruvate Kinase Deficiency"), thereby leading to metabolic failure and hemolysis. Large numbers of reticulocytes were found when specimens from the spleen of a patient with GPI deficiency were examined by transmission electron microscopy.[74] Furthermore, the reticulocyte count often increases after splenectomy.[65,74,80,82] Because hemoglobin levels also increase, this observation suggests survival of a population of reticulocytes that would otherwise be hemolyzed almost immediately after their release from bone marrow.

Genetics and Inheritance

Like most other glycolytic enzymopathies, GPI deficiency is inherited as an autosomal recessive trait. Heterozygotes are hematologically normal but exhibit reduced erythrocyte GPI activity (usually to about 50% of normal). They inherit one mutant and one normal GPI allele, which results in the synthesis of two unlike GPI subunits that may combine in one of three ways to form a normal homodimer, a mutant homodimer, or a heterodimer that contains both normal and mutant subunits. Electrophoresis of GPI from the erythrocytes of heterozygotes will demonstrate one to three bands, depending on the extent to which the charge or activity of the mutant subunit is altered. Post-translational events, such as oxidation of enzyme protein, may alter the electrophoretic pattern and confuse its interpretation.[106,107]

GPI mutations associated with hemolytic anemia are listed in Table 16-3. Of the 31 known mutations, 2 are splice site, 3 are nonsense, and 26 are missense mutations involving a single amino acid substitution.[61,108] The mutations are found in 12 of the 18 exons and are generally unique to one or at most a few families. The rarity of GPI deficiency and the heterogeneity of the mutations identified indicate that no selective advantage is conferred to affected individuals. Half of the homozygotes or compound heterozygotes for missense mutations have mild to moderate hemolytic anemia, and half have severe anemia. In contrast, all compound heterozygotes for missense mutations and either splice site or nonsense mutations have severe hemolytic anemia. Hemolytic anemia occurs in individuals when GPI activity drops below about 40% of the normal mean activity. Substrate kinetics and the optimal pH of mutant enzymes have almost always been normal, but most mutant enzymes have exhibited varying degrees of thermal instability. Short of direct detection of the mutation at the DNA level, the most useful means of classifying the numerous GPI variants reported has been on the basis of stability, electrophoretic mobility, or residual enzyme activity in red cells and leukocytes.[64,65,67-71,78-82,90-99,109-112] Until DNA mutation analysis has been completed on these variants, it will not be clear how many are truly unique. Immunologic titration of functionally inactive enzyme protein in red cells indicates that some mutant GPI alleles are "silent" and produce no detectable enzyme protein whereas

TABLE 16-3   **Mutations Associated with Glucose Phosphate Isomerase Deficiency and Hemolytic Anemia**

Variant	Ethnic Origin	Genotype	Exon	Amino Acid Change	Red Cell GPI Activity (IU/g Hb)
HOMOZYGOTES—MISSENSE MUTATIONS					
Matsumoto	Japanese	14C→T	1	Thr5Ile	27
	American Indian	247C→T	3	Arg83Trp	16.4
Sarsina	Italian	301G→A	4	Val101Met	7.2*
Iwate	Japanese	671C→T	7	Thr224Met	10.2
	Turkish	970G→A	12	Gly324Ser	49.7*
Morcone	Italian	1028A→G	12	Gln343Arg	7.2*
Narita	Japanese	1028A→G	12	Gln343Arg	32.4
Mount Scopus	Ashkenazi	1039C→T	12	Arg347Cys	14.8+*
	Spanish†	1040G→A	12	Arg347Hist	≈9*
	Hispanic	1415G→A	16	Arg472His	15.4
	Turkish	1415G→A	16	Arg472His	24.9
	? English	1574T→C	18	Ile525Thr	3*
Fukuoka	Japanese	1615G→A	18	Asp539Asn	6.4
COMPOUND HETEROZYGOTES—NONSENSE/MISSENSE MUTATIONS					
Stuttgart	German	43C→T/1028A→G	1, 12	Gln15Stop/Gln343Arg	27.9*
Elyria	Caucasian	223A→G/286C→T	3, 4	Arg75Gly/Arg96Stop	4*
Bari	Italian	286C→T/584C→T	4, 6	Arg96Stop/Thr196Ile	14.9*
	Russian	286C→T/1039C→T	4, 12	Arg96Stop/Arg347Cys	19
Zwickau	German	1039C→T/1538G→A	12, 17	Arg347Cys/Trp513Stop	21*
Catalonia	Spanish	1648A→G	18	Lys550Glu	<7*
COMPOUND HETEROZYGOTES—SPLICE SITE/MISSENSE MUTATIONS					
Mola	Italian	584C→T/del1473-IVS16(+2)	6, 16	Thr195Ile/splice site	12.9*
Nordhorn	German	1028A→G/IVS15(−2) A→C	12/IVS15	Gln343Arg/splice site	11.4*
COMPOUND HETEROZYGOTES—MISSENSE/MISSENSE MUTATIONS					
Homburg	German	59A→C/1016T→C	1, 12	His20Pro/Leu339Pro	3.5†*
Barcelona	Spanish	341A→T/663T→G	4, 7	Asp113Val/Asn220Lys	20
	? English	475G→A/1040G→A	5, 12	Gly159Ser/Arg347His	6*
	African American	671C→T/1483G→A	7, 17	Thr224Met/Glu495Lys	12.2
	African American	818G→A/1039C→T	10, 12	Arg273His/Arg347Cys	15.9
	Caucasian	833C→T/1459C→T	10, 16	Ser278Leu/Leu487Phe	9.8
	Hispanic	898G→C/1039C→T	11, 12	Ala300Pro/Arg347Cys	25.4*
Kinki	Japanese	1124C→G/1615G→A	13, 18	Thr375Arg/Asp539Asn	3.7*
Calden	German	1166A→G/1549→G	13, 18	His389Arg/Leu517Val	12*

*Severe disease (splenectomy, frequent red cell transfusions, and/or reticulocyte count >15%).
†The Spanish patients are described by Repiso and colleagues.[108,108a]
Adapted from data summarized by Kugler W, Lakomek M: Glucose-6-phosphate isomerase deficiency. Baillieres Clin Haematol. 2000;13:89-101.

others produce structurally altered protein with varying degrees of activity and stability in vivo.[109-111]

A single GPI isozyme is present in all human tissues.[84] GPI deficiency is usually less severe in nonerythroid tissues than in erythrocytes because nonerythrocytic tissues retain the ability to synthesize GPI subunits. Clinical abnormalities outside the hematopoietic system are rare and, if present, are neuromuscular in nature. Leukocytes are capable of normal phagocytosis and chemotaxis despite a reduction in GPI activity to 25%[90] to 73%[98] of normal, but if GPI activity is more severely depressed, granulocyte function is impaired.[71,112] Similarly, platelet GPI may be only 20% to 30% of normal; however, clot formation, platelet aggregation, and other clotting studies are normal.[90,98] Prenatal diagnosis is feasible by DNA analysis if the mutations are known or by measurement of GPI activity in amniotic fluid fibroblasts[63] or chorionic villus trophoblasts.[113]

Therapy

Transfusion requirements are usually eliminated by removal of the spleen, but the anemia persists.[65,74,80,98] The postsplenectomy hemoglobin levels of 6.7 to 10.3 g/dL and reticulocyte counts of 36% to 73% observed in three siblings by Paglia and co-workers[100] reflect the magnitude of the continued hemolysis that may be present. Attempts by Arnold and colleagues[98] to enhance glycolysis in a GPI-deficient patient by intravenous administration of methylene blue or inorganic phosphate (P_i) did not have a lasting benefit.

PHOSPHOFRUCTOKINASE DEFICIENCY

Clinical Manifestations

Inherited deficiency of PFK can involve erythrocytes, muscle, or both, depending on the PFK subunit affected and the nature of the biochemical defect (Table 16-4). Although low erythrocyte PFK activity and mild hemolytic anemia are commonly found in type VII glycogen storage disease (Tarui's syndrome), the dominant clinical feature of this disorder is exertional myopathy caused by deficient muscle PFK activity.[118,119] Physical activity is limited not by anemia but by weakness, easy fatigability, and severe muscle cramps associated with the myopathy. The disease may be evident at birth and cause death during infancy as a result of respiratory insufficiency and other complications,[120] or it may be so mild that it is not manifested until old age.[121] However, in most affected individuals the disorder is first detected during adolescence or young adulthood. The diagnosis may be suspected if no lactate is produced during an ischemic (anaerobic) forearm exercise test, but confirmation requires muscle biopsy for determination of PFK activity or noninvasive magnetic resonance imaging (MRI) studies of muscle carbohydrate metabolism.[122]

When PFK deficiency is confined to erythrocytes, there are no symptoms of myopathy, and the blood lactate response to anoxic exercise is normal.[123-125] Such patients may be hematologically normal[116,126,127] or exhibit mild to moderate hemolytic anemia.[123,127] In general, red cell morphologic characteristics are not strikingly abnormal, although prominent basophilic stippling has occasionally been noted.

Biochemistry

PFK is one of several glycolytic enzymes that reversibly bind to the inner aspect of the erythrocyte membrane. Binding, which is thought to occur between the amino-terminal position of the transmembrane protein band 3 and the adenine nucleotide binding site, located in a cleft between the two dimers that form the PFK tetramer, may serve to both activate the enzyme and protect it against proteolytic degradation during erythrocyte aging.[128]

The active form of human erythrocyte PFK is a tetramer (molecular weight, 380,000) composed in varying combinations of two different subunits, one identical to the M subunit found in muscle PFK and the other identical to the L subunit found in liver PFK.[129,130] The molecular weight of the M subunit is 85,000 and that of the L subunit is 80,000.[129] About 50% of the erythrocyte enzyme is formed from M subunits,[124,129] whereas muscle PFK is composed entirely of M subunits.[124,131] A deficiency in M subunits severely depresses muscle PFK activity and results in myopathy, but it has a lesser effect on erythrocyte PFK because residual L subunits, under separate genetic control, combine to form an active L4 tetramer of PFK. However, PFK formed entirely from L subunits is unstable to heat or dilution in vitro and is more sensitive to ATP inhibition than muscle (M4) PFK is.[123] At the in vivo concentrations of ATP that are present within normal erythrocytes, the enzyme activity of L4 PFK tetramers is severely inhibited, thus possibly explaining the presence of hemolytic anemia even when enzyme activity, as measured in vitro, is approximately 50% of normal. Most recognized examples of PFK deficiency are the result of either missing[116,118] or structurally altered[125] M subunits. An interesting exception was found in a clinically normal individual, fortuitously discovered when he volunteered to serve as a "control" during studies of red cell PFK carried out by Vora and colleagues.[116] Normal M subunits but mutant, unstable L subunits were found in his red cells. There was no myopathy, and although erythrocyte PFK was only 65% of normal, hemolytic anemia was not present, presumably because residual enzyme activity within the red cell was entirely

TABLE 16-4   Various Forms of Human Phosphofructokinase Deficiency

Type	No. of Patients	Affected PFK Subunit	RED BLOOD CELL		MUSCLE		Other
			Hemolysis	PFK Activity*	Myopathy	PFK Activity*	
I	18	M (absent or unstable)	Present	29-64	Present	0-5	Hyperuricemia, arthritis
II	3	NA	NA	17	Present	0-6	
III	3	M (unstable)	Present	8-62	Absent	100	
IVa	2	M (unstable)	Absent	28-50	Absent	78†	Asymptomatic
IVb	3	L (unstable)	Absent	60-65	Absent	NA	Asymptomatic
V	3	NA	NA	75†	Present	2-6	Arthritis

NA, data not available.
*Percentage of normal value.
†Studied in only one patient.
Data from Tani and associates[114,115] and Vora and co-workers.[116,117]
From Mentzer WC, Glader BE. Disorders of erythrocyte metabolism. In Mentzer WC, Wagner GM (eds). The Hereditary Hemolytic Anemias. New York, Churchill Livingstone, 1989, pp 269-319.

due to the presence of M4 tetramers of PFK. The relatively greater stability and lesser susceptibility to ATP inhibition of this form of PFK apparently allowed adequate enzyme activity under conditions normally found within the red cell in vivo.

Because of the central role of PFK in regulation of erythrocyte metabolism, it is not surprising to find that a deficiency of this important enzyme is associated with hemolysis, but the mechanism of hemolysis is not well understood. Erythrocyte sodium and potassium concentrations, sodium influx, and lactate production were normal in one patient.[122] Despite their normal glycolytic capability in vitro, deficient cells were incapable of maintaining normal ATP concentrations in vivo. The low (73% of normal) intracellular ATP concentration in these cells, though indicative of an abnormality in cellular metabolism, may also exert a positive influence by partially relieving the inhibitory influence of ATP on PFK. Extensive in vitro study of erythrocytes obtained from a Swedish family with Tarui's disease and mild compensated hemolytic anemia found elevated intraerythrocytic calcium levels associated with increased calcium permeability of the erythrocyte membrane. High intracellular calcium levels activated the Gardos channel with subsequent ATP depletion, potassium depletion, increased mean corpuscular hemoglobin concentration (MCHC), and diminished erythrocyte deformability. The authors point out that the PFK and Ca^{2+} channel genes are in close proximity to one another on chromosome 12q, but the reason for abnormal Ca homeostasis remains undefined.[132,133]

The complex interaction between metabolites that may dictate actual PFK activity in vivo is illustrated by physiologic studies performed on four individuals with Tarui's syndrome.[134] At usual levels of physical activity, the pattern of erythrocyte glycolytic intermediates clearly reflected inhibition at the PFK step, and the concentration of the important downstream metabolite 2,3-DPG was only 50% of the level found in normal red cells. After the patients had 2 days of bed rest, their red cell 2,3-DPG levels sank to just a third of normal. Subsequently, ergometric exercise on a bicycle eliminated the glycolytic intermediate pattern of PFK inhibition and allowed downstream intermediates, including 2,3-DPG, to increase toward normal. Release of large amounts of inosine and ammonia from enzymopathic muscle during exercise into plasma was observed in these patients. Ammonia is a powerful activator of PFK; inosine can be metabolized to lactate by glycolytic pathways (i.e, the HMP shunt) that bypass the PFK reaction. Thus, the muscle metabolic abnormalities created by PFK deficiency generate metabolites that alleviated the enzymopathy in erythrocytes. (Diversion of the flow of erythrocyte glycolysis through the HMP shunt by the block at PFK may also generate increased amounts of purines and pyrimidines from 5-phosphoribosylpyrophosphate [PRPP].) The hyperuricemia sometimes noted in individuals with PFK deficiency (see Table 16-4) may be explained on this basis.[117]

An inherited deficiency of PFK found in English springer spaniels allows interesting comparisons to be made with the human condition.[135-137] As in humans, canine PFK deficiency is an autosomal recessive disorder. Red cell PFK levels are only 7% to 22% of normal in homozygotes because the muscle subunit, which is lacking, accounts for the majority of the available subunits in normal dog red cells.[138] PFK deficiency in dogs is associated with severe hemolytic anemia. Newborn dogs are not anemic because there is a greater abundance of L subunits and thus of functional PFK enzymes in their red cells. The hemolytic anemia appears because the normal developmental pattern of replacement of L by M subunit synthesis occurs in a setting in which M subunits either are not synthesized or are defective.[139]

A unique feature of dog PFK deficiency is episodic hemolysis induced by hyperventilation during exercise, mating, barking, or other similar activities.[137] Dog red cells with high sodium levels exhibit spontaneous hemolysis at alkaline pH; even the small pH change induced by hyperventilation is sufficient to generate the effect in PFK-deficient animals. Underlying the susceptibility of PFK-deficient dog red cells to hyperventilation-induced hemolysis may be their low 2,3-DPG levels, which increase intracellular pH. Raising 2,3-DPG levels to normal in vitro normalizes the response to alkalinity.[140] In comparison to humans, there is less evidence of exertional myopathy, even though dog muscle PFK activity is nearly absent,[141] because dogs do not rely on anaerobic glycolysis for generation of energy during exercise.[142] During exercise, PFK-deficient dogs do exhibit less extraction of oxygen from hemoglobin than normal dogs do, either because the affinity of hemoglobin for oxygen is high (caused by low 2,3-DPG levels in their erythrocytes) or because oxidative metabolism is impaired.[143]

PFK activity in erythrocytes from newborn infants is about 50% to 60% of that in normal adult cells.[144] PFK deficiency is more evident in older cells made earlier in gestation, perhaps because of accelerated enzyme decay.[145] Vora and Piomelli[146] showed that 25% to 30% of newborn erythrocyte PFK consists of L4 isozyme, with the remainder being divided equally between three hybrid isozymes of L and M subunits (L1M3, L2M2, and L3M1). The L4 isozyme, not found in normal adult red cells, is unstable and presumably accounts for the reduced PFK activity of older cord red cells. The demonstration that PFK deficiency may result in hemolytic anemia in adults suggests that the enzyme deficiency characteristic of normal newborn red cells may contribute to their shortened survival.

Genetics and Inheritance

The gene locus for the L subunit of PFK has been assigned to chromosome 21, whereas the M subunit locus is on chromosome 12.[117,147] The erythrocytes, but not the leukocytes and platelets of individuals with trisomy 21, consistently contain increased PFK

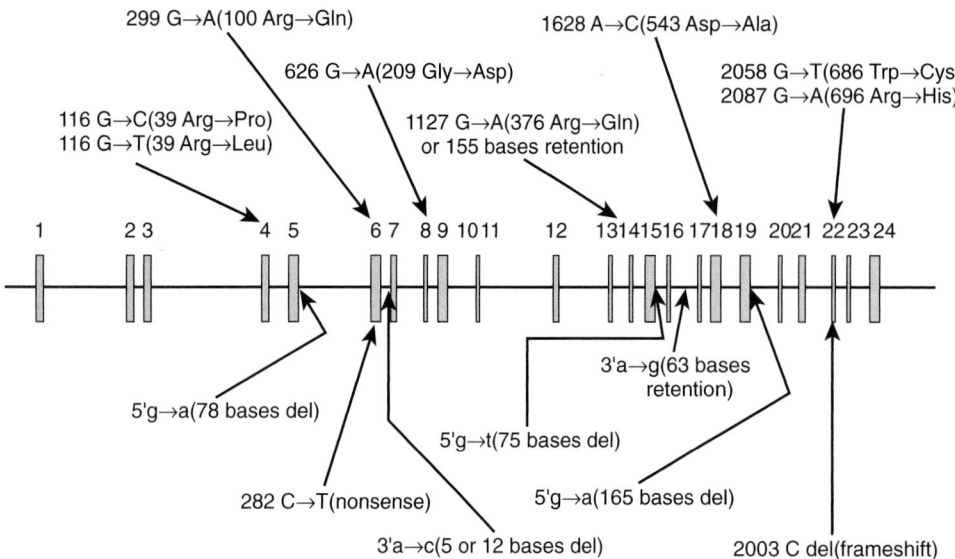

FIGURE 16-3. Mutations in the muscle phosphofructokinase gene. del, deletion. *(From Fujii H, Miwa S. Other erythrocyte enzyme deficiencies associated with non-haematological symptoms: Phosphoglycerate kinase and phosphofructokinase deficiency. Baillieres Clin Haematol 2000;13: 141-148. By copyright permission of Harcourt Publishers Ltd.)*

TABLE 16-5   Mutations Associated with Aldolase A Deficiency and Hemolytic Anemia

Ethnicity	Genotype	Amino Acid Change	Aldolase Activity in Erythrocytes	Aldolase Thermolability	Hemolytic Anemia	Myopathy	Mental Retardation	Reference
Jewish	*	Unknown	15	Not reported	Yes	No	Yes	154
Japanese	†	Unknown	7	Increased	Yes	No	No	155
Japanese	Homozygote	Asp128→Gly	5	Increased	Yes	No	No	155, 156
German	Homozygote	Glu206→Lys	4	Increased	Yes	Yes	No	157
Sicilian	Compound heterozygote	Cys338→Tyr Arg303→X	23	Increased	Yes	Yes	No	158, 159
Italian	Heterozygote	Gly346→Ser	Not reported	Normal	No	Yes	No	160, 161

*Presumed homozygote because the parents were first cousins.
†Homozygote or compound heterozygote.

---

activity.[148] Increased erythrocyte PFK activity is due to increased amounts of L subunit, consistent with a simple gene dosage effect.[117]

Inheritance is autosomal recessive. Type I PFK deficiency (Tarui's disease), which is found predominantly in Ashkenazi Jews and Japanese individuals, is the result of mutations involving the *PFKM* gene.[149,150] The 15 reported mutations[145] (5 splice site, 8 missense, 1 nonsense, and 1 frameshift) are shown in Figure 16-3.[151] The widely scattered location of the mutations makes it difficult to correlate genotype and phenotype. In PFK-deficient dogs, a missense mutation involving 120 nucleotides from the 3' end of the coding region produces a truncated mRNA and an unstable PFKM subunit tetramer with altered kinetic properties.[152,153]

Therapy

Supportive care with red cell transfusions as needed and daily folic acid supplementation are the mainstays of therapy for the hemolytic anemia.

ALDOLASE DEFICIENCY

Clinical Manifestations, Biochemistry, and Genetics

Aldolase A is found in erythrocytes, muscle, and the fetal brain. Only six individuals with CNSHA and erythrocyte aldolase deficiency have been reported. Their clinical course has varied, with one also exhibiting mental retardation, three an associated myopathy, and two no abnormalities other than hemolytic anemia (Table 16-5). Two members of a Japanese family who had a severe deficiency of red cell aldolase[155] exhibited severe chronic hemolytic anemia, sometimes exacerbated by infections. In vitro, red cell glycolysis and HMP shunt activity were depressed, thus indicating that the deficiency of aldolase was of functional significance. Both parents were hematologically normal but had intermediate reductions in red cell aldolase A activity. The mutant aldolase was strikingly thermolabile. A missense mutation (GAT→GGT) giving rise to a single amino acid substitution (Asp→Gly) at position 128 was present in the mutant enzyme.[156]

Transfection of *Escherichia coli* with an expression plasmid containing normal, mutant, or modified (by site-directed mutagenesis) aldolase A complementary DNA (cDNA) generated functional aldolase molecules that were used to confirm that the amino acid substitution at position 128, a site distant from the catalytic site but within an exposed hinge region, was responsible for the enzyme thermolability.[162]

In a German child, homozygosity for a point mutation at residue 206 (Glu→Lys) in the coding region of aldolase A also led to thermolability and severe enzyme deficiency in both erythrocytes and skeletal muscle.[157] Unlike the Japanese subjects, this child had a metabolic myopathy, as well as mild to moderate hemolytic anemia. The mutation at residue 206 would be predicted to disrupt the main subunit interface of the aldolase tetramer and cause thermolability. Why myopathy was noted in one setting but not in the other is unknown.

A girl of Sicilian ancestry whose red cell aldolase activity was less than a quarter of normal also exhibited myopathy and chronic hemolytic anemia.[158] Elevated plasma creatine phosphokinase activity was noted with febrile illnesses. She died at the age of 54 months of rhabdomyolysis and hyperkalemia during an acute febrile illness. Like the German patient, her aldolase A enzyme was thermolabile, which offered an explanation for the exacerbation of myopathy during fever.[159] DNA analysis revealed two mutations in the aldolase A gene in this patient: one was a premature stop codon mutation (931C→T) and the second was a missense mutation (1037G→A) that conferred thermolability on the enzyme.[158,159]

Another patient with aldolase deficiency exhibited CNSHA, mental retardation, mild glycogen storage disease, intestinal lactase deficiency, growth retardation, and peculiar facial features. Enzyme activity was approximately 15% of normal in erythrocytes and cultured skin fibroblasts.[154] No structural abnormality of residual erythrocyte aldolase was detected by electrophoresis, isoelectric focusing, heat stability studies, or kinetic examination. The patient was the offspring of a consanguineous marriage, but both parents were hematologically normal and had normal red cell aldolase activity.

A sixth patient, heterozygous for a thermostable mutation of aldolase A, had myopathy, arthrogryposis multiplex congenita, and hypopituitarism but normal IQ and no evidence of hemolytic anemia.[160,161] Because both parents were clinically normal, the aldolase mutation in the patient may have no relationship to his clinical abnormalities.

TRIOSE PHOSPHATE ISOMERASE DEFICIENCY

Clinical Manifestations

An association with TPI deficiency has been documented in approximately 50 patients with congenital hemolytic anemia.[163-178] In addition to chronic hemolysis, a severe neuromuscular disorder characterized initially by spasticity and psychomotor retardation and often progressing to weakness and hypotonia has been found in nearly all patients surviving beyond the neonatal period. Increased susceptibility to bacterial infection has also been noted. The neurologic abnormalities are not usually manifested before 6 to 12 months of age and are progressive, with death occurring before the age of 5 years. Occasionally, these abnormalities may stabilize during childhood[179] or adolescence.[164] In a Hungarian family, one adult son with severe TPI deficiency had extrapyramidal neurologic symptoms, whereas his older brother, who was equally TPI deficient, remained symptom free.[176,180] Further investigation has shown that these brothers have both inherited the same two TPI mutations (see later) but that levels of dihydroxyacetone phosphate (DHAP), methylglyoxal, and advanced glycation end products were much higher in the neurologiclly affected brother.[181] The basis for the prolonged survival of both brothers and their different neurologic status is unknown, but epigenetic factors are suspected.

Anemia is variable, but most patients require at least occasional blood transfusions. Macrocytosis and polychromatophilia are evident on the blood smear because of the presence of reticulocytosis, which may reach 50% on occasion. Aside from occasional small, dense spiculated cells, no striking changes in erythrocyte morphologic characteristics are present.

Biochemistry

TPI is a homodimer whose two subunits (molecular weight, 26,750[182]) are the product of a single locus on the short arm of chromosome 12.[183] Post-translational modification of one or both subunits may occur by deamidination of aspartines at positions 15 and 71, thereby resulting in multiple forms of the enzyme.[184,185] The 248–amino acid sequence of human (placental) TPI has been determined directly[182] and is nearly, but not completely identical to the sequence predicted by nucleotide analysis of adult human liver cDNA.[169]

TPI is a classic housekeeping gene, present in all tissues, whose amino acid sequence has been remarkably well conserved during evolution.[186] The eight-stranded $\alpha\beta$-barrel structure of the human enzyme has been confirmed at 2.8-nm resolution by x-ray crystallography.[186] TPI has no requirement for cofactors or metal ions, and there is no evidence of cooperativity or allosteric interactions between subunits.

When measured in vitro, erythrocyte TPI activity is approximately 1000 times that of HK, the least active glycolytic enzyme. Even TPI-deficient erythrocytes exhibiting only 2% to 35% of normal TPI activity in vitro possess far more TPI than HK activity. Not surprisingly, TPI-deficient erythrocytes are capable of normal glycolysis in vitro, even when compared with reticulocyte-rich normal blood.[164] Furthermore, mathematical modeling shows that increased activity of glycolytic kinases can lead to normal conversion of glucose to lactate in TPI-deficient cells.[187] Nonetheless, DHAP, the substrate for TPI, accumulates to high levels in TPI-deficient erythrocytes,[187] and the ATP concentration is usually low for cell age. These results indicate the presence of a substantial impairment in glycolysis in vivo. Reduction of residual TPI activity in deficient cells by binding to the red cell membrane or to brain microtubulin has been proposed to account for some of the differences between in vitro determinations of TPI activity and the evidence of a more severe impairment in enzyme function in vivo.[188-190] The defect can be partially bypassed by way of the HMP shunt, which generates glyceraldehyde 3-phosphate from glucose without the participation of TPI. Methylene blue stimulation of the shunt produces a lesser increase in glycolysis relative to baseline in TPI-deficient erythrocytes than in reticulocyte-rich control blood.[164] This has been interpreted as indicating a markedly greater "resting" shunt rate in the deficient cells, consistent with the proposed reliance of such cells on the shunt. Evidence indicates that TPI-deficient red cells are relatively deficient in antioxidant capabilities and that this deficiency may contribute to their shortened life span.[165,191]

Rare electrophoretic variants of TPI, not associated with reduced enzyme activity or hemolysis, have been described.[185,186,192,193] In anemic patients, enzyme kinetics and electrophoretic mobility are usually normal, but in vitro evidence of enzyme lability after heating is often obtained,[167-169,171] thus suggesting that instability and rapid loss of enzyme protein play an important role in the pathogenesis of hemolysis in vivo.[167,169] A single amino acid substitution (Glu→Asp) at position 104 has been identified in at least 17 geographically widely distributed families with clinically affected children and is the most commonly encountered mutation responsible for TPI deficiency.[173,178] Its relative rate of occurrence is thought to be due to a founder effect. The Glu104→Asp TPI gene product is thermolabile.[194] Computer modeling indicates that a substituted amino acid at position 104, which is buried in a hydrophilic side pocket of the normal enzyme, will reduce the stability of the pocket, promote unfolding, and enhance thermolability.[194]

Fourteen TPI mutations have been defined.[173] Most clinically affected individuals are homozygous for a single mutation or compound heterozygous for two different mutations. In the Hungarian pedigree mentioned earlier,[180] a point mutation at codon 240 (Phe→Leu) produced a moderately thermolabile TPI with abnormal substrate kinetics and electrophoretic migration.[195] Phe240 is near the active site of the enzyme and appears to be essential for maintaining its correct geometry.[186] Furthermore, both anemic brothers in this pedigree inherited a nonsense mutation at codon 145 that terminated TPI protein synthesis, thereby producing a truncated protein, and also reduced the output of TPI mRNA from the affected allele by 10- to 20-fold.[196] The red cells

of the brothers had less than 10% of the TPI activity found in normal cells.[180,195]

The enzyme deficiency is manifested not only in red cells but also in leukocytes, platelets, muscle, serum, and cerebrospinal fluid. Histologic examination of muscle from a girl with TPI deficiency and myopathy revealed marked degenerative changes of the contractile system, altered mitochondria, and absent TPI by histochemical staining.[197] Brain and nerve tissue have not yet been analyzed, but the cerebrospinal fluid deficiency suggests that deficient TPI activity in neural tissue is responsible for the neurologic abnormalities observed in enzymopenic patients. Although increased susceptibility to infection might be the consequence of defective function by TPI-deficient leukocytes,[170] functional studies carried out on such cells in vitro have often been normal.[166,179] A functional defect in TPI-deficient platelets has been described.[198]

Genetics and Inheritance

Several large pedigrees display an autosomal recessive mode of inheritance of TPI deficiency.[166,169,173] Obligate heterozygotes are clinically normal, but their erythrocytes contain only approximately half the TPI activity of control erythrocytes. As is often the case in other glycolytic enzymopathies, no clear boundary exists between heterozygous deficient and low-normal enzyme activity. Several upstream polymorphisms are found at a high rate of occurrence in African American populations.[173,199] Although they may be associated with mild reductions in erythrocyte TPI activity, they do not seem to be associated with clinical abnormalities, even in homozygotes.[173] At the other extreme, in mice the homozygous state for a TPI null allele is lethal early in embryogenesis.[200] Simultaneous heterozygous inheritance of TPI deficiency and either G6PD deficiency or sickle cell trait has not altered the typical clinical pattern of the disorders when either is present alone.[165] TPI deficiency can be diagnosed prenatally by analysis of fetal blood cells,[172] cultured amniocytes,[171] or trophoblastic cells[177] with suitable precautions.[201] If the mutation is known, mutation analysis can be performed directly on fetal DNA.[177,196]

Therapy

Transfusions and folic acid supplementation are the therapies presently available. Splenectomy in one patient did not alter the intensity of hemolysis.[166] In vitro studies point to the possibility of transfer of TPI enzyme protein from normal to deficient cells with transient improvement in enzyme activity and a reduction in DHAP levels.[202] There have been no attempts to deliver normal TPI enzyme to patient tissues, but in other disease settings direct enzyme transfer from normal hematopoietic stem cell–derived microglial cells to enzyme-deficient nervous tissue after allogeneic stem cell transplantation has been successful.[202]

GLYCERALDEHYDE-3-PHOSPHATE DEHYDROGENASE DEFICIENCY

Clinical Manifestations, Biochemistry, and Genetics

Study of a large kindred in which three members exhibited a reduction in erythrocyte G3PD activity to 50% of normal levels yet were hematologically normal have clearly established that G3PD deficiency need not result in hemolysis.[203] The clinical severity of hemolytic anemia in four members of this pedigree who inherited both hereditary spherocytosis and G3PD deficiency was no greater than that associated with spherocytosis alone. Affected members of this kindred were presumed to be heterozygotes because the amounts of both G3PD enzyme activity and enzyme protein were reduced equally to about 50% of normal and the amount of residual G3PD was qualitatively normal. Two of three anemic patients with G3PD deficiency in other kindreds had even lower levels of enzyme activity (20% to 30% of normal) and conceivably were either homozygotes or doubly heterozygous for two mutant G3PD genes.[204,205] However, as with the spherocytosis pedigree, a cause-and-effect relationship between hemolytic anemia and G3PD deficiency was not established.

PHOSPHOGLYCERATE KINASE DEFICIENCY

Clinical Manifestations

PGK deficiency is a sex-linked disorder that largely affects males. Nonspherocytic hemolytic anemia may occur alone or in combination with neurologic abnormalities ranging from emotional instability to seizures, movement disorders, psychomotor retardation, aphasia, or tetraplegia.[151,206] In a subset of individuals with PGK deficiency, myopathy is the dominant and sometimes the only clinical manifestation (Table 16-6). Individuals with one form of mild PGK deficiency (PGK München) exhibit no clinical abnormalities (Table 16-6). In females, erythrocyte PGK activity is less depressed than it is in males, hemolytic anemia is mild or absent, and neurologic and muscle abnormalities are not seen (see Table 16-6).

Hematologic findings in anemic individuals with PGK deficiency have been those customarily associated with hemolysis, namely, jaundice and reticulocytosis. Hemolytic episodes are often associated with acute febrile illnesses. No changes in erythrocyte morphologic characteristics have been seen, and osmotic fragility has usually been normal.

Biochemistry

PGK is a monomeric enzyme with a primary structure consisting of 417 amino acids.[238] Horse and pig muscle PGK has a primary structure that is highly homologous to that of human PGK.[239,240] Crystallographic studies show that its tertiary structure consists of two lobes (the C and N domains) connected by a hinge-like structure that allows considerable conformational change to occur during substrate binding (Fig. 16-4).[239,240] Because the nucleotide (adenosine diphosphate [ADP] and ATP) combining site is located within the C domain and the phosphoglycerate (1,3-DPG or 3-phosphoglyerate) binding site is within the N domain, bending of the enzyme is required to bring the several substrates required for the PGK reaction into close proximity.[240] Mutant PGKs often exhibit abnormal enzyme kinetics and diminished stability in vitro, properties that are likely to impair enzyme function in vivo (see Table 16-6).

PGK-deficient red cells are capable of normal glycolysis in vitro.[207,236] Intracellular ATP concentrations are normal or slightly low,[207,212,236] whereas the 2,3-DPG concentration is elevated, sometimes to two or three times the normal level.[207,212,217,222,236] These results reflect increased flow through the 2,3-DPG cycle (see Fig. 16-1) at the expense of the ATP-generating PGK reaction. Despite the availability of an alternative pathway (the Rapoport-Luebering shunt or the 2,3-DPG cycle) to bypass PGK, substantial accumulation of glycolytic intermediates proximal to the enzyme defect is found in fresh red cells, thus indicating that the normal flow of erythrocyte glycolysis is impeded in vivo.

Little is known about the mechanism of hemolysis of PGK-deficient red cells. Most PGK activity is membrane associated.[241] It has been suggested that the ATP for membrane adenosine triphosphatase (ATPase)-mediated cation transport is mostly (or entirely) generated by membrane-bound PGK. Indeed, ADP derived from membrane ATPase exerts an important regulatory influence on glycolysis by its participation in the PGK reaction.[242] However, the implication of a special role for PGK in cation transport has been challenged.[243] Active transport of Na⁺ and K⁺ by PGK-deficient red cells with residual PGK activity only 10% to 15% of normal was not impaired, even with the challenge of an increase in intracellular Na⁺ concentration.[244] Thus, it seems unlikely that hemolysis of PGK-deficient red cells is related to premature cation pump failure as a direct result of inadequate PGK activity.

PGK activity in leukocytes is consistently subnormal in affected males, but white cell function is not usually compromised.[218,245]

Genetics and Inheritance

The major structural gene for PGK, located on the long arm of the X chromosome, is 23 kb in size and composed of 11 exons and 10 introns.[246-249] PGK-deficient male hemizygotes demonstrate very little active enzyme and have more symptoms than heterozygous females do, who have higher levels of PGK activity (see Table 16-6). A second functional PGK gene, expressed only in

TABLE 16-6 Characteristics of Reported Cases of Phosphoglycerate Kinase Deficiency

References	Variant	Mutation*	RBC PGK Activity (% of Normal)	Stability In Vitro	Kinetic Abnormalities	Hemolytic Anemia	Neurologic Abnormalities	Myopathy
HEMIZYGOTES (MALE): HEMOLYTIC ANEMIA OR NO CLINICAL MANIFESTATIONS								
207-210	New York/Amiens	Asp164→Val	2-2.7	Normal		+	+	0
211	Alabama	Lys190 or 91 del	4			+	0	0
212-214	Matsue	Leu89→Pro	5	Low	+	+	+	0
215, 216	Uppsala	Arg206→Pro	5-10	Low	+	+	+	0
217, 218	Cincinnati		8-11			+	+	0
219	Tokyo	Val266→Met	10	Low	+	+	+	0
220	Michigan	Cys315→Arg	10	Low	+	+	+	0
221	Barcelona	Ile147→Asn	10			+	0	0
222	San Francisco		12			+	0	0
223, 224	München	Asp267→Asn	21	Normal	+	0	0	0
221	Murcia	Ser319→Asn	49.0	Low	0	+	+	0
225	Herlev	Asp285→Val	50			+	0	0
HEMIZYGOTES (MALE): MUSCLE DISEASE								
226	Shizuoka	Gly158→Asp	0.7	Normal	0	+	0	+
227	North Carolina	10-amino acid insert	3	Normal	+	0	+	+
228	Creteil	Asp315→Asn	3	Low	+	0	0	+
229	Trondheim		5			0	0	+
229	Antwerp	Glu252→Ala†	5.6			0	0	+
230	Fukui	4-bp del, exon 6‡	5.6			0	0	+
231	Kyoto	Ala354→Pro	6			+	+/-	+
232, 233	Hammamatsu	253Ile→Thr	8	Normal	0	0	+	+
234	New Jersey		18	Normal	+	0	0	+
235	Alberta		1.5 (muscle)	Normal	+	0	0	+
HETEROZYGOTES (FEMALE)								
236	Piedmont		27			+	0	0
237	Memphis		78			+	0	0
207-209	Amiens		77			+	0	0

*Mutation position as corrected by Beutler.[206]
†This mutation also adversely affects mRNA splicing efficiency to about 10% of normal.
‡Frameshift at codon 706-709 resulting in a stop codon truncating phosphoglycerate kinase to 231 amino acids in length.

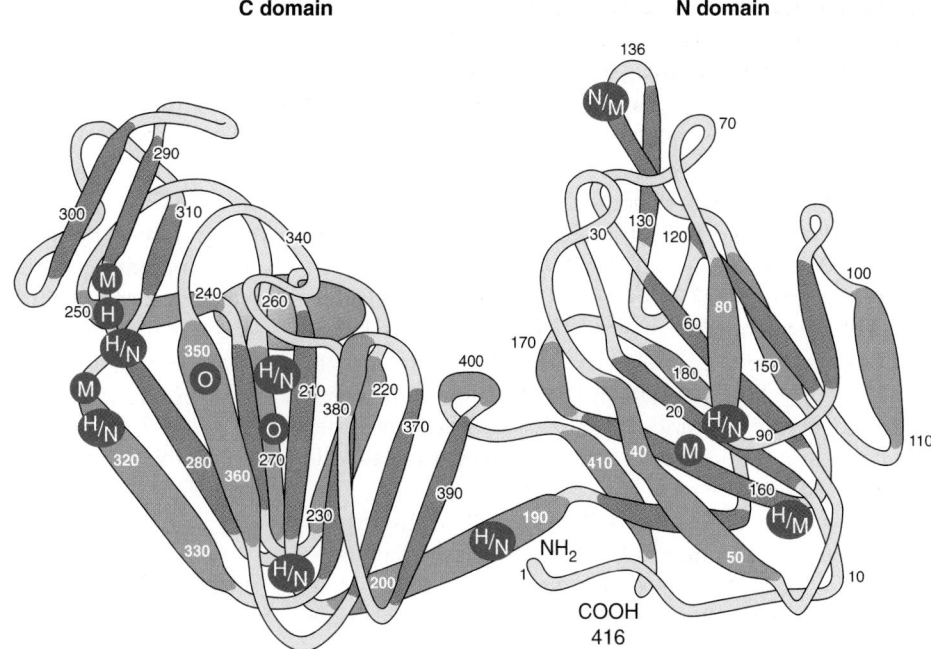

FIGURE 16-4. Three-dimensional model of human phosphoglycerate kinase (PGK). This figure is based on the three-dimensional model of horse PGK published by Banks et al.[240] Positions of the amino acid substitutions and the clinical features associated with 14 PGK point mutations are indicated by *filled circles* (H, hemolytic anemia; M, muscle disease; N, neurologic manifestations; O, no clinical abnormalities). The *shaded ellipse* in the C domain indicates the location of the adenosine triphosphate (ATP) and adenosine diphosphate (ADP) binding site. Random coil (*clear*), β strands (*solid*), and α helices (*striped*) are indicated by shading. (*Modified from Fujii H, Kanno H, Hironi A, et al: A single amino acid substitution [157 Gly→Val] in a phosphoglycerate kinase variant [PGK Shizuoka] associated with chronic hemolysis and myoglobinuria. Blood 1992;79:1582-1585.*)

spermatozoa, is found on chromosome 19.[250] This autosomal PGK gene lacks introns but is otherwise similar to the X-chromosomal PGK gene. A single isozyme of PGK is found in all human nonhematopoietic tissues except spermatozoa.[251] It is therefore not surprising that nonerythroid tissues may be compromised in patients with erythrocyte PGK deficiency.

In 1972, Yoshida and co-workers[252] succeeded in purifying and sequencing both normal erythrocyte PGK and a clinically normal but electrophoretically distinct human mutant PGK, the New Guinea variant. The mutant enzyme differed from normal PGK by the substitution of arginine for threonine at position 352.[238] Subsequently, the structure of 17 other PGK mutants, most associated with clinical manifestations, has been determined by peptide or nucleotide sequencing (see Table 16-6). Fifteen of these mutants involve only a single amino acid (14 missense mutations and 1 deletion). The 16th activates a cryptic splice site that leads to the insertion of 10 additional amino acids into the PGK polypeptide, and the 17th, a 4–amino acid deletion, also affects splicing and produces a truncated polypeptide. The majority of the mutants are found within the C domain, as shown in Figure 16-4. It is not clear how the particular spectrum of clinical abnormalities associated with each mutation is related to its position within the molecule. For example, PGK Michigan, a point mutation at amino acid 316, is associated with hemolytic anemia and neurologic abnormalities, whereas individuals with PGK Creteil, a point mutation of the adjacent amino acid at position 315, do not have anemia and neurologic abnormalities but exhibit rhabdomyolysis.[253] Both mutants are thermolabile and demonstrate kinetic abnormalities in vitro, and both have similarly reduced activity in erythrocytes (see Table 16-6). Random inactivation of the mutant

X chromosome may produce differing proportions of enzyme-deficient cells in female heterozygotes. Some may be anemic (see Table 16-6), whereas others are clinically and hematologically normal.[213] In the latter, the population of PGK-deficient red cells may be so small that erythrocyte PGK activity will be completely normal.[212]

Therapy

In one patient, splenectomy had no beneficial effect on anemia,[237] but in several others, surgery has decreased or eliminated the need for transfusions, reduced the degree of reticulocytosis, and sometimes resulted in an increase of several grams in the hemoglobin level.

2,3-BISPHOSPHOGLYCERATE MUTASE DEFICIENCY

Clinical Manifestations

Absence of erythrocyte 2,3-bisphosphoglycerate mutase (BPGM) activity does not affect red cell life span but may have other hematologic consequences. In one pedigree, four siblings who completely lacked functional red cell BPGM had polycythemia but were otherwise clinically and hematologically normal. All three children of these individuals had about 50% of the normal amount of red cell BPGM and were hematologically normal except for polycythemia.[254,255] In another patient with polycythemia, BPGM activity was only 4% of normal, 2,3-DPG was almost undetectable, and hemoglobin's oxygen affinity curve was shifted to the left. Despite the concomitant inheritance of severe erythrocyte G6PD deficiency, this individual did not have evidence of hemolytic anemia.[256]

Biochemistry

Human red cell BPGM is a homodimer whose identical subunits (molecular weight, 29,840) each consist of 258 amino acids.[257] Nearly all 2,3-bisphosphoglycerate phosphatase activity also resides in the BPGM molecule, so 2,3-DPG metabolism is controlled by a single, multifunctional enzyme. In fact, purified BPGM is also capable of performing as a monophosphoglycerate mutase (MPGM), though at a low rate of activity.[258] Considerable structural homology exists between red cell 2,3-DPG mutase and MPGM,[259,260] and the enzymes, to some extent, exhibit overlapping functions. However, both biochemical[259] and genetic[261] evidence indicates that they are each unique and under separate genetic control.

The BPGM molecule has been modified in vitro by site-directed mutagenesis in an attempt to model a potential therapeutic approach to sickle cell disease.[262] Replacement of Gly13 by Arg enhances phosphatase activity at the expense of the mutase. The effect of such an alteration in vivo, achieved by gene therapy or by pharmacologic means, would be to lower erythrocyte 2,3-DPG levels, increase the affinity of hemoglobin for oxygen, and in this way retard the polymerization of hemoglobin S.

BPGM deficiency results in reduced synthesis of 2,3-DPG. In complete BPGM deficiency, there is virtually no 2,3-DPG within the red cell.[254-256] The affinity of whole blood for oxygen is increased because of lack of 2,3-DPG, thereby accounting for the polycythemia noted in individuals with BPGM deficiency.[254-256] The pattern of glycolytic intermediates is disturbed,[241] with a crossover at PFK sometimes being exhibited,[255] which is consistent with relief of the inhibitory influence of 2,3-DPG on PFK. The erythrocyte ATP concentration is usually normal or slightly increased, compatible with diversion of 2,3-DPG into the PGK reaction as a consequence of reduced flow through BPGM. Erythrocyte glycolysis and pentose phosphate pathway activity have been normal in vitro.[254] Probably as a consequence of the large amount of 1,3-DPG present in BPGM-deficient red cells, hemoglobin A may undergo post-translational modification by glycerylation at $\alpha82$. The modified hemoglobin, about 3% of the total, has a lower isoelectric-electric point than hemoglobin A_{1C} does and is easily identified by isoelectric focusing.[263]

Genetics and Inheritance

The BPGM locus is on chromosome 7 (7q22-34).[264] The gene is fully expressed only in erythroid tissue.[255] BPGM deficiency has the expected autosomal recessive mode of inheritance.[254-256] Individuals from the large pedigree with polycythemia and virtually no red cell BPGM activity have been shown to be compound heterozygotes for two different BPGM mutations.[265] One, BPGM Creteil I, is a point mutation (Arg89→Cys) at or near the BPGM active site,[266] and the other, BPGM Creteil II, is a frame-shift mutation caused by a deletion of nucleotide 205 or 206.[267] Only BPGM Creteil I enzyme protein is found in red cells.[268] It is catalytically inactive and thermolabile in vitro and exhibits altered electrophoretic mobility.[268] Although BPGM and 2,3-bisphosphoglycerate phosphatase activity was virtually absent in compound heterozygotes, MPGM activity was nearly normal, thus illustrating the complex nature of this multifunctional enzyme.[266] The individual with severe BPGM and G6PD deficiency was homozygous for a missense mutation (185G→A; Arg 62→Gln) in exon 2.[256]

Therapy

Polycythemia, if symptomatic, may require phlebotomy.[255]

MONOPHOSPHOGLYCERATE MUTASE DEFICIENCY

Clinical Manifestations, Biochemistry, Genetics, and Therapy

A woman with hereditary spherocytosis whose erythrocyte MPGM activity was reduced to about 50% of normal was found to have inherited two copies of a missense mutation (230met→isol) in the MPGM-BB isoenzyme, which is the form that contributes most of the MPGM activity in erythrocytes.[269] The mutant enzyme exhibited reduced thermal stability but normal kinetics.[270] Family members who inherited a single copy of the mutation were healthy, and no evidence was presented to indicate that in homozygotes MPGM deficiency influences the hemolysis associated with hereditary spherocytosis.[271]

ENOLASE DEFICIENCY

Clinical Manifestations, Biochemistry, Genetics, and Therapy

A woman in whom red cell enolase activity was only 6% of normal exhibited a modest reduction in the survival of ^{51}Cr-labeled autologous erythrocytes (half-life of 18 days; normal, 25 to 30 days) but no overt chronic anemia.[272] A severe, life-threatening acute hemolytic episode occurred when nitrofurantoin was administered for the treatment of a urinary tract infection. Enzymes of the HMP shunt all exhibited normal or increased activity, and glutathione stability was normal. Such drug-induced hemolysis is distinctly uncommon in disorders of the Embden-Meyerhof pathway, although it is theoretically possible in enzyme-deficient reticulocytes.[273] In this patient, in whom sudden massive hemolysis involved predominantly mature red cells, no biochemical mechanism has yet been defined, and the association between enolase deficiency and hemolytic anemia may be coincidental. A sister was hematologically normal, even though her red cells were as deficient in enolase activity as those of the propositus.

Partial red cell enolase deficiency was inherited in an autosomal dominant manner by six members of a second pedigree that spanned four generations. With the exception of the propositus, a 13-day-old boy with profound hemolytic anemia, affected family members were not anemic and had little or no evidence of hemolysis. Spherocytes were present on the peripheral blood smear, and the MCHC was usually elevated.[274]

Therapy remains undefined, but avoidance of oxidant drugs would seem prudent.

PYRUVATE KINASE DEFICIENCY

Clinical Manifestations

PK deficiency is the most commonly encountered glycolytic enzymopathy associated with anemia. Its incidence has been estimated to be 51 cases per million in white individuals.[275] Of the approximately 500 human patients thus far reported,[6] the majority have been of Northern European extraction. Sporadic instances have been seen in other ethnic groups. A hemolytic anemia resembling that seen in human PK deficiency has also been described in basenji dogs,[276,277] beagles,[278] and inbred mice[279] that inherited mutant forms of erythrocyte PK with subnormal activity. Anemia, jaundice, and splenomegaly are regularly present in PK deficiency. The anemia may be profound, occurring in utero[280,281] or in early infancy,[62] and require regular blood transfusions for survival. Conversely, the anemia may be mild enough to evade discovery until adulthood. In a few patients, anemia is absent, hemolysis is fully compensated for, and jaundice may be the sole clinical abnormality. When present, anemia is a lifelong condition and its intensity usually varies little, although it may become more severe during pregnancy.[282,283] Exacerbations of anemia are uncommon and generally result from transient erythroid hypoplasia after infections[284] or, rarely, from increased hemolysis of unknown cause. Iron overload is an occasional problem. Transfusion, splenectomy, and coinheritance of hereditary hemochromatosis genes are factors that make iron overload more likely in PK deficiency.[285] Manifestations of PK deficiency outside the hematopoietic system are uncommon. In several pedigrees, chronic leg ulcers have been observed in family members with PK deficiency and hemolytic anemia.[286,287]

Hyperbilirubinemia is often encountered in newborns with PK deficiency, and these infants may require exchange transfusions.[62] Serum unconjugated bilirubin levels remain elevated in later life, and gallstones are common. Unconjugated bilirubin levels greater than 6 mg/dL are occasionally seen[288]; one brother and sister regularly had levels greater than 20 mg/dL.[289] These patients have abnormal hepatic function in addition to

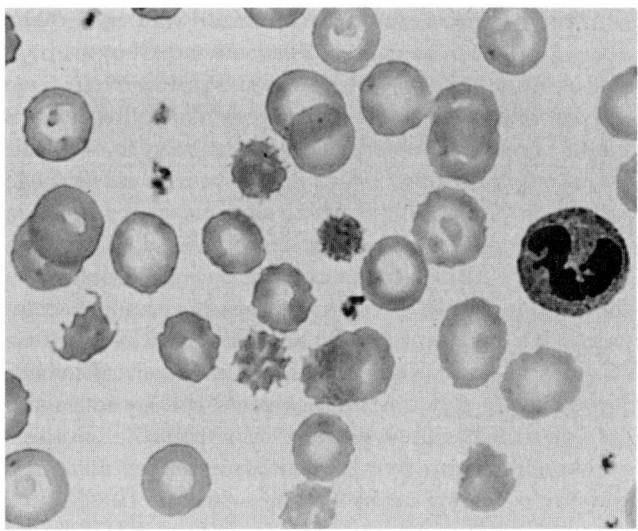

FIGURE 16-5. Postsplenectomy blood smear from a patient with severe pyruvate kinase deficiency. *(From Nathan DG, Oski FA, Sidel VW, Diamonk LK. Extreme hemolysis and red cell distortion in erythrocyte pyruvate kinase deficiency. I. Morphology, erythrokinetics, and family enzyme studies. N Engl J Med 1964;270:1023-1030. Reprinted by permission of the New England Journal of Medicine.)*

hemolysis. Whether abnormalities in liver PK contribute to hyperbilirubinemia is unknown.[290,291]

Macrocytosis, occasional shrunken, spiculated erythrocytes, and rarely, acanthocytes may be observed on examination of the blood smear; these changes may be accentuated by splenectomy. More extreme alterations in erythrocyte morphologic characteristics are sometimes encountered (Fig. 16-5).[292,293] Such abnormalities in shape may result from the inadequate ATP synthesis characteristic of PK-deficient erythrocytes.[294] A paradoxical increase in the reticulocyte count often follows splenectomy despite evidence of a beneficial reduction in the rate of hemolysis. Reticulocyte counts may exceed 90%, and in many patients counts of 40% to 70% are maintained for years. Conversely, in other patients the expected reduction in reticulocyte count is seen after splenectomy. The osmotic fragility of fresh and incubated erythrocytes is most often normal, although minor populations of fragile or resistant cells may be encountered in occasional patients after incubation. The results of an autohemolysis test are generally, but not invariably[295] abnormal, with hemolysis of as many as 50% of erythrocytes after 48 hours of incubation in saline. Prior addition of glucose may reduce the hemolysis in some instances, but glucose usually has little or no effect. In fact, if the reticulocyte count exceeds 25%, incubation with glucose regularly accentuates the hemolysis. This phenomenon has been attributed to inhibition of oxidative phosphorylation by glucose (the Crabtree effect), with unfavorable consequences in PK-deficient reticulocytes because of their reliance on oxidative phosphorylation for synthesis of ATP.[296]

Biochemistry

The active form of PK is a homotetramer formed from one of four different tissue-specific subunits. The R subunit is found in red cells; the L subunit in liver; the M1 subunit in muscle, heart, and brain; and the M2 subunit in all early fetal tissues and most adult tissues, including leukocytes and platelets.[297] The R and L subunits derive from a common gene (*PKLR*) located on chromosome 1 (1q21),[298] whereas the M1 and M2 subunits are generated by a second gene (*PKM*) located on chromosome 15 (15q22).[299] In the rat, the *PKM* gene is 20 kb long and consists of 12 exons and 11 introns.[300] M1- or M2-specific mRNA is formed from a common primary transcript by alternative spicing involving the removal of either exon 9 (M2) or exon 10 (M1).[301] Because human and rat M2 cDNA is highly homologous,[299] alternative splicing probably also accounts for the differences in M1 and M2 mRNA in humans. The *PKLR* gene also consists of 12 exons.[302] Tissue-specific expression of one of two different promoters generates a transcript containing either an R or an L exon at the 5' end.[303,304] The remaining 10 exons are identical. L-type cDNA encodes a polypeptide of 543 amino acids,[303] whereas R-type cDNA encodes a product that is longer by 31 amino acids.[305]

The three-dimensional structure of cat and rabbit muscle PK has been studied by x-ray crystallography.[306] There is extensive sequence homology among species and between M and R subunits, particularly in the vicinity of the active site,[307] thus indicating that the enzyme structure has been conserved during evolution. As shown in Figure 16-6, each muscle PK (M1) subunit consists of a short amino-terminal region and three distinct domains (A, B, and C). Domain A is cylindrical and formed by eight parallel strands of β sheet encased by an outer coaxial cylinder of eight α helices, domain B consists of a closed antiparallel β sheet, and domain C is a five-stranded β sheet connected by α helices. The active site lies in a pocket between domains A and B, the potassium and magnesium binding sites are in domain A, and allosteric modulation of PK function primarily involves interactions with domain C.

In erythroid cells, PK is a tetramer (molecular weight, 230,000[307]) whose subunits may vary in type. In erythroid precursors, M2 homotetramers are the predominant PK isoenzyme. With erythroid maturation, synthesis of M2 subunits declines and is replaced by production of R-type subunits.[308-310] The mature red cell enzyme may exist in either of two physical conformations, analogous to the R and T forms proposed by Monod and colleagues[311] for allosteric proteins. Partially purified enzyme preparations usually exhibit sigmoid kinetics in the presence of increasing concentrations of substrate (phosphoenolpyruvate). Small amounts of phospho*enol*pyruvate facilitate further binding of substrate by the enzyme in a manner analogous to that seen with heme-heme interactions. Fructose 6-diphosphate (FDP) induces a transition

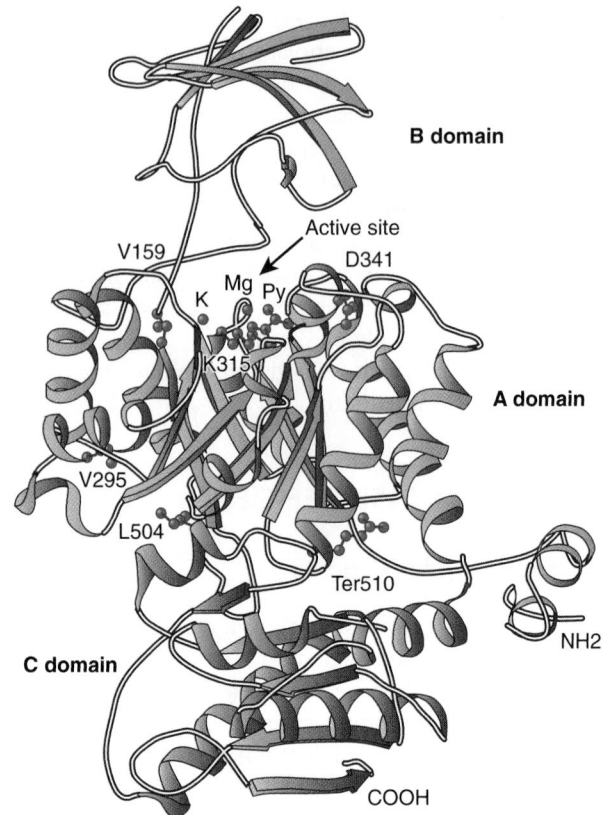

FIGURE 16-6. Ribbon representation of the structure of rabbit muscle pyruvate kinase (PK). The three domains (A, B, and C), the position of potassium (K) and magnesium (Mg) ions, and the location of the active catalytic site (Py) that binds pyruvate are indicated. Six point mutations that alter a single amino acid in the primary structure of R-type (erythrocyte) PK are indicated. V295 is an asymptomatic heterozygote. Ter510, which leads to the formation of a truncated PK enzyme that has lost 63 amino acids in the C domain, was found in the mother of a child with severe hemolytic anemia. L504, found in a homozygote with severe hemolytic anemia, is distant from the active binding site but interferes with a salt bridge that holds domain C to domain A. The remaining three mutations (V159, K315, D341) were found in subjects with hemolytic anemia who had also inherited a second PK mutation at another site and were compound heterozygotes. V159 affects the adenosine diphosphate binding site; K315, the Mg²⁺ binding site; and D341, a highly conserved region of the A domain. *(Modified from Demina A, Varughese KI, Barbot J, et al. Six previously undescribed pyruvate kinase mutations causing enzyme deficiency. Blood 1998; 92:647-652.)*

from sigmoid to hyperbolic kinetics, probably by acting directly at the phospho*enol*pyruvate binding site.[312]

A number of factors may result in post-translational modification of the enzyme. Transition between an FDP-sensitive conformation with sigmoid kinetics and an insensitive form with hyperbolic kinetics has been achieved by varying pH,[313] temperature,[313,314] and conditions of storage. Aging of the enzyme in vivo appears to favor the FDP-sensitive conformation.[315] These transitions may play a significant role in modulation of PK activity in vivo. Post-translational modification of enzyme properties mediated by oxidation of exposed thiol groups on the surface of the molecule may explain some abnormalities previously ascribed to genetic or acquired alterations in the primary structure of the enzyme.[315-320] In several instances it has been possible with the use of sulfhydryl reagents to restore to normal the altered stability and abnormal kinetics of mutant PK from individuals with hemolytic anemia.[316,321] On the other hand, it has often not been possible to implicate oxidation of enzyme thiol groups as a cause of abnormal enzyme properties.[322,323]

The enzyme is subject to numerous other regulatory influences. ATP is a competitive inhibitor ($K_i = 3.5 \times 10^{-4}$ mol/L)[324]; at physiologic ATP concentrations (approximately 1 mmol/L), erythrocyte PK activity should be significantly constrained by ATP. Both potassium[312,314] and magnesium[314,325] activate PK; rubidium (Rb^+) or ammonium (NH_4^+) substitute for potassium (K^+), whereas manganese (Mn^{2+}) or cobalt (Co^{2+}) can replace magnesium (Mg^{2+}).[318] Activation of purified PK by FDP has been demonstrated at concentrations normally found within the erythrocyte.[326] At a higher concentration (0.5 mmol/L), another glycolytic intermediate, glucose 6-phosphate, activates PK.[327] The glycolytic intermediate 2,3-DPG, of particular interest because of its high concentration in PK-deficient erythrocytes, has no influence on PK in hemolysates[328] but has variously been reported to inhibit[329] or activate[330] purified PK. Phosphorylation of PK, mediated by cyclic adenosine monophosphate, alters its kinetic properties and may regulate 2,3-DPG levels and thus oxygen transport by red cells.[330,331] It is clear that intracellular PK activity will be determined by the complex interplay of a number of regulatory factors and may bear little relationship to measures of activity determined in vitro under optimal conditions.

When erythrocyte PK (R homotetramer) is abnormal, hepatic PK (L homotetramer) may also be affected because the R and L subunits are derived from a common gene. In two anemic individuals with PK deficiency, liver PK was reduced to 59%[332] and 46%[333] of normal. Residual liver PK, measured in the latter patient, was mostly of the M2 type. No disorders of hepatic function appear to result from such partial deficiency of PK.[334] In another individual, total liver PK activity was only 22% of normal, virtually no L-type enzyme was detectable, and there were abnormalities in serum aminotransferases.[290] Paradoxically, in still another individual, liver L-type PK exhibited entirely normal activity and properties despite abnormalities in the supposedly identical isoenzyme in the red cells.[291]

The metabolic capabilities of PK-deficient erythrocytes in vitro vary considerably. Although resting HMP shunt activity may be slightly to moderately low for cell age,[335] no significant effect on either oxidized or reduced glutathione (GSH) levels has been observed,[336,337] even after incubation with acetylphenylhydrazine.[336,338,339] However, results of the ascorbate cyanide test are abnormal in patients with PK deficiency, and stimulated HMP shunt activity is modestly depressed.[337] In many instances, glycolysis, as measured by the glucose consumption or lactate production of incubated erythrocytes, is markedly subnormal.[289,296,335] Such diminished glycolysis is relative rather than absolute because the glycolytic rate of enzymopenic cells can be increased substantially by incubation in a high-P_i medium.[296,340] A reduction of residual PK activity within the erythrocyte to 10% of normal will still leave sufficient enzyme to support normal glycolysis if potential enzyme activity is fully used. Such considerations indicate that intracellular regulators of PK function must play an important role in the reduced glycolysis characteristic of enzymopenic cells. Frequently, particularly with kinetic variants of PK, glycolytic rates characteristic of mature normal erythrocytes are achieved.[341-344] However, such rates are clearly subnormal in comparison to those attained by reticulocyte-rich control blood of an equivalent mean cell age.[341] Furthermore, the glucose consumption of incubated normal hemolysate is unchanged when supplemental purified PK is added, whereas the addition of supplemental PK to hemolysate from PK-deficient erythrocytes produces a substantial rise in glucose consumption.[341]

Accumulation of glycolytic intermediates proximal to the enzyme defect has customarily,[341,344] though not invariably[341] been observed.[343] Detection of elevated 2,3-DPG or 3-phosphoglycerate levels in red cells may help confirm a clinical diagnosis of PK deficiency,[345,346] and the degree of elevation in 2,3-DPG or glucose 6-phosphate levels is directly correlated with clinical severity.[101,347] An alteration in the normal ratio of reduced nicotinamide adenine dinucleotide (NADH) to nicotinamide adenine dinucleotide (NAD), as well as complex changes in the substrates governing the rate of PK and 2,3-DPG mutase, appears to be responsible for triose phosphate accumulation when glycolysis is accelerated by P_i in normal red cells.[348] Such striking elevations in triose phosphate intermediates can be returned to normal in both control and PK-deficient red cells by the addition of exogenous pyruvate or another oxidant.[339] Concentrations of both NAD and NADH are low in PK-deficient erythrocytes,[334,349] or if the level of NAD is normal in fresh cells, it falls with undue rapidity on incubation in vitro.[340] The concentration of 2,3-DPG in PK-deficient erythrocytes may be greater than three times normal values, thereby leading to a rightward shift of the oxyhemoglobin dissociation curve.[50,51] The ability to extract a greater percentage of available oxygen from hemoglobin at any given P_{O_2} associated with such a right-shifted curve increases the exercise tolerance of patients with PK deficiency.[51] Such patients, though anemic, may exhibit none of the expected symptoms of fatigue and exercise intolerance.

The level of erythrocyte ATP and the formation of PRPP[350] are often abnormally low in PK deficiency, although patients with reticulocyte counts greater than 25% usually have normal ATP levels. In blood with such high reticulocyte counts, ATP is unstable on incubation with glucose, in contrast to normal reticulocyte-rich blood. When incubated without glucose, however, the PK-deficient reticulocyte conserves ATP more successfully than the normal cell does.[296] The reticulocyte, able to generate ATP from substrates other than glucose via oxidative phosphorylation, can circumvent its glycolytic defect. However, in a high-glucose environment, ATP levels plummet. The PK-deficient reticulocyte is thus exquisitely dependent on oxidative phosphorylation for maintenance of ATP, as was first shown by Keitt.[296] The greater oxygen consumption of PK-deficient reticulocytes than normal reticulocytes (3.75 ± 1.55 versus 0.56 ± 0.5 μL of $O_2/109$ reticulocytes/hr[289]) underscores the reliance of such cells on oxidative phosphorylation. Reticulocyte oxygen consumption is abolished by hypoxia in vitro at approximately venous PO_2 levels (Fig. 16-7). When exposed to prolonged periods of hypoxia in vivo, therefore, or on maturation with consequent loss of mitochondria, the PK-deficient immature erythrocyte will become reliant on its inadequate glycolytic apparatus, with loss of cell ATP being the inevitable consequence. In contrast, the reduced ATP needs of the mature erythrocyte may be marginally, but adequately served for a time by the diminished glycolytic activity of the PK-deficient cell.

ATP depletion greatly increases the cation permeability of PK-deficient erythrocytes.[289] In part, this is the consequence of failure of the ouabain-inhibitable ATPase cation pump, which transports approximately 1 to 2 mEq of K^+ per hour per liter of erythrocytes.[351] Although adequate membrane ATPase is present,[341,352] a net loss of 0.2 to 6.3 mEq of K^+ per hour per liter of cells occurs in freshly obtained PK-deficient blood.[294,341,351] After ATP depletion, net K^+ loss may exceed 20 mEq/hr/L of cells.[289] Failure of the cation pump cannot explain such large losses of K^+. The effect of ATP depletion on K^+ permeability, first described by Gardos and Straub,[353] is a feature of all metabolically depleted red cells and is not unique to PK deficiency. It is thought to be related to altered binding of membrane-associated Ca^{2+} and can be partially prevented by ethylenediaminetetraacetic acid or quinine, even though these agents have no direct influence on the rate or extent of ATP depletion.[289,354]

Initially, in the ATP-depleted cell, potassium loss exceeds sodium gain. The resultant net loss of cations is accompanied by an obligate osmotic loss of water and a reduction in cell volume. The shrunken, crenated cells produced by ATP depletion in PK-deficient reticulocytes are shown in Figure 16-8. These spiculated cells pass, with difficulty, through 8-μm Millipore filters, and cell suspensions demonstrate increased viscosity in the Wells-Brookfield viscometer.[289] The destiny of such ATP-depleted erythrocytes, then, is to become dehydrated, rigid "desicytes" or "xerocytes," whose unfavorable characteristics may well prematurely terminate their existence.[355] Membranes prepared from PK-deficient or normal ATP-depleted red cells are more dense than normal as a result of absorption of cytoplasmic components—in particular, an as yet unidentified 50,000-dalton protein—on the inner membrane surface.[356] Such changes in the cell membrane may contribute to the increased rigidity of these cells. There is evidence that membrane abnormalities not related to ATP depletion may also exist in PK-deficient red cells, but the role, if any, of such abnormalities

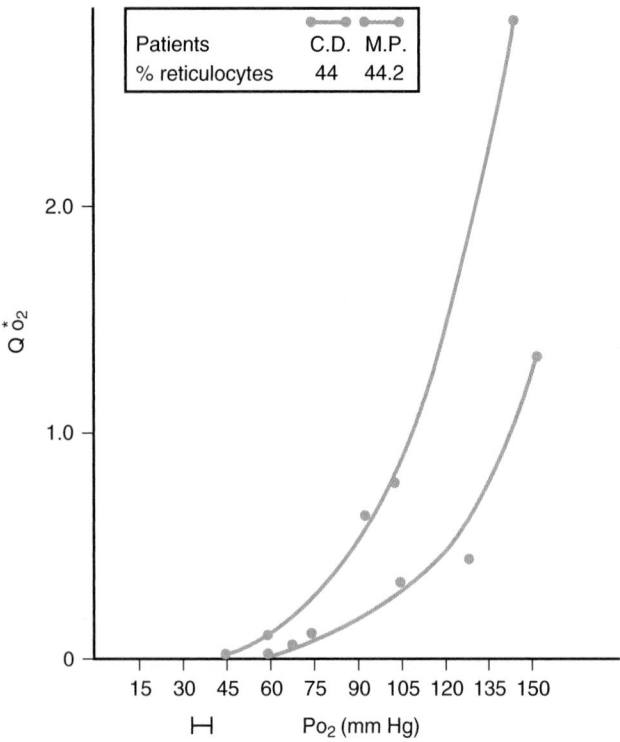

Patients	C.D.	M.P.
% reticulocytes	44	44.2

*Microliters O_2/hour/10^9 reticulocytes

FIGURE 16-7. Influence of PO_2 on oxygen consumption by pyruvate kinase–deficient reticulocytes. The normal range for venous PO_2 is indicated by the *solid bar*. *(From Mentzer WC, Baehner RL, Schmidt-Schonbein H, et al. Selective reticulocyte destruction in erythrocyte pyruvate kinase deficiency. J Clin Invest 1971;50:688-699, by copyright permission of the American Society for Clinical Investigation.)*

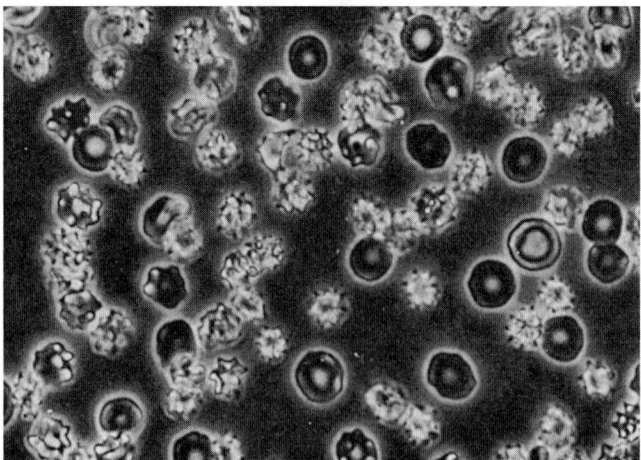

FIGURE 16-8. Phase-contrast micrograph of pyruvate kinase–deficient blood (patient C.D., whose anemia was severe after a 2-hour exposure to 5 mmol/L of cyanide to deplete adenosine triphosphate). The spiculated cells are, for the most part, reticulocytes (magnification ×6600). *(From Mentzer WC, Baehner RL, Schmidt-Schonbein H, et al. Selective reticulocyte destruction in erythrocyte pyruvate kinase deficiency. J Clin Invest 1971;50:688-699, by copyright permission of the American Society for Clinical Investigation.)*

in the hemolytic process is not established.[357] Not all workers have found abnormalities in the red cell membrane protein profile on sodium dodecyl sulfate–polyacrylamide gel electrophoresis,[358] and results of several other types of membrane analyses (spectrin extractability and membrane fluidity) have been normal.[359]

As enzyme-deficient erythrocytes age, a progressive reduction in glycolysis should accompany the inevitable gradual degradation of enzyme protein. Such deteriorating glycolysis will eventually result in ATP depletion and, subsequently, hemolysis. However, centrifuge studies have not revealed dramatic differences in the PK activity of enzymopenic young and old cells,[289] with the exception of one unstable PK variant[360] in which accelerated denaturation of enzyme protein was present in vivo, as well as in vitro. Deterioration in catalytic efficiency, reported to occur in both normal[315] and variant[361] enzymes on aging in vivo, may also hasten the demise of enzymopenic cells.

The normal or nearly normal survival of radiolabeled, severely PK-deficient erythrocytes reported by several investigators[289,342,343] indicates that diminished PK activity need not significantly curtail the life span of affected erythrocytes. Biphasic erythrocyte survival curves are sometimes obtained[362,363] and suggest that two populations of cells are present, one destined for almost immediate destruction and the other having a considerably better outlook for survival. Ferrokinetic studies[289,363] indicate that destruction of newly made erythrocytes in the bone marrow, spleen, or liver may be the major source of hemolysis in this disorder. Organ monitoring has shown that as reticulocytes are released from the marrow, some are almost immediately sequestered in the spleen. The paradoxical reticulocytosis that follows splenectomy is probably the consequence of improved survival of this population of reticulocytes.

Spleens removed from anemic patients with PK deficiency contain an unduly large number of reticulocytes.[338,364] Splenic histologic analysis shows the following results that contrast with those seen in hereditary spherocytosis: (1) the pulp spaces are empty rather than packed with erythrocytes; (2) erythrophagocytosis of reticulocytes and mature red cells by reticuloendothelial histiocytes is prominent in PK deficiency but rare in spherocytosis; and (3) many more crenated, deformed cells are seen in PK deficiency.[364,365] Studies of such cells obtained from peripheral blood have demonstrated them to be poorly deformable.[366] The hypoxic, acidic environment of the spleen would be expected to produce just such crenation in reticulocytes through the sequence of events outlined earlier—inhibition of oxidative phosphorylation, ATP depletion, selective K^+ leakage, loss of cell water, and resultant loss of cell volume. These rigid desicytes should negotiate the 3-μm fenestrations between the splenic cords and sinuses only with difficulty. Thus, they are doomed to a stay of uncertain duration in the metabolically unfavorable splenic environment, and further deterioration in cell capabilities would seem inevitable. Isotope studies show that the final coup de grace often occurs in the liver.[367,368]

Splenic destruction of reticulocytes is a variable feature of PK deficiency; in some instances, either bone marrow or liver destruction predominates. Why some reticulocytes are destroyed whereas others survive to reach maturity and thereafter have a nearly normal existence despite their enzyme defect is unclear. It is possible that chance determines which reticulocytes will be detained in unfavorable metabolic circumstances. On the other hand, there is some evidence for actual variation in PK activity among reticulocytes.[289] Those with the most PK activity would be more likely to survive.

Although cellular dehydration has been given a central mechanistic role in the destruction of PK-deficient human red cells, it appears to be unimportant in the hemolytic process in PK-deficient basenji dogs. When PK-deficient dog red cells with high sodium levels are exposed to cyanide in vitro, they rapidly lose ATP. However, the ensuing loss of K^+ is balanced by an equivalent gain in Na^+, so no cellular dehydration occurs. Other mechanisms must explain the hemolysis in this setting.[367] Of possible interest in this regard is the finding of apoptosis of erythroid progenitors within the spleen of PK-deficient mice, thus suggesting a role for ineffective erythropoiesis in the anemia seen in this species,[368] and perhaps in humans as well.[368a]

Genetics and Inheritance

Autosomal recessive transmission of the enzyme defect is usually observed in PK deficiency. Homozygotes and compound heterozygotes exhibit hemolytic anemia. Simple heterozygotes can be distinguished from compound heterozygotes or homozygotes by the degree of reticulocytosis, the extent of accumulation of red cell glucose 6-phosphate, and the in vitro properties of the mutant PK.[369,370] Although simple heterozygotes usually remain clinically normal despite an approximately 50% reduction in erythrocyte PK activity, some may exhibit evidence of mild hemolysis.[370,371] Population surveys in different ethnic groups based on assays of red cell PK activity have estimated the incidence of PK heterozygosity to be 0.14% to 6%.[372-376] Because activity assays may sometimes falsely identify heterozygotes as normal and vice versa, DNA analysis should provide a more accurate estimate of the prevalence of PK mutations. A survey based on DNA analysis reported the rate of occurrence of heterozygosity in white individuals for the 1456T mutation, the most common PK mutation in southern Europe, to be 3.5×10^{-3} and that for the 1529A mutation to be 2.03×10^{-3}. In African Americans, the rate of occurrence of heterozygosity was 3.90×10^{-3} for the 1456T mutation, and in Asians, it was 7.94×10^{-3} for the 1468T mutation.[275] Evidence in PK-deficient mice with chronic hemolytic anemia suggests that PK deficiency may play a protective role against malaria.[377] In vitro studies with *P. falciparum*–infected red cells from PK-deficient homozygotes and heterozygotes indicate that a similar protective effect may be present in humans.[377a]

There is little correlation between the severity of anemia in homozygotes and the level of erythrocyte PK activity as measured by the conventional in vitro assay system unless enzyme activity is corrected for the degree of reticulocytosis present.[347] Variable clinical severity is explained, at least in part, by the existence of numerous mutant forms of the enzyme whose differing properties result in variable degrees of hemolysis. Mutants are distinguishable in vitro on the basis of maximal activity, electrophoretic mobility, substrate kinetics, stability, immunologic properties, and response to the activator FDP. In general, mutants with unfavorable kinetics are usually associated with more severe hemolysis.[347,378,379] Diminished thermal stability of the enzyme in vitro also seems important in determining clinical severity.[380] Homozygous frameshift, promoter, or deletion mutations that greatly reduce or completely abolish PK activity generally lead to such severe phonotypes as intrauterine death or life-threatening neonatal anemia, as does inheritance of a single copy of such deleterious mutations along with another severe PK gene.[381-384,384a]

International standards for the characterization of mutant PK phenotypes have facilitated the comparison of mutants studied in different laboratories.[385] In compound heterozygotes, full characterization is difficult because tetramers formed from varying proportions of the two different mutant subunits are present, each with unique properties.[378] The best-defined phenotypes are those found in true homozygotes, who are usually the offspring of consanguineous matings. The kinetic and electrophoretic abnormalities characteristic of each variant PK reflect underlying structural changes in the enzyme secondary to point mutations or deletions. A total of 180 mutations in the *PKLR* gene associated with chronic hemolytic anemia have been defined at the nucleic acid level.[380,384a,386-388] Single-nucleotide missense mutations (including 2 in the promoter region) account for 124 of the total. The rest are splice site mutations (23), stop codon mutations (9), large deletions (3), and small deletions, frameshifts, or insertions (21). Additional PK mutations are known, but because they are present only as single copies in patients with chronic anemia, their role in the pathophysiology of hemolysis has not been defined.[380,386,387] In the basenji dog, PK deficiency is attributable to a frameshift mutation (deletion of C at nucleotide 433),[389] and in PK-deficient mice, a missense mutation in ribose-phosphate pyrophosphokinase (338Gly→Asp) is responsible for the enzymopathy.[279] Most PK mutations are extremely rare and usually limited to a single family. Exceptions are the 1529G→A and the 1456C→T substitutions, common in European patients with PK deficiency,[380,390-393] and the 1151C→T substitution, common in Japanese patients.[394] The majority of the mutations are located within exon 8 or 9 (A domain), where components of the active site and the K+ binding site are located, or in exons 10 or 11 (C domain),

a region responsible for the allosteric regulatory properties of the enzyme. Although important information about genotype-phenotype correlation has been developed,[347,380,384a,395-397] detailed analysis of the way in which each mutation disturbs the function of PK and produces the clinical phenotype observed has only recently become available after ascertainment of the crystalline structure of human R-type PK and the use of recombinant ribose-phosphate pyrophosphokinase generated in *E. coli* to study enzyme kinetics and stability.[380,398,399] For example, generation of the 1529G→A (510 Arg→Gln) mutant, the most common mutation found in northern Europe, by site-directed mutagenesis produced a recombinant enzyme with normal substrate kinetics and activation by FDP but with strikingly decreased stability.[399] These studies suggest that the hemolytic anemia seen in 1529G→A homozygotes, which can be moderate to severe, is the result of low PK activity caused by enzyme instability in vivo rather than unfavorable enzyme kinetics. The variable clinical severity seen in different 1529G→A homozygotes remains unexplained by these molecular studies and suggests a role for epigenetic or environmental factors.[380,384a] DNA analysis has indicated that several PK variants thought to be unique because of differing enzyme properties are in fact due to a single shared mutation. For example PK Maebashi, PK Fukushima, and PK Sendai are each the consequence of a substitution of A for C at nucleotide 1261.[380] DNA analysis has also made possible the prenatal diagnosis of PK-deficient fetuses.[400]

When kinetic abnormalities have been discovered in anemic patients, at least one parent has exhibited similar abnormalities. The other parent may also have kinetically aberrant PK[401] or is found to have a low-activity variant with normal kinetics.[402] Occasionally, it has not been possible to demonstrate an abnormality of erythrocyte PK in one[386] or both[360] parents of patients with PK activity in the homozygous deficient range. Staal and coworkers[360] have speculated that in some heterozygotes, a compensatory increase in synthesis of enzyme protein by the normal allele may result in enzyme activity indistinguishable from normal. The "classic" form of PK deficiency is associated with severe enzyme deficiency, persistence of the M2 isoenzyme in mature erythrocytes, and little or no R isozymes. The persistence of M2 isoenzyme may represent an attempt to compensate for the lack of R subunit–containing forms of PK.[293] An analogy to the persistence of fetal hemoglobin synthesis in β-thalassemia has been made by Miwa.[403] When M2 compensation is incomplete or absent,[383] PK activity in mature red cells is low, and hemolytic anemia ensues. When M2 isoenzyme is synthesized at a higher rate, greater than normal amounts of PK activity can accumulate in mature red cells.[310,404-407] Such patients do not have hemolytic anemia, and in fact the increased glycolytic flow through PK at the expense of the 2,3-DPG–generating pathway may lower 2,3-DPG levels, increase the affinity of hemoglobin for oxygen, and result in erythrocytosis. Similarly, mice bearing a mutant form of R-type

PK exhibit a delayed onset of hemolytic anemia after birth that coincides with delayed switching from the M2 isoenzyme to the mutant R isoenzyme.[408]

A kindred in which hemolytic anemia occurred in heterozygotes for PK mutants was studied by Etiemble and colleagues.[409] PK activity was well below (17% to 45%) the 50% activity usually encountered in the presence of one normal and one mutant PK allele. It was thought that perhaps the presence of only one mutant subunit in the PK tetramer might be sufficient to reduce its catalytic function, with greater impairment found in the presence of additional mutant subunits. Similar considerations were raised in another kindred (PK Greensboro), in which heterozygotes exhibited less than 50% of the normal red cell PK activity but no hemolytic anemia.[410] However, in neither kindred was the presence of multiple combinations of mutant and normal subunits (i.e., M4, M3N, M2N2, MN3, and N4, where M is the the mutant subunit and N is the normal subunit) actually confirmed.

To date, no evidence suggests interaction between PK deficiency and other disorders of the erythrocyte such as β-thalassemia minor,[411] band 3 deficiency,[412] or G6PD deficiency.[292] Reports of spherocytosis or paroxysmal nocturnal hematuria in heterozygotes for PK deficiency have not mentioned unusual features of either disease. Markedly increased involvement of the kidneys was noted at autopsy in a patient with Gaucher's disease who also exhibited hemolytic anemia and deficiency of erythrocyte PK. It was suggested that cerebroside production was enhanced as a result of hemolysis.[413]

Therapy

Although complete cure is not achieved by splenectomy, elimination or amelioration of transfusion requirements, a decrease in bilirubin level, and an increase in hemoglobin concentration are seen quite often. Even though splenectomy may be lifesaving in individuals with severe anemia,[338,343] the procedure may have no effect in individuals with mild anemia. When significant morbidity exists, it would seem reasonable to recommend splenectomy while bearing in mind the fact that the degree of benefit cannot be predicted with certainty.[414] The results of therapeutic intervention with agents that either circumvent the metabolic aberrations induced by the defective enzyme or directly modify enzyme activity have generally been disappointing.[321,360,415,416]

Although hemolytic crises are uncommon in patients with PK deficiency and have not been associated with drug ingestion, Glader[273] demonstrated a potential hazard with the use of large doses of salicylate in patients with severe PK deficiency. Salicylates inhibit oxidative phosphorylation and thus cause ATP depletion and cellular dehydration in severely PK-deficient reticulocytes in vitro. The salicylate doses used by Glader were high but were equivalent to serum levels achieved with chronic salicylate therapy for disorders such as rheumatoid arthri-tis. It is prudent to select alternative therapy for such patients when possible or to monitor them carefully for signs of increased hemolysis.

Bone marrow transplantation has permanently corrected the hemolytic anemia seen in PK-deficient basenji dogs,[417] in PK-deficient mice,[418,419] and in a single human with PK deficiency.[420] The potential feasibility of gene therapy has been demonstrated in PK-deficient mice.[421,421a]

LACTATE DEHYDROGENASE DEFICIENCY

Clinical Manifestations, Biochemistry, and Genetics

Partial or complete absence of the H subunit of lactate dehydrogenase (LDH) in erythrocytes, leukocytes, platelets, and serum is not associated with anemia or hemolysis.[422] M-subunit deficiency, though associated with exertional myoglobinuria and a characteristic skin eruption, also does not lead to hemolytic anemia.[423] In contrast to humans, mice homozygous for a low-activity mutation of the skeletal muscle subunit of LDH have less than 10% of normal enzyme activity in erythrocytes and exhibit severe lifelong hemolytic anemia.[424]

ABNORMALITIES OF ERYTHROCYTE NUCLEOTIDE METABOLISM

In individuals with CNSHA, low erythrocyte ATP levels often play a central role in the pathogenesis of hemolysis. Hemolytic anemia associated with an unusually high erythrocyte ATP level has also been described.[425] Red cell PK levels were normal in the affected pedigree, so the mechanism for ATP elevation would appear to differ from that found in other families with high red cell ATP levels, low 2,3-DPG, erythrocytosis, and a twofold or greater elevation in PK activity.[404-406] In yet another family, two infants with hemolytic anemia, high erythrocyte ATP levels, and low 2,3-DPG levels had reduced 2,3-DPG phosphatase activity.[426] The relationship of this enzyme abnormality to the unusual elevation in erythrocyte ATP level or to hemolysis is uncertain. In the three disorders of erythrocyte nucleotide metabolism to be described in the text that follows, evidence of a relationship between the abnormal enzyme and hemolytic anemia is more convincing, although even in these disorders much remains to be learned about the pathogenesis of hemolysis.

Pyrimidine 5'-Nucleotidase Deficiency

Clinical Manifestations

Deficiency of erythrocyte P-5'-N, the most common inherited abnormality of nucleotide metabolism causing hemolytic anemia, is associated with lifelong anemia of moderate severity.[9,427-437] Splenomegaly is usually present. Developmental delay is sometimes seen, but whether it is a direct result of P-5'-N deficiency has not been determined. Pronounced basophilic stippling, which may occur in as many as 5% of all erythrocytes, is an important and useful finding and an exception to the usual lack of distinguishing morphologic abnormalities in erythroenzymopathies. Definitive diagnosis requires assay of red cell P-5'-N activity.

Biochemistry

Reticulocyte maturation requires disposition of intraerythrocytic ribosomal RNA, which is no longer required for protein synthesis. The hydrolysis of pyrimidine nucleotides (cytidine monophosphate [CMP] and uridine monophosphate [UMP]) formed by the action of ribonucleases on ribosomal RNA, an essential step in RNA degradation, is catalyzed by P-5'-N. The cytidine and uridine formed can diffuse across the cell membrane, whereas the pyrimidine nucleotide substrates of the nucleotidase reaction are incapable of diffusion and accumulate within the cell when activity of the nucleotidase is subnormal.[9]

Hirono and associates[438] found two different isoenzymes of P-5'-N in hemolysates from normal subjects and those with P-5'-N deficiency. Only one isoenzyme, CMP responsive, was deficient in all five subjects evaluated with P-5'-N deficiency, whereas the other, deoxythymidine monophosphate (dTMP) responsive, was normal. Kinetic and thermostability abnormalities were seen in the CMP-responsive isoenzyme from subjects with P-5'-N deficiency but not in the dTMP-responsive isoenzyme. Apparently, the lack of overlapping substrate sensitivities makes it impossible for the residual normal isoenzyme to substitute for its deficient partner in enzymopenic individuals.

The amount of nucleotides in P-5'-N–deficient red cells is increased by 1.3 to 5.0 times, chiefly as a result of an increase in pyrimidine derivatives (CMP, cytidine diphosphate [CDP], cytidine triphosphate [CTP], UMP, uridine diphosphate, and uridine triphosphate [UTP]).[9,429,430,439,440] The most abundant derivatives are the diphosphodiesters CDP-choline and CDP-ethanolamine.[438] Accumulation of pyrimidine derivatives is undoubtedly due in part to RNA degradation,[430] but it may also reflect de novo synthesis of these compounds from the uridine and orotate transported into the red cell.[441] Classification of P-5'-N deficiency as a high-ATP syndrome was based on early observations of unusually high ATP levels in cells, as measured with an enzymatic assay of ATP content that also reflected the presence of other nucleotide triphosphates, notably CTP and UTP. More specific assays have subsequently shown that cell adenine nucleotide levels are normal or even low rather than elevated.[9,431,440]

The extraordinary accumulation of pyrimidine nucleotides within P-5'-N–deficient red cells is easily detected by subjecting cellular extracts to MRI[442] or to ultraviolet spectroscopy. Extracts from normal cells exhibit an absorbance peak at 255 to 260 nm (caused almost entirely by the presence of adenine nucleotides). In P-5'-N deficiency, a higher absorbance peak slightly shifted in position (266 to 270 nm) is observed as a result of the presence of large amounts of pyrimidine nucleotides and provides a relatively simple means of screening patients for the disorder.[9,430] The secondary effects of P-5'-N deficiency are complex. For example, the concentration of GSH is regularly increased by a factor of 1.5 to 2.3,[429] a finding that may help confirm the diagnosis in patient suspected of having P-5'-N deficiency. Red cell PRPP synthetase activity is markedly low (15% to 35% of normal) in P-5'-N–deficient red cells.[442,443] In fact, PRPP synthetase deficiency was originally thought to be the primary defect responsible for the hemolysis. It is now regarded as a secondary phenomenon.[436] Pyrimidine nucleotides have been shown to bind and sequester magnesium, a cofactor required for subunit aggregation and maximal activation of PRPP synthetase.[445] Magnesium depletion (by the addition of pyrimidine nucleotides) also inhibits PK and pentose phosphate pathway activity in hemolysates. On the other hand, red cell magnesium levels are normal or even elevated in P-5'-N–deficient red cells, and incubation of these cells with exogenous magnesium does not reduce their susceptibility to autohemolysis or to Heinz body formation.[446] The role of magnesium deficiency (or unavailability) in the central abnormalities that limit the life span of P-5'-N–deficient red cells is not clear.

In fact, it is not known why P-5'-N–deficient red cells are destroyed prematurely. Perhaps the pyrimidine nucleotides that accumulate interfere with the normal function of key glycolytic enzymes by competing for available binding sites with the adenine nucleotides that are the normal enzyme substrate. The possible importance of pyrimidine nucleotides in hemolysis is underscored by the report of an individual with chronic hemolysis, basophilic stippling, and normal P-5'-N activity, in whom the only biochemical abnormality detected was a striking elevation in erythrocyte CDP-choline.[447] Accumulation of pyrimidine nucleotide has been shown to lower red cell pH in P-5'-N–deficient red cells as a result of shifts in Donnan equilibrium caused by the increase in fixed intracellular anion.[434,439] This drop of 0.1 to 0.2 pH unit is sufficient to increase the red cell's oxygen affinity above the normal range[440] and may also explain the slightly subnormal glycolytic rate of P-5'-N–deficient red cells.[448] Tomoda and colleagues[434] demonstrated a moderate impairment in stimulated pentose phosphate pathway activity in P-5'-N–deficient erythrocytes, which they attributed to inhibition of G6PD by pyrimidine nucleotides. This impairment in shunt activity is noted in both light and dense red cells separated by centrifugation and is accompanied by a parallel decrease in G6PD activity.[449] It is hard to visualize how pentose phosphate pathway failure could result in the unusually high levels of GSH characteristic of P-5'-N deficiency because the opposite effect, a deficiency in GSH, would be predicted.[434]

Study of individuals with lead poisoning has confirmed the central role of P-5'-N deficiency in the origin of hemolytic anemia. P-5'-N is markedly inhibited in vitro by low concentrations of lead, and the red cells of patients with significant lead poisoning have depressed levels of P-5'-N activity.[450] The basophilic stippling that is present in some patients with lead poisoning has been attributed to nucleotidase deficiency.[451] Although accumulation of pyrimidine nucleotides within erythrocytes is not found in all patients with lead poisoning in which P-5'-N activity is reduced, it is regularly found in patients exhibiting acute lead-induced hemolytic anemia.[450,451] Perhaps because of the shorter duration or less severe character of the enzyme deficiency, the red cells of lead-poisoned individuals do not exhibit ribose phosphate pyrophosphokinase (RPPK) deficiency.[451] GSH levels are normal[451] or elevated.[430] Despite the less than perfect homology between congenital and acquired P-5'-N deficiency, study of the latter may be expected to provide important insight into the mechanisms of hemolysis in this disorder.

Genetics and Inheritance

The gene for P-5'-N is located on chromosome 7 and consists of 11 exons. Alternative splicing leads to the production of three proteins: one is 286 amino acids long (P-5'-N I), the second is 297 amino acids long, and the third, found only in reticulocytes, is 285 amino acids long.[452,453] P-5'-N I is the major isoenzyme expressed in erythrocytes. Twenty different mutations in P-5'-N I have been identified in patients with P-5'-N deficiency and chronic hemolytic anemia. Six are missense mutations, 2 are in-frame deletions that lead to loss of a single amino acid, and the remaining 12 are nonsense mutations, splice site alterations, insertions, or larger deletions.[437]

Sixty-six patients from 56 unrelated families with P-5'-N deficiency and hemolytic anemia have been described.[436,437,454] The disorder has been found in many ethnic groups.[437] Inheritance is autosomal recessive.[430,437] Nearly all P-5'-N–deficient patients who exhibit hemolytic anemia are homozygous for a single P-5'-N mutation; the remainder are compound heterozygotes for two different mutations.[437] Heterozygotes have no clinical manifestations but exhibit a reduction of about 50% in red cell P-5'-N activity.[9,430,436,437] The wide range of enzyme activity encountered in normal individuals makes detection of heterozygotes difficult in some families.[455] Variation in the severity of disease is, in part, due to heterogeneity in the molecular nature of the defective enzyme.[428,438,456] This has been shown most clearly by study of the biochemical properties of purified recombinant mutant P-5'-N.[457] These studies also revealed that despite profound abnormalities in P-5'-N kinetics or stability in vitro, erythrocytes containing certain P-5'-N mutations exhibited only a moderated reduction in P-5'-N activity, thus suggesting that other pathways or other

P-5'-N isoenzymes could compensate for P-5'-N I deficiency. P-5'-N has been found in the spleen,[456] kidney,[458,459] The presence of the enzyme in brain may be relevant to the mental retardation noted in several P-5'-N–deficient individuals with hemolytic anemia.[431]

Therapy

The congenital form of P-5'-N deficiency must be distinguished from the acquired form associated with lead poisoning because specific therapy is available for the latter. The benefit of splenectomy in congenital P-5'-N deficiency is limited.[436] Investigational therapeutic use of allopurinol in one affected individual had no effect on hemolysis and actually increased erythrocyte pyrimidine nucleotide levels.[441]

Adenylate Kinase Deficiency

Clinical Manifestations, Biochemistry, and Genetics

Controversy exists regarding the exact role of adenylate kinase (AK) deficiency in hemolytic anemia. Beutler and colleagues[460] studied two African American siblings whose red cells lacked measurable AK activity. One had hemolytic anemia, but the other did not. It was suggested that in this family the hemolysis was unrelated to AK deficiency or that another coexistent defect was required for hemolysis to occur. The latter seemed to be the case in an Arab family in which two siblings had severe red cell AK deficiency but only the sibling who had also inherited severe G6PD deficiency exhibited hemolysis.[461] However, further investigation of this large pedigree disclosed six more individuals with severe AK deficiency and mental retardation.[462] All had chronic nonspherocytic hemolytic anemia. Three had also inherited G6PD deficiency and were severely anemic, with red cell transfusions required 6 to 10 times annually. The other three, who did not have G6PD deficiency, were moderately anemic and only occasionally required transfusions. Family members who had carrier levels of red cell AK activity (50% of normal), either with or without G6PD deficiency, and individuals with G6PD deficiency alone did not have chronic hemolytic anemia. These results suggest that either AK deficiency has a direct role in hemolysis or the enzyme defect is a marker for another genetically linked but as yet unidentified defect that is the primary cause of the anemia.[463] Lachant and colleagues[463] found no AK activity in the red cells of a Syrian girl who had chronic hemolytic anemia. Only modest impairment in the formation of ADP from adenosine monophosphate was observed in intact cells, thus suggesting that alternative pathways might be available to substitute for the missing AK. Alternatively, it was proposed that AK itself might be present in intact cells but somehow became inactivated during preparation of a hemolysate for assay of enzyme activity. Eight additional patients with AK deficiency associated with hemolytic anemia have been reported in France,[464] Japan,[465,466] Spain,[467] and Italy.[468-470] Molecular study of these patients has defined three missense, two in-frame single-codon, and two nonsense mutations. Site directed mutagenesis of wild type AK1 cDNA followed by expression of mutant enzyme proteins in an *E. coli* system and purification of enzyme protein allowed characterization of five of these mutations. Marked abnormalities in enzyme stability and catalytic properties were found.[470a] Modeling studies using the structure of porcine AK, which is highly homologous to human AK, have begun to define the structural basis for mutation-associated defects in enzyme function.[467] The Japanese subject inherited a missense mutation (Arg128→Trp) in the coding region of the *AK1* gene from her mother and a normal *AK1* allele from her father. Although both mother and child were heterozygous for AK deficiency, only the child exhibited hemolytic anemia, and the mother was hematologically normal.[466] An Italian girl homozygous for a missense mutation at codon 164 had virtually undetectable erythrocyte AK activity and moderate hemolytic anemia.[468,469] Another Italian girl, who also had moderate hemolytic anemia, was homozygous for a deletion that created a frameshift with a premature stop codon. Even though no erythrocyte AK mRNA was detectable, thus implying rapid degradation of the truncated mRNA, a low level of AK enzyme activity was present in hemolysates from the propositus. Evidence of activity of other AK isozymes, not usually present in erythrocytes, was obtained, and this residual AK activity was thought to have mitigated the clinical severity of the enzymopathy.[470] Two siblings in a third Italian family who were homozygous for a nonsense mutation at codon 107 (CGA→TGA) had no detectable erythrocyte AK activity and mild to moderate chronic hemolytic anemia.[469] Both siblings also exhibited psychomotor retardation. Similar findings in other families[462,464] suggest that AK deficiency may be shared by the red cell and the brain.

Therapy

Splenectomy led to prompt disappearance of anemia and hemolysis in five of six Arab patients.[462]

Adenosine Deaminase Overproduction

Clinical Manifestations, Biochemistry, and Genetics

Fourteen individuals in three families have been found to have hereditary hemolytic anemia, sharply diminished amounts of intraerythrocytic adenosine nucleotides (to less than 50% of normal), and a remarkable 45- to 110-fold increase in red cell ADA activity.[471-474] In contrast to virtually all other erythroenzymopathies, ADA excess is transmitted as an autosomal dominant trait. Hemolysis is apparently the consequence of diminished red cell ATP content, which is caused by the diversion of nearly all adenosine metabolism through the unusually active ADA reaction at the expense of the competing adenosine kinase reaction. The former results in irreversible loss of adenosine nucleotides, whereas the latter conserves such nucleotides and preserves cell ATP stores. The finding of abnormalities of lesser magnitude in other enzymes of nucleotide metabolism in affected individuals suggests that the excess ADA activity may be caused by an as yet undefined primary defect. The physical properties of the mutant ADA are normal,[473,475] which indicates that the great excess of ADA activity is due to overproduction rather than an increase in catalytic efficiency. In one subject, an increase in red cell ADA protein equivalent to the striking increase in ADA activity was demonstrated by immunoblotting.[476] Synthesis of ADA by erythroid progenitors grown from bone marrow cells was 11-fold greater in an affected individual.[477] RNase mapping techniques and Northern blotting have revealed at least a 100-fold increase over normal in the ADA mRNA content of affected reticulocytes. Sequencing of ADA cDNA showed no abnormalities in the coding region and 5'- and 3'-untranslated regions of the parent mRNA. Examination of genomic DNA by Southern blotting did not disclose evidence of gene amplification, deletion, or gross rearrangements. Thus, although the basis for ADA excess appears to be an overabundance of apparently normal mRNA, the mechanism underlying this abnormality remains obscure.[478]

Linkage analysis with a polymorphic TAAA repeat located 1.1 kb upstream from the ADA gene strongly indicated that the mutation was located in *cis* rather than in *trans*.[479] DNA constructs containing 10.6 kb of 5'-flanking sequences and 12.3 kb of the first intron of the normal or mutant ADA gene were linked to a reporter gene (chloramphenicol acyltransferase) and used to study expression in transient transfection assays and in transgenic mice. No difference in expression between wild-type and mutant alleles was found. Therefore, the mutation is thought to reside at a more distant 5' site, within a different intron, or 3' to the coding region.[480]

Much lower increases in ADA activity (approximately fourfold) are seen in congenital hypoplastic anemia,[481,482] arthrogryposis multiplex congenita,[483] acquired immunodeficiency syndrome,[484] and cartilage-hair hypoplasia.[485] The origin and implications of these increases are obscure, but they are not associated with hemolysis.

ACQUIRED DISORDERS OF ERYTHROCYTE GLYCOLYSIS

Alterations in the external chemical milieu may profoundly influence erythrocyte metabolism. The rate of glycolysis, for example, is governed by the availability of P_i. High concentrations of P_i augment and low concentrations impede the glycolytic synthesis of ATP and 2,3-DPG. Erythrocytes from uremic patients with hyperphosphatemia contain an average of 70% more

ATP than normal erythrocytes do, and a lesser, but significant increase in 2,3-DPG concentration is also found in the hyperphosphatemic cell.[486] Conversely, hypophosphatemia induced by hyperalimentation with low-phosphate nutrients[487] or by anion resin therapy for hyperphosphatemia[488] is associated with a reduction in erythrocyte organic phosphates. The organic phosphate depletion resulting from hypophosphatemia may be sufficient to displace the oxyhemoglobin dissociation curve to the left, thereby unfavorably influencing tissue oxygenation. Profound hypophosphatemia may produce a spherocytic hemolytic anemia secondary to erythrocyte ATP deficiency.[488-490] Some investigators have found that experimental magnesium deficiency in the rat resembles hypophosphatemia in that erythrocyte glycolysis is inhibited, ATP and 2,3-DPG levels are subnormal, and red cell rigidity is increased. Spherocytes are evident on the blood smear, and red cell survival is reduced.[491] Magnesium is essential for the normal function of a variety of glycolytic and nonglycolytic enzymes. However, using a different diet to induce magnesium deficiency, Piomelli and co-workers[492] showed that although hemolytic anemia accompanies magnesium depletion in rats, erythrocyte glycolysis and the activity of red cell glycolytic enzymes remain normal. Magnesium deficiency also influences other red cell components, notably the membrane,[493] and the relative contribution of such abnormalities to shortened red cell life span remains undefined.

Iron deficiency not only decreases the production of red cells but also accelerates their destruction.[494] Studies of the metabolic properties of iron-deficient red cells have revealed several abnormalities that might reduce cell viability. Although erythrocyte glycolysis in vitro is normal for cell age,[495] cell ATP is unstable on incubation. The ATP concentration in freshly obtained red cells may be either normal[496] or low.[497] The spontaneous autohemolysis of iron-deficient red cells incubated at 37° C is increased.[498] The increased rigidity characteristic of an ATP-depleted cell is present in iron-deficient cells as well.[498] These findings suggest that a defect in energy metabolism may contribute to the shortened survival of iron-deficient red cells.

Alterations in erythrocyte enzyme activity are often found during the course of either acute or chronic leukemia,[499] nonmalignant pancytopenia,[499,500] congenital dyserythropoietic anemia,[501] acquired dyserythropoietic anemia,[499,502] myeloid metaplasia,[499] and polycythemia vera.[499] One, several, or many enzymes may be involved, and activity may be either increased or decreased. The unusual pattern of enzyme activity may, on occasion, be useful in diagnosis, for example, to distinguish congenital hypoplastic anemia from transient erythroblastopenia of childhood.[503]

Several quite different processes appear to be responsible for the development of acquired enzymopathies.[504] Reversion to fetal hematopoiesis may alter enzyme function.[505] Post-translational changes in normal enzyme protein have been demonstrated.[506] Synthesis of enzyme protein by developing erythroid cells may be impaired, perhaps as a result of alterations in chromosome number or disorderly and dyssynchronous nuclear maturation. Although some components of the abnormal pattern of enzymes (such as low PFK or high enolase activity) may suggest a reversion to fetal erythropoiesis, others do not. The possibility that these enzyme abnormalities may be familial and antedate the onset of an acquired blood disorder has not been fully explored.

REFERENCES

1. Dacie JV, Mollison PL, Richardson N, et al. Atypical congenital hemolytic anemia. Q J Med. 1953;22:79-98.
2. Valentine WN, Paglia DE. Erythrocyte enzymopathies, hemolytic anemia, and multisystem disease. An annotated review. Blood. 1984;64:583-591.
3. Selwyn JG, Dacie JV. Autohemolysis and other changes resulting from the incubation in vitro of red cells from patients with congenital hemolytic anemia. Blood. 1954;9:414-438.
4. Robinson MA, Loder PB, DeGruchy DE. Red cell metabolism in nonspherocytic congenital haemolytic anemia. Br J Haematol. 1961;7:327-339.
5. Valentine WN, Tanaka KR, Miwa S. A specific erythrocyte enzyme defect (pyruvate kinase) in three subjects with congenital non-spherocytic hemolytic anemia. Trans Assoc Am Physicians. 1961;74:100-110.
6. Jacobasch G. Biochemical and genetic basis of red cell enzyme deficiencies. Baillieres Clin Haematol. 2000;13:1-20.
7. Miwa S, Fujii H. Molecular basis of erythroenzymopathies associated with hereditary hemolytic anemia: tabulation of mutant enzymes. Am J Hematol. 1996;51:122-132.
8. van Wijk R, Solinge WW. The energy-less red blood cell is lost: erythrocyte enzyme abnormalities of glycolysis. Blood. 2005;106:4034-4042.
9. Valentine WN, Fink K, Paglia DE, et al. Hereditary hemolytic anemia with human erythrocyte pyrimidine-5'-nucleotidase deficiency. J Clin Invest. 1974;54:866-879.
10. Beutler E. Why has the autohemolysis test not gone the way of the cephalin flocculation test? Blood. 1978;51:109-11.
11. Keitt AS. Diagnostic strategy in a suspected red cell enzymopathy. Clin Haematol. 1981;10:3-30.
12. Beutler E, Blume KG, Kaplan JC, et al. International Committee for Standardization in Haematology: recommended methods for red-cell enzyme analysis. Br J Haematol. 1977;35:331-340.
13. Jansen G, Koenderman L, Rijksen G, et al. Characteristics of hexokinase, pyruvate kinase, and glucose-6-phosphate dehydrogenase during adult and neonatal reticulocyte maturation. Am J Hematol. 1985;20:203-215.
14. Beutler E. Biphasic loss of red cell enzyme activity during in vivo aging. Prog Clin Biol Res. 1985;195:317-333.
15. Lakomek M, Schroter W, De Maeyer G, Winkler H. On the diagnosis of erythrocyte defects in the presence of high reticulocyte counts. Br J Haematol. 1989;72:445-451.

16. Low PS, Rathinavelu P, Harrison M L. Regulation of glycolysis via reversible enzyme binding to the membrane protein, band 3. J Biol Chem. 1993;268:14627-14631.

17. Gilsanz F, Meyer E, Paglia DE, et al. Congenital hemolytic anemia due to hexokinase deficiency. Am J Dis Child. 1978;132:636-637.

18. Rijksen G, Staal GEJ. Human erythrocyte hexokinase deficiency: characterization of a mutant enzyme with abnormal regulatory properties. J Clin Invest. 1978;62: 294-301.

19. Valentine WN, Oski FA, Paglia DE, et al. Hereditary hemolytic anemia with hexokinase deficiency. N Engl J Med. 1967;276:1-11.

20. Kanno H: Hexokinase: Gene structure and mutations. Baillieres Clin Haematol. 2000;13:83-88.

21. Paglia DE, Shende A, Lanzkowsky P, et al. Hexokinase "New Hyde Park": a low activity erythrocyte isozyme in a Chinese kindred. Am J Hematol. 1981;10:107-117.

22. Magnani M, Stocchi V, Cucchiarini L, et al. Hereditary nonspherocytic hemolytic anemia due to a new hexokinase variant with reduced stability. Blood. 1985;66: 690-697.

23. Magnani M, Chiarantini L, Stocchi V, et al. Glucose metabolism in fibroblasts from patients with erythrocyte hexokinase deficiency. J Inherit Metab Dis. 1986;9: 129-139.

24. Rijksen G, Akkerman JWN, van den Wall Bake AWL, et al. Generalized hexokinase deficiency in the blood cells of a patient with nonspherocytic hemolytic anemia. Blood. 1983;61:12-18.

25. Board PG, Trueworthy R, Smith JE, et al. Congenital nonspherocytic hemolytic anemia with an unstable hexokinase variant. Blood. 1978;51:111-118.

26. Newman P, Muir A, Parker AC. Non-spherocytic haemolytic anaemia in mother and son associated with hexokinase deficiency. Br J Haematol. 1980;46:537-547.

27. Magnani M, Stocchi V, Canestrari F, et al. Human erythrocyte hexokinase deficiency: A new variant with abnormal kinetic properties. Br J Haematol. 1985;61:41-50.

28. Beutler E, Dyment PG, Matsumoto F. Hereditary nonspherocytic hemolytic anemia and hexokinase deficiency. Blood. 1978;51:935-940.

29. Goebel KM, Gassel WD, Goebel FD, et al. Hemolytic anemia and hexokinase deficiency associated with malformations. Klin Wochenschr. 1972;50:849-851.

30. Keitt AS. Hemolytic anemia with impaired hexokinase activity. J Clin Invest. 1969;48:1997-2007.

31. Moser K, Ciresa M, Schwarzmeier J. Hexokinasemangel bei hämolytischer Anämie. Med Welt. 1970;21: 1977-1981.

32. Semenuk M, Wicks T, Toews CJ, et al. Hexokinase Hamilton: an enzyme variant with abnormal K_m for adenosine triphosphate (ATP) in non-spherocytic hemolytic anemia. Clin Res. 1975;23:628a.

33. Siimes MA, Rahiala EL, Leisti J. Hexokinase deficiency in erythrocytes: a new variant in 5 members of a Finnish family. Scand J Haematol. 1979;22:214-218.

34. Necheles TF, Rai US, Cameron D. Congenital nonspherocytic hemolytic anemia associated with an unusual erythrocyte hexokinase abnormality. J Lab Clin Med. 1970;76:593-602.

35. Magnani M, Serafini G, Stocchi V. Hexokinase type I multiplicity in human erythrocytes. Biochem J. 1988;254: 617-620.

36. Murakami K, Blei F, Tilton W, et al. An isozyme of hexokinase specific for the human red blood cell (HKg). Blood. 1990;75:770-775.

37. Murakami K, Kanno H, Miwa S, et al. Human HKR isozyme: organization of the hexokinase I gene, the erythroid-specific promoter, and transcription initiation site. Mol Genet Metab. 1999;67:118-130.

38. Magnani M, Stocchi V, Chiarantini L, et al. Rabbit red blood cell hexokinase. Decay mechanism during reticulocyte maturation. J Biol Chem. 1986;261:8327-8333.

39. Murakami K, Piomelli S. The isoenzymes of mammalian hexokinase: tissue specificity and in vivo decline. In Magnani M, De Flora A (eds). Red Blood Cell Aging. New York, Plenum Press, 1991, pp 277-284.

40. Thorburn DR, Beutler E. Decay of hexokinase during reticulocyte maturation: is oxidative damage a signal for destruction? Biochem Biophys Res Commun. 1989;162: 612-618.

41. Fornaini G, Dacha M, Stocchi V, et al. Role of hexokinase in the regulation of glucose metabolism in human erythrocytes. Ital J Biochem. 1986;35:316-320.

42. Magnani M, Rossi L, Bianchi M, et al. Role of hexokinase in the regulation of erythrocyte hexose monophosphate pathway under oxidative stress. Biochem Biophys Res Commun. 1988;155:423-428.

43. Magnani M, Rossi L, Bianchi M, et al. Improved metabolic properties of hexokinase-overloaded human erythrocytes. Biochim Biophys Acta. 1988;972:1-8.

44. Magnani M, Rossi L, Bianchi M, et al. Human red blood cell loading with hexokinase-inactivating antibodies. An in vitro model for enzyme deficiencies. Acta Haematol. 1989;82:27-34.

45. Valentine WN, Oski FA, Paglia DE, et al. Erythrocyte hexokinase and hereditary hemolytic anemia. In Beutler E (ed). Hereditary Disorders of Erythrocyte Metabolism. New York, Grune & Stratton, 1968, pp 288-300.

46. Gerber GK, Schultze M, Rapoport SM. Occurrence and function of a high K_m hexokinase in immature red blood cells. Eur J Biochem. 1970;17:445-449.

47. Jandl JH, Aster RH. Increased splenic pooling and the pathogenesis of hypersplenism. Am J Med Sci. 1967;253: 383-398.

48. Rakitzis ET, Mills GC. Relation of red-cell hexokinase activity to extracellular pH. Biochim Biophys Acta. 1967;141:439-441.

49. Brewer GJ. Erythrocyte metabolism and function: Hexokinase inhibition by 2,3-diphosphoglycerate and interaction with ATP and Mg^{2+}. Biochim Biophys Acta. 1969;192:157-161.

50. Delivoria-Papadopoulos M, Oski FA, Gottlieb AJ. Oxygen hemoglobin dissociation curves: effect of inherited enzyme defects of the red cell. Science. 1969;165:601-602.

51. Oski FA, Marshall BE, Cohen PJ, et al. Exercise with anemia: the role of the left-shifted or right-shifted oxygen-hemoglobin equilibrium curve. Ann Intern Med. 1971;74:44-46.

52. Kosower NS, Vanderhoff GA, London IM. Hexokinase activity in normal and glucose-6-phosphate dehydrogenase deficient erythrocytes. Nature. 1964;201:684-685.

53. Bethenod M, Kissin C, Mathieu M, et al. Déficit en hexokinase intraérythrocytaire. Ann Pediatr. 1967;14: 826-828.

54. Bianchi M, Magnani M. Hexokinase mutations that produce nonspherocytic hemolytic anemia. Blood Cells Mol Dis. 1995;21:2-8.

55. Bianchi M, Crinelli R, Serafini G, et al. Molecular bases of hexokinase deficiency. Biochim Biophys Acta. 1997; 1360:211-221.

56. van Wijk R, Rijksen G, Huizinga, EG, et al. HK Utrecht: missense mutation in the active site of human hexokinase associated with hexokinase deficiency and severe non-spherocytic hemolytic anemia. Blood. 2003;101:345-347.

57. Rogers PA, Fisher RA, Harris H. An electrophoretic study of the distribution and properties of human hexokinases. Biochem Genet. 1975;13:857-866.

58. Povey S, Corney G, Harris H. Genetically determined polymorphism of a form of hexokinase, HK III, found in human leukocytes. Ann Hum Genet. 1975;38:407-415.

59. Akkerman JW, Rijksen G, Gorter G, Staal GE. Platelet function and energy metabolism in a patient with hexoki-nase deficiency. Blood. 1984;63:147-153.

60. Peters LL, Lane PW, Andrsen SG, et al. Downeast anemia (*dea*), a new mouse model of severe nonspherocytic hemo-lytic anemia caused by hexokinase (HK1) deficiency. Blood Cells Mol Dis. 2001;27:850-860.

61. Kugler W, Lakomek M: Glucose-6-phosphate isomerase deficiency. Baillieres Clin Haematol. 2000;13:89-101.

62. Matthay KK, Mentzer WC. Erythrocyte enzymopathies in the newborn. Clin Haematol. 1981;10:31-55.

63. Whitelaw AGL, Rogers PA, Hopkinson DA, et al. Con-genital haemolytic anaemia resulting from glucose phos-phate isomerase deficiency: Genetics, clinical picture, and prenatal diagnosis. J Med Genet. 1979;16:189-196.

64. Ravindranath Y, Paglia DE, Warrier I, et al. Glucose phos-phate isomerase deficiency as a cause of hydrops fetalis. N Engl J Med. 1987;316:258-261.

65. Hutton JJ, Chilcote RR. Glucose phosphate isomerase deficiency with hereditary nonspherocytic hemolytic anemia. J Pediatr. 1974;85:494-497.

66. Arnold H, Lohr GW, Hasslinger K, Ludwig R. Combined erythrocyte glucose-phosphate isomerase (GPI) and glucose-6-phosphate dehydrogenase (G6PD) deficiency in an Italian family. Hum Genet. 1981;57:226-229.

67. Schroter W, Brittinger G, Zimmerschmitt E, et al. Com-bined glucose-phosphate isomerase and glucose-6-phos-phate dehydrogenase deficiency of the erythrocytes: A new hemolytic syndrome. Br J Haematol. 1971;20: 249-261.

68. Kahn A, Bue HA, Girot R, et al. Molecular and functional anomalies in two new mutant glucose-phosphate isomer-ase variants with enzyme deficiency and chronic hemoly-sis. Hum Genet. 1978;40:293-304.

69. Van Biervliet JPGM. Glucose-phosphate isomerase defi-ciency in a Dutch family. Acta Paediatr Scand. 1975;64: 868-872.

70. Zanella A, Izzo C, Rebulla P, et al. The first stable variant of erythrocyte glucose-phosphate isomerase associated with severe hemolytic anemia. Am J Hematol. 1980; 9:1-11.

71. Schroter W, Eber SW, Bardosi A, et al. Generalised glucose-phosphate isomerase (GPI) deficiency causing haemolytic anaemia, neuromuscular symptoms and impairment of granulocytic function: A new syndrome due to a new stable GPI variant with diminished specific activity (GPI Homburg). Eur J Paediatr. 1985;144: 301-305.

72. Beutler E, West C, Britton HA, et al. Glucose-phosphate isomerase (GPI) deficiency mutations associated with hereditary nonspherocytic hemolytic anemia (HNSHA). Blood Cells Mol Dis. 1997;23:402-409.

73. Kugler W, Breme K, Laspe P, et al. Molecular basis of neurological dysfunction coupled with haemolytic anaemia in human glucose-6-phosphate isomerase (GPI) defi-ciency. Hum Genet. 1998;103:450-454.

74. Matsumoto N, Ishihara T, Oda E, et al. Fine structure of the spleen and liver in glucose-phosphate isomerase (GPI) deficiency hereditary nonspherocytic hemolytic anemia: Selective reticulocyte destruction as a mechanism of hemolysis. Acta Haematol Jpn. 1973;36:46-54.

75. Van Biervliet JPGM, Staal GE. Excessive hepatic glyco-gen storage in glucose-phosphate isomerase deficiency. Acta Paediatr Scand. 1977;66:311-315.

76. Merkle S, Pretsch W. Glucose-6-phosphate isomerase associated with nonspherocytic hemolytic anemia in the mouse: An animal model for the human disease. Blood. 1993;81:206-213.

77. Oski FA, Fuller E. Glucose-phosphate isomerase (GPI) deficiency associated with abnormal osmotic fragility and spherocytes. Clin Res. 1971;19:427.

78. Vives-Corrons JL, Carrera A, Triginer J, et al. Anemia hemolitica por deficit congenito en fosfohexaisomerasa. Sangre. 1975;20:197-206.

79. Blume KG, Hryniuk W, Powars D, et al. Characterization of two new variants of glucose-phosphate-isomerase defi-ciency with hereditary nonspherocytic hemolytic anemia. J Lab Clin Med. 1972;79:942-949.

80. Cayanis E, Penfold GK, Freiman I, MacDougall LG. Haemolytic anaemia associated with glucose-phosphate isomerase (GPI) deficiency in a black South African child. Br J Haematol. 1977;37:363-371.

81. Van Biervliet JP, Vlug A, Barstra H, et al. A new variant of glucose-phosphate isomerase deficiency. Humangene-tik. 1975;30:35-40.

82. Schroter W, Koch HH, Wonneberger B, et al. Glucose phosphate isomerase deficiency with congenital non-spherocytic hemolytic anemia; a new variant (type Nord-horn). I. Clinical and genetic studies. Pediatr Res. 1974;8:18-25.

83. Tilley BE, Gracy RW, Welch SG. A point mutation increas-ing the stability of human phosphoglucose isomerase. J Biol Chem. 1974;249:4571-4579.

84. McMorris FA, Chen TR, Ricciuti F. Chromosome assign-ments in man of the genes from two hexose-phosphate isomerases. Science. 1973;17:1129-1131.

85. Read J, Pearce J, Li X, et al. The crystal structure of human phosphoglucose isomerase at 1.6 A resolution: implications for catalytic mechanism, cytokine activity and haemolytic anaemia. J Mol Biol. 2001;309:447-463.

86. Chaput M, Claes V, Portetelle D, et al. The neurotrophic factor neuroleukin is 90% homologous with phospho-hexose isomerase. Nature. 1988;332:454-455.

87. Faik P, Walker JIH, Redmill AAM, Morgan MJ. Mouse glucose-6-phosphate isomerase and neuroleukin have identical 3' sequences. Nature. 1988;332:455-456.

88. Watanabe H, Takehana K, Date M, et al. Tumor cell auto-crine motility factor is the neuroleukin phosphohexose isomerase polypeptide. Cancer Res. 1996;56:2960-2963.

89. Xu W, Seiter K, Feldman E, et al. The differentiation and maturation mediator for human myeloid leukemia cells

shares homology with neuroleukin or phosphoglucose isomerase. Blood. 1996;87:4502-4506.

90. Helleman PW, Van Biervliet JPGM. Haematological studies in a new variant of glucose-phosphate isomerase deficiency (GPI Utrecht). Helv Paediatr Acta. 1975;30: 525-536.

91. Beutler E, Sigalove WH, Muir WA, et al. Glucose-phosphate-isomerase (GPI) deficiency: GPI Elyria. Ann Intern Med. 1974;80:730-732.

92. Miwa S, Nakashima K, Tajiri M, et al. Three cases in two families with congenital nonspherocytic hemolytic anemia due to defective glucose-phosphate isomerase: GPI Matsumoto. Acta Haematol Jpn. 1975;38:238-247.

93. Staal GE, Akkerman JW, Eggermont E, van Biervliet JP. A new variant of glucose-phosphate isomerase deficiency: GPI-Kortrijk. Clin Chim Acta. 1977;78:121-127.

94. Zanella A, Rebulla P, Izzo C, et al: A new mutant erythrocyte glucose-phosphate isomerase associated with GSH abnormality. Am J Hematol. 1978;5:11-23.

95. Arnold H, Hasslinger K, Witt I. Glucose-phosphate-isomerase type Kaiserslautern: A new variant causing congenital nonspherocytic hemolytic anemia. Blut. 1983;46: 271-277.

96. Paglia DE, Paredes R, Valentine WN, et al. Unique phenotypic expression of glucose-phosphate isomerase deficiency. Am J Hum Genet. 1975;27:62-70.

97. Arnold H, Engelhardt R, Lohr GW, et al. Glucose-phosphate-isomerase type Recklinghausen: Eine neue defekt-variante mit hämolytischer anamie. Klin Wochenschr. 1973;51:1198-1204.

98. Arnold H, Blume KG, Busch D, et al. Klinische und biochemische Untersuchungen zur Glucosephosphatisomerase normaler menschlicher Erythrocyten und bei Glucosephosphatisosmerase Mangel. Klin Wochenschr. 1970;21:1299-1308.

99. Baughan M, Valentine WN, Paglia DE, et al. Hereditary hemolytic anemia associated with glucose-phosphate isomerase (GPI) deficiency—a new enzyme defect of human erythrocytes. Blood. 1968;32:236-249.

100. Paglia DE, Holland P, Baughan MA, Valentine WN. Occurrence of defective hexose-phosphate isomerization in human erythrocytes and leukocytes. N Engl J Med. 1969;280:66-71.

101. Arnold H, Blume KG, Engelhardt R, Lohr GW. Glucose-phosphate isomerase deficiency: Evidence for in vivo instability of an enzyme variant with hemolysis. Blood. 1973;41:691-699.

102. Schroter W, Tillmann W. Decreased deformability of erythrocytes in haemolytic anaemia associated with glucose-phosphate isomerase deficiency. Br J Haematol. 1977;36:475-484.

103. Lakomek M, Winkler H. Erythrocyte pyruvate kinase and glucose phosphate isomerase deficiency: perturbation of glycolysis by structural defects and functional alterations of defective enzymes and its relation to the clinical severity of chronic hemolytic anemia. Biophys Chem. 1997;66: 269-284.

104. Goulding FJ. Priapism caused by glucose phosphate isomerase deficiency. J Urol. 1976;116:819-820.

105. Coetzer T, Zail SS. Erythrocyte membrane proteins in hereditary glucose phosphate isomerase deficiency. J Clin Invest. 1979;63:552-561.

106. Hopkinson DA. The investigation of reactive sulphydryls in enzymes and their variations by starch-gel electrophoresis: Studies on the human phosphohexose isomerase variant PH15-1. Ann Hum Genet. 1970;34:79-84.

107. Detter JC, Ways PO, Giblett ER, et al. Inherited variations in human phosphohexose isomerase. Ann Hum Genet. 1968;31:329-338.

108. Repiso A, Baldomero O, Vives Corrons J-L, et al. Glucose-phosphate isomerase deficiency: enzymatic and familial characterization of Arg 346His mutation. Biochim Biophysic Acta. 2005;1740:467-471.

108a. Repiso A, Oliva B, Vives-Corrons J-L, et al. Red cell glucose phosphate isomerase (GPI): a molecular study of three novel mutations associated with hereditary nonspherocytic hemolytic anemia. Hum Mutat 2006; online publication #937.

109. Arnold H, Seiberling M, Blume KG, Lohr GW. Immunological studies on glucose-phosphate isomerase deficiency: Instability and impaired synthesis of the defective enzyme. Klin Wochenschr. 1975;53:1135-1136.

110. Kahn A, Vives-Corrons JL, Bertrand O, et al. Glucose-phosphate isomerase deficiency due to a new variant (GPI Barcelona) and to a silent gene: biochemical, immunological and genetic studies. Clin Chim Acta. 1976;66: 145-155.

111. Kahn A, Van Biervliet JPGM, Vives-Corrons JL, et al. Genetic and molecular mechanisms of the congenital defects in glucose phosphate isomerase activity: studies of four families. Pediatr Res. 1977;11:1123-1129.

112. Neubauer BA, Eber SW, Lakomek M, et al. Combination of congenital nonspherocytic haemolytic anaemia and impairment of granulocyte function in severe glucose phosphate isomerase deficiency. A new variant enzyme designated GPI Calden. Acta Haematol. 1990;83: 206-210.

113. Dallapiccola BH, Novelli G, Gerranti G, et al. First trimester monitoring of a pregnancy at risk for glucose phosphate isomerase deficiency. Prenat Diagn. 1986;6: 101-107.

114. Tani K, Fujii H, Miwa S, et al. Phosphofructokinase deficiency associated with congenital nonspherocytic hemolytic anemia and mild myopathy: Biochemical and morphological studies on muscle. Tohoku J Exp Med. 1983;141:287-293.

115. Tani K, Fujii H, Takegawa S, et al. Two cases of phosphofructokinase deficiency associated with congenital hemolytic anemia found in Japan. Am J Hematol. 1983;14: 165-174.

116. Vora S, Davidson M, Seamon C, et al. Heterogeneity of the molecular lesions in inherited phosphofructokinase deficiency. J Clin Invest. 1983;72:1995-2006.

117. Vora S: Isozymes of phosphofructokinase. Isozymes. Curr Top Biol Med Res. 1982;6:119-167.

118. Tarui S, Okuno G, Ikura Y, et al. Phosphofructokinase deficiency in skeletal muscle: a new type of glycogenolysis. Biochem Biophys Res Commun. 1965;19: 517-523.

119. Layzer RB, Rowland LP, Ranney HM. Muscle phosphofructokinase deficiency. Arch Neurol. 1967;17:512-523.

120. Servidei S, Bonilla E, Diedrich RG, et al. Fatal infantile form of phosphofructokinase deficiency. Neurology. 1986;36:1465-1470.

121. Danon MJ, Servidei S, DiMauro S, Vora S. Late-onset muscle phosphofructokinase deficiency. Neurology. 1988; 38:956-960.

122. Duboc D, Jehenson P, Tran Dinh S, et al. Phosphorus NMR spectroscopy study of muscular enzyme deficiencies involving glycogenolysis and glycolysis. Neurology. 1987;37:663-671.

123. Miwa S, Sato T, Murao H, et al. A new type of phosphofructokinase deficiency: Hereditary nonspherocytic hemolytic anemia. Acta Haematol Jpn. 1972;35:113-118.

124. Waterbury L, Frenkel EP. Hereditary nonspherocytic hemolysis with erythrocyte phosphofructokinase deficiency. Blood. 1972;39:415-425.

125. Etiemble J, Kahn A, Boivin P, et al. Hereditary hemolytic anemia with erythrocyte phosphofructokinase deficiency. Hum Genet. 1975;31:83-91.

126. Boulard MR, Meienhofer MC, Bois M, et al. Red cell phosphofructokinase deficiency. N Engl J Med. 1974;291: 978-979.

127. Etiemble J, Picat C, Simeon J, et al. Inherited erythrocyte phosphofructokinase deficiency: molecular mechanism. Hum Genet. 1980;55:383-390.

128. Jenkins JD, Kezdy Fsteck TL. Mode of interaction of phosphofructokinase with the erythrocyte membrane. J Biol Chem. 1985;260:10426-10433.

129. Karadsheh NS, Uyeda K, Oliver RM. Studies on structure of human erythrocyte phosphofructokinase. J Biol Chem. 1977;252:3515-3524.

130. Vora S, Piomelli S. A fetal isozyme of phosphofructokinase in newborn erythrocytes. Pediatr Res. 1977;11: 483a.

131. Layzer RB, Rasmussen J. The molecular basis of muscle phosphofructokinase deficiency. Arch Neurol. 1974;31: 411-417.

132. Ronquist G, Rudolphi O, Engstrom I, Waldenstrom A. Familial phosphofructokinase deficiency is associated with a disturbed calcium homeostasis in erythrocytes. J Intern Med. 2001;249:85-95.

133. Waldenstrom A, Engstrom I, Ronquist G. Increased erythrocyte content of Ca^{2+} in patients with Tarui's disease. J Intern Med. 2001;249:97-102.

134. Shimizu T, Kono N, Kiyokawa H, et al. Erythrocyte glycolysis and its marked alteration by muscular exercise in type VII glycogenosis. Blood. 1988;71:1130-1134.

135. Giger U, Harvey JW. Hemolysis caused by phosphofructokinase deficiency in English springer spaniels: seven cases (1983-1986). J Am Vet Med Assoc. 1987;191: 453-459.

136. Giger U, Reilly MP, Asakura T, et al. Autosomal recessive inherited phosphofructokinase deficiency in English springer spaniel dogs. Anim Genet. 1986;17:15-23.

137. Giger U, Harvey JW, Yamaguchi RA, et al. Inherited phosphofructokinase deficiency in dogs with hyperventilation-induced hemolysis: increased in vitro and in vivo alkaline fragility of erythrocytes. Blood. 1985;65:345-351.

138. Vora S, Giger U, Turchen S, Harvey JW. Characterization of the enzymatic lesion in inherited phosphofructokinase deficiency in the dog: an animal analogue of human glycogen storage disease type VII. Proc Natl Acad Sci U S A. 1985;82:8109-8113.

139. Harvey JW, Reddy GR. Postnatal hematologic development in phosphofructokinase-deficient dogs. Blood. 1989;74:2556-2561.

140. Harvey JW, Sussman WA, Pate MG. Effect of 2,3-diphosphoglycerate concentration on the alkaline fragility of phosphofructokinase-deficient canine erythrocytes. Comp Biochem Physiol. 1988;89B:105-109.

141. Giger U, Kelly AM, Teno PS. Biochemical studies of canine muscle phosphofructokinase deficiency. Enzyme. 1988;40:25-29.

142. Giger U, Argov Z, Schnall M, et al. Metabolic myopathy in canine muscle-type phosphofructokinase deficiency. Muscle Nerve. 1988;11:1260-1265.

143. McCully K, Chance B, Giger U. In vivo determination of altered hemoglobin saturation in dogs with M-type phosphofructokinase deficiency. Muscle Nerve. 1999;22: 621-627.

144. Komazawa M, Oski FA. Biochemical characteristics of "young" and "old" erythrocytes of the newborn infant. J Pediatr. 1975;87:102-106.

145. Travis SF, Garvin JH Jr. In vivo lability of red cell phosphofructokinase in term infants: the possible molecular basis of the relative phosphofructokinase deficiency in neonatal red cells. Pediatr Res. 1977;11:1159-1161.

146. Vora S, Piomelli S. Multiple isozymes of human erythrocyte phosphofructokinase and their subunit structural characterization. Blood. 1977;50(Suppl 1):87a.

147. Nakajima H, Raben N, Hamaguchi T, Yamasaki T. Phosphofructokinase deficiency; past, present and future. Curr Mol Med. 2002;2:197-212.

148. Layzer RB, Epstein CJ. Phosphofructokinase and chromosome 2I. Am J Hum Genet. 1972;24:533-543.

149. Sherman JB, Raben N, Nicastri C, et al. Common mutations in the phosphofructokinase-M gene in Ashkenazi Jewish patients with glycogenesis VII and their population frequency. Am J Hum Genet. 1994;55:305-313.

150. Nakajima H, Kono N, Yamasaki T, et al. Genetic defect in muscle phosphofructokinase deficiency. J Biol Chem. 1990;265:9392-9395.

151. Fujii H, Miwa SI. Other erythrocyte enzyme deficiencies associated with non-haematological symptoms: Phosphoglycerate kinase and phosphofructokinase deficiency. Baillieres Clin Haematol. 2000;13:141-148.

152. Mhaskar Y, Giger U, Dunaway GA. Presence of a truncated M-type subunit and altered kinetic properties of 6-phosphofructo-1-kinase isozymes in the brain of a dog affected by glycogen storage disease type VII. Enzyme. 1991;45:137-144.

153. Smith BF, Stedman H, Rajpurohit Y, et al. Molecular basis of canine muscle type phosphofructokinase deficiency. J Biol Chem. 1996;271:20070-20074

154. Beutler E, Scott S, Bishop A, et al. Red cell aldolase deficiency and hemolytic anemia: a new syndrome. Trans Assoc Am Physicians. 1973;86:154-166.

155. Miwa S, Fujii H, Tani K, et al. Two cases of red cell aldolase deficiency associated with hereditary hemolytic anemia in a Japanese family. Am J Hematol. 1981;11:425-437.

156. Kishi H, Mukai T, Hirono A, et al. Human aldolase A deficiency associated with a hemolytic anemia: thermolabile aldolase due to a single base mutation. Proc Natl Acad Sci U S A. 1987;84:8623-8627.

157. Kreuder J, Borkhardt A, Repp R, et al. Brief report: inherited metabolic myopathy and hemolysis due to a mutation in aldolase A. N Engl J Med. 1996;334:1100-1104.

158. Yao DC, Tolan DR, Murray MF, et al. Hemolytic anemia and severe rhabdomyolysis caused by compound hetero-

zygous mutations of the gene for erythrocyte/muscle isozyme of aldolase, ALDOA (Arg303/Cys338Tyr). Blood. 2004;103:2401-2403.

159. Esposito G, Vitagliano L, Cevenini A, et al. Unraveling the structural and functional features of an aldolase A mutant involved in the hemolytic anemia and severe rhabdomyolysis reported in a child. Blood. 2005;105: 905-906.

160. Parano E, Trifiletti RR, Barone R, et al. Arthrogryposis multiplex congenital and pituitary ectopia. A case report. Neuropediatrics. 2000;31:325-327.

161. Esposito G, Vitagliano L, Costanzo P, et al. Human aldolase A natural mutants: relationship between flexibility of the C-terminal region and enzyme function. Biochem J. 2004;380:51-56.

162. Takasaki Y, Takahashi I, Mukai T, Hori K. Human aldolase A of a hemolytic anemia patient with Asp-128→Gly substitution: Characteristics of an enzyme generated in *E. coli* transfected with the expression plasmid pHAAD128G. J Biochem (Tokyo). 1990;108:153-157.

163. Schneider AS, Valentine WN, Baughan MA, et al: Triosephosphate isomerase deficiency. A multisystem inherited enzyme disorder: clinical and genetic aspects. In Beutler E (ed). Hereditary Disorders of Erythrocyte Metabolism. New York, Grune & Stratton, 1968, pp 265-272.

164. Schneider AS, Dunn I, Ibsen KH, Weinstein IM. Triosephosphate isomerase deficiency. B. Inherited triosephosphate isomerase deficiency. Erythrocyte carbohydrate metabolism and preliminary studies of the erythrocyte enzyme. In Beutler E (ed). Hereditary Disorders of Erythrocyte Metabolism. New York, Grune & Stratton, 1968, pp 273-279.

165. Valentine WN, Schneider AS, Baughan MA, et al. Hereditary hemolytic anemia with triosephosphate isomerase deficiency. Am J Med. 1966;41:27-41.

166. Schneider AS, Valentine WN, Hattori M, Heins HL Jr. Hereditary hemolytic anemia with triose phosphate isomerase deficiency. N Engl J Med. 1965;272:229-235.

167. Skala H, Dreyfus JC, Vives-Corrons JL, et al. Triose phosphate isomerase deficiency. Biochem Med. 1977;18: 226-234.

168. Maquat LE, Chilcote R, Ryan PM. Human triosephosphate isomerase cDNA and protein structure. Studies of triosephosphate isomerase deficiency in man. J Biol Chem. 1985;260:3748-3753.

169. Rosa R, Prehu MO, Calvin MC, et al. Hereditary triose phosphate isomerase deficiency: Seven new homozygous cases. Hum Genet. 1985;71:235-240.

170. Zanella A, Mariani M, Colombo MB, et al. Triosephosphate isomerase deficiency: 2 new cases. Scand J Haematol. 1985;34:417-424.

171. Clark ACL, Szobolotzky MA. Triose phosphate isomerase deficiency: Report of a family. Aust Paediatr J. 1986;22: 135-137.

172. Bellingham AJ, Lestas AN, Williams LH, Nicolaides KH. Prenatal diagnosis of a red cell enzymopathy: Triosephosphate isomerase deficiency. Lancet. 1989;2: 419-421.

173. Schneider AS. Triosephosphate isomerase deficiency: Historical perspectives and molecular aspects. Baillieres Clin Haematol. 2000;13:119-140.

174. Schneider A, Westwood B, Yim C, et al. Triosephosphate isomerase deficiency: repetitive occurrence of point mutation in amino acid 104 in multiple apparently unrelated families. Am J Hematol. 1995;50:263-268.

175. Pekrun A, Neubauer BA, Eber SW, et al. Triosephosphate isomerase deficiency: biochemical and molecular genetic analysis for prenatal diagnosis. Clin Genet. 1995;47: 175-179.

176. Valentin C, Pissard S, Martin J, et al. Triose phosphate isomerase deficiency in 3 French families: two novel null alleles, a frameshift mutation (TPI Alfortville) and an alteration in the initiation codon (TPI Paris). Blood. 2000;96:1130-1135.

177. Arya R, Lalloz MRA, Nicolaides KH, et al. Prenatal diagnosis of triosephosphate isomerase deficiency. Blood. 1996;87:4507-4509.

178. Arya R, Lalloz MRA, Bellingham AJ, Layton DM. Evidence for founder effect of the Glu104Asp substitution and identification of new mutations in triosephosphate isomerase deficiency. Hum Mutat. 1997;10:290-294.

179. Eber W, Pekrun A, Bardosi A, et al. Triosephosphate isomerase deficiency: Haemolytic anaemia, myopathy with altered mitochondria and mental retardation due to a new variant with accelerated enzyme catabolism and diminished specific activity. J Pediatr. 1991;150:761-766.

180. Hollan S, Fujii H, Hirono A, et al. Hereditary triosephosphate isomerase (TPI) deficiency: Two severely affected brothers, one with and one without neurological symptoms. Hum Genet. 1993;92:486-490.

181. Ahmed N, Battah S, Karachalias N, et al. Increased formation of methylglyoxal and protein glycation, oxidation and nitrosation in triosephosphate isomerase deficiency. Biochim Biophys Acta. 2003;1639:121-132.

182. Lu HS, Yuan PM, Gracy RW. Primary structure of human triosephosphate isomerase. J Biol Chem. 1984;259: 11958-11968.

183. Jongsma APM, Los WRT, Hagemeijer A. Evidence for synteny between the human loci for triose phosphate isomerase, lactate dehydrogenase-B, peptidase-B and the regional mapping of these loci on chromosome 12. Cytogenet Cell Genet. 1974;13:106-107.

184. Yuan PM, Talent JM, Gracy RW. Molecular basis for the accumulation of acidic isozymes of triosephosphate isomerase on aging. Mech Ageing Dev. 1981;17:151-162.

185. Peters J, Hopkinson DA, Harris H. Genetic and nongenetic variation of triose phosphate isomerase isozymes in human tissues. Ann Hum Genet. 1973;36:297-312.

186. Mande SC, Mainfroid V, Kalk H, et al. Crystal structure of recombinant human triosephosphate isomerase at 2.8 A resolution. Triosephosphate isomerase–related human genetic disorders and comparison with the trypanosomal enzyme. Protein Sci. 1994;3:810-821.

187. Olah J, Orosz F, Puskas LG, et al. Triosephosphate isomerase deficiency: consequences of an inherited mutation at mRNA, protein and metabolic levels. Biochem J. 2005;392:675-683.

188. Orosz F, Vertessy BG, Hollán S, et al: Triosephosphate isomerase deficiency: Predictions and facts. J Theor Biol. 1996;182:437-447.

189. Orosz F, Wagner G, Lilliom K, et al. Enhanced association of mutant triosephosphate isomerase to red cell membranes and to brain microtubules. Proc Natl Acad Sci U S A. 2000;97:1026-1031.

190. Orosz F, Olah J, Alvarez M, et al. Distinct behavior of mutant triosephosphate isomerase in hemolysate and in

isolated form: molecular basis of enzyme deficiency. Blood. 2001;98:3106-3112.

191. Karg E, Nemeth I, Horanyi M, et al. Diminished blood levels of reduced glutathione and α-tocopherol in two triosephosphate isomerase–deficient brothers. Blood Cells Mol Dis. 2000;26:91-100.

192. Asakawa J, Satoh C, Takahashi N, et al. Electrophoretic variants of blood proteins in Japanese. III. Triosephosphate isomerase. Hum Genet. 1984;68:185-188.

193. Perry BA, Mohrenweiser HW. Human triosephosphate isomerase: Substitution of Arg for Gly at position 122 in a thermolabile electromorph variant, TPI-Manchester. Hum Genet. 1992;88:634-638.

194. Daar IO, Artymiuk PJ, Phillips DC, Maquat LE. Human triosephosphate isomerase deficiency: a single amino acid substitution results in a thermolabile enzyme. Proc Natl Acad Sci U S A. 1986;83:7903-7907.

195. Chang ML, Artymiuk PJ, Wu X, et al. Human triosephosphate isomerase deficiency resulting from mutation of Phe-240. Am J Hum Genet. 1993;52:1260-1269.

196. Valentin C, Cohen-Solal M, Maquat L, et al. Identical germ-line mutations in the triosephosphate isomerase alleles of two brothers are associated with distinct clinical phenotypes. C R Acad Sci III. 2000;323:245-250.

197. Bardosi A, Eber SW, Hendrys M, Pekrun A. Myopathy with altered mitochondria due to a triosephosphate isomerase (TPI) deficiency. Acta Neuropathol. 1990;79:387-394.

198. Pogliani EM, Colombi M, Zanella A. Platelet function defect in triosephosphate isomerase deficiency. Haematologica. 1986;71:349-350.

199. Mohrenweiser HW, Fielek S. Elevated frequency of carriers for triosephosphate isomerase deficiency in newborn infants. Pediatr Res. 1982;16:960-963.

200. Merkle S, Pretsch W. Characterization of triosephosphate isomerase mutants with reduced enzyme activity in *Mus musculus*. Genetics. 1989;123:837-844.

201. Bellingham AJ, Lestas AN. Prenatal diagnosis of triose phosphate isomerase deficiency. Lancet. 1990;1:230.

202. Ationu A, Humphries A, Lalloz MR, et al. Reversal of metabolic block in glycolysis by enzyme replacement in triosephosphate isomerase–deficient cells. Blood. 1999;94:3193-3198.

203. McCann SR, Finkel B, Cadman S, Allen DW. Study of a kindred with hereditary spherocytosis and glyceraldehyde-3-phosphate dehydrogenase deficiency. Blood. 1976;47:171-181.

204. Harkness DR. A new erythrocytic enzyme defect with hemolytic anemia: glyceraldehyde-3-phosphate dehydrogenase deficiency. J Lab Clin Med. 1966;68:879-880.

205. Oski FA, Whaun J. Hemolytic anemia and red cell glyceraldehyde-3-phosphate dehydrogenase. Clin Res. 1969;17:427a.

206. Beutler E. PGK deficiency. Br J Haematol. 2007;136:3-11.

207. Valentine WN, Hsieh HS, Paglia DE. Hereditary hemolytic anemia associated with phosphoglycerate kinase deficiency in erythrocytes and leukocytes. N Engl J Med. 1969;280:528-534.

208. Turner G, Fletcher J, Elber J, et al: Molecular defect of a phosphoglycerate kinase variant associated with haemolytic anaemia and neurological disorders in a large kindred. Br J Haematol. 1995;91:60-65.

209. Dodgson SJ, Lee CS, Holland RA, et al. Erythrocyte phosphoglycerate kinase deficiency: Enzymatic and oxygen binding studies. N Z J Med. 1980;10:614-621.

210. Flanagan JM, Rhodes M, Wilson M, Beutler E. The identification of a recurrent phosphoglycerate kinase mutation associated with chronic haemolytic anaemia and neurological dysfunction in a family from USA. Br J Haematol. 2006;134:233-237.

211. Yoshida A, Twele TW, Dave V, Beutler E. Molecular abnormality of a phosphoglycerate kinase variant (PGK Alabama). Blood Cells Mol Dis. 1995;21:179-181.

212. Miwa S, Nakashima K, Oda S, et al. Phosphoglycerate kinase (PGK) deficiency hereditary nonspherocytic hemolytic anemia: Report of a case found in Japanese family. Acta Haematol Jpn. 1972;35:571-574.

213. Maeda M, Yoshida A. Molecular defect of a phosphoglycerate kinase variant (PGK Matsue) associated with hemolytic anemia: Leu→Pro substitution caused by T/A→C/G transition in exon 3. Blood. 1991;77:1348-1352.

214. Yoshida A, Miwa S. Characterization of a phosphoglycerate kinase variant associated with a hemolytic anemia. Am J Hum Genet. 1974;26:378-384.

215. Fujii H, Yoshida A. Molecular abnormality of phosphoglycerate kinase-Uppsala associated with chronic nonspherocytic hemolytic anemia. Proc Natl Acad Sci U S A. 1980;77:5461-5465.

216. Hjelm M, Wadam B, Yoshida A. A phosphoglycerate kinase variant, PGK Uppsala, associated with hemolytic anemia. J Lab Clin Med. 1980;96:1015-1021.

217. Konrad PN, McCarthy DJ, Mauer AM, et al. Erythrocyte and leukocyte phosphoglycerate kinase deficiency with neurologic disease. J. Pediatr. 1973;82:456-460.

218. Strauss RG, McCarthy DJ, Mauer AM. Neutrophil function in congenital phosphoglycerate kinase deficiency. J Pediatr. 1974;854:341-344.

219. Fujii H, Chen SH, Akasuka J, et al. Use of cultured lymphoblastoid cells for the study of abnormal enzymes: molecular abnormality of a phosphoglycerate kinase variant associated with hemolytic anemia. Proc Natl Acad Sci U S A. 1981;78:2587-2590.

220. Maeda M, Bawle EV, Kulkarni R, et al. Molecular abnormalities of a phosphoglycerate kinase variant generated by spontaneous mutation. Blood. 1992;79:2759-2762.

221. Noel N, Flanagan J, Kalko SG, et al. Two new phosphoglycerate kinase mutations associated with chronic haemolytic anaemia and neurological dysfunction in two patients from Spain. Br J Haematol. 2005;132:523-529.

222. Guis MS, Karadsheh N, Mentzer WC. Phosphoglycerate kinase San Francisco: a new variant associated with hemolytic anemia but not with neuromuscular manifestations. Am J Hematol. 1987;25:175-182.

223. Fujii H, Krietsch WKG, Yoshida A. A single amino acid substitution (Asp-Asn) in a phosphoglycerate kinase variant (PGK Munchen) associated with enzyme deficiency. J Biol Chem. 1980;255:6421-6423.

224. Kreitsch WKG, Eber SW, Haas B, et al. Characterization of a phosphoglycerate kinase deficiency variant not associated with hemolytic anemia. Am J Hum Genet. 1980;32:364-373.

225. Valentin C, Birgens H, Craescu CT, et al. A phosphoglycerate kinase mutant (PGK Herlev; D285V) in a Danish patient with isolated chronic hemolytic anemia: mecha-

nism of mutation and structure-function relationships. Hum Mutat. 1998;12:280-287.

226. Fujii H, Kanno H, Hirono A, et al. A single amino acid substitution (157 Gly→Val) in a phosphoglycerate kinase variant (PGK Shizuoka) associated with chronic hemolysis and myoglobinuria. Blood. 1992;79:1582-1585.

227. Tsujino S, Tonin P, Shanske S, et al. A splice junction mutation in a new myopathic variant of phosphoglycerate kinase deficiency (PGK North Carolina). Ann Neurol. 1994;35:349-353.

228. Rosa R, George C, Fardeau M, et al. A new case of phosphoglycerate kinase deficiency, PGK Creteil, associated with rhabdomyolysis and lacking hemolytic anemia. Blood. 1982;60:84-91.

229. Ookawara T, Dave V, Willems P, et al. Retarded and aberrant splicings caused by single exon mutation in a phosphoglycerate kinase variant. Arch Biochem Biophys. 1996;327:35-40.

230. Hamano T, Mutoh T, Sugie H, et al. Phosphoglycerate kinase deficiency: an adult myopathic form with a novel mutation. Neurology. 2000;54:1188-1190.

231. Morimoto A, Ueda I, Hirashima Y, et al. A novel missense mutation (1060G→C) in the *phosphoglycerate kinase* gene in a Japanese boy with chronic haemolytic anaemia, developmental delay and rhabdomyolysis. Br J Haematol. 2003;122:1009-1013.

232. Sugie H, Sugie Y, Nishida M, et al. Recurrent myoglobinuria in a child with mental retardation: phosphoglycerate kinase deficiency. J Child Neurol. 1989;4:95-99.

233. Sugie H, Sugie Y, Ito M, Fukuda T. A novel missense mutation (837T→C) in the phosphoglycerate kinase gene of a patient with a myopathic form of phosphoglycerate kinase deficiency. J Child Neurol. 1998;13:93-97.

234. DiMauro S, Dalakas M, Miranda AF. Phosphoglycerate kinase deficiency: another cause of recurrent myoglobinuria. Ann Neurol. 1983;13:11-19.

235. Tonin P, Shanske S, Miranda AF, et al. Phosphoglycerate kinase deficiency: Biochemical and molecular genetic studies in a new myopathic variant (PGK Alberta). Neurology. 1993;43:387-391.

236. Arese P, Bosai A, Gallo E, et al. Red cell glycolysis in a case of 3-phosphoglycerate kinase deficiency. Eur J Clin Invest. 1973;3:86-92.

237. Kraus AP, Langston MF, Lynch BL. Red cell phosphoglycerate kinase deficiency. Biochem Biophys Res Commun. 1968;30:173-177.

238. Huang IY, Fujii H, Yoshida A. Structure and function of normal and variant human phosphoglycerate kinase. Hemoglobin. 1980;4:601-609.

239. Flachner B, Kovari Z, Varga A, et al. Role of phosphate chain mobility of MgATP in completing the 3-phosphoglycerate kinase catalytic site: binding, kinetic, and crystallographic studies with ATP and MgATP. Biochemistry. 2004;43:3436-3449.

240. Banks RD, Blake CC, Evans PR, et al. Sequence, structure and activity of phosphoglycerate kinase: a possible hinge-bending enzyme. Nature. 1979;279:773-777.

241. Schrier SL, Ben-Bassat I, Junga I, et al. Characterization of erythrocyte membrane–associated enzymes (glyceraldehyde-3-phosphate dehydrogenase and phosphoglyceric kinase). J Lab Clin Med. 1975;85:797-810.

242. Parker JC, Hoffman JF. The role of membrane phosphoglycerate kinase in the control of glycolytic rate by active cation transport in human red cells. J Gen Physiol. 1967;50:893-916.

243. Chillar RK, Beutler E. Explanation for the apparent lack of ouabain inhibition of pyruvate production in hemolysates; the "backward" PGK reaction. Blood. 1976;47:507-512.

244. Segel GB, Feig SA, Glader BE, et al: Energy metabolism in human erythrocytes: the role of phosphoglycerate kinase in cation transport. Blood. 1975;46:271-278.

245. Boivin P, Hakim J, Mandereau J, et al. Erythrocyte and leucocyte 3-phosphoglycerate kinase deficiency. Studies of properties of the polymorphonuclear leucocytes and a review of the literature. Nouv Rev Fr Hematol. 1974;14:496-508.

246. Chen SH, Malcolm LA, Yoshida A, Giblett ER. Phosphoglycerate kinase: an X-linked polymorphism in man. Am J Hum Genet. 1971;23:87-91.

247. Michelson AM, Blake CC, Evans ST, Orkin SH. Structure of the human phosphoglycerate kinase gene and the intron-mediated evolution and dispersal of the nucleotide-binding domain. Proc Natl Acad Sci U S A. 1985;82:6965-6969.

248. Deys BF, Grzeschick KH, Grzeschick A, et al. Human phosphoglycerate kinase and inactivation of the X chromosome. Science. 1972;175:1002-1003.

249. Michelson AM, Markham AF, Orkin SH. Isolation and DNA sequence of a full-length cDNA clone for human X chromosome–encoded phosphoglycerate kinase. Proc Natl Acad Sci U S A. 1983;80:472-476.

250. Gartler SM, Riley DE, Lebo RV, et al. Mapping of human autosomal phosphoglycerate kinase sequence to chromosome 19. Somat Cell Mol Genet. 1986;12:395-401.

251. Beutler E. Electrophoresis of phosphoglycerate kinase. Biochem Genet. 1969;3:189-195.

252. Yoshida A, Watanabe S, Chen SH, et al. Human phosphoglycerate kinase II. Structure of a variant enzyme. J Biol Chem. 1972;247:446-449.

253. Cohen-Solal M, Valentin C, Plassa F, et al. Identification of new mutations in two phosphoglycerate kinase (PGK) variants expressing different clinical syndromes: PGK Créteil and PGK Amiens. Blood. 1994;84:898-903.

254. Galacteros F, Rosa R, Prehu MO, Calvin MC. Deficit en diphosphoglycerate mutase: Nouveaux cas associes a une polyglobulie. Nouv Rev Fr Hematol. 1984;26:69-74.

255. Rosa R, Prehu MO, Beuzard Y, Rosa J. The first case of a complete deficiency of diphosphoglycerate mutase in human erythrocytes. J Clin Invest. 1978;62:907-915.

256. Hoyer JD, Allen SL, Beutler E, et al. Erythrocytosis due to bisphosphoglycerate mutase deficiency with concurrent glucose-6-phosphate dehydrogenase (G-6-PD) deficiency. Am J Hematol. 2004;75:205-208.

257. Joulin V, Peduzzi J, Romeo PH. Molecular cloning and sequencing of the human erythrocyte 2,3-bisphosphoglycerate mutase cDNA: Revised amino acid sequence. EMBO J. 1986;5:2275-2283.

258. Kappel WK, Hass LF. The isolation and partial characterization of diphosphoglycerate mutase from human erythrocytes. Biochemistry. 1976;15:290-295.

259. Hass LF, Kappel WK, Miller KB, Engle RL. Evidence for structural homology between human red cell phosphoglycerate mutase and 2,3-biphosphoglycerate synthase. J Biol Chem. 1978;253:77-78.

260. Craescu CT, Schaad O, Garel MC, et al. Structural modeling of the human erythrocyte bisphosphoglycerate mutase. Biochimie. 1992;74:519-526.

261. Chen SH, Anderson JE, Giblett ER. Human red cell 2,3-diphosphoglycerate mutase and monophosphoglycerate mutase: Genetic evidence for two separate loci. Am J Hum Genet. 1977;29:405-407.

262. Garel MC, Arous N, Calvin MC, et al. A recombinant bisphosphoglycerate mutase variant with acid phosphatase homology degrades 2,3-diphosphoglycerate. Proc Natl Acad Sci U S A. 1994;91:3593-3597.

263. Blouquit Y, Rhoda MD, Delanoe-Garin J, et al. Glycerated hemoglobin in $\alpha_2\beta_2 82$ (EF6) N-ε-glyceryllysine: A new posttranslational modification occurring in erythrocyte bisphosphoglyceromutase deficiency. Biomed Biochim Acta. 1987;46:S202-S206.

264. Barichard F, Joulin V, Henry I, et al. Chromosomal assignment of the human 2,3-bisphosphoglycerate mutase gene (BPGM) to region 7q34-7q22. Hum Genet. 1987;77:283-285.

265. Joulin V, Garel MC, Le Boulch, P, et al. Isolation and characterization of the human 2,3-bisphosphoglycerate mutase gene. J Biol Chem. 1988;263:15785-15790.

266. Rosa R, Galacteros F, Prehu MO, Calvin MC. Inactive bisphosphoglycerate mutase variants: New data. Biomed Biochim Acta. 1987;46:S207.

267. Lemarchandel V, Joulin V, Valentin C, et al. Compound heterozygosity in a complete erythrocyte bisphosphoglycerate mutase deficiency. Blood. 1992;80:2643-2649.

268. Rosa R, Blouquit Y, Calvin MC, et al. Isolation, characterization, and structure of a mutant 89 Arg→Cys bisphosphoglycerate mutase. Implication of the active site in the mutation. J Biol Chem. 1989;264:7837-7843.

269. Repiso A, Perez de la Ossa P, Aviles X, et al. Red blood cell phosphoglycerate mutase. Description of the first human BB isoenzyme mutation. Haematologica. 2003;88:(3)ECR07.

270. De Atauri P, Repiso A, Oliva B, et al. Characterization of the first described mutation of human red blood cell phosphoglycerate mutase. Biochim Biophys Acta. 2005;1740:403-410.

271. Repiso A, Bajo MJR, Vives Corrons J-L, et al. Phosphoglycerate mutase BB isoenzyme deficiency in a patient with non-spherocytic anemia: familial and metabolic studies. Haematologica. 2005;90:257-259.

272. Stefanini M. Chronic hemolytic anemia associated with erythrocyte enolase deficiency exacerbated by ingestion of nitrofurantoin. Am J Clin Pathol. 1972;58:408-414.

273. Glader BE: Salicylate-induced injury of pyruvate-kinase deficient erythrocytes. N Engl J Med. 1976;294:916-918.

274. Lachant NA, Jennings MA, Tanaka KR. Partial erythrocyte enolase deficiency: a hereditary disorder with variable clinical expression. Blood. 1986;68:55A.

275. Beutler E, Gelbart T. Estimating the prevalence of pyruvate kinase deficiency from the gene frequency in the general white population. Blood. 2000;95:3585-3588.

276. Searcy GP, Miller DR, Tasker JB. Congenital hemolytic anemia in the basenji dog due to erythrocyte pyruvate kinase deficiency. Can J Comp Med. 1971;35:67-70.

277. Nakashima K, Miwa S, Shinohara K, et al. Electrophoretic, immunologic and kinetic characterization of erythrocyte pyruvate kinase in the basenji dog with pyruvate kinase deficiency. Tohoku J Exp Med. 1975;117:179-185.

278. Prasse KW, Crouser D, Beutler E, et al. Pyruvate kinase deficiency anemia with terminal myelofibrosis and osteosclerosis in a beagle. J Am Vet Med Assoc. 1975;166:1170-1175.

279. Kanno H, Morimoto M, Fujii H, et al. Primary structure of murine red blood cell–type pyruvate kinase (PK) and molecular characterization of PK deficiency identified in the CBA strain. Blood. 1995;86:3205-3210.

280. Ghidini A, Sirtori M, Romero R, et al. Hepatosplenomegaly as the only prenatal finding in a fetus with pyruvate kinase deficiency anemia. Am J Perinatol. 1991;8:44-46.

281. Hennekam RC, Beemer FA, Cats BP, et al. Hydrops fetalis associated with red cell pyruvate kinase deficiency. Genet Couns. 1990;1:75-79.

282. Fanning J, Hinkle RS. Pyruvate kinase deficiency hemolytic anemia: two successful pregnancy outcomes. Am J Obstet Gynecol. 1985;153:313-314.

283. Ghidini A, Korker VL. Severe pyruvate kinase deficiency anemia. A case report. J Reprod Med. 1998;43:713-715.

284. Duncan JR, Potter CB, Capellini MD, et al. Aplastic crisis due to parvovirus infection in pyruvate kinase deficiency. Lancet. 1983;2:14-16.

285. Zanella A, Bianchi P, Iurlo A, et al. Iron status and HFE genotype in erythrocyte pyruvate kinase deficiency: Study of Italian cases. Blood Cells Mol Dis. 2001;27:653-661.

286. Muller-Soyano A, de Roura ET, Duke PR, et al. Pyruvate kinase deficiency and leg ulcers. Blood. 1976;47:807-813.

287. Vives-Corrons JL, Marie J, Pujades MA, Kahn A. Hereditary erythrocyte pyruvate kinase (PK) deficiency and chronic hemolytic anemia: clinical, genetic and molecular studies in six new Spanish patients. Hum Genet. 1980;53:401-408.

288. Morisaki T, Tani K, Takahashi K, et al. Ten cases of pyruvate kinase (PK) deficiency found in Japan: enzymatic characterization of the patients' PK. Acta Haematol Jpn. 1988;51:1080-1085.

289. Mentzer WC Jr, Baehner RL, Schmidt-Schonbein H, et al. Selective reticulocyte destruction in erythrocyte pyruvate kinase deficiency. J Clin Invest. 1971;50:688-699.

290. Staal GE J, Rijksen G, Vlug AM, et al. Extreme deficiency of L-type pyruvate kinase with moderate clinical expression. Clin Chim Acta. 1982;118:241-253.

291. Etiemble J, Picat C, Boivin P. A red cell pyruvate kinase mutant with normal L-type PK in the liver. Hum Genet. 1982;61:256-258.

292. Oski FA, Nathan DG, Sidel VW, Diamond LK. Extreme hemolysis and red cell distortion in erythrocyte pyruvate kinase deficiency. I. Morphology, erythrokinetics, and family enzyme studies. N Engl J Med. 1964;270:1023-1030.

293. Leblond PF, Lyonnais J, Delage JM. Erythrocyte populations in pyruvate kinase deficiency anemia following splenectomy. I. Cell morphology. Br J Haematol. 1978;39:55-61.

294. Nathan DG, Oski FA, Sidel VW, et al. Studies of erythrocyte spicule formation in haemolytic anaemia. Br J Haematol. 1966;12:385-395.

295. Zanella A, Colombo MB, Miniero R, et al. Erythrocyte pyruvate kinase deficiency: 11 new cases. Br J Haematol. 1988;69:399-404.

296. Keitt AS. Pyruvate kinase deficiency and related disorders of red cell glycolysis. Am J Med. 1966;41:762-785.

297. Kanno H, Fujii H, Hirono A, Miwa S. cDNA cloning of human R-type pyruvate kinase and identification of a single amino acid substitution (Thr→Met) affecting enzymatic stability in a pyruvate kinase variant (PK Tokyo) associated with hereditary hemolytic anemia. Proc Natl Acad Sci U S A. 1991;88:8218-8221.

298. Tani K, Fujii H, Tsutsumi H, et al. Human liver type pyruvate kinase: cDNA cloning and chromosomal assignment. Biochem Biophys Res Commun. 1987;143:431-438.

299. Tani K, Yoshida MC, Satoh H, et al. Human M2-type pyruvate kinase: cDNA cloning, chromosomal assignment and expression in hepatoma. Gene. 1988;73:509-516.

300. Takenaka M, Noguchi T, Inoue H, et al. Rat pyruvate kinase M gene. Its complete structure and characterization of the 5'-flanking region. J Biol Chem. 1989;264:2363-2367.

301. Noguchi T, Inoue H, Tanaka T. The M1-and M2-type isozymes of rat pyruvate kinase are produced from the same gene by alternative RNA splicing. J Biol Chem. 1986;261:13807-13812.

302. Baronciani L, Beutler E. Analysis of pyruvate kinase deficiency mutations that produce nonspherocytic hemolytic anemia. Proc Natl Acad Sci U S A. 1993;90:4324-4327.

303. Marie J, Simon MP, Dreyfus JC, Kahn A. One gene, but two messenger RNAs encode liver L and red cell L' pyruvate kinase subunits. Nature. 1981;292:70-72.

304. Noguchi T, Yamada K, Inoue H, et al. The L- and R-type isozymes of rat pyruvate kinase are produced from a single gene by use of different promoters. J Biol Chem. 1987;262:14366-14377.

305. Tani K, Fujii H, Nagata S, Miwa S. Human liver type pyruvate kinase: Complete amino acid sequence and the expression in mammalian cells. Proc Natl Acad Sci U S A. 1988;85:1792-1795.

306. Muirhead H, Clayden DA, Barford D, et al. The structure of cat muscle pyruvate kinase. EMBO J. 1986;5:475-481.

307. Peterson JS, Chern CJ, Harkins RN, Black JA. The subunit structure of human muscle and human erythrocyte pyruvate kinase isozymes. FEBS Lett. 1974;49:73-77.

308. Takegawa S, Fujii H, Miwa S. Change of pyruvate kinase isozymes from M2- to L-type during development of the red cell. Br J Haematol. 1983;54:467-474.

309. Takegawa S, Miwa S. Change of pyruvate kinase (PK) isozymes in classical type PK deficiency and other PK deficiency cases during red cell maturation. Am J Hematol. 1984;16:53-58.

310. Max-Audit I, Kechemir D, Mitjavila MT, et al. Pyruvate kinase synthesis and degradation by normal and pathologic cells during erythroid maturation. Blood. 1988;72:1039-1044.

311. Monod J, Wyman J, Changeux JP. On the nature of allosteric transitions: A plausible model. J Mol Biol. 1965;12:88-118.

312. Koler RD, Vanbellinghen P. The mechanism of precursor modulation of human pyruvate kinase I by fructose diphosphate. Adv Enzyme Regul. 1968;6:127-142.

313. Koster JF, Staal GEJ, van Milligan-Boersma L. The effect of urea and temperature on red blood cell pyruvate kinase. Biochim Biophys Acta. 1971;236:362-365.

314. Lakomek M, Scharnetzky M, Tillmann W, et al. On the temperature and salt-dependent conformation change in human erythrocyte pyruvate kinase. Hoppe-Seylers Z Physiol Chem. 1983;364:787-792.

315. Paglia DE, Valentine WN. Evidence of molecular alteration of pyruvate kinase as a consequence of erythrocyte aging. J Lab Clin Med. 1970;76:202-212.

316. Van Berkel TJ, Staal GEJ, Koster JF. On the molecular basis of pyruvate kinase deficiency. II. Role of thiol groups in pyruvate kinase from pyruvate kinase–deficient patients. Biochim Biophys Acta. 1974;334:361-367.

317. Valentine WN, Toohey JI, Paglia DE, et al. Modification of erythrocyte enzyme activities by persulfides and methanethiol: possible regulatory role. Proc Natl Acad Sci U S A. 1987;84:1394-1398.

318. Solvonuk PF, Collier HB. The pyruvic phosphoferase of erythrocytes. I. Properties of the enzyme and its activity in erythrocytes of various species. Can J Biochem Physiol. 1955;33:38-45.

319. Valentine WN, Paglia DE. Studies with human erythrocyte pyruvate kinase (PK): effect of modification of sulfhydryl groups. Br J Haematol. 1983;53:385-398.

320. Badwey JA, Westhead EW. Post-translational modification of human erythrocyte pyruvate kinase. Biochem Biophys Res Commun. 1977;74:1326-1331.

321. Zanella A, Rebulla P, Giovanetti AM, et al. Effects of sulphydryl compounds on abnormal red cell pyruvate kinase. Br J Haematol. 1976;32:373-385.

322. Nakashima K. Further evidence of molecular alteration and aberration of erythrocyte pyruvate kinase. Clin Chim Acta. 1974;55:245-254.

323. Blume KG, Arnold H, Lohr GW, Scholz G. On the molecular basis of pyruvate kinase deficiency. Biochim Biophys Acta. 1974;370:601-604.

324. Koler RD, Bigley RH, Jones RT, et al. Pyruvate kinase: Molecular differences between human red cell and leukocyte enzyme. Symp Quant Biol. 1964;29:213-221.

325. Munro GF, Miller DR. Mechanism of fructose diphosphate activation of a mutant pyruvate kinase from human red cells. Biochim Biophys Acta. 1970;206:87-97.

326. Blume KG, Hoffbauer RW, Busch D, et al. Purification and properties of pyruvate kinase in normal and in pyruvate kinase–deficient human red blood cells. Biochim Biophys Acta. 1971;227:364-372.

327. Staal GEJ, Koster JF, Kamp H, et al. Human erythrocyte pyruvate kinase. Its purification and some properties. Biochim Biophys Acta. 1971;227:86-96.

328. Srivastava SK, Beutler E. The effect of normal red cell constituents on the activities of red cell enzymes. Arch Biochem Biophys. 1972;148:249-255.

329. Ponce J, Roth S, Harkness DR. Kinetic studies on the inhibition of glycolytic kinases of human erythrocytes by 2,3-diphosphoglycerate acid. Biochim Biophys Acta. 1971;250:63-74.

330. Westhead EW, Kiener PA, Carroll D, Gikner J. Control of oxygen delivery from the erythrocyte by modification of pyruvate kinase. Curr Top Cell Regul. 1984;24:21-34.

331. Fujii S, Nakashima K, Yanagihara T, et al. Cyclic AMP–dependent phosphorylation of erythrocyte variant pyruvate kinase. Biochem Med. 1984;31:47-53.

332. Brunetti P, Puxeddu A, Nenci G. Anemia emolitica congenita non sferocitica de carenza di piruvico-chinasi (PK). Haematologica. 1962;47:505-576.

333. Bigley RH, Koler RD. Liver pyruvate kinase (PK) isoenzymes in a PK-deficient patient. Ann Hum Genet. 1968;31:383-388.

334. Nakashima K, Miwa S, Fujii H, et al. Characterization of pyruvate kinase from the liver of a patient with aberrant erythrocyte pyruvate kinase, PK Nagasaki. J Lab Clin Med. 1977;90:1012-1020.

335. Grimes AJ, Meisler A, Dacie JV. Hereditary nonspherocytic haemolytic anaemia. A study of red-cell carbohydrate metabolism in twelve cases of pyruvate kinase deficiency. Br J Haematol. 1964;10:403-411.

336. Necheles TF, Finkel HE, Sheehan RG, Allen DM. Red cell pyruvate kinase deficiency. The effect of splenectomy. Arch Intern Med. 1966;118:75-78.

337. Tomoda A, Lachant NA, Noble NA, Tanaka KR. Inhibition of the pentose phosphate shunt by 2,3-diphosphoglycerate in erythrocyte pyruvate kinase deficiency. Br J Haematol. 1983;54:475-484.

338. Bowman HS, Procopio F. Hereditary nonspherocytic hemolytic anemia of the pyruvate-kinase deficient type. Ann Intern Med. 1963;58:567-591.

339. Oski FA, Diamond LK. Erythrocyte pyruvate kinase deficiency resulting in congenital nonspherocytic hemolytic anemia. N Engl J Med. 1963;269:763-770.

340. Rose IA, Warms JVB. Control of glycolysis in the human red blood cell. J Biol Chem. 1966;241:4848-4854.

341. Oski FA, Bowman H. A low K_m phosphoenolpyruvate mutant in the Amish with red cell pyruvate kinase deficiency. Br J Haematol. 1969;17:289-297.

342. Paglia DE, Valentine WN, Baughan MA, et al. An inherited molecular lesion of erythrocyte pyruvate kinase. Identification of a kinetically aberrant isoenzyme associated with premature hemolysis. J Clin Invest. 1968;47:1929-1946.

343. Zuelzer WW, Robinson AR, Hsu TH. Erythrocyte pyruvate kinase deficiency in nonspherocytic hemolytic anemia: a system of multiple genetic markers? Blood. 1968;32:33-48.

344. Miwa S, Nishina T, Kakehashi Y, Oyama H. Studies on erythrocyte metabolism in various hemolytic anemias: With special reference to pyruvate kinase deficiency. Acta Haematol Jpn. 1970;33:501-518.

345. Lestas AN, Kay LA, Bellingham AJ. Red cell 3-phosphoglycerate level as a diagnostic aid in pyruvate kinase deficiency. Br J Haematol. 1987;67:485-488.

346. Colombo MB, Zanella A, Sirchia G. 2,3-Diphosphoglycerate and 3-phosphoglycerate in red cell pyruvate kinase deficiency. Br J Haematol. 1988;68:423-424.

347. Lakomek M, Neubauer B, von der Luhe A, et al. Erythrocyte pyruvate kinase deficiency: relations of residual enzyme activity, altered regulation of defective enzymes and concentrations of high-energy phosphates with the severity of clinical manifestation. Eur J Haematol. 1992;49:82-92.

348. Rose IA, Warms JVB: Control of red cell glycolysis. The cause of triose phosphate accumulation. J Biol Chem. 1970;245:4009-4015.

349. Zerez CR, Tanaka KR. Impaired nicotinamide adenine dinucleotide synthesis in pyruvate kinase–deficient human erythrocytes: A mechanism for decreased total NAD content and a possible secondary cause of hemolysis. Blood. 1987;69:999-1005.

350. Zerez CR, Wong MD, Lachant NA, Tanaka KR. Impaired erythrocyte phosphoribosylpyrophosphate formation in hemolytic anemia due to pyruvate kinase deficiency. Blood. 1988;72:500-506.

351. Nathan DG, Oski FA, Sidel VW, Diamond LK. Extreme hemolysis and red cell distortion in erythrocyte pyruvate kinase deficiency. II. Measurements of erythrocyte glucose consumption, potassium flux and adenosine triphosphate stability. N Engl J Med. 1965;272:118-123.

352. Twomey JJ, O'Neal FB, Alfrey CP, Moser RH. ATP metabolism in pyruvate kinase deficient erythrocytes. Blood. 1967;30:576-586.

353. Gardos G, Straub FB. Über die rolle der adenosintriphosphor-säure (ATP) in der K-permeabilität der menschlichen roten Blutkörperchen. Acta Physiol Acad Sci Hung. 1957;12:1-8.

354. Koller CA, Orringer EP, Parker JC. Quinine protects pyruvate-kinase deficient red cells from dehydration. Am J Hematol. 1979;7:193-199.

355. Nathan DG, Shohet SB. Erythrocyte ion transport defects and hemolytic anemia: "hydrocytosis" and "desicytosis." Semin Hematol. 1970;7:381-408.

356. Allen DW, Groat JD, Finkel B, et al. Increased adsorption of cytoplasmic proteins to the erythrocyte membrane in ATP depleted normal and pyruvate kinase–deficient mature cells and reticulocytes. Am J Hematol. 1983;14:11-25.

357. Zanella A, Brovelli A, Mantovani A, et al. Membrane abnormalities of pyruvate kinase deficient red cells. Br J Haematol. 1979;42:101-108.

358. Marik T, Brabec V, Kselikova M, et al. Reticulocyte-dependent labeling alterations of red cell membrane in pyruvate kinase deficiency anemia. Biomed Biochim Acta. 1987;46:S192-S196.

359. Marik T, Brabec V, Kodicek M, Jarolim P. Pyruvate kinase–deficiency anemia: Membrane approach. Biochem Med Metab Biol. 1988;39:55-63.

360. Staal GEJ, Sybesma HB, Cameron AR, et al. Familial hemolytic anaemia due to pyruvate kinase deficiency. Folia Med Neerl. 1971;14:72-76.

361. Staal GEJ, Koster JF, Nijessen JG. A new variant of red blood cell pyruvate kinase deficiency. Biochim Biophys Acta. 1971;258:685-687.

362. Nathan DG, Oski FA, Miller DR, Gardner FH. Life-span and organ sequestration of the red cells in pyruvate kinase deficiency. N Engl J Med. 1968;278:73-81.

363. Najean Y, Dresch C, Bussel A. Étude de l'érythrocinétique dans 8 cas de déficit homozygote en pyruvate kinase. Nouv Rev Fr Hematol. 1969;9:850-859.

364. Bowman HS, Oski FA. Splenic macrophage interaction with red cells in pyruvate kinase deficiency and hereditary spherocytosis. Vox Sang. 1970;19:168-175.

365. Matsumoto N, Ishihara T, Nakashima K, et al. Sequestration and destruction of reticulocytes in the spleen in pyruvate kinase deficiency hereditary nonspherocytic hemolytic anemia. Acta Haematol Jpn. 1972;35:525-537.

366. Leblond PF, Coulombe L, Lyonais J. Erythrocyte populations in pyruvate kinase deficiency following splenectomy. II. Cell deformability. Br J Haematol. 1978;39:63-70.

367. Muller-Soyano A, Platt O, Glader BE. Pyruvate kinase deficiency in dog and human erythrocytes: Effects of

energy depletion on cation composition and cellular hydration. Am J Hematol. 1986;23:217-221.

368. Aizawa S, Harada T, Kanbe E, et al. Ineffective erythropoiesis in mutant mice with deficient pyruvate kinase activity. Exp Hematol. 2005;33:1292-1298.

368a. Aisaki K-I, Aizawa S, Fujii H, et al. Glycolytic inhibition by mutation of pyruvate kinase gene increases oxidative stress and causes apoptosis of a pyruvate kinase deficient cell line. Exp Hematol 2007;35:1190-1200.

369. Lakomek M, Winkler H, Linne S, Schroter W. Erythrocyte pyruvate kinase deficiency: A kinetic method for differentiation between heterozygosity and compound-heterozygosity. Am J Hematol. 1989;31:225-232.

370. Paglia DE, Valentine WN, Williams KO, Konrad PN. An isozyme of erythrocyte pyruvate kinase (PK-Los Angeles) with impaired kinetics corrected by fructose-1,6-diphosphate. Am J Clin Pathol. 1977;78:229-234.

371. Bossu M, Dacha M, Fornaini G. Neonatal hemolysis due to a transient severity of inherited pyruvate kinase deficiency. Acta Haematol. 1968;40:166-175.

372. el-Hazmi MAF, Al-Swailem AR, Al-Faleh FZ, Warsy AS. Frequency of glucose-6-phosphate dehydrogenase, pyruvate kinase and hexokinase deficiency in the Saudi population. Hum Hered. 1986;36:45-49.

373. Feng CS, Tsang SS, Mak YT. Prevalence of pyruvate kinase deficiency among the Chinese: Determination by the quantitative assay. Am J Hematol. 1993;43:271-273.

374. Wu ZL, Yu WD, Chen SC. Frequency of erythrocyte pyruvate kinase deficiency in Chinese infants. Am J Hematol. 1985;20:139-144.

374a. Ayi K, Min-Oo G, Serghides L, et al. Pyruvate kinase deficiency and malaria. N Engl J Med 2008;358: 1805-1810.

375. Blume KG, Lohr GW, Praetsch O, Rudiger HW. Beitrag sur Populationsgenetik der Pyruvat-kinase menshlicher Erythrocyten. Humangenetik. 1968;6:261-265.

376. Mohrenweiser HW. Frequency of enzyme deficiency variants in erythrocytes of newborn infants. Proc Natl Acad Sci U S A. 1981;78:5046-5050.

377. Min-Oo G, Fortin A, Tam M-F, et al. Phenotypic expression of pyruvate kinase deficiency and protection against malaria in a mouse model. Genes Immunity. 2004;5: 168-175.

378. Ishida Y, Miwa S, Fujii H, et al. Thirteen cases of pyruvate kinase deficiency found in Japan. Am J Hematol. 1981;10:239-250.

379. Kahn A, Marie J, Vives-Corrons JL, et al. Search for a relationship between molecular anomalies of the mutant erythrocyte pyruvate kinase variants and their pathological expression. Hum Genet. 1981;57:172-175.

380. Zanella A, Fermo E, Bianchi P, Valentini G. Red cell pyruvate kinase deficiency: molecular and clinical aspects. Br J Haematol. 2005;130:11-25.

381. Cotton F, Bianchi P, Zanella A, et al. A novel mutation causing pyruvate kinase deficiency responsible for a severe neonatal respiratory distress syndrome and jaundice. Eur J Pediatr. 2001;160:523-524.

382. van Wijk R, van Solinge WW, Nerlov C, et al. Disruption of a novel regulatory element in the erythroid-specific promoter of the human PKLR gene causes severe pyruvate kinase deficiency. Blood. 2003;101:1596-1602.

383. Diez A, Gilsanz F, Martinez J, et al. Life-threatening nonspherocytic hemolytic anemia in a patient with a null mutation in the PKLR gene and no compensatory PKM gene expression. Blood. 2995;106:1851-1856.

384. Sedano IB, Rothlisberger B, Deleze G, et al. PK Aarau: first homozygous nonsense mutation causing pyruvate kinase deficiency. Br J Haematol. 2004;127:360-369.

384a. Zanella A, Fermo E, Bianchi P, et al. Pyruvate kinase deficiency: the genotype-phenotype association. Blood Rev. 2007;21:217-231.

385. Miwa S. Recommended methods for the characterization of red cell pyruvate kinase variants. Br J Haematol. 1979;43:275-286.

386. Pissard S, Max-Audit I, Skopinski L, et al. Pyruvate kinase deficiency in France; a 3-year study reveals 27 new mutations. Br J Haematol. 2006;133:683-689.

387. van Wijk R, Rijksen G, van Solinge WW. Molecular characterization of pyruvate kinase deficiency—concerns about the description of mutant PKLR alleles. Br J Haematol. 1996;136:167-169.

388. Pissard S, Wajcman H. Molecular characterization of pyruvate kinase deficiency—concerns about the description of mutant PKLR alleles—response to van Wijk et al. Br J Haematol. 2006;136:169-170.

389. Whitney KM, Goodman SA, Bailey EM, Lothrop CD Jr. The molecular basis of canine pyruvate kinase deficiency. Exp Hematol. 1994;22:866-874.

390. Lenzner C, Nurnberg P, Thiele BJ, et al. Mutations in the pyruvate kinase L-gene in patients with hereditary hemolytic anemia. Blood. 1994;83:2817-2822.

391. Baronciani L, Beutler E. Molecular study of pyruvate kinase–deficient patients with hereditary nonspherocytic hemolytic anemia. J Clin Invest. 1995;95:1702-1709.

392. Lakomek M, Huppke P, Neubauer B, et al: Mutations in the R-type pyruvate kinase gene and altered enzyme kinetic properties in patients with hemolytic anemia due to pyruvate kinase deficiency. Ann Hematol. 1994;68: 253-260.

393. Zanella A, Bianchi P, Fermo E, et al. Molecular characterization of the PK-LR gene in sixteen pyruvate kinase–deficient patients. Br J Haematol. 2001;113:43-48.

394. Kanno H, Fujii H, Hirono A, et al. Identical point mutations of the R-type pyruvate kinase (PK) cDNA found in unrelated PK variants associated with hereditary hemolytic anemia. Blood. 1992;79:1347-1350.

395. Demina A, Varughese KI, Barbot J, et al. Six previously undescribed pyruvate kinase mutations causing enzyme deficiency. Blood. 1998;92:647-652.

396. van Solinge WW, Kraaijenhagen RJ, Rijksen G, et al. Molecular modelling of human red blood cell pyruvate kinase: Structural implications of a novel G1091 to A mutation causing severe nonspherocytic hemolytic anemia. Blood. 1997;90:4987-4995.

397. Pastore L, Della Morte R, Frisso G, et al. Novel mutations and structural implications in R-type pyruvate kinase–deficient patients from southern Italy. Hum Mutat. 1998;11:127-134.

398. Valentini G, Chiarelli LR, Fortin R, et al. Structure and function of human erythrocyte pyruvate kinase: Molecular basis of nonspherocytic hemolytic anemia. J Biol Chem. 2002;277:23807-23814.

399. Wang C, Chiarelli LR, Bianchi P, et al. Human erythrocyte pyruvate kinase: characterization of the recombinant enzyme and a mutant form (R510Q) causing nonspherocytic hemolytic anemia. Blood. 2001;98:3113-3120.

400. Baronciani L, Beutler E. Prenatal diagnosis of pyruvate kinase deficiency. Blood. 1994;84:2354-2356.

401. Sachs JR, Wicker DJ, Gilcher RO, et al. Familial hemolytic anemia resulting from an abnormal red blood cell pyruvate kinase. J Lab Clin Med. 1968;72:359-362.

402. Paglia DE, Valentine WN, Rucknagel DL. Defective erythrocyte pyruvate kinase with impaired kinetics and reduced optimal activity. Br J Haematol. 1972;221:651-665.

403. Miwa S. Hereditary disorders of red cell enzymes in the Embden-Meyerhof pathway. Am J Hematol. 1983;14:381-391.

404. Max-Audit I, Rosa R, Marie J. Pyruvate kinase hyperactivity genetically determined: Metabolic consequences and molecular characterization. Blood. 1980;56:902-909.

405. Rosa R, Max-Audit I, Izrael V, et al. Hereditary pyruvate kinase abnormalities associated with erythrocytosis. Am J Hematol. 1981;10:47-55.

406. Staal GE J, Jansen G, Roos D. Pyruvate kinase and the "high ATP syndrome." J Clin Invest. 1984;74:231-235.

407. Kechemir D, Max-Audit I, Rosa R. Comparative study of human M2-type pyruvate kinases isolated from human leukocytes and erythrocytes of a patient with red cell pyruvate kinase hyperactivity. Enzyme. 1989;41:121-130.

408. Tsujino K, Kanno H, Hashimoto K, et al. Delayed onset of hemolytic anemia in CBA-Pk-1slc/Pk1slc mice with a point mutation of the gene encoding red blood cell type pyruvate kinase. Blood. 1998;91:2169-2174.

409. Etiemble J, Picat C, Dhermy D, et al. Erythrocytic pyruvate kinase deficiency and hemolytic anemia inherited as a dominant trait. Am J Hematol. 1984;17:251-260.

410. Valentine WN, Herring WB, Paglia DE, et al. Pyruvate kinase Greensboro. A four-generation study of a high K0.5s (phosphoenolypyruvate) variant. Blood. 1988;72:1054-1059.

411. Baughan MA, Paglia DE, Schneider AS, Valentine WN. An unusual hematological syndrome with pyruvate kinase deficiency and thalassemia minor in the kindreds. Acta Haematol. 1968;39:345-358.

412. Branca R, Costa E, Rocha S, et al. Coexistence of congenital red cell pyruvate kinase and band 3 deficiency. Clin Lab Haematol. 2004;26:297-300.

413. Eulderink F, Cleton FJ. Gaucher's disease with severe renal involvement combined with pyruvate kinase deficiency. Pathol Eur. 1970;5:409-419.

414. Sandoval C, Stringel G, Weisberger J, Jayabose S. Failure of partial splenectomy to ameliorate the anemia of pyruvate kinase deficiency. J Pediatr Surg. 1997;32:641-642.

415. Blume KG, Busch D, Hoffbauer RW, et al. The polymorphism of nucleoside effect in pyruvate kinase deficiency. Humangenetik. 1970;9:257-259.

416. Staal GE J, Van Berkel TH, Nijessen JG, Koster JF. Normalization of red blood cell pyruvate kinase in pyruvate kinase deficiency by riboflavin treatment. Clin Chim Acta. 1975;60:323-327.

417. Weiden PL, Hackman RC, Deeg HJ, et al. Long-term survival and reversal of iron overload after marrow transplantation in dogs with congenital hemolytic anemia. Blood. 1981;57:66-70.

418. Morimoto M, Kanno H, Asai H, et al. Pyruvate kinase deficiency of mice associated with nonspherocytic hemolytic anemia and cure of the anemia by marrow transplantation without host irradiation. Blood. 1995;86:4323-4330.

419. Richard RE, Weinreich M, Chang K-H, et al. Modulating erythrocyte chimerism in a mouse model of pyruvate kinase deficiency. Blood. 2004;103:4432-4439.

420. Tanphaichitr VS, Suvatte V, Issaragrisil S, et al. Successful bone marrow transplantation in a child with red blood cell pyruvate kinase deficiency. Bone Marrow Transplant. 2000;26:689-690.

421. Tani K, Yoshikubo T, Ikebuchi K, et al. Retrovirus-mediated gene transfer of human pyruvate kinase (PK) cDNA into murine hematopoietic cells: Implications for gene therapy of human PK deficiency. Blood. 1994;83:2305-2310.

421a. Kanno H, Utsugisawa T, Aizawa S, et al. Transgenic rescue of hemolytic anemia due to red blood cell pyruvate kinase deficiency. Haematologica 2007;92:731-737.

422. Miwa S, Nishina T, Kakehashi Y, et al. Studies on erythrocyte metabolism in a case with hereditary deficiency of H-subunit of lactate dehydrogenase. Acta Haematol Jpn. 1971;34:228-232.

423. Kanno T, Maekawa M: Lactate dehydrogenase M-subunit deficiencies: Clinical features, metabolic background, and genetic heterogeneities. Muscle Nerve. 1995;(Suppl 3):S54-S60.

424. Kremer JP, Datta T, Pretsch W, et al. Mechanisms of compensation of hemolytic anemia in a lactate dehydrogenase mouse mutant. Exp Hematol. 1987;15:664-670.

425. Brewer GJ. A new inherited abnormality of human erythrocytes: Elevated erythrocyte adenosine triphosphate. Biochem Biophys Res Commun. 1965;18:430.

426. Jacobasch G, Syllm-Rappoport I, Roigas H, Rappoport S. 2,3PGase-Mangel als mögliche ursache erhöhten ATP-Gehaltes. Clin Chim Acta. 1964;10:477-478.

427. Ben-Bassat I, Brok-Simoni F, Kende G, et al. A family with red cell pyrimidine 5'-nucleotidase deficiency. Blood. 1976;47:919-922.

428. Rosa R, Rochant H, Dreyfus B, et al. Electrophoretic and kinetic studies of human erythrocytes deficient in pyrimidine-5'-nucleotidase. Hum Genet. 1977;38:209-215.

429. Miwa S, Nakashima K, Fujii H, et al. Three cases of hereditary hemolytic anemia with pyrimidine-5'-nucleotidase deficiency in a Japanese family. Hum Genet. 1977;37:361-364.

430. Paglia DE, Valentine WN: Haemolytic anaemia associated with disorders of the purine and pyrimidine salvage pathways. Clin Haematol. 1981;10:81-98.

431. Beutler E, Baranko PV, Feagler J, et al: Hemolytic anemia due to pyrimidine-5'-nucleotidase deficiency; report of eight cases in six families. Blood. 1980;56:251-255.

432. Miwa S, Ishida Y, Kibe A, et al. Two cases of hereditary hemolytic anemia with pyrimidine-5' nucleotidase deficiency. Acta Haematol Jpn. 1981;44:187-189.

433. Ozsoylu S, Gurgey A. A case of hemolytic anemia due to erythrocyte pyrimidine-5'-nucleotidase deficiency. Acta Haematol. 1981;66:56-58.

434. Tomoda A, Noble NA, Lachant NA, Tanaka KR. Hemolytic anemia in hereditary pyrimidine 5'-nucleotidase deficiency: Nucleotide inhibition of G6PD and the pentose phosphate shunt. Blood. 1982;60:1212-1218.

435. Hansen TW, Seip M, deVerdier CH, Ericson A. Erythrocyte pyrimidine-5'-nucleotidase deficiency. Scand J Haematol. 1983;31:122-128.

436. Vives I, Corrons J-L. Chronic non-spherocytic haemolytic anaemia due to congenital pyrimidine 5' nucleotidase deficiency: 25 years later. Baillieres Clin Haematol. 2000;13:103-118.

437. Zanella A, Bianchi P, Fermo E, Valentini G. Hereditary pyrimidine 5'-nucleotidase deficiency: from genetics to clinical manifestations. Bri J Haematol. 2006;133: 113-123.

438. Hirono A, Fujii H, Natori H, et al. Chromatographic analysis of human erythrocyte pyrimidine-5'-nucleotidase from five patients with pyrimidine-5'-nucleotidase deficiency. Br J Haematol. 1987;65:35-41.

439. Swanson MS, Angle CR, Stohs SJ, et al. ^{31}P NMR study of erythrocytes from a patient with hereditary pyrimidine-5'-nucleotidase deficiency. Proc Natl Acad Sci U S A. 1983;80:169-172.

440. Swanson MS, Markin RS, Stohs SJ, Angle CR. Identification of cytidine diphosphodiesters in erythrocytes from a patient with pyrimidine 5' nucleotidase deficiency. Blood. 1984;63:665-670.

441. Harley EH, Heaton A, Wicomb W. Pyrimidine metabolism in hereditary erythrocyte pyrimidine-5'-nucleotidase deficiency. Metabolism. 1978;27:1743-1754.

442. Kagimoto T, Shirono K, Higaki T, et al. Detection of pyrimidine-5'-nucleotidase deficiency using H- or P-nuclear magnetic resonance. Experientia. 1986;42: 69-72.

443. Valentine WN, Anderson HM, Paglia DE, et al. Studies on human erythrocyte nucleotide metabolism. II. Nonspherocytic hemolytic anemia, high red cell ATP, ribose-phosphate pyrophosphokinase (RPK, EC 2.7.6.1) deficiency. Blood. 1972;39:674-684.

444. Valentine WN, Bennett JM, Krivit W, et al. Nonspherocytic haemolytic anaemia with increased red cell adenine nucleotides, glutathione and basophilic stippling and ribose-phosphate pyrophosphokinase (RPK) deficiency: Studies on two new kindreds. Br J Haematol. 1973;24: 157-167.

445. Lachant NA, Zerez CR, Tanaka KR. Pyrimidine nucleotides impair phosphoribosylpyrophosphate (PRPP) synthetase subunit aggregation by sequestering magnesium. A mechanism for the decreased PRPP synthetase activity in hereditary erythrocyte pyrimidine-5'-nucleotidase deficiency. Biochem Biophys Acta. 1989; 994:81-88.

446. Lachant NA, Tanaka KR: Red cell metabolism in hereditary pyrimidine-5'-nucleotidase deficiency: Effect of magnesium. Br J Haematol. 1986;63:615-623.

447. Paglia DE, Valentine WN, Nakatani M, Rauth BJ. Cytosol accumulation of cytidine diphosphate (CDP)-choline as an isolated erythrocyte defect in chronic hemolysis. Proc Natl Acad Sci U S A. 1983;80:3081-3085.

448. Oda S, Tanaka KR. Metabolism studies in erythrocyte pyrimidine 5'-nucleotidase deficiency. Clin Res. 1976;34: 149A.

449. David O, Ramenghi U, Camaschella C, et al. Inhibition of hexose monophosphate shunt in young erythrocytes by pyrimidine nucleotides in hereditary pyrimidine-5' nucleotidase deficiency. Eur J Haematol. 1991;47:48-54.

450. Paglia DE, Valentine WN, Dahlgren JG. Effects of low-level lead exposure on pyrimidine-5'-nucleotidase and other erythrocyte enzymes. J Clin Invest. 1975;56: 1164-1169.

451. Valentine WN, Paglia DE, Fink K, Madokoro G. Lead poisoning. Association with hemolytic anemia, basophilic stippling erythrocyte pyrimidine-5'-nucleotidase deficiency, and intraerythrocytic accumulation of pyrimidines. J Clin Invest. 1976;58:926-932.

452. Marinaki AM, Escuredo E, Duley JA, et al. Genetic basis of hemolytic anemia caused by pyrimidine 5' nucleotidase deficiency. Blood. 2001;97:3327-3332.

453. Molecular basis of Japanese variants of pyrimidine 5'-nucleotidase deficiency. Br J Haematol. 2004;126: 265-271.

454. Chiarelli LR, Fermo E, Abrusci P, et al. Two new mutations of the P5'N-1 gene found in Italian patients with hereditary hemolytic anemia: the molecular basis of the red cell enzyme disorder. Haematologica. 2006;91: 1244-1247.

455. Torrance JD, Whittaker D, Jenkins T. Erythrocyte pyrimidine-5'-nucleotidase. Br J Haematol. 1980;45:585-597.

456. Li JY, Wan SD, Ma ZM, et al. A new mutant erythrocyte pyrimidine-5'-nucleotidase characterized by fast electrophoretic mobility in a Chinese boy with chronic hemolytic anemia. Clin Chim Acta. 1991;200:43-47.

457. Chiarelli LR, Bianchi P, Fermo E, et al. Functional analysis of pyrimidine 5'-nculeotidase mutants causing nonspherocytic hemolytic anemia. Blood. 2005;105:3340-3345.

458. Amici A, Ciccioli K, Naponelli V, et al. Evidence for essential catalytic determinants for human erythrocyte pyrimidine 5'-nucleotidase. Cell Mol Life Sci. 2005;62: 1613-1620.

459. Beutler E, West C. Tissue distribution of pyrimidine-5'-nucleotidase. Biochem Med. 1982;27:334.

460. Beutler E, Carson D, Dannawi H, et al. Metabolic compensation for profound erythrocyte adenylate kinase deficiency: A hereditary enzyme defect without hemolytic anemia. J Clin Invest. 1983;72:648-655.

461. Szeinberg A, Kahana D, Gavendo S, et al. Hereditary deficiency of adenylate kinase in red blood cells. Acta Haematol. 1969;42:111-126.

462. Toren A, Brok-Simoni F, Ben-Basset I, et al. Congenital haemolytic anaemia associated with adenylate kinase deficiency. Br J Haematol. 1994;87:376-380.

463. Lachant NA, Zerez CR, Barredo J, et al. Hereditary erythrocyte adenylate kinase deficiency: A defect of phosphotransferases. Blood. 1991;77:2774-2784.

464. Boivin P, Galand C, Hakim J, et al. Anémie hémolytique congénitale non sphérocytaire et déficit héréditaire en adenylate kinase érythrocytaire. Presse Med. 1971; 79:215-218.

465. Miwa S, Fujii H, Tani K, et al. Red cell adenylate kinase deficiency associated with hereditary nonspherocytic hemolytic anemia: Clinical and biochemical studies. Am J Hematol. 1983;14:325-333.

466. Matsuura S, Igarashi M, Tanizawa Y, et al. Human adenylate kinase deficiency associated with hemolytic anemia. A single base substitution affecting solubility and catalytic activity of the cytosolic adenylate kinase. J Biol Chem. 1989;264:10148-10155.

467. Vives Corrons J-L, Garcia E, Tusell JJ, et al. Red cell adenylate kinase deficiency: molecular study of 3 new mutations (118G→A, 190G→A, and GAC deletion) associated with hereditary nonspherocytic hemolytic anemia. Blood. 2003;102:353-356.

468. Qualtieri A, Pedace V, Bisconte MG, et al. Severe erythrocyte adenylate kinase deficiency due to homozygous ArG substitution at codon 164 of human AK gene associated with chronic haemolytic anemia. Br J Haematol. 1997;99:770-776.

469. Bianchi P, Zappa M, Bredi E, et al. A case of complete adenylate kinase deficiency due to a nonsense mutation in AK-1 gene (Arg 107→stop, CGA→TGA) associated with chronic haemolytic anaemia. Br J Haematol. 1999;105:75-79.

470. Ferma E, Bianchi P, Vercellati C, et al. A new variant of adenylate kinase (delG138) associated with severe hemolytic anemia. Blood Cells Mol Dis. 2004;33:146-149.

470a. Abrusci P, Chiarelli LR, Galizzi A, et al. Erythrocyte adenylate kinase deficiency: Characterization of recombinant mutant forms and relationship with nonspherocytic hemolytic anemia. Exp Hematol 2007;35:1182-1189.

471. Valentine WN, Paglia DE, Tartaglia AP, Gilsanz F. Hereditary hemolytic anemia with increased red cell adenosine deaminase (45- to 70-fold) and decreased adenosine triphosphate. Science. 1977;195:783-785.

472. Miwa S, Fujii H, Matsumoto N, et al. A case of red-cell adenosine deaminase overproduction associated with hereditary hemolytic anemia found in Japan. Am J Hematol. 1978;5:107-115.

473. Perignon JL, Hamet M, Buc HA, et al. Biochemical study of a case of hemolytic anemia with increased (85-fold) cell adenosine deaminase. Clin Chim Acta. 1982;124:205-212.

474. Kanno H, Tani K, Fujii H. Adenosine deaminase (ADA) overproduction associated with congenital hemolytic anemia: Case report and molecular analysis. Jpn J Exp Med. 1988;58:1-8.

475. Fujii H, Miwa S, Suzuki K. Purification and properties of adenosine deaminase in normal and hereditary hemolytic anemia with increased red cell activity. Hemoglobin. 1980;4:693-705.

476. Chottiner EG, Cloft HJ, Tartaglia AP, Mitchell BS. Elevated adenosine deaminase activity and hereditary hemolytic anemia. Evidence for abnormal translational control of protein synthesis. J Clin Invest. 1987;79:1001-1005.

477. Fujii H, Miwa S, Tani K, et al. Overproduction of structurally normal enzyme in man: Hereditary haemolytic anaemia with increased red cell adenosine deaminase activity. Br J Haematol. 1982;51:427-430.

478. Chottiner EG, Ginsburg D, Tartaglia AP, Mitchell BS. Erythrocyte adenosine deaminase overproduction in hereditary hemolytic anemia. Blood. 1989;74:448-453.

479. Chen EH, Tartaglia AP, Mitchell BS. Hereditary overexpression of adenosine deaminase in erythrocytes: Evidence for a cis-acting mutation. Am J Hum Genet. 1993;53:889-893.

480. Chen EH, Mitchell B. Hereditary overexpression of adenosine deaminase in erythrocytes: Studies in erythroid cell lines and transgenic mice. Blood. 1994;84:2346-2353.

481. Glader BE, Backer K, Diamond LK. Elevated erythrocyte adenosine deaminase activity in congenital hypoplastic anemia. N Engl J Med. 1983;309:1486-1490.

482. Glader BE, Backer K. Comparative activity of erythrocyte adenosine deaminase and orotidine decarboxylase in Diamond-Blackfan anemia. Am J Hematol. 1986;23:135-139.

483. Novelli G, Stocchi V, Giannotti A, et al. Increased erythrocyte adenosine deaminase activity without haemolytic anaemia. Hum Hered. 1986;36:37-40.

484. Cowan MJ, Brady RO, Widder KG. Elevated erythrocyte adenosine deaminase activity in patients with acquired immunodeficiency syndrome. Proc Natl Acad Sci U S A. 1986;83:1089-1091.

485. Sanchez-Corona J, Garcia-Cruz D, Medina C. Increased adenosine deaminase activity in a patient with cartilage-hair hypoplasia. Ann Genet. 1990;33:99-102.

486. Lichtman MA, Miller DR. Erythrocyte glycolysis, 2,3-diphosphoglycerate and adenosine triphosphate concentration in uremic subjects: Relationship to extracellular phosphate concentration. J Lab Clin Med. 1970;76:267.

487. Travis SF, Sugerman HJ, Ruberg RL, et al. Red cell metabolic alterations induced by intravenous hyperalimentation. N Engl J Med. 1971;285:763-768.

488. Lichtman MA, Miller DR, Weed RI. Energy metabolism in uremic red cells: Relationship of red cell adenosine triphosphate concentration to extracellular phosphate. Trans Assoc Am Physicians. 1969;82:331-343.

489. Jacob HS, Amsden T. Acute hemolytic anemia with rigid red cells in hypophosphatemia. N Engl J Med. 1971;285:1446-1450.

490. Weed RI, LaCelle PL, Merrill ET. Metabolic dependence of red cell deformability. J Clin Invest. 1969;48:795-809.

491. Oken MM, Lichtman MA, Miller DR, Leblond P. Spherocytic hemolytic disease during magnesium deprivation in the rat. Blood. 1971;38:468-478.

492. Piomelli S, Jansen V, Dancis J. The hemolytic anemia of magnesium deficiency in adult rats. Blood. 1973;41:451-459.

493. Elin RJ, Tan HK: Erythrocyte membrane plaques from rats with magnesium deficiency. Blood. 1977;49:657-664.

494. MacDougall LG, Judisch JM, Mistry SB. Red cell metabolism in iron deficiency anemia. II. The relationship between red cell survival and alterations in red cell metabolism. J Pediatr. 1970;76:660-675.

495. MacDougall LG. Red cell metabolism in iron deficiency anemia. J Pediatr. 1968;71:303-318.

496. Slawsky P, Desforge JF. Erythrocyte 2,3-diphosphoglycerate in iron deficiency. Arch Intern Med. 1972;129:914-917.

497. Brewer GJ: Metabolism of ATP in thalassemic and iron-deficient erythrocytes. J Lab Clin Med. 1967;70:1016a.

498. Card RT, Weintraub LR: Metabolic abnormalities of erythrocytes in severe iron deficiency. Blood. 1971;37:725-732.

499. Boivin P, Galand C, Hakim J, Kahn A. Acquired erythroenzymopathies in blood disorders: Study of 200 cases. Br J Haematol. 1975;31:531-543.

500. Lohr GW, Waller HD Anschutz F, Knopp A. Hexokinasemangel in Blutzellen bei einer Sippe mit familiarer Panmyelopathie (Typ Fanconi). Klin Wochenschr. 1965;43:870-875.

501. Valentine WN, Crookston JH, Paglia DE, Konrad PN. Erythrocyte enzymatic abnormalities in HEMPAS (hereditary erythroblastic multinuclearity with a positive acidified-serum test). Br J Haematol. 1972;23:107-112.

502. Valentine WN, Konrad PN, Paglia DE. Dyserythropoiesis, refractory anemia, and "preleukemia": Metabolic features of the erythrocytes. Blood. 1973;41:857-875.

503. Wang WC, Mentzer WC: Differentiation of transient erythroblastopenia of childhood from congenital hypoplastic anemia. J Pediatr. 1976;88:784-789.

504. Kahn A. Abnormalities of erythrocyte enzymes in dyserythropoiesis and malignancies. Clin Haematol. 1981;10:123-138.

505. Tani K, Fujii H, Takahashi K, et al. Erythrocyte activities in myelodysplastic syndromes: Elevated pyruvate kinase activity. Am J Hematol. 1989;30:97-103.

506. Kahn A, Marie J, Bernard JF, et al. Mechanisms of the acquired erythrocyte enzyme deficiencies in blood diseases. Clin Chim Acta. 1976;71:379-387.

17 Glucose-6-Phosphate Dehydrogenase Deficiency

Lucio Luzzatto and Vincenzo Poggi

Most hemolytic anemias can be categorized, at least at first approximation, as being either inherited or acquired, due to either intracorpuscular or extracorpuscular causes. Hemolytic anemia associated with deficiency of glucose-6-phosphate dehydrogenase (G6PD) glaringly defies this categorization. Indeed, the majority of persons with inherited G6PD deficiency have no anemia and almost no hemolysis. Both develop only as a result of challenge by exogenous agents. Because the metabolic role of G6PD in red blood cells is primarily related to its reductive potential, the threat to G6PD-deficient red cells is oxidative damage. Therefore, to understand hemolytic anemia associated with G6PD deficiency, we first need to define the physiologic role of G6PD[1-3] and pinpoint why the red cells are deficient in G6PD.[4-6]

G6PD IN RED CELL METABOLISM

In metabolic maps, G6PD is commonly referred to as the first enzyme of the hexose monophosphate shunt, or the pentose phosphate pathway (Fig. 17-1). Although these time-honored phrases persist in textbooks, it is now clear that the main role of G6PD is not glucose utilization (G6PD accounts for less than 10% of that); rather, it is production of the reduced form of nicotinamide adenine dinucleotide phosphate (NADPH). NADPH has a crucial role in preventing oxidative damage to proteins and to other molecules in all cells (Fig. 17-2).[7,8] This role is particularly crucial in red cells because being oxygen carriers par excellence, they have a literally built-in danger of damage by oxygen radicals generated continuously in the course of methemoglobin formation.[9] The highly reactive oxygen radicals either decay spontaneously or are converted by superoxide dismutase to hydrogen peroxide (H_2O_2), which is still highly toxic. Detoxification of H_2O_2 to H_2O is effected by catalase[10] and by glutathione peroxidase[11] (GSHPX). NADPH is crucial for the function of both these enzymes: it is a structural component of catalase,[12] and it is required as a substrate by glutathione reductase, which regenerates GSH when it has been oxidized to GSSG by GSHPX (see Fig. 17-2). G6PD-deficient red cells are highly vulnerable to oxidative damage (see later), even though G6PD deficiency is never complete in humans. When complete G6PD defi-

ciency was produced in mouse embryonic stem cells (ESCs) by targeted inactivation of the G6PD gene,[13] the G6PD-null cells thus obtained were viable, but they formed colonies only in a low-oxygen environment; even so, they had an impaired capacity to form erythroid colonies.[14] When G6PD-null ESCs were injected into mouse blastocysts, chimeric embryos were obtained, and germline transmission was achieved; however, only female heterozygous mice were obtained because hemizygous male embryos died.[15] Thus, a G6PD-null mutation is an embryonically lethal condition.

Structure and Biochemistry of G6PD

G6PD is a ubiquitous enzyme that must be quite ancient in evolution because it has been found in all organisms, from prokaryotes to yeasts, to protozoa, to plants and animals.[2,16,17] In mammals, G6PD is a good example of

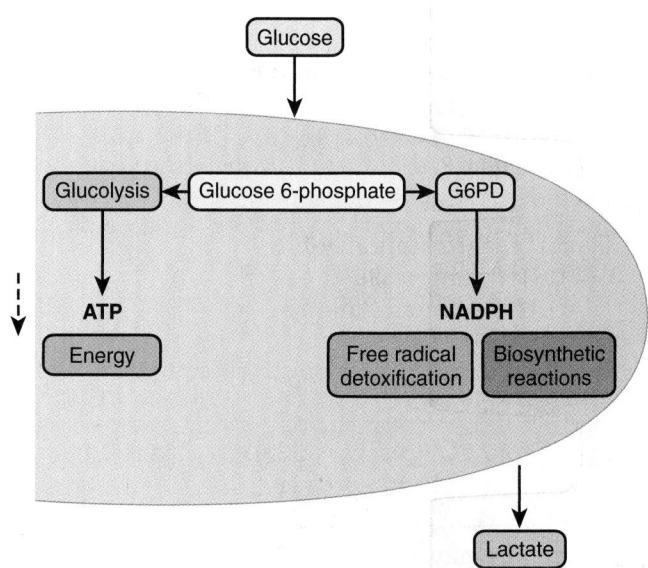

FIGURE 17-1. The role of G6PD in red blood cell metabolism. As a somewhat crude oversimplification, glucose can be visualized, after phosphorylation to glucose 6-phosphate (G6P), as being at the bifurcation between two major pathways: glycolysis, which produces adenosine triphosphate (ATP), and the pentose phosphate pathway, which generates reducing power (reduced nicotinamide adenine dinucleotide phosphate [NADPH]). Under "normal" conditions, probably less than 1% of G6P enters the pentose phosphate pathway; under maximal oxidative stress, the amount may reach 10%.

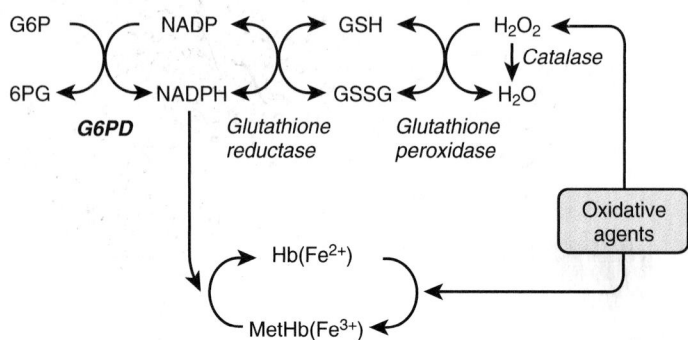

FIGURE 17-2. G6PD and the glutathione (GSH) cycle. The front-line defense against oxidative damage by hydrogen peroxide (H_2O_2) is GSH by means of GSH peroxidase (GSHPX). GSHPX uses up GSH, and its regeneration can be effected in the red blood cell only through GSH reductase (GSSGR) by NADPH, which is ultimately provided by G6PD. (*Redrawn from Luzzatto L, Mehta A, Vulliamy T. Glucose-6-phosphate dehydrogenase deficiency. In Scriver C, Beaudet A, Sly W, Valle D [eds]. The Metabolic & Molecular Bases of Inherited Disease, 8th ed. New York, McGraw-Hill, 2001, pp 4517-4553.*)

a housekeeping enzyme produced by a housekeeping gene; indeed, the gene is expressed in all cells of the body. G6PD is a typical cytoplasmic enzyme, although some G6PD activity is associated with peroxisomes in liver and kidney cells.[18] This is consistent with the view that these organelles have evolved as part of the need of early eukaryotes to defend against oxygen, which is germane to the role of G6PD today.

The enzymatically active form of G6PD is either a dimer or a tetramer (Fig. 17-3) of a single polypeptide subunit of about 59 kd.[19] The complete primary structure of the human enzyme has been deduced from the sequence of a full-length complementary DNA clone.[20] The amino acid sequence of rat liver G6PD shows 94% homology to the human sequence and provides evidence that the N-terminal amino acid is *N*-acetylalanine, which must result from post-translational cleavage of the N-terminal methionine. The same is probably true of the human enzyme.[21]

Extensive data are available on the kinetics of G6PD. Its coenzyme specificity is exquisite; human G6PD has practically no activity with nicotinamide adenine dinucleotide (NAD). Its substrate specificity is also very high because activity on other hexose phosphates (e.g., mannose 6-phosphate or galactose 6-phosphate) is negligible. The affinity for nicotinamide adenine dinucleotide phosphate (NADP) is about 1 order of magnitude higher than the affinity for glucose 6-phosphate (G6P).[2,16]

The tertiary structure of the molecule has been determined (see Fig. 17-3).[23] The G6P binding site is near K205, and the critical role of this amino acid in electron transfer[27] has been confirmed by showing that its replacement with threonine nearly abolishes catalytic activity.[28] The NADP binding site is located near a fan of β-sheet structures, with a critical G-X-X-G-X-X peptide motif corresponding to amino acids 38 to 43 encoded in exon 3.

Although many natural and non-natural substances can affect the activity of G6PD, it is not certain which ones may be important physiologically. NADPH, one product of the G6PD reaction, is a potent quasi-competitive inhibitor,[29] and since most of the coenzyme in cells is in the reduced form,[30] it can be assumed that G6PD is normally under strong inhibition. Because the K_m values for both G6P and NADP are higher than their normal respective intracellular concentrations, it is likely that these two substrates themselves are the main regulators of intracellular G6PD activity, together with NADPH. Any oxidative event affecting the cell will alter the NADPH/NADP ratio in favor of NADP. The simultaneous increase in NADP and decrease in NADPH act additively to increase G6PD activity by increasing the substrate drive on the reaction rate and decreasing

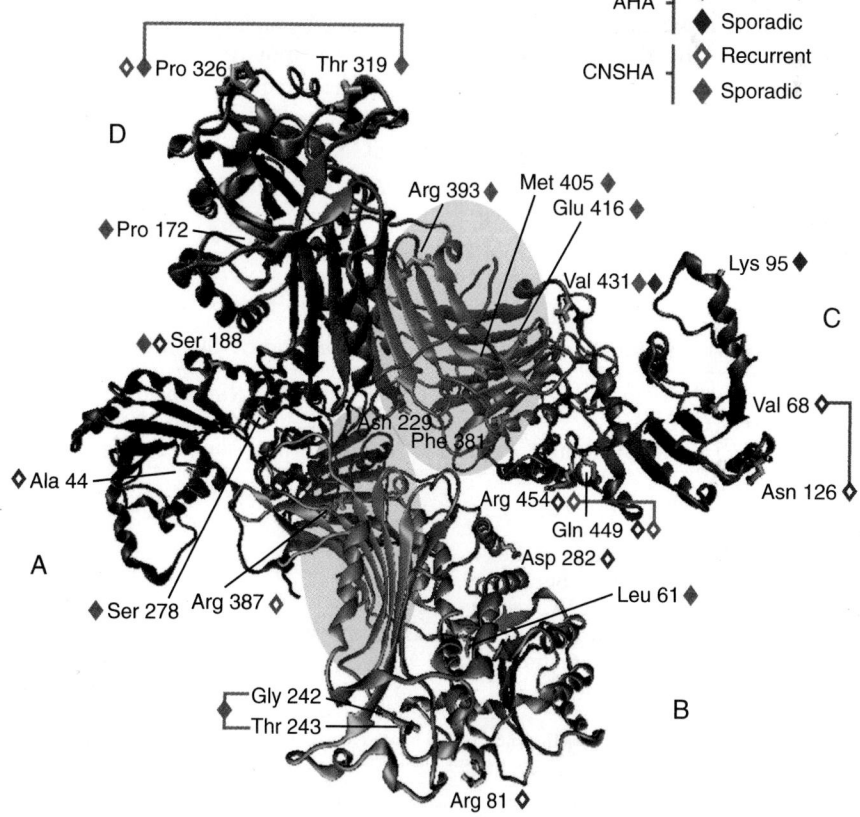

FIGURE 17-3. Three-dimensional structure of the human G6PD tetramer. The structure of the dimer was modeled first,[22] and then the tetramer structure was solved[23,24] and the details of substrate binding elucidated.[25,26] A to D are the four identical monomers. The tetramer is a dimer of a dimer, and both the dimer and the tetramer are enzymatically active, whereas the monomer is not. The monomer consists of two domains—a smaller coenzyme domain encompassing residues 1 to 198 and a larger β + α domain consisting of residues 199 to 514. The *gray background* outlines, within each dimer, the critical area of the monomer-monomer interface, in which 57 amino acid residues are involved. Only some of the many mutations known are indicated; most of those in the dimer interface cause severe G6PD deficiency with congenital nonspherocytic hemolytic anemia (CNSHA). AHA, acute hemolytic anemia (see Table 17-1). (*Redrawn from Mason PJ, Bautista JM, Gilsanz F. G6PD deficiency: the genotype-phenotype association. Blood Rev. 2007;21:267-283.*)

product inhibition.[8] Under most conditions this may be the most important short-term regulatory signal, although it is, of course, possible that other regulatory effects play a role as well.

Notes on Terminology

G6PD is the accepted abbreviation for the enzyme glucose-6-phosphate dehydrogenase (E.C. 1.1.1.49); the G6PD gene is designated *Gd*.[4,16] In this chapter the terms *G6PD normal* and *G6PD deficient* are used to designate the phenotypes of persons; G6PD(+) and G6PD(−) are used to designate the phenotypes of individual cells. Because *Gd* is X-linked (see later), males can be only normal hemizygotes (*Gd$^+$*) or deficient hemizygotes (*Gd$^-$*); females can be normal homozygotes (*Gd$^+$/Gd$^+$*), deficient homozygotes (*Gd$^-$/Gd$^-$*), or heterozygotes (*Gd$^+$/Gd$^-$*). The phenotype of the last group is often referred to as "intermediate" because their overall red cell G6PD level usually lies in between the normal and the deficient range; however, exceptions do occur (see later). Consequently, G6PD deficiency should not be regarded as a recessive but rather as a codominant trait. According to a classification introduced in 1966 (Table 17-1), G6PD-deficient variants that result in congenital nonspherocytic hemolytic anemia (CNSHA) are designated class I; G6PD-deficient variants that do not result in CNSHA are designated class II or class III, depending on the severity of the reduction in enzyme activity in red cells. The separation between class II and class III is blurred and probably no longer useful. Class IV variants are those with normal activity. Class V was reserved for variants with increased activity, but after an initial report (G6PD Hektoen[31]), none has been found. In practice, because the majority of G6PD-deficient persons are mostly asymptomatic, their G6PD deficiency is referred to as mild, simple, or common (corresponding to class II or III); the minority of persons who have CNSHA are referred to as having rare, sporadic, or severe G6PD deficiency (corresponding to class I).

When a diagnostic test for G6PD is carried out, the phrase "positive result" is sometimes used to indicate that the test has shown G6PD deficiency; this has caused confusion and should be avoided by saying that the test has shown either a *normal* result or a *deficient* result.

Genetics of G6PD

Gd, the G6PD gene, is located near the telomeric region of the long arm of the X chromosome[32-34] (band Xq28); historically, *Gd* has been a valuable X-linked genetic marker and a precious tool for studying the X-chromosome inactivation phenomenon[35,36] and clonal populations of somatic cells.[37-39] The *Gd* region was also one of the first regions of the human genome to be fully sequenced.[40]

X-linkage of *Gd* has three major consequences: (1) *Gd* mutations display the typical pattern of mendelian X-linked inheritance[41]; (2) severe G6PD deficiency is much more common in males than in females; and (3) as a result of X-chromosome inactivation, females heterozygous for two different *Gd* alleles exhibit somatic cell mosaicism.[35,42] This means that if one of the alleles entails enzyme deficiency, about half the cells will be G6PD(+) and the other half will be G6PD(−), although there is a large range of variation around that average[43,44] for various reasons, not all of them fully known. At first approximation it can be assumed that X-inactivation takes place at random, and therefore a binomial distribution would be expected; the width of this distribution depends on the number of cells in the embryo or in individual embryonic tissue at the time of X-inactivation. If this number is 32 to 64, a fraction of about 2% of women with an "extreme phenotype" is predicted, that is, with less than 5% of one of the two cell types; this is in good agreement with observation in an unselected sample of *Gd$^+$/Gd$^-$* heterozygotes,[44] although some studies have suggested an even larger proportion.[45]

TABLE 17-1	Heterogeneity and Clinical Expression of Glucose-6-Phosphate Dehydrogenase Deficiency				
Class*	Clinical Manifestations†	G6PD Activity (% of Normal)	Number of Known Mutant Alleles‡	Examples	Comments
IV	None	>85	2	A, B	G6PD B is the normal "wild type"
II + III	Asymptomatic in the steady state, but risk for NNJ, AHA, favism	<30	75	Med, A⁻, Orissa, Mahidol, Canton, Vanua Lava, Seattle	Most of these variants are known to be polymorphic
I	NNJ (severe), CNSHA, acute exacerbations	<10 in most cases	61	Sunderland, Nara, Guadalajara	Never polymorphic; but same mutation can recur

*The separation between class II and class III is blurred and, in the authors' opinion, no longer useful.
†In brief, variants in class II and III can be regarded as having a *mild* phenotype confined to *acute* episodes; variants in class I have a *severe* phenotype with *chronic* illness.
‡See Fig. 17-4B. We have counted only variants for which the mutation is known and the clinical expression clearly reported.
AHA, acute hemolytic anemia; CHSHA, congenital nonspherocytic hemolytic anemia; NNJ, neonatal jaundice.

Thus, in many cases unbalanced phenotypes may arise simply by chance, according to the laws of statistics. However, in certain cases there is evidence of selection at the somatic cell level after X-chromosome inactivation. This was first well established in women who are heterozygous for hypoxanthine phosphoribosyltransferase (HPRT) deficiency,[46] and it has also been observed in several women heterozygous for severely deficient G6PD variants.[47,48] In these cases one has to infer that the G6PD(–) state is a selective disadvantage for hematopoietic stem cells; interestingly, this disadvantage is cell lineage specific because it does not affect, for instance, fibroblasts.[47] Finally, because selection might take place at other X-linked loci,[49] heterozygotes exhibiting extreme phenotypes by analysis of G6PD may arise from selection acting on an allele at another locus (a "hitchhiking effect"), as has been suggested in a family with G6PD Ilesha.[50-52]

At the genomic level, the *Gd* gene (Fig. 17-4A) consists of 13 exons, the first of which is noncoding.[53] The total length of the gene is about 18.5 kilobases (kb), much of which (about 12 kb) consists of intron 2. The significance of this large intron is unknown; it may be important for efficient transcription or for processing because it is still the largest intron, even in the compressed version of the G6PD gene found in the puffer fish *Fugu rubripes*.[54] The promoter region is highly enriched in guanine and cytosine residues (i.e., GC rich), as found characteristically in other housekeeping genes.[55] Deletion analysis has revealed that the "essential" portion of the promoter is only about 150 bp long.[56] Within this

region, two Sp1 binding sites have been identified, either of which is essential for promoter activity.[57] This and other regions are highly conserved between human and mouse,[58] thus supporting the notion that they are important for gene regulation.

Features of G6PD in Red Cells

There is only one structural gene for G6PD, although a related autosomal hexose dehydrogenase also exists.[59,60] Biochemical evidence is in keeping with the notion that the G6PD protein in red cells is the same as that in other somatic cells; thus, when red cells are severely deficient in G6PD, this deficiency is also found to a greater or lesser degree in other somatic cells.[16] However, a significant difference in the metabolism of G6PD arises from the characteristic inability of mature red cells to synthesize protein. As a result, whereas in most somatic cells G6PD is subject to turnover, in red cells any G6PD molecule undergoing denaturation or proteolytic breakdown cannot be replaced (this is true, of course, not only for G6PD but also for most other red cell enzymes[61]). In normal red cells, the decay of G6PD approximates an exponential (see Fig. 17-6) with a half-life of about 60 days,[62] although it has been claimed that it may more closely approximate a two-slope curve with very fast breakdown when reticulocytes mature to erythrocytes and much slower breakdown subsequently.[63] The age dependence of red cell G6PD activity is so characteristic that it can almost be regarded as a marker of red cell age. In normal blood, reticulocytes have about five times more activity than the 10% oldest red cells.[64]

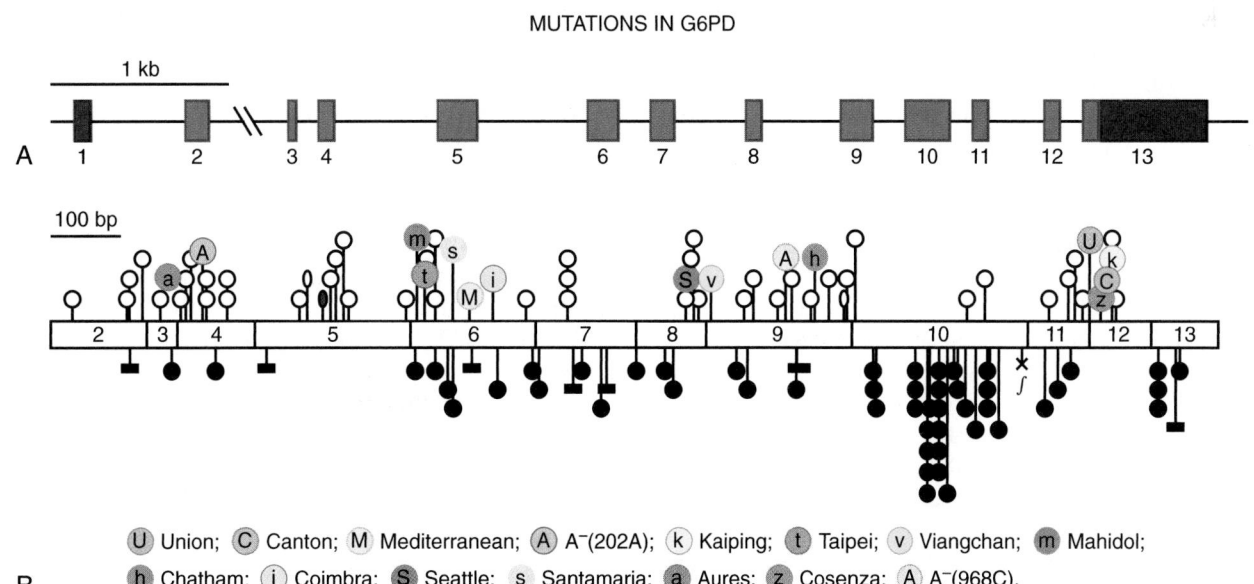

MUTATIONS IN G6PD

U Union; C Canton; M Mediterranean; A A⁻(202A); k Kaiping; t Taipei; v Viangchan; m Mahidol; h Chatham; i Coimbra; S Seattle; s Santamaria; a Aures; z Cosenza; A A⁻(968C).

FIGURE 17-4. The human G6PD genomic gene (**A**) showing exon-intron organization and a map of many of the known mutations (**B**). All variants shown, except G6PD A, are associated with enzyme deficiency. Below the diagram are mutations associated with a severe phenotype (class I), all of which are sporadic and rare. Above the diagram mutations are associated with a mild phenotype (class II or III), many of which are polymorphic, and some of those that have been more extensively investigated are shown by *initialed lollipop symbols*. A⁻ is heterogeneous because it can result from a combination of the N126D replacement with any of three additional mutations. However, in the large majority of instances (probably more than 90%), the second mutation of G6PD A⁻ is V68M.

Molecular Basis of G6PD Deficiency

In principle, genetically determined deficiency of G6PD, like that of any other protein, might be due either to quantitative changes, such as mutations that affect the amount of the enzyme but not its structure, or to qualitative changes, such as mutations that affect the structure of the enzyme and hence its stability or catalytic efficiency. Extensive investigations of G6PD from G6PD-deficient cells, mostly carried out before the sequence of G6PD was known, revealed that (1) enzyme activity, even when severely reduced (sometimes to less than 1% of normal), is never completely absent and (2) enzymic properties (K_m, K_i, activity on substrate analogues, thermostability, etc.) are often different from those of the normal enzyme[65] (i.e., G6PD deficiency is associated with qualitative abnormalities). These data are consistent with point mutations in the coding region. In fact, from a database[66] of nearly 150 mutant alleles now known a reasonably clear pattern has emerged.

1. In nearly all the G6PD variants there is a *single amino acid replacement* caused by a single missense point mutation.
2. In a few cases (namely, G6PD Santamaria, G6PD Mount Sinai, G6PD Akrokorinthos, and the three types of G6PD A⁻), *two amino acid replacements are found*; in all these cases one of the replacements is G6PD A (N126D). Because this nondeficient G6PD variant is polymorphic in Africa, the most likely explanation is that a second point mutation has taken place in a Gd^A gene. In another case, the two mutations G6PD Cassano (Q449H) and G6PD Union (R454C) are found in tandem in G6PD Hermoupolis; because both of the former are polymorphic, the latter night have arisen through intragenic recombination.[67]
3. Three small *in-frame deletions* have been discovered: one removes a single amino acid (G6PD Sunderland),[68] one removes two adjacent amino acids (G6PD Stonybrook),[69] and one removes eight adjacent amino acids (G6PD Nara).[70]
4. Only one mutation affecting *splicing*[71] has been discovered thus far.
5. The majority of the mutations (see Fig. 17-4B) in the database[66] are *sporadic*, and most of them have been detected because they result in G6PD deficiency and CNSHA by causing sufficient loss of activity in red cells to become limiting for their in vivo survival. Sporadic variants associated with CNSHA are not likely to spread by genetic drift. However, in several instances the same variant has been encountered recurrently (for instance, we have found G6PD Tokyo in Scotland,[72] G6PD Guadalajara has turned up in Japan[73] and in Belfast,[72,74] and G6PD Nara has been observed at least three times).[75] That the same mutation may be found recurrently in people who are almost certainly not ancestrally related is not trivial; these observations corroborate the notion that there must be specific subtle constraints whereby a particular G6PD variant has a distinctly severe clinical expression but remains compatible with life.
6. *Polymorphic mutations* (Fig. 17-5). The majority of known mutations in this category again are associated with G6PD deficiency, and there is overwhelming evidence that they have become polymorphic as a result of malaria selection (see later). For these mutations we can visualize more stringent constraints; indeed, though still causing deficiency in red cells, they must not affect them so severely that the advantage with respect to malaria is outweighed. Thus, it is not surprising that nearly all the polymorphic variants fall into classes II or III and none of them cause CNSHA (class I; see Table 17-1).
7. The *pattern of G6PD mutations*, whereby null mutations (such as nonsense mutations, frameshifts, or large deletions) are conspicuously absent, is in striking contrast to that seen in other inherited disorders, such as the thalassemias, hemophilia, and muscular dystrophy. An important functional difference between these conditions and G6PD deficiency is that the former result from mutations in tissue-specific genes whereas *Gd* is a housekeeping gene. When a tissue-specific gene is totally inactivated by a mutation, it may cause severe disease but will not necessarily have interfered with embryonic development. By contrast, we know that G6PD-null mutations are lethal to the mouse embryo[15]; they probably occur in humans, but we never see them because they must be lethal in the human embryo as well. Some clue regarding what mutation can cause G6PD deficiency has come from alignment of the amino acid sequence of G6PD from 42 different organisms; there was a striking correlation between the amino acid replacements that cause G6PD deficiency in humans and the sequence conservation of G6PD.[17] Interestingly two thirds of such replacements are in highly and moderately conserved (50% to 99%) amino acids; relatively few are in fully conserved amino acids (where they might be lethal) or in poorly conserved amino acids, where presumably they simply would not cause G6PD deficiency.
8. The *biochemical mechanism of G6PD deficiency* is strongly contingent on the fact that in normal red cells, G6PD decreases exponentially as red cells age, with a half-life of about 50 days (see earlier). Because G6PD is an oligomeric globular protein, it is not surprising that many point mutations producing replacement of individual amino acids can further decrease the stability of G6PD; in fact, for most mutants, enzyme instability is the main mechanism of enzyme deficiency[6,66,76] (Fig. 17-6). The instability is most extreme when the amino acid involved is at the interface between the two subunits of G6PD; in such cases the dimer does not form or falls apart.[24] This situation applies to G6PD mutants that cause the most severe clinical phenotypes (that of CNSHA; see later). In a few cases (e.g., G6PD Orissa), altered catalytic func-

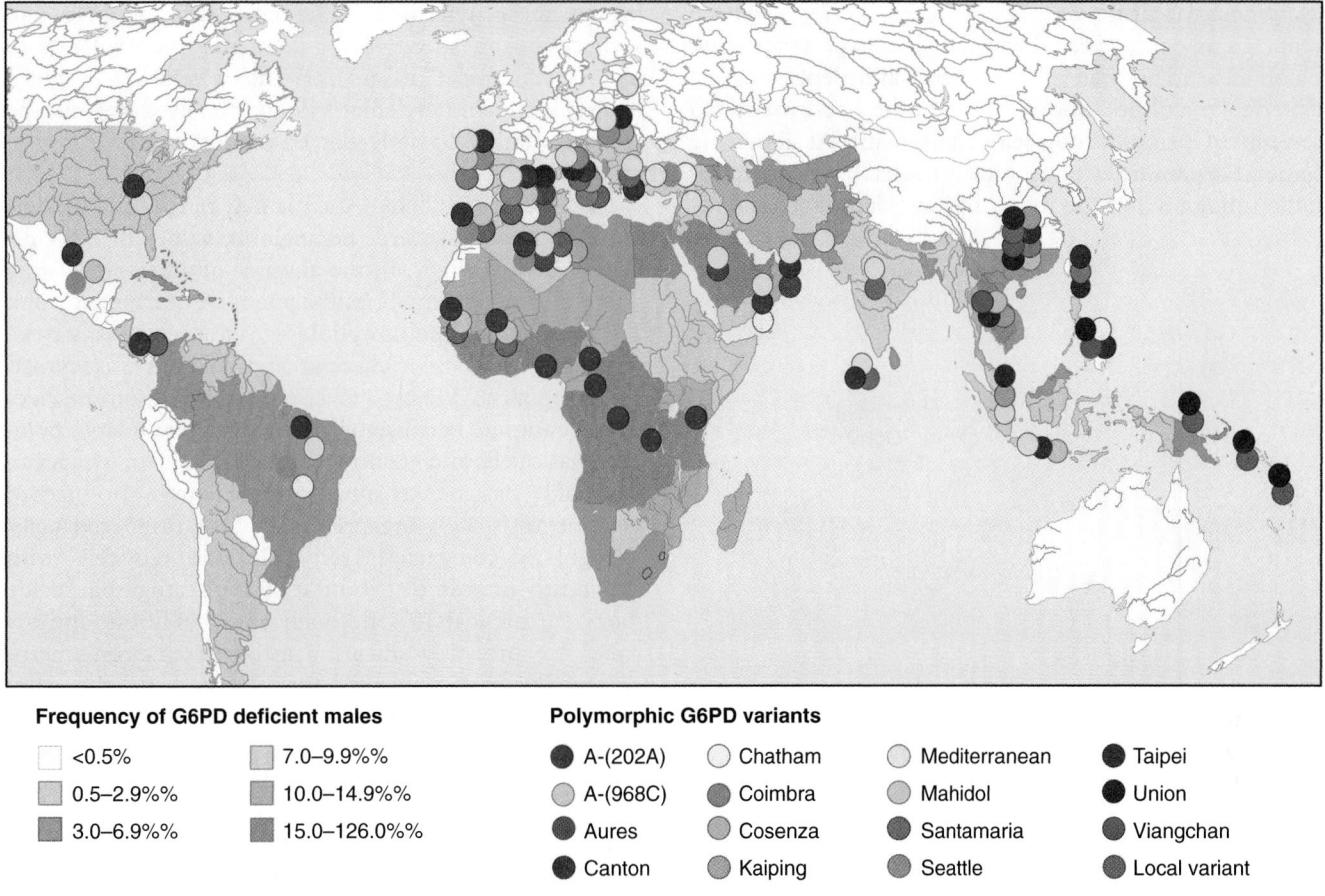

FIGURE 17-5. World map of G6PD deficiency. The *shadings* indicate the overall prevalence of G6PD deficiency in individual countries; the distribution of individual G6PD variants is shown by *colored symbols*. *(Redrawn from WHO Working Group. Glucose-6-phosphate dehydrogenase deficiency. Bull World Health Organ. 1989;67:601-611, and modified from Tan KL, Boey KW. Clinical experience with phototherapy. Ann Acad Med Singapore. 1989;18:43-48.)*

tion (instead of or in addition to protein instability) may be the main mechanism of G6PD deficiency.[77]

Epidemiology of G6PD Deficiency

The geographic distribution[78] of G6PD deficiency is rather extraordinary in two ways. First, it has a very high prevalence overall, with more than 500 million people estimated to be involved (most of them mostly asymptomatic); second, it has a high prevalence in many populations in most tropical and subtropical parts of the world because of malaria selection (see Fig. 17-5 and the last section in this chapter). Thus, G6PD is prevalent in all five continents; it has never been reported in Amerindians, and one might speculate that this is related to the fact that they have been exposed to malaria only over the past 3 centuries.

CLINICAL MANIFESTATIONS OF G6PD DEFICIENCY

The most classic manifestation of G6PD deficiency is acute hemolytic anemia (AHA); in children, however,

another syndrome of great clinical and public health importance is neonatal jaundice (NNJ). CNSHA is a much rarer manifestation of G6PD deficiency and a life-long hemolytic process. These different clinical manifestations are discussed in turn.

Acute Hemolytic Anemia

Clinical Picture. A child with G6PD deficiency is clinically and hematologically normal most of the time, and this can be designated as a steady-state condition. However, a rather dramatic clinical picture can develop upon ingestion of fava beans (favism),[79] during the course of infection, or after exposure to certain oxidative agents (see Table 17-3). With infection or drugs the clinical picture may be more complicated than with favism; therefore, here we will describe favism as a paradigm. After a lag of hours the child may become fractious and irritable or subdued and even lethargic. Within 24 to 48 hours the child's temperature is often moderately elevated. Nausea, abdominal pain, diarrhea, and rarely vomiting may be present. In striking contrast to these relatively nonspecific symptoms, the patient or a parent will observe, within 6 to 24 hours, the telltale and rather frightening event that the urine is discolored (Fig. 17-7). It will be reported as dark, as red, brown, or black, or as "passing blood instead of water;" it will be said, depending on experience, culture, and socioeconomic background, to resemble Coke or strong tea or port wine. At about the same time jaundice will become obvious. Physical examination may reveal little more than the signs corresponding to these symptoms. The child will be pale and tachycardic; in severe cases there may be evidence of hypovolemic shock or, less likely, heart failure. The spleen is usually moderately enlarged, and the liver may also be enlarged; either or both may be tender.

Laboratory Findings. Anemia may range from moderate to extremely severe (hemoglobin values of 2.5 g/dL have been recorded). In the absence of other preexisting hematologic abnormalities the anemia is normocytic and normochromic. The morphology of the red cells may be striking (Fig. 17-8A). There is often marked anisocytosis (reflected as a wide red cell size distribution on the electronic counter) because of the coexistence of large polychromatic cells and "contracted" cells, some of which can be frankly classified as spherocytes. There is also marked poikilocytosis with the presence of distorted red cells, "irregularly contracted" red cells, and red cells with apparently uneven distribution of the hemoglobin inside them (hemighosts).[80] Although some of these appearances are probably smearing artifacts, electron micrographic evidence suggests that in some of the cells, opposing surfaces of the membrane have become "crosslinked."[81] Probably the most characteristic poikilocytes are those in which the cell margin literally appears dented, as though a portion has been plucked out or bitten away ("bite cells"; see Fig. 17-8A). The reticulocyte count is increased and may reach peaks of 30% or greater (blood counters using immunofluorescent technology will show an elevated percentage of the immature reticulocyte fraction); this reflects a prompt and effective bone marrow response, which will take place provided that there is no preexisting or concomitant bone marrow pathology. Careful inspection of reticulocyte preparations may reveal inclusion bodies different from those normally seen in reticulocytes; these bodies are discrete, round, and 1 to 3 μm in diameter, and they usually appear to be leaning, from the interior, against the cell membrane. These inclusions are more clearly displayed by supravital staining with methyl violet and are referred to as *Heinz bodies* (see Fig. 17-8B). They consist of precipitates of denatured

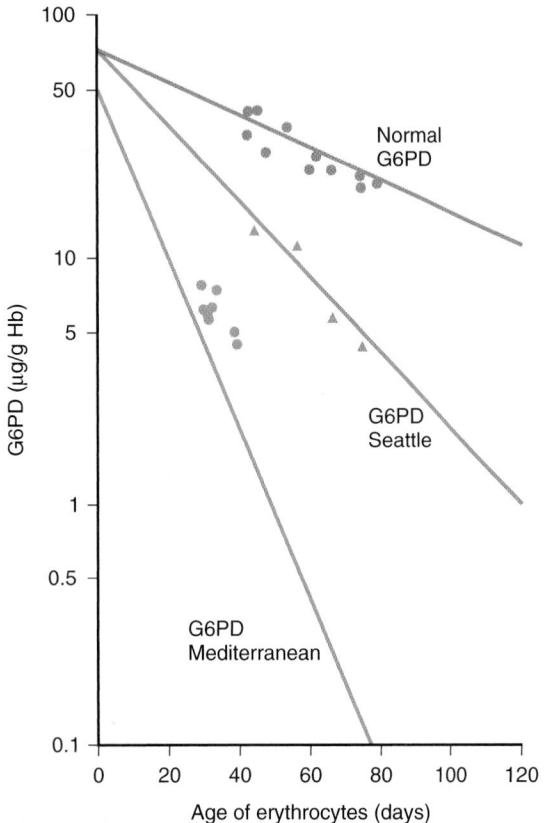

FIGURE 17-6. The main mechanism of G6PD deficiency in red cells is in vivo instability of mutant enzyme. For many G6PD variants, such as the two studied here, this is essentially acceleration of a process that takes place normally with the aging of red cells in the circulation. (*Redrawn from Morelli A, Benatti U, Gaetani GF, De Flora A. Biochemical mechanisms of glucose-6-phosphate dehydrogenase deficiency. Proc Natl Acad Sci U S A. 1978;75:1979-1983.*)

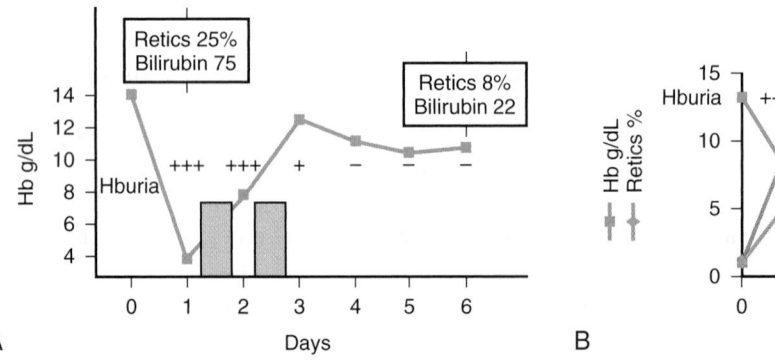

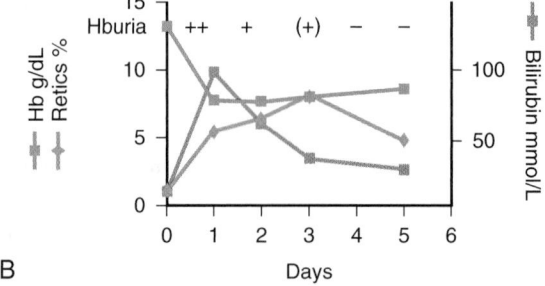

FIGURE 17-7. Clinical charts of children with acute favism. **A,** Severe attack in a 21-month-old boy, who required two blood transfusions (*hatched bars*) because of life-threatening anemia after the ingestion of fava beans. The second blood transfusion was administered because of persistent hemoglobinuria (Hburia). **B,** Milder attack in a 5-year-old boy. The mother, who is a physician and knows that she is G6PD deficient, reported that the child had eaten fava beans 2 days before admission. Both children had severe G6PD deficiency (red blood cell G6PD activity less than 3% of normal). The values on day 0 are presumed. Hb, hemoglobin; Retics, reticulocytes. (*Courtesy of Professor Tullio Meloni, Sassari, Sardinia.*)

TABLE 17-2	Hemoglobinuria in Children	
Condition	**Circumstances**	**Diagnostic Approach**
G6PD deficiency	Exposure to a trigger of hemolysis	Test for G6PD activity
Blackwater fever	Relatively rare complication of malaria	Blood slide for malaria parasites
Paroxysmal cold hemoglobinuria	Usually associated with viral infection	Test for Donath-Landsteiner antibody
Mismatched blood transfusion	Usually ABO incompatibility	Repeat crossmatch
Paroxysmal nocturnal hemoglobinuria	Tends to recur	Flow cytometry for CD59
Clostridium welchii septicemia	Burns, severe open trauma, transfusion of contaminated blood	Culture of blood or appropriate patient material

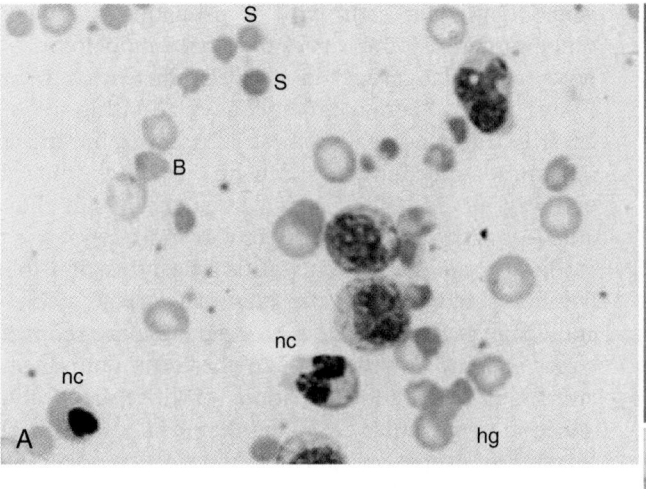
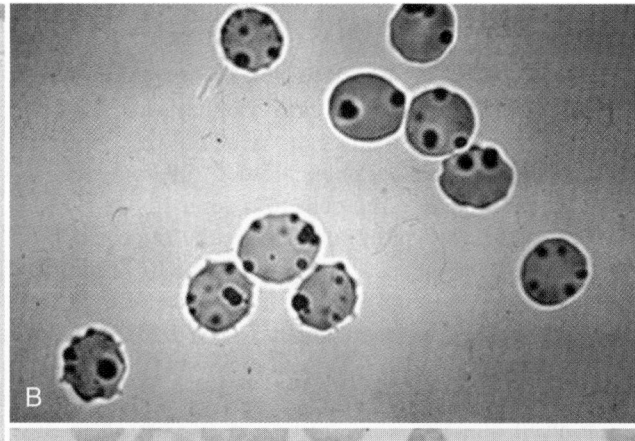
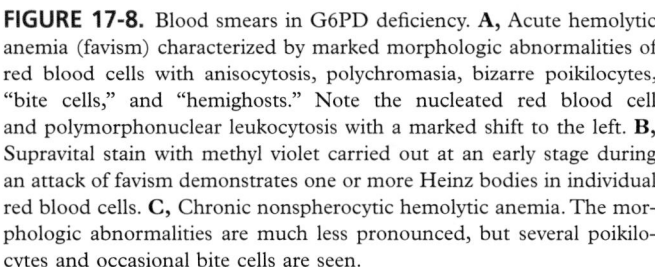
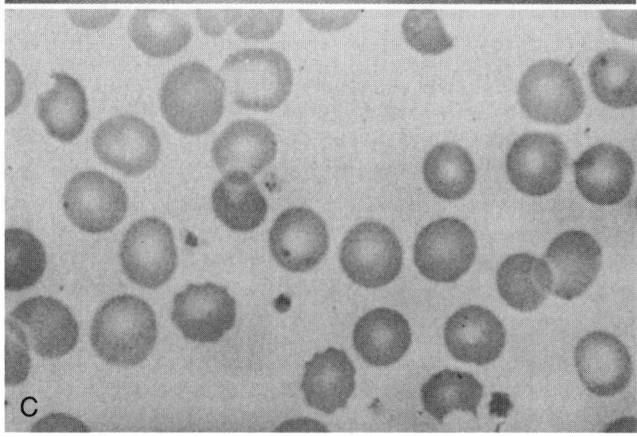

FIGURE 17-8. Blood smears in G6PD deficiency. **A,** Acute hemolytic anemia (favism) characterized by marked morphologic abnormalities of red blood cells with anisocytosis, polychromasia, bizarre poikilocytes, "bite cells," and "hemighosts." Note the nucleated red blood cell and polymorphonuclear leukocytosis with a marked shift to the left. **B,** Supravital stain with methyl violet carried out at an early stage during an attack of favism demonstrates one or more Heinz bodies in individual red blood cells. **C,** Chronic nonspherocytic hemolytic anemia. The morphologic abnormalities are much less pronounced, but several poikilocytes and occasional bite cells are seen.

hemoglobin, and they are the vivid manifestation of the oxidative insult that this protein and the cell itself has suffered. However, Heinz bodies are a very transient finding because they tend to be promptly "pinched off" by the spleen[82] (thus giving rise to bite cells) and the red cells containing them are very rapidly removed from the circulation. Haptoglobin is reduced to the point of being undetectable. In severe cases it is possible to demonstrate free hemoglobin in plasma (*hemoglobinemia*). The white blood cell count is usually moderately elevated, with a predominance of granulocytes. The platelet count may be normal, increased, or moderately decreased. The unconjugated bilirubin level is elevated, but "liver enzyme" levels are generally normal. The dark urine tests strongly positive for blood because of the presence of free hemoglobin (see the differential diagnosis of this sign in Table 17-2).

Clinical Course. In the majority of cases the hemolytic attack, even if severe, is self-limited and tends to resolve spontaneously (see Fig. 17-7B). Depending on the proportion of red cells that have been destroyed (as reflected by the severity of the anemia), the hemoglobin level may be back to normal in 3 to 6 weeks. Although the blood urea level may be transiently elevated, the development of renal failure in children is exceedingly rare, even in the presence of massive hemoglobinuria (see Fig. 17-7A).

Diagnosis. With a history of fava bean ingestion followed by hemoglobinuria (see Table 17-2), the diagnosis is almost always straightforward, and it can be made quite confidently even before obtaining the final proof that the patient is G6PD deficient (see later). If the hemoglobinuria has already subsided and the history is uncertain, one is faced instead with the much wider differential diagnosis of AHA. A negative direct antiglobulin test will militate against autoimmune hemolytic anemia. In endemic areas it will be important to exclude malaria or the much rarer babesiosis. In hemolytic-uremic syndrome, the red cell morphology is different and there will be evidence of impaired renal function. In all cases, demonstration of G6PD deficiency will be conclusive, and in uncertain cases it will be crucial.

Pathophysiology. The clinical picture of AHA in a G6PD-deficient child is a vivid expression of the fact that as we know already, hemolysis results from the action of an exogenous factor on intrinsically abnormal red cells. Hemoglobinemia and hemoglobinuria unambiguously indicate that the hemolysis is at least in part intravascular. At first approximation we can visualize the following sequence of events: (1) an oxidative agent causes conversion of GSH to GSSG; (2) because of the limited capacity of G6PD-deficient red cells to regenerate GSH, their GSH reserve is rapidly depleted; (3) once GSH is exhausted, the sulfhydryl groups of hemoglobin and probably other proteins are oxidized to disulfides or sulfoxides; and (4) coarse precipitates of denatured hemoglobin cause irreversible damage to the membrane, and the red cells lyse.

Not all of these steps from oxidative attack to final hemolysis have been fully documented in vivo, in part because of one major difficulty: in the course of AHA the red cells sampled from the patient are obviously, at any given stage, those that have not yet hemolyzed. However, GSH depletion is a most characteristic finding when red cells are subjected to oxidative challenge,[83,84] and in one careful study it has been demonstrated that during an attack of favism, the first measurable biochemical change is a fall in NADPH, followed by a fall in GSH,[85] in keeping with stages 1 and 2 described earlier. Heinz bodies (see Fig. 17-8B) are the visible expression of stage 3. Stage 4 is less clearly defined, although studies suggest that the abnormal proteolytic activity is associated with increased intracellular calcium,[86,87] as well as binding of hemichromes (arising from denaturation of hemoglobin) to band 3 molecules.[88]

Even though intravascular hemolysis in AHA associated with G6PD deficiency is important in pathophysiology and diagnosis, a substantial proportion of the hemolysis is extravascular (as shown by the enlarged spleen). Probably the most severely damaged red cells hemolyze in the bloodstream on their own, whereas less severely damaged red cells will be recognized as abnormal by macrophages and will undergo extravascular hemolysis in the reticuloendothelial system. This process has been referred to as an example of an "innocent bystander" phenomenon[89] (although the red cells, by virtue of being G6PD deficient, are not that innocent), in which complement and immunoglobulins may be involved.[90] Finally, it is important to remember that the red cell destruction in AHA associated with G6PD deficiency is an orderly function of red cell age (see Fig. 17-6). The oldest red cells with the least G6PD are the first to hemolyze, and the hemolytic process progresses upstream toward cells with more and more G6PD.[91] As a result, there is a selective enrichment in red cells that despite being genetically G6PD deficient, have relatively higher levels of G6PD. This phenomenon can be so marked with certain G6PD variants that patients in the post-hemolytic state are found to be relatively resistant to further challenge; thus, the patient may be in a state of compensated hemolysis.[92]

Triggers and Mechanism of Hemolysis. G6PD deficiency was first discovered by investigating a possible genetic basis for sensitivity to primaquine. Since that time, numerous other drugs have been reported as being potentially dangerous in G6PD-deficient individuals (Table 17-3). There is no obvious relationship in chemical structure among all of these substances, but they have in common the ability to stimulate the pentose phosphate pathway in red cells,[93] which must mean that they are able to oxidize NADPH, directly or indirectly. Extensive studies on the components of fava beans responsible for hemolysis have led to the identification of vicine and convicine, two β-glycosides that generate the redox aglycones divicine and isouramil.[94] These compounds, in the course of their auto-oxidation, produce free radicals, which in turn oxidize GSH and thereby activate the chain reaction of events previously outlined.[95] The drugs listed in Table 17-3, or their metabolites, act in a similar way. Cosmetic use of henna dyes in several populations, mainly in Asia, can also cause serious hemolysis.[96-99]

An intriguing feature of AHA associated with G6PD deficiency is its considerably erratic character, which is

TABLE 17-3	Drugs That Can Trigger Hemolysis in G6PD-Deficient Children*	
Category of Drug	**Definite Risk**	**Possible Risk**
Antimalarials	Primaquine Dapsone-containing combinations†	Chloroquine Quinine
Analgesics	Acetanilid	Aspirin
Sulfonamides/sulfones	Sulfamethoxazole/co-trimoxazole Dapsone†	Sulfasalazine Sulfadiazine
Quinolones	Nalidixic acid Ciprofloxacin Norfloxacin Moxifloxacin Ofloxacin	
Other antimicrobials	Nitrofurantoin Methylene blue	Chloramphenicol
Other	Niridazole	Vitamin K Rasburicase Ascorbic acid Glibenclamide

*For all drugs the risk of hemolysis is dose related, as well as the severity of hemolysis. For instance, aspirin up to 20 mg/kg is probably safe; three times that dose will almost certainly cause some hemolysis.
†Dapsone can cause hemolysis even in non–G6PD-deficient children.
Table modified from British National Formulary, 55th edition, March 2008.

more conspicuous with certain agents than with others. For instance, it is estimated that in adults, ingestion of fava beans does not trigger AHA in more than 25% of cases, and even in the same person favism may occur on one occasion but not on another.[90] One obvious factor must be the dosage, that is, the amount of fava beans ingested (in relation to body mass). Another is the quality, with raw fava beans being more likely to cause favism than cooked, frozen, or canned fava beans. Perhaps even more important is the finding that the glycoside content is a function of the maturity of the beans, with young, small beans being much richer (as well as more tasty!). With respect to drugs, primaquine causes hemolysis regularly but aspirin does so only sometimes[100]; once again, the dosage must be important, but additional genetic or acquired factors affecting metabolism of the drug may play a role. As regards infection, the best documented precipitants are hepatitis, pneumonia, and typhoid fever, but viral infections of the upper respiratory or gastrointestinal tract may also trigger hemolysis.[101] Recently it has been reported[102] that in a group of patients who suffered major trauma in road traffic accidents, the frequency and severity of infection were significantly higher in patients who were G6PD deficient; in addition, more severe anemia occurred in this group.

Release of peroxides during phagocytosis of bacteria by granulocytes might explain the hemolytic process in bacterial infections.[103] In this respect it is possible that hemolysis has sometimes been attributed to drugs used for treating infection when it should have been blamed on the infection itself.

Treatment. A child with AHA may be a diagnostic problem that once solved, does not require any specific treatment at all, or the child may be a medical emergency requiring immediate action. The most urgent question is whether a blood transfusion is needed. It is difficult to give absolute directives, but the following guidelines may be useful[104]:

1. If the hemoglobin level is below 7 g/dL, the child should be transfused forthwith.
2. If the hemoglobin level is below 9 g/dL and there is evidence of persistent brisk hemolysis (hemoglobinuria), immediate blood transfusion is also indicated.
3. If the hemoglobin level is above 9 g/dL but hemoglobinuria persists or if the hemoglobin level is between 7 and 9 g/dL but there is no hemoglobinuria, the child is kept under close observation for at least 48 hours and transfused if either condition 1 or 2 develops.

The most important complication that may require treatment is acute renal failure, which is exceedingly rare in children.

Neonatal Jaundice

From an *epidemiologic* point of view, it is noteworthy that the frequency of NNJ varies widely in different populations; in many populations in which G6PD deficiency is prevalent, the rate of pregnancies at risk for Rhesus incompatibility happens to be low.[105,106] In addition, as rhesus-related hemolytic disease of the newborn (HDN) is disappearing thanks to the implementation of appropriate prophylaxis, one can expect G6PD-related NNJ to be generally on the increase, at least in relative terms.

Clinical Features. NNJ related to G6PD deficiency is very rarely present at birth; it has a peak incidence between day 2 and day 3.[107] There is more jaundice than anemia, and the anemia is very rarely severe.[108] For this reason the terms *HDN* and *NNJ* cannot be regarded as interchangeable, at least in the context of G6PD deficiency. The severity of G6PD-related NNJ varies from being subclinical to imposing the threat of kernicterus if not treated. Thus, prompt recognition of the problem is extremely important to avoid crippling neurologic sequelae.[109-112]

Nature of the Association between G6PD Deficiency and Neonatal Jaundice. It is not fully explained why NNJ develops in some but not all G6PD-deficient newborns. Several clinical studies have established beyond any possible doubt that the association is statistically much higher than could be expected by chance (Table 17-4).[113] However, because not *all* G6PD-deficient newborns have NNJ (Table 17-5), it is likely that genetic or environmental factors (or both) are involved in addition to G6PD deficiency and that the same factors can also, if more extreme, make the NNJ more severe. NNJ is not the prerogative of some G6PD variant because it is prevalent in widely remote parts of the world (e.g., Nigeria,[113] Sardinia,[114] Singapore,[115] China[116]) in which the *Gd* alleles underlying G6PD deficiency are different; moreover, both within Sardinia[117] and within Taiwan,[118] NNJ has been found in babies with any of several different G6PD variants. The possibility that NNJ correlates with the quantitative level of residual G6PD activity is controversial.[119,120] Specific features of erythrocytes in newborns, such as elevated levels of ascorbic acid, depressed activity of glutathione reductase,[113] and low levels of vitamin E, GSHPX, and other enzymes,[121] could contribute to the degree of jaundice. It must be noted that there is a

TABLE 17-4	Association between G6PD Deficiency and Jaundice in Newborns	
	Number	% G6PD Deficient
Normal	500	22.5
Mild jaundice (bilirubin 150-200 µmol/L)	38	45
Severe jaundice (bilirubin >230 µmol/L)	70	60
Admitted with kernicterus	20	78

Data collected in Ibadan, Nigeria, on consecutive babies born in or admitted to a teaching hospital; see Bienzle U, Effiong CE, Luzzatto L. Erythrocyte glucose 6-phosphate dehydrogenase deficiency (G6PD type A⁻) and neonatal jaundice. Acta Paediatr Scand. 1976;65:701-704.

TABLE 17-5   Features of Neonatal Jaundice in 500 African American Male Babies

	G6PD Normal (*n* = 436)	G6PD Deficient (*n* = 64)
Plasma total bilirubin (PTB), mmol/L	139 ± 48	157 ± 43
Median end-tidal CO, ppm	2.1 (1.7-2.5)	2.4 (2.0-2.9)
Babies with PTB >75th percentile (%)	23.4	48
Babies with PTB >95th percentile (%)	6.7	22
Mean age at which the highest PTB occurs (hr)	64	55
Babies requiring phototherapy (%)	5.7	20.3

Data from Kaplan M, Herschel M, Hammerman C, et al. Hyperbilirubinemia among African American, glucose-6-phosphate dehydrogenase–deficient neonates. Pediatrics. 2004;114:e213-e219.

remarkable dissociation between hyperbilirubinemia and anemia in G6PD-deficient neonates.[108,114] Indeed, in one series there was no difference in the distribution of hematocrit values in cord blood and on day 3 between jaundiced and nonjaundiced G6PD-deficient newborns, thus suggesting that to a large extent this jaundice may be of hepatic origin rather than hemolytic. In keeping with this notion, measurements of the bilirubin production-conjugation index have demonstrated that the NNJ in otherwise healthy G6PD-deficient neonates depends more on inefficient bilirubin conjugation than on hemolysis.[122] The *UDPGT1* mutation characteristic of Gilbert's disease is associated with a much higher risk for NNJ and kernicterus in G6PD-deficient babies.[123,124] In addition, environmental factors can certainly exacerbate NNJ, in some cases by causing hemolysis in individual G6PD-deficient newborns; such factors include prematurity, breast-feeding,[125] naphthalene (camphor balls) inhalation, acidosis, hypoxia, infection such as viral hepatitis,[126] oxidant drugs, and ingestion of drugs[127] or fava beans (favism in utero[128]) by the mother before delivery.

In summary, there are probably two different types of NNJ associated with G6PD deficiency: (1) a more common type (see Table 17-5) can best be visualized as a marked exaggeration of "physiologic jaundice"; this type is usually clinical benign and not greatly influenced by the environment; and (2) a rarer, frankly hemolytic type, more severe, can be visualized as AHA occurring in a newborn baby because the baby happened to be exposed to one of the same agents that could cause AHA even in an adult.

Severe NNJ can occur in girls heterozygous for G6PD deficiency.[129] In addition, in geographic areas where G6PD deficiency is very common, female newborns might be homozygous for the trait, thus behaving like a hemizygous G6PD-deficient male newborn.

Treatment. Management of NNJ associated with G6PD deficiency does not differ from that recommended for other causes. Thus, mild cases do not require treatment; intermediate cases require phototherapy; and severe cases require exchange transfusion, just as in NNJ caused by "classic" HDN. Kernicterus is still an impending threat, especially when severe NNJ is associated with anemia, hypoxia, or infection. Clinical practice guidelines for the management of hyperbilirubinemia in newborns quote: "measurement of the glucose-6-phosphate dehydrogenase (G6PD) is recommended for a jaundiced infant who is receiving phototherapy and whose family history or ethnic or geographic origin suggest the likelihood of G6PD deficiency or for an infant in whom the response to the phototherapy is poor."[130] G6PD-deficient newborns must be considered as being "*at high risk*"[125] and therefore requiring greater surveillance and more intensive treatment of hyperbilirubinemia. Specifically, it is recommended that in full-term newborns, exchange transfusion be carried out if the serum bilirubin level exceeds 15 mg/dL in the first 2 days of life or 19 mg/dL at any time in the first week of life.

Congenital Nonspherocytic Hemolytic Anemia

A small minority of children with G6PD deficiency have hemolytic anemia not only when it is triggered by an exogenous factor but even in the steady state (Fig. 17-9). These children have special G6PD mutations (class I); all of them are rare, but they are scattered worldwide, regardless of whether G6PD deficiency is endemic in the region.

The patient is invariably male and in general is evaluated because of unexplained jaundice, frequently presenting at birth (NNJ). (The only known exception is a woman heterozygous for G6PD Volendam, who had an extremely skewed X-inactivation pattern favoring, paradoxically, the X chromosome with the abnormal G6PD allele.[132]) Unfortunately, anemia recurs and the jaundice fails to clear completely, thus requiring further investigation. In other cases, NNJ may have been overlooked or forgotten and the patient is reinvestigated only much later in life (e.g., because of gallstones in a boy or in a young adult). The severity of the anemia ranges from being borderline to being transfusion dependent in different patients (Table 17-6). The anemia is usually normochromic but somewhat macrocytic because a large proportion of reticulocytes (up to 20% or more) will cause an increased mean corpuscular volume and a shifted, wider than normal red cell size distribution curve. The red cell morphology is mostly not characteristic, and

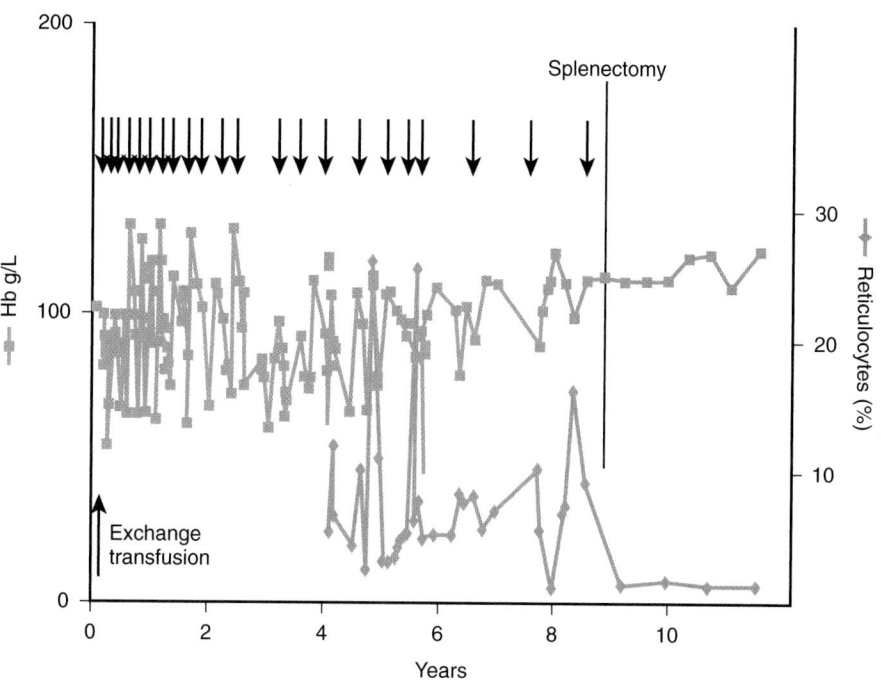

FIGURE 17-9. Clinical course of a boy with congenital nonspherocytic hemolytic anemia (CNSHA) caused by severe G6PD deficiency. Severe neonatal jaundice was the initial manifestation; subsequently, the child developed normally but required many blood transfusions. The transfusion dependence remitted after splenectomy. Currently, the patient, now in his early twenties, has had a cholecystectomy; he has moderate anemia and is still jaundiced. The patient's *Gd* mutation was characterized as G6PD Harilaou (F216L).[47,131]

TABLE 17-6	Clinical Spectrum of Chronic Nonspherocytic Hemolytic Anemia Caused by Severe G6PD Deficiency	
Patients studied		**25 (all male)**
% With neonatal jaundice		100
% Requiring exchange transfusion		24
% With splenomegaly		68
Steady-state hemoglobin, range (g/dL)		6-14
Lowest hemoglobin known, range (g/dL)		3.8-9.3
Reticulocytes, range (%)		3-51
% Requiring multiple blood transfusion		72

for this reason it is referred to in the negative as being "nonspherocytic." The bone marrow shows normoblastic hyperplasia, unless the increased requirement for folic acid associated with the high red cell turnover has caused it to become megaloblastic. There is chronic hyperbilirubinemia, decreased haptoglobin, and increased lactate dehydrogenase. Hemoglobinuria is rare, but hemosiderinuria may be detected sometimes. The spleen is usually moderately enlarged in small children, and subsequently it may increase in size sufficiently to cause mechanical discomfort, hypersplenism, or both.

Pathophysiology. The pattern of hemolysis in these patients is different from that described earlier for AHA associated with G6PD deficiency and instead more reminiscent of the chronic hemolysis seen in hereditary spherocytosis. However, oxidative stress caused by exposure to the same agents that cause AHA will cause acute exacerbation of hemolysis in CNSHA. Unlike the situation in thalassemia major, even in severe cases there is no

evidence of ineffective erythropoiesis. The fact that there is no hemoglobinuria, at least in the steady state, suggests that the hemolysis is mainly extravascular and therefore that its mechanism is different from that of AHA. Studies of red cell membrane proteins have revealed the presence of high-molecular-weight aggregates[133,134] consisting largely of spectrin, which seem to make the membrane abnormally susceptible to shear-induced fragmentation.[135] These abnormalities in the red cells of G6PD-deficient patients with CNSHA are not found in asymptomatic G6PD-deficient subjects, thus suggesting that whereas in the latter the reductive potential of residual G6PD is adequate in the steady state, in the former, continuous oxidation of sulfhydryl groups takes place, followed by irreversible changes in the configuration of membrane proteins. The reason why the severity of CNSHA associated with G6PD deficiency is so variable is that almost every case is due to a different mutation (see later) and each mutation will have a different effect on stability of the enzyme, on its kinetic properties, or on both.

Diagnosis. Laboratory diagnosis of G6PD deficiency is discussed next, but a special problem in relation to CNSHA is to firmly establish the causal link between the former and the latter. If the patient is, for example, a Swede of Swedish ancestry or a Japanese of Japanese ancestry, the link will be taken for granted, and this is generally justified, given the rarity of G6PD deficiency in these populations. On the other hand, if the patient is from a population in which G6PD deficiency is common, its presence in a patient with CNSHA might be a mere coincidence, and the cause of the CNSHA might be something else altogether. In such cases, while other causes of CNSHA are being ruled out, it becomes essential to characterize the G6PD of the patient. If it is a common variant known to be asymptomatic in other subjects, it can certainly be exonerated, whereas if it is a new unique variant, it is likely to be the culprit.

Treatment. In general terms, management of CNSHA associated with G6PD deficiency does not differ from that of CNSHA related to other causes (e.g., pyruvate kinase deficiency). If the anemia is not severe, regular folic acid supplements and regular hematologic surveillance suffice. It is important to avoid exposure to potentially hemolytic drugs, and blood transfusion may be indicated when exacerbations occur, mostly in concomitance with intercurrent infection. In rare patients, the anemia is so severe that it must be regarded as transfusion dependent. In these cases blood transfusion will probably be needed at approximately 2-month intervals to keep the hemoglobin in the 8- to 10-g/dL range. A hypertransfusion regimen aiming to maintain a normal hemoglobin level is not indicated (because there is no ineffective erythropoiesis in the bone marrow). However, depending on the extent of the blood transfusion requirement, appropriate iron chelation should be instituted from the age of 2 years onward and must be continued as long as transfusion treatment is necessary; sometimes the transfusion requirement may decrease after puberty.

A special problem is that of splenectomy.[72] There is no evidence of selective red cell destruction in the spleen, as in hereditary spherocytosis. However, the fact that the spleen is usually enlarged suggests that its role in hemolysis is not negligible. In practice, there are three indications for splenectomy: (1) if splenomegaly becomes a physical encumbrance; (2) if there is evidence of hypersplenism; and (3) if the anemia is severe, even in the absence of the first two indications. Splenectomy may reduce the overall rate of hemolysis (see Fig. 17-9) just enough to make a transfusion-dependent child become transfusion independent.[136] This is doubly important because it will make it possible to dispense with iron chelation. Active immunizations before splenectomy and penicillin prophylaxis after splenectomy must be started according to national guidelines such as that produced by the British Committee for the Standards in Haematology (http://www.bcshguidelines.com/pdf/SPLEEN21.pdf).

When a diagnosis of CNSHA is made, the family must be given genetic counseling, and it is advisable to establish whether the mother is a heterozygote. If she is, the chance of recurrence is 1:2 for every subsequent male pregnancy. Prenatal diagnosis should be offered; although it could be carried out on amniotic fluid cells, it would be much preferable[137] to determine the mutation involved and test for it on DNA from chorionic villi. G6PD-deficient patients with severe CNSHA (see Fig. 17-9), because its clinical manifestations are limited to blood cells, would in principle be good candidates for gene therapy by gene transfer into hematopoietic stem cells. This approach has not yet reached the stage of clinical application, but preclinical experiments have been carried out successfully in mice[138] and Rhesus monkeys.[139]

LABORATORY DIAGNOSIS OF G6PD DEFICIENCY

Although the clinical picture of favism and other forms of AHA associated with G6PD deficiency is characteristic, the final diagnosis must rely on direct demonstration of decreased activity of this enzyme in red cells. In NNJ and CNSHA, the differential diagnosis is much wider, and therefore this test is even more important. Fortunately, the enzyme assay is very easy, and numerous "screening tests" can be used as substitutes if a spectrophotometer is not available. However, a number of potential pitfalls and sources of error must be understood, and the use of commercial kits is not a substitute for such understanding. Here the value and limitations of the regular quantitative assay are discussed first, and then the use of alternatives is mentioned.

Tests for G6PD Deficiency

G6PD can be assayed by the classic spectrophotometric method,[140] which directly measures the rate of formation of NADPH through its characteristic absorption peak in the near ultraviolet spectrum at 340 nm. Red cell activity is expressed in international units (micromoles of NADPH produced per minute) per gram of hemoglobin; therefore, it is best to assay the enzyme activity and the hemoglobin concentration in the same hemolysate and work out the ratio. Because G6PD activity is much higher in leukocytes (particularly in granulocytes) than in erythrocytes, for accurate measurements it is essential to remove all leukocytes by the Ficoll-Hypaque method or by filtration through cellulose powder[141] rather than by the cruder approach of sucking off the buffy coat; however, for the purpose of clinical diagnosis of G6PD deficiency, this is not strictly necessary. In normal red cells the range of G6PD activity, measured at 30° C, is 7 to 10 IU/g of hemoglobin.

Several "screening tests" for G6PD deficiency are useful and reliable provided that they are run properly and their limitations are understood. The most popular are the dye decolorization tests,[142] the methemoglobin reduction test,[143] and the fluorescence spot test.[144] Recently, a formazan-based screening test has been developed[145] and field-tested.[146] All these methods are semiquantitative, and they are meant to classify a sample simply as "normal" or "deficient." The cutoff point can be set by following the appropriate instructions and by trial and error in the individual diagnostic laboratory; one should aim to classify as deficient any sample having less than 30% of normal activity because above this level one is unlikely to encounter clinical manifestations. Screening tests are of course especially useful for testing large numbers of samples. They are also perfectly adequate for diagnostic purposes in patients who are in the steady state but *not* for patients in the post-hemolytic period or with other complications; in addition, they cannot be expected to identify all heterozygotes. Finally, an ideal screening test ought not to give "false-negative" results

TABLE 17-7	Red Blood Cell G6PD Levels in Various Clinical Situations			
Clinical Condition	Gender	Result of Screening Test	Result of G6PD Assay	Interpretation
Normal	M or F	Normal	8.1	Normal
Normal	M	Abnormal	0.4	G6PD deficiency, steady state
Normal	F	Abnormal	2.1	Heterozygote for G6PD deficiency
Normal	F	Normal	4.9	Heterozygote for G6PD deficiency
Acute hemolysis	M	Abnormal	2.3	AHA in G6PD-deficient boy
Acute hemolysis	F	Normal	7.2	AHA in G6PD heterozygote girl
Chronic hemolysis	M	Normal	15.5	Hemolysis unrelated to G6PD deficiency
Chronic hemolysis	M	Abnormal	1.4	CNSHA, probably caused by G6PD deficiency

AHA, acute hemolytic anemia; CNSHA, congenital nonspherocytic hemolytic anemia; G6PD, glucose-6-phosphate dehydrogenase.

(i.e., it should not misclassify a G6PD-deficient subject as normal), but it can be allowed to give a few "false-positive" results (i.e., a G6PD-normal subject might be misclassified as being G6PD deficient). Ideally, every patient found to be G6PD deficient by screening should be confirmed by the spectrophotometric assay. For special purposes, formazan-based cytochemical methods are also available.[147,148]

The Effect of Red Cell Age and Selective Hemolysis. Because G6PD decreases gradually as red cells age,[61] any condition associated with reticulocytosis will entail an *increase* in G6PD activity (Table 17-7). This means that if a subject is genetically G6PD normal, in the course of hemolysis, red cell G6PD activity will now be *above* the normal range. This does not affect the diagnosis because G6PD deficiency will be correctly ruled out. However, if the subject is genetically G6PD deficient, red cell G6PD may now be raised to the extent of being near or even within the normal range, and the patient might therefore be misclassified as being G6PD normal[149] (even though at the onset of the attack the level may have been low).[150] Thus, after a hemolytic attack two circumstances concur to cause a risk of misdiagnosis: first, the older cells have been destroyed selectively; second, the marrow response has caused a sudden outpouring of young cells into the peripheral blood. (A third confusing factor may be admixture of G6PD-normal red cells if the patient has been transfused.) Although the reticulocyte count is a good warning to avoid this mistake, it must be realized that because reticulocytes turn into morphologically "mature" erythrocytes within 1 to 2 days, their count is not a sensitive index of mean red cell age; in other words, mean red cell age may be significantly younger than normal even when the reticulocyte count is normal. There are several ways to circumvent these problems. First, a G6PD level in the low-normal range (as opposed to higher than normal) in the presence of reticulocytosis is always suspicious; indeed, this finding suggests that the patient is actually G6PD deficient. Second, if the patient is suffering or is recovering from AHA, the suspicion generated from the finding just mentioned can be simply kept in store for a few weeks, when the situation will be evolving toward the steady state, and a repeat test will prove

whether the patient is indeed G6PD deficient. Third, if either the urgency of some clinical decision or academic curiosity demands a more prompt solution of the problem, the presence of severely G6PD-deficient red cells can be demonstrated either by enzyme assay of the oldest cells (fractionated by sedimentation) or by a cytochemical method (see earlier).

G6PD Deficiency in Heterozygotes. For hemolysis to be clinically significant in heterozygous girls, at least 50% of the red cells must be deficient, and therefore the G6PD level will be about 50% of normal or less. This level of deficiency can be diagnosed by a quantitative test; however, the problems associated with current or recent hemolysis outlined for male patients will be compounded in the case of heterozygous females, and they can usually be overcome by a similar approach, particularly with the use of a cytochemical test. A different matter is the biologic diagnosis of heterozygosity, regardless of immediate clinical implications, as may sometimes be required for appropriate genetic counseling. In cases of "extreme phenotypes" (sometimes referred to as arising from "imbalanced lyonization"), the G6PD-deficient red cells may be so few that the only way to identify heterozygous G6PD deficiency will be by DNA analysis, for which the underlying mutation must be known or identified for the purpose. A special situation involves heterozygotes for G6PD variants associated with CNSHA. In the authors' experience, the mothers of (male) patients with this condition are often G6PD normal, either because the variant in the offspring is due to a de novo mutation[151] or because the mother is a heterozygote but is phenotypically normal, presumably because somatic selection has favored the hematopoietic progenitor cells with the normal G6PD allele.[48]

Molecular Analysis of the G6PD Gene. In the vast majority of cases, the family history, the clinical course, and a G6PD assay are sufficient to establish the diagnosis of conditions associated with G6PD deficiency. In special cases (see the previous section for heterozygote diagnosis) and particularly in the case of CNSHA, identification of mutations in the G6PD gene can be carried out, with reference to the large numbers of mutations already known (see Human Gene Mutation Database, http://www.hgmd.cf.ac.uk/ac/gene.php?gene=G6PD). Furthermore, in this way new mutations are still likely to be discovered.

GENOTYPE-PHENOTYPE CORRELATIONS

A rigorous definition of a polymorphic allele is one with a frequency higher than can be accounted for by recurrent mutation; however, for convenience, a conservative practical criterion is any allele with a frequency of at least 1% in at least one population. By this criterion there are 26 well-mapped *Gd* polymorphic alleles (see Figs. 17-4B and 17-5) already known.[66] The ratio of subjects having G6PD deficiency associated with CNSHA to those having "simple" G6PD deficiency varies in different populations. For instance, in Japan, where G6PD deficiency is, on the whole, very rare, the majority of patients with G6PD deficiency have been reported to have CNSHA.[152] This suggests that CNSHA, caused by rare sporadic variants, many of which may result from recent mutations, reflects the intrinsic mutation rate of the human *Gd* gene, which is likely to be uniform throughout the world; in contrast, "simple" G6PD deficiency almost always results from common variants that have arisen many generations ago and spread through biologic selection.

The three variants mentioned previously, G6PD A⁻, G6PD Mediterranean, and G6PD Mahidol, are probably those for which clinical expression has best been characterized.[153] Although the former is often quoted as having fewer clinical manifestations than the others, the differences are marginal, and they are unlikely to be relevant with respect to patient management. The severity of hemolysis and whether it is "self-limited" depend on the offending agent, on its dose, and on the time course of exposure probably more than it depends on the G6PD variant involved. Notably, favism has been unambiguously documented with G6PD A⁻.[154-156]

In terms of clinical expression, the demarcation between class I variants and all others is, by definition, much more clear-cut. Indeed, one of the outstanding questions in the biochemical genetics of G6PD is why a particular variant can cause CNSHA rather than just AHA. In certain cases the level of residual enzyme activity is not the whole answer—qualitative differences are also important, as first suggested by Kirkman and Riley.[157] The most likely way in which a structural change can significantly alter the function of G6PD, *given the same level of deficiency*, is by affecting the binding of one of the main ligands (i.e., G6P, NADP, NADPH). For instance, G6PD Mediterranean and G6PD Coimbra both have mutations near the G6P binding site, and both have *increased* affinity for G6P. Perhaps because of this, although they are both severely deficient, they belong to class II and not to class I. G6PD Orissa, the main polymorphic variant in tribal Indian populations[158] also belongs to class II despite having *decreased* affinity for

NADP. Thus, the affinity for G6P appears to be of greater importance. Indeed, comparison of the distribution of K_m^{G6P} values of class I variants with that of class II and III variants shows that they are significantly lower in the latter group.[8]

However, in most cases the main factor responsible for causing CNSHA is a very low level of residual activity in red cells, which in turn is due to marked in vivo instability. It is quite remarkable that although G6PD mutations as a whole are evenly spread throughout the gene's coding sequence, the majority of class I mutations are clustered in exons 10 and 11 (see Fig. 17-4B). The three-dimensional model of the human G6PD dimer has, at long last, provided a reasonable explanation for this finding.[66,159] Indeed, these two exons encode the protein region that constitutes the interface between the two identical subunits of the enzyme. As a result, any mutation in this region causes the respective amino acid replacements in the two subunits to be quite near each other in the dimer structure, thus potentially increasing their deleterious effects. Even more important, because there is no covalent link between the subunits, it stands to reason that any interference in the shape of the interface surfaces may affect their mutual fit and therefore dramatically destabilize the active form of the enzyme. Defects in protein folding have been studied in detail for certain G6PD variants.[160,161]

G6PD DEFICIENCY AND PREVENTIVE MEDICINE

Because NNJ and AHA are the most common manifestations of G6PD deficiency, it is most important to consider how they can be prevented. The first step is to identify G6PD-deficient individuals, which is where screening is most pertinent. Of course, whether population-wide screening is both desirable and feasible depends primarily on the prevalence of G6PD deficiency in any particular community; this will determine the cost-benefit ratio. If screening is done at all, it is best done on cord blood. Once a subject is known to be G6PD deficient, the two main implications are the risk for NNJ and the importance of avoiding exposure to agents that can cause AHA. NNJ cannot be prevented as yet, but awareness of G6PD deficiency must entail surveillance for NNJ until at least day 4 and special recommendations with respect to factors, such as naphthalene, that can cause it or make it worse. By contrast, at least one type of AHA, namely, favism, is completely preventable (Fig. 17-10). Prevention of infection-induced hemolysis is obviously more difficult. Prevention of drug-induced hemolysis is possible in most cases by choosing alternative drugs, but it may be difficult when none are available. The most common problem is the need to administer primaquine for the eradication of malaria caused by *Plasmodium vivax* or *Plasmodium malariae*. In these cases, administration of a lower dosage for a longer time is the recommended

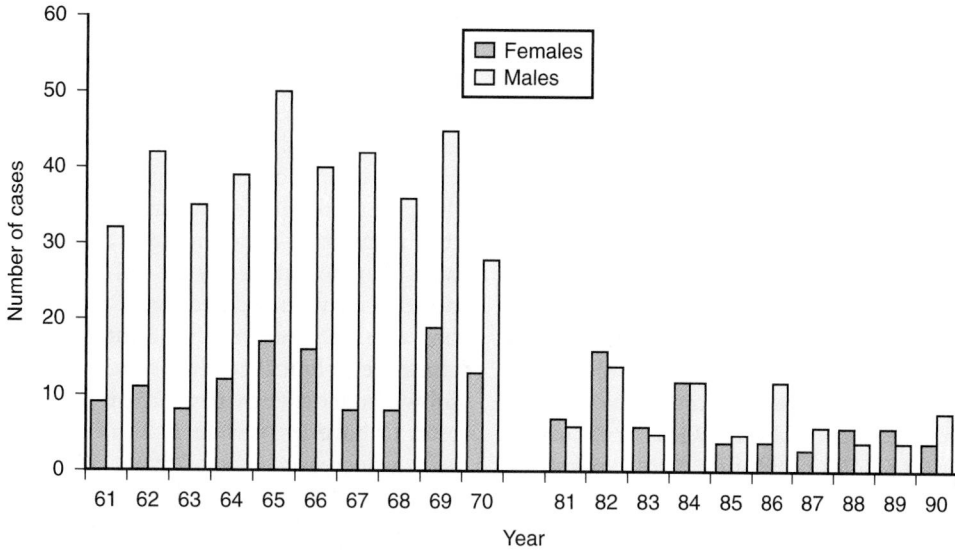

FIGURE 17-10. Control of favism in a community. The data show the decrease in the number of yearly admissions for favism in the children's department of the main city and university hospitals in Sassari, northern Sardinia. During the 10-year period intervening between the two sets of data, two preventive measures were adopted: (1) education through the media and (2) screening of all newborns for G6PD deficiency. Note the dramatic reduction in the incidence of favism in boys and the more modest decrease in girls. The data suggest that (1) preventive measures are effective; (2) the increased proportion of girls can be attributed to failure of the screening method used to pick out many of the heterozygotes; and (3) in view of (2), the dramatic reduction observed in boys can perhaps be credited to screening more than to the educational campaign. (*Courtesy of Professor Tullio Meloni, Sassari, Sardinia.*)

approach. Hemolysis will still occur, but under appropriate surveillance it will be of an acceptably mild degree.

A special problem in prevention is what to do about new drugs, the hemolytic potential of which is unknown. Although in vitro methods to test drugs in this respect do exist,[162,163] such tests are unfortunately not routinely carried out before drugs are released on the market, so their hemolytic potential will become apparent only from clinical observation. Recently, a combination of dapsone and chlorproguanil, used as an antimalarial in several African countries,[164,165] has been withdrawn from the market because of life-threatening hemolytic complications.

G6PD DEFICIENCY IN NONERYTHROID CELLS

As mentioned earlier, because nucleated somatic cells have the capability to synthesize G6PD constitutively, they are affected less than red cells by G6PD deficiency.[166] For instance, subjects with G6PD Mediterranean have less than 5% G6PD activity in red cells but about 30% of normal in granulocytes; subjects with G6PD A− have about 12% G6PD activity in red cells but nearly normal activity in granulocytes. On the other hand, if deficiency results from a drastic change in catalytic efficiency or in substrate affinity, deficiency may be more universal. In practice, the only well-documented pathologic effect is expressed in granulocytes. Very few of the class I G6PD variants cause not only CNSHA but also granulocyte dysfunction, mainly in the way of impaired killing of phagocytosed bacteria (an example is G6PD Barce-

lona).[167] Patients with these variants have increased susceptibility to bacterial infection, particularly with *Staphylococcus aureus*. Recently, in a group of patients who suffered major trauma in road traffic accidents, Spolarics and colleagues[102] made the interesting observation that the frequency and severity of infection were significantly higher in patients who were G6PD deficient; thus, neutrophil function may be affected in extreme situations, even in the common type of G6PD deficiency (the patients in the clinical study all had G6PD A−). The mechanism whereby G6PD deficiency impairs phagocytosis is a defect of the oxidative burst caused by a shortage in NADPH supply, similar to that observed in chronic granulomatous disease, in which one of the components of the cytochrome-b_{245} system is defective.[168] Functional abnormalities have also been demonstrated in macrophages from G6PD-deficient mice.[169]

Erythrocytes are not the only non-nucleated cells in the body. Another example is in the eye lens, and juvenile cataracts have been reported occasionally in subjects with G6PD deficiency.[170,171] Whether G6PD deficiency is more generally associated with a higher frequency or earlier onset of cataracts appears to still be controversial.[172-175]

G6PD DEFICIENCY COEXISTING WITH OTHER DISORDERS

In areas where G6PD deficiency is common, it is not infrequent that it may be encountered in the same patient together with another condition, whether a hematologic or a nonhematologic condition.

Association with Other Hematologic Diseases. The combination of G6PD deficiency with the sickle cell trait has been no more frequent than could be expected by chance.[176,177] Several studies have shown that there are no significant differences in a variety of clinical and hematologic parameters between two otherwise comparable groups of patients with sickle cell anemia, those with and without G6PD deficiency,[149,178-180] but it must be borne in mind that acute intravascular hemolysis superimposed on chronic severe extravascular hemolysis is an added risk with this association. The combination of G6PD deficiency with the β-thalassemia trait has been found to cause a significant increase in mean corpuscular volume,[181] which remains, however, below the normal range. Association of G6PD deficiency with thalassemia major is unlikely to be a problem because patients with the latter condition are treated with regular blood transfusions or with bone marrow transplantation. However, the association may be significant in patients with various forms of thalassemia intermedia syndromes (e.g., hemoglobin E–β-thalassemia).[182]

Occasionally, G6PD deficiency has been observed in association with much rarer red cell abnormalities, such as pyruvate kinase deficiency,[183,184] congenital dyserythropoietic anemia type II,[185-187] and hereditary elliptocytosis.[188] In these cases the two abnormalities seem to produce only additive clinical effects, but in at least one family G6PD deficiency was synergistic with hereditary spherocytosis in causing moderately severe chronic hemolytic anemia.[189]

Association with Nonhematologic Diseases. Several studies have reported variable degrees of association between diabetes and G6PD deficiency.[190-196] It now appears clear that diabetic ketoacidosis does not trigger hemolysis[197]; on the other hand, downregulation of G6PD has been reported in some West African patients with type 1 diabetes predisposed to ketoacidosis.[198] Apart from the fact that hepatitis can precipitate hemolysis in G6PD-deficient children, ribavirin, now much used in the treatment of hepatitis C, can itself cause hemolytic anemia (regardless of whether the patient is G6PD deficient). On the other hand, it has recently been shown that G6PD-deficient patients with hepatitis C can be treated safely with ribavirin and pegylated interferon.[199]

Trauma and G6PD Deficiency. Although G6PD deficiency protects against malaria, there are reports indicating that it worsens the clinical course of traumatic patients.[189] Altered cytokine response would be the underlying pathogenetic mechanism predisposing to infections in G6PD-deficient individuals.[200]

G6PD POLYMORPHISM AND MALARIA

The striking correlation between the worldwide distribution of G6PD deficiency (see Fig. 17-5) and that of *Plasmodium falciparum* prompted formulation of the "malaria hypothesis" nearly half a century ago.[201,202] Since that time, numerous more detailed epidemiologic studies, which can be referred to as "micromapping,"[203] as well as clinical studies,[204] have supported the notion that G6PD deficiency confers some degree of resistance to the potentially lethal malaria parasite *P. falciparum;* and that in malaria-endemic areas, G6PD alleles associated with enzyme deficiency have therefore been subjected to positive darwinian selection.[205-207] A geographic correlation certainly does not amount to proof, but three large controlled clinical studies, all carried out in Africa, have shown concordantly that children with G6PD deficiency tend to have less severe malaria and, therefore, presumably a decreased risk of dying of malaria. It is puzzling that in one of these studies (from Nigeria[208]), increased resistance to the parasite (relative to that in appropriate controls) was significant only in heterozygous females; in another study (from Gambia and Kenya[209]), a protective effect was seen in both males and females; and in the third study (from Mali[210]), a protective effect was noted only in males. These differences might result from genetic variations (other than G6PD) in different populations, from the use of different criteria to measure the severity of malaria, from different levels of statistical power, or from any combination of these factors. However, all three studies concur in supporting the notion of malaria selection for G6PD deficiency. A more difficult issue is understanding the mechanism of this phenomenon. In vitro studies have shown that invasion of G6PD-deficient red cells by *P. falciparum* takes place normally and the parasite can multiply efficiently in G6PD-deficient red cells, at least after several cycles.[211] On the other hand, in vitro experiments have shown that parasitized red cells are recognized more promptly by macrophages when they are G6PD deficient[212]; thus, accelerated removal of parasitized red cells (suicidal infection)[213] may be the most important mechanism of protection, as it is for subjects with the sickle cell trait.[214] An additional strong argument in favor of malaria selection is the genetic heterogeneity of polymorphic *Gd⁻* alleles in itself. Indeed, each one of these alleles, having arisen through an independent mutational event, must have increased in frequency on its own in a particular geographic area[215] where malaria was or still is endemic—a good example of convergent evolution driven by the same selective force.[216]

REFERENCES

1. Beutler E. Glucose 6-phosphate dehydrogenase deficiency. In Beutler E (ed). Hemolytic Anemia in Disorders of Red Cell Metabolism. New York, Plenum, 1978, pp 23-167.
2. Levy HR. Glucose 6-phosphate dehydrogenase. In Meister A (ed). Advances in Enzymology, vol 48. New York, Wiley, 1979, pp 97-192.
3. Arese P, Mannuzzu L, Turrini F. Pathophysiology of favism. Folia Haematol. 1989;116:745-752.

4. Beutler E. The genetics of glucose-6-phosphate dehydrogenase deficiency. Semin Hematol. 1990;27:137-164.

5. Beutler E. Glucose 6-phosphate dehydrogenase deficiency. N Engl J Med. 1991;324:169-174.

6. Luzzatto L, Mehta A, Vulliamy T. Glucose-6-phosphate dehydrogenase deficiency. In Scriver C, Beaudet A, Sly W, Valle D (eds). The Metabolic & Molecular Bases of Inherited Disease, 8th ed. New York, McGraw-Hill, 2001, pp 4517-4553.

7. Berg JM, Tymoczko JL, Stryer L. Biochemistry, 5th ed. New York, WH Freeman, 2002.

8. Luzzatto L, Testa U. Human erythrocyte glucose 6-phosphate dehydrogenase: structure and function in normal and mutant subjects. Curr Top Hematol. 1978;1:1-70.

9. Peisach J, Blumberg WE, Rachmielewicz EA. The demonstration of ferrihemochrome intermediates in Heinz body formation following the reduction of oxyhemoglobin A by acetylphenylhydrazine. Biochim Biophys Acta. 1975;393:404-418.

10. Gaetani GF, Kirkman HN, Mangerini R, Ferraris AM. Importance of catalase in the disposal of hydrogen peroxide within human erythrocytes. Blood. 1994;84:325-330.

11. Gaetani GF, Galiano S, Canepa L, et al. Catalase and glutathione peroxidase are equally active in detoxification of hydrogen peroxide in human erythrocytes. Blood. 1989;73:334-339.

12. Kirkman HN, Gaetani GF. Catalase: a tetrameric enzyme with four tightly bound molecules of NADPH. Proc Natl Acad Sci U S A. 1984;81:4343-4347.

13. Pandolfi PP, Sonati F, Rivi R, et al. Targeted disruption of the housekeeping gene encoding glucose 6-phosphate dehydrogenase (G6PD): G6PD is dispensable for pentose synthesis but essential for defense against oxidative stress. EMBO J. 1995;14:5209-5215.

14. Paglialunga F, Fico A, Iaccarino I, et al. G6PD is indispensable for erythropoiesis after the embryonic-adult hemoglobin switch. Blood. 2004;104:3148-3152.

15. Longo L, Vanegas OC, Patel M, et al. Maternally transmitted severe glucose 6-phosphate dehydrogenase deficiency is an embryonic lethal. EMBO J. 2002;21:4229-4239.

16. Luzzatto L, Battistuzzi G. Glucose 6-phosphate dehydrogenase. Adv Hum Genet. 1985;14:217-329.

17. Notaro R, Afolayan A, Luzzatto L. Human mutations in glucose 6-phosphate dehydrogenase reflect evolutionary history. FASEB J. 2000;14:485-494.

18. Antonenkov VD. Dehydrogenases of the pentose phosphate pathway in rat liver peroxisomes. Eur J Biochem. 1989;183:75-82.

19. Cohen P, Rosemeyer MA. Human glucose-6-phosphate dehydrogenase: purification of the erythrocyte enzyme and the influence of ions on its activity. Eur J Biochem. 1969;8:1-7.

20. Persico MG, Viglietto G, Martini G, et al. Isolation of human glucose-6-phosphate dehydrogenase (G6PD) cDNA clones: primary structure of the protein and unusual 5′ non-coding region. Nucleic Acids Res. 1986;14:2511-2522.

21. Jeffery J, Soderling-Barros J, Murray LA, et al. Glucose 6-phosphate dehydrogenase. Characteristics revealed by the rat liver enzyme. Eur J Biochem. 1989;186:551-556.

22. Rowland P, Basak A, Gover S, et al. The three-dimensional structure of glucose 6-phosphate dehydrogenase from *Leuconostoc mesenteroides* refined at 2.0 Å resolution. Structure. 1994;2:1073-1087.

23. Au SW, Naylor CE, Gover S, et al. Solution of the structure of tetrameric human glucose 6-phosphate dehydrogenase by molecular replacement. Acta Crystallogr. 1999;55:826-834.

24. Au SW, Gover S, Lam VM, Adams MJ. Human glucose-6-phosphate dehydrogenase: the crystal structure reveals a structural NADP(+) molecule and provides insights into enzyme deficiency. Structure. 2000;8:293-303.

25. Scopes DA, Bautista JM, Naylor CE, et al. Amino acid substitutions at the dimer interface of human glucose-6-phosphate dehydrogenase that increase thermostability and reduce the stabilising effect of NADP. Eur J Biochem. 1998;251:382-388.

26. Kotaka M, Gover S, Vandeputte-Rutten L, et al. Structural studies of glucose-6-phosphate and NADP$^+$ binding to human glucose-6-phosphate dehydrogenase. Acta Crystallogr. 2005;61:495-504.

27. Bautista JM, Mason PJ, Luzzatto L. Human glucose-6-phosphate dehydrogenase. Lysine 205 is dispensable for substrate binding but essential for catalysis. FEBS Lett. 1995;366:61-64.

28. Mason PJ, Vulliamy TJ, Foulkes NS, et al. The production of normal and variant human glucose-6-phosphate dehydrogenase in cos cells. Eur J Biochem. 1988;178:109-113.

29. Luzzatto L. Regulation of the activity of glucose-6-phosphate dehydrogenase by NADP$^+$ and NADPH. Biochim Biophys Acta. 1967;146:18-25.

30. Kirkman HN, Gaetani GD, Clemons EH, Mareni C. Red cell NADP and NADPH in glucose-6-phosphate dehydrogenase deficiency. J Clin Invest. 1975;55:875-880.

31. Dern RJ, McCurdy PR, Yoshida A. A new structural variant of glucose-6-phosphate dehydrogenase with a high production rate (G6PD Hektoen). J Lab Clin Med. 1969;73:283-290.

32. Pai GS, Sprenkle JA, Do TT, et al. Localization of the loci for hypoxanthine phosphoribosyltransferase and glucose-6-phosphate dehydrogenase and biochemical evidence of non-random X-chromosome expression from studies of human X-autosome translocation. Proc Natl Acad Sci U S A. 1980;77:2810-2813.

33. Szabo P, Purrello M, Rocchi M, et al. Cytological mapping of the human glucose-6-phosphate dehydrogenase gene distal to the fragile-X site suggests a high rate of meiotic recombination across this site. Proc Natl Acad Sci U S A. 1984;81:7855-7859.

34. Patterson M, Schwartz C, Bell M, et al. Physical mapping studies on the human X chromosome in the region Xq27-Zqter. Genomics. 1987;1:297-300.

35. Beutler E, Yeh M, Fairbanks VF. The normal human female as a mosaic of X-chromosome activity: studies using the gene for G6PD deficiency as a marker. Proc Natl Acad Sci U S A. 1962;48:9-16.

36. Migeon BR. Glucose 6-phosphate dehydrogenase as a probe for the study of X-chromosome inactivation in human females. In Rattazzi MC, Scandalios JC, Whitt GS (eds). Isozymes: Current Topics in Biological and Medical Research, vol 9. New York, Alan R Liss, 1983, pp 189-200.

37. Fialkow PJ, Gartler SM, Yoshida A. Clonal origin of chronic myelocytic leukaemia in man. Proc Natl Acad Sci U S A. 1967;58:1468-470.

38. Oni SB, Osunkoya BO, Luzzatto L. Paroxysmal nocturnal hemoglobinuria: evidence for monoclonal origin of abnormal red cells. Blood. 1970;36:145-152.

39. Gartler SM. X-chromosome inactivation and selection in somatic cells. Fed Proc. 1976;35:2191-2194.

40. Chen EY, Zollo M, Mazzarella R, et al. Long-range sequence analysis in Xq28: thirteen known and six candidate genes in 219.4 kb of high GC DNA between the RCP/GCP and G6PD loci. Hum Mol Genet. 1996;5:659-668.

41. Adam A. Linkage between deficiency of glucose 6-phosphate dehydrogenase and colour-blindness. Nature. 1961;189:686-688.

42. Gall JC, Brewer GJ, Dern RJ. Studies of glucose 6-phosphate dehydrogenase activity of individual erythrocytes. The methemoglobin elution test for the detection of females heterozygous for G6PD deficiency. Am J Hum Genet. 1965;17:359.

43. Nance WE. Genetic tests with a sex-linked marker: G-6-PD. Cold Spring Harbor Symp Quant Biol. 1964;29:415-425.

44. Rinaldi A, Filippi G, Siniscalco M. Variability of red cell phenotypes between and within individuals in an unbiased sample of 77 certain heterozygotes for G6PD deficiency in Sardinians. Am J Hum Genet. 1976;28:496-505.

45. Gale RE, Wheadon H, Linch DC. X-chromosome inactivation patterns using HPRT and PGK polymorphisms in haematologically normal and post-chemotherapy females. Br J Haematol. 1991;79:193-197.

46. Nyhan WL, Bakay B, Connor JD, et al. Hemizygous expression of glucose 6-phosphate dehydrogenase deficiency in erythrocytes of heterozygotes for the Lesch-Nyhan syndrome. Proc Natl Acad Sci U S A. 1970;65:214-218.

47. Town M, Athanasiou-Metaxa M, Luzzatto L. Intragenic interspecific complementation of glucose 6-phosphate dehydrogenase in human-hamster cell hybrids. Somat Cell Mol Genet. 1990;16:97-108.

48. Filosa S, Giacometti N, Wangwei C, et al. Somatic-cell selection is a major determinant of the blood-cell phenotype in heterozygotes for glucose 6-phosphate dehydrogenase mutations causing severe enzyme deficiency. Am J Hum Genet. 1996;59:887-895.

49. Puck JM, Willard HF. X inactivation in females with X-linked disease. N Engl J Med. 1998;338:325-328.

50. Luzzatto L, Usanga EA, Bienzle U, et al. Imbalance in X-chromosome expression: evidence for a human X-linked gene affecting growth of haemopoietic cells. Science. 1979;205:1418-1420.

51. Vulliamy TJ, D'Urso M, Battistuzzi G, et al. Diverse point mutations in the human glucose-6-phosphate dehydrogenase gene cause enzyme deficiency and mild or severe hemolytic anemia. Proc Natl Acad Sci U S A. 1988;85:5171-5175.

52. Luzzatto L, Martini G. X-linked Wiskott-Aldrich syndrome in a girl [letter]. N Engl J Med. 1998;338:1850-1851.

53. Martini G, Toniolo D, Vulliamy TJ, et al. Structural analysis of the X-linked gene encoding human glucose 6-phosphate dehydrogenase. EMBO J. 1986;5:1849-1855.

54. Mason PJ, Stevens DJ, Luzzatto L, et al. Genomic structure and sequence of the *Fugu rubripes* glucose-6-phosphate dehydrogenase gene (G6PD). Genomics. 1995;26:587-591.

55. Strachan TR, Read AP. Human Molecular Genetics, 2nd ed. New York, John Wiley, 1999.

56. Ursini MV, Scalera L, Martini G. High level of transcription driven by a 400 bp segment of the human G6PD promoter. Biochem Biophys Res Commun. 1990;170:1203-1209.

57. Philippe M, Larondelle Y, Lemaigre F, et al. Promoter function of the human glucose-6-phosphate dehydrogenase gene depends on two GC boxes that are cell specifically controlled. Eur J Biochem. 1994;226:377-384.

58. Rivella S, Tamanini F, Bione S, et al. A comparative transcriptional map of a region of 250 kb on the human and mouse X chromosome between the G6PD and the FLN1 genes. Genomics. 1995;28:377-382.

59. Hino Y, Minakami S. Hexose-6-phosphate dehydrogenase of rat liver microsomes. Isolation by affinity chromatography and properties. J Biol Chem. 1982;257:2563-2568.

60. Mason PJ, Stevens D, Diez A, et al. Human hexose-6-phosphate dehydrogenase (glucose 1-dehydrogenase) encoded at 1p36: coding sequence and expression. Blood Cells Mol Dis. 1999;25:30-37.

61. Beutler E. Haemolytic Anaemia in Disorders of Red Cell Metabolism (Topics in Haematology). New York, Plenum, 1978.

62. Piomelli S, Corash LM, Davenport DD, et al. In vivo lability of glucose-6-phosphate dehydrogenase in Gd A and Gd Mediterranean deficiency. J Clin Invest. 1968;47:940-948.

63. Beutler E. The relationship of red cell enzymes to red cell life-span. Blood Cells. 1988;14:69-91.

64. Marks PA, Johnson AB. Relationship between the age of human erythrocytes and their osmotic resistance: a basis for separating young and old erythrocytes. J Clin Invest. 1958;37:1542-1548.

65. Luzzatto L, Testa U. Human erythrocyte G6PD: structure and function in normal and mutant subjects. In Piomelli S, Yachnin S (eds). Current Topics in Hematology, vol 1. New York, Alan R Liss, 1978, pp 1-70.

66. Mason PJ, Bautista JM, Gilsanz F. G6PD deficiency: the genotype-phenotype association. Blood Rev. 2007;21:267-283.

67. Menounos P, Zervas C, Garinis G, et al. Molecular heterogeneity of the gluscose-6-phosphate dehydrogenase deficiency in the Hellenic population. Hum Hered. 2000;50:237-241.

68. MacDonald D, Town M, Mason PJ, et al. Deficiency in red blood cells. Nature. 1991;350:115.

69. Xu W, Westwood B, Bartsocas CS, et al. Glucose-6 phosphate dehydrogenase mutations and haplotypes in various ethnic groups. Blood. 1995;85:257-263.

70. Hirono A, Fujii H, Shima M, Miwa S. G6PD Nara: a new class I glucose 6-phosphate dehydrogenase variant with an eight amino acid deletion. Blood. 1993;82:3250-3252.

71. Sanders S, Smith DP, Thomas GA, Williams ED. A glucose-6-phosphate dehydrogenase (G6PD) splice site

consensus sequence mutation associated with G6PD enzyme deficiency. Mutat Res. 1997;374:79-87.

72. Mason PJ, Sonati MF, MacDonald D, et al. New glucose 6-phosphate dehydrogenase mutations associated with chronic anemia. Blood. 1995;85:1377-1380.

73. Ohga S, Higashi E, Nomura A, et al. Haptoglobin therapy for acute favism: a Japanese boy with glucose-6-phosphate dehydrogenase Guadalajara. Br J Haematol. 1995;89:421-423.

74. Mason PJ. New insights into G6PD deficiency. Br J Haematol. 1996;94:585-591.

75. Ainoon O, Boo NY, Yu YH, et al. G6PD deficiency with hemolytic anemia due to a rare gene deletion—a report of the first case in Malaysia. Hematology. 2006;11:113-118.

76. Morelli A, Benatti U, Gaetani GF, DeFlora A. Biochemical mechanisms of glucose-6-phosphate dehydrogenase deficiency. Proc Natl Acad Sci U S A. 1978;75:1979-1983.

77. Kaeda JS, Chootray GP, Ranjit MR, et al. A new glucose-6-phosphate dehydrogenase variant, G6PD Orissa (44 Ala→Gly), is the major polymorphic variant in tribal populations in India. Am J Hum Genet. 1995;57:1335-1341.

78. WHO Working Group. Glucose-6-phosphate dehydrogenase deficiency. Bull World Health Organ. 1989;67:601-611.

79. Fermi C, Martinetti P. Studio sul favismo. Annali di Igiene Sperimentale. 1905;15:76-112.

80. Chan TK, Chan WC, Weed RI. Erythrocyte hemighosts: a hallmark of severe oxidative injury in vivo. Br J Haematol. 1982;50:575-582.

81. Fischer TM, Meloni T, Pescarmona GP, et al. Membrane cross bonding in red cells in favic crisis: a missing link in the mechanism of extravascular hemolysis. Br J Haematol. 1985;59:159-169.

82. Rifkind RA. Heinz bodies anaemia: an ultrastructural study. II. Red cell sequestration and destruction. Blood. 1965;26:433-448.

83. Beutler E. The glutathione instability of drug-sensitive red cells. A new method for the in vitro detection of drug sensitivity. J Lab Clin Med. 1957;49:84-90.

84. Jollow DJ, McMillan DC. Oxidative stress, glucose-6-phosphate dehydrogenase and the red cell. Adv Exp Med Biol. 2001;500:595-605.

85. Gaetani GF, Mareni C, Salvidio E, et al. Favism: erythrocyte metabolism during haemolysis and reticulocytosis. Br J Haematol. 1979;43:39-48.

86. Morelli A, Grasso M, Meloni T, et al. Favism: impairment of proteolytic systems in red blood cells. Blood. 1987;69:1753-1758.

87. De Flora A, Benatti U, Guida L, et al. Favism: disordered erythrocyte calcium hemostasis. Blood. 1985;66:294-300.

88. Waugh SM, Walder JA, Low PS. Partial characterization of the copolymerization reaction of erythrocyte membrane band 3 with hemichrome. Biochemistry. 1987;26:1777-1783.

89. Kasper ML, Miller WJ, Jacob HS. G6PD deficiency infectious haemolysis: a complement dependent innocent bystander phenomenon. Br J Haematol. 1986;63:85-91.

90. Arese P, De Flora A. Pathophysiology of hemolysis in glucose 6-phosphate dehydrogenase deficiency. Semin Hematol. 1990;27:1-40.

91. Beutler E, Dern RJ, Alving AS. The hemolytic effect of primaquine. IV. The relationship of cell age to hemolysis. J Lab Clin Med. 1954;44:439-442.

92. Tarlov AR, Brewer GJ, Carson PE, Alving AS. Primaquine sensitivity. Glucose-6-phosphate dehydrogenase deficiency: an inborn error of metabolism of medical and biological significance. Arch Intern Med. 1962;109:209-234.

93. Szeinberg A, Marks PA. Substances stimulating glucose catabolism by the oxidative reactions of the pentose phosphate pathway in human erythrocytes. J Clin Invest. 1961;40:914-924.

94. Chevion M, Navok T, Glaser G, Mager J. The chemistry of favism-inducing compounds. The properties of isouramil and divicine and their reaction with glutathione. Eur J Biochem. 1982;127:405-409.

95. Winterbourn C, Cowden WB, Sutton HC. Autooxidation of dialuric acid, divicine and isouramil. Superoxide dependent and independent mechanisms. Biochem Pharmacol. 1989;38:611-618.

96. Zinkham WH, Oski FA. Henna: a potential cause of oxidative hemolysis and neonatal hyperbilirubinemia. Pediatrics. 1996;97:707-709.

97. Raupp P, Hassan JA, Varughese M, Kristiansson B. Henna causes life threatening haemolysis in glucose-6-phosphate dehydrogenase deficiency. Arch Dis Child. 2001;85:411-412.

98. Ozsoylu S. Henna intoxication [letter]. Lancet. 1996;348:1173.

99. Kandil HH, Al-Ghanem MM, Sarwat MA, Al-Thallab FS. Henna (*Lawsonia inermis* Linn.) inducing haemolysis among G6PD-deficient newborns. A new clinical observation. Ann Trop Paediatr. 1996;16:287-291.

100. Meloni T, Forteleoni G, Ogana A, Francavilla V. Aspirin-induced acute hemolytic anemia in glucose 6-phosphate dehydrogenase deficient children with systemic arthritis. Acta Haematol. 1989;81:208-209.

101. McCurdy PR. Discussion. In Yoshida A, Beutler E (eds). Glucose 6-Phosphate Dehydrogenase. New York, Academic Press, 1986, pp 273-278.

102. Spolarics Z, Siddiqi M, Siegel JH, et al. Increased incidence of sepsis and altered monocyte functions in severely injured type A⁻ glucose-6-phosphate dehydrogenase–deficient African American trauma patients. Crit Care Med. 2001;29:728-736.

103. Baehner RL, Nathan DG, Castle WB. Oxidant injury of Caucasian glucose-6-phosphate dehydrogenase deficient red blood cells by phagocytosing leukocytes during infection. J Clin Invest. 1971;50:2466-2473.

104. Luzzatto L, Meloni T. Hemolytic anemia due to glucose 6-phosphate dehydrogenase deficiency. In Brian MC, Carbone PP (eds). Current Therapy in Hematology-Oncology: 1985-1986. St. Louis, CV Mosby, 1985, pp 21-24.

105. Valaes T. Severe neonatal jaundice associated with glucose-6-phosphate dehydrogenase deficiency: pathogenesis and global epidemiology. Acta Paediatr. 1994;394(Suppl):58-76.

106. Worlledge S, Luzzatto L, Ogiemudia SE, et al. Rhesus immunization in Nigeria. Vox Sang. 1968;14:202-211.

107. Doxiadis SA, Valaes F. The clinical picture of glucose 6-phosphate dehydrogenase deficiency in early childhood. Arch Dis Child. 1964;39:545-553.

108. Meloni T, Costa S, Cutillo S. Haptoglobin, hemopexin, hemoglobin and hematocrit in newborns with erythrocyte glucose-6-phosphate dehydrogenase deficiency. Acta Haematol. 1975;54:284-290.

109. Singh A. Glucose 6-phosphate dehydrogenase deficiency: a preventable cause of mental retardation. BMJ. 1986;292:397-398.

110. Kaplan M, Hammerman C, Vreman HJ, et al. Acute hemolysis and severe neonatal hyperbilirubinemia in glucose-6-phosphate dehydrogenase–deficient heterozygotes. J Pediatr. 2001;139:137-140.

111. Kaplan M, Algur N, Hammerman C. Onset of jaundice in glucose-6-phosphate dehydrogenase–deficient neonates. Pediatrics. 2001;108:956-959.

112. Kaplan M, Hammerman C, Renbaum P, et al. Differing pathogenesis of perinatal bilirubinemia in glucose-6-phosphate dehydrogenase–deficient versus–normal neonates. Pediatr Res. 2001;50:532-537.

113. Bienzle U, Effiong C, Luzzatto L. Erythrocyte glucose 6-phosphate dehydrogenase deficiency (G6PD type A⁻) and neonatal jaundice. Acta Paediatr Scand. 1976;65:701-703.

114. Meloni T, Cagnazzo G, Dore A, Cutillo S. Phenobarbital for prevention of hyperbilirubinemia in glucose 6-phosphate dehydrogenase–deficient newborn infants. J Pediatr. 1973;82:1048-1051.

115. Tan KL, Boey KW. Clinical experience with phototherapy. Ann Acad Med Singapore. 1989;18:43-48.

116. Yu MW, Hsiao KJ, Wu KD, Chen CJ. Association between glucose-6-phosphate dehydrogenase deficiency and neonatal jaundice: interaction with multiple risk factors. Int J Epidemiol. 1992;21:947-952.

117. Testa U, Meloni T, Lania A, et al. Genetic heterogeneity of glucose 6-phosphate dehydrogenase deficiency in Sardinia. Hum Genet. 1980;56:99-105.

118. Huang MJ, Kua KE, Teng HC, et al. Risk factors for severe hyperbilirubinemia in neonates. Pediatr Res. 2004;56:682-689.

119. Meloni T, Cutillo S, Testa U, Luzzatto L. Neonatal jaundice and severity of glucose 6-phosphate dehydrogenase deficiency in Sardinian babies. Early Hum Dev. 1987;15:317-322.

120. Ho HY, Cheng ML, Chiu DT. Glucose-6-phosphate dehydrogenase—from oxidative stress to cellular functions and degenerative diseases. Redox Rep. 2007;12:109-118.

121. Gross S. Hemolytic anemia in premature infants: relationship to vitamin E, selenium, glutathione peroxidase and erythrocyte lipids. Semin Hematol. 1976;3:187-200.

122. Kaplan M, Muraca M, Vreman HJ, et al. Neonatal bilirubin production-conjugation imbalance: effect of glucose-6-phosphate dehydrogenase deficiency and borderline prematurity. Arch Dis Child. 2005;90:F123-F127.

123. Kaplan M, Renbaum P, Levy-Lahad E, et al. Gilbert syndrome and glucose-6-phosphate dehydrogenase deficiency: a dose-dependent genetic interaction crucial to neonatal hyperbilirubinemia. Proc Natl Acad Sci U S A. 1997;94:12128-12132.

124. Kaplan M, Hammerman C, Beutler E. Hyperbilirubinaemia, glucose-6-phosphate dehydrogenase deficiency and Gilbert syndrome. Eur J Pediatr. 2001;160:195.

125. Kaplan M, Herschel M, Hammerman C, et al. Studies in hemolysis in glucose-6-phosphate dehydrogenase–deficient African American neonates. Clin Chim Acta. 2006;365:177-182.

126. Mert A, Tabak F, Ozturk R, et al. Acute viral hepatitis with severe hyperbilirubinemia and massive hemolysis in glucose-6-phosphate dehydrogenase deficiency. J Clin Gastroenterol. 2001;32:461-462.

127. Ifekwunigwe AE, Luzzatto L. Kernicterus in G6PD deficiency. Lancet. 1966;i:667.

128. Corchia C, Balata A, Meloni GF, Meloni T. Favism in a female newborn infant whose mother ingested fava beans before delivery. J Pediatr. 1995;127:807-808.

129. Kaplan M, Vreman HJ, Hammerman C, et al. Contribution of haemolysis to jaundice in Sephardic Jewish glucose-6-phosphate dehydrogenase deficient neonates. Br J Haematol. 1996;93:822-827.

130. American Academy of Pediatrics Subcommittee on Hyperbilirubinemia. Management of hyperbilirubinemia in the newborn infant 35 or more weeks of gestation. Pediatrics. 2004;114:297-316.

131. Poggi V, Town M, Foulkes NS, Luzzatto L. Identification of a single base change in a new human mutant glucose-6-phosphate dehydrogenase gene by polymerase-chain-reaction amplification of the entire coding region from genomic DNA. Biochem J. 1990;271:157-160.

132. Roos D, van Zwieten R, Wijnen JT, et al. Molecular basis and enzymatic properties of glucose 6-phosphate dehydrogenase Volendam, leading to chronic nonspherocytic anemia, granulocyte dysfunction, and increased susceptibility to infections. Blood. 1999;94:2955-2962.

133. Allen DW, Johnson GJ, Cadman S, Kaplan ME. Membrane polypeptide aggregates in glucose-6-phosphate dehydrogenase deficient and in vitro aged red blood cells. J Lab Clin Med. 1978;91:321-327.

134. Johnson GJ, Allen DW, Cadman S, et al. Red cell membrane polypeptide aggregates in glucose-6-phosphate dehydrogenase mutants with chronic haemolytic disease: a clue to the mechanism of haemolysis. N Engl J Med. 1979;301:522-527.

135. Johnson RM, Ravindranath Y, El-Alfy M, Goyette GJ. Oxidant damage to erythrocyte membrane in glucose 6-phosphate dehydrogenase deficiency: correlation with in vivo reduced glutathione concentration and membrane protein oxidation. Blood. 1994;83:1117-1123.

136. Hamilton JW, Jones FG, McMullin MF. Glucose-6-phosphate dehydrogenase Guadalajara—a case of chronic non-spherocytic haemolytic anaemia responding to splenectomy and the role of splenectomy in this disorder. Hematology. 2004;9:307-309.

137. Beutler E, Kuhl W, Fox M, et al. Prenatal diagnosis of glucose 6-phosphate dehydrogenase deficiency. Acta Haematol. 1992;87:103-104.

138. Rovira A, De Angioletti M, Camacho-Vanegas O, et al. Stable in vivo expression of glucose-6-phosphate dehydrogenase (G6PD) and rescue of G6PD deficiency in stem cells by gene transfer. Blood. 2000;96:4111-4117.

139. Shi PA, De Angioletti M, Donahue RE, et al. In vivo gene marking of rhesus macaque long-term repopulating hematopoietic cells using a VSV-G pseudotyped versus amphotropic oncoretroviral vector. J Gene Med. 2004;6:367-373.

140. Horecker BL, Smyrniotis A. Glucose 6-phosphate dehydrogenase. In Colowick N, Kaplan NO (eds). Methods in Enzymology, vol 1. New York, Academic Press, 1955.

141. Morelli A, Benatti U, Lenzerini L, et al. The interference of leukocytes and platelets with measurement of glucose 6-phosphate dehydrogenase activity of erythrocytes with low activity variants of the enzyme. Blood. 1981;58:642-644.

142. Motulsky AG, Campbell-Kraut JM. Population genetics of glucose 6-phosphate dehydrogenase deficiency of the red cell. In Blumberg BS (ed). Proceedings of Conference on Genetic Polymorphisms and Geographic Variations in Disease. New York, Grune & Stratton, 1961, pp 159-180.

143. Brewer GJ, Tarlov AR, Alving AS. The methemoglobin reduction test for primaquine-type sensitivity of erythrocytes. A simplified procedure for detecting a specific hypersusceptibility to drug hemolysis. JAMA. 1962;180:386-388.

144. Morelli A, Benatti U, Lenzerini L, et al. The Interference of leukocytes and platelets with measurement of glucose-6-phosphate dehydrogenase activity of erythrocytes with low activity variants of the enzyme. Blood. 1981;58:642-644.

145. Tantular IS, Kawamoto F. An improved, simple screening method for detection of glucose-6-phosphate dehydrogenase deficiency. Trop Med Int Health. 2003;8:569-574.

146. Jalloh A, Tantular IS, Pusarawati S, et al. Rapid epidemiologic assessment of glucose-6-phosphate dehydrogenase deficiency in malaria-endemic areas in Southeast Asia using a novel diagnostic kit. Trop Med Int Health. 2004;9:615-623.

147. Fairbanks VF, Lampe LT. A tetrazolium-linked cytochemical method for estimation of glucose 6-phosphate dehydrogenase activity in individual erythrocytes: applications in the study of heterozygotes for glucose 6-phosphate dehydrogenase deficiency. Blood. 1968;31:589.

148. Van Noorden CJF, Vogels IMC. A sensitive cytochemical staining method for glucose-6-phosphate dehydrogenase activity in individual erythrocytes. Br J Haematol. 1985;60:57-60.

149. Bienzle U, Sodeinde O, Effiong CE, Luzzatto L. G6PD deficiency and sickle cell anemia: frequency and features of the association in an African community. Blood. 1975;46:591-597.

150. Herschel M, Beutler E. Low glucose-6-phosphate dehydrogenase enzyme activity level at the time of hemolysis in a male neonate with the African type of deficiency. Blood Cells Mol Dis. 2001;27:918-923.

151. Vulliamy TJ, D'Urso M, Battistuzzi G, et al. Diverse point mutations in the human glucose-6-phosphate dehydrogenase gene cause enzyme deficiency and mild or severe hemolytic anemia. Proc Natl Acad Sci U S A. 1988;85:5171-5175.

152. Miwa S, Fujii H. Glucose 6-phosphate dehydrogenase variants in Japan. In Yoshida A, Beutler E (eds). Glucose 6-Phosphate Dehydrogenase. New York, Academic Press, 1986, pp 261-272.

153. Luzzatto L. Inherited haemolytic states: glucose-6-phosphate dehydrogenase deficiency. Clin Haematol. 1975;4:83-108.

154. Calabrò V, Cascone A, Malaspina P, Battistuzzi G. Glucose-6-phosphate dehydrogenase (G6PD) deficiency in Southern Italy: a case of G6PD A(−) associated with favism. Haematologica. 1989;74:71-73.

155. Galiano S, Gaetani GF, Barabino A, et al. Favism in the African type of glucose-6-phosphate dehydrogenase deficiency (A⁻). BMJ. 1990;300:236.

156. Vives-Corrons JL, Pujades A. Heterogeneity of "Mediterranean type" glucose 6-phospahte dehydrogenase (G6PD) deficiency in Spain and description of two new variants associated with favism. Hum Genet. 1982;60:216-221.

157. Kirkman HN, Riley HD. Congenital non-spherocytic hemolytic anemia. Studies on a family with a qualitative defect in glucose-6-phosphate dehydrogenase. Am J Dis Child. 1961;102:313-320.

158. Kaeda JS, Chhotray GP, Ranjit MR, et al. A new glucose-6-phosphate dehydrogenase variant, G6PD Orissa (44 Ala→Gly), is the major polymorphic variant in tribal populations in India. Am J Hum Genet. 1995;57:1335-1341.

159. Naylor CE, Rowland P, Basak AK, et al. Glucose 6-phosphate dehydrogenase mutations causing enzyme deficiency in a model of the tertiary structure of the human enzyme. Blood. 1996;87:2974-2982.

160. Gomez-Gallego F, Garrido-Pertierra A, Mason PJ, Bautista JM. Unproductive folding of the human G6PD-deficient variant A⁻. FASEB J. 1996;10:153-158.

161. Huang Y, Choi MY, Au SW, et al. Purification and detailed study of two clinically different human glucose 6-phosphate dehydrogenase variants, G6PD(Plymouth) and G6PD(Mahidol): evidence for defective protein folding as the basis of disease. Mol Genet Metab. 2008;93:44-53.

162. Bloom KE, Brewer GJ, Magon AM, Wetterstroem N. Microsomal incubation test of potentially hemolytic drugs for glucose-6-phosphate dehydrogenase deficiency. Clin Pharmacol Ther. 1983;33:403-409.

163. Gaetani GD, Mareni C, Ravazzolo R, Salvidio E. Hemolytic effect of two sulphonamides evaluated by a new method. Br J Haematol. 1976;32:183-190.

164. Mutabingwa TK, Maxwell CA, Sia IG, et al. A trial of proguanil-dapsone in comparison with sulfadoxine-pyrimethamine for the clearance of *Plasmodium falciparum* infections in Tanzania. Trans R Soc Trop Med Hyg. 2001;95:433-438.

165. Alloueche A, Bailey W, Barton S, et al. Comparison of chlorproguanil-dapsone with sulfadoxine-pyrimethamine for the treatment of uncomplicated falciparum malaria in young African children: double-blind randomised controlled trial. Lancet. 2004;363:1843-1848.

166. Morellini M, Colonna-Romano S, Meloni T, et al. Glucose 6-phosphate dehydrogenase of leukocyte sub-populations in normal and enzyme-deficient individuals. Haematologica. 1985;70:390-395.

167. Vives Corrons JL, Feliu E, Pujades MA, et al. Severe-glucose-6-phosphate dehydrogenase (G6PD) deficiency associated with chronic hemolytic anemia, granulocyte dysfunction, and increased susceptibility to infections: description of a new molecular variant (G6PD Barcelona). Blood. 1982;59:428-434.

168. Roos D, deBoer M, Kuribayashi F, et al. Mutations in the X-linked and autosomal recessive forms of chronic granulomatous disease. Blood. 1996;87:1663-1681.

169. Wilmanski J, Siddiqi M, Deitch EA, Spolarics Z. Augmented IL-10 production and redox-dependent signaling pathways in glucose-6-phosphate dehydrogenase–deficient mouse peritoneal macrophages. J Leukoc Biol. 2005;78:85-94.

170. Westring DN, Pisciotta AV. Anemia, cataracts and seizures in a patient with glucose-6-phosphate dehydrogenase deficiency. Arch Intern Med. 1966;118:385-390.

171. Harley JD, Agar NS, Yoshida A. Glucose 6-phosphate dehydrogenase variants: Gd(+) Alexandra associated with neonatal jaundice and Gd(−) Camperdown in a young man with lamellar cataracts. J Lab Clin Med. 1978;91:295-300.

172. Meloni T, Carta F, Forteleoni G, et al. Glucose 6-phosphate dehydrogenase deficiency and cataract of patients in northern Sardinia. Am J Ophthalmol. 1990;110:661-664.

173. Orzalesi M, Fossarello M, Sarcinelli R, Schlich U. The relationship between glucose 6-phosphate dehydrogenase deficiency and cataracts in Sardinia. An epidemiological and biochemical study. Doc Ophthalmol. 1984;57:187-201.

174. Chen Y, Zeng L, Ma Q, et al. The study of G6PD in erythrocyte and lens in senile and presenile cataract. Yan Ke Xue Bao. 1992;8:12-15.

175. Assaf AA, Tabbara KF, el-Hazmi MA. Cataracts in glucose-6-phosphate dehydrogenase deficiency. Ophthalmic Paediatr Genet. 1993;14:81-86.

176. Luzzatto L, Allan NC. Relationship between the genes for glucose 6-phosphate dehydrogenase and haemoglobin in a Nigerian population. Nature. 1968;219:1041-1042.

177. Nieuwenhuis F, Wolf B, Bomba A, De Graaf P. Haematological study in Cabo Delgado province, Mozambique; sickle cell trait and G6PD deficiency. Trop Geogr Med. 1986;38:183-187.

178. Gibbs WN, Wardle J, Serjeant GR. Glucose 6-phosphate dehydrogenase deficiency and homozygous sickle cell disease in Jamaica. Br J Haematol. 1980;45:73-80.

179. Steinberg MH, West MS, Gallagher D, Mentzer W. Effects of glucose-6-phosphate dehydrogenase deficiency upon sickle cell anemia. Blood. 1988;71:748-752.

180. Bouanga JC, Mouele R, Prehu C, et al. Glucose-6-phosphate dehydrogenase deficiency and homozygous sickle cell disease in Congo. Hum Hered. 1998;48:192-197.

181. Piomelli S, Siniscalco M. The haematological effects of glucose 6-phosphate dehydrogenase deficiency and thalassaemia trait: interaction between the two genes at the phenotype level. Br J Haematol. 1969;16:537-549.

182. Carpentieri U, Haggard ME, Schneider RG, Hightower BJ. Hb E–beta thalassemia associated with G6PD deficiency. South Med J. 1980;73:518-520.

183. Vives Corrons JL, Garcia AM, Sosa AM, et al. Heterozygous pyruvate kinase deficiency and severe hemolytic anemia in a pregnant woman with concomitant, glucose-6-phosphate dehydrogenase deficiency. Ann Hematol. 1991;62:190-193.

184. Mahendra P, Dollery CT, Luzzatto L, Bloom SR. Pyruvate kinase deficiency: association with G6PD deficiency. BMJ. 1992;305:760-762.

185. Ventura A, Panizon F, Soranzo MR, et al. Congenital dyserythropoietic anaemia type II associated with a new type of G6PD deficiency (G6PD Gabrovizza). Acta Haematol. 1984;71:227-234.

186. Szeto SC, Ng CS. A case of congenital dyserythropoietic anemia in a male Chinese. Pathology. 1986;18:165-168.

187. Gangarossa S, Romano V, Miraglia del Giudice E, et al. Congenital dyserythropoietic anemia type II associated with G6PD Seattle in a Sicilian child. Acta Haematol. 1995;93:36-39.

188. Panich V, Na-Nakorn S, Wasi P. Hereditary elliptocytosis (the first report in Thailand) in association with erythrocyte glucose-6-phosphate dehydrogenase deficiency and hemoglobin E. J Med Assoc Thai. 1970;53:593-600.

189. Alfinito F, Calabrò V, Cappellini MD, et al. Glucose 6-phosphate dehydrogenase deficiency and red cell membrane defects: additive or synergistic interaction in producing chronic haemolytic anaemia. Br J Haematol. 1994;87:148-152.

190. Eppes RB, Lawrence AM, McNamara JV, et al. Intravenous glucose tolerance in negro men deficient in glucose-6-phosphate dehydrogenase. N Engl J Med. 1969;281:60-63.

191. Eppes RB, Brewer GJ, De Gowin RL, et al. Oral glucose tolerance in Negro men deficient in G6PD. N Engl J Med. 1966;275:855-860.

192. Billis AG, Xefteris ED, Ioannides PJ, Papastamatis SC. Abnormal glucose tolerance in favism. Diabetologia. 1970;6:425-429.

193. Saha N. Association of glucose-6-phosphate dehydrogenase deficiency with diabetes mellitus in ethnic groups of Singapore. J Med Genet. 1979;16:431-434.

194. Meloni T, Pacifico A, Forteleoni G, Meloni GF. G6PD deficiency and diabetes mellitus in northern Sardinian subjects [letter]. Haematologica. 1992;77:94-95.

195. Wan GH, Tsai SC, Chiu DT. Decreased blood activity of glucose-6-phosphate dehydrogenase associates with increased risk for diabetes mellitus. Endocrine. 2002;19:191-195.

196. Niazi GA. Glucose-6-phosphate dehydrogenase deficiency and diabetes mellitus. Int J Hematol. 1991;54:295-298.

197. Shalev O, Wollner A, Menczel J. Diabetic ketoacidosis does not precipitate haemolysis in patients with the Mediterranean variant of glucose-6-phosphate dehydrogenase deficiency. BMJ. 1984;288:179-180.

198. Sobngwi E, Gautier JF, Kevorkian JP, et al. High prevalence of glucose-6-phosphate dehydrogenase deficiency without gene mutation suggests a novel genetic mechanism predisposing to ketosis-prone diabetes. J Clin Endocrinol Metab. 2005;90:4446-4451.

199. Balestrieri C, Serra G, Cauli C, et al. Treatment of chronic hepatitis C in patients with glucose-6-phosphate dehydrogenase deficiency: is ribavirin harmful? Blood. 2006;107:3409-3410.

200. Meloni T, Forteleoni G, Meloni GF. Marked decline of favism after neonatal glucose-6-phosphate dehydrogenase screening and health education: the northern Sardinian experience. Acta Haematol. 1992;87:29-31.

201. Allison AC. Glucose 6-phosphate dehydrogenase deficiency in red blood cells of East Africans. Nature. 1960;186:531-532.

202. Motulsky AG. Metabolic polymorphisms and the role of infectious diseases in human evolution. Hum Biol. 1960;32:28-62.

203. Luzzatto L. Genetic factors in malaria. Bull World Health Organ. 1974;50:195-202.

204. Kar S, Seth S, Seth PK. Prevalence of malaria in Ao Nagas and its association with G6PD and HbE. Hum Biol. 1992;64:187-197.

204. Luzzatto L. Genetics of red cells and susceptibility to malaria. Blood. 1979;54:961-976.

205. Luzzatto L, O'Brien S, Usanga E, Wanachiwanawin W. Origin of G6PD polymorphism: malaria and G6PD deficiency. In Yoshida A, Beutler E, Orlando FL (eds). Glucose-6-Phosphate Dehydrogenase. New York, Academic Press, 1986, pp 181-193.

206. Miller LH. Genetically determined human resistance factors. In Wernsdorfer WH, McGregor I (eds). Malaria: Principles and Practice of Malariology. Edinburgh, Churchill-Livingstone, 1988, pp 487-500.

207. Bienzle U, Ayeni O, Lucas AO, Luzzatto L. Glucose-6-phosphate dehydrogenase deficiency and malaria. Greater resistance of females heterozygous for enzyme deficiency and of males with non-deficient variant. Lancet. 1972;1: 107-110.

208. Ruwende C, Khoo SC, Snow RW, et al. Natural selection of hemi- and heterozygotes for G6PD deficiency in Africa by resistance to severe malaria. Nature. 1995;376: 246-249.

210. Guindo A, Fairhurst RM, Doumbo OK, et al. X-linked G6PD deficiency protects hemizygous males but not heterozygous females against severe malaria. PLoS Med. 2007;4(3):e66.

211. Usanga EA, Luzzatto L. Adaptation of *Plasmodium falciparum* to glucose 6-phosphate dehydrogenase deficient host red cells by production of parasite-encoded enzyme. Nature. 1985;313:793-795.

212. Cappadoro M, Giribaldi G, O'Brien E, et al. Early phagocytosis of glucose-6-phosphate dehydrogenase (G6PD)-deficient erythrocytes parasitized by *Plasmodium falciparum* may explain malaria protection in G6PD deficiency. Blood. 1998;92:2527-2534.

213. Luzzatto L, Usanga FA, Reddy S. Glucose-6-phosphate dehydrogenase deficient red cells: resistance to infection by malarial parasites. Science. 1969;164:839-842.

214. Luzzatto L, Pinching AJ. Commentary to R Nagel—innate resistance to malaria: the intraerythrocytic cycle. Blood Cells. 1990;16:340-347.

215. Tishkoff SA, Varkonyi R, Cahinhinan N, et al. Haplotype diversity and linkage disequilibrium at human G6PD: recent origin of alleles that confer malarial resistance. Science. 2001;293:455-462.

216. Luzzatto L, Notaro R. Malaria. Protecting against bad air. Science. 2001;293:442-443.

VI Disorders of Hemoglobin

18 Hemoglobins: Normal and Abnormal

H. Franklin Bunn and Ronald L. Nagel

This chapter deals with the structure and properties of hemoglobin (Hb) and disorders stemming from structural abnormalities (mutations of the coding sequence) that lead to clinical manifestations. Not included are sickle cell disease and the thalassemias, which are covered in Chapters 19 and 20.

At last count (mid-2008), 983 human Hb mutations have been cataloged: 267 for the α1 gene, 314 for the α2 gene, 732 for the β gene, 79 for the δ gene, 50 for the [A]γ gene, and 56 for the [G]γ gene. Of these, 91 have high affinity for O_2 and 134 are unstable. (A list of the mutants can be found at the Globin Gene Server [http://globin.cse.psu.edu], a website founded by Ross Hardison and initially based on Titus Huisman's database.)

NORMAL HEMOGLOBIN A: STRUCTURE AND FUNCTION

Overall Hemoglobin Structure

The major Hb molecule in adults is a tetramer formed by four polypeptide chains, two α chains (141 amino acids long) and two β chains (146 amino acids long). The primary structure (amino acid sequence) is illustrated in Table 18-1. Each of these chains is attached to a prosthetic group heme formed by protoporphyrin IX and complexed with an iron molecule. All globins consist of eight helices and interconnecting loops (nonhelical), except for α Hb subunits, which lack the D helix because of deletion of five consecutive residues. Each chain is formed by helical regions and nonhelical regions (which allow for bending) that fold into a tightly globular protein.

α Chains of Hemoglobin (Tertiary Structure)

The α chains have the general architecture of myoglobin (Fig. 18-1) but are shorter and contain 141 rather than 153 amino acids as a result of the absence of six residues from the C-terminal portion and six from the D helix. The D helix in myoglobin and in the β subunit of Hb is required for retention of heme.[1]

The deletion of the D helix in the α chains has no explanation. Disappearance of the nonhelical C-terminal

TABLE 18-1	Primary Amino Acid Structure of the Hemoglobin Molecule*						
Helix	**α**	**ξ**	**Helix**	**β**	**δ**	**γ**	**ε**
NA1	1 Val	Ser	NA1	1 Val	Val	Gly	Val
			NA2	2 His	His	His	His
NA2	2 Leu	Leu	NA3	3 Leu	Leu	Phe	Phe
A1	3 Ser	Thr	A1	4 Thr	Thr	Thr	Thr
A2	4 Pro	Lys	A2	5 Pro	Pro	Glu	Ala
A3	5 Ala	Thr	A3	6 Glu	Glu	Glu	Glu
A4	6 Asp	Glu	A4	7 Glu	Glu	Asp	Glu
A5	7 Lys	Arg	A5	8 Lys	Lys	Lys	Lys
A6	8 Thr	Thr	A6	9 Ser	Thr	Ala	Ala
A7	9 Asn	Ile	A7	10 Ala	Ala	Thr	Ala
A8	10 Val	Ile	A8	11 Val	Val	Ile	Val
A9	11 Lys	Val	A9	12 Thr	Asn	Thr	Thr
A10	12 Ala	Ser	A10	13 Ala	Ala	Ser	Ser
A11	13 Ala	Met	A11	14 Leu	Leu	Leu	Leu
A12	14 Trp	Trp	A12	15 Trp	Trp	Trp	Trp
A13	15 Gly	Ala	A13	16 Gly	Gly	Gly	Ser
A14	16 Lys	Lys	A14	17 Lys	Lys	Lys	Lys
A15	17 Val	Ile	A15	18 Val	Val	Val	Met
A16	18 Gly	Ser					
AB1	19 Ala	Thr					
B1	20 His	Gln	B1	19 Asn	Asn	Asn	Asn
B2	21 Ala	Ala	B2	20 Val	Val	Val	Val
B3	22 Gly	Asp	B3	21 Asp	Asp	Glu	Glu
B4	23 Glu	Thr	B4	22 Glu	Ala	Asp	Glu
B5	24 Tyr	Ile	B5	23 Val	Val	Ala	Ala
B6	25 Gly	Gly	B6	24 Gly	Gly	Gly	Gly
B7	26 Ala	Thr	B7	25 Gly	Gly	Gly	Gly
B8	27 Glu	Glu	B8	26 Glu	Glu	Glu	Glu
B9	28 Ala	Thr	B9	27 Ala	Ala	Thr	Ala
B10	29 Leu	Leu	B10	28 Leu	Leu	Leu	Leu
B11	30 Glu	Glu	B11	29 Gly	Gly	Gly	Gly
B12	31 Arg	Arg	B12	30 Arg	Arg	Arg	Arg

TABLE 18-1	Primary Amino Acid Structure of the Hemoglobin Molecule*—cont'd						
Helix	**α**	**ξ**	**Helix**	**β**	**δ**	**γ**	**ε**
B13	32 Met	Leu	B13	31 Leu	Leu	Leu	Leu
B14	33 Phe	Phe	B14	32 Leu	Leu	Leu	Leu
B15	34 Leu	Leu	B15	33 Val	Val	Val	Val
B16	35 Ser	Ser	B16	34 Val	Val	Val	Val
C1	36 Phe	His	C1	35 Tyr	Tyr	Tyr	Tyr
C2	37 Pro	Pro	C2	36 Pro	Pro	Pro	Pro
C3	38 Thr	Gln	C3	37 Trp	Trp	Trp	Trp
C4	39 Thr	Thr	C4	38 Thr	Thr	Thr	Thr
C5	40 Lys	Lys	C5	39 Gln	Gln	Gln	Gln
C6	41 Thr	Thr	C6	40 Arg	Arg	Arg	Arg
C7	42 Tyr	Tyr	C7	41 Phe	Phe	Phe	Phe
CE1	43 Phe	Phe	CD1	42 Phe	Phe	Phe	Phe
CE2	44 Pro	Pro	CD2	43 Glu	Glu	Asp	Asp
CE3	45 His	His	CD3	44 Ser	Ser	Ser	Ser
CE4	46 Phe	Phe	CD4	45 Phe	Phe	Phe	Phe
			CD5	46 Gly	Gly	Gly	Gly
CE5	47 Asp	Asp	CD6	47 Asp	Asp	Asn	Asn
CE6	48 Leu	Leu	CD7	48 Leu	Leu	Leu	Leu
CE7	49 Ser	His	CD8	49 Ser	Ser	Ser	Ser
CE8	50 His	Pro	D1	50 Thr	Ser	Ser	Ser
			D2	51 Pro	Pro	Ala	Pro
			D3	52 Asp	Asp	Ser	Ser
			D4	53 Ala	Ala	Ala	Ala
			D5	54 Val	Val	Ile	Ile
			D6	55 Met	Met	Met	Leu
CE9	51 Gly	Gly	D7	56 Gly	Gly	Gly	Gly
E1	52 Ser	Ser	E1	57 Asn	Asn	Asn	Asn
E2	53 Ala	Ala	E2	58 Pro	Pro	Pro	Pro
E3	54 Gln	Gln	E3	59 Lys	Lys	Lys	Lys
E4	55 Val	Leu	E4	60 Val	Val	Val	Val
E5	56 Lys	Arg	E5	61 Lys	Lys	Lys	Lys
E6	57 Gly	Ala	E6	62 Ala	Ala	Ala	Ala
E7	58 His	His	E7	63 His	His	His	His
E8	59 Gly	Gly	E8	64 Gly	Gly	Gly	Gly
E9	60 Lys	Ser	E9	65 Lys	Lys	Lys	Lys
E10	61 Lys	Lys	E10	66 Lys	Lys	Lys	Lys
E11	62 Val	Val	E11	67 Val	Val	Val	Val
E12	63 Ala	Val	E12	68 Leu	Leu	Leu	Leu
E13	64 Asp	Ser	E13	69 Gly	Gly	Thr	Thr
E14	65 Ala	Ala	E14	70 Ala	Ala	Ser	Ser
E15	66 Leu	Val	E15	71 Phe	Phe	Leu	Phe
E16	67 Thr	Gly	E16	72 Ser	Ser	Gly	Gly
E17	68 Asn	Asp	E17	73 Asp	Asp	Asp	Asp
E18	69 Ala	Ala	E18	74 Gly	Gly	Ala	Ala
E19	70 Val	Val	E19	75 Leu	Leu	Ile, Thr	Ile
E20	71 Ala	Lys	E20	76 Ala	Ala	Lys	Lys
EF1	72 His	Ser	EF1	77 His	His	His	Asn
EF2	73 Val	Ile	EF2	78 Leu	Leu	Leu	Met
EF3	74 Asp	Asp	EF3	79 Asp	Asp	Asp	Asp
EF4	75 Asp	Asp	EF4	80 Asn	Asn	Asp	Asn
EF5	76 Met	Ile	EF5	81 Leu	Leu	Leu	Leu
EF6	77 Pro	Gly	EF6	82 Lys	Lys	Lys	Lys
EF7	78 Asn	Gly	EF7	83 Gly	Gly	Gly	Pro
EF8	79 Ala	Ala	EF8	84 Thr	Thr	Thr	Ala
F1	80 Leu	Leu	F1	85 Phe	Phe	Phe	Phe
F2	81 Ser	Ser	F2	86 Ala	Ser	Ala	Ala
F3	82 Ala	Lys	F3	87 Thr	Gln	Gln	Lys
F4	83 Leu	Leu	F4	88 Leu	Leu	Leu	Leu
F5	84 Ser	Ser	F5	89 Ser	Ser	Ser	Ser
F6	85 Asp	Glu	F6	90 Glu	Glu	Glu	Glu
F7	86 Leu	Leu	F7	91 Leu	Leu	Leu	Leu
F8	87 His	His	F8	92 His	His	His	His
F9	88 Ala	Ala	F9	93 Cys	Cys	Cys	Cys
FG1	89 His	Tyr	FG1	94 Asp	Asp	Asp	Asp

Continues

TABLE 18-1	Primary Amino Acid Structure of the Hemoglobin Molecule*—cont'd						
Helix	α	ξ	Helix	β	δ	γ	ε
FG2	90 Lys	Ile	FG2	95 Lys	Lys	Lys	Lys
FG3	91 Leu	Leu	FG3	96 Leu	Leu	Leu	Leu
FG4	92 Arg	Arg	FG4	97 His	His	His	His
FG5	93 Val	Val	FG5	98 Val	Val	Val	Val
G1	94 Asp	Asp	G1	99 Asp	Asp	Asp	Asp
G2	95 Pro	Pro	G2	100 Pro	Pro	Pro	Pro
G3	96 Val	Val	G3	101 Glu	Glu	Glu	Glu
G4	97 Asn	Asn	G4	102 Asn	Asn	Asn	Asn
G5	98 Phe	Phe	G5	103 Phe	Phe	Phe	Phe
G6	99 Lys	Lys	G6	104 Arg	Arg	Lys	Lys
G7	100 Leu	Leu	G7	105 Leu	Leu	Leu	Leu
G8	101 Leu	Leu	G8	106 Leu	Leu	Leu	Leu
G9	102 Ser	Ser	G9	107 Gly	Gly	Gly	Gly
G10	103 His	His	G10	108 Asn	Asn	Asn	Asn
G11	104 Cys	Cys	G11	109 Val	Val	Val	Val
G12	105 Leu	Leu	G12	110 Leu	Leu	Leu	Met
G13	106 Leu	Leu	G13	111 Val	Val	Val	Val
G14	107 Val	Val	G14	112 Cys	Cys	Thr	Ile
G15	108 Thr	Thr	G15	113 Val	Val	Val	Ile
G16	109 Leu	Leu	G16	114 Leu	Leu	Leu	Leu
G17	110 Ala	Ala	G17	115 Ala	Ala	Ala	Ala
G18	111 Ala	Ala	G18	116 His	Arg	Ile	Thr
G19	112 His	Arg	G19	117 His	Asn	His	His
GH1	113 Leu	Phe	GH1	118 Phe	Phe	Phe	Phe
GH2	114 Pro	Pro	GH2	119 Gly	Gly	Gly	Gly
GH3	115 Ala	Ala	GH3	120 Lys	Lys	Lys	Lys
GH4	116 Glu	Asp	GH4	121 Glu	Glu	Glu	Glu
GH5	117 Phe	Phe	GH5	122 Phe	Phe	Phe	Phe
H1	118 Thr	Thr	H1	123 Thr	Thr	Thr	Thr
H2	119 Pro	Ala	H2	124 Pro	Pro	Pro	Pro
H3	120 Ala	Glu	H3	125 Pro	Gln	Glu	Glu
H4	121 Val	Ala	H4	126 Val	Met	Val	Val
H5	122 His	His	H5	127 Gln	Gln	Gln	Gln
H6	123 Ala	Ala	H6	128 Ala	Ala	Ala	Ala
H7	124 Ser	Ala	H7	129 Ala	Ala	Ser	Ala
H8	125 Leu	Trp	H8	130 Tyr	Tyr	Trp	Trp
H9	126 Asp	Asp	H9	131 Gln	Gln	Gln	Gln
H10	127 Lys	Lys	H10	132 Lys	Lys	Lys	Lys
H11	128 Phe	Phe	H11	133 Val	Val	Met	Leu
H12	129 Leu	Leu	H12	134 Val	Val	Val	Val
H13	130 Ala	Ser	H13	135 Ala	Ala	Thr	Ser
H14	131 Ser	Val	H14	136 Gly	Gly	Gly, Ala	Ala
H15	132 Val	Val	H15	137 Val	Val	Val	Val
H16	133 Ser	Ser	H16	138 Ala	Ala	Ala	Ala
H17	134 Thr	Ser	H17	139 Asn	Asn	Ser	Ile
H18	135 Val	Val	H18	140 Ala	Ala	Ala	Ala
H19	136 Leu	Leu	H19	141 Leu	Leu	Leu	Leu
H20	137 Thr	Thr	H20	142 Ala	Ala	Ser	Ala
H21	138 Ser	Glu	H21	143 His	His	Ser	His
HC1	139 Lys	Lys	HC1	144 Lys	Lys	Arg	Lys
HC2	140 Tyr	Tyr	HC2	145 Tyr	Tyr	Tyr	Tyr
HC3	141 Arg	Arg	HC3	146 His	His	His	His

*The α and α-related (δ) subunits are shown at the left. The β and β-related (δ, γ, and ε) chains are at the right. The amino acids' relationship to the eight globin helices (A to H) is also shown. Thus, A16 is the 16th amino acid in the A helix. Interhelical elbows are named for the two adjacent helices (e.g., AB1 is the first amino acid between helices A and B). The N- and C-terminal residues are labeled NA and HC, respectively. The residues are aligned to maximize the homology between subunits, which causes some gaps.

Modified from Bunn HF, Forget BG. Hemoglobin: Molecular, Genetic, and Clinical Aspects. Philadelphia, WB Saunders, 1986.

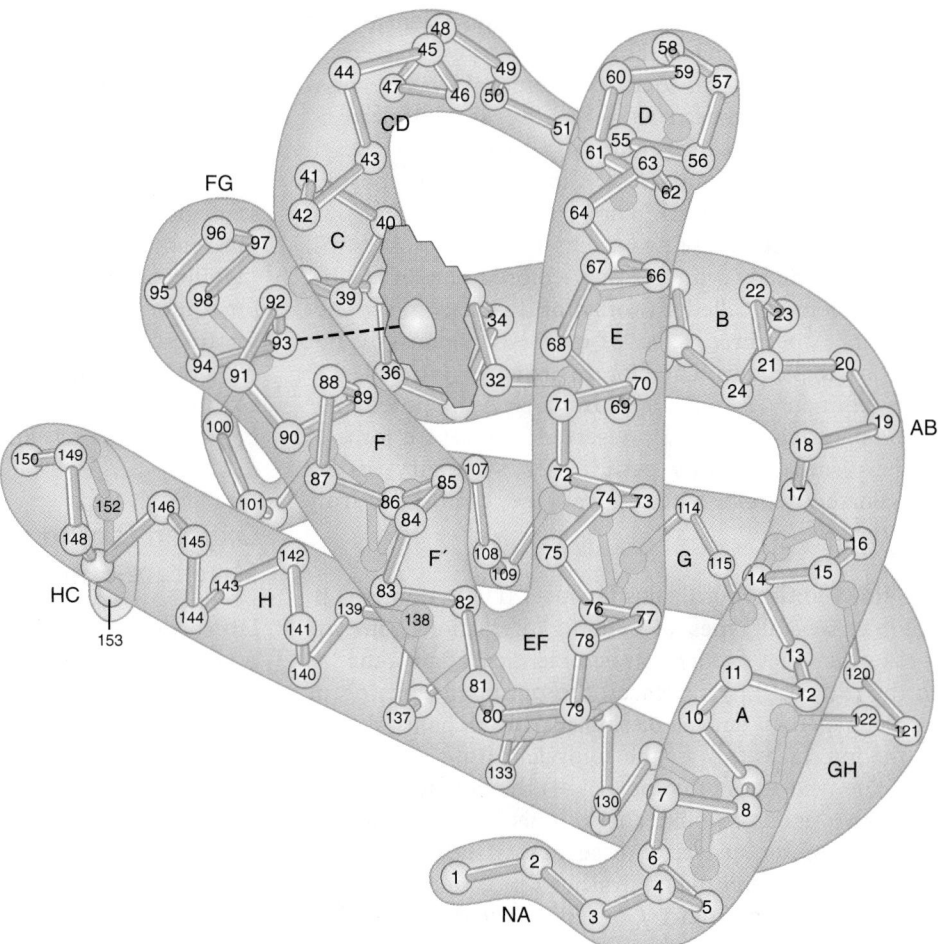

FIGURE 18-1. Myoglobin structure. The myoglobin molecule consists of eight stretches of helix that surround the heme group to form a pocket. Single letters signify a helix and double letters a corner or bend (nonhelical regions). The heme pocket is formed by helices E and F. Helices B, G, and H are at the bottom, and the CD corner closes the open end. Histidine side chains interact with the heme from both sides. *(From Dickerson RE, Geis I. Hemoglobin: Structure, Function, Evolution, and Pathology. Menlo Park, CA, Benjamin/Cummings, 1983, p 26.)*

residues could be related to the important bond between Arg-α141 and Tyr-α140 and the appropriate receptor, which are important for the conformational changes involved in the transformation from oxygenated (oxy) to deoxygenated (deoxy) forms (see later discussion), a central feature of the tetramer structure-function relationship. The additional C-terminal residues in myoglobin might strain these critical molecular interactions and make the conformational change impossible.

The differences between α chains and myoglobin could also be derived from the need for α chains to bind several different β-like chains (γ, δ, and ε), with varied requirements for generation of the quaternary structure. Specifically, generation of a quaternary structure implies changes in the character of the residues involved in subunit contact. That is, residues that are polar in myoglobin (because they are in direct contact with the solvent) might be buried in an intersubunit contact in several of the Hbs and hence have to be replaced by hydrophobic amino acids. For example, in residue B15, a lysine in myoglobin is a leucine in human α chains, whereas residue C1, a histidine in myoglobin, is a phenylalanine.[1,2]

β Chains of Hemoglobin (Tertiary Structure)

Human β chains, which contain 146 residues, are also shorter than myoglobin. The general architecture of the chain and its secondary and tertiary structure complies closely with the myoglobin fold.[3-5]

Two small structural differences with myoglobin are apparent: disappearance of two residues from the junction of the A and B helices, thereby making the AB elbow sharper, and six residues missing from the C-terminal sequence (as in the α chains). The reason for the change in the AB elbow is not understood. The critical bonds involving His-β142 and Tyr-β145 might be incompatible with the presence of the nonhelical terminal residues found in myoglobin. In the β chains, changes of charged to hydrophobic residues can also be observed in areas of the sequence involved in subunit interaction.

The Tetramer (Quaternary Structure)

The Hb molecule is a tetramer formed by two α chains and two β chains and has a total molecular mass of 64.5 kd.

How Do the Two Pairs of Chains Generate a Tetramer? The arrangement of the two types of chains in the tetramer conforms to a 222 symmetry. This designation means that the structure can be characterized by three twofold axes of symmetry perpendicular to each other (Fig. 18-2). To understand this symmetry, consider the upper half (the dark pair of chains) in the vertical axis. If you rotate these two chains 180 degrees, they will coincide perfectly with the light-colored pair of chains, an arrangement called a twofold or diad axis of symmetry, hence the three "2"s. Of course, α chains are not identical to β chains. Therefore, in an actual Hb molecule this symmetry is only approximate. A homotetramer of β chains (β_4 or HbH), observed in a severe form of α-thalassemia, exhibits perfect 222 symmetry in the oxygenated tetramer because all the chains are truly identical.

How Do the Four Chains Interact? The tetramer $\alpha_2\beta_2$ exhibits several types of subunit interactions, but the weakest contact occurs between identical chains, that is, in the $\alpha_1\alpha_2$ or $\beta_1\beta_2$ interfaces. Strong interactions occur in contacts between the dissimilar pair of chains, that is, in the interfaces $\alpha_1\beta_1$ or the equivalent $\alpha_2\beta_2$.

The next level of complexity is the contact between these two pairs of unlike chains. This contact occurs in two areas on the surface of these dimers: the $\alpha_1\beta_2$ contact (see Fig. 18-2) and the equivalent $\alpha_2\beta_1$ contact, which is called the sliding contact. Conversely, the $\alpha_1\beta_1$ dimer has

areas of interaction between the α and β chains that are called packing contacts. These dimers are strong and can be broken only with very high concentrations of urea or certain salts, and they remain as such throughout the conformational changes of Hb.

The sliding contact, in contrast, is weaker and has strategically located hydrogen (H^+) bonds and salt bridges that can be broken and reformed elsewhere to allow mobility of the two surfaces, a phenomenon indispensable for conformational changes (see next section). When the tetramer dissociates, $\alpha_1\beta_1$ dimers are generated. About 20% of the surface area of the subunits is consumed in subunit-subunit interactions, 60% of which are involved in packing contacts and 35% in sliding contacts.[6]

Oxygen Binding of Hemoglobin and Structure-Function Relationships

Hb carries O_2 from the lungs to the capillaries and carbon dioxide (CO_2) in the reverse direction. In addition, mammals need to adapt to sudden changes in oxygenation requirements; therefore, they require modulation of the O_2-carrying capacity of Hb. Functions of Hb are summarized as follows:

1. Cooperative O_2 binding that is allosterically regulated
2. pH-dependent oxygen binding (Bohr effect)

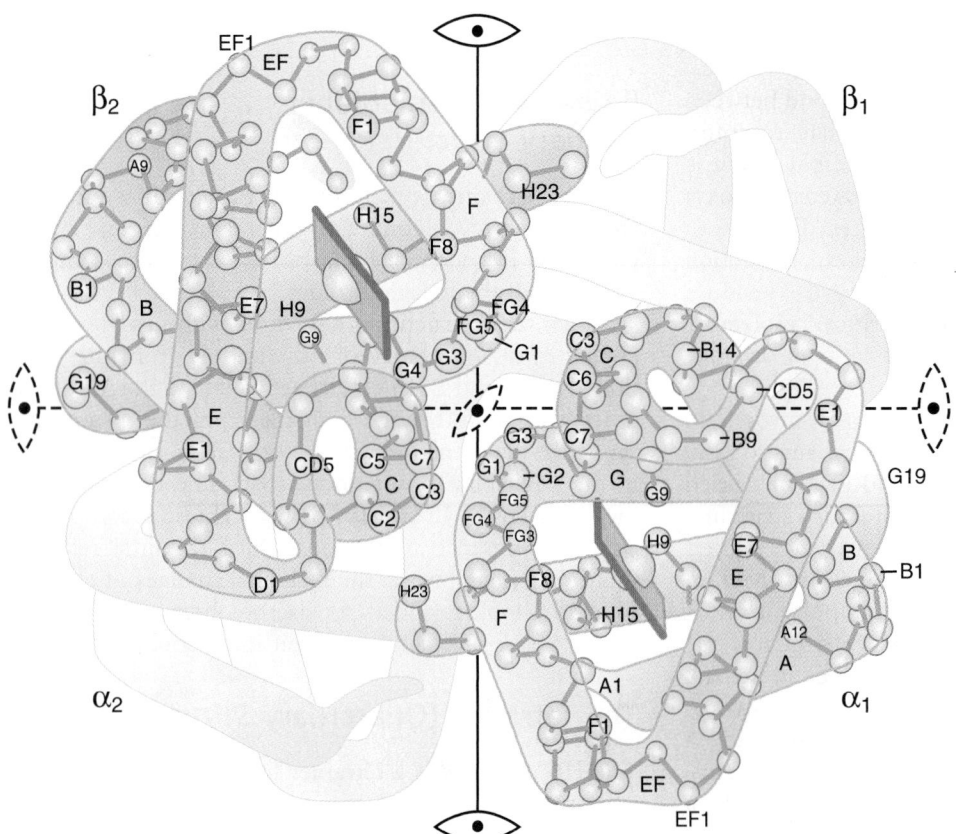

FIGURE 18-2. The four chains of hemoglobin, front view: $\alpha_1\beta_2$ contacts (the $\alpha_2\beta_1$ contacts are identical on the back side of the molecule). The perpendicular pseudoaxis is indicated by *dashes*. Only the carbons of the main chains are shown. The side chains involved in contact between subunits are indicated by *numbers* in large circles. *(From Dickerson RE, Geis I. Hemoglobin: Structure, Function, Evolution, and Pathology. Menlo Park, CA, Benjamin/Cummings, 1983, p 36.)*

3. Allosteric effectors (2,3-diphosphoglycerate [2,3-DPG], H^+, and CO_2) that modulate O_2 affinity

Allostery and Cooperativity

Hemoglobin Binds Oxygen Allosterically. The myoglobin molecule, being a monomer, binds O_2 as predicted by mass action; a plot of the partial pressure of O_2 (PO_2) versus O_2 saturation can be described as hyperbolic. In contrast, the Hb tetramer, with four hemes, binds O_2 with a sigmoidal curve (Fig. 18-3). Binding of O_2 by myoglobin can be described at equilibrium by the simple relationship

$$y = K_a PO_2 / (1 + K_a PO_2),$$

where y is the fractional saturation of the myoglobin molecule with O_2, K_a is the association constant, and PO_2 is the partial pressure of O_2.

For the Hb molecule, binding of O_2 is different, and at equilibrium this reaction can be described by the formula

$$y = K_a PO_2^n / (1 + K_a PO_2^n),$$

where n is the Hill coefficient, an empirical number that is an index of the sigmoidicity of the curve and an index of the extent of cooperativity. The Hill coefficient is approximately 3 for Hb, whereas it is equal to 1 for myoglobin.

What Is Cooperativity? Cooperativity underlies the sigmoid shape of the O_2 equilibrium curve of Hb. The initial portion of the curve has a low slope, which reflects a low affinity for O_2 by Hb at the beginning of the loading process. That is, when Hb is totally deoxygenated, it has rather poor avidity for O_2 (see Fig. 18-3). As loading proceeds and Hb binds more O_2 molecules, the slope of

the reaction begins to change rapidly and becomes steep. Hence, the affinity for O_2 becomes much higher. Thus, the initial molecules of O_2 that bind a deoxy-Hb tetramer change the avidity of the protein for O_2. This property, called cooperativity, ensures that the Hb tetramer, after it begins to accept O_2, promptly and readily binds the remaining heme groups. Consequently, if we measure the distribution of O_2 in all the Hb molecules in a solution that contains enough O_2 to oxygenate only half the hemes available, most Hb molecules would either not be oxygenated at all or would be entirely oxygenated, with a small compartment of partially oxygenated Hb.

The Molecular Basis of Cooperativity. The generally accepted basis of cooperativity is the two-state (or concerted) model of Monod, Wyman, and Changeaux[7] (the MWC model). The model is based on two fundamentally different conformations: one for oxygenated Hb and another for the deoxygenated molecule. In its strictest form, this model does not accept meaningful intermediate conformations, only two extreme ones. It predicts that the molecule of Hb will bind two or three molecules of O_2 at low affinity (deoxy conformation) and then, suddenly, the molecule will flip to the oxygenated conformation, thereby drastically increasing the O_2 affinity of the molecule as a whole. Perutz and colleagues[8-11] were very successful in accommodating the MWC model to their structural analyses (Fig. 18-4).

Formally, the two-state model can be defined by two quantities: c, which represents the difference in activity between the two enzyme states but, in the special case of Hb, corresponds to the ratio of the O_2 affinity constants between the two conformation states (K_a oxy/K_a deoxy = c). The second quantity, the allosteric constant L, is the fraction of Hb molecules in the T state. The rest are R structures. L defines the equilibrium constant for the conformational change itself between the two states: T

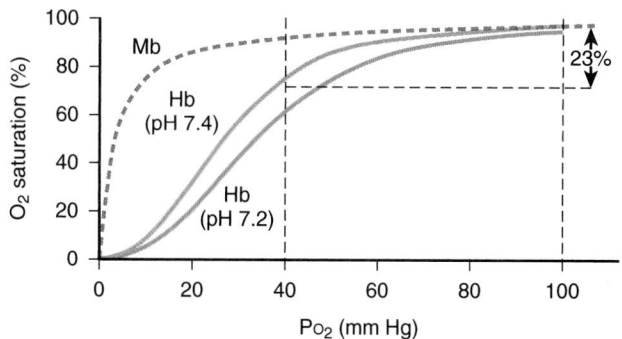

FIGURE 18-3. Oxygen equilibrium curves of sperm whale myoglobin (Mb) and hemoglobin (Hb) in human red cells. At pH 7.4 and 37° C, oxygen saturation of the red cells is 98% at the arterial blood partial pressure of O_2 (PO_2) (100 mm Hg) and 75% at mixed venous blood PO_2 (40 mm Hg), so oxygen corresponding to a saturation difference of 23% is transported by circulating red cells. *(After Imai K. Allosteric Effects in Haemoglobin. Cambridge, England, Cambridge University Press, 1982.)*

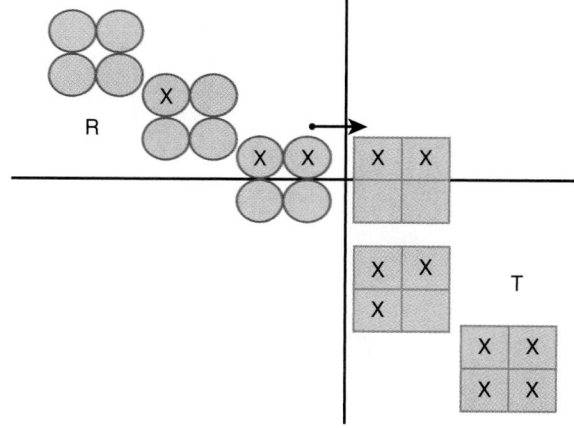

FIGURE 18-4. Two-state model of binding of oxygen and other ligands to hemoglobin. *R* stands for the relaxed or high-affinity conformer, and *T* stands for the tense or low-affinity conformer. *X* stands for the ligand. Each chain is in the R state *(sphere)* or the T state *(square)*. Notice that when the tetramer is liganded in two of the hemes, it tends to adopt (switches to) the T conformer.

for tense, the nonaccepting or low-affinity state (the deoxygenated conformer in the case of Hb), and R for relaxed, the accepting or high-affinity state (the oxygenated conformer in the case of Hb). The significant switch in conformation occurs in Hb somewhere between the binding of two and three molecules of O_2. Under physiologic conditions of pH, the presence of effectors, and osmolarity, at full saturation only 1 in 3 million Hb molecules has the T structure. The results of recent analyses argue convincingly that the two-state MWC model of Perutz defines the fundamental function of Hb and, in addition, casts doubt on the interpretation of some of the experiments that seem to contradict this model.[12,13]

Why Is the Hemoglobin Tetramer of Higher Organisms Allosteric?

Allosterism makes Hb a molecule with lower affinity for O_2 than for myoglobins or the isolated Hb chains. Allosteric effectors such as 2,3-DPG and H^+ ions modulate the reduced affinity by lowering K_T (the association constant for the T state) and raising the L constant. K_R (association constant of the R state) and L at full O_2 saturation are not modified.[8]

What Are the Structural Events Underlying Cooperativity?

The critical differences between the R and T conformers involve the areas of contact between the $\alpha_1\beta_1$ and $\alpha_2\beta_2$ dimers. The intersubunit areas of contact in the $\alpha_1\beta_1$ and $\alpha_2\beta_2$ dimers are essentially immobile during the conformational change because these dimers move as a unit. These events are pictured in Figure 18-5.

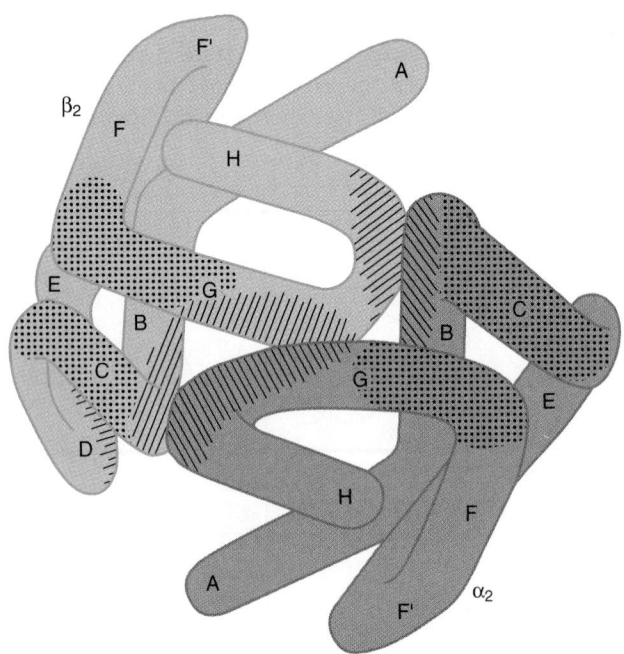

FIGURE 18-5. The $\alpha_2\beta_2$ dimer is seen in a side view. The *dotted areas* depict the packing contacts that hold the dimer together. The sliding contacts with the $\alpha_1\beta_1$ dimer are depicted by areas of *gray stippling*. (From Dickerson RE, Geis I. *Hemoglobin: Structure, Function, Evolution, and Pathology.* Menlo Park, CA, Benjamin/Cummings, 1983, p 38.)

Three regions sustain the major changes during the R-to-T conformational change, which consists of a 15-degree rotation of the $\alpha_1\beta_1$ dimer with respect to the $\alpha_2\beta_2$ dimer around a pivot passing through the terminal portions of the H helix in both chains. These movements exclusively involve the residues that touch each other in the $\alpha_1\beta_2$ areas of contact (Fig. 18-6). One movement involves pivotal sliding of the two dimers with respect to each other, with the contact involving the β FG corner moving farther away from the pivotal axis. This is called the switch region. Another movement involves the FG corner of the α chains contacting the C helix of the β chains, but the contact is less affected because the α FG corner is much closer to the pivotal axis. This is called the flexible joint. In addition, a change is seen in the set of salt bridges between the H helix (C-terminal portion of the β chain) and the C helix of the α chain and between the C-terminal portion of the α chains and the C helix of the β chain. These contact points have no particular name but are referred to here as the C-terminal changes. Detailed residue interactions are depicted in Figure 18-6.

All these H bonds and salt bridges are broken in the oxy conformer, thus providing one of the most important sources of the difference in free energy between the T and R states in Hb.

What Triggers the Conformation Change at the Level of the Heme Molecule?

The iron in deoxy-Hb is slightly out of the plane of the heme molecule (domed configuration) because the pyrrole rings are also slightly pyramidal. The angle between the heme plane and iron is 8 degrees in the α heme and 7 degrees in the β heme. The His F8 axis is 8 degrees off center, and the Val FG5 is in contact with the vinyl side chain of pyrrole 3 (Fig. 18-7). When the ligand binds the sixth coordinating position of the iron, significant steric stresses are introduced, particularly between the heme and the proximal histidine, the ligand and the heme, and the heme and Val FG5. To relieve this strain, the histidine moves 8 degrees to become perpendicular to the heme, thereby significantly decreasing doming of the iron (the angle between iron and the heme molecule falls to 4 degrees). In addition, FG5 is displaced in the direction of His F8. The configuration around the heme has now changed to the oxygenated or R state, and a chain of events involving the critical interactions in the $\alpha_1\beta_2$ area of contact follow.

What Is the Conformational Micropath between the Heme and the Globin?

In the α chain, displacement of His F8 to straighten up its 8-degree tilt in the liganded heme requires that the F helix move with it. This displacement of the F helix, along its axis, is accompanied by a shift downward, which moves it closer to the heme. The heme shifts toward the interior of the heme pocket. The changes in the F helix are propagated along the E and G helices, but the rest of the α chain is left unchanged. In the β subunit, the changes are similar, except that the

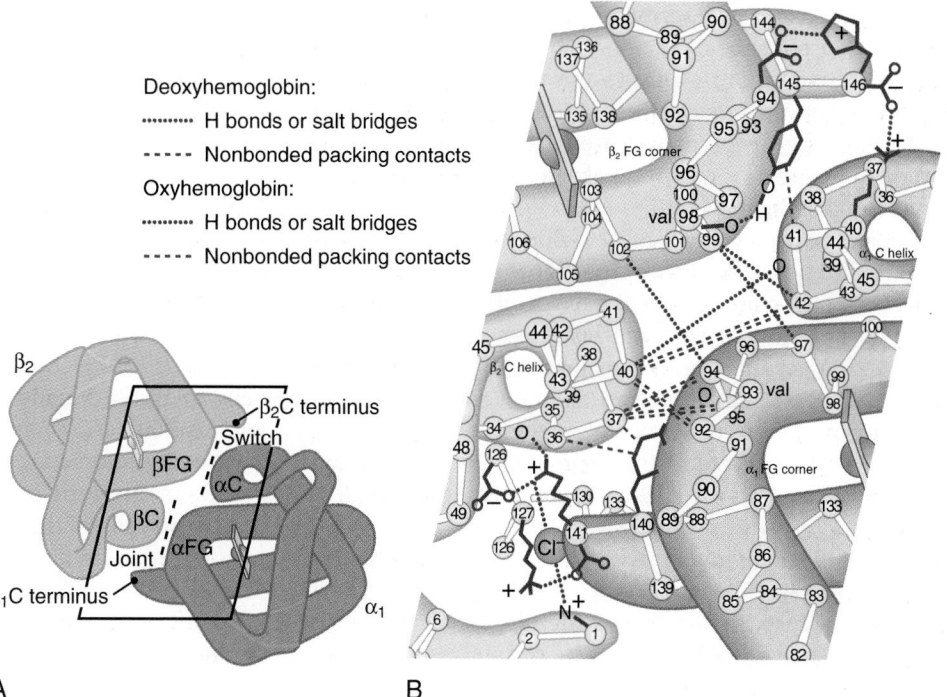

FIGURE 18-6. Front view of hemoglobin showing extensive subunit interactions between the FG corners and C helices in the $\alpha_1\beta_2$ contacts. The area outlined in **A** is enlarged in **B**. Important interaction regions from top to bottom are the β-chain C-terminal, the switch region, the flexible joint, and the β-chain terminal. *(From Dickerson RE, Geis I. Hemoglobin: Structure, Function, Evolution, and Pathology. Menlo Park, CA, Benjamin/Cummings, 1983, p 43.)*

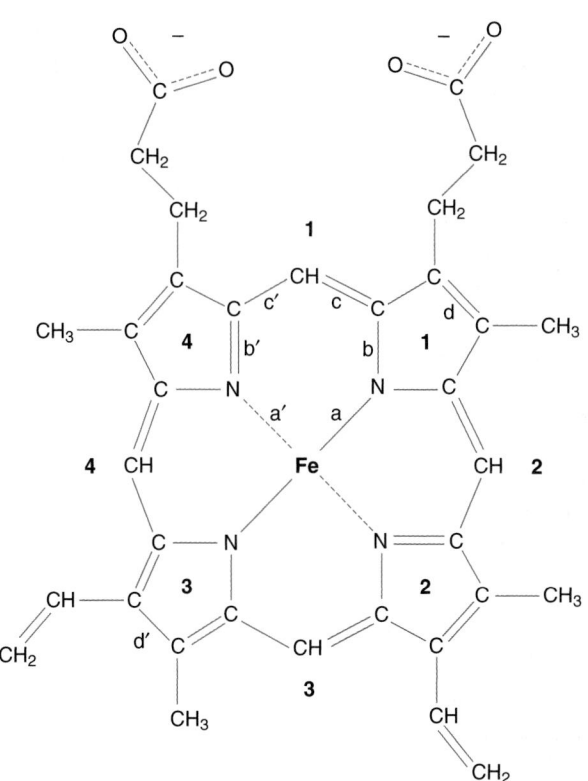

FIGURE 18-7. The protoporphyrin IX heme structure consists of four pyrrole rings with the following side chain replacements: two methyl and two propionic acids in pyrrole 1 and 4 and two methyl and two vinyls in pyrroles 2 and 3. Iron is tetracoordinated by the nitrogens of the pyrrole rings. *(From Dickerson RE, Geis I. Hemoglobin: Structure, Function, Evolution, and Pathology. Menlo Park, CA, Benjamin Cummings, 1983, p 55.)*

heme also tilts around a pyrrole 2-4 axis. In both heme niches, Val FG5 moves closer to the vinyl side chains; this van der Waals contact breaks the critical H bonds between Val98 and Tyr145 in the β chain and between Val98 and Tyr140 in the α chain. The rest of the H bonds and salt bridges described earlier for the C-terminals become weakened to the point of breakage, which releases the molecule from the T state (closed and low affinity) to the R state (open and high affinity).

Allosteric Effectors: Protons, 2,3-Diphosphoglycerate, and CO_2

Oxygen Binding Is pH Dependent. The Bohr effect describes pH-dependent changes in O_2 affinity. Within the physiologic range, the lower the pH, the lower the affinity or the higher the partial pressure of O_2 at which Hb is half saturated (P_{50}). That is, an increased concentration of protons favors a low-affinity state in Hb. Deoxy-Hb binds more protons than the oxy conformer does, which means that in the absence of a buffer, oxygenation is accompanied by a drop in pH (Haldane effect). The enhanced ability of deoxy-Hb to bind protons endows blood with very high buffering capacity. In the microcirculation, CO_2 from respiring tissue readily enters red cells and dissociates into bicarbonate anions and protons. The protons then bind to deoxy-Hb. When the blood reaches the lungs, Hb is reoxygenated and the Bohr protons are expelled; they recombine with bicarbonate, and CO_2 is exhaled.

All the features described in the previous paragraph are the consequence of H^+ ions acting as allosteric effectors: H^+ binds more avidly to the deoxy conformer (T state) than to the oxy conformer (R state). The so-called Bohr protons (protons released during oxygenation) originate primarily from breakage of the C-terminal bonds during ligand binding (see Fig. 18-6).

Seventy-five percent of the Bohr effect is derived from differences in the pK of the following residues when the molecule changes from the oxy to the deoxy conformation: (1) the two terminal histidines of the β chains (β146 His) account for approximately 40% of the Bohr protons as determined by Perutz and associates,[14-17] (2) the α amino groups of the two N-terminal residues (Val1) of the α chains account for approximately 25% of the Bohr proteins, and (3) α122 His contributes about 10% of the Bohr protons.[18]

Recently, individual pK values of the 24 histidyl residues of HbA have been measured.[19] Among these surface histidyl residues, β146 His has the biggest contribution to the physiologic Bohr effect. The sum of the contributions from 24 surface histidyl residues accounted for 86% of the alkaline Bohr effect at pH 7.4 and about 55% of the acid Bohr effect at pH 5.1. The results of this study support the presence of a global electrostatic network for regulation of the Bohr effect in the Hb molecule.

Hemoglobin Binds CO_2 While It Is Unloading O_2 and Releases CO_2 When It Is Binding O_2.

Hb is designed to bind CO_2 after delivering O_2 to tissues, thereby helping dissipate the increase in concentration of CO_2 by delivery of this metabolic end product to the lung alveoli. This exchange is facilitated because CO_2 is an allosteric inhibitor of Hb and thus decreases the O_2 affinity of the molecule.

CO_2 binds to Hb by forming carbamates with the α amino groups of the α chains. Through this new negative charge, CO_2 can bind Arg141 in the absence of Cl^- ions. This bond stabilizes the T conformer and decreases O_2 affinity of the molecule.[20] The reaction is

$$Hb—NH2 + CO_2 \rightarrow Hb—NH—COO^- + H^+.$$

Although CO_2 also binds the α amino groups of the β chains, thus helping transport more of this end product, the reaction does not contribute to allosterism. The β-chain carbamate reaction favors the deoxy conformer by the production of H^+, but this effect is counteracted by the reduction in positive charges in the central cavity, an event that favors the R state. Binding of CO_2 to hemoglobin contributes much less than the Bohr effect to the buffering capacity of blood.

Other Allosteric Effectors That Modulate the O_2 Affinity of Hemoglobin.

Benesch and Benesch[21] discovered the effects of 2,3-DPG on the function of Hb after they noticed, while examining tabular data in preparation for a lecture to medical students, that this intraerythrocytic organic phosphate was almost equimolar to the Hb tetramer (≈5 mM). Oxygen equilibrium measurements in the presence and absence of 2,3-DPG readily demonstrated that this effector drastically displaced the P_{50} of Hb to the right, thereby making Hb less avid for the ligand.

Independently and simultaneously, Chanutin and Curnish[22] realized that these substances have an important biologic effect on the red blood cell. Their discoveries were followed by the finding that inositol pentaphosphate, a higher-level polyphosphate than 2,3-DPG and a more powerful effector, has the same function as 2,3-DPG but at lower concentration in the red cells of birds. Finally, in some fish, red cell adenosine triphosphate (ATP) and guanosine triphosphate seem to be the physiologic O_2 modulators.

In an allosteric model, the effector must bind differentially to each of the conformational states. For an effector to be an inhibitor (a molecule that decreases the activity of the molecule—in this case O_2 affinity), it must bind more strongly to the T form. Biochemical[23] and crystallographic[24] studies have demonstrated that 2,3-DPG binds to the central cavity of Hb, that is, the space surrounding the true diad axis of symmetry between the two β chains (ββ) (Fig. 18-8). The displacement of the β chains away from each other by 7 Å in deoxy-Hb makes this single site in the tetramer capable of accommodating the highly negatively charged 2,3-DPG molecule, whereas the tighter ββ interaction in oxy-Hb does not allow the effector to penetrate the central cavity. The five negative charges of 2,3-DPG bind to complementary positive charges on the β chains to form salt bridges just under the edge of the ββ central cavity. The globin residues involved in the binding are the two N-terminals of the β chains, the two β143 histidines, and one of the two β82 lysines. The purpose of this effector is to modulate the O_2 equilibrium curve according to physiologic requirements. For example, in anemia, synthesis of 2,3-DPG increases, thereby favoring the release of O_2 and partially compensating for the decrease in the number of O_2 carriers.

Red Cell Oxygen Transport

The O_2 equilibrium of red cells depends on the following factors: (1) the intrinsic O_2 affinity of the Hb molecule (determined in solutions stripped of phosphate), (2) intraerythrocytic pH, (3) the intraerythrocytic concentration of 2,3-DPG, (4) temperature, and (5) the partial pressure of CO_2 (PCO_2).

Intraerythrocytic pH.

The Bohr effect of whole blood is essentially identical to that of Hb in solution. For normal blood (37° C and 40 mm Hg CO_2), the log P_{50}-to-pH ratio is close to 0.5. Intracellular pH is approximately 0.2 unit below extracellular pH, as determined by the concentration of permeant anions, chloride and bicarbonate, and the major impermeant anions, Hb itself and 2,3-DPG.

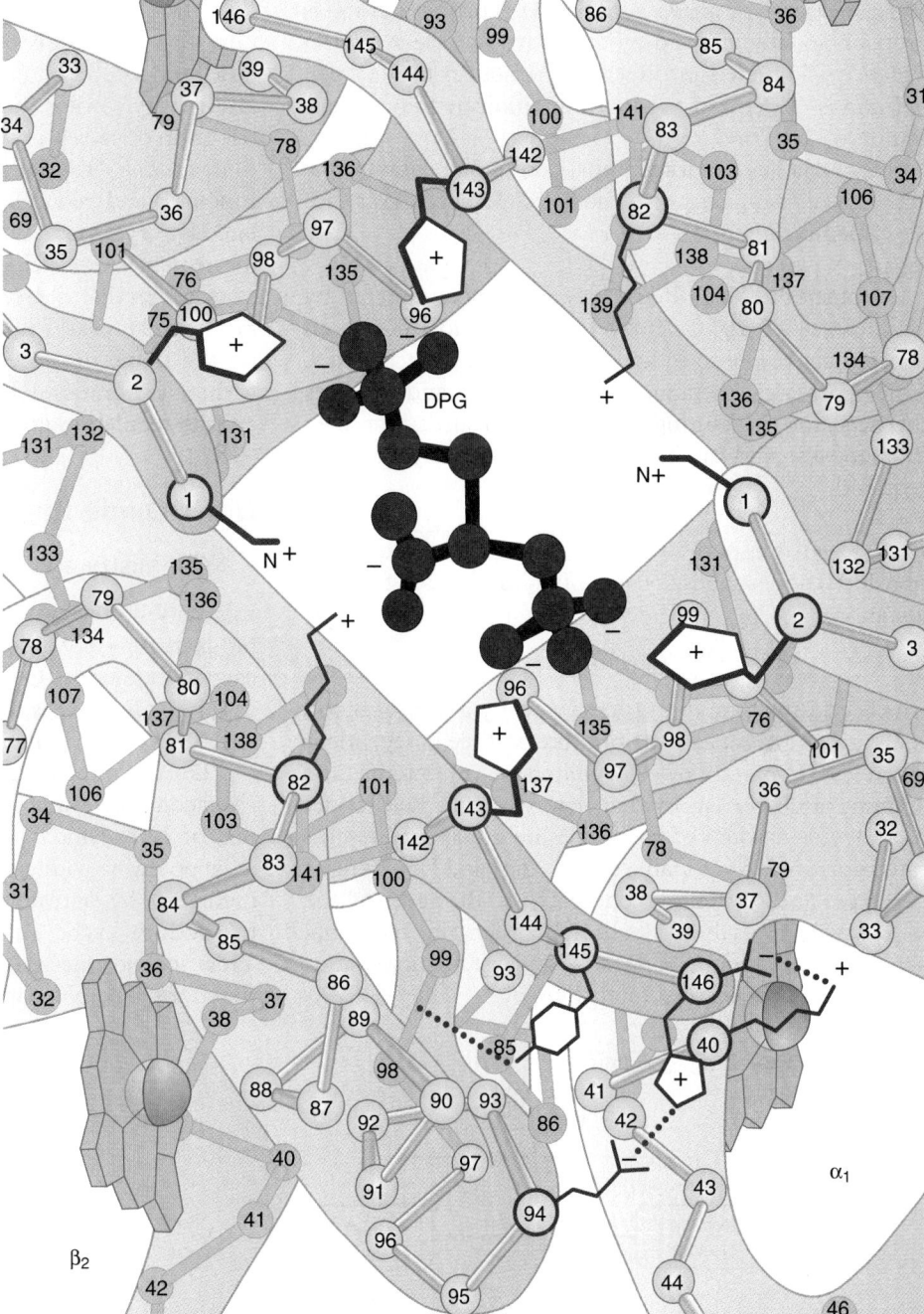

FIGURE 18-8. Amino acid side chains around the 2,3-diphosphoglycerate (DPG) binding site. This top view of the central cavity in human deoxyhemoglobin shows the positive charges lining the DPG site: two each from the N-terminal (Val-β1), from His-β2, from Lys-β82, and from His-β143. The DPG molecule, with its five negative charges, sits in the middle of this ring of positive charges. The fetal γ chain loses two of its eight positive charges by substituting Ser for His at β143, thereby decreasing the affinity for DPG. *(From Dickerson RE, Geis I. Hemoglobin: Structure, Function, Evolution, and Pathology. Menlo Park, CA, Benjamin/Cummings, 1983, p 44.)*

Concentrations of solutes inside and outside the red cell follow the Gibbs-Donnan relationship, which requires electroneutrality and due consideration of differences in activity coefficients in the two compartments. As Hb and 2,3-DPG, which are negatively charged at pH 7.4, are trapped inside the red cell, the erythrocyte Cl⁻ concentration has to be decreased, thus accounting for the 0.7 ratio between intracellular and extracellular Cl⁻. Calculation of the Gibbs-Donnan equilibrium predicts the observed 0.2-unit difference in pH between the inside and outside of the red cell, which suggests that no significant participant is missing in this phenomenon.

2,3-Diphosphoglycerate. The normal mean level of red cell 2,3-DPG is 12.8 μmol/g of Hb for males and 13.8 μmol/g of Hb for females.[25] Children younger than 5 years and elderly patients have increased and decreased levels, respectively.[26,27] This amount of 2,3-DPG makes organic phosphate almost equimolar with Hb in red cells, whereas in other cells it exists in very small concentrations.

Metabolically, 2,3-DPG is generated by the Rapoport-Luebering shunt from 1,3-DPG by 2,3-DPG synthase or mutase. Its level depends on its rates of synthesis and hydrolysis. The rate of synthesis is complex and depends on the amount of the substrate 1,3-DPG generated by glycolysis, which in turn increases directly with pH, and on the amount of 1,3-DPG entering the shunt. The alternative pathway for 1,3-DPG, and the most energetic, is conversion into 3-phosphoglycerate and generation of an ATP molecule. This alternative is probably greatly affected by the activity of the synthase, which is stimulated in direct proportion to the red cell pH and is under end-product inhibition by the concentration of 2,3-DPG.

Hypoxia has a marked impact on these relationships, and the consequences of acidosis and alkalosis are described in Figure 18-9.

Temperature. The P_{50} of blood is almost doubled by an increase of 10° C (between 20° C and 30° C), an appropriate response to hypothermia and hyperthermia. Cold decreases metabolic requirements and reduces the need for O_2. During fever, metabolism is increased dramatically, and an increase in the delivery of O_2 is required.

Oxygen Transport to Tissues. The fundamental relationship that describes delivery of O_2 to tissues is the Fick equation:

$$Vo_2 = 1.39(Q)(Hb)(Sao_2 - Svo_2)$$

where Vo_2, milliliters of O_2 delivered by a liter of blood to tissues per minute, is the product of three independent variables: (1) blood flow (Q) in liters per minute; (2) the amount of O_2 carried by that flow, which is the product of 1.39 (the amount of O_2 in milliliters that a fully saturated gram of Hb is capable of carrying) and Hb in grams per liter; and (3) extraction of O_2 at the level of the tissues, which is the difference between the fractional saturation of arterial blood (Sao_2) and the fractional saturation of mixed venous blood (Svo_2).

The consequence of this analysis is that when regulation of O_2 release is desired, it is done in the following independent ways: (1) *blood flow (Q)*—this in turn is affected by cardiac output and the luminal size and distribution of vessels in the microcirculation; (2) *hemoglobin concentration*—red cell mass is the balance between erythropoiesis and red cell destruction and is actively regulated by erythropoietin as a response to hypoxia detected in the postarterial side of the renal circulation by a detection system that is described in Chapter 6; and (3) *oxygen extraction by tissues* ($Sao_2 - Svo_2$)—this parameter depends on the shape of the O_2 equilibrium curve, as discussed earlier, and on tissue Po_2. The determinants of tissue Po_2 and its regulation are poorly understood.

Nitric Oxide Binding

Chemistry and Physiology

In addition to oxygen, heme in its reduced (ferrous) form binds readily to two other important gaseous ligands, carbon monoxide (CO) and nitric oxide (NO). The affinity of Hb for NO is 100 times higher than that for CO and 20,000 times higher than that for O_2.

During the past 2 decades there has been an explosive accumulation of information on the biologic properties of NO, which include, *primus inter pares*, its role as a potent vasodilator. The biologic activity of NO is mediated by activation of a soluble guanylyl cyclase to produce cyclic guanosine monophosphate (cGMP). This second messenger is involved in many cellular functions. The NO formed by the action of NO synthase

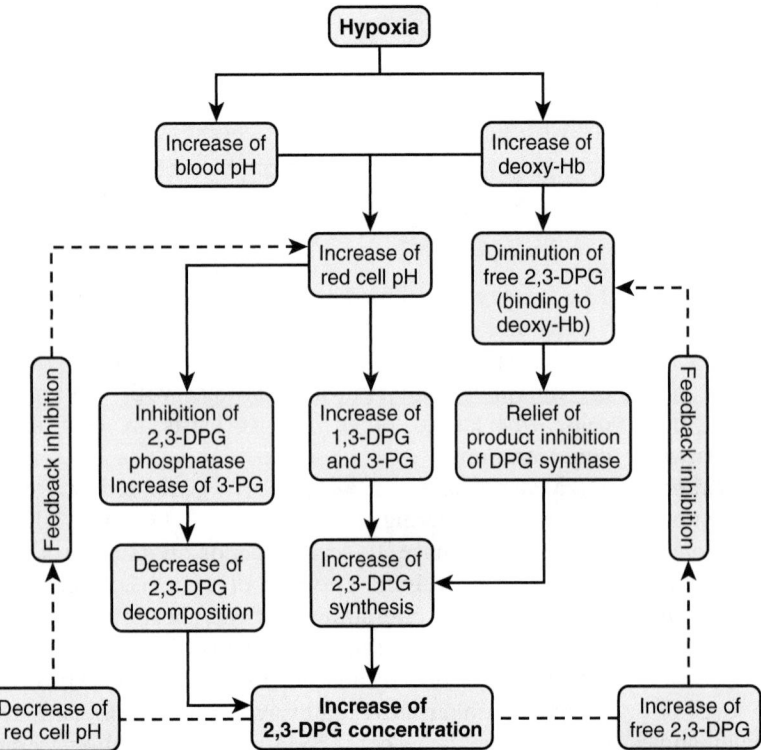

FIGURE 18-9. Effect of hypoxia on red cell pH and 2,3-diphosphoglycerate (2,3-DPG). *(After Bunn HF, Forget BG. Hemoglobin: Molecular, Genetic, and Clinical Aspects. Philadelphia, WB Saunders, 1986.)*

diffuses out of its cell of origin and affects only nearby target cells (because NO has a short half-life); it binds the heme group of cytosolic guanylate cyclase and activates this enzyme by breaking the iron–proximal histidine bond.

The steady-state level of blood NO reflects a balance between the production of NO by NO synthase and binding or scavenging of NO by Hb (bound at the heme level). It is likely that most NO bioactivity involves direct cell-to-cell interactions rather than mediation by blood NO. Nevertheless, two hypotheses have proposed in which Hb plays a central and catalytic role in the regulation of hypoxic vasodilation, an important adaptation against tissue ischemia. Stamler and colleagues[28] have shown that the oxidized nitrosyl derivative of NO (NO⁺) can form adducts with the sulfhydryl groups on cysteine residues, including the highly conserved β93 Cys on Hb, which lies in close proximity to the subunit's heme pocket. These investigators propose that the SNO adduct of Hb enables release of NO into the microcirculation, where it dilates blood vessels.[28-31] NO, produced in pulmonary arteries and arterioles, binds to the reactive β93 Cys in oxy-Hb to form the SNO derivative. As blood passes through the microcirculation, unloading of oxygen to tissues results in formation of the deoxy or T-state Hb, which precludes binding of NO to β93 Cys. The NO is thus ejected and diffuses out of the red cell into the lumen of the arteriolar and precapillary resistance vessels, where it functions as a vasodilator. The more hypoxic the tissue, the more NO that is released, thereby enhancing flow and maximizing oxygenation. As deoxygenated blood returns to the lungs, the increase in oxy-Hb allows re-formation of the SNO adducts, thus completing a dynamic and physiologically appropriate cycle. More recently, Stamler's group[32] has reported that the SNO-Hb generated from NO associates predominantly with the red blood cell membrane and principally with cysteine residues in the Hb binding, cytoplasmic domain of band 3, the anion channel in the red cell membrane. The authors postulate that the interaction with band 3 promotes the deoxygenated structure in SNO-Hb, which facilitates transfer of NO to the membrane. Although this model has enormous appeal, it remains highly controversial because of methodologic challenges in measuring extremely small in vivo levels of SNO-Hb and the rate of flow through the microcirculation, as well as difficulties reconciling the release and transit of NO or NO-like species from the red cell with what is currently known about the chemistry of Hb binding to NO.[33] Although the concept of SNO-Hb is attvactive, the in vivo significance of this phenomenon has been challenged by a recent report[34] showing that mice expressing human Hb in which β93 Cys has been mutated to alanine have normal circulatory dynamics and unimpaired vasodilation in response to hypoxia.

Gladwin and his group have proposed an alternative, but equally controversial model of how Hb may function catalytically in the mediation of hypoxic vasodilation.[35]

These investigators reason that plasma contains low to sub-micromolar concentrations of nitrite which could be a stable biologic reservoir of NO. They demonstrated a significant arterial-venous drop in the level of plasma nitrite in forearm blood flow studies even after abolishing endogenous production of NO, which is a known source of plasma nitrite.[36] These investigators went on to demonstrate that infusions of nitrite induce vasodilation along with binding of hemoglobin heme to NO.[37] The fact that this effect was maximal when red cell Hb was half saturated with oxygen led these investigators to conclude that an oxygen-dependent conformational change in Hb was required for maximal nitrite reductase activity[38] and that Hb may therefore mediate hypoxic vasodilation by serving as both the oxygen sensor and the requisite enzyme for regulated production of NO. This process apparently does not involve SNO-Hb because mutants with other residues replacing β93 Cys have even greater nitrite reductase activity.

Both the SNO model and the nitrite reductase model are heuristic but difficult to fully comprehend. The red cell is such a vast sink for NO that it is difficult to imagine how biologically significant amounts of NO or some other nitrogenous product can be released unless there is exquisite compartmentalization at the red cell membrane.

Clinical Relevance

In addition to red cell Hb, free Hb in plasma may also have an important impact on NO biology and pathogenesis of disease. Hb is released into plasma by both intravascular and extravascular hemolysis. Gladwin and colleagues at the National Institutes of Health have obtained results suggesting that sickle homozygotes with a relatively high degree of hemolysis appear to be more likely to have pulmonary hypertension, ankle ulcers, priapism, and early mortality.[39,40] In contrast, those with a comparatively low degree of hemolysis are more likely to have vaso-occlusive episodes, including acute pain crises. They hypothesize that enhanced hemolysis may have an impact on sickle cell pathogenesis by virtue of NO metabolism. Red cells that are prematurely destroyed in the circulation release arginase, which can lower the availability of arginine, a substrate required for the biosynthesis of NO via NO synthase. In addition, free Hb in plasma diffuses readily to the surface of endothelial cells and is capable of scavenging the NO that is released from these cells. These two processes can lead to a relative deficiency in NO that results in enhanced vasomotor tone, as well as activation of platelets that may independently accentuate vaso-occlusion.

The utility of the degree of hemolysis as an independent index of prognosis in sickle cell disease depends on how readily sickle homozygotes can be segregated into two groups of high versus low hemolytic rate. If these groups are readily separable, such laboratory assessment could be useful in helping assign prognostic risk to a given sickle patient. In a recent comparison of a group of 223 sickle cell patients with priapism and a group of 979 controls who lacked this complication, those with priapism indeed had a somewhat higher rate of hemolysis, but the difference between the two groups was small.[41] The laboratory parameter that was most statistically significant in distinguishing between those with and without priapism was the white blood cell count. However, in all these measurements there is a very high degree of overlap between the two groups. Results such as this suggest that hemolysis may not segregate sufficiently into discrete subgroups to make it useful for assessing prognosis.

OTHER NORMAL HEMOGLOBINS

Hemoglobin F

In 1866, Korber[42] discovered that the red cells of newborns are resistant to alkaline denaturation. This was the first suggestion that these cells contain Hb that is different from normal adult Hb. The composition of this fetal Hb (HbF) is $\alpha_2\gamma_2$.

The γ chains are different from the β chains in 39 or 40 positions in the sequence.[43] γ Chains are the product of two genes placed in tandem between the ε and pseudo-β genes in the β-like globin cluster on chromosome 11. The only difference between the two gene products is the presence of glycine in position $\gamma 136$ in the $^G\gamma$ gene, the left gene, and the presence of alanine in the same position in the $^A\gamma$ gene, to the right. A common polymorphism is found in the $^A\gamma$ gene, with threonine replacing isoleucine at position 75.[44] The striking similarities in the protein sequences are reflected at the nucleotide level, where the homology between the two genes is high. Smithies and associates[45] were the first to point out that this is a consequence of gene conversion, a mutational event in which sequences upstream replace sequences downstream, particularly in tandem genes, and homogenize them in the process. This phenomenon was demonstrated in the Bantu haplotype linked to the β^S gene.[46]

One interpretation of this phenomenon is that considerable selective value is placed on the sequence of γ chains and on the structure of HbF. This is not surprising because HbF is present throughout most of fetal life (though mostly during the last two trimesters), and abnormalities could easily cause fetal death.

Sequence Differences between γ and β Chains

The 39 differences include 22 on the surface of the molecule (see Table 18-1). Four critical substitutions are in the $\alpha_1\beta_1$ area of contact (the packing contact). This is the strong contact that dissociates only under extreme conditions such as very low or high pH.

Nevertheless, two of these substitutions, Thr112 and Try130, in the $\alpha_1\gamma_1$ contact could be involved in the alkaline resistance of HbF, as well as in its decreased

dissociation to monomers. In the β chains, position $\beta 112$ is a Cys and $\beta 130$ is a Tyr. Both these residues ionize at alkaline pH, which could promote dissociation of the dimer into monomers. Thr and Tyr are polar but not ionizable. No sequence changes affect the $\alpha_1\beta_2$ area of contact (sliding contact), which is critical for the ligand-dependent conformational changes.

Protein Conformation

Crystallographic studies of HbF at 2.5-Å resolution show almost complete isomorphism between HbA and HbF.[47] The only difference is in the N-terminal portion. This change increases the distance of 2,3-DPG from $\gamma 2$ His, which may contribute to the reduction of the effect of 2,3-DPG on HbF.

Ligand Binding

The red cells of newborns (containing mostly HbF) have higher O_2 affinity than adult red cells do (P_{50} of ≈ 15 mm Hg versus ≈ 26 mm Hg in adults), but the O_2 affinities of neonatal and adult red cell hemolysates are indistinguishable.[48] This finding suggests that HbF and HbA have identical O_2-binding properties but that the red cells contain effectors that interact differentially with HbF.

2,3-DPG exhibits decreased binding to HbF.[49] The structural basis for this finding is replacement of $\beta 143$ His (phosphate binding site in the central cavity) with a serine residue at $\gamma 143$. This substitution abolishes an important binding site. Secondary effects arise from displacement of the N-terminal portion of the γ chains, which inhibits the binding of phosphates with $\gamma 2$ His. In addition, HbF molecules that are acetylated at the γ-chain N-terminal are incapable of binding 2,3-DPG.[23]

The effect of Cl^- is also altered.[50] This anion binds at the 2,3-DPG site in the central cavity. At low NaCl concentrations (up to 0.05 mol/L), HbF has lower affinity for O_2 than HbA does. At higher Cl^- concentrations, the differences disappear. This effect is not well understood but might have to do with the diminution of positive charges in the central cavity; therefore, the binding affinity for anions and the destabilizing effect on the T state are reduced. The increased stability of the T state induced by the absence of anion-neutralizing positive charges would favor low ligand affinity.

Binding of CO_2 to HbF is drastically decreased.[51] Fewer carbamates are formed at the N-terminal over a range of P_{CO_2} values. The γ-chain N-terminal amino acid has a pK_a of 8.1, which is much higher than the pK_a of β chains (6.6). Under physiologic conditions, 90% of the γ sites are protonated and unable to bind CO_2.

The alkaline Bohr effect (relationship between high pH and ligand affinity) is increased by 20% in HbF-containing red cells.[52] This seems to be an effect of Cl^- because in isolated HbF at low anion concentrations, HbA and HbF have an identical Bohr effect and the Bohr effect of HbF increases pari passu with the Cl^- concentration. A plausible explanation is that binding of Cl^- at low pH to β143 His stabilizes the R state. The absence of this Cl⁻ site in γ chains would lower the low-pH Bohr effect because it is a situation that favors the T state. As a consequence, the alkaline Bohr effect is favored in HbF.

Physiology of Hemoglobin F–Containing Red Cells

How do the aforementioned properties of HbF benefit the fetus and newborn? Perhaps the main feature of the fetal circulation, as opposed to the circulation in postnatal life, is that O_2 loading is accomplished under more difficult circumstances in the fetus (liquid-liquid interface) than in the neonate (gas-liquid interface). On the positive side, the tissues of the fetus have a high metabolic rate; therefore, the limitation may be on loading sufficient O_2 rather than delivery of O_2 because a significant difference between the Po_2 of blood and that of tissue is likely to exist in the fetus. This explains why the O_2 affinity of HbF-containing red cells is increased, a situation that favors uptake of O_2 in the placenta. Indeed, in nearly all mammals, fetal red cells have higher O_2 affinity compared with maternal red cells.

The Bohr effect accounts for 40% of the normal fetal gas exchange.[52] In addition, in the fetus, an increased Bohr effect can modulate delivery of O_2 to tissues (if needed), even in the absence of 2,3-DPG. About 50% of the delivery to tissues is accounted for by the increased Bohr effect. Finally, the increased Bohr effect could also explain the paradox observed[53] in which mothers with high-affinity Hb variants do not have pregnancy complications or fetal morbidity. The advantage of HbF is not limited to the difference in P_{50} with HbA. If the difference in affinity is erased, as in patients with high-affinity Hb, the enhanced Bohr effect can make up at least some of the difference.

As noted earlier, γ chains are synthesized by two sequence-identifiable genes. Additional heterogeneity arises from N-terminal acetylation of 10% to 15% of the γ chains of newborns. Acetylation is common in proteins that have N-terminal alanine, serine, and to a lesser extent, glycine residues.[54] Hb needs to have its N-termini free for functional reasons; therefore, it is not surprising that acetylation has been largely excluded by selection. In the case of HbF, it contributes to the decrease in 2,3-DPG binding, apparently a welcome feature. Acetylation occurs after synthesis, probably early in the process, and involves catalytic transfer of the acetyl moiety from acetyl coenzyme A to the protein by acetyltransferase. Hb Raleigh (β1 [NA1] Val→acetylatable alanine) is 100% acetylated. Cat Hb, in which the β1 residue is serine, is also 100% acetylated (and does not interact with 2,3-DPG[55]).

Laboratory Determination of Hemoglobin F

The best methods of determining the level of HbF in the hemolysate depend on its concentration. For normal levels (0.1% to 1.5% of total Hb), immunologic assays are best. For levels between 1.5% and 40%, alkaline denaturation is accurate. For levels greater than 40%, high-performance liquid chromatography (HPLC) is probably the best method, although it can also be used at lower concentrations. A method of enriching HbF by chromatography or isoelectric focusing, followed by HPLC, allows this technique to be applied to all concentrations of HbF. Disposable columns for determination of HbF in hemolysates that contain no HbA (such as red cells from patients with HbSS or HbCC disease) are also available and produce reasonably accurate results.

HbF is unevenly distributed among red cells in normal subjects and in those with most medical conditions except for some forms of hereditary persistence of HbF.[56] Immunologic techniques that allow identification of red cells containing HbF (F cells and F reticulocytes) and measurement of the average amount of HbF per cell have become powerful tools for the study of HbF expression.[57-59] About 0.5% to 7% of red cells are F cells in normal adults.

Agar electrophoresis at pH 6.4 (available as a kit) offers an additional method to isolate or identify HbF. Hbs are subjected to a combination of chromatography and electrophoresis in agar. The agar matrix interacts with the central cavity of Hbs,[60] and Hbs with abnormalities in that region (such as HbF) tend to migrate faster (or slower) than their electrophoretic mobility would predict at pH 6.4. Therefore, when an Hb with anomalous electrophoretic mobility in agar is compared with cellulose acetate (pH 8.6), a mutation of the central cavity should be suspected. Hb Hope is an example of this phenomenon.

Medical Conditions Apart from Hemoglobinopathies Associated with High Hemoglobin F

Newborns have between 65% and 95% HbF. This amount decreases progressively during the first year of life. The normal adult level is approached by 1 year of age and is achieved by 5 years.

Pregnancy is accompanied by a modest increase in HbF in the second trimester. Hydatidiform moles are associated with particularly high HbF values. Although maternal pregnancy hormones have been implicated, the mechanism of this elevation is not clear.[61]

Some conditions (besides hemoglobinopathies) retard downregulation of HbF in the first 5 years of life. Such conditions include prematurity, trisomy 13, and maternal diabetes.[62] Acceleration of the decrease in HbF is observed in patients with Down syndrome and those with C/D translocations.

Hemolytic anemias, acute bleeding, and treatment with hydroxyurea or arabinocytidine can all be associated with higher than normal values of HbF. This phenomenon has been interpreted to mean that under these conditions, early progenitors are rushed through development while they retain their HbF program because the reduction in the number of cell divisions precludes their downregulation.

Invariably, juvenile chronic myeloid leukemia, Diamond-Blackfan anemia, and Fanconi's anemia are accompanied by significant elevations of HbF. Erythroleukemia, paroxysmal nocturnal hemoglobinuria, kala-azar, preleukemia, and recovery from marrow aplasia are also associated with variable elevations of HbF. The highest levels are found in patients with Di Guglielmo's disease (erythroleukemia). Many conditions, including solid tumors, occasionally cause increased levels of HbF.[62-64]

Mutations in the $^G\gamma$ Genes

Variants of the $^G\gamma$ Gene. Fifty-six variants with a single amino acid substitution in the $^G\gamma$ gene have been described. Of these, two are unstable: HbF Poole ($^G\gamma130$ [H8] Trp→Gly), which is significantly unstable, and HbF Xin Jin ($^G\gamma119$ [GH2] Gly→Arg).[65] A mutation at the same site, but not the same amino acid as in Hb Poole, has also been identified in β chains (Hb Wien [β130 Try→Asp]).

Also found in HbF is the equivalent of M Hbs in the β chains: HbF-M Fort Ripley, which has a cyanotic phenotype in the newborn and corresponds to substitution of the proximal histidine, γ92 (F8) His→Tyr. It is perfectly equivalent to Hb Hyde Park. The other mutation, HbF-M Osaka,[66] involves the distal histidine, γ63 (E7) His→Tyr, and is equivalent to HbM Saskatoon. Newborns with α-chain substitutions of the proximal or distal histidines have the same cyanotic phenotype as that of adults, with the cyanosis appearing early in the neonatal period.[67,68]

Finally, one high-affinity variant has been described: HbF Onoda[69] ($^G\gamma146$ [HC3] His→Tyr).

Hemoglobin A_2

HbA_2 is present both in the neonatal period and during the rest of an individual's life and is a product of the combination of α chains with δ chains ($\alpha_2\delta_2$). The δ gene is expressed at a very low level. HbA_2 represents about 2.4% of the Hbs present in normal hemolysates. The δ gene resides in the cluster of β-like genes between the pseudo-β gene and the β gene.

δ Gene

The δ gene arose from a duplication of the β gene about 40 million years ago (although one cannot exclude the possibility that gene conversion could have erased differences of an older gene). The δ gene also exists and is expressed at low levels in New World primates (1% to 6%). In some Old World primates, the δ gene is present but not expressed. The δ gene is absent in other mammals. In any case, the distribution among animals suggests that this was the last globin gene to emerge in the β-like gene cluster. Its relatively recent appearance (or recent gene conversion) explains why the δ chain exhibits only 10 sequence differences from the β gene.

The low level of transcription of the δ gene might be the consequence of changes in the 5′ flanking region. Of the three CCAAT box-like sequences, none is perfectly conserved. Instability of δ-mRNA may also contribute to poor expression of the δ gene.

Functional and Structural Aspects

HbA and HbA_2 have similar ligand-binding curves, although the latter has slightly higher O_2 affinity. The Bohr effect, cooperativity, and the response to 2,3-DPG are identical.

Among the differences are that the fact HbA_2 is more thermostable because of a change at Arg-δ116. This Arg forms a salt bridge with Pro-α114, thereby increasing the stability of the $\alpha_1\alpha_1$ packing contact even further. Another difference is that HbA_2 binds to the red cell membrane better than HbA does.[70]

The low levels of HbA_2 and the multiple functionally abnormal mutations found in primate δ-like genes have been suggested as reasons for the lack of functional importance of this minor component. According to this view, the δ gene is condemned to the biologic trash heap of history as a pseudogene. This conclusion presupposes that the only functional role of any Hb is to carry O_2. If so, HbA_2 is clearly useless. Alternatively, the increased binding of HbA_2 to the membrane could indicate another role for this Hb. It is necessary to know what proteins in addition to band 3 are capable of binding this Hb and whether such binding has any functional role. The finding of an HbA_2 polymorphism in the Dogon region of the Republic of Mali (see later) stimulates this thinking.

Mutational Events Involving the δ Gene

Nearly 80 amino acid substitutions, all resulting from single base changes, have been described in HbA_2. This might be the tip of the iceberg because these substitutions are difficult to detect. Two mutations, HbA_2 Wrens (δ98 [FG4] Val→Met)[71] and HbA_2 Manzanares (δ121 [GH4] Glu→Val),[72] are unstable. HbA_2 Canada (δ99 [G1] Asp→Asn)[73] has very high affinity for O_2, but because of its low level, no erythrocytosis is present.

A common mutation, found mostly among African Americans and Africans, is HbA'_2, also called HbB_2 (δ16 [A13] Gly→Arg). In Africa, it has been described in samples from different geographic locations, one of which is Ghana. HbA'_2 has been found at polymorphic rates in one of the castes in the Dogon region of the Republic of Mali. Haplotype analysis of the Mali β-like gene cluster demonstrates that all unrelated persons carrying this mutation have the same haplotype. Samples from unrelated African Americans with this mutation also demonstrate haplotype homogeneity. Hence, it is possible that HbA'_2 arose in Africa unicentrically and was distributed to other regions of Africa by gene flow.

An interesting set of mutational events involves unequal crossover between the δ gene and the β gene. Such crossover generates Hbs with portions of δ chains and portions of β chains. They are called Lepore-type Hbs after the first family described. The first three examples of this type of event were characterized in heterozygotes by low levels of the Lepore-type Hb (about 20%), electrophoretic migration similar to that of HbS, and a thalassemic phenotype (microcytosis, hypochromia, and hemolytic anemia). In homozygotes for this condition, severity varies from transfusion dependency to moderate anemia. Groups at risk are principally Italians, Greeks, and Yugoslavians (the latter being the most severely affected), but examples have been found in Turkish Cypriots, inhabitants of Papua New Guinea, African Americans, Indians, and Romanians.

Hb Lepore Hollandia, Hb Lepore Baltimore, and Hb Lepore Washington-Boston (the first described)[74-76] have different lengths of the δ sequence in the N-terminal portion of the hybrid chain and complementary portions of the β chains at the C-terminal end. All have a total of 146 amino acids. The more recently described Lepore-type Hb, Hb Parchman, is a patchwork in which a segment of the β sequence is located in the center of the chain. The location of the crossover is uncertain because with only 10 amino acid differences between the δ and β chains, there are too few informative sites.

If a Lepore-type unequal crossover occurs, an anti-Lepore Hb molecule is also generated, but finding it depends on its prevalence and luck. HbP Nilotic is the anti-Lepore of Lepore Hollandia. Hb Lincoln Park is probably the same with an added deletion at position δ137. Hb Miyada and HbP Congo could be anti-Lepores of Lepore Hbs that are yet to be found. Electrophoretically, HbP Congo, HbP Nilotic, and Hb Lincoln Park migrate like HbS, whereas Hb Miyada and Hb Parchman migrate like HbC.

Variation of Hemoglobin A₂ Levels with Other Clinical Conditions

Levels of HbA_2 are elevated in a number of conditions; in some instances this feature is of diagnostic value. The most common and important clinical instance is β-thalassemia (see Chapter 20). HbA_2 is also elevated in sickle trait, in blood from patients with SS disease, particularly SS disease with α-thalassemia, and in acquired conditions such as megaloblastic anemia and hyperthyroidism. HbA_2 may also be elevated in patients with malaria. Elevation of HbA_2 is not due to an increase in the synthesis of δ chains but is a consequence of the preferential assembly of δ with α chains, particularly if β chains are in short supply.[77] Decreased levels of HbA_2 are found in α-thalassemia, $\delta\beta$-thalassemia, and δ-thalassemia and in hereditary persistence of HbF, either because the δ gene is deleted or because the α chains are more avid for γ or β chains than for δ chains. A decrease in HbA_2 is also seen with iron deficiency, but it returns to normal after iron therapy.

Embryonic Hemoglobins

At 4 to 14 weeks of gestation, the human embryo synthesizes three distinct Hbs in yolk sac–derived primitive nucleated erythroid cells: $\zeta_2\varepsilon_2$ (Hb Gower-1), $\zeta_2\gamma_2$ (Hb Portland), and $\alpha_2\varepsilon_2$ (Hb Gower-2).[78] ζ- and ε-globin chains are expressed before the γ- and α-globin chains. After establishment of the placenta, at 14 days of development, embryonic Hbs are replaced by HbF, but ζ- and ε-globin chains can be found in definitive fetal erythrocytes.[79] At 15 to 22 weeks of gestation, 53% of fetal cells contained ζ-globin chains and 5% had ε-globin chains. At term, cord blood contained 34% and 0.6% of ζ- and ε-globin chain–positive cells, respectively. Erythrocytes from normal adults do not contain embryonic globins.

Developmental timing of the synthesis of embryonic Hbs has been studied in embryonic erythroid cells.[80] Embryonic, fetal, and adult globins are synthesized in vivo and in cultures of erythroid burst-forming units in the yolk sac (where primitive erythropoiesis occurs) and in liver cells (site of definitive erythropoiesis). Similarly, the adult α-globin gene and the corresponding embryonic α-like chains (ζ-globin gene) are coexpressed in the earliest murine erythrocyte progenitors.[81] From these studies and from the recent finding of embryonic Hb in cord blood, it appears that embryonic globin is expressed in both primitive and definitive erythroblasts, though in vastly different quantities. These results are compatible with the notion that the switch from embryonic to fetal globin synthesis represents a time-dependent change in programs of progenitor cells rather than a change in hemopoietic cell lineages.

Embryonic Hbs obtained from an in vitro expression system in the absence of any effector of Hb function, including Cl^-, all have O_2 affinity and ligand-binding rates similar to those of HbA.[82] In the presence of organic phosphates, the O_2 affinity of $\zeta_2\varepsilon_2$ and $\alpha_2\varepsilon_2$ is lowered, though to a lesser extent than for normal HbA. This demonstrates that ε-globin chains do bind 2,3-DPG, but less than β chains do. Hb Portland binds organic phosphates even less well, which is not surprising because its central cavity is formed by γ-globin chains (see earlier discussion).

Decreased rates of O_2 dissociation from embryonic Hbs appear to be responsible for the high O_2-binding affinity of the embryonic proteins.[83] The pH dependence of the O_2 dissociation rate constants also accounts for the rather unusual Bohr effects characteristic of embryonic Hbs. In $\alpha_2\varepsilon_2$ (Hb Gower-2),[84] the tertiary structure of the α-globin chain is unchanged from that of HbA and HbF.

Crystallographic data on the CO form are available for $\alpha_2\varepsilon_2$ (Hb Gower-2).[85] When compared with the structures of HbA and HbF, the tertiary structure of the α-globin chain is unchanged. The ε-globin chain has a structure very similar to that of the β-globin chain, with small differences in the N-terminal and A helix.

The most distinct difference in Hb Gower-2 and HbA is a shift of the N-terminal and the A helix, similar to that seen in HbF. The α helix moves into the central cavity as a consequence of complex disruption of the N-terminal region. This shift may explain the decrease in binding of 2,3-DPG to Hb Gower-2.

Finally, embryonic ζ- and ε-globin subunits assemble with each other and with adult α- and β-globin subunits into Hb heterotetramers in both primitive and definitive erythrocytes. The use of complex transgenic knockout mice that express these Hbs at high level has allowed functional characterizations of these hybrids.[86] The exchange of ζ chains for α chains increases P_{50} and decreases the Bohr effect, thereby increasing O_2 transport capacity. In comparison, the exchange of ε chains for β chains has little impact on these parameters. Hb Gower-1, assembled entirely from embryonic subunits, displays an elevated P_{50}, a reduced Bohr effect, and decreased 2,3-DPG binding in comparison to HbA. The data support the hypothesis that Hb Gower-2, assembled from reactivated ε-globin in individuals with hemoglobinopathies and thalassemias, would serve as a physiologically acceptable substitute for deficient or dysfunctional HbA. In addition, the unexpected properties of Hb Gower-1 make a primary role for it in embryonic development unlikely.

Mutations Affecting Embryonic Hemoglobins

The most common mutation producing lethal hydrops fetalis is the Southeast Asian (–/SEA) double α-globin gene deletion.[87] Erythrocytes from adults heterozygous for the (–/SEA) deletion have minute amounts of embryonic ζ-globin chains detectable by anti-ζ-globin monoclonal antibodies. The majority of subjects are of Chinese, Filipino, or Laotian ancestry. The (–/SEA) double α deletion was the only abnormality in two thirds of these individuals. In others, this deletion was combined with α-globin or β-globin mutations or coincidental iron deficiency. Four other samples from (–/SEA) heterozygotes produced negative results with this immunologic assay. Anti-ζ–negative samples included deletions of the total α-globin region (–/Tot), single α-globin deletions, and a variety of β-globin mutations; normocytic samples with normal α genes also produced negative results. Benign triplicated ζ-globin genes were detected as well. Anti-ζ immunobinding testing provides rapid, simple, and reliable screening for the (–/SEA) double α-globin deletion, although it does not detect the (–/Tot) total α-globin deletions.

PATHOPHYSIOLOGY OF HEMOGLOBIN ABNORMALITIES

Nearly 1000 mutant human hemoglobins have been reported. Those involving the δ and γ subunits have been mentioned in earlier sections of this chapter. Because HbA ($\alpha_2\beta_2$) constitutes about 97% of Hb within the red cell after infancy, the most common and most important human Hb mutants pertain to either the α or the β subunit.

Assembly of Mutant Hemoglobins

The composition of normal and mutant Hbs in the red cells of heterozygotes provides insight into the assembly of human Hbs.[88,89] The great majority of β-chain mutants are synthesized at the same rate as β^A and have normal stability. Therefore, heterozygotes would be expected to have equal amount of normal and mutant Hb. However, measurements of the proportion of normal and abnormal Hbs in heterozygotes have revealed unexpected variability. Figure 18-10 shows a comparison of stable β-chain mutants. Positively charged mutants, such as Hbs S, C, D Los Angeles, and E, account for significantly less than half of the total Hb in heterozygotes and are reduced further in the presence of α-thalassemia. In contrast, many of the negatively charged mutants are present in amounts exceeding that of HbA. In two heterozygotes who had a negatively charged mutant (HbJ Baltimore or HbJ Iran) in conjunction with α-thalassemia, the proportion of the mutant Hb was found to be increased further. Analysis of the proportion of β-chain mutant in heterozygotes suggests that alterations in surface charge contribute to different rates of assembly of the Hb tetramer. This hypothesis is supported by in vitro mixing experiments on normal and mutant subunits showing that when α chain is present in limiting amounts (mimicking α-thalassemia), negatively charged mutants are

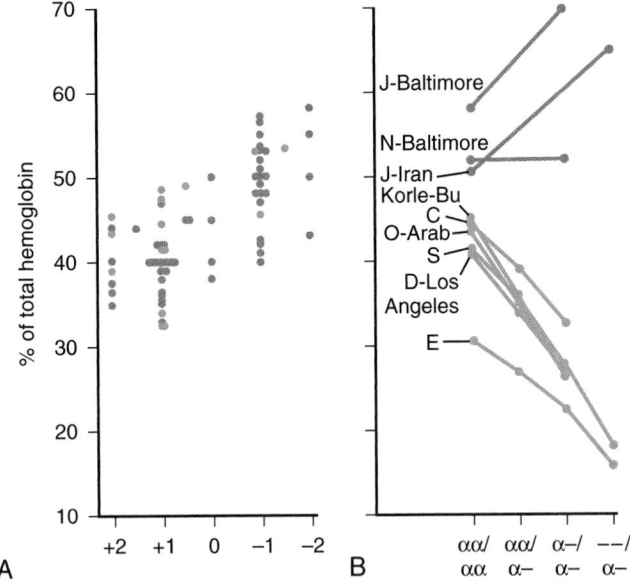

FIGURE 18-10. A, Effect of charge on the proportion of abnormal hemoglobin in individuals heterozygous for 72 stable β-globin variants. Each data point represents a mean value for a given variant. The *blue points* (•) denote measurements of Huisman[90] by high-resolution chromatography. Substitutions involving a histidine residue were scored as a change of one-half charge. The "–1" group differs significantly from the "+1" group ($P < .001$) and from the "0" group ($P < .05$). **B,** Effect of α-thalassemia on the proportion of six positively charged β-chain variants (*blue dots*) and three negatively charged variants (*orange dots*). (Data from Bunn HF, McDonald MJ. Electrostatic interactions in the assembly of haemoglobin. *Nature. 1983;306:498-500*; Rahbar S, Bunn HF: Association of hemoglobin H disease with Hb J-Iran (beta 77 His----Asp): impact on subunit assembly. *Blood 1987;70:1790-1791.*)

formed much more readily than positively charged mutants.[91,92] This electrostatic model of Hb assembly has clinical implications. Differences in rates of assembly explain not only the low proportion in HbS–sickle C (SC) disease (see later) but also the differences in levels of HbA₂[89] and HbF[93,94] that accompany certain hematologic disorders.

The majority of human Hb mutants were discovered as an incidental finding, unassociated with any hematologic or clinical phenotype. However, a number of α- and β-globin mutants are associated with distinct clinical phenotypes, which fall into four broad categories: mutants with high oxygen affinity resulting in erythrocytosis, unstable mutants causing congenital Heinz body hemolytic anemia, low–oxygen affinity mutants and the M Hbs causing cyanosis, and mutants associated with a thalassemia phenotype.

High–Oxygen Affinity Hemoglobins: Erythrocytosis

Structural Defects

Mutations resulting in changes in the primary structure of the α or β chains can lead to changes in oxygen affinity. An example is shown in Figure 18-11. Increases in the O_2 affinity of Hb result from various mechanisms. In most instances, the changes in O_2 affinity are in concordance with our understanding of the structure-function relationships of Hb. In a few instances, the known alterations in the primary structure are not sufficient to explain the observed effect, given the state of our knowledge.

The mutations that generate high-affinity Hbs can arise from single point substitutions, double point substitutions (although some of these substitutions could be crossover events between two mutated chains), deletions, additions, frameshift mutations, and fusion genes.

The molecular mechanisms of ligand high-affinity Hb mutants can be grouped into four categories. (For more detailed information, see the article by Wajcman and Galacteros[94]).

1. Alterations in the switch region, the flexible joint, or the C-terminus in the $\alpha_1\beta_2$ area of contact that favor the R (or oxy) state, either by stabilizing this conformer or by destabilizing the T (or deoxy) state; examples include Hb Bethesda (β145 [HC2] Tyr→His)[95] and Hb Kempsey (β99 [G1] Asp→Asn).[96]
2. Alteration of the $\alpha_1\beta_1$ area of contact with disruption of the overall architecture of Hb that favors the R state. Examples include Hb San Diego (β109 [G11] Val→Met)[97] and Hb Crete (β129 [H7] Ala→Pro).[98]
3. Reduction in heme-heme interaction by restraining of quaternary conformation because of a tendency to aggregate or polymerize. In Hb Porto Alegre (β9 [A6] Ser→Cys), the additional cysteine sulfhydryl results in disulfide cross-linking and increases oxygen affinity.[99,100]
4. Mutations that decrease the affinity of Hb for 2,3-DPG; examples include Hb Providence (β82 [EF6] Lys→Asn→Asp)[101] and Hb Old Dominion (β143 [H21] His→Tyr).[102]

Identification of High–Oxygen Affinity Hemoglobins

In 1966, an 81-year-old patient complaining of mild angina was found to have erythrocytosis, an abnormal band in his Hb on electrophoresis, and red cells with increased O_2 affinity.[103] The abnormal Hb proved to be a Leu→Arg substitution in residue 92 of the α chains. Discovery of the first carrier of Hb Chesapeake opened a new chapter in the study of hemoglobinopathies because it demonstrated that a variant of this molecule could generate a distinct clinical syndrome. Discovery of this and other high-affinity Hbs has been useful in elucidation of the molecular mechanisms underlying the function of normal Hb.

Is the mild angina seen in the Hb Chesapeake pedigree a characteristic of carriers of high-affinity Hbs? Other members of the same pedigree and a large number of carriers of high-affinity Hbs generally have had no clinical consequences.

Patients with high-affinity Hbs have normal white cell and platelet counts and do not have splenomegaly. They sometimes have a family history of "thick blood," but a significant number of high-affinity Hbs are new mutations; that is, no abnormal Hb is found in parents or siblings.

The differential diagnosis of erythrocytosis is outlined in Box 18-1. Erythrocytosis should not be confused with polycythemia, in which numbers of white cells and platelets are elevated and splenomegaly is usually present. Diagnosis of the conditions in Box 18-1

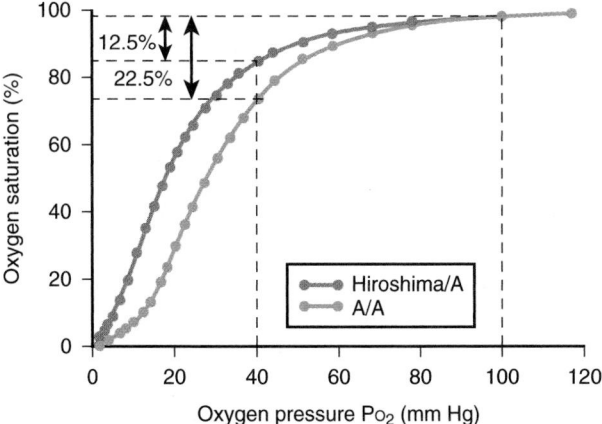

FIGURE 18-11. Oxygen equilibrium curves of red cells from a healthy person (A/A) and those from a person heterozygous for Hb Hiroshima (Hiroshima/A). Oxygen pressure is plotted against oxygen saturation. *Vertical dotted lines* mark the typical Po_2 of the lungs (100 mm Hg) and the tissues (40 mm Hg). *Horizontal dotted lines* mark oxygen extraction (lungs minus tissues) in normal red cells (22.5%) and the reduction observed in high-affinity red cells (12.5%).

Box 18-1	Differential Diagnosis of Erythrocytosis

A. Primary increase in erythropoiesis (low plasma erythropoietin levels)
   1. Polycythemia vera
   2. Mutations of the erythropoietin receptor
B. Secondary increase in erythropoiesis (appropriately high erythropoietin levels)
   1. Hypoxemia related to
      a. Chronic pulmonary disease
      b. Right-to-left cardiac shunts
      c. Sleep apnea
      d. Massive obesity (pickwickian syndrome)
      e. High altitude
   2. Red cell hemoglobin defects
      a. High–oxygen affinity hemoglobins
      b. Absence or decrease in 2,3-diphosphoglycerate mutase
      c. Some cases of congenital methemoglobinemia
      d. Chronic carbon monoxide poisoning (smoking and work-related exposure)
C. Secondary increase in erythropoiesis (inappropriately high erythropoietin levels)
   1. Erythropoietin-producing neoplasms
   2. Erythropoietin-producing renal lesions
   3. Defects in oxygen sensing
      a. von Hippel-Lindau mutant (Chuvash polycythemia)
      b. Prolyl hydroxylase 2 mutants
      c. Hypoxia-inducible transcription factor-2α mutants
D. Idiopathic familial erythrocytosis

---

is facilitated by measurement of blood erythropoietin levels. Hypoxia of pulmonary or cardiovascular origin can be excluded by analysis of arterial blood gases. Affected patients characteristically have low Po_2 values and low O_2 saturation. Patients with red cells that have an altered capacity to transport O_2 have normal arterial Po_2.

Individuals with increased O_2 affinity can be investigated further by comparing the oxygen binding of phosphate-free hemolysates at physiologic pH and temperature with that of the red cells. The hemolysates identify intrinsic defects in the Hb molecule; study of intact red cells identifies other red cell factors (such as 2,3-DPG) that alter the O_2 affinity of otherwise normal Hb. Deficiency of 2,3-DPG mutase results in red cells with high O_2 affinity, normal O_2 affinity of the red cell hemolysate, and a very low 2,3-DPG concentration.[104] In all these cases the absorption spectrum of the hemolysates is normal.

Methemoglobin (Met-Hb) (such as that seen in congenital or toxic methemoglobinemia) and carboxy-Hb (secondary to CO poisoning)[105] can be identified by spectrophotometric examination of the red cell hemolysate. Several gas-measuring apparatuses are available in hospitals (e.g., the IL CO oximeter) that can give an accurate reading of Met-Hb and carboxy-Hb concentrations in whole blood.

Finally, many individuals with familial erythrocytosis have normal O_2 affinity, regardless of whether red cells or hemolysate is used. The inheritance pattern may be either dominant or recessive. Affected individuals may exhibit clubbing.[106] Two interesting groups of patients have erythrocytosis unrelated to Hb variants or enzyme abnormalities: erythropoietin receptor mutations and erythrocytosis caused abnormal oxygen sensing.

Erythropoietin Receptor Mutations. A number of families have been encountered in which erythrocytosis is inherited in an autosomal dominant manner as a result of truncation of the cytosolic portion of the erythropoietin receptor, which eliminates the negative regulatory domain of the receptor. The truncation does not allow the physiologically appropriate shutoff of the signaling cascade induced by erythropoietin binding and receptor dimerization. This leads to inappropriate erythropoietin signaling, increased red cell formation relative to plasma levels of erythropoietin, and high Hb levels.

Oxygen Sensing Mutations. In addition to mutations of globin, red cell enzymes, and the erythropoietin receptor, familial erythrocytosis can also be caused by inherited defects in the oxygen-sensing pathway leading to enhanced production of erythropoietin. Normally, erythropoietin mRNA expression is driven by the hypoxia-inducible transcription factor (HIF). In normoxic cells, HIF is markedly suppressed by proline hydroxylation of the HIF α subunit, thereby enabling it to bind to von Hippel-Lindau (VHL) protein, which mediates ubiquitylation of HIF-α and destruction in the proteasome.[107] A sizable population living in the Chuvash district of central Russia has autosomal recessive erythrocytosis because of a mutation in the VHL gene.[108] In addition, familial erythrocytosis with increased expression of erythropoietin may also be due to mutations in the prolyl hydroxylase 2 gene[109,110] and the HIF-2α gene.[111,112]

To summarize, in the identification of high-affinity Hb variants, the following points should be remembered:

1. Normal results on electrophoresis do not exclude the diagnosis of a high-affinity Hb.
2. A P_{50} value useful for diagnosis of a high-affinity Hb cannot be a value "calculated" from Po_2 data. (One has to be able to directly measure Hb saturation and Po_2 to obtain a useful P_{50} value. Types of apparatus such as the Hem-o-Scan are adequate for this purpose.)
3. Plasma erythropoietin levels are diagnostically useful.

Pathophysiologic and Clinical Aspects of High–Oxygen Affinity Hemoglobins

Most patients with high-affinity Hbs and erythrocytosis have a benign clinical course and no apparent complications. Although the first high-affinity Hb was identified in the course of a workup for angina, this association was probably fortuitous.

Patients with Hb Moke have been reported to have symptoms and to have benefited from phlebotomy and the transfusion of normal blood, but this is the exception and not the rule.[113] In a significant number of these patients, erythrocytosis is diagnosed during routine hematologic examination or when the pedigree of a propositus is examined. There are generally no physical findings, except occasionally a ruddy complexion. Hb and hematocrit levels are only moderately increased.

The most pressing reason to identify these high-affinity Hbs early and accurately is to avoid submitting the patient to unnecessary invasive diagnostic procedures and inappropriate and often dangerous therapeutic interventions. Some have undergone several courses of radioactive phosphorus (^{32}P) treatment based on a mistaken diagnosis of polycythemia vera. As a general rule, any patient suspected of having polycythemia vera who is about to undergo a serious therapeutic intervention should have a whole blood O_2 equilibrium measurement.

In patients who have had a physiologically significant high-affinity Hb all their lives, reasonable compensation is probably present throughout their lives. The reduced delivery of O_2 to tissues is compensated for primarily by increases in erythropoietin-induced red cell mass and also probably by increases in blood flow and changes in perfusion patterns in selected regions.

Erythropoietin-mediated increases in red cell mass respond to hypoxic stimuli.[114-116] Patients with several high-affinity Hbs and erythrocytosis have had normal urinary erythropoietin levels that dramatically increased when they were phlebotomized to a normal red cell mass. This effect was not observed in patients with idiopathic familial erythrocytosis. Patients with high-affinity Hbs have normal O_2 consumption, normal arterial Po_2 values,[114] slightly reduced mixed venous Po_2 values in some instances, and slightly decreased resting cardiac output. More important, these numbers change significantly after phlebotomy or measured exercise, with marked increases in cardiac output and lowering of mixed venous Po_2. The compensatory mechanisms might include increased perfusion efficiency. For example, patients with Hb Malmo have been shown to have increased myocardial blood flow, and patients with Hb Yakima have increased cerebral blood flow.

Following childbirth of women with high affinity mutants, no increase in morbidity or mortality in the infant or mother is observed, thus suggesting that compensatory mechanisms other than the differences in O_2 affinity between HbF and HbA (the former has lower affinity) must operate in pregnancies in which the mother's Hb has higher O_2 affinity than that of HbF.[117]

Why do the levels of Hb vary among carriers of the same high-affinity Hb? Charache and colleagues[117] observed that carriers of Hb Osler had the same O_2 affinity as patients with Hb McKees Rocks but that Hb levels

were significantly higher (by more than 4 g/dL) in male carriers of the former. When O_2 transport was assessed in these two groups, only a small decrease in mixed venous Po_2 was observed. This could be a consequence of better O_2 extraction by carriers of Hb McKees Rocks; as a result, they do not require as much of an increase in red cell mass as needed for those with Hb Osler.

These results imply that epistatic (modifier) genetic effects might be operating, thus making the extent of increase in red cell mass variable according to a person's genetic makeup. Charache and colleagues[117] have pointed out that adaptation to hypoxia at high altitude is also different in different ethnic groups. Among the Sherpas of Nepal, a lower hematocrit value, no chronic mountain sickness, and a normal O_2 equilibrium curve are found, whereas in the populations adapted to the Andes (Quechuas and Aymaras), a higher hematocrit value, chronic mountain sickness, and right-shifted O_2 equilibrium curves are observed. These findings suggest that adaptation might involve a choice among several possible strategies (with potential differences in success) according to the different genetic background.

Should carriers of high-affinity Hbs undergo phlebotomy? The preceding discussion suggests that patients with high-affinity Hbs have a reasonable compensation for their abnormality with correction of O_2 delivery to tissues despite increases in blood viscosity; therefore, no intervention is needed. Results of exercise studies before and after phlebotomy in patients with Hb Osler showed no need for phlebotomy.[118] Nevertheless, as mentioned earlier, there are reports of individual patients who have benefited from the procedure. Perhaps, in some patients other factors interfere with the normal compensation for a high-affinity Hb and the increased viscosity may become a burden. These are exceptional patients, and prudence dictates a conservative approach and review of the patient's condition at 6-month intervals during the first few years after diagnosis. In older patients, attention to coronary status is recommended.

Conditions of low ambient Po_2 (e.g., unpressurized airplane cabins or living or climbing in mountains) do not represent a risk to patients with these high-affinity Hbs. In fact, they are better equipped than the average person to handle such situations because their Hbs bind O_2 avidly.[118a]

Low–Oxygen Affinity Hemoglobin Mutants: Cyanosis

Carriers of some low–O_2 affinity Hb variants have a slate gray color of their skin and other teguments. Cyanosis can be present from birth in the α-chain mutants and from the middle to the end of the first year of life in the β-chain mutants. This differential pattern results because α chains are expressed from the second trimester of fetal life whereas β chains begin to be synthesized in the perinatal period and do not reach significant levels until about 6 months of age. Cyanosis caused by abnormal Hbs has to be distinguished from other more common causes, particularly pulmonary and cardiac disorders.

Many fewer low-affinity than high-affinity Hbs are described. They can be classified as resulting from the following three structural perturbations, which are discussed at length later:

1. Alterations in the switch region, the flexible joint, or the C-terminal of the $\alpha_1\beta_2$ area of contact that favor the T state, either by stabilizing this conformer or by destabilizing the R state. Examples include Hb Kansas (β102 [G4] Asn→Thr), Hb Beth Israel (β102 [G4] Asn→Ser),[119] and Hb Bruxelles (β42 [CD1] Phe→0).[120,121]
2. Steric hindrance of the heme resulting in decreased affinity for ligands. An example is Hb Chico (β66 [E10] Lys→Thr).
3. Alteration of the $\alpha_1\beta_1$ area of contact with disruption of the overall architecture of the Hb that favors the T state. Examples include Hb Yoshizuka (β108 [G10] Asn→Asp) and Hb Presbyterian (β108 [G10] Asn→Lys). Affected carriers usually have mild anemia and no cyanosis.

Hb Beth Israel[119] was found in a person of Italian descent, but the abnormal Hb was not detected in his parents. The propositus exhibited clinically apparent cyanosis involving his fingers, lips, and nail beds.[119] He had been severely disciplined in the past for constantly having "dirty hands," and the abnormal skin color was not noticeable to him or his parents. The cyanosis was detected by a surgeon about to perform a herniorrhaphy. As shown in Figure 18-12, whole blood P_{50} was 88 mm Hg (normal is 26 mm Hg), and arterial blood was only 63% saturated despite a normal P_{O_2} of 97 mm Hg. Red cell 2,3-DPG was mildly elevated (20 mmol/L). The hemolysate showed low O_2 affinity and a normal Bohr effect. The molecular mechanism involved here is the same as that in Hb Kansas: the amino acid replacement at the $\alpha_1\beta_2$ interface destabilizes the R quaternary structure.

Pathophysiologic Considerations

Low-affinity Hbs generally deliver more O_2 to tissues. The difference between O_2 binding at 100 mm Hg (lungs) and 40 mm Hg (tissues) in a low-affinity curve can be twice as high as that of a normal O_2 equilibrium curve. However, the increase in oxygen extraction is not monotonic with the increase in P_{50}. Hence, patients with moderately right-shifted red cell O_2 equilibrium curves (P_{50} of 35 to 55 mm Hg) could be "anemic." Less oxygen-carrying capacity is needed because of the enhanced oxygen unloading (see the Fick equation, discussed earlier). However, no anemia should be expected in patients with severely right-shifted curves ($P_{50} \approx$ 80 mm Hg). Findings in patients with Hb Kansas, Hb Beth Israel, Hb Titusville, and Hb Seattle confirm this analysis. Clinically apparent cyanosis is observed in

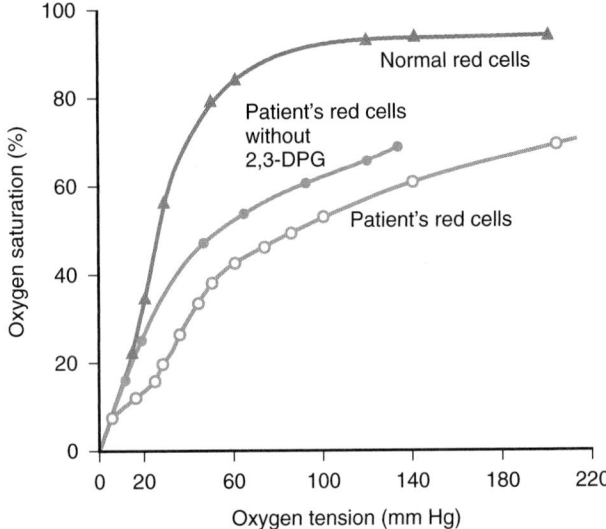

FIGURE 18-12. Oxygen equilibrium curves of normal red cells (*triangles*) and red cells from a patient heterozygous for Hb Beth Israel before (*open circles*) and after (*closed circles*) depletion of 2,3-diphosphoglycerate (2,3-DPG). The P_{50} for Hb Beth Israel–containing cells was 88 mm Hg (normal, 27 mm Hg). The patient's cells depleted of 2,3-DPG had a P_{50} of 55 mm Hg. Normal red cells subjected to the same procedure had a P_{50} of 16 mm Hg. The heterozygous patient's red cells have a biphasic or triphasic curve composed of the oxygen affinity curves of normal hemoglobin (particularly the bottom portion of the composite patient curve), the abnormal hemoglobin Beth Israel (top of the composite curve), and probably hybrid molecules containing one β Beth Israel chain and one normal β chain (intermediate portion of the curve). (*After Nagel RL, Joshua L, Johnson J, et al. Hemoglobin Beth Israel: a mutant causing clinically apparent cyanosis. N Engl J Med. 1976;295:125.*)

carriers with markedly right-shifted curves ($P_{50} >$ 50 mm Hg).

The effect of the right-shifted curve on the level of 2,3-DPG is of interest. In erythrocytes, 20% of the conversion of 1,3-DPG to 3-phosphoglycerate is done indirectly through the formation of 2,3-DPG. The level of red cell 2,3-DPG rises in conditions associated with hypoxia. This effect is related to the decrease in O_2 saturation of red cells and is independent of the presence of hypoxia per se; therefore, it applies to the low-affinity Hbs despite the absence of tissue hypoxia.

Desaturation increases intraerythrocytic pH as a result of deoxy-Hb binding more protons than oxy-Hb does (Bohr effect). This slight red cell alkalosis stimulates two enzymes involved in 2,3-DPG synthesis: phosphofructokinase, which controls the overall glycolytic rate, and 2,3-DPG mutase, which directly controls the rate of 2,3-DPG synthesis. In addition, high pH inhibits 2,3-DPG phosphatase. Hence, increased pH simultaneously increases the synthesis of 2,3-DPG and decreases its destruction. Finally, relief of end-product inhibition may also be involved. Red cells with low-affinity Hb have an increased proportion of deoxy-Hb and will bind more 2,3-DPG, thereby decreasing free 2,3-DPG and thus inhibiting 2,3-DPG mutase[25] (see Fig. 18-9).

Identification of Low–Oxygen Affinity Hemoglobin Variants

The presence of a low-affinity Hb should always be considered in patients with cyanosis, particularly when cardiopulmonary causes can be ruled out. In patients with cyanosis of unknown origin, it is advisable to perform electrophoresis of Hb and measure whole blood P_{50} before expensive or risky invasive diagnostic procedures are undertaken. The search for low-affinity Hbs as the explanation for anemia is less compelling because the yield is very low and the tests are not cost-effective. Nevertheless, if other investigations prove to be fruitless, unexplained normocytic anemias can be explored with the aforementioned tests.

A simple "bedside" test (even able to be performed at the bedside) to distinguish low-affinity Hbs and cardiopulmonary cyanosis from methemoglobinemia, the presence of M Hbs, and sulfhemoglobinemia is to expose blood from the patient to pure O_2. This will turn the purple deoxy-Hb in normal venous blood and that of patients with low-affinity Hbs to the bright red color of oxy-Hb. In contrast, the blood of patients with methemoglobinemia, sulfhemoglobinemia, or M Hbs retains its abnormal color despite exposure to O_2.

M Hemoglobins: Cyanosis

Description and Pathophysiologic Features of the M Hemoglobins

Horlein and Weber[122] described a family with congenital cyanosis caused by abnormal red cells 1 year before Pauling's discovery of HbS. The defect was autosomal dominant and was produced by red cells with an abnormal pigment that was similar to Met-Hb. The genetic defect resided in the globin and not in the heme, based on recombination experiments in which the patients' globin was bound to normal heme and the patients' heme to normal globin. The amino acid substitutions characterizing three of these M Hbs were determined by Gerald and Efron.[123] About the same time, the Japanese[124] solved the problem of hereditary nigremia (kuroko or "black child") observed in the Shiden village of the Iwate prefecture for more than 160 years. They found a brownish colored Hb in the hemolysate of a patient with this condition, which was later called Hb Iwate.

In the M Hbs, each mutated globin chain (α or β) creates an abnormal microenvironment for the heme iron in which the equilibrium is displaced toward the oxidized or ferric state. The combination of the iron (Fe^{3+}) and its abnormal coordination with the substituted amino acid generates an abnormal visible spectrum that resembles but is different from Met-Hb (oxidized heme iron in a normal globin chain). The strength at which the abnormal hemes are locked into this situation differs from one M Hb to another.

In four of the five known M Hbs, the distal or proximal histidine that interacts with the heme iron is replaced by tyrosine, either in the α chains or in the β chains. In the fifth, HbM Milwaukee-I, Val-β67 (E11) is replaced by a glutamic acid whose longer side chains can reach and perturb the heme iron.

Several molecular abnormalities are associated with the M Hbs. They can be classified into the following categories.

Weak Heme Attachment. X-ray crystallographic studies of deoxy-HbM Hyde Park (β92 [F8] His→Tyr) showed a loss of 20% to 30% of the heme.[125] Others detected a minor component (5%) in the hemolysate of these patients that migrated between HbA$_2$ and HbA Hyde Park.[126] The α chains of the abnormal component were normal, but only one of the two β^{HP} chains contained heme.

In this context, the mutation in Hb Auckland (α97 [F8] His→Asn) is particularly interesting.[127] This mutation, which involve the proximal histidine, does not lead to methemoglobinemia, as do other mutations of the proximal histidine, but to instability and accelerated heme loss. The clinical picture is a mild compensated hemolytic anemia but not methemoglobinemia.

Binding of the Iron to the Remaining Histidine and to the Newly Introduced Tyrosine. In β^M chains (Hb Hyde Park) and α^M chains (HbM Iwate), the proximal F8 histidine is replaced by tyrosine. Crystallographic analysis of HbM Hyde Park showed that the Tyr must be accommodated by movements of the F helix, which appears to be largely destabilized.[125]

The findings in HbM Iwate (α87 [F8] His→Tyr) are the opposite. Here, crystallographic studies[125] show that the E helix of the α chains is displaced toward the heme plane by about 2 Å, which enables the heme iron to bind to the distal histidine (α58 [E7]).[128-130]

The distal histidines (E7) are substituted by tyrosines in the β^M chain of HbM Saskatoon (β63 [E7] His→Tyr) and the α^M chain in HbM Boston (α58 [E7] His→Tyr). In HbM Boston, as illustrated in Figure 18-13, the tyrosine surprisingly fills the fifth coordinating position of the heme iron despite the presence of a normal proximal histidine.[131] This bond moves the plane of the heme sufficiently to make interaction between the proximal histidine and the heme iron impossible. No crystallographic data are available on HbM Saskatoon.

Finally, HbM Milwaukee-I is unique among the M Hbs in that it is not a mutation of the proximal or distal histidines but a mutation of a nearby residue (67Val [E11]). When substituted by Glu, it perturbs the heme iron and generates an M Hb (defined as a variant having an abnormal Met-Hb–like spectrum). Other mutations at that site, such as Hb Bristol (Asp) or Hb Sidney (Ala), are unstable or have low affinity but do not generate an abnormal ferric state of the heme iron. The carboxylic group of the new glutamate in β^M Milwaukee occupies

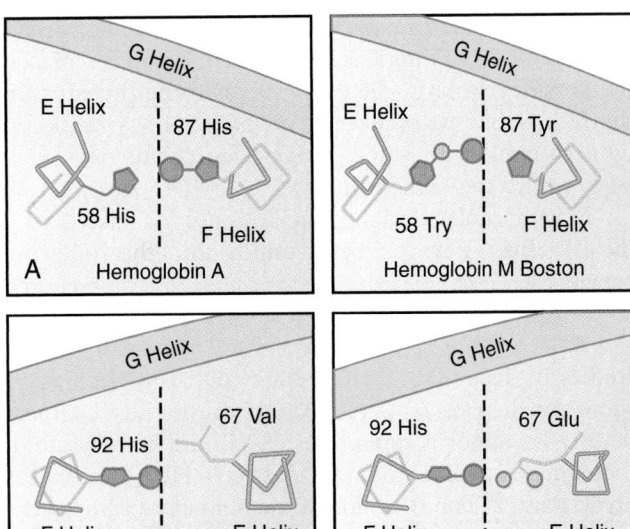

FIGURE 18-13. Schematic depiction of the crystallographic findings in HbM Boston (**A,** α58 [E7] His→Tyr) and HbM Milwaukee-I (**B,** β67 [E11] Val→Glu) versus those of normal hemoglobin. (*A, After Pulsinelli PD, Perutz MF, Nagel RL. Structure of hemoglobin M Boston, a variant with a five-coordinated ferric heme. Proc Natl Acad Sci U S A. 1973;70:3870. B, after Perutz MF, Pulsinelli PD, Ranney HM. Structure and subunit interaction of haemoglobin M-Milwaukee. Nature. 1972; 237:259.*)

the sixth coordination position of the iron, and the proximal histidine maintains its role in binding iron at the fifth coordinating position.[132] This situation, of course, stabilizes the abnormal ferric state of HbM Milwaukee-I.

Oxygen-Binding Properties and R→T Transition of M Hemoglobins. HbM Milwaukee-I, HbM Hyde Park, and HbM Boston all adopt a deoxy or deoxy-like conformation upon deoxygenation of the two normal chains (despite the fact that the abnormal chains cannot deoxygenate). This finding helps us understand the function of normal Hb; that is, after two hemes become deoxygenated, the molecule as a whole adopts a deoxy conformation (T state).

HbM Milwaukee-I, HbM Saskatoon, and HbM Hyde Park adopt the R state when the two normal chains are oxygenated. Nuclear magnetic resonance studies on HbM Milwaukee-I[133] also support a conformational change when the normal hemes are oxygenated. In contrast, HbM Iwate is in the crystallographic T-configuration state when the normal hemes are in the ferric state. This explains its decreased affinity. The molecule does not shift to the R state when the normal hemes are liganded and remains in the low-affinity T state. Similarly, in HbM Boston the deoxy-Hb crystal remains intact after oxygenation, thus suggesting that no conformational change has occurred.[131]

The reason that HbM Boston and HbM Saskatoon have different properties (despite their common substitution of the distal histidine) is that the former does not

change conformation when oxygenated and the latter does. Why β chains differ from α chains when their distal histidine is substituted has not been resolved.

Iron Oxidation and Spectral Characteristics. The fundamental characteristic of the M Hbs is that their hemes are stabilized in the abnormal ferric state. Hence, they exhibit an abnormal visible spectrum that can easily be distinguished from that of normal methemoglobin A. This characteristic separates these variants from Hb mutants that have a tendency to form normal Met-Hb, such as Hb Saint Louis,[134] Hb Bicêtre,[135] HbI Toulouse,[136] and Hb Seattle,[137] all of which are unstable.

Clinical Aspects and Diagnosis

The predominant clinical feature associated with M Hb carriers is cyanosis.[138-148] The skin and mucosal membranes may be brownish or slate colored, more like the coloration seen in methemoglobinemia, but not as blue-purple as the much more common cyanosis due to increased deoxyhemoglobin. The distinction is subtle and might not be apparent without contrasting the two conditions simultaneously. The reason for the difference is that the color of the skin is induced by Hb molecules that have an abnormal Met-Hb state rather than by the presence of more than 5 g/dL of deoxy-Hb. The cyanosis is present from birth in individuals with α-chain abnormalities and from the middle of the first year in those with β-chain mutants. In addition, a mixture of the abnormal pigment and increased desaturation of the normal chains are observed in the low-affinity M Hbs (HbM Boston and HbM Iwate).

Affected persons apparently have normal life expectancy and no dyspnea or clubbing. A mild hemolytic anemia (with an increased reticulocyte count) has been observed in HbM Hyde Park and can be explained by instability of the Hb induced by partial loss of the hemes.

The possibility of M Hb should be considered in all patients with abnormal homogeneous coloration of the skin and mucosa, particularly when pulmonary and cardiac function is normal. The diagnosis can be reinforced by observing an abnormal brown coloration of a blood sample. To distinguish this coloration from that caused by Met-Hb, the addition of potassium cyanide to the hemolysate is useful. Hemolysates containing Met-Hb turn red; those containing M Hb often change color more slowly. The rate of color conversion varies among the M Hbs. A recording spectrophotometer is required for definitive diagnosis.

Electrophoresis is of limited value because the oxy forms are not separable from normal Hb by cellulose acetate. Agar electrophoresis is preferable.

Perhaps the greatest hazard for carriers of M Hb is misdiagnosis and the risk of expensive and hazardous workups. A 1-week-old infant underwent a Blalock procedure because of misdiagnosis of pseudotruncus arteriosus. When the family study was completed many years later, the father and child were identified as carriers of HbM Boston.

Unstable Hemoglobin Variants: Congenital Heinz Body Hemolytic Syndrome

Some Hb mutants have substitutions that alter the solubility of the molecule in the red cell.[149] The intraerythrocytic precipitated material derived from the unstable abnormal Hb is detectable by a supravital stain as dark globular aggregates called Heinz bodies (HBs). These intracellular inclusions reduce the life span of the red cell and generate a hemolytic process of varied severity called congenital HB hemolytic anemia.

Structural Abnormalities Involved in Unstable Hemoglobins

Substitutions in the primary sequence can lead to alterations in the tertiary or quaternary structure and result in a globin polypeptide chain or a Hb tetramer that is relatively unstable and tends to precipitate inside the red cell. The structural alterations leading to this event can be classified as follows.

Mutations That Weaken or Modify Heme-Globin Interactions. Binding of heme to globin is important not only for the O_2-binding properties of the molecule but also for its stability and solubility. Such mutations include the following:

1. Substitutions that introduce a charged side chain into the heme pocket where a nonpolar side chain existed previously: examples are Hb Boras, Hb Bristol, Hb Olsted, Hb Himeji, and others
2. Deletions involving residues that directly interact with heme, such as Hb Gun Hill
3. Nontyrosine substitutions of the proximal histidine (F8), such as Hb Saint Etienne (also known as Hb Istanbul), HbJ Altgeld Gardens, Hb Mozhaisk, Hb Newcastle, Hb Iwata, and Hb Redondo (also known as Hb Ishehara)
4. Nontyrosine substitutions of the distal histidine (E7), such as Hb Zurich and Hb Bicêtre

Hb Zurich ($\beta63$ [E7] His→Arg) is an interesting mutation that deserves special mention.[150] Substitution of an arginine for the distal histidine in the β chains makes the space available for ligand binding around the iron much larger, thereby fundamentally changing some of its interactions with ligands.

Carriers of Hb Zurich exhibit an increased affinity for CO because of the increased space in the heme pocket. This is a protective mechanism of sorts. It does not allow the abnormal β chain to become ferric, which would increase its instability. Smokers with Hb Zurich have high levels of carboxy-Hb, but carriers who are nonsmokers also have abnormal carboxy-Hb levels. Because of the partially protective effect of carboxy-Hb

Zurich, hemolysis is less severe in smokers than in nonsmokers with this abnormal Hb.[150]

Carriers of Hb Zurich are especially susceptible to hemolytic crises induced by sulfanilamide. The increased aperture of the heme pocket also explains this phenomenon: sulfanilamide is capable of binding to the heme and producing Met-Hb directly. Again, CO has a protective effect.

Mutations That Interfere with the Secondary Structure of the Subunits. As previously mentioned, Hb is composed of more than 75% α-helical regions, and any disruption of this secondary structure reduces the solubility of the subunit. Unstable Hb mutants can result from introduction of proline into the helical structure or substitution of glycine by a mutation in invariant positions in the bands. About 15% of mutations responsible for unstable Hbs involve the introduction of a proline residue.

Hb Brockton ($\beta138$ [H16] Ala→Pro)[151] is associated with moderate anemia. It cannot be separated from HbA by standard electrophoretic procedures. Crystallography showed that the tertiary structure was disrupted in the vicinity of the mutated residue. Its molecular instability is probably the result of breakage of a buried hydrogen bond that normally links Ala-$\beta138$ with Val-$\beta134$, a task that the proline side chain cannot accomplish.

Hb Singapore ($\alpha141$ Arg→Pro) is an unusual exception in which the introduction of a proline is not accompanied by instability. The reason is that the substituted residue is the last amino acid of the α chain, Arg141, and no disruption of an α helix takes place.

Mutations That Interfere with the Tertiary Structure of the Subunits. Hb is a globular protein, quite tightly bound, which means that the α-helical regions must be folded into a solid sphere. This design places enormous constraints on its three-dimensional structure. Substitutions of the sequence can occur with no change in solubility as long as (1) no charged residues (hydrophilic) are allowed to point inward, (2) no bulky side chains are allowed to substitute for less bulky residues inside the molecule, and (3) loss of critical nonpolar residues from the surface of the subunit is avoided. The latter includes hydrophobic residues that are located on the surface and serve to prevent water from invading the interior of the molecule.

Mutations That Affect Subunit Interactions: Interference with the Quaternary Structure. These mutations involve the introduction of charged residues into the interior or the loss of intersubunit contact hydrogen bonds or salt bridges in the $\alpha_1\beta_1$ contact. Normal oxy-Hb tetramer readily dissociates at the $\alpha_1\beta_2$ interface into $\alpha\beta$ dimers. In contrast, breakdown of $\alpha_1\beta_1$ dimers normally occurs to a vanishingly small extent but is a great threat to the molecule because it generates Met-Hb and consequent instability. Dissociation of $\alpha_1\beta_1$ dimers generates monomeric α and β chains, which uncoil and loosen their heme-globin interaction, thereby favoring Met-Hb formation. Several unstable Hb mutations involve residues located in the $\alpha_1\beta_1$ area of contact: Hb Philly,[152] Hb Peterborough,[153] Hb Stanmore,[154] HbJ Guantanamo,[155] and Hb Khartoum.[156]

Hyperunstable Hemoglobins. This term was coined by Ohba[157,158] to characterize unstable Hbs that are either barely detectable or undetectable in hemolysates. These Hbs are presumably synthesized normally but are rapidly destroyed in bone marrow, thus creating a phenotype closer to thalassemia than to the hemolytic anemia normally associated with unstable Hbs. Hb mutants associated with a thalassemic phenotype are discussed in a later section.

Clinical Characteristics of the Congenital Heinz Body Hemolytic Anemias

Anemia is the centerpiece of the syndrome, but its intensity varies widely among patients, depending on the Hb variant.

Unstable Hbs are uncommon mutational events generally limited to a single pedigree. One exception is Hb Köln ($\beta98$ [FG5] Val$\rightarrow$Met), which has been detected in many different pedigrees and geographic locations. The time at which anemia appears depends on the chain affected. One of the α-chain mutants, Hb Hasharon ($\alpha47$ [CE5] Asp$\rightarrow$His), which is found predominantly among Ashkenazi Jews, produces significant hemolysis in newborns but is milder in adults.[159,160] In some carriers it produces a mild anemia, whereas no hemolysis is observed in other carriers within the same pedigree. Epistatic effects of other nonlinked genes are probably involved here.

Unstable γ-chain variants, such as HbF Poole, cause significant hemolysis in the first 3 months of life[65] that is ameliorated by the emergence of β chains at the end of the first year.

Patients with unstable Hb may have hemolytic crises associated with bacterial or viral infections or exposure to oxidants. Pyrexia and transient acidosis contribute to hemolysis because they increase Hb denaturation. Drugs (e.g., sulfonamides) have been directly implicated in hemolytic crisis associated with Hb Zurich, Hb Hasharon, Hb Shepards Bush, and Hb Peterborough. The crises are generally self-limited, and stopping the administration of all drugs is prudent. Patients are also susceptible to parvovirus B19–induced aplastic crises.

Patients with unstable Hbs can have characteristically dark urine or pigmenturia. The color change is not due to bilirubin but rather to the presence of dipyrrole methylenes of the mesobilifuscin group.[161] These compounds probably arise from nonenzymatic catabolism of heme. Fluorescent dipyrroles may also be present in HBs.[162]

The absence of pigmenturia does not exclude the diagnosis of unstable Hb because not all mutants exhibit pigmenturia. In addition, the extent of hemolysis does not correlate with pigmenturia because significant pigmenturia is seen with both Hb Köln (severe hemolytic anemia) and Hb Zurich (little hemolysis).

Congenital HB hemolytic anemias related to unstable Hbs are generally mild and do not require therapy except for supportive and preventive measures, including administration of folic acid to ensure that the overworked marrow does not become deficient in this nutrient, prevention and prompt treatment of infections, avoidance of pyrexia with the use of aspirin, and avoidance of oxidant drugs such as acetaminophen. In patients with more severe disease, hydroxyurea may be effective in lowering the hemolytic rate.[163]

The question of splenectomy arises for patients with more severe hemolysis. There is little doubt that the spleen plays an important pathophysiologic role in the destruction of HB-containing red cells. Nevertheless, this needs to be balanced with the role of the spleen in the susceptibility to pneumococcal infections early in life and the need to use antipneumococcal vaccines after splenectomy in childhood. There is additional concern that splenectomy may promote the development of thrombosis and pulmonary hypertension.[164] Splenectomy is beneficial, on balance, for patients with the most severe unstable hemoglobinopathies, and partial correction of the anemia has been achieved.[165] Nevertheless, the success of the splenectomy cannot be ensured.

Identification of Unstable Hemoglobins

Elements in the differential diagnosis of unstable Hbs consist of the following:

1. HBs spontaneously present in blood (less often) or induced by 24-hour incubation of a sterile sample in sterile saline and stained by supravital pigments
2. Abnormal Hb electrophoresis (sometimes a smeared band is observed); normal results are not diagnostically useful
3. Positive tests for heat or isopropanol stability

All these tests are useful and should be pursued because the results of any one of them could be negative. The heat and isopropanol stability tests are the least likely to be negative.

Because the spleen removes HBs efficiently, many patients with unstable Hbs lack HBs before splenectomy, and the differential diagnosis includes autoimmune hemolytic anemias and other disorders with nonspecific red cell morphology, such as glycolytic and other red cell enzyme defects, Wilson's disease, paroxysmal nocturnal hemoglobinuria, hereditary xerocytosis, and (very rarely) erythropoietic porphyria.

The differential diagnosis of an unstable hemoglobinopathy in an adult is the same as that for other causes of congenital HB hemolytic syndrome and acquired forms of HB hemolytic anemia (acquired methemoglobinemia, chemical and drug oxidants, and other conditions). In rare instances, several of these entities interact with each other to the detriment of the patient.[166]

Smear and Heinz Body Preparation. The blood smear reveals nonspecific abnormalities, including anisocytosis and sometimes hypochromia and microcytosis. Basophilic stippling is often prominent and is a useful clue to the diagnosis because it is uncommon in other hemolytic anemias, except for the rare pyridine 5′-nucleotidase deficiency. Howell-Jolly bodies and normoblasts may also be observed in the peripheral blood of splenectomized patients.

Detection of HBs requires the use of methyl blue or crystal violet supravital stains. HBs appear as irregular pale purple inclusions, singly or a few together. They are 2 μm in diameter or smaller and often appear to be attached to the membrane.[161] Sometimes HBs are apparent in fresh blood, but usually sterile incubation of the blood for 24 hours in the absence of glucose is required to elicit HBs. A sample of normal blood should always be run as a control. After splenectomy, red cells with HBs occur more often and are easier to detect. Indeed, in occasional patients HBs can be detected only after splenectomy.

Electrophoresis. Electrophoresis of Hb can demonstrate an abnormal component, but many times the unstable Hb appears as a diffuse band. This alteration is probably related to the partial denaturation of Hb molecules during electrophoresis (as a result of the heat generated) or during manipulations of the hemolysate. Occasionally, only precipitated material at the origin is observed. Many unstable Hbs are not detectable by electrophoresis.

Heat Stability Test. The heat denaturation test, which consists of incubation of a hemolysate for 1 or 2 hours at 50° C, is a simple and reliable procedure.[165,166] Normal hemolysates are stable under these conditions, and the presence of an unstable Hb is signaled by the appearance of a visible precipitate. Some abnormal Hbs, such as Hb Hasharon, precipitate at temperatures higher than 50° C. Irrespective of incubation temperature, controls are indispensable. Normal Hb begins to precipitate at about 55° C.

Other laboratory procedures are available. The isopropanol test[167] is used in many laboratories, but it gives false-positive results when the sample contains more than 5% HbF. HbF does not interfere with zinc acetate precipitation.[168] Mechanical agitation can also reveal the presence of unstable Hbs.[169]

Pathophysiology of the Heinz Body Hemolytic Syndrome Produced by Unstable Hemoglobins

Thermostability of Hemoglobins. When heat-unstable Hbs were related to the presence of an HB hemolytic anemia, the conceptual framework for understanding this syndrome was generated. Homeothermic mammals and birds have relatively thermostable Hbs. If a hemolysate is incubated for 1 or 2 hours at 50° C, little protein precipi-

tation occurs. This property is observed even among reptile Hb, though to a lesser degree. In amphibians and fish, the thermostability of Hb decreases substantially.

The molecular basis of thermostability is not clear. Perutz and Raidt[170] suggested that the thermostability of proteins, including Hb, is based on electrostatic interactions and salt bridge formations. Others[171] contend that hydrophobic interactions are critical, and some claim that both electrostatic and hydrophobic interactions are contributory.[172] Most of the evidence comes from structural analysis of proteins obtained from thermophilic and mesophilic bacteria[173] or from comparison of amino acid sequences in the Hbs of organisms living at different temperatures.[174]

Other contributions to thermostability come from the strength of the heme-globin bonds. Heme exchange between Hb and albumin and between Hbs decreases considerably when the Met-Hb heme is ligated with cyanide.[175] Cyanomethemoglobin has a stronger heme-globin attachment than Met-Hb does and is more similar to liganded Hb. Deoxy-Hb has an even tighter bond.

Denaturation of Hemoglobin and Hemichrome Formation. HBs, one of the hallmarks of the hemolytic syndrome generated by unstable Hbs, are the product of Hb denaturation. HBs probably contain a significant amount of heme-depleted globin chains.[172,176] The precipitated material is hemichromes.[177-180] As shown in Figure 18-14, these hemichromes are derivatives of the low-spin forms of ferric Hb that have the sixth coordination position occupied by a ligand provided by the globin: a hydroxyl group (—OH) or an unprotonated histidyl (reversible hemichrome) or a protonated histidyl (irreversible hemichrome).[181] Irreversible hemichromes seem to be an indispensable stage in the formation of HBs, and both α and β chains are present.[182]

Anemia with the Unstable Hemoglobins That Generate Heinz Body Hemolytic Syndrome. The primary cause of the anemia is the reduced life span of the red cells that contain HBs. Evidence indicates that HBs, at least in part, adhere to the cytosolic side of the membrane[183] by hydrophobic interactions and not through covalent bonds.[184,185]

Unstable Hbs generate considerable amounts of hemichromes, some of which bind to the negatively charged cytosolic domain of band 3,[186-189] a transmembrane protein that functions as the primary anion exchanger in the red cell. It is not surprising that these red cells exhibit decreased deformability, a characteristic that will condemn them to be preferentially trapped in the spleen, the organ that maintains red cell quality control.[190] It is possible that HB-containing red cells are pitted initially. The term *pitting* refers to the mechanism by which HBs and a portion of the overlying plasma membrane are excised from the cells during their passage through the spleen. This manipulation converts red cells

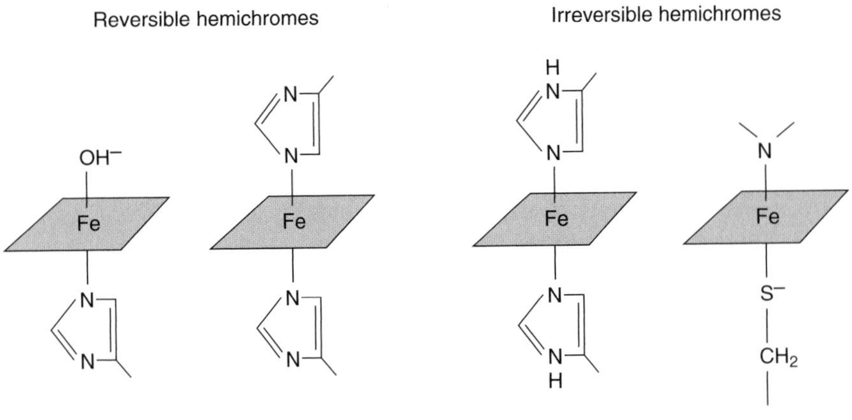

Reversible hemichromes

Irreversible hemichromes

FIGURE 18-14. Diagrammatic representation of the structure of hemichromes showing the proximal histidine below the plane of the heme and the distal histidine above the plane. One or both of the histidines can be substituted. *(After Peisach J, Blumberg WE, Rachmilewitz EA. The demonstration of ferrihemochrome intermediates in Heinz body formation following the reduction of oxyhemoglobin A by acetylphenylhydrazine. Biochim Biophys Acta. 1975;393:404.)*

progressively into spherocytes through loss of membrane, which produces a rigid remnant that will eventually be eliminated from the circulation.

Other sources of membrane damage come from peroxidation and cross-linking of membrane proteins. These are probably related to the presence of free heme and iron and to free radicals generated during the formation of Met-Hb and denaturation of Hb.[191-194] Other evidence of membrane alteration is the presence of abnormal potassium (K^+) efflux in some of these cells.[190,195]

Another determinant of the anemia in patients with unstable Hbs is the O_2 equilibrium curve. The level of 2,3-DPG is generally normal,[196] but some variants have high or low O_2 affinity. As discussed earlier, persons with high-affinity unstable Hbs tend to have less anemia than those with low-affinity unstable Hbs. Finally, several unstable Hbs coexist with α- or β-thalassemia: the α-chain mutants Hb Suan-Dok and Hb Petah Tikva coexist in *cis* with α-thalassemia, and the β-chain mutant Hb Leiden coexists in *cis* with β-thalassemia.

Hemoglobin Mutations with Abnormal Assembly: Dominant Thalassemia Syndrome

The dominant thalassemia syndrome includes mutations in the coding region of the globin genes that lead to a significant deficit in synthesis and that are clinically manifested as autosomal dominant thalassemia. Examples include Hb Indianapolis (β112 [G14] Cys→Arg)[197] and Hb Manhattan (β109 [G11] → −G→ frame shift).[197]

Clinical Picture and Diagnosis

The dominant thalassemia syndrome is characterized by significant anemia, often transfusion dependent, by splenomegaly, and by a blood smear with prominent hypochromia, microcytosis, and basophilic stippling.[198] The reticulocyte count is often high. Inclusion bodies are frequently observed in erythrocyte precursors with supravital staining, which is why some authors call this syndrome "inclusion body thalassemia." The bone marrow shows considerable erythroid hyperplasia and evidence

of ineffective erythropoiesis. Finally, the full-fledged thalassemic syndrome is found in members of different generations in the same pedigree, often in one of the parents or progeny of the propositus. Although the syndrome is similar to thalassemia intermedia, an astute clinician can exclude this diagnosis when the intensity of the disease in the parents or descendants is equal to that seen in the propositus. Thalassemia intermedia usually results from homozygosity or double heterozygosity for much milder defects; hence, the parents or progeny have much milder disease. Nevertheless, lack of parental involvement does not exclude the diagnosis because the mutation can arise de novo. A clinical picture of thalassemia in a patient with an ethnic origin not associated with β-thalassemia should also increase suspicion of the clinician for this syndrome.

Electrophoresis might not reveal an abnormal band because the abnormal Hb either is synthesized at an extremely low level, is rapidly catabolized, or both.

Highly unstable α-globin variants, in contrast to β-globin variants, are usually phenotypically apparent only when they interact with other α-thalassemia mutations. A child with clinical and hematologic features consistent with those of β-thalassemia intermedia nonetheless had a DNA analysis that excluded β-globin gene mutations. Instead, the propositus had a novel deletion (β37 [C2] Pro→0 [Hb Heraklion]) in the α_1-globin gene in *trans* to a common Mediterranean nondeletional α-thalassemia mutation.[199] This deletion results in severe instability of the variant Hb, which interacts with the α-thalassemia mutation and causes a relatively severe dyserythropoietic anemia—an alternative phenotype associated with the highly unstable α-chain variants. The dyserythropoietic marrow is due to the premature destruction of early red cell precursors.

Pathophysiology

The molecular basis of the dominant thalassemia syndrome involves several types of changes: (1) single point mutations (substitutions and deletions) affecting, in particular, exon 3; (2) exon 3 chain length shortening (premature termination) or elongation (frameshift mutation leading to an altered stop codon); and (3) amino acid replacements in α-globin that impair binding to α-globin stabilizing protein (AHSP). Such mutations include Hb Groene Hart (α119 [H2] Pro→Ser) and Hb Diamant (α119[H2]Pro→Leu).[200] For more information on AHSP, see Chapter 20.

What causes the severity of the phenotype of dominant thalassemia? The answer lies in the notion that in dominant thalassemia, the abnormal chain is synthesized at close to the normal rate but is rapidly destroyed because it cannot assemble into tetramers; inclusions are created and free radicals are generated as a result of oxidation of the heme groups to metheme.

Clinically Important Interactions among Mutant Hemoglobins

Hemoglobin C

HbS (β6 [A3] Glu→Val), HbC (β6 [A3] Glu→Lys), and HbE (β26 [B8] Glu→Lys) are the three most prevalent abnormal Hbs in humans. HbS and sickle cell disease are discussed in Chapter 19. HbE, which confers a mild thalassemia phenotype, is discussed in detail in Chapter 20.

The unique pathogenetic feature of HbC is its capacity to induce erythrocyte dehydration. In CC disease (homozygous state for the HbC gene), this pathologic change results only in mild hemolytic anemia. In SC disease, in which equal levels of HbS and HbC coexist, HbC accentuates the deleterious properties of HbS and produces a clinically significant disorder, though milder than sickle cell anemia.[201]

Origins, Selection, and Distribution of the Hemoglobin C Gene

HbC is the product of the β^C-globin gene generated by a GAG→AAG (Glu→Lys) substitution in codon 6 of the β-globin gene. The β^C mutation occurred originally among ethnic groups in Burkina Faso (previously Upper Volta). HbC reaches its highest rate of occurrence in central western Africa, and occurrence of the gene decreases concentrically outward from this region. It is also found in western Africa, west of the Niger River, and exclusively in areas where HbS is also present.[201]

The HbC gene exists at polymorphic rates (>1%), thus suggesting that its presence confers selective advantage to the carrier. Modiano and collaborators,[202] in a large case-control study performed in Burkina Faso on 4348 Mossi subjects, found that HbC is associated with a 29% reduction in the risk for clinical malaria in HbC heterozygotes (AC) (*P* = .0008) and a 93% reduction in HbC homozygotes (CC) (*P* = .0011). These findings establish the fact that HbC is selected for in malaria caused by *Plasmodium falciparum*. Balanced polymorphism[203] explains the selective advantage of the HbS trait and is based on the advantage of heterozygotes and the disadvantage of homozygotes. It does not seem to apply

to HbC because both heterozygotes and homozygotes have some level of advantage, and surprisingly, that of homozygotes is stronger. These findings, together with the limited pathologic changes in the AC and CC genotypes versus those of the severely affected SS and SC genotypes and the low occurrence of the β^S gene in the geographic epicenter of HbC, also support the hypothesis that in the long term and in the absence of malaria control, HbC interferes with the lysis of parasitized red cells in the late schizont state, thereby impairing the dispersion of merozoites.[204]

Properties of Hemoglobin C–Containing Erythrocytes

The erythrocytes of HbCC homozygotes have microcytic and hyperchromic target cells, microspherocytes, and cells with crystalline inclusions.[201] Target cells, a diagnostically useful feature, are presumably the consequence of the greater surface-to-volume ratio of HbCC red cells, which in turn is a consequence of their reduced water content (see later).

Red cell life span is shortened to approximately 40 days in HbCC disease. However, this is at least three times as long as the life span of cells in sickle cell anemia.[205]

Scanning electron microscopic examination of cells isolated from density gradients showed intracellular HbC crystals.[206] Freeze-fracture preparations, followed by electron microscopy, also showed intracellular crystals.[207] Circulating crystals can be detected in unperturbed wet preparations from individuals with HbC disease, but they are rare. Together, these observations are consistent with early reports of an increase in intraerythrocytic crystals in patients with HbC disease after splenectomy.[208]

Why do red cells that contain HbC crystals not induce vaso-occlusion? The answer to this riddle is that the crystal forms of oxy-HbC and deoxy-HbC differ. HbC crystals in the red cells of splenectomized patients with CC disease were found to be in the oxy state and melted after deoxygenation.[209] Moreover, when cells from venous and arterial blood were fixed and counted, there was a significant difference in the mean percentage of crystal-containing cells in the arterial circulation versus the venous circulation (1.6% ± 0.22% versus 1.1% ± 0.23%). Hence, the oxy-HbC crystals melt before they can do any damage to the microcirculation.

Effect of Hemoglobin C on Cell Density

A high mean corpuscular hemoglobin concentration (MCHC) and low intracellular water content are characteristics of HbC-containing cells. Red cell density is directly related to the MCHC. Cells in both HbC trait and HbC disease are denser than normal.[210,211] The average MCHC in CC disease, SC disease, HbC trait, and HbA cells is 38, 37, 34, and 33 g/dL, respectively. Cells in all four of these genotypes have a narrow density distribution such that the youngest and lightest cells differ from the oldest and most dense cells by only 3 to

4 g/dL. In contrast, cells in sickle cell anemia have a very wide density distribution. The reticulocytes of individuals with CC and SC disease and HbC trait are denser than normal reticulocytes. This implies either that these cells are denser than normal when they first enter the circulation or that their density changes within their first 24 hours in the circulation when they are still recognizable as reticulocytes.

Increased volume-regulated loss of red cell K^+ and water makes an HbC-containing cell dehydrated and more dense than normal.[210,211] This single feature may be responsible for all the abnormalities that have been detected in erythrocytes that contain high levels of this Hb.

Binding of Hemoglobin C to Cell Membranes

Like HbS, HbC interacts more strongly with the erythrocyte membrane than HbA does. This interaction has been studied by using changes in the fluorescence intensity of a membrane-embedded probe, the fluorescence of which is quenched when it is approached by Hb.[212-214] The cytoplasmic portion of band 3 was implicated as the binding site for both HbA and HbC.

In HbC, substitution of a charged lysine residue for β6 glutamic acid causes a very different pathophysiologic condition than the hydrophobic β6 valine present in HbS does. Whereas deoxy-HbS polymerizes, oxy-HbC has an increased tendency for intraerythrocytic crystallization, which along with cell dehydration caused by the HbC-induced loss of K^+ and water, is the basis of the pathophysiology of HbC disease, particularly the hemolytic process. As discussed later, similar mechanisms contribute to the pathologic changes in HbSC disease, with the addition that here, the presence of intraerythrocytic HbC induces a reduction in volume by loss of water and K^+, thereby increasing the tendency of HbS to polymerize.

HbC crystals are most likely to form in cells with low HbF content.[209] When the cells of individuals with CC disease are density fractionated, cells of the highest density have the lowest HbF content. In this dense cell fraction, no F cells contained HbC crystals. HbF inhibition of HbC crystallization might contribute to the potentially beneficial effects of hydroxyurea in HbSC disease in individuals who have an increase in HbF in response to treatment with this drug (see later).

Vaso-occlusive episodes are not a feature of HbC disease despite the presence of intraerythrocytic HbC crystals because as mentioned earlier, oxy-HbC crystals will melt when HbC cells approach the microcirculation in which P_{O_2} is low.

Pathophysiology of Hemoglobin SC Disease

Why is SC a "Disease"? Individuals who are compound heterozygotes for HbS and HbC have a disorder with clinical manifestations that are very similar to those of SS disease, though less severe. A critical question is why SC patients have significant morbidity whereas individuals with sickle trait have virtually no significant pathology. Three explanations have been proffered:

1. HbC enhances the polymerization of HbS (like HbO Arab, see later). Indeed, early in vitro studies suggested that this might be the case.[215-217] However rigorous mixing experiments of deoxygenated solutions of pure HbS and HbC under carefully controlled solvent conditions showed that the polymerization was identical to comparable mixtures of HbS and HbA.[218,219] Thus there must be another explanation for why HbSC is a disease whereas sickle trait is not.

2. The higher intracellular Hb concentration in SC red cells than in AS red cells leads to enhanced polymerization. As stressed in Chapter 19, the rate of polymerization of sickle Hb is exquisitely dependent on the intracellular Hb concentration. It has long been appreciated that SC red cells have a higher MCHC than AS red cells do. More recent studies of SC and CC cells by density gradients revealed that the presence of HbC results in dehydration, thus making red cells denser.[210,218]

3. SC red cell contain a higher proportion of HbS than HbAS red cells do. Patients with HbSC disease generally have about 50% HbS and 50% HbA. In contrast, individuals with sickle trait have about 35% to 40% HbS and 60% to 65% HbA. The higher amount of HbS in SC red cells can be explained by the importance of electrostatic attraction in the assembly of Hb tetramers within the developing red cell (see earlier, Assembly of Mutant Hemoglobins).[89] In AS cells, positively charged α subunits have a substantially higher rate of combination with $β^A$ subunits that have a strong negative charge than they do with $β^S$ subunits, which have a weaker negative charge. In contrast, in SC red cells the positively charged α subunits bind more readily to $β^S$ subunits than to $β^C$ subunits, which have an even weaker negative charge.[91]

Careful quantitative assessment of the second and third contributors, the intracellular Hb concentration and the fraction of HbS, indicated that they each contribute about equally to HbS polymerization and to the pathogenesis of HbSC disease.[218]

Cellular Factors Accounting for the Pathophysiology and Severity of SC Disease. Rarely, crystals may be observed in Wright- and vital dye–stained smears and in wet preparations from fingerstick blood samples.[210] When α-thalassemia is present with SC disease, the typical crystals are absent. The red cells of all patients with SC disease exhibit heavily stained conglomerations of Hb that appear marginated with rounded edges as opposed to the straight-edged crystals. Such cells have been called "billiard ball" cells. Both crystals and billiard ball cells are found in the densest fraction of cells from individuals with SC disease and represent aggregation of Hb distinct from the polymerization of HbS. An enlarged, infarcted, and perhaps abnormally functioning spleen might fail intermittently in its pitting function and thus allow Hb crystals and aggregates to remain in the cell.

Regardless of the α-globin gene haplotype, the blood of patients with SC disease has additional abnormally shaped cells that are strikingly apparent on scanning electron microscopic examination. Typical are "folded cells," some of which have a single fold and resemble—to the gastronomically inclined—pita bread or a taco. These are most likely the cells that Diggs called "fat cells" because in Wright-stained smears they appear as wide bipointed cells. Other misshapen cells are triconcave triangular cells with three dimples, very much like those seen in acute alcoholism that Bessis termed "knizocytes." One remarkable shape was the "triple-folded cells" that appeared as two pita breads stuck together. These bizarre shapes are the product of an increased surface-to-volume ratio, which provides an excess of surface for the cytosol volume. Excessive surface is resolved largely by membrane folding.

Cation Content. The cation content of SC disease red cells is intermediate between that of normal and that of CC disease cells.[211] Oxygenated SC disease cells exhibit a volume-stimulated potassium efflux similar to that observed in sickle cell anemia and CC disease.[211] This transporter appears to be chloride dependent and stimulated by *N*-ethylmaleimide[220]; it is found in the young cells of normal control subjects and individuals with sickle cell anemia and SC disease. It is inhibited by deoxygenation through modulation of cytosolic magnesium (Mg^{2+}).[221-223]

SC disease cells also exhibit a diminished change in cell volume in response to variations in the osmolarity of the suspending medium, which is likely to be due to the volume-regulated potassium efflux. Volume-regulated K^+ efflux should have an adverse impact on the pathophysiology of disease because any increase in MCHC will aggravate HbS polymerization.

Correction of SC Disease. SC disease cells share the increased red cell density characteristics of all cells containing HbC. Because of the increased MCHC, the intracellular HbS concentration is raised to a level at which polymerization occurs under physiologic conditions. Reducing the MCHC in individuals with SC disease to normal levels of 33 g/dL by osmotically swelling SC cells results in normalization of many of the polymerization-dependent abnormal properties of these cells[206]: increased Hb-oxygen affinity (reduced in SC disease), a reduction in the viscosity of deoxygenated erythrocyte suspensions (increased in SC disease), a decrease in the rate of sickling (similar to that in sickle cell anemia), and a reduction in the deoxygenation-induced K^+ leak (greater than that observed in sickle cell anemia). At an osmolarity of 240 mOsm/L, SC cells become biconcave discs. This is a welcome feature of the rehydration of SC disease cells

because the discoid shape is indispensable for normal deformation of red cells in the microcirculation.

Better knowledge of the transport physiology and genetics of red cells could reveal interventions that can cure SC disease by changing the hydration status of SC cells.[224]

Hemoglobins O Arab, S Oman, and S

HbO Arab (β121 [GH4] Glu→Lys) is of special interest because double heterozygotes for HbS and HbO Arab have significant hemolytic anemia and red cells denser than normal, with some as dense as the densest cells found in sickle cell anemia. As with HbD Los Angeles (D Punjab) (β121 [GH4] Glu→Gln), HbO Arab copolymerizes with HbS, and as a result, compound heterozygotes have clinical manifestations similar to those of HbS disease. HbO Arab, having the same charge as HbC, is more strongly bound than HbS and is even more tightly membrane bound than HbC.[225] This suggests that both electrostatic charge and the protein conformation in the vicinity of the charged groups play a role in membrane binding.

All red cells from patients homozygous for HbO Arab were denser than normal red cells, as is observed for patients homozygous for HbC, and red cell density was strongly influenced by the presence of α-thalassemia, which resulted in an average red cell density slightly greater than that of normal (HbAA) red cells. Patients heterozygous for HbO Arab but without α-thalassemia had denser red cells, similar to those seen in patients with sickle cell disease, with some cells of normal density but with most cells being very dense.

Reticulocytes in patients homozygous for HbO Arab were found in the densest density fraction. Cation transport in patients homozygous for HbO Arab is abnormal, with enhanced K^+-Cl^- cotransport activity leading to red cell dehydration. The similarity of the charge and consequences of the presence of both HbC and HbO Arab, which are the products of mutations at opposite ends of the β chain, raises the possibility that this pathologic change is the result of a charge-dependent interaction of these Hbs with the red cell membrane or its cytoskeleton and that this abnormality is present early in red cell development.[77]

HbS Oman has two mutations in the β chains. In addition to the classic β^S mutation, it contains a second mutation in the same chain (β121 [GH4] Glu→Lys) that is identical to the HbO Arab mutation. An informative pedigree of heterozygous carriers of HbS Oman segregates into two types of patients: those expressing about 20% HbS Oman and concomitant −α/α α-thalassemia and those with about 14% HbS Oman and concomitant −α/−α α-thalassemia.[225] Higher expressors of HbS Oman have a sickle cell anemia clinical syndrome of moderate intensity, whereas lower expressors have no clinical syndrome. In addition, higher expressors exhibit a unique form of irreversibly sickled cells shaped like a "yarn and knitting needle," in addition to folded and target cells. The C_{SAT} (solubility of the polymer) of HbS Oman is identical to that of HbS Antilles, another supersickling Hb whose carriers express the abnormal Hb at 40% to 50%, with a clinical picture very similar to that of HbS Oman. Because the level of expression is so different and the clinical picture is so similar and on the basis of C_{SAT} values of the hemolysates, it was concluded that HbS Oman produces pathologic changes beyond its sickling tendencies. There is increased association of HbS Oman with the red blood cell membrane, the presence of dense cells by isopyknic gradients, the presence of folded cells, and accelerated K^+-Cl^- cotransport in red cells expressing more than 20% HbS Oman. Hence, the pathologic effect of heterozygous HbS Oman is the product of the sickling properties of the Val-β6 mutation, which are enhanced by the second mutation at β121, in addition to further enhancement by a hemolytic anemia induced by the mutation at β121. It is likely that the additional hemolysis results from the abnormal association of the highly positively charged HbS Oman (three charges different from normal Hb) with the red cell membrane.

REFERENCES

1. Whitaker TL, Berry MB, Ho EL, et al. The D-helix in myoglobin and in the beta subunit of hemoglobin is required for the retention of heme. Biochemistry. 1995;34: 8221-8226.
2. Komiyama NH, Shih DT, Looker D, et al. Was the loss of the D helix in α-globin a functionally neutral mutation? Nature. 1991;352:349-351.
3. Perutz MF, Rossman MG, Cullis AF, et al. Structure of haemoglobin: a three-dimensional Fourier synthesis at 5.5 Å resolution, obtained by x-ray analysis. Nature. 1960; 185:416.
4. Baldwin JM. The structure of human carbonmonoxy haemoglobin at 2.7 Å resolution. J Mol Biol. 1980;136:103-128.
5. Fermi G, Perutz MF, Shaanan B, Fourme R. The crystal structure of human deoxyhaemoglobin at 1.7 Å resolution. J Mol Biol. 1984;175:159-174.
6. Chothia C, Wodak S, Janin J. Role of subunit interfaces in the allosteric mechanism of hemoglobin. Proc Natl Acad Sci U S A. 1976;73:3793-3797.
7. Monod J, Wyman J, Changeaux JP. On the nature of allosteric transition: a plausible model. J Mol Biol. 1967; 12:88.
8. Perutz MF, Sanders JKM, Chenery DH, et al. Interactions between the quaternary structure of the globin and the spin state of the heme in ferric mixed spin derivatives of hemoglobin. Biochemistry. 1978;17:3640-3652.
9. Perutz MF, Kilmartin JV, Nagai K, et al. Influence of globin structures on the state of the heme: ferrous low spin derivatives. Biochemistry. 1976;15:378-387.
10. Baldwin J, Chothia C. Haemoglobin: the structural changes related to ligand binding and its allosteric mechanism. J Mol Biol. 1979;129:175-220.
11. Perutz MF, Wilkinson AJ, Paoli M, Dodson GG. The stereochemical mechanism of the cooperative effects in

12. Eaton WA, Henry ER, Hofrichter J, et al. Is cooperative oxygen binding by hemoglobin really understood? Nat Struct Biol. 1999;351-358.
13. Henry ER, Jones CM, Hofrichter J, et al. Can a two-state MWC allosteric model explain hemoglobin kinetics? Biochemistry. 1997;3:6511-6528.
14. Perutz MF. Stereochemistry of the cooperative effects in haemoglobin. Nature. 1970;288:726-739.
15. Perutz MF, Gronenbom AM, Clore GM, et al. The pK_a values of two histidine residues in human haemoglobin, the Bohr effect, and the dipole moments of α-helices. J Mol Biol. 1985;183:491-498.
16. Perutz MF. Molecular anatomy and physiology of hemoglobin. In Steinberg MH, Forget BG, Higgs, Nagel RL (eds). Disorders of Hemoglobin: Genetics, Pathophysiology, Clinical Management. New York, Cambridge University Press, 2000.
17. Kilmartin JV, Fogg JH, Perutz MF. Role of C-terminal histidine in the alkaline Bohr effect of human hemoglobin. Biochemistry. 1980;19:3189-3183.
18. Russu IM, Ho NT, Ho C. Role of the β146 histidyl residue in the alkaline Bohr effect of hemoglobin. Biochemistry. 1980;19:1043-1052.
19. Fang TY, Zou M, Simplaceanu V, et al. Assessment of roles of surface histidyl residues in the molecular basis of the Bohr effect and of β143 histidine in the binding of 2,3-bisphosphoglycerate in human normal adult hemoglobin. Biochemistry. 1999;38:13423-13432.
20. Perrella M, Kilmartin JV, Fogg J, Rossi-Bernardi L. Identification of the high and low affinity CO_2 binding sites of human haemoglobin. Nature. 1975;256:759-761.
21. Benesch R, Benesch RE. The effect of organic phosphates from the human erythrocyte on the allosteric properties of hemoglobin. Biochem Biophys Res Commun. 1967; 26:162-167.
22. Chanutin A, Curnish RR. Effect of organic and inorganic phosphates on the oxygen equilibrium of human erythrocytes. Arch Biochem Biophys. 1967;121:96-102.
23. Bunn HF, Briehl RW. The interaction of 2,3-diphosphoglycerate with various human hemoglobins. J Clin Invest. 1970;49:1088-1095.
24. Arnone A. X-ray diffraction study of binding of 2,3-diphosphoglycerate to human deoxyhaemoglobin. Nature. 1972;237:146-149.
25. Rose ZB. The enzymology of 2,3-bisphosphoglycerate. Adv Enzymol Relat Areas Mol Biol. 1980;51:211-253.
26. Card R, Brain M. The "anemia" of childhood. N Engl J Med. 1973;288:388-392.
27. Purcell Y, Brozovic B. Red cell 2,3-diphosphoglycerate concentration in man decreases with age. Nature. 1974;251:511-512.
28. Jia L, Bonaventura C, Bonaventura J, Stamler JS. S-Nitrosohaemoglobin: a dynamic activity of blood involved in vascular control. Nature. 1996;380:221-226.
29. Stamler JS, Jia L, Eu JP, et al. Blood flow regulation by S-nitrosohemoglobin in the physiological oxygen gradient. Science. 1997;276:2034-2037.
30. Gow AJ, Stamler JS. Reactions between nitric oxide and haemoglobin under physiological conditions. Nature. 1998;391:169-173.

31. Singel DJ, Stamler JS. Chemical physiology of blood flow regulation by red blood cells: the role of nitric oxide and S-nitrosohemoglobin. Annu Rev Physiol. 2005;67:99-145.

32. Pabloski JR, Hess DT, Stamler JS. Export by red blood cells of nitric oxide bioactivity. Nature. 2001;409:622-626.

33. Isbell TS, Sun CW, Wu LC, et al. SNO-hemoglobin not essential for red blood cell dependent hypoxic vasodilation. Nat Med. 2008;14:773-777.

34. Yonetani T. Nitric oxide and hemoglobin. Nippon Yakurigaku Zasshi. 1998;112:155-160.

35. Kim-Shapiro DB, Gladwin MT, Patel RP, Hogg N. The reaction between nitrite and hemoglobin: the role of nitrite in hemoglobin-mediated hypoxic vasodilation. J Inorg Biochem. 2005;99:237-246.

36. Gladwin MT, Shelhamer JH, Schechter AN, et al. Role of circulating nitrite and S-nitrosohemoglobin in the regulation of regional blood flow in humans. Proc Natl Acad Sci U S A. 2000;97:11482-11487.

37. Cosby K, Partovi KS, Crawford JH, et al. Nitrite reduction to nitric oxide by deoxyhemoglobin vasodilates the human circulation. Nat Med. 2003;9:1498-1505.

38. Huang Z, Shiva S, Kim-Shapiro DB, et al. Enzymatic function of hemoglobin as a nitrite reductase that produces NO under allosteric control. J Clin Invest. 2005;115:2099-2107.

39. Rother RP, Bell L, Hillmen P, Gladwin MT. The clinical sequelae of intravascular hemolysis and extracellular plasma hemoglobin: a novel mechanism of human disease. JAMA. 2005;293:1653-1662.

40. Kato GJ, McGowan V, Machado RF, et al. Lactate dehydrogenase as a biomarker of hemolysis-associated nitric oxide resistance, priapism, leg ulceration, pulmonary hypertension, and death in patients with sickle cell disease. Blood. 2006;107:2279-2285.

41. Nolan VG, Adewoye A, Baldwin C, et al. Sickle cell leg ulcers: associations with haemolysis and SNPs in Klotho, TEK and genes of the TGF-beta/BMP pathway. Br J Haematol. 2006;133:570-578.

42. Korber E. Inaugural dissertation: uber Differenzen des Blutfarbstoffes. Dorpat, 1866.

43. Schroeder WA, Shelton JR, Shelton JB, et al. The amino acid sequence of the α-chain of human fetal hemoglobin. Biochemistry. 1963;2:992-1008.

44. Schroeder WA, Huisman THJ, Efremov GD, et al. Further studies on the frequency and significance of the Tα-chain of human fetal hemoglobin. J Clin Invest. 1979;63:268-275.

45. Slightom JL, Blechl AE, Smithies O. Human fetal $^Gγ$- and $^Aγ$-globin genes: complete nucleotide sequences suggest that DNA can be exchanged between these duplicated genes. Cell. 1980;21:627-638.

46. Bouhassira EE, Lachman H, Krishnamoorthy R, et al. A gene conversion located 5′ to the $^Aγ$ gene is in linkage disequilibrium with the Bantu haplotype in sickle cell anemia. J Clin Invest. 1989;83:2070-2073.

47. Frier JA, Perutz M. Structure of human foetal deoxyhemoglobin. J Mol Biol. 1977;112:97-112.

48. Allen DW, Wyman J, Smith CA. The oxygen equilibrium of foetal and adult human hemoglobin. J Biol Chem. 1953;203:81-87.

49. Tyuma I, Shamizu K. Different response to organic phosphates of human fetal and adult hemoglobins. Arch Biochem Biophys. 1969;129:404-405.

50. Poyart C, Burseaux E, Guesnon P, Teisseire B. Chloride binding and Bohr effect of human fetal erythrocytes and HbFII solutions. Pfluegers Arch. 1978;37:169-175.

51. Gros G, Bauer C. High pK value of the N-terminal amino group of the γ chains causes low CO_2 binding of human fetal hemoglobin. Biochem Biophys Res Commun. 1978;80:56-62.

52. Bursaux E, Poyart C, Guesnon P, Teisseire B. Comparative effects of CO_2 on the affinity for O_2 of fetal and adult hemoglobins. Pfluegers Arch. 1979;378:197-203.

53. Charache S, Catalano P, Burns S, et al. Pregnancy in carriers of high-affinity hemoglobins. Blood. 1985;65:713-718.

54. Boissel JP, Kasper T, Bunn HF. Cotranslational N-terminal processing of cytosolic proteins: cell free expression of site-directed mutants of human hemoglobin. J Biol Chem. 1988;263:8443-8449.

55. Bunn HF. Differences in the interaction of 2,3-diphosphoglycerate with certain mammalian hemoglobins. Science. 1971;172:1049-1050.

56. Kleihauer E, Braun H, Betke K. Demonstration of fetal hemoglobin in erythrocytes of a blood smear. Klin Wochenschr. 1957;35:637-638.

57. Dover GJ, Boyer SH, Bell WR. Microscopic method for assaying F cell production: illustrative changes during infancy and in aplastic anemia. Blood. 1978;52:664-672.

58. Dover GJ, Boyer SH, Pembrey ME. F cell production in sickle cell anemia: regulation by genes linked to β-hemoglobin locus. Science. 1981;211:1441-1444.

59. Dover GJ, Boyer SH, Charache S, Heintzelman K. Individual variation in the production and survival of F-cells in sickle cell disease. N Engl J Med. 1978;299:1428-1435.

60. Winter WP, Seale WR, Yodh J. Interaction of hemoglobin S with anionic polysaccharides. Am J Pediatr Hematol Oncol. 1984;6:77-81.

61. Pembrey ME, Weatherall DJ, Clegg JB. Maternal synthesis of haemoglobin F in pregnancy. Lancet. 1973;16:1351-1354.

62. Wood WG, Stamatoyannopoulos G, Lim G, Nute PE. F-cells in the adult: normal values and levels in individuals with hereditary and acquired elevations of Hb F. Blood. 1975;46:671-682.

63. Boyer SH, Belding TK, Margolet L, et al. Variations in the frequency of fetal hemoglobin–bearing erythrocytes (F-cells) in well adults, pregnant women, and adult leukemics. Johns Hopkins Med J. 1975;137:105-115.

64. Newman DR, Pierre RV, Linman JW. Studies on the diagnostic significance of hemoglobin F levels. Mayo Clin Proc. 1973;48:199-202.

65. Lee-Potter JP, Deacon-Smith RA, Simpkiss MJ, et al. A new cause of haemolytic anemia in the newborn: a description of an unstable fetal haemoglobin—F Poole $α_2$$^Gγ_2$ 130 tryptophan→glycine. J Clin Pathol. 1975;28:317-320.

66. Hayashi A, Fujita T, Fujimura M, Titani K. A new abnormal fetal hemoglobin, Hb FM-Osaka (alpha 2 gamma 2 63His replaced by Tyr). Hemoglobin. 1980;4:447-448.

67. Priest JR, Watterson J, Jones RT, et al. Mutant fetal hemoglobin causing cyanosis in a newborn. Pediatrics. 1989;83:734-736.

68. Glader BE. Hemoglobin FM-Fort Ripley: another lesson from the neonate. Pediatrics. 1989;83:792-793.

69. Harano T, Harano K, Doi K, et al. HbF-Onoda or $\alpha_2\gamma_2$G146(HC3) His→Tyr, a newly discovered fetal hemoglobin variant in a Japanese newborn. Hemoglobin. 1990;14:217-222.

70. Fischer S, Nagel RL, Bookchin RM, et al. The binding of hemoglobin to membranes of normal and sickle erythrocytes. Biochim Biophys Acta. 1975;375:422-433.

71. Codrington JF, Kutlar F, Harris HF, et al. Hb A_2-Wrens or $\alpha_2\gamma_2$G 98(FG5) Val→Met, an unstable chain variant identified by sequence analysis of amplified DNA. Biochim Biophys Acta. 1989;1009:87-89.

72. Garcia CR, Navarro JL, Lam H, et al. Hb A_2-Manzanares or $\alpha_2\gamma_2$G 121(GH4) Glu→Val, an unstable chain variant observed in a Spanish family. Hemoglobin. 1983;7:435-442.

73. Salkie ML, Gordon PA, Rigal WM, et al. Hb A_2-Canada or $\alpha_2\gamma_2$G 99(G1) Asp→Asn: a newly discovered chain variant with increased oxygen affinity occurring in *cis* to β-thalassemia. Hemoglobin. 1982;6:223-231.

74. Baglioni C. The fusion of two peptide chains in hemoglobin Lepore and its interpretation as a genetic deletion. Proc Natl Acad Sci U S A. 1962;48:1880-1886.

75. Flavell RA, Kooter JM, De Boer E, et al. Analysis of the β-δ-globin gene loci in normal and Hb Lepore DNA: direct determination of gene linkage and intergene distance. Cell. 1987;15:25-41.

76. Mears JG, Ramirez F, Leibowitz D, et al. Organization of human δ- and β-globin genes in cellular DNA and the presence of intragenic inserts. Cell. 1978;15:15-23.

77. Bunn HF. Subunit assembly of hemoglobin: an important determinant of hematologic phenotype. Blood. 1987;69:1-6.

78. Huehns ER, Dance N, Beaven GH, et al. Human embryonic hemoglobins. Cold Spring Harbor Symp Quant Biol. 1964;19:327-331.

79. Luo HY, Liang XL, Frye C, et al. Embryonic hemoglobins are expressed in definitive cells. Blood. 1999;94:359-361.

80. Stamatoyannopoulos G, Constantoulakis P, Brice M, et al. Coexpression of embryonic, fetal, and adult globins in erythroid cells of human embryos: relevance to the cell-lineage models of globin switching. Dev Biol. 1987;123:191-197.

81. Leder A, Kuo A, Shen MM, et al. In situ hybridization reveals co-expression of embryonic and adult α globin genes in the earliest murine erythrocyte progenitors. Development. 1992;116:1041-1049.

82. Hoffmann OM, Brittain T, Wells RM. The control of oxygen affinity in the three human embryonic haemoglobins by respiration linked metabolites. Biochem Mol Biol Int. 1997;42:553-566.

83. Hoffmann OM, Brittain T. Ligand binding kinetics and dissociation of the human embryonic haemoglobins. Biochem J. 1996;315:65-70.

84. Hoffman O, Currucan G, Robson N, et al. The chloride effect in the human embryonic haemoglobins. Biochem J. 1995;309:959-962.

85. Sutherland-Smith AJ, Baker HM, Hoffmann OM, et al. Crystal structure of human embryonic haemoglobin: the carbonmonoxide for Gower II ($\alpha_2\epsilon_2$) haemoglobin at 2.9 Å resolution. J Mol Biol. 1998;280:475-484.

86. He Z, Russell JE. Expression, purification, and characterization of human hemoglobins Gower-1 ($\zeta_2\epsilon_2$), Gower-2 ($\alpha_2\epsilon_2$), and Portland-2 ($\zeta_2\beta_2$) assembled in complex transgenic-knockout mice. Blood. 2001;97:1099-1105.

87. Ireland JH, Luo HY, Chui DH, et al. Detection of the (−SEA) double α-globin gene deletion by a simple immunologic assay for embryonic ζ-globin chains. Am J Hematol. 1993;44:22-28.

88. Bunn HF, McDonald MJ. Electrostatic interactions in the assembly of haemoglobin. Nature. 1983;306:498-500.

89. Mrabet NT, McDonald MJ, Turci S, et al. Electrostatic attraction governs the dimer assembly of human hemoglobin. J Biol Chem. 1986;261:5222-5228.

90. Huisman TH. Percentages of abnormal hemoglobins in adults with a heterozygosity for an alpha chain and/or a beta chain variant. Am J Hematol. 1983;14:393-404.

91. Adachi K, Yamaguchi T, Pang J, Surrey S. Effects of increased anionic charge in the β-globin chain on the assembly of human hemoglobin in vitro. Blood. 1998;91:1438-1445.

92. Adams JD, Coleman MB, Hayes J, et al. Modulation of fetal hemoglobin synthesis by iron deficiency. N Engl J Med. 1985;313:1402-1405.

93. Chui DH, Patterson M, Dowling CE, et al. Hemoglobin Bart's disease in an Italian boy. Interaction between alpha-thalassemia and hereditary persistence of fetal hemoglobin. N Engl J Med. 1990;323:179-182.

94. Wajcman H, Galacteros F. Hemoglobins with high oxygen affinity leading to erythrocytosis. New variants and new concepts. Hemoglobin. 2005;29:91-106.

95. Olson JS, Gibson QH. The functional properties of hemoglobin Bethesda ($\alpha_2\beta_2^{145His}$). J Biol Chem. 1972;247:3662-3670.

96. Bunn HF, Wohl RC, Bradley TB, et al. Functional properties of hemoglobin Kempsey. J Biol Chem. 1974;249:7402-7409.

97. Nute PE, Stamatoyannopoulos G, Hermodson MA, et al. Hemoglobinopathic erythrocytosis due to a new electrophoretically silent variant, hemoglobin San Diego (β 109 [Gil] Val→Met). J Clin Invest. 1974;53:320.

98. Maniatis A, Bousios T, Nagel RL, et al. Hemoglobin Crete (β 129 Ala→Pro): a new high-affinity variant interacting with β^0- and delta β^0-thalassemia. Blood. 1979;54:54.

99. Tondo C, Bonaventura J, Bonaventura C, et al. Functional properties of hemoglobin Porto Alegre ($\alpha_2\beta_2$ 9 Ser→Cys) and the reactivity of its extra cysteinyl residue. Biochim Biophys Acta. 1974;342:15-20.

100. Bonaventura J, Riggs A. Polymerization of hemoglobins of mouse and man: structural basis. Science. 1967;158:800-802.

101. Bonaventura J, Bonaventura C, Sullivan B, et al. Hemoglobin providence. Functional consequences of two alterations of the 2,3-diphosphoglycerate binding site at position beta 82. J Biol Chem. 1976;251:7563-7571.

102. Elder GE, Lappin TR, Horne AB, et al. Hemoglobin Old Dominion/Burton-upon-Trent, β 143 (H21) His→Tyr, codon 143 CAC→TAC—a variant with altered oxygen affinity that compromises measurement of glycated hemo-

globin in diabetes mellitus: Structure, function, and DNA sequence. Mayo Clin Proc. 1998;73:321-328.

103. Charache S, Weatherall DJ, Clegg JB. Polycythemia associated with a hemoglobinopathy. J Clin Invest. 1966;45:813-822.

104. Rosa R, Prehu MO, Beuzard Y, Rosa J. The first case of a complete deficiency of diphosphoglycerate mutase in human erythrocytes. J Clin Invest. 1978;62:907-915.

105. Kales SN. Carbon monoxide intoxication. Am Fam Physician. 1993;48:1100-1104.

106. Adamson JW. Familial polycythemia. Semin Hematol. 1975;12:383-396.

107. Semenza GL. Life with oxygen. Science. 2007;318:62-64.

108. Ang SO, Chen H, Hirota K, et al. Disruption of oxygen homeostasis underlies congenital Chuvash polycythemia. Nat Genet. 2002;32:614-621.

109. Percy MJ, Zhao Q, Flores A, et al. A family with erythrocytosis establishes a role for prolyl hydroxylase domain protein 2 in oxygen homeostasis. Proc Natl Acad Sci U S A. 2006;103:654-659.

110. Percy MJ, Furlow PW, Beer PA, et al. A novel erythrocytosis-associated PHD2 mutation suggests the location of a HIF binding groove. Blood. 2007;110:2193-2196.

111. Percy MJ, Furlow PW, Lucas GS, et al. A gain-of-function mutation in the HIF2A gene in familial erythrocytosis. N Engl J Med. 2008;358:162-168.

112. Percy M, Beer P, Campbell G, et al. A mutational hot spot in the HIF2A gene associated with erythrocytosis. Blood. 2008;111:5400-5402.

113. Grace RJ, Gover PA, Treacher DF, et al. Venesection in haemoglobin Yakima, a high oxygen affinity haemoglobin. Clin Lab Haematol. 1992;14:195-199.

114. Adamson JW, Finch CA. Erythropoietin and the polycythemias. Ann N Y Acad Sci. 1968;149:560-563.

115. Adamson JW, Hayashi A, Stamatoyannopoulos G, Burger WF. Erythrocyte function and marrow regulation in hemoglobin Bethesda (β 145 histidine). J Clin Invest. 1972;51:2883-2888.

116. Adamson JW, Finch CA. Hemoglobin function, oxygen affinity and erythropoietin. Annu Rev Physiol. 1975;37:351-369.

117. Charache S, Achuff S, Winslow R, et al. Variability of the homeostatic response to altered p50. Blood. 1978;52:1156-1162.

118. Butler WM, Spratling L, Kark JA, Schoomaker EB. Hemoglobin Osler: report of a new family with exercise studies before and after phlebotomy. Am J Hematol. 1982;13:293-301.

118a. Hebbel RP, Eaton JW, Kronenberg RS, et al. Human llamas: Adaptation to altitude in subjects with high hemoglobin oxygen affinity. J Clin Invest. 1978;62:593-600.

119. Nagel RL, Lynfield J, Johnson J, et al. Hemoglobin Beth Israel: a mutant causing clinically apparent cyanosis. N Engl J Med. 1976;295:125-130.

120. Blouquit Y, Bardakdjian J, Lena-Russo D, et al. Hb Bruxelles: α₂β₂ 41 or 42(C7 or CD1) Phe deleted. Hemoglobin 1989;13:465-474.

121. Griffon N, Badens C, Lena-Russo D, et al. Hb Bruxelles, deletion of Phe β42, shows a low oxygen affinity and low cooperativity of ligand binding. J Biol Chem. 1996;271:25916-25920.

122. Horlein H, Weber G. Uber chronisch familiare Methamoglobinanue und eine neue Modifikation des Methamoglobins. Dtsch Med Wochenschr. 1948;73:476-478.

123. Gerald DS, Efron ML. Chemical studies of several varieties of Hb M. Proc Natl Acad Sci U S A. 1961;47:1758-1767.

124. Shibata S, Tanuira A, Iuchi I. Hemoglobin M1 demonstration of a new abnormal hemoglobin in hereditary nigremia. Acta Haematol Jpn. 1960;23:96-105.

125. Greer J. Three dimension studies of abnormal human hemoglobins M Hyde Park and M Iwate. J Mol Biol. 1971;59:107-126.

126. Ranney HM, Nagel RL, Heller P, et al. Oxygen equilibrium of hemoglobin M-Hyde Park. Biochim Biophys Acta. 1968;160:112-115.

127. Brennan SO, Matthews JR. Hb Auckland [β87(F8) His→Asn]: a new mutation of the proximal histidine identified by electrospray mass spectrometry. Hemoglobin. 1997;21:393-403.

128. Feher G, Isaacson RA, Scholes CP. Endor studies on normal and abnormal hemoglobins. Ann N Y Acad Sci. 1973;222:86-101.

129. Peisach J, Gersonde K. Binding of CO to mutant chains of HbM Iwate: evidence for distal imidazole ligation. Biochemistry. 1977;16:2539-2545.

130. La Mar GR, Nagai K, Jue T, et al. Assignment of proximal histidyl imidazole exchangeable proton NMR resonances to individual subunits in HbA, Boston, Iwate and Milwaukee. Biochem Biophys Res Commun. 1980;96:1172-1177.

131. Pulsinelli PD, Perutz MF, Nagel RL. Structure of hemoglobin M Boston, a variant with a five-coordinated ferric heme. Proc Natl Acad Sci U S A. 1973;70:3870-3874.

132. Perutz MF, Pulsinelli PD, Ranney HM. Structure and subunit interaction of haemoglobin M Milwaukee. Nat New Biol. 1972;237:259-263.

133. Lindstrom TR, Ho C, Pisciotta AV. Nuclear magnetic resonance studies of haemoglobin M Milwaukee. Nat New Biol. 1972;237:263-264.

134. Thillet J, Cohen-Solal M, Seligmann M, Rosa J. Functional and physiochemical studies of hemoglobin St. Louis β 28 (B10) Leu→Gln. J Clin Invest. 1976;58:1098-1106.

135. Wajcman H, Krishnamoorthy R, Gacon G, et al. A new hemoglobin variant involving the distal histidine: Hb Bicetre (β63 (E7) His→Pro). J Mol Med. 1976;1:187.

136. Rosa J, Labie D, Wajcman H, et al. Haemoglobin I Toulouse: β66 (E10) Lys→Glu: a new abnormal haemoglobin with a mutation localized on the E10 porphyrin surrounding zones. Nature. 1969;223:190-191.

137. Kurachi S, Hermodson M, Hornung S, Stamatoyannopoulos G. Structure of haemoglobin Seattle. Nat New Biol. 1973;243:275-276.

138. Shibata S, Mijaji T, Iuchi I. Methemoglobin M's of the Japanese. Bull Yamaguchi Med Sch. 1967;14:141-147.

139. Shibata S. Hemoglobinopathies in Japan. Hemoglobin. 1981;5:509-515.

140. Hayashi A, Suzuki T, Shimizu A, Yamamura Y. Properties of hemoglobin M: unequivalent nature of the α and β subunits in the hemoglobin molecule. Biochim Biophys Acta. 1968;168:262-273.

141. Ranney HM, Nagel RL, Heller P, Udem L. Oxygen equilibrium of hemoglobin M (Hyde Park). Biochim Biophys Acta. 1968;160:112-115.

142. Suzuki T, Hayashi A, Shimizu A, Yamamura Y. The oxygen equilibrium of hemoglobin M Saskatoon. Biochim Biophys Acta. 1966;127:280-282.

143. Suzuki T, Hayashi A, Yamamura Y, et al. Functional abnormality of hemoglobin M. Biochem Biophys Res Commun. 1965;19:691-695.

144. Udem L, Ranney HM, Bunn HF, Pisciotta A. Some observations on the properties of hemoglobin M Milwaukee-1. J Mol Biol. 1970;48:489-498.

145. Hayashi A, Suzuki T, Imai K, et al. Properties of hemoglobin M Milwaukee I variant and its unique characteristics. Biochem Biophys Acta. 1969;194:6-15.

146. Nagel RL, Bookchin RM. Human hemoglobin mutants with abnormal oxygen binding. Semin Hematol. 1974;11:385-403.

147. Moo-Penn WF, Bechtel KC, Schmidt RM, et al. Hemoglobin Raleigh (β1 valine→acetylamine). Biochemistry. 1977;16:4872-4879.

148. Park CM, Nagel RL. Sulfhemoglobin: clinical and molecular aspects. N Engl J Med. 1984;310:1579-1584.

149. Cathie AB. Apparent idiopathic Heinz body anemia. Great Ormond St J. 1952;3:43-47.

150. Virshup DM, Zinkham WH, Sirota RL, Caughey WS. Unique sensitivity of Hb Zurich to oxidative injury by phenazopyridine: reversal of the effects by elevating carboxyhemoglobin in vivo and in vitro. Am J Hematol. 1983;14:315-324.

151. Moo-Penn WF, Jue DL, Johnson MH, et al. Hemoglobin Brockton [β 138 (H16) Ala→Pro]: an unstable variant near the C-terminus of the β-subunits with normal oxygen-binding properties. Biochemistry. 1988;27:7614-7619.

152. Reider RF, Oski FA, Clegg JB. Hemoglobin Philly (β35 tyrosine→phenylalanine): studies in the molecular pathology of hemoglobin. J Clin Invest. 1969;48:1627-1642.

153. King MAR, Wiltshire BG, Lehmann H, Morimoto H. An unstable haemoglobin with reduced oxygen affinity: haemoglobin Peterborough, β111 (G13) valine→phenylalanine, its interaction with normal haemoglobin and with haemoglobin Lepore. Br J Haematol. 1972;22:125-134.

154. Como PF, Wylie BR, Trent RJ, et al. A new unstable and low oxygen affinity hemoglobin variant: Hb Stanmore [β111(G13) Val→Ala]. Hemoglobin. 1991;15:53-65.

155. Martinez G, Lima F, Colombo B. Haemoglobin J Guantanamo (α2β2 128 (H6) Ala→Asp). A new fast unstable haemoglobin found in a Cuban family. Biochim Biophys Acta. 1977;491:1-6.

156. Clegg JB, Weatherall DJ, Boon WH, Mustafa D. Two new haemoglobin variants involving proline substitutions. Nature. 1969;22:379-380.

157. Ohba Y. Unstable hemoglobins. Hemoglobin. 1990;14:353-388.

158. Ohba Y, Yamamoto K, Hattori Y, et al. Hyperunstable hemoglobin Toyama α2136 (H19) Leu→Arg β2: Detection and identification by in vitro biosynthesis with radioactive amino acids. Hemoglobin. 1987;11:539-556.

159. Tatsis B, Dosik H, Rieder R, et al. Hemoglobin Hasharon: severe hemolytic anemia and hypersplenism associated with a mildly unstable hemoglobin. Birth Defects Orig Artic Ser. 1972;8:25-32.

160. Levine RL, Lincoln DR, Buchholz WM, et al. Hemoglobin Hasharon in a premature infant with hemolytic anemia. Pediatr Res. 1975;9:7-11.

161. Schmid R, Brecher G, Clemens T. Familial hemolytic anemia with erythrocyte inclusion bodies and a defect in pigment metabolism. Blood. 1959;14:991-1007.

162. Eisinger J, Flores J, Tyson JA, Shohet SB. Fluorescent cytoplasm and Heinz bodies of Köln erythrocytes: evidence for intracellular heme catabolism. Blood. 1985;65:886-893.

163. Rose C, Bauters F, Galacteros F. Hydroxyurea therapy in highly unstable hemoglobin carriers. Blood. 1996;88:2807-2808.

164. Beutler E, Lang A, Lehmann H. Hemoglobin Duarte: (alpha2beta2 62(E6)Ala leads to Pro): a new unstable hemoglobin with increased oxygen affinity. Blood. 1974;43:527-535.

165. Grimes AJ, Meisler A. Possible cause of Heinz bodies in congenital Heinz body anaemia. Nature. 1962;194:190-191.

166. Grimes AJ, Meisler A, Dacie JV. Congenital Heinz-body anaemia: further evidence on the cause of Heinz-body production in red cells. Br J Haematol. 1964;10:281-290.

167. Carrell RW, Kay R. A simple method for the detection of unstable hemoglobins. Br J Haematol. 1972;23:615-619.

168. Carrell RW, Lehmann H. Zinc acetate as a precipitant of unstable haemoglobins. J Clin Pathol. 1981;34:796-799.

169. Asakura T, Adachi K, Shapiro M, et al. Mechanical precipitation of hemoglobin Köln. Biochim Biophys Acta. 1975;412:197-201.

170. Perutz MF, Raidt H. Stereochemical bases of heat stability in bacterial ferredoxins and in hemoglobin A2. Nature. 1975;255:256-259.

171. Argos P, Rossman MG, Grau UM, et al. Thermal stability and protein structure. Biochemistry. 1979;18:5698-5703.

172. Rachmilewitz EA, Peisach J, Blumberg WE. Studies on the stability of oxyhemoglobin A and its constituent chains and their derivatives. J Biol Chem. 1971;246:3356-3366.

173. Argos P, Rossman MG, Grau UM, et al. Thermal stability and protein structure. Biochemistry. 1979;18:5698-5703.

174. Jacob HS, Winterhalter KH. The role of hemoglobin heme loss in Heinz body formation: studies with a partially heme-deficient hemoglobin and with genetically unstable hemoglobin. J Clin Invest. 1970;49:2008-2016.

175. Bunn FH, Jandl JH. Exchange of heme among hemoglobins and between hemoglobin and albumin. J Biol Chem. 1968;243:465-475.

176. Rachmilewitz EA, Harari E. Intermediate hemichrome formation after oxidation of three unstable hemoglobins (Freiburg, Riverdale-Bronx and Koln). Hamatol Bluttransfus. 1972;10:241-250.

177. Rachmilewitz EA, Peisach J, Blumberg WE. Studies on the stability of oxyhemoglobin A and its constituent chains and their derivatives. J Biol Chem. 1971;246:3356-3366.

178. Rachmilewitz EA, White JM. Haemichrome formation during the in vitro oxidation of haemoglobin Köln. Nat New Biol. 1973;241:115-117.

179. Rachmilewitz EA. Denaturation of the normal and abnormal hemoglobin molecule. Semin Hematol. 1974;11:441-462.

180. Peisach J, Blumberg WE, Rachmilewitz EA. The demonstration of ferrihemochrome intermediates in Heinz body formation following the reduction of oxyhemoglobin A by acetylphenylhydrazine. Biochim Biophys Acta. 1975; 393:404-418.

181. Winterbourn CC, Carrell RW. Studies of hemoglobin denaturation and Heinz body formation in the unstable hemoglobins. J Clin Invest. 1974;54:678-689.

182. Winterbourn CC, McGrath BM, Carrell RW. Reactions involving superoxide and normal and unstable haemoglobins. Biochem J. 1976;155:493-502.

183. Rifkind RA. Heinz body anemia: an ultrastructural study. II. Red cell sequestration and destruction. Blood. 1965;26: 433-448.

184. Schnitzer B, Rucknagel DL, Spencer HH, Aikawa M. Erythrocytes: pits and vacuoles as seen with transmission and scanning electron microscopy. Science. 1971;173:251-252.

185. Winterbourn CC, Carrell RW. Characterization of Heinz bodies in unstable haemoglobin haemolytic anaemia. Nature. 1972;240:150-152.

186. Low P. Interaction of native and denatured hemoglobins with band 3: consequences for erythrocyte structure and function. In Agre P, Parker JC (eds). Red Blood Cell Membranes. New York, Marcel Dekker, 1989.

187. Low PS, Westfall MA, Allen DP, Appell KC. Characterization of the reversible conformational equilibrium of the cytoplasmic domain of erythrocyte membrane band 3. J Biol Chem. 1984;259:13070-13076.

188. Waugh SM, Low PS. Hemichrome binding to band 3: nucleation of Heinz bodies on the erythrocyte membrane. Biochemistry. 1985;24:34-39.

189. Walder JA, Chatterjee R, Steck T, et al. The interaction of hemoglobin with the cytoplasmic domain of band 3 of the human erythrocyte membrane. J Biol Chem. 1984;259: 10238-10246.

190. Jandl JH, Simmons RL, Castle WB. Red cell filtration and the pathogenesis of certain hemolytic anemias. Blood. 1961;18:133-148.

191. Miller DR, Weed RI, Stamatoyannopoulos G, Yoshida A. Hemoglobin Köln disease occurring as a fresh mutation: erythrocyte metabolism and survival. Blood. 1971;38: 715-729.

192. Chou AC, Fitch CD. Mechanism of hemolysis induced by ferriprotoporphyrin IX. J Clin Invest. 1981;68:672-677.

193. Allen DW, Burgoyne CF, Groat JD, et al. Comparison of hemoglobin Köln erythrocyte membranes with malondialdehyde-reacted normal erythrocyte membranes. Blood. 1984;64:1263-1269.

194. Flynn TP, Allen DW, Johnson GJ, White JG. Oxidant damage of the lipids and proteins of the erythrocyte membranes in unstable hemoglobin disease: evidence for the role of lipid peroxidation. J Clin Invest. 1983;71:1215-1223.

195. Jacob HS, Brain MK, Dacie JV. Altered sulfhydryl reactivity of hemoglobins and red blood cell membranes in congenital Heinz body hemolytic anemia. J Clin Invest. 1968;47:2664-2677.

196. De Furia FG, Miller DR. Oxygen affinity in hemoglobin Köln disease. Blood. 1972;39:398-406.

197. Kazazian HH Jr, Dowling CE, Hurwitz RL, et al. Dominant thalassemia-like phenotypes associated with mutations in exon 3 of the β-globin gene. Blood. 1992;79: 3014-3018.

198. Thein SL. Dominant β thalassaemia: molecular basis and pathophysiology. Br J. Haematol. 1992;80:273-277.

199. Traeger-Synodinos J, Papassotiriou I, Metaxotou-Mavrommati A, et al. Distinct phenotypic expression associated with a new hyperunstable α globin variant (Hb Heraklion, α₁cd37(C2)Pro>0): Comparison to other α-thalassemic hemoglobinopathies. Blood Cells Mol Dis. 2000;26:276-284.

200. Vasseur-Godbillon C, Marden MC, Giordano P, et al. Impaired binding of AHSP to alpha chain variants: Hb Groene Hart illustrates a mechanism leading to unstable hemoglobins with alpha thalassemic like syndrome. Blood Cells Mol Dis. 2006;37:173-179.

201. Nagel RL, Steinberg MH. HbSC and HbC disease. In Steinberg MH, Forget BG, Higgs DR, Nagel RL (eds). Disorders of Hemoglobin: Genetics, Pathophysiology, Clinical Management. New York, Cambridge University Press, 2001.

202. Modiano D, Luoni G, Sirima BS, et al. Haemoglobin C protects against clinical *Plasmodium falciparum* malaria. Nature. 2001;414:305-308.

203. Haldane JBS. The rate of mutation of human genes. Hereditas. 1949;35(Suppl):267-273.

204. Olson JA, Nagel RL. Synchronized cultures of *P. falciparum* in abnormal red cells: the mechanism of the inhibition of growth in HbCC cells. Blood. 1987;67: 997-1000.

205. Prindle KH Jr, McCurdy PR. Red cell lifespan in hemoglobin C disorders (with special reference to hemoglobin C trait). Blood. 1970;36:14-19.

206. Lawrence C, Fabry ME, Nagel RL. The unique red cell heterogeneity of SC disease: crystal formation, dense reticulocytes, and unusual morphology. Blood. 1991;78: 2104-2112.

207. Hirsch RE, Raventos-Suarez C, Olson JA, et al. Ligand state of intraerythrocytic circulating HbC crystals in homozygote CC patients. Blood. 1985;66:775-777.

208. Nagel RL. Genetically Abnormal Red Cells. Boca Raton, FL, CRC Press, 1988.

209. Hirsch RE, Raventos-Suarez C, Olson JA, Nagel RL. Ligand state of intraerythrocytic circulating HbC crystals in homozygote CC patients. Blood. 1985;66:775-777.

210. Fabry ME, Kaul DK, Raventos C, et al. Some aspects of the pathophysiology of homozygous Hb CC erythrocytes. J Clin Invest. 1981;67:1284-1291.

211. Brugnara C, Kopin AS, Bunn HF, et al. Regulation of cation content and cell volume in hemoglobin erythrocytes from patients with homozygous hemoglobin C disease. J Clin Invest. 1985;75:1608-1617.

212. Reiss GH, Ranney HM, Shaklai N. Association of HbC with erythrocyte ghosts. J Clin Invest. 1982;70:946-952.

213. Ballas SK, Embi K, Goshar D, et al. Binding of β S, β C and β O Arab globins to the erythrocyte membrane. Hemoglobin. 1981;5:501-505.

214. Nagel RL, Krishnamoorthy R, Fattoum S, et al. The erythrocyte effects of haemoglobin O (Arab). Br J. Haematol. 1999;107:516-521.

215. Singer K, Singer L. Studies on abnormal hemoglobins. VIII. The gelling phenomenon of sickle cell hemoglobin: its biologic and diagnostic significance. Blood. 1953;8:1008-1023.

216. Allison AC. Properties of sickle-cell haemoglobin. Biochem J. 1957;65:212-219.

217. Charache S, Conley CL. Rate of sickling of red cells during deoxygenation of blood from persons with various sickling disorders. Blood. 1964;24:25-48.

218. Bunn HF, Noguchi CT, Hofrichter J, et al. Molecular and cellular pathogenesis of hemoglobin SC disease. Proc Natl Acad Sci U S A. 1982;79:7527-7531.

219. Bookchin RM, Balazs T. Ionic strength dependence of the polymer solubilities of deoxyhemoglobin S + C and S + A mixtures. Blood. 1986;67:887-892.

220. Canessa M, Spalvins A, Nagel RL. Volume-dependent and NEM-stimulated K^+,Cl^- transport is elevated in oxygenated SS, SC and CC human red cells. FEBS Lett. 1986;200:197-202.

221. Canessa M, Fabry ME, Blumenfeld N, Nagel RL. Volume-stimulated, Cl-dependent K^+ efflux is highly expressed in young human red cells containing normal hemoglobin or HbS. J Membr Biol. 1987;97:97-105.

222. Canessa M, Fabry ME, Spalvins A, et al. Activation of a K : Cl cotransporter by cell swelling in HbAA and HbSS red cells. Prog Clin Biol Res. 1987;240:201-115.

223. Canessa M, Fabry ME, Nagel FL. Deoxygenation inhibit the volume-stimulated, Cl- dependent K^+ efflux in SS and young AA cells: A cytosolic Mg^{2+} modulation. Blood. 1987;70:1861-1866.

224. Nagel RL, Lawrence C. The distinct pathobiology of sickle cell–hemoglobin C disease. Therapeutic implications. Hematol Oncol Clin North Am. 1991;5:433-551.

225. Nagel RL, Daar S, Romero JR, et al. HbS-Oman heterozygote: a new dominant sickle syndrome. Blood. 1998;92: 4375-4382.

19 Sickle Cell Disease

Matthew Heeney and George J. Dover

HISTORY

Sickle cell anemia was first described in a West Indian dentistry student, Walter Clement Noel, by Herrick and Irons in 1910.[1,2] Sydenstricker and colleagues described the first cases in children, recognized the association with hemolytic anemia, and introduced the term *crisis* to describe periodic acute episodes of pain.[3] The pathologic basis of the disorder and its relationship to the hemoglobin molecule were defined in 1927 by Hahn and Gillespie.[4] Shortly after the application of moving-boundary electrophoresis to the separation of sickle from normal hemoglobin by Pauling and co-workers,[5] Neel[6] defined the genetics of the disorder and clearly distinguished sickle trait—the heterozygous condition (AS)—from sickle cell anemia—the homozygous state (SS). Further understanding of the molecular basis of the disorder was made possible by the finding that normal human hemoglobin is composed of two pairs of globin subunits: one pair that is invariant, the α chain, and another pair that is variable, the ε, γ, δ, or β chain. The relative ease with which sickle hemoglobin (HbS) could be isolated by chromatography or zone electrophoresis techniques led to Ingram's application of tryptic digestion, high-voltage electrophoresis, and paper chromatography to isolated HbS, with the result that the amino acid substitution in HbS is now known to be a valine instead of a glutamic acid in the number 6 position of the β chain. The α chain is normal.[7] The chemical nomenclature for HbS is therefore $\alpha_2\beta_2^{Glu6\rightarrow Val}$. (See Fig. 19-1 for an overview of pathophysiology of the β^S mutation.) Excellent reviews of the history of sickle cell anemia are available.[8]

PATHOPHYSIOLOGY

Hemoglobin S Mutation

Origins. The sickle gene is a common mutant that in the heterozygous state provides some protection to infants who might otherwise succumb to cerebral falciparum malaria. The frequency of the sickle gene in a population parallels the historical incidence of malaria. Whereas the average incidence of the sickle gene among American blacks is approximately 8%,[9] its frequency is much higher in inhabitants of certain areas of Africa. Polymorphic sites around globin DNA and their linkages to the β^S gene indicate that this mutation may have developed independently and spontaneously at least five times.[10-12] However, analysis of nuclear and mitochondrial DNA from African populations suggests that a single mutation may have occurred 50,000 years ago.[13] In Africa, there are four major sickle haplotypes, each associated with a particular geographic region: "Senegal" (Atlantic West Africa), "Benin" (Central West Africa), "Bantu" (also called "CAR" for Central African Republic), and Cameroon.[11,14] The Benin type is found not only in Benin but also in Ibadan,[15] Algeria,[12] Sicily,[16] Turkey,[17] Greece, Yemen,

and southwest Saudi Arabia.[15] In North American sickle cell patients of African heritage, 50% to 70% of chromosomes are Benin, 15% to 30% are Bantu-CAR, and 5% to 15% are Senegal.[18,19] In Africa, virtually all patients in a region are homozygous for a given haplotype. Nagel and co-workers documented the different hematologic characteristics of the different homozygote groups.[20,21] Benin and Senegalese individuals have higher levels of fetal hemoglobin (HbF) and fewer dense cells than Bantu-CAR people do. The Senegalese have a high proportion of $^G\gamma$ HbF. In contrast to what is found among Africans in Africa, African Americans are mainly heterozygotes. Less common β^S-linked haplotypes are usually recombinations of the common haplotypes occurring 5′ to the β-globin gene.[22,23] When patients identified in hospital-based clinics are studied, these haplotypes may be associated with overall clinical severity—Bantu-CAR being the most severe and Senegalese the least.[24]

A different haplotype is found in India and parts of Saudi Arabia.[15] In the Eastern oases of Saudi Arabia, the African haplotypes are not seen, but a unique "Arabian-Indian" haplotype is found. This haplotype is also noted in patients from Orissa and Poona, India. Patients from these regions have long been recognized as having mild disease and elevated levels of HbF.[25-28] In contrast, in Riyadh, Saudi Arabia, all patients with sickle cell anemia are from southwest Saudi Arabia and Yemen and are homozygous Benin.

Interaction with Malaria. Heterozygotes with HbS, HbC, HbE, α- and β-thalassemia, and glucose-6-phosphate dehydrogenase (G6PD) deficiency are protected from malaria relative to the normal population.[29] The physiologic basis for the influence of malaria on the sickle gene (so-called balanced polymorphism) is not well understood. It may be due to increased phagocytosis of infected red blood cells (RBCs),[30,31] failure to grow within RBCs,[32] decreased RBC invasion of the parasite because of RBC rigidity,[33] or reduced bioavailability of nitric oxide (NO).[34] Transgenic mice expressing HbS are partially protected from malaria.[35] Interestingly, protection against *Plasmodium falciparum* in inhabitants of Kenya is lost with coinheritance of HbAS and α-thalassemia (negative epistasis).[36]

The Hemoglobin S Polymer

Polymer Structure. In 1927, Hahn and Gillespie[4] showed that sickling, the change from a biconcave disc to the sickle form, was dependent on deoxygenation. Harris[37] subsequently demonstrated that cellular sickling was associated with the formation of "tactoids" of HbS, which appeared as the hemoglobin became deoxygenated. Electron micrographs of sickled red cells[38-41] reveal long, thin bundles of HbS fibers that run parallel to the long axis of the cell or the abnormal protuberances. The ultrastructure of HbS fibers, as detailed by electron microscopy and image reconstruction, reveals a complex

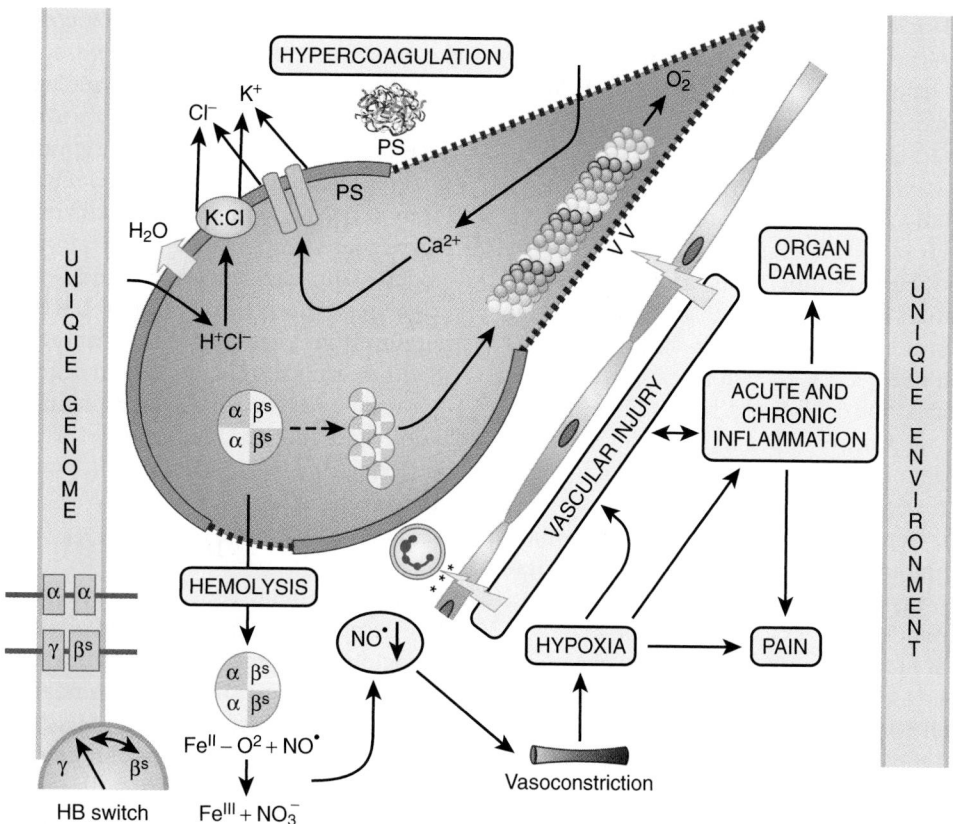

FIGURE 19-1. Pathophysiology of sickle cell disease. The β^S mutation, A→T in the sixth codon, results in an abnormal globin with valine instead of glutamic acid in the sixth position. That hydrophobic valine is exposed when the globin tetramer assumes the deoxy confirmation and tends to burrow into the hydrophobic pocket of nearby β chains. Polymerization of hemoglobin S tetramers occurs rapidly and leads to increased red rigidity. The inherent instability of the HbS polymer leads to oxidative damage (O_2^-) of the red cell membrane (*red dashed lines*). In the area of red cell membrane damage, phosphatidylserine (PS) becomes exposed on the outer surface of the membrane, which activates the coagulation system and leads to hypercoagulation. Membrane damage also leads to increased influx of Ca^{2+} into the cell, which activates the Gardos channel (*tan vertical bars*) and leads to the efflux of K^+ and Cl^-. To compensate for the loss of K^+ and Cl^-, water exits the cell and the cell becomes more acidic (influx of H^+Cl^-). Acidosis then activates the K^+-Cl^- cotransporter (K:Cl), thereby leading to further efflux of K^+ and Cl^- and more dehydration and intracellular acidosis. Some intravascular hemolysis occurs as a result of red blood cell (RBC) membrane damage, which leads to free hemoglobin tetramer binding to plasma nitric oxide (NO). Depletion of plasma NO leads to vasoconstriction, which along with increased RBC rigidity and increased adherence of sickled RBCs to vessel walls, leads to decreased blood flow, hypoxia, and vascular injury and localized damage to endothelial cells (lightning bolt). Endothelial damage leads to expression of adherent proteins on the surface of the endothelial cells (★★★, VV), thus increasing adherence of red and white blood cells to the vessel wall. Endothelial injury and hypoxia lead to vascular injury and acute and chronic inflammation. This ultimately results in organ damage. Each SS patient has a unique environment (e.g., exposure to infections) and unique genetic makeup (e.g., increase in fetal hemoglobin because of genetic modifiers of the hemoglobin switch) that can modify the severity of the disease and thereby make the clinical severity of SS disease extremely variable.

solid-core structure 21 nm in diameter and composed of 14 filaments arranged as seven pairs of double filaments[42,43]—an inner pair with six peripheral pairs.[44] Each filament pair is half-staggered along the fiber axis and has an inherent polarity (three pairs of one polarity and four pairs of the other polarity).[45-48] The radius of the HbS fibers are polymorphic and related to the helical pitch of the double filaments.[49]

The detailed crystal structure suggested by Wishner, Love, and colleagues[50,51] identified several critical intermolecular contact sites: Asp β73, and Glu β121. A topographic map of the HbS fiber at the level of specific amino acids was proposed by Edelstein.[52] Three classes of intermolecular contacts are evident in this model. Contacts along the axis of the filament are made by α and β chains and include the following residues in which mutants affect fiber formation: β121 (O Arab), β16 (J

Baltimore), β17 (J Amiens), β19 (D Ouled Rabah), β22 (G Coushatta), α16 (I), and α116 (O Indonesia). The lateral contacts between filaments of a pair are largely between β chains and include the primary sickle mutation β6. For each hemoglobin tetramer, one chain contributes the β6 mutation, whereas the other contributes a critical receptor region around the Phe β85 residue. In this critical receptor region lie residues where mutants affect fiber formation: β73 (Korle Bu), β66 (I Toulouse), β83 (Pyrgos), and β87 (D Ibadan). Within the acceptor pocket, the mutant valine closely contacts four different hydrophobic residues (β70, β73, β84, and β85), and in addition to the hydrophobic interaction, water molecules are present near the mutant valine and form hydrophilic interactions in the lateral contact region.[53] Contact between filament pairs is largely through α chains. α-Chain mutations (J Mexico α54, Sealy α47, Winnipeg α75, Stanleyville II α78, Sawara α6, Anantharaj α11, and G Philadelphia α68) that occur at sites critical for inter-pair associations also influence fiber formation. With resolution of the crystalline structure of HbS to 2.0 Å, this model has been confirmed.[54]

Polymer Formation. Polymerization of deoxy-HbS is a highly complex process that results in the formation of gelled, aggregated HbS tetramers in equilibrium with hemoglobin tetramers in solution. Pertubations in oxygen levels,[55,56] temperature,[57-59] pH,[60] ionic strength,[61] 2,3-diphosphoglycerate (2,3-DPG),[60,62] and carbon monoxide[63-65] affect the formation of HbS gels. This polymerization of HbS is the basic feature that leads to the viscosity changes, distortion of cell morphology, sludging, and organ infarction that are identified as the clinical manifestations of sickle cell disease (SCD). Although data from various techniques differ somewhat, a representative kinetic model was proposed by Hofrichter, Ross, and Eaton[57,63] and expanded by Ferrone[66] (Fig. 19-2).

The kinetics of HbS polymerization can be explained by a double-nucleation mechanism. Gelation is initiated by a process called "homogeneous nucleation" in which single deoxy-HbS molecules aggregate. Aggregation of a few molecules is thermodynamically unstable, but once a certain number of molecules aggregate, termed the *critical nucleus*, the addition of further molecules pro-duces a more stable aggregate or polymer. Thus, homogeneous nucleation is very highly dependent on the concentration of deoxy-HbS molecules. The second nucleation phase, termed *heterogeneous nucleation*, takes place on the surface of preexisting polymer. Recent data suggest that the same intermolecular contacts between the mutant valine and its receptor on the surface of the polymer are responsible for heterogeneous nucleation and cross-linking between strands.[67] As polymerization progresses, more surface area becomes available and therefore the reaction becomes autocatalytic.

The result of this double-nucleation mechanism is a measurable *delay time* between the initiation of polymerization and the exponential rise in polymer formation. The delay time varies as the 30th power of the hemoglobin concentration:

$$1/t_d = K(C/C_s)^n$$

in which t_d = delay time, C = hemoglobin concentration, C_s = hemoglobin solubility, and $n = 30$ (the number of hemoglobin tetramers in the "critical polymer"). Because n is so large, small changes in hemoglobin concentration have a profound effect on the delay time. For example, decreasing the mean corpuscular hemoglobin concentration (MCHC) from 32 to 30 g/dL will increase the delay time threefold.[68] Gelation is also exquisitely sensitive to changes in temperature and pH. A change from 38.5° C to 37° C or an increase in intracellular pH of 0.03 would also double the delay time.

The phenomenon of delayed gelling of HbS in solution is also seen in red cells containing HbS.[69,70] The distribution of observed delay times within intact RBCs is consistent with the distribution of MCHC in cells. The double-nucleation hypothesis provides for the formation of a network of polymers termed a *domain* that is non-uniformly distributed within the cell. Rapid deoxygenation leads to the formation of multiple small domains of polymer and little morphologic deformation of the cell. On the other hand, slow deoxygenation results in large, aligned polymers, which causes significant distortion of cell morphology.[71,72]

A kinetic model of HbS gelation that incorporates the concept of a critical delay time has led Eaton and co-workers to propose that polymerization kinetics plays an important role in the pathophysiology of SS disease.[73,74] Oxygenation and deoxygenation of cells in the circulation take place in a time frame that is of the same order of magnitude as the sickling and unsickling of HbS in vitro. Cells exposed to the high PO₂ of the lungs are quickly "degelled" because HbS gels melt in less than 0.5 second when exposed to oxygen. The cells contain little polymerized HbS while in the oxygenated environment of the arterial circulation. As the cells enter the capillary circulation, oxygen saturation decreases rapidly, as does hemoglobin solubility. The red cell spends an average of 1 second in the capillary circulation, although this is highly variable. If the delay time is less than 1 second, the cell will sickle and occlude the capillary. If the delay time is

← RATE-LIMITING HOMOGENEOUS NUCLEATION PHASE →
sensitive to: HgB concentration, pH, temperature, ionic strength

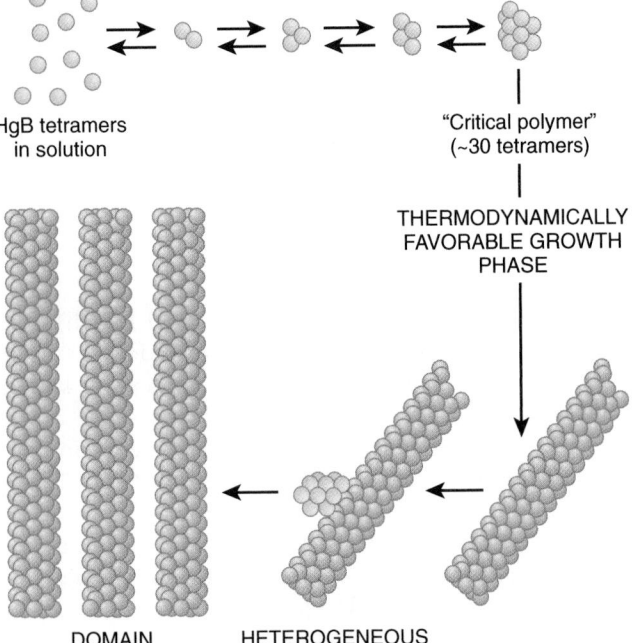

HgB tetramers
in solution

"Critical polymer"
(~30 tetramers)

THERMODYNAMICALLY
FAVORABLE GROWTH
PHASE

DOMAIN   HETEROGENEOUS
FORMATION   NUCLEATION

FIGURE 19-2. Model of the polymerization and alignment of deoxy-hemoglobin S. (*Adapted from Hofrichter J, Ross PD, Eaton WA. Super saturation in sickle cell hemoglobin solutions. Proc Natl Acad Sci U S A. 1976;73:3035-3039; and Ferrone FA, Hofrichter J, Eaton WA. Kinetics of sickle hemoglobin polymerization; II A double nucleation mechanism. J Mol Biol. 1985;183:611-631.*)

prolonged, sickling will not take place in the capillary and obstruction will not occur. If the transit time through the capillary is shortened and is less than the delay time, occlusion will not occur. This is presumably the situation in the myocardium, in which sickling and infarction do not occur because of the extremely short transit time despite the high oxygen extraction. Factors such as low pH, high hemoglobin concentration, and high ionic strength, which shorten the delay time in vitro, also affect in vivo sickling. Patients who become hypoxic, acidotic, dehydrated, and febrile are likely to experience vaso-occlusive episodes. The hypertonic renal medulla and the acidotic, high-hematocrit environment of the spleen make these organs prime targets for sickling.

Relatively little is know about the uniformity of the depolymerization process within RBCs. It is likely that depolymerization occurs from both the ends and sides of polymer fibers.[75] Failure of complete depolymerization in the passage through the oxygentated environment of the lungs (1 to 3 seconds) may lead to the residual polymer observed by Noguchi and associates.[76] Using nuclear magnetic resonance, they measured the quantity of HbS polymer in AS and SS red cells under varying conditions related to MCHC and oxygenation[77,78] and found polymer formation and impaired erythrocyte deformability at oxygen saturations above the level at which cells appear to morphologically sickle.[79] They proposed that the amount of HbS polymer present at equilibrium in SS patients is the major factor determining clinical severity[80,81]; however, this relationship was not confirmed by others.[82] Important variables that affect the HbS polymer fraction (HbF, 2,3-DPG levels, oxygen saturation, and pH) are heterogeneously distributed within subsets of red cells, and these factors along with other factors, such as membrane abnormalities and red cell–endothelial interactions, are likely to play a role in the variable clinical severity of SCD.

Interactions of Hemoglobin S with Hemoglobin A and Hemoglobin F. Study of the interaction with other hemoglobins supports a rational basis for understanding the clinical manifestations of the various sickle syndromes and provides a rationale for therapy. Investigators have extensively studied mixtures of HbS with HbF or HbA to determine the effects on gelation[83-88] and solubility.[89-91] In these studies the nonideal behavior of concentrated hemoglobin solutions[58,92] was considered—the bulky hemoglobin molecules take up much of the solution volume, thus making the *effective* concentration of hemoglobin higher than the *measured* concentration. Kinetic data show that HbA and HbF have a profound, dose-related effect in which delay time is increased and the HbS polymer content in cells is decreased (Fig. 19-3). The effect of HbF is considerably greater than the effect of HbA. Sunshine and others demonstrated that when compared with pure HbS solutions (as seen in sickle cell anemia), mixtures with 15% to 30% HbA (as found in S–β+-thalassemia) have delay times that are 10 to 10^2 times longer, mixtures with 20% to 30% HbF (as found in S–hereditary persistence of fetal hemoglobin [HPFH]) have delay times that are 10^3 to 10^4 times longer, and mixtures with 60% HbA (as found in sickle trait) have delay times that are 10^6 times longer.[83,85] HbA and HbF also increase the solubility of HbS, with HbF being more effective than HbA. Studies of the composition of the gels and supernatant of these mixtures demonstrate that asymmetric hybrids of HbS and HbA ($\alpha_2\beta^S\beta^A$) are readily incorporated into the gel. In mixtures of HbF and HbS in which the concentration of HbF is less than 40%, very little if any HbF is incorporated into polymer, thus suggesting that asymmetric hybrids of HbS and HbF ($\alpha_2\beta^S\gamma$) and HbF ($\alpha_2\gamma_2$) are not incorporated into polymer under most physiologic conditions.[84,86,89-91] HbA has a lesser effect on HbS solubility than HbF does because the asymmetric hybrids readily copolymerize with HbS.[93]

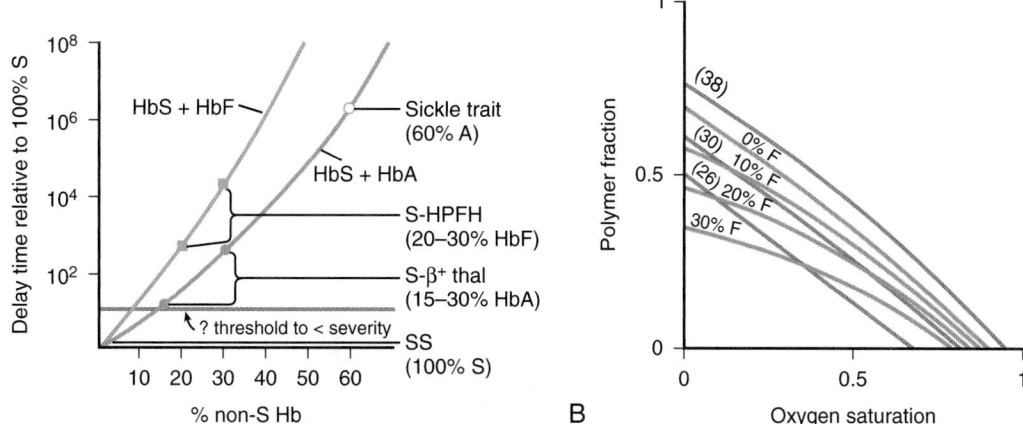

FIGURE 19-3. A, Effect of increase in concentrations of fetal hemoglobin (HbF) and adult hemoglobin (HbA) on delay time of polymerization of sickle hemoglobin (HbS). **B,** HbS polymer formation as a function of oxygen saturation for different levels of HbF (0%, 10%, 20%, 30%) at hemoglobin concentration of 34 g/dL and for concentrations of 26, 30, and 38 g/dL of pure HbS. S-HPFH, HbS and hereditary persistence of HbF; thal, thalassemia. (**A,** *Based on the work of Sunshine HR, Hofrichter J, Eaton WA. Requirement for therapeutic inhibition of sickle hemoglobin gelation. Nature. 1978;275:238-240;* **B,** *based on Noguchi DT, Torchia DA, Schechter AN. Intracellular polymerization of sickle hemoglobin. Effects of cell heterogeneity. J Clin Invest. 1983;72:846-852.*)

Crowding of hemoglobin molecules can reduce the effect of HbF replacement at hemoglobin concentrations higher than 30 g/dL.[94] Replacement of HbS by 20% HbF at hemoglobin concentrations above 30 g/dL will increase the delay time only by 10 times, *not* by the 1000 times predicted at concentrations of hemoglobin lower than 30 g/dL.

Membrane Damage

The basic pathophysiology of sickle cell anemia is directly related to polymerization of HbS. Secondary effects of the primary lesion may modulate clinical expression of the disease. Alterations in the red cell membrane because of structural damge from HbS polymerization or oxidative damage as a result of unstable HbS may be important determinants of disease severity for several reasons (see Fig. 19-1). First, the membrane is the structure most intimately associated with the abnormal gene product and is therefore vulnerable to damage. Second, the membrane is largely responsible for maintaining the environment in which this abnormal product resides. Third, the membrane is the face that the red cell presents and is recognized by proteins in plasma, by other cells in the circulation, by the vascular endothelium, and by the reticuloendothelium.

Mechanism of Membrane Damage.
In normal cells, HbA has been shown to bind to membranes[95,96] at or near the cytoplasmic portion of band 3 protein[97,98] and with relatively low affinity to phospholipids on the inner surface of the memebrane.[99] Hemoglobin at physiologic concentrations stabilizes the configuration of spectrin heterodimers.[100] HbS and β^S-globin bind to membranes more readily than HbA does.[101-103] Evans and Mohandas demonstrated that membrane-associated HbS was a major determinant of erythrocyte rigidity.[104] In these experiments, normal deformability was found when normal hemoglobin was reconstituted in sickle or normal membrane ghosts, but abnormal deformability was associated with reconstitution of sickle or normal red cell membranes with HbS. In one study, membrane rigidity was associated with the presence of a small amount of a high-molecular-weight spectrin-hemoglobin complex in the membrane.[105]

HbS is inherently unstable[106,107] and has an increased tendency to denature and form small aggregates— "micro–Heinz bodies." These bodies attach with high affinity to the cytoplasmic portion of band 3 protein at or near the HbA binding site.[108] Such binding on the inside surface of the membrane is translated into changes on the outside surface because both band 3 protein and glycophorin (the major bearers of the cell's antigens and charge) are found to be clustered above the micro–Heinz bodies.[109] Clustering of band 3 protein is associated with deposition of specific anti–band 3 protein antibodies on the cell,[108,110] a process linked to normal cell senescence[111,112] and perhaps contributing to the short life span of SS cells.[113] Ankyrin is also abnormally clustered around the denatured HbS and, like band 3 protein, may be damaged in the process.[109] In addition, the hydrophobic surface of the Heinz body sequesters lipid, spectrin, band 3, ankyrin, and protein 4.1 inside the cell and may contribute to the reduced surface area of such cells.[114]

HbS has an increased tendency to auto-oxidize and form methemoglobin, thereby generating superoxide and losing heme.[115] In fact, sickle cells generate twice the normal amount of the potent oxidants superoxide, peroxide, and hydroxyl radical.[116] Iron in different compartments (denatured hemoglobin, free heme, hemichromes, and nonheme iron) is found bound to various sites in the sickle red cell membrane. This iron serves as a catalyst for the production of highly reactive hydroxyl radicals, which leads to oxidative damage of the various components of the membrane.[117,118]

Membrane Deformability.
As sickle cells are deoxygenated and fill with polymerized hemoglobin, they become less deformable.[118-122] However, even fully oxygenated cells have abnormal rheologic properties.[123] Using the ektacytometer, Clark and colleagues studied the deformability of SS red cells and showed that decreased deformability was directly related to increased MCHC and that correcting the elevated MCHC restored normal deformability.[124] By means of a high-shear/hemolysis assay, normalization of the tendency to hemolyze was noted when MCHC was corrected, except in the most dense fraction, where normalization was incomplete.[125] This incomplete normalization suggests that severe cellular dehydration itself may contribute to the development of a membrane lesion. Using micropipette techniques to measure membrane deformability, two studies[126,127] have shown that MCHC is the major contributor to cell rigidity but that irreversible membrane changes as a result of dehydration also increase membrane rigidity.

Membrane rigidity is further evidence that a structural membrane lesion is present. The finding that the cytoskeleton of irreversibly sickled cells (ISCs) was permanently distorted led several investigators to analyze the various components. Abnormalities in the cytoskeleton of ISCs include aberrant cross-linking of actin,[128] dissociation of spectin tetramers,[129] and clustering of band 3 protein and glycophorin.[130] Disordered mobility of the cytoskeleton relative to the overlying membrane may relate to decreased binding of normal ankyrin to sickle protein 3[131] or to binding of normal spectrin to sickle ankyrin.[132] With the use of newer proteomic techniques, four groups of proteins appear to be increased in sickle RBC membranes: actin accessory proteins, components of lipid rafts, scavengers of oxygen radicals, and protein repair participants.[133] All these observations support the hypothesis that membrane rigidity is due to cytoskeletal damage associated with HbS polymer formation and oxidative damage.

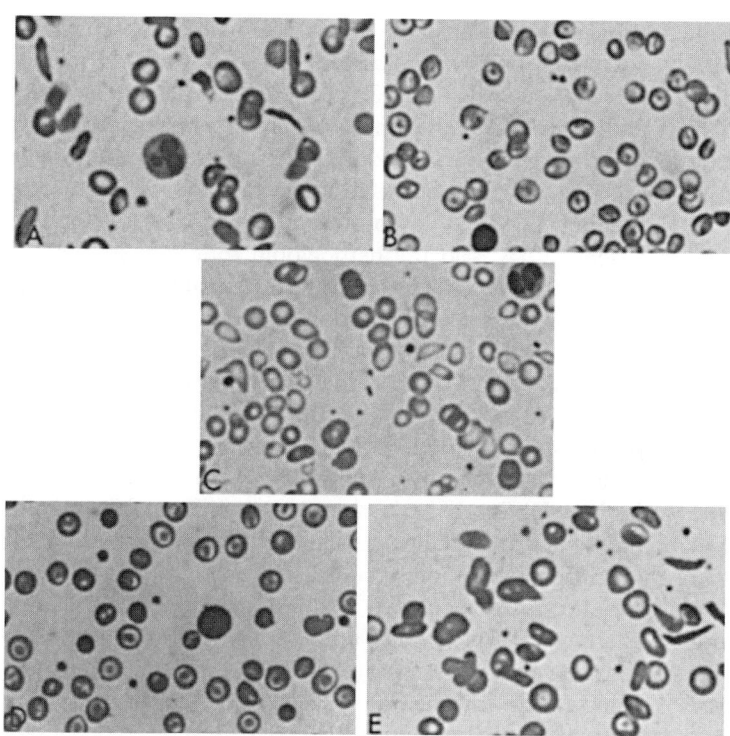

FIGURE 19-4. Oxygenated peripheral blood smears from individuals with sickle cell anemia (**A**), hemoglobin SC disease (**B**), sickle-β⁰-thalassemia (**C**), homozygous hemoglobin C (**D**), and hemoglobin SD disease (**E**).

Hemoglobin Concentration. Sickle cell individuals have more light cells (reticulocytes) and more dense cells (MCHC >37 mg/dL) than normal individuals do (Figs. 19-4 and 19-5). The vaso-occlusive nature of these dense cells was reported by Kaul and colleagues, who showed that cells separated by density (and therefore MCHC) from patients with sickle cell anemia obstruct flow in an artificially perfused capillary system in proportion to their MCHC.[134] Although early reports suggested that the percentage of dense cells decreases during vaso-occlusive crises,[135] there is no correlation between the percentage of dense cells and the frequency or onset of crises.[136] The decreased MCHC associated with α-thalassemia leads to a more uniform distribution of red cell densities and a decreased percentage of dense cells.[137,138] Paradoxically, individuals with HbSC have milder clinical disease but more dense cells than do individuals with homozygous sickle cell anemia (see Fig. 19-5).[139]

The heterogeneity of red cell shape and density in sickle cell anemia is due partially to the heterogeneous distribution of HbF in a subset of red cells called F cells.[140] Because HbF interferes with HbS polymerization, F cells survive longer in the circulation than do cells with no HbF,[141] and the relative proportion of F cells in the densest cell fractions is very low.[137,142] The densest cell fraction in SS contains the oldest non–HbF-containing RBCs, ISCs, and young reticulocytes poor in HbF that dehydrate rapidly.[143]

Shape Changes (Sickling) in Red Blood Cell. The time course of cellular events associated with oxygenation and deoxygenation has been investigated by Hahn and associates,[143a] who studied cells from patients with SS disease under physiologic time and oxygen conditions.

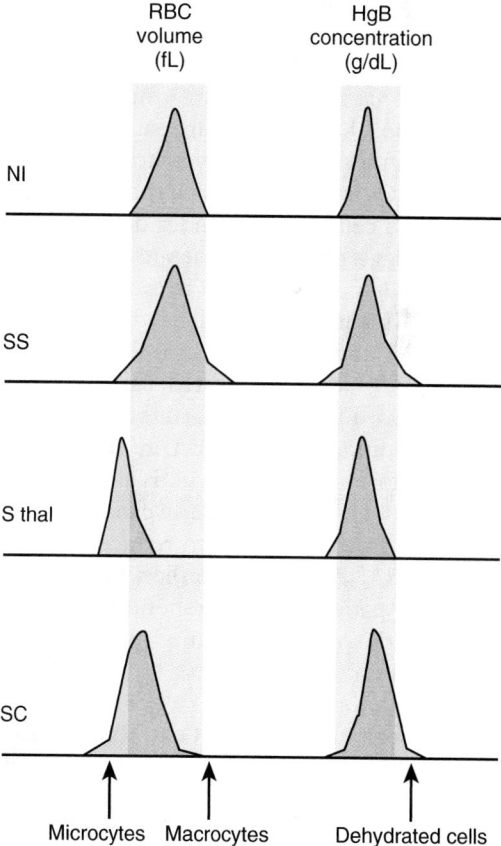

FIGURE 19-5. Typical distribution patterns of cell volume and hemoglobin concentration in different sickle syndromes. Note that in SS disease, the cells fall below and above the normal (*shaded*) range of both volume and concentration. The large (microcytic) cells are low-density reticulocytes. The dehydrated population is enriched in irreversibly sickled cells and is low in HbF. In S-thalassemia (S thal) syndromes, the entire volume curve is shifted toward the left, and few dense cells are seen. In SC disease, the microcytes are often spherocytic, very dehydrated cells. Nl, normal.

They described two categories of cells—a fraction of dense cells (MCHC >36 g/dL) that exhibited reversible polymerization and shape change (reversibly sickled cells [RSCs]) and a fraction of very dense cells (MCHC of 44 g/dL) that exhibited reversible polymerization but irreversible shape change (ISCs). Changes in the rheology of the cells paralleled the appearance of polymers in cytoplasm a considerable time before any detectable distortion of cell shape.

RSCs have normal shape and normal viscosity when oxygenated. The vaso-occlusive complications of SCD may be due to the "Trojan horse performance" of these RSCs, which are able to slip into the microvasculature because of their normal rheologic properties when oxygenated and then become distorted and viscous as they become deoxygenated in the vessel.

ISCs are slender, elongated cells with blunt ends that are visible on an oxygenated peripheral blood smear in SCD (see Fig. 19-4). These cells are extremely dense, have little HbF to dilute their concentrated HbS, and survive in the circulation for only a few days.[142] In 1968, Dobler and Bertles[143] demonstrated unpolymerized hemoglobin in an oxygenated ISC. In the Hahn studies,[143a] ISCs underwent hemoglobin polymerization and depolymerization upon deoxygenation and reoxygenation. When compared with the RSC fraction, however, polymerization took place sooner, was much more highly aligned, and took longer to disappear upon deoxygenation. Onishi and Horiuchi demonstrated that in vitro formation of ISCs is correlated with the maximum linear distortion of red cell diameter under deoxygenated conditions, thus suggesting that the length of HbS polymer fibers in SS cells contributes to irreversible membrane damage.[144] ISCs can be formed in vitro by prolonged deoxygenation,[145] by incubation of red cells in a high-calcium buffer,[146] and by repeated oxygenation-deoxygenation cycles.[122] Reversible oxidative damage to β-actin and loss of ubiquitination of α-spectrin lead to ISC membrane skeleton formation. The result is a membrane cytoskeleton that is "locked" because it cannot disassemble or reassemble.[147] Antioxidants can reduce the formation of ISCs in vitro.[148] As detailed earlier, ISCs vary widely from patient to patient and correspond well with hemolytic rate[149] and spleen size[150] but poorly with vaso-occlusive severity.

Ion Transport and Volume Control. The abnormal cation permeability of a sickled red cell is characterized by calcium loading, potassium depletion, increased acidosis, and dehydration, which enhances the tendency for HbS polymerization (see Fig. 19-1). In 1955, Tosteson and colleagues[151,152] showed that HbS polymer formation with deoxygenation causes reversible potassium loss and sodium gain in SS cells. Because this cation flux was reversible with reoxygenation, by itself it could not explain the dehydration associated with ISCs and other very dense SS red cells. The abnormal water and cation movement across the sickle cell membrane has been shown to be associated with a variety of pumps, channels, and leaks involving potassium (K^+), sodium (Na^+), chloride (Cl^-), calcium (Ca^{2+}), and magnesium (Mg^{2+}). Although the pathogenesis of these pathways remains incompletely understood, they are undoubtedly related to the physical distortion associated with sickling,[125-127,151-157] young cell age,[158-160] oxidant damage,[161-163] and the hemoglobin mutation itself.[164-166] At least two major channels are responsible for the dehydrating process: the Gardos channel and the K^+-Cl^- cotransporter (KCC). Several investigators noted that ISCs and other dense sickle RBCs had increased concentrations of Ca^{2+},[167,168] and this was later shown to be partially due to the high concentrations of Ca^{2+} found in endocytic vesicles in sickle RBCs.[169] The molecular basis for how HbS polymerization leads to influx of Ca^{2+} is still unknown. SS reticulocytes exposed to deoxygenation and HbS polymerization accumulate sufficient Ca^{2+} to activate the Gardos channel,[170] a Ca^{2+}-sensitive, K^+-selective channel. Cl^- and HCO_3^- are also lost via parallel voltage-sensitive pathways. Loss of KCl and $KHCO_3$ results in osmotically driven water loss. The activated Gardos channel leads to rapid RBC dehydration to a much greater extent than other transporters do. The Gardos channel has been shown to be inhibited by clotrimazole, an imidazole antimycotic agent in vitro,[171] in the SAD mouse model for SCD in vivo,[172] and in a short-term study in patients with SCD.[173]

A second pathway involved in RBC dehydration is the KCC. The KCC pathway is stimulated to lose K^+, Cl^-, and water when (predominantly young) sickle cells are exposed to a low pH environment, as might occur in areas of poor perfusion.[174] The KCC pathway is also activated by deoxygentation of hemoglobin[148,175] and by low levels of Mg^{2+}.[176,177] Acid activation of the KCC is exaggerated in SS reticulocytes and may be due to sulfhydyl oxidation.[178] Genes for four KCC isoforms have been identified. The 1, 3, and 4 isoforms of KCC are present in SS and normal RBCs, but SS RBCs may have N-terminal splicing variants of these isoforms.[179] The KCC pathway is inhibitable by magnesium in vivo,[176,177] and Mg^{2+} is depleted in sickle erythrocytes, possibly through abnormal Na/Mg exchange.[180] Two preliminary studies demonstrated the effectiveness of oral magnesium in the prevention of cellular dehydration in a mouse model of SCD[181] and in patients,[182,183] and clinical trials are under way.

Lew and Bookchin reviewed the evolution of our knowledge of ion transport pathology in SS dehydration and proposed a multistep dehydration model that leads to the formation of ISCs from SS reticulocytes.[184] HbS polymerization in SS reticulocyes distorts the RBC membrane, which results in the influx of Ca^{2+} sufficient to activate the Gardos channel, thereby leading to loss of K^+, Cl^-, and HCO_3^-. These losses result in dehydration and acidification predominantly through reentry of H^+ and Cl^-. Subsequently, acid-stimulated KCC channels lead to further loss of K^+ and Cl^- and acidification and dehydration of the cell. In the acidic state, the KCC pathway would remain active in both the oxygenated and deoxygenated state.[158] This model explains how reticulocytes may rapidly become ISCs.

External Membrane Interactions

Increased Red Cell Adhesion to Endothelium. More than 15 years ago, investigators first discovered that sickle erythrocytes have an abnormal propensity to stick to vascular endothelial cells,[185,186] an adhesive force that results from numerous attachment sites[187] that can withstand the detaching forces found in low-shear vascular beds.[188] This observation has taken on increased importance in conceptualizing the pathophysiology of SCD. As cells flow through vessels of critical dimension, an increased tendency to linger at the endothelial surface will increase the odds that polymerization and obstruction will occur (see Fig. 19-1). Support for this hypothesis comes from studies that suggest a correlation between adhesiveness and clinical severity.[189,190]

A variety of RBC adhesion molecules are found on SS RBCs, especially SS reticulocytes. The adhesion process can alter or even dislodge endothelial cells. Such circulating cells may have left behind areas of exposed subendothelium. SS RBCs bind to three subendothelial extracellular matrix proteins, laminin, thrombospondin, and fibronectin.[191] SS red cells show the highest affinity for laminin because of two isoforms of the protein that bear the Lutheran blood group antigens (B-CAM and LU).[192,193] Adhesion proteins to thrombospondin on SS reticulocytes include CD47 and VLA-4 (very late antigen 4). Mature SS RBCs retain CD47 receptors but not VLA-4. CD44 is the adhesion protein found on RBCs that binds to fibronectin. VLA-4 ($\alpha_4\beta_1$ integrin) also binds to the endothelial protein vascular cell adhesion molecule 1 (VCAM-1).[191]

Perhaps more significantly, a variety of agonists can activate SS RBC adhesion properties. Protein kinase C can activate adhesion to fibronectin and thrombospondin.[194,195] Activation of signaling pathways within the RBC involving adrenergic receptors, cyclic adenosine monophosphate (cAMP), and protein kinase A also increases RBC adhesion.[196-199] SS RBCs are more responsive than normal RBCs to these agonist, possibly because of higher levels of signaling transduction proteins found in younger RBCs. Endothelial cells differ in their repertoire of surface molecules—for example, CD36 is expressed on microvascular but not large vessel endothelium.[200] Endothelial cells also express differing amounts of surface molecules and become more or less adherent, depending on environmental stimuli. Cytokines such as interleukin-18 and tumor necrosis factor[201] promote endothelial adherence, largely as a result of upregulated VCAM-1 expression. Infected endothelial cells become adhesive by a variety of mechanisms. Herpesvirus-infected cells attract sickle red cells because of increased Fc receptor expression.[202] Endothelial cells exposed to Sendai viral double-stranded

RNA become adhesive through upregulated VCAM-1.[203] In transgenic sickle mice, the anti-inflammatory agent dexamethasone inhibited hypoxia-induced endothelial cell activation of NFκB, VCAM-1, and intercellular adhesion molecule 1 (ICAM-1), whereas blocking antibodies to VCAM-1 and ICAM-1 blocked RBC- and leukocyte-mediated vaso-occlusion.[204]

Circulating endothelial cells from patients with SCD exhibit an activated phenotype displaying ICAM-1, VCAM-1, E-selectin, P-selectin, and tissue factor.[205,206] Increased production of endothelial-derived adhesion molecules (VAM-1, ICAM-1, and E-selectin) was seen in 10 adult SS patients during acute sickle cell pain crises.[207] Furthermore, in a cohort of 160 adult patients in steady state, soluble levels of VCAM-1, ICAM-1, and E-selectin were elevated and independently associated with pulmonary hypertension (PHT) and mortality.[208]

Membrane Lipid Orientation and Coagulation Defects. Normally, the phospholipids of the red cell membrane are partitioned with amino phospholipids (phosphatidylserine [PS] and phosphatidylethanolamine [PE]) sequestered on the inner (cytoplasmic) surface and with sphingomyelin and phosphatidylcholine (PC) exposed on the outer surface (see Fig. 19-1). This asymmetry is not unique to the red cell and probably reflects a general structural pattern that keeps the amino phospholipids from activating soluble coagulation factors. This asymmetry is maintained by the interaction of spectrin[209] with the phospholipids and by a specific adenosine triphosphate (ATP)-dependent translocation process.[210] In RSCs, PS and PE flip back and forth from the inner leaflet to the outer leaflet during oxygenation and deoxygenation. Although early studies suggested that PS was permanently stuck to the outer leaflet in deoxygenated sickle cells,[211] later studies suggested that small amounts of PS accumulate on the outer surface of subpopulations of sickle cells[212] where the lipid bilayer is uncoupled from the cytoskeleton and when the cell is depleted of ATP.[213] Exposure of PS or PE on the outer surface during sickling may lead to increased phagocytosis by PS-binding proteins secreted by macrophages,[214] and these proteins may bind to specific PS receptors on certain enthothelial cells.[215] Alteration of the fatty acyl groups in PC results in changes in cell shape and deformability of SS cells, thus suggesting that the species composition of PC can affect membrane permeability and cellular deformability.[216] Both plasma and SS RBC membrane are deficient in certain long-chain polyunsaturated fatty acids. This deficiency is correlated with steady-state hemoglobin levels and may be affected by dietary intake.[217]

Abnormal lipid asymmetry accelerates clotting in vitro,[218] and PS-positive sickle RBCs (not PS-positive platelets) are correlated with markers of thrombin generation (prothrombin fragment F1.2, thrombin-antithrombin complexes) and fibrin degradation (D-dimers and plasmin-antiplasmin complexes).[219] Another marker of thrombophilia is the reduction in protein C and protein

S.[220] Platelet activation is also present in the steady state. In addition, microparticles from endothelial cells, platelets, monocytes, and red cells are seen in the steady state and increase during crises.[221] These microparticles are associated with increased hemolysis and activation of the procoagulant system.[222]

A growing body of evidence suggests that procoagulant and anticoagulant proteins and platelets play an important role in adhesion of sickle RBCs to endothelium. von Willebrand factor,[223-225] platelets,[226] and thrombospondin[227,228] increase RBC adhesiveness. Platelet-activating factor increases sickle red cell adherence to endothelium, and this interaction can be selectively blocked by an anti–$\alpha_V\beta_3$ integrin antibody, thus suggesting a potential therapeutic strategy.[229] Hence, abundant data support the view that SCD is a "hypercoagulable state."[230] It is unclear whether the hypercoagulable state is a consequence or a cause of vaso-occlusion, and large well-controlled trials of anticoagulants have not been conducted.[230]

Hemolysis

RBC life span is shortened in SS disesease to approximately 8 to 21 days. Hemolysis is both extravascular and intravascular. Extravascular hemolysis is enhanced by externalized PS on SS RBCs, which is recognized by macrophages with receptors specific for PS.[214] The membrane changes found in SS RBCs are similar to those seen in nucleated cells undergoing apoptosis (externalization of PS, annexin binding to and blebbing of the membrane along with cell shrinkage). These changes are accentuated by accumulation of intracellular Ca^{2+} secondary to oxidative stress.[231] Approximately 30% of the total hemoglobin is released intravascularly, with approximately 4 micromoles of plasma hemoglobin being present during steady state.[232]

Nitric Oxide Depletion. NO is produced by endothelial cells from L-arginine by isoforms of the enzyme NO synthetase (NOS). NO increases intracellular cyclic guanosine monophosphate (cGMP), which decreases smooth muscle calcium concentrations and leads to muscle relaxation, vasodilation, and increased regional blood flow.[233] NO also suppresses platelet aggregation,[234] reduces expression of endothelial cell adhesion molecules,[235] and reduces the secretion of procoagulant proteins.[236] NO levels may be depleted in patients with SCD for several reasons. Sickle cell patients have low arginine levels[237] and high plasma arginase levels.[238] NO reacts with oxyhemoglobin and deoxyhemoglobin to produce nitrate, methemoglobin, and iron nitrosylhemoglobin (reviewed by Reiter and colleagues[239]). Free plasma hemoglobin consumes NO 1000 times more rapidly than intracellular hemoglobin does.[240] Reiter and associates have shown that SS patients have elevated levels of plasma free hemoglobin, that plasma from SS patients consumes NO, and that SS patients with elevated plasma free hemoglobin

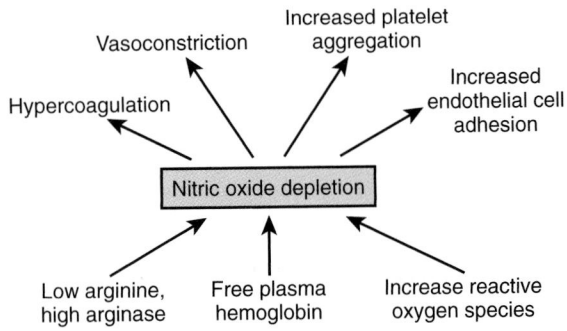

FIGURE 19-6. Factors leading to and the results of nitric oxide depletion. Intravascular hemolysis leads to elevated levels of plasma arginase and free plasma hemoglobin. Increased reactive oxygen species results from denatured HbS, oxidative damage to red cell membranes, tissue ischemia/reperfusion injury, and increase expression of endothelial xanthine oxidase, reduced endothelial nicotinamide adenine dinucleotide phosphate oxidase, and uncoupled endothelial nitric oxide synthetase.

have reduced forearm blood flow responses to infusion of an NO donor, nitroprusside[239] (see Fig. 19-1). The reactive oxygen species that are elevated in sickle cell patients for multiple reasons also reduce NO.[116,117,241] Work by Gladwin and co-workers has led to the hypothesis that SCD leads to depletion of NO and thereby a "hemolysis-induced endothelial dysfunction syndrome" characterized by PHT, priapism, leg ulcers, stroke, renal insufficiency, and esophageal dysmotility.[242,243] Furthermore, hemolysis-induced NO depletion may play a role in the SS metabolic hypercoagulable state[244] (Fig. 19-6).

Acute and Chronic Inflammation

Several lines of evidence suggest that the HbS mutation leads to an acute and chronic inflammatory state. Markers of inflammation, including increased levels of white blood cells (WBCs), platelets, C-reactive protein, and fibrinogen, all increased at steady state and during crises.[245,246] Increased adherence of SS RBCs, neutrophils, and platelets to vascular endothelium may initiate local inflammatory responses. Hypoxia, increased proinflammatory cytokines (interleukins 1, 2, 4, 6, and 8; tumor necrosis factor-α), and infections may activate vascular endothelium and leukocytes, which in turn can further increase adhesion molecules on both circulating cell surfaces and endothelial cell surfaces[246] (see Fig. 19-1).

White Blood Cells. There has been increasing evidence that circulating WBCs, particularly neutrophils, play a role in the pathogenesis of SS disease. Baseline WBC counts in SS individuals are elevated. The degree of elevation is directly related to early mortality[247] and an increased frequency of acute chest syndrome (ACS)[248] and is a predictor of clinical severity in infants.[249] Elevated WBCs in the normal population appear to be genetically determined,[250] but in SS patients it is also associated with elevated levels of granulocyte-macrophage colony-stimulating factor (GM-CSF).[251] Polymorphonuclear neutrophils (PMNs) show enhanced adhesion to endothelium during crises.[252] Activation of neutrophils is seen in the stready state and during vaso-occlusive crises.[253] In a transgenic sickle mouse model, PMNs are involved in reperfusion inflammation after hypoxia. This reperfusion injury can be abated by blocking PMN adherence with an antibody to P-selectin.[254] Thus, elevated level of PMNs in blood and the adhesiveness of PMNs to endothelium may reduce blood flow and, in association with sickled erythrocytes, can cause microvascular occlusion and crisis.[255]

Genetic Modifiers

Any analysis of the pathophysiology of SCD must address the remarkable heterogeneity in clinical severity that is observed in individuals homozygous for the sickle mutation. With completion of the human genome map, several important concepts have emerged. First, there is remarkable genomic heterogeneity between individuals, including single nucleotide polymorphisms (SNPs), varying length of tandem repeat sequences, and previously underappreciated structural variation in the genome.[256-258] Second, coexistence of the sickle mutation with variations in multiple genes whose interactions are associated with common complex disorders (stroke, hypertension) may be responsible for some variation in the severity of SCD. Third, known mutations in nonglobin genes associated with other single-gene disorders (G6PD gene in G6PD deficiency, uridine diphosphate-glucuronosyltransferase 1A [UGT1A] in Gilbert's disease) may explain some of the heterogeneity in the phenotype of SCD. New technology now allows scanning of the whole genome or large genomic regions in large numbers of SS individuals with and without common subphenotypes (stroke, ACS, elevated HbF levels), which has resulted in identification of genes that might contribute to that phenotype. Finally, newer appreciation of how the environment has led over evolutionary time to the selection of more favorable variations in proteins continues to enlighten our understanding of susceptibility to certain acquired diseases (malaria).

Glucose-6-Phosphate Dehydrogenase. G6PD deficiency is a single-gene variant common in black populations that also protects against malaria. There is no increased incidence of G6PD deficiency in SCD.[40,259,260] In a survey of 801 SS males, G6PD deficiency did not cause more hemolysis or increased anemic episodes.[259] Episodes of accelerated hemolysis of G6PD-deficient SS red cells have been described.[260] Because of the large population of very young G6PD-rich cells, this accelerated hemolysis is likely to be due to the enzyme abnormality only when the population is shifted toward the oldest cells, that is, during an aplastic episode. Recently, the common type A variant of G6PD deficiency has been associated with increased septic complications and anemia in African Americans trauma patients,[261] thus suggesting that individuals with SS disease and G6PD deficiency may have a poorer prognosis in this setting or with sepsis.

α-Thalassemia. Homozygous HbSS disease with accompanying α-thalassemia has been well described.[137,262-270] The diagnosis is based on the following criteria: (1) hemoglobin electrophoresis showing no HbA, normal HbA$_2$, and predominantly HbS; (2) microcytosis without iron deficiency; (3) both parents with the S trait, one with the typical AS α-thalassemia picture (microcytosis and HbS concentration <35%); (4) elevated Hb Bart's (γ$_4$) detectable in cord blood; and (5) α-gene mapping showing a total of two or three α genes. Approximately 30% of American blacks have three α genes, and approximately 2% only have two α genes. α-Thalassemia in U.S. SS disease patients is usually due to the α-thal-2 haplotype, a deletion of approximately 3.7 kilobases (kb) involving the entire α$_2$ gene.[269] There has been considerable interest in these patients because α-thalassemia has an effect on some of the hematologic features of sickle cell anemia and may provide insight into the pathophysiology of the disease. The primary effect of α-thalassemia is to decrease the cellular content of HbS, which increases the surface-to-volume ratio and results in a reduced MCHC that prolongs the delay time for HbS polymerization. Patients with α-thalassemia tend to have smaller, lighter cells with a higher hemoglobin level and fewer reticulocytes.[262,269-271] Although the hematologic parameters of sickle cell anemia are clearly improved by coexisting α-thalassemia, the vaso-occlusive severity is not obviously different. One study[262] indicated that leg ulcers and ACS were less frequent with α-thalassemia, but this finding was not confirmed by others.[267] Avascular necrosis (AVN) of the femoral head was increased in sickle cell anemia with α-thalassemia. α-Thalassemia does not protect children with SS disease from strokes.[272] Mears and co-workers have suggested that α-thalassemia is associated with increased life expectancy.[273] α-Thalassemia not only reduces mean corpuscular volume (MCV) and MCHC but also decreases the percentage of dense cells and ISCs.[137,274] The cells of patients with α-thalassemia and SS disease are more deformable and have fewer cation fluxes and a greater ratio of membrane surface area to volume.[264] Differences in hemoglobin values between children with SS disease with four and two genes is not apparent until after the age of 4 years,[275] but the microcytosis and elevated red cell counts are present at birth.[276] Steinberg has recently summarized the effects of α-thalassemia in SS disease.[277]

Hemoglobin F Production. HbF levels in sickle cell anemia may vary over a 60-fold range from 0.5% to 30%. Because of the known ameliorating effect of HbF in reducing HbS polymerization, the origin of this marked variability has been of great interest. Because HbF is heterogeneously distributed among the red cells of SS individuals, the percentage of HbF is the result of three independent processes: the number of cells produced that contain HbF (F cells), the amount of HbF per F cell, and the variable preferential survival of F cells over non-F cells in the circulation.[141] Early investigators suggested that different "threshold" levels of HbF (between 10% and 20%) were necessary to ameliorate the clinical severity of SS disease.[278,279] In a natural history study, Platt and co-workers showed that any increment in HbF above 4% was associated with reduced pain crises[280] and that HbF levels greater than 9% were associated with decreased mortality.[247]

Three broad categories of genetic mutations that increase HbF in association with HbS have been described. Large deletions of the γδβ-globin gene region resulting in δβ-thalassemia or pancellular HPFH are rare in the general sickle cell population (see Chapter 20 for more details on these deletions). HbS–pancellular HPFH patients represent a unique syndrome in which one finds between 24% and 34% HbF distributed in all red cells, no anemia, minimal microcytosis (MCV of 78.8 μm^3), and no clinical disease.[281-283]

A second group of mutations that increase HbF in SCD are linked to the β-globin gene region and are termed *nondeletion HPFH*.[284-287] Some linked mutations may be associated with single nucleotide substitutions in the promoter regions of the γ genes; however, such mutations are quite rare in the general SS population.[288] HbF is usually distributed heterogeneously in these disorders, but some have been associated with a pancellular distribution. Another type of linked nondeletion mutation that may increase HbF (^{G}γ-C158→T) is associated with the Senegal and Arab–Indian (Saudi) β-globin haplotypes.[20,25-28] These haplotypes are found commonly in genetic isolates in Western Africa, in Shiite Saudi Arabians, and in the Orissa region of India.[289-292] Among U.S. patients with sickle cell anemia, less than 10% have one chromosome with either of these haplotypes and less than 2% are homozygous for the Senegal haplotype.[18,19]

A third group of genetic disorders that influence HbF levels in patients with SS disease are not linked to the β-globin region.[293-295] A third of full siblings each with SS disease have significantly different genetic programs for production of HbF.[295] Because both siblings inherited the same γδβ-globin regions from their sickle trait parents, the HbF program must be separate from the γδβ-globin region. After Myoshi and associates[296] noted that HbF (defined by F-cell levels) in normal blood donors was inherited in an X-linked pattern, it was shown that F-cell production in sickle cell patients was inherited by a diallelic gene on the short arm of the X chromosome, Xp22-23, termed the F-cell production (FCP) locus.[297] The FCP locus accounted for 40% of the variation in HbF levels in sickle cell anemia patients and one form of β-thalassemia in Sicily.[298,299] However, twin studies of normal individuals by Thein and colleagues have not detected an X-linked locus[300] but suggested a locus on chromosome 8 that may interact with β-globin haplotypes. Thein has localized another genetic locus that controls F-cell levels in normal white individuals and in an Asian-Indian kindred to chromosome 6q22.3[301] and

recently has identified a potential role for the gene *cMYB* in regulation of HbF levels in this population.[302] Steinberg and colleagues, using haplotype mapping of SNPs, have recently shown in 1311 SS individuals that 6q22.3-23.2, the *TOX* gene on chromosome 8, and Xp22.2-22.3 are involved in baseline HbF levels.[303] They also showed that these same regions on chromosomes 6 and 8 and loci on chromosomes 1, 12, 13, and 14 were involved in the change in HbF levels in response of SS patients to hydroxyurea. BCL11A on chromosome 2, along with the C-MYB region on chromosome 6, has been associated with HbF levels in a genome-wide association study of thalassemia and SS patients in the Cooperative Study of Sickle Cell Disease (CSSCD).[304] In addition to these disorders, it has been shown that α-thalassemia is associated with decreased HbF levels in SS disease. The differences in HbF levels among SS patients with or without α–thalassemia may be indirectly related to the lowered MCHC of the SS-thalassemia red cells. Preferential survival of F cells over non-F cells is less in SS–α-thalassemia because the non-F cells in α-thalassemia have less cation loss and a lower MCHC, which reduces HbS polymerization and results in a longer life span.[137,263]

Genetic Modifiers of Clinical Subphenotypes. It is likely that networks of genes that respond to or modulate hemolysis, vasoregulation, inflammation, cell adhesion, hemostasis, and oxidative stress play roles in the severity of SS disease (Table 19-1; see also Fig. 19-1). As knowledge of the genes involved in these various pathways has increased, numerous investigators have used candidate gene approaches to study the association of genetic modifiers with clinical complications in SS disease. The studies published thus far on large cohorts of SS patients who have been rigorously phenotyped are most likely to yield the best evidence for genetic modifiers. However, by definition, the candidate gene approach will not identify unknown networks of genes or unknown genes in a defined pathway involved in the clinical phenotype. Association between a genetic variant and a phenotype does not necessarily mean causality. Association studies alone may identify SNPs within a gene, but this association may indicate that the gene is involved or that genes in linkage disequilibrium with the SNP are involved. In addition, studies that look at large number of genes or numerous polymorphisms in a single gene are likely to lead to false-positive associations. Finally, most associations, albeit statistically significant, have shown relatively small effects (<5% of the variation), thus suggesting that a large number of genes are likely to be involved in any one clinical subphenotype.

The hemolysis associated with the sickle mutation leads to release of free hemoglobin, scavenging of NO, and increased oxidative stress. Clinical phenotypes associated with increased hemolysis in SS disease include stroke, priapism, PHT, and leg ulcers.[317] Interestingly, priapism,[318,319] leg ulcers,[320,321] and PHT[322] are seen to a lesser extent in other hemolytic anemias. Among the so-called hemolytic phenotypes, certain common genetic

TABLE 19-1	Putative Genetic Modifiers Identified by Single Nucleotide Polymorphisms of Candidate Genes
Genetic Modifiers	**Clinical Subphenotype**
VCAM-1,[305] TGF-β/BMP,[306] SELP,[306] ANXA2,[306] BMP6,[306] ERG,[306] ILA4R,[307] TNF,[307] LDLR,[307] ADRB2[307]	Nonhemorrhagic stroke
BMPR2,[308] TGF-β/BMP,[308] ADCY6,[309] ADRB1[308]	Pulmonary hypertension
UGT1A[310]	Cholelithiasis/ hyperbilirubinemia
BMPR1B[311]	Renal failure
KL,[312] TGF-β/BMP,[312] ANXA2[312]	Osteonecrosis
KL[313]	Priapism
TGF-β/BMP,[314] IGF1R[314]	Bacteremia/sepsis
KL,[315] TGF-β/BMP,[315] TEK[315]	Leg ulcers
TOX,[316] AQP9,[316] MAP2K1,[316] HBS1l-MYB,[316] SMAD,[316] GPM6B,[316] BCL11A[304]★	Elevated hemoglobin F

*Performed by genome-wide association technology, not candidate gene analysis.

ADCY6, adenylate cyclase 6 gene; ADRB2, beta-adrenergic receptor gene; ANXA2, annexin A2; AQP9, aquaporin 9; BCL11A, B cell lymphoma 11A gene; BMP, bone morphogenetic protein; BMPR, bone morphogenetic protein receptor; ERG, Ets (transcription factor)–related gene; GPM6B, golli-myelin basic protein gene; HBS1l-MYB, intergenic region of the gene for HBS1L (a G-protein/elongation factor) and the *MYB* oncogene; IGF, insulin-like growth factor; IGFR1, insulin-like growth factor receptor gene; IL4HR, interleukin-4 receptor gene; KL, Klotho; LDLR, low-density lipoprotein receptor; MAP2K1, mitogen-activated protein kinase 2 gene; SELP, soluable P-selectin gene; SMAD, signaling mediators and antagonists of the transforming growth factor-beta (TGF-beta); TEK, tyrosine kinase receptor gene; TGF-β, transforming growth factor β; TNF, tumor necrosis factor; TOX, thymocyte selection–associated HMG box protein gene; UGT1A1, Uridine diphosphate-glucuronosyltransferase 1A1; VCAM-1, vascular cell adhesion molecule 1.

modifiers appear. Polymorphisms of Klotho (KL), a gene that encodes a membrane protein that regulates many vascular functions, including expression of vascular endothelial growth factor and release of NO by endothelium,[323] is associated with priapism[324] and leg ulcers.[315] KL may also participate in bone metabolism and is associated with an increase risk for osteonecrosis of the hip or the shoulder (or both) in SS patients.[312]

Several subphenotypes (stroke,[306] leg ulcers,[315] osteonecrosis,[312] PHT,[325] and bacteremia[314]) are associated with genes in the transforming growth factor β/bone morphogenic protein (TGF-β/BMP) pathway. BMPs, including *BMP6*, are pleiotropic secreted proteins structurally related to TGF-β and activins. BMP6 and SAND (a transcription factor activated by BMP6) are involved in inflammatory processes[326] and are important for bone formation.[327] The TGF-β/BMP pathway also consist of genes that play a role in cell proliferation, tissue repair, immune surveillance, and inflammation.[328,329]

Some genes have been implicated in similar disorders in the normal population and in patients with SCD: polymorphisms in P-selectin (SELP) are associated with an increased risk for stroke in the normal population[330] and in SCD patients,[306] BMPR2 is associated with both familial and sporadic PHT in normal individuals[331] and in SCD,[325] and polymorphisms of UGT1A are associated with hyperbilirubinemia in normal persons (Gilbert's syndrome)[332] and with higher bilirubin levels and gallstones in sickle cell patients.[310]

Ultimately, identification of genetic modifiers should lead to detection of sickle cell individuals at increased risk for a particular complication. Because it is likely that multiple factors are involved, few studies have been robust enough to test the predictability of their findings in a general SS population. Sebastiani and colleagues analyzed 114 individuals (7 with and 107 without stroke) not included in their original study of genetic modifiers of stroke in SS disease. The polymorphism associated with six SNPs in five genes (ANXA2, BMP6, SELP, TGF-β3, and ERG) gave an overall predicted accuracy of 98.2%.[306] Reproduction of these findings has not yet been performed.

DIAGNOSIS

The Fetus. The ability to perform prenatal diagnosis for sickle cell anemia has progressed rapidly in the past 3 decades. In 1978, Kan and Dozy[333] described DNA polymorphisms around the β-globin gene that were in linkage disequilibrium with the β^S gene, thereby leading to the first DNA-based method for prenatal diagnosis. Identification of the A→T substitution in codon 6 responsible for the glutamic acid–to-valine change in β-globin can be detected by alteration of a site of a specific restriction enzyme, by homologous synthetic oligonucleotides that detect a single base substitution, and by polymerase chain reaction amplification of DNA.[334-340] With the advent of polymerase chain reaction amplification of specific DNA sequences, sufficient DNA can be obtained from a very small number of fetal cells, thereby eliminating the necessity for culture of fetal fibroblasts.[341,342] Chorionic villus biopsy offers an alternative to amniocentesis for obtaining fetal cells as early as 8 to 10 weeks' gestation.[343,344] Preimplantation genetic diagnosis of single blastomeres by single-cell polymerase chain reaction followed by standard in vitro fertilization has led to the birth of unaffected twins to a couple both with sickle trait.[345]

The Newborn. A newborn with sickle cell anemia is not generally anemic and is asymptomatic because of the protective effect of HbF. The "sickle prep" and solubility tests are unreliable during the first few months of life. Because recognition of the disease in a newborn can lead to prevention of mortality and morbidity, it is now recommended that all newborns at risk be screened for sickle cell anemia. Screening combined with comprehensive follow-up care was first begun by Pearson in New Haven and Serjeant and colleagues in Jamaica in the 1970s.[346,347] Present screening methodologies include acid and alkaline electrophoresis, high-performance liquid chromatography, and isoelectric focusing. These tests can be performed on cord blood or on a dried blood specimen blotted on filter paper. False-negative screening results with these methods have been reported in infants who received perinatal transfusions before screening.[348] Diagnosis can also be performed by polymerase chain reaction amplification of DNA extracted from filter paper.[349] Universal screening versus targeted screening of newborns of parents "at risk" has been shown to identify more infants with disease and prevent more deaths and is cost effective in areas in which sickle trait occurs in 7 to 15 per 1000 births.[350,351]

The Older Child. After the first few months of life, as β^S-globin production increases and HbF declines, the clinical syndrome of sickle cell anemia emerges (Table 19-2). Although at 1 week of age the hemoglobin level of SS infants is statistically lower than that of AA infants, the overlap between the two groups is considerable and

does not diverge much before the second month of life.[346] Anemia and reticulocytosis are usually evident by 4 months of age.[346] ISCs are frequently absent from the peripheral blood of young children, and the morphology is typical of that of normal newborns—target cells, fragments, and poikilocytes. By 3 years of age, the typical peripheral blood smear is seen, including ISCs, target cells, spherocytes, fragments, biconcave discs, Howell-Jolly bodies, and nucleated red cells. The amount of HbF decreases with age, as in normal children, but it occurs much more slowly.[346,352]

CLINICAL MANIFESTATIONS

The clinical manifestations of SCD are extremely variable. Some patients are entirely asymptomatic, whereas others are constantly plagued by painful episodes. Most

TABLE 19-2   Hematology of Infants with SS Disease, SC Disease, and S–β⁺-Thalassemia

		AGE (mo)										
	Percentile	2-3	4-5	6-8	9-11	12-14	15-17	18-23	24-29	30-35	36-47	48-60
SS DISEASE												
Hemoglobin	5	7.0	7.0	7.1	7.2	7.2	7.2	7.1	6.9	6.7	6.4	6.6
level (g/dL)	50	9.3	9.2	9.2	9.2	9.1	9.0	8.9	8.6	8.3	8.1	8.3
	95	11.4	11.3	11.4	11.5	11.5	11.5	11.3	11.1	10.9	10.5	10.4
Mean	5	72	69	68	67	67	67	67	68	69	71	72
corpuscular	50	84	81	81	82	82	83	84	85	86	88	90
volume (fL)	95	96	94	94	95	96	96	96	97	97	98	100
Fetal	5	14.6	12.3	10.8	9.1	7.8	6.7	5.6	4.8	4.5	4.4	3.3
hemoglobin	50	43.5	34.1	29.1	24.3	20.6	17.7	14.8	12.8	12.4	12.4	9.0
level (%)	95	68.5	59.0	53.0	47.3	42.7	39.1	35.3	32.5	31.2	29.6	21.9
Reticulocyte	5	1.0	1.1	1.2	1.3	1.4	1.6	1.9	2.3	2.6	2.7	1.8
count (%)	50	4.0	5.1	5.9	6.7	7.4	8.0	8.7	9.3	9.8	10.4	11.8
	95	15.5	17.9	19.4	20.7	21.8	22.5	23.2	23.5	23.6	23.6	25.8
SC DISEASE												
Hemoglobin	5	8.0	8.2	8.6	8.9	9.2	9.3	9.5	9.5	9.4	9.3	9.6
level (g/dL)	50	9.7	9.8	10.1	10.3	10.5	10.6	10.7	10.8	10.7	10.6	10.6
	95	11.6	11.5	11.7	11.8	12.0	12.0	12.1	12.2	12.2	12.1	11.9
Mean	5	68	65	64	64	63	63	63	63	64	66	69
corpuscular	50	81	78	77	75	74	74	74	74	76	77	77
volume (fL)	95	91	88	86	85	84	84	84	84	86	88	87
Fetal	5	13.6	2.9	2.9	3.1	3.1	2.9	2.4	1.4	0.5	0.0	2.0
hemoglobin	50	31.6	17.9	14.5	11.6	9.3	7.4	5.5	4.2	3.9	4.4	4.2
level (%)	95	54.0	39.1	32.1	25.7	20.9	17.6	14.7	13.8	14.7	15.9	8.3
Reticulocyte	5	0.8	0.8	0.8	0.7	0.7	0.7	0.7	0.7	0.7	0.7	0.9
count (%)	50	2.8	2.8	2.7	2.6	2.5	2.5	2.5	2.6	2.7	2.9	2.8
	95	8.2	8.8	8.9	9.0	8.9	8.7	8.4	8.0	7.9	8.8	13.4
S–β⁺-THALASSEMIA												
Hemoglobin	5	9.2	9.4	9.1	8.5	9.1	9.1	9.9	10.0	9.8	9.3	10.0
level (g/dL)	50	10.8	10.9	11.0	10.8	10.6	11.2	10.9	11.0	10.7	10.6	10.8
	95	12.4	12.7	13.5	11.8	14.1	12.0	12.0	13.0	11.3	11.6	11.2
Mean	5	70	64	61	61	63	82	63	61	66	64	66
corpuscular	50	80	73	72	69	72	70	70	70	72	76	68
volume (fL)	95	88	83	84	75	84	73	77	79	76	76	76
Reticulocyte	5	1.1	0.0	1.1	0.9	0.8	0.9	0.7	1.5	1.2	1.0	3.0
count (%)	50	2.6	1.8	2.5	2.5	3.0	2.5	2.4	2.2	3.4	2.2	4.1
	95	8.5	6.4	2.5	4.6	5.9	7.4	5.1	6.2	7.4	7.6	5.7

Data from Brown AK, Sleeper LA, Miller ST, et al. Reference values and hematologic changes from birth to five years in patients with sickle cell disease. Arch Pediatr Adolesc Med. 1994;148:796-804.

patients fall between these extremes and have relatively long asymptomatic periods punctuated by occasional clinical crises. The complex nature of the clinical variability from patient to patient and from time to time in each patient has been prospectively studied on a large scale by the CSSCD under the auspices of the Sickle Cell Disease Branch of the National Heart, Lung, and Blood Institute (NHLBI).[353,354]

Sickle Cell Crisis

The term *sickle cell crisis* was defined by Diggs[355] as "any new syndrome that develops rapidly in patients with sickle cell disease due to the inherited abnormality." There are three categories of sickle crisis—vaso-occlusive, sequestration, and aplastic—and they are covered individually in the next few sections. The best perspective on how these acute events play out in a typical group of children comes from a report by Gill and colleagues describing the experience of almost 700 infants monitored for 10 years as part of the CSSCD.[356] The age at first event is displayed in Figure 19-7.

Vaso-occlusive Sickle Crises

Vaso-occlusive crises are acute, often painful episodes caused by intravascular sickling and tissue infarction. In a prospective study of children with SS disease moni-

tored since birth in Jamaica, painful crisis was the first symptom in more than a fourth of the patients and the most frequent symptom after the age of 2 years.[357] Painful episodes are such a prominent manifestation of the disease that African tribal names for SCD are onomatopoeic repetitive descriptions of pain, such as "chwech-weechwa" (Ga tribe), "nwiiwii" (Fante tribe), "nucdudui" (Ewe tribe), and "ahotutuo" (Twi tribe). Tribal names translate as "beaten up," "body biting," and "body chewing."[358] Vaso-occlusive episodes are the major clinical manifestations of SCD and occur most commonly in the bones, lungs, liver, spleen, brain, and penis. Frequently, the differential diagnosis is very difficult because there is no definitive objective hallmark of a vaso-occlusive crisis.

Painful Crisis. The most common acute vaso-occlusive crisis is acute pain. Virtually all patients with SS disease experience some degree of acute pain. For many, these episodes are mild and are handled entirely at home, school, or work. Little is known about the extent or nature of pain-coping activities that go on outside the medical environment, but diary studies suggest that it is enormous. The "tip" of the pain "iceberg" is made of episodes that drive patients to seek medical attention. These episodes vary widely among patients[280] (Fig. 19-8) and represent the most common reason for patients to

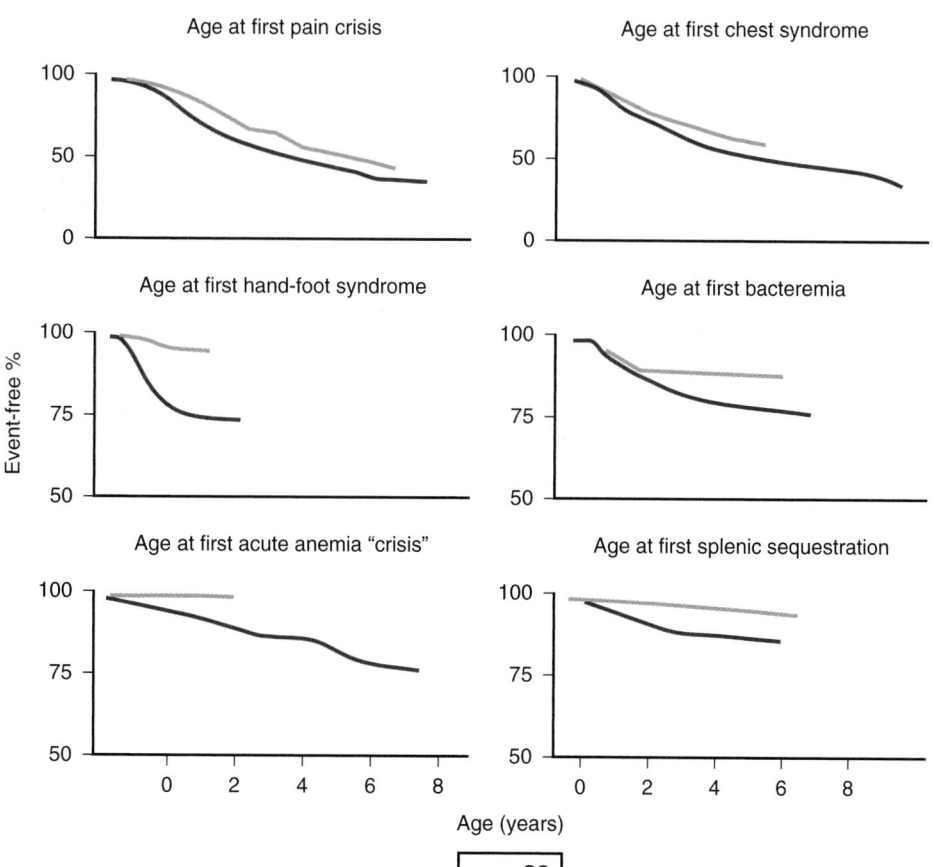

FIGURE 19-7. Age at first clinical event in patients with sicke cell disease, from birth to 10 years of age. **A,** Painful events. **B,** Acute chest syndrome. **C,** Hand-foot syndrome. **D,** Bacteremia. **E,** Acute anemic crisis. **F,** Splenic sequestration. *(Adapted from Gill FM, Sleeper LA, Weiner SJ, et al. Clinical events in the first decade in a cohort of infants with sickle cell disease. Cooperative Study of Sickle Cell Diseases. Blood. 1995;86: 776-783.)*

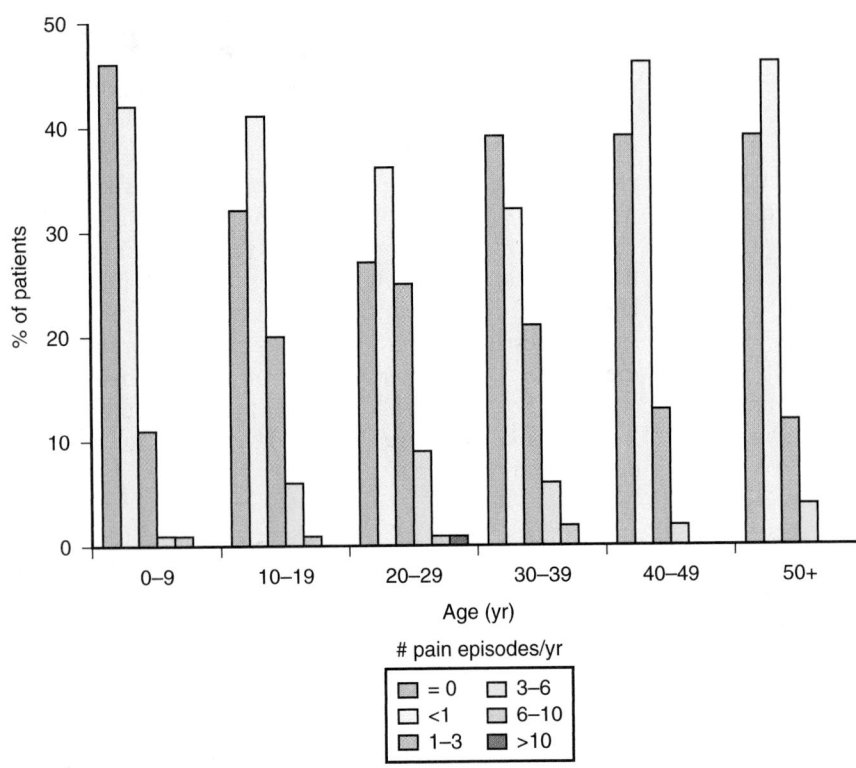

FIGURE 19-8. Distribution of pain rate in patients with SS disease. *(Data from Platt OS, Thorington BD, Brambilla DJ, et al. Pain in sickle cell disease. Rates and risk factors. N Engl J Med. 1991;325:11-16.)*

visit outpatient offices and emergency departments and be admitted for inpatient care. Despite the fact that there is variation in how or why individual patients decide to seek attention for a given episode of pain, epidemiologic evidence strongly indicates that patients with higher rates of medical attention for pain have lower levels of HbF, higher WBC counts, higher steady-state hemoglobin concentrations, and higher mortality.[247,280] Some studies have suggested that infections, changes in climate,[359,360] and psychological factors may precipitate pain episodes, although commonly no precipitating factors can be identified. These patients typically have a rapid onset of deep, gnawing, throbbing pain, usually without any abnormal physical or laboratory findings but sometimes accompanied by local tenderness, erythema, warmth, and swelling. The underlying pathology is bone marrow ischemia, sometimes leading to frank infarction with acute inflammatory infiltrates.[361-363] The most frequently involved areas are the lumbosacral spine, knee, shoulder, elbow, and femur. Less often, the sternum, ribs, clavicles, calcaneus, iliac crest, mandible, and zygoma are involved.[358] Joint effusions during acute episodes are particularly common in the knees and elbows. Typically, aspiration yields straw-colored fluid, usually with a "noninflammatory" profile. Rarely, sterile purulent exudates are found.[364] Given the range of marrow involvement and inflammatory response, it is not surprising that the patients with the most inflammation mimic the findings of osteomyelitis and those without findings are at risk of being considered malingerers.

Even in patients with measurable signs of inflammation, the diagnosis of infarction is favored over osteomyelitis. The results of one study suggest that acute long bone infarction is at least 50 times more common than osteomyelitis.[365] In this study of 41 acute long bone infarcts, 38% affected the humerus, 23% affected the tibia, and 19% affected the femur. All patients experienced local tenderness, with swelling in 85%, joint findings in 68%, and local heat in 65%. Fourteen percent appeared "toxic," 21% had a temperature higher than 39° C, and 43% had a temperature lower than 38° C. The total WBC count ranged between 7200 and 43,000 cells/mm^3, with a mean of 17,000. The mean sedimentation rate was 30.5 mm/hr, with a range of 3 to 66. Although various radionuclide scans have been suggested as a way of distinguishing between infarction and infection,[366-370] in many studies[371-373] such investigations were inconclusive. Magnetic resonance imaging (MRI) of patients with SS disease shows decreased intensity of short relaxation time/echo time pulse sequence imaging as a result of hyperplastic marrow that converts to high intensity on long relaxation time/echo time images in painful crises,[363] but no definitive series has compared infarction with infection. Therefore, despite the progress made in the development and use of imaging techniques, a definitive diagnosis of osteomyelitis in SCD still relies more on clinical assessment together with positive cultures from blood or bone obtained by aspiration or biopsy than on any single imaging modality.[374]

Except for a positive blood or tissue culture, no laboratory test can differentiate acute infection from a painful crisis.[362,375] Needle aspiration and culture of the highly suspicious area are critical in isolating the organism and should be done before initiating empirical antibiotic therapy. The aspirated fluid may be quite purulent, even in the patients with sterile infarcts. In most series, the most common organism causing osteomyelitis is *Salmonella*,[376] although *Staphylococcus*, *Streptococcus pneumoniae*, and gram-negative enteric bacilli are also common.[377] Initial empirical antibiotic therapy should be chosen to cover these possibilities. Treatment failures are seen when anything but the most aggressive antibiotic regimens are used.

As described earlier, episodes of acute bone pain and impressive signs of inflammation may be difficult to distinguish at outset from osteomyelitis. More common and just as challenging are the evaluation and management of severely painful episodes in patients without signs of inflammation. Some of these patients will show laboratory evidence of acute inflammation such as elevated C-reactive protein,[37] of fibrinolysis such as elevated D-dimers,[379,380] or of red cell trapping such as loss of dense cells.[381] These measurements are not helpful in the management of individual cases, nor should they be used in an attempt to "validate" an individual patient's report of symptoms. In a research setting, these measurements, done on large numbers of patients with and without symptoms, provide clues to potential innovative therapeutic interventions. For example, the common finding of elevated acute phase reactants stimulated a trial of methylprednisolone for treating acute bone pain.[382] This preliminary work showed that a short course of high-dose corticosteroid decreases the duration of severe pain but results in more "rebound" attacks after treatment is discontinued. Similarly, despite the fact that previous trials of aspirin therapy were not encouraging,[383] there is significant interest in the role of platelets,[384,385] soluble procoagulants,[206] anticoagulants,[386,387] and endothelial cells[254] in precipitation or propagation of vaso-occlusion to reopen this potential line of treatment.

In children younger than 5 years, the small bones of the hands and feet are frequently affected, and in contrast to most episodes of bone pain in older children, physical findings are common. This painful dactylitis ("hand-foot syndrome") is typically the first clinical manifestation of SCD. A young child cries with pain; refuses to bear weight; and has puffy, tender, and warm feet or hands, or both. The child may appear acutely ill, be febrile, and have an impressive leukocytosis. At the onset of soft tissue swelling, bony changes are not generally apparent on radiographs. After 1 to 2 weeks, subperiosteal new bone, irregular areas of radiolucency, cortical thinning, or complete destruction of bone can be seen. All the bone changes are usually reversible but may persist for as long as 8 months.[388,389] A rare complication, permanent shortening of the digits after hand-foot crisis, has been reported.[390] Dactylitis before 1 year of age is a strong predictor of overall severity (stroke, death, high pain rate, or recurrent ACS) by 10 years of age,[249] although recent single-institution evidence suggests that dactylitis is not a strong predictor of subsequent pain or ACS.[391] In addition to dactylitis, the risk for severe disease is further increased if the child has also experienced an episode in which the hemoglobin content dropped below 7 g/dL or the baseline WBC count is elevated (or both).[249]

Acute Chest Syndrome. ACS is an acute illness with lung injury characterized by any combination of chest pain, fever, or respiratory symptoms and accompanied by a new pulmonary infiltrate on a chest radiograph. The diagnostic criteria most commonly include radiographic evidence of a new segmental pulmonary infiltrate *and* one or more of the following: fever, tachypnea, cough, new-onset hypoxia, increased work of breathing (intercostal retractions, nasal flaring, accessory muscle use), or chest pain.[392] The term "acute chest syndrome" was introduced by Charache and co-workers[393]; it reflects the difficulty of establishing a definitive etiology and emphasizes the fact that in individual patients, knowing the specific etiology is less critical for management than being able to assess the magnitude and pace of the lung injury.

The critical pathophysiology is that only deoxygenated HbS polymerizes and that reoxygenation eradicates the polymer. The lung is the critical organ that protects the arterial side of the circulation from the sludge of sickle polymers. When the lung is injured, underventilated, or inflamed, protection is inadequate, and downstream tissues, including the injured lung itself, become increasingly susceptible to sickling and ischemia. In fact, when flow is eventually restored, reperfusion injury may occur, as suggested by the study by Kaul and Hebbel, who found that cycles of oxygenation/deoxygenation cause classic P-selectin–inhibitable movement of inflammatory cells to tissue in a sickle mouse model.[254]

Although some patients, particularly adults, are initially seen with a full-blown picture of chest pain, hypoxia, and abnormal x-ray findings, frequently the diagnosis becomes clear only days into an event that starts as a fever without source, abdominal pain, or extremity pain. The diagnosis of ACS can be very difficult to make. Children younger than 4 years often have few signs at initial evaluation: 35% to 40% have a normal lung examination, 30% to 40% have no tachypnea, and 30% to 50% have no tachycardia.[394] Radiographic evolution often lags behind clinical progression. In one series, only 36% of patients had abnormal radiographic findings on evaluation, although abnormal findings eventually developed in all.[395]

Vichinsky and associates demonstrated that almost half of all patients in whom ACS develops were initially admitted for other reasons, frequently with vaso-occlusive pain.[392] Opioid analgesics and pain in the spine, ribs, and abdomen can lead to hypoventilation with decreased tidal volume, development of atelectasis, and ventilation-perfusion (V/Q) mismatch. The subsequent hypoxemia results in further intrapulmonary sickling. Secretory phospholipase A_2 (sPLA2) and serum C-reactive protein have been proposed as possible laboratory predictors of the development of ACS.[396-398] Elevated sPLA2 as a trigger for simple transfusion appeared to reduce the risk of ACS developing in comparison to standard therapy in one small uncontrolled trial.[399]

ACS is a leading cause of morbidity and mortality. It represents the second most common acute complication (pain episode is first), with a rate of 12.8 cases per 100 patient-years,[248] and the most common condition at the time of death.[247,392] The highest incidence is found in children 2 to 4 years of age (25.3 per 100 patient-years in sickle cell anemia) and lowest in adults (8.8 per 100 patient-years in sickle cell anemia).[248] Patients who have not experienced an episode of ACS have longer life expectancy than do those who have, and those with a higher level of HbF and lower steady-state leukocyte count have a lower attack rate for ACS.[248] Hydroxyurea therapy lowers the attack rate in adults by about 50%.[400] Asthma appears to be a risk factor for ACS.[401-406]

Vichinsky and colleagues prospectively studied 671 episodes of ACS.[392,407] The most common causes were fat/bone marrow emboli and bacterial (Chlamydia, Mycoplasma), viral, or mixed infection. In contrast to patients with infection, those with bone marrow emboli were more likely to have an associated episode of bone pain, chest pain, abnormal neurologic symptoms, and fall in platelet count.[407]

Bacterial pneumonia was rare overall, but more common in children than adults, in whom it was associated with bacteremia in 58% of cases of *S. pneumoniae* and 18% of cases of *Haemophilus influenzae*.[394] Regardless of etiology, ACS is always accompanied by some degree of localized sickling and lung ischemia; in 16% of cases no precipitating embolus or pathogen was identified. Overall, the prognosis is poor. Thirteen percent of patients required mechanical ventilation, new abnormal neurologic findings developed in 11%, and 9% of patients who were 20 years or older died. In general, the death rate from ACS is four times higher in adults than children.[394]

There was a considerable change in blood counts at initial evaluation in patients with ACS. Hemoglobin dropped an average of 0.7 g/dL, and WBC counts increased an average of 69%. The mean Po_2 was 71 mm Hg, with a fifth of patients having a Po_2 of less than 60 mm Hg. Because the hemoglobin-oxygen dissociation curve varies among patients and because the shallow portion of the curve is between a Po_2 of 50 and 100 mm Hg, transcutaneous oxygen saturation measurements are not sufficient unless there are enough simultaneous direct measurements of arterial Po_2 to detect trends.[408] In one study, all children with SS disease and ACS had transcutaneous saturation measurements below 96% or only 3 points below their steady-state values.[409] Given that it is not unusual for a transcutaneous measurement to vary by as much as 3 points with slight differences in positioning of the probe, it is unwise to place too much reliance on single measurement in isolation. Unfortunately, no clinical findings are reliably predictive of the degree of hypoxia.[394]

Several important therapeutic principles emerged from the Vichinsky study.[392,394] First of all, bronchodilator therapy was remarkably effective in 20% of the patients with wheezing or pulmonary function tests indicating obstruction at initial evaluation (61% of all the patients). This is consistent with the observation that measurable airway hyperactivity has been documented in as many as 73% of children with SS, even without a history of asthma.[410] Second, red cell transfusion improved oxygenation. Simple transfusion was used in 68% of patients and appears to be as effective as exchange transfusion—although the study was not designed to test this hypothesis. It may be that the efficacy of simple transfusions relates to the fact that ACS is typically associated with a 0.5- to 1.0-g/dL decrease in hemoglobin at initial evaluation. Third, the prominence of *Chlamydia* and *Mycoplasma* underscores the importance of including macrolide antibiotics in the initial broad empirical therapy.

Optimal management of patients with ACS requires vigilant monitoring and considered judgment. A few guidelines are presented here, but they should not substitute for consultation and collaboration with a clinician experienced in managing this complex problem. All patients with ACS must be managed in the hospital, in a setting where they can have frequent monitoring of vital signs and arterial blood gases. Oxygen therapy is critically important in hypoxic patients. Broad-spectrum antibiotics, including a macrolide, should be used empirically after careful culturing while keeping in mind the prevalence of *Chlamydia*, *Mycoplasma*, *S. pneumoniae*, and *H. influenzae*. A trial of bronchodilator therapy should be instituted, especially in patients with a history of obstructive lung disease or those who exhibit wheezing on examination. A Po_2 of less than 75 mm (or a 25% decrease from baseline if the patient is chronically hypoxic) carries a poor prognosis.[386] Simple transfusion should be considered early for those with persistent or worsening hypoxia (Po_2 <75 mm Hg or a 25% decrease from baseline). Exchange transfusion is indicated if the hematocrit is high, the hypoxia is worsening, or the patient is deteriorating rapidly despite simple transfusion. Because the splinting and atelectasis associated with chest pain may exacerbate or even cause ACS, analgesic therapy should not be withheld from patients with chest pain but should titrated with extreme caution to analgesic effect. These patients may hover on the brink of hypoventilation from either too little or too much analgesia. Compulsive continuous monitoring of oxygen saturation and the respiratory rate monitoring and pain evaluation are critical. Fluid overload with pulmonary edema, congestive failure, or both is easy to achieve in the setting of ACS. Once normal hydration is attained, maintenance fluids should be given. Progression to respiratory failure is not uncommon if treatment is not early and aggressive, and mechanical ventilation is sometimes required. Both high-frequency ventilation[411] and extracorporeal membrane oxygenation[412,413] have been used successfully in severe cases of respiratory failure in ACS. In ventilated patients, bronchoscopy may have both diagnostic and therapeutic benefit by detection of plastic bronchitis and removal of branching bronchial casts that can exacerbate the hypoxemia and V/Q mismatch.[414,415] Alternatively, nebulized recombinant human DNase has shown some efficacy in plastic bronchitis.[416] Preliminary evidence suggests that inhaled NO, a selective pulmonary vasodilator, may be of benefit in severe cases.[417,418] However, there have been no controlled studies confirming a role of NO therapy in the treatment of ACS.

Although most patients with ACS recover uneventfully, the course is unpredictable, and rapid, unexpected deterioration is common. Most series of ACS include a section on autopsy findings. Pulmonary postmortem findings typically include areas of alveolar wall necrosis and focal parenchymal scars.[419] In one autopsy, multiple large infarcts but no accompanying occluded vessels were found, thus suggesting that severe vasospasm may play a role in some cases.[420]

Acute Abdominal Pain. Severe acute abdominal pain is a common event that often poses a difficult differential diagnosis. The cause of this syndrome is unknown, although mesenteric sickling and vertebral disease with nerve root compression have been suggested. This type of crisis can be accompanied by guarding, tenderness, rebound, fever, and leukocytosis that are indistinguishable from an acute surgical abdomen. Frequently, the patient is the best judge and is aware of whether the pain is characteristic of a "crisis."

These patients should receive the general supportive measures described later in this chapter, with the omission of high-dose analgesics. Patients should be given nothing by mouth and be monitored closely by both medical and surgical personnel. Abdominal films, including upright views, may be helpful in identifying a perforated viscus. Usually, a patient with vaso-occlusive pain will remain stable or improve slightly with hydration and mild sedation. In extreme cases in which the clinical situation is deteriorating, emergency surgical exploration may be necessary. Simple or exchange transfusion should be done if possible before surgery.

Acute right upper quadrant pain may be a result of acute cholecystitis or intrahepatic sickling.[421,422] Abdominal ultrasonography will indentify cholelithiasis and choledocholithiasis in the hands of a skilled operator. The presence of gallstones and a clinical syndrome characteristic of cholecystitis does not necessarily mean that the symptoms are due to the stones. Many patients and their physicians have been disappointed when their "cholecystitis" returned after cholecystectomy. In a retrospective study of acute abdomen in 28 patients with SS disease,[423] the presence of gallstones on ultrasound evaluation did not predict which patients could be managed without surgery. Sickle patients with acute cholecystitis should undergo surgery only after the gallbladder has had a chance to "cool down" because postoperative management can be fraught with complications.[424] (For further discussion, see the section on the hepatobiliary system.)

Intrahepatic sickling can result in acute right upper quadrant pain from acute sickle hepatic crisis, hepatic sequestration, or sickle cell intrahepatic cholestasis (or any combination of these conditions). Acute hepatic crisis occurs in approximately 10% of patients with sickle cell anemia[422] and is commonly manifested as acute right upper quadrant pain, tender hepatomegaly, nausea, low-grade fever, and jaundice. Transaminases are rarely greater than 300 IU/L, and serum bilirubin levels are usually less than 15 mg/dL.[422,425] The crisis generally resolves within 2 weeks with intravenous hydration and analgesia. Hepatic sequestration is also manifested as sudden tender hepatomegaly; however, in contrast, it is accompanied by acute anemia but without cholestasis or transaminitis.[426,427] Treatment is to replace circulating volume by crystalloid or simple transfusion. Transfusion must be undertaken judiciously because the liver may "release" the endogenous sickle erythrocytes, which can lead to an elevated hematocrit and subsequent problems secondary to hyperviscosity. Exchange transfusion should be considered. Sickle cell intrahepatic cholestasis is a severe syndrome consisting of right upper quadrant pain, nausea/vomiting, fever, tender hepatomegaly, leukocytosis, and extreme direct hyperbilirubinemia. The spectrum of this entity includes acute liver failure with bleeding diatheses, encephalopathy, renal failure, and progression to multiorgan failure, and it is associated with high mortality.[425,428,429] These hepatic complications are not to be confused with "benign hyperbilirubinema" described by Buchanan and Glader,[421] which is characterized by marked conjugated hyperbilirubinemia, only mild transaminitis, and no liver synthetic dysfunction. This entity resolves spontaneously within 2 to 8 weeks and may represent a very mild variant of intrahepatic cholestasis.

Acute Central Nervous System Event. Acute infarction of the brain can result in a devastating stroke, which occurs in approximately 7% of children with SCD.[430,431] The incidence is estimated to be 0.7% per year during the first 20 years of life, with the highest rates in children 5 to 10 years of age.[432] This disaster may occur as an isolated event but also appears in the setting of evolving ACS, aplastic crisis, viral illness, painful crisis, priapism, or dehydration.[430,431] The most common underlying lesion is an intracranial arterial stenosis or obstruction, usually in the internal carotid and often in the proximal middle cerebral or anterior cerebral arteries.[433-435] Pathologically, these vessels, whose endothelium has presumably been chronically injured by sickle erythrocytes, show heaped-up intima with proliferation of fibroblasts and smooth muscle.[436] The lumen may be narrowed or completely obliterated by the vascular lesion, thus suggesting that *acute* sickling may simply be the "last straw" causing acute infarction in the setting of a chronic vasculopathy. Hemiparesis, focal seizures, gait dysfunction, and speech defects are the most common signs.

A careful discussion of the evaluation of a child with new neurologic symptoms is provided by Adams.[437] As soon as cerebral ischemia is suspected and the patient is stabilized, the best initial diagnostic test is a non–contrast-enhanced computed tomography (CT) scan. Although CT may not be positive for infarction within the first 6 hours of ischemia, it can rule out hemorrhage or nonischemic causes. Diffusion-weighted MRI and fluid-attenuated inversion recovery (FLAIR) sequences are highly sensitive and provide better detail of the areas of ischemia within minutes of ischemia.[438-440] The typical findings are infarcts associated with obstruction of major vessels or distal obstruction of smaller vessels leading to infarction in the "border zone" area between the anterior cerebral and middle cerebral vessels.[441,442] Assessment of the intracranial and cervical artery vasculature by three-dimensional time-of-flight (TOF) magnetic resonance angiography (MRA) is becoming increasingly useful in the early evaluation of a patient with new symptoms[443] and is nearly as accurate as conventional cerebral angiography.[444]

The standard approach to treating a patient with acute infarction is immediate exchange transfusion (see the section on transfusion for details). If exchange transfusion is delayed, temporization by hydration with crystalloid and simple transfusion may be beneficial. There are no data on the use of recombinant tissue plasminogen activator (tPA) in sickle-associated cerebral ischemia. Patients treated by exchange transfusion usually show marked improvement in motor function, although the prognosis is considerably worse for those with multiple infarcts. After the initial exchange, a chronic maintenance transfusion program should be carried out (see "Transfusion"). In untreated patients, the mortality rate is approximately 20%, with about 70% of patients experiencing a recurrence within 3 years. In these untreated patients, more than 70% were left with permanent motor disabilities and a deficit in IQ.[430] A regular chronic maintenance transfusion program designed to keep HbS less than 30% reduces the incidence of stroke to 10% to 15%, which is a 90% reduction in stroke rate in comparison to no intervention.[434,445-448] Patients whose initial stroke was temporally unrelated to another medical event (e.g., ACS) are at higher risk for recurrent stroke while receiving regular transfusions.[449] Repeat arteriograms in patients maintained on transfusion generally, but not invariably show stabilization and smoothing of intimal lesions, whereas untransfused patients demonstrate progression of disease.[445] The appropriate duration of chronic erythrocyte transfusions for secondary stroke prophylaxis has not been firmly established. Two prospective studies documented a very high risk for recurrent stroke (60% to 70%) after discontinuation of either a short-term (1 to 2 years) or long-term (5 to 12 years) transfusion regimen.[434,450] Therefore, it is recommended that the maintenance transfusion program be continued indefinitely to prevent secondary stroke. In one informative series, liberalization of the transfusion regimen allowed the pretransfusion percentage of HbS to rise to 50% and effectively prevented recurrent infarction over 84 months

of follow-up.[451] Unfortunately, liberalization did not prevent hemorrhage—two patients died, one of intraventricular and one of subarachnoid bleeding. Though clearly beneficial, indefinite maintenance transfusion carries the risks of allosensitization,[452] autoantibody formation,[453] transfusion-borne infections, and the certain problem of iron overload. Bone marrow transplantation in patients with strokes can be curative,[454] although parenchymal brain disease may progress.[455] Hydroxyurea treatment to increase HbF and as an alternative to chronic transfusion[456] effectively prevented secondary stroke in a single institution,[457] and a prospective randomized trial is under way.[458]

Application of newer techniques for noninvasive assessment of the brain and its vasculature has focused attention on two new areas—identifying children at high risk for stroke and identifying children with "asymptomatic" brain disease. Adams and associates demonstrated that children with abnormally increased blood flow in their intracerebral arteries as measured by transcranial Doppler (TCD) had a relative risk of stroke of 44 (95% confidence interval, 5.5 to 346).[459] A systematic study of MRI findings in asymptomatic children with SCD revealed that unanticipated infarcts are highly predictive of subsequent clinical stroke.[460] However, in older children (mean age of 11 years) without evidence of previous central nervous system (CNS) disease, abnormal TCD and MRI findings are often discordant, thus indicating that these tests may be measuring different aspects of CNS pathology in these subjects.[461] MRI has revealed that as many as 17% of children older than 6 years have evidence of silent infarcts,[462] and in one study of 36 asymptomatic children 7 to 48 months of age, the incidence was 11%.[463] These silent infarcts are associated with impaired performance on psychometric tests that measure fine motor skills and cognitive ability.[464,465] Older children (>6 years) with silent infarcts were more likely to have a history of seizures, low hemoglobin level, and high WBC count (>11.8 × 10⁹/L).[462] In a study of 392 children monitored prospectively up to 10 years, an elevated WBC count, dactylitis, and low hemoglobin content (<7 g/dL) before the age of 2 years were associated with adverse outcomes, including strokes.[249] In other studies, low hematocrit,[466] ACS,[467] and hypertension[468] have been associated with silent infarcts, clinical strokes, or both. In the multicenter prospective Stroke Prevention Trial in Sickle Cell Anemia (STOP) of 130 asymptomatic children with abnormal Doppler flow measurements (>200 cm/sec), subjects were randomized to transfusions or standard care. The study was terminated early when it was shown that only 1 of 63 transfused children versus 11 of 67 had strokes, a 92% decrease in the relative stroke rate in the treated group.[469] The NHLBI issued a Clinical Alert suggesting that children between the ages of 2 and 16 years be screened with Doppler and that transfusion therapy be considered for those with abnormal Doppler studies. A second randomized, controlled clinical trial (STOP 2) tested whether chronic transfusions for primary stroke prevention based on abnormal TCD findings could be safely discontinued after at least 30 months in children who had not had an overt stroke and who exhibited reversion to low-risk TCD flow measurements (<170 cm/sec) with chronic transfusion therapy. After 79 of a planned 100 children were randomized, the trial was also terminated early because 16 of 41 subjects randomized to stop transfusion achieved an end point (14 reversions to high-risk TCD findings without stroke and 2 ischemic strokes) versus 0 of 38 in those maintained on chronic transfusion treatment.[470] The NHLBI issued another Clinical Alert recommending continuation of transfusion and acknowledging the need for alternative therapy to transfusion for primary stroke prophylaxis. These observations suggest that TCD or MRI (or both) should be used to screen older children with poor school performance or evidence of other risks factors. Clinical trials under consideration or under way include transfusions,[471,472] hydroxyurea,[456,473] and bone marrow transplantation[474] in younger children with MRI evidence of silent infarcts or abnormal intracranial Doppler flow measurements.

Not all acute focal neurologic events in patients with sickle cell anemia are infarcts. Intracranial hemorrhage is the other major category of sickle-related CNS events, although the incidence may be higher in adults than in children.[467] These events are manifested as a sudden severe headache, sometimes with neck pain, vertigo, syncope, nystagmus, ptosis, meningismus, or photophobia. Many of these episodes are subarachnoid hemorrhages from small bleeding aneurysms that probably arise as a result of intimal damage during childhood. Multiple aneurysms with extensive collaterals (similar to moyamoya disease) have been found incidentally during angiographic evaluation of children with stroke.[436] Many risk factors for hemorrhagic stroke have been proposed, but few have been rigorously evaluated exclusively in children. Risk factors include increasing age, low steady-state hemoglobin concentration, high steady-state leukocyte count,[467] previous ischemic stroke,[475] moyamoya,[476] cerebral aneurysms,[477] ACS,[150] acute hypertension, transfusion,[478] and recent corticosteroid use.[479] Although mortality in some series approaches 50%,[430] some describe more successful aggressive neurosurgical approaches to these bleeding lesions[480-482] and suggest that angiography should be performed to identify patients with surgically amenable lesions.

Priapism. Priapism occurs in males of all ages. In a Jamaican study of 104 males aged 10 to 62 years, 42% reported at least one episode of priapism, with a median age at onset of 21 years.[483] A long-term follow-up of patients in Los Angeles determined that priapism develops in about 7% of SS and approximately 2% of SC males, with a median age at onset of about 22 years.[24] A questionnaire survey administered to 98 patients younger than 20 years in Dallas found the mean age at the initial episode to be 12 years, with an average number of episodes per patient of 15.7 and an 89% actuarial probability of experiencing priapism by 20 years of age.[484] Prolonged sexual arousal, fever, cold exposure, nocturnal tumescence (rapid eye movement [REM] sleep), full bladder, dehydration, alcohol, cocaine, and testosterone therapy have all been implicated as triggers.[485-487] Several genetic polymorphisms[324,489] (see "Genetic Modifiers") and particularly high hemolytic rates[317,482] have also been associated with a risk for priapism. Because early intervention and treatment may prevent irreversible penile fibrosis and impotence, to prevent embarrassment, patients and parents should be educated in advance of its occurrence to treat prolonged priapism as a urologic emergency.

Four clinical entities are described: stuttering priapism, with short (less than 2 to 3 hours), often multiple episodes; acute prolonged priapism (more than 24 hours), which can persist for weeks; chronic priapism, a painless induration that may last for years; and acute-on-chronic priapism, with acute painful episodes complicating chronic induration. Sexual dysfunction was reported by 46% of patients with a history of priapism.[483] In general, young patients with brief episodes restricted to the corpora cavernosa ("bicorporal priapism") are less likely to become dysfunctional,[490,491] whereas adults with involvement of the corpora cavernosa and corpus spongiosum ("tricorporal priapism") tend to have prolonged episodes and a better than 50% chance of becoming impotent.[492] Urinary retention requiring catheterization may complicate such acute episodes. Patients with tricorporal involvement are also particularly susceptible to acute severe neurologic complications and overall increased morbidity—even those treated by exchange transfusion.[493,494] They should be monitored closely for early neurologic symptoms, especially headache.

Diagnostic studies such as technetium scans, MRI, Doppler flow studies, measurements of corporal pressure, hemoglobin electrophoresis, and blood gases are currently being used in a variety of settings to help define the anatomy and potential prognostic features of priapism. As yet, they have not had an impact on clinical decision making in individual patients.[495-497]

A consensus on treatment of priapism has not been reached; no controlled clinical trials have been conducted to guide therapy.[498] Short episodes of acute priapism usually occur on awakening and can be managed at home. Patients should be instructed to urinate frequently, perform some vigorous exercise, increase fluid intake, soak in a warm tub, and take analgesics. If the episode does not resolve within a few hours, the patient should appear for medical treatment with intravenous fluid and analgesics. If the episode persists beyond 4 hours, intracavernosal aspiration and instillation of an α-agonist should be performed and repeated.[499,500] Although the role of RBC transfusion is somewhat controversial,[501] priapism may respond to simple red cell transfusion.[490] Exchange transfusion may produce results in 6 to 8 hours,[502,502] but most do not show signs of detumescence for 24 to 48 hours and some do not respond at all.[504] Use of intracorporal and oral α-adrenergic agents has been tried successfully in a small experimental group in Paris in both the acute and chronic setting,[500] and in one group of patients with stuttering priapism in Jamaica, stilbestrol was helpful in preventing recurrences.[505] Numerous therapeutic options have been attempted, including diethylstilbestrol, gonadotropin-releasing hormone analogues, various adrenergic agonists, and hydroxyurea.[498,506]

Surgical shunting procedures should be considered for patients who have not shown any signs of detumescence 12 to 24 hours after corporal irrigation, transfusion, or both, particularly if they are postpubertal. Historically, these procedures have carried a high complication rate with subsequent penile deformities and impotence. In fairness, it is difficult to determine how much of any observed adverse effects are related to the procedure and how much to the priapism itself. The most conservative shunt is Winter's procedure or one of its modifications, whereby a needle or scalpel is inserted through the glans into one of the corpora and the viscous blood is aspirated. This temporarily allows drainage of cavernous blood into the systemic circulation and has been used successfully in SS disease patients.[507] Intermittent compression with a blood pressure cuff is critical to limit refilling. Anecdotal evidence suggests that penile implants to correct impotence may be more easily inserted soon after an impotence-causing episode.[508,509]

Splenic Sequestration

One of the leading causes of death in children with sickle cell anemia is an acute splenic sequestration crisis.[510] Children with SS disease who have not yet undergone autosplenectomy, as well as older patients with SC disease or S–β-thalassemia,[511] may have sudden, rapid, massive enlargement of the spleen with trapping of a considerable portion of the red cell mass. Patients suddenly become weak and dyspneic, with a rapidly distending abdomen, left-sided abdominal pain, vomiting, and shock. The tempo of this crisis may be so fast that the patient dies before reaching the hospital. On physical examination, there may be profound hypotension with cardiac decompensation and massive splenomegaly. The hemoglobin concentration is at least 2 g/dL lower than baseline and is accompanied by a brisk reticulocytosis with increased nucleated red cells and moderate to severe thrombocytopenia.[510] This complication has been described as early as 8 weeks of age.[512]

Emond and colleagues described the natural history of acute sequestration crisis in a cohort of 308 children with SS disease in Jamaica.[513] Eighty-nine patients experienced 113 attacks, with 67 children having their first attack before the age of 2 years. There were 13 fatalities, 10 of which occurred before the age of 2. The most frequently associated clinical problem was upper respiratory tract infection and ACS. Sixteen percent of the patients had positive blood cultures. Recurrences are frequent and develop in 49% of survivors of the first attack. A

parental education program directed toward teaching parents the technique of spleen palpation and the urgency of seeking medical attention for an enlarged spleen and pallor led to an increase in the incidence of cases (from 4.6 to 11.3 per 100 patient-years of observation) and a decrease in the fatality rate (from 29.4 to 3.1 per 100 events).

Therapy consists of emergency restoration of intravascular volume and oxygen-carrying capacity by the immediate transfusion of packed red cells. Once normal cardiovascular status is restored, patients improve rapidly. The spleen usually shrinks within a few days, and the thrombocytopenia resolves. Care must be taken to not transfuse to baseline hemoglobin levels because with improvement, the spleen releases the endogenous erythrocytes and a relative erythrocytosis with hyperviscosity may result. Recurrence of sequestration is common, usually within 4 months of the initial episode. To eliminate recurrence, some have recommended elective splenectomy after the first significant episode[514]; others, concerned with postsplenectomy sepsis, have suggested splenectomy after two episodes of sequestration.[510] Emergency splenectomy during acute sequestration is not indicated.

Kinney and co-workers' review of splenic sequestration from Duke University strengthens the position of those who favor elective splenectomy for children who have had one episode of acute sequestration.[515] In this series of 23 patients, 4 underwent early splenectomy, 7 were observed carefully, and 12 were placed on a maintenance transfusion program. Of those treated by transfusion, two were well and still receiving transfusions, three had recurrences while still receiving transfusions, four experienced recurrence within 3 months of the last transfusion, and only three remained well at 11 months (3.9 years after the last transfusion). Fourteen percent of children became alloimmunized, and non-A, non-B hepatitis developed in 1. Eventually, 14 of the 23 patients underwent splenectomy. All were immunized against pneumococcus and were prescribed penicillin for prophylaxis. None had experienced a life-threatening infection 65.6 patient-years later. Serjeant's group has demonstrated in a 22.5-year follow-up study that postspenectomy children in Jamaica are not at greater risk for infection than a matched control group of SS patients.[516]

Rao and Gooden described a subacute form of sequestration in 11 patients characterized by increased spleen size, a 25% drop in hematocrit, less than 100,000 platelets, and elevation in the reticulocyte count above the patient's baseline. All responded to chronic transfusion programs, but seven patients had recurrent episodes after transfusions were stopped and eventually required splenectomy.[517]

Sequestration can also take place in the liver. Tender hepatomegaly, increased anemia, reticulocytosis, and hyperbilirubinemia are the usual clinical features,[421,426,427] but because the liver is not as distensible as the spleen, there is rarely pooling of red cells significant enough to cause cardiovascular collapse.

Aplastic Crisis

The clinical characteristics of the aplastic crisis of SCD have been well characterized.[518-520] In the normal steady state, a patient with sickle cell anemia can compensate for the decreased red cell survival (15 to 50 days) by increasing bone marrow output sixfold to eightfold. Temporary cessation of bone marrow activity because of suppression by intercurrent viral or bacterial infection causes the hematocrit value to fall as much as 10% to 15% per day with no compensatory reticulocytosis. The short-lived HbF-poor cells are the first to disappear from the circulation, whereas the high-HbF–containing cells linger. This natural selection of HbF-containing cells accounts for the apparent increase in the percentage of HbF during aplastic episodes.

Patients usually exhibit pallor and fatigue but no jaundice and have laboratory evidence of severe anemia below baseline with associated reticulocytopenia. Spontaneous recovery is generally heralded by a markedly elevated nucleated RBC count, followed in 1 or 2 days by a brisk reticulocytosis. Spontaneous recovery usually occurs within 7 to 10 days and may require no therapy, but some patients are extremely ill when initially seen, and many require short-term hospitalization and erythrocyte transfusions. This recovery phase, with the characteristic anemia, nucleated red cells, reticulocytosis, and occasional hyperbilirubinemia, is probably responsible for most cases referred to as "hyperhemolytic crisis."

In 1981, two groups linked transient aplastic crisis to parvovirus.[521,522] The Jamaican group subsequently documented the epidemiology and follow-up of parvovirus in a cohort of infants identified at birth—308 with sickle cell anemia and 239 controls.[523,524] They made a number of important observations: (1) the frequency of infection (about 40%) did not differ between sickle and control groups, (2) 20% of infections in the sickle group did *not* result in significant aplasia, (3) 100% of aplastic episodes were associated with parvovirus, (4) no patient had recurrent aplasia, and (5) 45% of infected patients maintained elevated parvovirus-specific IgG after 5 years. In a more recent series of aplastic episodes, approximately 70% were associated with positive diagnostic tests for parvovirus.[525] The secondary attack rate of siblings with SCD is 50% to 60%, so siblings with SCD should be monitored for evolving aplastic crisis when acute parvovirus B19 infection is diagnosed in another sibling. Parvovirus B19 has also been implicated as the etiologic agent in erythema infectiosum (fifth disease),[526,527] although frequently the classic rash of fifth disease is absent.[527,528] Parvovirus B19 infection has been related to several other sickle cell complication as well, including acute splenic sequestration,[529] hepatic sequestration,[530,531] ACS,[392] glomerulonephritis,[532,533] and stroke.[534] Many sickle patients will be seropositive for parvovirus B19 without a history of an aplastic event, thus suggesting

that many infections are subclinical.[535] Since then, the relationship between parvovirus and erythropoiesis has been studied in detail. The virus specifically retards late erythroid precursor differentiation[536] and is responsible for temporary erythroid aplasia in a broad array of hemolytic anemias.[528]

Infections

Infection is the most common cause of death in children with sickle cell anemia.[537-539] In one study, the risk of acquiring sepsis or meningitis was greater than 15% in children younger than 5 years, with an associated mortality of approximately 30%.[540] In young children, the risk for pneumococcal sepsis appears to be 400 times greater than that of normal children, and *H. influenzae* sepsis appears to be two to four times as common.[541] These two reports date from the period before the licensing of conjugated vaccines for *S. pneumoniae* and *H. influenzae*. In general, the organisms responsible for infection are primarily encapsulated bacteria and are not unusual pathogens (Table 19-3), but the infections that they cause in such patients are more frequent and severe.

The major risk factor for this increased vulnerability to infection is splenic dysfunction. The spleen normally serves two separate immunologic functions: (1) clearance of particles from the intravascular space and (2) antibody synthesis. Both functions are impaired in sickle cell anemia.

During the first year of life, "functional asplenia," the inability to clear particulate matter from the blood, develops in patients with sickle cell anemia.[542] This is heralded by the appearance of red cells with Howell-Jolly bodies and irregular surface characteristics (pits). When the percentage of "pitted" red cells exceeds 3.5%, the spleen is generally considered nonfunctional.[543] Splenic dysfunction occurs early in life, with 50% of 2068 children with SS disease having greater than 3.5% "pitted" red cells by 2 years of age. Dysfunction occurred less rapidly and less commonly in children with HbSC and S–β-thalassemia. Despite palpable splenomegaly, children with elevated numbers of pitted RBCs have no splenic uptake of technetium 99m (^{99m}Tc) sulfur colloid and are susceptible to the most serious infectious complication of asplenia and pneumococcal sepsis.[544] Repeated infarction results in a nonpalpable, fibrotic, often calcified spleen that may be visualized on a ^{99m}Tc-diphosphonate bone scan.[545] Splenic infarction in young children with SS disease appears to be an insidious process—usually without much in the way of symptoms. In older children and adults, however, especially those with HbSC and S–β-thalassemia, severe left upper quadrant pain often accompanies the infarction. Transfusion,[546] hydroxyurea,[547,548] and bone marrow transplantation[549] can correct the splenic phagocytic defect, although these treatments are not indicated for splenic dysfunction per se.

Children with functional asplenia fail to respond to intravenously administered antigen,[550] even when phago-

TABLE 19-3 Bacteremia and Associated Acute Events in a Cohort of 694 Children with Sickle Cell Anemia (SS) and Hemoglobin SC Disease Monitored Prospectively from Infancy

Organism	Patient	Total No. Cases	Isolated Bacteremia	Acute Chest Syndrome	Meningitis	Bone/Joint
Streptococcus pneumoniae	SS	62	39 (5 dead)	14 (1 dead)	8 (2 dead)	1
	SC	12	9	3	0	0
Haemophilus influenzae	SS	10	6 (2 dead)	3	1	0
	SC	4	2	2	1	0
Staphylococcus aureus	SS	5	2	2	0	1
	SC	1	1	0	0	0
Viridans streptococci	SS	5	4	1	0	0
	SC	1	1	0	0	0
Escherichia coli	SS	5	3	1	0	1
	SC	2	0	1	0	1
Salmonella species	SS	3	2	0	0	1
	SC	2	1	0	0	1
Other	SS	2	1	1	0	0
	SC	0	0	0	0	0

Data from Gill FM, Sleeper LA, Weiner SJ, et al. Clinical events in the first decade in a cohort of infants with sickle cell disease. Blood. 1995;86:776.

cytic function of the spleen has been restored by transfusion. As in other asplenic individuals, however, these children do respond normally to intramuscularly administered polysaccharide and conjugated pneumococcal vaccine.[551-553]

Levels of serum immunoglobulins are normal or increased in children with sickle cell anemia.[552,554,555] However, the serum is deficient in heat-labile opsonizing activity[556] because of an abnormality in the properdin pathway[557,558] that is specific for the phagocytosis of pneumococci. There is increased activation of complement via the alternative pathway[559] and no intrinsic defect in the complement system.[560] Opsonic activity can be reconstituted in vitro by addition of only the F(ab')$_2$ fragments of capsular antibodies to *S. pneumoniae*.[561] This abnormal opsonic activity and associated functional asplenia may partially explain the propensity for pneumococcal infections.

Boggs and co-workers[562] have demonstrated that the chronic leukocytosis of SCD is a reflection of a shift of granulocytes from the marginating to the circulating pool with a high granulocyte turnover rate. Neutrophil chemotaxis is normal to slightly reduced, and no specific abnormality in neutrophil oxidative metabolism has been found in patients with SS disease.[563-565] There is evidence to suggest that the phagocytic function of neutrophils toward *Candida albicans* may be reduced in some individuals with sickle cell anemia and is correlated with the severity of SCD.[566] Epidemiologic studies have also shown a positive correlation between chronic leukocytosis and early mortality[247] and frequent chest syndromes.[248]

Recurrent pneumococcal infections have been described in sickle cell patients.[567] In one series, patients with serious invasive bacterial infections were 4.8 and 15.8 times more likely to have a second or third infection,

thus suggesting that a subgroup of SS patients have an increased susceptibility to infection.[568]

Treatment. Because of the increased incidence of serious bacterial infections in patients with sickle cell anemia, the index of suspicion for infection should always be high. In general, the higher the temperature[569] and leukocyte count,[570] the higher the probability of a serious bacterial infection. Unfortunately, however, the wide variability in the temperature and laboratory values of bacteremic children does not permit accurate prediction of whether an individual febrile child is bacteremic. The following are guidelines for empirical evaluation and treatment of a febrile child younger than 12 years:

- Perform a complete blood cell count, urinalysis, chest radiography, and cultures of blood, urine, and throat.
- "Toxic" children, or those with temperatures higher than 39.9° C, should be treated with parenteral antibiotics promptly, before radiographs are taken or the results of laboratory tests are available. These children should be admitted to the hospital.
- Lumbar puncture should be performed on "toxic" children and those with any signs of meningitis.
- Nontoxic children with temperatures below 40° C, but with infiltrates on the chest radiograph, a WBC count higher than 30,000/mm^3 or lower than 500/mm^3, a platelet count less than 100,000/mm^3, hemoglobin below 5 g/dL, or a history of sepsis should be treated parenterally and admitted to the hospital.
- Nontoxic children with temperatures below 40° C, a normal chest radiograph, normal leukocyte count, and reliable parents can be treated with a long-acting antibiotic (e.g., ceftriaxone, 50 to 75 mg/kg, parenterally),

observed over a period of hours, and be discharged home for follow-up evaluation the next day and a possible repeat empirical antibiotic dose.[571]

- Empirical antibiotic selection should be based on the ability to kill both pneumococcus and *H. influenzae* and to penetrate the CNS. In areas where β-lactamase–producing *H. influenzae* or penicillin- and cephalosporin-resistant pneumococci are regularly encountered, these issues should be factored into the choice of drug.
- If children do well and culture results remain negative after 24 to 48 hours, antibiotics can be discontinued.
- Documented sepsis should be treated parenterally for a minimum of 1 week.
- Bacterial meningitis should be treated for a minimum of 10 days parenterally or for at least 1 week after the cerebrospinal fluid has been sterilized.
- Patients with infiltrates on the chest radiograph should have cultures of sputum, blood, and stool and be treated as described for ACS. Because of the high incidence of pneumococcal, chlamydial, and mycoplasmal pneumonia, patients should be treated with an appropriate antipneumococcal agent and macrolide antibiotic. *M. pneumoniae* infection may be manifested as a lobar infiltrate,[572] and the presence of a positive cold agglutinin, albeit nonspecific, should be an indication for a macrolide. A stool culture positive for *Salmonella* may be the only evidence of *Salmonella* pneumonia. In most cases, no bacterial confirmation will be available, and the patient should receive at least a 1-week course of antibiotics to cover pneumococci, *H. influenzae*, and atypical organisms (e.g., *M. pneumoniae*).

Despite advances in laboratory and imaging techniques, the diagnosis of osteomyelitis in SCD is often very difficult to distinguish from aseptic bone infarct and still relies heavily on clinical assessment.[374] Patients with clinical findings that are highly suggestive of osteomyelitis should undergo needle aspiration and culture of the lesion. After obtaining material for culture, children who appear acutely ill should be started on antibiotics. The antibiotic regimen chosen should include agents effective against *Salmonella* and *Staphylococcus aureus*. Antibiotics should be discontinued or modified when culture reports are available.

Prevention. Attempts at preventing pneumococcal disease in patients with sickle cell anemia have focused on prophylactic antibiotics and vaccines. Prophylactic penicillin was first shown to be effective in the prevention of pneumococcal disease by John and associates,[573] who used monthly intramuscular injections of long-acting penicillin. However, if penicillin prophylaxis was discontinued after 3 years of age, an increase in pneumococcal infections was noted. Gaston and co-workers, in a blinded placebo-controlled clinical trial in the United States, showed that 84% of the pneumococcal infections in children younger than 5 years could be prevented with oral penicillin.[574] As a result of this landmark study, aggressive

universal newborn screening programs have been organized throughout the United States so that all children with sickle cell anemia can be identified and started on penicillin prophylaxis by 8 weeks of age. If penicillin is discontinued after 5 years, patients do not have a higher incidence of infections than those who remained on prophylaxis,[575] and there are conflicting data regarding the increased risk for penicillin-resistant pneumococcal colonization while on prophylaxis.[576,577] Our approach to prophylaxis is as follows:

- Give prophylaxis to all newborns with SS, S–β-thalassemia, and SC disease. (Some practitioners prefer not to treat infants with SC disease because their splenic dysfunction typically appears later in life.)
- Start as early as possible—optimally by 8 weeks of age.
- Prescribe penicillin, 125 mg orally twice a day, until 3 years of age. At age 3, increase the dose to 250 mg orally twice a day. Penicillin can be stopped after 5 years of age without resulting in an increased incidence of infection.
- Prescribe erythromycin ethyl succinate, 10 mg/kg orally twice a day, for patients allergic to penicillin.
- Educate families on the importance of compliance and early recognition of signs of infection.
- Polyvalent pneumococcal vaccine has been shown to be effective in eliciting a normal antibody response, increasing pneumococcal opsonizing activity, and reducing the incidence of pneumococcal disease.[553,559,578] Both heptavalent conjugated and 24-valent polysaccharide pneumococcal vaccines are commercially available. The 24-valent vaccine includes 90% of the common serotypes of pathogenic pneumococci. Children younger than 2 years respond relatively poorly in general to this vaccine,[579] and 2-year-old children respond poorly to two common pneumococcal serotypes, 6A and 19.[580] Revaccination after 4 years improved protective levels of antibody without serious adverse reactions in children.[581] The newer heptavalent vaccine, when given in repeated doses to children younger than 1 year, is effective in mounting antibody titers to the capsular antigens that it includes, increases opsonizing activity, and is recommended for all children, including sickle patients.[553,582,583] *H. influenzae* conjugated vaccine is immunogenic in children with SCD and should be given at the same schedule used for normal infants.[584,585]

Even though prophylactic penicillin and new vaccines are clearly effective in preventing some overwhelming infections, several children have been documented to have fatal pneumococcal sepsis who were vaccinated and had been prescribed oral penicillin.[586] Although penicillin-resistant pneumococci were not demonstrated in patients receiving prophylaxis, multidrug-resistant pneumococci appeared to emerge in patients treated for longer than 5 years.[576] These examples underscore the need for physicians to emphasize the importance of compliance and to continue to have a high index of suspicion of sepsis in a febrile child with SCD.

Chronic Organ Damage

Cardiovascular System. Abnormal cardiac findings are present in most patients with sickle cell anemia[587-590] and are primarily the result of chronic anemia and the compensatory increased cardiac output.[591] On physical examination, the most common findings are systolic ejection murmur, S_3, split S_1, suprasternal notch thrill, and diastolic murmur.[587] Cardiac findings may closely resemble the findings in rheumatic valvular disease or congenital cardiac anomalies. Frequently, echocardiography is necessary to diagnose abnormal cardiac structure. Cardiomegaly is present in most patients, with electrocardiographic findings of left ventricular hypertrophy seen in about 50% of patients.[588]

In view of the fact that the hallmark of SCD is vaso-occlusion, it is remarkable that myocardial infarction is an extremely rare event.[588,592,593] In one review of the postmortem literature in SCD, including examination of 153 hearts, only four infarcts were reported.[592] Despite the high oxygen extraction in the coronary circulation, blood in the coronary sinus contains no more sickled forms than blood in the general circulation does,[593] presumably because of the short transit time through the coronary vessels.[591] Atherosclerosis is virtually absent in this population, seen in one study in none of the 100 hearts of patients (55 of whom were 16 to 47 years old, with a median age of 30) examined at autopsy.[592] This is in marked contrast to a Vietnamese study,[595] in which atherosclerosis was found in 45% of 105 battle casualties. When injected at autopsy, a sickle cell heart has normal patent coronary arteries, frequently of larger caliber than seen in normal hearts.[596] The cause of this apparent protective effect against atherosclerosis is unknown but may involve genetic or dietary factors or anemia itself.

The most comprehensive prospective examination of cardiac function in an unselected population of patients with sickle cell anemia was done as part of the CSSCD.[597] One hundred ninety-one steady-state patients 13 years and older underwent echocardiography, and all of the measurements were done centrally by an investigator without access to other patient data. After appropriately adjusting for body surface area, the left and right ventricles, aortic root, and left atrium were noted to be larger than normal. Significant wall thickening was found only in the septum. The left ventricular dilation correlated with hemoglobin and age, thus suggesting that the major cardiac findings are indeed related to the years of increased stroke volume in compensation for the anemia and abnormal rheology. The finding of normal left and right ventricular function suggests that if a specific "sickle myocardiopathy" exists, it is rare. As discussed in the section on chronic lung disease, patients with cor pulmonale and right ventricular dysfunction have a high mortality rate.

PHT is a common complication in adult patients with SCD, with a reported prevalence of approximately 20% to 40%.[598-601] Multiple retrospective studies report significantly increased mortality in SCD patients with PHT when compared with those without PHT.[599,601,603] Castro and colleagues demonstrated that SCD patients with PHT confirmed by right heart catheterization had a median survival of 25.6 months whereas patients without PHT had greater than a 70% survival rate at the end of a 10-year observation period.[603] A more recent study of 195 SCD patients reported a significantly higher mortality rate in adult patients with PHT (defined as a tricuspid regurgitant jet velocity >2.5 m/sec on echocardiography) than in those with no PHT after a median follow-up of 18 months.[601] Markers of hemolysis (increased lactate dehydrogenase, bilirubin, reticulocyte count) resulted in increased risk for adult PHT.[601,604] Intravascular hemolysis leads to increased plasma hemoglobin and arginase and is associated with indicators of reduced NO bioavailability (also see the section on NO depletion), subsequent endothelial dysfunction, and PHT.[317] The prevalence of elevated TR jet velocity in children appears similar to that in adults[605-607]; however, the significance of the finding and the prognostic implications remain to be established in this age group.[608]

Arrhythmias are rare under usual conditions, although in one study, during the first hour of therapy for painful crisis, 80% of patients had arrhythmias—67% atrial and 60% ventricular. These arrhythmias were not clinically significant and probably represented response to pain.[609]

Blood pressure in steady-state patients with sickle cell anemia (and to a lesser extent, SC disease) is lower than in a race-, gender-, and age-matched normal population (Table 19-4).[468] This finding may be related to the tendency to lose sodium and water in urine. This study demonstrated that high blood pressure is a risk factor for stroke and early mortality and that the diagnosis of high blood pressure depends on knowing the "normal values" for this population (see Table 19-4). Blood pressures above the 90% percentile in this population overlap with the normal range in a normal population, and a steady-state blood pressure of 140/90 is ominous. Such patients should be considered candidates for antihypertensive therapy.

Renal System. Hyposthenuria, hematuria, nephrotic syndrome, and uremia are the major renal complications of SCD.[610] In addition, production of erythropoietin in response to anemia may be lower in older patients with SS disease, possibly because of primary renal disease.[611]

Hyposthenuria[612,613] develops early in childhood and, as is the case with functional asplenia, may be temporarily reversed by transfusion.[614,615] The hypertonic environment of the renal medulla promotes sickling even at normal Po_2,[616] which leads to decreased medullary blood flow and derangement of the countercurrent multiplier. Abnormality of the countercurrent multiplier may be the

TABLE 19-4	**Blood Pressure in Patients with Sickle Cell Anemia**												
		AGE (yr)											
	Percentile	2-3	4-5	6-7	8-9	10-11	12-13	14-15	16-17	18-24	25-34	35-44
FEMALES												
Systolic	50	90	95	96	96	104	106	110	110	110	110	110
	90	100	110	110	110	110	118	120	122	122	125	130
Diastolic	50	52	60	60	60	60	62	70	70	64	68	70
	90	62	70	70	70	74	74	80	78	80	80	84
MALES												
Systolic	50	90	95	100	100	100	110	108	112	112	114	110
	90	104	110	108	116	112	120	120	128	130	130	132
Diastolic	50	54	60	60	60	60	64	64	70	68	70	70
	90	66	68	68	70	70	72	78	80	80	80	84

Data from Pegelow CH, Colangelo L, Stunberg M, et al. Natural history of blood pressure in sickle cell disease. Am J Med. 1997;102:171-177.

mechanism for hyposthenuria, or as suggested by Buckalew and Someren,[610] it may be due to decreased flow to nephrons in patients with long loops of Henle and preservation of flow to nephrons with short loops. The obligatory water loss results in a tendency toward dehydration and invalidates the use of urine volume or concentration as an indicator of the patient's state of hydration. Nocturia and enuresis are common complaints of these patients, who excrete large volumes of dilute urine.[617] Urinary sodium losses may be high and result in significant hyponatremia.[618] A renal tubular acidification defect,[619,620] as well as hyporeninemic hypoaldosteronism[621] and impaired potassium excretion,[622] has been identified. In one review, de Jong and Statius van Eps emphasized that renal-vasodilating prostaglandins are increased in sickle cell patients, thereby leading to a compensatory increase in renal blood flow, glomerular filtration rate, and proximal tubular activity.[623]

Although hematuria is usually mild, bleeding is occasionally severe enough to cause significant blood loss.[624] Papillary necrosis is generally the underlying anatomic defect.[625] Maintenance of high urinary flow with increased fluid intake will eliminate clots from the bladder and decrease medullary osmolality. Urinary alkalinization and diuretics may be beneficial. ε-Aminocaproic acid has been suggested for stopping severe hematuria that is refractory to transfusion,[626] but it must be used cautiously because of the risk of ureteral or pelvic clotting and obstruction. In patients with long-standing hematuria, supplemental iron may be necessary to prevent iron deficiency. Hematuria may also be the initial symptom of a renal tumor. A surprisingly high incidence of renal medullary carcinoma has been reported in adults and children with sickle cell anemia and sickle trait.[627,628]

Uremia is a rare complication in children with SCD that may follow a symptom complex of nephrotic syndrome[629] and glomerulonephritis. The nature of the glomerular lesion is unknown but may represent a response to iron deposition,[630] an antigen-antibody complex,[631] or mesangial phagocytosis of fragmented sickled cells.[632,633]

Recently, parvovirus infection, with or without an antecedent aplastic crisis, has been associated with acute glomerulonephritis.[532,533] Proteinuria in SCD frequently progresses to nephrotic syndrome[634] and ultimately to renal failure,[633,635] which is a common cause of mortality in adults with SCA.[247,636] Microalbuminuria, as manifested by a ratio of albumin to creatinine of greater than 20, is seen in more than 40% of adults and in a similar percentage of children 10 to 18 years of age with SCD.[637] Recently, a study of 442 children with SCD monitored for 10 years showed that proteinuria occurred in 6.2% and increased to 12% in teenagers. Proteinuria was associated with lower hemoglobin levels, higher MCV, higher WBC counts, and more clinically severe disease.[638] A study of 381 adults with SCD demonstrated that 7% had elevated serum creatinine levels and 26% had proteinuria.[639] Ten patients with proteinuria underwent renal biopsy, and the glomerular lesions showed perihilar focal segmental sclerosis and glomerular enlargement, similar to findings in an animal model with glomerular hypertension and efferent arteriolar vasoconstriction. To test the animal analogy, these patients were treated with enalapril, an angiotensin-converting enzyme (ACE) inhibitor that has been shown to decrease efferent arteriolar constriction. In all treated patients, the level of proteinuria fell during treatment and returned toward abnormal after discontinuation.

The predictive value of microalbuminuria has not been fully elucidated in children but has been suggested by some.[637,640] Serum cystatin C may be a better screen for the glomerular filtration rate than creatinine is in sickle cell anemia because it appears to rise according to the degree of albuminuria and before significant elevation in serum creatinine is detected.[641]

Treatment of microalbuminuria[642] or proteinuria[639] with ACE inhibitors can be effective, but long-term therapeutic benefits for the prevention of progressive glomerular disease have not yet been demonstrated.[643] Addition of hydroxyurea to ACE inhibitors may further improve renal function.[644]

Bakir and associates estimated that nephrosis develops in 4% of adult SS patients and that in two thirds of these patients, renal failure eventually develops.[633] Renal failure can be managed by peritoneal dialysis, hemodialysis, and transplantation. Renal transplantation can be successful in patients with end-stage sickle nephropathy, but 3-year allograft and patient survival is significantly decreased when compared with other patient populations.[645]

Hepatobiliary System. Liver and biliary tract abnormalities are common in SCD[646,647] and are the result of cholelithiasis, hepatic infarction, and transfusion-related hepatitis.

Bilirubin stones are common.[648,649] Two large series have studied the incidence of gallstones as detected by ultrasound in children with SS disease.[650,651] The percentage of gallstones in 226 patients aged 5 to 13 selected randomly from a group of children with SS disease identified at birth was 13%,[646] a value lower than that found in a survey of clinic patients studied by Sarnaik and associates.[650] In this report, the incidence of gallstones was 12% by 2 to 4 years of age.[650] With advancing age, the incidence increased gradually and reached 42% in the 15- to 18-year-old age group. Fourteen of the 226 patients were noted to have "sludge" in the gallbladder and had ultrasonograms repeated up to 2 years later. Stones developed in four, four had no further evidence of sludge, and six remained unchanged. Comorbid Gilbert's syndrome (UGT1A genotype) significantly increases serum bilirubin levels in children with SCD and the likelihood of requiring early cholecystectomy.[310] Evidence is good that children tolerate elective cholecystectomy with little morbidity if they are prepared properly for surgery.[424,652,653] Laparoscopic cholecystectomy has been particularly effective in reducing postoperative hospital stay in children with SCD.[654] In contrast, operating during the acute phase carries a significant risk of complication.[424,655]

Intrahepatic sickling can result in massive hyperbilirubinemia,[421] elevated liver enzyme values, and a painful syndrome mimicking acute cholecystitis[422] or viral hepatitis[648] (see "Acute Abdominal Pain"). Fulminant hepatic failure with massive cholestasis and rapidly progressing hepatic encephalopathy and shock has been described as a rare, often fatal complication of SCD that may be amenable to exchange transfusion.[425,656,657]

A review of postmortem liver findings in 70 SCD patients examined at Johns Hopkins Hospital[658] revealed hepatic necrosis, portal fibrosis, regenerative nodules, and cirrhosis in adults, thought to be a consequence of recurrent vascular obstruction and repair. In contrast, 19 liver biopsy specimens from symptomatic patients with SS disease failed to show necrosis and more often showed evidence of acute or subacute infection.[659]

Eyes. Tortuosity and sacculation of conjunctival vessels are noted in more than 90% of patients with SCD.

These lesions are best seen in the lower temporal area, disappear after exchange transfusion, and are curiously related to the ISC count in peripheral blood.[660] They have no deleterious effect on the eye.

Retinopathy is classified as either proliferative or nonproliferative. Nonproliferative retinopathy probably results from retinal arteriolar infarction with adjacent hemorrhage and requires no therapy. Depending on the duration, layer, and extension of the hemorrhage, the result can be a salmon patch, schism cavity, vitreous hemorrhage, or black sunburst.[661] In two patients with documented acute arteriolar occlusion, salmon patches developed in a matter of hours to days, with atrophic schism cavities evolving in 3 to 4 months.[662] In older patients, angioid streaks are common, but the cause is unknown.[663,664]

The more serious complication is proliferative retinopathy, which has been classified by Goldberg[665] as stage 1, peripheral arteriolar occlusions; stage 2, arteriolar-venular anastomoses; stage 3, neovascularization; stage 4, vitreous hemorrhages; and stage 5, retinal detachment. Because these lesions may progress to blindness, laser therapy to occlude the feeding vessels of advanced proliferative lesions has been advocated. Unfortunately, photocoagulation carries the risk of neovascularization of the choroid[666] and retinal breaks,[667] complications that can result in blindness. The dilemma of choosing potentially blinding therapy for a potentially blinding lesion is complicated by the observation that some proliferative lesions heal spontaneously by autoinfarction. In one study of untreated retinopathy in Jamaica, 567 eyes were observed for 8 years.[668] Proliferative retinopathy was initially present in 12% of the eyes and developed in another 8% during follow-up. Blindness resulted in 12% of the eyes with retinopathy. In the original group of eyes with retinopathy, progressive retinopathy developed in 30%, 10% underwent spontaneous regression, and the remaining 30% showed a mix of regression and progression. In another prospective Jamaican study, treatment of retinopathy was compared with no treatment.[669] No statistical difference in visual acuity between the two groups was reported. Macular ischemia and color blindness have been reported to be prevalent in patients with SS disease without evidence of retinal lesions on ophthalmologic examination.[670,671]

Rarely, acute painless loss of vision is the result of central retinal artery occlusion. Although such lesions may resolve spontaneously, exchange transfusion has been recommended for bilateral disease.[672]

Blunt trauma to the eye may result in hyphema (bleeding into the anterior chamber). Because the conditions in this chamber overwhelmingly favor sickling, any hemoglobin-containing red cell will sickle and may cause obstructive glaucoma and blindness. Common medical treatments that might be considered in nonsickle patients may promote sickling and should be avoided (e.g., hyperosmotic/diuretic agents, carbonic anhydrase inhibitors). Initial topical β-adrenergic antagonists (e.g., timolol) or

α_2-adrenergic agonists (e.g., brimonidine) may be effective,[673] but a low threshold for surgical evacuation of anterior chamber blood should be observed so that vision is preserved.[674] This condition is one of the true ocular emergencies that occurs in patients with sickle trait or SCD.

Skin. Leg ulcers do not usually occur in childhood. In adolescence and adulthood, ulcers may constitute a crippling symptom. This skin lesion is seen with other chronic hemolytic anemias such as hereditary spherocytosis, thalassemia, elliptocytosis, and pyruvate kinase deficiency[675] and therefore may not represent vaso-occlusion. Ulceration may result from increased venous pressure in the legs caused by the expanded blood volume in the hypertrophied bone marrow.[676] In tropical areas in which shoes are not generally worn and insect bites are common, leg ulcers are frequent.[677] In Jamaica, leg ulcers typically start in the 10- to 20-year-old group and eventually appear in 75% of adults. Koshy and colleagues[678] reported data from the CSSCD regarding leg ulcers in sickle cell patients. Leg ulcers appear to be less frequent in individuals with two α genes than in those with three or four genes. Leg ulcer frequencies appear to decrease consistently with increases in HbF production.[678] Venous outflow is decreased in the lower extremities of patients with leg ulcers when compared with patients without ulcers, thus suggesting that venous incompetence may contribute to the development or failure of these lesions to heal.[679] In addition, low steady-state hemoglobin values and markers of a high hemolytic rate are associated with an increased incidence of leg ulcers and may be associated with decreased NO bioavailability and endothelial dysfunction.[315,680]

Chronic lesions become a major source of morbidity and have a profound negative impact on educational achievement and employment.[681] Usually present over the medial surface of the lower part of the tibia or just posterior to the medial malleolus, they begin as a small depression with central necrosis and, if unattended, widen to encircle the entire lower portion of the leg. Débridement, scrupulous hygiene, topical antibiotics, bed rest, and elevation of the leg are the mainstays of therapy. In some patients, protection of the ulcer by the application of a soft sponge-rubber doughnut and low-pressure elastic bandage seems to be beneficial. One report suggested that an RGD peptide matrix designed to mimic the normal matrix was beneficial.[682] Close attention to improved venous circulation with the use of above-the-knee elastic stockings may prevent ulceration. If ulcers persist despite optimal care, transfusion therapy may be implemented and consideration given to split-thickness skin grafts. Transfusion therapy is sometimes effective, but in many patients the ulcers either do not heal or recur after discontinuation of this therapy. Oral zinc sulfate may promote healing of leg ulcers,[683] and peripheral vasodilator therapy appears to be ineffective.[684]

Ears. Sensorineural hearing loss at both ends of the auditory spectrum was found in a substantial number of sickle cell patients in Jamaica.[685,686] In a U.S. study, 12% of children with SS disease had high-frequency sensorineural hearing loss.[687] Interestingly, although there was no increased otitis media or meningitis in the affected group, five of the six children with CNS disease had abnormal hearing. The pathology of the auditory apparatus appears to be sickling in the cochlear vasculature with destruction of hair cells.[688]

Skeleton. Skeletal changes in SCD are common[364,374,689,690] and are due to expansion of the marrow cavity and repeated bone infarction. The expanded marrow is best seen on radiographs of the thickened calvaria with a wide diploic space. Overgrowth of the anterior part of the maxilla may lead to severe orthodontic and cosmetic problems. Vertebrae are generally flattened, with a characteristic biconcave deformity called "codfish vertebrae." In older patients, vertebral disease may cause chronic back pain. These individuals need to be treated as other patients who have chronic back disease: appropriate exercises, braces, bed rest, muscle relaxants, and moral support.

The major chronic bone complication of SCD is AVN. Indeed, the most common cause of AVN of the femoral head in children is SCD. As shown in (Fig. 19-9), the incidence is relatively low in children, with an estimated prevalence of 3% in children younger than 15 years.[691] The incidence is remarkably increased in patients with SS disease and coexistent α-thalassemia.[692] Patients at highest risk for complications were those with the highest rates of painful crises and those with the highest hematocrits. The recent discovery of SNPs in several genes related to bone metabolism may affect the natural history of AVN.[312] The pathophysiology of AVN is unknown but is hypothesized to be related to sludging in marrow sinusoids, marrow necrosis, healing with increased intramedullary pressure, necrosis of the articular surface, bone resorption, and eventually, epiphyseal collapse.[692,693] The diagnosis is made radiographically, classically with a spectrum of findings from subepiphyseal lucency and a widened joint space to flattening or fragmentation and scarring of the epiphysis. Although roughly half of the patients in whom AVN was diagnosed on the basis of screening radiographs were asymptomatic, significant chronic pain and limited joint mobility plagued the others. MRI can identify changes of AVN earlier than conventional films can.[691,694] Managing osteonecrosis of the femoral head in young adults is a challenging problem with limited treatment options and often disappointing outcomes. Strict bed rest is helpful in a minority of patients,[695] with little or no evidence to support the use of chronic transfusion therapy. Injection of cement[696] and core decompression[697] have been used successfully in some series. It is possible that these procedures might be helpful in patients with very early disease. A randomized prospective study of hip core decompression versus phys-

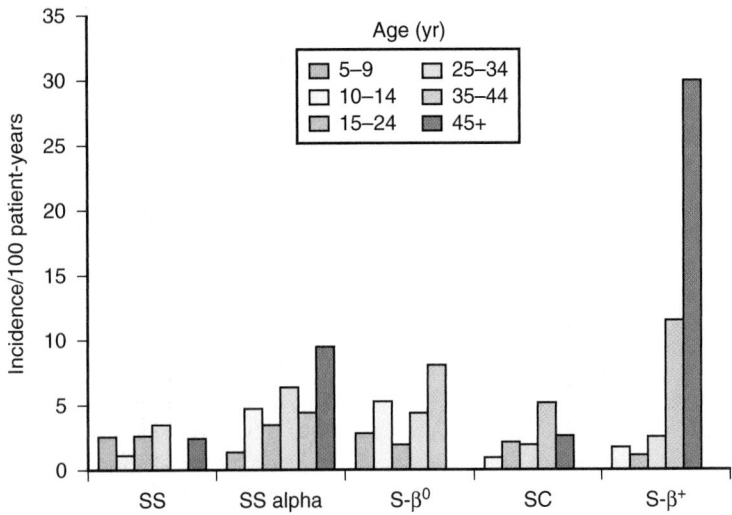

FIGURE 19-9. Incidence of osteonecrosis of the femoral head per 100 patient-years by genotype. (*Data from Milner PF, Kraus AP, Sebes JI, et al. Sickle cell disease as a cause of osteonecrosis of the femoral head. N Engl J Med. 1991;325: 1476-1481.*)

ical therapy for the treatment of early femoral head osteonecrosis revealed clinical improvement in both groups but one not more effective than the other.[698] Despite interventions to preserve the femoral head, progression is frequent and may result in the need for total hip replacement arthroplasty in severely compromised patients. In the study of Milner and colleagues, 17% of patients underwent hip replacement, 30% of replaced hips required surgical revision within 4.5 years, and more than 60% of patients continued to have pain and limited mobility postoperatively.[692] The epidemiology of AVN of the humeral head is virtually identical to that of the femur.[699] In general, however, patients are less symptomatic, and shoulder arthroplasty was exceedingly rare.

Lungs. In contrast to ACS, chronic lung disease has been difficult to define and quantitate. In older children, lung volumes are reduced[700,701] in comparison to those of the normal white population but are appropriate when compared with those of a black control population.[702] Others report an early restrictive and obstructive pulmonary function pattern in steady-state children with SCD.[703,704] Resting arterial PO_2 in asymptomatic children with SCD is typically 65 to 85 mm Hg (normal, >87 mm Hg). There are large alveolar-arterial PO_2 differences with room air (27 to 42 mm Hg; normal, <16 mm Hg) and on 100% O_2 (186 to 246 mm Hg; normal, <86 mm Hg). These values are consistent with increased pulmonary shunting of 12% to 16% (normal, <7%).[702] The decreased membrane-diffusing capacity observed can be explained on the basis of anemia alone and does not suggest a substantial element of pulmonary vascular occlusion. No definitive profile of pulmonary function in SCD has emerged, although 90% of adults from the CSSCD had abnormal pulmonary function test results, with 74% showing a restrictive pattern.[705] In one survey of adults, fatal progressive pulmonary disease may have been related to history of previous chest syndromes[706]; however, the relationship between acute episodes of chest syndrome and chronic lung disease has

been difficult to establish reproducibly. There appears to be an emerging link between obstructive lung disease and the pathogenesis of ACS, particularly in children.[404,410,707,708] An increase in obstructive lung disease was documented in adult patients who had two to four episodes of ACS versus patients with no history.[709] In another study, patients with SS disease were found to have abnormally small lungs, but this abnormality was not related to episodes of ACS.[710] In a study of infants 3 to 30 months of age, restrictive lung disease was present in 3 of 12 infants and was not related to a history of ACS.[711] These studies suggest that subtle subacute damage to the lungs proceeds even in the absence of acute disease. Hydroxyurea therapy[400] reduces the incidence of recurrent ACS but does not lead to improved pulmonary function. In 24 patients with a history of chest syndromes studied after bone marrow transplantation, 22 showed no improvement and 2 had worse pulmonary function after transplantation.[712]

Central Nervous System. Abnormal neurologic findings in SCD were discussed earlier. Kral and co-workers found that children with SCD perform more poorly on measures of neurocognitive functioning with increasing age or lower hematocrits.[713] In addition, TCD ultrasonography was the only radiologic measure that could predict neurocognitive outcome after controlling for age and hematocrit. Changes on CT and MRI may antedate the neurologic dysfunction and represent subclinical infarcts.[440,441,446,714] It is now clear that cognitive functioning and fine motor skills are impaired in sickle cell patients with silent infarcts as diagnosed by MRI.[464,715] Because abnormal Doppler or MRI studies, or both, can be seen in children with decreased neurocognitive performance, these radiologic studies are being considered as screening tools to select very young patients for experimental therapies that may prevent further CNS damage.

Growth and Development. The birth weight of infants with sickle cell anemia is normal.[716] Subsequently, a pattern of delayed growth emerges. Detailed anthropomorphic measurements of Jamaican children revealed decreased limb length, sitting height, and skinfold thickness, along with increased anteroposterior chest diameter,[717] possibly related to cardiomegaly.[718] Height and weight growth curves (Fig. 19-10) for individuals with SCD in the United States were generated as part of the CSSCD, sponsored by the Sickle Cell Disease Branch of the NHLBI.[719] The important features of these curves are that they are different from those for normal black controls, that weight is more affected than height, and that patients with sickle cell anemia and S–β⁰-thalassemia experience more delay in growth than do patients with HbSC disease and S–β⁺-thalassemia. In general, by the end of adolescence, patients with SCD have caught up with controls in height but not weight. The reason for this poor weight gain is not understood but is likely to represent increased caloric requirements of elevated resting energy expenditure related to anemia, increased bone marrow activity, and cardiovascular compensation.[720] In a second large prospective study in Jamaica, both height and weight were significantly lower than that of age- and sex-matched controls as early as 2 years of age.[721] Zinc deficiency has been suggested as a cause of poor growth in children with SS disease[722,723] but has not been confirmed.[724] Levels of vitamins A, B₆, and D have been discovered to be lower than those of ethnically matched children and may relate to morbidity.[725,726] Growth hormone deficiency is a rare and reversible cause of growth delay.[727] In general, growth hormone levels and growth hormone stimulation studies appear to be normal in children with SS disease who have impaired growth.[728] A review of nutritional studies in patients with SS disease is available,[729] and one study has suggested that hyperalimentation may be useful in some patients.[730]

Sexual development is also delayed in patients with SCD.[719] Such delay is found in both males and females and follows the same pattern as height and weight in other hemoglobinopathies. The estimated median age of attainment of Tanner stage for each hemoglobinopathy is

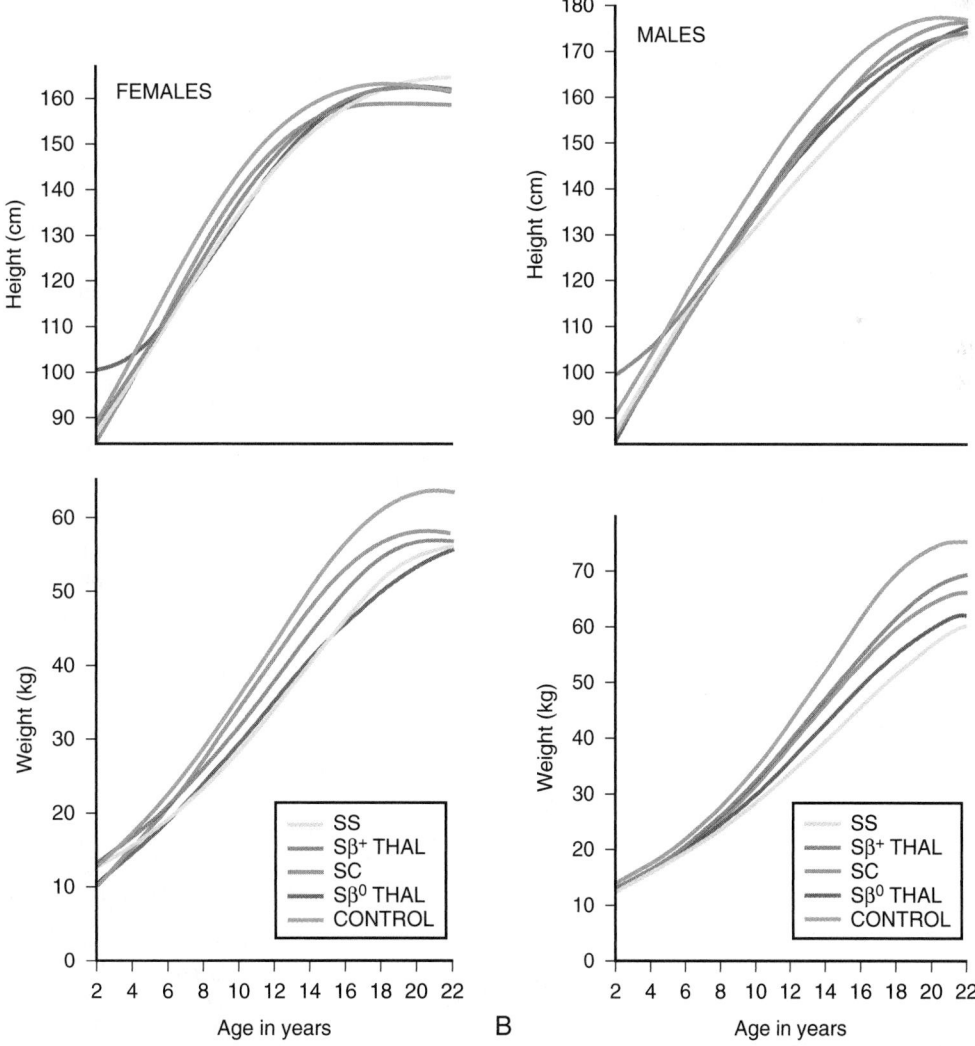

FIGURE 19-10. Height and weight growth curves for females (**A**) and males (**B**) 2 to 22 years of age according to type of hemoglobinopathy. Shown are the 50% curves. (*Redrawn from Platt OS, Rosenstock W, Espeland MA. Influence of sickle hemoglobinopathies on growth and development. N Engl J Med. 1984; 311:7-12. Reprinted by permission from The New England Journal of Medicine.*)

listed in Table 19-5. For females (regardless of hemoglobinopathy), menarche status is a function of age and weight. This normal relationship between menarche and weight suggests that in females, delayed sexual maturity is constitutional. This finding has been confirmed in a careful analysis of female fertility in Jamaica, which revealed no difference in the interval between sexual exposure and pregnancy between patients and controls.[731] Most males do undergo delayed sexual maturation, also suggesting constitutional delay. However, among males there does seem to be evidence of decreased fertility, with abnormal sperm motility, morphology, and number.[732] Transient primary hypogonadism[733] and hypothalamic hypogonadism responsive to clomiphene[734] have also been described.

Psychological Aspects. As in any chronic disease, patients require strong, sympathetic support. Most patients with sickle cell anemia handle their illness very well. In one study,[735] patients did not differ from controls in personal, social, or total adjustment. Interestingly, acute anxiety was less frequent in patients than in controls, although patients did demonstrate lower self-concept. Another study pointed out the pitfalls of interpreting excessive fatigue as depression in these children.[736] Problems of particular concern to patients are coping with chronic pain, inability to keep up with peers, fears of premature death, and delayed sexual maturity. Discussion of prenatal diagnosis and selective abortion, particularly in a patient's own family, increases doubt about self-worth. These issues need to be addressed openly and frankly and with appropriate psychological support. Self-help groups for patients and families are gaining in effectiveness and popularity throughout the country.

Mortality. Leikin and colleagues from the CSSCD examined mortality in children with SCD.[737] They found that the peak incidence of death was between 1 and 3 years of age and that it was generally due to infection. The overall mortality rate was 0.5 per 100 patient-years, and for patients with SS disease, the probability of surviving to 29 years of age was about 85%. For those with SC disease, the probability of surviving to 20 years was about 95%. Quinn and associates from the Dallas Newborn Cohort reported an overall survival rate of 86% and a death rate of 0.59 per 100 patient-years for children with SS disease monitored from birth through 18 years of age.[539] The Dallas cohort also showed trends of decreasing sickle-related mortality, increasing mean age at death, and a smaller proportion of deaths related to infection than noted in the CSSCD[356] and Jamaican[738] cohorts.

As shown in Figure 19-11, when the data on deaths in children from the CSSCD are combined with the data on adults, it appears that the median age at death was 42 years for males with SS disease, 48 years for females with SS disease, 60 years for males with SC disease, and 68 years for females with SC disease.[247] Among adults, those with the lowest levels of HbF, highest steady-state WBC counts, and highest rates of pain and chest syndrome had the highest risk of dying at an early age. There is an age-related pattern in mortality rates: a peak in patients younger than 5 years and a gradual increase starting in late adolescence. Younger patients die primarily of pneu-

TABLE 19-5	**Estimated Median Age at Attainment of Tanner Stages According to Hemoglobinopathy**			
	Tanner Stage	**MEDIAN AGE**		
		SS	**SC**	**S-β⁺**	**S-β⁰**
FEMALES					
Breasts	2	11.8	9.8	10.6	11.8
	3	13.5	11.9	12.6	12.8
	4	15	13.9	13.8	14.8
	5	17.3	16	16.5	17.2
Pubic hair	2	12	10.1	10	11.5
	3	13.5	11.8	11.2	12.8
	4	15.2	14	13.8	14.2
	5	19.2	17	17	20.8
MALES					
Penis	2	12	10.4	11.9	12.4
	3	14.2	13	13	13.2
	4	16	14.1	13.5	15.5
	5	17.6	16.6	16.6	18.8
Pubic hair	2	13.2	11.5	12	13.2
	3	14.8	13.2	13	13.9
	4	16.2	14.2	13.9	16.2
	5	17.9	16.6	17.1	18.5

Reprinted with permission from Platt OS, Rosenstock MSPH, Espeland MA. Influence of sickle hemoglobinopathies on growth and development. N Engl J Med. 1984;311:7.

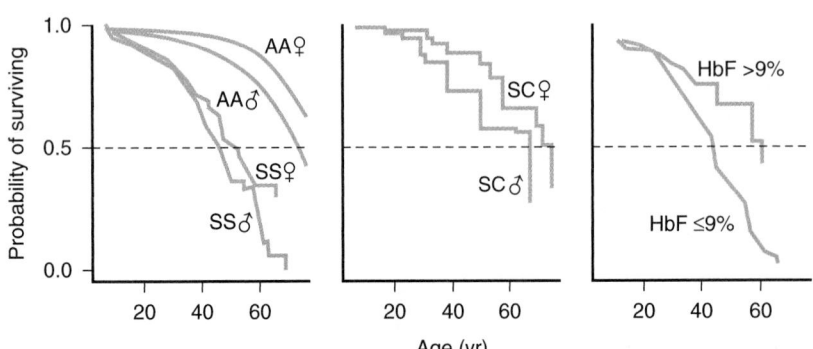

FIGURE 19-11. Survival of male and female patients with SS disease and SC disease. Those in the highest quartiles (>9%) of HbF level are compared with the others. African American (AA) controls are shown for comparison. *(Adapted from Platt OS, Brambilla DJ, Rosse WF, et al. Mortality in sickle cell disease. Life expectancy and risk factors for early death. N Engl J Med. 1994;330:1639-1644. Adapted by permission from the The New England Journal of Medicine.)*

mococcal disease and less often of acute splenic seques-tration, ACS, or stroke.[537,739] Older patients die of ACS, during pain crises, of chronic organ system failure from cancer and other specific diseases of adults, and suddenly without obvious cause.[247] It is encouraging that coincident with the widespread use of prophylactic penicillin in young children, aggressive treatment of pulmonary disease and infection, careful selection of patients for transfusion therapy, and thoughtful comprehensive care have led to improvement in survival.[740]

Much is known about the risk factors for early mortality in patients with sickle cell anemia. Those with a higher level of HbF have a longer life expectancy,[247] as do whose with a low rate of pain crisis,[247] low rate of ACS,[248] no hand-foot crisis before 1 year of age,[249] no severe anemia before 2 years of age,[247,249] low baseline WBC count,[249] and low blood pressure.[468]

APPROACHES TO THERAPY

Replacement of the Defective Gene

The most direct approach to reduction of HbS polymer is to replace the defective globin gene with a normal gene. Bone marrow transplants from sickle trait or normal siblings have been performed in more than 200 patients.[712,741-747] After preparation with various regimens and prophylactic treatment of graft-versus-host disease, the overall survival rate was 93%, the event-free survival rate was 82%, and SCD recurred in just 11% of 147 patients receiving HLA-identical sibling marrow transplants.[748] More recently, among 87 consecutive patients treated with myeloablative regimens, the addition of antithymocyte globulin reduced the rate of rejection from 23% to 3%.[746] Newer nonmyeloablative regimens have not yet proved successful in SS patients.[749] Transplant complications have included CNS hemorrhage (particularly in patients with a history of stroke), hypogonadal function, graft rejection, and acute or chronic graft-versus-host disease.[746,747,750,751] Prophylactic anticonvulsant treatment and maintenance of a high platelet count may result in reduced CNS morbidity. The restoration of splenic function in successful transplant recipients holds out hope that other chronic organ dysfunction may improve with this approach.[549,752] In a recent summary of 53 children with SS disease undergoing bone marrow transplantation, growth was not impaired in younger children, but diminished growth occurred in patients who received transplants near or during the adolescent growth spurt.[745] Selecting patients for this high-risk therapy is particularly problematic because of the unpredictability of the clinical course, the paucity of sibling matches,[753] and parental concern.[754] Availability of unrelated or sibling cord blood stem cells may offer an increased donor pool for transplantation.[755,756] More specific "gene therapy," such as random insertion of a normal β gene or "correction" of the abnormal gene product in hema-

topoietic stem cells, remains a long-term goal. However, awareness that random insertion of normal genes into donor stem cells might lead to insertional mutagenesis and malignant transformation has tempered enthusiasm for this approach.[757] Transplantation of embryonic stem cells or induction of pluripotent stem cells from donor fibroblasts after homologous recombination has replaced the human β[S] gene with a normal human β-globin gene has led to correction of the sickle mutation in transgenic mice.[758,759]

Reduction of Polymer Formation

Stimulation of Hemoglobin F Production. As noted in the section on interactions of HbS with HbF, increasing the amount of HbF will increase the delay time and solubility of HbS. In SCD, both 5-azacytidine[760-763] and hydroxyurea[764-767] have been used successfully to increase HbF in adult SS individuals. Recombinant erythropoietin with hydroxyurea has inconsistently increased HbF above levels obtained with hydroxyurea alone.[768,769] Butyric acid analogues also increase HbF production in sickle cell patients, some thalassemia patients, and normal individuals.[770-772] Charache and colleagues demonstrated that daily hydroxyurea treatment of adult sickle cell patients increases HbF levels from pretreatment mean levels of 4% to 16% without clinically significant bone marrow toxicity.[766] In addition to increasing HbF, hydroxyurea has been noted to reduce the proportion of dense cells and increase the MCV and mean corpuscular hemoglobin (MCH) of sickle cells.[760,763-765] On the basis of epidemiologic data that an increase in HbF from 4% to 16% could decrease vaso-occlusive crises by 50%,[280] a multicultured double-blind prospective clinical trial of daily hydroxyurea treatment of SS adults was undertaken.[400] This trial was terminated early when it was obvious that vaso-occlusive crisis, chest syndromes, and transfusions were reduced by almost 50% in the hydroxyurea-treated group versus controls. However, increases in HbF alone did not predict the decrease in painful crises seen in the controlled trial of hydroxyurea in adult SS patients.[400] Multiple factors such as perturbation of WBC or cytokine levels, changes in RBC adherence to vascular endothelium (see Fig. 19-1), or alteration of NO/intravascular hemoglobin equilibrium may also play a role in the hydroxyurea-related decrease in crises.[773,774]

A long-term follow-up of patients taking hydroxyurea revealed an impressive 40% reduction in mortality.[775] However, there has been variable acceptance of hydroxyurea therapy in adults with SS.[776] Hospitalization for neither pediatric (<18 years) nor adult (>18 years) sickle cell patients has decreased from 1996 to 2004, thus indicating that on a population basis, hydroxyurea has not reduced hospital admissions.[777]

Small-scale trials of hydroxyurea therapy in children demonstrated that the drug can be given safely,[456,778-781] and 5- and 10-year follow up studies in SS children continue to demonstrate its ability to increase HbF with minimal side effects.[782] It is noteworthy that in the only large study of 122 SS children in which maximum tolerated doses (MTDs) were obtained in the same fashion as in the adult MSH study,[400] very few if any nonresponders were noted. Hydroxyurea therapy at MTDs was well tolerated and demonstrated sustained hematologic efficacy with apparent long-term safety.[783]

Infants with SS diseases tolerate prolonged hydroxyurea therapy and exhibit sustained hematologic benefits, fewer ACS events, improved growth, and possibly preserved organ function.[548] However, previous data suggesting than an elevated WBC count, dactylitis, and anemia predicted more severe later outcomes in children younger than 4 years[249] was not confirmed in a second cohort of patients.[391] Thus, predicting clinical severity in very young children remains problematic. Recent data indicate that children taking hydroxyurea have decreased TCD velocities, which suggests that the drug may reduce the risk for stroke in young children.[784,785] These data leave open the possibility that the first efficacy trial of hydroxyrea in infants with SS disease should be directed toward prevention of CNS disease in this vulnerable age group.

Decreased Cell Hemoglobin S Concentration. Because polymerization of HbS is exquisitely concentration dependent, reduction of the MCHC by swelling the cell with water has been considered as a therapeutic maneuver. Two approaches have been tried: lowering plasma osmolarity and increasing intracellular cations. The first approach was used by Rosa and colleagues,[786] who successfully reduced the duration and frequency of painful crises by lowering the MCHC with dietary salt restriction and desmopressin. Subsequently, others have found this therapy too difficult to maintain, neurologically toxic, and ineffective.[787-789] The second approach has been used primarily in vitro and has focused on the property of various membrane-active agents to increase intracellular cations. Some of the interesting agents include the antibiotics monensin[790] and gramicidin[791]; the calcium channel blockers nitrendipine, nifedipine, and verapamil[792]; and the peripheral vasodilator cetiedil.[793] As discussed previously, preliminary evidence suggests that blocking the Gardos channel with oral clotrimazole[171] and blocking K$^+$-Cl$^-$ cotransport with oral magnesium[182,183] may decrease the HbS concentrations by preventing dehydration and could therefore prove to be useful therapies. Dipyridamole has been observed to block sickling-induced cation fluxes in vitro, but no trials have been reported.[794]

Increased Hemoglobin S Solubility. The most straightforward approach to preventing polymerization of HbS is to attack the β6 valine, the key to fiber formation. Unfortunately, this is an extremely unreactive residue, so efforts to increase the solubility of HbS have hinged on the importance of the other intermolecular contacts. Reagents that increase deoxy-HbS solubility by noncovalent interactions with HbS have been recognized. Chang

and colleagues[791] compared the effects of 15 antisickling agents on HbS solubility, oxygen affinity, and cell sickling. Urea is an effective agent but requires concentrations greater than 200 μM, too high for in vivo use. The best studied covalent modifier is cyanate, but clinical trials have not been promising. Unfortunately, despite the encouraging clinical and in vitro data, this compound is not usable because of significant neurotoxicity[795] and cataract formation.[796] A major problem with covalent reagents is that they interact with a wide variety of functional groups found in many molecules other than hemoglobin.

Decreased Dwell Time. Any manipulation that would allow a cell to traverse a vessel faster than its delay time will prevent occlusion of that vessel. Therapy aimed at reducing endothelial adherence has thus far not been successful.[797] Rodgers and co-workers[798] showed that microcirculatory flow in patients with SCD has an unusual periodic pattern indicative of abnormal vasomotor control. Recent work indicates that free plasma HbS binds NO, thereby reducing the ability of NO to maintain vasodilation.[242,243] Efforts to increase NO with hydroxyurea,[773,774,799] arginine therapy,[800,801] or inhaled NO[802] could possibly lead to less vasocontriction and increased dwell time (see Figs. 19-1 and 19-6).

Routine Health Maintenance

Patients with sickle cell anemia should be monitored on a routine basis (Table 19-6). Regular visits along with routine laboratory studies when the patient is well help establish both the individual's steady-state normal values (e.g., hemoglobin, reticulocytes, WBCs, differential, platelet count, erythrocyte sedimentation rate, chest film, electrocardiogram) and baseline physical findings (e.g., icterus, cardiomegaly, murmurs, organomegaly). These baseline data are extremely helpful in sorting out problems when the patient is ill.

Careful evaluation of the interval history may provide insight into factors that provoke painful crises. Continuing education of patients and families on how to avoid and treat painful episodes will reduce the morbidity and hospitalization rate and promote the patient's sense of independence. Education should also include genetic counseling of the parents so that they understand the risks of SCD in future pregnancies.

Careful attention is paid to routine immunization schedules; all patients should receive the complete schedule of conjugated pneumococcal, conjugated H. influenzae, and hepatitis B vaccines. Prophylactic penicillin should be given to all children younger than 5 years.[574] Most important, the patient and family should be educated about the importance of early detection and treatment of infection.

Although folic acid, 1 mg/day, is recommended for prevention of folate deficiency in adults, no definite advantage has been seen in children.[803] Iron deficiency is

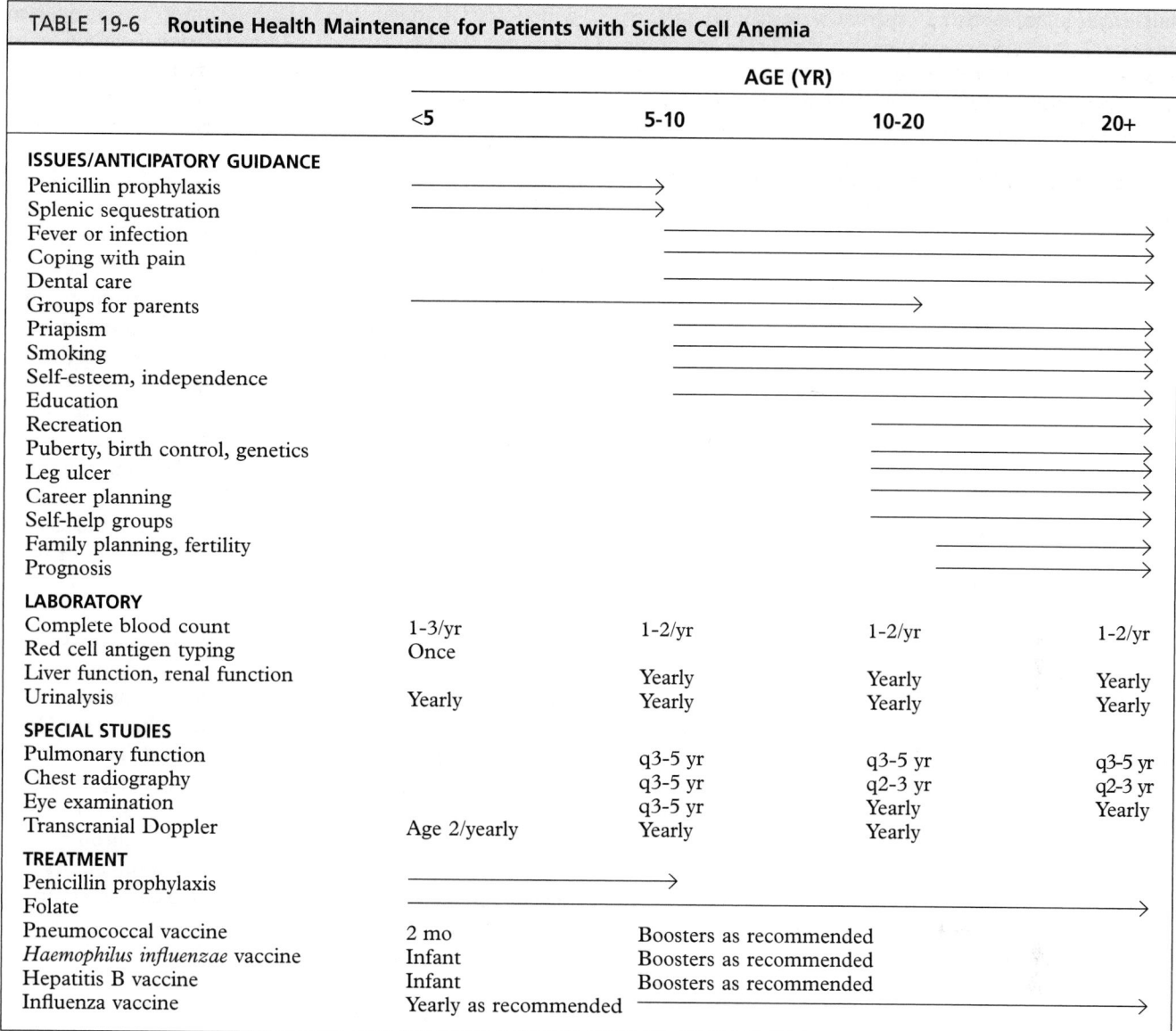

TABLE 19-6 **Routine Health Maintenance for Patients with Sickle Cell Anemia**

ISSUES/ANTICIPATORY GUIDANCE	<5	5-10	10-20	20+
Penicillin prophylaxis	——————————→			
Splenic sequestration	——————————→			
Fever or infection		——————————————————→		
Coping with pain		——————————————————→		
Dental care		——————————————————→		
Groups for parents	———————————————————→			
Priapism		——————————————→		
Smoking		——————————————→		
Self-esteem, independence		——————————————→		
Education		——————————————→		
Recreation		——————————————→		
Puberty, birth control, genetics			——————————→	
Leg ulcer			——————————→	
Career planning			——————————→	
Self-help groups			——————————→	
Family planning, fertility			——————————→	
Prognosis			——————————→	
LABORATORY				
Complete blood count	1-3/yr	1-2/yr	1-2/yr	1-2/yr
Red cell antigen typing	Once			
Liver function, renal function		Yearly	Yearly	Yearly
Urinalysis	Yearly	Yearly	Yearly	Yearly
SPECIAL STUDIES				
Pulmonary function		q3-5 yr	q3-5 yr	q3-5 yr
Chest radiography		q3-5 yr	q2-3 yr	q2-3 yr
Eye examination		q3-5 yr	Yearly	Yearly
Transcranial Doppler	Age 2/yearly	Yearly	Yearly	
TREATMENT				
Penicillin prophylaxis	——————————→			
Folate				——————→
Pneumococcal vaccine	2 mo	Boosters as recommended		
Haemophilus influenzae vaccine	Infant	Boosters as recommended		
Hepatitis B vaccine	Infant	Boosters as recommended		
Influenza vaccine	Yearly as recommended	——————————————→		

extremely rare because of the hemolysis-induced increased absorption of gastrointestinal iron. Iron supplements are used only when iron deficiency is documented or when blood loss is chronic (e.g., hematuria).

Specially trained ultrasonographers can use TCD according to the STOP criteria to screen children with sickle cell anemia and S–β⁰-thalassemia to identify those at increased risk for primary stroke. Children with internal carotid or middle cerebral blood flow greater than 200 cm/sec benefit from prophylactic maintenance transfusion to prevent stroke.[469] The ideal age range and frequency of TCD screening have not been determined yet[804]; however, the NHLBI recommends screening approximately every 6 months in patients 2 to 16 years of age, when the risk for stroke is highest.

Ophthalmologic examinations should be started at school age and repeated every few years unless retinopathy is discovered. For patients with retinopathy, more frequent follow-up and fluorescein angiography are nec-

essary to establish the tempo of the lesion and to determine appropriate therapy.

Regular dental care is critical in preventing the intraoral lesions that might predispose to infections such as mandibular osteomyelitis.[805]

Birth control options should be discussed as with any adolescent patient. Barrier methods and low-dose estrogen oral and depot injectable contraceptives can be used safely.[806,807]

Management of Painful Crises

Most painful crises can be successfully treated at home by increased fluid intake and oral analgesics. If the pain is too severe for oral analgesics or if the patient cannot maintain adequate fluid intake, the episode must be treated at the hospital. Hospital management of painful crisis includes hydration and analgesia. In dehydrated patients, the intravenous fluid rate is usually one and a half times maintenance; however, some cannot tolerate this expansion of intravascular volume. Frequent monitoring of vital signs during fluid administration is essential to prevent iatrogenic cardiac failure. Serum electrolyte levels must be checked early and intravenous solutions adjusted appropriately. Though theoretically sound, the use of intravenous bicarbonate has not been shown to be effective.[808] Face mask oxygen is of little therapeutic value unless the patient is hypoxic. Furthermore, Embury and colleagues have shown that continuous oxygen inhalation can suppress erythropoiesis, with reticulocyte counts falling within days.[809] In addition, painful crisis may result from rebound marrow activity after the abrupt discontinuation of oxygen therapy or cessation of transfusion programs.[810]

Analgesia must be sufficient to control the pain. Analgesics and other adjuvants may be combined to optimize efficacy/safety. "Standard doses" may not be adequate to "capture" an individual patient's pain, especially if not opioid naïve on initial evaluation, so dosing should be titrated to relief. Although opioid dependence or enhanced opioid-seeking behavior may be a problem for rare patients, overestimation of the incidence of this unusual situation must not affect the decision to control severe pain.[811] It is very unfortunate that subtle misconceptions interfere with providing appropriate pain relief. In one study, standardized patients with a chief complaint of pain who gave histories of frequent pain crises were given less opioid by nurses than were identical patients whose scripts included a history of infrequent pain episodes.[812]

One should choose opioids with side effects, drug interactions, serum half-lives, and previous efficacy in mind. Changes in the route of administration (intravenous, oral, transdermal) require adjustments for equianalgesic dosages. Serial intramuscular injections should be avoided because they can lead to the formation of sterile abscesses. High-dose meperidine may cause seizures, particularly in the setting of compromised renal function, in which toxic levels of normeperidine accumulate.[813] At the onset of inpatient therapy for severe pain, regular dosage intervals based on half-life should be used and not an "as-needed" dosage strategy. This approach may avoid the recurrence of pain and anxiety as a result of delay in obtaining the next dose of medicine after being requested. Continuous intravenous opioid therapy in children has been successfully used,[814] but ACS may be precipitated by respiratory depression.[815] Perhaps an optimal approach is the use of patient-controlled analgesia[816,817] initiated in the emergency department[818] to provide adequate pain relief at a lower total opioid dose.[819]

Hypoventilation is the most serious side effect of opioid therapy and must be carefully avoided by careful monitoring of oxygen saturation, aggressive use of incentive spirometry,[820] and use of oxygen when the patient is hypoxic. In one study, epidural anesthesia was successfully used to alleviate pain and maintain or improve oxygenation.[821] Constipation and urinary retention are common problems that should be remedied early. Sometimes it is virtually impossible to make a patient entirely comfortable with safe doses of opioids. This frustrating situation needs to be approached with care and sensitivity, with involvement of every member of the patient care team.[822,823] The addition of nonsteroidal anti-inflammatory agents is helpful to some patients. Others have benefitted from adjuncts such as acupuncture,[824] biofeedback, and hypnosis.[825] For the rare patient who is incapacitated by recurrent episodes of pain and who spends more time in the hospital than out, chronic outpatient opioid therapy may be useful.[826] Although transfusion (even exchange transfusion) is rarely effective for acute pain, a brief maintenance program may facilitate completion of a school year or an important project at work; however, this must be tempered by risks of allosensitization, iron overload, and blood-borne infection. Hydroxyurea is effective at decreasing the frequency of recurrent painful crises, but its favorable effect may be delayed by months or until MTDs are reached.[393]

Transfusion

Transfusions improve the oxygen-carrying capacity and decrease the proportion of erythrocytes that carry HbS. Although transfusion is typically not used for the treatment of chronic anemia or acute painful crises, it is often necessary for associated comorbid conditions.[827] Current transfusion practices include episodic or chronic regimens, depending on whether the reduction in risk for severe clinicopathologic sequelae from SCD (e.g., stroke or recurrent ACS) outweighs the risks inherent in a chronic transfusion regimen.

Episodic transfusions (simple or exchange) are used primarily to treat acute complications of SCD. Simple transfusion is possible when the anticipated post-transfusion hemoglobin level will not exceed 10 to 11 g/dL. Exchange transfusion (either by manual technique or automated erythrocytapheresis) is reserved for complications that are either life threatening or pose risk for irreversible tissue damage (e.g., stroke, severe ACS) or when initial simple transfusion was ineffective. The primary goal of exchange transfusion is to reduce the HbS concentration rapidly to less than 30% of the total hemoglobin content without increasing blood viscosity or expanding the blood volume, thereby reducing potential cardiovascular strain. In centers in which an automated cell separator is available, a two-volume exchange transfusion can be efficiently accomplished in less than 90 minutes.[502,503] Episodic transfusion is indicated for the management of symptomatic episodes of acute anemia (e.g., aplastic crisis triggered by parvovirus infection), severe/progressive ACS, acute stroke, splenic sequestration, and priapism unresponsive to medical therapy, as well as perioperatively. As discussed previously, simple transfusion is preferred instead of exchange transfusion in the preoperative setting.

Chronic transfusion therapy is implemented when the ongoing risk of morbidity from sickle cell complications outweighs the risks inherent in recurrent blood exposure. In a chronic regimen involving simple or exchange methods, transfusions are usually scheduled every 3 to 4 weeks, with the goal of maintaining the HbS level between 30% and 50%. Chronic transfusion therapy has been indicated for primary stroke prevention in high-risk children identified by TCD and for prevention of recurrent stroke in children who have already experienced an overt stroke. Limited-duration regular transfusions may be indicated for reducing the frequency and severity of ACS, complicated pregnancy, prolonged hematuria, and chronic vaso-occlusive complications (e.g., nonhealing leg ulcer). Sickle trait blood should not be used.

Chronic transfusion regimens in SCD may increase risk for the transfusion-associated complications of allosensitization, infection, and progressive iron overload. Transfusional iron accumulation is ultimately unavoidable, though often clinically undetected and undertreated. Excess iron is deposited in multiple organs, including the liver, heart, pancreas, endocrine glands, and skin, with potential for organ damage. There is no physiologic mechanism for iron removal, but fortunately, parenteral deferoxamine[828,829] and oral deferasirox[830] are effective chelators if adhered to chronically. Serial assessment of serum ferritin levels may provide insight into ongoing iron balance in SCD,[831,832] but because infections and vaso-occlusive crises also increase ferritin levels, it is a suboptimal predictor of liver iron burden and liver fibrosis. However, high liver iron levels were not associated with as much liver disease as expected from similar data in thalassemia.[833]

In children who have received multiple transfusions, the rate of alloimmunization is between 7% and 20%.[834-837] The likelihood of alloimmunization is related to the number of transfusions, racial differences between the common donor and recipient erythrocyte phenotype, and as yet unknown genetic factors that control the responsiveness of the recipient to transfused antigens.[452] Opinions and practices differ in regard to the utility of preventing sensitization with the use of expensive antigen-matched cells as opposed to providing these cells after sensitization occurs.[838,839] The most common antibody-provoking antigens are K, C, E, S, Fy^a, Fy^b, and Jk^b. Ideally, patients with SS SCD should receive antigen-matched red cells beyond ABO and D to include C, E, and Kell to reduce the hazard of sensitization,[839] and such a strategy has been demonstrated prospectively to reduce sensitization.[840] Some suggest further extension of phenotype matching,[841,842] but the added expense and relative scarcity of the required random donors make this impractical.[839] Potential benefits from attempting to prevent allosensitization include prevention of complications from the first delayed transfusion reaction and possibly the prevention of autoantibodies that appear in the same context. Clinically significant autoantibodies do occur in about 10% of patients with SCD, and the incidence appears to be higher in those with alloantibodies.[837,842,843] In 183 children the incidence of autoantibodies was 7.6%, and when associated with C3 on the red cells, the autoantibodies resulted in hemolysis.[453]

Preparation for Surgery

Children with SCD have an increased likelihood of undergoing surgical procedures, in particular, cholecystectomy, splenectomy, and joint replacement. The CSSCD found that 7% of all deaths in patients with sickle cell anemia were related to surgery.[247] In 1079 surgical procedures on 717 patients of all genotypes, the mortality within 30 days of the procedure was 1.1% (12 deaths); however, no deaths were reported in children younger than 14 years.[844] That same series illustrated comparable complication rates in the SS and SC groups and suggested that patients undergoing regional anesthesia were at higher risk for complications than those undergoing general anesthesia.[844]

The CSSCD "natural history" study did not definitively address the important question of the effectiveness of preoperative transfusion. In a review of records from Dallas Children's Hospital, pulmonary complications were particularly common in patients undergoing laparotomy, thoracotomy, or tonsillectomy and adenoidectomy who were not transfused preoperatively (9/29) when compared with those who underwent transfusion for these procedures (0/8).[845] More recently, Vichinsky and collaborators in the Preoperative Transfusion in Sickle Cell Disease Study Group reported the findings of a prospective, multi-institutional study that randomized more than 600 preoperative HbSS patients to receive either simple transfusion designed to increase the total hemoglobin concentration to 10 g/dL or exchange transfusion designed to decrease the HbS percentage to less than 30 and increase total hemoglobin to 10 g/dL.[846-850] Several key points emerged from that study:

- There was no significant difference between the two transfusion strategies in terms of complications; both strategies reported a high 30% postpartum complication rate. Transfusion-related complications were twice as common (14%) in the exchange transfusion arm as in the simple transfusion arm (7%).
- The most common and serious complication was ACS, which occurred in 10% of procedures in both arms. The average time at onset was postoperative day 3, the average length of the episode was 8 days, 11% of the patients required intubation, and two died.
- Those in a higher surgical risk category—history of pulmonary disease, occurrence of ACS, and increased frequency of hospitalization—were at higher risk for complications.

These data suggest that at minimum, a simple transfusion designed to raise the preoperative hemoglobin level to 10 g/dL should be administered to all patients with HbSS disease.

In addition to transfusion, perioperative morbidity can be minimized safely by careful collaboration between the hematologist, anesthesiologist, and surgeon during the perioperative period. Those with previous pulmonary dysfunction or a history of multiple hospital admissions should receive a minimum of overnight maintenance intravenous hydration and be monitored as high-risk patients. During the procedure and in the postoperative period, all patients should have compulsive attention paid to oxygenation, hydration, maintenance of warm body temperature, acid-base balance, and positioning that does not impair circulation.[844,851-856] Choice of an anesthetic agent is not as critical as the care with which it is delivered.[853]

Management of Pregnancy

Although many women with SCD have normal pregnancies, pregnancy can be associated with serious problems for both the mother and fetus. Pregnant women should be monitored closely and collaboratively by obstetricians and hematologists experienced in high-risk pregnancies. Maternal complications may include an increase in the frequency and severity of painful crises, an increase in the severity and frequency of chest syndrome, exaggeration of physiologic anemia of pregnancy, toxemia, and death.[857] Because of sickling in the placenta, fetal complications can include spontaneous abortion, prematurity, and intrauterine growth retardation. Some authors have suggested that pregnancy outcome could be improved further if mothers are prophylactically transfused,[858,859] but no significant benefit of transfusions to the mother or fetus during pregnancy was demonstrated in the only prospective trial.[860] Hepatitis, alloimmunization, and hemolytic transfusion reactions[860,861] have been reported in transfused pregnant sickle patients. Therefore, transfusion therapy is not recommended prophylactically and is reserved for acute, severe, or persistent complications.[862,863] With modern obstetric management, regular prenatal care, and better nutrition, maternal mortality has been reduced to less than 1% and perinatal deaths have declined to less than 15%.[864,865]

OTHER SICKLE SYNDROMES

Sickle Cell Trait: $\alpha_2\beta_2$, $\alpha_2\beta_2^{Val6}$

Sickle cell trait is a benign condition that is not associated with increased morbidity or mortality.[866-870] There is no associated anemia, abnormal morphology, or decreased red cell survival. Most individuals have approximately 40% HbS and 60% HbA. A population with 28% to 35% HbS has been identified and shown to have accompanying α-thalassemia.[871] Decreased levels of HbS can also be seen in patients with iron[872] and folate[873] deficiencies. Growth, behavior, educational achievement, and pregnancy risks in children with sickle trait are entirely normal.[874-876] Black American professional football players

have the same incidence of sickle trait as the general black population does.[877] In a retrospective study of sudden death during physical training in the U.S. Armed Forces, Kark and colleagues noted a 1 in 3200 incidence of sudden death among sickle trait recruits, a frequency 27 times greater than that in non-HbS controls.[878] All deaths were associated with strenuous physical exertion, and risks increased with age. After this report, modifications in basic training for all recruits have been recommended, but follow-up data are not yet available. A subsequent prospective study of 25 sickle trait recruits and non-HbS controls revealed no difference in exercise tolerance or physical conditioning after 7 weeks of basic training.[879] Several authors have stressed that these data do not justify restriction of sickle trait men from the armed services or organized sports.[880-882] Although anecdotal reports of various severe vaso-occlusive episodes in those with sickle trait appear in the literature, they are extremely rare and not clearly due to sickle trait. However, Eichner has reviewed the sudden death of nine college athletes with sickle trait and summarized findings that distinguished sickling from more common heat-related illnesses.[883] Postmortem findings of intravascular sickling are not evidence that the sickling had occurred before death. Under certain extreme conditions, however, sickling and even death may occur in individuals with sickle trait. Such conditions include severe pneumonia,[884] unpressurized flying, and exercise at high altitudes.[885,886] The risk associated with routine aviation in individuals with sickle trait has been overstated.[887] Careful general anesthesia does not carry great risk for a person with sickle trait,[888,889] but tourniquet surgery[853] and deep hypothermia should be avoided. The most consistent abnormality found in sickle trait is an inability to concentrate urine.[890] Persistent hematuria in sickle trait individuals has been associated with papillary necrosis of the kidney[891] and rarely renal medullary carcinoma.[627] Traumatic hyphema in sickle trait is a medical emergency because in the hypoxic conditions of the anterior chamber of the eye, HbAS red cells will sickle and lead to increased intraocular pressure.[892] Sickle trait women in one prospective study showed an increased risk for preeclampsia, and their infants had a minimal decrease in gestational age and birth weight but no increased infant mortality.[893] Previous retrospective and case-control studies have provided conflicting data regarding differences in birth weight or gestational age at birth.[894-897] Patients in whom sickle trait is diagnosed but a clinical and laboratory phenotype consistent with a sickling disorder develops should be considered for molecular globin diagnostics to ensure accuracy of the diagnosis.[898,899]

SC Disease: $\alpha_2\beta_2^{Val6}$, $\alpha_2\beta_2^{Lys6}$

Hemoglobin SC disease is a mild chronic hemolytic anemia associated with variable degrees of vaso-occlusive complications. As described in Table 19-2, the patient typically has a hemoglobin concentration of 10 to 12 g/

dL, a reticulocyte count of 1% to 13%, and a relative microcytosis for the degree of reticulocytosis. The peripheral blood smear (see Fig. 19-4) is more characteristic of HbC than HbS and reveals impressive target cells and rare, if any ISCs. The clinical course is quite variable, with some patients severely affected at an early age and others entirely asymptomatic and identified only as adults on routine screening. Hemolysis is less severe in SC disease than in SS disease[900] and therefore results in a higher hematocrit in patients with SC disease.

The major complications of HbSS disease are not as common in SC disease but have been reported to include recurrent painful bone crises, painful abdominal crises, gallstones, pulmonary infarction, priapism, and CNS infarction.[901-904] As shown in Figure 19-7, the pattern of clinical events is different in SC disease, with most events occurring not only less frequently but also later in life. Certain complications appear to be more common in the SC disease population: eye disease,[665,902,905-907] AVN of the femoral heads, renal papillary necrosis,[908] and pregnancy-related problems.[909] Splenomegaly is found in approximately 60% of patients with SC disease and has been associated with splenic infarction[910] and splenic sequestration,[911] particularly at high altitudes. Although infection is not as common in SC disease as in SS disease,[912] splenic hypofunction and an increased risk for pneumococcal and *H. influenzae* sepsis are found in SC disease.[913] Pneumococcal and *H. influenzae* vaccines are indicated in SC disease, and the use of prophylactic penicillin is recommended.

Patients with SC disease clearly have more sickling complications than do individuals with sickle trait, who are essentially free of sickling complications. One would therefore assume that mixtures of HbS and HbA are less likely to polymerize than mixtures of HbS and HbC. Interestingly, Bunn and associates[914] have shown that such is not the case because the kinetic and equilibrium behavior of mixtures of HbS and HbA is essentially identical to the behavior of mixtures of HbS and HbC. One can resolve this apparent paradox by considering how the hemoglobin mixtures are packaged in SC and AS cells. There are two major factors that explain why SC cells sickle more readily than AS cells do: (1) there is more HbS in an SC cell, and (2) an SC cell has a higher MCHC. Because the charge and affinity for β-globin differs between $β^S$-globin and $β^C$-globin, individuals with SC disease usually have 50% HbS and 50% HbC, whereas those with sickle trait typically have 60% HbA and 40% HbS.[908] The increased HbS content of SC cells results in an approximately sevenfold increase in the rate of polymerization.[915] The increase in MCHC in SC disease, which is quite obvious on density separation of SC red cells[139,914,916] (see Fig. 19-5) and even C trait red cells,[915] is probably due to activation of the KCC system by the positively charged HbC molecules.[917] The cellular dehydration and microcytosis associated with HbC has been well characterized by Brugnara and colleagues[918] and Ballas and associates.[916]

Hemoglobin SC and α-Thalassemia

One patient with HbSC and α-thalassemia trait has been described.[919] This 7-year-old child had the following laboratory values: hematocrit, 25.8%; hemoglobin, 7.9 g/dL; MCV, 53 μm³; MCH, 16.2 pg; MCHC, 30.6 g/dL; reticulocytes, 7.2%; HbS, 50.5%; HbC, 47.7%; and HbF, 1.8%. One parent had 27% HbS with an MCV of 71 μm³; the other had 24% HbC with an MCV of 57 μm³. This patient, like many patients with SC disease, was relatively asymptomatic. Of interest is that her hematocrit level and reticulocyte count are compatible with a considerable degree of hemolysis.

SO Arab: $α_2β_2{}^{Val6}$, $α_2β_2{}^{Lys121}$

SO_{Arab} double heterozygotes are quite rare and have a relatively severe disorder with chronic hemolytic anemia and vaso-occlusive episodes.[920] As seen in Figure 19-4, the O Arab mutation lies within the area critical to axial contact in the HbS fiber. Routine cellulose acetate electrophoresis at pH 8.6 does not distinguish between HbC and HbO_{Arab}. Citrate agar electrophoresis at pH 6 does separate HbC from HbO and should be performed for patients who appear to have HbSC disease on cellulose acetate electrophoresis but who have particularly severe symptoms.[921]

SD: $α_2β_2{}^{Val6}$, $α_2β_2{}^{Glu121}$

SD double heterozygotes have severe hemolytic anemia with a peripheral blood smear comparable to that seen in HbSS. These rare patients have severe vaso-occlusive complications,[922-924] thus illustrating, as in those with HbO_{Arab}, the critical nature of the β121 contact site. HbD migrates with HbS on cellulose acetate electrophoresis at alkaline pH and can be distinguished from HbS on citrate agar electrophoresis at acid pH. HbD is suspected when a hemoglobin appears to be HbS on cellulose acetate electrophoresis but gives a negative "sickle prep." Identification of a parent with HbD is important socially because it may become difficult to explain how a child has "SS disease" and only one parent has a positive sickle prep.

S Korle Bu: $α_2β_2{}^{Val6}$, $α_2β_2{}^{Asn73}$

Hemoglobin Korle Bu is a rare hemoglobin mutant.[925] It is mentioned here only because it illustrates an important pathophysiologic point. Korle Bu participates poorly in sickling.[926] This mutation interferes with lateral contact between HbS fibers by blocking the critical receptor area for $β^{Val6}$. S Korle Bu double heterozygotes are entirely symptom free.

Hemoglobin C Harlem (C Georgetown): $α_2β_2{}^{Val6, Asn73}$

Hemoglobin C_{Harlem} (also known as $C_{Georgetown}$) has two substitutions on the β chain: the sickle mutation $β^{Val6}$ and the Korle Bu mutation β^{Asn73}.[927] Patients with these mutations are asymptomatic. Patients doubly heterozygous for HbS and HbC$_{Harlem}$ have clinical crises resembling SS disease.[927,928]

Hemoglobin S Antilles: $\alpha_2\beta_2^{Val6, \, Ile23}$

HbS Antilles also has two substitutions on the β chain: the sickle mutation β^{Val6} and a second mutation β^{Ile23}.[929] This mutation results in hemoglobin with low oxygen affinity that in heterozygotes for HbA and HbS Antilles, results in mild hemolytic anemia and the presence of 5% to 7% ISCs. A transgenic mouse with HbS Antilles and the HbD mutations (see earlier) exhibits many of the clinical features of SS disease.[930]

Sickle–β-Thalassemia

Patients heterozygous for HbS and β-thalassemia have clinical severity that depends on the output of the thalassemic β gene.[511,931,932] If no HbA is produced ("S–β[0]-thalassemia"), the clinical course is comparable (see Table 19-2 and Fig. 19-9) to that of homozygous sickle cell anemia. Electrophoresis shows mostly HbS with slightly elevated HbA$_2$ and variable amounts of HbF. Features that distinguish these patients from those with sickle cell anemia are that they may be of Mediterranean origin, have microcytosis, and often have splenomegaly. One parent will have classic sickle trait, whereas the other will have β-thalassemia trait. The hemolytic rate is lower, and the patients tend to have a slightly higher hematocrit and lower reticulocyte count. Their peripheral blood morphology is notable for target cells, microcytosis, and generally fewer ISCs than in sickle cell anemia. If there is output from the β-thalassemia gene ("S–β[+]-thalassemia"), patients tend to have a milder clinical course, comparable to that of SC disease. Electrophoresis in these patients shows predominantly HbS, elevated HbA$_2$, variable amounts of HbF, and HbA. Features that distinguish these individuals from those with sickle cell anemia are HbA, microcytosis, splenomegaly, and a relatively benign clinical course. The ameliorative effects of HbA (see Table 19-2 and Figs. 19-5 and 19-9) are apparent. These patients can be distinguished from individuals with sickle trait because of a higher percentage of HbS than HbA, microcytosis, hemolytic anemia, abnormal peripheral morphology, and splenomegaly. α-Thalassemia with HbS–β[0]-thalassemia results in higher hemoglobin levels, lower reticulocyte counts, and increases in MCV and MCHC.[271]

Hemoglobin C Disease: $\alpha_2\beta_2^{Lys6}$

Homozygous HbC disease is a mild disorder characterized by hemolytic anemia, microcytosis, and splenomegaly.[933-938] The tendency of HbC to aggregate and crystallize[939-941] is probably responsible for the characteristic target morphology of the stained and dried red cell

in homozygous C disease and in HbC trait, although these crystals are not likely to be directly responsible for the hemolytic anemia. In HbC trait, target cell formation and mild microcytosis are the only manifestation of the anomaly. Hemolytic anemia is not present.

The basis of the aggregation and crystal formation of HbC cells is not precisely understood. It is thought that the substantial charge difference between HbC and HbA is in some way responsible for the tendency toward aggregation of C molecules, which leads to local increments in hemoglobin concentration in excess of its solubility.[938] The structure of these crystals has been examined by x-ray diffraction analysis.[939-941]

The hemolytic anemia of homozygous HbC disease is probably due to the fact that these cells are dehydrated. Brugnara and colleagues have demonstrated that CC red cells have decreased water and cation content associated with a large efflux of potassium.[918] As discussed in the previous section on membrane abnormalities, this volume-dependent potassium efflux is regulated by the KCC pathway.

REFERENCES

1. Herrick JB. Peculiar elongated and sickle-shaped corpuscles in a case of severe anemia. Arch Intern Med. 1910;6:517-521.
2. Savitt TL, Goldberg MF. Herrick's 1910 case report of sickle cell anemia. The rest of the story. JAMA. 1989;261:266-271.
3. Sydenstricked VP, Mulherin WA, Houseal RW. The AJDC archives. August 1923. Sickle cell anemia. Report of two cases in children, with necropsy in one case. By V. P. Sydenstricked [sic], W. A. Mulherin and R. W. Houseal. Am J Dis Child. 1987;141:612-615.
4. Hahn E, Gillespie E. Sickle cell anemia: report of a case greatly improved by splenectomy. Arch Intern Med. 1927;39:233.
5. Pauling L, Itano HA, Singer SJ, Wells IC. Sickle cell anemia, a molecular disease. Science. 1949;110:543-548.
6. Neel JV. The inheritance of the sickling phenomenon, with particular reference to sickle cell disease. Blood. 1951;6:389-412.
7. Ingram VM. Gene mutations in human haemoglobin: the chemical difference between normal and sickle cell haemoglobin. Nature. 1957;180:326-328.
8. Conley CL. Sickle cell anemia—the first molecular disease. In Wintrobe MM (ed). Blood, Pure and Eloquent. New York, McGraw-Hill, 1980.
9. Motulsky AG. Frequency of sickling disorders in U.S. blacks. N Engl J Med. 1973;288:31-33.
10. Kan YW, Dozy AM. Evolution of the hemoglobin S and C genes in world populations. Science. 1980;209:388-391.
11. Antonarakis SE, Boehm CD, Serjeant GR, et al. Origin of the beta S-globin gene in blacks: the contribution of recurrent mutation or gene conversion or both. Proc Natl Acad Sci U S A. 1984;81:853-856.

12. Pagnier J, Mears JG, Dunda-Belkhodja O, et al. Evidence for the multicentric origin of the sickle cell hemoglobin gene in Africa. Proc Natl Acad Sci U S A. 1984;81:1771-1773.

13. Stine OC, Dover GJ, Zhu D, Smith KD. The evolution of two west African populations. J Mol Evol. 1992;34:336-344.

14. Lapoumeroulie C, Dunda O, Ducrocq R, et al. A novel sickle cell mutation of yet another origin in Africa: the Cameroon type. Hum Genet. 1992;89:333-337.

15. Kulozik AE, Wainscoat JS, Serjeant GR, et al. Geographical survey of beta S-globin gene haplotypes: evidence for an independent Asian origin of the sickle-cell mutation. Am J Hum Genet. 1986;39:239-244.

16. Ragusa A, Lombardo M, Sortino G, et al. Beta S gene in Sicily is in linkage disequilibrium with the Benin haplotype: implications for gene flow. Am J Hematol. 1988;27:139-141.

17. Aluoch JR, Kilinc Y, Aksoy M, et al. Sickle cell anaemia among Eti-Turks: haematological, clinical and genetic observations. Br J Haematol. 1986;64:45-55.

18. Schroeder WA, Powars DR, Kay LM, et al. Beta-cluster haplotypes, alpha-gene status, and hematological data from SS, SC, and S-beta-thalassemia patients in southern California. Hemoglobin. 1989;13:325-353.

19. Hattori Y, Kutlar F, Kutlar A, et al. Haplotypes of beta S chromosomes among patients with sickle cell anemia from Georgia. Hemoglobin. 1986;10:623-642.

20. Nagel RL, Fabry ME, Pagnier J, et al. Hematologically and genetically distinct forms of sickle cell anemia in Africa. The Senegal type and the Benin type. N Engl J Med. 1985;312:880-884.

21. Nagel RL, Rao SK, Dunda-Belkhodja O, et al. The hematologic characteristics of sickle cell anemia bearing the Bantu haplotype: the relationship between G gamma and HbF level. Blood. 1987;69:1026-1030.

22. Srinivas R, Dunda O, Krishnamoorthy R, et al. Atypical haplotypes linked to the beta S gene in Africa are likely to be the product of recombination. Am J Hematol. 1988;29:60-62.

23. Antonarakis SE, Boehm CD, Giardina PJ, Kazazian HH Jr. Nonrandom association of polymorphic restriction sites in the beta-globin gene cluster. Proc Natl Acad Sci U S A. 1982;79:137-141.

24. Powars D, Chan LS, Schroeder WA. The variable expression of sickle cell disease is genetically determined. Semin Hematol. 1990;27:360-376.

25. Perrine RP, Brown MJ, Clegg JB, et al. Benign sickle-cell anaemia. Lancet. 1972;2:1163-1167.

26. Pembrey ME, Wood WG, Weatherall DJ, Perrine RP. Fetal haemoglobin production and the sickle gene in the oases of eastern Saudi Arabia. Br J Haematol. 1978;40:415-429.

27. Perrine RP, Pembrey ME, John P, et al. Natural history of sickle cell anemia in Saudi Arabs. A study of 270 subjects. Ann Intern Med. 1978;88:1-6.

28. Brittenham G, Lozoff B, Harris JW, et al. Sickle cell anemia and trait in southern India: further studies. Am J Hematol. 1979;6:107-123.

29. Min-Oo G, Gros P. Erythrocyte variants and the nature of their malaria protective effect. Cell Microbiol. 2005;7:753-763.

30. Luzzatto L, Nwachuku-Jarrett ES, Reddy S. Increased sickling of parasitised erythrocytes as mechanism of resistance against malaria in the sickle-cell trait. Lancet. 1970;1:319-321.

31. Roth EF Jr, Friedman M, Ueda Y, et al. Sickling rates of human AS red cells infected in vitro with *Plasmodium falciparum* malaria. Science. 1978;202:650-652.

32. Friedman MJ, Trager W. The biochemistry of resistance to malaria. Sci Am. 1981;244:154-155, 158-164.

33. Pasvol G, Weatherall DJ, Wilson RJ. Cellular mechanism for the protective effect of haemoglobin S against *P. falciparum* malaria. Nature. 1978;274:701-703.

34. Sobolewski P, Gramaglia I, Frangos J, et al. Nitric oxide bioavailability in malaria. Trends Parasitol. 2005;21:415-422.

35. Hood AT, Fabry ME, Costantini F, et al. Protection from lethal malaria in transgenic mice expressing sickle hemoglobin. Blood. 1996;87:1600-1603.

36. Williams TN, Mwangi TW, Wambua S, et al. Negative epistasis between the malaria-protective effects of alpha+-thalassemia and the sickle cell trait. Nat Genet. 2005;37:1253-1257.

37. Harris JW. Studies on the destruction of red blood cells. VIII. Molecular orientation in sickle cell hemoglobin solutions. Proc Soc Exp Biol Med. 1950;75:197-201.

38. Stetson CA Jr. The state of hemoglobin in sickled erythrocytes. J Exp Med. 1966;123:341-346.

39. Lessin LS. [Helicoidal polymerization of the hemoglobin molecules in sickle-shaped erythrocytes. Study by means of the frozen-etched method.] C R Acad Sci Hebd Seances Acad Sci D. 1968;266:1806-1808.

40. Beutler E, Johnson C, Powars D, West C. Prevalence of glucose-6-phosphate dehydrogenase deficiency in sickle-cell disease. N Engl J Med. 1974;290:826-828.

41. Finch JT, Perutz MF, Bertles JF, Dobler J. Structure of sickled erythrocytes and of sickle-cell hemoglobin fibers. Proc Natl Acad Sci U S A. 1973;70:718-722.

42. Dykes G, Crepeau RH, Edelstein SJ. Three-dimensional reconstruction of the fibres of sickle cell haemoglobin. Nature. 1978;272:506-510.

43. Garrell RL, Crepeau RH, Edelstein SJ. Cross-sectional views of hemoglobin S fibers by electron microscopy and computer modeling. Proc Natl Acad Sci U S A. 1979;76:1140-1144.

44. Dykes GW, Crepeau RH, Edelstein SJ. Three-dimensional reconstruction of the 14-filament fibers of hemoglobin S. J Mol Biol. 1979;130:451-472.

45. Edelstein SJ. Patterns in the quinary structures of proteins. Plasticity and inequivalence of individual molecules in helical arrays of sickle cell hemoglobin and tubulin. Biophys J. 1980;32:347-360.

46. Magdoff-Fairchild B, Chiu CC. X-ray diffraction studies of fibers and crystals of deoxygenated sickle cell hemoglobin. Proc Natl Acad Sci U S A. 1979;76:223-226.

47. Rodgers DW, Crepeau RH, Edelstein SJ. Pairings and polarities of the 14 strands in sickle cell hemoglobin fibers. Proc Natl Acad Sci U S A. 1987;84:6157-6161.

48. Carragher B, Bluemke DA, Becker M, et al. Structural analysis of polymers of sickle cell hemoglobin. III. Fibers within fascicles. J Mol Biol. 1988;199:383-388.

49. Makowski L, Magdoff-Fairchild B. Polymorphism of sickle cell hemoglobin aggregates: structural basis for limited radial growth. Science. 1986;234:1228-1231.

50. Wishner BC, Ward KB, Lattman EE, Love WE. Crystal structure of sickle-cell deoxyhemoglobin at 5 Å resolution. J Mol Biol. 1975;98:179-194.

51. Padlan EA, Love WE. Refined crystal structure of deoxyhemoglobin S. II. Molecular interactions in the crystal. J Biol Chem. 1985;260:8280-8291.

52. Edelstein SJ. Molecular topology in crystals and fibers of hemoglobin S. J Mol Biol. 1981;150:557-575.

53. Harrington JP, Elbaum D, Bookchin RM, et al. Ligand kinetics of hemoglobin S containing erythrocytes. Proc Natl Acad Sci U S A. 1977;74:203-206.

54. Harrington DJ, Adachi K, Royer WE Jr. The high resolution crystal structure of deoxyhemoglobin S. J Mol Biol. 1997;272:398-407.

55. Gill SJ, Spokane R, Benedict RC, et al. Ligand-linked phase equilibria of sickle cell hemoglobin. J Mol Biol. 1980;140:299-312.

56. Sunshine HR, Hofrichter J, Ferrone FA, Eaton WA. Oxygen binding by sickle cell hemoglobin polymers. J Mol Biol. 1982;158:251-273.

57. Ross PD, Hofrichter J, Eaton WA. Calorimetric and optical characterization of sickle cell hemoglobin gelation. J Mol Biol. 1975;96:239-253.

58. Ross PD, Hofrichter J, Eaton WA. Thermodynamics of gelation of sickle cell deoxyhemoglobin. J Mol Biol. 1977;115:111-134.

59. Magdoff-Fairchild B, Poillon WN, Li T, Bertles JF. Thermodynamic studies of polymerization of deoxygenated sickle cell hemoglobin. Proc Natl Acad Sci U S A. 1976; 73:990-994.

60. Briehl RW. Gelation of sickle cell hemoglobin. IV. Phase transitions in hemoglobin S gels: separate measures of aggregation and solution-gel equilibrium. J Mol Biol. 1978;123:521-538.

61. Poillon WN, Bertles JF. Deoxygenated sickle hemoglobin. Effects of lyotropic salts on its solubility. J Biol Chem. 1979;254:3462-3467.

62. Swerdlow PH, Bryan RA, Bertles JF, et al. Effect of 2, 3-diphosphoglycerate on the solubility of deoxy-sickle hemoglobin. Hemoglobin. 1977;1:527-537.

63. Hofrichter J, Ross PD, Eaton WA. Supersaturation in sickle cell hemoglobin solutions. Proc Natl Acad Sci U S A. 1976;73:3035-3039.

64. Hofrichter J, Ross PD, Eaton WA. A physical description of hemoglobin S gelation. In Hercules JI, Waterman MR, Schechter AN (eds). Proceedings of the Symposium on Molecular and Cellular Aspects of Sickle Cell Disease. Bethesda, MD, National Institutes of Health, Department of Health, Education and Welfare, 1976, pp 185-223.

65. Hofrichter J. Ligand binding and the gelation of sickle cell hemoglobin. J Mol Biol. 1979;128:335-369.

66. Ferrone FA, Hofrichter J, Eaton WA. Kinetics of sickle hemoglobin polymerization. II. A double nucleation mechanism. J Mol Biol. 1985;183:611-631.

67. Mirchev R, Ferrone FA. The structural link between polymerization and sickle cell disease. J Mol Biol. 1997; 265:475-479.

68. Eaton WA, Hofrichter J. Hemoglobin S gelation and sickle cell disease. Blood. 1987;70:1245-1266.

69. Rampling MW, Sirs JA. The rate of sickling of cells containing sickle-cell haemoglobin. Clin Sci Mol Med. 1973;45:655-664.

70. Coletta M, Hofrichter J, Ferrone FA, Eaton WA. Kinetics of sickle haemoglobin polymerization in single red cells. Nature. 1982;300:194-197.

71. Adachi K, Asakura T. Multiple nature of polymers of deoxyhemoglobin S prepared by different methods. J Biol Chem. 1983;258:3045-3050.

72. Asakura T, Mayberry J. Relationship between morphologic characteristics of sickle cells and method of deoxygenation. J Lab Clin Med. 1984;104:987-994.

73. Eaton WA, Hofrichter J, Ross PD. Delay time of gelation: a possible determinant of clinical severity in sickle cell disease [editorial]. Blood. 1976;47:621-627.

74. Mozzarelli A, Hofrichter J, Eaton WA. Delay time of hemoglobin S polymerization prevents most cells from sickling in vivo. Science. 1987;237:500-506.

75. Turner MS, Agarwal G, Jones CW, et al. Fiber depolymerization. Biophys J. 2006;91:1008-1013.

76. Noguchi CT, Torchia DA, Schechter AN. Intracellular polymerization of sickle hemoglobin. Effects of cell heterogeneity. J Clin Invest. 1983;72:846-852.

77. Noguchi CT, Torchia DA, Schechter AN. Determination of deoxyhemoglobin S polymer in sickle erythrocytes upon deoxygenation. Proc Natl Acad Sci U S A. 1980; 77:5487-5491.

78. Noguchi CT, Schechter AN. The intracellular polymerization of sickle hemoglobin and its relevance to sickle cell disease. Blood. 1981;58:1057-1068.

79. Green MA, Noguchi CT, Keidan AJ, et al. Polymerization of sickle cell hemoglobin at arterial oxygen saturation impairs erythrocyte deformability. J Clin Invest. 1988;81: 1669-1674.

80. Brittenham GM, Schechter AN, Noguchi CT. Hemoglobin S polymerization: primary determinant of the hemolytic and clinical severity of the sickling syndromes. Blood. 1985;65:183-189.

81. Keidan AJ, Sowter MC, Johnson CS, et al. Effect of polymerization tendency on haematological, rheological and clinical parameters in sickle cell anaemia. Br J Haematol. 1989;71:551-557.

82. Poillon WN, Kim BC, Castro O. Intracellular hemoglobin S polymerization and the clinical severity of sickle cell anemia. Blood. 1998;91:1777-1783.

83. Sunshine HR, Hofrichter J, Eaton WA. Requirement for therapeutic inhibition of sickle haemoglobin gelation. Nature. 1978;275:238-240.

84. Sunshine HR, Hofrichter J, Eaton WA. Gelation of sickle cell hemoglobin in mixtures with normal adult and fetal hemoglobins. J Mol Biol. 1979;133:435-467.

85. Behe MJ, Englander SW. Mixed gelation theory. Kinetics, equilibrium and gel incorporation in sickle hemoglobin mixtures. J Mol Biol. 1979;133:137-160.

86. Adachi K, Segal R, Asakura T. Nucleation-controlled aggregation of deoxyhemoglobin S. Participation of hemoglobin F in the aggregation of deoxyhemoglobin S in concentrated phosphate buffer. J Biol Chem. 1980;255: 7595-7603.

87. Adachi K, Matarasso SL, Asakura T. Nucleation-controlled aggregation of deoxyhemoglobin S. Effect of organic phosphates on the kinetics of aggregation of deoxyhemoglobin S in concentrated phosphate buffer. Biochim Biophys Acta. 1980;624:372-377.

88. Adachi K, Ozguc M, Asakura T. Nucleation-controlled aggregation of deoxyhemoglobin S. Participation of hemo-

globin A in the aggregation of deoxyhemoglobin S in concentrated phosphate buffer. J Biol Chem. 1980;255: 3092-3099.

89. Goldberg MA, Husson MA, Bunn HF. Participation of hemoglobins A and F in polymerization of sickle hemoglobin. J Biol Chem. 1977;252:3414-3421.

90. Benesch RE, Edalji R, Benesch R, Kwong S. Solubilization of hemoglobin S by other hemoglobins. Proc Natl Acad Sci U S A. 1980;77:5130-5134.

91. Jones MM, Steinhardt J. Evidence of the incorporation of normally nonaggregating hemoglobins into crystalline aggregates of deoxy hemoglobin S. J Biol Chem. 1982;257: 1913-1920.

92. Minton AP. Non-ideality and the thermodynamics of sickle-cell hemoglobin gelation. J Mol Biol. 1977;110: 89-103.

93. Sunshine HR. Effect of other hemoglobins on gelation of sickle cell hemoglobin. Tex Rep Biol Med. 1980;40: 233-250.

94. Rotter M, Aprelev A, Adachi K, Ferrone FA. Molecular crowding limits the role of fetal hemoglobin in therapy for sickle cell disease. J Mol Biol. 2005;347:1015-1023.

95. Shaklai N, Yguerabide J, Ranney HM. Classification and localization of hemoglobin binding sites on the red blood cell membrane. Biochemistry. 1977;16:5593-5597.

96. Eisinger J, Flores J, Salhany JM. Association of cytosol hemoglobin with the membrane in intact erythrocytes. Proc Natl Acad Sci U S A. 1982;79:408-412.

97. Cassoly R. Quantitative analysis of the association of human hemoglobin with the cytoplasmic fragment of band 3 protein. J Biol Chem. 1983;258:3859-3864.

98. Salhany JM, Cordes KA, Gaines ED. Light-scattering measurements of hemoglobin binding to the erythrocyte membrane. Evidence for transmembrane effects related to a disulfonic stilbene binding to band 3. Biochemistry. 1980;19:1447-1454.

99. Szundi I, Szelenyi JG, Breuer JH, Berczi A. Interactions of haemoglobin with erythrocyte membrane phospholipids in monomolecular lipid layers. Biochim Biophys Acta. 1980;595:41-46.

100. Liu SC, Palek J. Hemoglobin enhances the self-association of spectrin heterodimers in human erythrocytes. J Biol Chem. 1984;259:11556-11562.

101. Klipstein FA, Ranney HM. Electrophoretic components of the hemoglobin of red cell membranes. J Clin Invest. 1960;39:1894-1899.

102. Bank A, Mears G, Weiss R, et al. Preferential binding of beta S globin chains associated with stroma in sickle cell disorders. J Clin Invest. 1974;54:805-809.

103. Fung LW. Spin-label detection of hemoglobin-membrane interaction at physiological pH. Biochemistry. 1981;20: 7162-7166.

104. Evans EA, Mohandas N. Membrane-associated sickle hemoglobin: a major determinant of sickle erythrocyte rigidity. Blood. 1987;70:1443-1449.

105. Fortier N, Snyder LM, Garver F, et al. The relationship between in vivo generated hemoglobin skeletal protein complex and increased red cell membrane rigidity. Blood. 1988;71:1427-1431.

106. Asakura T, Agarwal PL, Relman DA, et al. Mechanical instability of the oxy-form of sickle haemoglobin. Nature. 1973;244:437-438.

107. Asakura T, Minakata K, Adachi K, et al. Denatured hemoglobin in sickle erythrocytes. J Clin Invest. 1977;59: 633-640.

108. Schluter K, Drenckhahn D. Co-clustering of denatured hemoglobin with band 3: its role in binding of autoantibodies against band 3 to abnormal and aged erythrocytes. Proc Natl Acad Sci U S A. 1986;83:6137-6141.

109. Waugh SM, Willardson BM, Kannan R, et al. Heinz bodies induce clustering of band 3, glycophorin, and ankyrin in sickle cell erythrocytes. J Clin Invest. 1986;78: 1155-1160.

110. Petz LD, Yam P, Wilkinson L, et al. Increased IgG molecules bound to the surface of red blood cells of patients with sickle cell anemia. Blood. 1984;64:301-304.

111. Kay MM. Mechanism of removal of senescent cells by human macrophages in situ. Proc Natl Acad Sci U S A. 1975;72:3521-3525.

112. Kay MM, Sorensen K, Wong P, Bolton P. Antigenicity, storage, and aging: physiologic autoantibodies to cell membrane and serum proteins and the senescent cell antigen. Mol Cell Biochem. 1982;49:65-85.

113. Hebbel RP, Miller WJ. Phagocytosis of sickle erythrocytes: immunologic and oxidative determinants of hemolytic anemia. Blood. 1984;64:733-741.

114. Liu SC, Yi SJ, Mehta JR, et al. Red cell membrane remodeling in sickle cell anemia. Sequestration of membrane lipids and proteins in Heinz bodies. J Clin Invest. 1996; 97:29-36.

115. Hebbel RP, Morgan WT, Eaton JW, Hedlund BE. Accelerated autoxidation and heme loss due to instability of sickle hemoglobin. Proc Natl Acad Sci U S A. 1988; 85:237-241.

116. Hebbel RP, Eaton JW, Balasingam M, Steinberg MH. Spontaneous oxygen radical generation by sickle erythrocytes. J Clin Invest. 1982;70:1253-1259.

117. Hebbel RP. The sickle erythrocyte in double jeopardy: autoxidation and iron decompartmentalization. Semin Hematol. 1990;27:51-69.

118. Browne P, Shalev O, Hebbel RP. The molecular pathobiology of cell membrane iron: the sickle red cell as a model. Free Radic Biol Med. 1998;24:1040-1048.

119. Itoh T, Chien S, Usami S. Deformability measurements on individual sickle cells using a new system with pO_2 and temperature control. Blood. 1992;79:2141-2147.

120. Mackie LH, Hochmuth RM. The influence of oxygen tension, temperature, and hemoglobin concentration on the rheologic properties of sickle erythrocytes. Blood. 1990;76:1256-1261.

121. Nash GB, Johnson CS, Meiselman HJ. Influence of oxygen tension on the viscoelastic behavior of red blood cells in sickle cell disease. Blood. 1986;67:110-118.

122. Sorette MP, Lavenant MG, Clark MR. Ektacytometric measurement of sickle cell deformability as a continuous function of oxygen tension. Blood. 1987;69:316-323.

123. Chien S, Usami S, Bertles JF. Abnormal rheology of oxygenated blood in sickle cell anemia. J Clin Invest. 1970;49:623-634.

124. Clark MR, Mohandas N, Shohet SB. Deformability of oxygenated irreversibly sickled cells. J Clin Invest. 1980;65:189-196.

125. Platt OS. Exercise-induced hemolysis in sickle cell anemia: shear sensitivity and erythrocyte dehydration. Blood. 1982;59:1055-1060.

126. Evans E, Mohandas N, Leung A. Static and dynamic rigidities of normal and sickle erythrocytes. Major influence of cell hemoglobin concentration. J Clin Invest. 1984;73:477-488.

127. Nash GB, Johnson CS, Meiselman HJ. Mechanical properties of oxygenated red blood cells in sickle cell (HbSS) disease. Blood. 1984;63:73-82.

128. Shartava A, Monteiro CA, Bencsath FA, et al. A posttranslational modification of beta-actin contributes to the slow dissociation of the spectrin–protein 4.1–actin complex of irreversibly sickled cells. J Cell Biol. 1995; 128:805-818.

129. Liu SC, Derick LH, Palek J. Dependence of the permanent deformation of red blood cell membranes on spectrin dimer-tetramer equilibrium: implication for permanent membrane deformation of irreversibly sickled cells. Blood. 1993;81:522-528.

130. Corbett JD, Golan DE. Band 3 and glycophorin are progressively aggregated in density-fractionated sickle and normal red blood cells. Evidence from rotational and lateral mobility studies. J Clin Invest. 1993;91:208-217.

131. Platt OS, Falcone JF. Membrane protein lesions in erythrocytes with Heinz bodies. J Clin Invest. 1988;82:1051-1058.

132. Platt OS, Falcone JF, Lux SE. Molecular defect in the sickle erythrocyte skeleton. Abnormal spectrin binding to sickle inside-out vesicles. J Clin Invest. 1985;75:266-271.

133. Kakhniashvili DG, Griko NB, Bulla LA Jr, Goodman SR. The proteomics of sickle cell disease: profiling of erythrocyte membrane proteins by 2D-DIGE and tandem mass spectrometry. Exp Biol Med (Maywood). 2005;230:787-792.

134. Kaul DK, Fabry ME, Windisch P, et al. Erythrocytes in sickle cell anemia are heterogeneous in their rheological and hemodynamic characteristics. J Clin Invest. 1983;72:22-31.

135. Billett HH, Fabry ME, Nagel RL. Hemoglobin distribution width: a rapid assessment of dense red cells in the steady state and during painful crisis in sickle cell anemia. J Lab Clin Med. 1988;112:339-344.

136. Billett HH, Kim K, Fabry ME, Nagel RL. The percentage of dense red cells does not predict incidence of sickle cell painful crisis. Blood. 1986;68:301-303.

137. Noguchi CT, Dover GJ, Rodgers GP, et al. Alpha thalassemia changes erythrocyte heterogeneity in sickle cell disease. J Clin Invest. 1985;75:1632-1637.

138. Baudin V, Pagnier J, Labie D, et al. Heterogeneity of sickle cell disease as shown by density profiles: effects of fetal hemoglobin and alpha thalassemia. Haematologia (Budap). 1986;19:177-184.

139. Fabry ME, Kaul DK, Raventos-Suarez C, et al. SC erythrocytes have an abnormally high intracellular hemoglobin concentration. Pathophysiological consequences. J Clin Invest. 1982;70:1315-1319.

140. Boyer SH, Belding TK, Margolet L, Noyes AN. Fetal hemoglobin restriction to a few erythrocytes (F cells) in normal human adults. Science. 1975;188:361-363.

141. Dover GJ, Boyer SH, Charache S, Heintzelman K. Individual variation in the production and survival of F cells in sickle-cell disease. N Engl J Med. 1978;299:1428-1435.

142. Bertles JF, Milner PF. Irreversibly sickled erythrocytes: a consequence of the heterogeneous distribution of hemoglobin types in sickle-cell anemia. J Clin Invest. 1968;47:1731-1741.

143. Dobler J, Bertles JF. The physical state of hemoglobin in sickle-cell anemia erythrocytes in vivo. J Exp Med. 1968;127:711-714.

143a. Hahn JA, Messer MJ, Bradley TB. Ultrastructure of sickling and unsickling in time-lapse studies. Br J Haematol. 1976;34:559-565.

144. Ohnishi ST, Horiuchi KY, Horiuchi K. The mechanism of in vitro formation of irreversibly sickled cells and modes of action of its inhibitors. Biochim Biophys Acta. 1986;886:119-129.

145. Jensen M, Shohet SB, Nathan DG. The role of red cell energy metabolism in the generation of irreversibly sickled cells in vitro. Blood. 1973;42:835-842.

146. Glader BE, Nathan DG. Cation permeability alterations during sickling: relationship to cation composition and cellular hydration of irreversibly sickled cells. Blood. 1978;51:983-989.

147. Ghatpande SS, Goodman SR. Ubiquitination of spectrin regulates the erythrocyte spectrin–protein 4.1–actin ternary complex dissociation: implications for the sickle cell membrane skeleton. Cell Mol Biol (Noisy-le-grand). 2004;50:67-74.

148. Gibson XA, Shartava A, McIntyre J, et al. The efficacy of reducing agents or antioxidants in blocking the formation of dense cells and irreversibly sickled cells in vitro. Blood. 1998;91:4373-4378.

149. Serjeant GR, Serjeant BE, Milner PF. The irreversibly sickled cell; a determinant of haemolysis in sickle cell anaemia. Br J Haematol. 1969;17:527-533.

150. Serjeant GR. Irreversibly sickled cells and splenomegaly in sickle-cell anaemia. Br J Haematol. 1970;19:635-641.

151. Tosteson DC. The effects of sickling on ion transport. II. The effect of sickling on sodium and cesium transport. J Gen Physiol. 1955;39:55-67.

152. Tosteson DC, Carlsen E, Dunham ET. The effects of sickling on ion transport. I. Effect of sickling on potassium transport. J Gen Physiol. 1955;39:31-53.

153. Mohandas N, Rossi ME, Clark MR. Association between morphologic distortion of sickle cells and deoxygenation-induced cation permeability increase. Blood. 1986;68:450-454.

154. Joiner CH. Deoxygenation-induced cation fluxes in sickle cells: II. Inhibition by stilbene disulfonates. Blood. 1990;76:212-220.

155. Joiner CH, Morris CL, Cooper ES. Deoxygenation-induced cation fluxes in sickle cells. III. Cation selectivity and response to pH and membrane potential. Am J Physiol. 1993;264:C734-C744.

156. Bookchin RM, Lew VL. Effects of a "sickling pulse" on the calcium and potassium permeabilities of intact, sickle trait red cells [proceedings]. J Physiol. 1978;284:93P-94P.

157. Etzion Z, Tiffert T, Bookchin RM, Lew VL. Effects of deoxygenation on active and passive Ca^{2+} transport and on the cytoplasmic Ca^{2+} levels of sickle cell anemia red cells. J Clin Invest. 1993;92:2489-2498.

158. Bookchin RM, Ortiz OE, Lew VL. Evidence for a direct reticulocyte origin of dense red cells in sickle cell anemia. J Clin Invest. 1991;87:113-124.

159. Fabry ME, Romero JR, Buchanan ID, et al. Rapid increase in red blood cell density driven by K:Cl cotransport in a

subset of sickle cell anemia reticulocytes and discocytes. Blood. 1991;78:217-225.

160. Sugihara T, Hebbel RP. Exaggerated cation leak from oxygenated sickle red blood cells during deformation: evidence for a unique leak pathway. Blood. 1992;80:2374-2378.

161. Hebbel RP, Mohandas N. Reversible deformation-dependent erythrocyte cation leak. Extreme sensitivity conferred by minimal peroxidation. Biophys J. 1991;60:712-715.

162. Hebbel RP, Shalev O, Foker W, Rank BH. Inhibition of erythrocyte Ca^{2+}-ATPase by activated oxygen through thiol- and lipid-dependent mechanisms. Biochim Biophys Acta. 1986;862:8-16.

163. Leclerc L, Girard F, Galacteros F, Poyart C. The calmodulin-stimulated $(Ca^{2+} + Mg^{2+})$-ATPase in hemoglobin S erythrocyte membranes: effects of sickling and oxidative agents. Biochim Biophys Acta. 1987;897:33-40.

164. Brugnara C, Bunn HF, Tosteson DC. Regulation of erythrocyte cation and water content in sickle cell anemia. Science. 1986;232:388-390.

165. Olivieri O, Vitoux D, Galacteros F, et al. Hemoglobin variants and activity of the (K^+Cl^-) cotransport system in human erythrocytes. Blood. 1992;79:793-797.

166. Canessa M, Spalvins A, Nagel RL. Volume-dependent and NEM-stimulated K^+,Cl^- transport is elevated in oxygenated SS, SC and CC human red cells. FEBS Lett. 1986;200:197-202.

167. Eaton JW, Skelton TD, Swofford HS, et al. Elevated erythrocyte calcium in sickle cell disease. Nature. 1973;246:105-106.

168. Palek J, Liu A, Liu D, et al. Effect of procaine HCl on ATP: calcium-dependent alterations in red cell shape and deformability. Blood. 1977;50:155-164.

169. Lew VL, Hockaday A, Sepulveda MI, et al. Compartmentalization of sickle-cell calcium in endocytic inside-out vesicles. Nature. 1985;315:586-589.

170. Tiffert T, Spivak JL, Lew VL. Magnitude of calcium influx required to induce dehydration of normal human red cells. Biochim Biophys Acta. 1988;943:157-165.

171. Brugnara C, de Franceschi L, Alper SL. Inhibition of Ca^{2+}-dependent K^+ transport and cell dehydration in sickle erythrocytes by clotrimazole and other imidazole derivatives. J Clin Invest. 1993;92:520-526.

172. De Franceschi L, Saadane N, Trudel M, et al. Treatment with oral clotrimazole blocks Ca^{2+}-activated K^+ transport and reverses erythrocyte dehydration in transgenic SAD mice. A model for therapy of sickle cell disease. J Clin Invest. 1994;93:1670-1676.

173. Brugnara C, Gee B, Armsby CC, et al. Therapy with oral clotrimazole induces inhibition of the Gardos channel and reduction of erythrocyte dehydration in patients with sickle cell disease. J Clin Invest. 1996;97:1227-1234.

174. Brugnara C, Van Ha T, Tosteson DC. Acid pH induces formation of dense cells in sickle erythrocytes. Blood. 1989;74:487-495.

175. Joiner CH, Jiang M, Franco RS. Deoxygenation-induced cation fluxes in sickle cells. IV. Modulation by external calcium. Am J Physiol. 1995;269:C403-C409.

176. Brugnara C, Tosteson DC. Inhibition of K transport by divalent cations in sickle erythrocytes. Blood. 1987;70:1810-1815.

177. Jennings ML. Volume-sensitive K^+/Cl^- cotransport in rabbit erythrocytes. Analysis of the rate-limiting activation

and inactivation events. J Gen Physiol. 1999;114:743-758.

178. Joiner CH, Rettig RK, Jiang M, et al. Urea stimulation of KCl cotransport induces abnormal volume reduction in sickle reticulocytes. Blood. 2007;109:1728-1735.

179. Crable SC, Hammond SM, Papes R, et al. Multiple isoforms of the KCl cotransporter are expressed in sickle and normal erythroid cells. Exp Hematol. 2005;33:624-631.

180. Rivera A, Ferreira A, Bertoni D, et al. Abnormal regulation of Mg^{2+} transport via Na/Mg exchanger in sickle erythrocytes. Blood. 2005;105:382-386.

181. De Franceschi L, Beuzard Y, Jouault H, Brugnara C. Modulation of erythrocyte potassium chloride cotransport, potassium content, and density by dietary magnesium intake in transgenic SAD mouse. Blood. 1996;88:2738-2744.

182. De Franceschi L, Bachir D, Galacteros F, et al. Oral magnesium supplements reduce erythrocyte dehydration in patients with sickle cell disease. J Clin Invest. 1997;100:1847-1852.

183. De Franceschi L, Bachir D, Galacteros F, et al. Oral magnesium pidolate: effects of long-term administration in patients with sickle cell disease. Br J Haematol. 2000;108:284-289.

184. Lew VL, Bookchin RM. Ion transport pathology in the mechanism of sickle cell dehydration. Physiol Rev. 2005;85:179-200.

185. Hoover R, Rubin R, Wise G, Warren R. Adhesion of normal and sickle erythrocytes to endothelial monolayer cultures. Blood. 1979;54:872-876.

186. Hebbel RP, Yamada O, Moldow CF, et al. Abnormal adherence of sickle erythrocytes to cultured vascular endothelium: possible mechanism for microvascular occlusion in sickle cell disease. J Clin Invest. 1980;65:154-160.

187. Mohandas N, Evans E. Adherence of sickle erythrocytes to vascular endothelial cells: requirement for both cell membrane changes and plasma factors. Blood. 1984;64:282-287.

188. Barabino GA, McIntire LV, Eskin SG, et al. Endothelial cell interactions with sickle cell, sickle trait, mechanically injured, and normal erythrocytes under controlled flow. Blood. 1987;70:152-157.

189. Smith BD, La Celle PL. Erythrocyte–endothelial cell adherence in sickle cell disorders. Blood. 1986;68:1050-1054.

190. Hebbel RP, Boogaerts MA, Eaton JW, Steinberg MH. Erythrocyte adherence to endothelium in sickle-cell anemia. A possible determinant of disease severity. N Engl J Med. 1980;302:992-995.

191. Telen MJ. Erythrocyte adhesion receptors: blood group antigens and related molecules. Transfus Med Rev. 2005;19:32-44.

192. Udani M, Zen Q, Cottman M, et al. Basal cell adhesion molecule/Lutheran protein. The receptor critical for sickle cell adhesion to laminin. J Clin Invest. 1998;101:2550-2558.

193. Lee SP, Cunningham ML, Hines PC, et al. Sickle cell adhesion to laminin: potential role for the alpha5 chain. Blood. 1998;92:2951-2958.

194. Kumar A, Eckmam JR, Swerlick RA, Wick TM. Phorbol ester stimulation increases sickle erythrocyte adherence to endothelium: a novel pathway involving alpha 4 beta 1

integrin receptors on sickle reticulocytes and fibronectin. Blood. 1996;88:4348-4358.

195. de Jong K, Rettig MP, Low PS, Kuypers FA. Protein kinase C activation induces phosphatidylserine exposure on red blood cells. Biochemistry. 2002;41:12562-12567.

196. Hines PC, Zen Q, Burney SN, et al. Novel epinephrine and cyclic AMP–mediated activation of BCAM/Lu-dependent sickle (SS) RBC adhesion. Blood. 2003;101:3281-3287.

197. Brittain JE, Mlinar KJ, Anderson CS, et al. Activation of sickle red blood cell adhesion via integrin-associated protein/CD47-induced signal transduction. J Clin Invest. 2001;107:1555-1562.

198. Sager G. Receptor binding sites for beta-adrenergic ligands on human erythrocytes. Biochem Pharmacol. 1982;31:99-104.

199. Zennadi R, Hines PC, De Castro LM, et al. Epinephrine acts through erythroid signaling pathways to activate sickle cell adhesion to endothelium via LW-$\alpha_v\beta_3$ interactions. Blood. 2004;104:3774-3781.

200. Swerlick RA, Lee KH, Wick TM, Lawley TJ. Human dermal microvascular endothelial but not human umbilical vein endothelial cells express CD36 in vivo and in vitro. J Immunol. 1992;148:78-83.

201. Vordermeier S, Singh S, Biggerstaff J, et al. Red blood cells from patients with sickle cell disease exhibit an increased adherence to cultured endothelium pretreated with tumour necrosis factor (TNF). Br J Haematol. 1992;81:591-597.

202. Hebbel RP, Visser MR, Goodman JL, et al. Potentiated adherence of sickle erythrocytes to endothelium infected by virus. J Clin Invest. 1987;80:1503-1506.

203. Smolinski PA, Offermann MK, Eckman JR, Wick TM. Double-stranded RNA induces sickle erythrocyte adherence to endothelium: a potential role for viral infection in vaso-occlusive pain episodes in sickle cell anemia. Blood. 1995;85:2945-2950.

204. Belcher JD, Mahaseth H, Welch TE, et al. Critical role of endothelial cell activation in hypoxia-induced vasoocclusion in transgenic sickle mice. Am J Physiol Heart Circ Physiol. 2005;288:H2715-H2725.

205. Solovey A, Lin Y, Browne P, et al. Circulating activated endothelial cells in sickle cell anemia. N Engl J Med. 1997;337:1584-1590.

206. Solovey A, Gui L, Key NS, Hebbel RP. Tissue factor expression by endothelial cells in sickle cell anemia. J Clin Invest. 1998;101:1899-1904.

207. Blum A, Yeganeh S, Peleg A, et al. Endothelial function in patients with sickle cell anemia during and after sickle cell crises. J Thromb Thrombolysis. 2005;19:83-86.

208. Kato GJ, Martyr S, Blackwelder WC, et al. Levels of soluble endothelium-derived adhesion molecules in patients with sickle cell disease are associated with pulmonary hypertension, organ dysfunction, and mortality. Br J Haematol. 2005;130:943-953.

209. Haest CW. Interactions between membrane skeleton proteins and the intrinsic domain of the erythrocyte membrane. Biochim Biophys Acta. 1982;694:331-352.

210. Seigneuret M, Devaux PF. ATP-dependent asymmetric distribution of spin-labeled phospholipids in the erythrocyte membrane: relation to shape changes. Proc Natl Acad Sci U S A. 1984;81:3751-3755.

211. Chiu D, Lubin B, Shohet SB. Erythrocyte membrane lipid reorganization during the sickling process. Br J Haematol. 1979;41:223-234.

212. Kuypers FA, Lewis RA, Hua M, et al. Detection of altered membrane phospholipid asymmetry in subpopulations of human red blood cells using fluorescently labeled annexin V. Blood. 1996;87:1179-1187.

213. Middelkoop E, Lubin BH, Bevers EM, et al. Studies on sickled erythrocytes provide evidence that the asymmetric distribution of phosphatidylserine in the red cell membrane is maintained by both ATP-dependent transloca-tion and interaction with membrane skeletal proteins. Biochim Biophys Acta. 1988;937:281-288.

214. Dasgupta SK, Thiagarajan P. The role of lactadherin in the phagocytosis of phosphatidylserine-expressing sickle red blood cells by macrophages. Haematologica. 2005;90:1267-1268.

215. Setty BN, Betal SG. Microvascular endothelial cells express a phosphatidylserine receptor: a functionally active receptor for phosphatidylserine-positive erythrocytes. Blood. 2008;111:905-914.

216. Kuypers FA, Chiu D, Mohandas N, et al. The molecular species composition of phosphatidylcholine affects cellular properties in normal and sickle erythrocytes. Blood. 1987;70:1111-1118.

217. Ren H, Obike I, Okpala I, et al. Steady-state haemoglobin level in sickle cell anaemia increases with an increase in erythrocyte membrane n-3 fatty acids. Prostaglandins Leukot Essent Fatty Acids. 2005;72:415-421.

218. Chiu D, Lubin B, Roelofsen B, van Deenen LL. Sickled erythrocytes accelerate clotting in vitro: an effect of abnormal membrane lipid asymmetry. Blood. 1981;58:398-401.

219. Setty BN, Rao AK, Stuart MJ. Thrombophilia in sickle cell disease: the red cell connection. Blood. 2001;98:3228-3233.

220. Schnog JB, Mac Gillavry MR, van Zanten AP, et al. Protein C and S and inflammation in sickle cell disease. Am J Hematol. 2004;76:26-32.

221. Shet AS, Aras O, Gupta K, et al. Sickle blood contains tissue factor–positive microparticles derived from endothelial cells and monocytes. Blood. 2003;102:2678-2683.

222. Piccin A, Murphy WG, Smith OP. Circulating micropar-ticles: pathophysiology and clinical implications. Blood Rev. 2007;21:157-171.

223. Wick TM, Moake JL, Udden MM, McIntire LV. Unusually large von Willebrand factor multimers preferentially promote young sickle and nonsickle erythrocyte adhesion to endothelial cells. Am J Hematol. 1993;42:284-292.

224. Brittain HA, Eckman JR, Wick TM. Sickle erythrocyte adherence to large vessel and microvascular endothelium under physiologic flow is qualitatively different. J Lab Clin Med. 1992;120:538-545.

225. Kaul DK, Nagel RL, Chen D, Tsai HM. Sickle erythrocyte-endothelial interactions in microcirculation: the role of von Willebrand factor and implications for vasoocclusion. Blood. 1993;81:2429-2438.

226. Antonucci R, Walker R, Herion J, Orringer E. Enhancement of sickle erythrocyte adherence to endothelium by autologous platelets. Am J Hematol. 1990;34:44-48.

227. Sugihara K, Sugihara T, Mohandas N, Hebbel RP. Thrombospondin mediates adherence of CD36$^+$ sickle reticulocytes to endothelial cells. Blood. 1992;80:2634-2642.

228. Brittain HA, Eckman JR, Swerlick RA, et al. Thrombospondin from activated platelets promotes sickle erythrocyte adherence to human microvascular endothelium under physiologic flow: a potential role for platelet activation in sickle cell vaso-occlusion. Blood. 1993;81:2137-2143.

229. Kaul DK, Tsai HM, Liu XD, et al. Monoclonal antibodies to $\alpha_V\beta_3$ (7E3 and LM609) inhibit sickle red blood cell–endothelium interactions induced by platelet-activating factor. Blood. 2000;95:368-374.

230. Ataga KI, Orringer EP. Hypercoagulability in sickle cell disease: a curious paradox. Am J Med. 2003;115:721-728.

231. Lang KS, Roll B, Myssina S, et al. Enhanced erythrocyte apoptosis in sickle cell anemia, thalassemia and glucose-6-phosphate dehydrogenase deficiency. Cell Physiol Biochem. 2002;12:365-372.

232. Naumann HN, Diggs LW, Barreras L, Williams BJ. Plasma hemoglobin and hemoglobin fractions in sickle cell crisis. Am J Clin Pathol. 1971;56:137-147.

233. Furchgott RF, Zawadzki JV. The obligatory role of endothelial cells in the relaxation of arterial smooth muscle by acetylcholine. Nature. 1980;288:373-376.

234. Jin RC, Voetsch B, Loscalzo J. Endogenous mechanisms of inhibition of platelet function. Microcirculation. 2005;12:247-258.

235. Space SL, Lane PA, Pickett CK, Weil JV. Nitric oxide attenuates normal and sickle red blood cell adherence to pulmonary endothelium. Am J Hematol. 2000;63:200-204.

236. Voetsch B, Jin RC, Loscalzo J. Nitric oxide insufficiency and atherothrombosis. Histochem Cell Biol. 2004;122:353-367.

237. Morris CR, Kuypers FA, Larkin S, et al. Patterns of arginine and nitric oxide in patients with sickle cell disease with vaso-occlusive crisis and acute chest syndrome. J Pediatr Hematol Oncol. 2000;22:515-520.

238. Morris CR, Kato GJ, Poljakovic M, et al. Dysregulated arginine metabolism, hemolysis-associated pulmonary hypertension, and mortality in sickle cell disease. JAMA. 2005;294:81-90.

239. Reiter CD, Wang X, Tanus-Santos JE, et al. Cell-free hemoglobin limits nitric oxide bioavailability in sickle-cell disease. Nat Med. 2002;8:1383-1389.

240. Liu X, Miller MJ, Joshi MS, et al. Diffusion-limited reaction of free nitric oxide with erythrocytes. J Biol Chem. 1998;273:18709-18713.

241. Aslan M, Freeman BA. Oxidant-mediated impairment of nitric oxide signaling in sickle cell disease—mechanisms and consequences. Cell Mol Biol (Noisy-le-grand). 2004;50:95-105.

242. Rother RP, Bell L, Hillmen P, Gladwin MT. The clinical sequelae of intravascular hemolysis and extracellular plasma hemoglobin: a novel mechanism of human disease. JAMA. 2005;293:1653-1662.

243. Mack AK, Kato GJ. Sickle cell disease and nitric oxide: a paradigm shift? Int J Biochem Cell Biol. 2006;38:1237-1243.

244. Ataga KI, Moore CG, Hillery CA, et al. Coagulation activation and inflammation in sickle cell disease–associated pulmonary hypertension. Haematologica. 2008;93:20-26.

245. Opkala I. Leucocyte adhesion and the pathophysiology of sickle cell disease. Curr Opin Hematol. 2006;13:40-44.

246. Hebbel RP, Osarogiagbon R, Kaul D. The endothelial biology of sickle cell disease: inflammation and a chronic vasculopathy. Microcirculation. 2004;11:129-151.

247. Platt OS, Brambilla DJ, Rosse WF, et al. Mortality in sickle cell disease. Life expectancy and risk factors for early death. N Engl J Med. 1994;330:1639-1644.

248. Castro O, Brambilla DJ, Thorington B, et al. The acute chest syndrome in sickle cell disease: incidence and risk factors. The Cooperative Study of Sickle Cell Disease. Blood. 1994;84:643-649.

249. Miller ST, Sleeper LA, Pegelow CH, et al. Prediction of adverse outcomes in children with sickle cell disease. N Engl J Med. 2000;342:83-89.

250. Garner C, Tatu T, Reittie JE, et al. Genetic influences on F cells and other hematologic variables: a twin heritability study. Blood. 2000;95:342-346.

251. Conran N, Saad ST, Costa FF, Ikuta T. Leukocyte numbers correlate with plasma levels of granulocyte-macrophage colony-stimulating factor in sickle cell disease. Ann Hematol. 2007;86:255-261.

252. Fadlon E, Vordermeier S, Pearson TC, et al. Blood polymorphonuclear leukocytes from the majority of sickle cell patients in the crisis phase of the disease show enhanced adhesion to vascular endothelium and increased expression of CD64. Blood. 1998;91:266-274.

253. Mollapour E, Porter JB, Kaczmarski R, et al. Raised neutrophil phospholipase A_2 activity and defective priming of NADPH oxidase and phospholipase A_2 in sickle cell disease. Blood. 1998;91:3423-3429.

254. Kaul DK, Hebbel RP. Hypoxia/reoxygenation causes inflammatory response in transgenic sickle mice but not in normal mice. J Clin Invest. 2000;106:411-420.

255. Platt OS. Sickle cell anemia as an inflammatory disease. J Clin Invest. 2000;106:337-338.

256. Kruglyak L, Nickerson DA. Variation is the spice of life. Nat Genet. 2001;27:234-236.

257. Redon R, Ishikawa S, Fitch KR, et al. Global variation in copy number in the human genome. Nature. 2006;444:444-454.

258. Mullally A, Ritz J. Beyond HLA: the significance of genomic variation for allogeneic hematopoietic stem cell transplantation. Blood. 2007;109:1355-1362.

259. Steinberg MH, Dreiling BJ. Glucose-6-phosphate dehydrogenase deficiency in sickle-cell anemia. A study in adults. Ann Intern Med. 1974;80:217-220.

260. Smits HL, Oski FA, Brody JI. The hemolytic crisis of sickle cell disease: the role of glucose-6-phosphate dehydrogenase deficiency. J Pediatr. 1969;74:544-551.

261. Wilmanski J, Villanueva E, Deitch EA, Spolarics Z. Glucose-6-phosphate dehydrogenase deficiency and the inflammatory response to endotoxin and polymicrobial sepsis. Crit Care Med. 2007;35:510-518.

262. Higgs DR, Aldridge BE, Lamb J, et al. The interaction of alpha-thalassemia and homozygous sickle-cell disease. N Engl J Med. 1982;306:1441-1446.

263. Dover GJ, Chang VT, Boyer SH, et al. The cellular basis for different fetal hemoglobin levels among sickle cell individuals with two, three, and four alpha-globin genes. Blood. 1987;69:341-344.

264. Embury SH, Dozy AM, Miller J, et al. Concurrent sickle-cell anemia and alpha-thalassemia: effect on severity of anemia. N Engl J Med. 1982;306:270-274.

265. Serjeant BE, Mason KP, Kenny MW, et al. Effect of alpha thalassaemia on the rheology of homozygous sickle cell disease. Br J Haematol. 1983;55:479-486.

266. Higgs DR, Pressley L, Serjeant GR, et al. The genetics and molecular basis of alpha thalassaemia in association with Hb S in Jamaican Negroes. Br J Haematol. 1981;47:43-56.

267. Steinberg MH, Rosenstock W, Coleman MB, et al. Effects of thalassemia and microcytosis on the hematologic and vasoocclusive severity of sickle cell anemia. Blood. 1984;63:1353-1360.

268. de Ceulaer K, Higgs DR, Weatherall DJ, et al. α-Thalassemia reduces the hemolytic rate in homozygous sickle-cell disease. N Engl J Med. 1983;309:189-190.

269. Steinberg MH, Embury SH. Alpha-thalassemia in blacks: genetic and clinical aspects and interactions with the sickle hemoglobin gene. Blood. 1986;68:985-990.

270. Milner PF, Garbutt GJ, Nolan-Davis LV, et al. The effect of Hb F and alpha-thalassemia on the red cell indices in sickle cell anemia. Am J Hematol. 1986;21:383-395.

271. Vyas P, Higgs DR, Weatherall DJ, et al. The interaction of alpha thalassaemia and sickle cell–beta zero thalassaemia. Br J Haematol. 1988;70:449-454.

272. Miller ST, Rieder RF, Rao SP, Brown AK. Cerebrovascular accidents in children with sickle-cell disease and alpha-thalassemia. J Pediatr. 1988;113:847-849.

273. Mears JG, Lachman HM, Labie D, Nagel RL. Alpha-thalassemia is related to prolonged survival in sickle cell anemia. Blood. 1983;62:286-290.

274. Fabry ME, Mears JG, Patel P, et al. Dense cells in sickle cell anemia: the effects of gene interaction. Blood. 1984;64:1042-1046.

275. Felice AE, McKie KM, Cleek MP, et al. Effects of alpha-thalassemia-2 on the developmental changes of hematological values in children with sickle cell disease from Georgia. Am J Hematol. 1987;25:389-400.

276. Stevens MC, Maude GH, Beckford M, et al. Alpha thalassemia and the hematology of homozygous sickle cell disease in childhood. Blood. 1986;67:411-414.

277. Steinberg MH. Predicting clinical severity in sickle cell anaemia. Br J Haematol. 2005;129:465-481.

278. Powars DR, Schroeder WA, Weiss JN, et al. Lack of influence of fetal hemoglobin levels or erythrocyte indices on the severity of sickle cell anemia. J Clin Invest. 1980;65:732-740.

279. Powars DR, Weiss JN, Chan LS, Schroeder WA. Is there a threshold level of fetal hemoglobin that ameliorates morbidity in sickle cell anemia? Blood. 1984;63:921-926.

280. Platt OS, Thorington BD, Brambilla DJ, et al. Pain in sickle cell disease. Rates and risk factors. N Engl J Med. 1991;325:11-16.

281. Charache S, Conley CL. Hereditary persistence of fetal hemoglobin. Ann N Y Acad Sci. 1969;165:37-41.

282. Jacob GF, Raper AB. Hereditary persistence of foetal haemoglobin production, and its interaction with the sickle-cell trait. Br J Haematol. 1958;4:138-149.

283. Murray N, Serjeant BE, Serjeant GR. Sickle cell–hereditary persistence of fetal haemoglobin and its differentia-tion from other sickle cell syndromes. Br J Haematol. 1988;69:89-92.

284. Old JM, Ayyub H, Wood WG, et al. Linkage analysis of nondeletion hereditary persistence of fetal hemoglobin. Science. 1982;215:981-982.

285. Milner PF, Leibfarth JD, Ford J, et al. Increased HbF in sickle cell anemia is determined by a factor linked to the beta S gene from one parent. Blood. 1984;63:64-72.

286. Stamatoyannopoulos G, Wood WG, Papayannopoulou T, Nute PE. A new form of hereditary persistence of fetal hemoglobin in blacks and its association with sickle cell trait. Blood. 1975;46:683-692.

287. Makler MT, Berthrong M, Locke HR, Dawson DL. A new variant of sickle-cell disease with high levels of foetal haemoglobin homogeneously distributed within red cells. Br J Haematol. 1974;26:519-526.

288. Economou EP, Antonarakis SE, Kazazian HH Jr, et al. Variation in hemoglobin F production among normal and sickle cell adults is not related to nucleotide substitutions in the gamma promoter regions. Blood. 1991;77:174-177.

289. Miller BA, Salameh M, Ahmed M, et al. Analysis of hemoglobin F production in Saudi Arabian families with sickle cell anemia. Blood. 1987;70:716-720.

290. Kar BC, Satapathy RK, Kulozik AE, et al. Sickle cell disease in Orissa State, India. Lancet. 1986;2:1198-1201.

291. Miller BA, Salameh M, Ahmed M, et al. High fetal hemoglobin production in sickle cell anemia in the eastern province of Saudi Arabia is genetically determined. Blood. 1986;67:1404-1410.

292. Kulozik AE, Kar BC, Satapathy RK, et al. Fetal hemoglobin levels and beta (s) globin haplotypes in an Indian populations with sickle cell disease. Blood. 1987;69:1742-1746.

293. Gianni AM, Bregni M, Cappellini MD, et al. A gene controlling fetal hemoglobin expression in adults is not linked to the non–alpha globin cluster. EMBO J. 1983;2:921-925.

294. Wood WG, Weatherall DJ, Clegg JB. Interaction of heterocellular hereditary persistence of foetal haemoglobin with beta thalassaemia and sickle cell anaemia. Nature. 1976;264:247-249.

295. Boyer SH, Dover GJ, Serjeant GR, et al. Production of F cells in sickle cell anemia: regulation by a genetic locus or loci separate from the beta-globin gene cluster. Blood. 1984;64:1053-1058.

296. Miyoshi K, Kaneto Y, Kawai H, et al. X-linked dominant control of F-cells in normal adult life: characterization of the Swiss type as hereditary persistence of fetal hemoglobin regulated dominantly by gene(s) on X chromosome. Blood. 1988;72:1854-1860.

297. Dover GJ, Smith KD, Chang YC, et al. Fetal hemoglobin levels in sickle cell disease and normal individuals are partially controlled by an X-linked gene located at Xp22.2. Blood. 1992;80:816-824.

298. Chang YC, Smith KD, Moore RD, et al. An analysis of fetal hemoglobin variation in sickle cell disease: the relative contributions of the X-linked factor, beta-globin haplotypes, alpha-globin gene number, gender, and age. Blood. 1995;85:1111-1117.

299. Chang YP, Littera R, Garau R, et al. The role of heterocellular hereditary persistence of fetal haemoglobin in

beta(0)-thalassaemia intermedia. Br J Haematol. 2001;
114:899-906.

300. Garner C, Silver N, Best S, et al. Quantitative trait locus on chromosome 8q influences the switch from fetal to adult hemoglobin. Blood. 2004;104:2184-2186.

301. Game L, Close J, Stephens P, et al. An integrated map of human 6q22.3-q24 including a 3-Mb high-resolution BAC/PAC contig encompassing a QTL for fetal hemoglobin. Genomics. 2000;64:264-276.

302. Jiang J, Best S, Menzel S, et al. cMYB is involved in the regulation of fetal hemoglobin production in adults. Blood. 2006;108:1077-1083.

303. Ma Q, Wyszynski DF, Farrell JJ, et al. Fetal hemoglobin in sickle cell anemia: genetic determinants of response to hydroxyurea. Pharmacogenomics J. 2007;7:386-394.

304. Uda M, Galanello R, Sanna S, et al. Genome-wide association study shows BCL11A associated with persistent fetal hemoglobin and amelioration of the phenotype of beta-thalassemia. Proc Natl Acad Sci U S A. 2008;105:1620-1625.

305. Taylor JGt, Tang DC, Savage SA, et al. Variants in the VCAM1 gene and risk for symptomatic stroke in sickle cell disease. Blood. 2002;100:4303-4309.

306. Sebastiani P, Ramoni MF, Nolan V, et al. Genetic dissection and prognostic modeling of overt stroke in sickle cell anemia. Nat Genet. 2005;37:435-440.

307. Hoppe C, Klitz W, Cheng S, et al. Gene interactions and stroke risk in children with sickle cell anemia. Blood. 2004;103:2391-2396.

308. Ashley-Koch AE, Elliott L, Kail ME, et al. Identification of genetic polymorphisms associated with risk for pulmonary hypertension in sickle cell disease. Blood. 2008;111:5721-5726.

309. Eyler CE, Jackson T, Elliott LE, et al. β₂-Adrenergic receptor and adenylate cyclase gene polymorphisms affect sickle red cell adhesion. Br J Haematol. 2008;141:105-108.

310. Passon RG, Howard TA, Zimmerman SA, et al. Influence of bilirubin uridine diphosphate-glucuronosyltransferase 1A promoter polymorphisms on serum bilirubin levels and cholelithiasis in children with sickle cell anemia. J Pediatr Hematol Oncol. 2001;23:448-451.

311. Nolan VG, Ma Q, Cohen HT, et al. Estimated glomerular filtration rate in sickle cell anemia is associated with polymorphisms of bone morphogenetic protein receptor 1B. Am J Hematol. 2007;82:179-184.

312. Baldwin C, Nolan VG, Wyszynski DF, et al. Association of klotho, bone morphogenic protein 6, and annexin A2 polymorphisms with sickle cell osteonecrosis. Blood. 2005;106:372-375.

313. Hoppe C, Klitz W, Noble J, et al. Distinct HLA associations by stroke subtype in children with sickle cell anemia. Blood. 2003;101:2865-2869.

314. Adewoye AH, Nolan VG, Ma Q, et al. Association of polymorphisms of IGF1R and genes in the transforming growth factor-beta/bone morphogenetic protein pathway with bacteremia in sickle cell anemia. Clin Infect Dis. 2006;43:593-598.

315. Nolan VG, Adewoye A, Baldwin C, et al. Sickle cell leg ulcers: associations with haemolysis and SNPs in Klotho, TEK and genes of the TGF-beta/BMP pathway. Br J Haematol. 2006;133:570-578.

316. Sebastiani P, Wang L, Nolan VG, et al. Fetal hemoglobin in sickle cell anemia: bayesian modeling of genetic associations. Am J Hematol. 2008;83:189-195.

317. Kato GJ, Gladwin MT, Steinberg MH. Deconstructing sickle cell disease: reappraisal of the role of hemolysis in the development of clinical subphenotypes. Blood Rev. 2007;21:37-47.

318. Macchia P, Massei F, Nardi M, et al. Thalassemia intermedia and recurrent priapism following splenectomy. Haematologica. 1990;75:486-487.

319. Andrieu V, Dumonceau O, Grange MJ. Priapism in a patient with unstable hemoglobin: hemoglobin Koln. Am J Hematol. 2003;74:73-74.

320. Stevens DM, Shupack JL, Javid J, Silber R. Ulcers of the leg in thalassemia. Arch Dermatol. 1977;113:1558-1560.

321. Giraldi S, Abbage KT, Marinoni LP, et al. Leg ulcer in hereditary spherocytosis. Pediatr Dermatol. 2003;20:427-428.

322. Verresen D, De Backer W, Van Meerbeeck J, et al. Spherocytosis and pulmonary hypertension coincidental occurrence or causal relationship? Eur Respir J. 1991;4:629-631.

323. Yamamoto M, Clark JD, Pastor JV, et al. Regulation of oxidative stress by the anti-aging hormone klotho. J Biol Chem. 2005;280:38029-38034.

324. Nolan VG, Baldwin C, Ma Q, et al. Association of single nucleotide polymorphisms in klotho with priapism in sickle cell anaemia. Br J Haematol. 2005;128:266-272.

325. Ashley-Koch A, De Castro L, Lennon-Graham F. Genetic polymorphisms associated with the risks for pulmonary hypertension and proteinuria in sickle cell disease. Blood. 2004;104:464a.

326. Rosendahl A, Pardali E, Speletas M, et al. Activation of bone morphogenetic protein/Smad signaling in bronchial epithelial cells during airway inflammation. Am J Respir Cell Mol Biol. 2002;27:160-169.

327. Jane JA Jr, Dunford BA, Kron A, et al. Ectopic osteogenesis using adenoviral bone morphogenetic protein (BMP)-4 and BMP-6 gene transfer. Mol Ther. 2002;6:464-470.

328. Eaves CJ, Cashman JD, Kay RJ, et al. Mechanisms that regulate the cell cycle status of very primitive hematopoietic cells in long-term human marrow cultures. II. Analysis of positive and negative regulators produced by stromal cells within the adherent layer. Blood. 1991;78:110-117.

329. Schmidt-Weber CB, Blaser K. Regulation and role of transforming growth factor-beta in immune tolerance induction and inflammation. Curr Opin Immunol. 2004;16:709-716.

330. Zee RY, Cook NR, Cheng S, et al. Polymorphism in the P-selectin and interleukin-4 genes as determinants of stroke: a population-based, prospective genetic analysis. Hum Mol Genet. 2004;13:389-396.

331. Machado RD, Pauciulo MW, Thomson JR, et al. BMPR2 haploinsufficiency as the inherited molecular mechanism for primary pulmonary hypertension. Am J Hum Genet. 2001;68:92-102.

332. Bosma PJ, Chowdhury JR, Bakker C, et al. The genetic basis of the reduced expression of bilirubin UDP-glucuronosyltransferase 1 in Gilbert's syndrome. N Engl J Med. 1995;333:1171-1175.

333. Kan YW, Dozy AM. Polymorphism of DNA sequence adjacent to human beta-globin structural gene: relationship to sickle mutation. Proc Natl Acad Sci U S A. 1978;75:5631-5635.

334. Chang JC, Kan YW. A sensitive new prenatal test for sickle-cell anemia. N Engl J Med. 1982;307:30-32.

335. Orkin SH, Little PF, Kazazian HH Jr, Boehm CD. Improved detection of the sickle mutation by DNA analysis: application to prenatal diagnosis. N Engl J Med. 1982;307:32-36.

336. Wallace RB, Johnson MJ, Hirose T, et al. The use of synthetic oligonucleotides as hybridization probes. II. Hybridization of oligonucleotides of mixed sequence to rabbit beta-globin DNA. Nucleic Acids Res. 1981;9:879-894.

337. Conner BJ, Reyes AA, Morin C, et al. Detection of sickle cell beta S-globin allele by hybridization with synthetic oligonucleotides. Proc Natl Acad Sci U S A. 1983;80:278-282.

338. Pirastu M, Kan YW, Cao A, et al. Prenatal diagnosis of beta-thalassemia. Detection of a single nucleotide mutation in DNA. N Engl J Med. 1983;309:284-287.

339. Saiki RK, Chang CA, Levenson CH, et al. Diagnosis of sickle cell anemia and beta-thalassemia with enzymatically amplified DNA and nonradioactive allele-specific oligonucleotide probes. N Engl J Med. 1988;319:537-541.

340. Chehab FF, Kan YW. Detection of sickle cell anaemia mutation by colour DNA amplification. Lancet. 1990;335:15-17.

341. Saiki RK, Scharf S, Faloona F, et al. Enzymatic amplification of beta-globin genomic sequences and restriction site analysis for diagnosis of sickle cell anemia. Science. 1985;230:1350-1354.

342. Embury SH, Scharf SJ, Saiki RK, et al. Rapid prenatal diagnosis of sickle cell anemia by a new method of DNA analysis. N Engl J Med. 1987;316:656-661.

343. Goossens M, Dumez Y, Kaplan L, et al. Prenatal diagnosis of sickle-cell anemia in the first trimester of pregnancy. N Engl J Med. 1983;309:831-833.

344. Old JM, Fitches A, Heath C, et al. First-trimester fetal diagnosis for haemoglobinopathies: report on 200 cases. Lancet. 1986;2:763-767.

345. Xu K, Shi ZM, Veeck LL, et al. First unaffected pregnancy using preimplantation genetic diagnosis for sickle cell anemia. JAMA. 1999;281:1701-1706.

346. Serjeant GR, Grandison Y, Lowrie Y, et al. The development of haematological changes in homozygous sickle cell disease: a cohort study from birth to 6 years. Br J Haematol. 1981;48:533-543.

347. Pearson HA. A neonatal program for sickle cell anemia. Adv Pediatr. 1986;33:381-400.

348. Reed W, Lane PA, Lorey F, et al. Sickle-cell disease not identified by newborn screening because of prior transfusion. J Pediatr. 2000;136:248-250.

349. Jinks DC, Minter M, Tarver DA, et al. Molecular genetic diagnosis of sickle cell disease using dried blood specimens on blotters used for newborn screening. Hum Genet. 1989;81:363-366.

350. Panepinto JA, Magid D, Rewers MJ, Lane PA. Universal versus targeted screening of infants for sickle cell disease: a cost-effectiveness analysis. J Pediatr. 2000;136:201-208.

351. Davies SC, Cronin E, Gill M, et al. Screening for sickle cell disease and thalassaemia: a systematic review with supplementary research. Health Technol Assess. 2000;4:i-v, 1-99.

352. O'Brien RT, McIntosh S, Aspnes GT, Pearson HA. Prospective study of sickle cell anemia in infancy. J Pediatr. 1976;89:205-210.

353. Gaston M, Smith J, Gallagher D, et al. Recruitment in the Cooperative Study of Sickle Cell Disease (CSSCD). Control Clin Trials. 1987;8:131S-140S.

354. Gaston M, Rosse WF. The cooperative study of sickle cell disease: review of study design and objectives. Am J Pediatr Hematol Oncol. 1982;4:197-201.

355. Diggs LW. Sickle cell crisis. Am J Clin Pathol. 1965;44:1-19.

356. Gill FM, Sleeper LA, Weiner SJ, et al. Clinical events in the first decade in a cohort of infants with sickle cell disease. Cooperative Study of Sickle Cell Disease. Blood. 1995;86:776-783.

357. Bainbridge R, Higgs DR, Maude GH, Serjeant GR. Clinical presentation of homozygous sickle cell disease. J Pediatr. 1985;106:881-885.

358. Konotey-Ahulu FI. The sickle cell diseases. Clinical manifestations including the "sickle crisis." Arch Intern Med. 1974;133:611-619.

359. Redwood AM, Williams EM, Desal P, Serjeant GR. Climate and painful crisis of sickle-cell disease in Jamaica. BMJ. 1976;1:66-68.

360. Ibrahim AS. Relationship between meteorological changes and occurrence of painful sickle cell crises in Kuwait. Trans R Soc Trop Med Hyg. 1980;74:159-161.

361. Milner PF, Brown M. Bone marrow infarction in sickle cell anemia: correlation with hematologic profiles. Blood. 1982;60:1411-1419.

362. Charache S, Page DL. Infarction of bone marrow in the sickle cell disorders. Ann Intern Med. 1967;67:1195-1200.

363. Mankad VN, Williams JP, Harpen MD, et al. Magnetic resonance imaging of bone marrow in sickle cell disease: clinical, hematologic, and pathologic correlations. Blood. 1990;75:274-283.

364. Diggs LW. Bone and joint lesions in sickle-cell disease. Clin Orthop Relat Res. 1967;52:119-143.

365. Keeley K, Buchanan GR. Acute infarction of long bones in children with sickle cell anemia. J Pediatr. 1982;101:170-175.

366. Sain A, Sham R, Silver L. Bone scan in sickle cell crisis. Clin Nucl Med. 1978;3:85-90.

367. Alavi A, Schumacher HR, Dorwart B, Kuhl DE. Bone marrow scan evaluation of arthropathy in sickle cell disorders. Arch Intern Med. 1976;136:436-440.

368. Hammel CF, DeNardo SJ, DeNardo GL, Lewis JP. Bone marrow and bone mineral scintigraphic studies in sickle cell disease. Br J Haematol. 1973;25:593-598.

369. Lutzker LG, Alavi A. Bone and marrow imaging in sickle cell disease: diagnosis of infarction. Semin Nucl Med. 1976;6:83-93.

370. Kahn CE Jr, Ryan JW, Hatfield MK, Martin WB. Combined bone marrow and gallium imaging. Differentiation of osteomyelitis and infarction in sickle hemoglobinopathy. Clin Nucl Med. 1988;13:443-449.

371. Rao S, Solomon N, Miller S, Dunn E. Scintigraphic differentiation of bone infarction from osteomyelitis in children with sickle cell disease. J Pediatr. 1985;107:685-688.

372. Kim HC, Alavi A, Russell MO, Schwartz E. Differentiation of bone and bone marrow infarcts from osteomyelitis

in sickle cell disorders. Clin Nucl Med. 1989;14: 249-254.

373. Guze BH, Hawkins RA, Marcus CS. Technetium-99m white blood cell imaging: false-negative result in salmonella osteomyelitis associated with sickle cell disease. Clin Nucl Med. 1989;14:104-106.

374. Almeida A, Roberts I. Bone involvement in sickle cell disease. Br J Haematol. 2005;129:482-490.

375. Cole TB, Smith SJ, Buchanan GR. Hematologic alterations during acute infection in children with sickle cell disease. Pediatr Infect Dis J. 1987;6:454-457.

376. Syrogiannopoulos GA, McCracken GH Jr, Nelson JD. Osteoarticular infections in children with sickle cell disease. Pediatrics. 1986;78:1090-1096.

377. Burnett MW, Bass JW, Cook BA. Etiology of osteomyelitis complicating sickle cell disease. Pediatrics. 1998;101: 296-297.

378. Stuart J, Stone PC, Akinola NO, et al. Monitoring the acute phase response to vaso-occlusive crisis in sickle cell disease. J Clin Pathol. 1994;47:166-169.

379. Devine DV, Kinney TR, Thomas PF, et al. Fragment D-dimer levels: an objective marker of vaso-occlusive crisis and other complications of sickle cell disease. Blood. 1986;68:317-319.

380. Francis RB Jr. Elevated fibrin D-dimer fragment in sickle cell anemia: evidence for activation of coagulation during the steady state as well as in painful crisis. Haemostasis. 1989;19:105-111.

381. Ballas SK, Smith ED. Red blood cell changes during the evolution of the sickle cell painful crisis. Blood. 1992;79:2154-2163.

382. Griffin TC, McIntire D, Buchanan GR. High-dose intravenous methylprednisolone therapy for pain in children and adolescents with sickle cell disease. N Engl J Med. 1994;330:733-737.

383. Greenberg J, Ohene-Frempong K, Halus J, et al. Trial of low doses of aspirin as prophylaxis in sickle cell disease. J Pediatr. 1983;102:781-784.

384. Villagra J, Shiva S, Hunter LA, et al. Platelet activation in patients with sickle disease, hemolysis-associated pulmonary hypertension, and nitric oxide scavenging by cell-free hemoglobin. Blood. 2007;110:2166-2172.

385. Wun T, Paglieroni T, Rangaswami A, et al. Platelet activation in patients with sickle cell disease. Br J Haematol. 1998;100:741-749.

386. Bashawri LA, Al-Mulhim AA, Ahmed MA, Bahnassi AA. Platelet aggregation and physiological anticoagulants in sickle-cell disease. East Mediterr Health J. 2007;13: 266-272.

387. Francis RB Jr. Protein S deficiency in sickle cell anemia. J Lab Clin Med. 1988;111:571-576.

388. Watson RJ, Burko H, Megas H, Robinson M. The hand-foot syndrome in sickle-cell disease in young children. Pediatrics. 1963;31:975-982.

389. Worrall VT, Butera V. Sickle-cell dactylitis. J Bone Joint Surg Am. 1976;58:1161-1163.

390. Serjeant GR, Ashcroft MT. Shortening of the digits in sickle cell anaemia: a sequela of the hand-foot syndrome. Trop Geogr Med. 1971;23:341-346.

391. Quinn CT, Shull EP, Ahmad N, et al. Prognostic significance of early vaso-occlusive complications in children with sickle cell anemia. Blood. 2007;109:40-45.

392. Vichinsky EP, Neumayr LD, Earles AN, et al. Causes and outcomes of the acute chest syndrome in sickle cell disease. National Acute Chest Syndrome Study Group. N Engl J Med. 2000;342:1855-1865.

393. Charache S, Scott JC, Charache P. "Acute chest syndrome" in adults with sickle cell anemia. Microbiology, treatment, and prevention. Arch Intern Med. 1979;139: 67-69.

394. Vichinsky EP, Styles LA, Colangelo LH, et al. Acute chest syndrome in sickle cell disease: clinical presentation and course. Cooperative Study of Sickle Cell Disease. Blood. 1997;89:1787-1792.

395. Davies SC, Luce PJ, Win AA, et al. Acute chest syndrome in sickle-cell disease. Lancet. 1984;1:36-38.

396. Ballas SK, Files B, Luchtman-Jones L, et al. Secretory phospholipase A_2 levels in patients with sickle cell disease and acute chest syndrome. Hemoglobin. 2006;30: 165-170.

397. Bargoma EM, Mitsuyoshi JK, Larkin SK, et al. Serum C-reactive protein parallels secretory phospholipase A_2 in sickle cell disease patients with vasoocclusive crisis or acute chest syndrome. Blood. 2005;105:3384-3385.

398. Styles LA, Aarsman AJ, Vichinsky EP, Kuypers FA. Secretory phospholipase A_2 predicts impending acute chest syndrome in sickle cell disease. Blood. 2000;96: 3276-3278.

399. Styles LA, Abboud M, Larkin S, et al. Transfusion prevents acute chest syndrome predicted by elevated secretory phospholipase A_2. Br J Haematol. 2007;136: 343-344.

400. Charache S, Terrin ML, Moore RD, et al. Effect of hydroxyurea on the frequency of painful crises in sickle cell anemia. Investigators of the Multicenter Study of Hydroxyurea in Sickle Cell Anemia. N Engl J Med. 1995;332:1317-1322.

401. Boyd JH, Moinuddin A, Strunk RC, DeBaun MR. Asthma and acute chest in sickle-cell disease. Pediatr Pulmonol. 2004;38:229-232.

402. Boyd JH, Macklin EA, Strunk RC, DeBaun MR. Asthma is associated with acute chest syndrome and pain in children with sickle cell anemia. Blood. 2006;108:2923-2927.

403. Bryant R. Asthma in the pediatric sickle cell patient with acute chest syndrome. J Pediatr Health Care. 2005;19: 157-162.

404. Knight-Madden JM, Forrester TS, Lewis NA, Greenough A. Asthma in children with sickle cell disease and its association with acute chest syndrome. Thorax. 2005;60: 206-210.

405. Sylvester KP, Patey RA, Broughton S, et al. Temporal relationship of asthma to acute chest syndrome in sickle cell disease. Pediatr Pulmonol. 2007;42:103-106.

406. Duckworth L, Hsu L, Feng H, et al. Physician-diagnosed asthma and acute chest syndrome: associations with NOS polymorphisms. Pediatr Pulmonol. 2007;42:332-338.

407. Vichinsky E, Williams R, Das M, et al. Pulmonary fat embolism: a distinct cause of severe acute chest syndrome in sickle cell anemia. Blood. 1994;83:3107-3112.

408. Pianosi P, Charge TD, Esseltine DW, Coates AL. Pulse oximetry in sickle cell disease. Arch Dis Child. 1993;68: 735-738.

409. Rackoff WR, Kunkel N, Silber JH, et al. Pulse oximetry and factors associated with hemoglobin oxygen desatura-

tion in children with sickle cell disease. Blood. 1993;81: 3422-3427.

410. Leong MA, Dampier C, Varlotta L, Allen JL. Airway hyperreactivity in children with sickle cell disease. J Pediatr. 1997;131:278-283.

411. Wratney AT, Gentile MA, Hamel DS, Cheifetz IM. Successful treatment of acute chest syndrome with high-frequency oscillatory ventilation in pediatric patients. Respir Care. 2004;49:263-269.

412. Pelidis MA, Kato GJ, Resar LM, et al. Successful treatment of life-threatening acute chest syndrome of sickle cell disease with venovenous extracorporeal membrane oxygenation. J Pediatr Hematol Oncol. 1997;19:459-461.

413. Trant CA Jr, Casey JR, Hansell D, et al. Successful use of extracorporeal membrane oxygenation in the treatment of acute chest syndrome in a child with severe sickle cell anemia. ASAIO J. 1996;42:236-239.

414. Moser C, Nussbaum E, Cooper DM. Plastic bronchitis and the role of bronchoscopy in the acute chest syndrome of sickle cell disease. Chest. 2001;120:608-613.

415. Raghuram N, Pettignano R, Gal AA, et al. Plastic bronchitis: an unusual complication associated with sickle cell disease and the acute chest syndrome. Pediatrics. 1997; 100:139-142.

416. Manna SS, Shaw J, Tibby SM, Durward A. Treatment of plastic bronchitis in acute chest syndrome of sickle cell disease with intratracheal rhDNase. Arch Dis Child. 2003;88:626-627.

417. Atz AM, Wessel DL. Inhaled nitric oxide in sickle cell disease with acute chest syndrome. Anesthesiology. 1997; 87:988-990.

418. Sullivan KJ, Goodwin SR, Evangelist J, et al. Nitric oxide successfully used to treat acute chest syndrome of sickle cell disease in a young adolescent. Crit Care Med. 1999;27:2563-2568.

419. Haupt HM, Moore GW, Bauer TW, Hutchins GM. The lung in sickle cell disease. Chest. 1982;81:332-337.

420. Athanasou NA, Hatton C, McGee JO, Weatherall DJ. Vascular occlusion and infarction in sickle cell crisis and the sickle chest syndrome. J Clin Pathol. 1985;38:659-664.

421. Buchanan GR, Glader BE. Benign course of extreme hyperbilirubinemia in sickle cell anemia: analysis of six cases. J Pediatr. 1977;91:21-24.

422. Sheehy TW. Sickle cell hepatopathy. South Med J. 1977;70:533-538.

423. Serafini AN, Spoliansky G, Sfakianakis GN, et al. Diagnostic studies in patients with sickle cell anemia and acute abdominal pain. Arch Intern Med. 1987;147:1061-1062.

424. Stephens CG, Scott RB. Cholelithiasis in sickle cell anemia: surgical or medical management. Arch Intern Med. 1980;140:648-651.

425. Schubert TT. Hepatobiliary system in sickle cell disease. Gastroenterology. 1986;90:2013-2021.

426. Hatton CS, Bunch C, Weatherall DJ. Hepatic sequestration in sickle cell anaemia. Br Med J (Clin Res Ed). 1985;290:744-745.

427. Hernandez P, Dorticos E, Espinosa E, et al. Clinical features of hepatic sequestration in sickle cell anaemia. Haematologia (Budap). 1989;22:169-174.

428. Banerjee S, Owen C, Chopra S. Sickle cell hepatopathy. Hepatology. 2001;33:1021-1028.

429. Shao SH, Orringer EP. Sickle cell intrahepatic cholestasis: approach to a difficult problem. Am J Gastroenterol. 1995;90:2048-2050.

430. Powars D, Wilson B, Imbus C, et al. The natural history of stroke in sickle cell disease. Am J Med. 1978;65: 461-471.

431. Balkaran B, Char G, Morris JS, et al. Stroke in a cohort of patients with homozygous sickle cell disease. J Pediatr. 1992;120:360-366.

432. Ohene-Frempong K. Stroke in sickle cell disease: demographic, clinical, and therapeutic considerations. Semin Hematol. 1991;28:213-219.

433. Stockman JA, Nigro MA, Mishkin MM, Oski FA. Occlusion of large cerebral vessels in sickle-cell anemia. N Engl J Med. 1972;287:846-849.

434. Wilimas J, Goff JR, Anderson HR Jr, et al. Efficacy of transfusion therapy for one to two years in patients with sickle cell disease and cerebrovascular accidents. J Pediatr. 1980;96:205-208.

435. Boros L, Thomas C, Weiner WJ. Large cerebral vessel disease in sickle cell anaemia. J Neurol Neurosurg Psychiatry. 1976;39:1236-1239.

436. Merkel KH, Ginsberg PL, Parker JC Jr, Post MJ. Cerebrovascular disease in sickle cell anemia: a clinical, pathological and radiological correlation. Stroke. 1978;9: 45-52.

437. Adams RJ. Neurologic complications. In Embury SH, Hebbel RP, Mohandas N, Steinberg MH (eds). Sickle Cell Disease: Basic Principles and Clinical Practice. New York, Raven Press, 1994, pp 599-621.

438. Gauvrit JY, Leclerc X, Girot M, et al. Fluid-attenuated inversion recovery (FLAIR) sequences for the assessment of acute stroke: inter observer and inter technique reproducibility. J Neurol. 2006;253:631-635.

439. Hacke W, Warach S. Diffusion-weighted MRI as an evolving standard of care in acute stroke. Neurology. 2000;54:1548-1549.

440. Pavlakis SG, Bello J, Prohovnik I, et al. Brain infarction in sickle cell anemia: magnetic resonance imaging correlates. Ann Neurol. 1988;23:125-130.

441. Adams RJ, Nichols FT, McKie V, et al. Cerebral infarction in sickle cell anemia: mechanism based on CT and MRI. Neurology. 1988;38:1012-1017.

442. Herold S, Brozovic M, Gibbs J, et al. Measurement of regional cerebral blood flow, blood volume and oxygen metabolism in patients with sickle cell disease using positron emission tomography. Stroke. 1986;17:692-698.

443. Zimmerman RA. MRI/MRA evaluation of sickle cell disease of the brain. Pediatr Radiol. 2005;35:249-257.

444. Kandeel AY, Zimmerman RA, Ohene-Frempong K. Comparison of magnetic resonance angiography and conventional angiography in sickle cell disease: clinical significance and reliability. Neuroradiology. 1996;38: 409-416.

445. Russell MO, Goldberg HI, Hodson A, et al. Effect of transfusion therapy on arteriographic abnormalities and on recurrence of stroke in sickle cell disease. Blood. 1984;63:162-169.

446. Russell MO, Goldberg HI, Reis L, et al. Transfusion therapy for cerebrovascular abnormalities in sickle cell disease. J Pediatr. 1976;88:382-387.

447. Lusher JM, Haghighat H, Khalifa AS. A prophylactic transfusion program for children with sickle cell anemia complicated by CNS infarction. Am J Hematol. 1976;1: 265-273.

448. Seeler RA, Royal JE. Commentary: sickle cell anemia, stroke, and transfusion. J Pediatr. 1980;96:243-244.

449. Scothorn DJ, Price C, Schwartz D, et al. Risk of recurrent stroke in children with sickle cell disease receiving blood transfusion therapy for at least five years after initial stroke. J Pediatr. 2002;140:348-354.

450. Wang WC, Kovnar EH, Tonkin IL, et al. High risk of recurrent stroke after discontinuance of five to twelve years of transfusion therapy in patients with sickle cell disease. J Pediatr. 1991;118:377-382.

451. Cohen AR, Martin MB, Silber JH, et al. A modified transfusion program for prevention of stroke in sickle cell disease. Blood. 1992;79:1657-1661.

452. Rosse WF, Gallagher D, Kinney TR, et al. Transfusion and alloimmunization in sickle cell disease. The Cooperative Study of Sickle Cell Disease. Blood. 1990;76:1431-1437.

453. Castellino SM, Combs MR, Zimmerman SA, et al. Erythrocyte autoantibodies in paediatric patients with sickle cell disease receiving transfusion therapy: frequency, characteristics and significance. Br J Haematol. 1999;104: 189-194.

454. Panepinto JA, Walters MC, Carreras J, et al. Matched-related donor transplantation for sickle cell disease: report from the Center for International Blood and Transplant Research. Br J Haematol. 2007;137:479-485.

455. Woodard P, Helton KJ, Khan RB, et al. Brain parenchymal damage after haematopoietic stem cell transplantation for severe sickle cell disease. Br J Haematol. 2005; 129:550-552.

456. Ware RE, Zimmerman SA, Schultz WH. Hydroxyurea as an alternative to blood transfusions for the prevention of recurrent stroke in children with sickle cell disease. Blood. 1999;94:3022-3026.

457. Ware RE, Zimmerman SA, Sylvestre PB, et al. Prevention of secondary stroke and resolution of transfusional iron overload in children with sickle cell anemia using hydroxyurea and phlebotomy. J Pediatr. 2004;145:346-352.

458. Heeney MM, Whorton MR, Howard TA, et al. Chemical and functional analysis of hydroxyurea oral solutions. J Pediatr Hematol Oncol. 2004;26:179-184.

459. Adams R, McKie V, Nichols F, et al. The use of transcranial ultrasonography to predict stroke in sickle cell disease. N Engl J Med. 1992;326:605-610.

460. Kugler S, Anderson B, Cross D, et al. Abnormal cranial magnetic resonance imaging scans in sickle-cell disease. Neurological correlates and clinical implications. Arch Neurol. 1993;50:629-635.

461. Wang WC, Gallagher DM, Pegelow CH, et al. Multicenter comparison of magnetic resonance imaging and transcranial Doppler ultrasonography in the evaluation of the central nervous system in children with sickle cell disease. J Pediatr Hematol Oncol. 2000;22:335-339.

462. Kinney TR, Sleeper LA, Wang WC, et al. Silent cerebral infarcts in sickle cell anemia: a risk factor analysis. The Cooperative Study of Sickle Cell Disease. Pediatrics. 1999;103:640-645.

463. Wang WC, Langston JW, Steen RG, et al. Abnormalities of the central nervous system in very young children with sickle cell anemia. J Pediatr. 1998;132:994-998.

464. Schatz J, Brown RT, Pascual JM, et al. Poor school and cognitive functioning with silent cerebral infarcts and sickle cell disease. Neurology. 2001;56:1109-1111.

465. Bernaudin F, Verlhac S, Freard F, et al. Multicenter prospective study of children with sickle cell disease: radiographic and psychometric correlation. J Child Neurol. 2000;15:333-343.

466. Steen RG, Langston JW, Reddick WE, et al. Quantitative MR imaging of children with sickle cell disease: striking T1 elevation in the thalamus. J Magn Reson Imaging. 1996;6:226-234.

467. Ohene-Frempong K, Weiner SJ, Sleeper LA, et al. Cerebrovascular accidents in sickle cell disease: rates and risk factors. Blood. 1998;91:288-294.

468. Pegelow CH, Colangelo L, Steinberg M, et al. Natural history of blood pressure in sickle cell disease: risks for stroke and death associated with relative hypertension in sickle cell anemia. Am J Med. 1997;102:171-177.

469. Adams RJ, McKie VC, Hsu L, et al. Prevention of a first stroke by transfusions in children with sickle cell anemia and abnormal results on transcranial Doppler ultrasonography. N Engl J Med. 1998;339:5-11.

470. Adams RJ, Brambilla D. Discontinuing prophylactic transfusions used to prevent stroke in sickle cell disease. N Engl J Med. 2005;353:2769-2778.

471. Kirkham FJ, Lerner NB, Noetzel M, et al. Trials in sickle cell disease. Pediatr Neurol. 2006;34:450-458.

472. Silent Cerebral Infarct Multi-Center Clinical Trial. National Institutes of Health. Vol 2008. Available at ClinicalTrialsgov.

473. Ferster A, Tahriri P, Vermylen C, et al. Five years of experience with hydroxyurea in children and young adults with sickle cell disease. Blood. 2001;97:3628-3632.

474. Hoppe CC, Walters MC. Bone marrow transplantation in sickle cell anemia. Curr Opin Oncol. 2001;13:85-90.

475. Powars D, Adams RJ, Nichols FT, et al. Delayed intracranial hemorrhage following cerebral infarction in sickle cell anemia. J Assoc Acad Minor Physicians. 1990;1:79-82.

476. Dobson SR, Holden KR, Nietert PJ, et al. Moyamoya syndrome in childhood sickle cell disease: a predictive factor for recurrent cerebrovascular events. Blood. 2002;99:3144-3150.

477. Diggs LW, Brookoff D. Multiple cerebral aneurysms in patients with sickle cell disease. South Med J. 1993;86: 377-379.

478. Royal JE, Seeler RA. Hypertension, convulsions, and cerebral haemorrhage in sickle-cell anaemia patients after blood-transfusions. Lancet. 1978;2:1207.

479. Strouse JJ, Hulbert ML, DeBaun MR, et al. Primary hemorrhagic stroke in children with sickle cell disease is associated with recent transfusion and use of corticosteroids. Pediatrics. 2006;118:1916-1924.

480. Oyesiku NM, Barrow DL, Eckman JR, et al. Intracranial aneurysms in sickle-cell anemia: clinical features and pathogenesis. J Neurosurg. 1991;75:356-363.

481. Anson JA, Koshy M, Ferguson L, Crowell RM. Subarachnoid hemorrhage in sickle-cell disease. J Neurosurg. 1991;75:552-558.

482. Schmugge M, Frischknecht H, Yonekawa Y, et al. Stroke in hemoglobin (SD) sickle cell disease with moyamoya:

successful hydroxyurea treatment after cerebrovascular bypass surgery. Blood. 2001;97:2165-2167.

483. Emond AM, Holman R, Hayes RJ, Serjeant GR. Priapism and impotence in homozygous sickle cell disease. Arch Intern Med. 1980;140:1434-1437.

484. Mantadakis E, Cavender JD, Rogers ZR, et al. Prevalence of priapism in children and adolescents with sickle cell anemia. J Pediatr Hematol Oncol. 1999;21:518-522.

485. Adeyoju AB, Olujohungbe AB, Morris J, et al. Priapism in sickle-cell disease; incidence, risk factors and complications—an international multicentre study. BJU Int. 2002;90:898-902.

486. Jiva T, Anwer S. Priapism associated with chronic cocaine abuse. Arch Intern Med. 1994;154:1770.

487. Conrad ME, Perrine GM, Barton JC, Durant JR. Provoked priapism in sickle cell anemia. Am J Hematol. 1980;9:121-122.

488. Elliott L, Ashley-Koch AE, De Castro L, et al. Genetic polymorphisms associated with priapism in sickle cell disease. Br J Haematol. 2007;137:262-267.

489. Nolan VG, Wyszynski DF, Farrer LA, Steinberg MH. Hemolysis-associated priapism in sickle cell disease. Blood. 2005;106:3264-3267.

490. Seeler RA. Priapism in children with sickle cell anemia. Clin Pediatr (Phila). 1971;10:418-419.

491. Chakrabarty A, Upadhyay J, Dhabuwala CB, et al. Priapism associated with sickle cell hemoglobinopathy in children: long-term effects on potency. J Urol. 1996;155:1419-1423.

492. Sharpsteen JR Jr, Powars D, Johnson C, et al. Multisystem damage associated with tricorporal priapism in sickle cell disease. Am J Med. 1993;94:289-295.

493. Rackoff WR, Ohene-Frempong K, Month S, et al. Neurologic events after partial exchange transfusion for priapism in sickle cell disease. J Pediatr. 1992;120:882-885.

494. Siegel JF, Rich MA, Brock WA. Association of sickle cell disease, priapism, exchange transfusion and neurological events: ASPEN syndrome. J Urol. 1993;150:1480-1482.

495. Dunn EK, Miller ST, Macchia RJ, et al. Penile scintigraphy for priapism in sickle cell disease. J Nucl Med. 1995;36:1404-1407.

496. Miller ST, Rao SP, Dunn EK, Glassberg KI. Priapism in children with sickle cell disease. J Urol. 1995;154:844-847.

497. Burnett AL, Allen RP, Tempany CM, et al. Evaluation of erectile function in men with sickle cell disease. Urology. 1995;45:657-663.

498. Maples BL, Hagemann TM. Treatment of priapism in pediatric patients with sickle cell disease. Am J Health Syst Pharm. 2004;61:355-363.

499. Mantadakis E, Ewalt DH, Cavender JD, et al. Outpatient penile aspiration and epinephrine irrigation for young patients with sickle cell anemia and prolonged priapism. Blood. 2000;95:78-82.

500. Virag R, Bachir D, Lee K, Galacteros F. Preventive treatment of priapism in sickle cell disease with oral and self-administered intracavernous injection of etilefrine. Urology. 1996;47:777-781; discussion 781.

501. Merritt AL, Haiman C, Henderson SO. Myth: blood transfusion is effective for sickle cell anemia–associated priapism. CJEM. 2006;8:119-122.

502. Rifkind S, Waisman J, Thompson R, Goldfinger D. RBC exchange pheresis for priapism in sickle cell disease. JAMA. 1979;242:2317-2318.

503. Walker EM Jr, Mitchum EN, Rous SN, et al. Automated erythrocytopheresis for relief of priapism in sickle cell hemoglobinopathies. J Urol. 1983;130:912-916.

504. McCarthy LJ, Vattuone J, Weidner J, et al. Do automated red cell exchanges relieve priapism in patients with sickle cell anemia? Ther Apheresis. 2000;4:256-258.

505. Serjeant GR, de Ceulaer K, Maude GH. Stilboestrol and stuttering priapism in homozygous sickle-cell disease. Lancet. 1985;2:1274-1276.

506. Saad ST, Lajolo C, Gilli S, et al. Follow-up of sickle cell disease patients with priapism treated by hydroxyurea. Am J Hematol. 2004;77:45-49.

507. Noe HN, Wilimas J, Jerkins GR. Surgical management of priapism in children with sickle cell anemia. J Urol. 1981;126:770-771.

508. Douglas L, Fletcher H, Serjeant GR. Penile prostheses in the management of impotence in sickle cell disease. Br J Urol. 1990;65:533-535.

509. Upadhyay J, Shekarriz B, Dhabuwala CB. Penile implant for intractable priapism associated with sickle cell disease. Urology. 1998;51:638-639.

510. Seeler RA, Shwiaki MZ. Acute splenic sequestration crises (ASSC) in young children with sickle cell anemia. Clinical observations in 20 episodes in 14 children. Clin Pediatr (Phila). 1972;11:701-704.

511. Pearson HA. Hemoglobin S–thalassemia syndrome in Negro children. Ann N Y Acad Sci. 1969;165:83-92.

512. Pappo A, Buchanan GR. Acute splenic sequestration in a 2-month-old infant with sickle cell anemia. Pediatrics. 1989;84:578-579.

513. Emond AM, Collis R, Darvill D, et al. Acute splenic sequestration in homozygous sickle cell disease: natural history and management. J Pediatr. 1985;107:201-206.

514. Jenkins ME, Scott RB, Baird RL. Studies in sickle cell anemia. XVI. Sudden death during sickle cell anemia crises in young children. J Pediatr. 1960;56:30-38.

515. Kinney TR, Ware RE, Schultz WH, Filston HC. Long-term management of splenic sequestration in children with sickle cell disease. J Pediatr. 1990;117:194-199.

516. Wright JG, Hambleton IR, Thomas PW, et al. Postsplenectomy course in homozygous sickle cell disease. J Pediatr. 1999;134:304-309.

517. Rao S, Gooden S. Splenic sequestration in sickle cell disease: role of transfusion therapy. Am J Pediatr Hematol Oncol. 1985;7:298-301.

518. Maciver JE, Parker-Williams EJ. The aplastic crisis in sickle-cell anaemia. Lancet. 1961;1:1086-1089.

519. Singer K, Motulsky AG, Wile SA. Aplastic crisis in sickle cell anemia; a study of its mechanism and its relationship to other types of hemolytic crises. J Lab Clin Med. 1950;35:721-736.

520. Leikin SL. The aplastic crisis of sickle-cell disease; occurrence in several members of families within a short period of time. AMA J Dis Child. 1957;93:128-139.

521. Serjeant GR, Topley JM, Mason K, et al. Outbreak of aplastic crises in sickle cell anaemia associated with parvovirus-like agent. Lancet. 1981;2:595-597.

522. Pattison JR, Jones SE, Hodgson J, et al. Parvovirus infections and hypoplastic crisis in sickle-cell anaemia. Lancet. 1981;1:664-665.

523. Goldstein AR, Anderson MJ, Serjeant GR. Parvovirus associated aplastic crisis in homozygous sickle cell disease. Arch Dis Child. 1987;62:585-588.

524. Serjeant GR, Serjeant BE, Thomas PW, et al. Human parvovirus infection in homozygous sickle cell disease. Lancet. 1993;341:1237-1240.

525. Rao SP, Desai N, Miller ST. B19 parvovirus infection and transient aplastic crisis in a child with sickle cell anemia. J Pediatr Hematol Oncol. 1996;18:175-177.

526. Plummer FA, Hammond GW, Forward K, et al. An erythema infectiosum–like illness caused by human parvovirus infection. N Engl J Med. 1985;313:74-79.

527. Chorba T, Coccia P, Holman RC, et al. The role of parvovirus B19 in aplastic crisis and erythema infectiosum (fifth disease). J Infect Dis. 1986;154:383-393.

528. Saarinen UM, Chorba TL, Tattersall P, et al. Human parvovirus B19–induced epidemic acute red cell aplasia in patients with hereditary hemolytic anemia. Blood. 1986;67:1411-1417.

529. Wethers DL, Grover R, Oyeku S. Aplastic crisis and acute splenic sequestration crisis. J Pediatr Hematol Oncol. 2000;22:187-188.

530. Koduri PR, Patel AR, Pinar H. Acute hepatic sequestration caused by parvovirus B19 infection in a patient with sickle cell anemia. Am J Hematol. 1994;47:250-251.

531. Lowenthal EA, Wells A, Emanuel PD, et al. Sickle cell acute chest syndrome associated with parvovirus B19 infection: case series and review. Am J Hematol. 1996;51:207-213.

532. Tolaymat A, Al Mousily F, MacWilliam K, et al. Parvovirus glomerulonephritis in a patient with sickle cell disease. Pediatr Nephrol. 1999;13:340-342.

533. Wierenga KJ, Pattison JR, Brink N, et al. Glomerulonephritis after human parvovirus infection in homozygous sickle-cell disease. Lancet. 1995;346:475-476.

534. Wierenga KJ, Serjeant BE, Serjeant GR. Cerebrovascular complications and parvovirus infection in homozygous sickle cell disease. J Pediatr. 2001;139:438-442.

535. Zimmerman SA, Davis JS, Schultz WH, Ware RE. Subclinical parvovirus B19 infection in children with sickle cell anemia. J Pediatr Hematol Oncol. 2003;25:387-389.

536. Mortimer PP, Humphries RK, Moore JG, et al. A human parvovirus-like virus inhibits haematopoietic colony formation in vitro. Nature. 1983;302:426-429.

537. Seeler RA. Deaths in children with sickle cell anemia. A clinical analysis of 19 fatal instances in Chicago. Clin Pediatr (Phila). 1972;11:634-637.

538. Barrett-Connor E. Bacterial infection and sickle cell anemia. An analysis of 250 infections in 166 patients and a review of the literature. Medicine (Baltimore). 1971;50:97-112.

539. Quinn CT, Rogers ZR, Buchanan GR. Survival of children with sickle cell disease. Blood. 2004;103:4023-4027.

540. Overturf GD, Powars D, Baraff LJ. Bacterial meningitis and septicemia in sickle cell disease. Am J Dis Child. 1977;131:784-787.

541. Powars D, Overturf G, Turner E. Is there an increased risk of *Haemophilus influenzae* septicemia in children with sickle cell anemia? Pediatrics. 1983;71:927-931.

542. Pearson HA, Spencer RP, Cornelius EA. Functional asplenia in sickle-cell anemia. N Engl J Med. 1969;281:923-926.

543. Pearson HA, McIntosh S, Ritchey AK, et al. Developmental aspects of splenic function in sickle cell diseases. Blood. 1979;53:358-365.

544. Seeler RA, Reddi CU, Kittams D. *Diplococcus pneumoniae* osteomyelitis in an infant with sickle cell anemia. Clin Pediatr (Phila). 1974;13:372-374.

545. Fischer KC, Shapiro S, Treves S. Visualization of the spleen with a bone-seeking radionuclide in a child with sickle-cell anemia. Radiology. 1977;122:398.

546. Pearson HA, Cornelius EA, Schwartz AD, et al. Transfusion-reversible functional asplenia in young children with sickle-cell anemia. N Engl J Med. 1970;283:334-337.

547. Claster S, Vichinsky E. First report of reversal of organ dysfunction in sickle cell anemia by the use of hydroxyurea: splenic regeneration. Blood. 1996;88:1951-1953.

548. Hankins JS, Ware RE, Rogers ZR, et al. Long-term hydroxyurea therapy for infants with sickle cell anemia: the HUSOFT extension study. Blood. 2005;106:2269-2275.

549. Abboud MR, Jackson SM, Barredo J, et al. Bone marrow transplantation for sickle cell anemia. Am J Pediatr Hematol Oncol. 1994;16:86-89.

550. Schwartz AD, Pearson HA. Impaired antibody response to intravenous immunization in sickle cell anemia. Pediatr Res. 1972;6:145-149.

551. Ammann AJ, Addiego J, Wara DW, et al. Polyvalent pneumococcal-polysaccharide immunization of patients with sickle-cell anemia and patients with splenectomy. N Engl J Med. 1977;297:897-900.

552. Overturf GD, Rigau-Perez JG, Selzer J, et al. Pneumococcal polysaccharide immunization of children with sickle cell disease. I. Clinical reactions to immunization and relationship to preimmunization antibody. Am J Pediatr Hematol Oncol. 1982;4:19-23.

553. O'Brien KL, Swift AJ, Winkelstein JA, et al. Safety and immunogenicity of heptavalent pneumococcal vaccine conjugated to CRM(197) among infants with sickle cell disease. Pneumococcal Conjugate Vaccine Study Group. Pediatrics. 2000;106:965-972.

554. Evans HE, Reindorf C. Serum immunoglobulin levels in sickle cell disease and thalassemia major. Am J Dis Child. 1968;116:586-590.

555. De Ceulaer K, Forbes M, Maude GH, et al. Complement and immunoglobulin levels in early childhood in homozygous sickle cell disease. J Clin Lab Immunol. 1986;21:37-41.

556. Winkelstein JA, Drachman RH. Deficiency of pneumococcal serum opsonizing activity in sickle-cell disease. N Engl J Med. 1968;279:459-466.

557. Johnston RB Jr, Newman SL, Struth AG. An abnormality of the alternate pathway of complement activation in sickle-cell disease. N Engl J Med. 1973;288:803-808.

558. Wilson WA, Hughes GR, Lachmann PJ. Deficiency of factor B of the complement system in sickle cell anaemia. BMJ. 1976;1:367-369.

559. Chudwin DS, Wara DW, Matthay KK, et al. Increased serum opsonic activity and antibody concentration in patients with sickle cell disease after pneumococcal polysaccharide immunization. J Pediatr. 1983;102:51-54.

560. Bjornson AB, Gaston MH, Zellner CL. Decreased opsonization for *Streptococcus pneumoniae* in sickle cell disease: studies on selected complement components and immunoglobulins. J Pediatr. 1977;91:371-378.

561. Bjornson AB, Lobel JS. Lack of a requirement for the Fc region of IgG in restoring pneumococcal opsonization via the alternative complement pathway in sickle cell disease. J Infect Dis. 1986;154:760-769.

562. Boggs DR, Hyde F, Srodes C. An unusual pattern of neutrophil kinetics in sickle cell anemia. Blood. 1973; 41:59-65.

563. Dimitrov NV, Douwes FR, Bartolotta B, et al. Metabolic activity of polymorphonuclear leukocytes in sickle cell anemia. Acta Haematol. 1972;47:283-291.

564. Strauss RG, Johnston RB Jr, Asbrock T, et al. Neutrophil oxidative metabolism in sickle cell disease. J Pediatr. 1976;89:391-394.

565. Boghossian SH, Wright G, Webster AD, Segal AW. Investigations of host defence in patients with sickle cell disease. Br J Haematol. 1985;59:523-531.

566. Anyaegbu CC, Okpala IE, Akren'Ova YA, Salimonu LS. Peripheral blood neutrophil count and candidacidal activity correlate with the clinical severity of sickle cell anaemia (SCA). Eur J Haematol. 1998;60:267-268.

567. Hongeng S, Wilimas JA, Harris S, et al. Recurrent *Streptococcus pneumoniae* sepsis in children with sickle cell disease. J Pediatr. 1997;130:814-816.

568. Magnus SA, Hambleton IR, Moosdeen F, Serjeant GR. Recurrent infections in homozygous sickle cell disease. Arch Dis Child. 1999;80:537-541.

569. McIntosh S, Rooks Y, Ritchey AK, Pearson HA. Fever in young children with sickle cell disease. J Pediatr. 1980;96: 199-204.

570. Buchanan GR, Glader BE. Leukocyte counts in children with sickle cell disease. Comparative values in the steady state, vaso-occlusive crisis, and bacterial infection. Am J Dis Child. 1978;132:396-398.

571. Wilimas JA, Flynn PM, Harris S, et al. A randomized study of outpatient treatment with ceftriaxone for selected febrile children with sickle cell disease. N Engl J Med. 1993;329:472-476.

572. Shulman ST, Bartlett J, Clyde WA Jr, Ayoub EM. The unusual severity of mycoplasmal pneumonia in children with sickle-cell disease. N Engl J Med. 1972;287: 164-167.

573. John AB, Ramlal A, Jackson H, et al. Prevention of pneumococcal infection in children with homozygous sickle cell disease. Br Med J (Clin Res Ed). 1984;288:1567-1570.

574. Gaston MH, Verter JI, Woods G, et al. Prophylaxis with oral penicillin in children with sickle cell anemia. A randomized trial. N Engl J Med. 1986;314:1593-1599.

575. Falletta JM, Woods GM, Verter JI, et al. Discontinuing penicillin prophylaxis in children with sickle cell anemia. Prophylactic Penicillin Study II. J Pediatr. 1995;127: 685-690.

576. Woods GM, Jorgensen JH, Waclawiw MA, et al. Influence of penicillin prophylaxis on antimicrobial resistance in nasopharyngeal *S. pneumoniae* among children with sickle cell anemia. The Ancillary Nasopharyngeal Culture Study of Prophylactic Penicillin Study II. J Pediatr Hematol Oncol. 1997;19:327-333.

577. Daw NC, Wilimas JA, Wang WC, et al. Nasopharyngeal carriage of penicillin-resistant *Streptococcus pneumoniae* in children with sickle cell disease. Pediatrics. 1997;99:E7.

578. Wong WY, Powars DR, Chan L, et al. Polysaccharide encapsulated bacterial infection in sickle cell anemia: a thirty year epidemiologic experience. Am J Hematol. 1992;39:176-182.

579. Buchanan GR, Schiffman G. Antibody responses to polyvalent pneumococcal vaccine in infants with sickle cell anemia. J Pediatr. 1980;96:264-266.

580. Kaplan J, Frost H, Sarnaik S, Schiffman G. Type-specific antibodies in children with sickle cell anemia given polyvalent pneumococcal vaccine. J Pediatr. 1982;100:404-406.

581. Kaplan J, Sarnaik S, Schiffman G. Revaccination with polyvalent pneumococcal vaccine in children with sickle cell anemia. Am J Pediatr Hematol Oncol. 1986;8: 80-82.

582. Nowak-Wegrzyn A, Winkelstein JA, Swift AJ, Lederman HM. Serum opsonic activity in infants with sickle-cell disease immunized with pneumococcal polysaccharide protein conjugate vaccine. The Pneumococcal Conjugate Vaccine Study Group. Clin Diagn Lab Immunol. 2000; 7:788-793.

583. Overturf GD. American Academy of Pediatrics. Committee on Infectious Diseases. Technical report: prevention of pneumococcal infections, including the use of pneumococcal conjugate and polysaccharide vaccines and antibiotic prophylaxis. Pediatrics. 2000;106:367-376.

584. Frank AL, Labotka RJ, Rao S, et al. *Haemophilus influenzae* type b immunization of children with sickle cell diseases. Pediatrics. 1988;82:571-575.

585. Gigliotti F, Feldman S, Wang WC, et al. Immunization of young infants with sickle cell disease with a *Haemophilus influenzae* type b saccharide-diphtheria CRM197 protein conjugate vaccine. J Pediatr. 1989;114:1006-1010.

586. Buchanan GR, Smith SJ. Pneumococcal septicemia despite pneumococcal vaccine and prescription of penicillin prophylaxis in children with sickle cell anemia. Am J Dis Child. 1986;140:428-432.

587. Lindsay J Jr, Meshel JC, Patterson RH. The cardiovascular manifestations of sickle cell disease. Arch Intern Med. 1974;133:643-651.

588. Shubin H, Kaufman R, Shapiro M, Levinson DC. Cardiovascular findings in children with sickle cell anemia. Am J Cardiol. 1960;6:875.

589. Batra AS, Acherman RJ, Wong WY, et al. Cardiac abnormalities in children with sickle cell anemia. Am J Hematol. 2002;70:306-312.

590. Chung EE, Dianzumba SB, Morais P, Serjeant GR. Cardiac performance in children with homozygous sickle cell disease. J Am Coll Cardiol. 1987;9:1038-1042.

591. Finch CA. Pathophysiologic aspects of sickle cell anemia. Am J Med. 1972;53:1-6.

592. Barrett O Jr, Saunders DE Jr, McFarland DE, Humphries JO. Myocardial infarction in sickle cell anemia. Am J Hematol. 1984;16:139-147.

593. Assanasen C, Quinton RA, Buchanan GR. Acute myocardial infarction in sickle cell anemia. J Pediatr Hematol Oncol. 2003;25:978-981.

594. Jensen WN, Rucknagel DL, Taylor WJ. In vivo study of the sickle cell phenomenon. J Lab Clin Med. 1960;56: 854-865.

595. McNamara JJ, Molot MA, Stremple JF, Cutting RT. Coronary artery disease in combat casualties in Vietnam. JAMA. 1971;216:1185-1187.

596. Gerry JL, Bulkley BH, Hutchins GM. Clinicopathologic analysis of cardiac dysfunction in 52 patients with sickle cell anemia. Am J Cardiol. 1978;42:211-216.

597. Covitz W, Espeland M, Gallagher D, et al. The heart in sickle cell anemia. The Cooperative Study of Sickle Cell Disease (CSSCD). Chest. 1995;108:1214-1219.

598. Simmons BE, Santhanam V, Castaner A, et al. Sickle cell heart disease. Two-dimensional echo and Doppler ultrasonographic findings in the hearts of adult patients with sickle cell anemia. Arch Intern Med. 1988;148:1526-1528.

599. Sutton LL, Castro O, Cross DJ, et al. Pulmonary hypertension in sickle cell disease. Am J Cardiol. 1994;74:626-628.

600. Ataga KI, Sood N, De Gent G, et al. Pulmonary hypertension in sickle cell disease. Am J Med. 2004;117:665-669.

601. Gladwin MT, Sachdev V, Jison ML, et al. Pulmonary hypertension as a risk factor for death in patients with sickle cell disease. N Engl J Med. 2004;350:886-895.

602. Collins FS, Orringer EP. Pulmonary hypertension and cor pulmonale in the sickle hemoglobinopathies. Am J Med. 1982;73:814-821.

603. Castro O, Hoque M, Brown BD. Pulmonary hypertension in sickle cell disease: cardiac catheterization results and survival. Blood. 2003;101:1257-1261.

604. Ataga KI, Moore CG, Jones S, et al. Pulmonary hypertension in patients with sickle cell disease: a longitudinal study. Br J Haematol. 2006;134:109-115.

605. Suell MN, Bezold LI, Okcu MF, et al. Increased pulmonary artery pressures among adolescents with sickle cell disease. J Pediatr Hematol Oncol. 2005;27:654-658.

606. Ambrusko SJ, Gunawardena S, Sakara A, et al. Elevation of tricuspid regurgitant jet velocity, a marker for pulmonary hypertension in children with sickle cell disease. Pediatr Blood Cancer. 2006;47:907-913.

607. Onyekwere OC, Campbell A, Teshome M, et al. Pulmonary hypertension in children and adolescents with sickle cell disease. Pediatr Cardiol. 2008;29:309-312.

608. Kato GJ, Onyekwere OC, Gladwin MT. Pulmonary hypertension in sickle cell disease: relevance to children. Pediatr Hematol Oncol. 2007;24:159-170.

609. Maisel A, Friedman H, Flint L, et al. Continuous electrocardiographic monitoring in patients with sickle-cell anemia during pain crisis. Clin Cardiol. 1983;6:339-344.

610. Buckalew VM Jr, Someren A. Renal manifestations of sickle cell disease. Arch Intern Med. 1974;133:660-669.

611. Sherwood JB, Goldwasser E, Chilcote R, et al. Sickle cell anemia patients have low erythropoietin levels for their degree of anemia. Blood. 1986;67:46-49.

612. Whitten CF, Younes AA. A comparative study of renal concentrating ability in children with sickel cell anemia and in normal children. J Lab Clin Med. 1960;55:400-415.

613. Hatch FE, Culbertson JW, Diggs LW. Nature of the renal concentrating defect in sickle cell disease. J Clin Invest. 1967;46:336-345.

614. Statius van Eps LW, Schouten H, La Porte-Wijsman LW, Struyker Boudier AM. The influence of red blood cell transfusions on the hyposthenuria and renal hemodynamics of sickle cell anemia. Clin Chim Acta. 1967;17:449-461.

615. Statius van Eps LW, Pinedo-Veels C, de Vries GH, de Koning J. Nature of concentrating defect in sickle-cell nephropathy. Microradioangiographic studies. Lancet. 1970;1:450-452.

616. Perillie PE, Epstein FH. Sickling phenomenon produced by hypertonic solutions: a possible explanation for the hyposthenuria of sicklemia. J Clin Invest. 1963;42:570-580.

617. Noll JB, Newman AJ, Gross S. Enuresis and nocturia in sickle cell disease. J Pediatr. 1967;70:965-967.

618. Radel EG, Kochen JA, Finberg L. Hyponatremia in sickle cell disease. A renal salt-losing state. J Pediatr. 1976;88:800-805.

619. Goossens JP, Statius van Eps LW, Schouten H, Giterson AL. Incomplete renal tubular acidosis in sickle cell disease. Clin Chim Acta. 1972;41:149-156.

620. Oster JR, Lee SM, Lespier LE, et al. Renal acidification in sickle cell trait. Arch Intern Med. 1976;136:30-35.

621. Yoshino M, Amerian R, Brautbar N. Hyporeninemic hypoaldosteronism in sickle cell disease. Nephron. 1982;31:242-244.

622. Oster JR, Lanier DC Jr, Vaamonde CA. Renal response to potassium loading in sickle cell trait. Arch Intern Med. 1980;140:534-536.

623. de Jong PE, Statius van Eps LW. Sickle cell nephropathy: new insights into its pathophysiology. Kidney Int. 1985;27:711-717.

624. Allen TD. Sickle cell disease and hematuria: report of 29 cases. J Urol. 1964;91:177-183.

625. Diggs LW. Anatomic lesions in sickle cell disease. In Abramson H, Bertles JF, Wethers DL (eds). Sickle Cell Disease; Diagnosis, Management, Education, and Research. St Louis, CV Mosby, 1973.

626. Bilinsky RT, Kandel GL, Rabiner SF. Epsilon aminocaproic acid therapy of hematuria due to heterozygous sickle cell diseases. J Urol. 1969;102:93-95.

627. Davis CJ Jr, Mostofi FK, Sesterhenn IA. Renal medullary carcinoma. The seventh sickle cell nephropathy. Am J Surg Pathol. 1995;19:1-11.

628. Wesche WA, Wilimas J, Khare V, Parham DM. Renal medullary carcinoma: a potential sickle cell nephropathy of children and adolescents. Pediatr Pathol Lab Med. 1998;18:97-113.

629. Nicholson GD, Amin UF, Alleyne GA. Proteinuria and the nephrotic syndrome in homozygous sickle cell anaemia. West Indian Med J. 1980;29:239-246.

630. McCoy RC. Ultrastructural alterations in the kidney of patients with sickle cell disease and the nephrotic syndrome. Lab Invest. 1969;21:85-95.

631. Pardo V, Strauss J, Kramer H, et al. Nephropathy associated with sickle cell anemia: an autologous immune complex nephritis. II. Clinicopathologic study of seven patients. Am J Med. 1975;59:650-659.

632. Elfenbein IB, Patchefsky A, Schwartz W, Weinstein AG. Pathology of the glomerulus in sickle cell anemia with and without nephrotic syndrome. Am J Pathol. 1974;77:357-374.

633. Bakir AA, Hathiwala SC, Ainis H, et al. Prognosis of the nephrotic syndrome in sickle glomerulopathy. A retrospective study. Am J Nephrol. 1987;7:110-115.

634. Pham PT, Pham PC, Wilkinson AH, Lew SQ. Renal abnormalities in sickle cell disease. Kidney Int. 2000;57:1-8.

635. Powars DR, Elliott-Mills DD, Chan L, et al. Chronic renal failure in sickle cell disease: risk factors, clinical course, and mortality. Ann Intern Med. 1991;115:614-620.

636. Abbott KC, Hypolite IO, Agodoa LY. Sickle cell nephropathy at end-stage renal disease in the United States: patient characteristics and survival. Clin Nephrol. 2002;58:9-15.

637. Dharnidharka VR, Dabbagh S, Atiyeh B, et al. Prevalence of microalbuminuria in children with sickle cell disease. Pediatr Nephrol. 1998;12:475-478.

638. Wigfall DR, Ware RE, Burchinal MR, et al. Prevalence and clinical correlates of glomerulopathy in children with sickle cell disease. J Pediatr. 2000;136:749-753.

639. Falk RJ, Scheinman J, Phillips G, et al. Prevalence and pathologic features of sickle cell nephropathy and response to inhibition of angiotensin-converting enzyme. N Engl J Med. 1992;326:910-915.

640. McBurney PG, Hanevold CD, Hernandez CM, et al. Risk factors for microalbuminuria in children with sickle cell anemia. J Pediatr Hematol Oncol. 2002;24:473-477.

641. Alvarez O, Zilleruelo G, Wright D, et al. Serum cystatin C levels in children with sickle cell disease. Pediatr Nephrol. 2006;21:533-537.

642. Foucan L, Bourhis V, Bangou J, et al. A randomized trial of captopril for microalbuminuria in normotensive adults with sickle cell anemia. Am J Med. 1998;104:339-342.

643. de Santis Feltran L, de Abreu Carvalhaes JT, Sesso R. Renal complications of sickle cell disease: managing for optimal outcomes. Paediatr Drugs. 2002;4:29-36.

644. Fitzhugh CD, Wigfall DR, Ware RE. Enalapril and hydroxyurea therapy for children with sickle nephropathy. Pediatr Blood Cancer. 2005;45:982-985.

645. Ojo AO, Govaerts TC, Schmouder RL, et al. Renal transplantation in end-stage sickle cell nephropathy. Transplantation. 1999;67:291-295.

646. Green TW, Conley CL, Berthrong M. [The liver in sickle cell anemia.] Bull Johns Hopkins Hosp. 1953;92:99-127.

647. Bogosh A, Casselman WGB, Margolies MP, Bockus HL. Liver disease in sickle cell anemia; a correlation of clinical, biochemical, histologic and histochemical observations. Am J Med. 1955;19:583-609.

648. Barrett-Connor E. Cholelithiasis in sickle cell anemia. Am J Med. 1968;45:889-898.

649. Rennels MB, Dunne MG, Grossman NJ, Schwartz AD. Cholelithiasis in patients with major sickle hemoglobinopathies. Am J Dis Child. 1984;138:66-67.

650. Sarnaik S, Slovis TL, Corbett DP, et al. Incidence of cholelithiasis in sickle cell anemia using the ultrasonic gray-scale technique. J Pediatr. 1980;96:1005-1008.

651. Webb DK, Darby JS, Dunn DT, et al. Gall stones in Jamaican children with homozygous sickle cell disease. Arch Dis Child. 1989;64:693-696.

652. Ware R, Filston HC, Schultz WH, Kinney TR. Elective cholecystectomy in children with sickle hemoglobinopathies. Successful outcome using a preoperative transfusion regimen. Ann Surg. 1988;208:17-22.

653. Malone BS, Werlin SL. Cholecystectomy and cholelithiasis in sickle cell anemia. Am J Dis Child. 1988;142:799-800.

654. Ware RE, Kinney TR, Casey JR, et al. Laparoscopic cholecystectomy in young patients with sickle hemoglobinopathies. J Pediatr. 1992;120:58-61.

655. Goers T, Panepinto J, Debaun M, et al. Laparoscopic versus open abdominal surgery in children with sickle cell disease is associated with a shorter hospital stay. Pediatr Blood Cancer. 2008;50:603-606.

656. Sheehy TW, Law DE, Wade BH. Exchange transfusion for sickle cell intrahepatic cholestasis. Arch Intern Med. 1980;140:1364-1366.

657. Klion FM, Weiner MJ, Schaffner F. Cholestasis in sickle cell anemia. Am J Med. 1964;37:829-832.

658. Bauer TW, Moore GW, Hutchins GM. The liver in sickle cell disease. A clinicopathologic study of 70 patients. Am J Med. 1980;69:833-837.

659. Omata M, Johnson CS, Tong M, Tatter D. Pathological spectrum of liver diseases in sickle cell disease. Dig Dis Sci. 1986;31:247-256.

660. Armaly MF. Ocular manifestations in sickle cell disease. Arch Intern Med. 1974;133:670-679.

661. Asdourian G, Nagpal KC, Goldbaum M, et al. Evolution of the retinal black sunburst in sickling haemoglobinopathies. Br J Ophthalmol. 1975;59:710-716.

662. Jampol LM, Condon P, Dizon-Moore R, et al. Salmon-patch hemorrhages after central retinal artery occlusion in sickle cell disease. Arch Ophthalmol. 1981;99:237-240.

663. Condon PI, Serjeant GR. Ocular findings of elderly cases of homozygous sickle-cell disease in Jamaica. Br J Ophthalmol. 1976;60:361-364.

664. Hamilton AM, Pope FM, Condon PI, et al. Angioid streaks in Jamaican patients with homozygous sickle cell disease. Br J Ophthalmol. 1981;65:341-347.

665. Goldberg MF. Natural history of untreated proliferative sickle retinopathy. Arch Ophthalmol. 1971;85:428-437.

666. Dizon-Moore RV, Jampol LM, Goldberg MF. Chorioretinal and choriovitreal neovascularization. Their presence after photocoagulation of proliferative sickle cell retinopathy. Arch Ophthalmol. 1981;99:842-849.

667. Jampol LM, Goldberg MF. Retinal breaks after photocoagulation of proliferative sickle cell retinopathy. Arch Ophthalmol. 1980;98:676-679.

668. Condon PI, Serjeant GR. Behaviour of untreated proliferative sickle retinopathy. Br J Ophthalmol. 1980;64:404-411.

669. Condon PI, Serjeant GR. Photocoagulation in proliferative sickle retinopathy: results of a 5-year study. Br J Ophthalmol. 1980;64:832-840.

670. Roy MS, Rodgers G, Gunkel R, et al. Color vision defects in sickle cell anemia. Arch Ophthalmol. 1987;105:1676-1678.

671. Lee CM, Charles HC, Smith RT, et al. Quantification of macular ischaemia in sickle cell retinopathy. Br J Ophthalmol. 1987;71:540-545.

672. Weissman H, Nadel AJ, Dunn M. Simultaneous bilateral retinal arterial occlusions treated by exchange transfusions. Arch Ophthalmol. 1979;97:2151-2153.

673. Walton W, Von Hagen S, Grigorian R, Zarbin M. Management of traumatic hyphema. Surv Ophthalmol. 2002;47:297-334.

674. Goldberg MF, Dizon R, Raichand M, et al. Sickled erythrocytes, hyphema, and secondary glaucoma: III. Effects of

sicle cell and normal human blood samples in rabbit anterior chambers. Ophthalmic Surg. 1979;10:52-61.

675. Peachey RD. Leg ulceration and haemolytic anaemia: an hypothesis. Br J Dermatol. 1978;98:245-249.

676. Thrall JH, Rucknagel DL. Increased bone marrow blood flow in sickle cell anemia demonstrated by thallium-201 and Tc-99m human albumin microspheres. Radiology. 1978;127:817-819.

677. Wolfort FG, Krizek TJ. Skin ulceration in sickle cell anemia. Plast Reconstr Surg. 1969;43:71-77.

678. Koshy M, Entsuah R, Koranda A, et al. Leg ulcers in patients with sickle cell disease. Blood. 1989;74:1403-1408.

679. Mohan JS, Vigilance JE, Marshall JM, et al. Abnormal venous function in patients with homozygous sickle cell (SS) disease and chronic leg ulcers. Clin Sci (Lond). 2000;98:667-672.

680. Kato GJ, McGowan V, Machado RF, et al. Lactate dehydrogenase as a biomarker of hemolysis-associated nitric oxide resistance, priapism, leg ulceration, pulmonary hypertension, and death in patients with sickle cell disease. Blood. 2006;107:2279-2285.

681. Alleyne SI, Wint E, Serjeant GR. Social effects of leg ulceration in sickle cell anemia. South Med J. 1977;70:213-214.

682. Wethers DL, Ramirez GM, Koshy M, et al. Accelerated healing of chronic sickle-cell leg ulcers treated with RGD peptide matrix. RGD Study Group. Blood. 1994;84:1775-1779.

683. Serjeant GR, Galloway RE, Gueri MC. Oral zinc sulphate in sickle-cell ulcers. Lancet. 1970;2:891-892.

684. Serjeant GR, Howard C. Isoxsuprine hydrochloride in the therapy of sickle cell leg ulceration. West Indian Med J. 1977;26:164-166.

685. Todd GB, Serjeant GR, Larson MR. Sensori-neural hearing loss in Jamaicans with SS disease. Acta Otolaryngol. 1973;76:268-272.

686. Serjeant GR, Norman W, Todd GB. The internal auditory canal and sensori-neural hearing loss in homozygous sickle cell disease. J Laryngol Otol. 1975;89:453-455.

687. Friedman EM, Herer GR, Luban NL, Williams I. Sickle cell anemia and hearing. Ann Otol Rhinol Laryngol. 1980;89:342-347.

688. Morgenstein KM, Manace ED. Temporal bone histopathology in sickle cell disease. Laryngoscope. 1969;79:2172-2180.

689. Bohrer SP. Acute long bone diaphyseal infarcts in sickle cell disease. Br J Radiol. 1970;43:685-697.

690. Reynolds J. Radiologic manifestations of sickle cell hemoglobinopathy. JAMA. 1977;238:247-250.

691. Gupta R, Adekile AD. MRI follow-up and natural history of avascular necrosis of the femoral head in Kuwaiti children with sickle cell disease. J Pediatr Hematol Oncol. 2004;26:351-353.

692. Milner PF, Kraus AP, Sebes JI, et al. Sickle cell disease as a cause of osteonecrosis of the femoral head. N Engl J Med. 1991;325:1476-1481.

693. Aguilar C, Vichinsky E, Neumayr L. Bone and joint disease in sickle cell disease. Hematol Oncol Clin North Am. 2005;19:929-941, viii.

694. Frush DP, Heyneman LE, Ware RE, Bissett GS 3rd. MR features of soft-tissue abnormalities due to acute marrow infarction in five children with sickle cell disease. AJR Am J Roentgenol. 1999;173:989-993.

695. Washington ER, Root L. Conservative treatment of sickle cell avascular necrosis of the femoral head. J Pediatr Orthop. 1985;5:192-194.

696. Hernigou P, Bachir D, Galacteros F. Avascular necrosis of the femoral head in sickle-cell disease. Treatment of collapse by the injection of acrylic cement. J Bone Joint Surg Br. 1993;75:875-880.

697. Hungerford DS. Response: the role of core decompression in the treatment of ischemic necrosis of the femoral head. Arthritis Rheum. 1989;32:801-806.

698. Neumayr LD, Aguilar C, Earles AN, et al. Physical therapy alone compared with core decompression and physical therapy for femoral head osteonecrosis in sickle cell disease. Results of a multicenter study at a mean of three years after treatment. J Bone Joint Surg Am. 2006;88:2573-2582.

699. Milner PF, Kraus AP, Sebes JI, et al. Osteonecrosis of the humeral head in sickle cell disease. Clin Orthop Relat Res. 1993;289:136-143.

700. Miller GJ, Serjeant GR. An assessment of lung volumes and gas transfer in sickle-cell anaemia. Thorax. 1971;26:309-315.

701. Femi-Pearse D, Gazioglu KM, Yu PN. Pulmonary function studies in sickle cell disease. J Appl Physiol. 1970;28:574-577.

702. Wall MA, Platt OS, Strieder DJ. Lung function in children with sickle cell anemia. Am Rev Respir Dis. 1979;120:210-214.

703. Bowen EF, Crowston JG, De Ceulaer K, Serjeant GR. Peak expiratory flow rate and the acute chest syndrome in homozygous sickle cell disease. Arch Dis Child. 1991;66:330-332.

704. Hijazi Z, Onadeko BO, Khadadah M, et al. Pulmonary function studies in Kuwaiti children with sickle cell disease and elevated Hb F. Int J Clin Pract. 2005;59:163-167.

705. Klings ES, Wyszynski DF, Nolan VG, Steinberg MH. Abnormal pulmonary function in adults with sickle cell anemia. Am J Respir Crit Care Med. 2006;173:1264-1269.

706. Powars D, Weidman JA, Odom-Maryon T, et al. Sickle cell chronic lung disease: prior morbidity and the risk of pulmonary failure. Medicine (Baltimore). 1988;67:66-76.

707. Koumbourlis AC, Zar HJ, Hurlet-Jensen A, Goldberg MR. Prevalence and reversibility of lower airway obstruction in children with sickle cell disease. J Pediatr. 2001;138:188-192.

708. Sylvester KP, Patey RA, Milligan P, et al. Pulmonary function abnormalities in children with sickle cell disease. Thorax. 2004;59:67-70.

709. Santoli F, Zerah F, Vasile N, et al. Pulmonary function in sickle cell disease with or without acute chest syndrome. Eur Respir J. 1998;12:1124-1129.

710. Pianosi P, D'Souza SJ, Charge TD, et al. Pulmonary function abnormalities in childhood sickle cell disease. J Pediatr. 1993;122:366-371.

711. Koumbourlis AC, Hurlet-Jensen A, Bye MR. Lung function in infants with sickle cell disease. Pediatr Pulmonol. 1997;24:277-281.

712. Walters MC, Storb R, Patience M, et al. Impact of bone marrow transplantation for symptomatic sickle cell disease: an interim report. Multicenter investigation of bone

marrow transplantation for sickle cell disease. Blood. 2000;95:1918-1924.

713. Kral MC, Brown RT, Connelly M, et al. Radiographic predictors of neurocognitive functioning in pediatric sickle cell disease. J Child Neurol. 2006;21:37-44.

714. Wiznitzer M, Ruggieri PM, Masaryk TJ, et al. Diagnosis of cerebrovascular disease in sickle cell anemia by magnetic resonance angiography. J Pediatr. 1990;117:551-555.

715. Armstrong FD, Thompson RJ Jr, Wang W, et al. Cognitive functioning and brain magnetic resonance imaging in children with sickle cell disease. Neuropsychology Committee of the Cooperative Study of Sickle Cell Disease. Pediatrics. 1996;97:864-870.

716. Booker CR, Scott RB, Ferguson AD. Studies in sickle cell anemia. XXII. Clinical manifestations of sickle cell anemia during the first two years of life. Clin Pediatr (Phila). 1964;3:111-115.

717. Stevens MC, Hayes RJ, Serjeant GR. Body shape in young children with homozygous sickle cell disease. Pediatrics. 1983;71:610-614.

718. Morais PV, Clarke WF, Hayes RJ, Serjeant GR. Heart size and chest shape in homozygous sickle cell disease. West Indian Med J. 1983;32:157-160.

719. Platt OS, Rosenstock W, Espeland MA. Influence of sickle hemoglobinopathies on growth and development. N Engl J Med. 1984;311:7-12.

720. Singhal A, Davies P, Sahota A, et al. Resting metabolic rate in homozygous sickle cell disease. Am J Clin Nutr. 1993;57:32-34.

721. Stevens MC, Maude GH, Cupidore L, et al. Prepubertal growth and skeletal maturation in children with sickle cell disease. Pediatrics. 1986;78:124-132.

722. Prasad AS, Cossack ZT. Zinc supplementation and growth in sickle cell disease. Ann Intern Med. 1984;100:367-371.

723. Phebus CK, Maciak BJ, Gloninger MF, Paul HS. Zinc status of children with sickle cell disease: relationship to poor growth. Am J Hematol. 1988;29:67-73.

724. Abshire TC, English JL, Githens JH, Hambidge M. Zinc status in children and young adults with sickle cell disease. Am J Dis Child. 1988;142:1356-1359.

725. Nelson MC, Zemel BS, Kawchak DA, et al. Vitamin B_6 status of children with sickle cell disease. J Pediatr Hematol Oncol. 2002;24:463-469.

726. Schall JI, Zemel BS, Kawchak DA, et al. Vitamin A status, hospitalizations, and other outcomes in young children with sickle cell disease. J Pediatr. 2004;145:99-106.

727. Nunlee-Bland G, Rana SR, Houston-Yu PE, Odonkor W. Growth hormone deficiency in patients with sickle cell disease and growth failure. J Pediatr Endocrinol Metab. 2004;17:601-606.

728. Oberfield SE, Wethers DL, Kirkland JL, Levine LS. Growth hormone response to growth hormone releasing factor in sickle cell disease. Am J Pediatr Hematol Oncol. 1987;9:331-334.

729. Reed JD, Redding-Lallinger R, Orringer EP. Nutrition and sickle cell disease. Am J Hematol. 1987;24:441-455.

730. Heyman MB, Vichinsky E, Katz R, et al. Growth retardation in sickle-cell disease treated by nutritional support. Lancet. 1985;1:903-906.

731. Alleyne SI, Rauseo RD, Serjeant GR. Sexual development and fertility of Jamaican female patients with homozygous sickle cell disease. Arch Intern Med. 1981;141:1295-1297.

732. Osegbe DN, Akinyanju O, Amaku EO. Fertility in males with sickle cell disease. Lancet. 1981;2:275-276.

733. Olambiwonnu NO, Penny R, Frasier SD. Sexual maturation in subjects with sickle cell anemia: studies of serum gonadotropin concentration, height, weight, and skeletal age. J Pediatr. 1975;87:459-464.

734. Landefeld CS, Schambelan M, Kaplan SL, Embury SH. Clomiphene-responsive hypogonadism in sickle cell anemia. Ann Intern Med. 1983;99:480-483.

735. Kumar S, Powars D, Allen J, Haywood LJ. Anxiety, self-concept, and personal and social adjustments in children with sickle cell anemia. J Pediatr. 1976;88:859-863.

736. Yang YM, Cepeda M, Price C, et al. Depression in children and adolescents with sickle-cell disease. Arch Pediatr Adolesc Med. 1994;148:457-460.

737. Leikin SL, Gallagher D, Kinney TR, et al. Mortality in children and adolescents with sickle cell disease. Cooperative Study of Sickle Cell Disease. Pediatrics. 1989;84:500-508.

738. Lee A, Thomas P, Cupidore L, et al. Improved survival in homozygous sickle cell disease: lessons from a cohort study. BMJ. 1995;311:1600-1602.

739. Thomas AN, Pattison C, Serjeant GR. Causes of death in sickle-cell disease in Jamaica. Br Med J (Clin Res Ed). 1982;285:633-635.

740. Davis H, Schoendorf KC, Gergen PJ, Moore RM Jr. National trends in the mortality of children with sickle cell disease, 1968 through 1992. Am J Public Health. 1997;87:1317-1322.

741. Johnson FL, Look AT, Gockerman J, et al. Bone-marrow transplantation in a patient with sickle-cell anemia. N Engl J Med. 1984;311:780-783.

742. Vermylen C, Cornu G. Bone marrow transplantation for sickle cell disease. The European experience. Am J Pediatr Hematol Oncol. 1994;16:18-21.

743. Johnson FL, Mentzer WC, Kalinyak KA, et al. Bone marrow transplantation for sickle cell disease. The United States experience. Am J Pediatr Hematol Oncol. 1994;16:22-26.

744. Walters MC, Patience M, Leisenring W, et al. Bone marrow transplantation for sickle cell disease. N Engl J Med. 1996;335:369-376.

745. Eggleston B, Patience M, Edwards S, et al. Effect of myeloablative bone marrow transplantation on growth in children with sickle cell anaemia: results of the multicenter study of haematopoietic cell transplantation for sickle cell anaemia. Br J Haematol. 2007;136:673-676.

746. Bernaudin F, Socie G, Kuentz M, et al. Long-term results of related myeloablative stem-cell transplantation to cure sickle cell disease. Blood. 2007;110:2749-2756.

747. Bhatia M, Walters MC. Hematopoietic cell transplantation for thalassemia and sickle cell disease: past, present and future. Bone Marrow Transplant. 2008;41:109-117.

748. Fixler J, Vichinsky E, Walters MC. Stem cell transplantation for sickle cell disease: can we reduce the toxicity? Pediatr Pathol Mol Med. 2001;20:73-86.

749. Horan JT, Liesveld JL, Fenton P, et al. Hematopoietic stem cell transplantation for multiply transfused patients with sickle cell disease and thalassemia after low-dose total body irradiation, fludarabine, and rabbit anti-

thymocyte globulin. Bone Marrow Transplant. 2005;35: 171-177.

750. Walters MC, Sullivan KM, Bernaudin F, et al. Neurologic complications after allogeneic marrow transplantation for sickle cell anemia. Blood. 1995;85:879-884.

751. Fitzhugh CD, Perl S, Hsieh MM. Late effects of myeloablative bone marrow transplantation (BMT) in sickle cell disease (SCD). Blood. 2008;111:1742-1743; author reply 1744.

752. Ferster A, Bujan W, Corazza F, et al. Bone marrow transplantation corrects the splenic reticuloendothelial dysfunction in sickle cell anemia. Blood. 1993;81:1102-1105.

753. Mentzer WC, Heller S, Pearle PR, et al. Availability of related donors for bone marrow transplantation in sickle cell anemia. Am J Pediatr Hematol Oncol. 1994;16: 27-29.

754. Kodish E, Lantos J, Stocking C, et al. Bone marrow transplantation for sickle cell disease. A study of parents' decisions. N Engl J Med. 1991;325:1349-1353.

755. Adamkiewicz TV, Boyer MW, Bray R, et al. Identification of unrelated cord blood units for hematopoietic stem cell transplantation in children with sickle cell disease. J Pediatr Hematol Oncol. 2006;28:29-32.

756. Walters MC, Quirolo L, Trachtenberg ET, et al. Sibling donor cord blood transplantation for thalassemia major: experience of the Sibling Donor Cord Blood Program. Ann N Y Acad Sci. 2005;1054:206-213.

757. Kohn DB, Sadelain M, Glorioso JC. Occurrence of leukaemia following gene therapy of X-linked SCID. Nat Rev Cancer. 2003;3:477-488.

758. Hanna J, Wernig M, Markoulaki S, et al. Treatment of sickle cell anemia mouse model with iPS cells generated from autologous skin. Science. 2007;318:1920-1923.

759. Wu LC, Sun CW, Ryan TM, et al. Correction of sickle cell disease by homologous recombination in embryonic stem cells. Blood. 2006;108:1183-1188.

760. Ley TJ, DeSimone J, Anagnou NP, et al. 5-Azacytidine selectively increases gamma-globin synthesis in a patient with beta+ thalassemia. N Engl J Med. 1982;307:1469-1475.

761. Charache S, Dover G, Smith K, et al. Treatment of sickle cell anemia with 5-azacytidine results in increased fetal hemoglobin production and is associated with nonrandom hypomethylation of DNA around the gamma-delta-beta-globin gene complex. Proc Natl Acad Sci U S A. 1983;80:4842-4846.

762. Ley TJ, DeSimone J, Noguchi CT, et al. 5-Azacytidine increases gamma-globin synthesis and reduces the proportion of dense cells in patients with sickle cell anemia. Blood. 1983;62:370-380.

763. Dover GJ, Charache SH, Boyer SH, et al. 5-Azacytidine increases fetal hemoglobin production in a patient with sickle cell disease. Prog Clin Biol Res. 1983;134:475-488.

764. Platt OS, Orkin SH, Dover G, et al. Hydroxyurea enhances fetal hemoglobin production in sickle cell anemia. J Clin Invest. 1984;74:652-656.

765. Dover GJ, Humphries RK, Moore JG, et al. Hydroxyurea induction of hemoglobin F production in sickle cell disease: relationship between cytotoxicity and F cell production. Blood. 1986;67:735-738.

766. Charache S, Dover GJ, Moyer MA, Moore JW. Hydroxyurea-induced augmentation of fetal hemoglobin production in patients with sickle cell anemia. Blood. 1987;69: 109-116.

767. Rodgers GP, Dover GJ, Noguchi CT, et al. Hematologic responses of patients with sickle cell disease to treatment with hydroxyurea. N Engl J Med. 1990;322:1037-1045.

768. Goldberg MA, Brugnara C, Dover GJ, et al. Treatment of sickle cell anemia with hydroxyurea and erythropoietin. N Engl J Med. 1990;323:366-372.

769. Rodgers GP, Dover GJ, Uyesaka N, et al. Augmentation by erythropoietin of the fetal-hemoglobin response to hydroxyurea in sickle cell disease. N Engl J Med. 1993;328: 73-80.

770. Perrine SP, Ginder GD, Faller DV, et al. A short-term trial of butyrate to stimulate fetal-globin-gene expression in the beta-globin disorders. N Engl J Med. 1993;328: 81-86.

771. Dover GJ, Brusilow S, Charache S. Induction of fetal hemoglobin production in subjects with sickle cell anemia by oral sodium phenylbutyrate. Blood. 1994;84:339-343.

772. Sher GD, Olivieri NF. Rapid healing of chronic leg ulcers during arginine butyrate therapy in patients with sickle cell disease and thalassemia. Blood. 1994;84:2378-2380.

773. Cokic VP, Beleslin-Cokic BB, Tomic M, et al. Hydroxyurea induces the eNOS-cGMP pathway in endothelial cells. Blood. 2006;108:184-191.

774. Iyamu EW, Cecil R, Parkin L, et al. Modulation of erythrocyte arginase activity in sickle cell disease patients during hydroxyurea therapy. Br J Haematol. 2005;131: 389-394.

775. Steinberg MH, Barton F, Castro O, et al. Effect of hydroxyurea on mortality and morbidity in adult sickle cell anemia: risks and benefits up to 9 years of treatment. JAMA. 2003;289:1645-1651.

776. Lanzkron S, Haywood C Jr., Segal JB, Dover GJ. Hospitalization rates and costs of care of patients with sickle-cell anemia in the state of Maryland in the era of hydroxyurea. Am J Hematol. 2006;81:927-932.

777. Steiner C, Miller J. Sickle Cell Disease Patients in U.S. Hospitals, 2004. HCUP Statistical Brief #21 2006. Rockville, MD, Agency for Healthcare Research and Quality, 2006.

778. Kinney TR, Helms RW, O'Branski EE, et al. Safety of hydroxyurea in children with sickle cell anemia: results of the HUG-KIDS study, a phase I/II trial. Pediatric Hydroxyurea Group. Blood. 1999;94:1550-1554.

779. Scott JP, Hillery CA, Brown ER, et al. Hydroxyurea therapy in children severely affected with sickle cell disease. J Pediatr. 1996;128:820-828.

780. Jayabose S, Tugal O, Sandoval C, et al. Clinical and hematologic effects of hydroxyurea in children with sickle cell anemia. J Pediatr. 1996;129:559-565.

781. de Montalembert M, Begue P, Bernaudin F, et al. Preliminary report of a toxicity study of hydroxyurea in sickle cell disease. French Study Group on Sickle Cell Disease. Arch Dis Child. 1999;81:437-439.

782. de Montalembert M, Brousse V, Elie C, et al. Long-term hydroxyurea treatment in children with sickle cell disease: tolerance and clinical outcomes. Haematologica. 2006;91: 125-128.

783. Zimmerman SA, Schultz WH, Davis JS, et al. Sustained long-term hematologic efficacy of hydroxyurea at maximum tolerated dose in children with sickle cell disease. Blood. 2004;103:2039-2045.

784. Gulbis B, Haberman D, Dufour D, et al. Hydroxyurea for sickle cell disease in children and for prevention of cerebrovascular events: the Belgian experience. Blood. 2005; 105:2685-2690.

785. Kratovil T, Bulas D, Driscoll MC, et al. Hydroxyurea therapy lowers TCD velocities in children with sickle cell disease. Pediatr Blood Cancer. 2006;47:894-900.

786. Rosa RM, Bierer BE, Thomas R, et al. A study of induced hyponatremia in the prevention and treatment of sickle-cell crisis. N Engl J Med. 1980;303:1138-1143.

787. Leary M, Abramson N. Induced hyponatremia for sickle-cell anemia. N Engl J Med. 1981;304:844-845.

788. Charache S, Walker WG. Failure of desmopressin to lower serum sodium or prevent crisis in patients with sickle cell anemia. Blood. 1981;58:892-896.

789. Charache S, Moyer MA, Walker WG. Treatment of acute sickle cell crises with a vasopressin analogue. Am J Hematol. 1983;15:315-319.

790. Clark MR, Mohandas N, Shohet SB. Hydration of sickle cells using the sodium ionophore monensin. A model for therapy. J Clin Invest. 1982;70:1074-1080.

791. Chang H, Ewert SM, Bookchin RM, Nagel RL. Comparative evaluation of fifteen anti-sickling agents. Blood. 1983;61:693-704.

792. Ohnishi ST, Horiuchi KY, Horiuchi K, et al. Nitrendipine, nifedipine and verapamil inhibit the in vitro formation of irreversibly sickled cells. Pharmacology. 1986;32:248-256.

793. Schmidt WF 3rd, Asakura T, Schwartz E. Effect of cetiedil on cation and water movements in erythrocytes. J Clin Invest. 1982;69:589-594.

794. Joiner CH, Jiang M, Claussen WJ, et al. Dipyridamole inhibits sickling-induced cation fluxes in sickle red blood cells. Blood. 2001;97:3976-3983.

795. Peterson CM, Tsairis P, Onishi A, et al. Sodium cyanate induced polyneuropathy in patients with sickle-cell disease. Ann Intern Med. 1974;81:152-158.

796. Charache S, Duffy TP, Jander N, et al. Toxic-therapeutic ratio of sodium cyanate. Arch Intern Med. 1975;135: 1043-1047.

797. Orringer EP, Casella JF, Ataga KI, et al. Purified poloxamer 188 for treatment of acute vaso-occlusive crisis of sickle cell disease: A randomized controlled trial. JAMA. 2001;286:2099-2106.

798. Rodgers GP, Schechter AN, Noguchi CT, et al. Microcirculatory adaptations in sickle cell anemia: reactive hyperemia response. Am J Physiol. 1990;258:H113-H120.

799. King SB. Nitric oxide production from hydroxyurea. Free Radic Biol Med. 2004;37:737-744.

800. Morris CR, Kuypers FA, Larkin S, et al. Arginine therapy: a novel strategy to induce nitric oxide production in sickle cell disease. Br J Haematol. 2000;111:498-500.

801. Morris CR. New strategies for the treatment of pulmonary hypertension in sickle cell disease: the rationale for arginine therapy. Treat Respir Med. 2006;5:31-45.

802. Montero-Huerta P, Hess DR, Head CA. Inhaled nitric oxide for treatment of sickle cell stroke. Anesthesiology. 2006;105:619-621.

803. Rabb LM, Grandison Y, Mason K, et al. A trial of folate supplementation in children with homozygous sickle cell disease. Br J Haematol. 1983;54:589-594.

804. Mazumdar M, Heeney MM, Sox CM, Lieu TA. Preventing stroke among children with sickle cell anemia: an analysis of strategies that involve transcranial Doppler testing and chronic transfusion. Pediatrics. 2007;120: e1107-e1116.

805. Sanger RG, Greer RO Jr, Averbach RE. Differential diagnosis of some simple osseous lesions associated with sickle-cell anemia. Oral Surg Oral Med Oral Pathol. 1977;43:538-545.

806. Freie HM. Sickle cell diseases and hormonal contraception. Acta Obstet Gynecol Scand. 1983;62: 211-217.

807. Manchikanti A, Grimes DA, Lopez LM, Schulz KF. Steroid hormones for contraception in women with sickle cell disease. Cochrane Database Syst Rev. 2007;2: CD006261.

808. Treatment of sickle cell crisis with urea in invert sugar. A controlled trial. Cooperative urea trials group. JAMA. 1974;228:1125-1128.

809. Embury SH, Garcia JF, Mohandas N, et al. Effects of oxygen inhalation on endogenous erythropoietin kinetics, erythropoiesis, and properties of blood cells in sickle-cell anemia. N Engl J Med. 1984;311:291-295.

810. Keidan AJ, Marwah SS, Vaughan GR, et al. Painful sickle cell crises precipitated by stopping prophylactic exchange transfusions. J Clin Pathol. 1987;40:505-507.

811. Shapiro BS, Benjamin LJ, Payne R, Heidrich G. Sickle cell–related pain: perceptions of medical practitioners. J Pain Symptom Manage. 1997;14:168-174.

812. Armstrong FD, Pegelow CH, Gonzalez JC, Martinez A. Impact of children's sickle cell history on nurse and physician ratings of pain and medication decisions. J Pediatr Psychol. 1992;17:651-664.

813. Szeto HH, Inturrisi CE, Houde R, et al. Accumulation of normeperidine, an active metabolite of meperidine, in patients with renal failure of cancer. Ann Intern Med. 1977;86:738-741.

814. Robieux IC, Kellner JD, Coppes MJ, et al. Analgesia in children with sickle cell crisis: comparison of intermittent opioids vs. continuous intravenous infusion of morphine and placebo-controlled study of oxygen inhalation. Pediatr Hematol Oncol. 1992;9:317-326.

815. Cole TB, Sprinkle RH, Smith SJ, Buchanan GR. Intravenous narcotic therapy for children with severe sickle cell pain crisis. Am J Dis Child. 1986;140:1255-1259.

816. Schechter NL, Berrien FB, Katz SM. The use of patient-controlled analgesia in adolescents with sickle cell pain crisis: a preliminary report. J Pain Symptom Manage. 1988;3:109-113.

817. Trentadue NO, Kachoyeanos MK, Lea G. A comparison of two regimens of patient-controlled analgesia for children with sickle cell disease. J Pediatr Nurs. 1998;13:15-19.

818. Melzer-Lange MD, Walsh-Kelly CM, Lea G, et al. Patient-controlled analgesia for sickle cell pain crisis in a pediatric emergency department. Pediatr Emerg Care. 2004;20: 2-4.

819. van Beers EJ, van Tuijn CF, Nieuwkerk PT, et al. Patient-controlled analgesia versus continuous infusion of morphine during vaso-occlusive crisis in sickle cell disease, a

randomized controlled trial. Am J Hematol. 2007;82:955-960.

820. Bellet PS, Kalinyak KA, Shukla R, et al. Incentive spirometry to prevent acute pulmonary complications in sickle cell diseases. N Engl J Med. 1995;333:699-703.

821. Yaster M, Tobin JR, Billett C, et al. Epidural analgesia in the management of severe vaso-occlusive sickle cell crisis. Pediatrics. 1994;93:310-315.

822. Vichinsky EP, Johnson R, Lubin BH. Multidisciplinary approach to pain management in sickle cell disease. Am J Pediatr Hematol Oncol. 1982;4:328-333.

823. Shapiro BS. The management of pain in sickle cell disease. Pediatr Clin North Am. 1989;36:1029-1045.

824. Co LL, Schmitz TH, Havdala H, et al. Acupuncture: an evaluation in the painful crises of sickle cell anaemia. Pain. 1979;7:181-185.

825. Zeltzer L, Dash J, Holland JP. Hypnotically induced pain control in sickle cell anemia. Pediatrics. 1979;64:533-536.

826. Portenoy RK. Chronic opioid therapy in nonmalignant pain. J Pain Symptom Manage. 1990;5:S46-62.

827. Ohene-Frempong K. Indications for red cell transfusion in sickle cell disease. Semin Hematol. 2001;38:5-13.

828. Cohen A, Schwartz E. Excretion of iron in response to deferoxamine in sickle cell anemia. J Pediatr. 1978;92:659-662.

829. Wang WC, Ahmed N, Hanna M. Non–transferrin-bound iron in long-term transfusion in children with congenital anemias. J Pediatr. 1986;108:552-557.

830. Vichinsky E, Onyekwere O, Porter J, et al. A randomised comparison of deferasirox versus deferoxamine for the treatment of transfusional iron overload in sickle cell disease. Br J Haematol. 2007;136:501-508.

831. Files B, Brambilla D, Kutlar A, et al. Longitudinal changes in ferritin during chronic transfusion: a report from the Stroke Prevention Trial in Sickle Cell Anemia (STOP). J Pediatr Hematol Oncol. 2002;24:284-290.

832. Olivieri NF. Progression of iron overload in sickle cell disease. Semin Hematol. 2001;38:57-62.

833. Harmatz P, Butensky E, Quirolo K, et al. Severity of iron overload in patients with sickle cell disease receiving chronic red blood cell transfusion therapy. Blood. 2000;96:76-79.

834. Davies SC, McWilliam AC, Hewitt PE, et al. Red cell alloimmunization in sickle cell disease. Br J Haematol. 1986;63:241-245.

835. Reisner EG, Kostyu DD, Phillips G, et al. Alloantibody responses in multiply transfused sickle cell patients. Tissue Antigens. 1987;30:161-166.

836. Sarnaik S, Schornack J, Lusher JM. The incidence of development of irregular red cell antibodies in patients with sickle cell anemia. Transfusion. 1986;26:249-252.

837. Vichinsky EP, Earles A, Johnson RA, et al. Alloimmunization in sickle cell anemia and transfusion of racially unmatched blood. N Engl J Med. 1990;322:1617-1621.

838. Osby M, Shulman IA. Phenotype matching of donor red blood cell units for nonalloimmunized sickle cell disease patients: a survey of 1182 North American laboratories. Arch Pathol Lab Med. 2005;129:190-193.

839. Castro O, Sandler SG, Houston-Yu P, Rana S. Predicting the effect of transfusing only phenotype-matched RBCs to patients with sickle cell disease: theoretical and practical implications. Transfusion. 2002;42:684-690.

840. Vichinsky EP, Luban NLC, Wright E, et al. Prospective RBC phenotype matching in a stroke-prevention trial in sickle cell anemia: a multicenter transfusion trial. Transfusion. 2001;41:1086-1092.

841. Tahhan HR, Holbrook CT, Braddy LR, et al. Antigen-matched donor blood in the transfusion management of patients with sickle cell disease. Transfusion. 1994;34:562-569.

842. Ambruso DR, Githens JH, Alcorn R, et al. Experience with donors matched for minor blood group antigens in patients with sickle cell anemia who are receiving chronic transfusion therapy. Transfusion. 1987;27:94-98.

843. Orlina AR, Unger PJ, Koshy M. Post-transfusion alloimmunization in patients with sickle cell disease. Am J Hematol. 1978;5:101-106.

844. Koshy M, Weiner SJ, Miller ST, et al. Surgery and anesthesia in sickle cell disease. Cooperative Study of Sickle Cell Diseases. Blood. 1995;86:3676-3684.

845. Griffin TC, Buchanan GR. Elective surgery in children with sickle cell disease without preoperative blood transfusion. J Pediatr Surg. 1993;28:681-685.

846. Vichinsky EP, Haberkern CM, Neumayr L, et al. A comparison of conservative and aggressive transfusion regimens in the perioperative management of sickle cell disease. The Preoperative Transfusion in Sickle Cell Disease Study Group. N Engl J Med. 1995;333:206-213.

847. Vichinsky EP, Neumayr LD, Haberkern C, et al. The perioperative complication rate of orthopedic surgery in sickle cell disease: report of the National Sickle Cell Surgery Study Group. Am J Hematol. 1999;62:129-138.

848. Haberkern CM, Neumayr LD, Orringer EP, et al. Cholecystectomy in sickle cell anemia patients: perioperative outcome of 364 cases from the National Preoperative Transfusion Study. Preoperative Transfusion in Sickle Cell Disease Study Group. Blood. 1997;89:1533-1542.

849. Neumayr L, Koshy M, Haberkern C, et al. Surgery in patients with hemoglobin SC disease. Preoperative Transfusion in Sickle Cell Disease Study Group. Am J Hematol. 1998;57:101-108.

850. Waldron P, Pegelow C, Neumayr L, et al. Tonsillectomy, adenoidectomy, and myringotomy in sickle cell disease: perioperative morbidity. Preoperative Transfusion in Sickle Cell Disease Study Group. J Pediatr Hematol Oncol. 1999;21:129-135.

851. Spigelman A, Warden MJ. Surgery in patients with sickle cell disease. Arch Surg. 1972;104:761-764.

852. Howells TH, Huntsman RG. Anaesthesia in sickle cell states. Anaesthesia. 1973;28:339-341.

853. Searle JF. Anaesthesia and sickle-cell haemoglobin. Br J Anaesth. 1972;44:1335-1336.

854. Burrington JD, Smith MD. Elective and emergency surgery in children with sickle cell disease. Surg Clin North Am. 1976;56:55-71.

855. Janik JS, Seeler RA. Surgical procedures in children with sickle hemoglobinopathy. J Pediatr. 1977;91:505-506.

856. Bentley PG, Howard ER. Surgery in children with homozygous sickle cell anaemia. Ann R Coll Surg Engl. 1979;61:55-58.

857. Freeman MG, Ruth GJ. SS disease, SC disease, and CC disease—obstetric considerations and treatment. Clin Obstet Gynecol. 1969;12:134-156.

858. Cunningham FG, Pritchard JA, Mason R. Pregnancy and sickle cell hemoglobinopathies: results with and without prophylactic transfusions. Obstet Gynecol. 1983;62:419-424.

859. Morrison JC, Morrison FS. Prophylactic transfusions in pregnant patients with sickle cell disease. N Engl J Med. 1989;320:1286-1287.

860. Koshy M, Burd L, Wallace D, et al. Prophylactic red-cell transfusions in pregnant patients with sickle cell disease. A randomized cooperative study. N Engl J Med. 1988;319:1447-1452.

861. Brumfield CG, Huddleston JF, DuBois LB, Harris BA Jr. A delayed hemolytic transfusion reaction after partial exchange transfusion for sickle cell disease in pregnancy: a case report and review of the literature. Obstet Gynecol. 1984;63:13S-15S.

862. Hassell K. Pregnancy and sickle cell disease. Hematol Oncol Clin North Am. 2005;19:903-916, vii-viii.

863. Lottenberg R, Hassell KL. An evidence-based approach to the treatment of adults with sickle cell disease. Hematology Am Soc Hematol Educ Program. 2005;58-65.

864. Charache S, Scott J, Niebyl J, Bonds D. Management of sickle cell disease in pregnant patients. Obstet Gynecol. 1980;55:407-410.

865. Smith JA, Espeland M, Bellevue R, et al. Pregnancy in sickle cell disease: experience of the Cooperative Study of Sickle Cell Disease. Obstet Gynecol. 1996;87:199-204.

866. Boyle E Jr, Thompson C, Tyroler HA. Prevalence of the sickle cell trait in adults of Charleston Charleston County, SC. An epidemiological study. Arch Environ Health. 1968;17:891-898.

867. Ashcroft MT, Miall WE, Milner PF. A comparison between the characteristics of Jamaican adults with normal hemoglobin and those with sickle cell trait. Am J Epidemiol. 1969;90:236-243.

868. Ashcroft MT, Desai P. Mortality and morbidity in Jamaican adults with sickle-cell trait and with normal haemoglobin followed up for twelve years. Lancet. 1976;2:784-786.

869. Sears DA. The morbidity of sickle cell trait: a review of the literature. Am J Med. 1978;64:1021-1036.

870. Kramer MS, Rooks Y, Pearson HA. Growth and development in children with sickle-cell trait. A prospective study of matched pairs. N Engl J Med. 1978;299:686-689.

871. Huisman TH. Trimodality in the percentages of beta chain variants in heterozygotes: the effect of the number of active Hbα structural loci. Hemoglobin. 1977;1:349-382.

872. Levere RD, Lichtman HC, Levine J. Effect of iron-deficiency anaemia on the metabolism of the heterogenic haemoglobins in sickle cell trait. Nature. 1964;202:499-501.

873. Heller P, Yakulis VJ, Epstein RB, Friedland S. Variation in the amount of hemoglobin S in a patient with sickle cell trait and megaloblastic anemia. Blood. 1963;21:479-483.

874. Ashcroft MT, Serjant GR. Growth, morbidity, and mortality in a cohort of Jamaican adolescents with homozygous sickle cell disease. West Indian Med J. 1981;30:197-201.

875. Kramer MS, Rooks Y, Pearson HA. Cord blood screening for sickle hemoglobins: evidence for female preponderance of hemoglobin S. J Pediatr. 1978;93:998-1000.

876. Blattner P, Dar H, Nitowsky HM. Pregnancy outcome in women with sickle cell trait. JAMA. 1977;238:1392-1394.

877. Murphy JR. Sickle cell hemoglobin (Hb AS) in black football players. JAMA. 1973;225:981-982.

878. Kark JA, Posey DM, Schumacher HR, Ruehle CJ. Sickle-cell trait as a risk factor for sudden death in physical training. N Engl J Med. 1987;317:781-787.

879. Weisman IM, Zeballos RJ, Martin TW, Johnson BD. Effect of Army basic training in sickle-cell trait. Arch Intern Med. 1988;148:1140-1144.

880. Charache S. Sudden death in sickle trait. Am J Med. 1988;84:459-461.

881. Sullivan LW. The risks of sickle-cell trait: caution and common sense. N Engl J Med. 1987;317:830-831.

882. Pearson HA. Sickle cell trait and competitive athletics: is there a risk? Pediatrics. 1989;83:613-614.

883. Eichner ER. Sickle cell trait. J Sport Rehabil. 2007;16:197-203.

884. Ober WB, Bruno MS, Weinberg SB, et al. Fatal intravascular sickling in a patient with sickle-cell trait. N Engl J Med. 1960;263:947-949.

885. Jones SR, Binder RA, Donowho EM Jr. Sudden death in sickle-cell trait. N Engl J Med. 1970;282:323-325.

886. O'Brien RT, Pearson HA, Godley JA, Spencer RP. Splenic infarct and sickle-(cell) trait. N Engl J Med. 1972;287:720.

887. Long ID. Sickle cell trait and aviation. Aviat Space Environ Med. 1982;53:1021-1029.

888. Atlas SA. The sickle cell trait and surgical complications. A matched-pair patient analysis. JAMA. 1974;229:1078-1080.

889. Metras D, Coulibaly AO, Ouattara K, et al. Open-heart surgery in sickle-cell haemoglobinopathies: report of 15 cases. Thorax. 1982;37:486-491.

890. Schlitt LE, Keitel HG. Renal manifestations of sickle cell disease: a review. Am J Med Sci. 1960;239:773-778.

891. Ataga KI, Orringer EP. Renal abnormalities in sickle cell disease. Am J Hematol. 2000;63:205-211.

892. Lai JC, Fekrat S, Barron Y, Goldberg MF. Traumatic hyphema in children: risk factors for complications. Arch Ophthalmol. 2001;119:64-70.

893. Larrabee KD, Monga M. Women with sickle cell trait are at increased risk for preeclampsia. Am J Obstet Gynecol. 1997;177:425-428.

894. Roopnarinesingh S, Ramsewak S. Decreased birth weight and femur length in fetuses of patients with the sickle-cell trait. Obstet Gynecol. 1986;68:46-48.

895. Anyaegbunam A, Langer O, Brustman L, et al. The application of uterine and umbilical artery velocimetry to the antenatal supervision of pregnancies complicated by maternal sickle hemoglobinopathies. Am J Obstet Gynecol. 1988;159:544-547.

896. Baill IC, Witter FR. Sickle trait and its association with birthweight and urinary tract infections in pregnancy. Int J Gynaecol Obstet. 1990;33:19-21.

897. Brown S, Merkow A, Wiener M, Khajezadeh J. Low birth weight in babies born to mothers with sickle cell trait. JAMA. 1972;221:1404-1405.

898. Geva A, Clark JJ, Zhang Y, et al. Hemoglobin Jamaica plain—a sickling hemoglobin with reduced oxygen affinity. N Engl J Med. 2004;351:1532-1538.

899. Tubman VN, Bennett CM, Luo HY, et al. Sickle cell disease caused by Hb S/Quebec-CHORI: treatment with hydroxyurea and response. Pediatr Blood Cancer. 2007;49:207-210.

900. McCurdy PR. Erythrokinetics in abnormal hemoglobin syndromes. Blood. 1962;20:686-699.

901. Tuttle AH, Koch B. Clinical and hematological manifestations of hemoglobin CS disease in children. J Pediatr. 1960;65:331-342.

902. Serjeant GR, Ashcroft MT, Serjeant BE. The clinical features of haemoglobin SC disease in Jamaica. Br J Haematol. 1973;24:491-501.

903. Rowley PT, Enlander D. Hemoglobin S-C disease presenting as acute cor pulmonale. Am Rev Respir Dis. 1968;98:494-500.

904. Fabian RH, Peters BH. Neurological complications of hemoglobin SC disease. Arch Neurol. 1984;41:289-292.

905. Ryan SJ, Goldberg MF. Anterior segment ischemia following scleral buckling in sickle cell hemoglobinopathy. Am J Ophthalmol. 1971;72:35-50.

906. Goldberg MF. Treatment of proliferative sickle retinopathy. Trans Am Acad Ophthalmol Otolaryngol. 1971;75:532-556.

907. Barton CJ, Cockshott WP. Bone changes in hemoglobin SC disease. Am J Roentgenol Radium Ther Nucl Med. 1962;88:523-532.

908. Kay CJ, Rosenberg MA, Fleisher P, Small J. Renal papillary necrosis in hemoglobin SC disease. Radiology. 1968;90:897-899.

909. Pritchard JA, Scott DE, Whalley PH, et al. The effects of maternal sickle cell hemoglobinopathies and sickle cell trait on reproductive performance. Am J Obstet Gynecol. 1973;117:662-670.

910. Yeung KY, Lessin LS. Splenic infarction in sickle cell–hemoglobin C disease. Demonstration by selective splenic arteriogram and scintillation scan. Arch Intern Med. 1976;136:905-911.

911. Githens JH, Gross GP, Eife RF, Wallner SF. Splenic sequestration syndrome at mountain altitudes in sickle/hemoglobin C disease. J Pediatr. 1977;90:203-206.

912. Barrett-Connor E. Infection and sickle cell–C disease. Am J Med Sci. 1971;262:162-169.

913. Buchanan GR, Smith SJ, Holtkamp CA, Fuseler JP. Bacterial infection and splenic reticuloendothelial function in children with hemoglobin SC disease. Pediatrics. 1983;72:93-98.

914. Bunn HF, Noguchi CT, Hofrichter J, et al. Molecular and cellular pathogenesis of hemoglobin SC disease. Proc Natl Acad Sci U S A. 1982;79:7527-7531.

915. Bunn HF, McDonald MJ. Electrostatic interactions in the assembly of haemoglobin. Nature. 1983;306:498-500.

916. Ballas SK, Larner J, Smith ED, et al. The xerocytosis of Hb SC disease. Blood. 1987;69:124-130.

917. Orringer EP, Brockenbrough JS, Whitney JA, et al. Okadaic acid inhibits activation of K-Cl cotransport in red blood cells containing hemoglobins S and C. Am J Physiol. 1991;261:C591-C593.

918. Brugnara C, Kopin AS, Bunn HF, Tosteson DC. Regulation of cation content and cell volume in hemoglobin erythrocytes from patients with homozygous hemoglobin C disease. J Clin Invest. 1985;75:1608-1617.

919. Honig GR, Gunay U, Mason RG, et al. Sickle cell syndromes. I. Hemoglobin SC–alpha-thalassemia. Pediatr Res. 1976;10:613-620.

920. Milner PF, Miller C, Grey R, et al. Hemoglobin O arab in four negro families and its interaction with hemoglobin S and hemoglobin C. N Engl J Med. 1970;283:1417-1425.

921. Charache S, Zinkham WH, Dickerman JD, et al. Hemoglobin SC, SS/G$_{Philadelphia}$ and SO$_{Arab}$ diseases: diagnostic importance of an integrative analysis of clinical, hematologic and electrophoretic findings. Am J Med. 1977;62:439-446.

922. Sturgeon P, Itano HA, Bergren WR. Clinical manifestations of inherited abnormal hemoglobins. I. The interaction of hemoglobin-S with hemoglobin-D. Blood. 1955;10:389-404.

923. Schneider RG, Ueda S, Alperin JB, et al. Hemoglobin D Los Angeles in two Caucasian families: hemoglobin SD disease and hemoglobin D thalassemia. Blood. 1968;32:250-259.

924. Cawein MJ, Lappat EJ, Brangle RW, Farley CH. Hemoglobin S-D disease. Ann Intern Med. 1966;64:62-70.

925. Konotey-Ahulu FI, Gallo E, Lehmann H, Ringelhann B. Haemoglobin Korle-Bu (beta 73 aspartic acid replaced by asparagine) showing one of the two amino acid substitutions of haemoglobin C Harlem. J Med Genet. 1968;5:107-111.

926. Bookchin RM, Nagel RL. Ligand-induced conformational dependence of hemoglobin in sickling interactios. J Mol Biol. 1971;60:263-270.

927. Bookchin RM, Nagel RL, Ranney HM. Structure and properties of hemoglobin C-Harlem, a human hemoglobin variant with amino acid substitutions in 2 residues of the beta-polypeptide chain. J Biol Chem. 1967;242:248-255.

928. Moo-Penn W, Bechtel K, Jue D, et al. The presence of hemoglobin S and C Harlem in an individual in the United States. Blood. 1975;46:363-367.

929. Monplaisir N, Merault G, Poyart C, et al. Hemoglobin S Antilles: a variant with lower solubility than hemoglobin S and producing sickle cell disease in heterozygotes. Proc Natl Acad Sci U S A. 1986;83:9363-9367.

930. Trudel M, De Paepe ME, Chretien N, et al. Sickle cell disease of transgenic SAD mice. Blood. 1994;84:3189-3197.

931. Weatherall DJ. Biochemical phenotypes of thalassemia in the American Negro population. Ann N Y Acad Sci. 1964;119:450-462.

932. Serjeant GR, Ashcroft MT, Serjeant BE, Milner PF. The clinical features of sickle-cell– thalassaemia in Jamaica. Br J Haematol. 1973;24:19-30.

933. Itano HA. A third abnormal hemoglobin associated with hereditary hemolytic anemia. Proc Natl Acad Sci U S A. 1951;37:775-784.

934. Thomas ED, Motulsky AG, Walters DH. Homozygous hemoglobin C disease; report of a case with studies on the pathophysiology and neonatal formation of hemoglobin C. Am J Med. 1955;18:832-838.

935. Agner R, Jensen WN, Schoefield RA. Clinical and necropsy findings in hemoglobin C disease. Blood. 1957;12:74-83.

936. Charache S, Conley CL, Waugh DF, et al. Pathogenesis of hemolytic anemia in homozygous hemoglobin C disease. J Clin Invest. 1967;46:1795-1811.

937. Kraus AP, Diggs LW. In vitro crystallization of hemoglobin occuring in citrated blood from patients with hemoglobin C. J Lab Clin Med. 1965;47:700-705.

938. Smith EW, Krevans JR. Clinical manifestations of hemoglobin C disorders. Bull Johns Hopkins Hosp. 1959;104:17-43.

939. Fitzgerald PM, Love WE. Structure of deoxy hemoglobin C (beta six Glu replaced by Lys) in two crystal forms. J Mol Biol. 1979;132:603-619.

940. Girling RL, Houston TE, Amma EL, Huisman TH. An X-ray determination of the molecular interactions in hemoglobin C: a disease characterized by intraerythrocytic crystals. Biochem Biophys Res Commun. 1979;88:768-773.

941. Houston TE, Girling RL, Amma EL, Huisman TH. Structure of human hemoglobin C: a disease with intraerythrocytic crystals. Biochim Biophys Acta. 1979;576:497-501.

20

The Thalassemias

Melody J. Cunningham, Vijay G. Sankaran, David G. Nathan, and Stuart H. Orkin

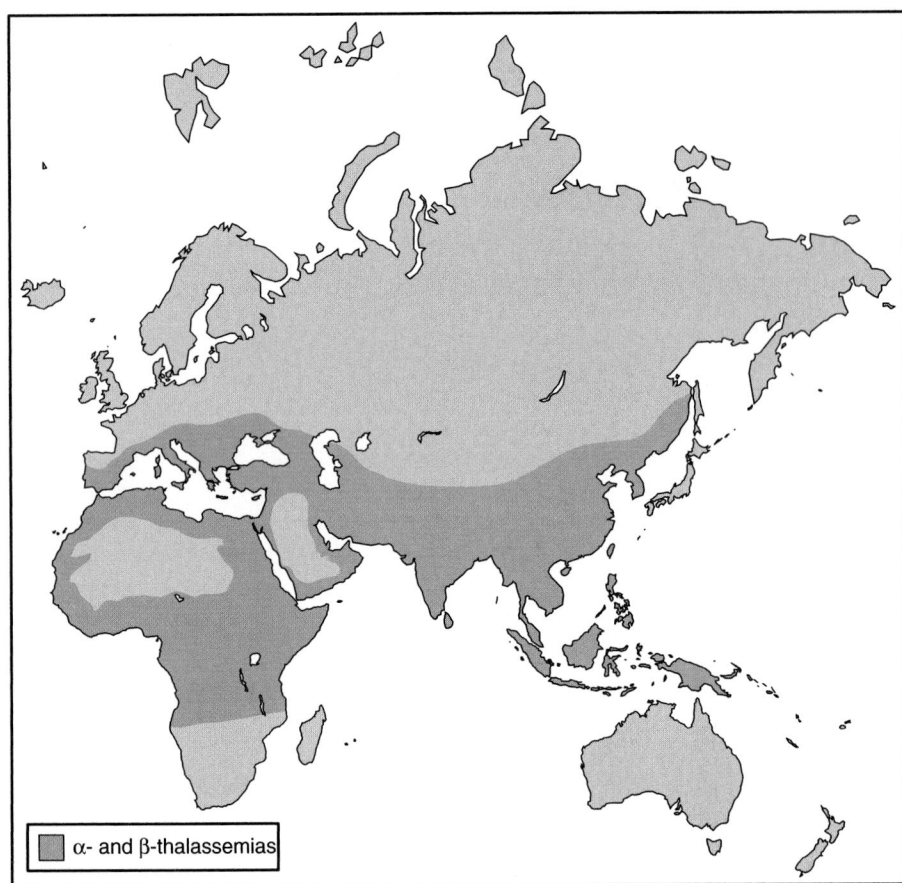

FIGURE 20-1. Geographic distribution of thalassemia.

α- and β-thalassemias

The thalassemias are a heterogeneous group of inherited anemias caused by mutations affecting the synthesis of hemoglobin.[1-3] Milder forms are among the most commonly seen genetic disorders, whereas the less often seen severe forms lead to significant morbidity and mortality worldwide (Fig. 20-1).

Study of the thalassemias traces the history of the application of recombinant DNA methods to analysis of inherited diseases and underscores how naturally occurring mutations in humans illuminate genetic principles. Here, the genetics of hemoglobin genes are reviewed as background for discussion of the molecular basis of the thalassemia syndromes, their clinical phenotypes, prenatal diagnosis, and current management.

HUMAN HEMOGLOBINS: COMPOSITION AND GENETICS

Normal hemoglobins are tetramers of two α-like and two β-like globin polypeptides. The predominant hemoglobin in normal adult red blood cells is hemoglobin A (HbA), $\alpha_2\beta_2$.[4,5] The α- and β-globins contain 141 and 146 amino acids, respectively. In addition to HbA, adult red cells normally contain two minor hemoglobins: HbA$_2$ ($\alpha_2\delta_2$) and fetal hemoglobin (HbF) ($\alpha_2\gamma_2$). The γ and δ polypeptides are related to β but differ in their primary amino acid sequences; hence they may be referred to as β-like

globins. HbA$_2$ normally accounts for 2% to 3.5% of the total hemoglobin. Though a minor component in adult red cells, HbF is the predominant hemoglobin in fetal red cells during the latter two trimesters of gestation. Because it does not bind 2,3-diphosphoglycerate, its affinity for oxygen is higher than that of HbA.[6] As such, HbF enhances the fetus' ability to extract oxygen from the placenta. HbF constitutes a small fraction of the total hemoglobin in adult red cells (0.3% to 1.2%), in which it is largely restricted to a small subset of circulating erythrocytes (0.2% to 7% of the total cells) referred to as F cells.[7,8] Production of HbF in normal adults appears to be largely genetically controlled as demonstrated by studies in twins and families.[9-13] During the first trimester in utero, embryonic hemoglobins with differing subunit composition are found in the yolk sac–derived macrocytic (or primitive) red cells.[1]

The genes that encode the globin polypeptides are organized into two small clusters.[2,4,5,14,15] The α-like genes are located near the telomere of the short arm of chromosome 16 (16p13.3), whereas the β-like genes reside on chromosome 11 at band 11p15.5.[16,17] A schematic diagram of the human globin genes and the composition of the various hemoglobins are shown in Figure 20-2.

The α-globin gene cluster contains three functional genes, ζ, α_2, and α_1, oriented in a 5′-to-3′ direction along the chromosome.[2,15,18,19] ζ-Globin, encoded by the ζ gene, is found in two embryonic hemoglobins, Hb

FIGURE 20-2. Chromosomal organization of the globin genes and their expression during development. The *blue boxes* indicate functional globin genes, whereas the *yellow boxes* indicate pseudogenes (see text). The Θ1 globin gene is depicted by a *brown box* and is expressed at very low levels compared with the adult α-globin genes. The scale of the depicted chromosomal segments is in kilobases of DNA. The switch from embryonic to fetal hemoglobin occurs between 6 and 10 weeks of gestation, and the switch from fetal to adult hemoglobin occurs at about the time of birth.

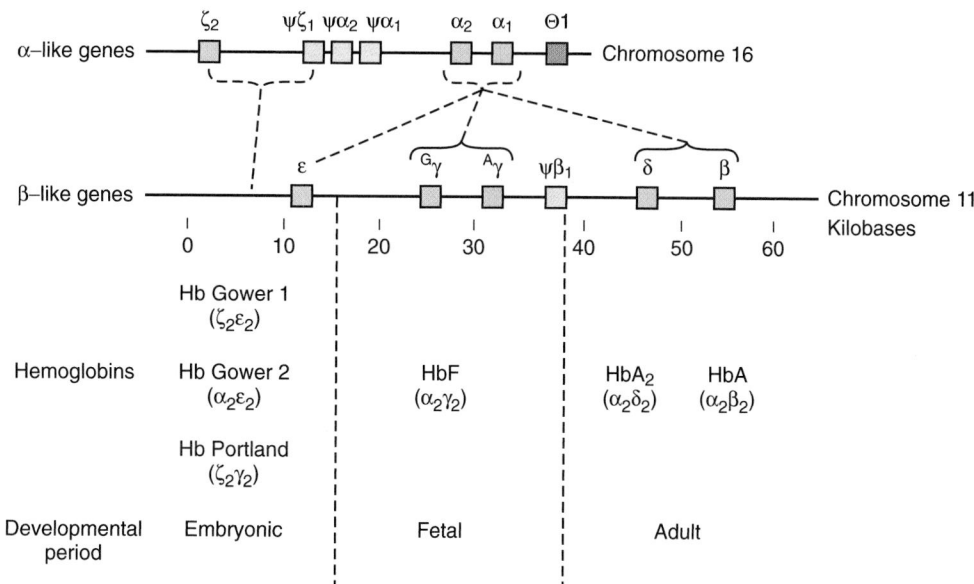

Gower-1 ($\zeta_2\varepsilon_2$) and Portland ($\zeta_2\gamma_2$).[20] The duplicated α-globin genes (α_1 and α_2) encode identical polypeptides. DNA sequence analysis has revealed three additional globin gene–like sequences in the cluster: pseudo-ζ (ζ_1), pseudo-α_1, and pseudo-α_2.[2,15] Although they resemble the functional genes, sequence differences in coding or critical regulatory regions render these genes inactive; hence they are referred to as pseudogenes.

Five functional genes, ε, $^G\gamma$, $^A\gamma$, δ, and β, are present within the β-like cluster and are arranged in a 5'-to-3' direction as they are expressed during development.[21-24] The product of the embryonic ε gene is found in the embryonic hemoglobins Hb Gower-1 ($\zeta_2\varepsilon_2$) and Hb Gower-2 ($\alpha_2\varepsilon_2$). The fetal γ genes are duplicated but encode globins differing only at amino acid 136; $^G\gamma$-globin and $^A\gamma$-globin contain a glycine or alanine residue, respectively. $^G\gamma$- and $^A\gamma$-globins are both found normally in HbF ($\alpha_2\gamma_2$). The δ-globin gene encodes a polypeptide differing in only 10 of 146 residues from β, and yet it is expressed at a very low level in adult red cells (<3% of β). The poor expression of δ-globin is attributed to differences in critical regulatory sequences[25] within the gene that appear to inhibit messenger RNA (mRNA) processing[26] and the inherent instability of δ mRNA.[27] Only a single functional β-globin gene is present in the cluster. β-Globin is the predominant β-like globin in adult red cells, in which HbA ($\alpha_2\beta_2$) accounts for more than 95% of the total hemoglobin.

The relative synthesis of individual globin chains and the major sites of erythropoiesis during development are depicted in Figure 20-3.[1,4,28-30] Embryonic hemoglobins are expressed nearly exclusively in primitive nucleated red cells differentiating in the yolk sac blood islands. HbF production commences during the next wave of erythropoiesis in the fetal liver. Fetal liver–derived red cells lose their nuclei as terminal maturation occurs, whereas the primitive, yolk sac–derived cells remain nucleated. The

transition from HbF to HbA coincides approximately with the switch from fetal liver to bone marrow erythropoiesis. Despite this correlation between the site of erythropoiesis and the hemoglobins expressed, careful analysis of tissues derived from experimental animals and human fetuses has shown that embryonic hemoglobins are synthesized in the liver as well as the yolk sac and HbFs are produced in the bone marrow as well as the liver. The developmental switches in hemoglobin expression are related to the time of gestation rather than the anatomic site of erythropoiesis per se.

Globin Gene Structure

The globin genes were among the first eukaryotic genes to be isolated by recombinant DNA cloning methods in the late 1970s. Subsequent work has provided the entire DNA sequences of the human α- and β-globin gene clusters and extensive sequences of other vertebrate globin complexes. These data have been invaluable in determining the mutations underlying thalassemia syndromes and in manipulating gene regulatory regions.

Intervening Sequences or Introns

A remarkable finding was made on initial study of the globin genes: the coding region, rather than being organized in a single continuous unit, is interrupted by noncoding DNA known as intervening sequences (IVSs), or introns. The majority of eukaryotic genes contain one or more introns. As indicated in Figure 20-4, globin genes are interrupted at two positions. The discontinuous nature of the coding region of globin genes poses a formidable problem for the formation of mRNA that must be translated into globin polypeptides on cytoplasmic ribosomes. Transcription of a globin gene generates a precursor mRNA containing introns. Formation of mature mRNA is accomplished by post-transcriptional

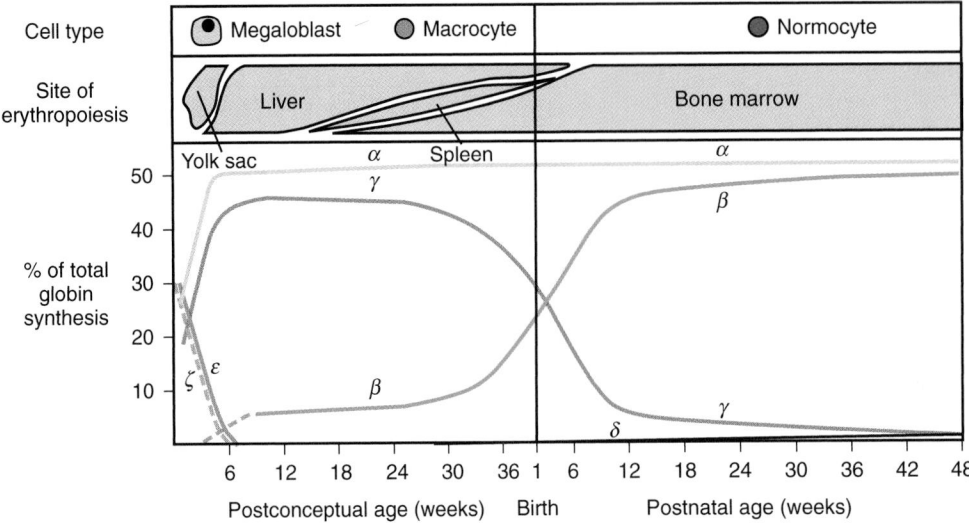

FIGURE 20-3. Sites of erythropoiesis and pattern of globin biosynthesis during development. Nucleated megaloblasts are produced predominantly in the yolk sac. They are replaced by macrocytic fetal red cells produced in the liver and subsequently in the spleen and bone marrow. The height of the *shaded area* approximates the proportion of circulating red cells produced by each organ. Globin biosynthetic measurements were made to obtain the data shown in the lower part of the figure through incubation of intact cells in the presence of radioactive amino acids followed by globin chain separation. (*Redrawn from Weatherall DG, Clegg JB. The Thalassemia Syndromes. Oxford, Blackwell Scientific, 1981, p 54.*)

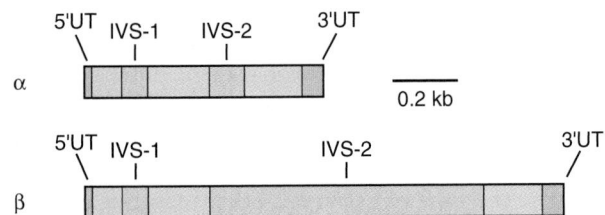

FIGURE 20-4. Structure of the human α- and β-globin genes. Untranslated (UT) regions, exon, and intervening sequences (IVS, introns) are depicted by green, salmon, and blue boxes, respectively.

processing, termed RNA splicing. The pathway of RNA processing is depicted in Figure 20-5.

RNA splicing must be executed with exquisite precision for functional mRNA to be generated. Because translation of mRNA proceeds by the reading of triplets (codons), excision of introns needs to be accurate to the nucleotide; otherwise, shifts in the reading frame of the translated polypeptide will result. RNA processing is guided by specific sequences, known as splice site consensus sequences, located at the 5′ and 3′ boundaries of the introns. The donor site, which marks the 5′ end of the intron, generally conforms to the sequence 5′ (C/A)AG′GT(A/G)AGT, where the prime sign indicates the position of splicing and GT is an essentially invariant dinucleotide at the 5′ end of the intron. The acceptor site, which defines the 3′ end of the intron, usually fits the consensus 5′ (T/C)$_n$N(C/T)AG′G, where *n* is 11 or greater, N is any nucleotide, the prime sign indicates the site of splicing, and AG is an essentially invariant dinucleotide. Excision of introns generally occurs between the dinucleotides GT and AG, the GT-AG rule.

Conserved Features of Mature Globin mRNA

Sequences of human globin genes represented in processed globin mRNA include additional segments located before (5′) and after (3′) the coding region. These untranslated regions are depicted in Figure 20-5. In addition, the mature mRNA is modified at both termini. At the 5′ end a methylated guanylic acid (m⁷G) cap structure is present. A variable number of adenylic acid residues are added at the 3′ end and constitute a poly(A) tail. The 5′ cap structure appears to be important for efficient initiation of mRNA translation, whereas the poly(A) tail contributes to mRNA stability. Overlapping the beginning of the mRNA sequence in genomic DNA are sequences that aid in directing the initiation of transcription to the proper site. In some eukaryotic genes these sequences conform to an initiator (Inr) consensus element.[31] The human β-globin gene has been shown to possess an Inr element that is functional in transcription reactions performed in vitro.[32]

Polyadenylation at the 3′ end of mRNA precursors depends on a signal in the 3′-untranslated region, generally AAUAAA (AATAAA in genomic DNA). The mechanism of modification of the 3′ end is complex and involves not only polyadenylation but also cleavage of the precursor RNA because the primary RNA transcript extends several hundred nucleotides past what becomes the position at which the poly(A) tail is added.

Translation of mRNA into a polypeptide proceeds by the reading of triplets (codons) on cytoplasmic ribosomes. The first AUG codon (specifying methionine) present in the mRNA specifies the start site for translation of the mRNA into protein and is embedded in a sequence context (the Kozak consensus sequence, typi-

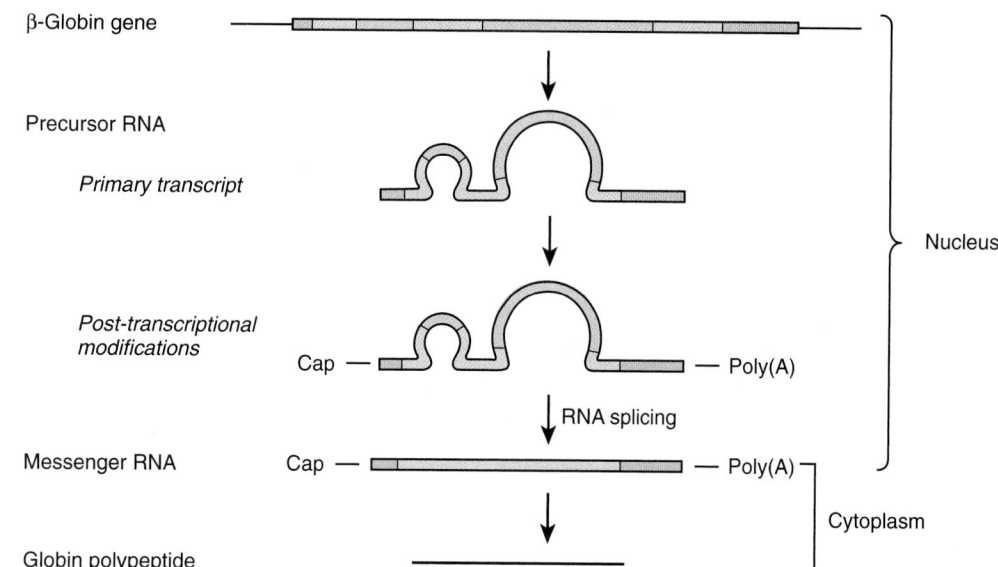

FIGURE 20-5. Expression of the β-globin gene. Transcription of the gene generates the precursor RNA, which is processed by RNA splicing to form messenger RNA.

cally CC[A/G]CC*ATG*G) that signals the binding of translation initiation factors and ribosomes to the RNA. Usually, the amino-terminal methionine residue is removed from the growing polypeptide chain even before its synthesis is completed. Termination of polypeptide chain translation is directed by the termination codons UAA, UAG, or UGA. Mutation of these codons allows continued translation into the 3′-untranslated sequences of mRNA, as occurs in selected α-globin chain variants associated with α-thalassemia (see later).

As briefly reviewed earlier, the formation of functional mature mRNA demands extraordinary precision and depends on highly conserved sequence elements. As exemplified by the thalassemia syndromes, point (or other) mutations in these signals lead to reduced or absent polypeptide chain synthesis, the hallmark of thalassemia. Mutations causing thalassemia involve all phases of gene expression, including gene transcription, RNA splicing, integrity of the coding sequence, 3′ polyadenylation, and translation initiation (see later).

Regulation of Globin Gene Expression

Globin genes in all vertebrates are expressed in a tissue-specific and developmentally programmed manner. Their transcription is activated only within developing erythroid precursor cells. Moreover, individual globin genes are expressed at different developmental stages. Hence, within the genes of the β cluster, globins are expressed at the embryonic (ε), fetal (γ), or adult (β and δ) stages, whereas within the α cluster, embryonic (ζ) and adult (α) chain expression is seen. A central problem posed by the organization of the globin gene clusters is how these patterns of tissue- and developmental-stage specificity are achieved. Current findings suggest that interactions between regulatory regions and their chromatin-bound proteins located near the genes (the proximal regulatory

elements) and more distant control regions provide the means by which transcription is orchestrated in globin gene clusters.

Proximal Regulatory Sequences and Transcription Factors

Several conserved sequence elements (motifs) in the 5′-flanking sequences of globin genes comprise the promoter, a region required for accurate and efficient transcription of genes by RNA polymerase II.[33-36] Promoters of vertebrate globin genes are similar in overall configuration and subset of motifs present but differ in their detailed organization and sequences. Promoters generally cooperate with more distant regulatory elements termed enhancers to stimulate transcription.[37-39] As discussed later, globin gene promoters appear to interact in a synergistic fashion with very powerful distant elements known as locus control regions (LCRs).

The TATA (or ATA) box is a motif seen in nearly all promoters, including those of the globin genes. The TATA box, typically located 20 to 30 base pairs (bp) upstream from the transcription start site, constitutes the binding site for a general transcription factor, the TATA-binding protein (TBP).[40-42] Binding of TBP to the TATA box is the first step in the assembly of a basal transcription complex (often termed TFIID) that includes many additional proteins (such as TFIIA, TFIIB, TFIIE/F, and TFIIH) and RNA polymerase II.[36] Mutations within the TATA box, as occur in some types of β-thalassemia,[43-49] decrease the binding of TBP to the promoter and decrease transcription.[40,41,50]

DNA sequence motifs located upstream of the TATA box bind proteins that interact with the general transcription machinery through protein-protein contacts with the TFIID complex and other associated proteins.[35,37,38,42] These promoter-bound proteins may either increase (activate) or decrease (repress) the rate of transcription.

A relatively small set of motifs are consistently present in globin gene promoters, including the CCAAT box, the CACC box, and GATA consensus sequences. Each motif may be viewed as a potential binding site for one or multiple transcription factors, which are either tissue restricted or ubiquitous in their cellular distribution.

Transcription factors are typically viewed as modular proteins made up of two domains that fulfill different functions: a DNA-binding domain responsible for sequence-specific DNA recognition and an activation (or repression) domain or domains that interact with components of the basal complex to modulate transcription. Additionally, some transcription factors may function to recruit activities that modify the histones around which DNA is wrapped to make chromatin. These modifications can indirectly alter the activity of the basal transcriptional complex. It is currently believed that transcriptional specificity is achieved by functional cooperation and interaction between cell-restricted and general transcription factors. As background for understanding globin gene control, the presently characterized erythroid-enriched transcription factors are reviewed here. For additional discussion of these proteins, readers are referred elsewhere.[51,52]

The consensus motif (A/T)GATA(A/G), the GATA motif, is found in the promoter region of most vertebrate globin genes and binds an abundant erythroid-restricted transcription factor, GATA-1. GATA motifs have been identified in the regulatory elements of virtually all erythroid-expressed genes, consistent with the notion that GATA-1 should serve a critical role in erythroid gene expression. As noted later, multiple GATA sites are also present within distant regulatory elements. The essential role of GATA-1 in erythroid development was formally demonstrated through gene targeting experiments in mouse embryonic stem cells. Disruption of the single X-chromosome GATA-1 gene in totipotent embryonic stem cells prevents their development into normal erythroid cells. Naturally occuring hypomorphic mutations of GATA-1 in humans have been shown to cause β-thalassemia or disrupt normal erythroid development.[53-58] The GATA-1 protein is a member of a small family of related "GATA factors" that are distinguished by a novel zinc-finger DNA-binding domain. In addition to merely specifying DNA recognition, this domain also mediates protein-protein interactions. Accordingly, GATA-1 is able to interact physically with other GATA-1 molecules or with other types of zinc-finger proteins, including the ubiquitous CACC- or GC-binding factor Sp1, the transcription factor erythroid Krüppel-like factor (EKLF), and a specific cofactor called FOG-1 (for friend of GATA-1)[59,60] (see later). It is envisioned that through its multiple physical interactions GATA-1 cooperates with other transcription factors, perhaps bound to DNA at distant sites, to program erythroid-specific transcription.

CACC motifs, which are represented by diverse sequences within globin and other gene promoters, bind a variety of transcription factors. Many CACC sequences are recognized by Sp1, a ubiquitous zinc-finger activator protein.[61] A particular CACC motif, CCACACCCT, is found in the adult β-globin gene promoter and is recognized with high affinity by the erythroid-specific protein EKLF. The functional relevance of this binding site has been established through naturally occurring mutations that lead to β-thalassemia (see later). In addition, gene targeting (or knockout) experiments in mice have formally established that EKLF is necessary for efficient β-globin transcription in vivo.[62]

A third erythroid transcription factor, known as NF-E2, binds to an extended motif—(T/C)TGCTGA(C/G)TCA(T/C)—that is found within some distant regulatory elements (see later) and a small subset of erythroid promoters, but not within globin gene promoters. NF-E2 is a heterodimer of two polypeptides of the basic domain–leucine zipper (or b-zip) class of transcription factors.[63,64] One subunit of NF-E2 is tissue restricted, whereas the other is ubiquitous. Although NF-E2 is essential for globin gene expression in mouse erythroleukemia cells in tissue culture,[65,66] its role in vivo appears to overlap that of one or more unknown factors that may act through the same target sites in DNA.[67]

Locus Control Regions and Chromatin Domains

How is globin gene transcription activated and developmentally controlled? Inspection of the DNA sequences of globin gene promoters in the early 1980s failed to provide substantive insight. Initial attempts to dissect control elements involved introducing globin genes into the germline of mice by oocyte injection but were plagued by low-level and erratic transgene expression. Nonetheless, it was possible to show that stage specificity was imparted by the human β- and γ-globin gene promoters. For example, when the human β-globin promoter is introduced into transgenic mice, it directs gene expression only in adult erythroid cells,[68-71] whereas the human γ-globin promoter is active only in embryonic erythroid cells (mice do not have an HbF stage).[72,73]

These early globin gene regulation studies suggested that critical regulatory elements required for high-level expression were missing from the immediate vicinity of the genes themselves. When sensitivity to digestion by the enzyme DNase I was used as an indicator of chromatin structure in the mid-1980s, regions of extreme sensitivity (hypersensitivity sites [HSs]) were identified far upstream (≈30 to 50 kilobases [kb]) of the adult human β-globin gene[74,75] (Fig. 20-6). Four subregions were delimited; they are present in the chromatin of erythroid but not nonerythroid cells. An additional site located even further upstream was found in all tissues. In a formal test of their functional relevance, the HSs were linked to a human β-globin and introduced into the germline of mice. Remarkably, transgenic mice then expressed the human β-globin gene at a level equivalent to that of the endogenous mouse β gene.[76] Further studies showed that the transgene is expressed not only in a tissue-specific manner but

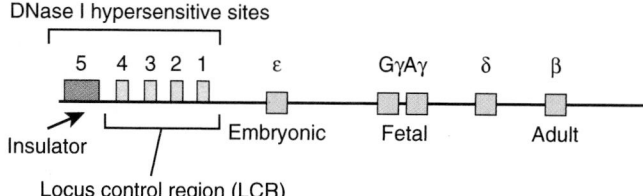

FIGURE 20-6. Schematic representation of the human β-globin gene locus. The *yellow boxes* depict the core DNase I hypersensitive subregions of the locus control region. The individual globin genes are indicated with their stage of expression.

also in a copy number–dependent fashion, independent of the chromosomal site of integration. These HSs comprise an essential distal regulatory domain, now referred to as the LCR (see elsewhere[51,52] for more detailed history and discussion).

Other globin gene clusters also contain erythroid-specific DNase I HSs. A segment of extreme DNase I hypersensitivity (known as HS-40) located far upstream of the human α-globin genes serves as an enhancer for the α locus. HS-40, however, does not display the full properties of an LCR because it does not direct copy number–dependent transgene expression.[77] Nonetheless, the in vivo relevance of both the β-LCR and HS-40 is underscored by the discovery of patients with thalassemia who have specific deletions in these regions (see later).

The human β-LCR, HS-40, and analogous regions studied in other species are composed of cores, each encompassing a DNase I HS. Cores are approximately 200 to 300 bp in length. Remarkably, within the cores three major protein-binding sites are consistently found: GATA, AP-1 (NF-E2), and CACC sequences. The position-independent activity of the β-LCR correlates best with the presence of GATA and CACC motifs, particularly within the subregion known as HS-3. Enhancer activity of the LCR, particularly within subregion HS-2, requires the NF-E2 motif. The protein-binding motifs within the LCR are also found in globin and other erythroid-expressed gene promoters. To date, no protein-binding sites unique to LCR elements have been identified. Hence, the distinctive properties of the LCR (or HS-40) appear to reflect the synergistic interactions of more typical transcription factors rather than the action of a new set of regulatory proteins.

The discovery of distant control elements, marked by DNase I hypersensitivity, emphasizes the relationship between chromatin structure and globin gene regulation, an association solidified by the unraveling of a rare syndrome, α-thalassemia with X-linked mental retardation.[78] This condition results from mutations in a gene designated *XH2* (or *ATR-X*) that encodes a member of the helicase superfamily.[79] Such proteins, which are often involved in DNA recombination and repair and in the regulation of transcription in *Drosophila*, yeast, and mammals, appear to influence transcription in a global manner by altering chromatin structure.

Regulation at a Distance: Globin Gene Switching

How do LCR sequences influence globin gene transcription over large distances (>50 kb)? How are the individual globin genes developmentally regulated? Two formal possibilities have been considered. On the one hand, the LCR might merely provide an environment conducive for activation of the downstream globin genes. The globin genes would be autonomously regulated; that is, the developmental profile of their expression would be intrinsic to the individual genes (and presumably determined by their promoters). The "influence" of the LCR is most simply viewed as reflecting physical association of the LCR with globin genes brought into apposition by chromosomal looping. On the other hand, sequential activation of the particular genes might depend (at least in part) on competition of each gene for influence of the LCR such that only one gene-LCR interaction would be productive on a single chromosome at any time. The outcome of the competition would be dependent on the array of proteins bound not only at each promoter but also at specific sites in the LCR. Data in favor of both autonomous and competitive mechanisms of regulation have been obtained (see Orkin[51] for detailed discussion).

The human embryonic ζ- and ε-globin genes appear to be largely autonomously regulated. LCR-containing transgenes are expressed during embryonic erythropoiesis (the yolk sac stage) and then extinguished during the fetal liver stage. The information required for shutoff is contained near the globin genes, and competition by adjacent globin genes is not required. Shutoff is hypothesized to reflect the action of repressors, or silencer proteins, that bind the gene promoters. Motifs within the human ε-globin promoter involved in silencing bind GATA-1 and a ubiquitous factor, YY1.[80]

The competitive model of gene regulation is based on experiments in chicken red blood cells that demonstrate competition between the chicken β- and ε-globin gene promoters for a single enhancer located between the genes.[81] In the chicken it has been proposed that an adult stage–specific factor (NF-E4) favors interaction of the β promoter with the enhancer to the exclusion of the ε promoter. In an analogous fashion, data suggest that the human β-globin gene may be negatively regulated in a competitive fashion by the γ-globin gene. Whereas the γ gene is largely autonomously regulated, the β-globin gene is silenced in the embryonic and early fetal stage by a linked γ gene (a γ gene in *cis* to β). Shutoff of the γ gene, presumably as a result of repressors (or silencers), allows the adult β-globin to be expressed. It has been suggested that a protein complex known as the stage-selector protein (SSP), which binds to a site in the proximal γ promoter, serves a function analogous to that proposed for chicken NF-E4 and tips the balance to γ-globin transcription at early stages.[82] Of interest, both NF-E4 and SSP complexes appear to contain the ubiquitous transcription factor CP2.[82] Although other models are theoretically possible, the capacity of the LCR to act at a distance in regulating activation of globin genes is most compatible with the formation of physical contacts between the LCR (or subregions thereof) and their associated proteins with regulatory elements neighboring the genes themselves. Stage-specific and competitive regulation would therefore reflect engagement of the LCR with genes one at a time. LCR-gene interactions probably have intrinsic stabilities and off-rates such that a single erythroid cell might express more than one globin over time, even from a single chromosome. Experiments examining nascent human globin RNA along the β-gene complex tend to support such models and lend credence to the notion that chromosomal looping brings the LCR and individual genes in apposition. Evidence for LCR interactions with the proximal promoter regions of both the β- and α-globin genes has recently been directly demonstrated by using novel in vivo biochemical approaches.[83-85] Dynamic interactions between the β-LCR and the γ- and β-globin genes appear to underlie the reciprocal expression of these genes in erythroid cells and provide hope that subtle alterations in the nuclear environment may facilitate reactivation of γ-globin genes in patients with hemoglobinopathies such as sickle cell anemia or β-thalassemia.

CLASSIFICATION OF THE THALASSEMIAS

The hallmark of thalassemia syndromes is decreased (or absent) synthesis of one or more globin chains. The designation α- and β-thalassemia refers to deficits in α- and β-globin production, respectively. The α- and β-thalassemias include clinical syndromes of varying severity (Table 20-1). Knowledge of molecular genetics provides a framework in which to consider their clinical heterogeneity.

TABLE 20-1	Clinical Classification of the Thalassemias
Silent carrier (α or β)	Hematologically normal
Thalassemia trait (α or β)	Mild anemia with microcytosis and hypochromia
HbH disease (α-thal)	Moderately severe hemolytic anemia, icterus, and splenomegaly
Hydrops fetalis (α-thal)	Death in utero caused by severe anemia
Severe β-thalassemia (Cooley's anemia)	Severe anemia, growth retardation, hepatosplenomegaly, bone marrow expansion, and bone deformities
Thalassemia major	Transfusion dependent
Thalassemia intermedia	No regular transfusion requirement

thal, thalassemia.

Because the structural gene for α-globin is duplicated on chromosome 16, each diploid cell contains four copies of the α-globin gene. The four α-thalassemia syndromes—silent carrier, α-thalassemia trait, HbH disease, and hydrops fetalis (see Table 20-1)—reflect the inheritance of molecular defects affecting the output of one, two, three, or four of the α-globin genes, respectively. More than 30 different mutations affecting one or both α-globin genes on a chromosome have been described. Some mutations abolish expression of an α-globin gene (α⁰), whereas others reduce expression of the gene to a variable degree (α⁺). Within the four general categories of α-thalassemia there is marked genetic and clinical heterogeneity. Heterogeneity arises because the syndrome in any given individual may represent a combination (or so-called interaction) of 2 of the 30 or more mutations that have been described.

The β-thalassemias also include four clinical syndromes of increasing severity—silent carrier, thalassemia trait, thalassemia intermedia, and thalassemia major (see Table 20-1).[1,3,86,87] In contrast to the α-thalassemias, the four classes of β-thalassemia are not correlated with the number of functioning genes. Because a single functional β-globin gene resides on each chromosome 11, a diploid cell normally has two β-globin genes. The clinical heterogeneity of the β-thalassemias represents the diversity of specific mutations that variably affect β-globin gene expression. Almost exclusively, these mutations involve the β-globin gene rather than an unlinked genetic determinant. Many mutations eliminate β-gene expression (β⁰), whereas others cause a variable decrease in the level of β-gene expression (β⁺).[3,87] The capacity of individual patients to synthesize γ-globin modulates the clinical severity. Such is the case because the severity of thalassemias is determined by the degree of globin chain imbalance rather than by the absolute level of either α- or β-globin synthesis per se.[88-92] Substantial synthesis of γ-globin in the marrow cells of individuals with β-thalassemia lessens the extent of chain imbalance and therefore improves red cell production.[93-95] Particular mutations of the β-globin gene in β-thalassemia appear to affect γ-globin gene expression directly. However, some individuals with otherwise severe β-thalassemia may coinherit additional genetic determinants that enhance the synthesis of HbF. Coincident inheritance of an α-thalassemia mutation also reduces chain imbalance in patients with homozygous or heterozygous β-thalassemia.[96] Clinical severity in any individual patient represents the outcome of these complex genetic interactions.

Origin of Thalassemia Mutations: The Influence of Malaria

Mutations causing thalassemia have arisen spontaneously. The nearly exclusive distribution of lethal red blood cell disorders, such as thalassemia, sickle cell disease, and glucose 6-phosphate deficiency, in tropical and subtropical regions led Haldane in 1949 to propose that the heterozygous carrier state for these conditions confers a selective advantage in locations where malaria is endemic.[97] The incidence of these genes in a population is determined by the balance between premature death of homozygotes and increased fitness of heterozygotes. The frequency of β-thalassemia mutations is high (>1%) in regions such as the Mediterranean basin, northern Africa, Southeast Asia, India, and Indonesia but uncommon in northern Europe, Korea, Japan, and northern China.[3,98,99] The incidence of β-thalassemia trait may exceed 20% in some villages in Greece.[100] α-Thalassemia is perhaps the most common single gene disorder in the world.[2] The frequency of α[+]-thalassemia alleles ranges from 5% to 10% in the Mediterranean basin,[101] 20% to 30% in portions of West Africa,[102] and 68% in the southwest Pacific.[103] The incidence of α-thalassemia is less than 1% in Britain, Iceland, and Japan.[104,105] Although the incidence of malaria and the rate of occurrence of thalassemia are not always inversely correlated, the anomalies and inconsistencies seem to be the result of genetic drift, migration, and demographic changes that have occurred in the last 10,000 years.[106]

Additional epidemiologic studies have provided further evidence for the validity of the "malaria hypothesis" in both α- and β-thalassemia.[103,107-114] Siniscalco and associates[107] showed that β-thalassemia is uncommon in inhabitants of the mountainous areas of Sardinia, where malaria is rare, as compared with the incidence in coastal populations. In Melanesia, α-thalassemia is correlated with malaria across both latitude and altitude.[103] β-Thalassemia in Melanesia is also associated with malarious coastal regions.[111] A study by Williams and colleagues found that children with α-thalassemia trait appear to have a higher incidence of malaria in childhood that appears to confer subsequent immunity to more severe malarial infections.[115] Follow-up studies in other populations have demonstrated that although α-thalassemia does not confer a reduced risk of malarial infection, it does dramatically reduce the incidence of severe malarial complications.[116,117]

The cellular mechanisms responsible for the selective advantage of thalassemia heterozygotes remain incompletely defined. Cultured erythrocytes containing high concentrations of HbF retard the growth and development of *Plasmodium falciparum*.[118] β-Thalassemia heterozygotes have a delayed disappearance of HbF in the first year of life.[1] This might provide protection from potentially fatal cerebral malaria early in life as the passive immunity acquired in utero wanes. Until recently, however, investigators were unable to document decreased invasion or growth of *P. falciparum* in red cells from thalassemia heterozygotes except under conditions of unusual oxidant stress.[99,119] Using modified tissue culture conditions, Brockelman and associates[120] and, more recently, Pattanapanyasat and colleagues[121] demonstrated decreased parasite multiplication in the red cells of β-thalassemia heterozygotes. They theorized that *P. falciparum* resistance

was a consequence of the inability of the parasite to acquire sufficient nutrients from the digestion of hemoglobin in thalassemic red cells. In one study, red cells with α- and β-thalassemia trait bound greater levels of antibody than control cells did. This could lead to greater removal of parasitized red cells and hence provide protection.[122] Recent studies have suggested that parasitized red cells from α-thalassemia heterozygotes may have altered membrane properties that more readily allow binding of antibody to the red cell and may promote more effective antimalarial immune responses.[123] Erythrocytes from individuals with HbH disease also appear to inhibit *P. falciparum* in vitro.[120,124] Recently, it has been suggested that rosette formation, the binding of uninfected red cells to *P. falciparum*–infected red cells, is decreased in thalassemia because of reduced red cell size and that such impaired rosette formation may hinder the development of cerebral malaria by lessening sequestration.[125]

The difficulty in documenting the cellular mechanism of *P. falciparum* resistance in thalassemic erythrocytes in vitro suggests that the heterozygote advantage may be small. The high mortality associated with malaria in endemic regions is a powerful selective force that may be sufficient to amplify a small increase in fitness.

Classes of Mutations That Cause Thalassemia

Thalassemia is the consequence of mutations that diminish (or abolish) production of either the α or β chain of hemoglobin. Molecular cloning, DNA sequencing, and functional analysis of cloned genes have provided the tools with which to dissect the thalassemia syndromes. This analysis has revealed remarkable heterogeneity in the specific alterations in DNA that lead to these clinical syndromes.

Typically, single nucleotide mutations associated with thalassemia interfere with one of the critical steps in mRNA production (Fig. 20-7 and Table 20-2). Base substitutions alter promoter function, RNA processing, or mRNA translation or modify a codon into a "nonsense codon" that leads to premature termination of translation or substitution of an incorrect amino acid. Insertion or deletion mutations within the coding region of the mRNA create "frameshifts" that prevent the synthesis of a complete, normal globin polypeptide. Large deletions within the α- or β-globin clusters may remove one or more genes and alter regulation of the remaining genes in the cluster. The phenotype that results from the diverse mutations found in thalassemia is determined by the degree of inactivation of the affected gene or genes and the extent of associated increases in expression of other genes within the cluster.

Mutations Affecting Gene Transcription

Point mutations within promoter sequences recognized by transcription factors tend to reduce the affinity with

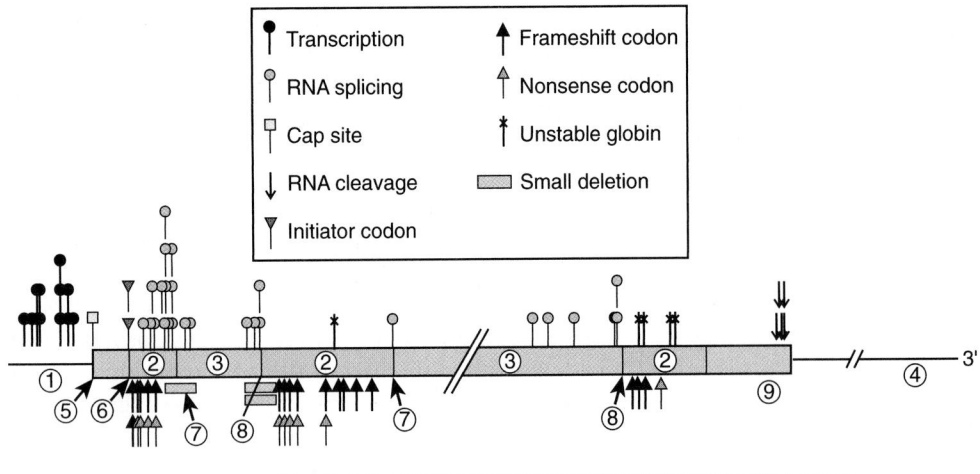

● Transcription	▲ Frameshift codon
○ RNA splicing	△ Nonsense codon
⊓ Cap site	‡ Unstable globin
↓ RNA cleavage	▭ Small deletion
▽ Initiator codon	

FIGURE 20-7. Location of various classes of point mutations that cause β-thalassemia with respect to important structural elements present in the β-globin gene. *(Adapted from Kazazian HH Jr, Boehm CD. Molecular basis and prenatal diagnosis of beta-thalassemia. Blood. 1988;72:1107-1116.)*

1. PROMOTER: DNA sequences required for accurate and efficient initiation of transcription.

2. EXONS: DNA that specifies the amino acid sequence of the polypeptide.

3. INTRONS: DNA that interrupts the coding sequence of the gene.

4. ENHANCER: DNA sequences that increase promoter activity at a distance and independent of orientation relative to coding sequence.

5. CAP SITE: Position where transcription of gene into RNA begins.

6. TRANSLATION INITIATION SITE: Position where translation of mRNA into protein begins.

7. SPLICE DONOR SITE } Sequences required for precise and efficient
8. SPLICE ACCEPTOR SITE } removal of RNA transcribed from introns.

9. RNA CLEAVAGE/POLYADENYLATION SIGNAL: Sequence that specifies the 3' end of the RNA transcript and the addition of the poly(A) tail.

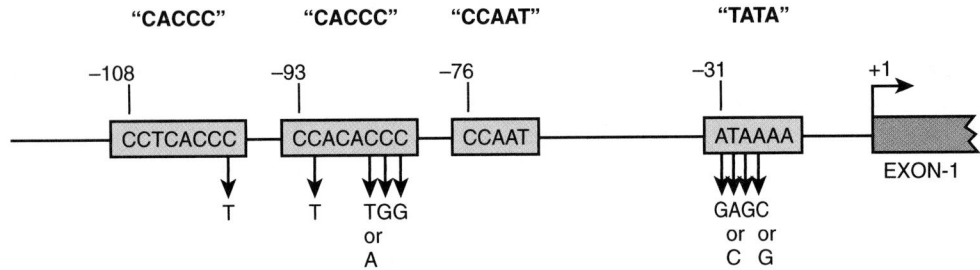

FIGURE 20-8. Point mutations in the β-globin gene promoter. The sequences of conserved motifs within the promoter and their distance from the transcription start site are indicated. A single base substitution at the indicated positions results in β+-thalassemia.

which these proteins bind. Typically, this leads to reduced gene transcription. Analysis of the promoter for the β-globin gene in patients with β-thalassemia has identified a variety of mutations clustered in the ATA and CACC motifs (Fig. 20-8; see also Table 20-2).[3,40-46,126-129] These mutations are associated with preservation of some β-globin expression and hence are customarily associated with the phenotype of thalassemia intermedia. The C→T substitution at position −101, which results in a particularly mild defect, is associated with the "silent carrier" phenotype in heterozygous carriers.[126,204] Although the CCAAT box is highly conserved in globin genes, no mutations within this motif have been identified in thalassemia. Rare mutations in transcription factors that result in thalassemia have been

detected, and exceedingly rare families have been identified in which a thalassemia mutation is unlinked to the globin clusters (see the section on mutations not linked to the globin gene clusters that alter globin gene expression).

Mutations of the ATA box presumably reduce binding of TBP and therefore lead to decreased transcription initiation. Substitutions in the CACC motifs decrease the affinity of binding by several transcription factors, including the erythroid-specific factor EKLF and the ubiquitous protein Sp1. Studies showing that mice engineered to lack EKLF suffer lethal β-thalassemia at the fetal liver stage have established EKLF as a β-globin activator protein in vivo.[62,205] Human β-thalassemias resulting from mutation of a single CACC motif are presumably mild

TABLE 20-2	**Point Mutations That Cause Thalassemia**					
Gene	Position*	Mutation	Classification	Ethnic Group†	Detection‡	References
A. TRANSCRIPTION MUTATIONS						
β	1 -101	C→T	β⁺	Turkish		126
				Bulgarian		
				Italian		
	2 -92	C→T	β⁺	Mediterranean		3
	3 -88	C→T	β⁺	American black	(+) *Fok*I	127
				Asian Indian		
	4 -88	C→A	β⁺	Kurdish		128
	5 -87	C→G	β⁺	Mediterranean	(−) *Avr*II	129
	6 -86	C→G	β⁺	Lebanese		3
	7 -31	A→G	β⁺	Japanese		43
	8 -30	T→A	β⁺	Turkish		44
				Bulgarian		
	9 -30	T→C	β⁺	Chinese		45
	10 -29	A→G	β⁺	American black	(+) *Nla*III	46
				Chinese		47
	11 -28	A→C	β⁺	Kurdish		48
	12 -28	A→G	β⁺	Chinese		49
B. CAP SITE MUTATION						
β	11	A→C	β⁺	Asian Indian		130
C. RNA SPLICING MUTATIONS						
1. Splice Junction Change in						
a. 5′ Donor Site						
α₂	1 IVS-1 n. 2-6	5-bp deletion	α⁰	Mediterranean		131, 132
β	1 IVS-1 n. 1	G→A	β⁰	Mediterranean	(−) *Bsp*M1	129
	2 IVS-1 n. 1	G→T	β⁰	Asian Indian	(−) *Bsp*M1	133
				Chinese		
	3 IVS-1 n. 2	T→G	β⁰	Tunisian		134
	4 IVS-1 n. 2	T→C	β⁰	Black		135
	5 IVS-1 5′ end	44-bp deletion	β⁰	Mediterranean		136
	6 IVS-2 n. 1	G→A	β⁰	Mediterranean	(−) *Hph*I	137
				Tunisian		134
				American black		138
b. 3′ Acceptor Site						
β	1 IVS-1 n. 130	G→C	β⁰	Italian		3
	2 IVS-1 n. 130	G→A	β⁰	Egyptian		3
	3 IVS-1 3′ end	17-bp deletion	β⁰	Kuwaiti		136
	4 IVS-1 3′ end	25-bp deletion	β⁰	Asian Indian		139
	5 IVS-2 n. 849	A→G	β⁰	American black		46
	6 IVS-2 n. 849	A→C	β⁰	American black		140
2. Splice Consensus Sequence Change in						
a. 5′ Donor Site						
β	1 IVS-1 n. −3 (codon 29)	C→T	?	Lebanese		133
	2 IVS 1 n. −1 (codon 30)	G→C	Hb Monroe	Tunisian		134
				American black		141
	3 IVS 1 n. −1 (codon 30)	G→A	?	Bulgarian		142
	4 IVS-1 n. 5	G→C	β⁺	Asian Indian		133
				Chinese		143
	5 IVS-1 n. 5	G→T	β⁺	Melanesian		111
				Mediterranean		144
				American black		145
	6 IVS-1 n. 5	G→A	β⁺	Algerian	(+) *Eco*RV	146
				Mediterranean		
	7 IVS-1 n. 6	T→C	β⁺	Mediterranean	(+) *Sfa*NI	129
B. 3′ Acceptor Site						
β	1 IVS-1 n. 128	T→G	β⁺	Saudi Arabian		147
	2 IVS-2 n. 843	T→G	β⁺	Algerian		148
	3 IVS-2 n. 848	C→A	β⁺	Iranian		147
				Egyptian		
				American black		145

Continues

TABLE 20-2	Point Mutations That Cause Thalassemia—cont'd					
Gene	**Position***	**Mutation**	**Classification**	**Ethnic Group†**	**Detection‡**	**References**
3. Mutations within Exons That Affect Processing						
β	1 Codon 19 (Asn-Ser)	A→G	Hb Malay	Malaysian		149
	2 Codon 24 (silent)	T→A	β+	American black		150
	3 Codon 26 (Glu-Lys)	G→A	Hb E	Southeast Asian	(−) *Mnl*I	87, 151
				European		
	4 Codon 27 (Ala-Ser)	G→T	Hb Knossos	Mediterranean		152
4. Internal IVS Change						
β	1 IVS-1 n. 110	G→A	β+	Mediterranean		153, 154
	2 IVS-1 n. 116	T→G	β0	Mediterranean		155
	3 IVS-2 n. 654	C→T	β0	Chinese		127
	4 IVS-2 n. 705	T→G	β+	Mediterranean		156
	5 IVS-2 n. 745	C→G	β+	Mediterranean	(+) *Rsa*I	129
D. RNA CLEAVAGE AND POLYADENYLATION MUTATIONS						
α2	1 Cleavage signal	AATAAA→ AATAAG	α+	Middle Eastern Mediterranean		157, 158
β	1 Cleavage signal	AATAAA→ AACAAA	β+	American black		159
	2 Cleavage signal	AATAAA→ AATAAG	β+	Kurdish		128
	3 Cleavage signal	AATAAA→ AATGAA	β+	Mediterranean		160
	4 Cleavage signal	AATAAA→ AATAGA	β+	Malaysian		160
	5 Cleavage signal	AATAAA→A (−AATAA)	β+	Arab		3
E. INITIATION CONSENSUS SEQUENCE MUTATIONS						
α2:	1 Initiation codon	ATG→ACG	α0	Mediterranean	(−) *Nco*I	161
α1:	2 Initiation codon	ATG→GTG	α0	Mediterranean	(−) *Nco*I	162
−α:	3 Initiation codon	ATG→GTG	α0	Black	(−) *Nco*I	163
−α3.7II	4 Initiation consensus	CCACCATGG→ CC . . . CATGG	α+	Algerian		164
				Mediterranean		165
β	1 Initiation codon	ATG→AGG	β0	Chinese		3
	2 Initiation codon	ATG→ACG	β0	Yugoslavian		160
	3 Initiation codon	ATG→ATA	β0	Swedish		
F. PREMATURE TERMINATION MUTATIONS						
1. Substitutions						
α2	1 Codon 116	GAC→TAG	α0	Black		166
β	1 Codon 15	G→A	β0	Asian Indian		133
	2 Codon 17	A→T	β0	Chinese	(+) *Mae*I	167
	3 Codon 35	C→A	β0	Thai		168
	4 Codon 37	G→A	β0	Saudi Arabian		169
	5 Codon 39	C→T	β0	Mediterranean	(+) *Mae*I	170
	6 Codon 43	G→T	β0	European		171
	7 Codon 61	A→T	β0	Chinese	(−) *Hinf*I	172
				Black		145
2. Frameshifts						
−a	1 Codons 30/31	−2 bp (−AG)	α0	Black		173
β	1 Codon 1	−1 bp (−G)	β0	Mediterranean		3
	2 Codon 5	−2 bp (−CT)	β0	Mediterranean		174
	3 Codon 6	−1 bp (−A)	β0	Mediterranean	(−) *Cvn*I	145
				American black		174
	4 Codon 8	−2 bp (−AA)	β0	Turkish		175
	5 Codon 8/9	+1 bp (+G)	β0	Asian Indian		133
	6 Codon 11	−1 bp (−T)	β0	Mexican		3
	7 Codons 14/15	+1 bp (+G)	β0	Chinese		176
	8 Codon 16	−1 bp (−C)	β0	Asian Indian		133
	9 Codons 27/28	+1 bp (+C)	β0	Chinese		3
	10 Codon 35	−1 bp (−C)	β0	Indonesian		150
	11 Codons 36/37	−1 bp (−T)	β0	Iranian		128
	12 Codon 37	−1 bp (−G)	β0	Kurdish		129

Continues

TABLE 20-2   Point Mutations That Cause Thalassemia—cont'd

Gene	Position*	Mutation	Classification	Ethnic Group†	Detection‡	References
	13 Codons 37-39	−7 bp (−GACCCAG)	β⁰	Turkish		177
	14 Codons 41/42		β⁰	Asian Indian		133
		−4 bp (−CTTT)		Chinese		178
	15 Codon 44	−1 bp (−C)	β⁰	Kurdish		179
	16 Codon 47	+1 bp (+A)	β⁰	Surinamese black		3
	17 Codon 64	−1 bp (−G)	β⁰	Swiss		180
	18 Codon 71	+1 bp (+T)	β⁰	Chinese		3
	19 Codons 71/72	+1 bp (+A)	β⁰	Chinese		143
	20 Codon 76	−1 bp (−C)	β⁰	Italian		181
	21 Codons 82/83	−1 bp (−G)	β⁰	Azerbaijani		3
	22 Codons 106/107	+1 bp (+G)	β⁰	American black		130
G. TERMINATION CODON MUTATIONS						
α₂	1 Codon 142 (ter-Gin)	TAA→CAA	Hb Constant Spring	Chinese		182, 183
	2 Codon 142 (ter-Lys)	TAA→AAA	Hb Icaria	Mediterranean		184
	3 Codon 142 (ter-Ser)	TAA→TCA	Hb Koya Dora	Indian		185
	4 Codon 142 (ter-Glu)	TAA→GAA	Hb Seal Rock	Black		186
β	1 Codon 147 (ter-Gin)		Hb Tak	Thai		187
H. UNSTABLE HEMOGLOBIN CHAINS						
1. Amino Acid Substitutions						
−α	1 Codon 14 (Trp-Arg)		Hb Evanston	Black		188
α₂	2 Codon 109 (Leu-Arg)	T→G	Hb Suan Dok	Southeast Asian		189, 190
α	3 Codon 110 (Ala-Asp)	T→C	Hb Petah Tikvah	Middle Eastern		191
α₂	4 Codon 125 (Leu-Pro)		Hb Quong Sze	Southeast Asian		192, 193
β	1 Codon 60	T→A	β⁺	Italian		194
	2 Codon 110 (Leu-Pro)	T→C	Hb Showa-Yakushiji	Japanese		195
	3 Codon 112 (Cys-Arg)		Hb Indianapolis	European		196
	4 Codon 127 (Gin-Pro)		Hb Houston	British		197
	5 Codons 127/128 (Gin, Ala-Pro)	−3 bp (−AGG)	β⁺	Japanese		198
2. Frameshift, Extended Chain						
β	1 Codon 94	+2 bp (+TG)	Hb Agnana (inclusion body)	Italian		199
	2 Codons 109/110	−1 bp (−G)	Hb Manhattan	Lithuanian		3, 197
	3 Codon 114	−2, +1 (−CT, + G)	Hb Geneva (inclusion body)	French-Swiss		200
	4 Codons 128-135	Net-10 bp	β⁺ (inclusion body)	Irish		201
3. Premature Termination						
β	1 Codon 121	G-T	β⁰ (inclusion body)	Greek-Polish French-Swiss British		201-203

*The position specifies the location in the gene at which the point mutation occurs. Positions are specified with reference to the start site for transcription (Cap site), the position within the intron (intervening sequence [IVS]), or the position of the codon.

†When more than one ethnic group is indicated, the mutation has had more than one origin.

‡Loss (−) or gain (+) of a restriction enzyme site with mutation is indicated; the remainder of the mutations can be detected with allele-specific oligonucleotides (see the section on direct detection of thalassemia mutations).

We are grateful to Drs. Halg Kazazian and Titus Huisman and colleagues for providing us with their detailed lists of β-thalassemia point mutations. (From Kazazian H. The thalassemia syndromes: molecular basis and prenatal diagnosis in 1990. Semin Hematol. 1990;27:209; and Huisman TH. Beta-thalassemia repository. Hemoglobin. 1990;14:661, by courtesy of Marcel Dekker, Inc.)

because of the presence of one normal CACC motif within the promoter.

In addition to the protein-binding sites in the promoter, proper transcription depends on sequences surrounding the start site of transcription (known as +1). These sequences often display functional activity in in vitro assays and herald the binding of specific protein complexes to this type of element, termed the Inr. Mild β-thalassemia has been associated with a base substitution (A→C) at +1. Recently, this substitution has been shown to impair the β-globin Inr.[32] The proteins that mediate this effect are unknown.

A novel mechanism by which transcription at the α-globin locus can be disrupted has recently been described and serves as a paradigm for a new class of mutations that can cause human disease. Higgs and colleagues found a variant single nucleotide change upstream of the α-globin genes that creates a binding site for the transcription factor GATA-1.[206] This in turn produces a novel promoter that competes with the endogenous α-globin promoters for interaction with upstream enhancer elements such as HS-40. As a result of this mutation, α-globin gene synthesis is reduced and α-thalassemia results. This mutation is present in approximately 4% of the Melanesian population.

RNA Processing Defects in Thalassemia

The importance of RNA splicing for the formation of functional mRNA cannot be overemphasized. As discussed earlier, removal of introns must be precise to the nucleotide for a continuous, translatable mRNA to be generated from an mRNA precursor. As soon as introns were discovered, it was hypothesized that mutations affecting RNA splicing would probably be involved in the thalassemia syndromes. Apart from its role in constructing a functional mRNA, RNA splicing also appears to be a determinant of mRNA stability[207,208] and is possibly coupled to RNA transport from the nucleus to the cytoplasm.[209]

Mutations That Alter Splice Junctions or Splice Consensus Sequences

Mutations at the 5′ donor site (GT)[129,131-138] or at the 3′ splice acceptor site (AG)[3,46,135,136,139,140,210] abolish proper splicing of the pre-mRNA transcript and result in α⁰- or β⁰-thalassemia (Fig. 20-9; see also Table 20-2). Substitutions at other sites within the splice junction consensus sequence have varied effects; because some correctly spliced RNA is produced, albeit a reduced amount, a β⁺-thalassemia phenotype ensues.[110,128,129,133,134,141-148,211]

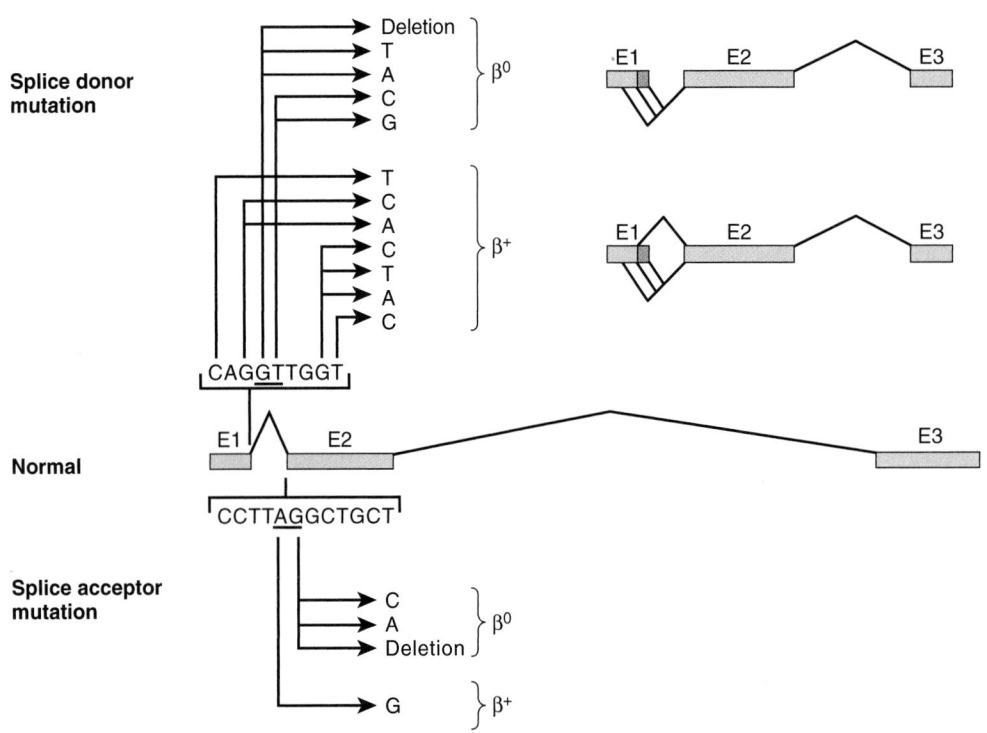

FIGURE 20-9. Examples of abnormal splicing that result from alterations in the splicing consensus sequences. The three β-globin gene exons are symbolized by *blue boxes*, the normal splicing pattern is illustrated by *lines* that project above the exons, and the splice donor and splice acceptor sequences of the first intron are shown. Mutations in the invariant GT dinucleotide of the splice donor site abolish normal splicing of the first intron and result in β⁰-thalassemia, whereas mutations elsewhere in the consensus sequence preserve some normal splicing and cause β⁺-thalassemia. Changes in the splice donor site are associated with abnormal splicing from three cryptic splice donors (*lines* that project below the exons); one site is within the first intron and results in the addition of intron sequences to exon 1 (*brown boxes*). Similarly, changes in the invariant AG dinucleotide of the splice acceptor sequence are associated with β⁰-thalassemia, whereas a mutation in an adjacent nucleotide causes β⁺-thalassemia.

Mutations within the splice site or the splice site consensus sequences favor improper processing of the mRNA precursor. These secondary splicing events, which are not seen under normal circumstances, occur at positions that resemble splice site consensus sequences. Splicing at these "cryptic" sites generates aberrantly processed, nonfunctional globin mRNA (see Fig. 20-9). Mutations within the β-globin IVS-1 splice donor site activate two cryptic donor sites in exon 1 and a third site in IVS-1,[129,136,212] whereas mutation in the IVS-2 splice donor activates a cryptic donor site in IVS-2.[137] Mutation of the IVS-2 splice acceptor site activates an upstream cryptic splice acceptor at position 579 in IVS-2.[46] These incorrectly spliced mRNA molecules suffer either insertions or deletions in the coding region and also shifts in the translational reading frame downstream of the cryptic splice site. The polypeptide synthesized beyond this point bears no resemblance to the globin chain and is often prematurely shortened by a termination codon encountered in the new reading frame.

Mutations within Exons That Create an Alternative Splice Site

RNA from β-thalassemia genes with mutations in the IVS-1 donor splice site may be processed via a cryptic splice donor site GTG*GT*GAGG in exon 1 (codons 24 through 27). Four independent mutations have been identified that activate this cryptic site in the presence of a normal IVS-1 splice donor site (Fig. 20-10; see also Table 20-2).[87,150-152] These mutations appear to enhance the ability of the cryptic site to compete with the normal site for binding of the splicing complex. A T→A mutation at codon 24 is "silent" at the translational level, yet approximately 80% of RNA transcripts are spliced at this incorrect site; hence, mild β+-thalassemia ensues. Two mutations—GAG→AAG in codon 26 and GCC→TCC in codon 27—lead to amino acid replacements that produce the hemoglobin variants HbE and Hb Knossos, respectively, in normally processed mRNA. Because a proportion of transcripts are aberrantly spliced, mild β+-thalassemia results. An analogous mutation in codon 19 produces β+-thalassemia with the hemoglobin variant Hb Malay.[149] These represent mutations that lead to thalassemic hemoglobinopathies.

Mutations within Introns That Create an Alternate Splice Site

Mutations within β-globin IVS-1 may create a new splice acceptor sequence (Fig. 20-11; see also Table 20-2).[153-155] In the first of this class of mutations to be characterized, a G→A substitution at position 110 (19 nucleotides upstream of the normal intron/exon boundary), the majority of globin mRNA precursors are spliced at this alternate site.[153,154,213,214] Because the incorrectly spliced mRNA contains 19 nucleotides from IVS-1, a shift in the reading frame leads to premature termination of translation. A T→G mutation at position 116 of IVS-1 creates a new acceptor site that is used exclusively, thereby leading to little or no normal β-globin mRNA production and to β0-thalassemia.[155]

Three mutations in IVS-2 create new donor sites and activate an upstream cryptic donor site located 579 nucleotides from the exon 2–IVS-2 boundary (see Table 20-2 and Fig. 20-11).[129,143,156] The consequence of these mutations is the insertion of a fourth "exon" derived from sequences within IVS-2. Although the normal donor and acceptor sites are unaffected, little or no correctly spliced β-globin mRNA may be produced.[129,143,156]

RNA Cleavage and Polyadenylation Defects

Proper cleavage at the 3′ end of the pre-mRNA and subsequent poly(A) addition depend on the integrity of the AAUAAA signal in the 3′-untranslated region. The importance of the polyadenylation signal for efficient production of globin mRNA was first demonstrated in α-thalassemia.[157,158,215] An AAUAAA→AAUAAG mutation in the α2 gene reduces the efficiency of cleavage-polyadenylation of precursor RNA and leads to "run-on" transcripts that terminate downstream of the gene (see Fig. 20-13). Mutations in the AAUAAA element have also been described in β-thalassemia,[128,159,160] in which the presence of elongated in vivo transcripts has been demonstrated.[159] The transcripts appear to terminate at the next AAUAAA signal, which is present approximately 900 nucleotides downstream of the normal cleavage site. These mutations lead to a moderate reduction in the level of β-globin mRNA and a β+ phenotype.

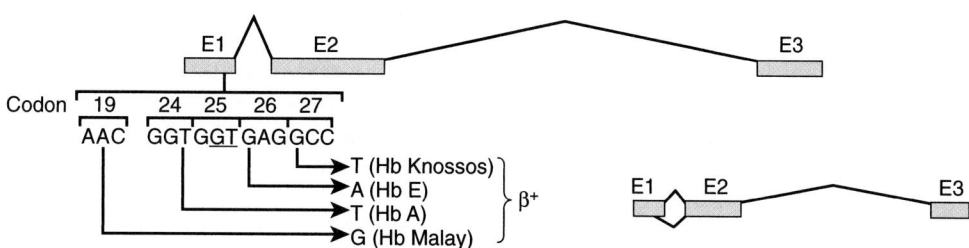

FIGURE 20-10. Mutations that create an alternate splice donor site in the first exon decrease but do not abolish the occurrence of normal splicing (pattern that projects above the exons) and are associated with splicing from the new site in the first exon (pattern that projects below the exons). Three of these mutations lead to the incorporation of a different amino acid into the β-globin chain derived from the decreased quantity of correctly spliced β-globin mRNA and generate variant hemoglobins.

Mutations Affecting mRNA Translation Initiation

Translation begins at an AUG codon that usually lies within the consensus sequence (GCC)GCC(A/G)CCATGG.[216] Substitutions within the AUG codon abolish translation, whereas those in other positions of the consensus often result in less efficient initiation of translation.

Four mutations in α-globin genes alter the consensus sequence and impair translation (see Table 20-2). Three of them affect the AUG initiator.[161-163] No globin polypeptide is produced because the next downstream initiator is in a different reading frame. The fourth α-globin mutation in this class, found on a chromosome in which one α-globin gene was deleted, alters the consensus sequence by the deletion of 2 bp and reduces mRNA translation to 50% of normal.[164,165] Two AUG initiator mutations of the β-globin gene have been described, and both are of the β[0] type (see Table 20-2).[3,160]

Premature Termination (Nonsense) Mutations

Nucleotide substitutions within the coding region are innocuous if they occur in the third position of a codon and do not alter the amino acid inserted during translation. Substitutions that alter codons from one amino acid to another lead to hemoglobin structural variants. Some substitutions change a triplet coding for an amino acid to a stop codon (UAG, UUA, or UGA). Such chain termination (or nonsense) mutations abort mRNA translation and lead to the synthesis of a truncated polypeptide. Moreover, nonsense mutations also reduce the amount of stable mRNA generated, which is a reflection of coupling between mRNA biogenesis and mRNA translation (Fig. 20-12).[217]

Chang and Kan[167] described the first nonsense mutation in β-thalassemia in which a lysine codon at amino acid position 17 was converted to a stop codon (AAG→UAG). Although no β-globin chains were produced in vivo, complete translation of the abnormal mRNA could be achieved in a cell-free extract capable of protein synthesis by the addition of a "suppressor" tRNA that inserts a serine at the UAG codon.[218] Several other nonsense mutations causing thalassemia have been described (Fig. 20-13; see also Table 20-2).[133,145,168-172] In addition, single or dinucleotide insertions or deletions have been observed that alter the translational reading frame and introduce a premature stop codon as a consequence.[3,128,143,146,149,173-180,219] Two termination mutations have been described in the α-globin genes, one that introduces a stop codon[166] and the other a frameshift.[172] In addition, frameshift mutations have been described that result in abnormal elongation of globin chains (see the section on unstable β-globin chains).

mRNA molecules with termination mutations often do not accumulate to a normal level in vivo.[215,220] The extent of this effect is variable and depends on the specific mutations; deletion of the third nucleotide (C) from codon 41 (Fig. 20-14) leads to complete absence of globin mRNA,[221] whereas a single substitution in the β39 codon allows the accumulation of roughly 5% to 10% of the normal amount of globin mRNA.[220] The basis for the quantitative deficiency in these mRNA species is of considerable interest. Some data suggest that such mutations lead to intranuclear degradation of abnormal globin RNA and suggest a link between mRNA translation and nuclear RNA processing or nuclear to cytoplasmic transport of mRNA.[222,223] Experimental studies in tissue culture systems have shown that the deficiency in β-globin mRNA accumulation is specific for nonsense mutations and is not observed with missense mutations[217]; a suppressor tRNA that allows the abnormal mRNA molecule to be translated completely will correct the quantitative deficiency in globin mRNA.[223] Recent work from a number of investigators has begun to unravel the molecular machinery that mediates this phenomenon, which has been termed nonsense-mediated decay and appears to play an important role in normal physiology, as well as pathologic states.[224]

Termination Codon Mutations

UAA is the normal termination codon for both α- and β-globin mRNA translation. The 3'-untranslated regions are 109 and 132 nucleotides for α- and β-globin mRNA, respectively. A single nucleotide substitution in the termination codon could either create another stop codon (UAG) or permit incorporation of an amino acid at this position and translation of the otherwise untranslated 3' sequences until the next in-frame stop codon. Four termination codon mutations involving the α₂ gene have been reported (see Table 20-2).[182-187] These mutants differ only in the specific amino acid incorporated at the terminator codon position (Fig. 20-14). Translation terminates in each instance at a UAA codon in the polyadenylation signal (AAUAAA) downstream, and a 172–amino acid polypeptide is produced. The first of these elongated α chains to be described was found in Hb Constant Spring.[182,183] The α chain in this hemoglobin has a glycine substituted at codon 142. Hb Constant Spring produces an associated thalassemia phenotype because of a marked reduction in α₂-globin mRNA stability.[225-227]

Mutations that give rise to elongated β-globin chains have also been described. Hb Tak is a 157–amino acid product of a β-globin mRNA molecule containing two inserted nucleotides in the terminator codon 147.[187] An analogous elongated β-globin with 157 amino acids found in Hb Cranston reflects a dinucleotide insertion in codon 147, but red cells containing Hb Cranston are morphologically normal.[228] The mechanism by which the β[Tak] mutation causes thalassemia has not been elucidated.

Mutations Affecting Globin Chain Stability

Hemoglobin Assembly

Shortly after synthesis is completed, α- and β-globin chains bind a heme moiety and rapidly associate into

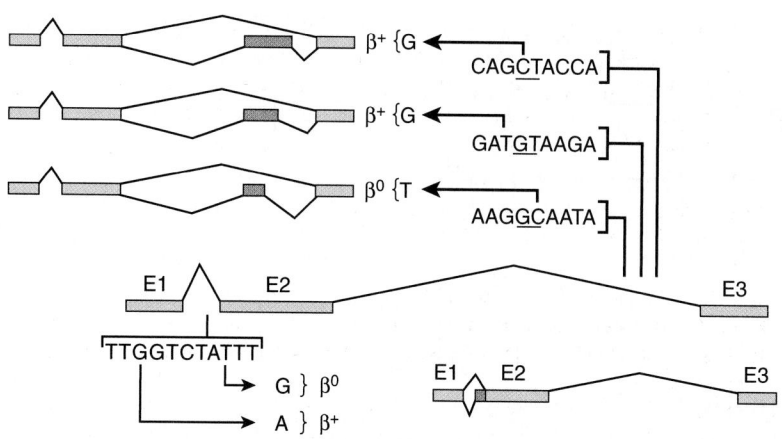

FIGURE 20-11. Mutations within introns that create a new splice site. Three mutations in the second intron create a new splice acceptor site (the invariant GT is underlined) and activate the identical cryptic splice donor site located just upstream. Abnormal splicing from these sites (pattern that projects below the exons) leads to the creation of a fourth exon (*brown boxes*) derived from sequences within the second intron. Two mutations in the first intron create a new splice acceptor site with the conserved AG dinucleotide, and abnormal splicing from this site (pattern that projects below the exons) adds sequences from the first intron to the beginning of the second exon.

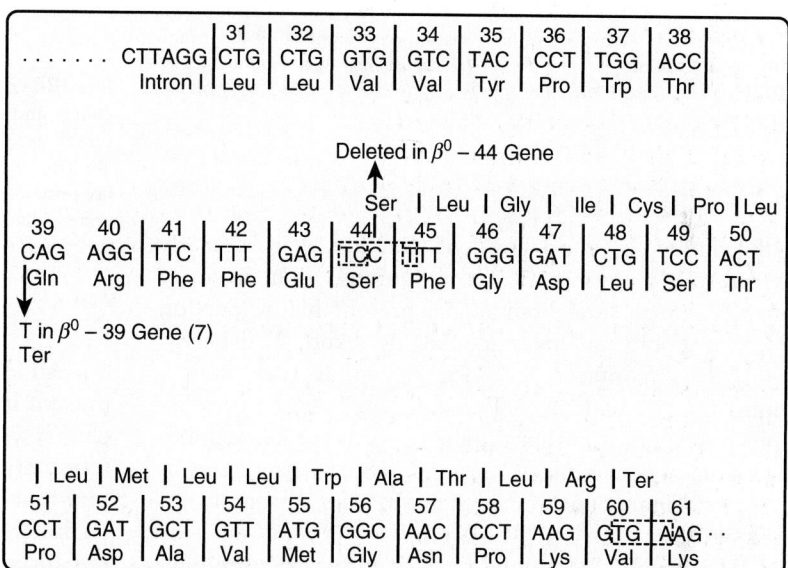

FIGURE 20-12. Two of the several thalassemia mutations that destroy gene function by the introduction of a premature translation termination codon in β-globin mRNA. The numbers above the individual codons refer to the position of the encoded amino acid in the β-globin. Replacement of C with T in codon 39 introduces the terminator UAG in β-globin mRNA. Another β⁰ gene has a deletion of the third nucleotide (C) in codon 41. This results in a shift in the reading frame of the mRNA; the new amino acid sequence is shown above the line. This new reading frame has an in-phase terminator (UGA) in a position corresponding to codon 60 to 61. (*Redrawn from Nienhuis AW, Anagnou NP, Ley TJ. Advances in thalassemia research. Blood. 1984;63: 738-758.*)

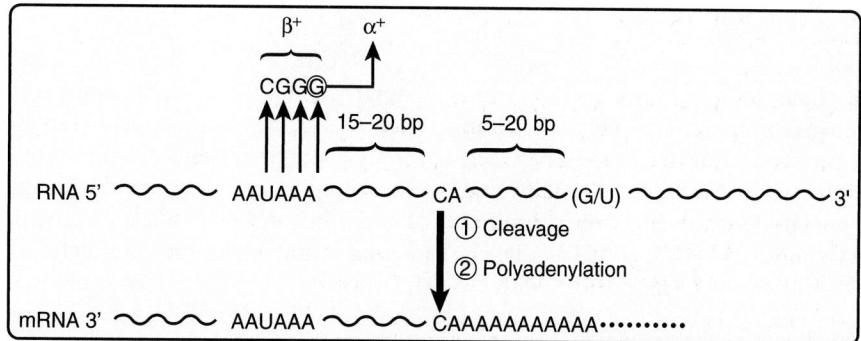

FIGURE 20-13. RNA cleavage and polyadenylation occur 15 to 20 bp downstream from the AAUAAA polyadenylation signal. Mutational analysis in the rabbit β-globin gene has established that sequences located downstream from the polyadenylation site, called the G/U cluster, are also required for efficient cleavage and polyadenylation. Individual point mutations at one of several nucleotides within the AAUAAA polyadenylation signal result in β⁺-thalassemia. The same A→G mutation in the last position that causes β-thalassemia has been observed in the α₂-globin gene and results in α⁺-thalassemia.

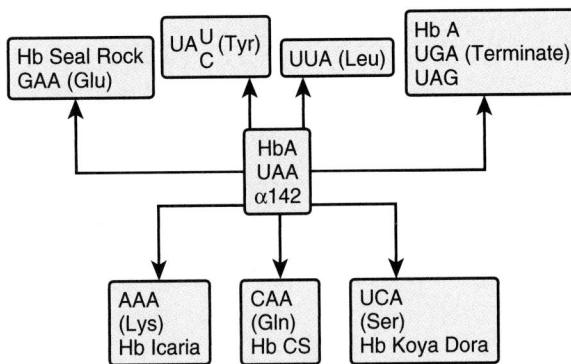

FIGURE 20-14. Point mutations in the terminator codon of the α-globin gene that lead to the synthesis of elongated α-globins. The normal terminator, UAA, of α-globin mRNA is shown in the *center*. Each of the nine possible single nucleotide substitutions is depicted; two would result in the formation of another terminator codon, whereas the other seven would lead to insertion of an amino acid at this position and continued synthesis of the globin chain. Four such mutations have been described; the mutation that causes the synthesis of Hb Constant Spring (CS) is the most common. *(Adapted from Weatherall DJ, Clegg JB. The Thalassemia Syndromes. Oxford, Blackwell Scientific, 1981, p 578.)*

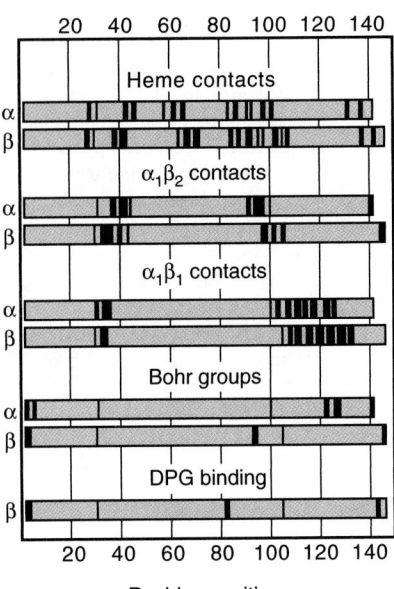

FIGURE 20-15. Schematic representation of the α- and β-globin chains and the location of residues involved in different hemoglobin functions (*black vertical bars*). Heme contact sites and α₁β₂ contacts are concentrated in the second exon (*blue*), whereas α₁β₁ contacts are principally located in the third exon (*salmon*). DGP, diphosphoglycerate. *(Adapted from Eaton WA. The relationship between coding sequences and function in haemoglobins. Nature. 1980;284:183-185. Reprinted by permission from Nature, copyright © 1980, Macmillan Magazines Limited.)*

α₁β₁ dimers in a noncovalent reaction that is nearly irreversible under physiologic conditions.[229] The majority of the heme contact points are present in the portion of the globin chains encoded by exon 2, whereas most α₁β₁ contacts are located within the exon 3 domain (Fig. 20-15).[6,230] These dimers may then reversibly associate with other dimers to form the hemoglobin tetramer. Formation of the α₁β₁ dimer, therefore, is the principal controlling step in the assembly of hemoglobin.

Hemoglobin assembly is an important determinant of the final hemoglobin composition of the erythrocyte.[229,231,232] The rate constant of dimer formation depends greatly on the surface electrostatic charge of the subunits.[229] α-Globin has a net positive surface charge, whereas β-globin has a net negative surface charge. The other normal β-like globin chains, γ-globin and δ-globin, dimerize with the α chain at a lower rate. δ-Globin has a lower net negative surface charge than β-globin does, and the significant structural differences between γ- and β-globin presumably account for the differing dimerization rates. When β-globin chains are in limited supply (i.e., β-thalassemia), HbA₂ and HbF levels may rise because of enhanced dimerization with α chains, independent of changes in the production of δ and γ chains. In α-thalassemia or iron deficiency, HbA₂ and HbF levels will fall because of competition with β chains for the limited number of α chains. Similarly, β-chain variants may have decreased (βˢ and βᴱ) or increased (β^Baltimore) affinity for α chains based on their net surface charge. The net hemoglobin composition of the cell is determined by these simple rules of competition based on the relative affinity of hemoglobin subunits.

An efficient, energy-dependent proteolytic system is present in erythrocytes that rapidly degrades free globin chains while leaving chains incorporated into dimers or tetramers unaffected.[229] Changes in globin chain structure that result from amino acid substitutions, premature chain termination, or chain elongation may slow or block the formation of stable α₁β₁ dimers and lead to rapid degradation of the globin chain. In some instances, as discussed later, mutations may also enhance association of the free globin chain with the cell membrane and thereby promote oxidative damage to the membrane and shortened red cell survival.

Recently, an erythroid-specific protein called AHSP (for α-hemoglobin–stabilizing protein) has been identified that appears to act as a chaperone for free α-globin chains. In the absence of this protein mice exhibit mild hemolytic anemia as a result of α-globin precipitation.[233] When this protein is absent in the presence of a β-thalassemia mutation in mice, a much more severe thalassemic phenotype occurs.[234] However, it is currently not clear whether variation in the structure or expression of this gene in humans causes phenotypic variability in patients with β-thalassemia. One study has suggested that this was not the case in patients with HbE–β-thalassemia in Thailand.[235] Another study has suggested that expression levels of this gene vary in humans and that such levels may correlate with the severity of β-thalassemia.[236] Further studies will need to be conducted to better understand whether AHSP plays a role as a modifier gene in β⁺-thalassemia.

During hemoglobin biosynthesis it is also important that the globin chains not be produced in excess of heme. A protein called heme-regulated inhibitor kinase (HRI) appears to mediate this function by inhibiting globin chain translation when an erythroid precursor is deficient in heme.[237] When HRI is absent in mice with a β-thalassemia mutation, the thalassemic phenotype is exacerbated and lethality of the mice results.[238]

Unstable α-Globin Chains

One such unstable variant was identified on sequencing of a mutant α-globin gene (see Table 20-2).[192] The α[Quong Sze] variant, which contains a Leu→Pro substitution at position 125, is so unstable that the mutant globin chain cannot be detected by biosynthetic studies in intact cells or by conventional hemoglobin electrophoresis.[193] The α[Quong Sze] chain appears to be stable once it is incorporated into the hemoglobin tetramer. Three other similar unstable α-globin chain mutations have been described (see Table 20-2).[188-191]

Unstable β-Globin Chains

Several unstable β-globin chains have been associated with thalassemia (see Table 20-2). Five mutations lead to amino acid substitutions in the β-globin chain.[194-198] Frameshift mutations in the third exon result in the synthesis of an elongated β-globin chain with a novel carboxy-terminal.[3,197,199-203] A premature termination mutation in exon 3 has also been described.[201-203] Many of the unstable β-globin chain mutations in exon 3 are associated with a dominantly inherited form of thalassemia (see the section on dominant β-thalassemia).[197,198] Thein and associates[201] proposed that alterations in β-globin structure in exon 3 interfere with $\alpha_1\beta_1$ dimer formation yet may permit binding of heme to the mutant globin chain through contacts in the exon 2 domain. These free, heme-associated β chains may be more resistant to proteolysis and associate with the cell membrane, where they form "inclusion bodies" and induce oxidative damage.

Thalassemic Hemoglobinopathies

The mutations described in this section, taken together with the RNA-processing mutants HbE, Hb Knossos, and Hb Malay and the termination mutant Hb Tak, include a distinctive set characterized by structural changes in the hemoglobin molecule and a thalassemia phenotype. These mutations are often referred to as "thalassemic hemoglobinopathies" (see the section on thalassemic hemoglobinopathies)[239] and are characterized clinically by a syndrome of ineffective erythropoiesis. Other globin variants may be associated with mild hypochromia, microcytosis, and chronic hemolysis because of instability and degradation of hemoglobin tetramers and are discussed in detail in Chapter 18. Because thalassemia is the consequence of an imbalance in α- and β-globin chains, these variants are not considered part of the spectrum of thalassemia.

Identification, Characterization, and Ethnic Distribution of β-Thalassemia Mutations

The hemoglobin disorders serve as a paradigm for the molecular analysis of genetic disease. Study of β-thalassemia was aided by the introduction of now widely used methods for identifying and characterizing mutant alleles. Accordingly, the identification of β-thalassemia mutations in many ethnic groups is nearly complete.[3,136]

In this section we briefly outline molecular techniques that have been applied to the characterization of β-thalassemia mutations. An understanding of these methods is important not only because they are broadly used in the study of other genetic diseases but also because they are directly relevant to strategies for genetic screening and prenatal diagnosis of β-thalassemia.

Haplotype Analysis

The first several β-thalassemia mutations were identified by cloning and sequencing β-globin genes isolated from individuals with β-thalassemia major.[130,137,153,154,167,170,219,240-243] Because certain mutations are extremely common, a nondirected strategy is inefficient since β genes with common mutations will be repeatedly studied. For example, 95% of the β-thalassemia alleles on the island of Sardinia contain the codon 39 nonsense mutation.[244]

To facilitate the search for new β-thalassemia mutations, Orkin, Kazazian, and their colleagues[129,245,246] introduced the concept of haplotype analysis to the study of thalassemia. Naturally occurring, genetically neutral, nonselected sequence differences among individuals constitute polymorphisms, which are estimated to occur roughly once every 100 bp.[247] These sequence differences are heritable, and those residing close to one another on a chromosome tend to be inherited together, a property known as *linkage*. A subset of polymorphisms will alter the cleavage site for a restriction enzyme or create a site where one did not exist. Therefore, when DNA from unrelated individuals is digested with a restriction enzyme and analyzed by Southern blotting, polymorphisms in the restriction enzyme digest pattern may be observed and are referred to as restriction fragment length polymorphisms (RFLPs).[248] Within the 60 kb of the human β-globin cluster, more than such 20 RFLPs are known[5,249]; at least 13 have been identified in the α cluster.[2,250] The pattern of these RFLPs (each based on the presence [+] or absence [−] of a restriction enzyme cutting site) along the chromosome defines a haplotype of associated or linked polymorphisms. Seven RFLPs were used initially to define nine distinct haplotypes (I through IX) of the β-gene cluster in the analysis of thalassemia mutations in Greek and Italian populations from the Mediterranean basin (Fig. 20-16).[129]

Close inspection of these haplotypes revealed a nonrandom association of restriction digest patterns within the β-gene cluster (Fig. 20-17).[245,251] The pattern of restriction sites 5′ of the δ-globin gene is inherited as a

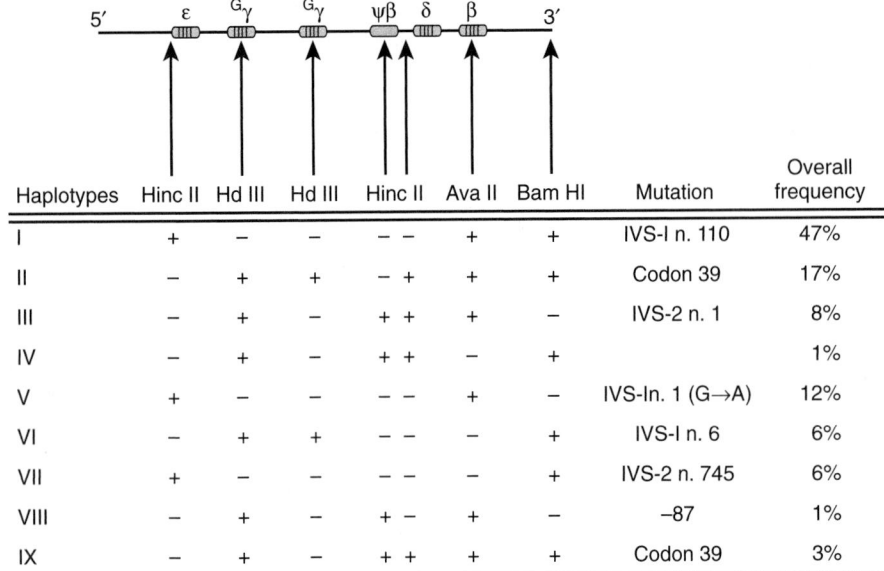

Haplotypes	Hinc II	Hd III	Hd III	Hinc II	Ava II	Bam HI	Mutation	Overall frequency
I	+	−	−	− −	+	+	IVS-I n. 110	47%
II	−	+	+	− +	+	+	Codon 39	17%
III	−	+	−	+ +	+	−	IVS-2 n. 1	8%
IV	−	+	−	+ +	−	+		1%
V	+	−	−	− −	+	−	IVS-In. 1 (G→A)	12%
VI	−	+	+	− −	−	+	IVS-I n. 6	6%
VII	+	−	−	− −	−	+	IVS-2 n. 745	6%
VIII	−	+	−	+ −	+	−	−87	1%
IX	−	+	−	+ +	+	+	Codon 39	3%

FIGURE 20-16. Linkage of chromosomal haplotypes to specific β-thalassemia mutations in Mediterranean populations. A haplotype is defined by the sequential pattern of restriction enzyme sites (present "+" or absent "−") along a chromosome. In this example, seven restriction enzyme sites were used to classify nine haplotypes. Overall frequency refers to the prevalence of the specific haplotype as found in all individuals, with or without thalassemia. IVS, intervening sequence. *(Adapted from Orkin SH, Kazazian HH Jr, Antonarkis SE, et al. Linkage of beta thalassemia mutations and beta-globin gene polymorphisms with DNA polymorphisms in the human beta-globin gene cluster. Nature. 1982;296:627-631. Reprinted by permission from Nature, copyright © 1982, Macmillan Magazines Limited.)*

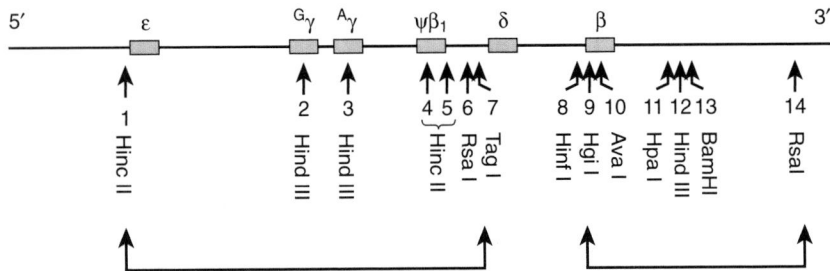

FIGURE 20-17. Restriction endonuclease sites for which restriction fragment length polymorphisms (RFLPs) have been identified in the β-globin gene cluster. A recombinational hot spot has been identified between the two brackets; the RFLP enclosed in each bracket must often remain associated during recombination (see text).

group, whereas restriction sites downstream (including the β-globin gene) track as another set. In all populations only a few haplotypes predominate.[252] The full spectrum of haplotypes is derived from random association over evolutionary time between the 5′ and the 3′ subhaplotypes, presumably reflecting the presence of a recombination "hot spot" lying between these regions.[137,251,253,254]

The generation of haplotypes appears to be an ancient event predating racial dispersion. Consequently, a specific haplotype may be found in diverse ethnic and racial groups from different geographic locations. The introduction of malaria as a selective pressure for certain random mutations is a more recent phenomenon. A mutation leading to thalassemia would be under positive selection and amplified within a population; accordingly, the mutation would be expected to be found on the haplotype background in which it originated in that ethnic group. Several conclusions can be derived from the study of different racial groups.[87] Within a single population both normal and thalassemia β-globin genes are found on the same haplotype, but specific thalassemia mutations tend to be linked to a single haplotype. Individual thalassemia mutations are generally restricted to a single population (see Table 20-2). In circumstances in which specific mutations are found in different populations, the identical thalassemia mutation may have occurred and

been selected for independently and will be found on a different haplotype background.[47,141,255] This observation has provided a sound genetic basis for the belief that thalassemia has had multiple distinct origins throughout the world. In circumstances in which a specific mutation is found on more than one haplotype within a population, the 3′ subhaplotypes (where the β-globin gene resides) may be identical, whereas the 5′ subhaplotypes differ because of recombination between the two subhaplotypes (for an example, see codon 39 mutation, see Fig. 20-16). By this mechanism, specific mutations can be distributed to new haplotypes within an ethnic group, and an independent origin of the mutation need not be invoked.

New thalassemia mutations were identified by cloning thalassemia β-globin genes from distinct haplotypes within a population, thereby avoiding the likelihood of repeated cloning of the same common mutation.[129] In this way, the great diversity of thalassemia mutations was elucidated.[139]

Direct Detection of Thalassemia Mutations

Restriction Enzyme Analysis

Several thalassemia mutations fortuitously result in the creation or destruction of a restriction enzyme cleavage site within the α- or β-globin gene. The change in the restriction digest pattern can be detected in a Southern blot of digested genomic DNA or can be visualized directly when the analysis is performed on DNA amplified by polymerase chain reaction (PCR) (see later).[256-258] A list of mutations that alter restriction enzyme sites is provided in Table 20-2. Although approximately 50% of the common thalassemia mutations in Mediterranean populations may be detected in this manner, this approach is of less utility in other groups.[3,139]

Allele-Specific Oligonucleotide Hybridization and Polymerase Chain Reaction

Specific synthetic oligonucleotide probes approximately 19 nucleotides in length extend the capacity to detect specific thalassemia mutations directly in genomic DNA or in DNA amplified by PCR.[258,259] Single nucleotide mismatches between a probe of this length and a target DNA sequence destabilize hybridization.[260] To study a given mutation or allele, two probes are generally used, one identical in sequence to the normal gene and the other identical to the mutant sequence. To facilitate detection of a mutation, probes are generally designed to position the difference in the center of the probe. In Southern blots, such probes can be shown to be highly specific for cloned DNA fragments containing particular mutations. When the target is DNA amplified by PCR, probes with low specific activity or nonradioactive probes can be used to detect the presence or absence of the mutation.[261-264] Although there are many β-thalassemia mutations, relatively few predominate in each ethnic group (see the section on ethnic distribution). Hence, a small panel of oligonucleotides can be used to identify the majority of potential mutations in any given population.[265,266]

The introduction of PCR in 1985[267] and subsequent modification of the procedure with the use of thermostable Taq polymerase[268] have revolutionized molecular biology and the ease with which specific mutations can be identified in DNA.[269,270] Application of PCR to the analysis of thalassemia facilitated the rapid identification of several new and quite rare mutations.[137] Several features of the PCR method are of particular relevance.[268-270] First, only minute quantities of relatively impure genomic DNA are required as starting material; in fact, the DNA of a single cell may be sufficient. Fragments ranging from 50 to several thousand base pairs can be rapidly amplified more than 10^6-fold in vitro. Second, the product of PCR, double-stranded DNA, can be readily subcloned, subjected to restriction enzyme analysis,[257,258] hybridized to allele-specific probes,[261,264] or directly sequenced.[130] As discussed earlier, the combination of PCR with restriction enzyme analysis or oligonucleotide hybridization lessens the need to work with high–specific activity radioactive probes to detect mutations. Third, the technique is easily automated. Finally, the analysis, including DNA sequencing if required, can be completed within several days of obtaining tissue for DNA preparation.

Ethnic Distribution

Determining the incidence of specific β-thalassemia mutations in different ethnic groups is particularly relevant to strategies for prenatal diagnosis of thalassemia.[3] Nearly complete surveys of thalassemia mutations have been performed in Greek and Italian,[246] Asian Indian,[208,271] American black,[43,145] Sardinian,[244] Chinese,[272,273] Lebanese,[209] Turkish,[274] Spanish,[275] Sicilian,[181] Thai,[168] Kurdish Jewish,[128] and Japanese[198] populations. From these studies, several general conclusions can be drawn. First, in each ethnic group a small subset of mutations (as few as four or six) constitute more than 90% of the mutant alleles. This is particularly striking on the island of Sardinia, where the codon 39 nonsense mutation accounts for 95% of the β-thalassemia genes and a codon 6 frameshift represents another 4%.[244] Second, the remaining 5% to 10% of mutant alleles in an ethic group are divided among a larger number of rarer alleles. For example, four alleles account for 90% of the β-thalassemia genes in Chinese, and 11 rare alleles account for the remaining 10%.[3,272] Third, several mutations appear to have originated independently in different ethnic groups and are present on different haplotype backgrounds as discussed earlier. For example, the IVS-2 no. 1 (G→A) mutation is present in Mediterranean, Tunisian, and American black populations[134,136,138]; the IVS-1 no. 5 (G→C) substitution is present in Asian Indians, Chinese, and Melanesians.[111,133,143] Finally, as a consequence of the large number of mutations present in each population, most individuals with severe β-thalassemia are genetic compound heterozygotes for two different thalassemia mutations.

Mutations That Affect β-Globin Gene Regulation

Deletions within the β-globin gene cluster often lead to thalassemia. Many of these deletions are associated with a significant increase in the level of HbF, a finding that distinguishes them from the common varieties of β-thalassemia. Ordinarily, heterozygous carriers of β-thalassemia have an increase in the level of HbA_2 (to >3% of total hemoglobin) and, at most, a slight increase in the level of HbF. Before detailed molecular analysis was available, these conditions were broadly grouped into two categories, hereditary persistence of fetal hemoglobin (HPFH) and δβ-thalassemia[4,276,277] (Table 20-3). HPFH heterozygotes have normocytic, normochromic red cells, whereas δβ-thalassemia heterozygotes have hypochromic and microcytic cells. Many HPFH heterozygotes have high levels of HbF (up to 30%) with a uniform or pancellular distribution in circulating erythrocytes, whereas in δβ-thalassemia heterozygotes, the amount of HbF is less abundant and it is present in an uneven or heterocellular distribution among red cells. In rare individuals homozygous for either condition, only HbF is found. HPFH homozygotes have normal or slightly elevated total hemoglobin concentrations, their red cells are slightly hypochromic and microcytic, and globin synthesis is modestly imbalanced.[278,279] Thus, these mutations are appropriately considered along with the thalassemia mutations.

Deletion mutations of the β-globin gene cluster represent in vivo experiments of nature useful in developing and validating experimental models of gene regulation. Multiple regulatory elements are present within the cluster, and the clinical phenotypes observed with specific deletions relate to removal of one or more such regulatory elements. More than 30 deletion mutations have been described (Table 20-4 and Fig. 20-18)[293]; they vary greatly in size from a few hundred base pairs of the β-globin gene to more than 100 kb with loss of the entire cluster. In addition to deletion mutations, significant elevations of HbF in adults may arise as a result of single base substitutions within the γ-globin gene promoters (Table 20-5). Such mutations, also classified as nondeletion HPFH, appear to enable the γ-globin genes to "capture" the influence of the LCR at the adult stage. Individuals with these HPFH mutations have HbF values ranging from only slightly elevated to more than 20%, which can be distributed in either a heterocellular or pancellular fashion.

HPFH and δβ-thalassemia mutations are uncommon, and individuals who inherit these mutations are asymptomatic or have mild disease. Their importance relates to the insight that they provide into globin gene regulation and the role of HbF in modulating disease severity in patients with severe β-thalassemia or sickle cell anemia.

Isolated point mutations of the δ-globin gene, similar to those in β-thalassemia, may lead to "δ-thalassemia." This is a benign condition with no clinical significance that when inherited with a β-thalassemia mutation may lead to a normal- or low-HbA₂ thalassemia phenotype in heterozygotes.[374,375]

Crossover Globins: Hemoglobin Lepore and Hemoglobin Kenya

Deletion mutations in the α- and β-globin gene clusters arise through unequal homologous recombination or through nonhomologous (illegitimate) recombination. In contrast to the α-globin cluster, in which there are blocks of tandem duplicated sequences (see later discussion), the only directly repeated homologous segments of DNA in the β cluster are the globin genes themselves. Hence, mutations arising from homologous, but unequal crossover in the β-globin cluster are relatively uncommon and usually involve two globin genes directly (Fig. 20-19).

TABLE 20-3	Phenotypes of ᴳγᴬγ Hereditary Persistence of Fetal Hemoglobin and ᴳγᴬγ (δβ)⁰-Thalassemia Heterozygotes	
	HPFH	δβ-Thalassemia
Red cell morphology	Normal	Abnormal
MCH	Nearly normal	Decreased
Hematocrit	Normal	Slightly decreased
HbF (%)	15-30	1-15
HbF distribution in red cells	Pancellular	Heterocellular

HPFH, hereditary persistence of fetal hemoglobin; MCH, mean corpuscular hemoglobin.

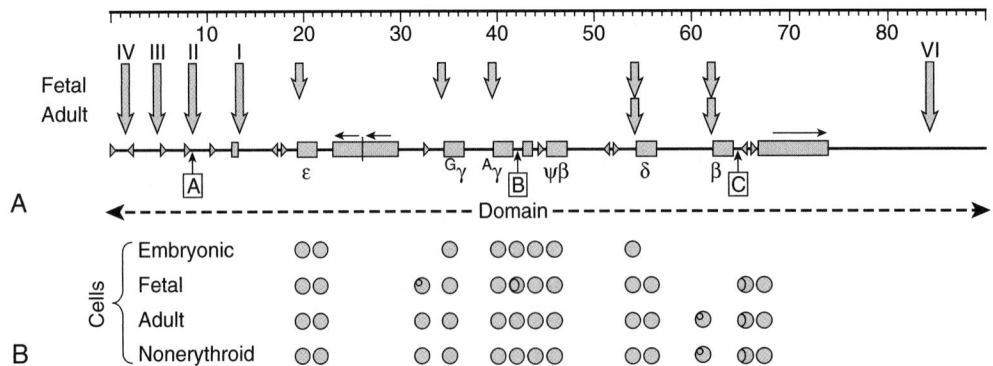

FIGURE 20-18. A, Organization and chromatin structure of the human β-globin cluster. The expressed genes are shown as *salmon boxes* and the single pseudogene in the cluster as a *blue box*. The *arrowheads* in the line figure indicate the location and orientation of Alu repetitive DNA sequences, whereas the *green boxes* represent members of the L1 family of repetitive DNA. The *salmon downward arrows* mark developmentally stable, erythroid-specific hypersensitive sites that constitute the locus-activating region (LAR) flanking the cluster. The true boundaries of the "active" chromatin domain established by these sites are unknown and extend beyond the cluster. Hypersensitive sites are also found over the promoters of the expressed genes (*blue downward arrows*). The location of the three enhancers in the cluster are marked by letters: A, hypersensitive site II enhancer; B, 3′ ᴬγ enhancer; C, 3′ β enhancer. **B,** The methylation pattern of the locus at different stages of ontogeny is depicted. *Blue circles* show an unmethylated site, *salmon circles* show a totally methylated site, and *circles with blue and salmon* show the degree of site methylation. The coordinates refer to distance in kilobases. *(Adapted from Stamatoyannopoulos G, Nienhuis AW. Hemoglobin switching. In Stamatoyannopoulos G, Nienhuis AW, Leder P, Majerus PW [eds]. The Molecular Basis of Blood Diseases. Philadelphia, WB Saunders, 1987, p 79.)*

TABLE 20-4	Deletion Mutations of the β-Globin Gene Cluster					
Type	Ethnic Group	Deletion Size (kb)	Deletion Coordinates	HbF Level in Heterozygotes (%)	Other Information	References
A. $^A\gamma^0$						
1		2.5	37.7-40.2	0.2	"Silent"	280
B. δ^0						
1	Corfu	7.20	48.9-56.1	1.1-1.6	δ^0-Thalassemia	281-283
C. β^0						
1	Indian	0.619	63.?-64.0	Normal	β^0-Thalassemia	133, 242, 245, 284
2	American black	1.393	61.6-63.0	7.0-7.9	β^0-Thalassemia	285, 286
3	Dutch	12.6	59.7-72.3	4-11	β^0-Thalassemia	287, 288
4	Turkish	0.29	62.1-62.4	2.7-3.3	β^0-Thalassemia	289, 290
	Jordanian			9.4	β^0-Thalassemia	291
5	Czech Canadian	4.237	58.9-63.1	3.3-5.7	β^0-Thalassemia	292
D. $(\delta\beta)^0$						
1	Sicilian	13.377	56.0-69.4	5-15		293-295
2	Spanish	≅114	52.2-?	5-15		296-298
3	American black	12.0	52.3-64.1	25	Pancellular*	299
4	Japanese	>130	43.1-?	5-7		300, 301
5	Laotian	12.5	56.0-68.5	11.5		302
6	Macedonian	18-23	54-74	7-14		303
7	Mediterranean	7.4	55.3-62.7	1-5	Hb Lepore	304-307
E. $^G\gamma^+(^A\gamma\delta\beta)^0$						
1	Indian	Total 8.3 kb	40.1-40.9	10-15		308, 309
	Iranian	Deleted	55.5-63.0			
	Kuwaiti	14.6 kb inverted	40.9-55.5			
2	American black	35.7	40.7-76.4	6-16		293, 310
3	Turkish American black	36.22	37.1-73.3	10-15		293, 311, 312
4	Malaysian (1)	>27	37.0-?	Unknown		313
5	Malaysian (2)	>40	39.1-?	Unknown		314
6	Chinese	≅100	40.5-?	10-15		313, 315
7	German	53.0	37.6-90.6	9.9-12.5		316
8	Cantonese	>43	37.0-?	20		309
F. $(\gamma\delta\beta)^0$						
1	Hispanic	39.5	-19.5-10.0			317
2	English	>100	?-35.9			318
3	Dutch	99.4	?-59.8			319-321
4	Anglo-Saxon	95.9	?-62.6			312, 320, 322
5	Mexican	>105	?-?			323
6	Scotch-Irish	>105	?-64-71			324
7	Yugoslavian	>148	?-?			325
8	Canadian	>185	?-?			325
G. HPFH						
1	American black	≅106	51.2-?	20-30 (5% G)†	HPFH-1	298, 312, 326, 327
2	Black (Ghana)	≅105	47-?	20-30 (30% G)†	HPFH-2	280, 298, 326-330
3	Indian	48.5	45.0-93.5	22-23 (70% G)†	HPFH-3	58, 298, 331
4	Italian	40.0	50.0-90.0	14-30	HPFH-4	332
5	Italian	12.9	51.6-64.5	16-20 (15% G)†		333
6	Kenyan	22.8	40.0-62.8	5-8	Hb Kenya	334-336

*In a compound δβ-thalassemia/HbS heterozygote.
†Percentage of $^G\gamma$ in total γ ($G\gamma/G\gamma + A\gamma$). Forty percent $^G\gamma$ is the normal value for an adult.
HPFH, hereditary persistence of fetal hemoglobin.

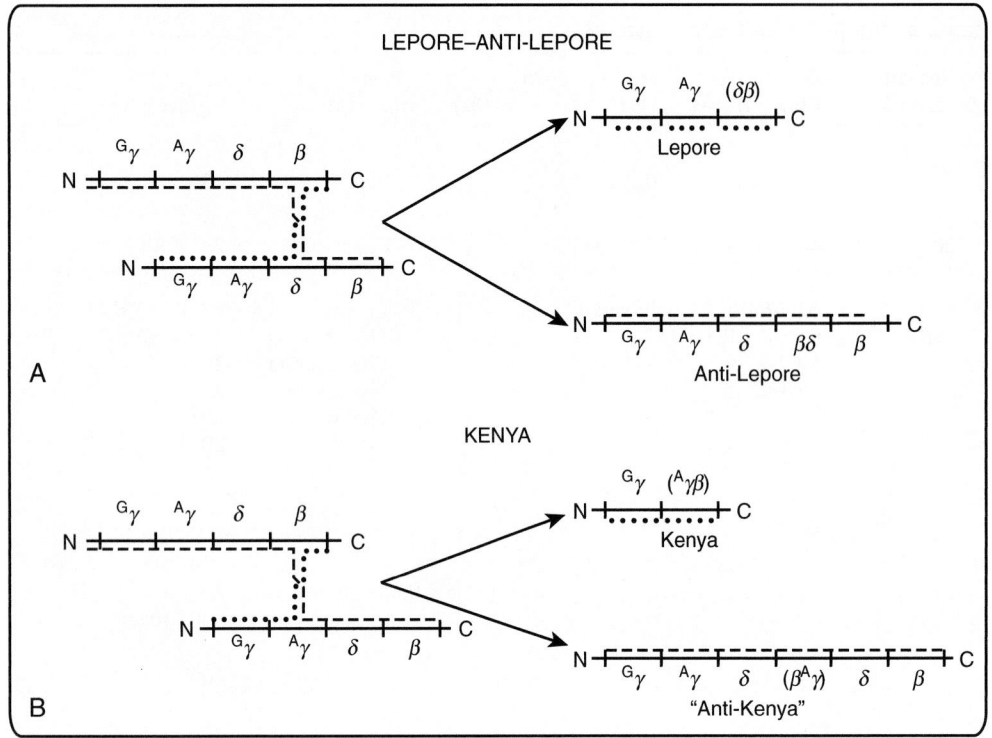

FIGURE 20-19. Schematic representation of the unequal crossover events that occur during meiosis and result in formation of the Lepore and anti-Lepore (**A**) and the Kenya (**B**) genes. *(Redrawn from Nienhuis AW, Benz EJ Jr. Regulation of hemoglobin synthesis during the development of the red cell. N Engl J Med. 1977;297:1318. Reprinted, by permission, from The New England Journal of Medicine.)*

Two crossover hemoglobins, Hb Lepore and Hb Kenya, are associated with thalassemia.

In 1958, Gerald and Diamond[376] identified a minor hemoglobin component by starch gel electrophoresis in the blood of parents of a patient with thalassemia major. Structural analysis revealed that the hemoglobin was composed of α-globin and a heretofore undescribed globin consisting of fusion of the 80 to 100 amino-terminal amino acids of δ-globin with the carboxyl portion of β-globin.[304,305,307,377] This "chimeric" globin polypeptide, named Lepore after the family in which it was first described, arose from an unequal, homologous recombination event between the δ-globin and β-globin genes (Fig. 20-19). It is poorly expressed because transcription of the fusion gene is under control of the γ-gene promoter. Other Lepore-type globins have been characterized in which the relative contribution of the δ and β genes to the fusion protein varies as a result of a different point of crossover. Homozygotes for Hb Lepore have 90% HbF and approximately 10% Hb Lepore, but no HbA or HbA_2, whereas heterozygotes have mainly HbA, 2% to 4% Hb Lepore, and 3% to 5% HbF.[378,379] In heterozygotes, red cells have a very heterogeneous HbF content. Anti-Lepore globins with the amino-terminal sequence of β-globin and the carboxyl sequence of δ-globin have also been described (see Fig. 20-19).[380-383] Individuals with anti-Lepore genes also have two normal δ- and two normal β-globin genes; consequently, their red cells lack any stigmata of thalassemia. The anti-Lepore globins are produced in very low amounts, perhaps because of sequences within the large intron

of the δ-globin gene that may reduce mRNA production.[26]

Hb Kenya, another important crossover hemoglobin, contains a non–α-globin composed of amino sequences of γ-globin and carboxyl sequences of β-globin[334-336,384] (see Fig. 20-19). Molecular analysis demonstrated that the ^Aγ-globin gene was involved in the crossover. The crossover occurred approximately at the position of amino acid codon 100. Hb Kenya was first observed in an individual who was heterozygous for a β^S gene. This patient had an increased level of HbF (up to 6%) that was uniformly distributed in all his red cells. The HbF was entirely of the ^Gγ type. Hb Kenya accounted for 17% to 20% of the total hemoglobin. Individuals who are heterozygous for Hb Kenya without HbS are clinically well. Approximately 10% Hb Kenya and 6% to 10% HbF of the ^Gγ type are found homogenously distributed in their red cells, in contrast to the distribution of HbF with the Lepore-type deletion.[336] It was originally hypothesized that the deletion removes a regulatory element that suppresses γ synthesis in adult life, thereby leading to a pancellular or uniform increase in HbF in the red cells of individuals with the Kenya fusion gene.[385] Even before discovery of the LCR and other regulatory elements within the β cluster, this hypothesis was disproved by analysis of several other deletion mutations (see later). Current models of hemoglobin switching posit that increased expression and pancellular distribution of the ^Aγβ fusion gene and the adjacent ^Gγ gene result from deletion of the adult-stage δ- and β-globin genes and their promoters, which serves to eliminate competition for the LCR. In addition, the deletion repositions an enhancer 3′ to the β-globin gene immediately downstream of the γ-globin genes and may also contribute to their increased expression.

Silent Deletions

Deletions that eliminate a single γ-globin gene or the δ-globin gene are unlikely to result in a phenotype that would be detected in hematologic screening. Thus, few of these mutations have been detected and described. A clinically silent deletion of the ^{A}γ-globin gene was identified through extensive molecular screening of chromosomes in Melanesians.[280] A 7.2-kb deletion involving the δ-globin gene but not the γ- or β-globin gene was reported in Corfu (δβ)^0-thalassemia in *cis* to the G→A substitution at IVS-1 position 5.[281] Homozygotes for the IVS-1 position 5 mutation ordinarily exhibit a mild β+-thalassemia intermedia phenotype with 10% to 20% HbA,[146] but homozygotes for Corfu (δβ)^0-thalassemia display the clinical phenotype of β^0-thalassemia intermedia with 100% HbF. This has been interpreted as evidence that sequences in the deleted region are important in activating the β-globin gene and potentially in suppressing γ-gene expression. Subsequently, however, the identical deletion was identified in *cis* to a normal β-globin gene.[282] In this circumstance, the deletion leads to failure of δ-globin gene expression but has no demonstrable effect on expression of the γ- and β-globin genes on the same chromosome. Recent work has suggested that this deletion may increase γ-gene expression in *cis* to the deletion but that translation of the γ gene may be limiting in certain settings, thus helping explain the discrepancy between carriers of the deletion and homozygotes.[283] Nonetheless, the basis for the lack of β-gene expression in Corfu (δβ)^0-thalassemia remains unresolved.

β^0-Thalassemia Deletion Mutations

Several deletions remove the β-globin gene and are associated with typical high-HbA$_2$ β^0-thalassemia (see Table 20-4). Interestingly, deletions that remove the promoter region are associated with somewhat higher HbF levels than usually seen in β^0-thalassemia heterozygotes (e.g., see Oner and colleagues[386]). The HbF is distributed in a heterocellular pattern. In contrast, a 0.6-kb deletion at the 3′ end of the β gene that spares the β-globin promoter, seen in Asian Indians, is not associated with an increased level of HbF in heterozygotes.[133,240-242,284] One explanation for the different phenotypes relates to the possibility that an intact β-gene promoter may interact productively with the LCR and thereby effectively compete with an incompletely silenced γ-globin gene at the adult stage. Removal of the promoter may alleviate competition and favor persistent γ-globin expression.

δβ-Thalassemia

Individuals heterozygous for these deletions generally have 5% to 15% HbF composed of both ^{G}γ- and ^{A}γ-globins and distributed in a heterocellular fashion (see Table 20-4). The erythrocytes are typically hypochromic and microcytic.[1] The level of HbA$_2$ is characteristically low in comparison to the modest elevations observed in most individuals with β-thalassemia trait. Homozygotes for these deletions produce only HbF yet exhibit a mild β^0-thalassemia intermedia phenotype with hemoglobin levels of approximately 10 g/dL. The most common of these deletions is referred to as the Sicilian type.[285,294,295,387] The deletion extends from within the δ-globin gene to just beyond the β-globin gene (see Table 20-4).

The 5′ breakpoint junctions of δβ-thalassemia deletions generally lie between the pseudo-β gene and the δ-globin gene. Located within this region are moderately repetitive sequences known as Alu sequences.[388] Although the function of such sequence elements is unknown, their preservation in δβ-thalassemia deletions and their deletion in HPFH encouraged speculation that the Alu elements might be involved in modulating HbF production during development.[308,385] Based on analysis of additional deletion mutations, this hypothesis may not be likely (see Table 20-4). For example, the 7.2-kb Corfu deletion removes both Alu elements and the δ-globin gene, but it has not been associated with increased γ-gene expression.[281,282] As described earlier (see the section on silent deletions), more recent work suggests that γ-gene transcription may be increased in *cis* to the deletion.[283] However, the Japanese type of deletion, which also removes the Alu elements, is associated with a heterocellular distribution of HbF and thalassemic red cell indices.[300,301] The increase in HbF expression may be more appropriately explained by the deletion of local δ- and β-globin gene regulatory elements, which leaves the γ-globin genes to interact with the LCR unopposed by competition from the adult genes.

^{A}γδβ-Thalassemia

The phenotype of these deletions in heterozygotes is identical to that of δβ-thalassemia: hypochromic microcytic red cells with low levels of HbA$_2$ and moderately increased ^{G}γ-HbF levels (5% to 15%) with a heterocellular distribution (see Table 20-4). Homozygotes have β^0-thalassemia intermedia with 100% ^{G}γ-HbF. The 5′ breakpoints in these instances lie between the two γ genes or within the body of the ^{A}γ gene, thereby resulting in silencing of the ^{A}γ gene together with the δ and β genes.[308-312,314-316,389,390] The 3′ end points of several of these deletions have been precisely mapped. Other deletions are very large and extend well beyond the boundary of the β-gene complex (see Table 20-4). One interesting mutation of this type, the Indian form (see Table 20-4), has two deletions, one involving the γ gene and the second involving a portion of the δ and β genes and intragenic DNA. The segment of DNA between the two deletions is inverted such that the 5′ ends of the γ and δ genes come to be adjacent but in an inverted orientation.[308,309]

γδβ-Thalassemia

The diagnosis of γδβ-thalassemia should be considered in newborns with hemolytic disease associated with hypochromic red cells. In adults, it is also a cause of normal-HbA$_2$, normal-HbF β-thalassemia trait. The syndrome was first identified in a newborn with microcytic, hemolytic anemia.[391] Heterozygous β-thalassemia associated with normal levels of HbA$_2$ and HbF was identified in the father and many relatives. Decreased γ- and β-chain synthesis was demonstrated in the infant's reticulocytes. The anemia was self-limited; as the baby grew older, the hemolytic anemia disappeared and the phenotype of simple heterozygous β-thalassemia developed in the child.

The syndrome of γδβ-thalassemia results from large deletions within the β-globin gene cluster (see Table 20-4). They can be divided into two categories: extremely large deletions that remove the entire β-globin gene cluster or all of the structural genes[323-325] and deletions such as the Hispanic, English, Dutch, and Anglo-Saxon forms in which the structural genes are left intact but the LCR elements are removed.[312,317-322] The remaining genes on the chromosome are not expressed and are found in inactive chromatin that is methylated and resistant to nuclease digestion. Study of these deletions has provided the most convincing evidence that the LCR is required in normal erythroid cells for transcription of the β-like globin genes in vivo. Homozygous γδβ-thalassemia is expected to be incompatible with survival and has not been observed.

β-Thalassemia Mutants Unlinked to the β-Globin Complex

Until recently, the mutations characterized in β-thalassemias resided within or near the β-globin gene itself or the β-globin locus. In principle, defects in trans-acting regulatory factors could lead to failure of proper β-globin gene expression. Two examples are now known.

Mutation of the xeroderma pigmentosum disease (XPD) helicase gene, which encodes a component of the general transcription factor TFIIH, results in β-thalassemia in association with trichothiodystrophy. Patients with specific mutations in *XPD* have typical features of β-thalassemia trait, including reduced levels of β-globin synthesis. Inadequate expression of diverse, highly expressed genes is presumed to be the direct consequence of an abnormality in TFIIH.[392]

Mild β-thalassemia trait in association with thrombocytopenia was reported as an X-linked trait in a rare family.[393] Linkage studies demonstrated that the gene mutated in this family resides on the short arm of the X chromosome, near the Wiskott-Aldrich syndrome (*WAS*) gene and the erythroid/megakaryocytic transcription factor GATA-1 gene.[331] Subsequently, it was shown that affected boys in this family have a specific amino acid substitution in the amino zinc finger of GATA-1 that subtly alters its interaction with DNA and leaves its physical interaction with the cofactor FOG-1 intact.[58] How this change in the properties of GATA-1 leads to a slight imbalance in globin gene expression is unknown. Presumably, interactions of the regulatory elements of the LCR and β-globin complex are affected by the manner by which GATA-1 binds to DNA. More recently, similar mutations have been found in other patients. In one case, β-thalassemia was present along with an elevation in HbF to nearly 60%.[56] This patient also had features of erythropoietic porphyria and mild thrombocytopenia. However, another patient with a similar mutation had features of only gray platelet syndrome, and β-thalassemia was not present.[57] These phenotypic differences may be due to modifier loci that vary with the genetic background of these different patients.

Hereditary Persistence of Fetal Hemoglobin

Individuals heterozygous or homozygous for mutations that enhance HbF are asymptomatic. They are identified incidentally in routine screening programs or during investigation of family members with hematologic disease because of interaction of these variants with other mutations in the β-globin gene cluster. Homozygotes for deletion forms of HPFH have normal hemoglobin concentrations, but their red cells are slightly hypochromic and microcytic.[278,279] Minimal globin chain biosynthetic imbalance may be seen. No symptoms or physiologic impairment has been associated with the exclusive production of HbF despite its high oxygen affinity.

Hereditary Persistence of Fetal Hemoglobin Deletion Mutations

Several deletions produce the HPFH phenotype of increased levels of HbF in otherwise normal red cells (Table 20-5).* The 5′ breakpoints lie between the ^{A}γ-globin gene and the δ-globin gene, and in all cases (with the exception of Hb Kenya), an enhancer 3′ to the ^{A}γ gene is unaffected by the mutation. Two of the deletions (HPFH-1 and HPFH-2) are very large and extend beyond the 3′ end of the cluster (see Table 20-4). The Kenya mutation is also included in this category because of the pancellular distribution of HbF that is characteristic of this mutation.

Heterozygotes for these deletions produce up to 30% HbF containing both ^{G}γ and ^{A}γ chains in a pancellular distribution. Differences in the relative percentages of ^{G}γ and ^{A}γ chains can be detected between different types of HPFH deletions (see Table 20-4). Heterozygotes have normocytic red cells. The red cells of homozygotes

---

*See references 58, 293, 298, 312, 326-330, 333-335, 337, 384, 394, 395.

				Percentage of HbF in Heterozygotes	Chains $^G\gamma$, $^A\gamma$	Distribution of HbF	
Type	**Molecular Defect**	**γ Gene**	**Ethnic Group**				**References**
1	C→G at −202	G	Black	15-20	G only	Pancellular	337-339
2	C→T at −202	A	Black	2-3	93% A	Heterocellular	340
3	+C insertion at −200	G	Tunisian	18-27	G only		341
4	T→C at −198	A	British★	4-12	90% A	Heterocellular	342-344
5	C→T at −196	A	Chinese	10-15	90% A	Heterocellular†	345, 346
			Italian‡	10-20	95% A	Pancellular	347, 348
7	T→C at −175	G	Italian	20-30	90% G		351
			Black	30†§	G only	Pancellular	353
8	T→C at −175	A	Black	35-40	80% A	Pancellular	354
9	G→A at −161	G	Black	1-2		Heterocellular	355
10	G→T at −158¶	G	Saudi#	2-4	G > A	Heterocellular	356-362
11	G→A at −117	A	Mediterranean★★	10-20	95% A	Pancellular	349, 350, 363
			Black	10-20	85% A	Pancellular	346
12	C→G at −114	G	Australian	8.5	90% G		364
13	C→T at −114	G	Japanese	11-14	G > A		365
14	C→T at −114	A	Black	3-5	90% A		366
15	Deletion −114 to −102	A	Black	30†§	85% A‡		367
16	X-Linked	G	"Swiss"‡‡	0.8-3.4		Heterocellular	368
17	Unknown‡	G	German	5-8	A and G	Heterocellular	369
18	Unknown	G	"Georgia"	2.6-6	G > A	Heterocellular	370, 371
19	Unknown	G	"Seattle"	3.7-7.8	G = A	Heterocellular	372, 373

★Also found in whites in North America.
†More than 80% of the red cells contain fetal hemoglobin.
‡Also found in *cis* to codon 39 mutation (Sardinian δβ-thalassemia).
§In a β-S heterozygote.
¶This determinant appears to increase HbF only in patients with erythropoietic stress.
#Identified in Greek and Sardinian families.
★★Also found in several other ethnic groups.
‡‡Ratio varies in different families.
‡‡Found in all ethnic groups.

contain HbF exclusively. The higher oxygen affinity of HbF may lead to slightly elevated hemoglobin levels in such individuals. Although homozygotes are clinically well, the α-globin–to–γ-globin chain biosynthetic ratio may be slightly imbalanced, and mild microcytosis and hypochromia may be observed. This suggests that γ-chain synthesis occurs at levels below the output of the normal β-globin gene on these chromosomes.

Several hypotheses have been put forward to account for the increased expression and pancellular distribution of HbF in the deletion HPFH syndromes, particularly when compared with the moderate increase and heterocellular distribution in δβ-thalassemia. Sequence analysis has confirmed that the γ-globin genes linked to the HPFH-1 deletion do not contain additional mutations responsible for the increased HbF expression.[396] As discussed earlier, deletion of postulated inhibitory sequences[297,385] has not been substantiated by the effects of other mutations that remove similar elements. Because several mutations extend far beyond the 3′ end of the β-globin cluster, it has been suggested that introduction of a distant enhancer into the locus might lead to activation of the γ genes. Some evidence is consistent with this

model. Sequences located immediately 3′ of the HPFH-1 deletion breakpoint and translocated into the cluster by the deletion event display transient enhancer activity when tested in erythroid cell lines.[298] In addition, the DNA in the vicinity of this enhancer is hypomethylated and nuclease sensitive in normal erythroid cells and contains a long open reading frame,[298,397] thus suggesting that the enhancer may belong to a distinct gene that is also transcribed in erythroid cells. RNA transcripts from this putative gene have been detected in erythroid cell lines.[398] In Spanish δβ-thalassemia, which exhibits a deletion nearly identical to that in HPFH-1, the 3′ breakpoint is located approximately 9 kb downstream of HPFH-1, and therefore the putative distant enhancer is not imported into the locus.[298]

In another type of deletion HPFH observed in an Italian family, a 12.9-kb deletion removes the δ- and β-globin genes and brings the enhancer 3′ of the β-globin gene closer to the γ-globin genes.[333] Analogous to the comparisons between HPFH-1 and Spanish δβ-thalassemia, deletions similar in size and location to the 12.9-kb Italian HPFH deletion that remove the 3′ β enhancer result in δβ-thalassemia rather than HPFH.[332] The

TABLE 20-6   α-Thalassemia Syndromes

Syndrome	Clinical Features	Hemoglobin Pattern	α-Globin Genes Affected by the Thalassemia Mutation
Silent carrier (α-thal-2)	No anemia, normal red cells	1-2% Hb Bart's (γ_4) at birth; may have 1-2% Hb Constant Spring; remainder HbA	1
Thalassemia trait (α-thal-1)	Mild anemia, hypochromic and microcytic red cells	5-10% Hb Bart's (γ_4) at birth; may have 1-2% Hb Constant Spring; remainder HbA	2
Hemoglobin H (HbH) disease	Moderate anemia; fragmented, hypochromic, and microcytic red cells; inclusion bodies may be demonstrated	5-30% HbH (β_4); may have 1-2% Hb Constant Spring; remainder HbA	3
Hydrops fetalis	Death in utero caused by severe anemia	Mainly Hb Bart's; small amounts of HbH and Hb Portland also present	4

Kenyan deletion also brings the 3′ β-globin gene enhancer closer to the γ-globin genes. Though distributed in a pancellular pattern, the level of HbF is lower in the Kenyan deletion than in the other HPFH syndromes. It is noteworthy that it is also the only deletion mutation that does not spare the 3′ $^A\gamma$-globin enhancer.

Nondeletion Hereditary Persistence of Fetal Hemoglobin Mutations

Individuals with these mutations exhibit elevated levels of HbF with normal red cell indices and are identified through hemoglobin screening programs or by study of families in which a segregating high-HbF allele modulates the severity of sickle cell disease or β-thalassemia.[93,94] (The role of nondeletion HPFH mutations in modifying the course of sickle cell disease is discussed in more detail in Chapter 19.[141]) In many instances, single base changes have been discovered within the promoter region of either the $^G\gamma$- or $^A\gamma$-globin gene.[338-340,342-350,352-363,367,399] These mutations are postulated to alter the binding of nuclear regulatory proteins and lead to a more favorable interaction of the promoter with the LCR at the adult stage.[349,350,400-405] Typically, only increased expression of the γ-globin gene in which the mutation is found occurs. In instances of the nondeletion HPFH syndrome, no mutation has been characterized. As discussed in a later section, the Swiss HPFH determinant may segregate with the X chromosome.[12]

The level of HbF observed in patients with this syndrome varies greatly and ranges from 1% to 4% in Swiss HPFH[12,368] to 30% in the −175 T→C substitution found in either the $^G\gamma$- or $^A\gamma$-globin gene.[352-354] Similar to the deletion forms of HPFH, the HbF may be found in either a heterocellular or a pancellular distribution (Table 20-6 and Fig. 20-20). The −158 C→T substitution in the $^G\gamma$-globin gene is associated with a normal level of HbF in otherwise normal heterozygotes but with a high level of HbF in the presence of erythropoietic stress.[356-362] For example, in Saudi Arabia, patients with sickle cell anemia

often have high HbF levels (25% or greater) and mild disease, whereas their parents with sickle cell trait have normal or only slightly elevated levels.[356] Identification of individuals with this mutation (or polymorphism) has been aided by the finding that it is linked to a rare subhaplotype.[357,358] The −158 HPFH substitution also improves the clinical course of β-thalassemia. A Chinese individual homozygous for the −29 promoter mutation has transfusion-dependent β-thalassemia,[47] yet black patients homozygous for the same mutation who coinherit the −158 HPFH mutation in the $^G\gamma$ promoter have mild β-thalassemia.[46,95]

Confirmation that the base substitutions in the promoter region are the cause of increased γ-chain synthesis rather than associated random DNA polymorphisms is based on several lines of evidence (reviewed by Ottolenghi and co-workers[406]). As mentioned earlier, they are generally associated with overexpression of the gene in which the mutation is found and typically represent the only sequence change. None of the mutations listed, with the exception of the −158 mutation, have been observed in individuals with normal HbF levels. Haplotype analysis in some pedigrees of patients with HPFH has demonstrated that the HPFH determinant is linked to the β-globin cluster. The British type of nondeletion HPFH is quite informative in this regard. The gene has been tracked through three generations, and three homozygous individuals have been observed.[342-344,407] Haplotype analysis using restriction enzyme polymorphisms has established linkage of the British HPFH phenotype to the β-globin gene locus.[343] More than 90% of the γ chains are of the $^G\gamma$ type, and there is an associated mutation at −198 of the $^G\gamma$ gene.[343] Even the three homozygotes, with approximately 20% HbF, have heterogeneous distribution of HbF among their red cells. Two homozygotes for −117 $^A\gamma$ HPFH have also been described, and they had 24% HbF in a pancellular pattern.[408] More recent transgenic experiments unequivocally demonstrate that the single base substitutions seen in

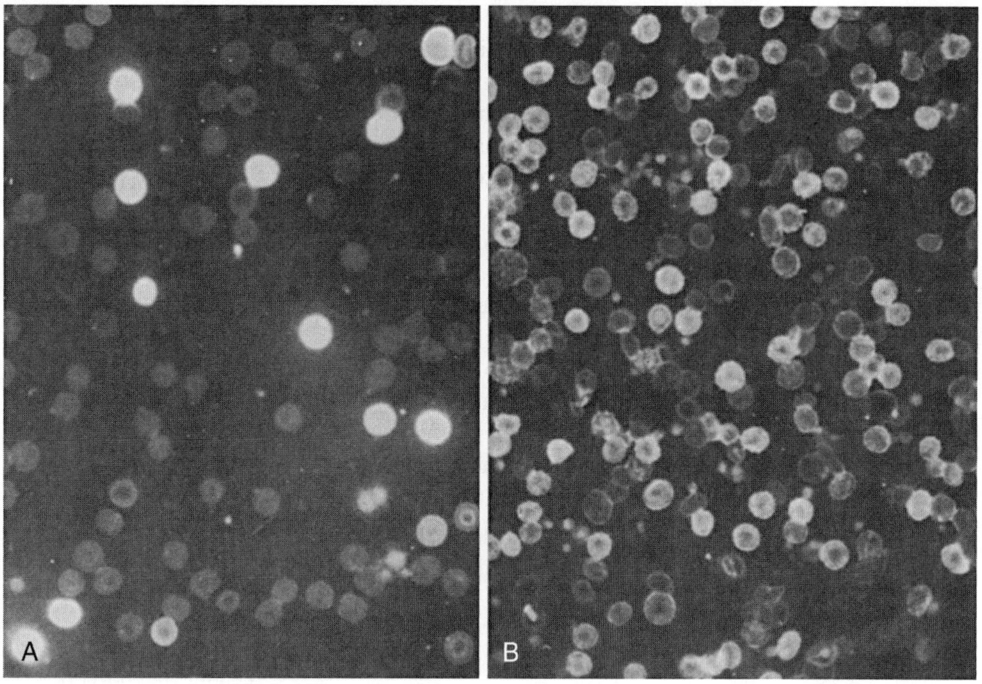

FIGURE 20-20. A, Immunofluorescent staining of erythrocytes with antibody directed against HbF shows the distribution of HbF in a heterocellular pattern. **B,** Immunofluorescent staining of erythrocytes with HbF distributed in a pancellular pattern. *(Courtesy of Dr. George Stamatoyannopoulos.)*

HPFH lead to enhanced γ-globin expression into adult life.

An interesting aspect of this syndrome is a balanced α-globin–to–non–α-globin chain synthetic ratio, even in homozygotes,[408] which implies that increased γ-globin synthesis is offset by decreased β-globin synthesis.[363] Expression of the β gene in *cis* to the mutation may be reduced by 20% to 30%.[338,353,354,367,409] It has also been observed that HbA$_2$ levels are uniformly low in the nondeletion HPFH syndromes and generally correlate inversely with HbF levels.[1] The reduction in δ- and β-globin gene expression in *cis* to the HPFH mutations is compatible with models of competitive regulation of β-globin expression by the linked γ-globin gene.

Mutations That Alter α-Globin Gene Regulation

In contrast to the β-globin cluster, in which single nucleotide substitutions are the most common cause of thalassemia, large deletions within the α-globin cluster are the predominant basis of α-thalassemia. The overall impairment in α-globin chain synthesis that results from defects in the α-globin cluster is determined by the number of genes inactivated (either by deletion or mutation), the type of lesion (deletion or mutation), and whether the lesion affects the α$_2$ or α$_1$ gene.

The α-globin cluster on chromosome 16[16,410,411] contains three functional genes (ζ, α$_2$, and α$_1$), an expressed gene of no apparent significance, and three pseudogenes[2,15] (see Fig. 20-2). Transcription of the genes depends on the integrity of the distant regulatory element

HS-40. An α-thalassemia deletion mutation (αα^{RA}) has been reported that removes a large segment of DNA upstream of the ζ$_2$ gene but spares the remainder of the cluster.[412] In heterozygotes, no expression of the ζ- or α-globin genes from this chromosome is detected in heterozygotes. These findings are formally analogous to those in Hispanic and English γδβ-thalassemias (see Table 20-4),[317,318] in which upstream LCR elements of the β-globin cluster are deleted.

The two human α-globin genes are thought to have been generated through a gene duplication event that occurred approximately 60 million years ago.[413] The nucleotide sequences of the α$_2$ and α$_1$ genes have remained remarkably similar and represent an example of concerted evolution[414-416] in which the two genes have exchanged genetic information through crossover fixation and gene conversion events. The coding regions of the two genes are virtually the same and encode identical polypeptides.[4149-417] The genes differ only in minor respects within IVS-2, whereas the sequences diverge significantly in the 3′-untranslated region.

The α-globin genes are expressed in embryonic, fetal, and adult-stage erythroid cells. Initially it was believed that the two α genes were expressed at similar levels, but subsequent RNA analysis relying on sequence differences in their 3′-untranslated regions revealed that α$_2$ RNA predominates over α$_1$ RNA by a ratio of 3:1.[225,418-420] Because the two α-globin mRNA molecules have the same intrinsic stability, the higher level of α$_2$ RNA reflects increased transcription of the α$_2$ gene. "Transcriptional interference" of the α$_1$ gene by the upstream α$_2$ gene has been proposed as an explanation for this observation.[421] Ribosome-loading studies suggest that α$_2$ and α$_1$ transcripts are translated at equivalent rates.[422] Systematic characterization of the expression of α-globin structural variants at both the α_2 and α_1 loci has confirmed that the α_2 gene has a predominant role in α-globin chain production.[418,419] A direct prediction of this model is that mutations altering the α_2 gene would result in a greater deficiency of α-globin chain production than would mutations of the α_1 gene. Clinical support for this prediction is provided by study of Sardinian patients with HbH disease who are heterozygous for one chromosome with a deletion of both α genes (−/) and a chromosome with a nondeletion mutation affecting the initiator codon of either the α_2 gene ($\alpha^T\alpha$/) or the α_1 gene ($\alpha\alpha^T$/).[162] Patients with the mutation in the α_2 gene (−/$\alpha^T\alpha$) have clinically more severe disease. Consistent with its predominance, the α_2 gene is involved in the majority of the reported mutations of the α-globin genes (see Table 20-2).

Deletion Mutations within the α-Globin Gene Cluster

Mutations That Remove One α-Globin Gene

The two α-globin genes are embedded in highly homologous, tandem repeated sequence blocks (called X, Y, and Z) that are separated by nonhomologous segments (Fig. 20-21).[18] Unequal, homologous recombination through the X and Z blocks generates a chromosome with a single α-globin gene and another with three α-globin genes. Homologous recombination in the small Y box has not been observed. The most common type of deletion in this class removes 3.7 kb as a result of misalignment of the Z boxes and is known as "rightward deletion." The products of this crossover are the (−$\alpha^{3.7}$/)[423,424] and ($\alpha\alpha\alpha^{anti-3.7}$/) haplotypes.[425,426] The −$\alpha^{3.7}$ products may be further subdivided into types I, II, and III by the precise location of recombination within the Z box.[416] Unequal crossover events through the X box leads to "leftward deletion" of 4.2 kb of DNA and the −$\alpha^{4.2}$ chromosome[406] and its triplicated antitype.[427,428] The incidence of the observed recombination products appears to reflect the size of the homologous target sequence within the boxes because −$\alpha^{3.7I}$ (1436 bp) is the most common, followed by −$\alpha^{4.2}$ (1339 bp), −$\alpha^{3.7II}$ (171 bp), and −$\alpha^{3.7III}$ (46 bp).[2,414,415,429] Unequal α-gene recombination through the X and Z boxes has been reproduced in both prokaryotic and eukaryotic experimental systems with episomal vectors.[18,430,431]

The −$\alpha^{3.7I}$ deletion is extremely common and is seen in all populations in which α-thalassemia is prevalent, whereas the −$\alpha^{4.2}$ deletion is most common in Asian populations.[2,15] Frequencies of up 80% to 90% for the single-deletion chromosome have been reported in some populations.[103] The association of these mutations with a variety of α-globin cluster haplotypes and α-globin variants in different populations suggests that they have arisen through numerous independent mutational events.[103,432]

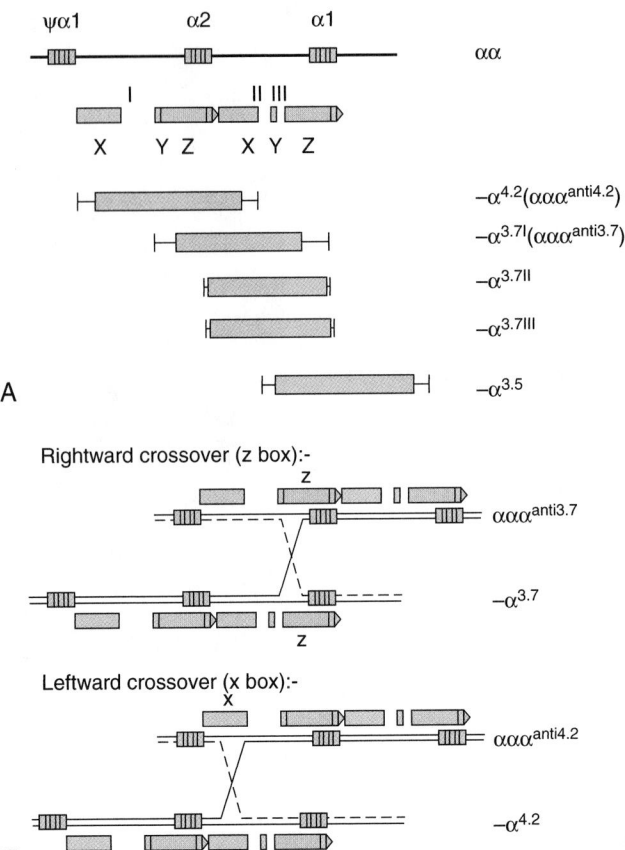

FIGURE 20-21. A, Deletion mutations that give rise to α-thalassemia. The two α-globin genes are embedded in a duplicated segment of DNA with homologous (X, Y, and Z boxes) and nonhomologous (I, II, and III) regions. The extent of specific mutations that delete a single α-globin gene are indicated by *salmon boxes* and the limits of the breakpoints as *solid lines*. These deletions and the reciprocal chromosomes containing three functional α-globin genes result from misalignment and unequal recombination mediated by the homologous blocks. **B,** Unequal crossover through the Z box deletes 3.7 kb of DNA and produces the $\alpha^{3.7}$ chromosome and its antitype, whereas recombination through the X box produces the −$\alpha^{4.2}$ chromosome and its antitype. The −$\alpha^{3.7}$ deletion can be further subdivided (I to III) by the exact location within the Z box where recombination occurs (see **A**). *(Redrawn from Higgs DR, Vickers MA, Wilkie AO, et al. A review of the molecular genetics of the human alpha-globin gene cluster. Blood. 1989;73:1081-1104.)*

Deletion of one α-globin gene does not affect expression of the ζ-globin gene[433] but has unanticipated consequences on expression of the remaining α-globin gene. The α_1 gene that remains on the −$\alpha^{3.7}$ chromosome is expressed approximately 1.8 times more often than the α_1 gene on a normal chromosome.[419] Individuals homozygous for the leftward deletion (−$\alpha^{4.2}$/−$\alpha^{4.2}$), who carry two copies of the α_1 gene, express more α-globin than the anticipated 25% of normal.[434] Homozygotes for the −$\alpha^{3.7III}$ deletion (−$\alpha^{3.7III}$/−$\alpha^{3.7III}$), who carry two α_2 genes, express less than the anticipated 75% of normal.[434] The increased expression of the α_1 gene on the −$\alpha^{3.7}$ and −$\alpha^{4.2}$ chromosomes may be secondary to release of transcriptional interference from the upstream α_2 gene,[421] whereas the lower expression of the α_2 gene in the $-\alpha^{3.7III}$ deletion remains to be explained. An important consequence of this observation, however, is that common mutations that delete the α_2 gene ($\alpha^{3.7I}$ and $\alpha^{4.2}$) may lead to increased expression of the remaining α_1 gene and to a less severe clinical phenotype than predicted from expression studies of the native α-globin genes.[434] Single nucleotide substitutions that inactivate the α_2 gene do not affect α_1 expression and consequently lead to a more severe clinical phenotype than single gene deletions do.[2,15]

Triplicated α-gene chromosomes are observed in populations in which the $\alpha^{3.7I}$ and $\alpha^{4.2}$ chromosomes are present. The third gene is expressed and leads to a slight increase in the α-chain–to–β-chain ratio in homozygotes for the triplication, but this is generally of no clinical consequence.[435,436] However, if a triplicated α-gene chromosome is coinherited with a β-thalassemia gene, thalassemia intermedia may be seen.[437,438] A unique deletion that removes the α_1 gene and some downstream sequence was recently described as a cause of α-thalassemia and appears to be due to a novel biologic mechanism.[439] As a result of the deletion, a promoter in the antisense orientation is brought into close proximity to the remaining α_2 gene. Antisense transcripts are created and appear to cause methylation of DNA and silencing of the chromatin in the region, thus attenuating transcription of the intact α_2 gene. Recent work in both yeast and human cells has begun to delineate the mechanisms that may be responsible for this phenomenon, which may normally play a major role in physiologic gene regulation.[440]

Mutations That Remove Both α-Globin Genes

Illegitimate, nonhomologous recombination within the α-globin cluster results in partial or complete deletion of both α-globin genes and generates an α^0 chromosome.[2,412,441-445] (Note that the term α^+ and α^0 may refer to the expression of α-globin from a single gene or may refer to the presence or absence of an intact α-globin gene on a chromosome.) In some circumstances, the ζ-globin gene may also be encompassed by the deletion. The boundaries of many of the deletions that have been characterized are summarized in Figure 20-22. The geographic distribution of these lesions is more restricted than that of the α^+-thalassemia deletions, the most common being the $-^{SEA}$ (Southeast Asia) and $-^{MED}$ (Mediterranean) deletions, thus suggesting that they are rare genetic events. Theories concerning the mechanisms of these deletions are summarized elsewhere.[2]

Homozygotes for α^0 chromosomes ($-/-$) suffer from hydrops fetalis, whereas individuals heterozygous for an α^+ chromosome and an α^0 chromosome ($-/-\alpha$ or $-/\alpha^T\alpha$) exhibit HbH disease. Increased expression of minute quantities of ζ-globin into adulthood may accompany some of the mutations in which the ζ gene is left intact by the deletion.[433] Sensitive radioimmunologic assays for the presence of ζ-globin chains in heterozygous adult carriers of these mutations have been devised,[446] and they may prove useful in areas such as Southeast Asia, where the incidence of the $-^{SEA}$ chromosome is as high as 3%.[447]

Mutations Not Linked to the Globin Gene Clusters That Alter Globin Gene Expression

Acquired Hemoglobin H Disease

A particularly severe, acquired form of HbH disease has been described in elderly men with clonal myeloproliferative disorders.[448-451] In this setting, levels of HbH approaching 60% may be seen.[426] Extremely low α-chain–to–β-chain synthesis ratios and low α-globin mRNA levels have been documented in bone marrow

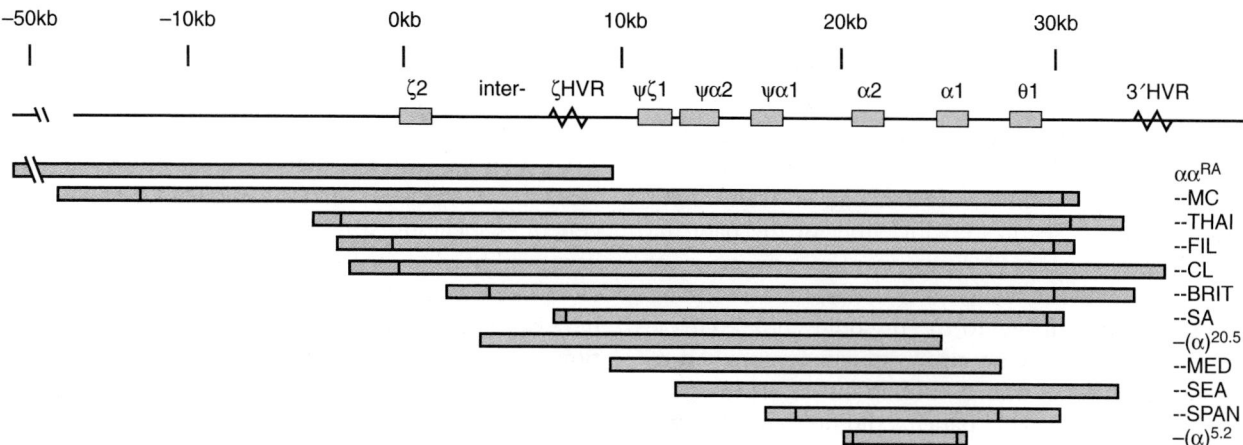

FIGURE 20-22. Deletion mutations that give rise to α^0-thalassemia. The organization of the α-globin cluster is shown. Expressed genes are represented by *salmon boxes*, whereas pseudogenes are shown as *blue boxes*. Two hypervariable regions (HVRs) are indicated as *zigzag lines*. Coordinates are in kilobase pairs (kb). The extent of each deletion is defined by a *salmon box* and the uncertainty of the breakpoints by *blue boxes*. The designation of the genotype is indicated to the right of each deletion. *(From Higgs DR, Vickers MA, Wilkie AO, et al. A review of the molecular genetics of the human alpha-globin gene cluster. Blood. 1989;73:1081-1104.)*

cells from affected individuals.[449,450] Residual α-globin mRNA expression may be derived from nonclonal erythroid cells. A bimorphic population of cells is present on examination of the peripheral blood smear. The manifestations of hemolytic disease caused by HbH may increase and decrease with the clinical course of the myeloproliferative disorder.[449]

Available evidence suggests that the absence of a positive regulatory factor in the clonal population or the presence of an inhibitory factor is responsible for the lack of α-globin gene expression. Extensive molecular analysis of the α-globin gene cluster in patients with acquired HbH disease indicates that it is structurally intact and hypomethylated in these individuals.[449,450] Human α-globin gene expression can be detected in somatic cell hybrids derived by fusion of bone marrow cells from patients with acquired HbH disease to murine erythroleukemia cells,[452] thus further suggesting that the transcriptional defect is not linked to the α-globin cluster. Additional study of this unusual condition may provide important information about factors regulating the α-globin gene cluster.

X-Linked α-Thalassemia Associated with Mental Retardation Syndrome

Rare instances of α-thalassemia occurring in individuals of Anglo-Saxon origin with phenotypically normal parents first drew attention to a new syndrome.[453] Further investigation revealed the commonly seen association of profound mental retardation, facial anomalies, and genital abnormalities.[78] Important recent studies demonstrated mutation of the *AH2* gene, a member of the DNA helicase superfamily and presumed global transcriptional regulator, as the underlying basis of this syndrome.[79]

Silent β-Thalassemia

Hematologically normal "silent carriers" of β-thalassemia are identified through family studies.[1,6,454-457] Some instances of "silent" β-thalassemia may be attributed to mutations that cause a very modest reduction in β-globin gene expression—the −101 promoter mutation[126,130] and the +1 cap site mutation[133]—or attributed to the inheritance of triplicated α-globin gene chromosomes.[437,438] In an Albanian family in which the father was a silent carrier, the mother had high-HbA$_2$ β-thalassemia trait, and two children had β-thalassemia, the silent carrier determinant did not appear to segregate with either of the paternal β-globin gene clusters.[458] Subsequently, a number of reports of families in which a β-thalassemia mutation appeared to be unlinked to the β-globin complex have been reported.[459-461] These rare instances of unlinked β-thalassemia may be due to mutations in *trans*-acting factors. However, all these patients did not have the syndromic features seen in those with the previously characterized *trans*-acting regulatory factor mutations (see the section on β-thalassemia mutants unlinked to the β-globin complex). Thus, new insight may be gained from genetic analysis of these rare cases.

Swiss Hereditary Persistence of Fetal Hemoglobin

Ordinarily, HbF constitutes less than 1% of the total hemoglobin in normal adult erythrocytes and is restricted to a subpopulation of erythrocytes (F cells) that represent between 3% and 7% of the total number of red cells.[7,8] Both the percentage of F cells present in the circulation and the amount of HbF per F cell are under genetic control, and evidence suggests that the determinants are not linked to the β-globin gene cluster.[462]

In the Swiss type of nondeletion HPFH (see Table 20-5), HbF is distributed in a heterocellular fashion with levels of HbF of 0.8% to 3.4% in heterozygotes.[1,12,93,368,462] Interpretation of earlier studies of Swiss HPFH was complicated by the small size of the pedigrees, overlap of HbF levels in heterozygotes and normal subjects, varying age of the research subjects (HbF levels tend to fall with age), and concomitant inheritance of β-globin gene alleles that can also influence HbF levels.

Several studies have been published in which linkage analysis clearly demonstrates that the HPFH determinant segregates independently from the β-globin gene cluster. In the first, a large Sardinian pedigree,[463,464] and the second, a large Asian Indian pedigree,[465] nondeletion HPFH and β^0-thalassemia genes were segregating in each family. Studies of normal individuals in Japan with Swiss HPFH in which the F-cell percentage rather than the HbF level was used to define HPFH have suggested that the "high–F-cell trait" segregates as an X-linked determinant.[12] A recent study has also localized a genetic determinant for HbF production to the long arm of chromosome 6 in a large HPFH pedigree.[13] An additional locus for HbF production has been found on chromosome 8 in the Asian Indian pedigree just described and also in a European twin study.[466] Further mapping of these HPFH determinants may provide important insight into the mechanisms regulating hemoglobin switching. There is substantial evidence from the results of twin and family studies that HbF and F-cell levels are genetically controlled.[9-11] Traditional approaches have used linkage analysis in an attempt to find genetic determinants that modulate HbF levels, but it is likely that complex trait analysis will be necessary to delineate putative common variants that have an effect on HbF.[467] Recently the analysis of HbF-regulating variants using genetic association studies has led to initial insight into genes unlinked to the β-globin locus that alter fetal hemoglobin levels. Two regions harboring genetic variants have been found in the course of whole-genome association studies in nonanemic Caucasian populations[467a,467b]. One region is found on chromosome 6 and is in an intergenic region between the genes *HBS1L* and *cMYB*.[467a-467c] The other region is found on chromosome 2 and is within an intron of the zinc-finger transcription factor *BCL11A*[467a,467b]. How these particular variants lead to changes in fetal hemoglobin levels remains to be uncovered. Interestingly, the variant in *BCL11A* on chromosome 2 also appears to ameliorate the severity of β-thalassemia in a cohort of patients from Sardinia.[467a]

CLINICAL HETEROGENEITY OF THALASSEMIA SECONDARY TO DIVERSITY OF MUTATIONS

In the previous sections, the extraordinary array of mutations associated with the clinical syndrome of thalassemia has been described. In populations in which thalassemia is prevalent, different types of mutations that affect genes of either the α-globin, β-globin, or both globin clusters may coexist. Frequently, patients are compound heterozygotes for these mutations. The relative degree to which globin chain synthesis is impaired reflects this genetic heterogeneity and determines the clinical phenotype. In the following clinical description of the thalassemia syndromes, we emphasize such genetic interrelationships.

α-Thalassemia

Nomenclature and Genetics of α-Thalassemia

α-Thalassemia is divided into four clinical subsets that reflect the extent of impairment in α-globin chain production: silent carrier (–α/αα), α-thalassemia trait (–α/–α or –/αα), HbH disease (–/–α), and hydrops fetalis (–/–) (see Table 20-6). Before the introduction of molecular analysis, these syndromes were classified on the basis of red blood cell parameters (hemoglobin level, mean corpuscular volume [MCV], mean corpuscular hemoglobin [MCH], globin biosynthetic ratio, presence of inclusions, and HbH [β4] levels), as well as the manner in which they interacted genetically to produce different phenotypes. Much of this early work relied on the study of Asian populations in which α-thalassemia is particularly common.[1]

The silent carrier state for α-thalassemia, in which a single α-globin gene on a chromosome is inactivated, has traditionally been designated α-thalassemia-2. Homozygosity for α-thalassemia-2 or heterozygosity for an allele causing more severe disease in which both α-globin genes are inactivated leads to α-thalassemia trait, also termed α-thalassemia-1. According to the historical nomenclature, HbH disease reflects heterozygosity for α-thalassemia-2 and α-thalassemia-1, whereas hydrops fetalis results from homozygosity for α-thalassemia-1.

Advances in molecular characterization of the α-globin gene cluster have clarified the genetic basis of these phenotypes. Weatherall and colleagues proposed a more informative nomenclature for these mutations.[1,2] Each chromosome may be designated as α^+ or α^0 to indicate the presence or absence of any α-globin chain production derived from that chromosome. This is referred to as a haplotype and should be distinguished from use of the term haplotype in describing the linkage of DNA polymorphisms on a chromosome. Haplotypes are further subdivided by the status of each α-globin gene

on a chromosome. As discussed previously, mutations may be of the deletion or nondeletion type. Normal individuals are designated (αα/αα) to indicate the presence of four active α genes, two on each chromosome 16, with the first position corresponding to the α_2 gene and the second position to the α_1 gene. Deletion of a single α-globin gene on a chromosome is designated (–α/), whereas deletion of both genes is indicated as (–/). Further refinement of this nomenclature includes a designation of the specific mutation; for example, ($-^{SEA}$/) signifies the α^0 deletion mutation that is common in Southeastern Asian populations (see Fig. 20-22), and ($-\alpha^{3.7}$/) symbolizes the α^+ rightward α-gene deletion that is extremely common in the American black population (see Fig. 20-22). Nondeletion mutations in a haplotype are designated in this scheme by a superscript T ($\alpha\alpha^T$) and can be more precisely described by symbols for the specific mutation and the gene affected. For example, ($\alpha^{CS}\alpha$) designates a chromosome bearing the Constant Spring chain termination mutation affecting the α_2 gene (see Table 20-2), and ($\alpha^{QS}\alpha$) designates a chromosome bearing the α gene with a substitution in codon 125 that leads to the synthesis of an unstable globin (see Table 20-2). This shorthand nomenclature is extremely useful when a patient's genotype is known in detail and has simplified description of the many genotypes that interact to generate the heterogeneous clinical syndromes.

At least 30 mutations that may inactivate one or both α-globin genes are known; thus, the different combinations of chromosomes bearing α-thalassemia mutations number more than 200. The number of occurrences of the different genotypes and haplotypes define the spectrum of disease observed in a given ethnic group. For example, severe forms of α-thalassemia (HbH disease and hydrops fetalis) are uncommon in blacks. In this group the single-deletion chromosome is very common,[468,469] whereas chromosomes with two defective α genes are quite rare. In some circumstances the phenotype of HbH disease is not readily related to genotype. Indeed, there is a significant spectrum of disease severity in individuals from the Southeast Asian area with the same genotype ($-\alpha^{3.7}/-^{SEA}$).[432] The observed phenotype may be further complicated by the inheritance of another hemoglobin disorder (β-thalassemia) or the influence of environmental factors such as iron or other nutritional deficiency.

Silent Carrier

The silent carrier state, or the α-thalassemia-2 defect, is due to the presence of a mutation affecting only one α-globin gene. Most often this occurs because of a deletion mutation (–α/αα). Patients who are silent carriers for α-thalassemia have three rather than four functional α-globin genes.[424,470] Thus, the impairment in α-globin synthesis is very mild. There is significant overlap of their globin biosynthetic ratio with both that of normal subjects and that of individuals with only two functional α-globin genes (Fig. 20-23). Similarly, the mean MCV of patients with three functional genes is slightly lower than

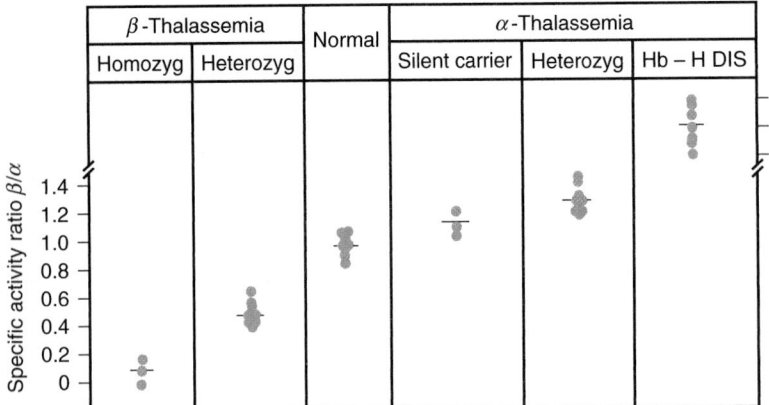

FIGURE 20-23. Biosynthetic α-globin–to–β-globin ratio in various forms of thalassemia. Peripheral blood cells were incubated with [^{14}C]leucine for 2 hours in autologous plasma. The globin chains were isolated by ion exchange chromatography. The specific activity of the chains and the ratio of their radioactivities were then calculated. *(Redrawn from Nathan DG. Thalassemia. N Engl J Med. 1972;286:586-594. Copyright 1972, Massachusetts Medical Society.)*

that in normal subjects, but significant overlap between the two groups exists.[2] Despite these differences that become apparent on comparison of groups with different numbers of α-globin genes, there is no reliable way to diagnose silent carriers of α-thalassemia by hematologic criteria. Diagnosis has been reported by detection of small amounts of Hb Bart's in cord blood,[1] but additional studies indicate that this approach is unreliable in ascertaining the presence of the silent carrier state.[471,472] However, a more recent U.K. study using high-performance liquid chromatography (HPLC) and genotyping to verify α-globin genotype on fresh cord blood samples demonstrated HPLC to be a reliable technique for determining the silent carrier state.

Silent Carrier Variant: Hemoglobin Constant Spring

Some silent carriers og α-thalassemia produce small quantities of slowly migrating hemoglobins (Fig. 20-24) that contain elongated α-globin chain variants resulting from termination codon mutations (see Table 20-2 and Fig. 20-14).[182-186] The original elongated α-chain variant, Hb Constant Spring, was named for the small Jamaican town in which the Chinese family in whom these hemoglobins were first discovered resided.[183] The family had three children with HbH disease; each had a small amount of the abnormal hemoglobins. One parent had typical thalassemia trait, whereas the other had normal red cells but, in addition, had approximately 1% of the abnormal hemoglobin. Similar slowly migrating hemoglobins have been found in other racial groups in Thailand and Greece.[473] Individuals homozygous for the α^{CS} mutation ($\alpha^{CS}\alpha/\alpha^{CS}\alpha$) have a clinical syndrome similar to HbH disease, although their erythrocytes contain Hb Bart's (γ_4) rather than HbH and the degree of anemia and the extent of abnormalities in red cell indices are milder than those in most patients with HbH disease.[474] Compound heterozygotes for the α^0 and α^{CS} haplotypes ($-/\alpha^{CS}\alpha$) exhibit typical HbH disease.

α-Thalassemia Trait

Two genotypes ($-/\alpha\alpha$ and $-\alpha/-\alpha$) that reflect inactivation of two α-globin genes are associated with α-thalassemia trait. Substitution mutations that affect the predominant α_2 gene ($\alpha^T\alpha/\alpha\alpha$) may also lead to α-thalassemia trait.

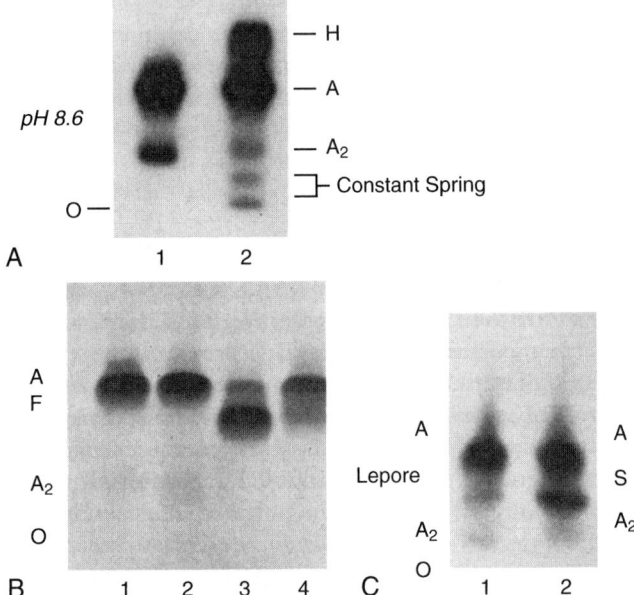

FIGURE 20-24. Hemoglobin electrophoresis. **A,** Starch gel electrophoresis at pH 8.6; 1, normal; 2, HbH disease with Hb Constant Spring. **B,** Agarose electrophoresis at pH 8.6; 1, normal; 2, β-thalassemia trait with increased HbA$_2$; 3 and 4, homozygous β-thalassemia with different relative amounts of HbA and HbF. **C,** Starch gel electrophoresis at pH 8.6; 1, Hb Lepore trait; 2, sickle cell trait. "O" indicates the origin. The anode is at the top of the figure.

The extent of the observed changes in red cell indices mirrors the reduction in α-globin production seen with each genotype, with the ($-\alpha/-\alpha$) genotype being less affected than the ($-/\alpha\alpha$) genotype. α-Thalassemia trait is characterized by marked microcytosis and hypochromia of red cells in conjunction with mild anemia and erythrocytosis (see Table 20-6). Levels of HbA$_2$ and HbF are generally normal or low. Diagnosis of this condition is typically made by family studies or by exclusion of iron deficiency and β-thalassemia trait. The incidence is particularly high in Asian populations and less in African, Mediterranean, and American black populations. Even in the neonatal period, the red cells appear hypochromic and microcytic. The proportion of Hb Bart's may be as high as 1% in the blood of normal newborns, but levels of 4% to 6% are attained in infants who are later shown to have α-thalassemia trait[1] (see Table 20-6). Beyond the neonatal period, biochemical markers such as HbA$_2$ and HbF in β-thalassemia are not particularly helpful in confirming the diagnosis of α-thalassemia trait. The one exception occurs in circumstances in which the expression of ζ-globin is increased because of deletion of both α-globin genes on a chromosome.[433,445,475] In Southeast Asia, where the $-^{SEA}$ allele is common, a sensitive radioimmunoassay allows detection of ζ-globin chains in adult carriers of this mutation.

Measurement of the β-to-α biosynthetic ratio has little place in the routine diagnosis of α-thalassemia trait. Although detection of impaired α-globin synthesis has been reported,[476,477] measurement is technically difficult because these individuals have a low reticulocyte count and the measured values overlap with those found in normal individuals (see Table 20-6). Iron deficiency may raise the measured β-to-α biosynthetic ratio, thus further complicating interpretation.[478-481] Consequently, in most patients the diagnosis of α-thalassemia trait is established by red cell morphology and parameters, coupled with exclusion of β-thalassemia trait and iron deficiency. Gene deletions responsible for deficient α-globin production can be demonstrated by restriction endonuclease mapping; this technique may be applied when an accurate diagnosis is critical. Newer technology allows PCR detection of deletion[482] and triplication[483] of α genes, and it has the same level accuracy as the more cumbersome Southern blotting and DNA hybridization with ϕζ-globin gene probe.

Hemoglobin H Disease

Genetics

HbH disease occurs in individuals who have only a single fully functional α-globin gene. the genotypes leading to HbH disease are diverse.[2] Most common is heterozygosity for the single- and double-deletion chromosomes (–/–α). As a result, HbH disease is observed most often in Southeast Asia ($-^{SEA}/-\alpha^{3.7}$) and the Mediterranean basin ($-^{MED}/-\alpha^{3.7}$), where the incidence of both the α$^+$ and α^0 haplotypes is significant. Nondeletion mutations may also interact to cause HbH disease. As discussed earlier, the α$_2$ genes are responsible for the production of approximately 75% of the total α-globin chains. Mutations that decrease expression from the α$_2$ gene (α^{T}α/) result in an α+ haplotype that produces fewer α-globin chains than a deletion α+ haplotype (–α/) does. Thus, homozygosity for mutations in both α$_2$ genes (α^{T}α/α^{T}α) is phenotypically equivalent to deletion of three genes and is associated with HbH disease and not α-thalassemia trait.[2,15] Consistent with this observation, nondeletion α+-thalassemia haplotypes that are paired with α^0-thalassemia haplotypes (–/α^{T}α) lead to more severe HbH disease than does the interaction of the deletion α+ haplotypes (–/–α).

Hemoglobin Pattern

Anemia of moderate severity characterized by hypochromia, microcytosis, striking red cell fragmentation (Fig. 20-25), and the presence of a fast migrating hemoglobin,

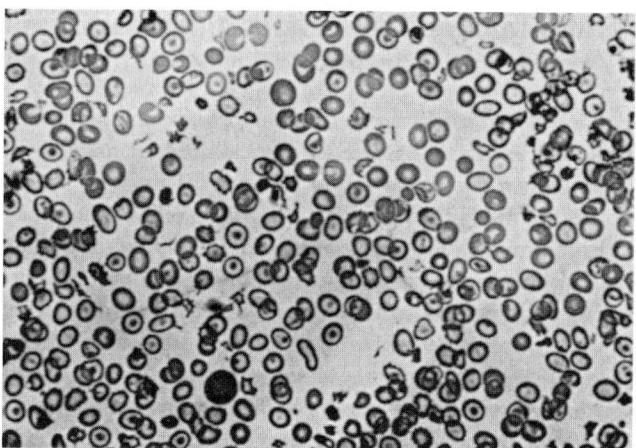

FIGURE 20-25. Peripheral blood smear from a patient with HbH disease.

HbH (β$_4$), on electrophoresis (see Fig. 20-24) may be shown to represent an α-thalassemia syndrome by measurement of the β-to-α biosynthetic ratio.[476,484,485] Incubation of peripheral blood reticulocytes with [^{3}H]leucine and subsequent chromatographic resolution of the globins indicate that such patients have a twofold to fivefold excess of β-chain synthesis (see Table 20-6 and Fig. 20-23). These excess β chains form HbH, which accounts for 5% to 30% of the total hemoglobin in patients with HbH disease.[486] In approximately 50% of individuals with HbH disease in Southeast Asia, small quantities of Hb Constant Spring are found (see Fig. 20-24). HbH disease may be suspected in anemic neonates in whom all the red cells are severely hypochromic. At birth, patients with HbH disease also have large amounts of Hb Bart's (γ$_4$). In patients with HbH disease and an intact spleen, incubation of peripheral blood cells in brilliant cresyl blue produces many small inclusions in most red cells (Fig. 20-26). The dye induces precipitation of HbH by a redox reaction. In contrast, large and usually single preformed inclusions (Heinz bodies) may be visualized with methyl violet in the red cells of splenectomized patients (see Fig. 20-26).[91,487] These inclusions are composed of precipitated β-globin rendered insoluble by hemichrome formation or by interaction of β-globin sulfhydryl groups with the red cell membrane.[91,488]

Pathophysiology

HbH exhibits no Bohr effect or heme-heme interaction and thus is not effective for oxygen transport under physiologic conditions.[489] Consequently, patients with appreciable amounts of HbH have a more severe deficit in functional hemoglobin and oxygen-carrying capacity than the measured hemoglobin concentration might suggest. Red cells containing HbH are sensitive to oxidative stress, thus accounting for the enhanced red cell destruction that may occur with the administration of oxidant drugs such as sulfonamides.[490] As erythrocytes age and lose their capacity to withstand oxidant stress, precipitation of HbH occurs and leads to premature destruction of circulating red cells.[91] Hence, HbH is primarily a hemolytic disorder.[487,491] Inclusions of HbH are

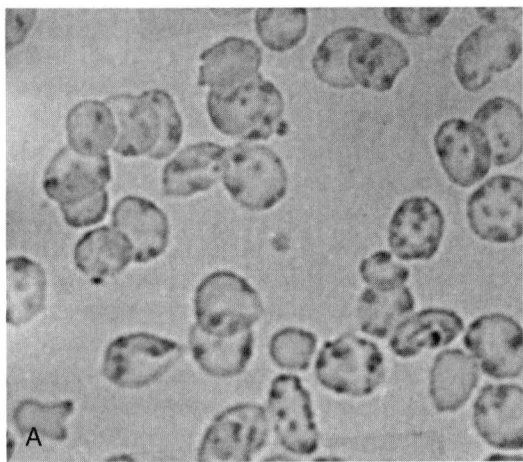 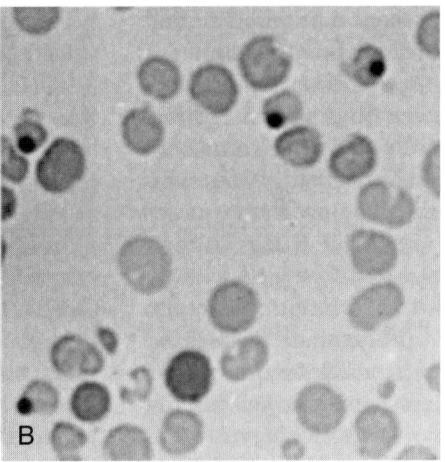

FIGURE 20-26. Red cell inclusions in HbH disease. **A,** Inclusions induced by incubation of peripheral blood in 1% brilliant cresyl blue and 0.4% citrate for 30 minutes at 37° C (patient not splenectomized). **B,** Preformed inclusions in the peripheral blood of a splenectomized patient stained by a new methylene blue reticulocyte stain.

rarely seen in bone marrow cells,[492] and erythropoiesis is fairly effective.[491]

Clinical Features

Typical patients with HbH disease live quite normally. Generally, the anemia is moderate with a hemoglobin concentration of 7 to 10 g/dL, although occasional patients may have hemoglobin levels as low as 3 to 4 g/dL.[1] The complications of HbH disease are related to chronic hemolysis. Jaundice and hepatosplenomegaly are commonly present. Folic acid deficiency, pigment gallstones, leg ulcers, and increased susceptibility to infection are also observed. Hemolytic episodes may be precipitated by drugs or infection. Iron overload is uncommon but may occur in patients receiving transfusions and those older than 45 years.[493] Development of the characteristic thalassemic facies, which reflects expansion of marrow space equivalent to that seen in patients with severe β-thalassemia, is rare. Usually, only moderate bone marrow erythroid hyperplasia is evident.[481]

Therapy

Consistent with the benign course of HbH disease, treatment is primarily supportive. Therapy includes supplementation with folic acid, avoidance of oxidant drugs and iron salts, prompt treatment of infectious episodes, and judicious use of transfusions. Splenectomy should be contemplated in patients with HbH disease only if hypersplenism is present as reflected by leukopenia, thrombocytopenia, and worsening anemia or the development of a transfusion requirement in a patient whose condition was previously stable. Thrombocytosis after splenectomy may be complicated by a clotting diathesis, recurrent pulmonary emboli, and pulmonary hypertension, particularly in patients with severe HbH disease and a fairly normal hematocrit.[493-495] The use of measurements of red cell survival and splenic sequestration by ^{51}Cr labeling of red cells is controversial in making a clinical decision regarding splenectomy because the label binds selectively to β-globin chains and may, by virtue of selective removal of HbH inclusions from red cells in the spleen, give a falsely high index of splenic destruction.[496] Other studies,

however, suggest that results from the ^{51}Cr technique may be valid.[497]

Other Hemoglobin H Syndromes

Syndrome of α-Thalassemia with Mental Retardation

Patients with a syndrome characterized by mental retardation and a form of α-thalassemia that cannot be explained by simple mendelian inheritance of an α-thalassemia gene have been described.[453,498] In rare patients, the mutation arises as a de novo event in a paternal germ cell. These patients can be divided into two distinct syndromes (deletion and nondeletion) on the basis of their clinical features and the results of molecular analysis of their α-globin gene clusters.

Patients have been described with extensive deletions involving chromosome band 16p3.3 or, alternatively, with deletions resulting from unbalanced chromosome translocations that also lead to aneuploidy in a second chromosome. Patients with deletion mutations exhibit mild to moderate mental retardation and a broad spectrum of dysmorphic features. Other rare patients are characterized by more severe mental retardation and a uniform pattern of dysmorphic features, including genital abnormalities, but no detectable deletions involving the α-globin gene cluster.[78] Such patients fall into the category of the syndrome of X-linked α-thalassemia with mental retardation. As noted earlier, the affected gene is a putative global regulator (XH2).[79]

Although these disorders are seen rarely, they may be under-recognized. This is particularly true of ethnic groups in which α-thalassemia is uncommon, and the mild hematologic findings in patients who do not inherit a second α-thalassemia gene might be overlooked. Infants with uncharacterized mental retardation should be studied with techniques suitable for detection of a deficiency in α-globin synthesis.

Acquired Hemoglobin H Disease

HbH is also found rarely in the red cells of patients with erythroleukemia or a myeloproliferative syndrome.[448-450]

The disorder may be clonal and displays a striking male predisposition (85% of confirmed instances).[453] The clinical features manifested by these patients are those of their primary disorder; the finding of HbH is incidental to the outcome of the disease, although striking red cell abnormalities and active hemolysis may be present. The genetic mechanism of this syndrome appears to involve abnormal regulation of α-gene expression because of a mutation affecting a distant genetic locus (see earlier).

Hydrops Fetalis

Genetics

Homozygosity for the α⁰ haplotype (–/–) leads to hydrops fetalis, a disorder that is particularly common in Southeast Asia where the α⁰ haplotype is seen frequently. In rare infants from Greece and Southeast Asia, hydrops fetalis has been shown to result from the interaction of α⁰ haplotypes with nondeletion α⁺ haplotypes.[499-501]

Hemoglobin Pattern

The birth of stillborn infants to parents with α-thalassemia trait reflects the most severe form of α-thalassemia.[502,503] Because of the inability to synthesize any α-globin, their blood contains only Hb Bart's (γ_4), HbH (β_4), and small amounts of Hb Portland ($\zeta_2\gamma_2$) within red cells displaying morphologic changes characteristic of severe thalassemia.[504,505]

Pathophysiology

Although the hemoglobin concentration averages 6.2 g/dL, both HbH and Hb Bart's have high oxygen affinity and no subunit cooperativity. Therefore, a hydropic infant has very little functional hemoglobin. Viability in utero is maintained by the presence of small quantities of Hb Portland 1 and 2.

Clinical Features

Generally, affected infants are delivered stillborn at 30 to 40 weeks' gestation or die shortly after delivery at term.[447,504] Infants are grossly edematous or hydropic as a result of congestive heart failure induced by severe anemia. The blood smear is characterized by large hypochromic macrocytes and numerous nucleated red cells. At autopsy, extensive extramedullary hematopoiesis and placental hypertrophy are seen. A high incidence of toxemia of pregnancy and postpartum hemorrhage is observed in mothers of hydropic infants,[481,506] presumably as a consequence of the massive placenta. Hence, early recognition of the disorder in at-risk pregnancies by prenatal diagnosis should lead to consideration of termination of the pregnancy.

Therapy

At least five infants born prematurely with hydrops fetalis have survived with the use of chronic transfusion regimens.[507,508] Intrauterine transfusion of fetuses with hydrops fetalis should also be considered if treatment after delivery is contemplated.[509] Marrow transplantation may be considered if the affected infant is delivered safely.

Mild β-Thalassemia

Silent Carrier

A silent carrier state for β-thalassemia was recognized through the study of families in which affected children had a more severe β-thalassemia syndrome than a parent with typical β-thalassemia trait.[1,6,454-457] A study of the "normal" parent often revealed mild microcytosis or a slight impairment in β-globin synthesis on radiolabeling of the globin chains in peripheral blood reticulocytes. Characteristically, silent carriers of β-thalassemia have normal levels of HbA_2. These silent carriers must be distinguished from individuals whose red cells have all the stigmata of β-thalassemia trait but have normal levels of HbA_2. Several patients who are homozygous for the silent carrier β-thalassemia gene have been described.[1] Anemia is moderate (hemoglobin concentration of 6 to 7.0 g/dL), and these patients rarely require transfusion. Hepatosplenomegaly may be significant. HbF values range from 10% to 15%, and the HbA_2 level is elevated to the range normally seen in individuals with thalassemia trait.

The silent carrier state of β-thalassemia appears to be a distinct clinical and biochemical entity. The underlying molecular defects cause only a modest reduction in β-globin synthesis. Two point mutations in the β-globin gene region have been linked to the silent carrier phenotype. The –101 promoter mutation appears to be a common cause of silent β-thalassemia in the Italian population[204] and has been observed in Bulgarian and Turkish individuals,[126] whereas the +1 cap site Inr mutation is associated with a silent carrier phenotype in an Indian family.[133] As noted earlier, rare instances of silent β-thalassemia secondary to mutations unlinked to the β-gene cluster have been reported.

β-Thalassemia Trait

Genetics

In 1925, Rietti[510] described Italian patients with mild anemia whose red cells exhibited increased resistance to osmotic lysis. A similar syndrome was later recognized in American patients of Italian descent by Wintrobe and co-workers,[511] who noted that both parents of a patient with Cooley's anemia also had this syndrome. Detailed analysis of several pedigrees by Valentine and Neel[512] and others[513,514] established the fact that this form of thalassemia occurs in individuals who are heterozygous for a mutation that affects β-globin synthesis. Expression of one β gene is impaired by mutation, whereas the other gene is normal.

Hemoglobin Pattern

Characteristically, HbA_2, HbF, or both are elevated in patients with β-thalassemia trait, although normal levels are observed occasionally. The relative amounts of HbA_2 or HbF have been used to classify thalassemia trait, which has relevance to the molecular lesion in certain instances and also to the severity of the disease in homozygous offspring.

Globin Biosynthetic Ratio

In peripheral blood reticulocytes, the measured β-to-α biosynthetic ratio varies from 0.5 to 0.7, as predicted for inactivation of a single β gene (see Fig. 20-23). However, when bone marrow cells are incubated with [³H]leucine, the measured β-to-α biosynthetic ratio is often 1:1 in patients with heterozygous β-thalassemia.[515-519] The capacity of bone marrow cells to degrade free α-globin by proteolysis may explain why it is difficult to demonstrate unbalanced synthesis of β- and α-globin chains in the marrow cells of heterozygotes. The measured β-to-α ratio is approximately 0.5 in pulses of 10 to 20 minutes, but if the incubation of bone marrow cells is prolonged, proteolysis apparently destroys the excess newly synthesized α-globin.[520,521] Fractionation of bone marrow cells after incubation in [³H]leucine demonstrated that proteolysis is most efficient in the earliest erythroid cels, namely, proerythroblasts and basophilic erythroblasts.[521] The impairment in β-globin synthesis becomes easier to detect as erythroid cells mature, thus accounting for the reduced β-to-α biosynthetic ratio that is usually found in peripheral blood reticulocytes.

δ-Globin Synthesis

Among inherited anemias, the elevation in HbA_2 level is unique to β-thalassemia. The absolute quantity of HbA_2 present in red cells is a complex function of the inherent capacity for δ-globin chain synthesis and factors regulating rates of hemoglobin dimer and tetramer assembly. As discussed earlier, δ-globin is normally expressed at a low level, approximately 2.5% that of β-globin. The level may be reduced further by mutations that affect δ-globin expression. Heterozygous[522,523] and homozygous[524] states have been described. δ-Thalassemias reflect point mutations that completely silence the already defective δ-globin genes.[282,374,375,457,525-527]

In heterozygous β-thalassemia, the observed increase in HbA_2 represents a relative as well as an absolute increase in the quantity of HbA_2 per red cell from the normal level of 0.6 to 0.7 pg to 1.0 pg.[1] The increased amount of HbA_2 contains δ-globin chains derived from the δ gene adjacent to the mutant β gene, as well as from the δ gene on the opposite chromosome. This has been inferred from the study of β-thalassemia heterozygotes who also have a variant δ chain.[528] The increase in the HbA_2 level can be accounted for by enhanced incorporation of δ-globin chains into hemoglobin dimers as a consequence of deficient β-globin chain production (see earlier discussion on hemoglobin assembly).[229]

Environmental factors also influence the absolute level of HbA_2. Iron deficiency leads to a decrease in the level of HbA_2, which may become normal in thalassemia

heterozygotes and therefore mask the diagnosis of β-thalassemia trait. In such instances, the level of HbA_2 becomes elevated with iron repletion.[529] An increase in the level of HbA_2 may be seen in acquired megaloblastic disorders associated with either folic acid or vitamin B_{12} deficiency.[529]

Clinical Features

Peripheral blood smears from patients with β-thalassemia trait are shown in Figure 20-27. Microcytosis, hypochromia, targeting, basophilic stippling, and elliptocytosis may be striking features, although the red cells may be nearly normal in occasional patients. The bone marrow is characterized by mild to moderate erythroid hyperplasia; red cell survival is modestly decreased, and slight ineffective erythropoiesis is present.[530] Inclusions in bone marrow cells and peripheral red cells are rare. Similar hematologic parameters appear to characterize Thai, Chinese, Greek, British, and Italian populations with β-thalassemia trait,[531-534] whereas African Americans appear to have a milder syndrome.[535] Hepatomegaly and spleno-

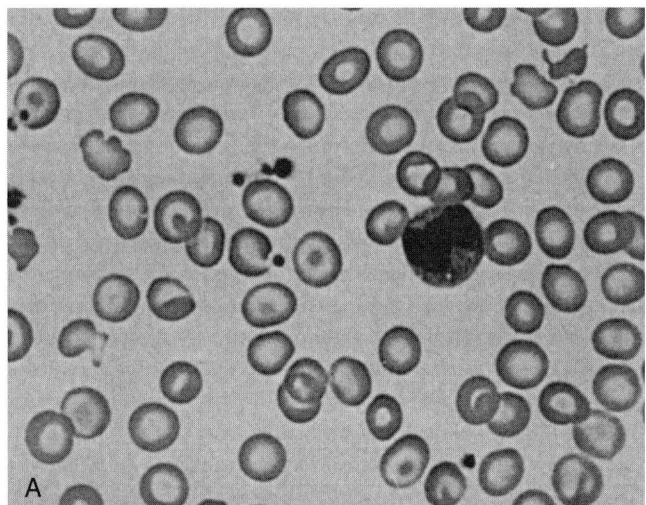

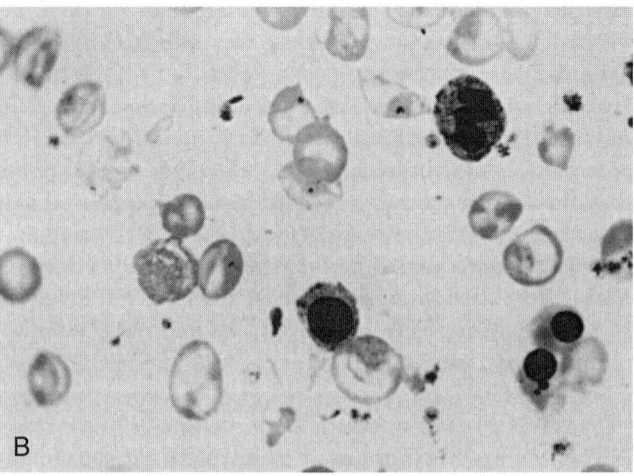

FIGURE 20-27. Peripheral blood smears from patients with heterozygous β-thalassemia (**A**) and homozygous β-thalassemia (**B**) after splenectomy.

megaly have been reported in 10% to 19% of Italian and Greek patients but are less common in other groups.[533,534] Iron or folic acid deficiency, pregnancy, or intercurrent illness may exacerbate the anemia in patients with thalassemia trait.

Therapy

No therapy is required for thalassemia trait, but genetic counseling is imperative. The homozygous offspring of two individuals with high-HbA₂ β-thalassemia trait usually have transfusion-dependent anemia and thalassemia major, but they may sometimes have a thalassemia intermedia phenotype. The precise nature of the mutation or mutations in homozygous individuals is one factor in determining the clinical phenotype.

β-Thalassemia Trait Phenotypes

High-A₂ β-Thalassemia

This is the most common form of β-thalassemia trait. HbA₂ levels vary from 3.5% to 8.0%, whereas the HbF level varies from less than 1% to 5%.[1,531-535] The vast majority of single base mutations resulting in β-thalassemia (see Table 20-2) lead to typical high-HbA₂ β-thalassemia trait. Although individual mutations variably reduce β-globin synthesis, efforts to differentiate the effect of specific mutations in heterozygous individuals have largely been unrewarding.[1,533,536,537] In blacks, β⁰ and β⁺ mutations can often be distinguished in individual families by the rate of occurrence of double heterozygotes for a β-thalassemia mutation and the βˢ mutation. In this population, MCV and MCH values are higher in β⁺ heterozygotes than in β⁰ heterozygotes, but circulating hemoglobin concentrations are nearly equivalent.[535,538] The common mutations found in American blacks, most notably residing in the ATA box of the promoter (see Table 20-2), only modestly impair β-globin gene expression,[46,146] which perhaps accounts for the relatively mild phenotype of many individuals with heterozygous or homozygous β⁺-thalassemia in this population.

δβ-Thalassemia

Individuals heterozygous for these mutations have increased levels of HbF (5% to 15%) and low HbA₂ levels. This phenotype is most often generated by deletions that remove most or all of the coding sequences of the δ- and β-globin genes (see Table 20-4). The propensity of these deletion mutations for enhancement of the expression of γ-globin genes contributes to a relatively mild phenotype in homozygous individuals or those in whom a δβ-thalassemia deletion is inherited along with a thalassemia allele with a typical substitution mutation.

High-A₂, High-F β-Thalassemia

A distinct variant of β-thalassemia trait has been described in which the level of HbA₂ is elevated and the level of HbF is also elevated (5% to 20%).[287,288,539] This form of thalassemia trait is associated with deletions of the β-globin gene that leave the δ and γ genes intact (see Table 20-4).

Normal-A₂ β-Thalassemia

This form of β-thalassemia trait should be distinguished from the silent carrier state. Although both are characterized by low or normal HbA₂ levels, the red cells in individuals with normal-HbA₂ β-thalassemia are characteristically hypochromic and microcytic,[456,540] in contrast to silent carriers, whose red cells appear near normal.[453,455] Individuals who coinherit this type of β-thalassemia allele from one parent along with a high-HbA₂ β-thalassemia allele from the other usually have severe transfusion-dependent β-thalassemia.

This phenotype is thought to represent coinheritance of mutations (usually deletions) that decrease β- and δ-gene function. The mutations in the δ-globin gene may be present on the same chromosome or on the opposite chromosome from the β-thalassemia gene.[282,374,3759,457,525-527]

Differential Diagnosis of Thalassemia Trait

In clinical practice, thalassemia trait must be distinguished from iron deficiency (see Chapter 12 for additional discussion of the differential diagnosis of microcytosis and iron deficiency). Frequently, the differential diagnosis may be suspected from red blood cell indices; mild erythrocytosis and marked microcytosis are characteristic of thalassemia trait (Table 20-7).[548-550] The red cell count is usually decreased in patients with iron deficiency, whereas red cell volume may be normal or decreased, depending on whether the iron deficiency anemia is acute or chronic,[551-554] but red cell volume is rarely as low as in thalassemia trait. The mean corpuscular hemoglobin concentration (MCHC) is usually normal in thalassemia trait, whereas the MCHC may be low in a subset of cells in iron deficiency; in both syndromes the hypochromic appearance of the red cells reflects their small size, diminished hemoglobin content, and high surface-to-volume ratio. The red cell distribution width (RDW), a parameter available in modern automated cell counters, was originally believed to distinguish between iron deficiency and other causes of microcytosis.[555,556] However, the RDW is also increased in the thalassemias and other hemoglobinopathies and is not a useful independent discriminator.[557-561] The absence of stainable iron in a bone marrow specimen is highly suggestive of iron deficiency, but the presence of iron does not necessarily exclude an iron-responsive anemia.

Several formulas have been developed to assist in the diagnosis of thalassemia trait during the assessment of microcytic hypochromic anemia (Table 20-8).[552,562,563] None of the discriminant functions are infallible. Nonetheless, the Mentzer index[552] is useful as an office screening test. More accuracy in separating thalassemia trait from iron deficiency may be achieved with the England and Fraser function,[563-565] but when both conditions exist

TABLE 20-7 Hematologic Parameters in Thalassemia Trait and Iron Deficiency

Parameter	α-Thal	β-Thal	Iron Deficiency
Hemoglobin concentration (g/dL)	12.6 ± 1.1 (541)* 12 ± 0.7	†M—12.6 ± 1.4 (542-545) F—10.8 ± 0.9 (542-545) C—11.3 ± 1 (542-545) Adults—12 ± 1.3	10.2 ± 1.6 (546)
Red cell count (×10⁶/μL)	5.6 ± 0.5	M—5.8 ± 0.6 (542-545) F—5.1 ± 0.9 (542-545) C—4.7 ± 0.6 (542-545) Adults—6 ± 0.48	4.67 ± 0.43 (546)
Mean corpuscular volume 88.7 ± 5.3 (677) 4 m³/red cell	72.2 ± 3.3 (541) 65.2 ± 3 (547)	64.7 ± 4.3 (541) 60.8 ± 5.6 (546)	67 ± 6.6 (546)
Mean corpuscular hemoglobin pg/red cell	23.2 ± 3.3 (541) 21 ± 1 (547)	20.3 ± 2.2 (541) 20.2 ± 1.9 (546)	21.8 ± 2.9 (546)
Hemoglobin A₂ (2-3.5%)	Normal or decreased	5.2 ± 0.8 (542-545)	Normal or decreased
Hemoglobin F (<1%)	<1%	2.1 ± 1.2 (542-545)	<1%

*Numbers in parentheses are reference citations.
C, children; F, females; M, males.

TABLE 20-8 Formulas for Differentiation of Thalassemia Trait from Iron Deficiency

	Thalassemia Trait	Iron Deficiency
Mentzer index (552)* MCV/RBC	<13	>13
Shine and Lal (562) (MCV) 2 × MCH	<1530	>1530
England and Fraser (563) MCV − RBC −(5 × Hb) − 8.4	Negative values	Positive values

*Numbers in parentheses are reference citations.
MCV, mean corpuscular volume; RBC, red blood cell.

simultaneously, all indices are subject to error. Additional discriminant functions and automated protocols have been proposed that may also prove useful.[566-568] Free erythrocyte protoporphyrin, often incorporated into the initial workup of hypochromic microcytic anemia in childhood to screen for lead exposure, is an additional useful test for patients suspected of having thalassemia trait.[569,570] This technique has been especially helpful in evaluating newly arrived Southeast Asian refugees to the United States.[571] Of course, measurement of transferrin saturation or ferritin may also be used to verify or exclude the diagnosis of iron deficiency. The ratio between microcytic (MCV <61 fL) and hypochromic (MCHC <28 g/dL) erythrocytes is a helpful parameter. A ratio greater than 1.0 is highly suggestive of thalassemic trait, whereas a ratio less than 1.0 is mostly associated with iron deficiency.

In office practice the distinction between thalassemia trait and iron deficiency generally depends on examination of peripheral blood smears and, above all, the patient's clinical history, as well as measurement of red cell indices in the parents. It is worth remembering that patients with thalassemia trait are not immune to iron deficiency. In these patients, iron deficiency may mask increases in the levels of HbA₂ and HbF that would otherwise suggest a diagnosis of β-thalassemia.

After iron deficiency is excluded, differential diagnosis between α- and β-thalassemia trait depends on measurement of HbA₂ and HbF levels (see Table 20-7) and rarely if ever on measurement of the α-to-β biosynthetic ratio in peripheral blood reticulocytes. In patients with microcytosis, hypochromia, and erythrocytosis but without evidence of iron deficiency or altered HbA₂ and HbF levels, α-thalassemia is the most probable diagnosis. When both α- and β-thalassemia coexist, changes in the levels of HbF and HbA₂ characteristic of β-thalassemia trait may not be present[96] (see later). Molecular genetic analysis and family studies are often necessary to define these complex interactions.

Severe β-Thalassemia

Historical Perspective

It was not until Thomas Cooley, a Detroit pediatrician, first described the clinical entity that was to bear his name that thalassemia major was recognized as a distinct disease.[572,573] Cooley recognized similarities in the appearance and clinical course of four children of Greek and Italian ancestry. These children exhibited severe anemia (hemoglobin concentration of 3 to 7 g/dL), massive hepatosplenomegaly, and severe growth retardation. In addition, bone deformities, such as frontal bossing and maxillary prominence, gave the patients a characteristic facies. Deformities of the long bones of the legs were also commonly seen and thought to reflect severe osteoporosis. Thalassemia major, or "Cooley's anemia," was and is far more common in Greece and Italy than in the United States, and descriptions of the disease in these countries soon followed Cooley's original report.[574]

Autopsy studies revealed extraordinary expansion of bone marrow at the expense of bony structures. Extramedullary hematopoiesis was often a striking feature and appeared as either isolated massive hepatosplenomegaly or hepatosplenomegaly in association with intrathoracic or intra-abdominal masses.[573-575] Children were also noted to have significant iron deposition in almost all organs, the significance of which was not initially appreciated.[575] Before regular blood transfusion regimens were used, these changes progressed inexorably and were invariably fatal during the first few years of life. Patients died of the effects of their anemia: congestive heart failure, intercurrent infection, or complications resulting from all too commonly seen pathologic fractures.

Initial transfusion regimens were mainly palliative; transfusions were recommended only when the anemia interfered significantly with a patient's ability to function on a daily basis. In defense of this regimen, we must realize that the pathophysiologic basis of the disease was not understood and that clinicians first attempted to minimize the transfusional iron administered because they feared that the iron, seen ubiquitously in these patients at autopsy, might itself be the cause of the disease.[575] Palliative transfusion therapy enabled affected individuals to live somewhat longer than patients not receiving transfusions, but the bone deformities and severe anemia forced them to lead markedly restricted lives.

In an attempt to improve the quality of life of these patients, trials using routine transfusion schedules to maintain hemoglobin levels of 8.5 g/dL or greater were initiated.[576-578] The condition of patients improved dramatically, with fewer overt side effects of anemia and more normal growth.[579,580] Clinical improvement proved transient, however, because regular transfusions led to the complications of chronic iron overload, including growth retardation from endocrine disturbances, diabetes mellitus, and delayed sexual maturation. Death invariably ensued in the second or early third decade of life, most often as a result of iron-induced cardiac arrhythmias or intractable congestive heart failure.[581]

Pathophysiology

Imbalance in Globin Biosynthesis

That severe β-thalassemia was caused by impaired production of β-globin was established in the mid-1960s by direct measurement of globin biosynthesis in reticulocytes.[582-586] Soon thereafter, impaired production of α chains was demonstrated in the α-thalassemia syn-

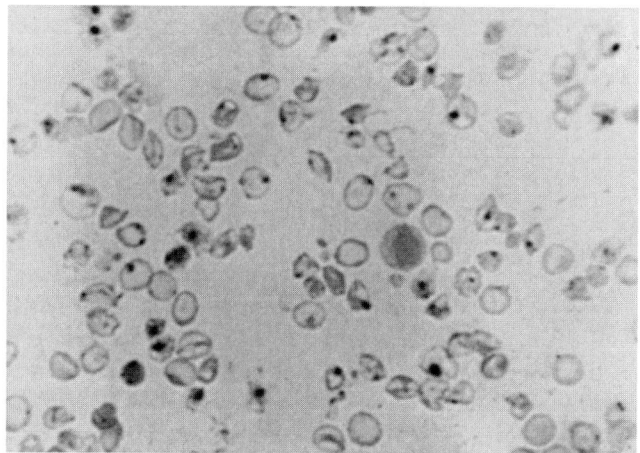

FIGURE 20-28. Supervital stain (methyl violet) of the peripheral blood cells from a patient with homozygous β-thalassemia after splenectomy.

dromes.[476] Decreased hemoglobin production is reflected in the peripheral blood smear by hypochromia, microcytosis, and target cells (which are a sign of the severe impairment in total hemoglobin production), as well as by teardrops, fragments, and microspherocytes (see Fig. 20-27). Red cell fragmentation is a direct consequence of unbalanced globin chain synthesis. Excess α chains, which have no complementary non–α chains with which to pair, form insoluble inclusions, demonstrable on methyl violet staining of the peripheral blood of asplenic patients with β-thalassemia (Fig. 20-28). In nonsplenectomized individuals, these inclusions are difficult to demonstrate because they are efficiently removed during the passage of red cells through the splenic sinusoids, where fragments and teardrops are generated (Fig. 20-29).

α-Globin inclusions in the erythrocytes and nucleated erythroid cells of patients with thalassemia major were first demonstrated by Fessas and associates[587-589] and by Nathan.[590] The incidence of the inclusions parallels the degree of impairment in β-globin synthesis. Inclusions have several deleterious effects on erythroid cells and are believed to lead to severe ineffective erythropoiesis. Intranuclear α-globin inclusions, visualized with electron microscopy, have been hypothesized to interfere with cell division.[591,592] Intracytoplasmic inclusions oxidize and mechanically damage cell membranes, interfere with mitochondrial function, and permit the ingress of calcium ions, which perturb the internal monovalent cationic environment and thereby contribute to the intramedullary death of erythroid cells. Moreover, α inclusions reduce red cell deformability and very likely interfere with egress from the bone marrow spaces, as well as from the tortuous vasculature of the spleen. The combined effects of ineffective erythropoiesis and severe anemia account for the extraordinary marrow expansion seen in patients with thalassemia major. In fact, these individuals have a nonfunctional cell mass that approximates the 10^{15} tumor cells present in patients with fatal leukemia and is associated with a profound hypermetabolic state that includes fever, wasting, and hyperuricemia.[590]

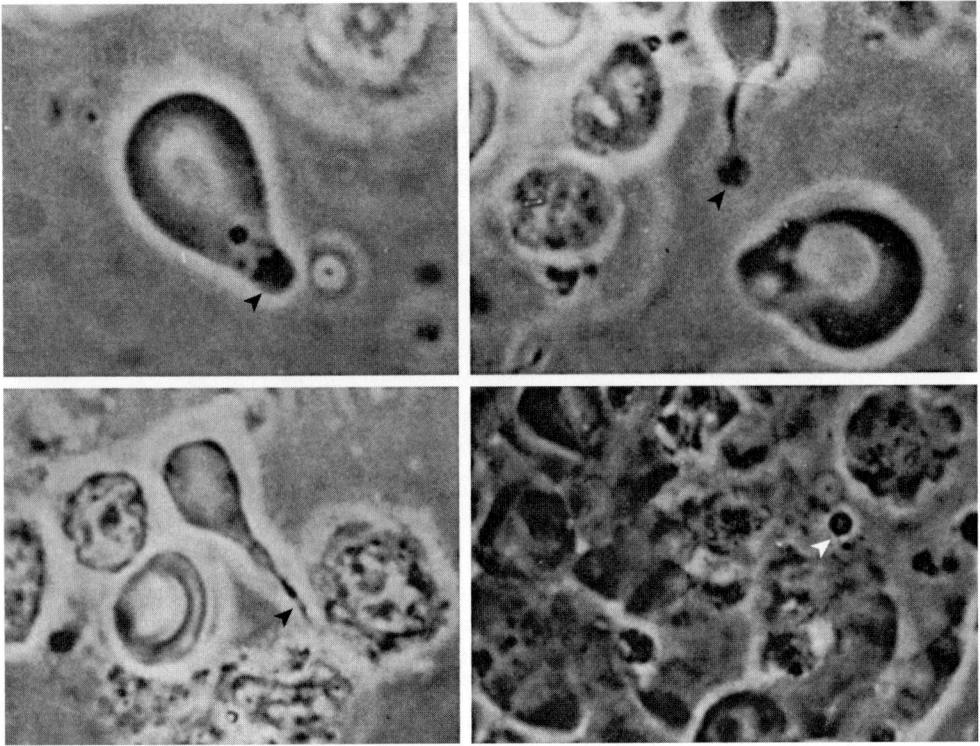

FIGURE 20-29. Phase-contrast microscopy of a wet preparation of scrapings from the spleen of a patient with homozygous β-thalassemia. Note the chain inclusion bodies (*black arrowheads*) within teardrop-shaped red cells, inclusions being pulled out, or "pitted," from the red cell by reticuloendothelial cell action (*lower left*), and inclusions free in the splenic pulp (*white arrowhead*).

The Red Cell Membrane

Numerous membrane abnormalities of thalassemic erythrocytes have been described.[488,490,593] Many are attributable to oxidative damage from excess globin chains and the association of heme and iron with the cell membrane after the degradation of precipitated hemoglobin chains.[488,594] Other abnormalities may result from selective interaction of excess α or β chains with the membrane cytoskeleton. After oxidation, globin chains, as well as trace metals such as iron and copper, generate free oxygen radicals that foster oxidative injury to the membrane.[595] Peroxidation of lipids in the red cell membrane is reflected by altered membrane lipid composition and distribution; polymerization of membrane components caused by lipid peroxidation leads to excessive calcium influx, monovalent cation loss and dehydration, decreased cell deformability, and increased rigidity of the phospholipid bilayer.[90,91,596] Similar changes are observed in normal red cells forced to engulf excess α chains.[597] The reductions observed in the level of serum and red cell vitamin E, a natural antioxidant, may result from accelerated consumption secondary to oxidant stress. The abnormal lipid distribution may contribute to enhanced clearance by macrophages. Increased binding of autologous immunoglobulin G (IgG) with an α-antigalactosyl specificity, originally proposed to reflect a decrease in sialic acid content of the membrane, may also promote clearance of thalassemic red cells from the circulation. The increased calcium content of thalassemic red cells is a hallmark of membrane damage.

Electrophoresis of red cell membrane proteins readily demonstrates an increased association of globin chains with the red cell membrane (up to 11% of total protein), and similar findings can be reproduced in nonthalassemic erythrocytes by exposure to experimental oxidative stress.[598] The α- and β-globin chains interact differently with components of the cytoskeleton.[599-601] The specificity of these interactions may contribute to the different phenotypic manifestations of the disorders. Membrane protein 4.1 of β-thalassemia erythrocytes has a diminished capacity to enhance the binding of spectrin to actin. In HbH disease, protein 4.1 appears to be normal, but binding of spectrin to inside-out vesicles is decreased, potentially because of oxidative damage to ankyrin promoted by binding of HbH to protein band 3, with which ankyrin interacts. Spectrin binding is normal in β-thalassemia erythrocytes.

Schrier and colleagues[602] reported differences in the rheologic properties of erythrocytes obtained from patients with HbH disease and β-thalassemia intermedia. Erythrocytes from both groups had a normal surface area but decreased cellular volume and increased membrane rigidity that resulted in decreased cellular deformability under conditions of hypertonic osmotic stress. Although HbH erythrocytes exhibit an increase in mechanical stability and a decrease in cell density, β-thalassemia erythrocytes are prone to cellular dehydration and have markedly decreased mechanical stability. In a murine model of β-thalassemia, these cellular abnormalities correlated with the extent of α-globin associated with the membrane; small increases in β-globin chain expression through the introduction of a β-globin transgene resulted in a marked decrease in membrane-associated globin and significant reversal of the rheologic abnormalities.[603] Thus, the slight improvements in chain synthetic balance that accompany increased expression of γ-globin or decreased expression of α-globin may result in dramatic improvements in membrane integrity in patients with β-thalassemia. More detailed understanding of the red cell membrane abnormalities in thalassemia may facilitate the development of novel therapies in the future.

Genetic Heterogeneity

In current hematologic parlance, the term *thalassemia major* refers to patients with severe β-thalassemia who require regular blood transfusions to sustain life. In the vast majority of such patients, both β-globin genes are affected by a thalassemia mutation; hence, they are described as homozygous β-thalassemics, although in the United States most are actually double heterozygotes. In other patients who also appear to be homozygous for β-thalassemia mutations based on family studies, a hemoglobin concentration of 6 to 10 g/dL is maintained without blood transfusions except during periods of infection, surgery, or other stress.[1,604] Such patients are said to have *thalassemia intermedia*. Thalassemia intermedia is a clinical term that describes the transfusion status of the patient. The term *Cooley's anemia* is still often used and applied somewhat indiscriminately to individual patients with either the major or intermedia clinical syndrome. Although other acquired and genetic modifiers exist, disease severity in the β-thalassemias is most directly related to the degree of imbalance between α- and total non–α-globin synthesis. Three major factors emerge as important determinants of the biosynthetic ratio in individual patients: the nature of the specific mutation or mutations, the presence of abnormalities in the α-globin cluster that increase or decrease α-globin expression, and the genetic capacity for synthesis of HbF. Proteolysis of excess α chains, evident on comparison of the α-to–non-α biosynthetic ratio by short- and long-term incubation of bone marrow cells[515-519] (see earlier), is also likely to modulate disease severity, although no meaningful quantitative studies of this mechanism have yet appeared. Recently, a chaperone of free α-globin chains has been described (see earlier discussion).

Nature of Specific Mutations

The capacity for production of β-globin chains in an individual with thalassemia is directly determined by the specific mutations involving the β-globin gene. Because several different mutations are commonly found in populations with a high incidence of β-thalassemia, most American patients with clinical homozygous β-thalassemia are heterozygous for two different mutations. The effect of specific mutations may range from total loss to only a mild impairment in β-globin synthesis, and thus the potential interactions based on the many different mutations are extraordinary. Indeed, disease severity may

be viewed as a continuum, the extremes of which have been shown to correlate with specific mutations.

Mutations in the IVS-1 splice donor site (see Table 20-2 and Fig. 20-11) provide a particularly illustrative example of the variable consequences of specific mutations on β-chain synthesis. These mutations lead to either a complete block in correct splicing of β-globin mRNA or merely a reduction in the abundance of normal mRNA. Patients homozygous for a mutation in the conserved GT splice junction dinucleotide and who have not coinherited an α-thalassemia gene or a determinant that increases HbF synthesis display severe transfusion-dependent β[0]-thalassemia.[129,133-135] Substitution of C or T at position 5 of the splice donor consensus sequence results in severe β[+]-thalassemia,[111,133,143-145] whereas substitution of A at the same position results in a more mild phenotype.[146] The T→C substitution at position 6 is also associated with mild β[+]-thalassemia.[129]

Dominant β-Thalassemia

In rare circumstances, the heterozygous state of β-thalassemia may be associated with severe disease rather than typical thalassemia trait. Several pedigrees with severe heterozygous β-thalassemia characterized by splenomegaly, cholelithiasis, and leg ulcers have been described.[605,606] A striking association has been noted between mutations involving exon 3 of the β-globin gene and these unusual cases of dominantly inherited β-thalassemia.[197,201] Third-exon mutations typically lead to the production of an unstable β-globin chain. A subset of third-exon β-thalassemia mutations are associated with the presence of inclusion bodies in the normoblasts of affected heterozygotes (see Table 20-2)[199-203] and were first reported as "inclusion-body β-thalassemia," originally defined as a dominantly inherited dyserythropoietic anemia.[607,608] The inclusion bodies, which may contain both α-globin and β-globin, represent an aggregation of precipitated α-globin and unstable β-globin chains with the cell membrane, where they presumably potentiate oxidative damage. The dominantly inherited β-thalassemias are relatively rare and are found in ethnic groups from nonmalarious regions.[197,201] Presumably, there is little selective pressure for these mutations because of the decreased fitness of heterozygous individuals.

Increased production of α-globin chains above normal levels may exacerbate the chain imbalance in β-thalassemia heterozygotes; coinheritance of triplicated α-globin gene chromosomes is another potential cause of severe heterozygous β-thalassemia, and patients usually have the phenotype of thalassemia intermedia.[437,438,6-9-611]

Interaction with Genetic Determinants That Increase Hemoglobin F Synthesis

Deletions within the β-globin gene cluster and mutations in the γ-globin promoters are sometimes associated with increased expression of γ-globin (see earlier discussion). Relatively small, genetically determined heterocellular increases in HbF ameliorate the clinical course of thalassemia,[93,94,343,356,463,539] thereby raising the prospect that pharmacologic augmentation of γ-chain production may be of particular benefit in the management of thalassemia (see later).

Readily demonstrated in thalassemic patients is an apparent amplification of the capacity for HbF synthesis during erythroid maturation. In the earliest erythroid precursor cells, γ-globin may be synthesized at a level less than that of β-globin and at only a small percentage of that of α-globin, yet the final proportion of HbF in patients not receiving transfusions may be quite high.[1,90] This occurs because the subset of cells expressing γ-globin have less overall globin chain imbalance and therefore preferentially survive in both bone marrow and peripheral blood. Hence, measurement of steady-state HbF levels provides an imperfect measure of the capacity for γ-globin synthesis in individual patients. More accurate assessment of the HbF program is achieved by measurement of the HbF accumulated in progenitor-derived erythroid colonies produced in vitro.[612]

Interaction of α- and β-Thalassemia Mutations

Because the clinical severity of α- and β-thalassemia correlates with the degree of imbalance in the production of α and non-α chains, coinheritance of α- and β-thalassemia mutations would be anticipated to yield syndromes of intermediate severity.[613-619] This principle has been validated by clinical experience.[96,620,621] One striking example is the influence of the number of functional α genes in individuals with β-thalassemia trait in Sardinia.[96] As shown in Table 20-9, MCV and MCH improve in a stepwise fashion as α-globin production decreases and the α-globin–to–β-globin ratio approaches 1, but they then deteriorate as the ratio decreases to less than 1. This analysis provides conclusive evidence that the degree of chain synthesis imbalance determines the red cell phenotype. Thus, a higher incidence of α-gene deletions (−α/αα or −α/−α) has been found in patients with thalassemia intermedia than in those with thalassemia. Further evidence for the effect of α-gene number on clinical phenotype is the occurrence of thalassemia intermedia in a subset of individuals doubly heterozygous for β-thalassemia and triplicated α genes (ααα/αα)[437,551,609-611] or severe β-thalassemia trait in individuals also heterozygous for triplicated α genes.[600,601,622-628] Individuals heterozygous for β-thalassemia but homozygous for triplicated α genes invariably have thalassemia intermedia.

Clinical Features and Laboratory Values on Initial Evaluation

Severe β-thalassemia is most often diagnosed between 6 months and 2 years of age when the normal physiologic anemia of the newborn fails to improve. γ-Globin production is not impaired in utero; therefore, only when β-globin becomes the predominant β-like globin does anemia ensue. Occasionally, the disease is not recognized until 3 to 5 years of age because prolonged HbF synthesis compensates for the lack of HbA. When first seen, affected infants usually display pallor, poor growth, and abdominal enlargement from hepatosplenomegaly.

Children with severe β-thalassemia are readily distinguished from those with other congenital hemolytic anemias. At initial evaluation, patients who have not received transfusions show 20% to 100% HbF, 2% to 7% HbA$_2$, and 0% to 80% HbA (see Fig. 20-24), depending on the precise genotype. Consistent with severe ineffective erythropoiesis and splenomegaly, the reticulocyte count is characteristically low (often<1%), whereas the nucleated red cell count is elevated. Erythrocytes are severely microcytic (MCV of 50 to 60 μm^3) with a hemoglobin content as low as 12 to 18 pg/cell. HbF can be shown to be heterogeneously distributed among the red cells either by the Betke-Kleihauer acid elution technique or by anti-HbF fluorescent staining (see Fig. 20-20).

Bone marrow examination reveals marked erythroid hyperplasia, often with an erythroid-to-myeloid cell ratio of 20:1 or greater. Before the onset of hypersplenism, the accelerated rate of hematopoiesis may also be reflected by elevated white cell and platelet counts in peripheral blood. The serum iron value is markedly elevated, but total iron-binding capacity is usually only slightly increased, thereby resulting in a transferrin saturation of 80% or greater. Serum ferritin levels are generally elevated for age.

If laboratory parameters fail to establish the diagnosis of thalassemia, demonstration of a mild microcytic and hypochromic anemia, indicative of the presence of thalassemia trait in both parents, will allow the diagnosis to be made with confidence. If the diagnosis remains in doubt, it can be confirmed by globin genotyping.

TABLE 20-9   **Effect of Successive α-Globin Gene Deletion on Hematologic Parameters in a Homogeneous Population with β-Thalassemia Trait**

Group/Genotype	Hb (g/dL)	MCV (mm³)	MCH (pg)	HbA₂ (%)	HbF (%)	Ratio
αα/αα (n = 20)	12.4 ± 1.2	66.2 ± 3.7	21.2 ± 1.2	4.8 ± 0.7	1.4 ± 1.3	2.2 ± 0.3
α−/αα (n = 12)	12.8 ± 1.3	67.3 ± 3.4	22.1 ± 1.1	5.2 ± 0.7	1 ± 0.3	1.3 ± 0.1
α−/α− (n = 4)	14.1 ± 1.1	76 + 3.4	24.8 ± 1.4	4.8 ± 0.6	1.3 ± 0.7	0.8 ± 0.1
α−/−− (n = 4)	11.7 ± 0.8	54.7 ± 2.5	18.4 ± 0.8	4.6 ± 0.2	—	0.5 ± 0.05

Adapted from Kanavakis K, Wainscoat JS, Wood WG, et al. The interaction of alpha thalassemia with beta thalassemia. Br J Haematol. 1982;52:465-473.

Complications

The etiology of the complications of thalassemia is multifactorial and variable and depends on the genotype, other known and unknown phenotypic modifiers, and availability and adherence to therapy. The pathophysiology of the complications stems from ineffective and extramedullary hematopoiesis and treatment-related side effects, including transfusional iron overload, transfusion-associated infections, and chelation. In addition, more recently recognized but not fully understood is the increased risk for clinically evident and silent thromboses leading to pulmonary hypertension and overt portal vein thromboses. The complications of thalassemia in a large group of North American patients have recently been reviewed.[629]

Bones

To appreciate the full spectrum of bone changes in severe β-thalassemia, one must examine patients who receive transfusions rarely.[572,573] Bone disease in such patients is primarily related to erythroid expansion and not to iron overload or abnormalities in vitamin D metabolism.[630,631] Maintenance of nearly normal hemoglobin levels results in suppression of erythropoiesis and tends to reverse the bone abnormalities,[600,601,622-628,632-634] but osteoporosis is common even in patients who receive regular transfusions.[635-638] Some clinics report a high incidence of vertebral compression fractures.[637] A recent review of more than 700 patients with thalassemia syndromes reported an overall fracture prevalence of 12.1% that ranged from 2.5% in very young patients to 23% in those older than 20 years. Therapy with excessively high doses and sometimes even standard doses of deferoxamine may also lead to metaphyseal dysplasia.[639-641]

Radiologic abnormalities may be present during the first 6 months of life but are not usually marked until about 1 year of age.[642] In the small bones of the hands and feet the trabecular pattern is coarse, cystic abnormalities are present, and the bones are tubular in appearance. The long bones of the extremities exhibit thinning of the cortices and marked dilation of the medullary cavities. Accordingly, they become extremely fragile and prone to pathologic fractures.[643] The skull is also classically involved, with marked widening of the diploic space and arrangement of the trabeculae in vertical rows, which tends to give a "hair on end" appearance to the skull radiograph (Fig. 20-30). Other radiologic abnormalities in the skull include failure of pneumatization of the maxillary sinuses and overgrowth of the maxilla. These changes lead to maxillary overbite, prominence of the upper incisors, and separation of the orbits—changes that contribute to the classic "thalassemic facies."

Other bone changes caused by medullary overgrowth include widening of the ribs with notching and the development of masses of extramedullary hematopoietic tissue, which may appear as tumors in the chest and mediastinum. The vertebrae are square with coarse trabeculae.

The aforementioned osteoporosis and associated bone pain may be relieved by calcitonin therapy,[644] but the role of vitamin D and calcium supplementation in the prevention of osteoporosis in patients with thalassemia has not been established. Controlled randomized studies have revealed the potential value of bisphosphonate therapy to improve bone denisty as measured with bone density scans.[645]

Gallbladder

Calcium bilirubinate gallstones secondary to excessive excretion of the products of heme catabolism are common in older patients.

Iron Deposition

Most longitudinal studies of iron overload have used serum iron, iron-binding capacity, and ferritin as noninvasive measures of stored iron. As mentioned earlier, these parameters are easily perturbed by the effects of other diseases (e.g., hepatitis) or are highly variable (iron/iron-binding capacity). Some clinics still rely on the measurement of ferritin.[646] The relationship between serum ferritin and body iron stores as measured by quantitative assay of liver iron remains poor. In a recent study using superconducting quantum interference device (SQUID) technology, only 25% of the variance in body iron could be explained by the variance in serum ferritin.[647] This confirms the earlier studies of Brittenham and co-workers.[648] The poor correlation between serum ferritin and total body iron in thalassemic patients receiving many transfusions[649] can perhaps be improved somewhat by measuring the glycosylated form.[650] Grading of stainable iron in liver biopsy samples also offers a rough assessment of parenchymal iron stores. Biopsy also provides a view of histology, as well as direct chemical measurement of iron. It should be mentioned that excessive fibrosis may cause a false reduction in tissue iron content as estimated by measurements on biopsy material. Thus, there is no true "gold standard" of liver iron content. Only serial measurements of ferritin and an imaging signal in which patients serve as their own control provide a practical approach to analysis of the course of treatment.

Computed tomography (CT) has been used to demonstrate iron overload in patients with thalassemia by detection of increased density of the liver.[651-654] CT scans have also shown increased density of the spleen, pancreas, adrenal glands, and lymph nodes in the abdomens of these patients[655] while also offering another assessment of extramedullary hematopoiesis[656-658] and bone abnormalities.[659] Repeated CT examinations involve substantial radiation doses. Magnetic resonance imaging (MRI) has become the favored repeated imaging approach for iron assessment in the liver because of x-ray dosage considerations. The procedure is not always suitable for small children because it requires cooperation, but recent applications have provided reproducible and clinically useful results within the range of hepatic iron content

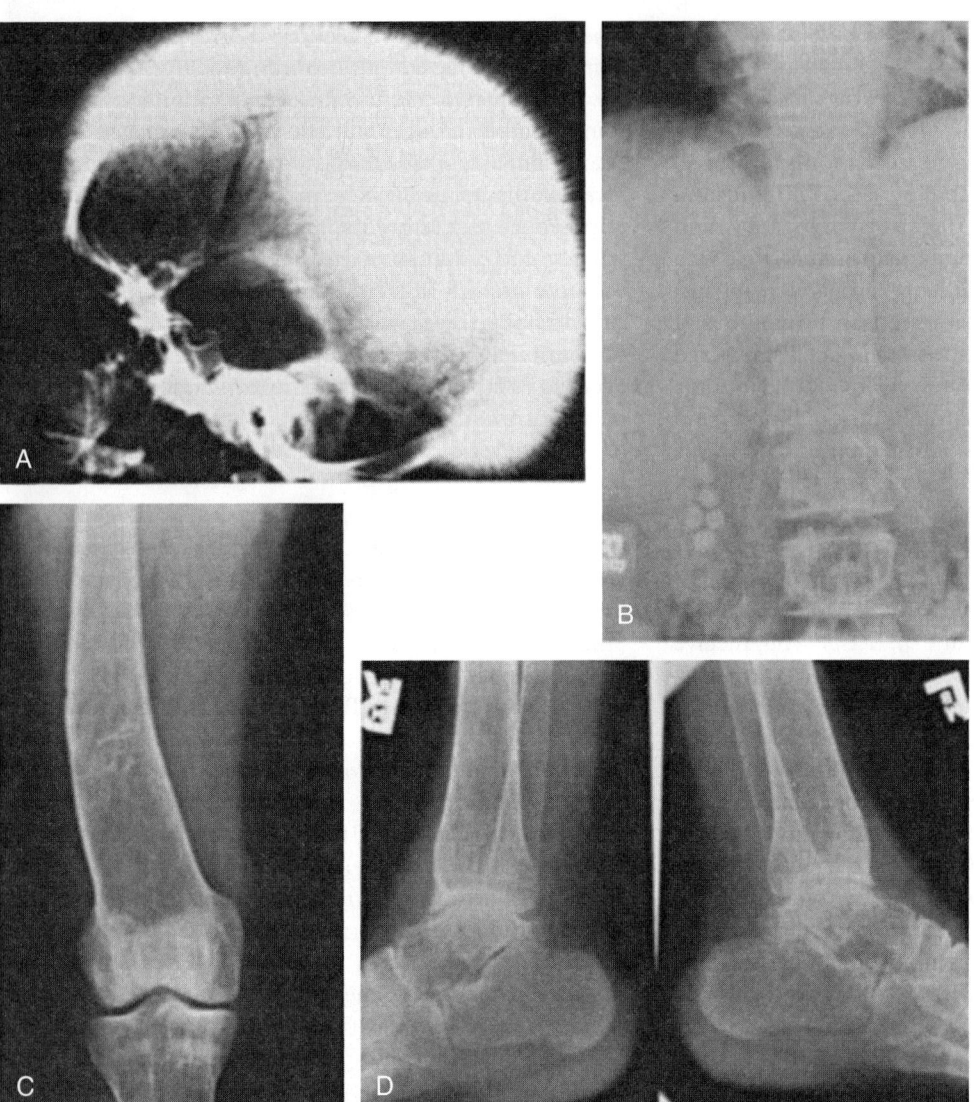

FIGURE 20-30. Radiologic abnormalities in a patient with homozygous β-thalassemia who receives blood transfusions rarely (thalassemia intermedia). **A,** Skull radiograph illustrating the typical "hair on end" appearance of the diploë and failure of pneumatization of the frontal sinus. **B,** Abdominal film illustrating the coarse trabeculation and osteoporosis within the vertebrae. Multiple calcified gallstones are also seen. **C,** Severe osteoporosis, pseudofractures, thinning of the cortex, and bowing of the femur. **D,** Degenerative arthritis affecting the tibiotalar joint in particular is reflected by loss of the cartilage space and sclerosis in the adjacent bone.

expected in thalassemic patients.[6592,660] T2* MRI is now used in thalassemia centers for assessment of cardiac iron content because it is a technique uniquely suited to capturing data from a moving organ. Though yet to be validated in patients by an independent measurement, it is useful clinically and in therapeutic research.[661,662] This technology has demonstrated that iron is removed more slowly from the heart than from the liver and has allowed enhanced chelation strategies to remove lethal iron from the heart.[663]

Determination of hepatic magnetic susceptibility with SQUID technology has been proved to have excellent correlation with direct measurement of hepatic iron by biopsy,[542,543] but it is very expensive, highly complex, generally unavailable, and poorly reproducible from center to center. It will probably be abandoned as a clinical tool.

Pathophysiology of Iron Deposition. The original pathologic description of thalassemia[544,575] was concerned

with conditions extant in the untreated state and is not relevant to conditions seen in patients today who receive transfusions chronically and thus become iron overloaded. In countries in which transfusion is widely available, patients demonstrate few of the stigmata that characterized the disease during the first few years of life in patients who do not receive transfusions. Depending on the level of hemoglobin maintained, most patients fortunately no longer have difficulty with the marked erythroid hyperplasia that causes extensive medullary expansion and its consequent pathologic changes.[576] However, patients are now confronted with consequences of the chronic iron overload that accompany routine transfusion therapy.[664] In a study of British Cypriot patients at autopsy, Modell[665] found evidence of marked iron deposition in the liver, pancreas, thyroid, parathyroid, adrenal zona glomerulosa, renal medulla, heart, bone marrow, and spleen. Such parenchymal iron loading and the accumulation of "free" or non–transferrin-bound iron in blood remain the major causes of morbidity and mortality in patients with severe β-thalassemia.

Although the contribution of transfusional iron to iron toxicity is easily appreciated, anemic thalassemic patients also have markedly enhanced gastrointestinal iron absorption,[666] particularly patients with thalassemia intermedia, such as those with HbE-β-thalassemia.[545,667] This seems paradoxical because one might expect suppression of iron absorption in the presence of iron overload. In normal individuals, a portion of dietary iron presented to the gut lumen is transported across the brush border of the gut epithelium and is available for transfer to the plasma iron transport protein transferrin. The individual's iron status should then determine the amount of iron eventually presented to the serum pool.[668] The observation that anemic patients with thalassemia major bypass the ferroportin mechanism in intestinal epithelial cells (see Chapter 12) and thereby display increased iron absorption is at least partially understood.

Calculations by Modell and Berdoukas[669] suggested that the kinetic requirement of the expanded bone marrow for iron to make new red cells exceeds the rate at which the reticuloendothelial system is able to salvage iron from senescent red cells and replenish the erythron with iron. On this basis they argue that the bone marrow is relatively iron deficient on a kinetic basis, thereby leading to enhanced gastrointestinal absorption. Increased absorption is variable[666] (range, 2% to 40%) and appears to be directly related to erythroid activity[670,671] measured by either morphologic observation of patient bone marrow[672] or enumeration of nucleated red cells in peripheral blood.[666] Experimental studies in animals suggest that hypoxia, even in the absence of increased erythropoiesis, may increase iron absorption.[673]

Hepcidin and ferroportin are pivotal to the increased iron absorption in the presence of ineffective erythropoiesis (see Chapter 12 for further details). It was first discovered that elevated hepcidin mediates iron retention by macrophages and causes internalization of ferroportin on the intestinal brush border, which leads to failure of intestinal absorption. Conversely, hepcidin levels fall in response to iron deficiency, hypoxia, erythropoietin, or ineffective erythropoiesis, thus explaining the increase in intestinal iron absorption in thalassemic syndromes.[674,675] That hepcidin remains inappropriately low suggests that the erythroid drive is a more potent regulator than the iron overload. A decrease in erythroid drive via transfusions upregulates hepcidin.[675,676] The signaling molecule between erythroid drive and down-regulation of hepcidin is being actively investigated. A recent study in the murine model demonstrated that inappropriately low hepcidin levels dominate the pathophysiology of iron loading early in life and upregulation of ferroportin mediates the absorption in later life.[676] This has yet to be studied in humans. Concomitant mutations in the *HFE* gene also increase iron overload in thalassemia.[677,678]

With most modern transfusion regimens, iron absorption is significantly decreased but iron loading is increased as transfused red cells become senescent and their iron is deposited in the reticuloendothelial system. Reticuloendothelial cells relinquish iron directly to transferrin. Although the erythron usually claims most of this circulating iron, a certain amount is also delivered to other cells according to their individual needs. Cellular uptake may normally depend on the number of transferrin receptors on the cell membrane.[679] As iron accumulates in the body, individual tissues, particularly the liver, accelerate their production of apoferritin molecules to store the iron in a nontoxic form as ferritin or hemosiderin.[680,681]

Apoferritin production can be monitored by measurement of the serum ferritin concentration via radioimmunoassay. In patients receiving multiple transfusions[682] and in patients with increased gastrointestinal iron absorption who do not receive transfusions,[683] serum ferritin levels correlate well with total body iron stores during the first several years of iron loading, but less well later.[684] Serum ferritin is an acute phase reactant, as well as a product of hepatocellular damage. Infection, congestive heart failure, and hepatitis may elevate serum ferritin levels. Thus, in patients with marked iron overload, the serum ferritin level correlates poorly with liver iron concentration. Patients with thalassemia intermedia have severe hepcidin deficiency, which leads to hyperabsorption of dietary iron, as well as depletion of iron in macrophages. It has been suggested that this is the basis of the lack of correlation between liver iron content and serum ferritin levels in thalassemia intermedia.[685]

The human body is extremely conservative in its handling of iron (see Chapter 12). Under normal conditions, iron is always found in the presence of a chelating protein with a high affinity constant. Serum transferrin binds iron with an association constant of 10 to 20 mol/L.[686-688] When transferrin arrives at its surface receptor, the complex is transferred to the "labile iron pool"[689] by receptor-mediated endocytosis.[541,688,690,691] This pool supplies iron to cytosolic proteins. The remaining iron is directed to apoferritin for storage as ferritin. When ferritin molecules accumulate, the protein moiety is apparently cleaved, with smaller hemosiderin granules remaining but with greater iron concentrations.[547] Theoretically, these storage forms of iron are inert and do not exert any pathologic damage. However, accumulated hemosiderin granules appear to cause release of hydrolytic enzymes from lysosomes that are toxic to the cell.[692,693]

As iron stores increase from both transfusions and gastrointestinal absorption, transferrin becomes saturated with iron to greater than 90%. In parallel, a circulating pool of non–transferrin-bound or free serum iron is found in iron-overloaded individuals.[546,694-698] Its source is uncertain but presumably reflects expansion of the intracellular labile iron pool, and it is thought to be particularly cardiotoxic.

Cell damage probably occurs as a result of iron-related catalysis leading to oxidation of membrane components.[699,700] Unbound iron induces lipid peroxidation in vitro.[701-703] Peroxidation of mitochondrial membranes and hepatocyte microsomes has been demonstrated in vivo in rats overloaded with iron by parenteral or oral administration[704] and in the spleens of thalassemic patients.[705] Lysosomal leakage of hemosiderin and hydrolytic enzymes may also occur.[706,707] Cultured rat myocardial cells have been used to study the effects of iron deposition.[708] Peroxidation of membrane lipids induces functional abnormalities in cultured myocardial cells that are exacerbated by ascorbic acid (see later), corrected in part by the antioxidant vitamin E, and markedly suppressed by chelation with deferoxamine.[709]

Further evidence in support of the free radical hypothesis stems from measurement of substances that defend against free radical attack. Vitamin E, a potent antioxidant, is decreased in the serum and red cells of iron-overloaded thalassemic patients.[488,710] Both vitamin E levels[711] and total serum antioxidant activity bear strong inverse correlations to the degree of iron overload.[712] Perhaps most intriguing is a correlation between superoxide production in resting neutrophils and serum ferritin in patients receiving multiple transfusions. The observed superoxide generation approaches five times normal in some patients.[713] It should be empahsized, however, that replacement therapy with vitamin E has little or no value in thalassemia. Elimination of iron by chelation is the only way to prevent iron-induced oxidative damage.

Indirect data also suggest that the route of accumulation (i.e., gastrointestinal absorption versus parenteral red cell transfusion) may be an important determinant of iron toxicity.[714,715] Attention must be paid to the contribution of gastrointestinal iron absorption.[666,672] Experiments in rats suggest that oral iron loading leads to more global hepatocyte damage than parenteral loading does.[704] Patients with hereditary hemochromatosis and thalassemia intermedia who do not receive transfusions sustain parenchymal damage entirely from gastrointestinal absorption.[672,716,717] On the other hand, extensive transfusion in patients with hypoplastic anemia is associated with a lower incidence of cirrhosis.[714] Nonetheless, the view that reticuloendothelial iron derived from transfused red cells is innocuous is overly simplistic. There are no reasons to believe that transfusion protocols, designed to maintain a normal hemoglobin level and reduce gastrointestinal iron absorption, will be free of the complications of iron overload.

Clinical Consequences of Iron Deposition. Patients with thalassemia major have traditionally died of the cardiac complications of iron overload.[581] Recurrent pericarditis, distinguished by characteristic pain, fever, and a friction rub, may be the initial manifestation of myocardial iron deposition and occasionally requires pericardectomy to relieve constriction. Ventricular tachycardia and fibrillation or severe refractory congestive heart failure are often fatal.[718]

Cardiac iron deposition has been studied in autopsies of patients with transfusional hemosiderosis and idiopathic hemochromatosis.[719,720] Patients with a history of transfusion of more than 100 units of red cells without chronic blood loss generally exhibit significant cardiac iron deposition. Cardiac hemosiderosis is not observed unless significant iron accumulation has occurred in other organs. Cardiac iron deposits that are grossly visible at autopsy indicate that the patient experienced cardiac dysfunction during life, but severe cardiac dysfunction may also occur in the absence of significant deposits of cardiac hemosiderin.[720,721] Therefore, iron toxicity must be due to a small, highly reactive intracellular iron pool or to the labile pool of non–transferrin-bound iron in plasma. Prevention of cardiac dysfunction therefore requires a reduction in the iron load and persistent presence of a chelator in the blood. Preliminary data suggest that deferiprone, a chelator approved in Europe but not in the United States, removes iron from the heart more effectively than deferoxamine does.[722] In vitro data demonstrate better access to and removal of iron from rat cardiac myocytes by both deferiprone and deferasirox than by deferoxamine.[723] In a gerbil model of iron overload, deferiprone and deferasirox have similar capacity to remove iron from myocytes.[724] The clinical significance of these observations remains to be confirmed.

Cardiac disease in thalassemia and particularly thalassemia intermedia after splenectomy may be unrelated to cardiac iron deposition but instead be due to pulmonary hypertension secondary to platelet activation together with the circulation of erythrocyte membrane fragments and the induction of an hypercoagulable state.[725-727]

Gross anatomic cardiac changes attributable to iron loading include dilation of the atrial and ventricular cavities and overall thickening of the muscle layer resulting in a twofold to threefold increase in heart weight. Microscopic evaluation suggests that iron is first deposited in the ventricular myocardium and later in conduction tissue.[719] Thus, intracavitary endomyocardial biopsy is not useful in these patients as a means of evaluating cardiac iron deposition.[728,729] Supraventricular arrhythmias correlate well with the extent of iron deposition in the atrial myocardium but may occur in its relative absence. Cardiac abnormalities seem to be a function of both the quantity of iron deposited per fiber and the absolute number of fibers affected. Link and colleagues[730] have shown that myocardial cells in culture take up iron if there is no physiologic or pharmacologic chelator present. As iron loading takes place, peroxidation products accumulate and contractility and rhythm are disturbed.[709] This in vitro model parallels concepts developed from clinical findings.

Noninvasive Studies of Cardiac Function. Echocardiography, radionuclide cineangiography, and 24-hour recording of cardiac rhythm have been used to assess the effects of iron deposition in the heart and evaluate the results of chelation therapy.[731] In general, echocardiography may reveal alterations in cardiac anatomy but little change in cardiac function until clinically evident cardiomyopathy develops.[732-734] Low-dose dobutamine echocardiography is thought by some to be more helpful.[735] Radionuclide cineangiography offers the ability to observe dynamic cardiac function during exercise and may reveal changes in function before the appearance of clinical disease.[734,736-738] Twenty-four-hour recordings of cardiac rhythm in patients with iron overload have demonstrated marked disturbances in most patients older than 12 years regardless of clinical symptoms.[731] As previosuly mentioned, T2* MRI can be used to assess cardiac iron. It demonstrates that patients with high cardiac iron content are at substantial risk for sudden cardiac decompensation. However, patients with high liver iron and low cardiac iron are also at risk, and liver and cardiac iron correlate poorly, largely because the kinetics of iron flux are different in the two organs. Serial MRI assessment of *both* liver and cardiac iron are required for careful follow-up of thalassemic patients. Box 20-1 summarizes the clinical course of patients before the onset of aggressive chelation programs. The efficacy of future transfusion and chelation programs must be assessed in this context. Considerable data have recently demonstrated the bene-fits of chelation therapy, both for prophylaxis and for treatment of cardiac disease in patients with iron overloading (see later).

Hepatic Abnormalities. Liver enlargement, long viewed as a hallmark of thalassemia, is prominent with contemporary transfusion regimens only in patients older than 10 years. Hepatomegaly is due to progressive engorgement of hepatic parenchymal and phagocytic cells with hemosiderin deposits rather than extramedullary hematopoiesis.[739] Hepatic iron stores correlate very well with total body iron stores.[740] In addition, iron deposition induces intralobular fibrosis.[741,742] Intercurrent episodes of hepatitis may lead to marked liver dysfunction and contribute to the development of fibrosis and cirrhosis.[743-745] Liver enzyme levels are rarely elevated in the absence of hepatitis. The concentration of total bilirubin in patients receiving adequate transfusion therapy is seldom greater than 2 mg/dL, 50% or less of which is typically indirect. Recent data clearly demonstrate that chelation therapy reduces the liver iron concentration[740,746-748] and forestalls iron-induced liver damage. Progressive liver disease in patients receiving appropriate therapy is often due to viral hepatitis.[749] A recent study demonstrated the value of interferon and ribavirin in the management of hepatitis C in patients with thalassemia.[749a] Despite expected increases in transfusion requirements because of ribavirin-induced hemolysis, patients tolerated the therapy, the degree of inflammation as measured by alanine transaminase and hepatic biopsy decreased, and the molar efficacy of deferoxamine improved.

Endocrine Abnormalities. Endocrine disorders commonly associated with thalassemia in the United States today are generally thought to be caused by chronic iron loading.[664,669,750,751] Most of the pathologic changes develop slowly and are not usually apparent until the second decade of life. In patients not receiving transfusions, these abnormalities develop more slowly.

Growth and Development. Growth retardation, historically considered a typical finding in thalassemia major,[750] is generally associated with moderate retardation in bone age. Patients undergoing chronic transfusion therapy may be spared growth retardation,[752] which is seen in more than 50% of patients and then not until the second decade of life.[669] Growth retardation is less evident in patients receiving chelation therapy,[752,753] although excessive amounts of deferoxamine can also impair growth.[754,755] Alternative causes should be sought in young thalassemic children who are receiving adequate transfusion therapy and still exhibit significant growth retardation.

Growth retardation may also be associated with evidence of endocrine dysfunction. Impaired growth hormone production has been reported in some patients[756-758] but not confirmed in others.[759] Treatment with growth hormone may accelerate the growth rate, but final height may not be changed.[760] A subset of patients

---

| BOX 20-1 | **Cardiac Disease in Patients with Iron Overload** |

STAGE I (<100 UNITS TRANSFUSED)

Asymptomatic
Echocardiogram: slight left ventricular wall thickening
Radionuclide cineangiogram: normal
24-Hour electrocardiogram: normal

STAGE II (100-400 UNITS TRANSFUSED)

Asymptomatic or mild fatigue
Echocardiogram: left ventricular wall thickening; left ventricular dilation but normal ejection fraction
Radionuclide cineangiogram: normal at rest but no increase or fall in ejection fraction with exercise
24-Hour electrocardiogram: atrial and ventricular premature beats

STAGE III

Palpitations and/or congestive heart failure
Echocardiogram: decreased ejection fraction
Radionuclide cineangiogram: normal or decreased ejection fraction at rest but a fall in ejection fraction during exercise
24-Hour electrocardiogram: atrial and ventricular premature beats, often in pairs or runs

Adapted from Nienhuis AW, Griffith P, Strawczynski H, et al. Evaluation of cardiac function in patients with thalassemia major. Ann N Y Acad Sci. 1980;344:384-396.

with normal growth hormone production have low serum levels of somatomedin,[761] a factor produced by the liver in response to growth hormone that promotes cartilage growth. Failure of adrenal androgen production may also contribute to growth failure.[762] Thyroid deficiency is an additional factor that may potentially contribute (see later). A thorough search for endocrine dysfunction is warranted in patients with growth retardation because a favorable response to specific replacement therapy may be anticipated.

Puberty. Puberty will occur normally in many patients with β-thalassemia who receive appropriate treatment and is typically seen in those with the least growth retardation. Sexual maturation is variably observed in other patients and is retarded in patients whose transfusion and chelation therapy is inadequate.[763] Failure of patients receiving transfusions to mature sexually may be the first indication of iron toxicity. Breast development in females tends to begin normally, but menarche is frequently delayed until the late teenage years. In many female patients who progress through puberty normally, secondary amenorrhea will develop as a result of progressive iron accumulation.

Failure of patients to develop sexually is not usually related to primary end-organ unresponsiveness.[764,765] Although males tend to have low baseline testosterone levels, the response to treatment with human chorionic gonadotropin is generally normal.[765] Moreover, spermatogenesis correlates directly with the stage of sexual maturation of the patient.[766] Gonadotropins, on the other hand, have been implicated in a number of studies as the primary cause of dysfunction in the hypothalamic-pituitary-gonadal axis.[765,767-770] Although defective ovarian function has been described in some patients,[771] patients who fail to attain puberty or who have experienced regression of secondary sexual characteristics demonstrate blunted responses to luteinizing hormone–releasing factor (LHRF) and follicle-stimulating hormone. Prolactin levels respond normally to thyroid-releasing factor stimulation. Failure of sexual maturation therefore appears to most often be related to hypothalamic-pituitary axis dysfunction, and the anterior pituitary is often loaded with iron.

Although one report suggested preservation of normal gonadotropin production in young patients receiving large amounts of chelation therapy,[766] modification of transfusion schedules and chelation therapy has not yet been found to preserve normal function in many patients. This is a problem of increasing severity as the long-term clinical prognosis for patients improves. In approaching such patients, Modell and Berdoukas[669] have likened the attainment of puberty as a trophy in a race between a patient's physical growth and iron overload. Patients with a constitution that favors tall stature and a rapid growth rate and whose transfusion programs and chelation regimens are adequate are likely to attain puberty. Those who do not require transfusion in the first year of life may also have an advantage. Constitutionally short children and those whose transfusion and chelation regimens are inadequate often fail to "win the race."

For patients with delayed puberty, initial efforts should be devoted to assessment of nutritional status, general health (i.e., presence of hepatitis), and the adequacy of transfusion and chelation therapy. In addition, attention should be paid to the availability of calcium for growth (see later). For those receiving maximal therapy who have delayed puberty and also biochemical evidence of hypothalamic-pituitary axis dysfunction,[772,773] pulsatile gonadotropin-releasing hormone infusions have been used to artificially induce puberty and growth (Chaterjee B: personal communication),[774] although this approach may or may not be successful.[769] More conventional treatment regimens include testosterone or estrogen supplementation after the age of 14 or 15 for those in whom puberty was not achieved or in whom secondary hypogonadism has developed, either clinically or based on loss of response to LHRF.

Thyroid Gland. Even though iron deposition in thyroid parenchymal tissue is often extensive, dysfunction is usually limited to primary subclinical hypothyroidism.[775] In one large series in which simultaneous serum thyroxine and thyroid-stimulating hormone (TSH) levels were obtained in 31 thalassemic patients, mean thyroxine levels were significantly lower (6.2 versus 9.5 µg/dL) and TSH levels were significantly higher (3.2 versus 1.0 µU/mL) than those in age-matched control subjects.[767] In a longitudinal study, serum thyroxine levels declined, whereas TSH secretion increased. Although the means were significantly different, individual patients with thalassemia could not be reliably distinguished from control subjects. Androgen replacement in males may correct abnormalities in thyroid function.[776]

Adrenal Gland. In the adrenal gland, pathologic changes in patients with thalassemia are historically characterized by iron deposition limited primarily to the zona glomerulosa,[544] the site of mineralocorticoid production. Iron deposition in the zona fasciculata may also occur.[669] In one series, normal aldosterone production in response to salt deprivation was achieved only at the expense of a marked increase in serum renin.[761] Basal morning adrenocorticotropic hormone (ACTH) levels measured in prepubertal thalassemic patients were 3 to 10 times normal.[777] Basal glucocorticoid production and response to ACTH and insulin provocation are generally normal in younger patients, although older patients often demonstrate a blunted provocative response.

Pancreas. Diabetes mellitus, a common and often under-recognized complication of thalassemia, is due to both pancreatic hypoproduction[778] and (at least in some patients) insulin resistance.[779] Even in patients between

5 and 10 years of age whose iron burden is approximately 5 to 20 g, fasting blood glucose levels are significantly elevated.[777] When glucose tolerance tests are performed, as many as 50% of thalassemic patients have "chemical diabetes"; the majority of these patients have normal or elevated circulating insulin levels.[779,780] Insulin resistance may predate the onset of glucose intolerance, as revealed by the euglycemic clamp method.[781] In contrast, thalassemic patients who have not received transfusions display accelerated insulin clearance and normal tissue sensitivity.[782] As symptoms of diabetes become evident, insulin output decreases, as occurs in most patients with juvenile diabetes. Glucose intolerance generally correlates with the number of transfusions received, age of the patient, and genetic predisposition.[783]

Parathyroid Glands. Symptomatic parathyroid disease manifested by classic tetany, hypocalcemia, and hyperphosphatemia is said to be an uncommon complication of iron overload.[767,778,783-785] However, the prevalence was 10% in one recent study. Affected patients had severe iron overloading.[786] Subclinical deficiency of parathyroid function is difficult to diagnose. The provocative use of calcium chelates to identify subclinical deficiency of parathormone has been described.[787] Patients with thalassemia major have been reported to show diminished response to a challenge. Although symptomatic parathyroid disease may be rare, more common defects may affect the mobilization of calcium for growth and the preservation of normal serum ionized calcium, which are important in patients with cardiomyopathy or arrhythmia. To complicate matters, deficiency of activated vitamin D may occur, perhaps partially as a consequence of parathormone deficiency. Symptoms of 25-hydroxytachysterol deficiency, which are relieved either by iron chelation therapy or by vitamin D supplementation, have been described in case reports.[788,789] Therefore, careful attention should be paid to calcium, phosphate, and vitamin D intake in patients with growth disturbances and cardiac disease.

Pulmonary Abnormalities

Arterial Hypoxemia and Pulmonary Hypertension. In 1981, Fucharoen and co-workers[790] reported significant arterial hypoxemia in patients with HbE–β-thalassemia, especially in those who had been splenectomized. These authors found circulating platelet aggregates in such patients and successfully used aspirin and dipyridamole to improve oxygenation. Other groups have reported hypoxemia in thalassemia major[791-800] but have related it to changes in ventilatory mechanics, obstructive airway disease, or iron deposition in the lungs. Pulmonary hypertension, possibly associated with thrombocytosis and a general hypercoagulable state,[801] may contribute to right ventricular dysfunction in these patients.[802-807] A more recent multivariate analysis demonstrated that splenectomy was significant correlated with pulmonary hypertension in patients with thalassemia syndromes. Further studies support the role of increased platelet activation as measured by P-selectin[727] and impaired nitric oxide.[808]

Therapy for β-Thalassemia

Transfusion

Choice of Transfusion Regimen. The mainstay of management of severe β-thalassemia remains blood transfusion.[809-816] Transfusion programs have several aims. By increasing the hemoglobin content, transfusions enhance the oxygen-carrying capacity of blood and thereby decrease tissue hypoxia. The concomitant fall in erythropoietin levels blunts the massive erythroid expansion associated with the anemia. Furthermore, improved tissue oxygenation and reversal of the hypercatabolic state promote more normal growth and development. Suppression of erythropoiesis is associated with decreased intestinal iron absorption. These benefits must be weighed against the prospects of excessive iron loading, particularly with more intensive transfusion protocols.

Transfusion management and the optimal maintenance level of hemoglobin have evolved. Wolman and associates[576,655] first recommended a pretransfusion hemoglobin level of 8.5 g/dL. This approach improved survival, but chronic illness, bone disease, and anemic cardiomyopathy persisted. To enhance quality of life, Piomelli and colleagues[580] suggested maintaining the hemoglobin level at greater than 10 g/dL with a mean of 12 g/dL. Such "hypertransfusion," if initiated in the first year of life, promotes normal initial growth and development, limits the development of hepatosplenomegaly, prevents disfiguring bone abnormalities, reduces intestinal iron absorption, and decreases cardiac workload.[817-820]

In 1980, Propper co-workers[821] proposed a "supertransfusion" program with a pretransfusion hemoglobin level greater than 12 g/dL and a mean of 14 g/dL to more effectively eliminate chronic tissue hypoxia. Initial studies reported that the quantity of blood required to maintain a higher hemoglobin level was no greater than that required for maintenance of a lower level because of a decrease in intravascular volume.[821-823] Further data, however, suggested that increasing the pretransfusion hemoglobin level may simply increase the quantity of transfused blood and thus increase iron loading,[669,824] and this regimen is no longer recommended.

Senescence in red cells is a function of cell age. Because the iron content of transfused erythrocytes is independent of cell age, attempts have been made to improve the "quality" of transfused blood by infusing the youngest third of red cells present in whole blood ("neocytes").[818,825] Administration of these cells would be predicted to decrease the transfusion requirement. Neocytes can be readily prepared with automated cell separators,[826-830] but 3 or more units is required to prepare the equivalent of 1 unit of blood, thus drastically increasing donor exposure for these patients. Although prolonged survival of neocytes has been documented in vivo, the observed sparing of transfusions with such therapy has been disappointing.[831-834] Similarly, methods to remove "gerocytes" (old red cells) from the recipient's circulation at the time of transfusion, though technically feasible, have not been widely applied.[833,835] These approaches should be considered experimental at present.

Although specific practices differ among clinical centers, transfusion is indicated both to correct anemia and to suppress erythropoiesis.[809] After diagnosis, a period of observation should be initiated to determine whether transfusion is required to maintain the hemoglobin level at 7 g/dL or greater. The condition of patients with thalassemia intermedia will be stable without transfusion. If the hemoglobin level falls to less than 7 g/dL, a transfusion program should be initiated to maintain the hemoglobin level at 9.5 to 11.5 g/dL. During the first decade of life, normal growth provides reassurance that the transfusion regimen is adequate. Because the rate of iron absorption parallels the number of nucleated red cells in peripheral blood,[666] adequate transfusion should suppress the nucleated cell count to less than 5 per 100 white blood cells[809]; however, in older patients who received inadequate transfusion therapy early in life, it may not be possible to achieve this level. During the teenage years, growth failure may reflect endocrine dysfunction rather than inadequate transfusions; laboratory investigation and appropriate replacement therapy are then indicated. After the epiphyses have fused and growth is complete, a hemoglobin level of 8.0 of 9.0 g/dL may be well tolerated. If the transfusion requirement exceeds 200 mL of packed red cells per kilogram per year, splenectomy should be considered (see further discussion later).[809] Our current transfusion procedure is outlined in Box 20-2.

Complications of Blood Transfusion. The primary long-term complication of blood transfusion is iron loading and the resultant parenchymal organ toxicity, as discussed earlier. Febrile reactions to leukocyte antigenic determinants and allergic reactions to plasma components are commonly encountered in patients receiving transfusions chronically. The use of prestorage leukoreduction filters has significantly decreased the rate of febrile reactions. Washing of red cells in saline to remove plasma proteins can be beneficial.[836]

Alloimmunization to minor blood group antigens occurs in 20% to 30% of patients[837-840] and may be manifested as delayed hemolysis. Rare circumstances of multiple alloantibodies may be a potentially life-threatening complication in patients with transfusion-dependent β-thalassemia because it may not be possible to find sufficient appropriately matched blood. Alloimmunization is frequently a less significant problem in patients in whom transfusion is initiated before the age of 3 years.[837-840] The

---

BOX 20-2	**Guidelines for Chronic Transfusions in Patients with Thalassemia**

1. Determine the blood type of the patient completely to identify minor red cell antigens before the first transfusion.
2. Keep the pretransfusion hemoglobin level between 9.5 and 11.5 mg/dL as needed for suppressing ineffective erythropoiesis and maintaining a reasonable sense of well-being.
3. Give 10 to 20 mL/kg of leukocyte-poor, washed, and filtered red blood cells at a maximum infusion rate of 10 mL/kg over a 2-hour period; transfuse more slowly in patients with heart disease.
4. Avoid raising the post-transfusion hemoglobin level to greater than 16 g/dL.
5. Choose a transfusion interval to maintain pretransfusion levels as outlined above (3 to 5 weeks, depending on individual patient needs). (*Comment*: Some patients tolerate slightly lower pretransfusion hemoglobin levels and need 5 weeks between transfusions, whereas others feel best coming every 4 weeks. Some prefer receiving fewer units and coming every 3 weeks. Some of the younger patients whose weight would require between 1 and 2 units receive a transfusion every 3 or 4 weeks and alternate between 1 and 2 units per transfusion.)
6. Pretransfusion laboratory tests include a complete blood cell count, differential, crossmatch, and red cell antibody screen.
7. Height and weight are recorded at least every 3 months.
8. Liver function (AST, ALT, bilirubin, and LDH) is evaluated every 3 months and serum ferritin every 3 to 6 months. A deferoxamine (Desferal) challenge test is performed at irregular intervals to measure the appropriate Desferal dosage and chelatable iron stores.

ALT, alanine transaminase; AST, aspartate transaminase; LDH, lactate dehydrogenase.

---

benefit of extended red cell phenotyping to minimize alloimmunization has been debated in the literature,[841,842] but crossmatching for the rhesus and Kell systems from the time of initial transfusion may decrease the incidence of alloimmunization.[839] Detailed red cell phenotyping should be performed in all patients with newly diagnosed thalassemia before transfusion. The average transfusion regimen in most centers is 12 to 15 mL of leukocyte-poor red cells per kilogram per month. Autoimmune hemolytic anemia is a rare but perilous complication of allosensitization. It must be managed aggressively to prevent dangerous iron overload.

Transmission of viral infections by transfusion remains a serious and significant problem in patients receiving transfusions chronically in countries in which the safety measures of volunteer donors, detailed donor questionnaires, and serologic and nucleic acid testing are not used. In one study, approximately 25% of transfusion-dependent patients with thalassemia had been exposed to hepatitis B, 80% of whom had clinical evidence of hepatitis.[843] Exposure to hepatitis C, with an incidence of approximately 6% per transfusion, was nearly inevitable in thalassemic patients receiving regular transfusions, and this agent accounts for the active hepatitis seen in many older patients. Identification of the hepatitis C agent and the development of a serologic test to screen donors have greatly minimized this risk,[844,845] but the infection can lead to fibrosis, cirrhosis, and hepatic carcinoma if untreated.[846-848] Treatment with interferon alfa and ribavirin is indicated and has now been demonstrated to be safe in patients with thalassemia despite the increased rate of hemolysis and transfusion secondary to ribavirin.[749a] Some studies have suggested that iron overload inhibits a therapeutic response,[849-852] but others have shown little or no such effect.[853,854] A minority of patients with thalassemia have become infected with human immunodeficiency virus, and the rate of progression to symptomatic acquired immunodeficiency syndrome has been proportionally lower than in most infected populations.[855] Although death and complications from these illnesses are uncommon in this patient population, it is prudent to exercise precautions. The most important consideration is the use of blood products screened for the presence of potential infectious agents. Patients should be immunized against hepatitis B upon diagnosis or if they have not acquired immunity. When practical, exposure to multiple donors or units of blood should be minimized. In this regard it is important to recognize that the use of washed or frozen red cells may lead to an increase in the number of transfused units.

Splenectomy

Splenectomy may be indicated in some patients in an attempt to decrease transfusion requirements. The role of the spleen must be carefully considered in patients who are treated with transfusion, iron chelation programs, or both. The spleen serves both as a scavenger by increasing red cell destruction and iron redistribution and as a storage depot by sequestration of the released iron in a potentially nontoxic pool. Unfortunately, splenic iron may equilibrate with other iron pools throughout the body. In one uncontrolled study, three splenectomized patients exhibited cirrhosis and massive iron deposition, whereas slightly younger patients with an intact spleen had only iron deposition.[856] Risdon and colleagues,[739] however, observed no difference between splenectomized and nonsplenectomized patients with regard to pathologic changes in the liver. If the spleen acts primarily as a storage depot for excess iron, premature removal could theoretically be detrimental. On the other hand, if the splenic pool is a particular target for deferoxamine, the beneficial effects of aggressive chelation therapy might be diminished by preferential removal of iron from this relatively innocuous pool. Perhaps most important is the

feasibility of achieving negative iron balance with conventional chelation regimens (see later). Eventually, an increased requirement for transfusion because of hypersplenism perturbs the balance and contributes to iron loading.[857]

Splenectomy may be indicated in the management of patients with severe β-thalassemia. Massive splenomegaly with hypersplenism causing leukopenia, thrombocytopenia, and an increasing transfusion requirement is often seen in young patients whose transfusion regimens are sporadic. Early splenectomy is often required. The development of splenomegaly is delayed in patients who are receiving a high number of transfusions.[858] Several factors should be considered in the decision to remove the spleen. Modell[669,859,860] carefully documented the annual blood requirement of splenectomized patients with thalassemia major and suggested that the spleen be removed if the observed requirement exceeds that predicted by 50%. Data from other investigators suggest that the benefits of splenectomy on iron balance are realized if the transfusion requirement exceeds 200 to 250 mL of packed red cells per kilogram per year with a minimum hemoglobin level of 10 g/dL.[857,861] Because a huge spleen, irrespective of functional hypersplenism, may account for a large fraction of the total blood volume, its removal often leads to a marked, though transient reduction in the patient's requirement for blood.[862,863] Most patients show a moderate, but significant reduction in their requirement for transfusion to the predicted 200 mL of packed red cells per kilogram per year,[859,860] and it remains stable for many years.[864]

The immediate surgical risk accompanying splenectomy is minimal for experienced practitioners, although reports of acute portal vein thrombosis are increasingly being recognized. There is some evidence that iron overload itself may inhibit the immune response.[865,866] Infections with *Yersinia* are sometimes observed in patients with iron overload.[867] The potential for overwhelming infection by *Diplococcus pneumoniae*, *Haemophilus influenzae*, or *Neisseria meningitidis*[868-870] should always be considered by the attending physician. Because removal of the spleen may blunt the primary immune response to encapsulated organisms, delay of splenectomy until after approximately 5 years of age is preferable. Patients should be immunized with polyvalent pneumococcal, meningococcal, and *H. influenzae* vaccines.[871-874] Supplemental prophylactic oral penicillin may also be used to prevent colonization by strains not covered by vaccines,[809] particularly in young children. Illnesses accompanied by high fever of uncertain cause should be treated aggressively with parenteral antibiotics until bacterial culture results are available. Patients in regions endemic for malaria should receive prophylactic treatment.[860] Infections appear to be significant causes of morbidity in HbE–β-thalassemia.[875]

Red cell survival usually increases immediately after splenectomy.[862] The peripheral blood smear may reveal increased numbers of hypochromic, microcytic, and nucleated red cells. Platelet counts greater than 10^6 are often seen, although correction of anemia by transfusion generally results in suppression of platelet production.[494] White blood cell counts of 15,000 to 20,000 are common; the differential is usually normal.

As discussed in more detail previously, arterial hypoxemia and evidence of pulmonary vascular disease have been reported in patients with thalassemia, and it has been suggested that splenectomy may exacerbate these problems.[790,802] Accordingly, splenectomized patients should be examined carefully for these findings. Because thrombocytosis may be an inciting factor,[802,876] prophylaxis with low-dose aspirin may be considered, although effective transfusion to correct anemia is probably the best form of preventive therapy.

Chelation Therapy

Progressive iron overload is the life-limiting complication of transfusion therapy. In the absence of adequate chelation, cardiac dysfunction ends the life of a thalassemic patient receiving transfusions during the teenage years. Regular chelation with the drug deferoxamine has proved remarkably effective in reducing the iron burden of patients receiving transfusions. Cardiac disease is delayed or prevented, susceptibility to infection is reduced,[876] and life expectancy is significantly extended; nonetheless, endocrine dysfunction may develop and persist. Unfortunately, effective use of deferoxamine requires strict compliance to subcutaneous administration via a mechanical pump. The lack of oral absorption of the drug and its short serum half-life dictate this cumbersome route of administration. Recently, two oral iron chelators have been studied. Deferiprone is approved in more than 40 countries but not approved by the Food and Drug Administration (FDA) in the United States. Deferasirox was approved in the United States and many other countries in 2004. Data on each of these chelators will be reviewed.

Deferoxamine. Deferoxamine has, until very recently, been the only approved iron chelator in the United States. The drug is a hexavalent hydroxylamine with a remarkable affinity for iron. It binds metal iron stoichiometrically with a binding ratio of deferoxamine to iron of approximately 1:1. Deferoxamine enters cells, chelates iron, and appears in serum and bile as the iron chelate product feroxamine.[699]

Humans have no intrinsic mechanism for excreting excess iron. Iron available for chelation is thought to be derived from the "labile iron pool"[689]; the size of this pool is directly related to the total body iron burden.[877,878] Non–transferrin-bound plasma iron should also be available for chelation.[695,696] A fraction of reticuloendothelial iron salvaged from red cells may likewise be chelated,[879] perhaps only when stored as ferritin.[880] Urinary iron excretion appears to be proportional to marrow erythroid activity and is diminished by transfusion.[881] Net iron loss, however, is not compromised because the diminution in urinary iron excretion is balanced by increased fecal excretion of iron.[880,881] In patients with primary hemochromatosis, in whom iron deposition is seen predominantly in parenchymal cells and erythropoiesis is normal, administration of deferoxamine results primarily in enhanced fecal iron excretion.[699] Thus, the site of iron removal is influenced by the transfusion schedule, but no data are available regarding the influence of hemoglobin level on prevention or removal of cardiac iron deposits. In brief, chelation from a small labile pool that is in equilibrium with a much larger storage pool in the organs eventually reduces stored iron, but at different rates from different organs because of variations in efflux rates.

Deferoxamine Chelation Regimens. Deferoxamine is active when administered by the intramuscular, subcutaneous, or intravenous routes. After its introduction in 1962, the drug was given by the intramuscular route until the late 1970s. This regimen was only partially successful because rapid clearance from plasma via metabolism and biliary and urinary excretion[699] led to insufficient iron removal to achieve a negative net iron balance in most patients.[882] Supplemental oral administration of ascorbic acid enhanced urinary excretion (see later),[883] but just 14 to 16 mg of iron could be removed per day, even from patients with severe hemosiderosis. Adults receiving full transfusion support require removal of more than 35 mg/day to have a negative net iron balance.[882] Continuous intravenous infusion significantly enhances iron excretion,[882,884] presumably because of exchange between deferoxamine and tissue iron pools. Substantial plasma and tissue drug concentrations can be attained by continuous subcutaneous administration via a pump mechanism.[885] Iron excretion is markedly enhanced in comparison to the intramuscular route,[882,885-887] and net negative iron balance can be achieved in most patients older than 3 or 4 years with an iron burden of 4 to 5 g.[817,824,885]

A typical regimen involves the administration of 30 to 40 mg/kg of drug overnight (8 to 12 hours) at least 5 to 6 nights per week; the patient thereby avoids the need to carry the pump during the daytime hours. Obviously, such a program is a compromise in that optimal management demands drug infusion every hour of every day, a schedule met with poor compliance, particularly among teenagers. Data now show that regular use of deferoxamine, if started by the age of 3 or 4, forestalls significant iron overload. It also promotes elimination of excess iron in patients if started after a substantial transfusional iron burden has already developed.[748,888-892] It is generally agreed that treatment should be initiated by 5 years in transfusion-dependent patients; some advocate treatment by the age of 3.[812,824,893-895] It has been argued that irreversible tissue damage, particularly to endocrine glands, occurs at a very low iron burden during the first years of life. However, the toxicity of deferoxamine is most significant in patients with a low iron burden (see later). Indeed, growth retardation and other toxic effects have been documented in children younger than 3 years who are given high doses of the drug.[664] A test infusion of deferoxamine may be used to determine whether mobilizable iron is present.[809,812]

Periodic intravenous administration allows the use of higher doses (6 to 10 g/day); local reactions at the site of administration limit the tolerable subcutaneous dose to 2.0 to 2.5 g/day. By extending the time of infusion and increasing the drug dose, iron removal can be greatly enhanced over that achievable with conventional subcutaneous therapy. Chelation with high drug doses by the intravenous route is capable of reversing established cardiac disease in some patients who continue to require transfusions (Nienhuis AW: unpublished observations, 1990).[737,813, 896,897] This regimen is most effective when instituted while the patient's heart is still compensating, either with or without cardiac medications.

Efficacy of Deferoxamine Chelation. Clinical experience has shown subcutaneous deferoxamine administration to be effective in preventing cardiac disease and prolonging the life of thalassemic patients receiving transfusions.[748,891,898-900] Life expectancy was previously approximately 16 years, with rare patients surviving into their mid-20s.[581,718,901] Since the introduction of subcutaneous deferoxamine therapy, the projected life expectancy extends into the middle of the fourth decade.[902] Several studies have also documented sparing of cardiac disease in patients receiving adequate chelation therapy.[748,891,903,904] Figure 20-31 shows a striking comparison between two groups of patients; one group received adequate chelation therapy, whereas the other group was poorly compliant. Onset of cardiac disease has been observed in the chelated group in whom negative iron balance was achieved,[903] but the dose of the drug used was relatively low.

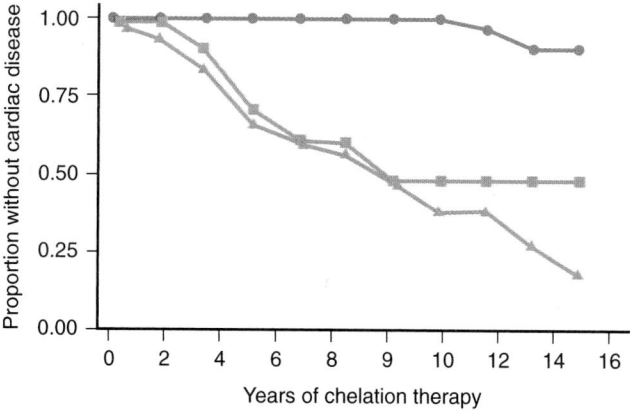

FIGURE 20-31. Cardiac disease–free survival of patients with respect to the serum ferritin level. The *circles* depict cardiac disease–free survival of patients with less than 33% of ferritin measurements greater than 2500 ng/mL; *squares*, patients with 33% to 67% of measurements greater than 2500 ng/mL; and *triangles*, patients with more than 67% of measurements greater than 2500 ng/mL. *(From Olivieri NF, Nathan DG, MacMillan JH, et al. Survival in medically treated patients with homozygous beta-thalassemia. N Engl J Med. 1994;331:574-578. Copyright 1994, Massachusetts Medical Society.)*

Unfortunately, the cohort of patients in whom subcutaneous administration of deferoxamine was initiated in their late first decade of life after significant iron deposits had accumulated continues to exhibit endocrine dysfunction and growth retardation.[892] Glucose intolerance and diabetes are observed even in patients receiving adequate chelation therapy,[905] although the incidence is reduced.[748] There is scant evidence that deferoxamine can reverse established endocrine dysfunction. It remains to be determined whether patients in whom a regimen of subcutaneous deferoxamine is started at a very young age will fare better with respect to growth, sexual development, and endocrine function. Because this cohort of patients is just now entering their teenage years, information on this point may become available in the near future.

Toxicity of Deferoxamine. At high doses of deferoxamine, significant side effects are seen.[699,809] Local erythema may occur at the site of infusion and contribute to an inflammatory response characterized by multiple subcutaneous nodules. These local reactions can be partially suppressed by the inclusion of 5 to 10 mg of hydrocortisone in the deferoxamine solution.

Of particular concern is neurosensory toxicity observed at high doses. Several large series report a 30% to 40% incidence of high-frequency hearing loss, which may become symptomatic.[906-910] Reversal with discontinuation of the drug has been reported, although other patients have experienced persistent hearing loss. Ocular toxicity has also been reported.[906,911] Progressive visual failure with night and color blindness and field loss has also been described[912] but may be not be related to chelation therapy.[913] In fact, in one study iron dysfunction was thought to be related to failure to take deferoxamine.[914] Reversal after discontinuation of deferoxamine has also been reported.

The neurosensory complications of deferoxamine are dose related and inversely correlated with the body iron burden. Patients with heavy iron loading are relatively protected, but those with lower iron burdens who receive aggressive chelation therapy may be more susceptible to these toxic effects.[909,915,916] Administration of deferoxamine to patients with rheumatoid arthritis and normal iron stores has induced neurologic deficits, including confusion, nausea and vomiting, and coma.[915,917] These findings suggest that the toxicity is caused by free drug, which may chelate other metal irons.[910] Alternatively, deferoxamine may reduce the concentration of iron in neurosensory cells below a threshold needed for normal function. These serious complications necessitate careful monitoring of patients receiving deferoxamine. Young children and individuals from whom the majority of iron has been removed by chelation are particularly susceptible to these effects. The occurrence of complications is most likely in patients receiving continuous intravenous infusions of more than 50 mg/kg/day. Formal audiometry and ophthalmologic examination should be performed at

6-month intervals. The use of a test infusion to assess the ability of deferoxamine to mobilize iron, as advocated by Fosburg and Nathan,[809] may help in avoiding toxicity.

Deferoxamine is normally used by microorganisms to facilitate iron uptake.[699,918] *Yersina enterocolitica*, for example, uses deferoxamine in this manner.[859] Although it is associated with low virulence in humans, serious *Y. enterocolitica* infections have been reported in treated patients.[919,920] Mucormycosis has also been reported in patients undergoing hemodialysis who receive deferoxamine.[921] Of interest is the observation that iron chelators have profound in vitro effects on T-lymphocyte function.[809,922-927] Whether these effects can be put to practical use is not known.[926]

Additional rare complications have been associated with high-dose deferoxamine. Pulmonary infiltrates and respiratory insufficiency have been reported in eight patients[928,929] and in iron-loaded mice.[930] Curiously, deferoxamine also protects the developing lung[931]; therefore, the view that deferoxamine causes pulmonary toxicity in the treatment of iron overload is controversial.[932] Indeed, iron overload is thought to contribute to pulmonary disease in thalassemia,[802] although the latter is complex and probably also related to pulmonary vascular obstruction associated with chronic thrombocytosis.[803,876] Acute and chronic renal decompensation has likewise been described.[803,876,933-935] Growth failure and skeletal changes have been reported as well.[936,937]

The array of potential side effects should not obscure the finding that deferoxamine has proved to be very safe in the vast majority of patients. Many of the side effects have been seen only at higher intravenous doses or in patients with a low iron burden. Although careful follow-up is warranted, patients can be reassured that deferoxamine therapy is both remarkably effective and generally quite safe. Indeed, methods have been designed to permit chronic intravenous infusion.[938-940] The major limitation of deferoxamine use is compliance and the serious problems faced by patients and their families as they deal with this lifesaving but onerous therapy.[941-943]

Deferiprone. Deferiprone, L-1-(1,2-dimethyl-3-hydroxy-pyridin-4-one), is a bivalent iron chelator initially synthesized by Hider and colleagues.[944] It was briefly licensed to Ciba-Geigy (now Novartis) but abandoned by the company in 1993 because of its low therapeutic index in non–iron-overloaded animals, its poor stoichiometry (three molecules of drug are required for binding of each iron atom),[945] and its rapid removal from the circulation.[946,947]

Efficacy of Deferiprone Chelation. Deferiprone was first investigated in uncontrolled clinical trials by a group at the Royal Free Hospital in London.[948] These trials were followed by two studies by Olivieri, Brittenham, and their colleagues,[949,950] who measured iron stores by liver biopsy and SQUID in patients treated with deferiprone. Their initial results, published in 1995, were encouraging.[949]

The drug appeared to reduce or maintain liver iron levels in patients with thalassemia who were receiving many transfusions.[951] In a second study, hepatic iron levels were not reduced below their starting points or actually increased to a value considerably above their starting points in a substantial fraction of deferiprone-treated patients.[950] In addition, increased hepatic fibrosis appeared to have developed in some of the deferiprone-treated patients but none of the deferoxamine-treated patients (who had much lower liver iron levels on average). Other studies have confirmed that iron stores, measured by liver biopsy, are not effectively reduced by deferiprone.[952,953] The influence of the drug on hepatic fibrosis remains uncertain.[952,954,955] Recent published studies of deferiprone have been based on the level of serum ferritin as an index of effectiveness, but such studies[956-958] are unreliable. Thus far the drug has been inadequately assessed.[959] Further studies of deferiprone are warranted. The drug may play a role in shuttling iron within membranes and within intracellular pools.[960,961] More recent studies, retrospective, prospective, and epidemiologic, provide some important data suggesting that deferiprone alone or in combination with deferoxamine may provide some important cardioprotective effect.

Toxicity of Deferiprone. Administration of deferiprone is associated with severe adverse side effects, including idiosyncratic agranulocytosis in 0.5% to 1% of patients and neutropenia in up to 5% of patients. Other complications include arthropathy, zinc deficiency, gastrointestinal symptoms, and abnormal liver function test results.[962,963] Until the risk-to-benefit ratio of deferiprone is established by additional clinical trials in which iron stores are measured, compliant patients should be advised to continue an effective deferoxamine chelation program.[697,963,964]

Deferasirox. Deferasirox, known in original studies as ICL670, produced promising results in early preclinical trials[965] and was approved by the FDA in 2004. Deferasirox is a tridentate chelator in a class of compounds known as 3,5-bis-(orthohydroxyphenyl)-1,2,4-triazoles. Therefore, two molecules of desferasirox are required to bind one molecule of iron. After an oral dose the drug is promptly absorbed, persists in blood with a half-time of 8 to 16 hours, and excretes iron largely in feces.

Efficacy of Deferasirox Chelation. In short-term dose-finding clinical trials, the drug removed an amount of iron that would be expected to be delivered in a standard transfusion regimen.[966] It has been extensively studied in preclinical[967] and phase I, II,[968,969] and III[970,971] studies. The phase III study in patients with thalassemia demonstrated no inferiority to deferoxamine at only at the higher deferasirox doses of 20 and 30 mg/kg/day. Further study has demonstrated that the efficacy of deferasirox is related to ongoing transfusional iron burden and that this factor should be carefully monitored in patients.

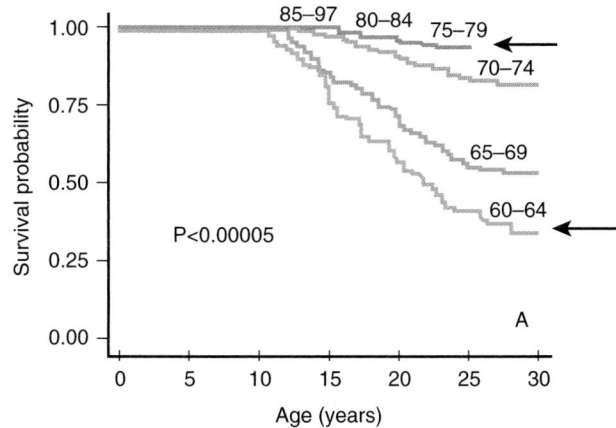

FIGURE 20-32. Kaplan-Meier survival curves, by birth cohort, of 977 patients from seven Italian centers participating in a natural history study by Borgna-Pignatti and colleagues. Statistically significant improvements in survival were demonstrated overall (*P* < .00005) and in later cohorts (*P* = .024). (*From Borgna-Pignatti C, Rugolotto S, De Stefano P, et al. Survival and complications in patients with thalassemia major treated with transfusion and deferoxamine. Haematologica. 2004;89:1187-1193.*)

Toxicity of Deferasirox. Deferasirox has generally been well tolerated in the clinical trial setting. Mild gastrointestinal adverse events and rashes were the most common toxicities, and discontinuation of the study drug because of adverse events was rare. Mild increases in creatinine occurred, and in a small number it increased above the upper limit of normal. There were no reports of progressive or severe renal failure. Of more than 800 patients treated, none have had significant myelosuppression.[967-969]

Survival

There has been a marked improvement in the survival of patients with thalassemia major. In a cohort of U.S. patients born from 1960 to 1976, the median survival was 17.1 years. In Italy, 50% of patients died before the age of 12 years in the late 1970s. Borgna-Pignatti and co-authors[972] reported on more than 1000 patients born since 1960 and demonstrated a statistically significant improvement in survival in each of the more contemporary cohorts (Fig. 20-32).

Vitamin Supplementation

Ascorbic Acid. The role of ascorbic acid in iron metabolism and chelation therapy is complex and controversial.[699,973] Tissue deficiency of vitamin C often develops in patients with hemosiderosis because of accelerated catabolism; frank scurvy is documented in individuals with marginal dietary intake.[974-977] Administration of vitamin C significantly augments iron excretion in response to deferoxamine, particularly in patients who have vitamin C deficiency. Serum iron and ferritin levels may also rise.[881,977,978] Ascorbic acid retards the rate of conversion of ferritin to hemosiderin[979,980] and presumably allows more iron to remain in a chelatable form.

Unfortunately, ascorbic acid also enhances iron-mediated peroxidation of membrane lipids[981,982] and has been shown to increase iron-induced membrane damage in cultured myocardial cells.[709] It has also been observed that patients with iron overloads who are receiving vitamin C may experience cardiac dysfunction that is reversed when the supplementation is discontinued.[983,984]

Some investigators have suggested giving low doses of ascorbic acid (3 mg/kg) at the start of each subcutaneous infusion of deferoxamine. The chelator should be able to block the deleterious effects of ascorbic acid on lipid peroxidation of cellular organelles in vitro. Others avoid using vitamin C in patients with iron overload and argue that iron depletion can be achieved without supplemental vitamin C. Patients with significant iron burdens should be cautioned against self-administration of substantial amounts of ascorbic acid because abrupt cardiac deterioration has been observed in this setting (Nienhuis AW: unpublished observations, 1990).

Vitamin E. Deficiency of vitamin E has been noted in many patients with thalassemia major receiving transfusions chronically.[711,712,884,985,986] It may contribute to hemolysis as a result of red cell membrane damage.[488,710] α-Tocopherol has long been considered to be a potent antioxidant that protects membrane lipids from attack by free radicals formed when excess iron is present. Deficiency in the neonatal period[987] or deficiency caused by malnutrition is associated with varying degrees of hemolysis. Hemolysis and the characteristic increased red cell susceptibility to in vitro hydrogen peroxide are readily reversed by the administration of supplemental vitamin E. Of interest, supplemental iron administration increases the hemolytic rate, even in nonthalassemic patients with vitamin E deficiency.[987] In patients with iron overload, supplemental vitamin E may lessen iron-mediated cellular toxicity. One study in experimental animals suggests that vitamin E may also inhibit deferoxamine-induced urinary iron excretion.[988] Although vitamin E is used clinically, the efficacy of this therapy remains to be demonstrated.

Folic Acid. Megaloblastic anemia, which is almost invariably due to folic acid deficiency, may occur in patients with severe β-thalassemia.[989-991] In contrast, vitamin B_{12} deficiency is extremely rare in thalassemic patients.[991] Folic acid deficiency is thought to develop as a result of decreased absorption, low dietary intake, and the enormous demand of bone marrow expansion. Most patients benefit from daily folic acid administration (1 mg), although patients receiving adequate transfusions to suppress erythropoiesis and those living in countries where folic acid is added to many breads and cereals probably do not require supplementation.

Trace Metals. Trace metal deficiency associated with thalassemia or aggressive chelation therapy is not commonly observed.[699,992] Zinc deficiency (acrodermatitis enteropathica) has been reported in a patient receiving diethylenetriaminepentaacetic acid for chelation.[993] The reversible toxic effects seen with high-dose deferoxamine chelation may reflect trace metal deficiency or intracellular chelation of a trace metal. Newer techniques to analyze trace metal concentrations may reveal subtle deficiencies; yearly screening for zinc deficiency is appropriate, but supplementation is not usually required.

Allogeneic Bone Marrow Transplantation

Successful cure of β-thalassemia by bone marrow transplantation was first reported by Thomas and associates in 1982.[994] Subsequently, a number of centers have explored the use of this modality as definitive therapy for β-thalassemia. The most extensive published experience with bone marrow transplantation in β-thalassemia is that of Lucarelli and co-workers in Italy.[995-999] The results of their early attempts to use transplantation in this patient population were discouraging.[996] The preparative regimens used were often ineffective and associated with graft failure, toxicity, and high mortality. Their recent experience is considerably more promising.[999] Patients were analyzed to identify clinically important variables predictive of transplant outcome. The probability of survival was decreased in patients with poor chelation status, hepatomegaly (>2 cm), and portal fibrosis. The probability of event-free survival was reduced in the presence of hepatomegaly. Risk factors for hepatomegaly and portal fibrosis were used to divide patients into three classes: class 1, absence of both risk factors; class 2, one risk factor; and class 3, both risk factors. However, such classification of patients may be difficult to reproduce (i.e., hepatomegaly of ≤2 cm and a history of adherence to chelation therapy). The most recent data from Lucarelli for class 3 patients younger than 17 years who received HLA-identical matched sibling donor transplants demonstrated significant improvement with the addition of hydroxyurea, azathioprine, and fludarabine to the previous regimen of cyclophosphamide and busulfan. In the 33 patients treated with the new protocol (protocol 26), the survival rate was increased to 93% and the rate of graft rejection decreased from 30% to 8%.[1000] Adults treated with protocol 26 demonstrated an improved thalassemia-free survival rate of 62% to 67%, and transplant-related mortality was decreased but still significant at 27%, down from 37%.

One of the major reasons for failure of bone marrow transplantation in patients with thalassemia may be the unpredictable pharmacologic effects of the busulfan used in most preparative regimens. Hyperabsorption of the drug is associated with hepatic veno-occlusive disease and hypoabsorption with recurrent thalassemia. Improved control of busulfan levels during induction may provide better clinical results.[1001] Whatever the event-free survival estimates, bone marrow transplantation is the only viable option for patients who cannot or refuse to adhere to a well-administered transfusion and chelation program.[1002]

On the basis of available data, bone marrow transplantation may be recommended to patients receiving adequate chelation with no evidence of liver disease. Many of these patients can be cured. Although most such patients are very young, age does not appear to be a significant variable in determining outcome. Chronic graft-versus-host disease is still a potential long-term complication of successful allogeneic transplantation. A current limitation to the general applicability of this therapy is the availability of a related, HLA-matched donor. Only one in four siblings on average will be HLA identical. Improved management of graft-versus-host disease and the development of technologies for bone marrow transplantation from unrelated donors may expand the pool of potential donors in the near future. Some encouraging results have recently been reported.[1003] The use of cord blood stem cells may also extend the donor pool.[1004,1005]

Pharmacologic Manipulation of Hemoglobin F Synthesis

The interaction between β-thalassemia and genetic syndromes that increase γ-globin synthesis has illustrated how even small increases in γ-globin production lead to a significant improvement in the effectiveness of red blood cell production in patients with thalassemia. Although steady-state production of HbF is a genetically determined trait,[12] perturbations in erythropoiesis may be associated with an increased capacity for HbF synthesis. Treatment of experimental animals or patients with a variety of cytoreductive agents, including 5-azacytidine (5-Aza), hydroxyurea, vinblastine, and cytosine arabinoside, leads to an increase in production of HbF.[1006-1016] Although the precise mechanism of action of these drugs remains incompletely defined, the increased capacity for γ-globin synthesis appears to be linked to rapid erythroid regeneration. Consistent with this hypothesis, hematopoietic growth factors that promote the expansion and maturation of erythroid precursors, including erythropoietin,[1017-1019] interleukin-3,[1018-1020] and granulocyte-macrophage colony-stimulating factor,[1018] have also been shown to enhance HbF synthesis in primate models. Of particular interest is the observation that infants delivered of diabetic mothers exhibit a delayed switch from γ- to β-globin.[1021] Levels of butyric acid derivatives are elevated in the serum of these mothers and their infants before birth. Similarly, patients with metabolic disorders associated with increased levels of short-chain fatty acids also have elevated HbF levels.[1022] Infusions of sodium butyrate or α-aminobutyric acid into fetal sheep markedly delay the perinatal switch,[1023] whereas infusions in primates lead to activation of the γ gene (McDonagh KT, Bodine DM, Nienhuis AW: unpublished observations).[1024,1025] It has been proposed that butyrate, propionate, or the metabolite acetate promotes increased γ-globin expression by acetylation of histones and alteration of chromatin structure, but other mechanisms cannot be excluded.[1026,1027] A flurry of articles have described the results of treatment of patients with sickle cell anemia with butyrate or its derivatives.[1028-1033] One patient[1029] had a sustained increase in hemoglobin, and healing of leg ulcers without an increment in circulating hemoglobin has also been observed.[1032] A recent report cited a sustained increase in HbF in sickle cell anemia.[1034,1035] Caution must be exercised, however, because high doses of butyrate are associated with neurotoxicity in simians.[1036]

The most extensive experience with pharmacologic manipulation of HbF synthesis in patients has involved administration of hydroxyurea to patients with sickle cell disease (Dover GJ: personal cummunication).[1012,1037-1041] In this population, the majority of patients appear to respond to the drug with a twofold or greater increase in HbF levels over their baseline. In many patients, HbF levels between 10% and 15% of total hemoglobin are seen. This increase reflects both augmented production and enhanced survival of HbF-containing cells. The clinical results in patients with sickle cell anemia are impressive as described in Chapter 19. However, the results in patients with thalassemia have been disappointing thus far.[1014]

A response to 5-Aza has been seen in several patients with thalassemia[1007,10427,1043] (Fig. 20-33). The dramatic increases in HbF levels associated with administration of this drug may result from a combination of cytotoxicity and inhibition of postsynthetic methylation of DNA.[1043-1047] Global demethylation of DNA, including the γ-globin gene, is observed after the administration of 5-Aza. Despite its effectiveness, the use of 5-Aza in the treatment of hemoglobinopathies has been limited by concerns about its known carcinogenic potential,[1048-1050] as well as the demonstrated effectiveness and safety of current treatment strategies involving transfusion and chelation. Because response to the drug is short-lived, chronic therapy would be required.

Treatment of β-thalassemia with busulfan (Myleran) has been reported in two patients in China.[1051] Combinations of agents, notably erythropoietin and hydroxyurea, often enhance HbF production in experimental animals[1019,1052] and have shown promise in preliminary trials in sickle cell patients (Rodgers GP: personal communication). Undoubtedly, the response of individual patients to these medications will be influenced by their endogenous, genetically determined capability for γ- and β-chain synthesis.[1053,1054]

Gene Therapy

As a result of advances in molecular biology, treatment of hematologic disease through the introduction of new genetic material into bone marrow stem cells is a goal for the foreseeable future.[1055-1058] Application of somatic gene therapy to the treatment of hematologic diseases requires improved efficiency of gene delivery, regulated and sustained expression of the introduced genes, and biologic studies demonstrating expression of the foreign gene. Although active research is ongoing, experimental shortcomings in all these aspects presently preclude the use of gene therapy for the management of thalassemia or sickle cell anemia.

Correction of thalassemia by gene transfer will necessitate the introduction of a normal β-globin gene into pluripotent hematopoietic stem cells.[1055-1057] Experimen-

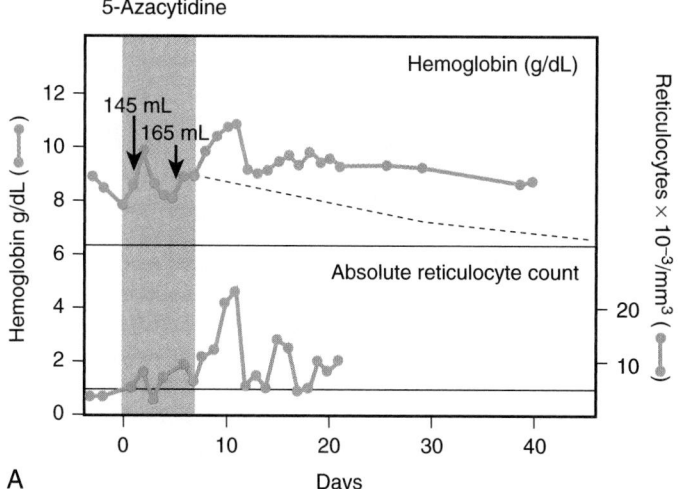
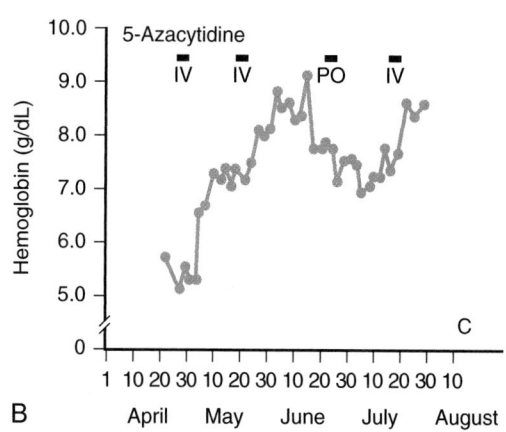

FIGURE 20-33. A, Effects of 5-azacytidine on erythropoiesis in a patient with severe homozygous β-thalassemia after a single administration of the drug by continuous infusion over a period of 7 days. Two small blood transfusions were administered on days 2 and 5. The *dashed line* indicates the projected hemoglobin concentration and reticulocyte count in this patient without treatment based on clinical records. **B,** Effects of sequential courses of treatment with 5-azacytidine in a patient with β-thalassemia who had severe cardiomyopathy and alloimmunization. *(A, Adapted from information appearing in Ley TJ, DeSimone J, Anagnou NP, et al. 5-Azacytidine selectively increases gamma-globin synthesis in a patient with beta thalassemia. N Engl J Med. 1982;307:1469-1475. Reprinted by permission from The New England Journal of Medicine; B, from Dunbar C, Travis W, Kan YW, Nienhuis A. 5-Azacytidine treatment in a beta zero-thalassaemic patient unable to be transfused due to multiple alloantibodies. Br J Haematol. 1989;72:467-468.)*

tal studies in mice have demonstrated that retroviral vectors are capable of transferring foreign sequences to hematopoietic stem cells.[1059,1060] Expression of transferred genes has been more problematic but has been improved with use of a new vector containing a portion of the LCR, which has led to 17% to 33% HbF.[1061] The efficiency with which primate (or human) stem cells are infected by retroviral vectors appears to be lower than that observed in murine cells. Nonetheless, transfer of foreign sequences to long-term repopulating hematopoietic cells of primates and humans has been demonstrated.[1062]

For treatment of β-thalassemia (or sickle cell anemia) it will be necessary to express the transferred gene at high levels in erythroid cells. This has been a challenge in the field, but vectors that incorporate elements of the LCR have recently been generated. Lentiviral vectors containing such elements have been constructed. Indeed, it has become possible to achieve long-term correction of both sickle cell anemia and β-thalassemia in mouse models with these viruses.[1063-1065] A phase I human gene therapy trial has been initiated in France for thalassemia and sickle cell disease, but clinical data are not yet available.[1066]

Interaction of Thalassemia with Globin Structural Variants

In geographic areas in which thalassemia mutations and structural variants of α- and β-globin genes are both commonly seen (such as Africa and Southeast Asia), compound heterozygotes with a thalassemia mutation and a structural variant are common.[1] In such double heterozygotes, disease may be more or less severe than that seen in individuals who are heterozygous for only the structural variant. For example, heterozygotes for a β^S gene have 30% to 45% HbS and are usually clinically well, whereas patients with a β^S gene and a β-thalassemia mutation (in the *trans* β gene) have 60% to 95% HbS and may have a severe sickling disorder. Individuals with a β^S gene and α-thalassemia trait generally have less HbS than those with sickle trait[1067,1068] and are asymptomatic.[1069,1070] The interaction of α- and β-thalassemia mutations and the HPFH mutations with the β^S gene are described in detail in Chapter 19.

Hemoglobin E–β-Thalassemia

This syndrome is particularly common in Southeast Asia, where as many as 4000 to 5000 patients may reside in Thailand alone.[1071,1072] As a result of immigration from Southeast Asia, HbE–β-thalassemia is now a commonly encountered form of transfusion-dependent thalassemia in certain areas of the United States.[1073,1074] Double heterozygotes not receiving transfusions have hemoglobin levels of 2.3 to 7 g/dL, depending primarily on the output of the β-thalassemia gene. Because α-thalassemia is common in Southeast Asia, more complex phenotypes may be observed.[1075] Nucleated red blood cells are found on the peripheral blood smear, whereas they are absent in patients homozygous for β^E. HbE and HbA$_2$ account for 50% to 70% of the total hemoglobin (5% HbA$_2$ by HPLC).[1074,1076] Small quantities of HbA are found in association with a β^+-thalassemia gene. Patients with HbE–β-thalassemia usually require transfusions and exhibit the clinical features of thalassemia major. In areas where intensive treatment is unavailable, the disease resembles classic thalassemia major, with patients exhibiting massive hepatosplenomegaly, hypersplenism, severe skeletal disease, and death from infection in childhood. Iron loading occurs as a result of either transfusion or enhanced intestinal absorption.[1077] Proper treatment is the same as that recommended for thalassemia major or intermedia, depending on the requirement for regular blood transfusion. Recent work has also suggested that there are different compensatory responses in HbE–β-thalassemia as patients get older, and this may have important implications in the management of this disease.[1078] These alterations in the compensatory responses of older patients are also likely to be applicable to patients with other forms of β-thalassemia.

Hemoglobin C–β-Thalassemia

The β^C gene, which encodes a variant β chain with a lysine→glutamic acid substitution at position 6,[1079] is common in blacks of West African origin. The only hematologic consequence of simple heterozygosity for the β^C gene is increased target cells on the peripheral smear. Double heterozygotes with a β^C gene and β-thalassemia genes exhibit moderately severe hemolytic anemia with splenomegaly. The peripheral blood smear reveals hypochromia and microcytosis with many target cells. HbC accounts for 65% to 95% of the total hemoglobin, depending on whether the thalassemia mutation is of the β^+ or β^0 variety. In the black population the disease is generally mild because of the prevalence of mild β-thalassemia genes (see earlier),[535] whereas in Italian,[1080] North African,[1081] and Turkish patients,[1082] the disease is more severe, particularly in those who have a β^0-thalassemia mutation.

Thalassemic Hemoglobinopathies

As discussed in detail in earlier sections, several variant polypeptides can be described as thalassemic hemoglobinopathies. With the exception of HbE and the elongated α-chain variants, these mutations are very uncommon. Interest in these mutations arises from the unique mechanisms by which they produce the thalassemia phenotype.[239,1083] The most common thalassemic hemoglobinopathy is HbE disease.

Hemoglobin E Disease

As described earlier, the β^E mutation activates a cryptic splice site in exon 1 (see Fig. 20-10). Because the correct splice site is less efficiently used, production of functional β-globin mRNA that codes for the variant decreases.[142] The incidence of the β^E gene is extraordinarily high in some populations (≈30% in Laos, Cambodia, and Thailand).[1071,1084] The occurrence of the gene in immigrants from Southeast Asia to the United States reflects these origins.[1074]

In the heterozygous form, patients are largely asymptomatic with a hemoglobin level of 12 g/dL or greater, no reticulocytosis, an MCV of 74 ± 10.6 μm³, and an MCH of 25 ± 2.5 pg. The peripheral blood smear is distinguished by mild microcytosis and occasional target cells. Hemoglobin electrophoresis reveals HbE comigrating with HbA₂ in the range of 19% to 34%. The α-to-β biosynthetic ratio is usually 0.8 or greater, hence the mild nature of HbE trait.

Patients with homozygous HbE disease are also asymptomatic.[1072,1076] The hemoglobin level is rarely less than 10 g/dL, and significant reticulocytosis is uncommon. The red cells, however, are markedly microcytic (MCV of 50 to 66 μm³) and hypochromic (MCH of 20.1 pg). Target cells and occasional coarse stippling are evident on the smear. HbE accounts for 90% or more of the total hemoglobin, with varying levels of HbF.

The differential diagnosis of microcytic anemia in the Southeast Asian population initially requires the exclusion of iron deficiency. When present, electrophoresis will identify HbE. However, its level may be diminished in the presence of α-thalassemia or iron deficiency because the affinity of normal β chains for α-globin exceeds that of β^E chains. Interaction of α-thalassemia mutations with the β^E gene is usually seen because of the high incidence of each in the Southeast Asian population.[1075]

PRENATAL DIAGNOSIS OF THALASSEMIA

The morbidity and mortality associated with severe forms of thalassemia prompted efforts to develop effective prenatal diagnosis more than 2 decades ago. For the vast majority of β-thalassemias, for which point mutations are usually responsible, early efforts focused on determination of globin chain synthesis in fetal blood cells obtained by aspiration of placental vessels or direct visualization of fetal vessels.[1085-1087] The risk associated with fetal blood sampling at 18 to 20 weeks' gestation proved to be acceptably low when performed by experienced personnel (fetal loss rate of ≈3%; error rate of <0.5%) such that between 1975 and 1985, more than 7900 pregnancies were studied.[1088] As molecular methods and the knowledge of mutations leading to thalassemia improved, strategies for prenatal detection of these conditions evolved.

Successful prenatal diagnosis of α-thalassemia of the hydrops fetalis variety by solution hybridization methods to detect deficiency of α-globin genes in amniotic fluid cell DNA was first reported by Kan and associates in 1975.[1089] Southern blot analysis rapidly supplanted this approach for the detection of gene deletion in either the α- or β-thalassemias.[1090,1091] Detection of mutations in DNA rapidly became the preferred strategy for prenatal diagnosis as mutations became defined in the β-thalassemias.[3] The introduction of PCR methods further facilitated the detection of mutations and also permitted the use of nonradioactive tests.[1092] Coupled with chorionic villus biopsy, accurate and safe diagnosis can be accomplished within the first trimester of pregnancy. More recently, noninvasive methods consisting of examination of fetal erythrocytes in maternal plasma[1093] and analysis of nucleic acids in maternal plasma[1094] have provided promise for detection of severe thalassemia syndromes, without risk to the fetus.

Besides molecular biology, prenatal diagnosis of thalassemia has relied on identification of couples at risk, widespread public education, and genetic counseling. In countries in which the incidence of β-thalassemia is high and the burden of disease to the overall population great,

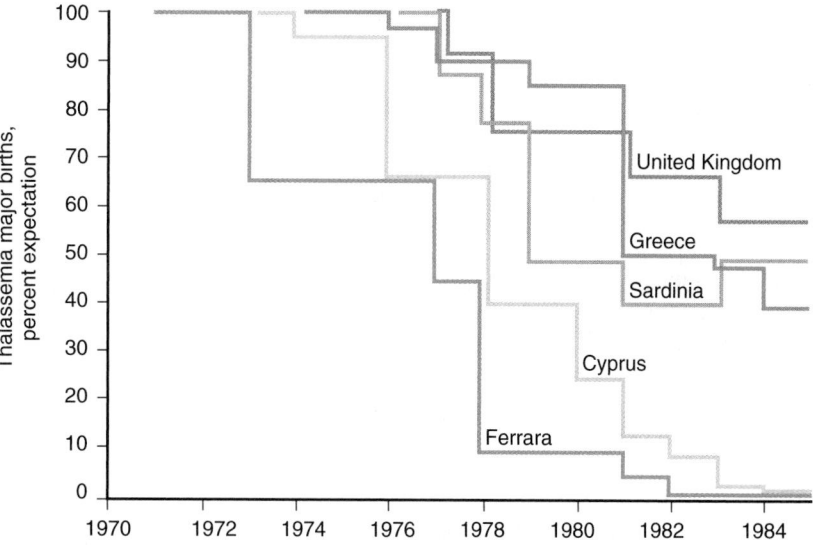

FIGURE 20-34. A decrease in the birth rate of infants with thalassemia major in Great Britain and several Mediterranean regions after the introduction of effective prenatal diagnosis. *(Adapted from Modell B, Bulyzhenkov V. Distribution and control of some genetic disorders. World Health Stat Q. 1988;41: 209-218. By permission of the World Health Organization.)*

such as on the island of Sardinia and in Greece, intensive prevention programs have been established and have proved to be extraordinarily successful. For example, the birth of children with β-thalassemia in these area has been reduced by more than 90% in recent years[1095-1100] (Fig. 20-34). These results represent major achievements in the prevention of genetic disease and paradigms for other disorders.*

REFERENCES

1. Weatherall DJ, Clegg JB. The Thalassaemia Syndromes, 4th ed. Oxford, Blackwell Scientific, 2001.
2. Higgs DR, Vickers MA, Wilkie AO, et al. A review of the molecular genetics of the human alpha-globin gene cluster. Blood. 1989;73:1081-1104.
3. Kazazian HH Jr. The thalassemia syndromes: molecular basis and prenatal diagnosis in 1990. Semin Hematol. 1990;27:209-228.
4. Karlsson S, Nienhuis AW. Developmental regulation of human globin genes. Annu Rev Biochem. 1985; 54:1071-1108.
5. Collins FS, Weissman SM. The molecular genetics of human hemoglobin. Prog Nucleic Acid Res Mol Biol. 1984;31:315-462.
6. Bunn HF, Forget BG. Hemoglobin: Molecular, Genetic and Clinical Aspects. Philadelphia, WB Saunders, 1986.
7. Boyer SH, Belding TK, Margolet L, Noyes AN. Fetal hemoglobin restricted to a few erythrocytes (F-cells) in normal human adults. Science. 1975;188:361-363.
8. Wood WG, Stamatoyannopoulos G, Lim G, Nute PE. F-cells in the adult: normal values and levels in individuals with hereditary and acquired elevations of Hb F. Blood. 1975;46:671-682.
9. Garner C, Tatu T, Reittie JE, et al. Genetic influences on F cells and other hematologic variables: a twin heritability study. Blood. 2000;95:342-346.
10. Weatherall MW, Higgs DR, Weiss H, et al. Phenotype/genotype relationships in sickle cell disease: a pilot twin study. Clin Lab Haematol. 2005;27:384-390.
11. Pilia G, Chen WM, Scuteru A, et al. Heritability of cardiovascular and personality traits in 6,148 Sardinians. PLoS Genet. 2006;2:e132.
12. Miyoshi K, Kaneto Y, Kawai H, et al. X-linked dominant control of F-cells in normal adult life: characterization of the Swiss type as hereditary persistence of fetal hemoglobin regulated dominantly by gene(s) on X chromosome. Blood. 1988;72:1854-1860.
13. Craig JE, Rochette J, Fisher CA, et al. Dissecting the loci controlling fetal haemoglobin production on chromosomes 11p and 6q by the regressive approach. Nat Genet. 1996;12:58-64.
14. Maniatis T, Fritsch EF, Lauer J, Lawn RM. The molecular genetics of human hemoglobins. Annu Rev Genet. 1980;14:145-178.
15. Liebhaber SA. Alpha thalassemia. Hemoglobin. 1989; 13:685-731.
16. Deisseroth A, Nienhuis AW, Turner P, et al. Localization of the human alpha-globin structural gene to chromosome 16 in somatic cell hybrids by molecular hybridization assay. Cell. 1977;12:205-218.
17. Deisseroth A, Nienhuis AW, Lawrence J, et al. Chromosomal localization of the human beta-globin gene on chromosome 11 in somatic cell hybrids. Proc Natl Acad Sci U S A. 1978;75:1459-1460.
18. Lauer J, Shen CKJ, Maniatis T, et al. The chromosomal arrangement of human alpha-like globin genes: sequence homology and alpha-globin gene deletions. Cell. 1980;20:119-130.
19. Liebhaber SA, Goossens M, Kan YW, et al. Homology and concerted evolution at the alpha-1 and alpha-2 loci of human alpha-globin. Nature. 1981;290:26-29.
20. Proudfoot NJ, Gil A, Maniatis T, et al. The structure of the human zeta-globin gene and a closely linked, nearly identical pseudogene. Cell. 1982;31:553-563.
21. Fritsch EF, Lawn RM, Maniatis T, et al. Molecular cloning and characterization of the human beta-like globin gene cluster. Cell. 1980;19:959-972.
22. Efstratiadis A, Posakony JW, Maniatis T, et al. The structure and evolution of the human beta-globin gene family. Cell. 1980;21:653-658.
23. Slightom JL, Blechl AE, Smithies O. Human fetal G gamma- and A gamma-globin genes: complete nucleotide sequences suggest that DNA can be exchanged between these duplicated genes. Cell 1980;21:627-638.
24. Baralle FE, Shoulders CC, Proudfoot NJ. The primary structure of the human epsilon-globin gene. Cell. 1980;21:621-626.
25. Humphries RK, Ley T, Turner P, et al. Differences in human alpha-, beta- and delta-globin gene expression in monkey kidney cells. Cell. 1982;30:173-183.
26. Kosche KA, Dobkin C, Bank A. DNA sequences regulating human beta globin gene expression. Nucleic Acids Res. 1985;13:7781-7793.
27. Ross J, Pizarro A. Human beta and delta globin messenger RNAs turn over at different rates. J Mol Biol. 1983;167:607-617.
28. Pataryas HA, Stamatoyannopoulos G. Hemoglobins in human fetuses: evidence for adult hemoglobin production after the 11th gestational week. Blood. 1972;39: 688-696.
29. Henri A, Testa U, Tonthat H, et al. Disappearance of the Hb F and i antigen during the first year of life. Am J Hematol. 1980;9:161-170.
30. Terrenato L, Bertilaccio C, Spinelli P, Columbo B. The switch from haemoglobin F to A: the time course of qualitative and quantitative variations of haemoglobins after birth. Br J Haematol. 1981;47:31-41.
31. Smale ST, Baltimore D. The "initiator" as a transcriptional control element. Cell. 1989;57:103-113.
32. Lewis BA, Orkin SH. A functional initiator element in the human β-globin promoter. J Biol Chem. 1995;270: 28139-28144.
33. Dynan WS, Tjian R. Control of eukaryotic messenger RNA synthesis by sequence-specific DNA-binding proteins. Nature. 1985;316:774-778.
34. McKnight S, Tjian R. Transcriptional selectivity of viral genes in mammalian cells. Cell. 1986;46:795-805.

*See references 280, 285, 286, 289-292, 296-299, 302, 303, 313, 369-373.

35. Maniatis T, Goodbourn S, Fischer JA. Regulation of inducible and tissue-specific gene expression. Science. 1987;236:1237-1245.

36. Saltzman AG, Weinmann R. Promoter specificity and modulation of RNA polymerase II transcription. FASEB J. 1989;3:1723-1733.

37. Dynan WS. Modularity in promoters and enhancers. Cell. 1989;58:1-4.

38. Guarente L. UASs and enhancers: common mechanism of transcriptional activation in yeast and mammals. Cell. 1988;52:303-305.

39. Müller MM, Gerster T, Schaffner W. Enhancer sequences and the regulation of gene transcription. Eur J Biochem. 1988;176:485-495.

40. Peterson MG, Tanese N, Pugh BF, Tjian R. Functional domains and upstream activation properties of cloned human TATA binding protein. Science. 1990;248:1625-1630.

41. Kao CC, Lieberman PM, Schmidt MC, et al. Cloning of a transcriptionally active human TATA binding factor. Science. 1990;248:1646-1650.

42. Lewin B. Commitment and activation at pol II promoters: a tail of protein-protein interactions. Cell. 1990;61:1161-1164.

43. Takihara Y, Nakamura T, Yamada H, et al. A novel mutation in the TATA box in a Japanese patient with beta+-thalassemia. Blood. 1986;67:547-550.

44. Fei YJ, Stoming TA, Efremov GD, et al. Beta-thalassemia due to a T→A mutation within the ATA box. Biochem Biophys Res Commun. 1988;153:741-747.

45. Cai SP, Zhang JZ, Doherty M, Kan YW. A new TATA box mutation detected at prenatal diagnosis for beta-thalassemia. Am J Hum Genet. 1989;45:112-114.

46. Antonarakis SE, Orkin SH, Chang T-C, et al. Beta thalassemia in American blacks: novel mutations in the TATA box and an acceptor splice site. Proc Natl Acad Sci U S A. 1984;81:1154-1158.

47. Huang S, Wong C, Antonarakis SE, et al. The same TATA box beta thalassemia mutation in Chinese and U.S. blacks: another example of independent origins of mutation. Hum Genet. 1986;74:162-164.

48. Poncz M, Ballantine M, Solowiejczyk D, et al. Beta thalassemia in a Kurdish Jew. J Biol Chem. 1983;257:5994-5996.

49. Orkin SH, Sexton JP, Cheng TC, et al. ATA box transcription mutation in beta-thalassemia. Nucleic Acids Res. 1983;11:4727-4734.

50. Hoey T, Dynlacht BD, Peterxson MG, et al. Isolation and characterization of the *Drosophila* gene encoding the TATA box binding protein, TFIID. Cell. 1990;61:1179-1186.

51. Orkin SH. Regulation of globin gene expression in erythroid cells. Eur J Biochem. 1995;231:271-281.

52. Li Q, Peterson KR, Fang X, Stamatoyannopoulos G. Locus control regions. Blood. 2002;100:3077-3086.

53. Nichols KE, Crispino JD, Poncz M, et al. Familial dyserythropoietic anaemia and thrombocytopenia due to an inherited mutation in GATA1. Nat Genet. 2000;24:266-270.

54. Freson KK, Devriendt K, Matthijs G, et al. Platelet characteristics in patients with X-linked macrothrombocytopenia because of a novel GATA1 mutation. Blood. 2001;98:85-92.

55. Mehaffey MG, Newton AL, Gandhi MJ, et al. X-linked thrombocytopenia caused by a novel mutation of GATA-1. Blood. 2001;98:2681-2688.

56. Phillips JD, Steensma DP, Pulsipher MA, et al. Congenital erythropoietic porphyria due to a mutation in GATA1: the first trans-acting mutation causative for a human porphyria. Blood. 2007;109:2618-2621.

57. Tubman VN, Levine JE, Campagna DR, et al. X-linked gray platelet syndrome due to a GATA1 Arg216Gln mutation. Blood. 2007;109:3297-3299.

58. Yu C, Niakan KK, Matsushita M, et al. X-linked thrombocytopenia with thalassemia from a mutation in the amino finger of GATA-1 affecting DNA binding rather than FOG-1 interaction. Blood. 2002;100:2040-2045.

59. Tsang AP, Visvader JE, Turner CA, et al. FOG, a multitype zinc finger protein acts as a cofactor for transcription factor GATA-1 in erythroid and megakaryocytic differentiation. Cell. 1997;90:109-119.

60. Crispino JD, Lodish MB, MacKay JP, Orkin SH. Use of altered specificity mutants to probe a specific protein-protein interaction in differentiation: the GATA-1:FOG comples. Mol Cell. 1999;3:219-228.

61. Kadonaga JT, Carner KR, Masiarz FR, Tjian R. Isolation of cDNA encoding transcription factor Sp1 and functional analysis of the DNA binding domain. Cell. 1987;51:1079-1090.

62. Perkins AC, Sharpe AH, Orkin SH. Lethal β-thalassaemia in mice lacking the erythroid CACCC-transcription factor EKLF. Nature. 1995;375:318-322.

63. Andrews NC, Erdjument-Bromage H, Davidson MB, et al. Erythroid transcription factor NF-E2 is a haematopoietic-specific basic-leucine zipper protein. Nature. 1993;362:722-728.

64. Andrews NC, Kotkow KJ, Ney PA, et al. The ubiquitous subunit of erythroid transcription factor NF-E2 is a small basic-leucine zipper protein related to the v-maf oncogene. Proc Natl Acad Sci U S A. 1993;90:11488-11492.

65. Lu SJ, Rowan S, Bani MR, Ben-David Y. Retroviral integration within the Fli-2 locus results in inactivation of the erythroid transcription factor NF-E2 in Friend erythroleukemias: evidence that NF-E2 is essential for globin expression. Proc Natl Acad Sci U S A. 1994;91:8398-8402.

66. Kotkow KJ, Orkin SH. Dependence of globin gene expression in mouse erythroleukemia cells on the NF-E2 heterodimer. Mol Cell Biol. 1995;15:4640-4647.

67. Shivdasani RA, Orkin SH. Erythropoiesis and globin gene expression in mice lacking the transcription factor NF-E2. Proc Natl Acad Sci U S A. 1995;92:8690-8694.

68. Chada K, Magram J, Raphael K, et al. Specific expression of a foreign beta-globin gene in erythroid cells of transgenic mice. Nature. 1985;314:377-380.

69. Magram J, Chada K, Constantini F. Developmental regulation of a cloned adult beta-globin gene in transgenic mice. Nature. 1985;315:338-340.

70. Townes TM, Lingrel JB, Chen HY, et al. Erythroid-specific expression of human beta-globin genes in transgenic mice. EMBO J. 1985;4:1715-1723.

71. Costantini F, Radice G, Magram J, et al. Developmental regulation of human globin genes in transgenic mice.

Cold Spring Harbor Symp Quant Biol. 1985;50: 361-370.

72. Chada K, Magram J, Constantini F. An embryonic pattern of expression of a human fetal globin gene in transgenic mice. Nature. 1986;319:685-689.

73. Kollias G, Wrighton N, Hurst J, Grosveld F. Regulated expression of human A gamma-, beta-, and hybrid gamma beta-globin genes in transgenic mice: manipulation of the developmental expression patterns. Cell. 1986;46:89-94.

74. Tuan D, Solomon W, Li Q, London IM. The "beta-like-globin" gene domain in human erythroid cells. Proc Natl Acad Sci U S A. 1985;82:6384-6388.

75. Tuan DY, Solomon WB, London IM, Lee DP. An erythroid-specific, developmental-stage–independent enhancer far upstream of the human "beta-like globin" genes. Proc Natl Acad Sci U S A. 1989;86:2554-2558.

76. Grosveld F, van Assendelft GB, Greaves DR, Kollias G. Position-independent, high-level expression of the human beta-globin gene in transgenic mice. Cell. 1987;51:975-985.

77. Higgs DR, Wood WG, Jarman AP, et al. A major positive regulatory region is located far upstream of the human α-globin gene locus. Genes Dev. 1990;4:1588-1601.

78. Gibbons RJ, Brueton L, Buckle VJ, et al. Clinical and hematologic aspects of the X-linked α-thalassemia/mental retardation syndrome (ATR-X). Am J Med Genet. 1995;55:288-299.

79. Gibbons RJ, Picketts DJ, Villard L, Higgs DR. Mutations in a putative global transcriptional regulator cause X-linked mental retardation with alpha-thalassemia (ATR-X syndrome). Cell. 1995;80:837-845.

80. Raich N, Clegg CH, Grofti J, et al. GATA1 and YY1 are developmental repressors of the human epsilon-globin gene. EMBO J. 1995;14:801-809.

81. Choi OR, Engel JD. Developmental regulation of beta-globin gene switching. Cell. 1988;55:17-26.

82. Jane SM, Ney PA, Vanin EF, et al. Identification of a stage selector element in the human γ-globin gene promoter that fosters preferential interaction with the 5′ HS2 enhancer when in competition with the β-promoter. EMBO J. 1992;11:2961-2999.

83. Palstra RJ, Tolhuis B, Splinter E, et al. The beta-globin nuclear compartment in development and erythroid differentiation. Nat Genet. 2003;35:190-194.

84. Vakoc CR, Letting DL, Gheldof N, et al. Proximity among distant regulatory elements at the beta-globin locus requires GATA-1 and FOG-1. Mol Cell. 2005;17: 453-462.

85. Vernimmen D, De Gobbi M, Sloane-Stanley JA, et al. Long-range chromosomal interactions regulate the timing of the transition between poised and active gene expression. EMBO J. 2007;26:2041-2051.

86. Nienhuis AW, Anagnou NP, Ley TJ. Advances in thalassemia research. Blood. 1984;63:738-758.

87. Orkin SH, Kazazian HH Jr. Mutation and polymorphism of the human beta-globin gene and its surrounding DNA. Annu Rev Genet. 1984;18:131-171.

88. Benz EJ Jr, Nathan DG. Pathophysiology of the anemia in thalassemia. In Weatherall DJ (ed). Congenital Disorders of Erythropoiesis. Amsterdam, Elsevier, 1976, p 205.

89. Fessas P, Loukopoulos D. The beta-thalassemias. Clin Haematol. 1974;3:411-420.

90. Nathan DG, Gunn RB. Thalassemia: the consequences of unbalanced hemoglobin synthesis. Am J Med. 1966;41:815-830.

91. Nathan DG, Stossel TB, Gunn RB, et al. Influence of hemoglobin precipitation on erythrocyte metabolism in alpha and beta thalassemia. J Clin Invest. 1969;48: 33-41.

92. Nathan DG. Thalassemia. N Engl J Med. 1972;286: 586-594.

93. Wood WG, Weatherall DJ, Clegg JB. Interaction of heterocellular hereditary persistence of fetal haemoglobin with beta thalassaemia and sickle cell anemia. Nature. 1976;264:247-249.

94. Prchal J, Stamatoyannopoulos G. Two siblings with unusually mild homozygous beta thalassemia: a didactic example of nonallelic modifier gene on the expressivity of a monogenic disorder. Am J Med Genet. 1981;10: 291-300.

95. Safaya S, Rieder RF, Dowling CE, et al. Homozygous beta-thalassemia without anemia. Blood. 1989;73: 324-328.

96. Kanavakis K, Wainscoat JS, Wood WG, et al. The interaction of alpha thalassemia with beta thalassemia. Br J Haematol. 1982;52:465-473.

97. Haldane JBS. The rate of mutation of human genes. In Proceedings of the VIII International Congress on Genetics and Heredity. 1949, p 267.

98. Livingstone FB. Frequency of Hemoglobin Variants. New York, Oxford University Press, 1985.

99. Weatherall DJ. Common genetic disorders of the red cell and the "malaria hypothesis." Ann Trop Med Parasitol. 1987;81:539-548.

100. Fraser GR, Stamatoyannopoulos G, Kattamis C, et al. Thalassemias, abnormal hemoglobins, and glucose-6-phosphate dehydrogenase deficiency in the Arta area of Greece: diagnostic and genetic aspects of complete village studies. Ann N Y Acad Sci. 1964;119:415-435.

101. Kanavakis E, Tzotzos S, Liapake K, et al. Molecular basis and prevalence of alpha-thalassemia in Greece. Birth Defects Orig Artic Ser. 1988;23:377-380.

102. Falusi AG, Esan GJ, Ayyub H, Higgs DR. Alpha-thalassaemia in Nigeria: its interaction with sickle-cell disease. Eur J Haematol. 1987;38:370-375.

103. Flint J, Hill AV, Bowden DK, et al. High frequencies of alpha-thalassaemia are the result of natural selection by malaria. Nature. 1986;321:744-750.

104. Flint J, Hill AV. Alpha globin genotypes in two North European populations [letter]. Br J Haematol. 1986; 63:796.

105. Shimizu K, Harano T, Harano K, et al. Abnormal arrangements in the alpha- and gamma-globin gene clusters in a relatively large group of Japanese newborns. Am J Hum Genet. 1986;38:45-58.

106. Flint J, Harding RM, Boyce AJ, Clegg JB. The population genetics of the haemoglobinopathies. Bailieres Clin Haematol. 1998;11:1-51.

107. Siniscalco M, Bernini L, Filippi G, et al. Population genetics of haemoglobin variants, thalassemia and glucose-6-phosphate dehydrogenase deficiency, with particular reference to malaria hypothesis. Bull WHO. 1966;34:379-393.

108. Willcox M, Bjorkman A, Brohult J. Falciparum malaria and beta-thalassaemia trait in northern Liberia. Ann Trop Med Parasitol. 1983;77:335-347.

109. Oppenheimer SJ, Higgs DR, Weatherall DJ, et al. Alpha thalassaemia in Papua New Guinea. Lancet. 1984;1:424-426.

110. Teo CG, Wong HB. The innate resistance of thalassemia to malaria: a review of the evidence and possible mechanisms. Singapore Med J. 1985;26:504-509.

111. Hill AV, Bowden DK, O'Shaughnessy DF, et al. Beta thalassemia in Melanesia: association with malaria and characterization of a common variant (IVS-1 nt 5 G→C). Blood. 1988;72:9-14.

112. Lell B, May J, Schmidt-Ott RJ, et al. The role of red blood cell polymorphisms in resistance and susceptibility to malaria. Clin Infect Dis. 1999;28:794-799.

113. Sakai Y, Kobayashi S, Shibata H, et al. Molecular analysis of alpha-thalassemia in Nepal: correlation with malaria endemicity. J Hum Genet. 2000;45:127-132.

114. Clegg JB, Weatherall DJ. Thalassemia and malaria: new insights into an old problem. Proc Assoc Am Physicians. 1999;111:278-282.

115. Williams TN, Maitland K, Bennett S, et al. High incidence of malaria in alpha-thalassaemic children. Nature. 1996;383:522-525.

116. Williams TN, Wambua S, Uyoga S, et al. Both heterozygous and homozygous alpha+ thalassemias protect against severe and fatal *Plasmodium falciparum* malaria on the coast of Kenya. Blood. 2005;106:368-371.

117. Wambua S, Mwangi TW, Kortok M, et al. The effect of alpha+ thalassaemia on the incidence of malaria and other diseases in children living on the coast of Kenya. PLoS Med. 2006;3:e158.

118. Pasvol G, Weatherall DJ, Wilson RJ. Effects of foetal haemoglobin on susceptibility of red cells to *Plasmodium falciparum*. Nature. 1977;270:171-173.

119. Nagel RL, Roth EF Jr. Malaria and red cell genetic defects. Blood. 1989;74:1213-1221.

120. Brockelman CR, Wongsattayanont B, Tan-ariya P, Fucharoen S. Thalassemic erythrocytes inhibit in vitro growth of *Plasmodium falciparum*. J Clin Microbiol. 1987;25:56-60.

121. Pattanapanyasat K, Yongvanitchit K, Tongtawe P, et al. Impairment of *Plasmodium falciparum* growth in thalassemic red blood cells: further evidence by using biotin labeling and flow cytometry. Blood. 1999;93:3116-3119.

122. Luzzi GA, Merry AH, Newbold CI, et al. Surface antigen expression on *Plasmodium falciparum*–infected erythrocytes is modified in alpha- and beta-thalassemia. J Exp Med. 1991;1991:785-791.

123. Williams TN, Weatherall DJ, Newbold CI. The membrane characteristics of *Plasmodium falciparum*–infected and –uninfected heterozygous alpha(0)thalassaemic erythrocytes. Br J Haematol. 2002;118:663-670.

124. Ifediba TC, Stern A, Ibrahim A, Rieder RF. *Plasmodium falciparum* in vitro: diminished growth in hemoglobin H disease erythrocytes. Blood. 1985;65:452-455.

125. Carlson J, Nash GB, Gabutti V, et al. Natural protection against severe *Plasmodium falciparum* malaria due to impaired rosette formation. Blood. 1994;84:3909-3914.

126. Gonzalez-Redondo JM, Stoming TA, Kutlar A, et al. A C→T substitution at nt-101 in a conserved DNA sequence of the promotor region of the beta-globin gene is associated with "silent" beta-thalassemia. Blood. 1989;73:1705-1711.

127. Orkin SH, Antonarakis SE, Kazaxian HH Jr. Base substitution at position -88 in a beta-thalassemic globin gene. Further evidence for the role of distal promoter element ACACCC. J Biol Chem. 1984;259:8679-8681.

128. Rund D, Filon D, Rachmilewitz EA, et al. Molecular analysis of beta thalassemia in Kurdish Jews: novel mutations and expression studies. Blood. 1989;74:821A.

129. Orkin SH, Kazazian HH Jr, Antonarkis SE, et al. Linkage of beta thalassaemia mutations and beta-globin gene polymorphisms with DNA polymorphisms in the human beta-globin gene cluster. Nature. 1982;296:627-631.

130. Wong C, Dowling CE, Saiki RK, et al. Characterization of beta-thalassaemia mutations using direct genomic sequencing of amplified single copy DNA. Nature. 1987;330:384-386.

131. Orkin SH, Goff SC, Hechtman RL. Mutation in an intervening sequence splice junction in man. Proc Natl Acad Sci U S A. 1981;78:5041-5045.

132. Felber BK, Orkin SH, Hamer DH. Abnormal RNA splicing causes one form of alpha thalassemia. Cell. 1982;29:895-902.

133. Kazazian HH Jr, Orkin SH, Antonarakis SE, et al. Molecular characterization of seven beta-thalassemia mutations in Asian Indians. EMBO J. 1984;3:593-596.

134. Chibani J, Vidaud M, Duquesnoy P, et al. The peculiar spectrum of beta-thalassemia genes in Tunisia. Hum Genet. 1988;78:190-192.

135. Gonzalez-Redondo JM, Stoming TA, Kutlar F, et al. Severe Hb S-beta zero-thalassemia with a T→C substitution in the donor splice site of the first intron of the beta-globin gene. Br J Haematol. 1989;71:113-117.

136. Kazazian HH Jr, Boehm CD. Molecular basis and prenatal diagnosis of beta-thalassemia. Blood. 1988;72:1107-1116.

137. Treisman R, Proudfoot NJ, Shander M, Maniatis T. A single base change at a splice site in a beta 0-thalassemia gene causes abnormal RNA splicing. Cell. 1982;29:903-911.

138. Wong C, Antonarakis SE, Goff SC, et al. On the origin and spread of beta-thalassemia: recurrent observation of four mutations in different ethnic groups. Proc Natl Acad Sci U S A. 1986;83:6529-6532.

139. Orkin SH, Sexton JP, Goff SC, Kazazian HH Jr. Inactivation of an acceptor RNA splice site by a short deletion in beta-thalassemia. J Biol Chem. 1983;258:7249-7251.

140. Atweh GF, Anagnou NP, Shearin J, et al. Beta-thalassemia resulting from a single nucleotide substitution in an acceptor splice site. Nucleic Acids Res. 1985;13:777-790.

141. Gonzalez-Redondo JM, Stoming TA, Kutlar F, et al. Hb Monroe or alpha$_2$beta$_2$ 30(B12)Arg→Thr, a variant associated with beta-thalassemia due to A G→C substitution adjacent to the donor splice site of the first intron. Hemoglobin. 1989;13:67-74.

142. Kalydjieva L, Eigel A, Horst J, et al. The molecular basis of thalassemia in Bulgaria. Paper presented at the 3rd

International Conference on Thalassemia and the Hemoglobinopathies, 1989, Sardinia.

143. Cheng TC, Orkin SH, Antonarakis SE, et al. Beta thalassemia in Chinese: use of in vivo RNA analysis and oligonucleotide hybridization in systematic characterization of molecular defects. Proc Natl Acad Sci U S A. 1984;81:2821-2825.

144. Atweh GF, Wong C, Reed R, et al. A new mutation in IVS-1 of the human beta globin gene causing beta thalassemia due to abnormal splicing. Blood. 1987;70:147-151.

145. Gonzalez-Redondo JM, Stoming TA, Lanclos DK, et al. Clinical and genetic heterogeneity in black patients with homozygous beta-thalassemia from the southeastern United States. Blood. 1988;72:1007-1014.

146. Lapoumeroulie C, Pagnier J, Bank A, et al. Beta thalassemia due to a novel mutation in IVS 1 sequence donor site consensus sequence creating a restriction site. Biochem Biophys Res Commun. 1986;139:709-713.

147. Wong C, Antonarakis SE, Goff SC, et al. Beta-thalassemia due to two novel nucleotide substitutions in consensus acceptor splice sequences of the beta-globin gene. Blood. 1989;73:914-918.

148. Beldjord C, Lapoumeroulie C, Pagnier J, et al. A novel beta thalassemia gene with a single base mutation in the conserved polypyrimidine sequence at the 3' end of IVS 2. Nucleic Acids Res. 1988;16:4927-4935.

149. Yang KG, Kutlar F, George E, et al. Molecular characterization of beta-globin gene mutations in Malay patients with Hb E–beta-thalassaemia and thalassaemia major. Br J Haematol. 1989;72:73-80.

150. Goldsmith ME, Humphries RK, Ley T, et al. "Silent" nucleotide substitution in a beta⁺-thalassemia globin gene activates splice site in coding sequence RNA. Proc Natl Acad Sci U S A. 1983;80:2318-2322.

151. Orkin SH, Kazazian HH Jr, Antonarakis SE, et al. Abnormal RNA processing due to the exon mutation of the beta E globin gene. Nature. 1982;300:768-769.

152. Orkin SH, Antonarakis SE, Loukopoulos D. Abnormal processing of beta Knossos RNA. Blood. 1984;64:311-313.

153. Spritz RA, Jagadeeswaran P, Choudary PV, et al. Base substitution in an intervening sequence of a beta⁺ thalassemic human globin gene. Proc Natl Acad Sci U S A. 1981;78:2455-2459.

154. Westaway D, Williamson R. An intron nucleotide sequence variant in a cloned beta⁺-thalassemia globin gene. Nucleic Acids Res. 1981;9:1777-1788.

155. Metherall JE, Collins FS, Pan J, et al. Beta zero thalassemia caused by a base substitution that creates an alternative splice acceptor site in an intron. EMBO J. 1986;5:2551-2557.

156. Dobkin C, Pergolizzi RG, Bahre P, Bank A. Abnormal splice in a mutant human beta-globin gene not at the site of a mutation. Proc Natl Acad Sci U S A. 1983;80:1184-1188.

157. Higgs DR, Goodbourn SE, Lamb J, et al. Alpha-thalassaemia caused by a polyadenylation signal mutation. Nature. 1983;306:398-400.

158. Thein SL, Wallace RB, Pressley L, et al. The polyadenylation site mutation in the alpha-globin gene cluster. Blood. 1988;71:313-319.

159. Orkin SH, Cheng TC, Antonarakis SE, Kazazian HH Jr. Thalassemia due to a mutation in the cleavage-polyadenylation signal of the human beta-globin gene. EMBO J. 1985;4:453-456.

160. Jankovic L, Efremov GD, Petkov G, et al. Three novel mutations leading to beta thalassemia. Blood. 1989;74:226A.

161. Pirastu M, Saglio G, Chang JC, et al. Initiation codon mutation as a cause of alpha thalassemia. J Biol Chem. 1984;259:12315-12317.

162. Moi P, Cash FE, Liebhaber SA, et al. An initiation codon mutation (AUG→GUG) of the human alpha 1-globin gene. Structural characterization and evidence for a mild thalassemic phenotype. J Clin Invest. 1987;80:1416-1421.

163. Olivieri NF, Chang LS, Poon AO, et al. An alpha-globin gene initiation codon mutation in a black family with HbH disease. Blood. 1987;70:729-732.

164. Morle F, Starck J, Godet J. Alpha-thalassemia due to the deletion of nucleotides -2 and -3 preceding the AUG initiation codon affects translation efficiency both in vitro and in vivo. Nucleic Acids Res. 1986;14:3279-3292.

165. Morle F, Lopez B, Henni T, Godet J. Alpha-thalassaemia associated with the deletion of two nucleotides at position -2 and -3 preceding the AUG codon. EMBO J. 1985;4:1245-1250.

166. Liebhaber SA, Coleman MB, Adams JG 3rd, et al. Molecular basis for nondeletion alpha-thalassemia in American blacks: alpha 2(116GAG→UAG). J Clin Invest. 1987;80:154-159.

167. Chang JC, Kan YW. Beta zero thalassemia, a nonsense mutation in man. Proc Natl Acad Sci U S A. 1979;76:2886-2889.

168. Fucharoen S, Fucharoen G, Fucharoen P, Fukumaki Y. A novel ochre mutation in the beta-thalassemia gene of a Thai. Identification by direct cloning of the entire β-globin gene amplified using polymerase chain reactions. J Biol Chem. 1989;264:7780-7783.

169. Boehm CD, Dowling CE, Wabner PG, et al. Use of oligonucleotide hybridization in the characterization of a beta zero-thalassemia gene (beta 37 TGG→TGA) in a Saudi Arabian family. Blood. 1986;67:1185-1188. [Published erratum appears in Blood. 1986;68:323.]

170. Trecartin RF, Liebhaber SA, Chang JC, et al. Beta zero thalassemia in Sardinia is caused by a nonsense mutation. J Clin Invest. 1981;68:1012-1017.

171. Chehab FF, Honig GR, Kan YW. Spontaneous mutation in beta-thalassaemia producing the same nucleotide substitution as that in a common hereditary form. Lancet. 1986;1:3-5.

172. Atweh GF, Brickner HE, Zhu XX, et al. New amber mutation in a beta-thalassemic gene with nonmeasurable levels of mutant messenger RNA in vivo. J Clin Invest. 1988;82:557-561.

173. Safaya S, Rieder RF. Dysfunctional alpha-globin gene in hemoglobin H disease in blacks. A dinucleotide deletion produces a frameshift and a termination codon. J Biol Chem. 1988;263:4328-4332.

174. Kollia P, Gonzalez-Redondo JM, Stoming TA, et al. Frameshift codon 5 [Fsc-5 (-CT)] thalassemia; a novel mutation detected in a Greek patient. Hemoglobin. 1989;13:597-604.

175. Kazazian HH Jr, Orkin SH, Boehm CD, et al. Beta thalassemia due to a deletion of the nucleotide which is substituted in the beta S-globin gene. Am J Hum Genet. 1983;35:1028-1033.

176. Chan V, Chan TK, Kan YW, Todd D. A novel beta-thalassemia frameshift mutation (codon 14/15), detectable by direct visualization of abnormal restriction fragment in amplified genomic DNA. Blood. 1988;72:1420-1430.

177. Schnee J, Griese EU, Eigel A, et al. Beta-thalassemia gene analysis in a Turkish family reveals a 7 BP deletion in the coding region [letter]. Blood. 1989;73:2224.

178. Kimura A, Matsunaga E, Takihara Y, et al. Structural analysis of a beta-thalassemia gene found in Taiwan. J Biol Chem. 1983;258:2748-2749.

179. Kinniburgh AJ, Maquat LE, Schedl T, et al. mRNA-deficient beta zero thalassemia results from a single nucleotide deletion. Nucleic Acids Res. 1982;10:5421-5427.

180. Chehab FF, Winterhalter KH, Kan YW. Characterization of a spontaneous mutation in beta-thalassemia associated with advanced paternal age. Blood. 1989;74:852-854.

181. DiMarzo R, Dowling CE, Wong C, et al. The spectrum of beta-thalassaemia mutations in Sicily. Br J Haematol. 1988;69:393-397.

182. Clegg JB, Weatherall DJ, Millner PF. Haemoglobin Constant Spring—a chain termination mutant? Nature. 1971;234:337-340.

183. Milner PF, Clegg JB, Weatherall DJ. Haemoglobin H disease due to a unique haemoglobin variant with an elongated alpha chain. Lancet. 1971;1:729-732.

184. Clegg JB, Weatherall DJ, Contopolou-Griva I, et al. Haemoglobin Icaria, a new chain termination mutant which causes alpha thalassemia. Nature. 1974;251:245-247.

185. De Jong WW, Meera Khan P, Bernini LF. Hemoglobin Koya Dora: high frequency of a chain termination mutant. Am J Hum Genet. 1975;27:81-90.

186. Bradley TB, Wohl RC, Smith GJ. Elongation of the alpha globin chain in a black family: interaction with Hb G Philadelphia [abstract]. Clin Res. 1975;23:1314.

187. Lehmann H, Casey R, Lang A, et al. Hemoglobin Tak: a beta chain elongation. Br J Haematol. 1975;31:119.

188. Honig GR, Shamsuddin M, Vida LN, et al. Hemoglobin Evanston (alpha 14 Trp→Arg): an unstable alpha-chain variant expressed as alpha-thalassemia. J Clin Invest. 1984;73:1740-1749.

189. Sanguansermsri T, Matragoon S, Changloah L, Flatz G. Hemoglobin Suan-Dok (alpha 2 109(G16) Leu-Arg beta 2): an unstable variant associated with alpha thalassemia. Hemoglobin. 1979;3:161-174.

190. Steinberg MH, Coleman MB, et al. Thalassemic expression of an alpha-2 globin structural mutant. Blood. 1987;70:80A.

191. Honig GR, Shamsuddin M, Zaizov R, et al. Hemoglobin Petah Tikvah (alpha110 Ala→Asp): a new unstable variant with alpha thalassemia like expression. Blood. 1981;57:705-711.

192. Goossens M, Lee KY, Liebhaber SA, Kan YW. Globin structural mutant alpha125 Leu→Pro is a novel cause of alpha thalassemia. Nature. 1982;296:864-865.

193. Liebhaber SA, Kan YW. Alpha thalassemia caused by an unstable alpha-globin mutant. J Clin Invest. 1983;71:461-466.

194. Podda A, Galanello R, et al. A new unstable hemoglobin variant producing a beta thalassemia like phenotype. Paper presented at the 3rd International Conference on Thalassemia and the Hemoglobinopathies, 1989, Sardinia.

195. Kobayashi Y, Fukumaki Y, Komatsu N, et al. A novel globin structural mutant, Showa-Yakushiji (beta 110 Leu-Pro) causing a beta-thalassemia phenotype. Blood. 1987;70:1688-1691.

196. Adams JG, Steinberg MH, Boxer LA, et al. The structure of hemoglobin Indianapolis (β^{112}(G14) arginine): an unstable variant detectable only by isotopic labelling. J Biol Chem. 1979;254:3479-3482.

197. Kazazian HH Jr, Dowling CE, Hurwitz RL, et al. Thalassemia mutations in exon 3 of the beta globin gene often cause a dominant form of thalassemia and show no predilection for malarial-endemic regions of the world [abstract]. Am J Hum Genet. 1989;45:A242.

198. Hattori Y, Yamane A, Yamashiro Y, et al. Characterization of beta-thalassemia mutations among the Japanese. Hemoglobin. 1989;13:657-670.

199. Ristaldi MS, Pirastu M, Murru S, et al. A spontaneous mutation produced a novel elongated beta-globin chain structural variant (Hb Agnana) with a thalassemia-like phenotype [letter]. Blood. 1990;75:1378-1379.

200. Beris P, Miescher PA, Siaz-Chico JC, et al. Inclusion body beta-thalassemia trait in a Swiss family is caused by an abnormal hemoglobin (Geneva) with an altered and extended beta chain carboxy-terminus due to a modification in codon beta 114. Blood. 1988;72:801-805.

201. Thein SL, Hesketh C, Taylor P, et al. Molecular basis for dominantly inherited inclusion body beta thalassemia. Proc Natl Acad Sci U S A. 1990;87:3924-3928.

202. Kazazian HH Jr, Orkin SH, Boehm CD, et al. Characterization of a spontaneous mutation to a beta-thalassemia allele. Am J Hum Genet. 1986;38:860-867.

203. Fei YJ, Stoming TA, Kutler A, et al. One form of inclusion body beta-thalassemia is due to a GAA→TAA mutation at codon 121 of the beta chain [letter]. Blood. 1989;73:1075.

204. Ristaldi MS, Murru S, Loudianos G, et al. The C-T substitution in the distal CACCC box of the beta-globin gene promoter is a common cause of silent beta thalassemia in the Italian population. Br J Haematol. 1990;74:480-486.

205. Nuez B, Michalovich D, Bygrave A, et al. Defective haematopoiesis in fetal liver resulting from inactivation of the EKLF gene. Nature. 1995;375:316-318.

206. De Gobbi M, Viprakasit V, Hughes JR, et al. A regulatory SNP causes a human genetic disease by creating a new transcriptional promoter. Science. 2006;312:1215-1217.

207. Brinster RL, Allen JM, Behringer RR, et al. Introns increase transcriptional efficiency in transgenic mice. Proc Natl Acad Sci U S A. 1988;85:836-840.

208. Buchman AR, Berg P. Comparison of intron-dependent and intron-independent gene expression. Mol Cell Biol. 1988;8:4395-4405.

209. Chang DD, Sharp PA. Messenger RNA transport and HIV rev regulation. Science. 1990;249:614-615.

210. Padanilam BJ, Huisman TH. The beta zero-thalassemia in an American black family is due to a single nucleotide substitution in the acceptor splice junction of the second intervening sequence. Am J Hematol. 1986;22:259-263.

211. Chehab FF, Der Kaloustian V, Khouri FI, et al. The molecular basis of beta-thalassemia in Lebanon: application to prenatal diagnosis. Blood. 1987;69:1141-1145.

212. Treisman R, Orkin SH, Miniatis T. Specific transcription and RNA splicing defects in five cloned beta-thalassaemia genes. Nature. 1983;302:591-596.

213. Busslinger M, Moschonas N, Flavell RA. Beta-thalassemia: aberrant splicing results from a single point mutation in an intron. Cell. 1981;27:289-298.

214. Fukumaki Y, Ghosh PK, Benz EJ Jr, et al. Abnormally spliced messenger RNA in erythroid cells from patients with beta thalassemia and monkey kidney cells expressing a cloned beta-thalassemia gene. Cell. 1982;28:585-593.

215. Whitelaw E, Proudfoot N. Alpha-thalassaemia caused by a poly(A) site mutation reveals that transcriptional termination is linked to 3′ end processing in the human alpha 2 globin gene. EMBO J. 1986;5:2915-2922.

216. Kozak M. An analysis of 5′-noncoding sequences from 699 vertebrate messenger RNAs. Nucleic Acids Res. 1987;15:8125-8148.

217. Baserga SJ, Benz EJ. Nonsense mutations in the human beta-globin gene affect mRNA metabolism. Proc Natl Acad Sci U S A. 1988;85:2056-2060.

218. Chang JC, Temple GF, Trecartin RF, Kan YW. Suppression of the nonsense mutation in homozygous beta thalassemia. Nature. 1979;281:602-603.

219. Orkin SH, Goff SC. Nonsense and frameshift mutations in β⁰-thalassemia detected in cloned β-globin genes. J Biol Chem. 1981;256:9782-9784.

220. Benz EJ Jr, Forget BG, Hillman DG, et al. Variability in the amount of beta-globin mRNA in beta thalassemia. Cell. 1978;14:299-312.

221. Maquat LE, Kinniburgh AJ, Rachmilewitz EA, Ross J. Unstable beta-globin mRNA in mRNA-deficient beta-thalassemia. Cell. 1981;27:543-553.

222. Humphries RK, Ley TJ, Anagnou NP, et al. Beta-39-thalassemia gene: a premature termination codon causes beta-mRNA deficiency without changing cytoplasmic beta-mRNA stability. Blood. 1984;64:23-32.

223. Takeshita K, Forget BG, Scarpa A, Benz EJ Jr. Intranuclear defect in beta-globin mRNA accumulation due to a premature translation termination codon. Blood. 1984;64:13-22.

224. Holbrook JA, Neu-Yilik G, Hentze MW, Kulozik AE. Nonsense-mediated decay approaches the clinic. Nat Genet. 2004;36:801-808.

225. Liebhaber SA, Kan YW. Differentiation of the mRNA transcripts originating from the alpha-1 and alpha-2 globin loci in normals and alpha thalassemics. J Clin Invest. 1981;68:439-446.

226. Hunt DM, Higgs DR, Winichagoon P, et al. Haemoglobin Constant Spring has an unstable alpha chain messenger RNA. Br J Haematol. 1982;51:405-413.

227. Derry S, Wood WG, Pippard M, et al. Hematologic and biosynthetic studies in homozygous hemoglobin Constant Spring. J Clin Invest. 1984;73:1673-1682.

228. Bunn HF, Schmidt GJ, Haney DN, Dluhy RG. Hemoglobin Cranston, an unstable variant having an elongated beta chain due to non-homologous cross over between two normal beta chain genes. Proc Natl Acad Sci U S A. 1975;72:3609-3613.

229. Bunn HF. Subunit assembly of hemoglobin: an important determinant of hematologic phenotype. Blood. 1987;69:1-6.

230. Eaton WA. The relationship between coding sequences and function in haemoglobins. Nature. 1980;284:183-185.

231. Adams JG III, Coleman MB, Hayes J, et al. Modulation of fetal hemoglobin synthesis by iron deficiency. N Engl J Med. 1985;313:1402-1405.

232. Chui DHK, Patterson M, Dowling CE, et al. Hemoglobin Bart's disease in an Italian boy. N Engl J Med. 1990;323:179-182.

233. Kihm AJ, Kong Y, Hong W, et al. An abundant erythroid protein that stabilizes free alpha-haemoglobin. Nature. 2002;417:758-763.

234. Kong Y, Zhou S, Kihm AJ, et al. Loss of alpha-hemoglobin–stabilizing protein impairs erythropiesis and exacerbates beta-thalassemia. J Clin Invest. 2004;114:1457-1466.

235. Viprakasit V, Tanphaichitr VS, Chinchang W, et al. Evaluation of alpha hemoglobin stabilizing protein (AHSP) as a genetic modifier in patients with beta thalassemia. Blood. 2004;103:3296-3299.

236. Lai MI, Jiang J, Silver N, et al. Alpha-haemoglobin stabilising protein is a quantitative trait gene that modifies the phenotype of beta-thalassaemia. Br J Haematol. 2006;133:675-682.

237. Chen JJ. Regulation of protein synthesis by the heme-regulated eIF2α kinase: relevance to anemias. Blood. 2007;109:2693-2699.

238. Han AP, Fleming MD, Chen JJ. Heme-regulated eIF2α kinase modifies the phenotypic severity of murine models of erythropoietic protoporphyria and beta-thalassemia. J Clin Invest. 2005;115:1562-1570.

239. Adams JG 3rd, Coleman MB. Structural hemoglobin variants that produce the phenotype of thalassemia. Semin Hematol. 1990;27:229-238.

240. Flavell RA, Bernards R, Kooter JM, et al. The structure of the human beta-globin gene in beta-thalassaemia. Nucleic Acids Res. 1979;6:2749-2760.

241. Orkin SH, Old JM, Weatherall DJ, Nathan DG. Partial deletion of beta-globin gene DNA in certain patients with beta-thalassemia. Proc Natl Acad Sci U S A. 1979;76:2400-2404.

242. Orkin SH, Kolodner R, Michelson A, Hussan R. Cloning and direct examination of a structurally abnormal human beta-thalassemia globin gene. Proc Natl Acad Sci U S A. 1980;77:3558-3562.

243. Moschonas N, deBoer E, Grosveld FG, et al. Structure and expression of a cloned beta thalassemia globin gene. Nucleic Acids Res. 1982;9:4391-4401.

244. Rosatelli C, Falchi AM, Tuveri T, et al. Prenatal diagnosis of beta-thalassaemia with the synthetic-oligomer technique. Lancet. 1985;1:241-243.

245. Antonarakis SE, Boehm CD, Giardina PJ, Kazazian HH Jr. Nonrandom associations of polymorphic restriction sites in the beta-globin gene cluster. Proc Natl Acad Sci U S A. 1982;79:137-141.

246. Kazazian HH Jr, Orkin SH, Markham AF, et al. Quantitation of the close association between DNA haplotypes and specific beta-thalassaemia mutations in Mediterraneans. Nature. 1984;310:152-154.

247. Jeffreys AJ. DNA sequence variants in the ^{G}gamma-, ^{A}gamma-, delta, and beta-globin genes of man. Cell. 1979;18:1-10.

248. Kan YW, Dozy AM. Polymorphism of DNA sequence adjacent to human beta-globin structural gene: relationship to sickle mutation. Proc Natl Acad Sci U S A. 1978;75:5631-5635.

249. Antonarakis SE, Kazazian HH Jr, Orkin SH. DNA polymorphism and molecular pathology of the human globin gene clusters. Hum Genet. 1985;69:1-14.

250. Higgs DR, Wainscoat JS, Flint J, et al. Analysis of the human alpha-globin gene cluster reveals a highly informative genetic locus. Proc Natl Acad Sci U S A. 1986;83:5165-5169.

251. Chakravarti A, Buetow KH, Antonarakis SE, et al. Nonuniform recombination within the human beta-globin gene cluster. Am J Hum Genet. 1984;36:1239-1258.

252. Wainscoat JS, Hill AVS, Boyce AL, et al. Evolutionary relationships of human populations from an analysis of nuclear DNA polymorphisms. Nature. 1986;319: 491-493.

253. Gerhard DS, Kidd KK, Kidd JR, et al. Identification of a recent recombination event within the human beta-globin gene cluster. Proc Natl Acad Sci U S A. 1984;81:7875-7879.

254. Old JM, Heath C, Fitches A, et al. Meiotic recombination between two polymorphic restriction sites within the beta globin gene cluster. J Med Genet. 1986;23:14-18.

255. Antonarakis SE, Orkin SH, Kazazian HH Jr, et al. Evidence for multiple origins of the beta E-globin gene in Southeast Asia. Proc Natl Acad Sci U S A. 1982; 79:6608-6611.

256. Chehab FF, Doherty M, et al. Detection of sickle cell anaemia and thalassaemias [letter]. Nature. 1987;329:293. [Published erratum appears in Nature. 1987;329:678.]

257. Kulozik AE, Lyons J, Kohne E, et al. Rapid and nonradioactive prenatal diagnosis of beta thalassaemia and sickle cell disease: application of the polymerase chain reaction (PCR). Br J Haematol. 1988;70:455-458.

258. Pirastu M, Ristaldi MS, Cao A. Prenatal diagnosis of beta thalassaemia based on restriction endonuclease analysis of amplified fetal DNA. J Med Genet. 1989; 26:363-367.

259. Orkin SH, Markham AF, Kazazian HH Jr. Direct detection of the common Mediterranean beta-thalassemia gene with synthetic DNA probes. An alternative approach for prenatal diagnosis. J Clin Invest. 1983;71:775-779.

260. Wallace RB, Schold M, Johnson MJ, et al. Oligonucleotide directed mutagenesis of the human beta-globin gene: a general method for producing specific point mutations in cloned DNA. Nucleic Acids Res. 1981;9: 3647-3656.

261. Saiki RK, Chang CA, Levenson CH, et al. Diagnosis of sickle cell anemia and beta-thalassemia with enzymatically amplified DNA and nonradioactive allele-specific oligonucleotide probes. N Engl J Med. 1988;319: 537-541.

262. Cai SP, Zhang JZ, Huang DH, et al. A simple approach to prenatal diagnosis of beta-thalassemia in a geographic area where multiple mutations occur. Blood. 1988;71: 1357-1360.

263. Cai SP, Chang CA, Zhang ZH, et al. Rapid prenatal diagnosis of beta thalassemia using DNA amplification and nonradioactive probes. Blood. 1989;73:372-374.

264. Ristaldi MS, Pirastu M, Rosatelli C, et al. Prenatal diagnosis of beta-thalassaemia in Mediterranean populations by dot blot analysis with DNA amplification and allele specific oligonucleotide probes. Prenat Diagn. 1989;9: 629-638.

265. Sutcharitchan P, Saiki R, Fucharoen S, et al. Reverse dot-blot detection of Thai beta-thalassaemia mutations. Br J Haematol. 1995;90:809-816.

266. Giambona A, Lo Gioco P, Marino M, et al. The great heterogeneity of thalassemia molecular defects in Sicily. Hum Genet. 1995;95:526-530.

267. Saiki RK, Scharf S, Faloona T, et al. Enzymatic amplification of beta-globin genomic sequences and restriction site analysis for diagnosis of sickle cell anemia. Science. 1985;230:1350-1354.

268. Saiki RK, Gelfand DH, Stoffel S, et al. Primer-directed enzymatic amplification of DNA with a thermostable DNA polymerase. Science. 1988;239:487-491.

269. Erlich HA, Gelfand DH, Saiki RK. Specific DNA amplification. Nature. 1988;331:461-462.

270. Eisenstein BI. The polymerase chain reaction: a new method of using molecular genetics for medical diagnosis. N Engl J Med. 1990;322:178-183.

271. Thein SL, Hesketh C, Wallace RB, Weatherall DJ. The molecular basis of thalassaemia major and thalassaemia intermedia in Asian Indians: application to prenatal diagnosis. Br J Haematol. 1988;70:225-231.

272. Kazazian HH Jr, Dowling CE, Waber PG, et al. The spectrum of beta-thalassemia genes in China and Southeast Asia. Blood. 1986;68:964-966.

273. Zhang JZ, Cai SP, He X, et al. Molecular basis of beta thalassemia in South China: strategy for DNA analysis. Hum Genet. 1988;78:37-40.

274. Diaz-Chico JC, Yang KG, Stoming TA, et al. Mild and severe beta-thalassemia among homozygotes from Turkey: identification of the types by hybridization of amplified DNA with synthetic probes. Blood. 1988;71: 248-251.

275. Amselem S, Nunes V, Vidaud M, et al. Determination of the spectrum of beta-thalassemia genes in Spain by use of dot-blot analysis of amplified beta-globin DNA. Am J Hum Genet. 1988;43:95-100.

276. Weatherall DJ, Clegg JB. The Thalassemia Syndromes, 3rd ed. Oxford, Blackwell Scientific, 1981.

277. Weatherall DJ, Wood WG, et al. The developmental genetics of human hemoglobin. In Stamatoyannopoulos G, Nienhuis AW (eds). Experimental Approaches for the Study of Hemoglobin Switching. New York, Alan R. Liss, 1985, p 3.

278. Charache S, Clegg JB, Weatherall DJ. The Negro variety of hereditary persistence of fetal hemoglobin is a model form of thalassemia. Br J Haematol. 1976;34:527-534.

279. Friedman S, Schwartz E, Ahern E, Ahern V. Variation in globin chain synthesis in hereditary persistence of fetal hemoglobin. Br J Haematol. 1976;32:357-364.

280. Tate VE, Hill AV, Bowden DK, et al. A silent deletion in the beta-globin gene cluster. Nucleic Acids Res. 1986;14:4743-4750.

281. Kulozik AE, Yarwood N, Jones RW. The Corfu delta beta zero thalassemia: a small deletion acts at a distance to selectively abolish beta globin gene expression. Blood. 1988;71:457-462. [Published erratum appears in Blood. 1988;71:1509.]

282. Galanello R, Podda A, Melis MA, et al. Interaction between deletion delta-thalassemia and beta zero-thalassemia (codon 39 nonsense mutation) in a Sardinian family. Prog Clin Biol Res. 1989;316B:113-121.

283. Chakalova L, Osborne CS, Dai YF, et al. The Corfu deltabeta thalassemia deletion disrupts gamma-globin gene silencing and reveals post-transcriptional regulation of HbF expression. Blood. 2005;105:2154-2160.

284. Spritz RA, Orkin SH. Duplication followed by deletion accounts for the structure of an Indian deletion beta thalassemia. Nucleic Acids Res. 1982;10:8025-8029.

285. Padanilam BJ, Felice AE, Huisman TH. Partial deletion of the 5′ beta-globin gene region causes beta zero-thalassemia in members of an American black family. Blood. 1984;64:941-944.

286. Anand R, Boehm CD, Kazazian HH Jr, Vanin EF. Molecular characterization of a beta zero-thalassemia resulting from a 1.4 kilobase deletion. Blood. 1988;72:636-641.

287. Gilman JG, Huisman TH, Abels J. Dutch beta⁰-thalassaemia: a 10 kilobase DNA deletion associated with significant gamma-chain production. Br J Haematol. 1984;56:339-348.

288. Gilman JG. The 12.6 kilobase DNA deletion in Dutch beta zero-thalassaemia. Br J Haematol. 1987;67:369-372.

289. Diaz-Chico JC, Yang KG, Kutlar A, et al. An approximately 300 bp deletion involving part of the 5′ beta-globin gene region is observed in members of a Turkish family with beta-thalassemia. Blood. 1987;70:583-586.

290. Spiegelberg R, Aulehla-Scholz C, Erlich H, Horst J. A beta-thalassemia gene caused by a 290–base pair deletion: analysis by direct sequencing of enzymatically amplified DNA. Blood. 1989;73:1695-1698.

291. Aulehla-Scholz C, Spiegelberg R, Horst J. A beta-thalassemia mutant caused by a 300-bp deletion in the human beta-globin gene. Hum Genet. 1989;81:298-299.

292. Popovich BW, Rosenblatt DS, Kendall AG, Nishioka Y. Molecular characterization of an atypical beta-thalassemia caused by a large deletion in the 5′ beta-globin gene region. Am J Hum Genet. 1986;39:797-810.

293. Henthorn PS, Smithies O, Mager DL. Molecular analysis of deletions in the human beta-globin gene cluster: deletion junctions and locations of breakpoints. Genomics. 1990;6:226-237.

294. Ottolenghi S, Comi P, Giglioni B, et al. Delta beta thalassemia is due to a gene deletion. Cell. 1976;9:71-80.

295. Bernards R, Kooter JM, Flavell RA. Physical mapping of the globin gene deletion in delta beta thalassemia. Gene. 1979;6:265-280.

296. Ottolenghi S, Giglioni B. The deletion in a type of delta⁰-beta⁰- thalassemia begins in an inverted Alu I repeat. Nature. 1982;300:770-771.

297. Ottolenghi S, Giglioni B, Tamarelli R, et al. Molecular comparison of delta beta thalassemia and hereditary persistence of fetal hemoglobin DNAs: evidence of a regulatory area? Proc Natl Acad Sci U S A. 1982;79:2347-2351.

298. Feingold EA, Forget BG. The breakpoint of a large deletion causing hereditary persistence of fetal hemoglobin occurs within an erythroid DNA domain remote from the beta-globin gene cluster. Blood. 1989;74:2178-2186.

299. Anagnou NP, Papayannopoulou T, Stamatoyannopoulos G, Nienhuis AW. Structurally diverse molecular deletions in the beta-globin gene cluster exhibit an identical phenotype on interaction with the beta S-gene. Blood. 1985;65:1245-1251.

300. Matsunaga E, Kimura A, Yamada H, et al. A novel deletion in delta beta-thalassemia found in Japan. Biochem Biophys Res Commun. 1985;126:185-191.

301. Shiokawa S, Yamada H, Takihara Y, et al. Molecular analysis of Japanese delta beta-thalassemia. Blood. 1988;72:1771-1776.

302. Zhang JW, Stamatoyannopoulos G, Anagnou NP. Laotian (delta-beta)⁰-thalassemia: molecular characterization of a novel deletion associated with increased production of fetal hemoglobin. Blood. 1988;72:983-988.

303. Efremov GD, Nikolov N, Hattori Y, et al. The 18- to 23-kb deletion of the Macedonian delta beta-thalassemia includes the entire delta and beta globin genes. Blood. 1986;68:971-974.

304. Baglioni C. The fusion of two peptide chains in hemoglobin Lepore and its interpretation as a genetic deletion. Proc Natl Acad Sci U S A. 1962;48:1880-1886.

305. Flavell RA, Kooter JM, De Boer E, et al. Analysis of the beta delta globin gene loci in normal and Hb Lepore DNA: direct determination of gene linkage and intergene distance. Cell. 1978;15:25-41.

306. Baird M, Schreiner C, Driscoll C, Bank A. Localization of the site of recombination in formation of the Lepore Boston globin gene. J Clin Invest. 1981;68:560-564.

307. Mavilio F, Giampaolo A, Caré A, et al. The delta-beta crossover region in Lepore Boston hemoglobinopathy is restricted to a 59 base pair region around the 5′ splice junction of the large globin gene intervening sequence. Blood. 1983;62:230-233.

308. Jones RW, Old JM, Trent RJ, et al. Major rearrangement in the human beta globin gene cluster. Nature. 1981;291:39-44.

309. Jennings MW, Jones RW, Wood WG, Weatherall DJ. Analysis of an inversion within the human beta globin gene cluster. Nucleic Acids Res. 1985;13:2897-2906.

310. Henthorn PS, Smithies O, Nakatsuji T, et al. (ᴬgamma delta beta)-Thalassaemia in blacks is due to a deletion of 34 kbp of DNA. Br J Haematol. 1985;59:343-356.

311. Orkin SH, Alter B, Altay C. Deletion of the ᴬgamma gene in ᴳgamma-delta-beta thalassemia. J Clin Invest. 1979;64:866-869.

312. Tuan D, Feingold E, Newman M, et al. Different 3′ end points of deletions causing δβ-thalassemia and hereditary persistence of fetal hemoglobin: implications for the

control of γ-globin gene expression in man. Proc Natl Acad Sci U S A. 1983;80:6937-6941.

313. Jones RW, Old JM, Trent RJ, et al. Restriction mapping of a new deletion responsible for ^Ggamma(delta-beta) thalassemia. Nucleic Acids Res. 1981;9:6813-6825.

314. George E, Faridah K, Trent RJ, et al. Homozygosity for a new type of ^Ggamma (^Agamma delta beta)⁰-thalassemia in a Malaysian male. Hemoglobin.1986;10:353-363.

315. Mager DL, Henthorn PS, Smithies O. A Chinese ^Ggamma⁺ (^Agamma delta beta)⁰ thalassemia deletion: comparison to other deletions in the human beta-globin gene cluster and sequence analysis of the breakpoints. Nucleic Acids Res. 1985;13:6559-6575.

316. Anagnou NP, Papayannopoulou T, Nienhuis AW, Stomatoyannopoulos G. Molecular characterization of a novel form of (^Agamma delta beta)⁰-thalassemia deletion with a 3′ breakpoint close to those of HPFH-3 and HPFH-4: insights for a common regulatory mechanism. Nucleic Acids Res. 1988;16:6057-6066.

317. Driscoll MC, Dobkin CS, Alter BP, et al. Gamma delta beta-thalassemia due to a de novo mutation deleting the 5′ beta-globin gene activation-region hypersensitive sites. Proc Natl Acad Sci U S A. 1989;86:7470-7474.

318. Curtin P, Pirastu M, Kan YW, et al. A distant gene deletion affects beta-globin gene function in an atypical gamma delta beta-thalassemia. J Clin Invest. 1985;76:1554-1558.

319. Kioussis D, Vanin E, deLange T, et al. Beta-globin gene inactivation by DNA translocation in gamma beta-thalassaemia. Nature. 1983;306:662-666.

320. Vanin EF, Henthorn PS, Kioussis D, et al. Unexpected relationships between four large deletions in the human beta-globin gene cluster. Cell. 1983;35:701-709.

321. Wright S, Taramelli R, Rosenthal A, et al. DNA sequences required for regulated expression of the human beta-globin gene. Prog Clin Biol Res. 1985;191:251-268.

322. Orkin SH, Goff SC, Nathan DG. Heterogeneity of the DNA deletion in gamma-delta-beta thalassemia. J Clin Invest. 1981;67:878-884.

323. Pirastu M, Kan YW, Lin CC, et al. Hemolytic disease of the newborn caused by a new deletion of the entire beta-globin cluster. J Clin Invest. 1983;72:602-609.

324. Fearon ER, Kazazian HH Jr, Waber PG, et al. The entire beta-globin gene cluster is deleted in a form of gamma delta beta-thalassemia. Blood. 1983;61:1269-1274.

325. Diaz-Chico JC, Huang HJ, Juricic D, et al. Two new large deletions resulting in epsilon gamma delta beta-thalassemia. Acta Haematol (Basel). 1988;80:79-84.

326. Fritsch EF, Lawn RM, Maniatis T. Characterization of deletions which affect the expression of fetal globin genes in man. Nature. 1979;279:598-603.

327. Tuan D, Murnane MJ, deRiel JL, Forget BG. Heterogeneity in the molecular basis of hereditary persistence of fetal hemoglobin. Nature. 1980;285:335-337.

328. Bernards R, Flavell RA. Physical mapping of the globin gene deletion in hereditary persistence of foetal hemoglobin (HPFH). Nucleic Acids Res. 1980;8:1521-1534.

329. Jagadeeswaran P, Tuan D, Forget BG, Weissman SM. A gene deletion ending at the midpoint of a repetitive DNA sequence in one form of hereditary persistence of fetal hemoglobin. Nature. 1982;296:469-470.

330. Kutlar A, Gardiner MB, Headlee MG, et al. Heterogeneity in the molecular basis of three types of hereditary persistence of fetal hemoglobin and the relative synthesis of the ^Ggamma and ^Agamma types of gamma chains. Biochem Genet. 1984;22:21-35.

331. Raskind W, Niakan KK, Wolff J, et al. Mapping of a syndrome of X-linked thrombocytopenia with thalassemia to band Xp11-12: further evidence of genetic heterogeneity of X-linked thrombocytopenia. Blood. 2000;95:2262-2268.

332. Saglio G, Camaschella C, Serra A, et al. Italian type of deletional hereditary persistence of fetal hemoglobin. Blood. 1986;68:646-651.

333. Camaschella C, Serra A, Gottardi E, et al. A new hereditary persistence of fetal hemoglobin deletion has the breakpoint within the 3′ beta-globin gene enhancer. Blood. 1990;75:1000-1005.

334. Huisman THJ, Wrightstone RN, Wilson JB, et al. Hemoglobin Kenya: the product of fusion of alpha- and beta-polypeptide chains. Arch Biochem Biophys. 1972;152:850-853.

335. Kendall AG, Ojwang PJ, Schroeder WA, Huisman TH. Hemoglobin Kenya, the product of a gamma-beta fusion gene: studies of the family. Am J Hum Genet. 1973;25:548-563.

336. Huisman THJ, Shroeder WA, et al. Hemoglobin Kenya, the product of non-homologous crossing-over of gamma and beta genes. Blood. 1972;40:947.

337. Nute PE, Wood WG, Stamatoyannopoulos G, et al. The Kenya form of hereditary persistence of fetal hemoglobin: structural studies and evidence for homogeneous distribution of haemoglobin F using fluorescent antihaemoglobin F antibodies. Br J Haematol. 1976;32:55-63.

338. Collins FS, Stoeckert CJ Jr, Serjeant GR, et al. ^Ggamma beta⁺ hereditary persistence of fetal hemoglobin: cosmid cloning and identification of a specific mutation 5′ to the ^Ggamma gene. Proc Natl Acad Sci U S A. 1984;81:4894-4898.

339. Collins FS, Boehm CD, Waber PG, et al. Concordance of a point mutation 5′ to the gamma globin gene with ^Ggamma beta hereditary persistence of fetal hemoglobin in the black population. Blood. 1984;64:1292-1296.

340. Gilman JG, Mishima N, Wen XJ, et al. Upstream promoter mutation associated with a modest elevation of fetal hemoglobin expression in human adults. Blood. 1988;72:78-81.

341. Pissard S, M'rad A, Beuzard Y, Romeo PH. A new type of hereditary persistence of fetal haemoglobin (HPFH): HPFH Tunisia beta + (+C-200)G gamma. Br J Haematol. 1996;95:67-72.

342. Weatherall DJ, Cartner R, Clegg JB, et al. A form of hereditary persistence of fetal haemoglobin characterized by uneven cellular distribution of haemoglobin F and the production of haemoglobins A and A₂ in homozygotes. Br J Haematol. 1975;29:205-220.

343. Old JM, Ayyub H, Wood WG, et al. Linkage analysis of nondeletion hereditary persistence of fetal hemoglobin. Science. 1982;215:981-982.

344. Tate VE, Wood WG, Weatherall DJ. The British form of hereditary persistence of fetal hemoglobin results from a single base mutation adjacent to an S1 hypersensitive site 5′ to the ^Agamma globin gene. Blood. 1986;68:1389-1393.

345. Farquhar M, Gelinas R, Tatsis B, et al. Restriction endonuclease mapping of gamma-delta-beta-globin region in

Ggamma (beta)+ HPFH and a Chinese Agamma HPFH variant. Am J Hum Genet. 1983;35:611-620.

346. Gelinas R, Bender M, Lotshaw C, et al. C to T at position -196 of the Agamma gene promoter. Blood. 1986;67: 1777-1779.

347. Giglioni B, Casini C, Mantovani R, et al. A molecular study of a family with Greek hereditary persistence of fetal hemoglobin and beta-thalassemia. EMBO J. 1984;3:2641-2645.

348. Ottolenghi S, Giglioni B, Pulazzini A, et al. Sardinian delta beta zero-thalassemia: a further example of a C to T substitution at position -196 of the Agamma globin gene promoter. Blood. 1987;69:1058-1061.

349. Collins FS, Metherall JE, Yamakawa M, et al. A point mutation in the Agamma-globin gene promoter in Greek hereditary persistence of fetal haemoglobin. Nature. 1985;313:325-326.

350. Gelinas R, Endlich B, Pfeiffer C, et al. G to A substitution in the distal CCAAT box of the Agamma-globin gene in Greek hereditary persistence of fetal haemoglobin. Nature. 1985;313:323-325.

351. Fessas P, Stamatoyannopoulos G. Hereditary persistence of fetal hemoglobin in Greece. A study and a comparison. Blood. 1964;24:223-240.

352. Ottolenghi S, Nicolis S, Taramelli R, et al. Sardinian Ggamma-HPFH: A T→C substitution in a conserved "octamer" sequence in the Ggamma-globin promoter. Blood. 1988;71:815-817.

353. Surrey S, Delgrosso K, Malladi P, Schwartz E. A single-base change at position -175 in the 5'-flanking region of the Ggamma-globin gene from a black with Ggamma-beta+ HPFH. Blood. 1988;71:807-810.

354. Stoming TA, Stoming GS, Lanclos KD, et al. An Agamma type of nondeletional hereditary persistence of fetal hemoglobin with a T→C mutation at position -175 to the cap site of the Agamma globin gene. Blood. 1989; 73:329-333.

355. Gilman JG, Kutlar F, Johnson ME, Huisman TH. A G to A nucleotide substitution 161 base pairs 5' of the Ggamma globin gene cap site (-161) in a high Ggamma non-anemic person. Prog Clin Biol Res. 1987;251: 383-390.

356. Pembrey ME, Wood WG, Weatherall DJ, Perrine RP. Fetal hemoglobin production and the sickle gene in the oases of Eastern Saudi Arabia. Br J Haematol. 1978;40:415-429.

357. Wainscoat JS, Thein SL, Higgs DR, et al. A genetic marker for elevated levels of hemoglobin F in homozygous sickle cell disease? Br J Haematol. 1985;60: 261-268.

358. Gilman JG, Huisman THJ. DNA sequence variation associated with elevated fetal Ggamma globin production. Blood. 1985;66:783-787.

359. Labie D, Pagnier J, Lapoumeroulie C, et al. Common haplotype dependency of high Ggamma-globin gene expression and high Hb F levels in beta-thalassemia and sickle cell anemia patients. Proc Natl Acad Sci U S A. 1985;82:2111-2114.

360. Labie D, Dunda-Belkhodja O, Rouabhi F, et al. The -158 site 5' to the Ggamma gene and Ggamma expression. Blood. 1985;66:1463-1465.

361. Miller BA, Salameh M, Ahmed M, et al. High fetal hemoglobin production in sickle cell anemia in the eastern province of Saudi Arabia is genetically determined. Blood. 1986;67:1404-1410.

362. Miller BA, Olivieri N, Salameh M, et al: Molecular analysis of the high-hemoglobin-F phenotype in Saudi Arabian sickle cell anemia. N Engl J Med. 1987;316: 244-250.

363. Ottolenghi S, Camaschella C, Comi P, et al. A frequent Agamma-hereditary persistence of fetal hemoglobin in northern Sardinia: its molecular basis and hematologic phenotype in heterozygotes and compound heterozygotes with beta-thalassemia. Hum Genet. 1988;79: 13-17.

364. Motum PI, Deng ZM, Huong L, Trent RJ. The Australian type of nondeletional G gamma-HPFH has a C→G substitution at nucleotode -114 of the G gamma gene. Br J Haematol. 1994;86:219-221.

365. Fucharoen S, Shimizu K, Fukumaki Y. A novel C-T transition within the distal CCAAT motif of the G gamma-globin gene in the Japanese HPFH: implication of factor binding in elevated fetal globin expression. Nucleic Acids Res. 1990;18:5245-5253.

366. Oner R, Kutlar F, Gu LH, Huisman TH. The Georgia type of nondeletional hereditary persistence of fetal hemoglobin has a C-T mutation at nucleotide -114 of the A gamma-globin Gene. Blood. 1991;77:1124-1125.

367. Gilman JG, Mishima N, Wen XJ, et al. Distal CCAAT box deletion in the Agamma globin gene of two black adolescents with elevated fetal Agamma globin. Nucleic Acids Res. 1988;16:10635-19642.

368. Marti HR. In Normale und Anormale Menschliche Hemoglobine. Berlin, Springer-Verlag, 1963, p 81.

369. Jensen M, Wirtz A, Walther JU, et al. Hereditary persistence of fetal haemoglobin (HPFH) in conjunction with a chromosomal translocation involving the haemoglobin beta locus. Br J Haematol. 1984;56:87-94.

370. Sukumaran PK, Huisman THJ, Schroeder WA, et al. A homozygote for the gamma type of fetal hemoglobin in India: a study of two Indians and four Negro families. Br J Haematol. 1972;23:403-417.

371. Boyer SH, Margolet L, Boyer ML, et al. Inheritance of F cell frequency in heterocellular hereditary persistence of fetal hemoglobin: an example of allelic exclusion. Am J Hum Genet. 1977;29:256-271.

372. Stamatoyannopoulos G, Wood WG, Papayannopoulou T, Nute PE. A new form of hereditary persistence of fetal hemoglobin in blacks and its association with sickle cell trait. Blood. 1975;46:683-692.

373. Gelinas RE, Rixon M, Magis W, Stamatopoulos G. Gamma gene promoter and enhancer structure in Seattle variant of hereditary persistence of fetal hemoglobin. Blood. 1988;71:1108-1112.

374. Oggiano L, Pirastu M, Moi P, et al. Molecular characterization of a normal Hb A2 beta-thalassaemia determinant in a Sardinian family. Br J Haematol. 1987;67: 225-229.

375. Moi P, Paglietti E, Sanna A, et al. Delineation of the molecular basis of delta- and normal HbA2 beta-thalassemia. Blood. 1988;72:530-532.

376. Gerald PS, Diamond LK. The diagnosis of thalassemia trait by starch block electrophoresis of the hemoglobin. Blood. 1958;13:61-69.

377. Mears JG, Ramirez F, Leibowitz D, et al. Changes in restricted human cellular DNA fragments containing

globin gene sequences in thalassemia and related disorders. Proc Natl Acad Sci U S A. 1978;75:1222-1226.

378. Fessas P, Karaklis A. Two-dimensional paper-agar electrophoresis of hemoglobin. Clin Chim Acta. 1962;7:133-138.

379. Duma H, Efremov G, Sadikario A, et al. Study of nine families with hemoglobin-Lepore. Br J Haematol. 1978;15:161-172.

380. Lehmann H, Charlesworth D. Observations on hemoglobin P (Congo type). Biochem J. 1970;119:43P.

381. Ohta Y, Yamaoka K, Sumida I, Yanase T. Hemoglobin Miyada, a beta-delta fusion peptide (anti-Lepore) type discovered in a Japanese family. Nat (New Biol). 1971;234:218-220.

382. Baird FM, Lorkin PA, Lehmann H. Hemoglobin P. Nilotic containing a beta-delta chain. Nat (New Biol). 1973;242:107-110.

383. Kimura A, Ohta Y, Fukumaki Y, Takagi Y. A fusion gene in man: DNA sequence analysis of the abnormal globin gene of hemoglobin Miyada. Biochem Biophys Res Commun. 1984;119:968-974.

384. Ojwang PJ, Nakatsuji T, Gardiner MB, et al. Gene deletion as the molecular basis for the Kenya-gamma-HPFH condition. Hemoglobin. 1983;7:115-123.

385. Huisman THJ, Schroeder WA, Efremov GD, et al. The present status of the heterogeneity of fetal hemoglobin in beta-thalassemia: an attempt to unify some observations in thalassemia and related conditions. Ann N Y Acad Sci. 1974;232:107-124.

386. Oner C, Oner R, Gürgey A, Altay C. A new Turkish type of beta-thalassemia major with homozygosity for two non-consecutive 7.6 kb deletions of the psi-beta and beta-genes and an intact delta gene. Br J Hematol. 1995;89:306-312.

387. Ramirez F, O'Donnell JV, Marks PA, et al. Abnormal or absent beta mRNA in beta Ferrara and gene deletion in delta beta thalassemia. Nature. 1976;263:471-475.

388. Schmid CW, Jelinek WR. The Alu family of dispersed repetitive sequences. Science. 1982;216:1065-1070.

389. Trent RJ, Jones RW, Clegg JB, et al. (^Agamma delta beta) thalassaemia: similarity of phenotype in four different molecular defects, including one newly described. Br J Haematol. 1984;57:279-289.

390. Zeng YT, Huang SZ, Chen B, et al. Hereditary persistence of fetal hemoglobin or (delta beta)^0-thalassemia: three types observed in South-Chinese families. Blood. 1985;66:1430-1435.

391. Kan YW, Forget BG, Nathan DG. Gamma-beta thalassemia: a cause of hemolytic disease of newborns. N Engl J Med. 1972;286:129-134.

392. Viprakasit V, Gibbons RJ, Broughton BC, et al. Mutations in the general transcription factor TFIIH result in beta-thalassemia in individuals with trichothiodystrophy. Hum Mol Genet. 2001;10:2797-2802.

393. Thompson AR, Wood WG, Stamatoyannopoulos G. X-linked syndrome of platelet dysfunction, thrombocytopenia, and imbalanced globin chain synthesis with hemolysis. Blood. 1977;50:303-216.

394. Wainscoat JS, Old JM, Wood WG, et al. Characterization of an Indian (delta beta)^0 thalassaemia. Br J Haematol. 1984;58:353-360.

395. Henthorn PS, Mager D, Huisman TH, Smithies O. A gene deletion ending within a complex array of repeated sequences 3' to the human beta-globin gene cluster. Proc Natl Acad Sci U S A. 1986;83:5194-5198.

396. Stolle CA, Penny LA, Ivory S, et al. Sequence analysis of the gamma-globin gene locus from a patient with the deletion form of hereditary persistence of fetal hemoglobin. Blood. 1990;75:499-504.

397. Elder JT, Forrester WC, Thompson C, et al. Translocation of an erythroid-specific hypersensitive site in deletion-type hereditary persistence of fetal hemoglobin. Mol Cell Biol. 1990;10:1382-1389.

398. Feingold EA, Forget BG. The breakpoint of a large deletion causing hereditary persistence of fetal hemoglobin occurs within an erythroid DNA domain remote from the beta-globin gene cluster. Blood. 1989;74:2178-2186.

399. Yang KG, Stoming TA, Fei YJ, et al. Identification of base substitutions in the promoter regions of the ^Agamma- and ^Ggamma-globin genes in ^Agamma- (or ^Ggamma-) beta^+-HPFH heterozygotes using the DNA-amplification–synthetic oligonucleotide procedure. Blood. 1988;71:1414-1417.

400. Gumucio DL, Rood KL, Gray TA, et al. Nuclear proteins that bind the human gamma-globin gene promoter: alterations in binding produced by point mutations associated with hereditary persistence of fetal hemoglobin. Mol Cell Biol. 1988;8:5310-5322.

401. Superti-Furga G, Barberis A, Schaffner G, Busslinger M. The -117 mutation in Greek HPFH affects the binding of three nuclear factors to the CCAAT region of the gamma-globin gene. EMBO J. 1988;7:3099-3107.

402. Martin DI, Tsai SF, Orkin SH. Increased gamma-globin expression in a nondeletion HPFH mediated by an erythroid-specific DNA-binding factor. Nature. 1989;338:435-438.

403. Mantovani R, Superti-Furga G, Gilman J, Ottolenghi S. The deletion of the distal CCAAT box region of the ^Agamma-globin gene in black HPFH abolishes the binding of the erythroid specific protein NFE3 and of the CCAAT displacement protein. Nucleic Acids Res. 1989;17:6681-6691.

404. Sykes K, Kaufman R. A naturally occurring gamma globin gene mutation enhances SP1 binding activity. Mol Cell Biol. 1990;10:95-102.

405. Ronchi A, Nicolis S, Santoro C, Ottolenghi S. Increased Sp1 binding mediates erythroid-specific overexpression of a mutated (HPFH) gamma-globulin promoter. Nucleic Acids Res. 1989;17:10231-10241.

406. Ottolenghi S, Mantovani R, Nicolis S, et al. DNA sequences regulating human globin gene transcription in nondeletional hereditary persistence of fetal hemoglobin. Hemoglobin. 1989;13:523-541.

407. Wood WG, MacRae IA, Darbre PD, et al. The British type of non-deletion HPFH: characterization of developmental changes in vivo and erythroid growth in vitro. Br J Haematol. 1982;30:401-414.

408. Camaschella C, Oggiano L, Sampietro M, et al. The homozygous state of G to A 117 ^Agamma hereditary persistence of fetal hemoglobin. Blood. 1989;73:1999-2002.

409. Friedman S, Schwartz E. Hereditary persistence of foetal haemoglobin with beta-chain synthesis in cis position (^Ggamma-beta^+-HPFH) in a Negro family. Nature. 1976;259:138-140.

410. Nicholls RD, Jonasson JA, McGee JO, et al. High resolution gene mapping of the human alpha globin locus. J Med Genet. 1987;24:39-46.

411. Simmers RN, Mulley JC, Hylund VJ, et al. Mapping the human alpha globin gene complex to 16p13.2-pter. J Med Genet. 1987;24:761-766.

412. Nicholls RD, Fischel-Ghodsian N, Higgs DR. Recombination at the human alpha-globin gene cluster: sequence features and topological constraints. Cell. 1987;49:369-378.

413. Sawada I, Schmid CW. Primate evolution of the alpha-globin gene cluster and its Alu-like repeats. J Mol Biol. 1986;192:693-709.

414. Michelson AM, Orkin SH. Boundaries of gene conversion within the duplicated human alpha-globin genes. Concerted evolution by segmental recombination. J Biol Chem. 1983;258:15245-15254.

415. Hess JF, Schmid CW, Shen CK. A gradient of sequence divergence in the human adult alpha-globin duplication units. Science. 1984;226:67-70.

416. Higgs DR, Hill AV, Bowden DK, et al. Independent recombination events between the duplicated human alpha globin genes; implications for their concerted evolution. Nucleic Acids Res. 1984;12:6965-6977.

417. Foldi J, Cohen-Solal M, Valentin C, et al. The human alpha-globin gene. The protein products of the duplicated genes are identical. Eur J Biochem. 1980;109:463-470.

418. Orkin SH, Goff SC. The duplicated human alpha-globin genes: their relative expression as measured by RNA analysis. Cell. 1981;24:345-351.

419. Liebhaber SA, Cash FE, Main DM. Compensatory increase in alpha 1-globin gene expression in individuals heterozygous for the alpha-thalassemia-2 deletion. J Clin Invest. 1985;76:1057-1064.

420. Liebhaber SA, Cash FE, Ballas SK. Human alpha-globin gene expression. The dominant role of the alpha 2-locus in mRNA and protein synthesis. J Biol Chem. 1986;261:15327-15333.

421. Proudfoot NJ. Transcriptional interference and termination between duplicated alpha-globin gene constructs suggests a novel mechanism for gene regulation. Nature. 1986;322:562-565.

422. Shakin SH, Liebhaber SA. Translational profiles of alpha 1-, alpha 2-, and beta-globin messenger ribonucleic acids in human reticulocytes. J Clin Invest. 1986;78:1125-1129.

423. Orkin SH, Old J, Lazarus H, et al. The molecular basis of alpha thalassemias: frequent occurrence of dysfunctional alpha loci among non-Asians with Hb H disease. Cell. 1979;17:33-42.

424. Embury SH, Miller JA, Doxy AM, et al. Two different molecular organizations account for the single alpha-globin gene of the alpha-thalassemia-2 genotype. J Clin Invest. 1980;66:1319-1325.

425. Goossens M, Dozy AM, Embury SH, et al. Triplicated alpha-globin loci in humans. Proc Natl Acad Sci U S A. 1980;77:518-521.

426. Higgs DR, Old JM, Pressley L, et al. A novel alpha-globin gene arrangement in man. Nature. 1980;284:632-635.

427. Lie-Injo LE, Herrera AR, Kan YW. Two types of triplicated alpha-globin loci in humans. Nucleic Acids Res. 1981;9:3707-3717.

428. Trent RJ, Higgs DR, Clegg JB, Weatherall DJ. A new triplicated alpha-globin gene arrangement in man. Br J Haematol. 1981;49:149-152.

429. Hess JF, Fox M, Schmid C, Shen CK. Molecular evolution of the human adult alpha-globin–like gene region: insertion and deletion of Alu family repeats and non-Alu DNA sequences. Proc Natl Acad Sci U S A. 1983;80:5970-5974.

430. Hu WS, Shen CK. Reconstruction of human alpha thalassemia-2 genotypes in monkey cells. Nucleic Acids Res. 1987;15:2989-3008.

431. Gomez-Pedrozo M, Hu WS, Shen CK. Recombinational resolution in primate cells of two homologous human DNA segments with a gradient of sequence divergence. Nucleic Acids Res. 1988;16:11237-11247.

432. Winichagoon P, Higgs DR, Goodbourn SE, et al. The molecular basis of alpha-thalassaemia in Thailand. EMBO J. 1984;3:1813-1818.

433. Chui DH, Wong SC, Chung SW, et al. Embryonic zeta-globin chains in adults: a marker for alpha-thalassemia-1 haplotype due to a greater than 17.5-kb deletion. N Engl J Med. 1986;314:76-79.

434. Bowden DK, Hill AV, Higgs DR, et al. Different hematologic phenotypes are associated with the leftward (-alpha 4.2) and rightward (-alpha 3.7) alpha⁺-thalassemia deletions. J Clin Invest. 1987;79:39-43.

435. Galanello R, Ruggeri R, Paglietti E, et al. A family with segregating triplicated alpha globin loci and beta thalassemia. Blood. 1983;62:1035-1040.

436. Trent RJ, Mickleson KN, Wilkinson T, et al. Alpha globin gene rearrangements in Polynesians are not associated with malaria. Am J Hematol. 1985;18:431-433.

437. Kulozik AE, Thein SL, Wainscoat JS, et al. Thalassaemia intermedia: interaction of the triple alpha-globin gene arrangement and heterozygous beta-thalassaemia. Br J Haematol. 1987;66:109-112.

438. Camaschella C, Bertero MT, Serra A, et al. A benign form of thalassaemia intermedia may be determined by the interaction of triplicated alpha locus and heterozygous beta-thalassaemia. Br J Haematol. 1987;66:103-107.

439. Tufarelli C, Stanley JA, Garrick D, et al. Transcription of antisense RNA leading to gene silencing and methylation as a novel cause of human genetic disease. Nat Genet. 2003;34:157-165.

440. Saetrom P, Snove O Jr, Rossi JJ. Epigenetics and microRNAs. Pediatr Res. 2007;61:17R-23R.

441. Fischel-Ghodsian N, Vickers MA, Seip M, et al. Characterization of two deletions that remove the entire human zeta-alpha globin gene complex (–/–THAI and –/–FIL). Br J Haematol. 1988;70:233-238.

442. Fortina P, Delgrosso K, Rappaport E, et al. A large deletion encompassing the entire alpha-like globin gene cluster in a family of northern European extraction. Nucleic Acids Res. 1988;16:11223-11235.

443. Drysdale HC, Higgs DR. Alpha-thalassaemia in an Asian Indian [letter]. Br J Haematol. 1988;68:264.

444. Gonzalez-Redondo JM, Diaz-Chico JC, Malcorra-Azpiazu JJ, Balda-Aguirre ML. Characterization of a newly discovered alpha-thalassaemia-1 in two Spanish patients with Hb H disease. Br J Haematol. 1988;70:459-463.

445. Gonzalez-Redondo JM, Gilsanz F, Ricard P. Characterization of a new alpha-thalassemia-1 deletion in a Spanish family. Hemoglobin. 1989;13:103-116.

446. Luo HY, Clarke BJ, Gauldie J, et al. A novel monoclonal antibody based diagnostic test for alpha-thalassemia-1 carriers due to the (-SEA/) deletion. Blood. 1988;72:1589-1594.

447. Liang ST, Wong VC, So WW, et al. Homozygous alpha-thalassaemia: clinical presentation, diagnosis and management. A review of 46 cases. Br J Obstet Gynaecol. 1985;92:680-684.

448. Kueh YK. Acute lymphoblastic leukemia with brilliant cresyl blue erythrocytic inclusions—acquired hemoglobin H? N Engl J Med. 1982;307:193-194.

449. Higgs DR, Wood WG, Clegg JB, Weatherall DJ. Clinical features and molecular analysis of acquired hemoglobin H disease. Am J Med. 1983;75:181-191.

450. Anagnou NP, Ley TJ, Chesbro B, et al. Acquired alpha-thalassemia in preleukemia is due to decreased expression of all four alpha-globin genes. Proc Natl Acad Sci U S A. 1983;80:6051-6055.

451. Abbondanzo SL, Anagnou NP, Sacher RA. Myelodysplastic syndrome with acquired hemoglobin H disease. Evolution through megakaryoblastic transformation into myelofibrosis. Am J Clin Pathol. 1988;89:401-406.

452. Helder J, Deisseroth A. S1 nuclease analysis of alpha-globin gene expression in preleukemic patients with acquired hemoglobin H disease after transfer to mouse erythroleukemia cells. Proc Natl Acad Sci U S A. 1987;84:2387-2390.

453. Wilkie AO, Zeitlin HC, Lindinbaum RH, et al. Clinical features and molecular analysis of the alpha thalassemia/mental retardation syndromes. II. Cases without detectable abnormality of the alpha globin complex. Am J Hum Genet. 1990;46:1127-1140.

454. Schwartz E. The silent carrier of beta thalassemia. N Engl J Med. 1969;281:1327-1333.

455. Aksoy M, Dincol G, Erdem S. Different types of beta-thalassemia intermedia. Acta Haematol (Basel). 1978;59:178-189.

456. Kattamis C, Metaxotou-Mavromati A, Wood WG, et al. The heterogeneity of normal Hb A₂ beta thalassemia in Greece. Br J Haematol. 1979;42:109-123.

457. Kanavakis E, Metaxotou-Mavromati A, Kattamis C, et al. Globin gene mapping in normal Hb A₂ types of beta thalassemia. Br J Haematol. 1982;51:59-64.

458. Semenza GL, Delgrosso K, Poncz M, et al. The silent carrier allele: beta thalassemia without a mutation in the beta-globin gene or its immediate flanking regions. Cell. 1984;39:123-128.

459. Murru S, Loudianos G, Porcu S, et al. A beta-thalassaemia phenotype not linked to the beta-globin cluster in an Italian family. Br J Haematol. 1992;81:283-287.

460. Thein SL, Wood WG, Wickramasinghe SN, Galvin MC. Beta-thalassemia unlinked to the beta-globin gene in an English family. Blood. 1993;82:961-967.

461. Faa V, Meloni A, Moi L, et al. Thalassaemia-like carriers not linked to the beta-globin gene cluster. Br J Haematol. 2006;132:640-650.

462. Boyer SH. The emerging complexity of genetic control of persistent fetal hemoglobin biosynthesis in adults. Ann N Y Acad Sci. 1989;565:23-36.

463. Cappellini MD, Fiorelli G, Bernini LF. Interaction between homozygous beta zero thalassemia and the Swiss type of hereditary persistence of fetal haemoglobin. Br J Haematol. 1981;48:561-572.

464. Gianni AM, Bregni M, Cappellini MD, et al. A gene controlling fetal hemoglobin expression in adults is not linked to the non–alpha globin cluster. EMBO J. 1983;2:921-925.

465. Thein SL, Weatherall DJ. A non-deletion hereditary persistence of fetal hemoglobin (HPFH) determinant not linked to the beta-globin gene complex. In Stamatoyannopoulos G, Nienhuis AW (eds). Hemoglobin Switching, Part B: Cellular and Molecular Mechanisms. New York, Alan R Liss, 1989, p 97.

466. Garner C, Silver N, Best S, et al. Quantitative trait locus on chromosome 8q influences the switch from fetal to adult hemoglobin. Blood. 2004;104:2184-2186.

467. Hirschhorn JN, Daly MJ. Genome-wide association studies for common diseases and complex traits. Nat Rev Genet. 2005;6:95-108.

467a. Uda M, Galanello R, Sanna S, et al. Genome-wide association study shows BCL11A associated with persistent fetal hemoglobin and amelioration of the phenotype of beta-thalassemia. Proc Natl Acad Sci U S A. 2008;105:1620-1625.

467b. Menzel S, Garner C, Gut I, et al. A QTL influencing F cell production maps to a gene encoding a zinc-finger protein on chromosome 2p15. Nat Genet. 2007;39:1197-1199.

467c. Thein SL, Menzel S, Peng X, et al. Intergenic variants of HBS1L-MYB are responsible for a major quantitative trait locus on chromosome 6p23 influencing fetal hemoglobin levels in adults. Proc Natl Acad Sci U S A. 2007;104:11346-11351.

468. Dozy AM, Kan YW, Embry SH, et al. Alpha-globin gene organization in blacks precludes the severe form of alpha-thalassemia. Nature. 1979;280:605-607.

469. Higgs DR, Pressley L, Clegg JB, et al. Alpha thalassemia in black populations. Johns Hopkins Med J. 1980;146:300-310.

470. Phillips JAI, Vik TA, Scott AF, et al. Unequal crossing-over: a common basis of single alpha-globin genes in Asians and American blacks with hemoglobin-H disease. Blood. 1980;55:1066-1069.

471. Galanello R, Maccioni L, Ruggeri R, et al. Alpha thalassaemia in Sardinian newborns. Br J Haematol. 1984;58:361-368.

472. Kanavakis E, Tzotzos S, Liapaki A, et al. Frequency of alpha-thalassemia in Greece. Am J Hematol. 1986;22:225-232.

473. Weatherall DJ, Clegg JB. The alpha-chain-termination mutants and their relation to the alpha thalassemias. Philos Trans R Soc Lond B Biol Sci. 1975;271:411-455.

474. Pootrakul P, Winichagoon P, Fucharoen S, et al. Homozygous haemoglobin Constant Spring: a need for revision of concept. Hum Genet. 1981;59:250-255.

475. Chui DH, Luo HY, Clarke BJ. Potential application of a new screening test for alpha-thalassemia-1 carriers. Hemoglobin. 1988;12:459-463.

476. Kan YW, Schwartz E, Nathan DG. Globin chain synthesis in alpha-thalassemia syndromes. J Clin Invest. 1968;47:2515-2522.

477. Pootrakul S, Sapprapa S, Wasi P, et al. Hemoglobin synthesis in 28 obligatory cases for alpha-thalassemia trait. Humangenetik. 1975;29:121-126.

478. Ben-Bassat I, Mozel M, Ramot B. Globin synthesis in iron-deficiency anemia. Blood. 1974;44:551-555.

479. El-Hazmi MAF, Lehmann H. Interaction between iron deficiency and alpha thalassemia: the in vitro effect of haemin on alpha chain synthesis. Acta Haematol (Basel). 1978;60:1-9.

480. Rigas DA, Koler RD, Osgood EE. New hemoglobin possessing a higher electrophoretic mobility than normal adult hemoglobin. Science. 1955;121:372.

481. Wasi P, Na-Nakorn S, Pootrakul S, et al. Alpha and beta-thalassemia in Thailand. Ann N Y Acad Sci. 1969;165:60-82.

482. Ko TM, Tseng LH, Hsieh FJ, et al. Carrier detection and prenatal diagnosis of alpha-thalassemia of Southeast Asian deletion by polymerase chain reaction. Hum Genet. 1992;88:245-248.

483. Chan V, Yip B, Lam YH, et al. Quantitative polymerase chain reaction for the rapid prenatal diagnosis of homozygous alpha-thalassaemia (Hb Barts hydrops fetalis). Br J Haematol. 2001;115:341-346.

484. Clegg JB, Weatherall DJ. Hemoglobin synthesis in alpha-thalassemia (hemoglobin H disease). Nature. 1967;215:1241-1243.

485. Benz EJ Jr, Swerdlow PS, Forget BG. Globin messenger RNA in Hb H disease. Blood. 1973;42:825-833.

486. Jones RT, Schroeder WA. Chemical characterization and subunit hybridization of human hemoglobin H and associated compounds. Biochemistry. 1963;2:1357-1367.

487. Rigas DA, Koler RD. Decreased erythrocyte survival in hemoglobin H disease as a result of the abnormal properties of hemoglobin H: the benefit of splenectomy. Blood. 1961;18:1-17.

488. Rachmilewitz E, Shinar E, Shaley O, et al. Erythrocyte membrane alterations in beta-thalassemia. Clin Hematol. 1985;14:163-182.

489. Benesch RE, Ranney HM, Benesch R, Smith GM. The chemistry of the Bohr effect: II. Some properties of hemoglobin H. J Biol Chem. 1961;236:2926-2929.

490. Shinar E, Rachmilewitz EA. Oxidative denaturation of red blood cells in thalassemia. Semin Hematol. 1990;27:70-82.

491. Pearson HA, McFarland W. Erythrokinetics in thalassemia. II. Studies in Lepore trait and hemoglobin H disease. J Lab Clin Med. 1962;59:147-157.

492. Fessas P, Yataganas X. Intra-erythroblastic instability of hemoglobin beta (HbH). Blood. 1968;31:323-331.

493. Tso SC, Loh TT, Todd D. Iron overload in patients with haemoglobin H disease. Scand J Haematol. 1984;32:391-394.

494. Hirsh J, Dacie JV. Persistent post-splenectomy thrombocytosis and thromboembolism: a consequence of continuing anemia. Br J Haematol. 1966;12:45-53.

495. Tso SC, Chan TK, Todd D. Venous thrombosis in haemoglobin H disease after splenectomy. Aust N Z J Med. 1982;12:635-638.

496. Gabuzda TC, Nathan DG, Gardner FH. The metabolism of the individual C[14] labeled hemoglobins in patients with H-thalassemia; with observations on radiochromate binding to the hemoglobins during red cell survival. J Clin Invest. 1961;44:315-325.

497. Tso SC. Red cell survival studies in hemoglobin H disease using [51Cr]chromate and [32P]di-isopropyl phosphofluoridate. Br J Haematol. 1972;23:621-629.

498. Wilkie AOM, Buckle VJ, Harris PC, et al. Clinical features and molecular analysis of the alpha thalassemia/mental retardation syndromes. I. Cases due to deletions involving chromosome band 16p13.3. Am J Hum Genet. 1990;46:1112-1126.

499. Sharma RS, Yu V, Walters WA. Haemoglobin Bart's hydrops fetalis syndrome in an infant of Greek origin and prenatal diagnosis of alpha thalassemia. Med J Aust. 1979;2:433-434.

500. Trent RJ, Wilkinson T, Yakas J, et al. Molecular defects in 2 examples of severe Hb H disease. Scand J Haematol. 1986;36:272-279.

501. Chan V, Chan TK, Liang ST, et al. Hydrops fetalis due to an unusual form of Hb H disease. Blood. 1985;66:224-228.

502. Lie-Injo LE, Jo BH. A fast-moving hemoglobin in hydrops fetalis. Nature. 1960;185:698.

503. Kan YW, Allen A, Lowenstein L. Hydrops fetalis with alpha thalassemia. N Engl J Med. 1967;276:18-23.

504. Weatherall DJ, Clegg JB, Boon WH. The hemoglobin constitution of infants with haemoglobin Bart's hydrops foetalis syndrome. Br J Haematol. 1970;18:357-367.

505. Todd D, Lai MCS, Beaven GH, Huehns ER. The abnormal hemoglobins in homozygous alpha thalassaemia. Br J Haematol. 1970;19:27-31.

506. Wasi P, Na-Nakorn S, Pootrakul SN. The alpha thalassemias. Clin Haematol. 1974;3:383-410.

507. Beaudry MA, Ferguson DJ, Pearse K, et al. Survival of a hydropic infant with homozygous alpha-thalassemia-1. J Pediatr. 1986;108:713-716.

508. Bianchi DW, Beyer EC, Stark AR, et al. Normal long-term survival with alpha-thalassemia. J Pediatr. 1986;108:716-718.

509. Carr S, Rubin L, Dixon D, et al. Intrauterine therapy for homozygous alpha-thalassemia. Obstet Gynecol. 1995;85:876-879.

510. Rietti F. Ittero emolitico primitivo. Atti Accad Sci Med Nat Ferrara. 1925;2:14-19.

511. Wintrobe MM, Mathews E, Pollack R, Dobyns BM. Familial hemopoietic disorder in Italian adolescents and adults resembling Mediterranean disease (thalassemia). JAMA. 1940;114:1530-1538.

512. Valentine WN, Neel JV. Hematologic and genetic study of transmission of thalassemia (Cooley's anemia: Mediterranean anemia). Arch Intern Med. 1944;74:185-196.

513. Smith CH. Detection of mild types of Mediterranean (Cooley's anemia). Am J Dis Child. 1948;75:505-527.

514. Silvestroni E, Bianco I. Microcytemia, constitutional microcytic anemia and Cooley's anemia. Am J Hum Genet. 1949;1:83-93.

515. Braverman AS, Bank A. Changing rates of globin chain synthesis during erythroid cell maturation in thalassemia. J Mol Biol. 1969;42:57-64.

516. Schwartz E. Heterozygous beta-thalassemia: balanced globin synthesis in bone marrow cells. Science. 1970;167:1513-1514.

517. Kan YW, Nathan DG, Lodish HF. Equal synthesis of alpha- and beta-globin chains in erythroid precursors in heterozygous beta-thalassemia. J Clin Invest. 1972;51:1906-1909.

518. Freidman S, Oski FA, Schwartz E. Bone marrow and peripheral blood globin synthesis in an American black family with beta thalassemia. Blood. 1972;39:785-793.

519. Nienhuis AW, Canfield PH, Anderson WF. Hemoglobin messenger RNA from human bone marrow: Isolation and translation in homozygous and heterozygous beta thalassemia. J Clin Invest. 1973;52:1735-1745.

520. Chalevelakis G, Clegg JB, Weatherall DJ. Imbalanced globin synthesis in heterozygous beta-thalassemia bone marrow. Proc Natl Acad Sci U S A. 1975;72:3853-3857.

521. Wood W, Stamatoyannopoulos G. Globin synthesis in fractionated normoblasts of beta thalassemia heterozygotes. J Clin Invest. 1975;55:567-578.

522. Fessas P, Stamatoyannopoulos G. Absence of haemoglobin A_2 in an adult. Nature. 1962;195:1215-1216.

523. Thompson RB, Odom J, Warrington R, Bell WN. Thalassemia with complete absence of hemoglobin A_2 in adult. Acta Haematol. 1965;33:186-190.

524. Ohta Y, Yamaoka K, Sumida I, et al. Homozygous delta-thalassemia first discovered in a Japanese family with hereditary persistence of fetal hemoglobin. Blood. 1971;37:706-715.

525. Kimura A, Matsunaga E, Ohta Y, et al. Structure of cloned delta-globin genes from a normal subject and a patient with delta-thalassemia: sequence polymorphisms found in the delta-globin gene region of Japanese individuals. Nucleic Acids Res. 1982;10:5725-5732.

526. Taramelli R, Giglioni B, Comi P, et al. Delta thalassemia: a non-deletion defect. Eur J Biochem. 1983;129:589-592.

527. Pirastu M, Galanello R, Melis MA, et al. Delta$^+$-thalassemia in Sardinia. Blood. 1983;62:341-345.

528. Huisman TJH, Punt K, Shoad JD. Thalassemia minor associated with hemoglobin B heterozygosity. A family report. Blood. 1961;17:747-757.

529. Alperin JB, Dow PA, Petteway MB. Hemoglobin A levels in health and various hematologic disorders. Am J Clin Pathol. 1977;67:219-226.

530. Pearson HA, McFarland W, King ER. Erythrokinetic studies in thalassemia trait. J Lab Clin Med. 1960;56:866-872.

531. Mazza U, Saglio G, Cappio FC, et al. Clinical and hematological data on 254 cases of beta-thalassemia trait in Italy. Br J Haematol. 1976;33:91-99.

532. Malamos B, Fessas P, Stamatoyannopoulos G. Types of thalassemia-trait carriers as revealed by a study of their incidence in Greece. Br J Haematol. 1962;8:5-14.

533. Pootrakul P, Wasi P, Na-Nakorn S. Hematological data in 312 cases of beta-thalassemia trait in Thailand. Br J Haematol. 1973;24:703-712.

534. Knox-Macaulay HH, Weatherall DJ, Clegg JB, Pembrey ME. Thalassaemia in the British. BMJ. 1973;3:150-155.

535. Weatherall DJ. Biochemical phenotypes of thalassemia in the American Negro population. Ann N Y Acad Sci. 1964;119:450-462.

536. Pootrakul S, Assayamunkong S, Na-Nakorn S. Beta-thalassemia trait: hematologic and hemoglobin synthesis studies. Hemoglobin. 1976;1:75-83.

537. Agraphiotis A, Fessas P, et al. Hematological, biochemical and biosynthetic differences between beta and beta thalassemia heterozygotes. In Proceedings of the XVII Congress of the International Society of Hematology, Paris, 1978.

538. Millard DP, Mason K, Serjeant BE, Serjeant GR. Comparison of hematological features of the beta and beta thalassemia traits in Jamaican Negroes. Br J Haematol. 1977;36:161-170.

539. Schokler RC, Went LN, Bok J. A new genetic variant of beta-thalassemia. Nature. 1966;209:44-46.

540. Kalpsoya-Tassopoulos A, Zoumbos N, Loukopoulos D, et al. "Silent" beta thalassemia and normal HbA_2 beta thalassemia. Br J Haematol. 1980;45:177-178.

541. Dautry-Varsat A, Ciechanover A, Lodish HF. pH and the recycling of transferrin during receptor-mediated endocytosis. Proc Natl Acad Sci U S A. 1983;80:2258-2262.

542. Brittenham G, Sheth S, Allen CJ, Farrell DE. Noninvasive methods for quantitative assessment of transfusional iron overload in sickle cell disease. Semin Hematol. 2001;38(1 Suppl 1):37-56.

543. Fischer R, Tiemann CD, Englehardt R, et al. Assessment of iron stores in children with transfusion siderosis by biomagnetic liver susceptometry. Am J Hematol. 1999;60:289-299.

544. Ellis JT, Schulman I, Smith CH. Generalized siderosis with fibrosis of liver and pancreas in Cooley's (Mediterranean) anemia with observations on the pathogenesis of the siderosis and fibrosis. Am J Pathol. 1954;30:287-309.

545. Olivieri NF, De Silva S, Premawardena A, et al. Iron overload and iron-chelating therapy in hemoglobin E–beta thalassemia. J Pediatr Hematol Oncol. 2000;22:593-597.

546. Breuer W, Ronson A, Slotki IN, et al. The assessment of serum nontransferrin-bound iron in chelation therapy and iron supplementation. Blood. 2000;95:2975-2982.

547. Seligman PA. The biochemistry of proteins involved in iron transport and storage. In Stamatoyannopoulos G, Nienhuis AW, Leder P, Majerus PW (eds). The Molecular Basis of Blood Diseases. Philadelphia, WB Saunders, 1987.

548. Pearson HA, O'Brien RT, McIntosh S. Screening for thalassemia trait by electronic measurement of means corpuscular volume (MCV). N Engl J Med. 1973;288:351-353.

549. Torlontano G, Tata A, Camagna A. A rapid screen test for thalassemia trait. Acta Haematol. 1972;48:234-238.

550. Hegde UM, White JM, Hart GH, Marsh GW. Diagnosis of alpha thalassemia trait from Coulter counter "S" indices. J Clin Pathol. 1977;30:884-889.

551. Conrad ME, Crosby WH. The natural history of iron deficiency induced by phlebotomy. Blood. 1962;20:173-185.

552. Mentzer WC. Differentiation of iron deficiency from thalassemia trait. Lancet. 1973;1:882.

553. England JM, Fraser PM. Differentiation of iron deficiency from thalassemia trait by routine blood count. Lancet. 1973;I:449-452.

554. England JM, Ward SM, Down MC. Microcytosis, anisocytosis, and the red cell indices in iron deficiency. Br J Haematol. 1976;34:589-597.

555. Bessman JD, Gilmer PR Jr, Gardner FH. Improved classification of anemias by MCV and RDW. Am J Clin Pathol. 1983;80:322-326.

556. McClure S, Custer E, Bessman JD. Improved detection of early iron deficiency in nonanemic subjects. JAMA. 1985;253:1021-1023.

557. Ghionni A, Miotti TC, Camandona U. Differential erythrocyte parameters in thalassemia minor and hyposideremic syndromes. Minerva Med. 1985;76:1143-1148.

558. Roberts GT, El-Badawi SB. Red blood cell distribution width in some hematologic diseases. Am J Clin Pathol. 1985;83:222-226.

559. Flynn MM, Reppun TS, Bhagavan NV. Limitations of red blood cell distribution width (RDW) in evaluation of microcytosis. Am J Clin Pathol. 1986;85:445-449.

560. Marti HR, Fischer S, Killer D, Bürgi W. Can automated haematology analysers discriminate thalassaemia from iron deficiency? Acta Haematol (Basel). 1987;78:180-183.

561. Miguel A, Linares M, Miguel A, Miguel-Borja JM. Red cell distribution width analysis in differentiation between iron deficiency and thalassemia minor. Acta Haematol (Basel). 1988;80:59.

562. Shine I, Lal S. A strategy to detect beta-thalassaemia minor. Lancet. 1977;1:692-694.

563. England JM, Fraser P. Discrimination between iron deficiency and heterozygous-thalassemia syndromes in the differential diagnosis of microcytosis. Lancet. 1979;1:145-148.

564. Rowley PT. The diagnosis of beta thalassemia trait: A review. Am J Hematol. 1976;1:129-137.

565. Chalevelakis G, Tsiroyannis K, Hatziioannou J, Arapakis G. Screening for thalassemia and/or iron deficiency. Scand J Clin Lab Invest. 1984;44:1-6.

566. Bessman JD, McClure S, Bates J. Distinction of microcytic disorders: comparison of expert, numerical-discriminant, and microcomputer analysis. Blood Cells 1989;15:533-540.

567. Green R, King R. A new red cell discriminant incorporating volume dispersion for differentiating iron deficiency anemia from thalassemia minor. Blood Cells. 1989;15:481-491; discussion 492-495.

568. Makris PE. Utilization of a new index to distinguish heterozygous thalassemic syndromes: comparison of its specificity to five other discriminants. Blood Cells. 1989;15:497-506; discussion 507.

569. Piomelli S, Brickman A, Carlos E. Rapid diagnosis of iron deficiency by measurement of free erythrocyte porphyrins and hemoglobins: the FEP/hemoglobin ratio. Pediatrics. 1976;57:136-141.

570. Meloni T, Gallisai D, Demontis M, Erre S. Free erythrocyte porphyrin (REP) in the diagnosis of beta thalassemia trait and iron deficiency anemia. Haematologica. 1982;67:341-348.

571. Hurst D, Tittle B, Kleman KM, et al. Anemia and hemoglobinopathies in Southeast Asian refugee children. J Pediatr. 1983;102:692-697.

572. Cooley TB, Witwer ER, Lec P. Anemia in children with splenomegaly and peculiar changes in the bones. Report of cases. Am J Dis Child. 1927;34:347-363.

573. Cooley TB, Lee P. Series of cases of splenomegaly in children with anemia and peculiar bone changes. Trans Am Pediatr Soc. 1925;37:29-33.

574. Castagnari G. Intorno ad una particolare sindrome osteopatica diffusa in una caso di anemia eritroblastica dell'infanzia. Boll Sci Med (Bologna). 1933;1:399.

575. Whipple GH, Bradford WL. Racial or familial anemia of children associated with fundamental disturbances of bone and pigment metabolism (Cooley-von Jaksch). Am J Dis Child. 1932;44:336-365.

576. Wolman LJ. Transfusion therapy in Cooley's anemia: growth and health as related to long-range hemoglobin levels. A progress report. Ann N Y Acad Sci. 1964;119:736-747.

577. Schorr JB, Radel E. Transfusion therapy and its complications in patients with Cooley's anemia. Ann N Y Acad Sci. 1964;119:703-708.

578. Modell CB. High transfusion treatment of a case of thalassemia major. Trans R Soc Trop Med Hyg. 1967;61:174-177.

579. Beard ME, Necheles TF, et al. Intensive transfusion therapy in thalassemia major. Pediatrics. 1967;40:911-915.

580. Piomelli S, Danoff SJ, Becker MH, et al. Prevention of bone malformation and cardiomegaly in Cooley's anemia by early hypertransfusion regimen. Ann N Y Acad Sci. 1969;165:427-436.

581. Engle MA. Cardiac involvement in Cooley's anemia. Ann N Y Acad Sci. 1964;119:694-702.

582. Heywood JD, Karon M, Weissman S. Amino acid incorporation into alpha- and beta-chains of hemoglobin by normal and thalassemic reticulocytes. Science. 1964;146:530-531.

583. Heywood JD, Karon M, Weissman S. Asymmetric incorporation of amino acids into alpha and beta chains of hemoglobin synthesized in thalassemic reticulocytes. J Lab Clin Med. 1965;66:476-482.

584. Weatherall DJ, Clegg JB, Naughton MA. Globin synthesis in thalassemia: An in vitro study. Nature. 1965;208:1061-1065.

585. Bank A, Marks PA. Excess alpha chain synthesis relative to beta chain synthesis in thalassemia major and minor. Nature. 1966;212:1198-1200.

586. Bargellesi A, Pontremoli S, Conconi F. Absence of beta-globin synthesis in homozygous beta thalassemia. Eur J Biochem. 1967;1:73-79.

587. Fessas P. Inclusions of hemoglobin in erythroblasts and erythrocytes of thalassemia. Blood. 1963;21:21-32.

588. Fessas P, Loukopoulos D, Thorell B. Absorption spectra of inclusion bodies in beta-thalassemia. Blood. 1965;25:105-109.

589. Fessas P, Loukopoulos D, Kaltsoya A. Peptide analysis of the inclusions of erythroid cells in beta thalassemia. Biochim Biophys Acta. 1966;124:430-432.

590. Nathan DG. Thalassemia as a proliferative disorder. Medicine (Baltimore). 1964;43:779-782.

591. Polliack A, Yataganas P, Thorell B, Rachmilewitz EA. An electron microscopic study of the nuclear abnormalities and erythroblasts in beta-thalassemia major. Br J Haematol. 1974;26:201-204.

592. Wichramsinghe SN. The morphology and kinetics of erythropoiesis in homozygous beta thalassemia. In Weatherall DJ (ed). Congenital Disorders of Erythropoiesis. Amsterdam, Elsevier, 1975, p 221.

593. Shinar E, Rachnilewitz EA. Haemoglobinopathies and red cell membrane function. Baillieres Clin Haematol. 1993;6:357-369.

594. Schrier SL. Thalassemia: pathophysiology of red cell changes. Annu Rev Med. 1994;45:211-218.

595. Yuan J, Bunyaratvej A, Fucharoen S, et al. The instability of the membrane skeleton in thalassemic red blood cells. Blood. 1995;86:3945-3950.

596. Gaguzda TG, Nathan DG, Gardner FH. The metabolism of the individual C[14]-labelled hemoglobins in patients with H-thalassemia, with observations on radiochromate binding to the hemoglobins during red cell survival. J Clin Invest. 1965;44:315-325.

597. Scott MD. Entrapment of purified alpha-hemoglobin chains in normal erythrocytes as a model for human beta thalassemia. Adv Exp Med Biol. 1992;326:139-148.

598. Shinar E, Shalev O, Rachmilewitz EA, Schrier SL. Erythrocyte membrane skeleton abnormalities in severe beta-thalassemia. Blood. 1987;70:158-164.

599. Shinar E, Rachmilewitz EA, Lux SE. Differing erythrocyte membrane skeletal protein defects in alpha and beta thalassemia. J Clin Invest. 1989;83:404-410.

600. Advani R, Rubin E, Mohandas N, Schrier SL. Oxidative red blood cell membrane injury in the pathophysiology of severe mouse beta-thalassemia. Blood. 1992;79:1064-1067.

601. Olivieri O, DeFranceschi L, Capellini MD, et al. Oxidative damage and erythrocyte membrane transport abnormalities in thalassemias. Blood. 1994;84:315-320.

602. Schrier SL, Rachmilewitz E, Mohandas N. Cellular and membrane properties of alpha and beta thalassemic erythrocytes are different: implication for differences in clinical manifestations. Blood. 1989;74:2194-2202.

603. Sorensen S, Rubin E, Polster H, et al. The role of membrane skeletal-associated alpha-globin in the pathophysiology of beta-thalassemia. Blood. 1990;75:1333-1336.

604. Wainscoat JS, Thein SL, Weatherall DJ. Thalassaemia intermedia. Blood Rev. 1987;1:273-279.

605. McCarthy GM, Temperley IJ, Clegg JB, Weatherall DJ. Thalassemia in an Irish family. Irish J Med Sci. 1968;l:303-309.

606. Friedman S, Ozsoylu S, Luddy R, Schwartz E. Heterozygous beta-thalassemia of unusual severity. Br J Haematol. 1976;32:65-77.

607. Weatherall DJ, Clegg JB, Knox-Macauley HH, et al. A genetically determined disorder with features both of thalassaemia and congenital dyserythropoietic anaemia. Br J Haematol. 1973;24:681-702.

608. Stamatoyannopoulos G, Woodson R, Papayannopoulou T, et al. Inclusion-body–beta-thalassemia trait. A form of thalassemia producing clinical manifestations in simple heterozygotes. N Engl J Med. 1974;290:939-943.

609. Kanavakis E, Metaxotou A, Kattamis C, et al. The triplicated alpha gene locus and beta thalassaemia. Br J Haematol. 1983;54:201-207.

610. Sampietro M, Cazzola M, Cappellini MD, Fiorelli G. The triplicated alpha-gene locus and heterozygous beta thalassaemia: a case of thalassaemia intermedia. Br J Haematol. 1983;55:709-710.

611. Thein SL, Al-Hakim I, Hoffbrand AV. Thalassaemia intermedia: a new molecular basis. Br J Haematol. 1984;56:333-337.

612. Friedman AD, Linch DC, Miller B, et al. Determination of the hemoglobin F program in human progenitor-derived erythroid cells. J Clin Invest. 1985;75:1359-1368.

613. Pearson HA. Alpha-beta thalassemia disease in a Negro family. N Engl J Med. 1966;275:176-181.

614. Kan YW, Nathan DG. Mild thalassemia: the result of interactions of alpha and beta thalassemia genes. J Clin Invest. 1970;49:635-642.

615. Knox-Macaulay HH, Weatherall DJ, Clegg JB, et al. The clinical and biosynthetic characterization of alpha beta-thalassemia. Br J Haematol. 1972;22:497-512.

616. Ozsoylu S, Hiçsönmez C, Altay C. Hemoglobin H-beta-thalassemia. Acta Haematol. 1973;50:184-190.

617. Altay C, Say B, Yetgin S, Huisman TH. Alpha-thalassemia and beta-thalassemia in a Turkish family. Am J Hematol. 1977;2:1-15.

618. Bate CM, Humphries G. Alpha-beta thalassemia. Lancet. 1977;1:1031-1034.

619. Furbetta M, Galanello R, Ximenes A, et al. Interaction of alpha and beta thalassemia genes in two Sardinian families. Br J Haematol. 1979;41:203-210.

620. Wainscoat JS, Kanavakis E, Wood WG, et al. Thalassaemia intermedia in Cyprus: the interaction of alpha and beta thalassaemia. Br J Haematol. 1983;53:411-416.

621. Winichagoon P, Fucharoen S, Weatherall D, Wisi P. Concomitant inheritance of alpha-thalassemia in beta-thalassemia/Hb E disease. Am J Hematol. 1985;20:217-222.

622. Villegas A, López Rubio M, Sánchez J, et al. Primer caso de talasemia intermedia descrito en Espana debido a la interaccion de tres gene alpha con beta talasemia minor. Rev Clin Esp. 1993;192:268-270.

623. Camaschella C, Cappellini MD. Thalassemia intermedia. Haematologica. 1995;80:58-68.

624. Oron V, Filon D, Oppenheim A, Rund D. Severe thalassaemia intermedia caused by interaction of homozygosity for alpha-globin gene triplication with heterozygosity for beta zero-thalassemia. Br J Haematol. 1994;86:377-379.

625. Garewal G, Fearon CW, Warren TC, et al. The molecular basis of beta thalassaemia in Punjabi and Maharashtran Indians includes a multilocus aetiology involving triplicated alpha-globin loci. Br J Haematol. 1994;86:372-376.

626. Oggiano L, Rimini E, Frogheri L, et al. Haematological phenotypes in a family with triplicated alpha-globin gene, beta zero 39 and delta[+] 27 thalassaemia mutations. Clin Lab Haematol. 1992;14:289-292.

627. Villegas A, Perez-Clausell C, Sanchez J, Sal del Rio E. A new case of thalassemia intermedia: interaction of a triplicated alpha-globin locus and beta-thalassemia trait. Hemoglobin. 1992;16:99-101.

628. Leoni GB, Rosatelli C, Vitucci A, et al. Molecular basis of beta-thalassemia intermedia in a southern Italian (Puglia). Acta Haematol. 1991;86:174-178.

629. Cunningham, MJ, Macklin EA, Neufeld EJ, Cohen AR. Thalassemia Clinical Research Network. Complications of beta-thalassemia major in North America. Blood. 2004;104:34-39.

630. Dandona P, Menon RK, Houlder S, et al. Serum 1,25 dihydroxyvitamin D and osteocalcin concentrations in thalassaemia major. Arch Dis Child. 1987;62:474-477.

631. Rioja L, Girot R, Garabédian M, Cournot-Witmer G. Bone disease in children with homozygous beta-thalassemia. Bone Miner. 1990;8:69-86.

632. Lawson JP, Ablow RC, Pearson HA. The ribs in thalassemia. I. The relationship to therapy. Radiology. 1981;140:663-672.

633. Williams BA, Morris LL, Toogood IR, et al. Limb deformity and metaphyseal abnormalities in thalassaemia major. Am J Pediatr Hematol Oncol. 1992;14:197-201.

634. Orvieto R, Leichter I, Rachmilewitz EA, Margulies JY. Bone density, mineral content, and cortical index in patients with thalassemia major and the correlation to their bone fractures, blood transfusions, and treatment with desferrioxamine. Calcif Tissue Int. 1992;50: 397-399.

635. Wonke B, Hottbrand AV, Bouloux P, et al. New approaches to the management of hepatitis and endocrine disorders in Cooley's anemia. Ann N Y Acad Sci. 1998;850:232-241.

636. Jensen CE, Tuck SM, Agnew JE, et al. High incidence of osteoporosis in thalassemia major. J Pediatr Endocrinol Metab. 1998;3:975-977.

637. Giardina PJ, Schneider R, Lesser M, et al. Abnormal bone metabolism in thalassemia. In Ando S, Brancati C (eds). Endocrine Disorders in Thalassemia. Berlin, Springer-Verlag, 1995. p 39.

638. Lala R, Chiabotto P, Di Stefano M, et al. Bone density and metabolism in thalassemia. J Pediatr Endocrinol Metab. 1998;11(11 Suppl 3):785-790.

639. Brill PW, Winchester P, Giardina PJ, et al. Deferoxamine-induced bone dysplasia in patients with thalassemia major. AJR Am J Roentgenol. 1991;156:561-565.

640. de Virgiliis S, Congia M, Frau F, et al. Deferoxamine-induced growth retardation in patients with thalassemia major. J Pediatr 1988;113:661-669.

641. Chan YL, Li CK, Pang LM, Chik KW. Desferrioxamine-induced long bone changes in thalassaemic patients—radiographic features, prevalence and relations with growth. Clin Radiol. 2000;55:610-614.

642. Baker DH. Roentgen manifestations of Cooley's anemia. Ann N Y Acad Sci. 1964;119:641-661.

643. Michelson J, Cohen A. Incidence and treatment of fractures in thalassemia. J Orthop Trauma. 1988;2:29-32.

644. Canatan D, Akar N, Arcasoy A. Effects of calcitonin therapy on osteoporosis in patients with thalassemia. Acta Haematol. 1995;93:20-24.

645. Gilfillan CP, Strauss BJ, Rodda CP, et al. A randomized, double-blind, placebo-controlled trial of intravenous zoledronic acid in the treatment of thalassemia-associated osteopenia. Calcif Tissue Int. 2006;79:138-144.

646. Telfer PT, Prestcott E, Holden S, et al. Hepatic iron concentration combined with long-term monitoring of serum ferritin to predict complications of iron overload in thalassemia major. Br J Haematol. 2000;110: 971-977.

647. Nielsen P, Gunther U, Dürken M, et al. Serum ferritin iron in iron overload and liver damage: correlation to body iron stores and diagnostic relevance. J Lab Clin Med. 2000;135:413-418.

648. Brittenham GM, Cohen AR, McLaren CE, et al. Hepatic iron stores and plasma ferritin concentration in patients with sickle cell anemia and thalassemia major. Am J Hematol. 1993;42:81-85.

649. de Virgiliis S, Sanna G, Cornacchia G, et al. Serum ferritin, liver iron stores, and liver histology in children with thalassemia. Arch Dis Child. 1980;55:43-45.

650. Worwood M, Cragg SJ, Jacobs A, et al. Binding of serum ferritin to concanavalin A: patients with homozygous beta thalassemia and transfusional iron overload. Br J Haematol. 1980;46:409-411.

651. Houang MTW, Skalicka A, Arozena X, et al. Correlation between computed tomographic values and liver iron content in thalassemia major with iron overload. Lancet. 1979;1:1322-1323.

652. Mills SR, Doppman, JL, Nienhuis AW. Computed tomography in the diagnosis of disorders of excessive iron storage of the liver. J Comput Assist Tomogr. 1977;1:101-104.

653. Babiker MA, Patel PJ, Karrer ZA, Hateez MH. Comparison between serum ferritin and computed tomographic densities of liver, spleen, kidney and pancreas in beta-thalassaemia major. Scand J Clin Lab Invest. 1987;47:715-718.

654. Olivieri NF, Grisaru D, Daneman A, et al. Computed tomography scanning of the liver to determine efficacy of iron chelation therapy in thalassemia major. J Pediatr. 1989;114:427-430.

655. Long JA Jr, Doppmann JL, Nienhuis AW, Mills SR. Computed tomographic analysis of beta-thalassemic syndromes with hemochromatosis: pathologic findings with clinical and laboratory correlations. J Comput Assist Tomogr. 1980;4:159-165.

656. Long JA Jr, Doppman JL, Nienhuis AW. Computed tomographic studies of thoracic extramedullary hematopoiesis. J Comput Assist Tomogr. 1980;4:67-70.

657. Papavasiliou C, Gouliamos A, Ardreou J. The marrow heterotopia in thalassemia. Eur J Radiol. 1986;6:92-96.

658. Singcharoen T: Unusual long bone changes in thalassaemia: findings on plain radiography and computed tomographpy. Br J Radiol. 1989;62:168-171.

659. St Pierre TG, Clark PR, Chua-anusorn W, et al. Noninvasive measurement and imaging of liver iron concentrations using proton magnetic resonance. Blood. 2005;105:855-861.

660. Wood JC, Enriquez C, Ghugre N, et al. MRI R2 and R2* mapping accurately estimates hepatic iron concentration in transfusion-dependent thalassemia and sickle cell disease patients. Blood. 2005;106:1460-1465.

661. Ghugre NR, Enriquez CM, Gonzalez I, et al. MRI detects myocardial iron in the human heart. Magn Reson Med. 2006;56:681-686.

662. Tanner MA, Galanello R, Dessi C, et al. Myocardial iron loading in patients with thalassemia major on deferoxamine chelation. J Cardiovasc Magn Reson. 2006;8: 5543-5547.

663. Christoforidis A, Haritandi A, Tsitouridis I, et al. Correlative study of iron accumulation in liver, myocardium, and pituitary assessed with MRI in young thalassemic patients. J Pediatr Hematol Oncol. 2006;28:311-315.

664. Fink H. Transfusion hemochromatosis in Cooley's anemia. Ann N Y Acad Sci. 1964;119:680-685.

665. Modell B. A guide to the management of thalassemia. Paper presented at the European Molecular Biology Organization Conference on Thalassemia, 1978.

666. de Alarcon PA, Donovan ME, Forbes GB, et al. Iron absorption in the thalassemia syndromes and its inhibition by tea. N Engl J Med. 1979;300:5-8.

667. Fucharoen S, Ketvichit P, Pootrakul P, et al. Clinical manifestation of beta-thalassemia/hemoglobin E disease. J Pediatr Hematol Oncol. 2000;22:552-557.

668. Worwood M. The clinical biochemistry of iron. Semin Hematol. 1977;14:3-30.

669. Modell B, Berdoukas V. The Clinical Approach to Thalassemia. New York, Grune & Stratton, 1984.

670. Cazzola M, Finch CA. Iron balance in thalassemia. Prog Clin Biol Res. 1989;309:93-100.

671. Cazzola M, Beguin Y, Bergamaschi G, et al. Soluble transferrin receptor as a potential determinant of iron loading in congenital anaemias due to ineffective erythropoiesis. Br J Haematol. 1999;106:752-755.

672. Pippard MJ, Weatherall DJ. Iron absorption in non-transfused iron loading anemias: prediction of risk for iron loading and response to iron chelation treatment in beta thalassemia intermedia and congenital sideroblastic anemias. Haematologica. 1984;17:17-24.

673. Peters TJ, Raja KB, Simpson RJ, Snape S. Mechanisms and regulation of intestinal iron absorption. Ann N Y Acad Sci. 1988;526:141-147.

674. Papanikolaou G, Tzilianos M, Christakis JI, et al. Hepcidin in iron overload disorders. Blood. 2005;105:4103-4105.

675. Kearney SL, Nemeth E, Neufeld JE, et al. Urinary hepcidin in congenital chronic anemias. Pediatr Blood Cancer. 2007;48:57-63.

676. Gardenghi S, Marongiu MF, Ramos P, et al. Ineffective erythropoiesis in beta-thalassemia is characterized by increased iron absorption mediated by down-regulation of hepcidin and up-regulation of ferroportin. Blood. 2007;109:5027-5035.

677. Melis MA, Cau M, Deidda F, et al. H63D mutation in the HFE gene increases iron overload in beta-thalassemia carriers. Haematologica. 2002;87:242-245.

678. Piperno A, Mariani R, Arosio C, et al. Haemochromatosis in patients with beta-thalassaemia trait. Br J Haematol. 2000;111:908-914.

679. Bridges K, Cudkowicz A. Effect of iron chelators on the transferrin receptor in K562 cells. J Biol Chem. 1984;259:12970-12977.

680. Harrison PM. Ferritin: an iron storage molecule. Semin Hematol. 1977;14:55-70.

681. Drysdale JW, Adelman TG, Arosio P, et al. Human isoferritins in normal and disease states. Semin Hematol. 1977;14:71-88.

682. Letsky EA, Miller F, Wormwood M, Flynn DM. Serum ferritin in children with thalassemia regularly transfused. J Clin Pathol. 1974;27:652-655.

683. Lagos P, Lagona E, Kattamis C, Matsaniotis N. Serum ferritin in beta-thalassemia intermedia. Lancet. 1980;1:204-205.

684. Kaltwasser T, Werner E. Assessment of iron burden. Baillieres Clin Haematol. 1989;2:363-389.

685. Origa R, Galanello R, Ganz T, et al. Liver iron concentrations and urinary hepcidin in beta-thalassemia. Haematologica. 2007;92:583-588.

686. Morgan EH. Transferrin biochemistry, physiology and clinical significance. Mol Aspects Med. 1981;4:1-123.

687. Aisen P. The role of transferrin in iron transport. Br J Haematol. 1974;26:159-163.

688. Huebers HA, Finch CA. Transferrin: physiological behaviour and clinical implications. Blood. 1984;64:763-767.

689. Jacobs A. Low molecular weight intracellular iron transport compounds. Blood. 1977;50:433-439.

690. van Renswonde J, Bridges KR, Harford JB, Klausner RD. Receptor-mediated endocytosis of transferrin and the uptake of Fe in K562 cells: identification of a non-lysosomal acidic compartment. Proc Natl Acad Sci U S A. 1982;79:6186-6190.

691. Klausner RD, Ashwell G, van Renswoude J, et al. Binding of apo transferrin to K562 cells: explanation of the transferrin cycle. Proc Natl Acad Sci U S A. 1983;80:2263-2266.

692. Seymour CA, Peters TJ. Organelle pathology in primary and secondary hemochromatosis with special reference to lysosomal changes. Br J Haematol. 1978;40:239-253.

693. Roifman CM, Eytan GD, Iancu JC. Ferritin-phospholipid interaction: a model system for intralysosomal ferritin segregation in iron-overloaded hepatocytes. J Ultrastruct Res. 1982;79:307-313.

694. Richter GW. The iron-loaded cell—the cytopathology of iron storage: a review. Am J Pathol. 1978;91:362-404.

695. Hershko C, Graham G, Bates GW, Rachmilewitz EA. Non-specific serum iron fraction of potential toxicity. Br J Haematol. 1978;40:255-263.

696. Anuwajanakulchai M, Pootrakul P, Thuvasethakul P, Wasi P. Non-transferrin plasma iron in beta-thalassemia/Hb E and hemoglobin H diseases. Scand J Haematol. 1984;32:153-158.

697. Porter J. Practical management of iron overload. Br J Haematol. 2001;115:239-252.

698. Breuer W, Ermers MJ, Pootrakul P, et al. Desferrioxamine-chelatable iron, a component of serum non–transferrin-bound iron, used for assessing chelation therapy. Blood. 2001;97:792-798.

699. Hershko C, Weatherall DJ. Iron-chelating therapy. Crit Rev Clin Lab Sci. 1988;26:303-345.

700. Herbert V, Shaw S, Jayatilleke E, Stopler-Kasdan T. Most free-radical injury is iron-related: it is promoted by iron, hemin, holoferritin and vitamin C, and inhibited by desferoxamine and apoferritin. Stem Cells. 1994;12:289-303.

701. Willis ED. Effects of iron overload on lipid peroxide formation and oxidative demethylation by the liver endoplasmic reticulum. Biochem Pharmacol. 1972;21:239-247.

702. Tong Mak I, Weglicki WB. Characterization of iron-mediated peroxidative injury in isolated hepatic lysosomes. J Clin Invest. 1985;75:58-63.

703. Bacon BR, Park CH, Brittenham GM, et al. Hepatic mitochondrial oxidative metabolism in rats with chronic dietary iron overload. Hepatology. 1985;5:789-797.

704. Bacon BR, Tavill AS, Brittenham GM, et al. Hepatic lipid peroxidation in vivo in rats with chronic iron overload. J Clin Invest. 1983;71:429-439.

705. Heys AD, Dormandy TL. Lipid peroxidation in iron-overloaded spleens. Clin Sci (Lond). 1981;60:295-301.

706. Peters TJ, Seymour CA. Acid hydrolase activities and lysosomal integrity in liver biopsies from patients with iron overload. Clin Sci Mol Med. 1978;50:75-78.

707. O'Connell MJ, Ward RJ, Baum H, Peters TJ. The role of iron in ferritin- and haemosiderin-mediated lipid peroxidation in liposomes. Biochem J. 1985;229:135-139.

708. Hershko C, Link G, Pinson A. Modification of iron uptake and lipid peroxidation by hypoxia, ascorbic acid, and alpha-tocopherol in iron-loaded rat myocardial cell cultures. J Lab Clin Med. 1987;110:355-361.

709. Link G, Athias P, Grynberg A, et al. Effect of iron loading on transmembrane potential, contraction, and automaticity of rat ventricular muscle cells in culture. J Lab Clin Med. 1989;113:103-111.

710. Rachmilewitz EA, Shohet SB, Lubin BH. Lipid membrane peroxidation in beta-thalassemia major. Blood. 1976;47:495-505.

711. Miniero R, Piga A, Luzzatto L, Gabutti V. Vitamin E and beta thalassemia. Haematologica. 1983;68:562-563.

712. Cranfield M, Gollan JL, et al. Serum antioxidant activity in normal and abnormal subjects. Ann Clin Biochem. 1979;16:299-306.

713. de Martino M, Rossi ME, Resti M, et al. Change in superoxide anion production in neutrophils from multiply transfused beta thalassemia patients. Acta Haematol. 1984;71:289-298.

714. Bothwell TJ, Finch CA. Iron Metabolism. Boston, Little, Brown, 1962.

715. Fawwaz RA, Winchell HS, Pollycove M, Sargent T. Hepatic iron deposition in humans. I. First-pass hepatic deposition of intestinally absorbed iron in patients with low plasma latent iron-binding capacity. Blood. 1967;30:417-424.

716. Buonanno G, Valente A, Gonnella F, et al. Serum ferritin in beta thalassemia intermedia. Scand J Haematol. 1984;32:83-87.

717. Pippard MJ, Callender ST, Warner GT, Weatherall DJ. Iron absorption and loading in beta thalassemia intermedia. Lancet. 1979;2:819-821.

718. Engle MA, Erlandson M, Smith CH. Late cardiac complications of chronic, severe, refractory anemia with hemochromatosis. Circulation. 1964;30:698-705.

719. Buja LM, Roberts WC. Iron in the heart. Etiology and clinical signficance. Am J Med. 1971;51:209-221.

720. Sonakul D, Pacharee P, Thakerngpol K. Pathologic findings in 76 autopsy cases of thalassemia. Birth Defects Orig Artic Ser. 1988;23:157-176.

721. Finazzo M, Midiri M, D'Angelo P, et al. [The heart of the patient with beta thalassemia major. Study with magnetic resonance.] Radiol Med. 1998;96:462-465.

722. Borgna-Pignatti C, Cappellini MD, DeStefano P, et al. Cardiac morbidity and mortality in deferoxamine- or deferiprone-treated patients with thalassemia major. Blood. 2006;107:3733-3737.

723. Glickstein H, El RB, Link G, et al. Action of chelators in iron-loaded cardiac cells: accessibility to intracellular labile iron and functional consequences. Blood. 2006;108:3195-3203.

724. Wood JC, Otto-Duessel M, Gonzalez I, et al. Deferasirox and deferiprone remove cardiac iron in the iron-overloaded gerbil. Transl Res. 2006;148:272-280.

725. Hagar RW, Morris CR, Vichinsky EP. Pulmonary hypertension in thalassemia major patients with normal left ventricular systolic function. Br J Haematol. 2006;133:433-435.

726. Phrommintikul A, Sukonthasarn A, Kanjanavanit R, Nawarawong W. Splenectomy: a strong risk factor for pulmonary hypertension in patients with thalassaemia. Heart. 2006;92:1467-1472.

727. Singer, ST, Kuypers FA, Styles L, et al. Pulmonary hypertension in thalassemia: association with platelet activation and hypercoagulable state. Am J Hematol. 2006;81:670-675.

728. Lixi M, Montaldo P. Cardiological aspects and thalassemia syndrome in the past pediatric age: instrumental findings, intracavitary cardiac biopsy reports and autopsy findings. Boll Soc Ital Cardiol. 1979;24:637-648.

729. Fitchett DH, Coltart DJ, Littler WA, et al. Cardiac involvement in secondary hemochromatosis: a catheter biopsy study and analysis of myocardium. Cardiovasc Res. 1980;14:719-724.

730. Link G, Pinson A, Hershko C, et al. Heart cells in culture: a model of myocardial iron overload and chelation. J Lab Clin Med. 1985;106:147-153.

731. Nienhuis AW, Griffith P, Strawczynski H, et al. Evaluation of cardiac function in patients with thalassemia major. Ann N Y Acad Sci. 1980;344:384-396.

732. Henry WL, Nienhuis AW, Wiener M, et al. Echocardiographic abnormalities in patients with transfusion-dependent anemia and secondary myocardial iron deposition. Am J Med. 1978;64:547-555.

733. Valdez-Cruz LM, Reinecke C, Rutkowski M, et al. Preclinical abnormal segmental cardiac manifestations of thalassemia major in children on transfusion-chelation therapy: echographic alterations of left ventricular posterior wall contraction and relaxation patterns. Am Heart J. 1982;103:505-511.

734. Kremastinos DT, Toutouzas PK, Vyssoulis GP, et al. Iron overload and left ventricular performance in beta thalassemia. Acta Cardiol. 1984;39:29-40.

735. Mariotti E, Agostini A, Angelucci E, et al. Reduced left ventricular contractile reserve identified by low dose dobutamine echocardiography as an early marker of cardiac involvement in asymptomatic patients with thalassemia major. Echocardiography. 1996;13:463-472.

736. Leon MB, Borer JS, Bacharach SL, et al. Detection of early cardiac dysfunction in patients with severe beta-thalassemia and chronic iron overload. N Engl J Med. 1979;301:1143-1148.

737. Freeman AP, Giles RW, Berdoukas VA, et al. Early left ventricular dysfunction and chelation therapy in thalassemia major. Ann Intern Med. 1983;99:450-454.

738. Canale C, Terrachini V, Vallebona A, et al. Thalassemic cardiomyopathy: echocardiographic difference between major and intermediate thalassemia at rest and during isometric effort: yearly follow-up. Clin Cardiol. 1988;11:563-571.

739. Risdon RA, Barry M, Flynn DM. Transfusional iron overload: the relationship between tissue iron concentration and hepatic fibrosis in thalassemia. J Pathol. 1975;116:83-95.

740. Angelucci E, Brittenham GM, McLaren CE, et al. Hepatic iron concentration and total body iron stores in thalassemia major. N Engl J Med. 2000;343:327-331.

741. Iancu TL, Neustein HB. Ferritin in human liver cells of homozygous beta thalassemia: ultrastructural observations. Br J Haematol. 1977;37:527-535.

742. Weintraub LR, Goral A, Grasso J, et al. Pathogenesis of hepatic fibrosis in experimental iron overload. Br J Haematol. 1985;59:321-331.

743. Masera G, Jean G, Gazzola G, Novakova M. Role of chronic hepatitis in development of thalassemic liver disease. Arch Dis Child. 1976;51:680-685.

744. Masera G, Jean G, Conter V, et al. Sequental study of liver biopsy in thalassaemia. Arch Dis Child. 1980;55:800-802.

745. de Virgiliis S, Cornacchia G, Sanna G, et al. Chronic liver disease in transfusion-dependent thalassemia: liver iron quantitation and distribution. Acta Haematol. 1981;65:32-39.

746. Barry M, Flynn DM, Letsky EA, Risdon RA. Long-term chelation therapy in thalassemia major: effect on liver iron concentration, liver histology, and clinical progress. BMJ. 1974;2:16-20.

747. Cohen A. Current status of iron chelation therapy with deferoxamine. Semin Hematol. 1990;27:86-90.

748. Brittenham GM, Griffith PM, Nienhuis AW, et al. Efficacy of deferoxamine in preventing complications or iron overload in patients with thalassemia major. N Engl J Med. 1994;331:567-573.

749. Aldouri MA, Wonke B, Hoffbrand AV, et al. Iron state and hepatic disease in patients with thalassaemia major, treated with long term subcutaneous desferrioxamine. J Clin Pathol. 1987;40:1353-1359.

749a. Butensky E, Pakbaz Z, Foote D, et al. Treatment of hepatitis C virus infection in thalassemia. Ann NY Acad Sci. 2005;1054:290-299.

750. Wolman IJ, Ortalani M. Some clinical features of Cooley's anemia patients as related to transfusion schedules. Ann NY Acad Sci. 1969;105:407-414.

751. De Sanctis V, Vullo C, Katz M, et al. Endocrine complications in thalassaemia major. Prog Clin Biol Res. 1989;309:77-83.

752. Viprakasit V, Tanphaichitr VS, Mahasandana C, et al. Linear growth in homozygous beta-thalassemia and beta-thalassemia/hemoglobin E patients under different treatment regimens. J Med Assoc Thai. 2001;84:929-941.

753. García-Mayor RV, Andrade Olivie A, Fernández Catalina P, et al. Linear growth in thalassemic children treated with intensive chelation therapy. A longitudinal study. Horm Res. 1993;40:189-193.

754. Benso L, Gambotto S, Pastorin L, et al. Growth velocity monitoring of the efficacy of different therapeutic protocols in a group of thalassaemic children. Eur J Pediatr. 1995;154:205-208.

755. Caruso-Nicoletti M, De Sanctis V, Capra M, et al. Short stature and body proportion in thalassemia. J Pediatr Endocrinol Metab. 1998;11(Suppl 3):811-816.

756. Pintor C, Cella SG, Manso P, et al. Impaired growth hormone (GH) response to GH-releasing hormone in thalassemia major. J Clin Endocrinol Metab. 1986;62:263-267.

757. De Sanctis V, Stea S, Savarino L, et al. Growth hormone secretion and bone histomorphometric study in thalassaemic patients with acquired skeletal dysplasia secondary to desferrioxamine. J Pediatr Endocrinol Metab. 1998;11(Suppl 3):827-833.

758. Chatterjee R, Katz M. Evaluation of gonadotrophin insufficiency in thalassemic boys with pubertal failure: spontaneous versus provocative test. J Pediatr Endocrinol Metab. 2001;14:301-312.

759. Leheup BP, Cisternino M, Bozzola M, et al. Growth hormone response following growth hormone releasing hormone injection in thalassemia major: influence of pubertal development. J Endocrinol Invest. 1991;14:37-40.

760. Cavallo L, Gurrado R, Zecchino C, et al. Short-term therapy with recombinant growth hormone in polytransfused thalassaemia major patients with growth deficiency. J Pediatr Endocrinol Metab. 1998;11(Suppl 3):845-849.

761. Saenger D, Schwartz E, Markenson AL, et al. Depressed serum somatomedin activity in beta-thalassemia. J Pediatr. 1980;96:214-218.

762. Sklar CA, Lew LQ, Yoon DJ, David R. Adrenal function in thalassemia major following long-term treatment with multiple transfusions and chelation therapy. Evidence for dissociation of cortisol and adrenal androgen secretion. Am J Dis Child. 1987;141:327-330.

763. George A, Bhaduri A, Choudhry VP. Development of secondary sex characteristics in multitransfused thalassemic children. Indian J Pediatr. 1997;64:855-859.

764. Anoussakis CH, Alexiou D, Abatzis D, Bechrakis G. Endocrinological investigation of pituitary gonadal axis in thalassemia major. Acta Paediatr Scand. 1977;66:49-51.

765. Nienhuis AW, Peterson DT, Henry W. Evaluation and treatment of chronic iron overload. In Zaino EC, Roberts RH (eds). Chelation Therapy in Chronic Iron Overload. Miami, Symposia Specialists, 1977, p 1.

766. Masala A, Meloni T, Gallisai D, et al. Endocrine functioning in multi-transfused prepubertal patients with homozygous beta thalassemia. J Clin Endocrinol Metab. 1984;58:667-670.

767. Flynn DM, Fairney A, Jackson D, Clayton BE. Hormonal changes in thalassaemia major. Arch Dis Child. 1976;51:828-836.

768. De Sanctis V, Vullo C, Katz M, et al. Hypothalamic-pituitary-gonadal axis in thalassemic patients with secondary amenorrhea. Obstet Gynecol. 1988;72:643-647.

769. Wang C, Tso SC, Todd D. Hypogonadotropic hypogonadism in severe beta-thalassemia: effect of chelation and pulsatile gonadotropin-releasing hormone therapy. J Clin Endocrinol Metab. 1989;68:511-516.

770. Valenti S, Giusti M, McGuinness D, et al. Delayed puberty in males with beta-thalassemia major: pulsatile gonadotropin-releasing hormone administration induced changes in gonadotropin isoform profiles and an increase in sex steroids. Eur J Endocrinol. 1995;133:48-56.

771. De Sanctis V, Vullo C, Katz M, et al. Gonadal function in patients with beta thalassaemia major. J Clin Pathol. 1988;41:133-137.

772. Berkovitch M, Bistritzer T, Milone SD, et al. Iron deposition in the anterior pituitary in homozygous beta-thalassemia. J Pediatr Endocrinol Metab. 2000;13:179-184.

773. Argyropoulou MI, Metafratzi Z, Kiortsis DN, et al. T2 relaxation rate as an index of pituitary iron overload in patients with beta-thalassemia major. AJR Am J Roentgenol. 2000;175:1567-1569.

774. Chatterjee R, Katz M. Reversible hypogonadotrophic hypogonadism in sexually infantile male thalassaemic patients with transfusional iron overload. Clin Endocrinol. 2000;53:33-42.

775. Zervas A, Katopodi A, Protonotariou A, et al. Assessment of thyroid function in two hundred patients with beta-thalassemia major. Thyroid. 2002;12:151-154.

776. Spitz IM, Hirsch HJ, Landau H, et al. TSH secretion in thalassemia. J Endocrinol Invest. 1984;7:495-499.

777. McIntosh N. Endocrinopathy in thalassemia major. Arch Dis Child. 1976;51:195-201.

778. Saudek CD, Hemm RM, Peterson CM. Abnormal glucose tolerance in beta-thalassaemia major. Metabolism. 1977;26:43-52.

779. Lassman MN, Genel M, Wise JK, et al. Carbohydrate homeostasis and pancreatic islet function in thalassemia. Ann Intern Med. 1974;80:65-69.

780. Chern JP, Lin KH, Lu MY, et al. Abnormal glucose tolerance in transfusion-dependent beta-thalassemic patients. Diabetes Care. 2001;24:850-854.

781. Merkel PA, Simonson DC, Amiel SA, et al. Insulin resistance and hyperinsulinemia in patients with thalassemia major treated by hypertransfusion. N Engl J Med. 1988;318:809-814.

782. Brianda S, Maioli M, Frulio T, et al. The euglycemic clamp in patients with thalassaemia intermedia. Horm Metab Res. 1987;19:319-322.

783. Lassman MN, O'Brien RT, Pearson HA, et al. Endocrine evaluation in thalassemia major. Ann NY Acad Sci. 1974;232:226-237.

784. Christenson RA, Pootrakul P, Burnell JM, et al. Patients with thalassemia develop osteoporosis, osteomalacia, and hypoparathyroidism, all of which are corrected by transfusion. Birth Defects Orig Artic Ser. 1987;23:409-416.

785. DeSanctis V, Vullo C, Bagni B, Chiccoli L. Hypoparathyroidism in beta-thalassemia major. Acta Haematol. 1992;88:105-108.

786. Chern JP, Lin KH. Hypoparathyroidism in transfusion-dependent patients with beta-thalassemia. J Pediatr Hematol Oncol. 2002;24:291-293.

787. Gertner J, Boadus A, Anast CS, et al. Impaired parathyroid response to induced hypocalcemia in thalassemia major. J Pediatr. 1979;95:210-213.

788. Mautalen CA, Kuicala R, Perriard D, et al. Hypoparathyroidism and iron storage disease. Am J Med Sci. 1979;276:363-368.

789. Aloia JF, Ostuni JA, Yeh JK, Zaino EC. Combined vitamin D parathyroid defect in thalassemia major. Arch Intern Med. 1982;142:831-832.

790. Fucharoen S, Youngchaiyud P, Wasi P. Hypoxaemia and the effect of aspirin in thalassemia. Southeast Asian J Med Public Health. 1981;12:90-93.

791. Keens T, O'Neal M, Ortega JA, et al. Pulmonary function abnormalities in thalassemia patients on a hypertransfusion program. Pediatrics. 1981;65:1013-1017.

792. Cooper D, Mangell A, Werner MA, et al. Low lung capacity and hypoxemia in children with thalassemia major. Am Rev Respir Dis. 1980;121:639-646.

793. Grant GP, Mansell AL, Graziano JH, Mellins RB. The effect of transfusion on lung capacity, diffusing capacity, and arterial oxygen saturation in patients with thalassemia major. Pediatr Res. 1986;20:20-23.

794. Hoyt RW, Scarpa N, Wilmott RW, et al. Pulmonary function abnormalities in homozygous beta-thalassemia. J Pediatr. 1986;109:452-455.

795. Fung KP, Chow OK, So SY, Yuen PM. Pulmonary function in thalassemia major. J Pediatr. 1987;111:534-537.

796. Songkhla SN, Fucharoen S, Wasi, Bovornkitti S. Lung perfusion in thalassemia. Birth Defects Orig Artic Ser. 1987;23:371-374.

797. Youngchaiyud P, Suthamsmai T, Fucharoen S, et al. Lung function tests in splenectomized beta-thalassemia/ Hb E patients. Birth Defects Orig Artic Ser. 1987;23:361-370.

798. Piatti G, Allegra L, Ambrosetti U, et al. Beta-thalassemia and pulmonary function. Haematologica. 1999;84:804-808.

799. Filosa A, Esposito V, Meoli I, et al. Evidence of a restrictive spirometric pattern in older thalassemic patients. Respiration. 2001;68:273-278.

800. Zakynthinos E, Vassilakopoulos T, Kaltsas P, et al. Pulmonary hypertension, interstitial lung fibrosis, and lung iron deposition in thalassaemia major. Thorax. 2001;56:737-739.

801. Eldor A, Rachmilewitz EA. The hypercoagulable state in thalassemia. Blood. 2002;99:36-41.

802. Factor JM, Pottipati SR, Rappoport I, et al. Pulmonary function abnormalities in thalassemia major and the role of iron overload. Am J Respir Crit Care Med. 1994;149:1570-1574.

803. Eldor A, Maclouf J, Lellouche F, et al. A chronic hypercoagulable state and life-long platelet activation in beta thalassemia major. Southeast Asian J Trop Med Public Health. 1993;24(Suppl 1):92-95.

804. Koren A, Garty I, Antonelli D, Katzuni E. Right ventricular cardiac dysfunction in beta-thalassemia major. Am J Dis Child. 1987;141:93-96.

805. Giardini C, Angelucci E, Lucarelli G, et al. Bone marrow transplantation for thalassemia. Experience in Pesaro, Italy. Am J Pediatr Hematol Oncol. 1994;16:6-10.

806. Giardini C, Galimberti M, Lucarelli G, et al. Bone marrow transplantation in thalassemia. Annu Rev Med. 1995;46:319-330.

807. Lucarelli G, Galimberti M, Polchi P, et al. Bone marrow transplantation in thalassemia. Hematol Oncol Clin North Am. 1991;5:549-556.

808. Morris CR, Kuypers FA, Kato GJ, et al. Hemolysis-associated pulmonary hypertension in thalassemia. Ann NY Acad Sci. 2005;1054:481-485.

809. Fosburg MT, Nathan DG. Treatment of Cooley's anemia. Blood. 1990;76:435-444.

810. Giardina PJ, Hilgartner MW. Update on thalassemia. Pediatr Rev. 1992;13:55-62.

811. Dover GJ, Valle D. Therapy for beta-thalassemia—a paradigm for the treatment of genetic disorders. N Engl J Med. 1994;331:609-610.

812. Piomelli S, Loew T. Management of thalassemia major (Cooley's anemia). Hematol Oncol Clin North Am. 1991;5:557-569.

813. Olivieri NF. Thalassaemia: clinical management. Baillieres Clin Haematol. 1998;11:147-162.

814. Olivieri NF. The beta-thalassemias. N Engl J Med. 1999;341:99-109.

815. Borgna-Pignatti C, Rugolotto S, De Stefano P, et al. Survival and disease complications in thalassemia major. Ann NY Acad Sci. 1998;850:227-231.

816. Rebulla P, Modell B. Transfusion requirements and effects in patients with thalassaemia major. Lancet. 1991;337:277-280.

817. Weiner M, Kartpatkin M, Hart D, et al. Cooley anemia: high transfusion regimen and chelation therapy. Results and perspective. J Pediatr. 1978;92:653-658.

818. Necheles TF, Chung S, Sabbah R, Whitten D. Intensive transfusion therapy in thalassemia major: an eight year follow-up. Ann NY Acad Sci. 1974;232:179-185.

819. Brook CG, Thompson EN, Marshall WC, Whitehyouse RH. Growth in children with thalassemia major—an

effect of two different transfusion regimens. Arch Dis Child. 1969;44:612-616.

820. Kattamis C, Touliatds N, Haidas S, Matsoniatis N. Growth of children with thalassemia: effect of different transfusion regimens. Arch Dis Child. 1970;45:502-509.

821. Propper RD, Vutton LN, Nathan DG. New approaches to the transfusion management of thalassemia. Blood. 1980;55:55-60.

822. Masera G, Terzoli S, Avanzini A, et al. Evaluation of the supertransfusion regimen in homozygous beta-thalassaemia children. Br J Haematol. 1982;52:111-113.

823. Gabutti V, Piga A, Nicola P, et al. Hemoglobin levels and blood requirement in thalassemia. Arch Dis Child. 1982;57:156-158.

824. Piomelli S, Graziano J, Karpatkin M, et al. Chelation therapy, transfusion requirement and iron balance in young thalassemia patients. Ann N Y Acad Sci. 1980;344:409-417.

825. Piomelli S, Seaman C, Reibman J, et al. Separation of younger red cells with improved survival in vivo. An approach to chronic transfusion therapy. Proc Natl Acad Sci U S A. 1978;75:3474-3478.

826. Graziano JH, Piomelli S, Seaman C, et al. A simple technique for preparation of young red cells for transfusion from ordinary blood units. Blood. 1982;59:865-868.

827. Bracey AW, Klein HG, Chanbers S, Corash L. Ex-vivo selective isolation of young red blood cells using the IBM-2991 cell washer. Blood. 1983;61:1068-1071.

828. Hogan VA, Blanchette VS, Rock G. A simple method for preparing neocyte-enriched leukocyte poor blood for transfusion dependent patients. Transfusion. 1986;26:253-257.

829. Kevy SV, Jacobson MS, Fosburg M, et al. A new approach to neocyte transfusion: preliminary report. J Clin Apheresis. 1988;4:194-197.

830. Simon TL, Sohmer P, Nelson EJ. Extended survival of neocytes produced by a new system. Transfusion. 1989;29:221-225.

831. Cohen AR, Schmidt JM, Martin MB, et al. Clinical trial of young red cell transfusions. J Pediatr. 1984;104:865-868.

832. Marcus RE, Wonke B, Bantock HM, et al. A prospective trial of young red cells in 48 patients with transfusion-dependent thalassaemia. Br J Haematol. 1985;60:153-159.

833. Wolfe L, Sallan D, Nathan DG. Current therapy and new approaches to the treatment of thalassemia major. Ann N Y Acad Sci. 1985;45:248-255.

834. Piomelli S, Hart D, Graziano J, et al. Current strategies in the management of Cooley's anemia. Ann N Y Acad Sci. 1985;445:256-267.

835. Propper RD. Neocytes and neocyte-gerocyte exchange. Prog Clin Biol Res. 1982;88:227-233.

836. Meryman HT, Hornblower M. The preparation of red cells depleted of leukocytes. Transfusion. 1986;26:101-106.

837. Piomelli S, Karpatkin MH, Arzanian M, et al. Hyper-transfusion regimen in patients with Cooley's anemia. Ann N Y Acad Sci. 1974;232:186-192.

838. Coles SM, Klein HG, Holland PV. Alloimmunization in two multitransfused patient populations. Transfusion. 1981;21:462-466.

839. Michail-Merianou V, Pamphili-Panousopoulou L, Piperi-Lowes L, et al. Alloimmunization to red cell antigens in thalassemia: comparative study of usual versus better-match transfusion programmes. Vox Sang. 1987;52:95-98.

840. Spanos T, Karageorga M, Ladis V, et al. Red cell alloantibodies in patients with thalassemia. Vox Sang. 1990;58:50-55.

841. Diamond WJ, Brown FL, Bitterman P, et al. Delayed hemolytic transfusion reaction presenting a sickle cell crisis. Ann Intern Med. 1980;93:231-234.

842. Blumberg N, Ross K, Avila E, Peck K. Should chronic transfusion be matched for antigens other than ABO and Rh(o)D? Vox Sang. 1984;47:205-208.

843. Moroni GA, Piacentini G, Terzoli S, et al. Hepatitis B or non-A, non-B virus infection in multitransfused thalassaemic patients. Arch Dis Child. 1984;59:1127-1130.

844. Choo Q, Kuo G, Weiner AJ, et al. Isolation of a cDNA clone derived from a blood-borne non-A non-B hepatitis genome. Science. 1989;244:359-362.

845. Kuo G, Choo Q, Weiner AJ, et al. An assay for circulating antibodies to a major etiologic virus of human non-A non-B hepatitis. Science. 1989;244:359-362.

846. Alter MJ. Epidemiology of hepatitis C. Hepatology. 1997;26(3 Suppl 1):62S-65S.

847. Darby S, Ewart DW, Giangrande PL, et al. Mortality from liver cancer and liver disease in hemophiliac men and boys in UK given blood products contaminated with hepatitis C. Lancet. 1997;250:1425-1431.

848. Jonas MM. Hepatitis C infection in children. N Engl J Med. 1999;341:912-913.

849. Barton AL, Banner BF, Cable EE, Bonkovsky HL. Distribution of iron in the liver predicts the response of chronic hepatitis C infection to interferon therapy. Am J Clin Pathol. 1995;103:419-424. [Published erratum Am J Cln Pathol. 1995;104:232.]

850. Fargion S, Fracanzani AL, Sampietro M, et al. Liver iron influences the response to interferon alpha therapy in chronic hepatitis C. Eur J Gastroenterol Hepatol. 1997;9:497-503.

851. Haque S, Chandra B, Gerber MA, Lok AS. Iron overload in patients with chronic hepatitis C: a clinicopathologic study. Hum Pathol. 1996;27:1277-1281.

852. Olynyk JK, Reddy KR, Di Bisceglie AM, et al. Hepatic iron concentration as a predictor of response to interferon alfa therapy in chronic hepatitis C. Gastroenterology. 1995;108:1104-1109.

853. Riggio O, Montagnese F, Fiori P, et al. Iron overload in patients with chronic viral hepatitis: how common is it? Am J Gastroenterol. 1997;92:1298-1301.

854. Sievert W, Pianko S, Warner S, et al. Hepatic iron overload does not prevent a sustained virological response to inferferon-alpha therapy: a long term follow-up study in hepatitis C–infected patients with beta thalassemia major. Am J Gastroenterol. 2002;97:982-987.

855. Manconi PE, Dessi C, Sanna G, et al. Human immunodeficiency virus infection in multi-transfused patients with thalassaemia major. Eur J Pediatr. 1988;147:304-307.

856. Okon E, Levij S, Rachmilewitz EA. Splenectomy, iron overload, and liver cirrhosis in beta-thalassemia major. Acta Haematol. 1976;56:142-150.

857. Graziano JH, Piomelli S, Hilgartner M, et al. Chelation therapy in beta-thalassemia major. III. The role of splenectomy in achieving iron balance. J Pediatr. 1981;99: 695-699.

858. al-Salem AH, al-Dabbous I, Bhamidibati P. The role of partial splenectomy in children with thalassemia. Eur J Pediatr Surg. 1998;8:334-338.

859. Modell B. Management of thalassemia major. Br Med Bull. 1976;32:270-276.

860. Modell B. Total management of thalassaemia major. Arch Dis Child. 1977;52:489-500.

861. Cohen A, Markenson AL, Schwartz E. Transfusion requirements and splenectomy in thalassemia major. J Pediatr. 1980;97:100-102.

862. Blendis LM, Modell CB, Bowdler AJ, Williams R. Some effects of splenectomy in thalassemia major. Br J Haematol. 1974;28:77-87.

863. Engelhard D, Cividalli G, Rachmilewitz EA. Splenectomy in homozygous beta-thalassemia: a retrospective study of thirty patients. Br J Haematol. 1975;31: 391-403.

864. Cohen A, Gayer R, Mizanin J. Long-term effect of splenectomy on transfusion requirements in thalassemia major. Am J Hematol. 1989;30:254-256.

865. Cunningham-Rundles S, Giardina PJ, Grady RW, et al. Effect of transfusional iron overload on immune response. J Infect Dis. 2000;182(Suppl 1):S115-S121.

866. Walker EM Jr, Walker SM. Effects of iron overload on the immune system. Ann Clin Lab Sci. 2000;30: 354-365.

867. Green NS. *Yersinia* infections in patients with homozygous beta-thalassemia associated with iron overload and its treatment. Pediatr Hematol Oncol. 1992;9:247-254.

868. Eraklis AJ, Kevy SV, Diamond LK, Gross RE. Hazard of overwhelming infection after splenectomy in childhood. N Engl J Med. 1967;276:1225-1229.

869. Erickson WD, Burgert EO Jr, Lynn HB. The hazard of infection following splenectomy in children. Am J Dis Child. 1968;116:1-12.

870. Ein SH, Shandling V, Stephens CA, et al. The morbidity and mortality of splenectomy in childhood. Ann Surg. 1977;185:307-310.

871. Aommann AJ, Addiego J, Wara DW, et al. Polyvalent pneumococcal polysaccharide immunization of patients with sickle cell anemia and patients with splenectomy. N Engl J Med. 1977;297:897-900.

872. Kafidi KT, Rotschafer JC. Bacterial vaccines for splenectomized patients. Drug Intell Clin Pharm. 1988;22: 192-197.

873. Centers for Disease Control and Prevention (CDC). Recommendations of the Advisory Committee on Immunization Practices (ACIP). Use of vaccines and immune globulins in persons with altered immunocompetence. MMWR Recomm Rep. 1993;42(RR-4):1-18.

874. Ambrosino DM, Molrine DC. Critical appraisal of immunization strategies for prevention of infection in the immunocompromised host. Hematol Oncol Clin North Am. 1993;7:1027-1050.

875. Wanachiwanawin W. Infections in E-beta thalassemia. J Pediatr Hematol Oncol. 2000;22:581-587.

876. Rostagno C, Prisco D, Abbate R, Poggesi L. Pulmonary hypertension associated with long-standing thrombocytosis. Chest. 1991;99:1303-1305.

877. Karabus C, Fielding J. Desferroxamine chelatable iron in hemolytic, megaloblastic and sideroblastic anemia. Br J Haematol. 1967;13:924-933.

878. White GP, Bailey-Wood R, Jacobs A. The effect of chelating agents on cellular iron metabolism. Clin Sci Mol Med. 1976;50:145-152.

879. Hershko C, Rachmilewitz EA. Mechanism of deferrioxamine-induced iron excretion in thalassemia. Br J Haematol. 1979;42:125-132.

880. Bianco I, Graziani B, Lerone M, et al. A study of the mechanisms and sites of action of deferrioxamine in thalassemia major. Acta Haematol (Basel). 1984;71: 100-105.

881. Pippard M, Callendar ST, Finch CA. Ferrioxamine excretion in iron-loaded man. Blood. 1982;60:288-294.

882. Propper RD, Shurin SB, Nathan DG. Reassessment of the use of desferrioxamine B in iron overload. N Engl J Med. 1976;294:1421-1423.

883. O'Brien RT. Ascorbic acid enhancement of desferrioxamine-induced urinary iron excretion in thalassemia major. Ann N Y Acad Sci. 1974;232:221-225.

884. Modell CB, Beck J. Long-term desferrioxamine therapy in thalassemia. Ann N Y Acad Sci. 1974;232:201-210.

885. Propper RD, Cooper B, Rufo RR, et al. Continuous subcutaneous administration of desferrioxamine in patients with iron overload. N Engl J Med. 1977;297: 418-423.

886. Hussain MAM, Green N, Flynn DM, et al. Subcutaneous infusion and intramuscular injection of desferrioxamine in patients with transfusional iron overload. Lancet. 1976;2:1278-1280.

887. Graziano JH, Markenson A, Miller DR, et al. Chelation therapy in beta-thalassemia major. I. Intravenous and subcutaneous desferrioxamine. J Pediatr. 1978;92: 648-652.

888. Hoffbrand AV, Gorman A, Laulicht M, et al. Improvement in iron status and liver function in patients with transfusional iron overload with long-term subcutaneous desferrioxamine. Lancet. 1979;I:947-949.

889. Cohen A, Martin M, Schwartz E. Response to long-term deferoxamine therapy in thalassemia. J Pediatr. 1981;99: 689-694.

890. Modell B, Letsky E, Flynn DM, et al. Survival and desferrioxamine in thalassemia major. BMJ. 1982;284: 1081-1084.

891. Wolfe L, Olivieri N, Sallan D, et al. Prevention of cardiac disease by subcutaneous deferoxamine in patients with thalassemia major. N Engl J Med. 1985;312: 1600-1603.

892. Maurer HS, Lloyd-Still JD, Ingrisano C, et al. A prospective evaluation of iron chelation therapy in children with severe beta-thalassemia. A six-year study. Am J Dis Child. 1988;142:287-292.

893. de Virgiliis S, Cossu P, Toccatondi C, et al. Effect of subcutaneous desferrioxamine on iron balance in young thalassemia patients. Am J Pediat Hematol Oncol. 1983;5:73-77.

894. Fargion S, Taddei MT, Gabutti V, et al. Early iron overload in beta thalassemia major. When to start chelation therapy. Arch Dis Child. 1982;57:929-933.

895. Russo G, Romeo MA, Musumeci S, et al. Early iron chelation therapy in thalassemia major. Haematologica. 1983;68:69-73.

896. Davis BA, Porter JB. Long-term outcome of continuous 24-hour deferoxamine infusion via indwelling intravenous catheters in high-risk beta-thalassemia. Blood. 2000;95:1229-1236.

897. Marcus RE, Davies SC, Bantock HM, et al. Desferrioxamine to improve cardiac function in iron overloaded patients with thalassemia major. Lancet. 1984;1: 392-393.

898. Freeman AP, Giles RW, Berdoukas VA, et al. Sustained normalization of cardiac function by chelation therapy in thalassaemia major. Clin Lab Haematol. 1989;11: 299-307.

899. Olivieri NF, Nathan DG, MacMillan JH, et al. Survival in medically treated patients with homozygous beta-thalassemia. N Engl J Med. 1994;331:574-578.

900. Ehlers KH, Giardina PJ, Lesser ML, et al. Prolonged survival in patients with beta-thalassemia major treated with deferoxamine. J Pediatr. 1991;118:540-545.

901. Ehlers KH, Levin AR, Markenson AL, et al. Longitudinal study of cardiac function in thalassemia major. Ann N Y Acad Sci. 1980;344:397-404.

902. Matthew R, Brain M, et al. Thalassemia. In Current Therapy in Hematology/Oncology-3. Philadelphia, Decker, 1988, p 39.

903. Giardina PJ, Ehlers KH, Engle MA, et al. The effect of subcutaneous deferoxamine on the cardiac profile of thalassemia major: a five-year study. Ann N Y Acad Sci. 1985;445:282-292.

904. Lerner N, Blei F, Bierman F, et al. Chelation therapy and cardiac status in older patients with thalassemia major. Am J Pediatr Hematol Oncol. 1990;12:56-60.

905. De Sanctis V, D'Ascola G, Wonke B. The development of diabetes mellitus and chronic liver disease in long term chelated beta thalassaemic patients. Postgrad Med J. 1986;62:831-836.

906. Olivieri NF, Buncic JR, Chew E, et al. Visual and auditory neurotoxicity in patients receiving subcutaneous deferoxamine infusions. N Engl J Med. 1986;314: 869-873.

907. Barratt PS, Toogood IR. Hearing loss attributed to desferrioxamine in patients with beta-thalassaemia major. Med J Aust. 1987;147:177-179.

908. Albera R, Pia F, Lacilla M, et al. Hearing loss and desferrioxamine in homozygous beta-thalassemia. Audiology. 1988;27:207-214.

909. Porter JB, Jaswon MS, Huehns ER, et al. Desferrioxamine ototoxicity: evaluation of risk factors in thalassaemic patients and guidelines for safe dosage. Br J Haematol. 1989;73:403-409.

910. de Virgiliis S, Congia M, Turco MP, et al. Depletion of trace elements and acute ocular toxicity induced by desferrioxamine in patients with thalassaemia. Arch Dis Child. 1988;63:250-255.

911. Davies SC, Marcus RE, Hungerford JL, et al. Ocular toxicity of high-dose intravenous desferrioxamine. Lancet. 1983;2:181-184.

912. Marciani MG, Cianciulli P, Stefani N, et al. Toxic effects of high-dose deferoxamine treatment in patients with iron overload: an electrophysiological study of cerebral and visual function. Haematologica. 1991;76:131-134.

913. Rinaldi M, Della Corte M, Ruocco V, et al. Ocular involvement correlated with age in patients affected by major and intermedia beta-thalassemia treatment or not with desferrioxamine. Metab Pediatr Syst Ophthalmol. 1993;16:23-25.

914. Jiang C, Hansen RM, Gee BE, et al. Rod and rod mediated function in patients with beta-thalassemia major. Doc Ophthalmol. 1998;96:333-345.

915. Polson RJ, Jawed A, Bomford A, et al. Treatment of rheumatoid arthritis with desferrioxamine: relation between stores of iron before treatment and side effects. BMJ. 1985;291:448.

916. Bentur Y, Koren G, Tesoro A, et al. Comparison of deferoxamine pharmacokinetics between asymptomatic thalassemic children and those exhibiting severe neurotoxicity. Clin Pharmacol Ther. 1990;47:478-482.

917. Blake DR, Winyard P, Lunec J, et al. Cerebral and ocular toxicity induced by desferrioxamine. Q J Med. 1985;56:345-355.

918. Peto TEA, Hershko C. Iron and infection. Baillieres Clin Haematol. 1989;2:435-458.

919. Robins-Browne RM, Prpic JK. Effects of iron and desferrioxamine on infections with *Yersinia enterocolitica.* Infect Immun. 1985;47:774-779.

920. Gallant T, Freedman MH, Vellend H, Francombe WH. *Yersinia* sepsis in patients with iron overload treated with deferoxamine. N Engl J Med. 1986;314:1643.

921. Goodill JJ, Abuelo JG. Mucormycosis—a new risk of deferoxamine therapy in dialysis patients with aluminum or iron overload? N Engl J Med. 1987;317:54.

922. Bowern N, Ramshaw IA, Badenoch-Jones P, Doherty PC. Effect of an iron-chelating agent on lymphocyte proliferation. Aust J Exp Biol Med Sci. 1984;62: 743-754.

923. Bowern N, Ramshaw IA, Clark IA, Doherty R. Inhibition of autoimmune neuropathological process by treatment with an iron-chelating agent. J Exp Med. 1984;160: 1532-1543.

924. Bierer BE, Nathan DG. The effect of desferrithiocin, an oral iron chelator, on T cell function. Blood. 1990;76:2052-2059.

925. Carotenuto P, Pontesilli O, Cambier JC, Hayward AR. Desferoxamine blocks IL 2 receptor on T lymphocytes. J Immunol. 1986;136:2342-2347.

926. Estrov Z, Tawa A, Wang XH, et al. In vitro and in vivo effects of deferoxamine in neonatal acute leukemia. Blood. 1987;69:757-761.

927. Lederman HM, Cohen A, Lee JW, et al. Deferoxamine: a reversible S-phase inhibitor of human lymphocyte proliferation. Blood. 1984;64:748-753.

928. Freedman MH, Grisaru D, Olivieri N, et al. Pulmonary syndrome in patients with thalassemia major receiving intravenous deferoxamine infusions. Am J Dis Child. 1990;144:565-569.

929. Tenenbein M, Kowalski S, Sienko A, et al. Pulmonary toxic effects of continuous desferrioxamine administration in acute iron poisoning. Lancet. 1992;339: 699-701.

930. Adamson IY, Sienko A, Tenenbein M. Pulmonary toxicity of deferoxamine in iron-poisoned mice. Toxicol Appl Pharmacol. 1993;120:13-19.

931. Frank L. Hyperoxic inhibition of newborn rat lung development: protection by deferoxamine. Free Radic Biol Med. 1991;11:341-348.

932. Shannon M. Desferrioxamine in acute iron poisoning. Lancet. 1992;339:1601.

933. Koren G, Bentur Y, Strong D, et al. Acute changes in renal function associated with deferoxamine therapy. Am J Dis Child. 1989;143:1077-1080.

934. Koren G, Kochavi-Atiya Y, Bentur Y, Olivieri NF. The effects of subcutaneous deferoxamine administration on renal function in thalassemia major. Int J Hematol. 1991;54:371-375.

935. Cianciulli P, Sollecito D, Sorrentino F, et al. Early detection of nephrotoxic effects in thalassemic patients receiving desferrioxamine therapy. Kidney Int. 1994;46:467-470.

936. Hartkamp MJ, Babyn PS, Olivieri F. Spinal deformities in deferoxamine-treated homozygous beta-thalassemia major patients. Pediatr Radiol. 1993;23:525-528.

937. Olivieri NF, Koren G, Harris J, et al. Growth failure and bony changes induced by deferoxamine. Am J Pediatr Hematol Oncol. 1992;14:48-56.

938. Olivieri NF, Koren G, Matsui D, et al. Reduction of tissue iron stores and normalization of serum ferritin during treatment with the oral iron chelator L1 in thalassemia intermedia. Blood. 1992;79:2741-2748.

939. Tamary H, Goshen J, Carmi D, et al. Long-term intravenous deferoxamine treatment for noncompliant transfusion-dependent beta-thalassemia patients. Isr J Med Sci. 1994;30:658-664.

940. deMontalembert M, Jan D, Clairicia M, et al. Intensification du traitement chelateur du fer par la desferrioxamine a l'aide d'une chambre implantable d'acces veineux (Port-A-Cath). Arch Fr Pediatr. 1992;49:159-163.

941. Ward A, Caro JJ, Green TC, et al. An international survey of patients with thalassemia major and their views about sustaining life-long desferrioxamine use. BMC Clin Phamacol. 2002;2:3.

942. Caro JJ, Ward A, Green TC, et al. Impact of thalassemia major on patients and their families. Acta Haematol. 2002;107:150-157.

943. Treadwell MJ, Weissman L. Improving adherence with deferoxamine regimens for patients receiving chronic transfusion therapy. Semin Hematol. 2001;38(Suppl 1):77-81.

944. Hider RC, Singh S, Porter JB, Huehns ER. The development of hydroxypyridin-4-ones as orally active iron chelators. Ann Clin Lab Sci. 1990;612:327-338.

945. Berdoukas V, Bentley P, Frost H, et al. Toxicity of oral iron chelator L1 [letter]. Lancet. 1993;341:1088.

946. Singh S, Epemolu RO, Dobbins PS, et al. Urinary metabolic profiles in human and rat of 1,2-dimethyl- and 1,2-diethyl–substituted 3-hydroxypyridin-4-ones. Drug Metab Dispos. 1992;20:256-261.

947. Choudhury R, Singh S. Effect of iron overload on the metabolism and urinary recovery of 3-hydroxypyridin-4-one chelating agents in the rat. Drug Metab Dispos. 1995;23:314-320.

948. Kontoghiorghes GJ, Aldouri MA, Hoffbrand AV, et al. Effective chelation of iron in beta thalassemia with the oral chelator 1,2-dimethyl-3-hydroxypyrid-4-one. Br Med J (Clin Res Ed). 1987;295:1509-1512.

949. Olivieri NF, Brittenham GM, Matsui D, et al. Iron-chelation therapy with oral deferipronein patients with thalassemia major. N Engl J Med. 1995;332:918-922.

950. Olivieri NF, Brittenham GM, McLaren CE, et al. Long-term safety and effectiveness of iron-chelation therapy with deferiprone for thalassemia major. N Engl J Med. 1998;339:417-423.

951. Olivieri NF, Brittenham GM. Iron-chelation therapy and the treatment of thalassemia. Blood. 1997;89:739-761.

952. Töndury P, Zimmermann A, Nielsen P, Hirt A. Liver iron and fibrosis during long-term treatment with deferiprone in Swiss thalassaemic patients. Br J Haematol. 1998;101:413-415.

953. Del Vecchio GC, Crollo E, Schettini F, et al. Factors influencing effectiveness of deferiprone in a thalassaemia major clinical setting. Acta Haematol. 2000;104:99-102.

954. Wanless IR, Sweeney G, Dhillon AP, et al. Lack of progressive hepatic fibrosis during long-term therapy with deferiprone in subjects with transfusion-dependent beta-thalassemia. Blood. 2002;100:1566-1569.

955. Kowdley KV, Kaplan MM. Iron-chelation therapy with oral deferiprone—toxicity or lack of efficacy [editorial]? N Engl J Med. 1998;339:468.

956. Taher A, Sheikh-Taha M, Koussa S, et al. Comparison between deferoxamine and deferiprone (L1) in iron loaded thalassemia patients. Eur Haematol. 2001;67:30-34.

957. Barman Balfour JA, Foster RH. Deferiprone: a review of its clinical potential in iron overload in beta-thalassemia major and other transfusion-dependent diseases. Drugs. 1999;58:553-578.

958. Taher A, Chamoun FM, Koussa S, et al. Efficacy and side effects of deferiprone (L1) in thalassemia patients not compliant with desferrioxamine. Acta Haematol. 1999;101:173-177.

959. Deferiprone: new preparation. Poorly assessed. Prescrire Int. 2000;9:131-135.

960. de Franceschi L, Shalev O, Piga A, et al. Deferiprone therapy in homozygous human beta-thalassemia removes erythrocyte membrane free iron and reduces KCl cotransport activity. J Lab Clin Med. 1999;133:64-69.

961. Giardina PJ, Grady RW. Chelation therapy in beta-thalassemia: an optimistic update. Semin Hematol. 2001;38:360-366.

962. Hoffbrand AV. Oral iron chelation. Semin Hematol. 1996;33:1-6.

963. Pippard MJ, Weatherall DJ. Oral iron chelation therapy for thalassemia: an uncertain scene. Br J Haematol. 2000;111:2-5.

964. Naylor CD. The deferiprone controversy: time to move on. Can Med Assoc J. 2002;166:452-453.

965. Nick HP, Acklin P, et al. A new, potent, orally active iron chelator. In Badman BR, Brittenham GM (eds). Iron Chelators: New Development Strategies. Ponte Verde Beach, FL, Saratoga Group, 2000.

966. Nisbet-Brown E, Olivieri NF, Giardina PJ, et al. Effectiveness and safety of ICL670 in iron-loaded patients with thalassaemia: a randomised, double-blind placebo-controlled, dose-escalation trial. Lancet. 2003;361:1597-1602.

967. Hershko C, Konijn AM, Nick HP, et al. ICL670A: a new synthetic oral chelator: evaluation in hypertransfused rats with selective radioiron probes of hepatocellular and reticuloendothelial iron stores and in iron-loaded rat heart cells in culture. Blood. 2001;97:1115-1122.

968. Galanello R, Piga A, Forni GL, et al. Phase II clinical evaluation of deferasirox, a once-daily oral chelating

agent, in pediatric patients with beta-thalassemia major. Haematologica. 2006;91:1343-1351.

969. Piga A, Galanello R, Forni GL, et al. Randomized phase II trial of deferasirox (Exjade, ICL670), a once-daily, orally-administered iron chelator, in comparison to deferoxamine in thalassemia patients with transfusional iron overload. Haematologica. 2006;91:873-880.

970. Cappellini MD, Cohen A, Piga A, et al. A phase 3 study of deferasirox (ICL670), a once-daily oral iron chelator, in patients with beta-thalassemia. Blood. 2006;107:3455-3462.

971. Vichinsky E, Onyekwere O, Porter J, et al. A randomised comparison of deferasirox versus deferoxamine for the treatment of transfusional iron overload in sickle cell disease. Br J Haematol. 2007;136:501-508.

972. Borgna-Pignatti C, Rugolotto S, DeStefano P, et al. Survival and complications in patients with thalassemia major treated with transfusion and deferoxamine. Haematologica. 2004;89:1187-1193.

973. Roesner HP. The role of ascorbic acid in the turnover of storage iron. Semin Hematol. 1983;20:91-100.

974. Lynch SR, Seftel HC, Torrance JD, et al. Accelerated oxidative catabolism of ascorbic acid in siderotic Bantu. Am J Clin Nutr. 1967;20:641-647.

975. Lipschitz DA, Bothwell TH, Seftel HC, et al. The role of ascorbic acid in the metabolism of storage iron. Br J Haematol. 1972;20:155-163.

976. Wapnick AA, Bothwell TH, Seftel H. The relationship between serum iron levels and ascorbic acid stores in siderotic Bantu. Br J Haematol. 1970;19:271-276.

977. Cohen A, Cohen IJ, Schwartz E. Scurvy and altered iron stores in thalassemia major. N Engl J Med. 1981;304:158-160.

978. Nienhuis AW, Delea C, Aamodt R, et al. Evaluation of desferrioxamine and ascorbic acid for the treatment of chronic iron overload. Birth Defects Orig Artic Ser. 1976;12:177-185.

979. Bridges KR, Hoffman KE. The effects of ascorbic acid on the intracellular metabolism of iron and ferritin. J Biol Chem. 1986;261:14273-14277.

980. Bridges KR. Ascorbic acid inhibits lysosomal autophagy of ferritin. J Biol Chem. 1987;262:14773-14778.

981. Miller DM, Aust SD. Studies of ascorbate-dependent, iron-catalyzed lipid peroxidation. Arch Biochem Biophys. 1989;271:113-119.

982. Burkitt MJ, Gilbert BC. The control of iron-induced oxidative damage in isolated rat-liver mitochondria by respiration state and ascorbate. Free Radic Res Commun. 1989;5:333-334.

983. Nienhuis AW, Bern EJ, Propper R, et al. Thalassemia major: molecular and clinical aspects. Ann Intern Med. 1979;91:883-897.

984. Nienhuis AW. Vitamin C and iron. N Engl J Med. 1981;304:170-171.

985. Hyman CB, Landing B, Alfin-Slater R, et al. dl-α-Tocopherol, iron, and lipofuscin in thalassemia. Ann N Y Acad Sci. 1974;232:211-220.

986. Zannos-Mariolea L, Papagregoriou-Theodoridou M, Costantzas N, Matsaniotis N. Relationship between tocopherols and serum lipid levels in children with beta-thalassemia major. Am J Clin Nutr. 1978;31:259-263.

987. Oski FA, Barnes LA. Vitamin E deficiency: a previously unrecognized cause of hemolytic anemia in the premature infant. J Pediatr. 1967;70:211-220.

988. Hershko C, Rachmilewitz EA. The inhibitory effect of vitamin E on desferrioxamine-induced iron excretion in rats. Proc Soc Exp Biol Med. 1976;152:249-252.

989. Luhby AL, Cooperman JM, Feldman R, et al. Folic acid deficiency as a limiting factor in the anemia of thalassemia major. Blood. 1961;18:786.

990. Robinson MG, Watson RJ. Megaloblastic anemia complicating thalassemia major. Am J Dis Child. 1963;105:275-280.

991. Luhby AL, Cooperman JM, Lopez R, Giorgio AJ. Vitamin B_{12} metabolism in thalassemia major. Ann N Y Acad Sci. 1969;165:443-460.

992. Zaino E. Deferoxamine and trace metal excretion. In Zaino EC, Roberts RH (eds). Chelation Therapy in Chronic Iron Overload. Miami, FL, Symposium Specialists, 1977, p 95.

993. Ridley CM. Zinc deficiency developing in treatment for thalassemia. J R Soc Med. 1982;75:38-39.

994. Thomas ED, Buckner CD, Sanders JE, et al. Marrow transplantation for thalassaemia. Lancet. 1982;2:227-229.

995. Lucarelli G, Polchi P, Izzi T, et al. Allogeneic marrow transplantation for thalassemia. Exp Hematol. 1984;12:676-681.

996. Piomelli S, Lerner N, Cohen A, et al. Bone marrow transplantation for thalassemia [letter]. N Engl J Med. 1987;317:964.

997. Lucarelli G, Polchi P, Galimberti M, et al. Marrow transplantation for thalassaemia following busulphan and cyclophosphamide. Lancet. 1985;1:1355-1357.

998. Lucarelli G, Galimberti M, Polchi P, et al. Marrow transplantation in patients with advanced thalassemia. N Engl J Med. 1987;316:1050-1055.

999. Lucarelli G, Galimberti M, Polchi P, et al. Bone marrow transplantation in patients with thalassemia. N Engl J Med. 1990;322:417-421.

1000. Sodani P, Gaziev D, Polchi P, et al. New approach for bone marrow transplantation in patients with class 3 thalassemia aged younger than 17 years. Blood. 2004;104:1201-1203.

1001. Shulman HM, Hinterberger W. Hepatic veno-occlusive disease–liver toxicity syndrome after bone marrow transplantation. Bone Marrow Transfus. 1992;10:197-214.

1002. Apperley JF. Bone marrow transplant for the haemoglobinopathies: past, present and future. Baillieres Clin Haematol. 1993;6:299-325.

1003. La Nasa G, Giardini C, Argiolu F, et al. Unrelated donor bone marrow transplantation for thalassemia: the effect of extended haplotypes. Blood. 2002;99:4350-4356.

1004. Miniero R, Rocha V, Saracco P, et al. Cord blood transplantation in hemoglobinopathies. Bone Marrow Transplant. 1999;22(Suppl 1):S78-S79.

1005. Gluckman E, Rocha V, Chastang C. Cord blood stem cell transplantation. Best Pract Res Clin Haematol. 1999;12:279-292.

1006. DeSimone J, Heller P, Hall L, Zwiers D. 5-Azacytidine stimulates fetal hemoglobin synthesis in anemia baboons. Proc Natl Acad Sci U S A. 1982;79:4428-4431.

1007. Ley TJ, DeSimone J, Anagnou NP, et al. 5-Azacytidine selectively increases gamma-globin synthesis in a patient with beta thalassemia. N Engl J Med. 1982;307: 1469-1475.

1008. Charache S, Dover G, Smith K, et al. Treatment of sickle cell anemia with 5-azacytidine results in increased fetal hemoglobin production and is associated with nonrandom hypomethylation of DNA around the gamma-delta-beta-globin gene complex. Proc Natl Acad Sci U S A. 1983;80:4842-4846.

1009. Ley TJ, DeSimone J, Noguchi CT, et al. 5-Azacytidine increases gamma-globin synthesis and reduces the proportion of dense cells in patients with sickle cell anemia. Blood. 1983;62:370-380.

1010. Letvin NL, Linch DC, Beardsley GP, et al. Augmentation of fetal-hemoglobin production in anemic monkeys by hydroxyurea. N Engl J Med. 1984;310:869-873.

1011. Papayannopoulou T, Torrealha de Ron AT, Veith R, et al. Arabinosylcytosine induces fetal hemoglobin in baboons by perturbing erythroid cell differentiation kinetics. Science. 1984;224:617-619.

1012. Platt O, Orkin SH, Dover G, et al. Hydroxyurea enhances fetal hemoglobin production in sickle cell anemia. J Clin Invest. 1984;74:652-656.

1013. Lavelle D, DeSimone J, Heller P. Fetal hemoglobin reactivation in baboon and man: a short perspective. Am J Hematol. 1993;42:91-95.

1014. Hajjar FM, Pearson HA. Pharmacologic treatment of thalassemia intermedia with hydroxyurea. J Pediatr. 1994;125:490-492.

1015. Swank RA, Stamatoyannopoulos G. Fetal gene reactivation. Curr Opin Genet Dev. 1998;8:366-370.

1016. Olivieri NF, Weatherall DJ. The therapeutic reactivation of fetal haemoglobin. Hum Mol Genet. 1998;7: 1655-1658.

1017. Al-Khatti A, Veith RW, Papayannopoulou T, et al. Stimulation of fetal hemoglobin synthesis by erythropoietin in baboons. N Engl J Med. 1987;317:415-420.

1018. McDonagh KT, Dover GJ, Donahue R, et al. Manipulation of HbF production with hematopoietic growth factors. In Stamatoyannopoulos G, Nienhuis AW (eds). Hemoglobin Switching, Part B: Cellular and Molecular Mechanisms. New York, Alan R Liss, 1989, p 307.

1019. McDonagh KT, Dover GJ, Donohue RE, et al. Hydroxyurea-induced HbF production in anemic primates: augmentation by erythropoietin, hematopoietic growth factors, and sodium butyrate. Exp Hematol. 1992;20: 1156-1164.

1020. Umemura T, al-Khatti A, Donahue RE, et al. Effects of interleukin-3 and erythropoietin on in vivo erythropoiesis and F-cell formation in primates. Blood. 1989;74: 1571-1576.

1021. Perrine SP, Greene MF, Faller DV. Delay in the fetal globin switch in infants of diabetic mothers. N Engl J Med. 1985;312:334-338.

1022. Little JA, Dempsey NJ, Tuchman M, Ginder GD. Metabolic persistance of fetal hemoglobin. Blood. 1995;75:1712-1718.

1023. Perrine SP, Rudolph A, Faller DV, et al. Butyrate infusions in the ovine fetus delay the biologic clock for globin gene switching. Proc Natl Acad Sci U S A. 1988;85: 8540-8542.

1024. Constantoulakis P, Papayannopoulou T, Stamatoyannopoulos G. α-Amino-N-butyric acid stimulates fetal hemoglobin in the adult. Blood. 1988;72:1961-1967.

1025. Constantoulakis P, Knitter G, Stamatoyannopoulos G. On the induction of fetal hemoglobin by butyrates: in vivo and in vitro studies with sodium butyrate and comparison of combination treatments with 5-AzaC and AraC. Blood. 1989;74:1963-1971.

1026. Burns LJ, Glauber JG, Ginder GD. Butyrate induces selective transcriptional activation of a hypomethylated embryonic globin gene in adult erythroid cells. Blood. 1988;72:1536-1542.

1027. Stamatoyannopoulos G, Blau CA, Nakamoto B, et al. Fetal hemoglobin induction by acetate, a product of butyrate catabolism. Blood. 1994;84:3198-3204.

1028. Dover GJ, Brusilow S, Charache S. Induction of fetal hemoglobin production in subjects with sickle cell anemia by oral sodium phenylbutyrate. Blood. 1994;84: 339-343.

1029. Perrine SP, Ginder GD, Faller DV, et al. A short-term trial of butyrate to stimulate fetal-globin-gene expression in the beta-globin disorders. N Engl J Med. 1993; 328:81-86.

1030. Perrine SP, Olivieri NF, Faller DV, et al. Butyrate derivatives. New agents for stimulating fetal globin production in the beta-globin disorders. Am J Pediatr Hematol Oncol. 1994;16:67-71.

1031. Collins AF, Pearson HA, Giardina P, et al. Oral sodium phenylbutyrate therapy in homozygous beta thalassemia: a clinical trial. Blood. 1995;85:43-49.

1032. Sher GD, Olivieri NF. Rapid healing of chronic leg ulcers during arginine butyrate therapy in patients with sickle cell disease and thalassemia. Blood. 1994;84: 2378-2380.

1033. Sher GD, Ginder GD, Little J, et al. Extended therapy with intravenous arginine butyrate in patients with beta-hemoglobinopathies. N Engl J Med. 1995;332: 1606-1610.

1034. Atweh GF, Sutton M, Nassif I, et al. Sustained induction of fetal hemoglobin by pulse butyrate therapy in sickle cell disease. Blood. 1999;93:1790-1797.

1035. Bunn HF. Induction of fetal hemoglobin in sickle cell disease. Blood. 1999;93:1787-1789.

1036. Blau CA, Constantoulakis P, Shaw CM, Stamatoyannopoulos G. Fetal hemoglobin induction with butyric acid: efficacy and toxicity. Blood. 1993;81:529-537.

1037. Veith R, Galanelo R, Papayannopoulou T, Stamatoyannopoulos G. Stimulation of F-cell production in patients with sickle-cell anemia treated with cytarabine or hydroxyurea. N Engl J Med. 1985;313:1571-1575.

1038. Dover GJ, Humphries RK, Moore JG, et al. Hydroxyurea induction of hemoglobin F production in sickle cell disease: relationship between cytotoxicity and F-cell production. Blood. 1986;67:735-738.

1039. Charache S, Dover GJ, Moyer MA, Moore JW. Hydroxyurea-induced augmentation of fetal hemoglobin production in patients with sickle cell anemia. Blood. 1987; 69:109-116.

1040. Rodgers GP, Dover GJ, Noguchi CT, et al. Hematologic responses of patients with sickle cell disease to treatment with hydroxyurea. N Engl J Med. 1990;322: 1037-1045.

1041. Saxon BR, Rees D, Olivieri NF. Regression of extramedullary haemopoiesis and augmentation of fetal haemoglobin concentration during hydroxyurea therapy in beta thalassaemia. Br J Haematol. 1998;101:416-419.

1042. Dunbar C, Travis W, Kan YW, Nienhuis A. 5-Azacytidine treatment in a beta zero-thalassaemic patient unable to be transfused due to multiple alloantibodies. Br J Haematol. 1989;72:467-468.

1043. Lowrey CH, Nienhuis AW. Brief report: treatment with azacytidine of patients with end-stage beta-thalassemia. N Engl J Med. 1993;329:845-848.

1044. Riggs AD, Jones PA. 5-Methylcytosine, gene regulation, and cancer. Adv Cancer Res. 1983;40:1-30.

1045. Santi DV, Garrett CE, Barr PJ. On the mechanism of inhibition of DNA-cytosine methyltransferases by cytosine analogs. Cell. 1983;33:9-10.

1046. Cooper DN. Eukaryotic DNA methylation. Hum Genet. 1983;64:315-333.

1047. Jones PA. Altering gene expression with 5-azacytidine. Cell. 1985;40:485-486.

1048. Landolph JR, Jones PA. Mutagenicity of 5-azacytidine and related nucleosides in C3H/10T1/a clone 8 and V79 cells. Cancer Res. 1982;42:817-823.

1049. Harrison JJ, Anisowicz A, Gadi IK, et al. Azacytidine-induced tumorigenesis of CHEF/18 cells: correlated DNA methylation and chromosome changes. Proc Natl Acad Sci U S A. 1983;80:6606-6610.

1050. Darmon M, Nicolas J-F, Lamblin D. 5-Azacytidine is able to induce the conversion of teratocarcinoma-derived mesenchymal cells into epithelial cells. EMBO J. 1984;3:961-967.

1051. Liu DP, Liang CC, Ao ZH, et al. Treatment of severe beta-thalassemia (patients) with Myleran. Am J Hematol. 1990;33:50-55.

1052. Al-Khatti A, Papayannopoulou T, Knitter G, et al. Cooperative enhancement of F-cell formation in baboons treated with erythropoietin and hydroxyurea. Blood. 1988;72:817-819.

1053. Stamatoyannopoulos JA. Future prospects for treatment of hemoglobinopathies. West J Med. 1992;157:631-636.

1054. Maragoudaki E, Kanavakis E, Traeger-Synodinos J, et al. Molecular, haematological and clinical studies of the -101 C→T substitution of the beta-globin gene promoter in 25 beta thalassaemia intermedia patients and 45 heterozygotes. Br J Haematol. 1999;108:699-706.

1055. Anderson WF. Prospects for human gene therapy. Science. 1984;226:409.

1056. Friedmann T. Progress toward human gene therapy. Science. 1989;244:1275-1281.

1057. Cournoyer D, Caskey CT. Gene transfer into humans: a first step. N Engl J Med. 1990;323:601-603.

1058. Persons DA, Nienhuis AW. Gene therapy for the hemoglobin disorders: past, present, and future. Proc Natl Acad Sci U S A. 2000;97:5022-5024.

1059. Nienhuis AW, McDonagh KT, Bodine DM. Gene transfer into hematopoietic stem cells. Cancer. 1991;67(Suppl): 2700-2704.

1060. Friedmann T. The promise and overpromise of human gene therapy. Gene Ther. 1994;1:217-218.

1061. Hanawa H, Hargrove PW, Kepes S, et al. Extended beta-globin locus control region elements promote consistent therapeutic expression of a gamma-globin lentiviral vector in murine beta-thalassemia. Blood. 2004;104: 2281-2290.

1062. Brenner MK, Rill DR, Moen RC, et al. Gene-marking to trace origin of relapse after autologous bone-marrow transplantation. Lancet. 1993;341:85-86.

1063. May C, Rivella S, Chadburn A, Sadelain M. Successful treatment of murine beta-thalassemia intermedia by transfer of the human beta-globin gene. Blood. 2002;99: 1902-1908.

1064. May C, Rivella MC, Collegari J, et al. Therapeutic haemoglobin synthesis in beta-thalassaemic mice expressing lentivirus-encoded human beta-globin. Nature. 2000;406: 82-86.

1065. Pawliuk R, Westermark KA, Fabry ME, et al. Correction of sickle cell disease in transgenic mouse models by gene therapy. Science. 2001;294:2368-2371.

1066. Sadelain M, Lisowski L, Samakoglu S, et al. Progress toward the genetic treatment of the beta-thalassemias. Ann N Y Acad Sci. 2005;1054:78-91.

1067. Huisman THJ. Trimodality in the percentages of beta chain variants in heterozygotes. The effect of the number of active Hb alpha structural loci. Hemoglobin. 1977;1: 239-282.

1068. Higgs DR, Pressley L, Serjeant GR, et al. The genetics and molecular basis of alpha thalassemia in association with HbS in Jamaican Negroes. Br J Haematol. 1981;47:43-56.

1069. Steinberg MH, Adams JG 3rd, Dreiling BJ. Alpha thalassemia in adults with sickle-cell trait. Br J Haematol. 1975;30:31-37.

1070. Shaeffer JR, DeSimone J, Kleve LJ. Hemoglobin synthesis in a family with alpha-thalassemia trait and sickle cell trait. Biochem Genet. 1975;13:783-788.

1071. Wasi P. Hemoglobinopathies including thalassemia. Part I: Tropical Asia. Clin Haematol. 1981;10:707-729.

1072. Cunningham TM. Hemoglobin E in Indochinese refugees. West J Med. 1982;137:186-190.

1073. Monzon CM, Fairbanks VF, Burgert EO Jr, et al. Hereditary red cell disorders in Southeast Asian refugees and the effect on the prevalence of thalassemia disorders in the United States. Am J Med Sci. 1986;292:147-151.

1074. Anderson HM, Ranney HM. Southeast Asian immigrants: the new thalassemias in Americans. Semin Hematol. 1990;27:239-246.

1075. Sicard D, Lieurzou Y, Lapoumeroulie C, Labie D. High genetic polymorphism of hemoglobin disorders in Laos; complex phenotypes due to associated thalassemic syndromes. Hum Genet. 1979;50:327-336.

1076. Marsh WL, Rogers ZR, Nelson DP, Vedvick TS. Hematologic findings in Southeast Asian immigrants with particular reference to hemoglobin E. Ann Clin Lab Sci. 1983;13:299-306.

1077. Bhamarapravati N, Na-Nakorn S, Wasi P, Tuchinda S. Pathology of abnormal hemoglobin diseases seen in Thailand: I. Pathology of beta-thalassemia hemoglobin E disease. Am J Clin Pathol. 1967;47:745-758.

1078. O'Donnell A, Premawardhena A, Arambepola M, et al. Age-related changes in adaptation to severe anemia in childhood in developing countries. Proc Natl Acad Sci U S A. 2007;104:9440-9444.

1079. Itano HA, Neel JV. A new inherited abnormality of human hemoglobin. Proc Natl Acad Sci U S A. 1950;36: 613-617.

1080. Perosa L, Manganelli G, Dalfino G. Il primo caso di Hb C–thalassemia descritto in Italia. Haematologica. 1961; 46:211-272.

1081. Portier A, de Traverse P, Duzer A, et al. L'hemoglobinose C–thalassemia. Presse Med. 1960;68:1760-1763.

1082. Goksel V, Tartaroglu N. Haemoglobin-C–thalassemia bei zwei Geschwistern von weisser Rasse. In Lehmann H, Betke K (eds). Haemoglobin Colloquium. Stuttgart, Germany, Georg Thieme, 1961, p 55.

1083. Steinberg MH, Adams JG. Thalassemic hemoglobinopathies. Am J Pathol. 1983;113:396-409.

1084. Flatz G. Hemoglobin E: distribution and population genetics. Human Genet. 1967;3:189-234.

1085. Kan YW, Valenti C, Carnazza V, et al. Fetal blood-sampling in utero. Lancet. 1974;1:79-80.

1086. Rodeck C. Fetoscopy guided by real-time ultrasound for pure fetal blood samples, fetal skin samples, and examination of the fetus in utero. Br J Obstet Gynaecol. 1980; 87:449-456.

1087. Daffos F, Capella-Pavlovsky M, Forestier F. Fetal blood sampling via the umbilical cord using a needle guided by ultrasound. Prenat Diagn. 1983;3:271-277.

1088. Alter BP. Prenatal diagnosis: general introduction, methodology, and review. Hemoglobin. 1988;12:763-772.

1089. Kan YW, Golbus MS, Klein P, Dozy AM. Successful application of prenatal diagnosis in a pregnancy at risk for homozygous beta-thalassemia. N Engl J Med. 1975;292:1096-1099.

1090. Orkin SH, Alter BP, Altay C, et al. Application of endonuclease mapping to the analysis and prenatal diagnosis of thalassemias caused by globin-gene deletion. N Engl J Med. 1978;299:166-172.

1091. Dozy AM, Forman EN, Abuelo DN, et al. Prenatal diagnosis of homozygous alpha thalassemia. JAMA. 1979;241: 1610-1612.

1092. Saiki RK, Walsh PS, Levenson CH, Erlich HA. Genetics analysis of amplified DNA with immobilized sequence-specific oligonucleotide probes. Proc Natl Acad Sci U S A. 1989;86:6230-6234.

1093. Lau ET, Kwok YK, Luo HY, et al. Simple non-invasive prenatal detection of Hb Bart's disease by analysis of fetal erythrocytes in maternal blood. Prenat Diagn. 2005;25:123-128.

1094. Ding C, Chiu RW, Lau TK, et al. MS analysis of single-nucleotide differences in circulating nucleic acids: application to noninvasive prenatal diagnosis. Proc Natl Acad Sci U S A. 2004;101:10762-10767.

1095. Cao A, Galanello RM, Rosatelli MC, et al. Clinical experience of management of thalassemia: the Sardinian experience. Semin Hematol. 1996;33:66-75.

1096. Modell B, Petrou M, Ward RH, et al. Effect of fetal diagnostic testing on birth-rate of thalassaemia major in Britain. Lancet. 1984;2:1383-1386.

1097. Loukopoulos D. Prenatal diagnosis of thalassemia and of the hemoglobinopathies; a review. Hemoglobin. 1985;9:435-459.

1098. Modell B, Bulyzhenkov V. Distribution and control of some genetic disorders. World Health Stat Q. 1988;41: 209-218.

1099. Cao A, Rosatelli C, Galanello R, et al. The prevention of thalassemia in Sardinia. Clin Genet. 1989;36: 277-285.

1100. Loukopoulos D. Current status of thalassemia and the sickle cell syndromes in Greece. Semin Hematol. 1996;33:76-86.

VII The Phagocyte System

The Phagocyte System and Disorders of Granulopoiesis and Granulocyte Function

21

The Phagocyte System and Disorders of Granulopoiesis and Granulocyte Function

Mary C. Dinauer and Peter E. Newburger

Phagocytic leukocytes are bone marrow–derived cells that have the capacity to engulf and digest particulate matter. Phagocytes are essential for the host response to infection and injury and are equipped with specialized machinery enabling them to seek out, ingest, and kill microorganisms. Other functions include the synthesis and secretion of cytokines, pyrogens, and other inflammatory mediators, as well as the digestion of senescent cells and debris. These functions are important for resolution of injury and wound repair, as well as for linking innate to adaptive immunity.

The phagocyte system has two principal limbs: granulocytes (neutrophils, eosinophils, and basophils) and mononuclear phagocytes (monocytes and tissue macrophages). Both limbs participate in innate immunity and initiation of acquired immune responses. Neutrophils, the rapid effector cells of the innate immune system, circulate in the bloodstream until encountering specific chemotactic signals that promote adhesion to the vascular endothelium, diapedesis into tissues, and migration to sites of microbial invasion or tissue injury, where they release chemotactic signals to attract and activate inflammatory monocytes, dendritic cells, and lymphocytes. Mononuclear phagocytes also function as resident cells in certain tissues, such as the lung, liver, spleen, and peritoneum, where they perform a surveillance role. Both granulocytes and mononuclear phagocytes dispose of target cells and particles by engulfment and sequestration within intracellular vacuoles, followed by the release of digestive lysosomal enzymes and bactericidal antibiotic proteins from storage granules and the generation of highly reactive oxidants from the respiratory burst pathway.

This chapter is divided into three major sections. The first describes the normal distribution, structure, and function of granulocytes and mononuclear phagocytes. The second section reviews the clinical disorders associated with deficient or excessive phagocytic number. The third focuses on disorders of phagocyte function, including both intrinsic phagocyte defects and conditions secondary to other disease processes.

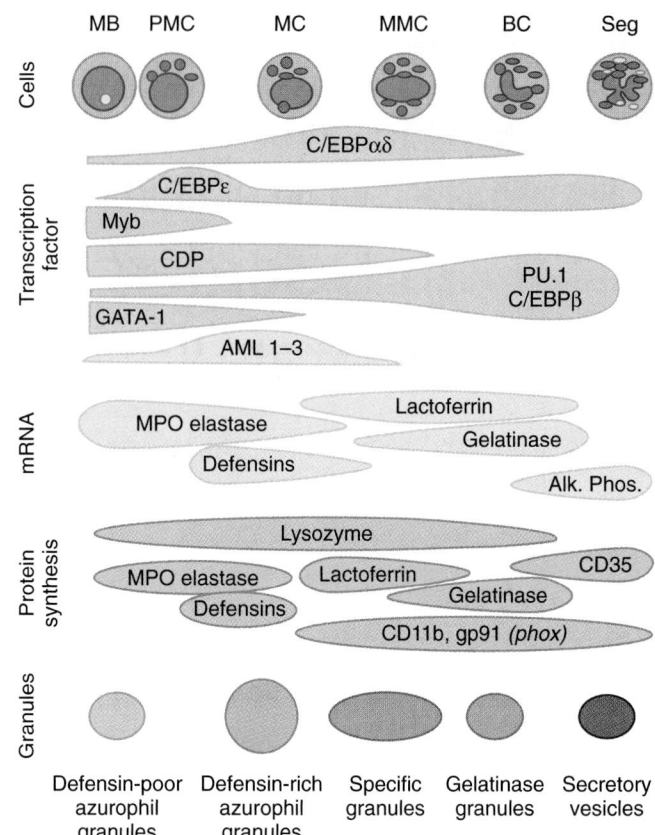

FIGURE 21-1. Neutrophil maturation. Neutrophil maturation and control of granule protein biosynthesis are achieved by the sequential and combined action of specific transcription factors, including PU.1, the CCAAT/enhancer-binding protein (C/EBP) and acute myelogenous leukemia (AML) families, CDP, Myb, and GATA-1. The granules formed at any given stage of maturation will be composed of the granule proteins synthesized at that time. The different subsets of neutrophil granules are the result of differences in the biosynthetic windows during maturation and not the result of specific sorting between individual granule subsets. When the formation of granules ceases, it is believed that secretory vesicles will form. It cannot be ruled out that post-transcriptional control occurs, so biosynthesis of proteins may not always be a precise reflection of the corresponding mRNA levels. BC, band cell; MB, myeloblast; MC, myelocyte; MMC, metamyelocyte; MPO, myeloperoxidase; PMC, promyelocyte; Segm., segmented cell (mature neutrophil). *(Adapted with permission from Borregaard N, Cowland JB. Granules of the human neutrophilic polymorphonuclear leukocyte. Blood. 1997;89:3503-3521.)*

PHAGOCYTE DISTRIBUTION AND STRUCTURE

Regulation of Myelopoiesis

Granulocytes and monocytes are produced in the bone marrow in a complex, highly regulated, dynamic process that requires both specific hematopoietic growth factors and an appropriate bone marrow microenvironment. As reviewed in Chapter 6, multipotent, self-renewing hematopoietic stem cells give rise to lineage-restricted progenitor cells that divide and further differentiate in bone marrow before release into the intravascular compartment. Transcription factors of the PU.1 and CCAAT/enhancer-binding protein (C/EBP) families play promi-

nent roles in normal myelopoiesis (Fig. 21-1). PU.1 is important for the development of early myeloid precursors and is absolutely essential for subsequent differentiation of the monocyte/macrophage lineage.[1,2] Early steps in the differentiation of granulocytes are dependent on C/EBPα, whereas C/EBPε activity is required for terminal maturation beyond the metamyelocyte stage.[2] Cytokines that promote the proliferation and differentiation of neutrophils and monocytes from primitive precursor cells include interleukin-3 (IL-3), IL-6, granulocyte-macrophage colony-stimulating factor (GM-CSF), macrophage colony-stimulating factor (M-CSF), and granulocyte colony-stimulating factor (G-CSF).[3-5] The latter two cytokines are relatively specific for the monocyte and neutrophil lineages, respectively. During infection, activated macrophages release cytokines, such as IL-1, IL-6, and tumor necrosis factor (TNF), that activate stromal cells and T lymphocytes to produce additional amounts of colony-stimulating factors and increase the production of myeloid cells. IL-5 plays an important role in inducing eosinophil differentiation,[6-8] and IL-3 is the principal cytokine inducing human basophil growth and differentiation.[9] In addition to their regulatory role in hematopoiesis, hematopoietic growth factors can act on mature myeloid cells and stimulate their functional activities. For example, circulating phagocytes become "primed" to undergo an enhanced respiratory burst on exposure to GM-CSF.[10]

Myeloid differentiation also appears to be modulated by transcriptional repressors such as Gfi 1 and retinoic acid receptors.[11-14] The participation of retinoic acid in myeloid development was originally surmised from its ability to induce differentiation of myeloid leukemia cell lines and leukemic promyelocytes in patients with acute promyelocytic leukemia[15] (see Chapter 11, Myeloid Leukemia, Myelodysplasia and Myeloproliferative Disease in Children, in *Oncology of Infancy and Childhood*).

Granulocytes

Neutrophils

The neutrophil life span is traditionally divided into the bone marrow, circulating, and tissue phases. Approximately 14 days are spent in the bone marrow, where proliferation and the early stages of neutrophil differentiation are followed by the final stages of maturation and retention in a large, nonmitotic storage pool that is manyfold larger than the circulating and tissue neutrophil populations (Table 21-1).[16-19] Once released into the bloodstream, neutrophils have a half-life of 6 to 10 hours and move between the circulating and marginated pools in a reversible fashion. Neutrophils then exit by diapedesis between endothelial cells into tissue sites of infection or inflammation. Once in tissues, neutrophils are believed to live for another 1 to 2 days before undergoing apoptosis and engulfment by macrophages.[20-22]

Myeloblasts are the earliest morphologically recognizable granulocyte precursor in marrow and are identified by their relatively undifferentiated appearance consisting of a large, oval nucleus, several prominent nucleoli, and few or no granules in gray-blue cytoplasm on Wright-stained preparations. This stage of neutrophil differentiation is followed by the promyelocyte and myelocyte stages, which are distinguished by the appearance of distinct neutrophil granule populations[23] (Table 21-2). Azurophilic, or primary, granules are formed during the promyelocyte stage and contain myeloperoxidase (MPO), bactericidal peptides, and lysosomal enzymes. The subsequent myelocyte stage is distinguished by the formation of peroxidase-negative specific, or secondary, granules containing lactoferrin. No further cell divisions occur after the myelocyte stage. The metamyelocyte, band, and mature neutrophil exhibit progressive nuclear condensation, accumulation of glycogen, and accumulation of tertiary gelatinase-rich granules and secretory vesicles marked by alkaline phosphatase.[24,25]

TABLE 21-1 Neutrophil and Monocyte Kinetics		
	Transit Time Range (hr)	**Total Cells (× 10⁹/kg)**
NEUTROPHILS		
Marrow mitotic compartment		
Myeloblast	23	0.14
Promyelocyte	26-78	0.51
Myelocyte	17-1266	1.95
Postmitotic marrow maturation and storage compartment		
Metamyelocyte	8-108	2.7
Band	12-96	3.6
Neutrophil	0-120	<u>2.5</u>
Total storage		8.8
Vascular compartment		
Circulating neutrophils	4-10	0.3
Marginated neutrophils	4-10	<u>0.4</u>
Total blood neutrophils		0.7
Tissue compartments	0-3 days (?)	Not known
Neutrophil turnover rate	1.6×10^6/kg/day	
MONOCYTES		
Marrow mitotic compartment: promonocyte	≈160	0.006
Postmitotic marrow compartment: monocyte	24	0.10
Vascular compartment	36-104	0.024
Tissue compartment	Days-months	Not known
Blood monocyte turnover rate	6×10^6/kg/day	

Neutrophil and monocyte kinetics based on references in the text.

TABLE 21-2   **Content of Human Neutrophil Granules and Secretory Organelles**

Primary: Azurophil Granules	Secondary: Specific Granules	Tertiary: Gelatinase Granules	Secretory Vesicles
MEMBRANE	**MEMBRANE**	**MEMBRANE**	**MEMBRANE**
CD63	CD11b/CD18 (Mac-1)	CD11b/CD18 (Mac-1)	Alkaline phosphatase
CD68	CD15 antigens (Lewis X)	CD67	CD10
Presenilin-1	CD66	Cytochrome b_{558}	CD11b/CD18 (Mac-1)
Stomatin	CD67	Diacylglycerol-deacylating enzyme	CD13
V-type H$^+$-ATPase	Cytochrome b_{558}	Formyl peptide receptor	CD14
	Formyl peptide receptor	Leukolysin (MMP-25)	CD16 (FcγIIIR)
	Fibronectin receptor	NRAMP-1	CD35 (complement receptor type 1)
	G protein α subunit	SCAMP	CD45
	Laminin receptor	SNAP-23, -25	CD67
	NB-1 antigen (CD177)	Tumor necrosis factor receptor	Chemokine receptors
	Rap1, Rap2	Urokinase-type plasminogen activator (uPA) receptor	Cytochrome b_{558}
	SCAMP	V-type H$^+$-ATPase	Decay-accelerating factor
	SNAP-23, -25	VAMP-2	Ig (G, A, E) FcR
	Stomatin		Formyl peptide receptor
MATRIX	Thrombospondin receptor		Leukolysin (MMP-25)
Acid β-glycerophosphatase	Tumor necrosis factor receptor		SNAP-23, -25
Acid mucopolysaccharide	Urokinase-type plasminogen activator (uPA) receptor		Tumor necrosis factor receptor
α_1-Antitrypsin	VAMP-2		V-type H$^+$-ATPase
α-Mannosidase	Vitronectin		VAMP-2
Azurocidin/CAP37/ heparin-binding protein			
Bactericidal/permeability-increasing protein (BPI)			
	MATRIX	**MATRIX**	**MATRIX**
β-Glycerophosphatase	β_2-Microglobulin	Acetyltransferase	Plasma proteins
β-Glucuronidase	Collagenase (MMP-8)	β_2-Microglobulin	
Cathepsins	Gelatinase (MMP-9)	Gelatinase (MMP-9)	
Defensins	hCAP-18	Lysozyme	
Elastase	Heparanase		
Lysozyme	Histaminase		
Myeloperoxidase	Lactoferrin		
N-acetyl-β-glucosaminidase	Lipocalin (NGAL)		
Proteinase-3	Lysozyme		
Sialidase	Plasminogen activator		
Ubiquitin-protein conjugate	Vitamin B$_{12}$–binding protein (transcobalamin I)		

See text for references.
Adapted with permission from Borregaard N, Cowland JB: Granules of the human polymorphonuclear leukocyte. Blood 1997;10:3503-3521.

On Wright-stained blood smears, a mature neutrophil is 10 to 15 mm in size and has a multilobed, polymorphic nucleus with highly condensed chromatin and yellow-pink cytoplasm containing numerous granules, as well as clumps of glycogen. The mean lobe count is usually slightly less than three. Circulating neutrophils appear round with some cytoplasmic projections and surface ruffling. A scaffold of cytoskeletal filaments, composed of largely actin microfilaments and microtubules, plays a key role in mediating neutrophil locomotion on surfaces, phagocytosis, and exocytosis.[26-28] Microtubules radiate from the centriole in the perinuclear cytoplasm near the Golgi region, whereas actin tends to be located more peripherally, where it forms an organelle-excluding meshwork. Actin is associated with a variety of actin-binding proteins (ABPs) that regulate the structure of this meshwork and link the actin cytoskeleton to the plasma membrane.[27]

The morphologic changes seen with neutrophil differentiation are accompanied by temporally coordinated changes in gene expression and protein synthesis (see Fig. 21-1).[29-31] Transcription and translation of mRNA for MPO and cathepsin, which are both primary granule constituents, are restricted to myeloblasts and promyelocytes.[31-34] In contrast, expression of secondary granule proteins, such as lactoferrin and transcobalamin I, occurs in myelocytes and metamyelocytes.[33,34] Gelatinase expression occurs even later in maturation and is first detected in bands and bone marrow neutrophils.[34] The leukocyte β integrin subunit CD11b is first detectable in myelocytes and increases throughout the later stages of neutrophil differentiation.[31] The gp91*phox* subunit of the respiratory burst oxidase complex is expressed relatively late in neutrophil maturation,[24] consistent with the observation that respiratory burst activity is not detected until the metamyelocyte stage.[35]

A mature neutrophil, previously thought of as an "end-stage" cell, retains the capacity for inducible gene expression and protein synthesis even after release from the marrow cavity.[36-39] For example, cytokines induce neutrophil expression of mRNA transcripts encoding respiratory burst oxidase components, Toll-like receptor 2 (TLR2), and IL-8.[40,41] Mature neutrophils also synthesize and secrete a variety of cytokines, including IL-1, IL-6, TNF-α, GM-CSF, M-CSF, and IL-8, which may promote recruitment and activation of both phagocyte and lymphocyte populations in the inflammatory response.[39,42] In some cases, increased cytokine synthesis is regulated by activating translation of preformed mRNA transcripts.[43]

Abnormalities in Neutrophil Morphology

Upon neutrophil activation by inflammatory signals, granule fusion can result in vacuolization and toxic granulation (prominent azurophilic granules). These morphologic changes reflect a nonspecific response to inflammation and do not necessarily indicate the presence of bacterial infection. Large azurophilic granules are also seen in the Alder-Reilly anomaly, an autosomal recessive trait, but neutrophil function does not appear to be affected. Döhle bodies can be seen in normal neutrophils at times of infection. These inclusions represent strands of rough endoplasmic reticulum that are retained from a more immature stage and stain bluish because of their high content of RNA and ribosomes. Döhle bodies in granulocytes and monocytes, in combination with leukopenia, giant platelets, and variable thrombocytopenia, characterize the May-Hegglin anomaly. This autosomal dominant syndrome, like the very similar Fechtner and Sebastian syndromes, is caused by mutations in the gene encoding nonmuscle myosin heavy chain-9.[44]

Neutrophil hypersegmentation can be a sign of vitamin B$_{12}$ or folate deficiency. Hypersegmented neutrophils, with a mean of four lobes, also occur as a rare autosomal dominant trait that is not associated with disease. Nuclear hyposegmentation is seen in Pelger-Huët anomaly, an autosomal dominant trait caused by mutations in the gene encoding the lamin B receptor, an integral protein of the nuclear envelope.[45] Typically, the nucleus is bilobed (often described as pince-nez) but has mature, coarse, densely clumped chromatin. The nucleus remains round in the rare homozygote. Pelger-Huët anomaly must be distinguished from neutrophil band forms and from the acquired or "pseudo"–Pelger-Huët anomaly, which can be seen in myeloproliferative disorders. Bilobed neutrophil nuclei are also seen in a rare functional disorder of neutrophil maturation—specific granule deficiency (SGD). In this disorder the pink-staining specific granules are absent in peripheral blood neutrophils. Giant granules representing defective membrane targeting of proteins in secretory lysosomes are seen in the neutrophils of patients with Chédiak-Higashi syndrome (CHS), most prominently in the bone marrow. SGD and CHS are discussed in more detail in the section "Disorders of Granulocyte and Mononuclear Phagocyte Function" later in this chapter.

Neutrophil Granule Biosynthesis and Classification

The numerous intracellular granules and vesicles in a neutrophil's cytoplasm function as storage pools for cell surface receptors and as reservoirs of sequestered digestive and microbicidal proteins. Many compounds are multifunctional. For example, cathepsin G, defensins, and azurocidin are both antimicrobial and chemotactic for monocytes and T cells, which helps amplify the inflammatory response and link innate to adaptive immunity. The older classification of granules as either peroxidase positive (azurophilic or primary) and peroxidase negative (specific or secondary) has proved to be too simplistic.[24,38,39,46] A current classification of neutrophil granules is shown in Table 21-2, which summarizes the composition of their membranes and luminal (matrix) contents.

Azurophilic (primary) granules are defined histochemically by the presence of MPO, an enzyme in the oxygen-dependent killing pathway. This green heme enzyme lends its color to collections of mature neutrophils (pus) or myeloid leukemia cells in the bone marrow or extramedullary tumors ("chloromas"). Azurophilic granules also contain defensins and bactericidal/permeability-increasing (BPI) protein, cytotoxic polypeptides that participate in oxygen-independent killing of microbes. Other components of the azurophilic granule matrix include neutral serine proteases, such as cathepsin and elastase, and other digestive enzymes.

Specific (secondary) granules, which are uniquely found in neutrophils, are classically identified by their content of lactoferrin, an iron-binding protein that also has direct bactericidal activity. Specific granules contain additional antibiotic substances as well, including lysozyme, lipocalin (also known as neutrophil gelatinase–associated lipocalin [NGAL]), a bacterial siderophore–binding protein, and the metalloproteinases collagenase and gelatinase. The membranes of secondary granules contain a major proportion of the neutrophil's supply of flavocytochrome b_{558}, the electron carrier of the respiratory burst oxidase.[47,48] Specific granule membranes also contain a pool of receptors for adhesive proteins, TNF, and chemotactic formyl peptides.

Although specific granules contain collagenase and some gelatinase, most of the neutrophil's store of gelatinase is localized to the matrix of gelatinase (tertiary) granules, which also contain the membrane-associated metalloproteinase leukolysin (MMP-25). Tertiary granules are formed relatively late in neutrophil differentiation and are smaller and more easily mobilized for exocytosis than secondary granules are. Secretory vesicles are formed in bands and mature neutrophils by endocytosis of the plasma membrane and serve as an important store of leukolysin, as well as the adhesive protein Mac-1 (CD11b/CD18) and many other membrane receptors (see Table 21-2).

The generation of different classes of granules largely reflects the sequential synthesis of granule proteins during granulopoiesis ("targeting by timing") (see Fig. 21-1).[24,38,39,46] As mentioned earlier, expression of primary, or azurophilic, granule proteins is restricted to myeloblasts and promyelocytes.[31-34] Expression of specific and gelatinase granule matrix proteins occurs later in granulopoiesis and requires the transcription factor C/EBPε. Specific and gelatinase granules are absent in neutrophils from C/EBPε-nullizygous mice generated by gene targeting.[49] The phenotype of C/EBPε-nullizygous mice is similar to that seen in the rare inherited disorder SGD, and mutations in the C/EBPε coding sequence have been reported in several affected patients (see later in this chapter).[50,51]

Neutrophil Cell Surface Receptors

The primary function of a mature neutrophil is to move rapidly into tissue sites to destroy invading microbes and clear inflammatory debris. To respond to inflammatory stimuli, the neutrophil is equipped with an array of cell surface receptors for adhesive ligands, chemoattractants, and cytokines that can be divided into groups based on their structure and major intracellular signaling pathway to which they are linked (Table 21-3). Many of these surface proteins are pattern recognition molecules such as TLRs and formyl peptide receptor,[52,53] a reflection of the neutrophil's role in the innate immune response. The signal transduction cascades triggered upon binding of ligand to neutrophil receptors are complex and probably redundant.[54-56] A common early event downstream of neutrophil receptor binding is activation of phospholipase C, which hydrolyzes the membrane phospholipid phosphatidylinositol 4,5-bisphosphate (PIP_2) to generate two important second messengers, diacylglycerol and 1,4,5-inositol triphosphate (IP_3),[57,58] which in turn cause the release of calcium from intracellular stores and activate protein kinase C. Changes in intracellular calcium concentration are important for neutrophil degranulation and secretion and for phagolysosome fusion during phagocytosis.[59] Activation of phosphatidylinositol 3'-kinase (PI3K) is another common early event that catalyzes the phosphorylation of PIP_2 to generate a third important lipid messenger, phosphatidylinositol 3,4,5-

TABLE 21-3	Receptors in Neutrophils	
Receptor Grouping	**Examples**	**Structural Characteristics**
G protein linked	fMLP, C5a, PAF, LTB, IL-8, chemokines	Seven-transmembrane–spanning domains (serpentine); linked to heterotrimeric GTP-binding proteins
Membrane tyrosine kinases	PDGF	Integral membrane protein, intrinsic tyrosine kinase activity; ligation leads to receptor dimerization and cross ("auto") phosphorylation
Tyrosine kinase linked	FcγRIIA, GM-CSF	FcγRII is a member of the immunoglobulin family of receptors The GM-CSF receptor is an 84-kd transmembrane protein related to receptors for IL-2 and IL-6 Ligation of receptor activates cytosolic tyrosine kinases
GPI linked	FcγRIIIB, DAF, CD14	Receptors with no transmembrane or intracellular domains. May associate with a partner receptor to mediate signal transduction
Adhesion molecules	β₂ Integrins L-selectin	β-Integrins are heterodimers with relatively long cytoplasmic tails L-selectin has an extracellular lectin-binding domain and a very short cytoplasmic tail Ligation results in potentiation of the oxidative burst and phagocytosis in adherent cells, calcium signaling, actin cytoskeletal changes, and upregulation of gene expression
Ceramide linked	TNF	Single-membrane-spanning glycoproteins; ligation activates membrane-bound sphingomyelinase with generation of ceramide, which in turn activates a 96-kd protein kinase

DAF, decay-accelerating factor; fMLP, N-formyl-methionyl-leucyl-phenylalanine (formyl peptide); GM-CSF, granulocyte-macrophage colony-stimulating factor; GPI, glycosylphosphatidylinositol; IL, interleukin; LTB₄, leukotriene B₄; PAF, platelet-activating factor; PDGF, platelet-derived growth factor; SH2, src homology 2; TNF, tumor necrosis factor.

Adapted with permission from Downey GP, Fukushima T, Fialkow L. Signaling mechanisms in human neutrophils. Curr Opin Hematol. 1995;2:76-88.

triphosphate (PIP$_3$). Neutrophil activation is also accompanied by alterations in the phosphorylation status of intracellular proteins, as regulated by protein kinase C, tyrosine kinases and phosphatases, and serine/threonine kinases of the mitogen-activated protein kinase (MAPK) family.[59-63] Guanine nucleotide–binding proteins play important roles in neutrophil signal transduction. Such proteins include the heterotrimeric guanosine triphosphate (GTP)-binding proteins, which are coupled to the seven-transmembrane–spanning domain (7-TMS; serpentine or heptahelical) receptors for chemokines and other chemoattractants,[64-66] and the low-molecular-weight guanosine triphosphatases (GTPases) of the Ras superfamily.[67] The latter category includes p21Ras itself, which can be activated via chemoattractant receptors,[68] and the Rho family GTPases Rho, Rac, and Cdc42, which are involved in the regulation of many neutrophil responses, including adhesion, the respiratory burst reduced nicotinamide adenine dinucleotide phosphate (NADPH) oxidase, and actin remodeling during migration and phagocytosis.[54] A dominant-negative form of the Rac2 GTPase has been identified in an infant with recurrent deep-seated bacterial infections and leads to multiple defects in phagocyte function.[69,70]

Eosinophils

Like neutrophils, eosinophils are compartmentalized in the bone marrow into mitotic and storage pools; they usually constitute no more than 0.3% of the nucleated bone marrow cells.[71] Eosinophils arise from a progenitor cell, the eosinophil colony-forming cell (CFC-Eo), that is committed at a relatively early stage to differentiate into eosinophils instead of neutrophils and monocytes. GATA-1 plays a critical role in the transcriptional regulation of eosinophil lineage commitment and differentiation.[72,73] Morphologic differentiation and maturation of the eosinophil parallel that of the neutrophil series, and the characteristic eosin-staining specific granules of this granulocyte lineage are prominent by the myelocyte stage. IL-3, IL-5, and GM-CSF mediate eosinophil production in the bone marrow; IL-5, IL-13, chemokines (such as eotaxins [CCL11] and RANTES [CCL5]), and leukotrienes (such as leukotriene B$_4$ [LTB$_4$]) play key roles in regulating eosinophil differentiation, chemotaxis, and functional activation.[6-8,74,75]

Once released from bone marrow, eosinophils have a half-life in the bloodstream similar to that of neutrophils.[76] After leaving the circulation, eosinophils typically localize in areas exposed to the external environment, such as the tracheobronchial tree, gastrointestinal tract, mammary glands, and vagina and cervix.[77] They are also found in connective tissue immediately below the epithelial layer. As discussed in a later section, eosinophils have both immunoenhancing and immunosuppressive functions and play a role in helminthic infection, allergy, and the response to certain tumors.[6,7,74,78] The majority of mature eosinophils reside in tissues, with an estimated blood-to-tissue ratio of 1 : 300 to 1 : 500. The life span of

tissue eosinophils is not known but may be several weeks.[77] The number of circulating eosinophils tends to be highest late at night, decreases during the morning, and begins to rise at mid-afternoon. These changes correlate inversely with the diurnal variation in adrenal glucocorticoid levels, to which circulating eosinophils are very sensitive.[79]

A mature eosinophil is slightly larger than a neutrophil, with a diameter of 12 to 17 μm. The nucleus is characteristically bilobed, although multiple lobes can be seen in patients with eosinophilia of diverse causes. The cytoplasm has prominent and morphologically distinctive granules that stain strongly with acid aniline dyes because of their high content of basic proteins.

Like the neutrophil, a mature eosinophil is endowed with the capacity for chemotaxis, phagocytosis, degranulation, and the synthesis of reactive oxidants and arachidonate metabolites.[7,77,80,81] Eosinophil cell surface membranes express a wide variety of molecules, including receptors for immunoglobulin and members of the immunoglobulin superfamily; cytokine receptors; adhesion molecules; chemokine, complement, and other chemotactic receptors; and major histocompatibility complex (MHC) class I and II and costimulatory molecules.[7,77,80]

The distinctive mature eosinophil granules are membrane-bound organelles 0.15 to 1.5 μm in length and 0.3 to 1.0 μm in width that contain a variety of enzymes and cytotoxic proteins.[7,80] These small granules are round and homogeneous by electron microscopy and include the primary granules, which develop early in eosinophilic maturation,[82] and a smaller population appearing in late eosinophils that contain arylsulfatase and other enzymes.[83] The more numerous eosin-staining secondary (specific) granules are large ovoid bodies that contain an electron-dense crystalloid core surrounded by a less dense matrix. The eosinophil major basic protein (MBP) makes up about 50% of the dense crystalloid core of the eosinophilic specific granule, along with other basic proteins rich in lysine, arginine, and phospholipids.[84,85] MBP strongly absorbs to membranes, precipitates DNA, and neutralizes heparin.[86] MBP is toxic to the schistosomules of *Schistosoma mansoni* and larvae of *Trichinella spiralis*[87] and induces the release of histamine from basophils and mast cells.[88] Hydrolytic enzymes, cathepsin, and an eosinophil-specific peroxidase are located in the matrix. Eosinophil peroxidase plays an important role in the anthelmintic function of eosinophils[89,90] and uses bromate to generate hypobromous acid from hydrogen peroxide.[91] The specific granule matrix also contains eosinophilic cationic protein and eosinophil-derived neurotoxin, two cationic proteins with ribonuclease activity.[77]

Eosinophil granule products—particularly MBP, eosinophil peroxidase, and eosinophil neurotoxin—are toxic to tissues, including the heart, lung, and brain.[7,80] These substances mediate many of the adverse clinical complications of eosinophilia and hypereosinophilic syndrome (HES), such as Löffler's endocarditis and pneumonia.[92,93]

Both eosinophils and basophils contain a lysophospholipase in the plasma membrane and primary granules that can polymerize to form the bipyramidal hexagons known as Charcot-Leyden crystals (CLCs).[94,95] CLCs are typically found in areas of eosinophil degeneration, such as sputum from asthmatic patients, nasal mucus of patients with allergies, stool of patients with parasitic infections, and pleural fluid of patients with pulmonary eosinophilic infiltrates. The CLC lysophospholipase, whose protein sequence is distinct from that of other eukaryotic or prokaryotic lysophospholipases,[96] catalyzes the hydrolysis and inactivation of lysophospholipids generated by phospholipase A_2 and thereby prevents the generation of proinflammatory arachidonic acid metabolites. The CLC protein constitutes about 5% of the total protein in eosinophils.[77]

Basophils

Basophils, like other granulocytes, differentiate and mature in the bone marrow over a period of 7 days before their release into the bloodstream; they are not normally found in connective tissue.[97] Basophils account for approximately 0.5% of the total circulating leukocytes and 0.3% of nucleated marrow cells.[98] Mature basophils have a bilobed nucleus and contain prominent metachromatic granules that stain purple or bluish with Wright stain because of their high content of sulfated glycosaminoglycans. These granules are rich in heparin, chondroitin sulfate, histamine, and kallikrein but lack acid hydrolases, alkaline phosphatase, and peroxidase.[94,99] The heparin of basophils appears to have poor anticoagulant activity. Basophil granules also contain small amounts of MBP, as well as serine proteases. Receptors expressed on the plasma membrane of basophils include a high-affinity receptor for the Fc portion of IgE, which is an important trigger for the release of granule contents and the production of arachidonic acid metabolites in anaphylactic degranulation.[100] Hence, basophils are key effector cells in certain hypersensitivity reactions.[99] Basophils synthesize and secrete IL-4 and IL-13 and may thus mediate a link between the innate and adaptive immune systems for the generation of T_H2 responses.[99,101]

Basophils share certain morphologic and functional features with mast cells, which appear to be derived from a common marrow progenitor.[102,103] However, mast cells and basophils are distinct terminally differentiated cell lineages.[9,104] Similar to basophils, mast cells contain histamine-laden metachromatic granules, express high-affinity IgE receptors, and participate in immediate and cutaneous hypersensitivity.[94,102,105,106] However, mast cells lack receptors for IL-2, IL-3, and CD11b/CD18, which are present on basophils.[9] The c-kit receptor for stem cell factor is present on mast cells but absent on the majority of basophils.[105,107] Murine mast cells can secrete a wide variety of mitogenic or inflammatory cytokines, including many interleukins (IL-1, IL-3, IL-4, IL-5, and IL-6),

chemokines, GM-CSF, and TNF-α, that are likely to play an important role in leukocyte recruitment and inflammation.[105]

Mast cells are ordinarily distributed throughout normal connective tissue, where they are often situated adjacent to blood and lymphatic vessels, near or within nerve sheaths, and beneath epithelial surfaces that are exposed to environmental antigens, such as the respiratory and gastrointestinal tracts.[106] Mature mast cells do not circulate in the blood, although circulating mast cell progenitors have been described[102] and retain a limited proliferative capacity in the tissue compartment.[108] In contrast to monocytes and macrophages, a transformation between the circulating and tissue forms of basophils and mast cells has not been observed. The fate of basophils in tissues is unknown.

Mononuclear Phagocytes

The blood monocyte is derived from a bone marrow progenitor cell (colony-forming unit–granulocyte-macrophage [CFU-GM]) that is shared with the neutrophil and undergoes differentiation through stages as monoblasts and promonocytes in the marrow cavity. The transit time of monocytes in the marrow compartment is briefer than that of neutrophils, and the mature monocyte is released into the circulation only 24 hours after the last mitosis (see Table 21-1).[109-111] Consequently, a relative monocytosis in peripheral blood commonly precedes the return of granulocytes during recovery from bone marrow aplasia or hypoplasia. Monocyte production and differentiation are regulated by IL-3, IL-6, GM-CSF, and the more lineage-specific cytokine M-CSF.[3-5,112,113]

The monocyte may spend several days in the intravascular compartment in either circulating or marginated pools.[114] Monocytes then migrate into tissues and body cavities to participate in inflammatory processes as exudate macrophages and to replenish the resident tissue macrophages, which have a relatively long life span. At least two subsets of circulating monocytes are present in humans.[115-119] The majority are $CD14^+CD16^-$ and are recruited into inflamed sites. A second subset is $CD14^+CD16^+$ and also expresses high levels of CX_3CR1, a receptor for fraktalkine, which is a transmembrane chemokine found on endothelial cells (see later in this chapter). This subset is proposed to be a source of resident macrophages in noninflamed tissue. In patients receiving allogeneic bone marrow transplants, host tissue macrophages disappear gradually and are replaced by donor macrophages approximately 3 months after transplantation.[120]

Circulating monocytes in Wright-stained blood smears are 10 to 18 μm in diameter with a convoluted surface, gray-blue cytoplasm, and an indented or kidney-shaped, foamy nucleus. However, some monocytes can be as small as 7 μm in diameter and may be difficult to distinguish morphologically from lymphocytes.[109] In contrast to neutrophils, monocytes contain a single class of granules with lysosomal characteristics.[121] After leaving the circulation, monocytes become larger and take on the appearance of tissue macrophages characteristic of the organ in which they reside. The nucleus of macrophages is typically oval with more prominent nucleoli, and the cytoplasm stains blue because of an increase in RNA content. Monocytes and macrophages are distinguished histochemically by the presence of a fluoride-inhibitable nonspecific esterase and can be identified immunohistologically by a variety of monoclonal antibodies such as F4/80 in the mouse and anti-CD68 in human tissue.[122,123]

Monocytes and macrophages share many structural and functional features with neutrophils and are capable of sensing chemotactic gradients, migrating to inflamed sites, ingesting microorganisms, and killing them with a variety of cytocidal products. However, when compared with neutrophils, mononuclear phagocytes have a large and diverse developmental potential.[115,119,124] In addition to their protective function as phagocytic cells in host defense, mononuclear phagocytes play a central role in the adaptive immune response by presenting antigens to lymphocytes; elaborating growth factors and cytokines important for lymphocyte function, wound repair, and hematopoiesis; and participating in a variety of scavenger and homeostatic pathways.

Factors modifying the enzymatic, antigenic, and functional profile of mononuclear phagocytes are incompletely understood and involve a combination of tissue-specific signals and release of inflammatory cytokines and toxins.[115,125-127] Mononuclear phagocytes at inflammatory sites become "activated" and display morphologic alterations and a variety of enhanced functions, including more pronounced ruffling of the plasma membrane and pseudopod formation, increased capacity for adherence and migration to chemotactic factors, increased microbicidal and tumoricidal activity, and enhanced ability to release cytokines.[128]

In keeping with their broad range of activities, mononuclear phagocytes possess an assortment of cell surface receptors not found in neutrophils, including receptors for the coagulation factors VII, VIIa, and thrombin[129,130] and receptors for low-density (LDL) and very-low-density (VLDL) lipoprotein.[131] Macrophages and monocytes are also active secretory cells capable of secreting more than a hundred defined substances,[132] many of which are listed in Box 21-1. These substances include molecules important in control of microbial pathogens, such as lysozyme, neutral proteases, acid hydrolases and reactive oxidants, components of the complement cascade, and coagulation factors. Mononuclear phagocytes secrete a large array of cytokines and hormones that regulate the proliferation and function of other cells that participate in the immune response, inflammation, wound repair, and hematopoiesis. Tissue macrophages also play an important role in the clearance of apoptotic cells during embryogenesis, tissue homeostasis, and resolution of inflammation.[23,133]

Monocytes and tissue macrophages are considered to make up a "mononuclear-phagocyte system," a term that has replaced the "reticuloendothelial system." Resident tissue macrophages were formerly referred to as histiocytes, an imprecise and often loosely applied term. Tissue macrophages are widely distributed and perform specialized functions at portals of entry, such as the pulmonary alveoli, and in sterile sites, such as the bone marrow.[115]

Spleen. Macrophages are distributed in all parts of the spleen, including the germinal centers, where they are associated with lymphocytes. Splenic macrophages located in the red pulp and sinuses serve a clearance function, where sluggish blood circulation maximizes the interaction between blood elements and macrophages lining the sinus walls.

Liver. The portal circulation percolates through a labyrinthine system, the spaces of Disse, before exiting via the hepatic venous system. This hepatic circulation, though less sluggish than that of the spleen, provides considerable contact between blood and the resident liver macrophages, known as Kupffer cells, that reside within these vascular sinuses.

Lymph Nodes. As in the spleen, macrophages are present throughout all regions of peripheral lymph nodes. They are most abundant in the medullary zone close to efferent lymphatic and blood capillaries. This location is probably related to the important role that macrophages play in the presentation of antigens to T lymphocytes.[127,134]

Lungs. Pulmonary macrophages reside both in the interstitium of alveolar sacs and free within the air spaces, where they participate in the clearance of inhaled microorganisms and particulate matter. The number of lung macrophages increases in many chronic pulmonary inflammatory disorders. Pulmonary macrophages are easily seen in the lungs of smokers, where black inclusions mark the macrophage vacuoles.[135] Hemosiderin-laden alveolar macrophages can be indicative of recurrent pulmonary hemorrhage, such as seen in idiopathic hemosiderosis or Goodpasture's syndrome. Gastric aspiration to detect ingested iron-laden macrophages is a useful test for these disorders.

Bone Marrow. Macrophages are found throughout the bone marrow cavity. They are particularly abundant within hematopoietic islands and on the walls of the marrow sinuses.[136] Bone marrow macrophages may have a clearance function in normal or pathologic states of ineffective hematopoiesis.[137] The clearance function of marrow macrophages is dramatically illustrated by lysosomal storage diseases such as Gaucher's disease.[138] Large inclusions build up within marrow macrophages (as well as hepatic and splenic macrophages) because of

Box 21-1	Products Secreted by Mononuclear Phagocytes

ENZYMES

Acid ceramidase, lipase, phosphatase, DNAase, RNAase

α-Iduronidase, α-L-fucosidase, α-mannosidase, α-neuraminidase

α-Naphthylesterase

Angiotensin-converting enzyme

Arginase

Aspartyglycosaminidase

β-Glucuronidase, β-glucosidase, β-galactosidase

Cathepsins, collagenase, elastase

Leucine-2-naphthylaminidase

Lipoprotein lipase

Lysozyme

N-acetyl-β-galactosaminidase, N-acetyl-β-glucosaminidase

Phospholipase A_2

Sphingomyelinase

Sulfatases

OXIDANTS

Hydroxyl radical, hydrogen peroxide, hypohalous acids, nitric oxide, peroxynitrate, superoxide anion

BINDING PROTEINS

Avidin, apolipoprotein E, acidic isoferritins, gelsolin, haptoglobin, transcobalamin II, transferrin

COAGULATION SYSTEM PROTEINS

Factors V, VII, IX, X, XIII

Tissue factor/procoagulant activity (PCA), plasminogen activator, urokinase, thrombospondin, plasminogen activator inhibitors, plasmin inhibitors

LIPID METABOLITES

Prostaglandins E_2, F_2, I; thromboxane A_2; leukotrienes B, C, D, E; malonyldialdehyde; mono-diHETEs; platelet-activating factor

COMPLEMENT SYSTEM PROTEINS

C1, 2, 3, 4, 5; factors B, D, H; properidin; C3b inactivator

CYTOKINES AND GROWTH FACTORS

Interferons α, β, γ

Interleukin 1α, 1β, 6, 8

Tumor necrosis factor (TNF)-α

Fibroblast growth factor (FGF), platelet-derived growth factor (PDGF), transforming growth factor-β (TGF-β)

Colony-stimulating factors (CSFs) G (granulocyte), GM (granulocyte/monocyte), M (monocyte)

Macrophage inflammatory proteins (MIP) 1α, 1β, 2

Monocyte chemoattractent proteins (MCP) 1, 2, 3

Thymosin B_4

MATRIX PROTEINS

Fibronectin, proteoglycans, thrombospondin

OTHER METABOLITES, PEPTIDES, AND PROTEINS

Glutathione, purines, pyrimidines

Sterol hormones, including 1α-25-dihydroxyvitamin D_3

Adapted from Nathan C. Secretory products of mononuclear phagocytes. J Clin Invest. 1987;79:319. Reproduced from the Journal of Clinical Investigation, 1987, vol. 79, pp. 319-326, by copyright permission of the American Society for Clinical Investigation.

the inability of these cells to break down lysosomal contents.[139]

Other Sites. Mononuclear phagocytes associated with lymphoid cells reside throughout the alimentary tract, particularly in submucosal tissue and small intestinal villi. They are present as microglial cells in the central nervous system (CNS), where their numbers increase after injury as monocytes emigrate across the blood-brain barrier,[140] and they may contribute to the pathogenesis of the CNS manifestations of human immunodeficiency virus (HIV) infection.[141] Mammary gland macrophages released into milk during lactation have been implicated as a potential source of postnatal transmission of HIV.[142]

Dendritic Cells. Dendritic cells are specialized antigen-presenting cells with long cytoplasmic processes and are located in tissues throughout the body, except for the brain.[143] They include the Langerhans cells of the epidermis, the veiled cells in lymph, and interdigitating cells in lymph nodes. Many dendritic cells have some of the antigenic characteristics of mononuclear phagocytes and share a common progenitor cell with granulocytes and monocytes/macrophages.[119,124,143,144] Monocytes can give rise to dendritic cells in various in vitro culture systems.[143-145] Some dendritic cells are also derived from the lymphoid lineage.[119,146] Antigen presentation by dendritic cells, which have a high density of MHC class II molecules, is a particularly potent stimulus for T-cell mediation of the primary immune response.[143,146,147]

Osteoclasts. Osteoclasts are large, multinucleated mononuclear phagocytes that resorb mineralized cartilage and bone.[148,149] Rodent transplantation studies have shown that osteoclasts can be derived from granulocyte-macrophage progenitor cells.[150] Defects in osteoclast function result in osteopetrosis, a genetically heterogeneous group of disorders characterized by defective bone resorption.[149,151] The *op/op* osteopetrotic mouse mutant lacks M-CSF, which results in deficiencies of both osteoclasts and tissue macrophages.[152] However, M-CSF levels and osteoclast numbers are normal in human infantile ("malignant") osteopetrosis,[153] an autosomal recessive disorder characterized by progressive obliteration of the marrow space.[149,151] This severe form of osteopetrosis is caused by mutations in genes encoding a vacuolar proton pump or the ClC-7 chloride channel[154,155] and is correctable by bone marrow transplantation.[151,156] Gene therapy targeting hematopoietic stem cells has shown promising results in the mouse model of the disease.[157] Administration of recombinant interferon-γ (IFN-γ), a major activator of macrophage function, can produce a clinically significant increase in bone resorption in children with infantile osteopetrosis.[158]

FUNCTION OF PHAGOCYTES

Phagocytic leukocytes play a central role in the acute phases of the inflammatory response, where they are rapidly mobilized into sites of tissue infection or injury and release an array of cytotoxic molecules to quickly eliminate the offending substance or microbe, as well as mediators that initiate an adaptive immune response. Phagocytes are also essential for normal repair of tissue injury, as evidenced by the impairment in wound healing in patients with deficits in leukocyte function or number.

The classic signs of the inflammatory response were described by the Roman writer Celsus as "rubor et tumor, cum calore et delore," redness and swelling with heat and pain.[159] However, it was not until the late 19th century that the cellular events associated with these signs were studied by Virchow and by Cohnheim.[159] The beneficial role of phagocytes in the inflammatory process for host defense and wound healing was championed by Metchnikov. Much of his work, for which he received a Nobel prize,[159,160] involved studies on the wandering ameboid mesenchymal cells of marine organisms such as the larval starfish, for which he coined the term "phagocyte" after the Greek word *phagein*, "to eat."

In this section the principal functions of granulocytes and mononuclear phagocytes in the inflammatory process are reviewed. Although these functions will be discussed as individual components, it is important to recognize that many occur either simultaneously or in rapid succession. Moreover, many of the cellular structures or secreted molecules participating in the inflammatory process have multiple and redundant functions. For example, phagocyte cell surface proteins that act as adhesive ligands for receptors on the vascular endothelium can also trigger phagocytosis and activation of the phagocyte respiratory burst. An overview of early events in the inflammatory process and crosstalk between different leukocyte populations is shown in Figure 21-2. Note that the proinflammatory events that are critical for the response to tissue injury and effective elimination of microbial challenge also set into motion the generation of counter-regulatory signals leading to resolution of the inflammatory response.[161,162]

Humoral Mediators of the Inflammatory Response

The acute inflammatory response reflects an ongoing collaboration between tissue macrophages and mast cells, vascular endothelial cells, and circulating phagocytes.[162,163] The release of soluble inflammatory mediators plays a

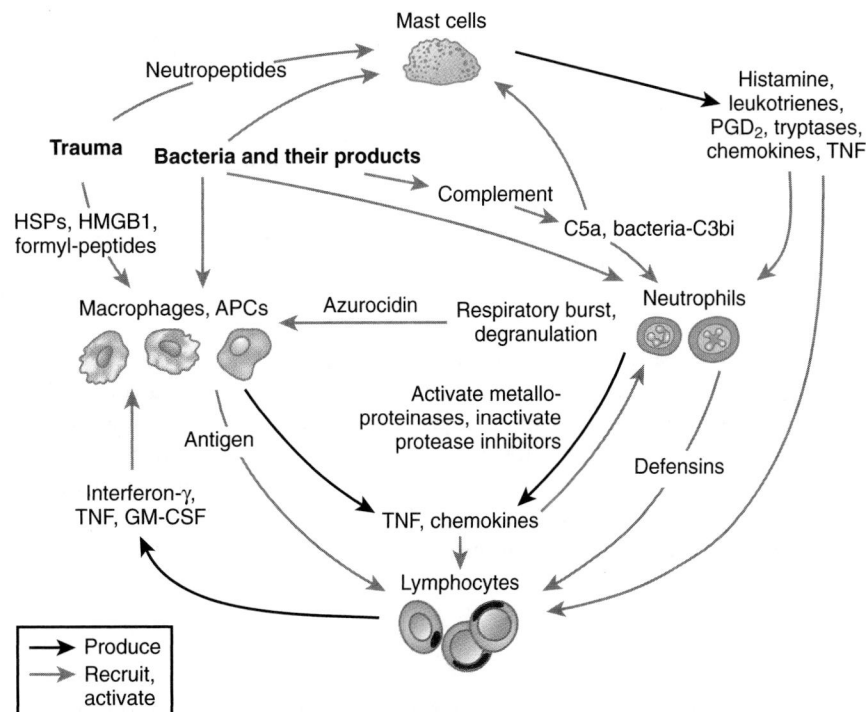

FIGURE 21-2. Early events in the response to infection accompanied by mild tissue injury. During the early inflammatory response, a variety of soluble inflammatory mediators are involved in crosstalk between different leukocyte populations and lead to their recruitment and activation. Multiple signals, generally requiring evidence of both injury and infection, are required before each population fully joins in to amplify the inflammatory process. Not shown are interactions among leukocytes, the endothelium, and the coagulation system; the generation of counter-regulatory signals that dampen the inflammatory response; and signals that regulate the subsequent transition to wound healing. APCs, antigen-presenting cells; GM-CSF, granulocyte-macrophage colony-stimulating factor; HMGB1, high–molecular group box 1 protein; HSPs, heat shock proteins; PDG₂, prostaglandin G₂; TNF, tumor necrosis factor. (*Reprinted with permission from Nathan C. Points of control in inflammation. Nature. 2002;420:846-852.*)

crucial role in activating and coordinating this process. These molecules can be generated from serum proteins (e.g., the complement-derived protein fragment C5a), secreted by endothelial cells or inflammatory leukocytes (e.g., lipid metabolites, histamine, cytokines, S100 protein), derived from invading microbes (e.g., endotoxin or formylated chemotactic peptides), or released from damaged cells (e.g., heat shock proteins [HSPs], the nuclear high–molecular group box 1 protein [HMGB1]) (see Fig. 21-2).[162,164-166]

The proinflammatory cytokines TNF-α and IL-1 have a broad range of activities in the acute inflammatory response.[55,167] Both IL-1 and TNF can cause fever and muscle breakdown and are involved in the cachexia associated with chronic infection and malignancy. The synthesis of acute phase reactants by the liver is induced by IL-6, whose synthesis and secretion are stimulated by IL-1. Proinflammatory cytokines also induce a proadhesive state on the surface of endothelium and increase the production of chemotactic cytokines (chemokines). IFN-γ is another important proinflammatory mediator that enhances the responsiveness of phagocytes to inflammatory stimuli.[126,168,169] Counterbalancing the activities of these polypeptides are IL-4, IL-10, and transforming growth factor β (TGF-β), which tend to downregulate the acute inflammatory response.[170-172]

Vasodilation and increased vascular permeability are two early responses to an inflammatory insult that are elicited, in large part, by products secreted by granulocytes and mononuclear phagocytes. Activated basophils and tissue mast cells release histamine, which leads to vasodilation of tissue arterioles and microvascular beds through H_1-type receptors.[173,174] The lipid metabolite platelet-activating factor (PAF), secreted by activated macrophages, mast cells, and endothelial cells, induces platelet degranulation and the release of additional histamine, as well as serotonin, another vasoactive amine.[175,176] Prostaglandin E and other arachidonic acid metabolites secreted by activated neutrophils and macrophages are another group of potent vasodilators.[161,175,177] Finally, vasodilation can be triggered by the release of nitric oxide (NO) from endothelial and smooth muscle cells, as well as perhaps activated macrophages, which may be particularly important in the hypotension seen in patients with gram-negative septicemia.[178,179] The increased vascular permeability that produces the edema of acute inflammation allows plasma proteins such as immunoglobulins and complement to enter tissues to promote phagocyte activation and opsonize microbes. Agents that increase vascular permeability include histamine, serotonin, PAF, and the leukotrienes LTC_4, LTD_4, and LTE_4.[175,176] Bradykinin, which is generated as a result of cleavage of Hageman factor (factor XII), also induces enhanced vascular permeability.

Chemokines and Other Chemoattractants

A wide variety of chemoattractants for neutrophils and other circulating phagocytes are generated at sites of inflammation (Table 21-4).[68,180-183] These molecules are chemically diverse and derived from many different sources in response to bacterial products and inflammatory mediators released as a result of tissue necrosis. This diversity provides functional redundancy and ensures that leukocytes will be attracted to sites of injury or infection. In addition to molecules generated by the activation of complement (C5a) or bacteria themselves (formylated peptides), many are secreted by activated phagocytes, which acts as a positive feedback loop for additional recruitment and activation of inflammatory cells.

The phospholipid PAF, released by both activated phagocytes and endothelial cells, triggers platelet activation and release of granules, in addition to being a potent chemoattractant for neutrophils and eosinophils.[175,176] Activation of phagocytes also stimulates phospholipase A_2–mediated cleavage of membrane phospholipids to generate arachidonic acid, which is then converted into a variety of eicosanoid metabolites, including the chemoattractant LTB_4.[161,184] Lipid mediators synthesized at later time points retard the accumulation of neutrophils and other leukocytes, which plays an important role in resolution of the inflammatory response. Such mediators include lipoxins, another class of eicosanoids derived from arachidonic acid, as well as the resolvins and protectins, two newly discovered families of lipid mediators generated from ω-3 polyunsaturated fatty acids.[161]

Chemokines (named for their combined *chemo*tactic and cyto*kine* properties), a family of small (8 to 10 kd) basic heparin-binding proteins, are an important group of phagocyte chemoattractants.[68,181-183,185,186] Chemokines were first discovered in the late 1980s as molecules that interact relatively specifically with subsets of inflammatory leukocytes and therefore help orchestrate the sequential influx of neutrophils, monocytes, and finally lymphocytes into an inflamed tissue site. The heparin-binding sites on chemokines can bind to negatively charged proteoglycans on endothelial cells or in the subendothelial matrix to produce locally high chemokine concentrations at an inflamed site.[180,187,188] As additional chemokines and their receptors have been identified, many other functions have emerged, including regulation of lymphoid homeostasis, hematopoiesis, and angiogenesis.[68,182,183,185] Of note, stromal cell–derived factor 1 (SDF-1, CXCl2) provides a key retention signal for neutrophils in the marrow through its interaction with the CXCR4 receptor, and mutations in the CXCR4 receptor account for myelokathexis syndrome, an inherited neutropenia (see the later section Myelokathexis and the WHIM Syndrome).[189]

Members of the chemokine family, which have a conserved structure containing two cysteine pairs, have been divided into two groups based on their disulfide sequence pattern. The CXC family, in which the first cysteine pair is separated by an intervening amino acid, include IL-8 (CXCL8), the GRO peptides (CXCL1,

TABLE 21-4   Granulocyte and Monocyte Chemoattractants in Humans

Chemoattractant	Receptor(s)	Source	Upregulators	Target Cells
LIPIDS				
PAF	PAFR	N, E, B, P, M, endothelium (phosphatidylcholine metabolism)	Calcium ionophores	N, E
LTB$_4$	B-LTR	N, M (arachidonate metabolism)	Microbial pathogens, *N*-formyl peptides	N, M, E
12-HETE	P (arachidonate metabolism)	Platelet activation		E
CXC CHEMOKINES				
IL-8 (CXCL8)	CXCR1, 2	M, N, endothelium, many other cells	LPS, IL-1, TNF, IL-3	N, B
GRO α, β, γ (CXCL1, 2, 3)	CXCR2, 1	M, endothelium, many other cells	IL-1, TNF	N, B
NAP-2 (CXCL7)	CXCR2	P*	Platelet activators	N
PF4 (CXCL4)	CXCR3B	P	Platelet activators	N, M, E
SDF-1 (CXCL12)	CXCR4	Marrow stroma, other		N, M, B, T
Fractalkine (CX$_3$CL1)	CX$_3$CRI	M, endothelium, other	IL-1, TNF, LPS, IFN-γ	M, T, NK
CC CHEMOKINES				
MCP-1, 2, 3, 4	CCR2, 3 (CCL2, 8, 7, 13)	M, endothelium, many other cells	IL-1, TNF, LPS, PDGF	M, B, E, T
RANTES (CCL5)	CCR1, 3, 5	M, E	IL-1, TNF, anti-CD3	M, B, E, T
Eotaxin (CCL11)	CCR3	M, endothelium, other	Allergens	E, B, T$_H$2
OTHER				
N-formyl peptides	fMLPR	Bacteria, mitochondria	—	N, M, E, B
C5a	C5aR	Plasma complement	Complement activation	N, M, E, B
PDGF	PDGFR	P	Platelet activation	M
TGF-β	TGFR	P, other	Platelet activation	N, M

*Platelets, when activated, secrete platelet basic protein (PBP) and connective tissue–activating peptide III (CTAP-III), which are cleaved to NAP-2 by cathepsin.

B, basophil; E, eosinophil; F, fibroblast; IL-1, interleukin-1; K, keratinocyte; LPS, lipopolysaccharide; LTB$_4$, leukotriene B$_4$; M, monocyte; MCAF, monocyte chemotactic and activating factor; MCP-1, monocyte chemoattractant protein 1; N, neutrophil; NAP-2, neutrophil-activating peptide 2; NK, natural killer; P, platelet; PAF, platelet-activating factor; PDGF, platelet-derived growth factor; RANTES, regulated upon activation, normal T cell expressed and presumably secreted; SDF-1, stromal cell–derived factor; T, T lymphocyte; T$_H$2 = T$_H$2 lymphocyte; TNF, tumor necrosis factor.

Adapted with permission from from Curnutte J, Orkin S, Dinauer M. Genetic disorders of phagocyte function. In Stamoyannopoulos G (ed). The Molecular Basis of Blood Diseases, 2nd ed. Philadelphia, WB Saunders, 1994, p 493-522. See text for additional references.

CXCL2, CXCL3), and NAP-2 (CXCL7), which are all potent neutrophil activators and chemoattractants. NAP-2 is generated from the peptide CTAP-III released from platelets by proteolytic cleavage mediated by cathepsin G, a protease released from monocytes and neutrophils.[190] The IL-8 and GRO chemokines are secreted by phagocytes and mesenchymal cells (including endothelial cells) in response to inflammatory mediators such as IL-1 and TNF.[68,182,185] Fraktalkine (CX$_3$CL1) is unique in having three intervening amino acids between the first two cysteine residues. In addition, rather than being soluble, fraktalkine is expressed on the cell surface because it is linked via a mucin-like stalk to a transmembrane domain.[191] The other major family of chemokines is called the "CC" family because the first two cysteines are adjacent to each other. CC chemokines include two important inducers of mononuclear phagocyte migration, monocyte chemoattractant protein 1 (MCP-1, CCL2) and RANTES (CCL5).[192-194] MCP-1 is produced by a wide variety of cells, whereas RANTES is secreted by macrophages and eosinophils.[68] RANTES is chemotactic for eosinophils, basophils, memory T cells, and

monocytes,[193] and both MCP-1 and RANTES induce the release of histamine from basophils.[173,174,193]

Chemokine receptors belong to the 7-TMS, G protein–coupled receptor family, with 6 receptors for CXC chemokines and 10 receptors for CC chemokines identified to date.[68,181,183,185] Most chemokines bind to more than one receptor, and most chemokine receptors, particularly those for CC chemokines, recognize more than one chemokine. Neutrophils, monocytes/macrophages, eosinophils, basophils, dendritic cells, lymphocytes, and T cells each express a distinctive subset of chemokine receptors. According to one model, specific receptors are used sequentially in successive gradients of chemoattractants. Some transmit desensitizing rather than activating signals or even fail to signal and act instead as "decoy" receptors to downregulate inflammatory reactions.[181,183] Of note, a number of chemokine receptors are coreceptors for HIV-1, including CCR5 and CCR3, whose ligands include RANTES, and CXCR4, the major receptor for SDF-1, which is a chemoattractant for T lymphocytes, CD34$^+$ hematopoietic progenitor cells, and neutrophils.[68,189]

In addition to their role as chemoattractants, the molecules listed in Table 21-4 induce the activation of other many other phagocyte functions on binding to their cognate cell surface receptors. Such functions include the upregulation and increased affinity of leukocyte integrin adhesion receptors to promote firm attachment to the endothelium, degranulation, and activation of the phagocyte respiratory burst.[180,182,185] The latter two responses generally require higher ligand concentrations than those that elicit chemotaxis, which can be as low as 10^{-9} mol/L.[195] Strong attachment of leukocytes to the endothelium can also be mediated by the membrane-tethered chemokine fraktalkine.

Despite the diverse chemical structures of the phagocyte chemoattractants listed in Table 21-4, all of the corresponding receptors that have been cloned to date belong to the 7-TMS family of receptors, also known as heptahelical or serpentine receptors.[67,196,197] The transduction of signals through chemoattractant receptors is mediated by binding of heterotrimeric G proteins to specific intracellular domains of the receptor.[198] Binding of ligand to the receptor promotes the exchange of GTP for guanosine diphosphate (GDP) bound to the G-protein α subunit, which in turns leads to dissociation of the β-γ subunits and their interaction with downstream signaling effectors, including enzymes that catalyze the production of important phospholipid second messengers at the cell membrane.[63] Phospholipase C generates diacylglycerol and IP_3 from PIP_2, which then activate protein kinase C and induce the release of intracellular calcium stores. PI3K is another key target of activated heterotrimeric G proteins and catalyzes the phosphorylation of PIP_2 to form PIP_3. Binding of formylated peptides to neutrophils also activates the p21ras-MAPK pathway and the Rho GTPases Cdc42 and Rac, with the latter known to play important roles in regulating the actin cytoskeleton and oxidant production [54,199-202] Certain Gα subunits are expressed preferentially in leukocytes and are important in signaling through the phagocyte 7-TMS receptors.[203,204]

Adhesion and Migration into Tissues

The discovery that leukocytes migrate from the bloodstream into extravascular sites of inflammation, described by Cohnheim in 1867, was a major milestone in the conceptualization of the inflammatory process.[159] Cohnheim, who used intravital microscopy to study the microvasculature in the frog tongue and mesentery after tissue injury, also first proposed that inflammatory stimuli induce a molecular change in the blood vessel wall that promotes increased adherence of leukocytes, a concept that was finally proved a century later.

To move from the bloodstream into inflamed sites, leukocytes must attach to the vascular endothelium, migrate between adjacent endothelial cells in a process referred to as diapedesis, and penetrate the basement membrane. The molecular mechanisms underlying these events involve a series of sequential adhesive interactions between chemoattractant-activated leukocytes and endothelial cells that are activated by inflammatory mediators (Fig. 21-3).[6,116,180,205,206]

Leukocyte Adhesion and Migration into Tissues

The initial step in emigration from postcapillary venules is a low-affinity interaction between the neutrophil and

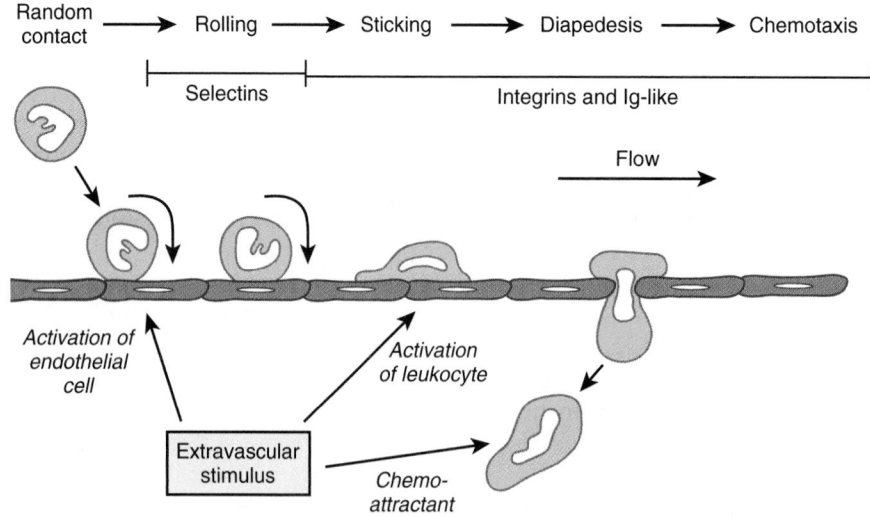

FIGURE 21-3. Adhesive interactions during phagocyte emigration. Under conditions of flow within postcapillary venules, leukocytes are first observed to roll along the endothelium adjacent to the extravascular site of inflammation. Subsequently, some of the rolling leukocytes adhere firmly, pass between endothelial cells by diapedesis, and then migrate into subendothelial tissue. Leukocyte rolling is mediated by multiple low-affinity interactions between selectin receptors and carbohydrate counter-receptors, and firm adhesion and diapedesis are largely mediated by integrin and immunoglobulin (Ig)-like adhesion proteins. Chemokines or other chemoattractants are important for both upregulating the cell surface expression of leukocyte integrins and triggering inside-out signaling to increase their avidity for endothelial ligands. *(Adapted with permission from Carlos TM, Harlan JM. Leukocyte-endothelial adhesion molecules. Blood. 1994;84:2068-2101.)*

the endothelium that is often referred to as "rolling" based on its appearance on intravital microscopy. This transient adherence, also called "tethering," is mediated by the upregulation of selectin expression on endothelial cells. The selectin family of adhesion molecules consists of membrane-spanning glycoproteins (Fig. 21-4) that bind to fucosylated structures such as Lewis X (Galβ1→4[Fucα1→3]GlcNac→R), sialyl-Lewis X, and other specific carbohydrates.[205,207-209] P-selectin is important for the initial steps of neutrophil adhesion to the endothelium and is stored in the Weibel-Palade bodies and alpha granules of endothelial cells and platelets, respectively. Upon endothelial cell activation by histamine, thrombin, and other inflammatory molecules, these cytoplasmic storage granules fuse with the cell membrane to rapidly increase the surface expression of P-selectin. E-selectin is expressed on endothelial cells at low levels but is upregulated by transcriptional activation and de novo protein synthesis in response to inflammatory cytokines.[210] E-selectin binds to three different ligands on neutrophils, P-selectin glycoprotein ligand 1 (PSGL-1), E-selectin ligand 1 (ESL-1), and CD44.[211] These ligands allow endothelial cells to capture neutrophils by mediating tethering, rolling, and slowing of neutrophil velocity, respectively. L-selectin is expressed constitutively on the surface of neutrophils, mononuclear phagocytes, and lymphocytes and is shed within minutes of leukocyte activation by a proteolytic cleavage event near the external membrane surface insertion site.[212,213] Circulating L-selectin may modulate leukocyte adhesion during inflammation.[214]

Rolling neutrophils can detach and return to the circulation. Others will come to a halt and, within seconds, adopt a flattened, adherent morphology and attach firmly to the vessel wall.[205] This firm attachment appears to be mediated in large part by binding of leukocyte integrin adhesion receptors to intercellular adhesion molecules (ICAMs) on the endothelium.[205,206] In addition, complement fragments are found on the endothelial surface at inflamed sites and may also function as integrin-binding sites. Activation of leukocytes by chemoattractants and other inflammatory mediators is critical to the development of these strong adhesive interactions because it leads to upregulation of the number and avidity of cell surface integrins ("inside-out signaling"). Exposure to locally high concentrations of chemoattractants may be enhanced by selectin-mediated tethering and by retention of chemokines on the extracellular matrix.[187,188]

The integrins, a large family of adhesion proteins that are glycosylated heterodimers of a noncovalently linked α and β chain, are classified into subfamilies according to the type of β subunit.[205-207,215] Many integrins mediate attachment to extracellular matrices by serving as receptors for matrix proteins. Others are involved in hemostasis, such as glycoprotein IIb/IIIa on platelets. Neutrophil β₂ and β₁ integrins appear to be involved in regulating neutrophil retention and release, respectively, from the bone marrow storage pool into the circulation.[189]

Leukocyte β₂ integrins (Fig. 21-5) play a critical role in mediating adhesive interactions in inflammation, including attachment of leukocytes to endothelial cells, and are also opsonic receptors for complement fragment C3bi-coated particles. There are four different leukocyte β₂ integrins, each with a common 95-kd β subunit (CD18) but different α subunits: CD11a (177 kd), CD11b (165 kd), CD11c (150 kd), and CD11d (160 kd) (Fig. 21-5). Lymphocyte function antigen 1 (LFA-1) is

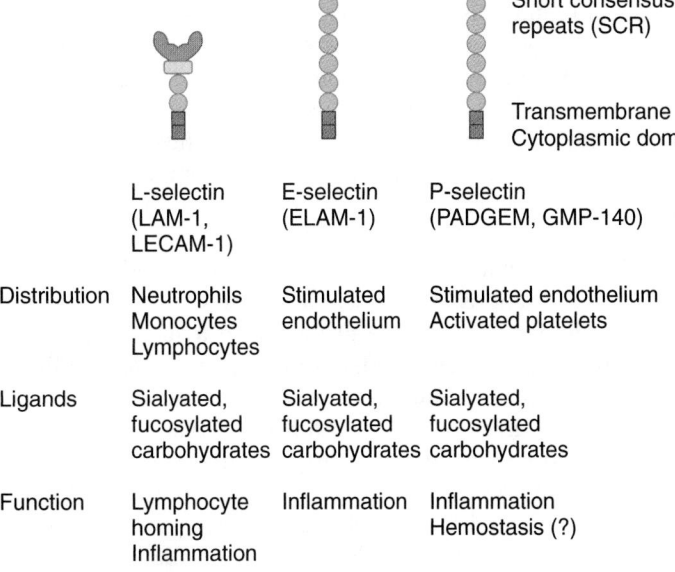

FIGURE 21-4. Selectin family of adhesion molecules. EGF, epidermal growth factor. *(Adapted with permission from Kishimoto TK, Rothlein R. Integrins, ICAMs, and selectins: role and regulation of adhesion molecules in neutrophil recruitment to inflammatory sites. Adv Pharm. 1994;25: 117-169.)*

	L-selectin (LAM-1, LECAM-1)	E-selectin (ELAM-1)	P-selectin (PADGEM, GMP-140)
Distribution	Neutrophils Monocytes Lymphocytes	Stimulated endothelium	Stimulated endothelium Activated platelets
Ligands	Sialyated, fucosylated carbohydrates	Sialyated, fucosylated carbohydrates	Sialyated, fucosylated carbohydrates
Function	Lymphocyte homing Inflammation	Inflammation	Inflammation Hemostasis (?)

Lectin domain
EGF domain
Short consensus repeats (SCR)
Transmembrane domain
Cytoplasmic domain

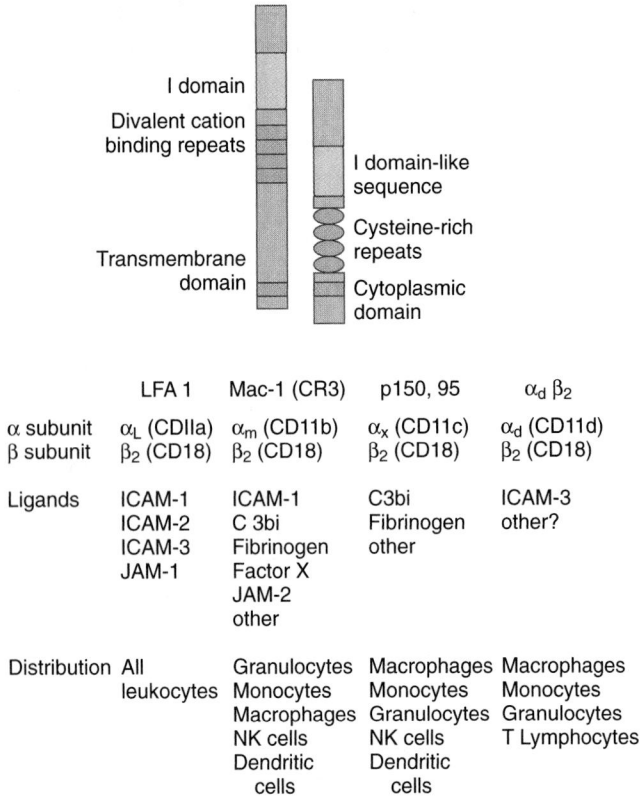

	LFA 1	Mac-1 (CR3)	p150, 95	$\alpha_d \, \beta_2$
α subunit	α_L (CDIIa)	α_m (CD11b)	α_x (CD11c)	α_d (CD11d)
β subunit	β_2 (CD18)	β_2 (CD18)	β_2 (CD18)	β_2 (CD18)
Ligands	ICAM-1 ICAM-2 ICAM-3 JAM-1	ICAM-1 C 3bi Fibrinogen Factor X JAM-2 other	C3bi Fibrinogen other	ICAM-3 other?
Distribution	All leukocytes	Granulocytes Monocytes Macrophages NK cells Dendritic cells	Macrophages Monocytes Granulocytes NK cells Dendritic cells	Macrophages Monocytes Granulocytes T Lymphocytes

FIGURE 21-5. The β_2 (CD18) family of leukocyte integrins. ICAM, intercellular adhesion molecule; JAM-1, junctional adhesion molecule 1; NK, natural killer. See text for additional details and references.

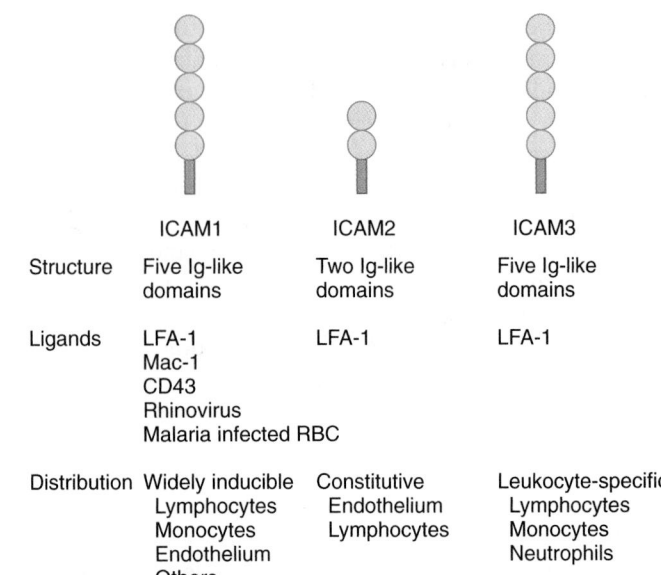

	ICAM1	ICAM2	ICAM3
Structure	Five Ig-like domains	Two Ig-like domains	Five Ig-like domains
Ligands	LFA-1 Mac-1 CD43 Rhinovirus Malaria infected RBC	LFA-1	LFA-1
Distribution	Widely inducible Lymphocytes Monocytes Endothelium Others	Constitutive Endothelium Lymphocytes	Leukocyte-specific Lymphocytes Monocytes Neutrophils

FIGURE 21-6. Intercellular adhesion molecules (ICAMs). Ig, immunoglobulin. LFA-1, lymphocyte function antigen 1; RBC, red blood cell. *(Adapted with permission from Kishimoto TK, Rothlein R. Integrins, ICAMs, and selectins: role and regulation of adhesion molecules in neutrophil recruitment to inflammatory sites. Adv Pharm. 1994;25:117-169.)*

expressed by all leukocytes, including lymphocytes. Mac-1 and p150,95 are expressed by granulocytes, mononuclear phagocytes, some activated T lymphocytes, and large granular lymphocytes.[205-207,215] Mac-1 is the most prominent β_2 integrin on neutrophils, whereas $\alpha_d \, \beta_2$ is expressed particularly in tissue macrophages. Mutations in the common β subunit result in an inherited defect in phagocyte function—leukocyte adhesion deficiency type I (LAD I), as discussed in a later section. All β_2 integrins are absent in LAD I, thus indicating that the stability of each α subunit requires association with the β chain. The β subunit has a large, glycosylated extracellular domain, a single transmembrane-spanning domain, and a short cytoplasmic tail.[216] The extracellular domain has two regions that are conserved among other β subunits.[215] There are four cysteine-rich tandem repeats that appear to be important for the tertiary structure of the β subunit. Another conserved region, located near the N-terminal, is critical for maintenance of the α/β heterodimer and may bind divalent cations as well. The α subunit is also a glycosylated integral membrane protein with a single membrane-spanning segment and a short cytoplasmic tail. The external domain contains three divalent cation-binding motifs that must be occupied for ligand binding to occur. A second important extracellular domain, the I domain (for inserted or interactive domain), can coordinate divalent cations and is likewise thought to be involved in ligand binding. The intracellular domain of the α

subunit includes a conserved sequence that is critical for the modulation of integrin avidity (see later).[217] The cytoplasmic tails of both the α and β integrin subunits also interact with cytoskeletal proteins.[207,215] The endoparasite hookworm *Ancylostoma caninum* produces a heavily glycosylated protein called NIF that binds to CD11b/CD18 to inhibit neutrophil spreading and attachment to the endothelium.[218,219]

Although β_2 integrins are constitutively expressed on the neutrophil cell surface, a large pool is stored in intracellular secretory vesicles (see Table 21-2). These vesicles are rapidly mobilized upon neutrophil activation by chemoattractants and fuse with the membrane to increase the cell surface expression of β_2 integrins by about 10-fold.[180,220] Signaling through chemoattractant receptors also markedly increases the avidity of β_2 integrins for their ligands, which plays an even more important role in rapidly upregulating integrin activity and promoting firm attachment to the blood vessel wall.[205,206,215] The increased adhesiveness of the β_2 integrins appears to involve a conformational change in integrin structure upon cellular activation.

The major counter-receptors for the β_2 integrins are the ICAMs (Fig. 21-6), which are members of the immunoglobulin superfamily.[205,206,215] These transmembrane proteins contain anywhere from two to six immunoglobulin domains and are present on endothelial cells, T cells, and a variety of other cell types. ICAM-1 and ICAM-2 are of particular importance in mediating binding of neutrophils and other leukocytes to the endothelium. Endothelial cell expression of ICAM-1, which promotes increased cell-cell interactions with leukocytes at inflamed sites, increases in response to inflammatory cytokines.

Vascular cell adhesion molecule 1 (VCAM-1) is another immunoglobulin superfamily member expressed on endothelial cells that can be induced by cytokines.[206,221] VCAM-1 is the counter-receptor for the β_1 integrin very late antigen 4 (VLA-4) and appears to be important in promoting the adherence of monocytes and eosinophils during inflammation. The β_2 integrin Mac-1 (CD11b/CD18) also has an important role as an opsonic receptor for the complement fragment C3bi, as discussed later.

In addition to their role in adhesion, β_2 integrins play an important role in leukocyte activation.[222,223] Binding of ligand to integrins results in their clustering and activation of tyrosine kinase and other signaling cascades,[224] which provides costimulatory signals to enhance migration, the respiratory burst, Fcγ-mediated phagocytosis, and degranulation.

Although leukocyte β_2 integrin–mediated adhesion is clearly important for recruitment of neutrophils from the systemic microvasculature into inflammatory sites, emigration of neutrophils out of the pulmonary circulation can also be mediated by alternative pathways, depending on the inflammatory stimulus.[225] Whether the alternative pathway in pulmonary capillaries involves selectins or other adhesion molecules remains to be defined.

The final steps in emigration of neutrophils from the blood vessel lumen into inflamed tissue involves squeezing between adjacent endothelial cells (diapedesis) and penetrating the basement membrane (see Fig. 21-3). The presence of a chemotactic gradient is required to induce the directional migration of neutrophils.[187,226,227] Adhesive interactions between the β_2 integrins and endothelial cell ICAM-1 are essential for neutrophil diapedesis, whereas VCAM-1 and E-selectin can mediate the transmigration of monocytes and eosinophils.[6,116] Junctional adhesion molecule 1 (JAM-1), an immunoglobulin superfamily protein expressed at the tight junctions of resting endothelial cells and epithelial cells, facilitates leukocyte transmigration via binding to LFA-1 (CD11a/CD18).[228] Transendothelial migration of neutrophils is also dependent on homologous binding between neutrophil and endothelial cell platelet–endothelial cell adhesion molecule 1 (PECAM-1, CD31), another immunoglobulin superfamily member expressed on the surface of leukocytes, platelets, and endothelial cells, where it is localized at the junctions between cells.[229,230] Migrating neutrophils induce increases in endothelial intracellular calcium levels and changes in the actin cytoskeleton that facilitate transmigration.[231,232] Finally, chemoattractant-induced neutrophil degranulation results in the release of digestive enzymes, including collagenase, elastase, and gelatinase, which facilitate penetration of the basement membrane.[46,233]

Chemotaxis

Chemotaxis is the directional movement of a cell along a concentration gradient.[26,28,31,234,235] Defects in neutrophil cellular motility or other steps in chemotaxis can result in decreased resistance to bacterial and fungal infections, as discussed later in this chapter. The neutrophil chemotactic response occurs at chemoattractant concentrations that approximate the dissociation constants of the chemotactic factors for their receptors, which are much lower than those that elicit degranulation and activation of the respiratory burst.[29,195] Cells respond to a chemotactic gradient by constantly sensing across their surface, and bound chemotactic receptors are continuously internalized. A migrating neutrophil has a polarized appearance, with pseudopodia or lamellipodia, thin structures rich in actin filaments and lacking intracellular organelles, extending at the leading edge.[29,31] The pseudopods appear to glide forward and pull the cell body behind them. The nucleus tends to remain in the posterior half of the moving leukocyte. Migration also requires the formation of a uropod at the "tail" of the leukocyte that deattaches from the underlying matrix and retracts the rear of the cell as it moves forward.[236] Rho GTPases play an important role in establishing chemoattractant-induced polarization and migration.[54,202]

Neutrophil movement is dependent on the dynamic assembly and disassembly of filamentous actin, coordinated by various ABPs whose activity is regulated by intracellular signaling molecules.[26,28,234,235,237,238] Leukocyte motility is inhibited by the cytochalasins, which block actin assembly. Actin can exist either as a soluble monomer (globular actin) or in needle-like helical filaments (filamentous actin). Actin filaments align spontaneously in parallel bundles, but in the cell they are organized into a branching network because of the presence of actin filament cross-linkers such as ABP.[239,240] Another class of actin regulatory proteins sequesters actin monomers and can thus control the availability of globular actin for filament formation. Prophyllin and thymosin B$_4$ are two major actin monomer–binding proteins in neutrophils.[241] Other ABPs, such as gelsolin, cap the fast-growing barbed end of the actin filament or sever filamentous actin into shorter pieces, or both.[29,31]

Agonists acting via receptors on the cell membrane trigger the generation of second messengers that interact with ABPs to control dynamic local cycles of filamentous actin assembly.[31] For example, increased local calcium concentrations activate gelsolin, which promotes actin disassembly by cleaving actin filaments and capping its barbed ends. On the other hand, actin assembly is stimulated by the accumulation of phosphoinositols liberated from membrane phospholipids around an activated receptor. Phosphoinositols such as PIP$_2$ interact both with actin-sequestering proteins to liberate actin monomers and with gelsolin to uncap the barbed ends of filamentous actin. The Rho GTPases Cdc42 and Rac are important regulators of actin remodeling and are activated by binding of ligand to chemoattractant receptors.[54,201,202,234,242] Cdc42 activates proteins of the Wiskott-Aldrich syndrome protein (WASP) family, which then bind to a complex of seven proteins known as the Arp2/3 complex to nucleate assembly of new actin filaments at the leading edge of migrating cells.[234,237,243] Activation of Rac appears to be important both for de novo actin nucleation by the Arp2/3 complex and for stimulating uncapping of existing actin filament barbed ends.[199]

During pseudopod extension in chemoattractant-activated neutrophils, new actin polymerization occurs at the site of membrane protrusion while the filamentous actin in the rear of the cell disassembles.[28,235,244] How actin assembly-disassembly results in membrane extension and the formation of pseudopodia is not fully understood but may involve localized changes in osmotic pressure as a result of alterations in actin polymerization.[29,31] Membrane movement and retraction of the rear of the cell are mediated in part by Rho GTPase–regulated contractile proteins such as myosin 1.[235,245,246]

Recognition, Opsonization, and Phagocytosis

Recognition, ingestion, and disposal of microbes, foreign particulate matter, and damaged cells constitute a major aspect of phagocyte function. To facilitate their recognition by phagocytes, these targets are coated with serum opsonins (from the Greek word meaning "to prepare for dining") that include proteolytic fragments derived from the complement cascade, as well as specific immunoglobulins. The key humoral opsonins are the proteolytic cleavage products of C3 (C3b and C3bi), which can be generated in the absence of specific immunity by the alternative and mannose-binding lectin (MBL) pathways (see later), and the opsonic antibodies IgM, IgG1, and IgG3. Targets are opsonized by the deposition of C3b and C3bi or IgG onto their surfaces via the specific (Fab) portion of the antibody. Antibacterial IgM antibodies, though not opsonic by themselves, play an important role in phagocytosis by activating complement. Opsonins are recognized by phagocyte cell surface glycoprotein receptors for immunoglobulin and C3 cleavage products, as described later. Inherited deficiencies of opsonization can result in increased susceptibility to bacterial infections, as discussed in a following section. In contrast, primary defects in phagocyte receptors for these opsonins appear to be an uncommon cause of recurrent infections.[247]

Phagocytes also have cell surface receptors capable of recognizing targets even in the absence of opsonins. These members of the "pattern recognition receptor" (PRR) family recognize broad classes of macromolecules.[248-250] PRRs include scavenger receptors that have broad binding specificity for polyanionic ligands and participate in the clearance of diverse material, including modified LDL and apoptotic cells.[248] Many PRRs detect conserved molecular structures unique to microbes that are referred to as pathogen-associated molecular patterns (PAMPs).[248-251] The mannose receptor recognizes carbohydrate structures present in a range of cells infected by bacteria, fungi, viruses, and parasites, whereas the β-glucan receptor (dectin-1) binds to β-glucan structures in zymosan and other yeast-derived particles. Mamma-

lian TLRs are an important group in the PRR family.[249,250,252] At least 12 different TLRs have been described; they recognize conserved peptide, lipid, carbohydrate, and nucleic acid structures expressed by different groups of microbes. For example, peptidoglycan and lipopolysaccharide are PAMPs associated with gram-positive and gram-negative bacteria and are recognized by TLR2 and TLR4, respectively. Binding to PRRs, which often occurs in a combinatorial fashion, activates an array of proinflammatory responses, including expression of proinflammatory cytokines and release of oxidants and reactive nitrogen intermediates. TLR signaling activates the NF-κβ and interferon regulatory factor (IRF)-dependent pathways, and genetic defects in the protein that couples TLRs to NF-κβ lead to recurrent bacterial infections.[253] Some PRRs, including the mannose receptor, scavenger receptors, and β-glucan receptor, also trigger phagocytosis.[251]

In addition to cell surface PRRs, soluble PRRs present in serum or tissues serve important roles in alerting phagocytes to the presence of microbes.[254,255] Such PRRs include the collectins (calcium-dependent lectins), which bind to oligosaccharide or lipid moieties of microorganisms to enhance their opsonization and efficiently activate phagocytes. Members of the collectin family include the lung alveolar surfactant proteins A and D and the MBL, also known as MBP.[255-257] Binding of MBL to mannose residues initiates a third pathway of complement activation (in addition to the classical and alternative pathways) by interacting with the serine proteases MASP1 and MASP2 and thereby generating opsonic C3 fragments.[254,258] MBL itself can also function as an opsonin for promoting uptake by the complement receptor CR1.[255,258]

Complement Receptors

Activation of complement C3 to generate the cleavage fragments C3b and C3bi is the dominant source of opsonins in the absence of antibodies. Four C3 fragment receptors have been described on phagocytic leukocytes (Table 21-5). The human phagocyte C3b receptor (CR1, CD35) is a high-molecular-weight, single-subunit glycoprotein that shows substantial heterogeneity in size because of the presence of four distinct alleles in the human population that encode proteins ranging in size from 160 to 250 kd. CR1 is responsible for the binding of C3b-opsonized particles and for initiating their ingestion.[258,259] CR1 also recognizes microbes opsonized with MBL.[255,256,258] The other major opsonic receptor, CR3, recognizes particles opsonized with C3bi. This receptor is the same as the β_2 integrin Mac-1 (CD11b/CD18) discussed in detail in an earlier section (see Fig. 21-5). Binding of C3bi-opsonized particles to CD11b/CD18 triggers both phagocytosis and, in neutrophils, the respiratory burst. The CR4 receptor is the same as the β_2 integrin CD11c/CD18 and, on macrophages, can also initiate phagocytosis of C3bi-coated targets. Finally, a newly discovered receptor that binds the complement

TABLE 21-5	Human Phagocyte Receptors for Complement C3 Fragment			
	CR1 (CD35)	**CR3 (CD11b/CD18; Mac-1)**	**CR4 (CD11d/CD18)**	**CRIg**
Cell distribution	Neutrophils Monocytes B lymphocytes	Neutrophils Monocytes Macrophages NK cells	Macrophages Dendritic cells	Kupffer cells, certain other resident tissue macrophages
Structure	Transmembrane protein	Transmembrane, two subunits	Transmembrane, two subunits	Transmembrane protein
Ligands	C3b C4b C3bi C1q Mannose-binding lectin (mannose-binding protein)	C3bi ICAM-1, 2 Fibrinogen Factor X	C3bi Fibrinogen	C3b C3bi
Function	Phagocytosis	Phagocytosis Respiratory burst (neutrophils) Adhesion Activation	Phagocytosis Adhesion	Phagocytosis

See text for references.

CR, complement receptor; ICAM, intracellular adhesion molecule; NK, natural killer.

fragments C3b and C3bi, termed CRIg (complement receptor of the immunoglobulin superfamily) is expressed primarily in resident macrophages of the liver (Kupffer cells).[260] CRIg appears to play a critical role in mediating phagocytosis and clearance of C3 fragment–opsonized bacteria from the circulation, at least in mice.[260]

Immunoglobulin Receptors

Immunoglobulins are recognized by Fc receptors, which are members of the immunoglobulin gene superfamily. Fc receptors bind to the "constant domain" of the antibody molecule, these being specific to each class of immunoglobulin (IgA, IgE, IgG, and IgM).[247,261-263] The most important from the standpoint of microbial opsonization are Fc receptors that recognize IgG (Table 21-6). The Fcγ receptors include three distinct classes, FcγRI, FcγRII, and FcγRIII, which are encoded by at least eight genes that have evolved through gene duplication and alternative splicing, although not all give rise to detectable mRNA or protein.[264] The low-affinity FcγR genes (FcγRII and FcγIII families) and two of the genes for the high-affinity IgE receptor are clustered on chromosome 1q22. The high-affinity IgG Fc receptors map to other sites on chromosome 1.

Except for FcγRIIIb, which is anchored in the membrane by a glycosylphosphatidylinositol (GPI) moiety, the FcγR proteins have a single transmembrane domain. FcγRI and FcγRIIIa exist as oligomeric complexes with γ (in phagocytes) or ζ (in lymphocytes) chains that are important for both their stable expression and signaling functions.[264] These accessory chains contain YXXL immunoreceptor tyrosine activation motifs (ITAMs), which become tyrosine-phosphorylated upon receptor cross-linking to initiate downstream signaling cas-

cades.[247,261-263] The cytoplasmic tail of FcγRIIa contains variant ITAMs, and hence this receptor does not require accessory chains for its function. There is no murine equivalent to FcγRIIa.[263] The GPI-linked FcγRIIIb must be colligated to either FcγRIIa or the β₂ integrin CR3 (Mac-1) to initiate signaling functions upon ligation.[247,261-263] FcγRIIb, expressed on monocytes/macrophages, mast cells, and lymphocytes, contains immunoreceptor tyrosine inhibition motif (ITIM) sequences and instead inhibits cellular activation upon immunoglobulin cross-linking.[261-263]

Each FcγR is expressed at different levels, depending on the type of phagocytic cell (see Table 21-6), and some FcγRII and FcγRIII family members are also expressed on lymphocytes, platelets, thymocytes, natural killer (NK) cells, and mast cells.[263,264] The FcγRI class includes the products of three highly homologous genes, denoted A, B, and C, although the protein products of the latter two have not been detected in vivo. FcγRIa receptors are expressed by monocytes and neutrophils or eosinophils stimulated by IFN-γ or G-CSF and have high affinity for monomeric IgG.[247,262,263] Members of the FcγRII and FcγRIII families have low affinity for monomeric IgG, but high affinity for clusters of IgG (e.g., several antibodies bound to the same particle) and immune complexes. Only neutrophils and IFN-γ–stimulated eosinophils appear to express FcγRIIIb, and polymorphisms in this receptor correspond to the serologically defined NA1/NA2 antigen system, which is a common antibody target in autoimmune and alloimmune neutropenia.[265,266] Polymorphisms in FcγRIIa, FcγRIIIa, and FcγRIIIb are associated with an increased incidence or severity of various autoimmune or infectious diseases.[267] For example, the 131H allele of FcγRIIa, which is the only FcγR that

---

TABLE 21-6 Human Phagocyte Fcγ Receptors

	FcγRIa (CD64)	FcγRIIa (CD32)	FcγRIIIa, b (CD16)
Polymorphisms		131R/H	IIIa: 48L/R/H, 158F/V IIIb: NA-1, NA-2
Cell distribution	Monocytes Macrophages IFN-γ– or G-CSF–treated neutrophils IFN-γ–treated eosinophils	Monocytes Neutrophils Macrophages Eosinophils Basophils Platelets	IIIa: macrophages, monocytes (some), T cells, NK cells IIIb: neutrophils, IFN-γ–treated eosinophils
Protein size, type	72 kd, transmembrane	40 kd, transmembrane	50-90 kd IIIa: transmembrane IIIb: GPI anchored
Associated proteins	FcRγ homodimer	—	IIIa: FcRγ homodimer (macrophage, monocyte) IIIb: colligation with FcγRIIa or CR3
Ligands	Monomeric IgG (G1 = G3 > G4 >> G2)	Complexed IgG (G1 = G3 >> G2, G4) (FcγRIIa 131H-G2)	Complexed IgG (G1 = G3 >> G2, G4)
Affinity Function	High Phagocytosis Respiratory burst Endocytosis of IC ADCC Antigen presentation	Low Phagocytosis Respiratory burst Exocytosis Endocytosis of IC ADCC Antigen presentation	Low Phagocytosis Exocytosis Endocytosis of IC ADCC (IIIa) Antigen presentation (IIIa)

See text for references.
ADCC, antibody-dependent cellular cytotoxicity; G-CSF, granulocyte colony stimulating factor; IFN-γ, interferon-γ; FcγR, Fc receptor for IgG; GPI, glycosylphosphatidylinositol; IC, immune complexes; NK, natural killer.

---

mediates efficient phagocytosis of IgG2-opsonized bacteria, has been linked to a lower incidence of infections with encapsulated bacteria.[247]

Cross-linking of FcγRs can trigger a wide range of functional responses, including phagocytosis of IgG-coated microbes, blood cells, or tumor cells; ingestion of immune complexes; release of inflammatory mediators; activation of the respiratory burst; and antibody-dependent cellular cytotoxicity (ADCC). The relative roles of different phagocyte FcγR classes have not been clearly delineated, although all can function as receptors for opsonized particles or immune complexes. Binding of IgG to FcγRI and FcγRIIa activates the respiratory burst, whereas secretion of granular contents is a prominent response on binding to FcγRII and FcγRIIIb.[247,261] Although the ligand-binding domains of different FcγRs all bind IgG, the specificity of the cellular response may be governed by the unique transmembrane and cytoplasmic domains of a particular Fc receptor subtype.[261-263]

Ligation and cross-linking of FcγRs induce a cascade of biochemical signals that are initiated by activation of nonreceptor protein tyrosine kinases of the Src family, which phosphorylate ITAMs in the FcRγ chain and in FcγRIIa to recruit and activate the Syk tyrosine kinase and further amplify ITAM phosphorylation.[261,268-270] Subsequent activation of several parallel pathways, including activation of phospholipase C, PI3K, MAPK-related pathways, and other targets, leads to various cellular responses, such as actin and membrane remodeling for ingestion of particles, activation of NADPH oxidase, and release of cytokine.

Opsonization of microbes with secretory IgA antibodies is likely to be important in the clearance of microbes from the mucosal surfaces of the respiratory, gastrointestinal, and urogenital tracts. Neutrophils and monocytes have an Fc receptor for IgA (FcRα) that has close structural similarities with other members of the Fc receptor family.[271] Ligation of phagocyte FcRα can trigger phagocytosis, degranulation, and release of superoxide.[272,273] IgE antibodies can activate eosinophils and mast cells through the high-affinity FcεRI receptors.

Phagocytosis

Engagement of any of the opsonic receptors initiates phagocytosis of an opsonized particle by forming a phagocytic vacuole to enclose the particle. The molecular details of this process are incompletely understood but involve membrane remodeling and regulated assembly and disassembly of the actin cytoskeleton, in a fashion analogous to the mechanisms that result in cell movement when chemotactic receptors are engaged. FcγR-mediated phagocytosis triggers the extension of long pseudopodia that attach in a zipper-like fashion around the particle and then fuse to form the phagosome, which is then drawn into the cell.[268-270] In contrast, complement-opsonized particles attach to the cell surface only at limited points and "sink" into the cytoplasm in the absence of any pseudopod extension.[269] These morphologic differences are associated with differences in the underlying biochemical pathways. FcR-mediated phagocytosis is sensitive to inhibitors of tyrosine kinases and requires the Rac and Cdc42 GTPases, whereas CR3-mediated phagocytosis is dependent on protein kinase C and the Rho GTPase.

Microorganisms can also enter phagocytes by nonopsonic routes, which enables them to evade the cytocidal weapons that are otherwise activated upon phagocytosis. For example, after binding to the macrophage cell surface, *Salmonella typhimurium* induces extensive membrane ruffling that leads to internalization of the bacterium into a macropinisome, or "spacious phagosome."[274] Attachment of *Legionella pneumophila* to macrophages induces the formation of a pseudopod that spirals around the bacterium to form a "coiling phagosome" that does not acidify or fuse with lysosomes. [274]

Cytocidal and Digestive Activity

Binding of ligands to phagocyte chemoattractant and opsonic receptors ultimately leads to the mobilization of phagocyte granules that contain cytotoxic and hydrolytic proteins and to the activation of enzymatic reactions that generate toxic oxygen metabolites (see Fig. 21-8). These complementary processes are designed to modify or destroy the inciting object and are often classified as oxygen-independent and oxygen-dependent pathways.

Neutrophil granules are secretory organelles that can be divided into four general classes, as discussed in a preceding section (see Table 21-2). Degranulation (also referred to as exocytosis or mobilization), or the fusion of granule membranes with the plasma or phagosome membrane, results in the transfer of granule membrane constituents to a new membrane compartment and discharge of the granule contents into the extracellular fluid or phagocytic vacuole. Microtubules and microfilaments are involved in granule translocation. Degranulation is triggered by increases in calcium concentration when neutrophils are activated through chemoattractant and other receptors. Different neutrophil granule populations have marked differences in expression of VAMP-2, a fusogenic protein involved in exocytosis; expression is highest in secretory vesicles, less in gelatinase granules, and still lower in specific granules.[39] Thus, different granule classes vary in their responsiveness to calcium, which leads to the mobilization of different granule classes, depending on the calcium concentration, which in turn is proportion to the concentration of the chemoattractant or other activating signal.[24,46,275] Secretory vesicles, whose membranes are storage pools for β_2 integrin adhesion proteins and other receptors, are mobilized with relatively low concentrations of calcium. Fusion of secretory vesicles with the plasma membrane provides a rapid means of upregulating the cell surface expression of these receptors, along with the metalloproteinase leukolysin (MMP-25), another membrane constituent of secretory vesicles. Gelatinase (tertiary) granules are also easily mobilized for exocytosis at the cell surface to release gelatinase (MMP-9). These metalloproteinases are stored as inactive proforms and become activated by proteolysis after exocytosis to facilitate the breakdown of extracellular matrix during the early phases of neutrophil migration.[25,233] At the opposite end of the spectrum, azurophilic (primary) granules, which contain cytotoxic proteins and hydrolytic enzymes, undergo only limited exocytosis and fuse primarily with phagocytic vacuoles to deliver their contents into a sequestered compartment.

Monocytes and macrophages do not have populations of cytoplasmic storage granules and secretory vesicles equivalent to those found in neutrophils. Instead, internalized phagosomes fuse sequentially with endocytic vesicles and subsequently lysosomes to form a phagolysosome, which has a highly acidic interior rich in hydrolases.[121,268,269]

Certain microorganisms can become intracellular parasites because they have developed mechanisms to prevent fusion of granules with the phagocytic vacuole or otherwise evade the phagocyte digestive and oxidative armamentarium. For example, although mycobacteria exist intracellularly within a phagosome, they produce compounds that inhibit their fusion with lysosomes.[276] *L. pneumophila* and *Toxoplasma* may inhibit acidification and lysosomal fusion.[274] Virulent strains of *Salmonella* engulfed by macrophages produce compounds that prevent translocation of the respiratory burst oxidase to the phagosomal membrane.[277] *Listeria monocytogenes* escapes the phagocytic vacuole altogether to avoid attack by lysosomal products and can survive in the cytoplasm of relatively quiescent macrophages and hepatocytes.[274] *Yersinia*, group A streptococci, *Helicobacter*, *Ehrlichia*, and *Francisella* are examples of microbes that have developed similar strategies to survive in neutrophils.[278]

In addition to delivering their antimicrobial granule contents to the interior of phagosomes, dying neutrophils are also capable of extruding web-like extracellular structures, termed neutrophil extracellular traps (NETs), composed of chromatin and granule proteins that can bind and kill microbes.[279] The formation of NETs appears to involve a novel process of cell death that is dependent on oxidants generated from neutrophil NADPH oxidase.[280]

Oxygen-Independent Toxicity

Phagocyte granules supply preformed cytotoxic and digestive compounds that play a key role in oxygen-independent killing and digestion of microbes, senescent cells, and particulate debris. In neutrophils, azurophilic (primary) and specific (secondary) granules serve as the main storage reservoir of these compounds. Oxygen-independent pathways complement those dependent on the respiratory burst (see the following section) and are also important for phagocyte antimicrobial activity under the adverse conditions of hypoxia and acidosis often encountered locally at the site of infection.

Numerous cationic antimicrobial proteins are contained within neutrophil azurophilic granules.[46,275,281,282] Defensins are small (29- to 25–amino acid residue) basic peptides that constitute more than 5% of the total cellular protein of human neutrophils, although they are absent in murine neutrophils. These peptides exert antimicrobial effects against a broad range of gram-positive and gram-negative organisms, fungi, mycobacteria, and some enveloped viruses. Defensins are also cytotoxic to mammalian cells. Defensins kill target cells by insertion into the cellular membrane and formation of voltage-regulated channels. Defensin-like peptides have also been found in small intestinal Paneth cells and in tracheal epithelium.[281,282] BPI is a 55-kd cationic protein that has potent cytotoxic effects on gram-negative bacteria.[283] BPI binds avidly to lipopolysaccharide, which leads both to bacterial killing by damaging the cell membrane and to neutralization of the endotoxin associated with the bacterial cell wall and in serum. Serpocidins are a family of 25- to 29-kd glycoproteins that are homologous to members of the serine protease superfamily; they include azurocidin (CAP37) and three serine proteases (cathepsin G, elastase, and proteinase-3).[282,284] In human neutrophils, serpocidins are even more potent than defensins in antimicrobial activity and have a broad spectrum of cytotoxicity that is, with few exceptions, unrelated to proteolytic activity. Cathepsin G, elastase, and proteinase-3 are often referred to as neutral proteases because the optimal pH for their proteolytic activity is approximately 7. Azurocidin can bind to endotoxin, which appears to account for its activity against gram-negative bacteria.[285] Azurocidin is also a potent chemoattractant for monocytes, as well as fibroblasts and T cells.[285] Exogenous administration of antimicrobial peptides is being studied as an adjunctive or alternative therapy to conventional antibiotics in a number of settings.[286]

Both azurophilic and specific granules contain lysozyme, which hydrolyzes the cell wall of saprophytic gram-positive organisms and may also assist in the nonlytic killing of other organisms.[46] hCAP-18, a member of the cathelicidin family of antimicrobial peptides, is cleaved by proteinase-3 after exocytosis. Its N-terminal region is homologous to that of other cathelicidins, whereas its 37–amino acid C-terminal fragment, termed LL-37, has additional activities, including acting as chemoattractant, as well as effects on apoptosis.[39] Specific granules also contain the iron-binding glycoprotein lactoferrin, which has direct bactericidal activity both related and unrelated to the chelation of iron compounds required for bacterial metabolism. Lactoferrin may also catalyze the nonenzymatic formation of OH· radicals during the respiratory burst (see the following section). Vitamin B_{12} (cobalamin) binding–protein has been proposed to bind an analogous family of compounds found in bacteria to exert an antimicrobial effect.[287] Lipocalin, also known as NGAL, interferes with bacterial iron utilization by binding to bacterial ferric-siderophore complexes.[46]

Azurophilic granules contain a variety of hydrolases (see Table 21-2) that have a lower optimal pH (<6), consistent with the lysosomal character of these granules. Studies using indicator dyes and biochemical techniques suggest that after a transient rise, the pH of the phagocytic vacuole falls below 6, which would enhance the activity of these enzymes upon their discharge into the vacuole.[288,289] The acid hydrolases serve primarily a digestive rather than a microbicidal function.[290] Azurophilic granules also contain MPO, which is an important enzyme in the microbicidal oxygen-dependent reactions that are described in the following section.

Inherited partial or complete deficiency of MPO, which occurs in 0.05% of the population, can occasionally result in increased susceptibility to infection (see later in this chapter). Deficiencies in other individual neutrophil granule proteins have not yet been described in humans, but gene-targeted mice lacking the neutrophil granule serine proteases elastase or cathepsin G have impaired host defense against gram-negative sepsis and fungal infections.[291,292] A few rare disorders involving defects in granule formation (SGF) or degranulation (CHS) are associated with recurrent bacterial infections. Inherited mutations in neutrophil elastase have recently been identified in patients with cyclic neutropenia and severe congenital neutropenia (SCN).[293,294] The mutant forms of elastase may have abnormal properties that exert a toxic effect on granulopoiesis.

Oxygen-Dependent Toxicity

The resting neutrophil relies primarily on glycolysis for energy and hence consumes relatively little oxygen.[295] However, within seconds after contacting opsonized microbes or high concentrations of chemoattractants, oxygen consumption increases dramatically, often by more than 100-fold. This "extra respiration of phagocytosis" was first observed in 1933,[296] but it was almost 30 years before it was appreciated that this process was insensitive to mitochondrial poisons and thus not related to increased energy demands.[297] The enzyme complex responsible for this phenomenon, referred to as the NADPH or respiratory burst oxidase, is associated with the plasma and phagolysosomal membranes and catalyzes the transfer of an electron from NADPH to molecular oxygen, thereby forming the superoxide radical (O_2^-) (Fig. 21-7).[298-301] Superoxide, though itself a relatively weak microbicidal agent, is the precursor to a family of potent oxidants that are essential for the killing of many microorganisms (Fig. 21-8; also see Fig. 21-7).[298,299,302,303] The importance of the respiratory burst to normal host defense is underscored by the recurrent and often life-threatening infections seen in patients with chronic granulomatous disease (CGD); such patients are genetically deficient in respiratory burst oxidase activity.

The respiratory burst oxidase is a multi-subunit enzyme complex assembled from membrane-bound and soluble proteins upon phagocyte activation (Fig. 21-9). Identification of the components of this enzyme has ben-

FIGURE 21-7. Reactions of the respiratory burst pathway. The enzymes responsible for reactions 1 to 9 are as follows: (1) the respiratory burst oxidase (reduced nicotinamide adenine dinucleotide phosphate [NADPH] oxidase); (2) superoxide dismutase or spontaneous; (3) nonenzymatic, Fe²⁺ catalyzed; (4) myeloperoxidase; (5) spontaneous; (6) glutathione peroxidase; (7) glutathione reductase; (8) glucose-6-phosphate dehydrogenase; (9) glutathione synthetase. GSH, reduced glutathione; GSSG, oxidized glutathione. *(Adapted with permission from Curnutte J, Orkin S, Dinauer M. Genetic disorders of phagocyte function. In Stamoyannopoulos G [ed]. The Molecular Basis of Blood Diseases, 2nd ed. Philadelphia, WB Saunders, 1994, p 493.)*

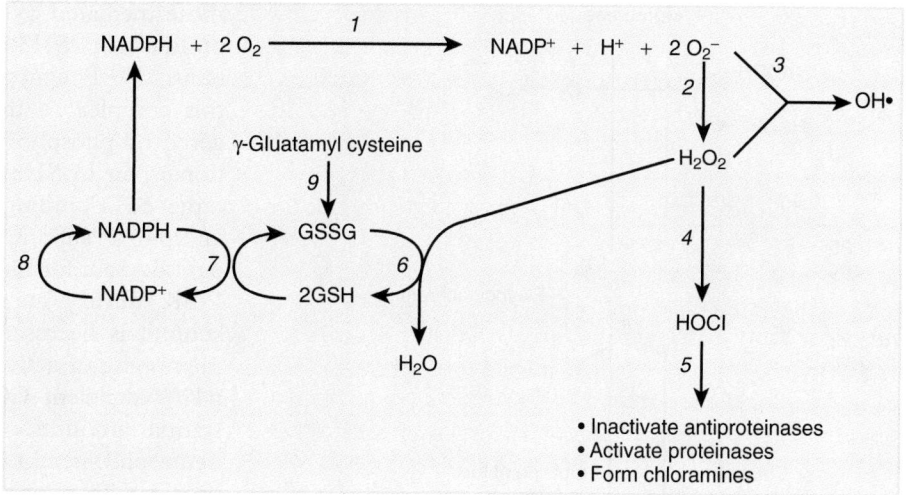

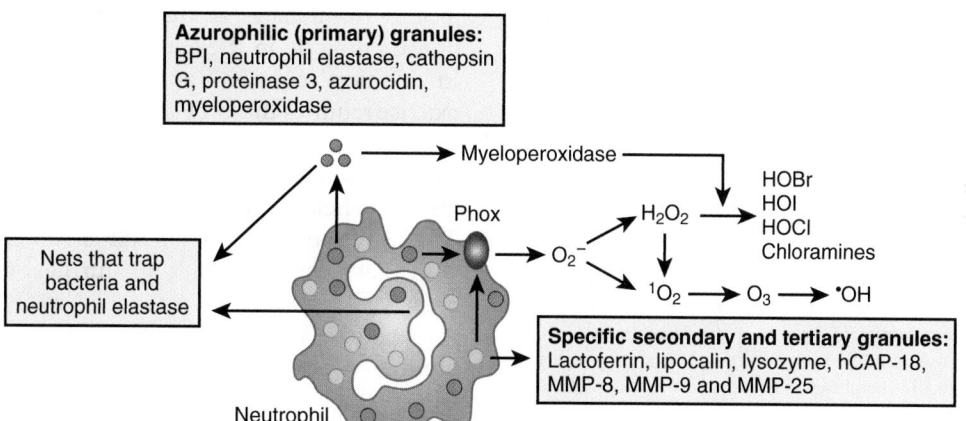

FIGURE 21-8. Neutrophils deliver multiple antimicrobial molecules. Microbicidal products arise from most compartments of the neutrophil: azurophilic granules (also known as primary granules), specific granules (also known as secondary granules), tertiary granules, plasma and phagosomal membranes, the nucleus, and the cytosol. BPI, bactericidal/permeability-increasing protein; H_2O_2, hydrogen peroxide; HOBr, hypobromous acid; HOCl, hypochlorous acid; HOI, hypoiodous acid; MMP, matrix metalloproteinase; $^1O_2$, singlet oxygen; O_2^-, superoxide; O_3, ozone; ·OH, hydroxyl radical; phox, phagocyte oxidase. *(Adapted with permission from Nathan C. Neutrophils and immunity: challenges and opportunities. Nat Rev Immunol. 2006;6:173-182.)*

efited greatly from the biochemical and molecular genetic analysis of patients with CGD. Four polypeptides, gp91^{phox}, p22^{phox}, p47^{phox}, and p67^{phox}, that are essential for respiratory burst function have been identified (Table 21-7), and mutations in the corresponding genes are responsible for the four different genetic subgroups of CGD. The oxidase subunits have been given the designation "*phox*" for *ph*agocyte *ox*idase. A fifth *phox* protein, p40^{phox}, exists in a complex with p47^{phox} and p67^{phox},[301] and though not required for enzyme activity, is important for high levels of superoxide production during phagocytosis.[304-306]

An unusual *b*-type flavocytochrome, located in the plasma membranes and specific granules of resting neutrophils, mediates electron transfer in the oxidase complex. This flavocytochrome is a heterodimer that contains a 91-kd glycosylated protein, gp91^{phox}, and a nonglycosylated subunit, p22^{phox}.[307-310] The gene for gp91^{phox}, which is the site of mutations in the X-linked form of CGD, was one of the first human disease–associated genes to be identified by positional cloning.[310]

The respiratory burst oxidase flavocytochrome has been referred to as flavocytochrome b_{558} for its spectral peak of light absorbance at 558 nm or as flavocytochrome b_{-245} in reference to its midpoint potential of −245 mV, which is the lowest reported for any mammalian cytochrome[311] gp91^{phox} in the redox center of the oxidase; it contains two heme prosthetic groups embedded within the membrane in the hydrophobic amino-terminal of the protein and a flavoprotein domain in the carboxy-terminal with binding sites for flavin and NADPH.[300,301] The p22^{phox} subunit is also an integral membrane protein and provides an important docking site for p47^{phox} during the assembly of NADPH oxidase.[312] Heterodimer formation with gp91^{phox} is essential for heme incorporation and intracellular stability of both flavocytochrome subunits.[313,314]

Based on the redox properties of flavocytochrome b_{558}, the following pathway has been proposed for transfer of electrons from NADPH to O_2 in the respiratory burst (reaction 1 in Fig. 21-7):

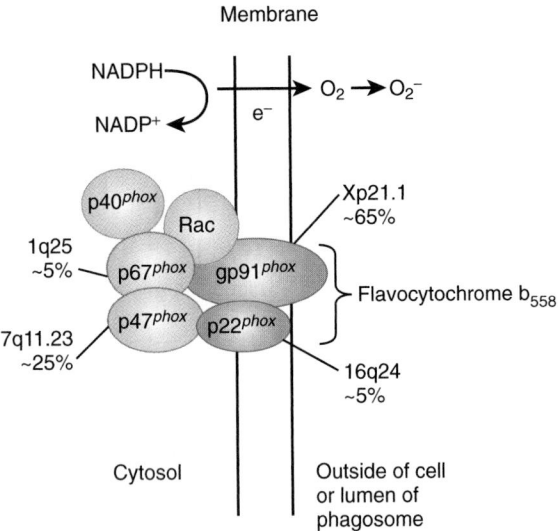

FIGURE 21-9. Activation of reduced nicotinamide adenine dinucleotide phosphate (NADPH) oxidase. Shown is the assembled form of the enzymatically active NADPH oxidase, along with subunits affected in the four different genetic subgroups of chronic granulomatous disease (CGD), the approximate incidence, and the chromosomal location of the corresponding gene. Flavocytochrome b_{558}, the redox center of the enzyme, is located in plasma, specific granule, and phagolysosomal membranes. This heterodimer is composed of gp91^{phox} and p22^{phox}, which are affected in X-linked and an autosomal recessive form of CGD, respectively. Mutations in the genes encoding two soluble regulatory proteins, p47^{phox} and p67^{phox}, account for two autosomal recessive forms of CGD. These subunits, along with a fifth *phox* protein, p40^{phox}, are found in the cytosol until phagocyte activation, after which they move as a complex to the membrane to assemble the active NADPH oxidase complex. Membrane translocation of the p47^{phox}-p67^{phox}-p40^{phox} complex is mediated by binding domains on 47^{phox} that are exposed by activation-induced p47^{phox} phosphorylation. Another essential regulatory component of NADPH oxidase is the small guanosine triphosphatase Rac, which in its active guanosine triphosphate–bound state becomes membrane bound and associates with p67^{phox}. By a mechanism that involves an activation domain on p67^{phox}, binding of these multiple regulatory subunits activates the flavocytochrome to catalyze the transfer of electrons from cytosolic NADPH across the membrane via the flavin adenine dinucleotide and heme redox centers to molecular oxygen, thereby forming superoxide in the extracellular or intraphagosomal compartment. No cases of CGD have been reported to result from mutations in p40^{phox} or Rac. *(Adapted with permission from Dinauer MC. Chronic Granulomatous Disease and Other Disorders of Phagocyte Function. Washington, DC, American Society of Hematology, 2005, pp 83-89.)*

$$\text{NADPH} \xrightarrow[-330\,\text{mV}]{} \text{flavin} \xrightarrow[-256\,\text{mV}]{} \text{heme} \xrightarrow[-245\,\text{mV}]{} \text{O}_2 \xrightarrow[-160\,\text{mV}]{} \text{O}_2^-$$

The flavocytochrome spans the membrane, with NADPH being oxidized at the cytoplasmic surface and oxygen being reduced to form O_2^- on the outer surface of the plasma membrane (or the inner surface of the phagosomal membrane).[298]

The p47^{phox} and p67^{phox} subunits, along with the Rac GTPase, regulate NADPH binding and electron transfer in the flavocytochrome. The p47^{phox}, p67^{phox}, and p40^{phox} subunits are found in the cytosol as a complex that is stabilized by intermolecular interactions that include

those mediated by Src homology domain 3 (SH3) and proline-rich SH3-binding motifs within these proteins.[300,301] Phagocyte activation induces translocation of this complex to the membrane flavocytochrome, triggered by phosphorylation of p47^{phox} to expose an additional pair of SH3 domains that bind to a proline-rich target SH3-binding sequence in p22^{phox}.[301,312] The p47^{phox} and p40^{phox} subunits also contain a PX (for *phox* homology) domain for binding phosphoinositides generated by PI3K during neutrophil activation.[315-317] The p47^{phox} subunit is necessary for translocation of p67^{phox} to the membrane of activated neutrophils based on studies of p47^{phox}-deficient CGD neutrophils.[300,318] However, substantial amounts of superoxide can be generated from neutrophil membranes in vitro in the absence of p47^{phox}, provided that high concentrations of p67^{phox} and Rac-GTP are supplied.[300] Hence, p47^{phox} acts as an "adaptor" protein to mediate the translocation of p67^{phox} and position it correctly in the active NADPH oxidase complex. In addition to p47^{phox} and p67^{phox}, the active NADPH oxidase requires the GTP-bound form of the Rho GTPase Rac.[54,202,300,301] The main target of Rac-GTP is the p67^{phox} subunit, which contains a Rac-binding domain created by four α-helical tetratricopeptide repeat (TPR) motifs.[319] The GTP-bound form of Rac also appears to interact with flavocytochrome *b* to further regulate enzyme activity.[320]

Oxidase assembly is triggered by receptor-mediated binding of many soluble chemoattractants (see Table 21-4), which requires higher concentrations of these molecules than needed for the initiation of chemotaxis. Binding of opsonized microbes to Fcγ and complement receptors is another major physiologic trigger of the respiratory burst that is activated at sites of microbial contact.[321,322] The specific pathways in the signal transduction cascade leading to oxidase assembly and activation are still incompletely defined, but the two critical downstream events are phosphorylation of p47^{phox} and activation of Rac to its GTP-bound state.[202,300,301] The functional oxidase complex is assembled at the plasma membrane in response to soluble agonists. During phagocytosis, additional flavocytochrome *b* for assembly of NADPH oxidase is delivered to the phagosome by the membrane fusion of specific granules, which contain the majority of the neutrophil's supply of flavocytochrome *b*.[24,46,275] Because release of O_2^- occurs largely at the extracellular side of the membrane, oxidants are released at sites of microbial contact or within the phagocytic vacuole, where they can interact with granule contents to potentiate their microbicidal effects.

Once formed, the O_2^- radical is first converted, either spontaneously or by means of superoxide dismutase, into H_2O_2 (reaction 2 in Fig. 21-7). Azurophilic granule–derived MPO, in the presence of halides, catalyzes the conversion of H_2O_2 to hypochlorous acid (HOCl), the active agent in household bleach (reaction 4 in Fig. 21-7). Hydrogen peroxide may also be converted to hydroxyl radical (OH·) in a nonenzymatic reaction with

TABLE 21-7   Properties of the Phagocyte Respiratory Burst Oxidase (*phox*) Components

	gp91*phox*	p22*phox*	p47*phox*	p67*phox*	p40*phox*
Synonyms	β Chain Heavy chain	α Chain Light chain	NCF-1 SOC II	NCF-2 SOC III	NCF-4
Amino acids	570	195	390	526	339
Gene locus	*CYBB* Xp21.1	*CYBA* 16q24	*NCF1* 7q11.23	*NCF2* 1q25	*NCF4* 22q.13.1
Cellular location in resting neutrophil	Specific granule and secretory vesicle membranes Plasma membrane	Specific granule and secretory vesicle membranes Plasma membrane	Cytosol	Cytosol	Cytosol
Tissue specificity	N, M/M, E B lymphocytes	mRNA in all cells tested; protein only in myeloid and B cells	N, M/M, E B lymphocytes	N, M/M, E B lymphocytes	N, M/M, E Other leukocytes
Functional domains	Binding sites for heme and FAD NADPH binding sites for cytosolic oxidase components	Proline-rich domain in carboxy-terminal that binds p47*phox*	9 potential serine phosphorylation sites SH3 domains Proline-rich domains PX domain	SH3 domains Proline-rich domains TPR repeats that bind Rac-GTP PB1 domain	SH3 domain PX domain PB1 domain
Homologies	NOX protein family Ferredoxin-NADP$^+$ reductase (FNR) Yeast ferric iron reductase	Polypeptide I of cytochrome *c* oxidase (weak homology)	NOXO1 Interacts with other NOXs	NOXA1 Interacts with other NOXs	

E, eosinophils; FAD, flavin adenine dinucleotide; GTP, guanosine triphosphate; M/M, monocyte/macrophages; N, neutrophils; NADPH, reduced nicotinamide adenine dinucleotide phosphate; NCF, neutrophil cytosol factor; NOX, NADPH oxidase; *phox*, phagocyte oxidase component; PX, *phox* homology; SH3, src homology domain 3; SOC, soluble oxidase component; TPR, tetratricopeptide repeat.

Modified with permission from Curnutte JT. Molecular basis of the autosomal recessive forms of chronic granulomatous disease. Immunodefic Rev. 1992;3:149-172.

O_2^- catalyzed by either iron or copper ions (reaction 3 in Fig. 21-7). Hydrogen peroxide, HOCl, and OH· are all strong oxidants that participate in microbial killing within the phagocytic vacuole.[303,323] Reactive oxidants also regulate phagocyte proteolytic activity by activating latent phagocyte metalloproteinases (such as collagenase and gelatinase) and inactivating plasma antiproteinases.[46,233] Enhanced phagocyte proteolysis at localized sites may be important for facilitating cellular migration into inflamed tissues, destruction of microbes, and removal of cellular debris.

Other enzymatic pathways related to oxidant generation include the detoxification of H_2O_2 by glutathione peroxidase and reductase (reactions 6 and 7, Fig. 21-7).[323] Glutathione is produced from γ-glutamylcysteine by the enzyme glutathione synthetase (reaction 9, Fig. 21-7). Other important antioxidant systems in phagocytes and other tissues include catalase, which catalyzes the conversion of H_2O_2 to oxygen and water, ascorbic acid, and α-tocopherol (vitamin E).[324] Generation of NADPH is important for providing a source of reducing equivalents for the glutathione detoxification pathway, as well as the respiratory burst itself. NADPH is replenished from NADP$^+$ by leukocyte glucose-6-phosphate dehydrogenase (G6PD; reaction 8, Fig. 21-7) in the hexose monophosphate shunt.

A second oxygen-dependent pathway with antimicrobial effects involves the generation of NO from the oxidation of L-arginine to L-citrulline. This reaction is catalyzed by nitric oxide synthase (NOS), with molecular oxygen supplying the oxygen in NO.[325-327] There are three different NOS isoforms, two of which are constitutively expressed in a variety of tissues, including the endothelium, brain, and neutrophils. Expression of a third, high-output isoform of inducible NOS (iNOS) is mediated by inflammatory stimuli in a variety of cells, including macrophages and neutrophils, where it has a wide spectrum of antitumor and antimicrobial activity against bacteria, parasites, helminths, viruses, and tumor cells.[325-327] NO can also interact with superoxide to form peroxynitrite, which mediates tyrosine nitration of cellular and bacterial proteins.[302] High levels of iNOS-catalyzed NO production are readily elicited in normal mouse macrophages by exposure, for example, to IFN-γ and endotoxin. In human monocytes and macrophages, IFN-α/β, IL-4 plus anti-CD23, or chemokines can induce iNOS expression.[326] Expression of iNOS has been detected in a variety of inflammatory and infectious diseases in humans, including malaria, hepatitis C, tuberculosis, tuberculoid leprosy, and the dementia associated with acquired immunodeficiency syndrome (AIDS).[326] Cytokine-activated human neutrophils also exhibit inducible production of NO, which leads to the nitration of ingested bacteria.[328]

Nonphagocyte NADPH Oxidases

The gp91^{phox}, p22^{phox}, p67^{phox}, and p47^{phox} subunits of the phagocyte respiratory burst oxidase have also been detected in endothelial cells and smooth muscle cells.[329] Expression of these components, as well as oxidant production, appears to be much lower than in phagocytic leukocytes. The physiologic significance of *phox* expression in nonphagocytic cells is controversial, but it has been speculated to play a role in intracellular signaling. Because there are many other potential sources of reactive oxidants, such as from xanthine oxidase, mitochondria, or other NAD(P)H oxidases, it has been difficult to ascribe any specific functions to vascular *phox* protein expression. However, recent studies in CGD knockout mice suggest that endothelial cell expression of these *phox* subunits may play a role in regulating inflammatory cell recruitment.[330,331]

Close homologues of the gp91^{phox} flavocytochrome subunit have recently been discovered.[332-334] This family is known as the NOX (NAD(P)H oxidase) proteins, of which there are six members in mammalian cells, in addition to gp91^{phox}, which is designated NOX2 in this classification. All NOX proteins share a similar protein structure, with transmembrane domains for heme binding and an intracellular flavoprotein domain. The other NOX proteins are expressed in various cell types, including the epithelium, smooth muscle cells, and gut, and appear capable of generating superoxide, generally at much lower levels than the phagocyte enzyme. At least some appear to be located in intracellular membranes rather than at the plasma membrane. Homologues of p67^{phox} (NOXA1) and p47^{phox} (NOXO1) that regulate several of the nonphagocyte NOXs have also been identified. The biologic functions of the nonphagocyte NOXs are under investigation and may include epithelial host defense, intracellular signaling for the regulation of cell growth and differentiation, and post-translational modification of proteins.

Specialized Functions of Mononuclear Phagocytes

Mononuclear phagocytes, particularly tissue macrophages, participate in a broad range of activities important for tissue homeostasis and repair, as well as in host defense against viruses, bacteria, fungi, and protozoa (Box 21-2).[115,126,133,134,168] From the standpoint of antimicrobial function, activated macrophages play a key role in the ingestion and killing of intracellular parasites such as mycobacteria, *Listeria*, *Leishmania*, *Toxoplasma*, and some fungi,[335] although various intracellular organisms have evolved specialized evasion mechanisms.[336] Both oxygen-dependent and oxygen-dependent systems are involved in this process, as described earlier. When

---

Box 21-2   Functions of Mononuclear Phagocytes

INFLAMMATORY RESPONSE AND PATHOGEN CONTROL

Antimicrobial activity
Antiviral activity
Antitumor activity
Secretion of cytokines, eicosanoids, proteases, coagulation factors, etc.
Granuloma formation

IMMUNE REGULATION

Antigen processing and presentation
Secretion of cytokines and chemokines

TISSUE HOMEOSTASIS AND REPAIR

Scavenger function
   Removal of apoptotic, senescent, or necrotic cells
   Phagocytosis of debris
Wound repair
   Débridement and phagocytosis
   Secretion of growth factors for endothelial cells and fibroblasts
Hematopoiesis
   Secretion of growth factors
Iron metabolism
Lipid metabolism

---

microbes (most characteristically mycobacteria, but any other organism or particle) cannot be fully ingested or killed, macrophages fuse in a cytokine-mediated process to form giant cells and granulomas.[337,338]

Activated macrophages also exhibit cytotoxicity against tumor cells, although the importance of this process in vivo remains to be determined.[339,340] Tumor cell killing can be mediated by antibody-dependent and antibody-independent processes that are highly dependent on macrophage activation. On the other hand, macrophage-mediated inflammation can contribute to tumorigenesis,[341] and tumor-associated macrophages can participate in tumor angiogenesis, invasion, and metastasis.[342,343] Osteoclasts, a specialized form of bone macrophage, cause bone resorption in osteolytic tumor metastases.[344]

IFN-γ, one of the principal macrophage-activating factors, is secreted by T lymphocytes, as well as by macrophages and neutrophils.[126,134,168,169] The cytokine induces changes in macrophage gene expression through the JAK (Janus kinase)-STAT (signal transducer and activator of transcription) pathway, elements of which are shared by many other cytokines, including IL-2, IL-6, and G-CSF.[29,345,346] Endotoxin, the bacterial lipopolysaccharide derived from gram-negative bacteria, is another important trigger of macrophage activation through pathways involving CD14 and TLRs.[126,347]

Interactions of macrophages with T and B cells are essential for the development of cellular and humoral immunity.[147,348,349] Macrophages, particularly the specialized form of dendritic cells, are professional antigen-presenting cells that initiate and regulate NK-, T-, and B-cell responses. Macrophage production of IL-1, as well as subsequent interactions between stimulated T and B cells, leads to B-cell production of antigen-specific immunoglobulins.[349] Macrophages are also major physiologic sources of cytokines and chemokines that regulate both the innate and the adaptive immune systems.[127,147,348,350] As a source of "endogenous pyrogens," they are responsible for the production of fever in response to infection or inflammation.[351]

Macrophages participate in many aspects of wound repair.[352,353] The early phases of this process are dominated by an influx of neutrophils, followed by the migration of monocytes that differentiate into activated macrophages and, finally, the appearance of T lymphocytes. Proliferating fibroblasts secrete collagen and other matrix proteins important for wound closure and tissue remodeling, and migrating keratinocytes regenerate the epithelial surface. Both neutrophils and macrophages protect against infection and dispose of phagocytosed debris. Mononuclear phagocytes also elaborate fibroblast, epithelial, and angiogenic growth factors (see Box 21-1) that stimulate the normal progression of tissue repair and neovascularization that characterize the later phases of wound healing.[132,352,353]

Macrophages ingest and dispose of apoptotic and necrotic cells.[133,354,355] This function not only contributes to cellular processing for antigen presentation but also plays a critical role in tissue remodeling and homeostasis, embryologic development, and resolution of inflammation. A redundant and promiscuous system of receptors, including integrins, scavenger receptors, complement receptors, calreticulin, CD14, and Mer receptor, recognize and effect the uptake of apoptotic cells. Resident tissue macrophages, particularly those lining the sinusoids of the spleen and liver (formerly known as the "reticuloendothelial system"), clear senescent and antibody-bound blood cells from the circulation.[356-358]

Iron from the catabolism of hemoglobin in aged erythrocytes is incorporated into ferritin and hemosiderin, where it accounts for about two thirds of the body's store of reserve iron. Iron in this macrophage storage pool turns over and returns in a transferrin-bound form to the bone marrow for new red blood cell synthesis (see Chapter 12).[359] Sequestration of iron in macrophages leads to the anemia of chronic disease.[360]

Monocytes and macrophages contribute to the pathophysiology of atherosclerosis through the uptake, metabolism, and oxidation of LDL and VLDL by receptor-mediated endocytosis.[131,361] Macrophages in blood vessel walls that are exposed to sufficient quantities of cholesterol develop into the foam cells characteristic of atherosclerotic plaque[362] and contribute to the important inflammatory component of plaque formation and destabilization.[363]

Specialized Functions of Eosinophils and Basophils

Eosinophils and basophils, though sharing many of the functional characteristics of neutrophils and mononuclear phagocytes, participate in distinctive aspects of the inflammatory response and interact with each other in the context of certain allergic reactions. Eosinophils and mast cells are often situated beneath epithelial surfaces exposed to environmental antigens, such as the respiratory and gastrointestinal tracts, where they may be actively involved in mucosal immune responses. However, the role of eosinophils, basophils, and mast cells is better known in pathologic settings than in normal homeostasis.

Eosinophils appear to have both immunoenhancing and immunosuppressive functions (Table 21-8).[6,7,74,75] Though capable of ingesting and killing bacteria, eosinophils are not particularly efficient at this task. Rather, they possess an unusual ability to destroy invasive metazoan parasites, especially helminthic parasites. Eosinophils bind to the surface of both adult and larval helminths and inflict damage through the release of cationic granule proteins and the generation of reactive oxidants, including the eosinophil peroxidase–catalyzed formation of hypohalous acids via the action of the respiratory burst and eosinophil peroxidase.[6,7]

Eosinophil production of the lipid inflammatory mediators LTC_4 and PAF plays a role in the pathogenesis of allergic diseases.[7] PAF and LTC_4 can induce smooth muscle contraction and promote the secretion of mucus, and PAF itself is a potent activator of eosinophils. The

TABLE 21-8	Eosinophil Function
Function	**Mechanism**
Defense against helminths (both larval and adult forms)	Binding of eosinophils to surface
	Peroxidation of larval surface mediated by eosinophil peroxidase
	Toxicity to larval surface by released major basic protein
Immunosuppression of immediate hypersensitivity reactions	Engulfment of most cell granules
	Release of prostaglandin E_1/E_2 to suppress basophil degranulation
	Release of histaminase
	Oxidation of slow-reacting substance of anaphylaxis
	Release of phospholipase D to inactive mast cell platelet-activating factor
	Release of major basic protein for binding of mast cell heparin
	Release of plasminogen to reduce local thrombus formation

release of eosinophil granule contents may also contribute to localized tissue damage. Purified eosinophil MBP, for example, can cause cytopathic changes in tracheal epithelium in vitro that are similar to the changes observed in asthmatic patients.

Eosinophils may also perform an immunosuppressive function in immediate hypersensitivity reactions (see Table 21-8). IgE-activated basophils or mast cells release eosinophilic chemotactic factor of anaphylaxis, which recruits eosinophils to the site. Subsequent eosinophil degranulation releases products that can inactivate inflammatory mediators. For example, histaminase inactivates histamine, phospholipase B inactivates PAF, MBP inactivates mast cell heparin, and lysophospholipase prevents the generation of arachidonic acid metabolites.

Basophils and mast cells are central participants in a variety of inflammatory and immunologic disorders, particularly immediate hypersensitivity diseases, and may also play a role in host defense against bacterial infections. Basophils and mast cells express plasma membrane receptors that specifically bind with high affinity the Fc portion of the IgE antibody (Fcε receptors).[264] After active or passive sensitization with IgE, exposure to specific multivalent antigen triggers an almost immediate release of granule contents (anaphylactic degranulation) and the synthesis and release of newly generated chemical mediators such as LTC_4, which stimulates smooth muscle contraction, secretion of mucus, and vasoactive changes.[364] Degranulation can also be triggered in response to insect venom, radiocontrast dye, and other nonspecific agents. Recent studies on mutant mice engineered by gene targeting to lack Fcγ or Fcε receptors (or both) have shown that mast cell FcγRIII receptors are essential in activating the inflammatory response to IgG immune complexes (Arthus reaction), heretofore an unrecognized role for the mast cell.[365] Mast cells can secrete numerous mitogenic or inflammatory cytokines, including many interleukins (1, 3, 4, 5, and 6), chemokines, GM-CSF, and TNF-α, that are also likely to regulate leukocyte recruitment and inflammation in IgE-dependent reactions and immune complex injury.[107,366,367] The inflammatory cytokines and leukotrienes released from tissue mast cells have recently been recognized to play an important role in neutrophil recruitment during the acute response to bacterial infection.[368-370]

Pathologic Consequences of Phagocyte Activation and Inflammatory Response

Though normally serving a protective function, the inflammatory response can also result in damage to host tissues. The release of proteases, oxygen radicals, and proinflammatory cytokines by activated phagocytes appears to play a major role in the generation of tissue injury in a wide variety of pathologic inflammatory processes (Box 21-3).[162,233,371-373] For example, neutrophil

---

Box 21-3 | **Selected Pathologic Inflammatory Reactions Associated with Phagocyte-Induced Tissue Injury**

Arthus reaction
Systemic inflammatory response syndrome
Nephrotoxic and immune complex nephritis
Postischemic myocardial damage
Adult respiratory distress syndrome
Atherosclerosis
Bronchiectasis
Acute and chronic allograft rejection
Malignant transformation with chronic inflammation
Rheumatoid arthritis

See text for references.

---

elastase has been implicated in the pathogenesis of emphysema in both adult smokers and individuals with α_1-antitrypsin deficiency. Neutrophil granule proteases may contribute to the joint destruction in rheumatoid arthritis and other chronic arthropathies. Neutrophils are also believed to play a key role in the systemic inflammatory response syndrome, a term that has been created to encompass the host response to both infectious (e.g., gram-negative sepsis) and noninfectious (e.g., pancreatitis, trauma) causes and can lead to organ dysfunction and tissue damage.[372] Sequestration of activated neutrophils in the pulmonary capillary bed along with subsequent release of tissue-damaging agents is an important component in the development of adult respiratory distress syndrome. Activation of the complement cascade by artificial membrane surfaces during hemodialysis and cardiopulmonary bypass can also result in neutrophil activation, intrapulmonary sequestration, and lung injury. Macrophages are integral to the pathophysiology of atherosclerosis by uptake of serum lipoproteins and contribute an important inflammatory component that influences the development and rupture of atherosclerotic plaque.[361-363] In addition to their cytotoxic effects, the oxidative products released by activated phagocytes are also mutagenic, as documented by plasmid mutagenesis, sister chromatid exchange, and transformation of cells in culture.[374] Hence, the increased risk for malignancy observed with certain chronic inflammatory states, such as ulcerative colitis or chronic hepatitis, has been postulated to be in part related to oxidant-induced carcinogenesis.

The development of anti-inflammatory interventions based on agents that block leukocyte adhesion or inhibit the action of specific proinflammatory agents has been an area of intense interest. TNF-α antagonists are now widely used for the treatment of rheumatoid arthritis, and IL-1 receptor antagonists also have efficacy in this disease.[375] Antagonists of leukocyte integrins have shown benefit in phase II and III studies for inflammatory bowel disease, psoriasis, and multiple sclerosis.[206] However, although protective effects of monoclonal antibodies directed against either β_2 integrins, ICAM-1, or selectins were found in various animal models of inflammation, including ischemia-reperfusion injury, endotoxic shock, and acute arthritis, the results of clinical trials failed to show significant benefit.[206] The contributions of non-phagocytic cells to inflammatory tissue injury must also be kept in mind. For example, adult respiratory distress syndrome can occur in the presence of severe neutropenia.[376] Moreover, despite the adverse consequences of the acute inflammatory process, these events are also important for normal healing. For instance, the use of anti-inflammatory agents in myocardial infarction, which can decrease infarct size acutely, results in impaired healing of the myocardium and the formation of fragile scar tissue.[371] Finally, the impact of the new anti-inflammatory biologic agents on host defense must be kept in mind, particularly if being used in combination with other immunosuppressive drugs such as steroids. For example, patients receiving TNF-α antagonists have increased rates of tuberculosis and infection with endemic mycotic or intracellular bacterial pathogens.[377]

QUANTITATIVE GRANULOCYTE AND MONONUCLEAR PHAGOCYTE DISORDERS

This section reviews clinical disorders associated with disturbances in granulocyte number, with particular emphasis on syndromes in which the granulocyte abnormality is a central feature. Several disorders have now been associated with specific genetic defects, although the molecular pathophysiology leading from the gene to the phenotype often remains obscure. This section of the chapter is organized by clinical characteristics of the disorders, with genetic and functional laboratory data provided when available.

Neutropenia

Definition and Classification

Neutropenia is defined as an absolute decrease in the number of circulating neutrophils in blood. Normal neutrophil levels should be stratified for age, race, and other factors. For whites, the lower limit for normal neutrophil counts (neutrophils and bands) is 1000 cells/μL in infants between 2 weeks and 1 year of age; after infancy it rises to 1500 cells/μL. Blacks have somewhat lower neutrophil counts, with counts of less than 1500 cells/μL in 4.5% of black participants in the 1999-2004 National Health and Nutrition Examination Survey.[378] The lower limits of normal are generally considered to be 200 to 600/μL less than those in whites. This difference probably derives from a relative decrease in neutrophil release from the bone marrow storage compartment.[379-381] Falsely low white blood cell counts can result when counts are performed long after blood is drawn, after leukocyte clump-

ing in small clots, or in the presence of certain paraproteins.

Neutropenia can represent disturbances in production, shifts of neutrophils from the circulating to the marginated or tissue pools, increased peripheral utilization or destruction, or combinations of these causes. However, assays of leukokinetics and myelopoiesis are not routinely available, so mechanisms may be hard to identify. Classifications based on biochemical or functional studies are also difficult because of the paucity of neutrophils in the circulation of neutropenic patients. In general, neutropenic syndromes are broadly classified as intrinsic, or caused by defects in myelopoiesis, or as acquired and caused by extrinsic factors such as drugs, infections, or autoantibodies (Box 21-4).

The clinical significance of neutropenia depends on the level of depression of the absolute neutrophil count (ANC). Mild neutropenia, with neutrophil counts of 1000 to 1500 cells/μL, and moderate neutropenia, with counts of 500 to 1000 cells/μL, are not generally clinically significant with respect to host defense but may warrant evaluation to determine the underlying cause. Severe neutropenia refers to ANCs below 500 cells/μL, with the term "agranulocytosis" usually reserved for counts below 200 cells/μL. Children with severe chronic neutropenia can be registered with the Severe Chronic

---

Box 21-4	Classification of Neutropenia

NEUTROPENIA CAUSED BY INTRINSIC DEFECTS IN GRANULOCYTES OR THEIR PROGENITORS

Reticular dysgenesis
Cyclic neutropenia
Severe congenital neutropenia (including Kostmann's syndrome)
Myelokathexis/WHIM syndrome
Shwachman-Diamond syndrome
Albinism/neutropenia syndromes (including Chédiak-Higashi)
Familial benign neutropenia
Bone marrow failure syndromes (congenital and acquired)

NEUTROPENIA CAUSED BY EXTRINSIC FACTORS

Infection
Drug-induced neutropenia
Autoimmune neutropenia
Chronic benign neutropenia (including chronic autoimmune neutropenia of childhood)
Neonatal immune neutropenia
Neutropenia associated with immune dysfunction
Neutropenia associated with metabolic diseases
Nutritional deficiencies
Reticuloendothelial sequestration
Bone marrow infiltration
Chronic idiopathic neutropenia (may also be intrinsic)

Types of neutropenia are listed in order of discussion in the text.
WHIM, warts, hypogammaglobulinemia, infections, myelokathexis.

Neutropenia International Registry (SCNIR; http://depts.washington.edu/registry/).

Symptoms of Neutropenia

The hallmark of neutropenia is increased susceptibility to bacterial and fungal infection; neutropenia by itself does not diminish host defense against viral or parasitic infections. The most frequent types of pyogenic infections in patients with significant neutropenia are cellulitis, furunculosis, superficial or deep cutaneous abscesses, pneumonia, and septicemia.[382-386] Stomatitis, gingivitis, and periodontitis may be initial signs of neutropenia that develops into chronic problems. Perirectal inflammation and otitis media (especially in younger children) occur as well. Endogenous bacteria are the most frequent cause of infections, but colonization or infection may occur with a variety of nosocomial and opportunistic organisms. The most commonly isolated organisms from neutropenic patients are *Staphylococcus aureus* and gram-negative bacteria, but almost any organisms can be isolated, particularly in hospitalized patients or those receiving frequent or prolonged courses of antibiotics. The usual symptoms and signs of local infection—such as exudates, fluctuation, ulceration, and regional adenopathy—may be less evident in neutropenic patients than in normal individuals.[387]

Susceptibility to bacterial infection, even with severe neutropenia, can be quite variable, depending on the underlying cause. For example, some patients with chronic neutropenia secondary to autoantibodies do not experience serious infections over a period of many years, even with neutrophil counts as low as 200 cells/μL, most likely because these individuals have rapid production and transit of normal neutrophils, with relative preservation of neutrophil delivery to tissues.[388] Many patients with chronic neutropenia also have normal to increased numbers of circulating monocytes, an alternative phagocyte.[389] However, the recruitment of monocytes to inflammatory sites is delayed relative to neutrophils, and monocytes are not as efficient as neutrophils in ingesting bacteria.[390,391] Thus, monocytes appear to provide only marginal protection against pyogenic organisms in severely neutropenic patients. It is likely that the humoral, cell-mediated, and tissue macrophage immune systems also play important alternative or compensatory roles preventing infection in these individuals.

Neutropenia Caused by Intrinsic Defects in Granulocytes or Their Progenitors

These disorders are also discussed in detail, with more emphasis on molecular pathogenesis, in Chapter 8.

Reticular Dysgenesis

The selective failure of stem cells committed to myeloid and lymphoid development leads to reticular dysgenesis, one of the rarest and most severe forms of combined immunodeficiency.[392-397] It is characterized by severe leukopenia, including both agranulocytosis and lymphopenia; defective cellular and humoral immunity; and absence of lymph nodes, tonsils, Peyer's patches, and splenic follicles. Erythroid and megakaryocyte development is normal. Most patients have been male, but two females and several nontwin males have been reported, thus suggesting autosomal inheritance. All reported infants have died of bacterial or viral infections within the first weeks of life, except a few treated by hematopoietic stem cell transplantation (HSCT).[395,398,399]

Cyclic Neutropenia

Cyclic neutropenia is a sporadic or autosomal dominant disorder characterized by regular periodic oscillations approximately every 21 days in the number of peripheral blood neutrophils, with a nadir of less than 200 cells/μL (Fig. 21-10).[400,401] In most typical cases, reticulocytes, platelets, and other leukocytes also cycle. The frequency of occurrence of cyclic neutropenia has been estimated at 0.5 to 1 case per million population.[402] During the neutropenic nadir of each cycle, patients may suffer malaise, fever, oral ulcers, gingivitis, periodontitis, and pharyngitis associated with lymph node enlargement. Symptoms typically begin during the first year of life but may not commence until adulthood. More serious complications can occur occasionally, including mastoiditis, pneumonia, or ulceration of vaginal or intestinal mucosa. The severity of the infections tends to parallel the depth of the neutropenia, but some patients escape infections entirely during the neutropenic period. Many patients experience improvement in symptoms as they grow older. In these individuals, the cycles tend to become less noticeable as the neutrophil nadir rises to a more functionally adequate level. Although cyclic neutropenia is frequently viewed as a benign condition, 10% of patients in historical reviews have died of infectious complications.[401,403] Pneumonia and peritonitis, the latter complicated by clostridial sepsis, have been the most frequent causes of death.[400,401]

Oscillations in the rate of bone marrow production of neutrophils result in neutropenia with nadirs at intervals of 21 ± 3 days in the majority of patients, although the cycles can be as long as 28 to 36 days and as short as 14 days.[403] Neutrophil counts often fall to 0 at some time during the nadir and remain below 200 cells/μL for at least 3 to 5 days. In most patients, monocytosis occurs when neutrophil counts are at their lowest. In the recovery phase, neutrophil counts rise, often into the low-normal range, and monocyte counts drop. Oscillations are subtle in some individuals, particularly older patients, who instead have a pattern more consistent with chronic neutropenia. Oscillations in reticulocyte and platelet counts may parallel those seen for neutrophils,[401,404] hence the alternative term "cyclic hematopoiesis," but these other cell numbers range between normal and elevated levels and thus have no clinical impact. Marrow aspirates show highly variable morphology, depending on the phase of the cycle. The myeloid series may show hypoplasia with "maturation arrest" at the myelocyte

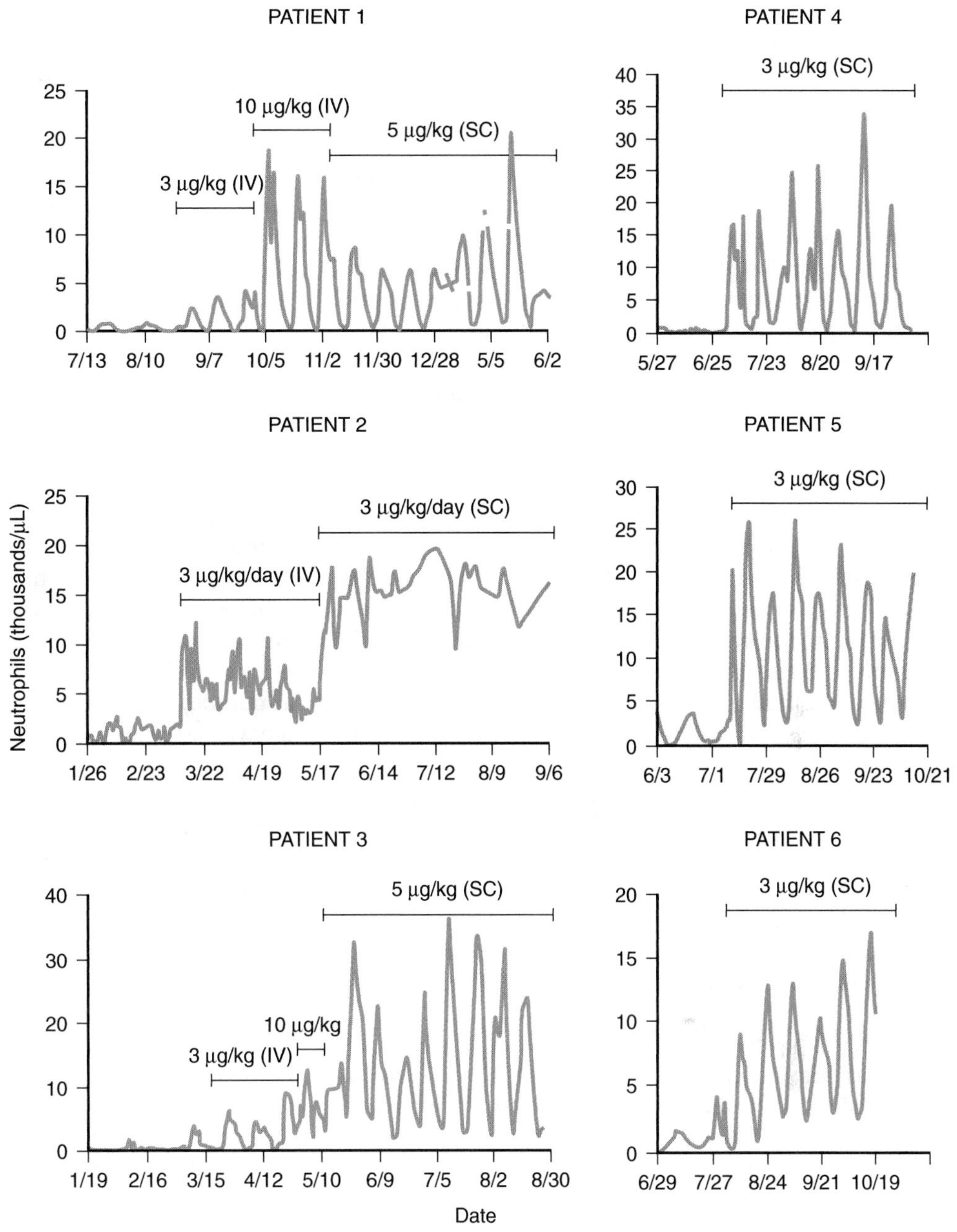

FIGURE 21-10. Cyclic neutropenia and the response to clinical administration of granulocyte colony-stimulating factor (G-CSF) in six patients. The cycling of neutrophil counts before and during therapy with various doses of G-CSF is shown. The *rectangles* represent the duration of G-CSF treatment, with the corresponding dose shown above each rectangle. Note the approximately 21-day cycle before therapy in patients 1, 5, and 6, which is characteristic of cyclic neutropenia. The cycle shortened to approximately 14 days during G-CSF therapy, whereas the peak neutrophil counts increased approximately 10-fold. (*Reprinted with permission from Hammond WP, Price TH, Souza LM, Dale DC. Treatment of cyclic neutropenia with granulocyte colony-stimulating factor. N Engl J Med. 1989;320:1306-1311.*)

stage during the declining phase of neutrophil oscillation, but normal or hyperplastic myelopoiesis during neutrophil recovery. The marrow stem cell defect in cyclic neutropenia has been demonstrated by transfer of the disorder via allogeneic bone marrow transplantation from a child with cyclic neutropenia to a sibling undergoing treatment of leukemia.[405]

Patients with both sporadic and autosomal dominant forms of cyclic neutropenia have been shown to have coding sequence mutations in the *ELA2* gene encoding neutrophil elastase, a serine protease synthesized at the promyelocyte-myelocyte stage.[293,294] This gene was discovered by linkage analysis of families with autosomal dominant cyclic neutropenia, but mutations in *ELA2* have now also been identified in approximately 60% to 80% of kindreds with SCN (see later and Chapter 8).

How mutations in neutrophil elastase result in the cyclic production of neutrophils and other blood cells is not currently well understood. Bone marrow samples from both cyclic neutropenia and SCN patients demonstrate increased apoptosis of neutrophil precursors.[406-409] Thus, expression of mutant neutrophil elastase may induce excessive apoptosis through either aberrant subcellular targeting of the protein or induction of a strong unfolded protein response.[407,408,410,411] Cycling may occur as a result of partial recovery of myelopoiesis via G-CSF production at the nadir, but with oscillation rather than homeostasis taking place because of the abnormal kinetics of the feedback loop.[412,413]

Cyclic neutropenia must be distinguished from cyclic fever without neutropenia[414] and from other causes of neutropenia. To establish the diagnosis of cyclic neutropenia, neutrophil counts should be monitored twice or at least once a week for 6 to 8 weeks. The genetic diagnosis can be confirmed by sequencing of the *ELA2* gene.

Management of patients with cyclic neutropenia includes careful attention to identification and treatment of infections acquired when these patents are neutropenic. In general, fevers, upper respiratory symptoms, and cervical lymphadenopathy occurring during neutropenic episodes require no specific therapy. However, the physician must remain alert to symptoms suggesting a specific infection, particularly the sometimes fatal abdominal complications. Careful attention to oral and dental hygiene is important to minimize periodontal disease and ameliorate the discomfort of mouth sores. To prevent the development of severe dental complications and because of the risk of life-threatening infections, prophylactic G-CSF (filgrastim) therapy is recommended for patients with cyclic neutropenia with nadirs consistently below 500 cells/μL. G-CSF has been very effective in improving peripheral blood neutrophil counts in this disorder, along with the signs and symptoms associated with neutropenic nadirs.[415-418] Most patients still experience cycles, and in fact the amplitude of the cycling may increase, but with shortened cycle periods and increased neutrophil counts at the nadir (see Fig. 21-8).[412,418] The dose of G-CSF required to maintain peripheral neutrophil counts in the normal range in most patients with cyclic neutropenia is usually 2 to 4 μg/kg/day, administered either daily or on alternate days.[415,417,418] Cases of myelodysplastic syndrome (MDS) or acute myelogenous leukemia (AML) have not been reported in cyclic neutropenia patients, including those treated with G-CSF.[386,406,417]

Severe Congenital Neutropenia

SCN was first described by Kostmann in 1956 as an autosomal recessive disorder associated with severe neutropenia that was identified in the population of an isolated northern parish of Sweden.[419] Other forms of SCN have since been identified with sporadic occurrence or with historical or genetic evidence of autosomal recessive or autosomal dominant inheritance.[382,417,420,421] This disorder is also discussed in detail, with emphasis on the genetics and molecular pathogenesis, in Chapter 8. Although the nomenclature is still in flux, we suggest that the term SCN (Online Mendelian Inheritance in Man [OMIM] 202700) be used to refer to the entire disorder regardless of inheritance or genotype and that Kostmann's disease (OMIM 610738) be used to refer to the autosomal recessive subtype, caused in all or most cases by mutations in the *HAX1* gene[422] (see later).

The incidence of SCN is approximately two cases per million population.[402] Affected patients generally maintain ANCs of less than 200 cells/μL, which has been documented on the first day of life in several cases.[423] Frequent episodes of fever, skin infections (including omphalitis), stomatitis, pneumonia, and perirectal abscesses typically appear during the first months of life. Infections often disseminate to the blood, meninges, and

peritoneum and are usually caused by *S. aureus*, *Escherichia coli*, and *Pseudomonas* species. Before the current era of G-CSF therapy, most patients died in the first 1 to 2 years of life,[417,424] and survivors were known to be at risk for the development of MDS and AML.[424-426]

Peripheral blood counts generally show, in addition to agranulocytosis, moderate to marked monocytosis, mild to moderate eosinophilia, and secondary changes such as anemia and thrombocytosis. G-CSF production in SCN patients appears to be normal, if not elevated.[427,428] Antineutrophil antibodies may be present, and a positive test should not be used to rule out SCN.[429]

Bone marrow examination characteristically shows a myeloid "maturation arrest" at the myelocyte stage of development, with normal to increased numbers of promyelocytes but few if any more mature forms.[382,402] The promyelocytes may have dysplastic morphology, including large size, atypical nuclei, and vacuolated cytoplasm. Marrow eosinophilia and monocytosis are common and do not change during treatment. Cellularity is usually normal or slightly decreased. Megakaryocytes are normal in number and morphology. The in vitro growth of granulocyte colonies from SCN bone marrow is defective, with few colonies formed, but most patients' bone marrow produces colonies with some capability for full maturation to neutrophils in the presence of exogenous G-CSF, thus indicating that the "arrest" is intrinsic but incomplete.[430-432]

The genetic basis of 60% to 80% of SCN cases derives from mutations in the *ELA2* gene,[293,294,433] which encodes neutrophil elastase and is also responsible for the related but distinct disorder cyclic neutropenia (discussed earlier). *ELA2*-related SCN may be sporadic or inherited in an autosomal dominant mendelian pattern, as dramatically illustrated by a series of five affected children from four families, all conceived by sperm from the same anonymous donor.[420] An additional, recently identified case of cyclic neutropenia with the identical S97L missense mutation from the same sperm donor not only confirms the autosomal dominant inheritance of *ELA2*-related disorders but also indicates that genetic background can result in the same genotype being expressed phenotypically as either SCN or cyclic neutropenia. Additional, rare cases of autosomal dominant SCN appear to arise from mutations in the *Gfi1* gene,[434] which encodes a transcriptional repressor that inhibits multiple genes involved in neutrophil maturation, including *ELA2*.[11,12]

Similar to cyclic neutropenia, the bone marrow of SCN patients shows evidence of accelerated apoptosis of neutrophil precursors.[435] As noted earlier, expression of mutant neutrophil elastase or other aberrant proteins may induce excessive apoptosis through either aberrant subcellular targeting of the protein or induction of a strong unfolded protein response.[407,408,410,411]

Mutations in most autosomal recessive SCN kindreds, including several originally studied by Kostmann, have been identified in the *HAX1* gene,[422] which encodes a mitochondrial protein with putative functions in signal transduction and cytoskeletal control. Other rare mutations responsible for an SCN phenotype include defects in the Wiskott-Aldrich syndrome (WAS) gene[436,437] and constitutional defects (as opposed to acquired mutations—see later) in the gene encoding the G-CSF receptor.[407,438]

G-CSF, the standard treatment modality for SCN, has greatly improved both life span and quality of life for these patients.[416,417,439] Until the availability of this cytokine in the 1980s, severe neutropenia would inevitably lead to fatal infections in the majority of patients despite supportive care with prophylactic trimethoprim-sulfamethoxazole, aggressive use of antibiotics at the time of documented infections, and scrupulous attention to oral hygiene. More than 95% of SCN patients respond to G-CSF treatment with an increase in the ANC to greater than 1000/μL, along with a documented reduction in infections.[416,417,439] There is often a delay of 7 to 10 days before the rise of peripheral blood neutrophil counts at the start of treatment. In patients enrolled in the SCNIR between 1993 and 1999, more than 90% of congenital neutropenia patients responded to G-CSF treatment with rises in the ANC to greater than 1.0×10^9/L and required significantly less antibiotic therapy and less frequent hospitalization.[421] SCN patients required G-CSF doses ranging from 0.56 to 190 μg/kg/day, with mean of 10.2 and standard deviation of 19.0 μg/kg/day.[417] These doses are significantly higher than those needed for cyclic or idiopathic neutropenia.[417] The percentage of maturing neutrophils in bone marrow increases with G-CSF, although morphologically abnormal promyelocytes with vacuolized and asynchronous nuclear-cytoplasmic maturation can persist, and the number of monocytes and eosinophils in marrow and peripheral blood may remain high.[402]

Based on data from the SCNIR, a starting daily dose of G-CSF of 5 μg/kg/day is recommended, increasing gradually, if necessary, to as high as 100 μg/kg/day for at least 14 days to achieve a neutrophil count of 1000 to 2000/μL.[440] The drug is generally administered subcutaneously, but it may be given intravenously at equal dosage if clinical conditions warrant or if vehicle volumes are too high to permit comfortable subcutaneous injection. In G-CSF–refractory patients, combination therapy with stem cell factor has been reported to be effective,[402] but rarely used, because it also leads to mast cell activation with the release of histamine and anaphylactoid reactions. GM-CSF treatment results in large increases in eosinophils and monocytes, but not neutrophils.[441]

Side effects of G-CSF treatment are usually mild and include bone pain, headache, and rashes. Other common, but often asymptomatic findings include splenomegaly and osteopenia.[415,417] Splenomegaly has been reported in patients with SCN before and during G-CSF therapy.[415,417] Palpable splenomegaly, with a median spleen measurement of 2 cm below the costal margin, was recorded in 18.2% of untreated patients registered in the SCNIR. During the first year of G-CSF therapy, the incidence increased to 38.2% and remained at this level (26.7% to 44.7%) through 10 years of therapy, with no trend to progression in spleen size during therapy.[417] Of 731 SCNIR patients analyzed in 2003, osteopenia or osteoporosis was reported in 127, including 93 with SCN. Findings included abnormal bone density only (46), abnormal bone density and clinical problem (67), and clinical problem only (14). G-CSF doses in the patient group in whom osteopenia/osteoporosis developed ranged from 0.3 to 240 μg/kg/day, and there was no correlation with the dose of G-CSF, duration of treatment, or patient age or sex.[417,442] The SCNIR recommends regular monitoring of bone density. Rare patients were also found to have vasculitis or glomerulonephritis, both before and during G-CSF therapy.[417]

The SCNIR has reported thrombocytopenia (platelet count $<50 \times 10^3$/μL) in 26 patients, including 17 with SCN.[417] Seven were not receiving G-CSF, and among the 19 treated patients, 7 became thrombocytopenic concurrent with conversion to MDS/AML. Thus, development of thrombocytopenia in SCN patients requires thorough evaluation as a possible heralding sign of disease progression.

Conversion to MDS/AML and bacterial sepsis remain the most serious complications of SCN. The predilection to acute leukemia was recognized before the availability of G-CSF,[424,425] but most affected children probably died of severe infections. Now, longer survivors appear to be at increased risk for the development of MDS, which almost invariably progresses to AML,[443] whereas death from sepsis has become rarer but can still occur in G-CSF–responsive patients.

During long-term G-CSF therapy, some SCN patients acquire mutations in the G-CSF receptor gene (*GCSFR*), then myelodysplasia characterized by monosomy 7, and finally myeloid leukemia.[406,443-445] Acquired mutations in *GCSFR* have been detected in approximately 80% of SCNIR patients in whom MDS/AML developed, whereas mutations in the *FLT3*, *KIT*, and *JAK2* tyrosine kinase genes, frequently found in de novo AML, are uncommon.[445-448] Some SCN patients with *GCSFR* mutations have not progressed, including some who lost the mutated clone after discontinuation of G-CSF therapy and reacquired it upon resumption of treatment.[445-447] Cytogenetic abnormalities, particularly monosomy 7, also precede and predict leukemic conversion. For this reason, the SCNIR recommends yearly bone marrow surveillance, including karyotyping and chromosome 7 fluorescence in situ hybridization (FISH) for all SCN patients. Although clonal cytogenetic abnormalities may spontaneously remit, their appearance should be considered a strong indication for HSCT, including the use of a matched unrelated donor if necessary, because transplantation is more likely to be successful when undertaken before progression to MDS/AML.[449,450]

Recent studies by the SCNIR and the French Severe Chronic Neutropenia Study Group[386,444] have shed light on the incidence and some of the risk factors for sepsis and MDS/AML. In the SCNIR analysis of 374 SCN patients, many monitored for 10 or more years, the cumulative incidence of death from sepsis was 8% after 10 years of G-CSF therapy, and the cause-specific hazard of death from sepsis was stable over time at 0.9% per year.[386] In contrast, the cumulative incidence of MDS/AML was 21% after 10 years of G-CSF therapy and 36% after 12 years, with the cause-specific hazard of MDS/AML increasing over time from 2.9% per year at 6 years up to 8% per year after 11.7 years of therapy. Thus, there is an increasing risk for MDS/AML as patients receive G-CSF for longer periods.

Importantly, the SCNIR analysis also identified a subgroup of SCN patients at greatest risk for MDS/AML.[386,451] The "worst responder" group, which received a G-CSF dose of 8 µg/kg/day or greater and had an ANC of less than 2188 cells/µL, had relative hazards of 3.1-fold for MDS/AML and 5.6-fold for sepsis. In the worst responder group, the cumulative incidence at 10 years was 40% for MDS/AML and 14% for death from sepsis versus 11% and 4%, respectively, for the best responder group (G-CSF dose <8 µg/kg/day and ANC ≥2188 cells/µL). However, it is notable that even the best responders were not free of the risk of MDS/AML or even death from sepsis. Although data were not available for blood counts at the time of onset of sepsis, these patients were considered G-CSF responders, generally with an ANC of greater than 1000 cells/µL, thus suggesting that granulocytes from such patients, though seemingly adequate in number, may still be limited in function.[452] For patients in the "worst responder" category—high G-CSF dose requirements and low ANC during therapy—early transplantation should be considered, depending on donor availability, but the indication is not as strong as for those already showing abnormal cytogenetics.

Notably, multiple studies have shown a higher risk for MDS/AML in patients with Shwachman-Diamond syndrome than in those with SCN, but no progression to MDS or leukemia in cyclic neutropenia.[386,443,444] The latter finding is particularly striking because as discussed earlier, most cases of cyclic neutropenia and SCN derive from mutations in the same gene, *ELA2*.

Myelokathexis and WHIM Syndrome

Myelokathexis is an uncommon form of moderate to severe chronic neutropenia characterized by granulocyte hyperplasia in the bone marrow, which contains degenerating neutrophils with cytoplasmic vacuoles, prominent granules, and nuclear hypersegmentation with very thin filaments connecting pyknotic-appearing nuclear lobes.[453-455] Comparable abnormalities can be seen in the majority of peripheral blood neutrophils. Eosinophils exhibit similar abnormal morphology, but lymphocytes, monocytes, and basophils appear normal,[454] although relative lymphopenia has been noted in some patients.[454]

Recurrent warts and hypogammaglobulinemia (low IgG and occasionally low IgM and IgA) have often been reported in patients in whom myelokathexis has been diagnosed; hence, the acronym WHIM refers to warts, hypogammaglobulinemia, infections, and myelokathexis.[456]

The recurrent sinopulmonary infections and other bacterial infections in WHIM syndrome probably reflect increased susceptibility as a result of both neutropenia and hypogammaglobulinemia. However, early deaths related to infection have not been reported, and affected patients are capable of mobilizing increased numbers of neutrophils into peripheral blood during infectious episodes.[455] Neutrophil function has generally been reported to be normal. Since the description of first patient in 1964, more than 25 cases have been reported,[455,457-459] including a kindred of six affected individuals in three generations[454] and dizygotic twin sisters.[460] The sex ratio among reported patients has a female preponderance.

The genetic basis of WHIM syndrome was discovered by analysis of four WHIM kindreds in which affected members all carried a truncating mutation in the cytoplasmic tail domain of the gene encoding chemokine receptor 4 (CXCR4),[461] a G protein–coupled receptor with a unique ligand, CXCL12, also known as SDF-1. This work indicated autosomal dominant inheritance of the WHIM syndrome. However, in other kindreds with wild-type CXCR4 genes and probably autosomal recessive inheritance, patients' lymphocytes and neutrophils displayed similar marked enhancement of G protein–dependent responses to CXCR4 ligands.[462,463] Therefore, aberrant dysfunction of the CXCR4-mediated signaling constitutes a common biologic trait of WHIM syndrome with different causative genetic anomalies. Because the interaction between CXCR4 and CXCL12 provides a key retention signal for neutrophils in bone marrow,[189] myelokathexis has been suggested to result from retention of neutrophils in the marrow ("kathexis" = retention), where they eventually undergo apoptosis, evident in their diminished expression of the antiapoptotic factor bcl-x.[458]

The neutropenia and excessive granulocyte apoptosis associated with WHIM syndrome are partially corrected by G-CSF or GM-CSF therapy, with responses typically seen within 4 to 8 hours of administration.[455,458] Immunoglobulin levels also return to normal in patients treated with G-CSF.[455]

Shwachman-Diamond Syndrome

Shwachman-Diamond syndrome, a rare multiorgan disease inherited as an autosomal recessive trait, includes clinical findings of neutropenia, pancreatic exocrine insufficiency, short stature, and metaphyseal chondrodysplasia.[464-466] The pancreatic acini are largely replaced by fatty tissue with relative sparing of the pancreatic ducts and islets.[465,466] Patients are at risk for the development of progressive bone marrow failure and eventual conversion to MDS/AML.[464] Growth failure and short stature are usually noted during the first or second year of life, and puberty is often delayed.

Patients may be seen in infancy because of eczema, skin infections, and otitis media; pneumonia, osteomyelitis, and sepsis can also be present. Pancreatic insufficiency is typically manifested in early infancy as steatorrhea, weight loss, and failure to thrive. Later in childhood, pancreatic function may improve, thus rendering the clinical diagnosis elusive.[467] Serum levels of trypsinogen or pancreatic isoamylase are generally low, but not specifically diagnostic. Mild abnormalities of the liver, including hepatomegaly or elevated serum liver enzymes, are seen in 50% to 75% of younger patients but are usually mild and tend to resolve with age.

Common skeletal abnormalities include metaphyseal dysostosis in about 50% of affected children, most often involving the femoral head but generally asymptomatic.[465] Other anomalies include rib cage defects (shortened ribs with flared ends, costochondral thickening, and a narrow rib cage), clinodactyly, syndactyly, pes cavus, kyphosis, scoliosis, osteopenia, vertebral collapse, slipped femoral epiphysis, and supernumerary digits.[465] Skeletal radiologic findings can include "cup" deformation of the ribs, metaphyseal widening and hypoplasia of the iliac bones, and extremity shortening,[468] but these abnormalities may not be detectable until after 12 months or even several years of age.[465]

Neutropenia is the most common hematologic manifestation of the syndrome, although anemia or thrombocytopenia can also occur.[465,467,469] Neutrophil counts fall below 1000 cells/μL in approximately two thirds of patients, with no reciprocal monocytosis, but the neutropenia may be intermittent. Some patients also have a defect in chemotaxis that may contribute to the increased susceptibility to pyogenic infection.[470,471] Anemia is also seen frequently, and a fourth of patients have mild to moderate thrombocytopenia.[465,467,469] Bone marrow studies have generally shown some degree of myeloid hypoplasia,[465,467,469] but this finding is not diagnostic.

Evaluation of immune function in 11 patients with Shwachman-Diamond syndrome[472] identified varying degrees of impairment in the number or function of B cells (including low IgG or IgG subclasses, low percentage of circulating B cells, decreased in vitro proliferative responses, and diminished antibody or isohemagglutinin production), T cells (low circulating total CD3$^+$ cells or CD3$^+$/CD4$^+$ ratio, inverse CD4/CD8 ratios, and low mitogen responses), and NK cells.

The diagnosis of Shwachman-Diamond syndrome may be based on a combination of neutropenia, possibly other types of cytopenia, pancreatic insufficiency, and skeletal anomalies.

Around 90% of patients who meet the clinical criteria harbor mutations in the Shwachman-Bodian-Diamond syndrome gene *SBDS*.[469,473] The majority of mutations appear to arise from gene conversion events, with an adjacent pseudogene producing a protein with diminished expression or function.[474] The SBDS protein is localized throughout the cell but shuttles into the nucleolus, the major cellular site of ribosome biogenesis, in a cell cycle–dependent manner.[475] Studies in yeast indicate that the protein may function in ribosomal RNA maturation, thus suggesting that Shwachman-Diamond syndrome may share some ribosomal pathobiologic mechanisms with other bone marrow failure syndromes.[467,469]

Treatment includes pancreatic enzyme replacement, which does not improve the neutropenia or dwarfism. Steatorrhea tends to diminish with time, although the pancreatic insufficiency persists.[476] The frequency of bacterial infections can vary between patients, but they generally respond to appropriate antibiotics. Administration of G-CSF increases the neutrophil count to the normal range[465,469] and should used in patients with persistently severe neutropenia and recurrent or life-threatening infections. However, aplastic anemia or MDS develops in up to a fourth to a third of patients, often with the acquisition of a structural chromosomal abnormality.[465,469,474] Hence, regular blood counts are recommended and bone marrow examination should be performed annually—or even more frequently in the face of evolving peripheral blood findings.[465] As is the case for SCN and other congenital bone marrow failure syndromes, there is a high risk of subsequent leukemic transformation if MDS develops. However, cytogenetic abnormalities, particularly i(7q), may be transient or unaccompanied by marrow dysplasia. Thus, criteria for HSCT in this disease remain unclear at the present time.

Albinism-Neutropenia Syndromes

This group of rare primary immunodeficiency syndromes derives from autosomal recessive defects in the biogenesis or trafficking of lysosomes and related late endosomal organelles.[477] As a result, they share varying degrees of overlap in phenotype, including defects in the formation of melanosomes (hence partial albinism), abnormal platelet function, and immunologic defects involving not only neutrophil number but also the function of neutrophils, B lymphocytes, and cytotoxic T lymphocytes.

CHS is a rare genetic disorder characterized by partial oculocutaneous albinism, giant lysosomes in many cell types, including granulocytes, and neuropathy.[478-485] Most patients have moderate neutropenia, apparently caused by ineffective granulopoiesis, and are at high risk for the development of hemophagocytic lymphohistiocytosis (HLH). CHS is described in detail in a later section of this chapter.

Hermansky-Pudlak syndrome, another rare autosomal recessive disease characterized by oculocutaneous albinism, is best known for associated platelet defects (see Chapter 29). One subtype, Hermansky-Pudlak syndrome type 2, also includes neutropenia and decreased numbers of NK cells and therefore leads to increased susceptibility to infections.[486] The *AP3B1* gene responsible for this disorder,[487] as well as for cyclic neutropenia in gray collie dogs,[488] encodes an adapter protein involved in shuttling granule proteins, including neutrophil elastase, and thus may provide a connection to the molecular pathology of SCN.[407,488]

Griscelli's syndrome type 2 falls within the spectrum of Griscelli syndrome subtypes that share a phenotype of hypomelanosis with varying degrees of neurologic impairment and immunodeficiency.[489] The type 2 variant is characterized by neutropenia, hypogammaglobulinemia, partial albinism, and (like CHS) a predisposition to terminal lymphohistiocytic proliferation with hemophagocytosis.[490] It is caused by mutations in the *RAB27A* gene,[491] which encodes a small GTPase that serves as a key effector of granule exocytosis.[492]

Cohen's syndrome is an autosomal recessive condition that includes neutropenia, pigmentary retinopathy, developmental delay, and facial dysmorphism.[493] The gene responsible for Cohen's syndrome, *COH1*, shares homology to a yeast protein that functions in vesicular sorting and intracellular protein trafficking.

A single Mennonite family has been described with severe chronic neutropenia combined with short stature, albinism, coarse facial features, and recurrent bronchopulmonary infections with *Streptococcus pneumoniae*.[494] This syndrome is caused by defects in the endosomal adaptor protein p14, which is involved in MAPK signaling to late endosomes.[477]

Familial Benign Neutropenia

Familial benign neutropenia is characterized by mild neutropenia and no tendency for increased infections. Autosomal dominant transmission has been identified in some familial cases.[495] Familial benign neutropenia has been described in Yemenite Jews,[496] American and African blacks,[497] and Germans, French, Americans, and South Africans.[498]

Other Causes of Neutropenia Resulting from Intrinsic Defects in Myelopoiesis

Congenital or acquired bone marrow failure syndromes, including Fanconi's anemia, dyskeratosis congenita, aplastic anemia, and MDS, can occasionally be manifested as isolated neutropenia. Fanconi's anemia and dyskeratosis congenita should usually be easily recognized by other features associated with these disorders (see Chapter 8).[499]

Schimke's Immuno-osseous Dysplasia

This rare autosomal recessive syndrome with variable expressivity is characterized by spondyloepiphyseal dysplasia, focal segmental glomerulosclerosis leading to steroid-resistant nephritic syndrome and renal failure, lymphopenia with defective cellular immunity, neutropenia, and other types of cytopenia.[500,501] Vaso-occlusive processes, including cerebral and generalized atherosclerosis, are a life-limiting complication in the more severely affected patients.[502] The disorder is associated with mutations in the gene *SMARCAL1*, which encodes the swi/snf-related matrix-associated actin-dependent regulator of chromatin, subfamily a–like 1 protein,[503] although the genetics may be heterogeneous.[504] The immunodeficiency and cytopenia can be treated with HSCT[505]; neutropenia, seen in a few patients, responds to G-CSF or GM-CSF therapy.[501]

Neutropenia Caused by Extrinsic Factors

Infection

The most common cause of transient neutropenia in childhood is viral infection. Viruses commonly causing neutropenia include cytomegalovirus, Epstein-Barr virus, hepatitis A and B, HIV, influenza A and B, measles, respiratory syncytial virus, parvovirus B19, rubella, and varicella.[506-513] Neutropenia develops during the first 24 to 48 hours of the illness and may persist for 3 to 6 days. This period usually corresponds to the time of acute viremia and may relate to virus-induced redistribution of neutrophils from the circulating to the marginated granulocyte pool, sequestration, or increased neutrophil utilization after tissue damage by the viruses.[514,515] Several human viruses, including measles and herpes simplex virus, have been demonstrated to replicate in human endothelial cells and lead to the expression of receptors on endothelium for immune complexes containing IgG and C3, which might potentially promote enhanced neutrophil adhesion to the endothelium.[516,517] Acute transient neutropenia often occurs during the early stages of infectious mononucleosis[518,519] and may be related to both direct infection of progenitors[507] and accelerated destruction of neutrophils by antineutrophil antibodies.[520,521] Parvovirus B19 can cause transient neutropenia and can also be associated with prolonged neutropenia with or without the development of antineutrophil antibodies.[506,522-524]

Leukopenia is commonly seen in patients with AIDS.[508,525,526] In the pediatric AIDS population, neutropenia can be caused by antiviral drugs, vitamin B$_{12}$ or folate deficiency, or cellular immune dysfunction.[527] Neutropenia in HIV infection can also be associated with hypersplenism and antineutrophil antibodies.[528,529]

Significant neutropenia may occur during typhoid, paratyphoid, tuberculosis, brucellosis, tularemia, and rickettsial infections.[512,513,530-532] The mechanisms responsible for neutropenia in these conditions remain ill defined. During periods of relapsing fever caused by acute vivax malaria, the apparent neutropenia may be secondary to increased neutrophil margination in the intravascular compartment.[533]

Sepsis is one of the more serious causes of neutropenia. The neutropenia in patients with bacteremia and endotoxemia may result from excessive destruction of neutrophils and depletion of the bone marrow reserve pool. This consumption can occur after the phagocytosis of microbes, from the release of metabolites of arachidonic acid, or as a result of activation of the complement system through either the alternative or classical pathway.

The resultant generation of the chemoattractant C5a induces neutrophil aggregation and leads to the formation of leukoemboli, which adhere to and damage endothelial surfaces in the pulmonary capillary bed. Complement-mediated neutropenia may also occur transiently during hemodialysis, during continuous-flow leukapheresis, and after burn injury.[534-537]

Significant neutropenia occurs most commonly in neonatal bacterial sepsis. Newborns can exhaust their neutrophil reserves during overwhelming bacterial infection because their neutrophil storage pool is small and neutrophil production is already near a maximum.[538] Septic newborns may benefit from granulocyte transfusion[539-542] or G-CSF,[543-547] but clinical trials have not yet provided compelling evidence for benefit from either modality.

Drug-Induced Neutropenia

Drug-induced neutropenia is a disorder characterized by a severe and selective reduction in levels of circulating blood neutrophils (usually to levels of less than 200 cells/µL) and is due to an idiosyncratic reaction to the offending drug (Table 21-9).[548-562] This definition thus excludes disorders in which other cell lines are perturbed (such as aplastic anemia), those in which drug administration is not a feature, and the predictable neutropenia observed with anticancer therapy. Implicit in this definition is the unpredictability of the condition. Although the majority of patients will recover, drug-induced neutropenia is a serious disorder with high morbidity (e.g., deep tissue infection and sepsis) and recent mortality rates of 5%, but most deaths occur in patients who are elderly or have metabolic complications such as shock or renal failure.[548]

Idiosyncratic reactions tend to develop more frequently in women than in men and more often in older than in younger persons.[552] Drugs reported to have been associated with agranulocytosis have been extensively reviewed.[548,549,551,554,556,560,561] The most common drug classes include antimicrobial agents, particularly sulfonamides and penicillins; antithyroid drugs; antipsychotics such as phenothiazines and clozapine; antipyretics, particularly aminopyrine; antirheumatics, including gold, levamisole, and penicillamine; and sedatives, including barbiturates and benzodiazepines (see Table 21-9).

Although the underlying mechanisms for most drug-induced neutropenia are unknown, most studies suggest that they can be classified as leading to toxic suppression of neutrophil formation or immune destruction of mature cells.[551,553,560,561] First, differences in drug pharmacokinetics can lead to toxic levels of the drug or metabolites in the marrow microenvironment. An example is the neutropenia induced by sulfasalazine. Although neutropenia can be observed in any patient taking this drug, individuals who are slow acetylators show much greater toxicity than do those who are fast acetylators.[559] Second, a susceptible patient's myeloid precursors may be abnormally sensitive to typical drug concentrations. Phenothiazines induce neutropenia by this mechanism in that myeloid precursors in the marrow are particularly sensitive to these agents.[551,561,563] The toxic damage induced by phenothiazines is manifested as a neutropenia that appears 20 to 40 days after the patient has started taking the drug. Neutropenia secondary to drug-induced myelosuppression is usually insidious in onset and may be asymptomatic. Oral mucositis may be the first clinical sign before infectious complications occur.

Drugs can also induce immune-mediated peripheral destruction of neutrophils by alternative mechanisms. In one, the drug serves as a hapten in promoting the synthesis of antibodies that are capable of destroying mature neutrophils. Aminopyrine, penicillin, propylthiouracil, and gold can cause neutropenia by this mechanism.[551,555,558,561] Alternatively, the drug can elicit the formation of circulating immune complexes that attach to the surface of the neutrophil and lead to its destruction, as in the case of quinidine. In addition, immunologic changes induced by drugs can suppress granulopoiesis. For example, activation of both cellular and humoral immune responses has been reported to impair myelopoiesis after therapy with quinidine and phenytoin, respectively.[553,561] Drug-induced immune neutropenia is characterized by an abrupt onset—often with fever, chills, and prostration—7 to 14 days after the first exposure to the drug or immediately after re-exposure.

The duration of drug-induced neutropenia is highly variable. Acute idiosyncratic drug reactions may last only a few days, whereas chronic idiosyncratic reactions may persist for months or years. By contrast, immune-mediated neutropenia usually lasts for 6 to 8 days. Once neutropenia occurs, the most important therapeutic action is, of course, to withdraw all drugs that are not absolutely essential, particularly those suspected of being myelotoxic. During recovery from drug-induced neutropenia, rebound leukocytosis accompanied by a left-shifted marrow and circulating immature leukocytes can occur. G-CSF therapy may hasten neutrophil recovery slightly, but evidence-based data to justify its routine use are lacking,[407,564,565] so the clinical indication is questionable unless the patient has a severe infection.

Autoimmune Neutropenia

Autoimmune neutropenia (AIN) can be seen as an isolated phenomenon, in association with other autoimmune diseases, or as a secondary manifestation of infection, drugs, or malignancy.[382,564,566] Many cases of chronic idiopathic neutropenia in children and adults are now recognized as being secondary to autoimmunity directed against neutrophils. In primary AIN, low circulating neutrophil counts are the only hematologic finding, and associated diseases or other factors that cause neutropenia are absent. The peak incidence of AIN occurs in infants and young children,[567,568] where it is generally a benign disorder that remits spontaneously, as discussed in the following section. Immune-mediated neutropenia

TABLE 21-9   Partial List of Drugs Causing Idiosyncratic Drug-Induced Neutropenia

Drug	POSSIBLE MECHANISM		
	Direct Suppression	Metabolite Suppression	Immune Destruction
ANTI-INFLAMMATORY AGENTS			
Aminopyrine			X
Ibuprofen			X
Indomethacin	X		
Phenylbutazone	X		
Sulfasalazine	X		
ANTIBIOTICS			
Chloramphenicol	X		
Dapsone		X	
Penicillins	X		X
Sulfonamides	X		
Trimethoprim/sulfamethoxazole	X		
ANTICONVULSANTS			
Phenytoin			X
Carbamazepine		X	
Valproic acid	X		
ANTITHYROID AGENTS			
Methimazole			X
Propylthiouracil			X
CARDIOVASCULAR AGENTS			
Hydralazine			X
Procainamide			X
Quinidine			X
PSYCHOTROPIC AGENTS			
Chlorpromazine	X		
Phenothiazines	X		
Clozapine	X		
OTHER			
Chlorpropamide			X
Cimetidine, ranitidine	X		
Levamisole			X
Ticlopidine			

Underlining indicates drugs with the highest relative risk for neutropenia and agranulocytosis. See text for references.

is also seen in association with other disorders (Box 21-5), where it is often referred to as secondary AIN.

Patients with AIN may have highly—and rapidly—varying neutrophil counts ranging from mild neutropenia (ANC < 1000 cells/μL) to agranulocytosis (ANC < 200 cells/μL). Monocytosis is common. Bone marrow examination generally shows normal to increased cellularity with myeloid hyperplasia and normal to increased numbers of mature neutrophils, although diminished neutrophils or maturation arrest at earlier stages of differentiation can also be seen.[382,564,566] Mild splenomegaly is occasionally present. The incidence of pyogenic infection is not always related to the degree of neutropenia,[382,388] and it is usually limited to cutaneous and respiratory infections. Serious infections are generally uncommon. Spontaneous remission resolves the process in most infants but occurs less commonly in older children (see the following section).

Neutrophil-specific cell surface antigens identified as targets of autoantibodies include NA1 and NA2, NB1,

ND1, and NE1.[265,266] The NA1 and NA2 antigens are glycosylated isoforms of the neutrophil immunoglobulin receptor FcγRIIIb (CD16) (see Table 21-6), and the NB1 antigen is a 58- to 64-kd GPI-anchored membrane glycoprotein found on the plasma membrane and secondary granules.[569] Then mechanisms that trigger autoantibody production are unknown. In children, primary AIN is usually associated with NA allele–specific antibodies, but secondary AIN is associated with pan-FcγRIIIb antibodies.[570]

To detect antineutrophil antibodies, a combination of an indirect granulocyte immunofluorescence test (GIFT) and granulocyte agglutination test (GAT) appears to result in optimal sensitivity and specificity.[265,266,571] These assays detect IgG and IgM antibodies, both of which been identified in AIN. In the GIFT assay, a panel of heterologous donor granulocytes is incubated with serum or plasma from patients and controls, and bound immunoglobulins are detected by a fluorescent dye–labeled antihuman immunoglobulin antibody and

Box 21-5	Disorders Associated with Immune-Mediated Neutropenia

AUTOIMMUNE DISORDERS

Autoimmune cytopenias (hemolytic anemia, immune thrombocytopenia purpura, Evans' syndrome)
Autoimmune lymphoproliferative syndrome
Felty's syndrome (arthritis, splenomegaly, leukopenia)
Primary biliary cirrhosis
Sjögren's syndrome
Scleroderma
Systemic lupus erythematosus

INFECTION

Infectious mononucleosis
HIV infection

MALIGNANCY

Leukemia
Lymphoma
Hodgkin's disease

HYPOGAMMAGLOBULINEMIAS, DYSGAMMAGLOBULINEMIAS

Common variable immunodeficiency
Hyper-IgM syndrome
IgA deficiency
X-linked agammaglobulinemia

ANGIOIMMUNOBLASTIC LYMPHADENOPATHY (CASTLEMAN'S DISEASE)

DRUG REACTION

quantitated by fluorescence microscopy or flow cytometry. The GIFT assay is analogous to the indirect antiglobulin (Coombs) test for erythrocyte antibodies. It is subject to false-positive results from anti-HLA antibodies unless they are specifically absorbed before testing. The analogous direct antineutrophil antibody test can be performed by detection of immunoglobulin bound to patient neutrophils, similarly detected by microscopy or flow cytometry. Importantly, the standard laboratory test for antineutrophil cytoplasmic antibody (ANCA) does *not* detect the antibodies responsible for AIN.

The GAT is less sensitive but is useful for detecting a subgroup of antibodies against antigens other than CD16, although these are not typical of AIN.[265,266,571] Neutrophil-binding immune complexes may also give positive results in these assays and may be important in the pathogenesis of neutropenia in Felty's syndrome.[572] Confirmatory testing of autoantibody specificity can be done by assay involving monoclonal antibody immobilization of granulocyte antigens, in which binding of patient sera to a panel of donor neutrophils is compared with binding of monoclonal antibodies of defined specificity.[571,573] Sera containing HLA antibodies requires preabsorption or other controls to determine whether there is specific antineutrophil activity. Because of the limited

sensitivity and specificity of these assays, even in combination, laboratory demonstration of antineutrophil antibodies may not always be necessary to make the diagnosis of AIN, and their interpretation depends on the specific clinical setting.

The neutropenia of AIN is presumed to primarily be due to peripheral destruction of antibody-coated neutrophils, which may be also be augmented by the deposition of C3. Phagocytosis of neutrophils in the spleens of AIN patients has been observed.[574] In some cases, antineutrophil antibodies also appear to interfere with myelopoiesis.[572,575,576] Impairment of phagocytosis, respiratory burst activity, and adhesion by neutrophil-directed antibodies has likewise been observed and may contribute to the risk of infection in AIN.[572,575,577]

Treatment of patients with immune neutropenia includes the judicious use of appropriate antibiotics for bacterial infections and antimicrobial mouthwashes and regular dental hygiene for mouth sores or gingivitis. Infections tend to be less frequent in patients with immune neutropenia than in those with the corresponding degree of neutropenia from other causes, probably because granulopoiesis is intact in most cases. Prophylactic administration of trimethoprim-sulfamethoxazole may be also helpful in the management of recurrent minor infections, although no controlled studies have addressed the efficacy of this approach.

For definitive therapy, administration of G-CSF, starting at low doses of 1 to 2 µg/kg/day, has been successful in increasing the neutrophil count to the normal range or even higher in patients with primary AIN, including secondary immune neutropenia and Felty's syndrome.[566,567,578,579] The initial response may be apparent within days of starting therapy, but up to 2 weeks may be required. Patients with a normal or high ANC during therapy may be weaned to very-low-dose or alternate-day administration of G-CSF. The incidence of bone pain appears to be higher in AIN than in hypoproductive neutropenia, probably as a result of expansion of the already hyperplastic bone marrow. Because most patients with immune neutropenia do not suffer serious infectious complications, G-CSF therapy should be reserved for those with serious or recurrent infections or multiple hospitalizations for febrile neutropenia.

Administration of intravenous immunoglobulin can result in normalization of the neutrophil count, but its efficacy is variable and often short lived.[566,567,578] Corticosteroids can raise the neutrophil count but may actually increase the risk for serious infection. Similarly, splenectomy can provide transient benefit that is offset by the risk for sepsis.

Chronic Benign Neutropenia and Autoimmune Neutropenia of Childhood

Most cases of what was termed chronic benign neutropenia of infancy and childhood are now believed to represent an AIN that has parallels to childhood idiopathic thrombocytopenic purpura.[566,567,578,580] The handful of

TABLE 21-10	Summary of Autoimmune Neutropenia of Childhood
Incidence	Most common cause of chronic neutropenia in infancy and childhood; incidence ≥1 per 100,0000 children per year
Clinical features	Median age at diagnosis, 8-11 months (range, 3-38 months). Slight female preponderance (56% F, 44% M)
	Relatively minor infections (otitis media, gingivitis, upper respiratory tract, skin) occur with increased frequency in some patients and respond well to antimicrobial therapy. Rare patients (usually young infants) have pneumonia or sepsis
Laboratory evaluation	Median ANC at time of diagnosis ≈200 neutrophils/μL (range, 0-500 cells/μL). Hemoglobin, platelet count generally normal. Antineutrophil antibodies can be detected in majority of patients and are often directed to the NA1 antigen (neutrophil FcγIII receptor). Bone marrow evaluation (if performed) shows normal to increased myelopoiesis, sometimes with a decrease in mature neutrophils or maturation arrest at earlier stages
Therapy	Antibiotics for acute infection; prophylactic antibiotics may be helpful in some patients with recurrent otitis media. Consider use of G-CSF in the event of serious infection or very high frequency of minor infections
Prognosis	Excellent. Although the ANC often remains below 500 cells/μL for 12 or more months, spontaneous remission occurs in almost all patients (median, 20 months; range, 6-54 months)

ANC, absolute neutrophil count; G-CSF, granulocyte colony-stimulating factor.

cases reported as "lazy leukocyte syndrome," characterized by profound neutropenia, normal-appearing bone marrow, and little increase in the peripheral blood neutrophil count in response to steroids or epinephrine,[581] are also likely to have been AIN of childhood.

AIN of childhood occurs predominantly in children younger than 3 years (Table 21-10). The median age at diagnosis is 8 to 11 months, with a range of 2 to 54 months.[566,567,578,580] There is a slight female preponderance. Although AIN of childhood is the most common cause of chronic neutropenia in the pediatric age group, it is still a relatively infrequent diagnosis, with an incidence of approximately 1 in 100,000 children per year.[385,582] However, this figure is probably an underestimate because of the generally benign course of the disorder.

The initial ANC is often in the severe range (<200 cells/μL) and may approach zero, usually with a relative monocytosis or eosinophilia, or both. Transient increases in circulating neutrophil counts can occur in response to infection. Other peripheral counts are normal for age, although mild thrombocytopenia (≥100,000 cells/μL) has been reported.[583] There is usually no family history of neutropenia.

Antineutrophil antibodies can be detected in almost all patients when a combination of immunofluorescence and agglutination assays are used, with repeated testing if necessary.[571,573,578,580] However, absence of detectable antibody does not exclude the diagnosis, and a positive result does not exclude SCN.[429] As in AIN in adults, antibodies are typically directed against neutrophil-specific antigens of the NA, NB, and ND loci. Antibody specificity to NA1, an allele of the neutrophil immunoglobulin FcγRIII receptor, is seen most commonly.[571,573,578,580] Some, but not all studies report a correlation between the strength of the antibody and the severity of clinical manifestations.[571,573,578,580] As the neutropenia resolves, antibodies gradually become undetectable. Bone marrow examination generally shows normal

to increased cellularity with myeloid hyperplasia and normal to increased numbers of mature neutrophils, although some patients with intramedullary destruction of neutrophils or their precursors may show a "maturation arrest." Some, but not all patients will manifest an increase in the peripheral neutrophil count in response to hydrocortisone or prednisone.

Bacterial infections in AIN of childhood are often increased in frequency but are mild (e.g., skin infections, upper respiratory infections, otitis media, gingivitis) and responsive to standard antibiotics.[385,575,584] Cellulitis involving the labia majora was seen in 23% of 26 girls with AIN in one series, often caused by *Pseudomonas aeruginosa*.[385] Pneumonia, sepsis, and meningitis have been reported only occasionally in infants with AIN.[575] Spontaneous remission occurs in almost all patients, with neutropenia persisting for a median duration of 20 months.[584] Children younger than 9 months at the time of diagnosis may recover normal peripheral neutrophil counts more rapidly.[583] With increasing age, spontaneous remission becomes less likely.

The diagnosis of AIN of childhood is generally straightforward if the signs and symptoms occur within the first 2 years of life, there is no history of serious infections over a period of several months of observation, and neutrophil morphology and other peripheral counts are otherwise normal. Demonstration of antineutrophil antibody is not necessary for diagnosis in a patient with the typical clinical features of childhood AIN (see Table 21-10). Because of the association of AIN with immunodeficiency syndromes (see later in this section), evaluation of immunoglobulin levels should be performed to exclude dysgammaglobulinemia or hypogammaglobulinemia. If lymphopenia or clinical signs of cell-mediated immunodeficiency are present, T-cell function should also be studied. Bone marrow examination should always be performed if hematologic abnormalities other than neutropenia are present, if the child's age falls outside the usual range for AIN of infancy, or if the patient has an unusual or deep-seated infection suggesting poor marrow neutrophil reserve. Other laboratory tests to consider are outlined later in this section.

Febrile episodes should be managed aggressively, including the use of broad-spectrum parenteral antibiotics, in the initial period before the diagnosis of childhood AIN is established. However, once the diagnosis is definite and the patient has had no serious infections, subsequent febrile illnesses can be managed more conservatively if clinically warranted. Prophylactic trimethoprim-sulfamethoxazole can be helpful in children with recurrent otitis media and other minor infections. Administration of G-CSF results in an increased peripheral neutrophil count in childhood AIN and is the treatment of choice for the rare child with AIN who manifests very severe or recurrent major infections.[566,567,578,580] G-CSF doses of 1 to 2 μg/kg/day or less are usually effective, and responses are typically seen within days. Steroids and intravenous gamma globulin have also been used but have limited efficacy, as discussed earlier.

Neonatal Immune Neutropenia

Immune-mediated neutropenia in the newborn may be alloimmune and be due to maternal immune response to fetal alloantigens or may be isoimmune and be due to passive transfer of maternal autoantibody.

Neonatal alloimmune neutropenia, an immunologic disorder analogous to Rh hemolytic disease, results from maternal sensitization to fetal neutrophils bearing antigens that differ from the mother's. Maternal IgG antibodies cross the placenta and result in an immune-mediated neutropenia that can be severe and last from several weeks to as long as 6 months.[266,568,585] During the neutropenic phase, the infant's bone marrow demonstrates myeloid hyperplasia, usually with depletion of mature neutrophil forms.

Neutrophil antibodies are found in the serum of the mother and the infant and are frequently directed to the neutrophil-specific NA antigen system. The NA1 and NA2 antigens are two isotypes of the neutrophil FcγRIII receptor (see Table 21-6). Affected infants may be asymptomatic or can exhibit omphalitis, cutaneous infections, pneumonia, sepsis, and meningitis. Because neonatal sepsis can itself be associated with profound neutropenia, the underlying immune-mediated neutrophil destruction may not be appreciated immediately in affected newborns with sepsis.

The initial management of neonatal alloimmune neutropenia should include parenteral antibiotics, even if signs of infection are absent, because of the association of neutropenia with neonatal sepsis. Intravenous gamma globulin may sometimes be effective in increasing neutrophil counts.[586,587] Treatment with G-CSF, starting at 5 to 10 μg/kg/day intravenously, should be considered for very profound neutropenia or when serious infections develop in infants with alloimmune neutropenia.[568,588,589]

Neonatal immune neutropenia can also occur in infants of mothers with AIN. Transplacental passage of an IgG antineutrophil antibody can react with the infant's neutrophils bearing the inciting antigen and result in a profound neutropenia lasting 2 to 4 weeks.[568,590] Treatment is similar to that for isoimmune neutropenia. Leukoagglutinating antibodies directed against HLA antigens are frequently found in multiparous women and their newborn children's sera[591,592]; these antibodies are not associated with neutropenia and thus need to be distinguished from neutrophil-specific antibodies in laboratory assays.[571,585]

Neutropenia Associated with Immune Dysfunction

Primary disorders of immunoglobulin production have been associated with neutropenic syndromes.[593-595] A third of males with X-linked agammaglobulinemia have neutropenia at some time during the course of their disease.[593,595] Persistent or cyclic neutropenia is common in patients with the hyper-IgM immunodeficiency syndrome, which in many instances appears to be secondary to the formation of autoantibodies.[593,595] Immunoglobulin replacement therapy abolished the neutropenia in some, but not all of these patients.[596] AIN and other autoimmune cytopenias can also be seen in common variable immunodeficiency and isolated IgA deficiency.[593,594]

Autoimmune lymphoproliferative syndrome (ALPS), which reflects a family of defects in lymphocyte apoptosis, is characterized by lymphadenopathy, splenomegaly, and a variety of autoimmune disorders, including immune thrombocytopenia, anemia, and neutropenia.[597,598] The neutropenia associated with ALPS tends to be chronic and, because of the unique pathophysiology of the underlying disorder, represents one of the few forms of neutropenia treated by immunosuppression with corticosteroids or mycophenolate mofitil.[598,599]

Cartilage-hair hypoplasia, an autosomal recessive disorder found frequently in the Amish population, is characterized by short-limbed dwarfism, fine hair, moderate neutropenia (100 to 2000 cells/μL), and impaired cell-mediated immunity.[600,601] The disorder arises from mutations in the noncoding RNA gene *RMRP*,[602] which provides the RNA subunit of the RNase mitochondrial RNA-processing enzyme, a complex involved in multiple cellular RNA-processing events.[603] G-CSF therapy has been reported to be effective in a single patient who also had an antineutrophil antibody[604]; bone marrow transplantation has corrected both the immunologic defects and the neutropenia.[605]

Neutropenia can be seen as part of a broader spectrum of disease in a variety of other disorders of the immune system. Autoimmune disorders such as systemic lupus can be associated with antibody- or immune complex–mediated destruction of neutrophils or their precursors, as discussed earlier. G-CSF therapy is effective but may precipitate flares of the underlying disease.[606,607] Finally, in patients with HIV infection, neutropenia is common and has multiple causes, including antiretroviral drugs, cellular immune dysfunction, ineffective hematopoiesis, antineutrophil antibodies, and hypersplenism.[526-529]

T-cell large granular lymphocyte leukemia (LGL), a clonal disorder of cytotoxic T lymphocytes most common in the elderly, is often manifested as severe chronic neutropenia, with or without accompanying anemia.[407,608] LGL-associated neutropenia, which overlaps clinically with Felty's syndrome, may derive from either immune complex– or cell-mediated mechanisms and generally responds to a combination of immunosuppressive and cytotoxic therapy for the underlying disease and G-CSF for the neutropenia.[407]

Neutropenia Associated with Metabolic Diseases

Significant neutropenia, often with a relative monocytosis, occurs in Barth's syndrome, a distinctive X-linked disorder also associated with dilated cardiomyopathy, growth retardation, and 3-methylglutaconic aciduria.[609,610] Symptoms develop in infancy or childhood in affected boys, and neutropenia can precede the development of cardiac abnormalities. Children suffering from hyperglycinemia, isovaleric acidemia, propionic acidemia, methylmalonic acidemia, and tyrosinemia may also have significant neutropenia, although clinically it is not as consequential as other features of the disorders.[611-618] The mechanisms underlying the neutropenia associated with disorders of organic acid metabolism are not known, but the finding that propionate and isovalerate impair the development of myeloid colonies in vitro suggests that altered levels of metabolites may suppress myelopoiesis in vivo.[619]

Neutrophils in patients with glycogen storage disease type IB are not only diminished in number, with neutrophil counts commonly less than 500 cells/µL,[611,612,620,621] but also functionally defective, with abnormalities reported in chemotaxis, respiratory burst activity, and bacterial killing.[612,614] There is no correlation between a given mutation in the microsomal glucose-6-phosphate gene and the clinical severity of neutropenia or systemic complications of the enzyme deficiency, thus indicating that other genes can modify the phenotype.[622] Recombinant G-CSF has been effective in correcting the neutropenia and reducing serious infections in glycogen storage disease type IB.[623] Prolonged use of G-CSF has not been associated with any increased risk for MDS/AML in this disease.[444]

Macrocytic anemia, often accompanied by neutropenia or thrombocytopenia, is a hematologic hallmark of Pearson's syndrome, a rare and fatal congenital disorder involving not only the hematopoietic system but also the exocrine pancreas, liver, and kidneys.[624] The bone marrow shows normal cellularity, but striking abnormalities include vacuolization of erythroid and myeloid precursors, hemosiderosis, and ringed sideroblasts. A mitochondrial defect related to large deletions in mitochondrial DNA, whose integrity depends on a specific DNA polymerase, probably leads to impaired hematopoiesis.[625]

Nutritional Deficiencies

Ineffective granulopoiesis is part of the megaloblastic marrow pathology observed in patients with nutritional deficiencies of vitamin B_{12} or folic acid.[626] As a reflection of the increased neutrophil turnover secondary to ineffective myelopoiesis, serum muramidase levels are often elevated.[626] Neutropenia also occurs with starvation in such conditions as anorexia nervosa[627] and marasmus in infants, as well as occasionally in patients maintained by parenteral feeding. In addition, neutropenia and marrow megaloblastosis have been observed in patients thought to have copper deficiency because these patients responded promptly to copper replacement.[628] Notably, these nutritional deficiencies do not cause isolated neutropenia; anemia is virtually universal and thrombocytopenia is an occasional additional finding.

Reticuloendothelial Sequestration

Splenic enlargement as a result of portal hypertension, intrinsic splenic disease, or splenic hyperplasia can lead to neutropenia. The usual picture is one of moderate neutropenia, usually accompanied by similar degrees of thrombocytopenia and anemia. The reduced neutrophil survival corresponds with the size of the spleen, and the extent of neutropenia is proportional to bone marrow compensatory mechanisms.[629] The neutropenia is usually mild and may be ameliorated by successful treatment of the underlying disease. Bed rest alone may lead to restoration of the neutrophil counts because of a reduction in portal pressure. In selected situations, splenectomy may be necessary to restore the neutrophil count to normal. Histiocytic disorders (see Chapter 24, Histiocytosis, in *Oncology of Infancy and Childhood*) may also cause reticuloendothelial hyperplasia leading to neutropenia and anemia secondary to the ingestion of neutrophils and red cells.[549]

Bone Marrow Infiltration

Malignancies—including leukemia, lymphoma, and solid tumors—that infiltrate the bone marrow result in a myelophthisic picture characterized by leukoerythroblastic peripheral blood smears with neutropenia, usually accompanied by other cytopenias. Tumor-induced myelofibrosis may further reduce the peripheral blood neutrophil count.[630] Neutropenia can also result from bone marrow involvement in granulomatous infections, lysosomal storage disease, or osteopetrosis.[631-633]

Chronic Idiopathic Neutropenia

Chronic idiopathic neutropenia represents a group of disorders that by definition, are poorly understood and cannot be placed in any of the aforementioned categories.[407,634] Investigation of the mechanism of neutropenia has suggested that in some cases, decreased or ineffective production of neutrophils may be the result of excessive apoptosis, as in congenital neutropenia.[635] Overall, the clinical features, bone marrow findings, and natural history of chronic idiopathic neutropenia are variable but generally milder than those of congenital neutropenia; it is likely that many of the patients described in older studies had antibody-mediated neutrophil destruction and normal bone marrow reserve.[634,636] Treatment, when necessary, should be based on the severity of symptoms; G-CSF has proved effective at lower doses than needed for SCN and without any reported increase in risk for MDS/AML.[417]

Evaluation of Patients with Neutropenia

The basic approach to a patient with neutropenia includes a history and physical examination with emphasis on (1) related phenotypic abnormalities; (2) determination of whether bacterial infection is present (including evaluation of the gingiva and perineum); (3) evaluation of lymphadenopathy, hepatosplenomegaly, and any other signs of an underlying associated chronic illness; and (4) a history of recent infection and drug exposure. The frequency and duration of symptoms are important, and a history of periodontitis, dental abscesses, or tooth loss is particularly suspicious for significant chronic or recurrent neutropenia. The family history may reveal other individuals with recurrent infection. Unexplained deaths in children younger than 1 year and the race and ethnic background of each patient should be noted.

The duration and severity of the neutropenia and the presence or absence of significant other symptoms or physical findings greatly influence the speed and extent of laboratory evaluation. If the patient has isolated neutropenia and is asymptomatic and if other findings are absent, clinical observation for several weeks is usually the best approach. Any medications known or suspected to be associated with neutropenia should be discontinued. Any signs of an acute bacterial infection in a patient with moderate to severe neutropenia and fever call for prompt evaluation and treatment, including the use of intravenous broad-spectrum antibiotics.

Patients with persistent neutropenia should have white blood and differential counts obtained twice weekly for 6 to 8 weeks to evaluate for periodicity suggestive of cyclic neutropenia. Direct and indirect antiglobulin (Coombs) tests should be performed to evaluate for the presence of red cell autoantibodies, and serum immunoglobulins (IgG, IgA, and IgM, but not IgE) should be measured to detect associated immunoglobulin abnormalities. HIV testing is also indicated in chronic cases. Antineutrophil antibody testing, though technically imperfect, is generally included in an initial evaluation because of the frequency of AIN.

Bone marrow aspiration and biopsy with cytogenetics should be part of the initial evaluation if leukoerythroblastosis, anemia, macrocytosis, or thrombocytopenia is present and should be performed eventually if the diagnosis remains obscure despite initial testing. If SCN is suspected, bone marrow analysis with cytogenetic screening for monosomy 7 should be performed both to establish the diagnosis and to provide a baseline before G-CSF therapy. Other laboratory tests that should be considered, depending on the clinical situation, include evaluation for collagen vascular disease, exocrine pancreatic insufficiency, and metabolic disorders (e.g., organic acidurias), as well as measurement of vitamin B_{12}, folate, and copper levels. Radiographic studies of the femoral heads, rib cage, and spine may be useful in the diagnosis of Shwachman-Diamond syndrome. Assessing the response of the peripheral neutrophil count to a single dose of corticosteroid may be useful for assessment of bone marrow reserves and, if normal, may indicate a more benign course[637] but should not relax clinical vigilance for febrile neutropenia.

Principles of Therapy for Neutropenia

Management of neutropenia depends on the underlying cause and severity of the neutropenia. The major concern in neutropenic patients is the development of serious pyogenic infection. Patients with severe neutropenia (ANC ≤ 500 cells/μL) and poor marrow reserves are at highest risk for progressive infection and septicemia. Fever may often be the only indication of infection inasmuch as local signs and symptoms of inflammation may be diminished in the face of neutropenia. Organisms involved are usually from the skin or gastrointestinal tract. Thus, febrile patients with severe neutropenia secondary to poor marrow function should be treated promptly with broad-spectrum antimicrobials after blood and other appropriate samples are obtained for culture. If the patient defervesces and blood cultures do not reveal any growth, the antibiotics should be continued for at least 2 to 3 days after the patient is afebrile. However, if the patient continues to have fevers of 38°C or higher, antimicrobial therapy should be continued despite negative blood cultures. Neutropenic patients who are febrile for more than 4 days while receiving broad-spectrum antibacterial antibiotics are at risk for fungal infection, so empirical treatment with antifungal antibiotics should be considered in this setting.[638] Neutropenic patients with documented fungal infection or gram-negative bacterial sepsis who have not responded to appropriate therapy are candidates for granulocyte transfusions.[539,639,640]

Neutropenic patients with normal to increased marrow cellularity, such as in the setting of AIN, often have a minimally increased risk of pyogenic infection and respond more briskly to appropriate antibiotics. A less aggressive course may be a reasonable approach to a febrile illness in such patients who clinically look well, even if the ANC is below 500 cells/μL. A child in whom the diagnosis of AIN of childhood has been established and fever or infection develops can generally be managed as an outpatient, unless the infection is severe.

An important component in the management of all patients with chronic or cyclic neutropenia is close attention to oral hygiene. Chronic gingivitis and periodontitis can be a persistent source of morbidity and result in tooth loss. All patients should receive regular dental care, along with regular use of antibiotic mouthwash.

The advent of recombinant G-CSF and other hematopoietic growth factors has revolutionized the treatment of neutropenia.[407,416,417,439,564,579] As discussed in previous sections, G-CSF has been successfully used to increase the neutrophil count in a wide variety of conditions, including SCN, cyclic neutropenia, and immune-mediated neutropenia. In some cases, chronic prophylactic use of G-CSF is recommended, such as in SCN, in which patients have poor marrow production of neutrophils and a high risk for the development of serious infection. For other causes of neutropenia in which patients tend to have fewer problems with infection, such as AIN, G-CSF therapy should be reserved for specific clinical indications such as repeated or progressive infection.

Antibiotic prophylaxis, usually with trimethoprim-sulfamethoxazole, may be useful in some neutropenic patients with normal to increased myelopoiesis who do not meet the criteria for G-CSF therapy.[579] There are no evidence-based data to indicate the effectiveness of reverse precautions or neutropenic diets in chronic neutropenia patients without concurrent immunosuppression, but careful hand washing is clearly indicated (as for all patients), and common sense suggests that avoidance of environmental mold exposure[638,641] might reduce the risk for invasive fungal infection.

Neutrophilia

Neutrophilia refers to an alteration in the total number of blood neutrophils that is in excess of about 7500 cells/μL in adults (Box 21-6). During the first few days of life the upper limit of the normal neutrophil count ranges from 7000 to 13,000 cells/μL for neonates born prematurely and at term gestation, respectively.[642] A decrease to adult levels occurs within the first few weeks of life and is maintained thereafter. An increase in circulating neutrophils is the result of a disturbance in the normal equilibrium involving neutrophil bone marrow production, movement in and out of the marrow compartments into the circulation, and neutrophil destruction (see Box 21-6). Three mechanisms, either alone or in combination, largely account for neutrophilia.[17,643] First, increased numbers of neutrophils may be mobilized from either the bone marrow storage compartment or the peripheral marginating pools into the circulating pool. Second, blood neutrophil survival may be increased because of impaired neutrophil egress into tissue. Finally, the circulating neutrophil pool might be expanded as a result of (1) increased progenitor cell proliferation and terminal differentiation through the neutrophilic series, (2) increased mitotic activity of neutrophilic cell precursors, or (3) shortening of the cell mitotic cycle in neutrophil precursors. Acute neutrophilia occurs rapidly within minutes in response to exercise or epinephrine-induced reactions and has been attributed to mobilization of the marginating pool of neutrophils into the circulating

Box 21-6	**Classification of Neutrophilia**

INCREASED PRODUCTION

Chronic infection
Chronic inflammation
    Ulcerative colitis
    Rheumatoid arthritis
Tumors (perhaps with necrosis)
Postneutropenia rebound
Myeloproliferative disease
Drugs (lithium; rarely ranitidine, quinidine)
Chronic idiopathic neutrophilia
Familial cold urticaria
Leukemoid reactions

ENHANCED RELEASE FROM MARROW STORAGE POOL

Corticosteroids
Stress
Hypoxia
Acute infection
Endotoxin

DECREASED EGRESS FROM CIRCULATION

Corticosteroids
Splenectomy
Leukocyte adhesion deficiency

REDUCED MARGINATION

Stress
Infection
Exercise
Epinephrine

pool.[644,645] Slower onset of acute neutrophilia can occur after glucocorticoid administration or with inflammation or infection associated with the generation of endotoxin, TNF, IL-1, and a cascade of growth factors.[4,5,646,647] Maximal response usually occurs within 4 to 24 hours after exposure to these agents and is probably due to release of neutrophils from the marrow storage compartment into the circulation. Mechanisms that underlie release from the marrow pool involve interactions between neutrophils and the bone marrow stroma mediated by adhesion molecules such as β_2 integrins and by chemokines such as SDF-1 and its receptor CXCR4.[189] Glucocorticoids may also slow the egress of neutrophils from the circulation into tissue.[648] Less well understood mechanisms leading to delayed-onset acute neutrophilia have been reported after electric shock trauma, anesthesia, and surgery.[649-651]

Chronic neutrophilia is usually associated with continued stimulation of neutrophil production, possibly through perturbation of marrow feedback mechanisms. Chronic neutrophilia may accompany the prolonged administration of glucocorticoids, persistent inflammatory reactions, infection, chronic blood loss, or chronic anxiety.[652-656] Infections with pyogenic microorganisms, leptospira, and certain viruses (including herpes simplex, varicella, rabies, and poliomyelitis) may all produce neutrophilia.[657] Significant neutrophilic leukocytosis has also been reported with both Kawasaki's disease and infectious mononucleosis.[658,659] Occasionally, extreme neutrophilia has been observed in tuberculosis, generally in seriously ill patients with widespread necrotizing inflammatory disease.[660] Chronic inflammation is frequently responsible for persistent neutrophilia, especially in patients with juvenile rheumatoid arthritis.[661] Marked neutrophilia is a hallmark of functional disorders of neutrophils caused by impaired adhesion or motility, as in patients with LAD or actin dysfunction (see later). Sustained moderate neutrophilia invariably follows either surgical or functional asplenia,[662] probably because of decreased clearance of circulating neutrophils.[18]

Congenital primary neutrophilia is rare. In a single reported family with autosomal dominant hereditary neutrophilia, affected individuals maintained absolute granulocyte counts between 14,000 and 164,000 cells/µL, along with increased leukocyte alkaline phosphatase, hepatosplenomegaly, and Gaucher-type histiocytes.[663] Neutrophilia also occurs in familial cold urticaria, in which cold exposure elicits, after about 7 hours, elevated neutrophil counts, fever, urticaria, and a rash characterized histologically by a neutrophil infiltrate.[664,665]

Leukemoid Reactions

The elevation of normal leukocytes to counts greater than 50×10^3 cells/µL is referred to as a leukemoid reaction.[666] The peripheral blood may show small proportions of immature myeloid cells, including occasional myeloblasts and promyelocytes. Leukemoid reactions need to be distinguished from chronic myelogenous leukemia (CML), which features a more extreme "left shift" and basophilia in the peripheral blood differential count, as well as the characteristic clinical, laboratory, and cytogenetics signs of a myeloproliferative disorder (see Chapter 11, Myeloid Leukemia, Myelodysplasia and Myeloproliferative Disease in Children, in *Oncology of Infancy and Childhood*). Chronic neutrophilic leukemia is a distinct, extremely rare malignant cause of mature neutrophilia, with a mean age at diagnosis of 62.5 years (range, 15 to 86) in 33 reported cases.[667]

Leukemoid reactions can be triggered by pyogenic infections, especially those secondary to *S. aureus* or *S. pneumoniae*. Leukemoid reactions can also occur with tuberculosis, brucellosis, toxoplasmosis, and inflammatory syndromes such as acute glomerulonephritis, acute rheumatoid arthritis, liver failure, and diabetic acidosis.[666] A transient myeloid myeloproliferative disorder that can be difficult to distinguish from a leukemoid reaction may develop in infants with Down syndrome[668,669] (see Chapter 11, Myeloid Leukemia, Myelodysplasia and Myeloproliferative Disease in Children, in *Oncology of Infancy and Childhood*). However, more often there is marked leukoerythroblastosis, and large numbers of circulating blast cells can be present. Although the syndrome is transient, it portends a high risk for subsequent leukemia.[670] Leukemoid reactions have also been identified in neonates with thrombocytopenia–absent radius syndrome, but without any subsequent increased risk for leukemia.[671]

Clinical States Associated with Alterations in Eosinophil Number

Eosinophilia

Eosinophil stimulation most commonly occurs after repetitive or prolonged antigen exposure, especially when the antigens are deposited in tissues and elicit hypersensitivity reactions, whether of the immediate (IgE-mediated) or delayed (T lymphocyte–mediated) type. Stimulation of eosinophilia is T lymphocyte dependent and underlies the immune response to metazoan parasites.[6,7] A very broad range of conditions can elicit an eosinophilic response (Box 21-7).

Allergy is the most common cause of eosinophilia in children in the United States.[672] Acute allergic reactions may cause leukemoid eosinophilic responses, with eosinophil counts exceeding 20,000 cells/µL, whereas chronic allergy is rarely associated with eosinophil counts of greater than 2000 cells/µL.[673] A variety of skin diseases have been associated with eosinophilia,[674] the best documented being atopic dermatitis, eczema, pemphigus, acute urticaria, and toxic epidermal necrolysis. Drug reactions often elicit eosinophilia,[675] including the potentially fatal disorder "drug rash with eosinophilia and systemic symptoms" (DRESS syndrome).[676]

Outside the United States and hence also in immigrants and returning travelers, parasitic infections are the most common causes of eosinophilia.[677-679] Infestations by certain parasites, including helminths, induce greater degrees of eosinophilia than protozoan infestations do.[7,672,674] Although some parasite antigens appear to be potent immunogens, the eosinophilia resulting from parasitic infection is not due to some unique component of the parasites themselves but rather to a tissue granulomatous response requiring the participation of intact parasites. Other parasites, such as *Giardia lamblia*, *Enterobius vermicularis*, and *Trichuris trichiura*, fail to elicit an eosinophilic response, probably because they remain localized to the intestinal tract and do not enter the systemic circulation. When parasites invade systemic organs, they may incite clinical symptoms and signs related to the involved organs, such as hepatomegaly and pulmonary infiltrates.

These features are further associated with eosinophilic leukocytosis, anemia, and hyperglobulinemia, as commonly seen in visceral larva migrans from *Toxocara canis*. The patient may be brought for medical attention because of fever, cough, and wheezing. Complications include seizures, encephalitis, myocarditis, retinal lesions (which are often difficult to distinguish from retinoblastoma), and skin nodules on the palms of the hands and

Box 21-7	**Causes of Eosinophilia**

ALLERGIC DISORDERS

Acute urticaria
Allergic bronchopulmonary aspergillosis
Asthma
Atopic rhinitis
Drug reaction

DERMATITIS

Atopic dermatitis
Pemphigus, pemphigoid

PARASITES AND INFECTIONS

Amebiasis
Coccidioidomycosis
Fungal rhinosinusitis
Helminths (particularly if invasive)
Malaria
Scabies
Scarlet fever
Toxoplasmosis
Tuberculosis

GASTROINTESTINAL DISORDERS

Eosinophilic gastroenteritis
Food allergy

HEREDITARY DISORDERS

Familial eosinophilia
Hereditary angioedema

Hyper-IgE syndrome
Omenn's syndrome
Severe congenital neutropenia
Thrombocytopenia with absent radius
Wiskott-Aldrich syndrome

NEOPLASMS

Acute lymphoblastic leukemia
Lymphoma (Hodgkin's and non-Hodgkin's)
Metastatic cancer
Myeloproliferative disorders

RHEUMATOLOGIC DISORDERS

Eosinophilic fasciitis
Polyarteritis nodosa
Scleroderma

MISCELLANEOUS

Adrenal insufficiency
Graft-versus-host disease
Peritoneal dialysis or hemodialysis
Sarcoidosis
Toxins (eosinophilia/myalgia, toxic oil syndromes)

HYPEREOSINOPHILIC SYNDROME

Clonal HES
Idiopathic HES

soles of the feet. Leukocyte counts may exceed 100,000 cells/μL, with marked eosinophilia persisting from months to years after resolution of the symptoms. Polyclonal hypergammaglobulinemia is frequent. Increased anti-A and anti-B titers are commonly observed because of cross-reactivity between red cell and parasitic antigens.

In contrast to viral exanthems, scarlet fever is frequently associated with modest degrees of eosinophilia. Eosinophilia is also observed in cytomegalovirus pneumonia of infancy, cat-scratch disease, infectious lymphocytosis, and occasionally, infectious mononucleosis. Many patients with acute pulmonary tuberculosis show decreased numbers of circulating eosinophils followed by an increase in eosinophils during the convalescent phase, but rare patients exhibit marked eosinophilia at diagnosis.

In general, fungal diseases do not cause eosinophilia, but important exceptions are allergic and nonallergic fungal sinusitis and rhinosinusitis, coccidioidomycosis, and allergic bronchopulmonary aspergillosis.[674,680-682] The latter two diagnoses fit into the spectrum of pulmonary eosinophilic syndromes, which also include idiopathic eosinophilic pneumonia, Churg-Strauss syndrome (a form of vasculitis), tropical pulmonary eosinophilia (caused by microfilariae and other parasites), and drug- and radiation-induced pulmonary eosinophilia.[674,683,684]

Gastrointestinal disorders may also be associated with eosinophilia.[672,685] Primary eosinophil-mediated disorders usually involve the esophagus and stomach, but they can affect any or all segments of the gastrointestinal tract. Eosinophilia can also be a secondary sign of food allergy.[686] Inflammatory bowel disease and gluten enteropathy may involve large numbers of tissue eosinophils but show little or no elevation in blood eosinophil numbers.[685,687,688] Eosinophilia is a prominent feature of several immunodeficiency disorders, especially hyper-IgE (Job's) syndrome (see later), WAS, and Omenn's syndrome.[437,689] It can also be associated with hereditary angioedema, a defect in the complement C1 inhibitor.[690,691] In approximately 10% of patients with rheumatoid arthritis, mild eosinophilia develops during the course of their disease.

Autosomal dominant familial eosinophilia has been reported in several families in which individuals displayed marked eosinophilia, but few had pulmonary, cardiac, or neurologic involvement.[692,693] The disorder has been mapped to chromosome 5q31-q33, a region that contains a cytokine cluster that includes genes encoding IL-3, IL-5, and GM-CSF.[694] However no mutations or functional polymorphisms have been identified within the promoter, exons, or introns of any of these genes, thus suggesting that the primary defect in familial eosinophilia is located in another gene in the cluster. The disorder can be distinguished from HES (see later) by the relative absence of eosinophil activation markers and the rarity of end-organ damage.[693]

Marked eosinophilia can accompany or precede the diagnosis of malignancies, including Hodgkin's and non-Hodgkin's lymphoma, acute lymphoblastic leukemia, and a variety of solid tumors.[674,695,696] Excessive numbers of normal eosinophils may also be produced in response to the production of cytokines, primarily IL-5, by abnormal (but only sometimes clonal) T cells with aberrant immunophenotypic markers.[697] In about a third of patients undergoing chronic hemodialysis, blood eosinophilia develops without apparent cause.[698] Similarly, chronic peritoneal dialysis may cause an eosinophilic peritoneal effusion and occasionally an elevated number of eosinophils in blood.[699]

Eosinophilia can produce organ damage—particularly to the heart, lungs, and gastrointestinal tract—by infiltration and deposition of toxic granule proteins. If treatment of the underlying infection or disease is not sufficient to reduce the eosinophil count, steroid therapy generally produces a rapid decline in eosinophil production and circulating cell numbers. More recently, anti–IL-5 antibody therapy has shown promise as an alternative.[700]

Hypereosinophilic Syndrome

HES is defined as persistent eosinophilia in patients who meet the following criteria: (1) absolute eosinophil count of 1500 cells/μL or higher for longer than 6 months (or fatal termination within 6 months), (2) lack of other diagnoses to explain secondary eosinophilia, and (3) signs and symptoms of organ involvement by infiltrating eosinophils.[701] Clinical manifestations result from tissue infiltration by eosinophils and from tissue damage caused by the release of eosinophil granule products. Symptoms include nonspecific findings of fever, weight loss, and fatigue. Cardiac damage is the major cause of morbidity and mortality in HES and includes endocardial fibrosis and the formation of mural thrombi with infiltrating eosinophils (Löffler's endocarditis).[672,674,702-705] These findings can also be seen with eosinophilia of multiple other causes, including parasitic infection, drug reactions, and malignancies. Hepatosplenomegaly, pulmonary infiltrates, and skin involvement with urticarial or nodular lesions are common; neuropathies, encephalopathy, and CNS thromboembolism can also occur.

There is still controversy on the proper classification of HES in relation to chronic eosinophilic leukemia and idiopathic HES. One proposed subdivision, after elimination of reactive eosinophilias, classifies HES into clonal eosinophilias and idiopathic HES (i.e., everything else).[674,702] The clonal forms of HES can be further classified—and in many cases treatment guided—by identification of specific gene rearrangements.[674,702,703,706] The most common involve the gene encoding platelet-derived growth factor receptor α, *PDGFRA*, which forms

fusion products that generate constitutively active tyrosine kinase molecules.[706,707] Fusion partners include the Fip1-like 1 gene *FIP1L1* and, less commonly, *BCR* or *CDK5RAP2*, which encodes CDK5 regulatory subunit–associated protein 2. The *FIP1L1-PDGFRA* fusion results from an interstitial chromosome 4q12 deletion that is not cytogenetically detectable. This rearrangement results in HES with a marked male preponderance and a phenotype that includes splenomegaly, elevated serum vitamin B_{12} and tryptase levels, and hypercellular bone marrow with fibrosis and increased eosinophils and mast cells. Other patients with clonal HES have rearrangements of the gene encoding the platelet-derived growth factor receptor β, *PDGFRB*, and rare cases have been reported with rearrangements of *FGFR1* and other genes.[674,702] Most importantly, patients with either of the PDGFR fusion products are likely to respond to imatinib therapy, sometimes at doses lower than those used for CML.[702,704,707]

HES can generally be distinguished from the M4Eo variant of AML (see Chapter 11, Myeloid Leukemia, Myelodysplasia and Myeloproliferative Disease in Children, in *Oncology of Infancy and Childhood*), which is characterized by myelomonocytic blasts with eosinophilia and has been referred to in the past as eosinophilic leukemia.[708] In acute leukemia, there is typically a marked increase in the number of immature eosinophils in blood or marrow (or both), infiltration of tissue by immature cells of predominantly an eosinophilic type, and secondary anemia and thrombocytopenia. The eosinophils in M4Eo leukemia have an additional granule population that stains with periodic acid–Schiff and chloroacetate esterase. Almost all patients in the M4Eo leukemia subgroup have inversion or another cytogenetically detectable abnormality in chromosome 16.[709]

Eosinopenia

Eosinopenia is not uncommon but is seldom recognized clinically because its precise diagnosis requires an absolute eosinophil count.[710] Eosinopenia may be produced by at least two mechanisms: (1) acute stress, with resultant stimulation of adrenal corticoids or release of epinephrine (or both), and (2) acute inflammatory states. The immediate eosinopenia after the administration of glucocorticoids reflects the destabilization of mRNA encoding cytokines such as eotaxins and inhibition of the cytokine-dependent survival of eosinophils.[7,711] Glucocorticoids also suppress the transcription of a number of factors involved in eosinophil production and trafficking, including IL-3, IL-4, IL-5, and GM-CSF.[7] Acute inflammation is associated with alterations in eosinophil distribution and production that resemble those observed after corticosteroid administration. At least part of this response occurs independent of adrenal corticoid release. Acute infections associated with a marked inflammatory response, including invasive bacterial and most acute viral infections, may be accompanied by eosinopenia throughout the period of the fever. Chronic infections cause a less predictable eosinophil reaction.

Basophilia and Basophilopenia

Basophils are associated with hypersensitivity reactions of the immediate type[99,101,712] (Box 21-8). Basophil levels may be elevated in allergic responses, helminth infections, and chronic inflammatory diseases.[101,713,714] Most importantly, basophil levels are increased in myeloproliferative disorders such as CML (see Chapter 11, Myeloid Leukemia, Myelodysplasia and Myeloproliferative Disease in Children, in *Oncology of Infancy and Childhood*). Basophil counts exceeding 30% can occur during the course of CML; marked basophilia often heralds a poor prognosis,[715,716] and the cells may be morphologically and functionally abnormal.[717,718] Patients with marked basophilia may have symptoms attributable to the release of biogenic amines or heparin-like material from degranulated basophils[718,719] and may benefit from the administration of antihistamines. Increased numbers of marrow basophils may occur in MDS and sideroblastic anemia.[720,721] Peripheral blood or bone marrow basophilia may also be seen with AML, usually in association with 6p or 12p chromosomal abnormalities,[722] or juvenile myelomonocytic leukemia.[718] Basophilopenia occurs in conditions that are associated with eosinophilopenia, such as during acute infection or after the administration of glucocorticoids.[723-725] Basophil counts are diminished in thyrotoxicosis and after treatment with thyroid hormones, and conversely they may be increased in myxedema.[724]

Monocytosis and Monocytopenia

The normal absolute blood monocyte count varies with the age of the patient, and this variation must be taken into account when assessing monocytosis. During the first 2 weeks of life, the absolute monocyte count is greater than 1000 cells/μL.[726] With increasing age there is a gradual decline in the monocyte count until it reaches a plateau of 400 cells/μL in adulthood. Monocytosis may therefore be defined as a total monocyte count of greater than 500 cells/μL. Given the widespread importance of monocytes, as previously described, it is not surprising that many clinical disorders give rise to monocytosis (Box 21-9). Typically, monocytosis is associated with bacterial, protozoan, and rickettsial infections; examples include subacute bacterial endocarditis, tuberculosis, syphilis, Rocky Mountain spotted fever, and kala-azar.[114,727] Monocytosis is a hallmark of juvenile myelomonocytic leukemia (see Chapter 11, Myeloid Leukemia, Myelodysplasia and Myeloproliferative Disease in Children, in *Oncology of Infancy and Childhood*) and can also be observed in malignant disorders such as preleukemia, AML, CML, lymphomas, and advanced-stage carcinomas.[727,728] Approximately 25% of all patients with Hodgkin's disease have monocytosis, although its presence does not correlate with prognosis.[726] Monocytosis has also been noted in a wide variety of inflammatory and immune disorders, including lupus, rheumatoid arthritis, sarcoidosis, and inflammatory bowel disease.[727] Finally, as discussed earlier, both relative and absolute

---

Box 21-8 **Disorders Associated with Basophilia**

MILD BASOPHILIA

Hypersensitivity reactions
    Drug and food hypersensitivity
    Urticaria
Infection
    Helminths
    Chickenpox
    Influenza
    Smallpox
    Tuberculosis
Inflammation
    Rheumatoid arthritis
    Ulcerative colitis
Hypothyroidism (severe)

MARKED BASOPHILIA

Chronic myelogenous leukemia
Myelodysplastic syndrome
Acute myeloid leukemia (rare)

Box 21-9 **Disorders Associated with Monocytosis**

INFECTION

Subacute bacterial endocarditis
Tuberculosis
Syphilis
Protozoal and rickettsial infections (e.g., Rocky Mountain spotted fever, kala-azar)
Fever of unknown origin

MALIGNANCY

Preleukemia
Juvenile myelomonocytic leukemia
Acute myelogenous leukemia
Chronic myelogenous leukemia
Lymphoma (Hodgkin's and non-Hodgkin's)
Solid tumors (usually advanced carcinoma)

RHEUMATOLOGIC DISORDERS

System lupus erythematosus
Rheumatoid arthritis
Myositis

GRANULOMATOUS DISEASE

Ulcerative colitis
Crohn's disease
Sarcoidosis

MISCELLANEOUS DISORDERS

Severe chronic neutropenia
Recovery from transient neutropenia
Postsplenectomy status
Tetrachlorethane poisoning

monocytosis occurs in some forms of severe chronic neutropenia and in patients recovering from myelosuppressive chemotherapy. Monocytopenia has been observed after glucocorticoid administration and in infections associated with endotoxemia.[729,730] In the latter case, systemic activation of complement and deposition of C5a on the surface of monocytes lead to their aggregation and clearance. In contrast to the profound granulocytopenia and lymphopenia associated with irradiation or cytotoxic chemotherapy, noncirculating monocytes and tissue macrophages are relatively resistant to these agents.[731] Decreased monocyte superoxide production, chemotaxis, and microbial killing have been reported in Gaucher's disease, which possibly contributes to the risk of infection in patients with this disease.[732-734] The defects are reversed at least partially by enzyme replacement therapy.[732]

Infantile (malignant) osteopetrosis is an autosomal recessive disease caused by failure of bone resorption and remodeling by osteoclasts, a form of specialized tissue macrophage.[148,149,151] This disorder arises in infancy and is characterized by progressive obliteration of the bone marrow space by bone and leads to progressive loss of marrow function, hepatosplenomegaly, growth retardation, and compression of cranial nerves. Autosomal recessive osteopetrosis is caused by mutations in genes encoding a vacuolar proton pump or the ClC-7 chloride channel.[154,155] Autosomal dominant osteopetrosis, a less severe form, is also caused by ClC-7 gene mutations, probably with a dominant-negative phenotype.[735] Generation of superoxide by peripheral blood leukocytes is defective in patients with autosomal recessive (malignant) osteopetrosis,[736] and recombinant IFN-γ (also used for CGD; see later) has been shown to increase bone resorption and improve hematopoietic marrow function in children with infantile osteopetrosis.[158] Infantile osteopetrosis has been treated by bone marrow transplantation,[151,156] and promising studies in a mouse model of the disease suggest that gene therapy targeted at hematopoietic stem cells might be a future therapeutic approach.[157]

DISORDERS OF GRANULOCYTE AND MONONUCLEAR PHAGOCYTE FUNCTION

Abnormalities in one or more steps of phagocyte function—adhesion, chemotaxis, ingestion, degranulation, and oxidative metabolism—are causes of inherited and acquired clinical disorders, which can be classified on the basis of the function primarily affected. Consistent with the critical role of phagocyte function in host defense, patients afflicted with these disorders often suffer recurrent, difficult-to-treat bacterial and fungal infections in the skin or mucosa, lungs, lymph nodes, or deep tissue (abscesses). Many of these disorders have characteristic clinical and microbiologic features related to the particular functional defect. As will be seen, some of the disorders manifest abnormalities in several phagocyte functions. In these instances, the primary defect is used

to classify the disorder. Finally, inherited disorders involving cytokine receptors and their signal transduction are increasingly being recognized,[737] many of which affect phagocyte function and result in recurrent infections. These disorders are described near the end of this chapter.

During the past 25 years, numerous papers have been published that describe abnormalities in phagocyte function, often associated with other diseases. In many of these reports, marginal abnormalities were noted with the use of in vitro phagocyte assays, with little evidence that the observed defects were responsible for the clinical predisposition to infection. In this section, disorders in which good correlations exist between the phagocyte abnormality and the clinical condition will be emphasized. In several of these disorders, particularly LAD and CGD, the molecular basis for the functional abnormality is well understood. Because these conditions serve as prototypes for understanding the less well characterized phagocyte disorders, the underlying biochemical and molecular genetic aspects of these conditions will be reviewed in some depth.

One final point should be emphasized. In clinical practice, most physicians encounter a number of patients who experience recurrent bacterial infections. Although it is true that nearly all patients with well-characterized phagocyte abnormalities have recurrent infections, the converse is seldom the case. Most patients with impressive histories of persistent and repeated infections do not have identifiable qualitative or quantitative phagocyte abnormalities. Therefore, the major disorders described in this section account for only a fraction of the patients with recurrent infections. This point will be discussed further in the final section describing the laboratory evaluation of phagocyte function.

Disorders of Adhesion

Leukocyte Adhesion Deficiency Type I

LAD I is a rare, autosomal recessive disorder in which phagocyte adhesion, chemotaxis, and ingestion of C3bi-opsonized microbes are impaired because of mutations in the gene for CD18, β subunit of the β₂ integrins. As a result, expression of β₂ integrins on leukocyte cell surfaces is reduced or absent.[738-741] More than 100 patients with this disorder have been described in the literature. The hallmark of LAD I is the occurrence of repeated, frequently severe bacterial and fungal infections without the accumulation of pus despite a persistent granulocytosis (Table 21-11). The clinical syndrome is heterogeneous and related to the severity of the reduction in β₂ integrin expression. A severe clinical phenotype is seen when less than 0.3% of the normal amount of β₂ integrins is present, whereas a more moderate phenotype is observed at levels of 2.5% to 11% of normal. Patients with the severe form of LAD I, which is more common, are generally seen in early infancy with neutrophilia,

TABLE 21-11 Clinical Features of Leukocyte Adhesion Deficiency Type I

Chronic Conditions	Acute Infections	Infecting Organisms	Other
Persistent granulocytosis(12,000-100,000 cells/mm³)	Omphalitis	*Staphylococcus aureus*	Delayed umbilical cord separation
Gingivitis	Cutaneous abscesses and cellulitis (possibly invasive)	*Escherichia coli*	
Periodontitis	Perirectal abscesses and cellulitis (possibly invasive)	*Pseudomonas aeruginosa*	
Stomatitis	Facial cellulitis	*Pseudomonas* species	
Impaired wound healing	Sepsis	*Proteus*	
	Pneumonia	*Klebsiella*	
	Laryngotracheitis	*Candida albicans*	
	Peritonitis	*Aspergillus* species	
	Necrotizing enterocolitis	Viral (slightly increased risk)	
	Sinusitis		
	Esophagitis		
	Erosive gastritis		
	Appendicitis		
	Otitis media		

Each list is arranged in approximate order of frequency based on reviews summarizing various series of patients with leukocyte adhesion deficiency (see text for references).

omphalitis, and delayed separation of the umbilical cord. Recurrent necrotic and indolent infections of the skin, mucous membranes, and gastrointestinal tract also occur, including perirectal abscesses, which often heal poorly. An aggressive form of gingivitis and periodontitis is characteristic, and ulcerative lesions of the tongue and pharynx can be seen. Otitis media and pneumonia are also often encountered. The majority of infections are caused by *S. aureus* and gram-negative enteric bacteria. Fungal infections occur as well, particularly *Candida albicans* and *Aspergillus* infection.

The molecular basis for LAD I was first suggested by Crowley and colleagues,[742] who found that neutrophils from a patient with this clinical syndrome lacked a high-molecular-weight membrane glycoprotein. Because the patient's neutrophils neither adhered to plastic surfaces nor underwent an oxidative burst when exposed to serum-opsonized particles, it was hypothesized that the missing glycoprotein was responsible for both adhesion and cell-particle interactions. A similar glycoprotein was also found to be missing in several other patients,[743,744] which proved to be the α subunit (CD11b) of the Mac-1 β_2 integrin (CD11b/CD18).[745] It was subsequently recognized that leukocyte β_2 integrins (see Fig. 21-5) were absent or severely deficient in LAD I.[738,739]

Deficient β_2 integrin expression impairs a variety of leukocyte adhesion-dependent activities, with neutrophil function being the most significantly affected.[739-743,746] In addition to their role in mediating adhesive interactions during neutrophil emigration and phagocytosis, signaling through β_2 integrins potentiates virtually all functional responses of adherent neutrophils, including the production of reactive oxidants and degranulation.[747] Hence, LAD I neutrophils have a profound defect in their ability to become fully activated.

One of the striking findings in LAD I is the failure of neutrophils to migrate to sites of inflammation. The initial phase of neutrophil adhesion to the endothelium (see Fig. 21-3), which is mediated by selectins and their sialylated counter-receptors, is normal in LAD. However, because of the absence or a marked deficiency of Mac-1 (CD11b/CD18) expression, LAD I neutrophils are neither able to attach firmly to the endothelium nor undergo transendothelial migration.[748] Neutrophil intravascular survival is prolonged,[749] presumably related to deficient adhesion and migration. In vitro assays of neutrophil adhesion to glass or cultured endothelial cells and neutrophil chemotaxis also exhibit marked abnormalities. An exception to these observations is neutrophil adhesion and emigration in the pulmonary capillary bed, which can be mediated by CD11/CD18-independent mechanisms under some circumstances.[225] In autopsy tissue from a patient with severe LAD I, no neutrophils were observed in infected appendiceal and skin lesions, whereas many neutrophils were seen within the alveolar spaces.[225] In contrast to neutrophils, other leukocytes (monocytes, eosinophils, and lymphocytes) express the β_1 integrin VLA-4 and are able to use this adhesion molecule to emigrate into inflammatory sites throughout the body.

Another major defect in LAD I is the inability of neutrophils and monocytes to recognize microorganisms coated with the opsonic complement fragment C3bi because Mac-1 is a major C3bi receptor.[742,746,750] Binding of C3bi normally triggers neutrophil degranulation, phagocytosis, and activation of the respiratory burst, but these responses are diminished or absent in neutrophils from patients with LAD I. Controlled experiments have consistently demonstrated, however, that these responses can be at least partially activated in LAD I neutrophils by opsonins (e.g., IgG, C3b) that have different cell surface receptors or by soluble agonists that bypass Mac-1.[742,747]

Defects in lymphocyte functions dependent on LFA-1 (CD11a/CD18) have been observed in many LAD I patients in vitro. Such defects include proliferative responses to mitogens, NK cell function, and lymphocyte-mediated killing.[751-753] Nevertheless, most patients with LAD I manifest few, if any problems related to lymphocyte dysfunction in vivo. Cutaneous hypersensitivity reactions are normal, and patients are not generally unusually susceptible to viral infections, including varicella. However, one patient has died of an overwhelming respiratory infection with picornavirus, and one or more episodes of aseptic meningitis have been reported in three patients.[754]

Molecular Basis of Leukocyte Adhesion Deficiency

That LAD I involves a deficiency of all leukocyte CD11/CD18 integrins focused attention on the common β_2 chain (CD18) of this integrin family as the site of the molecular defect. This hypothesis has proved to be correct. Expression of leukocyte integrin α subunits is normal in LAD I, but these subunits are not transported to the cell surface because the β_2 chain is absent or contains mutations that disrupt the β_2 structure or its interaction with the α subunit.[755] More than 30 different mutations have now been characterized at the molecular genetic level in over 35 patients with LAD I, and all involve mutations in the β_2 gene, which is located on chromosome 21q22.3. A computerized database is available: http://bioint.uta.fi.[756] The mutations are heterogeneous. Many patients are compound heterozygotes for two different mutant alleles, whereas others are homozygous for a single mutant allele. About half of LAD I patients with characterized genetic defects have point mutations that result in single–amino acid substitutions in CD18, almost invariably between amino acids 111 to 361.[757,758] This protein domain is highly conserved among all β subunits and appears to be important for interaction with the α subunit. In this LAD I subgroup, approximately half exhibit a low level of CD11/CD18 cell surface expression and moderate disease, with the remainder having absent expression and the severe phenotype. mRNA splicing abnormalities resulting in either deletion or insertion of amino acids in the conserved extracellular domain of CD18 have also been described, as well as small deletions within CD18 coding sequences or nucleotide substitutions resulting in a premature termination signal.

There are several animal models of LAD I,[741] including the occurrence of a severe form of the disease in an Irish setter born of a mother-son mating[759,760] and in Holstein cattle.[761,762] In the latter case, affected calves could be traced to a common sire and have been shown to be homozygous for a point amino acid substitution in the conserved extracellular domain of CD18.[763] Finally, CD18-deficient mice have produced by gene targeting.[740,741]

Diagnosis and Treatment of LAD I

The diagnosis of LAD I should be suspected in any infant or child with unusually severe or recurrent infections or periodontitis accompanied by persistently elevated peripheral blood neutrophil counts (see Table 21-11). Although this laboratory finding may simply represent a leukemoid reaction in an otherwise immunologically normal infant, the diagnosis of LAD I should nonetheless be considered, particularly if there is a paucity of neutrophils at affected sites or delayed separation of the umbilical cord. A well infant with delayed separation of the umbilical cord and normal blood counts is very unlikely to have LAD I. Although the mean age at cord separation has been reported to be 7 to 15 days, 10% of healthy infants can exhibit cord separation at 3 weeks of age or later.[764,765] A rare cause of recurrent, deep-seated tissue infections in association with neutrophilia and poor formation of pus is mutations in the Rac2 GTPase, which leads to neutrophil signaling defects affecting chemotaxis and adhesion (see "Disorders of Chemotaxis" later in this chapter).[71,766,767]

The diagnosis of LAD I is established by flow cytometric analysis to assess cell surface expression of any of the β_2 integrin α (CD11) subunits or the shared CD18 subunit. Monoclonal antibodies to each are commercially available. Neutrophil Mac-1 deficiency is more dramatic if neutrophils are first stimulated, which normally upregulates Mac-1 cell surface expression. Though not necessary to establish the diagnosis of LAD I, in vitro functional assays of neutrophils obtained from these patients demonstrate striking defects in adherence, chemotaxis, and C3bi-mediated phagocytosis and activation of the respiratory burst. Carriers of LAD I can also generally be identified by flow cytometry because they typically express approximately 50% of the normal level of β_2 integrins on leukocyte cell surfaces.[738,768] For prenatal diagnosis of LAD I in families in which the mutations in the two CD18 alleles are known, chorionic villus or amniocyte DNA can be analyzed, and commercial testing is available. Flow cytometry on fetal blood granulocytes, which express Mac-1 by 20 weeks' gestation, has been used for prenatal diagnosis.[769,770]

Treatment of LAD I depends on the clinical severity of the disorder. In patients with the moderate clinical phenotype, who typically have some residual β_2 integrin expression, cutaneous and oral infections should be treated aggressively as they occur. The use of prophylactic trimethoprim-sulfamethoxazole appears to be beneficial. Aggressive prophylactic treatment of periodontal disease is also advisable in the form of frequent dental cleaning and the use of antimicrobial oral rinses such as chlorhexidine gluconate. Clinical management of patients with a moderate phenotype should be guided by the observation that these patients are still at risk of dying of overwhelming infection, with 75% succumbing between the ages of 12 and 32 years.[769] Patients with severe LAD I have an even grimmer prognosis, with a high incidence of death secondary to infection before the age of 2 years, and therefore bone marrow transplantation is recommended for this group of patients.[738,771-776] Graft rejection or graft-versus-host disease can be problematic with partially compatible HLA matching.[773-775] Nonmyeloablative bone marrow transplantation for LAD I has also been reported.

Because LAD I is caused by a defect in a single gene, transfer of a normal CD18 sequence into a patient's hematopoietic stem cells via retroviral or other vectors should, in principle, correct the defect. High-level expression of the transferred CD18 sequence may not be necessary to confer substantial clinical benefits based on the observed milder course of patients with some residual β_2 integrin expression. Studies in canine LAD I suggest that restoring CD18 expression to even 10% of leukocytes will result in clinical improvement.[771,777] At present, a major obstacle in applying this approach to clinical use is the development of techniques that achieve high-level gene transfer into human hematopoietic stem cells.[771,778]

Leukocyte Adhesion Deficiency Type II

LAD II is a very rare autosomal recessive clinical syndrome similar to LAD I but is associated with defective selectin-mediated adhesion because of deficiency of sialyl-Lewis X ligands.[779-783] This autosomal recessive disease was first described by Etzioni and colleagues[779] and since reported in a total of five kindreds (four Arab and one Turkish). As in CD11/CD18-deficient LAD, these children suffered from periodontitis, recurrent cellulitis, otitis media, and pneumonia without the formation of pus despite peripheral leukocyte counts of 30,000 to 150,000 cells/μL. However, neutrophils had normal levels of CD18, and infectious symptoms were not as serious as in LAD I. Also in distinction from classic LAD I, affected children had short stature, a distinctive facial appearance consisting of a flat face and depressed nasal bridge, and severe mental retardation. All had the rare Bombay (hh) blood phenotype, a clue to the molecular defect, in which red cells express a nonfucosylated variant of the H antigen. Red cells were also secretor negative and Lewis antigen negative. The Bombay and nonsecretor phenotypes are caused by deficient formation of Fucα1→2 Gal linkages in ABO blood group core antigens, whereas the Lewis antigen–negative phenotype is due to failure to synthesize Fucα1→4 GlcNAc and Fucα1→3 GlcNAc moieties. The defect in fucose metabolism in LAD II cells results from point mutations in the Golgi GDP-fucose transporter,[782,783] which leads to generalized loss of fucosylated glycans on cell surfaces, particularly the sialylated and fucosylated tetrasaccharide SleX (CD15a) on the neutrophil. As a result, LAD II neutrophils cannot bind to E- and P-selectin receptors. The early step of neutrophil rolling on activated endothelial cells is defective in LAD II,[748,779] consistent with the role of selectin-mediated adhesion in this process (see Fig. 21-3). However, chemoattractant-induced tight adhesion and emigration of LAD II neutrophils are

normal, both of which are severely impaired in LAD I.[748]

All of the Arab patients have the same nucleotide substitution in the Golgi GDP-fucose transporter mRNA, which alters an amino acid in a transmembrane domain, whereas the Turkish patient has a different nucleotide alteration that results in an amino acid substitution in a different transmembrane domain of the transporter.[782,783] The different mutations may explain why the Turkish patient had some response to oral fucose therapy consisting of increased expression of certain fucosylated ligands and improved clinical symptoms except mental retardation but the Arab children did not.[780,784,785] It is speculated that the mutation in the Turkish child leads to a decrease in transport affinity for GDP-fucose, which can be overcome by higher concentrations of fucose, whereas the mutant protein in Arab children has normal affinity for GDP-fucose but decreased transport activity.[781]

Leukocyte Adhesion Deficiency Type III

LAD III is a newly described subgroup of LAD that has been reported in a handful of patients with severe, recurrent infections similar to LAD I, as well as a severe bleeding tendency similar to Glanzmann's thrombasthenia.[786-790] First described in 1997 by Kuijpers and colleagues, almost a dozen patients have now been reported in the literature, most of whom are descendents of Turkish ancestors.[786-792] The disorder has also been termed LAD-1/variant syndrome.[791] Inheritance appears to be autosomal recessive, and it is associated with functional defects in the "inside-out" activation of multiple classes of integrins in response to G protein–coupled receptor stimulation; the defects appear to be restricted to the hematopoietic cell lineage. In addition to abnormalities in cell adhesion and platelet activation, stimulation of the respiratory burst by unopsonized zymosan is markedly reduced as a result of the integrin activation defect.[791] Rap1 GTPase is implicated in integrin activation, and a decreased level of the active form of Rap1 was reported in several LAD III kindreds.[792,793] A mouse genetically engineered to lack a blood cell–specific guanine nucleotide exchange factor, CalDAG-GEFI, which catalyzes the formation of Rap-GTP, had defective β integrin activation and manifestations similar to those of LAD III.[794] Two LAD III patients from the same region of Turkey exhibited decreased expression of CalDAG-GEFI in association with a homozygous mRNA splice junction mutation in the corresponding gene.[792] However, Rap1 activation was normal in other LAD III patients, thus suggesting that genetic defects in other signaling proteins can also be responsible for LAD III.[791] Because the clinical manifestations are typically severe, early bone marrow transplantation may be indicated for patients with LAD III.[786,790]

Acquired Disorders of Adherence

Neutrophils may exhibit decreased adhesiveness after exposure to a variety of drugs, the most common being corticosteroids and epinephrine.[645,795,796] Clinically, the diminished adhesiveness induced by these drugs is manifested by a dramatic rise in the total neutrophil count in blood as cells from the marginated pool are quickly released into the circulating pool. Although the mechanisms by which corticosteroids alter adherence are probably complex,[797] epinephrine and other β-adrenergic agonists exert their effect indirectly by causing endothelial cells to release cyclic AMP (cAMP), which in turn impairs the ability of neutrophils to adhere.[645,798]

Adhesiveness of neutrophils can be dramatically increased in a variety of clinical conditions that have in common the formation of biologically active complement fragments: gram-negative bacterial sepsis, severe thermal injury, pancreatitis, trauma, and exposure of neutrophils to artificial membrane surfaces during hemodialysis and cardiopulmonary bypass.[799] In these various conditions, generation of complement fragments leads to activation of neutrophils and enhanced adhesiveness, possibly as a result of enhanced expression of β_2 integrins. Under these conditions, neutrophils exhibit increased aggregation with each other and become trapped within capillary beds, such as those in the lungs.[800] It is believed that the aggregated neutrophils then generate toxic oxygen radicals and release proteases that conspire to damage structural protein such as collagen and elastin.[233] Binding of viral proteins to neutrophils can depress adhesion and other neutrophil functions in influenza or HIV infection.[799]

Amphotericin B has been associated with increased neutrophil aggregation, particularly when administered in conjunction with transfusions of neutrophils that have been harvested by filtration (rather than by centrifugation).[801,802] It is possible that the enhanced aggregation is mediated by upregulation of surface β_2 integrins induced both by the amphotericin B and by the filters used to harvest the cells. Liposomal amphotericin causes substantially less in vitro aggregation of mobilized neutrophils and may therefore be easier to use in patients being treated for fungal infections who are also receiving allogeneic neutrophil transfusions.[803]

Disorders of Chemotaxis

Directed migration into sites of infection and inflammation involves a complex series of events. As reviewed in the beginning of this chapter, the generation of chemotactic signals and their binding to specific receptors on the phagocyte surface lead to the generation of intracellular second messengers. These intracellular signals, in turn, trigger changes in adhesiveness and in the actin cytoskeleton that result in adhesion to the endothelium and chemotaxis to the inflamed tissue site. Given the numerous cellular functions involved in chemotaxis, it is perhaps not surprising that impaired phagocyte chemotaxis is observed in a large number of clinical conditions.[799,804] Some of the more important syndromes are listed in Box 21-10. These disorders are classified according to the mechanisms thought to be responsible for the

| Box 21-10 | Clinical Conditions Associated with Impaired Neutrophil Chemotaxis |

DEFECT IN GENERATION OF CHEMOTACTIC AGENTS

Familial deficiency of C1r, C2, C4
Familial deficiency of C3, C5
Other abnormalities of complement pathways (e.g., systemic lupus erythematosus, immature complement system in neonates, diabetes mellitus, C5 dysfunction, chronic hemodialysis, glomerulonephritis)

EXCESSIVE PRODUCTION OF NORMAL CHEMOTACTIC FACTOR INACTIVATORS

Hodgkin's disease
Cirrhosis of the liver
Sarcoidosis
Lepromatous leprosy

INHIBITORS OF THE NEUTROPHIL RESPONSE TO CHEMOTACTIC FACTORS

Hyperimmunoglobulin E syndrome
Localized juvenile periodontitis
Immune complex diseases (rheumatoid arthritis, systemic lupus erythematosus)
Influenza virus
HIV
IgA paraproteinemia states
Solid tumors
Bone marrow transplantation
Drugs (ethanol, antithymocyte globulin, interleukin-2)

DEACTIVATION (DOWNREGULATION) BY INCREASED LEVELS OF CHEMOTACTIC FACTORS

Wiskott-Aldrich syndrome
C5a generation in plasma (hemodialysis)
Bacterial sepsis

PHAGOCYTE DEFECTS

Neutrophil actin dysfunction
Rac2 mutation
Localized juvenile periodontitis
Neonatal neutrophils
Leukocyte adhesion deficiency
Chédiak-Higashi syndrome
Specific granule deficiency

MISCELLANEOUS DEFECTS

Hypophosphatemia
Shwachman-Diamond syndrome
Burn patients

defective chemotaxis, which are related either to abnormalities in the production or inhibition of chemotactic factors or to defects in the phagocyte itself involving adhesiveness and locomotion. In some cases, abnormal chemotaxis is one component of a disorder that involves multiple defects.

It is worth noting that in many of the reports describing defective in vitro chemotaxis of neutrophils from various clinical conditions, it is not clear whether the increased number of infections observed clinically is due to the observed chemotactic abnormality or to medical complications of the underlying disorder (such as malnutrition or exposure to nosocomial infection). Further complicating the interpretation of these reports is that in vitro assays for chemotaxis are subject to laboratory artifacts and may not accurately reflect the in vivo extracellular environment.[805-807] Phagocyte migration to an inflamed site in vivo can be measured by the skin window technique of Rebuck and Crowley, in which a superficial dermal abrasion is produced in the patient and the appearance of inflammatory cells in the lesion is monitored over a 24-hour period.[808] Because of difficulties in standardizing the dermal lesion, variable results may be obtained with this method. Moreover, the assay can measure only the response of phagocytes to the chemotactic signals generated by this type of sterile injury.

As outlined in Box 21-10, several of the conditions associated with impaired neutrophil chemotaxis are due to complement deficiencies and other immunodeficiency syndromes (e.g., WAS). These disorders are discussed elsewhere in this text. In addition, several disorders of phagocyte function (LAD, CHS, and SGD) are reviewed in other sections of this chapter. This section focuses on clinical conditions in which there is evidence that a chemotactic defect plays a major contribution to the decreased resistance to bacterial and fungal infections.

Hyperimmunoglobulin E Syndrome

The hyperimmunoglobulin E syndrome (HIES) (see Chapter 5 in *Oncology of Infancy and Childhood*) is a relatively rare disorder characterized by markedly elevated serum levels of IgE (often greater than 2000 IU/mL), serious recurrent staphylococcal infections of the skin and lower respiratory tract, pneumatoceles, chronic pruritic dermatitis, and skeletal and dental abnormalities.[809-814] The key features of HIES are summarized in Table 21-12. Neutrophils from patients with this syndrome exhibit a variable, but at times severe, chemotactic defect.[810,815,816] This syndrome was originally known as "Job's syndrome" when it was first reported in 1966 in two red-haired, fair-skinned females who had hyperextensible joints and "cold" abscesses that lacked the usual characteristics of inflammation.[809] It is now appreciated that only a small fraction of patients with HIES have red hair or hyperextensible joints, and it may be that Job's syndrome is a variant subset of HIES. The disease can occur in both males and females and in all ethnic groups, including blacks and Asians. The mode of inheritance is variable. Many cases are sporadic. Familial patterns suggest autosomal dominant inheritance with variable expressivity, as well as, rarely, autosomal recessive inheritance.[812,813,817]

The clinical manifestations of HIES are often severe and usually become apparent during infancy. Staphylococcal furuncles on the head and neck, as well as chronic dermatitis, are seen most frequently in younger patients. The skin abscesses in HIES typically lack erythema (cold abscesses). Chronic candidiasis of the mucosa and nail beds is also frequent and can occur in children. Recurrent staphylococcal pneumonia is a common problem as patients grow older and can be complicated by the formation of persistent pneumatoceles that can become superinfected with *Haemophilus influenzae*, gram-negative

TABLE 21-12	Summary of Hyperimmunoglobulin E Syndrome
Incidence	More than 200 cases reviewed in the literature
Inheritance	Autosomal dominant with variable expressivity, sporadic forms, autosomal recessive (rare)
Molecular defect	Dominant-negative mutations in STAT3 (autosomal dominant and sporadic cases), Tyk2 kinase (autosomal recessive)
Clinical manifestations	"Cold" cutaneous skin abscesses and furuncles
	Chronic eczematoid dermatitis
	Mucocutaneous candidiasis
	Staphylococcal pneumonia, pneumatoceles
	Fungal superinfection of lung cysts
	Coarse facies
	Delayed shedding of primary teeth
	Scoliosis
	Recurrent fractures
	Hyperextensible joints
Laboratory evaluation	Serum IgE > 2500 IU/mL
	Peripheral blood eosinophilia
Differential diagnosis	Atopic dermatitis
	Wiskott-Aldrich syndrome, DiGeorge's syndrome
	Hypergammaglobulinemia
	Chronic granulomatous disease
Therapy	Prophylactic antibiotics for *Staphylococcus aureus*
	Aggressive treatment of acute infections with parenteral antibiotics
	Surgical drainage of deep infections and resection of lung cysts
	Monitoring for scoliosis and fractures
Prognosis	Generally good if managed aggressively

bacteria, or *Aspergillus*. Chronic infections of the ears, sinuses, and eyes (keratoconjunctivitis) are seen, and septic arthritis and osteomyelitis have been observed. Dental and bone abnormalities are also common features of HIES. Delayed shedding or failure to shed primary teeth occurs in the majority. Hyperextensible joints and scoliosis are frequent. Osteopenia of unknown etiology is observed many patients, and there is also an increased risk for fractures of the long bones and vertebral bodies, even in the absence of osteopenia.[812] Coarse facial features characterized by a broad nasal bridge and a prominent nose are evident in the majority of patients by the time that they reach the teen-age years. Craniosynostosis can also occur.

There is a subgroup of HIES with autosomal recessive inheritance, with 13 reported patients from six consanguineous families.[817] In addition to high IgE, eosinophilia, eczema, and recurrent pneumonia and abscesses, many patients had recurrent or chronic viral infections, including molluscum contagiosum, herpes simplex, and varicella, as well as increased susceptibility to atypical mycobacterial infection.[817,818] Pneumatoceles were not seen, in contrast to autosomal dominant HIES, nor were skeletal abnormalities, dental problems, or the characteristic facies. Significant neurologic symptoms were often present and ranged from partial facial paralysis to hemiplegia.

The molecular basis of HIES and how the immunologic abnormalities relate to the dental and skeletal defects that are the other hallmarks of this disorder have been puzzling. It has been proposed that the immunologic manifestations may reflect an underlying T helper 1 cell (T_H1)/T_H2 imbalance in T lymphocytes.[819] Skewing toward a T_H2 response might lead to abnormal regulation of IgE production and greatly reduced production of IFN-γ and TNF.[813,820,821] This putative T-cell defect may also explain the abnormal antibody responses that have recently been documented in some patients in response to various vaccines.[822] Patients with HIES produce excessive amounts of IgE directed against *S. aureus* at the expense of protective antistaphylococcal IgG.[823,824] The recurrent bacterial infections in HIES may also be aggravated by the chemotactic defect that is periodically observed in these patients.

Recent breakthrough studies have identified genetic defects in the JAK-STAT pathways in all three forms of HIES, which helps explain the pathogenesis of HIES and its multisystem manifestations. Thus, HIES can be considered a disorder of cytokine signaling. A patient with autosomal recessive HIES exhibited defects in IL-6, IL-10, IL-12, and IFN-α signaling associated with a homozygous frameshift mutation in the tyrosine kinase 2 (Tyk2) JAK family member.[818] This is consistent with the broader spectrum of infections seen in autosomal recessive HIES. In contrast, mutations in STAT3 itself account for a large proportion of autosomal dominant and sporadic forms of HIES. Missense mutations and single-codon in-frame deletions in STAT3 were identi-

fied in autosomal dominant and sporadic cases of HIES.[825,826] Many affect the DNA-binding and Src homology 2 (SH2) domains. Mutations in the DNA-binding domain can have dominant-negative effects on STAT3 signaling, which in turn interferes with cytokine signaling by the IL-6 and IL-10 pathways, but not with IL-12 and IFN-α responses.[826] Defective responses to the proinflammatory cytokine IL-6 may account for the minimal inflammatory response characteristic of HIES, and the enhanced IgE production may reflect dysregulated immune responses secondary to defects in signaling by IL-10, a negative regulator. STAT3 also influences lymphocyte IL-17 production, which is important for host defense against extracellular bacteria and may predispose to staphylococcal infections. The dental and skeletal abnormalities may be related to defects in STAT3-dependent cytokine responses in osteoblasts and osteoclasts.

The diagnosis of HIES should be considered in any child with the aforementioned clinical history. Almost all patients have peripheral eosinophilia. Markedly elevated polyclonal serum IgE, or at least a value of 2500 IU/mL, is a constant laboratory finding, although IgE levels can fluctuate over time and occasional decrease to the normal range.[812,814] Despite the impressive elevations in serum IgE (up to 150,000 IU/mL), this laboratory finding alone is not diagnostic in that comparably high serum levels of IgE can be seen in patients with atopic dermatitis. Because many patients with atopic dermatitis suffer from superficial skin infections and eczema, this disorder must be considered in the differential diagnosis of HIES. The two can be distinguished from each other by the severe and recurrent nature of the staphylococcal furuncles and the pneumonia seen in patients with HIES.

Treatment of HIES is largely supportive.[813,814] One of the mainstays of therapy for HIES is the use of prophylactic antibiotics such as dicloxacillin or trimethoprim-sulfamethoxazole. These drugs can help prevent staphylococcal infections and should be prescribed at the time of diagnosis. Pneumonia and other deep-seated infections should be treated aggressively with parenteral antibiotics. Patients with HIES are unusually predisposed to the development of pneumatoceles as a result of staphylococcal lung infections. If these lesions persist, they should be surgically resected to prevent superinfection by fungal and gram-negative organisms. Plasmapheresis has been reported to be effective in patients who are responding poorly to the aforementioned therapies. Cyclosporine or intravenous IgG infusions have also shown some success in the management of HIES.[813] Dermatitis can be treated with topical steroids. Delayed shedding of primary teeth may necessitate extraction. Patients should be carefully monitored for scoliosis, and skeletal fractures can occur after even minor trauma. If infections and their complications are managed aggressively, the prognosis for patients with HIES is good. Recombinant human IFN-γ (rIFN-γ) has been used with inconsistent results.[813]

Neutrophil Actin Dysfunction

Primary defects in neutrophil actin polymerization are exceedingly rare. The first such case, described by Boxer and colleagues in 1974, was a male infant who suffered from recurrent *S. aureus* skin infections and a cutaneous-cecal fistula complicated by *Streptococcus faecalis* sepsis.[827] Despite marked neutrophilia, sites of infections were devoid of neutrophils and healed slowly. The patient's neutrophils showed markedly diminished chemotaxis and a decreased capacity to ingest serum-opsonized particles. He underwent bone marrow transplantation with transient engraftment of normally functioning neutrophils but succumbed to infectious complications. The underlying defect in this patient appeared to involve neutrophil actin or an ABP. Neutrophils from his parents and a sibling exhibited decreased actin polymerization in vitro. Neutrophils from family members also had intermediate levels and decreased expression of the Mac-1 integrin (CD11b/CD18),[828,829] thus raising the question of whether the neutrophil actin dysfunction in the proband was a variant of LAD I. However, actin filament assembly is normal in LAD I patients.[829] Alternatively, a primary actin-associated defect might alter cell surface expression of the integrins, which have binding sites in their cytoplasmic domains for cytoskeletal proteins.[790]

Coates and co-workers reported a male infant of Tongan descent who was afflicted with severe skin and mucosal infections.[830] At the age of 2 months he was found to have hepatosplenomegaly, moderate thrombocytopenia, recurrent pulmonary infiltrates, and a lingual ulcer that grew *Candida tropicalis*. Two siblings had previously died in infancy with a similar clinical picture. Neutrophils from this patient, which had normal cell surface expression of CD11b, exhibited abnormalities in a wide range of motile behavior, including chemotaxis, phagocytosis, and spreading on glass. Morphologically, the neutrophils had thin, filamentous projections of membrane with an underlying abnormal cytoskeletal structure. Biochemical studies revealed markedly defective actin polymerization and severe deficiency of an 89-kd protein, along with a markedly elevated level of a 47-kd protein. Hence, this disorder has been referred to as neutrophil actin dysfunction with 47- and 89-kd protein abnormalities (NAD 47/89). The 47-kd protein has recently been identified as LSP1 (lymphocyte-specific protein 1),[831] which is an ABP present in normal neutrophils. Neutrophils from the patient's parents showed a partial defect in actin polymerization and intermediate abnormalities in levels of LSP1 and the 89-kd protein. These observations, along with the history of previously affected siblings, suggest that NAD 47/89 is an autosomal recessive disorder. The patient underwent allogeneic bone marrow transplantation at the age of 7 months and no longer suffers from thrombocytopenia or the neutrophil motility disorder.

Markedly impaired neutrophil chemotaxis associated with a heterozygous point mutation in β-actin was reported by Nunoi and colleagues in a female patient with recurrent infections, stomatitis, photosensitivity, and mental retardation.[832] The defect lies within a domain that binds to profilin and other actin regulatory molecules, and the mutant β-actin may interfere with normal actin function in a dominant-negative manner. Interestingly, formyl peptide–induced superoxide production was also decreased in the patient's neutrophils, thus suggesting that actin function is important for normal NADPH oxidase assembly.

Localized Juvenile Periodontitis

Localized juvenile periodontitis (LJP) is a group of disorders of unknown etiology characterized by severe alveolar bone loss localized to the first molars and incisors, with an onset around the time of puberty.[833-836] LJP appears to be an acquired disorder in some patients and a genetic disorder in others. Defective neutrophil chemotaxis has been identified in vitro in approximately 70% of LJP patients and may be due to the intrinsic variability present in in vitro chemotaxis assays (see earlier) or to a fundamental heterogeneity in this disorder.[834,837-841] For example, whereas most individuals with LJP have defective chemotaxis in response to both formyl peptides and C5a, others may have an abnormality in response to only formyl peptides.[838] Further support for the heterogeneity of LJP is provided by studies showing that factors elaborated by periodontopathic bacteria may secondarily alter leukocyte function and depress chemotaxis (e.g., *Capnocytophaga* species, *Actinobacillus actinomycetemcomitans*, and *Bacteroides* species).[842-844] Whether these factors are the same as the chemotactic inhibitors identified in the sera of some patients with LJP remains to be determined.[839,845] In the subset of patients with LJP who have abnormal chemotaxis, phagocytosis has generally been found to be abnormal, whereas degranulation (of specific granules) and superoxide generation are unaltered.[846]

The observations that LJP tends to cluster in families and that the neutrophil chemotactic activity is not restored in vitro or after the patient is treated for periodontal infection lend support to the hypothesis that some LJP patients may have an inherited disorder affecting chemotactic receptors. A 40% to 50% decrease in the total number of receptors for formyl peptides and C5a has been reported for some patients with LJP.[838,847] Preliminary studies have identified point mutations in the ligand-binding domain of the formyl peptide receptor in a few LJP patients.[836]

The diagnosis of LJP should be suspected in any adolescent with unusually severe and destructive alveolar bone loss involving the first molars and incisors. From a diagnostic point of view, it is important to bear in mind that many qualitative and quantitative neutrophil disorders are associated with periodontal disease that, at times, may be severe.[833] The differential diagnosis should include LAD, CGD, CHS, leukemia, chronic neutropenia, and cyclic neutropenia.

Neonatal Neutrophilia

Although most infants are able to defend themselves successfully against microbial challenges, they are nonetheless at increased risk for the development of severe bacterial infections—particularly sepsis, pneumonia, and meningitis caused by group B streptococci.[848] The risk of infection and the rate of mortality from pyogenic infections are even greater in premature infants. As a result, the development of innate immunity in neonates has been the subject of intense investigation for many years.[848-850] It is generally agreed that neonates have defects in various aspects of specific immunity (immune cellular cytotoxic mechanisms and cytokine generation). Defects in neutrophil adherence, chemotaxis, phagocytosis, and bacterial killing have all been reported.[849,850] Compounding these functional defects in neonates is a deficiency of antibodies directed against organisms that typically infect infants. Furthermore, neonates can easily exhaust bone marrow reserves of granulocytes and exhibit neutropenia in the midst of severe pyogenic infections, as discussed in the previous section.

The most important of the functional defects, at least from a clinical point of view, appears to be the depressed chemotactic ability of neonatal neutrophils. When compared with adult cells, directed migration of neonatal neutrophils toward a variety of chemotactic agents (C5a, formyl peptides, and bacterial extracts) is reduced by approximately 50% for the first several weeks of life.[849,851-853] The biochemical basis for the diminished chemotaxis does not appear to be related to abnormalities in the number or affinity of either the C5a or formyl peptide receptor.[849,853] Instead, there appears to be a defect in the chemotaxis-induced upregulation of cell adhesion molecules. Cell surface expression of the two subunits of the β_2 integrin Mac-1 (CD11b and CD18) was found to be normal in neonatal neutrophils but failed to increase normally after exposure to chemotactic concentrations of C5a and formyl peptides.[854,855] Fetal, preterm, and term infant neutrophils expressed levels of Mac-1 in stimulated neutrophils that were only 40% to 60% of those seen in adult cells. Total cellular Mac-1 is decreased in neonatal neutrophils.[856] Because internal membrane stores serve as an intracellular pool for Mac-1 (see Table 21-3), the overall reduction in cellular Mac-1 could explain the diminished upregulation of Mac-1 seen in neonatal cells after stimulation. Another underlying biochemical abnormality that may contribute to the chemotaxis defect is diminished polymerization of F-actin in neonatal neutrophils after stimulation.[857] Finally, Hill[849] reported that neonatal neutrophils fail to increase the intracellular concentration of free calcium to normal levels in response to chemotactic factors.

Other Disorders of Neutrophil Chemotaxis

A new syndrome of severe neutrophil dysfunction caused by a dominant-negative mutation in the small GTPase Rac2 has recently been described in a male infant born to unrelated parents. This child had recurrent, rapidly progressive soft tissue infections, including perirectal abscesses and a necrotic periumbilical infection, associated with poor formation of pus and neutrophilia.[71,766,767] Although the clinical manifestation was suggestive of LAD, expression of β_2 integrins and fucosylated cell surface proteins was normal. Marked abnormalities were seen in chemoattractant-induced neutrophil function, including F-actin formation, chemotaxis, degranulation, and the respiratory burst, along with defects in phagocytosis and L-selectin–mediated adhesion.[71,767] Responses to other agonists were normal, thus suggesting a selective defect in signal transduction. This constellation of functional abnormalities resembled those described for gene-targeted mice lacking the hematopoietic-specific GTPase Rac2.[200,201] Analysis of the Rac2 gene in this patient identified a point mutation that affects the guanine nucleotide–binding pocket. The patient was heterozygous for this mutation, which apparently exerts a dominant-negative effect on wild-type Rac2 that interferes with normal signal transduction.[71,767] Neither parent had the mutant Rac2 allele. The patient was successfully treated by HLA-matched bone marrow transplantation from a sibling. The clinical history, neutrophilia, and functional neutrophil defects in this patient are very similar to those seen in another infant described in an earlier report.[858] This patient, a female, was the first child of nonconsanguineous healthy parents, both originating from India; she suffered from chronic omphalitis and otitis media secondary to *S. aureus*, buccal candidiasis, and internal cecal fistulation that ultimately led to death from gram-negative sepsis at 8 months of age.

A recent study of 240 patients with a significant history of recurrent infection, generally requiring at least one hospitalization, identified 10 patients, all children, with consistently markedly reduced chemotactic activity in vitro that was not associated with any other neutrophil abnormalities.[859] In six of these patients, partial reduction in chemotactic activity was also seen in either the mother or a sibling. However, other than for the disorders discussed earlier, well-defined clinical entities in which defective neutrophil chemotaxis plays a predominant role in impaired host resistance to bacteria and fungi have not been established or the underlying mechanisms identified. In part, this is related to the difficulty of performing and interpreting in vitro assays of adhesion and chemotaxis, except in specialized research settings. Biochemical approaches to delineating a specific abnormality are also difficult because of the complex nature of the chemotactic response.

Disorders of Opsonization and Ingestion

Clinical disorders of recognition fall into two major categories: humoral and cellular. In the former, deficient or absent plasma-derived opsonins result in incomplete opsonization. In contrast, the cellular disorders are characterized by defective receptors for opsonins or by abnormalities in the actin cytoskeletal system responsible for ingestion of microbes.

Humoral Disorders of Opsonization

Primary B-cell deficiencies result in decreased or absent production of immunoglobulins, most commonly IgG. Patients afflicted with these antibody deficiency syndromes suffer from recurrent infections with pyogenic bacteria such as *S. aureus*, pneumococci, and *H. influenzae*. One of the major functional abnormalities in these disorders is defective opsonization of pathogenic microorganisms. As a result, these microbes are not efficiently cleared by the host phagocytic system. A variety of clinical disorders may lead to antibody deficiency, including deficiencies in specific IgG subclasses; such disorders are discussed elsewhere in this text.

Complement deficiencies can also result in recurrent infections, particularly when they involve factors shared by both the classical and the alternative pathways. Therefore, patients with deficiencies of C1, C2, or C4 have relatively minor problems with infections because the alternative pathway remains intact. In the case of C3, on the other hand, recurrent infections are much more common because this protein is the direct precursor of two major complement opsonins—C3b and C3bi. Two forms of C3 deficiency have been described, and both are quite rare. In one, congenital deficiency of C3 is inherited in an autosomal recessive manner and has been described in around 20 patients.[860-864] Heterozygotes contain half the normal levels of C3 but do not suffer from infections. The molecular genetic basis of the C3 deficiency has been identified in several families, and the mutations are heterogeneous.[863,864] A second type of C3 deficiency is caused by unchecked catabolism of C3 as a result of the absence of a C3 protease inhibitor.[865] In both types of C3 deficiency, the majority of patients experience recurrent pyogenic infections caused by encapsulated bacteria such as pneumococci. Patients with deficiencies of the terminal complement components (C5, C6, C7, C8, or C9) are particularly susceptible to infections with meningococci or gonococci. Infections in complement-deficient individuals should be treated aggressively with antibiotics, and immunization against *H. influenzae*, *S. pneumoniae*, and *Neisseria meningitidis* may be helpful.

Approximately 5% of the population have low serum levels of MBL, also known as MBP. MBL is a serum lectin secreted by the liver and functions as a soluble PRR by binding to mannose sugars present on the surface of bacteria, fungi, and some viruses.[254,256,257] Bound MBL activates the complement cascade to mediate opsonization of a broad range of microbes with C3 cleavage products. The incidence of MBL deficiency is higher in infants with frequent unexplained infections, chronic diarrhea, and otitis media. It has been proposed that MBL serves as a primitive antibody of broad specificity to provide an important defense mechanism during the period when maternal "antibody" levels have waned yet the antibody repertoire of the infant is still immature.[254,256,257] MBL deficiency is associated with autosomal dominant inheritance of point mutations in a collagen-like domain of the MBL polypeptide.[866-868] These mutations decrease MBL levels by interfering with normal polymerization of the MBL subunits to form the oligomeric structure required for complement activation. A polymorphism in the promoter of the MBL gene has also been described that can influence MBL levels.[254] Clinical illness associated with MBL deficiency may not be limited to infants. In a recent report, MBL deficiency was the only identifiable immune defect in four adults with recurrent infections, as well as in one patient who also had IgA deficiency.[869] The spectrum of illness included recurrent skin abscesses, chronic cryptosporidial diarrhea, meningococcal meningitis with recurrent herpes simplex, and fatal *Klebsiella* pneumonia. Three of the five adults were homozygotes for mutant MBL alleles. Decreased MBL levels are seen in some populations, such as in sub-Saharan Africa, thus suggesting that low levels of this protein may be beneficial in certain settings. For example, low levels of MBL may partially protect against mycobacterial infections.[254]

Cellular Disorders of Ingestion

Patients with LAD I show a marked abnormality in the phagocytosis of C3bi-opsonized particles because the Mac-1 β_2 integrin (CD11b/CD18) that is deficient in LAD I functions as the C3bi receptor (see Tables 21-2 and 21-4). Patients with neutrophil actin dysfunction also show abnormal ingestion because actin assembly plays a critical role in the formation of phagosomes.

A deficiency in FcγRIa has been described in four members of a Dutch family.[870] The monocytes from the affected family members did not bind IgG with high affinity. However, these individuals did not have increased susceptibility to infection despite this receptor deficiency. There is an incidence of 4 in 3377 in the French population for complete absence of FcγRIIIb, and neutrophils from affected individuals type as NA-null.[871] None of these individuals exhibit any increased incidence of infection, although infants of women with the NA-null phenotype are susceptible to alloimmune neutropenia because of placental transmission of anti-FcγRIIIb antibodies. Similar findings were also reported in a study of 21 individuals from 14 families with FcγRIIIb deficiency in the Netherlands.[247] Complete absence of the FcγRIIIb gene was found in all kindreds studied. Three of the women who had multiple pregnancies lacked antineutrophil antibodies, thus suggesting that neonatal alloimmune neutropenia does not always develop in this setting. Marked deficiency in neutrophil FcγRIIIb has also been observed in patients with paroxysmal nocturnal hemoglobinuria (PNH),[872] an acquired stem cell disorder caused by a defect in the biosynthesis of GPI membrane anchors. Because neutrophil FcγRIIIb is linked to the plasma membrane by means of a GPI anchor,[873] this receptor is unable to insert in the cell membranes in patients with PNH. Decay-accelerating factor and acetylcholinesterase are likewise deficient in the membranes of patients with PNH because these two proteins are also anchored by GPI moieties. Neutrophils from patients with PNH undergo a normal oxidative burst in response to IgG-coated latex particles.[873] Hence, there appears to be sufficient redundancy in the function of Fc and complement receptors to permit normal phagocyte function in these cases of FcγRI and FcγRIIIb deficiency.

Allelic polymorphisms in FcγRIIa (131H versus 131R) and in FcγRIIIb (NA1 versus NA2) may each contribute to a subtle defect in the host response to encapsulated microorganisms. The polymorphism in amino acid 131 in FcγRIIa affects binding to IgG2, with "H" referring to "high" responder and the ability to bind to this IgG subclass. The 131H versus 131R polymorphism is seen in about equal frequencies in the white population, but it is distributed in a 3:1 ratio in Japanese and Chinese populations.[247] The FcγRIIa 131H allele is the only FcγR able to mediate efficient phagocytosis of IgG2-opsonized bacteria, and the FcγRIIa 131H/131H genotype in children was associated with a lower incidence of infections with encapsulated bacteria.[247] The NA1 polymorphism in FcγRIIIb, which affects receptor glycosylation, is associated with more efficient phagocytosis of IgG-opsonized particles than the NA2 allele is.[247,874] The allelic frequency of NA1 is approximately 0.33 versus about 0.64 for the NA2 allele in whites, but this ratio is reversed in Japanese and Chinese populations. Patients who are homozygous for both the FcγRIIa 131R and the FcγRIIIb NA2 alleles appear to be at higher risk for meningococcal meningitis.[875]

Disorders of Neutrophil Granules

Phagocytes kill microorganisms with a variety of cytotoxic compounds, as reviewed earlier in this chapter, including a host of preformed antimicrobial polypeptides that are stored within intracellular granules and released into the phagocytic vacuole upon phagocytosis. The importance of granule contents in host defense is attested to by two clinical syndromes associated with disorders of neutrophil granules, CHS and SGD.

Chédiak-Higashi Syndrome

CHS, a rare, autosomal recessive, multiorgan disease resulting from defects in granule morphogenesis, is characterized by partial oculocutaneous albinism, frequent bacterial infections, giant lysosomes in granulocytes, and (in some patients) a mild bleeding diathesis, as well as peripheral and cranial neuropathies associated with decussation defects at the optic chiasm[478-485] (Table 21-13). Ten types of oculocutaneous albinism have been described in humans, and CHS is one of the tyrosinase-positive forms that has been designated type VIB. Because granule defects also affect cytotoxic T-cell and NK-cell function, CHS is associated with HLH in the "accelerated" phase of the disease that often develops after the first or second decade of life.[482-485,876,877]

CHS is caused by a fundamental defect in granule morphogenesis that results in abnormally large granules in multiple tissues. The most extensively studied of the affected cells are neutrophils. In the early stages of myelopoiesis, some of the normally sized azurophilic granules

---

TABLE 21-13	**Summary of Chédiak-Higashi Syndrome**
Incidence	More than 200 cases described
Inheritance	Autosomal recessive
Molecular defect	Defect in granule morphogenesis in multiple tissues as a result of mutations in the *CHS1* gene, which encodes a lysosomal trafficking protein
Pathogenesis	Giant coalesced azurophilic/specific granules in neutrophils resulting in ineffective granulopoiesis and neutropenia, delayed and incomplete degranulation, and defective chemotaxis
Clinical manifestations	Partial oculocutaneous albinism
	Recurrent severe bacterial infections (usually *Staphylococcus aureus*)
	Gingivitis and periodontitis
	Cranial and peripheral neuropathies (muscle weakness, ataxia, sensory loss, nystagmus)
	HLH (accelerated phase)
Laboratory evaluation	Giant granules in peripheral blood granulocytes and in bone marrow myeloid progenitor cells
	Widespread lymphohistiocytic infiltrates in accelerated phase
Prenatal diagnosis	Demonstration of giant granules in fetal blood neutrophils or cultured amniotic cells
Differential diagnosis	Other genetic forms of oculocutaneous albinism
	Giant granules can be seen in acute and chronic myelogenous leukemia
Therapy	Prophylactic trimethoprim-sulfamethoxazole
	Parenteral antibiotics for acute infections
	Ascorbic acid (200 mg/day for infants; 6 g/day for adults)
	Steroids, cyclosporine, etoposide for HLH
	Bone marrow transplantation before or at beginning of HLH
Prognosis	Most patients die of infection or complications of HLH in the accelerated phase during the first or second decade of life unless transplantation performed. A few patients have survived into their thirties

HLH, hemophagocytic lymphohistiocytosis.

coalesce to form giant granules that later fuse with some of the specific granules to form huge secondary lysosomes containing constituents of both granule types.[878-880] In addition to this uncontrolled fusion of granules, CHS neutrophils are markedly deficient in neutral proteases,[881] including two azurophilic granule enzymes, cathepsin G and elastase.[882] In melanocytes, there are giant melanosomes that prevent the even distribution of melanin and result in hypopigmentation of the hair, skin, iris, and ocular fundus. Giant granules are also seen in other leukocytes, Schwann cells, and certain cells in the liver, spleen, pancreas, gastric mucosa, kidney, adrenal gland, and pituitary gland.[483,485] In addition, disorders similar to human CHS have been described in many mammalian species, including Aleutian mink, *beige* mice, blue foxes, cats, killer whales, and Hereford cattle.[479,480,483,484,883]

Mutations in the *CHS1* gene, believed to normally regulate lysosome biogenesis, account for most cases of CHS.[884-886] *CHS1* is located on the long arm of chromosome 1 and is homologous to the *bg* locus responsible for the granule defect in *beige* mice.[887] The *beige* gene was positionally cloned and termed LYST for its presumed function as a lysosomal trafficking regulatory protein.[884,886] The encoded CHS/LYST protein is a very large (3801 amino acids) polypeptide, and at least one of its functions may be to inhibit lysosome fusion with other intracellular membrane vesicles.[888] Frameshift and nonsense mutations have been identified in the *CHS1* gene in patients with CHS and result in truncated forms of the protein.[482,884-886,889] Patients with clinically typical CHS who lack identifiable mutations in *CHS1* have been reported, thus suggesting that additional genetic loci may be affected in some cases.[890]

Some of the most dramatic examples of the granule defect in CHS are manifested in the various blood cells and are summarized in Box 21-11. A few to a large majority of circulating neutrophils contain giant coalesced azurophil/specific granules. These giant granules are often more prominent in bone marrow than in peripheral blood because many of the abnormal myeloid precursors are destroyed before they ever leave the marrow.[891] Extensive myeloid cell vacuolization, enhanced marrow cellularity, and elevated levels of serum lysozyme all reflect this process of intramedullary granulocyte destruction. As a result, most patients with CHS have moderate neutropenia with ANCs ranging between 500 and 2000 cells/mm[3].[478,481] Monocytes are also affected in CHS and have similar, but not identical cytoplasmic inclusions that appear to be ring-shaped lysosomes.[892] Lymphocytes can also contain giant cytoplasmic granules that contribute to abnormal cytotoxic T-cell and NK-cell function (see later). Finally, CHS platelets have a decreased number of dense granules and a storage pool deficiency of adenosine diphosphate and serotonin.[893-896] This abnormality leads to a defect in platelet aggregation and an increased bleeding time manifested clinically as easy bruising, intestinal bleeding, and epistaxis. Most patients with

---

Box 21-11	Hematologic Manifestations of Chédiak-Higashi Syndrome

STABLE PHASE

Neutrophils
Giant, coalesced azurophilic specific granules
Vacuolization of marrow neutrophils (ineffective myelopoiesis)
Neutropenia (intramedullary destruction)
Decreased bactericidal activity
    Decreased chemotaxis in vivo and in vitro
    Delayed and incomplete degranulation

Monocytes/Macrophages
Ring-shaped lysosomes
Decreased chemotaxis

Lymphocytes/Natural Killer Cells
Giant cytoplasmic granules
Diminished natural killer function
Diminished antibody-dependent cell-mediated cytolysis

Platelets
Giant cytoplasmic granules may be seen
Normal platelet count
Increased bleeding time because of abnormal aggregation caused by storage pool deficiency of adenosine diphosphate and serotonin

ACCELERATED PHASE (HEMOPHAGOCYTIC LYMPHOHISTIOCYTOSIS)

Hepatosplenomegaly
Bone marrow infiltration
Hemophagocytosis by histiocytes
Worsening neutropenia, thrombocytopenia, and anemia as a result of the first three manifestations

---

CHS do not have thrombocytopenia until they enter the accelerated phase of the disease (see later).

The infections usually encountered with CHS involve the skin, respiratory tract, and mucous membranes and are caused by both gram-positive and gram-negative bacteria, as well as by fungi. The most common organism is *S. aureus*. These infections are often recurrent and can be fatal. Gingivitis and periodontitis are common. The skin is also susceptible to severe sunburn, and photosensitivity in bright light is common.

The neutrophil defects are primarily responsible for the propensity to bacterial infection. In addition to the moderate neutropenia, several defects in neutrophil function lead to impaired bactericidal activity. First, chemotaxis is markedly depressed, whether measured in vivo by the Rebuck skin window or in vitro by chemotaxis assays.[481,897] The large granules appear to interfere with the ability of neutrophils to travel through narrow passages, such as those between endothelial cells. Second, degranulation is delayed and incomplete in CHS neutrophils.[898,899] Third, the marked deficiency of antimicrobial proteins such as cathepsin G probably contributes to the diminished bactericidal potency of CHS neutrophils.[899] Finally, decreased expression of Mac-1 (CD11b/CD18) in CHS neutrophils may also play a role.[900]

Contributing to the enhanced susceptibility to infection are abnormalities in monocytes, lymphocytes, and NK cells. Monocytes, like neutrophils, exhibit decreased chemotaxis.[901] Peripheral blood CHS lymphocytes demonstrate diminished ADCC of tumor cells.[902] Perhaps most important, cytotoxic T-cell and NK-cell cytolytic function is profoundly abnormal in CHS.[877,902-904] This defect may not only contribute to the recurrent bacterial infections but also lead to the development of HLH in the "accelerated phase" of CHS, which is sometimes precipitated by a herpes-type virus such as Epstein-Barr virus or varicella.[876,877,905-907]

Patients who survive the infectious and neurologic problems of the stable phase of CHS have a high risk of progressing to the accelerated phase of the disease, now recognized to be a genetic form of HLH.[478,876,877] HLH results from uncontrolled hyperinflammation and multiorgan dysfunction and can be triggered by viral infections or other stimuli; it typically develops during the first or second decade of life in patients with CHS.[478,906] The accelerated phase is characterized pathologically by diffuse lymphohistiocytic infiltration of the liver, spleen, lymph nodes, and bone marrow, and the outcome for the patient is uniformly fatal if not treated.[906] The accelerated phase is heralded by hepatosplenomegaly, bone marrow infiltration, and hemophagocytosis leading to worsening of the neutropenia and an ever-increasing risk for infection. Thrombocytopenia likewise develops and intensifies the bleeding disorder already present in the platelets.

The diagnosis of CHS should be suspected in any child with one or more of the following findings: (1) recurrent bacterial infections of unknown etiology; (2) hypopigmentation of the hair, skin, and eyes; a white forelock can be present; (3) the presence of giant peroxidase-positive lysosomal granules in granulocytes from peripheral blood or bone marrow; (4) mild to moderate neutropenia; (5) easy bruising or nose bleeding despite a normal platelet count; and (6) unexplained hepatosplenomegaly (associated with the accelerated phase of the disease). CHS is usually manifested in infancy or early childhood but may become evident later when the child is in the accelerated phase. In some patients, the disease may be suspected on the basis of neurologic abnormalities, including ataxia, muscle weakness, decreased deep tendon reflexes, sensory loss, a diffusely abnormal electroencephalogram, and abnormal visual and auditory evoked potentials.[908,909] The physician should not be dissuaded from considering the diagnosis of CHS if the patient does not have clear-cut oculocutaneous albinism. Depending on the skin coloration in the family, the only manifestations of the albinism may be a metallic sheen in the hair (which can vary from blond to dark brown) and a lighter skin color than seen in siblings. In younger patients, there is likely to be a cartwheel distribution of pigment in the iris and an abnormal red reflex.

The diagnosis of CHS is made by finding giant peroxidase-positive lysosomal granules in blood or bone marrow myeloid cells. In some cases, relatively few abnormal granulocytes will be seen in peripheral blood, presumably because of extensive intramedullary destruction of myeloid precursors, and a bone marrow aspirate may be necessary to identify the large lysosomes. Microscopic examination of the hair reveals giant melanin granules. In the accelerated phase, biopsy of the liver, spleen, and lymph nodes reveals diffuse infiltrates of lymphohistiocytic cells. An affected fetus with CHS diagnosed by fetal blood sampling, which showed large abnormal granules in neutrophils, was also found to have significantly larger than normal acid phosphatase lysosomes in cultured amniotic and chorionic villus cells.[910] Microscopic examination of fetal hair shafts for prenatal diagnosis has also been reported.[911] This suggests that prenatal diagnosis of CHS might be accomplished with these latter techniques, which is less risky than fetal blood sampling.

The differential diagnosis for CHS includes other genetic forms of partial albinism.[477] One condition characterized by partial albinism is Griscelli's syndrome,[490] which is distinguished from CHS by the lack of giant cytoplasmic granules in neutrophils, the presence of large pigment clumps in hair shafts, and accumulation of mature melanosomes in melanocytes. HLH also typically develops in patients with Griscelli's syndrome, again secondary to defective cytolytic T-cell and NK-cell function.[877,912] Hermansky-Pudlak syndrome is another disorder marked by partial albinism, but it is characterized by platelet function defects and an associated bleeding diathesis. Giant granules resembling those in CHS can be seen in both AML and CML[913-915] and should not be confused with those seen in CHS.

Management of the stable phase of CHS primarily involves the treatment of infectious complications. Prophylactic trimethoprim-sulfamethoxazole may be beneficial. Infections should be treated vigorously with appropriate intravenous antibiotics. Treatment with high doses of ascorbic acid (20 mg/kg/day) has been reported to result in clinical improvement, as well as improved function of neutrophils in vitro (neutrophil chemotaxis or bactericidal function, or both).[916,917] Although there is some disagreement in the literature regarding the efficacy of ascorbic acid,[918] it seems reasonable to try this medication given its safety in moderate doses. NK cell function appears to remain abnormal even after ascorbate therapy.

Treatment of HLH (accelerated phase) has improved in recent years with the use of combinations of drugs that suppress the function of activated macrophages and T cells, followed by allogeneic HSCT. Regimens for HLH include corticosteroids, cyclosporine, and etoposide, and they are recommended for the accelerated phase of CHS.[876,877] In patients with moderate symptoms, corticosteroids and immunoglobulin infusions may be sufficient to induce an initial remission, although the use of etoposide should not be delayed if symptoms progress.[877]

Active therapy should be maintained until bone marrow transplantation can be performed. The only curative therapy is bone marrow transplantation with matched related or unrelated donor grafts.[876,919-925] This procedure is ideally performed before onset of the accelerated phase. Transplantation does not prevent the progressive neuropathy associated with CHS.[921]

Specific (Secondary) Granule Deficiency

SGD is an extremely rare congenital disorder of neutrophil function characterized by recurrent bacterial infections and multiple abnormalities in neutrophil structure and composition, including absent specific granules and bilobed nuclei.[926,927] Despite its rarity, SGD is an important part of the differential diagnosis in patients with suspected phagocyte immunodeficiencies and provides important insight into the transcriptional regulation of granule biogenesis and the functional roles of lactoferrin, vitamin B_{12}–binding protein, and other specific granule constituents of host defense. To date, five patients have been reported with SGD.[431,882,928-941] Inheritance appears to be autosomal recessive.[938,939,942]

The key features of SGD are summarized in Table 21-14. Clinically, patients with this disorder suffer from indolent, smoldering cutaneous infections punctuated by episodes (sometimes prolonged) of severe infections involving the lungs, ears, lymph nodes, and deeper structures of the skin. Lung abscesses and mastoiditis have been reported as complications of these infections. *S. aureus*, *P. aeruginosa*, *Proteus* species, other enteric gramnegative bacteria, and *C. albicans* appear to be the major pathogens. Further complicating the clinical course in some patients is the presence of neutropenia that is either intermittent and mild[928,930] or prolonged and severe.[431]

The clinical picture of SGD is consistent with the functional defects identified in patient neutrophils. There is a marked abnormality in chemotaxis that can be observed in vivo by the Rebuck skin window technique.[928,930,931,939] The indolent nature of some infections in SGD may be attributable to this chemotactic defect. In vitro measurements of neutrophil killing of *E. coli* and *S. aureus* show a moderate impairment despite the presence of a normal respiratory burst.[928-931,939,941] Patient neutrophils adhere normally to plastic surfaces[929,939] but exhibit slightly diminished sticking to nylon fibers and endothelial cells.[931] Degranulation of both azurophilic and (to the extent that they are present) specific granules also appears to be normal.[929,931,939]

At least three cellular compartments are affected by the underlying molecular defect or defects in SGD: the nucleus, specific granules, and azurophilic granules. Approximately half or more of the peripheral blood neutrophils in SGD have nuclei that resemble those seen in the Pelger-Huët anomaly. The nucleus has a kidney-shaped, bilobed configuration that is flawed by a series of microlobulations and clefts apparent on electron microscopy.[930,931,939] On a Wright stain of peripheral blood, neutrophils appear to be devoid of the pink-staining specific granules. By electron microscopic analysis, however, it is apparent that the specific granules are not actually absent but instead are present as empty, elongated vesicles that retain their characteristic trilamellar membrane structure and positive staining for complex carbohydrates.[930,932,934,938] Biochemical measurements of specific granule contents parallel the morphologic studies. Lactoferrin, vitamin B_{12}–binding protein, and gelatinase[943] are present at levels that are only 3% to 10% of normal.[929,931,939] Thus, there appears to be an abortive

TABLE 21-14	Summary of Neutrophil Specific Granule Deficiency
Incidence	Five cases reported
Inheritance	Autosomal recessive
Molecular defect	Protein deficiencies in azurophilic granules (defensins), specific granules (lactoferrin, vitamin B_{12}–binding protein, gelatinase), and secretory vesicles (alkaline phosphatase) suggest a common defect in regulation of the production of these proteins in myeloid cells. Eosinophil specific granules also deficient in protein contents. Mutations in the myeloid transcription factor C/EPBε identified in several patients
Pathogenesis	Recurrent infections result from the combined effect of deficiencies in microbicidal granule protein (e.g., defensins and lactoferrin) and abnormal chemotaxis, perhaps as a result of failure to upregulate surface β_2 integrins and chemotactic peptide receptors from granule stores
Clinical manifestations	Recurrent (sometimes indolent) pyogenic infections of the skin, ears, lungs, and lymph nodes that may have diminished neutrophil infiltration; onset usually during infancy
Laboratory evaluation	Absent or empty specific granule vesicles in neutrophils by electron microscopy (by light microscopy, granules appear absent)
	Bilobed nuclei resembling the Pelger-Huët anomaly are frequently seen in neutrophils
	Severe deficiency of neutrophil lactoferrin, vitamin B_{12}–binding protein, defensins, and alkaline phosphatase (by histochemical assay)
Differential diagnosis	Acquired specific granule deficiency (e.g., thermal burns or myeloproliferative syndromes)
Therapy	Prophylactic antibiotics
	Parenteral antibiotics for acute infections
	Surgical drainage or resection of refractory infections
Prognosis	With appropriate medical management, patients can survive into their adult years

and incomplete formation of normal specific granules. Azurophilic (primary) granules in this disorder are also strikingly abnormal. Although they contain a normal (if not slightly elevated) amount of MPO and are present in normal numbers, they are severely deficient in defensins.[882] In addition, there is a severe deficiency of alkaline phosphatase activity in peripheral blood neutrophils,[928,930,939] which is normally localized to secretory vesicles, and its deficiency probably represents yet another organelle abnormality in this disorder.[934] Finally, granule formation also appears to be abnormal in eosinophils. These cells are deficient in three eosinophil-specific granule proteins (eosinophil cationic protein, MBP, and eosinophil-derived neurotoxin), although the corresponding mRNA transcripts are present.[944]

In view of the multiple deficits in granule matrix contents produced after the promyelocyte stage, it had long been speculated that SGD is due to an abnormality in biosynthetic regulation of granule (and probably non-granule) proteins during granulopoiesis. This mechanism is also consistent with the observation that the SGD neutrophils are severely deficient in defensins, which are stored in azurophilic granules. In contrast to other azurophilic granule proteins that are synthesized at the promyelocyte stage, defensins are produced during the subsequent myelocyte stage, along with the specific granule matrix proteins (see Fig. 21-1).

At least some cases of SGD result from autosomal recessive mutations in a transcription factor that regulates gene expression during granulocyte differentiation. Serendipitously, mice generated with a targeted deletion in the myeloid transcription factor C/EBPε exhibit absence of neutrophil secondary granules and their matrix proteins, bilobed neutrophil nuclei, impaired chemotaxis, and increased susceptibility to bacterial infection.[49,945,946] Mutations in the C/EBPε gene have been identified in two SGD patients to date. In one case, a 5–base pair (bp) deletion resulted in a truncated, nonfunctional protein,[947] whereas a second, unrelated patient was homozygous for a nucleotide insertion in the coding sequence that also leads to the synthesis of a truncated and nonfunctional form of C/EBPε.[59] However, DNA sequencing of the C/EBPε gene in several other SGD patients has not revealed abnormalities, which suggests that SGD is a genetically heterogeneous disorder.[948]

The cellular defects just described can explain, at least in part, the clinical problems observed in SGD. The markedly abnormal specific granules and secretory vesicles, which contain intracellular stores of both β_2 integrins[949-951] and a chemotactic peptide receptor,[952] fail to support normal upregulation of these two types of receptors[936,939] and may thereby contribute to the chemotactic defect. Furthermore, the severe deficiency of key bactericidal proteins such as lactoferrin and the defensins renders the cell less efficient in killing bacteria and *Candida*. Neutropenia, when it does occur, also impairs host defense and appears to be caused by intramedullary

destruction of the abnormal neutrophils, as evidenced by their ingestion by marrow macrophages.[938]

The diagnosis of SGD can be made by light microscopic examination of Wright-stained peripheral blood neutrophils. Electron microscopic studies can confirm the presence of empty specific granule vesicles. Bilobed nuclei and greatly diminished levels of alkaline phosphatase by histochemical analysis also support the diagnosis. In conjunction with these morphologic studies, biochemical and immunologic measurements of lactoferrin, vitamin B_{12}–binding protein, and defensins can be made. As discussed previously, all three of these granule proteins are severely deficient in this disorder. Acquired SGD is observed in myeloproliferative syndromes and after thermal burns.[926,953] In these acquired disorders, however, at least a few intact specific granules are still observed microscopically, and the deficiencies of the various granule enzymes are less profound.

As with other neutrophil disorders, prophylactic antibiotics appear to be beneficial based on anecdotal experience. Parenteral antibiotics should be used aggressively for acute infections. With appropriate medical management, patients can survive into their adult years. Malignant transformation of the dysmorphic myeloid cells in this disorder has not been reported.

Disorders of Oxidative Metabolism

The elimination of many pathogens requires oxygen-derived microbicidal compounds generated by the phagocyte respiratory burst pathway in response to inflammatory stimuli (see Fig. 21-7). Five clinically recognized defects have been identified in this series of reactions, including deficiencies in NADPH oxidase (reaction 1 in Fig. 21-7), G6PD, (reaction 8), MPO (reaction 4), glutathione reductase (reaction 7), and glutathione synthetase (reaction 9).

Chronic Granulomatous Disease

CGD is an inherited disorder of phagocyte function in which generation of superoxide by the respiratory burst oxidase (see Fig. 21-9) in neutrophils, monocytes, macrophages, and eosinophils is absent or markedly deficient.[771,954-959] The disorder occurs at an estimated minimum incidence of approximately 1 in 200,000 to 250,000 individuals, thus making it the most common clinically significant disorder of phagocyte function that is inherited.[957] CGD is due to mutations in any one of four essential subunits of the respiratory burst oxidase (Table 21-15; also see Fig. 21-9 and Table 21-7). Though originally described as an X-linked recessive disorder affecting boys,[957,960-964] approximately a third of CGD cases are inherited as an autosomal recessive trait[965,966] (see Table 21-15). In more than 90% of patients, superoxide production by activated phagocytes is undetectable. A respiratory burst 1% to 10% of normal is observed in the remaining patients, who are often referred to as having "variant" CGD.[966-969] Other aspects of phagocyte

TABLE 21-15 **Classification of Chronic Granulomatous Disease**

Component Affected	Inheritance	Subtype*	Cytochrome *b* Spectrum	NBT Score (% Positive)	Frequency (% of Cases)	PROTEIN EXPRESSION			
						gp91*phox*	p22*phox*	p47*phox*	p67*phox*
gp91*phox*	X	X91^0	0	0	60	0	0-trace	N	N
		X91$^-$	Low	80-100 (weak)	5	Low	Low	N	N
		X91$^-$	Low	5-10	<1	Low	Low	N	N
		X91$^+$	0	0	1	N	N	N	N
p22*phox*	A	A22^0	0	0	4	0	0	N	N
		A22$^+$	N	0	<1	N	N	N	N
p47*phox*	A	A47^0	N	0	25	N	N	0	N
p67*phox*	A	A67^0	N	0	5	N	N	N	0
		A67$^+$	N	0	<1	N	N	N	N

*In this nomenclature, the first letter represents the mode of inheritance (X-linked [X] or autosomal recessive [A]), whereas the number indicates the *phox* component that is genetically affected. The superscript symbols indicate whether the level of protein of the affected component is undetectable (^{0}), diminished ($^-$), or normal ($^+$) as measured by immunoblot analysis. NBT, nitroblue tetrazolium.

function are normal in CGD, including adherence, ingestion, and degranulation.[970-972]

Clinical Manifestations

CGD is associated with a distinctive clinical syndrome that provides clear evidence for the importance of the phagocyte respiratory burst in host defense and the inflammatory response (for reviews, see elsewhere[957,973-981]). Patients suffer from recurrent, often severe purulent bacterial and fungal infections, often caused by organisms not ordinarily considered pathogens. The other and distinctive hallmark of this disorder is a propensity for the development of chronic inflammatory granulomas that can be widely distributed in tissues. This feature of the disease, at least in part, reflects a role for NADPH oxidase–derived superoxide as a cofactor in the oxidative cleavage of tryptophan to L-kynurenine by indolamine 2,3-dioxygenase (IDO), an important immunomodulatory pathway that otherwise downregulates inflammation.[982,983] The majority of patients with CGD manifest symptoms within the first year of life,[957,977] although some may remain relatively symptom free until later in childhood or even adult life.[984-990]

Table 21-16 summarizes the types of infections and infecting organisms most frequently encountered in CGD.[957,974,975,977-979,991,992] The major sites of infection are those that come into contact with the external environment—the lungs, skin, gastrointestinal tract, and lymph nodes draining these organs. Hematogenous seeding can lead to liver abscesses or osteomyelitis. The most common pathogens include *S. aureus*, *Aspergillus* species (most often *A. fumigatus* but occasionally *A. nidulans*),[992-994] and a variety of gram-negative bacilli, including *Serratia marcescens* and various *Salmonella* species. Members of the *Burkholderia cepacia* complex are aggressive and potentially lethal pathogen in CGD.[957,995,996] *Burkholderia* species that cause infection in CGD include *B. cenocepa-*

cia, *B. gladioli*, and *B. mallei*, which causes melioidosis in East Asian countries.[995,996] In many febrile illnesses, no organism can be identified despite extensive culturing. In such cases it is important to look carefully for the presence of unusual microbes that can occasionally cause serious infections in CGD (see Table 21-16 and references).[985,992,997-1004] Of note, disseminated *Mycobacterium bovis* infection has been reported after bacille Calmette-Guérin (BCG) vaccination in CGD,[1005] and infections with other atypical mycobacteria are also reported in CGD.[1006] A newly identified member of the gram-negative Acetobacteraceae family named *Granulobacter bethesdensis*, heretofore not associated with human disease, was identified in a CGD patient with recurrent fever and a chronic necrotizing deep lymphatic infection.[1007]

Pneumonia is most frequently caused by *S. aureus*, *Aspergillus* species, and enteric bacteria. It is common for an organism to not be identified even in lung biopsy specimens. Complications of pneumonia include empyema or lung abscess. Suppurative lymphadenitis, usually involving the cervical nodes, is especially common in younger patients and is typically caused by *S. aureus* and enteric bacilli such as *Serratia* and *Klebsiella*. Staphylococcal skin infections are also common. Hepatic and perihepatic abscesses, usually caused by *S. aureus*, are surprisingly frequent and should suggest the diagnosis of CGD if it has not already been made.[1008-1010] Bone infections can be particularly problematic in CGD and are caused by either direct spread of infection from contiguous sites or hematogenous spread from more distant locations.[957,1011] The former type of osteomyelitis is usually seen in the ribs and vertebral bodies as a result of invasion by pulmonary *Aspergillus*.[1011] The latter type is more frequently seen in peripheral long and small bones and is typically caused by *S. marcescens*, *Nocardia* species, and *S. aureus*.[1011] Perirectal infections are extremely difficult to treat in CGD and can lead to fistula formation.[1008] The

TABLE 21-16	Infections in Chronic Granulomatous Disease		
Infections	**% of Infections**	**Infecting Organisms**	**% of Isolates**
Pneumonia	70-80	*Staphylococcus aureus*	30-50
Lymphadenitis*	60-80	*Aspergillus* species	10-20
Cutaneous infections/impetigo*	60-70	*Escherichia coli*	5-10
Hepatic/perihepatic abscesses*	30-40	*Klebsiella* species	5-10
Osteomyelitis	20-30	*Salmonella* species	5-10
Perirectal abscesses/fistulas*	15-30	*Burkholderia cepacia*	5-10
Septicemia	10-20	*Serratia marcescens*	5-10
Otitis media*	≈20	*Staphylococcus epidermidis*	5
Conjunctivitis	≈15	*Streptococcus* species	4
Enteric infections	≈10	*Enterobacter* species	3
Urinary tract infections/pyelonephritis	5-15	*Proteus* species	3
Sinusitis	<10	*Candida albicans*	3
Renal/perinephric abscesses	<10	*Nocardia* species	2
Brain abscesses	<5	*Haemophilus influenzae*	1
Pericarditis	<5	*Pneumocystis carinii*	<1
Meningitis	<5	*Mycobacterium fortuitum*	<1
		Chromobacterium violaceum	<1
		Francisella philomiragia	<1
		Torulopsis glabrata	<1

The relative frequencies of different types of infections in CGD are estimated from data pooled from several large series of patients in the United States, Europe, and Japan. See text for references. These series encompass approximately 550 patients with CGD after accounting for overlap between reports. The list of infecting organisms is also arranged according to the data in these reports and is not paired with the entries in the first column.

*Infections most frequently seen at initial evaluation.

rare pathogen *Chromobacterium violaceum* is found in brackish waters and is an uncommon but potentially serious cause of soft tissue infection, pneumonia, or sepsis in CGD patients in the southern part of the United States.[999,1000,1012] *C. violaceum* infection in northern areas has also been reported.

It has long been recognized that patients with CGD are particularly susceptible to organisms that contain catalase, which prevents the CGD phagocyte from scavenging microbially generated H_2O_2 for phagosomal killing.[1013] Thus, infections with streptococci or *Haemophilus* species, which are typically catalase negative, are not problematic in CGD. Another possible link among the organisms with increased virulence in CGD is that they are resistant to the nonoxidative killing mechanisms of the phagocyte mediated by antibiotic proteins contained within the various granule compartments.[282,1014,1015]

The chronic conditions associated with CGD are responsible for many of the major complications seen with this disorder and are summarized in Table 21-17. This includes the formation of granulomas, which are believed to reflect a chronic inflammatory response to inadequate phagocyte killing or digestion and are a distinctive feature of CGD. These lesions contain a mixture of lymphocytes and inflammatory macrophages, some of which may have a foamy lipoid cytoplasm that has a characteristic yellow-brown color. Though not pathognomonic of CGD, the presence of such macrophages in granulomas or other tissue sites should suggest the diagnosis of CGD.[961,962,964,1016] The tendency toward granulomatous inflammation is believed to reflect in part a dysregulated inflammatory response in the absence of

TABLE 21-17	Chronic Conditions Associated with Chronic Granulomatous Disease
Condition	**% of Cases**
Lymphadenopathy	98
Hypergammaglobulinemia	60-90
Hepatomegaly	50-90
Splenomegaly	60-80
Anemia of chronic disease	Common*
Underweight	70
Chronic diarrhea	20-60
Short stature	50
Gingivitis	50
Dermatitis	35
Hydronephrosis	10-25
Ulcerative stomatitis	5-15
Pulmonary fibrosis	<10*
Esophagitis	<10*
Gastric antral narrowing	<10
Granulomatous ileocolitis	<10
Granulomatous cystitis	<10
Chorioretinitis	<10
Glomerulonephritis	<10
Discoid lupus erythematosus	<10

*The relative frequencies of the chronic conditions associated with CGD were estimated from the series of reports listed in Table 22-16. See text for additional references.

respiratory burst–derived oxidants; it leads to abnormally high level of cytokines and other proinflammatory mediators, in addition to delayed neutrophil apoptosis at inflammatory sites.[1017-1019] These abnormalities have recently been linked to defective superoxide-dependent cleavage of tryptophan to L-kynurenine by IDO.[983] Proinflammatory stimuli upregulate IDO expression in dendritic cells and phagocytes, and IDO-catalyzed tryptophan metabolism then downregulates the inflammation by suppressing γδ T-cell activity and mediating the production of IL-17 after initial activation of the innate immune response.[982] Inefficient degradation of debris in the absence of oxidants is also likely to be a contributing factor to the chronic inflammation in CGD.[1019-1021] Granulomatous inflammation can develop independent of active infection.[1019]

Granuloma formation can lead to obstructive symptoms in the upper gastrointestinal tract, including gastric outlet obstruction that can be confused clinically with pyloric stenosis.[1008,1009,1022-1024] A chronic ileocolitis syndrome resembling Crohn's disease is seen in approximately 5% to 10% of patients and can lead to a debilitating syndrome of diarrhea and malabsorption.[1009,1024,1025] Chronic inflammatory lesions have been identified in the urinary bladder walls of some patients and can cause a chronic cystitis that can be manifested as dysuria, penile pain, and decreased urine volume.[1026-1030] In one study of 60 CGD patients, 11 cases of granulomatous inflammation of the bladder wall, ureters, or urethra were seen, accompanied by stricture formation in the latter two sites.[1031] Hydronephrosis can occur as a complication of obstruction.

Other chronic inflammatory complications of CGD include lymphadenopathy, hepatosplenomegaly, and an eczematoid dermatitis,[975,977,1032] along with hypergammaglobulinemia, anemia of chronic disease, and short stature (see Table 21-17). Gingivitis and ulcerative stomatitis can occur.[1033] Chorioretinitis[1034,1035] and destructive white matter lesions in the brain have also been described.[1036,1037] Glomerulonephritis has been reported.[1038,1039] Occasionally, either discoid or systemic lupus erythematosus, juvenile rheumatoid arthritis, or sarcoidosis may develop.[1040-1045] Subtle defects in CGD memory B cells[1046,1047] may influence the development of autoimmune disease in CGD.

The severity and pattern of complications of CGD are heterogeneous, which may partly reflect the heterogeneity of molecular defects (see later) and whether any residual respiratory burst oxidase function is present. However, a severe clinical course can occur in some patients in the latter "variant" category that is indistinguishable from what is observed in patients with complete absence of phagocyte superoxide production.[969,1048] On the other hand, some individuals with undetectable levels of respiratory burst activity can experience relatively few symptoms and have intervals of years between severe infections. Hence, polymorphisms in oxygen-independent antimicrobial systems or other components regulating the innate immune response are likely to play an important role in modifying disease severity in CGD. Specific polymorphisms in the MPO, MBL, and FcγRIIa genes are associated with a higher risk for granulomatous or autoimmune/rheumatologic complications in CGD.[1049] Patients with p47[phox] deficiency overall tend to have milder disease, possibly because of very small but detectable levels of superoxide production.[957,1050]

Heterozygous carriers of the CGD trait are generally asymptomatic, but there are several important exceptions. Carriers of the autosomal recessive forms of CGD have a normal phagocyte respiratory burst and are free from infection. Carriers of X-linked CGD, on the other had, typically have two populations of circulating neutrophils and monocytes—some with normal respiratory burst activity and others with none[1051-1057]—because of random X-chromosome inactivation.[1058,1059] In most X-linked carriers, these two populations are approximately equal in number, but occasionally individuals have an unusually small percentage of either abnormal or normal cells. If the number of functioning neutrophils is less than 10% to 15%, the carrier often suffers from some of the infectious complications of CGD.[969,986,1051,1060] Clinical problems more commonly seen in female carriers of X-linked CGD are aphthous ulcers or discoid lupus erythematosus.[1042,1061] In a 1991 review of the literature,[1042] 22 cases were summarized from 11 reports. Clinically, the carriers had discoid-like skin lesions (13 of 22 patients), photosensitivity (13 patients), and recurrent aphthous stomatitis (12 patients). In a few, polyarthritis, arthralgia, and Raynaud's phenomenon were also observed. Serologic testing for lupus was generally negative, as were immunofluorescence studies of biopsied lesions. Interestingly, all the reported cases were carriers of X-linked CGD. Discoid lupus–like lesions have also been reported in five autosomal recessive CGD patients.[1040,1041,1062] Because the lupus skin lesions typically do not appear to develop unless there is at least a subpopulation of nonfunctioning phagocytes, it has been hypothesized that autoantibodies to antigens from incompletely destroyed microbes may be responsible for the syndrome.[1042]

Molecular Basis of CGD

CGD is classified according to the respiratory burst oxidase subunit that is affected (see Table 21-15). Nomenclature has also been adopted for an abbreviated designation within each major genetic subgroup that includes the mode of inheritance and level of *phox* protein expression. The genes or corresponding cDNA (or both) of all four subunits have been cloned and their chromosomal locations mapped (see Fig. 21-9 and Table 21-7).[310,719,955,1063,1064] In two large studies of 140 pedigrees in the United States and Europe, defects in the X-linked gene for the gp91[phox] subunit of flavocytochrome *b* accounted for approximately two thirds of cases, with the remainder being due to autosomal recessive inheritance of defects in p47[phox] (25%), p67[phox] (5%), and p22[phox] (5%).[957,965,966] However, deficiency of p47[phox] has been reported to account for only 7% of cases of CGD in Japan.[1065]

Mutations in Flavocytochrome *b*. That CGD might result from a genetic defect in an electron-transporting cytochrome was first suspected from reports that neutrophils obtained from the majority of CGD patients lacked a low-potential cytochrome *b*.[725,1066,1067] It is now known that the respiratory burst cytochrome is a flavocytochrome composed of two subunits and contains both flavin and heme groups that mediate the transfer of electrons from NADPH to molecular oxygen to generate superoxide.[301,1068] The cytochrome has two subunits, a 91-kd glycoprotein (gp91[phox]) that is the site of mutations in X-linked CGD and a 22-kd polypeptide (p22[phox]) that is defective in a rare subgroup of patients with autosomal recessive inheritance of CGD. Formation of the gp91[phox]/ p22[phox] heterodimer appears to be important to stabilize each subunit within the phagocyte, and absent expression of both subunits is typically seen in both forms of cytochrome-negative CGD.[308,1069,1070]

The gene encoding gp91[phox] was mapped to Xp21.1 by its linkage to the X-linked form of CGD.[1071] It was the first human gene to be cloned on the basis of its chromosomal location,[310] an approach referred to as positional cloning or "reverse genetics." The gp91[phox] gene (termed *CYBB*) contains 13 exons and spans approximately 30 kilobases (kb) in the Xp21.1 region of the X chromosome.[310,1071,1072] Mechanisms that regulate phagocyte-specific transcription of this gene include a repressor protein, known as CCAAT displacement protein (CDP), that binds to DNA sites upstream of the promoter to block transcription in nonphagocytic or undifferentiated myeloid cells.[1072] Some regulatory elements appear to be located relatively long distances from the coding portion of the gp91[phox] gene.[1072,1073]

Defects in the gene for gp91[phox] X-linked CGD are very heterogeneous[956,958,1065,1074,1075] and, with few exceptions, are associated with absence of both the flavocytochrome heterodimer (X91⁰) and respiratory burst activity. Mutations in the gp91[phox] gene have been identified in more than 400 patients with X-linked CGD. An international registry, CYBBbase, is accessible at http://bioinf. uta.fi.[756,1076] In general, each mutation is unique to a given kindred, although some have been seen in several unrelated pedigrees. The overall heterogeneity of mutations and lack of any predominant genotype indicate that CGD is due to many different mutational events without any founder effect, as expected for a formerly lethal disorder. Approximately 10% to 15% of cases of X-linked CGD are caused by new germline mutations.[1074]

The majority of X-linked CGD patients have mutations limited to only one or several nucleotides, which results in missense, mRNA splicing site, frameshift, or nonsense mutations. A small percentage of patients with X-linked CGD express a small amount of residual flavocytochrome *b* (X91⁻) associated with low levels of superoxide production. In addition, individuals have been reported who have normal levels of a dysfunctional flavocytochrome *b* (X91⁺). Some of the mutations that result in normal levels of a dysfunctional flavocytochrome affect gp91[phox] domains that either participate in oxidase assembly[1077,1078] or are involved in its redox function.[955,956,958,988,1075,1079-1081]

Relatively large deletions in Xp21.1 involving *CYBB* and adjacent loci have been described in a few rare patients.[310,1071,1082-1085] These individuals have complex phenotypes that include CGD and McLeod's syndrome (mild hemolytic anemia with acanthocytosis associated with depressed levels of Kell antigens because of defects in the red cell antigen Kˣ), with or without concomitant Duchenne's muscular dystrophy and retinitis pigmentosa. Patients with the McLeod phenotype may develop anti-Kell antibodies when transfused with red blood cells, which can make future transfusion very difficult. Nerve and muscle disorders related to Kell expression in nonerythroid tissues can also develop in these patients.[1086,1087] Smaller deletions of the gp91[phox] gene have been reported as well.[1075]

Mutations affecting the regulation of gp91[phox] transcription are rare and have been identified in two unusual phenotypes. In one type, described in two unrelated kindreds, affected males have two distinct populations of neutrophils.[1048] One population has normal respiratory burst activity and accounts for 5% to 15% of the circulating phagocytes and myeloid progenitor cells, whereas the other population, which accounts for the remainder of the cells, lacks a respiratory burst entirely. Affected males had a severe clinical course.[1048] Sequencing of the gp91[phox] gene identified a point mutation in the promoter sequence that was located 57 bp upstream of the normal transcription initiation site in one kindred and 54 bp upstream in the other.[1060] Another unusual patient with X-linked CGD had normal levels of gp91[phox] expression and function in circulating eosinophils, but this patient's neutrophils, monocytes, and B lymphocytes had markedly reduced levels of gp91[phox].[1088] Molecular analysis identified a mutation 53 bp upstream of the transcription start site in this kindred.[1089] These mutations disrupt the binding of several transcriptions important for normal expression of the *CYBB* gene,[1089,1090] thus suggesting that gp91[phox] gene expression is dependent on this region of the promoter in all but a subset of granulocytes.

Mutations in the gene for the p22[phox] subunit of flavocytochrome *b*, designated *CYBA*, are an uncommon cause of autosomal recessive CGD (see Table 21-15). The *CYBA* locus resides at 16q24 and contains six exons that span 8.5 kb.[1063] The genetic defects that have been identified in this flavocytochrome subunit are heterogeneous and range from a large interstitial gene deletion[1063] to point mutations associated with missense, frameshift, or RNA-splicing defects.[776,958] In all but one case, p22[phox] is not expressed (A22⁰ CGD). A proline-to-glutamine substitution in a cytoplasmic domain of p22[phox] is associated with normal levels of flavocytochrome *b* and a nonfunctional oxidase (A22⁺ CGD).[1079] This mutation disrupts a proline-rich docking sequence in p22[phox] that binds to a pair of SH3 domains in the p47[phox] domains and is required for assembly of the active oxidase complex.[301,1068] The proline substitution in p22[phox] is the one example of a genetic disease caused by disruption of protein-protein interactions mediated via SH3 domains. A kindred with X-linked agammaglobulinemia caused by deletion of the SH3 region of Bruton's tyrosine kinase has also been reported.[1091]

Mutations in Cytosolic Factors. A key discovery in unraveling the molecular basis of the different genetic subgroups in CGD was the observation that both the plasma membrane and the cytosol were required to reconstitute a catalytically active oxidase in a cell-free assay.[1092-1095] Complementation analysis using this assay identified two different subgroups of CGD in which the defect involved a cytosolic protein rather than the membrane-bound flavocytochrome *b*.[1096,1097] Mutations in the gene encoding a cytosolic phosphoprotein, p47*phox*, account for approximately a fourth of all cases of CGD in the United States and Europe, whereas in Japan the incidence is only approximately 7%.[724,1065] Inherited defects in the p67*phox* gene also account for a small subgroup of autosomal recessive CGD (see Table 21-15). Neither p47*phox* nor p67*phox* appear to participate directly in electron transfer but act in a regulatory role. The p47*phox* subunit is believed to function as an "adaptor" protein important for efficient recruitment of p67*phox* translocation to the flavocytochrome. Consistent with this role, substantial amounts of superoxide can be generated from neutrophil membranes in vitro, even in the absence of p47*phox*, provided that high concentrations of p67*phox* and Rac-GTP are supplied.[300]

The gene for p47*phox*, termed *NCF1* (for neutrophil cytosolic factor 1), resides on chromosome 7[1098] and contains nine exons spanning 18 kb.[1099] In contrast to other forms of CGD, the majority of p47*phox*-deficient CGD is due to a single type of mutation, a GT deletion at the beginning of exon 2 that results in a frameshift and premature translational termination.[1099,1100] Most patients are homozygous for this mutation without any history of consanguinity, although a few compound heterozygotes have been described with a missense mutation accompanying the GT deletion.[1101] The high frequency of the GT deletion appears to reflect the fact that humans have highly and closely linked conserved pseudogenes for p47*phox* that contain the GT deletion.[1102] Some individuals also have a gene-pseudogene-pseudogene chimera.[1103] Recombination or gene conversion events between the authentic p47*phox* gene and its pseudogene or pseudogenes lead to a nonfunctional p47*phox* allele containing the GT deletion.[1104] All reported patients with p47*phox* gene mutations do not express this protein (A47⁰). Perhaps because p47*phox* is an adaptor protein rather than directly involved in activating electron transport, A47⁰ neutrophils can still generate very small but detectable amounts of superoxide, which may account for the overall milder course of this genetic subgroup.[957,1050]

The gene for p67*phox*, *NCF2*, which has been mapped to the long arm of chromosome 1,[1105] spans 37 kb and contains 16 exons.[1106] Mutations identified in p67*phox*-deficient CGD are heterogeneous and typically result in absent p67*phox* expression (A67⁰ CGD).[1107-1111] In one patient, in whom a triplet nucleotide deletion resulted in

an in-frame deletion of lysine 58, a nonfunctional form of p67*phox* was expressed that failed to translocate and was unable to bind to Rac.[1112]

Diagnosis

A diagnosis of CGD is suggested by the characteristic clinical features (see Tables 21-16 and 21-17) or by a family history of the disease. Because the severity and onset of the disease can vary considerably among patients, CGD should still be considered in adolescents and adults with an unusual site of infection or organism typical of CGD (see Table 21-16). The diagnosis of CGD is established by demonstrating an absent or greatly diminished neutrophil respiratory burst. It is important to have testing performed on appropriately handled blood samples and by experienced laboratories to avoid inconclusive or false-normal results.

Many different methods have been used to monitor respiratory burst activity. Assays include those that monitor chemiluminescence or fluorescence when superoxide is released from activated phagocytes.[1054,1055,1113,1114] One of the simplest and most accurate techniques is the nitroblue tetrazolium (NBT) test, in which neutrophils in freshly isolated blood are stimulated to undergo a respiratory burst in the presence of NBT.[1052,1053,1115,1116] When reduced by electrons donated from superoxide, the water-soluble, yellow tetrazolium dye is converted to deep blue, insoluble formazan deposits that precipitate on any cell that undergoes a respiratory burst. NBT reduction can be evaluated quantitatively on cells in suspension[1115] or, preferably, by examination of neutrophils and monocytes that have adhered to a microscope slide (the NBT slide test).[1052,1053] As shown in the NBT slide test in Figure 21-11, stimulated neutrophils and monocytes are normally strongly stained with NBT formazan deposits (panel B). Cells from patients with X91⁰, A22⁰, A47⁰, and A67⁰ CGD fail to stain with NBT (an X91⁰ patient is shown in panel C), whereas patients with variant forms of the disease show light staining (an X91⁻ patient is shown in panel E). In addition to X91⁻ CGD neutrophils, weak staining in the NBT test and a small but measurable level of dihydroxyrhodamine 123 (DHR 123) fluorescence (see later) can be seen in A47⁰ cells and reflects a small amount of residual oxidant production. The NBT slide test can also diagnose the carrier states of either X91⁰ or X91⁻ CGD because a mixed population of NBT-positive and NBT-negative (or weakly NBT stained) cells is observed (Fig. 21-11D and F). Failure to detect a mixed population of formazan-staining cells does not necessarily rule out the X-linked carrier state because nonrandom inactivation of cells with the mutant X chromosome can occur by chance. A normal maternal NBT test may also indicate that there has been a de novo mutation in the germline of a parent[1074,1098] or that the patient has one of the autosomal recessive forms of CGD. Intermediate levels of NBT reduction are not seen in the phagocytes of autosomal recessive carriers. Flow cytometric assays of oxidase activity, such as those

FIGURE 21-11. Evaluation of chronic granulomatous disease (CGD) with the nitroblue tetrazolium (NBT) test. Photomicrographs are shown of NBT tests performed on normal cells (at rest and after stimulation with phorbol myristate acetate [PMA]) and on PMA-stimulated cells from X91⁰ and X91⁻ CGD patients and their mothers (who are carriers). Dense formazan crystals are seen in all the normal phagocytes after stimulation (**B**) but are absent from resting cells (**A**). The CGD patients are seen to have homogeneous populations of cells that either do not respond (X91⁰, **C**) or respond only minimally (X91⁻, **E**) to PMA. In contrast, NBT tests on CGD carriers show heterogeneous populations of cells that respond either normally or in a fashion similar to that of the abnormal cells from their offspring (**D** and **F**). In the case of the maternal carrier shown in **F**, the cells with normal deposits of formazan (*arrow*) are intermixed with cells containing minimal amounts of formazan (*arrowheads*) identical to those seen in her affected male child (**E**). (*Reprinted from Smith RM, Curnutte JT. Molecular basis of chronic granulomatous disease. Blood. 1991;77:673–686.*)

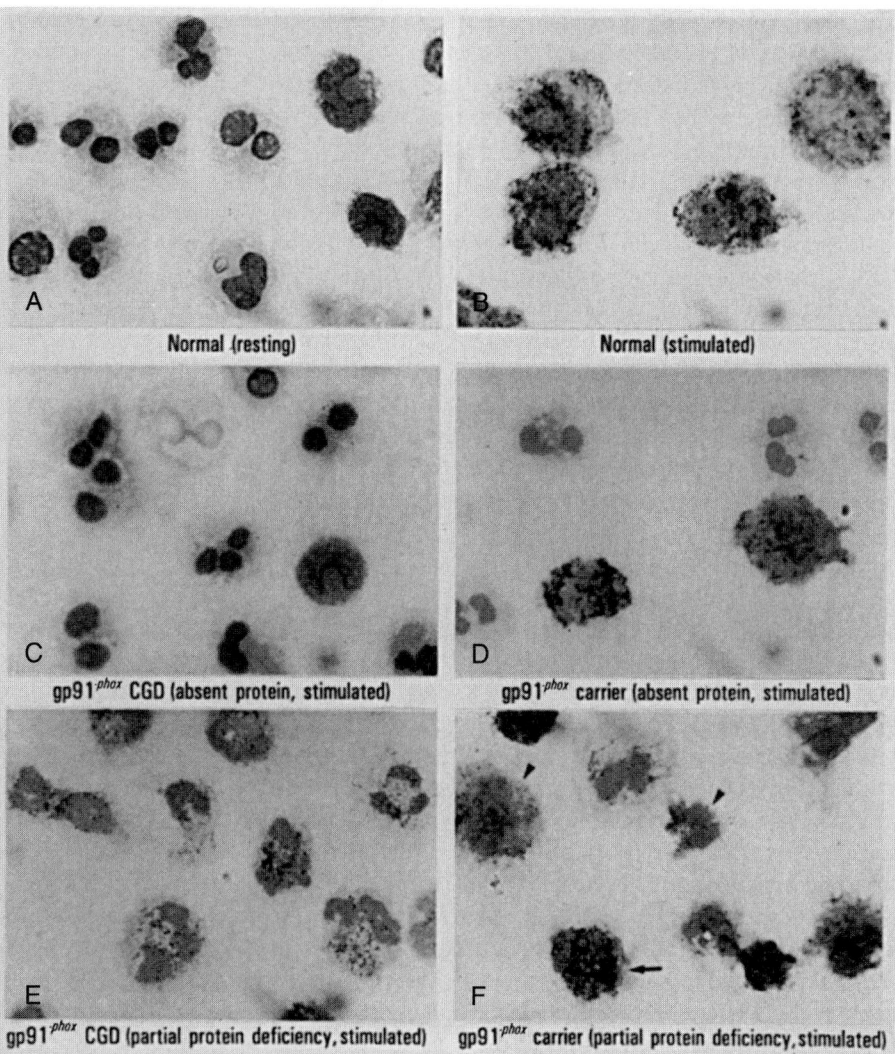

A — Normal (resting)
B — Normal (stimulated)
C — gp91^phox CGD (absent protein, stimulated)
D — gp91^phox carrier (absent protein, stimulated)
E — gp91^phox CGD (partial protein deficiency, stimulated)
F — gp91^phox carrier (partial protein deficiency, stimulated)

based on the conversion of DHR 123 to rhodamine 123,[1113,1114] are increasing in use for the diagnosis of CGD and, like the NBT test, provide both quantitative measurements of oxidant generation and cell-by-cell distribution of activity. The DHR 123 assay for neutrophil respiratory burst activity is available in many referral centers and reference laboratories and can be performed on blood collected in heparin and stored overnight.

With the exception of classic X-linked disease in a male whose mother is a carrier, determining the specific oxidase gene affected in a given CGD patient (see Table 21-15) requires additional studies. Genetic (DNA) testing for all four subgroups of CGD is now available commercially. Other assays, available in research laboratories, include immunoblot analysis of *phox* protein expression in neutrophil extracts, flavocytochrome *b* spectroscopy, and functional analysis of membrane and cytosol fractions in the cell-free oxidase assay. In a male with absent flavocytochrome *b* without clear evidence of a maternal carrier, it is necessary to search for the mutation in both the gp91^phox and p22^phox genes by DNA sequencing or another method of analysis. Identification of the specific genetic subgroup of a patient is useful primarily for purposes of genetic counseling and prenatal diagnosis. In prenatal testing for suspected X-linked CGD, further analysis is not necessary if the fetus is determined to be a 46,XX female.

Prognosis and Treatment

The prognosis for patients afflicted with CGD has continued to improve since the disorder was first described in the 1950s, at which time almost all patients died in childhood.[960-962] In one retrospective review of 38 patients monitored between 1964 and 1989, actuarial analysis showed a 50% survival rate through the third decade of life.[1117] In another retrospective study of 48 patients monitored between 1969 and 1985 in Paris, the actuarial survival rate was 50% at 10 years of age, with a prolonged plateau thereafter.[978] Further refinements in treatment and the use of prophylactic antimicrobials, coupled with the introduction of IFN-γ therapy, have continued to improve the prognosis for CGD.[1118,1119] Despite the lack of prospective data examining the long-term impact of these newer management strategies, it is generally agreed that a large majority of patients should survive well into their adult years. The overall mortality for all patients with CGD in the United States, including adults, was estimated to be 5% per year for X-linked CGD and 2% per year for autosomal recessive CGD in a recent retrospective analysis.[957] The most common causes of death were pneumonia or sepsis (or both) as a result of infection with *Aspergillus* species or *B. cepacia*.[957,980] A single-institution study involving 76 younger patients reported an overall mortality of 1.5% per year.[1119] As already noted, patients with a deficiency of p47[phox] have often been noted to exhibit milder disease than those with flavocytochrome-negative CGD, possibly because of small amounts of residual superoxide produced.[1050,1120]

A multifaceted therapeutic approach has been responsible for the greatly improved prognosis in CGD. The cornerstones of current management include (1) prevention and early treatment of infections; (2) use of prophylactic antibacterial and antifungal therapy; (3) early use of parenteral antibiotics, including antifungal drugs, augmented by surgical drainage or resection of recalcitrant abscesses; and (4) the use of prophylactic rIFN-γ.

Several approaches can be used to prevent infections. Patients with CGD should receive all routine immunizations (including live virus vaccines) on schedule and an influenza vaccine yearly. Cuts and skin abrasions should be promptly cleaned with soap and water and rinsed with a 2% solution of hydrogen peroxide. The frequency and severity of rectal infections can be greatly reduced by avoiding constipation and soaking early lesions in warm, soapy water. Flossing and professional dental cleaning can help prevent gingivitis and periodontitis. The risk of *Aspergillus* infection can be decreased by avoiding marijuana smoke[1121] and decaying plant material (e.g., rotting wood, mulch, hay), both of which often contain numerous *Aspergillus* spores.[1122]

The prophylactic use of antibiotics for bacterial and fungal infections is another important component in the management of CGD. Retrospective studies showed that chronic prophylaxis with trimethoprim-sulfamethoxazole (5 mg/kg/day of trimethoprim given in one or two doses) can decrease the number of bacterial infections in patients with CGD without increasing rates of fungal infection or infection with pathogens resistant to trimethoprim-sulfamethoxazole.[978,1120] Dicloxacillin (25 to 50 mg/kg/day) can be used in sulfa-allergic patients, although there are relatively few data documenting its efficacy. Itraconazole is used for prophylaxis against fungal disease. A prospective study found an incidence of 3.4 *Aspergillus* infections (lung) per 100 patient-years as compared with 11.5 in a historical control group that did not receive any prophylaxis.[1123] A subsequent randomized, double-blind, placebo-controlled study further documented the efficacy of itraconazole for prophylaxis of fungal infections in CGD.[1124] Daily itraconazole is therefore now recommended for all CGD patients (200 mg daily if 13 years or older or if weighing at least 50 kg or 100 mg daily if younger than 13 years or weighing less than 50 kg). Liver function tests should be monitored in patients receiving itraconazole.

rIFN-γ is another cornerstone of current management that reduces the frequency of serious infection in patients with CGD.[1119,1125-1127] rIFN-γ enhances many aspects of normal phagocyte function, including nonoxidative microbial killing. The recommended dose of rIFN-γ in CGD is 0.05 mg (50 μg)/m² or 0.0015 mg/kg if less than 0.05 m², given three times a week subcutaneously. A multicenter double-blinded, placebo-controlled phase III trial first established that rIFN-γ was an effective and well-tolerated treatment that reduces the infectious complications of CGD in all four genetic subgroups,[1128] a result that has continued to be supported by longer follow-up phase IV studies.[1119,1126,1127] The main conclusions of the original study are summarized in Table 21-18. Patients receiving rIFN-γ had a 70% reduction in the number of serious infections during the study period. These beneficial effects were independent of age, mode of inheritance, and concomitant use of prophylactic antibiotics. The most common side effects were mild fever, headache, and other flu-like symptoms. No additional adverse effects, including any increased incidence of chronic inflammatory complications, have been noted with longer periods of prophylactic rIFN-γ (>10 years).[1119] On average, these patients are averaging one serious infection per patient every 4 to 5 years.

The beneficial effect of rIFN-γ in most CGD patients is not fully understood but appears to be achieved by enhancing nonoxidative antimicrobial pathways and other phagocyte functions. For example, administration of rIFN-γ to normal volunteers increases expression of FcγR1 and enhances phagocytosis.[1129] Overall, no difference was found in neutrophil superoxide production and killing of *S. aureus* in CGD patients receiving either rIFN-γ or placebo.[1128,1130] However, because rIFN-γ increases levels of gp91[phox] mRNA expression,[1131] increased superoxide production and bacterial killing can be seen in some patients with variant X-linked CGD (see X91⁻ in Table 21-15).[1131-1134] One site of action of rIFN-γ, at least in X91⁻ patients, appears to be granulocyte-monocyte precursor cells in the bone marrow.[1132,1134]

A frequent shortcoming in the treatment of patients with CGD is failure to treat potentially serious infections promptly or long enough with the appropriate parenteral antibiotics. CGD patients do not always have typical symptoms and signs, even with serious infections, and fever and leukocytosis can be absent. An elevated sedimentation rate is often present and can be very useful both as a clue to the presence of significant infection and for monitoring the response to therapy.[991] Therapy should be directed initially at characteristic pathogens. In the absence of a diagnostic culture, a broad-spectrum gram-negative antibiotic effective against *B. cepacia* should be administered in conjunction with a potent antistaphylococcal agent (e.g., a combination of nafcillin and ceftazidime). If the site of infection, the offending pathogen, or both are not known and the patient is severely ill and not responding to the initial therapy within 24 to 48 hours, an aggressive search for the underlying infection should

TABLE 21-18 **Summary of the Phase III Study Establishing the Efficacy of Recombinant Interferon-γ for Infection Prophylaxis in Chronic Granulomatous Disease**

Variable	TREATMENT GROUP		P Value
	Interferon	Placebo	
Number of patients	63	65	
Patient years on study	52.1	50.9	
Age ± SD (yr)	14.3 ± 10.1	15.0 ± 9.6	
Number of patients with at least one serious infection	14 (22%)	30 (46%)	.0006
Serious infections per patient-year	0.38	1.1	
Total number of serious infections	20	56	<.0001
Number of hospital days per patient-year	8.6	28.2	
	Percentage without Serious Infection*		
Age			
<10 yr (52 patients)	81	20	
≥10 yr (76 patients)	73	34	
Inheritance			
X-linked (86 patients)	79	33	
Autosomal (42 patients)	71	39	
Prophylactic antibiotics			
Yes (111 patients)	78	33	
No (17 patients)	69	28	

The table shows a summary of the final results of a phase III randomized, double-blind, placebo-controlled study in which 128 patients with CGD received either recombinant interferon-γ (50 mg/m² per dose) or placebo by subcutaneous injections three times per week for an average duration of 8.9 months (a controlled trial of interferon gamma to prevent infection in chronic granulomatous disease. The International Chronic Granulomatous Disease Cooperative Study Group. N Engl J Med. 1991;324:509-516). The major end points of the study were time to the first serious infection and the number of such infections. A serious infection was defined as an event requiring hospitalization and parenteral antibiotics.

*The bottom portion of the table shows the Kaplan-Meier estimates of the cumulative proportion of patients free from serious infections for 12 months (after randomization) with adjustment for stratification factors.

be conducted, including bronchoscopy or open biopsy, if indicated. In ill patients, therapy for fungi, *Nocardia* species, and *B. cepacia* may have to be given empirically. *B. cepacia* is notorious for causing persistent fevers followed by bloodstream dissemination from the lung or other sites that results in sudden septic shock. *B. cepacia* generally responds to ceftazidime or meropenem,[995] which are most effective if given before dissemination into the bloodstream. Proven or suspected fungal infections have been treated with amphotericin B in the past, although its use is being replaced with newer azole antifungal agents such as voriconazole.[1135-1137] Even when appropriate antibiotics are used, infections often respond slowly and should generally be treated with an antibiotic course that is more prolonged than for a patient with normal neutrophil function. Some infections may require many months of therapy, particularly *Aspergillus*, but staphylococcal infections as well. Surgical drainage or resection can play a key role in the management of lymphadenitis, osteomyelitis, and abscesses of the liver, lungs, kidney, brain, and rectum. Finally, granulocyte transfusions may be helpful in the treatment of recalcitrant or life-threatening infections.[991,1138,1139]

Granulomatous inflammation in the esophagus, gastric antrum, and bladder can result in symptoms of obstruction, and in the bowel wall, a syndrome resembling inflammatory bowel disease can occur. These complications can cause considerable morbidity in some patients with CGD and are generally managed with a combination of antibiotics and steroids.[1023,1029,1119,1140-1143] Although the anti-inflammatory effects of steroids are often beneficial in this setting, even at low oral doses (1 mg/kg/day of prednisone),[1143] their use should be carefully monitored because of the additional immunosuppression associated with them. Cyclosporine has also been used to successfully treat a case of intractable gastrointestinal disease, although a serious fungal pneumonia secondary to *Paecilomyces variotii* did develop while taking cyclosporine.[1025] IFN-γ has had no clear role in management of the chronic inflammatory complications of CGD; however, anecdotal reports suggest that it may be beneficial in some patients. A recent study in a mouse model of CGD suggested that combining IFN-γ with L-kynurenine may be beneficial in counteracting the dysregulated inflammatory response in CGD.[983] NADPH oxidase–derived superoxide appears to be an important cofactor in the oxidative cleavage of tryptophan to L-kynurenine by IDO, which is an important immunomodulatory pathway that otherwise downregulates inflammation.[983]

Allogeneic bone marrow transplantation can be used to treat CGD.[398,772,1144-1150] Because of the risks associated with this procedure, marrow transplantation is generally considered only for patients who have frequent and severe infections despite aggressive medical management and also have a fully HLA-matched sibling donor. Nonmyeloablative conditioning regimens for allogeneic transplantation have also been used successfully in CGD, including several cases with ongoing fungal infections, although graft-versus-host disease can be a significant problem in adult patients.[1148,1150,1151] Cord blood transplants have been reported as well.[1152,1153]

Because CGD results from single-gene defects in proteins expressed in myeloid cells, this disorder is considered to be an excellent candidate for gene replacement therapy targeted at hematopoietic stem cells. Based on the lack of symptoms observed in female carriers of X-linked CGD with as few as 10% to 20% NBT-positive neutrophils, significant clinical benefit may result even if a minority of the phagocyte population is successfully corrected.[959] Studies of bone marrow transplantation and gene therapy in murine CGD have been useful in evaluating the level of correction required to prevent symptoms and have generally confirmed the clinical observations in female X-linked CGD carriers and variant X-linked CGD.[1154-1157] Thus, genetic modification of marrow stem cells may be a useful future therapeutic modality for CGD if obstacles in achieving safe and effective gene delivery can be overcome.[771,1030,1158,1159] Early phase I clinical trials using retroviral vectors for gene therapy for CGD showed "proof of concept" in that oxidase-positive peripheral blood neutrophils were detected, though at very low levels (<0.5%) and disappearing within 9 months.[771,1160] This was not surprising because patients did not receive any preparative regimen and there is no intrinsic selection for gene-corrected cells in CGD. A subsequent clinical trial in Germany for X-linked CGD used a gamma-retroviral vector with a more potent viral long terminal repeat driving expression of the X-linked CGD protein, as well as partially ablative busulfan conditioning.[1161] In the first two patients reported, much higher numbers of oxidase-positive neutrophils (20% to 50%) were seen, along with resolution of chronic infectious complications. However, this high level of correction resulted from expansion of myeloid precursors that harbored vector insertions in genes that are master regulators of myeloid cell growth.[1161] Current efforts at gene therapy for CGD are focused on the development of gamma-retroviral and lentiviral vectors that lack strong viral enhancer sequences to reduce the potential for insertional mutagenesis as a result of activation of neighboring genes.[771,1159]

Glucose-6-Phosphate Dehydrogenase Deficiency

The substrate for the respiratory burst oxidase, NADPH, is generated by the first two reactions of the hexose monophosphate shunt: G6PD (see Fig. 21-7, reaction 8) and 6-phosphogluconate dehydrogenase (6PGD). Because G6PD is the first enzyme in this pathway, its absence results in greatly diminished shunt activity and thus a severe decrease in the availability of NADPH. Consequently, severe G6PD deficiency in neutrophils results in an attenuated respiratory burst and, in some cases, a clinical picture somewhat similar to that observed in CGD.[1162-1165] The key features of G6PD deficiency are summarized in Table 21-19. The organisms causing infection in severely deficient patients are similar to those observed in CGD and are predominately catalase-positive bacteria.

In light of the relatively high frequency of G6PD mutations in the American black and Mediterranean populations,[1166] as well as the fact that leukocyte and erythrocyte G6PD is encoded by the same gene, it might

TABLE 21-19	**Summary of Neutrophil Glucose-6-Phosphate Dehydrogenase Deficiency**
Incidence	Extremely rare
Inheritance	X-linked
Molecular defect	Poorly characterized family of mutations that cause CNSHA in erythrocytes and functional failure of G6PD in neutrophils (possibly kinetic mutants); other rare mutants may also be responsible
Pathogenesis	Severe functional failure of neutrophil G6PD (<5% of normal) leading to an extremely low steady-state concentration of NADPH, which serves as the substrate for NADPH oxidase
Clinical manifestations	CNSHA (hemolytic anemia that occurs even in the absence of redox stress)
	CGD-like syndrome with recurrent bacterial infections
Laboratory evaluation	Neutrophil C6PD activity < 5% of normal
	Severely diminished respiratory burst and abnormal nitroblue tetrazolium test
	Associated CNSHA with elevated reticulocyte count and diminished erythrocyte G6PD activity
Differential diagnosis	CGD
	Glutathione reductase or synthetase deficiency
Therapy	Prophylactic trimethoprim-sulfamethoxazole
	Aggressive use of parenteral antibiotics
	Transfusion support for severe anemia
Prognosis	Not clear because too few patients have been reported
	May be as severe as CGD

CGD, chronic granulomatous disease; CNSHA, congenital nonspherocytic hemolytic anemia; G6PD, glucose-6-phosphate dehydrogenase; NADPH, reduced nicotinamide adenine dinucleotide phosphate.

Reprinted from Curnutte JT. Disorders of phagocyte function. In Hoffman R, Benz EF, Shattil S, et al (eds). Hematology: Basic Principles and Practice. New York, Churchill Livingstone, 1991, p 577.

be expected that clinically significant neutrophil G6PD deficiency would occur more often than it does (fewer than 10 cases have been reported in the literature). One of the reasons that it does not is that neutrophils must have a severe deficiency (<5% of normal G6PD levels) before respiratory burst function is adversely affected. Even low levels of G6PD are apparently sufficient to recycle NADP$^+$ back to NADPH at a rate that permits reasonable levels of respiratory burst activity. Furthermore, studies on patients with variant CGD indicate that surprisingly low levels of respiratory burst activity (5% to 10% of normal) can still provide adequate protection against microbial infection (see earlier). Therefore, clinically significant decreases in levels of neutrophil G6PD are rarely encountered. In most types of G6PD deficiency, neutrophil levels are in the range of 20% to 75% of normal.[1167,1168] Because most G6PD mutations cause the enzyme to decay over a period of days and weeks, levels in the short-lived neutrophil do not usually become critically low, even in some of the more unstable G6PD variants. Hence, it appears that only a rare (and poorly understood) group of mutations cause extremely low levels of G6PD in neutrophils.

The diagnosis of G6PD deficiency should be considered in any patient with congenital nonspherocytic hemolytic anemia (CNSHA) in whom the erythrocyte G6PD level is unusually low or the frequency of infections is high. The diagnosis is established by measuring the level of G6PD activity in neutrophil homogenates. Though not necessary for the diagnosis, neutrophil function tests show a diminished respiratory burst (5% to 30% of normal).[1164,1169] Treatment of neutrophil G6PD deficiency is similar to that of CGD except that efficacy of rIFN-γ has not been demonstrated in the former. In general, G6PD deficiency appears to be somewhat milder than CGD, although recurrent pneumonia and a fatal infection with *C. violaceum* have been described.[1164,1169]

Myeloperoxidase Deficiency

MPO deficiency is the most common inherited disorder of phagocytes but is rarely associated with clinical symptoms. Although only 17 known cases had been collected up to 1979, the diagnosis is now easily made with the widespread use of automated flow cytochemistry in clinical hematology laboratories to enumerate peripheral blood neutrophils with peroxidase activity. In the United States and Europe, complete deficiency is seen in approximately 1 in 4000 individuals, and partial deficiencies occur in 1 in 2000 people, whereas MPO deficiency is uncommon in Japan.[1170-1172] MPO deficiency is seen in neutrophils and monocytes. Peroxidase levels in eosinophils, on the other hand, are normal because eosinophil peroxidase is encoded by a different gene.

MPO plays a pivotal role in amplifying the toxicity of hydrogen peroxide generated by the respiratory burst, and it catalyzes the formation of HOCl from chloride and hydrogen peroxide (see Fig. 21-7, reaction 4).[303,1171] HOCl, in turn, reacts with a variety of primary and sec-

ondary amines to form chloramines, some of which can be toxic.[233] Moreover, HOCl is capable of activating latent metalloproteinases. Based on these considerations, one would expect that severe MPO deficiency should attenuate important antimicrobial reactions catalyzed by HOCl. MPO-deficient mice have impaired host defense against *Candida* and *Klebsiella*.[1173,1174] Neutrophils from MPO-deficient patients show markedly abnormal in vitro killing of *C. albicans* and hyphal forms of *A. fumigatus*.[1171,1172] Curiously, however, these abnormalities are rarely reflected in an increased incidence of infection in patients, except for rare individuals who also suffer from diabetes mellitus.[1170,1172] In these individuals, disseminated candidiasis can be seen (Table 21-20). Several studies have suggested that MPO deficiency may also be associated with an increased susceptibility to malignancy.[1170,1175,1176]

Congenital MPO deficiency is inherited in an autosomal recessive manner,[1171,1172] and variable expression of the defect has been reported.[1176] The gene for MPO has been localized to the long arm of chromosome 17 at position q22-q23 near the breakpoint for the 15;17 translocation of promyelocytic leukemia.[1177,1178] The primary translation product is a 80-kd protein that undergoes cotranslational glycosylation and subsequent proteolytic cleavage to heavy and light chains, which oligomerize to form a tetramer composed of two heavy and two light chains.[1171] The molecular basis of congenital MPO deficiency reflects defects affecting MPO processing and heme incorporation. A variety of mutations have been reported.[1171] One common cause of complete absence of immunoreactive MPO is a point mutation that results in an arginine-to-tryptophan substitution at codon 569 (R569W).[1179,1180] The R569W mutation results in maturation arrest of the MPO apoprotein, which fails to incorporate heme.[1181]

In addition to inherited MPO deficiency, secondary or acquired MPO deficiency can occur. MPO-deficient cells can be seen in the M2, M3, and M4 forms of AML, as well as in approximately 25% of patients with MDS and CML.[1182,1183] Other clinical situations in which secondary MPO deficiency can occur include pregnancy, iron deficiency, lead poisoning, ceroid lipofuscinosis, and Hodgkin's disease.[1170]

There are several possible reasons for the surprisingly mild clinical phenotype of MPO deficiency. First, neutrophils contain such a large amount of MPO that appreciable levels may be left in the cell even in cases of severe deficiency. These residual stores, coupled with normal levels of eosinophil peroxidase, may provide at least some degree of peroxidative activity at sites of infection. Second, the respiratory burst in MPO-deficient neutrophils is substantially augmented in terms of velocity and duration.[1184,1185] This may be due to the enhanced stability of the respiratory burst oxidase made possible by the absence of HOCl, which normally inactivates the oxidase.[1186] Finally, other oxidants produced by the respiratory burst may work together with the various granule

TABLE 21-20   **Summary of Myeloperoxidase Deficiency**

Incidence	1 in 2000 (partial deficiency) 1 in 4000 (total deficiency)
Inheritance	Autosomal recessive with variable expression; myeloperoxidase gene on chromosome 17 at q22-q23
Molecular defect	Defective post-translational processing of an abnormal myeloperoxidase precursor polypeptide because of a variety of mutations; eosinophil peroxidase encoded by different gene, and levels normal
Pathogenesis	Partial or complete myeloperoxidase deficiency leads to diminished production of HOCl and HOCl-derived chloramines; myeloperoxidase products are necessary for rapid killing of microbes (especially *Candida*) but not absolutely required
Clinical manifestations	Usually clinically silent Rarely disseminated candidiasis/fungal disease (usually in conjunction with diabetes mellitus) May be increased risk of malignancy
Laboratory findings	Deficiency of neutrophil/monocyte peroxidase by histochemical analysis (eosinophil peroxidase normal) Delayed, but eventually normal killing of bacteria in vitro Failure to kill *Candida albicans* and hyphal forms of *Aspergillus fumigatus* in vitro
Differential diagnosis	Acquired partial myeloperoxidase deficiency seen in acute myelocytic leukemia (M2, M3, and M4), myelodysplastic syndromes, iron deficiency, or pregnancy
Therapy	None in asymptomatic patients Aggressive treatment of fungal infections when they occur Control of blood glucose levels in diabetes
Prognosis	Usually excellent

Modified from Curnutte JT. Disorders of phagocyte function. In Hoffman R, Benz EJ, Shattil S, et al (eds). Hematology: Basic Principles and Practice. New York, Churchill Livingstone, 1991, p 578.

antimicrobial proteins to provide sufficient protection against most microorganisms.

Given the mild clinical nature of MPO deficiency, no treatment is generally required. When they occur, infections are treated as in normal individuals. It is important for the clinician to be aware of the increased risk for *Candida* infections in MPO-deficient patients and to treat them aggressively when they do occur.

Disorders of Glutathione Metabolism

As shown in Figure 21-7 (reaction 6), glutathione peroxidase protects neutrophil proteins (including NADPH oxidase) from the harmful effects of the hydrogen peroxide generated in the course of the respiratory burst by degrading it to water. The reducing equivalents for this reaction are carried by the reduced form of glutathione (GSH), intracellular levels of which are maintained by recycling oxidized glutathione (GSSG) back to GSH by means of glutathione reductase (Fig. 21-7, reaction 7). Glutathione levels are also maintained through de novo synthesis catalyzed by glutathione synthetase (Fig. 21-7, reaction 9). Severe deficiencies of glutathione reductase and glutathione synthetase in neutrophils have been reported and found to cause moderately severe abnormalities in the respiratory burst.[1187-1191] The key features of each of these extremely rare disorders are summarized in Table 21-21.

Glutathione reductase deficiency has been reported in one family in which three siblings were found to have a marked deficiency of this enzyme in their neutrophils (10% to 15% of normal).[1187,1189] The inheritance appeared

to be autosomal recessive inasmuch as the parents of the children were first cousins and their neutrophils contained 50% of the normal levels of glutathione reductase. The mutation responsible for the enzyme deficiency in this family has not been reported yet. It is known that the gene for glutathione reductase is located on chromosome 8 at position p21.1.[1192]

Clinically, none of the affected patients showed signs of increased infection. Their erythrocytes were also deficient in glutathione reductase and therefore were prone to hemolysis in the face of oxidant stress. Two siblings did suffer from juvenile cataracts and deafness. In vitro studies of neutrophil function were normal except for premature termination of the respiratory burst after about 5 minutes.[1187] The probable reason for this defect is that NADPH oxidase is inactivated by products of the MPO reaction.[1186] If glutathione reductase is deficient, the neutrophils cannot maintain a level of GSH sufficient to detoxify hydrogen peroxide. After several minutes of the respiratory burst, toxic levels of hydrogen peroxide accumulate and lead to deactivation of the oxidase. This explanation is supported by experiments showing that glutathione reductase–deficient neutrophils pre-exposed to exogenous hydrogen peroxide fail to undergo even an abbreviated respiratory burst. One important insight gained from the study of these patients is that only a brief respiratory burst appears to be necessary for adequate microbial killing.

The diagnosis of glutathione reductase deficiency is made by measuring levels of this enzyme in neutrophil homogenates. The finding of a truncated respiratory

TABLE 21-21	Disorders of Glutathione Metabolism	
Disease Aspect	**Glutathione Reductase Deficiency**	**Glutathione Synthetase Deficiency**
Incidence	One family, three siblings	Several reported cases
Inheritance	Autosomal recessive	Autosomal recessive
Molecular defect	Diminished glutathione reductase levels in neutrophils (10-15% of normal) and erythrocytes; mutation not known	Severe deficiency of glutathione synthetase activity (5-10% of normal); mutation(s) not know
Pathogenesis	Brief respiratory burst truncated by toxic accumulation of H_2O_2 by glutathione	Same as with glutathione reductase deficiency except that the respiratory burst is normal; elevated 5-oxoproline levels because of lack of feedback inhibition by glutathione
Clinical manifestations	No history of repeated infection Hemolysis with oxidant stress	Metabolic acidosis caused by elevated 5-oxoproline Otitis media Intermittent neutropenia Hemolysis with oxidant stress Severe decrease in glutathione synthetase level
Laboratory evaluation	Glutathione reductase level diminished	Normal respiratory burst
Differential diagnosis	Premature cessation of O_2^- production by neutrophils Chronic granulomatous disease Glucose-6-phosphate dehydrogenase deficiency	Glutathione reductase deficiency
Therapy	None required	Vitamin E for hemolysis and infections Treatment of metabolic acidosis
Prognosis	Benign disorder	Relatively benign disorder

Reprinted with permission from Curnutte JT. Disorders of phagocyte function. In Hoffman R, Benz EJ, Shattil S, et al (eds). Hematology: Basic Principles and Practice. New York, Churchill Livingstone, 1991, p 578.

burst provides supporting evidence, although a similar abnormality can be seen in G6PD deficiency. No therapy is required, but avoiding foods and drugs containing potent oxidants will decrease the chance of depleting intracellular glutathione.

Several forms of congenital glutathione synthetase deficiency have been described, all of which are inherited in an autosomal recessive fashion. Specific mutations have not been reported. Only in cases in which glutathione synthetase activity is severely deficient in neutrophils (5% to 10% of normal) is a phagocytic abnormality detected.[1188,1190,1191] In contrast to glutathione reductase deficiency, neutrophils deficient in glutathione synthetase have a normal respiratory burst.[1188,1191] For reasons that are uncertain, in vitro bacterial killing is decreased. Despite this in vitro microbicidal defect, patients with glutathione synthetase deficiency have only a relatively mild problem resolving infections. They do suffer from a severe metabolic acidosis resulting from elevated levels of 5-oxoproline, a metabolite formed in one of the early steps in the pathway of glutathione synthesis. This acidosis may be responsible for the intermittent neutropenia observed in glutathione synthetase–deficient patients.[1188] Because these patients' erythrocytes are also deficient in glutathione synthetase, a hemolytic anemia brought on by oxidant stress is seen. Therapy with vitamin E (400 IU/day) has been found to be beneficial in patients who suffer from hemolysis and infection.[1188]

Glutathione peroxidase (see Fig. 21-7, reaction 6) was found to be decreased to levels 25% of normal in three unrelated patients with a clinical syndrome resembling CGD.[1193,1194] Although this enzyme plays an important role in removing hydrogen peroxide, it has not been established whether the degree of deficiency seen in these patients is sufficient to cause functional abnormalities in neutrophils. Two of the affected kindreds have recently been restudied, and a severe deficiency of the respiratory burst oxidase flavocytochrome *b* has been identified in affected members of each.[1060] It thus appears that in at least two of these previously reported cases, CGD is the underlying problem, not glutathione peroxidase deficiency.

Disorders of Cytokines and Impaired Phagocyte Function

Inherited defects in the production and response to inflammatory cytokines by phagocytes or other cells of the immune system can be manifested as recurrent infections.[737] All of these disorders are rare. In addition to the disorders described later in this section, HIES is also due to defects in cytokine signaling. Sporadic and autosomal dominant cases of HIES result from mutations in STAT3, and autosomal aggressive HIES can result from defects in Tyk2, a JAK kinase family member.[818,825,826] HIES is discussed earlier in this chapter.

Defects in a group of genes regulating the production and macrophage response to IFN-γ are associated with recurrent and severe atypical mycobacterial infections, as well as *Salmonella* and viral infections in some subgroups.[737,1195-1197] The phenotype of this group of disorders is also referred to as mendelian susceptibility to mycobacterial diseases (MSMD). The distinctive and limited spectrum of infections in affected patients results from defects in the IFN-γ pathway. IFN-γ is secreted by NK and T cells in response to IL-12 and IL-23 released by macrophages and dendritic cells. Some patients have autosomal recessive mutations in the p40 subunit of the IL-12 and IL-23 cytokines that lead to decreased expression of these cytokines, and another subgroup of patients have mutations in the β1 subunit of the receptor for IL-12 and IL-23; in both these groups, levels of IFN-γ are abnormally low. Other patients have autosomal recessive mutations affecting the IFN-γ receptor that lead to either

loss of receptor expression or complete or partial loss of IFN-γ binding. Dominant IFN-γ receptor mutations resulting in partial IFN-γ receptor deficiency are also described. The phenotype is milder in patients with partial defects. Very rarely, patients have partial or complete deficiency of the STAT1 protein, which is critical for transduction of IFN-γ–mediated signals.

Recurrent pyogenic infections are characteristic of a group of genetic disorders involving the NF-κB signaling pathway. Included in this group are patients with autosomal recessive mutations in interleukin-1 receptor–associated kinase-4 (IRAK-4), a kinase in the Toll and IL-1 receptor signaling pathway.[737,1198,1199] Affected chil-

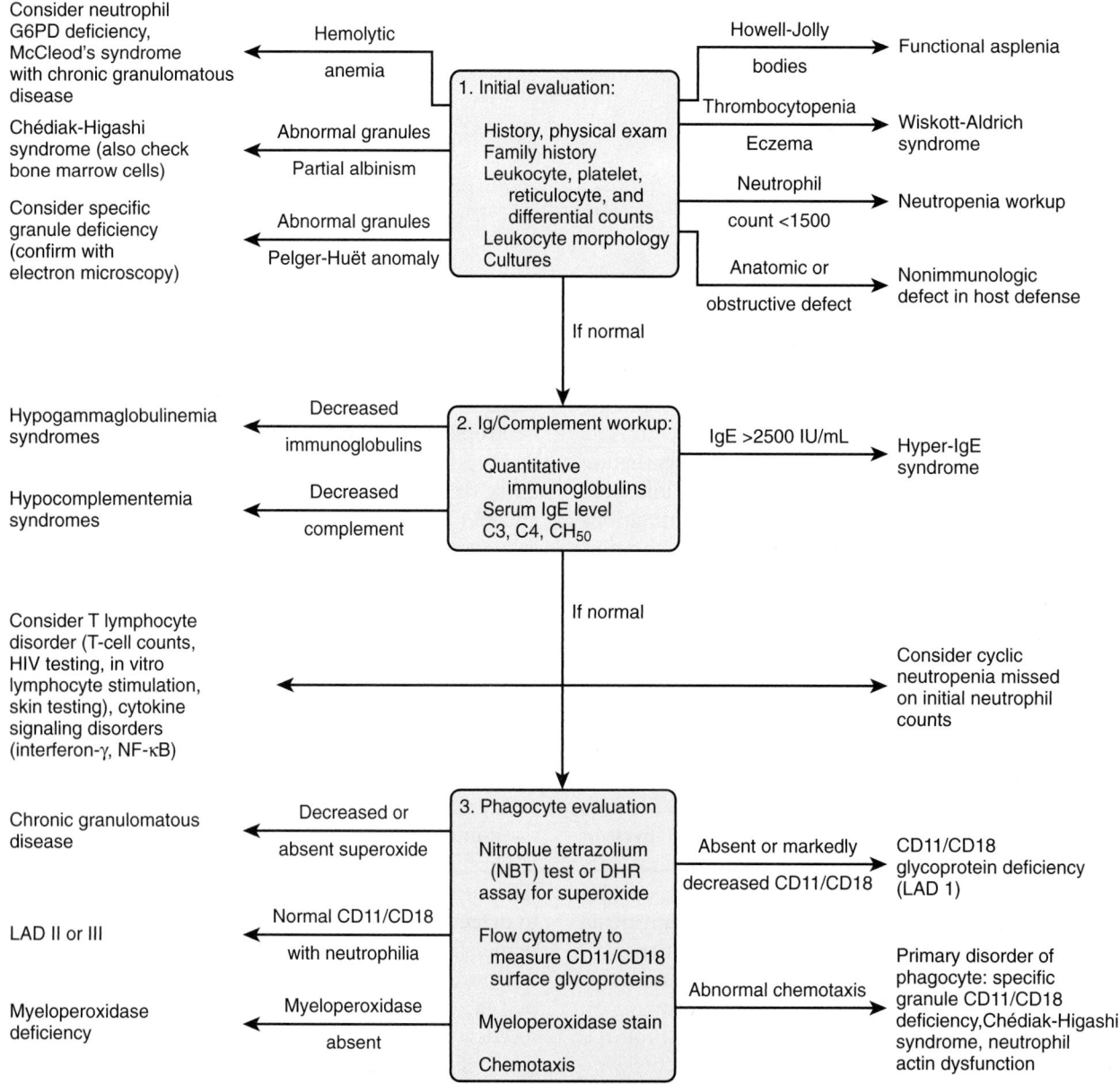

FIGURE 21-12. Algorithm for the workup of a patient with recurrent infections. The various tests are described in the appropriate sections of the chapter. G6PD, glucose-6-phosphate dehydrogenase; HIV, human immunodeficiency syndrome; Ig, immunoglobulin; LAD, leukocyte adhesion deficiency; NBT, nitroblue tetrazolium; O_2^-, superoxide. Units for the neutrophil count (box 1) are neutrophils/mm³. *(Adapted with permission from Lehrer RI, Ganz T, Selsted ME, et al. Neutrophils and host defense. Ann Intern Med. 1988;109:127-142.)*

dren have recurrent and sometimes fatal infections with *S. pneumoniae* and *S. aureus*, along with low or absent fever and inflammatory responses. Patients with the syndrome of anhidrotic ectodermal dysplasia with immunodeficiency (EDA-ID) have either X-linked recessive mutations in the gene encoding NEMO, a regulatory protein that activates NF-κB, or much less commonly, an autosomal dominant defect in IκBA, an NF-κB inhibitor. In addition to widely spaced abnormal teeth, hypohidrosis, and hypotrichosis, children with EDA-ID have recurrent pyogenic infections with a minimal systemic inflammatory response, and opportunistic infections with atypical mycobacteria, viruses, or *Pneumocystis carinii* can also develop.

Evaluation of Patients with Recurrent Infections

Patients with recurrent infections can be a diagnostic challenge. Many of the phagocyte disorders have similar clinical manifestations, which can overlap those seen in inherited or acquired disorders of lymphocyte function. Furthermore, the majority of patients with recurrent infections do not have an identifiable granulocyte or monocyte defect. Given this low yield and the lack of ability to characterize many aspects of phagocyte function in routine laboratory studies, physicians are faced with the difficult question of which patients merit a complete evaluation. Those who have at least one of the following clinical features are more likely to have a phagocyte defect: (1) an unusually high frequency of bacterial and fungal infections, (2) the presence of an infection at an unusual site (e.g., a hepatic or brain abscess), (3) infections with atypical pathogens (e.g., *Aspergillus* pneumonia, disseminated candidiasis, lymphadenitis secondary to *Serratia* or *Klebsiella*, disseminated mycobacterial infection), (4) infections of exceptional severity, and (5) childhood periodontal disease. Certain other clinical findings can also be helpful. For example, a child with nystagmus, fair skin, and recurrent staphylococcal infections should be evaluated for CHS, whereas an infant with neutrophilia, bacterial infections, and delayed separation of the umbilical cord should be tested for LAD. Once the physician has decided that a phagocyte evaluation is warranted, the algorithm presented in Figure 21-12 may be helpful in organizing the workup. When coupled with a thorough clinical history and physical examination, the laboratory tests outlined in Figure 21-12 should help the physician establish the diagnosis and formulate an appropriate therapeutic plan.

REFERENCES

1. Gangenahalli GU, Gupta P, Saluja D, et al. Stem cell fate specification: role of master regulatory switch transcription factor PU.1 in differential hematopoiesis. Stem Cells Dev. 2005;14:140-152.

2. Koschmieder S, Rosenbauer F, Steidl U, et al. Role of transcription factors C/EBPα and PU.1 in normal hematopoiesis and leukemia. Int J Hematol. 2005;81:368-377.

3. Lieschke GJ, Burgess AW. Granulocyte colony-stimulating factor and granulocyte-macrophage colony-stimulating factor (part II). N Engl J Med. 1992;327:99-106.

4. Metcalf D. The molecular control of cell division, differentiation commitment and maturation of hematopoietic stem cells. Blood. 1989;339:27-33.

5. Sieff CA. Hematopoietic growth factors. J Clin Invest. 1987;79:1549-1551.

6. Lampinen M, Carlson M, Hakansson LD, Venge P. Cytokine-regulated accumulation of eosinophils in inflammatory disease. Allergy. 2004;59:793-805.

7. Rothenberg ME, Hogan SP. The eosinophil. Annu Rev Immunol. 2006;24:147-174.

8. Warren DJ, Moore MA. Synergism among interleukin 1, interleukin 3, and interleukin 5 in the production of eosinophils from primitive hematopoietic stem cells. J Immunol. 1988;140:94-98.

9. Denburg JA. Basophil and mast cell lineages in vitro and in vivo. Blood. 1992;79:846-860.

10. Wittmann S, Rothe G, Schmitz G, Frohlich D. Cytokine upregulation of surface antigens correlates to the priming of the neutrophil oxidative burst response. Cytometry A. 2004;57:53-62.

11. Dahl R, Iyer SR, Owens KS, et al. The transcriptional repressor GFI-1 antagonizes PU.1 activity through protein-protein interaction. J Biol Chem. 2007;282:6473-6483.

12. Hock H, Orkin SH. Zinc-finger transcription factor Gfi-1: versatile regulator of lymphocytes, neutrophils and hematopoietic stem cells. Curr Opin Hematol. 2006;13:1-6.

13. Jacobsen SEW, Fahlman C, Blomhoff HK, et al. All-trans- and 9-cis-retinoic acid: Potent direct inhibitors of primitivie murine hematopoietic progenitors in vitro. J Exp Med. 1994;179:1665-1670.

14. Tsai S, Collins SJ. A dominant negative retinoic acid receptor blocks neutrophil differentiation at the promyelocyte stage. Proc Natl Acad Sci U S A. 1993;90:7153-7157.

15. Lo Coco F, Avvisati G, Diverio D, et al. Molecular evaluation of response to all-trans retinoic acid therapy in patients with acute promyelocytic leukemia. Blood. 1991;77:1657-1659.

16. Athens JW, Haab OP, Raab SO, et al. Leukokinetic studies. IV. The total blood, circulating and marginal granulocyte pools and the granulocyte turnover rate in normal subjects. J Clin Invest. 1961;40:989-995.

17. Cronkite EP. Kinetics of granulopoiesis. Clin Haematol. 1979;8:351-370.

18. Dancey JT, Deubelbeiss KA, Harker LA, Finch CA. Neutrophil kinetics in man. J Clin Invest. 1976;58:705-715.

19. Donohue DM, Reiff RH. Quantitative measurement of the erythrocytic and granulocytic cells of the marrow and blood. J Clin Invest. 1958;37:1571-1576.

20. Fadok VA, Savill JS, Haslett C, et al. Different populations of macrophages use either the vitronectin receptor or the phosphatidylserine receptor to recognize and

remove apoptotic cells. J Immunol. 1992;149:4029-4035.

21. Klebanoff SJ, Durack DT. Functional studies on human peritoneal eosinophils. Infect Immun. 1977;17:167-173.

22. Van Furth R, Raeburn JA. Characteristics of human mononuclear phagocytes. Blood. 1979;54:485-490.

23. Savill J. Apoptosis in resolution of inflammation. J Leukoc Biol. 1997;61:375-380.

24. Borregaard N, Cowland JB. Granules of the human neutrophilic polymorphonuclear leukocyte. Blood. 1997;89:3503-3521.

25. Savill JS, Wyllie AH, Henson JE, et al. Macrophage phagocytosis of aging neutrophils in inflammation. Programmed cell death in the neutrophil leads to recognition by macrophages. J Clin Invest. 1989;83:865-875.

26. Parent CA. Making all the right moves: chemotaxis in neutrophils and *Dictyostelium*. Curr Opin Cell Biol. 2004;16:4-13.

27. Stossel TP. The E. Donnall Thomas Lecture, 1993. The machinery of blood cell movements. Blood. 1994;84:367-379.

28. Van Haastert PJ, Devreotes PN. Chemotaxis: signalling the way forward. Nat Rev Mol Cell Biol. 2004;5:626-634.

29. Howard TH, Watts RG. Actin polymerization and leukocyte function. Curr Opin Hematol. 1994;1:61-68.

30. Shapiro LH, Look AT. Transcriptional regulation in myeloid cell differentiation. Curr Sci. 1995;2:3-11.

31. Stossel TP. On the crawling of animal cells. Science. 1993;260:1086-1094.

32. Berliner N, Hsing A, Graubert T, et al. Granulocyte colony-stimulating factor induction of normal human bone marrow progenitors results in neutrophil-specific gene expression. Blood. 1995;85:799-803.

33. Tenen DG, Hromas R, Licht JD, Zhang DE. Transcription factors, normal myeloid development, and leukemia. Blood. 1997;90:489-519.

34. Shivdasani RA, Orkin SH. The transcriptional control of hematopoiesis. Blood. 1996;87:4025-4039.

35. Grisolano JL, Sclar GM, Ley TJ. Early myeloid-specific expression of the human cathepsin G gene in transgenic mice. Proc Natl Acad Sci U S A. 1994;91:8989-8995.

36. Kobayashi SD, Voyich JM, Buhl CL, et al. Global changes in gene expression by human polymorphonuclear leukocytes during receptor-mediated phagocytosis: cell fate is regulated at the level of gene expression. Proc Natl Acad Sci U S A. 2002;99:6901-6906.

37. Zhang X, Kluger Y, Nakayama Y, et al. Gene expression in mature neutrophils: early responses to inflammatory stimuli. J Leukoc Biol. 2004;75:358-372.

38. Theilgaard-Monch K, Porse BT, Borregaard N. Systems biology of neutrophil differentiation and immune response. Curr Opin Immunol. 2006;18:54-60.

39. Borregaard N, Sorensen OE, Theilgaard-Monch K. Neutrophil granules: a library of innate immunity proteins. Trends Immunol. 2007;28:340-345.

40. Kurt-Jones EA, Mandell L, Whitney C, et al. Role of toll-like receptor 2 (TLR2) in neutrophil activation: GM-CSF enhances TLR2 expression and TLR2-mediated interleukin 8 responses in neutrophils. Blood. 2002;100:1860-1868.

41. Orkin SH. Molecular genetics of chronic granulomatous disease. Annu Rev Immunol. 1989;7:277-307.

42. Newburger PE, Dai Q, Whitney C. In vitro regulation of human phagocyte cytochrome *b* heavy and light chain gene expression by bacterial lipopolysaccharide and recombinant human cytokines. J Biol Chem. 1991;266:16171-16177.

43. Lindemann SW, Yost CC, Denis MM, et al. Neutrophils alter the inflammatory milieu by signal-dependent translation of constitutive messenger RNAs. Proc Natl Acad Sci U S A. 2004;101:7076-7081.

44. Seri M, Cusano R, Gangarossa S, et al. Mutations in MYH9 result in the May-Hegglin anomaly, and Fechtner and Sebastian syndromes. The May-Hegglin/Fechtner Syndrome Consortium. Nat Genet. 2000;26:103-105.

45. Hoffmann K, Dreger CK, Olins AL, et al. Mutations in the gene encoding the lamin B receptor produce an altered nuclear morphology in granulocytes (Pelger-Huët anomaly). Nat Genet. 2002;31:410-414.

46. Faurschou M, Borregaard N. Neutrophil granules and secretory vesicles in inflammation. Microbes Infect. 2003;5:1317-1327.

47. Borregaard N, Kjeldsen L, Lollike K, Sengelov H. Granules and secretory vesicles of the human neutrophil. Clin Exp Immunol. 1995;101(Suppl 1):6-9.

48. Liu CH, Lehan C, Speer ME, et al. Degenerative changes in neutrophils: An indicator of bacterial infection. Pediatrics. 1984;74:823-827.

49. Yamanaka R, Barlow C, Lekstrom-Himes J, et al. Impaired granulopoiesis, myelodysplasia, and early lethality in CCAAT/enhancer binding protein epsilon–deficient mice. Proc Natl Acad Sci U S A. 1997;94:13187-13192.

50. Borregaard N, Tauber AI. Subcellular localization of the human neutrophils NADPH oxidase, *b*-cytochrome and associated flavoprotein. J Biol Chem. 1984;259:47-52.

51. Jesaitis AJ, Buescher ES, Harrison D, et al. Ultrastructural localization of cytochrome *b* in the membranes of resting and phagocytosing human granulocytes. J Clin Invest. 1990;85:821-835.

52. Sabroe I, Dower SK, Whyte MK. The role of Toll-like receptors in the regulation of neutrophil migration, activation, and apoptosis. Clin Infect Dis. 2005;41(Suppl 7):S421-S426.

53. Triantafilou M, Brandenburg K, Gutsmann T, et al. Innate recognition of bacteria: engagement of multiple receptors. Crit Rev Immunol. 2002;22:251-268.

54. Bokoch GM. Regulation of innate immunity by Rho GTPases. Trends Cell Biol. 2005;15:163-171.

55. Kato T, Kitagawa S. Regulation of neutrophil functions by proinflammatory cytokines. Int J Hematol. 2006;84:205-209.

56. Niggli V. Signaling to migration in neutrophils: importance of localized pathways. Int J Biochem Cell Biol. 2003;35:1619-1638.

57. Bokoch GM. Chemoattractant signaling and leukocyte activation. Blood. 1995;86:1649-1660.

58. Downey GP, Fukushima T, Fialkow L. Signaling mechanisms in human neutrophils. Curr Opin Hematol. 1995;2:76-88.

59. Gombart AF, Shiohara M, Kwok SH, et al. Neutrophil specific granule deficiency: homozygous recessive inheritance of a frameshift mutation in the gene encoding

transcription factor CCAAT/enhancer binding protein-epsilon. Blood. 2001;97:2561-2567.

60. Berkow RI, Dodson RW. Tyrosine-specific protein phosphorylation during activation of human neutrophils. Blood. 1990;75:2445-2452.

61. Grinstein S, Furuya W, Butler JR, Tseng J. Receptor-mediated activation of multiple serine/threonine kinases in human leukocytes. J Biol Chem. 1993;268:20223-20231.

62. Thelen M, Wirthmueller U. Phospholipases and protein kinases during phagocyte activation. Curr Opin Immunol. 1994;6:106-112.

63. Wu D, Huang CK, Jiang H. Roles of phospholipid signaling in chemoattractant-induced responses. J Cell Sci. 2000;113:2935-2940.

64. Herlaar E, Brown Z. p38 MAPK signalling cascades in inflammatory disease. Mol Med Today. 1999;5:439-447.

65. Rollet E, Caon AC, Roberge CJ, et al. Tyrosine phyosphorylation in activated nehuman neutrophils: Comparison of the effects of different classes of agonists and identification of signalling pathways involved. J Immunol. 1994;153:353-363.

66. Kunkel SL, Lukacs N, Strieter RM. Expression and biology of neutrophil and endothelial cell–derived chemokines. Semin Cell Biol. 1995;6:327-336.

67. Perez HD. Chemoattractant receptors. Curr Opin Hematol. 1994;1:40-44.

68. Rollins BJ. Chemokines. Blood. 1997;90:909-928.

69. Benard V, Bohl BP, Bokoch GM. Characterization of rac and cdc42 activation in chemoattractant-stimulated human neutrophils using a novel assay for active GTPases. J Biol Chem. 1999;274:13198-13204.

70. Benard V, Bokoch GM, Diebold BA. Potential drug targets: small GTPases that regulate leukocyte function. Trends Pharmacol Sci. 1999;20:365-370.

71. Williams DA, Tao W, Yang F, et al. Dominant negative mutation of the hematopoietic-specific Rho GTPase, Rac2, is associated with a human phagocyte immunodeficiency. Blood. 2000;96:1646-1654.

72. Hirasawa R, Shimizu R, Takahashi S, et al. Essential and instructive roles of GATA factors in eosinophil development. J Exp Med. 2002;195:1379-1386.

73. Yu C, Cantor AB, Yang H, et al. Targeted deletion of a high-affinity GATA-binding site in the GATA-1 promoter leads to selective loss of the eosinophil lineage in vivo. J Exp Med. 2002;195:1387-1395.

74. Mattes J, Foster PS. Regulation of eosinophil migration and Th2 cell function by IL-5 and eotaxin. Curr Drug Targets Inflamm Allergy. 2003;2:169-174.

75. Yang M, Hogan SP, Mahalingam S, et al. Eotaxin-2 and IL-5 cooperate in the lung to regulate IL-13 production and airway eosinophilia and hyperreactivity. J Allergy Clin Immunol. 2003;112:935-943.

76. Carlson M, Peterson C, Venge P. The influence of IL-3, IL-5, and GM-CSF on normal human eosinophil and neutrophil C3b-induced degranulation. Allergy. 1993;48:437-442.

77. Enokihara H, Furusawa S, Nakakabo H, et al. T cells from eosinophilic patients produce interleukin-5 with interleukin-2 stimulation. Blood. 1989;73:1809-1813.

78. Munitz A, Levi-Schaffer F. Eosinophils: "new" roles for "old" cells. Allergy. 2004;59:268-275.

79. Rothenberg ME. Eosinophilia. N Engl J Med. 1998;338:1592-1600.

80. Kariyawasam HH, Robinson DS. The eosinophil: the cell and its weapons, the cytokines, its locations. Semin Respir Crit Care Med. 2006;27:117-127.

81. Thevathason OI, Gordon AS. Adrenocorticomedullary interactions on the blood eosinophils. Acta Haematol. 1958;19:162-170.

82. Dvorak AM, Ackerman SJ, Weller PF. Subcellular morphology and biochemistry of eosinophils. In Harris JR (ed). Blood Cell Biochemistry, vol. 2. London, Plenum Publishing, 1990, pp 237-344.

83. Bainton D, Farquhar MG. Segregation and packaging of granule enzymes in eosinophilic leukocytes. J Cell Biol. 1970;45:54-73.

84. Weiss SJ, Test ST, Eckmann CM, et al. Brominating oxidants generated by human eosinophils. Science. 1986;234:200-203.

85. Weller PF. The immunobiology of eosinophils. N Engl J Med. 1991;324:1110-1118.

86. Temkin V, Aingorn H, Puxeddu I, et al. Eosinophil major basic protein: first identified natural heparanase-inhibiting protein. J Allergy Clin Immunol. 2004;113:703-709.

87. Olsson I, Venge P. Arginine-rich cationic proteins of human eosinophil granules. Comparison of the constituents of eosinophilic and neutrophilic leukocytes. Lab Invest. 1977;36:493-501.

88. Butterworth AE, Wassom DL, Gleich GJ, et al. Damage to schistosomula of Schistosoma mansoni induced idrectly by eosinophil major basic protein. J Immunol. 1979;122:221-229.

89. Jong EC, Henderson WR, Klebanoff SR. Bactericidal activity of eosinophil peroxidase. J Immunol. 1980;124:1378-1386.

90. Parmley RT, Spicer SS. Cytochemical and ultrastructural identification of a small type granule in human late eosinophils. Lab Invest. 1974;30:557-567.

91. Magler R, DeChatelet LR, Bass DA. Human eosinophil peroxidase: Role in bactericidal activity. Blood. 1978;51:445-453.

92. Corssmit EP, Trip MD, Durrer JD. Löffler's endomyocarditis in the idiopathic hypereosinophilic syndrome. Cardiology. 1999;91:272-276.

93. Loffler W. Transient lung infiltrations with blood eosinophilia. Int Arch Allergy Appl Immunol. 1956;8:54-59.

94. Dvorak AM. Ultrastructural studies of human basophils and mast cells. J Histochem Cytochem. 2005;53:1043-1070.

95. O'Donnell MC, Ackerman SJ, Gleich GJ, et al. Activation of basophil and mast cell histamine release by eosinophil major basic protein. J Exp Med. 1983;257:1981-1990.

96. Ackerman SJ, Corrette SE, Rosenberg HF, et al. Molecular cloning and characterization of human eosinophil Charcot-Leyden crystal protein (lysophospholipase). Similarities to IgE binding proteins and the S-type animal lectin superfamily. J Immunol. 1993;150:456-468.

97. Weller PF, Bach D, Austen KF. Human eosinophil lysophospholipase: the sole protein component of Charcot-Leyden crystals. J Immunol. 1982;128:1346-1349.

98. Murakami I, Ogawa M, Amo H, Ota K. [Studies on kinetics of human leukocytes in vivo with ^{3}H-thymidine autoradiography II. Eosinophils and basophils.] Nippon Ketsueki Gakki Zashi. 1969;32:384-390.

99. Gibbs BF. Human basophils as effectors and immunomodulators of allergic inflammation and innate immunity. Clin Exp Med. 2005;5:43-49.

100. MacGlashan D Jr. IgE and FcεRI regulation. Clin Rev Allergy Immunol. 2005;29:49-60.

101. Min B, Le Gros G, Paul WE. Basophils: a potential liaison between innate and adaptive immunity. Allergol Int. 2006;55:99-104.

102. Gurish MF, Boyce JA. Mast cells: ontogeny, homing, and recruitment of a unique innate effector cell. J Allergy Clin Immunol. 2006;117:1285-1291.

103. Seder RA, Paul WE, Dvorak AM, et al. Mouse splenic and bone marrow cell populations that express high-affinity Fcε receptors and produce interleukin-4 are highly enriched in basophils. Proc Natl Acad Sci U S A. 1991;88:2835-2839.

104. Hatanaka K, Kitamura Y, Nishimune Y. Local development of mast cells from bone marrow–derived precursors in the skin of mice. Blood. 1979;53:142-147.

105. Galli SJ, Hammel I. Mast cell and basophil development. Curr Opin Hematol. 1994;1:33-39.

106. Agis H, Fureder W, Bankl HC, et al. Comparative immunophenotypic analysis of human mast cells, blood basophils and monocytes. Immunology. 1996;87:535-543.

107. Galli SJ. New concepts about the mast cell. N Engl J Med. 1993;328:257-265.

108. Columbo M, Horowitz EM, Botana LM, et al. The human recombinant c-kit receptor ligand, rhSCF, induces mediator release from human cutaneous mast cells and enhances IgE-dependent mediator release from both skin mast cells and peripheral blood basophils. J Immunol. 1992;149:599-608.

109. Kuriu A, Sonoda S, Kanakura Y, et al. Proliferative potential of degranulated murine peritoneal mast cells. Blood. 1989;74:925-929.

110. Whitelaw DM. Observations on human monocyte kinetics after pulse labeling. Cell Tissue Kinet. 1972;5:311-317.

111. Whitelaw DM. The intravascular lifespan of monocytes. Blood. 1966;28:445-464.

112. Fixe P, Praloran V. M-CSF: haematopoietic growth factor or inflammatory cytokine? Cytokine. 1998;10:32-37.

113. Friedman AD. Transcriptional regulation of granulocyte and monocyte development. Oncogene. 2002;21:3377-3390.

114. van Furth R. Origin and turnover of monocytes and macrophages. Curr Top Pathol. 1989;79:125-150.

115. Gordon S, Taylor PR. Monocyte and macrophage heterogeneity. Nat Rev Immunol. 2005;5:953-964.

116. Imhof BA, Aurrand-Lions M. Adhesion mechanisms regulating the migration of monocytes. Nat Rev Immunol. 2004;4:432-444.

117. Geissmann F, Jung S, Littman DR. Blood monocytes consist of two principal subsets with distinct migratory properties. Immunity. 2003;19:71-82.

118. Passlick B, Flieger D, Ziegler-Heitbrock HW. Identification and characterization of a novel monocyte subpopulation in human peripheral blood. Blood. 1989;74:2527-2534.

119. Grage-Griebenow E, Flad HD, Ernst M. Heterogeneity of human peripheral blood monocyte subsets. J Leukoc Biol. 2001;69:11-20.

120. Thomas ED, Ramberg RE, Sale GE, et al. Direct evidence for a bone marrow origin of the alveolar macrophage in man. Science. 1976;192:1016-1018.

121. Tapper H. The secretion of preformed granules by macrophages and neutrophils. J Leukoc Biol. 1996;59:613-622.

122. McKnight AJ, Macfarlane AJ, Dri P, et al. Molecular cloning of F4/80, a murine macrophage-restricted cell surface glycoprotein with homology to the G-protein–linked transmembrane 7 hormone receptor family. J Biol Chem. 1996;271:486-489.

123. Pulford KA, Sipos A, Cordell JL, et al. Distribution of the CD68 macrophage/myeloid associated antigen. Int Immunol. 1990;2:973-980.

124. Hume DA. The mononuclear phagocyte system. Curr Opin Immunol. 2006;18:49-53.

125. Linehan SA, Martinez-Pomares L, Gordon S. Macrophage lectins in host defence. Microbes Infect. 2000;2:279-288.

126. Ma J, Chen T, Mandelin J, et al. Regulation of macrophage activation. Cell Mol Life Sci. 2003;60:2334-2346.

127. Taylor PR, Martinez-Pomares L, Stacey M, et al. Macrophage receptors and immune recognition. Annu Rev Immunol. 2005;23:901-944.

128. Johnston R Jr. Current concepts: immunology. Monocytes and macrophages. N Engl J Med. 1988;318:747-752.

129. Bar-Shavit R, Kahn A, Wilner GD, Fenton JW II. Monocyte chemotaxis: stimulation by specific exosite region in thrombin. Science. 1983;220:728-731.

130. Broze G. Binding of human factor VII and VIIa to monocytes. J Clin Invest. 1982;70:526-532.

131. Brown MS, Goldstein JL. Lipoprotein metabolism in the macrophage: implications for cholesterol deposition in atherosclerosis. Annu Rev Biochem. 1983;52:223-261.

132. Nathan CF. Secretory products of macrophages. J Clin Invest. 1987;79:319-326.

133. Geske FJ, Monks J, Lehman L, Fadok VA. The role of the macrophage in apoptosis: hunter, gatherer, and regulator. Int J Hematol. 2002;76:16-26.

134. Fujiwara N, Kobayashi K. Macrophages in inflammation. Curr Drug Targets Inflamm Allergy. 2005;4:281-286.

135. Hocking WG, Golde DW. The pulmonary alveolar macrophage (first of two parts). N Engl J Med. 1979;301:580-587.

136. Hanspal M, Hanspal JS. The association of erythroblasts with macrophages promotes erythroid proliferation and maturation: a 30-kD heparin-binding protein is involved in this contact. Blood. 1994;84:3494-3504.

137. Tavassoli M. Intravascular phagocytosis in the rabbit bone marrow: a possible fate of normal senescent red cells. Br J Haematol. 1977;36:323-330.

138. Beutler E. Gaucher disease: multiple lessons from a single gene disorder. Acta Paediatr Suppl. 2006;95:103-109.

139. Bussink AP, van Eijk M, Renkema GH, et al. The biology of the Gaucher cell: the cradle of human chitinases. Int Rev Cytol. 2006;252:71-128.

140. Gordon S. The macrophage. Bioessays. 1995;17:977-986.

141. Ho D, Pomerantz R, Kaplan JC. Pathogenesis of infection with human immunodeficiency virus. N Engl J Med. 1987;317:278-286.

142. Friedland GH, Klein RS. Transmission of the human immunodeficiency virus. N Engl J Med. 1987;317:1125-1130.

143. Banchereau J, Steinman RM. Dendritic cells and the control of immunity. Nature. 1998;392:245-252.

144. Spits H, Lanier LL. Natural killer or dendritic: what's in a name? Immunity. 2007;26:11-16.

145. Randolph GJ, Beaulieu S, Lebecque S, et al. Differentiation of monocytes into dendritic cells in a model of transendothelial trafficking. Science. 1998;282:480-483.

146. Liu YJ, Kanzler H, Soumelis V, Gilliet M. Dendritic cell lineage, plasticity and cross-regulation. Nat Immunol. 2001;2:585-589.

147. Foti M, Granucci F, Pelizzola M, et al. Dendritic cells in pathogen recognition and induction of immune responses: a functional genomics approach. J Leukoc Biol. 2006;79:913-916.

148. Teitelbaum SL. Bone resorption by osteoclasts. Science. 2000;289:1504-1508.

149. Teitelbaum SL, Ross FP. Genetic regulation of osteoclast development and function. Nat Rev Genet. 2003;4:638-649.

150. Schneider GB, Relfson M. The effects of transplantation of granulocyte-macrophage progenitors on bone resorption in *ia* osteopetrotic rats. J Bone Miner Res. 1988;3:225-232.

151. Tolar J, Teitelbaum SL, Orchard PJ. Osteopetrosis. N Engl J Med. 2004;351:2839-2849.

152. Suda T, Takahashi N, Martin TJ. Modulation of osteoclast differentiation. Endocr Rev. 1992;13:66-80.

153. Orchard PJ, Dahl N, Aukerman SL, et al. Circulating macrophage colony-stimulating factor is not reduced in malignant osteopetrosis. Exp Hematol. 1992;20:103-105.

154. Frattini A, Orchard PJ, Sobacchi C, et al. Defects in TCIRG1 subunit of the vacuolar proton pump are responsible for a subset of human autosomal recessive osteopetrosis. Nat Genet. 2000;25:343-346.

155. Kornak U, Kasper D, Bosl MR, et al. Loss of the ClC-7 chloride channel leads to osteopetrosis in mice and man. Cell. 2001;104:205-215.

156. Coccia PF, Krivit W, Cervenka J, et al. Successful bone-marrow transplantation for infantile malignant osteopetrosis. N Engl J Med. 1980;302:701-708.

157. Johansson MK, de Vries TJ, Schoenmaker T, et al. Hematopoietic stem cell–targeted neonatal gene therapy reverses lethally progressive osteopetrosis in *oc/oc* mice. Blood. 2007;109:5178-5185.

158. Key LL, Rodriguiz RM, Willi SM, et al. Long-term treatment of osteopetrosis with recombinant human interferon gamma. N Engl J Med. 1995;332:1594-1595.

159. Plytycz B, Seljelid R. From inflammation to sickness: historical perspective. Arch Immunol Ther Exp (Warsz). 2003;51:105-109.

160. Metchnikov I. Immunity in Infective Diseases. New York, Dover, 1968.

161. Serhan CN, Savill J. Resolution of inflammation: the beginning programs the end. Nat Immunol. 2005;6:1191-1197.

162. Nathan C. Points of control in inflammation. Nature. 2002;420:846-852.

163. Nathan C. Neutrophils and immunity: challenges and opportunities. Nat Rev Immunol. 2006;6:173-182.

164. Bianchi ME. DAMPs, PAMPs and alarmins: all we need to know about danger. J Leukoc Biol. 2007;81:1-5.

165. Oppenheim JJ, Yang D. Alarmins: chemotactic activators of immune responses. Curr Opin Immunol. 2005;17:359-365.

166. Yang H, Wang H, Czura CJ, Tracey KJ. The cytokine activity of HMGB1. J Leukoc Biol. 2005;78:1-8.

167. Dinarello CA. The IL-1 family and inflammatory diseases. Clin Exp Rheumatol. 2002;20:S1-13.

168. Mosser DM. The many faces of macrophage activation. J Leukoc Biol. 2003;73:209-212.

169. Schroder K, Hertzog PJ, Ravasi T, Hume DA. Interferon-gamma: an overview of signals, mechanisms and functions. J Leukoc Biol. 2004;75:163-189.

170. Kulkarni AB, Huh CG, Becker D, et al. Transforming growth factor beta-1 null mutation in mice causes excessive inflammatory response and early death. Proc Natl Acad Sci U S A. 1993;90:770-774.

171. Moore KW, O'Garra A, de Waal Maalefyt R, et al. Interleukin-10. Annu Rev Immunol. 1993;11:165-190.

172. Wahl SM. Transforming growth factor-beta: innately bipolar. Curr Opin Immunol. 2007;19:55-62.

173. Alam R, Lett-Brown MA, Forsythe PA, et al. Monocyte chemotactic and activating factor is a potent histamine-releasing factor for basophils. J Clin Invest. 1992;89:723-728.

174. Kuna P, Reddigari SR, Schall TJ, et al. RANTES, a monocyte and T lymphocyte chemotactic cytokine releases histamine from human basophils. J Immunol. 1992;149:636-642.

175. Christie PE, Henderson WR Jr. Lipid inflammatory mediators: leukotrienes, prostaglandins, platelet-activating factor. Clin Allergy Immunol. 2002;16:233-254.

176. Stafforini DM, McIntyre TM, Zimmerman GA, Prescott SM. Platelet-activating factor, a pleiotrophic mediator of physiological and pathological processes. Crit Rev Clin Lab Sci. 2003;40:643-672.

177. Louis NA, Hamilton KE, Colgan SP. Lipid mediator networks and leukocyte transmigration. Prostaglandins Leukot Essent Fatty Acids. 2005;73:197-202.

178. Lowenstein CJ, Snyder SH. Nitric oxide, a novel biologic messenger. Cell. 1992;70:705-707.

179. Nathan C. Nitric oxide as a secretory product of mammalian cells. FASEB J. 1992;6:3051-3064.

180. Springer TA. Traffic signals for lymphocyte recirculation and leukocyte emigration: the multistep paradigm. Cell. 1994;76:310-314.

181. Locati M, Murphy PM. Chemokines and chemokine receptors: biology and clinical relevance in inflammation and AIDS. Annu Rev Med. 1999;50:425-440.

182. Gillitzer R, Goebeler M. Chemokines in cutaneous wound healing. J Leukoc Biol. 2001;69:513-521.

183. Mantovani A, Bonecchi R, Locati M. Tuning inflammation and immunity by chemokine sequestration: decoys and more. Nat Rev Immunol. 2006;6:907-918.

184. Peters-Golden M, Canetti C, Mancuso P, Coffey MJ. Leukotrienes: underappreciated mediators of innate immune responses. J Immunol. 2005;174:589-594.

185. Baggiolini M. Chemokines and leukocyte traffic. Nature. 1998;392:565-568.

186. Charo IF, Ransohoff RM. The many roles of chemokines and chemokine receptors in inflammation. N Engl J Med. 2006;354:610-621.

187. Huber AR, Kunkel SL, Todd RF, Weiss SL. Regulation of transendothelial neutrophil migration by endogenous interleukin-8. Science. 1991;254:99-102.

188. Tanaka Y, Adams DH, Hubscher S, et al. T-cell adhesion induced by proteoglycan-immobilized cytokine MIp-1b. Nature. 1993;361:79-82.

189. Christopher MJ, Link DC. Regulation of neutrophil homeostasis. Curr Opin Hematol. 2007;14:3-8.

190. Walz A, Baggiolini M. Generation of the neutrophil-activating peptide NAP-2 from platelet basic protein or connective tissue–activating peptide III through monocyte proteases. J Exp Med. 1990;171:449-454.

191. Bazan JF, Bacon KB, Hardiman G, et al. A new class of membrane-bound chemokine with a CX3C motif. Nature. 1997;385:640-644.

192. Rollins BJ, Walz A, Baggiolini M. Recombinant human MCP-1/JE induces chemotaxis, calcium flux, and the respiratory burst in human monocytes. Blood. 1991;78:1112-1116.

193. Schall TJ, Bacon K, Toy KJ, Goeddel D. Selective attraction of monocytes and T lymphocytes of the memory phenotype by cytokines RANTES. Nature. 1990;347:669-671.

194. Zachaiae CO, Anderson AO, Thompson HL, et al. Properties of monocyte chemotactic and activating factor (MCAF) purified from a human fibrosarcoma cell line. J Exp Med. 1990;171:2177-2182.

195. Zigmond S. The ability of polymorphonuclear leukocytes to orient in gradients of chemotactic factors. J Cell Biol. 1977;117:606-613.

196. Gerard C, Gerard NP. The pro-inflammatory seven-transmembrane segment receptors of the leukocyte. Curr Opin Immunol. 1994;6:140-145.

197. Murphy PM. The molecular biology of leukocyte chemoattractant receptors. Annu Rev Immunol. 1994;12:593-633.

198. Polakis PG, Uhing RJ, Snyderman R. The formylpeptide chemoattractant receptor copurifies with a GTP-binding protein containing a distinct 40 kDa pertussis toxin substrate. J Biol Chem. 1988;263:4969-4976.

199. Glogauer M, Hartwig J, Stossel T. Two pathways through Cdc42 couple the N-formyl receptor to actin nucleation in permeabilized human neutrophils. J Cell Biol. 2000;150:785-796.

200. Kim C, Dinauer M. Rac2 is an essential regulator of neutrophil nicotinamide adenine dinucleotide phosphate oxidase activation in response to specific signaling pathways. J Immunol. 2001;166:1223-1232.

201. Roberts AW, Kim C, Zhen L, et al. Deficiency of the hematopoietic cell–specific Rho family GTPase Rac2 is characterized by abnormalities in neutrophil function and host defense. Immunity. 1999;10:183-196.

202. Dinauer MC. Regulation of neutrophil function by Rac GTPases. Curr Opin Hematol. 2003;10:8-15.

203. Amatruda TT, Steele DA, Slepak VZ, Simon MI. G alpha 16, a G protein alpha subunit specifically expressed in hematopoietic cells. Proc Natl Acad Sci U S A. 1991;88:5587-5591.

204. Davignon I, Catalina MD, Smith D, et al. Normal hematopoiesis and inflammatory responses despite discrete signaling defects in Gα15 knockout mice. Mol Cell Biol. 2000;20:797-804.

205. McIntyre TM, Prescott SM, Weyrich AS, Zimmerman GA. Cell-cell interactions: leukocyte-endothelial interactions. Curr Opin Hematol. 2003;10:150-158.

206. Yonekawa K, Harlan JM. Targeting leukocyte integrins in human diseases. J Leukoc Biol. 2005;77:129-140.

207. Kishimoto TK, Rothlein R. Integrins, ICAMS, and selectins: role and regulation of adhesion molecules in neutrophil recruitment to inflammatory sites. Adv Pharm. 1994;25:117-169.

208. McEver RP. Selectins. Curr Opin Immunol. 1994;6:75-84.

209. Rosen SD. Ligands for L-selectin: homing, inflammation, and beyond. Annu Rev Immunol. 2004;22:129-156.

210. Bevilacqua MP, Stengelin S, Gimbrone MA Jr, Seed B. Endothelial leukocyte adhesion molecule 1: an inducible receptor of neutrophils related to complement regulatory proteins and lectins. Science. 1989;243:1160-1165.

211. Hidalgo A, Peired AJ, Wild MK, et al. Complete identification of E-selectin ligands on neutrophils reveals distinct functions of PSGL-1, ESL-1, and CD44. Immunity. 2007;26:477-489.

212. Jung TM, Dailey MO. Rapid modulation of homing receptors (gp90MEL-14) induced by activators of protein kinase C. Receptor shedding due to accelerated proteolytic cleavage at the cell surface. J Immunol. 1990;144:3130-3136.

213. Kishimoto TK, Jutila MA, Berg EL, Butcher EC. Neutrophil Mac-1 and MEL-14 adhesion proteins inversely regulated by chemotactic factors. Science. 1989;245:1238-1241.

214. Smalley DM, Ley K. L-selectin: mechanisms and physiological significance of ectodomain cleavage. J Cell Mol Med. 2005;9:255-266.

215. Harris ES, McIntyre TM, Prescott SM, Zimmerman GA. The leukocyte integrins. J Biol Chem. 2000;275:23409-23412.

216. Kishimoto TK, O'Connor K, Lee A, et al. Cloning of the b subunit of the leukocyte adhesion proteins: homology to an extracellular matrix receptor defines a novel supergene family. Cell. 1987;48:681-690.

217. O'Toole TE, Katagiri Y, Faull RJ, et al. Integrin cytoplasmic domains mediate inside-out signal transduction. J Cell Biol. 1994;124:1047-1059.

218. Moyle M, Foster DL, McGrath DE, et al. A hookworm glycoprotein that inhibits neutrophil function is a ligand of the integrin CD11b/CD18. J Biol Chem. 1994;269:10008-10015.

219. Rieu P, Ueda T, Haruta I, et al. The A-domain of β2 integrin CR3 (CD11b/CD18) is a receptor for the hookworm-derived neutrophil adhesion inhibitor NIF. J Cell Biol. 1994;127:2081-2091.

220. Sengeløv H, Kjeldsen L, Diamond MS, et al. Subcellular localization and dynamics of Mac-1 (amb2) in human neutrophils. J Clin Invest. 1993;92:1467-1476.

221. Galkina E, Ley K. Vascular adhesion molecules in atherosclerosis. Arterioscler Thromb Vasc Biol. 2007;27:2292-2301.

222. Brown E. Neutrophil adhesion and the therapy of inflammation. Semin Hematol. 1997;34:319-326.

223. Abram CL, Lowell CA. Convergence of immunoreceptor and integrin signaling. Immunol Rev. 2007;218:29-44.

224. Berton G, Mocsai A, Lowell CA. Src and Syk kinases: key regulators of phagocytic cell activation. Trends Immunol. 2005;26:208-214.

225. Doerschuk CM, Winn RK, Coxson HO, et al. CD18-dependent and independent mechanisms of neutrophil adherence in the pulmonary and systemic microvasculature of rabbits. J Immunol. 1990;144:2327-2333.

226. Hechtman DH, Cybulsky MI, Fuchs HJ, et al. Intravascular IL-8: inhibitor of polymorphonuclear leukocyte accumulation at sites of acute inflammation. J Immunol. 1991;147:883-892.

227. Rosengren S, Olofsson AM, von Andrian UH, et al. Leukotriene B$_4$–induced neutrophil-mediated endothelial leakage in vitro and in vivo. J Appl Physiol. 1991;71:1322-1330.

228. Ostermann G, Weber KS, Zernecke A, et al. JAM-1 is a ligand of the β$_2$ integrin LFA-1 involved in transendothelial migration of leukocytes. Nat Immunol. 2002;3:151-158.

229. Muller WA, Weigl SA, Deng X, Phillips DM. PECAM-1 is required for transendothelial migration of leukocytes. J Exp Med. 1993;178:449-460.

230. Vaporciyan AA, DeLisser HM, Yan HC, et al. Involvement of platelet–endothelial cell adhesion molecule-1 in neutrophil recruitment in vivo. Science. 1993;262:1580-1582.

231. Hordijk PL. Endothelial signalling events during leukocyte transmigration. FEBS J. 2006;273:4408-4415.

232. Wang Q, Doerschuk CM. The signaling pathways induced by neutrophil–endothelial cell adhesion. Antioxid Redox Signal. 2002;4:39-47.

233. Weiss SJ. Tissue destruction by neutrophils. N Engl J Med. 1989;320:365-376.

234. Jones GE. Cellular signaling in macrophage migration and chemotaxis. J Leukoc Biol. 2000;68:593-602.

235. Bagorda A, Mihaylov VA, Parent CA. Chemotaxis: moving forward and holding on to the past. Thromb Haemost. 2006;95:12-21.

236. Ridley AJ, Schwartz MA, Burridge K, et al. Cell migration: integrating signals from front to back. Science. 2003;302:1704-1709.

237. Bi E, Zigmond SH. Actin polymerization: where the WASP stings. Curr Biol. 1999;9:R160-R163.

238. Wu D. Signaling mechanisms for regulation of chemotaxis. Cell Res. 2005;15:52-56.

239. Hartwing JH, Shevlin P. The architecture of actin filaments and the ultrastructural location of actin-binding protein in the periphery of lung macrophages. J Cell Biol. 1986;103:1007-1018.

240. Cicchetti G, Allen PG, Glogauer M. Chemotactic signaling pathways in neutrophils: from receptor to actin assembly. Crit Rev Oral Biol Med. 2002;13:220-228.

241. Cassimeris L, Safer D, Nachmias VT, Zigmond SH. Thymosin B$_4$ sequesters the majority of G-actin in resting human polymorphonuclear leukocytes. J Cell Biol. 1992;119:1261-1270.

242. Ridley A, Hall A. The small GTP-binding protein Rac regulates growth factor–induced membrane ruffling. Cell. 1992;70:401-410.

243. Machesky LM, Insall RH. Signaling to actin dynamics. J Cell Biol. 1999;146:267-272.

244. Coates TD, Watts RG, Hartman R, Howard TH. Relationship of F-actin distribution to development of polar shape in human polymorphonuclear neutrophils. J Cell Biol. 1992;117:765-774.

245. Pestonjamasp KN, Forster C, Sun C, et al. Rac1 links leading edge and uropod events through Rho and myosin activation during chemotaxis. Blood. 2006;108:2814-2820.

246. Worthylake RA, Lemoine S, Watson JM, Burridge K. RhoA is required for monocyte tail retraction during transendothelial migration. J Cell Biol. 2001;154:147-160.

247. de Haas M, Kleijer M, van Zwieten R, et al. Neutrophil FcγRIIIb deficiency, nature, and clinical consequences: a study of 21 individuals from 14 families. Blood. 1995;86:2403-2413.

248. Gordon S. Pattern recognition receptors: doubling up for the innate immune response. Cell. 2002;111:927-930.

249. Medzhitov R, Janeway CA Jr. Decoding the patterns of self and nonself by the innate immune system. Science. 2002;296:298-300.

250. Trinchieri G, Sher A. Cooperation of Toll-like receptor signals in innate immune defence. Nat Rev Immunol. 2007;7:179-190.

251. Brown GD. Dectin-1: a signalling non-TLR pattern-recognition receptor. Nat Rev Immunol. 2006;6:33-43.

252. Netea MG, van der Graaf C, Van der Meer JW, Kullberg BJ. Toll-like receptors and the host defense against microbial pathogens: bringing specificity to the innate-immune system. J Leukoc Biol. 2004;75:749-755.

253. Picard C, Puel A, Bonnet M, et al. Pyogenic bacterial infections in humans with IRAK-4 deficiency. Science. 2003;299:2076-2079.

254. Walport MJ. Complement. First of two parts. N Engl J Med. 2001;344:1058-1066.

255. van de Wetering JK, van Golde LM, Batenburg JJ. Collectins: players of the innate immune system. Eur J Biochem. 2004;271:1229-1249.

256. Dommett RM, Klein N, Turner MW. Mannose-binding lectin in innate immunity: past, present and future. Tissue Antigens. 2006;68:193-209.

257. Takahashi K, Ip WE, Michelow IC, Ezekowitz RA. The mannose-binding lectin: a prototypic pattern recognition molecule. Curr Opin Immunol. 2006;18:16-23.

258. Gasque P. Complement: a unique innate immune sensor for danger signals. Mol Immunol. 2004;41:1089-1098.

259. Sengelov H. Complement receptors in neutrophils. Crit Rev Immunol. 1995;15:107-131.

260. Helmy KY, Katschke KJ Jr, Gorgani NN, et al. CRIg: a macrophage complement receptor required for phagocytosis of circulating pathogens. Cell. 2006;124:915-927.

261. McKenzie SE, Schreiber AD. Fc gamma receptors in phagocytes. Curr Opin Hematol. 1998;5:16-21.

262. Ravetch JV, Bolland S. IgG Fc receptors. Annu Rev Immunol. 2001;19:275-290.

263. Takai T. Fc receptors and their role in immune regulation and autoimmunity. J Clin Immunol. 2005;25:1-18.

264. Ravetch JV. Fc receptors: rubor redux. Cell. 1994;78:553-560.

265. Bux J. Molecular nature of antigens implicated in immune neutropenias. Int J Hematol. 2002;76(Suppl 1):399-403.

266. Stroncek D. Neutrophil alloantigens. Transfus Med Rev. 2002;16:67-75.

267. van Sorge NM, van der Pol WL, van de Winkel JG. FcγR polymorphisms: implications for function, disease susceptibility and immunotherapy. Tissue Antigens. 2003;61:189-202.

268. Lee WL, Harrison RE, Grinstein S. Phagocytosis by neutrophils. Microbes Infect. 2003;5:1299-1306.

269. Swanson JA, Hoppe AD. The coordination of signaling during Fc receptor–mediated phagocytosis. J Leukoc Biol. 2004;76:1093-1103.

270. Greenberg S. Modular components of phagocytosis. J Leukoc Biol. 1999;66:712-717.

271. Maliszewski CR, March CJ, Schoenborn MA, et al. Expression cloning of a human Fc receptor for IgA. J Exp Med. 1990;172:1665-1672.

272. Albrechtsen M, Yeaman GR, Kerr MA. Characterization of the IgA receptor from human polymorphonuclear leucocytes. Immunology. 1988;64:201-205.

273. Kerr MA. The structure and function of human IgA. Biochem J. 1990;271:285-296.

274. Aderem A, Ulevitch RJ. Toll-like receptors in the induction of the innate immune response. Nature. 2000;406:782-787.

275. Lacy P. The role of Rho GTPases and SNAREs in mediator release from granulocytes. Pharmacol Ther. 2005;107:358-376.

276. Deretic V, Singh S, Master S, et al. *Mycobacterium tuberculosis* inhibition of phagolysosome biogenesis and autophagy as a host defence mechanism. Cell Microbiol. 2006;8:719-727.

277. Vazquez-Torres A, Xu Y, Jones-Carson J, et al. *Salmonella* pathogenicity island 2–dependent evasion of the phagocyte NADPH oxidase. Science. 2000;287:1655-1658.

278. Allen LA. Mechanisms of pathogenesis: evasion of killing by polymorphonuclear leukocytes. Microbes Infect. 2003;5:1329-1335.

279. Brinkmann V, Reichard U, Goosmann C, et al. Neutrophil extracellular traps kill bacteria. Science. 2004;303:1532-1535.

280. Fuchs TA, Abed U, Goosmann C, et al. Novel cell death program leads to neutrophil extracellular traps. J Cell Biol. 2007;176:231-241.

281. Ganz T. Defensins: antimicrobial peptides of innate immunity. Nat Rev Immunol. 2003;3:710-720.

282. Ganz T, Weiss J. Antimicrobial peptides of phagocytes and epithelia. Semin Hematol. 1997;34:343-354.

283. Elsbach P. The bactericidal/permeability-increasing protein (BPI) in antibacterial host defense. J Leukoc Biol. 1998;64:14-18.

284. Pham CT. Neutrophil serine proteases: specific regulators of inflammation. Nat Rev Immunol. 2006;6:541-550.

285. Pereira HA. CAP37, a neutrophil-derived multifunctional inflammatory mediator. J Leukoc Biol. 1995;57:805-812.

286. Cole AM, Waring AJ. The role of defensins in lung biology and therapy. Am J Respir Med. 2002;1:249-259.

287. Murphy MF, Sourial NA, Burman JF, et al. Megaloblastic anemia due to vitamin B$_{12}$ deficiency caused by small intestinal bacterial overgrowth: possible role of vitamin B$_{12}$ analogues. Br J Haematol. 1986;62:7-12.

288. Cech P, Lehrer RI. Phagolysosomal pH of human neutrophils. Blood. 1984;63:88-95.

289. Segal AW, Geisow M, Garcia R, et al. The respiratory burst of phagocytic cells is associated with a rise in vacuolar pH. Nature. 1981;290:406-409.

290. Welsh IRH, Spitznagel JK. Distribution of lysosomal enzymes, cationic proteins, and bactericidal substances and subcellular fractions of human polymorphonuclear leukocytes. Infect Immun. 1971;4:97-102.

291. Belaaouaj A, McCarthy R, Baumann M, et al. Mice lacking neutrophil elastase reveal impaired host defense against gram negative bacterial sepsis. Nat Med. 1998;4:615-618.

292. Tkalcevic J, Novelli M, Phylactides M, et al. Impaired immunity and enhanced resistance to endotoxin in the absence of neutrophil elastase and cathepsin G. Immunity. 2000;12:201-210.

293. Dale DC, Person RE, Bolyard AA, et al. Mutations in the gene encoding neutrophil elastase in congenital and cyclic neutropenia. Blood. 2000;96:2317-2322.

294. Horwitz M, Benson KF, Person RE, et al. Mutations in ELA2, encoding neutrophil elastase, define a 21-day biological clock in cyclic haematopoiesis. Nat Genet. 1999;23:433-436.

295. Babior BM. Oxygen-dependent microbial killing by phagocytes. N Engl J Med. 1978;298:659.

296. Baldridge CW, Gerard RW. The extra respiration of phagocytosis. Am J Physiol. 1933;103:235-236.

297. Sbarra AJ, Karnovsky ML. The biochemical basis of phagocytosis. I. Metabolic changes during the ingestion of particles by polymorphonuclear leukocytes. J Biol Chem. 1959;234:1355-1362.

298. Cross AR, Jones OTG. Enzymic mechanisms of superoxide production. Biochim Biophys Acta. 1991;1057:281-298.

299. Babior BM, Kipnes RS, Curnutte JT. Biological defense mechanisms: the production by leukocytes of superoxide, a potential bactericidal agent. J Clin Invest. 1973;52:741-745.

300. Babior BM. NADPH oxidase: an update. Blood. 1999;93:1464-1476.

301. Nauseef WM. Assembly of the phagocyte NADPH oxidase. Histochem Cell Biol. 2004;122:277-291.

302. Fang FC. Antimicrobial reactive oxygen and nitrogen species: concepts and controversies. Nat Rev Microbiol. 2004;2:820-832.

303. Hampton MB, Kettle AJ, Winterbourn CC. Inside the neutrophil phagosome: oxidants, myeloperoxidase, and bacterial killing. Blood. 1998;92:3007-3017.

304. Ellson C, Davidson K, Anderson K, et al. PtdIns3P binding to the PX domain of p40^{phox} is a physiological signal in NADPH oxidase activation. EMBO J. 2006;25:4468-4478.

305. Ellson CD, Davidson K, Ferguson GJ, et al. Neutrophils from p40^{phox}–/– mice exhibit severe defects in NADPH oxidase regulation and oxidant-dependent bacterial killing. J Exp Med. 2006;203:1927-1937.

306. Suh CI, Stull ND, Li XJ, et al. The phosphoinositide-binding protein p40^{phox} activates the NADPH oxidase during FcγIIA receptor–induced phagocytosis. J Exp Med. 2006;203:1915-1925.

307. Parkos CA, Allen RA, Cochrane CG, Jesaitis AJ. Purified cytochrome *b* from human granulocyte plasma membrane is comprised of two polypeptides with relative molecular weights of 91,000 and 22,000. J Clin Invest. 1987;80:732-742.

308. Dinauer MC, Orkin SH, Brown R, et al. The glycoprotein encoded by the X-linked chronic granulomatous disease locus is a component of the neutrophil cytochrome *b* complex. Nature. 1987;327:717-720.

309. Teahan C, Rowe P, Parker P, et al. The X-linked chronic granulomatous disease gene codes for the beta-chain of cytochrome *b*-245. Nature. 1987;327:720-721.

310. Royer-Pokora B, Kunkel LM, Monaco AP, et al. Cloning the gene for an inherited human disorder—chronic granulomatous disease—on the basis of its chromosomal location. Nature. 1986;322:32-38.

311. Cross AR, Jones OTG, Harper AM, Segal AW. Oxidation-reduction properties of the cytochrome *b* found in the plasma-membrane fraction of human neutrophils. Biochem J. 1981;194:599-606.

312. McPhail LC. SH3-dependent assembly of the phagocyte NADPH oxidase. J Exp Med. 1994;180:2011-2015.

313. Parkos CA, Dinauer MC, Walker LE, et al. Primary structure and unique expression of the 22-kilodalton light chain of human neutrophil cytochrome *b*. Proc Natl Acad Sci U S A. 1988;85:3319-3323.

314. Yu L, Quinn MT, Cross AR, Dinauer MC. Gp91^{phox} is the heme binding subunit of the superoxide-generating NADPH oxidase. Proc Natl Acad Sci U S A. 1998;95:7993-7998.

315. Wishart MJ, Taylor GS, Dixon JE. Phoxy lipids: revealing PX domains as phosphoinositide binding modules. Cell. 2001;105:817-820.

316. Kanai F, Liu H, Field SJ, et al. The PX domains of p47^{phox} and p40^{phox} bind to lipid products of PI$_3$K. Nat Cell Biol. 2001;3:675-678.

317. Ellson CD, Anderson KE, Morgan G, et al. Phosphatidylinositol 3-phosphate is generated in phagosomal membranes. Curr Biol. 2001;11:1631-1635.

318. Heyworth PG, Curnutte JT, Nauseef WM, et al. Neutrophil nicotinamide adenine dinucleotide phosphate oxidase assembly. Translocation of p47-*phox* and p67-*phox* requires interaction between p47-*phox* and cytochrome *b*$_{558}$. J Clin Invest. 1991;87:352-356.

319. Lapouge K, Smith SJ, Walker PA, et al. Structure of the TPR domain of p67^{phox} in complex with Rac-GTP. Mol Cell. 2000;6:899-907.

320. Diebold BA, Bokoch GM. Molecular basis for Rac2 regulation of phagocyte NADPH oxidase. Nat Immunol. 2001;2:211-215.

321. Ohno YI, Hirai KI, Kanoh T, et al. Subcellular localization of hydrogen peroxide production in human polymorphonuclear leukocytes stimulated with lectins, phorbol myristate acetate, and digitonin: an electron microscope study using CeCl$_3$. Blood. 1982;60:1195-1202.

322. Robinson JM, Badwey JA. The NADPH oxidase complex of phagocytic leukocytes: a biochemical and cytochemical view. Histochemistry. 1995;103:163-180.

323. Klebanoff SJ. Oxygen metabolites from phagocytes. In Gallin JI, Goldstein IM, Snyderman R (eds). Inflammation: Basic Principles and Clinical Correlates. New York, Raven Press, 1992, pp 541-588.

324. Bast A, Haenen GRMM, Doelman CJA. Oxidants and antioxidants: state of the art. Am J Med. 1991;91(Suppl 3C):2S-13S.

325. Marletta MA. Nitric oxide synthase: aspects concerning structure and catalysis. Cell. 1994;78:927-930.

326. Bogdan C. Nitric oxide and the immune response. Nat Immunol. 2001;2:907-916.

327. MacMicking J, Xie QW, Nathan C. Nitric oxide and macrophage function. Annu Rev Immunol. 1997;15:323-350.

328. Evans TJ, Buttery LD, Carpenter A, et al. Cytokine-treated human neutrophils contain inducible nitric oxide synthase that produces nitration of ingested bacteria. Proc Natl Acad Sci U S A. 1996;93:9553-9558.

329. Griendling KK. Novel NAD(P)H oxidases in the cardiovascular system. Heart. 2004;90:491-493.

330. Wood KC, Hebbel RP, Granger DN. Endothelial cell NADPH oxidase mediates the cerebral microvascular dysfunction in sickle cell transgenic mice. FASEB J. 2005;19:989-991.

331. Abdala-Valencia H, Earwood J, Bansal S, et al. Nonhematopoietic NADPH oxidase regulation of lung eosinophilia and airway hyperresponsiveness in experimentally induced asthma. Am J Physiol Lung Cell Mol Physiol. 2007;292:L1111-L1125.

332. Bedard K, Lardy B, Krause KH. NOX family NADPH oxidases: not just in mammals. Biochimie. 2007;89:1107-1112.

333. Geiszt M, Leto TL. The Nox family of NAD(P)H oxidases: host defense and beyond. J Biol Chem. 2004;279:51715-51718.

334. Lambeth JD. NOX enzymes and the biology of reactive oxygen. Nat Rev Immunol. 2004;4:181-189.

335. Sharma SD, Remington JS. Macrophage activation and resistance to intracellular infection. Lymphokines. 1981;3:181-212.

336. Denkers EY, Butcher BA. Sabotage and exploitation in macrophages parasitized by intracellular protozoans. Trends Parasitol. 2005;21:35-41.

337. Anderson JM. Multinucleated giant cells. Curr Opin Hematol. 2000;7:40-47.

338. Co DO, Hogan LH, Kim SI, Sandor M. Mycobacterial granulomas: keys to a long-lasting host-pathogen relationship. Clin Immunol. 2004;113:130-136.

339. Bingle L, Brown NJ, Lewis CE. The role of tumour-associated macrophages in tumour progression: implications for new anticancer therapies. J Pathol. 2002;196:254-265.

340. Dunn GP, Old LJ, Schreiber RD. The immunobiology of cancer immunosurveillance and immunoediting. Immunity. 2004;21:137-148.

341. Mantovani A. Cancer: inflammation by remote control. Nature. 2005;435:752-753.

342. Condeelis J, Pollard JW. Macrophages: obligate partners for tumor cell migration, invasion, and metastasis. Cell. 2006;124:263-266.

343. Lewis CE, Pollard JW. Distinct role of macrophages in different tumor microenvironments. Cancer Res. 2006; 66:605-612.

344. Guise TA, Mohammad KS, Clines G, et al. Basic mechanisms responsible for osteolytic and osteoblastic bone metastases. Clin Cancer Res. 2006;12:6213s-6216s.

345. Darnell JE Jr, Kerr IM, Stark GR. Jak-STAT pathways and transcriptional activation in response to IFNs and other extracellular signaling proteins. Science. 1994;264: 1415-1421.

346. Ihle JN, Kerr IM. Jaks and Stats in signaling by the cytokine receptor superfamily. Trends Genet. 1995;11: 69-74.

347. Aderem A. Role of Toll-like receptors in inflammatory response in macrophages. Crit Care Med. 2001;29: S16-S18.

348. Kabelitz D, Medzhitov R. Innate immunity—cross-talk with adaptive immunity through pattern recognition receptors and cytokines. Curr Opin Immunol. 2007;19: 1-3.

349. Unanue ER, Allen PM. The basis for the immunoregulatory role of macrophages and other accessory cells. Science. 1987;236:551-557.

350. Iwasaki A, Medzhitov R. Toll-like receptor control of the adaptive immune responses. Nat Immunol. 2004;5: 987-995.

351. Romanovsky AA, Steiner AA, Matsumura K. Cells that trigger fever. Cell Cycle. 2006;5:2195-2197.

352. Martin P, Leibovich SJ. Inflammatory cells during wound repair: the good, the bad and the ugly. Trends Cell Biol. 2005;15:599-607.

353. Tsirogianni AK, Moutsopoulos NM, Moutsopoulos HM. Wound healing: immunological aspects. Injury. 2006;37(Suppl 1):S5-S12.

354. Krysko DV, D'Herde K, Vandenabeele P. Clearance of apoptotic and necrotic cells and its immunological consequences. Apoptosis. 2006;11:1709-1726.

355. Xu W, Roos A, Daha MR, van Kooten C. Dendritic cell and macrophage subsets in the handling of dying cells. Immunobiology. 2006;211:567-575.

356. Arese P, Turrini F, Bussolino F, et al. Recognition signals for phagocytic removal of favic, malaria-infected and sickled erythrocytes. Adv Exp Med Biol. 1991;307: 317-327.

357. Halma C, Daha MR, van Es LA. In vivo clearance by the mononuclear phagocyte system in humans: an overview of methods and their interpretation. Clin Exp Immunol. 1992;89:1-7.

358. Semple JW. Immune pathophysiology of autoimmune thrombocytopenic purpura. Blood Rev. 2002;16:9-12.

359. Anderson GJ, Darshan D, Wilkins SJ, Frazer DM. Regulation of systemic iron homeostasis: how the body responds to changes in iron demand. Biometals. 2007;20: 665-674.

360. Andrews NC. Anemia of inflammation: the cytokine-hepcidin link. J Clin Invest. 2004;113:1251-1253.

361. Choudhury RP, Lee JM, Greaves DR. Mechanisms of disease: macrophage-derived foam cells emerging as therapeutic targets in atherosclerosis. Nat Clin Pract Cardiovasc Med. 2005;2:309-315.

362. Rader DJ, Pure E. Lipoproteins, macrophage function, and atherosclerosis: beyond the foam cell? Cell Metab. 2005;1:223-230.

363. Stoll G, Bendszus M. Inflammation and atherosclerosis: novel insights into plaque formation and destabilization. Stroke. 2006;37:1923-1932.

364. Marone G, Casolaro V, Cirillo R, et al. Pathophysiology of human basophils and mast cells in allergic disorders. Clin Immunol Immunopathol. 1989;50:S24-S40.

365. Sylvestre DL, Ravetch JV. Fc receptors initiate the Arthus reaction: redefining the inflammatory cascade. Science. 1994;265:1095-1098.

366. Ramos BF, Qureshi R, Olsen KM, Jakschik BA. The importance of mast cells for the neutrophil influx in immune complex–induced peritonitis in mice. J Immunol. 1990;145:1868-1873.

367. Ramos BF, Zhang Y, Qureshi R, Jakschik BA. Mast cells are critical for the production of leukotrienes responsible for neutrophil recruitment in immune complex–induced peritonitis in mice. J Immunol. 1991;147:1636-1641.

368. Galli SJ, Wershil BK. The two faces of the mast cell. Nature. 1996;381:21-22.

369. Malaviya R, Ikeda T, Ross E, Abraham SN. Mast cell modulation of neutrophil influx and bacterial clearance at sites of infection through TNF-alpha. Nature. 1996; 381:77-80.

370. Echtenacher B, Mannel DN, Hultner L. Critical protective role of mast cells in a model of acute septic peritonitis. Nature. 1996;381:75-77.

371. Lehr HA, Arfors KE. Mechanisms of tissue damage by leukocytes. Curr Opin Hematol. 1994;1:92-99.

372. American College of Chest Physicians/Society of Critical Care Medicine Consensus Conference: definitions for sepsis and organ failure and guidelines for the use of innovative therapies in sepsis. Crit Care Med. 1992;20: 864-867.

373. Matzner Y. Acquired neutrophil dysfunction and diseases with an inflammatory component. Semin Hematol. 1997;34:291-302.

374. Weitzman SA, Gordon LI. Inflammation and cancer: role of phagocyte-generated oxidants in carcinogenesis. Blood. 1990;76:655-663.

375. Nurmohamed MT, Dijkmans BA. Efficacy, tolerability and cost effectiveness of disease-modifying antirheumatic drugs and biologic agents in rheumatoid arthritis. Drugs. 2005;65:661-694.

376. Ognibene FP, Martin SE, Parker MM, et al. Adult respiratory distress syndrome in patients with severe neutropenia. N Engl J Med. 1986;315:547-551.

377. Crum NF, Lederman ER, Wallace MR. Infections associated with tumor necrosis factor-alpha antagonists. Medicine (Baltimore). 2005;84:291-302.

378. Hsieh MM, Everhart JE, Byrd-Holt DD, et al. Prevalence of neutropenia in the U.S. population: age, sex, smoking status, and ethnic differences. Ann Intern Med. 2007;146:486-492.

379. Haddy TB, Rana SR, Castro O. Benign ethnic neutropenia: what is a normal absolute neutrophil count? J Lab Clin Med. 1999;133:15-22.

380. Mason BA, Lessin L, Schechter GP. Marrow granulocyte reserves in black Americans. Hydrocortisone-induced granulocytosis in the "benign" neutropenia of the black. Am J Med. 1979;67:201-205.

381. Shoenfeld Y, Modan M, Berliner S, et al. The mechanism of benign hereditary neutropenia. Arch Intern Med. 1982;142:797-799.

382. Boxer L, Dale DC. Neutropenia: causes and consequences. Semin Hematol. 2002;39:75-81.

383. Dale DC, Guerry D 4th, Wewerka JR, et al. Chronic neutropenia. Medicine (Baltimore). 1979;58:128-144.

384. Howard MW, Strauss RG, Johnston RB. Infections in patients with neutropenia. Am J Dis Child. 1977;131: 788-790.

385. Jonsson OG, Buchanan GR. Chronic neutropenia during childhood. A 13-year experience in a single institution. Am J Dis Child. 1991;145:232-235.

386. Rosenberg PS, Alter BP, Bolyard AA, et al. The incidence of leukemia and mortality from sepsis in patients with severe congenital neutropenia receiving long-term G-CSF therapy. Blood. 2006;107:4628-4635.

387. Sickles EA, Greene WH, Wiernik PH. Clinical presentation of infection in granulocytopenic patients. Arch Intern Med. 1975;135:715-719.

388. Wright DG, Meierovics AI, Foxley JM. Assessing the delivery of neutrophils to tissues in neutropenia. Blood. 1986;67:1023-1030.

389. Pincus SH, Boxer LA, Stossel TP. Chronic neutropenia in childhood. Analysis of 16 cases and a review of the literature. Am J Med. 1976;61:849-861.

390. Baehner RL, Johnston RB Jr. Monocyte function in children with neutropenias and chronic infections. Blood. 1972;40:31-41.

391. Greenwood MF, Jones EA Jr, Holland P. Monocyte functional capacity in chronic neutropenia. Am J Dis Child. 1978;132:131-135.

392. Alonso K, Dew JM, Starke WR. Thymic alymphoplasia and congenital aleukocytosis (reticular dysgenesis). Arch Pathol. 1972;94:179-183.

393. De Vaal OM, Seynhaeve V. Reticular dysgenesia. Lancet. 1959;2:1123-1125.

394. Gitlin D, Vawter G, Craig JM. Thymic alymphoplasia and congenital aleukocytosis. Pediatrics. 1964;33:184-192.

395. Levinsky RJ, Tiedeman K. Successful bone-marrow transplantation for reticular dysgenesis. Lancet. 1983;1: 671-673.

396. Ownby DR, Pizzo S, Blackmon L, et al. Severe combined immunodeficiency with leukopenia (reticular dysgenesis) in siblings: immunologic and histopathologic findings. J Pediatr. 1976;89:382-387.

397. Roper M, Parmley RT, Crist WM, et al. Severe congenital leukopenia (reticular dysgenesis). Immunologic and morphologic characterizations of leukocytes. Am J Dis Child. 1985;139:832-835.

398. Fischer A, Griscelli C, Friedrich W, et al. Bone-marrow transplantation for immunodeficiencies and osteopetrosis: European survey, 1968-1985. Lancet. 1986;1:1080-1084.

399. Knutsen AP, Wall DA. Umbilical cord blood transplantation in severe T-cell immunodeficiency disorders: two-year experience. J Clin Immunol. 2000;20:466-476.

400. Dale DC, Hammond WP. Cyclic neutropenia: a clinical review. Blood Rev. 1988;2:178-185.

401. Wright DG, Dale DC, Fauci AS, Wolff SM. Human cyclic neutropenia: clinical review and long-term follow-up of patients. Medicine (Baltimore). 1981;60:1-13.

402. Welte K, Boxer LA. Severe chronic neutropenia: pathophysiology and therapy. Semin Hematol. 1997;34:267-278.

403. Lange RD. Cyclic hematopoiesis: human cyclic neutropenia. Exp Hematol. 1983;11:435-451.

404. Engelhard D, Landreth KS, Kapoor N, et al. Cycling of peripheral blood and marrow lymphocytes in cyclic neutropenia. Proc Natl Acad Sci U S A. 1983;80:5734-5738.

405. Krance RA, Spruce WE, Forman SJ, et al. Human cyclic neutropenia transferred by allogeneic bone marrow grafting. Blood. 1982;60:1263-1266.

406. Aprikyan AA, Kutyavin T, Stein S, et al. Cellular and molecular abnormalities in severe congenital neutropenia predisposing to leukemia. Exp Hematol. 2003;31: 372-381.

407. Berliner N, Horwitz M, Loughran TP Jr. Congenital and acquired neutropenia. Hematology Am Soc Hematol Educ Program. 2004:63-79.

408. Massullo P, Druhan LJ, Bunnell BA, et al. Aberrant subcellular targeting of the G185R neutrophil elastase mutant associated with severe congenital neutropenia induces premature apoptosis of differentiating promyelocytes. Blood. 2005;105:3397-3404.

409. Aprikyan AA, Liles WC, Rodger E, et al. Impaired survival of bone marrow hematopoietic progenitor cells in cyclic neutropenia. Blood. 2001;97:147-153.

410. Kollner I, Sodeik B, Schreek S, et al. Mutations in neutrophil elastase causing congenital neutropenia lead to cytoplasmic protein accumulation and induction of the unfolded protein response. Blood. 2006;108:493-500.

411. Grenda DS, Murakami M, Ghatak J, et al. Mutations of the *ELA2* gene found in patients with severe congenital neutropenia induce the unfolded protein response and cellular apoptosis. Blood. 2007;110:4179-4187.

412. Migliaccio AR, Migliaccio G, Dale DC, Hammond WP. Hematopoietic progenitors in cyclic neutropenia: effect of granulocyte colony-stimulating factor in vivo. Blood. 1990;75:1951-1959.

413. von Schulthess GK, Mazer NA. Cyclic neutropenia (CN): a clue to the control of granulopoiesis. Blood. 1982;59:27-37.

414. Simon A, van der Meer JW. Pathogenesis of familial periodic fever syndromes or hereditary autoinflammatory syndromes. Am J Physiol Regul Integr Comp Physiol. 2007;292:R86-R98.

415. Bonilla MA, Dale D, Zeidler C, et al. Long-term safety of treatment with recombinant human granulocyte colony-stimulating factor (r-metHug-CSF) in patients with severe congenital neutropenias. Br J Haematol. 1994;88:723-730.

416. Dale DC, Bonilla MA, Davis MW, et al. A randomized controlled phase III trial of recombinant human granulocyte colony-stimulating factor (filgrastim) for treatment of severe chronic neutropenia. Blood. 1993;81: 2496-2502.

417. Dale DC, Cottle TE, Fier CJ, et al. Severe chronic neutropenia: treatment and follow-up of patients in the Severe Chronic Neutropenia International Registry. Am J Hematol. 2003;72:82-93.

418. Hammond WP, Price TH, Souza LM, Dale DC. Treatment of cyclic neutropenia with granulocyte colony-stimulating factor. N Engl J Med. 1989;320:1306-1311.

419. Kostmann R. Infantile genetic agranulocytosis; agranulocytosis infantilis hereditaria. Acta Paediatr Suppl. 1956;45:1-78.

420. Boxer LA, Stein S, Buckley D, et al. Strong evidence for autosomal dominant inheritance of severe congenital neutropenia associated with *ELA2* mutations. J Pediatr. 2006;148:633-636.

421. Welte K, Zeidler C, Dale DC. Severe congenital neutropenia. Semin Hematol. 2006;43:189-195.

422. Klein C, Grudzien M, Appaswamy G, et al. HAX1 deficiency causes autosomal recessive severe congenital neutropenia (Kostmann disease). Nat Genet. 2007;39: 86-92.

423. Kostmann R. Infantile genetic agranulocytosis. A review with presentation of ten new cases. Acta Paediatr Scand. 1975;64:362-368.

424. Gilman PA, Jackson DP, Guild HG. Congenital agranulocytosis: prolonged survival and terminal acute leukemia. Blood. 1970;36:576-585.

425. Rosen RB, Kang SJ. Congenital agranulocytosis terminating in acute myelomonocytic leukemia. J Pediatr. 1979;94:406-408.

426. Wong W-Y, Williams D, Slovak ML, et al. Terminal acute myelogenous leukemia in a patient with congenital agranulocytosis. Am J Hematol. 1993;43:133-138.

427. Mempel K, Pietsch T, Menzel T, et al. Increased serum levels of granulocyte colony-stimulating factor in patients with severe congenital neutropenia. Blood. 1991;77:1919-1922.

428. Pietsch T, Buhrer C, Mempel K, et al. Blood mononuclear cells from patients with severe congenital neutropenia are capable of producing granulocyte colony-stimulating factor. Blood. 1991;77:1234-1237.

429. Boxer LA, Bolyard AA, Schwinzer B, et al. Antineutrophil antibodies lead to mistaken identity in severe congenital neutropenia [abstract]. Blood. 2005;106: 385.

430. Coulombel L, Morardet N, Veber F, et al. Granulopoietic differentiation in long-term bone marrow cultures from children with congenital neutropenia. Am J Hematol. 1988;27:93-98.

431. Parmley RT, Ogawa M, Darby CP Jr, Spicer SS. Congenital neutropenia: neutrophil proliferation with abnormal maturation. Blood. 1975;56:723-734.

432. Zucker-Franklin D, L'Esperance P, Good RA. Congenital neutropenia: an intrinsic cell defect demonstrated by electron microscopy of soft agar colonies. Blood. 1977; 49:425-436.

433. Bellanne-Chantelot C, Clauin S, Leblanc T, et al. Mutations in the *ELA2* gene correlate with more severe expression of neutropenia: a study of 81 patients from the French Neutropenia Register. Blood. 2004;103: 4119-4125.

434. Person RE, Li FQ, Duan Z, et al. Mutations in proto-oncogene GFI1 cause human neutropenia and target ELA2. Nat Genet. 2003;34:308-312.

435. Dinauer MC, Lekstrom-Himes JA, Dale DC. Inherited neutrophil disorders: molecular basis and new therapies. Hematology Am Soc Hematol Educ Program. 2000: 303-318.

436. Ancliff PJ, Blundell MP, Cory GO, et al. Two novel activating mutations in the Wiskott-Aldrich syndrome protein result in congenital neutropenia. Blood. 2006; 108:2182-2189.

437. Ochs HD, Thrasher AJ. The Wiskott-Aldrich syndrome. J Allergy Clin Immunol. 2006;117:725-738.

438. Ward AC, van Aesch YM, Gits J, et al. Novel point mutation in the extracellular domain of the granulocyte colony-stimulating factor (G-CSF) receptor in a case of severe congenital neutropenia hyporesponsive to G-CSF treatment. J Exp Med. 1999;190:497-507.

439. Bonilla MA, Gillio AP, Ruggeiro M, et al. Effects of recombinant human granulocyte colony-stimulating factor on neutropenia in patients with congenital agranulocytosis. N Engl J Med. 1989;320:1574-1580.

440. Bolyard M, Bonilla L, Boxer S. Algorithm for the management of Kostmann's neutropenia based on data from the Severe Chronic Neutropenia International Registry. Blood. 1999;94:174b.

441. Welte K, Zeidler C, Reiter A, et al. Differential effects of granulocyte-macrophage colony-stimulating factor and granulocyte colony-stimulating factor in children with severe congenital neutropenia. Blood. 1990;75:1056-1063.

442. Yakisan E, Schirg E, Zeidler C, et al. High incidence of significant bone loss in patients with severe congenital neutropenia (Kostmann's syndrome). J Pediatr. 1997; 131:592-597.

443. Freedman MH, Bonilla MA, Fier C, et al. Myelodysplasia syndrome and acute myeloid leukemia in patients with congenital neutropenia receiving G-CSF therapy. Blood. 2000;96:429-436.

444. Donadieu J, Leblanc T, Bader Meunier B, et al. Analysis of risk factors for myelodysplasias, leukemias and death from infection among patients with congenital neutropenia. Experience of the French Severe Chronic Neutropenia Study Group. Haematologica. 2005;90: 45-53.

445. Germeshausen M, Ballmaier M, Welte K. Incidence of CSF3R mutations in severe congenital neutropenia and relevance for leukemogenesis: Results of a long-term survey. Blood. 2007;109:93-99.

446. Jeha S, Chan KW, Aprikyan AG, et al. Spontaneous remission of granulocyte colony-stimulating factor–associated leukemia in a child with severe congenital neutropenia. Blood. 2000;96:3647-3649.

447. Skokowa J, Germeshausen M, Zeidler C, Welte K. Severe congenital neutropenia: inheritance and pathophysiology. Curr Opin Hematol. 2007;14:22-28.

448. Link DC, Kunter G, Kasai Y, et al. Distinct patterns of mutations occurring in de novo AML versus AML arising in the setting of severe congenital neutropenia. Blood. 2007;110:1648-1655.

449. Choi SW, Boxer LA, Pulsipher MA, et al. Stem cell transplantation in patients with severe congenital neutropenia with evidence of leukemic transformation. Bone Marrow Transplant. 2005;35:473-477.

450. Zeidler C, Welte K, Barak Y, et al. Stem cell transplantation in patients with severe congenital neutropenia without evidence of leukemic transformation. Blood. 2000;95:1195-1198.

451. Newburger PE. Disorders of neutrophil number and function. Hematology Am Soc Hematol Educ Program. 2006:104-110.

452. Donini M, Fontana S, Savoldi G, et al. G-CSF treatment of severe congenital neutropenia reverses neutropenia but does not correct the underlying functional deficiency of the neutrophil in defending against microorganisms. Blood. 2007;109:4716-4723.

453. Latger-Cannard V, Bensoussan D, Bordigoni P. The WHIM syndrome shows a peculiar dysgranulopoiesis: myelokathexis. Br J Haematol. 2006;132:669.

454. Gorlin RJ, Gelb B, Diaz GA, et al. WHIM syndrome, an autosomal dominant disorder: clinical, hematological, and molecular studies. Am J Med Genet. 2000;91: 368-376.

455. Hord JD, Whitlock JA, Gay JC, Lukens JN. Clinical features of myelokathexis and treatment with hematopoietic cytokines: a case report of two patients and review of the literature. J Pediatr Hematol Oncol. 1997;19:443-448.

456. Wetzler M, Talpaz M, Kleinerman ES, et al. A new familial immunodeficiency disorder characterized by severe neutropenia, a defective marrow release mechanism, and hypogammaglobulinemia. Am J Med. 1990;89:663-672.

457. Zuelzer WW. Myelokathexis—a new form of chronic granulocytopenia. Report of a case. N Engl J Med. 1964;270:699-704.

458. Aprikyan AA, Liles WC, Park JR, et al. Myelokathexis, a congenital disorder of severe neutropenia characterized by accelerated apoptosis and defective expression of bcl-x in neutrophil precursors. Blood. 2000;95:320-327.

459. Krill CE Jr, Smith HD, Mauer AM. Chronic idiopathic granulocytopenia. N Engl J Med. 1964;270:973-979.

460. Taniuchi S, Yamamoto A, Fujiwara T, et al. Dizygotic twin sisters with myelokathexis: mechanism of its neutropenia. Am J Hematol. 1999;62:106-111.

461. Hernandez PA, Gorlin RJ, Lukens JN, et al. Mutations in the chemokine receptor gene CXCR4 are associated with WHIM syndrome, a combined immunodeficiency disease. Nat Genet. 2003;34:70-74.

462. Balabanian K, Lagane B, Pablos JL, et al. WHIM syndromes with different genetic anomalies are accounted for by impaired CXCR4 desensitization to CXCL12. Blood. 2005;105:2449-2457.

463. Sanmun D, Garwicz D, Smith CI, et al. Stromal-derived factor-1 abolishes constitutive apoptosis of WHIM syndrome neutrophils harbouring a truncating CXCR4 mutation. Br J Haematol. 2006;134:640-644.

464. Dror Y, Durie P, Ginzberg H, et al. Clonal evolution in marrows of patients with Shwachman-Diamond syndrome: a prospective 5-year follow-up study. Exp Hematol. 2002;30:659-669.

465. Dror Y, Freedman MH. Shwachman-Diamond syndrome. Br J Haematol. 2002;118:701-713.

466. Shwachman H, Diamond LK, Oski FA, Khaw KT. The syndrome of pancreatic insufficiency and bone marrow dysfunction. J Pediatr. 1964;65:645-663.

467. Shimamura A. Inherited bone marrow failure syndromes: molecular features. Hematology Am Soc Hematol Educ Program. 2006:63-71.

468. Berrocal T, Simon MJ, al-Assir I, et al. Shwachman-Diamond syndrome: clinical, radiological and sonographic findings. Pediatr Radiol. 1995;25:356-359.

469. Shimamura A. Shwachman-Diamond syndrome. Semin Hematol. 2006;43:178-188.

470. Aggett PJ, Harries JT, Harvey BAM, Soothill JF. An inherited defect of neutrophil mobility in Shwachman's syndrome. J Pediatr. 1979;94:391-394.

471. Smith OP, Hann IM, Chessells JM, et al. Haematological abnormalities in Shwachman-Diamond syndrome. Br J Haematol. 1996;94:279-284.

472. Dror Y, Ginzberg H, Dalal I, et al. Immune function in patients with Shwachman-Diamond syndrome. Br J Haematol. 2001;114:712-717.

473. Boocock GR, Morrison JA, Popovic M, et al. Mutations in SBDS are associated with Shwachman-Diamond syndrome. Nat Genet. 2003;33:97-101.

474. Shammas C, Menne TF, Hilcenko C, et al. Structural and mutational analysis of the SBDS protein family. Insight into the leukemia-associated Shwachman-Diamond Syndrome. J Biol Chem. 2005;280:19221-19229.

475. Austin KM, Leary RJ, Shimamura A. The Shwachman-Diamond SBDS protein localizes to the nucleolus. Blood. 2005;106:1253-1258.

476. Hill RE, Durie PR, Gaskin KJ, et al. Steatorrhea and pancreatic insufficiency in Shwachman syndrome. Gastroenterology. 1982;83:22-27.

477. Dell'Angelica EC. Bad signals jam organelle traffic. Nat Med. 2007;13:31-32.

478. Blume RS, Wolff SM. The Chédiak-Higashi syndrome: studies in four patients and a review of the literature. Medicine (Baltimore). 1972;51:247-280.

479. Windhorst DB, Padgett G. The Chédiak-Higashi syndrome and the homologous trait in animals. J Invest Dermatol. 1973;60:529-537.

480. Witkop CJ Jr, Quevedo WC Jr, Fitzpatrick TB, King RA. Albinism. New York, McGraw-Hill, 1989.

481. Wolff SM, Dale DC, Clark RA, et al. The Chédiak-Higashi syndrome: studies of host defenses. Ann Intern Med. 1972;76:293-306.

482. Huizing M, Anikster Y, Gahl WA. Hermansky-Pudlak syndrome and Chédiak-Higashi syndrome: disorders of vesicle formation and trafficking. Thromb Haemost. 2001;86:233-245.

483. Spritz RA. Genetic defects in Chédiak-Higashi syndrome and the beige mouse. J Clin Immunol. 1998;18: 97-105.

484. Ward DM, Shiflett SL, Kaplan J. Chédiak-Higashi syndrome: a clinical and molecular view of a rare lysosomal storage disorder. Curr Mol Med. 2002;2:469-477.

485. Introne W, Boissy RE, Gahl WA. Clinical, molecular, and cell biological aspects of Chédiak-Higashi syndrome. Mol Genet Metab. 1999;68:283-303.

486. Kotzot D, Richter K, Gierth-Fiebig K. Oculocutaneous albinism, immunodeficiency, hematological disorders, and minor anomalies: a new autosomal recessive syndrome? Am J Med Genet. 1994;50:224-227.

487. Jung J, Bohn G, Allroth A, et al. Identification of a homozygous deletion in the AP3B1 gene causing Hermansky-Pudlak syndrome, type 2. Blood. 2006;108:362-369.

488. Horwitz M, Benson KF, Duan Z, et al. Hereditary neutropenia: dogs explain human neutrophil elastase mutations. Trends Mol Med. 2004;10:163-170.

489. Bahadoran P, Busca R, Chiaverini C, et al. Characterization of the molecular defects in Rab27a, caused by RAB27A missense mutations found in patients with Griscelli syndrome. J Biol Chem. 2003;278:11386-11392.

490. Griscelli C, Durandy A, Guy-Grand D, et al. A syndrome associating partial albinism and immunodeficiency. Am J Med. 1978;65:691-702.

491. Menasche G, Pastural E, Feldmann J, et al. Mutations in *RAB27A* cause Griscelli syndrome associated with

haemophagocytic syndrome. Nat Genet. 2000;25:173-176.

492. Munafo DB, Johnson JL, Ellis BA, et al. Rab27a is a key component of the secretory machinery of azurophilic granules in granulocytes. Biochem J. 2007;402:229-239.

493. Kolehmainen J, Wilkinson R, Lehesjoki AE, et al. Delineation of Cohen syndrome following a large-scale genotype-phenotype screen. Am J Hum Genet. 2004; 75:122-127.

494. Bohn C, Rigoulay C, Bouloc P. No detectable effect of RNA-binding protein Hfq absence in *Staphylococcus aureus*. BMC Microbiol. 2007;7:10.

495. Cutting HO, Lang JE. Familial benign chronic neutropenia. Ann Intern Med. 1964;61:876-887.

496. Mintz U, Sachs L. Normal granulocyte-forming cells in the bone marrow of Yemenite Jews with genetic neutropenia. Blood. 1973;41:745-751.

497. Shaper AG, Lewis P. Genetic neutropenia in people of African origin. Lancet. 1971;1:1021-1023.

498. Jacobs P. Familial benign chronic neutropenia. S Afr Med J. 1975;49:692.

499. Sieff CA, Nisbet-Brown E, Nathan DG. Congenital bone marrow failure syndromes. Br J Haematol. 2000; 111:30-42.

500. Clewing JM, Antalfy BC, Lucke T, et al. Schimke immuno-osseous dysplasia: a clinicopathological correlation. J Med Genet. 2007;44:122-130.

501. Boerkoel CF, O'Neill S, Andre JL, et al. Manifestations and treatment of Schimke immuno-osseous dysplasia: 14 new cases and a review of the literature. Eur J Pediatr. 2000;159:1-7.

502. Lucke T, Tsikas D, Kanzelmeyer NK, et al. Vaso-occlusion in Schimke immuno-osseous dysplasia: is the NO pathway involved? Horm Metab Res. 2006;38:678-682.

503. Boerkoel CF, Takashima H, John J, et al. Mutant chromatin remodeling protein SMARCAL1 causes Schimke immuno-osseous dysplasia. Nat Genet. 2002;30:215-220.

504. Clewing JM, Fryssira H, Goodman D, et al. Schimke immunoosseous dysplasia: suggestions of genetic diversity. Hum Mutat. 2007;28:273-283.

505. Petty EM, Yanik GA, Hutchinson RJ, et al. Successful bone marrow transplantation in a patient with Schimke immuno-osseous dysplasia. J Pediatr. 2000;137:882-886.

506. Lehmann HW, von Landenberg P, Modrow S. Parvovirus B19 infection and autoimmune disease. Autoimmun Rev. 2003;2:218-223.

507. Savard M, Gosselin J. Epstein-Barr virus immunosuppression of innate immunity mediated by phagocytes. Virus Res. 2006;119:134-145.

508. Sloand E. Hematologic complications of HIV infection. AIDS Rev. 2005;7:187-196.

509. Nagaraju M, Weitzman S, Baumann G. Viral hepatitis and agranulocytosis. Am J Dig Dis. 1973;18:247-252.

510. Benjamin B, Ward SM. Leukocytic responses to measles. Am J Dis Child. 1932;44:921-963.

511. Holbrook AA. The blood picture in chicken pox. Arch Intern Med. 1941;68:294.

512. Horsfall FL, Tamm L. Viral and Rickettsial Infections of Man, 4th ed. Philadelphia, JB Lippincott, 1965.

513. Murdoch JM, Smith CC. Infection. Clin Haematol. 1972;1:619-643.

514. Downie AW. Pathway of virus infection. In Smith E (ed). Mechanisms of Virus Infection. New York, Academic Press, 1963.

515. MacGregor RR, Friedman HM, Macarak EJ, Kafalides NA. Virus infection of endothelial cells increased granulocyte adherence. J Clin Invest. 1980;65:1469-1477.

516. Cines DB, Lyss AP, Bina M, et al. Fc and C3 receptors induced by herpes simplex virus on cultured human endothelial cells. J Clin Invest. 1982;69:123-128.

517. Ryan US, Schultz DR, Ruan JW. Fc and C3b receptors on pulmonary endothelial cells: induction by injury. Science. 1981;214:557-558.

518. Habib MA, Babka JC, Burningham RA. Profound granulocytopenia associated with infectious mononucleosis. Am J Med Sci. 1973;265:339-346.

519. Hammond WP, Harlan JM, Steinberg SE. Severe neutropenia in infectious mononucleosis. West J Med. 1979;131:92-97.

520. Schooley RT, Densen P, Harmon D, et al. Antineutrophil antibodies in infectious mononucleosis. Am J Med. 1984;76:85-90.

521. Stevens DL, Everett ED, Boxer LA, Landefeld RA. Infectious mononucleosis with severe neutropenia and opsonic antineutrophil activity. South Med J. 1979;72: 519-521.

522. McClain K, Estrov Z, Chen H, Mahoney DH Jr. Chronic neutropenia of childhood: frequent association with parvovirus infection and correlations with bone marrow culture studies. Br J Haematol. 1993;85:57-62.

523. Mustafa MM, McClain KL. Diverse hematologic effects of parvovirus B19 infection. Pediatr Clin North Am. 1996;43:809-821.

524. Scheurlen W, Ramasubbu K, Wachowski O, et al. Chronic autoimmune thrombopenia/neutropenia in a boy with persistent parvovirus B19 infection. J Clin Virol. 2001;20: 173-178.

525. Moses A, Nelson J, Bagby GC Jr. The influence of human immunodeficiency virus-1 on hematopoiesis. Blood. 1998;91:1479-1495.

526. Zon LI, Groopman JE. Hematologic manifestations of the human deficiency virus (HIV). Semin Hematol. 1988;25:208-218.

527. Israel DS, Plaisance KI. Neutropenia in patients infected with human immunodeficiency virus. Clin Pharmacol. 1991;10:268-279.

528. Fronteira M, Myers AM. Peripheral blood and bone marrow abnormalities in the acquired immunodeficiency syndrome. West J Med. 1987;147:157-160.

529. McCance-Katz EF, Hoecker JL, Vitale NB. Severe neutropenia associated with anti-neutrophil antibody in a patient with acquired immunodeficiency syndrome-related complex. Pediatr Infect Dis. 1987;6:417-418.

530. Ball K, Jones H. Acute tuberculosis septicemia with leukopenia. BJM. 1951;2:869.

531. Dietrich HS. Typhoid fever in children. A study of 60 cases. J Pediatr. 1937;10:191.

532. Pullen RL, Stuart BM. Tularemia. JAMA. 1945;129:495-500.

533. Dale DC, Wolff SM. Studies of the neutropenia of acute malaria. Blood. 1973;41:197-206.

534. Chenoweth DE, Cooper SW, Hugli TE, et al. Complement activation during cardiopulmonary bypass: evidence for generation of C3a and C5a anaphylatoxins. N Engl J Med. 1981;304:497-503.

535. Craddock PR, Hammerschmidt DE, Moldow DF, et al. Granulocyte aggregation as a manifestation of membrane interactions with complement: possible role in leukocyte margination, microvascular occlusion, and endothelial damage. Semin Hematol. 1979;16:140-147.

536. Ivanovich P, Chenoweth DE, Schmidt R, et al. Symptoms of activation of granulocytes and complement with two dialysis membranes. Kidney Int. 1983;24:758-763.

537. Wolach B, Coates TD, Hugli TE, et al. Plasma lactoferrin reflects granulocyte activation via complement in burn patients. J Lab Clin Med. 1984;103:284-293.

538. Strauss RG. Granulopoiesis and neutrophil function in the neonate. In Stockman JA, Pochedley C (eds). Developmental and Neonatal Hematology. New York, Raven Press, 1988.

539. Sachs UJ, Reiter A, Walter T, et al. Safety and efficacy of therapeutic early onset granulocyte transfusions in pediatric patients with neutropenia and severe infections. Transfusion. 2006;46:1909-1914.

540. Cairo M. The use of granulocyte transfusions in neonatal sepsis. Transfus Med Rev. 1990;4:14-22.

541. Christensen RD, Bradley PP, Rothstein G. The leukocyte left shift in clincal and experimental neonatal sepsis. Fetal Neonatal Med. 1981;98:101-105.

542. Christensen RD, Rothstein G, Anstall HB, Bybee B. Granulocyte transfusions in neonates with bacterial infection, neutropenia, and depletion of mature marrow neutrophils. Pediatrics. 1982;70:1-6.

543. Ahmad A, Laborada G, Bussel J, Nesin M. Comparison of recombinant granulocyte colony-stimulating factor, recombinant human granulocyte-macrophage colony-stimulating factor and placebo for treatment of septic preterm infants. Pediatr Infect Dis J. 2002;21:1061-1065.

544. Juul SE, Christensen RD. Effect of recombinant granulocyte colony-stimulating factor on blood neutrophil concentrations among patients with "idiopathic neonatal neutropenia": a randomized, placebo-controlled trial. J Perinatol. 2003;23:493-497.

545. Cairo M. Review of G-CSF and GM-CSF. Effects on neonatal neutrophil kinetics. Am J Pediatr Hematol Oncol. 1989;11:238-244.

546. Gillan E, Christensen R, Suen Y, et al. A randomized, placebo-controlled trial of recombinant human granulocyte colony-stimulating factor administration in newborn infants with presumed sepsis: significant induction of peripheral and bone marrow neutrophilia. Blood. 1994; 84:1427-1433.

547. Roberts RL, Szelc CM, Scates SM, et al. Neutropenia in an extremely premature infant treated with recombinant human granulocyte colony-stimulating factor. Am J Dis Child. 1991;145:808-812.

548. Andersohn F, Konzen C, Garbe E. Systematic review: agranulocytosis induced by nonchemotherapy drugs. Ann Intern Med. 2007;146:657-665.

549. Risks of agranulocytosis and aplastic anemia: a first report of their relation to drug use and special reference to analgesics. The International Agranulocytosis and Aplastic Anemia Study. JAMA. 1986;256:1749.

550. Mamus SW, Burton JD, Groate JD, et al. Ibuprofen-associated pure white-cell aplasia. N Engl J Med. 1986;314:624-625.

551. Pisciotta AV. Drug induced agranulocytosis peripheral destruction of polymorphonuclear leukocytes and their marrow precursors. Blood Rev. 1990;4:226-237.

552. Pisciotta AV. Immune and toxic mechanisms in drug-induced agranulocytosis. Semin Hematol. 1973;10:291-310.

553. Salama A, Schutz B, Kiefel V, et al. Immune-mediated agranulocytosis related to drugs and their metabolites: mode of sensitization and heterogeneity of antibodies. Br J Haematol. 1989;72:127-132.

554. Vincent PC. Drug-induced aplastic anemia and agranulocytosis: incidence and mechanisms. Drugs. 1986;31:52-63.

555. Weitzman SA, Stossel TP. Drug-induced immunological neutropenia. Lancet. 1978;1:1068-1072.

556. Hartl PW. Drug-induced agranulocytosis. In Girdwood RH (ed). Blood Disorders Due to Drugs and Other Agents. Amsterdam, Excerpta Medica, 1973, p 147.

557. Heit WFW. Hematologic effects of antipyretic analgesics. Drug induced agranulocytosis. Am J Med. 1983; 74(5A):65-69.

558. Murphy MF, Riordon T, Minchinton RM, et al. Demonstration of an immune-mediated mechanism of penicillin-induced neutropenia and thrombocytopenia. Br J Haematol. 1983;55:155-160.

559. Schröder H, Evans DAP. Acetylator phenotype and adverse effects of sulfasalazine in healthy subjects. Gut. 1972;13:278-284.

560. Uetrecht J. Drug metabolism by leukocytes and its role in drug-induced lupus and other idiosyncratic drug reactions. CRC Crit Rev Toxicol. 1990;20:213-235.

561. Young GA, Vincent PC. Drug-induced agranulocytosis. Clin Haematol. 1980;9:438-504.

562. van der Klauw MM, Wilson JH, Stricker BH. Drug-associated agranulocytosis: 20 years of reporting in The Netherlands (1974-1994). Am J Hematol. 1998;57:206-211.

563. Nitrous oxide and the bone-marrow [editorial]. Lancet. 1978;2:613.

564. Palmblad JE, von dem Borne AE. Idiopathic, immune, infectious, and idiosyncratic neutropenias. Semin Hematol. 2002;39:113-120.

565. Sprikkelman A, de Wolf JT, Vellenga E. The application of hematopoietic growth factors in drug-induced agranulocytosis: a review of 70 cases. Leukemia. 1994;8:2031-2036.

566. Capsoni F, Sarzi-Puttini P, Zanella A. Primary and secondary autoimmune neutropenia. Arthritis Res Ther. 2005;7:208-214.

567. Bruin M, Dassen A, Pajkrt D, et al. Primary autoimmune neutropenia in children: a study of neutrophil antibodies and clinical course. Vox Sang. 2005;88:52-59.

568. Maheshwari A, Christensen RD, Calhoun DA. Immune-mediated neutropenia in the neonate. Acta Paediatr Suppl. 2002;91:98-103.

569. Stroneck DF, Skubitz KM, Shanker RA, et al. Biochemical characterization of the neutrophil specific antigen NB1. Blood. 1990;75:744-755.

570. Bruin MC, von dem Borne AE, Tamminga RY, et al. Neutrophil antibody specificity in different types of childhood autoimmune neutropenia. Blood. 1999;94:1797-1802.

571. Lucas G, Rogers S, de Haas M, et al. Report on the Fourth International Granulocyte Immunology Workshop: progress toward quality assessment. Transfusion. 2002;42:462-468.

572. Shastri KA, Logue GL. Autoimmune neutropenia. Blood. 1993;81:1984-1995.

573. Manny N, Zelig O. Laboratory diagnosis of autoimmune cytopenias. Curr Opin Hematol. 2000;7:414-419.

574. Boxer LA, Greenberg MS, Boxer GJ, et al. Autoimmune neutropenia. N Engl J Med. 1975;293:748-753.

575. Bux J, Mueller-Eckhardt C. Autoimmune neutropenia. Semin Hematol. 1992;29:45-53.

576. Duckham DJ, Rhyne RL Jr, Smith FE, Williams RC Jr. Retardation of colony growth of in vitro bone marrow culture using sera from patients with Felty's syndrome, disseminated lupus erythematosus (DLE), rheumatoid arthritis and other disease states. Arthritis Rheum. 1975;18:323-333.

577. Hartman KR, Wright DG. Identification of autoantibodies specific for the neutrophil adhesion glycoproteins CD11b/CD18 in patients with autoimmune neutropenia. Blood. 1991;78:1096-1104.

578. Bux J, Behrens G, Jaeger G, Welte K. Diagnosis and clinical course of autoimmune neutropenia in infancy: analysis of 240 cases. Blood. 1998;91:181-186.

579. Smith MA, Smith JG. The use of granulocyte colony-stimulating factor for treatment of autoimmune neutropenia. Curr Opin Hematol. 2001;8:165-169.

580. Kobayashi M, Nakamura K, Kawaguchi H, et al. Significance of the detection of antineutrophil antibodies in children with chronic neutropenia. Blood. 2002;99:3468-3471.

581. Miller ME, Oski FA, Harris MB. Lazy-leucocyte syndrome: a new disorder of neutrophil function. Lancet. 1971;1:665-669.

582. Lyall EGH, Lucas GF, Eden OB. Autoimmune neutropenia of infancy. J Clin Pathol. 1992;45:431-434.

583. Neglia JP, Watterson J, Clay M, et al. Autoimmune neutropenia of infancy and early childhood. Pediatr Hematol Oncol. 1993;10:369-376.

584. Lalezari P, Khorshidi M, Petrosova M. Autoimmune neutropenia in infancy. J Pediatr. 1986;109:764-769.

585. McFarland JG. Platelet and neutrophil alloantigen genotyping in clinical practice. Transfus Clin Biol. 1998;5:13-21.

586. Cartron J, Tchernia G, Cleton J, et al. Alloimmune neonatal neutropenia. Am J Pediatr Hematol Oncol. 1991;13:21-25.

587. Gilmore M, Stroncek D, Korones D. Treatment of alloimmune neonatal neutrophenia with granulocyte colony-stimulating factor. J Pediatr. 1994;125:948-951.

588. Calhoun DA, Christensen RD, Edstrom CS, et al. Consistent approaches to procedures and practices in neonatal hematology. Clin Perinatol. 2000;27:733-753.

589. Rodwell RL, Gray PH, Taylor KM, Minchinton R. Granulocyte colony stimulating factor treatment for alloimmune neonatal neutropenia. Arch Dis Child Fetal Neonatal Ed. 1996;75:F57-F58.

590. Van Leeuwen EF, Roord JJ, DeGast GC, et al. Neonatal neutropenia due to maternal autoantibodies against neutrophils. Br Med J (Clin Res Ed). 1983;287:94.

591. Abilgaard H, Jensen KG. The influence of maternal leukocyte antibodies in infants. Scand J Haematol. 1964;1:47-62.

592. Payne R. Neonatal neutropenia and leukoagglutinins. Pediatrics. 1964;33:194-204.

593. Cham B, Bonilla MA, Winkelstein J. Neutropenia associated with primary immunodeficiency syndromes. Semin Hematol. 2002;39:107-112.

594. Ogershok PR, Hogan MB, Welch JE, et al. Spectrum of illness in pediatric common variable immunodeficiency. Ann Allergy Asthma Immunol. 2006;97:653-656.

595. Winkelstein JA, Marino MC, Lederman HM, et al. X-linked agammaglobulinemia: report on a United States registry of 201 patients. Medicine (Baltimore). 2006;85:193-202.

596. Winkelstein JA, Marino MC, Ochs H, et al. The X-linked hyper-IgM syndrome: clinical and immunologic features of 79 patients. Medicine (Baltimore). 2003;82:373-384.

597. Kwon SW, Procter J, Dale JK, et al. Neutrophil and platelet antibodies in autoimmune lymphoproliferative syndrome. Vox Sang. 2003;85:307-312.

598. Rao VK, Straus SE. Causes and consequences of the autoimmune lymphoproliferative syndrome. Hematology. 2006;11:15-23.

599. Rao VK, Dugan F, Dale JK, et al. Use of mycophenolate mofetil for chronic, refractory immune cytopenias in children with autoimmune lymphoproliferative syndrome. Br J Haematol. 2005;129:534-538.

600. Lux SE, Johnston RB Jr, August CS, et al. Chronic neutropenia and abnormal cellular immunity in cartilage-hair hypoplasia. N Engl J Med. 1970;282:231-236.

601. McKusick VA, Eldridge R, Hostetler JA, et al. Dwarfism in the Amish. II. Cartilage-hair hypoplasia. Bull Johns Hopkins Hosp. 1965;116:285-328.

602. Hermanns P, Tran A, Munivez E, et al. RMRP mutations in cartilage-hair hypoplasia. Am J Med Genet A. 2006;140:2121-2130.

603. Martin AN, Li Y. RNase MRP RNA and human genetic diseases. Cell Res. 2007;17:219-226.

604. Ammann RA, Duppenthaler A, Bux J, Aebi C. Granulocyte colony-stimulating factor–responsive chronic neutropenia in cartilage-hair hypoplasia. J Pediatr Hematol Oncol. 2004;26:379-381.

605. Guggenheim R, Somech R, Grunebaum E, et al. Bone marrow transplantation for cartilage-hair-hypoplasia. Bone Marrow Transplant. 2006;38:751-756.

606. Starkebaum G. Chronic neutropenia associated with autoimmune disease. Semin Hematol. 2002;39:121-127.

607. Vasiliu IM, Petri MA, Baer AN. Therapy with granulocyte colony-stimulating factor in systemic lupus erythematosus may be associated with severe flares. J Rheumatol. 2006;33:1878-1880.

608. Lamy T, Loughran TP Jr. Clinical features of large granular lymphocyte leukemia. Semin Hematol. 2003;40:185-195.

609. Barth PG, Valianpour F, Bowen VM, et al. X-linked cardioskeletal myopathy and neutropenia (Barth syndrome): an update. Am J Med Genet A. 2004;126:349-354.

610. Bione S, D'Adamo P, Maestrini E, et al. A novel X-linked gene, G4.5, is responsible for Barth syndrome. Nat Genet. 1996;12:385-389.

611. Ambruso DR, McCabe ERB, Anderson D, et al. Infectious and bleeding complications in patients with glycogenosis Ib. Am J Dis Child. 1985;139:691-697.

612. Beaudet AL, Anderson DC, Michels VV, et al. Neutropenia and impaired neutrophil migration in type 1B glycogen storage disease. J Pediatr. 1980;97:906-910.

613. Childs B, Nyhan WL, Borden M, et al. Idiopathic hyperglycinuria and hperglycinuria: a new disorder of amino acid metabolism. I Pediatrics. 1961;27:522-538.

614. Couper R, Kapelushnik J, Griffiths AM. Neutrophil dysfunction in glycogen storage disease Ib: association with Crohn's-like colitis. Gastroenterology. 1991;100:549-554.

615. Rosenberg LE, Fenton WA. Disorders of propionate and methylmalonate metabolism. In Scriver CR, Beaudet AL, Sly WS, Valle D (eds). The Metabolic Basis of Inherited Disease. New York, McGraw-Hill, 1989, pp 821-844.

616. Soriano JR, Taitz LS, Finberg L, Edelmann CM. Hyperglycinemia with ketacidosis and leukopenia: metabolic studies on the nature of the defect. Pediatrics. 1967;39:818-828.

617. Sweetman L. Branched chain organic acidurias. In Scriver CR, Beaudet AL, Sly WS, Valle D (eds). The Metabolic Basis of Inherited Disease. New York, McGraw-Hill, 1989, pp 791-819.

618. Lindstedt S, Holme E, Lock EA, et al. Treatment of hereditary tyrosinaemia type I by inhibition of 4-hydroxyphenylpyruvate dioxygenase. Lancet. 1992;340:813-817.

619. Hutchinson RJ, Bunnell K, Thoene JG. Suppression of granulopoietic progenitor cell proliferation by metabolites of the branched chain amino acids. J Pediatr. 1985;106:62-65.

620. Schroten H, Wendel U, Burdach S, et al. Colony-stimulating factors for neutropenia in glycogen storage disease Ib. Lancet. 1991;337:736-737.

621. Wang WC, Crist WM, Ihle JN, et al. Granulocyte colony-stimulating factor corrects the neutropenia associated with glycogen storage disease type 1b. Leukemia. 1991;5:347-349.

622. Melis D, Fulceri R, Parenti G, et al. Genotype/phenotype correlation in glycogen storage disease type 1b: a multicentre study and review of the literature. Eur J Pediatr. 2005;164:501-508.

623. Calderwood S, Kilpatrick L, Douglas SD, et al. Recombinant human granulocyte colony-stimulating factor therapy for patients with neutropenia and/or neutrophil dysfunction secondary to glycogen storage disease type 1b. Blood. 2001;97:376-382.

624. Pearson HA, Lobel JS, Kocoshis SA, et al. A new syndrome of refractory sideroblastic anemia with vacuolization of marrow precursors and exocrine pancreatic dysfunction. J Pediatr. 1979;95:976-984.

625. Inoue S, Yokota M, Nakada K, et al. Pathogenic mitochondrial DNA–induced respiration defects in hematopoietic cells result in anemia by suppressing erythroid differentiation. FEBS Lett. 2007;581:1910-1916.

626. Perillie PE, Kaplan SS, Finch SC. Significance of changes in serum muramidase activity in megaloblastic anemia. N Engl J Med. 1967;277:10-12.

627. Pearson HA. Marrow hypoplasia in anorexia nervosa. J Pediatr. 1967;71:211-215.

628. Huff JD, Keung YK, Thakuri M, et al. Copper deficiency causes reversible myelodysplasia. Am J Hematol. 2007;82:625-630.

629. Natelson EA, Lynch EC, Hettig RA, Alfrey CP Jr. Histiocytic medullary reticulosis: the role of phagocytosis in pancytopenia. Arch Intern Med. 1968;122:223-229.

630. Boxer LA, Camitta BM, Berenberg W, Fanning JP. Myelofibrosis-myeloid metaplasia in childhood. Pediatrics. 1975;55:861-865.

631. Goldblatt J. Type I Gaucher disease. J Med Genet. 1988;25:415-418.

632. Loria-Cortes R, Quesada-Calvo E, Cordero-Chaverri C. Osteopetrosis in children: a report of 26 cases. J Pediatr. 1977;91:43-47.

633. Wessels G, Schaaf HS, Beyers N, et al. Haematological abnormalities in children with tuberculosis. J Trop Pediatr. 1999;45:307-310.

634. Greenburg PL, Mara B, Steed S, Boxer L. The chronic idiopathic neutropenia syndrome: correlation of clinical features with in vitro parameters of granulocytopoiesis. Blood. 1980;55:915-921.

635. Papadaki HA, Eliopoulos AG, Kosteas T, et al. Impaired granulocytopoiesis in patients with chronic idiopathic neutropenia is associated with increased apoptosis of bone marrow myeloid progenitor cells. Blood. 2003;101:2591-2600.

636. Logue GL, Shastri KA, Laughlin M, et al. Idiopathic neutropenia: antineutrophil antibodies and clinical correlations. Am J Med. 1991;90:211-216.

637. De Alarcon PA, Goldberg J, Nelson DA, Stockman JA III. Chronic neutropenia: diagnostic approach and prognosis. Am J Pediatr Hematol Oncol. 1983;5:3-9.

638. Segal BH, Almyroudis NG, Battiwalla M, et al. Prevention and early treatment of invasive fungal infection in patients with cancer and neutropenia and in stem cell transplant recipients in the era of newer broad-spectrum antifungal agents and diagnostic adjuncts. Clin Infect Dis. 2007;44:402-409.

639. Dale DC, Liles WC, Llewellyn C, et al. Neutrophil transfusions: kinetics and functions of neutrophils mobilized with granulocyte-colony-stimulating factor and dexamethasone. Transfusion. 1998;38:713-721.

640. Einsele H, Northoff H, Neumeister B. Granulocyte transfusion. Vox Sang. 2004;87(Suppl 2):205-208.

641. Carreras E. Preventing exposure to moulds. Clin Microbiol Infect. 2006;12:77-83.

642. Coulombel L, Dehan M, Tchernia G, et al. The number of polymorphonuclear leukocytes in relation to gestational age in the newborn. Acta Paediatr Scand. 1979;68:709-711.

643. Cartwright GE, Athens JW, Haab OP, et al. Blood granulocyte kinetics in conditions associated with granulocytosis. Ann NY Acad Sci. 1964;113:963-973.

644. Athens JW. Leukocyte physiology. JAMA. 1966;198:38.

645. Boxer LA, Allen JM, Baehner RL. Diminished polymorphonuclear leukocyte adherence. Function dependent on release of cyclic AMP by endothelial cells after stimulation of beta-receptors by epinephrine. J Clin Invest. 1980;66:268-274.

646. Dale DC, Fauci AS, Guerry D IV, Wolff SM. Comparison of agents producing a neutrophilic leukocytosis in man. Hydrocortisone, prednisone, endotoxin, and etiocholanolone. J Clin Invest. 1975;56:808-813.

647. Ostlund RE, Bishop CR, Athens JW. Evaluation of non–steady-state neutrophil kinetics during endotoxin-induced granulocytosis. Proc Soc Exp Biol Med. 1971;137:763-767.

648. Bishop CR, Athens JW, Boggs DR, et al. Leukokinetic studies. XIII. A non–steady-state evaluation of the mechanism of cortisone-induced granulocytosis. J Clin Invest. 1968;47:249-260.

649. Rey JJ, Wolf PL. Extreme leukocytosis in accidental electric shock. Lancet. 1968;1:18-19.

650. Ryhanen P. Effects of anaesthesia and operative surgery on the immune response of patients of different ages. Ann Clin Res. 1977;9(Suppl 19):7.

651. Watkins J, Ward AM, Appleyard TM. Changes in peripheral blood leukocytes following i.v. anaesthesia and surgery. Br J Anaesthesiol. 1977;49:953.

652. Craddock CG, Perry S, Lawrence JS. Dynamics of leukopoiesis and leukocytosis, as studied by leukapheresis and isotopic techniques. J Clin Invest. 1956;35:285-296.

653. Milhorat AT, Small SM. Leukocytosis during various emotional states. Arch Neurol Psychiatry. 1942;47:779-792.

654. Peterson LA, Hrisinko MA. Benign lymphocytosis and reactive neutrophilia. Clin Lab Med. 1993;13:863-877.

655. Shoenfeld Y, Gurewich Y, Gallant LA, Pinkhas J. Prednisone-induced leukocytosis. Influence of dosage, method, and duration of administration on the degree of leukocytosis. Am J Med. 1981;71:773-778.

656. Walker RI, Willemze R. Neutrophil kinetics and the regulation of granulopoiesis. Rev Infect Dis. 1980;2:282-292.

657. Holland P, Mauer AM. Myeloid leukemoid reactions in children. Am J Dis Child. 1963;105:568-575.

658. Calabro JJ, Williamson P, Love ES, et al. Kawasaki syndrome. N Engl J Med. 1982;306:237-238.

659. Finch SC. Laboratory findings in infectious mononucleosis. In Carter RL, Penman HG (eds). Infectious Mononucleosis. Oxford, Blackwell Scientific, 1969, p 57.

660. Skårberg KO, Lagerlöf B, Reizenstein P. Leukaemia, leukaemoid reaction and tuberculosis. Acta Med Scand. 1967;182:427-432.

661. Schaller J, Wedgewood RJ. Juvenile rheumatoid arthritis: a review. Pediatrics. 1970;50:940-953.

662. McBride JA, Dacie JV, Shapely R. The effect of splenectomy on the leukocyte count. Br J Haematol. 1968;14:225-231.

663. Herring WB, Smith LB, Walker RI, Herion JC. Hereditary neutrophilia. Am J Med. 1974;56:729-734.

664. Doeglas HM, Bleumink E. Familial cold urticaria. Clinical findings. Arch Dermatol. 1974;110:382-388.

665. Tindall JP, Beeker SK, Rosse WF. Familial cold urticaria. A generalized reaction involving leukocytosis. Arch Intern Med. 1969;124:129-134.

666. Sakka V, Tsiodras S, Giamarellos-Bourboulis EJ, Giamarellou H. An update on the etiology and diagnostic evaluation of a leukemoid reaction. Eur J Intern Med. 2006;17:394-398.

667. Reilly JT. Chronic neutrophilic leukaemia: a distinct clinical entity? Br J Haematol. 2002;116:10-18.

668. Henry E, Walker D, Wiedmeier SE, Christensen RD. Hematological abnormalities during the first week of life among neonates with Down syndrome: data from a multihospital healthcare system. Am J Med Genet A. 2007;143:42-50.

669. Vyas P, Crispino JD. Molecular insights into Down syndrome–associated leukemia. Curr Opin Pediatr. 2007;19:9-14.

670. Vyas P, Roberts I. Down myeloid disorders: a paradigm for childhood preleukaemia and leukaemia and insights into normal megakaryopoiesis. Early Hum Dev. 2006;82:767-773.

671. Hedberg VA, Lipton JM. Thrombocytopenia with absent radii. A review of 100 cases. Am J Pediatr Hematol Oncol. 1988;10:51-64.

672. Wagelie-Steffen A, Aceves SS. Eosinophilic disorders in children. Curr Allergy Asthma Rep. 2006;6:475-482.

673. Lowell FC. Clinical aspects of eosinophilia in atopic diseases. JAMA. 1967;202:875-878.

674. Tefferi A, Patnaik MM, Pardanani A. Eosinophilia: secondary, clonal and idiopathic. Br J Haematol. 2006;133:468-492.

675. Roujeau JC. Clinical heterogeneity of drug hypersensitivity. Toxicology. 2005;209:123-129.

676. Tas S, Simonart T. Management of drug rash with eosinophilia and systemic symptoms (DRESS syndrome): an update. Dermatology. 2003;206:353-356.

677. Caruana SR, Kelly HA, Ngeow JY, et al. Undiagnosed and potentially lethal parasite infections among immigrants and refugees in Australia. J Travel Med. 2006;13:233-239.

678. Gyawali P, Whitty CJ. Investigating eosinophilia in patients returned from the tropics. Hosp Med. 2001;62:25-28.

679. Hochberg N, Ryan ET. Medical problems in the returning expatriate. Clin Occup Environ Med. 2004;4:205-219.

680. Carney AS, Tan LW, Adams D, et al. Th2 immunological inflammation in allergic fungal sinusitis, nonallergic eosinophilic fungal sinusitis, and chronic rhinosinusitis. Am J Rhinol. 2006;20:145-149.

681. Harley WB, Blaser MJ. Disseminated coccidioidomycosis associated with extreme eosinophilia. Clin Infect Dis. 1994;18:627-629.

682. Moss RB. Pathophysiology and immunology of allergic bronchopulmonary aspergillosis. Med Mycol. 2005;43(Suppl 1):S203-S206.

683. Chitkara RK, Krishna G. Parasitic pulmonary eosinophilia. Semin Respir Crit Care Med. 2006;27:171-184.

684. Sharma OP, Bethlem EP. The pulmonary infiltration with eosinophilia syndrome. Curr Opin Pulm Med. 1996;2:380-389.

685. Lee JJ, Furuta GT. Upper gastrointestinal tract eosinophilic disorders: pathobiology and management. Curr Gastroenterol Rep. 2006;8:439-442.

686. Assa'ad AH. Gastrointestinal food allergy and intolerance. Pediatr Ann. 2006;35:718-726.

687. Benfield GF, Asquith P. Blood eosinophilia and ulcerative colitis—influence of ethnic origin. Postgrad Med J. 1986;62:1101-1105.

688. D'Arienzo A, Manguso F, Astarita C, et al. Allergy and mucosal eosinophil infiltrate in ulcerative colitis. Scand J Gastroenterol. 2000;35:624-631.

689. Omenn GS. Familial reticuloendotheliosis with eosinophilia. N Engl J Med. 1965;273:427-432.

690. Cicardi M, Igarashi T, Rosen FS, Davis AE 3rd. Molecular basis for the deficiency of complement 1 inhibitor in type I hereditary angioneurotic edema. J Clin Invest. 1987;79:698-702.

691. Gleich GJ, Schroeter AL, Marcoux JP, et al. Episodic angioedema associated with eosinophilia. N Engl J Med. 1984;310:1621-1626.

692. Naiman JL, Oski FA, Allen FH Jr, Diamond LK. Hereditary eosinophilia. Report on a family and review of literature. Am J Hum Genet. 1964;16:195-203.

693. Klion AD, Law MA, Riemenschneider W, et al. Familial eosinophilia: a benign disorder? Blood. 2004;103:4050-4055.

694. Rioux JD, Stone VA, Daly MJ, et al. Familial eosinophilia maps to the cytokine gene cluster on human chromosomal region 5q31-q33. Am J Hum Genet. 1998;63:1086-1094.

695. Tancrede-Bohin E, Ionescu MA, de La Salmoniere P, et al. Prognostic value of blood eosinophilia in primary cutaneous T-cell lymphomas. Arch Dermatol. 2004;140:1057-1061.

696. Wilson F, Tefferi A. Acute lymphocytic leukemia with eosinophilia: two case reports and a literature review. Leuk Lymphoma. 2005;46:1045-1050.

697. Simon HU, Plotz SG, Simon D, et al. Clinical and immunological features of patients with interleukin-5–producing T cell clones and eosinophilia. Int Arch Allergy Immunol. 2001;124:242-245.

698. Hoy WE, Castero RVM. Eosinophilia in maintenance hemodialysis patients. J Dialysis. 1979;3:73-87.

699. Lee S, Schoen I. Eosinophilia and peritoneal fluid and peripheral blood associated with chronic peritoneal dialysis. Am J Clin Pathol. 1967;47:638-640.

700. Simon D, Braathen LR, Simon HU. Anti–interleukin-5 antibody therapy in eosinophilic diseases. Pathobiology. 2005;72:287-292.

701. Chusid MJ, Dale DC, West BC, Wolff SM. The hypereosinophilic syndrome: analysis of fourteen cases with review of the literature. Medicine (Baltimore). 1975;54:1-27.

702. Fletcher S, Bain B. Diagnosis and treatment of hypereosinophilic syndromes. Curr Opin Hematol. 2007;14:37-42.

703. Gleich GJ, Leiferman KM. The hypereosinophilic syndromes: still more heterogeneity. Curr Opin Immunol. 2005;17:679-684.

704. Klion AD, Bochner BS, Gleich GJ, et al. Approaches to the treatment of hypereosinophilic syndromes: a workshop summary report. J Allergy Clin Immunol. 2006;117:1292-1302.

705. Benezet-Mazuecos J, de la Fuente A, Marcos-Alberca P, Farre J. Loeffler endocarditis: what have we learned? Am J Hematol. 2007;82:861-862.

706. Gotlib J, Cools J, Malone JM 3rd, et al. The FIP1L1-PDGFRα fusion tyrosine kinase in hypereosinophilic

707. Cools J, DeAngelo DJ, Gotlib J, et al. A tyrosine kinase created by fusion of the PDGFRA and FIP1L1 genes as a therapeutic target of imatinib in idiopathic hypereosinophilic syndrome. N Engl J Med. 2003;348:1201-1214.

708. Bennett J, Catovsky D, Daniel M. Proposed revised criteria for the classification of acute myeloid leukemia. A report of the French-American-British Cooperative Group. Ann Intern Med. 1985;103:620-625.

709. Liu PP, Hajra A, Wijmenga C, Collins FS. Molecular pathogenesis of the chromosome 16 inversion in the M4Eo subtype of acute myeloid leukemia. Blood. 1995;85:2289-2302.

710. Bass DA. Eosinopenia. In Mahmoud AAF, Austen KF (eds). The Eosinophil in Health and Disease. New York, Grune & Stratton, 1980, p 275.

711. Schleimer RP, Bochner BS. The effects of glucocorticoids on human eosinophils. J Allergy Clin Immunol. 1994;94:1202-1213.

712. Shelley WB, Parnes HM. The absolute basophil count. JAMA. 1965;192:368-370.

713. Falcone FH, Zillikens D, Gibbs BF. The 21st century renaissance of the basophil? Current insights into its role in allergic responses and innate immunity. Exp Dermatol. 2006;15:855-864.

714. Mitre E, Nutman TB. Basophils, basophilia and helminth infections. Chem Immunol Allergy. 2006;90:141-156.

715. Denburg JA, Browman G. Prognostic implications of basophil differentiation in chronic myeloid leukemia. Am J Hematol. 1988;27:110-114.

716. Hasford J, Pfirrmann M, Hehlmann R, et al. Prognosis and prognostic factors for patients with chronic myeloid leukemia: nontransplant therapy. Semin Hematol. 2003;40:4-12.

717. Lett-Brown MA, Juneja HS. Basophil function in patients with chronic myelogenous leukaemia. Br J Haematol. 1985;61:621-626.

718. Rothenberg ME, Caulfield JP, Austen KF, et al. Biochemical and morphological characterization of basophilic leukocytes from two patients with myelogenous leukemia. J Immunol. 1987;138:2616-2625.

719. Leto TL, Lomax KJ, Volpp BD, et al. Cloning of a 67-kDa neutrophil oxidase factor with similarity to a non-catalytic region of p60[c-src]. Science. 1990;248:727-730.

720. Matsushima T, Handa H, Yokohama A, et al. Prevalence and clinical characteristics of myelodysplastic syndrome with bone marrow eosinophilia or basophilia. Blood. 2003;101:3386-3390.

721. Weiss S, Gafter U, van der Lyn E, Dialdetti M. Congenital dyserythropoietic anaemia with peculiar nuclear abnormality. Scand J Haematol. 1975;15:261-271.

722. Hoyle CF, Sherrington PD, Fischer P, Hayhoe FG. Basophils in acute myeloid leukaemia. J Clin Pathol. 1989;42:785-792.

723. Fredericks RE, Moloney WC. The basophilic granulocyte. Blood. 1959;14:571-583.

724. Iwata M, Nunoi H, Yamazaki H, et al. Homologous dinucleotide (GT or TG) deletion in Japanese patients with chronic granulomatous disease with p47-phox

deficiency. Biochem Biophys Res Commun. 1994;199: 1372-1377.

725. Segal AW, Jones OTG, Webster D, Allison AC. Absence of a newly described cytochrome *b* from neutrophils of patients with chronic granulomatous disease. Lancet. 1978;2:446-449.

726. Juhlin L. Basophil leukocyte differential in blood and bone marrow. Acta Haematol. 1963;29:89-95.

727. Koster E, Lennert K, Martin H. [Mastell leukemia.] Acta Haematol. 1956;16:255-272.

728. Johnson RA, Roodman GD. Hematologic manifestations of malignancy. Dis Mon. 1989;35:721-768.

729. Kato K. Leukocytes in infancy and childhood: a statistical analysis of 1,081 total and differential counts from birth to fifteen years. J Pediatr. 1935;7:7-15.

730. Maldonado JE, Hanlon DG. Monocytosis: a current appraisal. Mayo Clin Proc. 1965;40:248-259.

731. Koeffler HP, Golde DW. Human preleukemia. Ann Intern Med. 1980;93:347-353.

732. Marodi L, Kaposzta R, Toth J, Laszlo A. Impaired microbicidal capacity of mononuclear phagocytes from patients with type I Gaucher disease: partial correction by enzyme replacement therapy. Blood. 1995;86:4645-4649.

733. Aker M, Zimran A, Abrahamov A, et al. Abnormal neutrophil chemotaxis in Gaucher disease. Br J Haematol. 1993;83:187-191.

734. Liel Y, Rudich A, Nagauker-Shriker O, et al. Monocyte dysfunction in patients with Gaucher disease: evidence for interference of glucocerebroside with superoxide generation. Blood. 1994;83:2646-2653.

735. Cleiren E, Benichou O, Van Hul E, et al. Albers-Schonberg disease (autosomal dominant osteopetrosis, type II) results from mutations in the ClCN7 chloride channel gene. Hum Mol Genet. 2001;10:2861-2867.

736. Beard CJ, Key L, Newburger PE, et al. Neutrophil defect associated with malignant infantile osteopetrosis. J Lab Clin Med. 1986;108:498-505.

737. Picard C, Casanova JL. Inherited disorders of cytokines. Curr Opin Pediatr. 2004;16:648-658.

738. Arnaout MA. Structure and function of the leukocyte adhesion molecules CD11/CD18. Blood. 1990;75:1037-1050.

739. Anderson D, Smith C. Leukocyte adhesion deficiency. In Scriver C, Beaudet A, Sly W, Valle D (eds). The Metabolic & Molecular Basis of Inherited Disease, 8th ed. New York, McGraw-Hill, 2001, pp 4829-4856.

740. Gu YC, Bauer TR Jr, Ackermann MR, et al. The genetic immunodeficiency disease, leukocyte adhesion deficiency, in humans, dogs, cattle, and mice. Comp Med. 2004;54:363-372.

741. Bauer TR Jr, Gu YC, Creevy KE, et al. Leukocyte adhesion deficiency in children and Irish setter dogs. Pediatr Res. 2004;55:363-367.

742. Crowley CA, Curnutte JT, Rosin RE, et al. An inherited abnormality of neutrophil adhesion: its genetic transmission and its association with a missing protein. N Engl J Med. 1980;302:1163-1168.

743. Arnaout MA, Pitt J, Cohen HJ, et al. Deficiency of a granulocyte-membrane glycoprotein (gp150) in a boy with recurrent bacterial infections. N Engl J Med. 1982;306:693-699.

744. Bowen TJ, Ochs HD, Altman LC, et al. Severe recurrent bacterial infections associated with defective adherence and chemotaxis in two patients with neutrophils deficient in a cell-associated glycoprotein. J Pediatr. 1982; 101:932-940.

745. Dana N, Todd RF III, Pitt J, et al. Deficiency of a surface membrane glycoprotein (Mo1) in man. J Clin Invest. 1984;73:153-159.

746. Arnaout MA. Leukocyte adhesion molecules deficiency: its structural basis, pathophysiology and implications for modulating the inflammatory response. Immunol Rev. 1990;114:145-180.

747. Lowell CA, Berton G. Integrin signal transduction in myeloid leukocytes. J Leukoc Biol. 1999;65:313-320.

748. von Andrian UH, Berger EM, Ramezani L, et al. In vivo behavior of neutrophils from two patients with distinct inherited leukocyte adhesion deficiency syndromes. J Clin Invest. 1993;91:2893-2897.

749. Davies KA, Toothill VJ, Savill J, et al. A 19-year-old man with leukocyte adhesion deficiency. In vitro and in vivo studies of leucocyte function. Clin Exp Immunol. 1991;84:223-231.

750. Beller DI, Springer TA, Schreiber RD. Anti-Mac 1 selectively inhibits the mouse and human type three complement receptor. J Exp Med. 1982;156:1000-1009.

751. Kohl S, Springer TA, Schmalstieg FC, et al. Defective natural killer cytotoxicity and polymorphonuclear leukocyte antibody-dependent cellular cytotoxicity in pateints with LFA-1/OKM-1 deficiency. J Immunol. 1984;133: 2972-2978.

752. Kohl S, Loo LS, Schmalstieg FC, Anderson DC. The genetic deficiency of leukocyte surface glycoprotein Mac-1, LFA-1, p150,95 in humans is associated with defective antibody-dependent cellular cytotoxicity in vitro and defective protection against herpes simplex virus infection in vivo. J Immunol. 1986;137:1688-1694.

753. Krensky AM, Sanchez-Madrid F, Robbins E, et al. The functional significance, distribution, and structure of LFA-1, LFA-2, LFA-3: cell surface antigens associated with CTL-target interactions. J Immunol. 1983;131: 611-616.

754. Anderson DC, Schmalstieg FC, Finegold MJ, et al. The severe and moderate phenotypes of heritable Mac-1, LFA-1 deficiency: their quantitative definition and relation to leukocyte dysfunction and clinical features. J Infect Dis. 1985;152:668-689.

755. Hibbs ML, Wardlaw AJ, Stacker SA, et al. Transfection of cells from patients with leukocyte adhesion deficiency with an integrin β subunit (CD18) restores lymphocyte function–associated antigen-1 expression and function. J Clin Invest. 1990;85:674-681.

756. Piirila H, Valiaho J, Vihinen M. Immunodeficiency mutation databases (IDbases). Hum Mutat. 2006;27:1200-1208.

757. Roos D, Law SK. Hematologically important mutations: leukocyte adhesion deficiency. Blood Cells Mol Dis. 2001;27:1000-1004.

758. Hogg N, Bates PA. Genetic analysis of integrin function in man: LAD-1 and other syndromes. Matrix Biol. 2000; 19:211-222.

759. Giger U, Boxer LA, Simpson PJ, et al. Deficiency of leukocyte surface glycoproteins Mo1, LFA-1, and Leu M5 in a dog with recurrent bacterial infections: an animal model. Blood. 1987;69:1622-1630.

760. Renshaw HW, Davis WC. Canine granulocytopathy syndrome: an inherited disorder of leukocyte function. Am J Pathol. 1979;95:731-744.

761. Hagemoser WA, Roth JA, Lofstedt J, Fagerland JA. Granulocytopathy in a Holstein heifer. J Am Vet Med Assoc. 1983;183:1093-1094.

762. Kehrli ME Jr, Schmalstieg FC, Anderson DC, et al. Molecular definition of the bovine granulocytopathy syndrome: identification of deficiency of the Mac-1 (CD11b/CD18) glycoprotein. Am J Vet Res. 1990;51: 1826-1836.

763. Shuster DE, Kehrli ME Jr, Ackermann MR, Gilbert RO. Identification and prevalence of a genetic defect that causes leukocyte adhesion deficiency in Holstein cattle. Proc Natl Acad Sci U S A. 1992;89:9225-9229.

764. Oudesluys-Murphy AM, Eilers GA, de Groot CJ. The time of separation of the umbilical cord. Eur J Pediatr. 1987;146:387-389.

765. Wilson CB, Ochs HD, Almquist J, et al. When is umbilical cord separation delayed? J Pediatr. 1985;107:292-294.

766. Kurkchubasche AG, Panepinto JA, Tracy TF Jr, et al. Clinical features of a human Rac2 mutation: a complex neutrophil dysfunction disease. J Pediatr. 2001;139: 141-147.

767. Ambruso DR, Knall C, Abell AN, et al. Human neutrophil immunodeficiency syndrome is associated with an inhibitory Rac2 mutation. Proc Natl Acad Sci U S A. 2000;97:4654-4659.

768. Arnaout MA, Spits H, Terhorst C, et al. Deficiency of a leukocyte surface glycoprotein (LFA-1) in two patients with Mo1 deficiency. Effects of cell activation on Mo1/LFA-1 surface expression in normal and deficient leukocytes. J Clin Invest. 1984;74:1291-1300.

769. Fischer A, Lisowska-Grospierre B, Anderson DC, Springer TA. Leukocyte adhesion deficiency: molecular basis and functional consequences. Immunodefic Rev. 1988;1:39-54.

770. Weisman SJ, Mahoney MJ, Anderson DC, et al. Prenatal diagnosis for Mo1 (CDw18) deficiency [abstract]. Clin Res. 1987;35:435a.

771. Malech HL, Hickstein DD. Genetics, biology and clinical management of myeloid cell primary immune deficiencies: chronic granulomatous disease and leukocyte adhesion deficiency. Curr Opin Hematol. 2007;14: 29-36.

772. Horwitz ME. Stem-cell transplantation for inherited immunodeficiency disorders. Pediatr Clin North Am. 2000;47:1371-1387.

773. Thomas C, Le Deist F, Cavazzana-Calvo M, et al. Results of allogeneic bone marrow transplantation in patients with leukocyte adhesion deficiency. Blood. 1995;86:1629-1635.

774. Mancias C, Infante AJ, Kamani NR. Matched unrelated donor bone marrow transplantation in leukocyte adhesion deficiency. Bone Marrow Transplant. 1999;24: 1261-1263.

775. Farinha NJ, Duval M, Wagner E, et al. Unrelated bone marrow transplantation for leukocyte adhesion deficiency. Bone Marrow Transplant. 2002;30:979-981.

776. Rae J, Noack D, Heyworth PG, et al. Molecular analysis of 9 new families with chronic granulomatous disease caused by mutations in CYBA, the gene encoding p22^{phox}. Blood. 2000;96:1106-1112.

777. Bauer TR Jr, Hai M, Tuschong LM, et al. Correction of the disease phenotype in canine leukocyte adhesion deficiency using ex vivo hematopoietic stem cell gene therapy. Blood. 2006;108:3313-3320.

778. Larochelle A, Dunbar CE. Genetic manipulation of hematopoietic stem cells. Semin Hematol. 2004;41: 257-271.

779. Etzioni A, Frydman M, Pollack S, et al. A syndrome of leukocyte adhesion deficiency (LAD II) due to deficiency of sialyl-Lewis-X, a ligand for selectins. N Engl J Med. 1992;327:1789-1792.

780. Marquardt T, Luhn K, Srikrishna G, et al. Correction of leukocyte adhesion deficiency type II with oral fucose. Blood. 1999;94:3976-3985.

781. Hirschberg CB. Golgi nucleotide sugar transport and leukocyte adhesion deficiency II. J Clin Invest. 2001; 108:3-6.

782. Lubke T, Marquardt T, Etzioni A, et al. Complementation cloning identifies CDG-IIc, a new type of congenital disorders of glycosylation, as a GDP-fucose transporter deficiency. Nat Genet. 2001;28:73-76.

783. Luhn K, Wild MK, Eckhardt M, et al. The gene defective in leukocyte adhesion deficiency II encodes a putative GDP-fucose transporter. Nat Genet. 2001;28:69-72.

784. Sturla L, Puglielli L, Tonetti M, et al. Impairment of the Golgi GDP–L-fucose transport and unresponsiveness to fucose replacement therapy in LAD II patients. Pediatr Res. 2001;49:537-542.

785. Etzioni A, Doerschuk CM, Harlan JM. Similarities and dissimilarities between humans and mice looking at adhesion molecules defects. Adv Exp Med Biol. 2000; 479:147-161.

786. McDowall A, Inwald D, Leitinger B, et al. A novel form of integrin dysfunction involving β_1, β_2, and β_3 integrins. J Clin Invest. 2003;111:51-60.

787. Etzioni A, Alon R. Leukocyte adhesion deficiency III: a group of integrin activation defects in hematopoietic lineage cells. Curr Opin Allergy Clin Immunol. 2004; 4:485-490.

788. Alon R, Aker M, Feigelson S, et al. A novel genetic leukocyte adhesion deficiency in subsecond triggering of integrin avidity by endothelial chemokines results in impaired leukocyte arrest on vascular endothelium under shear flow. Blood. 2003;101:4437-4445.

789. Kuijpers TW, Van Lier RA, Hamann D, et al. Leukocyte adhesion deficiency type 1 (LAD-1)/variant. A novel immunodeficiency syndrome characterized by dysfunctional β_2 integrins. J Clin Invest. 1997;100:1725-1733.

790. Harris ES, Shigeoka AO, Li W, et al. A novel syndrome of variant leukocyte adhesion deficiency involving defects in adhesion mediated by β_1 and β_2 integrins. Blood. 2001;97:767-776.

791. Kuijpers TW, van Bruggen R, Kamerbeek N, et al. Natural history and early diagnosis of LAD-1/variant syndrome. Blood. 2007;109:3529-3537.

792. Pasvolsky R, Feigelson SW, Kilic SS, et al. A LAD-III syndrome is associated with defective expression of the Rap-1 activator CalDAG-GEFI in lymphocytes, neutrophils, and platelets. J Exp Med. 2007;204:1571-1582.

793. Kinashi T, Aker M, Sokolovsky-Eisenberg M, et al. LAD-III, a leukocyte adhesion deficiency syndrome

associated with defective Rap1 activation and impaired stabilization of integrin bonds. Blood. 2004;103:1033-1036.

794. Bergmeier W, Goerge T, Wang HW, et al. Mice lacking the signaling molecule CalDAG-GEFI represent a model for leukocyte adhesion deficiency type III. J Clin Invest. 2007;117:1699-1707.

795. Oseas RS, Allen J, Yang HH, et al. Mechanism of dexamethasone inhibition of chemotactic factor–induced granulocyte aggregation. Blood. 1982;59:265-269.

796. Skubitz KM, Craddock PR, Hammerschmidt DE, August JT. Corticosteroids block binding of chemotactic peptide to the receptor on granulocytes and cause disaggregation of granulocyte aggregates in vitro. J Clin Invest. 1981;68:13-20.

797. Caramori G, Adcock I. Anti-inflammatory mechanisms of glucocorticoids targeting granulocytes. Curr Drug Targets Inflamm Allergy. 2005;4:455-463.

798. Bryant RE, Sutcliff MC. The effect of 3′, 5′-adenosine monophosphate on granulocyte adhesion. J Clin Invest. 1974;54:1241-1244.

799. Engelich G, Wright DG, Hartshorn KL. Acquired disorders of phagocyte function complicating medical and surgical illnesses. Clin Infect Dis. 2001;33:2040-2048.

800. Ware LB. Pathophysiology of acute lung injury and the acute respiratory distress syndrome. Semin Respir Crit Care Med. 2006;27:337-349.

801. Wright DG, Robichaud KJ, Pizzo PA, Deisseroth AB. Lethal pulmonary reactions associated with the combined use of amphotericin B and leukocyte transfusions. N Engl J Med. 1981;304:1185-1189.

802. Boxer LA, Ingraham LM, Allen J, et al. Amphotericin-B promotes leukocyte aggregation of nylon wool fiber–treated polymorphonuclear leukocytes. Blood. 1981;58:518-523.

803. Sulis ML, Van de Ven C, Henderson T, et al. Liposomal amphotericin B (AmBisome) compared with amphotericin B +/− FMLP induces significantly less in vitro neutrophil aggregation with granulocyte-colony-stimulating factor/dexamethasone-mobilized allogeneic donor neutrophils. Blood. 2002;99:384-386.

804. Brown CC, Gallin JI. Chemotactic disorders. Hematol Oncol Clin North Am. 1988;2:61-79.

805. Boyden S. The chemotactic effect of mixtures of antibody and antigen on polymorphonuclear leukocytes. J Exp Med. 1962;115:453-466.

806. Smith CW, Hollers JC, Patrick RA, Hassett C. Motility and adhesiveness in human neutrophils: effects of chemotactic factors. J Clin Invest. 1979;63:221-229.

807. Nelson RD, Quie PG, Simmons RL. Chemotaxis under agarose: a new and simple method for measuring chemotaxis and spontaneous migration of human polymorphonuclear leukocytes and monocytes. J Immunol. 1975;115:1650-1656.

808. Rebuck JW, Crowley JH. A method of studying leukocytic functions in vivo. Ann NY Acad Sci. 1955;59:757-805.

809. Davis SD, Schaller J, Wedgwood RJ. Job's syndrome: reccurent, "cold," staphylococcal abscesses. Lancet. 1966;1:1013-1015.

810. Donabedian H, Gallin JI. The hyperimmunoglobulin E recurrent-infection (Job's) syndrome. A review of the NIH experience and the literature. Medicine (Baltimore). 1983;62:195-208.

811. Buckley RH, Wray BB, Belmaker EZ. Extreme hyperimmunoglobulinemia E and undue susceptibility to infection. Pediatrics. 1972;49:59-69.

812. Grimbacher B, Holland SM, Gallin JI, et al. Hyper-IgE syndrome with recurrent infections—an autosomal dominant multisystem disorder. N Engl J Med. 1999; 340:692-702.

813. Grimbacher B, Holland SM, Puck JM. Hyper-IgE syndromes. Immunol Rev. 2005;203:244-250.

814. Erlewyn-Lajeunesse MD. Hyperimmunoglobulin-E syndrome with recurrent infection: a review of current opinion and treatment. Pediatr Allergy Immunol. 2000; 11:133-141.

815. Hill HR, Estensen RD, Hogan NA, Quie PG. Severe staphylococcal disease associated with allergic manifestation, hyperimmunoglobulinemia E, and defective neutrophil chemotaxis. J Lab Clin Med. 1976;88:796-806.

816. Hill HR, Ochs HD, Qioe PG, et al. Defect in neutrophil granulocyte chemotaxis in Job's syndrome of recurrent "cold" staphylococcal abscesses. Lancet. 1974;2:617-619.

817. Renner ED, Puck JM, Holland SM, et al. Autosomal recessive hyperimmunoglobulin E syndrome: a distinct disease entity. J Pediatr. 2004;144:93-99.

818. Minegishi Y, Saito M, Morio T, et al. Human tyrosine kinase 2 deficiency reveals its requisite roles in multiple cytokine signals involved in innate and acquired immunity. Immunity. 2006;25:745-755.

819. Geha RS, Reinherz E, Leung D, et al. Deficiency of suppressor T cells in hyperimmunoglobulin E syndrome. J Clin Invest. 1981;68:783-791.

820. Matricardi PM, Capobianchi MR, Paganelli R, et al. Interferon production in primary immunodeficiencies. J Clin Immunol. 1984;4:388-394.

821. Del Prete G, Tiri A, Maggi E, et al. Defective in vitro production of gamma interferon and tumor necrosis factor-alpha by circulating T cells from patients with the hyper-immunoglobulin E syndrome. J Clin Invest. 1989;84:1830-1835.

822. Sheerin KA, Buckley RH. Antibody responses to protein, polysaccharide, and phi X174 antigens in the hyperimmunoglobulinemia E (hyper-IgE) syndrome. J Allergy Clin Immunol. 1991;87:803-811.

823. Ruoslahti E. Integrins. J Clin Invest. 1991;87:1-5.

824. Leung DYM, Geha RS. Clinical and immunologic aspects of the hyperimmunoglobulin E syndrome. Hematol Oncol Clin North Am. 1988;2:81-100.

825. Holland SM, DeLeo FR, Elloumi HZ, et al. STAT3 mutations in the hyper-IgE syndrome. N Engl J Med. 2007;357:1608-1619.

826. Minegishi Y, Saito M, Tsuchiya S, et al. Dominant-negative mutations in the DNA-binding domain of STAT3 cause hyper-IgE syndrome. Nature. 2007;448:1058-1062.

827. Boxer LA, Hedley-Whyte ET, Stossel TP. Neutrophil actin dysfunction and abnormal neutrophil behavior. N Engl J Med. 1974;291:1093-1099.

828. Southwick FS, Dabiri GA, Stossel TP. Neutrophil actin dysfunction is a genetic disorder associated with partial impairment of neutrophil actin assembly in

three family members. J Clin Invest. 1988;82:1525-1531.

829. Southwick FS, Howard TH, Holbrook T, et al. The relationship between CR3 deficiency and neutrophil actin assembly. Blood. 1989;73:1973-1979.

830. Coates TD, Torkildson JC, Torres M, et al. An inherited defect of neutrophil motility and microfilamentous cytoskeleton associated with abnormalities in 47-Kd and 89-Kd proteins. Blood. 1991;78:1338-1346.

831. Howard T, Li Y, Torres M, et al. The 47-kD protein increased in neutrophil actin dysfunction with 47- and 89-kD protein abnormalities is lymphocyte-specific protein. Blood. 1994;83:231-241.

832. Nunoi H, Iwata M, Tatsuzawa S, et al. AG dinucleotide insertion in a patient with chronic granulomatous disease lacking cytosolic 67-kD protein. Blood. 1995;86:329-333.

833. Van Dyke TE, Vaikuntam J. Neutrophil function and dysfunction in periodontal disease. Curr Opin Periodontol. 1994:19-27.

834. Van Dyke TE, Schweinebraten M, Cianciola LJ, et al. Neutrophil chemotaxis in families with localized juvenile periodontitis. J Periodont Res. 1985;20:503-514.

835. Donly KJ, Ashkenazi M. Juvenile periodontitis: a review of pathogenesis, diagnosis and treatment. J Clin Pediatr Dent. 1992;16:73-78.

836. De Nardin E. The molecular basis for neutrophil dysfunction in early-onset periodontitis. J Periodontol. 1996;67:345-354.

837. Cianciola LJ, Genco RJ, Patters MR, et al. Defective polymorphonuclear leukocyte function in a human periodontal disease. Nature. 1977;265:445-447.

838. Perez HD, Kelly E, Elfman F, et al. Defective polymorphonuclear leukocyte formyl peptide receptor(s) in juvenile periodontitis. J Clin Invest. 1991;87:971-976.

839. Clark RA, Page RC, Wilde G. Defective neutrophil chemotaxis in juvenile periodontitis. Infect Immun. 1977;18:694-700.

840. Van Dyke TE, Horoszewicz HU, Cianiola LJ, Genco RJ. Neutrophil chemotaxis dysfunction in human periodontitis. Infect Immun. 1980;27:124-132.

841. Suzuki JB, Colison BC, Falker WF Jr, Nauman RK. Immunologic profile of juvenile periodontitis. II. Neutrophil chemotaxis, phagocytosis and spore germination. J Periodont. 1984;55:461-467.

842. Anderson DC, Smith CW, Springer TA. Leukocyte adhesion deficiency and other disorders of leukocyte motility. In Scriver CR, Beaudet AL (eds). The Metabolic Basis of Inherited Disease. New York, McGraw-Hill, 1989, pp 2751-2777.

843. Shurin SB, Socransky SS, Sweeney E, Stossel TP. A neutrophil disorder induced by capnocytophaga, a dental micro-organism. N Engl J Med. 1979;301:849-859.

844. Tsai C-C, McArthur WP, Baehni PC, et al. Extraction and partial characterization of a leukotoxin from a plaque-derived gram-negative microorganism. Infect Immun. 1979;25:427-439.

845. Agarwal S, Suzuki JB. Altered neutrophil function in localized juvenile periodontitis: intrinsic cellular defect or effect of immune mediators? J Periodont Res. 1991;26:276-278.

846. Van Dyke TE, Zinney W, Winkel K, et al. Neutrophil function in localized juvenile periodontitis. Phagocytosis, superoxide production and specific granule release. J Periodont. 1986;57:703-708.

847. Van Dyke TE. Role of the neutrophil in oral disease: receptor deficiency in leukocytes from patients with juvenile periodontitis. Rev Infect Dis. 1985;7:419-425.

848. Wilson CB. Immunologic basis for increased susceptibility of the neonate to infection. J Pediatr. 1986;108:1-12.

849. Hill HR. Biochemical, structural, and functional abnormalities of polymorphonuclear leukocytes in the neonate. Pediatr Res. 1987;22:375-382.

850. Koenig JM, Yoder MC. Neonatal neutrophils: the good, the bad, and the ugly. Clin Perinatol. 2004;31:39-51.

851. Hill HR, Augustin NH, Jaffe HS. Human recombinant interferon gamma enhances neonatal polymorphonuclear leukocyte activation and movement, and increases free intracellular calcium. J Exp Med. 1991;173:767-770.

852. Klein RB, Fischer TJ, Gard SE, et al. Decreased mononuclear and polymorphonuclear chemotaxis in human newborns, infants, and young children. Pediatrics. 1977;60:467-472.

853. Anderson DC, Hughes BJ, Smith CW. Abnormal motility of neonatal polymorphonuclear leukocytes: relationship to impaired redistribution of surface adhesion sites by chemotactic factor or colchicine. J Clin Invest. 1981;68:863-874.

854. Anderson DC, Freeman KL, Heerdt B, et al. Abnormal stimulated adherence of neonatal granulocytes: impaired induction of surface MAC-1 by chemotactic factors or secretagogues. Blood. 1987;70:740-750.

855. Smith JB, Campbell DE, Ludomirsky A, et al. Expression of the complement receptors CR1 and CR3 and the type III Fc-gamma receptor on neutrophils from newborn infants and from fetuses with Rh disease. Pediatr Res. 1990;28:120-126.

856. Abughali N, Berger M, Tosi MF. Deficient total cell content of CR3 (CD11b) in neonatal neutrophils. Blood. 1994;83:1086-1092.

857. Sacchi F, Rondini G, Mingrat G, et al. Different maturation of neutrophil chemotaxis in term and preterm newborn infants. J Pediatr. 1982;101:273-274.

858. Roos D, Kuijpers TW, Mascart-Lemone F, et al. A novel syndrome of severe neutrophil dysfunction: unresponsiveness confined to chemotaxin-induced functions. Blood. 1993;81:2735-2743.

859. Brenneis H, Schmidt A, Blaas-Mautner P, et al. Chemotaxis of polymorphonuclear neutrophils (PMN) in patients suffering from recurrent infection. Eur J Clin Invest. 1993;23:693-698.

860. Alper CA, Colten HR, Rosen FS, et al. Homozygous deficiency of C3 in a patient with repeated infections. Lancet. 1972;2:1179-1181.

861. Botto M, Fong KY, So AK, et al. Molecular basis of hereditary C3 deficiency. J Clin Invest. 1990;86:1158-1163.

862. Roord JJ, Daha M, Kuis W, et al. Inherited deficiency of the third component of complement associated with recurrent pyogenic infections, circulating immune complexes, and vasculitis in a Dutch family. N Engl J Med. 1983;71:81-87.

863. Matsuyama W, Nakagawa M, Takashima H, et al. Molecular analysis of hereditary deficiency of the third com-

ponent of complement (C3) in two sisters. Intern Med. 2001;40:1254-1258.

864. Singer L, Colten HR, Wetsel RA. Complement C3 deficiency: human, animal, and experimental models. Pathobiology. 1994;62:14-28.

865. Alper CA, Abramson N, Johnston RB Jr, et al. Studies in vivo and in vitro on an abnormality in the metabolism of C3 in a patient with increased susceptibility to infection. J Clin Invest. 1970;49:1975-1985.

866. Sumiya M, Super M, Tabona P, et al. Molecular basis of opsonic defect in immunodeficient children. Lancet. 1991;337:1569-1570.

867. Turner MW, Lipscombe RJ, Levinsky RJ, et al. Mutations in the human mannose binding protein gene: their frequencies in three distinct populations and relationship to serum levels of the protein. Immunodeficiency. 1993;4:285-287.

868. Madsen HO, Garred P, Kurtzhals JA, et al. A new frequent allele is the missing link in the structural polymorphism of the human mannan-binding protein. Immunogenetics. 1994;40:37-44.

869. Summerfield JA, Ryder S, Sumiya M, et al. Mannose binding protein gene mutations associated with unusual and severe infections in adults. Lancet. 1995;345:886-889.

870. Ceuppens JL, Bloemmen FJ, Van Wauwe JP. T-cell unresponsiveness to the mitogenic activity of OKT3 antibody results from a deficiency of the monocyte Fc gamma receptors for murine IgG2a and inability to cross-link the T3-Ti complex. J Immunol. 1985;135:3882-3886.

871. Fromont P, Bettaib A, Skouri H, et al. Frequency of the polymorphonuclear neutrophil Fc-gamma receptor III deficiency in the French population and its involvement in the development of neonatal alloimmune neutropenia. Blood. 1992;79:2131-2134.

872. Selvaraj P, Rosse WF, Silber R, Springer TA. The major Fc receptor in blood has a phosphatidylinositol anchor and is deficient in paroxysmal nocturnal haemoglobinuria. Nature. 1988;333:565-567.

873. Huizinga TW, van der Schoot CE, Jost C, et al. The PI-linked receptor FcR III is released on stimulation of neutrophils. Nature. 1988;333:667-669.

874. Gessner JE, Heiken H, Tamm A, Schmidt RE. The IgG Fc receptor family. Ann Hematol. 1998;76:231-248.

875. Van De Winkel JGJ, Capel PJA. Human IgG Fc receptor heterogeneity: molecular aspects and clinical implications. Immunol Today. 1993;14:215-221.

876. Filipovich AH. Hemophagocytic lymphohistiocytosis and related disorders. Curr Opin Allergy Clin Immunol. 2006;6:410-415.

877. Janka G, Zur Stadt U. Familial and acquired hemophagocytic lymphohistiocytosis. Hematology Am Soc Hematol Educ Program. 2005;82-88.

878. White JG, Clawson CC. The Chédiak-Higashi syndrome: the nature of the giant neutrophil granules and their interactions with cytoplasm and foreign particulates. I. Progressive enlargement of the massive inclusions in mature neutrophils. II. Manifestations of cytoplasmic injury and sequestration. III. Interactions between giant organelles and foreign particulates. Am J Pathol. 1980;98:151-196.

879. Rausch PG, Pryzwansky KB, Spitznagel JK. Immunocytochemical identification of azurophilic and specific

880. Davis WC, Spicer SS, Greene WB, Padgett GA. Ultrastructure of cells in bone marrow and peripheral blood of normal mink and mink with the homologue of the Chédiak-Higashi trait of humans. II. Cytoplasmic granules in eosinophils, basophils, mononuclear cells and platelets. Am J Pathol. 1971;63:411-432.

881. Vassali JD, Piperno-Granelli A, Griscelli C, Reich E. Specific protease deficiency in polymorphonuclear leukocytes of Chédiak-Higashi syndrome and beige mice. J Exp Mice. 1978;149:1285-1290.

882. Ganz T, Metcalf JA, Gallin JI, et al. Microbicidal/cytotoxic proteins of neutrophils are deficient in two disorders: Chédiak-Higashi syndrome and "specific" granule deficiency. J Clin Invest. 1988;82:552-556.

883. Sjaastad OV, Blom AK, Stormorken H, Nes N. Adenine nucleotides, serotonin and aggregation properties of the platelets of blue foxes (Alopex lagopus) with the Chédiak-Higashi syndrome. Am J Med Genet. 1990;35:373-378.

884. Barbosa MD, Nguyen QA, Tchernev VT, et al. Identification of the homologous beige and Chédiak-Higashi syndrome genes. Nature. 1996;382:262-265.

885. Nagle DL, Karim MA, Woolf EA, et al. Identification and mutation analysis of the complete gene for Chédiak-Higashi syndrome. Nat Genet. 1996;14:307-311.

886. Perou CM, Moore KJ, Nagle DL, et al. Identification of the murine beige gene by YAC complementation and positional cloning. Nat Genet. 1996;13:303-308.

887. Jenkins NA, Justice MJ, Gilbert DJ, et al. Nidogen/entactin (Nid) maps to the proximal end of mouse chromosome 13 linked to beige (bg) and identifies a new region of homology between mouse and human chromosomes. Genomics. 1991;9:401-403.

888. Kypri E, Schmauch C, Maniak M, Lozanne AD. The BEACH protein LvsB is localized on lysosomes and postlysosomes and limits their fusion with early endosomes. Traffic. 2007;8:774-783.

889. Certain S, Barrat F, Pastural E, et al. Protein truncation test of LYST reveals heterogenous mutations in patients with Chédiak-Higashi syndrome. Blood. 2000;95:979-983.

890. Fukai K, Oh J, Karim MA, et al. Homozygosity mapping of the gene for Chédiak-Higashi syndrome to chromosome 1q42-q44 in a segment of conserved synteny that includes the mouse beige locus (bg). Am J Hum Genet. 1996;59:620-624.

891. Blume RS, Bennett JM, Yankee RA, Wolff SM. Defective granulocyte regulation in the Chédiak-Higashi syndrome. N Engl J Med. 1968;279:1009-1015.

892. White JG, Clawson CC. The Chédiak-Higashi syndrome. Ring-shaped lysosomes in circulating monocytes. Am J Pathol. 1979;96:781-798.

893. Buchanan GB, Handin RI. Platelet function in the Chédiak-Higashi syndrome. Blood. 1976;47:941-948.

894. Boxer GJ, Holmsen H, Robkin L, et al. Abnormal platelet functions in Chédiak-Higashi syndrome. Br J Haematol. 1977;35:521-533.

895. Novak EK, McGarry MP, Swank RT. Correction of symptoms of platelet storage pool deficiency in animal models for Chédiak-Higashi syndrome and Hermansky-Pudlak syndrome. Blood. 1985;66:1196-1201.

896. Bell TG, Meyers KM, Prieur DJ, et al. Decreased nucleotide and serotonin storage associates with defective function in Chédiak-Higashi syndrome cattle and human platelets. Blood. 1976;48:175-184.

897. Clark RA, Kimball HR. Defective granulocyte chemotaxis in the Chédiak-Higashi syndrome. J Clin Invest. 1971;50:2645-2652.

898. Clawson CC, Repine JE, White JG. Chédiak-Higashi syndrome: quantitative defect in bactericidal capacity. Blood. 1971;38:814.

899. Root RK, Rosenthal AS, Balestra DJ. Abnormal bactericidal, metabolic, and lysosomal functions of Chédiak-Higashi syndrome leukocytes. J Clin Invest. 1972;51:649-665.

900. Cairo MS, Vandeven C, Toy C, et al. Fluorescent cytometric analysis of polymorphonuclear leucocytes in Chédiak-Higashi syndrome: diminished C3bi receptor expression (OKM-1) with normal granular cell density. Pediatr Res. 1988;24:673-676.

901. Boxer LA, Smolen JE. Neutrophil granule constituents and their release in health and disease. Hematol Oncol North Am. 1988;2:101-134.

902. Klein M, Roder J, Haliotis T, et al. Chédiak-Higashi gene in humans. II. The selectivity of the defect in natural-killer and antibody-dependent cell-mediated cytotoxicity function. J Exp Med. 1980;151:1049-1058.

903. Abo T, Roder JC, Abo W, et al. Natural killer (HNK-1⁺) cells in Chédiak-Higashi patients are present in normal numbers but are abnormal in function and morphology. J Clin Invest. 1982;70:193-197.

904. Haliotis T, Roder J, Klein M, et al. Chédiak-Higashi gene in humans. I. Impairment of natural-killer function. J Exp Med. 1980;151:1039-1048.

905. Merino F, Henle W, Ramirez-Duque P. Chronic active Epstein-Barr virus infection in patients with Chédiak-Higashi syndrome. J Clin Immunol. 1986;6:299-305.

906. Rubin CM, Burke BA, McKenna RW, et al. The accelerated phase of Chédiak-Higashi syndrome. An expression of the virus-associated hemophagocytic syndrome? Cancer. 1985;56:524-530.

907. Okano M, Gross TG. A review of Epstein-Barr virus infection in patients with immunodeficiency disorders. Am J Med Sci. 2000;319:392-396.

908. Pettit RE, Berdal KG. Chédiak-Higashi syndrome: neurologic appearance. Arch Neurol. 1984;41:1001-1002.

909. Creel D, Boxer LA, Fauci AS. Visual and auditory anomalies in Chédiak-Higashi syndrome. Electroencephalogr Clin Neurophysiol. 1983;55:252-257.

910. Diukman R, Tanigawara S, Cowan MJ, Golbus MS. Prenatal diagnosis of Chédiak-Higashi syndrome. Prenat Diagn. 1992;12:877-885.

911. Durandy A, Breton-Gorius J, Guy-Grand D, et al. Prenatal diagnosis of syndromes associating albinism and immune deficiencies (Chédiak-Higashi syndrome and variant). Prenat Diagn. 1993;13:13-20.

912. Kumar M, Sackey K, Schmalstieg F, et al. Griscelli syndrome: rare neonatal syndrome of recurrent hemophagocytosis. J Pediatr Hematol Oncol. 2001;23:464-468.

913. Van Slyck E, Rebuck JW. Pseudo–Chédiak-Higashi anomaly in acute leukemia. Am J Clin Pathol. 1974;62:673-678.

914. Gorman AM, O'Connell LG. Letter: pseudo–Chédiak-Higashi anomaly in acute leukemia. Am J Clin Pathol. 1976;65:1030-1031.

915. Tulliez M, Vernant JP, Breton-Gorius J, et al. Pseudo–Chédiak-Higashi anomaly in a case of acute myeloid leukemia: electron microscopic studies. Blood. 1979;54:863-871.

916. Weening RS, Schoorel EP, Roos D, et al. Effect of ascorbate on abnormal neutrophil, platelet, and lymphocyte function in a patient with the Chédiak-Higashi syndrome. Blood. 1981;57:856-865.

917. Boxer LA, Watanabe AM, Rister M, et al. Correction of leukocyte function in Chédiak-Higashi syndrome by ascorbate. N Engl J Med. 1976;295:1041-1045.

918. Gallin JI, Elin RJ, Hubert RT, et al. Efficacy of ascorbic acid in Chédiak-Higashi syndrome (CHS): studies in humans and mice. Blood. 1979;53:226-234.

919. Gordon N, Mullen CA, Tran H, et al. Fludarabine and once-daily intravenous busulfan for allogeneic bone marrow transplantation for Chédiak-Higashi syndrome. J Pediatr Hematol Oncol. 2003;25:824-826.

920. Haddad E, Le Deist F, Blanche S, et al. Treatment of Chédiak-Higashi syndrome by allogeneic bone marrow transplantation: report of 10 cases. Blood. 1995;85:3328-3333.

921. Tardieu M, Lacroix C, Neven B, et al. Progressive neurologic dysfunctions 20 years after allogeneic bone marrow transplantation for Chédiak-Higashi syndrome. Blood. 2005;106:40-42.

922. Trigg ME, Schugar R. Chédiak-Higashi syndrome: hematopoietic chimerism corrects genetic defect. Bone Marrow Transplant. 2001;27:1211-1213.

923. Sakata N, Kawa K, Kato K, et al. Unrelated donor marrow transplantation for congenital immunodeficiency and metabolic disease: an update of the experience of the Japan Marrow Donor Program. Int J Hematol. 2004;80:174-182.

924. Mottonen M, Lanning M, Saarinen UM. Allogeneic bone marrow transplantation in Chédiak-Higashi syndrome. Pediatr Hematol Oncol. 1995;12:55-59.

925. Ouachee-Chardin M, Elie C, de Saint Basile G, et al. Hematopoietic stem cell transplantation in hemophagocytic lymphohistiocytosis: a single-center report of 48 patients. Pediatrics. 2006;117:e743-e750.

926. Gallin JI. Neutrophil specific granule deficiency. Annu Rev Med. 1985;36:263-274.

927. Gombart AF, Koeffler HP. Neutrophil specific granule deficiency and mutations in the gene encoding transcription factor C/EBPε. Curr Opin Hematol. 2002;9:36-42.

928. Komiyama A, Morosawa H, Nakahata T, et al. Abnormal neutrophil maturation in a neutrophil defect with morphologic abnormality and impaired function. J Pediatr. 1979;94:19-25.

929. Ambruso DR, Sasada M, Nishiyama H, et al. Defective bactericidal activity and absence of specific granules in neutrophils from a patient with recurrent bacterial infections. J Clin Immunol. 1984;4:23-30.

930. Strauss RG, Bove KE, Jones JF, et al. An anomaly of neutrophil morphology with impaired function. N Engl J Med. 1974;290:278-284.

931. Boxer LA, Coates TD, Haak RA, et al. Lactoferrin deficiency associated with altered granulocyte function. N Engl J Med. 1982;307:404-410.

932. Parmley RT, Tzeng DY, Baehner RL, Boxer LA. Abnormal distribution of complex carbohydrates in neutrophils of a patient with lactoferrin deficiency. Blood. 1983;62:538-548.

933. Borregaard N, Boxer LA, Smolen JE, Tauber AI. Anomalous neutrophil granule distribution in a patient with lactoferrin deficiency: pertinence to the respiratory burst. Am J Hematol. 1985;18:255-260.

934. Parmley RT, Gilbert CS, Boxer LA. Abnormal peroxidase-positive granules in "specific granule" deficiency. Blood. 1989;73:838-844.

935. Lomax KJ, Leto TL, Nunoi H, et al. Recombinant 47-kD cytosol factor restores NADPH oxidase in chronic granulomatous disease. Science. 1989;245:409-412.

936. Petty HR, Francis JW, Todd RF III, et al. Neutrophil C3bi receptors: formation of membrane clusters during cell triggering requires intracellular granules. J Cell Physiol. 1987;133:235-242, 256.

937. Lomax KJ, Gallin JI, Rotrosen D, et al. Selective defect in myeloid cell lactoferrin gene expression in neutrophil specific granule deficiency. J Clin Invest. 1989;83:514-519.

938. Breton-Gorius J, Mason DY, Buriot D, et al. Lactoferrin deficiency as a consequence of a lack of specific granules in neutrophils from a patient with recurrent infections. Detection by immunoperoxidase staining for lactoferrin and cytochemical electron microscopy. Am J Pathol. 1980;99:413-428.

939. Gallin JI, Fletcher MP, Seligmann BE, et al. Human neutrophil-specific granule deficiency: a model to assess the role of neutrophil-specific granules in the evolution of the inflammatory response. Blood. 1982;59:1317-1329.

940. O'Shea JJ, Brown EJ, Seligmann BE, et al. Evidence for distinct intracellular pools of receptors for C3b and C3bi in human neutrophils. J Immunol. 1985;134:2580-2587.

941. Spitznagel JK, Cooper MR, McCall AE, et al. Selective deficiency of granules associated with lysozyme and lactoferrin in human polymorphs (PMN) with reduced microbicidal capacity. J Clin Invest. 1972;51:92a.

942. Tamura A, Agematsu K, Mori T, et al. A marked decrease in defensin mRNA in the only case of congenital neutrophil-specific granule deficiency reported in Japan. Int J Hematol. 1994;59:137-142.

943. Hibbs MS, Bainton DF. Human neutrophil gelatinase is a component of specific granules. J Clin Invest. 1989;84:1395-1402.

944. Rosenberg HF, Galin JI. Neutrophil-specific granule deficiency includes eosinophils. Blood. 1993;82:268-273.

945. Lekstrom-Himes J, Xanthopoulos KG. CCAAT/enhancer binding protein epsilon is critical for effective neutrophil-mediated response to inflammatory challenge. Blood. 1999;93:3096-3105.

946. Verbeek W, Lekstrom-Himes J, Park DJ, et al. Myeloid transcription factor C/EBPε is involved in the positive regulation of lactoferrin gene expression in neutrophils. Blood. 1999;94:3141-3150.

947. Lekstrom-Himes JA, Dorman SE, Kopar P, et al. Neutrophil-specific granule deficiency results from a novel mutation with loss of function of the transcription factor CCAAT/enhancer binding protein epsilon. J Exp Med. 1999;189:1847-1852.

948. Khanna-Gupta A, Zibello T, Sun H, et al. C/EBP epsilon mediates myeloid differentiation and is regulated by the CCAAT displacement protein (CDP/cut). Proc Natl Acad Sci U S A. 2001;98:8000-8005.

949. Todd RF III, Arnaout MA, Rosin RE, et al. Subcellular localization of the large subunit of Mo1 (Mo1; formerly gp110), a surface glycoprotein associated with adhesion. J Clin Invest. 1984;74:1280-1290.

950. Miller LJ, Bainton DF. Stimulated mobilization of monocyte Mac-1 and p150,95 adhesion proteins from an intracellular vesicular compartment to the cell surface. J Clin Invest. 1987;80:535-544.

951. Petrequin PR, Todd RF III, Devall LJ, et al. Association between gelatinase release and increased plasma membrane expression of the Mo1 glycoprotein. Blood. 1987;69:605-610.

952. Fletcher MP, Gallin JI. Human neutrophils contain an intracellular pool of putative receptors for the chemoattractant N-formyl-methionyl-leucyl-phenylalanine. Blood. 1983;62:792-799.

953. Kuriyama K, Tomonaga M, Matsuo T, et al. Diagnostic significance of detecting pseudo–Pelger-Huët anomalies and micro-megakaryocytes in myelodysplastic syndrome. Br J Haematol. 1986;63:665-669.

954. Dinauer MC. The phagocyte system and disorders of granulopoiesis and granulocyte function. In Nathan DG, Orkin SH, Ginsburg D, Look AT (eds). Nathan and Oski's Hematology of Infancy and Childhood, 6th ed. Philadelphia, WB Saunders, 2003, pp 923-1010.

955. Segal BH, Leto TL, Gallin JI, et al. Genetic, biochemical, and clinical features of chronic granulomatous disease. Medicine (Baltimore). 2000;79:170-200.

956. Roos D, de Boer M, Kuribayashi F, et al. Mutations in the X-linked and autosomal recessive forms of chronic granulomatous disease. Blood. 1996;87:1663-1681.

957. Winkelstein JA, Marino MC, Johnston RB Jr, et al. Chronic granulomatous disease. Report on a national registry of 368 patients. Medicine (Baltimore). 2000;79:155-169.

958. Heyworth PG, Cross AR, Curnutte JT. Chronic granulomatous disease. Curr Opin Immunol. 2003;15:578-584.

959. Dinauer MC. Chronic granulomatous disease and other disorders of phagocyte function. Hematology Am Soc Hematol Educ Program. 2005:89-95.

960. Berendes H, Bridges RA, Good RA. Fatal granulomatosis of childhood: clinical study of new syndrome. Minn Med. 1957;40:309-312.

961. Landing BH, Shirkey HS. Syndrome of recurrent infection and infiltration of viscera by pigmented lipid histiocytes. Pediatrics. 1957;20:431-438.

962. Bridges RA, Berendes H, Good RA. A fatal granulomatous disease of childhood. The clinical, pathological, and laboratory features of a new syndrome. Am J Dis Child. 1959;97:387-408.

963. Windhorst DB, Holmes B, Good RA. A newly defined X-linked trait in man with demonstration of the Lyon effect in carrier females. Lancet. 1967;1:737-739.

964. Johnston RB Jr, McMurry JS. Chronic familial granulomatosis: report of five cases and the literature. Am J Dis Child. 1967;114:370-378.

965. Clark RA, Malech HL, Gallin JI, et al. Genetic variants of chronic granulomatous disease: prevalence of deficiencies of two cytosolic components of the NADPH oxidase system. N Engl J Med. 1989;321:647-652.

966. Casimir C, Chetty M, Bohler M-C, et al. Identification of the defective NADPH-oxidase component in chronic granulomatous disease: A study of 57 European families. Eur J Clin Invest. 1992;22:403-406.

967. Curnutte JT. Molecular basis of the autosomal recessive forms of chronic granulomatous disease. Immunodefic Rev. 1992;3:149-172.

968. Newburger PE, Luscinskas FW, Ryan T, et al. Variant chronic granulomatous disease: modulation of the neutrophil by severe infection. Blood. 1986;68:914-919.

969. Roos D, de Boer M, Borregard N, et al. Chronic granulomatous disease with partial deficiency of cytochrome *b*558 and incomplete respiratory burst: variants of the X-linked, cytochrome *b*558–negative form of the disease. J Leukoc Biol. 1992;51:164-171.

970. Stossel TP, Root RK, Vaughan M. Phagocytosis in chronic granulomatous disease and the Chédiak-Higashi syndrome. N Engl J Med. 1972;286:120-123.

971. Gaither TA, Medley SR, Gallin JI, Frank MM. Studies of phagocytosis in chronic granulomatous disease. Inflammation. 1987;11:211-227.

972. Hasui M, Hirabayashi Y, Hattori K, Kobayashi Y. Increased phagocytic activity of polymorphonuclear leukocytes of chronic granulomatous disease as determined with flow cytometric assay. J Lab Clin Med. 1991;117:291-298.

973. Bohler MC, Seger RA, Mouy R, et al. A study of 25 patients with chronic granulomatous disease: a new classification by correlating respiratory burst, cytochrome *b*, and flavoprotein. J Clin Immunol. 1986;6:136-145.

974. Tauber AI, Borregaard N, Simons E, Wright J. Chronic granulomatous disease: a syndrome of phagocyte oxidase deficiencies. Medicine (Baltimore). 1983;62:286-309.

975. Forrest CB, Forehand JR, Axtell RA, et al. Clinical features and current management of chronic granulomatous disease. Hematol Oncol Clin North Am. 1988;2:253-266.

976. Babior BM, Woodman RC. Chronic granulomatous disease. Semin Hematol. 1990;27:247-259.

977. Johnston RB Jr, Newman SL. Chronic granulomatous disease. Pediatr Clin North Am. 1977;24:365-376.

978. Mouy R, Fischer A, Vilmer E, et al. Incidence, severity, and prevention of infections in chronic granulomatous disease. J Pediatr. 1989;114:555-560.

979. Hayakawa H, Kobayashi N, Yata J. Chronic granulomatous disease in Japan: a summary of the clinical features of 84 registered patients. Acta Paediatr Jpn. 1985;27:501-510.

980. Liese J, Kloos S, Jendrossek V, et al. Long-term follow-up and outcome of 39 patients with chronic granulomatous disease. J Pediatr. 2000;137:687-693.

981. Agudelo-Florez P, Prando-Andrade CC, Lopez JA, et al. Chronic granulomatous disease in Latin American patients: clinical spectrum and molecular genetics. Pediatr Blood Cancer. 2006;46:243-252.

982. Mellor AL, Munn DH. IDO expression by dendritic cells: tolerance and tryptophan catabolism. Nat Rev Immunol. 2004;4:762-774.

983. Romani L, Fallarino F, De Luca A, et al. Defective tryptophan catabolism underlies inflammation in mouse chronic granulomatous disease. Nature. 2008;451:211-215.

984. Styrt B, Klempner MS. Late-presenting variant of chronic granulomatous disease. Pediatr Infect Dis. 1984;3:556-559.

985. Chusid MJ, Parrillo JE, Fauci AS. Chronic granulomatous disease: diagnosis in a 27-year-old man with *Mycobacterium fortuitum*. JAMA. 1975;233:1295-1296.

986. Cazzola M, Sacchi F, Pagani A, et al. X-linked chronic granulomatous disease in an adult woman. Evidence for a cell selection favoring neutrophils expressing the mutant allele. Haematologica. 1985;70:291-295.

987. Dilworth JA, Mandell GL. Adults with chronic granulomatous disease of "childhood." Am J Med. 1977;63:233-243.

988. Schapiro BL, Newburger PE, Klempner MS, Dinauer MC. Chronic granulomatous disease presenting in a 69-year-old man. N Engl J Med. 1991;325:1786-1790.

989. Liese JG, Jendrossek V, Jansson A, et al. Chronic granulomatous disease in adults. Lancet. 1996;347:220-223.

990. Ramanuja S, Wolf KM, Sadat MA, et al. Newly diagnosed chronic granulomatous disease in a 53-year-old woman with Crohn disease. Ann Allergy Asthma Immunol. 2005;95:204-209.

991. Gallin JI, Buescher ES, Seligmann BE, et al. Recent advances in chronic granulomatous disease. Ann Intern Med. 1983;99:657-674.

992. Cohen MS, Isturiz RE, Malech HL, et al. Fungal infection in chronic granulomatous disease. The importance of the phagocyte in defense against fungi. Am J Med. 1981;71:59-66.

993. Almyroudis NG, Holland SM, Segal BH. Invasive aspergillosis in primary immunodeficiencies. Med Mycol. 2005;43(Suppl 1):S247-S259.

994. Segal BH, DeCarlo ES, Kwon-Chung KJ, et al. *Aspergillus nidulans* infection in chronic granulomatous disease. Medicine (Baltimore). 1998;77:345-354.

995. Bylund J, Campsall PA, Ma RC, et al. *Burkholderia cenocepacia* induces neutrophil necrosis in chronic granulomatous disease. J Immunol. 2005;174:3562-3569.

996. Renella R, Perez JM, Chollet-Martin S, et al. *Burkholderia pseudomallei* infection in chronic granulomatous disease. Eur J Pediatr. 2006;165:175-177.

997. Phillips P, Forbes JC, Speert DP. Disseminated infection with *Pseudallescheria boydii* in a patient with chronic granulomatous disease: response to gamma-interferon plus antifungal chemotherapy. Pediatr Infect Dis. 1991;10:536-539.

998. Schwartz DA. Sporothrix tenosynovitis—differential diagnosis of granulomatous inflammatory disease of the joints. J Rheumatol. 1989;16:550-553.

999. Sorensen RU, Jacobs MR, Shurin SB. *Chromobacterium violaceum* adenitis acquired in the northern United States as a complication of chronic granulomatous disease. Pediatr Infect Dis. 1985;4:701-702.

1000. Macher AM, Casale TB, Fauci AS. Chronic granulomatous disease of childhood and *Chromobacterium violaceum* infections in the southeastern United States. Ann Intern Med. 1982;97:51-55.

1001. Wenger JD, Hollis DG, Weaver RE, et al. Infection caused by *Francisella philomiragia* (formerly *Yersinia philomiragia*). A newly recognized human pathogen. Ann Intern Med. 1990;110:888-892.

1002. Kenney RT, Kwon-Chung KJ, Witebsky FG, et al. Invasive infection with *Sarcinosporon inkin* in a patient with chronic granulomatous disease. Am J Clin Pathol. 1990;94:344-350.

1003. Pedersen FK, Johansen KS, Rosenkvist J, et al. Refractory *Pneumocytis carinii* infection in chronic granulomatous disease: successful treatment with granulocytes. Pediatrics. 1979;64:935-938.

1004. Adinoff AD, Johnston RB Jr, Dolen J, South MA. Chronic granulomatous disease and *Pneumocytis carinii* pneumonia. Pediatrics. 1982;69:133-134.

1005. Jacob CM, Pastorino AC, Azevedo AM, et al. *Mycobacterium bovis* dissemination (BCG strain) among immunodeficient Brazilian infants. J Invest Allergol Clin Immunol. 1996;6:202-206.

1006. Ohga S, Ikeuchi K, Kadoya R, et al. Intrapulmonary *Mycobacterium avium* infection as the first manifestation of chronic granulomatous disease. J Infect. 1997;34:147-150.

1007. Greenberg DE, Ding L, Zelazny AM, et al. A novel bacterium associated with lymphadenitis in a patient with chronic granulomatous disease. PLoS Pathog. 2006;2:e28.

1008. Mulholland MW, Delaney JP, Simmons RL. Gastrointestinal complications of chronic granulomatous disease of childhood: surgical implications. Surgery. 1983;94:569-575.

1009. Barton LL, Moussa SL, Villar RG, Hulett RL. Gastrointestinal complications of chronic granulomatous disease: case report and literature review. Clin Pediatr (Phila). 1998;37:231-236.

1010. Lublin M, Bartlett DL, Danforth DN, et al. Hepatic abscess in patients with chronic granulomatous disease. Ann Surg. 2002;235:383-391.

1011. Sponseller PD, Malech HL, McCarthy EF Jr, et al. Skeletal involvement in children who have chronic granulomatous disease. J Bone Joint Surg Am. 1991;73:37-51.

1012. Sirinavin S, Techasaensiri C, Benjaponpitak S, et al. Invasive *Chromobacterium violaceum* infection in children: case report and review. Pediatr Infect Dis J. 2005;24:559-561.

1013. Mandell GL, Hook EW. Leukocyte bactericidal activity in chronic granulomatous disease: correlation of bacterial hydrogen peroxide production and susceptibility in intracellular killing. J Bacteriol. 1969;100:531-532.

1014. Gabay JE, Scott RW, Campanelli D, et al. Antibiotic proteins of human polymorphonuclear leukocytes. Proc Natl Acad Sci U S A. 1989;86:5610-5614.

1015. Odell EW, Segal AW. Killing of pathogens associated with chronic granulomatous disease by the non-oxidative microbicidal mechanisms of human neutrophils. J Med Microbiol. 1991;34:129-135.

1016. Johnston RB Jr, Baehner RL. Chronic granulomatous disease: correlation between pathogenesis and clinical findings. Pediatrics. 1971;48:730-739.

1017. Kobayashi SD, Voyich JM, Braughton KR, et al. Gene expression profiling provides insight into the pathophysiology of chronic granulomatous disease. J Immunol. 2004;172:636-643.

1018. Lekstrom-Himes JA, Kuhns DB, Alvord WG, Gallin JI. Inhibition of human neutrophil IL-8 production by hydrogen peroxide and dysregulation in chronic granulomatous disease. J Immunol. 2005;174:411-417.

1019. Morgenstern DE, Gifford MA, Li LL, et al. Absence of respiratory burst in X-linked chronic granulomatous disease mice leads to abnormalities in both host defense and inflammatory response to *Aspergillus fumigatus*. J Exp Med. 1997;185:207-218.

1020. Gallin JI, Buescher ES, Seligmann BE, et al. NIH conference. Recent advances in chronic granulomatous disease. Ann Intern Med. 1983;99:657-674.

1021. Segal AW. The NADPH oxidase and chronic granulomatous disease. Mol Med Today. 1996;2:129-135.

1022. Renner WR, Johnson JF, Lichtenstein JE, Kirks DR. Esophageal inflammation and stricture: complication of chronic granulomatous disease of childhood. Radiology. 1991;178:189-191.

1023. Hiller N, Fisher D, Abrahamov A, Blinder G. Esophageal involvement in chronic granulomatous disease. Pediatr Radiol. 1995;25:308-309.

1024. Marciano BE, Rosenzweig SD, Kleiner DE, et al. Gastrointestinal involvement in chronic granulomatous disease. Pediatrics. 2004;114:462-468.

1025. Rosh JR, Tang HB, Mayer L, et al. Treatment of intractable gastrointestinal manifestations of chronic granulomatous disease with cyclosporine. J Pediatr. 1995;126:143-145.

1026. Aliabadi H, Gonzalez R, Quie PG. Urinary tract disorders in patients with chronic granulomatous disease. N Engl J Med. 1989;321:706-708.

1027. Bauer SB, Kogan SJ. Vesical manifestations of chronic granulomatous disease in children. Its relation to eosinophilic cystitis. Urology. 1991;37:463-466.

1028. Cyr WL, Johnson H, Balfour J. Granulomatous cystitis as a manifestation of chronic granulomatous disease of childhood. J Urol. 1973;110:357-359.

1029. Southwick FS, Van der Meer JWM. Recurrent cystitis and bladder mass in two adults with chronic granulomatous disease. Ann Intern Med. 1988;109:118-121.

1030. Barese CN, Goebel WS, Dinauer MC. Gene therapy for chronic granulomatous disease. Exp Opin Biol Ther. 2004;4:1423-1434.

1031. Walther MM, Malech H, Berman A, et al. The urological manifestations of chronic granulomatous disease. J Urol. 1992;147:1314-1318.

1032. Windhorst DB, Good RA. Dermatologic manifestations of fatal granulomatous disease of childhood. Arch Dermatol. 1971;103:351-357.

1033. Cohen MS, Leong PA, Simpson DM. Phagocytic cells in periodontal defense: periodontal status of patients with chronic granulomatous disease of childhood. J Periodontol. 1985;56:611-617.

1034. Martyn LJ, Lischner HW, Pileggi AJ, Harley RD. Chorioretinal lesions in familial chronic granulomatous disease of childhood. Am J Ophthalmol. 1972;73:403-418.

1035. Valluri S, Chu FC, Smith ME. Ocular pathologic findings of chronic granulomatous disease of childhood. Am J Ophthalmol. 1995;120:120-123.

1036. Hadfield MG, Ghatak NR, Laine FJ, et al. Brain lesions in chronic granulomatous disease. Acta Neuropathol. 1991;81:467-470.

1037. Walker DH, Okiye G. Chronic granulomatous disease involving the central nervous system. Pediatr Pathol. 1983;1:159-167.

1038. Van Rhenen DJ, Koolen MI, Feltkamp-Vroom TM, Weening RS. Immune complex glomerulonephritis in chronic granulomatous disease. Case report of an eighteen-year-old girl. Acta Med Scand. 1979;206:233-237.

1039. Frifelt JJ, Schonheyder H, Valerius NH, et al. Chronic granulomatous disease associated with chronic glomerulonephritis. Acta Paediatr Scand. 1985;74:152-157.

1040. Stalder JF, Dreno B, Bureau B, Hakim J. Discoid lupus erythematosus–like lesions in an autosomal form of chronic granulomatous disease. Br J Dermatol. 1986;114:251-254.

1041. Smitt JHS, Bos JD, Weening RS, Krieg SR. Discoid lupus erythematosus–like skin changes in patients with autosomal recessive chronic granulomatous disease. Arch Dermatol. 1990;126:1656-1657.

1042. Manzi S, Urbach AH, McCune AB, et al. Systemic lupus erythematosus in a boy with chronic granulomatous disease: case report and review of the literature. Arthritis Rheum. 1991;34:101-105.

1043. Schmitt CP, Scharer K, Waldherr R, et al. Glomerulonephritis associated with chronic granulomatous disease and systemic lupus erythematosus. Nephrol Dial Transplant. 1995;10:891-895.

1044. Lee BW, Yap HK. Poly arthritis resembling juvenile rheumatoid arthritis in a girl with chronic granulomatous disease. Arthritis Rheum. 1994;37:773-776.

1045. De Ravin SS, Naumann N, Robinson MR, et al. Sarcoidosis in chronic granulomatous disease. Pediatrics. 2006;117:e590-e595.

1046. Bleesing JJ, Souto-Carneiro MM, Savage WJ, et al. Patients with chronic granulomatous disease have a reduced peripheral blood memory B cell compartment. J Immunol. 2006;176:7096-7103.

1047. Jackson SH, Devadas S, Kwon J, et al. T cells express a phagocyte-type NADPH oxidase that is activated after T cell receptor stimulation. Nat Immunol. 2004;5:818-827.

1048. Woodman RC, Newburger PE, Anklesaria P, et al. A new X-linked variant of chronic granulomatous disease characterized by the existence of a normal clone of respiratory burst–competent phagocytic cells. Blood. 1995;85:231-241.

1049. Foster CB, Lehrnbecher T, Mol F, et al. Host defense molecule polymorphisms influence the risk for immune-mediated complications in chronic granulomatous disease. J Clin Invest. 1998;102:2146-2155.

1050. Weening RS, Corbeel L, De Boer M, et al. Cytochrome *b* deficiency in an autosomal form of chronic granulomatous disease. A third form of chronic granulomatous disease recognized by monocyte hybridization. J Clin Invest. 1985;75:915-920.

1051. Johnston RB, Harbecker RJ, Johnston RB Jr. Recurrent severe infections in a girl with apparently variable expression of mosaicism for chronic granulomatous disease. J Pediatr. 1985;106:50-55.

1052. Ochs HD, Igo RP. The NBT slide test: a simple screening method for detecting chronic granulomatous disease and female carriers. J Pediatr. 1973;83:77-82.

1053. Meerhof LJ, Roos D. Heterogeneity in chronic granulomatous disease detected with an improved nitroblue tetrazolium slide test. J Leukoc Biol. 1986;39:699-711.

1054. Roesler J, Hecht M, Freihorst J, et al. Diagnosis of chronic granulomatous disease and of its mode of inheritance by dihydrorhodamine 123 and flow microcytofluorometry. Eur J Pediatr. 1991;150:161-165.

1055. Rothe G, Emmendorffer A, Oser A, et al. Flow cytometric measurements of the respiratory burst activity of phagocytes using dihydrorhodamine 123. J Immunol Methods. 1991;138:133-135.

1056. Hassan NF, Campbell DE, Douglas SD. Phorbol myristate acetate induced oxidation of 2′,7′-dichlorofluorescein by neutrophils from patients with chronic granulomatous disease. J Leukoc Biol. 1988;43:317-322.

1057. Windhorst DB, Page AR, Holmes B, et al. The pattern of genetic transmission of the leukocyte defect in fatal granulomatous disease of childhood. J Clin Invest. 1968;47:1026-1034.

1058. Lyon MF. Sex chromatin and gene action in the mammalian X-chromosome. Am J Hum Genet. 1962;14:135-148.

1059. Beutler E, Yeh M, Fairbans VF. The normal human female as a mosaic of X-chromosome activity: studies using the gene for G-6-PD deficiency as a marker. Proc Natl Acad Sci U S A. 1962;48:9-16.

1060. Newburger PE, Malawista SE, Dinauer MC, et al. Chronic granulomatous disease and glutathione peroxidase deficiency, revisited. Blood. 1994;84:3861-3869.

1061. Rupec RA, Petropoulou T, Belohradsky BH, et al. Lupus erythematosus tumidus and chronic discoid lupus erythematosus in carriers of X-linked chronic granulomatous disease. Eur J Dermatol. 2000;10:184-189.

1062. Strate M, Brandup F, Wang P. Discoid lupus erythematosus–like skin lesions in a patient with autosomal recessive chronic granulomatous disease. Clin Genet. 1986;30:184-190.

1063. Dinauer MC, Pierce EA, Bruns GAP, et al. Human neutrophil cytochrome *b* light chain (p22-*phox*): gene structure, chromosomal location, and mutations in cytochrome-negative autosomal recessive chronic granulomatous disease. J Clin Invest. 1990;86:1729-1737.

1064. Volpp BD, Nauseef WM, Donelson JE, et al. Cloning of the cDNA and functional expression of the 47-kilodalton cytosolic component of the human neutrophil respiratory burst oxidase. Proc Natl Acad Sci U S A. 1989;86:7195-7199.

1065. Ishibashi F, Nunoi H, Endo F, et al. Statistical and mutational analysis of chronic granulomatous disease in Japan with special reference to gp91-phox and p22-phox deficiency. Hum Genet. 2000;106:473-481.

1066. Borregaard N, Staehr-Johansen K, Taudorff E, Wandall JH. Cytochrome *b* is present in neutrophils from patients with chronic granulomatous disease. Lancet. 1979;1:949-951.

1067. Segal AW, Cross AR, Garcia RC, et al. Absence of cytochrome *b*-245 in chronic granulomatous disease: a multicenter European evaluation of its incidence and relevance. N Engl J Med. 1983;308:245-251.

1068. Groemping Y, Rittinger K. Activation and assembly of the NADPH oxidase: a structural perspective. Biochem J. 2005;386:401-416.

1069. Segal AW. Absence of both cytochrome *b*-245 subunits from neutrophils in X-linked chronic granulomatous disease. Nature. 1987;326:88-92.

1070. Parkos CA, Dinauer MC, Jesaitis AJ, et al. Absence of both the 91-kD and 22-kD subunits of human neutrophil cytochrome *b* in two genetic forms of chronic granulomatous disease. Blood. 1989;73:1416-1420.

1071. Baehner RL, Kunkel LM, Monaco AP, et al. DNA linkage analysis of X chromosome–linked chronic granulomatous disease. Proc Natl Sci Acad U S A. 1986;83:3398-3401.

1072. Skalnik DG, Strauss EC, Orkin SH. CCAAT displacement protein as a repressor of the myelomonocytic-specific gp91-*phox* gene promoter. J Biol Chem. 1991;266:16736-16744.

1073. Lien LL, Lee Y, Orkin SH. Regulation of the myeloid-cell–expressed human gp91-phox gene as studied by transfer of yeast artificial chromosome clones into embryonic stem cells: suppression of a variegated cellular pattern of expression requires a full complement of distant cis elements. Mol Cell Biol. 1997;17:2279-2290.

1074. Rae J, Newburger PE, Dinauer MC, et al. X-Linked chronic granulomatous disease: mutations in the *CYBB* gene encoding the gp91-phox component of respiratory-burst oxidase. Am J Hum Genet. 1998;62:1320-1331.

1075. Heyworth PG, Curnutte JT, Rae J, et al. Hematologically important mutations: X-linked chronic granulomatous disease (second update). Blood Cells Mol Dis. 2001;27:16-26.

1076. Roos D. X-CGDbase: a database of X-CGD–causing mutations. Immunol Today. 1996;17:517-521.

1077. Azuma H, Oomi H, Sasaki K, et al. A new mutation in exon 12 of the gp91-phox gene leading to cytochrome *b*–positive X-linked chronic granulomatous disease. Blood. 1995;85:3274-3277.

1078. Leusen JHW, Bolscher GJM, Hilarius PM, et al. 156Pro → Gln substitution in the light chain of cytochrome. J Exp Med. 1994;180:2011-2015.

1079. Dinauer MC, Pierce EA, Erickson RW, et al. Point mutation in the cytoplasmic domain of the neutrophil p22-*phox* cytochrome *b* subunit is associated with a nonfunctional NADPH oxidase and chronic granulomatous disease. Proc Natl Acad Sci U S A. 1991;88:11231-11235.

1080. Cross AR, Curnutte JT. The cytosolic activating factors p47^{phox} and p67^{phox} have distinct roles in the regulation of electron flow in NADPH oxidase. J Biol Chem. 1995;270:6543-6548.

1081. Dinauer MC, Curnutte JT, Rosen H, Orkin SH. A missense mutation in the neutrophil cytochrome *b* heavy chain in cytochrome-positive X-linked chronic granulomatous disease. J Clin Invest. 1989;84:2012-2016.

1082. Francke U, Ochs HD, DeMartinville B, et al. Minor Xp21 chromosome deletion in a male associated with expression of Duchenne muscular dystrophy, chronic granulomatous disease, retinitis pigmentosa, and McLeod syndrome. Am J Hum Genet. 1985;37:250-267.

1083. Kousseff B. Linkage between chronic granulomatous disease and Duchenne's muscular dystrophy. Am J Dis Child. 1981;135:1149.

1084. Frey D, Machler M, Seger R, et al. Gene deletion in a patient with chronic granulomatous disease and McLeod syndrome: fine mapping of the Xk gene locus. Blood. 1988;71:252-255.

1085. De Saint-Basile G, Bohler MC, Fischer A, et al. Xp21 DNA microdeletion in a patient with chronic granulomatous disease, retinitis pigmentosa, and McLeod phenotype. Hum Genet. 1988;80:85-89.

1086. Marsh WL, Redman CM. The Kell blood group system: a review. Transfusion. 1990;30:158-167.

1087. Russo D, Wu X, Redman CM, Lee S. Expression of Kell blood group protein in nonerythroid tissues. Blood. 2000;96:340-346.

1088. Kuribayashi F, Kumatori A, Suzuki S, et al. Human peripheral eosinophils have a specific mechanism to express gp91-phox, the large subunit of cytochrome b$_{558}$. Biochem Biophys Res Commun. 1995;2009:146-152.

1089. Suzuki S, Kumatori A, Haagen IA, et al. PU.1 as an essential activator for the expression of gp91^{phox} gene in human peripheral neutrophils, monocytes, and B lymphocytes. Proc Natl Acad Sci U S A. 1998;95:6085-6090.

1090. Eklund EA, Skalnik DG. Characterization of a gp91-phox promoter element that is required for interferon gamma–induced transcription. J Biol Chem. 1995;270:8267-8273.

1091. Zhu Q, Zhang M, Rawlings DJ, et al. Detection within the Src homology domain 3 of Bruton's tyrosine kinase resulting in X-linked agammaglobulinemia (XLA). J Exp Med. 1994;180:461-470.

1092. Bromberg Y, Pick E. Unsaturated fatty acids stimulate NADPH-dependent superoxide production by cell-free system derived from macrophages. Cell Immunol. 1984;88:213-221.

1093. Heyneman RA, Vercauteren RE. Activation of a NADPH oxidase from horse polymorphonuclear leukocytes in a cell-free system. J Leukoc Biol. 1984;36:751-759.

1094. Curnutte JT. Activation of human neutrophil nicotinamide adenine dinucleotide phosphate, reduced (triphosphopyridine nucleotide, reduced) oxidase by arachidonic acid in a cell-free system. J Clin Invest. 1985;75:1740-1743.

1095. McPhail LC, Shirley PS, Clayton CC, Snyderman R. Activation of the respiratory burst enzyme from human neutrophils in a cell-free system. J Clin Invest. 1985;75:1735-1739.

1096. Nunoi H, Rotrosen D, Gallin JI, Malech HL. Two forms of autosomal chronic granulomatous disease lack distinct neutrophil cytosol factors. Science. 1988;242:1298-1301.

1097. Curnutte JT, Scott PJ, Mayo LA. Cytosolic components of the respiratory burst oxidase: resolution of four components, two of which are missing in complementing types of chronic granulomatous disease. Proc Natl Acad Sci U S A. 1989;86:825-829.

1098. Francke U, Ochs HD, Darras BT, Swaroop A. Origin of mutations in two families with X-linked chronic granulomatous disease. Blood. 1990;76:602-606.

1099. Chanock SJ, Barrett DM, Curnutte JT, Orkins SH. Gene structure of the cytosolic component, phox-47 and mutations in autosomal recessive chronic granulomatous disease. Blood. 1991;78:165a.

1100. Casimir CM, Bu-Ghanim HN, Rodaway ARF, et al. Autosomal recessive chronic granulomatous disease caused by deletion at a dinucleotide repeat. Proc Natl Acad Sci U S A. 1991;88:2753-2757.

1101. Noack D, Rae J, Cross AR, et al. Autosomal recessive chronic granulomatous disease caused by defects in NCF-1, the gene encoding the phagocyte p47-phox: mutations not arising in the NCF-1 pseudogenes. Blood. 2001;97:305-311.

1102. Gorlach A, Lee PL, Roesler J, et al. A p47-phox pseudogene carries the most common mutation causing p47-phox–deficient chronic granulomatous disease. J Clin Invest. 1997;100:1907-1918.

1103. Heyworth PG, Noack D, Cross AR. Identification of a novel NCF-1 (p47-phox) pseudogene not containing the signature GT deletion: significance for A47⁰ chronic granulomatous disease carrier detection. Blood. 2002; 100:1845-1851.

1104. Roesler J, Curnutte JT, Rae J, et al. Recombination events between the p47-phox gene and its highly homologous pseudogenes are the main cause of autosomal recessive chronic granulomatous disease. Blood. 2000;95: 2150-2156.

1105. Francke U, Hsieh CL, Foellmer BE, et al. Genes for two autosomal recessive forms of chronic granulomatous disease assigned to 1q25 (NCF2) and 7q11.23 (NCF1). Am J Hum Genet. 1990;47:483-492.

1106. Kenney RT, Malech HL, Leto TL. Structural characterization of the p67-*phox* gene [abstract]. Clin Res. 1992; 40:261a.

1107. De Boer M, Bolscher BGJM. Splice site mutations are a common cause of X-linked chronic granulomatous disease. Blood. 1992;80:1553-1558.

1108. Tanugi-Cholley LC, Issartel JP, Lunardi J, et al. A mutation located at the 5′ splice junction sequence of intron 3 in the p67^phox gene causes the lack of p67^phox mRNA in a patient with chronic granulomatous disease. Blood. 1995;85:242-249.

1109. Patino PJ, Rae J, Noack D, et al. Molecular characterization of autosomal recessive chronic granulomatous disease caused by a defect of the nicotinamide adenine dinucleotide phosphate (reduced form) oxidase component p67-phox. Blood. 1999;94:2505-2514.

1110. Noack D, Rae J, Cross AR, et al. Autosomal recessive chronic granulomatous disease caused by novel mutations in NCF-2, the gene encoding the p67-phox component of phagocyte NADPH oxidase. Hum Genet. 1999;105:460-467.

1111. Bonizzato A, Russo MP, Donini M, Dusi S. Identification of a double mutation (D160V-K161E) in the p67^phox gene of a chronic granulomatous disease patient. Biochem Biophys Res Commun. 1997;231:861-863.

1112. Leusen JH, de Klein A, Hilarius PM, et al. Disturbed interaction of p21-rac with mutated p67-phox causes chronic granulomatous disease. J Exp Med. 1996;184: 1243-1249.

1113. Vowells SJ, Sekhsaria S, Malech HL, et al. Flow cytometric analysis of the granulocyte respiratory burst: a comparison study of fluorescent probes. J Immunol Methods. 1995;178:89-97.

1114. Vowells SJ, Fleisher TA, Sekhsaria S, et al. Genotype-dependent variability in flow cytometric evaluation of reduced nicotinamide adenine dinucleotide phosphate oxidase function in patients with chronic granulomatous disease. J Pediatr. 1996;128: 104-107.

1115. Baehner RL, Nathan DG. Quantitative nitroblue tetrazolium test in chronic granulomatous disease. N Engl J Med. 1968;278:971-976.

1116. Segal AW. Nitroblue-tetrazolium tests. Lancet. 1974;2: 1248-1252.

1117. Finn A, Hadzic N, Morgan G, et al. Prognosis of chronic granulomatous disease. Arch Dis Child. 1990;65:942-945.

1118. Cale CM, Jones AM, Goldblatt D. Follow up of patients with chronic granulomatous disease diagnosed since 1990. Clin Exp Immunol. 2000;120:351-355.

1119. Marciano BE, Wesley R, De Carlo ES, et al. Long-term interferon-gamma therapy for patients with chronic granulomatous disease. Clin Infect Dis. 2004;39:692-699.

1120. Margolis DM, Melnic DA, Alling DW, Gallin JI. Trimethoprim-sulfamethoxazole prophylaxis in the management of chronic granulomatous disease. J Infect Dis. 1990;162:723-726.

1121. Chusid MJ, Gelfand JA, Nutter C, Fauci AS. Pulmonary aspergillosis, inhalation of contaminated marijuana smoke, chronic granulomatous disease. Ann Intern Med. 1975;82:682-683.

1122. Conrad DJ, Warnock M, Blanc P, et al. Microgranulomatous aspergillosis after shoveling wood chips: report of a fatal outcome in a patient with chronic granulomatous disease. Am J Ind Med. 1992;22:411-418.

1123. Mouy R, Veber F, Blanche S, et al. Long-term itraconazole prophylaxis against *Aspergillus* infections in thirty-two patients with chronic granulomatous disease. J Pediatr. 1994;125:998-1002.

1124. Gallin JI, Alling DW, Malech HL, et al. Itraconazole to prevent fungal infections in chronic granulomatous disease. N Engl J Med. 2003;348:2416-2422.

1125. Gallin JI, Malech HL, Weening RS, et al. A controlled trial of interferon gamma to prevent infection in chronic granulomatous disease. N Engl J Med. 1991;324: 509-516.

1126. Weening RS, Leitz GJ, Seger RA. Recombinant human interferon-gamma in patients with chronic granulomatous disease—European follow up study. Eur J Pediatr. 1995;154:295-298.

1127. Bemiller LS, Roberts DH, Starko KM, Curnutte JT. Safety and effectiveness of long-term interferon gamma therapy in patients with chronic granulomatous disease. Blood Cells Mol Dis. 1995;21:239-247.

1128. A controlled trial of interferon gamma to prevent infection in chronic granulomatous disease. The International Chronic Granulomatous Disease Cooperative Study Group. N Engl J Med. 1991;324:509-516.

1129. Schiff DE, Rae J, Martin TR, et al. Increased phagocyte Fc gammaRI expression and improved Fc gamma-receptor–mediated phagocytosis after in vivo recombinant human interferon-gamma treatment of normal human subjects. Blood. 1997;90:3187-3194.

1130. Woodman RC, Erickson RW, Rae J, et al. Prolonged recombinant interferon-gamma therapy in chronic granulomatous disease: evidence against enhanced neutrophil oxidase activity. Blood. 1992;79:1558-1562.

1131. Ezekowitz RAB, Orkin SH, Newburger PE. Recombinant interferon gamma augments phagocyte superoxide production and X-chronic granulomatous disease gene expression in X-linked variant chronic granulomatous disease. J Clin Invest. 1987;80:1009-1016.

1132. Ezekowitz RB, Dinauer MC, Jaffe HS, et al. Partial correction of the phagocyte defect in patients with X-linked chronic granulomatous disease by subcutaneous interferon gamma. N Engl J Med. 1988;319:146-151.

1133. Sechler JMG, Malech HL, White CJ, Gallin JI. Recombinant human interferon-gamma reconstitutes defective phagocyte function in patients with chronic granulomatous disease. Proc Natl Acad Sci U S A. 1988;85:4374-4878.

1134. Ezekowitz RAB, Sieff CA, Dinauer MC, et al. Restoration of phagocyte function by interferon-gamma in X-linked chronic granulomatous disease occurs at the level of a progenitor cell. Blood. 1990;76:2443-2448.

1135. Johnson LB, Kauffman CA. Voriconazole: a new triazole antifungal agent. Clin Infect Dis. 2003;36:630-637.

1136. Herbrecht R, Denning DW, Patterson TF, et al. Voriconazole versus amphotericin B for primary therapy of invasive aspergillosis. N Engl J Med. 2002;347:408-415.

1137. Spanakis EK, Aperis G, Mylonakis E. New agents for the treatment of fungal infections: clinical efficacy and gaps in coverage. Clin Infect Dis. 2006;43:1060-1068.

1138. Emmendorffer A, Lohmann-Mathes ML, Roesler J. Kinetics of transfused neutrophils in peripheral blood and BAL fluid of a patient with variant X-linked chronic granulomatous disease. Eur J Haematol. 1991;47:246-252.

1139. Bielorai B, Toren A, Wolach B, et al. Successful treatment of invasive aspergillosis in chronic granulomatous disease by granulocyte transfusions followed by peripheral blood stem cell transplantation. Bone Marrow Transplant. 2000;26:1025-1028.

1140. Chin TW, Stiehm ER, Falloon J, Gallin JI. Corticosteroids in treatment of obstructive lesions of chronic granulomatous disease. J Pediatr. 1987;111:349-352.

1141. Quie PG, Belani KK. Corticosteroids for chronic granulomatous disease. J Pediatr. 1987;111:393-394.

1142. Fischer A, Segal AW, Weening RS. The management of chronic granulomatous disease. Eur J Pediatr. 1993;152:896-899.

1143. Danziger RN, Goren AT, Becker J, et al. Outpatient management with oral corticosteroid therapy for obstructive conditions in chronic granulomatous disease. J Pediatr. 1993;122:303-305.

1144. Schettini F, De Mattia D, Manzionna MM, et al. Bone marrow transplantation for chronic granulomatous disease associated with cytochrome b deficiency [letter]. Pediatr Hematol Oncol. 1987;4:277-279.

1145. Kamani N, August CS, Campbell DE, et al. Marrow transplantation in chronic granulomatous disease: An update, with 6-year follow-up. J Pediatr. 1988;113:697-700.

1146. O'Reilly RJ, Brochstein J, Dinsmore R, Kirkpatrick D. Marrow transplantation for congenital disorders. Semin Hematol. 1984;21:188-221.

1147. Del Giudice I, Iori AP, Mengarelli A, et al. Allogeneic stem cell transplant from HLA-identical sibling for chronic granulomatous disease and review of the literature. Ann Hematol. 2003;82:189-192.

1148. Sastry J, Kakakios A, Tugwell H, Shaw PJ. Allogeneic bone marrow transplantation with reduced intensity conditioning for chronic granulomatous disease complicated by invasive Aspergillus infection. Pediatr Blood Cancer. 2006;47:327-329.

1149. Seger RA, Gungor T, Belohradsky BH, et al. Treatment of chronic granulomatous disease with myeloablative conditioning and an unmodified hemopoietic allograft: a survey of the European experience, 1985-2000. Blood. 2002;100:4344-4350.

1150. Horwitz ME, Barrett AJ, Brown MR, et al. Treatment of chronic granulomatous disease with nonmyeloablative conditioning and a T-cell–depleted hematopoietic allograft. N Engl J Med. 2001;344:881-888.

1151. Gungor T, Halter J, Klink A, et al. Successful low toxicity hematopoietic stem cell transplantation for high-risk adult chronic granulomatous disease patients. Transplantation. 2005;79:1596-1606.

1152. Bhattacharya A, Slatter M, Curtis A, et al. Successful umbilical cord blood stem cell transplantation for chronic granulomatous disease. Bone Marrow Transplant. 2003;31:403-405.

1153. Suzuki N, Hatakeyama N, Yamamoto M, et al. Treatment of McLeod phenotype chronic granulomatous disease with reduced-intensity conditioning and unrelated-donor umbilical cord blood transplantation. Int J Hematol. 2007;85:70-72.

1154. Mardiney M 3rd, Jackson SH, Spratt SK, et al. Enhanced host defense after gene transfer in the murine p47^{phox}-deficient model of chronic granulomatous disease. Blood. 1997;89:2268-2275.

1155. Dinauer MC, Gifford MA, Pech N, et al. Variable correction of host defense following gene transfer and bone marrow transplantation in murine X-linked chronic granulomatous disease. Blood. 2001;97:3785-3745.

1156. Bjorgvinsdottir H, Ding C, Pech N, et al. Retroviral-mediated gene transfer of gp91^{phox} into bone marrow cells rescues defect in host defense against Aspergillus fumigatus in murine X-linked chronic granulomatous disease. Blood. 1997;89:41-48.

1157. Goebel WS, Mark LA, Billings SD, et al. Gene correction reduces cutaneous inflammation and granuloma formation in murine X-linked chronic granulomatous disease. J Invest Dermatol. 2005;125:705-710.

1158. Kohn DB. Gene therapy using hematopoietic stem cells. Curr Opin Mol Ther. 1999;1:437-442.

1159. Stein S, Siler U, Ott MG, et al. Gene therapy for chronic granulomatous disease. Curr Opin Mol Ther. 2006;8:415-422.

1160. Malech HL, Maples PB, Whiting-Theobald, N, et al. Prolonged production of NADPH oxidase-corrected granulocytes after gene therapy of chronic granulomatous disease. Proc Natl Acad Sci U S A. 1997;94:12133-12138.

1161. Ott MG, Schmidt M, Schwarzwaelder K, et al. Correction of X-linked chronic granulomatous disease by gene therapy, augmented by insertional activation of MDS1-EVI1, PRDM16 or SETBP1. Nat Med. 2006;12:401-409.

1162. Gray GR, Stamatoyannopoulos G, Naiman SC, et al. Neutrophil dysfunction, chronic granulomatous disease, and non-spherocytic haemolytic anaemia caused by complete deficiency of glucose-6-phosphate dehydrogenase. Lancet. 1973;2:530-534.

1163. Baehner RL, Johnston RB, Nathan DG. Comparative study of the metabolic and bactericidal characteristics of severely glucose-6-phosphate dehydrogenase deficient polymorphonuclear leukocytes and leukocytes from children with chronic granulomatous disease. J Reticuloendothel Soc. 1972;12:150-169.

1164. Vives Corrons JL, Feliu E, Pujades MA, et al. Severe glucose-6-phosphate dehydrogenase (G6PD) deficiency associated with chronic hemolytic anemia, granulocyte dysfunction, and increased susceptibility to infections: description of a new molecular variant (G6PD Barcelona). Blood. 1982;59:428-434.

1165. Cooper MR, Dechatelet LR, McCall CE, et al. Leukocyte G-6-PD deficiency. Lancet. 1970;2:110.

1166. Beutler E. G6PD deficiency. Blood. 1994;84:3613-3636.

1167. Justice P, Shih L-Y, Gordon J, et al. Characterization of leukocyte glucose-6-phosphate dehydrogenase in normal and mutant human subjects. J Lab Clin Med. 1966;68:552-559.

1168. Ramot B, Fisher S, Szeinberg A, et al. A study of subjects with erythrocyte glucose-6-phosphate dehydrogenase deficiency. II. Investigation of leukocyte enzymes. J Clin Invest. 1959;38:2234-2237.

1169. Mamlok RJ, Mamlok V, Mills GC, et al. Glucose-6-phosphate dehydrogenase deficiency, neutrophil dysfunction and *Chromobacterium violaceum* sepsis. J Pediatr. 1987;111:852-854.

1170. Lanza F. Clinical manifestation of myeloperoxidase deficiency. J Mol Med. 1998;76:676-681.

1171. Hansson M, Olsson I, Nauseef WM. Biosynthesis, processing, and sorting of human myeloperoxidase. Arch Biochem Biophys. 2006;445:214-224.

1172. Nauseef WM. Myeloperoxidase deficiency. Hematol Pathol. 1990;4:165-178.

1173. Aratani Y, Koyama H, Nyui S, et al. Severe impairment in early host defense against *Candida albicans* in mice deficient in myeloperoxidase. Infect Immun. 1999;67:1828-1836.

1174. Hirche TO, Gaut JP, Heinecke JW, Belaaouaj A. Myeloperoxidase plays critical roles in killing *Klebsiella pneumoniae* and inactivating neutrophil elastase: effects on host defense. J Immunol. 2005;174:1557-1565.

1175. Parry MF, Root RK, Metcalf JA, et al. Myeloperoxidase deficiency: prevalence and clinical significance. Ann Intern Med. 1981;95:293-301.

1176. Kitahara M, Eyre HJ, Simonian Y, et al. Hereditary myeloperoxidase deficiency. Blood. 1981;57:888-893.

1177. Chang KS, Schroeder W, Siciliano MJ, et al. The localization of the human myeloperoxidase gene is in close proximity to the translocation breakpoint in acute promyelocytic leukemia. Leukemia. 1987;1:458-462.

1178. van Tuinen P, Johnson KR, Ledbetter SA, et al. Localization of myeloperoxidase to the long arm of human chromosome 17: relationship to the 15,17 translocation of acute promyelocytic leukemia. Oncogene. 1987;1:319-322.

1179. Kizaki M, Miller CW, Selsted ME, Koeffler HP. Myeloperoxidase (MPO) gene mutation in hereditary MPO deficiency. Blood. 1994;83:1935-1940.

1180. Nauseef WM, Brigham S, Cogley M. Hereditary myeloperoxidase deficiency due to a missense mutation of arginine 569 to tryptophan. J Biol Chem. 1994;269:1212-1216.

1181. Nauseef WM, Cogley M, McCormick S. Effect of the R569W missense mutation on the biosynthesis of myeloperoxidase. J Biol Chem. 1996;271:9546-9549.

1182. Bendix-Hansen K, Kerndrup G. Myeloperoxidase-deficient polymorphonuclear leukocytes (V): relation to FAB classification and neutrophil alkaline phosphatase activity in primary myelodysplastic syndromes. Scand J Haematol. 1985;35:197-200.

1183. Bendix-Hansen K, Kerndrup G, Pedersen B. Myeloperoxidase-deficient polymorphonuclear leukocytes (VI): relation to cytogenetic abnormalities in primary myelodysplastic syndromes. Scand J Haematol. 1986;36:3-7.

1184. Stendahl O, Coble B-I, Dahlgren C, et al. Myeloperoxidase modulates the phagocytic activity of polymorphonuclear leukocytes. Studies with cells from a myeloperoxidase-deficient patient. J Clin Invest. 1984;73:366-373.

1185. Rosen H, Klebanoff SJ. Chemiluminescence and superoxide production by myeloperoxidase-deficient leukocytes. J Clin Invest. 1976;58:50-60.

1186. Jandl RC, André-Schwartz J, Borges-DuBois L, et al. Termination of the respiratory burst in human neutrophils. J Clin Invest. 1978;61:1176-1185.

1187. Roos D, Weening RS, Voetman AA, et al. Protection of phagocytic leukocytes by endogenous glutathione: studies in a family with glutathione reductase deficiency. Blood. 1979;53:851-866.

1188. Boxer LA, Oliver JM, Spielberg SP, et al. Protection of granulocytes by vitamin E in glutathione synthetase deficiency. N Engl J Med. 1979;301:901-905.

1189. Loos H, Roos D, Weening R, Houwerzijl J. Familial deficiency of glutathione reductase in human blood cells. Blood. 1976;48:53-62.

1190. Spielberg SP, Kramer LI, Goodman SI, et al. 5-Oxoprolinuria: Biochemical observations and case report. J Pediatr. 1977;91:237-241.

1191. Spielberg SP, Boxer LA, Oliver JM, et al. Oxidative damage to neutrophils in glutathione synthetase deficiency. Br J Haematol. 1979;42:215-223.

1192. Nevin NC, Morrison PJ, Jones J, Reid MM. Inverted tandem duplication of 8p12-p23.1 in a child with increased activity of glutathione reductase. J Med Genet. 1990;27:135-136.

1193. Holmes B, Park BH, Malawista SE, et al. Chronic granulomatous disease in females: a deficiency of leukocyte glutathione peroxidase. N Engl J Med. 1970;283:217-221.

1194. Matsuda I, Oka Y, Taniguchi N, et al. Leukocyte glutathione peroxidase deficiency in a male patient with chronic granulomatous disease. J Pediatr. 1976;88:581-583.

1195. Rosenzweig SD, Holland SM. Congenital defects in the interferon-gamma/interleukin-12 pathway. Curr Opin Pediatr. 2004;16:3-8.

1196. Ottenhoff TH, Verreck FA, Lichtenauer-Kaligis EG, et al. Genetics, cytokines and human infectious disease: lessons from weakly pathogenic mycobacteria and salmonellae. Nat Genet. 2002;32:97-105.

1197. Casanova JL, Abel L. Genetic dissection of immunity to mycobacteria: the human model. Annu Rev Immunol. 2002;20:581-620.

1198. Ku CL, Yang K, Bustamante J, et al. Inherited disorders of human Toll-like receptor signaling: immunological implications. Immunol Rev. 2005;203:10-20.

1199. Puel A, Picard C, Ku CL, et al. Inherited disorders of NF-κB–mediated immunity in man. Curr Opin Immunol. 2004;16:34-41.

VIII The Immune System

The Immune Response

Primary Immunodeficiency Diseases

22 The Immune Response

Sung-Yun Pai and Barbara Bierer

The immune system is a complex network of cells that serve to discriminate "self" from "nonself," that is, to recognize one cell as one's own and another cell as foreign or infected. This capacity helps protect the organism from infection by foreign pathogens (bacteria, viruses, and parasites) and from malignant degeneration. In addition, the cells involved in the immune response mediate rejection of foreign allografts. Although immune cells recognize and respond to all manner of foreign elements, at the same time they must not respond inappropriately to self-antigen. Education of immune cells results in a state of immunologic tolerance, that is, the absence of destructive antiself immune responses. Failure of self versus nonself discrimination, or failure of immunologic tolerance, may result in autoimmunity.

Whereas collectively a number of different kinds of cells are involved in the response to infection, the cells involved in mediating adaptive immunity are lymphocytes (Table 22-1). The adaptive immune response is broadly classified into two categories: (1) humoral immunity, mediated by antibodies produced by B lymphocytes and their progeny; and (2) cell-mediated immunity, dependent on cell-cell interactions and mediated by T lymphocytes. Both T and B lymphocytes are derived from early hematopoietic stem cells (HSCs) and are distinguished not by morphology but by rearrangement of their antigen-specific receptors, by function, and by the expression of different cell surface molecules. In addition to adaptive immunity, natural or innate immune mechanisms also work to defend an individual from pathogens (see Table 22-1). Natural killer (NK) cells, also derived from bone marrow progenitors, serve as principal components of innate immunity and are discussed briefly later in this chapter. In addition, polymorphonuclear leukocytes (neutrophils), eosinophils, macrophages, and other myeloid cells are important components of the body's early defense against microorganisms and are discussed in Chapter 21.

The acquired or adaptive immune response is mediated in large part by the recognition of a variety of cell surface proteins encoded by genes of the major histocompatibility complex (MHC). The MHC, located in the human genome on the short arm of chromosome 6, encodes two classes of proteins, MHC class I and MHC class II, that are highly polymorphic within the population and involved in the immune response. In humans, these genes are termed human leukocyte antigens (HLA

class I and HLA class II), as defined further later. In addition to HLA determinants, the MHC also encodes several secreted proteins of the complement system, selected immune modulators such as tumor necrosis factor (TNF), and specific proteins required for proper processing of antigen.

In addition to self-nonself discrimination, the adaptive immune response is further characterized by immunologic specificity and by memory. Acquired resistance to one antigen does not confer resistance to another unrelated (non–cross-reactive) antigen. The immune response must be capable of eliminating a foreign pathogen and developing mechanisms so that a second exposure to the same agent results not in worse disease but in more rapid elimination of the foreign agent. Cells previously exposed to and specific for one foreign protein or antigen respond more rapidly and more effectively to subsequent exposure to that same antigen, thereby leading to an anamnestic or secondary immune response. The immune response is highly regulated; cooperativity between different cellular elements and between cells and soluble mediators leads to modulation (i.e., amplification or suppression) of the immune response.

Technical advances, including single-cell cloning, monoclonal antibody production, generation of transgenic and knockout animals, and sequencing of the genome, have led to a veritable explosion in the number of cell surface proteins, cytokines, and chemokines discovered. The nomenclature has evolved and can be confusing. Cell surface proteins are generally named by a cluster of differentiation (CD) assignment; the website http://mpr.nci.nih.gov/prow/ is continuously updated with an annotated description of each CD and links to other relevant sites. Interleukins, the name given to soluble factors secreted by leukocytes or that act on leukocytes, or both, are named by the International Union of Immunologic Societies and can be found along with their receptors at http://www.genenames.org/genefamily/il.php. This chapter will focus on specific or acquired immunity and principally on the differentiation and function of B and T lymphocytes.

LYMPHOCYTE DEVELOPMENT

All B cells, T cells, and NK cells derive from pluripotent HSCs that arise first in fetal liver and then postnatally in

TABLE 22-1	Innate versus Acquired Immunity	
	Innate Immunity	**Acquired Immunity**
Specificity	Nonself	Random (in the context of self)
Effector cell type	Polymorphonuclear leukocytes (PMNs, neutrophils), natural killer cells, macrophages, eosinophils, etc.	Lymphocytes: B and T cells
Cell surface receptors	Germline	Rearranged
Distribution	Nonclonal	Clonal
Kinetics of the initial response	Rapid and immediate	Slow

the bone marrow. HSCs differentiate in the bone marrow and migrate to the appropriate lymphoid organs. These HSCs express cell surface CD34, a heavily glycosylated protein of 105 to 120 kd.[1] Although CD34 serves as a marker for hematopoietic progenitors, its expression is not limited to these cells alone. CD34 is also expressed on early lymphoid (but not pluripotent) progenitors, endothelial cells in small vessels, some embryonic fibroblasts, and some cells in the nervous system.[2] CD34 may be involved in cell-cell adhesion[3] and may be important for inhibition of hematopoietic differentiation.[4] CD34+ hematopoietic precursors give rise to both myeloid and lymphoid early progenitors. Early myeloid differentiation derives from common myeloid progenitors (CMPs), which can give rise to common granulocyte/monocyte precursors (GMPs) or megakaryocyte/erythroid precursors (MEPs). The common lymphoid progenitor (CLP) differentiates into cells of the T (and NK) and B lineage. Dendritic cells can be generated in vitro from CD34+ bone marrow cells exposed to certain cytokines, but the relevant in vivo precursor population remains controversial,[5] with the most recent data showing that CLP, CMP, and GMP all contain dendritic cell potential.[6-8] T-lymphocyte differentiation occurs largely in the thymus and is discussed in detail later. B-cell maturation occurs in the bone marrow and peripheral lymphoid organs.

Naïve B and T cells released into the peripheral blood have exquisite specificity. These resting B and T cells circulate in a quiescent state and function only after encountering cognate antigen (i.e., the specific substance that the lymphocyte recognizes). Recognition of antigen alone is generally insufficient to trigger lymphocyte activation; both B and T cells require other so-called costimulatory signals, in the form of cell surface receptor engagement or soluble factors, for effector function. Recognition of antigen by T cells and the costimulatory

signals for both B and T cells are typically mediated by accessory cells of the innate immune system termed antigen-presenting cells (APCs). Lymphocytes activated by specific antigen in the appropriate costimulatory context proliferate and mature into effector cells, a portion of which eventually differentiate into long-lived memory cells. The specifics of peripheral maturation, costimulation, and function of B and T cells are detailed in later sections.

LYMPHOCYTE SPECIFICITY

Immunologic specificity is conferred by antigen-specific receptors expressed on the surface of B and T lymphocytes and by specific antibodies (immunoglobulins [Igs]) secreted by B cells and plasma cells (Fig. 22-1). Individual lymphocytes have only one specific antigen to which it can respond. Each T cell expresses a unique T-cell receptor (TCR) and each B cell a unique Ig that can either be displayed on the surface (B-cell receptor [BCR]) or be secreted. The membrane BCR and secreted Ig of the B cell interact with epitopes expressed by naïve antigens, largely protein and nonprotein antigens such as complex epitopes of glycoproteins, lipids, and nucleic acids. Unlike Ig, the TCR recognizes small (9 to 20 amino acids) processed oligopeptides bound within the cleft of an MHC molecule on the surface of an accessory cell termed an APC. Dendritic cells, B cells, monocytes/macrophages, epithelial Langerhans cells, and in humans, endothelial cells function efficiently as APCs. These APCs bear costimulatory molecules on their cell surface (see later), secrete cytokines, and process antigen; it is the complex formed between the processed peptide fragment of antigen and MHC proteins that interacts with the TCR. Exposure to antigen induces activation of only

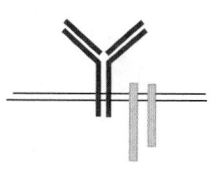

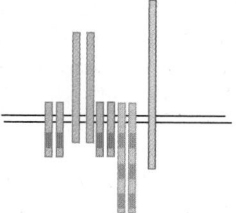

FIGURE 22-1. Characteristics of B and T lymphocytes. Both B and T lymphocytes have rearranged immune system receptors. Immunoglobulin (Ig) molecules are expressed on the surface of cells, whereas T cells are characterized by expression of the clonotypic T-cell receptor complexed to CD3 chains. Other important differences are listed.

	B lymphocyte	T lymphocyte
Antigen-specific receptor	Surface immunoglobulin (IgM, IgD)	T cell receptor (αβ or γδ)
Surface signaling molecules	Ig-α, Ig-β	CD3, ζ family
Surface molecules	CD19, CD22, FcR	CD4, CD8, CD2, CD28
Principal site of development	Bone marrow	Thymus
Effector function	Humoral immunity: antibody secretion	Cell-mediated immunity: cytokine production, cytolysis regulatory role

lymphocytes that bear Ig receptors or TCRs specific for that antigen. Any individual, however, has approximately 10^7 different T-cell and 10^7 to 10^9 different B-cell specificities. It is this clonal variability and diversity of the lymphocyte repertoire that maintain effective protection against foreign invasion.

B-CELL ONTOGENY

The first phase of B-cell maturation occurs in the bone marrow, where HSCs committed to B-lymphoid lineage develop into immature IgM^+ IgD^- B cells. The immature B cells exit the bone marrow, circulate in peripheral tissues, and mature further (Fig. 22-2). The most critical steps in B-cell development at this stage involve the expression of Ig molecules on the surface as BCR, whose specificity is the same as the antibody that will ultimately be secreted by activated mature B-cell progeny. The diversity of the B-cell repertoire is due in large part to random rearrangement of multiple germline genes for Ig that are spliced to encode a unique Ig molecule for each cell. Highly regulated checkpoints ensure that only B cells that successfully rearrange Ig genes are selected for survival.[9-11] Elimination of B cells whose receptors have high affinity for self-antigens is important to prevent autoreactivity. Finally, immature B cells released from the bone marrow complete their development in the spleen and differentiate into at least two distinct lineages of mature naïve B cells: follicular B cells and marginal-zone B cells.

Immunoglobulin Structure

The structures of antibody molecules all share remarkable conservation of secondary conformation. The Ig-like fold is a domain shared among diverse proteins, each with signature hydrophobic common cores and common disulfide bridges. The antibody molecule is the prototype member of the Ig supergene family, a group that includes not only Ig but also TCR, the MHC, and a number of costimulatory molecules. Each Ig molecule is composed of two light chains of approximately 25 kd and two heavy chains of approximately 50 or 70 kd (Fig. 22-3); each chain is composed of multiple Ig domains. B-cell antibodies can be subdivided by heavy-chain isotype and further subdivided by subclass (Table 22-2).

There are five classes of antibodies—IgM, IgG, IgA, IgD, and IgE—defined by expression of the heavy chain: μ, γ, α, δ, and ϵ. The Ig heavy chains contain sites for binding of Fc receptor (FcR) and complement, and each subtype appears to have a particular role in immune defense. The first class of antibody to be produced during development is IgM, which is expressed on the surface as a monomer and secreted as a pentamer. B cells that have undergone class switching (see later) express IgG, IgA, IgD, or IgE on the surface as the BCR or secrete a splice form of the Ig with the same heavy-chain isotype and specificity but lacking a transmembrane region (or both). The function of IgD in humans is not clear, although its expression is a marker for later B-cell development. IgA is secreted as a dimer and is found at mucosal surfaces such as the intestine. The bulk

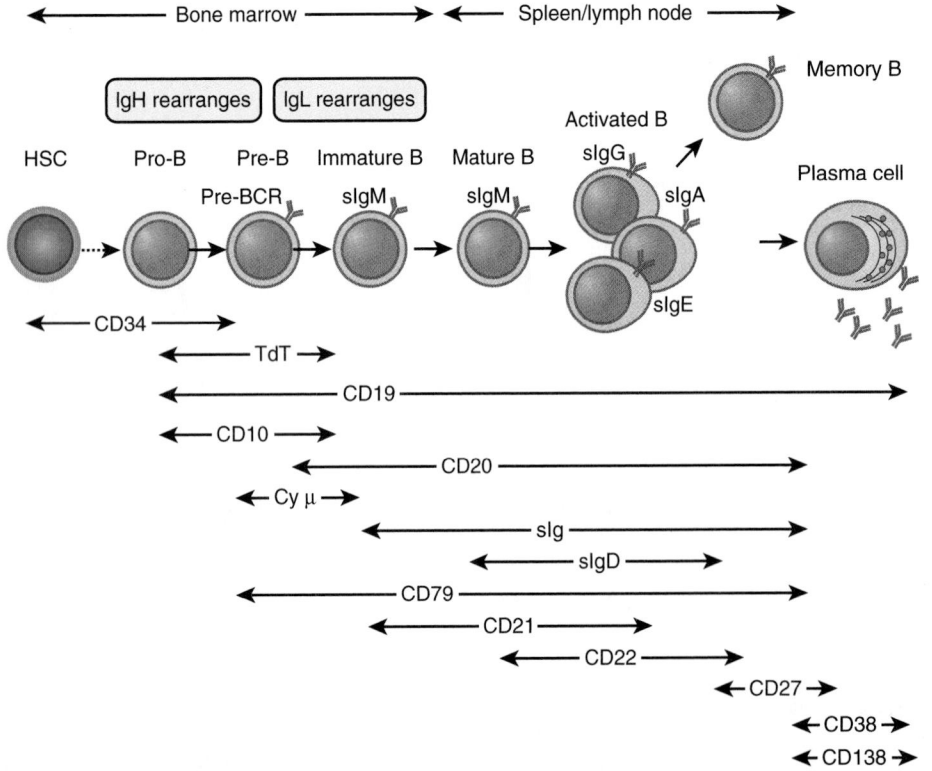

FIGURE 22-2. Overview of B-cell development. Pro-B cells develop from pluripotent hematopoietic stem cells (HSC) in bone marrow and acquire cell surface markers such as the pan-B-cell marker CD19, CD10, and terminal deoxynucleotidyl transferase (TdT). Serial rearrangement of the heavy and light chain loci drives expression of first the pre-B-cell receptor (pre-BCR) and later the B-cell receptor or surface IgM (sIgM). Downregulation of early markers at the pre-B stage gives way to expression of markers of immature and mature B cells, such as CD20, CD21, and CD22. Activation of the B cell with appropriate T-cell help leads to isotype switching and the expression of either IgA, IgG, or IgE. Switched B cells that form memory cells are characterized by expression of CD27 and downregulation of IgD, whereas activated B cells that proceed to the plasma cell stage lose most B-cell markers, upregulate CD38 and CD138, and secrete high levels of soluble specific antibody.

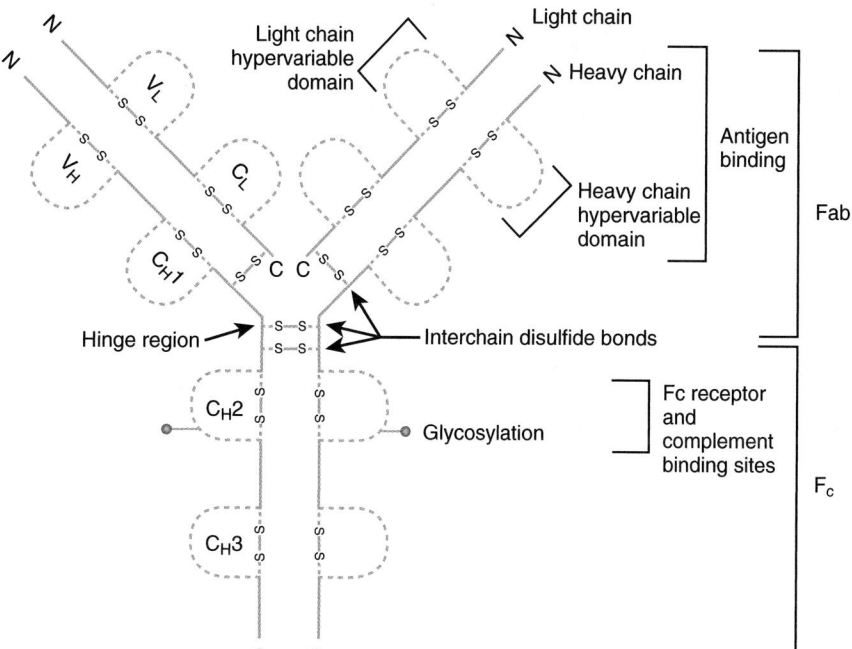

FIGURE 22-3. Diagrammatic representation of the immunoglobulin (Ig) molecule. The Ig molecule has two light chains of approximately 25 kd, each with two Ig domains (C_L and V_L), and two heavy chains of 50 to 70 kd, each composed of four Ig domains (C_H1, C_H2, C_H3, and V_H). The antigen binding region is defined by the variable regions of the heavy and light chains (V_H and V_L). There are five subclasses of the heavy chain: IgG, IgA, IgM, IgD, and IgE.

of circulating Ig is in the form of IgG, which is monomeric and further subdivided into four subclasses: IgG1, IgG2, IgG3, and IgG4. Persistently low serum levels of one or more IgG subclasses,[12,13] in the presence or absence of IgA deficiency,[14] may cause individuals to be susceptible to recurrent infections.[15] Though controversial, prophylactic use of intravenous Ig has been suggested.[16,17]

There are two subclasses of light chains: κ and λ (see Fig. 22-3). Both subclasses appear to serve similar functions. Monoclonal disorders of terminally differentiated mature B cells or plasma cells (e.g., multiple myeloma) express cells of a given light chain, that is, either κ or λ but not both.

The structure of each Ig molecule is determined by hydrophobic interactions and disulfide bridges between the two heavy chains and two light chains (see Fig. 22-3). For each chain the N-terminal domain has a variable or polymorphic amino acid structure (V_H for heavy chain, V_L for light chain), whereas the C-terminal portions are constant within each heavy-chain or light-chain class (termed C_H1, C_H2, C_H3 for heavy chain and C_L for light chain). These domains form pairs, V_H with V_L, C_H1 with C_L, and C_H3 with C_H3. Proteolytic digestion of Ig by papain results in two Fab fragments, each composed of the V_H/V_L, C_H1/C_L domains, and an Fc fragment composed of the two C_H2 and two C_H3 domains. The binding region of Ig that recognizes antigen is composed of portions of the V_H and V_L domains. Within each variable region there are three portions with increased amino acid variation, called hypervariable regions (HV1, HV2, HV3) or complementarity-determining regions (CDR1, CDR2, CDR3). The highest variability is found in CDR3, and all three CDRs from both chains participate in the

binding of antigen. Variability within each variable region and each CDR and pairing of a unique heavy chain with a unique light chain all contribute to the combinatorial diversity of Ig specificity.

Immunoglobulin Rearrangement and B-Cell Maturation in Bone Marrow

The genes encoding the heavy chains of Ig are located on human chromosome 14, whereas the genes encoding κ and λ light chains are located on chromosomes 2 and 22, respectively. The heavy- and light-chain loci are each composed of variable (V), diversity (D), and joining (J) gene segments that recombine to yield the V_H and V_L domains, which in turn form the antigen contact surface of the antibody molecule and confer specificity. In addition, the heavy-chain locus contains nine heavy-chain constant (C) region genes (μ, δ, γ1, γ2, γ3, γ4, α1, α2, and ε constant regions) that define the mature Ig isotype.

Ig rearrangement occurs serially, and cells failing to rearrange the Ig genes successfully are eliminated and do not develop further (Fig. 22-4). B-cell maturation also results in cell surface protein expression patterns that are used to define the pro-B-cell, pre-B-cell, and immature B-cell stages of development. CD34+ CD19– CD10– progenitors that have not yet committed to the B lineage have Ig genes in the germline configuration. The earliest B-cell precursors express the pan-B-cell marker CD19 and the early marker CD10. They also express components of the rearrangement machinery such as recombination-activating genes (RAGs) and thus have early gene rearrangements detectable. Rearrangement begins with

TABLE 22-2   Immunoglobulin Subclass Definition

Class	Isotype	Heavy Chain	Molecular Formula	Molecular Mass (kd)	Plasma Concentration (mg/mL)*	Cross Placenta	Fix Complement	Biologic Functions
IgG								Complement activation, opsonization for Fc receptor
	IgG1	$\gamma1$	$\gamma1_2\kappa_2$ $\gamma1_2\lambda_2$	150	7-9	+	+	Antitoxins, antibody to most bacterial antigens
	IgG2	$\gamma2$	$\gamma2_2\kappa_2$ $\gamma2_2\lambda_2$	150	2-3	+	+	Antipolysaccharide antibodies to bacterial capsules
	IgG3	$\gamma3$	$\gamma3_2\kappa_2$ $\gamma3_2\lambda_2$	150	0.7-1	+	+	Cytophilic antibodies, e.g., to Rh antigens
	IgG4	$\gamma4$	$\gamma4_2\kappa2$ $\gamma4_2\lambda_2$	150	0.3-0.5	+	−	Anticoagulants, such as anti–factor VIII in hemophiliacs
IgM		μ	$(\mu_2\kappa_2)_5$ $(\mu_2\lambda_2)_5$	950	1.5	−	+	Receptor in B-lymphocyte membrane, antibodies to lipopolysaccharides, complement activation, natural antibody
IgA				150 or 300				Present in external secretions, alternative complement activation (?)
	IgA1	$\alpha1$	$\alpha1_2\kappa_2$ $\alpha1_2\lambda_2$		1-3	−	−	Virus-neutralizing antibody
	IgA2	$\alpha2$	$(\alpha2_2\kappa_2)_2$		0.5-0.7	−	−	Principal secretory antibody
IgD		δ	$\delta_2\lambda_2$ $\delta_2\kappa_2$	180	0.3	−	−	Unknown, receptor in B lymphocyte membrane
IgE		ε	$\varepsilon_2\lambda_2$ $\varepsilon_2\kappa_2$	190	0.0005[†]	−	−	Anaphylactic antibodies or "reagins," binds to mast cells, mediator of release

*Plasma concentrations of the immunoglobulins vary significantly with age in pediatric populations. Adult norms are given here. IgG at birth reflects maternally transferred immunoglobulin and wanes over several months, with a nadir at approximately 4 months and rising thereafter as the infant's own production takes over. IgM and IgA levels rise with age during infancy and childhood.

[†]Usually expressed as international units; up to 200 IU is considered normal.

one heavy-chain allele; one of the 29 D_H exons is spliced to one of the 6 J_H exons, the intervening D and J sequences are eliminated, and a DJ segment is produced. The pro-B cell then splices one of the approximately 50 V_H exons to the DJ segment to form a V(D)J segment. Finally, the μ constant region of the heavy chain (C_μ) is spliced onto the V(D)J segments.

Differentiation to the pre-B stage is triggered by expression of intact μ heavy-chain protein or cytoplasmic μ, which occurs only in cells that bear in-frame productive V(D)J-C_μ rearrangements. If rearrangement of the first heavy-chain locus is unsuccessful, the second allele undergoes rearrangement. Because the light-chain genes have not yet been expressed, cytoplasmic μ complexes instead with the nonpolymorphic surrogate light-chain proteins $\lambda5$ and VpreB. Cytoplasmic μ, surrogate light

chain, and the accessory signaling molecules Ig-α (CD79a) and Ig-β (CD79b) together form the pre-B-cell receptor. Ensuing signals induce proliferation and instruct the cell to begin rearrangement of one of the κ light-chain loci. Pre-B cells lose CD34 expression, continue to express CD19 and CD10, and additionally upregulate CD20. The signaling cascade downstream of the pre-B-cell receptor is highly analogous to that of the mature BCR and activates a number of critical kinases, including Bruton's tyrosine kinase (Btk) (see later). Boys born with mutations in Btk, manifested as X-linked agammaglobulinemia, have normal numbers of pro-B cells but lack pre-B cells and their progeny.[18] Thus, formation of the pre-B-cell receptor along with activation of downstream signaling is a critical checkpoint in this stage of maturation.

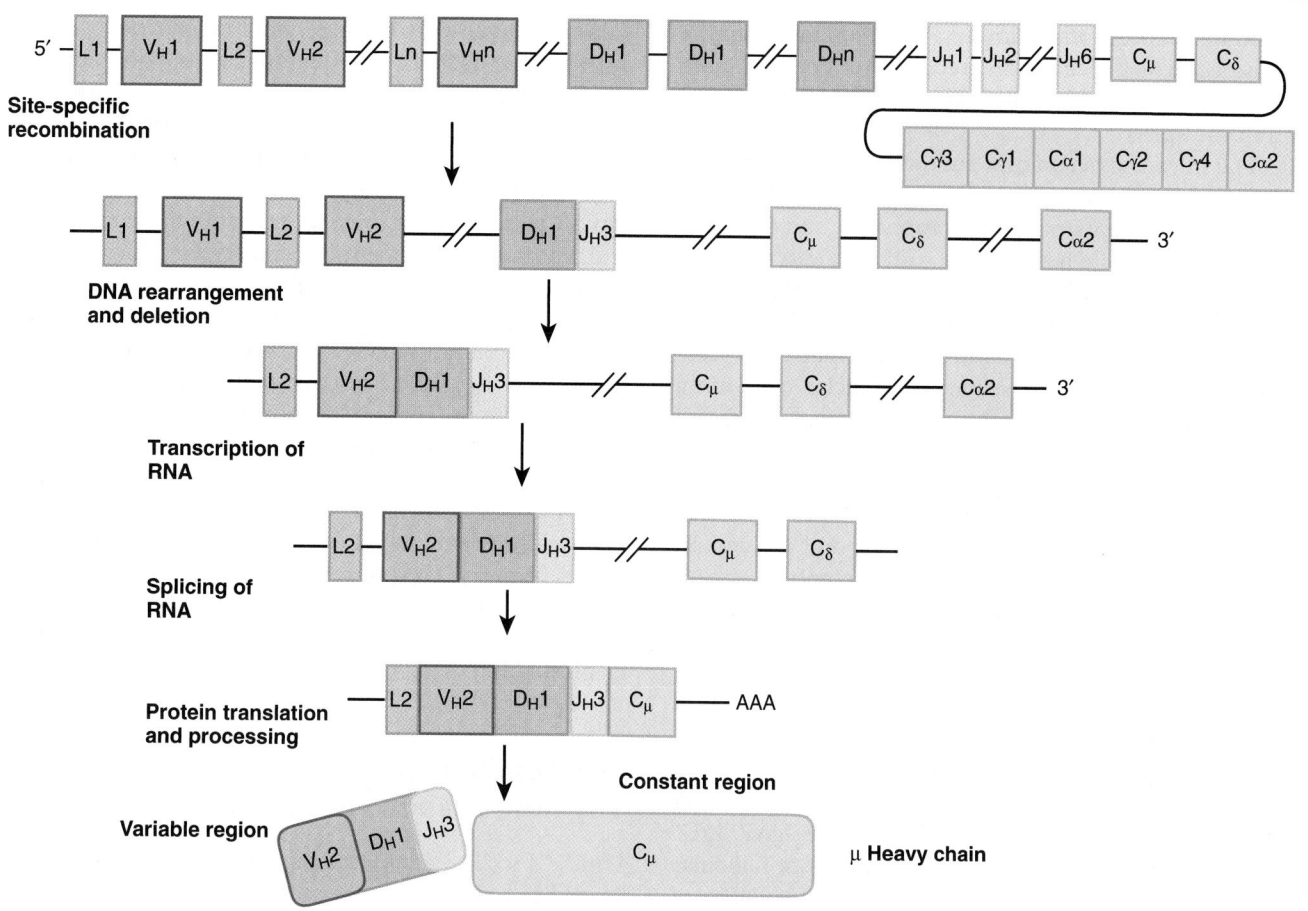

FIGURE 22-4. Immunoglobulin rearrangement. Immunoglobulin genes are encoded on human chromosome 14. Approximately 100 variable (V) genes, 50 diversity (D) genes, and 4 to 6 joining (J) genes make up the heavy-chain variable locus. The constant region consists of nine constant (C) genes. During immunoglobulin gene rearrangement, gene segments are deleted so that specific regions are joined to form one of many individual and characteristic genes.

Light-chain genes rearrange by a process similar to the recombination of heavy-chain genes. The variable region of the κ gene, located on chromosome 2, is spliced to the J gene segment to produce a VJ region, which then splices to the one constant region ($C_κ$). If nonproductive, the second κ locus will rearrange. If both attempts to rearrange the κ locus are unsuccessful, the λ locus, located on chromosome 22, will begin to rearrange. Productive rearrangement of any light-chain locus prevents further B-cell rearrangement and also generates survival signals. Pre-B cells that successfully rearrange a light-chain gene will then express mature IgM protein, which appears as surface IgM (sIgM) complexed to Ig-α and Ig-β, thus forming the BCR. Immature B cells are sIgM+, CD79+, CD19+, CD10+, and CD20+ but have not acquired IgD expression, which occurs after peripheral maturation.

Expression of the tissue-specific recombination-activating genes RAG-1 and RAG-2 is required for recombination.[19,20] In addition, diversity is enhanced by the fact that the junctions between the D and J regions and the V and DJ regions are not precise; not only can the nucleotides vary, but one or more nucleotides (termed N regions), not encoded in the genome, may also be randomly inserted (N-region diversification). The nuclear

enzyme terminal deoxyribonucleotidyl transferase (TdT) is the polymerase that adds random nucleotides to recombination junctions[21] and may have other roles.[22] Recruitment of TdT to the junctions appears to depend on the Ku molecule (specifically Ku80), a heterodimer that binds DNA ends and is required for V(D)J recombination and DNA double-stranded break repair.[23,24] Other proteins critical for nonhomologous end rejoining include Ku70, DNA-dependent protein kinase, DNA ligase IV, XRCC4, and the recently cloned protein Artemis.[25] Defects in the recombination machinery in genes such as RAG1, RAG2, DNA ligase IV, and Artemis all result in severe combined immunodeficiency (see Chapter 23).[26-28]

Peripheral B-Cell Maturation and Differentiation

Immature B cells must undergo further maturation in the spleen before acquiring the phenotype and functions of a naïve mature B cell. Naïve mature B cells are resting cells in G_0 phase; express the pan-B-cell marker CD19, the marker CD20, and sIgM; and in contrast to immature bone marrow B cells, have lost CD10 expression and gained IgD expression. A similar population in the mouse is believed to be the common precursor for both follicular and marginal-zone B cells, named for their location within the spleen.[29]

The spleen has a complex architecture divided grossly into red pulp and white pulp. The red pulp contains the sinusoids, which are lined by macrophages, and the cords of Billroth, which lie between the sinusoids and are composed of connective tissue, epithelial cells, monocytes, and macrophages. The white pulp is composed of primary follicles containing naïve mature B cells that co-express IgM and IgD, as well as secondary follicles containing activated B cells within its germinal center (GC), all termed follicular B cells. Naïve follicular B cells in the primary follicle are CD27⁻, in contrast to memory B cells, discussed later, which express CD27.[30,31]

In the mouse, T cells congregate around the central arteriole in the so-called periarteriolar lymphoid sheath (PALS) studded by follicles and GCs containing B cells; the marginal zone delineates the white pulp from the red and surrounds both the follicles and PALS. In humans, by contrast, T cells and B cells tend to interdigitate, and the follicles are encompassed within the PALS. The marginal zone in humans is positioned around the follicles, does not envelop the PALS, and is not in direct contact with red pulp.[32] Marginal zone B cells are IgM⁺ IgD⁻ CD1c⁺ CD23⁻ and thus are distinguished from follicular B cells (IgM⁻ IgD⁺ CD1c⁻ CD23⁺).[29] Additionally, marginal-zone B cells express high levels of CD21 and as a result are highly responsive to complement. Finally, in contrast to rodent marginal-zone B cells, which are sessile, marginal-zone B cells in humans can circulate in blood and have a memory phenotype, being IgM⁺ IgD⁺ CD27⁺.[33]

The development of early B precursors into immature B cells is a process that requires Ig rearrangement and expression of the pre-B-cell receptor and BCR, but it does not require recognition of antigen. Maturation to the naïve resting B cell involves selection of B cells that recognize antigen (positive selection) while eliminating B cells whose BCR recognize self-antigens with high affinity (negative selection). It has been proposed, based on murine data, that determination of mature B-cell fate relies on the relative signal strength and specificity of the BCR, with higher and lower signal strength driving to the follicular and marginal-zone lineages, respectively.[29] Negative selection in particular is important for the deletion of potentially autoreactive clones and induction of B-cell tolerance. Indeed, it is estimated that 55% to 75% of immature B cells in humans recognize self-antigens,[34] and thus a minority of developing B cells pass the negative-selection test.

B-CELL ACTIVATION AND FUNCTION

An appropriately diverse population of naïve B cells should collectively be capable of responding to any soluble antigen that the individual encounters, yet there are very few naïve B cells that are capable of recognizing any given antigen. B-cell activation that occurs in the appropriate costimulatory context is the trigger for clonal expansion of the responding B cell. A portion of these activated B cells differentiate into memory cells, which rapidly respond upon re-encounter with the same antigen, and another portion into plasma cells, which continuously secrete antibodies (see Fig. 22-2). In addition, activated B cells undergo isotype switching from low-affinity IgM to high-affinity IgG, IgA, or IgE and somatic hypermutation, also called affinity maturation, thus further ensuring that the humoral response is exquisitely specific, effective, and long lasting. Recognition of antigen by the BCR occurs with or without T-cell help, depending on the type of antigen, so-called thymus-dependent (TD) or thymus-independent (TI) antigens. BCR signals that occur during TD responses are modulated and enhanced by cell-cell contact with T cells via critical costimulatory molecules, discussed further in the section on T-cell costimulation.

Thymus-Dependent versus Thymus-Independent B-Cell Responses

Unlike T cells, which recognize either short peptides or small lipid molecules that must be presented in the cleft of an MHC or MHC-like molecule, the BCR is capable of binding a variety of antigens, including soluble proteins and polysaccharides. Recognition of protein antigen generally requires cooperation with T cells, or T-cell help, and thus such antigens are TD antigens. Naïve follicular B cells in lymph node follicles or the spleen recognize their cognate antigen while contacting a helper T cell specific for the same antigen; linked T-B interaction then fuels the formation of a key structure, the GC, where isotype switching, somatic hypermutation, memory cell generation, and plasma cell differentiation occur.

TI antigens are classified as type 1 or type 2 (TI-1 and TI-2).[35] TI-1 antigens are bacterial components that can trigger B-cell activation regardless of Ig specificity and thus lead to polyclonal activation. These components fall into the general category of pathogen-associated molecular pattern (PAMP) molecules, the canonic example being lipopolysaccharide (LPS). PAMP molecules activate B cells by binding to a distinct family of receptors, the Toll-like receptors (TLRs), thereby accounting for their independence from Ig. The Ig secreted in response to TI-1 antigens is typically low-affinity IgM because TI-1 antigen binding does not induce class switching.[36]

TI-2 antigens, in contrast, are molecules that have a repetitive structure and activate B cells by cross-linking of multiple BCRs on a single cell, hence leading to specific clonal antibody production. These antigens are typically bacterially derived polysaccharides, such as those found in the coating of encapsulated organisms. Marginal-zone B cells are important for responses to TI-2 antigens, and the fact that marginal-zone B cells typically take years to mature in children probably underlies the lack of response of children younger than 2 years to polysaccharides.[29] The spleen is the major site of TI-2 antigen recognition, and the antibody produced again is often IgM, although IgG responses also clearly occur. Class switching in this instance does not depend on cognate T-cell help but probably is enhanced by noncontact T-cell factors such as the cytokine interleukin-4 (IL-4).[35]

B-Cell Receptor Triggering and Signaling

B-cell activation involves a complex array of molecular signaling events. The signaling cascades that emanate from the BCR are highly analogous to those triggered in T cells by the TCR and involve a host of kinases, adaptor proteins, and other enzymes.

In brief, B-cell activation commences with engagement of surface Ig, which initiates receptor oligomerization, an event that depends on B-cell coreceptors such as

the stimulatory CD19 and CD21 receptors and the inhibitory low-affinity FcR.[37-40] In addition, aggregation of Ig receptors takes place in specialized membrane microdomains, termed lipid rafts, that are characterized by their cholesterol- and sphingolipid-rich content.[41-44] In cellular systems, lipid rafts have been postulated to function in intracellular trafficking, apical sorting, and signal transduction.[45,46] In both T and B lymphocytes, lipid raft components may function as a potential signaling platform to foster the aggregation and colocalization of signaling proteins.[41,47-49]

Within the lipid raft, the Ig molecule transmits signals through the associated Ig-α and Ig-β molecules (Fig. 22-5), together termed the BCR; the BCR, like other members of the immune recognition receptors, has no intrinsic tyrosine kinase activity. Upon oligomerization, the cytoplasmic domains of Ig-α and Ig-β become tyrosine phosphorylated on so-called immunoreceptor tyrosine–based activation motifs (ITAMs) with the amino acid consensus sequence D/ExxYxxL/Ix7YxxL/I. Phosphorylation of ITAMs is mediated by Src kinase family members, notably Fyn, Blk, and Lyn (see Fig. 22-5).[49-51]

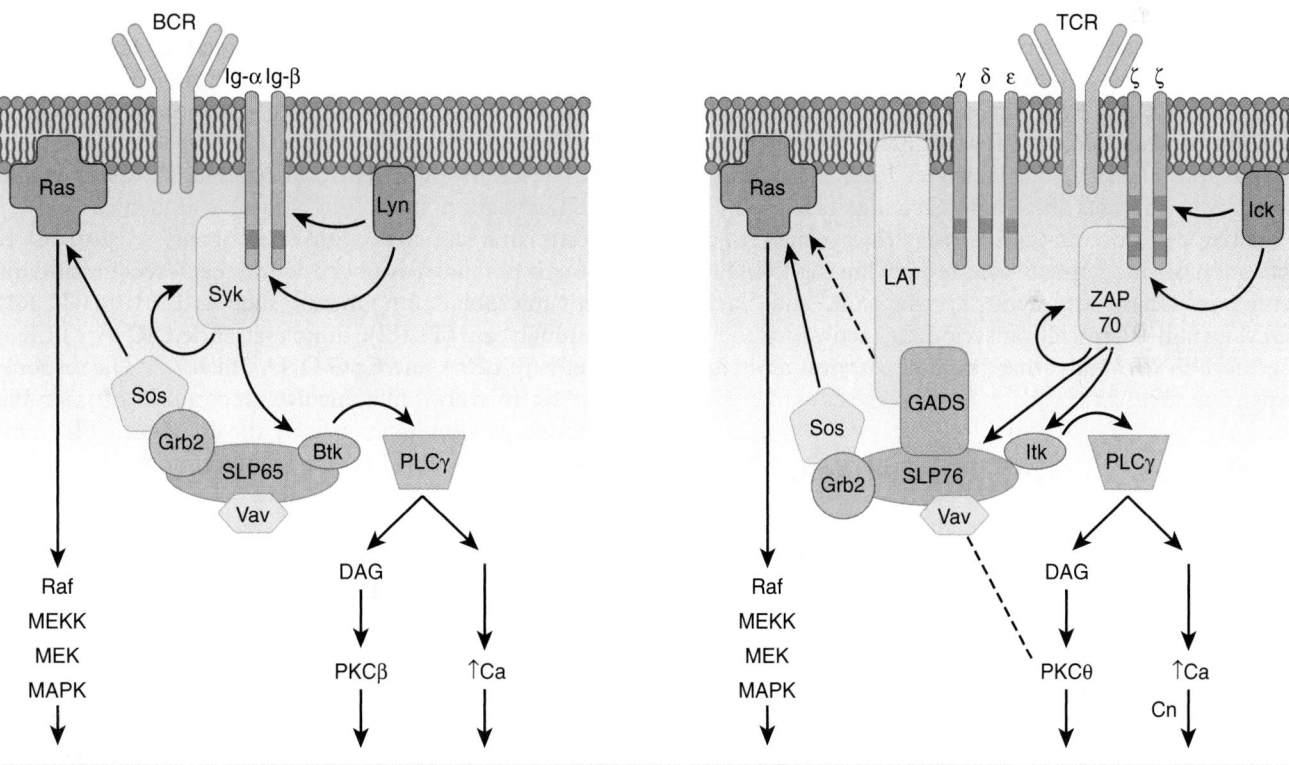

FIGURE 22-5. Schematic of B- and T-cell signaling pathways. Signaling cascades that emanate after engagement of antigen-specific receptors, the B-cell receptor (BCR) in B cells (*left*) and the T-cell receptor (TCR) in T cells (*right*), are depicted. Each receptor has short cytoplasmic tails that do not themselves signal; the receptors signal instead via a complex of associated transmembrane molecules (Ig-α, Ig-β for B cells and the CD3 γ, δ, ε, and ζ proteins for T cells) that have immunoreceptor tyrosine–based activation motifs (ITAMs, depicted as *blue boxes*). Phosphorylation of ITAMs by early protein tyrosine kinases such as Lyn and Lck is critical for recruitment of Syk in B cells and ZAP70 in T cells, which go on to trigger the rest of the cascade. Adaptor proteins such as SLP65 and SLP76 nucleate a host of signaling molecules to activate Ras and protein kinase C (PKC) and increase intracellular calcium (Ca). The final effects of proliferation, cytoskeletal reorganization, and transcriptional activation ensue. B and T cells share a number of intermediates such as phospholipase C γ (PLCγ), Grb2, Sos, Ras, and Vav. Related molecules specific to B or T cells are depicted with similar shapes (e.g., SLP65/SLP76, Btk/Itk). DAG, diacylglycerol; MAPK, mitogen-activated protein kinase; MEK, MAPK kinase; MEKK, MEK kinase.

which then recruit the critical tyrosine kinase Syk via its Src homology 2 (SH2) domains. Syk itself, when bound, requires activation either by autophosphorylation or phosphorylation by Src kinases, and thus clustering of multiple ITAM-bearing BCRs, Src kinases, and Syk is required to achieve a threshold of activation that initiates downstream cascades.[52]

Activation of Syk, similar to activation of ZAP70 in T cells (see later), is a crucial lynchpin in BCR signaling. Syk itself functions as a tyrosine kinase and is capable of phosphorylating key substrates, which then activate three main signals, the protein kinase C (PKC), intracellular calcium, and Ras pathways. Activation of these pathways occurs by assembly of a macromolecular complex of critical signaling molecules clustered on an adaptor protein known as the B-cell linker protein (BLNK) or SLP65.[51] Recruitment of a member of the Tec kinase family, Btk, to SLP65 via the SH2 and Src homology 3 (SH3) domains and to the membrane by the Pleckstrin homology (PH) domain activates Btk.[53] The critical nature of Btk activation in BCR signaling is underscored again by its role as the gene responsible for X-linked agammaglobulinemia. Btk in turn activates an isoform of phospholipase C (PLCγ2) that hydrolyzes inositol phosphates to generate diacylglycerol (DAG) and inositol 1,4,5-trisphosphate (IP$_3$). DAG activates both an isoform of PKC (PKCβ) and Ras, whereas IP$_3$ induces an increase in intracellular calcium. Recruitment of Sos via the adaptor protein Grb2 also activates the Ras pathway, as does Vav, a guanine nucleotide exchange factor for Rac. Together, activation of these three pathways then triggers activation of mitogen-activated protein kinases (MAPKs), reorganization of the actin cytoskeleton, and nuclear translocation of critical transcriptional activators, including the NF-κB family, that promote survival and clonal expansion (Fig. 22-5).[50,52]

Coreceptors Involved in B-Cell Activation

Three important coreceptors for B-cell activation are CD21 (also called complement receptor 2 [CR2]), CD19, and CD81. Antigens derived from bacteria or other extracellular microorganisms are more efficiently cleared when opsonized or bound by complement components, a mechanism that links the early innate immune response elicited by activation of complement to the adaptive humoral B-cell response. Binding of C3b to CD21 coclusters CD21, CD19, and CD81 with the BCR within lipid rafts.[39,49,54] Phosphorylation of CD19 by proximity to the activated BCR complex in turn generates docking sites for phosphatidylinositol 3′-kinase (PI3K), for Vav, and for Lyn. PI3K generates phospholipid intermediates that recruit Btk as described earlier. Vav activates Rac, thereby activating MAPKs and inducing cytoskeletal reorganization. The response to opsonized antigens recognized by the BCR via its specific epitope is thus greatly enhanced by the binding of C3b to CD21.[55] CD81 appears to function primarily as an adaptor and is criti-

cally required for BCR and CD21/CD19 to associate with lipid rafts.[56,57]

Stimulation via the antigen receptor alone is insufficient to activate B or T cells, and in fact, binding of receptor-ligand pairs between B and T cells is critical for activation of both. Many costimulatory pathways are shared between B and T cells and are discussed further later; binding of CD40 to its ligand CD40L (CD154) is the most crucial of these pathways for B-cell activation. CD40 is a 48-kd member of the TNF receptor superfamily that is expressed on B cells and other APCs constitutively, whereas CD40L is a 33-kd transmembrane protein with homology to TNF upregulated on activated CD4$^+$ T cells. CD40/CD40L binding has been shown to be essential for B-cell growth and differentiation.[58] In vitro stimulation of B cells by cross-linking via monoclonal antibodies is sufficient to promote growth and class switching and is synergized by BCR stimulation or treatment with IL-4, or both. Engagement of CD40 with trimeric CD40L and clustering of the cytoplasmic tails lead to recruitment of a class of adaptor proteins, the TNF receptor–associated factors (TRAFs), which in turn activate a variety of kinases that ultimately culminates in activation of MAPK and NF-κB.[59] In addition to clonal expansion and survival, CD40 signaling also leads to upregulation of other costimulatory molecules such as CD80 (B7) and CD54 (intercellular adhesion molecule 1 [ICAM-1]).[59]

The relatively recently discovered TLR can trigger B-cell activation alone (see earlier) and also can serve a costimulatory function with BCR signals.[36,60] At least 11 TLRs in humans have been found, each recognizing different microbial components, such as LPS (via TLR4), peptidoglycan (TLR2), double-stranded RNA (TLR3), flagellin (TLR5), and CpG DNA (TLR9).[61] The response to intact microbes may involve recognition of microbial components simultaneously by the BCR and TLR, and interestingly, BCR-TLR corecognition may play a role in the generation of autoantibodies.[62,63]

Follicular B-Cell Differentiation: The Germinal Center

Activation of B cells and differentiation into memory and plasma cells have become increasingly well understood in the context of cellular trafficking and the complex architecture of the specialized anatomic site, the GC.[64,65] B cells, T cells, and specialized follicular dendritic cells (FDCs) must interact via costimulatory contact and soluble factors to generate a long-lasting humoral response.

In the early stages of infection, innate immune cells such as dendritic cells and macrophages capture antigen, migrate to lymph nodes, and present peptides in the cleft of class II MHC to CD4$^+$ T cells. Simultaneously, naïve B cells that recognize the same pathogen can internalize complex protein particles by receptor-mediated internalization of Ig, with the protein fragments being broken down and displayed as peptides by class II MHC. Naïve B cells that encounter their cognate antigen and become activated then migrate through the T-cell zone and contact T cells stochastically during the journey.[66] When T and B cells that recognize the same antigen interact via TCR-MHC interactions, costimulatory signals, namely, CD40-CD40L interactions, enhance the interaction and result in clonal expansion of both T and B cells. These activated "helped" B cells then travel to the follicle and infiltrate a network of FDCs. FDCs are thought to have a specialized function consisting of capture of immune complexes and simultaneous binding of FcR to antibody and complement receptor 3 (CR3) to components of complement.[67] The antigen component of the immune complex can then be displayed to passing B cells via the BCR. Activated B cells that recognize antigen displayed on FDCs proliferate rapidly after further costimulation by CD4[+] T cells and become the centroblasts and centrocytes that form the GC.

Somatic hypermutation is thought to occur at the centroblast stage and further diversifies the overall antibody pool by introducing mutations in the V_H and V_L regions of Ig in B cells involved in a GC response.[68,69] Nucleotides are thought to be mutated in a somewhat random fashion, in both the rearranged and non-rearranged V regions, but ultimately, survival of B cells that have undergone hypermutation is dictated by positive and negative selection based on the affinity of the expressed Ig. In other words, mutations that disrupt affinity to the antigen to which the animal is responding will be selected against, whereas those that enhance affinity will be selected for, hence the term *affinity maturation*.

Isotype or class switching is thought to occur at the centrocyte stage. Because all naïve B cells express IgM, a low-affinity antibody, inducing activated B cells to produce high-affinity IgG or IgA significantly enhances the functional humoral immune response to specific antigen at the time of infection and requires splicing of the V(D)J regions to the C_γ or C_α region. CD40-CD40L interactions are critical for this process, and T-cell–derived cytokines enhance class switching while influencing the Ig class or subclass.[70-72] In the mouse, T-B interactions in the context of interferon-γ (IFN-γ) tend to promote switching to IgG2a and IgG3, whereas IL-4 directs switching to IgG1 and IgE (see Table 22-2).

GC B cells then differentiate into either plasma cells or switched memory B cells. How GC B cells "choose" between the plasma cell and memory B-cell fate remains unclear.[73] Plasma cells are terminally differentiated B cells found primarily in bone marrow and are specialized for high-level secretion of IgG, IgM, and IgA. They have a characteristic histologic appearance with so-called clockwork chromatin, eccentric nuclei, and markedly expanded endoplasmic reticulum and can be identified by expression of CD138 (also called syndecan-1). Class-switched memory B cells, which generally can be identi-

fied by virtue of the loss of IgD and gain of CD27 surface expression,[30] are able to circulate back to bone marrow and secondary lymphoid organs and, like memory T cells discussed later, are responsible for the rapid and effective anamnestic immune response characteristic of acquired immunity. A number of congenital deficiencies that affect T-cell–dependent B-cell maturation are characterized by a lack of GC formation and switched memory B cells; such conditions include CD40L deficiency (later), X-linked lymphoproliferative disease (caused by mutation in SH2D1A or SLAM-associated protein [SAP]), and two molecules recently shown when mutated in humans to cause common variable immunodeficiency, ICOS (inducible T-cell costimulator) and TACI (transmembrane activator and calcium modulator and cyclophilin ligand interactor).[74-78] More recently, both somatic hypermutation and class switch recombination have been found to require a newly discovered activation-induced deaminase (AID) that deaminates deoxycytidine to form deoxyuridine; subsequent repair of the deoxyuracil-deoxyguanosine mismatch triggers nucleotide substitution or excision, thereby generating diversity and also joining VDJ regions to a different constant region class.[69,79] Humans born with defects in the AID gene have failure of both processes that results in a hyper-IgM phenotype.[80-82]

B-Cell Tolerance

Like T-cell tolerance (discussed later), B-cell tolerance is essential to prevent autoimmune reactions. Immature B cells can be made tolerant in the bone marrow to antigens expressed by the host (i.e., self-antigens) through clonal deletion.[83] If the sIgM expressed on an immature B cell binds with high avidity to a self-antigen, the cell will be stimulated to undergo apoptosis, a form of cell death characterized by chromosomal fragmentation and membrane blebbing. The B cell may also undergo receptor editing, a process whereby that B cell's Ig gene will further rearrange to express a different, nonautoreactive Ig molecule.[84] The few B cells that escape central deletion may be rendered anergic in the periphery, a state in which the B cell expresses a gene that encodes a self-reactive antibody yet is unable to respond to antigen. The molecular mechanisms responsible for anergy are incompletely understood but may involve alternative signaling when the BCR is activated in the presence or absence of costimulation. For instance, BCR triggering in the context of concurrent TLR signaling (secondary to microbial products in addition to the BCR-specific antigen) leads to upregulation of CD86, which engages CD28 on T cells and recruits T-cell help. In the absence of TLR signals, the upregulation of CD86 is not sustained, and the BCR signals are attenuated.[85] A group of TNF and TNF receptor family members, including BAFF (TNFSF13B) and APRIL (TNFSF13A), whose receptors include TACI (TNFRSF13B, CD267), BCMA (TNFRSF17, CD269) and BAFF-R (TNFRSF13C, CD268), have been shown to be important in B-cell homeostasis and autoimmunity. Interestingly, mice that overexpress BAFF exhibit autoimmunity,[86,87] and humans with a variety of rheumatologic diseases have been shown to have high BAFF serum levels.[88] The increasing use of rituximab, humanized anti-CD20 antibody, for the treatment of autoimmune disease and, recently, chronic graft-versus-host disease underscores the importance of dysregulated humoral immunity in human disease.

Function of Secreted Immunoglobulin

Secretion of a diverse repertoire of Ig is essential for protection of the host from infection and for neutralization of toxin. Once formed, binding of specific antibodies to microorganisms, virally infected cells, toxins, or other pathogens is essential for complement-mediated lysis, antibody-dependent cellular cytotoxicity (ADCC), opsonization, phagocytosis, and neutralization of toxins and viruses (see Table 22-2). Different heavy-chain isotypes perform different functions preferentially. IgM, IgG1, IgG2, and IgG3 activate the complement cascade, whereas only IgG1 and IgG3 bind effectively to phagocytic Fcγ receptors. IgE is able to bind to the Fcγ receptors expressed on mast cells and eosinophils. In addition, secreted IgA antibodies play a role in protection from invasion through mucosal surfaces.

Different classes of antibodies not only have different functions but also predominate in different compartments in the body. IgA is predominantly secreted, IgM is primarily intravascular, and IgG is generally the major antibody found in tissues and peripheral blood. IgG is able to cross the placenta to provide some protective immunity to the fetus; passive protection from long-lived IgG molecules confers postnatal immunity. However, although the function and location of the antibody classes differ, subpopulations of B cells are able to migrate and home to specific regions of antigen presentation. Therefore, generalized B-cell immunity may result from localized antigen presentation, as paradigmatically demonstrated by the efficacy of successful vaccination programs.

T-CELL ONTOGENY

T lymphocytes, like B lymphocytes and all other blood cells, are derived from self-renewing pluripotent HSCs. T cells are unique, however, in that their development also requires passage through a specific organ, the thymus. Indeed, the absolute requirement for the thymus is made clear by human congenital immunodeficiency states such as the DiGeorge syndrome, in which thymic organogenesis and therefore T-cell development are absent (see Chapter 23). Similar to B-cell ontogeny, the generation of millions of diverse T cells is accomplished by serial rearrangement of germline genes encoding the receptor for antigen recognition, the TCR. The bulk of peripheral

T cells are either of the CD4[+] helper or CD8[+] cytolytic lineages.

T-Cell Receptor Subtypes and Specificity

The TCR is a cell surface receptor capable of recognizing discrete antigens bound to the MHC or to MHC-related molecules expressed on the surface of APCs. TCRs are disulfide-linked heterodimers of either αβ or γδ proteins.[89] TCR αβ–bearing T cells constitute the vast majority of circulating T cells, most of which recognize peptide antigens bound to polymorphic MHC class I or class II molecules. A subset of TCR αβ T cells, representing approximately 1% of all T cells in humans, in contrast recognize lipid antigens bound to the MHC class I–related nonpolymorphic molecule CD1 and are termed CD1-restricted or NKT cells, discussed in a later section. TCR γδ–bearing T cells account for a tiny fraction of the circulating T cells in humans but are very prevalent in intestinal tissue and are thought to recognize nonpeptide antigens (see later). The functions of CD1-restricted TCR αβ T cells and TCR γδ T cells are somewhat distinct from those of conventional TCR αβ T cells. The discussion of intrathymic T-cell development below will focus on the major conventional subset of T cells.

Early T-Cell Commitment and Seeding

The molecular events associated with and responsible for commitment to the T lineage have been increasingly elucidated in both mouse and human models over the last 10 years. The question of whether T-lineage commitment occurs within the thymus or the bone marrow has been actively investigated. In addition to pluripotent CD34[+] HSCs, a number of other more committed progenitors in bone marrow with specific cell surface marker characteristics have been identified with T-lymphoid potential, primarily in the mouse, but these progenitors in general also retain the capacity to differentiate into other lymphoid lineages, including the B and NK lineages.[90] That various subsets identified in the human thymus similarly retain bilineage potential (i.e., NK/T potential or NK/dendritic cell potential) has led to the notion that the final steps in T-cell commitment occur in the thymus rather than the bone marrow.[91]

In addition to losing the capacity to differentiate into non–T-lineage cells in vitro, T-lineage commitment is characterized by the upregulation of certain cell surface markers (Fig. 22-6) and T-cell–specific genes important for the execution of downstream developmental programs. CD34[+] cells in human thymus can be further subdivided by the expression of CD38 and the MHC-like molecule CD1a, with progression from the CD34[+] CD38[−] CD1a[−] stage to the CD34[+] CD38[+] CD1a[−] stage to the CD34[+] CD38[+] CD1a[+] stage. Acquisition of CD1a[+] is largely associated with the loss of NK, dendritic cell, and plasmacytoid dendritic cell differentiation in vitro.[91] Likewise, CD1a[+] cells express the recombinase-activating

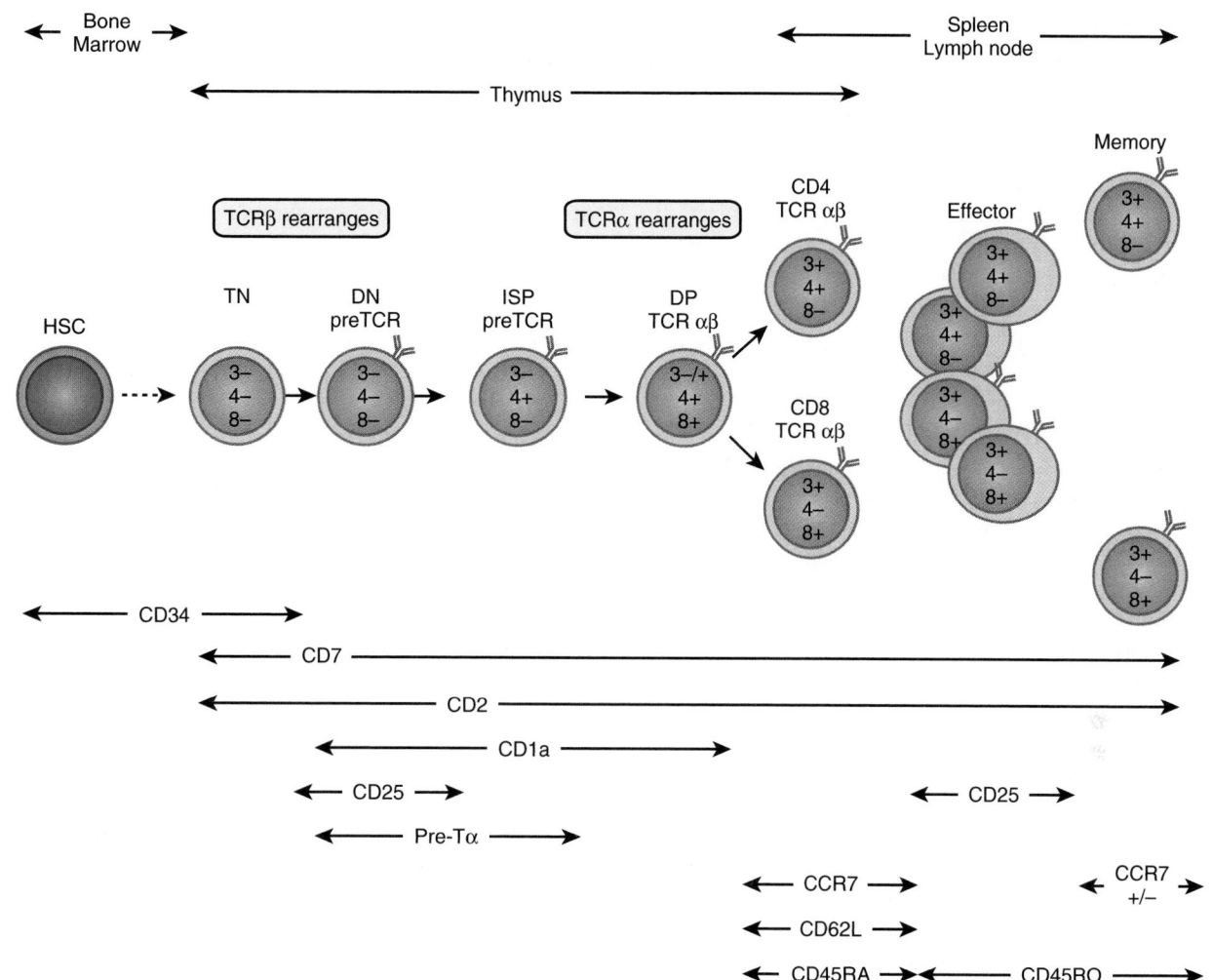

FIGURE 22-6. Overview of T-cell development. Pluripotent hematopoietic stem cells (HSC) in bone marrow commit to the T lineage, seed the thymus as early triple-negative CD3⁻ CD4⁻ CD8⁻ (TN) thymocytes, and express the T-cell markers CD7 and CD2. T-cell receptor genes rearrange serially (TCRβ then TCRα), which leads to expression of the first pre-T-cell receptor (pre-TCR) and then the mature TCR αβ complex. Double-negative CD4⁻ CD8⁻ (DN) thymocytes upregulate both CD4 and CD8 after passing through an intermediate single-positive (ISP) stage to become double-positive CD4⁺ CD8⁺ (DP) thymocytes, which undergo positive and negative selection. During lineage commitment, either CD4 or CD8 is downregulated, thereby resulting in the formation of single-positive (SP) thymocytes with CD4⁺ thymocytes restricted to major histocompatibility (MHC) class II and CD8⁺ thymocytes restricted to MHC class I. Mature T cells in the spleen and lymph node that have not encountered cognate antigen express markers associated with the naïve state such as CD45RA and CD62L, and the pattern of surface markers changes with activation, acquisition of effector function, and further differentiation into memory T cells.

gene products RAG1 and RAG2, and early TCR rearrangements are detectable after the acquisition of CD38 and CD1a. Transcription factors upregulated during these stages of early human T-cell commitment, whose requirement for T-cell development have also been demonstrated in gene-deficient mice, include GATA3 and NOTCH.[92-95]

Interactions between thymocytes and epithelial cells are critical for events in later thymic development, such as positive and negative selection, as detailed later, as well as for early commitment and development. The so-called nude mouse, which lacks expression of the epithelial transcription factor Foxn1, is born athymic, and humans lacking Foxn1 have severe T-cell deficiency, alopecia, and nail dystrophy.[96,97] Unlike B cells, which can be induced in vitro to mature from precursors by coculture on bone

marrow stromal cells, T cells generally cannot be differentiated in vitro by this means, only when seeded into a three-dimensional source of primary thymic stroma, such as whole thymic organ culture. This distinction implies that specific soluble or cell-cell contact factors present only in the three-dimensional primary organ are required to engage developing thymocytes and induce their differentiation. The Notch signaling pathway, which is activated by the interaction of Notch ligands on epithelial cells and Notch family members on thymocytes, has emerged as one such factor.[98,99] Expression of activated Notch1 in human HSCs is sufficient to induce T-cell development in vitro and in immunodeficient mice,[100] and deletion of Notch1 from mouse thymocytes severely impairs early T-cell development.[101] Interestingly, primary three-dimensional thymic stroma expresses Notch ligands such as Delta-like 1, and this expression is lost when the architecture is disrupted.[102] Indeed, expression of Delta-like 1 in the OP9 bone marrow stromal cell line is capable of directing mouse and human uncommitted HSCs and even embryonic stem cells into the T lineage when cocultured in a two-dimensional format in vitro.[99,103,104] This powerful system raises the intriguing possibility of differentiating and expanding T cells in vitro for use in human therapeutics[105] and underscores the importance of thymocyte-epithelial interactions during intrathymic development.

Stages of Intrathymic TCR αβ T-Cell Development and Spatial Considerations

T-lymphoid precursors that enter the thymus from the blood mature through a series of ordered developmental stages characterized by changes in cell surface markers, sequential expression of the TCR genes, and predictable migration from the cortex to the medulla (see Fig. 22-6). The earliest thymocytes reside in the cortex, are CD34+, express pan-T-cell markers such as CD2 and CD7, but lack TCR, the TCR-associated CD3 complex, and the helper and cytotoxic mature T-cell coreceptors CD4 and CD8 and hence are CD3− CD4− CD8−, or triple negative. During αβ T-cell development, triple-negative thymocytes that succeed in rearranging a functional TCRβ chain express TCRβ complexed to the invariant pre-TCRα protein. TCR signaling in thymocytes, similar to what occurs upon engagement of the TCR in peripheral mature T cells, promotes rapid expansion and differentiation into double-positive (DP) thymocytes expressing both the CD4 and CD8 coreceptors and initiates rearrangement of the TCRα gene. In humans, in contrast to mice, there is an additional intermediate stage

in which thymocytes express only CD4 and not CD8 (intermediate single positive [ISP]). DP thymocytes account for approximately 80% to 90% of the total thymocyte number and can be found at the corticomedullary junction. Although the majority of DP thymocytes die by apoptosis, those that successfully undergo positive and negative selection survive, commit to either the CD4/helper or CD8/cytotoxic lineage, and migrate to the thymic medulla before terminal maturation and export to the periphery.

T-Cell Recognition of Peptide-MHC Complexes

A hallmark of the cellular immune response is antigen specificity, which is conferred by the rearranged and selected TCR on the surface of T lymphocytes. The TCR recognizes processed fragments of foreign proteins embedded in MHC molecules. There are two forms of MHC molecules: MHC class I (the major determinants are HLA-A, HLA-B, and HLA-C in humans) and MHC class II (the major determinants are HLA-DR, HLA-DQ, and HLA-DP in humans) (Fig. 22-7).[106] MHC class I molecules are composed of a 42-kd transmembrane, polymorphic α chain encoded in the MHC and noncovalently associated with a 12-kd soluble, nonpolymorphic (non-MHC) β chain termed β2-microglobulin. X-ray crystallographic analysis of HLA molecules in which peptide was embedded[106] has demonstrated that the first two domains of the α chain both form α helices that together form a cleft (Fig. 22-8).[107] This cleft forms the binding domain for peptide antigen and accommodates a 9- to 11–amino acid fragment in an extended conformation; residues that interact with the MHC and those that interact with the TCR can be defined.[108,109] Polymor-

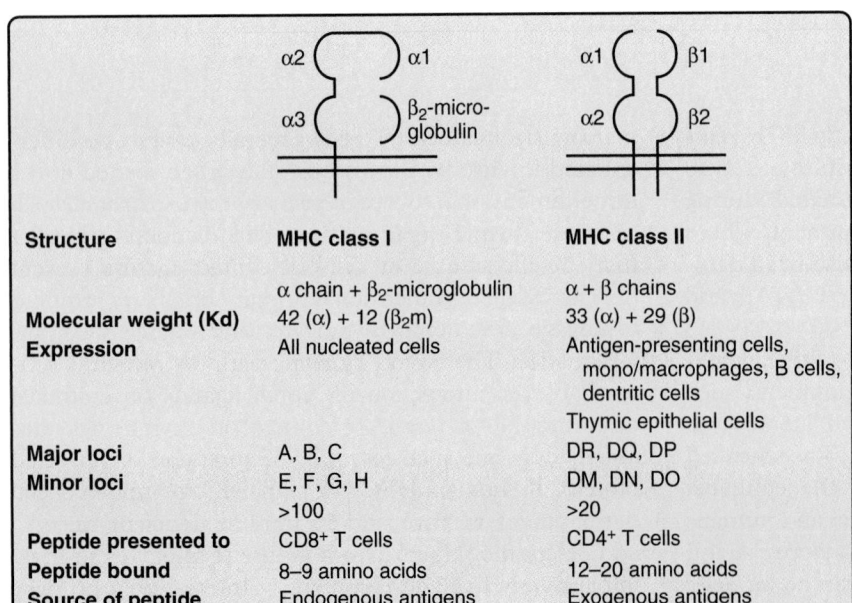

Structure	MHC class I	MHC class II
	α chain + β2-microglobulin	α + β chains
Molecular weight (Kd)	42 (α) + 12 (β2m)	33 (α) + 29 (β)
Expression	All nucleated cells	Antigen-presenting cells, mono/macrophages, B cells, dentritic cells
		Thymic epithelial cells
Major loci	A, B, C	DR, DQ, DP
Minor loci	E, F, G, H	DM, DN, DO
	>100	>20
Peptide presented to	CD8+ T cells	CD4+ T cells
Peptide bound	8–9 amino acids	12–20 amino acids
Source of peptide	Endogenous antigens	Exogenous antigens

FIGURE 22-7. Characteristics of major histocompatibility (MHC) class I and class II molecules. MHC class I molecules are single transmembrane molecules noncovalently associated with β2-microglobulin, whereas MHC class II molecules exist as heterodimers. CD8+ T cells recognize 8 to 9 amino acids, endogenous processed peptides embedded in the MHC class I groove, whereas CD4+ T cells recognize 12 to 20 amino acids, exogenous peptides embedded in the groove formed by MHC class II molecules. The major and minor loci are listed, as are important differences between the two classes.

phism within the MHC itself serves to ensure variation in the affinity of peptide binding; the extraordinary MHC polymorphism within the species further ensures that any single microbe is unlikely to mutate such that it is unable to bind all MHC molecules in the population and therefore escape T-cell recognition.[110-113]

MHC class II molecules are formed by the noncovalent association of two transmembrane glycoproteins, αβ, both of which are polymorphic and encoded in the MHC.[106,114] Solution of the structure of MHC class II molecules has shown that a peptide-binding cleft is formed by the first domains of each of the αβ chains; however, the ends of the cleft are open, unlike the situation in MHC class I molecules (see Fig. 22-8).[106] The peptide-binding cleft of MHC class II accommodates processed peptides that are 10 to 30 (mean of 14) amino acids in length.[115,116] As with MHC class I, the genetic polymorphism of MHC class II determines the affinity and specificity of peptide binding and T-cell recognition.[114-116] Although MHC class I molecules are expressed constitutively on all human nucleated cells, MHC class II molecules are constitutively expressed only on B cells, monocyte/macrophages, and dendritic cells. Expression of MHC class II proteins may be induced on the surface of monocyte/macrophages, fibroblasts, endothelial cells, and certain mesenchymal and epidermal cells by a variety of inflammatory mediators and cytokines such as IL-1. In humans but not in mice, MHC class II proteins can be inducibly expressed on T lymphocytes as well, thus rendering T cells capable of antigen presentation to other T cells. These two classes of MHC proteins generally interact with different classes of T lymphocytes: CD4+ T cells recognize peptide antigen in association with MHC

class II molecules, whereas CD8+ T cells recognize peptide antigen in association with MHC class I molecules, in part because CD8 binds to invariant portions of the α3 domain of MHC class I.

T-Cell Receptor Rearrangement and Selection in the Thymus

Effective adaptive immunity relies on the random generation of a diverse repertoire of antigen-specific T cells, along with appropriate quality control measures to ensure that nonfunctional T cells are not needlessly allowed to mature fully. To achieve this goal, the TCR genes undergo somatic rearrangement in a serial fashion, and the growth and proliferation of developing T cells are tightly linked to signaling and transcriptional events downstream of functional TCR or TCR intermediates.

The four TCR gene clusters, α, β, γ, δ, are each composed of germline genes encoding discontinuous variable regions ($V_α, V_β, V_γ, V_δ$), diversity regions ($D_β, D_δ$), joining regions ($J_α, J_β, J_γ, J_δ$), and constant regions ($C_α, C_β, C_γ, C_δ$).[117] The TCRγ locus is situated on human chromosome 7, and the remaining three are located on human chromosome 14, with the TCRδ locus embedded between the $V_α$ and $J_α$ regions of the TCRα locus. The TCRβ germline genes consist of around 50 $V_β$, 2 $D_β$, 13 $J_β$, and 2 $C_β$ genes, whereas the TCRα germline genes consists of at least 70 $V_α$, 60 $J_α$, and a single $C_α$ gene. The TCRβ and TCRα loci have many more genes than the TCRδ or TCRγ loci do; however, the diversity of TCR γδ T cells is increased by the splicing of 2 $D_δ$ regions to each other (VDDJ). Similar to the Ig genes in B cells, rear-

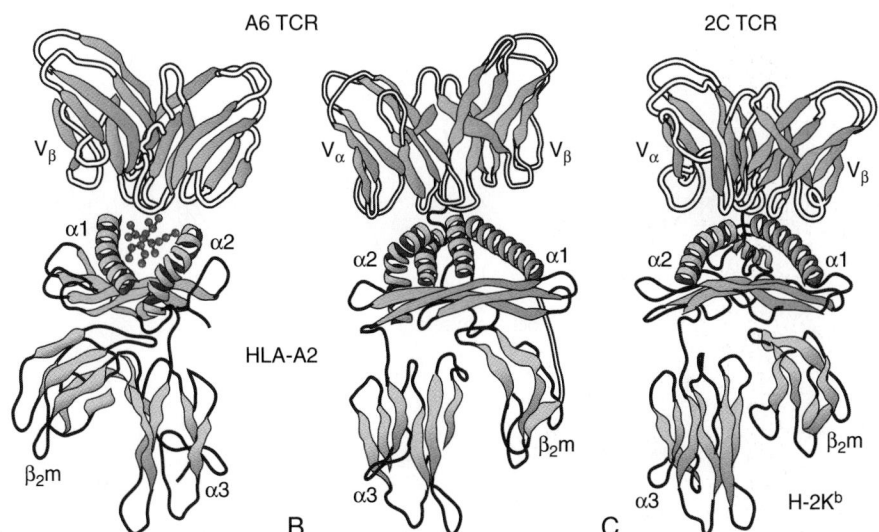

FIGURE 22-8. Peptide bound within the antigen-binding cleft of MHC class I molecules. **A,** Schematic representation of the structure of HLA-A2. **B,** Solution of the crystallographic structure of an influenza peptide bound within the peptide-binding groove of HLA-Aw68. The first α1 and α2 domains of the major histocompatibility (MHC) class I protein each form an a helix that together form a cleft. This cleft, or "groove," is the binding domain for the peptide antigen, here represented by amino acids 91 to 99 of influenza nucleoprotein. The T cell recognizes peptide plus MHC class I determinants. T cells become tolerant to self-peptides bound to MHC class I and class II proteins but retain the ability to respond to foreign or viral peptides bound to self-MHC class I or class II proteins. *(Reproduced From Bjorkman PJ. MHC restriction in three dimensions: a view of T cell receptor/ligand interactions. Cell. 1997;89:167-170.)*

rangement of the TCR genes is carried out by the RAG1 and RAG2 proteins, with serial somatic rearrangements between the V, D, J, and C regions. Although N-region diversification is found in both the TCRα and TCRβ genes, T cells do not undergo somatic mutation as readily as B cells do and instead undergo limited further rearrangements after emerging from the thymus.[84]

Several major checkpoints regulate the development of TCR αβ and TCR γδ thymocytes.[117-120] First, serial rearrangement of the TCR gene clusters in an ordered fashion ensures that the TCRβ and TCRα genes are not rearranged in developing TCR γδ T cells. Thus, in human thymocytes, TCRγ and TCRδ loci rearrange first, during the triple-negative stage.[95] That human TCR γδ T cells generally have unrearranged TCRβ genes and that TCR αβ T cells generally have nonproductively rearranged TCRδ genes imply that only thymocytes that do not generate a functional γδ TCR go on to rearrange the TCRβ gene.[121] The molecular mechanisms controlling this process are still being elucidated. The second or so-called beta selection checkpoint occurs after TCRβ rearrangement. Cells that undergo productive rearrangement of the TCRβ locus express functional TCRβ protein that complexes to the invariant pre-TCRα protein and CD3 signaling complex, thereby resulting in the expression of pre-TCR. In gene-deficient mice, where beta selection is known to occur during a precise phase of the triple-negative stage of development, loss of a number of signal-ing molecules or transcription factors downstream of pre-TCR results in defective beta selection, failure of differentiation into DP stage, and lack of proliferation or apoptosis (or both).[122] Beta selection in humans begins during the CD34+ CD38+ CD1a+ stage and continues through the CD4 ISP and early DP stage of development (see Fig. 22-6).[95,121] Thus, only thymocytes that express functional TCRβ are allowed to proliferate and proceed to TCRα locus rearrangement.

Before TCRα gene rearrangement, the TCRδ locus is excised by a nonproductive rearrangement between the δRec and ΨJα regions[123] that generates an episomal circle of DNA or T-cell receptor excision circle (TREC), which is increasingly being used on a research basis to quantify thymic activity (Fig. 22-9).[124,125] Unlike the TCRβ locus, rearrangement of the TCRα locus occurs processively; that is, V_α-J_α recombination of 5′ J segments that are nonproductive or out of frame is followed by further rearrangement on the same allele to more 3′ J segments.[126] This process increases the chances of generating a complete TCR αβ protein from any single developing DP thymocyte. Successful rearrangement of the TCRα gene results in expression of the mature TCR αβ and CD3 signaling complex during the late DP stage. These cells then undergo positive and negative selection (see the next section) and simultaneously commit to either the CD4 or the CD8 lineage to generate CD4 single-positive (SP) and CD8 SP thymocytes.

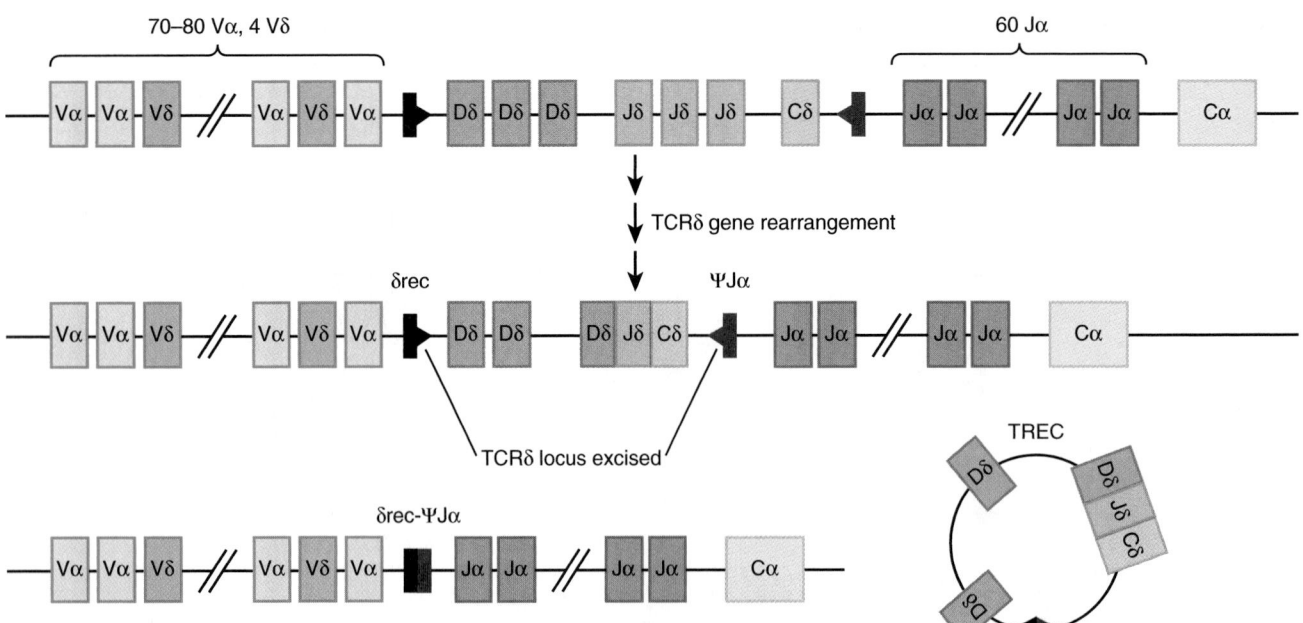

FIGURE 22-9. Formation of T-cell receptor excision circles (TRECs). The T-cell receptor α and δ (TCRα, TCRδ) loci are schematically depicted to show the basic rearrangement of variable (V), diversity (D), joining (J) and constant (C) regions. V_δ regions are interspersed between V_α regions, whereas the remainder of the TCRδ locus (D_δ, J_δ, C_δ) is embedded within the TCRα locus between the V_α and J_α regions. The *black box* and *red box* represent the δrec and ΨJα sequences, whereas the *black* and *white triangles* represent recombination signal sequences (RSSs) that recombina-tion-activating gene (RAG) products recognize. The *first line* depicts the locus in the germline configuration. After TCRδ rearrangement, the D_δ, J_δ, and C_δ segments are randomly recombined. Thereafter, if the cell undergoes TCRβ and TCRα rearrangement, joining of δrec to ΨJα excises the TCRδ locus and results in an episomal circle of DNA containing the fusion of RSS signals. Polymerase chain reaction primers specific for this joining region can thus be used to detect the presence of the excision circle, an indicator of active rearrangement and T-cell neogenesis.

Positive Selection, Negative Selection, and CD4/CD8 Lineage Commitment

The massive proliferation of DP thymocytes results in TCR αβ thymocytes with an immense range of specificities, including many that are incapable of binding host MHC, cannot recognize host MHC complexed to endogenous peptide ligands, or have inappropriately high affinity for MHC–self-peptide and hence are autoreactive. Selecting only thymocytes with intermediate MHC–self-peptide affinity (so-called Goldilocks or just-right conditions) is critical for maintaining diversity of the repertoire, conserving the energy of the animal, and promoting self-tolerance.[127]

Positive selection is the term used to describe the process of selecting thymocytes capable of recognizing host MHC complexed to self-peptides generated from the processing of endogenous proteins. DP thymocytes are exquisitely prone to cell death in response to γ-irradiation, corticosteroids, exposure to TCR or CD3 cross-linking antibodies, or simply removal of the thymus from the body, and thus a positive signal via TCR-MHC/peptide interactions is required to rescue the small number of DP thymocytes destined to become SP thymocytes from cell death. Gene-deficient mouse experiments have demonstrated that multiple elements of TCR signaling are required for optimal positive selection, including TCR components (TCRα, CD3δ), early signaling molecules (GADs, ZAP70), late signaling proteins (RasGRP, calcineurin, ERK), and transcription factors (nuclear factor of activated T cells [NF-AT], Egr family members).[126,128-130] Interestingly, humans deficient in CD3δ and ZAP70 have been described who have discrepant development when compared with the knockout mouse counterparts. Deficiency of CD3δ in humans causes an earlier block in development at the CD4⁻ CD8⁻ stage, well before the development of DP thymocytes.[131,132] ZAP70 deficiency results in selective deficiency of CD8 SP thymocytes and mature CD8⁺ T cells.[133-135] Likewise, although in the mouse interaction of DP thymocytes with MHC on radioresistant cortical thymic epithelium is probably the dominant requirement for positive selection, the source of MHC and the relative contributions of MHC from thymic epithelium, thymic dendritic cells, or other thymic APCs to positive selection in humans are less clear.

Negative selection is the term used to describe the process of removing thymocytes that are self-reactive, also termed "central tolerance," by clonal deletion.[136,137] This is the first and major mechanism for control of autoimmunity, although clones that escape deletion in the thymus are subject to peripheral tolerizing influences (discussed later). In mice, negative selection can be mediated by cortical epithelium, medullary epithelium, and medullary dendritic cells. However, it was never clear how thymocytes reactive against self-antigens expressed only in peripheral tissues, such as islet cells, were selected against in the thymus. In other words, how are these tissue-specific proteins expressed in the thymus? More recently, mouse and human studies have revealed that all three cell types, medullary thymic epithelial cells (mTECs) in particular, exhibit promiscuous gene expression and transcribe a broad range of tissue-specific, nonthymic antigens.[138] This insight helps explain how developing thymocytes reactive against nonthymic proteins can be centrally deleted during negative selection. A newly discovered gene, *AIRE* (autoimmune regulator), is a factor shown to control the transcription of tissue-specific antigen expression in murine mTECs.[139] Simultaneously, this gene was shown to be responsible for the autoimmune polyendocrinopathy–candidiasis–ectodermal dystrophy (APECED) syndrome, characterized by chronic mucocutaneous candidiasis, hypoparathyroidism, adrenal insufficiency, and other organ-specific autoimmune manifestations.[140,141] Thus, this disease may be the first example of failure of negative selection underpinning a human monogenic autoimmune disorder.

Maturation of CD4 and CD8 SP thymocytes from DP thymocytes occurs concurrently with positive selection and results in "matching" of coreceptor to MHC restriction with downregulation of the opposite coreceptor. The mechanisms controlling the CD4/CD8 lineage decision are separable from those governing positive selection[142] and have been the subject of active investigation in murine models.[143-146] Expression of class I and class II MHC in the thymus is not surprisingly required for SP thymocyte development.[147-149] Indeed, patients with defects in a number of genes that control MHC class II expression, including *RFXANK*, *RFX5*, *RFXAP* and *CIITA*, all manifest the so-called bare lymphocyte syndrome, a rare autosomal recessive disorder characterized by decreased numbers of CD4⁺ T cells, deficient helper function, and absence of specific antibody production because of lack of CD4-mediated B-cell maturation.[150]

T-CELL ACTIVATION AND FUNCTION

CD4⁺ and CD8⁺ TCR αβ T cells exported from the thymus circulate in a naïve or resting state in the blood and lymphoid organs but are poised to be activated by cognate antigen presented by MHC on the surface of APCs. CD8⁺ cytolytic T cells induce the lysis of foreign cells, such as infected, malignant, or allogeneic cells. CD4⁺ helper T cells interact with B cells via cell-cell and soluble factors to induce class switching and the generation of antigen-specific antibodies. They also provide "help" to CD8⁺ cytolytic T cells. Activation of resting T cells not only relies on signaling cascades downstream of the TCR-MHC interaction (signal 1) but also requires or is enhanced by the binding of a variety of T-cell surface molecules to their ligands on APCs (signal 2). The lack of a second signal generally results in nonresponsiveness or anergy of the T cell and serves to ensure that activation of the naïve T cell is not only antigen specific but regulated as well. The affinity of the cognate antigen, the engagement of specific costimulatory molecules, and the cytokine milieu collectively influence and modulate the outcome of T-cell activation and thereby result in the generation of distinct effector cell subsets. Although most effector T cells perform their function and expire, a subset of activated cells differentiate into long-lived memory cells capable of rapid anamnestic responses.

T-Cell Receptor Triggering and Activation

The accessibility of T cells from human blood, the development of transgenic and knockout murine models, the availability of agonistic and antagonistic antibodies to T-cell surface proteins, and live cell imaging with fluorescent confocal microscopy have made the study of T-cell signaling highly tractable.

In contrast to the highly polymorphic and critical extracellular domain of TCR, the intracellular domains of αβ and γδ TCR are short and do not have intrinsic signaling function. Rather, antigen recognition of sufficient density on the cell surface to cross-link and cluster the TCR triggers modification of the CD3 complex of proteins, which are noncovalently associated with the TCR's cytoplasmic domains. The CD3 family of proteins in humans consists of γ, δ, ε, and ζ subunits, all transmembrane proteins with conserved ITAMs, similar to those found in the accessory Ig-α and Ig-β proteins complexed to BCR (see earlier and Fig. 22-10).[151] The CD3 γδε subunits have similar structure with a single extracellular Ig domain and a single cytoplasmic ITAM and are encoded by closely linked genes on human chromosome 11q23. The CD3 ζ subunit, on the other hand, has a very short extracellular domain with a longer intracellular domain bearing three ITAMs and is encoded on human chromosome 1. In the mouse, an additional CD3 η subunit is generated by alternative splicing of the CD3 ζ gene; no CD3 η transcripts can be detected, however, in humans.[152] Complete assembly of TCR αβ, CD3 γ, δ, ε, and ζ in the endoplasmic reticulum is required for stability of the complex, which is then exported to the cell membrane in toto.[153] The CD3 ζ proteins exist as a homodimer linked by disulfides in the extracellular domain. The exact stoichiometry of the TCR-CD3 complex remains controversial.[154]

Our understanding of the signaling cascades downstream of the TCR has become increasingly complete and complex. Five major signal transduction pathways are triggered by TCR engagement: phosphotyrosine kinase (PTK) activation, plasma membrane phosphatidylinositol hydrolysis, changes in intracellular calcium concentration $[Ca^{2+}]_i$, RAS/MAPK, and PKC pathways (see Fig. 22-5). In recent years a variety of adaptor molecules and other families of proteins, including small Rho guanosine triphosphatases (GTPases), have been implicated in these pathways. Thus, there is much crosstalk between the main pathways, which then converge on the activation of nuclear transcription factors critical for the expression of T-cell effector molecules, namely, the cytokine genes,

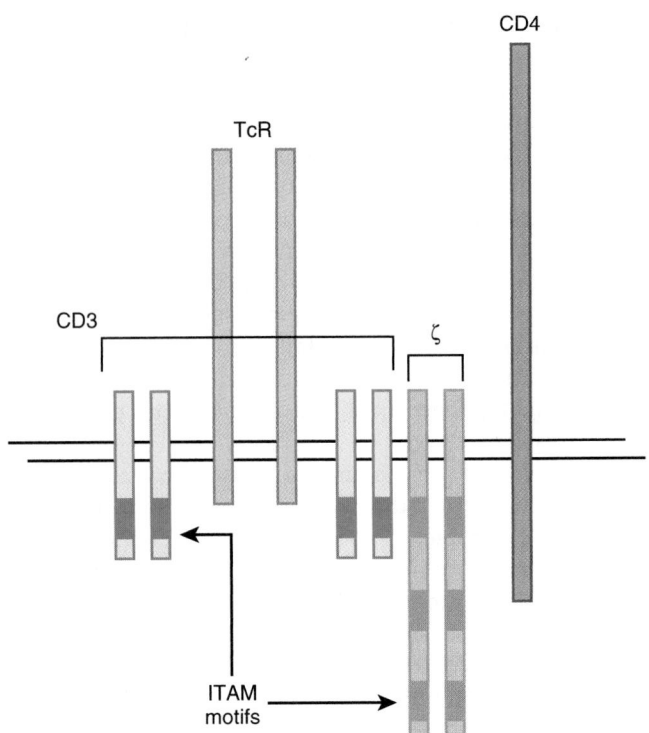

FIGURE 22-10. The T-cell receptor (TCR)-CD3 complex. The TCR is a covalently linked heterodimer composed generally of an α and β subunit and more rarely of a γ and δ subunit. The TCR is noncovalently complexed on the cell surface to a family of invariant proteins known as CD3 and to the ζ family, which together are thought to transduce activating signals from the TCR to the cytoplasm of the cell. The ζ subunit exists primarily as a homodimer of ζ-ζ in the TCR-CD3 complex but can be complexed to η or the FcR γ chain as heterodimers. Each of the CD3 and ζ chains has one and three intracellular activation motifs (ITAMs), respectively, which are important for initiation of signaling pathways in the cell. The physical association of CD3 and ζ with the TCR is required for proper assembly of the TCR-CD3 complex, for cell surface expression, and for signal transduction.

particularly IL-2. Finally, the spatial organization of the TCR signaling complex in ordered lipid microdomains, in which an "immune synapse" is formed at the point of contact between the T cell and APC, is thought to enhance T cell–APC interaction and allow directed secretion of cytokines locally to the contacting APC.[155,156]

On a macromolecular level, TCR signaling begins when recognition of cognate antigen clusters the TCR molecules to the site of T cell–APC contact. The exact mechanism of how TCR occupancy induces the allosteric changes in CD3 necessary to transmit a signal is unclear, but within seconds to minutes of engagement, PTKs such as Lck and Fyn are activated and phosphorylate the ITAMs on CD3 subunits, particularly CD3 ζ (see Fig. 22-5). The physical association of Lck with the CD4 and CD8 coreceptor molecules, recruitment to the membrane by myristoylation and other modifications, and the multiplicity of Lck molecules in close proximity when the TCR-coreceptor complex is cross-linked are thought to promote and amplify its rapid activation.[157] Phosphorylated ITAM on CD3 ζ in turn recruits ZAP70, a 70-kd protein kinase whose homologue in B cells is Syk, via the phosphotyrosine binding SH2 domain.[158] ZAP70 is phosphorylated by Lck, is activated, and then phosphorylates two key substrates, LAT (linker for activation of T cells) and SLP76 (SH2 domain–containing leukocyte protein of 76 kd). A host of downstream proteins, including Grb2, SOS, ITK, PLCγ, GADS, and VAV1, then converge on LAT and SLP76 to activate the phosphoinositol, calcium, and RAS/MAPK pathways.[51]

Recruitment of PLCγ to LAT and SLP76 catalyzes the hydrolysis of phosphatidylinositol 4,5-biphosphate to generate IP$_3$ and DAG, which in turn promote the increase in [Ca^{2+}]$_i$ and activation of the T-cell–specific isoform PKC θ, respectively (see Fig. 22-5).[159,160] The critical downstream effect of the rise in [Ca^{2+}]$_i$ is activation of the calcium- and calmodulin-dependent serine/threonine phosphatase calcineurin, whose key direct substrates in T cells are members of the NF-AT family.[161-163] Dephosphorylation of NF-AT allows translocation of it from the cytoplasm to the nucleus, where it binds, often in the presence of AP-1 elements, to the transcriptional regulatory sequences of IL-2 and other cytokine genes. The immunosuppressant agents cyclosporine and tacrolimus (FK506) function by forming macromolecular complexes with intracellular binding proteins (cyclophilins and FK-binding proteins [FKBPs], respectively), which in turn inhibit the phosphatase activity of calcineurin, thereby abrogating the early cytokine elaboration critical for T-cell expansion and function.[162,164,165]

Activation of the RAS pathway primarily occurs by the recruitment of the adaptor proteins Grb2 and Shc to phosphorylated LAT, which leads to recruitment of the guanine nucleotide exchange protein Sos (see Fig. 22-5). Sos catalyzes the conversion of inactive guanosine diphosphate (GDP)-bound RAS to active guanosine triphosphate (GTP)-bound RAS and activates a series of MAPKs.[166] Activation of PKCθ in response to PLCγ described earlier can crosstalk with this pathway and induce increases in RAS and MAPK activity, although the mechanisms and relative contributions are still unclear. Major downstream effects of PKCθ activation include stimulation of AP-1 nuclear activity, regulation of JNK (the upstream kinase of AP-1), and activation of NF-κB.[160] Induction of these and other transcription factors, which cooperate with NF-AT translocation in response to rises in [Ca^{2+}]$_i$, strongly stimulates production of IL-2.

The transcriptional program executed in response to TCR stimulation includes the major T-cell cytokine IL-2; other cytokines, including IFN-γ and IL-4, the canonic T-helper type 1 and type 2 cytokines (discussed later); proliferative factors, including c-myc and c-fos; a variety of activation markers such as CD69, CD45RO, CD44; and growth factor receptors, most prominently the high-affinity IL-2 receptor subunit IL2Rα, also called CD25.[167] Binding of IL-2 to its receptor, in both autocrine and paracrine fashion, results in a growth factor–induced signal to the cell and induces the transition from G$_1$ to S phase of the cell cycle. Interestingly, in recent years,

CD25 has been found not only to mark activated T cells but also to be expressed on naturally occurring T-regulatory cells, discussed later. The role of IL-2 in expanding activated effector cells and simultaneously its requirement for development and maintenance of the T-regulatory population result in pleiotropic effects of IL-2 in vivo and has complicated the potential use of IL-2 in the clinical setting.[168] The high-affinity IL-2 receptor is composed of IL-2Rα, IL-2Rβ (CD122), and IL2Rγ (γ$_c$, CD132), this last a common signaling component of the cytokine receptors for IL-2, IL-4, IL-7, IL-9, IL-15, and IL-21. Mutations in the IL2Rγ gene and the downstream factor JAK3 (Janus kinase 3) result in X-linked and autosomal recessive forms of severe combined immunodeficiency (SCID), respectively. In contrast to the inhibition of early signals downstream of [Ca^{2+}]$_i$ by cyclosporine and tacrolimus, the late proliferative response of T cells to binding of IL-2 to its receptor are abrogated by the immunosuppressant sirolimus (rapamycin), which complexes with FKBP to inhibit mTOR (mammalian target of rapamycin). All three of these agents have been used in the prevention and treatment of graft-versus-host disease and solid organ graft rejection, and the actions of calcineurin inhibitors and rapamycin on serial events in T-cell activation have encouraged their use in combination therapy.

Coreceptors Involved in T-Cell Activation and the Immune Synapse

Because the affinity of the TCR for cognate antigen–MHC complexes and the density of TCRs on the naïve T cell are both relatively low, activation of the T cell depends on augmentation of the TCR signal by a complex combination of TCR-associated coreceptors, adhesion molecules, and other costimulatory molecules that transduce distinct signals (Fig. 22-11). Recent techniques that visualize the distribution of TCR and these affiliated molecules in relation to the site of T cell–APC contact have led to a model in which the immune synapse segregates into central and peripheral supramolecular activation clusters (c-SMAC and p-SMAC, respectively). The functional relevance of different synapse morphologies and the dynamics of formation and disassembly of the synapse are just being investigated.[155,156,169]

The CD4 and CD8 glycoprotein coreceptors bind to class II and class I MHC molecules, respectively, and are used to classify T cells into helper and cytolytic subtypes. The proximity of CD4 and CD8 coreceptors to the TCR-MHC complex and the association of both CD4 and CD8 intracellular domains with the Src family tyrosine kinase p56lck are thought to increase avidity of the T cell for the APC and bring p56lck into close association with its target CD3 ζ.[170,171] CD4 and CD8 coreceptors are generally found in the c-SMAC with TCR.

CD2 is a T-cell–specific glycoprotein receptor that binds to several ligands on the APC, including CD58

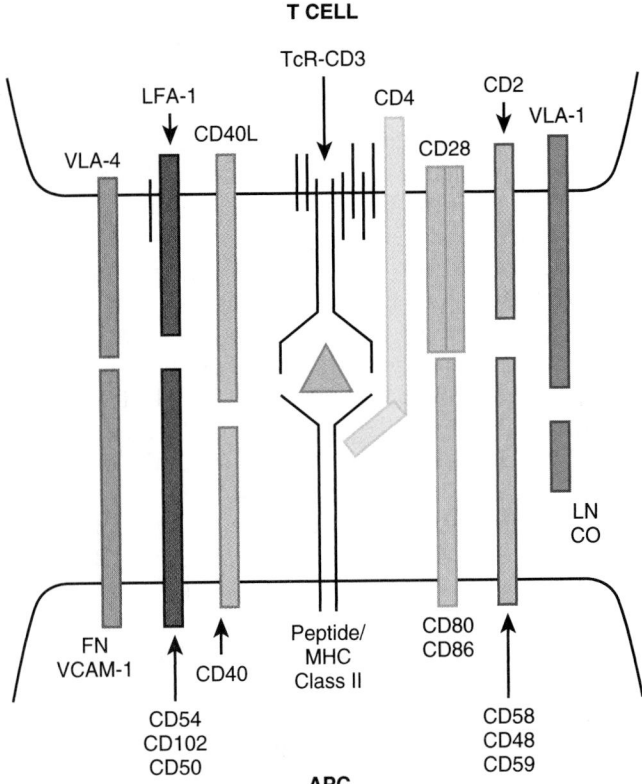

FIGURE 22-11. Receptor-ligand interactions important for T-cell adhesion and activation. The interaction of representative T-cell surface receptors with their ligands is shown. The T-cell receptor (TCR)-CD3 complex interacts with a specific antigen in association with major histocompatibility (MHC) class II (or class I) proteins. CD4 (or CD8) binds to monomorphic determinants on MHC class II (or MHC class I) proteins. The CD2 receptor binds to its principal ligand CD58 (shown). Two additional ligands, CD48 and CD59, have been identified. The ligands for CD28 and CD40L are CD80/CD86 and CD40, respectively, and are expressed on activated B cells. The ligands for CD26, CD43, and CD7 (not shown), among other molecules, are unknown. LFA-1 (CD11a/CD18, $\alpha_L\beta_2$) interacts with its ligands CD54, CD102, CD50, and perhaps others. Fibronectin (FN) and CD106 (vascular endothelial adhesion molecule 1[VCAM-1]) are two ligands for VLA-4 (CD49d/CD29, $\alpha_4\beta_1$). Two ligands for CD44 exist: hyaluronidate and osteopontin (Eta-1). The ligands for other lymphocyte homing receptors are shown in Table 22-3. APC, antigen-presenting cell; CO, collagen; Ln, laminin.

(LFA-3), CD59, and CD48 (see Fig. 22-11). Binding of CD2 to its ligand on the APC serves to improve adhesion and the strength of the TCR-MHC interaction, whereas the cytoplasmic region associates with p56lck and thus augments TCR-induced early signals. In turn, TCR signaling itself modifies the cytoplasmic tail via a critical asparagine residue and thereby induces conformational changes that improve CD2-ligand binding, an example of so-called inside-out signaling.[172] CD2 is generally found in the c-SMAC.

CD45, also known as leukocyte common antigen, is a phosphotyrosine phosphatase. It is generally excluded from the immune synapse in a manner that suggests that the size of the ectodomain of a given receptor determines its presence or absence in the synapse.[155] The major substrate of CD45 is thought to be p56lck, as well as possibly

JAK/STATs, CD3 ζ, and ZAP70[173]; it is suggested that the dynamic repositioning of CD45 during synapse formation and disruption alters its substrate specificity.[174] Deficiency of CD45 has been studied in mice and humans and results in defects in thymic T-cell development, T-cell function, and autoimmunity.[173,175,176] Alternative splicing of the CD45 message results in multiple isoforms, most notably CD45RA, expressed in naïve or resting T cells, and CD45RO, characteristic of activated or previously activated T cells.

Costimulation of T Cells

TCR ligation (signal 1), even in the presence of CD4 or CD8 engagement, is insufficient for activation of resting T cells. In the absence of appropriate costimulation, TCR occupancy alone can result in T-cell unresponsiveness (T-cell clonal anergy, ignorance, or tolerance) on subsequent exposure to antigen. Tolerance is characterized by the inability to proliferate or secrete cytokines in response to secondary stimulation by the same antigen. Anergy is classically defined as this same failure, but it can be rescued or reversed by exogenous IL-2 in vitro.[177] Costimulation (signal 2) typically is mediated by receptors on T cells recognizing ligands on activated APCs (see Fig. 22-11).

CD28, the first discovered costimulatory molecule that prevents the induction of anergy, is a member of a growing family of related molecules. Human CD28, a homodimer of two 44-kd glycoproteins, is expressed on essentially all CD4+ cells and approximately 50% of CD8+ cells. CD28 interacts with the B7 family members CD80 (B7-1) and CD86 (B7-2). Interaction of CD28 with CD80 or CD86 increases, quantitatively, the amount of IL-2 produced by both transcriptional and posttranscriptional mechanisms,[178] augments T-cell proliferative responses, and enhances T-cell survival by induction of the anti-apoptotic protein Bcl-X_L.[179] Notably, CD28-dependent costimulation appears to be resistant to inhibition by the immunosuppressants cyclosporine and tacrolimus (FK506), inhibitors of the serine/threonine phosphatase calcineurin, thus suggesting that this pathway uses a different cascade of biochemical signals than the calcineurin-sensitive TCR-CD3 complex.[180-182]

Structurally similar to CD28, CD152 (cytotoxic T-lymphocyte antigen 4, CTLA-4) is a second CD28 family member that also binds to CD80 and CD86. CD152 is expressed only minimally on resting T cells but is induced on recently activated T cells. Mice rendered genetically deficient in CD152 expression die postnatally with progressive lymphoproliferation[183,184]; it is now clear that the endogenous function of CD152 is to downregulate T-cell activation to terminate T-cell responses.[182,185]

CD278 (inducible costimulator [ICOS]) is another member of the CD28 family that was cloned by generating monoclonal antibodies directed against activated T cells.[186] Like CD152, ICOS is expressed on activated T cells. ICOS does not bind CD80 or CD86 but instead

TABLE 22-3   CD28/B7 Superfamily Interactions

Receptor	Mass (kd)	Molecular Chromosome	Human Ligands	Expression	Function
CD28	44-90	2q33	CD80, CD86	CD4+ T cells 50% CD8+ T cells	Activation: costimulation of cytokine production, particularly IL-2; prevention of induction of anergy
CD152 (CTLA-4)	35-80	2q33	CD80, CD86	Activated T cells	Inhibition: negative regulator of T-cell activation and proliferation
ICOS	55-60	ND	B7h/ICOSL	Thymocytes, activated T cells	Activation: costimulation of IL-10 > IL-4, IL-5, IFN-β, TNF-α; enhancement of CD40L expression; regulation of T-cell hemostasis
PD-1	55	2q37	PD-L1 or B7-H1	Activated T and B cells, myeloid cells	Inhibition: decreases T-cell proliferation, decreases IFN-γ and IL-10 production
Unknown			B7-H3	Activated T cells	Activation: increases IFN-γ production

CTLA-4, cytotoxic T-lymphocyte antigen 4; ICOS, inducible T-cell costimulator; IFN, interferon; IL, interleukin; ND, not determined; PD-1, programmed death 1; TNF, tumor necrosis factor.

binds to a novel, TNF-α–inducible adhesion molecule, CD275 (inducible costimulator ligand [ICOSL], B7h, B7-H2, B7RP-1).[187] Importantly, engagement of ICOS appears to affect T-helper differentiation by favoring IL-10 and IFN-γ production (see later). ICOS appears to be a key regulatory molecule for T-cell help, essential for normal humoral responses and B-cell heavy-class switching.

The number of CD28/B7 family members that function as costimulatory molecules continues to grow (Table 22-3). Expressed on thymocytes and activated immune cells, programmed death 1 (PD-1) is a CD152-like molecule that also functions as an important negative regulator of immune responses.[188-190] An autoimmune disorder resembling systemic lupus erythematosus develops in PD-1–deficient mice. The molecular mechanism of negative regulation by PD-1, like that by CD152, appears to be recruitment of a phosphotyrosine phosphatase (SHP-2) to the signaling receptor.[191] Two PD-1 ligands have been isolated; both are posited to play a role in the induction and maintenance of peripheral tolerance.[188,192,193] Finally, B7-H3, a distinct B7 family member important for costimulation of IFN-γ production, has been isolated[194]; B7-H3 binds a counter-receptor on activated T cells distinct from any CD28 family member heretofore characterized.

In addition to CD28/B7 family members, members of the TNF family function as important costimulatory molecules involved in T-cell effector and T-cell–dependent B-cell responses. Interaction of CD154 (CD40L) with CD40 is essential for B-cell activation, Ig production, and heavy-chain isotype differentiation, as discussed earlier. The interaction of CD154 with CD40 also upregulates CD80 expression on APCs and is thus important for sustaining a T-helper precursor cell (T$_H$1) response.[195] X-linked hyper-IgM syndrome is an autoso-

mal recessive disorder characterized by a deficiency of CD4+ T-cell function and T-cell–dependent antibody responses; it is caused by mutation in the CD154 gene located on human chromosome X.[196] Affected patients have normal or increased IgM levels and very low to undetectable IgG and IgA levels and are susceptible to opportunistic infections such as *Pneumocystis jiroveci* because of intrinsic CD4+ T-helper dysfunction.[197,198] Allogeneic stem cell transplantation offers a curative therapy for patients with an appropriate donor.[199] Murine models of X-linked hyper-IgM syndrome have been developed by genetic disruption of either the CD40 or CD154 genes, which mimics the phenotype of the human disorder.[200-203]

Other TNF family molecules that are important for costimulation include CD70 (CD27L/TNFSF7) and CD252 (OX40L/TNFSF4). CD70, a ligand of approximately 50 kd that is transiently expressed on recently activated T and B lymphocytes, binds CD27, a homodimer expressed on the surface of naïve CD4+ and CD8+ T cells.[204,205] CD27/CD70 interactions promote TNF-α but not IL-2 production from T cells, as well as expression of CD154 on the T-cell surface. This receptor-ligand interaction also appears to induce B-cell terminal differentiation to plasma cells.[31] Expression of CD134 (OX40), a glycoprotein of approximately 48 kd, depends on TCR signaling on CD4+ activated cells. CD134/CD252 costimulation enhances T-cell proliferation and cytokine production at limiting antigenic densities, enhances B-cell and dendritic cell function, and modulates T-cell migration to B-cell follicular areas.[206,207] Thus, CD134/CD252 interactions have been suggested to prolong and enhance clonal expansion and immune responses at sites of infection and inflammation.

Manipulation of costimulation by soluble receptors, ligands, or antibody-mediated blockade is of increasing interest in the treatment of autoimmunity, cancer, and solid organ rejection.[208-210] More recently, the discovery that regulatory T cells (see later) are also exquisitely sensitive to costimulatory signals has complicated the potential outcome of such therapeutics. The pleiotropic effects in vivo of our current armamentarium are underscored by the sobering case of six patients in England who suffered life-threatening cytokine storm within hours of receiving an anti-CD28 antibody agonist intended to expand regulatory T cells.[211]

PERIPHERAL T-CELL MATURATION

A hallmark of adaptive immunity is the generation of an antigen-specific response that can be rapidly recalled upon re-exposure to the same antigen at a later time. Naïve T cells released from the thymus have a broad range of TCR specificities, with few clones that recognize any given antigen, and they generally do not proliferate in the absence of cognate antigen. Exposure to antigen results in differentiation and rapid proliferation of the specific naïve precursor population into effector T cells that either kill targets bearing cognate antigen in the case of CD8+ T cells or produce polarized sets of effector cytokines in the case of CD4+ T cells. The expansion of effector cells is rapid and brief, with the majority dying by activation-induced cell death. Long-lived memory T cells that survive after the effector response serve to increase the precursor frequency in the periphery and thus arm the organism for a more rapid and efficient response on subsequent exposure to the same antigen.

Naïve T-Cell Differentiation to Effector and Memory T Cells

Circulating naïve, effector (activated), and memory T cells can be differentiated by phenotypic differences, as well as by genetic changes (Fig. 22-12). With T-cell activation, a number of cell surface receptors, including CD2, CD58, LFA-1, CD29, and CD44, are upregulated and increase the avidity of the interaction between the T cell and the antigen-bearing APC. CD45RA, which is constitutively expressed on naïve T cells, is downregulated and replaced by the CD45RO isoform.[212]

More recently, human T-cell memory populations have been further characterized by the expression of CD62L (L-selectin) and the chemokine receptor CCR7 as either effector memory (CCR7−) or central memory (CCR7+) subsets. CCR7 is a lymph node–homing receptor that interacts with its ligand SLC on endothelial cells.[213] It is proposed that differential CCR7 expression serves to segregate effector memory cells to tissues, where they rapidly release cytokines and kill targets, and central memory cells to lymph nodes, where interactions with dendritic cells and B cells orchestrate effective T-cell help and secondary proliferation.[214,215] In addition to these cell surface markers, tetramer-based technology now allows identification of antigen-specific CD8+ memory cells on a research basis.[216] Four MHC molecules are bound covalently and tagged with fluorescent marker and then loaded with specific cognate peptide.[217] T cells that recognize that MHC-peptide complex bind the tetramer and can be identified by flow cytometry. This technology is currently restricted by the number of MHC specificities and known peptides available and generally has been developed only for the more common HLA haplotypes in the white population.

Helper T-Cell Differentiation and Function

Effector helper T cells differentiate from naïve CD4+ T-helper precursors (T_Hp) into two main classes of T_H cells with distinct functional properties.[218,219] A panoply of factors in the microenvironment where antigen recognition occurs have been shown to influence the differentiation of T_H cells, including the nature and density of ligand, the strength of TCR ligation, the presence and kinds of costimulatory molecules, and the differentiation state of the APC.[220] The cytokines in the immediate milieu are thought to be critical and result in vitro and in vivo in the early upregulation of canonic transcription factors that drive the T_H cell to one lineage while suppressing the transcriptional program characteristic of the opposite lineage (Fig. 22-13).[221,222] For instance, under the influence of IL-12 and IFN-γ, the transcription factor T-bet is upregulated and drives the cell to the so-called T-helper type 1 (T_H1) lineage, which is characterized by production of the inflammatory cytokines IL-2, IFN-γ, and TNF-α.[223] These cytokines drive paracrine expansion of T cells and activation of macrophages and other innate cells, thus providing help to CD8+ T cells and promoting cell-based immune responses. IL-4 in the environment, in contrast, upregulates the transcription factor GATA-3, thereby directing the cell to a T-helper type 2 (T_H2) cell fate.[224,225] The elaboration of T_H2 cytokines such as IL-4 promotes class switching of B cells, important for T-cell–mediated help for humoral responses. IL-4 and other T_H2 cytokines such as IL-5 and IL-13 also promote eosinophil differentiation, IgE production, and the expulsion and control of parasites. Imbalance of T_H1 and T_H2 cell responses is thought to play a role in the development of autoimmunity, allergy, and asthma.

Cytotoxic T-Cell Differentiation and Function

The primary function of effector CD8+ T cells is direct killing of APCs infected by virus or other intracellular organisms. Cytotoxicity is antigen dependent, is contact dependent, and does not result in destruction of the cytotoxic T cell itself, which can kill multiple targets serially. At least two mechanisms of cytolysis are now recog-

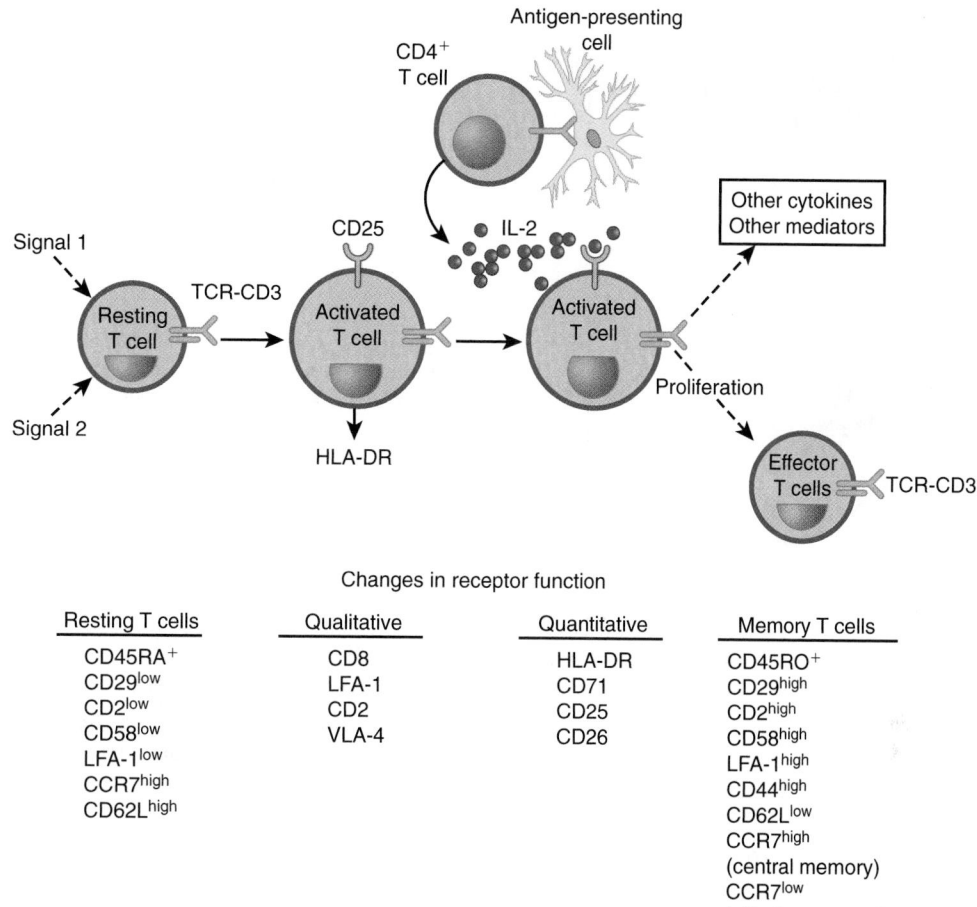

FIGURE 22-12. T-cell activation resulting in proliferation, acquisition of immunocompetence, and memory. Resting T cells are stimulated by antigen/major histocompatibility complex (MHC) molecules in the presence of a number of secondary signals. Appropriate activation results in an increase in both cell size and entry into the cell cycle. The high-affinity interleukin-2 (IL-2) receptor is expressed on the cell surface. Other activation antigens, such as transferrin receptor (CD71) and HLA-DR, are also expressed on the cell surface. The T cell is stimulated to produce cytokines (e.g., IL-2) that act in an autocrine and paracrine fashion on the T cell to promote cell replication and maturation to effector cells. CD4+ T cells generally differentiate to become helper T cells that are able to secrete IL-2 and other cytokines in response to peptide antigen in the context of MHC class II proteins. Helper T cells secrete cytokines, which in turn help B cells and other T cells to proliferate and differentiate. T lymphocytes that express CD8 on their cell surface generally function as cytotoxic T lymphocytes (CTLs) and are able to kill target cells that express a foreign peptide antigen or viral product in the context of MHC class I proteins. In addition, a certain proportion of CD8+ T cells function as suppressor T cells and inhibit the ability of B cells to secrete immunoglobulin, the generation of CTLs, or the production of cytokines by CD4+ cells. A small proportion of circulating, stimulating T cells become immunocompetent memory T cells that are able to respond to antigen exposure in a secondary immune response. The phenotype of resting T cells changes upon T-cell activation, transcriptional activation, and acquisition of the memory phenotype. Certain cell surface receptors are upregulated quantitatively as shown, within days after activation. Although the level of expression of the TCR-CD3 complex remains constant, that of CD2, CD58, CD29, and CD44 increases. L-selectin expression decreases, and CD45RA expression fails. Expression of CD45RO is characteristic of the memory phenotype. In addition to early (e.g., CD2) and late (e.g., VLA-1) quantitative changes in receptor expression, the avidity of a number of T-cell surface receptors is changed quantitatively after T-cell triggering. The avidity of LFA-1 (CD11a/CD18) for its ligands is upregulated after T-cell stimulation, as is CD8 for MHC class I proteins, CD2 for CD58, and VLA-β_1 receptors for their ligands. The specific and dynamic regulation of T-cell avidity may impart sensitivity and plasticity to the immune response.

nized, cytotoxic granules and the Fas-Fas ligand pathway. Effector CD8+ T cells release the contents of cytotoxic granules into the immune synapse after contact with an infected cell. The main components of these granules are perforin and the serine esterases granzyme A and granzyme B.[226] Perforin molecules form multimerized pores in the target cell and are classically thought to mediate delivery of granzymes into the cytoplasm. Targets then die by a combination of osmotic swelling and proteolytic damage. The importance of perforin in both responses to infection and immunoregulation is apparent by the study

of patients with congenital mutations in both alleles of perforin, which results in congenital hemophagocytic lymphohistiocytosis.[227,228] Because perforin is also produced by NK cells (see later), this disease is characterized by deficiencies in both CD8 and NK cytotoxic function. The second mechanism is induction of caspase-mediated apoptosis by engagement of CD95 (Fas, Apo-1) on target cells with its ligand CD95L (Fas ligand, CD178) on effector CD8+ T cells. CD95L is not constitutively expressed on naïve T cells and is upregulated on activation of T cells and NK cells. That this pathway also has

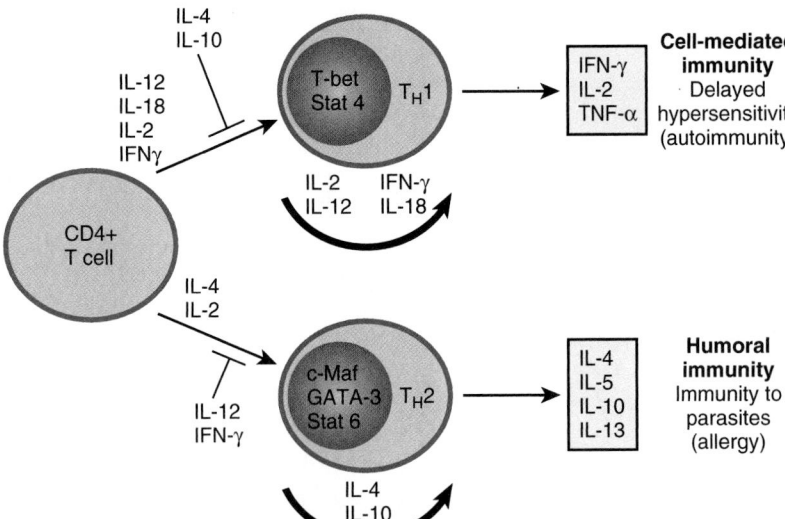

FIGURE 22-13. Differentiation of naïve CD4+ cells to T-helper precursor cells (T_H1 and T_H2). Naïve CD4+ cells, stimulated by ligation of the T-cell receptor and costimulatory molecules, differentiate into two classes of helper T cells. T_H1 cells produce inflammatory cytokines, characterized by interferon-γ (IFN-γ) and interleukin-2 (IL-2), that are capable of activating macrophages and promoting the further expansion of T cells; they appear to be the principal effectors of cell-mediated immunity. T_H2 cells produce IL-4, IL-10, and IL-5, among others, important for IgE production by B cells and differentiation of eosinophils, and thus are the principal effectors of humoral immunity. The cytokines produced by T_H1 cells (IL-2, IFN-γ, and IL-12) inhibit the induction of T_H2 differentiation, whereas the cytokines produced by T_H2 cells (IL-4 and IL-10) reciprocally inhibit the differentiation of T_H1 cells. TNF-α, tumor necrosis factor α.

important immunoregulatory function is implied by the fact that mutations in CD95 or CD95L typically cause not overwhelming infection but generalized lymphoproliferation and autoimmunity in humans.[229-231]

Control of the Immune Response: Regulation and Termination of T-Cell Activation

Maintaining a state of unresponsiveness to self-antigens, or self-tolerance, is as important for a healthy immune system as recognition of non-self, or foreign, antigens from infectious agents or tumors. Failure of self-tolerance can lead to autoimmunity. The main mechanisms of tolerance include central or clonal deletion (deletion by negative selection in the thymus, discussed earlier), anergy, activation-induced cell death (AICD; termination of T-cell activation), and cell-mediated suppression or regulation.

A productive T-cell response requires stimulation by antigen-MHC complexes via the T-cell receptor (signal 1) and appropriate costimulation (signal 2). T cells that encounter antigen in the absence of costimulation enter a state of anergy. Anergy is generally defined as the inability to proliferate when rechallenged with the same antigen while maintaining the ability to proliferate in response to cytokine (i.e., IL-2).[177,232] Anergy is also antigen specific, which means that an anergized cell can respond to other antigens if appropriately costimulated. Anergy ensures that autoreactive T cells that encounter peripherally expressed antigens in a noninflamed environment, where costimulatory molecules on APCs have not been upregulated, are not activated. AICD is important to ensure that the robust clonal expansion of antigen-specific T cells is short-lived. T cells exposed to foreign antigen or autoreactive T cells that escape thymic deletion and encounter self-antigen in the periphery can be killed by the CD95-CD95L pathway, which activates caspases and other

death signals. The importance of the CD95-CD95L pathway for control of lymphoproliferation in humans is demonstrated by the autoimmune lymphoproliferative syndrome (ALPS). Patients with ALPS have mutations in CD95 or more rarely CD95L or caspases, which leads to uncontrolled lymphoproliferation and autoimmunity.[231]

T cells that mediate suppression or regulation of other T cells have long been purported to exist. They were formerly thought to be a subset of CD8+ T cells, so-called suppressor cells, but in recent years a distinct population of CD4+ T cells with regulatory properties have emerged as important effectors of cell-based regulation. This population of so-called naturally occurring T-regulatory cells can be distinguished from other CD4+ T cells by the expression of certain cell surface receptors, most commonly CD25,[233] and more recently by expression of a key transcription factor, FoxP3.[234-236] FoxP3+ CD4+ CD25+ T cells develop in the thymus and in murine models require IL-2 for development and maintenance.[237] Humans deficient in FOXP3 have the immune dysregulation, polyendocrinopathy, enteropathy, X-linked (IPEX) syndrome, which is characterized by autoimmune diabetes and thyroiditis, inflammatory bowel disease, allergy, and other organ-specific autoimmunity.[238-240] In vitro, suppressive activity of these cells is defined by the ability to depress proliferation by lymphocytes stimulated via the TCR.[241-243] In vivo depletion of these cells in mice leads to spontaneous autoimmunity, whereas cotransfer suppresses autoimmunity in various models.[237]

NONCONVENTIONAL T-CELL SUBTYPES

In addition to conventional TCR αβ–bearing T cells that recognize peptide antigens, other nonconventional smaller populations of T cells exist. The function of these cells is less well characterized, but their conservation through evolution implies nonredundant roles in the immune system. Both populations share the ability to bind to the nonclassic MHC molecules and have restricted TCR diversity. They are generally believed to have functions during the innate immune response.

Development and Function of CD1-Restricted T Cells or Invariant Natural Killer T Cells

A subset of T cells that bear αβ TCR but recognize lipid antigens rather than peptide antigens has been defined in several ways over the past couple of decades. These cells were first characterized in the mouse as TCR αβ T cells that co-expressed cell surface markers also found on NK cells such as NK1.1 (CD161) and therefore were termed NK T cells.[244] When it was found that a subset of NK T cells recognize the CD1 family of nonclassic MHC molecules,[245] the term CD1-restricted T cells has been used as a more precise functional definition; conversely, not all CD1-restricted T cells express NK1.1. CD1 is a family of proteins with one isoform in the mouse, CD1d, and five isoforms in humans, CD1a, CD1b, CD1c, CD1d, CD1e, the last of which is not expressed on the cell surface.[246] These MHC class I–like proteins are generally expressed in a complex with β_2-microglobulin. The diversity of TCRα rearrangements used by CD1d-restricted T cells is limited, with many bearing $V_\alpha24$-$J_\alpha18$ rearranged TCRα protein, preferentially complexed to a $V_\beta11$ TCRβ protein. Thus, the term invariant NK T cells is also used to distinguish this main population from those with diverse αβ TCR restricted by CD1 molecules, and most studies have focused on the invariant CD1d-restricted subset.

Invariant NK T cells develop in the thymus, arise from the DP stage of development, and in mouse models are selected by other DP thymocytes that express CD1d rather than by thymic stroma.[247] In contrast to conventional T cells, invariant NK T cells recognize lipid presented by CD1.[248] A number of foreign lipids and glycolipids have been identified that are recognized by invariant NK T cells, although the discovery of self-antigens has been more elusive.[249] In the laboratory, α-galactosylceramide, derived from marine sponge, is a highly potent agonist for invariant NK T cells[250] and can be loaded onto tetramers of CD1d molecules tagged to fluorescent molecules to identify human or mouse invariant NK T cells by flow cytometry, similar to MHC tetramer technology.[251,252] About half of these cells do not express either CD4 or CD8 and half express CD4 in humans.[253] Invariant NK T cells produce cytokines, such as IL-4 and IFN-γ, more rapidly than conventional TCR αβ T cells do, within hours in mice after in vivo injection with antigen.[254] This early secretion has been proposed to function as bridge between innate and adaptive immunity in diverse processes, including the response to infection, antitumor immunity, autoimmune disease, and asthma.[255]

DEVELOPMENT AND FUNCTION OF TCR γδ T CELLS

TCR γδ T cells can be identified in mammals, chickens, and even cartilaginous fish, though not in jawless fish.[256] Although they develop in the thymus alongside TCR αβ T cells, in contrast to conventional T cells, the variety of γδ receptors is highly restricted, with 6 V_γ genes used (5 $V_\gamma1$ and 1 $V_\gamma2$) and 8 to 10 V_δ genes, 3 of which are commonly used in humans.[256,257] TCR γδ T cells make up a very small percentage of cells in the thymus or lymph node, on the order of 1% to 2%, but are much more abundant in mucosal surfaces, particularly the human gastrointestinal tract. Interestingly, the distribution of human TCR γδ T cells is skewed toward particular γδ combinations: peripheral blood contains a preponderance of $V_\gamma9V_\delta2^+$ T cells, whereas TCR γδ T cells found in intestinal epithelium often bear $V_\delta1^+$ or $V_\delta3^+$ TCR.[257] Most of these cells do not express either the CD4 or CD8 coreceptor. Although it is known that γδ rearrangement precedes αβ rearrangement and that γδ development occurs early during embryonic life, whether γδ development depends on ligand binding is unclear. Indeed, the natural ligands of TCR γδ T cells remain poorly defined but can be nonpeptides, as shown for circulating human TCR γδ T cells that recognize mycobacterial antigens.[258-260] $V_\gamma9V_\delta2^+$ T cells can generally recognize various types of phosphoantigens, whereas non-$V_\delta2^+$ T cells have more diverse ligands, including MHC class I–like molecules such as CD1. TCR γδ T cells can be expanded during responses to a variety of infections and tumors.[257]

NATURAL KILLER CELL DEVELOPMENT AND FUNCTION

In the peripheral blood of all individuals are circulating lymphocytes that morphologically resemble large granular lymphocytes and have distinctive physical characteristics that allow separation of them on a Percoll density gradient *in vitro*. These cells are termed NK cells and consist of a distinct subset of lymphocytes that unlike T lymphocytes, do not rearrange the T-cell antigen receptor genes (see Table 22-1).[261] These cells have the capacity to mediate the spontaneous lysis of sensitive target cells, including certain tumor cells, virus-infected cells, and hematopoietic cells, and to mediate ADCC.[262,263] NK cells appear to lyse their targets by pathways similar to those used by cytotoxic T lymphocytes.[262-264] NK cells have been shown to have a role in allograft rejection and tumor surveillance. Despite the relative homogenicity of morphologic appearance and function, NK cells are clearly a heterogeneous population of cells. NK cells are derived from a common lymphoid precursor cell. Peripheral blood NK cells may be derived directly from precursors in the bone marrow or may transit through the thymus, although the thymus is not required for their development. Phenotypic and functional NK cells may arise from immature CD7$^+$ CD1$^-$ TCR$^-$ CD3$^-$ CD4$^-$ CD8$^-$ prothymocyte precursors,[265,266] and they express CD2. Recent data indicate that Flt3L, IL-15, and IL-21, a cytokine closely related to IL-2 and IL-15, are all involved in NK hematopoietic development and expansion.[267] More recently, there is evidence that NK cells in humans can also mature in secondary lymphoid tissue.[268]

In addition to a role in immune surveillance, a role has been documented for NK cells in protection from viral infections, which is particularly important in the early phases of an immune response before T-cell recruitment. Indeed, NK cells are critical for protection against latent DNA viruses of the herpes family inasmuch as individuals with a deficiency in NK cell number or function typically have overwhelming herpesvirus infections.[264] Viral infection can trigger NK cell activity in several ways. First, elaboration of cytokines such as IFN-α, IFN-β, and IL-12 by infected cells, particularly monocytes, macrophages, and dendritic cells, induces NK cells to produce IFN-γ.[269] Second, cells expressing viral antigens that are then coated with specific Ig can bind to FcR on the surface of NK cells and trigger ADCC. Finally, NK cell surface receptors that usually recognize MHC class I and class I–like molecules mediate so-called missing self recognition.

NK cells interact with and are regulated by nonclassic MHC class I molecules. The killer cell Ig-like receptors (KIRs) recognize HLA class Ia and class Ib proteins, including HLA-G.[270] Members of a related family, termed Ig-like transcripts or leukocyte Ig-like receptors (LIRs), also recognize HLA class I proteins and are expressed not only by NK cells but also by cells of the myelomonocytic lineage.[271] These families of receptors act as inhibitory receptors that downregulate NK cell activity upon recognition of ligand by recruiting negative regulatory signaling proteins (e.g., tyrosine phosphatases) to the receptor complex.[272,273] Thus, NK cells can be activated or inhibited by HLA class I–like molecules; net activity depends on expression of these receptors and expression of MHC class I molecules on the target cells. Viruses may use the ability to downregulate MHC class I expression as a means of subverting the immune response; cells with low class I MHC expression are, however, targets of NK cytotoxicity. Importantly, human cytomegalovirus expresses an MHC class I homologue, UL18, that associates with β$_2$-microglobulin and endogenous host peptides. UL18 binds with high affinity to LIR-1 and related NK molecules, thereby effectively competing with host class I molecules, and escapes immune recognition.[274-276]

CONCLUSIONS

T and B cells play a central role in the acquired immune response, and NK cells are an early and critical effector of the innate immune response. The evolution of an adaptive immune response with the capacity for long-lived anamnestic responses affords exquisite specificity and adaptability to higher animals such that novel infections or arising malignancy can be both cleared initially and protected against upon re-exposure. Indeed, the requirement for T-cell function in normal homeostasis is exemplified by the consequences of its suppression. Deficiency of T-cell function associated with acquired immunodeficiency syndrome (AIDS), allogeneic stem cell transplantation, or T-cell–directed immunosuppressive therapy places patients at risk for herpes family viral reactivation (herpes simplex, herpes zoster, and cytomegalovirus) and lymphoproliferation (particularly Epstein-Barr virus–transformed B-cell lymphomas). As the mechanisms of immune control of nascent malignant degeneration become better understood, strategies to improve control of cancer by immunomodulatory therapy may become more tractable.

The same acquired immune response that gives higher animals an advantage in control of infection conversely predisposes these same species to the unique problems of autoimmunity. Failure of self-tolerance may result from the dysregulation of host T-cell responses after exposure to specific antigens in the setting of specific MHC molecules. Self-reactive B-cell clones may also mediate autoimmunity through inappropriate production of self-antigen–specific antibodies directed against a variety of tissue-specific targets. That enhancement of immune responses can precipitate autoimmunity is exemplified by the development of autoimmunity in melanoma patients who experienced tumor regression after peptide vaccination in the context of immunostimulatory anti–CTLA-4 antibody.[277] Greater understanding of antigen-specific activation and tolerance should open the way to the development of targeted immunomodulation and carry the field beyond global suppression of T-cell responses.

REFERENCES

1. Krause DS, Fackler MJ, Civin CI, May WS. CD34: structure, biology, and clinical utility. Blood. 1996;87:1-13.
2. Lin G, Finger E, Gutierrez-Ramos J. Expression of CD34 in endothelial cells, hematopoietic progenitors and nervous cells in fetal and adult mouse tissues. Eur J Immunol. 1995;25:1508-1516.
3. Baumheter S, Singer MS, Henzel W, et al. Binding of L-selectin to the vascular sialomucin CD34. Science. 1993;262:436-438.
4. Fackler MJ, Krause DS, Smith OM, et al. Full-length but not truncated CD34 inhibits hematopoietic cell differentiation of M1 cells. Blood. 1995;85:3040-3047.
5. Shortman K, Naik SH. Steady-state and inflammatory dendritic-cell development. Nat Rev Immunol. 2007;7:19-30.
6. Banchereau J, Briere F, Caux C, et al. Immunobiology of dendritic cells. Annu Rev Immunol. 2000;18:767-811.
7. Manz MG, Traver D, Miyamoto T, et al. Dendritic cell potentials of early lymphoid and myeloid progenitors. Blood. 2001;97:3333-3341.

8. Chicha L, Jarrossay D, Manz G. Clonal type I interferon-producing and dendritic cell precursors are contained in both human lymphoid and myeloid progenitor populations. J Exp Med. 2004;200:1519-1524.

9. Fugmann SD, Lee AI, Shockett PE, et al. The RAG proteins and V(D)J recombination: complexes, ends, and transposition. Annu Rev Immunol. 2000;18:495-527.

10. Gellert M. Recent advances in understanding V(D)J recombination. Adv Immunol. 1997;64:39-64.

11. Oettinger M. V(D)J recombination: on the cutting edge. Curr Opin Cell Biol. 1999;11:325-329.

12. Preud'homme J, Hanson L. IgG subclass deficiency. Immunodeficiency Rev. 1990;2:129-149.

13. Smith T. IgG subclasses. Adv Pediatr. 1992;39:101-126.

14. Hanson LA, Söderström R, Nilssen DE, et al. IgG subclass deficiency with or without IgA deficiency. Clin Immunol Immunopathol. 1991;61:S70-S77.

15. Kuijpers T, Weening R, Out T. IgG subclass deficiencies and recurrent pyogenic infections, unresponsiveness against bacterial polysaccharide antigens. Allergol Immunopathol (Madr). 1992;20:28-34.

16. Read G, Williams P. Evaluation of assays of serum IgG subclasses and IgG antigen–specific antibodies in the investigation of recurrent infection. Ann Clin Biochem. 2000;37:326-329.

17. Söderström T, Söderström R, Enskog A. Immunoglobulin subclasses and prophylactic use of immunoglobulin in immunoglobulin G subclass deficiency. Cancer. 1991;68(6 Suppl):1426-1429.

18. Gaspar HB, Conley ME. Early B cell defects. Clin Exp Immunol 2000;119:383-389.

19. Melek M, Gellert M, van Gent D. Rejoining of DNA by the RAG1 and RAG2 proteins. Science. 1998;280:301-303.

20. Sadofsky M. The RAG proteins in V(D)J recombination: more than just a nuclease. Nucleic Acids Res. 2001;29:1399-1409.

21. Benedict CL, Gilfillan S, Thai TH, Kearney JF. Terminal deoxynucleotidyl transferase and repertoire development. Immunol Rev. 2000;175:150-157.

22. Tuaillon N, Capra J. Evidence that terminal deoxynucleotidyltransferase expression plays a role in Ig heavy chain gene segment utilization. J Immunol. 2000;164:6387-6397.

23. Mahajan KN, Gangi-Peterson L, Sorscher DH, et al. Association of terminal deoxynucleotidyl transferase with Ku. Proc Natl Acad Sci U S A. 1999;96:13926-13931.

24. Purugganan MM, Shah S, Kearney JF, Roth DB. Ku80 is required for addition of N nucleotides to V(D)J recombination junctions by terminal deoxynucleotidyl transferase. Nucleic Acids Res. 2001;29:1638-1646.

25. Rooney S, Chaudhuri J, Alt FW. The role of the non-homologous end-joining pathway in lymphocyte development. Immunol Rev. 2004;200:115-131.

26. O'Driscoll M, Cerosaletti KM, Girard PM, et al. DNA ligase IV mutations identified in patients exhibiting developmental delay and immunodeficiency. Mol Cell. 2001;8:1175-1185.

27. Schwarz K, Gauss GH, Ludwig L, et al. RAG mutations in human B cell–negative SCID. Science. 1996;274:97-99.

28. Moshous D, Callebaut I, de Chasseval R, et al. Artemis, a novel DNA double-strand break repair/V(D)J recombination protein, is mutated in human severe combined immune deficiency. Cell. 2001;105:177-186.

29. Pillai S, Cariappa A, Moran ST. Marginal zone B cells. Annu Rev Immunol. 2005;23:161-196.

30. Klein U, Rajewsky K, Küppers R. Human immunoglobulin (Ig)M+IgD+ peripheral blood B cells expressing the CD27 cell surface antigen carry somatically mutated variable region genes: CD27 as a general marker for somatically mutated (memory) B cells. J Exp Med. 1998;188:1679-1689.

31. Agematsu K, Hokibara S, Nagumo H, Komiyama A. CD27: a memory B-cell marker. Immunol Today. 2000;21:204-206.

32. Steiniger B, Timphus EM, Barth PJ. The splenic marginal zone in humans and rodents: an enigmatic compartment and its inhabitants. Histochem Cell Biol. 2006;126:641-648.

33. Weller S, Braun MC, Tan BK, et al. Human blood IgM "memory" B cells are circulating splenic marginal zone B cells harboring a prediversified immunoglobulin repertoire. Blood. 2004;104:3647-3654.

34. Wardemann H, Yurasov S, Schaefer A, et al. Predominant autoantibody production by early human B cell precursors. Science. 2003;301:1374-1377.

35. Mond J, Lees A, Snapper C. T cell–independent antigens type 2. Annu Rev Immunol. 1995;13:655-692.

36. Iwasaki A, Medzhitov R. Toll-like receptor control of the adaptive immune responses. Nat Immunol. 2004;5:987-995.

37. Fearon DT, Carroll MC. Regulation of B lymphocyte responses to foreign and self-antigens by the CD19/CD21 complex. Annu Rev Immunol. 2000;18:393-422.

38. Fujimoto M, Fujimoto Y, Poe JC, et al. CD19 regulates intrinsic B lymphocyte signal transduction and activation through a novel mechanism of processive amplification. Immunol Res. 2000;22:281-298.

39. Rickert RC. Regulation of B lymphocyte activation by complement C3 and the B cell coreceptor complex. Curr Opin Immunol. 2005;17:237-243.

40. Ravetch J, Lanier L. Immune inhibitory receptors. Science. 2000;290:84-89.

41. Aman M, Ravichandran K. A requirement for lipid rafts in B cell receptor induced Ca(2+) flux. Curr Biol. 2000;10:393-396.

42. Brown R. Sphingolipid organization in biomembranes: what physical studies of model membranes reveal. J Cell Sci. 1998;111:1-9.

43. Cherukuri A, Dykstra M, Pierce S. Floating the raft hypothesis: lipid rafts play a role in immune cell activation. Immunity. 2001;14:657-660.

44. Simons K, Ikonen E. Functional rafts in cell membranes. Nature 1997;387:569-572.

45. Brown D, London E. Functions of lipid rafts in biological membranes. Annu Rev Cell Dev Biol. 1998;14:111-136.

46. Jacobson K, Dietrich C. Looking at lipid rafts? Trends Cell Biol. 1999;9:87-91.

47. Dykstra M, Cherukuri A, Pierce S. Floating the raft hypothesis for immune receptors: access to rafts controls receptor signaling and trafficking. Traffic. 2001;2:160-166.

48. Germain R, Stefanová I. The dynamics of T cell receptor signaling: complex orchestration and the key roles of

tempo and cooperation. Annu Rev Immunol. 1999;17: 467-522.

49. Gupta N, DeFranco AL. Lipid rafts and B cell signaling. Semin Cell Dev Biol. 2007;18:616-626.

50. DeFranco A, Chan V, Lowell C. Positive and negative roles of the tyrosine kinase Lyn in B cell function. Semin Immunol. 1998;10:299-307.

51. Koretzky G, Abtahian F, Silverman M. SLP76 and SLP65: complex regulation of signalling in lymphocytes and beyond. Nat Rev Immunol. 2006;6:67-78.

52. Bolen J. Protein tyrosine kinases in the initiation of antigen receptor signaling. Curr Opin Immunol. 1995;7:306-311.

53. Rawlings DJ, Scharenberg AM, Park H, et al. Activation of BTK by a phosphorylation mechanism initiated by SRC family kinases. Science. 1996;271:822-825.

54. Fearon D, Carter R. The CD19/CR2/TAPA-1 complex of B lymphocytes: linking natural to acquired immunity. Annu Rev Immunol. 1995;13:127-149.

55. Dempsey PW, Allison ME, Akkaraju S, et al. C3d of complement as a molecular adjuvant: bridging innate and acquired immunity. Science., 1996;271:348-350.

56. Cherukuri A, Carter RH, Brooks S, et al. B cell signaling is regulated by induced palmitoylation of CD81. J Biol Chem. 2004;279:31973-31982.

57. Cherukuri A, Shoham T, Sohn HW, et al. The tetraspanin CD81 is necessary for partitioning of coligated CD19/CD21–B cell antigen receptor complexes into signaling-active lipid rafts. J Immunol. 2004;172:370-380.

58. Foy TM, Aruffo A, Bajorath J, et al. Immune regulation by CD40 and its ligand GP39. Annu Rev Immunol. 1996;14:591-617.

59. Bishop GA, Hostager BS. The CD40-CD154 interaction in B cell–T cell liaisons. Cytokine Growth Factor Rev. 2003;14:297-309.

60. Lanzavecchia A, Sallusto F. Toll-like receptors and innate immunity in B-cell activation and antibody responses. Curr Opin Immunol. 2007;19:268-274.

61. Takeda K, Kaisho T, Akira S. Toll-like receptors. Annu Rev Immunol. 2003;21:335-376.

62. Leadbetter EA, Rifkin IR, Hohlbaum AM, et al. Chromatin-IgG complexes activate B cells by dual engagement of IgM and Toll-like receptors. Nature. 2002;416:603-607.

63. Leadbetter EA, Rifkin IR, Marshak-Rothstein A. Toll-like receptors and activation of autoreactive B cells. Curr Dir Autoimmun. 2003;6:105-122.

64. MacLennan I. Germinal centers. Annu Rev Immunol 1994;12:117-139.

65. Allen CD, Okada T, Cyster JG. Germinal-center organization and cellular dynamics. Immunity. 2007;27:190-202.

66. von Andrian UH, Mempel TR. Homing and cellular traffic in lymph nodes. Nat Rev Immunol. 2003;3: 867-878.

67. Kosco-Vilbois MH. Are follicular dendritic cells really good for nothing? Nat Rev Immunol. 2003;3:764-769.

68. Jacobs H, Bross L. Towards an understanding of somatic hypermutation. Curr Opin Immunol. 2001;13:208-218.

69. Di Noia JM, Neuberger MS. Molecular mechanisms of antibody somatic hypermutation. Annu Rev Biochem. 2007;76:1-22.

70. Kinoshita K, Lee C-G, Tashiro J, et al. Molecular mechanism of immunoglobulin class switch recombination. Cold Spring Harbor Symp Quant Biol. 1999;64:217-226.

71. Snapper C, Marcu K, Zelazowski P. The immunoglobulin class switch: beyond "accessibility." Immunity. 1997;6: 217-223.

72. Stavnezer J. Antibody class switching. Adv Immunol. 1996;61:79-146.

73. Tarlinton D. B-cell memory: are subsets necessary? Nat Rev Immunol. 2006;6:785-790.

74. Nichols KE, Harkin DP, Levitz S, et al. Inactivating mutations in an SH2 domain–encoding gene in X-linked lymphoproliferative syndrome. Proc Natl Acad Sci U S A. 1998;95:13765-13770.

75. Coffey AJ, Brooksbank RA, Brandau O, et al. Host response to EBV infection in X-linked lymphoproliferative disease results from mutations in an SH2-domain encoding gene. Nat Genet. 1998;20:129-135.

76. Sayos J, Wu C, Morra M, et al. The X-linked lymphoproliferative-disease gene product SAP regulates signals induced through the co-receptor SLAM. Nature. 1998; 395:462-469.

77. Grimbacher B, Hutloff A, Schlesier M, et al. Homozygous loss of ICOS is associated with adult-onset common variable immunodeficiency. Nat Immunol. 2003;4:261-268.

78. Castigli E, Wilson SA, Garibyan L, et al. TACI is mutant in common variable immunodeficiency and IgA deficiency. Nat Genet. 2005;37:829-834.

79. Longerici S, Basu U, Alt F, Storb U. AID in somatic hypermutation and class switch recombination. Curr Opin Immunol. 2006;18:164-174.

80. Muramatsu M, Kinoshita K, Fagarasan S, et al. Class switch recombination and hypermutation require activation-induced cytidine deaminase (AID), a potential RNA editing enzyme. Cell. 2000;102:553-563.

81. Notarangelo LD, Lanzi G, Peron S, Durandy A. Defects of class-switch recombination. J Allergy Clin Immunol. 2006;117:855-864.

82. Revy P, Muto T, Levy Y, et al. Activation-induced cytidine deaminase (AID) deficiency causes the autosomal recessive form of the hyper-IgM syndrome (HIGM2). Cell. 2000;102:565-575.

83. Brink R. Regulation of B cell self-tolerance by BAFF. Semin Immunol. 2006;18:276-283.

84. Nemazee D. Receptor editing in lymphocyte development and central tolerance. Nat Rev Immunol. 2006;6: 728-740.

85. Gauld SB, Merrell KT, Cambier JC. Silencing of autoreactive B cells by anergy: a fresh perspective. Curr Opin Immunol. 2006;18:292-297.

86. Khare SD, Sarosi I, Xia XZ, et al. Severe B cell hyperplasia and autoimmune disease in TALL-1 transgenic mice. Proc Natl Acad Sci U S A. 2000;97:3370-3375.

87. Mackay F, Woodcock SA, Lawton P, et al. Mice transgenic for BAFF develop lymphocytic disorders along with autoimmune manifestations. J Exp Med. 1999;190: 1697-1710.

88. Mackay F, Silveira PA, Brink R. B cells and the BAFF/APRIL axis: fast-forward on autoimmunity and signaling. Curr Opin Immunol. 2007;19:327-336.

89. Davis M, Bjorkman P. T-cell antigen receptor genes and T-cell recognition. Nature. 1988;334:395-402.

90. Bhandoola A, Sambandam A. From stem cell to T cell: one route or many? Nat Rev Immunol. 2006;6:117-126.

91. Spits H. Development of alphabeta T cells in the human thymus. Nat Rev Immunol. 2002;2:760-772.

92. Ting CN, Olson MC, Barton KP, Leiden JM. Transcription factor GATA-3 is required for development of the T-cell lineage. Nature. 1996;384:474-478.

93. Radtke F, Wilson A, Stark G, et al. Deficient T cell fate specification in mice with an induced inactivation of Notch1. Immunity. 1999;10:547-558.

94. Wilson A, MacDonald HR, Radtke F. Notch 1–deficient common lymphoid precursors adopt a B cell fate in the thymus. J Exp Med. 2001;194:1003-1012.

95. Dik WA, Pike-Overzet K, Weerkamp F, et al. New insights on human T cell development by quantitative T cell receptor gene rearrangement studies and gene expression profiling. J Exp Med. 2005;201:1715-1723.

96. Frank J, Pignata C, Panteleyev AA, et al. Exposing the human nude phenotype. Nature. 1999;398:473-474.

97. Pignata C, Fiore M, Guzzetta V, et al. Congenital alopecia and nail dystrophy associated with severe functional T-cell immunodeficiency in two sibs. Am J Med Genet. 1996; 65:167-170.

98. Zúñiga-Pflücker JC. T-cell development made simple. Nat Rev Immunol. 2004;4:67-72.

99. Schmitt TM, Zúñiga-Pflücker JC. Induction of T cell development from hematopoietic progenitor cells by delta-like-1 in vitro. Immunity. 2002;17:749-756.

100. De Smedt M, Reynvoet K, Kerre T, et al. Active form of Notch imposes T cell fate in human progenitor cells. J Immunol. 2002;169:3021-3029.

101. Wolfer A, Wilson A, Nemir M, et al. Inactivation of Notch1 impairs VDJbeta rearrangement and allows pre-TCR–independent survival of early alpha beta lineage thymocytes. Immunity. 2002;16:869-879.

102. Mohtashami M, Zúñiga-Pflücker JC. Three-dimensional architecture of the thymus is required to maintain delta-like expression necessary for inducing T cell development. J Immunol. 2006;176:730-734.

103. La Motte-Mohs RN, Herer E, Zúñiga-Pflücker JC. Induction of T-cell development from human cord blood hematopoietic stem cells by Delta-like 1 in vitro. Blood. 2005;105:1431-1439.

104. Schmitt TM, de Pooter RF, Gronski MA, et al. Induction of T cell development and establishment of T cell competence from embryonic stem cells differentiated in vitro. Nat Immunol. 2004;5:410-417.

105. Awong G, La Motte-Mohs RN, Zúñiga-Pflücker JC. Generation of pro-T cells in vitro: potential for immune reconstitution. Semin Immunol. 2007;19:341-349.

106. Bjorkman P. MHC restriction in three dimensions: a view of T cell receptor/ligand interactions. Cell. 1997;89: 167-170.

107. Bjorkman P, Saper MA, Samraoui B, et al. Structure of the human class I histocompatibility antigen, HLA-A2. Nature. 1987;329:506-512.

108. Madden D. The three-dimensional structure of peptide-MHC complexes. Annu Rev Immunol. 1995;13:587-622.

109. Engelhard V. Structure of peptides associated with class I and class II MHC molecules. Annu Rev Immunol. 1994; 12:181-207.

110. Pamer E, Cresswell P. Mechanisms of MHC class I–restricted antigen processing. Annu Rev Immunol. 1998; 16:323-358.

111. Wills C, Green D. A genetic herd-immunity model for the maintenance of MHC polymorphism. Immunol Rev. 1995;143:263-292.

112. Potts W, Slev P. Pathogen-based models favoring MHC genetic diversity. Immunol Rev. 1995;143:181-197.

113. Germain R. MHC-dependent antigen processing and peptide presentation: providing ligands for T lymphocyte activation. Cell. 1994;76:287-299.

114. Unanue E. Cellular studies on antigen presentation by class II MHC molecules. Curr Opin Immunol. 1992; 4:63-69.

115. Wolf P, Ploegh H. How MHC class II molecules acquire peptide cargo: biosynthesis and trafficking through the endocytic pathway. Annu Rev Cell Dev Biol. 1995;11: 267-306.

116. Cresswell P. Assembly, transport, and function of MHC class II molecules. Annu Rev Immunol 1994;12: 259-293.

117. Bentley G, Mariuzza R. The structure of the T cell antigen receptor. Annu Rev Immunol. 1996;14:563-590.

118. Haynes B, Denning SM, Le PT, Singer KH. Human intrathymic T cell differentiation. Semin Immunol. 1990;2:67-77.

119. Kruisbeek A. Development of alpha beta T cells. Curr Opin Immunol. 1993;5:227-234.

120. Shortman K. Cellular aspects of early T-cell development. Curr Opin Immunol. 1992;4:140-146.

121. Joachims M, Chain JL, Hooker SW, et al. Human alpha beta and gamma delta thymocyte development: TCR gene rearrangements, intracellular TCR beta expression, and gamma delta developmental potential—differences between men and mice. J Immunol. 2006;176:1543-1552.

122. Michie AM, Zúñiga-Pflücker JC. Regulation of thymocyte differentiation: pre-TCR signals and beta-selection. Semin Immunol. 2002;14:311-323.

123. de Villartay JP, Hockett RD, Coran D, et al. Deletion of the human T-cell receptor delta-gene by a site-specific recombination. Nature. 1988;335:170-174.

124. Douek DC, McFarland RD, Keiser PH, et al. Changes in thymic function with age and during the treatment of HIV infection. Nature. 1998;396:690-695.

125. Hazenberg MD, Verschuren MC, Hamann D, et al. T cell receptor excision circles as markers for recent thymic emigrants: basic aspects, technical approach, and guidelines for interpretation. J Mol Med. 2001;79:631-640.

126. Starr TK, Jameson SC, Hogquist KA. Positive and negative selection of T cells. Annu Rev Immunol. 2003;21: 139-176.

127. Yun TJ, Bevan MJ. The Goldilocks conditions applied to T cell development. Nat Immunol. 2001;2:13-14.

128. Canté-Barrett K, Winslow MM, Crabtree GR. Selective role of NFATc3 in positive selection of thymocytes. J Immunol. 2007;179:103-110.

129. Gallo EM, Winslow MM, Canté-Barrett K, et al. Calcineurin sets the bandwidth for discrimination of signals during thymocyte development. Nature. 2007;450:731-735.

130. Neilson JR, Winslow MM, Hur EM, Crabtree GR. Calcineurin B1 is essential for positive but not negative selection during thymocyte development. Immunity. 2004;20: 255-266.

131. Dadi HK, Simon AJ, Roifman CM. Effect of CD3delta deficiency on maturation of alpha/beta and gamma/delta T-cell lineages in severe combined immunodeficiency. N Engl J Med. 2003;349:1821-1828.

132. Dave VP, Cao Z, Browne C, et al. CD3 delta deficiency arrests development of the alpha beta but not the gamma delta T cell lineage. EMBO J. 1997;16:1360-1370.

133. Arpaia E, Shahar M, Dadi H, et al. Defective T cell receptor signaling and CD8+ thymic selection in humans lacking zap-70 kinase. Cell. 1994;76:947-958.

134. Chan A, Kadlecek TA, Elder ME, et al. ZAP-70 deficiency in an autosomal recessive form of severe combined immunodeficiency. Science. 1994;264:1599-1601.

135. Elder M, Lin D, Clever J, et al. Human severe combined immunodeficiency due to a defect in ZAP-70, a T cell tyrosine kinase. Science. 1994;264:1596-1599.

136. Kappler J, Roehm N, Marrack P. T cell tolerance by clonal elimination in the thymus. Cell. 1987;49:273-280.

137. Nossal G. Negative selection of lymphocytes. Cell. 1994;76:229-239.

138. Gill J, Malin M, Sutherland J, et al. Thymic generation and regeneration. Immunol Rev. 2003;195:28-50.

139. Anderson MS, Venanzi ES, Klein L, et al. Projection of an immunological self shadow within the thymus by the aire protein. Science. 2002;298:1395-1401.

140. Nagamine K, Peterson P, Scott HS, et al. Positional cloning of the APECED gene. Nat Genet. 1997;17:393-398.

141. Consortium F-GA. An autoimmune disease, APECED, caused by mutations in a novel gene featuring two PHD-type zinc-finger domains. Nat Genet. 1997;17:399-403.

142. Keefe R, Dave V, Allman D, et al. Regulation of lineage commitment distinct from positive selection. Science. 1999;286:1149-1153.

143. He X, Kappes DJ. CD4/CD8 lineage commitment: light at the end of the tunnel? Curr Opin Immunol. 2006;18:135-142.

144. Laky K, Fleischacker C, Fowlkes BJ. TCR and Notch signaling in CD4 and CD8 T-cell development. Immunol Rev. 2006;209:274-283.

145. Aliahmad P, Kaye J. Commitment issues: linking positive selection signals and lineage diversification in the thymus. Immunol Rev. 2006;209:253-273.

146. Bosselut R. CD4/CD8-lineage differentiation in the thymus: from nuclear effectors to membrane signals. Nat Rev Immunol. 2004;4:529-540.

147. Grusby MJ, Johnson RS, Papaioannou VE, Glimcher LH. Depletion of CD4+ T cells in major histocompatibility complex class II–deficient mice. Science. 1991;253:1417-1420.

148. Koller BH, Marrack T, Kappler JW, Smithies O. Normal development of mice deficient in beta 2M, MHC class I proteins, and CD8+ T cells. Science. 1990;248:1227-1230.

149. Zijlstra M, Bix M, Simister NE, et al. Beta 2-microglobulin deficient mice lack CD4-8+ cytolytic T cells. Nature. 1990;344:742-746.

150. Reith W, Mach B. The bare lymphocyte syndrome and the regulation of MHC expression. Annu Rev Immunol. 2001;19:331-373.

151. Cambier J. Signal transduction by T- and B-cell antigen receptors: converging structures and concepts. Curr Opin Immunol. 1992;4:257-264.

152. Lerner A, Diener AC, Reinherz EL, Clayton LK. Human genomic sequences corresponding to murine CD3 eta–related transcripts: lack of conservation or expression of homologous human products. Eur J Immunol. 1992;22:2135-2140.

153. Exley M, Terhorst C, Wileman T. Structure, assembly and intracellular transport of the T cell receptor for antigen. Semin Immunol. 1991;3:283-297.

154. Call ME, Wucherpfennig KW. Molecular mechanisms for the assembly of the T cell receptor–CD3 complex. Mol Immunol. 2004;40:1295-1305.

155. Cemerski S, Shaw A. Immune synapses in T-cell activation. Curr Opin Immunol. 2006;18:298-304.

156. Dustin M. A dynamic view of the immunological synapse. Semin Immunol. 2005;17:400-410.

157. Zamoyska R, Basson A, Filby A, et al. The influence of the src-family kinases, Lck and Fyn, on T cell differentiation, survival and activation. Immunol Rev. 2003;191:107-118.

158. Straus D, Weiss A. The CD3 chains of the T cell antigen receptor associate with the ZAP-70 tyrosine kinase and are tyrosine phosphorylated after receptor stimulation. J Exp Med. 1993;178:1523-1530.

159. Weiss A, Littman D. Signal transduction by lymphocyte antigen receptors. Cell. 1994;76:263-274.

160. Isakov N, Altman A. Protein kinase C(theta) in T cell activation. Annu Rev Immunol. 2002;20:761-794.

161. Wesselborg S, Fruman DA, Sagoo JK, et al. Identification of a physical interaction between calcineurin and nuclear factor of activated T cells (NFATp). J Biol Chem. 1996;271:1274-1277.

162. Rao A. NF-ATp: a transcription factor required for the co-ordinate induction of several cytokine genes. Immunol Today. 1994;15:274-281.

163. Clipstone NA, Crabtree GR. Identification of calcineurin as a key signalling enzyme in T-lymphocyte activation. Nature. 1992;357:695-697.

164. Bierer B, Hollander G, Fruman D, Burakoff SJ. Cyclosporin A and FK506: molecular mechanisms of immunosuppression and probes for transplantation biology. Curr Opin Immunol. 1993;5:763-773.

165. Klee C, Draetta G, Hubbard M. Calcineurin. Adv Enzymol Relat Areas Mol Biol. 1988;61:149-200.

166. Zhang L, Lorenz U, Ravichandran KS. Role of Shc in T-cell development and function. Immunol Rev. 2003;191:183-195.

167. Crabtree G, Clipstone N. Signal transmission between the plasma membrane and nucleus of T lymphocytes. Annu Rev Biochem. 1994;63:1045-1083.

168. Lohr J, Knoechel B, Abbas AK. Regulatory T cells in the periphery. Immunol Rev. 2006;212:149-162.

169. Bromley S, Burack WR, Johnson KG, et al. The immunological synapse. Annu Rev Immunol. 2001;19:375-396.

170. Miceli M, Parnes J. Role of CD4 and CD8 in T cell activation and differentiation. Adv Immunol. 1993;53:59-122.

171. Davis M, Boniface JJ, Reich Z, et al. Ligand recognition by alpha beta T cell receptors. Annu Rev Immunol. 1998;16:523-544.

172. Bierer B, Hahn W. T cell adhesion, avidity regulation and signaling: a molecular analysis of CD2. Semin Immunol. 1993;5:249-261.

173. Hermiston M, Xu Z, Weiss A. CD45: a critical regulator of signaling thresholds in immune cells. Annu Rev Immunol. 2003;21:107-137.

174. Zhang M, Moran M, Round J, et al. CD45 signals outside of lipid rafts to promote ERK activation, synaptic raft clustering, and IL-2 production. J Immunol. 2005;174:1479-1490.

175. Tchilian EZ, Wallace DL, Wells RS, et al. A deletion in the gene encoding the CD45 antigen in a patient with SCID. J Immunol. 2001;166:1308-1313.

176. Kung C, Pingel JT, Heikinheimo M, et al. Mutations in the tyrosine phosphatase CD45 gene in a child with severe combined immunodeficiency disease. Nat Med. 2000;6:343-345.

177. Schwartz R. Models of T cell anergy: is there a common molecular mechanism? J Exp Med. 1996;184:1-8.

178. Lindstein T, June CH, Ledbetter JA, et al. Regulation of lymphokine messenger RNA stability by a surface-mediated T cell activation pathway. Science. 1989;244:339-343.

179. Lenschow D, Walunas T, Bluestone J. CD28/B7 system of T cell costimulation. Annu Rev Immunol. 1996;14:233-258.

180. Bierer B, Schreiber S, Burakoff S. The effect of the immunosuppressant FK-506 on alternate pathways of T cell activation. Eur J Immunol. 1991;21:439-445.

181. June C, Ledbetter JA, Gillespie MM, et al. T-cell proliferation involving the CD28 pathway is associated with cyclosporine-resistant interleukin 2 gene expression. Mol Cell Biol. 1987;7:4472-4481.

182. Alegre ML, Frauwirth KA, Thompson CB. T-cell regulation by CD28 and CTLA-4. Nat Rev Immunol. 2001;1:220-228.

183. Waterhouse P, Penninger JM, Timms E, et al. Lymphoproliferative disorders with early lethality in mice deficient in Ctla-4. Science. 1995;270:985-988.

184. Tivol EA, Borriello F, Schweitzer AN, et al. Loss of CTLA-4 leads to massive lymphoproliferation and fatal multiorgan tissue destruction, revealing a critical negative regulatory role of CTLA-4. Immunity. 1995;3:541-547.

185. Chambers CA, Kuhns MS, Egen JG, Allison JP. CTLA-4-mediated inhibition in regulation of T cell responses: mechanisms and manipulation in tumor immunotherapy. Annu Rev Immunol. 2001;19:565-594.

186. Hutloff A, Dittrich AM, Beier KC, et al. ICOS is an inducible T-cell co-stimulator structurally and functionally related to CD28. Nature. 1999;397:263-266.

187. Sharpe AH, Freeman GJ. The B7-CD28 superfamily. Nat Rev Immunol. 2002;2:116-126.

188. Freeman G, Long AJ, Iwai Y, et al. Engagement of the PD-1 immunoinhibitory receptor by a novel B7 family member leads to negative regulation of lymphocyte activation. J Exp Med. 2000;192:1027-1034.

189. Nishimura H, Minato N, Nakano T, Honjo T. Immunological studies on PD-1 deficient mice: implication of PD-1 as a negative regulator for B cell responses. Int Immunol. 1998;10:1563-1572.

190. Ishida Y, Agata Y, Shibahara K, Honjo T. Induced expression of PD-1, a novel member of the immunoglobulin gene superfamily, upon programmed cell death. EMBO J. 1992;11:3887-3895.

191. Lee K, Chuang E, Griffin M, et al. Molecular basis of T cell inactivation by CTLA-4. Science. 1998;282:2263-2266.

192. Latchman Y, Wood CR, Chernova T, et al. PD-L2 is a second ligand for PD-1 and inhibits T cell activation. Nat Immunol. 2001;2:261-268.

193. Dong H, Zhu G, Tamada K, Chen L. B7-H1, a third member of the B7 family, co-stimulates T-cell proliferation and interleukin-10 secretion. Nat Med. 1999;5:1365-1369.

194. Chapoval A, Ni J, Lau JS, et al. B7-H3: a costimulatory molecule for T cell activation and IFN-gamma production. Nat Immunol. 2001;2:269-274.

195. Howland K, Aushubel LJ, London CA, Abbas AK. The roles of CD28 and CD40 ligand in T cell activation and tolerance. J Immunol. 2000;164:4465-4470.

196. Korthäuer U, Graf D, Mages HW, et al. Defective expression of T-cell CD40 ligand causes X-linked immunodeficiency with hyper-IgM. Nature. 1993;361:539-541.

197. Uronen H, Callard R. Absence of CD40-CD40 ligand interactions in X-linked hyper-IgM syndrome does not affect differentiation of T helper cell subsets. Clin Exp Immunol. 2000;121:346-352.

198. Winkelstein JA, Marino MC, Ochs H, et al. The X-linked hyper-IgM syndrome: clinical and immunologic features of 79 patients. Medicine (Baltimore). 2003;82:373-384.

199. Thomas C, de Saint Basile G, Le Deist F, et al. Brief report: correction of X-linked hyper-IgM syndrome by allogeneic bone marrow transplantation. N Engl J Med. 1995;333:426-429.

200. Castigli E, Alt FW, Davidson L, et al. CD40-deficient mice generated by recombination-activating gene-2-deficient blastocyst complementation. Proc Natl Acad Sci U S A. 1994;91:12135-12139.

201. Kawabe T, Naka T, Yoshida K, et al. The immune responses in CD40-deficient mice: impaired immunoglobulin class switching and germinal center formation. Immunity. 1994;1:167-178.

202. Renshaw BR, Fanslow WC 3rd, Armitage RJ, et al. Humoral immune responses in CD40 ligand-deficient mice. J Exp Med. 1994;180:1889-1900.

203. Xu J, Foy TM, Laman JD, et al. Mice deficient for the CD40 ligand. Immunity. 1994;1:423-431.

204. Jacquot S, CD27/CD70 interactions regulate T dependent B cell differentiation. Immunol Res 2000;21:23-30.

205. Hamann D, Kostense S, Wolthers KC, et al. Evidence that human CD8+CD45RA+CD27− cells are induced by antigen and evolve through extensive rounds of division. Int Immunol. 1999;11:1027-1033.

206. Walker L, Gulbranson-Judge A, Flynn S, et al. Compromised OX40 function in CD28-deficient mice is linked with failure to develop CXC chemokine receptor 5-positive CD4 cells and germinal centers. J Exp Med. 1999;190:1115-1122.

207. Brocker T, Gulbranson-Judge A, Flynn S, et al. CD4 T cell traffic control: in vivo evidence that ligation of OX40 on CD4 T cells by OX40-ligand expressed on dendritic cells leads to the accumulation of CD4 T cells in B follicles. Eur J Immunol. 1999;29:1610-1616.

208. Vincenti F. Costimulation blockade in autoimmunity and transplantation. J Allergy Clin Immunol. 2008;121:299-306; quiz 307-308.

209. Bashyam H. CTLA-4: From conflict to clinic. J Exp Med. 2007;204:1243.

210. Matthews JB, Ramos E, Bluestone JA. Clinical trials of transplant tolerance: slow but steady progress. Am J Transplant. 2003;3:794-803.

211. Suntharalingam G, Perry MR, Ward S, et al. Cytokine storm in a phase 1 trial of the anti-CD28 monoclonal antibody TGN1412. N Engl J Med. 2006;355:1018-1028.

212. Michie C, McLean A, Alcock C, Beverly PC. Lifespan of human lymphocyte subsets defined by CD45 isoforms. Nature. 1992;360:264-265.

213. Gunn MD, Tangamann K, Tam C, et al. A chemokine expressed in lymphoid high endothelial venules promotes the adhesion and chemotaxis of naive T lymphocytes. Proc Natl Acad Sci U S A. 1998;95:258-263.

214. Lanzavecchia A, Sallusto F. Understanding the generation and function of memory T cell subsets. Curr Opin Immunol. 2005;17:326-332.

215. Sallusto F, Lenig D, Förster R, et al. Two subsets of memory T lymphocytes with distinct homing potentials and effector functions. Nature. 1999;401:708-712.

216. Ogg GS, jin X, Bonhoeffers S, et al. Quantitation of HIV-1–specific cytotoxic T lymphocytes and plasma load of viral RNA. Science. 1998;279:2103-2106.

217. Altman JD, Moss PA, Goulder PJ, et al. Phenotypic analysis of antigen-specific T lymphocytes. Science. 1996;274:94-96.

218. Mosmann T, Coffman R. TH1 and TH2 cells: different patterns of lymphokine secretion lead to different functional properties. Annu Rev Immunol. 1989;7:145-173.

219. Mosmann TR, Cherwinski H, Bond MW, et al. Two types of murine helper T cell clone. I. Definition according to profiles of lymphokine activities and secreted proteins. J Immunol. 1986;136:2348-2357.

220. Heath W, Carbone F. Cross-presentation, dendritic cells, tolerance and immunity. Annu Rev Immunol. 2001;19:47-64.

221. Glimcher LH, Murphy KM. Lineage commitment in the immune system: the T helper lymphocyte grows up. Genes Dev. 2000;14:1693-1711.

222. Murphy KM, Reiner SL. The lineage decisions of helper T cells. Nat Rev Immunol, 2002;2:933-944.

223. Szabo SJ, Kim ST, Costa GL, et al. A novel transcription factor, T-bet, directs Th1 lineage commitment. Cell. 2000;100:655-669.

224. Zhang DH, Cohn L, Ray P, et al. Transcription factor Gata-3 is differentially expressed murine Th1 and Th2 cells and controls Th2-specific expression of the interleukin-5 gene. J Biologic Chem. 1997;272:21597-21603.

225. Zheng WP, Flavell RA. The transcription factor Gata-3 is necessary and sufficient for Th2 cytokine gene expression in CD4 T cells. Cell. 1997;89:587-596.

226. Peters PJ, Borst J, Oorschot V, et al. Cytotoxic T lymphocyte granules are secretory lysosomes, containing both perforin and granzymes. J Exp Med. 1991;173:1099-1109.

227. Janka GE. Hemophagocytic syndromes. Blood Rev. 2007;21:245-253.

228. Stepp SE, Dufourcq-Lagelous R, Le Deist F, et al. Perforin gene defects in familial hemophagocytic lymphohistiocytosis. Science. 1999;286:1957-1959.

229. Fisher GH, Rosenberg FJ, Straus SE, et al. Dominant interfering Fas gene mutations impair apoptosis in a human autoimmune lymphoproliferative syndrome. Cell. 1995;81:935-946.

230. Rieux-Laucat F, Le Deist F, Hivroz C, et al. Mutations in Fas associated with human lymphoproliferative syndrome and autoimmunity. Science. 1995;268:1347-1349.

231. Worth A, Thrasher AJ, Gaspar HB. Autoimmune lymphoproliferative syndrome: molecular basis of disease and clinical phenotype. Br J Haematol. 2006;133:124-140.

232. Schwartz RH. A cell culture model for T lymphocyte clonal anergy. Science. 1990;248:1349-1356.

233. Sakaguchi S, Sakaguchi N, Asano M, et al. Immunologic self-tolerance maintained by activated T cells expressing IL-2 receptor alpha-chains (CD25). Breakdown of a single mechanism of self-tolerance causes various autoimmune diseases. J Immunol. 1995;155:1151-1164.

234. Hori S, Nomura T, Sakaguchi S. Control of regulatory T cell development by the transcription factor Foxp3. Science. 2003;299:1057-1061.

235. Khattri R, Cox T, Yasayko SA, Ransdell F. An essential role for Scurfin in CD4$^+$CD25$^+$ T regulatory cells. Nat Immunol. 2003;4:337-342.

236. Fontenot JD, Gavin MA, Rudensky AY. Foxp3 programs the development and function of CD4$^+$CD25$^+$ regulatory T cells. Nat Immunol. 2003;4:330-336.

237. Sakaguchi S. Naturally arising Foxp3-expressing CD25$^+$CD4$^+$ regulatory T cells in immunological tolerance to self and non-self. Nat Immunol. 2005;6:345-352.

238. Wildin RS, Ramsdell F, Peake J, et al. X-linked neonatal diabetes mellitus, enteropathy and endocrinopathy syndrome is the human equivalent of mouse scurfy. Nat Genet. 2001;27:18-20.

239. Bennett CL, Christie J, Ramsdell F, et al. The immune dysregulation, polyendocrinopathy, enteropathy, X-linked syndrome (IPEX) is caused by mutations of FOXP3. Nat Genet. 2001;27:20-21.

240. Chatila TA, Blaeser F, Ho N, et al. JM2, encoding a fork head-related protein, is mutated in X-linked autoimmunity-allergic disregulation syndrome. J Clin Invest. 2000;106:R75-R81.

241. Thornton AM, Shevach EM. CD4$^+$CD25$^+$ immunoregulatory T cells suppress polyclonal T cell activation in vitro by inhibiting interleukin 2 production. J Exp Med. 1998;188:287-296.

242. Takahashi T, Kuniyasu Y, Toda M, et al. Immunologic self-tolerance maintained by CD25$^+$CD4$^+$ naturally anergic and suppressive T cells: induction of autoimmune disease by breaking their anergic/suppressive state. Int Immunol. 1998;10:1969-1980.

243. Read S, Mauze S, Asseman C, et al. CD38$^+$ CD45RB(low) CD4$^+$ T cells: a population of T cells with immune regulatory activities in vitro. Eur J Immunol. 1998;28:3435-3447.

244. Godfrey D, MacDonald HR, Kronenberg M, et al. NKT cells: what's in a name? Nat Rev Immunol. 2004;4:231-237.

245. Bendelac A, Lantz O, Quimby ME, et al. CD1 recognition by mouse NK1$^+$ T lymphocytes. Science. 1995;268:863-855.

246. Brigl M, Brenner M. CD1: antigen presentation and T cell function. Annu Rev Immunol. 2004;22:817-890.

247. Godfrey DI, Berzins SP. Control points in NKT-cell development. Nat Rev Immunol. 2007;7:505-518.

248. Beckman EM, Porcelli SA, Morita CT, et al. Recognition of a lipid antigen by CD1-restricted alpha beta⁺ T cells. Nature. 1994;372:691-694.

249. Bendelac A, Savage PB, Teyton L. The biology of NKT cells. Annu Rev Immunol. 2007;25:297-336.

250. Kawano T, Cui J, Koezuka Y, et al. CD1d-restricted and TCR-mediated activation of valpha14 NKT cells by gly-cosylceramides. Science. 1997;278:1626-1629.

251. Benlagha K, Weiss A, Beavis A, et al. In vivo identification of glycolipid antigen–specific T cells using fluorescent CD1d tetramers. J Exp Med. 2000;191:1895-1903.

252. Matsuda JL, Naidenko OV, Gapin L, et al. Tracking the response of natural killer T cells to a glycolipid antigen using CD1d tetramers. J Exp Med. 2000;192:741-754.

253. Gumperz J, Miyake S, Yamamura T, Brenner MB. Functionally distinct subsets of CD1d-restricted natural killer T cells revealed by CD1d tetramer staining. J Exp Med. 2002;195:625-636.

254. Chen H, Paul WE. Cultured NK1.1⁺ CD4⁺ T cells produce large amounts of IL-4 and IFN-gamma upon activation by anti-CD3 or CD1. J Immunol. 1997;159:2240-2249.

255. Godfrey DI, Kronenberg M. Going both ways: immune regulation via CD1d-dependent NKT cells. J Clin Invest. 2004;114:1379-1388.

256. Hayday A. γδ cells: a right time and a right place for a conserved third way of protection. Annu Rev Immunol. 2000;18:975-1026.

257. Thedrez A, Sabourin C, Gertner J, et al. Self/non-self discrimination by human gammadelta T cells: simple solutions for a complex issue? Immunol Rev. 2007;215:123-135.

258. Tanaka Y, Morita CD, Tanaka Y, et al. Natural and synthetic non-peptide antigens recognized by human gamma delta T cells. Nature. 1995;375:155-158.

259. Sieling PA, Chatterjee D, Porcelli SA, et al. CD1-restricted T cell recognition of microbial lipoglycan antigens. Science. 1995;269):227-230.

260. Constant P, Davodeau F, Peyrat MA, et al. Stimulation of human gamma delta T cells by nonpeptidic mycobacterial ligands. Science. 1994;2646):267-270.

261. Lanier LL, Cwirla S, Federspiel N, Phillips JH. Human natural killer cells isolated from peripheral blood do not rearrange T cell antigen receptor beta chain genes. J Exp Med. 1986;163:209-214.

262. Henkart P. Lymphocyte-mediated cytotoxicity: two pathways and multiple effector molecules. Immunity. 1994;1:343-346.

263. Herberman R, Reynolds C, Ortaldo J. Mechanism of cytotoxicity by natural killer (NK) cells. Annu Rev Immunol. 1986;4:651-680.

264. Orange J, Ballas Z. Natural killer cells in human health and disease. Clin Immunol. 2006;118:1-10.

265. Rodewald H, Moingeon P, Lucich JL, et al. A population of early fetal thymocytes expressing Fc gamma RII/III contains precursors of T lymphocytes and natural killer cells. Cell. 1992;69:139-150.

266. Sánchez M, Spits H, Lanier LL, Phillips JH. Human natural killer cell committed thymocytes and their relation to the T cell lineage. J Exp Med. 1993;178:1857-1866.

267. Parrish-Novak J, Dillon SR, Nelson A, et al. Interleukin 21 and its receptor are involved in NK cell expansion and regulation of lymphocyte function. Nature. 2000;408:57-63.

268. Freud AG, Caligiuri MA. Human natural killer cell development. Immunol Rev. 2006;214:56-72.

269. Biron CA, Brossay L. NK cells and NKT cells in innate defense against viral infections. Curr Opin Immunol. 2001;13:458-464.

270. Parham P. Immunogenetics of killer cell immunoglobulin-like receptors. Mol Immunol. 2005;42:459-462.

271. Colonna M, Nakajima H, Navarro F, López-Botet M. A novel family of Ig-like receptors for HLA class I molecules that modulate function of lymphoid and myeloid cells. J Leukoc Biol. 1999;66:375-381.

272. Long E. Regulation of immune responses through inhibitory receptors. Annu Rev Immunol. 1999;17:875-904.

273. López-Botet M, Bellón T. Natural killer cell activation and inhibition by receptors for MHC class I. Curr Opin Immunol. 1999;11:301-307.

274. Chapman T, Heikema AP, West AP Jr, Bjorkman PJ. Crystal structure and ligand binding properties of the D1D2 region of the inhibitory receptor LIR-1 (ILT2). Immunity. 2000;13:727-736.

275. Cosman D, Fanger N, Borges L, et al. A novel immunoglobulin superfamily receptor for cellular and viral MHC class I molecules. Immunity. 1997;7:273-282.

276. López-Botet M, Llano M, Ortega M. Human cytomegalovirus and natural killer–mediated surveillance of HLA class I expression: a paradigm of host-pathogen adaptation. Immunol Rev. 2001;181:193-202.

277. Phan GQ, Yang JC, Sherry RM, et al. Cancer regression and autoimmunity induced by cytotoxic T lymphocyte–associated antigen 4 blockade in patients with metastatic melanoma. Proc Natl Acad Sci U S A. 2003;100:8372-8377.

23 Primary Immunodeficiency Diseases

Francisco A. Bonilla and Raif S. Geha

TABLE 23-1	Internet Sites with Information Relevant to Primary Immunodeficiency Diseases
URL	**Name/Description**
http://www.aaaai.org	American Academy of Allergy, Asthma, and Immunology (AAAAI)
http://F.webring.com/hub? ring=pidring	Primary Immune Deficiency WebRing
http://www.info4pi.org	Primary Immunodeficiency Resource Center
http://www.jmfworld.org	Jeffrey Modell Foundation (JMF)
http://www.primaryimmune.org	Immune Deficiency Foundation (IDF)
http://www.uta.fi/imt/bioinfo	University of Tampere, Institute of Medical Mutation Databases (links to many sites)

Immune compromise arises either as a heritable genetic defect (primary disease) or as a consequence of (secondary to) another pathologic process such as infection, malignancy, or iatrogenic immunosuppression. Immune system dysfunction is most often manifested as recurrent and chronic infections. Malignancy and autoimmunity also occur in certain syndromes. In most instances, symptoms and signs of immunodeficiency develop soon after birth. However, onset may be delayed into childhood, and milder variants may not be diagnosed until adulthood. Even though many patients with severe immunodeficiency suffer dramatic morbidity and mortality in infancy and early childhood, the majority of patients with immunodeficiency have milder forms that permit survival into adulthood, but often with reduced longevity because of infection, autoimmune disease, or constitutional debility. Health-related quality of life is significantly impaired in children with primary immunodeficiency.[1] The challenge to clinicians is to recognize and intervene aggressively in these "milder" forms to maximize quality of life for these patients.

Immunodeficiencies may be classified with respect to the specific immune effector mechanisms disrupted.[2,3] In broadest terms, one may distinguish cellular and humoral components of both specific immunity (T-cell cytotoxicity and B-cell antibody production) and nonspecific immunity (phagocytosis and the complement system). Discussed here are selected syndromes of immunodeficiency arising from aberrant development and function of T and B cells, as well as the complement system. Phagocytic disorders are the subject of Chapter 21. Table 23-1 lists several Internet sites with information relevant to primary immunodeficiencies.

COMBINED IMMUNODEFICIENCIES

Severe Combined Immunodeficiency

The term severe combined immunodeficiency (SCID) designates a genetically heterogeneous group of syndromes having in common a profound disturbance in the development and function of both T and B cells.[4] In Figure 23-1 the development of lymphocytes is outlined. In some instances, the molecular defect leading to SCID prevents only T-cell function, and B cells are normal. However, because T cells play a role in most B-cell responses, serious T-cell dysfunction precludes effective humoral immunity. Not surprisingly, complete absence of specific cellular and humoral immunity leads to an extreme infectious diathesis. Mucocutaneous candidiasis is a common early finding. Infections with common viral pathogens (e.g., varicella, herpes simplex, measles, adenoviruses, respiratory syncytial virus, influenza, and parainfluenza) are often fatal. Patients are also susceptible to opportunistic infections with commensal organisms that are normally nonpathogenic, such as *Pneumocystis jiroveci*. Even attenuated vaccine organisms such as oral polio vaccine virus and bacille Calmette-Guérin (BCG) can cause severe or fatal infection. Transfusion of blood products containing viable lymphocytes may lead to fatal graft-versus-host disease. The few patients who do not die of infection during childhood have an increased risk for malignancy.

Typical symptoms of SCID are recurrent severe infections, chronic diarrhea, and failure to thrive.[2,4] Symptoms are often seen in the newborn period but may be delayed by several months. Antibodies derived from the mother by transfer across the placenta provide some early protection. Physical examination may reveal foci of infection (e.g., thrush) and the absence of discernible lymphoid tissue. Hypogammaglobulinemia is often present but is not universal. Specific antibody responses are almost always severely impaired.

Abnormalities in lymphocyte populations vary, depending on the specific molecular defect. T cells are almost always absent or their numbers are very low, and they do not function. SCID is most often classified according to the peripheral blood lymphocyte phenotype, that is, absence or presence of the major lymphocyte types. T cells are absent (or very low) in all classic forms of SCID, a phenotype designated "T⁻." The presence or absence of B cells is indicated by adding "B⁺" or "B⁻," respectively. The same pattern applies for natural killer (NK) cells. Table 23-2 lists the various lymphocyte phenotypes of SCID and the molecular defects associated with them. Some syndromes classified as SCID have phenotypes that do not fall easily into any of these principal groups and are listed individually. Figure 23-2 shows the relative frequency of SCID secondary to some

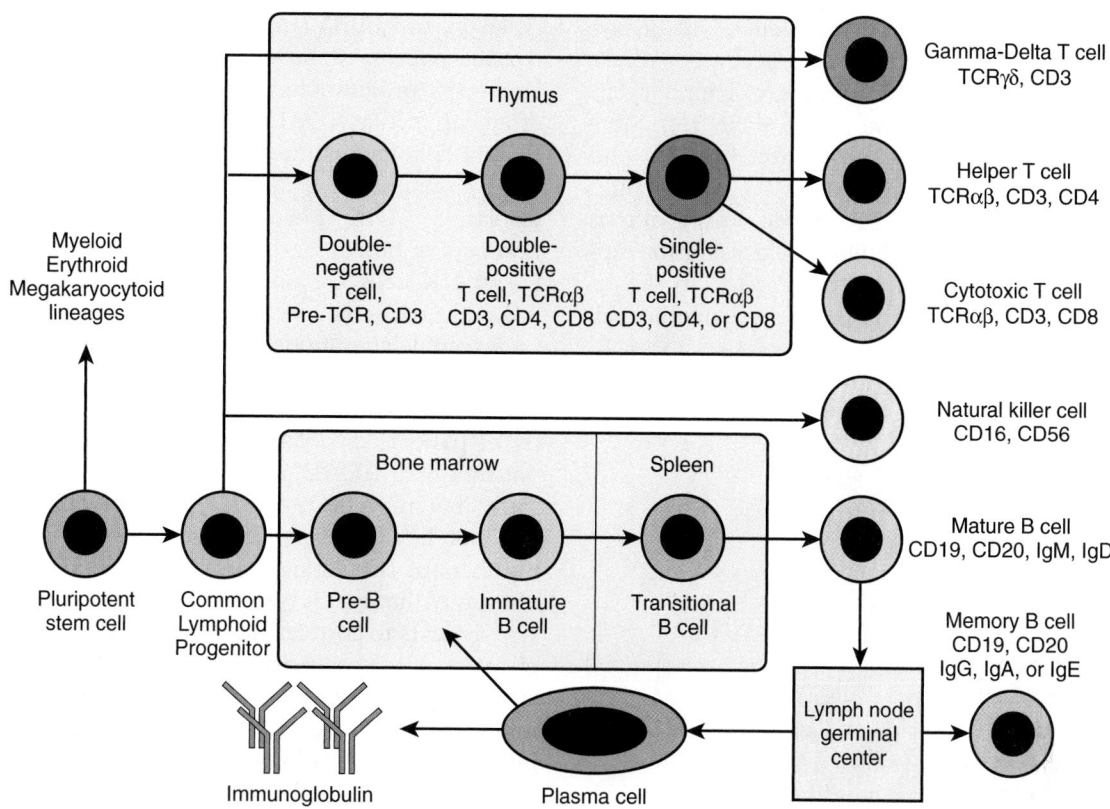

FIGURE 23-1. Diagram of lymphocyte development. Pluripotent stem cells give rise to all cellular blood elements. The common lymphoid progenitor gives rise to the three principal lineages of lymphocytes: T cells, B cells, and natural killer cells. T cells develop in the thymus. Most peripheral T cells express the αβ form of the T-cell antigen receptor (TCR) and develop through distinct stages in the thymus. Mature helper T cells express the CD3 antigen coreceptor complex along with the major histocompatibility complex (MHC) class II receptor CD4, whereas cytotoxic cells express the MHC class I receptor CD8. A minority (1% to 5%) of peripheral T cells express the γδ form of the TCR along with CD3, but without CD4 or CD8; less is known about their development. B cells develop initially in the bone marrow and pass through several stages before exiting to complete development in the spleen. Mature B cells express distinct markers (CD19 and CD20) along with surface immunoglobulin M (IgM) and IgD. B cells are activated in germinal centers to undergo class switching and become either memory B cells expressing IgG, IgA, or IgE or Ig-secreting plasma cells. Most IgG-producing plasma cells reside in the bone marrow. Natural killer cells are a distinct lineage of cytotoxic cells; little is known regarding their development from lymphoid precursors.

TABLE 23-2	Lymphocyte Phenotype Classification of Severe Combined Immunodeficiency and Associated Gene Defects
Lymphocyte Phenotype	**Genes**
T⁻B⁻NK⁻	*ADA, NP*
T⁻B⁻NK⁺	*RAG1, RAG2, DCLRE1C* (Artemis), *NHEJ1* (Cernunnos), *LIG4*
T⁻B⁺NK⁻	*IL2RG, JAK3, IL2RA* (CD25)
T⁻B⁺NK⁺	*IL7RA, PTPRC* (CD45), *CD3D, CD3Z*
CD4 deficiency	*MHCIITA, RFXANK, RFX5, RFXAP*
CD8 deficiency	*ZAP70, TAP1, TAP2, TAPBP, CD8A*

of these defined genetic lesions. Approximately 10% of SCID cases result from unknown genetic lesions. In as many as 40% of patients with SCID, maternal T cells may have engrafted in the fetus during gestation, and this situation may occasionally confuse the diagnostic picture.[5]

Maternally derived T cells tend to be anergic, but they may also be associated with clinical manifestations similar to those of graft-versus-host disease, such as eczematous rash, eosinophilia, and splenomegaly. In rare circumstances, maternal engraftment may lead to even more unusual clinical findings, such as IgA monoclonal gammopathy in an infant.[6]

T⁻B⁻NK⁻ Severe Combined Immunodeficiency

Adenosine Deaminase and Purine Nucleoside Phosphorylase Deficiencies

Figure 23-3 shows the salvage pathway of purine nucleotide synthesis. The enzymes adenosine deaminase (ADA) and purine nucleoside phosphorylase (PNP) are the only known defects of nucleotide synthesis associated with immunodeficiency.[7,8] ADA deficiency (ADAD), which has an incidence of 1 in 200,000 live births, accounts for approximately 15% of all patients with SCID (see Fig. 23-2), or approximately a third of SCID cases with autosomal recessive inheritance. PNP deficiency (PNPD) is quite rare (30+ patients described). Absence of ADA or

PNP leads to intracellular accumulation of deoxyadenosine and deoxyguanosine, respectively. These molecules are not themselves toxic to lymphocytes. However, when they are converted to their 5'-triphosphates (deoxyadenosine triphosphatase [dATP] and deoxyguanosine triphosphatase [dGTP]), they inhibit ribonucleotide reductase and prevent de novo synthesis of deoxynucleotides. Without building blocks for the replication and repair of DNA, the cells cease to divide. Lymphocytes die to a much greater extent than other cell

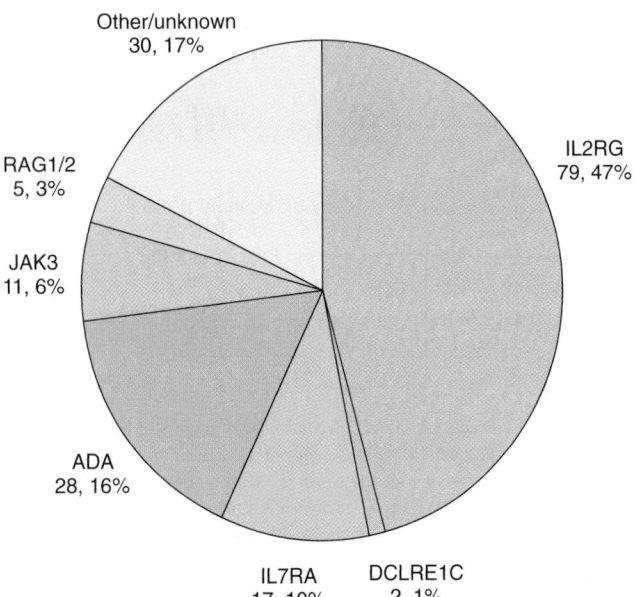

FIGURE 23-2. Relative occurrence of severe combined immunodeficiency (SCID) syndromes. The category labeled "Other/unknown" contains a few patients with some of the less common genetic mutations associated with SCID, along with some whose causes have yet to be determined. *(Adapted from Buckley RH. A historical review of bone marrow transplantation for immunodeficiencies. J Allergy Clin Immunol. 2004;113:793-800.)*

types do. In ADAD and PNPD, T-cell precursors in the thymus appear to be especially sensitive to death by apoptosis (programmed cell death).[9-12] B cells are more often depleted in ADAD than in PNPD. In the latter, the B-cell phenotype is more variable.

Approximately 85% of individuals with ADAD will display a SCID phenotype with markedly reduced numbers of both T and B cells and low serum antibody levels. NK cells are only rarely found in patients with ADAD. Additional clinical manifestations may include radiographic alterations of the ribs, vertebral bodies, and iliac crests, as well as cognitive impairment later in life.[7,13] Without bone marrow transplantation (BMT), the majority of patients die of infection. Ten percent to 15% of patients with ADAD may have a delayed or late-onset form that may be manifested in late infancy or early childhood.[12] These patients may initially have variable numbers of circulating lymphocytes and some humoral immunity that quickly wanes. The severity of the phenotype appears to correlate to some degree with the amount of residual ADA activity. As little as 3% to 5% residual enzyme activity may be sufficient to maintain normal immune function even into adulthood, at which time infectious complications may arise.[14] ADAD has also been described in a few adult patients with "idiopathic" CD4 lymphocytopenia (see later).[15]

PNPD is mainly expressed as a somewhat selective defect in cellular immunity, although it is usually discussed together with ADAD because of similarities in their biochemical pathophysiology. Patients are extremely susceptible to viral and fungal infections. They have decreased numbers of circulating T cells, often initially with normal numbers of B cells and normal serum immunoglobulin (Ig) levels. With time, humoral immunity usually deteriorates. Analysis of a murine model of PNPD suggests that accumulation of dGTP inhibits mitochondrial DNA repair and leads to increased T-cell apoptosis.[11] Approximately 50% of children with PNPD have

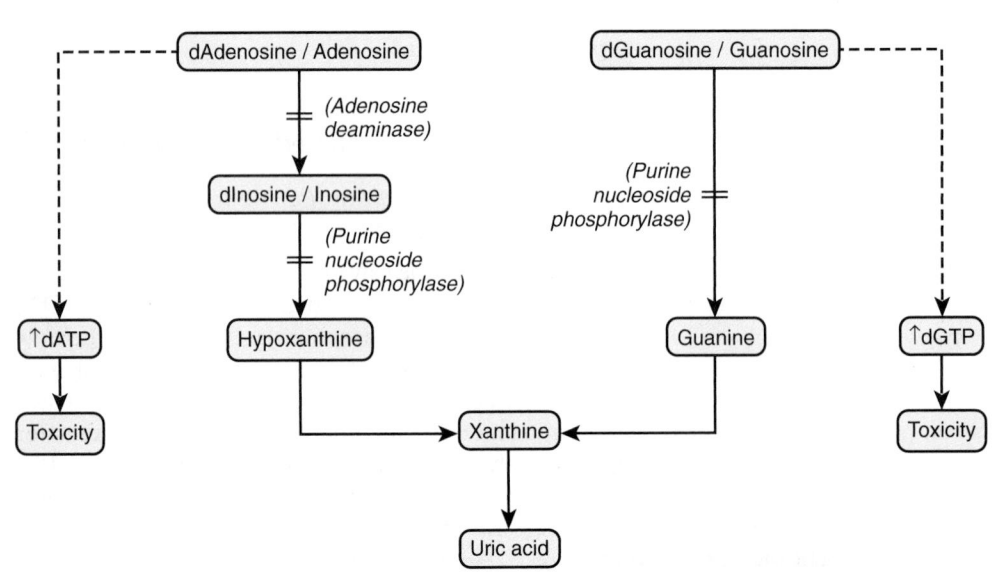

FIGURE 23-3. Salvage pathway of purine nucleotide biosynthesis. d, deoxy; dATP, deoxyadenosine triphosphatase; dGTP, deoxyguanosine triphosphatase.

neurologic complications such as spasticity, diplegia, paresis, and other motor disorders, as well as cognitive impairment.[16]

After clinical suspicion is aroused, diagnosis of ADAD or PNPD is not difficult. Both ADA and PNP activity is readily measurable in red blood cell (RBC) or leukocyte lysates. In symptomatic patients, activity is usually 1% or less of that in normal subjects. These methods may be applied for screening of in utero cord blood samples or cultured amniotic or chorionic villus cells. PNP is required for the production of hypoxanthine, a precursor of uric acid (see Fig. 23-3). Thus, individuals with PNPD will have reduced serum and urine urate levels. Such is not the case for patients with ADAD.

ADAD is amenable to enzyme replacement therapy. RBCs contain high levels of ADA, and RBC transfusions can ameliorate the enzyme defect.[17] Such treatment is effective in approximately 50% of patients, mainly those with evidence of some residual immune function. However, these patients have a risk of complications after chronic RBC transfusions, such as iron overload and transfusion-associated infections. An alternative therapy is infusion of polyethylene glycol–conjugated bovine ADA (PEG-ADA or pegademase).[9,18] This treatment is generally well tolerated, but immune reconstitution is incomplete. Infectious complications may occur occasionally during therapy with PEG-ADA, and malignancies such as cerebral Epstein-Barr virus (EBV)-positive lymphoma have also been observed.[19] RBC transfusions have not benefited patients with PNPD. Other forms of enzyme replacement have not been explored.

BMT is curative of the immunodeficiency associated with ADAD and PNPD (see later). Other features, such as neurologic impairment, are not improved after BMT. ADAD has also been cured by gene therapy (see later).

T⁻B⁻NK⁺ Severe Combined Immunodeficiency

Defects of Recombinase-Activating Genes 1 and 2

Patients have very low numbers of T and B lymphocytes, and NK cells are found in about 75% of these patients. This form of SCID results from mutations in one of two DNA-binding proteins, the products of recombinase-activating genes 1 or 2 (*RAG1* or *RAG2*).[20] These proteins have critical roles in directing the somatic recombination of Ig and T-cell antigen receptor (TCR) genes. RAG1 and RAG2 proteins bind to specific recognition sequences flanking gene segments and participate in cutting and splicing of the DNA that assembles mature Ig or TCR genes (Fig. 23-4). B- and T-cell precursors are

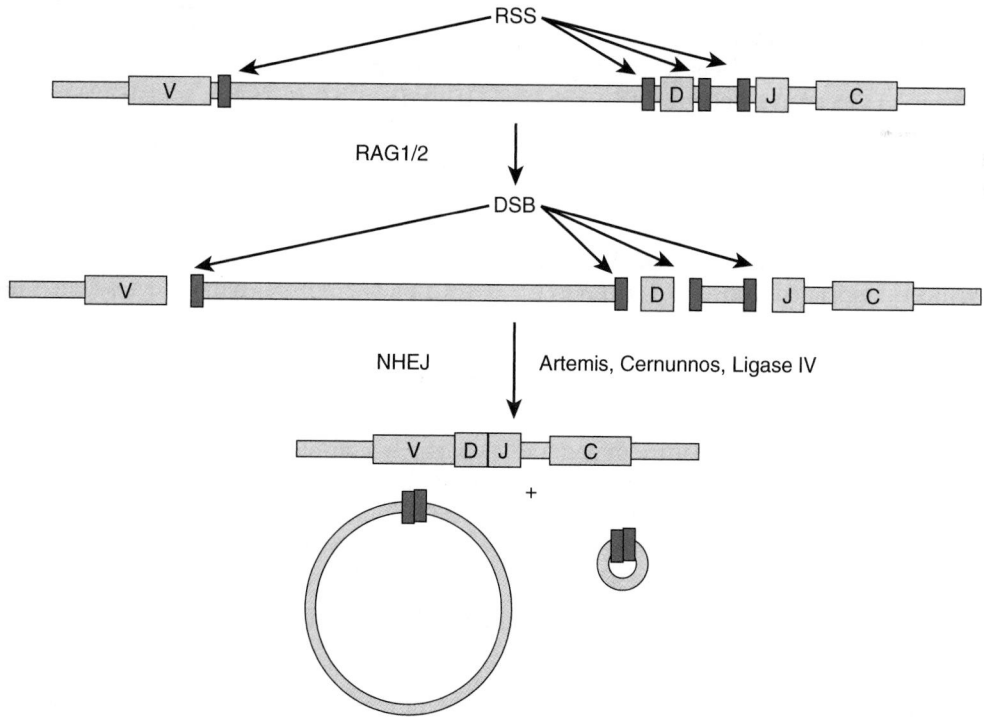

FIGURE 23-4. Gene defects affecting lymphocyte antigen receptor gene rearrangement and causing T⁻B⁻NK⁺ severe combined immunodeficiency. The genes that encode immunoglobulin and T-cell antigen receptors are assembled from subunit segments that are separated in the germline and undergo assembly or somatic rearrangement during lymphocyte development. In the figure, a TCR or Ig heavy chain is shown. The heavy chains are composed of four distinct segments: V, variable; D, diversity; J, joining; C, constant. Some of the segments are flanked by recombination signal sequences (RSS). RAG1 and RAG2 initiate the process that leads to double-strand breaks (DSB) in DNA. The DNA in between coding segments is looped out and forms circles, with the coding sequences joining to one another. In the case of T cells, the larger DNA circle is referred to as a T-cell receptor excision circle. All these DNA joints are made by a group of molecules that together subserve the function of nonhomologous end joining (NHEJ).

present, but they are arrested at an early stage of development. Some patients with *RAG1* or *RAG2* mutations have variable degrees of immune deficiency and atypical lymphocyte phenotypes (limited development of small numbers of B or T lymphocytes, or both).[20] Mutations in these genes should be sought in individuals with partial combined immunodeficiency without other specific molecular diagnoses.

A distinct SCID phenotype known as Omenn's syndrome (OS) also results from *RAG1* or *RAG2* mutations.[21] OS has similar manifestations as acute graft-versus-host disease. Symptoms include recurrent severe infections, failure to thrive, chronic severe diarrhea, and erythroderma with exfoliation and exudation. Examination may reveal hepatosplenomegaly and lymphadenopathy. Laboratory studies show anemia, hypogammaglobulinemia with an elevated IgE level, a decrease in the number of peripheral B cells and poor antibody responses to antigen, appearance of immature CD4+CD8+ T cells ("double-positive" T cells) in the circulation, and absence of T-cell function in vitro. Patients exhibit infiltration of the skin, intestinal mucosa, liver, and spleen with histiocytes and oligoclonal populations of T cells and lymphocyte depletion in the thymus, spleen, and other peripheral lymphoid tissues. It has been proposed that mutations in *RAG1* or *RAG2* that permit partial function (so-called hypomorphic mutations) result in the OS phenotype rather than "classic" SCID. However, recent observations of similar mutations in patients with these two disorders suggest that other factors also play a role in determining the phenotype.[22] In at least one case, progression to OS was observed in a patient with a *RAG2* mutation after infection with parainfluenza virus type 3.[23] Occasionally, somatic mutations may become superimposed on null or "amorphic" mutations and yield mosaicism with revertant or hypomorphic populations of lymphocytes and resultant OS.[24] Additional genetic defects have also been associated with OS (*DCLRE1C*, or Artemis, and *IL7RA*, see later).

Mutations of DCLRE1C (Artemis)

A form of autosomal recessive SCID with the classic T−B−NK+ phenotype has an associated feature of general radiation sensitivity not seen with *RAG1* or *RAG2* mutations and is caused by mutations in the gene *DCLRE1C* (DNA cross-link repair enzyme 1C), whose protein product is called Artemis.[25] Artemis has a critical role in the function of nonhomologous end joining (NHEJ), or the repair of double-stranded DNA breaks (see Fig. 23-4).[26] Absence or impaired function of Artemis blocks lymphocyte development in the same manner as mutations in *RAG1* and *RAG2* do, by preventing proper assembly of mature Ig and TCR genes through somatic recombination. Artemis is ubiquitously expressed, and the generalized radiation sensitivity phenotype in these patients results from loss of its function in nonhematopoietic tissue. OS has been observed in some patients with Artemis defects.[27]

DNA Ligase IV Defects

Mutations in the DNA ligase IV gene (*LIG4*) lead to a form of T−B−NK+ SCID and radiosensitivity very similar to Artemis deficiency, with the added features of microcephaly and cognitive impairment.[28-30] Ligase IV is also required for NHEJ. Fewer than 10 patients have been described thus far. The severity of the immunologic and neurologic features is variable. Some patients have pancytopenia, and two patients have had leukemia.

Cernunnos Deficiency

Five patients have recently been described with another form of T−B−NK+ SCID, very similar to ligase IV deficiency, that is due to mutations in the *NHEJ1* (nonhomologous end joining 1) gene.[31] The protein product has been called Cernunnos. Clinical features include lymphopenia, radiation sensitivity, growth retardation, microcephaly, and developmental delay.

T−B+NK− Severe Combined Immunodeficiency

X-Linked Severe Combined Immunodeficiency, Mutations of the Cytokine Receptor Common γ Chain

Slightly less than half of all patients with SCID are males with an X-linked form of the disease, referred to simply as X-linked SCID (XSCID), that is due to mutations in the cytokine receptor common γ chain (γc).[32] This molecule is shared by no less than six different cytokine receptor complexes, including those for interleukin-2 (IL-2), IL-4, IL-7, IL-9, IL-15, and IL-21 (Fig. 23-5). Thus, a defect in a single molecule interrupts several cytokine pathways, thereby severely disrupting immune function. One patient with this disease received intense media attention ("the boy in the bubble").[33] These patients have a classic SCID phenotype: T cells are absent, and the thymus is empty of lymphocytes. The number of B cells is normal or increased; however, Ig is virtually nonexistent. This deficiency results largely from the absence of T-cell help for antibody production. However, B cells are not completely normal. Their function can be only partially complemented by normal T cells. NK cells are found in about 10% of patients. Some patients with XSCID may have variable numbers of their own T cells or B cells and partial immune function.[34] In addition, maternal T cells may enter the fetus's circulation during gestation and subsequently expand.[35] Thus, the diagnosis of γc deficiency should at least be considered in all males with SCID.

T lymphocytes of female carriers of XSCID show a highly skewed pattern of lyonization, or nonrandom X-chromosome inactivation.[36] This may be studied with DNA probes specific for highly polymorphic repetitive sequence regions, some of which may be associated with specific genetic loci, such as monoamine oxidase, or with the androgen receptor. Female carriers express a single allele at a polymorphic locus of the X chromosome in

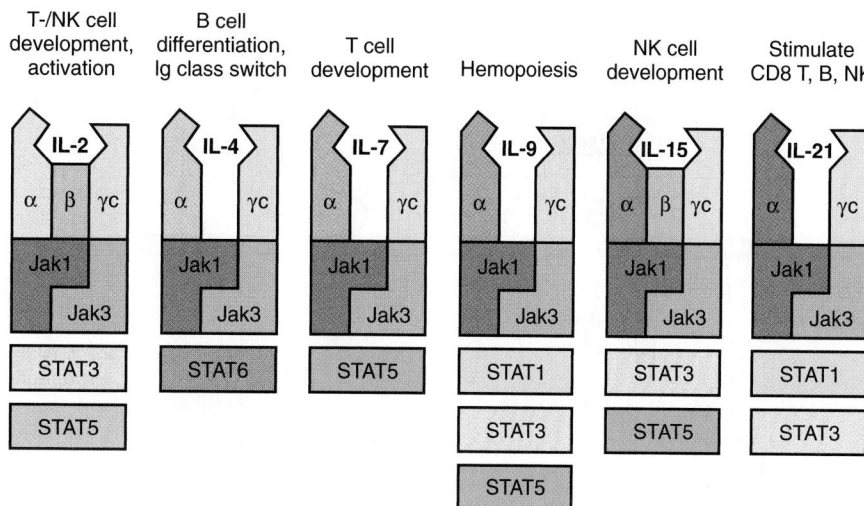

FIGURE 23-5. Cytokine receptors and signaling via γ_c and Jak3. The γ_c chain participates in signaling via all of these cytokine receptors; it associates with the Jak3 kinase in every case. The α chains of each receptor are distinct; receptors for interleukin-2 (IL-2) and IL-15 also share a β chain. The α or β chains or both associate with Jak1. After cytokine binding, Jak kinases recruit STAT (signal transducer and activator of transcription) proteins. These molecules dimerize and then translocate to the nucleus, where they associate with other transcriptional regulators and alter gene expression. NK, natural killer.

more than 95% of T lymphocytes. This represents the preferential survival of cells retaining the functional gene on the active X chromosome. The expression of alleles in other tissues is less unequal. Similar analyses are useful with other X-linked immunodeficiency disorders, such as Wiskott-Aldrich syndrome (WAS) and X-linked agammaglobulinemia (XLA).

Urgent BMT is the standard therapy for all forms of SCID, including XSCID. In some patients, B cells may fail to engraft after BMT (see later), thus leaving patients with their own B cells and residual humoral immunodeficiency despite normal T-cell function. Gene therapy has also been successful in the treatment of XSCID (see later).

Jak3 Deficiency

A form of T⁻B⁺NK⁻ SCID phenotypically very similar to XSCID is associated with defects in the tyrosine kinase Jak3.[37,38] The similarity with XSCID is easily understood because Jak3 is a critical signal-transducing molecule associated with the γ_c chain (see Fig. 23-5). Oligoclonal and poorly functional T cells may develop in some of these patients, but NK cells are not generally found. Because of the variable immunologic phenotype, the diagnosis should be considered in patients with combined immunodeficiency and B cells. One patient displayed highly unusual functional maternal engraftment that provided partial immune protection, and the diagnosis was made at 8 years of age.[39]

CD25 Deficiency

A male infant was reported to have a form of SCID caused by mutation of the gene encoding the α chain of the IL-2 receptor (also called CD25, the signaling chain for this receptor is γ_c; see Fig. 23-5).[40] This child was seen at 6 months of age with oral and esophageal candidiasis, chronic diarrhea, failure to thrive, chronic lung disease, and autoimmunity with lymphadenopathy and splenomegaly. He had a reduced number of CD4⁺ T cells and NK cells and poor in vitro T-cell function that could not

be corrected with exogenous IL-2. B-cell number and function were normal. CD25 is important in T-cell development. The finding of reduced apoptosis of thymocytes in this patient suggested that they were resistant to negative selection and that this resistance permitted many autoreactive T-cell clones to reach the periphery and expand.

T⁻B⁺NK⁺ Severe Combined Immunodeficiency

Defects of the Interleukin-7 Receptor α Chain

Between 10 and 20 patients with a T⁻B⁺NK⁺ SCID phenotype have been found to have mutations in the gene encoding the α chain of the IL-7 receptor (IL-7Rα, also called CD127; the signaling chain for this receptor is γ_c; see Fig. 23-5).[41] This molecule is also a component of the receptor for thymic stromal lymphopoietin, a member of the IL-2 family of cytokines. In one review of 16 patients, BMT was successful in 13.[41] At least one patient with IL-7Rα defects was found to have OS at initial evaluation.[42]

Mutations Affecting Components of the T-Cell Antigen Receptor Complex

The TCR is made up of several different polypeptides (Fig. 23-6),[43] including the TCRα and TCRβ (or TCRγ and TCRδ) chains of the receptor making contact with major histocompatibility antigen-peptide complexes, as well as components of the CD3 signal-transducing complex: CD3γ, CD3δ, and CD3ε and a ζ₂ dimer or a ζ-η heterodimer.

Defects in CD3δ lead to a T⁻B⁺NK⁺ SCID phenotype.[44-47] Of the nine patients (four kindreds) described, all had varying degrees of panhypogammaglobulinemia and disseminated viral infections (except one in whom the defect was diagnosed at birth because of a family history). Three patients had thymus glands of normal size, in marked contrast to almost all other forms of SCID, in which the thymus is absent or extremely hypoplastic.[46] One other patient had a small thymus, thus

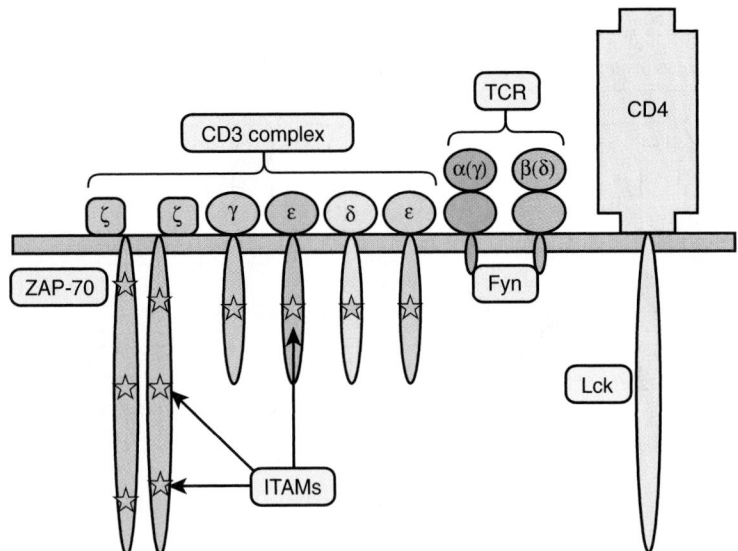

FIGURE 23-6. Components of the T-cell antigen receptor. The actual receptor making contact with a major histocompatibility complex (MHC)-peptide complex is a heterodimer of α and β (or γ and δ) chains. This heterodimer sits in the cell membrane in association with the signal-transducing CD3 complex. This complex contains two heterodimers, one γε and one δε, and one ζ dimer. Also shown is the MHC class II coreceptor molecule CD4. Tyrosine kinases Lck, Fyn, and ZAP-70 associate with components of the receptor complex via immunoreceptor tyrosine-based activating motifs (ITAMs) and transduce signals after interaction of the receptor with peptide/MHC.

suggesting that a normal-size thymus may not be a consistent feature of this form of SCID.[44] Three patients (one kindred) with deficiency of CD3ε leading to a similar phenotype have been described.[45,47] Finally, one patient with a similar phenotype and germline and mosaic partial revertant mutations of the gene encoding the CD3γ chain has also been described.[48]

One family has been identified in which two sibling boys had mutations in the genes encoding the γ chain of the CD3 complex.[49] One sibling had a SCID phenotype with a normal number of lymphocytes and a selective deficiency of IgG2. He died of parainfluenza 3 pneumonia at 31 months of age. His brother had a similar laboratory profile; however, he was healthy and did not have recurrent infections. The reason for the differential phenotypic expression of the same defect in these brothers is not known.

CD45 Deficiency

A few patients have been found to have a form of SCID resulting from mutations in the gene encoding the protein tyrosine phosphatase CD45.[50-52] This molecule plays an important role in T-cell activation. These patients have a SCID phenotype with diminished numbers of poorly functional T cells and normal numbers of B cells and NK cells.

Severe Combined Immunodeficiency with Selective Deficiency of CD4+ T Cells

Mutations Affecting the HLA Class II Gene Transcription Complex

The major histocompatibility complex (MHC) in humans is called the human leukocyte antigen (HLA) complex. The class I and class II HLA molecules expressed on cell surfaces are critical for practically all mechanisms of specific immune activation. Class I molecules are present on most cells of the body. They present antigenic peptides derived principally from intracellular sources to the antigen receptors of T cells expressing CD8. Class II HLA molecules are generally restricted to specialized antigen-presenting cells (APCs), including monocytes and macrophages, dendritic cells, and B cells. HLA class II molecules mainly present peptides imported from outside the cell to antigen receptors of T cells bearing CD4. Defects in the synthesis, expression, or function of HLA molecules may be expected to have profound consequences on immune competence.

More than 50 patients with HLA class II deficiency have been described to date.[53] Most children who have this disorder are seen within the first weeks of life with a classic SCID phenotype. Lymphocyte numbers tend to be normal, but all forms of MHC class II (DP, DQ, and DR) are not expressed. Most patients have profound hypogammaglobulinemia, no delayed hypersensitivity responses, and decreased numbers of circulating CD4+ T cells. Some patients have normal serum Ig levels; however, specific antibody responses are not elicited. Alloreactivity in mixed lymphocyte culture is preserved to a large extent. As a rule, these children do not survive without BMT. For reasons that are not clear, however, BMT in these patients has not been consistently successful.[54]

MHC class II deficiency results from defective regulation of gene transcription.[53] Four complementation groups (A through D) are recognized, each corresponding to a component of the HLA class II transcription complex (Fig. 23-7). Mutations in *CIITA* (class II transactivator) correspond to group A, mutations in *RFXANK* (the B subunit of the regulatory factor X complex) to group B, mutations in *RFX5* (encoding another subunit of RFX) to group C, and mutations in *RFXAP* to group D. Without a complete transcription complex, no mRNA is produced, and class II proteins cannot be synthesized. The same complex activates transcription at all HLA class II gene promoters.

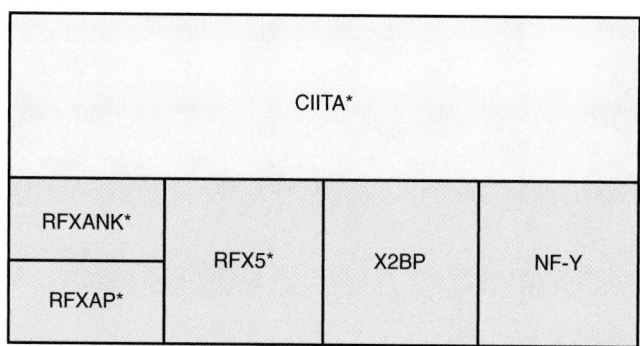

FIGURE 23-7. Transcription complex for major histocompatibility complex (MHC) class II genes. Shown are the known components of the complex of proteins that regulates transcription of MHC class II genes. Mutations of the genes encoding the components indicated by asterisks lead to MHC class II–deficient severe combined immunodeficiency (see text).

Partial MHC class II deficiency has also been reported in male twins.[55] These children had trace amounts of HLA-DR α and β protein detected by immunoblotting techniques. Interestingly, one twin was hypogammaglobulinemic and suffered from recurrent infections; he showed a good response to replacement therapy with intravenous immunoglobulin (IVIG). The other twin was completely asymptomatic and had normal serum antibody levels and immune responses, although he had no more DR expression than his brother did. The molecular defect in these children is not known.

Selective Deficiency of CD8⁺ T Cells

ZAP-70 Deficiency

Several patients with mutations in the gene encoding the ZAP-70 (TCRζ-associated protein of 70 kd) tyrosine kinase (see Fig. 23-6) have been described.[56] The ZAP-70 tyrosine kinase has a critical role in signals transmitted via the TCR. Individuals with ZAP-70 deficiency have a classic SCID phenotype. They may exhibit somewhat elevated total lymphocyte counts with a high number of CD4⁺ T cells and almost complete absence of CD8⁺ T cells. Although circulating CD4⁺ cells appear normal, they fail to respond to signals delivered via the TCR. These characteristics suggest that ZAP-70 kinase is critical for normal thymic development of CD8⁺ cells and not for the CD4⁺ subset. However, mature CD4⁺ T cells depend on ZAP-70 for activation.

Defective Expression of HLA Class I

Several patients with defective expression of HLA class I molecules have been described.[57,58] These patients have mutations in one of two genes encoding either TAP1 or TAP2 (transporter associated with antigen processing 1 or 2). The TAP1/TAP2 heterodimer is required for shuttling of cytosolic peptides across the endoplasmic reticulum to load onto nascent HLA class I molecules for eventual expression at the cell surface and presentation to TCRs (Fig. 23-8). HLA class I molecules are highly unstable without a peptide in their binding cleft, and they are not transported to the cell surface. Another patient has been described with reduced MHC class I expression because of a mutation affecting the molecular chaperone TAP-binding protein, also called tapasin.[59] These entities are frequently categorized as forms of SCID, although patients with defective expression of HLA class I appear to suffer mainly upper and lower respiratory tract bacterial infections and bronchiectasis. A few patients may exhibit granulomatous skin inflammation. Occasional asymptomatic individuals have also been described. The main immunologic abnormality is low peripheral blood CD8⁺ T cells; antibody responses may be normal.

Severe Combined Immunodeficiency with Normal Lymphocyte Populations

Defect in Orai1

After lymphocyte receptor engagement and costimulation by cytokines and other intercellular contacts, mobilization of calcium from both intracellular and extracellular sources is absolutely necessary for downstream signaling, activation, and proliferation. Two patients from a single kindred have been found to have a form of SCID caused by an impairment in this critical calcium flux.[60] The defective protein has been called Orai1, and its function is required for operation of the calcium release–activated calcium (CRAC) channel. These two males had essentially normal peripheral blood lymphocyte phenotypes with normal or elevated Ig levels.[61] However, T cells did not respond to stimulation in vitro, and no specific antibody was produced. One patient died of disseminated BCG infection. The other survived BMT but has persistent anhidrotic ectodermal dysplasia and myopathy.[60]

Griscelli's Syndrome

Griscelli's syndrome (GS) is one of a group of diseases of "pigmentary dilution" whereby abnormalities in melanosome trafficking within cells lead to characteristic pale skin and silvery-gray or ashen hair. In GS, this may be associated with a profound cellular immunodeficiency and neurologic abnormalities (seizures, ataxia, oculomotor and reflex abnormalities).[62,63] Screening studies of immune function may be normal. Patients may have lymphadenopathy and hepatosplenomegaly at initial evaluation. Infections consist principally of bacterial infections of the respiratory tract, skin, and other organs. Without BMT, fulminant and fatal lymphoproliferation with hemophagocytosis ultimately develops.

The full spectrum of symptoms in GS is referred to as GS type 2, and it results from mutations in *RAB27A*.[62,63] The *RAB27A* gene product plays an important role in transporting cytotoxic T-cell granules to the site of contact with a target cell. Lack of Rab27a protein impedes this process and diminishes the ability of cytotoxic T cells to kill their targets. Patients with GS type 1 exhibit

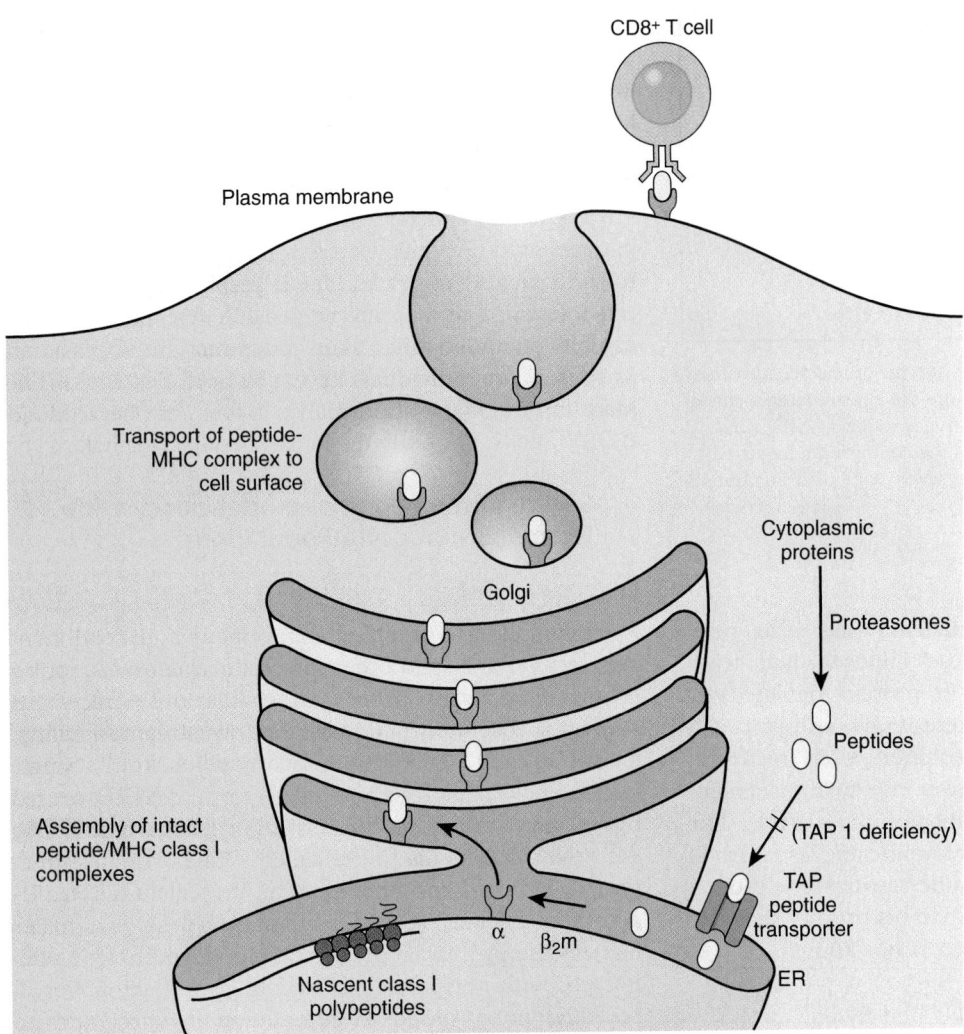

FIGURE 23-8. Synthesis and assembly of major histocompatibility complex (MHC) class I molecules. ER, endoplasmic reticulum; β_2m, β_2-microglobulin; TAP, transporter associated with antigen processing.

pigmentary changes and neurologic symptoms without immunodeficiency and have mutations in the *MYO5A* gene that encodes the myosin Va protein. Myosin Va binds to actin and hydrolyzes adenosine triphosphate. It also has a role in vesicle transport within cells. GS type 3 consists of only pigmentary change and is associated with defects in the melanin chaperone melanophilin.

Therapy for Severe Combined Immunodeficiency

Bone Marrow Transplantation

Identification of a patient with SCID is an immunologic "emergency."[64] Children with this disorder are so prone to infections that extreme measures must be taken to protect them from microbial invasion. Most patients are already infected when initially evaluated and require aggressive interventions to keep their clinical course from running inexorably downhill. After full immunologic evaluation has been performed (as expeditiously as possible), these patients should begin receiving IVIG infusions. Prophylaxis for *P. jiroveci* pneumonia is indicated for all patients.

Although alternative therapies may work for some patients (e.g., PEG-ADA for ADAD), the definitive treatment for the great majority of patients with SCID is BMT. A variety of sources have been used for stem cells, including HLA-identical sibling donors, haploidentical related donors (usually parents), HLA-matched unrelated donors, and partially matched umbilical cord blood.[65-70] Pretransplant conditioning with chemotherapy, radiation therapy, or both may be indicated, depending on the particular form of SCID and the relatedness of the donor. After BMT, patients have variable patterns of leukocyte chimerism. Almost universal reconstitution with donor T cells is seen. B-cell engraftment is less reliable, but its likelihood may be increased in some forms of SCID with prior myeloablation. Humoral immunity is generally intact if engraftment of donor B cells takes place. However, if it does not, lifelong replacement therapy with IVIG is required. The origins of NK and myeloid populations are unpredictable.

The best outcomes are obtained with BMT from HLA-identical related donors in the first 1 to 3 months of life in the absence of any infections. After BMT, thymic output of T cells may be measured by determining the number of T cells that bear T-cell receptor gene excision circles (TRECs).[71-73] TRECs are episomal DNA circles composed of the DNA segment between TCR variable region and D region gene segments that are excised in the process of somatic recombination during thymic T-cell development (see Fig. 23-4). The largest and earliest increases in TRECs predict the most robust T-cell reconstitution after BMT. However, more than 10 years after BMT, levels of TRECs fall more rapidly than in normal individuals, and the diversity of the T-cell repertoire is diminished.

TRECs can be measured in dried blood spots, such as those obtained in the course of newborn screening for a variety of inherited disorders.[74,75] In the vast majority of forms of SCID, TRECs are very low in number as a result of the absence of significant thymic T-cell output. Methods for detecting TRECs will probably soon be applied in pilot studies of newborn screening for SCID.

Gene Therapy

Gene therapy for the treatment of human disease was first attempted in patients with ADAD.[76] A functional copy of the ADA gene in a retroviral vector was transduced into populations of hematopoietic cells or mature T cells. Transduced cells expressed normal levels of ADA and showed normal function in vitro. However, clinical efficacy was difficult to assess in these early attempts because adjunctive therapy with PEG-ADA was considered to be mandated on ethical grounds, even after the reintroduction of transduced cells into patients. As the therapy developed, eventual complete immune reconstitution was achieved, even after discontinuation of PEG-ADA.[77,78] In some cases, myeloablative therapy was also administered.

The earliest "complete" success of gene therapy is considered to have occurred with XSCID.[79,80] Hematopoietic stem cells were transduced ex vivo with a retroviral vector carrying a functional copy of the γ_c gene and then infused into patients. Between 10 and 15 patients have been treated in this manner thus far in several trials in different locations. Most patients have exhibited rapid reconstitution of T cells. B-cell numbers are low, but Ig levels and antibody responses are adequate to permit cessation of IVIG replacement therapy. The therapy appears to work only early in development (within the first year of life) because of deterioration of the thymic rudiment over time.[81] Attempts at transduction in older patients after failed BMT have not succeeded.

Unfortunately, at least three late (>2 years after therapy) occurrences of T-cell leukemia in recipients of transduced cells have tempered the early enthusiasm.[82,83] The leukemias appear to have arisen after insertion of the vector into a leukemogenic site, the *LMO2* gene locus.[84] The *LMO2* gene product appears to modify the activities of several transcription factors; it is itself inappropriately transcribed in certain leukemogenic chromosomal translocations. Insertion of the γ_c vector had the same leukemogenic effect in these patients. It is likely that alterations in the vector and transduction methods will be required to avoid similar complications in the future.

Combined Immunodeficiency Associated with Other Syndromes

Wiskott-Aldrich Syndrome

These disorders and the selective cellular deficiencies, together with their associated gene defects, are listed in Table 23-3. Wiskott-Aldrich syndrome (WAS) is an X-linked disease, the classic manifestations of which include eczema, immunodeficiency, and thrombocytopenia.[85,86] Bloody diarrhea is often seen and may be the initial feature. Eczema may be mild or exuberant; staphylococcal superinfection is common. Recurrent otitides and sinopulmonary infections occur frequently, and opportunistic infections are also seen. In addition, autoimmune vasculitis and glomerulonephritis, as well as other autoimmune processes, have been observed in WAS. Patients most often die of overwhelming infection or massive hemorrhage. Those who avoid these complications have a greatly increased risk for lymphoma, many of which are

TABLE 23-3 Combined Immunodeficiencies, Cellular Deficiencies, and Associated Gene Defects

Syndrome	Gene
COMBINED IMMUNODEFICIENCIES	
Wiskott-Aldrich syndrome	*WAS*
Ataxia-telangiectasia	*ATM*
DiGeorge's syndrome	del22q11, *TBX1*
Hyper-IgM syndromes	
X-linked, CD40 ligand deficiency (HIM1)	*TNFSF5*
Activation-induced cytidine deaminase deficiency (HIM2)	*AICDA*★
CD40 deficiency (HIM3)	*TNFRSF5*
Defect in class switch recombination (HIM4)	Unknown
Uracil nucleoside glycosylase deficiency (HIM5)	*UNG*★
Mutations of the NF-κB pathway	*NEMO, IKKA*
Defect in toll-like receptor signaling	*IRAK4*
WHIM syndrome	*CXCR4*
X-linked lymphoproliferative syndrome	*SH2D1A*
Autoimmune polyglandular syndrome type 1	*AIRE*
CELLULAR IMMUNODEFICIENCIES	
Defects in the interferon-γ receptor and signal transduction	*IFNGR1, IFNGR2, STAT1*
Defects in interleukin-12/23 and receptors	*IL12B, IL12RB1*

★Strictly speaking, these are selective humoral immune defects (see text). They are listed here because of the common use of "HIM + number" abbreviations in the literature.
NF-κB, nuclear factor κB; WHIM, warts, hypogammaglobulinemia, infections, myelokathexis.

EBV positive. Atypical nonmalignant lymphoproliferation may also occur.[87]

Platelets are small, do not function normally, and are also cleared more rapidly and produced more slowly than normal (although the number of bone marrow megakaryocytes is normal or even increased).[85,86] In the appropriate clinical context, measurement of platelet size confirms the diagnosis. In normal individuals, platelet volume is 7.1 to 10.5 fL, with a diameter of 2.3 ± 0.12 µm, whereas platelets from patients with WAS have volumes ranging from 3.8 to 5.0 fL with diameters of 1.82 ± 0.12 µm. Small platelet size is occasionally seen in immune thrombocytopenias, but WAS can be distinguished by its other manifestations. However, immune thrombocytopenia may develop in as many as 20% of patients with WAS, either before or after splenectomy.

The only available cure for WAS is BMT.[88,89] Without BMT, survival beyond early childhood is uncommon. In general, BMT from a matched sibling donor is highly successful and considered the treatment of choice for WAS. To date, the results of BMT from an unmatched donor have been disappointing. Pretransplant morbidity and mortality may be reduced with regular infusions of IVIG, antibiotic prophylaxis, and blood component replacement.[85,86] Splenectomy often lessens the requirement for platelet transfusions, although immune thrombocytopenia may later supervene. Splenectomy alone increases the median survival in patients with WAS from 5 to 25 years.

The immune defects in WAS are variable.[85,86] Immune function may be normal in early infancy but gradually wanes. T-cell numbers may be decreased, and there may be inversion of the CD4/CD8 ratio. Cutaneous delayed hypersensitivity responses are often absent. T cells have diminished, but not absent responses to mitogens and antigens in vitro. T cells in WAS will also proliferate in response to nonspecific activating stimuli such as phorbol esters and calcium ionophores but show a striking absence of reactivity to antibodies directed against the CD3 complex of the TCR. The diversity of the T-cell repertoire appears normal throughout childhood, but it may become more restricted with consequent worsening immunodeficiency in adulthood.[90]

The level of IgM is diminished early in the course of the disease, whereas levels of IgG, IgA, and IgE may be elevated initially and then gradually decline. Isohemagglutinins and specific antibody responses are also elicited in young patients with WAS. This responsiveness likewise diminishes with time. Although the frequency of class-switched B cells (i.e., those not expressing IgM) appears to be normal, there are fewer memory B cells expressing CD27, thus indicating some alteration in B-cell activation in germinal centers that could underlie or contribute to the humoral immunodeficiency.[91]

The gene defective in WAS has been identified; its official name is *WAS* and its product is designated the WAS protein (WASP). One group recently studied descendants of the original patients reported by Dr. Wiskott to demonstrate the *WAS* mutation in this kindred.[92] The same gene is defective in the syndrome known as X-linked thrombocytopenia, as well as in X-linked congenital severe neutropenia.[85,86] WASP interacts with several intracellular partners, including the WASP-interacting protein (WIP), Rho family guanosine triphosphatases, and the Arp2/3 complex, which leads to reorganization of the actin cytoskeleton.[93] These processes recruit the additional internal and external membrane-associated molecules needed for full execution of the signaling programs after ligation of the TCR (and other receptors, such as NK receptors for HLA class I). Even though it is clear that WASP has direct and indirect relationships with various components of the cytoskeletal machinery, it also appears to have roles in activating nuclear factor of activated T cells (NF-AT) and nuclear factor κB (NF-κB) transcription factors after receptor engagement, independently of actin polymerization.[94] Although biochemical and cytoskeletal abnormalities have been observed in platelets, no clear defects in structure (other than size) or in function (e.g., aggregation) have been demonstrated.

The best clinical correlations with WASP mutation have come from careful analysis of WASP expression in lymphocytes with various *WAS* mutations.[95] This study has raised important challenges to assumptions regarding the consequences of genetic lesions for protein expression. In particular, missense mutations may lead to absence of protein rather than expression of mutant protein because of a failed stabilizing interaction with another partner. On the other hand, supposed null nonsense or frameshift *WAS* mutations may permit the expression of partially functional truncated forms of WASP. Splice site mutations may also lead to small amounts of normal protein or absence of protein. In general, the more severe phenotypes are associated with complete absence of protein and milder types with the presence of at least partially functioning protein. However, it is necessary to correlate the functional consequences of particular genetic lesions at the protein level directly rather than attempting to predict them.

WAS may be diagnosed in many patients by demonstration of the absence of WASP in Western blots of cytoplasmic lysates probed with specific antisera.[85,86] Intracellular flow cytometric analysis may yield the same finding. DNA-based methods may be used as well. Determination of maternal carrier status may also aid in diagnosis. Female carriers of WAS are generally asymptomatic and have normal platelet counts but show nonrandom X-chromosome inactivation in lymphocytes and granulocytes. One female with WAS has been reported; she is a carrier and her disease is expressed because of extreme nonrandom X-chromosome inactivation.[96] In a different consanguineous kindred, a female exhibited X-linked thrombocytopenia as a result of homozygous *WAS* mutations. Apparent spontaneous reversion of the WASP mutation has been observed in some populations of T cells in at least one patient.[97]

Ataxia-Telangiectasia

Ataxia-telangiectasia (AT) is an autosomal recessive disorder with an estimated incidence of 1 in 20,000 U.S. white births (95% confidence interval, 1 in 2,500 to 700,000).[98] AT is characterized by progressive cerebellar ataxia, oculocutaneous telangiectasia, and immunodeficiency.[99] Associated features are an increased incidence of lymphoma and sensitivity to radiation. Impairment in motor development may be noted early in the disease course and is progressive. Walking may be delayed until 16 to 18 months of age or later. Telangiectases of conjunctival and cutaneous vessels do not appear until children are 3 to 5 years of age. The cutaneous lesions are found mainly on the pinnae and in skin creases. Immunodeficiency will occur in approximately 70% of patients. Manifestation of the immunodeficiency is quite varied, but it is often seen as recurrent sinopulmonary bacterial infections. Growth retardation is a prominent feature in many patients and has been associated with decreases in insulin-like growth factor I and its binding protein; the mechanism is unknown.[100]

The median age at death in patients with AT is approximately 19 to 25 years.[101] Many patients die of progressive pulmonary disease caused by repeated infection. Possibly, noninfectious and ultimately fatal interstitial lung disease may also occur in approximately 25% of patients.[102] Beyond 10 years of age, the incidence of cancer in patients with AT is 1% per year; 85% of the cancers are acute leukemias or lymphomas.[103] Serum levels of oncofetoproteins such as α-fetoprotein and carcinoembryonic antigen are markedly elevated in about 95% of patients with AT.[99] In the appropriate clinical context, an elevated serum level of α-fetoprotein is diagnostic.

Numbers of circulating T and B cells are often normal. T cells bearing the γ-δ form of the TCR constitute up to 50% or more of the total number of T cells in patients with AT.[104] These cells make up only 1% to 5% of peripheral T cells in normal individuals. Cutaneous delayed hypersensitivity responses, as well as results of in vitro assays of T-cell function, are often depressed. Some suggest that T-cell dysfunction may not be as impaired as is often thought in this disease.[105] However, it is difficult to generalize from the small number (four) of patients studied in this report. Varying degrees of deficiency of particular antibody isotypes are common. IgA deficiency occurs in two thirds of patients. Decreased levels of IgG2, IgG4, and IgE are also common. Hypergammaglobulinemia occurs in about 40% of patients with AT.[106] It is usually of the IgM isotype, although elevated levels of IgG and IgA have also been observed. In about a fifth of these cases, the elevated Igs are oligoclonal or monoclonal. Impaired specific antibody responses, particularly to pneumococcal polysaccharide antigens, have also been noted in AT patients.[107]

The gene that is defective in AT is designated *ATM* (AT mutated).[99] ATM has critical roles in regulation of the cell cycle: it is involved in the detection of DNA damage and in the initiation of repair. There is a marked delay in induction of the tumor suppressors p53 and BRCA1 after exposure of AT cells to radiation. Even low-dose radiation leads to significantly greater DNA damage in AT fibroblasts and lymphoblasts than in normal individuals.[108]

Lymphocyte activation is linked to proliferation (i.e., induction of cell division), which also proceeds abnormally without functional ATM.[99] For example, defective activation of protein kinase C has been observed in T cells in AT, although the role of ATM here is not yet known. Lymphocytes of patients with AT also show a remarkable number of chromosomal translocations and inversions. These changes predominantly involve the loci that rearrange to generate mature Ig (2p12, 22q12, and 14q32) and TCR (7p15, 7q35, and 14q11) genes and reflect defective repair of the double-stranded breaks produced as part of the physiologic gene rearrangement process during lymphocyte development.

Whether pathologic changes result from the heterozygous carrier state of AT remains a subject of controversy. Carriers heterozygous for AT have none of the classic clinical manifestations of AT; however, the sensitivity of their DNA to radiation is increased, and they may have a higher incidence of malignancy. Several reports suggest that AT heterozygotes have an increased rate of a variety of malignancies, such as breast cancer.[109,110] Polymorphisms of AT may also affect the expression of malignancies such as lung cancer.[111]

The Nijmegen breakage syndrome is a disorder of chromosome fragility with autosomal recessive inheritance.[112] The phenotype is similar to that of AT and consists of growth retardation, microcephaly, immunodeficiency, sensitivity to radiation, and a high rate of lymphoma. The affected gene is called *NBS1*. Nibrin, its protein product, is another substrate of ATM in the cellular response to ionizing radiation. Absence of nibrin function leads to disruption of mechanisms of DNA repair, but it does not appear to result in abnormal function of cell cycle check points. Another similar syndrome called "AT-like disorder" results from mutations of the gene *MRE11*, which encodes another ATM substrate.[113] Polymorphisms of *MRE11* may be associated with the development of non-Hodgkin's lymphoma; however, this was not found for *NBS1*.[113]

DiGeorge's Syndrome

DiGeorge's syndrome (DGS) arises as a result of a failure of migration of neural crest cells into the third and fourth pharyngeal pouches. Patients display a characteristic facies, cardiac defects, parathyroid hormone deficiency, and varied immune defects.[114,115] The facies consists of hypertelorism, micrognathia, short philtrum, and low-set, posteriorly rotated ears with small pinnae. Cardiac defects are varied. Type B interrupted aortic arch is the most common and is associated with DGS in 50% of patients with this defect. Truncus arteriosus and other conotruncal anomalies are also common. Structural anomalies of the airways have likewise been found in some patients, as well as dysphagia secondary to laryngoesophageal dysmotility. The bilateral paired parathyroid glands are normally adherent to the thymus. Thus, these organs are affected together in this disease. The parathyroid deficiency is often more pronounced than the thymic defect; hypocalcemic tetany is one of the more common initial symptoms of DGS. Even small islands of ectopic thymus tissue permit the development of sufficient T cells for immune competence. Some degree of cognitive impairment is seen in many patients.

Partial and complete forms of DGS have been distinguished on the basis of clinical and immunologic characteristics.[114,115] In the complete form, the thymus is absent or weighs less than 1 g.[116] These patients have no or markedly decreased numbers of oligoclonal T cells that function poorly. B cells are present and their number may even be increased, but little if any antibody is produced. Complete DGS is usually fatal in early childhood; patients die of hypocalcemia, cardiac complications, infection, or a combination of these causes. However, rare patients may not exhibit hypocalcemia and dysmorphism, and their condition may be manifested as T$^-$B$^+$NK$^+$ SCID.[117] Though not seen as commonly as in SCID, engraftment of maternal T cells with a graft-versus-host reaction has also been reported.[118] In addition, patients may have features similar to those of OS.[116] In the largest series of patients with complete DGS reported (54 individuals), only half had a 22q11 deletion or structural heart disease, thus suggesting that there may be significant differences in the genetic makeup of the complete and partial forms.[116] An OS-like picture developed in a third of patients.

The occurrence of partial forms of DGS outnumbers that of the complete form by about 10:1. T-cell number and function in most patients are varied and presumably correlate with the amount of ectopic thymus tissue present. Immune function in patients with complete DGS does not improve; patients with partial DGS may have less immunodeficiency as they get older. In some cases the diagnosis has been made in adults being evaluated for hypoparathyroidism and hypocalcemia.[119] Most patients, despite having reduced numbers of T cells, have a normal or perhaps slightly diminished repertoire of expressed TCR V$_\beta$ genes and in vitro response to T-cell mitogens.[120,121] T-cell numbers are lowest in infancy and rise through the first years of life.[122] A relatively high prevalence (5% to 15%) of IgA deficiency has been reported.[123,124] Patients may also exhibit impaired responses to vaccine antigens (although this is not a consistent finding), as well as decreased peripheral memory (CD27$^+$) B cells.[123] Atopy, manifested as atopic dermatitis and asthma, may be increased in individuals with 22q11 deletion.[125]

Approximately 80% to 90% of patients with DGS have 2- to 3-megabase (Mb) deletions involving chromosome 22q11.2.[126] Deletions in the same region are found in patients with velocardiofacial syndrome and conotruncal anomaly–face syndrome and in some patients with isolated cardiac defects. There is heterogeneity in expression of the DGS phenotype, even in monozygotic twins. Approximately 40 genes are present in the deleted regions in DGS, and the contributions of each to the phenotype are only beginning to be understood.[127] TBX1 encodes a member of a family (T-box) of transcription factors. Mice that are heterozygous for deletion of this gene have a phenotype very similar to that of humans with DGS, including thymic and parathyroid hypoplasia, cardiac outflow tract abnormalities, and abnormal facial structure.[127] Point mutations in TBX1 have been found in six Japanese patients (four kindreds) with DGS or velocardiofacial syndrome.[128] Some patients with DGS have deletions on chromosome 10p.[129] Further genetic information relevant to DGS regarding this region does not yet exist. Additional genetic loci may also be responsible for the DGS phenotype. Thus far, major clinical distinctions between patients with and without 22q11 deletions have not been seen.

Most patients with partial DGS do not have significant difficulty with infections, and even live viral vaccines may be administered safely.[130-132] IVIG replacement or antibiotic prophylaxis may be helpful in patients with the more immunodeficient partial forms of DGS. Complete DGS has been treated very successfully by thymus transplantation, with 75% of the 44 most recent transplant recipients surviving up to 13 years.[116]

X-Linked Immunodeficiency with Normal or Elevated IgM

As its name implies, X-linked immunodeficiency with normal or elevated IgM (XHIM, also HIM1) denotes a form of selective hypogammaglobulinemia G and A, together with normal or elevated amounts of IgM. Approximately 200 patients have been described.[133] These patients are seen in the first 1 or 2 years of life with the recurrent bacterial infections often found in those with hypogammaglobulinemia, together with opportunistic infections by organisms such as P. jiroveci, Cryptosporidium, and Histoplasma. Affected patients are also prone to the development of neutropenia, anemia secondary to parvovirus, stomatitis, sclerosing cholangitis, and liver and hematologic malignancies. The number of circulating B cells is normal, but they express IgM exclusively (in association with IgD) on their surface. Immune responses are varied. Isohemagglutinins are often present, and vaccination may elicit specific IgM responses. No other isotypes are produced; there is no B-cell memory. Secondary lymphoid tissues are sparsely populated and do not contain germinal centers. Patients should be maintained on gamma globulin replacement therapy, as well as prophylaxis for P. jiroveci pneumonia. The disease is curable by BMT. Successful use of sequential liver transplantation and BMT has also been reported.[133,134]

The genetic lesion in XHIM is in TNFSF5 (tumor necrosis factor superfamily member 5), also known as

T-B Cell Interactions

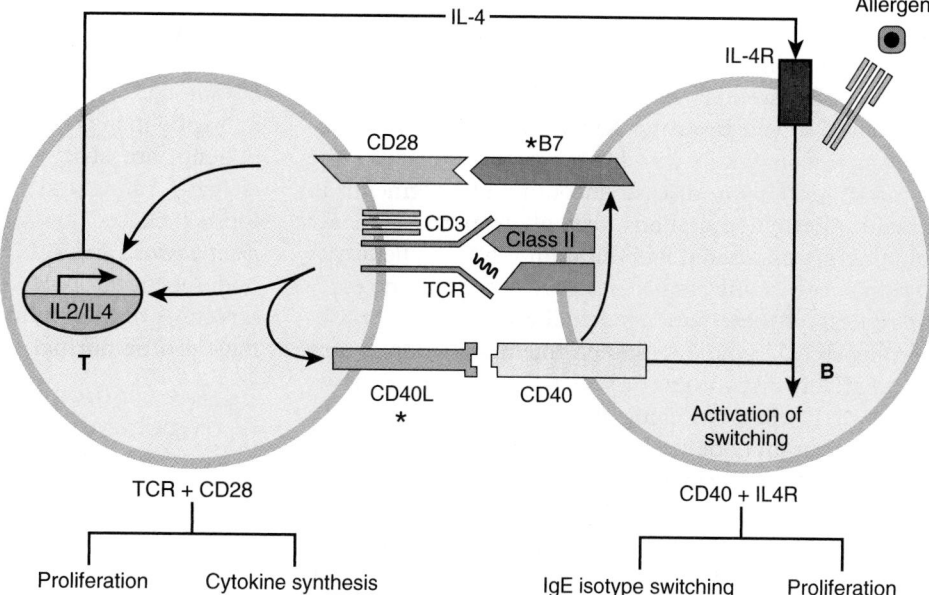

FIGURE 23-9. Signals required for T-cell activation by antigen-presenting cells, B-cell activation by the T cell, and B-cell immunoglobulin class switching. CD40L, CD40 ligand; IL-4R, interleukin-4 receptor; TCR, T-cell antigen receptor.

CD40 ligand (CD40L) and CD154.[133] This is an integral membrane protein that is mainly expressed on T cells after an activating stimulus, such as interaction of the TCR with an MHC-peptide complex on the surface of a B cell or APC (Fig. 23-9). The signal delivered via T-cell CD40L to CD40 is critical for Ig class switching (the production of isotypes other than IgM or IgD), the development of B-cell memory, affinity maturation of the antibody response (somatic hypermutation of Ig V regions), and the expression of important costimulatory molecules such as those of the B7 family by B cells and APCs (see Fig. 23-9).[135]

The CD40 system has additional roles in the interaction of T cells with monocytes. Several T-cell–derived cytokines (granulocyte-macrophage colony-stimulating factor, IL-3, and interferon-γ [IFN-γ]) induce the expression of CD40 on monocytes. Furthermore, engagement of monocyte CD40 induces cytokine synthesis and activates tumoricidal mechanisms.[136] These phenomena suggest an important interaction, the lack of which may underlie the predisposition to opportunistic infection and malignancy seen in patients with XHIM. One male patient has been described with a form of HIM associated with growth hormone deficiency.[137] Although the gene defect was not determined, it is most likely to have been the X-linked form because the association with growth hormone deficiency has been seen with other immunodeficiencies such as X-linked lymphoproliferative disease (XLPD) and XLA (see later).

Perhaps not too surprisingly, a clinically and immunologically identical immunodeficiency syndrome arises from mutations in the gene *TNFRSF5*, which encodes CD40.[138,139] Only a few patients with this defect have been found so far.

Other Forms of Hyperimmunoglobulin M Syndrome

Mutations in Activation-Induced Cytidine Deaminase and Uracil Nucleoside Glycosylase

Strictly speaking, activation-induced cytidine deaminase (AID) and uracil nucleoside glycosylase (UNG) deficiencies are best considered as humoral immunodeficiencies because these defects exclusively affect B-cell function and T-cell number and function are completely normal. They are included here because they have originally been defined in the medical literature as forms of hyper-IgM syndrome. They may be abbreviated as HIM2 (AID)[140-146] and HIM5 (UNG; see Table 23-3).[144,147,148] The AID and UNG enzymes are RNA modifiers expressed in B cells that act during class-switch recombination. In the absence of their activity, B cells cannot switch from production of IgM and IgD to production of downstream Ig isotypes (see Fig. 23-11). Somatic hypermutation is also affected. These processes occur normally during B-cell activation in germinal centers.

Another form of hyper-IgM syndrome with an unknown gene defect leads to impaired Ig class–switching recombination.[142,144,149] This has been called HIM4. All these disorders are very similar clinically and immunologically. Patients suffer mainly from respiratory tract bacterial infections and lymphadenopathy, and cellular immunodeficiency is not seen. IgG, IgA, and IgE are all low or absent; IgM levels tend to be higher than in the X-linked HIM syndrome. Patients tend to do well with IVIG replacement.

Mutations of the Nuclear Factor κB Pathway

NF-κB is a transcription factor that is critical for the activation of numerous genes upon leukocyte stimulation.[150] Activity of this factor is regulated by an inhibitor known as IκB. Phosphorylation of IκB by IκB kinase (IKK) liberates active NF-κB. IKK is composed of three subunits, α, β, and γ; the latter is also known as the NF-κB essential modulator (NEMO). The gene encoding NEMO is on the X chromosome. Null mutations are incompatible with life for males and lead to the X-linked dominant disease incontinentia pigmenti in females. Certain mutations that allow partial NEMO function are associated with an immunologic phenotype that may have some similarities to hyper-IgM. The earliest reports of these patients actually used the abbreviation hyper-IgM type 4, although this designation is now reserved for a syndrome associated with an unknown defect of Ig class switching (see earlier). Along with a combined immunodeficiency, these patients may exhibit hypohidrotic ectodermal dysplasia and lymphedema with osteopetrosis.[150-157]

Patients may suffer opportunistic-type disseminated viral infections and *P. jiroveci* pneumonia and are also highly susceptible to atypical mycobacterial infections. Most are hypogammaglobulinemic and have impaired vaccine responses (especially to polysaccharide antigens). In many patients, either elevated serum IgA or IgM may develop, but not both. Peripheral blood lymphocyte subsets and in vitro measures of lymphocyte function may be unremarkable or variably diminished; NK cell cytotoxicity may be impaired. Signaling via toll-like receptors (TLRs) is also affected. Therapy with gamma globulin and antibiotic prophylaxis is essential. Despite these measures, infections may still occur. A few patients have been successfully reconstituted by BMT,[158] but experience is limited.

A few patients have been found to have a similar phenotype as a result of a so-called hypermorphic (gain of function) function mutation of the IKK α chain.[150,152,159] In this situation, the IKK kinase is resistant to phosphorylation and cannot be dissociated, degraded, and induced to release NF-κB so that it may translocate to the nucleus to activate transcription.

Defects in Toll-Like Receptor Signaling

TLRs are a family of transmembrane molecules with a characteristic structure that bind to so-called pathogen-associated molecular patterns (PAMPs).[160,161] PAMPs are pathogenic microbial macromolecules consisting of repeating units such as lipoproteins, lipopolysaccharide, RNA, DNA, flagellin, and other constituents. TLRs are expressed variably by hematopoietic and other cell types; their ligation may promote the production of inflammatory cytokines such as tumor necrosis factor, IL-1β, IL-6, IL-8, and IL-12. Some TLRs also activate the production of type 1 (α and β) interferons by inducing the transcription factors interferon regulatory factors 3 and 7. TLRs influence many aspects of innate nonspecific inflammation, as well as the initiation and execution of adaptive immune responses. TLRs activate several signaling pathways, chief among them being the NF-κB pathway described earlier.

Recently, patients have been described with mutations of the interleukin-1 receptor–associated kinase 4 (IRAK-4).[150,162-166] Deficiency of this kinase impedes signaling by many of the TLRs and the IL-1 receptor. These patients are susceptible to severe infections (cellulitis, arthritis, meningitis, osteomyelitis, organ abscesses, and sepsis) caused by *Staphylococcus aureus*, *Streptococcus pneumoniae*, and other bacteria. Antibody responses to pneumococcal polysaccharides may be impaired, but screening tests of humoral and cellular immune function may also be normal.

The Syndrome of Warts, Hypogammaglobulinemia, Infections, and Myelokathexis

The WHIM (warts, hypogammaglobulinemia, infections, myelokathexis) syndrome is named for its major clinical manifestations.[167-172] This disorder is caused by defects in the chemokine receptor CXCR4. The chemokines are a large cytokine family that share a structural motif of conserved cysteine residues.[173,174] Many chemokines have important roles in activating leukocytes and directing homing or migration of cells in blood and lymph and in tissues in inflammation or immune responses. The infections usually seen in these patients are those most characteristic of hypogammaglobulinemia, generally respiratory tract bacterial infections. As the name suggests, verrucosis is also common and is indicative of an important component of impaired cellular immunity. One of the more common features of this disorder is myelokathexis, or retention of mature neutrophils in the bone marrow with resultant peripheral neutropenia. Although Ig levels are low, specific antibody formation may be normal. Gamma globulin replacement therapy generally reduces the rate of infection. There are no characteristic alterations in lymphocyte subsets, but in vitro (mitogen and antigen stimulation) and in vivo (cutaneous anergy) T-cell function may be impaired. Neutrophil counts are generally lower than 0.5×10^9 cells/L. Both granulocyte and granulocyte-macrophage colony-stimulating factors have been used to raise neutrophil counts.[175]

X-Linked Lymphoproliferative Disease

The "classic" manifestation of XLPD is fulminant, often fatal acute infectious mononucleosis secondary to EBV infection.[176] Additional clinical findings may include lymphoid necrosis, lymphoma, aplastic anemia, and pulmonary lymphoid granulomatosis with vasculitis. The diagnosis of XLPD is made in most patients before 10 years of age, but rare cases occur in adults.[177] Patients often have completely normal measures of humoral and cellular immune function; some may have impaired NK cell cytotoxicity.[178] Interestingly, NK T cells (NKT cells, or T cells that also express certain NK cell surface markers such as CD56) are absent in individuals with XLPD.[179]

NKT cells have important roles in regulating the immune response to infection, and their absence is likely to have a prominent role in the pathophysiology of the clinical manifestations of XLPD. Some patients show dysgammaglobulinemia with high levels of IgA or IgM and low levels of IgG1, IgG3, or both. A number of patients also have recurrent viral and bacterial infections. Some patients may have a clinical and laboratory phenotype consistent with common variable immunodeficiency (CVID).[180,181] One patient has been described with XLPD and growth hormone deficiency.[182] This association has previously been reported only with XLA (see later).

XLPD results from mutations in the gene encoding the SLAM (signaling lymphocyte activation molecule)-associated protein (SAP).[176] This molecule is also known as SH2D1A (SH2 [Src homology domain 2]-containing protein 1A).[183] SLAM is a member of the CD2 family of adhesion molecules that have roles in leukocyte-membrane interactions. SAP is also a member of a family of adapter proteins that link CD2 family members to downstream cytoplasmic signaling pathways. Another CD2 family member that signals through SAP is 2B4, a molecule important in triggering NK cell cytotoxicity. EBV-infected B cells express high levels of the 2B4 ligand CD48. Normal NK cells are activated by this interaction, whereas NK cells from patients with SAP mutations are strongly inhibited. The absence of the SAP interaction appears to lead to the constitutive association of 2B4 with the inhibitory tyrosine phosphatase SHP2.

Mononucleosis in XLPD can be treated with antiinflammatory and chemotherapeutic regimens; BMT may be curative. Recently, several patients with XLPD-associated hemophagocytic syndrome have been successfully treated with the monoclonal anti–B-cell antibody rituximab.[184] This therapy may be effective through the elimination of a large reservoir of EBV antigenic stimulus.

Autoimmune Polyglandular Syndrome Type 1

A heterogeneous group of disorders characterized by recurrent and severe skin and mucous membrane infections with *Candida albicans* are referred to as syndromes of chronic mucocutaneous candidiasis (CMC). In these individuals, cellular immunity to *Candida* is selectively impaired, whereas other aspects of cellular and humoral immunity are usually normal. Occasional patients exhibit more profound suppression of cellular immunity, variable defects such as a relative decrease in NK cells, or abnormalities in Igs, IgG subclasses, or specific antibody production.[185-187] The genetic defects in these patients have yet to be identified.

One particular form of CMC is autoimmune polyglandular syndrome type 1 (APS-1), also called autoimmune polyendocrinopathy–candidiasis–ectodermal dystrophy (APECED).[188-192]

In addition to *Candida* infection, patients with APS-1 have high levels of a variety of organ-specific autoanti-bodies (e.g., thyroid, ovary, testis, and adrenal gland), as well as non–organ-specific autoantibodies. The gene responsible for this disorder has been named autoimmune regulator (*AIRE*).[193] AIRE is a transcription factor expressed in thymic epithelium that directs the expression of an array of endocrine-related genes. When developing thymocytes that are specific for these antigens encounter them, they are deleted by a process of negative selection. In this way, the mature T-cell pool that leaves the thymus is depleted of cells with these self-reactivities. In the absence of functional AIRE, these clones are not deleted; they exit the thymus and are then activated when they encounter these antigens in endocrine tissues and cause autoimmune responses.

Hyperimmunoglobulin E Syndromes

The first or "classic" form of hyper-IgE syndrome (HIES) described, which has also been known by the eponym "Job's syndrome," consists of severe sinopulmonary bacterial infections, severe skin superinfections with *S. aureus* on a chronic eczematous eruption, and susceptibility to *Aspergillus fumigatus* pneumonitis with pneumatocele formation.[194-196] Inheritance is autosomal dominant; the defective gene has not yet been identified. Additional manifestations include asymmetric or coarse facial features, delayed shedding of primary teeth, bone fragility and fractures, scoliosis, and keratoconjunctivitis. *P. jiroveci* infection may complicate some cases,[197] and malignancies such as Hodgkin's lymphoma and T-cell lymphoma have been reported as well.[198,199] A few patients have also recently been reported to have associated cardiovascular anomalies such as patent ductus venosus,[200] thoracic aortic aneurysm,[201] and coronary artery aneurysms.[202] The major immunologic findings are elevated serum levels of IgE (3000 to >50,000 IU/mL) and, occasionally, impaired neutrophil chemotaxis (some classify HIES among the neutrophil disorders). Additional features include eosinophilia and the presence of *Staphylococcus*-binding IgE in serum. Note that these two findings are often likewise seen in patients with severe atopic dermatitis. Some patients with HIES also show evidence of reduced T-cell function in vitro. In particular, the lymphocyte response to IL-12 is abnormal, and IFN-γ production is reduced. The diagnosis is established on clinical and laboratory grounds; a scoring system has been developed that may be helpful.[203] Management of autosomal dominant HIES is mainly by prevention and treatment of infectious complications. One patient was treated with BMT and exhibited successful donor engraftment with resolution of disease, only to later suffer a relapse.[204] Other patients have been treated with interferon gamma or intravenous gamma globulin infusions. Neither of these therapies has been shown to have consistent benefit for patients.[205-208] Chronic molluscum contagiosum in one patient was successfully treated with systemic interferon alfa.[209]

At least one autosomal recessive form of HIES has also been characterized clinically; the gene defect is unknown, however.[194,210] This form of HIES has many similarities with the autosomal dominant form described earlier. Patients with the recessive type do not have skeletal or dental abnormalities, and pneumatoceles do not develop. This group of patients has the additional feature of autoimmune vasculopathy with central nervous system involvement.

A single patient with an autosomal recessive deficiency of the Tyk2 kinase and a phenotype similar to HIES has been reported.[211,212] It may be distinct from that just described, but this is not yet known. The patient with Tyk2 deficiency had recurrent respiratory tract and skin bacterial infections, molluscum contagiosum, oral thrush, cutaneous herpes simplex, and BCG infection. He had severe eczematous dermatitis and an IgE level of 2100 U/mL. Lymphocyte populations were normal. The Tyk2 kinase is required for signaling of receptors for IFN-α/β, IL-6, IL-10, IL-12, and IL-23.

CELLULAR IMMUNODEFICIENCY

Defects of the Interferon-γ/Interleukin-12/23 Pathway

IL-12 is a monocyte/macrophage product that is the principal stimulus for IFN-γ production by NK cells. Mononuclear cells rely on IFN-γ for activation of full microbicidal capacity for intracellular killing. Patients with defective response to IFN-γ have exquisite susceptibility to mycobacterial infection, especially atypical species.[213-216] Other types of infections may also occur, such as disseminated histoplasmosis.[217] The genetic lesions described include both chains of the IFN-γ receptor (*IFNGR1*, *IFNGR2*) and the gene encoding the STAT1 (signal transducer and activator of transcription 1) signaling molecule. Defects of *IFNGR1* include a "complete" (absent function) autosomal recessive form, as well as "partial" (partial function) autosomal dominant and recessive forms.[215,218] In at least one patient with a partial recessive form, disseminated *Mycobacterium avium-intracellulare* infection was diagnosed in adulthood after previously being healthy.[218] Patients with defects in the IL-12/23 pathway appear to have greater susceptibility to severe infections with *Salmonella* species.[213,214,219-222] These defects include the gene encoding the IL-12 receptor β₁ chain (*IL12RB1*), which is shared by the receptors for IL-12 and IL-23, as well as the gene encoding the IL-12 p40 subunit, which is also shared by IL-23. A similar patient with an IL-12 signaling defect and unknown genetic lesion has also been reported.[223] Most patients with these defects in IFN-γ and IL-12/23 signaling have normal lymphocyte subsets and in vitro T-cell responses to mitogens and antigens, together with normal Ig levels and antibody responses. These disorders are curable by BMT.[224] The phenotypes of patients with these genetic defects underscore the importance of these

pathways for the control of infections with microbes that replicate intracellularly.

SYNDROMIC IMMUNODEFICIENCY

The term syndromic immunodeficiency has been coined to describe the occurrence of a component of immune compromise and susceptibility to infection or malignancy (or both) in the setting of a genetically determined disorder with characteristic features of altered development or function of other organ systems or the body as a whole. Included are syndromes of large-scale chromosomal anomalies (monosomies, trisomies, translocations, etc.), as well as monogenic disorders of metabolism or other maldevelopment, in addition to "acquired" congenital diseases secondary to teratogen exposure. Space does not permit even a cursory description of the tremendous variety of syndromes that have been consistently or occasionally associated with immunodeficiency. Interested readers are referred to an excellent recent review.[225]

HUMORAL IMMUNODEFICIENCY

The humoral immunodeficiencies and their associated gene defects are listed in Table 23-4. These disorders are characterized by relative deficiency of antibody responses to various forms of antigenic challenge.[2,3] Cellular immunity is generally intact. Humoral immunodeficiency is most commonly manifested as recurrent bacterial infections of the upper and lower respiratory tract. Pyogenic skin infections, as well as meningitis, osteomyelitis, and other foci of infection, are also seen frequently. These infections are generally caused by the same organisms

TABLE 23-4	Humoral Immunodeficiencies and Associated Gene Defects	
Syndrome	**Gene**
The agammaglobulinemias	
X-linked (Bruton's)	*BTK*
IgM heavy-chain deficiency	*IGHM*
Surrogate light-chain deficiency	*IGLL1*
Ig-α deficiency	*IGA**
B-cell linker protein deficiency	*BLNK*
Leucine-rich repeat–containing 8 defect (hemizygous)	*LRRC8*
Common variable immunodeficiency	*ICOS*, *TACI*,[†] *CD19*
Selective IgA deficiency	Undefined
IgG subclass deficiency	Undefined
Specific antibody deficiency	Undefined
Transient hypogammaglobulinemia of infancy	Undefined

*Note that this is the gene designation for the Ig-α signal-transducing component of the B-cell antigen receptor. The designation for the gene encoding the immunoglobulin A (IgA) heavy chain is *IGHA*.
[†]A role for *TACI* mutation in common variable immunodeficiency has not yet been conclusively established.

that are virulent in immunocompetent hosts—predominantly encapsulated bacteria such as *S. pneumoniae*, *Haemophilus influenzae*, *S. aureus*, and *Neisseria meningitidis*. Viral infections usually resolve normally in these patients, although a higher rate of recurrence with the same agent may be seen because there is no production of neutralizing antibodies or B-cell memory. The results of physical examination are not specific and show only the presence or sequelae of microbial infections. A relative paucity of peripheral lymphoid tissue may be noted in some patients, especially areas rich in B cells (e.g., tonsils). Studies of peripheral blood lymphocyte subsets are often normal; the number of B cells may be reduced in certain syndromes.

The amounts of one or more antibody isotypes are reduced in many of these diseases.[2,3] The severity of the phenotype often correlates with the degree of hypogammaglobulinemia. The predisposition that patients have to particular types of infections may also depend on the affected isotypes (see later). Antibody titers to specific antigens may be measured before or after immunization. The specific antibodies most commonly assayed for protein antigens are tetanus toxoid and the capsular polysaccharide (polyribosylribitol phosphate) of *H. influenzae* type B (HiB). With respect to polysaccharide antigens, measurement of antibodies to pneumococcal serotypes is frequently undertaken. If a child has had a particular illness (e.g., varicella), a specific viral antibody titer may be useful. Note that the HiB vaccines and newer pneumococcal vaccines (e.g., Prevnar) currently in use for primary immunization in children are protein conjugates. Thus, measuring a polyribosylribitol phosphate or pneumococcal titer in children who have received these vaccines does not necessarily reflect a polysaccharide antibody response. The adequacy of carbohydrate responses may be tested by challenge with 23-valent pneumococcal polysaccharide vaccines (e.g., Pneumovax or Pnu-Imune) or meningococcal vaccines. In children who are not fully immunized, isohemagglutinins may be measured.

A high index of suspicion for antibody deficiency should be maintained in patients with recurrent, refractory, or severe infections.[2,3] One study in the United Kingdom of the delay in diagnosis of primary antibody deficiency found that the median delay was 2 years (mean, 4.4 years) after the onset of symptoms, even after the introduction of a set of national guidelines intended to reduce this delay.[226]

The mainstay of therapy for significantly impaired ability to produce antibody is gamma globulin replacement.[2,227] As has already been mentioned several times earlier, this therapy is also important for the treatment of any combined immunodeficiency in which defective antibody production may occur. In most countries, gamma globulin replacement is administered predominantly via the intravenous route every 3 to 4 weeks. However, IgG can also be administered by subcutaneous infusion.[228-231] Smaller doses are given weekly or twice weekly. Intravenous infusion is generally well tolerated but requires intravenous access and is associated with frequent mild (10% to 20% of patients) or moderate (5%) side effects. Subcutaneous infusions may be administered by patients themselves at their own convenience with a much lower rate of systemic effects at the cost of generally mild and transient (24-hour) local irritation. The general efficacy of intravenous versus subcutaneous administration appears to be equivalent. It is likely that subcutaneous infusions will become increasingly popular.

The Agammaglobulinemias

X-Linked Agammaglobulinemia

XLA is also known as "Bruton's agammaglobulinemia" because Bruton provided the classic description of the disease in 1952.[232] Affected males are often asymptomatic during the first months of life while they are protected by transplacentally acquired maternal antibodies. These antibodies fall to low levels by 6 to 9 months of age, and patients begin to experience recurrent bacterial infections.[233,234] Physical examination at any age often reveals a striking absence of tonsils and palpable lymphoid tissue. Serum Ig is absent or the level is extremely low; in addition, no B cells are found or their numbers are extremely low. Cellular immunity is completely intact. However, these patients are prone to the development of chronic enteroviral meningoencephalitis and vaccine-associated paralytic poliomyelitis, which suggests an important role for humoral immunity in the control of these infections. Moreover, patients may have arthropathy resembling rheumatic disease, which may be due to infection with *Mycoplasma* or *Ureaplasma* organisms. Other opportunistic infections such as *P. jiroveci* pneumonia are seen only rarely.[235]

XLA is another example of an immunodeficiency caused by a defect in a signal transduction molecule. In fact, this protein tyrosine kinase is now known as Bruton's tyrosine kinase (Btk, Fig. 23-10).[233,236] It is expressed in B cells at all stages of development, as well as in cell lines derived from monocytes, macrophages, mast cells, and erythroid cells. A variety of *BTK* gene defects such as point mutations, deletions, and insertions have been described in patients with XLA.[236-239] In most patients, B-cell development is impeded at an early stage (the pro-B-cell–pre-B-cell transition).

BTK mutations account for approximately 85% of all cases of agammaglobulinemia.[233] *BTK* mutations have also been described in patients with "atypical" XLA who have low numbers of B cells and low-level antibody production.[240,241] In some patients with atypical XLA, CVID was misdiagnosed (see later) before discovery of the Btk defect.[242] In general, *BTK* mutations that permit the expression of small amounts of functional or partially functional Btk protein are associated with milder clinical phenotypes and slightly higher numbers of B cells in the circulation.[233,236-239] However, even siblings with identical

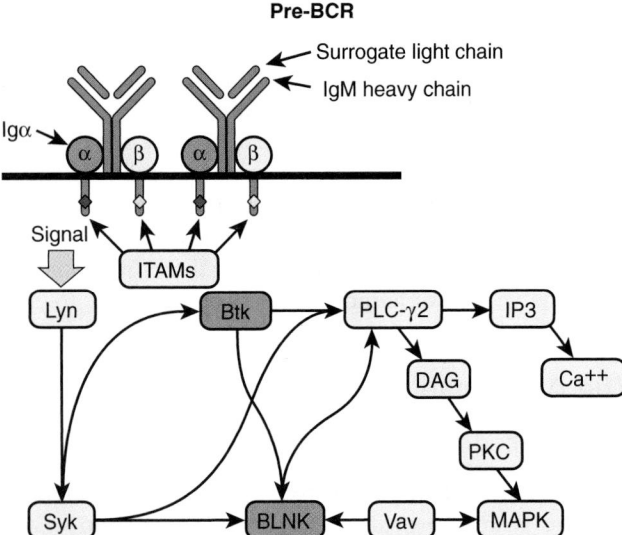

Pre-BCR

FIGURE 23-10. Signaling via the pre–B-cell receptor (Pre-BCR). The Pre-BCR is composed of an IgM heavy chain with a surrogate light-chain heterodimer (VpreB + λ5), along with a signaling heterodimer of Igα + Igβ. The immunoreceptor tyrosine-based activating motifs (ITAMs) (see Fig. 23-6) recruit tyrosine kinases (Lyn, Syk, Btk) that initiate downstream signaling. The adapter proteins BLNK and Vav recruit additional signaling intermediates. DAG, diacylglycerol; IP3, inositol triphosphate; PKC, protein kinase C; PLC, phospholipase C; MAPK, mitogen-activated protein kinase. Defects in components shown in blue lead to agammaglobulinemia by blocking pre-BCR signaling and interrupting B-cell development.

mutations may show quite divergent phenotypes. Female carriers of XLA show nonrandom X-chromosome inactivation in their B cells.[243]

Patients with XLA were the first to receive human gamma globulin therapy. The effect of intramuscular injections of gamma globulin was prompt and dramatic, with a reduction in the occurrence of infections. A retrospective study of bacterial infections in patients with XLA showed a reduction in incidence from 0.4 to 0.06 per patient per year with IVIG therapy.[244] Some viral infections, including enteroviral meningoencephalitis, occurred in patients while they were receiving IVIG. At present, administration of IVIG provides these patients with an almost normal lifestyle.[245]

A very small number of patients have been described with a distinct syndrome of XLA and growth hormone deficiency.[246-248] The clinical manifestation is similar to that of XLA described earlier, with the added feature of low growth hormone levels. In one patient a possible mutation in the transcription factor myeloid Elf-like 1 has been suggested but not clearly established.[246]

Autosomal Recessive Agammaglobulinemias

Female patients with agammaglobulinemia and no B cells and males with a similar phenotype lacking *BTK* mutations have been described. These patients have forms of agammaglobulinemia with autosomal recessive inheritance that result from several distinct molecular defects,[233] including mutations of the Ig μ heavy-chain

locus, which prevents formation of the IgM heavy chain required for formation of the Ig receptors on pre-B cells and mature B cells (see Fig. 23-10). Defects of λ5 (surrogate light chain) prevent formation of the pre-B-cell Ig receptor required for B-cell development. Igα (CD79a) is a transmembrane molecule required for signal transduction via the pre-B-cell and mature B-cell Ig receptors. Lesions in this gene prevent Ig receptor signaling and B-cell development. Defects in the signal transduction adapter protein BLNK (B-cell linker protein) have also been found; absence of BLNK function prevents signaling after ligation of the B-cell receptor. All these mutations arrest B-cell development at early stages in bone marrow.

One patient has been described with an apparent dominantly expressed translocation abrogating the function of the *LRRC8* (leucine-rich repeat–containing 8) gene.[249-251] The function of the LRRC8 protein is not yet known; it is a member of a growing family of proteins of unknown function called the LRRC8 family, within the much larger and very diverse superfamily of leucine-rich repeat proteins. The female patient has agammaglobulinemia with arrest of B-cell development in bone marrow.

Other Predominantly Antibody Deficiency Syndromes

Common Variable Immunodeficiency

The diagnostic label of CVID encompasses an unknown number of conditions that are genetically and etiologically distinct but have in common late-onset humoral immunodeficiency, most often in the first or third decades of life.[252,253] Hypogammaglobulinemia and impaired specific antibody production are universal by definition. Patients with CVID resemble individuals with XLA (and other humoral immunodeficiencies) because they also have recurrent sinopulmonary bacterial infections. Chronic enteroviral infections, including meningoencephalitis, may also be seen in CVID. A form of granulocytic/lymphocytic interstitial lung disease occurs in a subset of patients and has been linked to human herpesvirus 8 infection.[254] Additional manifestations include asthma, chronic rhinitis, chronic giardiasis, and recurrent or chronic arthropathy. The apparent "atopic" symptoms occur in the absence of allergen-specific IgE. Malabsorptive inflammatory bowel disease may occur. A broad spectrum of autoimmune diseases may be associated, including a variety of cytopenias, arthritides, and vasculitides.[255,256] Noncaseating granulomatous disease resembling sarcoidosis may be encountered in the skin or viscera. It often responds well to steroid therapy.[257,258] Widespread lymphoproliferation may cause splenomegaly, adenopathy, and intestinal lymphonodular hyperplasia. Patients with CVID also have a higher incidence of gastrointestinal and lymphoid malignancies. The relative risk for lymphoma has been estimated to be as much as 30- to 400-fold greater than that in the general population.[259]

Deficiency of IgA is very common in CVID.[253] IgM is also frequently affected; the pattern varies from one individual to another. The levels of particular isotypes in any patient are often static over time, but fluctuations may occur. B cells appear to be normal in many patients and produce antibody on stimulation in vitro, whereas others may have low numbers of poorly functional B cells. A reduction of the ratio of CD4⁺ to CD8⁺ T cells is common. A plethora of additional immunologic abnormalities have been reported in at least a fraction of patients with CVID. There are no single unifying immunologic features beyond those that are used to build the clinical definition. It is not useful to discuss most of these in detail here because their relationship to the pathogenesis of the disorder is not known. "Abnormalities" reported include altered thymic development,[260] cytokine production,[261-265] surface marker expression,[265-269] signal transduction,[270] and apoptosis[271] of T cells; altered surface marker expression on B cells[269,272]; altered development of plasma cells[273]; altered cytokine production by monocytes[264]; defective maturation,[274] altered distribution,[275] and altered cytokine production[276,277] of dendritic cells; and impaired signaling via TLR9.[278] Some authors have suggested that nutritional or biochemical imbalances such as vitamin A deficiency[279] or hypoleptinemia and insulin resistance[280,281] may even contribute to the immunodeficiency of CVID.

Memory B-cell subpopulations may be useful diagnostic and potentially prognostic markers in CVID.[282-285] Memory B cells express the CD27 (TNFRSF7) molecule. Naïve B cells express IgM and IgD. So-called unswitched memory B cells express IgM, some IgD, and CD27. After class switching in germinal centers, B cells cease expressing IgM and IgD, as well as "downstream" Ig isotypes such as IgG, IgA, and IgE (Fig. 23-11). Memory B cells after class switching ("switched" memory B cells) are CD27⁺ and IgM⁻IgD⁻. Some authors have devised classification schemes for CVID patients based on these markers (low switched memory B cells, in particular) that correlate at least partially with clinical characteristics (Table 23-5).[284-286] At least one study suggests that the number of memory B cells correlates better with infection, lymphoproliferation, and autoimmunity than serum Ig levels or specific antibody responses do.[287] Other authors have reported that low levels of unswitched (IgM) memory B cells correlate with impaired pneumococcal polysaccharide antibody responses and with chronic lung disease and bronchiectasis in CVID.[288] Classifications of CVID based on memory B-cell phenotypes are summarized in Table 23-5.

Most patients with CVID should be treated with IVIG infusions.[289] Antibiotic prophylaxis may also be required. Therapy for autoimmune or inflammatory complications in CVID generally follows regimens

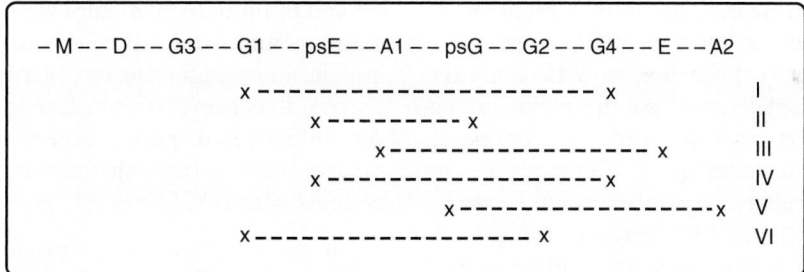

FIGURE 23-11. Immunoglobulin heavy-chain gene deletion haplotypes. The *top line* shows the order of the immunoglobulin constant region genes (e.g., M = IgM, etc.). The letters "ps" designate a pseudogene that is not expressed; numbers indicate subclasses. Six haplotypes have been defined (roman numerals). In each haplotype, the entire region indicated by the X's is missing. *(Data from Lefranc MP, Hammarstrom L, Smith CI, Lefranc G. Gene deletions in the human immunoglobulin heavy chain constant region locus: molecular and immunological analysis. Immunodefic Rev. 1991;2:265-281.)*

TABLE 23-5	**Classification of Common Variable Immunodeficiency Based on Memory B-Cell Phenotype**						
Memory B-Cell Phenotype	**CLASSIFICATION SCHEME**		**CLINICAL FEATURE/COMPLICATION**				
	Piqueras et al.[285]	Warnatz et al.[286]	SM/LPD	GR	AI	Ig	Vac. Ab
↓ Mem (CD27⁺)	MB0		↑	↑	+		
↓ Sw Mem (IgM⁻IgD⁻CD27⁺)	MB1	Group Ia (↓ CD21)	↑	↑	+	↓↓	↓↓
		Group Ib (NL CD21)		↑	+	↓↓	↓↓
NL Mem.	MB2	Group II			+	↓	↓

AI, autoimmunity; GR, granulomas; Ig, serum immunoglobulin level; Mem, memory; SM/LPD, splenomegaly/lymphoproliferative disease; NL, normal; Sw Mem, switched memory; Vac. Ab, vaccine-specific antibody responses; ↑, increased; ↓, decreased; +, present.

applied in similar situations in the absence of the immunodeficiency.[255,256,290-294] However, patients with CVID are even more at risk for infectious complications from such immunomodulation or immunosuppression.

The genetic heterogeneity of CVID is beginning to yield to molecular biologic analysis. Several single-gene defects have been found in varying (small) proportions of patients with CVID and are described in more detail later. It may also occur that individuals classified as having CVID (or a phenotype consistent with CVID) on clinical and laboratory grounds may be found to have mutations in genes characteristically associated with other primary immunodeficiencies. Such has been the case with some individuals with mutations in *BTK* (XLA),[242,295] *SH2D1A* (XLPD),[181] and *TNFSF5* (XHIM).[296]

Among the majority of CVID patients and in IgA deficiency, where immunologically relevant point mutations are still generally unknown, there is evidence for linkage to loci within the HLA complex on chromosome 6.[297-299] Both syndromes tend to occur in families, and it is possible for IgA deficiency to sometimes evolve into CVID. Some families have pedigrees that suggest an autosomal dominant pattern of inheritance. Study of one large kindred indicated linkage to a region of chromosome 4q.[300] Candidate genes in these regions are yet to be identified.

Deficiency of Inducible T-Cell Costimulator

The inducible T-cell costimulator (ICOS) is expressed on T cells after stimulation. It interacts with a member of the B7 family of molecules known as ICOS ligand. A total of nine patients have been found to have CVID associated with ICOS deficiency.[301] All these individuals have the same founder mutation and have ancestral origins in the Black Forest region of Germany. These patients may manifest recurrent respiratory and gastrointestinal infections in adulthood, panhypogammaglobulinemia and impaired vaccine responses, autoimmune disease (neutropenia), lymphoproliferation, and cancer (carcinoma of the vulva). Lymphoid tissues exhibit poorly formed germinal centers, and circulating switched memory B cells are markedly reduced.[302] To date, mutations of ICOS ligand have not been found in CVID patients.

Deficiency of Transmembrane Activator and Calcium Modulator and Cyclophilin Ligand Interactor

Defects of the transmembrane activator and calcium modulator and cyclophilin ligand interactor (TACI; official designation, TNFRSF13B) have been associated with CVID in approximately 10% of patients studied to date.[303-306] However, its pathogenic role is not yet clear. Some patients are homozygous or compound heterozygous for *TACI* mutations, whereas other patients are hemizygous. Furthermore, "deleterious" *TACI* mutations occur at a rate of 1% in the general population. It is possible that

other genes modify expression of *TACI* mutations or that *TACI* mutations predispose to pathology triggered by other infectious or environmental exposure (or both). To date, mutations in either of the TACI ligands α-proliferation–inducing ligand (APRIL; TNFSF13) and B-cell–activating factor (BAFF; TNFSF13B) have not been found in any CVID patients.[305-307]

TACI is expressed on B cells and interacts with the ligands BAFF and APRIL expressed on macrophages and dendritic cells. These interactions have important roles in B-cell activation and Ig class switching. CVID patients with *TACI* mutations have recurrent infections, autoimmunity (cytopenia, positive antinuclear antibody), lymphoproliferation and lymphoma, low IgG with or without low IgA, poor responses to vaccines (particularly pneumococcal polysaccharides), low B-cell number, and low switched memory B cells.

CD19 Deficiency

CD19 is expressed on B cells and is a component of a receptor complex that contains CD21, a receptor for the complement fragment C3dg (it is also called complement receptor 2, and it is the receptor for EBV). Simultaneous cross-linking of CD21 and the B-cell Ig receptor lowers the threshold for B-cell activation. Four patients in two kindreds have been found to have mutations in CD19.[308] They exhibit recurrent infections, hypogammaglobulinemia, and low levels of switched memory B cells.

The occurrence of thymoma in the context of a clinical and immunologic picture very similar to that of CVID with low numbers of B cells and generally more severely impaired T-cell function has been designated Good's syndrome. It is not clear whether these patients exhibit as yet undiscovered specific genetic or immunologic abnormalities that distinguish them from the larger group of patients with CVID.

Immunoglobulin A Deficiency

There are two subclasses of human IgA: IgA1 and IgA2. They are encoded by separate genes on the heavy-chain C region locus on chromosome 14 (see Fig. 23-11). IgA1 predominates in serum (80% to 90%), whereas IgA1 and IgA2 are equally prevalent in secretions. Both subclasses are equally affected in IgA deficiency (IGAD). Selective IGAD is defined as a serum IgA level of less than 0.07 g/L with normal serum IgG and IgM in a child older than 4 years of age in whom other causes of hypogammaglobulinemia have been excluded.[2] Note that this definition is restricted to the absence of serum IgA. There is no known clinical association with IgA levels between the lower limit of detection and the lower limit of the normal range. It is not appropriate to refer to patients with these nonzero low IgA values as being IgA deficient.

Failure to produce normal levels of IgA is seen in about 1 in 700 white individuals.[309] In contrast, its incidence among Japanese is only 1 in 18,500.[310] This presumably reflects population genetic differences, possibly related to the HLA complex. IGAD has been associated with extended HLA haplotypes similar to those observed in CVID.[298,299] The majority of individuals with IGAD are completely asymptomatic. Some may have a clinical course similar to that seen in CVID or in IgG subclass deficiency (see later). The proportion of patients with IGAD is increased in a population of people with chronic lung disease, and 20 years of observation of blood donors with IGAD has documented an increased incidence of respiratory infections and autoimmune disease.[311]

IGAD is also associated with an increased incidence of autoimmune syndromes, as with CVID.[312] In addition, atopic diseases appear to be more prevalent among those with IGAD, and some have noted an increased incidence of the type of malignancies encountered in CVID. In rare patients IGAD has evolved into CVID or levels of IgA have increased over time.[313,314] Treatment of IGAD has generally focused on management of complications as they occur. In some instances, gamma globulin infusions may be helpful, especially if an associated IgG subclass or specific antibody deficiency is present (see later). However, one study did not find an association between a history of infections and lower antibody responses to pneumococcal polysaccharides.[315] Some studies do show an association of increased infections if there is an IgG subclass deficiency or mannose-binding lectin (MBL) deficiency together with IGAD.[316]

Molecular genetic defects have not been described in IGAD. Lesions in IgA C region genes are not found, except in rare instances associated with other deletions (see later). IGAD and CVID have been associated with the HLA haplotype A1, B8, DR3 in whites.[299,317] An IGAD susceptibility locus (IGAD1) has been mapped to the boundary region between HLA class II and class III.[318-320] A more detailed analysis identified a positive association of IGAD with HLA-DRB1*0301, DQB1*02 and a negative association with DRB1*1501, DQB1*0602. Another study identified an association of IGAD with DRB1*0102, DQB1*0501.[321] The significance of these associations requires clarification.

IGAD may occur as a drug side effect, as has been reported with phenytoin, carbamazepine, valproic acid, zonisamide, sulfasalazine, gold, penicillamine, hydroxychloroquine, and nonsteroidal anti-inflammatory drugs.[322] The IgA level may normalize after cessation of use of the drug.

Immunoglobulin G Subclass Deficiency

Four subclasses of IgG exist in humans: IgG1, IgG2, IgG3, and IgG4. Their designations order their prevalence in serum, with each constituting roughly 67%, 23%, 7%, and 3% of the total, respectively. A different gene encodes the heavy-chain constant region of each subclass (see Fig. 23-11). Each subclass has unique structural properties and probably plays a different role in immune responses as a result of different interactions with the complement system and with receptors for IgG on phagocytic cells and lymphocytes. In addition, IgG

subclasses are produced in different relative amounts depending on the antigenic stimulus.[323] Mainly IgG1 is produced in response to soluble protein antigens. Viral antigens also elicit predominantly IgG1 responses and often significant amounts of IgG3 as well. Particular viruses (e.g., hepatitis, herpes simplex, and varicella) also elicit IgG4. The pneumococcal capsular polysaccharide response is almost exclusively of the IgG2 subclass, whereas HIB polysaccharide elicits mainly IgG2, with some IgG1 (the latter is found in younger children particularly). Note that the current HIB and new pneumococcal (Prevnar) vaccines are protein conjugates and elicit responses characteristic of protein antigens.

IgG subclass deficiency is defined as the relative lack of one or more IgG subclasses with a normal total level of IgG. If the level of total IgG is low, the diagnosis should usually be CVID.[2] Precise criteria for diagnosis are difficult to establish because of variability in Ig measurements by various techniques (e.g., nephelometry and radial immunodiffusion) and the wide variability in normal ranges with respect to age and ethnicity. The significance of decreased levels of IgG subclasses in patients with recurrent infections is further clouded by the fact that the majority of individuals with isolated subclass deficiencies are asymptomatic (see later). Assessing the response to antigen challenge is the most important element in evaluation of these patients. Most children have been immunized with tetanus toxoid and HIB, and antibody titers may be determined at the first visit. If titers are low, response to booster immunization may be assessed. Patients may also be immunized with 23-valent pneumococcal or meningococcal vaccines for rigorous assessment of polysaccharide responses. However, the latter vaccines produce unreliable results in normal children younger than 2 years, and negative responses in these patients should be interpreted with caution. Assessment of memory B-cell subsets may become a useful diagnostic tool; one study suggests that reduced switched memory B cells have better a correlation with risk for infection than antibody responses do.[287]

Patients with IgG subclass deficiency are commonly seen with recurrent sinopulmonary infections of varying severity caused by common respiratory bacterial pathogens.[324] Some may also have recurrent diarrhea, often of infectious origin. Furthermore, atopic diseases such as asthma and allergic rhinitis are more prevalent in patients with IgG subclass deficiency. Deficiency of the IgG2 subclass is detected most commonly in symptomatic patients. It may occur in isolation but is also usually associated with deficiency of IgG4, IgA, or both.[315,325,326] Selective deficiency of IgG3 alone is likewise observed (most often in adult females) and is associated with the same clinical picture described earlier.[325,327] The lowest IgG4 levels are usually associated with IgG2 deficiency. Recurrent infections have been described in some patients with only IgG4 deficiency.[328]

The C region genes determining antibody classes and subclasses are arranged in the same transcriptional orientation on chromosome 14 (see Fig. 23-11). As with IGAD, only rarely is clinically significant IgG subclass deficiency associated with genetic lesions of IgG C region genes. This has been observed in a single reported patient with IgG2 deficiency, in whom mutation prevented expression of cell surface IgG2.[329] In fact, large deletions of Ig C region genes are surprisingly common; six multigene deletion haplotypes have been identified (see Fig. 23-11).[330] In one population with a high degree of consanguinity, individuals were found to be homozygous for one haplotype or heterozygous for two different haplotypes. Fifteen of 16 people with deletions on both chromosomes were entirely healthy despite a complete lack of one or more IgG subclasses or IgA1; one person had recurrent infections. Similarly, two healthy siblings have been described, each having homozygous deletions of IgA1, IgG2, IgG4, and IgE.[331] Furthermore, an analysis of the Ig heavy-chain loci of 33 patients with CVID revealed only 2 patients who were heterozygous for C gene deletions.[332]

Specific Antibody Deficiency with Normal Immunoglobulins

A population of patients with recurrent infections and poor antibody responses (mainly to polysaccharide antigens) have completely normal levels of antibody classes and subclasses. This condition has been called "specific antibody deficiency with normal immunoglobulins" or "functional antibody deficiency."[333-336] In one recent retrospective compilation of 90 patients in a tertiary care institution in whom immunodeficiency was diagnosed, specific antibody deficiency with normal Igs was the most common diagnosis, made in 23% of patients.[333] Several studies have shown an increased proportion of individuals with subclass deficiencies among patients with recurrent infections. Not all of these patients have demonstrably impaired responses to vaccines, however. Thus, the relationship between lack of an antibody isotype and susceptibility to infection is far from straightforward. Measurement of memory B-cell populations may correlate better with infection risk in these patients, although further study is required.[287] IGAD, IgG subclass deficiency, and a subset of CVID may be entities in a spectrum with similar pathophysiologic characteristics.

Patients with recurrent infections, regardless of antibody class or subclass levels, should receive prophylactic antibiotic therapy initially and undergo thorough evaluation to rule out other potential predisposing factors (e.g., anatomic defects or environmental allergies).[2] Repeated immunization may lead to measurable antibody responses, although even protein conjugate pneumococcal polysaccharide vaccines may not be as effective as in healthy individuals.[337] If infections are recurrent and unacceptably severe and antibody responses to immunization are poor, gamma globulin replacement is indicated. Most children have a good response and a decreased incidence of infections.[2,334,335,338] The natural history of IgG subclass deficiency and specific antibody deficiency is usually slow spontaneous resolution. Most children have a greatly reduced incidence of infections by late childhood.

Transient Hypogammaglobulinemia of Infancy

Transient hypogammaglobulinemia of infancy (THI) is, as its name suggests, an antibody deficiency beginning in infancy that resolves spontaneously, usually by 4 to 5 years of age.[339-343] It is defined as the occurrence of an IgG level more than 2 SD below the mean for age. Many patients also have low IgA, and some also have low IgM. Vaccine antibody responses are usually intact, but this is not always the case. Peripheral lymphoid tissue is sparsely populated with small or no germinal centers and markedly reduced plasma cell contents. Numbers of circulating B and T cells are generally normal, as are in vitro assays of lymphocyte function (e.g., mitogen response). One recent study documented higher B-cell counts than in an age-matched group.[340]

Ig levels in THI gradually increase over time, and the majority of patients have normal levels by the age of 4 or 5. Thus, the diagnosis can be confirmed only after Ig levels normalize. Recent prospective studies show a preponderance of the diagnosis in males and normalization of Ig levels at a median of around 2 years with an upper limit of approximately 5 years.[339-341] Patients with lower IgG levels tend to take longer to normalize. One study showed a significantly longer time until normalization in females.[339]

The chain of recurrent infections in THI may often be broken with antibiotic prophylaxis. Particularly severe or recurrent infections may warrant a period of gamma globulin replacement.[2] After 6 to 12 months, infusions should be stopped and antibody production evaluated. For children in whom antibody levels increase sluggishly, the clinical course is particularly difficult, or a response to gamma globulin therapy is not seen, immune function should be thoroughly evaluated.

COMPLEMENT DEFICIENCIES

The complement system is composed of some 20 serum proteins, 5 complement receptors with varied distribution among leukocytes, and several integral membrane regulators found on most cells of the body.[344,345] The latter group of molecules limit cell damage as a result of a low constitutive level of complement activation. There are three distinct modes of complement activation: the classical pathway, the alternative pathway, and the lectin pathway. These pathways are shown in Figure 23-12. Soluble or surface-bound antigen-antibody complexes initiate the classical pathway; the alternative pathway is activated when complexes of properdin, factor B, and C3b are deposited on bacterial surfaces or extracellular matrix components. The lectin pathway is initiated by binding of MBL to mannose-containing microbial

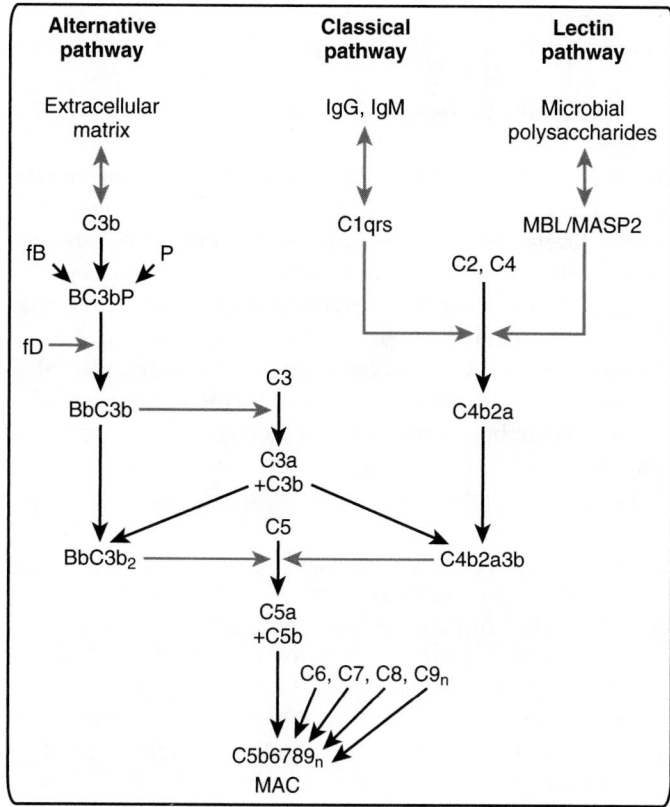

Alternative pathway

Extracellular matrix

C3b

fB, P

BC3bP

fD →

BbC3b — C3

C3a +C3b

BbC3b₂ — C5 — C4b2a3b

Classical pathway

IgG, IgM

C1qrs

C2, C4

C4b2a

Lectin pathway

Microbial polysaccharides

MBL/MASP2

C5a +C5b

C6, C7, C8, C9ₙ

C5b6789ₙ
MAC

FIGURE 23-12. Complement activation pathways. The alternative pathway is initiated when the C3b fragment with factor B (fB) and properdin (P) bind to the extracellular matrix or some microbial polysaccharides. Factor D (fD) cleaves fB to yield the C3 convertase BbC3b. Addition of C3b creates the C5 convertase BbC3b₂. The classical pathway begins when IgG or IgM bound to a surface forms a complex with C1qrs. The lectin pathway is initiated when mannose-binding lectin (MBL) and MBL-associated serine protease 2 (MASP2) bind to microbial polysaccharides. Activated C1qrs and MBL/MASP2 are both capable of cleaving C2 and C4 to yield the C3 convertase C4b2a. Addition of C3b to this complex yields the C5 convertase C4b2a3b. The C5 convertases generate C5b, the nucleus for the membrane attack complex (MAC), which is formed by the addition of one each of C6, C7, and C8 and several molecules of C9.

polysaccharides. All pathways consist of sequential proteolytic interactions having a common outcome: cleavage (activation) of the C3 complement component to yield the anaphylatoxin C3a and the C3b fragment. C3b attaches to cell membranes (e.g., bacteria) and is the principal opsonin for phagocytosis. After cleavage of the C5 component, additional reactions are nonenzymatic aggregation of C6, C7, C8, and C9 to form the macromolecular membrane attack complex. The membrane attack complex is an amphiphilic cylinder; its hydrophobic end inserts into target cell membranes and permits free flow of ions and other solutes, which leads to metabolic derangement or lysis. Genetic defects of almost all complement components are known.[346] The clinical manifestations of these defects are categorized in Table 23-6. Complement deficiencies are among the rarest of primary immunodeficiencies. Altogether, they account for less than 1% of all patients diagnosed.

TABLE 23-6 Clinical Associations with Complement Deficiencies

Component	Symptoms/Syndrome Associated with Deficiency
C1q, C1r	Systemic lupus erythematosus–like syndrome
C2	Systemic lupus erythematosus–like syndrome, vasculitis, polymyositis
C4	Systemic lupus erythematosus–like syndrome
C3	Recurrent pyogenic infections
C5, C6, C7, C8, C9	Neisserial infection, systemic lupus erythematosus–like syndrome
C1-INH	Hereditary angioedema
Factor I, factor H	Recurrent pyogenic infections
Factor D, properdin	Neisserial infections
MBL, MASP-2	Recurrent pyogenic infections

C1-INH, C1 esterase inhibitor; MASP, MBL-associated serine proteases; MBL, mannose-binding lectin.

Deficiency of Classical Complement Pathway Components

C1 Deficiency

C1 is a large complex multimer consisting of three major subunits: C1q, C1r, and C1s. C1q is itself a complex of 18 separate polypeptides, 6 molecules each of C1qA, C1qB, and C1qC. The C1 complex is completed by the addition of two molecules each of C1r and C1s, which brings the total to 22 polypeptides. Patients with defects in any of the major subunits of C1 have a syndrome resembling systemic lupus erythematosus (SLE) and susceptibility to recurrent infections.[347] Deficiency of C1q may be due to antigenically normal nonfunctional protein or complete absence of C1q.[348] The C1qA, C1qB, and C1qC genes are closely linked on chromosome 1; defects in the C1qB and C1qC genes have been described. The genes encoding C1r and C1s are closely linked on chromosome 12, and mutations of both C1r and C1s have also been described.[349-351]

C2 Deficiency

The monomeric C2 component of complement is the substrate for the activated C1s component of the C1q complex. Two fragments are generated in this reaction: the C2a fragment associates with C4b on a cell surface and becomes an activator for C3 ("C3 convertase"). The C2b fragment is a substrate for plasmin and releases a vasoactive peptide that may play a role in hereditary angioedema (HAE, see later). Approximately 50% of individuals with C2 deficiency are asymptomatic. The rest have one or more of the following: various forms of vasculitis such as discoid or systemic lupus erythematosus, chronic Henoch-Schönlein purpura, polymyositis, or recurrent pyogenic infections.[352-355] Only approximately

25% of C2-deficient patients are prone to infections.[352] C2 deficiency is associated with low levels of IgG subclasses, and low levels of IgG4 and IgA may play a role in determining susceptibility to infection.

The gene encoding C2 resides in the class III region of the HLA complex on chromosome 6. Between 1% and 1.5% of whites are heterozygous for a null C2 allele (*C2Q0*). Thus, about 1 in 10,000 will be homozygous for *C2Q0* and have a complete deficiency of C2. Two forms of C2 deficiency independent of *C2Q0* have been identified. In type I, a mutation results in loss of a mRNA splice site and C2 cannot be translated. In type 2 deficiency, C2 is not secreted, but the basis for this is unknown.

C4 Deficiency

The C4 component is another substrate for activated C1s. The C4a fragment is a very weak anaphylatoxin, and the C4b fragment associates with C2a on a cell membrane to constitute C3 convertase. Complete deficiency of C4 is rare. Virtually all such individuals with C4 deficiency have SLE and severe glomerulonephritis.[356-358] Renal failure and infection are the leading causes of death. The genes encoding C4 are also located in the class III region of the HLA complex. There are two copies on each chromosome, *C4A* and *C4B*. Each encodes proteins that differ in structure only minimally, although their biologic activities are distinct. Null alleles at these loci occur frequently; 35% of people have one copy of either *C4AQ0* or *C4BQ0*. Ten percent of the population have two null alleles, and 1% have three.[359] The presence of four null alleles (complete C4 deficiency) is rare. All of these partial deficiency states are often asymptomatic. However, HLA haplotypes containing null alleles are frequently found in patients with SLE, CVID, or IGAD.[360,361] One study has found an association of *C4B* null alleles with Henoch-Schönlein purpura.[362] The relatively high rate of occurrence of C2 and C4 null alleles leads to combined heterozygous partial deficiencies of both in about 1 in 1000 whites. Around a third of these patients have SLE and other autoimmune diseases.[347,363,364]

C3 Deficiency

The C3 component sits at the confluence of the classical and alternative pathways of complement activation. The various fragments of C3 generated through the action of C3 convertases (C4b2a and C3b2Bb), as well as other serum proteases, have diverse influences within the immune system. C3a is a potent anaphylatoxin, whereas C3b is the principal opsonin for phagocytosis and is a component of enzyme complexes in the alternative pathway of complement activation. Additional C3 fragments influence lymphocyte function. For example, C3d is an important regulator of B-cell activation.[365] Patients with C3 deficiency are susceptible to recurrent pyogenic infections, and this condition is often clinically indistinguishable from hypogammaglobulinemia. These patients may also exhibit skin, kidney, and joint inflammation caused by immune complex deposition.[366-369]

Deficiency of Alternative Complement Pathway Components

Properdin Deficiency

Properdin stabilizes the alternative pathway C3 convertase. The properdin gene is located on the X chromosome. Lack of properdin does not cause any changes in serum levels of complement components; activation through the alternative pathway is inefficient. Susceptibility to meningococcal infection and discoid lupus erythematosus has been associated with properdin deficiency.[347,364,370,371] One patient found to have coincidental deficiency of both properdin and C2 suffered recurrent *S. pneumoniae* bacteremia.[372] Concomitant deficiency of properdin and MBL may also lead to increased susceptibility to infection (meningitis).[373]

Factor D Deficiency

Factor D cleaves factor B after it associates with C3b. Only a handful of patients with factor D deficiency have been described. Three with complete deficiency had recurrent neisserial infections.[374,375] Another with partial deficiency had recurrent respiratory tract infections.[376] An additional patient was seen with neonatal pneumococcal sepsis.[377]

Deficiency of Lectin Pathway Complement Components

Mannose-Binding Lectin Deficiency

MBL is a member of the collectin protein family, which also includes lung surfactant proteins A and D.[378] MBL has a structure similar to C1q and interacts with polysaccharides containing mannose, glucose, and fucose, as well as acetylated derivatives of these sugars. Thus, MBL may interact with members of virtually all classes of infectious microbes. Three proteins called MBL-associated serine proteases (MASP) 1 to 3 are similar to C1r and C1s.[379] MASP-2 may have the most important role in catalyzing cleavage of C2 and C4 in a manner analogous to C1s. Once this is accomplished, the classical pathway C3 convertase has been created and further reactions are identical to the classical pathway. There are polymorphisms of the gene encoding MBL that affect both structure and expression.[380,381] Structural polymorphisms may impair the ability of MBL to form functional oligomers that bind effectively to carbohydrates and may also impair the association with MASP-2 and subsequent activation of the remainder of the classical pathway.[382] Promoter polymorphisms lead to variation in blood MBL levels of greater than 1000-fold from 5 ng up to 10 g/mL. The "cutoff" for clinical deficiency is not well established. Many studies use values of approximately 100 to 200 ng/mL, although slightly different values are occasionally used. Low MBL levels vary among ethnic groups. The genotype or functional tests may be more informative than the serum level alone because it is possible to have normal serum levels of a nonfunctional protein.[381]

Low blood MBL level or function does not by itself predispose to disease, except possibly during infancy, when it may be associated with a higher rate of bacterial respiratory tract infections.[380,381,383] In the setting of other disease processes or "stresses" on the immune system, MBL deficiency may predispose to a higher rate of a variety of infectious complications. Examples include the administration of chemotherapy and the development of systemic inflammatory response syndrome, sepsis, or adult respiratory distress syndrome after admission to an intensive care unit.[381,384] Low blood MBL levels may also increase the severity of the immunodeficiency occurring via other principal mechanisms, such as in CVID or with IgA/IgG subclass deficiencies or properdin deficiency.[316,373,385,386] In addition, MBL deficiency may predispose to or worsen autoimmune or inflammatory diseases such as rheumatoid arthritis, SLE, and celiac disease.[381] Recombinant human MBL is under development as a therapeutic agent; one phase I trial has shown no adverse effects of administration to healthy MBL-deficient individuals.[387]

MASP-2 Deficiency

The gene frequency of mutant *MASP2* is 3.6% among white individuals.[388] Abrogation of MASP-2 function is expected to have the same consequence as the absence of MBL function: failure to activate complement via the lectin pathway.[388,389] Patients homozygous for *MASP2* mutations who have recurrent respiratory bacterial infections and autoimmune disease have been described.[388,390]

Deficiency of Terminal Complement Components

Recurrent neisserial and pneumococcal infections and rheumatic disease have been reported in patients with C5,[391,392] C6,[393,394] and C7[395-398] deficiencies. In two families, patients with deficiency of both C6 and C7 have been identified.[399] C6 deficiency has been found in approximately 1 in 1600 African Americans in the southeastern United States in association with a higher incidence of meningococcal meningitis.[400] Molecular lesions have been defined in several patients.[401] A 1.1% incidence of a mutant C7 allele has been found in a large cohort of healthy people of Moroccan Jewish descent.[402] The C8 molecule is a heterotrimer of chains designated α, β, and γ. The α and β genes are on chromosome 1, whereas the γ gene resides on chromosome 9. C8 deficiency is also associated with recurrent neisserial infection; patients have been identified with lack of α and γ together or β alone.[403,404] Patients with lesions in C8 α genes also lack C8 γ protein, even though the latter genes are normal, because C8 α and γ are normally covalently linked. C9 deficiency is usually asymptomatic; a few patients with

recurrent neisserial infections have been described.[405-407] One patient with IgA nephropathy associated with C9 deficiency has been reported.[408] C9 deficiency has also been found in one patient with dermatomyositis.[409] Allotypy at IgG Fc receptor gene loci may have an impact on the susceptibility to infection in patients with deficiencies of terminal complement components.[410]

Deficiency of Complement Regulatory Factors

C1 Inhibitor Deficiency (Hereditary Angioedema)

HAE exhibits autosomal dominant inheritance. The symptoms of this disease are unpredictable recurrences of acute and profound subepithelial edema in a variety of locations.[411] Physical trauma may be a precipitating factor. The distal ends of the extremities, face, intestines, and pharynx are often affected. Extremity edema is painless but impedes function. Intestinal edema causes excruciating pain and is associated with abdominal distention, vomiting, and diarrhea. Pharyngeal edema may lead to fatal airway obstruction. Attacks evolve over a period of about 12 hours and resolve in 24 to 48 hours. Attacks in childhood are not uncommon but occur less frequently than in adulthood. An increase in incidence and severity often occurs during puberty and is sustained thereafter. Attacks may be associated with menses in females. Patients may become symptomatic or may have more frequent symptoms when receiving estrogen replacement or contraceptive therapy.[412]

C1 esterase inhibitor (C1-INH) is a serum serine protease inhibitor (serpin) that limits activities of the complement proteases C1r and C1s, as well as those of kallikrein, coagulation factors XIa and XIIa, and plasmin.[413,414] In type I HAE (about 85% of patients), levels of C1-INH are less than 30% of normal. In type II HAE, patients have normal levels of a mutated (nonfunctional) protein. There is at least one additional form of HAE with autosomal dominant inheritance and completely normal C1-INH function. It is designated HAE type III. In HAE I and II, the unopposed activities of C1r, C1s, and kallikrein lead to consumption of C2, C4, and bradykinin.[415] Diminished levels of these proteins are highly characteristic of HAE. Peptides derived from C2 and bradykinin cause an increase in vascular permeability and edema.

The C1-INH gene is located on chromosome 11. A variety of genetic lesions have been identified in patients with HAE.[416] Despite having one normal copy of the gene, patients have inadequate levels of C1-INH, well below the 50% one would expect to be due to a simple gene dosage effect. This may be attributable to a *trans*-inhibitory effect of the mutant allele, which leads to inhibition of transcription of the normal gene. Although inheritance is autosomal dominant, as many as 10% to

25% of patients may express new mutations. Only one patient with homozygous HAE has been reported.[417]

In managing acute attacks in patients with HAE, medications such as epinephrine, antihistamines, and corticosteroids, used to treat angioedema subsequent to hypersensitivity reactions, are entirely useless because the mechanism of swelling in HAE is unrelated.[418-421] Analgesia is indicated for painful abdominal crises. Airway protection is vital and may require a tracheostomy. Fresh frozen plasma has been used in attempts to replace C1-INH, but this is dangerous because fresh frozen plasma also contains C2 and bradykinin and may add fuel to the reaction. Intravenous infusion of purified human C1-INH from human plasma can immediately halt the progression of an HAE attack. This therapy may even be administered at home.[422] Unfortunately, despite more than a decade of experience worldwide indicating its safety and efficacy, a human C1-INH product has not yet been approved in the United States. In addition to replacement therapy for HAE, purified C1-INH may be useful in limiting the complement activation associated with sepsis, cytokine-induced vascular leak syndrome, acute myocardial infarction, or other diseases. Impeded androgens such as danazol, stanozolol, and oxandrolone are useful for reducing the rate of occurrence of attacks. These hormones act to increase expression of the normal C1-INH gene. Their use in children is limited by their tendency to promote epiphyseal closure; use in females is limited by their undesirable virilizing effects. Note that these drugs would not be effective in the very rare individuals with two mutant alleles. New small-molecule therapeutics are in development,[423] including a kallikrein inhibitor and a bradykinin receptor antagonist.

Acquired forms of HAE have also been described. In acquired angioedema (AAE) type 1, C1-INH levels decrease by an unknown mechanism, usually as a paraneoplastic process associated with lymphoma and lymphoproliferative disorders.[424] In AAE type 2, autoantibodies against C1-INH deplete it from serum.[425,426] These antibodies may arise sporadically or in association with lymphoproliferation.

Factor I Deficiency

Also known as C3 inactivator, the disulfide-linked heterodimeric complement regulatory molecule factor I cleaves C3b. Deficiency of factor I leads to increased degradation of C3 (and factor B), principally because of the inability to control constitutive low-level activity of the alternative pathway of activation. These patients have manifestations of C3 deficiency such as recurrent infections, urticaria, and immune complex disease.[427-431]

Factor H Deficiency

Factor H cooperates with factor I in the inactivation of C3b; its absence leads to reduced C3 and factor B and a syndrome of recurrent infections with *Neisseria meningitidis* and membranoproliferative glomerulonephritis.[432,433] Both familial and sporadic relapsing hemolytic-uremic syndromes have been associated with mutations in factor H.[434-436]

THE FUTURE

The diagnosis of disease, in general, may undergo significant transformation in the years ahead. This is no less true of primary immunodeficiency than it is of any other subspecialty in medicine. The refinement of a host of molecular methods that permit high-throughput analysis of gene structure and expression at all levels (RNA, protein, biochemistry, cell, and tissue/organ function) may bring definitive diagnosis into clear focus much more easily than is now possible.[437] Of course, much work is still needed to bring such techniques to fruition.

Study of patients who have the syndromes described in this chapter has provided a wealth of information about the physiology of the immune system. Each patient with one of these conditions—or with immune defects yet to be defined—presents a unique opportunity to gain further insight. As we continue to refine our understanding of the pathophysiology of these disorders, our therapies are increasingly able to compensate for these defects and help these patients lead productive lives.

REFERENCES

1. Zebracki K, Palermo TM, Hostoffer R, et al. Health-related quality of life of children with primary immunodeficiency disease: A comparison study. Ann Allergy Asthma Immunol. 2004;93:557-561.
2. Bonilla FA, Bernstein IL, Khan DA, et al. Practice parameter for the diagnosis and management of primary immunodeficiency. Ann Allergy Asthma Immunol. 2005;94:S1-S63.
3. Notarangelo L, Casanova JL, Conley ME, et al. Primary immunodeficiency diseases: An update from the international union of immunological societies primary immunodeficiency diseases classification committee meeting in Budapest, 2005. J Allergy Clin Immunol. 2006;117:883-896.
4. Fischer A, Le Deist F, Hacein-Bey-Abina S, et al. Severe combined immunodeficiency. A model disease for molecular immunology and therapy. Immunol Rev. 2005;203:98-109.
5. Muller SM, Ege M, Pottharst A, et al. Transplacentally acquired maternal T lymphocytes in severe combined immunodeficiency: A study of 121 patients. Blood. 2001;98:1847-1851.
6. Kobrynski LJ, Abramowsky C. Monoclonal IgA gammopathy due to maternal B cells in an infant with severe combined immunodeficiency (SCID) prior to hematopoietic stem cell transplantation. J Pediatr Hematol Oncol. 2006;28:53-56.
7. Hershfield MS. Adenosine deaminase deficiency: clinical expression, molecular basis, and therapy. Semin Hematol. 1998;35:291-298.

8. Markert ML, Finkel BD, McLaughlin TM, et al. Mutations in purine nucleoside phosphorylase deficiency. Hum Mutat. 1997;9:118-121.

9. Malacarne F, Benicchi T, Notarangelo LD, et al. Reduced thymic output, increased spontaneous apoptosis and oligoclonal B cells in polyethylene glycol–adenosine deaminase–treated patients. Eur J Immunol. 2005;35:3376-3386.

10. Blackburn MR, Kellems RE. Adenosine deaminase deficiency: Metabolic basis of immune deficiency and pulmonary inflammation. Adv Immunol. 2005;86:1-41.

11. Arpaia E, Benveniste P, Di Cristofano A, et al. Mitochondrial basis for immune deficiency. Evidence from purine nucleoside phosphorylase–deficient mice. J Exp Med. 2000;191:2197-2208.

12. Aldrich MB, Blackburn MR, Kellems RE. The importance of adenosine deaminase for lymphocyte development and function. Biochem Biophys Res Commun. 2000;272:311-315.

13. Rogers MH, Lwin R, Fairbanks L, et al. Cognitive and behavioral abnormalities in adenosine deaminase deficient severe combined immunodeficiency. J Pediatr. 2001;139:44-50.

14. Arredondo-Vega FX, Santisteban I, Daniels S, et al. Adenosine deaminase deficiency: genotype-phenotype correlations based on expressed activity of 29 mutant alleles. Am J Hum Genet. 1998;63:1049-1059.

15. Fairbanks LD, Simmonds HA, Webster AD, et al. Adenosine deaminase (ADA) deficiency as the unexpected cause of CD4⁺ T-lymphocytopenia in two HIV-negative adult female siblings. Adv Exp Med Biol. 1994;370:471-474.

16. Markert ML. Purine nucleoside phosphorylase deficiency. Immunodefic Rev. 1991;3:45-81.

17. Pulmar SH. Red cell therapy: its clinical and immunological efficacy in ADA deficiency. In Pollara B, Meuwisen HJ, Pickering RJ (eds). Inborn Errors of Specific Immunity. New York, Academic Press, 1979, p 343.

18. Chan B, Wara D, Bastian J, et al. Long-term efficacy of enzyme replacement therapy for adenosine deaminase (ADA)-deficient severe combined immunodeficiency (SCID). Clin Immunol. 2005;117:133-143.

19. Kaufman DA, Hershfield MS, Bocchini JA, et al. Cerebral lymphoma in an adenosine deaminase–deficient patient with severe combined immunodeficiency receiving polyethylene glycol–conjugated adenosine deaminase. Pediatrics. 2005;116:e876-e879.

20. Sobacchi C, Marrella V, Rucci F, et al. RAG-dependent primary immunodeficiencies. Hum Mutat. 2006;27:1174-1184.

21. Villa A, Sobacchi C, Notarangelo LD, et al. V₍δ₎j recombination defects in lymphocytes due to RAG mutations: Severe immunodeficiency with a spectrum of clinical presentations. Blood. 2001;97:81-88.

22. Corneo B, Moshous D, Gungor T, et al. Identical mutations in RAG1 or RAG2 genes leading to defective V₍δ₎j recombinase activity can cause either T-B-severe combined immune deficiency or Omenn syndrome. Blood. 2001;97:2772-2776.

23. Dalal I, Tabori U, Bielorai B, et al. Evolution of a T-B-SCID into an Omenn syndrome phenotype following parainfluenza 3 virus infection. Clin Immunol. 2005;115:70-73.

24. Wada T, Toma T, Okamoto H, et al. Oligoclonal expansion of T lymphocytes with multiple second-site mutations leads to Omenn syndrome in a patient with RAG1-deficient severe combined immunodeficiency. Blood. 2005;106:2099-2101.

25. Moshous D, Callebaut I, de Chasseval R, et al. Artemis, a novel DNA double-strand break repair/V₍δ₎j recombination protein, is mutated in human severe combined immune deficiency. Cell. 2001;105:177-186.

26. Le Deist F, Poinsignon C, Moshous D, et al. Artemis sheds new light on V₍δ₎j recombination. Immunol Rev. 2004;200:142-155.

27. Ege M, Ma Y, Manfras B, et al. Omenn syndrome due to artemis mutations. Blood. 2005;105:4179-4186.

28. van der Burg M, van Veelen LR, Verkaik NS, et al. A new type of radiosensitive T-B-NK⁺ severe combined immunodeficiency caused by a LIG4 mutation. J Clin Invest. 2006;116:137-145.

29. Enders A, Fisch P, Schwarz K, et al. A severe form of human combined immunodeficiency due to mutations in DNA ligase IV. J Immunol. 2006;176:5060-5068.

30. Buck D, Moshous D, de Chasseval R, et al. Severe combined immunodeficiency and microcephaly in siblings with hypomorphic mutations in DNA ligase IV. Eur J Immunol. 2006;36:224-235.

31. Buck D, Malivert L, de Chasseval R, et al. Cernunnos, a novel nonhomologous end-joining factor, is mutated in human immunodeficiency with microcephaly. Cell. 2006;124:287-299.

32. Kovanen PE, Leonard WJ. Cytokines and immunodeficiency diseases: Critical roles of the γ_c-dependent cytokines interleukins 2, 4, 7, 9, 15, and 21, and their signaling pathways. Immunol Rev. 2004;202:67-83.

33. Shearer WT, Ritz J, Finegold MJ, et al. Epstein-Barr virus–associated B cell proliferations of diverse clonal origins after bone marrow transplantation in a 12 year-old patient with severe combined immunodeficiency. N Engl J Med. 1985;312:1151-1159.

34. Somech R, Roifman CM. Mutation analysis should be performed to rule out γ_c deficiency in children with functional severe combined immune deficiency despite apparently normal immunologic tests. J Pediatr. 2005;147:555-557.

35. Plebani A, Stringa M, Prigione I, et al. Engrafted maternal T cells in human severe combined immunodeficiency: evidence for a T_H2 phenotype and a potential role of apoptosis on the restriction of T-cell receptor variable beta repertoire [published erratum appears in J Allergy Clin Immunol 1998 Aug;102(2):214]. J Allergy Clin Immunol. 1998;101:131-134.

36. Li SL, Ting SS, Lindeman R, et al. Carrier identification in X-linked immunodeficiency diseases. J Paediatr Child Health. 1998;34:273-279.

37. Roberts JL, Lengi A, Brown SM, et al. Janus kinase 3 (JAK3) deficiency: clinical, immunologic, and molecular analyses of 10 patients and outcomes of stem cell transplantation. Blood. 2004;103:2009-2018.

38. Notarangelo LD, Mella P, Jones A, et al. Mutations in severe combined immune deficiency (SCID) due to JAK3 deficiency. Hum Mutat. 2001;18:255-263.

39. Tezcan I, Ersoy F, Sanal O, et al. Long-term survival in severe combined immune deficiency: the role of persistent maternal engraftment. J Pediatr. 2005;146:137-140.

40. Roifman CM. Human IL-2 receptor alpha chain deficiency. Pediatr Res. 2000;48:6-11.

41. Giliani S, Mori L, de Saint Basile G, et al. Interleukin-7 receptor alpha (IL-7Rα) deficiency: cellular and molecular bases. Analysis of clinical, immunological, and molecular features in 16 novel patients. Immunol Rev. 2005;203:110-126.

42. Giliani S, Bonfim C, de Saint Basile G, et al. Omenn syndrome in an infant with IL7Rα gene mutation. J Pediatr. 2006;148:272-274.

43. Germain RN, Stefanova I. The dynamics of T cell receptor signaling: complex orchestration and the key roles of tempo and cooperation. Annu Rev Immunol. 1999;17:467-522.

44. Takada H, Nomura A, Roifman CM, Hara T. Severe combined immunodeficiency caused by a splicing abnormality of the CD3δ gene. Eur J Pediatr. 2005;164:311-314.

45. Fischer A, de Saint Basile G, Le Deist F. CD3 deficiencies. Curr Opin Allergy Clin Immunol. 2005;5:491-495.

46. Dadi HK, Simon AJ, Roifman CM. Effect of cd3δ deficiency on maturation of α/β and γ/δ T-cell lineages in severe combined immunodeficiency. N Engl J Med. 2003;349:1821-1828.

47. de Saint Basile G, Geissmann F, Flori E, et al. Severe combined immunodeficiency caused by deficiency in either the δ or the ε subunit of CD3. J Clin Invest. 2004;114:1512-1517.

48. Rieux-Laucat F, Hivroz C, Lim A, et al. Inherited and somatic CD3ζ mutations in a patient with T-cell deficiency. N Engl J Med. 2006;354:1913-1921.

49. Arnaiz-Villena A, Timon M, Corell A, et al. Primary immunodeficiency caused by mutations in the gene encoding the CD3-γ subunit of the T-lymphocyte receptor. N Engl J Med. 1992;327:529-533.

50. Tchilian EZ, Wallace DL, Wells RS, et al. A deletion in the gene encoding the CD45 antigen in a patient with SCID. J Immunol. 2001;166:1308-1313.

51. Kung C, Pingel JT, Heikinheimo M, et al. Mutations in the tyrosine phosphatase CD45 gene in a child with severe combined immunodeficiency disease. Nat Med. 2000;6:343-345.

52. Cale CM, Klein NJ, Novelli V, et al. Severe combined immunodeficiency with abnormalities in expression of the common leucocyte antigen, CD45. Arch Dis Child. 1997;76:163-164.

53. Krawczyk M, Reith W. Regulation of mhc class II expression, a unique regulatory system identified by the study of a primary immunodeficiency disease. Tissue Antigens. 2006;67:183-197.

54. Renella R, Picard C, Neven B, et al. Human leucocyte antigen–identical haematopoietic stem cell transplantation in major histocompatiblity complex class II immunodeficiency: reduced survival correlates with an increased incidence of acute graft-versus-host disease and pre-existing viral infections. Br J Haematol. 2006;134:510-516.

55. Wolf HM, Hauber I, Gulle H, et al. Twin boys with major histocompatibility complex class II deficiency but inducible immune responses. N Engl J Med. 1995;332:86-90.

56. Sharfe N, Arpaia E, Roifman CM. CD8 lymphocytopenia caused by ZAP-70 deficiency. Immunol Allergy Clin North Am. 2000;20:77-95.

57. Zimmer J, Andres E, Donato L, et al. Clinical and immunological aspects of HLA class I deficiency. QJM. 2005;98:719-727.

58. Gadola SD, Moins-Teisserenc HT, Trowsdale J, et al. TAP deficiency syndrome. Clin Exp Immunol. 2000;121:173-178.

59. Yabe T, Kawamura S, Sato M, et al. A subject with a novel type I bare lymphocyte syndrome has tapasin deficiency due to deletion of 4 exons by Alu-mediated recombination. Blood. 2002;100:1496-1498.

60. Feske S, Gwack Y, Prakriya M, et al. A mutation in ORAI1 causes immune deficiency by abrogating CRAC channel function. Nature. 2006;441:179-185.

61. Feske S, Muller JM, Graf D, et al. Severe combined immunodeficiency due to defective binding of the nuclear factor of activated T cells in T lymphocytes of two male siblings. Eur J Immunol. 1996;26:2119-2126.

62. Menasche G, Ho CH, Sanal O, et al. Griscelli syndrome restricted to hypopigmentation results from a melanophilin defect (GS3) or a MYO5a F-exon deletion (GS1). J Clin Invest. 2003;112:450-456.

63. Sanal O, Ersoy F, Tezcan I, et al. Griscelli disease: genotype-phenotype correlation in an array of clinical heterogeneity. J Clin Immunol. 2002;22:237-243.

64. Rosen FS. Severe combined immunodeficiency: a pediatric emergency. J Pediatr. 1997;130:345-346.

65. Slatter MA, Gennery AR. Umbilical cord stem cell transplantation for primary immunodeficiencies. Exp Opin Biol Ther. 2006;6:555-565.

66. Grunebaum E, Mazzolari E, Porta F, et al. Bone marrow transplantation for severe combined immune deficiency. JAMA. 2006;295:508-518.

67. Veys P, Rao K, Amrolia P. Stem cell transplantation for congenital immunodeficiencies using reduced-intensity conditioning. Bone Marrow Transplant. 2005;35(Suppl 1):S45-S47.

68. Bhattacharya A, Slatter MA, Chapman CE, et al. Single centre experience of umbilical cord stem cell transplantation for primary immunodeficiency. Bone Marrow Transplant. 2005;36:295-299.

69. Myers LA, Patel DD, Puck JM, Buckley RH. Hematopoietic stem cell transplantation for severe combined immunodeficiency in the neonatal period leads to superior thymic output and improved survival. Blood. 2002;99:872-878.

70. Knutsen AP, Wall DA. Umbilical cord blood transplantation in severe T-cell immunodeficiency disorders: Two-year experience. J Clin Immunol. 2000;20:466-476.

71. Patel DD, Gooding ME, Parrott RE, et al. Thymic function after hematopoietic stem-cell transplantation for the treatment of severe combined immunodeficiency. N Engl J Med. 2000;342:1325-1332.

72. Sarzotti M, Patel DD, Li X, et al. T cell repertoire development in humans with SCID after nonablative allogeneic marrow transplantation. J Immunol. 2003;170:2711-2718.

73. Borghans JA, Bredius RG, Hazenberg MD, et al. Early determinants of long-term T-cell reconstitution after hematopoietic stem cell transplantation for severe combined immunodeficiency. Blood. 2006;108:763-769.

74. McGhee SA, Stiehm ER, Cowan M, et al. Two-tiered universal newborn screening strategy for severe combined

immunodeficiency. Mol Genet Metab. 2005;86: 427-430.

75. Chan K, Puck JM. Development of population-based newborn screening for severe combined immunodeficiency. J Allergy Clin Immunol. 2005;115:391-398.

76. Onodera M, Sakiyama Y. Adenosine deaminase deficiency as the first target disorder in gene therapy. Exp Opin Investig Drugs. 2000;9:543-549.

77. Gaspar HB, Bjorkegren E, Parsley K, et al. Successful reconstitution of immunity in ADA-SCID by stem cell gene therapy following cessation of PEG-ADA and use of mild preconditioning. Mol Ther. 2006;14:505-513.

78. Aiuti A, Slavin S, Aker M, et al. Correction of ADA-SCID by stem cell gene therapy combined with non-myeloablative conditioning. Science. 2002;296:2410-2413.

79. Hacein-Bey-Abina S, Le Deist F, Carlier F, et al. Sustained correction of X-linked severe combined immunodeficiency by ex vivo gene therapy. N Engl J Med. 2002;346:1185-1193.

80. Cavazzana-Calvo M, Hacein-Bey S, de Saint Basile G, et al. Gene therapy of human severe combined immunodeficiency (SCID)-X1 disease. Science. 2000;288: 669-672.

81. Thrasher AJ, Hacein-Bey-Abina S, Gaspar HB, et al. Failure of SCID-X1 gene therapy in older patients. Blood. 2005;105:4255-4257.

82. Puck JM, Malech HL. Gene therapy for immune disorders: Good news tempered by bad news. J Allergy Clin Immunol. 2006;117:865-869.

83. Check E. Gene therapy put on hold as third child develops cancer. Nature. 2005;433:561.

84. Chinen J, Puck JM. Successes and risks of gene therapy in primary immunodeficiencies. J Allergy Clin Immunol. 2004;113:595-603; quiz 604.

85. Ochs HD, Thrasher AJ. The Wiskott-Aldrich syndrome. J Allergy Clin Immunol. 2006;117:725-738; quiz 739.

86. Notarangelo LD, Notarangelo LD, Ochs HD. WASP and the phenotypic range associated with deficiency. Curr Opin Allergy Clin Immunol. 2005;5:485-490.

87. Ma YC, Shyur SD, Ho TY, et al. Wiskott-Aldrich syndrome complicated by an atypical lymphoproliferative disorder: A case report. J Microbiol Immunol Infect. 2005;38:289-292.

88. Kobayashi R, Ariga T, Nonoyama S, et al. Outcome in patients with Wiskott-Aldrich syndrome following stem cell transplantation: an analysis of 57 patients in Japan. Br J Haematol. 2006;135:362-366.

89. Filipovich AH, Stone JV, Tomany SC, et al. Impact of donor type on outcome of bone marrow transplantation for Wiskott-Aldrich syndrome: Collaborative study of the International Bone Marrow Transplant Registry and the National Marrow Donor Program. Blood. 2001;97:1598-1603.

90. Wada T, Schurman SH, Garabedian EK, et al. Analysis of T-cell repertoire diversity in Wiskott-Aldrich syndrome. Blood. 2005;106:3895-3897.

91. Park JY, Shcherbina A, Rosen FS, et al. Phenotypic perturbation of B cells in the Wiskott-Aldrich syndrome. Clin Exp Immunol. 2005;139:297-305.

92. Binder V, Albert MH, Kabus M, et al. The genotype of the original Wiskott phenotype. N Engl J Med. 2006;355: 1790-1793.

93. Ochs HD, Notarangelo LD. Structure and function of the Wiskott-Aldrich syndrome protein. Curr Opin Hematol. 2005;12:284-291.

94. Huang W, Ochs HD, Dupont B, Vyas YM. The Wiskott-Aldrich syndrome protein regulates nuclear translocation of NFAT2 and NF-κB (RELA) independently of its role in filamentous actin polymerization and actin cytoskeletal rearrangement. J Immunol. 2005;174: 2602-2611.

95. Lutskiy MI, Rosen FS, Remold-O'Donnell E. Genotype-proteotype linkage in the Wiskott-Aldrich syndrome. J Immunol. 2005;175:1329-1336.

96. Parolini O, Ressmann G, Haas OA, et al. X-linked Wiskott-Aldrich syndrome in a girl. N Engl J Med. 1998;338:291-295.

97. Ariga T, Kondoh T, Yamaguchi K, et al. Spontaneous in vivo reversion of an inherited mutation in the Wiskott-Aldrich syndrome. J Immunol. 2001;166: 5245-5249.

98. Swift M, Morrell D, Cromartie E, et al. The incidence and gene frequency of ataxia-telangiectasia in the United States. Am J Hum Genet. 1986;39:573-583.

99. Taylor AM, Byrd PJ. Molecular pathology of ataxia telangiectasia. J Clin Pathol. 2005;58:1009-1015.

100. Schubert R, Reichenbach J, Zielen S. Growth factor deficiency in patients with ataxia telangiectasia. Clin Exp Immunol. 2005;140:517-519.

101. Crawford TO, Skolasky RL, Fernandez R, et al. Survival probability in ataxia telangiectasia. Arch Dis Child. 2006;91:610-611.

102. Schroeder SA, Swift M, Sandoval C, Langston C. Interstitial lung disease in patients with ataxia-telangiectasia. Pediatr Pulmonol. 2005;39:537-543.

103. Morrell D, Cromartie E, Swift M. Mortality and cancer incidence in 263 patients with ataxia telangiectasia. J Natl Cancer Inst. 1986;77:87-92.

104. Carbonari M, Cherchi M, Paganelli R, et al. Relative increase of T cells expressing the γ/δ rather than the α/β receptor in ataxia-telangiectasia. N Engl J Med. 1990;322: 73-76.

105. Pashankar F, Singhal V, Akabogu I, et al. Intact T cell responses in ataxia telangiectasia. Clin Immunol. 2006; 120:156-162.

106. Sadighi Akha AA, Humphrey RL, Winkelstein JA, et al. Oligo-/monoclonal gammopathy and hypergammaglobulinemia in ataxia-telangiectasia. A study of 90 patients. Medicine (Baltimore). 1999;78:370-381.

107. Guerra-Maranhao MC, Costa-Carvalho BT, Nudelman V, et al. Response to polysaccharide antigens in patients with ataxia-telangiectasia. J Pediatr (Rio J). 2006;82: 132-136.

108. Nakamura H, Yasui Y, Saito N, et al. DNA repair defect in at cells and their hypersensitivity to low-dose-rate radiation. Radiat Res. 2006;165:277-282.

109. Hall J. The ataxia-telangiectasia mutated gene and breast cancer: gene expression profiles and sequence variants. Cancer Lett. 2005;227:105-114.

110. Renwick A, Thompson D, Seal S, et al. ATM mutations that cause ataxia-telangiectasia are breast cancer susceptibility alleles. Nat Genet. 2006;38:873-875.

111. Kim JH, Kim H, Lee KY, et al. Genetic polymorphisms of ataxia telangiectasia mutated affect lung cancer risk. Hum Mol Genet. 2006;15:1181-1186.

112. Frappart PO, Tong WM, Demuth I, et al. An essential function for NBS1 in the prevention of ataxia and cerebellar defects. Nat Med. 2005;11:538-544.

113. Rollinson S, Kesby H, Morgan GJ. Haplotypic variation in MRE11, RAD50 and NBS1 and risk of non-Hodgkin's lymphoma. Leuk Lymphoma. 2006;47:2567-2583.

114. Oskarsdottir S, Persson C, Eriksson BO, Fasth A. Presenting phenotype in 100 children with the 22q11 deletion syndrome. Eur J Pediatr. 2005;164:146-153.

115. Goldmuntz E. DiGeorge syndrome: new insights. Clin Perinatol. 2005;32:963-978, ix-x.

116. Markert ML, Devlin BH, Alexieff MJ, et al. Review of 54 patients with complete DiGeorge anomaly enrolled in protocols for thymus transplantation: outcome of 44 consecutive transplants. Blood. 2007;109:4539-4547.

117. Al-Tamemi S, Mazer B, Mitchell D, et al. Complete DiGeorge anomaly in the absence of neonatal hypocalcemia and velofacial and cardiac defects. Pediatrics. 2005;116:e457-e460.

118. Markert ML, Alexieff MJ, Li J, et al. Complete DiGeorge syndrome: development of rash, lymphadenopathy, and oligoclonal T cells in 5 cases. J Allergy Clin Immunol. 2004;113:734-741.

119. Kar PS, Ogoe B, Poole R, Meeking D. Di-George syndrome presenting with hypocalcaemia in adulthood: two case reports and a review. J Clin Pathol. 2005;58:655-657.

120. Cancrini C, Romiti ML, Finocchi A, et al. Post-natal ontogenesis of the T-cell receptor CD4 and CD8 vbeta repertoire and immune function in children with DiGeorge syndrome. J Clin Immunol. 2005;25:265-274.

121. Pierdominici M, Marziali M, Giovannetti A, et al. T cell receptor repertoire and function in patients with DiGeorge syndrome and velocardiofacial syndrome. Clin Exp Immunol. 2000;121:127-132.

122. Chinen J, Rosenblatt HM, Smith EO, et al. Long-term assessment of T-cell populations in DiGeorge syndrome. J Allergy Clin Immunol. 2003;111:573-579.

123. Finocchi A, Di Cesare S, Romiti ML, et al. Humoral immune responses and CD27+ B cells in children with DiGeorge syndrome (22q11.2 deletion syndrome). Pediatr Allergy Immunol. 2006;17:382-388.

124. Smith CA, Driscoll DA, Emanuel BS, et al. Increased prevalence of immunoglobulin A deficiency in patients with the chromosome 22q11.2 deletion syndrome (DiGeorge syndrome/velocardiofacial syndrome). Clin Diagn Lab Immunol. 1998;5:415-417.

125. Staple L, Andrews T, McDonald-McGinn D, et al. Allergies in patients with chromosome 22q11.2 deletion syndrome (DiGeorge syndrome/velocardiofacial syndrome) and patients with chronic granulomatous disease. Pediatr Allergy Immunol. 2005;16:226-230.

126. McDonald-McGinn DM, Kirschner R, Goldmuntz E, et al. The Philadelphia story: the 22q11.2 deletion: report on 250 patients. Genet Couns. 1999;10:11-24.

127. Driscoll DA. Molecular and genetic aspects of DiGeorge/velocardiofacial syndrome. Methods Mol Med. 2006;126:43-55.

128. Yagi H, Furutani Y, Hamada H, et al. Role of TBX1 in human del22q11.2 syndrome. Lancet. 2003;362:1366-1373.

129. Van Esch H, Groenen P, Daw S, et al. Partial DiGeorge syndrome in two patients with a 10p rearrangement. Clin Genet. 1999;55:269-276.

130. Azzari C, Gambineri E, Resti M, et al. Safety and immunogenicity of measles-mumps-rubella vaccine in children with congenital immunodeficiency (DiGeorge syndrome). Vaccine. 2005;23:1668-1671.

131. Moylett EH, Wasan AN, Noroski LM, Shearer WT. Live viral vaccines in patients with partial DiGeorge syndrome: clinical experience and cellular immunity. Clin Immunol. 2004;112:106-112.

132. Perez EE, Bokszczanin A, McDonald-McGinn D, et al. Safety of live viral vaccines in patients with chromosome 22q11.2 deletion syndrome (DiGeorge syndrome/velocardiofacial syndrome). Pediatrics. 2003;112:e325.

133. Bonilla FA, Geha RS. CD154 deficiency and related syndromes. Immunol Allergy Clin North Am. 2001;21:65-89.

134. Tomizawa D, Imai K, Ito S, et al. Allogeneic hematopoietic stem cell transplantation for seven children with X-linked hyper-IgM syndrome: A single center experience. Am J Hematol. 2004;76:33-39.

135. van Kooten C, Banchereau J. CD40-CD40 ligand. J Leukoc Biol. 2000;67:2-17.

136. Wagner DH Jr, Stout RD, Suttles J. Role of the CD40-CD40 ligand interaction in CD4+ T cell contact–dependent activation of monocyte interleukin-1 synthesis. Eur J Immunol. 1994;24:3148-3154.

137. Ohzeki T, Hanaki K, Motozumi H, et al. Immunodeficiency with increased immunoglobulin M associated with growth hormone insufficiency. Acta Paediatr. 1993;82:620-623.

138. Lougaris V, Badolato R, Ferrari S, Plebani A. Hyper immunoglobulin M syndrome due to CD40 deficiency: clinical, molecular, and immunological features. Immunol Rev. 2005;203:48-66.

139. Ferrari S, Giliani S, Insalaco A, et al. Mutations of CD40 gene cause an autosomal recessive form of immunodeficiency with hyper IgM. Proc Natl Acad Sci U S A. 2001;98:12614-12619.

140. Notarangelo LD, Lanzi G, Peron S, Durandy A. Defects of class-switch recombination. J Allergy Clin Immunol. 2006;117:855-864.

141. Durandy A, Peron S, Taubenheim N, Fischer A. Activation-induced cytidine deaminase: structure-function relationship as based on the study of mutants. Hum Mutat. 2006;27:1185-1191.

142. Lee WI, Torgerson TR, Schumacher MJ, et al. Molecular analysis of a large cohort of patients with the hyper immunoglobulin M (IgM) syndrome. Blood. 2005;105:1881-1890.

143. Imai K, Zhu Y, Revy P, et al. Analysis of class switch recombination and somatic hypermutation in patients affected with autosomal dominant hyper-IgM syndrome type 2. Clin Immunol. 2005;115:277-285.

144. Durandy A, Revy P, Imai K, Fischer A. Hyper-immunoglobulin M syndromes caused by intrinsic B-lymphocyte defects. Immunol Rev. 2005;203:67-79.

145. Quartier P, Bustamante J, Sanal O, et al. Clinical, immunologic and genetic analysis of 29 patients with autosomal recessive hyper-IgM syndrome due to activation-induced cytidine deaminase deficiency. Clin Immunol. 2004;110:22-29.

146. Kasahara Y, Kaneko H, Fukao T, et al. Hyper-IgM syndrome with putative dominant negative mutation in activation-induced cytidine deaminase. J Allergy Clin Immunol. 2003;112:755-760.

147. Kavli B, Andersen S, Otterlei M, et al. B cells from hyper-IgM patients carrying UNG mutations lack ability to remove uracil from ssDNA and have elevated genomic uracil. J Exp Med. 2005;201:2011-2021.

148. Imai K, Slupphaug G, Lee WI, et al. Human uracil-DNA glycosylase deficiency associated with profoundly impaired immunoglobulin class-switch recombination. Nat Immunol. 2003;4:1023-1028.

149. Imai K, Catalan N, Plebani A, et al. Hyper-IgM syndrome type 4 with a B lymphocyte–intrinsic selective deficiency in Ig class-switch recombination. J Clin Invest. 2003;112:136-142.

150. Puel A, Picard C, Ku CL, et al. Inherited disorders of NF-κB–mediated immunity in man. Curr Opin Immunol. 2004;16:34-41.

151. Uzel G. The range of defects associated with nuclear factor κB essential modulator. Curr Opin Allergy Clin Immunol. 2005;5:513-518.

152. Orange JS, Levy O, Geha RS. Human disease resulting from gene mutations that interfere with appropriate nuclear factor-κB activation. Immunol Rev. 2005;203:21-37.

153. Orange JS, Levy O, Brodeur SR, et al. Human nuclear factor κB essential modulator mutation can result in immunodeficiency without ectodermal dysplasia. J Allergy Clin Immunol. 2004;114:650-656.

154. Orange JS, Jain A, Ballas ZK, et al. The presentation and natural history of immunodeficiency caused by nuclear factor κB essential modulator mutation. J Allergy Clin Immunol. 2004;113:725-733.

155. Jain A, Ma CA, Liu S, et al. Specific missense mutations in nemo result in hyper-IgM syndrome with hypohydrotic ectodermal dysplasia. Nat Immunol. 2001;2:223-228.

156. Doffinger R, Smahi A, Bessia C, et al. X-linked anhidrotic ectodermal dysplasia with immunodeficiency is caused by impaired NF-κB signaling. Nat Genet. 2001;27:277-285.

157. Zonana J, Elder ME, Schneider LC, et al. A novel X-linked disorder of immune deficiency and hypohidrotic ectodermal dysplasia is allelic to incontinentia pigmenti and due to mutations in IKK-γ (NEMO). Am J Hum Genet. 2000;67:1555-1562.

158. Dupuis-Girod S, Cancrini C, Le Deist F, et al. Successful allogeneic hemopoietic stem cell transplantation in a child who had anhidrotic ectodermal dysplasia with immunodeficiency. Pediatrics. 2006;118:e205-e211.

159. Courtois G, Smahi A, Reichenbach J, et al. A hypermorphic IκBα mutation is associated with autosomal dominant anhidrotic ectodermal dysplasia and T cell immunodeficiency. J Clin Invest. 2003;112:1108-1115.

160. Lee MS, Kim YJ. Signaling pathways downstream of pattern-recognition receptors and their cross talk. Annu Rev Biochem. 2007;76:447-480.

161. Kaisho T, Akira S. Toll-like receptor function and signaling. J Allergy Clin Immunol. 2006;117:979-987; quiz 988.

162. Cardenes M, von Bernuth H, Garcia-Saavedra A, et al. Autosomal recessive interleukin-1 receptor–associated kinase 4 deficiency in fourth-degree relatives. J Pediatr. 2006;148:549-551.

163. Puel A, Yang K, Ku CL, et al. Heritable defects of the human TLR signalling pathways. J Endotoxin Res. 2005;11:220-224.

164. Ku CL, Yang K, Bustamante J, et al. Inherited disorders of human toll-like receptor signaling: immunological implications. Immunol Rev. 2005;203:10-20.

165. Currie AJ, Davidson DJ, Reid GS, et al. Primary immunodeficiency to pneumococcal infection due to a defect in toll-like receptor signaling. J Pediatr. 2004;144:512-518.

166. Picard C, Puel A, Bonnet M, et al. Pyogenic bacterial infections in humans with IRAK-4 deficiency. Science. 2003;299:2076-2079.

167. Latger-Cannard V, Bensoussan D, Bordigoni P. The WHIM syndrome shows a peculiar dysgranulopoiesis: myelokathexis. Br J Haematol. 2006;132:669.

168. Tarzi MD, Jenner M, Hattotuwa K, et al. Sporadic case of warts, hypogammaglobulinemia, immunodeficiency, and myelokathexis syndrome. J Allergy Clin Immunol. 2005;116:1101-1105.

169. Diaz GA, Gulino AV. WHIM syndrome: a defect in CXCR4 signaling. Curr Allergy Asthma Rep. 2005;5:350-355.

170. Diaz GA. CXCR4 mutations in WHIM syndrome: a misguided immune system? Immunol Rev. 2005;203:235-243.

171. Hernandez PA, Gorlin RJ, Lukens JN, et al. Mutations in the chemokine receptor gene CXCR4 are associated with WHIM syndrome, a combined immunodeficiency disease. Nat Genet. 2003;34:70-74.

172. Gorlin RJ, Gelb B, Diaz GA, et al. WHIM syndrome, an autosomal dominant disorder: clinical, hematological, and molecular studies. Am J Med Genet. 2000;91:368-376.

173. Allen SJ, Crown SE, Handel TM. Chemokine:receptor structure, interactions, and antagonism. Annu Rev Immunol. 2007;25:787-820.

174. Rot A, von Andrian UH. Chemokines in innate and adaptive host defense: basic chemokinese grammar for immune cells. Annu Rev Immunol. 2004;22:891-928.

175. Hord JD, Whitlock JA, Gay JC, Lukens JN. Clinical features of myelokathexis and treatment with hematopoietic cytokines: a case report of two patients and review of the literature. J Pediatr Hematol Oncol. 1997;19:443-448.

176. Nichols KE, Ma CS, Cannons JL, et al. Molecular and cellular pathogenesis of X-linked lymphoproliferative disease. Immunol Rev. 2005;203:180-199.

177. Hoshino T, Kanegane H, Doki N, et al. X-linked lymphoproliferative disease in an adult. Int J Hematol. 2005;82:55-58.

178. Benoit L, Wang X, Pabst HF, et al. Defective NK cell activation in X-linked lymphoproliferative disease. J Immunol. 2000;165:3549-3553.

179. Nichols KE, Hom J, Gong SY, et al. Regulation of NKT cell development by SAP, the protein defective in XLP. Nat Med. 2005;11:340-345.

180. Soresina A, Lougaris V, Giliani S, et al. Mutations of the X-linked lymphoproliferative disease gene SH2D1A mimicking common variable immunodeficiency. Eur J Pediatr. 2002;161:656-659.

181. Morra M, Silander O, Calpe S, et al. Alterations of the X-linked lymphoproliferative disease gene SH2D1A in

common variable immunodeficiency syndrome. Blood. 2001;98:1321-1325.

182. Alangari A, Abobaker A, Kanegane H, Miyawaki T. X-linked lymphoproliferative disease associated with hypogammaglobulinemia and growth-hormone deficiency. Eur J Pediatr. 2006;165:165-167.

183. Ma CS, Nichols KE, Tangye SG. Regulation of cellular and humoral immune responses by the SLAM and SAP families of molecules. Annu Rev Immunol. 2007;25:337-379.

184. Milone M, Tsai DE, Hodinka RL, et al. Treatment of primary Epstein-Barr virus infection in patients with X-linked lymphoproliferative disease using B-cell directed therapy. Blood. 2005;105:994-996.

185. Kalfa VC, Roberts RL, Stiehm ER. The syndrome of chronic mucocutaneous candidiasis with selective antibody deficiency. Ann Allergy Asthma Immunol. 2003;90:259-264.

186. Lilic D. New perspectives on the immunology of chronic mucocutaneous candidiasis. Curr Opin Infect Dis. 2002;15:143-147.

187. Palma-Carlos AG, Palma-Carlos ML, da Silva SL. Natural killer (NK) cells in mucocutaneous candidiasis. Allerg Immunol (Paris). 2002;34:208-212.

188. Vogel A, Strassburg CP, Obermayer-Straub P, et al. The genetic background of autoimmune polyendocrinopathy–candidiasis–ectodermal dystrophy and its autoimmune disease components. J Mol Med. 2002;80:201-211.

189. Meloni A, Perniola R, Faa V, et al. Delineation of the molecular defects in the AIRE gene in autoimmune polyendocrinopathy–candidiasis–ectodermal dystrophy patients from southern Italy. J Clin Endocrinol Metab. 2002;87:841-846.

190. Kumar PG, Laloraya M, She JX. Population genetics and functions of the autoimmune regulator (AIRE). Endocrinol Metab Clin North Am. 2002;31:321-338, vi.

191. Heino M, Peterson P, Kudoh J, et al. Apeced mutations in the autoimmune regulator (AIRE) gene. Hum Mutat. 2001;18:205-211.

192. Obermayer-Straub P, Strassburg CP, Manns MP. Autoimmune polyglandular syndrome type 1. Clin Rev Allergy Immunol. 2000;18:167-183.

193. Rizzi M, Ferrera F, Filaci G, Indiveri F. Disruption of immunological tolerance: Role of AIRE gene in autoimmunity. Autoimmun Rev. 2006;5:145-147.

194. Grimbacher B, Holland SM, Puck JM. Hyper-IgE syndromes. Immunol Rev. 2005;203:244-250.

195. Buckley RH. The hyper-IgE syndrome. Clin Rev Allergy Immunol. 2001;20:139-154.

196. Grimbacher B, Holland SM, Gallin JI, et al. Hyper-IgE syndrome with recurrent infections—an autosomal dominant multisystem disorder. N Engl J Med. 1999;340:692-702.

197. Freeman AF, Davis J, Anderson VL, et al. *Pneumocystis jiroveci* infection in patients with hyper-immunoglobulin E syndrome. Pediatrics. 2006;118:e1271-e1275.

198. Kashef MA, Kashef S, Handjani F, Karimi M. Hodgkin lymphoma developing in a 4.5-year-old girl with hyper-IgE syndrome. Pediatr Hematol Oncol. 2006;23:59-63.

199. Onal IK, Kurt M, Altundag K, et al. Peripheral T-cell lymphoma and Job's syndrome: a rare association. Med Oncol. 2006;23:141-144.

200. Sagiv-Friedgut K, Witzling M, Dalal I, et al. Congenital patent ductus venosus: An association with the hyper IgE syndrome. J Pediatr. 2007;150:210-212.

201. Van der Meer JW, Weemaes CM, van Krieken JH, et al. Critical aneurysmal dilatation of the thoracic aorta in young adolescents with variant hyperimmunoglobulin E syndrome. J Intern Med. 2006;259:615-618.

202. Ling JC, Freeman AF, Gharib AM, et al. Coronary artery aneurysms in patients with hyper IgE recurrent infection syndrome. Clin Immunol. 2007;122:255-258.

203. Grimbacher B, Schaffer AA, Holland SM, et al. Genetic linkage of hyper-IgE syndrome to chromosome 4. Am J Hum Genet. 1999;65:735-744.

204. Gennery AR, Flood TJ, Abinun M, Cant AJ. Bone marrow transplantation does not correct the hyper IgE syndrome. Bone Marrow Transplant. 2000;25:1303-1305.

205. Wakim M, Alazard M, Yajima A, et al. High dose intravenous immunoglobulin in atopic dermatitis and hyper-IgE syndrome. Ann Allergy Asthma Immunol. 1998;81:153-158.

206. Pung YH, Vetro SW, Bellanti JA. Use of interferons in atopic (IgE-mediated) diseases. Ann Allergy. 1993;71:234-238.

207. King CL, Gallin JI, Malech HL, et al. Regulation of immunoglobulin production in hyperimmunoglobulin E recurrent-infection syndrome by interferon gamma. Proc Natl Acad Sci U S A. 1989;86:10085-10089.

208. Kimata H. High-dose intravenous gamma-globulin treatment for hyperimmunoglobulinemia E syndrome. J Allergy Clin Immunol. 1995;95:771-774.

209. Kilic SS, Kilicbay F. Interferon-alpha treatment of molluscum contagiosum in a patient with hyperimmunoglobulin E syndrome. Pediatrics. 2006;117:e1253-e1255.

210. Renner ED, Puck JM, Holland SM, et al. Autosomal recessive hyperimmunoglobulin E syndrome: a distinct disease entity. J Pediatr. 2004;144:93-99.

211. Watford WT, O'Shea JJ. Human TYK2 kinase deficiency: another primary immunodeficiency syndrome. Immunity. 2006;25:695-697.

212. Minegishi Y, Saito M, Morio T, et al. Human tyrosine kinase 2 deficiency reveals its requisite roles in multiple cytokine signals involved in innate and acquired immunity. Immunity. 2006;25:745-755.

213. Doffinger R, Patel SY, Kumararatne DS. Host genetic factors and mycobacterial infections: lessons from single gene disorders affecting innate and adaptive immunity. Microbes Infect. 2006;8:1141-1150.

214. Rosenzweig SD, Holland SM. Defects in the interferon-gamma and interleukin-12 pathways. Immunol Rev. 2005;203:38-47.

215. Dorman SE, Picard C, Lammas D, et al. Clinical features of dominant and recessive interferon gamma receptor 1 deficiencies. Lancet. 2004;364:2113-2121.

216. Remus N, Reichenbach J, Picard C, et al. Impaired interferon gamma–mediated immunity and susceptibility to mycobacterial infection in childhood. Pediatr Res. 2001;50:8-13.

217. Zerbe CS, Holland SM. Disseminated histoplasmosis in persons with interferon-gamma receptor 1 deficiency. Clin Infect Dis. 2005;41:e38-e41.

218. Remiszewski P, Roszkowska-Sliz B, Winek J, et al. Disseminated *Mycobacterium avium* infection in a 20-year-old

female with partial recessive IFNγR1 deficiency. Respiration. 2006;73:375-378.

219. Rosenzweig SD, Holland SM. Congenital defects in the interferon-gamma/interleukin-12 pathway. Curr Opin Pediatr. 2004;16:3-8.

220. van de Vosse E, Lichtenauer-Kaligis EG, van Dissel JT, Ottenhoff TH. Genetic variations in the interleukin-12/interleukin-23 receptor (β1) chain, and implications for IL-12 and IL-23 receptor structure and function. Immunogenetics. 2003;54:817-829.

221. Picard C, Fieschi C, Altare F, et al. Inherited interleukin-12 deficiency: IL12β genotype and clinical phenotype of 13 patients from six kindreds. Am J Hum Genet. 2002; 70:336-348.

222. Sakai T, Matsuoka M, Aoki M, et al. Missense mutation of the interleukin-12 receptor β1 chain–encoding gene is associated with impaired immunity against *Mycobacterium avium* complex infection. Blood. 2001;97:2688-2694.

223. Gollob JA, Veenstra KG, Jyonouchi H, et al. Impairment of STAT activation by IL-12 in a patient with atypical mycobacterial and staphylococcal infections. J Immunol. 2000;165:4120-4126.

224. Reuter U, Roesler J, Thiede C, et al. Correction of complete interferon-gamma receptor 1 deficiency by bone marrow transplantation. Blood. 2002;100:4234-4235.

225. Ming JE, Stiehm ER, Graham JM Jr. Syndromic immunodeficiencies: genetic syndromes associated with immune abnormalities. Crit Rev Clin Lab Sci. 2003;40:587-642.

226. Seymour B, Miles J, Haeney M. Primary antibody deficiency and diagnostic delay. J Clin Pathol. 2005;58:546-547.

227. Orange JS, Hossny EM, Weiler CR, et al. Use of intravenous immunoglobulin in human disease: a review of evidence by members of the Primary Immunodeficiency Committee of the American Academy of Allergy, Asthma and Immunology. J Allergy Clin Immunol. 2006;117:S525-S553.

228. Berger M. Subcutaneous immunoglobulin replacement in primary immunodeficiencies. Clin Immunol. 2004;112:1-7.

229. Gardulf A, Nicolay U, Asensio O, et al. Rapid subcutaneous IgG replacement therapy is effective and safe in children and adults with primary immunodeficiencies—a prospective, multi-national study. J Clin Immunol. 2006;26:177-185.

230. Gardulf A, Nicolay U, Math D, et al. Children and adults with primary antibody deficiencies gain quality of life by subcutaneous IgG self-infusions at home. J Allergy Clin Immunol. 2004;114:936-942.

231. Nicolay U, Kiessling P, Berger M, et al. Health-related quality of life and treatment satisfaction in North American patients with primary immunodeficiency diseases receiving subcutaneous IgG self-infusions at home. J Clin Immunol. 2006;26:65-72.

232. Bruton OC. Agammaglobulinemia. Pediatrics. 1952;9:722-728.

233. Conley ME, Broides A, Hernandez-Trujillo V, et al. Genetic analysis of patients with defects in early B-cell development. Immunol Rev. 2005;203:216-234.

234. Stewart DM, Lian L, Nelson DL. The clinical spectrum of Bruton's agammaglobulinemia. Curr Allergy Asthma Rep. 2001;1:558-565.

235. Alibrahim A, Lepore M, Lierl M, et al. *Pneumocystis carinii* pneumonia in an infant with X-linked agammaglobulinemia. J Allergy Clin Immunol. 1998;101:552-553.

236. Lindvall JM, Blomberg KE, Valiaho J, et al. Bruton's tyrosine kinase: cell biology, sequence conservation, mutation spectrum, siRNA modifications, and expression profiling. Immunol Rev. 2005;203:200-215.

237. Valiaho J, Smith CI, Vihinen M. Btkbase: the mutation database for X-linked agammaglobulinemia. Hum Mutat. 2006;27:1209-1217.

238. Broides A, Yang W, Conley ME. Genotype/phenotype correlations in X-linked agammaglobulinemia. Clin Immunol. 2006;118:195-200.

239. Lopez-Granados E, Perez de Diego R, Ferreira Cerdan A, et al. A genotype-phenotype correlation study in a group of 54 patients with X-linked agammaglobulinemia. J Allergy Clin Immunol. 2005;116:690-697.

240. Kaneko H, Kawamoto N, Asano T, et al. Leaky phenotype of X-linked agammaglobulinaemia in a Japanese family. Clin Exp Immunol. 2005;140:520-523.

241. Shinomiya N, Kanegane H, Watanabe A, et al. Point mutation in intron 11 of Bruton's tyrosine kinase in atypical X-linked agammaglobulinemia. Pediatr Int. 2000;42:689-692.

242. Stewart DM, Tian L, Nelson DL. A case of X-linked agammaglobulinemia diagnosed in adulthood. Clin Immunol. 2001;99:94-99.

243. Allen RC, Nachtman RG, Rosenblatt HM, Belmont JW. Application of carrier testing to genetic counseling for X-linked agammaglobulinemia. Am J Hum Genet. 1994;54:25-35.

244. Quartier P, Debre M, De Blic J, et al. Early and prolonged intravenous immunoglobulin replacement therapy in childhood agammaglobulinemia: a retrospective survey of 31 patients. J Pediatr. 1999;134:589-596.

245. Howard V, Greene JM, Pahwa S, et al. The health status and quality of life of adults with X-linked agammaglobulinemia. Clin Immunol. 2006;118:201-208.

246. Stewart DM, Tian L, Notarangelo LD, Nelson DL. Update on X-linked hypogammaglobulinemia with isolated growth hormone deficiency. Curr Opin Allergy Clin Immunol. 2005;5:510-512.

247. Arslan D, Patiroglu T, Kendirci M, Kurtoglu S. X-linked agammaglobulinemia and isolated growth hormone deficiency. Turk J Pediatr. 1998;40:609-612.

248. Fleisher TA, White RM, Broder S, et al. X-linked hypogammaglobulinemia and isolated growth hormone deficiency. N Engl J Med. 1980;302:1429-1434.

249. Kubota K, Kim JY, Sawada A, et al. LRRC8 involved in B cell development belongs to a novel family of leucine-rich repeat proteins. FEBS Lett. 2004;564:147-152.

250. Sawada A, Takihara Y, Kim JY, et al. A congenital mutation of the novel gene LRRC8 causes agammaglobulinemia in humans. J Clin Invest. 2003;112:1707-1713.

251. Smits G, Kajava AV. LRRC8 extracellular domain is composed of 17 leucine-rich repeats. Mol Immunol. 2004;41:561-562.

252. Castigli E, Geha RS. Molecular basis of common variable immunodeficiency. J Allergy Clin Immunol. 2006;117:740-746; quiz 747.

253. Cunningham-Rundles C, Bodian C. Common variable immunodeficiency: Clinical and immunological features of 248 patients. Clin Immunol. 1999;92:34-48.

254. Wheat WH, Cool CD, Morimoto Y, et al. Possible role of human herpesvirus 8 in the lymphoproliferative disorders in common variable immunodeficiency. J Exp Med. 2005;202:479-484.

255. Knight AK, Cunningham-Rundles C. Inflammatory and autoimmune complications of common variable immune deficiency. Autoimmun Rev. 2006;5:156-159.

256. Brandt D, Gershwin ME. Common variable immune deficiency and autoimmunity. Autoimmun Rev. 2006;5:465-470.

257. Morimoto Y, Routes JM. Granulomatous disease in common variable immunodeficiency. Curr Allergy Asthma Rep. 2005;5:370-375.

258. Bates CA, Ellison MC, Lynch DA, et al. Granulomatous-lymphocytic lung disease shortens survival in common variable immunodeficiency. J Allergy Clin Immunol. 2004;114:415-421.

259. Cunningham-Rundles C, Lieberman P, Hellman G, Chaganti RS. Non-Hodgkin lymphoma in common variable immunodeficiency. Am J Hematol. 1991;37:69-74.

260. De Vera MJ, Al-Harthi L, Gewurz AT. Assessing thymopoiesis in patients with common variable immunodeficiency as measured by T-cell receptor excision circles. Ann Allergy Asthma Immunol. 2004;93:478-484.

261. Sneller MC, Strober W. Abnormalities of lymphokine gene expression in patients with common variable immunodeficiency. J Immunol. 1990;144:3762-3769.

262. Fischer MB, Hauber I, Vogel E, et al. Defective interleukin-2 and interferon-gamma gene expression in response to antigen in a subgroup of patients with common variable immunodeficiency. J Allergy Clin Immunol. 1993;92:340-352.

263. Eisenstein EM, Jaffe JS, Strober W. Reduced interleukin-2 (IL-2) production in common variable immunodeficiency is due to a primary abnormality of CD4+ T cell differentiation. J Clin Immunol. 1993;13:247-258.

264. Zhou Z, Huang R, Danon M, et al. IL-10 production in common variable immunodeficiency. Clin Immunol Immunopathol. 1998;86:298-304.

265. Serrano D, Becker K, Cunningham-Rundles C, Mayer L. Characterization of the T cell receptor repertoire in patients with common variable immunodeficiency: Oligoclonal expansion of CD8+ T cells. Clin Immunol. 2000;97:248-258.

266. Farrington M, Grosmaire LS, Nonoyama S, et al. CD40 ligand expression is defective in a subset of patients with common variable immunodeficiency. Proc Natl Acad Sci U S A. 1994;91:1099-1103.

267. Vlkova M, Thon V, Sarfyova M, et al. Age dependency and mutual relations in T and B lymphocyte abnormalities in common variable immunodeficiency patients. Clin Exp Immunol. 2006;143:373-379.

268. Viallard JF, Blanco P, Andre M, et al. CD8+HLA-DR+ T lymphocytes are increased in common variable immunodeficiency patients with impaired memory B-cell differentiation. Clin Immunol. 2006;119:51-58.

269. Moratto D, Gulino AV, Fontana S, et al. Combined decrease of defined B and T cell subsets in a group of common variable immunodeficiency patients. Clin Immunol. 2006;121:203-214.

270. Paccani SR, Boncristiano M, Patrussi L, et al. Defective VAV expression and impaired F-actin reorganization in a subset of patients with common variable immunodefi-

ciency characterized by T-cell defects. Blood. 2005;106:626-634.

271. Iglesias J, Matamoros N, Raga S, et al. CD95 expression and function on lymphocyte subpopulations in common variable immunodeficiency (CVID); related to increased apoptosis. Clin Exp Immunol. 1999;117:138-146.

272. Denz A, Eibel H, Illges H, et al. Impaired up-regulation of CD86 in B cells of "type a" common variable immunodeficiency patients. Eur J Immunol. 2000;30:1069-1077.

273. Taubenheim N, von Hornung M, Durandy A, et al. Defined blocks in terminal plasma cell differentiation of common variable immunodeficiency patients. J Immunol. 2005;175:5498-5503.

274. Scott-Taylor TH, Green MR, Raeiszadeh M, et al. Defective maturation of dendritic cells in common variable immunodeficiency. Clin Exp Immunol. 2006;145:420-427.

275. Viallard JF, Camou F, Andre M, et al. Altered dendritic cell distribution in patients with common variable immunodeficiency. Arthritis Res Ther. 2005;7:R1052-R1055.

276. Cunningham-Rundles C, Radigan L. Deficient IL-12 and dendritic cell function in common variable immune deficiency. Clin Immunol. 2005;115:147-153.

277. Bayry J, Lacroix-Desmazes S, Kazatchkine MD, et al. Common variable immunodeficiency is associated with defective functions of dendritic cells. Blood. 2004;104:2441-2443.

278. Cunningham-Rundles C, Radigan L, Knight AK, et al. TLR9 activation is defective in common variable immune deficiency. J Immunol. 2006;176:1978-1987.

279. Kilic SS, Kezer EY, Ilcol YO, et al. Vitamin A deficiency in patients with common variable immunodeficiency. J Clin Immunol. 2005;25:275-280.

280. Ferraroni NR, Geloneze B, Mansour E, et al. Severe hypoleptinaemia associated with insulin resistance in patients with common variable immunodeficiency. Clin Endocrinol (Oxf). 2005;63:63-65.

281. Goldberg AC, Eliaschewitz FG, Montor WR, et al. Exogenous leptin restores in vitro T cell proliferation and cytokine synthesis in patients with common variable immunodeficiency syndrome. Clin Immunol. 2005;114:147-153.

282. Agematsu K, Nagumo H, Shinozaki K, et al. Absence of IgD-CD27+ memory B cell population in X-linked hyper-IgM syndrome. J Clin Invest. 1998;102:853-860.

283. Ferry BL, Jones J, Bateman EA, et al. Measurement of peripheral B cell subpopulations in common variable immunodeficiency (CVID) using a whole blood method. Clin Exp Immunol. 2005;140:532-539.

284. Ko J, Radigan L, Cunningham-Rundles C. Immune competence and switched memory B cells in common variable immunodeficiency. Clin Immunol. 2005;116:37-41.

285. Piqueras B, Lavenu-Bombled C, Galicier L, et al. Common variable immunodeficiency patient classification based on impaired B cell memory differentiation correlates with clinical aspects. J Clin Immunol. 2003;23:385-400.

286. Warnatz K, Denz A, Drager R, et al. Severe deficiency of switched memory B cells (CD27+IgM-IgD-) in subgroups of patients with common variable immunodeficiency: a new approach to classify a heterogeneous disease. Blood. 2002;99:1544-1551.

287. Alachkar H, Taubenheim N, Haeney MR, et al. Memory switched B cell percentage and not serum immunoglobulin concentration is associated with clinical complications in children and adults with specific antibody deficiency and common variable immunodeficiency. Clin Immunol. 2006;120:310-318.

288. Carsetti R, Rosado MM, Donnanno S, et al. The loss of IgM memory B cells correlates with clinical disease in common variable immunodeficiency. J Allergy Clin Immunol. 2005;115:412-417.

289. Busse PJ, Razvi S, Cunningham-Rundles C. Efficacy of intravenous immunoglobulin in the prevention of pneumonia in patients with common variable immunodeficiency. J Allergy Clin Immunol. 2002;109:1001-1004.

290. Swierkot J, Lewandowicz-Uszynska A, Chlebicki A, et al. Rheumatoid arthritis in a patient with common variable immunodeficiency: difficulty in diagnosis and therapy. Clin Rheumatol. 2006;25:92-94.

291. Medlicott SA, Coderre S, Horne G, Panaccione R. Multimodal immunosuppressant therapy in steroid-refractory common variable immunodeficiency sprue: a case report complicating cytomegalovirus infection. Int J Surg Pathol. 2006;14:101-106.

292. Lin JH, Liebhaber M, Roberts RL, et al. Etanercept treatment of cutaneous granulomas in common variable immunodeficiency. J Allergy Clin Immunol. 2006;117:878-882.

293. Wang J, Cunningham-Rundles C. Treatment and outcome of autoimmune hematologic disease in common variable immunodeficiency (CVID). J Autoimmun. 2005;25:57-62.

294. Thatayatikom A, Thatayatikom S, White AJ. Infliximab treatment for severe granulomatous disease in common variable immunodeficiency: a case report and review of the literature. Ann Allergy Asthma Immunol. 2005;95:293-300.

295. Kanegane H, Tsukada S, Iwata T, et al. Detection of Bruton's tyrosine kinase mutations in hypogammaglobulinaemic males registered as common variable immunodeficiency (CVID) in the Japanese immunodeficiency registry. Clin Exp Immunol. 2000;120:512-517.

296. de Saint Basile G, Tabone MD, Durandy A, et al. CD40 ligand expression deficiency in a female carrier of the X-linked hyper-IgM syndrome as a result of X chromosome lyonization. Eur J Immunol. 1999;29:367-373.

297. Schroeder HW Jr, Schroeder HW 3rd, Sheikh SM. The complex genetics of common variable immunodeficiency. J Investig Med. 2004;52:90-103.

298. Vorechovsky I, Cullen M, Carrington M, et al. Fine mapping of IGAD1 in IgA deficiency and common variable immunodeficiency: identification and characterization of haplotypes shared by affected members of 101 multiple-case families. J Immunol. 2000;164:4408-4416.

299. Schroeder HW. Genetics of IgA deficiency and common variable immunodeficiency. Clin Rev Allergy Immunol. 2000;19:127-140.

300. Finck A, Van der Meer JW, Schaffer AA, et al. Linkage of autosomal-dominant common variable immunodeficiency to chromosome 4q. Eur J Hum Genet. 2006;14:867-875.

301. Salzer U, Maul-Pavicic A, Cunningham-Rundles C, et al. ICOS deficiency in patients with common variable immunodeficiency. Clin Immunol. 2004;113:234-240.

302. Warnatz K, Bossaller L, Salzer U, et al. Human ICOS deficiency abrogates the germinal center reaction and provides a monogenic model for common variable immunodeficiency. Blood. 2006;107:3045-3052.

303. Salzer U, Grimbacher B. Common variable immunodeficiency: The power of co-stimulation. Semin Immunol. 2006;18:337-346.

304. Rachid R, Castigli E, Geha RS, Bonilla FA. TACI mutation in common variable immunodeficiency and IgA deficiency. Curr Allergy Asthma Rep. 2006;6:357-362.

305. Salzer U, Chapel HM, Webster AD, et al. Mutations in TNFRSF13B encoding TACI are associated with common variable immunodeficiency in humans. Nat Genet. 2005;37:820-828.

306. Castigli E, Wilson SA, Garibyan L, et al. TACI is mutant in common variable immunodeficiency and IgA deficiency. Nat Genet. 2005;37:829-834.

307. Losi CG, Salzer U, Gatta R, et al. Mutational analysis of human BLYS in patients with common variable immunodeficiency. J Clin Immunol. 2006;26:396-399.

308. van Zelm MC, Reisli I, van der Burg M, et al. An antibody-deficiency syndrome due to mutations in the CD19 gene. N Engl J Med. 2006;354:1901-1912.

309. Ropars C, Muller A, Paint N, et al. Large scale detection of IgA deficient blood donors. J Immunol Methods. 1982;54:183-189.

310. Kanoh T, Mizumoto T, Yasuda N, et al. Selective IgA deficiency in Japanese blood donors: frequency and statistical analysis. Vox Sang. 1986;50:81-86.

311. Koskinen S, Tolo H, Hirvonen M, Koistinen J. Long-term follow-up of anti-IgA antibodies in healthy IgA-deficient adults. J Clin Immunol. 1995;15:194-198.

312. Cunningham-Rundles C. Physiology of IgA and IgA deficiency. J Clin Immunol. 2001;21:303-309.

313. Johnson ML, Keeton LG, Zhu ZB, et al. Age-related changes in serum immunoglobulins in patients with familial IgA deficiency and common variable immunodeficiency (CVID). Clin Exp Immunol. 1997;108:477-483.

314. Espanol T, Catala M, Hernandez M, et al. Development of a common variable immunodeficiency in IgA-deficient patients. Clin Immunol Immunopathol. 1996;80:333-335.

315. Edwards E, Razvi S, Cunningham-Rundles C. IgA deficiency: clinical correlates and responses to pneumococcal vaccine. Clin Immunol. 2004;111:93-97.

316. Santaella ML, Peredo R, Disdier OM. IgA deficiency: clinical correlates with IgG subclass and mannan-binding lectin deficiencies. P R Health Sci J. 2005;24:107-110.

317. Schroeder HW Jr, Zhu ZB, March RE, et al. Susceptibility locus for IgA deficiency and common variable immunodeficiency in the HLA-DR3, -B8, -A1 haplotypes. Mol Med. 1998;4:72-86.

318. Alper CA, Marcus-Bagley D, Awdeh Z, et al. Prospective analysis suggests susceptibility genes for deficiencies of IgA and several other immunoglobulins on the [HLA-B8, SC01, DR3] conserved extended haplotype. Tissue Antigens. 2000;56:207-216.

319. Vorechovsky I, Webster AD, Plebani A, Hammarstrom L. Genetic linkage of IgA deficiency to the major histocompatibility complex: evidence for allele segregation distortion, parent-of-origin penetrance differences, and the role of anti-IgA antibodies in disease predisposition. Am J Hum Genet. 1999;64:1096-1109.

320. Reil A, Bein G, Machulla HK, et al. High-resolution DNA typing in immunoglobulin A deficiency confirms a positive association with DRB1*0301, DQB1*02 haplotypes. Tissue Antigens. 1997;50:501-506.

321. Fiore M, Pera C, Delfino L, et al. DNA typing of DQ and DR alleles in IgA-deficient subjects. Eur J Immunogenet. 1995;22:403-411.

322. Hammarstrom L, Vorechovsky I, Webster D. Selective IgA deficiency (SIGAD) and common variable immunodeficiency (CVID). Clin Exp Immunol. 2000;120:225-231.

323. Ferrante A, Beard LJ, Feldman RG. IgG subclass distribution of antibodies to bacterial and viral antigens. Pediatr Infect Dis J. 1990;9:S16-S24.

324. Umetsu DT, Ambrosino DM, Geha RS. Children with selective IgG subclass deficiency and recurrent sinopulmonary infection: impaired response to bacterial capsular polysaccharide antigens. Monogr Allergy. 1986;20:57-61.

325. De Gracia J, Rodrigo MJ, Morell F, et al. IgG subclass deficiencies associated with bronchiectasis. Am J Respir Crit Care Med. 1996;153:650-655.

326. Masin JS, Hostoffer RW, Arnold JE. Otitis media following tympanostomy tube placement in children with IgG2 deficiency. Laryngoscope. 1995;105:1188-1190.

327. Barlan IB, Geha RS, Schneider LC. Therapy for patients with recurrent infections and low serum IgG3 levels. J Allergy Clin Immunol. 1993;92:353-355.

328. Schur PH. IgG human subclasses—a review. Ann Allergy. 1987;58:89-96, 99.

329. Tashita H, Fukao T, Kaneko H, et al. Molecular basis of selective IgG2 deficiency. The mutated membrane-bound form of γ2 heavy chain caused complete IgG2 deficiency in two Japanese siblings. J Clin Invest. 1998;101:677-681.

330. Lefranc MP, Hammarstrom L, Smith CI, Lefranc G. Gene deletions in the human immunoglobulin heavy chain constant region locus: molecular and immunological analysis. Immunodefic Rev. 1991;2:265-281.

331. Plebani A, Ugazio AG, Meini A, et al. Extensive deletion of immunoglobulin heavy chain constant region genes in the absence of recurrent infections: When is IgG subclass deficiency clinically relevant? Clin Immunol Immunopathol. 1993;68:46-50.

332. Olsson PG, Hofker MH, Walter MA, et al. Ig h chain variable and c region genes in common variable immunodeficiency. Characteristics of two new deletion haplotypes. J Immunol. 1991;147:2540-2546.

333. Javier FC 3rd, Moore CM, Sorensen RU. Distribution of primary immunodeficiency diseases diagnosed in a pediatric tertiary hospital. Ann Allergy Asthma Immunol. 2000;84:25-30.

334. Chapel HM, Spickett GP, Ericson D, et al. The comparison of the efficacy and safety of intravenous versus subcutaneous immunoglobulin replacement therapy. J Clin Immunol. 2000;20:94-100.

335. Ortigas AP, Leiva LE, Moore C, et al. Natural history of specific antibody deficiency after IgG replacement therapy. Ann Allergy Asthma Immunol. 1999;82:71.

336. Sorensen RU, Leiva LE, Javier FC 3rd, et al. Influence of age on the response to *Streptococcus pneumoniae* vaccine in patients with recurrent infections and normal immunoglobulin concentrations. J Allergy Clin Immunol. 1998;102:215-221.

337. Shrimpton A, Duddridge M, Ziegler-Heitbrock L. Vaccination with polysaccharide-conjugate-vaccines in adult patients with specific antibody deficiency. Vaccine. 2006;24:3574-3580.

338. Schwartz HJ, Hostoffer RW, McFadden ER Jr, Berger M. The response to intravenous immunoglobulin replacement therapy in patients with asthma with specific antibody deficiency. Allergy Asthma Proc. 2006;27:53-58.

339. Whelan MA, Hwan WH, Beausoleil J, et al. Infants presenting with recurrent infections and low immunoglobulins: characteristics and analysis of normalization. J Clin Immunol. 2006;26:7-11.

340. Dorsey MJ, Orange JS. Impaired specific antibody response and increased B-cell population in transient hypogammaglobulinemia of infancy. Ann Allergy Asthma Immunol. 2006;97:590-595.

341. Kidon MI, Handzel ZT, Schwartz R, et al. Symptomatic hypogammaglobulinemia in infancy and childhood—clinical outcome and in vitro immune responses. BMC Fam Pract. 2004;5:23.

342. Kilic SS, Tezcan I, Sanal O, et al. Transient hypogammaglobulinemia of infancy: clinical and immunologic features of 40 new cases. Pediatr Int. 2000;42:647-650.

343. Dalal I, Reid B, Nisbet-Brown E, Roifman CM. The outcome of patients with hypogammaglobulinemia in infancy and early childhood. J Pediatr. 1998;133:144-146.

344. Walport MJ. Complement. First of two parts. N Engl J Med. 2001;344:1058-1066.

345. Walport MJ. Complement. Second of two parts. N Engl J Med. 2001;344:1140-1144.

346. Wen L, Atkinson JP, Giclas PC. Clinical and laboratory evaluation of complement deficiency. J Allergy Clin Immunol. 2004;113:585-593; quiz 594.

347. Pickering MC, Walport MJ. Links between complement abnormalities and systemic lupus erythematosus. Rheumatology (Oxf). 2000;39:133-141.

348. Hannema AJ, Kluin-Nelemans JC, Hack CE, et al. SLE-like syndromes and functional deficiency of C1q in members of a large family. Clin Exp Immunol. 1984;55:106-114.

349. Endo Y, Kanno K, Takahashi M, et al. Molecular basis of human complement C1s deficiency. J Immunol. 1999;162:2180-2183.

350. Inoue N, Saito T, Masuda R, et al. Selective complement C1s deficiency caused by homozygous four-base deletion in the C1s gene. Hum Genet. 1998;103:415-418.

351. Loos M, Heinz H. Component deficiencies. I. The first component: C1q, C1r, C1s. Prog Allergy. 1986;39:212-231.

352. Alper CA, Xu J, Cosmopulos K, et al. Immunoglobulin deficiencies and susceptibility to infection among homozygotes and heterozygotes for C2 deficiency. J Clin Immunol. 2003;23:297-305.

353. Antolin SC, Del Rey Cerros MJ, Sierra EM, et al. Frequency in Spanish population of familial complement factor 2 type I deficits and associated HLA haplotypes. Hum Immunol. 2005;66:1093-1098.

354. Jonsson G, Truedsson L, Sturfelt G, et al. Hereditary C2 deficiency in Sweden: frequent occurrence of invasive infection, atherosclerosis, and rheumatic disease. Medicine (Baltimore). 2005;84:23-34.

355. Litzman J, Freiberger T, Bartonkova D, et al. Early manifestation and recognition of C2 complement deficiency in the form of pyogenic infection in infancy. J Paediatr Child Health. 2003;39:274-277.

356. Lhotta K, Wurzner R, Rumpelt HJ, et al. Membranous nephropathy in a patient with hereditary complete complement C4 deficiency. Nephrol Dial Transplant. 2004;19:990-993.

357. Yang Y, Chung EK, Zhou B, et al. The intricate role of complement component C4 in human systemic lupus erythematosus. Curr Dir Autoimmun. 2004;7:98-132.

358. Yang Y, Lhotta K, Chung EK, et al. Complete complement components C4a and C4b deficiencies in human kidney diseases and systemic lupus erythematosus. J Immunol. 2004;173:2803-2814.

359. Hauptmann G, Tappeiner G, Schifferli JA. Inherited deficiency of the fourth component of human complement. Immunodef Rev. 1988;1:3-22.

360. Fielder AHL, Walport MJ, Batchelor HR, et al. Family study of the major histocompatibility complex in patients with systemic lupus erythematosus: importance of null alleles of C4a and C4b in determining disease susceptibility. BMJ. 1983;286:425-428.

361. Schaffer FM, Palermos J, Zhu ZB, et al. Individuals with IgA deficiency and common variable immunodeficiency share polymorphisms of major histocompatibility complex class III genes. Proc Natl Acad Sci U S A. 1989;86:8015-8019.

362. Stefansson Thors V, Kolka R, Sigurdardottir SL, et al. Increased frequency of C4b*q0 alleles in patients with Henoch-Schönlein purpura. Scand J Immunol. 2005;61:274-278.

363. Hartmann D, Fremeaux-Bacchi V, Weiss L, et al. Combined heterozygous deficiency of the classical complement pathway proteins C2 and C4. J Clin Immunol. 1997;17:176-184.

364. Pickering MC, Botto M, Taylor PR, et al. Systemic lupus erythematosus, complement deficiency, and apoptosis. Adv Immunol. 2000;76:227-324.

365. Fearon DT, Carroll MC. Regulation of B lymphocyte responses to foreign and self-antigens by the CD19/CD21 complex. Annu Rev Immunol. 2000;18:393-422.

366. Katz Y, Singer L, Wetsel RA, et al. Inherited complement C3 deficiency: a defect in C3 secretion. Eur J Immunol. 1994;24:1517-1522.

367. Singer L, Van Hee ML, Lokki ML, et al. Inherited complement C3 deficiency: reduced C3 mRNA and protein levels in a Laotian kindred. Clin Immunol Immunopathol. 1996;81:244-252.

368. Singer L, Whitehead WT, Akama H, et al. Inherited human complement C3 deficiency. An amino acid substitution in the beta-chain (Asp549 to Asn) impairs C3 secretion. J Biol Chem. 1994;269:28494-28499.

369. Winkelstein JA, Childs B. Why do some individuals have more infections than others? JAMA. 2001;285:1348-1349.

370. Fijen CA, van den Bogaard R, Schipper M, et al. Properdin deficiency: molecular basis and disease association. Mol Immunol. 1999;36:863-867.

371. Genel F, Atlihan F, Gulez N, et al. Properdin deficiency in a boy with fulminant meningococcal septic shock. Acta Paediatr. 2006;95:1498-1500.

372. Gelfand EW, Rao CP, Minta JO, Ham T. Inherited deficiency of properdin and C2 in a patient with recurrent bacteremia. Am J Med. 1987;82:671-675.

373. Bathum L, Hansen H, Teisner B, et al. Association between combined properdin and mannose-binding lectin deficiency and infection with *Neisseria meningitidis*. Mol Immunol. 2006;43:473-479.

374. Hiemstra PS, Langeler E, Compier N, et al. Complete and partial deficiencies of complement factor D in a Dutch family. J Clin Invest. 1989;84:1957-1961.

375. Sprong T, Roos D, Weemaes C, et al. Deficient alternative complement pathway activation due to factor D deficiency by 2 novel mutations in the complement factor D gene in a family with meningococcal infections. Blood. 2006;107:4865-4870.

376. Kluin-Nelemans HC, van VelzenBlad H, van Helden HP, Daha MR. Functional deficiency of complement factor d in a monzygous twin. Clin Exp Immunol. 1984;58:724-730.

377. Weiss SJ, Ahmed AE, Bonagura VR. Complement factor D deficiency in an infant first seen with pneumococcal neonatal sepsis. J Allergy Clin Immunol. 1998;102:1043-1044.

378. Sim RB, Clark H, Hajela K, Mayilyan KR. Collectins and host defence. Novartis Found Symp. 2006;279:170-181; discussion 181-176, 216-179.

379. Thiel S, Vorup-Jensen T, Stover CM, et al. A second serine protease associated with mannan-binding lectin that activates complement. Nature. 1997;386:506-510.

380. Turner MW, Hamvas RM. Mannose-binding lectin: structure, function, genetics and disease associations. Rev Immunogenet. 2000;2:305-322.

381. Thiel S, Frederiksen PD, Jensenius JC. Clinical manifestations of mannan-binding lectin deficiency. Mol Immunol. 2006;43:86-96.

382. Wallis R, Lynch NJ, Roscher S, Reid KB and Schwaeble WJ. Decoupling of carbohydrate binding and MASP-2 autoactivation in variant mannose-binding lectins associated with immunodeficiency. J Immunol. 2005;175:6846-6851.

383. Cedzynski M, Szemraj J, Swierzko AS, et al. Mannan-binding lectin insufficiency in children with recurrent infections of the respiratory system. Clin Exp Immunol. 2004;136:304-311.

384. Gong MN, Zhou W, Williams PL, et al. Polymorphisms in the mannose binding lectin-2 gene and acute respiratory distress syndrome. Crit Care Med. 2007;35:48-56.

385. Fevang B, Mollnes TE, Holm AM, et al. Common variable immunodeficiency and the complement system; low mannose-binding lectin levels are associated with bronchiectasis. Clin Exp Immunol. 2005;142:576-584.

386. Mulligan CG, Marshall SE, Welsh KI. Mannose binding lectin polymorphisms are associated with early age of disease onset and autoimmunity in common variable immunodeficiency. Scand J Immunol. 2000;51:111-122.

387. Petersen KA, Matthiesen F, Agger T, et al. Phase I safety, tolerability, and pharmacokinetic study of recombinant human mannan-binding lectin. J Clin Immunol. 2006;26:465-475.

388. Sorensen R, Thiel S, Jensenius JC. Mannan-binding-lectin–associated serine proteases, characteristics and disease associations. Springer Semin Immunopathol. 2005;27:299-319.

389. Thiel S, Steffensen R, Christensen IJ, et al. Deficiency of mannan-binding lectin associated serine protease-2 due to missense polymorphisms. Genes Immun. 2007;8:154-163.

390. Stengaard-Pedersen K, Thiel S, Gadjeva M, et al. Inherited deficiency of mannan-binding lectin–associated serine protease 2. N Engl J Med. 2003;349:554-560.

391. Asghar SS, Venneker GT, van Meegen M, et al. Hereditary deficiency of C5 in association with discoid lupus erythematosus. J Am Acad Dermatol. 1991;24:376-378.

392. Delgado-Cervino E, Fontan G, Lopez-Trascasa M. C5 complement deficiency in a Spanish family. Molecular characterization of the double mutation responsible for the defect. Mol Immunol. 2005;42:105-111.

393. Ikinciogullari A, Tekin M, Dogu F, et al. Meningococcal meningitis and complement component 6 deficiency associated with oculocutaneous albinism. Eur J Pediatr. 2005;164:177-179.

394. Orren A, Potter PC. Complement component C6 deficiency and susceptibility to Neisseria meningitidis infections. S Afr Med J. 2004;94:345-346.

395. Barroso S, Rieubland C, Jose Alvarez A, et al. Molecular defects of the C7 gene in two patients with complement C7 deficiency. Immunology. 2006;118:257-260.

396. Barroso S, Sanchez B, Alvarez AJ, et al. Complement component C7 deficiency in two Spanish families. Immunology. 2004;113:518-523.

397. Behar D, Schlesinger M, Halle D, et al. C7 complement deficiency in an Israeli Arab village. Am J Med Genet. 2002;110:25-29.

398. Kang HJ, Ki CS, Kim YS, et al. Two mutations of the C7 gene, C.1424g → a and C.281-1g → t, in two Korean families. J Clin Immunol. 2006;26:186-191.

399. Morgan BP, Vora JP, Bennett JA, et al. A case of hereditary combined deficiency of complement components C6 and C7 in man. Clin Exp Immunol. 1989;83:43-47.

400. Zhu Z, Atkinson TP, Hovanky KT, et al. High prevalence of complement component C6 deficiency among African-Americans in the south-eastern USA. Clin Exp Immunol. 2000;119:305-310.

401. Orren A. Molecular mechanisms of complement component C6 deficiency; a hypervariable exon 6 region responsible for three of six reported defects [editorial]. Clin Exp Immunol. 2000;119:255-258.

402. Halle D, Elstein D, Geudalia D, et al. High prevalence of complement C7 deficiency among healthy blood donors of Moroccan Jewish ancestry. Am J Med Genet. 2001;99:325-327.

403. Rosa DD, Pasqualotto AC, de Quadros M, Prezzi SH. Deficiency of the eighth component of complement associated with recurrent meningococcal meningitis—case report and literature review. Braz J Infect Dis. 2004;8:328-330.

404. Tedesco F. Component deficiencies 8: the eighth component. Prog Allergy. 1986;39:295-306.

405. Kang HJ, Kim HS, Lee YK, Cho HC. High incidence of complement C9 deficiency in Koreans. Ann Clin Lab Sci. 2005;35:144-148.

406. Khajoee V, Ihara K, Kira R, et al. Founder effect of the C9 R95X mutation in Orientals. Hum Genet. 2003;112:244-248.

407. Orren A, O'Hara AM, Morgan BP, et al. An abnormal but functionally active complement component C9 protein found in an Irish family with subtotal C9 deficiency. Immunology. 2003;108:384-390.

408. Kanda E, Shimamura H, Tamura H, et al. IgA nephropathy with complement deficiency. Intern Med. 2001;40:52-55.

409. Ichikawa E, Furuta J, Kawachi Y, et al. Hereditary complement (C9) deficiency associated with dermatomyositis. Br J Dermatol. 2001;144:1080-1083.

410. Fijen CA, Bredius RG, Kuijper EJ, et al. The role of Fcγ receptor polymorphisms and C3 in the immune defence against Neisseria meningitidis in complement-deficient individuals. Clin Exp Immunol. 2000;120:338-345.

411. Frank MM. Hereditary angioedema: The clinical syndrome and its management in the United States. Immunol Allergy Clin North Am. 2006;26:653-668.

412. Visy B, Fust G, Varga L, et al. Sex hormones in hereditary angioneurotic oedema. Clin Endocrinol (Oxf). 2004;60:508-515.

413. Cicardi M, Zingale L, Zanichelli A, et al. C1 inhibitor: molecular and clinical aspects. Springer Semin Immunopathol. 2005;27:286-298.

414. Davis AE 3rd. The pathophysiology of hereditary angioedema. Clin Immunol. 2005;114:3-9.

415. Davis AE 3rd. Mechanism of angioedema in first complement component inhibitor deficiency. Immunol Allergy Clin North Am. 2006;26:633-651.

416. Roche O, Blanch A, Duponchel C, et al. Hereditary angioedema: the mutation spectrum of SERPIN1/C1NH in a large Spanish cohort. Hum Mutat. 2005;26:135-144.

417. Blanch A, Roche O, Urrutia I, et al. First case of homozygous C1 inhibitor deficiency. J Allergy Clin Immunol. 2006;118:1330-1335.

418. Bowen T, Cicardi M, Farkas H, et al. Canadian 2003 international consensus algorithm for the diagnosis, therapy, and management of hereditary angioedema. J Allergy Clin Immunol. 2004;114:629-637.

419. Boyle RJ, Nikpour M, Tang ML. Hereditary angio-oedema in children: A management guideline. Pediatr Allergy Immunol. 2005;16:288-294.

420. Gompels MM, Lock RJ, Abinun M, et al. C1 inhibitor deficiency: consensus document. Clin Exp Immunol. 2005;139:379-394.

421. Zuraw BL. Diagnosis and management of hereditary angioedema: an American approach. Transfus Apher Sci. 2003;29:239-245.

422. Longhurst HJ, Carr S, Khair K. C1-inhibitor concentrate home therapy for hereditary angioedema: a viable, effective treatment option. Clin Exp Immunol. 2007;147:11-17.

423. Zuraw BL. Novel therapies for hereditary angioedema. Immunol Allergy Clin North Am. 2006;26:691-708.

424. Zingale LC, Castelli R, Zanichelli A, Cicardi M. Acquired deficiency of the inhibitor of the first complement component: presentation, diagnosis, course, and conventional management. Immunol Allergy Clin North Am. 2006;26:669-690.

425. Bouillet-Claveyrolas L, Ponard D, Drouet C, Massot C. Clinical and biological distinctions between type I and type II acquired angioedema. Am J Med. 2003;115:420-421.

426. Ponce IM, Caballero T, Reche M, et al. Polyclonal auto-antibodies against C1 inhibitor in a case of acquired

angioedema. Ann Allergy Asthma Immunol. 2002;88: 632-637.

427. Genel F, Sjoholm AG, Skattum L, Truedsson L. Complement factor I deficiency associated with recurrent infections, vasculitis and immune complex glomerulonephritis. Scand J Infect Dis. 2005;37:615-618.

428. Gonzalez-Rubio C, Ferreira-Cerdan A, Ponce IM, et al. Complement factor I deficiency associated with recurrent meningitis coinciding with menstruation. Arch Neurol. 2001;58:1923-1928.

429. Grumach AS, Leitao MF, Arruk VG, et al. Recurrent infections in partial complement factor I deficiency: evaluation of three generations of a Brazilian family. Clin Exp Immunol. 2006;143:297-304.

430. Sadallah S, Gudat F, Laissue JA, et al. Glomerulonephritis in a patient with complement factor I deficiency. Am J Kidney Dis. 1999;33:1153-1157.

431. Teisner B, Brandslund I, Folkerson J, et al. Factor I deficiency and C3 nephritic factor: Immunochemical findings and association with *Neisseria meningitidis* infection in two patients. Scand J Immunol. 1984;20:291-297.

432. Levy M, Halbwachs-Mecarelli L, Gubler M-C, et al. H deficiency in two brothers with atypical dense intramembranous deposit disease. Kidney Int. 1986;30:949-956.

433. Nielsen HE, Christensen KC, Koch C, et al. Hereditary, complete deficiency of complement factor H associated with recurrent meningococal disease. Scand J Immunol. 1989;30:711-718.

434. Buddles MR, Donne RL, Richards A, et al. Complement factor H gene mutation associated with autosomal recessive atypical hemolytic uremic syndrome. Am J Hum Genet. 2000;66:1721-1722.

435. Landau D, Shalev H, Levy-Finer G, et al. Familial hemolytic uremic syndrome associated with complement factor H deficiency. J Pediatr. 2001;138:412-417.

436. Warwicker P, Goodship TH, Donne RL, et al. Genetic studies into inherited and sporadic hemolytic uremic syndrome. Kidney Int. 1998;53:836-844.

437. Costabile M, Quach A, Ferrante A. Molecular approaches in the diagnosis of primary immunodeficiency diseases. Hum Mutat. 2006;27:1163-1173.

IX Storage Diseases

Storage Diseases of the Reticuloendothelial System

24 Storage Diseases of the Reticuloendothelial System

Alessandra d'Azzo, Edwin H. Kolodny, Erik Bonten, and Ida Annunziata

Lysosomal storage disease (LSDs) comprise a large group of congenital disorders of metabolism caused by impaired lysosomal function. These diseases are heterogeneous in nature and have a broad range of clinical manifestations that affect systemic organs and the nervous system to a different extent. At the cellular level, dramatic morphologic changes can be readily identified in circulating blood and the reticuloendothelial system. Such changes include pancytopenia, vacuolization of mononuclear cells, storage of foam cells, and enlargement of the liver, spleen, and lymph nodes.

The majority of the LSDs are caused by deficiency of a single lysosomal hydrolase, which underscores the lack of redundancy for these enzymes and their importance in maintaining cell homeostasis. Consequently, products of cellular metabolism that are ordinarily degraded by these enzymes remain undigested, overload the lysosomes, and cause severe disruption of cellular architecture.

LSDs have been the object of intensive study by clinician, biochemists, geneticists, and molecular biologists. Their investigations have established the following for each disease: mode of inheritance, histologic and ultrastructural features, chemical structure of the stored materials, and properties of the missing enzyme and its molecular genetics. In recent years, the generation of small laboratory animal models that closely recapitulate the corresponding human conditions has facilitated studies of disease pathogenesis and the implementation of various therapeutic modalities. Simple definitive laboratory methods have been developed that permit accurate prenatal and postnatal diagnosis of these diseases. As a result, many of them are now being diagnosed in many more patients, including individuals with perplexing clinical manifestations representing variant forms of LSDs.

A hematologic perspective is particularly pertinent to the diagnosis of inherited storage diseases. Circulating leukocytes have not only a rapid metabolic rate but also the capacity to phagocytize nondegradable materials. Therefore, these cells are doubly vulnerable, and thus it is not surprising that various morphologic changes are observed in leukocytes from patients with storage diseases and used as diagnostic tools. The same holds true for the bone marrow–derived monocytes and macrophages that become engorged with lysosomes full of undegraded metabolites. Consequently, bone marrow and other tissues of the hematopoietic system reflect the storage phenomenon, and examination of such tissues is often diagnostic of the disease.

Biochemical studies are usually required for a definitive diagnosis, and there too, peripheral blood may serve an important function. Serum, plasma, and mixed leukocyte fractions provide a rich and readily available source of material for substrate analysis and enzymatic assays. Enzyme testing in blood samples is also helpful for screening relatives who are heterozygous for the mutated allele. The incidence of some LSDs, such as the Tay-Sachs variant of G_{M2}-gangliosidosis, has actually been reduced by large-scale screening programs for testing serum and leukocytes in at-risk populations. If both members of a couple are discovered to be carriers of a disease allele and therefore at risk for bearing affected children, they can elect to have amniocentesis performed for prenatal diagnosis and, if the fetus is affected, can choose termination of the pregnancy. Through the use of more efficient and economical testing methods, this prototype program for prevention of genetic disease may become applicable to other storage diseases that are fatal in early childhood. In some clinical centers, neonatal screening for LSDs has recently been established. However, for now, we can still reduce the burden of these diseases by properly testing and counseling family members of individuals known to have these disorders. Such counseling should include full disclosure of the option for prenatal diagnosis as soon as possible after an LSD has been diagnosed.

Considerable phenotypic heterogeneity characterizes each of the storage diseases. The development of DNA-based methods for molecular diagnosis now makes possible improved genotype-phenotype correlations. Different mutations within the same gene appear to account for clinical variations within superficially similar diseases. Therefore, physicians faced with a perplexing occurrence of a suspected storage disease should not exclude otherwise similar conditions because of a few phenotypic dissimilarities. Although blood enzyme assays will remain a cornerstone in the classification of these diseases, greater diagnostic specificity is now possible by direct analysis of individual mutations in genomic DNA.

Therapies for LSDs pose a great challenge, given the systemic nature of most of these disorders and the involvement of the nervous system, which is invariably present, especially in patients with an early onset of symptoms. However, during the last decades, new or improved therapeutic approaches have been and continue to be tested for the treatment of LSDs, including enzyme replacement therapy (ERT) with genetically engineered recombinant enzymes, substrate reduction therapy (SRT) with specific inhibitors of the synthesis of target natural substrates, chaperone-mediated enzyme enhancement with synthetic sugar nucleotides, hematopoietic stem cell (HSC) transplantation, and ex vivo and in vivo gene therapy. Some of these therapeutic modalities are currently available to patients or are in clinical trials, whereas others have been tested only in animal models.

The emphasis here is on LSDs with manifestations in the reticuloendothelial system. One of the purposes of this chapter is to guide the reader through some of the complex chemical pathways involved in these diseases. The references provided at the end of the chapter reflect the most recent findings in this rapidly developing field of medicine, and they should be consulted for further clinical and biochemical information on the storage diseases.

GENERAL CONCEPTS

Lysosomes and Lysosomal Enzymes

Morphology and Physiology. Lysosomes are membrane-bound, specialized organelles that constitute up to 5% of the intracellular volume and are heterogeneous in size, morphology, and content. Lysosomes are found in basically all cells, with the exclusion of mature erythrocytes. Among hematopoietic cells, they account for the characteristic azurophilic-staining granules in polymorphonuclear leukocytes and eosinophils and are numerous in reticulocytes, especially after splenectomy.[1] Electron microscopic studies reveal that lysosomes are delineated by a single membrane that may fuse with pinocytic or phagocytic vesicles containing ingested foreign material (heterophagy) or with vacuoles containing cellular constituents or metabolites destined for further catabolism (autophagy).[2] The secondary lysosomes formed during the processes of heterophagy and autophagy are polymorphic in size. The undigested material remaining in secondary lysosomes after digestion coalesces into a residual body that can be extruded from the cell via an excretory pathway, for example, in bile from the liver and in urine from the kidney.

Biosynthesis. The lysosomal system represents the major site of intracellular compartmentalized degradation. With their complement of more than 70 hydrolytic enzymes, lysosomes regulate the turnover of many cellular constituents; proteins, glycoproteins, nucleic acids, polysaccharides, glycolipids, phospholipids, and neutral lipids are the enzymes' natural substrates.[3,4] Most of the lysosomal enzymes are soluble, whereas a few are membrane associated. Soluble enzyme precursors are specialized forms of secretory proteins. As the latter, they are synthesized on membrane-bound polysomes and gain access to the lumen of the endoplasmic reticulum (ER) via a conventional signal sequence; once in the ER, they are cotranslationally glycosylated on specific asparagine residues[5] and fold in their native tertiary structure with the aid of folding catalysts or assemble into multiprotein complexes. Partial modification of their sugar chains in the ER allows transfer of the enzyme precursors to the Golgi and trans-Golgi network. At this site they undergo further processing of their glycans and acquire a key determinant, the mannose 6-phosphate (M6P) recognition marker, that ensures segregation of the enzyme precursors from the bulk of secretory proteins by interaction with the M6P receptor and finally correct compartmentalization of them in endosomes/lysosomes.[6-8] In some instances, soluble enzyme precursors can reach the lysosomes in an M6P-independent manner.[9] Membrane-bound lysosomal enzymes use different receptors for reaching their final destination; such is the case for the enzyme glucocerebrosidase or β-glucosidase (see later), which is transported to lysosomes via interaction with the lysosomal integral membrane protein Limp-2.[10] Once in the acidic endosomal/lysosomal environment, most lysosomal enzyme precursors undergo partial proteolysis, which renders them fully mature and catalytically active. By default, a small percentage of the precursor proteins may escape to the exterior of the cell, but these secreted forms retain the capacity to be reinternalized via M6P receptor–mediated endocytosis and to be efficiently targeted to the lysosome, where they function normally.[11,12] This secretion and recapture mechanism of lysosomal enzymes may occur between cells[13] or between cells and the extracellular environment. Such exchange is readily demonstrable in skin fibroblast cultures. Release of enzyme from the cell can be demonstrated in culture media that do not initially contain any activity of the relevant enzyme. Cellular uptake of enzyme from nutrient media has been shown to restore enzyme activity in genetically deficient cells. This mode of cross-correction has served as the paradigm for the treatment of LSDs (see later). Release of lysosomal enzyme activity may also occur during phagocytosis or exocytosis, on exposure to membrane-disruptive agents or immune complexes,[14] or during treatment with acetylcholine and cyclic guanosine monophosphate in the presence of calcium.[15] In many hematopoietic cells, such as platelets, neutrophils, eosinophils, mast cells, macrophages, and cytotoxic T cells, a cohort of organelles with the characteristics of lysosomes have been shown to release their secretory products via calcium-dependent fusion of the lysosomal membrane with the plasma membrane, a process termed *lysosomal exocytosis*.[16] These observations gave rise to the concept of "secretory lysosomes,"[3,17] which was thought to be confined to specialized secretory cells. It is now apparent that the process of lysosomal exocytosis also plays the general role of membrane repair in nonsecretory cells such as fibroblasts.[18,19] Drugs such as epinephrine, isoproterenol, cyclic adenosine monophosphate,[15] and anti-inflammatory drugs[20] inhibit the release of lysosomal enzymes. Some of these factors could be involved in regulating levels of lysosomal enzyme activity in body fluids such as plasma, urine, and tears.

Enzyme Activity. Lysosomal enzymes are hydrolases that have maximal activity in an acidic pH environment and are specific with respect to the chemical linkage and structure of the monomeric unit that they hydrolyze. Small synthetic substrates can often substitute for more complex natural products in assays of lysosomal enzyme activity in vitro. Complex isozyme systems exist in which two or more enzymes act on a single substrate. The β-*N*-acetylhexosaminidases, arylsulfatases, α-galactosidases, α-mannosidases, and neuraminidases are examples. The specificity of lysosomal enzymes is reflected in the wide range of glycosidases and proteases, which represent the largest classes of these enzymes. Glycosidases bring about the catabolism of specific sugar chains on glycoconjugates in a stepwise and concerted fashion. If any of these enzymes is deficient or functionally defective, the process of degradation is halted at the level of the missing enzyme.

Such blockage leads first to the progressive intralysosomal accumulation of partially degraded metabolites and, subsequently, to the cellular and organ dysfunction associated with LSDs.[12,21] Not surprisingly, genetic lesions that result in faulty enzyme function are heterogeneous, given the numerous modifications that must occur with some precision between the site of synthesis of a lysosomal protein and its final sequestration and full activation within the lysosome. The genotype and familial history of the disease may eventually have an impact on the response to treatment.

Pathogenesis

Based on his studies of type II glycogen storage disease (Pompe's disease), Hers[22] proposed the concept of inborn lysosomal disease in 1965. He concluded that deficiency of a single lysosomal enzyme (α-glucosidase) results in the accumulation of its substrate (glycogen) within membrane-bound vesicles of lysosomal origin. According to this concept, progressive lysosomal accumulation of nonmetabolized material leads to abnormal expansion of the number of lysosomes within cells, disruption of normal cell functions, and possibly cell death.

The signs and symptoms produced by each of the storage diseases primarily reflect the pattern of distribution of the nondegradable natural products. In Gaucher's disease and Niemann-Pick disease, turnover of erythrocyte and leukocyte membranes leads to the formation of lipids that become trapped within the visceral organs principally involved in their metabolism. However, in disorders of ganglioside metabolism, the principal pathologic changes occur in the central nervous system (CNS) because ganglioside concentrations in this tissue under normal circumstances are much greater than those in extraneural tissues. Glycoproteins are abundant in nearly all tissues, both inside and outside the CNS. Therefore, diseases caused by the storage of mucopolysaccharides and other complex carbohydrates derived from glycoproteins affect a variety of different organ systems.

Natural materials with apparently intact pathways for their metabolism sometimes accumulate as secondary products in some of the LSDs. For example, cholesterol is closely associated with sphingomyelin in membranes and apparently for this reason also accumulates in Niemann-Pick disease (sphingomyelin lipidosis). High concentrations of mucopolysaccharide can inhibit β-galactosidase, so patients with mucopolysaccharidoses may secondarily accumulate not only mucopolysaccharide but also gangliosides in their brain tissue.

Genetics

Nearly all the LSDs are transmitted as autosomal recessive traits. Two exceptions, Fabry's disease (α-galactosidase deficiency) and Hunter's disease (iduronate sulfatase deficiency), follow an X-linked pattern of inheritance. During the seventies, interspecies somatic cell hybrids were widely used in gene-mapping experiments to make specific chromosome assignments for genes that code for lysosomal hydrolases. In situ hybridization of the cloned genes later provided additional information on their subchromosomal localization. With advent of the human genome project, lysosomal genes have been accurately mapped and their genomic organization established.[23] Knowledge of the gene and its genomic structure has enabled identification of disease-causing mutations in each of the LSDs and correlation between genotype and phenotype in patients with different clinical phenotypes (Table 24-1). Recombinant DNA technology has facilitated studies of the molecular basis of these diseases and has provided tools for more precise diagnosis, as well as the potential for definitive therapy through gene transfer.

Two or more enzyme activities can be affected by a single mutation in a particular gene locus. One explanation is that under ordinary circumstances, the gene involved in such situations regulates the synthesis of a subunit that is shared by more than one enzyme. For example, in Sandhoff's disease, failure to properly code for the β subunit shared by both the hexosaminidase A (Hex-A) and B (Hex-B) isozymes accounts for deficiencies in both these enzymes. Alternatively, the mutation could affect a post-translational event, such as attachment or removal of carbohydrate residues during conversion of the enzyme to its final glycoprotein form, which could result in an enzyme molecule that is catalytically active but can be neither retained nor selectively taken up by the cell. This type of defect occurs in mucolipidoses II and III and probably accounts for the altered electrophoretic properties of lysosomal enzymes in these diseases. In several LSDs, catalytically inactive enzyme protein can be detected by using antibodies to normal purified enzyme. Although the substrate binding or catalytic sites of this cross-reacting material may be altered, its antigenic sites are intact. Immunoassays for cross-reacting material are therefore an additional means of classifying variants of individual LSDs.

A number of heat-stable activator proteins, including the G_{M2} activator protein ($G_{M2}A$) and the saposins (SAP-A to SAP-D), have been shown to function either as natural detergents to stimulate the enzymatic hydrolysis of individual hydrophobic substrates or as cofactors of the enzyme.[24-26] Saposins are derived from proteolytic cleavage of a single, one-chain precursor, prosaposin.[27] Defects in these activator proteins are associated with variant forms of LSDs (see later). For example, in patients with a deficiency of SAP-C, a clinical condition resembling non-neuropathic Gaucher's disease develops.[28] Deficiency of $G_{M2}A$ has been implicated in the pathogenesis of the AB variant of G_{M2}-gangliosidosis.[29] In Morquio's disease type B, SAP-A works as cofactor of the mutant β-galactosidase in the degradation of G_{M1}-ganglioside (G_{M1}).[29] These various mechanisms allow enormous genetic heterogeneity and are, in fact, reflected

TABLE 24-1   Chromosome Assignment of Genes Coding for Certain Lysosomal Enzyme Activities

Enzyme	Disease	OMIM	Gene Map Locus
β-Mannosidase	β-Mannosidosis	248510	4q22-q25
α-L-Fucosidose	Fucosidosis	230000	1p34
Glucocerebrosidase	Gaucher's disease types 1, 2, and 3	230800, 230900, 231000	1q21
β-Galactosidase	G_{M1}-gangliodidosis	230500	3p21.33
α-L-Iduronidase	Hurler's disease type I, Scheie's disease	252800	4p16.3
UDP-N-acetylglucosamine : lysosomal enzyme N-Acetylglucosamine-1-phosphotransferase	I-cell disease, pseudo-Hurler polydystrophy, mucolipidosis type III	252500, 252600, 252605	16p; 12q23.3
Aspartylglucosaminidase	Aspartylglucosaminuria	208400	4q32-q33
Arylsulfatase B	Maroteaux-Lamy disease type IV	253200	5q11-q13
G_{M2}-ganglioside activator protein	Tay-Sachs disease, AB variant	272750	5q31.3-q33.1
Hexosaminidase B	Sandhoff's disease	268800	5q13
β-Glucuronidase	Sly's disease	253220	7q21.11
Cerebroside sulfate activator	Saposin B deficiency	249900	10q22.1
α-Neuraminidase	Sialidosis	256550	6p21.3
Acid lipase	Wolman's disease, cholesteryl ester storage disease	278000	10q24-q25
Sphingomyelinase	Niemann-Pick disease type A	257200	11p15.4-p15.1
N-Acetylglucosamine-6-sulfatase	Sanfilippo's disease type IIID	252940	12q14
Galactocerebrosidase	Krabbe's disease	245200	14q31
Hexosaminidase A (α chain only)	Tay-Sachs disease type B/B1	272800	15q23-q24
N-Acetylgalactosamine-6-sulfatase	Morquio's disease type A	253000	16q24.3
α-N-Acetylglucosaminidase	Sanfilippo's disease type IIIB	252920	17q21
α-Glucosidase	Pompe's disease	232300	17q25.2-q25.3
Heparan sulfamidase	Sanfilippo's disease type IIIA	252900	17q25.3
α-Mannosidase	α-Mannosidosis	248500	19cen-q12
Protective protein/cathepsin A (PPCA)	Galactosialidosis type 1	256540	20q13.1
α-N-Acetylgalactosaminidase	Schindler's disease types I and III	104170	22q11
Arylsulfatase A	Metachromatic leukodystrophy	250100	22q13.31-qter
α-Galactosidase A	Fabry's disease	301500	Xq22
Iduronate-2-sulfatase	Hunter's disease type II	309900	Xq28
SUMF1	Multiple sulfatase deficiency	272200	3p26
Mucolipin I	Mucolipidosis type IV	252650	19p13.3-p13.2

OMIM, Online Mendelian Inheritance in Man.

in the marked phenotypic variations that distinguish many of the storage diseases.

Clinical Diagnosis

The undigested products found in the lysosomes of patients with LSDs are not uniformly distributed in all organs. Instead, they accumulate preferentially in certain tissues or cell types where under normal conditions, they are actively metabolized or recycled. The distribution of the storage material reflects the pattern of expression of the involved lysosomal enzyme and the specific function or metabolic need of any given cell. The involvement of specific tissues and organs thus determines the manner of clinical expression of each of the storage diseases (Table 24-2).

Dysmorphic facial features and hepatomegaly are two common features. The former occurs in type 1 G_{M1}-gangliosidosis, the mucopolysaccharidoses, mucolipidoses II and III, α-mannosidosis, galactosialidosis, and

fucosidosis. Many of these diseases also display evidence of connective tissue infiltration, such as joint contractures, skeletal dysplasia, and corneal clouding. Some degree of liver enlargement also occurs in most of these disorders, including Gaucher's disease, Niemann-Pick disease, galactosialidosis, sialidosis type II, and Wolman's disease. Splenomegaly is also a common initial sign in Gaucher's disease, Niemann-Pick disease, galactosialidosis, sialidosis type II, and Wolman's disease. Lymphadenopathy and granulomatous joint deposits are characteristic of Farber's disease.

Signs of CNS dysfunction occur in most patients, particularly those with an early onset of signs of the disease. Slowed development, hypotonia, and excessive startle response in an infant may suggest a gangliosidosis. Actual regression in neurologic functioning with loss of previously acquired developmental milestones eventually occurs not only in the gangliosidoses but also in Niemann-Pick disease type A and several of the mucopolysaccharidoses. Seizures, megalencephaly, and blindness result

TABLE 24-2 Storage Diseases of the Reticuloendothelial System	
Age at Onset	**Initial Signs**
FIRST YEAR	
Niemann-Pick disease, type A	Slow development, hepatosplenomegaly
Gaucher's disease, type 2	Failure to thrive, hepatosplenomegaly, brainstem signs
Farber's disease	Hoarseness, vomiting, swollen joints, lymphadenopathy
G_{M1}-gangliosidosis, type 1	Slow development, increased startle, hepatosplenomegaly
G_{M2}-gangliosidosis, Sandhoff variant	Slow development, increased startle, cherry-red macula
Hurler's disease	Coarse facies, stiff joints
Hunter's disease	Coarse facies, stiff joints
Sanfilippo's disease	Coarse facies, stiff joints, severe mental retardation
Mucosulfatidosis	Slow development, coarse facies
Sialidosis, type II (infantile/congenital)	Fetal hydrops, coarse facies, hepatosplenomegaly, mental retardation
Galactosialidosis, early infantile	Fetal hydrops, coarse facies, hepatosplenomegaly, mental retardation
Mucolipidosis II	Wizened face at birth, gingival hyperplasia, stiff joints
Mucolipidosis IV	Slow development, corneal clouding
Sialic acid storage disease	Slow development, coarse facies, hepatosplenomegaly
Fucosidosis, type 1	Slow development, coarse facies
α-Mannosidosis	Slow development, coarse facies, hepatosplenomegaly
Wolman's disease	Vomiting, diarrhea, hepatosplenomegaly, calcified adrenals
Neuronal ceroid lipofuscinosis, infantile type	Slow development, poor vision
SECOND YEAR	
Niemann-Pick disease, type B	Hepatosplenomegaly
G_{M1}-gangliosidosis, type 2	Slow development, increased startle
Galactosialidosis, late infantile	Coarse facies, hepatospenomegaly, cherry-red macula, cardiac abnormalities
Morquio's syndrome	Dwarfism, skeletal abnormalities, loose joints
Maroteaux-Lamy syndrome	Coarse facies, stiff joints, corneal clouding
Mucolipidosis III	Stiff hands and shoulders
Fucosidosis, type 2	Slow neurologic deterioration
Aspartylglucosaminuria	Slow development, coarse facies, aggressive behavior
Neuronal ceroid lipofuscinosis, late infantile type	Seizures, myoclonus, decreased vision, decreased intellect
CHILDHOOD	
Niemann-Pick disease, chronic neuropathic form	Tetraparesis, hepatomegaly, decreased intellect
Gaucher's disease, type 1	Splenomegaly, anemia, thrombocytopenia
Scheie's disease	Clawhands
Cholesteryl ester storage disease	Hepatomegaly, increased plasma cholesterol and triglycerides
Neuronal ceroid lipofuscinosis, juvenile type	Blindness, seizures, decreased intellect
ADOLESCENCE	
Gaucher's disease, type 3	Splenomegaly, seizures, myoclonus
Sialidosis, type I	Unexpected falls, myoclonus, seizures, cherry-red macula
Galactosialidosis, juvenile/adult	Corneal clouding, coarse facies, seizures, cherry-red macula, mental retardation

later in the course of the ganglioside storage diseases. Vomiting may be an initial sign in Niemann-Pick disease type A and Wolman's disease.

Generally, the later clinical signs appear, the slower the progression of the disease and the less severe the disease process. In contrast to the severely retarded epileptic infant with a gangliosidosis and life expectancy measured in months, a patient who is seen in late childhood or early adolescence with seizures as a result of juvenile Gaucher's disease (type 3) or the cherry-red macula/myoclonus forms of sialidosis (type I) may survive 10 or more years without loss of intellect. Although mental retardation does occur in aspartylglucosaminuria, fucosidosis, the mannosidoses, and the less severe form of Hunter's disease, these diseases progress slowly, and patients survive into adulthood. In the adult form of Gaucher's disease (type 1) and Niemann-Pick disease type B, splenic lipid storage may build up very slowly, no mental deficiency occurs, and a normal life span is possible.

Knowledge of the patient's family history is often helpful in determining a diagnosis. Patients with adult Gaucher's disease and type A Niemann-Pick disease are very often of northeastern European Jewish ancestry. A Scandinavian background is common in patients with aspartylglucosaminuria, and many patients with fucosidosis are of Italian extraction. Therefore, in the clinical evaluation of patients suspected of having a storage disease, particular attention should be devoted to review of the chronology of the disease and the family background, and careful assessment should be made of the neurologic, visceral, and skeletal manifestations. However, because of considerable genetic heterogeneity, the physical signs and severity of the LSDs vary considerably. For this reason, laboratory studies play an important role in the diagnosis of these conditions.

Laboratory Diagnosis

Morphologic Findings

The histologic changes observed in the storage diseases are especially pronounced in organs with a significant reticuloendothelial component, such as the liver, spleen, lymph nodes, and bone marrow. The accumulations of natural products form inclusions that display specific staining characteristics and a defined ultrastructure. They may be readily observed in easily accessible tissues such as peripheral blood, bone marrow, liver, and skin (Table 24-3).

Peripheral Blood. Vacuolated lymphocytes are a common finding in the storage diseases (Fig. 24-1A through D).[30-37] They can be readily recognized in blood smears because they contain vacuoles that stain positively with periodic acid–Schiff (PAS). At the electron microscopic level, these vacuoles generally appear as dense cytoplasmic bodies or lamellar arrays surrounded by a single limiting membrane. In Wolman's disease, both intracytoplasmic and intranuclear lymphocytic vacuoles may occur. Other types of circulating monocytes, in addition to lymphocytes, may also form vacuoles. This change occurs, for example, in sialidosis, galactosialidosis, and mucolipidosis II. Excessive granulation of circulating neutrophils helps distinguish several of the storage diseases. In the mucopolysaccharidoses and mucosulfatidosis, metachromatic granules known as Alder-Reilly bodies are present (see Fig. 24-1B).[38] Azurophilic hypergranulation of neutrophils is a characteristic feature in many

---

TABLE 24-3 Laboratory Findings in the Storage Diseases: Presence of Inclusions in Readily Accessible Tissues

Disease	PERIPHERAL BLOOD		BONE MARROW	LIVER		SKIN	
	Vacuolated Lymphocytes	Granulated Neutrophils*	Foam Cells	Kupffer Cells	Hepatocytes	Biopsy	Culture
Gaucher's			Gaucher cell	Gaucher cell	Gaucher cell		+
Niemann-Pick	Nova	Scotia variant	+	+	+		+
Farber's			+	+	+	+	+
G$_{M1}$-gangliosidosis	+		+	+	+	+	+
Sandhoff variant of G$_{M2}$-gangliosidosis	+		+	+	+	+	+
Hurler's		+		+	+	+	+
Hunter's				+	+	+	+
Sanfilippo's, type A	+			+		+	+
Sanfilippo's, type B						+	+
Morquio's syndrome				+	+	+	+
Maroteaux-Lamy syndrome		+		+	+		+
β-Glucuronidase deficiency		+					+
Mucosulfatidosis	+	+	Granulated myeloid cells	+	+		+
Galactosialidosis	+		+	+	+		+
Sialidosis I	+		+		+		+
Sialidosis II, late infantile type	+	+	+	+	+		+
Mucolipidosis II	+		+				+
Mucolipidosis III			Vacuolated plasma cells				+
Mucolipidosis IV			+; vacuolated plasma cells	+	+		+
Sialic acid storage	+		+	+	+	+	+
Fucosidosis	+		+	+	+	+	+
Mannosidosis	+	+	+				+
Aspartylglucosaminuria	+				+		
Wolman's	+		+	+	+		
Neuronal ceroid lipofuscinosis	+	+	+			+	+

*Coarse granulations characteristic of Alder-Reilly bodies are seen in the granulocytes of patients with a mucopolysaccharidosis. In sialidosis II, fine granulations are present in granulocytes, lymphocytes, and monocytes. Leukocytes in neuronal ceroid lipofuscinosis show azurophilic granulation.

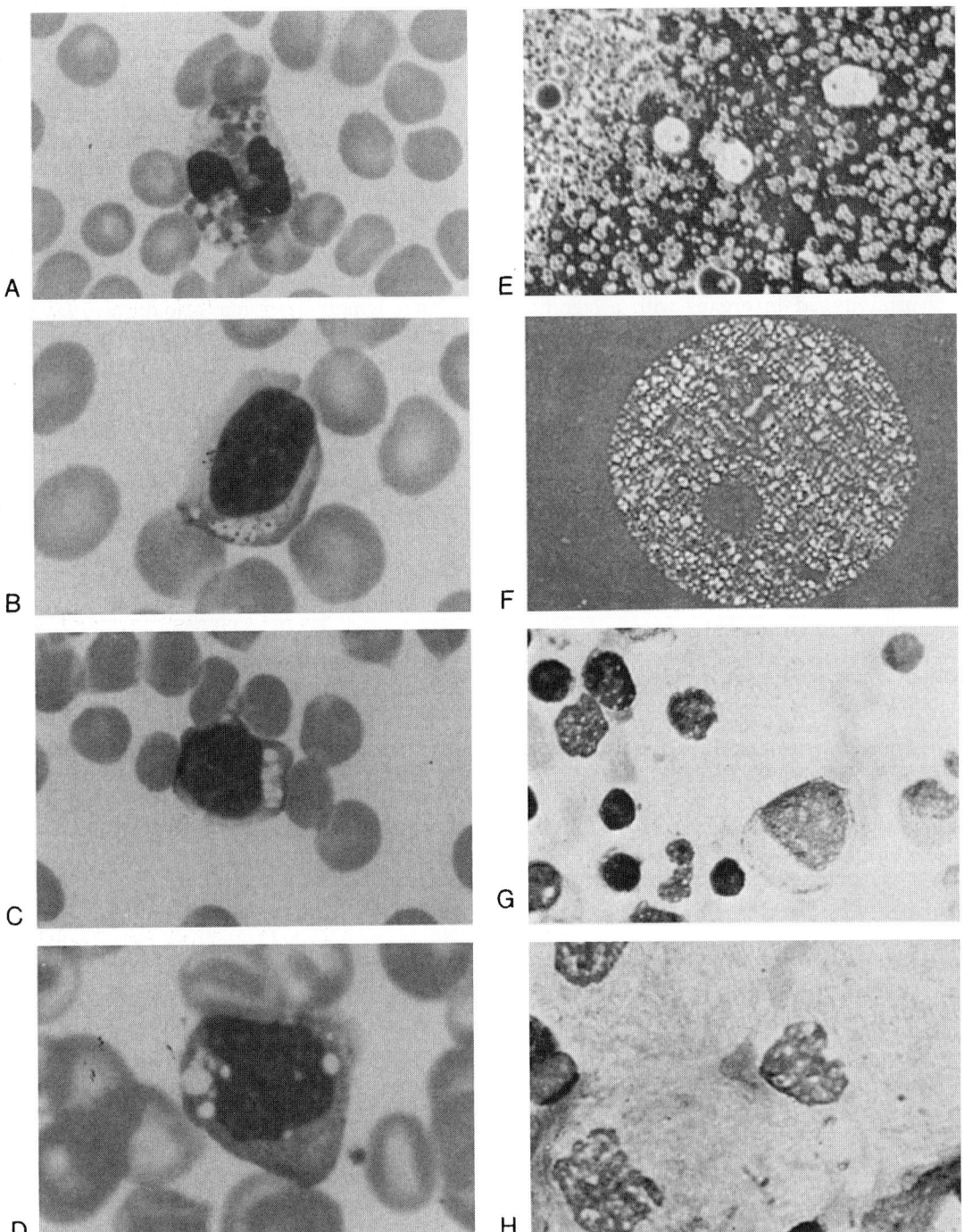

FIGURE 24-1. Photomicrographs of storage cells in peripheral blood (**A** through **D**) and in bone marrow (**E** through **H**). **A,** Eosinophil—G$_{M1}$-gangliosidosis; **B,** lymphocyte—Hunter's disease; **C,** lymphocyte—α-mannosidosis; **D,** monocyte—Niemann-Pick disease type C; **E,** foam cells—Niemann-Pick disease type B, darkfield; **F,** foam cell—Niemann-Pick disease type A, polarization; **G,** foam cell—Giemsa stain, Niemann-Pick disease type B; **H,** Gaucher cell—Giemsa stain, Gaucher's disease type 1. (*A through D, Courtesy of J. Alroy, Department of Pathology, Tufts New England Medical Center.*)

patients with the neuronal ceroid lipofuscinoses. Ultra-structural studies of buffy coat preparations from the peripheral blood of these patients can be used to detect the abnormal intracytoplasmic inclusions typical of these diseases.[39,40]

Bone Marrow. The foam cell, a lipid-laden macro-phage often called a histiocyte, provides perhaps the most

dramatic and convincing histologic evidence of a storage disease. It may be easily recognized in unstained prepara-tions of bone marrow aspirate as a round or oval cell measuring 20 to 90 µm in diameter. It generally has a single eccentric nucleus with a prominent nucleolus. Under darkfield microscopy, these cells appear as large, white spheres on a dark background (see Fig. 24-1E). They may be distinguished on phase-contrast microscopy as large, glittering cells with numerous cytoplasmic droplets or particles. These droplets are fairly uniform in size and, when viewed under polarization microscopy, are often birefringent (see Fig. 24-1F). They impart a mulberry- or honeycomb-like appearance to the cell and have a finely reticulated cytoplasmic web that is better seen in stained preparations (see Fig. 24-1G). Under the electron microscope, the droplets appear as polymorphic lipid vacuoles ranging from less than 1 μm to greater than 5 μm in diameter and consisting of both concentrically laminated myelin-like membranous arrays and dense homogeneous residual bodies.

The staining properties of foam cells in each of the storage diseases may differ. They often stain red with oil red O and black with Sudan black B, thus indicating that sudanophilic material is present. The PAS reaction may be weakly positive. The presence of lipofuscin is indicated by the appearance of autofluorescence under ultraviolet light. These histochemical reactions may be lost if alcohol or other lipid solvents are used to fix the bone marrow smears or tissue sections before staining. Therefore, for examining the staining properties of biopsy specimens from patients with storage diseases, formalin-fixed frozen sections are preferable to alcohol-treated paraffin-embedded material.

Occasionally, sea-blue histiocytes[41] are noted in the bone marrow preparations of patients with Niemann-Pick disease[42] and other systemic lipidoses.[43] These large cells measure up to 60 μm in diameter and contain several large, homogeneous granules that display a blue or blue-green color with Giemsa or Wright stains. Their major chemical constituent was believed to be ceroid, but increased levels of phospholipids and glycolipids are likely to occur. The Gaucher cell is sometimes mistakenly identified as a foam cell. It is also a large histiocyte that measures 20 to 100 μm in diameter, but instead of lipid droplets, its cytoplasm contains striated rod-shaped inclusion bodies that give it a wrinkled tissue paper or crumpled silk appearance (see Fig. 24-1H). The Gaucher cell stains pale pink with hematoxylin-eosin and stains only slightly with oil red O and Sudan black B. The inclusions are autofluorescent and PAS positive.

Electron microscopic studies indicate that these deposits consist of hollow tubules contained within a limiting membrane. Analysis of purified preparations of these deposits by freeze-fracture and x-ray diffraction techniques suggests that they exist as a series of gradually twisting membranous bilayers 3 to 6 nm thick.[44] They are composed of glucocerebroside (66%), phospholipid (17%), cholesterol (6%), and protein and glycoprotein (11%).[45] Strong acid phosphatase activity[46] and iron deposition[47] have also been demonstrated in Gaucher cells with the use of histochemical staining methods. Unlike the foam cell, which is found in many lipid storage diseases, the Gaucher cell is unique to the Gaucher form of inherited lipidosis. However, it cannot be regarded as being entirely specific for Gaucher's disease because it has also been observed in the bone marrow of some

patients with certain blood disorders, including chronic myelogenous leukemia[48] and thalassemia[49] and in one patient who had both Gaucher's disease and coexistent Philadelphia chromosome–positive chronic granulocytic leukemia.[50] Presumably, Gaucher cells can form when the breakdown of blood cells exceeds the capacity of macrophages to metabolize the effete lipids.

Careful examination of the bone marrow smear is therefore an essential part of the diagnosis of a storage disease. In addition to the foam cell, sea-blue histiocyte, and Gaucher cell, other abnormal structures can be detected in the bone marrow, such as the Alder-Reilly bodies characteristic of Hurler's disease and multiple sulfatase deficiency and the vacuolated plasma cells associated with mucolipidoses III and IV.

Liver. In many storage diseases, an enlarged liver provides a tempting target for diagnostic biopsy despite the fact that many of the cellular changes occurring in the liver are similar to those present in the bone marrow. A liver biopsy has the added advantage of allowing access to a solid tissue for biochemical analysis. Needle biopsy can yield 10 to 25 mg of fresh tissue that could be divided equally between the biochemistry and pathology laboratories. The specimen for biochemical studies must be preserved frozen in a sealed container, preferably one flushed with nitrogen gas before sealing to displace oxygen and prevent oxidation and dehydration during storage. One segment of the tissue destined for the pathology laboratory is immediately immersed in buffered glutaraldehyde for electron microscopic studies. The remainder is fixed in formalin and further subdivided into two specimens. Half of the specimen is routinely processed and embedded in paraffin. The other half of the formalin-fixed material is used to prepare frozen sections, with care taken to avoid exposure to alcohol or other lipid solvents.

Liver involvement may be reflected in changes in tissue macrophages (Kupffer cells), hepatocytes, and endothelial cells. Kupffer cells are enlarged and contain membrane-limited vacuoles of various size. Electron microscopic studies of their ultrastructure demonstrate cytoplasmic bodies ranging from membranous and granuloreticular lamellar structures to more polymorphous and homogeneous dense bodies. Vacuolated histiocytes may infiltrate the sinuses, where they appear as discrete islands of light-staining cells in routinely stained sections. Hepatic parenchymal cell involvement is variable. A mild vacuolar change may be noticed, or more extensive infiltration can occur in these cells, as indicated by obvious enlargement and foamy metamorphosis. On electron microscopic examination, dense bodies and osmophilic bodies are present. Vascular endothelial cells in the liver may also contain inclusions, and in some specimens the lobular architecture of the liver itself is disturbed. The typical appearance of the Gaucher cell in liver specimens from patients with Gaucher's disease and the presence of both intralysosomal and cytoplasmic glycogen in Pompe's disease distinguish these conditions from other forms of storage disease. In all other instances, the histologic changes in the liver are not distinctive enough to permit the diagnosis of a specific storage disease.

Skin. Many different types of cells are present in skin, including epithelial cells, hair follicles, fibroblasts, eccrine sweat glands, smooth muscle cells, sebaceous glands, vascular cells, and nerve bundles, thus making skin biopsy an extremely useful technique for the histologic diagnosis of storage diseases.[51] Vacuoles may be found in the secretory coils of eccrine sweat glands, the bulbs of hair follicles, fibroblasts, and Schwann cells in a number of diseases. Biopsy specimens from patients with the ganglioside storage diseases contain complex osmophilic lipid deposits in axons, Schwann cells, and nerve fascicles, whereas similar deposits in both neural and extraneural dermal elements characterize mucolipidosis IV. Study of skin ultrastructure is particularly helpful for diagnosis of the neuronal ceroid lipofuscinoses because the same distinctive pattern of inclusions present in the nervous system may be evident in skin[34,51-54] and enzymatic diagnosis of all forms of these diseases is not yet possible.

Cultured skin fibroblasts are less informative, but ultrastructural changes have also been noted in these cells.[55] The membrane-bound, electron-dense inclusions of mucolipidosis II[56] and IV[57] and the curvilinear profiles of neuronal ceroid lipofuscinoses[58] are examples of this phenomenon. However, not all storage diseases produce histologic changes in the skin; for example, none has been found in Gaucher's disease.[34] Nevertheless, as electron microscopists have become more proficient in examining this type of tissue and cell culture and specialists and biochemists have recognized the usefulness of cultured skin fibroblasts for metabolic studies, the popularity of diagnostic skin biopsy has increased. Other extracerebral tissues, including conjunctiva, skeletal muscle, and rectal tissue, may also provide useful samples for biopsy.[51]

Biochemical and Molecular Studies

Storage Substances. The results of morphologic studies suggest the presumptive diagnosis of a storage disease, but biochemical studies are required for a specific diagnosis (Table 24-4). For the majority of the storage diseases, structural identification of the major substances that accumulate preceded elucidation of the enzyme defects. Characterization of these compounds is generally more difficult than assaying the relevant enzyme, so for diagnostic purposes, determination of enzyme activity is preferred. However, a number of laboratory techniques have been developed that facilitate screening for storage products in readily available tissue and fluid specimens.

The urine of patients with sphingolipidoses, mucopolysaccharidoses, mucolipidoses, and other oligosaccharidoses is a rich source of storage material.[59] The sphingolipids present in a filtered 24-hour urine specimen can be extracted from the filter paper, separated from other lipids on a silicic acid column, and quantitated by a combination of thin-layer and gas-liquid chromatography.[60] An excess of mucopolysaccharides is recognized in urine by positive results on the Berry spot test,[61] and these substances can be isolated by precipitation with quaternary ammonium salts and fractionated into separated species by electrophoresis.[62] Complexing of urinary mucopolysaccharides with 1,9-dimethylmethylene blue simplifies their quantification.[63] Simple thin-layer chromatographic methods using microliter quantities of whole desalted urine have been described as a means of separating the oligosaccharides excreted in fucosidosis,[59,64] mannosidosis,[65] G_{M1}-gangliosidosis,[64] and the sialidoses[66,67] into patterns distinctive for each disease. The presence of aspartylglucosamine on a urinary amino acid chromatogram aids in the diagnosis of aspartylglucosaminuria. More recently, new detection methods have been applied to the diagnosis of LSDs, including a filter paper method for mass and high-risk urinary screening for Fabry's disease[68] and mass spectrometry.[69]

Sphingoglycolipids present in plasma can be quantitated by high-performance liquid chromatography.[70,71] The procedure requires less than 1 mL of plasma and permits detection of elevated ceramide, cerebroside, and globoside levels in Farber's disease,[70] Gaucher's disease,[71] and the Sandhoff variant of G_{M2}-gangliosidosis, respectively. The high-performance liquid chromatographic technique has also been used to demonstrate elevated sphingomyelin levels in cultured skin fibroblasts from patients with Niemann-Pick disease type A.[72]

In other storage diseases as well, cultured skin fibroblasts provide an opportunity for biochemical analysis of storage material. The kinetics of $^{35}SO_4$ accumulation has been used as an indicator of defective degradation of polysaccharides in the mucopolysaccharidoses[73] and mucolipidoses.[74,75] In Gaucher disease cells, metabolic utilization of radioactively labeled glucocerebroside is reduced,[76] and in vivo studies of Farber disease cells reveal a defect in their ability to metabolize the ceramide portion of a fatty acid–labeled precursor.[77] Fucosidosis fibroblasts store abnormal quantities of tritiated fucose,[78] and Wolman disease cell lines incorporate increased amounts of ^{14}C-mevalonate into cholesterol.[79] In certain instances, solid tissues may need to be analyzed. This step is required when a strong clinical presumption of storage disease exists, but studies of body fluids and more readily accessible tissues such as leukocytes and cultured fibroblasts disclose neither the nature of the stored substance nor the presence of a deficient enzyme. Biopsy of cerebral tissue is no longer warranted except in very rare instances of neurodegenerative disease without extraneural morphologic or biochemical stigmata.

Deficient Enzyme Activity. Specific enzyme defects have been established for all the LSDs, and in the majority of cases, enzymatic assays are an especially convincing means for confirming the diagnosis. These assays can be

TABLE 24-4 Laboratory Findings in the Storage Diseases: Biochemistry

Disease	Stored Material	Enzyme Deficiency	Substrates Used in Enzyme Assays	
			Natural	Artificial
SPHINGOLIPIDOSES				
Gaucher's	Glucocerebroside	Glucocerebrosidase	Glucocerebroside	4-MU-β-glucoside
Niemann-Pick	Sphingomyelin	Sphingomyelinase	Sphingomyelin	2-N-Hexadecanoyl-amino-4-nitrophenyl-phosphorylcholine monohydrate
Farber's	Ceramide	Ceramidase	Ceramide	
G_{M1}-gangliosidosis	G_{M1}-ganglioside, glycoprotein	G_{M1}-ganglioside, β-galactosidase	G_{M1}-ganglioside, asialo-G_{M2}-ganglioside, globoside	pNP-β-galactoside, 4-MU-β-galactoside
G_{M2}-gangliosidosis, Sandhoff variant	G_{M2}-ganglioside, globoside	Hexosaminidase A + B		pNP-β-N-acetylglucosamine, 4-MU-β-N-acetylglucosamine
MUCOPOLYSACCHARIDOSES				
Hurler's and Scheie's	Dermatan sulfate, heparan sulfate	α-Iduronidase		4-MU-α-L-iduronide
Hunter's	Dermatan sulfate, heparan sulfate	Iduronate sulfatase	^{35}S-heparin	Disulfated ^{3}H-disaccharide
Sanfilippo's				
Type A	Heparan sulfate	Heparan-N-sulfatase	Unacetylated trisaccharide isolated from heparin	4-MU-α-D-N-sulfoglucosamide
Type B	Heparan sulfate	N-Acetyl-α-glucosaminidase	[u-^{14}C]Glucosamine + acetyl CoA	pNP-α-N-acetylglucosaminide, 4-MU-α-N-acetylglucosaminide
Type C	Heparan sulfate	Acetyl CoA:α-glucosaminide acetyltransferase		4-MU-β-D-glucosaminide + acetyl CoA
Type D	Heparan sulfate	N-Acetyl-α-glucosamine-6-sulfatase	N-Acetylglucosamine 6-sulfate	4-MU-α-N-acetylglucosamine 6-sulfate
Morquio's syndrome				
Type A	Keratan sulfate	Galactosamine 6-sulfatase	Disulfated ^{3}H-trisaccharide	
Type B	Keratan sulfate	β-Galactosidase		4-MU-β-galactoside

Continues

TABLE 24-4   Laboratory Findings in the Storage Diseases: Biochemistry—cont'd

Disease	Stored Material	Enzyme Deficiency	SUBSTRATES USED IN ENZYME ASSAYS	
			Natural	Artificial
Maroteaux-Lamy syndrome	Dermatan sulfate	Galactosamine-4-sulfatase (arylsulfatase B)	Chondroitin 4-sulfate	p-Nitrocatechol sulfate, 4-MU-sulfate
β-Glucuronidase deficiency	Dermatan sulfate, heparan sulfate	β-Glucuronidase		pNP-glucuronide, 4-MU-glucuronide
Mucosulfatidosis	Sulfatides, mucopolysaccharides	Arysulfatase A, B, and C; other sulfatases	Disulfated disaccharide, heparan, sulfatide	p-Nitrocatechol sulfate, 4-MU-sulfate
MUCOLIPIDOSES/GLYCOPROTEINOSES				
Sialidosis (mucolipidosis I)	Sialyloligosaccharides, glycopeptides	NEU1		4-MU-α-D-N-acetylneuraminide
Galactosialidosis	Sialyloligosaccharides, glycopeptides	PPCA	Bioactive peptides	
Mucolipidosis II	Sialyloligosaccharides, glycoproteins, glycolipids	High serum, low fibroblast enzymes; N-acetylglucosamine-1-phosphate transferase		4-MU-glycosides, UDP-N-acetylglucosamine, α-methylmannoside
Mucolipidosis III	Glycoproteins, glycolipids	Same as above		Same as above
Mucolipidosis IV	Glycolipids, glycoproteins	Mucolipin I		
OTHER DISEASES OF COMPLEX CARBOHYDRATE METABOLISM				
Sialic acid storage disease	Free sialic acid	Sialin		
Fucosidosis	Fucoglycolipids, fucosyloligosaccharides	α-Fucosidase		pNP-α-L-fucoside, 4-MU-α-fucoside
Mannosidosis	Mannosyloligosaccharides	α-Mannosidase		pNP-α-mannoside, 4-MU-α-mannoside
Aspartylglucosaminuria	Aspartylglucosamine	Aspartylglucosamine amidase		1-Aspartamido-β-N-acetylglucosamine
Wolman's	Cholesteryl esters, triglycerides	Acid lipase	Glyceryl tripalmitate	pNP-palmitate, 4-MU-oleate
Neuronal ceroid lipofuscinoses	Ceroid lipofuscin pigments	CLN-1: palmitoyl-protein thioesterase CLN-2 to CLN-5: unknown		

CoA, coenzyme A; 4-MU, 4-methylumbelliferyl; pNP, nitrophenol.

performed in vitro on readily accessible patient material such as serum, plasma, leukocytes, lymphocytes, cultured skin fibroblasts, and tears.

As mentioned earlier, artificial substrates can substitute for natural substrates for measuring enzyme activity. The chromogenic *p*-nitrophenyl and fluorogenic 4-methylumbelliferyl derivatives are commonly used for this purpose because they are more easily cleaved in vitro than the natural substrates are and the aglycone product of their hydrolysis can readily be quantitated by colorimetry or fluorometry. When natural substrates are used, they generally carry a radioactive label. Assays with these compounds are processed by separating the reaction products and quantitating the labeled component in a liquid scintillation spectrometer. Reviews are available that describe the methodology used in assaying most of the enzymes shown in Table 24-4.[80,81] These techniques are usually beyond the scope of a routine clinical chemistry laboratory and are most competently performed in a research laboratory setting, preferably one devoted to lysosomal enzymology. It is fortunate that most lysosomal enzymes are quite stable on freezing (α-neuraminidase is an exception); so if necessary, enzyme preparations can be shipped to distant localities for assay.

A leukocyte pellet sufficient for multiple assays can be isolated from 10 mL of fresh, whole heparinized blood by the dextran sedimentation procedure.[82] A repeat sedimentation step can double the yield of leukocytes, an especially valuable consideration when the amount of blood is limited because of the size, age, or medical condition of the patient (usually a child). If molecular DNA analyses are to be performed, ethylenediaminetetraacetic acid is the preferred anticoagulant because heparin can inhibit the polymerase chain reaction (PCR) assay. Specimens of blood should also be obtained from the child's parents to be used for confirmation of any enzyme defect discovered in the child's blood. When tested for activity of the relevant enzyme, the parents' specimens should demonstrate intermediate levels of enzyme activity, indicative of their heterozygous status.

Molecular Analysis. Detection of heterozygotes in X-linked conditions, such as Hunter's disease, by enzyme assay is more difficult because of the overlap with normal values that can occur as a result of mosaicism in expression of the X chromosome in females,[83] and therefore DNA techniques[84] have proved to be more reliable for detection of carriers in this disease.[85,86] For each lysosomal enzyme gene that has been cloned, a multiplicity of mutant alleles have been discovered. Although a number of these mutations may be common in patients with the same LSDs, many are sporadic and specific to individual families. Therefore, it is not practical to use mutation analysis only as a marker for a particular disease or to screen for carriers of the gene for this disease. However, within a research laboratory setting, genomic DNA or total mRNA can be isolated from peripheral lymphocytes or cultured fibroblasts and pro-

cessed further for nucleotide base sequencing. For genomic DNA, single-strand conformational polymorphism is used to locate fragments with an anomalous migration pattern on a gel, possibly indicative of an abnormal sequence. With the use of primers specific to this fragment, it can be amplified by PCR and sequenced to find the error. Alternatively, PCR of sequences encompassing the exon/intron boundaries may help identify splicing variants. Such molecular analysis is especially useful when the clinical phenotype is severe and residual enzyme activity is very low or absent and thus suggests the possibility of no transcription to mRNA.

In later-onset forms of disease with a less severe phenotype, mRNA may be detectable. It can be reverse-transcribed to complementary DNA (cDNA) and the specific disease-related cDNA amplified by PCR and cloned so that its nucleotide base sequence can be determined. This method is likely to reveal point mutations causing primarily amino acid substitutions but may also reveal splicing errors, as well as small insertions and duplications. To distinguish polymorphic changes from true disease-causing mutations, transient enzyme expression studies can be done with a culture system such as the COS cell, a strain of monkey cells. For more accurate detection of mutant enzymes that have only low residual enzyme activity, transient expression studies should be performed on patient fibroblasts that have no endogenous enzyme activity.[87] Only alterations resulting in partial or complete loss of enzyme activity can be relied on as markers for the carrier state in relatives of an affected patient and for prenatal diagnosis.

In families in which specific molecular defects in DNA have been detected, enzyme analysis can be supplemented by mutation analysis. This approach is not only useful for carrier testing and prenatal diagnosis but can also be extended to retrospective diagnosis for an affected family member who died without a specific biochemical diagnosis. This option is available through PCR amplification of genomic DNA extracted from paraffin-embedded biopsy or autopsy material originally prepared for histologic study.

Animal Models

Although the common macroscopic evidence of LSD in tissues is the presence of vacuolated cells, the cellular and molecular consequences of the intralysosomal accumulation of various metabolites are still largely unknown. Given the complexity of these disorders, this information will prove crucial for addressing the feasibility and limitations of therapy for neurodegenerative LSDs, analysis of which is often impossible in affected children. Studies are currently beginning to emerge that will help relate storage of potentially toxic metabolites to cell dysfunction and cell death.[88,89] Many LSDs have now been genetically engineered in small laboratory animals or have been diagnosed in spontaneously occurring animal models. In most instances, these models closely recapitulate the corresponding human diseases and are therefore important tools for studies of disease pathogenesis and treatment of these disorders.[90,91]

Treatment

Symptomatic Treatment

After the diagnosis of a storage disease is made, the physician often believes that the family must be given a prognosis. Because none of the storage diseases can be cured and their progressive course cannot usually be halted, a bleak outlook is presented and the distraught family leaves without a clear understanding of how to manage their child's illness. Actually, the clinical state is quite stable in a number of the storage diseases (e.g., adult Gaucher's disease; type B Niemann-Pick disease, α-mannosidosis, aspartylglucosaminuria, and the cherry-red spot/myoclonus variant of sialidosis). Moreover, the same storage disease does not follow the same timetable of clinical signs in any two patients. Instead of prognostication, attention should be focused on alleviating or ameliorating existing signs and symptoms.

Feeding problems may arise because of bulbar paralysis, and hence changes in the consistency of the child's food and in feeding techniques might be required. Consultation with a nutritionist may be needed to ensure that the child continues to receive adequate fluid and caloric intake. Chronic constipation must be managed, the skin surface must be protected from ulcerations, and dental hygiene must be maintained to prevent caries. Seizures occurring in the course of gray matter storage disease of the brain generally respond to combinations of certain drugs, including diazepam (Valium), carbamazepine (Tegretol), valproic acid (Depakene), clonazepam (Klonopin), and lamotrigine (Lamictal). To prevent joint contractures, a regular program of physical therapy should be established. Orthopedic corrective procedures, otorhinolaryngologic surgery, and other types of operative intervention should not be withheld if they will make nursing care easier or bring relief to a child who has a clinically vexing problem.

The child's education is also important. Infant stimulation programs in daycare centers and special nursery school and kindergarten programs are available for handicapped children through the Easter Seals Society, United Cerebral Palsy, and similar organizations. By taking advantage of these resources, the family and child can feel that they are not missing out on opportunities for self-expression and achievement available to other children.

Enzyme Replacement Therapy

The lysosomal enzyme precursors secreted into the extracellular milieu are usually completely poised to be reinternalized by the same cell or neighboring cells via receptor-mediated endocytosis. Most cell types express the M6P receptor, which accommodates efficient uptake of mannose-6-phosphorylated lysosomal enzymes.[6]

However, Kupffer cells in the liver, microglia in the brain, and resident macrophages in other tissues express mannose receptors that allow uptake of mannosylated enzymes. Specific overexpression systems are currently used to achieve the desired modification of the overexpressed enzyme, such as CHO cells for M6P and yeast, plant, or insect cells for mannosylated enzymes.[92-95] Alternatively, the complex carbohydrates on CHO-expressed enzymes are enzymatically remodeled to the mannose core type to facilitate uptake by the mannose receptor.[96]

The unique capacity of most lysosomal enzyme to be released and recaptured by different cell types has formed the basis of ERT.[97] This therapeutic approach has been shown to be extraordinarily effective for patients with the non-neuropathic form of Gaucher's disease, the most prevalent metabolic storage disorder in humans and the first to be treated by this approach. Demonstration of the benefit of ERT in this disorder led eventually to extension of this therapeutic modality to the treatment of other LSDs.[98] The results of ERT in clinical trials of Pompe's disease,[99] Fabry's disease[100,101] and mucopolysaccharidosis I and VI (MPS I and VI),[102] as well as in numerous animal models,[102-105] have demonstrated that this procedure could be effective against some non-neuropathic LSDs. However, ERT alone is unlikely to ameliorate the more severe neuropathic forms of LSDs unless it is combined with other treatments.[106] The presence of the blood-brain barrier, which effectively prevents most soluble molecules from entering the CNS, hampers the applicability of this approach for the cure of neuropathic patients, so different therapies should be sought.

Substrate Reduction Therapy

Glycosphingolipids (GSLs) are components of the outer leaflet of plasma membranes in most eukaryotic cells. They are present in cell-specific patterns and are composed of a hydrophobic ceramide moiety that is linked to a hydrophilic glycan chain of variable length and structure. GSLs have been implicated in a variety of functions ranging from cellular differentiation to intracellular signaling. They are synthesized de novo, beginning with the rate-limiting step of ceramide formation by glycosyltransferase and the subsequent addition of glycan chains to this glycosylceramide core. Upon exerting their metabolic actions, they are eventually degraded in lysosomes via an endocytic process.[107]

Imino sugars such as N-butyldeoxygalactonojirimycin (NB-DGJ), one of the early GSL synthesis inhibitors to be studied, was initially investigated as an antiviral agent for patients with acquired immunodeficiency syndrome, but its use was abandoned when other antiviral agents became available.[108] However, further research into the biology of GSLs showed that inhibition of their synthesis may play a role in the treatment of some LSDs. The rationale behind this principle is that by reducing the amount of available substrate, a decrease in the degree of their deposition in affected cells should be expected.

It is also hypothesized that in certain LSD variants, the presence of residual enzymatic activity may be enough to control the signs and symptoms of disease if synthesis of GSLs is concomitantly decreased. This would therefore lead to a certain degree of "metabolic balance." One of the potential additional advantages of this approach is that these compounds cross the blood-brain barrier, in contrast to ERT, which is restricted to act outside the CNS and thus cannot aid in clearing lysosomal storage from neurons.

The first published suggestion for using this approach to treating the LSDs came from Radin.[109] Since then, several studies have been performed in vitro and in various animal models for these conditions and in at least one clinical trial.[110] In the latter, several patients with the non-neuronopathic variant of Gaucher's disease (type 1 β-glucocerebrosidase deficiency) were treated with *N*-butyldeoxynojirimycin (miglustat), a potent inhibitor of glucosylceramide synthase, which is a glucosyltransferase enzyme responsible for the first step in the synthesis of most GSLs; such treatment resulted in decreased visceral volumes and improved hematologic parameters after 1 year. Further studies in other animal models for LSDs, such as Fabry's disease[111] and G_{M2}-gangliosidosis,[112,113] have shown additional promising effects. Side effects often encountered include diarrhea, weight loss, a reversible peripheral neuropathy, and at least in mice, lymphoid organ acellularity.[114-117] In 2003, miglustat was approved by the Food and Drug Administration for the treatment of symptoms in Gaucher type 1 patients who were not treated with Cerezyme (see later). Miglustat is now commercially available as Zavesca (Actelion Pharmaceuticals) and may be administered in combination with Cerezyme. In addition, the therapeutic effects of miglustat in patients with type C Niemann-Pick disease have been evaluated in a clinical trial (see later). The therapeutic benefits were consistent with previous trials in type 1 Gaucher patients, and miglustat improved or stabilized multiple clinically relevant markers of Niemann-Pick disease type C.[118]

Chaperone-Mediated Enzyme Enhancement

Chaperone-mediated therapy is a new therapeutic approach that is being developed for the treatment of selected patients with LSDs.[117] This method is based on the use of small sugar nucleotides that function as pharmacologic chaperones by specifically binding to and stabilizing misfolded mutant proteins in the ER. Binding of the chaperone molecule to the nascent mutant enzyme helps it fold into its correct three-dimensional shape and to be transported out of the ER and routed to the lysosome. The end result is an increase in residual enzyme activity of the mutant protein, an increase that can be sufficient to clear storage products in lysosomes and to correct the disease phenotype. This therapeutic approach has proved beneficial for some of the disease-causing mutations in patients with Gaucher's disease.[119] Though very promising, the caveats of this strategy are that (1)

only patients with single point mutations and residual enzyme activity will be potentially responsive to treatment and (2) not all the amino acid substitutions on a given enzyme may be corrected by the chaperones.

Hematopoietic Stem Cell Transplantation

More than 25 years has passed since the first report of bone marrow transplantation (BMT) being used to treat an LSD, namely, Hurler's disease.[120] Subsequent studies have proved its efficacy for some, but not all of the LSDs (Table 24-5). However, many questions remain, including proper selection of candidates, expected final outcome, and the appropriate time to perform BMT. Furthermore, great advances have been made in understanding the cellular and biochemical mechanisms that underlie engraftment or rejection processes, yet the overall mortality rate associated with this procedure remains relatively high, between 5% and 15%, depending on the institution and type of underlying disease. Nevertheless, BMT is increasingly being used for a wider range of disorders, both genetic and acquired, and with fewer associated complications than before. Finally, ethical issues (including exposure of asymptomatic children to the morbidity associated with BMT) and the futile prolongation of a life without consciousness of existence are beginning to emerge, and it is likely that they will become more urgent with the use of stem cells in the near future.

Because autologous BMT is not yet a therapeutic option for patients with LSDs, allogeneic (either related or unrelated) donors are the usual source of hematopoietic progenitors for these patients.[133,148] Donors who were identical human leukocyte antigen (HLA) matches have been used, preferably not those who are heterozygous carriers for the condition, with good results; however, this situation is not a common one. Therefore, either distant relatives (partial HLA matches) or unrelated donors are still the most common sources of HSCs. This fact increases the likelihood of not only rejection but also graft-versus-host disease, a significant source of both morbidity and mortality in recipients of bone marrow transplants.

Besides BMT, umbilical cord blood from unrelated donors who are not HLA identical with the recipient has been applied to the treatment of pediatric LSDs and been shown to restore hematopoiesis after myeloablative therapy.[149] Although immunologic rejection can be avoided with this therapeutic approach, the amount of these cells that is commonly obtained is rate limiting, and therefore only infants are likely to benefit from this procedure.[150] Nonetheless, use of these immunologically privileged cells as an alternative to BMT has given promising results in eliminating graft-versus-host disease in the majority of treated patients.[149] Survival rates associated with this procedure can be expected to be at least similar to those seen when transplants from HLA-identical donors are used. Rates have been as high as 73% at 1 year after umbilical cord blood stem cell

TABLE 24-5	Bone Marrow Transplantation for Lysosomal Storage Diseases		
	CLINICAL RESPONSE		
Disease	**Effective***	**Not Effective**	**References**
Aspartylglucosaminuria		+	121, 122
Farber's disease	Reduction in nodule size		121, 123, 124
Fucosidosis	+		121, 125, 126
Gaucher's disease			
Type 1	+ (enzyme replacement therapy preferred)		121, 127, 128
Type 2		+	
Type 3	+		
Hunter's disease (MPS type II)	+ (effective for later-onset mild cases only)		129, 130
			131, 132
Hurler's syndrome (MPS type I)	+ (visceral effects improved)		121, 133
			134-138
Mannosidosis	+ (probable, if performed early)		121[†]
Maroteaux-Lamy syndrome (MPS type VI)	+ (cardiac improvement, prolonged survival)		139, 140
Neuronal ceroid lipofuscinosis		+	141, 142
Niemann-Pick disease			
Type A		+	143
Type B	+		144
Type C	+ (liver disease improved, but not CNS involvement)		145
Sanfilippo's disease (MPS type III), all variants		+	146
Sly's disease (MPS type VII)	+		121[†]
Wolman's disease	+		147[†]

*Effective if transplantation is performed early in the clinical course.
[†]Krivit W: Personal communication.
CNS, central nervous system, MPS, mucopolysaccharidoses.

transplantation.[149,150] However, it is not yet clear to what extent stem cells from umbilical cord blood can provide an adequate source of enzyme to correct the respective deficiency in the long term because many of these precursor cells may not be fully differentiated and able to degrade excess intracellular macromolecules.

Although data on the actual percentage of successful engraftment are quite encouraging, with values of up to 90% attained in patients with adrenoleukodystrophy (for both related and unrelated donors as a whole),* there is no evidence that enzymes circulating in blood can reach the brain parenchyma. Instead, the efficacy of this procedure is due to the entry of marrow-derived cells that can cross the blood-brain barrier. In several of the inherited leukodystrophies, neurologic progression has been halted by BMT,[133] possibly through the appearance of a new population of macrophage-derived microglia and perhaps even astrocytes.[151,152] In animal models, BMT has been particularly successful in improving or delaying the advent of CNS disease.[91,153] However, patients with diseases in which neuronal storage occurs (such as G_{M1}-gangliosidosis, Pompe's disease, acute neuronopathic Gaucher's disease, and Niemann-Pick disease type A) have not benefitted from BMT.

In summary, HSC transplantation is most likely to succeed when an HLA-identical donor is available, when the disease to be treated is not associated with gross nerve cell storage, and when the disease is treated before severe structural damage has occurred.[129,154] It seems very likely that with recent advances in understanding the molecular biology of the immune mechanisms underlying donor cell rejection and other associated complications, use of this procedure will become an acceptable means of treating patients with LSDs for which no additional therapy is yet available. Finally, the possibility of using minimal myeloablation in small infants to obtain initial engraftment with less associated morbidity is slowly becoming an additional option. However, it is important to keep in mind that response to HSC transplantation may also be influenced by the following variables that could have a different impact on the therapeutic outcome in different LSDs: (1) the type and number of engrafted donor cells; (2) the biochemical and physical properties of the secreted, correcting enzyme; (3) the efficiency of secretion and extracellular stability of the correcting enzyme; (4) the extent of uptake by target cells; and (5) the characteristics of the affected cells, as well as the level of cell degeneration.

Gene Therapy

Ex Vivo. Somatic gene therapy could be the treatment of choice for LSDs if the patient's own cells could

---

*Peters C: Personal communication.

be genetically modified in vitro or in vivo to constitutively express and secrete the correcting enzyme and thus become the source of the correcting enzyme in the patient. Both ex vivo and in vivo gene transfer methods have been tested for somatic gene therapy for LSDs. Delivery systems include gated vectors containing partial sequences from retroviruses, adenoviruses, adeno-associated viruses (AAVs), herpes simplex viruses, lentiviruses, and others, as well as nonviral systems. Although these methods have proved efficient for the transfer of genetic material into deficient cells in culture and for correction of the deficient enzyme activity,[155-150] the same gene transfer systems applied to humans or animal models have shown inconsistent results, the bases for which are not yet fully understood.

Retroviral vectors have thus far been the most exploited gene transfer vehicles[160] for the treatment of LSDs because they have the advantage of stably integrating at random sites into the host genome, thereby potentially affording long-term expression. However, their use is limited by the fact that they target only dividing cells, they are difficult to produce at high titer for in vivo application, and depending on their integration site, they can permanently alter the expression of neighboring genes. Nevertheless, numerous studies describing the use of retroviral-mediated gene therapy in animal models of LSDs are reported in the literature.[161-166]

The overall outcome of these studies points to the potential of retroviral-mediated gene transfer to HSCs for improving systemic disease in small laboratory animals, but again, use of this procedure for the treatment of CNS pathology has yielded inconsistent results in different animal models. Once more, the time of treatment seems to be the rate-limiting step in these therapeutic procedures, especially if we attempt to prevent or delay progression or even reverse CNS pathology. Despite the limitations encountered so far, ex vivo studies in animal models have helped set the stage for trials of human stem cell gene therapy in patients with Gaucher's disease.[167-169] HSCs from patients' peripheral blood or bone marrow were transduced with a retrovirus expressing human glucocerebrosidase cDNA and infused into nonablated recipients. Although transduction efficiency was low, gene-marked cells persisted for about 3 months, but the number of corrected cells was too low to afford any increase in enzyme activity and therapeutic benefit. To circumvent the problems of low transduction efficiency and expression, alternative gene therapy approaches are being developed that make use of vectors based on lentiviruses, including human immunodeficiency virus type 1 (HIV-1).[170] These vectors have a broader host range than retroviral vectors do because they transduce both dividing and nondividing cells and have been shown to effectively target human CD34+ cells.[171] In addition, treatment of the CNS pathology in LSDs remains a challenging issue that is specifically being addressed in many of the gene transfer studies currently pursued.

In Vivo. In vivo gene therapy refers to the injection of a gene transfer vector directly into a tissue or into the circulation. There are a number of preclinical studies in small and large animal models of LSD in which this procedure has been tested, with variable outcome. Although these have been useful, proof-of-principle experiments, expression of the gene of interest was often transient because of the severe immune reactions directed against the vector.[172]

Intravenous delivery of AAV-based vectors has resulted in biochemical, histologic, and clinical improvement in several murine models of LSD. Robust expression plus a reduction in lysosomal storage was observed in many tissues after AAV injection in young adult animals with MPS VII or Fabry's disease.[173,174] Even more convincing results, such as improved bone or skeletal development, retinal function, and auditory function, were observed in MPS VII and MPS I mice injected during the neonatal period.[175-177] Studies in neonates demonstrate the utility of early (disease prevention) rather than delayed (disease reversal) intervention for these progressive disorders. Lentiviral gene transfer vectors have also been tested for direct in vivo gene therapy applications. Intravenous injections of either a feline immunodeficiency viral vector in the MPS VII mouse or an HIV-based vector in MPS I and MPS IIIB mice resulted in persistent high-level expression of the respective enzymes and reduction of lysosomal storage in multiple tissues.[178-180]

Partial biochemical and histologic correction has been achieved in the mouse model of Fabry's disease after either hydrodynamic delivery of naked plasmid DNA or plasmid DNA complexed to cationic lipids.[181] Although these approaches reduce some of the concerns surrounding the use of viral vectors, expression is transient and repeated administration will be required.

Regardless of the delivery system, some diseases may be more resilient to treatment than others. In such instances, we might approach therapy from the standpoint of the accumulated products rather the enzyme deficiency. As discussed earlier, inhibition of substrate synthesis, as opposed to supplementation of the missing enzyme, has already been investigated for the treatment of glycolipid storage diseases with promising results.[110,115] Combining substrate inhibitors and BMT was found to be synergistic in correcting pathologic signs in the Sandhoff mouse model.[182] Last but not least, early treatment may be the only approach for early-onset patients, who are often devoid of residual enzyme. Ultimately, a combination of different therapies may be the method of choice for neurologic LSDs that require both systemic and CNS correction. Behind the relatively simple concept of cross-correction that makes LSDs particularly amenable models for gene therapy trials lies the complexity and diversity of these diseases, which must be addressed and carefully evaluated because they are likely to influence the response to treatment. It is clear that many limitations and pitfalls still need to be overcome to make the transition of gene therapy from animal models to the clinic an educated and judicious approach.

Prevention

In most instances, the amount of lysosomal enzyme activity correlates with the level of the wild-type gene present. For example, enzyme levels in carriers of an abnormal allele (heterozygotes) are approximately half those in normal individuals. Thus, heterozygotes for specific recessive disease traits can in principle be identified by enzyme assay, provided that there is no overlap between enzyme levels in heterozygotes and those in normal or diseased individuals. In actual practice, this is rarely, if ever achieved.

Detection of heterozygotes by enzyme assay serves several functions. The finding of heterozygosity in the parents of an individual with a storage disease helps confirm the diagnosis in that individual. This method of testing is particularly valuable when the propositus has died without enzymatic confirmation of a diagnosis. Siblings, cousins, and other close relatives of a patient with a storage disease can be told specifically whether there is a chance that they can pass the abnormal gene to their offspring. Relatives who have the abnormal gene and who are married will probably also want their spouses tested to assess their joint risk of having an affected child.

In families in which specific molecular defects in genomic DNA have been detected, enzyme analysis can be complemented by mutation analysis. This approach not only is useful for carrier testing and prenatal diagnosis but can also be extended to retrospective diagnosis for an affected family member who has died without a specific biochemical diagnosis. This option is available through PCR amplification of genomic DNA extracted from paraffin-embedded biopsy or autopsy material originally prepared for histologic study.

In the rare instances in which both spouses are heterozygotes, the risk with each pregnancy of producing an affected offspring is 25%. In these circumstances, chorionic villus biopsy performed at about the 8th to 9th week or amniocentesis at the 14th to 16th week of gestation permits biochemical determinations to be made on cells of fetal origin. In this way, a prenatal diagnosis can be made early enough so that a pregnancy can be terminated if the fetus is affected. Families previously affected by the tragedy of an infant with a fatal form of a storage disease may thus be spared the burden of additional progeny having the same disease and can anticipate having healthy children without fear. Happily, the outcome for the majority (75%) of prenatal diagnoses in these high-risk families is a clinically unaffected child. This reduces the incidence of abortion in families who are determined to avoid having an affected child because without this assurance, such families may otherwise elect to terminate all pregnancies.

Prenatal diagnosis has been accomplished or is theoretically possible for each of the storage diseases.[183] An abnormality often reported in these conditions is the presence of hydrops fetalis or unexplained fetal death. In these instances, examination of tissue morphology should be performed carefully.[184] Parents of a child with a sphingolipidosis, mucopolysaccharidosis, or oligosaccharidosis are advised to consult a genetic counselor as soon as possible after the diagnosis is made in their child to be judiciously informed about the availability of prenatal diagnosis for future pregnancies. Otherwise, one or both parents may choose to undergo a sterilization procedure in the mistaken belief that all their subsequent offspring will be similarly affected. In addition, the mother might already be pregnant or might become pregnant and be unaware of the prenatal diagnostic option until after the optimal time for conducting such studies has passed. Frequently, one of the factors motivating parents to obtain a specific diagnosis in their young child with a storage disease is a current pregnancy. This circumstance may place a severe time constraint on the laboratory by requiring diagnosis of the affected child before the pregnancy passes the midtrimester point, after which prenatal diagnostic amniocentesis is no longer practical.

Screening of large populations for heterozygotes has been accomplished most successfully for Tay-Sachs disease. The circumstances that have made this practicable are a high incidence of the gene in a small subgroup of the population (Ashkenazic Jews) and the availability of a simple, dependable, and economical test for heterozygotes. These conditions have not been met for massive screening of other storage diseases, either because the disease trait is very rare and distributed equally throughout the general population or because the enzyme assay for heterozygotes is complicated and cannot be automated or in some other way performed inexpensively. In addition, without knowledge of an index case in the family, interpretation of enzyme tests for heterozygotes may be difficult because carriers of two diseases with a different clinical prognosis, such as Hurler's disease and Scheie's disease, may be indistinguishable. Molecular probes should help clarify the exact genotype in such circumstances. Finally, because trace amounts of fetal DNA can be detected in the maternal circulation,[185] it is entirely possible that affected pregnancies will be identified at early stages of gestation and could then be analyzed for known or suspected mutations.

Preimplantation genetic diagnosis represents an alternative to prenatal diagnosis in couples in whom in vitro fertilization is an acceptable option. It involves the molecular analysis of embryonic cells that are removed at very early stages of development, usually polar bodies from the oocyte/zygote state or blastomeres.[186,187] After a diagnosis is made, the healthy embryos are then implanted, thereby avoiding the ethical and medical dilemmas that are commonly associated with termination of pregnancy.[188] However, at present, prevention of the storage diseases relies on the concepts of early case identification, screening of close relatives for heterozygosity, and prenatal diagnosis during pregnancies in which both spouses carry the same recessive trait.

GLYCOSPHINGOLIPIDOSES

The glycosphingolipidoses account for 10 categories of storage disease, each characterized by the accumulation of a particular sphingolipid in either neural or extraneural tissues, or both. The basic unit of the stored material, ceramide, is composed of the long-chain amino alcohol sphingosine joined to a fatty acid of 16 to 26 carbon atoms by an amide linkage at the nitrogen atom on carbon 2 of sphingosine (Fig. 24-2).

Individual sphingolipids belong to one of four subgroups, depending on the types of substituents joined to the primary alcohol on carbon 1 of sphingosine (i.e., sphingomyelin, neutral GSLs, sulfatoglycosphingolipids, and gangliosides). Sphingomyelin is a phospholipid component of cell membranes. The neutral GSLs are found in many body tissues, with normally high concentrations of globoside in red blood cell membranes and ceramide trihexoside in the kidney. The sulfolipids and galactolipids are important in the formation of myelin. Gangliosides are abundant in the nervous system.

Catabolism of the sphingolipids occurs by the stepwise hydrolysis of linkages joining the various components of the molecule. The sequence of cleavage is from the terminal nonreducing hydrophilic end of the molecule toward the hydrophobic sphingosine portion. The structure of the individual sphingolipids, their degradative pathway, and the reactions blocked in each of the sphingolipidoses are shown in Figure 24-3.

Not all the glycosphingolipidoses cause lipid storage in cells of the reticuloendothelial system. The pathologic findings in metachromatic leukodystrophy and Krabbe's disease are confined to the nervous system and consist of severe myelin destruction and a segmental peripheral neuropathy. Clinically, blindness, long-tract signs, and loss of reflexes occur. Elevated spinal fluid protein concentrations and delayed nerve conduction velocities are early diagnostic findings.

Tay-Sachs disease, the most common form of G_{M2}-gangliosidosis, results in ballooning of nerve cells throughout the neuraxis. Psychomotor retardation and a cherry-red spot in the macula are early signs. Eventually, seizures, megacephaly, blindness, and flaccid quadripare-

sis develop before the affected child dies, usually between 3 and 5 years of age. Before heterozygote testing for the Tay-Sachs trait became widely available, the majority of cases were found in the offspring of Ashkenazic Jews. As a result of carrier testing and prenatal diagnosis in this population, the number of patients with Tay-Sachs disease has since declined, with a much greater proportion now being observed in children of non-Jewish parentage.

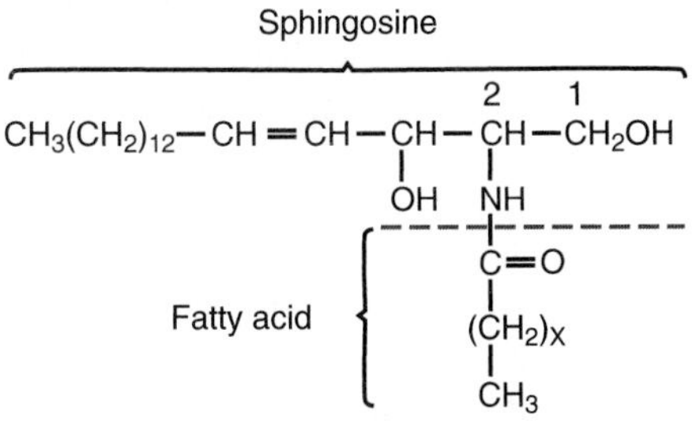

The lesions in Fabry's disease are predominantly extraneural, located primarily in the vascular endothelium and kidneys. It is an X-linked disease that is usually recognized in early adolescent boys by the onset of intermittent pain in the hands and feet and the appearance of clusters of purple punctate angiokeratomas. The presence of feathery corneal opacities on slit-lamp examination helps establish the diagnosis in hemizygotes and confirm heterozygosity in their mothers and sisters.

Another of the sphingolipidoses, fucosidosis, is discussed with the oligosaccharidoses.

Gaucher's Disease (Glucosylceramide Lipidosis)

Gaucher's disease is the oldest known and most often encountered type of inherited lipidosis. Large lipid-filled macrophages, known as Gaucher cells, accumulate within the bone marrow, spleen, liver, and other components of the reticuloendothelial system. It was first reported in 1882 by Philippe C. E. Gaucher, who described it as an epithelioma of the spleen without leukemia.[189] The degree of clinical involvement differs greatly in individual patients, even those harboring the same genotype and those affected within the same family. The major storage product is glucocerebroside, catabolism of which is blocked by a deficiency of the lysosomal enzyme glucocerebroside β-glucosidase (glucocerebrosidase). The glucocerebroside is derived from three compounds commonly present in senescent blood cells: (1) lactosylceramide, the major glycolipid of leukocytes; (2) globoside, the principal red blood cell glycolipid; and (3) the blood group GSLs. Gaucher's disease is also important from a historical perspective in the study of LSDs in that it was the first of such conditions in which identification of the accumulated product led to isolation and purification of the enzyme and eventual therapy for patients with these disorders. The success was such that it has become the prototype for research and therapeutic efforts in this field.

Gaucher's disease is a relatively common disorder. The three clinical forms of this condition (see later) are pan-ethnic. However, the incidence of type 1 is increased in Ashkenazic Jews to approximately 1 in 350 to 450 live births. In the general population the incidence of type 1 is 1 in 40,000 to 60,000 live births. The respective incidence of carriers is 1 in 8 to 10 for Ashkenazic Jews and 1 in 100 for non-Jews. Types 2 and 3 are much rarer, with an estimated incidence of about 1 in 500,000 and 1 in

Sphingosine

$$CH_3(CH_2)_{12}-CH = CH - \overset{2}{CH} - \overset{1}{CH} - CH_2OH$$

OH   NH

C=O

Fatty acid { $(CH_2)_x$

CH_3

FIGURE 24-2. Chemical structure of ceramide.

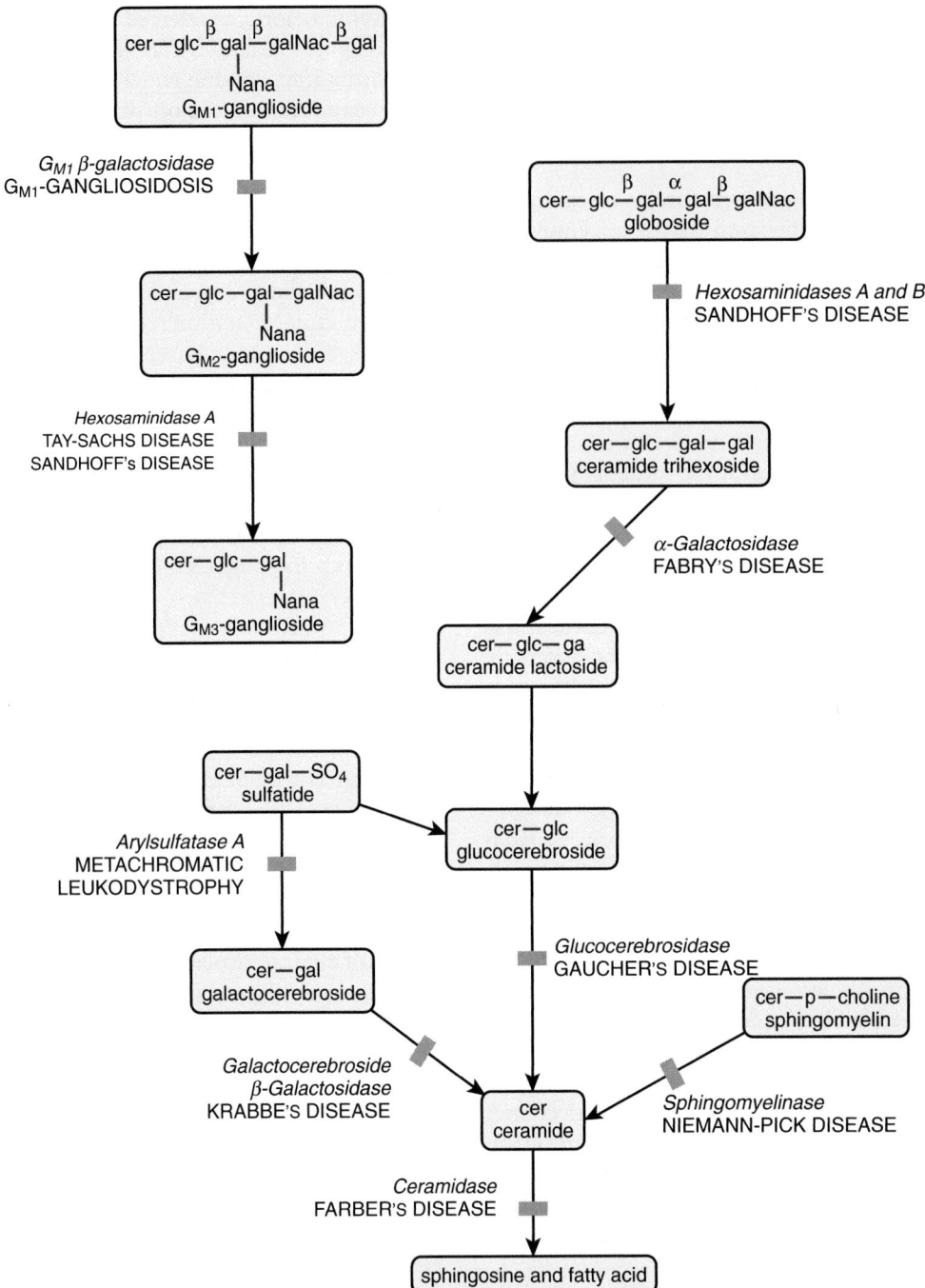

FIGURE 24-3. Pathways and diseases of sphingolipid metabolism. The enzymes involved are shown in *italics*. Listed below each enzyme is the disease that results from deficiency of that enzyme. cer, ceramide; gal, galactose; galNAC, *N*-acetylgalactosamine; glc, glucose; Nana, *N*-acetylneuraminic acid; p, phosphoryl.

50,000 live births, respectively, although an isolate of type 3 is present in the population of northern Sweden (Norbottnian). The comparable incidence of carriers is 1 in 150 and 1 in 100.

Gaucher's disease has been classified on the basis of CNS involvement into three types. Type 1, the most common form, has no primary CNS involvement. Types 2 and 3 both affect the CNS, but they do so at different rates. Type 2 is the so-called acute neuronopathic type, whereas type 3 has a more protracted course. However,

some investigators have recently challenged this classification[190] and believe that the distinction between type 2 and type 3 is probably artificial. They propose only two variants: the non-neuronopathic and the neuronopathic forms. Further discussion on this issue is likely to occur in the coming years because this distinction may have important implications for treatment and prognosis.

In addition, four other rare neuronopathic variants have been reported in infancy: one in which calcification of the aortic arch and valves is the prominent feature[191];

one in which nonimmune hydrops fetalis dominates the clinical picture[192]; one in which the neuronopathic findings are associated with hydrocephalus, corneal opacities, and deformed toes[193]; and one in which acute neuronopathic features are associated with congenital ichthyosis.[194,195] Interestingly, this fulminant form of the disease was identified after similar dermatologic findings were reported in the knockout mouse model for Gaucher's disease.[196] In this latter model death occurs within a few hours of birth.

Type 1: Chronic Non-neuronopathic (Adult) Gaucher's Disease

The great majority of occurrences of Gaucher's disease are type 1, the chronic non-neuronopathic form of the disease. Hematologic findings dominate the clinical picture of patients with this form of the disease, although osseous complications may on occasion be the initial feature. The spleen is usually enlarged from an early age and, in some patients, can become so large that it causes abdominal distention and pain. Anemia is generally present because of decreased red blood cell survival, although bone marrow infiltration may also be a contributing factor. The anemia may be either normocytic or microcytic and hypochromic and is probably due to hypersplenism rather than crowding out of erythropoietic activity in the bone marrow by Gaucher's cells. Although iron therapy may temporarily help the anemia, it is not recommended because Gaucher cells avidly take up iron, thereby reducing its availability for erythropoiesis and leading to secondary hemochromatosis.

A tendency toward bleeding as a result of thrombocytopenia and coagulation factor abnormalities is a more serious consequence of the hypersplenism and liver involvement that occurs in this form of Gaucher's disease. Easy bruising and epistaxis are also common complaints in childhood. Trauma to the enlarged spleen is a special danger because of the possibility of rupture and hemorrhage. This hazard also exists when a patient with Gaucher's disease and hypersplenism contracts an infection in which splenic involvement is common, such as acute mononucleosis. Bleeding into other organs and metrorrhagia may also occur. In one patient with portal hypertension, hematemesis occurred as a result of rupture of esophageal varices.[197] As mentioned earlier, various coagulation defects, including deficiencies of factors VIII, IX, and XI and von Willebrand factor antigen, probably contribute to the tendency for bleeding in this condition. These deficiencies are variable and not consistently demonstrable in all patients,[198-200] but they can become a source for concern in patients who will be subjected to either surgical or extensive dental procedures. In the past, splenectomy was performed because of thrombocytopenia with recurrent bleeding or because of marked abdominal pain and discomfort produced by the large spleen. Although platelet counts increase after splenectomy and episodes of bleeding no longer occur, this radical surgical approach is rarely recommended now because of its

inherent complications, including high susceptibility to infections. Fluctuations in spleen size can occur in Gaucher's disease as a result of intercurrent infection or pregnancy.[201] Additional hematologic complications include mild megaloblastic anemia secondary to vitamin B_{12} deficiency and monoclonal gammopathies. A few individuals with coexistent multiple myeloma have been reported.[202-204] As mentioned earlier, there is also a slightly increased incidence of malignancies, especially of the hematopoietic system,[204] such as leukemia[205] and Hodgkin's disease.[206] This increase in lymphoid neoplasia could result from the reduction in natural killer cells reported to occur in Gaucher's disease.[207] Finally, there is a general increase in activity of the immune system as manifested by hypergammaglobulinemia and a significant increase in the incidence of autoantibodies.[208] These most likely result from increased levels of cytokines. Commonly used serum inflammatory markers such as transferrin and angiotensin-converting enzyme are often elevated.

Bone complications are common. As Gaucher cells infiltrate the medullary cavity, there is loss of bone density, thinning of the cortex, loss of the normal trabeculations, patchy myelosclerosis, and bone infarcts and the resulting osteonecrosis. At least half of all patients show an "Erlenmeyer flask" deformity, in which the midshaft of the femur has a tapered appearance and the distal end is widened because of failure of trabeculation. This same change may also be seen in the proximal ends of the tibia and fibula. In addition, aseptic necrosis of the head and neck of the femur can occur and cause disability and pain that may require surgical arthroplasty. Other forms of pathologic fractures are also seen, as well as bone infarcts that cause episodes of severe incapacitating bone and joint pain.[209] In children with this condition, growth failure is commonly found. Such failure could be related to the anemia or to the reported increase in resting energy expenditure in patients with this condition.[210] Furthermore, although they may eventually reach their final predicted height late in life, there are serious concerns about the final quality of the bone and the possibility of early osteoporosis.

Most patients have some degree of hepatosplenomegaly, and portal hypertension sometimes occurs, but liver failure is rare, although mild abnormalities in liver function test results are commonly encountered. Rare patients in whom liver failure or cirrhosis has developed have a concomitant history of infection with hepatitis C virus, probably caused by previous transfusion of contaminated blood.

The onset of puberty may be delayed and heavy menstrual bleeding can occur. During pregnancy, anemia and thrombocytopenia may worsen and bone crises can develop. However, most women with Gaucher's disease successfully complete their pregnancies without complications from the disease.[211]

Diffuse pulmonary infiltration develops in a few patients, although this serious complication seems to occur more often in children with severe disease. Pulmonary hypertension is another rarely reported complication.[212] Renal disease is unusual. Finally, indirect neurologic involvement can also occur, such as spinal cord compression secondary to vertebral fractures or peripheral nerve injuries associated with long bone fractures or bleeding into a nerve sheath.

As mentioned earlier, approximately 60% of patients with type 1 Gaucher's disease are of Ashkenazic Jewish ancestry. In this particular population, the rate of occurrence of the gene may be as high as 8% or greater.[209] However, the actual incidence of disease is much less than expected because the clinical spectrum includes many mildly affected individuals in whom the condition remains undiagnosed until late in life[213] or who may never become symptomatic. This latter category has been grossly estimated to include up to 25% of all patients. The variability in clinical expression is evident in families in which several members are affected; one family member may have severe incapacitating bone disease, whereas another has only mild hypersplenism and occasional joint pain. A particularly malignant form of the disease is seen primarily in non-Jewish children, in whom substantial splenomegaly develops by age 3 and portal hypertension by age 10. These patients have massive abdominal swelling and stunted linear growth and tend to have severe bone involvement as well. In this group of patients there is always the question of whether their disease may actually represent an early form of the chronic neuronopathic variant usually associated with lower levels of enzyme activity.

Laboratory diagnosis depends on the presence of Gaucher cells in bone marrow and the demonstration of a deficiency in lysosomal β-glucosidase activity measured in leukocytes or cultured skin fibroblasts. Conventional radiographs are used to determine the extent and pattern of bone involvement but are not helpful for determination of disease activity.[214] Dual-energy radiographic and quantitative computed tomographic methods permit evaluation of osteoporosis. The use of abdominal magnetic resonance imaging allows volumetric determinations to be made of the spleen and liver. It can disclose the presence of splenic nodules and infarcts and zones of ischemia within the liver. Magnetic resonance imaging is also used for quantitative imaging of bone to measure the marrow fat fraction. Nuclear bone scanning with ^{99m}Tc-methylenediphosphonate is a sensitive tool for examining active bone disease.[215] Ancillary findings in serum include elevations in activities of non–tartrate-inhibitable acid phosphatase (isoenzyme 5B), angiotensin 1–converting enzyme,[216] and transcobalamin II.[217] Plasma chitotriosidase may be elevated more than several hundred–fold above normal and can serve as a useful parameter for monitoring the treatment of patients.[218]

Type 2: Acute Neuronopathic (Infantile) Gaucher's Disease

A child with the acute neuronopathic variety of Gaucher's disease (type 2) is seen between birth and 6 months of age with failure to thrive, hepatosplenomegaly, muscular hypertonicity, and signs of brainstem dysfunction, including strabismus and retroflexion of the head. Other nervous system signs include dysphagia, laryngospasm, dyspnea, vomiting, and generalized spasticity. In addition, there are feeding difficulties, inanition, and weight loss. Death is inevitable before 2 years of age. A later-onset form has also been recognized in which strabismus develops during the first year but the child is otherwise normal until the second or third year of age.

Perivascular accumulations of Gaucher cells are found in the brains of these children, and their nerve cells are swollen by a PAS-positive, weakly sudanophilic material.[219] Brain specimens from patients with type 2 Gaucher's disease contain the highest concentrations of glucocerebroside and psychosine (sphingosine glucose)[220] and the most pronounced deficiency of acid β-glucosidase activity.[221] Psychosine (lysosphingosine) is believed to be neurotoxic. Interestingly, the degree of substrate accumulation in the brain is not as extensive as suspected from the biochemical findings alone, and the presence of neuronal death (which can be extensive at the cerebellar level) is probably more of a contributing factor than the accumulation of glycolipid by itself. Clearly, other factors, which may include increased apoptosis or dysregulated cell growth, may contribute to the pathophysiologic course of this condition and somehow explain the lack of definitive clinical response to ERT in these patients. Because of the early onset and fatal outcome of type 2 Gaucher's disease, prenatal diagnosis provides a feasible alternative to families at risk for having additional children with this disorder. Unfortunately, no therapeutic modality has proved to be effective in patients with this type of Gaucher's disease.

Type 3: Subacute Neuronopathic (Juvenile) Gaucher's Disease

In rare instances, nervous system involvement has occurred in older children and adults with Gaucher's disease. Neurologic findings have included decreased mental ability, seizures, oculomotor apraxia, poor coordination, and an increase in muscle tone. In some patients the condition most closely resembles the acute neuronopathic variety of Gaucher's disease,[222] whereas in others the clinical course is similar in many respects to the more common adult non-neuronopathic variety of the disease.[223] In a subset of these patients, a relatively stable clinical course is suddenly altered by the appearance of myoclonic epilepsy; the prognosis for these patients is poor. Electrophysiologic studies, which include measurement of brainstem auditory evoked responses, are a monitoring tool for the development of neurologic disease.[224]

Genetically, this particular condition is distinct from type 1 adult Gaucher's disease. It has been identified in several related patients from the Norbottnian region of northern Sweden but has not been reported in Ashkenazic Jews because genotype/phenotype correlations have demonstrated that the presence of only one N370S allele protects against the neuronopathic forms of the disease. This type 3 variant is also more commonly seen in patients exhibiting the L444P homozygous allele.[225] After splenectomy, the neurologic symptoms and mental retardation worsen, possibly as a result of increased levels of glucocerebroside in blood and perivascular Gaucher cells in the brain.[226] Because of the relentlessly progressive neurologic deterioration, these patients have been prime candidates for therapeutic experimentation such as enzyme replacement,[227] organ transplantation,[228] and bone marrow replacement.[229-232] Fortunately, in at least a subset of these patients, a response or stabilization of their condition has been seen after the administration of high doses of ERT (see later).

Molecular and Genetic Aspects

The mature enzyme, glucocerebroside β-glucosidase, is a glycosylated polypeptide of 497 amino acids. Binding studies with conduritol-β-epoxide have identified Asp443 as the active amino acid residue site.[233] Its structural gene, which contains 11 exons and 10 introns, maps to the human chromosome locus 1q21[234] and consists of 7604 nucleotides.[235,236] Interestingly, a pseudogene has also been identified within a single 32-kilobase (kb) fragment of genomic DNA. This pseudogene is 96% homologous with the active gene, but it contains four large deletions and numerous point substitutions. Both structures map to the same chromosomal locus; thus, great care must be exercised when mutation analysis is performed for these patients because the pseudogene normally contains sequences that are pathologic if present in the functional gene. This duplicate mapping could potentially lead to substantial diagnostic errors. It has also been hypothesized that the proximity between these two structures somehow increases the chance of abnormal recombination events during DNA replication.

In close proximity to these two genes reside several other genes that could, at least theoretically, influence the phenotype of the disease: the metaxin (*MTX*) gene (which also has a nearby pseudogene) and the thrombospondin 3 gene.[237,238] Metaxin is a mitochondrial import protein[239] that seems to be required for embryonic development in the mouse.[237] The second closely located gene (thrombospondin 3) codes for a protein that is probably involved in a variety of cellular regulatory processes and has been linked to large cell lymphoma.[240] Tissue-specific expression of glucocerebroside β-glucosidase is suggested by the presence of high steady-state levels of acid β-glucosidase mRNA in epithelial cells, intermediate levels in skin fibroblasts and promyelocytes, low levels in macrophages, and barely detectable levels in B cells. In Gaucher's disease these levels are increased, indicative of possible feedback regulation of acid β-glucosidase expression.[241]

More than 200 mutations in the glucocerebrosidase gene are now known to cause Gaucher's disease.[242,243] The majority are missense mutations resulting in substi-

tution of one amino acid for another. There are also insertions and deletions, as well as recombination events caused by crossing over with the pseudogene. Four are "public" mutations in that they account for more than 96% of type 1 alleles in Ashkenazic Jews and 61% of type 1 alleles in non-Jews. The remainder are "private" mutations in that they are uncommon or rare and occur in only a single family or a few individuals.

The most common mutation, present in 6% of Ashkenazic Jews, results in an Asn370Ser amino acid substitution and is associated with about 7% to 12% residual enzyme activity and a generally milder phenotype. It is not present in either of the neuronopathic forms of Gaucher's disease. The second most common allele, found in 0.6% of the Jewish population, is the 84GG nucleotide insertion, which results in a frameshift that causes loss of all enzyme activity.[244]

Much rarer are the Leu444Pro and His409Asp amino acid substitutions and IVS2(+1) nucleotide insertion. The Leu444Pro change is close to the active site of the enzyme and results in severe loss of enzyme activity. Homozygotes for this mutation generally have neuronopathic disease, either type 2 or type 3.[243] Rarely, this mutation may also be found in patients with type 1 disease, who are usually compound heterozygotes and have more severe and earlier involvement than do type 1 patients with the Asn370Ser mutation. Eye movement abnormalities and calcifications of the aortic or mitral valves, or both, develop in patients with the His409Asp substitution.[191,245] Interestingly, this is the only genotypic variant in which close correlation with phenotype can be made. The IVS2(+1) mutation results in aberrant splicing of the mRNA.[246,247]

Finally, the activator protein SAP-C is required by β-glucosidase to exert its activity.[26] Two patients with deficiency of SAP-C have been described, both with the clinical course of type 3 Gaucher's disease.[28]

Treatment

The advent of ERT with macrophage-targeted α-mannosyl–terminated placental glucocerebrosidase has dramatically altered the approach to therapy for Gaucher's disease. In patients with type 1 and type 3 Gaucher's disease, ERT is efficacious,[190,224] whereas in patients with type 2 disease, it may slow but does not prevent the occurrence of lethal CNS disease.[248] Pulmonary disease also appears to be resistant to imiglucerase (Cerezyme) treatment, although some researchers have reported good results.[249] Various schedules of dosing ranging from 1 to 120 U/kg body weight infused intravenously every other day to once a month have been tried.[250,251] Currently, the usual starting dose ranges from 30 to 60 U/kg given by the intravenous route every 2 weeks. Within a few months there is an increase in hemoglobin concentration, and by 1 year, 60% to 70% of patients have a normal hemoglobin concentration and improved sense of well-being. Platelet counts rise, but the response is not as rapid as that for the anemia. A decrease in spleen and liver size correlates with the improvement in hemoglobin concentration. Skeletal responses to ERT occur more slowly, and usually a high-dose regimen (30 to 60 U/kg) is required for major improvements to be noted in cortical and trabecular bone mass.[252] However, a reduction in bone pain and a growth spurt in children who have short stature may be observed early during treatment. Allergic reactions occur in less than 0.1% of patients. The lack of reaction could be related to the presence of minimal amounts of residual enzymatic activity in these patients, which probably makes their immune systems more tolerant. Although IgG antibodies are commonly seen in up to 13% of patients undergoing ERT, they are generally of the non-neutralizing variant and are therefore not clinically relevant.[253,254]

ERT for Gaucher's disease has given patients with this condition the option of a nearly normal life if therapy is started at the appropriate time. Although questions remain about whether some of the CNS signs and symptoms respond to this therapy, the vast majority of patients (i.e., those with type 1 disease) experience a substantial improvement in hematologic parameters, bone quality, and overall quality of life. Splenectomy is now rarely necessary, and recurrent episodes of bone crisis have become a rarity. However, management of the complications that could already be present is mandatory because they still contribute to morbidity in these patients.

Alternative therapeutic strategies for patients with Gaucher's disease are also being studied. Gene therapy approaches have been applied to restore β-glucosidase activity in cultured human hematopoietic cells. Promising results were obtained, albeit in vitro, with enriched populations of these cells transduced with retroviral or AAV vectors containing normal β-glucosidase cDNA to promote long-term expression of enzyme activity.[255-257] An ex vivo gene therapy trial was performed in four human subjects[258]; however, gene expression was transient and lasted for only a few months but was accompanied by a modest degree of clinical improvement. The ultimate goal of these studies is to reintroduce into patients with Gaucher's disease autologous HSCs that have been transduced with the β-glucosidase gene and are capable of high levels of enzyme expression.

Another therapeutic modality, which involves the administration of miglustat, has shown promise in clinical trials in patients with Gaucher's disease.[259] This substance is a potent inhibitor of the enzyme glycosyltransferase and apparently also functions as a chemical chaperone by improving the activity of mutated β-glucosidase.[260] Side effects associated with the administration of miglustat to patients with Gaucher's disease have included persistent diarrhea, weight loss, and peripheral neuropathy, but they may be obviated in the future by the use of other pharmacologic chaperones (see earlier) that have recently been shown to increase the enzyme activity of some β-glucosidase mutant proteins in vitro.[261]

Symptomatic care is an important aspect of the management of patients with Gaucher's disease.[262] To coun-

teract the diffuse osteopenia, administration of vitamin D, calcium supplements, and aminohydroxypropylidene biphosphonate has been tried. Biphosphonate appears to diminish the incidence of traumatic bone fractures, normalize bone density, and encourage positive calcium balance.[263] Organ transplantation has been effective in a small number of patients. However, the inherent morbidity and mortality associated with this method make this option obsolete. The beneficial results achieved by successful allogeneic BMT in patients with Gaucher's disease[148,264] augurs well for the future of gene therapy trials. For patients with severe liver failure, liver transplantation has been a lifesaving procedure.

Finally, significant advances have been made in the field of prenatal diagnosis, and the choice of early detection of affected fetuses is now available for couples with a history of a previously affected child. Presumably, this option would be considered primarily in families who have members with type 2 or type 3 (i.e., CNS) variants. Preimplantation genetic diagnosis is also possible.[265]

Niemann-Pick Disease (Sphingomyelin Lipidosis)

Niemann-Pick disease (NPD) comprises a group of disorders in which the reticuloendothelial system is infiltrated by foam cells containing either sphingomyelin or unesterified cholesterol and other cell membrane lipids. The eponym refers to Albert Niemann, the German pediatrician who published the first clinical description in 1914,[266] and Ludwig Pick, whose histologic studies published in 1922 and 1927 differentiated this condition from Gaucher's disease.[267,268] The proposed division of NPD into four clinical subtypes by Crocker in 1961[269] and the later addition of a fifth (adult non-neuronopathic) form was based mainly on clinical and preliminary biochemical data. However, additional studies carried out since then suggest that this classification should be modified. Currently, two major patient groups are distinguished. Patients in whom the underlying metabolic defect is a deficiency of acid sphingomyelinase (ASM) activity with subsequent sphingomyelin accumulation in lysosomes have type A (NPD-A) and type B (NPD-B). The clinical spectrum of this disorder ranges from the early-onset, neurologic form, which results in death by 3 years of age (type A), to the non-neurologic form (type B), which is associated with survival into adulthood.[270] Patients with defective intracellular processing and transport of low-density lipoprotein–derived cholesterol have NPD-C and NPD-D.[271] It is now believed that the modest decrease in ASM activity levels in patients with the latter types is probably related more to a secondary disturbance in intracellular lipid metabolism than to a primary defect in the degradation of sphingomyelin.[272] All types of the disease share clinical involvement of the reticuloendothelial system and the presence of lipid-filled macrophages in pathologic studies.

Sphingomyelin is both a phospholipid and a sphingolipid. Its two major components are ceramide and phosphorylcholine, which are linked by a phosphodiester bond to the first carbon atom of sphingosine. The ASM gene has been mapped to an imprinted region on chromosome 11 (11p15.1-15.4).[273,274] More than 100 mutations have been identified in patients with type A and type B disease.[275-277] Of these, three (L302P, fsP330, and R496L) account for 92% of the mutant alleles in Ashkenazic Jewish patients with NPD-A,[278] and one, ΔR608, has a high prevalence in patients with type B disease who originate from northern Africa.[279]

Mouse models of NPD-A/B have also been created by gene targeting.[280,281] These ASM-deficient mice have been used to study disease pathogenesis and investigate different therapeutic modalities.[272,282,283] Based on these studies, an ERT clinical trial has recently begun in adult patients with non-neurologic sphingomyelinase-deficient NPD.

Though clinically similar, the underlying metabolic defect in NPD-C is quite different from that for classic NPD and primarily involves abnormal intracellular trafficking of cholesterol. It is caused by mutations in at least two unrelated genes named *NPC1* and *HE1* (see later). NPD-D is mostly a geographic variant of type C and occurs mainly in persons residing in Nova Scotia. However, it differs from the latter in that it tends to have a prominent degree of dystonia. Thus far it has been found to cosegregate with a mutation found in NPD-C, probably the result of a founder effect.[284] Therefore, the different forms of NPD are grouped together because of similarities in clinical features, including hepatosplenomegaly and foam cell infiltration of the bone marrow, rather than because each variant shares the same enzyme deficiency.

Acute Neuronopathic Form (Type A)

Patients with the classic infantile form of NPD are seen at 2 to 4 months of age with feeding difficulties, liver and spleen enlargement, and developmental delay. Periorbital puffiness, pulmonary infiltration, and lymphadenopathy may occur, and in most patients a cherry-red macula is noted on funduscopic examination. During the succeeding months, neurodevelopmental arrest occurs and is followed by regression, the abdomen becomes protuberant, intermittent jaundice may be noted, and general inanition is seen with wasting of the extremities and recurrent infections. Death occurs by 2 to 3 years of age. On postmortem examination, ascitic fluid is found in the abdomen; the liver, spleen, and lymph nodes are enlarged, yellow, and fatty; and foam cells are present in many different tissues. The brain is atrophic with widespread nerve cell loss and gliosis, and a profound lack of myelin lipids can be observed in the white matter.[285,286] Accumulation of the compound sphingosylphosphorylcholine has been seen in the brains of patients with this variant of NPD but not in the brains of those with the non-neuronopathic variants,[285] thus suggesting that this lyso-somal substance could play a role in the pathophysiologic process of brain dysfunction. Because sphingomyelin contents are normal in the brains of newborns affected with NPD-A, an alternative degradation pathway probably exists for this lipid, possibly through neutral sphingomyelinase, which is not defective in this disease.[286]

Many of these patients are of Ashkenazic Jewish heritage, but this disease is considerably less common than Tay-Sachs or adult (type 1) Gaucher's disease, two other sphingolipidoses that occur more often among Ashkenazim.

Chronic Form without Central Nervous System Involvement (Type B)

Patients with NPD-B are usually seen in early childhood with abdominal distention secondary to liver and spleen enlargement. Foam cell infiltration of the lungs may occur,[287] but survival with preservation of intellect for many years is common. The massive enlargement of the spleen in these patients may necessitate splenectomy, but curiously, plasma sphingomyelin levels are not elevated. Bone pathologic changes of the type seen in Gaucher's disease do not occur; however, osteoporosis, widening of the medullary cavities, and modeling defects can be demonstrated radiologically. There is periorbital fullness and a macular halo may be found in the fundus,[288] but vision is not disturbed. Growth retardation as a result of polyglandular involvement has also been reported.[289] Caution has been recommended by some researchers because increased levels of glycogen may be found in hepatic biopsy specimens and lead to the incorrect diagnosis of a glycogen storage disease.[290] Sea-blue histiocytes are present in the bone marrow of some patients. The bluish cast revealed by the Giemsa stain results from the accumulation of ceroid within these cells. The presence of residual sphingomyelinase activity in the brains of patients with type B probably protects their CNS from accumulation of sphingomyelin.[291] Life expectancy is still affected, and patients usually survive into their 30s.

Chronic Neuronopathic Form (Types C and D)

This category probably includes the largest group of patients with sphingomyelin-related lipidoses. In some patients, developmental delay and psychomotor retardation are present in the first year, whereas other children experience a period of normal early development followed by mild, but progressive intellectual impairment at a later age.[292] Those in the first group usually die at 5 to 6 years of age, whereas those in the second group survive into adulthood. Ataxia, progressive tetraparesis, loss of speech, and deterioration of mental function develop in affected children. Vertical gaze paresis, dysarthria, dysphagia, seizures, and dystonic posturing are also common.[293] Pyramidal tract signs and abnormal brainstem auditory evoked responses occur at a later stage, and finally the patient becomes nonambulatory and enters a vegetative state.[294] The initial manifestation in a patient with adult onset of the disease may be an atypical progressive dementia or a psychosis.[295,296] Rarely, a peripheral neuropathy may occur in patients with this clinically heterogeneous form of NPD.[297] Brain magnetic resonance imaging may show symmetrical cerebral and cerebellar atrophy, hypoplasia of the corpus callosum, and high signal intensity in the central white matter.[298] Approximately half of the patients with type C disease are seen in the newborn period with clinical features suggesting neonatal cholestatic hepatitis, including jaundice, hepatosplenomegaly, and the liver biopsy appearance of chronic hepatitis with giant cells. The cholestasis and hepatomegaly subside in most of these infants, but the splenomegaly can persist and serial liver biopsy specimens show hepatic fibrosis with progression to cirrhosis in some.[299] Patients with the Crocker-type C and D disease and some patients with the sea-blue histiocyte syndrome are included in this category. An in utero manifestation consisting of fetal ascites also occurs.[300] Interestingly, faster neurologic deterioration can be noticed in these patients as soon as puberty begins, a finding that has prompted therapeutic approaches in which onset of puberty is delayed.

Recent advances in the elucidation of intracellular cholesterol trafficking and metabolism have shed further light on the pathogenesis of this disorder. It is now known that in patients with NPD-C, incorporation of cholesterol into the lysosome is normal; however, proper processing and trafficking to the ER are abnormal.[301] This has led to the current concept of NPD-C as a disorder in which "exogenous cholesterol is trapped in traffic."[302] The fact that only exogenously derived cholesterol but no endogenously synthesized cholesterol accumulates in lysosomes is also part of the mystery surrounding the pathophysiologic features of NPD-C.[303]

Accumulation of low-density lipoprotein cholesterol has been demonstrated in all patients,[304] and in more than 90% a defect in intracellular cholesterol esterification is found when tests with a nonlipoprotein source of cholesterol are performed.[305] Cholesterol ester synthesis is partially reduced in cultured cells from heterozygotes. Positive filipin staining of the large amount of free cholesterol within cultured cells provides a useful diagnostic marker for NPD-C.

As mentioned earlier, this variant of NPD is caused by mutations in at least two genes, *NPC1*[306,307] and *HE1*.[308] *NPC1* maps to chromosome 18q11, and its product is a protein of the permease family with five transmembrane domains.[309] Genotype-to-phenotype correlations are now possible because mutations involving the coding sequence for the sterol-sensing domain seem to be present in patients with more severe and early-onset neurologic disease. The NPC1 protein shares structural homology with sterol-sensing domains and other enzymes involved in cellular cholesterol homeostasis, and mutations in this gene result in severe disruption of intracellular trafficking of cholesterol and trapping of low-density lipoprotein cholesterol and other lipids in lysosomes. The second gene, *HE1*, maps to chromosome 14q24.3,[308] and

mutations in this gene have been found in patients with NPD-C whose genetic defect did not involve the former gene. By subcellular fractionation methods, the protein product HE1 was localized to lysosomes.

Neurofibrillary tangles consisting of paired helical filaments strongly reactive to antibody to τ protein are present in many regions of the brain. They are ultrastructurally identical to those of Alzheimer's disease and are not associated with β-amyloid deposits. Their distribution corresponds fairly closely to that of the abnormal storage material, thus suggesting that they may be a reaction to the accumulating cytoplasmic material.[310-312]

Cholesterol-lowering agents will decrease hepatic and plasma cholesterol levels, but there is little evidence that this treatment can ameliorate the CNS complications of the disease.[313] One infant with NPD-C and an abnormal lipid signal on magnetic resonance spectroscopy at 9 months of age showed normal spectra 4 and 10 months after treatment with cholestyramine and lovastatin was begun.[314] Several reports have mentioned the need to avoid neuroleptic medications, mostly those of the hydrophobic amine type such as thioridazine, when one attempts to control behavioral disturbances in these patients. Although few other drugs are available (i.e., clozapine), experimental evidence suggests that such medications may worsen intracellular cholesterol accumulation, at least in vitro.[315]

Prenatal diagnosis of NPD-C has been successfully done numerous times.[316-318] The existence of various naturally occurring animal models for type C disease[319-321] should assist researchers in developing a better understanding of the molecular cause and pathogenesis of this disease. BMT has been attempted with promising results on liver enlargement, but the neurologic deterioration was not halted.[322]

Adult Non-neuronopathic Form

These patients have normal sphingomyelinase activity but store sphingomyelin in organs of the reticuloendothelial system. They usually have no neurologic involvement, and several have survived to old age. NPD must be suspected in infants and children with hepatosplenomegaly and bone marrow findings of enlarged foamy or sea-blue histiocytes. The diagnosis may be confirmed by the use of leukocytes or cultured skin fibroblasts to assay sphingomyelinase activity and cholesterol ester synthesis. Another useful finding is the presence of lymphocytic vacuolization in peripheral blood smears.

Heterozygotes for the A and B types can be identified by the reduced levels of sphingomyelinase activity present in their leukocytes or cultured skin fibroblasts, with ^{14}C-sphingomyelin used as substrate.

Treatment

BMT in one presymptomatic infant with NPD-A normalized his leukocyte sphingomyelinase activity. However, visceral storage increased and neurologic impairment progressed, though less rapidly than in his untreated sibling, and he died at 30 months of age.[143] Currently, there is no therapy available for this severe condition.

Preclinical studies involving the administration of recombinant ASM to knockout mice have shown promise in that treated animals exhibited striking improvements in histologic and biochemical parameters in their reticuloendothelial systems.[161] Unfortunately, neither prolonged life expectancy nor improvement in the neurologic compromise was seen. Phase I clinical trials are expected to begin soon.

More recently, implantation of neural stem cells in NPD-C mice was shown to extend the life span of these animals.[323] However, this procedure was found to be only partially therapeutic inasmuch as the overall clinical condition of the treated mutant animals was not significantly different from that of the untreated controls.[323] Because of their secondary ganglioside accumulation, NPD-C mice were treated with miglustat, which resulted in a reduction in ganglioside accumulation, delayed onset of neurologic symptoms, and increased survival.[324] Based on these positive effects, a randomized, controlled clinical trial was performed in NPD-C patients.[118] Twelve months after treatment, positive neurologic effects were observed only in the miglustat-treated group, thus suggesting that ganglioside accumulation rather than cholesterol storage is responsible for the neurologic symptoms of these patients.[325] These results encourage the use of SRT to treat the neurologic signs in patients with NPD-C.

Farber's Disease (Lipogranulomatosis)

To date, more than 70 cases of this autosomal recessive disease have been reported since Farber and colleagues' original description in 1957.[326] Death generally occurs before 2 years of age, but some patients with onset in the second year survive until the second decade.

In its most typical variant, the clinical manifestations of this rare disorder consist of painful swelling in the hands and feet, hoarseness, and recurrent vomiting. These difficulties may be present as early as a few weeks after birth. As the disease progresses, subcutaneous and periarticular nodules develop, especially near the interphalangeal, ankle, wrist, and elbow joints, and lead to flexion contractures. Swelling and granuloma formation in the epiglottis and larynx cause hoarseness or swallowing and respiratory disturbances. Foam cell infiltration and granulomatous deposits in the lungs further complicate the pulmonary problems. The tongue, heart, and liver may become enlarged, and granulomatous lesions of the heart valves also develop. Seven subtypes have been described, each with differing severity and sites of tissue involvement. A neonatal form has been observed that is characterized by massive hepatosplenomegaly but no subcutaneous nodules,[327] and in at least one patient the disease was manifested as nonimmune hydrops fetalis.[328]

Despite involvement of the degradative pathways of ceramide, there are few CNS signs in the clinical course

of some of the variants of Farber's disease, a finding that is somehow surprising because of the pivotal role that this compound plays in the biochemistry of the mammalian CNS. Ceramide and its intermediate breakdown product sphingosine have been shown to mediate many cellular events, including growth arrest, stress responses, and apoptosis.[329] In addition to CNS involvement, a peripheral neuropathy consisting of a decrease in response of the deep tendon reflexes and electromyographic signs of denervation occurs in some patients. Seizures have been reported in two patients.

The principal finding in pathologic studies is the presence of granulomatous infiltrates composed of foam cells containing a PAS-positive material that is extractable with lipid solvents. Comma-shaped curvilinear tubular structures (Farber bodies) are a characteristic feature of this disease. Analysis of this material by electron microscopy suggests a heterogeneous ultrastructure consisting principally of membrane-bound inclusions. Despite the absence of gross neurologic involvement, neuronal cytoplasm is also filled with PAS-positive storage material.

Chemical studies of the subcutaneous nodules indicate that ceramides account for 10% to 20% of the total lipids present. Increased ceramide concentrations in the urine, brain, and other organs have also been demonstrated.

Two enzymes, one with acid and another one with alkaline pH optima, have been described that are capable of catalyzing ceramide hydrolysis. Leukocytes, cultured skin fibroblasts, and solid tissue specimens from patients with Farber's disease are deficient in acid ceramidase. The first human alkaline ceramidase has recently been characterized and cloned[330] but to date has not been linked to any particular metabolic disorder. In addition, a novel ceramidase enzyme that is limited only to mitochondrial membranes has been described,[331] thus suggesting a topologically restricted pathway in sphingolipid metabolism.

Because acid ceramidase (together with glucosylceramidase and galactosylceramidase) also needs activation by the saposin family of proteins, it is not surprising that a patient with type 7 Farber's disease was found to have a mutation in the prosaposin gene.[332] The clinical features were very similar to those for Gaucher's disease type 2 (i.e., the acute neuronopathic form). That child had neonatal seizures, hepatosplenomegaly, and foamy macrophages. However, there were no joint deformities, subcutaneous nodules, or hoarseness. The child died at 16 weeks of age. Autopsy demonstrated an abnormal accumulation of ceramide, glucosylceramide, and lactosylceramide. Biochemical studies demonstrated diminished ceramidase activity.

Little is known about the pathophysiologic features of this condition, but clearly, recent advances in understanding the biologic roles of ceramide will shed light on the pathophysiology of Farber's disease.[333] In the meantime, the possible role of ceramide in the intracellular signaling cascade as a second messenger[334] and as a mediator in cellular apoptosis[329] may eventually give further insight on the molecular mechanisms of toxicity in this disease.

Human acid ceramidase has been characterized and purified,[335] and its gene has been cloned.[336] It maps to chromosome 8p22-21.2 and consists of 14 exons and 13 introns spanning approximately 26.5 kb of genomic DNA. To date, at least 10 different mutations have been reported.[337,338] Acid ceramidase activity can be measured in both cultured chorionic villus and amniotic fluid cells, thus allowing prenatal diagnosis of affected pregnancies.

No therapy is available for this condition, except for palliative management of its complications. Tracheostomy may be useful in managing upper airway obstruction, and some relief of joint pain may be obtained with the administration of corticosteroids. Resection of granulomas in the oral cavity was reported to improve upper airway obstruction.[339] Allogenic BMT was attempted in a presymptomatic infant at 9.5 months of age.[340] It resulted in reversal of the peripheral abnormalities (lipogranulomas, pain on joint motion, and hoarseness), but her neurologic deterioration progressed relentlessly. She died of pulmonary complications at 37 months of age. Correction of the metabolic defect in cultured Farber disease cells was achieved by retroviral vector–mediated transfection,[341] but no clinical reports on gene therapy are available to date. Current management of these patients has therefore focused on pain therapy, physical therapy, surgical correction of severe contractures, and anti-inflammatory medication.

G$_{M1}$-Gangliosidosis

G$_{M1}$-gangliosidosis was first defined clinically and pathologically by Landing and associates[342] as a familial neurovisceral lipidosis. Biochemical analysis demonstrated generalized accumulation of G$_{M1}$-ganglioside (G$_{M1}$) in the brain and visceral organs and led to designation of this disease as generalized gangliosidosis.[343] Shortly thereafter, deficient activity of the lysosomal acid β-D-galactosidase (β-gal) was found to be the primary defect in this disease.[344] G$_{M1}$-gangliosidosis is currently the third most frequently diagnosed LSD, and the incidence of specific allelic mutations is particularly high in certain geographic regions, such as Cyprus and southern Brazil.[345,346] The disease is transmitted as an autosomal recessive trait. The causative gene (GLB1), located on chromosome 3 (3p21-33),[347] codes for two distinct proteins derived from two alternatively spliced β-gal mRNA molecules.[348,349] The first is the canonic lysosomal β-gal enzyme; the second is an enzymatically inactive, functionally distinct product named the elastin-binding protein (EBP).[349,350] The latter protein controls early stages of elastogenesis and also contains a galactolectin domain that binds galactosugar-bearing molecules.[351] The EBP functions as a molecular chaperone that protects tropoelastin from premature intracellular degradation and hence facilitates assembly of the appropriately folded elastic fibers after deposition in the extracellular matrix.[352] A total of 99 mutations have been reported thus far in the GLB1 gene that alter lysosomal β-gal, EBP, or both, to a different extent.[353]

Gangliosides are acidic, sialic acid–containing GSLs that are found on the surface of essentially all mammalian cells but are particularly abundant on neuronal membranes. G$_{M1}$ accounts for 5% to 10% of the lipid mass of the plasma membrane of neurons.[354] Gangliosides are synthesized in the ER, Golgi, and trans-Golgi network by adding carbohydrate residues in a stepwise manner to the lipid membrane anchor ceramide.[355] De novo synthesized gangliosides are then transferred via vesicular transport mostly to the outer leaflet of the plasma membrane, where they distribute asymmetrically or segregate into unique membrane microdomains (e.g., caveolae and lipid rafts).[356] They are degraded in the endosomal/lysosomal compartment via the sequential removal of individual sugars; exoglycosidases or membrane sialidases work in concert with activator proteins to hydrolyze these compounds, and the products are either recycled or degraded.[26]

β-Gal is the primary enzyme involved in the degradation of GM1, for which it has the highest affinity. However, the enzyme can also remove β-linked galactosyl moieties from keratan sulfate, a mucopolysaccharide that belongs to an important group of extracellular proteins in bone and connective tissue. Although G$_{M1}$-gangliosidosis is clinically distinct from the mucopolysaccharidosis type B Morquio's disease, or MPS IVB (see later), they both result from deficiency of the same enzyme and are therefore allelic variants of the same gene defect.[357] The fact that G$_{M1}$-gangliosidosis is primarily a CNS condition whereas Morquio type B disease is primarily a disease of connective tissues reflects the relative tissue distribution of the main storage products G$_{M1}$ and keratan sulfate. This also explains why patients with these disorders may share some of their clinical manifestations; for instance, skeletal and connective tissue abnormalities and urinary excretion of keratan sulfate have been observed in some patients with G$_{M1}$-gangliosidosis.[358] Functional analysis of the different mutations affecting the GLB1 gene has explained at least in part why loss of activity of the same enzyme could lead to such different clinical outcome. It is now apparent that the diverse amino acid substitutions in β-gal found in either G$_{M1}$-gangliosidosis or Morquio B patients alter in a different way the enzyme's catalytic site and in turn its kinetic properties toward one or the other of the substrates.[359] In addition, because β-gal is part of a lysosomal multienzyme complex composed of at least two other enzymes—the protective protein/cathepsin A and neuraminidase (see galactosialidosis)—required for compartmentalization of β-gal and lysosomal stability, different β-gal mutations may impair the way that the enzyme is post-translationally regulated by the other two interacting proteins.[360] Finally, patients carrying mutations that affect both β-gal and EBP have impaired assembly and deposition of the elastic fibers.[351,352,361,362] Thus, impaired elastogenesis could contribute to the development of connective tissue abnormalities in patients with type B Morquio's disease and G_{M1}-gangliosidosis.

G_{M1}-gangliosidosis has a broad range of clinical manifestations that suggests a continuum of disease severity. Based on the age at onset and severity of symptoms, patients have been classified as having the early infantile (type 1), the late infantile (type 2), and the adult (type 3) form of the disease. The gray matter in the brain accumulates approximately 10 times the normal amount of G_{M1} because of a deficiency in G_{M1} β-gal. Therefore, the CNS is the primary affected site, which accounts for the severe neurologic signs characteristic of this disease. However, as discussed earlier, β-gal deficiency in extraneural tissues may also lead to accumulation of keratan sulfate in the liver, spleen, and bone and cause the typical subcutaneous and osseous features of this disease.[358] In general, higher residual enzyme activity is found in patients with type 2 and the adult form of G_{M1}-gangliosidosis than in patients with type 1 disease. In Morquio's disease, the residual β-gal is more active toward G_{M1} than toward keratan sulfate or oligosaccharide, and therefore patients are neurologically normal but display connective tissue and skeletal abnormalities. However, a more severe form of the disease may also occur (see MPS IVB).

Early Infantile G_{M1}-Gangliosidosis (Type 1)

Symptoms of early infantile G_{M1} (the most severe subtype, with onset shortly after birth) may include neurodegeneration, seizures, liver and spleen enlargement, coarsening of facial features, skeletal irregularities, joint stiffness, distended abdomen, muscle weakness, exaggerated startle response to sound, and problems with gait. A case of fetal hydrops has also been reported.[363] Cherry-red spots in the eye develop in about half of affected patients. Children may be deaf and blind by 1 year of age and often die by age 3 of cardiac complications or pneumonia.[359]

G_{M1}-gangliosidosis type 1 is the most common and severe subtype. The age at onset varies from birth to 6 to 7 months. Infants with early severe disease may be edematous at birth (nonimmune hydrops fetalis) with weak sucking, poor feeding, and slow weight gain. Developmental arrest typically occurs between 3 and 6 months of age. Hypotonia and an increased startle response may be the initial findings. CNS involvement is progressive, and spastic quadriplegia, decerebrate rigidity, clonic-tonic seizures, deafness, nystagmus, esotropia, and blindness ultimately develop. These children are born with or in their first few months exhibit coarse facial features with frontal bossing and a depressed nasal bridge. Bony deformities include stubby hands, broad wrists, anterior beaking of the lumbar vertebrae, thickening of the midshaft of the humerus, and spatulate ribs. A cherry-red macula occurs in half the infants with type 1 disease. In at least one infant, bilateral calcification of the basal

ganglia was noted as well.[364] Isolated cardiomyopathy has also been described in an infantile form of the disease.[361,365] Death usually results from bronchopneumonia between 1 and 2 years of age.

Late Infantile/Juvenile G_{M1}-Gangliosidosis (Type 2)

The early development of a patient with type 2 G_{M1}-gangliosidosis may be normal, but careful review of the history usually discloses an exaggerated startle response and hypotonia from an early age. The onset of symptoms, including locomotor ataxia, which ultimately leads to a state of decerebration with epileptic seizures, varies from 7 months to 3 years of age. The viscera are only slightly affected. Toward the end of the first year, the child may lose the ability to crawl, sit, and stand, and language development ceases. The plantar responses become extensor, and seizures develop. Some pallor of the optic discs may be noted, but a cherry-red spot is not usually present. Corneal clouding and rotatory nystagmus may occur. In most patients the liver is not enlarged and there are no skeletal abnormalities. These children may survive for 3 to 10 years after onset of the disease.[334]

Adult/Chronic Form (Type 3)

In the adult form (type 3), or chronic G_{M1}-gangliosidosis, the age at onset may be as early as 3 years to as late as 30 years; sometimes symptoms have already occurred in adolescence but the diagnosis is not made until adulthood. Clinical signs are variable and often resemble those found in juvenile forms of Parkinson's disease. Some patients have only focal neurologic signs, such as atypical spinocerebellar degeneration or dystonia, whereas others have a chronic and progressive disease with pyramidal and extrapyramidal signs and mental retardation. The degree of CNS involvement is not as extensive as in the other types. Skeletal changes are minimal, and visceromegaly and cherry-red spots do not occur.[358]

Pathologic and Molecular Aspects

Gross morphologic changes consisting of atrophy of the gray matter and cerebellum are evident in the type 1 and type 2 forms of G_{M1}-gangliosidosis. Autopsy and radiographic examination of the brain reveal delay[366,367] or even arrest[368] of myelination. The cortical architecture is severely altered by substantial neuronal cell loss.[358] Neurons appear distended with an expanded number of lysosomes often containing membranous material. The reticuloendothelial system contains foamy histiocytes filled with strongly PAS-positive granular material. Vacuolated lymphocytes can readily be recognized in peripheral blood and bone marrow smears, where sea-blue histiocytes may also be distinguished.[369] Tissue macrophages (histiocytes) with grossly distended cytoplasm filled with storage lysosomes can be identified in most of the organs, such as the liver, kidney, spleen, lymph nodes, thymus, lung, intestine, pancreas, and skeletal muscle.[370] Marked hepatosplenomegaly is usually detected in the early-onset cases, but it is less prominent or absent in late-onset patients. Storage of G_{M1} may occur in the liver of patients with type 1 but not type 2 G_{M1}-gangliosidosis. Accumulations of other galactose-containing oligosaccharides have been found to various degrees in the viscera and urine of individuals with all forms of the disease.[371] Several of these oligosaccharides appear to be derived from the incomplete degradation of certain erythrocyte glycoproteins and plasma immunoglobulins.[372]

The diagnosis of G_{M1}-gangliosidosis may be confirmed by assay of β-gal activity in plasma, leukocytes, or cultured fibroblasts.[373] Molecular analysis has demonstrated a wide variety of mutations associated with this disorder.[353,374] Common mutations that segregate with different forms of the disease have also been identified. For example, the mutations R201C and I51T have been found in Japanese patients with late infantile/juvenile G_{M1}-gangliosidosis and in white patients with adult/chronic G_{M}-gangliosidosis, respectively,[375] whereas the W273L mutation is found in patients with type B Morquio's syndrome.[376] A polymorphism has been shown to have a modulating effect on a mutation present in a patient with type 2 G_{M1}-gangliosidosis.[377]

Further studies on the molecular biology of β-gal have also led to important clues about post-translational processing and distribution of this lysosomal enzyme.[360] Zhang and associates[359] described patients with either G_{M1}-gangliosidosis or type B Morquio's disease who share the same two mutations. They suggested that although the missense mutations described in G_{M1}-gangliosidosis have little effect on catalytic activity, they nevertheless do affect protein conformation in such a way that the resulting protein cannot be transported out of the ER and fails to reach the lysosome. Stimulation of β-gal by SAP-A results in the hydrolysis of sulfatide and globotriaosylceramide.[25,378] Sulfatide but not G_{M1} accumulates in patients with SAP-A deficiency.[378]

The precise mechanism by which accumulation of ganglioside induces cellular dysfunction is not yet fully elucidated, but recent studies on the G_{M1}-gangliosidosis mouse model[379-381] have identified molecular pathways that are altered or activated as a consequence of the accumulation of G_{M1}. The G_{M1}-gangliosidosis mouse model closely recapitulates the clinical features of the human disease. A generalized nervous system condition characterized by tremors, ataxia, and abnormal gait develops in these mice and culminates in rigidity and paralysis of the hind limbs.[380] This phenotype is accompanied by gradual deterioration of motor function, progressive neurodegeneration, and neuroinflammation.[382]

Cell-specific morphologic and biochemical changes have been mapped in the CNS and the visceral organs of β-gal$^{-/-}$ mice with the use of light and electron microscopic and immunohistochemical methods. Both neurons and astroglia show extensive and progressive vacuolization of their cytosol as the animal ages. Lysosomes appear to be filled with heterogeneous membranous material, and neuronal cell death is a consistent feature that

accounts for the extensive neurodegenerative characteristic of the disease.[89] Neuronal apoptosis is accompanied by activation and upregulation of an inflammatory response consisting of increased levels of cytokines and chemokines in various regions of the brain and spinal cord.[165,382] Recent studies on the pathophysiology underlying the CNS phenotype in this model have begun to identify the molecular pathways that are deregulated by abnormal buildup of G_{M1} in lysosomes and other subcellular sites. Although the precise mechanism by which G_{M1} induces cellular dysfunction is not yet fully elucidated, it has been shown that impaired lysosomal degradation of this ganglioside leads to its accumulation at the ER membrane. Given the important role of gangliosides in calcium homeostasis and signaling,[383] increases in the local concentration of G_{M1} at the ER membrane have indeed been shown to provoke calcium imbalance through depletion of ER calcium stores.[89] Disruption of intracellular calcium levels induces the activation of an ER stress response or unfolded protein response (UPR).[384] Upregulation of folding catalysts and transcription factors and activation of specific kinases and caspases were found to occur in the brain and spinal cord of mice with G_{M1}-gangliosidosis and culminated in neuronal apoptosis. Remarkably, activation of the UPR pathway does not occur in mice doubly deficient in β-gal and ganglioside synthase, one of the enzymes responsible for the synthesis of G_{M1}; such mice do not accumulate G_{M1}. These observations directly implicate G_{M1} in causing ER stress and present a novel mechanism of neuronal apoptosis in an LSD.[89] In addition, they give new prospective on the role of GSLs, specifically gangliosides, in normal cell metabolism and disease pathogenesis. Investigation of the cellular events underlying these complex disorders will provide more insight into lysosomal function in normal cell physiology and prove crucial to the development of tailored or alternative therapies for neurodegenerative LSDs.

Treatment

No effective therapy is currently available for G_{M1}-gangliosidosis, but several therapeutic modalities have been tested both in vitro and in vivo. Retroviral vector–mediated gene transfer has corrected β-gal deficiency in human fibroblasts.[155] More recently, use of an amplicon hybrid vector containing sequences of herpes simplex virus type 1 and AAV for expression of the entire human *GLB1* gene has led to temporary expression and functional activity of β-gal in human deficient cells.[385] BMT in a presymptomatic juvenile-onset patient resulted in complete normalization of β-gal enzyme levels in white blood cells but did not improve the long-term clinical outcome.[386]

Encouraging results have recently been obtained in mouse models of G_{M1}-gangliosidosis. Knockout mice transplanted with bone marrow progenitor cells transduced ex vivo with a retroviral vector expressing murine β-gal cDNA have shown a remarkable increase in β-gal activity in different brain regions and reduction of lysosomal storage of G_{M1}. These surprising results were explained by the increased levels of chemokines in specific brain nuclei of the β-gal$^{-/-}$ mice that probably create a microenvironment within the CNS favoring the response to bone marrow–mediated therapy.[165] Indeed, these authors demonstrated that that β-gal–expressing bone marrow–derived monocytes selectively migrate to the CNS under a gradient of chemokines and become a source of enzyme for correction of deficient neurons, thereby resulting in reversion of the enzyme defect and restoration of neurologic function. These findings suggest that a condition such G_{M1}-gangliosidosis, which is characterized by neurodegeneration and neuroinflammation, may influence the response of the CNS to ex vivo gene therapy.[165]

Administration of low-molecular-weight substrate analogues, or chemical chaperones, has also been investigated for the treatment of murine G_{M1}-gangliosidosis.[387] These chemical chaperones act as both in vitro competitive inhibitors and intracellular enhancers by stabilizing the mutant enzyme. The compound *N*-octyl-4-epi-β-valienamine was administered orally to deficient mice expressing the R201C mutant human β-gal and shown to be delivered rapidly to the brain with no adverse effect. Treatment resulted in increased brain activity of β-gal, decreased G_{M1} storage, and prevention of neurologic deterioration during a treatment period of a few months.[387] These studies are supportive of the use of chemical chaperone therapy for G_{M1}-gangliosidosis. SRT has been tested in knockout mice and shown to result in reduced accumulation of GSLs in the cerebrum, brainstem, and cerebellum.[388]

G_{M2}-Gangliosidosis, Sandhoff Variant

The G_{M2}-gangliosidoses consist of a group of six GSL storage diseases that are of interest to the pediatric hematologist because of a mild to moderate degree of visceral involvement seen in one of its variants, Sandhoff's disease. These conditions are caused by impaired degradation of G_{M2}-ganglioside (G_{M2}), a minor brain acidic GSL,[26] as a result of deficiency of one of the isozymes Hex-A or Hex-B or their activator protein G_{M2}A.[389]

The hexosaminidases are two related dimeric enzymes that catalyze the removal of hexoses (both glucose and galactose) from complex molecules in the body, including gangliosides. Hex-A results from the dimerization of one α and one β subunit, whereas Hex-B is made up of two β subunits.[390,391] The Hex-S isozyme consists of an α-subunit homodimer and is thought to catabolize glycosaminoglycans (GAGs). These subunits are coded for by genes located on chromosomes 15 (α subunit) and 5 (β subunit).[390] Both hexosaminidases need the activator protein G_{M2}A to make their liposoluble substrates more accessible.

In the classic and most common form, Tay-Sachs disease, Hex-A is deficient. Hex-A activity is also reduced or absent in the juvenile and adult variants of G_{M2}-gangliosidosis, the so-called late-onset Tay-Sachs disease. In each of these variants, mutations have been found within the gene encoding the α subunit of this enzyme.[392] A fourth form of the disease known as the B1 variant also results from mutations within the α-subunit gene.[390] However, the Hex-A deficiency in this disorder becomes evident only when the enzyme assay is performed with a sulfated derivative of the artificial compound generally used for determination of Hex-A activity. Patients with the much rarer AB variant lack the G_{M2}A activator. G_{M2} and smaller amounts of its asialo derivative G_{A2} accumulate in the brain and, to a considerably lesser extent, in the visceral organs of patients with each of these diseases. Consequently, the clinical signs in these diseases are confined to the CNS, and obvious infiltration of the reticuloendothelial system has not been noted.

Considerable involvement of extraneural tissues does, however, occur in the Sandhoff variant of G_{M2}-gangliosidosis.[393] Sandhoff provided the first description of this neurodegenerative disorder that bears his name. This variant is due to mutations in the gene encoding the β subunit of hexosaminidase. Both Hex-A and Hex-B contain β subunits, so the activity of both enzymes is lacking in Sandhoff's disease. It is associated with more marked accumulation of G_{A2}-ganglioside in both the brain and viscera than in any of the other variants. In addition, levels of globoside, the major red blood cell glycolipid, are markedly elevated, particularly in the liver, spleen, and kidney.[391] Consequently, signs of involvement of the reticuloendothelial system emerge, including foam cells in the bone marrow and other organs. In all other respects, Sandhoff's disease in an infant is clinically indistinguishable from Tay-Sachs disease.

An infant with Tay-Sachs or Sandhoff's disease may appear normal at birth, but an alert parent or an experienced professional can detect hypotonia and an exaggerated startle response within the first 2 months. Between 3 and 6 months of age, motor weakness and then listlessness become evident. The child may roll from side to side but cannot turn over completely, slumps forward when placed in a sitting position, and cannot crawl or stand. There is poor visual fixation with roving eye movements. Quite early in the course of the disease and definitely by 4 months, a cherry-red spot with a white perimacular halo can be observed in both fundi. Weakness, spasticity, and increased deep tendon reflexes develop, and feeding difficulties with associated gagging become a concern.

At approximately 1 year of age, seizures are first noted, excessive drooling begins, and bouts of unmotivated laughter occur. During the second year, the head begins enlarging disproportionately. The optic discs become pale and atrophic, and cortical blindness ensues. After 2 years of age, there are episodes of autonomic dysfunction with unexplained temperature elevations; spells of rubor, pallor, or cyanosis; and irregular breathing. Although visceral lipid storage occurs in Sandhoff's disease, the liver and spleen are not clinically enlarged, and there are no obvious skeletal changes. Great effort must be expended to maintain hydration and nutrition, control constipation and seizures, and prevent infection. These children rarely survive beyond 3 or 4 years of age.

Sandhoff's disease can be distinguished from other forms of G_{M2}-gangliosidosis by the presence of foam cells in bone marrow and the total absence of β-N-acetylhexosaminidase in serum, leukocytes, cultured fibroblasts, tears, and urine.[391]

Individuals heterozygous for the gene for Sandhoff's disease can usually be identified by a reduced level of total serum hexosaminidase (A and B forms) and a higher than normal percentage (>70%) of the Hex-S isoform. The same test used to screen for carriers of the Tay-Sachs trait can be used to detect carriers of Sandhoff's disease. No instances of Sandhoff's disease have been recorded in children of Jewish parents, in contrast to Tay-Sachs disease, which until population screening became popular, was seen much more often in the offspring of Ashkenazic Jews.

Molecular Aspects

Recent advances in determining the neuropathophysiologic mechanisms in Sandhoff's disease have been made on the mouse model of this disease.[394-396] Genetically engineered mice with disruption of both Hex-A and Hex-B genes lack both the α and β subunits of hexosaminidase and display a total deficiency of all forms of lysosomal hexosaminidase, including the small amount of Hex-S (α-α homodimer). These mice exhibit the phenotypic, pathologic, and biochemical features of the mucopolysaccharidoses (see later), LSDs caused by the accumulation of GAGs (mucopolysaccharides). The mucopolysaccharidosis phenotype is not seen in the Tay-Sachs or Sandhoff mice disease model or in the corresponding human patients.[391,394,397] These findings demonstrate that GAGs are crucial substrates for β-hexosaminidase and that functional redundancy appears to exist, at least in mice, in the hexosaminidase enzyme system.

As is the case for G_{M1}-gagliosidosis, the pathogenesis of G_{M2}-gangliosidosis relates at least in part to massive accumulation of G_{M2} in the brain and other tissues. In the Sandhoff disease mouse model, abnormal buildup of G_{M2} alters the Vmax of the ER calcium pump, sarcoplasmic/endoplasmic reticulum Ca^{2+}-ATPase (SERCA), thereby inhibiting calcium uptake into the ER and increasing cytosolic calcium levels.[398,399] Investigators have recently shown a mechanistic link between G_{M2} accumulation, neuronal cell death, reduced activity, and axonal outgrowth in the Sandhoff mice and could demonstrate reversal of these phenotypes in embryonic hippocampal neurons transduced with a bicistronic lentiviral vector (SIV.ASB) encoding both the α and β chains of hexosaminidase. This transfer vector has previously been shown to correct the hexosaminidase deficiency and to reduce G_{M2} levels in both transduced and cross-corrected human Sandhoff fibroblasts. Normal axonal growth

rates were restored, as were the rate of Ca^{2+} uptake via the SERCA and the sensitivity of the neurons to thapsigargin-induced cell death, concomitant with a decrease in G_{M2} and G_{A2} levels. These data demonstrated that the bicistronic vector can reverse the biochemical defects and downstream consequences in Sandhoff neurons, thus reinforcing its potential for in vivo gene treatment of Sandhoff's disease.[399]

Treatment

Currently, no treatment is available for the G_{M2}-gangliosidoses, although recent animal studies involving inhibition of GSL synthesis seem promising.[115] Administration of miglustat to Sandhoff mice has delayed the onset of symptoms and disease progression and significantly increased life expectancy.[400] Combined treatment with miglustat and BMT was found to have a synergistic effect.[182] Based on these preclinical findings, clinical trials of miglustat are currently in progress for patients with late-onset G_{M2}-gangliosidosis. Although BMT has been shown to prolong life and ameliorate neurologic manifestations in animal models,[401] we are not aware of any reports involving human subjects.

Another approach based on the use of cationic liposome-mediated plasmid gene therapy has been evaluated in the Sandhoff mouse model.[402] The mice received a single intravenous injection of two plasmids encoding the human α and β subunits of hexosaminidase. As a result, 10% to 35% of normal levels of hexosaminidase expression, theoretically therapeutic levels, were achieved in most visceral organs, but not in the brain, 3 days after injection, with decreased levels evident by day 7. Histochemical staining confirmed widespread enzyme activity in visceral organs. Both G_{M2} and G_{A2} were reduced by almost 10% and 50%, respectively, on day 3 and by 60% and 70% on day 7 in comparison to untreated age-matched mice. Consistent with the biochemical results, a reduction in G_{M2} was observed in liver cells as well.[378]

Adenovirus-mediated transfer of the β subunit of β-hexosaminidase was shown to restore Hex-A and Hex-B activity after infection of Sandhoff fibroblasts. After direct intracerebral injection of this recombinant adenoviral vector into Sandhoff mice, nearly normal levels of enzymatic activity were demonstrated in the entire brain at the different doses tested. The addition of hyperosmotic concentrations of mannitol to the adenoviral vector resulted in enhanced diffusion of the vector in the injected hemisphere. Although adenoviral-induced lesions were found in brains injected with a high dose of the vector, they were not detected in brains injected with 100-fold lower doses, even in the presence of mannitol, thus suggesting the potential of this approach in achieving efficient vector transduction without viral cytotoxicity.[403] In another recent study, Sandhoff mice were treated by stereotactic intracranial inoculation of recombinant AAV vectors encoding the complementing human β-hexosaminidase α- and β-subunit genes and elements, including an HIV tat sequence, to enhance protein expression and distribution. The animals survived longer than 1 year with sustained, widespread, and abundant delivery of enzyme to the nervous system. Onset of the disease was delayed with preservation of motor function; inflammation and storage of G_{M2}-ganglioside in the brain and spinal cord were reduced. This study demonstrates that gene delivery of β-Hex-A via AAV vectors has realistic potential for treating the human Tay-Sachs–related diseases.[404]

MUCOPOLYSACCHARIDOSES

The mucopolysaccharidoses are a group of inherited disorders that result from deficiency of one or more of the lysosomal enzymes required for GAG or mucopolysaccharide catabolism. GAGs, which are a major constituent of connective tissue such as cartilage and bone, are long-chain complex carbohydrates that are usually linked to proteins to form proteoglycans, including chondroitin 4-sulfate, chondroitin 6-sulfate, heparan sulfate, dermatan sulfate, keratan sulfate, and hyaluronic acid. Patients with mucopolysaccharidosis typically display coarse facial features, skeletal dysplasia, and limitation of joint motion. These features, which dominate the clinical picture of the mucopolysaccharidoses, set this group of LSDs apart from the glycosphingolipidoses, although overlapping phenotypes are present. The urine of

these patients contains excessive amounts of mucopolysaccharides.[405]

The occurrence of this group of disorders is relatively rare. Nelson[406] in Northern Ireland found an overall incidence of approximately 1 in 25,000 live births, with MPS I occurring in approximately 1 in 76,000 live births. Some of these disorders occur even more rarely. For instance, the incidence of MPS I of the Hurler/Scheie variant is 1 in 280,000. MPS III may be as rare as 1 in 280,000 live births, although the incidence may be underreported. A total of seven variants have been described.

The typical mucopolysaccharide contains a core polypeptide to which a number of polysaccharide chains are attached by a xylose link. Each polysaccharide chain may contain 100 or more sugar residues joined together in repeating disaccharide units consisting of a uronic acid (glucuronic or L-iduronic acid) alternating with a sulfated hexosamine (glucosamine or galactosamine) (Fig. 24-4). The hexosamine in dermatan sulfate is N-acetyl-α-D-galactosamine; in heparan sulfate, it is N-acetyl-α-D-glucosamine. Iduronic acid is occasionally sulfated, but glucuronic acid is not. Fragments from one or both of these mucopolysaccharides accumulate in each of the mucopolysaccharidoses (Table 24-6) because of a block in their sequential hydrolysis as a result of a lysosomal enzyme deficiency (see Fig. 24-4). An exception is Morquio's syndrome, which is characterized by the accumulation of two other mucopolysaccharides, chondroitin 6-sulfate and keratan sulfate, with galactose substituting for the uronic acid moiety (Fig. 24-5).

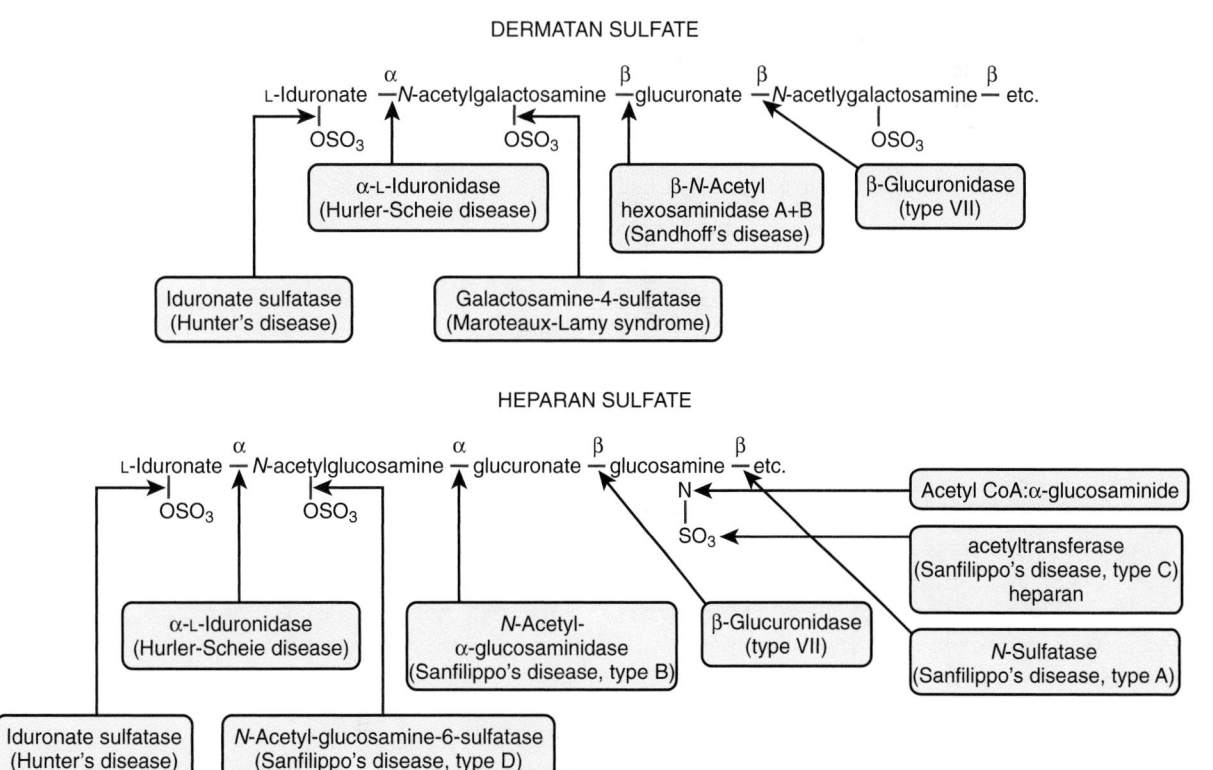

FIGURE 24-4. Pathways for the enzymatic degradation of dermatan sulfate and heparan sulfate. Deficiencies of each of the enzyme activities shown are correlated with specific mucopolysaccharidoses.

TABLE 24-6   The Mucopolysaccharidoses

Class	Eponym	Enzyme Defect	Urinary Mucopolysaccharides	Mental Retardation	Corneal Clouding	Skeletal Dysplasia	Life Expectancy (yr)
I H	Hurler's disease	α-L-Iduronidase	DS, HS	++	+	+++	<10
I S	Scheie's disease	α-L-Iduronidase	DS, HS	–	+	+	Normal
I H/S	Hurler-Scheie compound	α-L-Iduronidase	DS, HS	+	+	++	20s
II severe	Hunter's disease	Iduronate sulfatase	DS, HS	++	–	++	<15
II mild	Hunter's disease	Iduronate sulfatase	DS, HS	+/–	–	+	Adulthood
IIIA	Sanfilippo's disease	Heparan-N-sulfatase	HS	+++	–	+	<20
IIIB	Sanfilippo's disease	N-Acetyl-α-glucosaminidase	HS	+++	–	+	<20
IIIC	Sanfilippo's disease	Acetyl CoA:α-glucosaminide transferase	HS	++	–	+	Adulthood
IIID	Sanfilippo's disease	N-Acetylglucosamine-6-sulfatase	HS	++	–	+	<20
IVA	Morquio's syndrome	Galactosamine-6-sulfatase	KS, CS	–	+	+++	20-40
IVB	Morquio's syndrome	β-Galactosidase	KS	–	+	+++	20-40
VI	Maroteaux-Lamy syndrome	Galactosamine-4-sulfatase (arylsulfatase B)	DS	–	+	++	20s
VII	Sly's disease	β-Glucuronidase	DS, HS	+	+/–	+	<1-40
Mucosulfatidosis		Multiple sulfatases	DS, HS, Cholesterol S sulfatide	++	–	+	3-12

Cholesterol S, cholesterol sulfate; CS, chondroitin 6-sulfate; DS, dermatan sulfate; HS, heparan sulfate; KS, keratan sulfate.

KERATAN SULFATE

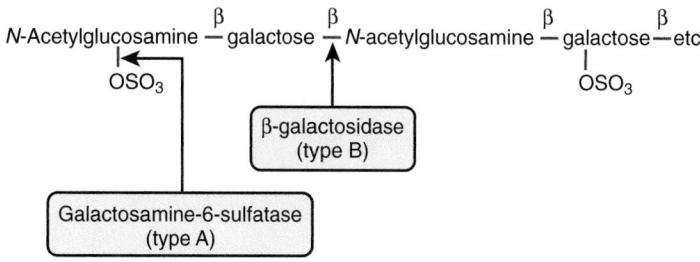

FIGURE 24-5. Glycosaminoglycans stored in Morquio's disease and sites for the probable action of the enzyme deficiencies in this disease.

CHONDROITIN-6-SULFATE

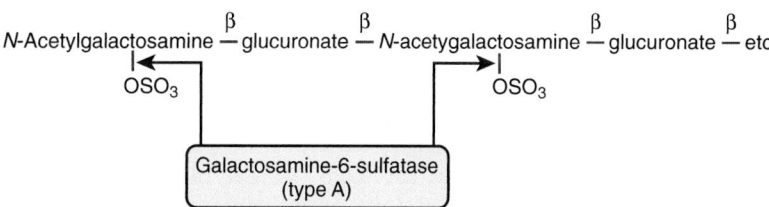

Mucopolysaccharide storage leads to several alterations in cell morphology in blood and bone marrow. Azurophilic granulations are present in polymorphonuclear leukocytes and lymphocytes (Alder-Reilly bodies) (see Fig. 24-1B).[38] Vacuoles with basophilic granulations are also found in circulating lymphocytes, bone marrow reticulocytes (Gasser cells), and bone marrow plasma cells (Buhot cells). Circulating lymphocytes may also contain metachromatic vacuoles without granulation (Mittwoch cells).

Other cells also manifest changes associated with excessive tissue mucopolysaccharide content. Coarse hair and skin, clouding of the cornea, thickening of the leptomeninges with hydrocephalus, alterations in bone architecture, thickening of heart valves, hepatic fibrosis, ballooning of neurons, and infiltration of the reticuloendothelial system by foam cells are some of the changes observed. Progressive narrowing of the trachea in these patients creates difficulty maintaining an adequate airway during and after surgical anesthesia. Operations for median nerve compression related to carpal tunnel syndrome and for compressive myelopathy have been especially useful in patients with normal intelligence. Abnormal binding of elastin to fibroblasts has been reported in MPS I, which could be related to inactivation of molecular chaperons and may somehow be related to the clinical involvement of connective tissue that is so prominent in these diseases.[407,408] In addition, an excess of intracellular amyloid-β peptide (Aβ [1-40]) has been reported in brains from patients with mucopolysaccharidosis, a finding that might help explain part of the CNS involvement that is commonly seen in some of these conditions.[408] The salient clinical and biochemical features of each type of mucopolysaccharidosis are presented in Table 24-6.

Mucopolysaccharidosis Type I (Hurler, Scheie, and Hurler-Scheie Syndromes)

MPS I is one of the most rare of these disorders. There are three variants that differ widely in severity, with Hurler's syndrome being the most severe, Scheie's syndrome the mildest, and Hurler-Scheie syndrome generating an intermediate phenotype.

These three autosomal recessive syndromes result from deficiency of the acid hydrolase α-L-iduronidase (IDUA). The clinical phenotype of type I is a continuum between the severe form, as found in Hurler's syndrome, and a mild form, as seen with Scheie's syndrome.

Infants with the Hurler phenotype usually appear to be normal at birth, although some have inguinal or umbilical hernias. These infants may seem to be unusually large, but by 6 to 18 months of age there is a deceleration in growth and they ultimately become dwarfed. Seven infants with type I were described who initially were seen with acute cardiomyopathy associated with endocardial fibroelastosis.[409,410] The diagnosis is usually made by the age of 6 to 24 months when coarse facial features, corneal opacities, chronic hearing loss, an enlarged tongue, a prominent forehead, hepatosplenomegaly, skeletal deformities, and joint stiffness become evident. Some may have glaucoma,[411] and communicating hydrocephalus with increased intracranial pressure develops. These children are severely developmentally delayed with limited language skills. They often have recurring upper respiratory tract and ear infections, stertorous breathing, and persistent rhinorrhea.

Skull radiographs may demonstrate a large thickened calvaria, premature closure of the sutures, poorly developed sinuses, shallow orbits, and a J-shaped sella turcica. Other radiologic signs include oar-shaped ribs, rounding and anterior beaking of the vertebrae, anterior hypoplasia of the lumbar vertebrae with kyphosis, and shortening of the metacarpals and phalanges. These skeletal abnormalities are known as dysostosis multiplex. Death usually occurs by 10 years of age. Cardiac disease with valvular involvement and cardiomegaly develops and contributes to the premature death of these patients. Other causes of death are obstructive airway disease and respiratory infections.

Patients with Hurler-Scheie syndrome are usually seen between the ages of 3 and 8 years with progressive corneal clouding, deafness, hepatosplenomegaly, joint stiffness, valvular heart disease, and dysostosis multiplex. They are less retarded, and some have nearly normal intellect. A receding chin and arachnoid cyst formation in the region of the sella turcica have been reported in several of these patients. GAGs may be deposited on the cervical dura (pachymeningitis cervicalis) and result in myelopathy. These patients may live well into their 20s; however, cardiac involvement and upper airway obstruction can result in early death.[405]

Scheie's syndrome is less common than Hurler's syndrome. Patients are generally seen after 5 years of age with joint stiffness and clawhand and clawfoot deformities. Intelligence and height are normal. These patients survive well into adulthood. They eventually suffer from visual disturbances such as glaucoma and retinal degeneration, in addition to the corneal opacities. Some patients have hearing loss. Aortic valvular disease may develop, and their facial features eventually become coarse. Sleep apnea can occur and is usually relieved with a tracheostomy. Classification in some patients may be rather difficult because there can be overlapping symptoms among the three phenotypes.[405]

Distinction among these three clinical phenotypes cannot be made by routine biochemical analysis. Most patients are subclassified solely on a clinical basis. Large amounts of partially degraded heparan sulfate and dermatan sulfate are stored and excreted in all three conditions. However, heparan sulfate is excreted in greater amounts in patients with Hurler's syndrome than in those with the Scheie and Hurler-Scheie syndromes.[412] Diagnosis of these syndromes plus detection of carriers is ultimately achieved by the demonstration of markedly reduced IDUA activity in cultured fibroblasts, leukocytes, plasma, or serum. Chromogenic (p-nitrophenyl) or fluorogenic (4-methylumbelliferyl) derivatives are commonly used as substrates in these assays. However, with desulfated heparan as the sulfate, enzymatic differences can be demonstrated in the different clinical phenotypes. Fibroblasts of patients with Hurler's disease cannot degrade this substrate, whereas this same substrate is effectively hydrolyzed by cells from patients with Hurler-Scheie and Scheie's disease.

The gene for IDUA has been localized to chromosome 4p16.3. Of the more than 30 mutations thus far described, most have been associated with the Hurler phenotype.[413,414] The two most common mutations,

Q70X and W402X, result in chain termination of the α-iduronidase protein and are therefore associated with a severe form of Hurler's disease. A recently described mutation (P533R) seems to be common in northern Africa.[415] Although most occurrences of the Hurler-Scheie phenotype are due to compound heterozygosity for two different mutant alleles, some patients have been reported with homozygosity for a single mutation.[414] Prenatal diagnosis has been successfully performed.[416] The biochemical diagnosis can also be confirmed by measuring deficient IDUA levels on filter paper obtained at birth during routine neonatal screening.[417]

Treatment

Successful engraftment after BMT has resulted in overall improvement of the facial features typically seen in patients with Hurler's syndrome. Urinary GAG excretion has returned to normal, metachromatic inclusions have disappeared, and clearing of lysosomal inclusions in the liver and improvement in corneal clouding have also been noted.[121] The skeletal anomalies are not reversed, except perhaps odontoid dysplasia.[418] Hydrocephalus does not appear to resolve, nor does it develop after BMT. Factors affecting the outcome include the child's age at the time of transplantation, the clinical phenotype, the defined genotype,[419] and the donor type.

Based on promising results of trials of ERT in animal models of MPS I,[420,421] clinical trials were performed in selected patients. Phase III clinical trials of recombinant IDUA therapy have been performed in patients with the Hurler/Scheie variant of MPS I.[102] Marked reductions in liver and spleen size were reported, together with improved joint range of motion and exercise tolerance. Moreover, there was a clear decrease in the amount of GAGs in the urine of these patients. Phase I/II and phase III clinical trials have recently been conducted and have demonstrated that this therapy is effective in treating patients with the attenuated forms of MPS I (i.e., little or no neuronal involvement).[422] A mild degree of humoral hypersensitivity reaction developed in about 50% of the patients, but almost all were managed conservatively, and the reactions eventually disappeared despite continuous exposure to the enzyme.

Gene therapy by means of AAV vectors containing human cDNA for IDUA has resulted in enzymatic correction and cellular cross-correction of affected cells.[423] In contrast to intravenous administration,[424] intrathecal injection of AAV vectors carrying the IDUA sequence into cerebrospinal fluid was reported.[425] This procedure was successful in restoring enzyme activity in the brain. In general, IDUA activity correlated with vector dose. High doses of vector resulted in enzyme levels close to normal in the brain. Histopathologic analysis revealed that the number of cells with storage vacuoles was reduced. Thus far, no human trials have been reported with this approach in MPS I.

Finally, the finding that treatment of human cells carrying stop codon mutations in the IDUA gene with gentamicin increases protein production has led to the proposal of a novel therapeutic approach. This antibiotic suppresses stop mutations within certain genes, and therefore it would be expected that protein production could be restored to a certain extent. At least in morphologic studies of such cells, lysosomal accumulation of mucopolysaccharides was quickly reduced after treatment with this substance.[426] Enhanced stop codon readthrough will be a potential treatment strategy for a large subgroup of MPS I patients.

Mucopolysaccharidosis Type II (Hunter's Syndrome)

Hunter's syndrome is an X-linked recessive disorder that has a broad spectrum of clinical phenotypes ranging from a mild to a severe form. All forms of the syndrome result from a deficiency of the lysosomal enzyme iduronate-2-sulfatase (IDS). The severe type has many features similar to those of Hurler's syndrome. These patients are characteristically seen between 2 and 4 years of age with coarse facial features, progressive mental retardation, progressive deafness, short stature, dysostosis multiplex, stiff joints, and hepatosplenomegaly. Atypical retinitis pigmentosa or retinal degeneration may occur, but unlike patients with Hurler's syndrome, the corneas remain clear. These patients are hirsute and may have white nodular skin lesions on the posterior of the thorax and upper part of the arms. Cardiac involvement is also common and may be manifested as aortic valve stenosis or mitral insufficiency, which could be severe and life threatening. Isolated mitral valve prolapse has also been reported.[427] The presence or absence of these lesions does not necessarily correlate with the severity of the disease. Survival beyond adolescence is rare.

In the mild form of Hunter's syndrome, minimal to no CNS involvement is characteristically seen, and patients survive into adult life. Some of the somatic features described in the severe form of Hunter's syndrome also develop in these patients, but at a slower rate of progression. Hearing impairment, carpal tunnel syndrome, joint stiffness, degenerative arthritis of the hips, heart disease, and hepatosplenomegaly may occur. Older adult patients have rosy cheeks and a hoarse voice.

The human *IDS* gene has been isolated, cloned, and sequenced.[428] It is a large gene that spans about 24 kb and contains nine exons. It is located on the Xq27-28 boundary.[429] Because IDS is deficient in all forms of Hunter's disease, it has been difficult to distinguish the clinical phenotypes biochemically. The clinical heterogeneity is believed to be a result of the different mutations found on the *IDS* gene. Thus far, 319 mutations have been described, including deletions, major rearrangements, and missense and nonsense point mutations (Human Gene Mutation Database).[86,430] In some very severe cases with unusual features, complete deficiency of the gene may be associated with loss of adjacent loci, suggestive of a contiguous

gene syndrome. Mutation analysis may help identify the various forms of Hunter's disease. A 140-kb pseudogene-like structure (*IDS2* gene) has been identified that is 20 kb distal to the active *IDS* gene.[431] The protein that it codes is identical to IDS except for absence of the 207–amino acid carboxyl-terminal domain.[432] Further studies will probably clarify its contribution to the clinical heterogeneity seen in Hunter's syndrome.

The diagnosis of Hunter's syndrome is occasionally considered in females with deficiency of IDS. However, on further study, some of these patients have been determined to have mucosulfatidosis (multiple sulfatase deficiency). One female patient with Hunter's disease was found to have a mutation on the paternal IDS locus that resulted in both a deficiency of IDS and inactivation of the maternal, structurally normal X chromosome.[433] Determination of heterozygosity is valid only when enzyme activity is reduced to levels less than 50% of normal. Normal levels of IDS activity in females with relatives who have Hunter's syndrome do not rule out heterozygosity. One method for carrier diagnosis uses ^{35}S-labeled sulfate incorporated into fibroblasts in the presence of fructose 1-phosphate. In the cell population, uptake of IDS produced by the normal cells in culture is prevented, and ^{35}S-labeled acid mucopolysaccharide therefore accumulates.[434]

Prenatal diagnosis has been accomplished with specimens from a variety of sources, including chorionic villi[435] and fetal plasma.[436]

Treatment

At present, the therapeutic approaches for MPS II are ERT and BMT, although these therapies have some limitations. Successful transfection of affected human cells has been achieved with specially designed retroviral vectors, which led to an increase in enzymatic activity of up to 49%.[437] A phase II/III clinical study of ERT was reported.[438] Although recombinant human IDS (idursulfase) was generally well tolerated, antibodies against the recombinant enzyme were found in almost 50% of patients during the study. Recently, an approach to gene therapy involving the use of AAV vectors for the treatment of MPS II in mice has been described. Viral particles were administrated to adult mice with MPS II.[439] IDS activity was completely restored in the plasma and tissue of all the treated mice and resulted in complete clearance of the accumulated GAGs in all tissues analyzed, normalization of GAG levels in urine, and correction of the skeletal abnormalities. These results suggest that this approach could be promising for the systemic treatment of patients with Hunter's syndrome.

Mucopolysaccharidosis Type III (Sanfilippo's Syndrome Types A, B, C, and D)

Patients with Sanfilippo's syndrome characteristically have progressive CNS disease but only mild physical stigmata typically associated with the mucopolysaccharidoses. This feature makes Sanfilippo's disease a very difficult entity to diagnose unless a high level of suspicion exists. In fact, it has been suggested that MPS III is probably more common than expected in institutions for the mentally handicapped. The mental retardation is usually extreme, although survival to adulthood is possible. Affected children are typically seen between 2 and 6 years of age with delayed development, marked hyperactivity with aggressive behavior, sleep disorders, and hirsutism. Joint stiffness and, in some patients, mild hepatosplenomegaly and hearing loss may be present. There is minimal skeletal involvement with mild dysostosis multiplex and usually normal stature for age. Radiologic signs include thickening of the calvaria and a biconvex configuration of the dorsolumbar vertebral bodies. The diagnosis may be delayed in these patients because of the mild somatic and radiographic features and a high incidence of false-negative results in the urinary screening test for mucopolysaccharides. Corneal opacities are absent.[405]

It is not clear why the selective CNS degeneration occurs in this variant of mucopolysaccharidosis. Recent studies have suggested that in addition to abnormal accumulation of mucopolysaccharide, excessive GSL deposits are also present.[440,441] G_{M3}, G_{D3}, and lactosyl ceramide were the principal GSLs accumulated in MPS IIID caprine brain specimens. These changes were attributed, in part, to the reduction in sialidase and UDP-N-acetylgalactosamine: G_{M3} N-acetylgalactosaminyltransferase (GalNAc-T) activities in MPS IIID caprine brain. Pathologic accumulation of subunit c of mitochondrial ATP synthase has been identified in the neuronal lysosomes of the MPS IIIB mouse model.[442]

All patients with Sanfilippo's syndrome seem to conform to a single phenotype, yet four forms can be distinguished enzymatically; all of them are transmitted in an autosomal recessive fashion. In the type A variant, an N-sulfatase also known as sulfamidase (heparan-N-sulfatase) is deficient. Its gene localizes to chromosome 17q25.3,[443] and about 62 different mutations have been described.[444]

The other variants are caused by deficiencies in O-sulfatases. In the type B variant, an α-N-acetylglucosaminidase is absent. This variant is particularly important in Sanfilippo's disease because a murine model is available and trials of ERT have been attempted with promising results.[445] Recently, the gene for the type C variant has been discovered, an acetyl coenzyme A (CoA)/acetyltransferase. It is a transmembrane protein 76 gene (*TMEM76*) that encodes a 73-kd protein with predicted multiple transmembrane domains and glycosylation sites.[446] In the type D variant, the deficient enzyme is N-acetylglucosaminide-6-sulfatase.

Although the type A variant can cause the most severe effects of the four variants, with an earlier onset, rapid progression of symptoms, and shorter survival, patients with mild disease have been reported.[447] Type B

is believed to have milder features, whereas type C may be intermediate between types A and B. Overall, the ultimate factor differentiating among the variants is biochemical analysis. Carriers of these diseases can be distinguished by enzyme assay, and prevention of each type is possible through prenatal diagnosis.

Treatment

Different therapeutic approaches have been tested in the animal models available for MPS III. MPS IIIA mice treated at birth with recombinant sulfamidase demonstrated a reduction in storage material in cells of the CNS and general improvement in body weight, behavior, and ability to learn.[448] In another trial, injection of recombinant human sulfamidase into cerebrospinal fluid via the cisterna magna in the CNS was shown to reduce lysosomal storage in different neural cells. An immune response to the recombinant protein was observed.[449] A substrate inhibitor, rhodamine B, has been shown to suppress GAG chain synthesis by inhibiting the formation of sugar precursors or the activity of glycosyltransferases, or both. Use of rhodamine B has been shown to diminish visceral symptoms and improve the behavioral aspects of murine MPS IIIA without causing any apparent side effects.[450] A gene therapy approach involving intraventricular injection of recombinant AAV in a mouse model of MPS IIIA was recently reported. Treatment with a recombinant AAV vector resulted in a visible reduction in lysosomal storage and inflammatory markers in transduced brain regions in the treated animals and general improvement in both motor and cognitive function. These results suggest that early treatment of CNS lesions by AAV-mediated intraventricular injection may be a feasible therapy for MPS IIIA.[451]

Gene therapy with genetically modified bone marrow transduced with human NAGLU cDNA in a mouse knockout model for MPS IIIB showed that genetically modified cells of hematopoietic origin can reduce the pathologic manifestations of MPS IIIB.[452] Transplanted human umbilical cord blood was used in another therapeutic approach and demonstrated that umbilical cord blood cells are able to survive long-term, migrate into the CNS and peripheral organs, and reduce GAGs in the livers of treated mutant mice.[453] A combined approach involving intravenous and intracisternal injection was used to achieve CNS delivery of an AAV vector for treating MPS IIIB in young adult mice. This treatment resulted in a significantly prolonged life span of the treated mice and variable correction of lysosomal storage pathology in the CNS and different visceral organs.[453]

Lentiviral-mediated gene transfer via systemic injections has been tested on an MPS IIIB mouse model. Long-term analysis has demonstrated that integration of the viral genome persists in target tissues and is accompanied by a decrease in GAG levels in several visceral tissues.[180]

Finally, a spontaneous caprine model for MPS IIID was used to evaluate the potential efficacy of ERT.

Recombinant caprine enzyme was administered systemically to one MPS IIID goat kid at different weeks of age. A significant reduction in lysosomal storage material in the hepatic cells of the treated animal was detected, but ERT had no effect on the CNS lesions.[455]

Mucopolysaccharidosis Type IV (Morquio's Syndrome [Types IVA and IVB])

Children with Morquio's syndrome usually have normal intelligence and a generalized skeletal dysplasia. MPS IVA and IVB result from two different enzyme deficiencies. MPS IVA is associated with a deficiency of the lysosomal enzyme *N*-acetylgalactosamine-6-sulfatase (GALNS, galactosamine-6-sulfatase), whereas MPS IVB is caused by a deficiency of lysosomal β-gal (see "G_{M1}-Gangliosidosis" earlier). Both variants result in a defect in the degradation of keratan sulfate. Therefore, excessive keratan sulfate is excreted in the urine of the patients.

Based on age at onset and severity of the bone dysplasia, type A is subdivided into three clinical subtypes (severe, intermediate, and mild forms). In the severe form, skeletal deformities begin to appear between 1 and 2 years of age. These children have a short neck and trunk, a prominent sternum, kyphosis, a waddling gait, bowed knees, and excessive excretion of keratan sulfate and chondroitin 6-sulfate. Absence or severe hypoplasia of the odontoid process of the second cervical vertebra results in atlantoaxial subluxation and subsequent cervical myelopathy. The maxilla is broad, and the dental enamel is abnormally thin. The joints are loose and hypermobile. The facial features become coarse, and deafness and mild corneal clouding develop. The major medical problem in adult life is cardiorespiratory insufficiency secondary to valvular heart disease and restrictions in size and motion of the thoracic cage.

In the mild phenotypic form, the disease progresses slowly, and patients are less severely affected. The broad spectrum of clinical phenotypes seen in MPS IVA correlates with different mutations of the *GALNS* gene, localized to chromosome 16q24.[456-458] Specific DNA analysis and polymorphic markers for carrier detection and prenatal diagnosis are available for families at risk for the disease.[459]

MPS IVB was initially thought to be a mild form of Morquio's syndrome because the symptoms were less pronounced than those in MPS IVA. However, ensuing reports have described patients with MPS IVB whose clinical symptoms were as severe as those seen in the severe form of MPS IVA.[460,461] Children with MPS IVB demonstrate a variety of bone and connective tissue abnormalities without major neurologic impairment. A variety of mutations of the *GLB1* gene have been found to cause different phenotypic expressions. Some mutations may affect the catabolism of both G_{M1} and keratan sulfate and cause a phenotype overlapping between that of G_{M1}-gangliosidosis and Morquio IVB, with both neurologic and skeletal manifestations.[462,463] Other amino acid changes only impair the activity of β-gal toward keratan sulfate. However, as discussed earlier, the β-gal precursor mRNA can give rise to an alternative spliced transcript that encodes EBP.[349] Mutations that affect both β-gal and EBP are believed to cause abnormal elastin fiber assembly and deposition in the extracellular matrix and to worsen the connective tissue and bone abnormalities characteristic of this disease.

Treatment

Except for management of its skeletal and spinal complications, no therapy is available for this condition.

Mucopolysaccharidosis Type VI (Maroteaux-Lamy Syndrome)

MPS VI is a clinically heterogeneous syndrome with severe, intermediate, and mild forms. Many of the signs and symptoms of Hurler's syndrome are also present in children with Maroteaux-Lamy syndrome, including short stature, clawhand deformities, coarse facies, umbilical or inguinal hernias, marked corneal clouding, and deafness. Sleep apnea may occur. These children may require shunting for progressive hydrocephalus. Contractions of the knees, hips, and elbows cause the children to assume a crouched stance. Involvement of the heart valves with associated murmurs and heart disease is common. Acute infantile cardiomyopathy has been reported as an initial symptom in Maroteaux-Lamy syndrome.[464] The preservation of intellect in this syndrome clearly differentiates it from Hurler's syndrome. Like Morquio's syndrome, there is hypoplasia of the odontoid process with subluxation of the C1 vertebra onto C2. Diffuse thickening of the dura and ligaments covering the spinal cord can cause chronic nerve root entrapment and myelopathy and necessitate laminectomy and opening of the dural sac.[465] Female patients with the mild variant require cesarean section to deliver a child because of involvement of their pelvic ligaments in the disease process.

Leukocytes from patients with Maroteaux-Lamy syndrome present a more striking picture of metachromatic inclusions than do leukocytes in most other mucopolysaccharidoses.

The lysosomal enzyme arylsulfatase B (ARSB, galactosamine-4-sulfatase) is deficient in this syndrome. Deficiency of the enzyme results in the accumulation of dermatan sulfate in tissues, primarily connective tissue, and in reticuloendothelial lysosomes and urine. The *ARSB* gene has been sequenced and cloned, and many mutations have been identified, with some exhibiting genotype/phenotype correlation.[466] Mutation analysis has demonstrated broad molecular heterogeneity in this syndrome, which should be expected because of the associated clinical heterogeneity.[467]

Treatment

BMT in several patients resulted in restitution of ARSB levels in both circulating leukocytes and the liver. At 1 to 9 years of follow-up, clinical improvement with regression of hepatosplenomegaly and improved joint mobility was noted. This treatment has been shown to prolong survival and improve quality of life.[139]

ERT with the recombinant product has been successfully attempted in the feline model of this condition,[103] and phase I and II human clinical trials are currently under study.* On the basis of the phase I/II results, a phase II study in patients with severe disease was initiated primarily to evaluate efficacy. ERT was shown to improve mobility and joint function and reduce urinary excretion of GAGs.[468] Cultured fibroblast ARSB mutant protein and residual activity were determined for each patient and, together with genotype information, used to predict the expected clinical severity of each patient.[469]

Gene therapy has also been attempted in the same feline animal model.[470] After gene transfer, muscle or liver can theoretically be converted into factories for systemic secretion of ARSB, thereby leading to uptake by nontransduced cells. In a recent study, newborn MPS VI rats and cats were injected with AAV vectors expressing ARSB under the control of liver-specific, muscle-specific, or universally active promoters. Systemic or intramuscular injection of AAV resulted in curative levels of ARSB that improved the skeletal abnormalities and significantly reduced GAG storage, inflammation, and apoptosis. This study suggests that AAV-mediated expression of ARSB from the liver could represent a potential therapeutic approach for MPS VI.[471]

Mucopolysaccharidosis Type VII (Sly's Syndrome)

More than 30 cases of mucopolysaccharidosis with β-glucuronidase deficiency have been observed since the publication of Sly and colleagues' original case report in 1973.[472] The clinical manifestation, however, has been quite varied. The original patient exhibited slowing of development at 2 to 3 years of age, coarse facial features, anterior chest deformity, hepatosplenomegaly, bilateral inguinal hernias, and clear corneas. He died at 19 years of age. At the time of his death he had dysostosis multiplex and extensive cardiovascular lesions, including arterial stenosis and marked fibrous thickening of the atrioventricular and aortic valves. There were only trace amounts of β-glucuronidase in multiple tissues postmortem. Various tissues demonstrated accumulation of chondroitin 4- and 6-sulfate.[473]

Other patients have had onset in infancy, clouding of the corneas, and dysostosis multiplex. Hydrops fetalis

was described in two infants; one died less than an hour after delivery and the other died at 6 months of age.[474] Patients with onset after 4 or 5 years of age are less likely to have cloudy corneas, pectus carinatum, hernia, short stature, or developmental delay.[475] Characteristics common to all patients with this syndrome are recurrent bouts of pneumonia during infancy and the abundant coarse granulations characteristic of Alder-Reilly bodies in their granulocytes. The excessive excretion of mucopolysaccharides may not be present in some patients.[476]

The gene encoding β-glucuronidase (*GUSB*)[477] has been localized to chromosome 7q21.1-q22.[478] Mutational analysis of the original patient with Sly's syndrome demonstrated a compound heterozygote with a missense mutation in exon 12 and a nonsense mutation in exon 7. Several other mutations have been described, among them the A354V and R611W substitutions identified in the first reported occurrence of nonimmune hydropic MPS VII.[479] These mutations correlate with the severe form of the syndrome. Prenatal diagnosis is available with chorionic villus and amniotic fluid sampling.[480]

Treatment

Naturally occurring dog and mouse models of β-glucuronidase deficiency were identified in the eighties.[481,482] Because the clinical manifestations are quite similar to the corresponding human conditions, these animals, in particular the mouse model, have been extensively exploited for testing numerous therapeutic protocols, including BMT, ERT, and ex vivo and in vivo gene therapy.[405] Neural progenitor cells have been transplanted into the CNS of newborn mice with the enzyme deficiency. β-Glucuronidase activity was found to be expressed along the entire neuraxis, which resulted in correction of the storage disease in the neurons and glia of the affected mice.[483] BMT has also been attempted in the mouse with some success.[484] ERT studies in the mouse model suggested that therapeutic enzyme can be delivered across the blood-brain barrier in adult mice if administered at higher doses than conventionally used in ERT trials.[485] A gene therapy study involving a murine model of MPS VII has been reported. Injection of AAV vectors containing β-glucuronidase into different regions of the brain was able to correct LSDs. The treated MPS VII mice showed improvement in spatial learning and memory, thus suggesting that this therapy could be effective in curing the CNS pathology.[486]

Mucosulfatidosis (Multiple Sulfatase Deficiency)

The clinical phenotype of patients with mucosulfatidosis (multiple sulfatase deficiency) combines the features of late infantile metachromatic leukodystrophy with those of a mucopolysaccharidosis.[487] Metachromatic leukodystrophy alone does not affect the reticuloendothelial system. It results from failure to degrade cerebroside

---

*Kakkis E: Personal communication, BioMarin Corp.

sulfate because of deficiency of arylsulfatase A. Metachromatic leukodystrophy leads to widespread degeneration of both central and peripheral myelin and subsequent spastic tetraparesis, blindness, peripheral neuropathy, and an elevation in cerebrospinal fluid protein content.

Neonatal, late infantile, and juvenile forms of multiple sulfatase deficiency have been described. In the early-onset form, facial dysmorphism, a short neck, hepatomegaly, vertebral hypoplasia, and epiphyseal dysplasia are present from birth. The early development of children with the late infantile form is usually less advanced than that of children with late infantile metachromatic leukodystrophy. The child may learn to sit and stand but does not develop speech and regresses after the second year, with previously acquired skills being lost. The forehead is prominent and the nasal bridge flattened. There may be an excessive startle reaction, spasticity, and extensor plantar responses. Seizures eventually appear. Hepatosplenomegaly has been reported in some patients. Many have had ichthyosis. The corneas are clear, and the maculae are abnormally gray. The skeletal changes are similar to those found in the mucopolysaccharidoses and include lumbar kyphosis, a prominent sternum, broad phalanges, and a J-shaped sella turcica. A less severe form beginning after 5 years of age with survival into the third decade has also been described.

A child with multiple sulfatase deficiency accumulates not only cerebroside sulfate but also cholesterol sulfate and sulfated mucopolysaccharides because of deficiencies of 17 different sulfatases, including arylsulfatases A and B, steroid sulfatase, heparan-*N*-sulfatase, iduronate sulfatase, and galactosamine-6-sulfatase. In tissue culture, these deficiencies can be partially corrected by maintaining the cells in a medium at high pH (pH 7.4) or by the addition of sodium thiosulfate. Laboratory tests for this disease should include a search for Alder-Reilly bodies in circulating granulocytes and bone marrow, a Berry spot test for mucopolysacchariduria, and determination of arylsulfatase A and B activity in leukocytes. Prenatal diagnosis may be achieved by chorionic villus sampling and detection of specific mutant alleles.[488]

In two of the sulfatases, structural analysis has indicated that in place of a cysteine residue normally expected on the basis of their cDNA sequence, a 2-amino-3-oxopropionic acid residue appears. However, in the sulfatases derived from cells with multiple sulfatase deficiency, the cysteine residue is retained. This suggests that the defect in multiple sulfatase deficiency is failure of the cotranslational or post-translational conversion of a cysteine to 2-amino-3-oxopropionic acid or α-formylglycine.[489] The gene mutated in multiple sulfatase deficiency has been identified by different approachs[490,491] and has been named sulfatase-modifying factor 1 (*SUMF1*). SUMF1 is responsible for conversion of the cysteine residue located in the active site of all the sulfatases to α-formylglycine. Recently, a mouse line carrying a mouse model for multiple sulfatase deficiency has been generated. Similar to patients with multiple sulfatase deficiency, the mouse model deficient in Sumf1 displays frequent early mortality, congenital growth retardation, skeletal abnormalities, and neurologic defects.[492]

GLYCOPROTEINOSES AND MUCOLIPIDOSES

In 1970, Spranger and Wiedemann[493] established a new category of storage diseases for patients who exhibited the clinical features of Hurler's disease (the so-called "mucopolysaccharidosis phenotype") without an excess of urinary mucopolysaccharides. The term *mucolipidosis* was selected to indicate the coexistence in these patients of signs and symptoms typical of both the mucopolysaccharidoses and the sphingolipidoses. Although excretion of mucopolysaccharides is not seen, the urine of these patients contains large quantities of oligosaccharides identical in structure to the carbohydrate side chains in glycoproteins. Therefore, the name glycoproteinoses more appropriately refers to this group of LSDs, whose common hallmark is the genetic defect of a lysosomal protein involved in the catabolic pathway of glycoproteins (Fig. 24-6; also see Table 24-4). The deficient protein may be a glycosidase, a protease, or a lysosomal mem-

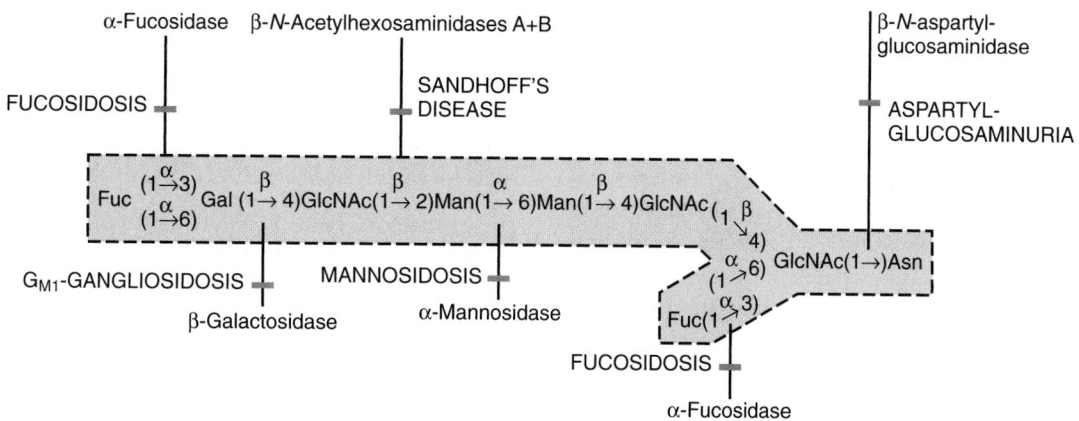

FIGURE 24-6. Fucosyloligosaccharide unit of a hypothetical glycoprotein indicating the sites of catabolic block in fucosidosis, G_{M1}-gangliosidosis, Sandhoff's disease, mannosidosis, and aspartylglucosaminuria. Asn, asparagine; Fuc, fucose; Gal, galactose; GlcNAc, *N*-acetylglucosamine; Man, mannose.

brane carrier that expels catabolic products into the cytosol. Degradation of glycoproteins begins with the action of exoglycosidases, which degrade the glycan portion of these substrates in a stepwise manner starting at their nonreducing end. The lack of a single enzyme leads to complete blockage of the catabolic chain and results in the accumulation of undegraded oligosaccharides and glycopeptides in lysosomes. Elevated urinary excretion of oligosaccharides is also diagnostic of these diseases.[494] The oligosaccharides are of two types: sialyloligosaccharides and neutral oligosaccharides.

High sialyloligosaccharide concentrations correlate with a primary or secondary deficiency of the acid lysosomal neuraminidase 1 (NEU1, sialidase), which is associated with sialidosis and galactosialidosis, two autosomal recessive LSDs primarily affecting the reticuloendothelial system.[495,496] The early infantile variant of sialidosis was known as mucolipidosis I in the past. Similar findings occur secondarily in mucolipidosis II and III. In these LSDs, which are two phenotypic variants of the same enzyme deficiency, the primary defect is in posttranslational modification of the carbohydrate unit that is common to most lysosomal enzymes (i.e., the M6P recognition marker). This is required for uptake of these enzymes from the cell surface. The latter is not formed because of a deficiency of N-acetylglucosamine phosphotransferase, and consequently the intracellular content of several soluble lysosomal enzymes (including neuraminidase) is reduced.

Laboratory screening for these diseases is accomplished by thin-layer chromatographic analysis of urine for oligosaccharides and sialyloligosaccharides and by quantitation of free sialic acid in urine.[67] In these conditions, mucopolysaccharides are not present in excess in the urine. On the basis of these tests, the activities of the relevant lysosomal enzymes are then examined in leukocytes or fibroblasts.

Sialidosis

Sialidosis (formerly mucolipidosis I) is caused by deficiency of NEU1 (sialidase).[496] The enzyme is encoded by the NEU1 gene on chromosome 6p21.3 and is genomically positioned inside the major histocompatibility complex.[497] In mammalian tissues, three additional neuraminidases—NEU2, NEU3, and NEU4—have been identified that differ in their subcellular distributions, pH optimum, kinetic properties, response to ions and detergents, and substrate specificity.[498,499] Of the four, only NEU1 is expressed in all tissues, albeit at different levels,[500,501] and is the only mammalian sialidase that is clinically relevant. The importance of these enzymes in normal cellular physiology is illustrated by the numerous metabolic processes that they control, including cellular proliferation and differentiation, cell adhesion, membrane fusion and fluidity, immunocyte function, and receptor modification.[499]

NEU1 initiates the intralysosomal hydrolysis of sialo-oligosaccharides and sialoglycoproteins by removing their terminal sialic acid residues. In both human and murine tissue, lysosomal neuraminidase forms a complex with at least two other proteins, β-gal and the protective protein/cathepsin A (PPCA).[495,502] By virtue of their association with PPCA, NEU1 and β-gal acquire their active and stable conformation in lysosomes. However, NEU1 strictly depends on PPCA for correct compartmentalization in lysosomes, which makes it unique among other mammalian sialidases. This is because the protein is poorly mannose-6-phosphorylated and requires PPCA for transport through the biosynthetic pathway and to remain catalytically active once in lysosomes.[503] Thus, PPCA appears to function as a chaperone/transport protein that is crucial to NEU1 both in route to and within the lysosome. Only a small amount of PPCA and β-gal activity is consistently found in the NEU1/PPCA/β-gal complex, which contains all of the neuraminidase activity. This finding further supports the notion that NEU1 is not active outside the protein complex.

Genetic evidence of the dependence of NEU1 on its interaction with PPCA to remain catalytically active is illustrated by the LSD galactosialidosis (discussed later). The latter condition is caused by a primary defect in the PPCA gene, but the clinical manifestations in patients are mostly attributed to the secondary deficiencies of NEU1 and β-gal. Therefore, sialidosis and galactosialidosis patients share many of their clinical and biochemical features. However, differences in onset, severity, and range of symptoms are associated with both diseases.

In addition to its known lysosomal activity, NEU1 may be involved in releasing sialic acids from cell surface glycoconjugates of neutrophils and monocytes during inflammatory or immune responses, as indicated by increasing evidence.[504,505] NEU1 may also regulate sialylation at the surface of immature thymocytes and, in turn, control T-cell response during development and differentiation.[506] Thus, NEU1 has a potential role in processes that influence the functional capacity of cells in the hematopoietic and immune systems.

Correct diagnosis of either sialidosis or galactosialidosis can be achieved by measuring the catalytic activity of cathepsin A, NEU1, and β-gal. To date, more than 20 unique mutations have been identified, most of which are missense mutations that result in single amino acid substitutions and involve conserved amino acids or are located within conserved regions of the enzyme.[497,507-512]

Sialidosis Type I (Normomorphic Sialidosis, Cherry-Red Spot/Myoclonus Syndrome)

Type I sialidosis is also referred to as "cherry-red spot–myoclonus" syndrome and is the attenuated form of this disease. Generally, patients have no obvious physical features, and their intelligence is normal or only slightly impaired. The disease is recognized in the second or third decade of life with the onset of gait abnormalities, decreased visual acuity, or both.[513-517] The visual loss is progressive and associated with bilateral macular cherry-red spots that may fade later in the course of the disease. In some patients, small punctate opacities occur in the lens.

The most striking clinical feature is myoclonus, which may be precipitated by voluntary movements, the thought of movement, passive joint movements, or light touch or sound stimuli. Initially there are intention tremors and difficulty with fine motor movements, but eventually the myoclonus becomes so disabling that despite continued normal muscle strength, patients cannot speak, feed themselves, walk, or even roll over in bed. The deep tendon reflexes are increased. Leg tremors and generalized seizures may occur in the early morning before awakening. Myoclonic jerking is more severe in the premenstrual phase of the monthly cycle. As the disease progresses, the patient is confined to a wheelchair and is helped by passive restraints on the limbs. Anticonvulsants suppress the convulsions but do not decrease the myoclonus dramatically. A significant reduction in action myoclonus has occurred in a few patients with the use of 5-hydroxytryptophan, with the best response noted in combination with carbidopa.[518] However, the disease has an inexorable and relentlessly progressive course.

Though disabled, patients have continued to be intellectually active. Sensation is normal, and there are no Hurler disease–like features such as corneal cloudiness, hepatomegaly, or bone or joint abnormalities. In a few patients, scoliosis has developed late in the course of the disease. Some patients have complained of severe pain in the hands and feet during hot weather of the type observed in Fabry's disease.

A few vacuolated lymphocytes may be seen in the peripheral blood smear, and foamy histiocytes have been described in the bone marrow. Nerve cells contain PAS-positive material that can be removed with alcohol fixation. Electron microscopic examination discloses vacuoles in the abnormal bone marrow cells and in Kupffer cells. Most of these vacuoles are empty, but some contain fine fibrillar material or electron-dense bodies. The sialic acid content of cultured fibroblasts may be normal or elevated,[517] but there is an increase in sialic acid–containing compounds in the urine.

Sialidosis Type II (Dysmorphic Sialidosis)

The type II form of sialidosis can be subdivided into congenital, infantile, and juvenile types, all of which feature dysmorphic facies and complete absence of NEU1 activity.[496,508,519] More than 10 patients with congenital sialidosis type II have been reported; 2 were stillborn infants with hydrops fetalis, ascites, hepatosplenomegaly, stippling of the epiphyses, and periosteal cloaking of the long bones.[520] Patients in this group were reported to also have severely reduced β-gal activity (5% to 10%), which may mean that many of the patients in this subgroup may actually suffer from early infantile galactosialidosis.

When the disease is manifested at birth, the infants have coarse puffy facies, a depressed nasal bridge, and a broad maxilla. Development is slow, but by 2 years of age the child can walk and speak single words. Many skeletal abnormalities are found, and radiologic examination reveals findings typical of dysostosis multiplex. The trunk is short and the extremities are relatively long. There may be a thoracic deformity of either the pectus excavatum or carinatum type, and thoracic kyphosis is present. Joint mobility is mildly restricted. Radiographic signs include stippled epiphyses, ovoid vertebral bodies, and thickened calvaria. Eye examination discloses punctate lens opacities and a macular cherry-red spot. Other signs include inner ear hearing loss, mild gingival hyperplasia, widely spaced teeth, and hepatomegaly.

Mental retardation is evident from an early age, and progressive neurologic deterioration occurs during childhood. Initially, the gait is broad based and waddling, but as muscle wasting and weakness develop, the patient exhibits further unsteadiness and then is unable to walk. Slowing of nerve conduction velocity suggests that these neurologic difficulties may be due to a degenerative neuropathy. Gross myoclonus and a tonic-clonic seizure disorder may develop, and death occurs later in childhood or adolescence.

In peripheral blood smears, a small number of lymphocytes and monocytes may contain large cytoplasmic vacuoles. Fine abnormal granulations may also be present in these cell types and granulocytes. Foam cells are found in the bone marrow. These cells contain vacuoles of different size that appear under the electron microscope as single membrane-bound clear inclusions. Similar cytoplasmic inclusions have also been found in liver, cartilage, and cultured fibroblasts. Neuronal storage has been demonstrated, and sural nerve biopsy has revealed myelin and axonal degeneration.

The quantity of bound sialic acid in the leukocytes and fibroblasts of these patients is increased severalfold, whereas the sialyloligosaccharide content of their urine is several hundred times greater than normal.[521,533] Thin-layer chromatographic analysis of urine is therefore a very useful diagnostic test. There is a marked deficiency of NEU1 activity in fibroblasts and a partial deficiency of this enzyme in obligate heterozygotes. The juvenile form of sialidosis type II is manifested as mild developmental delay and disproportionate stature with relatively long legs. Coarse facies are evident by 10 years of age, and radiographs reveal dysostosis multiplex. Intellect declines in adolescence. The patient becomes severely disabled, with death occurring in the second decade of life.

Galactosialidosis

Galactosialidosis is a neurosomatic disorder caused by mutation of the PPCA gene[495,523,524] and is the only LSD that is associated with deficiency of one of the lysosomal cathepsins. The physiologic consequences of total deficiency of cathepsin A are still unclear, given that most phenotypic abnormalities characteristic of the disease have been attributed to the secondary, profound loss of NEU1 activity. The PPCA gene maps to chromosome 20q13.1 and overlaps with two other genes: with the phospholipid transfer protein (PLTP) gene at the 3′ end[525] and with the gene encoding the neutralized-like protein OZZ at the 5′ end.[526,527] The PPCA gene is transcribed in the opposite orientation with respect to the OZZ gene, and the two genes share a minimal promoter; this rather unique genomic organization is conserved in the mouse and human. However, whereas PPCA is differentially but ubiquitously expressed in all tissues and cell types, OZZ expression is restricted to skeletal muscle and the heart. The OZZ protein is a component of a RING-type ubiquitin ligase complex that is involved in muscle development, differentiation, and regeneration.[527] It is therefore conceivable that mutations affecting the PPCA gene may influence expression of OZZ and account for some of the phenotypes observed in galactosialidosis patients.

The PPCA transcript encodes a 480–amino acid serine carboxypeptidase that is structurally similar to yeast and plant serine carboxypeptidases.[528] However, its protective function toward NEU1 and β-gal is unique to higher eukaryotic species, including fish, birds, and mammals. The 54-kd PPCA zymogen carries two N-glycans and is conventionally routed to the endosomal/lysosomal compartment via the M6P receptor. There is evidence in support of the view that both NEU1 and β-gal are poorly mannose-6-phosphorylated and depend at least in part on interaction with PPCA for correct lysosomal routing. Once in the lysosome, the PPCA precursor is activated by partial trypsin-like proteolysis of a short internal peptide that covers the catalytic pocket.[529] In lysosomes, the mature and active two-chain enzyme remains in complex with the other two glycosidases, which is essential for activation of NEU1 and stabilization of β-gal. In the absence of functional PPCA, the enzyme complex is not formed and NEU1 looses its catalytic activity. In vitro mutagenesis experiments have demonstrated that the cathepsin A activity of PPCA is apparently not needed for formation of the multienzyme complex and the activities of NEU1 and β-gal.[87,503,530,531]

Besides its acidic carboxypeptidase activity, at neutral pH PPCA functions as a deamidase and esterase toward a selected number of neuropeptides, such as substance P and neurokinin, and can hydrolyze the C-terminal amino acid from oxytocin-free acid, bradykinin, and endothelin I. In addition, catalytically active cathepsin A was shown to be released from thrombin-stimulated platelets and from ionophore B–stimulated natural killer cells and was also detected in granules of human interleukin-2–activated killer cells. All PPCA's catalytic properties were severely reduced in lymphoblastoid cells and fibroblasts from galactosialidosis patients. Together, these findings show that PPCA may be important in metabolic processes such as inactivation of bioactive peptides or granzyme-mediated cellular cytotoxicity.[532,533]

Eleven amino acid substitutions identified in mutant PPCAs from clinically different galactosialidosis patients have been modeled in a three-dimensional structure of the wild-type precursor form of PPCA.[531,534-536] Nine of the mutations were located in positions that appeared to drastically influence folding and stability of the mutant protein. Two other mutations had a less disruptive effect on the protein structure. None of the mutations involved the active site or were located at the surface, where they could have disrupted the protective functions toward NEU1 and β-gal. Close correlation was noted between the clinical severity of the patient and the effect of the corresponding mutation on the structure of PPCA. The most plausible reason for the many mutations that affect the overall folding of the protein is that no single mutation is likely to disrupt PPCA's protective properties toward both NEU1 and β-gal.

The secondary severe loss of NEU1 activity probably accounts for most of the overt clinical manifestations in galactosialidosis patients and for the pathogenesis of the disease, which in many respects is similar to that of sialidosis. Light microscopy revealed the presence of foam cells in bone marrow and vacuolated lymphocytes in the peripheral blood of patients with galactosialidosis. Sialyloligosacchariduria is also diagnostic of the disease, although it is indistinguishable from that measured in sialidosis patients. More than 20 different sialyloligosaccharides have been isolated from the urine of patients with galactosialidosis.[537] Autopsy studies have shown the presence of fibroblasts and macrophages containing cytoplasmic vacuoles limited by a unit membrane in the lymph nodes, liver, and spleen. The brainstem nuclei and anterior horn cells were swollen with Sudan black B–positive granular material. Ultrastructurally, these inclusions consisted of membranous lamellar structures and multilamellar arrangements mixed with vacuole-like granules of low electron density.[538]

Early Infantile Galactosialidosis

The most severe form of the disease has been reported in 19 patients and is manifested between birth and 3 months of age as fetal hydrops, neonatal edema, coarse facies, proteinuria, inguinal hernias, and telangiectases.[495,539-541] Other common features may include enlargement of the spleen and liver, kidney involvement, skeletal dysplasia most prominently in the spine, psychomotor delay, and severe neurodegeneration. Eye abnormalities such as corneal clouding and a cherry-red macula have been described in several infant patients. Cardiomegaly, a thickened septum, and cardiac failure have also been reported in several patients. Patients die on average at the early age of 7 months, probably as a result of renal or cardiac failure (or both).

Late Infantile Galactosialidosis

Thirteen patients have been reported with the late infantile form of galactosialidosis.[495,536,542,543] They are generally seen in the first months of life with coarse facies, hepatosplenomegaly, and dysostosis multiplex, again affecting the spine in particular. Ocular abnormalities such as cherry-red spots and corneal clouding were observed in several patients, whereas others had no ocular symptoms toward the end of their second decade of life. In addition, hearing loss has also been reported in several patients. Severe neurologic manifestations such as myoclonus and ataxia are absent in most patients, but very mild mental retardation has been reported in about 50% of cases. Progressive valvular heart disease characterized by thickened mitral and aortic valves develops in most patients. One of the reported patients died at the age of 15; all others are alive, some into their second decade of life.

Juvenile/Adult Galactosialidosis

The juvenile/adult form of galactosialidosis comprises the largest group of patients.[495,544,545] It owes its dual designation to the broad spectrum of clinical severity, symptoms, and age at onset, which varies from 1 to 40 years with an average of 16 years. Patients in this group are predominantly of Japanese descent, and parental consanguinity has been reported frequently. Patients have coarse facies but less pronounced than in most of the other LSDs. General myoclonus is rare, but some patients have spinal abnormalities. The most common symptoms include a cherry-red macula and corneal clouding with loss of visual acuity, cerebellar ataxia, and angiokeratoma. Neurologic symptoms include myoclonus, cerebellar ataxia, seizures, and progressive mental retardation. Remarkably, unlike the other two galactosialidosis groups, nearly all patients with the juvenile/adult form have no visceromegaly.

Molecular Aspects

In-depth understanding of the mechanisms of pathogenesis in sialidosis and galactosialidosis is likely to come from analysis of the corresponding animal models of these two LSDs. There are currently three mouse models with either primary or secondary neu1 deficiency and the clinical manifestation of sialidosis and galactosialidosis. Neu1- and ppca-deficient mice were generated by targeted disruption of the neu1 and ppca genes.[546,547]

Though viable and fertile, ppca$^{-/-}$ mice have clinical, biochemical, and pathologic manifestations reminiscent of early-onset galactosialidosis early in life.[548] As in affected children, massive oligosacchariduria is diagnostic of the disease. In knockout mice, cells of the reticuloendothelial system are primarily affected. Extensive lysosomal storage is present in these cells of most organs, particularly the kidney, spleen, bone marrow, liver, intestine, heart, and brain. Affected mice progressively deteriorate, with severe nephropathy and ataxia developing, and they succumb to the disease at around 10 months of age. The distribution of lysosomal ppca mRNA and ppca protein in normal adult mouse tissues coincides with the occurrence of lysosomal storage in ppca$^{-/-}$ mice.[501] The distribution of affected cells is particularly complex in the brain, where only selected neurons become affected,

most notably those of the limbic system and cerebellum. The most overt morphologic changes are seen in the cerebellum, where loss of Purkinje cells starts to occur at approximately 2.5 months of age and progresses throughout the life of the animal.

Neu1$^{-/-}$ mice display clinical abnormalities reminiscent of early-onset sialidosis in children. These homozygous mice are infertile and die between the age of 6 and 9 months. As is the case for galactosialidosis, the primary target of the disease is the reticuloendothelial system. Severe nephropathy, progressive edema, splenomegaly, kyphosis, and urinary excretion of sialylated oligosaccharides are the main pathologic features. Although the sialidosis mouse model shares clinical and histopathologic features with galactosialidosis mice, some phenotypic abnormalities seem to be specific for sialidosis mice, including progressive deformity of the spine, a high incidence of premature death, age-related extramedullary hematopoiesis, and lack of early degeneration of cerebellar Purkinje cells. The differences and similarities identified in these mouse models have helped investigators better understand the pathophysiology of these diseases in children and identify more targeted therapies for each of these diseases.

SM/J mice exhibit partial deficiency of neu1 activity. This naturally occurring strain is homozygous for a point mutation that alters the affinity of neu1 for its natural substrates and results in a mild sialidosis phenotype.[501] SM/J mice cannot elicit a T_H2-mediated immune response because they cannot stimulate naïve T cells to become T_H2 lymphocytes.[548] These immunologic aberrations reiterate a potential role of Neu1 in the processing of sialoglycoconjugates at the plasma membrane.

Treatment

BMT in ppca$^{-/-}$ mice was performed with transgenic bone marrow overexpressing the corrective enzyme in either erythroid cells or monocytes/macrophages.[546,549] This strategy effectively improved the phenotype and encouraged the use of genetically modified bone marrow cells for ex vivo gene therapy for galactosialidosis. Knockout mice that received hematopoietic progenitors transduced with a murine stem cell virus (MSCV)-based, bicistronic retroviral vector overexpressing ppca afforded stable donor hematopoiesis. Complete correction of the disease phenotype in systemic organs was achieved up to 10 months after transplantation.[163] ppca$^+$ hematopoietic and nonhematopoietic cells were detected in all tissues, with the highest expression in the liver, spleen, bone marrow, thymus, and lung, thus indicating efficient uptake of the corrective protein and cross-correction. ppca expression in the brain occurred throughout the parenchyma but was localized mainly in perivascular areas; however, expression was apparently sufficient to delay the onset of Purkinje cell degeneration and correct the ataxia.

Short-term ERT with mannosylated insect cell–produced enzymes has been investigated in both ppca-

and neu1-deficient mice.[95,550] This therapeutic strategy resulted in successful clearance of lysosomal storage in systemic organs. However, neu1 null mice died as a result of a rapid and severe immunologic response to the recombinant protein.

Mucolipidoses

Mucolipidosis Type II (I-Cell Disease)

Mucolipidosis II (or I-cell disease) is a rare autosomal recessive LSD caused by UDP-*N*-acetylglucosamine: lysosomal-enzyme *N*-acetylglucosamine-1-phosphotransferase (GNPT) deficiency. This enzyme catalyzes the initial step in synthesis of the M6P determinant required for intracellular lysosomal targeting of newly synthesized lysosomal hydrolases. GNPT catalyzes the formation of M6P markers on high-mannose–type oligosaccharides in the Golgi apparatus. M6P residues are required to bind to the M6P receptors (MPRs), which mediate the vesicular transport of lysosomal enzymes to the endosomal/prelysosomal compartment. Because of the low pH in these organelles, the lysosomal enzyme–MPR complex dissociates, upon which the enzyme is delivered to the lysosome.[551] GNPT is an $\alpha_2\beta_2\gamma_2$ hexameric complex[552] encoded by two separate genes.[9] It has been proposed that the α or the β subunit (or both) contains the catalytic portion of the enzyme and that the γ subunit is involved in recognition of the lysosomal enzymes.[553] The α and β subunits are encoded by the *GNPTAB* gene on chromosome 12q23.2, and the γ subunit is encoded by the *GNPTG* gene on chromosome 16p.[553] Both I-cell disease and pseudo-Hurler polydystrophy (mucolipidosis III) are caused by mutations in the *GNPTAB* gene, which leads to defective lysosomal targeting of many lysosomal enzymes. The clinical and radiologic signs are similar to those in Hurler's disease, albeit with earlier onset during the first months of life and sometimes before birth.

Although there are reports of patients surviving into their teens, death usually occurs between 5 and 8 years of age. Other distinguishing features of this disorder are striking gingival hyperplasia, less apparent corneal clouding, and hearing impairment in some. As in other mucolipidoses, these patients lack mucopolysaccharides in their urine. Birth weight and length are often less than normal, and the clinical features may be evident from birth. Neonates may be seen with coarse facial features, tight hip muscles with dislocation of the hip, joint stiffness, hernias, severe skeletal dysplasia, downy hirsutism, and a tight, thickened skin. Psychomotor delay is usually obvious by 6 months of age. Linear growth decelerates and stops by the second year of life.

Children with I-cell disease are often recognized after 6 months of age by an abnormal low-pitched cry, small triangular head, hypertrophied maxillary alveolar ridge, enlarged tongue, kyphoscoliosis, protuberant abdomen, hepatomegaly, and hypotonia with poor head control. Patients are able to sit but cannot walk. They often have systolic murmurs and recurrent respiratory tract infections. Death usually results from cardiopulmonary complications.

In a study of nine patients from eight families, both interfamilial and intrafamilial variability was described. Marked variability in age at onset, organ manifestation, and radiologic findings was noted, even among siblings.[554]

I-cell disease has been found in association with nonimmune hydrops fetalis and elevated amniotic fluid optical density (ΔOD450), thus indicating the possibility of fetal blood hemolysis in this disease.[555] Fetal ultrasonographic studies have shown abnormally short femurs and intrauterine growth retardation.[556] Radiographs of an affected fetus demonstrate deficient endosteal bone formation, small epiphyses, and poorly developed intervertebral discs. Skeletal lesions in infants with the disease are characterized by delayed conversion of cartilage to bone; diffuse periosteal new bone formation in the long bones and ribs; marked osteopenia; resorption of the scapula, clavicle, and mandible; and irregular demineralization of the metaphyses of long tubular bones.[557]

Among the many radiographic signs of skeletal dysplasia in this disease are thickening of the calvaria, cone-shaped phalanges, proximal pointing of metacarpals, V-shaped deformity of the wrist joint, short rounded vertebral bodies with anteroinferior beaking of T12 or L1, broad ribs, flaring of the iliac wing, dysplasia of the acetabulum, and cortical thickening in the diaphyses of long bones. Bone encroachment in the region of the foramen magnum causes significant brainstem and upper cervical cord compression. Neurologic consequences include respiratory impairment and obstruction of cerebrospinal fluid outflow from the fourth ventricle. The internal hydrocephalus produced may require a shunting procedure, and cervical laminectomy may be needed to prevent cord paralysis.

Vacuolated lymphocytes are abundant in circulating blood,[33] but no foam cells are seen in the bone marrow. The dense cytoplasmic inclusions in cultured fibroblasts stain positively with PAS and Sudan black but negatively with Alcian blue, which indicates that glycolipids but not mucopolysaccharides are stored in these cells. These inclusions are characteristic of this disease, hence the name inclusion cell (I-cell) disease. Foam cells staining positively with PAS are found in various tissues, including the spleen and portal spaces of the liver, but storage in Kupffer cells and neurons is variable.

M6P is a recognition marker needed for internalization of acid hydrolases into lysosomes[5] and acts as a "ZIP code" during intracellular trafficking. Patients with I-cell disease have a defect in synthesis of this marker. Under normal conditions, the enzyme GNPT phosphorylates the oligosaccharide portion of lysosomal enzymes to produce M6P. Patients with I-cell disease have a phosphotransferase deficiency that results in a defect in incorporation of M6P. Because M6P is the marker ultimately responsible for transfer of the various acid hydrolases into lysosomes, the deficiency explains the discrepancy in acid hydrolase activity between sera and fibroblasts. The gene for the phosphotransferase has been mapped to chromosome 4q21-q23.[558]

As a result of the primary underlying metabolic defect, a variety of acid hydrolases are deficient in the fibroblasts of these patients, including α-neuraminidase, β-hexosaminidase, iduronate sulfatase, and arylsulfatase A. However, β-glucosidase and acid phosphatase activities are not affected. The various acid hydrolase activities in serum, on the other hand, are far above normal levels. Leukocyte enzyme activity is generally normal.

The diagnosis of I-cell disease can be confirmed by measuring and comparing the activity of various lysosomal enzymes in serum and cultured fibroblasts. It can also be ascertained by measuring phosphotransferase activity within fibroblasts or leukocytes.[559]

Carrier detection is possible with the use of cultured fibroblasts and artificial substrates (α-methylmannoside). Prenatal diagnosis has been successfully achieved by assaying amniotic fluid cells for multiple deficiencies of lysosomal enzymes and for deficiency of phosphotransferase.[560] It has been reported that phosphotransferase assays may be performed on chorionic villi obtained at 9 weeks of gestation.[561]

Successful engraftment of bone marrow from a heterozygous sibling into an 8-month-old patient has resulted in a 50% to 80% reduction in plasma lysosomal enzyme activity and increases in lymphocytic and hepatic phosphotransferase activity. In addition, pulmonary function has improved, hepatomegaly has subsided, and no further progression of corneal clouding has been seen. However, mental and growth retardation, dysostosis multiplex, and gingival hyperplasia have persisted to age 4.[562]

Mucolipidosis Type III (Pseudo-Hurler Polydystrophy)

Mucolipidosis III is an attenuated form of I-cell disease that is caused by mutations in the α subunit of the *GNTPAB* gene. However, unlike I-cell disease, the age at onset is later and the course is slowly progressive. These patients can survive well into adulthood. Many clinical features of this autosomal recessive disease are reminiscent of those of MPS I (Hurler) and VI (Maroteaux-Lamy). However, patients with mucolipidosis III lack mucopolysaccharides in their urine. They are seen between 2 and 4 years of age with stiffness of the hands and shoulders, which initially may suggest a diagnosis of rheumatoid arthritis.[563] Coarsening of facial features, short stature, and scoliosis become noticeable by 6 years of age. The joint stiffness is progressive and ultimately results in restriction of joint mobility. Destruction of the hip joints produces a waddling gait. As the disease progresses, a clawhand deformity and carpal tunnel syndrome usually appear before 12 years of age. Other clinical features may include mild mental retardation, mild corneal clouding, retinal and optic nerve abnormalities,[564] cardiac murmurs of aortic or mitral

valvular disease, short stature, and progressive skeletal dysplasia, particularly of the spine and pelvis. Patients surviving into the 30s and as late as the 60s have been described.

Peripheral leukocytes in this disease are normal, but vacuolated plasma cells are found in bone marrow specimens. Cultured skin fibroblasts manifest the same phase-dense inclusions as seen in I-cell disease, although the findings are not always as prominent.

As in mucolipidosis II, these patients also have multiple acid hydrolase deficiencies in cultured fibroblasts and markedly elevated lysosomal enzyme activity in serum. They also have a deficiency of phosphotransferase in fibroblasts and leukocytes, although there is some residual activity in patients with mucolipidosis III.[565] Carrier detection has been described.[566]

Complementation studies of cultured mucolipidosis III fibroblasts have demonstrated genetic heterogeneity. Two different functions of *N*-acetylglucosamine-1-phosphotransferase have been identified. One is associated with its catalytic activity and the other with the specific site of recognition of the lysosomal enzymes. A less common variant of mucolipidosis III (group C of the complementation groups) has a mutation at the recognition site but normal enzymatic activity toward artificial substrates. Patients with this uncommon variant and heterozygotes will show normal phosphotransferase activity when α-methylmannoside is used as the acceptor substrate in the assay mixture.

Mucolipidosis Type IV

In 1974, this autosomal recessive disorder was first described in children of Ashkenazic Jewish parentage whose ancestry was traced to southern Poland.[567] Since then, a few more cases have been described in other ethnic groups.[568] Mucolipidosis type IV is characterized by a variety of neurologic and ophthalmologic abnormalities, including motor and language delay, and patients with this disease do not usually progress beyond the 12- to 15-month level developmentally. These children do not have coarse facial features, skeletal deformities, or hepatosplenomegaly, and mucopolysaccharides and oligosaccharides are not evident in urine. Other possible signs include short stature; normal tone or hypotonia; hyperreflexia; a small head, often below the third percentile; and a full face. More recently, constitutive achlorhydria and hypergastrinemia have been reported as almost pathognomonic findings for this condition.[569] Although most of these patients are described as being profoundly retarded, patients have been reported with minimal retardation.[570,571] These patients can survive well into adulthood.

Corneal clouding develops in nearly all patients, but the age at onset varies. It may remain static or lessen with time. The use of contact lenses has been associated with clearing of the cornea. In one patient who received a corneal transplant, the clouding subsequently returned. Other ophthalmologic manifestations include a pigmentary retinopathy, cataract formation, and optic atrophy. Bouts of tearing and conjunctival injection with photophobia have been troublesome in a few patients.

The original report of this disease described numerous large histiocyte-like cells in the bone marrow that contained small sudanophilic, weakly PAS-positive vacuoles. These cells also showed weak metachromasia after staining with toluidine blue.[567] However, bone marrow studies in another patient did not reveal storage cells. Blood smears from this patient were also normal when examined by light microscopy, but under the electron microscope, dense lamellar inclusion bodies were observed in lymphocytes of the buffy coat.[572] Ultrastructural changes have also been observed in various other tissues, including the brain, conjunctiva, and cultured fibroblasts.[573,574] These changes consist of concentric laminated lipid-like bodies and vacuoles containing amorphous, sparse fibrillogranular material. In the liver, multilamellar cytosomes are present in hepatocytes, whereas clear vacuoles are seen in Kupffer cells. Both types of inclusions appear in the epithelial and stromal cells of the conjunctiva, which may be sampled to aid in the diagnosis.[575]

The gene for mucolipidosis type IV (named *MCOLN1*) maps to chromosome 19p13.3-p13.2, and several mutations have been identified.[576] A founder effect was discovered in approximately 95% of affected Ashkenazic patients. The *MCOLN1* gene encodes a transmembrane protein called mucolipin that appears to regulate calcium influx in excitable and nonexcitable cells.[576] The protein belongs to the "transient receptor potential" family of proteins and functions as a nonselective cation channel whose activity is modulated by pH. Two defects have been described in patient fibroblasts: hyperacidification of lysosomes and a delay in the exit of lipids from lysosomes. It is plausible that the protein is involved in the endocytic process during lysosomal function because patients' cells display abnormal incorporation of lipids and abnormally large vesicles.[577]

A complete autopsy study was performed on a patient with mucolipidosis type IV. The results demonstrated that the storage material in neurons differed from that in non-neural cells. Neuronal inclusions stained with Sudan black but not with Luxol fast blue, thus suggesting that the stored material was a nonpolar lipid. In contrast, the storage material in hepatocytes, kidneys, and myocytes stained intensely with Luxol fast blue, thus suggesting that the accumulations were polar lipids. Inclusion material in all cells stained positively with PAS because of the accumulation of carbohydrates.[578,579]

Prenatal diagnosis has been accomplished by demonstration of abnormal storage bodies in cultured amniotic fluid cells[580] and cultured chorionic cells.[581] It is hoped that with elucidation of the underlying genetic defect in this condition, more accurate prenatal diagnosis will now be possible. Other than symptomatic treatment of its complications, no therapy is available for this condition.

Fucosidosis

Fucosidosis is a rare autosomal recessive disorder caused by deficient activity of the enzyme α-L-fucosidase. This disorder is due to faulty degradation of both sphingolipids and oligosaccharides. Fucose-containing oligosaccharides, glycopeptides, and glycolipids accumulate in both tissues and urine. The main storage material in the brain is oligosaccharides.[582,583] Glycolipids accumulate predominantly in the liver but are only a minor storage component in the brain.[584]

The clinical picture consists of progressive mental and motor deterioration. Three types of fucosidosis have been described on the basis of the initial findings and severity of the disease. Willems and associates[585] suggested that the disease exhibits a wide and continuous clinical spectrum with a rapidly progressive type 1 at one extreme and a slowly progressive type 2 at the other. At the DNA level, several mutations in the α-fucosidosis gene have been identified, but such genotypic differences do not explain the observed phenotypic differences.

Type 1 is recognized by a delay in psychomotor development between 6 and 18 months of age. Hypotonia rapidly progresses to hypertonia, then to severe spasticity, and finally to decerebrate rigidity. Thick skin, coarse facial features, skeletal abnormalities, and growth retardation develop. Other signs are a nonfunctioning ("strawberry") gallbladder and hyperhidrosis with a marked increase in the sodium chloride content of sweat. Patients have also had seizures, cardiomegaly, hepatomegaly, and corneal opacities. Respiratory tract infections are common, with most patients surviving only to 4 or 5 years of age.

Most patients with fucosidosis, however, experience a slower course of degeneration. Type 2 is a milder variant manifested at 2 or 3 years of age by slow neurologic deterioration. There are no corneal opacities, and the optic fundi are normal. Patients have coarse facies, growth retardation, dysostosis multiplex, and neurologic signs similar to those seen in type 1, except that they are slightly milder. Type 3 develops in the first few years of life and progresses slowly to a state of severe mental and motor deterioration by adolescence or adulthood. The major distinguishing features of type 2 are the presence of angiokeratoma corporis diffusum, more normal sodium chloride values in sweat, and longer survival. Telangiectatic lesions are seen in the mouth. Tortuosity of conjunctival vessels and pigmentary degeneration of the retina have been reported. Different forms of the disease may exist in the same family.[586]

Vacuoles are present in the cells of most tissues, including neurons, hepatocytes, Kupffer cells, and cells of the spleen, lung, kidney, heart, and skin. Electron microscopic studies demonstrate vacuoles with a heterogeneous content; some appear empty, some have a reticular pattern,[587,588] and others display a lamellar structure. There is vacuolization of the epithelial cells of the sweat glands and conjunctiva.[589] Peripheral lymphocytes contain vacuoles and granular inclusions. Histiocytes with inclusions surrounded by vacuoles have been reported in bone marrow smears.

The diagnosis is ultimately determined by the demonstration of low α-fucosidase activity in either leukocytes or fibroblasts. Because the residual activity of this enzyme may be relatively high, it is always necessary to carry out thin-layer chromatographic analysis for oligosaccharides. Quantitative differences in urinary excretion patterns were described between a patient with type 1 and a patient with type 2 disease.[590] Lewis blood group activity is increased in fucosidosis tissues, and elevated levels of Le[a] and Le[b] activity have been found in the sera, erythrocytes, and saliva of patients with fucosidosis.[591]

The gene encoding lysosomal α-fucosidase (*FUCA1*) has been mapped to the short arm of chromosome 1p34.1-p36.1. Both *FUCA1* and a pseudogene (*FUCA1P*) have been sequenced. The gene consists of eight exons spanning 23 kb. At least 22 different mutations have been identified among the different exons.[592-597] The pseudogene is 80% identical to that of fucosidase cDNA but does not contain an open reading frame.[598] *FUCA1P* has been mapped to chromosome 2q31-q32 by in situ hybridization.[599] A second gene (*FUCA2*) has been mapped to chromosome 6q25. This gene is not involved in α-fucosidosis but influences the activity of plasma α-fucosidase. It may be a regulatory gene rather than a structural gene. This is important to note because *FUCA2* is associated with low α-fucosidase activity in plasma, which is found in 6% to 11% of the normal population.[600] Plasma is not an appropriate source for testing the activity of this enzyme. Carrier testing is now possible, and prenatal diagnosis has been successfully performed.

Prospects for the use of BMT in this disease have received mild encouragement from studies performed in dogs with fucosidosis; these dogs exhibited improvements in visceral lesions and a more gradual improvement in CNS pathologic changes.[601] At least three patients with human α-fucosidosis have also received transplants, with some success in two of these patients.[125] In addition, both human and canine fibroblasts in α-L-fucosidase can be corrected by retroviral vector–mediated gene transfer.[602-604] The authors are not aware of an attempt to use ERT in patients with fucosidosis.

α-Mannosidosis

This autosomal recessive disease results from a deficiency of α-D-mannosidase activity. It was first described in 1967 by Ockerman.[605] Clinically and biochemically, α-mannosidosis conforms to the stereotype of an oligosaccharide storage disease. There is an accumulation of mannose-rich glycoconjugates in tissues and body fluids. Excessive amounts of mannose-rich oligosaccharides are also excreted in urine. As in fucosidosis and aspartylglucosaminuria, patients exhibit skeletal changes, a dysmorphic facial appearance, moderate to severe mental retardation, hepatomegaly, hernias, recurrent bacterial infections, lenticular or corneal opacities, lymphocytic vacuoles, foam cell infiltration of the bone marrow, and an absence of mucopolysacchariduria.[606-608]

Two distinct clinical phenotypes are described in the literature. Type I is the severe infantile phenotype, whereas type II is a milder juvenile-adult form. As for fucosidosis, it is more likely that there is a continuum of clinical expression rather than clear separation into two phenotypes. The type I variant is characterized by rapid mental deterioration, coarse facial features, hepatosplenomegaly, severe dysostosis multiplex, and frequently, death between 3 and 10 years of age. In patients with type II disease, early development may be normal or slightly delayed. The mental retardation may be varied and may not be apparent until childhood or adolescence. Hearing loss is a particularly prominent feature. The skeletal abnormalities may be mild, but more severe manifestations (including deforming arthropathy) have been reported in this latter variant.[609] Destructive synovitis,[610-612] gingival hyperplasia, hydrocephalus, spastic paraplegia, and pancytopenia have been reported.[613-616] Radiographic studies of the brain show thickened diploic spaces and enlargement of the Virchow-Robin spaces.[617] In one 3-year-old boy with α-mannosidase deficiency, macrocephaly and intracranial hypertension developed in conjunction with synostosis of multiple sutures.[618] Patients with this form of the disease may survive into adulthood.

Between 20% and 90% of the lymphocytes in the peripheral blood contain translucent vacuoles, and a proportion of the polymorphonuclear leukocytes are coarsely granulated. The vacuoles remain PAS positive after fixation with alcohol. They have also been found in hepatocytes and Kupffer cells, and in the nervous system they are associated with widespread ballooning of nerve cell cytoplasm in the cerebral cortex, brainstem, spinal medulla, and pituitary gland.[608,619] Abnormalities in the chemotactic function of neutrophils may account for the increased susceptibility of these patients to infection. Hypogammaglobulinemia has been described as well.

Thin-layer chromatographic analysis of urine easily discloses a pattern of glycoconjugates that is distinctive for this particular type of oligosacchariduria. The major oligosaccharide excreted is a trisaccharide. A defect in hydrolysis of this compound has been demonstrated in an enzyme preparation from the liver of a patient with α-mannosidosis. The deficient enzyme, lysosomal acid α-mannosidase, may be assayed with leukocytes or cultured fibroblasts as the enzyme source. Although this enzyme is not a major component of serum or plasma, careful adjustment of reaction conditions will allow detection of α-mannosidase deficiency in patient sera.[620] Heterozygote detection is available,[621] and prenatal diagnosis has been performed successfully.[622]

The gene for α-mannosidase (also named *LAMAN*) has been isolated and sequenced,[623] and it maps to 19cen-q12. More than 20 mutations, most of them private, have been reported.[624] In these studies no correlation between specific mutations and the clinical spectrum of the disease was found.

The residual α-mannosidase activity in mannosidosis can be stimulated and stabilized by zinc ions,[612,625] but long-term therapy with oral zinc sulfate has failed in several patients inasmuch as it caused no change in clinical status or biochemical findings.[626-629] In one patient who died 18 weeks after successful engraftment following BMT, the somatic effects of the disease were reversed, but lysosomal storage within the brain did not appear to be altered.[630]

Human recombinant α-mannosidase has been successfully synthesized and purified by expressing its cloned gene in Chinese hamster ovary cells.[631] Correction of affected human fibroblasts has been achieved by transfection with human cDNA via a retroviral vector.[632] This, together with the availability of animal models for this condition,[633,634] establishes the grounds for trials with either ERT or gene therapy. A guinea pig model of α-mannosidosis is available. Disease in this model resembles the clinical, histopathologic, biochemical, and molecular features of the human disease. In a recent study, the efficacy of ERT for α-mannosidosis was investigated in this model. Intravenous administration of human recombinant enzyme resulted in a significant increase in α-mannosidase activity (1.4 times normal levels) that was detected in the circulation 1 week after injection. By monitoring clearance of storage products with tandem mass spectrometry, this therapeutic approach was found to be effective in reducing accumulated metabolites in peripheral tissues and in brain in comparison to untreated controls. Reductions of up to 60% of urinary mannose containing oligosaccharides were also observed. No histologic improvement was observed in the brain, but a decrease in lysosomal vacuolation was seen in the liver, kidney, spleen, endocrine pancreas, and trigeminal ganglion neurons.[635]

BMT may be effective in controlling some manifestations of the disease if performed early in its course. Thus far, no clinical trials have been reported in the literature.

β-Mannosidosis

Since first described in humans in 1986, 11 cases of β-mannosidosis deficiency have been reported. All patients with this rare autosomal recessive disease are mentally retarded, but their other clinical findings have differed. The most severe phenotype described involved status epilepticus at 12 months of age, severe quadriplegia, and death by 15 months of age. The mildest phenotype described involved two adult brothers, one of whom was 50 years old with mental retardation, angiokeratomas, and few other phenotypic features.[636] Most patients were normal in the first few months of life, but mental retardation eventually developed in all. Other findings described included mild facial dysmorphism, hearing loss, speech impairment, seizures, angiokeratomas, aggressive behav-

ior, hypotonia, spastic quadriplegia, peripheral neuropathy, and rarely, skeletal abnormalities.[637] Interpretation of the clinical features has been complicated in some patients because one patient was coincidentally affected with type A Sanfilippo's disease[638] and another with ethanolaminuria.[639] A 14-year-old black African boy with severely deficient β-mannosidase activity was described who had bilateral thenar and hypothenar amyotrophy, electrophysiologically demonstrable demyelinating peripheral neuropathy, and cytoplasmic vacuolation of skin fibroblasts and lymphoid cells.[640] Hepatomegaly has not been described.

The enzymatic defect in this condition involves deficient removal of the innermost mannosyl residue in the N-linked oligosaccharide side chain, which is a β-linkage. As a result, there is excessive urinary excretion and tissue accumulation of oligosaccharides, particularly mannosyl-β-1,4-glucosamine. The specific deficiency of β-mannosidase can be demonstrated in leukocytes, cultured fibroblasts, and plasma. Parents are clinically unaffected but have reduced levels of β-mannosidase activity.

The gene for human β-mannosidase is located on chromosome 4q22-25.[641] Mutations in this gene have been identified in a pair of affected siblings, and prenatal diagnosis has been accomplished.[642]

A β-mannosidase knockout mouse was produced. Homozygous mutant mice have undetectable β-mannosidase activity. The general appearance and growth of the knockout mice are similar to that of their wild-type littermates. When older than 1 year, these mice exhibited no dysmorphology or overt neurologic problems. The mutant animals have consistent cytoplasmic vacuolation in the CNS and minimal vacuolation in most visceral organs. Thin-layer chromatography demonstrated an accumulation of disaccharide in the epididymis and brain. Because this mouse model closely resembles human β-mannosidosis, and it will provide a useful tool for studying the phenotypic variation in different species and facilitate the study of potential therapies for LSDs.[643]

Aspartylglucosaminuria

Aspartylglycosaminuria is a recessively inherited oligosaccharide storage disease that occurs primarily in the Finnish population. The carrier incidence of this disease was determined to be 1 in 36 in a sample of control individuals from the capital area of Finland.[644] Rare isolated instances have been reported in other countries, including Canada, Europe, Japan, Puerto Rico, Turkey, and the United States.[645-650] It is caused by a deficiency of the lysosomal enzyme aspartylglucosaminidase (N-aspartyl-β-glucosaminidase), which cleaves the bond between asparagine and N-acetylglucosamine during the lysosomal degradation of N-linked glycoproteins. Aspartylglucosamine accumulates in tissues, particularly the liver, spleen, and thyroid gland, with moderate increases in the kidney and brain.[651] Large amounts of aspartylglucosamine are excreted in urine.

The clinical features of the Finnish type appear to be consistent[652,653] in that the children are healthy for the first few months of life and then begin to have recurrent infections, diarrhea, and hernias during the rest of the first year of life. Some children have a history of muscular hypotonia and weak sucking as babies.[654] Short stature, microcephaly, and rarely, hepatomegaly develop in some. By the age of 10 there is coarsening of the facies and sagging skinfolds. Some of the other features noted are an increased incidence of acne, large nevi, sun sensitivity, angiokeratoma (seen in one patient), crystal-like lens opacification, macroglossia, hoarse voice, brachycephaly, and joint laxity. Macro-orchidism and subnormal excretion of 17-ketosteroids occur in some men, and menstrual abnormalities have been noted in some of the affected women. Reactive overgrowth of the oral mucosa and facial skin has recently been reported.[655] Cardiac valvular insufficiency is not common, but cardiac murmurs may be heard.

Progressive mental retardation is the main clinical symptom in aspartylglucosaminuria. Gradual loss of skills occurs after 13 to 16 years of age, and a rapid decline is noted after 25 to 28 years of age.[654] Intelligence quotient values are usually less than 40 in adults. Speech is delayed and remains poor or is never acquired. Behavioral abnormalities, such as excitability, hyperactivity, and at times, periods of apathy, are seen. The behavioral problems appear to become worse with age and could be related to the delayed myelination reported in patients with this condition, which is commonly seen in neuroradiologic studies.

Vacuolated lymphocytes and neutropenia are observed frequently. Many patients have a decrease in the prothrombin time. The radiographic findings may demonstrate very mild dysostosis multiplex with wedge-shaped vertebral bodies, spondylolisthesis, or spondylolysis. There is thickening of the calvaria with underdeveloped cranial sinuses. The non-Finnish children with aspartylglucosaminuria have all demonstrated mental retardation and skeletal dysplasia. The disease follows an insidious course, and many patients may live well into adulthood.

Aspartylglucosylamine may be detected in urine by chromatography. Because this compound serves as a link between the carbohydrate group and the peptide chain in glycoproteins and keratan sulfate, lesser amounts of other glycoasparagines containing galactose, N-acetylneuraminic acid, and additional *N*-acetylglucosamine residues have also been isolated from urine. Ultimately, the diagnosis is made by measuring aspartylglucosaminidase activity in an easily obtained tissue source, such as sonicates of white blood cells, fibroblasts, or amniotic fluid cells.[656,657] Serum, fibroblasts, and leukocytes of affected patients show less than 10% enzyme activity. The condition is best diagnosed in heterozygotes by using fibroblasts or lymphocytes.[658] Prenatal diagnosis is possible within the first trimester of pregnancy by enzyme analysis of direct chorionic villus biopsy material.[659,660]

The gene has been mapped to chromosome 4q32-q33 and has been cloned and sequenced. Currently, more than 20 different mutations have been reported.[661] In the most common form (the Finnish population), a double point mutation has been identified. Each results in an amino acid substitution: Arg161→Gln and Cys163→Ser. The first of these base changes is a polymorphism; the second is the disease-causing mutation. They occur together in 98% of Finnish patients with aspartylglucosaminuria. These mutations affect a critical region of the protein that triggers its autocatalytic processing before entering the ER. To screen for aspartylglucosaminuria carriers among the Finnish, a DNA-based test that can detect both mutations has been developed.[662] An improved screening method involving a PCR/oligonucleotide ligation assay is now available for the Finnish population; it is rapid, reliable, and nonisotopic.[663]

Two reports have described treatment of this condition with BMT.[664,665] In both, correction was seen only in the liver and not in the CNS.

The three-dimensional structure of *N*-aspartyl-β-glucosaminidase was used to predict the structural consequences of several mutations on intracellular stability, maturation, transport, and enzyme activity. Most mutations were amino acid substitutions that replaced the original amino acid with a bulkier residue. Mutations at the dimer interface prevented dimerization of the enzyme in the ER, whereas active-site mutations destroyed its catalytic activity and affected maturation of the precursor. Depending on their effects on stability of the enzyme, the authors categorized mutations as mild, moderate, or severe.[661]

An aspartylglycosaminuria mouse model was generated by targeted disruption of the mouse *N*-aspartyl-β-glucosaminidase gene. Homozygous mice had massive accumulation of aspartylglucosamine, extensive lysosomal vacuolization, and axonal swelling in the gracile nucleus and displayed impaired neuromotor coordination at 5 to 10 months of age. Older null mice (>10 months) showed progressive motor impairment and had impaired bladder function. The oldest surviving mice (20 months old) showed a dramatic loss of Purkinje cells, intensive astrogliosis, and vacuolation of neurons in the deep cerebellar nuclei leading to a severe ataxic gait. These findings are consistent with the pathogenesis of aspartylglycosaminuria in patients, and the knockout mice may be a suitable animal model for testing therapeutic modalities.[666,667]

ACID LIPASE DEFICIENCY

Wolman's disease and cholesteryl ester storage disease are autosomal recessive disorders that result in the massive accumulation of both cholesteryl ester and triglycerides in cells and tissues throughout the body. Both diseases are characterized by a defective lysosomal acid lipase, also known as acid esterase. Lysosomal acid lipase is found in fibroblasts, macrophages, lymphocytes, and hepatocytes. The full-length cDNA encoding acid lipase has been isolated and sequenced[668] and may provide tools for DNA diagnosis and possibly enzyme therapy in the future. The gene has been mapped to chromosome 10q23.2-q23.[669] It consists of 10 exons dispersed over 36 kb.[670] Several mutations have been reported.[671] One mutation in the last nucleotide of exon 8 has been found in 11 of 17 patients with cholesteryl ester storage disease.

Extracts of normal cultured fibroblasts contain at least three electrophoretically dissimilar acid lipase components: A, B, and C. The least anodal band, A, is most prominent but is reduced in heterozygotes with Wolman's disease and is undetectable in both Wolman's disease and cholesteryl ester storage disease cells. This isoenzyme pattern is also seen in amniotic fluid cells, chorionic villus cells, lymphocytes, and several other tissues.[672] Diagnosis of both disorders is determined by the clinical picture and demonstration of decreased acid lipase activity and band A in cultured skin fibroblasts, lymphocytes, or other tissues. Prenatal diagnosis is now possible by identifying a deficiency of both acid lipase and band A in amniotic and chorionic villus cells.[673]

A diet low in cholesterol and triglycerides and the use of both cholestyramine (0.22 g/kg twice daily) and simvastatin (0.28 mg/kg each evening), which is a 3-hydroxy-3-methylglutaryl CoA reductase inhibitor, with lipophilic vitamins (A, D, E, and K) has resulted in clinical improvement[674,675] in some patients with cholesteryl ester storage disease. Although these diseases share a common enzyme defect, they differ considerably in their clinical expression.

BMT has been attempted in a child with Wolman's disease with apparently good results.[676] The neurologic performance of this patient, who received a transplant at 5 months of age, has been good, and no deterioration has been seen. The procedure had been attempted previously in four other patients who died of complications of the BMT procedure. It seems that when the disease appears so early in life and tends to occur with such severity, BMT should be performed as soon as possible, probably in the first 2 weeks of life, even before signs or symptoms develop. It should be done with minimal myeloablation and a goal of partial but not full engraftment, which may minimize the incidence of complications at this early age.

More recently, trials of ERT in animal models of this condition[677] and gene transfer in affected cells[678] have been performed with good results.

Wolman's Disease

Wolman's disease is the more severe of the two conditions. Symptoms can begin as early as during the first few weeks of life.[679] The major clinical signs and symptoms are severe vomiting, failure to thrive, abdominal distention, massive hepatosplenomegaly, which has been reported in patients as young as 4 days of age,[680] and foul-smelling, watery stools. Jaundice or persistent low-grade fever develops in a few infants. A prominent feature, though not necessarily pathognomonic, is grossly symmetrically enlarged, calcified adrenal glands.[681] Radiographic examination demonstrates extensive, stippled, or punctuate calcific deposits.

By the sixth week of life, anemia usually develops and becomes progressively worse. Lymphocytes contain both intracytoplasmic and intranuclear lipid vacuoles. In contrast to other diseases characterized by vacuolated cells, the vacuoles in Wolman's disease are strongly sudanophilic. They also stain positively with oil red O, Nile red, and stains for cholesterol. Their lysosomal origin is indicated by a strong reaction to staining for acid phosphatase activity. Lipid droplets are also present in neutrophils and monocytes. Foam cells (lipid-laden histiocytes) are seen in the bone marrow, in the peripheral blood, and in all organs.[680] Thrombocytopenia has not been reported.

The vomiting, diarrhea, and inanition result from severe damage to the microvilli and the accumulation of foam cells in the intestinal mucosa. Abdominal ultrasonography may demonstrate the thickened bowel walls.[682] Enteral nutrition is not possible, and therefore nutritional care must be given by intravenous hyperalimentation, even if it is only palliative.[683] The disease progresses rapidly, and death usually occurs before 1 year of age.

The diagnosis is determined by the clinical findings and deficient activity of acid lipase in cultured fibroblasts or circulating leukocytes. Routine laboratory observations often demonstrate abnormal liver function test results and plasma lipid levels in the low end of the normal range. Calcifications of the adrenal glands may be seen in Addison's disease, adrenal teratomas, neuroblastoma, and other conditions, but the presence of bilateral adrenal calcification associated with hepatosplenomegaly and gastrointestinal symptoms strongly suggests the diagnosis of Wolman's disease. Atypical forms without adrenal calcifications have been described.[684]

Cholesteryl Ester Storage Disease

Cholesteryl ester storage disease has a variable phenotype. It can be benign and may be undetected until adulthood.[685] Hepatomegaly, a prominent sign, may be evident at birth, during early childhood, or occasionally in the second decade of life. It results from the fatty infiltration of foam cells and ultimately progresses to hepatic fibrosis. Alcohol has been known to accelerate the process and therefore should be avoided. Other possible signs and symptoms include splenomegaly, esophageal varices, a decreased concentration of blood clotting factor V,[686] recurrent abdominal pain, delayed puberty, recurrent epistaxis, and jaundice. Calcified adrenal glands are rarely present. Unlike the case in Wolman's disease, malabsorption and malnutrition have not been described in patients with cholesteryl ester storage disease.

Plasma levels of cholesterol, triglyceride, and low-density lipoproteins are elevated, and the plasma high-density lipoprotein concentration is reduced. No other abnormal results are noted on routine laboratory tests. Lymphocytes and monocytes are the only blood cells affected in cholesteryl ester storage disease. Bone marrow aspirates may demonstrate large macrophages filled with birefringent droplets. Cultured skin fibroblasts of patients with cholesteryl ester storage disease demonstrate birefringence in plain polarized light and absence of lysosomal acid lipase, thereby establishing the diagnosis. Hepatic acid esterase activity is reduced but detectable and is substantially greater than such activity in the liver of patients with Wolman's disease.[687]

In some patients, treatment with the 3-hydroxy-3-methylglutaryl CoA reductase inhibitor lovastatin has resulted in significant reductions in plasma cholesterol, triglyceride, and low-density lipoprotein cholesterol levels.[688] Two patients with cholesteryl ester storage disease received liver transplants and are reported to be doing well.[675,689]

A null-mutant mouse model of lysosomal acid lipase appeared normal at birth and developed normally into adulthood. However, massive accumulation of triglycerides and cholesteryl esters (30-fold increase in comparison to normal) occurred in several organs, and at 3 weeks of age the liver appeared yellow-orange and up to two times larger than normal. This mouse model is a phenocopy of cholesteryl ester storage disease and a biochemical and histopathologic mimic of human Wolman's disease.[690] ERT with recombinant acid lipase resulted in nearly complete resolution of the hepatic yellow color and a decrease in hepatic weight. Histologic analysis of tissues from ERT-treated mice showed a reduction in macrophage lipid storage and a 50% to 70% decrease in triglyceride and cholesterol levels in the liver, spleen, and small intestine. ERT with recombinant enzyme for human Wolman disease patients and patients with cholesteryl ester storage disease may be feasible.[677,678]

NEURONAL CEROID LIPOFUSCINOSES

Lysosomal accumulation of lipopigments is characteristic of the neuronal ceroid lipofuscinoses, a group of neurodegenerative conditions whose biochemical bases have only recently begun to be understood. The stored material consists of autofluorescent lipopigments resembling lipofuscin, the material that accumulates in neurons in normal aging. However, the storage material related to neuronal ceroid lipofuscinoses is less sharply outlined and more faintly stained by aldehyde fuchsin than the normal lipofuscin deposits.[691]

The accumulations present in brain lysosomes include glycoconjugates consisting primarily of dolichol pyrophosphate-linked oligosaccharides and proteins, the major component being subunit c (unit 9) of mitochondrial adenosine triphosphate (ATP) synthase. By immunohistochemistry, this excess of subunit c can be identified in skin fibroblasts[692] and in urine.[693] In infantile-onset disease, the major storage protein is not subunit c but the sphingolipid activator proteins A and D. Furthermore, two GSLs have also been identified in the stored lipids of infants with neuronal ceroid lipofuscinosis.[694]

On electron microscopy, the residual bodies have a heterogeneous ultrastructural appearance. They are present in all tissues but are particularly abundant in the neuronal perikaryon and axon hillock, where they continue to accumulate until the nerve cell degenerates. The various types of deposits found include curvilinear bodies, zebra bodies, fingerprint profiles, homogeneous osmiophilic bodies, and osmiophilic granular deposits.

Clinically, the neuronal ceroid lipofuscinoses represent a broad spectrum of diseases with an overall incidence of 1 in 12,500 to 25,000 births.[695] The age at onset; visual, mental, and motor signs; and types of inclusions present vary in the different forms of the disease. At least eight major forms of the disease have been identified (Table 24-7). These forms show a consistent clinical, pathologic, and genetic picture. The classic forms are infantile (CLN-1), late infantile (CLN-2), and juvenile (CLN-3) neuronal ceroid lipofuscinosis. These forms are inherited in an autosomal recessive pattern and have different genetic bases. An adult-onset variant without vision loss (CLN-4) also occurs. Most patients demonstrate autosomal recessive inheritance, but an autosomal dominant pattern has also been found in a few patients. Three additional variants (Gypsy/Indian or type 6, Turkish or type 7, and northern epilepsy with mental retardation or type 8) have thus far been restricted to specific ethnic groups. Their phenotypes resemble that for type 2, and only one of their genes has been identified (in type 8), in which a missense mutation has been found in all affected patients.

With only rare exceptions, patients who show symptoms before adulthood become blind, and for this reason older texts usually grouped these diseases among the familial amaurotic idiocies. However, the absence of ganglioside storage and the marked brain atrophy that occur in the neuronal ceroid lipofuscinoses clearly set these diseases apart from the classic forms of gangliosidoses, that is, Tay-Sachs disease, Sandhoff's disease, and the G_{M1}-gangliosidoses. Seizures, another common sign in neuronal ceroid lipofuscinoses, may be related to selective loss of inhibitory synapses within the axon hillock and initial segment of pyramidal cells. Their presence could lead to confusion with other causes of progressive myoclonic epilepsy, such as Unverricht-Lundborg disease, the myoclonus-epilepsy–ragged red fiber syndrome, Lafora body disease, and the sialidoses. Each variant of the neuronal ceroid lipofuscinoses, in contrast to these other disorders, is associated with the accumulation of autofluorescent material.

TABLE 24-7   Phenotypic/Genotypic Correlations of Neuronal Ceroid Lipofuscinoses

Form	Genetic Symbol	Age at Onset, Range (yr)	Initial Symptoms	EM	Enzyme Activity Assay	Gene Location	OMIM	DNA Testing (Common Mutation)
INCL	CLN1	Birth-37*	Seizures, cognitive/motor decline, visual loss	GROD	PPT1	1p32	256730	223A→G451C→T
Classic late-infantile NCL	CLN2	2-8	Seizures, cognitive/motor decline, visual loss	CV/mixed	TPPI	11p15.5	204500	T523-1G→ C636C→T
Juvenile NCL	CLN3	4-10	Visual loss, cognitive/motor decline, seizures	FP/mixed, vacuolated lymphocytes	TM	16p12.1	204200	1.02-kb deletion
Adult NCL	CLN4	15-50	A: seizures and cognitive/motor decline; B: abnormal behavior; cognitive, motor decline	Mixed	NA	NA	204300/162350	NA
Finnish-variant LINCL	CLN5	4-7	Cognitive/motor decline, seizures, visual loss	FP/CV/RL	TM	13q21.1-q32	256731	Tyr392STOP
Gypsy/Indian, early juvenile variant LINCL	CLN6	1.5-8	Cognitive/motor decline, seizures, visual loss	CV/FP/RL	NA	15q21-q23	601780	NA
Turkish-variant LINCL	CLN7	1-6	Seizures, motor decline, visual loss	FP/mixed	NA	4q28.1-q28.2	610951	NA
Northern epilepsy	CLN8	5-10	Seizures and cognitive decline	CV- or GROD-like structures	TM	8pter-p22	600143	Arg24Gly

*INCL has various phenotypes that overlap with onset of the other forms.

CV, curvilinear profiles; EM, electron microscopy; FP, fingerprint profiles; GROD, granular osmiophilic deposits; INCL, infantile NCL; LINCL, late infantile NCL; mixed, CV, FP, RL; NA, not available (unknown); NCL, neuronal ceroid lipofuscinosis; Northern epilepsy, progressive epilepsy with mental retardation (website: http://www.ucl.ac.uk/ncl); OMIM, Online Mendelian Inheritance in Man; PPT1, palmitoyl protein thioesterase 1; RL, rectilinear complex; TM, transmembrane protein; TPPI, tripeptidyl peptidase 1.

From Wisniewski KE. Pheno/genotypic correlations of neuronal ceroid lipofuscinoses. Neurology. 2001;57:576.

Retinal degeneration can be monitored with electro-retinography. With complete degeneration of the outer retinal layer, the electroretinographic response is totally abolished. Another useful test is electroencephalography, the results of which may be abnormal even before the development of dementia. Subtle electro-ophthalmologic findings have been reported in heterozygotes. Radiographic studies such as computed tomography and magnetic resonance imaging have been useful in the early diagnosis of infantile neuronal ceroid lipofuscinosis.[696] Measurements of mitochondrial ATP synthase subunit c may help in diagnosis of the late infantile and juvenile variants, but quantitative analysis of urinary dolichols is no longer considered a reliable biochemical marker for the disease because elevated urinary dolichol levels can also be detected in other degenerative neurologic diseases. It is not clear why these conditions involve the CNS almost exclusively because the proteins affected are also found in many extraneural tissues.[697]

Diagnosis of these relatively common disorders depends primarily on the clinical features, but examination of a skin biopsy specimen by electron microscopy also helps greatly. Lymphocyte vacuolization and azurophilic hypergranulation of neutrophils are often found in the peripheral blood smear, except in the infantile form of the disease. Electron microscopic studies of these blood elements and urinary sediment, conjunctiva, liver, skeletal muscle, and sural nerve have also aided in the diagnosis. In juvenile neuronal ceroid lipofuscinosis, fingerprint lipopigments may appear on electron micrographs of lymphocytes in the absence of vacuoles. More recently, molecular diagnosis has become available for some of the most common forms of neuronal ceroid lipofuscinosis.

Prenatal diagnosis of the infantile and juvenile forms has been accomplished through ultrastructural studies of chorionic villus biopsy specimens, and late infantile neuronal ceroid lipofuscinosis has been diagnosed by similar examination of uncultured amniotic fluid cells.[698] With prior knowledge of the individual mutations involved in a family, rapid and specific diagnosis can now be accomplished for the majority of these disorders.

Clinical, pathologic, and biochemical changes similar to those seen in humans with neuronal ceroid lipofuscinosis have been detected in several animal species.[699-702] These naturally occurring animal models provide important clues to the pathogenesis of neuronal ceroid lipofuscinoses and offer investigators the opportunity to study potential treatments of these disorders. Bone marrow and liver transplantation in English setter dogs did not succeed, nor have treatments with vitamin E, selenium, levodopa, or glutathione or peroxidase enzyme. Addition of 20% Maizena oil to their diet did improve their quality of life[700] but did not alter the natural history of the condition.

The only treatment currently available is symptomatic. Baclofen (15 to 25 mg/day, increasing to as much as 200 mg/day) and tizanidine (1 to 9 mg/day, later 20 to 60 mg/day) have been helpful for the irritability, choreoathetotic behavior, and sleep disturbances. Levomepromazine (5 to 20 mg/day) or benzodiazepines may also be beneficial.[703]

Infantile Type (Haltia-Santavuori Syndrome, CLN-1)

This is the most common progressive encephalopathy in Finnish children younger than 2 years, with an incidence of 1 in 20,000.[704] Early psychomotor development is normal until 6 to 12 months of age (stage 1), although some children have microcephaly at that time. Subsequently, development is slowed, with hypotonia, motor clumsiness, slight irritability, and sleeping problems (stage 2). Between 12 and 20 months there is rapid deterioration of the child's condition, with truncal ataxia, hyperkinesis of the upper extremities, dystonia, myoclonic jerks, and loss of vision (stage 3). The optic discs are pale, the retinal vessels are narrowed, and the retina itself is hypopigmented. By 24 to 36 months of age affected children are no longer able to sit (stage 4). A prolonged stationary burnt-out phase precedes death, which may not occur until 9 or 10 years of age.

The early stages of CLN-1 resemble those of Rett's syndrome, but sphingolipidoses and even less common disorders have to be considered. Severe neuronal destruction occurs, with almost total loss of cortical and subcortical neurons and cerebellar Purkinje cells resulting in severe brain atrophy and subsequent microcephaly. Magnetic resonance imaging can facilitate early diagnosis even before the appearance of clinical symptoms, with signal loss found in the thalami in children by 1 year of age. By 17 months of age, the basal ganglia look hypointense in comparison to the hyperintense white matter. Hyperintensity around the lateral ventricles is marked. Electroencephalographic findings consist of missing or abnormally slow sleep spindles during sleep, which begin to disappear by the age of 13 months, are absent by 2 years of age, and become isoelectric by 2.7 years.[705] Abnormal visual evoked potentials and electroretinograms are late manifestations and are clearly evident by stage 4. The diagnosis is ultimately confirmed by electron microscopic examination. The electron micrograph demonstrates membrane-bound irregular granular bodies, with the major storage material consisting of sphingolipid activator proteins A and D.

The gene for CLN-1 has been mapped to chromosome 1p32 and codes for palmitoyl-protein thioesterase (PPT1), a small glycoprotein that removes palmitate groups from cysteine residues in lipid-modified proteins.[706] The two most common mutations are 223A→G and 451C→T. The normal protein is transported to synaptosomes and is likely to be involved in early neuronal development.[707,708] Mutations in this gene can produce several phenotypes, including congenital, infantile, late infantile, juvenile, or even adult-onset variants.[709] These different phenotypes could be related to different degrees of disruption in intracellular trafficking of the mutant protein.[708] More than 39 mutations in this gene have been delineated, and a website has been developed for updating the mutations database in this group of conditions: http://www.ucl.ac.uk/ncl/.

Homologous cDNA to PPT1 was identified in the expressed sequence tags (EST) database.[710] The cDNA was derived from another gene that localizes to chromosome 6p21 and encodes a protein (PPT2) that shares 18% amino acid identity with PPT1. Recombinant PPT2, like PPT1, had thioesterase activity and localized to the lysosome. However, PPT2 could not substitute for PPT1 in correcting the metabolic defect in PPT1-deficient cells and was unable to remove palmitate groups from the palmitoylated proteins routinely used as substrates for PPT1.[710]

The three-dimensional structure of PPT1 was solved, with and without bound palmitate, by multiwavelength anomalous diffraction phasing. The structure showed an α/β-hydrolase fold with a catalytic triad consisting of Ser115-His289-Asp233. This has given insight into the structural basis for the phenotypes associated with PPT1 mutations.[711]

Ppt1 and Ppt2 null mice were generated that were deficient in either enzyme.[712] Mice from both knockout lines were viable and fertile, but spasticity developed at a median age of 21 weeks and 29 weeks, respectively. Myoclonic jerking and seizures were prominent in the Ppt1 mice, and motor abnormalities were progressive and caused death by 10 months of age. In contrast, Ppt2 homozygous mice were less affected and survived longer (>12 months). Neuronal loss and apoptosis were most prominent in the brains of Ppt1-deficient mice; however, autofluorescent storage material was prominent throughout the brains of both knockout mouse strains. These studies provided a mouse model for infantile neuronal ceroid lipofuscinosis and further suggested that PPT2 serves a role in the brain that is not carried out by PPT1.

Late Infantile Type (Jansky-Bielschowsky Syndrome, CLN-2)

This type is the second most common variant encountered in the United States. Onset occurs between 2 and 4 years of age. The earliest and most prominent symptoms are motor seizures of various types (myoclonic jerks, absence attacks, and atonic seizures) and truncal ataxia. The children are often described as being awkward, clumsy, tremulous, and dysarthric. The initial hypotonia progresses to spasticity with hyperactive reflexes, painful flexor spasms, and severe flexion contractures. By 5 years of age there is loss of intellect, inability to walk and talk, loss of vision, difficulty swallowing and clearing secretions, and incontinence. Death usually occurs between 10 and 15 years of age.

Eye examination reveals optic atrophy and granular or pigmentary degeneration of the macula. Initially, the visual evoked potentials are enlarged, but over the course of the disease both the visual evoked potentials and the electroretinogram signal become small and then absent. The electroencephalogram may show positive spikes during low-frequency photic stimulation.[713] The earliest radiographic findings demonstrate a large fourth ventricle and cerebellar atrophy,[714] with eventual progression to severe cortical atrophy.

Electron microscopic studies demonstrate the presence of curvilinear bodies. Large spheroidal lysosomal inclusion bodies, called protein-type myoclonus bodies, have also been identified. Their incidence, significance, and biochemical composition have not been determined. Unlike the curvilinear bodies, the majority of these inclusions were nonreactive to antibodies for subunit c.[715] Autopsy studies have disclosed storage material involving both neural cells and visceral cells such as the bone marrow parenchyma, spleen, Kupffer cells of the liver, lymph nodes, and renal parenchyma.

The CLN-2 gene encodes tripeptidyl peptidase 1, a lysosomal enzyme acting as an aminopeptidase that removes tripeptides from the free amino-terminals of proteins, and it maps to chromosome 11p15.[716] As in CLN-1, mutations in the same gene can also produce juvenile-onset disease.[709] At least 43 mutations have been identified. The diagnosis is confirmed by measuring tripeptidyl peptidase 1 activity in cells, most commonly fibroblasts. Because similar phenotypes can be produced in other variants of neuronal ceroid lipofuscinosis, enzymatic confirmation is recommended to corroborate the diagnosis.[709]

Early Juvenile Type (Variant Jansky-Bielschowsky Disease, Finnish Variant CLN-5)

Manifestations of this subtype begin at about the same age as those of the juvenile variant, but the course and neurophysiologic pattern are similar to those of the late infantile variant. Early psychomotor development is essentially normal up until 4 to 6 years of age, when motor clumsiness, epilepsy, and some visual difficulties begin to appear. The disease progresses in a subacute fashion, and by 9 to 10.5 years of age there is marked cognitive decline, ataxia with difficulty walking, dysarthria, and athetosis. Death occurs between 10 and 30 years of age. The characteristic electroencephalographic abnormalities seen in the late infantile type are also present in this variant. Visual evoked potentials and electroretinogram signals are abolished by 4 to 5 years of age. The characteristic abnormal early radiographic findings seen in the late infantile type are also seen in this variant. Unlike the juvenile variant, vacuolated lymphocytes have not been observed. Skin and rectal biopsy specimens are the preferred tissues for diagnosis. Electron microscopy demonstrates both the curvilinear and fingerprint patterns.

The CLN-5 gene localizes to chromosome 13q21-32[717] and encodes a putative 407–amino acid transmembrane protein.[718] The 60-kd glycoprotein is expressed in lysosomes in all human tissues, with up to a fivefold variation in levels of expression.[718,719] Glycosylated polypeptides were also present in the media of cultured cells, thus suggesting that the CLN5 protein may be a soluble lysosomal protein rather than an integral transmembrane protein as predicted previously.

To date, four mutations have been identified in the CLN-5 gene, including "Fin-major," a 2-bp deletion in exon 4, being the most common and two other isolated mutations that were found in non-Finnish patients (Dutch and Columbian).[720,721]

A knockout mouse model of CLN-5 was generated by targeted deletion of exon 3 of the mouse Cln5 gene.[722] Homozygous knockout mice had loss of vision and accumulation of autofluorescent storage material in the CNS and peripheral tissues, but no prominent brain atrophy. Profiling of brain transcripts in Cln5-deficient mice showed altered expression of several genes that are known to be involved in neurodegeneration, as well as genes involved in defense and immune response, findings typical of age-associated changes in the CNS. In addition, downregulation of structural components of myelin was detected, which was consistent with hypomyelination occurring in human CLN-5 patients. It was proposed that this mouse model may serve as a model for studying molecular processes associated with advanced aging.

Juvenile Type (Spielmeyer-Sjögren Syndrome, Batten's Disease, CLN-3)

This form is the most common variant seen in the United States. It has a chronic course, with the initial manifestations beginning between the ages of 4 and 6. The earliest symptoms are a decline in central visual acuity and retinitis pigmentosa. The disease course is insidious; it is slowly progressive and eventually leads to blindness, which is seldom detected before 7 or 8 years of age.[723] Formed and unformed visual hallucinations unrelated to seizures have been described.[724] By 10 to 12 years of age, only light perception remains, and low-frequency nystagmus is present. At about this same age, convulsions first appear and mental capacity declines. Thereafter, memory, school performance, and behavior steadily deteriorate. The behavioral problems may range from angry outbursts to depression. By the midteens these patients are moderately mentally retarded, and bouts of uncontrollable positional myoclonic jerking develop in some. Their speech is slurred and monotonous, with stammering, perseveration, and echolalia, and their thoughts become incoherent. An extrapyramidal syndrome consisting of a dull facial expression, peculiar postures, paratonic rigidity, and a parkinsonian-like gait can develop. Cerebellar

disturbances are also noticed, including clumsiness in all movements, progressive ataxia, and compulsive, monotonous, dysarthric speech. Patients become mute by their mid to late 20s and become bedridden in a semiflexed posture with recurrent seizures. These seizures are difficult to control and may be accompanied by opisthotonic posturing and prolonged spells of apnea. The early radiologic picture can be completely normal in 25% of patients, but by the late teens there is severe diffuse cerebral cortical, subcortical, and cerebellar atrophy. The visual evoked potentials and electroretinogram signal are initially abnormal but eventually are absent. The electroencephalogram is abnormal, and motor nerve conduction velocities are often decreased.

Twenty percent of the circulating lymphocytes in CLN-3 patients contain vacuoles. Microscopic examination has shown intracytoplasmic autofluorescent lipopigments in the nerve cells throughout the CNS and viscera. The reactive astrocytes are enlarged mainly in the superficial layers of the cerebral cortex. Calcifications have also been noted along the outer and inner brain surfaces.[725] The ultrastructural appearance of the lipopigments is predominantly a fingerprint-like profile. Treatment with polyunsaturated fatty acids may be of some benefit.[726]

The defective gene in CLN-3 is localized to chromosome 16p12.1 and encodes a deduced 438–amino acid hydrophobic transmembrane protein (battenin), which may be involved in the endocytosis/exocytosis pathway of vesicle-secreting cells.[727,728] In addition, battenin appears to contain a putative mitochondrial targeting site and has four predicted *N*-glycosylation sites. A yeast homologue of battenin was identified with 36% amino acid identity,[729] and it was reported that all known point mutations of *CLN3* concerned residues identical between the human and yeast protein. Of the more than 30 mutations that have been identified, one is especially common, a 1.02-kb deletion that involves exons 7 and 8.

Adult Type (Kufs' Disease, CLN-4)

The adult-type variant may represent up to 10% of all cases of neuronal ceroid lipofuscinosis.[730] Inheritance of CLN-4 is autosomal recessive or sporadic and occasionally dominant. The clinical course is chronic, insidious, and highly varied, beginning at between 20 and 60 years of age. Unlike the childhood forms, these patients do not have loss of vision or retinal degeneration. They may be seen with either myoclonic seizures (type A) or behavioral abnormalities (type B). Dementia, ataxia, and pyramidal and extrapyramidal signs are also present in both types. As with the progressive myoclonic epilepsies, the electroretinogram may show an intense photoparoxysmal response to low-frequency photic stimulation. Lafora's disease, myoclonus-epilepsy–ragged red fiber syndrome, G_{M2}-gangliosidosis, galactosialidosis, and other storage disorders should be considered, but enzymatic assays and ultrastructural findings in skin and muscle biopsy specimens help differentiate these diseases from CLN-4. Skin, muscle, rectal, or even brain biopsy may be necessary to confirm the diagnosis. Electron microscopic studies may show various types of abnormal profiles, for example, a combination of distorted curvilinear profiles and fingerprint and rectilin ear profiles in membrane-bound vacuoles. Lipofuscin pigments may be seen with normal aging, but not the characteristic profile of neuronal ceroid lipofuscinoses. Immunostaining with antibodies against β-amyloid protein and subunit c of mitochondrial ATP synthetase may also be useful in distinguishing these variants from Alzheimer's disease. Autofluorescent lipopigments have been demonstrated in the neuronal perikaryon and axonal hillocks of the isocortex, allocortex, basal ganglia, thalamus, brainstem nuclei, cerebellum, and neurons of the anterior horns in the spinal cord. Cerebellar atrophy is present. CLN-4 has not been mapped to any genetic locus, and the cause of the disease remains unknown.

REFERENCES

1. Kornfeld S, Gregory W. The identification and partial characterization of lysosomes in human reticulocytes. Biochim Biophys Acta. 1969;177:615-624.
2. Luzio JP, Pryor PR, Bright NA. Lysosomes: fusion and function. Nat Rev Mol Cell Biol. 2007;8:622-632.
3. Cuervo AM, Dice JF. Lysosomes, a meeting point of proteins, chaperones, and proteases. J Mol Med. 1998; 76:6-12.
4. Winchester B. Lysosomal metabolism of glycoproteins. Glycobiology. 2005;15(6):1R-15R.
5. Goldberg DE, Kornfeld S. Evidence for extensive subcellular organization of asparagine-linked oligosaccharide processing and lysosomal enzyme phosphorylation. J Biol Chem. 1983;258:3159-3165.
6. Sly WS, Fischer HD. The phosphomannosyl recognition system for intracellular and intercellular transport of lysosomal enzymes. J Cell Biochem. 1982;18:67-85.
7. Kornfeld S, Mellman I. The biogenesis of lysosomes. Annu Rev Cell Biol. 1989;5:483-525.
8. Hille-Rehfeld A. Mannose 6-phosphate receptors in sorting and transport of lysosomal enzymes. Biochim Biophys Acta. 1995;1241:177-194.
9. Kornfeld S, Sly WS. I-cell disease and pseudo-Hurler polydystrophy: disorders of lysosomal enzyme phosphorylation and localization. In Scriver CR, Sly WS, Childs B, et al (eds). The Metabolic and Molecular Bases of Inherited Disease, 8th ed. New York, McGraw-Hill, 2001, pp 3421-3452.
10. Reczek D, Schwake M, Schröder J, et al. LIMP-2 is a receptor for lysosomal mannose-6-phosphate–independent targeting of beta glucocerebrosidase. Cell. 2007; 131:770-783.
11. Neufeld EF, Fratantoni JC. Inborn errors of mucopolysaccharide metabolism. Science. 1970;169:141-146.
12. Neufeld EF. Lysosomal storage diseases. Annu Rev Biochem. 1991;60:257-280.
13. Kornfeld S. Trafficking of lysosomal enzymes in normal and disease states. J Clin Invest. 1986;77:1-6.
14. Weissmann G, Zurier RB, Spieler PJ, Goldstein IM. Mechanisms of lysosomal enzyme release from leukocytes exposed to immune complexes and other particles. J Exp Med. 1971;134:149s-165s.
15. Smith RJ, Ignarro LJ. Bioregulation of lysosomal enzyme secretion from human neutrophils: roles of guanine 3′,5′-monophosphate and calcium in stimulus-secretion coupling. Proc Natl Acad Sci U S A. 1975;72:108-112.
16. Andrews NW. Regulated secretion of conventional lysosomes. Trends Cell Biol. 2000;10:316-321.
17. Holt OJ, Gallo F, Griffiths GM. Regulating secretory lysosomes. J Biochem. 2006;140:7-12.
18. McNeil PL. Repairing a torn cell surface: make way, lysosomes to the rescue. J Cell Sci. 2002;115:873-879.
19. Gerasimenko JV, Gerasimenko OV, Petersen OH. Membrane repair: Ca(2+)-elicited lysosomal exocytosis. Curr Biol. 2001;11:R971-R974.
20. Smith RJ, Sabin C, Gilchrest H, Williams S. Effect of antiinflammatory drugs on lysosomes and lysosomal enzymes from rat liver. Biochem Pharmacol. 1976;25:2171-2177.
21. Scriver CR, Sly WS, Childs B, et al (eds). The Metabolic and Molecular Bases of Inherited Disease, 8th ed. New York, McGraw-Hill, 2001.
22. Hers HG. Inborn lysosomal diseases. Gastroenterology. 1965;48:625-633.
23. McPherson JD, Mara M, Hillier, et al., for the International Human Genome Mapping Consortium. A physical map of the human genome. Nature. 2001;409:934-941.
24. Conzelmann E, Sandhoff K. AB variant of infantile G_{M2} gangliosidosis: deficiency of a factor necessary for stimulation of hexosaminidase A–catalyzed degradation of ganglioside G_{M2} and glycolipid G_{A2}. Proc Natl Acad Sci U S A. 1978;75:3979-3983.
25. O'Brien JS, Kretz KA, Dewji N, et al. Coding of two sphingolipid activator proteins (SAP-1 and SAP-2) by same genetic locus. Science. 1988;241:1098-1101.
26. Kolter T, Sandhoff K. Principles of lysosomal membrane digestion: stimulation of sphingolipid degradation by sphingolipid activator proteins and anionic lysosomal lipids. Annu Rev Cell Dev Biol. 2005;21:81-103.
27. Vaccaro AM, Ciaffoni F, Tatti M, et al. pH-dependent conformational properties of saposins and their interactions with phospholipid membranes. J Biol Chem. 1995;270:30576-30580.
28. Tylki-Szymanska A, Czartoryska B, Vanier MT, et al. Non-neuronopathic Gaucher disease due to saposin C deficiency. Clin Genet. 2007;72:538-542.
29. Paschke E, Kresse H. Morquio disease, type B: activation of G_{M1}-β-galactosidase by G_{M1}-activator protein. Biochem Biophys Res Commun. 1982;109:568-575.
30. Lazarus SS, Vethamany VG, Schneck L, Volk BW. Fine structure and histochemistry of peripheral blood cells in Niemann-Pick disease. Lab Invest. 1967;17:155-170.
31. Vethamany VG, Welch JP, Vethamany SK. Type D Niemann-Pick disease (Nova Scotia variant). Ultrastructure of blood, skin fibroblasts, and bone marrow. Arch Pathol. 1972;93:537-543.
32. Belcher RW. Ultrastructure and cytochemistry of lymphocytes in the genetic mucopolysaccharidoses. Arch Pathol. 1972;93:1-7.
33. Rapola J, Autio S, Aula P, Nanto V. Lymphocytic inclusions in I-cell disease. J Pediatr. 1974;85:88-90.

34. Dolman CL, MacLeod PM, Chang E. Skin punch biopsies and lymphocytes in the diagnosis of lipidoses. Can J Neurol Sci. 1975;2:67-73.

35. Noonan SM, Weiss L, Riddle JM. Ultrastructural observations of cytoplasmic inclusions in Tay-Sachs lymphocytes. Arch Pathol Lab Med. 1976;100:595-600.

36. Schwendemann G. Lymphocyte inclusions in the juvenile type of generalized ceroid-lipofuscinosis. An electron microscopic study. Acta Neuropathol. 1976;36:327-338.

37. Stekhoven JHS, van Haelst UJGM. Ultrastructural study of so-called curvilinear bodies and fingerprint structures in lymphocytes in late-infantile amaurotic idiocy. Acta Neuropathol. 1976;35:295-306.

38. Reilly WA. The granules in the leukocytes in gargoylism. Am J Dis Child. 1941;62:489-491.

39. Curless RG, Parker JC Jr, Flynn JT. Neuronal ceroid lipofuscinosis. Diagnosis by semi-thin plastic-embedded sections of peripheral blood lymphocytes from a patient with a normal blood smear. Arch Neurol. 1982;39:308-310.

40. Anderson GW, Smith VV, Brooke I, et al. Diagnosis of neuronal ceroid lipofuscinosis (Batten disease) by electron microscopy in peripheral blood specimens. Ultrastruct Pathol. 2006;30:373-378.

41. Silverstein MN, Ellefson RD, Ahem EJ. The syndrome of the sea-blue histiocyte. N Engl J Med. 1970;282:1-4.

42. Elleder M, Hrodek J, Cihula J. Niemann-Pick disease: lipid storage in bone marrow macrophages. Histochem J. 1983;15:1065-1077.

43. Smith H. Sea-blue histiocytes in marrow in Batten-Spielmeyer-Vogt disease. Pathology. 1974;6:323-327.

44. Naito M, Takahashi K, Hojo H. An ultrastructural and experimental study on the development of tubular structures in the lysosomes of Gaucher cells. Lab Invest. 1988;58:590-598.

45. Glew RH, Lee RE. Composition of the membranous deposits occurring in Gaucher's disease. Arch Biochem Biophys. 1973;156:626-639.

46. Hibbs RG, Ferrans VJ, Cipriano PR, Tardiff KJ. A histochemical and electron microscopic study of Gaucher cells. Arch Pathol. 1970;89:137-153.

47. Lorber M. Iron distribution in adult-type Gaucher's disease [letter]. N Engl J Med. 1975;292:110.

48. Lee RE, Ellis LD. The storage cells of chronic myelogenous leukemia. Lab Invest. 1971;24:261-264.

49. Zaino EC, Rossi MB, Pham TD, Azar HA. Gaucher's cells in thalassemia. Blood. 1971;38:457-462.

50. Shinar E, Gershon ZL, Leiserowitz R, et al. Coexistence of Gaucher disease and Philadelphia-positive chronic granulocytic leukemia. Am J Hematol. 1982;12:199-202.

51. Prasad A, Kaye EM, Alroy J. Electron microscopic examination of skin biopsy as a cost-effective tool in the diagnosis of lysosomal storage diseases. J Child Neurol. 1996;11:301-308.

52. Carpenter S. Skin biopsy for diagnosis of hereditary neurologic metabolic disease. Arch Dermatol. 1987;123:1618-1621.

53. Kaesgen U, Goebel HH. Intraepidermal morphologic manifestations in lysosomal diseases. Brain Dev. 1989;11:338-341.

54. Boustany RM, Alroy J, Kolodny EH. Clinical classification of neuronal ceroid-lipofuscinosis subtypes. Am J Med Genet Suppl. 1988;5:47-58.

55. Takahashi K, Naito M, Suzuki Y. Genetic mucopolysaccharidoses, mannosidosis, sialidosis, galactosialidoses and I-cell disease. Ultrastructural analysis of cultured fibroblasts. Acta Pathol Jpn. 1987;37:385-400.

56. Nanai J, Leroy J, O'Brien JS. Ultrastructure of cultured fibroblasts in I-cell disease. Am J Dis Child. 1971;122:34-38.

57. Berman ER, Livni N, Shapira E, et al. Congenital corneal clouding with abnormal systemic storage bodies: A new variant of mucolipidosis. J Pediatr. 1974;84:519-526.

58. Miley CE 3rd, Gilbert EF, France TD, et al. Clinical and extraneural histologic diagnosis of neuronal ceroid-lipofuscinosis. Neurology. 1978;28:1008-1012.

59. Sewell AC. Urinary screening for disorders of heteroglycan metabolism. Klin Wochenschr. 1988;66:48-53.

60. Desnick RJ, Dawson G, Desnick SJ, et al. Diagnosis of glycosphingolipidoses by urinary-sediment analysis. N Engl J Med. 1971;284:739-744.

61. Berry HK. Screening for mucopolysaccharide disorders with the Berry spot test. Clin Biochem. 1987;20:365-371.

62. Cappelletti R, Del Rosso M, Chiarugi VP. A new electrophoretic method for the complete separation of all known animal glycosaminoglycans in a monodimensional run. Anal Biochem. 1979;99:311-315.

63. Whitley CB, Ridnour MD, Draper KA, et al. Diagnostic test for mucopolysaccharidosis. I. Direct method for quantifying excessive urinary glycosaminoglycan excretion. Clin Chem. 1989;35:374-379.

64. Humbel R, Collart M. Oligosaccharides in urine of patients with glycoprotein storage diseases. I. Rapid detection by thin-layer chromatography. Clin Chim Acta. 1975;60:143-145.

65. Friedman RB, Williams MA, Maser HW, Kolodny EH. Improved thin-layer chromatographic method in the diagnosis of mannosidosis. Clin Chem. 1978;24:1576-1577.

66. O'Brien JS. The cherry red spot–myoclonus syndrome: a newly recognized inherited lysosomal storage disease due to acid neuraminidase deficiency. Clin Genet. 1978;14:55-60.

67. Carroll JE, Roesel RA, DuRant RH, et al. Urinary sialic acid screening in neurologic disorders. Pediatr Neurol. 1986;2:67-71.

68. Auray-Blais C, Cyr D, Mills K, et al. Development of a filter paper method potentially applicable to mass and high-risk urinary screenings for Fabry disease. J Inherit Metab Dis. 2007;30:106.

69. Meikle PJ, Fuller M, Hopwood JJ. Mass spectrometry in the study of lysosomal storage disorders. Cell Mol Biol (Noisy-le-grand). 2003;49:769-777.

70. Sugita M, Iwamori M, Evans J, et al. High-performance liquid chromatography of ceramides: application to analysis in human tissues and demonstration of ceramide excess in Farber's disease. J Lipid Res. 1974;15:223-226.

71. Ullman MD, McCluer RH. Quantitative analysis of plasma neutral glycosphingolipids by high-performance liquid chromatography of their perbenzoyl derivatives. J Lipid Res. 1977;18:371-378.

72. Jungalwala FB, Milunsky A. High-performance liquid chromatography for the detection of homozygotes and heterozygotes of Niemann-Pick disease. Pediatr Res. 1978;12:655-659.

73. Fratantoni JC, Hall CW, Neufeld EF. The defect in Hurler's and Hunter's syndromes: faulty degradation of mucopolysaccharides. Proc Natl Acad Sci U S A. 1968;60: 699-706.

74. Schmickel RD, Distler JJ, Jourdian GW. Accumulation of sulfate containing acid mucopolysaccharides in I-cell fibroblasts. J Lab Clin Med. 1975;86:672-682.

75. Bach G, Ziegler M, Kohn G, Cohen MM. Mucopolysaccharide accumulation in cultured skin fibroblasts derived from patients with mucolipidosis IV. Am J Hum Genet. 1977;29:610-618.

76. Barton NW, Rosenberg A. Metabolism of glucosyl [³H]ceramide by human skin fibroblasts from normal and glucosylceramidotic subjects. J Biol Chem. 1975;250:3966-3971.

77. Kudoh T, Wenger DA. Diagnosis of metachromatic leukodystrophy, Krabbe disease and Farber disease after uptake of fatty acid–labeled ceramide sulfate into cultured skin fibroblasts. J Clin Invest. 1982;70:89-97.

78. Wood S. Cultured fucosidosis fibroblasts: a simple technique demonstrating storage of tritiated-fucose–labeled material. Clin Genet. 1976;10:183-186.

79. Kyriakides EC, Filippone N, Paul B, et al. Lipid studies in Wolman's disease. Pediatrics. 1970;46:431-436.

80. Glew RH, Peters SP (eds). Practical Enzymology of the Sphingolipidoses. New York, Alan R Liss, 1977.

81. Ginsburg V. Complex carbohydrates, part C. Methods Enzymol. 1978;50:1.

82. Kolodny EH. General principles and techniques of case identification, carrier testing and prenatal diagnosis. In Glew RH, Peters SP (eds). Practical Enzymology of the Spingolipidoses. New York, Alan R Liss, 1977, pp 18-20.

83. Froissart R, Maire I, Bonnet V, et al. Germline and somatic mosaicism in a female carrier of Hunter disease. J Med Genet. 1997;34:137-140.

84. Schröder W, Petruschka L, Wehnert M, et al. Carrier detection of Hunter syndrome (MPS II) by biochemical and DNA techniques in families at risk. J Med Genet. 1993;30:210-213.

85. Lualdi S, Regis S, Di Rocco M, et al. Characterization of iduronate-2-sulfatase gene-pseudogene recombinations in eight patients with mucopolysaccharidosis type II revealed by a rapid PCR-based method. Hum Mutat. 2005;25: 491-497.

86. Filocamo M, Bonuccelli G, Corsolini F, et al. Molecular analysis of 40 Italian patients with mucopolysaccharidosis type II: new mutations in the iduronate-2-sulfatase (IDS) gene. Hum Mutat. 2001;18:164-165.

87. Bonten EJ, d'Azzo A. Lysosomal neuraminidase. Catalytic activation in insect cells is controlled by the protective protein/cathepsin A. J Biol Chem. 2000;275:37657-37663.

88. Wada R, Tifft CJ, Proia RL. Microglial activation precedes acute neurodegeneration in Sandhoff disease and is suppressed by bone marrow transplantation. Proc Natl Acad Sci U S A. 2000;97:10954-10959.

89. Tessitore A, del P Martin M, Sano R, et al. G$_{M1}$-ganglioside–mediated activation of the unfolded protein response causes neuronal death in a neurodegenerative gangliosidosis. Mol Cell. 2004;15:753-766.

90. Suzuki K, Proia RL, Suzuki K. Mouse models of human lysosomal diseases. Brain Pathol. 1998;8:195-215.

91. d'Azzo A. Gene transfer strategies for correction of lysosomal storage disorders. Acta Haematol. 2003;110: 71-85.

92. Du H, Levine M, Ganesa C, et al. The role of mannosylated enzyme and the mannose receptor in enzyme replacement therapy. Am J Hum Genet. 2005;77:1061-1074.

93. Chiba Y, Sakuraba H, Kotani M, et al. Production in yeast of alpha-galactosidase A, a lysosomal enzyme applicable to enzyme replacement therapy for Fabry disease. Glycobiology. 2002;12:821-828.

94. Shaaltiel Y, Bartfeld D, Hashmueli S, et al. Production of glucocerebrosidase with terminal mannose glycans for enzyme replacement therapy of Gaucher's disease using a plant cell system. Plant Biotechnol J. 2007;5:579-590.

95. Bonten EJ, Wang D, Toy JN, et al. Targeting macrophages with baculovirus-produced lysosomal enzymes: implications for enzyme replacement therapy of the glycoprotein storage disorder galactosialidosis. FASEB J. 2004;18:971-973.

96. Van Patten SM, Hughes H, Huff MR, et al. Effect of mannose chain length on targeting of glucocerebrosidase for enzyme replacement therapy of Gaucher disease. Glycobiology. 2007;17:467-478.

97. Beck M. New therapeutic options for lysosomal storage disorders: enzyme replacement, small molecules and gene therapy. Hum Genet. 2007;121:1-22.

98. Brady RO. Enzyme replacement for lysosomal diseases. Annu Rev Med. 2006;57:283-296.

99. Van den Hout H, Reuser AJ, Vulto AG, et al. Recombinant human alpha-glucosidase from rabbit milk in Pompe patients. Lancet. 2000;356:397-398.

100. Eng CM, Banikazemi M, Gordon RE, et al. A phase 1/2 clinical trial of enzyme replacement in Fabry disease: pharmacokinetic, substrate clearance, and safety studies. Am J Hum Genet. 2001;68:711-722.

101. Schiffmann R, Kopp JB, Austin HA 3rd, et al. Enzyme replacement therapy in Fabry disease: a randomized controlled trial. JAMA. 2001;285:2743-2749.

102. Kakkis ED, Muenzer J, Tiller GE, et al. Enzyme-replacement therapy in mucopolysaccharidosis I. N Engl J Med. 2001;344:182-188.

103. Byers S, Crawley AC, Brumfield LK, et al. Enzyme replacement therapy in a feline model of MPS VI: modification of enzyme structure and dose frequency. Pediatr Res. 2000;47:743-749.

104. Yu WH, Zhao KW, Ryazantsev S, et al. Short-term enzyme replacement in the murine model of Sanfilippo syndrome type B. Mol Genet Metab. 2000;71:573-580.

105. Geel TM, McLaughlin PM, de Leij LF, et al. Pompe disease: current state of treatment modalities and animal models. Mol Genet Metab. 2007;92:299-307.

106. Sands M, Vogler C, Torrey A, et al. Murine mucopolysaccharidosis type VII: long term therapeutic effects of enzyme replacement and enzyme replacement followed by bone marrow transplantation. J Clin Invest. 1997;99: 1596-1605.

107. Tifft CJ, Proia RL. Stemming the tide: glycosphingolipid synthesis inhibitors as therapy for storage diseases. Glycobiology. 2000;10:1249.

108. Fleet GW, Karpas A, Dwek RA, et al. Inhibition of HIV replication by amino-sugar derivatives. FEBS Lett. 1988;237:128-132.

109. Radin NS. Treatment of Gaucher disease with an enzyme inhibitor. Glycoconj J. 1996;13:153-157.

110. Cox T, Lachmann R, Hollak C, et al. Novel oral treatment of Gaucher's disease with N-butyldeoxynojirimycin (OGT 918) to decrease substrate biosynthesis. Lancet. 2000;355: 1481-1485.

111. Asano N, Ishii S, Kizu H, et al. In vitro inhibition and intracellular enhancement of lysosomal alpha-galactosidase A activity in Fabry lymphoblasts by 1-deoxygalactonojirimycin and its derivatives. Eur J Biochem. 2000; 267:4179-4186.

112. Platt FM, Neises GR, Reinkensmeier G, et al. Prevention of lysosomal storage in Tay-Sachs mice treated with N-butyldeoxynojirimycin. Science. 1997;276:428-431.

113. Jeyakumar M, Butters TD, Cortina-Borja M, et al. Delayed symptom onset and increased life expectancy in Sandhoff disease mice treated with N-butyldeoxynojirimycin. Proc Natl Acad Sci U S A. 1999;96:6388-6393.

114. Lachmann RH. Miglustat: substrate reduction therapy for glycosphingolipid lysosomal storage disorders. Drugs Today (Barc). 2006;42:29-38.

115. Platt FM, Jeyakumar M, Andersson U, et al. Inhibition of substrate synthesis as a strategy for glycolipid lysosomal storage disease therapy. J Inherit Metab Dis. 2001;24: 275-290.

116. Pastores GM, Barnett NL. Substrate reduction therapy: miglustat as a remedy for symptomatic patients with Gaucher disease type 1. Expert Opin Investig Drugs. 2003;12:273-281.

117. Pastores GM, Sathe S. A chaperone-mediated approach to enzyme enhancement as a therapeutic option for the lysosomal storage disorders. Drugs R D. 2006;7:339-348.

118. Patterson MC, Vecchio D, Prady H, et al. Miglustat for treatment of Niemann-Pick C disease: a randomised controlled study. Lancet Neurol. 2007;6:765-772.

119. Fan JQ. A counterintuitive approach to treat enzyme deficiencies: use of enzyme inhibitors for restoring mutant enzyme activity. Biol Chem. 2008;389:1-11.

120. Hobbs JR, Hugh-Jones K, Barrett AJ. Reversal of clinical features of Hurler's disease and biochemical improvement after treatment by bone-marrow transplantation. Lancet. 1981;8249:709-712.

121. Krivit W, Peters C, Shapiro EG. Bone marrow transplantation as effective treatment of central nervous system disease in globoid cell leukodystrophy, metachromatic leukodystrophy, adrenoleukodystrophy, mannosidosis, fucosidosis, aspartylglucosaminuria, Hurler, Maroteaux-Lamy, and Sly syndromes, and Gaucher disease type III. Curr Opin Neurol. 1999;12:167-176.

122. Arvio M, Sauna-Aho O, Peippo M. Bone marrow transplantation for aspartylglucosaminuria: follow-up study of transplanted and non-transplanted patients. J Pediatr. 2001;138:288.

123. Koga M. Farber's lipogranulomatosis. Nippon Rinsho. 1995;53:3009.

124. Yeager AM, Uhas KA, Coles CD, et al. Bone marrow transplantation for infantile ceramidase deficiency (Farber disease). Bone Marrow Transplant. 2000;26:357-363.

125. Miano M, Lanino E, Gatti R, et al. Four year follow-up of a case of fucosidosis treated with unrelated donor bone marrow transplantation. Bone Marrow Transplant. 2001; 27:747-751.

126. Vellodi A, Cragg H, Winchester B, et al. Allogeneic bone marrow transplantation for fucosidosis. Bone Marrow Transplant. 1995;15:153-158.

127. Hoogerbrugge PM, Brouwer OF, Bordigoni P, et al. Allogeneic bone marrow transplantation for lysosomal storage diseases. The European Group for Bone Marrow Transplantation. Lancet. 1995;345:1398-1402.

128. Ringdén O, Groth CG, Erikson A, et al. Ten years' experience of bone marrow transplantation for Gaucher disease. Transplantation. 1995;59:864-870.

129. Vellodi A, Young E, Cooper A, et al. Long-term follow-up following bone marrow transplantation for Hunter disease. J Inherit Metab Dis. 1999;29:638-648.

130. Peters C, Krivit W. Hematopoietic cell transplantation for mucopolysaccharidosis IIB (Hunter syndrome). Bone Marrow Transplant. 2000;25:1097.

131. McKinnis EJ, Sulzbacher S, Rutledge JC, et al. Bone marrow transplantation in Hunter syndrome. J Pediatr. 1996;129:145-148.

132. Coppa GV, Gabrielli O, Zampini L, et al. Bone marrow transplantation in Hunter syndrome (mucopolysaccharidosis type II): two-year follow-up of the first Italian patient and review of the literature. Pediatr Med Chir. 1995;17: 227-235.

133. Krivit W, Aubourg P, Shapiro E, Peters C. Bone marrow transplantation for globoid cell leukodystrophy, adrenoleukodystrophy, metachromatic leukodystrophy, and Hurler syndrome. Curr Opin Hematol. 1999;6:377-382.

134. Braunlin EA, Rose AG, Hopwood JJ, et al. Coronary artery patency following long-term successful engraftment 14 years after bone marrow transplantation in the Hurler syndrome. Am J Cardiol. 2001;88:1075-1077.

135. Hite SH, Peters C, Krivit W. Correction of odontoid dysplasia following bone-marrow transplantation and engraftment (in Hurler syndrome MPS 1H). Pediatr Radiol. 2000;30:464.

136. Guffon N, Souillet G, Maire I, et al. Follow-up of nine patients with Hurler syndrome after bone marrow transplantation. J Pediatr. 1998;133:119-125.

137. Vellodi A, Young EP, Cooper A, et al. Bone marrow transplantation for mucopolysaccharidosis type I: Experience of two British centres. Arch Dis Child. 1997;76:92-99.

138. Peters C, Shapiro EG, Krivit W. Neuropsychological development in children with Hurler syndrome following hematopoietic stem cell transplantation. Pediatr Transplant. 1998;2:250.

139. Herskhovitz E, Young E, Rainer J, et al. Bone marrow transplantation for Maroteaux-Lamy syndrome (MPS VI): long-term follow-up. J Inherit Metab Dis. 1999; 22:50-62.

140. Lee V, Li CK, Shing MM, et al. Umbilical cord blood transplantation for Maroteaux-Lamy syndrome (mucopolysaccharidosis type VI). Bone Marrow Transplant 2000;26:455-458.

141. Lake BD, Steward CG, Oakhill A, et al. Bone marrow transplantation in late infantile Batten disease and juvenile Batten disease. Neuropediatrics. 1997;28:80-81.

142. Lake BD, Henderson DC, Oakhill A, Vellodi A. Bone marrow transplantation in Batten disease (neuronal ceroid-lipofuscinosis). Will it work? Preliminary studies on coculture experiments and on bone marrow transplant in

late infantile Batten disease. Am J Med Genet. 1995;57: 369-373.

143. Bayever E, Kamani N, Ferreira P, et al. Bone marrow transplantation for Niemann-Pick type IA disease. J Inherit Metab Dis. 1992;15:919-928.

144. Vellodi A, Hobbs JR, O'Donnell NM, et al. Treatment of Niemann-Pick disease type B by allogeneic bone marrow transplantation. Br Med J (Clin Res Ed). 1987;295: 1375-1376.

145. Hsu YS, Hwu WL, Huang SF, et al. Niemann-Pick disease type C (a cellular cholesterol lipidosis) treated by bone marrow transplantation. Bone Marrow Transplant. 1999;24:103-107.

146. Vellodi A, Young E, New M, et al. Bone marrow transplantation for Sanfilippo disease type B. J Inherit Metab Dis. 1992;15:911-918.

147. Krivit W, Peters C, Dusenbery K, et al. Wolman disease successfully treated by bone marrow transplantation. Bone Marrow Transplant. 2000;26:567-570.

148. Hoogerbrugge PM, Brouwer OF, Bordigoni P, et al. Allogeneic bone marrow transplantation for lysosomal storage diseases. The European Group for Bone Marrow Transplantation. Lancet. 1995;345:1398-1402.

149. Martin PL, Carter SL, Kernan NA, et al. Results of the cord blood transplantation study (COBLT): outcomes of unrelated donor umbilical cord blood transplantation in pediatric patients with lysosomal and peroxisomal storage diseases. Biol Blood Marrow Transplant. 2006;12: 184-194.

150. Cord blood banking for potential future transplantation: subject review. American Academy of Pediatrics. Work Group on Cord Blood Banking. Pediatrics. 1999;104: 116-118.

151. Meletis K, Frisen J. Have the bloody cells gone to our heads? J Cell Biol. 2001;155:699-702.

152. Kennedy D, Abkowitz J. Kinetics of central nervous system microglial and macrophage engraftment: analysis using a transgenic bone marrow transplantation model. Blood. 1997;90:986-993.

153. Shull RM, Hastings NE, Selcer RR, et al. Bone marrow transplantation in canine mucopolysaccharidosis I. J Clin Invest. 1987;79:435-443.

154. Krivit W, Shapiro E, Peters C, et al. Hematopoietic stem-cell transplantation in globoid-cell leukodystrophy. N Engl J Med. 1998;338:1119-1126.

155. Sena-Esteves M, Camp SM, Alroy J, et al. Correction of acid beta-galactosidase deficiency in G_{M1} gangliosidosis human fibroblasts by retrovirus vector–mediated gene transfer: higher efficiency of release and cross-correction by the murine enzyme. Hum Gene Ther. 2000;11: 715-727.

156. Luddi A, Volterrani M, Strazza M, et al. Retrovirus-mediated gene transfer and galactocerebrosidase uptake into twitcher glial cells results in appropriate localization and phenotype correction. Neurobiol Dis. 2001;8:600-610.

157. Pan D, Aronovich E, McIvor RS, Whitley CB. Retroviral vector design studies toward hematopoietic stem cell gene therapy for mucopolysaccharidosis type I. Gene Ther. 2000;7:1875-1883.

158. Tsutsudaasano A, Migita M, Takahashi K, Shimada T. Transduction of fibroblasts and CD34+ progenitors using a selectable retroviral vector containing cDNAs encoding arylsulfatase A and CD24. J Hum Genet. 2000;45: 18-23.

159. Yogalingam G, Muller V, Hopwood JJ, Anson DS. Regulation of N-acetylgalactosamine 4-sulfatase expression in retrovirus-transduced feline mucopolysaccharidosis type VI muscle cells. DNA Cell Biol. 1999;18:187-195.

160. Persons D, Allay J, Allay E, et al. Retroviral-mediated transfer of the green fluorescent protein gene into murine hematopoietic cells facilitates scoring and selection of transduced progenitors in vitro and identification of genetically modified cells in vivo. Blood. 1997;90:1777-1786.

161. Miranda SR, Erlich S, Friedrich VL Jr, et al. Hematopoietic stem cell gene therapy leads to marked visceral organ improvements and a delayed onset of neurological abnormalities in the acid sphingomyelinase deficient mouse model of Niemann-Pick disease. Gene Ther. 2000;20: 1768-1776.

162. Ohashi T, Yokoo T, Iizuka S, et al. Reduction of lysosomal storage in murine mucopolysaccharidosis type VII by transplantation of normal and genetically modified macrophages. Blood. 2000;95:3631-3633.

163. Leimig T, Mann L, Martin MDP, et al. Functional amelioration of murine galactosialidosis by genetically modified bone marrow hematopoietic progenitor cells. Blood. 2002;99:3169-3178.

164. Takenaka T, Murray GJ, Qin G, et al. Long-term enzyme correction and lipid reduction in multiple organs of primary and secondary transplanted Fabry mice receiving transduced bone marrow cells. Proc Natl Acad Sci U S A. 2000;97:7515-7520.

165. Sano R, Tessitore A, Ingrassia A, d'Azzo A. Chemokine-induced recruitment of genetically modified bone marrow cells into the CNS of G_{M1}-gangliosidosis mice corrects neuronal pathology. Blood. 2005;106:2259-2268.

166. Matzner U, Harzer K, Learish RD, et al. Long-term expression and transfer of arylsulfatase A into brain of arylsulfatase A–deficient mice transplanted with bone marrow expressing the arylsulfatase A cDNA from a retroviral vector. Gene Ther. 2000;7:1250-1257.

167. Rosenberg SA, Blaese RM, Brenner MK, et al. Human gene marker/therapy clinical protocols. Hum Gene Ther. 2000;11:919-979.

168. Schuening F, Longo W, Atkinson M, et al. Retrovirus-mediated transfer of the cDNA for human glucocerebrosidase into peripheral blood repopulation cells of patients with Gaucher's disease. Hum Gene Ther. 1997;8: 2143-2160.

169. Dunbar C, Kohn D, Schiffmann R, et al. Retroviral transfer of the glucocerebrosidase gene into CD34+ cells from patients with Gaucher disease: in vivo detection of transduced cells without myeloablation. Hum Gene Ther. 1998;9:2629-2640.

170. Richter J, Karlsson S. Clinical gene therapy in hematology: past and future. Int J Hematol. 2001;73:162-169.

171. Luther-Wyrsch A, Costello E, Thali M, et al. Stable transduction with lentiviral vectors and amplification of immature hematopoietic progenitors from cord blood of preterm human fetuses. Hum Gene Ther. 2001;12: 377-338.

172. Sands MS, Davidson BL. Gene therapy for lysosomal storage diseases. Mol Ther. 2006;13:839-849.

173. Watson GL, Sayles JN, Chen C, et al. Treatment of lysosomal storage disease in MPS VII mice using a recombinant adeno-associated virus. Gene Ther. 1998;5: 1642-1649.

174. Jung SC, Han IP, Limaye A, et al. Adeno-associated viral vector–mediated gene transfer results in long-term enzymatic and functional correction in multiple organs of Fabry mice. Proc Natl Acad Sci U S A. 2001;98: 2676-2681.

175. Daly T, Vogler C, Levy B, et al. Neonatal gene transfer leads to widespread correction of pathology in a murine model of lysosomal storage disease. Proc Natl Acad Sci U S A. 1999;96:2296-2300.

176. Daly TM, Ohlemiller KK, Roberts MS, et al. Prevention of systemic clinical disease in MPS VII mice following AAV-mediated neonatal gene transfer. Gene Ther. 2001;8:1291-1298.

177. Hartung SD, Frandsen JL, Pan D, et al. Correction of metabolic, craniofacial, and neurologic abnormalities in MPS I mice treated at birth with adeno-associated virus vector transducing the human alpha-L-iduronidase gene. Mol Ther. 2004;9:866-875.

178. Stein CS, Kang Y, Sauter SL, et al. In vivo treatment of hemophilia A and mucopolysaccharidosis type VII using nonprimate lentiviral vectors. Mol Ther. 2001;3: 850-856.

179. Kobayashi H, Carbonaro D, Pepper K, et al. Neonatal gene therapy of MPS I mice by intravenous injection of a lentiviral vector. Mol Ther. 2005;11: 776-789.

180. Di Natale P, Di Domenico C, Gargiulo N, et al. Treatment of the mouse model of mucopolysaccharidosis type IIIB with lentiviral-NAGLU vector. Biochem J. 2005;388:639-646.

181. Przybylska M, Wu IH, Zhao H, et al. Partial correction of the alpha-galactosidase A deficiency and reduction of glycolipid storage in Fabry mice using synthetic vectors. J Gene Med. 2004;6:85-92.

182. Jeyakumar M, Norflus F, Tifft CJ, et al. Enhanced survival in Sandhoff disease mice receiving a combination of substrate deprivation therapy and bone marrow transplantation. Blood. 2001;97:327.

183. Lake BD, Young EP, Winchester BG. Prenatal diagnosis of lysosomal storage diseases. Brain Pathol. 1998;8: 133-149.

184. Soma H, Yamada K, Osawa H, et al. Identification of Gaucher cells in the chorionic villi associated with recurrent hydrops fetalis. Placenta. 2000;21:412-416.

185. Bianchi D. Fetal DNA in maternal plasma: the plot thickens and the placental barrier thins. Am J Hum Genet. 1998;62:763-764.

186. Kanavakis E, Traeger-Synodinos J. Preimplantation genetic diagnosis in clinical practice. J Med Genet. 2002; 39:6-11.

187. Elias S. Preimplantation genetic diagnosis by comparative genomic hybridization. N Engl J Med. 2001;345:1569-1570.

188. Lissens W, Sermon K, Staessen C, et al. Review: preimplantation diagnosis of inherited disease. J Inherit Metab Dis. 1996;19:709-723.

189. Gaucher PCE. De l'Epithelioma Primitif de la Rate [thesis]. Paris, 1882.

190. Vellodi A, Bembi B, de Villemeur TB, et al. Management of neuronopathic Gaucher disease: a European consensus. J Inherit Metab Dis. 2001;24:319-327.

191. Chabás A, Cormand B, Grinberg D, et al. Unusual expression of Gaucher's disease: cardiovascular calcifications in three sibs homozygous for the D409H mutation. J Med Genet. 1995;32:740-742.

192. Stone DL, Sidransky E. Hydrops fetalis: lysosomal storage disorders in extremis. Adv Pediatr. 1999;46:409-440.

193. Inui K, Yanagihara K, Otani K, et al. A new variant neuropathic type of Gaucher's disease characterized by hydrocephalus, corneal opacities, deformed toes, and fibrous thickening of spleen and liver capsules. J Pediatr 2001; 138:137-139.

194. Sidransky E, Sherer DM, Ginns EI. Gaucher disease in the neonate: a distinct Gaucher phenotype is analogous to a mouse model created by targeted disruption of the glucocerebrosidase gene. Pediatr Res. 1992;32:494-498.

195. Stone DL, Carey WF, Christodoulou J, et al. Type 2 Gaucher disease: the collodion baby phenotype revisited. Arch Dis Child Fetal Neonatal. 2000;2:F163-F166.

196. Tybulewicz VL, Tremblay ML, LaMarca ME, et al. Animal model of Gaucher's disease from targeted disruption of the mouse glucocerebrosidase gene. Nature. 1992;357: 407-410.

197. Kozower M, Kaplan MM, Kanfer JN, et al. Esophageal varices in a 60-year-old man with Gaucher's disease. Am J Dig Dis. 1974;19:565-570.

198. Boklan BF, Sawitsky A. Factor IX deficiency in Gaucher disease. Arch Intern Med. 1976;136:489-492.

199. Berrebi A, Malnick SD, Vorst EJ, Stein D. High incidence of factor XI deficiency in Gaucher's disease. Am J Hematol. 1992;40:153.

200. Billett HH, Rizvi S, Sawitsky A. Coagulation abnormalities in patients with Gaucher's disease: effect of therapy. Am J Hematol. 1996;51:234-236.

201. Young KR, Payne MJ. Reversible splenic enlargement associated with pregnancy in a patient with Gaucher's disease. J R Army Med Corps. 1986;132:157-158.

202. Shoenfeld Y, Berliner S, Pinkhas J, Beutler E. The association of Gaucher's disease and dysproteinemias. Acta Haematol. 1980;64:241-243.

203. Gal R, Gukovsky-Oren S, Floru S, et al. Sequential appearance of breast carcinoma, multiple myeloma and Gaucher's disease. Haematologica. 1988;76:63-65.

204. Shiran A, Brenner B, Laor A, Tatarsky I. Increased risk of cancer in patients with Gaucher disease. Cancer. 1993;72:219-224.

205. Krause JR, Bures C, Lee RE. Acute leukemia and Gaucher's disease. Scand J Haematol. 1979;23:115-118.

206. Bruckstein AH, Karanas A, Di Re JJ. Gaucher's disease associated with Hodgkin's disease. Am J Med. 1980;68: 610-613.

207. Burstein Y, Zakuth V, Rechavi G, Spirer Z. Abnormalities of cellular immunity and natural killer cells in Gaucher's disease. J Clin Lab Immunol. 1987;23:149-151.

208. Shoenfeld Y, Beresovski A, Zharhary D, et al. Natural autoantibodies in sera of patients with Gaucher's disease. J Clin Immunol. 1995;15:363-372.

209. Kolodny EH, Ullman MD, Mankin HJ, et al. Phenotypic manifestations of Gaucher disease: clinical features in 48 biochemically verified type 1 patients and comment on type 2 patients. In Desnick RJ, Gatt S, Grabowski GA

(eds). Gaucher Disease: A Century of Delineation and Research. New York, Alan R Liss, 1982, pp 33-65.

210. Barton DJ, Ludman MD, Benkov K, et al. Resting energy expenditure in Gaucher's disease: assessment, monitoring and expectations. Metabolism. 1989;38:1238-1243.

211. Granovsky-Grisaru S, Aboulafia Y, Diamant YZ, et al. Gynecologic and obstetric aspects of Gaucher's disease: a survey of 53 patients. Am J Obstet Gynecol. 1995;172:1284-1290.

212. Bakst AE, Gaine SP, Rubin LJ. Continuous intravenous epoprostenol therapy for pulmonary hypertension in Gaucher's disease. Chest. 1999;116:1127-1129.

213. Berrebi A, Wishnitzer R, Von-der-Walde V. Gaucher's disease: unexpected diagnosis in three patients over seventy years old. Nouv Rev Fr Hematol 1984;26:201-203.

214. Hermann G, Shapiro RS, Abdelwahab IF, Grabowski G. MR imaging in adults with Gaucher disease type I: evaluation of marrow involvement and disease activity. Skeletal Radiol. 1993;22:247-251.

215. Hermann G, Goldblatt J, Levy RN, et al. Gaucher's disease type 1: assessment of bone involvement by CT and scintigraphy. AJR Am J Roentgenol. 1986;147:943-948.

216. Lieberman I, Beutler E. Elevation of serum angiotensin-converting enzyme in Gaucher's disease. N Engl J Med. 1976;294:1442-1444.

217. Gilbert HS, Weinreb N. Increased circulating levels of transcobalamin II in Gaucher's disease. N Engl J Med. 1976;295:1096-1101.

218. Den Tandt WR, Van Hoof F. Plasma methylumbelliferyl-tetra-N-acetyl-β-D-chitotetraoside hydrolase as a parameter during treatment of Gaucher patients [letter]. Biochem Mol Med. 1996;57:71-72.

219. Grafe M, Thomas C, Schneider J, et al. Infantile Gaucher's disease: a case with neuronal storage. Ann Neurol. 1988;28:300-303.

220. Kaye EM, Ullman MD, Wilson ER, Barranger JA. Type 2 and type 3 Gaucher disease: a morphological and biochemical study. Ann Neurol. 1986;20:223-230.

221. Svennerholm L, Mansson J, Rosengren B. Cerebroside-β-glucosidase activity in Gaucher brain. Clin Genet. 1986;30:131-135.

222. Grover WD, Tucker SH, Wenger DA. Clinical variation in 2 related children with neuronopathic Gaucher's disease. Ann Neurol. 1978;3:281-283.

223. Miller JD, McCluer R, Kanfer JN. Gaucher's disease: neurologic disorder in adult siblings. Ann Intern Med. 1973;78:883-887.

225. Garvey MA, Toro C, Goldstein S, et al. Somatosensory evoked potentials as a marker of disease burden in type 3 Gaucher disease. Neurology. 2001;56:391-394.

225. Stone DL, Tayebi N, Orvisky E, et al. Glucocerebrosidase gene mutations in patients with type 2 Gaucher disease. Hum Mutat. 2000;15:181-188.

226. Conradi NG, Kalimo H, Sourander P. Reactions of vessel walls and brain parenchyma to the accumulation of Gaucher cells in the Norrbottnian type (type III) of Gaucher disease. Acta Neuropathol. 1988;75:385-390.

227. Erikson A, Astrom M, Mansson JE. Enzyme infusion therapy of the Norrbottnian (type 3) Gaucher disease. Neuropediatrics. 1995;26:203-207.

228. Groth CG, Blomstrand R, Hagenfeldt L, et al. Metabolic changes following splenic transplantation in a case of Gaucher's disease. In Volk BW, Aronson SM (eds). Sphingolipids, Sphingolipidoses and Allied Disorders. New York, Plenum Press, 1972, pp 633-639.

229. Ringdén O, Groth CG, Erikson A, et al. Long-term follow-up of the first successful bone marrow transplantation in Gaucher disease. Transplantation. 1988;46:66-70.

230. Erikson A, Groth CG, Månsson JE, et al. Clinical and biochemical outcome of marrow transplantation for Gaucher disease of the Norrbottnian type. Acta Paediatr Scand. 1990;79:680-685.

231. Svennerholm L, Erikson A, Groth CG, et al. Norrbottnian type of Gaucher disease—clinical, biochemical and molecular biology aspects: successful treatment with bone marrow transplantation. Dev Neurosci. 1991;13:345-351.

232. Tsai P, Lipton JM, Sahdev I, et al. Allogenic bone marrow transplantation in severe Gaucher disease. Pediatr Res. 1992;31:503-507.

233. Dinur T, Osiecki KM, Legler G, et al. Human acid β-glucosidase: isolation and amino acid sequence of a peptide containing the catalytic site. Proc Natl Acad Sci U S A. 1986;83:1660-1664.

234. Horowitz M, Wilder S, Horowitz Z, et al. The human glucocerebrosidase gene and pseudogene: structure and evolution. Genomics. 1989;4:87-96.

235. Barneveld RA, Keijzer W, Tegelaers FP, et al. Assignment of the gene coding for human β-glucocerebrosidase to the region of q21Bq31 of chromosome 1 using monoclonal antibodies. Hum Genet. 1983;64:227-231.

236. Ginns EI, Choudary PV, Tsuji S, et al. Gene mapping and leader polypeptide sequence of human glucocerebrosidase: Implications for Gaucher disease. Proc Natl Acad Sci U S A. 1985;82:7101-7105.

237. Bornstein P, McKinney CE, LaMarca ME, et al. Metaxin, a gene contiguous to both thrombospondin 3 and glucocerebrosidase, is required for embryonic development in the mouse: implications for Gaucher disease. Proc Natl Acad Sci U S A. 1995;92:4547-4551.

238. Adolph KW, Bornstein P. The human thrombospondin 3 gene: analysis of transcription initiation and an alternatively spliced transcript. Mol Cell Biol Res Commun. 1999;2:47-52.

239. Abdul KM, Terada K, Yano M, et al. Functional analysis of human metaxin in mitochondrial protein import in cultured cells and its relationship with the Tom complex. Biochem Biophys Res Commun. 2000;276:1028-1034.

240. Rutella S, Rumi C, Di Mario A, Leone G. Expression of thrombospondin receptor (CD36) in chronic B-cell lymphoproliferative disorders: a role in tumor metastasis? Eur J Histochem. 1997;41(Suppl 2):53-54.

241. Reiner O, Wilder S, Givol D, Horowitz M. Efficient in vitro and in vivo expression of human glucocerebrosidase cDNA. DNA. 1987;6:101-108.

242. Sidransky E. Gaucher disease: complexity in a "simple" disorder. Mol Genet Metab. 2004;83:6-15.

243. Hruska KS, Lamarca ME, Scott CR, Sidransky E. Gaucher disease: mutation and polymorphism spectrum in the glucocerebrosidase gene (GBA). Hum Mutat. 2008;29:567-583.

244. Horowitz M, Tzuri G, Eyal N, et al. Prevalence of nine mutations among Jewish and non-Jewish Gaucher disease patients. Am J Hum Genet. 1993;53:921-930.

245. Abrahamov A, Elstein D, Gross-Tsur V, et al. Gaucher's disease variant characterized by progressive calcification of heart valves and unique genotype. Lancet. 1995;346:1000-1003.

246. Eyal N, Wilder S, Horowitz M. Prevalent and rare mutations among Gaucher patients. Gene. 1990;96:277-283.

247. Zimran A, Sorge J, Gross E, et al. A glucocerebrosidase fusion gene in Gaucher disease. Implications for the molecular anatomy, pathogenesis and diagnosis of this disorder. J Clin Invest. 1990;83:219-222.

248. Bove KE, Daugherty C, Grabowski GA. Pathological findings in Gaucher disease type 2 patients following enzyme therapy. Hum Pathol. 1995;26:1040-1045.

249. Goitein O, Elstein D, Abrahamov A, et al. Lung involvement and enzyme replacement therapy in Gaucher's disease. Q J M. 2001;94:407-415.

250. Charrow J, Esplin JA, Gribble TJ, et al. Gaucher disease: recommendations on diagnosis, evaluation, and monitoring. Arch Intern Med. 1998;16:1754-1760.

251. Tanaka N, Saito H, Ito T, et al. Initiation of enzyme replacement therapy for an adult patient with asymptomatic type 1 Gaucher's disease. Intern Med. 2001;40:716-721.

252. Sims KB, Pastores GM, Weinreb NJ, et al. Improvement of bone disease by imiglucerase (Cerezyme) therapy in patients with skeletal manifestations of type 1 Gaucher disease: results of a 48-month longitudinal cohort study. Clin Genet. 2008;73:430-440.

253. Richards SM, Olson TA, McPherson JM. Antibody response in patients with Gaucher disease after repeated infusion with macrophage-targeted glucocerebrosidase. Blood. 1993;82:1402-1409.

254. Grabowski GA, Barton NW, Pastores G, et al. Enzyme therapy in type 1 Gaucher disease: comparative efficacy of mannose-terminated glucocerebrosidase from natural and recombinant sources. Ann Intern Med. 1995;122:33-39.

255. Baudard M, Flotte TR, Aran JM, et al. Expression of the human multidrug resistance and glucocerebrosidase cDNAs from adeno-associated vectors: efficient promoter activity of AAV sequences in in vivo delivery via liposomes. Hum Gene Ther. 1996;7:1309-1322.

256. Bahnson AB, Nimgaonkar M, Fei Y, et al. Transduction of CD34+ enriched cord blood and Gaucher bone marrow cells of a retroviral vector carrying the glucocerebrosidase gene. Gene Ther. 1994;1:176-184.

257. Nimgaonkar MT, Bahnson AB, Boggs SS, et al. Transduction of mobilized peripheral blood CD34+ cells with the glucocerebrosidase cDNA. Gene Ther. 1994;1:201-207.

258. Barranger JA, Rice EO, Dunigan J, et al. Gaucher's disease: studies of gene transfer to haematopoietic cells. Baillieres Clin Haematol. 1997;10:765-778.

259. Cox T, Lachmann R, Hollak C, et al. Novel oral treatment of Gaucher's disease with N-butyldeoxynojirimycin (OGT 918) to decrease substrate biosynthesis. Lancet. 2000;355:1481-1485.

260. Alfonso P, Pampin S, Estrada J, et al. Miglustat (NB-DNJ) works as a chaperone for mutated acid beta-glucosidase in cells transfected with several Gaucher disease mutations. Blood Cells Mol Dis. 2005;35:268-276.

261. Steet RA, Chung S, Wustman B, et al. The iminosugar isofagomine increases the activity of N370S mutant acid beta-glucosidase in Gaucher fibroblasts by several mechanisms. Proc Natl Acad Sci U S A. 2006;103:13813-13818.

262. Zimran A, Kay A, Gelbart T, et al. Gaucher disease. Clinical, laboratory, radiologic, and genetic features of 53 patients. Medicine (Baltimore). 1992;71:337-353.

263. Samuel R, Katz K, Papapoulos SE, et al. Aminohydroxy propylidene bisphosphonate (APD) treatment improves the clinical skeletal manifestations of Gaucher's disease. Pediatrics. 1994;94:385-389.

264. Ringdén O, Groth CG, Erikson A, et al. Ten years' experience of bone marrow transplantation for Gaucher disease. Transplantation. 1995;59:864-870.

265. Rechitsky S, Strom C, Verlinsky O, et al. Accuracy of preimplantation diagnosis of single-gene disorders by polar body analysis of oocytes. J Assist Reprod Genet. 1999;16:192-198.

266. Niemann A. Ein unbekanntes Krankheitsbild. Jahrb Kinderheilkd. 1914;79:1-10.

267. Pick L. Zur pathologischen Anatomie des Morbus Gaucher. Med Klin. 1922;18:1408.

268. Pick L. Uber die lipoidzellige Splenohepatomegalie Typus Niemann-Pick als Stoffwechselerktankung. Med Klin. 1927;23:1483.

269. Crocker AC. The cerebral defect in Tay-Sachs disease and Niemann-Pick disease. J Neurochem. 1961;7:69-80.

270. Schuchman EH. The pathogenesis and treatment of acid sphingomyelinase–deficient Niemann-Pick disease. J Inherit Metab Dis. 2007;30:654-663.

271. Sidhu HS, Rastogi SA, Byers DM, et al. Regulation of low density lipoprotein receptor and 3-hydroxy-3-methyl-glutaryl-CoA reductase activities are differentially affected in Niemann-Pick type C and type D fibroblasts. Biochem Cell Biol. 1993;71:467-474.

272. Graber D, Salvayre R, Levade T. Accurate differentiation of neuronopathic and nonneuronopathic forms of Niemann-Pick disease by evaluation of the effective residual lysosomal sphingomyelinase activity in intact cells. J Neurochem. 1994;63:1060-1068.

273. da Veiga Pereira L, Desnick RJ, Adler DA, et al. Regional assignment of the human acid sphingomyelinase gene (SMPD 1) by PCR analysis of somatic cell hybrids and in situ hybridization to 11p15-p15.4. Genomics. 1991;9:229-234.

274. Simonaro CM, Park JH, Eliyahu E, et al. Imprinting at the SMPD1 locus: implications for acid sphingomyelinase–deficient Niemann-Pick disease. Am J Hum Genet. 2006;78:865-780.

275. Schuchman EH. Two new mutations in the acid sphingomyelinase gene causing type A Niemann-Pick disease: N389T and R441X. Hum Mutat. 1995;6:352-354.

276. Ferlinz K, Hurwitz R, Weiler M, et al. Molecular analysis of the acid sphingomyelinase deficiency in a family with an intermediate form of Niemann-Pick disease. Am J Hum Genet. 1995;56:1343-1349.

277. Ida H, Rennert OM, Maekawa K, Eto Y. Identification of three novel mutations in the acid sphingomyelinase gene of Japanese patients with Niemann-Pick disease type A and B. Hum Mutat. 1996;7:65-67.

278. Schuchman EH, Desnick RJ. Niemann-Pick disease types A and B: acid sphingomyelinase deficiencies. In Scriver

CR, Beaudet AL, WS Sly WS, Valle D (eds). The Metabolic and Molecular Bases of Inherited Disease. New York, McGraw-Hill, 1995, pp 2601-2624.

279. Vanier MT, Ferlinz K, Rousson R, et al. Deletion of arginine (608) in acid sphingomyelinase is the prevalent mutation among Niemann-Pick disease type B patients from northern Africa. Hum Genet. 1993;92:325-330.

280. Horinouchi K, Erlich S, Perl DP, et al. Acid sphingomyelinase deficient mice: a model of types A and B Niemann-Pick disease. Nat Genet. 1995;10:288-293.

281. Otterbach B, Stoffel W. Acid sphingomyelinase–deficient mice mimic the neurovisceral form of human lysosomal storage disease (Niemann-Pick disease). Cell. 1995;81:1053-1061.

282. Barbon CM, Ziegler RJ, Li C, et al. AAV8-mediated hepatic expression of acid sphingomyelinase corrects the metabolic defect in the visceral organs of a mouse model of Niemann-Pick disease. Mol Ther. 2005;12:431-440.

283. Passini MA, Bu J, Fidler JA, et al. Combination brain and systemic injections of AAV provide maximal functional and survival benefits in the Niemann-Pick mouse. Proc Natl Acad Sci U S A. 2007;104:9505-9510.

284. Greer WL, Riddell DC, Murty S, et al. Linkage disequilibrium mapping of the Nova Scotia variant of Niemann-Pick disease. Clin Genet. 1999;55:248-255.

285. Rodriguez-Lafrasse C, Vanier MT. Sphingosylphosphorylcholine in Niemann-Pick disease brain: accumulation in type A but not in type B. Neurochem Res. 1999;24:199-205.

286. Schuchman EH, Desnick RJ. Types A and B Niemann-Pick disease: deficiencies of acid sphingomyelinase activity. In Scriver CR, Sly WS, Childs B, et al. (eds). The Metabolic and Molecular Bases of Inherited Disease, 8th ed. New York, McGraw Hill, 2001, pp 3589-3610.

287. Niggemann B, Rebien W, Rahn W, Wahn U. Asymptomatic pulmonary involvement in 2 children with Niemann-Pick disease type B. Respiration. 1994;61:55-57.

288. Filling-Katz MR, Fink JK, Gorin MB, et al. Ophthalmologic manifestations of type B Niemann-Pick diseases. Metab Pediatr Syst Ophthalmol. 1992;15:16-20.

289. Strisciuglio P, DiMayo S, Parenti G, et al. Evidence of polyglandular involvement in Niemann-Pick disease type B. Eur J Pediatr. 1987;146:431-433.

290. Smith WE, Kahler SG, Frush DP, et al. Hepatic storage of glycogen in Niemann-Pick disease type B. J Pediatr. 2001;138:946-948.

291. Besley GT, Elleder M. Enzyme activities and phospholipid storage patterns in brain and spleen samples from Niemann-Pick disease variants: a comparison of neuropathic and non-neuropathic forms. J Inherit Metab Dis. 1986;9:59-71.

292. Breen L, Morris HH, Alperin JB, Schochet SS Jr. Juvenile Niemann-Pick disease with vertical supranuclear ophthalmoplegia. Arch Neurol. 1981;38:388-390.

293. Higgins JJ, Patterson MC, Dambrosia JM, et al. A clinical staging classification for type C Niemann-Pick disease. Neurology. 1992;42:2286-2290.

294. Hulette CM, Earl NL, Anthony DC, Crain BJ. Adult onset Niemann-Pick disease type C presenting with dementia and absent organomegaly. Clin Neuropathol. 1992;11:293-297.

295. Lanska DJ, Lanska MJ. Niemann-Pick disease type C in a middle-aged woman. Neurology. 1993;43:1435-1436.

296. Shulman LM, David NJ, Weiner WJ. Psychosis as the initial manifestation of adult-onset Niemann-Pick disease type C. Neurology. 1995;45:1739-1743.

297. Hahn AF, Gilbert JJ, Gillett J, et al. Nerve biopsy findings in Niemann-Pick type II (NPC). Acta Neuropathol. 1994;87:149-154.

298. Palmeri S, Battisti C, Federico A, Guazzi GC. Hypoplasia of the corpus callosum in Niemann-Pick type C disease. Neuroradiology. 1994;36:20-22.

299. Kelly DA, Portmann B, Mowat AP, et al. Niemann-Pick disease type C: diagnosis and outcome in children, with particular reference to liver disease. J Pediatr. 1993;123:242-247.

300. Manning DJ, Price WI, Pearse RG. Fetal ascites: an unusual presentation of Niemann-Pick disease type C. Arch Dis Child. 1990;3:335-336.

301. Marx J. Cell biology. Disease genes clarify cholesterol trafficking. Science. 2000;290:2227-2229.

302. Liscum L. Niemann-Pick type C mutations cause lipid traffic jam. Traffic. 2000;3:218-225.

303. Patterson MC, Pentchev PG. Niemann-Pick type C. Neurology. 1996;46:1785-1786.

304. Butler JD, Comly ME, Kruth HS, et al. Niemann-Pick variant disorders: comparison of errors of cellular cholesterol homeostasis in group D and group C fibroblasts. Proc Natl Acad Sci U S A. 1987;84:556-560.

305. Vanier MT, Wenger DA, Comly ME, et al. Niemann-Pick disease type C: clinical variability and diagnosis based on defective cholesterol esterification. Clin Genet. 1988;33:331-348.

306. Morris JA, Zhang D, Coleman KG, et al. The genomic organization and polymorphism analysis of the human Niemann-Pick C1 gene. Biochem Biophys Res Commun. 1999;261:493-498.

307. Millat G, Marcais C, Tomasetto C, et al. Niemann-Pick C1 disease: correlations between NPC1 mutations, levels of NPC1 protein, and phenotypes emphasize the functional significance of the putative sterol-sensing domain and of the cysteine-rich luminal loop. Am J Hum Genet. 2001;68:1373-1385.

308. Naureckiene S, Sleat DE, Lackland H, et al. Identification of HE1 as the second gene of Niemann-Pick C disease. Science. 2000;290:2298-2301.

309. Davies JP, Chen FW, Ioannou YA. Transmembrane molecular pump activity of Niemann-Pick C1 protein. Science. 2000;290:2295-2298.

310. Love S, Bridges LR, Case CP. Neurofibrillary tangles in Niemann-Pick disease type C. Brain. 1995;118:119-129.

311. Suzuki K, Parker CC, Pentchev PG, et al. Neurofibrillary tangles in Niemann-Pick disease type C. Acta Neuropathol. 1995;89:227-238.

312. Auer IA, Schmidt ML, Lee VM, et al. Paired helical filament tau (PHFt) in Niemann Pick type C disease is similar to PHFt in Alzheimer's disease. Acta Neuropathol 1995;90:547-551.

313. Patterson MC, Di Bisceglie AM, Higgins JJ, et al. The effect of cholesterol-lowering agents on hepatic and plasma cholesterol in Niemann-Pick disease type C. Neurology. 1993;43:61-64.

314. Sylvain M, Arnold DL, Scriver CR, et al. Magnetic resonance spectroscopy in Niemann-Pick disease type C: correlation with diagnosis and clinical response to

cholestyramine and lovastatin. Pediatr Neurol. 1994;10: 228-232.

315. Liscum L, Faust JR. The intracellular transport of low density lipoprotein–derived cholesterol is inhibited in Chinese hamster ovary cells cultured with 3-β-[2-(diethylamino)ethoxy]androst-5-en-17-one. J Biol Chem. 1989;264:11796-11806.

316. Vanier MT, Rodriguez-Lafrasse C, Rousson R, et al. Prenatal diagnosis of Niemann-Pick type C disease: current strategy from an experience of 37 pregnancies at risk. Am J Hum Genet. 1992;51:111-122.

317. de Winter JM, Janse HC, van Diggelen OP, et al. Prenatal diagnosis of Niemann-Pick disease type C. Clin Chim Acta. 1992;208:173-181.

318. Dumontel C, Girod C, Dijoud F, et al. Fetal Niemann-Pick disease type C: ultrastructural and lipid findings in liver and spleen. Virchows Arch. 1993;422:253-259.

319. Kuwamura M, Awakura T, Shimada A, et al. Type C Niemann-Pick disease in a boxer dog. Acta Neuropathol. 1993;85:345-348.

320. Muñana KR, Luttgen PJ, Thrall MA, et al. Neurological manifestations of Niemann-Pick disease type C in cats. J Vet Intern Med. 1994;8:117-121.

321. Higashi Y, Murayama S, Pentchev PG, Suzuki K. Peripheral nerve pathology in Niemann-Pick type C mouse. Acta Neuropathol. 1995;90:158-163.

322. Hsu YS, Hwu WL, Huang SF, et al. Niemann-Pick disease type C (a cellular cholesterol lipidosis) treated by bone marrow transplantation. Bone Marrow Transplant. 1999; 24:103-107.

323. Ahmad I, Hunter RE, Flax JD, et al. Neural stem cell implantation extends life in Niemann-Pick C1 mice. J Appl Genet. 2007;48:269-272.

324. Zervas M, Somers KL, Thrall MA, Walkley SU. Critical role for glycosphingolipids in Niemann-Pick disease type C. Curr Biol. 2001;11:1283-1287.

325. Erickson RP. A first therapy for Niemann-Pick C. Lancet Neurol. 2007;6:748-749.

326. Farber S, Cohen J, Uzman LL. Lipogranulomatosis. A new lipoglycoprotein "storage" disease. J Mt Sinai Hosp N Y. 1957;24:816-837.

327. van Lijnschoten G, Groener JE, Maas SM, et al. Intrauterine fetal death due to Farber disease: case report. Pediatr Dev Pathol. 2000;3:597-602.

328. Stone DL, Sidransky E. Hydrops fetalis: lysosomal storage disorders in extremis. Adv Pediatr. 1999;46:409-440.

329. Farina F, Cappello F, Todaro M, et al. Involvement of caspase-3 and G_{D3} ganglioside in ceramide-induced apoptosis in Farber disease. J Histochem Cytochem. 2000; 48:57-62.

330. Mao C, Xu R, Szulc ZM, et al. Cloning and characterization of a novel human alkaline ceramidase. J Biol Chem. 2001;276:26577-26588.

331. El Bawab S, Roddy P, Qian T, et al. Molecular cloning and characterization of a human mitochondrial ceramidase. J Biol Chem. 2000;275:21508-21513.

332. Kishimoto Y, Hiraiwa M, O'Brien JS. Saposins: structure, function, distribution, and molecular genetics. J Lipid Res. 1992;33:1255-1267.

333. Hannun YA, Luberto C, Argraves KM. Enzymes of sphingolipid metabolism: from modular to integrative signaling. Biochemistry. 2001;24:4893-4903.

334. Liu B, Obeid LM, Hannun YA. Sphingomyelinases in cell regulation. Semin Cell Dev Biol. 1997;8:311-322.

335. Bernardo K, Hurwitz R, Zenk T, et al. Purification, characterization, and biosynthesis of human acid ceramidase. J Biol Chem 1995;270:11098-11102.

336. Koch J, Gartner S, Li CM, et al. Molecular cloning and characterization of a full-length complementary DNA encoding human acid ceramidase. Identification of the first molecular lesion causing Farber disease. J Biol Chem. 1996;271:33110-33115.

337. Zhang Z, Mandal AK, Mital A, et al. Human acid ceramidase gene: novel mutations in Farber disease. Mol Genet Metab. 2000;70:301-309.

338. Bar J, Linke T, Ferlinz K, et al. Molecular analysis of acid ceramidase deficiency in patients with Farber disease. Hum Mutat. 2001;17:199-209.

339. Haraoka G, Muraoka M, Yoshioka N, et al. First case of surgical treatment of Farber's disease. Ann Plast Surg. 1997;39:405-410.

340. Yeager AM, Uhas KA, Coles CD, et al. Bone marrow transplantation for infantile ceramidase deficiency (Farber disease). Bone Marrow Transplant. 2000;26:357-363.

341. Medin JA, Takenaka T, Carpentier S, et al. Retrovirus-mediated correction of the metabolic defect in cultured Farber disease cells. Hum Gene Ther. 1999;10: 1321-1329.

342. Landing BH, Silverman FN, Craig JM, et al. Familial neurovisceral lipidosis. An analysis of eight cases of a syndrome previously reported as "Hurler-variant," "pseudo-Hurler disease" and "Tay-Sachs disease with visceral involvement." Am J Dis Child. 1964;108:503-522.

343. O'Brien JS, Stern MB, Landing BH, et al. Generalized gangliosidosis: another inborn error of ganglioside metabolism? Am J Dis Child. 1965;109:338-346.

344. Okada S, O'Brien JS. Generalized gangliosidosis: beta-galactosidase deficiency. Science. 1968;160:1002-1004.

345. Georgiou T, Stylianidou G, Anastasiadou V, et al. The Arg482His mutation in the beta-galactosidase gene is responsible for a high frequency of G_{M1} gangliosidosis carriers in a Cypriot village. Genet Test. 2005;9:126-132.

346. Severini MH, Silva CD, Sopelsa A, et al. High frequency of type 1 G_{M1} gangliosidosis in southern Brazil. Clin Genet. 1999;56:168-169.

347. Takano T, Yamanouchi Y. Assignment of human beta-galactosidase-A gene to 3p21.33 by fluorescence in situ hybridization. Hum Genet. 1993;92:403-404.

348. Oshima A, Tsuji A, Nagao Y, et al. Cloning, sequencing, and expression of cDNA for human β-galactosidase. Biochem Biophys Res Commun. 1988;157:238-244.

349. Morreau H, Galjart NJ, Gillemans N, et al. Alternative splicing of beta-galactosidase mRNA generates the classic lysosomal enzyme and a beta-galactosidase–related protein. J Biol Chem. 1989;264:20655-20663.

350. Privitera S, Prody CA, Callahan JW, Hinek A. The 67-kDa enzymatically inactive alternatively spliced variant of beta-galactosidase is identical to the elastin/laminin-binding protein. J Biol Chem. 1998;273:6319-6326.

351. Hinek A, Zhang S, Smith AC, Callahan JW. Impaired elastic-fiber assembly by fibroblasts from patients with either Morquio B disease or infantile G_{M1}-gangliosidosis is linked to deficiency in the 67-kD spliced variant of beta-galactosidase. Am J Hum Genet. 2000;67:23-36.

352. Hinek A. Nature and the multiple functions of the 67-kD elastin-/laminin binding protein. Cell Adhes Commun. 1994;2:185-193.

353. Brunetti-Pierri N, Scaglia F. G_{M1}-gangliosidosis: review of clinical, molecular and therapeutic aspects. Mol Genet Metab. 2008;94:391-396.

354. Huwiler A, Kolter T, Pfeilschifter J, Sandhoff K. Physiology and pathophysiology of sphingolipid metabolism and signaling. Biochim Biophys Acta. 2000;1485:63-99.

355. Tettamanti G. Ganglioside/glycosphingolipid turnover: new concepts. Glycoconj J. 2004;20:301-317.

356. Pike LJ. Growth factor receptors, lipid rafts and caveolae: an evolving story. Biochim Biophys Acta. 2005;1746: 260-273.

357. Callahan JW. Molecular basis of G_{M1} gangliosidosis and Morquio disease, type B. Structure-function studies of lysosomal beta-galactosidase and the non-lysosomal beta-galactosidase–like protein. Biochim Biophys Acta. 1999; 1455:85-103.

358. Suzuki Y, Oshima A, Nanba E. β-Galactosidase deficiency (β-galactosidosis): G_{M1} gangliosidosis and Morquio B disease. In Scriver CR, Sly WS, Childs B, et al (eds). The Metabolic and Molecular Bases of Inherited Disease, 8th ed. New York, McGraw-Hill, 2001, pp 3775-3810.

359. Zhang S, Bagshaw R, Hilson W, et al. Characterization of beta-galactosidase mutations Asp332→Asn and Arg148→ Ser, and a polymorphism, Ser532→Gly, in a case of G_{M1} gangliosidosis. Biochem J. 2000;348:621-632.

360. van der Spoel A, Bonten E, d'Azzo A. Processing of lysosomal beta-galactosidase. The C-terminal precursor fragment is an essential domain of the mature enzyme. J Biol Chem. 2000;275:10035-10040.

361. Morrone A, Bardelli T, Donati MA, et al. β-Galactosidase gene mutations affecting the lysosomal enzyme and the elastin binding protein in G_{M1}-gangliosidosis patients with cardiac involvement. Hum Mutat. 2000;15:354-366.

362. Caciotti A, Donati MA, Boneh A, et al. Role of beta-galactosidase and elastin binding protein in lysosomal and nonlysosomal complexes of patients with G_{M1}-gangliosidosis. Hum Mutat. 2005;25:285-292.

363. Sinelli MT, Motta M, Cattarelli D, et al. Fetal hydrops in GM(1) gangliosidosis: a case report. Acta Paediatr. 2005;94:1847-1849.

364. Chen CC, Chiu PC, Shieh KS. Type 1 G_{M1} gangliosidosis with basal ganglia calcification: a case report. Zhonghua Yi Xue Za Zhi (Taipei). 1999;62:40-45.

365. Lin HC, Tsai FJ, Shen WC, et al. Infantile form G_{M1} gangliosidosis with dilated cardiomyopathy: a case report. Acta Paediatr. 2000;89:880-883.

366. Al-Essa MA, Bakheet SM, Patay ZJ, et al. Cerebral fluorine-18 labeled 2-fluoro-2-deoxyglucose positron emission tomography (FDG PET), MRI, and clinical observations in a patient with infantile G_{M1} gangliosidosis. Brain Dev. 1999;21:559-562.

367. Folkerth RD, Alroy J, Bhan I, Kaye EM. Infantile G_{M1} gangliosidosis: complete morphology and histochemistry of two autopsy cases, with particular reference to delayed central nervous system myelination. Pediatr Dev Pathol. 2000;3:73-86.

368. Shen WC, Tsai FJ, Tsai CH. Myelination arrest demonstrated using magnetic resonance imaging in a child with type I G_{M1} gangliosidosis. J Formos Med Assoc. 1998;97:296-299.

369. Gascon GG, Ozand PT, Erwin RE. G_{M1} gangliosidosis type 2 in two siblings. J Child Neurol. 1992;7(Suppl): S41-S50.

370. Suzuki K, Chen GC. G_{M1} gangliosidosis (generalized gangliosidosis). Morphology and chemical pathology. Pathol Eur. 1968;3:389-408.

371. Takahashi Y, Orii T. Severity of G_{M1} gangliosidosis and urinary oligosaccharide excretion. Clin Chim Acta. 1989;179:153-162.

372. Ng-Ying-Kin NMK, Wolfe LS. Characterization of oligosaccharides and glycopeptides excreted in the urine of G_{M1}-gangliosidosis patients. Biochem Biophys Res Commun. 1975;66:123-130.

373. Raghavan S, Gajewski A, Kolodny EH. G_{M1}-ganglioside β-galactosidase in leukocytes and cultured fibroblasts. Clin Chim Acta. 1977;81:47-56.

374. Caciotti A, Donati MA, Procopio E, et al. G_{M1} gangliosidosis: molecular analysis of nine patients and development of an RT-PCR assay for GLB1 gene expression profiling. Hum Mutat. 2007;28:204.

375. Nishimoto J, Nanba E, Inui K, et al. G_{M1}-gangliosidosis (genetic beta-galactosidase deficiency): identification of four mutations in different clinical phenotypes among Japanese patients. Am J Hum Genet. 1991;49:566-574.

376. Oshima A, Yoshida K, Shimmoto M, et al. Human beta-galactosidase gene mutations in Morquio B disease. Am J Hum Genet. 1991;49:1091-1093.

377. Caciotti A, Bardelli T, Cunningham J, et al. Modulating action of the new polymorphism L436F detected in the GLB1 gene of a type-II G_{M1} gangliosidosis patient. Hum Genet. 2003;113:44-50.

378. Vogel A, Fürst W, Abo-Hashish MA, et al. Identity of the activator proteins for the enzymatic hydrolysis of sulfatide, ganglioside G_{M1} and globotriosylceramide. Arch Biochem Biophys. 1987;259:627-638.

379. Matsuda J, Suzuki O, Oshima A, et al. Beta-galactosidase–deficient mouse as an animal model for G_{M1}-gangliosidosis. Glycoconj J. 1997;14:729-736.

380. Hahn C, Martin M, Schröder M, et al. Generalized CNS disease and massive G_{M1}-ganglioside accumulation in mice defective in lysosomal acid β-galactosidase. Hum Mol Gen. 1997;6:205-211.

381. Itoh M, Matsuda J, Suzuki O, et al. Development of lysosomal storage in mice with targeted disruption of the beta-galactosidase gene: a model of human G(M1)-gangliosidosis. Brain Dev. 2001;23:379-384.

382. Jeyakumar M, Thomas R, Elliot-Smith E, et al. Central nervous system inflammation is a hallmark of pathogenesis in mouse models of G_{M1} and G_{M2} gangliosidosis. Brain. 2003;126:974-987.

383. Ledeen RW, Wu G. Ganglioside function in calcium homeostasis and signaling. Neurochem Res. 2002;27:637-647.

384. Patil C, Walter P. Intracellular signaling from the endoplasmic reticulum to the nucleus: the unfolded protein response in yeast and mammals. Curr Opin Cell Biol. 2001;13:349-355.

385. Oehmig A, Cortés ML, Perry KF, et al. Integration of active human beta-galactosidase gene (100 kb) into genome using HSV/AAV amplicon vector. Gene Ther. 2007;14:1078-1091.

386. Shield JP, Stone J, Steward CG. Bone marrow transplantation correcting beta-galactosidase activity does not

influence neurological outcome in juvenile G$_{M1}$-gangliosidosis. J Inherit Metab Dis. 2005;28:797-798.

387. Suzuki Y, Ichinomiya S, Kurosawa M, et al. Chemical chaperone therapy: clinical effect in murine G(M1)-gangliosidosis. Ann Neurol. 2007;62:671-675.

388. Kasperzyk JL, d'Azzo A, Platt FM, et al. Substrate reduction reduces gangliosides in postnatal cerebrum-brainstem and cerebellum in G$_{M1}$ gangliosidosis mice. J Lipid Res. 2005;46:744-751.

389. Neufeld EF. Natural history and inherited disorders of a lysosomal enzyme, beta-hexosaminidase. J Biol Chem. 1989;264:10927-10930.

390. Neufeld EF, d'Azzo A. Biosynthesis of normal and mutant beta-hexosaminidases. Adv Genet. 2001;44:165-171.

391. Gravel RA, Kaback MM, Proia RL, et al. The G$_{M2}$ gangliosidoses. In Scriver CR, Sly WS, Childs B, et al. (eds). The Metabolic and Molecular Bases of Inherited Disease, 8th ed. New York, McGraw-Hill, 2001, pp 2839-2879.

392. Kolodny EH. The G$_{M2}$-gangliosidoses. In Rosenberg RN, Prusiner SB, Dimauro S, Barchi RL (eds). The Molecular and Genetic Basis of Neurological Disease. Boston, Butterworth-Heinemann, 1966.

393. Sandhoff K, Harzer K, Jatzkewitz H. Densitometric microdetermination of gangliosides from total lipid extract following thin layer chromatography. Hoppe Seylers Z Physiol Chem. 1968;349:283-287.

394. Sango K, Yamanaka S, Hoffmann A, et al. Mouse models of Tay-Sachs and Sandhoff diseases differ in neurologic phenotype and ganglioside metabolism. Nat Genet. 1995;11:170-176.

395. Sango K, McDonald MP, Crawley JN, et al. Mice lacking both subunits of lysosomal beta-hexosaminidase display gangliosidosis and mucopolysaccharidosis. Nat Genet. 1996;14:348-352.

396. Proia RL. Targeting the hexosaminidase genes: mouse models of the G$_{M2}$ gangliosidoses. Adv Genet. 2001;44:225-231.

397. Yamanaka S, Johnson MD, Grinberg A, et al. Targeted disruption of the Hexa gene results in mice with biochemical and pathologic features of Tay-Sachs disease. Proc Natl Acad Sci U S A. 1994;91:9975-9979.

398. Pelled D, Lloyd-Evans E, Riebeling C, et al. Inhibition of calcium uptake via the sarco/endoplasmic reticulum Ca^{2+}-ATPase in a mouse model of Sandhoff disease and prevention by treatment with *N*-butyldeoxynojirimycin. J Biol Chem. 2003;278:29496-29501.

399. Arfi A, Zisling R, Richard E, et al. Reversion of the biochemical defects in murine embryonic Sandhoff neurons using a bicistronic lentiviral vector encoding hexosaminidase alpha and beta. J Neurochem. 2006;96:1572-1579.

400. Jeyakumar M, Butters TD, Cortina-Borja M, et al. Delayed symptom onset and increased life expectancy in Sandhoff disease mice treated with *N*-butyldeoxynojirimycin. Proc Natl Acad Sci U S A. 1999;96:6388-6393.

401. Norflus F, Tifft CJ, McDonald MP, et al. Bone marrow transplantation prolongs life span and ameliorates neurologic manifestations in Sandhoff disease mice. J Clin Invest. 1998;101:1881-1888.

402. Yamaguchi A, Katsuyama K, Suzuki K, et al. Plasmid-based gene transfer ameliorates visceral storage in a mouse model of Sandhoff disease. J Mol Med. 2003;81:185-193.

403. Bourgoin C, Emiliani C, Kremer EJ, et al. Widespread distribution of beta-hexosaminidase activity in the brain of a Sandhoff mouse model after coinjection of adenoviral vector and mannitol. Gene Ther. 2003;10:1841-1849.

404. Cachón-González MB, Wang SZ, Lynch A, et al. Effective gene therapy in an authentic model of Tay-Sachs–related diseases. Proc Natl Acad Sci U S A. 2006;103:10373-10378.

405. Neufeld EF, Muenzer J. The mucopolysaccharidoses. In Scriver CR, Sly WS, Childs B, et al. (eds). The Metabolic and Molecular Bases of Inherited Disease, 8th ed. New York, McGraw-Hill, 2001.

406. Nelson J. Incidence of the mucopolysaccharidoses in Northern Ireland. Hum Genet. 1997;101:355-358.

407. Hinek A, Wilson SE. Impaired elastogenesis in Hurler disease: dermatan sulfate accumulation linked to deficiency in elastin-binding protein and elastic fiber assembly. Am J Pathol. 2000;156:925-938.

408. Ginsberg SD, Galvin JE, Lee VM, et al. Accumulation of intracellular amyloid-β peptide (Aβ 1-40) in mucopolysaccharidosis brains. J Neuropathol Exp Neurol. 1999;58:815-824.

409. Donaldson MD, Pennock CA, Berry PJ, et al. Hurler syndrome with cardiomyopathy in infancy. J Pediatr. 1989;114:430-432.

410. Stephan MJ, Stevens EL Jr, Wenstrup RJ, et al. Mucopolysaccharidosis I presenting with endocardial fibroelastosis of infancy. Am J Dis Child. 1989;143:782-784.

411. Nowaczyk MJ, Clarke JT, Morin JD. Glaucoma as an early complication of Hurler's disease. Arch Dis Child. 1988;63:1091-1093.

412. Matalon R, Deanching M, Omura K. Hurler, Scheie, and Hurler-Scheie "compound": residual activity of α-L-iduronidase toward natural substrates suggesting allelic mutations. J Inherit Metab Dis. 1983;6(Suppl 2):133-134.

413. Tieu PT, Bach G, Matynia A, et al. Four novel mutations underlying mild or intermediate forms of α-L-iduronidase deficiency (MPS IS and MPS IH/S). Hum Mutat. 1995;6:55-59.

414. Bunge S, Kleijer WJ, Steglich C, et al. Mucopolysaccharidosis type I: identification of 13 novel mutations of the α-L-iduronidase gene. Hum Mutat. 1995;6:91-94.

415. Alif N, Hess K, Straczek J, et al. Mucopolysaccharidosis type I: characterization of a common mutation that causes Hurler syndrome in Moroccan subjects. Ann Hum Genet. 1999;63:9-16.

416. Kleijer WJ, Thompson EJ, Niermeijer MF. Prenatal diagnosis of the Hurler syndrome: report on 40 pregnancies at risk. Prenat Diagn. 1983;3:179-186.

417. Chamoles NA, Blanco M, Gaggioli D. Diagnosis of alpha-L-iduronidase deficiency in dried blood spots on filter paper: the possibility of newborn diagnosis. Clin Chem. 2001;47:780-781.

418. Hite SH, Peters C, Krivit W. Correction of odontoid dysplasia following bone-marrow transplantation and engraftment (in Hurler syndrome MPS 1H). Pediatr Radiol. 2000;30:464-470.

419. Hopwood JJ, Vellodi A, Scott HS, et al. Long-term clinical progress in bone marrow transplanted mucopolysaccharidosis type I patients with a defined genotype. J Inherit Metab Dis. 1993;16:1024-1033.

420. Kakkis ED, Schuchman E, He X, et al. Enzyme replacement therapy in feline mucopolysaccharidosis I. Mol Genet Metab. 2001;72:199-208.

421. Turner CT, Hopwood JJ, Brooks DA. Enzyme replacement therapy in mucopolysaccharidosis I: altered distribution and targeting of α-L-iduronidase in immunized rats. Mol Genet Metab. 2000;69:277-285.

422. Brooks DA. Alpha-L-iduronidase and enzyme replacement therapy for mucopolysaccharidosis I. Expert Opin Biol Ther. 2002;2:967-976.

423. Hartung SD, Reddy RG, Whitley CB, McIvor RS. Enzymatic correction and cross-correction of mucopolysaccharidosis type I fibroblasts by adeno-associated virus–mediated transduction of the α-L-iduronidase gene. Hum Gene Ther. 1999;10:2163-2172.

424. Lutzko C, Omori F, Abrams-Ogg AC, et al. Gene therapy for canine α-L-iduronidase deficiency: in utero adoptive transfer of genetically corrected hematopoietic progenitors results in engraftment but not amelioration of disease. Hum Gene Ther. 1999;10:1521-1532.

425. Watson G, Bastacky J, Belichenko P, et al. Intrathecal administration of AAV vectors for the treatment of lysosomal storage in the brains of MPS I mice. Gene Ther. 2006;13:917-925.

426. Keeling KM, Brooks DA, Hopwood JJ, et al. Gentamicin-mediated suppression of Hurler syndrome stop mutations restores a low level of α-iduronidase deficiency activity and reduces lysosomal glycosaminoglycan accumulation. Hum Mol Genet. 2001;10:291-299.

427. Sonino V, Sekarski N, Matthieu JM, Payot M. Mitral valve prolapse and type II mucopolysaccharidosis. Report of two familial cases. Arch Mal Coeur Vaiss. 2001;94:518-522.

428. Wilson PJ, Morris CP, Anson DS, et al. Hunter syndrome: isolation of an iduronate-2-sulfatase cDNA clone and analysis of patient DNA. Proc Natl Acad Sci U S A. 1990;87:8531-8535.

429. Wilson PJ, Suthers GK, Callen DF, et al. Frequent deletions at Xq28 indicate genetic heterogeneity in Hunter syndrome. Hum Genet. 1991;86:505-508.

430. Bunge S, Steglich C, Zuther C, et al. Iduronate-2-sulfatase gene mutations in 16 patients with mucopolysaccharidosis type II (Hunter syndrome). Hum Mol Genet. 1993;2:1871-1875.

431. Bondeson ML, Malmgren H, Dahl N, et al. Presence of an IDS-related locus (IDS2) in Xq28 complicates the mutational analysis of Hunter syndrome. Eur J Hum Genet. 1995;3:219-227.

432. Malmgren H, Carlberg BM, Pettersson U, Bondeson ML. Identification of an alternative transcript from the human iduronate-2-sulfatase (IDS) gene. Genomics. 1995;29:291-293.

433. Tuschl K, Gal A, Paschke E, et al. Mucopolysaccharidosis type II in females: case report and review of literature. Pediatr Neurol. 2005;32:270-272.

434. Tonnesen T, Guttler F, Lykkelund C. Reliability of the use of fructose-1-phosphate to detect Hunter cells in fibroblast-cultures of obligate characters of the Hunter syndrome. Hum Genet. 1983;64:371-375.

435. Pannone N, Gatti R, Lombardo C, Di Natale P. Prenatal diagnosis of Hunter syndrome using chorionic villi. Prenat Diagn. 1986;6:207-210.

436. Lissens W, Van Lierde M, Decaluwe J, et al. Prenatal diagnosis of Hunter syndrome using fetal plasma. Prenat Diagn. 1988;8:59-62.

437. Pan D, Jonsson JJ, Braun SE, et al. "Supercharged cells" for delivery of recombinant human iduronate-2-sulfatase. Mol Genet Metab. 2000;70:170-178.

438. Muenzer J, Wraith JE, Beck M, et al. A phase II/III clinical study of enzyme replacement therapy with idursulfase in mucopolysaccharidosis II (Hunter syndrome). Genet Med. 2006;8:465-473.

439. Cardone M, Polito VA, Pepe S, et al. Correction of Hunter syndrome in the MPSII mouse model by AAV2/8-mediated gene delivery. Hum Mol Genet. 2006;15:1225-1236.

440. Liour SS, Jones MZ, Suzuki M, et al. Metabolic studies of glycosphingolipid accumulation in mucopolysaccharidosis IIID. Mol Genet Metab. 2001;72:239-247.

441. Walkley SU. Secondary accumulation of gangliosides in lysosomal storage disorders. Semin Cell Dev Biol. 2004;15:433-444.

442. Ryazantsev S, Yu WH, Zhao HZ, et al. Lysosomal accumulation of SCMAS (subunit c of mitochondrial ATP synthase) in neurons of the mouse model of mucopolysaccharidosis III B. Mol Genet Metab. 2007;90:393-401.

443. Scott HS, Blanch L, Guo XH, et al. Cloning of the sulphamidase gene and the identification of mutations in Sanfilippo A syndrome. Nat Genet. 1995;11:465-467.

444. Yogalingam G, Hopwood JJ. Molecular genetics of mucopolysaccharidosis type IIIA and IIIB: diagnostic, clinical, and biological implications. Hum Mutat. 2001;18:264-281.

445. Yu WH, Zhao KW, Ryazantsev S, et al. Short-term enzyme replacement in the murine model of Sanfilippo syndrome type B. Mol Genet Metab. 2000;71:573-580.

446. Hrebícek M, Mrázová L, Seyrantepe V, et al. Mutations in TMEM76* cause mucopolysaccharidosis IIIC (Sanfilippo C syndrome). Am J Hum Genet. 2006;79:807-819.

447. Lindor NM, Hoffman A, O'Brien JF, et al. Sanfilippo syndrome type A in two adult sibs. Am J Med Genet. 1994;53:241-244.

448. Gliddon BL, Hopwood JJ. Enzyme-replacement therapy from birth delays the development of behavior and learning problems in mucopolysaccharidosis type IIIA mice. Pediatr Res. 2004;56:65-72.

449. Hemsley KM, King B, Hopwood JJ. Injection of recombinant human sulfamidase into the CSF via the cerebellomedullary cistern in MPS IIIA mice. Mol Genet Metab. 2007;90:313-328.

450. Roberts AL, Rees MH, Klebe S, et al. Improvement in behaviour after substrate deprivation therapy with rhodamine B in a mouse model of MPS IIIA. Mol Genet Metab. 2007;92:115-121.

451. Fraldi A, Hemsley K, Crawley A, et al. Functional correction of CNS lesions in a MPS-IIIA mouse model by intracerebral AAV-mediated delivery of sulfamidase and SUMF1 genes. Hum Mol Genet. 2007;16:2693-2702.

452. Zheng Y, Ryazantsev S, Ohmi K, et al. Retrovirally transduced bone marrow has a therapeutic effect on brain in the mouse model of mucopolysaccharidosis IIIB. Mol Genet Metab. 2004;82:286-295.

453. Garbuzova-Davis S, Willing AE, Desjarlais T, et al. Transplantation of human umbilical cord blood cells benefits

an animal model of Sanfilippo syndrome type B. Stem Cells Dev. 2005;14:384-394.

454. Fu H, Kang L, Jennings JS, et al. Significantly increased lifespan and improved behavioral performances by rAAV gene delivery in adult mucopolysaccharidosis IIIB mice. Gene Ther. 2007;14:1065-1077.

455. Downs-Kelly E, Jones MZ, Alroy J, et al. Caprine mucopolysaccharidosis IIID: a preliminary trial of enzyme replacement therapy. J Mol Neurosci. 2000;15:251-262.

456. Tomatsu S, Fukuda S, Masue M, et al. Morquio disease: isolation, characterization and expression of full-length cDNA for human *N*-acetylgalactosamine-6-sulfate sulfatase. Biochem Biophys Res Commun. 1991;181:677-683.

457. Masuno M, Tomatsu S, Nakashima Y, et al. Mucopolysaccharidosis IV A: assignment of the human *N*-acetylgalactosamine-6-sulfate sulfatase (GALNS) gene to chromosome 16q24. Genomics. 1993;16:777-778.

458. Ogawa T, Tomatsu S, Fukuda S, et al. Mucopolysaccharidosis IVA: screening and identification of mutations of the *N*-acetylgalactosamine-6-sulfate sulfatase gene. Hum Mol Genet. 1995;4:341-349.

459. Iwata H, Tomatsu S, Fukuda S, et al. Mucopolysaccharidosis IVA: polymorphic haplotypes and informative RFLPs in the Japanese population. Hum Genet. 1995;95:257-264.

460. van Gemund JJ, Giesberts MA, Eerdmans RF, et al. Morquio-B disease, spondyloepiphyseal dysplasia associated with acid β-galactosidase deficiency: report of three cases in one family. Hum Genet. 1983;64:50-54.

461. van der Horst GT, Kleijer WJ, Hoogeveen AT, et al. Morquio B syndrome: a primary defect in β-galactosidase. Am J Med Genet. 1983;16:261-275.

462. Ishii N, Oohira T, Oshima A, et al. Clinical and molecular analysis of a Japanese boy with Morquio B disease. Clin Genet. 1995;48:103-108.

463. Suzuki Y, Oshima A. A beta-galactosidase gene mutation identified in both Morquio B disease and infantile G_{M1}-gangliosidosis [letter]. Hum Genet. 1993;91:407.

464. Hayflick S, Rowe S, Kavanaugh-McHugh A, et al. Acute infantile cardiomyopathy as a presenting feature of mucopolysaccharidosis VI. J Pediatr. 1992;120:269-272.

465. Tamaki N, Kojima N, Tanimoto M, et al. Myelopathy due to diffuse thickening of the cervical dura mater in Maroteaux-Lamy syndrome: report of a case. Neurosurgery. 1987;21:416-419.

466. Voskoboeva E, Isbrandt D, von Figura K, et al. Four novel mutant alleles of the arylsulfatase B gene in two patients with intermediate form of mucopolysaccharidosis VI (Maroteaux-Lamy syndrome). Hum Genet. 1994;93:259-264.

467. Isbrandt D, Arlt G, Brooks DA, et al. Mucopolysaccharidosis VI (Maroteaux-Lamy syndrome): six unique arylsulfatase B gene alleles causing variable disease phenotypes. Am J Hum Genet. 1994;54:454-463.

468. Harmatz P, Ketteridge D, Giugliani R, et al. Direct comparison of measures of endurance, mobility, and joint function during enzyme-replacement therapy of mucopolysaccharidosis VI (Maroteaux-Lamy syndrome): results after 48 weeks in a phase 2 open-label clinical study of recombinant human *N*-acetylgalactosamine 4-sulfatase. Pediatrics. 2005;115:e681-e689.

469. Karageorgos L, Brooks DA, Harmatz P, et al. Mutational analysis of mucopolysaccharidosis type VI patients undergoing a phase II trial of enzyme replacement therapy. Mol Genet Metab. 2007;90:164-170.

470. Yogalingam G, Crawley A, Hopwood JJ, Anson DS. Evaluation of fibroblast-mediated gene therapy in a feline model of mucopolysaccharidosis type VI. Biochim Biophys Acta. 1999;1453:284-296.

471. Tessitore A, Faella A, O'Malley T, et al. Biochemical, pathological, and skeletal improvement of mucopolysaccharidosis VI after gene transfer to liver but not to muscle. Mol Ther. 2008;16:30-37.

472. Sly WS, Quinton BA, McAlister WH, Rimoin DL. Beta-glucuronidase deficiency: report of clinical, radiologic, and biochemical features of a new mucopolysaccharidosis. J Pediatr. 1973;82:249-257.

473. Vogler C, Levy B, Kyle JW, et al. Mucopolysaccharidosis VII: postmortem biochemical and pathological findings in a young adult with beta-glucuronidase deficiency. Mod Pathol. 1994;7:132-137.

474. Irani D, Kim HS, El-Hibri H, et al. Postmortem observations on beta-glucuronidase deficiency presenting as lethal hydrops fetalis. Ann Neurol. 1983;14:486-490.

475. Lee JE, Falk R, Ng WG, Donnell JN. β-Glucuronidase deficiency. Am J Dis Child. 1958;139:57.

476. de Kremer RD, Givogri I, Argaraña CE, et al. Mucopolysaccharidosis type VII (β-glucuronidase deficiency): a chronic variant with an oligosymptomatic severe skeletal dysplasia. Am J Med Genet. 1992;44:145-152.

477. Oshima A, Kyle JW, Miller RD, et al. Cloning, sequencing and expression of cDNA for human β-glucuronidase. Proc Natl Acad Sci U S A. 1987;84:685-689.

478. Miller R, Hoffmann J, Powell PP, et al. Cloning and characterization of the human β-glucuronidase gene. Genomics. 1990;7:280-283.

479. Wu BM, Sly WS. Mutational studies in a patient with the hydrops fetalis form of mucopolysaccharidosis type VII. Hum Mutat. 1993;2:446.

480. Chab's A, Guardiola A: β-Glucuronidase deficiency: identification of an affected fetus with simultaneous sampling of chorionic villus and amniotic fluid. Prenat Diagn. 1993;13:429.

481. Birkenmeier EH, Davisson MT, Beamer WG, et al. Murine mucopolysaccharidosis type VII. Characterization of a mouse with beta-glucuronidase deficiency. J Clin Invest. 1989;83:1258-1266.

482. Schuchman EH, Toroyan TK, Haskins ME, Desnick RJ. Characterization of the defective beta-glucuronidase activity in canine mucopolysaccharidosis type VII. Enzyme. 1989;42:174-180.

483. Snyder EY, Taylor RM, Wolfe JH. Neural progenitor cell engraftment corrects lysosomal storage throughout the MPS VII mouse brain. Nature. 1995;374:367.

484. Poorthuis BJ, Romme AE, Willemsen R, Wagemaker G. Bone marrow transplantation has a significant effect on enzyme levels and storage of glycosaminoglycans in tissues and in isolated hepatocytes of mucopolysaccharidosis type VII mice. Pediatr Res. 1994;36:187-193.

485. Vogler C, Levy B, Grubb JH, et al. Overcoming the blood-brain barrier with high-dose enzyme replacement therapy in murine mucopolysaccharidosis VII. Proc Natl Acad Sci U S A. 2005;102:14777-14782.

486. Liu G, Chen YH, He X, et al. Adeno-associated virus type 5 reduces learning deficits and restores glutamate receptor subunit levels in MPS VII mice CNS. Mol Ther. 2007; 15:242-247.

487. Guerra W, Verity MA, Fluharty AL, et al. Multiple sulfatase deficiency: clinical, neuropathological, ultrastructural and biochemical studies. J Neuropathol Exp Neurol. 1990;49:406-423.

488. Polten A, Fluharty AL, Fluharty CB, et al. Molecular basis of different forms of metachromatic leukodystrophy. N Engl J Med. 1991;324:18-22.

489. Schmidt B, Selmer T, Ingendoh A, von Figura K. A novel amino acid modification in sulfatases that is defective in multiple sulfatase deficiency. Cell. 1995;82:271-278.

490. Dierks T, Schmidt B, Borissenko LV, et al. Multiple sulfatase deficiency is caused by mutations in the gene encoding the human C(alpha)-formylglycine generating enzyme. Cell. 2003;113:435-444.

491. Cosma MP, Pepe S, Annunziata I, et al. The multiple sulfatase deficiency gene encodes an essential and limiting factor for the activity of sulfatases. Cell. 2003;113:445-456.

492. Settembre C, Annunziata I, Spampanato C, et al. Systemic inflammation and neurodegeneration in a mouse model of multiple sulfatase deficiency. Proc Natl Acad Sci U S A. 2007;104:4506-4511.

493. Spranger JW, Wiedemann HR. The genetic mucolipidoses: diagnosis and differential diagnosis. Hum Genet. 1970;9:113.

494. Michalski JC, Klein A. Glycoprotein lysosomal storage disorders: alpha- and beta-mannosidosis, fucosidosis and alpha-N-acetylgalactosaminidase deficiency. Biochim Biophys Acta. 1999;1455:69-84.

495. d'Azzo A, Andria G, Strisciuglio P, Galjaard H. Galactosialidosis. In Scriver CR, Sly WS, Childs B, et al (eds). The Metabolic and Molecular Bases of Inherited Disease, 8th ed. New York, McGraw-Hill, 2001, pp 3811-3826.

496. Thomas GH. Disorders of glycoprotein degradation and structure: α-mannosidosis, β-mannosidosis, fucosidosis, and sialidosis. In Scriver CR, Sly WS, Childs B, et al (eds). The Metabolic and Molecular Bases of Inherited Disease, 8th ed. New York, McGraw-Hill, 2001, pp 3507-3534.

497. Bonten E, van der Spoel A, Fornerod M, et al. Characterization of human lysosomal neuraminidase defines the molecular basis of the metabolic storage disorder sialidosis. Genes Dev. 1996;10:3156-3169.

498. Saito M, Yu RK. Biochemistry and function of sialidases. In Rosenberg A (ed). Biology of the Sialic Acids. New York, Plenum Press, 1995, pp 261-313.

499. Achyuthan KE, Achyuthan AM. Comparative enzymology, biochemistry and pathophysiology of human exo-alpha-sialidases (neuraminidases). Comp Biochem Physiol B Biochem Mol Biol. 2001;129:29-64.

500. Igdoura SA, Gafuik C, Mertineit C, et al. Cloning of the cDNA and gene encoding mouse lysosomal sialidase and correction of sialidase deficiency in human sialidosis and mouse SM/J fibroblasts. Hum Mol Genet. 1998;7:115-121.

501. Rottier RJ, Hahn CN, Mann LW, et al. Lack of PPCA expression only partially coincides with lysosomal storage in galactosialidosis mice: indirect evidence for spatial requirement of the catalytic rather than the protective function of PPCA. Hum Mol Genet. 1998;7:1787-1794.

502. d'Azzo A. Protective protein cathepsin A (PPCA). In Wiley Encyclopedia of Molecular Medicine. Hoboken, NJ, John Wiley, 2002, pp 2624-2628.

503. van der Spoel A, Bonten E, d'Azzo A. Transport of human lysosomal neuraminidase to mature lysosomes requires protective protein/cathepsin A. EMBO J. 1998;17:1588-1597.

504. Stamatos NM, Curreli S, Zella D, Cross AS. Desialylation of glycoconjugates on the surface of monocytes activates the extracellular signal–related kinases ERK 1/2 and results in enhanced production of specific cytokines. J Leukoc Biol. 2004;75:307-313.

505. Cross AS, Sakarya S, Rifat S, et al. Recruitment of murine neutrophils in vivo through endogenous sialidase activity. J Biol Chem. 2003;278:4112-4120.

506. Starr TK, Daniels MA, Lucido MM, et al. Thymocyte sensitivity and supramolecular activation cluster formation are developmentally regulated: a partial role for sialylation. J Immunol. 2003;171:4512-4520.

507. Pshezhetsky AV, Richard C, Michaud L, et al. Cloning, expression and chromosomal mapping of human lysosomal sialidase and characterization of mutations in sialidosis. Nat Genet. 1997;3:316-320.

508. Bonten EJ, Arts WF, Beck M, et al. Novel mutations in lysosomal neuraminidase identify functional domains and determine clinical severity in sialidosis. Hum Mol Genet. 2000;18:2715-2725.

509. Lukong KE, Elsliger MA, Chang Y, et al. Characterization of the sialidase molecular defects in sialidosis patients suggests the structural organization of the lysosomal multienzyme complex. Hum Mol Genet. 2000;9:1075-1085.

510. Naganawa Y, Itoh K, Shimmoto M, et al. Molecular and structural studies of Japanese patients with sialidosis type 1. J Hum Genet. 2000;45:241-249.

511. Seyrantepe V, Poupetova H, Froissart R, et al. Molecular pathology of NEU1 gene in sialidosis. Hum Mutat. 2003; 22:343-352.

512. Loren DJ, Campos Y, d'Azzo A, et al. Sialidosis presenting as severe nonimmune fetal hydrops is associated with two novel mutations in lysosomal alpha-neuraminidase. J Perinatol. 2005;25:491-494.

513. Palmeri S, Villanova M, Malandrina A, et al. Type I sialidosis: a clinical, biochemical and neuroradiological study. Eur Neurol. 2000;43:88-94.

514. Goldstein ML, Kolodny EH, Gascon CG, Gilles FH. Macular cherry-red spot, myoclonic epilepsy and neurovisceral storage in a 17-year-old girl. Trans Am Neurol Assoc. 1974;99:110-112.

515. Durand P, Gatti R, Cavalieri S, et al. Sialidosis (mucolipidosis 1). Helv Paediatr Acta. 1977;32:391-400.

516. Rapin I, Goldfischer S, Katzman R, et al. The cherry-red spot myoclonus syndrome. Ann Neurol. 1978;3:234-242.

517. Thomas GH, Tipton RE, Ch'ien LT, et al. Sialidase (α-N-acetyl-neuraminidase) deficiency: the enzyme defect in an adult with macular cherry-red spots and myoclonus without dementia. A new autosomal recessive disorder. Clin Genet. 1978;13:369-379.

518. Gascon G, Wallenberg B, Daif AK, Ozand P. Successful treatment of cherry-red spot myoclonus syndrome with 5-hydroxytryptophan. Ann Neurol. 1988;24:453-458.

519. Young ID, Young EP, Mossman J, et al. Neuraminidase deficiency: case report and review of the phenotype. J Med Genet. 1987;24:283-290.

520. Laver J, Fried K, Beer SI, et al. Infantile lethal neuraminidase deficiency (sialidosis). Clin Genet. 1983;23:97101.

521. van Pelt J, Kamerling JP, Vliegenthart JF, et al. A comparative study of the accumulated sialic acid–containing oligosaccharides from cultured human galactosialidosis and sialidosis fibroblasts. Clin Chim Acta. 1988;174:325-335.

522. van Pelt J, Kamerling JP, Vliegenthart JF, et al. Isolation and structural characterization of sialic acid–containing storage material from mucolipidosis I (sialidosis) fibroblasts. Biochim Biophys Acta. 1988;965:36-45.

523. d'Azzo A, Hoogeveen A, Reuser AJ, et al. Molecular defect in combined beta-galactosidase and neuraminidase deficiency in man. Proc Natl Acad Sci U S A. 1982;79:4535-4539.

524. d'Azzo A. Defects in lysosomal enzyme protection: galactosialidosis. In Platt F, Walkley S (eds). Lysosomal Disorders of Brain: Recent Advances in Molecular and Cellular Pathogenesis and Treatment. London, Oxford University Press, 2004, pp 170-185.

525. Day JR, Albers JJ, Lofton-Day CE, et al. Complete cDNA encoding human phospholipid transfer protein from human endothelial cells. J Biol Chem. 1994;269:9388-9391.

526. Wiegant J, Galjart NJ, Raap AK, d'Azzo A. The gene encoding human protective protein (PPGB) is on chromosome-20. Genomics. 1991;10:345-349.

527. Nastasi T, Bongiovanni A, Campos Y, et al. Ozz-E3, a muscle-specific ubiquitin ligase, regulates beta-catenin degradation during myogenesis. Dev Cell. 2004;2:269-282.

528. Galjart NJ, Gillemans N, Harris A, et al. Expression of cDNA encoding the human "protective protein" associated with lysosomal beta-galactosidase and neuraminidase: homology to yeast proteases. Cell. 1988;54:755-764.

529. Rudenko G, Bonten E, d'Azzo A, Hol WGJ. Three-dimensional structure of the human "protective protein": structure of the precursor form suggests a complex activation mechanism. Structure. 1995;3:1249-1259.

530. Galjart NJ, Gillemans N, Meijer D, d'Azzo A. Mouse "protective protein." cDNA cloning, sequence comparison, and expression. J Biol Chem. 1990;265:4678-4684.

531. Galjart NJ, Morreau H, Willemsen R, et al. Human lysosomal protective protein has cathepsin A–like activity distinct from its protective function. J Biol Chem. 1991;266:14754-14762.

532. Jackman HL, Morris PW, Deddish PA, et al. Inactivation of endothelin I by deamidase (lysosomal protective protein). J Biol Chem. 1992;267:2872-2875.

533. Jackman HL, Tan FL, Tamei H, et al. A peptidase in human platelets that deamidates tachykinins. Probable identity with the lysosomal "protective protein." J Biol Chem. 1990;265:11265-11272.

534. Rudenko G, Bonten E, Hol W, d'Azzo A. The atomic model of the human protective protein/cathepsin A suggests a structural basis for galactosialidosis. Proc Natl Acad Sci U S A. 1998;95:621-625.

535. Zhou XY, Galjart NJ, Willemsen R, et al. A mutation in a mild form of galactosialidosis impairs dimerization of the protective protein and renders it unstable. EMBO J. 1991;10:4041-4048.

536. Zhou X-Y, van der Spoel A, Rottier R, et al. Molecular and biochemical analysis of protective protein/cathepsin A mutations: correlation with clinical severity in galactosialidosis. Hum Mol Genet. 1996;5:1977-1987.

537. Van Pelt J, Hård K, Kamerling JP, et al. Isolation and structural characterization of twenty-one sialyloligosaccharides from galactosialidosis urine. Biol Chem Hoppe Seyler. 1989;370:191-203.

538. Sakuraba H, Suzuki Y, Akagi M, et al. α-Galactosidase-neuraminidase deficiency (galactosialidosis): clinical, pathological, and enzymatic studies in a postmortem case. Ann Neurol. 1983;13:497-503.

539. Kleijer WJ, Hoogeveen A, Verheijen FW, et al. Prenatal diagnosis of sialidosis with combined neuraminidase and β-galactosidase deficiency. Clin Genet. 1979;16:60-61.

540. Gravel R, Lowden J, Callahan J, et al. Infantile sialidosis: a phenocopy of type 1 G_{M1} gangliosidosis distinguished by genetic complementation and urinary oligosaccharides. Am J Hum Genet. 1979;31:669.

541. Zammarchi E, Donati MA, Marrone A, et al. Early infantile galactosialidosis: clinical, biochemical, and molecular observations in a new patient. Am J Med Genet. 1996;64:453-458.

542. Pinsky L, Miller J, Shanfield B, et al. G_{M1} gangliosidosis in skin fibroblast culture: enzymatic difference between types 1 and 2 and observations on a third variant. Am J Hum Genet. 1974;26:563-577.

543. Andria G, Strisciuglio P, Pontarelli G, et al. Infantile neuraminidase and β-galactosidase deficiencies (galactosialidosis) with mild clinical courses. In Durand P, Tettamanti G, DiDonato S (eds). Sialidases and Sialidoses. Milan, Italy, Edi Ermes, 1981, pp 379-395.

544. Orii T, Minami R, Sukegawa K, et al. A new type of mucolipidosis with β-galactosidase deficiency and glycopeptiduria. Tohoko J Exp Med. 1972;107:303.

545. Wenger DA, Tarby TJ, Wharton C. Macular cherry-red spots and myoclonus with dementia: coexistent neuraminidase and β-galactosidase deficiencies. Biochem Biophys Res Commun. 1978;82:589-595.

546. Zhou XY, Morreau H, Rottier R, et al. Mouse model for the lysosomal disorder galactosialidosis and correction of the phenotype with over-expressing erythroid precursor cells. Genes Dev. 1995;9:2623-2634.

547. De Geest N, Bonten E, Mann L, et al. Systemic and neurologic abnormalities distinguish the lysosomal disorders sialidosis and galactosialidosis in mice. Hum Mol Genet. 2002;11:1455-1464.

548. Chen XP, Enioutina EY, Daynes RA. The control of IL-4 gene expression in activated murine T lymphocytes: a novel role for neu-1 sialidase. J Immunol. 1997;158:3070-3080.

549. Hahn CN, del Pilar Martin M, Zhou XY, et al. Correction of murine galactosialidosis by bone marrow–derived macrophages overexpressing human protective protein/cathepsin A under control of the colony-stimulating factor-1 receptor promoter. Proc Natl Acad Sci U S A. 1998;95:14880-14885.

550. Wang D, Bonten EJ, Yogalingam G, et al. Short-term, high dose enzyme replacement therapy in sialidosis mice. Mol Genet Metab. 2005;85:181-189.

551. Tiede S, Muschol N, Reutter G, et al. Missense mutations in *N*-acetylglucosamine-1-phosphotransferase alpha/beta subunit gene in a patient with mucolipidosis III and a mild clinical phenotype. Am J Med Genet A. 2005;137: 235-240.

552. Bao M, Booth JL, Canfield WM. Bovine UDP-*N*-acetylglucosamine: lysosomal-enzyme *N*-acetylglucosamine-1-phosphotransferase. I. Purification and subunit structure. J Biol Chem. 1996;271:31437-31445.

553. Raas-Rothschild A, Cormier-Daire V, Bao M, et al. Molecular basis of variant pseudo-Hurler polydystrophy (mucolipidosis IIIC). J Clin Invest. 2000;105:673-681.

554. Beck M, Barone R, Hoffmann R, et al. Inter- and intrafamilial variability in mucolipidosis II (I-cell disease). Clin Genet. 1995;47:191-191.

555. Appelman Z, Blumberg B, Golabi M, Golbus MS. Nonimmune hydrops fetalis may be associated with an elevated δOD450 in the amniotic fluid. Obstet Gynecol. 1988;71:1005-1008.

556. Babcock DS, Bove KE, Hug G, et al. Fetal mucolipidosis II (I-cell disease): radiologic and pathologic correlation. Pediatr Radiol. 1986;16:32-39.

557. Pazzaglia UE, Beluffi G, Campbell JB, et al. Mucolipidosis II: correlation between radiological features and histopathology of the bones. Pediatr Radiol. 1989;19: 406-413.

558. Mueller OT, Wasmuth JJ, et al. Chromosomal assignment of *N*-acetylglucosaminylphosphotransferase, the lysosomal targeting enzyme deficient in mucolipidosis II and III [abstract]. Cytogenet Cell Genet. 1987;46: 664.

559. Ben-Yoseph Y, Baylerian MS, Nadler HL. Radiometric assays of *N*-acetylglucosaminylphosphotransferase and *N*-acetylglucosaminyl phosphodiesterase with substrates labeled in the glucosamine moiety. Anal Biochem. 1984; 142:297-304.

560. Parvathy MR, Mitchell D, Ben-Yoseph Y. Prenatal diagnosis of I-cell disease in the first and second trimester. Am J Med Sci. 1989;296:361-364.

561. Ben-Yoseph Y, Mitchell DA, Nadler HL. First trimester prenatal evaluation for I-cell disease by *N*-acetylglucosamine 1-phosphotransferase assay. Clin Genet. 1988;33:38-43.

562. Kurobane I, Aikawa J, et al. Bone marrow transplantation in I-cell disease. In Hobbs JR (ed). Correction of Certain Genetic Diseases by Transplantation. London, Cogent, 1989, p 132.

563. Brik R, Mandel H, Aizin A, et al. Mucolipidosis III presenting as a rheumatological disorder. J Rheumatol. 1993;20:133-136.

564. Traboulosi E, Maumenee I. Ophthalmologic findings in mucolipidosis III (pseudo-Hurler polydystrophy). Am J Ophthalmol. 1986;120:592.

565. Hasilik A, Waheed A, Cantz M, von Figura K. Impaired phosphorylation of lysosomal enzymes in fibroblasts of patients with mucolipidosis III. Eur J Biochem. 1982; 122:119-123.

566. Mueller O, Little L, Miller AL, et al. I-cell disease and pseudo-Hurler polydystrophy: heterozygote detection and characteristics of the altered *N*-acetyl-glucosamine-phosphotransferase in genetic variants. Clin Chim Acta. 1985;150:175-183.

567. Berman ER, Livni N, Shapira E, et al. Congenital corneal clouding with abnormal systemic storage bodies: a new variant of mucolipidosis. J Pediatr. 1974;84:519-526.

568. Crandell BF, Philippart M, Brown WJ, Bluestone DA. Review article: mucolipidosis IV. Am J Med Genet. 1982;12:301-308.

569. Lubensky IA, Schiffmann R, Goldin E, Tsokos M. Lysosomal inclusions in gastric parietal cells in mucolipidosis type IV: a novel cause of achlorhydria and hypergastrinemia. Am J Surg Pathol. 1999;23:1527-1531.

570. Lake BD, Milla PJ, Taylor DS, Young EP. A mild variant of mucolipidosis type 4 (ML4). Birth Defects. 1982;18:391-404.

571. Reis S, Sheffer RH, Merin S, et al. Mucolipidosis type IV: a mild form with late onset. Am J Med Genet. 1993; 47:392.

572. Tellez-Nagel I, Rapin I, Iwamoto T, et al. Mucolipidosis IV. Clinical, ultrastructural, histochemical, and chemical studies of a case, including a brain biopsy. Arch Neurol. 1976;33:828-835.

573. Merin S, Livni N, Berman ER, Yatziv S. Mucolipidosis IV: ocular, systemic and ultrastructural findings. Invest Ophthalmol. 1975;14:437-448.

574. Goutieres F, Arsenio-Nunes ML, Aicardi J, et al. Mucolipidosis IV. Neuropaediatrics. 1979;10:321-331.

575. Bargal R, Avidan N, Ben-Asher E, et al. Identification of the gene causing mucolipidosis type IV. Nat Genet. 2000;26:118-123.

576. Sun M, Goldin E, Stahl S, et al. Mucolipidosis type IV is caused by mutations in a gene encoding a novel transient receptor potential channel. Hum Mol Genet. 2000;9: 2471-2478.

577. Thompson EG, Schaheen L, Dang H, Fares H. Lysosomal trafficking functions of mucolipin-1 in murine macrophages. BMC Cell Biol. 2007;21:54.

578. Bach G, Desnick R. Lysosomal accumulation of phospholipids in mucolipidosis IV–cultured fibroblasts. Enzyme. 1988;40:40.

579. Folkerth RD, Alroy J, Lomakina I, et al. Mucolipidosis IV: morphology and histochemistry of an autopsy case. J Neuropathol Exp Neurol. 1995;54:154-164.

580. Kohn G, Livni N, Ornoy A, et al. Prenatal diagnosis of mucolipidosis IV by electron microscopy. J Pediatr. 1977;90:62-66.

581. Ornoy A, Arnon J, Grebner EE, et al. Early prenatal diagnosis of mucolipidosis IV. Am J Med Genet. 1987;27: 983-985.

582. Tsay GG, Dawson G. Oligosaccharide storage in brains from patients with fucosidosis, G_{M1}-gangliosidosis and G_{M2}-gangliosidosis (Sandhoff's disease). J Neurochem. 1976;27:733.

583. Tsay GC, Dawson G, Sung S-SJ. Structure of the accumulating oligosaccharide in fucosidosis. J Biol Chem. 1976;251:5852.

584. Dawson G, Spranger JW. Fucosidosis: a glycosphingolipidosis. N Engl J Med. 1971;285:122.

585. Willems PJ, Gatti R, Darby JK, et al. Fucosidosis revisited: a review of 77 patients. Am J Med Genet. 1991;38: 111-113.

586. Willems PJ, Garcia C, De Smedt MC, et al. Intrafamilial variability in fucosidosis. Clin Genet. 1988;34:7-14.

587. Loeb H, Tondeur M, Jonniarx G, et al. Biochemical and ultrastructural studies in a case of mucopolysaccaridosis

"F" (fucosidosis). Helv Paediatr Acta. 1969;24:519-537.

588. Freitag F, Küchemann K, Blümcke S. Hepatic ultrastructure in fucosidosis. Virchows Arch B Cell Pathol. 1971;7:99-113.

589. Libert J, Van Hoof F, Tondeur M. Ultrastructural study of conjunctiva and skin and enzyme analysis of tears. Invest Ophthalmol. 1976;15:626-639.

590. Ng Ying Kin NMK. Comparison of the urinary glycoconjugates excreted by patients with type I and type II fucosidosis. Clin Chem. 1987;33:44.

591. Alhadeff JA, O'Brien JS. Fucosidosis. In Glew RH, Peters SP (eds). Practical Enzymology of the Sphingolipidoses. New York, Alan R Liss, 1977, p 427.

592. Willems PJ, Seo HC, Coucke P, et al. Spectrum of mutations in fucosidosis. Eur J Hum Genet. 1999;1:60-67.

593. Willems PJ, Darby JK, DiCioccio RA, et al. Identification of a mutation in the structural α-L-fucosidase gene in fucosidosis. Am J Hum Genet. 1988;43:756-763.

594. Yang M, Allen H, DiCiccio RA. A mutation generating a stop codon in the α-L-fucosidase gene of a fucosidosis patient. Biochem Biophys Res Commun. 1992;189:1063-1068.

595. Yang M, Allen H, DiCiccio RA. Pedigree analysis of α-L-fucosidase gene mutations in a fucosidosis family. Biochim Biophys Acta. 1993;1182:245-249.

596. Seo HC, Willems PJ, Kretz KA, et al. Fucosidosis: four new mutations and a new polymorphism. Hum Mol Genet. 1993;2:423-429.

597. Willems PJ, Seo HC, O'Brien JS. Six additional mutations in fucosidosis: three nonsense mutations and three frameshift mutations. Hum Mol Genet. 1993;2:1205-1208.

598. Kretz KA, Cripe D, Carson GS, et al. Structure and sequence of the human α-L-fucosidase gene and pseudogene. Genomics. 1992;12:276-280.

599. Coucke P, Mangelschots K, Speleman F, et al. Assignment of the fucosidase pseudogene FUCA1P to chromosome region 2q31-q32. Cytogenet Cell Genet. 1991;57:120-122.

600. Carritt B, Welch HM. An α-fucosidase pseudogene on human chromosome 2. Hum Genet. 1987;3:248.

601. Taylor RM, Farrow BR, Stewart GJ. Amelioration of clinical disease following bone marrow transplantation in fucosidase-deficient dogs. Am J Med Genet. 1992;42:628-632.

602. Occhiodoro T, Hopwood JJ, Morris CP, Anson DS. Correction of α-L-fucosidase deficiency in fucosidosis fibroblasts by retroviral vector–mediated gene transfer. Hum Gene Ther. 1992;3:365-369.

603. Ferrara ML, Occhiodoro T, Fuller M, et al. Canine fucosidosis: a model for retroviral gene transfer into haematopoietic stem cells. Neuromuscul Disord. 1997;7:361-366.

604. Estruch EJ, Hart SL, Kinnon C, Winchester BG. Nonviral, integrin-mediated gene transfer into fibroblasts from patients with lysosomal storage diseases. J Gene Med. 2001;3:488-497.

605. Ockerman PA. A generalised storage disorder resembling Hurler syndrome. Lancet. 1967;2:239-241.

606. Kjellman B, Gamstorp I, Brun A, et al. Mannosidosis: a clinical and histopathologic study. J Pediatr. 1969;75:366-373.

607. Desnick RJ, Sharp HL, Grabowski GA, et al. Mannosidosis: clinical, morphologic, immunologic, and biochemical studies. Pediatr Res. 1976;10:985-996.

608. Kistler JP, Lott IT, Kolodny EH, et al. Mannosidosis. New clinical presentation, enzyme studies and carbohydrate analysis. Arch Neurol. 1977;34:45-51.

609. DeFriend DE, Brown AE, Hutton CW, Hughes PM. Mannosidosis: an unusual cause of a deforming arthropathy. Skeletal Radiol. 2000;29:358-361.

610. Patton MA, Barnes IC, Young ID, et al. Mannosidosis in two brothers: prolonged survival in the severe phenotype. Clin Genet. 1982;22:284-289.

611. Weiss SW, Kelly WD. Bilateral destructive synovitis associated with alpha mannosidase deficiency. Am J Surg Pathol. 1983;7:487.

612. Krishnan B, Mody DR, Ramzy I. α-Mannosidosis. Report of a case with morphologic, cytologic and immunohistochemical considerations. Acta Cytol. 1994;38:441-445.

613. Bartold PM. Biochemical and immunohistochemical studies on overgrown gingival tissues associated with mannosidosis. Virchows Arch. 1992;62:391.

614. Halperin JJ, Landis DMD, Weinstein LA, et al. Communicating hydrocephalus and lysosomal inclusions in mannosidosis. Arch Neurol. 1984;41:777-779.

615. Kawai H, Nishino H, Nishida Y, et al. Skeletal muscle pathology of mannosidosis in two siblings with spastic paraplegia. Acta Neuropathol. 1985;68:201-204.

616. Press OW, Fingert H, Lott IT, Dickerson CR. Pancytopenia in mannosidosis. Arch Intern Med. 1986;143:1266-1268.

617. Patlas M, Shapira MY, Nagler A, et al. MRI of mannosidosis. Neuroradiology. 2001;43:941-943.

618. Grabb PA, Albright AL, Zitelli BJ. Multiple suture synostosis, macrocephaly, and intracranial hypertension in a child with α-D-mannosidase deficiency. Case report. J Neurosurg. 1995;82:647-649.

619. Sung JH, Hayano M, Desnick RJ. Mannosidosis: pathology of the nervous system. J Neuropathol Exp Neurol. 1977;36:807.

620. Prence EM, Natowicz MR. Diagnosis of α-mannosidosis by measuring α-mannosidase in plasma. Clin Chem. 1992;38:501.

621. Masson PK, Lundblad A. Mannosidosis: detection of the disease and of heterozygotes using serum and leucocytes. Biochem Biophys Res Commun. 1974;56:296.

622. Poenaru L, Gerard S, Thepot F, et al. Antenatal diagnosis in three pregnancies at risk for mannosidosis. Clin Genet. 1979;16:428-432.

623. Nebes VL, Schmidt MC. Human lysosomal α-mannosidase: isolation and nucleotide sequence of the full-length cDNA. Biochem Biophys Res Commun. 1994;200:239.

624. Berg T, Riise HM, Hansen GM, et al. Spectrum of mutations in α-mannosidosis. Am J Hum Genet. 1999;64:77-88.

625. Hultberg B, Masson PK. Activation of residual acidic α-mannosidase activity in mannosidosis tissues by metal ions. Biochem Biophys Res Commun. 1975;67:1473.

626. Jansen PH, Schoonderwaldt HC, Renier WO, et al. Mannosidosis: a study of two patients presenting clinical heterogeneity. Clin Neurol Neurosurg. 1987;89:185-192.

627. Dickersin GR, Lott IT, Kolodny EH, Dvorak AM. A light and electron microscopic study of mannosidosis. Hum Pathol. 1980;11:245-256.

628. Grabowski GA, Walling LL, et al. Enzyme manipulations: evaluation of oral ZnSO₄ supplementation in mannosidosis type II. Pediatr Res. 1977;11:456.

629. Worg LTK, Vallance H, Savage A, et al. Oral zinc therapy in the treatment of α-mannosidosis. Am J Med Genet. 1993;46:410-414.

630. Will A, Cooper A, Hatton C, et al. Bone marrow transplantation in the treatment of α-mannosidosis. Arch Dis Child. 1987;62:1044-1049.

631. Berg T, King B, Meikle PJ, et al. Purification and characterization of recombinant human lysosomal α-mannosidase. Mol Genet Metab. 2001;73:18-29.

632. Sun H, Yang M, Haskins ME, et al. Retrovirus vector–mediated correction and cross-correction of lysosomal α-mannosidase deficiency in human and feline fibroblasts. Hum Gene Ther. 1999;10:1311-1319.

633. Crawley AC, Jones MZ, Bonning LE, et al. α-Mannosidosis in the guinea pig: a new animal model for lysosomal storage disorders. Pediatr Res. 1999;46:501-509.

634. Stinchi S, Lullmann-Rauch R, Hartman D, et al. Targeted disruption of the lysosomal α-mannosidase gene results in mice resembling a mild form of human α-mannosidosis. Hum Mol Genet. 1999;8:1365-1372.

635. Crawley AC, King B, Berg T, et al. Enzyme replacement therapy in alpha-mannosidosis guinea-pigs. Mol Genet Metab. 2006;89:48-57.

636. Cooper A, Sardharwalla IB, Roberts MM. Human β-mannosidase deficiency. N Engl J Med. 1986;315:1231.

637. Kleijer WJ, Hu P, Thoomes R, et al. β-Mannosidase deficiency: heterogeneous manifestation in the first female patient and her brother. J Inherit Metab Dis. 1990;13:867-872.

638. Wenger DA, Sujansky E, Fennessey PV, Thompson JN. Human β-mannosidase deficiency. N Engl J Med. 1986;315:1201-1205.

639. Wijburg H, de Jong J, Wevers R, et al. β-Mannosidosis and ethanolaminuria in a female patient. Eur J Pediatr. 1992;151:311.

640. Levade T, Graber D, Flurin V, et al. Human β-mannosidase deficiency associated with peripheral neuropathy. Ann Neurol. 1994;35:116-119.

641. Alkhayat AH, Kraemer SA, Leipprandt JR, et al. Human β-mannosidase cDNA characterization and first identification of a mutation associated with human beta-mannosidosis. Hum Mol Genet. 1998;7:75-83.

642. Kleijer WJ, Geilen GC, Van Diggelen OP, et al. Prenatal analyses in a pregnancy at risk for β-mannosidosis. Prenat Diagn. 1992;12:841-843.

643. Zhu M, Lovell KL, Patterson JS, et al. Beta-mannosidosis mice: a model for the human lysosomal storage disease. Hum Mol Genet. 2006;15:493-500.

644. Syvänen A-C, Ikonen E, Manninen T, et al. Convenient and quantitative determination of the frequency of a mutant allele using solid-phase minisequencing: application to aspartylglucosaminuria in Finland. Genomics. 1992;12:590-595.

645. Chitayat D, Nakagawa S, Marion RW, et al. Aspartylglucosaminuria in a Puerto Rican family: additional features of a panethnic disorder. Am J Med Genet. 1988;31:527-532.

646. Schmidt H, Ziegler R, et al. Skelettveranderungen bei zwei deutschen Kindern mit Aspartylglucosaminurie. Fortschr Geb Rontgenstr Nuklearmed. 1988;149:153.

647. Yoshida K, Ikeda S, Yanagisawa N, et al. Two Japanese cases with aspartylglycosaminuria: clinical and morphological features. Clin Genet. 1991;40:318-325.

648. Mononen IT, Kaartinen VM, Williams JC. A fluorometric assay for glycosylasparaginase activity and detection of aspartylglycosaminuria. Anal Biochem. 1993;208:372-374.

649. Tollersrud OK, Nilssen O, Tranebjaerg L, Borud O. Aspartylglucosaminuria in northern Norway: a molecular and genealogical study. J Med Genet. 1994;31:360-363.

650. Peltola M, Chiatayat D, Peltonen L, Jalanko A. Characterization of a point mutation in aspartylglucosaminidase gene: evidence for a readthrough of a translational stop codon. Hum Mol Genet. 1994;3:2237-2242.

651. Maury CP, Palo J. N-Acetylglucosamine-asparagine levels in tissues of patients with aspartylglycosaminuria. Clin Chim Acta. 1981;108:293.

652. Aula P, Autio S, Raivio KO, Rapola J. Aspartylglucosaminuria. In Durand P, O'Brien JS (eds). Genetic Errors of Glycoprotein Metabolism. Berlin, Springer Verlag, 1982, pp 122-152.

653. Autio S. Aspartylglycosaminuria: analysis of thirty-four patients. J Ment Defic Res. 1972;1:1.

654. Arvio M, Autio S, Louhiala P. Early clinical symptoms and incidence of aspartylglucosaminuria in Finland. Acta Paediatr. 1993;82:587-589.

655. Arvio P, Arvio M, Kero M, et al. Overgrowth of oral mucosa and facial skin, a novel feature of aspartylglucosaminuria. J Med Genet. 1999;36:398-404.

656. Aula P, Raivio K, Autio S, et al. Enzymatic diagnosis and carrier detection of aspartylglucosaminuria using blood samples. Pediatr Res. 1976;10:625-629.

657. Voznyi Y, Keulemans JL, Kleijer WJ, et al. Applications of a new fluorimetric enzyme assay for the diagnosis of aspartylglucosaminuria. J Inherit Metab Dis. 1993;16:929-934.

658. Aula P, Autio S, Ravio K, Nänö V. Detection of heterozygotes for aspartylglucosaminuria (AGU) in cultured fibroblasts. Humangenetik. 1974;25:307-314.

659. Aula P, Rapola J, von Koskull H, Ammälä P. Prenatal diagnosis and fetal pathology of aspartylglucosaminuria. Am J Med Genet. 1984;19:359-367.

660. Aula P, Mattila K, Piiroinen O, et al. First-trimester prenatal diagnosis of aspartylglucosaminuria. Prenat Diagn. 1989;9:617-620.

661. Saarela J, Laine M, Oinonen C, et al. Molecular pathogenesis of a disease: structural consequences of aspartylglucosaminuria mutations. Hum Mol Genet. 2001;10:983-995.

662. Ikonen E, Syvänen A-C, Peltonen L. Dissection of the molecular pathology of aspartylglucosaminuria provides the basis for DNA diagnostics and future therapeutic interventions. Scand J Clin Lab Invest. 1993;53:19.

663. Delahunty CM, Ankener W, Brainerd S, et al. Finnish-type aspartylglucosaminuria detected by oligonucleotide ligation assay. Clin Chem. 1995;41:59-61.

664. Arvio M, Sauna-Aho O, Peippo M. Bone marrow transplantation for aspartylglucosaminuria: follow-up study of transplanted and non-transplanted patients. J Pediatr. 2001;138:288.

665. Autti T, Rapola J, Autti T, et al. Bone marrow transplantation in aspartylglucosaminuria—histopathological and MRI study. Neuropediatrics. 1999;30:283-288.

666. Kaartinen V, Mononen I, Voncken JW, et al. A mouse model for the human lysosomal disease aspartylglycosaminuria. Nat Med. 1996;2:1375-1378.

667. Gonzalez-Gomez I, Mononen I, Heisterkamp N, et al. Progressive neurodegeneration in aspartylglycosaminuria mice. Am J Pathol. 1998;153:1293-1300.

668. Anderson RA, Sando GN. Cloning and expression of cDNA encoding human lysosomal acid lipase/cholesteryl ester hydrolase: similarities to gastric and lingual lipases. J Biol Chem. 1991;266:22479.

669. Anderson RA, Rao N, Byrum RS, et al. In situ localization of the genetic locus encoding the lysosomal acid lipase/cholesteryl esterase (LIPA) deficient in Wolman disease to chromosome 10q23.2Bq23.3. Genomics. 1993;15:245-247.

670. Anderson RA, Byrum RS, Coates PM, Sando GM. Mutations at the lysosomal acid cholesteryl ester hydrolase gene locus in Wolman disease. Proc Natl Acad Sci U S A. 1994;91:2718-2722.

671. Lohse P, Maas S, Sewell AC, et al. Molecular defects underlying Wolman disease appear to be more heterogeneous than those resulting in cholesteryl ester storage disease. J Lipid Res. 1999;40:221-228.

672. Cortner JA, Coates PM, Swoboda E, Schnatz JD. Genetic variation of lysosomal acid lipase. Pediatr Res. 1976;10:927-932.

673. Desai PK, Astrin KH, Thung SN, et al. Cholesteryl ester storage disease: pathologic changes in an affected fetus. Am J Med Genet. 1987;26:689-698.

674. Leone L, Ippoliti PF, Antonicelli R, et al. Use of simvastatin plus cholestyramine in the treatment of lysosomal acid lipase deficiency. J Pediatr. 1991;119:1008-1009.

675. Leone L, Ippoliti PF, Antonicelli R, et al. Treatment and liver transplantation for cholesterol ester storage disease. J Pediatr. 1995;127:509-510.

676. Krivit W, Peters C, Dusenbery K, et al. Wolman disease successfully treated by bone marrow transplantation. Bone Marrow Transplant. 2000;26:567-570.

677. Du H, Schiavi S, Levine M, et al. Enzyme therapy for lysosomal acid lipase deficiency in the mouse. Hum Mol Genet. 2001;10:1639-1648.

678. Tietge UJ, Sun G, Czarnecki S, et al. Phenotypic correction of lipid storage and growth arrest in Wolman disease fibroblasts by gene transfer of lysosomal acid lipase. Hum Gene Ther. 2001;12:279-289.

679. Marshall WC, Ockenden BG, Fosbrooke AS, Cumings JN. Wolman's disease: a rare lipidosis with adrenal calcification. Arch Dis Child. 1968;44:331-341.

680. Lough J, Fawcett J, Wiegensberg B. Wolman's disease: an electron microscopic, histochemical and biochemical study. Arch Pathol. 1970;89:103.

681. Wolman M, Sterk VV, Gatt S, Frenkel M. Primary familial xanthomatosis with involvement and calcification of the adrenals: report of two more cases in siblings of a previously described infant. Pediatrics. 1961;28:742-757.

682. Ozmen MN, Aygün N, Kiliç I, et al. Wolman's disease: ultrasonographic and computed tomographic findings. Pediatr Radiol. 1992;22:541-542.

683. Kikuchi M, Igarashi K, Noro T, et al. Evaluation of jejunal function in Wolman's disease. J Pediatr Gastroenteral Nutr. 1991;12:65-69.

684. Schaub J, Janka GE, Christomanou H, et al. Wolman's disease: clinical, biochemical and ultrastructural studies in an unusual case without striking adrenal calcification. Eur J Pediatr. 1980;135:45-53.

685. Elleder M, Ledvinová J, Cieslar P, Kuhn R. Subclinical course of cholesterol ester storage disease diagnosed in adulthood. Report on two cases with remarks on the nature of the liver storage process. Virchows Arch. 1990;416:357-365.

686. Pfeiffer U, Jeschke R. Cholesterylester-Speicherkrankheit. Virchows Arch. 1980;33:17.

687. Hoeg JM, Demosky SJ Jr, Peskovitz OH, Brewer HB Jr. Cholesteryl ester storage disease and Wolman disease: phenotype variants of lysosomal acid cholesteryl ester hydrolase deficiency. Am J Hum Genet. 1984;36:1190-1203.

688. Ginsberg HN, Le N-A, Short MP, et al. Suppression of apolipoprotein B production during treatment of cholesterol ester storage disease with lovastatin. J Clin Invest. 1987;80:1692-1697.

689. Ferry GD, Whisennand HH, Finegold MJ, et al. Liver transplantation for cholesteryl ester storage disease. J Pediatr Gastroenterol Nutr. 1991;12:376-378.

690. Du H, Duanmu M, Witte D, Grabowski GA. Targeted disruption of the mouse lysosomal acid lipase gene: long-term survival with massive cholesteryl ester and triglyceride storage. Hum Mol Genet. 1998;7:1347-1354.

691. Braak H, Braak E. Pathoarchitectonic pattern of iso- and allocortical lesions in juvenile and adult neuronal ceroid-lipofuscinosis. J Inherit Metab Dis. 1993;16:259.

692. Hosain S, Kaufmann WE, Negrin G, et al. Diagnosis of neuronal ceroid-lipofuscinosis by immunochemical methods. Am J Med Genet. 1995;57:239-245.

693. Wisniewski KE, Wojociech K, Golabek AA, Kida E. Rapid detection of subunit c of mitochondrial ATP synthase in urine as a diagnostic screening method for neuronal ceroid-lipofuscinoses. Am J Med Genet. 1995;57:246-249.

694. Tyynelä J, Baumann M, Henseler M, et al. Sphingolipid activator proteins (SAPs) are stored together with glycosphingolipids in the infantile neuronal ceroid-lipofuscinoses. Am J Med Genet. 1995;57:294-297.

695. Rider JA, Rider DL. Batten disease: past, present, and future. Am J Med Genet Suppl. 1988;5:21.

696. Vanhanen SL, Raininko R, Santavuori P. Early differential diagnosis of infantile neuronal ceroid lipofuscinosis, Rett syndrome, and Krabbe disease by CT and MR. Am J Neurol Radiol. 1994;15:1443-1453.

697. Chattopadhyay S, Pearce DA. Neural and extraneural expression of the neuronal ceroid lipofuscinoses genes CLN1, CLN2, and CLN3: functional implications for CLN3. Mol Genet Metab. 2000;71:207.

698. Goebels HH. Prenatal ultrastructural diagnosis in the neuronal ceroid-lipofuscinoses. Pathol Res Pract. 1994;190:728.

699. Koppang N. The significance of animal models for human ceroid-lipofuscinosis. J Inherit Metab Dis. 1993;16:272.

700. Jolly RD. Round table discussion of animal models of ceroid-lipofuscinosis (Batten disease). J Inherit Metab Dis. 1993;16:278.

701. Faust JR, Rodman JS, Daniel PF, et al. Two related proteolipids and dolichol linked oligosaccharides accumulate in motor neuron degeneration mice (mmd/mnd), a model of neuronal ceroid lipofuscinosis. J Biol Chem. 1994;269: 10150-10155.

702. Edwards JF, Storts RW, Joyce JR, et al. Juvenile-onset neuronal ceroid-lipofuscinosis in Rambouillet sheep. Vet Pathol. 1994;31:48-54.

703. Santavuori P, Linnankivi T, eJaeken J, t al. Psychological symptoms and sleep disturbances in neuronal ceroid-lipofuscinoses (NCL). J Inherit Metab Dis. 1993;16:245-248.

704. Santavuori P, Vanhanen SL, Sainio K, et al. Infantile neuronal ceroid-lipofuscinosis: diagnostic criteria. J Inherit Metab Dis. 1993;16:227-229.

705. Santavuori P, Jarvela I, Haltia M, et al. Update on infantile neuronal ceroid-lipofuscinosis (INCL). Brain Dev. 1990;12:661.

706. Schriner JE, Yi W, Hofmann SL. cDNA and genomic cloning of human palmitoyl-protein thioesterase (PPT), the enzyme defective in infantile neuronal ceroid lipofuscinosis. Genomics. 1996;34:317.

707. Lehtovirta M, Kyttälä A, Eskelinen EL, et al. Palmitoyl protein thioesterase (PPT) localizes into synaptosomes and synaptic vesicles in neurons: Implications for infantile neuronal ceroid lipofuscinosis (INCL). Hum Mol Genet. 2001;10:69-75.

708. Salonen T, Heinonen-Kopra O, Vesa J, Jalanko A. Neuronal trafficking of palmitoyl protein thioesterase provides an excellent model to study the effects of different mutations which cause infantile neuronal ceroid lipofuscinocis. Mol Cell Neurosci. 2001;18:131-140.

709. Wisniewski KE, Zhong N, Philippart M. Pheno/genotypic correlations of neuronal ceroid lipofuscinoses. Neurology. 2001;57:576-581.

710. Soyombo AA, Hofmann SL. Molecular cloning and expression of palmitoyl-protein thioesterase 2 (PPT2), a homolog of lysosomal palmitoyl-protein thioesterase with a distinct substrate specificity. J Biol Chem. 1997;272: 27456-27463.

711. Bellizzi J Jr, Widom J, Kemp C, et al. The crystal structure of palmitoyl protein thioesterase 1 and the molecular basis of infantile neuronal ceroid lipofuscinosis. Proc Natl Acad Sci U S A. 2000;97:4573-4578.

712. Gupta P, Soyombo AA, Atashband A, et al. Disruption of PPT1 or PPT2 causes neuronal ceroid lipofuscinosis in knockout mice. Proc Natl Acad Sci U S A. 2001;98: 13566-13571.

713. Autti T, Raininko R, Launes J, et al. Jansky-Bielschowsky variant disease: CT, MRI, and SPECT findings. Pediatr Neurol. 1992;8:121-126.

714. Dunn DW. CT in ceroid lipofuscinosis. Neurology. 1987; 37:1025.

715. Kida E, Wisniewski KE, Connell F. Topographic variabilities of immunoreactivity to subunit c of mitochondrial

716. Rawlings ND, Barrett AJ. Tripeptidyl-peptidase I is apparently the CLN2 protein absent in classical late-infantile neuronal ceroid lipofuscinosis. Biochim Biophys Acta. 1999;1429:496-500.

717. Savukoski M, Kestilä M, Williams R, et al. Defined chromosomal assignment of CLN5 demonstrates that at least four genetic loci are involved in the pathogenesis of human ceroid lipofuscinoses. Am J Hum Genet. 1994;55:695-701.

718. Savukoski M, Klockars T, Holmberg V, et al. CLN5, a novel gene encoding a putative transmembrane protein mutated in Finnish variant late infantile neuronal ceroid lipofuscinosis. Nat Genet. 1998;19:286-288.

719. Isosomppi J, Vesa J, Jalanko A, Peltonen L. Lysosomal localization of the neuronal ceroid lipofuscinosis CLN5 protein. Hum Mol Genet. 2001;11:885-891.

720. Zhong N. Neuronal ceroid lipofuscinoses and possible pathogenic mechanism. Mol Genet Metab. 2000;71: 195.

721. Pineda-Trujillo N, Cornejo W, Carrizosa J, et al. A CLN5 mutation causing an atypical neuronal ceroid lipofuscinosis of juvenile onset. Neurology. 2005;64:740-742.

722. Kopra O, Vesa J, von Schantz C, et al. A mouse model for Finnish variant late infantile neuronal ceroid lipofuscinosis, CLN5, reveals neuropathology associated with early aging. Hum Mol Genet. 2004;13:2893-2906.

723. Boustany R. Neurology of the neuronal ceroid-lipofuscinoses: Late infantile and juvenile types. Am J Med Genet. 1992;42:533.

724. Lanska DJ, Lanska M. Visual "release" hallucinations in juvenile neuronal ceroid-lipofuscinosis. Pediatr Neurol. 1993;9:316.

725. Bruun I, Reske-Nielsen E, Oster S, et al. Juvenile ceroid lipofuscinosis and calcifications of the CNS. Acta Neurol Scand. 1991;83:1-8.

726. Bennett MJ, Gayton AR, Rittey CD, Hosking GP. Juvenile neuronal ceroid-lipofuscinosis: developmental progress after supplementation with polyunsaturated fatty acids. Dev Med Child Neurol. 1994;36:630-638.

727. The International Batten Disease Consortium. Isolation of a novel gene underlying Batten disease, CLN3. Cell. 1995;82:949-957.

728. Janes RW, Munroe PB, Mitchison HM, et al. A model for Batten disease protein CLN3: functional implications from homology and mutations. FEBS Lett. 1996;399: 75-77.

729. Munroe PB, Mitchison HM, O'Rawe AM, et al. Spectrum of mutations in the Batten disease gene, CLN3. Am J Hum Genet. 1997;61:310-316.

730. Martin JJ. Adult type of neuronal ceroid lipofuscinosis. J Inherit Metab Dis. 1993;16:237.

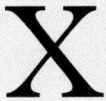

X Hemostasis

25

Platelets and the Vessel Wall

Peter J. Newman and Debra K. Newman

In a 1881 communication to the Turin Royal Academy of Medicine, the Italian physician Giulio Bizzozero disclosed the presence in circulating human blood of discrete elements that he termed "*piastrine*" ("*blutplättchen*" in a 1882 publication in a German journal and "*petites plaques*" in a communication in French).[1] Previously speculated to be merely nonphysiologic "*granular aggregates*," blood platelets have since become central to our understanding of thrombosis and hemostasis, and detailed understanding of their participation in cardiovascular disease, stroke, and even cancer has led to remarkable progress in the rational treatment of these disorders.

Although platelets are most often studied in the context of their ability to form a hemostatically effective plug, it is now widely recognized that their influence extends far beyond this process to all aspects of hemostasis, as well as to wound healing and vascular remodeling. For example, platelets generate or secrete biologically active mediators such as thromboxane A_2 (TXA_2) and serotonin, which not only amplify platelet activation responses but also modulate vascular tone. In addition, platelets secrete a broad array of granule constituents that stimulate vessel repair, induce megakaryocytopoiesis, promote coagulation, and limit fibrinolysis.

The same pathways that lead to platelet plug formation can also produce pathologic thrombosis, a process that has been described as hemostasis occurring at the wrong time or in the wrong place. Platelets are particularly important for hemostasis on the arterial side of the circulation, where blood flows under higher pressure and experiences greater shear force. As a result, platelet function is generally considered to be critical to the pathogenesis of arterial thrombosis and less so for venous thrombosis, and antiplatelet drugs are most widely used in the former setting. However, this distinction between the mechanisms underlying arterial and venous thrombosis is not absolute, and the spectrum of thrombotic disorders should be considered a continuum.

Arterial thrombosis is a particularly common problem in middle-aged and older adults and is a major cause of morbidity and mortality in developed countries. The thrombi that arise in atherosclerotic vessels are predominantly platelet in origin and are the proximate cause of myocardial infarction and most cerebrovascular accidents. Although arterial thrombosis is considerably less common in children than adults, it may contribute to major morbidity in patients with sickle cell disease, as well as complications of some childhood infections, Kawasaki's syndrome, and various forms of arteritis, autoimmune disorders, hemolytic-uremic syndrome, and thrombotic thrombocytopenic purpura (see Chapter 33).

In this chapter we review platelet structure and function, with special emphasis on the cell surface glycoproteins that function as sentries for areas of vascular damage and the signal transduction events that both amplify and limit platelet responsiveness. The information provided here should be helpful in understanding subsequent chapters that describe inherited and acquired platelet disorders (see Chapters 29 and 33) and the role of the adhesive protein von Willebrand factor (VWF) (see Chapter 30) in hemostasis. Finally, there is growing appreciation of the role that platelets play in inflammation and the pathogenesis of atherothrombosis, which is briefly discussed at the end of the chapter.

PLATELET MORPHOLOGY AND SUBCELLULAR ORGANIZATION

Platelets are adhesion and signaling machines that circulate as small, disc-shaped cellular fragments in the whole blood of healthy individuals at a concentration of approximately 150,000 to 300,000/μL. Early studies suggested that platelets might be produced via cytoplasmic fragmentation along a network of internal demarcation membranes that were observed in large, polyploid megakaryocytes.[2,3] More recent studies,[4-6] however, support the notion that proplatelets are assembled and packaged with their various constituents at the ends of long cytoplasmic extensions of differentiated megakaryocytes that have migrated from the proliferative osteoblastic niche to the capillary-rich vascular niche of the bone marrow microenvironment,[7] with the invaginated demarcation membrane system serving simply as a reservoir of internal membrane used for proplatelet extension.[8,9] Once adjacent to the adluminal face of the endothelium, proplatelets are released into the bloodstream, where they circulate as mature platelets for approximately 7 to 10 days before being cleared by the liver and spleen[10]—their life span being controlled, at least in part, by an antagonistic balance between the apoptotic proteins Bcl-xL and Bak.[11]

The size of resting platelets is somewhat variable, averaging approximately 1.5 μm in diameter and 0.5 to 1 μm in thickness. Platelet size is undoubtedly regulated by numerous factors during their biogenesis, but both the 224-kd nonmuscle myosin heavy chain IIA (MYHIIA) and the cell surface glycoprotein Ib (GPIb) complex appear to play critical roles. Thus, mutations in the *MYH9* gene predominantly interfere with contractile events important for platelet formation,[12] whereas failure to express GPIb—the molecular basis for the platelet disorder known as Bernard-Soulier syndrome[13,14]—disrupts critical associations with the cytoskeletal protein filamin[15,16] that play an essential role in both platelet formation and platelet compliance.[17] In both these inherited platelet disorders, platelets can appear as large as lymphocytes (see Chapter 29). Correction of GPIb expression in GPIb-deficient (Bernard-Soulier) mice has been shown to restore platelets to their normal size.[18]

The volume of a platelet (mean platelet volume) normally ranges from 6 to 10 fL (1 fL = 10^{-15} L). Platelet density is also variable,[19] and the issue of whether young platelets are more[20,21] or less[22] dense as they gain versus lose content during their circulating lifetime has never been satisfactorily resolved. Because platelets retain most species of messenger RNA (mRNA) for a short period after their release from bone marrow megakaryocytes,[23] young platelets can be distinguished from older ones by their RNA content.[24]

As shown in Figure 25-1A and C, resting platelets are discoid in shape, largely because of the presence of a circumferential coil of microtubules,[25,26] and they are packed with numerous electron-opaque alpha granules, a few dense granules (granule contents and their functions are discussed later), several mitochondria, and lysosomes.[27] Platelets also retain a few Golgi remnants, as well as occasional vestiges of rough endoplasmic reticulum—the exception being platelets from patients with rapid platelet turnover, in whom very young platelets containing more abundant protein synthesis machinery are readily observed in the circulation. Platelets also contain two highly specialized membrane systems not found in other cells of the body: the surface-connected open canalicular system (OCS) (see Fig. 25-1B and C) and the dense tubular system (DTS). The OCS is a series of tortuous invaginations of the plasma membrane that appear to tunnel throughout the cytoplasm of the cell[28] and serve as an internal reservoir of plasma membrane that is called upon when platelets round up, extend lamellipods and filopods (see Fig. 25-1B and D), and spread during platelet activation—a process that can increase the surface area of exposed plasma membrane by more than 400%.[29] Because

OCS channels are proximal to internal granules, they also probably function as a conduit for the rapid expulsion of alpha and dense granule contents during platelet activation.[30] The DTS, on the other hand, is a remnant of the smooth endoplasmic reticulum[31] and is found randomly dispersed throughout the cytoplasm. The DTS appears to be one of several organelles within the platelet known to harbor high concentrations of calcium,[32,33] and it is thought to contain a 100-kd calcium adenosine triphosphatase (ATPase) known as SERCA2b[34] that functions to sequester and store cytosolic calcium in resting cells. Recent evidence suggests that adenosine diphosphate (ADP) is able to induce selective release of calcium from the DTS[35] whereas activation of the GPIb/V/IX receptor for VWF releases calcium primarily from a poorly defined acidic compartment[36] within the cell.[35] Thrombin, a strong platelet agonist, appears to elicit release of calcium from both stores on binding to the platelet thrombin receptor PAR1.[35]

The platelet cytoskeleton is composed of a single rigid, but dynamic microtubule approximately 100 μm in length that is coiled about 8 to 12 times around the equatorial plane of the cell.[37-39] This marginal band of microtubules is largely responsible for maintaining the discoid shape of the resting cell, as illustrated by the observations that (1) incubation of platelets with colchicine—an agent that dissolves microtubules—results in their rounding,[40] (2) platelets from mice lacking

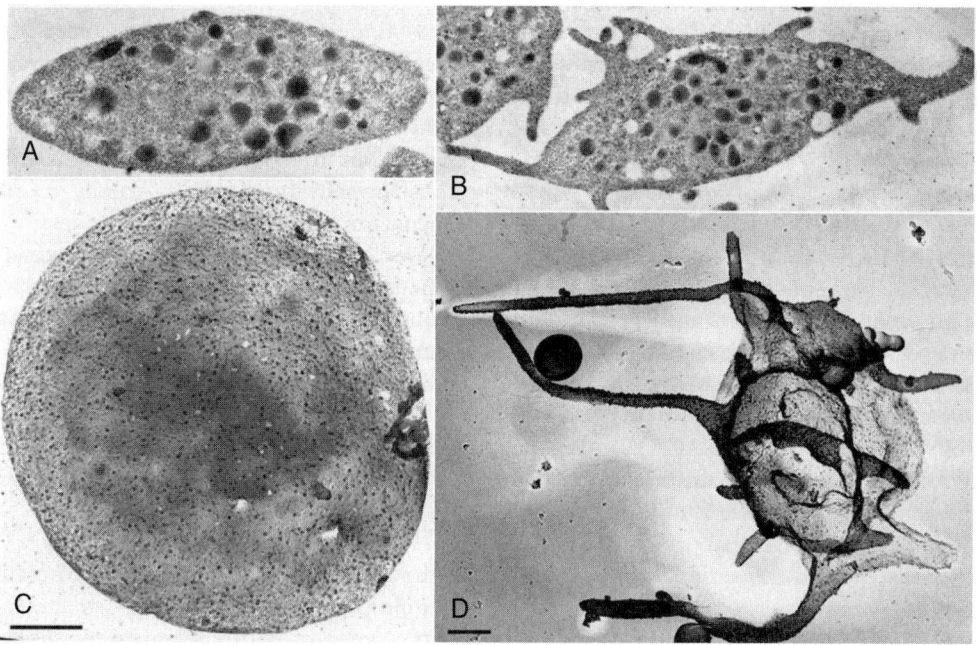

FIGURE 25-1. Platelet morphology. Resting platelets (shown in thin section in **A** and from a scanning electron micrograph of a flash-frozen, freeze-dried platelet in **C**) are shaped like a disc and contain numerous electron-opaque alpha granules, a few dense granules, and several mitochondria and lysosomes. A circumferential coil of microtubules (mc—highlighted with an *oval*) is responsible for maintaining their discoid shape. Platelets also contain a number of cytoplasmic membrane systems that subserve specialized functions, including vestiges of the smooth endoplasmic reticulum that sequester calcium and tortuous invaginations of the plasma membrane that form a surface-connected open canalicular system (OCS). When platelets become activated (**B** and **D**), they rapidly round up, extend lamellipodia (lam) and filopodia (fil), and release the contents of their granules, often into the nearby OCS. *(Photographs generously provided by John H. Hartwig and used with permission.)*

β_1-tubulin remain largely spherical,[41] and (3) *"platelet spherocytosis"* in humans results when tubulin fails to polymerize normally into microtubules.[42] Directly underneath the plasma membrane lies an intricate, two-dimensional, tightly woven membrane skeleton[43] composed of nonerythroid spectrin,[44,45] a network of actin filaments,[43,45] vinculin,[46] and the actin-binding protein filamin,[47] which itself is tethered to the inner face of the plasma membrane via linkages with the cytoplasmic domain of GPIb.[15,47] The membrane skeleton, because of its location, serves as a scaffold that links elements of the plasma membrane with contractile elements of the cytoskeleton and cytosolic signaling proteins and thereby regulates such diverse functions as receptor mobility,[48,49] receptor clustering,[50-52] and signal transduction.[53] Finally, the platelet is filled with an extensive cytoplasmic network of actin filaments[45,54] organized by the actin-binding proteins filamin[55,56] and α-actinin[57] that constitute its cytoskeleton.

When platelets become exposed to components of the extracellular matrix[58] or to soluble agonists such as ADP[59] or thrombin,[60,61] they undergo dramatic changes in their morphology.[62,63] The marginal band of microtubules disappears,[54] which allows the platelet to transform from a disc to an irregular sphere. At nearly the same time, the actin filament–capping protein α-adducin becomes phosphorylated and dissociates from existing F-actin filaments,[64] thereby exposing the barbed end of the filament to cytosolic actin monomers and driving rapid polymerization of actin into microfilaments.[62] This has the dual effect of driving the extension of lamellipodia and filopodia and forcing granules toward the center of the platelet, where they can fuse with membranes of the OCS and release their contents to the exterior of the cell. Phosphorylation of myosin additionally induces contractile events that facilitate centralization of the granules.[65]

PLATELET GENOMICS AND PROTEOMICS

Though anucleate, platelets contain measurable and manipulable levels of megakaryocyte-derived mRNA,[23] at least some of which is capable of being synthesized into small, but detectable amounts of protein.[66,67] Both serial analysis of gene expression (SAGE) and gene microarray analysis have been used to estimate the size and composition of the platelet transcriptome.[68-70] A consistent finding of all genomic analyses performed to date is that mitochondrially derived transcripts dominate the platelet transcriptome—presumably because of persistent transcription of the mitochondrial genome after platelet release from the bone marrow. This problem has recently been addressed by analyzing the transcriptome of cultured megakaryocytes derived from cord blood stem cells.[71] Of the 20,488 genes present in the human genome, 2000 to 3000 distinct transcripts have been identified in unstimulated platelets—considerably fewer

than normally found in a nucleated cell, but perhaps more than one might have expected from an anucleate circulating cellular fragment. One of the more surprising findings in recent years has been the identification of heterogeneous nuclear RNA (hnRNA) in the platelet cytosol, as well as all of the spliceosome components necessary to splice the hnRNA into mature message that can thereafter be translated into protein.[72] Enlisted during the activation process, signal-dependent protein translation has thus far been demonstrated for mRNA molecules encoding interleukin-1β (IL-1β),[72] tissue factor,[73] and Bcl-3,[74] the protein products of which have the potential to influence inflammation, thrombosis, and wound repair.

The platelet proteome appears to be equally complex and diverse and, unlike the transcriptome, reports both the breadth and relative amounts of protein products actually present in the cell. Obtained by refined two-dimensional gel electrophoretic techniques that were originally developed in the 1970s[75,76] or by liquid chromatographic separation, proteins are fragmented and separated via a combination of proteolytic and ionization techniques and then analyzed by mass spectrometry. Such analysis has allowed the identification of dozens of proteins present in complex cellular lysates or subcellular fractions (see elsewhere[77,78] for recent reviews of this topic). In addition to yielding the expected menu of major plasma membrane glycoprotein receptors, one of the more complete global profiling analyses to date[79] identified a core platelet proteome composed of 641 proteins, including an abundance of molecules involved in signal transduction, cytoskeletal change, and metabolism—understandable given the importance of cellular activation and its control in platelet function. By combining prefractionation methods with suitable separation techniques, proteomic analysis has also been used to compile an inventory of proteins that are either (1) posttranslationally modified (normally by phosphorylation) during the platelet activation process[80-82] or (2) present at low abundance in the total platelet proteome but enriched within various subcellular compartments, including the platelet cytoskeleton,[83] alpha granules,[81,84,85] membrane fraction,[86] membrane rafts,[87] and microparticles.[88]

ANTITHROMBOTIC COMPONENTS OF THE VESSEL WALL

Although hundreds of thousands of platelets per microliter circulate in blood, under normal conditions very few, if any, interact with the intact vessel wall because the endothelial lining of the blood vessel presents an excellent nonthrombogenic surface. In fact, this property of the vessel wall has not yet been duplicated in any prosthetic or extracorporeal device. Healthy endothelium not only provides an effective barrier between blood components and the highly thrombogenic components of the subendothelium (see later) but also actively produces both membrane-bound and secretory products that limit fibrin generation and promote clot dissolution. For example, heparin-like glycosaminoglycans present on the luminal side of the endothelial cell surface recruit plasma antithrombin, which effects a conformational change that promotes binding and neutralization of thrombin and other serine proteases.[89] Thrombin, when bound to the endothelial cell surface receptor thrombomodulin, takes on anticoagulant properties via its cleavage and activation of protein C, which in turn cleaves coagulation factors V and VIII, thereby further suppressing thrombin generation.[90] Endothelial cells also express a specific receptor for activated protein C that serves to concentrate the protein on the endothelial surface (see Chapter 26).[91] Finally, endothelial cells synthesize, secrete, and rebind tissue plasminogen activator,[92,93] which activates plasminogen to facilitate fibrin dissolution (see Chapter 27). These activities are summarized in schematic form in Figure 25-2.

The endothelial cell also produces two important inhibitors of platelet activation: prostacyclin (PGI$_2$)[94-96] and nitric oxide (NO).[97-99] A labile oxygenated metabolite of arachidonic acid generated by endothelial cell cyclooxygenase-2 (COX-2), PGI$_2$ diffuses out of the cell and binds to a platelet G$_s$ protein–coupled receptor (GPCR)

known as the isoprostenoid (IP) receptor.[100,101] Such binding stimulates adenylate cyclase to increase cytosolic cyclic adenosine monophosphate (cAMP) levels, which (1) activates a pump in the DTS that decreases cytosolic Ca^{2+}, thereby helping keep platelets quiescent, and (2) activates protein kinase A (PKA), the actions of which will be discussed later. PGI$_2$ also has potent vasodilatory effects by binding to IP on arterial smooth muscles cells to effect vessel relaxation.[94] The PGI$_2$ produced by vascular endothelium thus serves to counterbalance the proaggregatory and vasoconstrictor activities of the platelet-derived prostanoid TXA$_2$, the biology of which is discussed later. In fact, upsetting the delicate balance between COX-1–derived TXA$_2$ and COX-2–derived PGI$_2$ has been shown to increase the risk for adverse cardiovascular events.[102]

Whereas PGI$_2$ stimulates adenylate cyclase to produce cAMP, NO, a product of L-arginine generated by endothelial nitric oxide synthase (eNOS),[103] directly activates platelet guanylate cyclase, which results in increased cytosolic levels of cyclic guanosine monophosphate (cGMP). Although platelet responses to low levels of this cyclic nucleotide can at first be mildly stimulatory,[104] cGMP, largely via its activation of protein kinase G (PKG), has the overall effect of dampening platelet responses, inhibiting platelet adhesion[105,106] and aggregation,[107-110] and

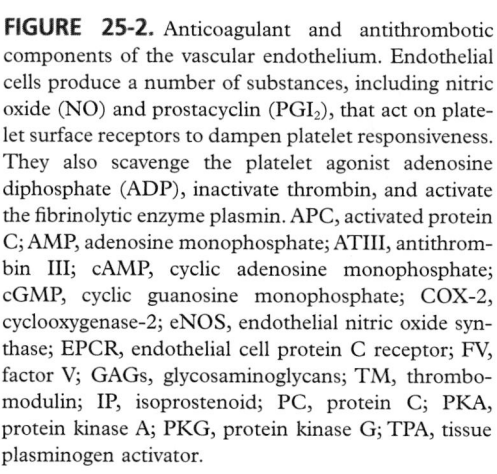
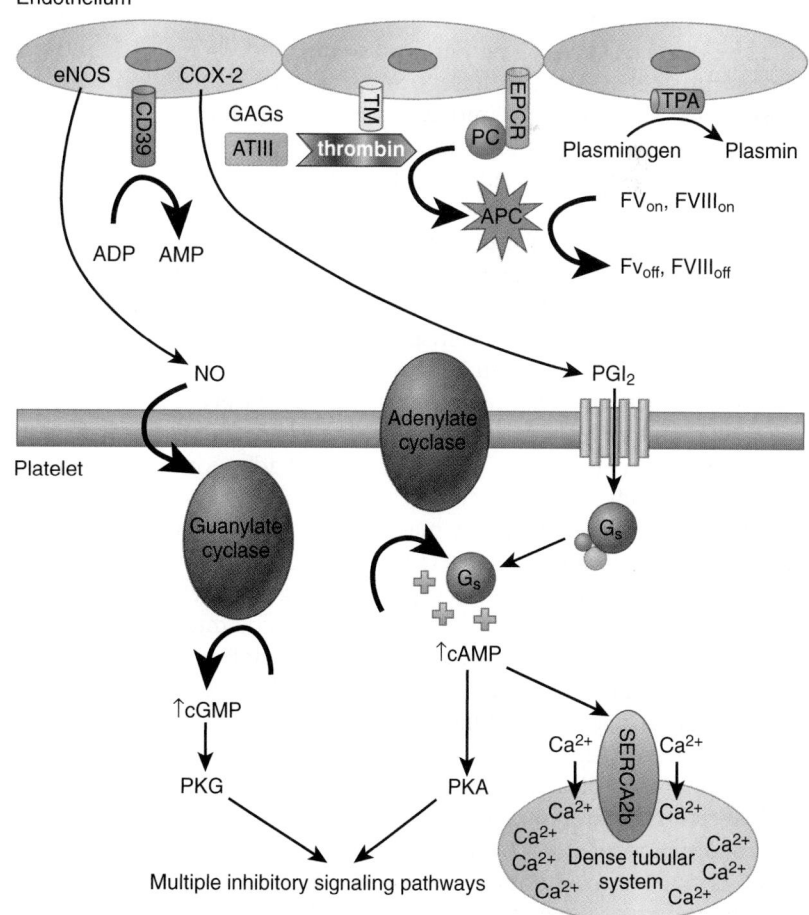

FIGURE 25-2. Anticoagulant and antithrombotic components of the vascular endothelium. Endothelial cells produce a number of substances, including nitric oxide (NO) and prostacyclin (PGI$_2$), that act on platelet surface receptors to dampen platelet responsiveness. They also scavenge the platelet agonist adenosine diphosphate (ADP), inactivate thrombin, and activate the fibrinolytic enzyme plasmin. APC, activated protein C; AMP, adenosine monophosphate; ATIII, antithrombin III; cAMP, cyclic adenosine monophosphate; cGMP, cyclic guanosine monophosphate; COX-2, cyclooxygenase-2; eNOS, endothelial nitric oxide synthase; EPCR, endothelial cell protein C receptor; FV, factor V; GAGs, glycosaminoglycans; TM, thrombomodulin; IP, isoprostenoid; PC, protein C; PKA, protein kinase A; PKG, protein kinase G; TPA, tissue plasminogen activator.

impeding platelet-mediated recruitment of leukocytes during the inflammatory response.[111] Its mechanism of action is discussed in more detail later.

In addition to the soluble metabolites PGI₂ and NO, endothelial cells also express on their surface a potent adenosine diphosphatase (ADPase) known as CD39 that scavenges plasma ADP to prevent platelet aggregation.[112,113] Finally, it is important to note that inflammatory cytokines, oxidized lipids, and immune complexes can, under pathologic conditions, inhibit these protective biochemical pathways and impair the antithrombotic state of the endothelial cell. The latter changes permit unrestrained formation of platelet- and fibrin-containing thrombi, as well as thrombus formation beyond sites of vascular injury, and can thus contribute to atherothrombosis—a topic that is discussed more extensively at the end of this chapter.

REACTING TO THE BREACH—CELL SURFACE RECEPTORS THAT MEDIATE TETHERING AND ADHESION AND TRANSMIT EARLY ACTIVATION SIGNALS

As antithrombotic as the endothelial lining is, the underlying extracellular matrix consists of a rich mixture of glycosaminoglycans into which are embedded an abundance of highly concentrated prothrombotic proteins, including structural components such as collagen and elastin (which constitute ≈30% of body weight) and adhesive proteins such as laminin, fibronectin, and VWF. Not surprisingly, platelets have evolved receptors for most of these proteins and initiate a series of rapid biochemical events both on the surface and inside the cell when exposed to them. As a result, adhesion is an activating event!

The large number of circulating red blood cells serve to marginate platelets, and when the vessel wall is breached, either by mechanical injury or after rupture of atherosclerotic plaque, the first layer of platelets to encounter exposed matrix undergoes a series of sequential events similar to what leukocytes experience during the inflammatory response—namely, tethering, initial signaling to the cell interior, integrin-mediated adhesion, and cytoskeletally directed cell spreading. Whereas leukocyte tethering is mediated by members of the selectin family, the first layer of platelets become tethered on VWF,[114] which is sprinkled on exposed collagen fibers. VWF interacts with a high-affinity, platelet-specific multisubunit receptor known as the GPIb/V/IX complex.[115] This latter complex, which is expressed at approximately 25,000 copies per cell,[116] binds to the A1 domain of VWF[117] with high-enough affinity to tether platelets even under conditions of arterial shear.[118] Loss of the GPIB/V/IX receptor in both humans and mice results in a clinical condition known as Bernard-Soulier syndrome,[13,14] which is characterized not only by an increase in platelet size but also by prolonged bleeding caused, in large part,

by the inability of platelets to adhere to the vessel wall. After engagement with its ligand, GPIb acts through membrane-proximal Src family kinases,[119] through adapter molecules,[120] and to a lesser extent, via its association with immunoreceptor tyrosine–based activation motif (ITAM)-bearing subunits[121,122] to transmit early activation signals[123,124] that together result in the recruitment and activation by tyrosine phosphorylation of phospholipase Cγ2 (PLCγ2),[125,126] a key enzymatic component of platelet amplification that is required to achieve thrombus growth and stability (Fig. 25-3).[127]

Once tethered, two different platelet integrins—each of which exists in a low-affinity state on the platelet surface—begin to engage specific extracellular matrix components and, together with the small calcium transients and kinase-generated signals emanating from the GPIb complex and from the mechanical shear force generated by the flowing blood,[128] initiate the reciprocal processes of platelet adhesion and activation. Thus, the α₂β₁ integrin binds to exposed collagen fibrils,[129] whereas the integrin receptor α₆β₁ engages laminin.[130] Both these integrins "hand off" to a member of the immunoglobulin superfamily, GPVI,[131,132] which via its noncovalent association in the plane of the plasma membrane with the ITAM-bearing Fc receptor γ chain dimer[131,133] elicits strong PLCγ2-dependent events that (1) begin the process of cytoskeletally directed shape change and cell spreading (discussed earlier); (2) initiate signal transduction pathways (illustrated in Fig. 25-3) that cause dramatic structural changes in platelet integrins and thereby result in their adopting a high-affinity, ligand-binding–competent conformation[134]—a process known as *"inside-out"* signal transduction (to be described in more detail later); and (3) facilitate fusion of alpha and dense granules with the OCS and underlying plasma membrane.

PLATELET GRANULES AND THEIR ROLE IN HEMOSTASIS

Platelet-specific granules are synthesized, assembled, and packaged during megakaryocyte biogenesis, and at later stages of maturation they appear to come into contact with microtubules, which then transport them, via the microtubule motor protein kinesin, along the shafts of proplatelets until they reach the proplatelet tips.[135] Once inside a mature platelet, platelet granules remain relatively evenly dispersed throughout the cytoplasm, their contents awaiting threshold signals for cellular activation, at which time their membranes fuse with the plasma membrane or, more likely, the invaginated subdomains of the plasma membrane known as the OCS[136] (see earlier). The regulated secretion of granule contents ensures that hemostasis remains highly localized—an event that has recently been exploited to deliver non–platelet-derived procoagulant proteins such as factor VIII to sites of vascular injury.[137,138]

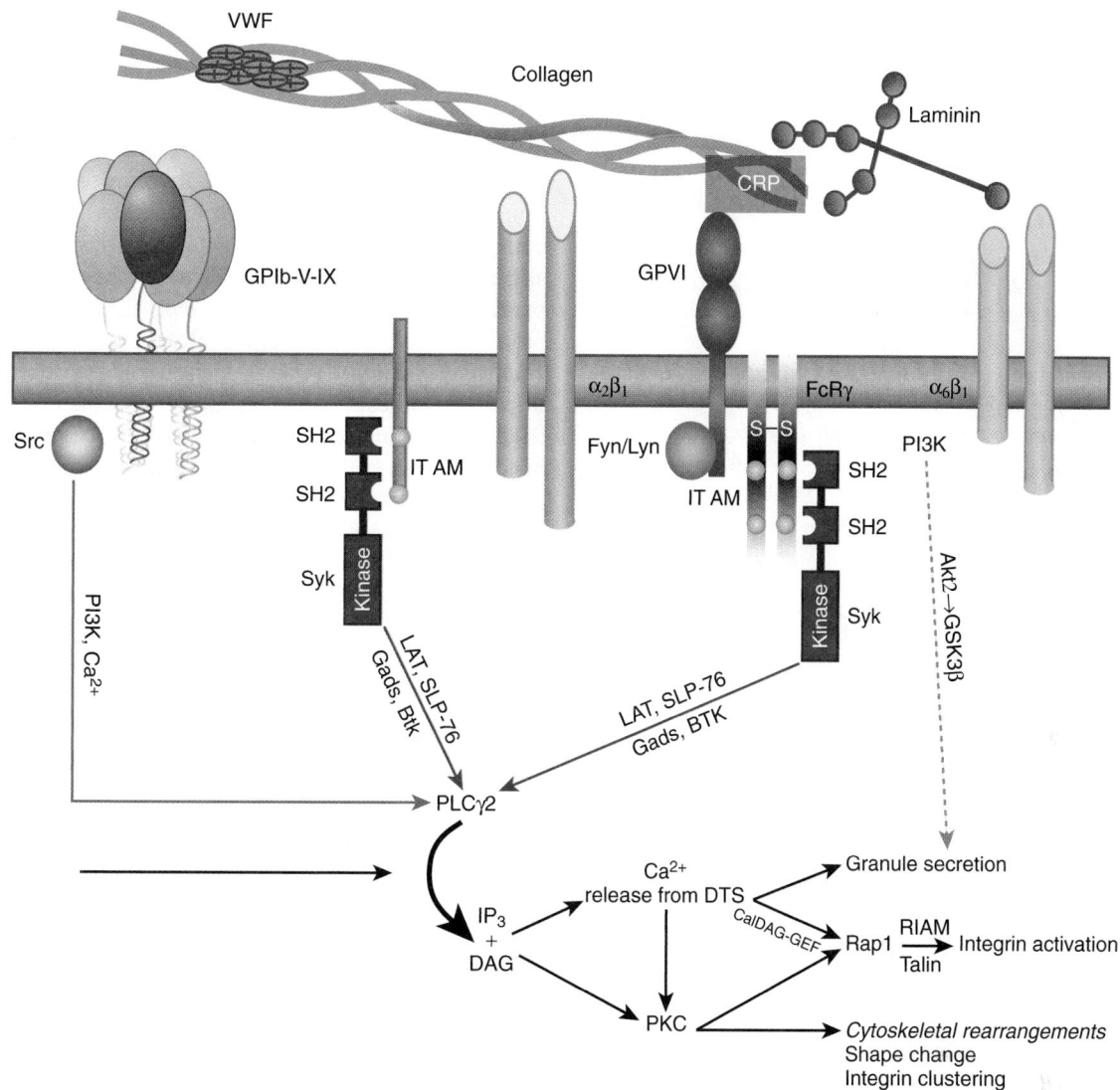

FIGURE 25-3. Platelet adhesion receptors that signal through phospholipase Cγ2 (PLCγ2). Each of the cell surface receptors shown recognizes different component of the extracellular matrix and thus works in coordinated fashion to send early activation signals into the cell. Binding of platelets to von Willebrand factor (VWF) slows platelets down so that integrins can associate productively with matrix collagen and laminin. Signals emanating from each of these events are transmitted into the cell interior, in part via the action of receptor-associated Src family kinases (Src, Fyn, Lyn), which phosphorylate tyrosine residues within nearby immunoreceptor tyrosine–based activation motifs (ITAMs), thus forming a nucleation point for the assembly of miniature organelles sometime referred to as signalosomes. Signalosomes are themselves composed of the adaptor proteins LAT, SLP-76, and Gads and the receptor tyrosine kinase Btk and function to localize, phosphorylate, and then activate PLCγ2, which coordinates all these responses by generating the classic signaling molecules 1,4,5-inositol triphosphate (IP$_3$) and diacylglycerol (DAG). Details regarding the molecular events that take place after the generation of IP$_3$ and DAG are shown in Figures 25-4 and 25-6. Btk, Bruton's tyrosine kinase; CRP, C-reactive protein; DTS, dense tubular system; GP1b, glycoprotein Ib; GSK3β, glycogen synthase kinase 3β; PI3K, posphatidylinositol-3′-kinase; PKC, protein kinase C; RIAM, Rap1$_{GTP}$-interacting adaptor molecule; SH2, Src homology domain 2.

Platelets harbor three distinct types of granules (Box 25-1). Two—alpha and dense granules—are found only in platelets, whereas lysosomes are present in nearly all cell types. Alpha granules are by far the most numerous, with as many as 40 to 80 per cell, and they contain a wide array of proteins and bioactive peptides. For ease of discussion, Box 25-1 classifies alpha granule proteins as those that reside within the alpha granule membrane (P-selectin being the most diagnostic), those pinocytosed from plasma and packaged (IgG, fibrinogen, albumin),[139] and those synthesized by megakaryocytes and stored (VWF,

platelet factor 4, thrombospondin). mRNA molecules encoding the latter group have all been identified in the platelet cytoplasm. Upon platelet activation, granules become redistributed toward the center of the cell,[136] at which time SNARE (soluble *N*-ethylmaleimide–sensitive attachment protein receptor) proteins within the alpha granule membrane facilitate fusion,[140] with members of the Rab family of low-molecular-weight guanosine triphosphatases (GTPases) playing a prominent role in vesicle docking and exocytosis.[141,142] After membrane fusion, P-selectin[143-145] and alpha granule membrane–

| Box 25-1 | **Platelet Granules and Their Contents** |

ALPHA GRANULES

Membrane proteins enriched in the granule membrane: P-selectin, TLT-1, CD40 ligand (which is cleaved after exposure on the platelet surface to release soluble CD40L), and tissue factor.

Membrane proteins present at similar concentrations as they are in the plasma membrane: GPIIb-IIIa, GPIb, PECAM-1, and perhaps many others

Granule contents:

Synthesized by megakaryocytes: Thrombospondin, VWF, platelet factor 4, β-thromboglobulin, PDGF

Endocytosed from plasma or origin not determined: Albumin, fibrinogen, fibronectin, IgG, Gas6, coagulation factor V, and many chemokines and growth factors, including RANTES, bFGF, EGF, TGF-β, and VEGF

DENSE GRANULES

ADP, ATP, 5′-HT, Ca^{2+}, polyphosphate

LYSOSOMES

Acid hydrolases, elastase, cathepsins, and other degradative enzymes

---

ADP, adenosine diphosphate; ATP, adenosine triphosphate; bFGF, basic fibroblast growth factor; EGF, epidermal growth factor; Gas6, growth arrest–specific gene 6; GP, glycoprotein; 5′-HT, 5′-hydroxytryptamine; PDGF, platelet-derived growth factor; PECAM-1, platelet endothelial cell adhesion molecule-1; RANTES, regulated on activation, T cell expressed and secreted; TGF-β, transforming growth factor β; TLT-1, TREM (triggering receptor expressed on myeloid cells)-like transcript-1; VEGF, vascular endothelial growth factor; VWF, von Willebrand factor.

---

specific proteins such as TLT-1[146] become expressed on the platelet surface, and the contents of the granule are released into the plasma milieu. Exposed P-selectin, diagnostic of an activated platelet,[147,148] serves to recruit leukocytes to the site of injury,[149] one of a number of important links between thrombosis and inflammation[150] (discussed at the end of this chapter). Proteins secreted from platelets include the adhesive ligands VWF and fibrinogen, which serve to support platelet-platelet interactions; growth factors and cytokines, which promote cell migration[151] and wound healing[152] and maintain vascular integrity[153]; and autocrine factors such as growth arrest–specific gene 6 (*Gas6*)[154] and CD40L,[155] which are released and rebind platelet receptors to help amplify platelet responsiveness. Finally, alpha granules and their contents are a source of procoagulant proteins, with release of factor V[156] and exposure of tissue factor[73,157] promoting localized fibrin deposition at sites of vascular injury. Platelet alpha granules, or at least their contents,[158] are severely reduced in an inherited bleeding disorder known as gray platelet syndrome (GPS) (see Chapter 29).[159]

Dense granules (four to eight per platelet) are morphologically distinct, electron-opaque storage organelles that contain the vasoconstrictive substance serotonin,[160-162] adenine and guanine nucleotides such as ADP and ATP, inorganic pyrophosphates[163] and polyphosphates,[164] and the divalent cation calcium.[165] Complexes of the latter two are probably responsible for the dark appearance of these bodies on thin-section electron microscopy.[166] Dense granule membranes contain a few components in common with lysosomal membranes, such as granulophysin (CD63, lysosome-associated membrane protein-3 [LAMP-3])[167] and LAMP-2,[168] as well as membrane proteins also present in alpha granule membranes, such as P-selectin,[167] thus suggesting a common origin during biogenesis. Like their alpha granule counterparts, these dense granule membrane proteins become expressed on the platelet cell surface after granule fusion and secretion and can be used as platelet activation markers. Curiously, a number of plasma membrane glycoproteins, including GPIb and GPIIb-IIIa, have also been reported in dense granule membranes.[169] Dense granule contents, especially ADP,[170] play a physiologically important role in hemostasis, as evidenced by characteristic platelet function defects in patients whose platelets lack dense granules or their contents,[171] collectively known as storage pool disorders.[172-174] Chédiak-Higashi and Hermansky-Pudlak[175] syndromes are two such examples of autosomal recessive dense granule defects that lead to platelet dysfunction and bleeding, the former being associated with immunodeficiency and the latter with albinism (see Chapter 29).

Primary lysosomes are the third organelle whose contents are secreted upon platelet activation, but only three or fewer per cell are normally identifiable.[176] Although a clear role for lysosomes in platelet function has not been identified, they do contain more than a dozen different acid hydrolases, cathepsins D and E, and other degradative enzymes that can be secreted if platelets are subjected to strong agonist stimulation. Their contents have been shown to be mildly reduced in the platelets of individuals with GPS,[177] in keeping with the notion that the latter disorder is caused by a defect in packaging. The membrane proteins on platelet lysosomes are typical of lysosomes in other cells and include LAMP-1,[178] LAMP-2,[168] and LAMP-3.[167]

FEED-FORWARD AMPLIFICATION PATHWAYS INVOLVED IN PLATELET RECRUITMENT AND THROMBUS STABILITY

Although platelet adhesion, early activation signals, and granule release are prerequisites for thrombus formation, *efficient* recruitment of additional platelets to the site of the vascular lesion to yield a stable platelet plug requires a host of additional receptor/ligand interactions—each of which results in signal transmission and subsequent biochemical and cell biologic changes that help sustain platelet activation. Among the most important of these is the binding of released ADP to one of its two platelet G protein–coupled receptors, P_2Y_{12}.[179,180] Like the α_2 receptor for epinephrine, P_2Y_{12} is coupled to an inhibitory G protein that slows down the activity of adenylate cyclase, thus lowering cytosolic levels of cAMP (Fig. 25-4). This greatly potentiates platelet responses by other agonists because it allows calcium ions—released from the DTS

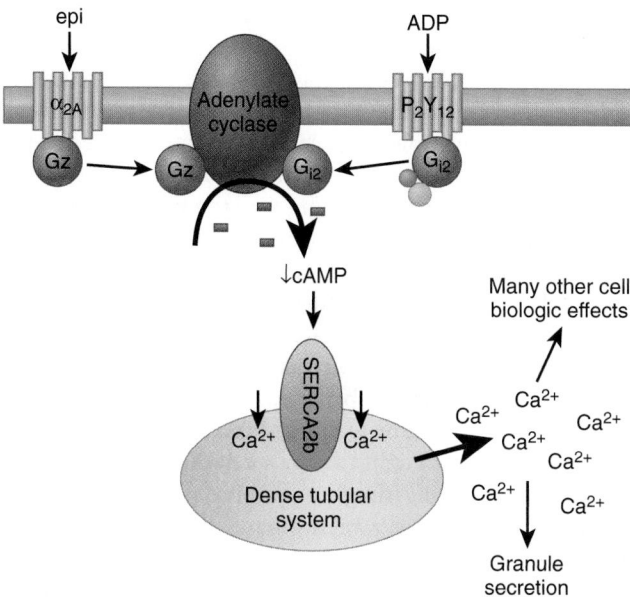

FIGURE 25-4. $G_\alpha i$ protein–coupled receptors on platelets inhibit adenylate cyclase and lower cyclic adenosine monophosphate (cAMP) levels. Shown are the two major receptors responsible for dampening the activity of adenylate cyclase. As cAMP levels drop, the ability of the SERCA2b calcium pump to sequester cytosolic calcium ions is impaired, thereby allowing calcium-mediated activation events to occur more readily.

as a result of the action of phospholipase-generated 1,4,5-inositol triphosphate (IP_3, discussed in more detail later)—to remain cytosolic. "Bioavailable" calcium ions, in turn, support a host of additional cellular events, including more robust granule secretion, activation of metal ion–dependent proteases, and activation of cell surface integrins. The importance of ADP in amplifying platelet responses is illustrated by the clinical effectiveness of ticlopidine and clopidogrel—widely used pharmacologic agents that antagonize the activity of P_2Y_{12}—in pacifying platelet reactivity and inhibiting platelet aggregation.[181]

In addition to ADP-induced, P_2Y_{12}-mediated signaling, nearly a dozen other soluble ligands are either generated or released at sites of vascular injury and function in signal amplification and platelet activation. These ligands can, for the sake of simplicity, be broken into three classes according to the type of platelet receptor to which they bind (Fig. 25-5). The first class of ligands is composed of ADP, thrombin, TXA_2, and serotonin (5′-hydroxytryptamine [5-HT]), each of which binds to a specific GPCR that is coupled to the heterotrimeric α subunit, G_q. Thus, ADP binds to P_2Y_1,[182-185] thrombin to the protease-activated receptors PAR1 and PAR4,[186,187] TXA_2 to the thromboxane receptor,[188,189] and serotonin to 5-HT_{2A}.[190] When released as a consequence of ligand binding to any of these GPCRs, the G_q subunit binds to the β isoform of phospholipase C (PLC). PLCs are lipid hydrolases that act on membrane-associated phosphatidylinositol 4,5-diphosphate (PIP_2) to produce the second messengers IP_3 and diacylglycerol (DAG). IP_3 binds and opens calcium channels, whereas DAG activates the most abundant forms of protein kinase C (PKC), thereby

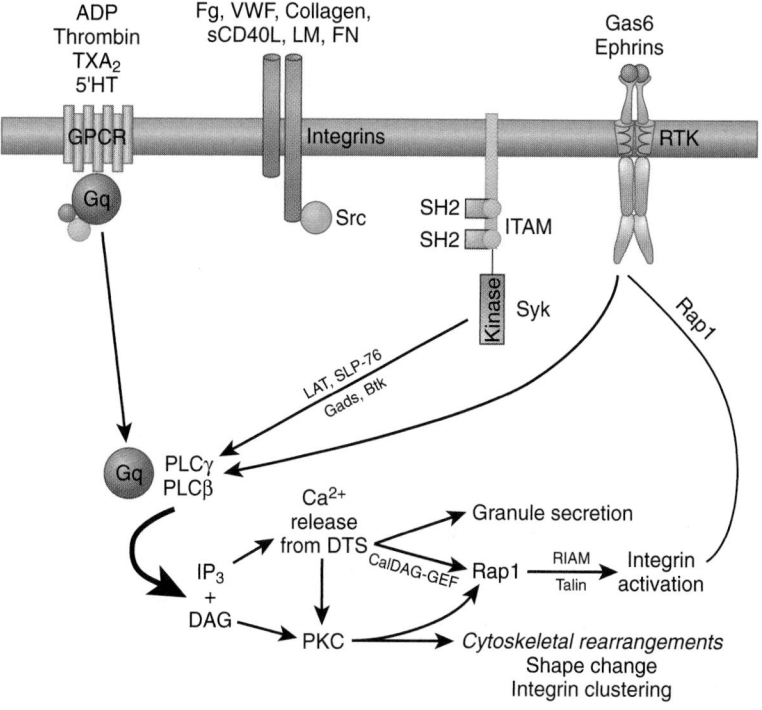

FIGURE 25-5. Agonist receptors that initiate or amplify platelet activation responses (or both). Three different families of receptors are involved in signal amplification pathways: G_q-coupled GPCRs, integrins, and receptor tyrosine kinases (RTKs). Note how each activates either the γ or β isoform of phospholipase C (PLC). The sum total of PLC-generated products serves to determine the activation state of the platelet, its ability to respond to vascular injury, and its participation in thrombus growth. ADP, adenosine triphosphate; Btk, Bruton's tyrosine kinase; DAG, diacylglycerol; DTS, dense tubular system; GPCR, G_s protein–coupled receptor; 5-HT, 5′-hydroxytryptamine; IP_3, 1,4,5-inositol triphosphate; ITAM, immunoreceptor tyrosine–based activation motif; PKC, protein kinase C; RIAM, $Rap1_{GTP}$-interacting adaptor molecule; SH2, Src homology domain 2; TXA_2, thromboxane A_2; VWF, von Willebrand factor.

initiating additional signaling cascades downstream of this serine/threonine kinase. As shown in Figure 25-5, it is the sum of these products—generated by the γ2 isoform of PLC in response to adhesion and by the β isoform of PLC in response to ligand-GPCR interactions—that the platelet integrates when deciding whether to become fully activated. This concept is important in the context of designing pharmacologic strategies to inhibit platelet function because blocking adhesion and its consequent activation of PLCγ2 leaves PLCβ-mediated platelet activation largely intact, and vice versa.

The second class of signal amplifiers consists of the cell surface integrins themselves.[191] As illustrated in the middle section of Figure 25-5, when ligands bind to integrins, the Src family kinases associated with integrin cytoplasmic tails[192] trigger a series of incompletely understood amplification events[193] that have been collectively termed "*outside-in*" signaling.[194-196] Although this has best been demonstrated after interaction of the major platelet integrin $\alpha_{IIb}\beta_3$ with its ligand fibrinogen, signals also probably emanate from $\alpha_2\beta_1$[134,197,198] and $\alpha_6\beta_1$[132] upon engaging collagen and laminin, respectively. Activation signals from the latter two may be relatively weak by comparison because of the fact that only a few thousand of each are expressed on each platelet as compared with 50,000 to 80,000 $\alpha_{IIb}\beta_3$ receptors per cell.[199,200] The protein kinases Syk and FAK have been shown to become activated downstream of $\alpha_{IIb}\beta_3$ engagement, as has activation of PLCγ2.[201] However, the details of these events remain to be worked out. Finally, there is at least one autocrine loop that uses integrin-mediated outside-in signal amplification—that being cleavage and rebinding of soluble CD40L after alpha granule fusion and secretion.[155]

The third class of feed-forward amplification reactions is mediated by ligand-activated plasma membrane receptor tyrosine kinases. The first of these to be described were receptors for Gas6, a vitamin K–dependent protein related to the anticoagulant protein S. Gas6 is thought to reside in platelet alpha granules[202,203] and, like other alpha granule proteins, becomes secreted upon platelet activation. Interestingly, platelets have three different receptors for Gas6—Axl, Sky, and Mer—all of which have active cytoplasmic tyrosine kinase activity (see Fig. 25-5). Upon engagement, Gas6 receptors appear to be able to trigger tyrosine phosphorylation of the β_3 integrin cytoplasmic domain and thereby support outside-in integrin signaling, as well as activate phosphatidylinositol-3'-kinase (PI3K) to further sustain granule secretion.[154] Platelets also express two members of the Eph receptor tyrosine kinase family, EphA4 and EphB1, which when in contact with their membrane-bound counter-receptor Ephrin B1, stimulate tyrosine phosphorylation of the integrin β_3 tail and activate the integrin activator Rap1b.[204] Like Gas6 signaling,[154,205,206] genetic loss or pharmacologic blockade of Ephrin/Eph kinase interactions results in decreased ability to form a stable thrombus or retract a fibrin clot.[207]

ACTIVATION OF THE MAJOR PLATELET INTEGRIN $\alpha_{IIb}\beta_3$ (GPIIB-IIIA COMPLEX)—THE FINAL COMMON END POINT OF PLATELET ACTIVATION

Human platelets express at least five different members of the 24-member integrin family,[196,208] including three β_1 integrins ($\alpha_2\beta_1$, $\alpha_5\beta_1$, and $\alpha_6\beta_1$—specific for collagen, fibronectin, and laminin, respectively) and two β_3 integrins—$\alpha_v\beta_3$ and its close relative $\alpha_{IIb}\beta_3$ (also known as the GPIIb-IIIa complex). $\alpha_{IIb}\beta_3$ is by far the most abundant and well studied. This section focuses on our current understanding of how $\alpha_{IIb}\beta_3$ becomes transformed from a resting to an active ligand-binding–competent conformation, with the understanding that the biochemical and cell biologic principles described for this integrin may well apply to the others.

As shown in schematic form on the left side of Figure 25-6, $\alpha_{IIb}\beta_3$ exists on the platelet surface in a bent-over conformation that is unable to associate effectively with its major soluble ligands fibrinogen, VWF, and fibronectin.[209,210] Though relatively short, the cytoplasmic domains of α_{IIb} and β_3 are thought to play a key role in maintaining the "off" state of this integrin complex as a result of weak charge interactions between them[211,212] that allow the hydrophobic transmembrane domain helices of each subunit to interact and maintain the integrin in a low-affinity state.[213,214] When platelets become activated—either by adhesion- or soluble agonist-mediated events—calcium and DAG, generated as a result of the actions of PLCγ2 and PLCβ (see Figs. 25-3 and 25-5), bind to and activate PKC and the guanine exchange factor CalDAG-GEF1. As illustrated in Figure 25-6, each of these can independently activate Rap1[215-219]—a low-molecular-weight GTPase that has been implicated in integrin activation.[220-222] Rap1 appears to activate integrins via an effector molecule known as RIAM (Rap1$_{GTP}$-interacting adaptor molecule), which recruits the highly abundant cytosolic protein talin to the inner face of the plasma membrane to form an integrin activation complex. Binding of RIAM-associated talin to the β_3 integrin subunit represents the final common step in integrin activation[223-225] because it disrupts the weak ionic clasp between the $\alpha_{IIb}\beta_3$ tails and thereby allows tail separation and a dramatic, rapid unfolding of the extracellular domain.[210] Simultaneous conformational changes in the integrin head[226,227] result in the formation of an integrin receptor with high affinity for its soluble adhesive ligands. Finally, clustering of integrins occurs[228] and ensures that bound ligands effectively broker with high avidity the platelet-platelet interactions that permit thrombus growth and stabilization.

CELL SURFACE AND CYTOSOLIC PROTEINS THAT LIMIT PLATELET RESPONSES

As anyone who has suffered a myocardial infarction or thrombotic stroke can attest to, unrestrained thrombus

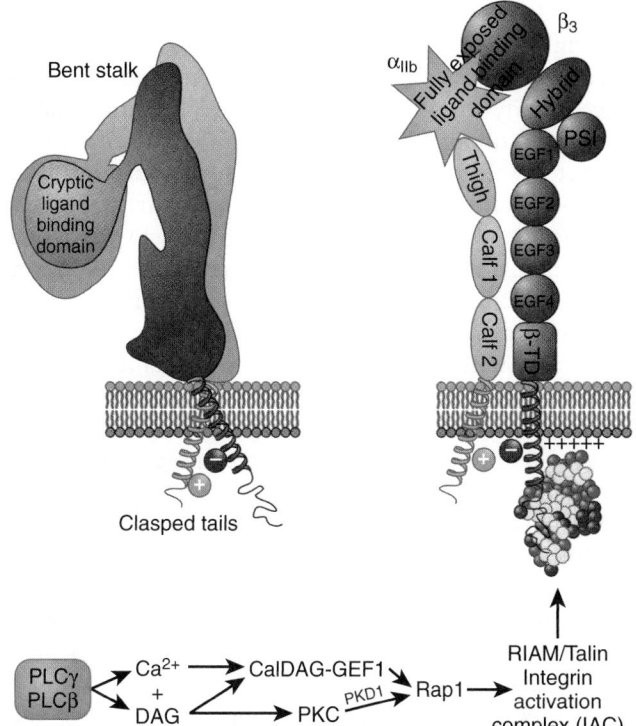

FIGURE 25-6. Integrin activation. As shown in the schematic at the *bottom*, calcium and diacylglycerol (DAG), generated as a result of the combined actions of phospholipase γ (PLCγ) and PLCβ, activate two proteins: (1) protein kinase C (PKC) and (2) the Rap guanine exchange factor CalDAG-GEF1. Each of these is able to independently activate the small guanosine triphosphates (GTPase) Rap1. In its GTP-bound form, Rap1 binds to and activates one of its effector molecules, Rap1$_{GTP}$-interacting adaptor molecule (RIAM), which then binds talin to form an integrin activation complex (IAC). When the IAC binds specific sites within the β$_3$ cytoplasmic domain, the clasp breaks, thereby destabilizing transmembrane domain helix associations that are thought to maintain the integrin in its low-affinity state (shown on the *left*). Breaking the hinge causes extensive conformational changes in the extracellular domain and produces a high-affinity, ligand-binding–competent integrin (shown on the *right*). EGF, epidermal growth factor; PSI, plexin-semiphorin-integrin; β-TD, beta terminal domain. *(Portions adapted from Wegener KL, Partridge AW, Han J, et al: Structural basis of integrin activation by talin. Cell 2007;128:171, with permission.)*

growth at inappropriate sites can be as harmful as excessive bleeding because it can result in vessel occlusion, ischemia, and tissue damage. Numerous active processes are therefore in place to limit platelet responsiveness in healthy vessels so that thrombus growth is kept localized to specific sites of vascular injury and dissolution of the platelet plug during recovery is facilitated.

As discussed earlier, healthy endothelium contributes to platelet passivation via rather continuous generation of PGI$_2$ and NO, which act on platelets by activating adenylate and guanylate cyclases to increase intracellular levels of cAMP and cGMP. These messengers activate PKA and PKG, respectively (illustrated in Fig. 25-2). PKG controls the threshold for platelet activation primarily by phosphorylating the IP$_3$ receptor–associated cGMP kinase substrate IRAG,[229] a protein that associates

with PKG and IP$_3$ receptor type I to inhibit IP$_3$-induced calcium release from intracellular stores.[230,231] Both PKA and PKG interfere with platelet activation by phosphorylating and inactivating VASP (vasodilator-stimulated phosphoprotein),[232] a molecule with anticapping activity that is important for the processes of actin polymerization and filopod formation.[233-237] PKCδ can also bind VASP and interfere with its ability to promote filopodia formation, although this pathway is unique to collagen-stimulated platelets and does not involve regulation of PKA- or PKG-mediated VASP phosphorylation.[238]

One of the better characterized inhibitory receptors in platelets is platelet endothelial cell adhesion molecule-1 (PECAM-1)—a cell surface molecule composed of six extracellular immunoglobulin domains, the most amino-terminal of which engages in homophilic interactions with PECAM-1 molecules on other cells, and two cytoplasmic immunoreceptor tyrosine–based inhibitory motifs (ITIMs) that upon phosphorylation, recruit and activate the cytosolic SH2 domain–containing protein tyrosine phosphatase-2 (SHP-2).[239,240] PECAM-1 has been shown to negatively regulate both GPVI- and GPIb/V/IX-mediated platelet activation[241-243]—perhaps by controlling the phosphorylation state of these two ITAM-bearing signaling receptors—and appears to be one of several inhibitory receptors that control the rate and extent of platelet thrombus formation in vivo.[244] Platelets have also recently been found to express two other immunoglobulin/ITIM-containing molecules: triggering receptor expressed on myeloid (TREM) cells–like transcript-1 (TLT-1) and products of the *G6b* gene. TLT-1 is contained within platelet alpha granules and is expressed on the platelet surface in an activation-dependent manner.[146,245] Although the two cytoplasmic ITIMs of TLT-1 are capable of becoming phosphorylated and recruiting SHP-2,[146] the extent to which TLT-1/SHP-2 complexes regulate platelet function is not yet known. The *G6b* gene, which is located within the class III region of the human major histocompatibility complex,[246] gives rise to multiple alternatively spliced transcripts (G6b-A through G6b-G).[247] Platelets contain at least two (G6b-A and G6b-B)[71,86,248] and possibly four (G6b-A, G6b-B, G6b-D, and G6b-E)[249] of these transcripts, and the G6b-B isoform contains cytoplasmic ITIMs that are capable of becoming tyrosine-phosphorylated and recruiting SHP-1 and SHP-2.[247] In platelets, the G6b-B isoform has been shown to be tyrosine-phosphorylated in resting and activated platelets, but to associate with SHP-1 only upon platelet activation.[248] Cross-linking of antibodies specific for *G6b* gene products has been shown to inhibit platelet aggregation in response to multiple stimuli[249]; however, whether these effects are due to the inhibitory function of G6b-B remains to be determined.

Several inhibitory pathways have been identified in platelets that either regulate or are regulated by PI3K—a lipid kinase that phosphorylates the 3′ position of PIP$_2$ to generate phosphatidylinositol 3,4,5-triphoshate (PIP$_3$), thereby creating docking sites on the inner face of the plasma membrane for Pleckstrin homology (PH) domain–containing molecules.[250] The actions of PI3K are opposed by the lipid phosphatase SHIP1 (SH2 domain–containing inositol 5′-phosphatase 1, which hydrolyzes the 5′-phosphate of PIP_3).[251,252] In platelets, SHIP1 has been shown to downregulate PIP_3 generation after $\alpha_{IIb}\beta_3$-mediated outside-in signaling[253] and thus may interfere with the feed-forward amplification pathways that increase the efficiency with which platelets are recruited to growing thrombi. Interestingly, the 5′-inositol phosphatase activity of SHIP1 appears to be enhanced, at least in part, by the actions of the Src family tyrosine kinase Lyn,[254-256] which itself has been shown to limit platelet aggregation in response to GPVI-specific stimuli[257] and after platelet spreading on immobilized fibrinogen.[253]

Akt (also known as protein kinase B) is a PH domain–containing serine/threonine kinase that is a well-characterized effector of PI3K.[258,259] Akt contributes positively to platelet activation in multiple ways, one of which appears to be by inactivating the serine/threonine kinase glycogen synthase kinase 3 (GSK3). The GSK3 family is composed of three isoforms (α, β, β_2) that are constitutively active in resting cells but become inactivated in activated cells by Akt-mediated phosphorylation.[260] Platelets express two isoforms of GSK3 (α and β), both of which become phosphorylated and inactivated after exposure of the platelet to multiple agonists that activate PI3K and Akt.[261] Whereas initial studies reported that specific inhibitors of GSK3 activity block rather than enhance platelet responses to agonist stimulation,[261] a recent report suggest that as in other cells, the β isoform of GSK3 acts as a negative regulator of platelet function both in vitro and in vivo.[262]

ADDITIONAL ROLES FOR PLATELETS IN VASCULAR PHYSIOLOGY: VESSEL REPAIR (ANGIOGENESIS), INFLAMMATION, AND ATHEROTHROMBOSIS

In addition to being essential for primary hemostasis, activated platelets and their secreted products have the ability to influence a broad array of pathophysiologic processes, including leukocyte trafficking and inflammation, tissue regeneration and angiogenesis, and both the beginning and end stages of atherosclerosis.

Activated platelets that become spread on components of the extracellular matrix, or on each other, display an altered surface phenotype—the most prominent of which is exposure of several thousand copies of the alpha granule–derived membrane protein P-selectin. P-selectin is also expressed on cytokine-activated endothelial cells. Thus, after either a thrombotic or inflammatory event, P-selectin appears on the luminal face of the vessel wall, where it serves to recruit monocytes and neutrophils into the underlying tissue by binding PSGL-1—a constitutively expressed counter-receptor for P-selectin that is

present on most leukocytes. In vivo, mice lacking P-selectin exhibit greatly diminished leukocyte rolling, delayed recruitment into sites of inflammation, and increased susceptibility to infection.[263,264] Although endothelial P-selectin no doubt has a major role in leukocyte capture, platelet P-selectin probably plays a prominent role in "secondary capture."[265,266] As in platelets, tethering also initiates activation of leukocyte integrins, which are then able to mediate cell spreading and transendothelial migration. P-selectin/PSGL-1 interactions therefore constitute an important link between thrombosis and inflammation.[150,267] Other platelet/leukocyte receptor/counter-receptor pairs have also been shown to facilitate the inflammatory response, including binding of platelet-associated fibrinogen to the leukocyte integrin MAC-1[268] and platelet JAM-3 binding to MAC-1 on monocytes[269] and dendritic cells.[270]

In addition to forming a platform for leukocyte recruitment during acute inflammation, platelets also deliver to the vessel wall proinflammatory chemokines that are thought to play a role in the development of atherosclerosis by promoting further chemoattraction of leukocytes and stimulating proliferation of vessel wall smooth muscle cells and fibroblasts. Such secreted factors include the C-X-C chemokine platelet factor 4, macrophage inflammatory protein 1a (MIP-1a), the C-C chemokine RANTES (regulated on activation, T cell expressed and secreted), CD40 ligand, platelet-derived growth factor (PDGF), and transforming growth factor β (TGF-β).[150,267,271,272] Activated platelets also synthesize de novo IL-1β,[273,274] a potent stimulator of endothelial cells and monocytes that upregulates adhesion molecule expression. Thus, platelets appear to contribute in a number of ways to the development and progression of atherosclerotic lesions.

Finally, so that one is not left with the impression that platelets only exacerbate chronic human disease, it should be noted that platelets and their secreted products were shown as early as 1969[153] to be able to "nurture" the vascular endothelium, and they have recently been proposed as a source of biologic response modifiers for a plethora of uses, including organ preservation, gum restoration after dental procedures, and tissue repair after surgery.[152] Their ability to adhere at sites of vascular injury and secrete both degradative enzymes and at the same time growth-promoting factors such as vascular endothelial growth factor (VEGF), PDGF, fibroblast growth factor (FGF), epidermal growth factor (EGF), and angiopoietin 1 allows them to play a uniquely supportive role in endothelial cell migration and survival during the process of wound healing and angiogenesis.[151]

Acknowledgment

The authors thank Robert I. Handin for valuable insights gleaned from versions of this chapter that appeared in earlier editions of this book. Research in the authors' laboratories is supported by grants from the American Heart Association and the National Heart, Lung, and Blood Institute of the National Institutes of Health.

REFERENCES

1. de Gaetano G. A new blood corpuscle: an impossible interview with Giulio Bizzozero. Thromb Haemost. 2001; 86:973-979.

2. Yamada E. The fine structure of the megakaryocyte in the mouse spleen. Acta Anat (Basel). 1957;29:267-290.

3. Shaklai M, Tavassoli M. Demarcation membrane system in rat megakaryocyte and the mechanism of platelet formation: a membrane reorganization process. J Ultrastruct Res. 1978;62:270-285.

4. Italiano JE, Lecine P, Shivdasani RA, Hartwig JH. Blood platelets are assembled principally at the ends of proplatelet processes produced by differentiated megakaryocytes. J Cell Biol. 1999;147:1299-1312.

5. Italiano JE Jr, Shivdasani RA. Megakaryocytes and beyond: the birth of platelets. J Thromb Haemost. 2003;1: 1174-1182.

6. Patel SR, Hartwig JH, Italiano JE Jr. The biogenesis of platelets from megakaryocyte proplatelets. J Clin Invest. 2005;115:3348-3354.

7. Avecilla ST, Hattori K, Heissig B, et al. Chemokine-mediated interaction of hematopoietic progenitors with the bone marrow vascular niche is required for thrombopoiesis. Nat Med. 2004;10:64-71.

8. Radley JM, Haller CJ. The demarcation membrane system of the megakaryocyte: a misnomer? Blood. 1982;60: 213-219.

9. Schulze H, Korpal M, Hurov J, et al. Characterization of the megakaryocyte demarcation membrane system and its role in thrombopoiesis. Blood. 2006;107:3868-3875.

10. Aster RH. Platelet sequestration studies in man. Br J Haematol. 1972;22:259-263.

11. Mason KD, Carpinelli MR, Fletcher JI, et al. Programmed anuclear cell death delimits platelet life span. Cell. 2007; 128:1173-1186.

12. Franke JD, Dong F, Rickoll WL, et al. Rod mutations associated with MYH9-related disorders disrupt nonmuscle myosin-IIA assembly. Blood. 2005;105:161-169.

13. Caen JP, Nurden AT, Jeanneau C, et al. Bernard-Soulier syndrome: a new platelet glycoprotein abnormality. Its relationship with platelet adhesion to the subendothelium and with the factor VIII von Willebrand protein. J Lab Clin Med. 1976;87:586-596.

14. Jenkins CS, Phillips DR, Clemetson KJ, et al. Platelet membrane glycoproteins implicated in ristocetin-induced aggregation. Studies of the proteins on platelets from patients with Bernard-Soulier syndrome and von Willebrand's disease. J Clin Invest. 1976;57:112-124.

15. Okita JR, Pidard D, Newman PJ, et al. On the association of glycoprotein Ib and actin-binding protein in human platelets. J Cell Biol. 1985;100:317-321.

16. Fox JE. Linkage of a membrane skeleton to integral membrane glycoproteins in human platelets. Identification of one of the glycoproteins as glycoprotein Ib. J Clin Invest. 1985;76:1673-1683.

17. White JG, Burris SM, Hasegawa D, Johnson M. Micropipette aspiration of human blood platelets: a defect in Bernard-Soulier's syndrome. Blood. 1984;63:1249-1252.

18. Ware J, Russell S, Ruggeri ZM. Generation and rescue of a murine model of platelet dysfunction: the Bernard-Soulier syndrome. Proc Natl Acad Sci U S A. 2000;97: 2803-2808.

19. Corash L, Tan H, Gralnick HR. Heterogeneity of human whole blood platelet subpopulations. I. Relationship between buoyant density, cell volume, and ultrastructure. Blood. 1977;49:71-87.

20. Karpatkin S. Heterogeneity of rabbit platelets. VI. Further resolution of changes in platelet density, volume, and radioactivity following cohort labelling with ^{75}Se-selenomethione. Br J Haematol. 1978;39:459-469.

21. Corash L, Costa JL, Shafer B, et al. Heterogeneity of human whole blood platelet subpopulations. III. Density-dependent differences in subcellular constituents. Blood. 1984;64:185-193.

22. Mezzano D, Hwang K, Catalano P, Aster RH. Evidence that platelet buoyant density, but not size, correlates with platelet age in man. Am J Hematol. 1981;11:61-76.

23. Newman PJ, Gorski J, White GC, et al. Enzymatic amplification of platelet-specific messenger RNA using the polymerase chain reaction. J Clin Invest. 1988;82:739-743.

24. Kienast J, Schmitz G. Flow cytometric analysis of thiazole orange uptake by platelets: a diagnostic aid in the evaluation of thrombocytopenic disorders. Blood. 1990;75: 116-121.

25. White JG, Krivit W. An ultrastructural basis for the shape changes induced in platelets by chilling. Blood. 1967;30: 625-635.

26. Kenney DM, Linck RW. The cystoskeleton of unstimulated blood platelets: structure and composition of the isolated marginal microtubular band. J Cell Sci. 1985; 78:1-22.

27. Bentfeld ME, Bainton DF. Cytochemical localization of lysosomal enzymes in rat megakaryocytes and platelets. J Clin Invest. 1975;56:1635-1649.

28. Behnke O. Electron microscopic observations on the membrane systems of the rat blood platelet. Anat Rec. 1967;158:121-137.

29. Escolar G, Leistikow E, White JG. The fate of the open canalicular system in surface and suspension-activated platelets. Blood. 1989;74:1983-1988.

30. White JG, Escolar G. The blood platelet open canalicular system: a two-way street. Eur J Cell Biol. 1991;56: 233-242.

31. Gerrard JM, White JG, Peterson DA. The platelet dense tubular system: its relationship to prostaglandin synthesis and calcium flux. Thromb Haemost. 1978;40:224-231.

32. Papp B, Enyedi A, Pászty K, et al. Simultaneous presence of two distinct endoplasmic-reticulum–type calcium-pump isoforms in human cells. Characterization by radio-immunoblotting and inhibition by 2,5-di-(t-butyl)-1,4-benzohydroquinone. Biochem J. 1992;288:297-302.

33. Wuytack F, Papp B, Verboomen H, et al. A sarco/endoplasmic reticulum Ca^{2+}-ATPase 3–type Ca^{2+} pump is expressed in platelets, in lymphoid cells, and in mast cells [published erratum appears in J Biol Chem. 1994;269(17):13056]. J Biol Chem. 1994;269:1410-1416.

34. Enouf J, Bredoux R, Papp B, et al. Human platelets express the SERCA2-b isoform of Ca²⁺-transport ATPase. Biochem J. 1992;286:135-140.

35. Jardin I, Ben-amor N, Bartegi A, et al. Differential involvement of thrombin receptors in Ca²⁺ release from two different intracellular stores in human platelets. Biochem J. 2007;401:167-174.

36. Lopez JJ, Camello-Almaraz C, Pariente JA, et al. Ca²⁺ accumulation into acidic organelles mediated by Ca²⁺- and vacuolar H⁺-ATPases in human platelets. Biochem J. 2005;390:243-252.

37. Haydon GB, Taylor DA. Microtubules in hamster platelets. J Cell Biol. 1965;26:673-676.

38. Behnke O. Further studies on microtubules. A marginal bundle in human and rat thrombocytes. J Ultrastruct Res. 1965;13:469-477.

39. White JG, Krumwiede M. Isolation of microtubule coils from normal human platelets. Blood. 1985;65:1028-1032.

40. White JG. Effects of colchicine and vinca alkaloids on human platelets. I. Influence on platelet microtubules and contractile function. Am J Pathol. 1968;53:281-291.

41. Schwer HD, Lecine P, Tiwari S, et al. A lineage-restricted and divergent beta-tubulin isoform is essential for the biogenesis, structure and function of blood platelets. Curr Biol. 2001;11:579-586.

42. White JG, de Alarcon PA. Platelet spherocytosis: a new bleeding disorder. Am J Hematol. 2002;70:158-166.

43. Fox JE, Boyles JK, Berndt MC, et al. Identification of a membrane skeleton in platelets. J Cell Biol. 1988;106:1525-1538.

44. Fox JE, Reynolds CC, Morrow JS, Phillips DR. Spectrin is associated with membrane-bound actin filaments in platelets and is hydrolyzed by the Ca²⁺-dependent protease during platelet activation. Blood. 1987;69:537-545.

45. Hartwig JH, DeSisto M. The cytoskeleton of the resting human blood platelet: structure of the membrane skeleton and its attachment to actin filaments. J Cell Biol. 1991;112:407-425.

46. Asijee GM, Sturk A, Bruin T, et al. Vinculin is a permanent component of the membrane skeleton and is incorporated into the (re)organising cytoskeleton upon platelet activation. Eur J Biochem. 1990;189:131-136.

47. Fox JEB. Identification of actin-binding protein as the protein linking the membrane skeleton to glycoproteins on platelet plasma membranes. J Biol Chem. 1985;260:11970-11977.

48. Loftus JC, Choate J, Albrecht RM. Platelet activation and cytoskeletal reorganization: high voltage electron microscopic examination of intact and Triton-extracted whole mounts. J Cell Biol. 1984;98:2019-2025.

49. Newman PJ, Hillery CA, Albrecht R, et al. Activation-dependent changes in human platelet PECAM-1: phosphorylation, cytoskeletal association, and surface membrane redistribution. J Cell Biol. 1992;119:239-246.

50. Bennett JS, Zigmond S, Vilaire G, et al. The platelet cytoskeleton regulates the affinity of the integrin $\alpha_{IIb}\beta_3$ for fibrinogen. J Biol Chem. 1999;274:25301-25307.

51. Hato T, Pampori N, Shattil SJ. Complementary roles for receptor clustering and conformational change in the adhesive and signaling functions of integrin $\alpha_{IIb}\beta_3$. J Cell Biol. 1998;141:1685-1695.

52. Fox JEB, Shattil SJ, Kinlough-Rathbone RL, et al. The platelet cytoskeleton stabilizes the interaction between $\alpha_{IIb}\beta_3$ and its ligand and induces selective movement of ligand-occupied integrin. J Biol Chem. 1996;271:7004-7011.

53. Fox JE, Lipfert L, Clark EA, et al. On the role of the platelet membrane skeleton in mediating signal transduction. Association of GP IIb-IIIa, pp60c-src, pp62c-yes, and the p21ras GTPase-activating protein with the membrane skeleton. J Biol Chem. 1993;268:25973-25984.

54. Nachmias VT. Cytoskeleton of human platelets at rest and after spreading. J Cell Biol. 1980;86:795-802.

55. Phillips DR, Jennings LK, Edwards HH. Identification of membrane proteins mediating the interaction of human platelets. J Cell Biol. 1980;86:77-86.

56. Rosenberg S, Stracher A, Lucas RC. Isolation and characterization of actin and actin-binding protein from human platelets. J Cell Biol. 1981;91:201-211.

57. Rosenberg S, Stracher A, Burridge K. Isolation and characterization of a calcium-sensitive alpha-actinin–like protein from human platelet cytoskeletons. J Biol Chem. 1981;256:12986-12991.

58. Kroll MH, Harris TS, Moake JL, et al. von Willebrand factor binding to platelet GPIb initiates signals for platelet activation. J Clin Invest. 1991;88:1568-1573.

59. White JG. Fine structural alterations induced in platelets by adenosine diphosphate. Blood. 1968;31:604-622.

60. Carlsson L, Markey F, Blikstad I, et al. Reorganization of actin in platelets stimulated by thrombin as measured by the DNase I inhibition assay. Proc Natl Acad Sci U S A. 1979;76:6376-6380.

61. Jennings LK, Fox JE, Edwards HH, Phillips DR. Changes in the cytoskeletal structure of human platelets following thrombin activation. J Biol Chem. 1981;256:6927-6932.

62. Fox JE, Phillips DR. Polymerization and organization of actin filaments within platelets. Semin Hematol. 1983;20:243-260.

63. Hartwig JH. Mechanisms of actin rearrangements mediating platelet activation. J Cell Biol. 1992;118:1421-1442.

64. Barkalow KL, Italiano JE Jr, Chou DE, et al. α-Adducin dissociates from F-actin and spectrin during platelet activation. J Cell Biol. 2003;161:557-570.

65. Fox JE, Phillips DR. Role of phosphorylation in mediating the association of myosin with the cytoskeletal structures of human platelets. J Biol Chem. 1982;257:4120-4126.

66. Booyse F, Rafelson ME Jr. In vitro incorporation of amino-acids into the contractile protein of human blood platelets. Nature. 1967;215:283-284.

67. Kieffer N, Guichard J, Farcet JP, et al. Biosynthesis of major platelet proteins in human blood platelets. Eur J Biochem. 1987;164:189-195.

68. Gnatenko DV, Dunn JJ, McCorkle SR, et al. Transcript profiling of human platelets using microarray and serial analysis of gene expression. Blood. 2003;101:2285-2293.

69. McRedmond JP, Park SD, Reilly DF, et al. Integration of proteomics and genomics in platelets: a profile of platelet proteins and platelet-specific genes. Mol Cell Proteomics. 2004;3:133-144.

70. Dittrich M, Birschmann I, Pfrang J, et al. Analysis of SAGE data in human platelets: features of the transcrip-

tome in an anucleate cell. Thromb Haemost. 2006;95: 643-651.

71. Macaulay IC, Tijssen MR, Thijssen-Timmer DC, et al. Comparative gene expression profiling of in vitro differentiated megakaryocytes and erythroblasts identifies novel activatory and inhibitory platelet membrane proteins. Blood. 2007;109:3260-3269.

72. Denis MM, Tolley ND, Bunting M, et al. Escaping the nuclear confines: signal-dependent pre-mRNA splicing in anucleate platelets. Cell. 2005;122:379-391.

73. Schwertz H, Tolley ND, Foulks JM, et al. Signal-dependent splicing of tissue factor pre-mRNA modulates the thrombogenicity of human platelets. J Exp Med. 2006;203: 2433-2440.

74. Weyrich AS, Denis MM, Schwertz H, et al. mTOR-dependent synthesis of Bcl-3 controls the retraction of fibrin clots by activated human platelets. Blood. 2007;109: 1975-1983.

75. O'Farrell PH. High resolution two-dimensional electrophoresis of proteins. J Biol Chem. 1975;250:4007-4021.

76. Ames GF, Nikaido K. Two-dimensional gel electrophoresis of membrane proteins. Biochemistry. 1976;15: 616-623.

77. Macaulay IC, Carr P, Gusnanto A, et al. Platelet genomics and proteomics in human health and disease. J Clin Invest. 2005;115:3370-3377.

78. Dittrich M, Birschmann I, Stuhlfelder C, et al. Understanding platelets. Lessons from proteomics, genomics and promises from network analysis. Thromb Haemost. 2005;94:916-925.

79. Martens L, Van DP, Van DJ, et al. The human platelet proteome mapped by peptide-centric proteomics: a functional protein profile. Proteomics. 2005;5:3193-3204.

80. Marcus K, Moebius J, Meyer HE. Differential analysis of phosphorylated proteins in resting and thrombin-stimulated human platelets. Anal Bioanal Chem. 2003;376: 973-993.

81. Maguire PB, Fitzgerald DJ. Platelet proteomics. J Thromb Haemost. 2003;1:1593-1601.

82. Garcia A, Senis YA, Antrobus R, et al. A global proteomics approach identifies novel phosphorylated signaling proteins in GPVI-activated platelets: involvement of G6f, a novel platelet Grb2-binding membrane adapter. Proteomics. 2006;6:5332-5343.

83. Gevaert K, Eggermont L, Demol H, Vandekerckhove J. A fast and convenient MALDI-MS based proteomic approach: identification of components scaffolded by the actin cytoskeleton of activated human thrombocytes. J Biotechnol. 2000;78:259-269.

84. Maguire PB, Moran N, Cagney G, Fitzgerald DJ. Application of proteomics to the study of platelet regulatory mechanisms. Trends Cardiovasc Med. 2004;14:207-220.

85. Coppinger JA, Cagney G, Toomey S, et al. Characterization of the proteins released from activated platelets leads to localization of novel platelet proteins in human atherosclerotic lesions. Blood. 2004;103:2096-2104.

86. Moebius J, Zahedi RP, Lewandrowski U, et al. The human platelet membrane proteome reveals several new potential membrane proteins. Mol Cell Proteomics. 2005;4:1754-1761.

87. Maguire PB, Foy M, Fitzgerald DJ. Using proteomics to identify potential therapeutic targets in platelets. Biochem Soc Trans. 2005;33:409-412.

88. Garcia BA, Smalley DM, Cho H, et al. The platelet microparticle proteome. J Proteome Res. 2005;4:1516-1521.

89. Damus PS, Hicks M, Rosenberg RD. Anticoagulant action of heparin. Nature. 1973;246:355-357.

90. Esmon CT. The roles of protein C and thrombomodulin in the regulation of blood coagulation. J Biol Chem. 1989;264:4743-4746.

91. Fukudome K, Esmon CT. Identification, cloning, and regulation of a novel endothelial cell protein C/activated protein C receptor. J Biol Chem. 1994;269:26486-26491.

92. Levin EG. Latent tissue plasminogen activator produced by human endothelial cells in culture: evidence for an enzyme-inhibitor complex. Proc Natl Acad Sci U S A. 1983;80:6804-6808.

93. Hajjar KA, Hamel NM, Harpel PC, Nachman RL. Binding of tissue plasminogen activator to cultured human endothelial cells. J Clin Invest. 1987;80:1712-1719.

94. Bunting S, Gryglewski R, Moncada S, Vane JR. Arterial walls generate from prostaglandin endoperoxides a substance (prostaglandin X) which relaxes strips of mesenteric and coeliac arteries and inhibits platelet aggregation. Prostaglandins. 1976;12:897-913.

95. Gryglewski RJ, Bunting S, Moncada S, et al. Arterial walls are protected against deposition of platelet thrombi by a substance (prostaglandin X) which they make from prostaglandin endoperoxides. Prostaglandins. 1976;12:685-713.

96. Moncada S, Gryglewski R, Bunting S, Vane JR. An enzyme isolated from arteries transforms prostaglandin endoperoxides to an unstable substance that inhibits platelet aggregation. Nature. 1976;263:663-665.

97. Furchgott RF, Zawadzki JV. The obligatory role of endothelial cells in the relaxation of arterial smooth muscle by acetylcholine. Nature. 1980;288:373-376.

98. Ignarro LJ, Buga GM, Wood KS, et al. Endothelium-derived relaxing factor produced and released from artery and vein is nitric oxide. Proc Natl Acad Sci U S A. 1987;84:9265-9269.

99. Palmer RM, Ferrige AG, Moncada S. Nitric oxide release accounts for the biological activity of endothelium-derived relaxing factor. Nature. 1987;327:524-526.

100. Boie Y, Rushmore TH, Darmon-Goodwin A, et al. Cloning and expression of a cDNA for the human prostanoid IP receptor. J Biol Chem. 1994;269:12173-12178.

101. Namba T, Oida H, Sugimoto Y, et al. cDNA cloning of a mouse prostacyclin receptor. Multiple signaling pathways and expression in thymic medulla. J Biol Chem. 1994; 269:9986-9992.

102. Cheng Y, Austin SC, Rocca B, et al. Role of prostacyclin in the cardiovascular response to thromboxane A_2. Science. 2002;296:539-541.

103. Pollock JS, Forstermann U, Mitchell JA, et al. Purification and characterization of particulate endothelium-derived relaxing factor synthase from cultured and native bovine aortic endothelial cells. Proc Natl Acad Sci U S A. 1991; 88:10480-10484.

104. Li Z, Xi X, Gu M, et al. A stimulatory role for cGMP-dependent protein kinase in platelet activation. Cell. 2003;112:77-86.

105. Radomski MW, Palmer RM, Moncada S. Endogenous nitric oxide inhibits human platelet adhesion to vascular endothelium. Lancet. 1987;2:1057-1058.

106. Sneddon JM, Vane JR. Endothelium-derived relaxing factor reduces platelet adhesion to bovine endothelial cells. Proc Natl Acad Sci U S A. 1988;85:2800-2804.

107. Azuma H, Ishikawa M, Sekizaki S. Endothelium-dependent inhibition of platelet aggregation. Br J Pharmacol. 1986;88:411-415.

108. Radomski MW, Palmer RM, Moncada S. The anti-aggregating properties of vascular endothelium: interactions between prostacyclin and nitric oxide. Br J Pharmacol. 1987;92:639-646.

109. Macdonald PS, Read MA, Dusting GJ. Synergistic inhibition of platelet aggregation by endothelium-derived relaxing factor and prostacyclin. Thromb Res. 1988;49:437-449.

110. Stamler J, Mendelsohn ME, Amarante P, et al. N-acetylcysteine potentiates platelet inhibition by endothelium-derived relaxing factor. Circ Res. 1989;65:789-795.

111. Michelson AD, Benoit SE, Furman MI, et al. Effects of nitric oxide/EDRF on platelet surface glycoproteins. Am J Physiol. 1996;270:H1640-H1648.

112. Kaczmarek E, Koziak K, Sevigny J, et al. Identification and characterization of CD39/vascular ATP diphosphohydrolase. J Biol Chem. 1996;271:33116-33122.

113. Marcus AJ, Broekman MJ, Drosopoulos JH, et al. The endothelial cell ecto-ADPase responsible for inhibition of platelet function is CD39. J Clin Invest. 1997;99:1351-1360.

114. Dopheide SM, Maxwell MJ, Jackson SP. Shear-dependent tether formation during platelet translocation on von Willebrand factor. Blood. 2002;99:159-167.

115. Lopez JA, Berndt MC. The GPIb-IX-V Complex. Platelets. San Diego, CA, Academic Press, 2002, pp 85-97.

116. Coller BS, Peerschke EL, Scudder IE, Sullivan CA. Studies with a murine monoclonal antibody that abolishes ristocetin-induced binding of von Willebrand factor to platelets: additional evidence in support of GPIb as a platelet receptor for von Willebrand factor. Blood. 1983;61:99-110.

117. Lankhof H, Wu YP, Vink T, et al. Role of the glycoprotein Ib-binding A1 repeat and the RGD sequence in platelet adhesion to human recombinant von Willebrand factor. Blood. 1995;86:1035-1042.

118. Savage B, Saldivar E, Ruggeri ZM. Initiation of platelet adhesion by arrest onto fibrinogen or translocation on von Willebrand factor. Cell. 1996;84:289-297.

119. Kasirer-Friede A, Cozzi MR, Mazzucato M, et al. Signaling through GP Ib-IX-V activates alpha IIb beta 3 independently of other receptors. Blood. 2004;103:3403-3411.

120. Kasirer-Friede A, Moran B, Nagrampa-Orje J, et al. ADAP is required for normal $\alpha_{IIb}\beta_3$ activation by VWF/GP Ib-IX-V and other agonists. Blood. 2007;109:1018-1025.

121. Sullam PM, Hyun WC, Szollosi J, et al. Physical proximity and functional interplay of the glycoprotein Ib-IX-V complex and the Fc receptor FcγRIIA on the platelet plasma membrane. J Biol Chem. 1998;273:5331-5336.

122. Falati S, Edmead CE, Poole AW. Glycoprotein Ib-V-IX, a receptor for von Willebrand factor, couples physically and functionally to the Fc receptor γ-chain, fyn, and lyn to activate human platelets. Blood. 1999;94:1648-1656.

123. Nesbitt WS, Kulkarni S, Giuliano S, et al. Distinct glycoprotein Ib/V/IX and integrin $\alpha_{IIb}\beta_3$-dependent calcium signals cooperatively regulate platelet adhesion under flow. J Biol Chem. 2002;277:2965-2972.

124. Mazzucato M, Pradella P, Cozzi MR, et al. Sequential cytoplasmic calcium signals in a 2-stage platelet activation process induced by the glycoprotein Ibα mechanoreceptor. Blood. 2002;100:2793-2800.

125. Jackson SP, Nesbitt WS, Kulkarni S. Signaling events underlying thrombus formation. J Thromb Haemost. 2003;1:1602-1612.

126. Mangin P, Yuan Y, Goncalves I, et al. Signaling role for PLCγ2 in platelet glycoprotein Ibα calcium flux and cytoskeletal reorganization involvement of a pathway distinct from FcRγ-chain and FcγRIIA. J Biol Chem. 2003;278:32880-32891.

127. Rathore V, Wang D, Newman DK, Newman PJ. Phospholipase Cγ2 contributes to stable thrombus formation on VWF. Febs Lett. 2004;573:26-30.

128. Goncalves I, Nesbitt WS, Yuan Y, Jackson SP. Importance of temporal flow gradients and integrin $\alpha_{IIb}\beta_3$ mechanotransduction for shear activation of platelets. J Biol Chem. 2005;280:15430-15437.

129. Staatz WD, Rajpara SM, Wayner EA, et al. The membrane glycoprotein Ia-IIa (VLA-2) complex mediates the Mg^{2+}-dependent adhesion of platelets to collagen. J Cell Biol. 1989;108:1917-1924.

130. Sonnenberg A, Modderman PW, Hogervorst F. Laminin receptor on platelets is the integrin VLA-6. Nature. 1988;336:487-489.

131. Gibbins JM, Okuma M, Farndale R, et al. Glycoprotein VI is the collagen receptor in platelets which underlies tyrosine phosphorylation of the Fc receptor γ-chain. Febs Lett. 1997;413:255-259.

132. Inoue O, Suzuki-Inoue K, McCarty OJ, et al. Laminin stimulates spreading of platelets through integrin $\alpha_6\beta_1$-dependent activation of GPVI. Blood. 2006;107:1405-1412.

133. Tsuji M, Ezumi Y, Arai M, Takayama H. A novel association of Fc receptor γ-chain with glycoprotein VI and their co-expression as a collagen receptor in human platelets. J Biol Chem. 1997;272:23528-23531.

134. Chen H, Kahn ML. Reciprocal signaling by integrin and nonintegrin receptors during collagen activation of platelets. Mol Cell Biol. 2003;23:4764-4777.

135. Richardson JL, Shivdasani RA, Boers C, et al. Mechanisms of organelle transport and capture along proplatelets during platelet production. Blood. 2005;106:4066-4075.

136. Stenberg PE, Shuman MA, Levine SP, Bainton DF. Redistribution of alpha-granules and their contents in thrombin-stimulated platelets. J Cell Biol. 1984;98:748-760.

137. Yarovoi HV, Kufrin D, Eslin DE, et al. Factor VIII ectopically expressed in platelets: efficacy in hemophilia A treatment. Blood. 2003;102:4006-4013.

138. Shi Q, Wilcox DA, Fahs SA, et al. Factor VIII ectopically targeted to platelets is therapeutic in hemophilia A with high-titer inhibitory antibodies. J Clin Invest. 2006;116:1974-1982.

139. Handagama PJ, George JN, Shuman MA, et al. Incorporation of a circulating protein into megakaryocyte and

platelet granules. Proc Natl Acad Sci U S A. 1987;84: 861-865.

140. Reed GL. Platelet secretory mechanisms. Semin Thromb Hemost. 2004;30:441-450.

141. Swank RT, Jiang SY, Reddington M, et al. Inherited abnormalities in platelet organelles and platelet formation and associated altered expression of low molecular weight guanosine triphosphate–binding proteins in the mouse pigment mutant gunmetal. Blood. 1993;81:2626-2635.

142. Shirakawa R, Yoshioka A, Horiuchi H, et al. Small GTPase Rab4 regulates Ca^{2+}-induced alpha-granule secretion in platelets. J Biol Chem. 2000;275:33844-33849.

143. Stenberg PE, McEver RP, Shuman MA, et al. A platelet alpha-granule membrane protein (GMP-140) is expressed on the plasma membrane after activation. J Cell Biol. 1985;101:880-886.

144. Berman CL, Yeo EL, Wencel-Drake JD, et al. A platelet alpha granule membrane protein that is associated with the plasma membrane after activation. J Clin Invest. 1986;78:130-137.

145. Beckstead JH, Stenberg PE, McEver RP, et al. Immuno-histochemical localization of membrane and alpha-granule proteins in human megakaryocytes: application to plastic-embedded bone marrow biopsy specimens. Blood. 1986;67:285-293.

146. Washington AV, Schubert RL, Quigley L, et al. A TREM family member, TLT-1, is found exclusively in the alpha-granules of megakaryocytes and platelets. Blood. 2004; 104:1042-1047.

147. Ruf A, Patscheke H. Flow cytometric detection of activated platelets: comparison of determining shape change, fibrinogen binding, and P-selectin expression. Semin Thromb Hemost. 1995;21:146-151.

148. Michelson AD, Furman MI. Laboratory markers of platelet activation and their clinical significance. Curr Opin Hematol. 1999;6:342-348.

149. Palabrica T, Lobb R, Furie BC, et al. Leukocyte accumulation promoting fibrin deposition is mediated in vivo by P-selectin on adherent platelets. Nature. 1992;359: 848-851.

150. Wagner DD, Burger PC. Platelets in inflammation and thrombosis. Arterioscler Thromb Vasc Biol. 2003;23:2131-2137.

151. Kisucka J, Butterfield CE, Duda DG, et al. Platelets and platelet adhesion support angiogenesis while preventing excessive hemorrhage. Proc Natl Acad Sci U S A. 2006; 103:855-860.

152. Anitua E, Andia I, Ardanza B, et al. Autologous platelets as a source of proteins for healing and tissue regeneration. Thromb Haemost. 2004;91:4-15.

153. Gimbrone MA Jr, Aster RH, Cotran RS, et al. Preservation of vascular integrity in organs perfused in vitro with a platelet-rich medium. Nature. 1969;222:33-36.

154. Angelillo-Scherrer A, Burnier L, Flores N, et al. Role of Gas6 receptors in platelet signaling during thrombus stabilization and implications for antithrombotic therapy. J Clin Invest. 2005;115:237-246.

155. Prasad KS, Andre P, He M, et al. Soluble CD40 ligand induces β_3 integrin tyrosine phosphorylation and triggers platelet activation by outside-in signaling. Proc Natl Acad Sci U S A. 2003;100:12367-12371.

156. Camire RM, Pollak ES, Kaushansky K, Tracy PB. Secretable human platelet-derived factor V originates from the plasma pool. Blood. 1998;92:3035-3041.

157. Panes O, Matus V, Saez CG, et al. Human platelets synthesize and express functional tissue factor. Blood. 2007;109:5242-5250.

158. Rosa JP, George JN, Bainton DF, et al. Gray platelet syndrome. Demonstration of alpha granule membranes that can fuse with the cell surface. J Clin Invest. 1987;80: 1138-1146.

159. Raccuglia G. Gray platelet syndrome. A variety of qualitative platelet disorder. Am J Med. 1971;51:818-828.

160. Da Prada M., Pletscher A, Tranzer JP, Knuchel H. Subcellular localization of 5-hydroxytryptamine and histamine in blood platelets. Nature. 1967;216:1315-1317.

161. White JG. The dense bodies of human platelets. Origin of serotonin storage particles from platelet granules. Am J Pathol. 1968;53:791-808.

162. Davis RB, White JG. Localization of 5-hydroxytryptamine in blood platelets: an autoradiographic and ultrastructural study. Br J Haematol. 1968;15:93-99.

163. Silcox DC, Jacobelli S, McCarty DJ. Identification of inorganic pyrophosphate in human platelets and its release on stimulation with thrombin. J Clin Invest. 1973;52: 1595-1600.

164. Ruiz FA, Lea CR, Oldfield E, Docampo R. Human platelet dense granules contain polyphosphate and are similar to acidocalcisomes of bacteria and unicellular eukaryotes. J Biol Chem. 2004;279:44250-44257.

165. Lages B, Scrutton MC, Holmsen H, et al. Metal ion contents of gel-filtered platelets from patients with storage pool disease. Blood. 1975;46:119-130.

166. Gerrard JM, Rao GH, White JG. The influence of reserpine and ethylenediaminetetraacetic acid (EDTA) on serotonin storage organelles of blood platelets. Am J Pathol. 1977;87:633-646.

167. Israels SJ, Gerrard JM, Jacques YV, et al. Platelet dense granule membranes contain both granulophysin and P-selectin (GMP-140). Blood. 1992;80:143-152.

168. Israels SJ, McMillan EM, Robertson C, et al. The lysosomal granule membrane protein, LAMP-2, is also present in platelet dense granule membranes. Thromb Haemost. 1996;75:623-629.

169. Youssefian T, Masse JM, Rendu F, et al. Platelet and megakaryocyte dense granules contain glycoproteins Ib and IIb-IIIa. Blood. 1997;89:4047-4057.

170. Lages B, Holmsen H, Weiss HJ, Dangelmaier C. Thrombin and ionophore A23187–induced dense granule secretion in storage pool deficient platelets: evidence for impaired nucleotide storage as the primary dense granule defect. Blood. 1983;61:154-162.

171. Weiss HJ, Ames RP. Ultrastructural findings in storage pool disease and aspirin-like defects of platelets. Am J Pathol. 1973;71:447-466.

172. Holmsen H, Weiss HJ. Hereditary defect in the release reaction caused by a deficiency in the storage pool of platelet adenine nucleotides. Br J Haematol. 1970;19: 643-649.

173. Weiss HJ, Witte LD, Kaplan KL, et al. Heterogeneity in storage pool deficiency: Studies on granule-bound substances in 18 patients including variants deficient in alpha-granules, platelet factor 4, β-thromboglobulin and

platelet-derived growth factor. Blood. 1979;54:1296-1319.

174. Weiss HJ, Hawiger J, Ruggeri ZM, et al. Fibrinogen-independent platelet adhesion and thrombus formation on subendothelium mediated by glycoprotein IIb-IIIa complex at high shear rate. J Clin Invest. 1989;83:288-297.

175. Hermansky F, Pudlak P. Albinism associated with hemorrhagic diathesis and unusual pigmented reticular cells in the bone marrow: report of two cases with histochemical studies. Blood. 1959;14:162-169.

176. Bentfeld-Barker ME, Bainton DF. Identification of primary lysosomes in human megakaryocytes and platelets. Blood. 1982;59:472-481.

177. Srivastava PC, Powling MJ, Nokes TJ, et al. Grey platelet syndrome: studies on platelet alpha granules, lysosomes and defective response to thrombin. Br J Haematol. 1987;65:441-446.

178. Febbraio M, Silverstein RL. Identification and characterization of LAMP-1 as an activation-dependent platelet surface glycoprotein. J Biol Chem. 1990;265:18531-18537.

179. Jantzen HM, Gousset L, Bhaskar V, et al. Evidence for two distinct G-protein–coupled ADP receptors mediating platelet activation. Thromb Haemost. 1999;81:111-117.

180. Murugappan S, Shankar H, Kunapuli SP. Platelet receptors for adenine nucleotides and thromboxane A_2. Semin Thromb Hemost. 2004;30:411-418.

181. Conley PB, Delaney SM. Scientific and therapeutic insights into the role of the platelet P_2Y_{12} receptor in thrombosis. Curr Opin Hematol. 2003;10:333-338.

182. Leon C, Hechler B, Vial C, et al. The P_2Y_1 receptor is an ADP receptor antagonized by ATP and expressed in platelets and megakaryoblastic cells. FEBS Lett. 1997;403:26-30.

183. Hechler B, Leon C, Vial C, et al. The P_2Y_1 receptor is necessary for adenosine 5′-diphosphate–induced platelet aggregation. Blood. 1998;92:152-159.

184. Jin J, Daniel JL, Kunapuli SP. Molecular basis for ADP-induced platelet activation. II. The P_2Y_1 receptor mediates ADP-induced intracellular calcium mobilization and shape change in platelets. J Biol Chem. 1998;273:2030-2034.

185. Leon C, Hechler B, Freund M, et al. Defective platelet aggregation and increased resistance to thrombosis in purinergic P_2Y_1 receptor-null mice. J Clin Invest. 1999;104:1731-1737.

186. Vu T-KH, Hung DT, Wheaton VI, Coughlin SR. Molecular cloning of a functional thrombin receptor reveals a novel proteolytic mechanism of receptor activation. Cell. 1991;64:1057-1068.

187. Kahn ML, Nakanishi-Matsui M, Shapiro MJ, et al. Protease-activated receptors 1 and 4 mediate activation of human platelets by thrombin. J Clin Invest. 1999;103:879-887.

188. Shenker A, Goldsmith P, Unson CG, Spiegel AM. The G protein coupled to the thromboxane A_2 receptor in human platelets is a member of the novel G_q family. J Biol Chem. 1991;266:9309-9313.

189. Kinsella BT, O'Mahony DJ, Fitzgerald GA. The human thromboxane A_2 receptor alpha isoform (TP alpha) functionally couples to the G proteins G_q and G_{11} in vivo and is activated by the isoprostane 8-epi prostaglandin F_2 alpha. J Pharmacol Exp Ther. 1997;281:957-964.

190. Hourani SM, Cusack NJ. Pharmacological receptors on blood platelets. Pharmacol Rev. 1991;43:243-298.

191. Du XP, Plow EF, Frelinger AL, et al. Ligands "activate" integrin $\alpha_{IIb}\beta_3$ (platelet GPIIb- IIIa). Cell. 1991;65:409-416.

192. Shattil SJ. Integrins and Src: dynamic duo of adhesion signaling. Trends Cell Biol. 2005;15:399-403.

193. Obergfell A, Eto K, Mocsai A, et al. Coordinate interactions of Csk, Src, and Syk kinases with $\alpha_{IIb}\beta_3$ initiate integrin signaling to the cytoskeleton. J Cell Biol. 2002;157:265-275.

194. Law DA, Nanniaai-Alaimo L, Phillips DR. Outside-in integrin signal transduction. $\alpha_{IIb}\beta_3$ (GPIIb-IIIa) tyrosine phosphorylation induced by platelet aggregation. J Biol Chem. 1996;271:10811-10815.

195. Shattil SJ. Signaling through platelet integrin $\alpha_{IIb}\beta_3$: inside-out, outside-in, and sideways. Thromb Haemost. 1999;82:318-325.

196. Shattil SJ, Newman PJ. Integrins: dynamic scaffolds for adhesion and signaling in platelets. Blood. 2004;104:1606-1615.

197. Keely PJ, Parise LV. The $\alpha_2\beta_1$ integrin is a necessary co-receptor for collagen-induced activation of syk and the subsequent phosphorylation of phospholipase Cγ2 in platelets. J Biol Chem. 1996;271:26668-26676.

198. Inoue O, Suzuki-Inoue K, Dean WL, et al. Integrin $\alpha_2\beta_1$ mediates outside-in regulation of platelet spreading on collagen through activation of Src kinases and PLCγ2. J Cell Biol. 2003;160:769-780.

199. Newman PJ, Allen RW, Kahn RA, Kunicki TJ. Quantitation of membrane glycoprotein IIIa on intact human platelets using the monoclonal antibody, AP-3. Blood. 1985;65:227-232.

200. Wagner CL, Mascelli MA, Neblock DS, et al. Analysis of GPIIb/IIIa receptor number by quantification of 7E3 binding to human platelets. Blood. 1996;88:907-914.

201. Goncalves I, Hughan SC, Schoenwaelder SM, et al. Integrin $\alpha_{IIb}\beta_3$-dependent calcium signals regulate platelet-fibrinogen interactions under flow: involvement of PLCγ2. J Biol Chem. 2003;278:34812-34822.

202. Angelillo-Scherrer A, de Frutos P, Aparicio C, et al. Deficiency or inhibition of Gas6 causes platelet dysfunction and protects mice against thrombosis. Nat Med. 2001;7:215-221.

203. Balogh I, Hafizi S, Stenhoff J, et al. Analysis of Gas6 in human platelets and plasma. Arterioscler Thromb Vasc Biol. 2005;25:1280-1286.

204. Prevost N, Woulfe DS, Tognolini M, et al. Signaling by ephrinB1 and Eph kinases in platelets promotes Rap1 activation, platelet adhesion, and aggregation via effector pathways that do not require phosphorylation of ephrinB1. Blood. 2004;103:1348-1355.

205. Gould WR, Baxi SM, Schroeder R, et al. Gas6 receptors Axl, Sky and Mer enhance platelet activation and regulate thrombotic responses. J Thromb Haemost. 2005;3:733-741.

206. Saller F, Burnier L, Schapira M, Angelillo-Scherrer A. Role of the growth arrest-specific gene 6 (gas6) product in thrombus stabilization. Blood Cells Mol Dis. 2006;36:373-378.

207. Prevost N, Woulfe DS, Jiang H, et al. Eph kinases and ephrins support thrombus growth and stability by regulating integrin outside-in signaling in platelets. Proc Natl Acad Sci U S A. 2005;102:9820-9825.

208. Hynes RO. Integrins: bidirectional, allosteric signaling machines. Cell. 2002;110:673-687.

209. Xiong JP, Stehle T, Diefenbach B, et al. Crystal structure of the extracellular segment of integrin $\alpha_V\beta_3$. Science. 2001;294:339-345.

210. Takagi J, Petre BM, Walz T, Springer TA. Global conformational rearrangements in integrin extracellular domains in outside-in and inside-out signaling. Cell. 2002;110:599-611.

211. Vinogradova O, Velyvis A, Velyviene A, et al. A structural mechanism of integrin $\alpha_{IIb}\beta_3$ "inside-out" activation as regulated by its cytoplasmic face. Cell. 2002;110:587-597.

212. Vinogradova O, Vaynberg J, Kong X, et al. Membrane-mediated structural transitions at the cytoplasmic face during integrin activation. Proc Natl Acad Sci U S A. 2004;101:4094-4099.

213. Luo BH, Springer TA, Takagi J. A specific interface between integrin transmembrane helices and affinity for ligand. PLoS Biol. 2004;2:e153.

214. Partridge AW, Liu S, Kim S, et al. Transmembrane domain helix packing stabilizes integrin $\alpha_{IIb}\beta_3$ in the low affinity state. J Biol Chem. 2005;280:7294-7300.

215. Medeiros RB, Dickey DM, Chung H, et al. Protein kinase D_1 and the β_1 integrin cytoplasmic domain control β_1 integrin function via regulation of Rap1 activation. Immunity. 2005;23:213-226.

216. Ebinu JO, Bottorff DA, Chan EY, et al. RasGRP, a Ras guanyl nucleotide–releasing protein with calcium- and diacylglycerol-binding motifs. Science. 1998;280:1082-1086.

217. Eto K, Murphy R, Kerrigan SW, et al. Megakaryocytes derived from embryonic stem cells implicate CalDAG-GEFI in integrin signaling. Proc Natl Acad Sci U S A. 2002;99:12819-12824.

218. Crittenden JR, Bergmeier W, Zhang Y, et al. CalDAG-GEFI integrates signaling for platelet aggregation and thrombus formation. Nat Med. 2004;10:982-986.

219. Han J, Lim CJ, Watanabe N, et al. Reconstructing and deconstructing agonist-induced activation of integrin $\alpha_{IIb}\beta_3$. Curr Biol. 2006;16:1796-1806.

220. Bertoni A, Tadokoro S, Eto K, et al. Relationships between Rap1b, affinity modulation of integrin $\alpha_{IIb}\beta_3$, and the actin cytoskeleton. J Biol Chem. 2002;277:25715-25721.

221. de Bruyn KM, Zwartkruis FJ, de Rooij J, et al. The small GTPase Rap1 is activated by turbulence and is involved in integrin $\alpha_{IIb}\beta_3$ -mediated cell adhesion in human megakaryocytes. J Biol Chem. 2003;278:22412-22417.

222. Bos JL, de Bruyn K, Enserink J, et al. The role of Rap1 in integrin-mediated cell adhesion. Biochem Soc Trans. 2003;31:83-86.

223. Tadokoro S, Shattil SJ, Eto K, et al. Talin binding to integrin beta tails: a final common step in integrin activation. Science. 2003;302:103-106.

224. Wegener KL, Partridge AW, Han J, et al. Structural basis of integrin activation by talin. Cell. 2007;128:171-182.

225. Petrich BG, Fogelstrand P, Partridge AW, et al. The antithrombotic potential of selective blockade of talin-dependent integrin $\alpha_{IIb}\beta_3$ (platelet GPIIb-IIIa) activation. J Clin Invest. 2007;117:2250-2259.

226. Xiao T, Takagi J, Coller BS, et al. Structural basis for allostery in integrins and binding to fibrinogen-mimetic therapeutics. Nature. 2004;432:59-67.

227. Zhu J, Boylan B, Luo BH, et al. Tests of the extension and deadbolt models of integrin activation. J Biol Chem. 2007;282:11914-11920.

228. Buensuceso C, de Virgilio M, Shattil SJ. Detection of integrin $\alpha_{IIb}\beta_3$ clustering in living cells. J Biol Chem. 2003;278:15217-15224.

229. Antl M, von Bruhl ML, Eiglsperger, C et al. IRAG mediates NO/cGMP-dependent inhibition of platelet aggregation and thrombus formation. Blood. 2007;109:552-559.

230. Schlossmann J, Ammendola A, Ashman K, et al. Regulation of intracellular calcium by a signalling complex of IRAG, IP$_3$ receptor and cGMP kinase Ib. Nature. 2000;404:197-201.

231. Ammendola A, Geiselhoringer A, Hofmann F, Schlossmann J. Molecular determinants of the interaction between the inositol 1,4,5-trisphosphate receptor–associated cGMP kinase substrate (IRAG) and cGMP kinase Ib. J Biol Chem. 2001;276:24153-24159.

232. Butt E, Abel K, Krieger M, et al. cAMP- and cGMP-dependent protein kinase phosphorylation sites of the focal adhesion vasodilator-stimulated phosphoprotein (VASP) in vitro and in intact human platelets. J Biol Chem. 1994;269:14509-14517.

233. Lambrechts A, Kwiatkowski AV, Lanier LM, et al. cAMP-dependent protein kinase phosphorylation of EVL, a Mena/VASP relative, regulates its interaction with actin and SH3 domains. J Biol Chem. 2000;275:36143-36151.

234. Bachmann C, Fischer L, Walter U, Reinhard M. The EVH2 domain of the vasodilator-stimulated phosphoprotein mediates tetramerization, F-actin binding, and actin bundle formation. J Biol Chem. 1999;274:23549-23557.

235. Svitkina TM, Bulanova EA, Chaga OY, et al. Mechanism of filopodia initiation by reorganization of a dendritic network. J Cell Biol. 2003;160:409-421.

236. Mejillano MR, Kojima S, Applewhite DA, et al. Lamellipodial versus filopodial mode of the actin nanomachinery: pivotal role of the filament barbed end. Cell. 2004;118:363-373.

237. Barzik M, Kotova TI, Higgs HN, et al. Ena/VASP proteins enhance actin polymerization in the presence of barbed end capping proteins. J Biol Chem. 2005;280:28653-28662.

238. Pula G, Schuh K, Nakayama K, et al. PKCδ regulates collagen-induced platelet aggregation through inhibition of VASP-mediated filopodia formation. Blood. 2006;108:4035-4044.

239. Newman PJ. Switched at birth: a new family for PECAM-1. J Clin Invest. 1999;103:5-9.

240. Newman PJ, Newman DK. Signal transduction pathways mediated by PECAM-1. New roles for an old molecule in platelet and vascular cell biology. Arterioscler Thromb Vasc Biol. 2003;23:953-964.

241. Patil S, Newman DK, Newman PJ. Platelet endothelial cell adhesion molecule-1 serves as an inhibitory receptor that modulates platelet responses to collagen. Blood. 2001;97:1727-1732.

242. Jones KL, Hughan SC, Dopheide SM, et al. Platelet endothelial cell adhesion molecule-1 is a negative regulator of platelet-collagen interactions. Blood. 2001;98: 1456-1463.

243. Rathore V, Stapleton MA, Hillery CA, et al. PECAM-1 negatively regulates GPIb/V/IX signaling in murine platelets. Blood. 2003;102:3658-3664.

244. Falati S, Patil S, Gross PL, et al. Platelet PECAM-1 inhibits thrombus formation in vivo. Blood. 2006;107: 535-541.

245. Barrow AD, Astoul E, Floto A, et al. Cutting edge: TREM-like transcript-1, a platelet immunoreceptor tyrosine–based inhibition motif encoding costimulatory immunoreceptor that enhances, rather than inhibits, calcium signaling via SHP-2. J Immunol. 2004;172:5838-5842.

246. Ribas G, Neville M, Wixon JL, et al. Genes encoding three new members of the leukocyte antigen 6 superfamily and a novel member of Ig superfamily, together with genes encoding the regulatory nuclear chloride ion channel protein (hRNCC) and an $N\omega$-$N\omega$-dimethylarginine dimethylaminohydrolase homologue, are found in a 30-kb segment of the MHC class III region. J Immunol. 1999; 163:278-287.

247. de Vet EC, Aguado B, Campbell RD. G6b, a novel immunoglobulin superfamily member encoded in the human major histocompatibility complex, interacts with SHP-1 and SHP-2. J Biol Chem. 2001;276:42070-42076.

248. Senis YA, Tomlinson MG, Garcia A, et al. A comprehensive proteomics and genomics analysis reveals novel transmembrane proteins in human platelets and mouse megakaryocytes including G6b-B, a novel immunoreceptor tyrosine–based inhibitory motif protein. Mol Cell Proteomics. 2007;6:548-564.

249. Newland SA, Macaulay IC, Floto AR, et al. The novel inhibitory receptor G6B is expressed on the surface of platelets and attenuates platelet function in vitro. Blood. 2007;109:4806-4809.

250. Cantley LC. The phosphoinositide 3-kinase pathway. Science. 2002;296:1655-1657.

251. Lioubin MN, Algate PA, Tsai S, et al. p150Ship, a signal transduction molecule with inositol polyphosphate-5-phosphatase activity. Genes Dev. 1996;10:1084-1095.

252. Damen JE, Liu L, Rosten P, et al. The 145-kDa protein induced to associate with Shc by multiple cytokines is an inositol tetraphosphate and phosphatidylinositol 3,4,5-triphosphate 5-phosphatase. Proc Natl Acad Sci U S A. 1996;93:1689-1693.

253. Maxwell MJ, Yuan Y, Anderson KE, et al. SHIP1 and Lyn kinase negatively regulate integrin $\alpha_{IIb}\beta_3$ signaling in platelets. J Biol Chem. 2004;279:32196-32204.

254. Gardai S, Whitlock BB, Helgason C, et al. Activation of SHIP by NADPH oxidase–stimulated Lyn leads to enhanced apoptosis in neutrophils. J Biol Chem. 2002; 277:5236-5246.

255. Baran CP, Tridandapani S, Helgason CD, et al. The inositol 5′-phosphatase SHIP-1 and the Src kinase Lyn negatively regulate macrophage colony-stimulating factor-induced Akt activity. J Biol Chem. 2003;278: 38628-38636.

256. Phee H, Jacob A, Coggeshall KM. Enzymatic activity of the Src homology 2 domain–containing inositol phosphatase is regulated by a plasma membrane location. J Biol Chem. 2000;275:19090-19097.

257. Quek LS, Pasquet JM, Hers I, et al. Fyn and Lyn phosphorylate the Fc receptor gamma chain downstream of glycoprotein VI in murine platelets, and Lyn regulates a novel feedback pathway. Blood. 2000;96:4246-4253.

258. Kandel ES, Hay N. The regulation and activities of the multifunctional serine/threonine kinase Akt/PKB. Exp Cell Res. 1999;253:210-229.

259. Scheid MP, Woodgett JR. PKB/AKT: functional insights from genetic models. Nat Rev Mol Cell Biol. 2001;2: 760-768.

260. Kim L, Kimmel AR. GSK3 at the edge: regulation of developmental specification and cell polarization. Curr Drug Targets. 2006;7:1411-1419.

261. Barry FA, Graham GJ, Fry MJ, Gibbins JM. Regulation of glycogen synthase kinase 3 in human platelets: a possible role in platelet function? FEBS Lett. 2003;553: 173-178.

262. Woulfe DS, August S, Li D. GSK3b is a negative regulator of platelet function in vitro and in vivo [abstract]. Blood. 2006;108:395.

263. Mayadas TN, Johnson RC, Rayburn H, et al. Leukocyte rolling and extravasation are severely compromised in P selectin–deficient mice. Cell. 1993;74:541-554.

264. Frenette PS, Mayadas TN, Rayburn H, et al. Susceptibility to infection and altered hematopoiesis in mice deficient in both P- and E-selectins. Cell. 1996;84:563-574.

265. Diacovo TG, Roth SJ, Buccola JM, et al. Neutrophil rolling, arrest, and transmigration across activated, surface-adherent platelets via sequential action of P-selectin and the β_2-integrin CD11b/CD18. Blood. 1996;88: 146-157.

266. Kuijper PH, Gallardo Torres HI, van der Linden JA, et al. Platelet-dependent primary hemostasis promotes selectin- and integrin-mediated neutrophil adhesion to damaged endothelium under flow conditions. Blood. 1996;87:3271-3281.

267. Gawaz M, Langer H, May AE. Platelets in inflammation and atherogenesis. J Clin Invest. 2005;115:3378-3384.

268. Weber C, Springer TA. Neutrophil accumulation on activated, surface-adherent platelets in flow is mediated by interaction of Mac-1 with fibrinogen bound to $\alpha_{IIb}\beta_3$ and stimulated by platelet-activating factor. J Clin Invest. 1997;100:2085-2093.

269. Santoso S, Sachs UJ, Kroll H, et al. The junctional adhesion molecule 3 (JAM-3) on human platelets is a counter-receptor for the leukocyte integrin Mac-1. J Exp Med. 2002;196:679-691.

270. Langer HF, Daub K, Braun G, et al. Platelets recruit human dendritic cells via Mac-1/JAM-C interaction and modulate dendritic cell function in vitro. Arterioscler Thromb Vasc Biol. 2007;27:1463-1470.

271. von HP, Weber KS, Huo Y, et al. RANTES deposition by platelets triggers monocyte arrest on inflamed and atherosclerotic endothelium. Circulation. 2001;103:1772-1777.

272. Huo Y, Ley KF. Role of platelets in the development of atherosclerosis. Trends Cardiovasc Med. 2004;14:18-22.

273. Hawrylowicz CM, Santoro SA, Platt FM, Unanue ER. Activated platelets express IL-1 activity. J Immunol. 1989;143:4015-4018.

274. Lindemann S, Tolley ND, Dixon DA, et al. Activated platelets mediate inflammatory signaling by regulated interleukin 1b synthesis. J Cell Biol. 2001;154:485-490.

26 Blood Coagulation

Kenneth G. Mann and Kathleen Brummel-Ziedins

OVERVIEW OF COAGULATION

Generation of the enzyme thrombin from its precursor prothrombin is the central event in the blood coagulation process, essential for hemostasis and the culprit in thrombosis. Blood loss through lack of hemorrhage control has captured the attention of individuals from many walks of life throughout history. At the end of the 19th century, the role of thrombin in the clotting of fibrinogen was accurately described by Schmitt.[1] Since that time hemostasis has been synonymous with blood clotting. Congenital diseases associated with absence or reduced production of thrombin (the hemophilias) represent important clinical problems (see Chapters 30 and 31). In contrast, the unregulated production of thrombin in an inappropriate location leads to another series of diseases associated with thrombotic occlusion (see Chapter 32).

The development of plasma clot–based assays in vitro has played a central role in establishing the logical relationships between the reactants and reactions of hemostasis (Fig. 26-1). The prothrombin time (PT) and the activated partial thromboplastin time (APTT) both rely on the end point of fibrin formation (clotting), which occurs with the generation of less than 5% of the thrombin ultimately produced. The primary pathway leading to hemostatic and thrombotic pathology appears to be associated with the tissue factor (TF)-initiated, "extrinsic" coagulation pathway. In contrast, components unique to the "intrinsic" or contact pathway (factor XII, prekallikrein, high-molecular-weight kininogen [HMWK]) do not appear to be essential to hemostasis.

The observation that tissue extracts added to plasma initiated clotting led Quick to develop the PT assay.[2] This assay is still used extensively in the management of warfarin anticoagulant therapy and establishes the continuity of components in the *extrinsic pathway*. The tissue preparations (thromboplastin) contain the protein TF and phospholipids, with plasma contributing factor VIIa and calcium to form the *extrinsic factor Xase*, which converts plasma factor X to factor Xa (see Fig. 26-1). Factor Xa subsequently combines with plasma factor Va, phospholipids, and calcium to activate prothrombin to thrombin, the latter serving as the catalyst that cleaves fibrinogen to produce fibrin, the clotting end point.

Langdell and colleagues[3] subsequently explored the spontaneous clotting of recalcified citrate plasma and developed the APTT, thus providing the tool that defined the *intrinsic pathway* of coagulation (see Fig. 26-1). This pathway, dependent only on the protein components present in blood plasma, was formalized by the cascade/waterfall hypotheses of MacFarlane[4] and Davie and Ratnoff.[5] The APTT assay involves the addition of an artificial surface, phospholipids, and calcium chloride to blood plasma. Initiation of this contact pathway begins with the surface-dependent activation of factor XII to factor XIIa; this leads to activation of prekallikrein to kallikrein, which, together with HMWK, provides a self-amplifying catalytic system that results in rapid activation of factor XI to factor XIa. Factor XIa, together with HMWK, phospholipid, and metal ions, catalyzes the activation of factor IX to factor IXa. Factor IXa, with factor VIIIa and a membrane surface, form the *intrinsic factor*

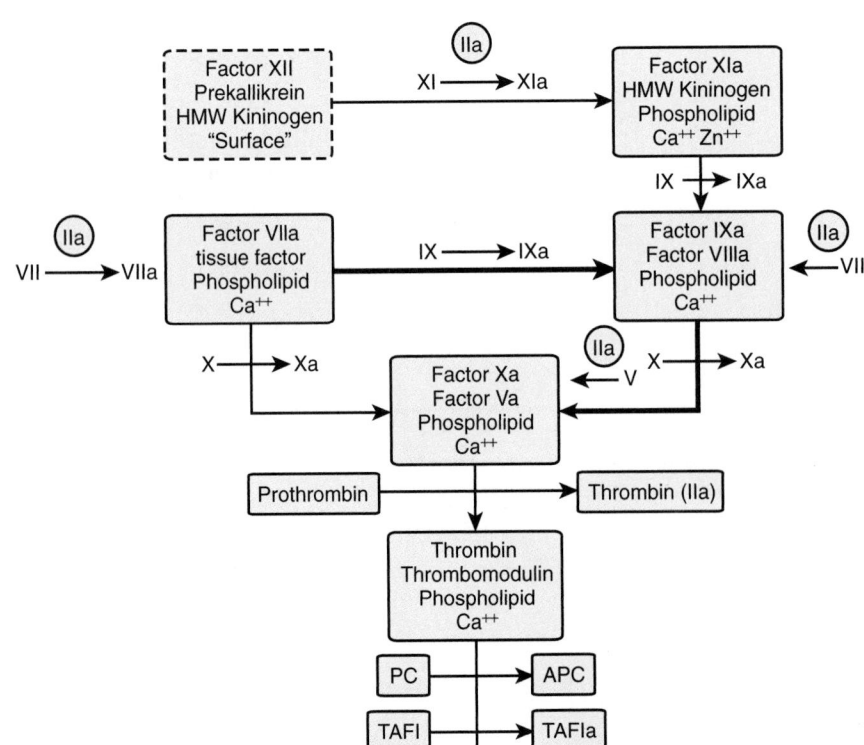

FIGURE 26-1. Schematic of the catalysts of the hemostatic system. The outline of the "contact catalyst" of the intrinsic pathway is *dashed* because of its uncertain contributions to hemostasis. The contribution of the contact catalyst to thrombosis is unresolved. The various points at which thrombin catalyzes its own generation by the conversion of zymogens and procofactors to the active species required for catalyst formation are illustrated by *circles* (IIa). APC, activated protein C; HMW, high molecular weight; PC, protein C; TAFI, thrombin-activatable fibrinolysis inhibitor.

Xase, which activates factor X to factor Xa as illustrated in Figure 26-1.

By the mid-1980s, the conclusion that TF was probably the principal initiator of the hemostatic process[6] and the absence of bleeding associated with deficiencies of the contact pathway initiators (factor XII, prekallikrein, and HMWK) presented a significant conundrum for the scientific community. This was accentuated by the absence of linkage between hemophilia A and B and the extrinsic pathway as evaluated by the PT assay. Subsequently, the intersections between intrinsic and extrinsic and the reactions linking these two "classical" pathways were identified.[7-9]

Of equal importance to the procoagulant process is its regulation by stoichiometric and dynamic inhibitory systems. Antithrombin (AT)[10] and tissue factor pathway inhibitor (TFPI)[11] are the primary stoichiometric inhibitors, whereas the thrombin-thrombomodulin–protein C system is dynamic in its inhibitory function. The latter catalyst activates protein C to activated protein C (APC), which proteolytically destroys the cofactors factor Va and factor VIIIa, thereby eliminating the intrinsic factor Xase and prothrombinase. TFPI blocks the factor VIIa–TF–factor Xa product complex,[12] thus effectively neutralizing the extrinsic factor Xase (Fig. 26-2). However, TFPI is present in low abundance ($\approx$2.5 nM) in blood and can only delay the hemostatic reaction.[13] AT, normally present in plasma at twice the concentration (~3.2 μM) of any potential coagulation enzyme, neutralizes all the procoagulant serine proteases, primarily in the uncomplexed state.[10]

The dynamic protein C system is activated by binding of thrombin to vascular thrombomodulin, with this complex (Fig. 26-3) converting protein C to its activated species APC.[14] APC proteolytically inactivates factors Va and VIIIa.[15] The protein C system, TFPI, and AT cooperate to produce steep TF concentration thresholds that act like a digital "switch" to allow or block thrombin formation.

Thus, there are three membrane-associated procoagulant complexes[16] (corresponding to the proteases factor IXa, factor Xa, and factor VIIa), each interacting with a cofactor protein (factor VIIIa, factor Va, TF). An analogous anticoagulant complex is composed of thrombin-thrombomodulin (see Fig. 26-3). Each complex involves a vitamin K–dependent serine protease, phospholipid, and an associated cofactor protein assembled on a membrane surface provided by an exposed, activated or damaged cell.

The membrane-binding properties of the vitamin K–dependent proteins (VKDPs) are the consequence of post-translational γ-carboxylation of these macromolecules. The cofactor proteins are either membrane-binding proteins (factor Va, factor VIIIa) recruited from plasma as procofactors or intrinsic membrane proteins (TF, thrombomodulin) regulated by presentation. Each complex catalyst is orders of magnitude (10^3- to 10^6-fold) more efficient than the individual serine protease acting on its substrate in solution.[17-19] When considered on a temporal scale, the amount of thrombin produced by prothrombinase in 1 minute would be produced by factor Xa acting alone in 6 months. As a consequence, factor Xa is ineffective in hemostasis without the presentation of both factor Va and the platelet membrane binding sites on which prothrombinase is formed. The blood coagulation reaction can be described as occurring in three overlapped phases: initiation, propagation, and termination.

FIGURE 26-2. Points of regulation of the catalyst of Figure 26-1 by tissue factor pathway inhibitor (TFPI), antithrombin (AT), and activated protein C (APC) are illustrated. HMW, high molecular weight; PC, protein C; TAFI, thrombin-activatable fibrinolysis inhibitor.

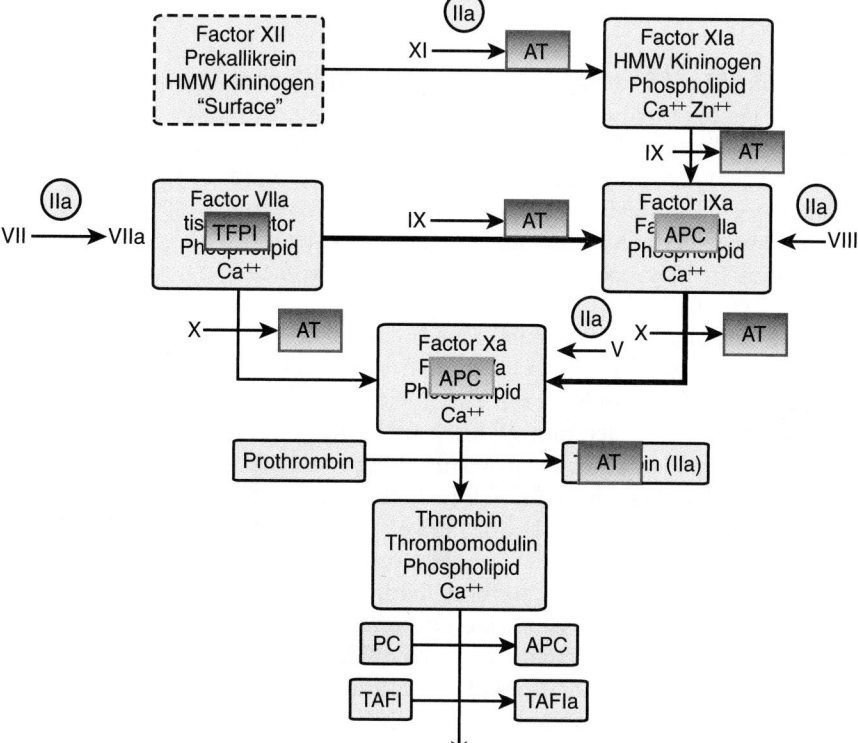

Extrinsic factor Xase   Intrinsic factor Xase

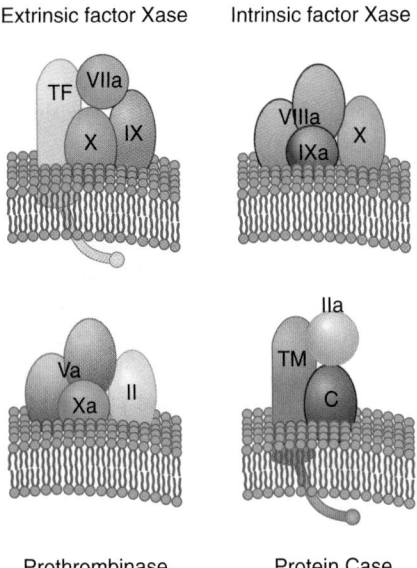

Prothrombinase   Protein Case

FIGURE 26-3. Vitamin K–dependent complexes. Three procoagulant complexes (extrinsic factor Xase, intrinsic factor Xase, and prothrombinase) and one anticoagulant complex (protein Case) are illustrated. Each membrane complex consists of a vitamin K–dependent serine protease (factor VIIa, factor IXa, prothrombin [II], or protein C [C]) and a soluble or cell surface–associated cofactor (factor VIIIa [heavy and light chain factor VIII$_H$ and factor VIII$_L$], factor Va [heavy- and light-chain factor V$_H$ and factor V$_L$], tissue factor [TF], or thrombomodulin [TM]). Each serine protease is shown in association with the appropriate cofactor protein and zymogen substrate or substrates (factors X, IX, and II and protein C) on the membrane surface. The membrane serves as a scaffold for the coagulation reactants and enhances reaction rates by 10^5- to 10^6-fold. (*Redrawn with permission from Mann KG. Dynamics of Hemostasis. Essex Junction, VT, Haematologic Technologies, 2002.*)

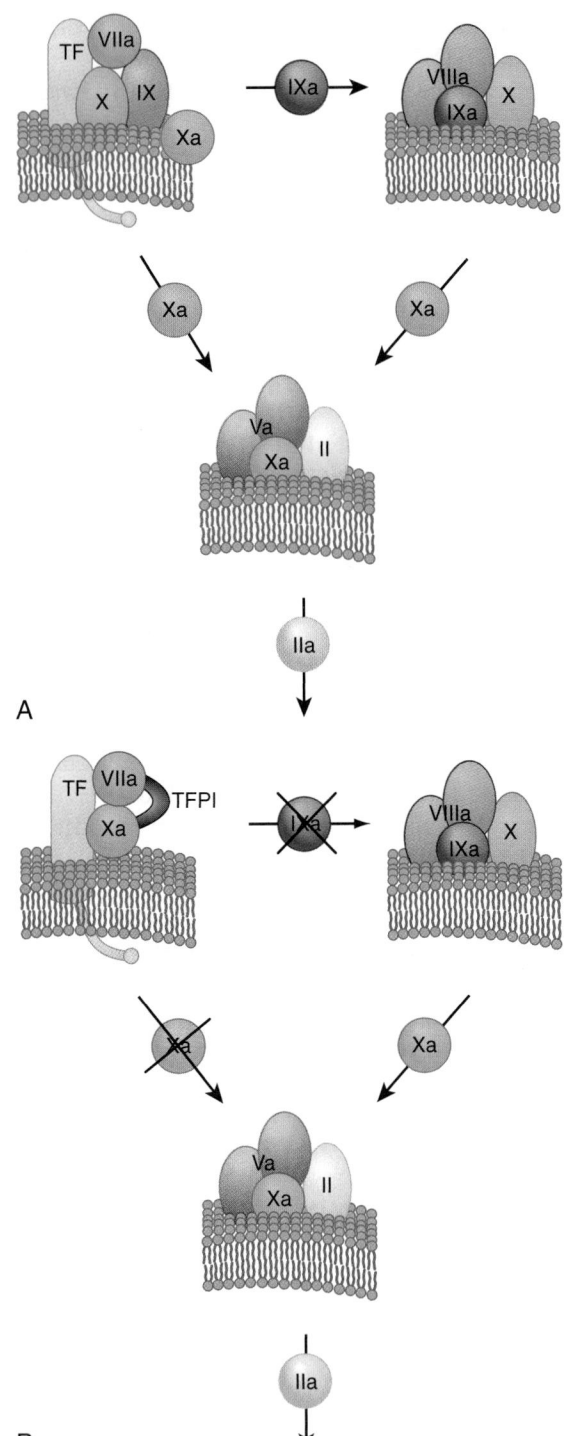

FIGURE 26-4. A, The factor Xa generated by the factor VIIa–tissue factor (TF) complex catalyzes the formation of a small amount of thrombin, which activates factors V and VIII and leads to the presentation of the intrinsic factor Xase (factor IXa-VIIIa) and prothrombinase (factor Xa-Va). At this point in the reaction, generation of factor IXa is cooperatively catalyzed by membrane-bound factor Xa and by factor VIIa–TF. The *thick arrow* representing generation of factor Xa by the intrinsic factor Xase illustrates the more efficient generation of factor Xa by this catalyst. **B,** The tissue factor pathway inhibitor (TFPI) interacts with the factor VIIa–TF–factor Xa product complex to block TF-initiated activation of both factor IX and X, thus leaving the factor IXaβ-VIIIa complex as the only viable catalyst for activation of factor X. (*Redrawn with permission from Mann KG. Dynamics of Hemostasis. Essex Junction, VT, Haematologic Technologies, 2002.*)

Initiation

The factor VIIa–TF–membrane complex (extrinsic factor Xase) (Fig. 26-4A; also see Fig. 26-3) catalyzes the activation of both factor IX and factor X, the latter being the more efficient substrate.[7] Thus, the initial product formed is factor Xa. Feedback cleavage of factor IX by membrane-bound factor Xa enhances the rate of generation of factor IXa in a cooperative process with the factor VIIa–TF complex.[9]

The initially formed, membrane-bound factor Xa activates small amounts of prothrombin to thrombin.[20] This initial activation of prothrombin provides the thrombin essential for acceleration of the hemostatic process by serving as the activator for platelets and the procofactors factor V[15] and factor VIII (see Fig. 26-1). Once factor VIIIa is formed, the factor IXa generated by the factor VIIa–TF complex combines with factor VIIIa on the activated platelet membrane to form the intrinsic factor Xase (Figs. 26-3 and 26-4A), which becomes the major activator of factor X. The factor IXa–factor VIIIa complex is 10^6-fold more active as a factor X activator and 50 times more efficient than the factor VIIa–TF complex in catalyzing activation of factor X (thus, the bulk of factor Xa is ultimately produced by the factor IXa–factor VIIIa complex).

Propagation

As the reaction progresses, generation of factor Xa by the more active intrinsic factor Xase exceeds that of the extrinsic factor Xase complex.[21] In addition, the extrinsic factor Xase complex is subject to inhibition by TFPI[11] (Fig. 26-4B). As a consequence, most (>90%) of factor Xa is ultimately produced by the factor VIIIa–factor IXa complex. In hemophilia A and hemophilia B, this amplification of factor Xa generation does not occur.[22] Factor Xa combines with factor Va on the activated platelet membrane receptors, and this factor Va–factor Xa prothrombinase catalyst (see Figs. 26-3 and 26-4) converts most prothrombin to thrombin. Prothrombinase is 300,000-fold more active than factor Xa alone in catalyzing activation of prothrombin.[17]

Termination

The same hemostatic process required for preventing leaks from the vasculature may also be life threatening when responsible for intravascular occlusion. Thus, equally important to the hemostatic process are the stoichiometric and dynamic inhibitory systems, which block the presentation of thrombin. The sum of inhibitory functions is far in excess of the potential coagulant response. These inhibitory processes governed by TFPI, AT, and the protein C pathway act in synergy to provide activation thresholds, for which a minimum level of TF stimulation must be achieved before significant thrombin generation can occur.[23] The termination phase thus occurs throughout the reaction process.

Flow Regulation

Current data are consistent with the concept of a two-compartment model for regulation of the procoagulant response to a breach in a blood vessel (Fig. 26-5). Regulation of clotting in the extravascular space, apart from providing the initiating TF, is primarily passive and controlled by the availability of fresh blood, whereas regulation in the intravascular compartment is dynamic. Mechanical disruption of a blood vessel results in the movement of blood to an environment where TF is exposed and platelets bind and are activated (see Fig. 26-5, stage 1). These events localize the initiating procoagulant reactions to blood now outside the vasculature, with adhesion and activation of platelets in this extravascular blood providing sufficient receptors and surfaces to support the propagation phase of thrombin generation (see Fig. 26-5, stage 2). This extravascular process rapidly becomes independent of TF as generation of thrombin becomes supplied by the intrinsic factor Xase and prothrombinase complexes. As long as new blood flows into

this space, and fibrin formation and platelet aggregation have not achieved a sufficient barrier to stop flow, the system is open and the propagation phase of thrombin generation will continue. If blood ceases to move into the extravascular compartment, the system becomes closed, available prothrombin is consumed, and the complex enzymes are ultimately destroyed or sequestered into inactive complexes (see Fig. 26-5, stage 3). However, the stability of the prothrombin activating potential incorporated into the platelet-rich thrombus and its localization in the extravascular space ensure that if the barrier springs a leak, robust generation of thrombin will begin immediately on contact and continue until consequent platelet activation and fibrin deposition re-establish a secure barrier.

Three mechanisms act to limit clot growth into the intravascular space (see Fig. 26-5, stage 4): thrombomodulin-dependent activation of protein C,[14] the presence of abundant AT, and the actively nonthrombogenic and nonadhesive surface of the vascular endothelium. Thus, thrombin generation with consequent ongoing fibrin deposition and platelet activation is suppressed at the extravascular-intravascular boundary by these processes. In contrast, complexes at the extravascular side will remain relatively protected from APC and AT by the forming barrier and are therefore ready to respond to any leakage of blood.

The general properties of proteins of the blood coagulation proteome are summarized in Table 26-1 and discussed in the following text.

THE VITAMIN K–DEPENDENT PROTEIN FAMILY

The Nobel Prize was awarded to Dam and Doisy in 1941 for their discovery of the fat-soluble vitamin K. Nearly simultaneously with the discovery of vitamin K, a naturally occurring antagonist, bishydroxycoumarin (dicumarol), was described. This antagonist was identified as a toxic agent in spoiled sweet clover that caused hemorrhage in cattle because of decreased thrombin formation. This agent was introduced as an anticoagulant in humans in 1941.[24]

Vitamin K, essential for the biosynthesis of clotting factors, contributes to the conversion of 10 to 13 glutamate residues to γ-carboxyglutamate residues (Gla). This post-translational modification endows the VKDP with Ca^{2+}- and membrane-binding qualities.[25] Gla formation is decreased or absent after treatment with coumarin derivatives.

The VKDPs (Fig. 26-6) can be divided into two classes: procoagulant (factors II, VII, IX, X) and anticoagulant (protein C, protein S, and protein Z). The homology among these proteins is probably due to a common ancestral gene.[26] Each VKDP is composed of discreet domains characterized by highly conserved regions. The NH$_2$-terminal "Gla" domains (see Fig. 26-6) are fol-

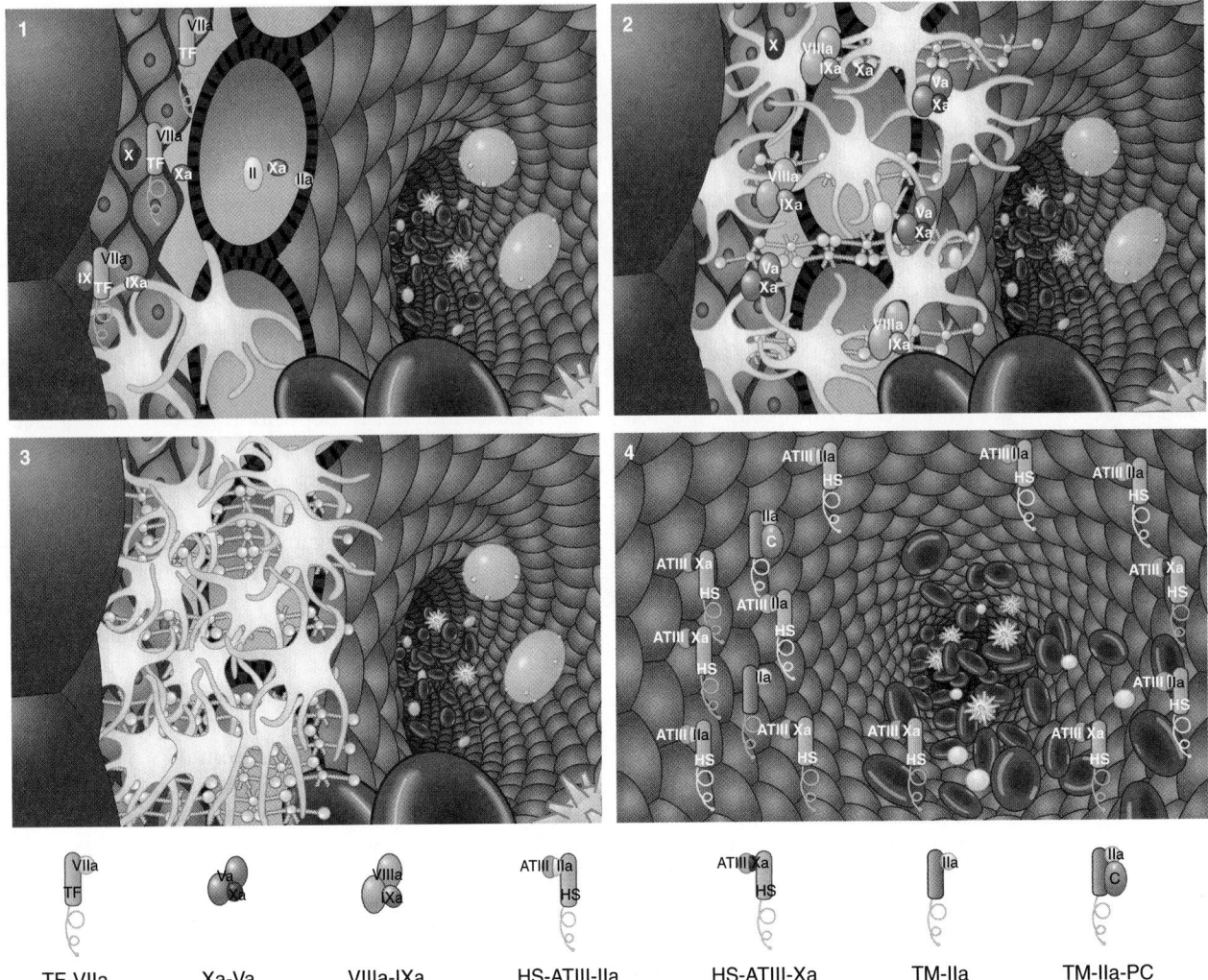

FIGURE 26-5. Schema of a two-compartment model of the regulation of tissue factor (TF)-initiated blood coagulation. A cross section of a blood vessel showing the luminal space, endothelial cell layer, and extravascular region is presented at the site of a perforation. The blood coagulation process in response is depicted in four stages. TF–factor VIIa complex, TF-VIIa; prothrombinase complex, Xa-Va; intrinsic factor Xase, VIIIa-IXa; antithrombin III (ATIII)–endothelial cell heparan sulfate (HS) proteoglycan complex bound to thrombin or factor Xa, HS-ATIII-(IIa or Xa); protein C (PC) bound to thrombomodulin-thrombin, TM-IIa-PC. **Stage 1.** Perforation results in delivery of blood and, with it, circulating factor VIIa and platelets to an extravascular space rich in membrane-bound TF. Platelets adhere to collagen and von Willebrand factor associated with the extravascular tissue, and TF binds factor VIIa , thereby initiating the process of activation of factor IX and X. Factor Xa activates small amounts of prothrombin to thrombin, which in turn activates more platelets and converts factors V and VIII to factors Va and VIIIa. **Stage 2.** The reaction is propagated by platelet-bound intrinsic factor Xase and prothrombinase, with the former being the principal generator of factor Xa. Initial clotting occurs and fibrin begins to fill in the void in cooperation with activated platelets. **Stage 3.** A barrier composed of activated platelets laden with procoagulant complexes and enmeshed in fibrin scaffolding is formed. The reaction in the now-filled perforation is terminated by consumption of reagent, which attenuates further generation of thrombin, but functional procoagulant enzyme complexes persist because they are protected from the dynamic inhibitory processes found on the intravascular face. **Stage 4.** View downstream of the perforation. Enzymes escaping from the plugged perforation are captured by antithrombin-heparan complexes, and the protein C system is activated by binding of residual thrombin to endothelial cell thrombomodulin, thereby initiating the dynamic anticoagulant system. These intravascular processes work against occlusion of the vessel despite continuous resupply of reactants across the intravascular face of the thrombus. (*From Orfeo T, Butenas S, Brummel-Ziedens KE, Mann KG. The tissue factor requirement in blood coagulation. J Biol Chem. 2005;280:42887-42896.*)

lowed by either kringle domains in prothrombin or epidermal growth factor (EGF)-like domains in factor VII, factor IX, factor X, protein C, protein S, and protein Z. Protein S contains four EGF domains followed by a sex hormone–binding domain (SHD). The serine protease domain for prothrombin, factor VII, factor IX, factor X, and protein C becomes functional after cleavage of specific peptide bonds. Protein S is not a serine protease precursor but is sensitive to thrombin cleavage. Protein

Z contains a "pseudocatalytic domain" in the COOH-terminal but cannot function as a serine protease.

Synthesis of these proteins occurs primarily in the liver, although synthesis in other tissue has been reported. The plasma concentration of circulating VKDP varies 200-fold from approximately 100 µg/mL for prothrombin to 0.5 µg/mL for factor VII (see Table 26-1). Clearance rates of the VKDPs vary with their half-lives, from 6 hours (factor VII) to 2.5 days (prothrombin; see Table 26-1).

TABLE 26-1 General Properties of Blood Coagulation Proteins

Protein	Molecular Weight	Plasma Concentration nmol/L	Plasma Concentration µg/mL	Plasma t$_{1/2}$ (Days)	Chromosome* (Gene Location)	Functional Classification
INTRINSIC PATHWAY PROTEINS						
Factor XII	80,000	500 (265)	40 (21)	2-3	Chr 5 (176 Mb)	Zymogen
Factor XI	160,000	30 (11)	4.8 (2)	2.5-3.3	Chr 4 (187 Mb)	Zymogen
Prekallikrein	85/88,000	486 (180)	42 (16)		Chr 4 (187 Mb)	Zymogen
HMW kininogen	120,000	670 (362)	80 (43)		Chr 3 (188 Mb)	Cofactor
LMW kininogen	66,000	1300	90		Chr 3 (188 Mb)	Cofactor
EXTRINSIC PATHWAY PROTEINS						
Prothrombin (factor II)	72,000	1400 (672)	100 (48)	2.5	Chr 11 (47 Mb)	VKD zymogen
α-Thrombin	37,000					Serine protease
Factor VII	50,000	10 (7)	0.5 (0.3)	0.25	Chr 13 (113 Mb)	VKD zymogen
Factor IX	55,000	90 (48)	5 (3)	1	X Chr (138 Mb)	VKD zymogen
Factor X	59,000	170 (68)	10 (4)	1.5	Chr 13 (113 Mb)	VKD zymogen
Protein C	62,000	65 (23)	4 (1)	.33	Chr 2 (128 Mb)	VKD zymogen
Protein S	69,000	300 (108)	20 (7)	1.75	Chr 3 (95 Mb)	VKD protein
Protein Z	62,000	47	3	2.5	Chr 13 (113 Mb)	VKD protein
Factor V	330,000	20 (14)	6.6 (5)	0.5	1q21-q25	Procofactor
Factor VIII	285,000	0.7 (0.7)	0.2 (0.2)	0.3-0.5	X Chr (154 Mb)	Procofactor
VWF	255,000 (monomer)	Varies	10		Chr 12 (6 Mb)	Platelet adhesion, factor VIII carrier
Tissue factor	44,000	—	—	—	Chr 1 (9 Mb)	Cell-associated cofactor
Thrombomodulin	100,000	—	—	—	Chr 20 (23 Mb)	Cofactor
Fibrinogen	340,000	7400 (8380)	2500 (2830)	3-5	Chr 4 (156 Mb)	Structural protein cell adhesion
Aα	66,500					
Bβ	52,000					
γ	46,500					
Factor XIII	320,000	94 (72)	30 (23)	9-10		Transglutaminase zymogen
A chain	83,200				Chr 6 (6 Mb)	
B chain	79,700				Chr 1 (195 Mb)	
Tissue factor pathway inhibitor	40,000	1-4	0.1	$6.4 \times 10^{-4} - 1.4 \times 10^{-3}$	Chr 2 (188 Mb)	Kunitz inhibitor
Antithrombin	58,000	2400 (1510)	140 (88)	2.5-3	Chr 1 (172 Mb)	Serpin inhibitor
Heparin cofactor II	66,000	950 (408)	62 (26)	2.5	Chr 22 (19 Mb)	Serpin inhibitor
Protein C inhibitor	57,000	90	5	1	Chr 14 (94 Mb)	Serpin inhibitor

*Chromosome number. Numbers in parentheses are approximate positions in megabases (from human genome build 36.2 www.ncbi.nlm.nih.gov).
HMW, high molecular weight; LMW, low molecular weight; VKD, vitamin K dependent; VWF, von Willebrand factor.

The VKDPs are synthesized as preproteins and are modified post-translationally at specific glutamates (γ-carboxylation) to form γ-carboxyglutamic acid (Gla).[25] Other modifications include β-hydroxylation at select aspartate and asparagine residues, tyrosine sulfation, and glycosylation. After synthesis of the single-chain precursors, the hydrophobic signal peptide directs each polypeptide to the endoplasmic reticulum. The propeptides, which play a role in docking vitamin K–dependent carboxylase,[27] are removed by an endoproteinase. For factor X and protein C, removal of an internal dipeptide or tripeptide converts them to their mature plasma two-chain zymogen forms.

The Gla domains constitute the first approximately 50 residues of the VKDPs (Fig. 26-6). The negative charge elicited from the string of Gla residues (9 to 13) contributes to the binding of Ca^{2+} and generation of the conformation required for binding to anionic phospholipid membranes. In vivo, this surface is supplied by activated platelets or other blood cells in response to vascular damage through exposure of the phosphatidylserine-rich internal face of their cell membranes. Without vitamin K, or in the presence of vitamin K antagonists, the coagulation protein precursors are synthesized but not γ-carboxylated. In this form they are still secreted into plasma but display diminished function. The γ-carboxylation reaction is catalyzed by the enzyme γ-glutamyl carboxylase. This enzyme is located in the rough endoplasmic reticulum and requires the reduced form of vitamin K, oxygen, and carbon dioxide[25] to convert glutamic acid residues to γ-carboxyglutamic acid.

Vitamin K_1 (phylloquinone) is primarily found in leafy green vegetables and vegetable oil. Additional K activity may be provided by vitamin K_2 (menaquinones) synthesized by intestinal gram-negative bacteria. Synthetic vitamin K_3 (menadione) has no intrinsic activity until it undergoes in vivo modification to the active

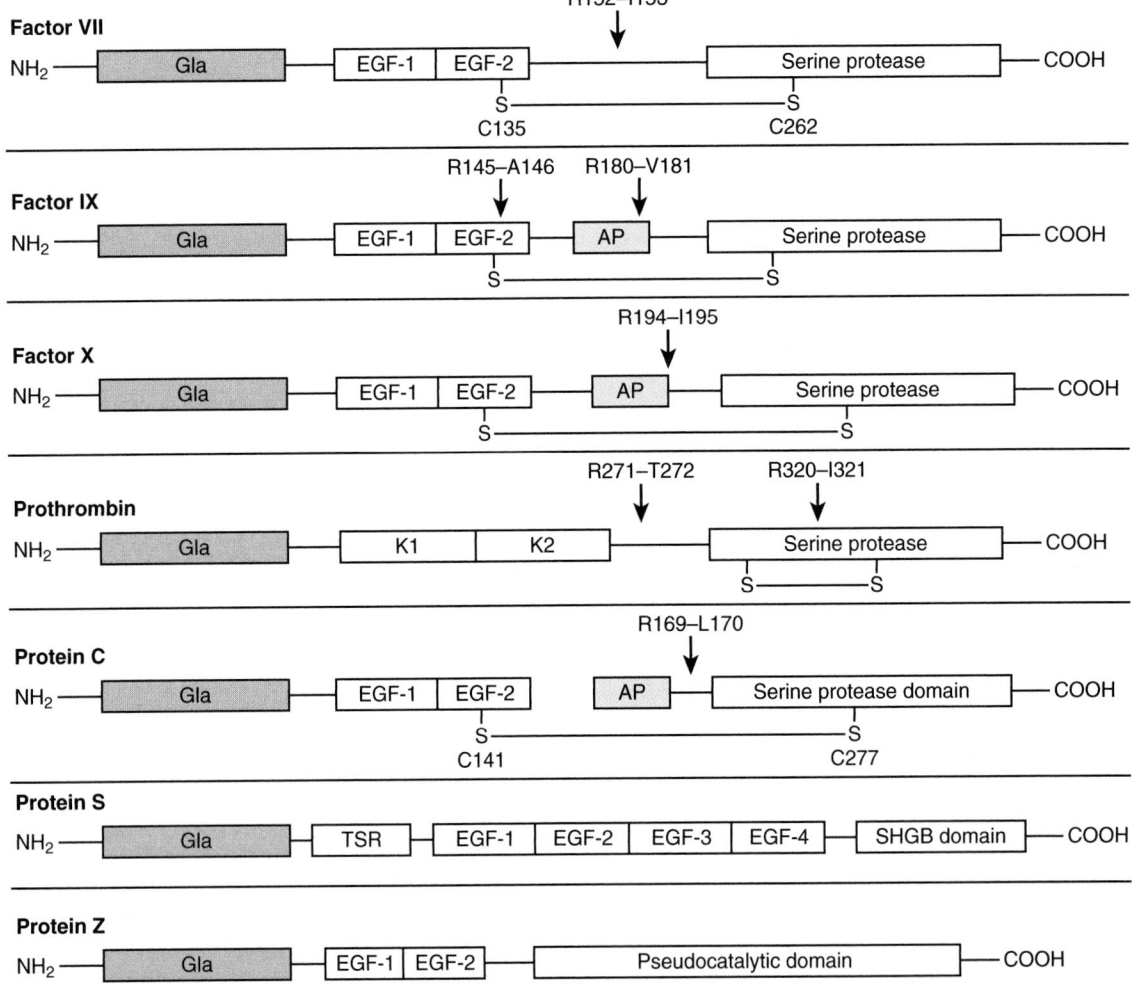

FIGURE 26-6. Schematic representation of the vitamin–K dependent proteins. The building blocks for these proteins are composed of Gla domains (9 to 13 Gla residues), followed by either kringle domains (K) in prothrombin or epidermal growth factor–like domains (EGF) in factors VII, IX, and X, protein C, protein S, and protein Z. Protein S contains a thrombin-sensitive region (TSR) before the EGF domain. The active site is contained within the serine protease domain for prothrombin, factors VII, IX, and X, and protein C and is functional upon cleavage at the activation site. Protein S is not a serine protease precursor and instead contains a sex hormone globulin binding–like domain (SHGB) in the COOH-terminal. Protein Z contains a "pseudocatalytic domain" in the COOH-terminal and does not function as a serine protease enzyme. For reference, the molecular weight for each protein is listed under its name, and disulfide bonds are illustrated as (-S-S-).

menaquinone form. In vivo, vitamin K is recycled in a microsomal oxidation-reduction system for continued use in the γ-carboxylation reaction.[28,29] In order to perform the γ-carboxylation reaction, vitamin K has to be present in its reduced hydroquinone form. As the precursor proteins are carboxylated, vitamin K is oxidized to the epoxide. The epoxide in the presence of 2,3-epoxide reductase, with thiols being used as the reducing agent, yields the quinone form of vitamin K.[30] A subsequent reduced nicotinamide adenine dinucleotide phosphate (NADPH) or NADH-dependent quinone reductase reaction resynthesizes the hydroquinone form. The cycle can thus continue. Warfarin anticoagulant therapy blocks the process required for the regeneration of reduced hydroquinone vitamin K.[28,29] Because warfarin and other coumarin derivative drugs indirectly affect carboxylation, they can be overcome with excess vitamin K.

The Gla domain is followed by two tandem EGF domains (EGF-1 and EGF-2) in factor VII, factor IX, factor X, and protein C and four EGF domains (EGF-1 to EGF-4) in protein S[31] (see Fig. 26-6). Each EGF-like domain consists of 40 to 50 amino acids, including six cysteine residues involved in disulfide bond formation. These domains are found widely distributed in extracellular and membrane proteins. Proteins containing these EGF-like domains are involved in blood coagulation, fibrinolysis, complement activation, connective tissue microfibril formation, and signal transduction.[32] The function of the EGF domain is still unclear. One hypothesis is that it serves as a spacer. There is a consistent elongation of the molecules of factors VII, IX, and X, protein C, and protein S. The distance between the membrane-binding Gla domain and the serine protease domain is crucial to placement of the active site in an appropriate position relative to the target peptide bond in its substrate.[33]

The serine protease domains (see Fig. 26-6) account for approximately half the mass of each protein. Peptide bond cleavage at specific sites converts the vitamin K–dependent zymogens to their active, chymotrypsin-like, serine protease forms. The mechanism of proteolysis by chymotrypsin involves a catalytic triad composed of Asp102, His57, and Ser195 (chymotrypsin numbering). The serine protease domains of all the Gla-containing factors are homologous members of the chymotrypsin family but cleave almost specifically at arginyl residues. However, unlike trypsin, which shows little specificity beyond the requirement for arginyl or lysyl residues at the cleavage site, the activated coagulation factors have extended substrate specificity pockets whereby only selected amino acid sequences are recognized by each protease. Thus, despite the high degree of homology between the protease domains of protein C and factors II, VII, IX, and X, each of these factors has a highly specific function in coagulation. Some of this discrimination is mediated by surface loops, along with other domains distant from the substrate binding pocket termed exosites.

Factor VII (Proconvertin, Convertin)

The single-chain factor VII zymogen is activated to its two-chain protease form by cleavage of a single peptide bond between Arg152 and Ile153 (see Fig. 26-6). The mechanism for the initial activation of this zymogen is unclear. The resulting protease consists of an NH₂-terminal light chain linked by a single disulfide bond to a COOH-terminal heavy chain containing the catalytic domain. Factor VIIa has very poor catalytic efficiency without the presence of its cofactor TF.[34,35] Cleavage of factor VII to factor VIIa can be catalyzed by several proteases, including α-thrombin,[36] factor IXa,[37] factor Xa,[36] factor XIIa,[38] and factor VII–activating protease,[39] as well as by auto-activation by factor VIIa.[40] The active factor VIIa serine protease bound to TF forms the extrinsic factor Xase complex (see Fig. 26-3).

Factor VIIa, unlike other serine proteases of the coagulation cascade,[35] is not readily inhibited by circulating protease inhibitors, including the AT-heparin complex, unless bound to TF.[41,42] Thus, regulation of TF expression is the primary means of controlling factor VIIa activity. Paradoxically, the zymogen factor VII (10 nM) is an effective competitor of factor VIIa (0.1 nM) for binding to TF. This competition downregulates the level of enzymatically active complex (factor VIIa–TF), thereby suppressing initiation of the clotting cascade. Once the extrinsic tenase complex activates factor X to factor Xa, TFPI can form a quaternary complex (factor VIIa–TF–factor Xa–TFPI) with no enzymatic activity[43] (see Fig. 26-4). Thus, once assembled and functioning, the extrinsic tenase, along with its substrate factor Xa, is a target for inactivation through the action of TFPI.

Factor IX (Plasma Thromboplastin Component, Christmas Factor, Hemophilia B Factor)

Factor IX is a single-chain zymogen consisting of 415 amino acids organized with a Gla domain (12 Gla residues), two tandem EGF domains, an activation peptide region, and a serine protease domain (see Fig. 26-6). Glycosylation in the form of O-linked and N-linked oligosaccharides makes up 17% of the factor IX protein by weight.[44] Activation of factor IX is a two-stage process that requires cleavage at Arg145 and Arg180 and results in the release of a 35-residue activation peptide[45] (see Fig. 26-6). The physiologic activators of factor IX are either TF–factor VIIa (extrinsic tenase complex)[7] or factor XIa. The first cleavage at Arg145-Ala146 results in factor IXα. This cleavage has been shown to be important in its affinity for its cofactor factor VIIIa.[46] The second cleavage occurs at Arg180-Val181 and results in factor IXαβ, the active form, also referred to as factor IXa. Both cleavages are required for the biologic activity of factor IXa.[45] Plasma factor IXa is primarily inhibited by AT[47] (see Fig. 26-2). In vitro experiments conducted on phospholipid vesicles and cell membranes showed that protease nexin-2/amyloid β-protein precursor (PN2/APP) can also inhibit factor IXa.[48]

Factor X (Stuart Factor)

Factor X is synthesized in the liver and circulates as a two-chain molecule linked by a disulfide bond. The NH$_2$-terminal light chain consists of a Gla domain and two EGF-like domains (Fig. 26-6). The COOH-terminal heavy chain consists of an activation peptide region and a catalytic (serine protease) domain. Factor X is activated by both the intrinsic and extrinsic factor Xases (see Figs. 26-1 and 26-3) by cleavage at Arg194-Ile195 (see Fig. 26-6). A 52–amino acid activation peptide is released. The resulting catalytic serine protease, factor Xa, is composed of a light chain and a disulfide-linked heavy chain. Factor X has to be bound to the membrane before activation.[19] Factor Xa participates in forming the prothrombinase complex (see Fig. 26-4).[17] The propagation phase of thrombin generation is catalyzed principally by factor Xa generated via the intrinsic tenase complex (see Fig. 26-3), which activates factor X at a 50- to 100-fold higher rate than the extrinsic tenase complex does.[9] The factor Xa active site associates with the COOH-terminal of TFPI.[49] The factor Xa–TFPI complex rapidly inactivates TF–factor VIIa to form a stable quaternary complex, TF–factor VIIa–TFPI–factor Xa.[49] Factor Xa is inhibited by AT[50] but only poorly when in the prothrombinase complex.[51]

Factor II (Prothrombin)

Prothrombin is the single-chain precursor of factor IIa (thrombin), the key enzyme in blood coagulation. The zymogen prothrombin is the most abundant of the plasma VKDPs and circulates in plasma at a mean concentration of 1.4 μM, or 100 μg/mL[52] (see Table 26-1). Prothrombin is synthesized primarily in the liver. Low levels of prothrombin expression have also been identified in other tissues, including the brain, diaphragm, stomach, kidney, spleen, intestine, uterus, placenta, and adrenal gland. Removal of the 43–amino acid propeptide generates the mature protein of 579 amino acids. An NH$_2$-terminal Gla domain is followed by two kringle domains and the serine protease precursor domain (see Fig. 26-6). Kringles have been identified as common motifs in many plasma proteins, including prothrombin, plasminogen, tissue plasminogen activator, urokinase, factor XII, and apolipoprotein(a).[53] The kringle 1 domain may interact with factor Va,[54] although kringle 2 appears to be the primary region mediating interaction with factor Va to form the prothrombinase complex.[55] This latter interaction may initiate conformational changes that make reaction sites accessible for enzymatic cleavage of prothrombin.[56] The NH$_2$-terminal Gla domain and the first kringle domain together are referred to as prothrombin fragment 1, with the kringle 2 domain being located in

prothrombin fragment 2. The sequence of the enzyme α-thrombin is contained within prethrombin 2.

Activation of prothrombin by prothrombinase proceeds through an initial cleavage of prothrombin at Arg320-Ile321, which gives rise to meizothrombin, a two-chain disulfide-linked molecule (see Fig. 26-6). Meizothrombin expresses some of the activities of α-thrombin. However, the fibrinogen clotting ability of meizothrombin is impaired in comparison to that of α-thrombin.[57] Meizothrombin is subsequently cleaved at Arg271-Thr272 to yield the NH$_2$-terminal half of the molecule (prothrombin fragment 1.2) and α-thrombin. α-Thrombin consists of an NH$_2$-terminal 49-residue A-chain disulfide linked to a COOH-terminal 259-residue B chain containing the catalytic triad.

An alternative cleavage pathway occurs when factor Xa independently acts on prothrombin. In the presence of factor Xa and Ca^{2+}, the initial cleavage occurs at Arg271-Thr272 and gives rise to prothrombin fragment 1.2 and prethrombin 2. Subsequent cleavage at Arg320 in prethrombin 2 yields α-thrombin. Prothrombin fragment 1.2 remains noncovalently associated with α-thrombin.[58] In contrast to other VKDPs, the phospholipid-binding Gla region is not covalently attached to the serine protease domain after cleavage of prothrombin to thrombin.

α-Thrombin is the central enzyme in blood coagulation in that it contributes to reactions at all levels, thereby allowing overall maintenance of vascular integrity. Its premier role in hemostasis results in platelet-fibrin clot formation.[59] However, the events that lead up to and beyond fibrin formation also involve protein cleavage by α-thrombin, as well as activating platelets,[60,61] factor VII,[36] factor V,[15] factor VIII,[62] factor XI,[8] and factor XIII. The contributions of α-thrombin also extend to anticoagulant and fibrinolytic reactions, including activation of protein C and thrombin-activatable fibrinolysis inhibitor (TAFI).[63]

The stable form of human α-thrombin possesses at least five distinct binding sites for substrates, inhibitors, cofactors, apolar molecules, and sodium ions (Na$^+$).[64] Exosite I, the fibrinogen binding site, is an electropositive anion binding site distinct from, but acting in concert with, the active site of the α-thrombin molecule. In addition to fibrinogen, exosite I also recognizes the COOH-terminal domain of hirudin, the hirudin-like region of PAR-1, and the fifth and sixth EGF-like domains of thrombomodulin.[64]

Many of the effects of α-thrombin on platelets and cells are elicited through the interaction of α-thrombin with receptor molecules, with α-thrombin binding to a receptor and initiating a signal transduction mechanism. The interaction between α-thrombin and the human platelet thrombin receptor PAR-1, however, is characterized by a more unusual mechanism in which the receptor is also a substrate for α-thrombin.[65] α-Thrombin cleaves the extracellular region of the receptor and produces a "tethered ligand." The new NH$_2$-terminal binds back to and activates the receptor.[65,66] Two additional α-thrombin receptors homologous to PAR-1, PAR-3 and PAR-4, have been identified. α-Thrombin's role continues beyond hemostasis into the realm of tissue repair and the remodeling phase necessary to regenerate damaged vascular tissue. α-Thrombin is a potent mitogen[67] and stimulates cell division in macrophages,[68] smooth muscle cells,[69] and endothelial cells.[70]

Protein C (Autoprothrombin II-A)

Protein C circulates as a heterodimer consisting of disulfide-linked heavy and light chains[71] (see Fig. 26-6). However, approximately 5% to 10% of circulating protein C is in the single-chain form. The NH_2-terminal light chain contains the Gla domain and a hydrophobic region that connects the Gla domain to two EGF domains. The COOH-terminal heavy chain contains the serine protease domain.[72] Cleavage at Arg169-Leu170 releases the activation peptide from the heavy chain to generate the enzyme. Although the α-thrombin–thrombomodulin complex is probably the major physiologic activator of protein C,[73] other potential activators include plasmin and factor Xa.[72] The half-life of protein C (8 to 10 hours; see Table 26-1) is markedly shorter than the half-life of other members of the VKDP family, which is probably the basis of the transient hypercoagulable state that may occur subsequent to the administration of coumarin-based anticoagulants.

The anticoagulant role of the dynamic protein C inhibitory pathway is proteolytic inactivation of factor Va. APC inactivates factor Va via a sequential series of proteolytic cleavages and thus inhibits the generation of α-thrombin.[74] APC also cleaves and inactivates factor VIIIa, although the spontaneous dissociation/inactivation of factor VIIIa is probably the physiologic regulator of factor Xa generation.[75] Complete inactivation of factor Va by APC requires an anionic phospholipid surface, and rates of inactivation of factors Va and VIIIa by APC have been reported to be enhanced by protein S.[76,77] APC also has profibrinolytic effects associated with decreased activation of TAFI. TAFI is activated by the α-thrombin–thrombomodulin complex and acts to prolong clot lysis. Cleavage of factor Va by APC inhibits α-thrombin generation, thus reducing α-thrombin–thrombomodulin–mediated TAFI activation.[78]

Protein C activation and APC activity are controlled on several levels. The endothelial cell protein C receptor (EPCR) provides cell-specific binding sites for both protein C and APC.[79] Inflammatory agents such as endotoxin, interleukin-1β (IL-1β), tumor necrosis factor-β (TNF-β), and TNF-α upregulate protein C activation on endothelial cells.[80-82] TNF-α downregulates thrombomodulin on the endothelial cell surface.[82] There are multiple other factors that downregulate thrombomodulin as well. APC activity is further regulated by the protein C inhibitor plasminogen activator inhibitor 3 (PAI-3).[83]

Protein S

Protein S is a VDKP that is not a serine protease precursor. Approximately 40% of protein S circulates in the free form, and the remaining 60% circulates as a 1:1 complex with C4b-binding protein (C4bBP), a regulatory protein of the complement system.[84] The precise function of protein S in the protein C inhibitory pathway is controversial. Protein S is thought to function as a cofactor for APC in the inactivation of factors Va and VIIIa.[85-87] Protein S has also been reported to bind to factor Xa,[88] factor VIII,[89] and factor Va[90] and compete for prothrombinase binding sites on the membrane surface.[91] The C4bBP–protein S complex may inhibit factor X activation as well.[92] Protein S may have other roles apart from anticoagulation.[93] α-Thrombin cleavage of protein S inhibits the ability of protein S to act as a cofactor for APC.[94] The anticoagulant activity of protein S is also neutralized when bound to C4bBP.[84,92]

Protein Z

Protein Z is an enzymatically inactive homologue of factors VII, IX, and X and protein C.[95,96] Protein Z circulates in plasma in a complex with protein Z–dependent protease inhibitor (ZPI). ZPI is a 72-kd member of the serpin superfamily. However, like protein S, protein Z does not function as a protease. Although the COOH-terminal contains a homologue to the catalytic domains present in serine protease zymogens, the catalytic triad is not present.[96] The function of protein Z in vivo is unclear. Even though protein Z–deficient mice appear normal, severe thrombosis is observed when combined in mice with factor V Leiden.[97]

FACTOR XI, THE CONTACT PATHWAY CROSSOVER (PLASMA THROMBOPLASTIN ANTECEDENT)

Factor XI is a substrate for thrombin (see Fig. 26-1) and, when cleaved to factor XIa, activates factor IX.[8] Factor XI circulates as a homodimer in complex with HMWK[98] (see Table 26-1) and is also found in platelets.[99] Unlike other members of the accessory or contact pathway, factor XIa has a role in coagulation as part of a positive feedback loop that enhances the generation of α-thrombin.[8] Plasma factor XI accounts for most of the factor XI activity in humans and is a disulfide-linked homodimer (see Table 26-1). The NH_2-terminal contains four tandem sequences termed Apple domains (Apple 1 to Apple 4), followed by the COOH-terminal catalytic domain. The Apple domains are homologous to the Apple domains in human plasma prekallikrein.[100] The Apple domains mediate factor XI dimerization, as well as binding to its various cofactors and substrates.[98,101]

Plasma factor XI is cleaved at an internal Arg369-Ile370 bond to yield a disulfide-linked two-chain activated serine protease. The factor XI homodimer yields two disulfide-linked heavy chains containing the Apple domains and two light chains containing the active sites.[102,103] Activation of factor XI can be accomplished by factor XIIa and α-thrombin and by autoactivation by factor XIa itself. Activation of factor XI by factor XIIa requires HMWK and an anionic surface. However, deficiencies of factor XII and HMWK do not result in bleeding diatheses, whereas factor XI deficiency is associated with hemorrhage. This suggests that factor XIIa–dependent activation of factor XI as part of the contact pathway is not likely to be the primary route of factor XIa generation in hemostasis. The physiologically relevant pathway for activation of factor XI in coagulation is believed to involve α-thrombin.[8,104] Subsequent to activation, factor XIa remains bound to the surface. Factor XIa is a trypsin-like serine protease that cleaves and activates factor IX in a Ca^{2+}-dependent fashion.[105,106] Factor IXa is the enzyme component of the intrinsic tenase complex that provides the burst of factor Xa needed for normal coagulation. As part of a positive feedback loop, α-thrombin activates factor XI. In turn, factor XIa generates factor IXa, which leads to the high levels of factor Xa that ensure efficient generation of α-thrombin.[8]

Factor XIa is regulated by four serine protease inhibitors: AT, α_1-protease inhibitor, C1 inhibitor, and α_2-antiplasmin.[107-109] Factor XIa is also reported to be inhibited by PAI-1 and protein C inhibitor.[110] In addition, platelets secrete several factor XIa inhibitors,[111] including PN2.[112]

COFACTOR PROTEINS

There are two categories of procoagulant cofactor proteins: the plasma-derived soluble procofactors factor V and factor VIII (the latter in complex with its circulating carrier von Willebrand factor [VWF]) and the cell-associated cofactors TF and thrombomodulin. Factors V and VIII are highly homologous (40% identity). The cell-associated cofactors are single-chain transmembrane proteins, each composed of extracellular, transmembrane, and cytoplasmic domains, but they do not share homology in primary structure.

Factor V (Labile Factor)

The procofactors factors VIII and V are organized into discrete structural domains (Fig. 26-7). Factor V was initially recognized as an unstable plasma component necessary for the generation of α-thrombin.[113] Most factor V circulates in plasma (see Table 26-1), but 18% to 25% of the total factor V is present in platelet alpha granules.[114]

The intron-exon structure of the factor V and factor VIII genes are quite similar, and the genes probably evolved from a common ancestor. The liver appears to be the primary site of factor V biosynthesis. Although human megakaryocytes have also been reported to express factor V,[115] platelet factor V appears to be primarily derived from plasma factor V.[116] Human factor V is composed of A1-A2 domains, a central B domain, and a COOH-terminal light-chain precursor (A3-C1-C2 domains). The A domains are homologous to those found in factor VIII and ceruloplasmin; the C domains are homologous to the slime mold protein discoidin. Like factor VIII and ceruloplasmin, factor V is a copper-binding protein.[117]

Factor V undergoes extensive post-translational modification, including phosphorylation, sulfation, and glycosylation. Phosphorylation at Ser692 affects the rate of inactivation of factor Va by APC.[118] The tyrosine sulfation status of factor V has also been related to its function.[119]

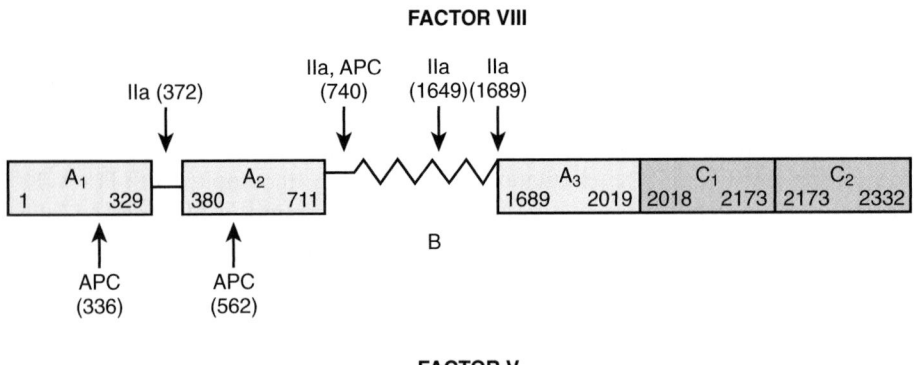

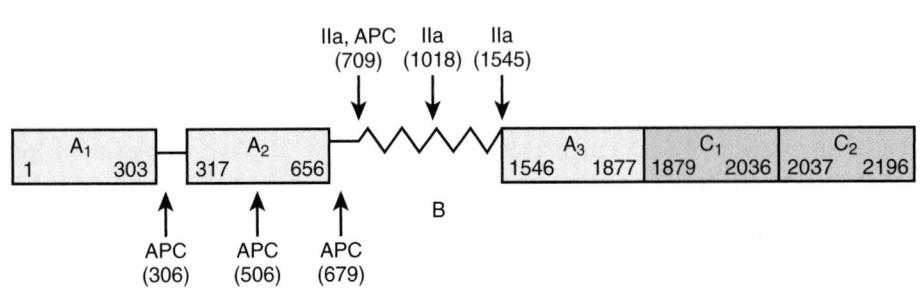

FIGURE 26-7. Soluble cofactor domain structures (factors VIII and V). The domain structures (A1-A2-A3-B-C1-C2) are bracketed by the beginning and ending amino acid residue. α-Thrombin (IIa) and activated protein C (APC)/factor Xa cleavage sites are shown with *vertical arrows*.

Carbohydrate accounts for 13% to 25% of the mass of factor V and about 50% of the mass of the B region.[120] Differential glycosylation of Asn2182 in the C2 domain is reported to be responsible for the factor V1 and factor V2 variants observed in plasma.[121] Factors Va1 and Va2 appear to also be distinguished by functional differences.

The procofactor factor V does not bind factor Xa and is essentially completely inactive.[17] Limited proteolysis of the factor V molecule yields the active cofactor. α-Thrombin cleaves factor V at Arg709, Arg1018, and Arg1545 (see Fig. 26-7). The α-thrombin–generated form of factor Va is a heterodimer consisting of an NH_2-terminal heavy chain (A1-A2 domains) linked noncovalently to a COOH-terminal light chain (A3-C1-C2 domains).[122-125] The B domain is excised during proteolytic activation.[126] Factor Xa also cleaves factor V to produce a molecule similar to the factor Va produced by α-thrombin cleavage.[127] In addition, other enzymes may fully or partially activate factor V.[128] Factor Va functions both as a receptor for factor Xa and as a positive modulator of the catalytic potential of factor Xa in the prothrombinase complex. The cofactor forms at least part of the receptor for factor Xa on platelets and serves to anchor factor Xa to the membrane surface.[15,16,62]

Factor Va is downregulated via proteolytic inactivation by APC. APC cleaves factor Va at three sites: Arg506, Arg306, and Arg679. Initial factor Va cleavage occurs at Arg506. Subsequently, the membrane-dependent cleavage at Arg306 results in dissociation of the A2 domain as two fragments and complete loss of factor Va cofactor activity. An additional APC-mediated cleavage of factor Va fragments occurs at Arg679. The importance of this regulatory mechanism is demonstrated by the "APC resistance" syndrome associated with factor V Leiden.[129,130] The factor V Leiden Arg506→Gln mutation eliminates the first and most rapid of the sequential inactivating cleavages by APC. Factor Va Leiden thus retains cofactor activity and continues to promote α-thrombin generation for an extended period. Ultimately, inactivation of factor Va Leiden by cleavage of the Arg306 bond does occur, but at a markedly slower rate.[131]

Factor VIII (Antihemophilic Factor, Factor VIII:C)

Factor VIII circulates in plasma in complex with the large multimeric protein VWF. The ratio of factor VIII to VWF is in the range of 1 molecule of factor VIII to 50 to 100 molecules of VWF monomeric units. VWF acts to transport and stabilize plasma factor VIII. Factor VIII in complex with VWF has a plasma half-life of approximately 12 hours, whereas factor VIII alone undergoes rapid clearance and has a half-life of approximately 2 hours.[132,133] The liver and spleen are thought to be the primary sites of factor VIII biosynthesis.[134]

Though synthesized as a 2351–amino acid single-chain protein, human plasma factor VIII undergoes significant proteolytic processing that results in a heterogenous collection of forms. The heterogeneity in molecular weight is due to proteolysis of the protein in circulation or processing before secretion (or both). The initial synthesized product is composed of three A domains, two C domains, and a connecting B domain (see Fig. 26-7). The secreted factor VIII molecule is a two-chain heterodimer as a result of intracellular proteolysis at the B-A3 junction. Additional cleavages within the B chain yield a heavy chain of A1-A2 domains linked to B fragments of variable length.[135] The B domain is highly glycosylated and contains 18 of the 25 potential N-linked glycosylation sites in factor VIII. Activation by α-thrombin involves cleavage at Arg372 (the A1-A2 junction), Arg740 (the A2-B junction), and Arg1689 in the light chain (the B-A3 junction) and excision of the remnant of the B domain. The resulting molecule contains three separate polypeptide chains: a light chain (A3-C1-C2) bound to the NH_2-derived heavy chain and the noncovalently associated A2 region of the heavy chain. Factor VIIIa is an unstable molecule, with dissociation of the A2 domain leading to spontaneous inactivation.[136] Factor VIII shares homology with the copper ion–binding protein ceruloplasmin and contains a reduced copper ion (Cu^+) binding site in the A1 domain that is important for function.[137] A specific VWF binding site has been identified between residues 1673 and 1684 of the factor VIII light chain.[138] The VWF binding site is removed from factor VIII during activation by α-thrombin cleavage at Arg1689. High-affinity factor IXa binding is observed for the factor VIIIa light-chain A3 domain.[139] Sulfation of several tyrosine residues in factor VIII is also important for function.[140]

The cofactor factor VIIIa binds factor IXa with Ca^{2+} (and membrane) to form the intrinsic factor Xase complex (see Fig. 26-3). The intrinsic factor Xase complex catalyzes the activation of factor X at a rate orders of magnitude greater than the enzyme factor IXa alone[18] (see Fig. 26-4). Factor Xa generated via the intrinsic factor Xase complex is the primary contributor of the factor Xa required for the propagation phase of thrombin generation.[21] In hemophilia A or B the intrinsic factor Xase complex cannot be formed, and the factor Xa levels required to induce the propagation phase of thrombin generation are not produced,[22] thereby resulting in lethargic thrombin formation and poor clot formation (see Fig. 26-5).

The spontaneous loss of factor VIIIa function is primarily a consequence of dissociation of the A2 subunit from the heterotrimer. Once the A2 subunit is displaced, factor VIIIa loses cofactor function. Dissociation occurs rapidly under physiologic conditions. The factor IXa–membrane complex interactions stabilize factor VIIIa and thus delay dissociation of the heterotrimer and prolong the transient activity of factor VIIIa.[141] Factor VIIIa is also regulated by limited proteolysis. Factor IXa cleaves the A1 subunit of factor VIIIa at Arg336 and eliminates factor VIIIa function.[142] APC is a key anticoagulant enzyme that likewise cleaves the A1 subunit at Arg336. APC also cleaves the A2 subunit of factor VIIIa at Arg562.[143] These APC cleavages occur sequentially, with the A1 cleavage occurring first and the A2 cleavage second.[144] Factor IXa protects factor VIIIa from APC cleavage at Arg562; however, protein S blocks the protective effect.[145] Although factor VIIIa is proteolytically inactivated by a number of enzymes, spontaneous dissociation appears to be the key regulator of cofactor function.

von Willebrand Factor (Ristocetin Cofactor)

VWF is a multifunctional protein with several key roles in coagulation. VWF circulates in plasma and is also contained in the alpha granules of human platelets.[146] In addition, it is known for its role in ristocetin-induced platelet aggregation (see Chapters 25 and 30). VWF is expressed by endothelial cells and megakaryocytes and is stored in Weibel-Palade bodies in endothelial cells and in alpha granules in platelets.[147,148] VWF is a large adhesive glycoprotein that circulates in plasma as a heterogeneous mixture of disulfide-linked multimers (Chapter 30). The disulfide-linked multimers range in size from dimers, M_r = 600,000, to extremely large multimers consisting of greater than 20 million Daltons. VWF has binding sites for factor VIII, heparin, collagen, platelet glycoprotein Ib and platelet glycoprotein IIb-IIIa.[149] Plasma VWF transports and stabilizes factor VIII and protects it from

inactivation by APC,[87] thus significantly prolonging the half-life of factor VIII in circulation.[133] VWF also acts as a bridge between platelets and promotes platelet aggregation. The primary platelet binding site for VWF is the glycoprotein Ib-IX-V receptor complex (Chapters 25 and 30). Endothelial cells secrete VWF multimers that are larger than those found circulating in plasma. The function of these large multimeric forms of VWF is to bind to and agglutinate blood platelets under high shear rates. These large multimers of VWF are degraded by a specific metalloproteinase, ADAMTS-13.[150]

Tissue Factor (Tissue Thromboplastin CD142 and Coagulation Factor III)

TF and thrombomodulin (Fig. 26-8) are intrinsic membrane proteins that are essential cofactors for factor VIIa and thrombin, respectively. They share no homology at the molecular level. TF is a transmembrane protein that functions as a cofactor for factor VIIa in the extrinsic factor Xase complex. In the absence of injury or stimulation, active TF is not ordinarily expressed on cellular surfaces in direct contact with circulating blood. Presentation of TF to the circulation is the event that triggers the primary procoagulant pathway of coagulation (see Fig. 26-1). Expression of TF can be induced in a number of cultured cell types. Monocytic cells and monocytes

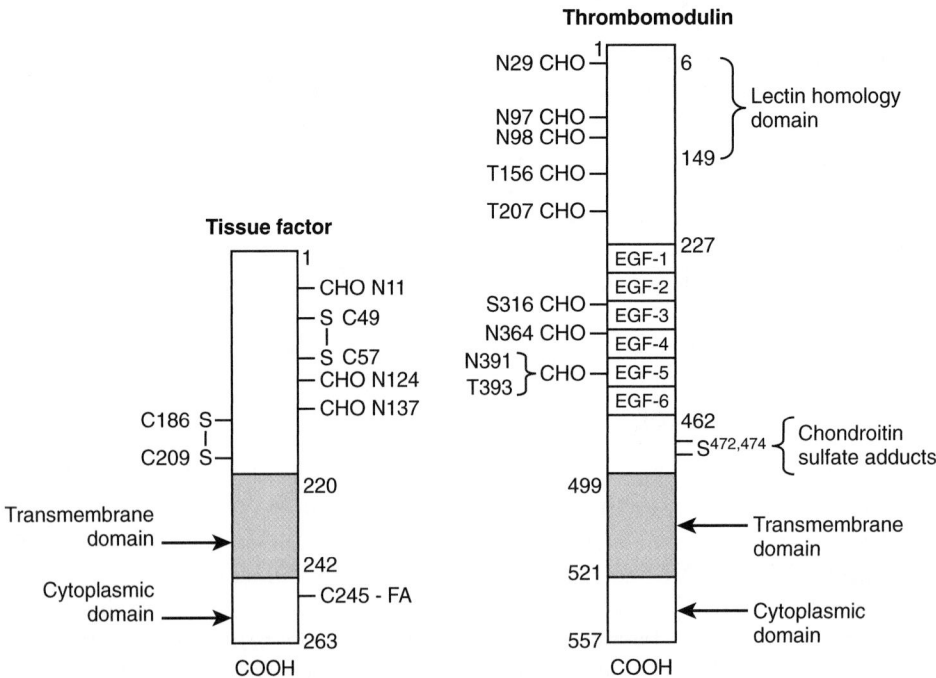

FIGURE 26-8. Transmembrane cofactors. Tissue factor is composed of an extracellular domain (residues 1 to 219), a transmembrane domain (residues 220 to 242), and a cytoplasmic domain (residues 243 to 263). Two disulfide bonds (S-S) and the sites of the three carbohydrate moieties (CHO) are identified by amino acid residue. One cysteine (C245) contains a thiol ester linkage to a fatty acid. Thrombomodulin is composed of five distinct domains. The domain structures are a lectin-like domain (residues 6 to 149), a domain containing six epidermal growth factor (EGF)-like (EGF) regions (residues 227 to 462), a small extracellular domain rich in threonine and serine residues (two have been identified as sites of chondroitin sulfate adducts: S472 and S474), a membrane-spanning region (residues 499 to 521), and a cytoplasmic tail (residues 522 to 557). There are nine known glycosylation sites (CHO) on the thrombomodulin molecule.

isolated from peripheral blood also express TF when stimulated by bacterial endotoxin or other proinflammatory agents. There is little or no detectable TF expression on unstimulated endothelial cells in vivo, although certain conditions such as sepsis, placental villitis, and graft rejection induce endothelial TF expression.[151] The mechanism governing TF expression under nonpathologic conditions is unknown.

TF is a member of the class 2 cytokine receptor superfamily and a type I integral membrane protein. The NH_2-terminal of TF (residues 1 to 219) is extracellular, whereas the COOH-terminal of the protein is intracellular (residues 243 to 263). TF also contains a hydrophobic membrane-spanning domain (see Fig. 26-8). This domain appears to function as an anchor for TF in the membrane.[152] The NH_2-terminal domain of TF is composed of two fibronectin type III domains and is glycosylated. The COOH-terminal cytoplasmic domain is quite short, and its function is unclear because deletion of this domain has no significant effect on TF procoagulant activity.[152]

TF can bind either factor VII or factor VIIa to form a high-affinity 1:1 complex. Once bound to TF, the zymogen factor VII may be converted to factor VIIa via limited proteolysis.[153,154] The TF–factor VIIa or extrinsic tenase complex activates both factor IX and factor X. When TF is exposed or expressed subsequent to vascular perturbation, the low levels of circulating factor VIIa bind to TF, and the extrinsic factor Xase complex triggers the procoagulant cascade (see Fig. 26-4A).[9,155]

In the absence of TF, factor VIIa is relatively inert. TF alters the active site of factor VIIa, thus functioning as an allosteric activator of the enzyme.[40,155] Although the cofactor is necessary for enzymatic activity, formation of the TF–factor VIIa complex does not require an anionic phospholipid membrane surface as do the other procoagulant complexes. The membrane dependency of the extrinsic factor Xase complex function in factor X and factor IX activation arises from membrane-mediated substrate delivery. Both factors X and IX bind to the membrane surface for efficient two-dimensional transfer to the extrinsic factor Xase complex.

TF is primarily regulated through availability. In normal hemostasis, the commonly accepted source of functional TF is through exposure of the subendothelium after vascular perforation. However, controversy has arisen regarding the sources and presentation of active TF and whether functional TF circulates in blood.[156,157] Once the TF–factor VIIa complex is formed in the vicinity of an injury, the extrinsic tenase activity is then modulated by TFPI and AT.

Thrombomodulin

Thrombomodulin is a type 1 transmembrane protein that is constitutively expressed on the surface of vascular endothelial cells (see Fig. 26-8). Thrombomodulin is a high-affinity receptor for α-thrombin and acts as a cofactor for the α-thrombin–dependent activation of protein

C and TAFI. Thrombomodulin expression has been reported in a variety of cell types, including vascular endothelial cells.[158] The activity of thrombomodulin on the surface of endothelial cells is decreased by inflammatory cytokines, which may contribute to the hypercoagulation characteristic of inflammatory states. Homozygous thrombomodulin-deficient mice die in utero before formation of the cardiovascular system, thus suggesting a potential role for thrombomodulin in mammalian development.[159]

The domain structure of thrombomodulin is depicted in Figure 26-8. The fifth and sixth EGF domains support α-thrombin association.[160] The presence of chondroitin sulfate increases the affinity for α-thrombin 10-fold.[161] The chondroitin sulfate moiety also enhances inactivation of α-thrombin by AT[162] and modulates protein C activation.[161,162] The O-linked sugar domain of thrombomodulin is required for generation of APC on cellular surfaces. This domain is extended and rigid and probably functions to elevate α-thrombin from the membrane surface.

Production of APC by the α-thrombin–thrombomodulin complex is approximately 1000 times faster than equivalent concentrations of protein C and α-thrombin. Once bound to thrombomodulin, α-thrombin's procoagulant activities are neutralized. The high-affinity α-thrombin–thrombomodulin interaction is mediated mainly by exosite I on the α-thrombin molecule. Exosite I also binds fibrinogen, and interaction of α-thrombin with thrombomodulin therefore blocks fibrinogen binding and cleavage. In addition, thrombomodulin induces conformational changes in α-thrombin.[163,164] The changes that occur upon interaction of α-thrombin with thrombomodulin reduce the ability of α-thrombin to generate fibrin, activate factor V, or activate platelets[165] and increase the inactivation of α-thrombin by AT.[165] Thus, the α-thrombin–thrombomodulin complex, or protein Case (see Fig. 26-3), functions in an anticoagulant and antifibrinolytic capacity.

THE INTRINSIC (ACCESSORY) PATHWAY FACTORS

The procoagulant proteins that make up the intrinsic or accessory pathway consist of factor XII, plasma prekallikrein, HMWK, and factor XI. These proteins are responsible for the contact (intrinsic) activation of blood coagulation (see Fig. 26-1).

Factor XII (Hageman Factor, Contact Factor)

Factor XII plays a primary role in initiation of the contact or intrinsic pathway of coagulation upon binding with substances such as glass or kaolin. The contact pathway is the basis for the APTT clotting assay. Deficiency of factor XII is not associated with bleeding abnormalities, and therefore the precise role of factor XII in hemostasis is unclear, although the components of the contact pathway may provide a link between coagulation and inflammation.

The factor XII molecule is composed of two domains: a NH_2-terminal heavy chain and a COOH-terminal light chain. The heavy chain contains fibronectin type I and type II domains, two EGF-like domains, a kringle domain, and a proline-rich region. The light chain contains the serine protease catalytic domain, a region homologous to the B chain of the enzyme plasmin.

Factor XII undergoes autoactivation upon interaction with negatively charged surfaces such as glass, kaolin, dextran sulfate, ellagic acid, celite, or bismuth subgallate.[166] These are probably artifactual triggers and the physiologic activator is unknown. Although factor XII associates with many physiologically relevant anionic surfaces, including negatively charged phospholipids, the autoactivation of factor XII induced by these surfaces in vitro does not appear to represent the mechanism of factor XII activation in vivo.[167]

Factor XIIa, prekallikrein, and HMWK form a complex on anionic phospholipids of the cell membrane, and prekallikrein is cleaved to kallikrein. Kallikrein activates factor XII by cleavage at Arg353-Val354 to generate an 80-kD two-chain enzyme, α-factor XIIa (factor XIIa). This cleavage is essential for exposure of the active site in factor XIIa.[168]

Factor XIIa activates factor XI and prekallikrein by mechanisms dependent on anionic surfaces and the cofactor HMWK. Factor XIIa also activates the C1 component of the complement system,[169] downregulates the Fc receptor on monocytes and macrophages,[170] and stimulates neutrophils.[171] Although these roles have no apparent impact on normal coagulation, factor XII/XIIa may be an important link between coagulation and inflammation. Factor XIIa also activates plasminogen to plasmin, thereby linking the contact pathway to fibrinolysis.[172]

Plasma Prekallikrein (Fletcher Factor)

Plasma prekallikrein deficiency is rare and not associated with a hemostatic defect. Approximately 75% of plasma prekallikrein circulates in a noncovalent complex with HMWK,[173] and the remaining 25% circulates as free prekallikrein. Prekallikrein contains four tandemly repeated Apple domains in the NH_2-terminal portion of the molecule that are highly homologous to the Apple domains of factor XI. Prekallikrein is activated by factor XIIa in complex with the cofactor HMWK on an anionic surface (see Fig. 26-1). The enzyme kallikrein is a two-chain molecule composed of an NH_2-terminal heavy chain containing the four Apple domains and a COOH-terminal light chain containing the active site.[174]

Kallikrein is a member of the trypsin family of serine proteases. In the presence of an appropriate anionic surface and the cofactor HMWK, kallikrein activates factor XII to factor XIIa and proteolyses factor XIIa to β-factor XIIa. Kallikrein also undergoes autoproteolysis

to yield β-kallikrein.[175] Enzyme activity is significantly reduced upon conversion of kallikrein to β-kallikrein. Kallikrein cleaves HMWK at two sites to generate the vasoactive nonapeptide bradykinin, a potent vasodilator. Kallikrein is also an activator of fibrinolytic zymogens and converts both plasminogen to plasmin and pro–urokinase plasminogen activator (pro-uPA) to uPA.[176] In addition, kallikrein has been reported to activate neutrophils and stimulate release of elastase as part of the hemostatic and inflammatory responses.[177] C1 inhibitor and α_2-macroglobulin are the major inhibitors of kallikrein.[178]

High-Molecular-Weight Kininogen (Fitzgerald Factor, Williams Factor)

HMWK acts as a cofactor for the activation of factor XII and prekallikrein and is the precursor of the vasoactive peptide bradykinin. A second form of kininogen, low-molecular-weight (LMWK), is also found in plasma. LMWK can be cleaved to yield bradykinin but has no procoagulant activity. Deficiencies of HMWK and LMWK are rare and not associated with bleeding diatheses.[179] The major established function of the kininogens is to serve as a source of bradykinin and thereby contribute to a number of vascular events regulated by bradykinin.

The two forms of kininogen, HMWK and LMWK, are the products of a single gene and are produced by alternative splicing.[180] The NH_2-terminal heavy chains of the two forms are identical and contain potent inhibitors of cysteine proteases such as calpain.[181] The central domain of both kininogens is the bradykinin region. The two forms of kininogen have different COOH-terminal light-chain regions. The light chain of HMWK contains binding sites for prekallikrein and factor XI.[182] Kallikrein, factor XIIa, and factor XIa cleave HMWK to release bradykinin. Kallikrein will also cleave LMWK to release bradykinin.

As noted earlier, the biologic significance of the contact pathway of coagulation is not established. In hemostasis, generation of factor XIa most likely proceeds via an α-thrombin–dependent pathway, and any factor XIa generated by the contact pathway would not have a measurable impact on coagulation. Release of bradykinin as a consequence of these activation events, however, does provide a key vasoactive agent with a variety of roles and directly links the contact pathway to vascular repair processes.

STOICHIOMETRIC INHIBITORS

In vivo, the hemostatic reaction is tightly regulated to ensure that adequate but limited levels of α-thrombin are generated. Two systems, one stoichiometric and one proteolytic, regulate the generation of thrombin. In the proteolytic system (described earlier), α-thrombin participates in its downregulation by binding to thrombomodulin on the vascular cell surface and converting protein C to APC. This anticoagulant serine protease cleaves factors Va and VIIIa, thereby eliminating thrombin generation. The stoichiometric inhibitors consist of the AT-heparin complex, which inhibits virtually all the procoagulant serine proteases, and TFPI, which targets the factor VIIa–TF–factor Xa complex and principally regulates the initiation phase of the blood coagulation process (see Fig. 26-2).

Tissue Factor Pathway Inhibitor (Extrinsic Pathway Inhibitor, Lipoprotein-Associated Coagulation Inhibitor)

TFPI is a multivalent protein that modulates TF-dependent coagulation by inhibiting the extrinsic tenase complex.[183] TFPI is expressed constitutively by cultured endothelial cells and consists of an acidic NH_2-terminal region, three tandem Kunitz-like serine protease inhibitor domains (K1 to K3), and a positively charged COOH-terminal region. The tandem Kunitz domains are essential for function.[184] Two variants of TFPI (isoforms α and β) are generated by alternative splicing. A significant proportion of TFPI molecules in blood are truncated to a variable extent at the COOH-terminal end, with resultant compromised inhibitory activity. The inhibitory activity of TFPI is enhanced by heparin. Upon heparin administration, TFPI is released from endothelial cells, with a 2- to 10-fold increase in circulating levels being achieved. Release of TFPI with heparin therapy is responsible for a portion of the observed elevation in PT and raises the possibility that part of the antithrombotic effect of heparin may be mediated by release of TFPI. A minor pool of TFPI (approximately 10% of the total TFPI in blood) is located within platelets.[185] Transgenic mice with complete TFPI deficiency do not survive.[186] There are no known human TFPI-deficient individuals.

TFPI is the principal stoichiometric inhibitor of the extrinsic pathway (see Figs. 26-2 and 26-4B). The TFPI mechanism allows the factor VIIa–TF complex to initiate factor Xa formation, but it suppresses the generation of high levels of factor Xa product formation by binding the enzyme-product complex (see Fig. 26-4B). The inhibitor mechanism involves rapid interaction between the second Kunitz domain of TFPI with the active site of factor Xa; localization of the complex to the membrane surface is mediated by the Gla domain of factor Xa.[49] Once surface bound, the factor Xa–TFPI complex rapidly inactivates TF–factor VIIa. This complex formation depends on binding of the first Kunitz domain of TFPI to the active site of factor VIIa. These interactions together form a stable quaternary complex, TF–factor VIIa–TFPI–factor Xa. The factor IXa–TFPI complex can also inhibit factor VIIa–TF, although the physiologic relevance of this route of inhibition is unclear because high plasma concentrations of TFPI are required. At normal plasma concentrations, this multicomponent interaction of TFPI allows basal function of the factor VIIa–TF complex but inhibits it after more extensive activation takes place.

When combined with the stoichiometric inhibitor AT, a synergistic regulatory effect of blood coagulation occurs by inducing kinetic "thresholds" such that the initiating TF stimulus must achieve a significant magnitude to propel thrombin generation.[187] TF concentrations below the threshold concentration are ineffective in promoting robust generation of thrombin because of the cooperative influence of the inhibitors; concentrations in excess of the threshold yield robust and almost equivalent thrombin generation. TFPI and the dynamic protein C–thrombomodulin-thrombin system also cooperate to provide threshold-limited, synergistic inhibition of thrombin production. In this instance, TFPI slows the initiation phase while the APC system reduces the availability of the cofactors factors Va and VIIIa, thereby shutting down the propagation phase of thrombin generation.

Antithrombin

AT is a member of the serpin proteinase inhibitor family and circulates in blood as a single-chain glycoprotein. Despite its name, AT inhibits not only thrombin but also most of the proteases in the coagulation pathway. Human AT circulates as two glycoforms, the α and β variants, that contain identical polypeptide backbones but differ in both carbohydrate content and heparin affinity. AT-β binds heparin more tightly than AT-α and is observed to preferentially accumulate on the vessel wall where heparan sulfate proteoglycans are exposed.[188]

AT has a broad spectrum of inhibitory activity, with most of its target proteases participating in the coagulation cascade. It is primarily an inhibitor of thrombin, factor Xa, factor IXa, factor VIIa–TF, factor XIa, factor XIIa, and plasma kallikrein[10,189] (see Fig. 26-2). AT also displays antiproliferative and anti-inflammatory properties that may derive from its ability to inhibit thrombin. Heparin and heparan sulfate potentiate these reactions and are used in the treatment of thrombosis. When AT is complexed with heparin, its rate of binding to thrombin increases 1000-fold. The general mechanism of inhibition involves reaction of the active site of the enzyme with a peptide loop structure of the serpin to form a tight, equimolar (1:1) complex, followed by inactivating structural rearrangements of both AT and the protease.

Heparin Cofactor II (Leuserpin 2)

Heparin cofactor II is another member of the serpin family and is uniquely stimulated by the proteoglycan dermatan sulfate. The only coagulation enzyme inhibited by heparin cofactor II appears to be thrombin.[190] However, the rate of thrombin inhibition by heparin cofactor II in the absence or presence of glycosaminoglycans is significantly slower than inhibition by AT under similar conditions. In view of the fact that the plasma concentration of heparin cofactor II is 25% to 50% that of AT and that low levels of heparin cofactor II are not strongly associated with thrombosis, the physiologic role of heparin cofactor II as a systemic thrombin inhibitor has been questioned.

Protein C Inhibitor (Plasminogen Activator Inhibitor 3)

Protein C inhibitor is a member of the serine proteinase inhibitor family. Its targets range from the procoagulant, anticoagulant, and fibrinolytic enzymes to plasma and tissue kallikreins, the sperm protease acrosin, and prostate-specific antigen. Hereditary or acquired protein C inhibitor deficiency has not been documented. Protein C inhibitor–deficient mice show impaired spermatogenesis and male infertility.[191] The importance of the regulation of APC by protein C inhibitor in humans is suggested by the use of this complex as a marker for detection of deep vein thrombosis by immunofluorometric assay measurements.[192]

PROTEINS OF CLOT FORMATION

The central event in blood coagulation is the conversion of soluble fibrinogen (factor I) to insoluble cross-linked fibrin. This conversion is accomplished when thrombin removes small polar peptides (termed fibrinopeptides A and B) from the fibrinogen molecule forming fibrin. These fibrin molecules noncovalently interact with each other to form a fibrin web. Fibrin stabilization is accomplished by the action of a second coagulation enzyme (factor XIIIa) that introduces numerous covalent cross-links between these fibrin molecules. The resulting fibrin web is able to capture platelets and red blood cells, thus effectively sealing the wound and stemming plasma loss.

Factor XIII (Fibrin-Stabilizing Factor)

Factor XIII is a protransglutaminase that when proteolytically activated, can form cross-linked amide bonds between glutamyl and lysinyl residues. The zymogen circulates in plasma as a tetramer composed of two A and two B subunits. It plays an important role in hemostasis and thrombosis, as well as participates in the physiologic processes of cell proliferation and cell migration. The product enzyme factor XIII(a) has multiple substrates, including fibrin/fibrinogen, fibronectin, α_2-plasmin inhibitor, collagen, vitronectin, VWF, actin, myosin, factor V, and thrombospondin.[193-196]

Factor XIII is distributed into plasma and platelet pools. Plasma factor XIII circulates as a 320-kD A_2B_2 heterotetramer composed of two identical A chains and two B chains associated noncovalently.[197] The A subunit

is the procatalyst and contains three important functional sites: the catalytic site, a calcium binding site, and the activation peptide.[198,199] The activation peptide of one A subunit limits access to the active site cysteine of the other A subunit of the dimer. The B chain has no enzymatic activity and has been thought to function as a carrier of the A subunit.[200]

Bone marrow is the prime site of synthesis of the A chain of plasma factor XIII,[201] which is also present intracellularly as a 160-kd A_2 homodimer in platelets, megakaryocytes, and monocytes.[202,203] How the A_2 dimer is transferred out of the cell and which cell types are the primary sources of plasma A_2 are not understood. Approximately 50% of the total potential factor XIII A chain activity in human blood is found in platelets.[202] The B subunit is synthesized in hepatocytes and secreted as a monomer.[204] After being secreted, the A and B subunits associate and become an A_2B_2 tetrameric molecule in plasma.

Plasma factor XIII is activated by cleavage of thrombin at the NH_2-terminal of the A chains, with release of a 36–amino acid activation peptide. Catalytic activity is expressed only after the A chain dimer is dissociated from the B chain. Fibrin/fibrinogen plays an important role as a cofactor in dissociation of the B chains from thrombin-cleaved factor XIII.[201] The intracellular form of factor XIII contains only the A chain and thus does not require dissociation of the B chain.

Activation of factor XIII during blood clotting is tightly correlated with fibrin formation.[205] This creates a regulated system in which cross-linked polymers occur coincident with fibrin being formed. The rate of thrombin cleavage of plasma factor XIII has been shown to be greatly accelerated by the presence of fibrin polymers.[206] This positive feedback network between thrombin, fibrin/fibrinogen, and factor XIIIa ensures that a stable clot can form rapidly to maintain hemostasis. To date, no known endogenous inhibitor has been described that regulates this important enzyme.[193-196] Fibrin is the main physiologic substrate for factor XIIIa.

Fibrinogen (Factor I) and Fibrin

Fibrinogen is composed of six polypeptide chains (two $A\alpha$ chains, two $B\beta$ chains, and two γ chains); after post-translational modification, the mature protein circulates in blood with an average molecular weight of 340,000 D (see Table 26-1).[207,208] The polypeptide chains are distributed into two symmetrical half molecules, each containing one $A\alpha$, one $B\beta$, and one γ chain, with the NH_2-terminals oriented toward each other (Fig. 26-9). The half molecules are linked by noncovalent and disulfide bonds near their NH_2-terminals to yield a linear arrangement of three nodular structures. The outside two domains, formed by the carboxyl-terminal regions of the $B\beta$ and γ chains of fibrinogen, are designated "D," whereas the central domain, which contains the amino-terminals of all the chains, is designated "E." Between 1.7 and 5.0 g

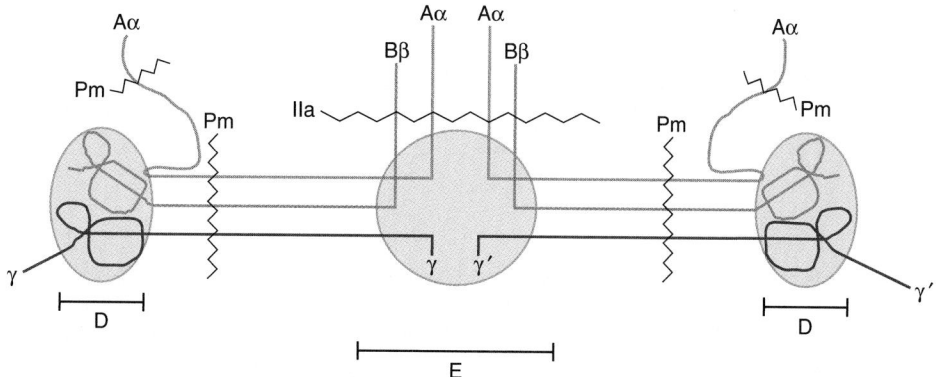

FIGURE 26-9. Schematic representation of fibrinogen to illustrate thrombin and plasmin cleavage sites in the intact molecule. The six polypeptide chains, $A\alpha_2B\beta_2\gamma_2$ are folded into three globular structures, two "D" and one "E," which are connected by "coiled-coil" segments. The NH_2-terminal regions of the $A\alpha$, $B\beta$ chains extend from the central "E" domain and, when cleaved by thrombin, yield fibrinopeptide A and fibrinopeptide B. The macromolecular product fibrin is then referred to as $\alpha_2\beta_2\gamma_2$. A small fraction of fibrinogen contains a COOH-terminal extension of the γ chain that is referred to as γ'.

of fibrinogen is synthesized per day by the liver, with approximately 75% of this fibrinogen being secreted into plasma and the remainder being distributed between the lymph and interstitial fluids.[209] Fibrinogen is an acute phase reactant and is upregulated 2- to 10-fold in response to a variety of physiologic stresses, including trauma, pregnancy, and tissue inflammation.

The fibrinogen locus is composed of three closely linked genes (specifying the polypeptides $A\alpha$, $B\beta$, and γ) found as single copies in a region of approximately 50 kilobases. The three fibrinogen genes most likely evolved from a common ancestor through a series of duplications that began approximately 1 billion years ago.[210] Expression of the three chains is coordinately controlled and, at least for the hepatocyte, results in almost equal levels of mRNA for each chain in the cell.[211] Although most γ chains end at γ-Val411 (human numbering), approximately 10% of the time during splicing the last intron is retained, which resulting in a new chain, γ', that ends at γ-Leu427.[212] A less common variant of the α chain adds a 236–amino acid extension at the C-terminal.[213] After synthesis but before secretion, a number of post-translational modifications occur, including glycosylation and phosphorylation. Factor XIIIa cross-linking occurs between sites on the $A\alpha$ and γ but not on the $B\beta$ chain.

Thrombin catalyzes the hydrolysis of Arg-Gly bonds, with small, polar amino-terminal pieces (fibrinopeptides) being removed from the α and β chains[207,208,214] (see Fig. 26-9). Cleavage of $A\alpha$-Arg16 by thrombin releases fibrinopeptide A (FPA) and forms fibrin I. The release of two FPA peptides exposes a site in the E domain that aligns with a complementary site in the D domain to form overlapping fibrils. Subsequent cleavage by thrombin at $B\beta$-Arg14 releases fibrinopeptide B (FPB) and leads to the formation of fibrin II, which presumably increases lateral aggregation of the protofibrils. FPA and FPB vary in length, between 13 and 21 amino acids in various mammals, and constitute less than 2% of the total mass.

Release of fibrinopeptides from fibrinogen results in the formation of an intermediate termed the fibrin monomer, which is all but indistinguishable from fibrinogen. In purified systems, removal of either FPA or FPB leads to formation of the fibrin dimer through noncovalent (i.e., charge-charge [salt links]) and hydrogen bond interactions. As fibrin monomers continue to be generated, the dimer elongates from both ends as a two-stranded molecule until it reaches approximately 30 monomers, at which point it becomes a protofibril. The second step in fibrin assembly is lateral association of the protofibrils into thicker fibrin fibers. These fibers are formed from the association of between 14 and 22 protofibrils. Because protofibrils, not dimers, are required for this step, it is believed that the forces involved in lateral association are weak and therefore become "strong" only in large numbers. Clots are known to branch, although how branching is accomplished is not clear.

The description of fibrinogen activation and fibrin assembly has been based on studies involving the use of citrated plasma or purified proteins, or both. To understand the in vivo process of fibrin formation, a system with nonanticoagulated blood has been used; in this experimental model the pattern of fibrin formation based on release of fibrinopeptide is different from systems using citrated plasma or purified fibrinogen.[205] In this study, most cleavage of FPA and subsequent clot formation take place just before the propagation phase of thrombin generation (Fig. 26-10). At the point of visual clot formation, virtually all fibrinogen (and some product already cross-linked) disappears from the fluid phase of the reaction. Thus, the "clot" appears to be a mixture composed of fibrin I and fibrinogen. The insoluble material present in the fibrin clot is virtually all cross-linked by factor XIIIa, whose activation occurs nearly simultaneously with removal of FPA[205] (see Fig. 26-10). It has been proposed that as many as six cross-links can form between a fibrin monomer and its neighbors and that the presence of these

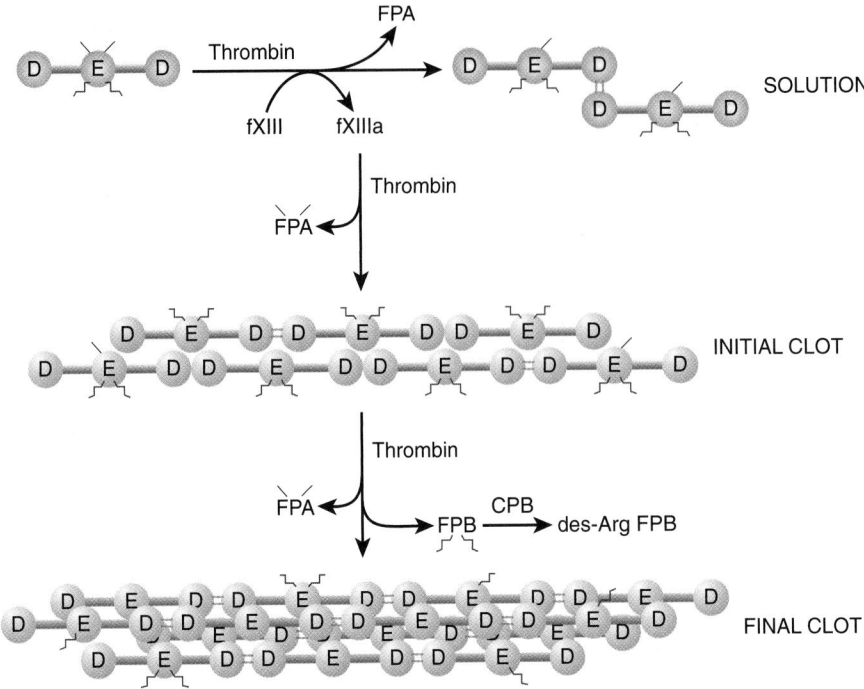

FIGURE 26-10. Schematic representation of whole blood fibrin formation. Thrombin at the beginning of clot formation simultaneously acts on fibrinogen (D-E-D) and factor XIII (fXIII). A portion (≈40%) of fibrinopeptide A (FPA) is released from fibrinogen, and an initial clot is formed from the complementary overlap of the exposed sites between the E and D domains of adjacent molecules. Activated factor XIII (fXIIIa) simultaneously cross-links adjacent D domains (D = D). Thus, the initial soluble fibrin clot is composed of fibrinogen, fibrin, and γ-γ dimers with fibrinopeptide B (FPB) still attached. The initial clot is continuously acted on by thrombin, which releases the remaining FPA and some of the FPB to yield a final clot with the majority of FPB still attached. The FPB released is selectively acted on by a carboxypeptidase B–like enzyme (CPB) to cleave the carboxyl-terminal arginine and produce des-Arg FPB. The significance of this cleavage is still unclear. *(Redrawn with permission from Brummel KE, Butenas S, Mann KG. An integrated study of fibrinogen during blood coagulation. J Biol Chem. 1999;274:22862-22870.)*

cross-links increases the strength, chemical resistance to urea, and lysis by plasmin.[207,208,215]

CONCLUSION

As the result of molecular investigation of blood coagulation for more than 100 years, the components of the blood coagulation system and their connections are well understood. Critical insights into this process and its regulation have often come from the study of patients with mutations in the genes encoding the relevant coagulation factors. It is only fitting that this knowledge has formed the basis for the development of reliable diagnostic tools and effective therapies for patients with both inherited and acquired disorders of hemostasis, as detailed in the ensuing chapters.

REFERENCES

1. Schmidt A. Zur Blutlehre. Leipzig, Germany, FCW Vogel, 1892.
2. Quick AJ. The prothrombin time in haemophilia and in obstructive jaundice. J Biol Chem. 1935;109:73-74.
3. Langdell RD, Wagner RH, Brinkhous KM. Effect of antihemophilic factor on one-stage clotting tests: a presumptive test of hemophilia and a single one-stage anti-hemophilic factor assay procedure. J Lab Clin Med. 1953;41:7637-7647.
4. MacFarlane RG. An enzyme in the blood clotting mechanism and its function as a biochemical amplifier. Nature. 1964;202:498-499.
5. Davie EW, Ratnoff OD. Waterfall sequence for intrinsic blood clotting. Science. 1964;145:1310-1312.
6. Nemerson Y. Tissue factor and hemostasis [published erratum appears in Blood. 1988;71(4):1178]. Blood. 1988;71:1-8.
7. Osterud B, Rapaport SI. Activation of factor IX by the reaction product of tissue factor and factor VII: additional pathway for initiating blood coagulation. Proc Natl Acad Sci U S A. 1977;74:5260-5264.
8. Gailani D, Broze GJ Jr. Factor XI activation in a revised model of blood coagulation. Science. 1991;253:909-912.
9. Lawson JH, Mann KG. Cooperative activation of human factor IX by the human extrinsic pathway of blood coagulation. J Biol Chem. 1991;266:11317-11327.
10. Olson ST, Bjork I, Shore JD. Kinetic characterization of heparin-catalyzed and uncatalyzed inhibition of blood coagulation proteinases by antithrombin. Methods Enzymol. 1993;222:525-559.
11. Girard TJ, Warren LA, Novotny WF, et al. Functional significance of the Kunitz-type inhibitory domains of lipoprotein-associated coagulation inhibitor. Nature. 1989;338:518-520.

12. Baugh RJ, Broze GJ Jr, Krishnaswamy S. Regulation of extrinsic pathway factor Xa formation by tissue factor pathway inhibitor. J Biol Chem. 1998;273:4378-4386.

13. Novotny WF, Brown SG, Miletich JP, et al. Plasma antigen levels of the lipoprotein-associated coagulation inhibitor in patient samples. Blood. 1991;78:387-393.

14. Esmon CT. The protein C pathway. Chest. 2003;124(3 Suppl):26S-32S.

15. Mann KG, Kalafatis M. Factor V: a combination of Dr Jekyll and Mr Hyde. Blood. 2003;101:20-30.

16. Mann KG, Nesheim ME, Church WR, et al. Surface-dependent reactions of the vitamin K–dependent enzyme complexes. Blood. 1990;76:1-16.

17. Nesheim ME, Taswell JB, Mann KG. The contribution of bovine factor V and factor Va to the activity of prothrombinase. J Biol Chem. 1979;254:10952-10962.

18. van Dieijen G, Tans G, Rosing J, Hemker HC. The role of phospholipid and factor VIIIa in the activation of bovine factor X. J Biol Chem. 1981;256:3433-3442.

19. Krishnaswamy S, Field KA, Edgington TS, et al. Role of the membrane surface in the activation of human coagulation factor X. J Biol Chem. 1992;267:26110-26120.

20. Butenas S, DiLorenzo ME, Mann KG. Ultrasensitive fluorogenic substrates for serine proteases. Thromb Haemost. 1997;78:1193-1201.

21. Hockin MF, Jones KC, Everse SJ, Mann KG. A model for the stoichiometric regulation of blood coagulation. J Biol Chem. 2002;277:18322-18333.

22. Cawthern KM, van't Veer C, Lock JB, et al. Blood coagulation in hemophilia A and hemophilia C. Blood. 1998;91:4581-4592.

23. van't Veer C, Golden NJ, Kalafatis M, Mann KG. Inhibitory mechanism of the protein C pathway on tissue factor–induced thrombin generation. Synergistic effect in combination with tissue factor pathway inhibitor. J Biol Chem. 1997;272:7983-7994.

24. Owen CA, Bowie EWJ. The history of the development of oral anticoagulant drugs. In Poller L, Hirsch J (eds). Oral Anticoagulants. London, Arnold, 1996, pp 1-8.

25. Stenflo J, Ferlund P, Egan W, Roepstorff P. Vitamin K dependent modifications of glutamic acid residues in prothrombin. Proc Natl Acad Sci U S A. 1974;71:2730-2733.

26. Patthy L. Evolutionary assembly of blood coagulation proteins. Semin Thromb Hemost. 1990;16:245-259.

27. Bristol JA, Ratcliffe JV, Roth DA, et al. Biosynthesis of prothrombin: intracellular localization of the vitamin K–dependent carboxylase and the sites of gamma-carboxylation. Blood. 1996;88:2585-2593.

28. Furie B, Furie BC. Molecular basis of vitamin K–dependent gamma-carboxylation. Blood. 1990;75:1753-1762.

29. Stafford DW. The vitamin K cycle. J Thromb Haemost. 2005;3:1873-1878.

30. Gardill SL, Suttie JW. Vitamin K epoxide and quinone reductase activities. Evidence for reduction by a common enzyme. Biochem Pharmacol. 1990;40:1055-1061.

31. Doolittle RF, Feng DF, Johnson MS. Computer-based characterization of epidermal growth factor precursor. Nature. 1984;307:558-560.

32. Campbell ID, Downing AK. Building protein structure and function from modular units. Trends Biotechnol. 1994;12(5):168-172.

33. Husten EJ, Esmon CT, Johnson AE. The active site of blood coagulation factor Xa. Its distance from the phospholipid surface and its conformational sensitivity to components of the prothrombinase complex. J Biol Chem. 1987;262:12953-12961.

34. Neuenschwander PF, Fiore MM, Morrissey JH. Factor VII autoactivation proceeds via interaction of distinct protease-cofactor and zymogen-cofactor complexes. Implications of a two-dimensional enzyme kinetic mechanism. J Biol Chem. 1993;268:21489-21492.

35. Lawson JH, Krishnaswamy S, Butenas S, Mann KG. Extrinsic pathway proteolytic activity. Methods Enzymol. 1993;222:177-195.

36. Radcliffe R, Nemerson Y. Activation and control of factor VII by activated factor X and thrombin. Isolation and characterization of a single chain form of factor VII. J Biol Chem. 1975;250:388-395.

37. Seligsohn U, Osterud B, Brown SF, et al. Activation of human factor VII in plasma and in purified systems: roles of activated factor IX, kallikrein, and activated factor XII. J Clin Invest. 1979;64:1056-1065.

38. Kisiel W, Fujikawa K, Davie EW. Activation of bovine factor VII (proconvertin) by factor XIIa (activated Hageman factor). Biochemistry. 1977;16:4189-4194.

39. Romisch J. Factor VII activating protease (FSAP): a novel protease in hemostasis. Biol Chem. 2002;383:1119-1124.

40. Lawson JH, Butenas S, Mann KG. The evaluation of complex-dependent alterations in human factor VIIa. J Biol Chem. 1992;267:4834-4843.

41. Rao LV, Nordfang O, Hoang AD, Pendurthi UR. Mechanism of antithrombin III inhibition of factor VIIa/tissue factor activity on cell surfaces. Comparison with tissue factor pathway inhibitor/factor Xa–induced inhibition of factor VIIa/tissue factor activity. Blood. 1995;85:121-129.

42. Lawson JH, Butenas S, Ribarik N, Mann KG. Complex-dependent inhibition of factor VIIa by antithrombin III and heparin. J Biol Chem. 1993;268:767-770.

43. Rapaport SI, Rao LV. Initiation and regulation of tissue factor–dependent blood coagulation. Arterioscler Thromb. 1992;12:1111-1121.

44. Kuraya N, Omichi K, Nishimura H, et al. Structural analysis of O-linked sugar chains in human blood clotting factor IX. J Biochem (Tokyo). 1993;114:763-765.

45. Griffith MJ, Breitkreutz L, Trapp H, et al. Characterization of the clotting activities of structurally different forms of activated factor IX. Enzymatic properties of normal human factor IXa alpha, factor IXa beta, and activated factor IX Chapel Hill. J Clin Invest. 1985;75:4-10.

46. Lenting PJ, ter Maat H, Clijsters PP, et al. Cleavage at arginine 145 in human blood coagulation factor IX converts the zymogen into a factor VIII binding enzyme. J Biol Chem. 1995;270:14884-14890.

47. Rsoenberg J, McKenna PW, Rosenberg RD. Inhibition of human factor IXa by human antithrombin. J Biol Chem. 1975;250:8883-8888.

48. Schmaier AH, Dahl LD, Hasan AA, et al. Factor IXa inhibition by protease nexin-2/amyloid beta-protein precursor on phospholipid vesicles and cell membranes. Biochemistry. 1995;34:1171-1178.

49. Huang ZF, Wun TC, Broze GJ Jr. Kinetics of factor Xa inhibition by tissue factor pathway inhibitor. J Biol Chem. 1993;268:26950-26955.

50. Gitel SN, Medina VM, Wessler S. Inhibition of human activated factor X by antithrombin III and alpha 1-proteinase inhibitor in human plasma. J Biol Chem. 1984;259:6890-6895.

51. Miletich JP, Jackson CM, Majerus PW. Properties of the factor Xa binding site on human platelets. J Biol Chem. 1978;253:6908-6916.

52. Lundblad RL, Kingdon HS, Mann KG. Thrombin. Methods Enzymol. 1976;45:156-176.

53. Patthy L. Evolution of the proteases of blood coagulation and fibrinolysis by assembly from modules. Cell. 1985; 41:657-663.

54. Deguchi H, Takeya H, Gabazza EC, et al. Prothrombin kringle 1 domain interacts with factor Va during the assembly of prothrombinase complex. Biochem J. 1997; 321:729-735.

55. Kotkow KJ, Deitcher SR, Furie B, Furie BC. The second kringle domain of prothrombin promotes factor Va–mediated prothrombin activation by prothrombinase. J Biol Chem. 1995;270:4551-4557.

56. Krishnaswamy S, Walker RK. Contribution of the prothrombin fragment 2 domain to the function of factor Va in the prothrombinase complex. Biochemistry. 1997;36: 3319-3330.

57. Doyle MF, Mann KG. Multiple active forms of thrombin. IV. Relative activities of meizothrombins. J Biol Chem. 1990;265:10693-10701.

58. Nesheim ME, Abbott T, Jenny R, Mann KG. Evidence that the thrombin-catalyzed feedback cleavage of fragment 1.2 at Arg154-Ser155 promotes the release of thrombin from the catalytic surface during the activation of bovine prothrombin. J Biol Chem. 1988;263:1037-1044.

59. Mosesson MW. The roles of fibrinogen and fibrin in hemostasis and thrombosis. Semin Hematol. 1992;29:177-188.

60. Davey MG, Luscher EF. Actions of thrombin and other coagulant and proteolytic enzymes on blood platelets. Nature. 1967;216:857-858.

61. Kahn ML, Zheng YW, Huang W, et al. A dual thrombin receptor system for platelet activation. Nature 1998; 394:690-694.

62. Mann KG, Jenny RJ, Krishnaswamy S. Cofactor proteins in the assembly and expression of blood clotting enzyme complexes. Annu Rev Biochem. 1988;57:915-956.

63. Bajzar L, Manuel R, Nesheim ME. Purification and characterization of TAFI, a thrombin-activatable fibrinolysis inhibitor. J Biol Chem. 1995;270:14477-14484.

64. Tulinsky A. Molecular interactions of thrombin. Semin Thromb Hemost. 1996;22:117-124.

65. Vu TK, Wheaton VI, Hung DT, et al. Domains specifying thrombin-receptor interaction. Nature. 1991;353:674-677.

66. Vu TK, Hung DT, Wheaton VI, Coughlin SR. Molecular cloning of a functional thrombin receptor reveals a novel proteolytic mechanism of receptor activation. Cell. 1991; 64:1057-1068.

67. Fenton JW. Regulation of thrombin generation and functions. Semin Thromb Hemost. 1988;14:234-240.

68. Bar-Shavit R, Kahn AJ, Mann KG, Wilner GD. Identification of a thrombin sequence with growth factor activity on macrophages. Proc Natl Acad Sci U S A. 1986;83: 976-980.

69. McNamara CA, Sarembock IJ, Gimple LW, et al. Thrombin stimulates proliferation of cultured rat aortic smooth muscle cells by a proteolytically activated receptor. J Clin Invest. 1993;91:94-98.

70. Sago H, Iinuma K. Cell shape change and cytosolic Ca^{2+} in human umbilical-vein endothelial cells stimulated with thrombin. Thromb Haemost. 1992;67:331-334.

71. Stenflo J. Structure and function of protein C. Semin Thromb Hemost. 1984;10:109-121.

72. Castellino FJ. Human protein C and activated protein C. Trends Cardiovasc Med. 1995;5:55-62.

73. Weiler-Guettler H, Christie PD, Beeler DL, et al. A targeted point mutation in thrombomodulin generates viable mice with a prethrombotic state. J Clin Invest. 1998;101: 1983-1991.

74. Kalafatis M, Rand MD, Mann KG. The mechanism of inactivation of human factor V and human factor Va by activated protein C. J Biol Chem. 1994;269:31869-31880.

75. Lollar P, Parker CG. pH-dependent denaturation of thrombin-activated porcine factor VIII. J Biol Chem. 1990;265:1688-1692.

76. Norstrom EA, Steen M, Tran S, Dahlback B. Importance of protein S and phospholipid for activated protein C–mediated cleavages in factor Va. J Biol Chem. 2003;278: 24904-24911.

77. Rosing J, Hoekema L, Nicolaes GA, et al. Effects of protein S and factor Xa on peptide bond cleavages during inactivation of factor Va and factor VaR506Q by activated protein C. J Biol Chem. 1995;270:27852-27858.

78. Bajzar L, Nesheim ME, Tracy PB. The profibrinolytic effect of activated protein C in clots formed from plasma is TAFI-dependent. Blood. 1996;88:2093-2100.

79. Fukudome K, Esmon CT. Identification, cloning, and regulation of a novel endothelial cell protein C/activated protein C receptor. J Biol Chem. 1994;269:26486-26491.

80. Moore KL, Andreoli SP, Esmon NL, et al. Endotoxin enhances tissue factor and suppresses thrombomodulin expression of human vascular endothelium in vitro. J Clin Invest. 1987;79:124-130.

81. Nawroth PP, Handley DA, Esmon CT, Stern DM. Interleukin 1 induces endothelial cell procoagulant while suppressing cell-surface anticoagulant activity. Proc Natl Acad Sci U S A. 1986;83:3460-3464.

82. Lentz SR, Tsiang M, Sadler JE. Regulation of thrombomodulin by tumor necrosis factor-alpha: comparison of transcriptional and posttranscriptional mechanisms. Blood. 1991;77:542-550.

83. Heeb MJ, Espana F, Geiger M, et al. Immunological identity of heparin-dependent plasma and urinary protein C inhibitor and plasminogen activator inhibitor-3. J Biol Chem. 1987;262:15813-15816.

84. Dahlback B. Purification of human C4b-binding protein and formation of its complex with vitamin K–dependent protein S. Biochem J. 1983;209:847-856.

85. Walker FJ. Protein S and the regulation of activated protein C. Semin Thromb Hemost. 1984;10:131-138.

86. Solymoss S, Tucker MM, Tracy PB. Kinetics of inactivation of membrane-bound factor Va by activated protein C. Protein S modulates factor Xa protection. J Biol Chem. 1988;263:14884-14890.

87. Koedam JA, Meijers JC, Sixma JJ, Bouma BN. Inactivation of human factor VIII by activated protein C. Cofactor activity of protein S and protective effect of von Willebrand factor. J Clin Invest. 1988;82:1236-1243.

88. Heeb MJ, Rosing J, Bakker HM, et al. Protein S binds to and inhibits factor Xa. Proc Natl Acad Sci U S A. 1994;91:2728-2732.

89. Koppelman SJ, Hackeng TM, Sixma JJ, Bouma BN. Inhibition of the intrinsic factor X activating complex by protein S: evidence for a specific binding of protein S to factor VIII. Blood. 1995;86:1062-1071.

90. Heeb MJ, Mesters RM, Tans G, et al. Binding of protein S to factor Va associated with inhibition of prothrombinase that is independent of activated protein C. J Biol Chem. 1993;268:2872-2877.

91. Butenas S, van't Veer C, Mann KG. "Normal" thrombin generation. Blood. 1999;94:2169-2178.

92. Koppelman SJ, van't Veer C, Sixma JJ, Bouma BN. Synergistic inhibition of the intrinsic factor X activation by protein S and C4b-binding protein. Blood. 1995;86:2653-2660.

93. Smiley ST, Stitt TN, Grusby MJ. Cross-linking of protein S bound to lymphocytes promotes aggregation and inhibits proliferation. Cell Immunol. 1997;181:120-126.

94. Dahlback B. Purification of human vitamin K–dependent protein S and its limited proteolysis by thrombin. Biochem J. 1983;209:837-846.

95. Broze GJ Jr, Miletich JP. Human protein Z. J Clin Invest. 1984;73:933-938.

96. Broze GJ Jr. Protein Z–dependent regulation of coagulation. Thromb Haemost. 2001;86:8-13.

97. Yin ZF, Huang ZF, Cui J, et al. Prothrombotic phenotype of protein Z deficiency. Proc Natl Acad Sci U S A. 2000;97:6734-6738.

98. Thompson RE, Mandle R Jr, Kaplan AP. Association of factor XI and high molecular weight kininogen in human plasma. J Clin Invest. 1977;60:1376-1380.

99. Hsu TC, Shore SK, Seshsmma T, et al. Molecular cloning of platelet factor XI, an alternative splicing product of the plasma factor XI gene. J Biol Chem. 1998;273:13787-13793.

100. Fujikawa K, Chung DW, Hendrickson LE, Davie EW. Amino acid sequence of human factor XI, a blood coagulation factor with four tandem repeats that are highly homologous with plasma prekallikrein. Biochemistry. 1986;25:2417-2424.

101. Sun MF, Zhao M, Gailani D. Identification of amino acids in the factor XI apple 3 domain required for activation of factor IX. J Biol Chem. 1999;274:36373-36378.

102. Kurachi K, Davie EW. Activation of human factor XI (plasma thromboplastin antecedent) by factor XIIa (activated Hageman factor). Biochemistry. 1977;16:5831-5839.

103. Bouma BN, Griffin JH. Human blood coagulation factor XI. Purification, properties, and mechanism of activation by activated factor XII. J Biol Chem. 1977;252:6432-6437.

104. Broze GJ Jr, Gailani D. The role of factor XI in coagulation. Thromb Haemost. 1993;70:72-74.

105. DiScipio RG, Kurachi K, Davie EW. Activation of human factor IX (Christmas factor). J Clin Invest. 1978;61:1528-1538.

106. Sinha D, Seaman FS, Walsh PN. Role of calcium ions and the heavy chain of factor XIa in the activation of human coagulation factor IX. Biochemistry. 1987;26:3768-3775.

107. Walsh PN, Sinha D, Kueppers F, et al. Regulation of factor XIa activity by platelets and alpha 1-protease inhibitor. J Clin Invest. 1987;80:1578-1586.

108. Meijers JC, Vlooswijk RA, Bouma BN. Inhibition of human blood coagulation factor XIa by C-1 inhibitor. Biochemistry. 1988;27:959-963.

109. Scott CF, Colman RW. Factors influencing the acceleration of human factor XIa inactivation by antithrombin III. Blood. 1989;73:1873-1879.

110. Berrettini M, Schleef RR, Espana F, et al. Interaction of type 1 plasminogen activator inhibitor with the enzymes of the contact activation system. J Biol Chem. 1989;264:11738-11743.

111. Smith RP, Higuchi DA, Broze GJ Jr. Platelet coagulation factor XIa-inhibitor, a form of Alzheimer amyloid precursor protein. Science. 1990;248:1126-1128.

112. Zhang Y, Scandura JM, Van Nostrand WE, Walsh PN. The mechanism by which heparin promotes the inhibition of coagulation factor XIa by protease nexin-2. J Biol Chem. 1997;272:26139-26144.

113. Quick AJ. On the constitution of prothrombin. Am J Physiol. 1943;140:212-214.

114. Tracy PB, Eide LL, Bowie EJ, Mann KG. Radioimmunoassay of factor V in human plasma and platelets. Blood. 1982;60:59-63.

115. Gewirtz AM, Shapiro C, Shen YM, et al. Cellular and molecular regulation of factor V expression in human megakaryocytes. J Cell Physiol. 1992;153:277-287.

116. Camire RM, Pollak ES, Kaushansky K, Tracy PB. Secretable human platelet–derived factor V originates from the plasma pool. Blood. 1998;92:3035-3041.

117. Mann KG, Lawler CM, Vehar GA, Church WR. Coagulation factor V contains copper ion. J Biol Chem. 1984;259:12949-12951.

118. Kalafatis M. Identification and partial characterization of factor Va heavy chain kinase from human platelets. J Biol Chem. 1998;273:8459-8466.

119. Pittman DD, Tomkinson KN, Kaufman RJ. Posttranslational requirements for functional factor V and factor VIII secretion in mammalian cells. J Biol Chem. 1994;269:17329-17337.

120. Fernandez JA, Hackeng TM, Kojima K, Griffin JH. The carbohydrate moiety of factor V modulates inactivation by activated protein C. Blood. 1997;89:4348-4354.

121. Nicolaes GA, Villoutreix BO, Dahlback B. Partial glycosylation of Asn2181 in human factor V as a cause of molecular and functional heterogeneity. Modulation of glycosylation efficiency by mutagenesis of the consensus sequence for N-linked glycosylation. Biochemistry. 1999;38:13584-13591.

122. Esmon CT. The subunit structure of thrombin-activated factor V. Isolation of activated factor V, separation of subunits, and reconstitution of biological activity. J Biol Chem. 1979;254:964-973.

123. Guinto ER, Esmon CT. Formation of a calcium-binding site on bovine activated factor V following recombination of the isolated subunits. J Biol Chem. 1982;257:10038-10043.

124. Kane WH, Majerus PW. The interaction of human coagulation factor Va with platelets. J Biol Chem. 1982;257:3963-3969.

125. Laue TM, Johnson AE, Esmon CT, Yphantis DA. Structure of bovine blood coagulation factor Va. Determination of the subunit associations, molecular weights, and asymmetries by analytical ultracentrifugation. Biochemistry. 1984;23:1339-1348.

126. Suzuki K, Dahlback B, Stenflo J. Thrombin-catalyzed activation of human coagulation factor V. J Biol Chem. 1982;257:6556-6564.

127. Thorelli E, Kaufman RJ, Dahlback B. Cleavage requirements for activation of factor V by factor Xa. Eur J Biochem. 1997;247:12-20.

128. Kalafatis M, Mann KG. The role of the membrane in the inactivation of factor Va by plasmin. Amino acid region 307-348 of factor V plays a critical role in factor Va cofactor function. J Biol Chem. 2001;276:18614-18623.

129. Dahlback B, Carlsson M, Svensson PJ. Familial thrombophilia due to a previously unrecognized mechanism characterized by poor anticoagulant response to activated protein C: prediction of a cofactor to activated protein C. Proc Natl Acad Sci U S A. 1993;90:1004-1008.

130. Bertina RM, Koeleman BP, Koster T, et al. Mutation in blood coagulation factor V associated with resistance to activated protein C. Nature. 1994;369:64-67.

131. Kalafatis M, Bernardi F, Simioni P, et al. Phenotype and genotype expression in pseudohomozygous factor V LEIDEN: the need for phenotype analysis. Arterioscler Thromb Vasc Biol. 1999;19:336-342.

132. Over J, Sixma JJ, Bruine MH, et al. Survival of ^{125}iodine-labeled factor VIII in normals and patients with classic hemophilia. Observations on the heterogeneity of human factor VIII. J Clin Invest. 1978;62:223-234.

133. Weiss HJ, Sussman II, Hoyer LW. Stabilization of factor VIII in plasma by the von Willebrand factor. Studies on posttransfusion and dissociated factor VIII and in patients with von Willebrand's disease. J Clin Invest. 1977;60:390-404.

134. Bontempo FA, Lewis JH, Gorenc TJ, et al. Liver transplantation in hemophilia A. Blood. 1987;69:1721-1724.

135. Andersson LO, Forsman N, Huang K, et al. Isolation and characterization of human factor VIII: molecular forms in commercial factor VIII concentrate, cryoprecipitate, and plasma. Proc Natl Acad Sci U S A. 1986;83:2979-2983.

136. Lollar P, Parker ET. Structural basis for the decreased procoagulant activity of human factor VIII compared to the porcine homolog. J Biol Chem. 1991;266:12481-12486.

137. Tagliavacca L, Moon N, Dunham WR, Kaufman RJ. Identification and functional requirement of Cu(I) and its ligands within coagulation factor VIII. J Biol Chem. 1997;272:27428-27434.

138. Saenko EL, Scandella D. The acidic region of the factor VIII light chain and the C2 domain together form the high affinity binding site for von Willebrand factor. J Biol Chem. 1997;272:18007-18014.

139. Lenting PJ, van de Loo JW, Donath MJ, et al. The sequence Glu1811-Lys1818 of human blood coagulation factor VIII comprises a binding site for activated factor IX. J Biol Chem. 1996;271:1935-1940.

140. Michnick DA, Pittman DD, Wise RJ, Kaufman RJ. Identification of individual tyrosine sulfation sites within factor VIII required for optimal activity and efficient thrombin cleavage. J Biol Chem. 1994;269:20095-20102.

141. Lollar P, Knutson GJ, Fass DN. Stabilization of thrombin-activated porcine factor VIII:C by factor IXa phospholipid. Blood. 1984;63:1303-1308.

142. Fay PJ, Beattie TL, Regan LM, et al. Model for the factor VIIIa–dependent decay of the intrinsic factor Xase. Role of subunit dissociation and factor IXa–catalyzed proteolysis. J Biol Chem. 1996;271:6027-6032.

143. Fay PJ, Smudzin TM, Walker FJ. Activated protein C–catalyzed inactivation of human factor VIII and factor VIIIa. Identification of cleavage sites and correlation of proteolysis with cofactor activity. J Biol Chem. 1991;266: 20139-20145.

144. Lu D, Kalafatis M, Mann KG, Long GL. Comparison of activated protein C/protein S–mediated inactivation of human factor VIII and factor V. Blood. 1996;87:4708-4717.

145. Regan LM, Lamphear BJ, Huggins CF, et al. Factor IXa protects factor VIIIa from activated protein C. Factor IXa inhibits activated protein C–catalyzed cleavage of factor VIIIa at Arg562. J Biol Chem. 1994;269:9445-9452.

146. Koutts J, Walsh PN, Plow EF, et al. Active release of human platelet factor VIII–related antigen by adenosine diphosphate, collagen, and thrombin. J Clin Invest. 1978;62:1255-1263.

147. Sporn LA, Chavin SI, Marder VJ, Wagner DD. Biosynthesis of von Willebrand protein by human megakaryocytes. J Clin Invest. 1985;76:1102-1106.

148. Wagner DD, Olmsted JB, Marder VJ. Immunolocalization of von Willebrand protein in Weibel-Palade bodies of human endothelial cells. J Cell Biol. 1982;95:355-360.

149. Sadler JE. Biochemistry and genetics of von Willebrand factor. Annu Rev Biochem. 1998;67:395-424.

150. Chung DW, Fujikawa K. Processing of von Willebrand factor by ADAMTS-13. Biochemistry. 2002;41:11065-11070.

151. Morrissey JH. Tissue factor and factor VII initiation of coagulation. In Colman RW, Hirsh J, Marder VJ, Clowes AW, George JN (eds). Hemostasis and Thrombosis. Philadelphia, Lippincott Williams & Wilkins, 2001, pp 89-101.

152. Paborsky LR, Caras IW, Fisher KL, Gorman CM. Lipid association, but not the transmembrane domain, is required for tissue factor activity. Substitution of the transmembrane domain with a phosphatidylinositol anchor. J Biol Chem. 1991;266:21911-21916.

153. Nemerson Y, Repke D. Tissue factor accelerates the activation of coagulation factor VII: the role of a bifunctional coagulation cofactor. Thromb Res. 1985;40:351-358.

154. Williams EB, Krishnaswamy S, Mann KG. Zymogen/enzyme discrimination using peptide chloromethyl ketones. J Biol Chem. 1989;264:7536-7545.

155. Butenas S, Mann KG. Kinetics of human factor VII activation. Biochemistry. 1996;35:1904-1910.

156. Giesen PL, Rauch U, Bohrmann B, et al. Blood-borne tissue factor: another view of thrombosis. Proc Natl Acad Sci U S A. 1999;96:2311-2315.

157. Santucci RA, Erlich J, Labriola J, et al. Measurement of tissue factor activity in whole blood. Thromb Haemost. 2000;83:445-454.

158. Maruyama I, Bell CE, Majerus PW. Thrombomodulin is found on endothelium of arteries, veins, capillaries, and

lymphatics, and on syncytiotrophoblast of human placenta. J Cell Biol. 1985;101:363-371.

159. Healy AM, Rayburn HB, Rosenberg RD, Weiler H. Absence of the blood-clotting regulator thrombomodulin causes embryonic lethality in mice before development of a functional cardiovascular system. Proc Natl Acad Sci U S A. 1995;92:850-854.

160. Kurosawa S, Stearns DJ, Jackson KW, Esmon CT. A 10-kDa cyanogen bromide fragment from the epidermal growth factor homology domain of rabbit thrombomodulin contains the primary thrombin binding site. J Biol Chem. 1988;263:5993-5996.

161. Ye J, Rezaie AR, Esmon CT. Glycosaminoglycan contributions to both protein C activation and thrombin inhibition involve a common arginine-rich site in thrombin that includes residues arginine 93, 97, and 101. J Biol Chem. 1994;269:17965-17970.

162. He X, Ye J, Esmon CT, Rezaie AR. Influence of arginines 93, 97, and 101 of thrombin to its functional specificity. Biochemistry. 1997;36:8969-8976.

163. Vindigni A, White CE, Komives EA, Di Cera E. Energetics of thrombin-thrombomodulin interaction. Biochemistry. 1997;36:6674-6681.

164. Ye J, Esmon NL, Esmon CT, Johnson AE. The active site of thrombin is altered upon binding to thrombomodulin. Two distinct structural changes are detected by fluorescence, but only one correlates with protein C activation. J Biol Chem. 1991;266:23016-23021.

165. Esmon NL, Carroll RC, Esmon CT. Thrombomodulin blocks the ability of thrombin to activate platelets. J Biol Chem. 1983;258:12238-12242.

166. Tankersley DL, Finlayson JS. Kinetics of activation and autoactivation of human factor XII. Biochemistry. 1984;23:273-279.

167. Schmaier A. Contact activation. In Loscalzo J, Schafer AI (eds). Thrombosis and Hemorrhage. Baltimore, Williams & Wilkins, 1998, pp 105-127.

168. Hovinga JK, Schaller J, Stricker H, et al. Coagulation factor XII Locarno: the functional defect is caused by the amino acid substitution Arg 353→Pro leading to loss of a kallikrein cleavage site. Blood 1994;84:1173-1181.

169. Kaplan AP, Silverberg M, Ghebrehiwet B. The intrinsic coagulation/kinin pathway—the classical complement pathway and their interactions. Adv Exp Med Biol. 1986;198:11-25.

170. Chien P, Pixley RA, Stumpo LG, et al. Modulation of the human monocyte binding site for monomeric immunoglobulin G by activated Hageman factor. J Clin Invest. 1988;82:1554-1559.

171. Wachtfogel YT, Pixley RA, Kucich U, et al. Purified plasma factor XIIa aggregates human neutrophils and causes degranulation. Blood. 1986;67:1731-1737.

172. Mandle R Jr, Kaplan AP. Hageman factor substrates. Human plasma prekallikrein: mechanism of activation by Hageman factor and participation in Hageman factor–dependent fibrinolysis. J Biol Chem. 1977;252:6097-6104.

173. Scott CF, Colman RW. Function and immunochemistry of prekallikrein–high molecular weight kininogen complex in plasma. J Clin Invest. 1980;65:413-421.

174. Chung DW, Fujikawa K, McMullen BA, Davie EW. Human plasma prekallikrein, a zymogen to a serine protease that contains four tandem repeats. Biochemistry. 1986;25:2410-2417.

175. Burger D, Schleuning WD, Schapira M. Human plasma prekallikrein. Immunoaffinity purification and activation to alpha- and beta-kallikrein. J Biol Chem. 1986;261:324-327.

176. Loza JP, Gurewich V, Johnstone M, Pannell R. Platelet-bound prekallikrein promotes pro-urokinase–induced clot lysis: a mechanism for targeting the factor XII dependent intrinsic pathway of fibrinolysis. Thromb Haemost. 1994;71:347-352.

177. Wachtfogel YT, Kucich U, James HL, et al. Human plasma kallikrein releases neutrophil elastase during blood coagulation. J Clin Invest. 1983;72:1672-1677.

178. van der Graaf F, Koedam JA, Bouma BN. Inactivation of kallikrein in human plasma. J Clin Invest. 1983;71:149-158.

179. Cheung PP, Kunapuli SP, Scott CF, et al. Genetic basis of total kininogen deficiency in Williams' trait. J Biol Chem. 1993;268:23361-23365.

180. Kitamura N, Kitagawa H, Fukushima D, et al. Structural organization of the human kininogen gene and a model for its evolution. J Biol Chem. 1985;260:8610-8617.

181. Bradford HN, Schmaier AH, Colman RW. Kinetics of inhibition of platelet calpain II by human kininogens. Biochem J. 1990;270:83-90.

182. Tait JF, Fujikawa K. Identification of the binding site for plasma prekallikrein in human high molecular weight kininogen. A region from residues 185 to 224 of the kininogen light chain retains full binding activity. J Biol Chem. 1986;261:15396-15401.

183. Schwartz AL, Broze GJ Jr. Tissue factor pathway inhibitor. Trends Cardiovasc Med. 1997;7:234-239.

184. Broze GJ Jr. Tissue factor pathway inhibitor and the revised theory of coagulation. Annu Rev Med. 1995;46:103-112.

185. Novotny WF, Girard TJ, Miletich JP, Broze GJ Jr. Platelets secrete a coagulation inhibitor functionally and antigenically similar to the lipoprotein associated coagulation inhibitor. Blood. 1988;72:2020-2025.

186. Huang ZF, Higuchi D, Lasky N, Broze GJ Jr. Tissue factor pathway inhibitor gene disruption produces intrauterine lethality in mice. Blood. 1997;90:944-951.

187. van't Veer C, Mann KG. Regulation of tissue factor initiated thrombin generation by the stoichiometric inhibitors tissue factor pathway inhibitor, antithrombin-III, and heparin cofactor-II. J Biol Chem. 1997;272:4367-4377.

188. Turk B, Brieditis I, Bock SC, et al. The oligosaccharide side chain on Asn-135 of alpha-antithrombin, absent in beta-antithrombin, decreases the heparin affinity of the inhibitor by affecting the heparin-induced conformational change. Biochemistry. 1997;36:6682-6691.

189. Olson ST, Shore JD. Demonstration of a two-step reaction mechanism for inhibition of alpha-thrombin by antithrombin III and identification of the step affected by heparin. J Biol Chem. 1982;257:14891-14895.

190. Parker KA, Tollefsen DM. The protease specificity of heparin cofactor II. Inhibition of thrombin generated during coagulation. J Biol Chem. 1985;260:3501-3505.

191. Uhrin P, Dewerchin M, Hilpert M, et al. Disruption of the protein C inhibitor gene results in impaired spermatogenesis and male infertility. J Clin Invest. 2000;106:1531-1539.

192. Strandberg K, Astermark J, Bjorgell O, et al. Complexes between activated protein C and protein C inhibitor measured with a new method: comparison of performance with other markers of hypercoagulability in the diagnosis of deep vein thrombosis. Thromb Haemost. 2001;86:1400-1408.

193. Chen R, Doolittle RF. Cross-linking sites in human and bovine fibrin. Biochemistry. 1971;10:4487-4491.

194. Mosher DF. Cross-linking of fibronectin to collagenous proteins. Mol Cell Biochem. 1984;58:63-68.

195. Lynch GW, Slayter HS, Miller BE, McDonagh J. Characterization of thrombospondin as a substrate for factor XIII transglutaminase. J Biol Chem. 1987;262:1772-1778.

196. Lowey AG, McDonagh J, Mikkola H, et al. Structure and function of factor XIII. In Colman RW, Hirsh J, Marder VJ, et al (eds). Hemostasis and Thrombosis. Philadelphia, Lippincott Williams & Wilkins, 2001, pp 233-247.

197. Radek JT, Jeong JM, Wilson J, Lorand L. Association of the A subunits of recombinant placental factor XIII with the native carrier B subunits from human plasma. Biochemistry. 1993;32:3527-3534.

198. Takahashi N, Takahashi Y, Putnam FW. Primary structure of blood coagulation factor XIIIa (fibrinoligase, transglutaminase) from human placenta. Proc Natl Acad Sci U S A. 1986;83:8019-8023.

199. Ichinose A, Hendrickson LE, Fujikawa K, Davie EW. Amino acid sequence of the a subunit of human factor XIII. Biochemistry. 1986;25:6900-6906.

200. Lorand L, Jeong JM, Radek JT, Wilson J. Human plasma factor XIII: subunit interactions and activation of zymogen. Methods Enzymol. 1993;222:22-35.

201. Poon MC, Russell JA, Low S, et al. Hemopoietic origin of factor XIII A subunits in platelets, monocytes, and plasma. Evidence from bone marrow transplantation studies. J Clin Invest. 1989;84:787-792.

202. McDonagh J, McDonagh RP Jr, Delage JM, Wagner RH. Factor XIII in human plasma and platelets. J Clin Invest. 1969;48:940-946.

203. Henriksson P, Becker S, Lynch G, McDonagh J. Identification of intracellular factor XIII in human monocytes and macrophages. J Clin Invest. 1985;76:528-534.

204. Nagy JA, Kradin RL, McDonagh J. Biosynthesis of factor XIII A and B subunits. Adv Exp Med Biol. 1988;231:29-49.

205. Brummel KE, Butenas S, Mann KG. An integrated study of fibrinogen during blood coagulation. J Biol Chem. 1999;274:22862-22870.

206. Naski MC, Lorand L, Shafer JA. Characterization of the kinetic pathway for fibrin promotion of alpha-thrombin–catalyzed activation of plasma factor XIII. Biochemistry. 1991;30:934-941.

207. Lord ST. Fibrinogen and fibrin: scaffold proteins in hemostasis. Curr Opin Hematol. 2007;14:236-241.

208. Mosesson MW. Fibrinogen and fibrin structure and functions. J Thromb Haemost. 2005;3:1894-1904.

209. Takeda Y. Studies of the metabolism and distribution of fibrinogen in healthy men with autologous ^{125}I-labeled fibrinogen. J Clin Invest. 1966;45:103-111.

210. Kant JA, Fornace AJ Jr, Saxe D, et al. Evolution and organization of the fibrinogen locus on chromosome 4: gene duplication accompanied by transposition and inversion. Proc Natl Acad Sci U S A. 1985;82:2344-2348.

211. Crabtree GR, Kant JA. Molecular cloning of cDNA for the alpha, beta, and gamma chains of rat fibrinogen. A family of coordinately regulated genes. J Biol Chem. 1981;256:9718-9723.

212. Francis CW, Mosesson MW. Terminology for fibrinogen gamma-chains differing in carboxyl terminal amino acid sequence. Thromb Haemost. 1989;62:813-814.

213. Fu Y, Weissbach L, Plant PW, et al. Carboxy-terminal–extended variant of the human fibrinogen alpha subunit: a novel exon conferring marked homology to beta and gamma subunits. Biochemistry. 1992;31:11968-11972.

214. Bailey K, Bettelheim FR, Lorand L, Middlebrook WR. Action of thrombin in the clotting of fibrinogen. Nature. 1951;167:233-234.

215. Francis CW, Marder VJ. Increased resistance to plasmic degradation of fibrin with highly crosslinked alpha-polymer chains formed at high factor XIII concentrations. Blood. 1988;71:1361-1365.

27 The Molecular Basis of Fibrinolysis

Katherine Amberson Hajjar

Fibrinolysis is the process by which the insoluble protein fibrin is converted to a defined set of soluble degradation products. It occurs in both intravascular and extravascular locations and is essential to human health and survival. Modern molecular biologic techniques have identified the major fibrinolytic genes, the mechanisms regulating their expression, and the consequences of their deficiency or overexpression in genetically engineered mice. In many cases these experiments have yielded surprising and instructive data that have revealed physiologic and pathophysiologic roles for the fibrinolytic system that are much more extensive than originally thought. Furthermore, with the dawn of the genomic age, molecular analysis of human syndromes has identified specific mutations that result in either thrombosis secondary to fibrinolytic deficiency or hemorrhage secondary to fibrinolytic excess. In this chapter the molecular basis of fibrinolysis, as well as its physiologic role in human health and disease, is reviewed.

BASIC CONCEPTS OF FIBRINOLYSIS

In response to vascular injury and activation of the coagulation cascade, thrombin induces polymerization of the soluble plasma protein fibrinogen, thereby producing an insoluble, cross-linked end product called fibrin (see Chapter 26). Once the flow of blood has been stemmed and vascular integrity restored, fibrin, which is found in both intravascular and extravascular sites, is cleared by a process known as fibrinolysis (Fig. 27-1A). Normally, the fibrinolytic process is tightly regulated by a series of activators, inhibitors, cofactors, and receptors.[1] In the presence of fibrin, which serves as a cofactor for its own destruction, tissue plasminogen activator (tPA) is released from endothelial cells and possibly other cell types and interacts with the circulating zymogen plasminogen. tPA, plasminogen, and fibrin form a ternary complex that accelerates the catalytic efficiency of plasmin generation by approximately 500-fold. Urokinase is also an efficient plasminogen activator (uPA), but its action is only minimally enhanced by fibrin. The action of plasmin on fibrin generates soluble fibrin degradation products, which have their own unique biologic properties.

The dynamic regulation of plasmin generation is complex. On the surface of a fibrin-containing thrombus, tPA and plasmin are protected from their major circulating inhibitors plasminogen activator inhibitor 1 (PAI-1) and α_2-antiplasmin (α_2-AP), respectively. On release into the circulation, however, plasmin and tPA are rapidly neutralized by these inhibitors and cleared by the liver. Because uPA and the nonenzymatic plasminogen activator streptokinase do not use fibrin as a cofactor, they function well in the fluid phase. Plasminogen may also be activated, albeit rather inefficiently, by proteases of the contact system such as kallikrein, factor XIa, and factor XIIa (Chapter 26).

Cell surfaces represent protected environments in which plasmin can be generated without the risk of neutralization by fluid-phase inhibitors (Fig. 27-1B).[2] Endothelial cells, platelets, monocytes, macrophages, and some tumor cells all express protein receptor sites for plasminogen, tPA, or uPA.[3] The broad substrate specificity of plasmin observed in vitro may relate to its generation in nonvascular sites through fibrin-independent mechanisms. Plasmin may thus play an important role in extravascular events such as the modification of growth and differentiation factors, processing of matrix proteins, and activation of procoagulant molecules.

COMPONENTS OF THE FIBRINOLYTIC SYSTEM

Plasminogen

Synthesized primarily in the liver,[4,5] plasminogen is a single-chain proenzyme with a molecular weight (M_r) of approximately 92,000 that circulates in plasma at a concentration of approximately 1.5 μmol/L (Table 27-1).[6] The plasma half-life of plasminogen in humans is approximately 2 days.[7] Its 791 amino acids are cross-linked by 24 disulfide bridges, 16 of which yield five homologous triple-loop structures called *kringles*[8] (Fig. 27-2). The first (K1) and fourth (K4) of these 80–amino acid structures with an M_r of 10,000 impart high- and low-affinity lysine binding, respectively.[9] The lysine-binding domains of plasminogen appear to mediate its specific interactions with fibrin, cell surface receptors, and other proteins, including its circulating inhibitor α_2-AP.[10-14]

Post-translational modification of plasminogen results in two glycosylation variants (forms 1 and 2)[15-17] (see Table 27-1). An *O*-linked oligosaccharide on Thr345 is common to both forms. Only form 2, however, contains an *N*-linked oligosaccharide on Asn288. The carbohydrate portion of plasminogen appears to regulate its affinity for cellular receptors and may also specify its physiologic degradation pathway.

Activation of plasminogen results from cleavage of a single Arg-Val peptide bond at position 560 to 561,[18] which produces the active protease plasmin (see Table 27-1). Plasmin contains a typical serine protease catalytic triad[6] but exhibits broad substrate specificity in comparison to other proteases of this class.[19] The circulating form of plasminogen, amino-terminal glutamic acid plasminogen (Glu-Plg), is readily converted by limited proteolysis to several modified forms known collectively as lysine plasminogen (Lys-Plg).[20,21] Hydrolysis of the Lys77-Lys78 peptide bond results in an altered conformation that more readily binds fibrin, displays twofold to threefold higher avidity for cellular receptors, and is activated 10 to 20 times more rapidly than Glu-Plg is.[12,18,22] Lys-Plg does not normally circulate in plasma[18] but has been identified on cell surfaces.[23]

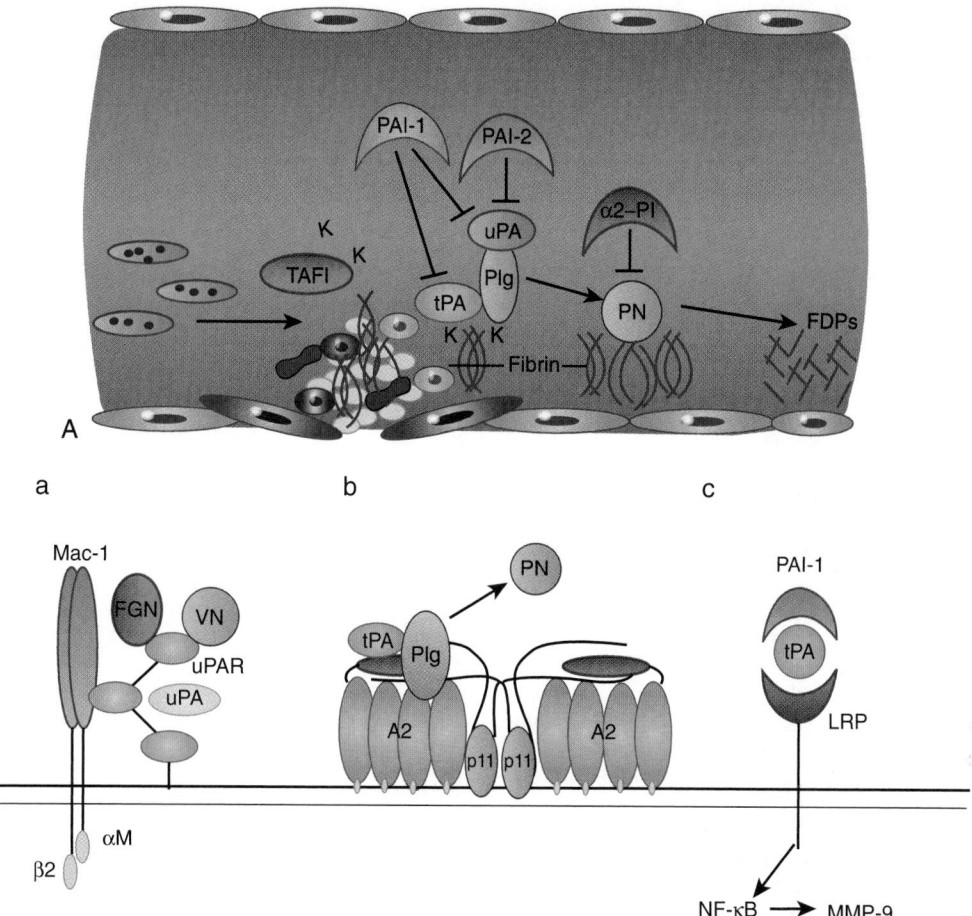

FIGURE 27-1. Overview of the fibrinolytic system. **A,** Fibrin-based plasminogen activation. The zymogen plasminogen (Plg) is converted to the active serine protease plasmin (PN) through the action of tissue plasminogen activator (tPA) or urokinase (uPA). The activity of tPA is greatly enhanced by its assembly with Plg through lysine residues (K) on a fibrin-containing thrombus. uPA acts independently of fibrin. Both tPA and uPA can be inhibited by plasminogen activator inhibitor 1 (PAI-1), which is released by endothelial cells and activated platelets. PAI-2, on the other hand, neutralizes uPA more efficiently than it does tPA. By binding to fibrin, plasmin is protected from its major inhibitor α_2-antiplasmin (α_2-AP). Bound plasmin degrades cross-linked fibrin, which gives rise to soluble fibrin degradation products (FDPs). **B,** Some cell surface fibrinolytic receptors. **a,** Endothelial cells, monocytes, and macrophages express the uPA receptor (uPAR), which can interact with both uPA, thereby preserving its activity, and adhesive glycoproteins, such as fibrinogen (FGN) and vitronectin (VN). uPAR association with Mac-1 appears to facilitate adhesive interactions, whereas its interaction with uPA has a negative impact on adhesion. **b,** Endothelial cells, monocytes, and macrophages also express annexin A2 (A2), a coreceptor for tPA and Plg that augments the efficiency of plasmin generation. A2 forms a heterotetramer with protein p11, a member of the S100 family, which accentuates the efficiency of plasmin generation. **c,** Low-density lipoprotein receptor–related protein (LRP) is expressed by macrophages and smooth muscle cells. It binds a wide variety of ligands, including α_2-macroglobulin (α_2-MG) and uPA or tPA in complex with PAI-1. Originally thought to function as a clearance receptor, LRP appears to signal to activate NF-κB and augment expression of downstream effectors such as metalloproteinase 9 (MMP-9). *(Adapted from Ragno P. The urokinase receptor: a ligand or a receptor? Cell Mol Life Sci. 2006;63:1028-1037.)*

Spanning 52.5 kilobases (kb) of DNA on chromosome 6q26-27, the plasminogen gene consists of 19 exons[24,25] and directs expression of a 2.7-kb messenger RNA (mRNA)[8] (see Fig. 27-2). Plasminogen gene activity is stimulated by the acute phase mediator interleukin-6, both in vitro and in vivo.[26] The gene is closely linked and structurally related to that of apolipoprotein(a), an apoprotein associated with the highly atherogenic low-density lipoprotein–like particle lipoprotein(a)[27] and more distantly related to other kringle-containing proteins such as tPA, uPA, hepatocyte growth factor, and macrophage-stimulating protein.[28-32] The significance of the latter two proteins to the fibrinolytic system remains to be determined.

Plasminogen Activators

Tissue Plasminogen Activator

One of the two major endogenous plasminogen activators, tPA is a 527–amino acid glycoprotein with an M_r of approximately 72,000[33] (see Table 27-1). tPA contains five structural domains, including a fibronectin-like "finger," an epidermal growth factor–like domain, two kringle structures homologous to those of plasminogen, and a serine protease domain (see Fig. 27-2). Cleavage of the Arg275-Ile276 peptide bond by plasmin converts tPA to a disulfide-linked, two-chain form.[33] Although single-chain tPA is less active than two-chain tPA in the

TABLE 27-1   Fibrinolytic Proteins

PROTEASES

Property	Plasminogen	tPA	uPA
Molecular mass (d)	92,000	72,000	54,000
Amino acids	791	527	411
Chromosome	6	8	10
Site of synthesis	Liver Neuronal cells Glial cells	Endothelium Neuronal cells Glial cells	Endothelium Kidney
Plasma concentration			
nmol/L	1500	0.075	0.150
µg/mL	140	0.005	0.008
Plasma half-life	48 hr	5 min	8 min
N-Glycosylation (%)	2	13	7
Form 1	—	Asn117, Asn184, Asn448	Asn302
Form 2	Asn288	Asn117, Asn448	—
O-Glycosylation			
α-Fucose	—	Thr61	Thr18
Complex	Thr345	—	—
Two-chain cleavage site	Arg560-Val561	Arg275-Ile276	Lys158-Ile159
Heavy-chain domains			
Finger	No	Yes	No
Growth factor	No	Yes	Yes
Kringles (no.)	5	2	1
Light-chain catalytic triad	His602, Asp645, Ser740	His322, Asp371, Ser478	His204, Asp255, Ser356

MAJOR SERPIN INHIBITORS

Property	α_2-AP	PAI-1	PAI-2
Molecular mass (d)	70,000	52,000	60,000 (glycosylated) 47,000 (nonglycosylated)
Amino acids	452	402	393
Chromosome	18	7	18
Sites of synthesis	Kidney, liver	Endothelium Monocytes/macrophages Hepatocytes Adipocytes	Placenta Monocytes/macrophages Tumor cells
Plasma concentration			
nmol/L	900	0.1-0.4	ND
µg/mL	50	0.02	ND
Serpin reactive site	Arg364-Met365	Arg346-Met347	Arg358-Thr359
Specificity	Plasmin	uPA = tPA	uPA > tPA

NONSERPIN INHIBITORS

Property	TAFI	α_2-MG
Molecular mass (d)	45,000	725,000 (monomer ≈180,000)
Amino acids	423	1451
Chromosome	13	12
Sites of synthesis	Liver	Liver Endothelium Macrophages Fibroblasts
Plasma concentration		
nmol/L	≈75	≈2000-5000
µg/mL	4	≈1450-3625
Activators	Plasmin >> thrombin	—
Specificity	C-terminal Lys and Arg	Broad spectrum

TABLE 27-1 Fibrinolytic Proteins—cont'd

SOME PROPOSED RECEPTORS				
Property	**uPAR**	**Annexin A2**	**LRP**	**Mannose Receptor**
Molecular mass (d)	55-60,000	36,000	600,000	175,000
Amino acids	313	339	4544	1456
Chromosome	19	15	12	10
Source	Endothelial cells	Endothelial cells	Hepatocytes	Macrophages
	Monocytes	Monocytes	Monocytes	
	Macrophages	Macrophages	Macrophages	
	Fibroblasts	Myeloid cells	Fibroblasts	
	Tumor cells			
Ligand(s)	uPA	tPA, Plg	uPA/PAI-1	tPA
			uPA/PAI-2	
			tPA/PAI-1	
			PN/α_2-AP	

α_2-AP, α_2-antiplasmin; LRP, low-density lipoprotein receptor–like protein; α_2-MG, α_2-macroglobulin; PAI, plasminogen activator inhibitor; ND, not determined; PN, plasmin; TAFI, thrombin-activatable fibrinolysis inhibitor; tPA, tissue plasminogen activator; uPA, urokinase plasminogen activator; uPAR, urokinase plasminogen activator receptor.

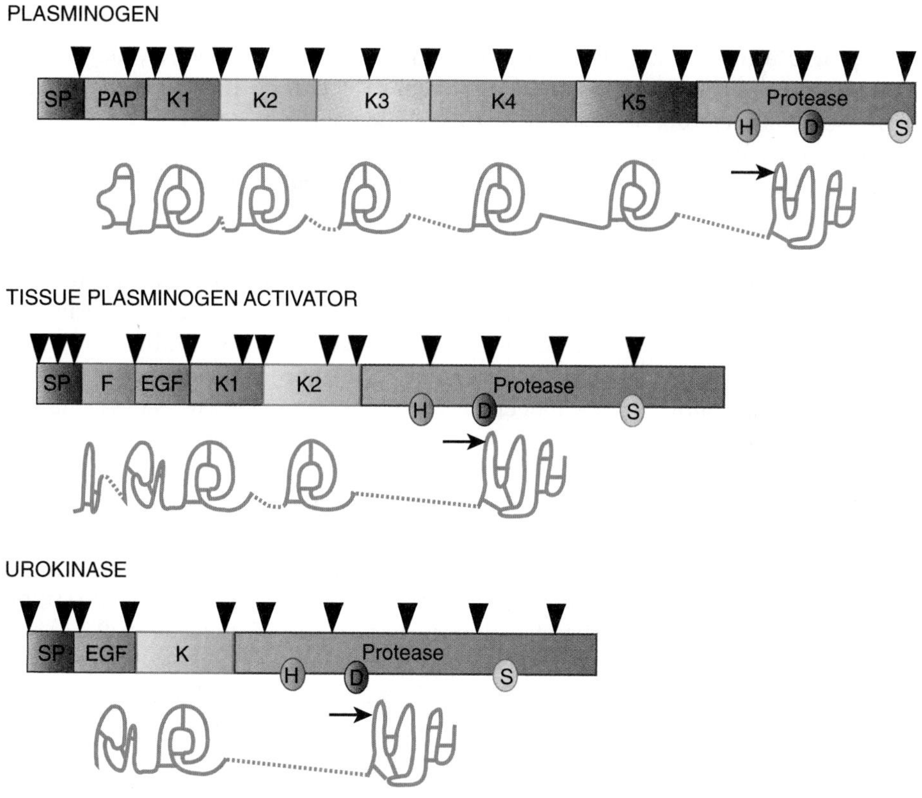

PLASMINOGEN

TISSUE PLASMINOGEN ACTIVATOR

UROKINASE

FIGURE 27-2. Structure-function relationships of plasminogen, tissue plasminogen activator (tPA), and urokinase (uPA) and alignment of the intron-exon structure of the plasminogen, tPA, and uPA genes with functional protein domains. Protein domains are labeled signal peptide (SP), preactivation peptide (PAP), kringle domains (K), fibronectin-like "finger" (F), epidermal growth factor–like domain (EGF), and protease. The position of the catalytic triad of amino acids histidine (H), aspartic acid (D), and serine (S) are shown within individual protease domains. The positions of individual introns relative to amino acid–encoding exons are indicated with *inverted triangles*.

fluid phase, both forms demonstrate equivalent activity when bound to fibrin.[34]

The two glycosylation forms of tPA are distinguishable by the presence (type 1) or absence (type 2) of a complex *N*-linked oligosaccharide moiety on Asn184 (see Table 27-1).[35,36] Both types, however, contain a high-mannose carbohydrate on Asn117, a complex oligosaccharide on Asn448, and an *O*-linked α-fucose residue on Thr61.[37] The carbohydrate moieties of tPA may modulate its functional activity, regulate its binding to cell surface receptors, and specify degradation pathways.

Located on chromosome 8p12-q11.2, the gene for human tPA is encoded by 14 exons spanning a total of 36.6 kb (see Fig. 27-2).[38-40] Most of the structural domains of tPA are encoded by one or two exons, and the organization of these exons is similar across related domains of tPA and the other fibrinolytic proteases (see Fig. 27-2). This observation suggests that the tPA gene arose by an evolutionary process called "exon shuffling," whereby functionally related genes are generated through rearrangement of exons encoding autonomous domains. Consistent with this hypothesis, various functions of tPA can be localized to specific domains. For example, deletion of the fibronectin-like finger or kringle 2, but not kringle 1, results in a tPA resistant to the cofactor activity of fibrin, whereas catalytic activity in the absence of fibrin remains intact.[41]

The proximal promoter of the human tPA gene contains binding sequences for potentially important transcriptional factors, including AP1, NF1, SP1, and AP2,[42,43] as well as a potential cyclic adenosine monophosphate (cAMP)-responsive element.[44] In vitro, many agents have been shown to exert small effects on the expression of tPA mRNA, but relatively few enhance tPA synthesis without augmenting PAI-1 synthesis as well. Agents that regulate tPA gene expression independently of PAI-1 include arterial shear stress, thrombin, endotoxin, histamine, butyrate, retinoids, and dexamethasone.[45-50] Forskolin, which increases intracellular cAMP levels, has been reported to decrease the synthesis of both tPA and PAI-1.[43,51]

tPA is synthesized and secreted primarily by endothelial cells, and its release is governed by a variety of stimuli such as shear stress, butyrate, thrombin, histamine, bradykinin, epinephrine, acetylcholine, arginine vasopressin, gonadotropins, exercise, and venous occlusion.[45,47,52,53] Its circulating half-life is exceedingly short ($\approx$5 minutes). By itself, tPA is a poor activator of plasminogen. However, in the presence of fibrin, the catalytic efficiency of tPA-dependent plasmin generation (k_{cat}/K_m) increases by at least 2 orders of magnitude[22] because of a dramatic increase in affinity (decreased Michaelis constant [K_m]) between tPA and its substrate plasminogen in the presence of fibrin. Although it is expressed by extravascular cells, tPA appears to represent the major intravascular activator of plasminogen.[19]

Urokinase

The second endogenous plasminogen activator, single-chain uPA or prourokinase, is a glycoprotein with an M_r of approximately 54,000 and consists of 411 amino acids (see Table 27-1). uPA contains an epidermal growth factor–like domain and a single plasminogen-like kringle and possesses a classic catalytic triad within its serine protease domain[54] (see Fig. 27-2). Cleavage of the Lys158-Ile159 peptide bond by plasmin or kallikrein converts single-chain uPA to a disulfide-linked two-chain derivative.[55] Located on chromosome 10, the human uPA gene is encoded by 11 exons spanning 6.4 kb and expressed by endothelial cells, macrophages, renal epithelial cells, and some tumor cells.[56,57] As noted earlier, its intron-exon structure is closely related to that of the tPA gene.

There is circumstantial evidence that uPA may be induced during neoplastic transformation, possibly through a mechanism involving the transcription factors AP1 and AP2.[58] Other agents that appear to induce expression of uPA in vitro include hormones, growth factors, and cAMP.[49] Inflammatory cytokines such as interleukin-1 and lipopolysaccharide induce only small increments in uPA expression, whereas tumor necrosis

factor and transforming growth factor β (TGF-β) have a more dramatic (5- to 30-fold) effect.[59-61]

Two-chain uPA occurs in both high-molecular-weight (M_r of 54,000) and low-molecular-weight (M_r of 33,000) forms that differ by the presence or absence, respectively, of a 135-residue amino-terminal fragment released by plasmin cleavage between Lys135 and Lys136.[62,63] Although both forms are capable of activating plasminogen, only the high-molecular-weight form binds to the uPA receptor (uPAR). uPA has much lower affinity for fibrin than tPA does and is an effective plasminogen activator both in the presence and in the absence of fibrin.[64,65] The extent to which prourokinase possesses intrinsic plasminogen-activating capacity is an area of controversy.[66,67]

Accessory Plasminogen Activators

Under certain conditions, proteases traditionally classified within the intrinsic arm of the coagulation cascade (see Chapter 26) have been shown to be capable of activating plasminogen directly. Such proteases include kallikrein, factor XIa, and factor XIIa.[68-70] Normally, however, they account for no more than 15% of the total plasmin-generating activity in plasma.

Inhibitors of Fibrinolysis

Plasmin Inhibitors

The action of plasmin is negatively modulated by a family of serine protease inhibitors called serpins[71] (see Table 27-1). All serpins share a common mechanism of action by forming an irreversible complex with the active-site serine of the target protease after proteolytic cleavage of the inhibitor by the target protease. Within such a complex, both protease and inhibitor lose their activity.

A single-chain glycoprotein with an M_r of approximately 70,000, α_2-AP circulates in plasma at relatively high concentrations ($\approx$0.9 μmol/L) and has a plasma half-life of 2.4 days[72] (see Table 27-1). This serpin contains about 13% carbohydrate by mass and consists of 452 amino acids with two disulfide bridges.[73] In humans, the gene is located on chromosome 18 and contains 10 exons distributed over 16 kb of DNA.[74] The promoter region of the α_2-AP gene contains a hepatitis B–like enhancer element that directs tissue-specific expression in the liver.[74] α_2-AP is also a constituent of platelet alpha granules.[75] Plasmin released into flowing blood or in the vicinity of a platelet-rich thrombus is immediately neutralized on forming an irreversible 1:1 stoichiometric, lysine binding site–dependent complex with α_2-AP. Interaction with plasmin is accompanied by cleavage of the Arg364-Met365 peptide bond, and the resulting covalent complexes are cleared in the liver.

Several other proteins appear to inhibit the activity of fibrinolytic serine proteases (see Table 27-1). α_2-Macroglobulin (α_2-MG) is a tetrameric protein with an M_r of

725,000 that is synthesized by the liver, endothelial cells, macrophages, and fibroblasts and is found in platelet alpha granules. The gene for α_2-MG, which consists of 36 exons distributed over 48 kb of DNA on chromosome 12, directs the expression of a 1451–amino acid polypeptide.[76-78] As a generic inhibitor of all four classes of proteases (serine, cysteine, aspartyl, and metallo), α_2-MG is a nonserpin that inhibits plasmin with approximately 10% of the efficiency exhibited by α_2-AP by forming a noncovalent complex.[79] C1 esterase inhibitor can also serve as an inhibitor of tPA in plasma.[80] The protease nexin may function as a noncirculating cell surface inhibitor[81] of trypsin, thrombin, factor Xa, urokinase, or plasmin and result in protease-inhibitor complexes that are endocytosed via a specific nexin receptor.[82]

Thrombin-activatable fibrinolysis inhibitor (TAFI) is a plasma carboxypeptidase that acts as a potent inhibitor of fibrinolysis.[83] Identical to the previously cloned carboxypeptidase B[84] and the previously isolated carboxypeptidase U,[85] this single-chain polypeptide with an M_r of 45,000 circulates in plasma at concentrations of about 75 nmol/L and undergoes limited proteolysis in the presence of plasmin or thrombin, which leads to its activation.[86] Carboxypeptidase B–like molecules remove carboxyl-terminal lysine or arginine residues from fibrin and other proteins, thereby reducing binding of plasminogen to fibrin and cell surfaces and limiting plasmin generation.[87] The potentially antifibrinolytic effect of thrombin appears to be mediated through its ability to activate TAFI in the presence of thrombomodulin.[83,88] Anticoagulation by inhibition of factor XI also appears to have an antifibrinolytic effect in vivo by downregulation of thrombin-mediated activation of TAFI.[89] In a system of purified components, TAFI has been shown to reduce tPA-induced fibrinolysis half-maximally at approximately 1 nmol/L, which is well below its concentration in plasma.[90]

Plasminogen Activator Inhibitors

Plasminogen Activator Inhibitor 1

Of the two major plasminogen activator inhibitors[91] (see Table 27-1), PAI-1 is the most ubiquitous. This single-chain cysteine-less glycoprotein with an M_r of approximately 52,000 is released by endothelial cells, monocytes, macrophages, hepatocytes, adipocytes, and platelets.[92-94] Release of PAI-1 is stimulated by many cytokines, growth factors, and lipoproteins common to the global inflammatory response.[60,95-97] The PAI-1 gene consists of nine exons spanning 12.2 kb on chromosome 7q21.3-q22.[98] The serpin reactive site is located at Arg346-Met347, and activity of this labile serpin is stabilized upon complex formation with vitronectin, a component of plasma and the pericellular matrix.[99,100]

Regulation of PAI-1 gene expression is complex.[101-104] Agents that have been shown to enhance expression of PAI-1 at the message level, the protein level, or both without affecting the synthesis of tPA include the inflammatory cytokines lipopolysaccharide, interleukin-1, tumor necrosis factor α,[60,61,95,97,105-107] TGF-β and basic fibroblast growth factor,[59,95,102,104] very-low-density lipoprotein and lipoprotein(a),[108,109] angiotensin II,[110] thrombin,[106,111] and phorbol esters.[112] In addition, endothelial cell PAI-1 is downregulated by forskolin[42,51] and by endothelial cell growth factor in the presence of heparin.[113]

Plasminogen Activator Inhibitor 2

Originally purified from human placenta,[91,114] PAI-2 is a 393–amino acid member of the serpin family whose reactive site is the Arg358-Thr359 peptide bond[114] (see Table 27-1). The gene encoding PAI-2 is located on chromosome 18q21-23, spans 16.5 kb, and contains eight exons.[115] PAI-2 exists as both a nonglycosylated intracellular form with an M_r of 47,000 and a glycosylated form with an M_r of 60,000 secreted primarily by macrophages and keratinocytes. Functionally, PAI-2 inhibits both two-chain tPA and two-chain uPA with comparable efficiency (second-order rate constants of 10^5 mmol/L/sec). However, it is less effective in inhibiting single-chain tPA (second-order rate constant of 10^3 mol/L/sec) and does not inhibit prourokinase.

Significant levels of PAI-2 are found in human plasma only during pregnancy but can be markedly enhanced in vitro by the inflammatory mediator tumor necrosis factor.[116] Regulation of PAI-2 gene expression is modulated by a variety of factors, including a number of inflammatory mediators.[117-120] In macrophages in vitro, secretion of PAI-2 is enhanced by endotoxin and phorbol esters.[120,121]

Cellular Receptors in Fibrinolysis

Though structurally diverse, cell surface fibrinolytic receptors can be classified into two groups whose integrated actions are likely to be essential for homeostatic control of plasmin activity[3] (see Table 27-1). Activation receptors localize and potentiate plasminogen activation, whereas clearance receptors eliminate plasmin and plasminogen activators from the blood or focal microenvironments.

Activation Receptors

Plasminogen Receptors

Plasminogen receptors are a diverse group of proteins expressed on a wide array of cell types.[3] Receptors reported include α-enolase, glycoprotein IIb-IIIa complex, the Heymann nephritis antigen, amphoterin, and annexin A2 (A2)/p11 and have been found to be expressed primarily on monocytoid cells,[122] platelets,[123] renal epithelial cells,[124] neuroblastoma cells,[125] and endothelial cells,[126-128] respectively. These binding proteins commonly interact with the kringle structures of plasminogen through carboxyl-terminal lysine residues.

The Urokinase Receptor

uPAR is expressed on monocytes, macrophages, fibroblasts, endothelial cells, and a variety of tumor cells[3] (see Table 27-1). uPAR complementary DNA (cDNA) was cloned and sequenced from a human fibroblast cDNA library[129] and encodes a protein of 313 amino acids with a 21-residue signal peptide. The gene structure consists of seven exons distributed over 23 kb of genomic DNA, which places this glycoprotein within the Ly-1/elapid venom toxin superfamily of cysteine-rich proteins.[130-132] uPAR is anchored to the plasma membrane through glycosylphosphatidylinositol linkages.[133] uPA bound to its receptor maintains its activity and susceptibility to PAI-1.[134] Formation of uPA–PAI-1 complexes appears to hasten clearance of uPA by hepatic or monocytoid cells.[135-137]

High-resolution (1.9 to 2.7 Å) analysis of the crystal structure of a complex formed by various amino-terminal uPA peptides and a soluble form of uPAR reveals that uPA engages a central cone-shaped cavity in uPAR formed by its three-finger motif. This arrangement leaves surface residues of uPAR available for binding of other proteins such as integrins and vitronectin. It is therefore postulated that these interactions may be regulated by binding of uPA itself.[138-140]

Aside from a potential role in fibrinolysis, uPAR appears to play a novel role in cellular signaling and adhesion events.[141] uPAR binds to the adhesive glycoprotein vitronectin at a site distinct from the uPA-binding domain,[142,143] and uPAR-transfected renal epithelial cells acquire enhanced adhesion to vitronectin and lose their adhesion to fibronectin.[144] Furthermore, uPAR colocalizes with integrins in focal contacts and at the leading edge of migrating cells[145] and also associates with caveolin, a major component of caveolae, structures abundant in endothelial cells and thought to participate in signaling events.[146-148] Thus, integrin function may be regulated by uPAR, an association signifying an integrated relationship between cellular adhesion and proteolysis.

These findings have important implications for the behavior of malignant cells, in which uPAR is frequently overexpressed.[149] High-level uPAR expression also appears to be an indicator of a poor prognosis in breast, lung, colon, esophageal, and gastric cancer.[149] uPA has been identified by protease activity profiling as being important in intravasation of fibrosarcoma,[150] and RNA interference–mediated "knockdown" of uPA and uPAR seems to block the in vivo invasiveness of highly malignant cells.[150,151]

Annexin A2

A2 is a widely distributed, highly conserved, peripheral membrane protein with an M_r of 36,000 that is expressed abundantly on endothelial cells,[128,146,148,152-154] monocyte/macrophages,[155,156] myeloid cells,[157] and some tumor cells.[158-160] It belongs to a more than 60-member superfamily of calcium-dependent, phospholipid-binding proteins[161,162] that have in common a conserved carboxyl-terminal "core" region preceded by a more variable amino-terminal "tail."[163] The human A2 gene consists of 13 exons distributed over 40 kb of genomic DNA on chromosome 15 (15q21).[164]

In vitro, A2 possesses the unique property of binding both plasminogen (K_d of 114 nmol/L)[127] and tPA (K_d of 30 nmol/L),[165] but not uPA.[126] Purified native human A2 stimulates the catalytic efficiency of tPA-dependent plasminogen activation by 60-fold in the fluid phase.[166] This effect is completely inhibited in the presence of lysine analogues or upon treatment of A2 with carboxypeptidase B, an agent that removes basic carboxyl-terminal amino acids. Although it lacks a classic signal peptide, A2 is constitutively translocated to the endothelial cell surface within 16 hours of its biosynthesis, where it binds phospholipid via core repeat 2.[167] Translocation of A2 requires association with protein p11, tyrosine phosphorylation by an src-like kinase, and a stimulus such as heat stress or thrombin stimulation.[168,169] The A2 heterotetramer, composed of two annexin monomers and two p11 subunits, may have even greater stimulatory effects on tPA-dependent plasmin generation.[170]

Lipoprotein(a), an atherogenic low-density lipoprotein–like particle, competes with plasminogen for binding to A2[171,172] and reduces cell surface plasmin generation. Lipoprotein(a) contains an apoprotein called apoprotein(a) that contains kringle structures highly homologous to those of plasminogen.[27] This mechanism may contribute to atherogenesis by reducing fibrinolytic surveillance at the blood vessel wall.

Binding of tPA to A2 requires residues 8 to 13 (LCKLSL) within the amino-terminal "tail" domain of the receptor.[173] This sequence is a target for homocysteine (HC), a thiol-containing amino acid that accumulates in association with nutritional deficiencies of vitamin B_6, vitamin B_{12}, or folic acid or in inherited abnormalities of cystathionine β-synthase, methylenetetrahydrofolate reductase, or methionine synthase; it is associated with atherothrombotic disease.[174-176] In vitro, HC impairs the intrinsic fibrinolytic system of the endothelial cell by approximately 50%[177] by forming a covalent derivative with Cys9 of A2, thereby preventing its interaction with tPA.[173] The half-maximal dose of HC for inhibition of binding of tPA to A2 is approximately 11 μmol/L HC, a value close to the upper limit of normal for HC in plasma (14 μmol/L).

There is now clear evidence that A2 contributes to intravascular fibrin balance in vivo. Homozygous A2-null mice display microvascular fibrin deposition, reduced clearance of arterial thrombi, and markedly deficient microvascular endothelial cell surface plasmin generation.[178] In addition, pretreatment of the rat carotid artery with A2 prevents vessel thrombosis in response to injury.[179] Furthermore, overexpression of A2 by acute promyelocytic leukemia cells appears to correlate with the severity of the hemorrhagic state seen at initial evaluation.[157] In addition, patients with antiphospholipid syndrome and anti-A2 antibodies have a significantly higher risk for clinical thrombosis than do those who lack this antibody.[180] There is also evidence that polymorphisms in A2 may correlate with a higher incidence of vaso-occlusive stroke in patients with sickle cell disease.[181]

Clearance Receptors

Both uPA and tPA are cleared from the circulation via the liver.[182] In vitro, clearance of tPA–PAI-1 complexes also appears to be mediated by a large two-chain receptor called the low-density lipoprotein receptor–related protein (LRP).[183-185] This complex interaction requires both the growth factor and finger domains of tPA. An additional "receptor-associated protein" with an M_r of 39,000 copurifies with LRP and may regulate the binding and uptake of LRP ligands.[186] Interestingly, LRP-knockout embryos undergo developmental arrest by 13.5 days after conception, thus suggesting that regulation of serine protease activity may be crucial for early embryogenesis.[187,188] Although several PAI-1–independent clearance pathways for tPA involving the large LRP subunit,[189] the mannose receptor,[190] or an α-fucose–specific receptor[191] have been proposed, in vivo studies in mice suggest that

LRP and the mannose receptor play a dominant role in clearance of tPA.[187]

THE FIBRINOLYTIC ACTIONS OF PLASMIN

Fibrinogen

Fibrinogen possesses distinct proteolytic cleavage sites for plasmin and thrombin (Fig. 27-3). Whereas plasmin cleaves carboxyl-terminal Aα and amino-terminal fibrinopeptide B moieties, thrombin primarily releases fibrinopeptide A, which exposes the Gly-Pro-Arg tripeptide sequence and allows fibrinogen to polymerize and form insoluble fibrin[192] (see Chapter 26). Cleavage of fibrinogen (M_r of 340,000) by plasmin initially produces carboxyl-terminal fragments from the α chain within the D domain of fibrinogen (Aα fragment).[193-196] Simultaneously but more slowly, the amino-terminal segments of the β chains are cleaved, with release of a peptide containing fibrinopeptide B. The resulting molecule with an M_r of approximately 250,000 is termed fragment X and represents a clottable form of fibrinogen.

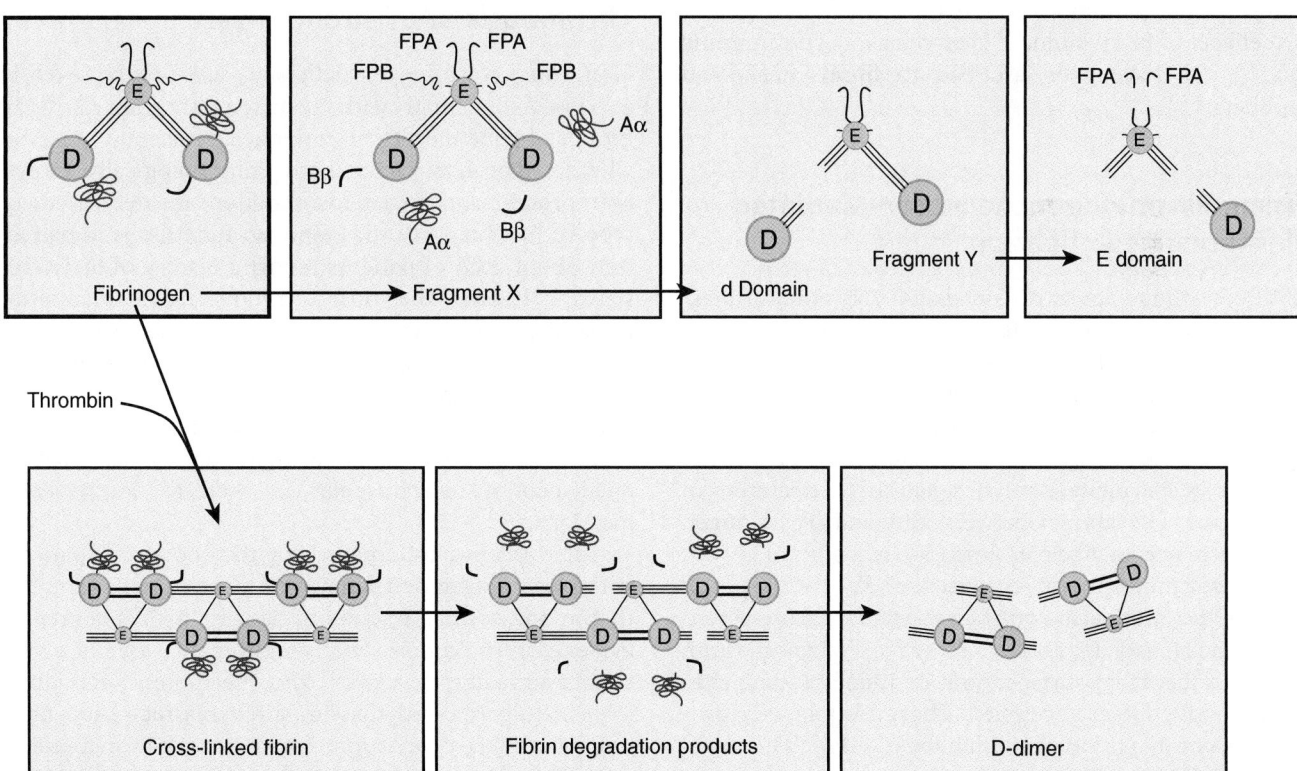

FIGURE 27-3. Degradation of fibrinogen and cross-linked fibrin by plasmin. **Top panel,** Plasmin initially cleaves the carboxyl-terminal regions of the α and β chains within the D domain of fibrinogen, thereby releasing the Aα and Bβ fragments. In addition, a fragment containing fibrinopeptide B (FPB) from the amino-terminal region of the β chain is released, with the intermediate fragment known as fragment X being produced. Subsequently, plasmin cleaves the three polypeptide chains connecting the D and E domains, which produces fragments D, E, and Y. **Bottom panel,** Fibrinogen can also be polymerized by thrombin to form fibrin. When degrading cross-linked fibrin, plasmin initially cleaves the carboxyl-terminal region of the α and β chains within the D domain. Subsequently, some of the connecting regions between the D and E domains are severed. Fibrin is ultimately solubilized upon hydrolysis of additional peptide bonds within the central portions of the coiled-coil connectors and gives rise to fibrin degradation products such as D-dimer.

Additional cleavage events may release the Bβ fragment from the carboxyl-terminal of the β chain, and in a series of subsequent reactions, plasmin cleaves the three polypeptide chains that connect the D and E domains to produce a free D domain (M_r of ≈100,000) plus the binodular D-E fragment known as fragment Y (M_r of ≈150,000). Finally, domains D and E are separated from each other, and some of the amino-terminal fibrinopeptide A sites on domain E are also modified. Although fragment X can be converted to fibrin by thrombin, the fragments Y, D, and E are all nonclottable and may in fact inhibit the spontaneous polymerization of fibrinogen.[197]

Fibrin

Degradation of fibrin by plasmin leads to a distinct set of molecular products.[198] Species similar to fragments Y, D, and E but lacking fibrinopeptide sites are released from non–cross-linked fibrin. If fibrin has been extensively cross-linked by factor XIII, however, the resulting D fragments are cross-linked to an E domain fragment. An assay of cross-linked D-dimer fragments is used clinically to identify disseminated intravascular coagulation–like states associated with excessive plasmin-mediated fibrinolysis. Several biologic activities, including inhibition of platelet function,[199] potentiation of the hypotensive effects of bradykinin,[200] chemotaxis,[201] and immune modulation, have been ascribed to fibrin breakdown products.[202]

Tissue Plasminogen Activator–Mediated Plasminogen Activation

With or without fibrin, tPA-mediated activation of plasminogen follows Michaelis-Menten kinetics.[22] In the absence of fibrin, tPA is a weak activator of plasminogen. However, in the presence of fibrin, the catalytic efficiency (k_{cat}/K_m) of tPA-dependent plasminogen activation is enhanced by at least 2 orders of magnitude. This is the basis for its specificity as a lytic agent in the treatment of thrombosis. The affinity between tPA and plasminogen in the absence of fibrin is low (K_m of 65 μmol/L) but increases significantly in its presence (K_m of 0.16 μmol/L), even though the catalytic rate constant remains essentially unchanged (k_{cat} of ≈0.05 sec^{-1}). When plasmin forms on the fibrin surface, both its lysine binding sites and its active site are occupied. Thus, it is relatively protected from its physiologic inhibitor α_2-AP.[203] The interaction of tPA with fibrin is probably initiated by its finger domain. However, once fibrin is modified by plasmin, carboxyl-terminal lysine residues are generated, and these residues become binding sites for kringle 2 of tPA and kringles 1 and 4 of plasminogen.[204] Therefore, fibrin accelerates its own destruction by (1) enhancing the catalytic efficiency of plasmin formation by tPA, (2) protecting plasmin from its physiologic inhibitor α_2-AP, and (3)

providing new binding sites for plasminogen and tPA once its degradation has begun.

Urokinase-Mediated Plasmin Generation

For activation of Glu-Plg by uPA in a fibrin-free system, reported K_m values vary from 1.4 to 200 μmol/L, whereas k_{cat} values range from 0.26 to 1.48 sec^{-1}. Interestingly, activation of Glu-Plg by two-chain uPA is increased in the presence of fibrin by about 10-fold even though uPA does not bind to fibrin.[205] In contrast, single-chain uPA has considerable fibrin specificity. This may reflect neutralization by fibrin of components in plasma that impair plasminogen activation.[206] It may also reflect a conformational change in plasminogen upon binding to fibrin.[207] It is important to recognize, however, that the intrinsic plasminogen-activating potential of single-chain uPA is less than 1% that of two-chain uPA. Two-chain uPA has been used effectively as a thrombolytic agent for many years.[208]

PHYSIOLOGIC FUNCTIONS OF THE FIBRINOLYTIC SYSTEM

Thrombosis and Thrombolysis

Congenital plasminogen deficiency was first reported in a 31-year-old man with recurrent thrombosis.[209] In groups of patients with plasminogen deficiency, however, whether type I, in which both immunologically detectable protein and enzymatic function are decreased, or type II, in which just plasminogen function is impaired, only about 25% of patients report a history of thrombosis.[210-212] Indeed, the most common clinical manifestations of plasminogen deficiency, occurring in 80% and 34% of patients, respectively, are ligneous conjunctivitis and ligneous gingivitis, disorders characterized by the deposition of fibrin-rich pseudomembranes on mucosal surfaces.[213] These findings strongly suggest that plasminogen acts in extravascular as well as intravascular locations.[214-216]

The relative infrequency of thrombosis in patients with plasminogen deficiency may, in part, reflect the fact that in only a small fraction of patients with sonographic evidence of thrombosis does symptomatic vascular occlusion eventually develop.[217] Furthermore, although a recent study showed that impaired plasma-based fibrinolysis conferred an approximately twofold increase in the risk for deep venous thrombosis,[218] the prevalence of plasminogen deficiency in consecutive patients with thrombophilia was only 1.9%.[219] Together, these data suggest that measurement of plasma plasminogen, tPA, or PAI-1 in patients with thrombophilia is likely to be a low-yield procedure[220,221] and that the physiologic roles of plasmin and plasminogen may be much broader than originally thought.

Although congenital deficiencies of plasminogen activators (tPA and uPA) have not been linked specifically to thrombophilia in humans,[220] elevated levels of fibrinolytic inhibitors appear to increase the risk for thrombosis. Increased levels of PAI-1 were prevalent in young survivors of myocardial infarction,[222] and TAFI levels above the 90th percentile in a case-control study approximately doubled the risk for venous thrombosis.[223] As one might expect, congenital deficiency of either α_2-AP or PAI-1 is generally associated with delayed rebleeding at sites of trauma or wound healing.[224,225] To date, no human disorders reflecting primary deficiencies of fibrinolytic receptors have been reported.

In general, analyses of genetically engineered mice support the hypothesis that the fibrinolytic system functions to regulate fibrin balance in both the intravascular and extravascular compartments (Table 27-2). That fibrinogen is central to hemostasis is underscored by findings of postnatal bleeding at multiple sites in fibrinogen-null mice,[226] similar to that seen in human patients with afibrinogenemia. Similarly, although mice deficient in plasminogen have normal embryogenesis, survive to adulthood, and can sire offspring, they display significant runting, spontaneous thrombi develop in multiple tissues, and extravascular fibrin accumulates in the liver (see Table 27-2).[227,228] Ulcerative lesions are observed in the gastrointestinal tract, particularly the rectum, where prolapse is also seen. Plg$^{-/-}$ mice also clear induced thrombi much less readily than wild-type mice do,[229] and this defect is reversed by bolus injection of exogenous plasminogen.[230] Because the spontaneous thrombosis observed in plasminogen-deficient mice is completely reversed when fibrinogen is also deleted, it is clear that the thrombosis observed in plasminogen deficiency is related to failure of intravascular fibrin clearance.[231] Plasminogen-deficient mice also display ligneous conjunctivitis, a disorder similar to that observed in humans with plasminogen deficiency.[232]

Because no examples of complete deficiency of tPA or uPA have been documented in humans, the most compelling evidence for their role in fibrin balance derives from gene-knockout experiments in the mouse (see Table 27-2).[233] Both uPA- and tPA-null mice exhibit normal fertility and embryonic development. Although little spontaneous thrombosis is seen in either genotype, uPA$^{-/-}$ mice exhibit occasional fibrin deposition and tPA-deficient mice display impaired lysis of artificially induced pulmonary thrombi. In contrast, doubly deficient (tPA$^{-/-}$, uPA$^{-/-}$) mice exhibit extensive spontaneous fibrin accumulation in multiple organs, rectal prolapse, runting, and cachexia, all reminiscent of the phenotype seen in Plg$^{-/-}$ mice. These findings demonstrate that tPA and uPA are not essential for normal embryologic development, but they do play crucial roles in the activation of plasminogen, in the lysis of spontaneous and induced thrombi, and in fibrinolytic surveillance.

Although complete PAI-1 deficiency in humans is associated with a moderately severe bleeding tendency,[224]

mice deficient in PAI-1 exhibit normal development, survival, and fertility, with no evidence of spontaneous hemorrhage[234] (see Table 27-2). PAI-1–deficient mice do, however, exhibit resistance to thrombosis after injury[235] and enhanced sensitivity to thrombolytic therapy.[236] On the other hand, in transgenic mice that overexpress human PAI-1, a dramatic vascular occlusive process develops in the tail and hind limbs.[237] This finding may be due to unique effects of human PAI-1 in the mouse in that mice overexpressing murine PAI-1 do not exhibit this abnormality.[238]

Deficiency of α_2-AP, the major serpin directly blocking plasmin activity, is a rare cause of bleeding disorder in humans.[239] Although no overt bleeding is seen in α_2-AP–deficient mice, increased lysis of artificially induced thrombi has been reported.[240] PAI-2–deficient mice exhibit no obvious phenotype even when PAI-1 is also absent in doubly deficient animals.[241] Complete TAFI deficiency in mice is fully compatible with life and does not appear to alter the response to vascular injury, artificially induced thrombosis, or endotoxin-induced disseminated intravascular coagulation.[242]

Mice transgenic for the catalytically inactive plasminogen analogue apolipoprotein(a) are subject to atherosclerosis and resistant to tPA-induced lysis of experimental pulmonary emboli.[243] The accelerated atherosclerosis observed in these mice is blunted under conditions of concomitant fibrinogen deficiency.[244] These data suggest that apolipoprotein(a)-associated atherosclerosis may be rooted in functional plasminogen deficiency and accumulation of intravascular fibrin.

Whereas complete deficiency of uPAR is associated with normal lysis of intravenously injected plasma clots in mice,[245] A2-deficient mice have impaired lysis of experimentally induced thrombi, and fibrin accumulates in both intravascular and extravascular locations.[178] In addition, A2-deficient microvascular endothelial cells lack tPA cofactor activity and migrate slowly through fibrin and collagen matrices. Interestingly, A2-deficient mice also display significant impairment of postnatal angiogenesis in a variety of experimental models.

Wound Healing and Tissue Fibrosis

As discussed earlier, extravascular fibrin deposition is a hallmark of plasminogen deficiency in both mice and humans.[227,228] Plasminogen-deficient mice, as well as uPA$^{-/-}$/tPA$^{-/-}$ but not uPAR$^{-/-}$/tPA$^{-/-}$ mice, also exhibit defective wound healing characterized by impaired keratinocyte migration despite abundant neovascularization and granulation tissue within experimental wounds.[246,247] Although fibrinogen-deficient mice exhibit subtle histologic defects in wound repair,[248] the impaired healing in plasminogen-deficient mice disappears when fibrinogen is also absent.[231] Consistent with the hypothesis that plasmin is necessary for clearance of extravascular fibrin, deficiency of either PAI-1 or α_2-AP in mice is associated with accelerated cutaneous wound healing.[249,250] In

TABLE 27-2 Fibrinolytic Gene Deletion Models

Genotype	PLASMINOGEN AND FIBRIN			PLASMINOGEN ACTIVATORS			RECEPTORS		INHIBITORS			
	Plg⁻/⁻	FgnA⁻/⁻	Plg⁻/⁻ FgnA⁻/⁻	tPA⁻/⁻	uPA⁻/⁻	tPA⁻/⁻ uPA⁻/⁻	A2⁻/⁻	uPAR⁻/⁻	PAI-1⁻/⁻	PAI-2⁻/⁻	α₂-AP⁻/⁻	TAFI⁻/⁻
GENERAL CONSEQUENCES												
Development	nl	nl	nl	nl	nl	nl	nl	nl	nl	nl	nl	nl
Fertility	♀→	♀→	♀→	nl	nl	nl	nl→	nl	nl	nl	nl	nl
Physical growth	→	nl	nl	nl	nl	→	nl	nl	nl	nl	nl	nl
Survival	→	↓/nl	nl	nl	nl	→	nl	nl	nl	nl	nl	nl
HEMOSTASIS AND THROMBOSIS												
Spontaneous thrombosis	+	–	–	–	–	+	+	–	–	–	–	–
Induced thrombosis	ND	–	ND	→	→	←	ND	ND	→	ND	→	nl
Lysis of artificial thrombi	‡	ND	ND	–	+	‡	‡	–	–	–	←	ND
Fibrin deposition	‡	–	–	–	+	‡	–	–	–	–	–	–
Spontaneous hemorrhage	–	‡	+	–	–	–	–	–	–	–	–	–
WOUND HEALING AND FIBROSIS												
Cutaneous wound healing	→	→	→	nl	nl	→	ND	nl	←	nl	←	nl→
Bleomycin-induced pulmonary fibrosis	←	nl	←	←	←	ND	ND	nl	→	ND	ND	
ATHEROSCLEROSIS AND CARDIOVASCULAR REMODELING												
Apolipoprotein E induced	←	nl							↓/nl			
Transplant induced	→								→			
Neointima formation	→			nl	→			nl				
Aneurysm	→			nl	→	→		nl				
TUMOR BIOLOGY												
Lewis lung carcinoma metastasis	nl											nl
Polyoma middle T mammary metastasis	→	→		nl	→	→						nl
Cutaneous sarcoma					→				→			
Metastatic melanoma implantation	nl	→			→				nl			nl
MICROBIAL VIRULENCE												
Borrelia burgdorferi	→											
Group A streptococci	→											
Yersinia pestis	→	←										

For references, see text.

A2, annexin A2; α₂-AP, α₂-antiplasmin; FgnA, fibrinogen A; nl, normal; PAI-1, plasminogen activator inhibitor 1; PAI-2, plasminogen activator inhibitor 2; Plg, plasminogen; TAFI, thrombin-activatable fibrinolysis inhibitor; uPA, urokinase; uPAR, urokinase receptor.

addition, sciatic nerve regeneration after crush injury also appears to require tPA/plasmin-mediated clearance of fibrin to protect against axonal degeneration and demyelination.[251] Surprisingly, TAFI deficiency seems to be associated with impaired, rather than accelerated healing of cutaneous wounds.[252]

Although extravascular fibrin commonly forms in response to injury, its exact role in tissue fibrosis is unclear. In a well-established model of bleomycin-induced pulmonary fibrosis, plasminogen[-/-], tPA[-/-], and uPA[-/-] mice but neither uPAR[-/-] nor fibrinogen[-/-] mice have increased deposition of both fibrin and collagen after injury.[253-255] Similarly, PAI-1–deficient mice exhibit less bleomycin-induced pulmonary fibrosis than wild-type animals do.[256] Surprisingly, however, fibrin does not seem to be a prerequisite for the induction of pulmonary fibrosis in this model because mice deficient in fibrinogen were susceptible to fibrosis to the same degree as wild-type animals.[256] Thus, the mechanism by which fibrinolytic proteins regulate fibrosis may relate to modulation of adhesive interactions that promote leukocyte adherence rather than plasmin catalytic activity.

Atherosclerosis and Cardiovascular Remodeling

Atherosclerosis is thought to represent a response to vascular injury that leads to atheromatous plaque formation and vascular remodeling.[257] In the setting of apolipoprotein E deficiency, simultaneous plasminogen deficiency accelerates vessel wall disease.[258] In this model, fibrin is not strictly required for the development of atherosclerotic lesions, thus suggesting that the role of plasmin may relate to its ability to remove one or more nonfibrin substrates.[259] Interestingly, although plasminogen deficiency accelerates hyperlipidemic atherosclerosis, the same mice are relatively resistant to transplant-associated atherosclerosis.[260]

Plasmin appears to promote the pathologic response to vascular and myocardial injury.[261] After induction of myocardial infarction in plasminogen-null mice, myocardial healing was markedly inhibited inasmuch as inflammatory cells failed to appear at the wound site, necrotic cardiomyocytes failed to disappear, and granulation and fibrous tissue failed to develop.[262] Similarly, healing of electrically injured femoral arteries, arteries treated with a flexible cuff, or arteries undergoing guidewire endothelial denudation was impaired in plasminogen-null mice, with reduced infiltration of inflammatory and smooth muscle cells and decreased neointima formation.[229,263,264] All these processes require cellular migration, which may entail plasmin-dependent matrix remodeling through activation of downstream matrix metalloproteinase 1 (MMP-1) and MMP-3.[265-267]

Plasmin may play a role in the activation of growth factors and in the proliferative response to blood vessel injury. Macrophages cultured on labeled matrices release both basic fibroblast growth factor and TGF-β into the medium in a plasminogen-dependent fashion.[268] TGF-β, a homodimeric polypeptide with an M_r of 25,000 whose effects on vascular cell growth and differentiation are pleiomorphic,[269] also appears to be converted from a latent to an active form by cell-associated plasmin. The latter process can be blocked by the presence of plasmin inhibitors such as aprotinin or α₂-AP and appears to involve alteration of its tertiary structure upon cleavage of an amino-terminal glycopeptide.[270]

uPA but neither tPA nor uPAR appears to be required for vascular cell migration and pericellular plasmin formation in some injured vessels.[271,272] uPA appears to mediate the activation of MMPs in both atherosclerotic aortic aneurysm[273] and postinfarction cardiac rupture,[274] presumably through its activation of plasmin rather than direct cleavage of pro-MMPs. Together, these data suggest a unique role for uPA in postinjury vascular remodeling.

Tumor Biology

Tumor cells may use the fibrinolytic system for local invasion and metastasis. Although plasminogen-deficient mice display normal growth of both primary and metastatic tumors in the Lewis lung carcinoma model,[275] pulmonary metastases from a polyoma middle T antigen–induced mammary cancer were significantly reduced in plasminogen-null animals.[276] Fibrinogen-null mice exhibited normal growth of implanted Lewis lung carcinoma, whereas lymph node and hematogenous lung metastases were markedly reduced in both Lewis lung carcinoma and melanoma.[277,278] These data suggest that plasmin-mediated fibrin clearance is required for tumor cell invasion and metastasis in these specific settings.

Analysis of tumor behavior in mice with genetic alterations in other components of the fibrinolytic system has produced a spectrum of results. uPA-deficient mice displayed markedly diminished murine sarcoma cell proliferation and tumor-associated angiogenesis when compared with wild-type animals.[279] These mice also failed to support local progression of cutaneous melanoma,[280] as well as polyoma middle T antigen–induced vascular tumors.[281] The absence of TAFI, on the other hand, does not appear to alter the progression of primary Lewis lung carcinoma, B16 melanoma, or T241 sarcoma tumors or their metastases.[282]

PAI-1 has a surprising stimulatory effect on the growth and invasiveness of murine tumors derived from malignant keratinocytes. In PAI-1–deficient mice, these tumors are subject to loss of local invasion and tumor vascularity,[283] thus suggesting that PAI-1 may play an adhesive rather than an anticatalytic role in this system. Similarly, murine fibrosarcoma cells implanted in PAI-1[-/-] mice display reduced tumor cell proliferation and neovascularization.[279] On the other hand, neither tumor cell burden nor overall host survival were affected by the absence of PAI-1 in a murine model of metastatic melanoma.[238] Thus, the precise role of PAI-1 in tumor biology may depend critically on the specific context.

Microbial Virulence and Host Defense Mechanisms

There is increasing evidence that pathogenic bacteria can usurp elements of the host fibrinolytic system to enhance their own virulence.[284,285] In Lyme disease, for example, dissemination of *Borrelia burgdorferi* in both the tick vector and the mammalian host requires that the spirochete bind host plasminogen and use host plasminogen activator.[286] Similarly, *Borrelia* species use host plasminogen for heart and brain invasion in relapsing fever.[287] Plasminogen-deficient mice also appear to be remarkably resistant to *Yersinia pestis*, whose own plasminogen activator (Pla) is required for the rapid progression of primary pneumonic plague.[287-289] Expression of human plasminogen in mice overrides their natural resistance to invasive infection with group A β-hemolytic streptococci.[290]

Components of the fibrinolytic system are required for the recruitment of host cells to sites of inflammation. In plasminogen-null mice, for example, the influx of neutrophils to the peritoneum in response to thioglycolate is normal, whereas recruitment of lymphocytes and monocytes is significantly impaired.[291] In the murine lung, similarly, recruitment of phagocytes and lymphocytes in response to *Cryptococcus neoformans*[292] and *Pneumocystis carinii*[293] requires uPA. Recruitment of neutrophils in response to *Pseudomonas aeruginosa*, on the other hand, depends on uPAR but not on uPA, thus suggesting a nonfibrinolytic, possibly adhesive role for this receptor.[294]

Neurologic Plasticity

tPA appears to play a relatively unique role in modulating plasticity and cell death within the central nervous system. tPA, which is stored within neuronal cells, is released upon calcium-mediated membrane depolarization[295] and participates in the immediate early response after electrical or pharmacologic stimulation of hippocampal neurons.[295,296] tPA expression is induced in Purkinje neurons after cerebellar motor learning,[297] and excessive tPA-related proteolytic activity in granule neurons may contribute to neuronal death in the weaver mouse cerebellum.[298] tPA-deficient mice do not display discernible motor or sensory deficiencies but do exhibit a mild defect in long-term potentiation.[299,300] These animals are resistant to excitotoxic neuronal degeneration in the hippocampus, in which plasmin-catalyzed degradation of laminin is blocked both by tPA deficiency and by infusion of a plasmin inhibitor.[301]

Neuronal migration within the cerebellum of the developing mouse brain is reduced by approximately 50% in tPA-deficient mice,[302] and these animals exhibit increased sensitivity to the locomotor effects of cocaine.[303]

During the remodeling of neuronal connections that occurs in response to seizure activity in the hippocampus, mice lacking either tPA or plasminogen show decreased mossy fiber outgrowth in this region and accumulate an extracellular matrix component known as DSD-1-PG/phosphacan. These data suggest both plasmin-dependent and plasmin-independent roles for tPA in neuronal plasticity.[304]

In both ischemic and hemorrhagic stroke, infusion of tPA can have a major effect on clinical outcome. After ischemic stroke in mice, tPA increases infarct size in both wild-type and tPA-null animals,[305] and smaller infarcts are observed in untreated tPA-deficient animals than in uPA-deficient or wild-type mice. Interestingly, the largest infarcts in the latter study were found in PAI-1[-/-] mice.[306] In a thrombotic stroke model, on the other hand, deficiency of tPA leads to more extensive vascular fibrin deposition and cerebrovascular thrombosis and consequently a sixfold to eightfold increase in infarct volume.[307]

Engagement of LRP by the tPA–PAI-1 complex may regulate the vascular response to injury by triggering NF-κB–mediated release and activation of MMP-9, which may lead to weakening of the blood-brain barrier and catastrophic hemorrhage. In a mouse model, this process was inhibited by concomitant infusion of activated protein C, which by interacting with endothelial protein C receptor or protease activated receptor 1, or both, blocked the activation of NF-κB and hence release of metalloproteinase.[308] Together, these data suggest that the actions of tPA in the central nervous system extend beyond the activation of plasmin.

NON–PLASMIN-MEDIATED FIBRINOLYSIS

There is accumulating evidence that proteases other than the traditional members of the fibrinolytic family may participate in fibrinolysis. Fibrin appears to be subject to degradation by activated monocytoid cells that express cathepsins.[309] In addition, MMP-3, MMP-7, and membrane type 1 MMP may cleave fibrinogen and cross-linked fibrin into fragments similar to those produced by plasmin.[310] Matrix MMPs have been shown to act as pericellular fibrinolysins, thereby providing an alternative pathway for fibrin-based angiogenesis in a plasminogen-free milieu.[311] In particular, membrane-type matrix MMPs appear to function in this way within a three-dimensional fibrin meshwork.[312]

REFERENCES

1. Hajjar KA, Francis CW. Fibrinolysis and thrombolysis. In Lichtman MA, Beutler E, Kipps TJ, et al (eds). Williams Hematology. New York, McGraw-Hill, 2006, pp 2089-2115.
2. Hajjar KA, Nachman RL. The human endothelial cell plasmin-generating system. In Colman RW, Marder VJ,

Clowes AW, et al (eds). Hemostasis and Thrombosis. Philadelphia, Lippincott Williams & Wilkins, 2006, pp 409-418.

3. Hajjar KA. Vascular biology. In Young NS, Gerson SL, High KA (eds). Clinical Hematology. Philadelphia, Mosby Elsevier, 2006, pp 123-133.

4. Bohmfalk J, Fuller G. Plasminogen is synthesized by primary cultures of rat hepatocytes. Science. 1980;209: 408-410.

5. Raum D, Marcus D, Alper CA, et al. Synthesis of human plasminogen by the liver. Science. 1980;208:1036-1037.

6. Castellino FJ. Biochemistry of human plasminogen. Semin Thromb Hemost. 1984;10:18-23.

7. Collen D, Tytgat G, Claeys H, et al. Metabolism of plasminogen in healthy subjects: effect of tranexamic acid. J Clin Invest. 1972;51:1310-1318.

8. Forsgren M, Raden B, Israelsson M, et al. Molecular cloning and characterization of a full-length cDNA clone for human plasminogen. FEBS Lett. 1987;213:254-260.

9. Miles LA, Dahlberg CM, Plow EF. The cell-binding domains of plasminogen and their function in plasma. J Biol Chem. 1988;263:11928-11934.

10. Hajjar KA, Harpel PC, Jaffe EA, Nachman RL. Binding of plasminogen to cultured human endothelial cells. J Biol Chem. 1986;261:11656-11662.

11. Markus G, De Pasquale JL, Wissler FC. Quantitative determination of the binding of epsilon-aminocaproic acid to native plasminogen. J Biol Chem. 1978;253: 727-732.

12. Markus G, Priore RL, Wissler FC. The binding of tranexamic acid to native (glu) and modified (lys) human plasminogen and its effect on conformation. J Biol Chem. 1979;254:1211-1216.

13. Miles LA, Plow EF. Cellular regulation of fibrinolysis. Thromb Haemost. 1991;66:32-36.

14. Rakoczi I, Wiman B, Collen D. On the biologic significance of the specific interaction between fibrin, plasminogen, and antiplasmin. Biochim Biophys Acta. 1978;540: 295-300.

15. Hayes ML, Castellino FJ. Carbohydrate of the human plasminogen variants. I. Carbohydrate composition, glycopeptide isolation, and characterization. J Biol Chem. 1979;254:8768-8771.

16. Hayes ML, Castellino FJ. Carbohydrate composition of the human plasminogen variants. II. Structure of the asparagine-linked oligosaccharide unit. J Biol Chem. 1979;254:8772-8776.

17. Hayes ML, Castellino FJ. Carbohydrate of the human plasminogen variants. III. Structure of the O-glycosidically-linked oligosaccharide unit. J Biol Chem. 1979;254: 8777-8780.

18. Holvoet P, Lijnen HR, Collen D. A monoclonal antibody specific for lys-plasminogen. J Biol Chem. 1985;260: 12106-12111.

19. Saksela O. Plasminogen activation and regulation of proteolysis. Biochim Biophys Acta. 1985;823:35-65.

20. Wallen P, Wiman B. Characterization of human plasminogen. I. On the relationship between different molecular forms of plasminogen demonstrated in plasma and found in purified preparations. Biochim Biophys Acta. 1970;221: 20-30.

21. Wallen P, Wiman B. Characterization of human plasminogen. II. Separation and partial characterization of different

molecular forms of human plasminogen. Biochim Biophys Acta. 1972;157:122-134.

22. Hoylaerts M, Rijken DC, Lijnen HR, Collen D. Kinetics of the activation of plasminogen by human tissue plasminogen activator: role of fibrin. J Biol Chem. 1982;257: 2912-2929.

23. Hajjar KA, Nachman RL. Endothelial cell–mediated conversion of glu-plasminogen to lys-plasminogen: further evidence for assembly of the fibrinolytic system on the endothelial cell surface. J Clin Invest. 1988;82:1769-1778.

24. Murray JC, Buetow KH, Donovan M, et al. Linkage disequilibrium of plasminogen polymorphisms and assignment of the gene to human chromosome 6q26-6q27. Am J Hum Genet. 1987;40:338-350.

25. Petersen TE, Martzen MR, Ichinose A, Davie EW. Characterization of the gene for human plasminogen, a key proenzyme in the fibrinolytic system. J Biol Chem. 1990;265:6104-6111.

26. Jenkins GR, Seiffert D, Parmer RJ, Miles LA. Regulation of plasminogen gene expression by interleukin-6. Blood. 1997;89:2394-2403.

27. McLean JW, Tomlinson JE, Kuang WJ, et al. cDNA sequence of human apolipoprotein(a) is homologous to plasminogen. Nature. 1987;330:132-137.

28. Byrne CD, Schwartz K, Meer K, et al. The human apolipoprotein(a)/plasminogen gene cluster contains a novel homologue transcribed in liver. Arterioscler Thromb. 1994;14:534-541.

29. Ichinose A. Multiple members of the plasminogen-apolipoprotein(a) gene family associated with thrombosis. Biochemistry. 1992;31:3113-3118.

30. Nakamura T, Nishizawa T, Hagiya M, et al. Molecular cloning and expression of human hepatocyte growth factor. Nature. 1989;342:440-443.

31. Weissbach L, Treadwell BV. A plasminogen-related gene is expressed in cancer cells. Biochem Biophys Res Commun. 1992;186:1108-1114.

32. Yoshimura T, Yuhki N, Wang MH, et al. Cloning, sequencing, and expression of human macrophage stimulating protein (MSP, MST 1) confirms MSP as a member of the family of kringle proteins and locates the MSP gene on chromosome 3. J Biol Chem. 1993;268:15461-15468.

33. Pennica D, Holmes WE, Kohr WJ, et al. Cloning and expression of human tissue-type plasminogen activator cDNA in E. coli. Nature. 1983;301:214-221.

34. Tate KM, Higgins DL, Holmes WE, et al. Functional role of proteolytic cleavage at arginine-275 of human tissue plasminogen activator as assessed by site-directed mutagenesis. Biochemistry. 1987;26:338-343.

35. Pohl G, Kenne L, Nilsson B, Einarsson M. Isolation and characterization of three different carbohydrate chains from melanoma tissue type plasminogen activator. Eur J Biochem. 1987;170:69-75.

36. Spellman MW, Basa LJ, Leonard CK, Chakel JA. Carbohydrate structures of tissue plasminogen activator expressed in Chinese hamster ovary cells. J Biol Chem. 1989;264:14100-14111.

37. Harris RJ, Leonard CK, Guzzetta AW. Tissue plasminogen activator has an O-linked fucose attached to threonine-61 in the epidermal growth factor domain. Biochemistry. 1991;30:2311-2314.

38. Browne MJ, Tyrrell AWR, Chapman CG, et al. Isolation of a human tissue-type plasminogen activator genomic clone and its expression in mouse L cells. Gene. 1985;33:279-284.

39. Degen SJF, Rajput B, Reich E. The human tissue plasminogen activator gene. J Biol Chem. 1986;261:6872-6885.

40. Ny T, Elgh F, Lund B. Structure of the human tissue-type plasminogen activator gene: correlation of intron and exon structures to functional and structural domains. Proc Natl Acad Sci U S A. 1984;81:5355-5359.

41. Van Zonnefeld A-J, Veerman H, Pannekoek H. Autonomous functions of structural domains on human tissue-type plasminogen activator. Proc Natl Acad Sci U S A. 1986;83:4670-4674.

42. Feng P, Ohlsson M, Ny T. The structure of the TATA-less rat tissue-type plasminogen activator gene. J Biol Chem. 1990;265:2022-2027.

43. Kooistra T, Bosma PJ, Toet K, et al. Role of protein kinase C and cyclic adenosine monophosphate in the regulation of tissue-type plasminogen activator, plasminogen activator inhibitor-1, and platelet-derived growth factor mRNA levels in human endothelial cells. Possible involvement of proto-oncogenes c-jun and c-fos. Arterioscler Thromb. 1991;11:1042-1052.

44. Medcalf RL, Ruegg M, Schleuning WD. A DNA motif related to the cAMP-responsive element and an exon-located activator protein-2 binding site in the human tissue-type plasminogen activator gene promoter cooperate in basal expression and convey activation by phorbol ester and cAMP. J Biol Chem. 1990;265:14618-14626.

45. Diamond SL, Eskin SG, McIntire LV. Fluid flow stimulates tissue plasminogen activator secretion by cultured human endothelial cells. Science. 1989;243:1483-1485.

46. Hanss M, Collen D. Secretion of tissue-type plasminogen activator and plasminogen activator inhibitor by cultured human endothelial cells: modulation by thrombin, endotoxin, and histamine. J Lab Clin Med. 1987;109:97-104.

47. Kooistra T, Van den Berg J, Tons A, et al. Butyrate stimulates tissue type plasminogen activator synthesis in cultured human endothelial cells. Biochem J. 1987;247:605-612.

48. Kooistra T, Opdenberg JP, Toet K, et al. Stimulation of tissue-type plasminogen activator synthesis by retinoids in cultured human endothelial cells and rat tissue in vivo. Thromb Haemost. 1991;65:565-572.

49. Medcalf RL, Van den Berg E, Schleuning WD. Glucocorticoid-modulated gene expression of tissue- and urinary-type plasminogen activator and plasminogen activator inhibitor-1 and 2. J Cell Biol. 1988;106:971-978.

50. Thompson EA, Nelles L, Collen D. Effect of retinoic acid on the synthesis of tissue-type plasminogen activator and plasminogen activator inhibitor 1 in human endothelial cells. Eur J Biochem. 1991;201:627-632.

51. Santell L, Levin EG. Cyclic AMP potentiates phorbol ester stimulation of tissue plasminogen activator release and inhibits secretion of plasminogen activator inhibitor-1 from human endothelial cells. J Biol Chem. 1988;263:16802-16808.

52. Dichek D, Quertermous T. Thrombin regulation of mRNA levels of tissue plasminogen activator inhibitor-1 in cultured human umbilical vein endothelial cells. Blood. 1989;74:222-228.

53. Levin EG, Marotti KR, Santell L. Protein kinase C and the stimulation of tissue plasminogen activator release from human endothelial cells. J Biol Chem. 1989;264:16030-16036.

54. Kasai S, Arimura H, Nishida M, Suyama T. Primary structure of single-chain pro-urokinase. J Biol Chem. 1985;260:12382-12389.

55. Gunzler WA, Steffens GJ, Otting F, et al. Structural relationship between high and low molecular mass urokinase. Physiol Chem. 1982;363:133-141.

56. Holmes WE, Pennica D, Blaber M, et al. Cloning and expression of the gene for pro-urokinase in *Escherichia coli*. Biotechnology. 1985;3:923-929.

57. Riccio A, Grimaldi G, Verde P, et al. The human urokinase-plasminogen activator gene and its promoter. Nucleic Acids Res. 1985;13:2759-2771.

58. Schmitt M, Wilhelm O, Janicke F, et al. Urokinase-type plasminogen activator (uPA) and its receptor (CD87): a new target in tumor invasion and metastasis. J Obstet Gynaecol. 1995;21:151-165.

59. Gerwin BI, Keski-Oja J, Seddon M, et al. TGF beta 1 modulation of urokinase and PAI-1 expression in human bronchial epithelial cells. Am J Pathol. 1990;259:262-269.

60. Medina R, Socher SH, Han JH, Friedman PA. Interleukin-1, endotoxin, or tumor necrosis factor/cachectin enhance the level of plasminogen activator inhibitor messenger RNA in bovine aortic endothelial cells. Thromb Res. 1989;54:41-52.

61. Van Hinsbergh VWM, Van den Berg EA, Fiers W, Dooijewaard G. Tumor necrosis factor induces the production of urokinase-type plasminogen activator by human endothelial cells. Blood. 1990;75:1991-1998.

62. Steffens GJ, Gunzler WA, Olting F, et al. The complete amino acid sequence of low molecular mass urokinase from human urine. Physiol Chem. 1982;363:1043-1058.

63. Stump DC, Lijnen HR, Collen D. Purification and characterization of a novel low molecular weight form of single-chain urokinase-type plasminogen activator. J Biol Chem. 1986;261:17120-17126.

64. Gurewich V, Pannell R, Louie S, et al. Effective and fibrin-specific clot lysis by a zymogen precursor from urokinase (pro-urokinase). A study in vitro and in two animal species. J Clin Invest. 1984;73:1731-1739.

65. Lijnen HR, Zamarron C, Blaber M, et al. Activation of plasminogen by pro-urokinase. J Biol Chem. 1986;261:1253-1258.

66. Lijnen HR, Van Hoef B, DeCock F, Collen D. The mechanism of plasminogen activation and fibrin dissolution by single chain urokinase-type plasminogen activator in a plasma milieu in vitro. Blood. 1989;73:1864-1872.

67. Petersen LC, Lund LR, Nielsen LS, et al. One-chain urokinase-type plasminogen activator from human sarcoma cells is a precursor with little or no intrinsic activity. J Biol Chem. 1988;263:11189-11195.

68. Colman RW. Activation of plasminogen by human plasma kallikrein. Biochem Biophys Res Commun. 1968;35:273-279.

69. Goldsmith GH, Saito H, Ratnoff OD. The activation of plasminogen by Hageman factor (factor XII) and

Hageman factor fragments. J Clin Invest. 1978;62: 54-60.

70. Mandle RJ, Kaplan AP. Hageman factor–dependent fibrinolysis: generation of fibrinolytic activity by the interaction of human activated factor XI and plasminogen. Blood. 1979;54:850-862.

71. Travis J, Salvesan GS. Human plasma proteinase inhibitors. Annu Rev Biochem. 1983;52:655-709.

72. Aoki N. Genetic abnormalities of the fibrinolytic system. Semin Thromb Hemost. 1984;10:42-50.

73. Holmes WE, Nelles L, Lijnen HR. Primary structure of human alpha2-antiplasmin, a serine protease inhibitor (serpin). J Biol Chem. 1987;262:1659-1664.

74. Hirosawa S, Nakamura Y, Miura O, et al. Organization of the human alpha2-antiplasmin inhibitor gene. Proc Natl Acad Sci U S A. 1988;85:6836-6840.

75. Plow EF, Collen D. The presence and release of alpha-2-antiplasmin from human platelets. Blood. 1981;58:1069-1074.

76. Bell GI, Rall LB, Sanchez-Pascador R, et al. Human α_2-macroglobulin gene is located on chromosome 12. Som Cell Mol Genet. 1985;11:285-289.

77. Matthus G, Devriendt K, Cassiman JJ, et al. Structure of the human alpha2-macroglobulin gene and its promoter. Biochem Biophys Res Commun. 1992;184:596-603.

78. Sottrup-Jensen L, Stepanik TM, Kristensen T, et al. Primary structure of human α_2-macroglobulin. V. The complete structure. J Biol Chem. 1984;259:8318-8327.

79. Aoki N, Moroi M, Tachiya K. Effects of alpha-2-plasmin inhibitor on fibrin clot lysis. Its comparison with alpha-2-macroglobulin. Thromb Haemost. 1978;39:22-31.

80. Huisman LG, Van Griensven JM, Kluft C. On the role of C1-inhibitor as inhibitor of tissue-type plasminogen activator in human plasma. Thromb Haemost. 1995;73:466-471.

81. Scott RW, Bergman BL, Bajpai A, et al. Protease nexin: properties and a modified purification procedure. J Biol Chem. 1985;260:7029-7034.

82. Cunningham DD, Van Nostrand WE, Farrell DH, Campbell CH. Interactions of serine proteases with cultured fibroblasts. J Cell Biochem. 1986;32:281-291.

83. Nesheim M, Wang W, Boffa M, et al. Thrombin, thrombomodulin and TAFI in the molecular link between coagulation and fibrinolysis. Thromb Haemost. 1997;78: 386-391.

84. Eaton DL, Malloy BE, Tsai SP, et al. Isolation, molecular cloning, and partial characterization of a novel carboxypeptidase B from plasma. J Biol Chem. 1991;269: 21833-21834.

85. Wang W, Hendriks DF, Scharpe SS. Carboxypeptidase U, a plasma carboxypeptidase with high affinity for plasminogen. J Biol Chem. 1994;269:15937-15944.

86. Bajzar L, Manuel R, Nesheim M. Purification and characterization of TAFI, a thrombin activatable fibrinolysis inhibitor. J Biol Chem. 1995;270:14477-14484.

87. Redlitz A, Tan AK, Eaton D, Plow EF. Plasma carboxypeptidases as regulators of the plasminogen system. J Clin Invest. 1995;96:2534-2538.

88. Bajzar L, Nesheim ME, Tracy PB. The profibrinolytic effect of activated protein C in clots formed from plasma is TAFI-dependent. Blood. 1996;88:2093-2100.

89. Bajzar L, Morser J, Nesheim M. TAFI, or plasma procarboxypeptidase B, couples the coagulation and fibrinolytic

cascades through the thrombin-thrombomodulin complex. J Biol Chem. 1996;271:16603-16608.

90. Minnema MC, Friederich PW, Levi M, et al. Enhancement of rabbit jugular vein thrombolysis by neutralization of factor XI: in vivo evidence for a role of factor XI as an anti-fibrinolytic factor. J Clin Invest. 1998;101:10-14.

91. Sprengers ED, Kluft D. Plasminogen activator inhibitors. Blood. 1987;69:381-387.

92. Kruithof EKO. Plasminogen activator inhibitor type 1: biochemical, biological, and clinical aspects. Fibrinolysis. 1988;2:59-70.

93. Ny T, Sawdey M, Lawrence D, et al. Cloning and sequence of a cDNA coding for the human beta-migrating endothelial-cell–type plasminogen activator inhibitor. Proc Natl Acad Sci U S A. 1986;83:6776-6780.

94. Samad F, Yamamoto K, Loskutoff DJ. Distribution and regulation of plasminogen activator inhibitor-1 in murine adipose tissue in vivo. J Clin Invest. 1996;97:37-46.

95. Sawdey M, Podor TJ, Loskutoff DJ. Regulation of type-1 plasminogen activator inhibitor gene expression in cultured bovine aortic endothelial cells. J Biol Chem. 1989; 264:10396-10401.

96. Van den Berg EA, Sprengers ED, Jaye M, et al. Regulation of plasminogen activator inhibitor-1 mRNA in human endothelial cells. Thromb Haemost. 1988;60:63-67.

97. Van Hinsbergh VWM, Kooistra T, Van den Berg EA, et al. Tumor necrosis factor increases the production of plasminogen activator inhibitor in human endothelial cells in vitro and in rats in vivo. Blood. 1988;72:1467-1473.

98. Loskutoff DJ, Linders M, Keijer J, et al. Structure of the human plasminogen activator inhibitor-1 gene: nonrandom distribution of introns. Biochemistry. 1987;26: 3763-3768.

99. Declerck PJ, De Mol M, Alessi MC, et al. Purification and characterization of a plasminogen activator inhibitor-1 binding protein from human plasma. Identification as multimeric form of S protein (vitronectin). J Biol Chem. 1988;263:15454-15461.

100. Mottonen J, Strand A, Symersky J, et al. Structural basis of latency in plasminogen activator inhibitor-1. Nature. 1992;355:270-273.

101. Bosma PJ, Van den Berg EA, Kooistra T, et al. Human plasminogen activator inhibitor-1 gene: promoter and structural nucleotide sequences. J Biol Chem. 1988;263: 9129-9141.

102. Keeton MR, Curriden SA, Van Zonneveld AJ, Loskutoff DJ. Identification of regulatory sequences in the type 1 plasminogen activator inhibitor gene responsive to transforming growth factor. J Biol Chem. 1991;266:23048-23052.

103. Van Zonnefeld AJ, Curriden SA, Loskutoff DJ. Type 1 plasminogen activator inhibitor gene: functional analysis and glucocorticoid regulation of its promoter. Proc Natl Acad Sci U S A. 1988;85:5525-5529.

104. Westerhausen DR, Hopkins WE, Billadello JJ. Multiple transforming growth factor beta–inducible elements regulate expression of the plasminogen activator inhibitor type-1 gene in HepG2 cells. J Biol Chem. 1991;266: 1092-1100.

105. Emeis JJ, Kooistra T. Interleukin 1 and lipopolysaccharide induce an inhibitor of tissue-type plasminogen activator in vivo and in cultured endothelial cells. J Exp Med. 1986;163:1260-1266.

106. Gelehrter TD, Scyncer-Laszuk R. Thrombin induction of plasminogen activator-inhibitor synthesis in vitro. J Clin Invest. 1986;77:165-169.

107. Schleef RR, Bevilacqua MP, Sawdey M, et al. Cytokine activation of vascular endothelium: effects on tissue-type plasminogen activator and type 1 plasminogen activator inhibitor. J Biol Chem. 1988;263:5797-5803.

108. Etingin OR, Hajjar DP, Hajjar KA, et al. Lipoprotein(a) regulates plasminogen activator inhibitor-1 expression in endothelial cells. J Biol Chem. 1990;266:2459-2465.

109. Stiko-Rahm A, Wiman B, Hamsten A, Nilsson J. Secretion of plasminogen activator inhibitor-1 from cultured human umbilical vein endothelial cells is induced by very low density lipoprotein. Arteriosclerosis. 1990;10:1067-1073.

110. Vaughan DE, Shen C, Lazo S. Angiotensin II induces plasminogen activator inhibitor synthesis in vitro. Circulation. 1992;86:I-557.

111. Van Hinsbergh VWM, Sprengers ED, Kooistra T. Effect of thrombin on the production of plasminogen activators and PA inhibitor-1 by human foreskin microvascular endothelial cells. Thromb Haemost. 1987;57:148-153.

112. Scarpati EM, Sadler JE. Regulation of endothelial cell coagulant properties. Modulation of tissue factor, plasminogen activator inhibitors, and thrombomodulin by phorbol 12-myristate 13-acetate and tumor necrosis factor. J Biol Chem. 1989;264:20705-20713.

113. Konkle BA, Kollros PR, Kelly MD. Heparin-binding growth factor-1 modulation of plasminogen activator inhibitor-1 expression. J Biol Chem. 1990;265:21867-21873.

114. Ye RD, Wun T-C, Sadler JE. cDNA cloning and expression in *Escherichia coli* of a plasminogen activator inhibitor from human placenta. J Biol Chem. 1987;262:3718-3725.

115. Ye RD, Aherns SM, Le Beau MM, et al. Structure of the gene for human plasminogen activator inhibitor-2. The nearest mammalian homologue of chicken ovalbumin. J Biol Chem. 1989;264:5495-5502.

116. Dear AE, Shen Y, Ruegg M, Medcalf RL. Molecular mechanisms governing tumor-necrosis-factor–mediated regulation of plasminogen-activator inhibitor type-2 expression. Eur J Biochem. 1996;241:93-100.

117. Antalis TM, Clok MA, Barnes T, et al. Cloning and expression of a cDNA coding for a human monocyte-derived plasminogen activator inhibitor. Proc Natl Acad Sci U S A. 1988;85:985-989.

118. Antalis TM, Costelloe E, Muddiman J, et al. Regulation of the plasminogen activator inhibitor type 2 gene in monocytes: localization of an upstream transcriptional silencer. Blood. 1996;88:3686-3697.

119. Mahony D, Kalionis B, Antalis TM. Plasminogen activator inhibitor type-2 (PAI-2) gene transcription requires a novel NF-κB–like transcriptional regulatory motif. Eur J Biochem. 1999;263:765-772.

120. Schleuning WD, Medcalf RL, Hession C, et al. Plasminogen activator inhibitor 2: regulation of gene transcription during phorbol ester–mediated differentiation of U-937 human histicytic lymphoma cells. Mol Cell Biol. 1987;7:4564-4567.

121. Chapman HA, Stone OL. A fibrinolytic inhibitor of human alveolar macrophages. Induction with endotoxin. Am Rev Respir Dis. 1985;132:569-575.

122. Miles LA, Dahlberg CM, Plescia J, et al. Role of cell surface lysines in plasminogen binding to cells: identification of alpha-enolase as a candidate plasminogen receptor. Biochemistry. 1991;30:1682-1691.

123. Miles LA, Ginsberg MA, White JG, Plow EF. Plasminogen interacts with platelets through two distinct mechanisms. J Clin Invest. 1986;77:2001-2009.

124. Kanalas JJ, Makker SP. Identification of the rat Heymann nephritis autoantigen (GP330) as a receptor site for plasminogen. J Biol Chem. 1991;266:10825-10829.

125. Parkkinen J, Rauvala H. Interactions of plasminogen and tissue plasminogen activator (t-PA) with amphoterin. J Biol Chem. 1991;266:16730-16735.

126. Hajjar KA, Hamel NM. Identification and characterization of human endothelial cell membrane binding sites for tissue plasminogen activator and urokinase. J Biol Chem. 1990;265:2908-2916.

127. Hajjar KA. The endothelial cell tissue plasminogen activator receptor: specific interaction with plasminogen. J Biol Chem. 1991;266:21962-21970.

128. Kassam G, Choi KS, Ghuman J, et al. The role of annexin II tetramer in the activation of plasminogen. J Biol Chem. 1998;273:4790-4799.

129. Roldan AL, Cubellis MV, Masucci MT, et al. Cloning and expression of the receptor for human urokinase plasminogen activator, a central molecule in cell surface, plasmin-dependent proteolysis. EMBO J. 1990;9:467-474.

130. Behrendt N, Ronne E, Ploug M, et al. The human receptor for urokinase plasminogen receptor. J Biol Chem. 1990;265:6453-6460.

131. Behrendt N, Ronne E, Dano K. The structure and function of the urokinase receptor, a membrane protein governing plasminogen activation on the cell surface. Biol Chem Hoppe-Seyler. 1995;376:269-279.

132. Casey JR, Petranka JG, Kottra J, et al. The structure of the urokinase-type plasminogen activator receptor gene. Blood. 1994;84:1151-1156.

133. Ploug M, Ronne E, Behrendt N, et al. Cellular receptor for urokinase plasminogen activator. Carboxyl-terminal processing and membrane anchoring by glycosylphosphatidylinositol. J Biol Chem. 1991;266:1926-1933.

134. Cubellis MV, Andreasson P, Ragno P, et al. Accessibility of receptor-bound urokinase to type-1 plasminogen activator inhibitor. Proc Natl Acad Sci U S A. 1989;86:4828-4832.

135. Cubellis MV, Wun TC, Blasi F. Receptor-mediated internalization and degradation of urokinase is caused by its specific inhibitor PAI-1. EMBO J. 1990;9:1079-1085.

136. Ellis V, Wun TC, Behrendt N, et al. Inhibition of receptor-bound urokinase by plasminogen activator inhibitor. J Biol Chem. 1990;265:9904-9908.

137. Ellis V, Behrendt N, Dano K. Plasminogen activation by receptor-bound urokinase. J Biol Chem. 1991;266:12752-12758.

138. Barinka C, Parry G, Callahan J, et al. Structural basis of interaction between urokinase-type plasminogen activator and its receptor. J Mol Biol. 2006;363:482-495.

139. Huai Q, Mazar AP, Kuo A, et al. Structure of human urokinase plasminogen activator in complex with its receptor. Science. 2006;311:656-659.

140. Llinas P, Le Du MH, Gardsvoll H, et al. Crystal structure of the human urokinase plasminogen activator receptor

bound to an antagonist peptide. EMBO J. 2006;24:1655-1663.

141. Chapman HA. Plasminogen activators, integrins, and the coordinated regulation of cell adhesion and migration. Curr Opin Cell Biol. 1997;9:714-724.

142. Waltz DA, Chapman HA. Reversible cellular adhesion to vitronectin linked to urokinase receptor occupancy. J Biol Chem. 1994;269:14746-14750.

143. Wei Y, Waltz DA, Rao N, et al. Identification of the urokinase receptor as an adhesion receptor for vitronectin. J Biol Chem. 1994;269:32380-32388.

144. Wei Y, Lukashev M, Simon DI, et al. Regulation of integrin function by the urokinase receptor. Science. 1996;273:1551-1555.

145. Xue W, Kindzelskii AL, Todd RF, Petty HR. Physical association of complement receptor type 3 and urokinase-type plasminogen activator in neutrophil membranes. J Immunol. 1994;152:4630-4640.

146. Anderson RG. Caveolae: where incoming and outgoing messengers meet. Proc Natl Acad Sci U S A. 1993;90:10909-10913.

147. Okamoto T, Schlegel A, Scherer PE, Lisanti MP. Caveolins, a family of scaffolding proteins for organizing "preassembled signaling complexes" at the plasma membrane. J Biol Chem. 1998;273:5419-5422.

148. Stahl A, Mueller BM. The urokinase-type plasminogen activator receptor, a GPI-linked protein, is localized in caveolae. J Cell Biol. 1995;129:335-344.

149. Laufs S, Schumacher J, Allgayer H. Urokinase-receptor (u-PAR): An essential player in multiple games of cancer. Cell Cycle. 2006;5:1760-1771.

150. Madsen MA, Deryugina EI, Niessen S, et al. Activity-based protein profiling indicates urokinase activation as a key step in human fibrosarcoma intravasation. J Biol Chem. 2006;281:15997-16005.

151. Pulukuri SM, Gondi CS, Lakka SS, et al. RNA interference–directed knockdown of urokinase plasminogen activator and urokinase plasminogen activator receptor inhibits prostate cancer cell invasion, survival, and tumorigenicity in vivo. J Biol Chem. 2006;280:36529-36540.

152. Chung CY, Erickson HP. Cell surface annexin II is a high affinity receptor for the alternatively spliced segment of tenascin-C. J Cell Biol. 1994;126:539-548.

153. Siever DA, Erickson HP. Extracellular annexin II. Int J Biochem Cell Biol. 1997;29:1219-1223.

154. Wright JF, Kurosky A, Wasi S. An endothelial cell-surface form of annexin II binds human cytomegalovirus. Biochem Biophys Res Commun. 1994;198:983-989.

155. Brownstein C, Deora AB, Jacovina AT, et al. Annexin II mediates plasminogen-dependent matrix invasion by human monocytes: enhanced expression by macrophages. Blood. 2004;103:317-324.

156. Falcone DJ, Borth W, Faisal Khan KM, Hajjar KA. Plasminogen-mediated matrix invasion and degradation by macrophages is dependent on surface expression of annexin II. Blood. 2001;97:777-784.

157. Menell JS, Cesarman GM, Jacovina AT, et al. Annexin II and bleeding in acute promyelocytic leukemia. N Engl J Med. 1999;340:994-1004.

158. Tressler RJ, Nicolson GL. Butanol-extractable and detergent-solubilized cell surface components from murine large cell lymphoma cells associated with adhesion to organ microvessel endothelial cells. J Cell Biochem. 1992;48:162-171.

159. Tressler RJ, Updyke TV, Yeatman TJ, Nicolson GL. Extracellular annexin is associated with divalent cation-dependent tumor cell adhesion of metastatic RAW 117 large-cell lymphoma cells. J Cell Biochem. 1993;53:265-276.

160. Yeatman TJ, Updyke TV, Kaetzel MA, et al. Expression of annexins on the surfaces of non-metastatic human and rodent tumor cells. Clin Exp Metastasis. 1993;11:37-44.

161. Gerke V, Moss SE. Annexins: from structure to function. Physiol Rev. 2002;82:331-371.

162. Gerke V, Creutz CE, Moss SE. Annexins: linking Ca^{++} signalling to membrane dynamics. Nat Rev Mol Cell Biol. 2005;6:449-461.

163. Swairjo MA, Seaton BA. Annexin structure and membrane interactions: a molecular perspective. Annu Rev Biophys Biomol Struct. 1994;23:193-213.

164. Spano F, Raugei G, Palla E, et al. Characterization of the human lipocortin-2–encoding multigene family: its structure suggests the existence of a short amino acid unit undergoing duplication. Gene. 1990;95:243-251.

165. Hajjar KA, Jacovina AT, Chacko J. An endothelial cell receptor for plasminogen and tissue plasminogen activator: I. Identity with annexin II. J Biol Chem. 1994;269:21191-21197.

166. Cesarman GM, Guevara CA, Hajjar KA. An endothelial cell receptor for plasminogen/tissue plasminogen activator: II. Annexin II–mediated enhancement of t-PA–dependent plasminogen activation. J Biol Chem. 1994;269:21198-21203.

167. Hajjar KA, Guevara CA, Lev E, et al. Interaction of the fibrinolytic receptor, annexin II, with the endothelial cell surface: essential role of endonexin repeat 2. J Biol Chem. 1996;271:21652-21659.

168. Deora AB, Kreitzer G, Jacovina AT, Hajjar KA. An annexin 2 phosphorylation switch mediates its p11-dependent translocation to the cell surface. J Biol Chem. 2004;279:43411-43418.

169. Petersen EA, Sutherland MR, Nesheim ME, Pryzdial EL. Thrombin induces endothelial cell-surface exposure of the plasminogen receptor annexin 2. J Cell Sci. 2003;116:2399-2408.

170. Kassam G, Le BH, Choi KS, et al. The p11 subunit of the annexin II tetramer plays a key role in the stimulation of t-PA–dependent plasminogen activation. Biochemistry. 1998;37:16958-16966.

171. Hajjar KA, Gavish D, Breslow J, Nachman RL. Lipoprotein(a) modulation of endothelial cell surface fibrinolysis and its potential role in atherosclerosis. Nature. 1989;339:303-305.

172. Miles LA, Fless GM, Levin EG, et al. A potential basis for the thrombotic risks associated with lipoprotein(a). Nature. 1989;339:301-303.

173. Hajjar KA, Mauri L, Jacovina AT, et al. Tissue plasminogen activator binding to the annexin II tail domain: direct modulation by homocysteine. J Biol Chem. 1998;273:9987-9993.

174. Boushey CJ, Beresford SAA, Omenn GS, Motulsky AG. A quantitative assessment of plasma homocysteine as a risk factor for vascular disease. JAMA. 1995;274:1049-1057.

175. Kraus JP. Molecular basis of phenotype expression in homocystinuria. J Inherit Metab Dis. 1994;17:383-390.

176. Refsum H, Ueland PM, Nygard O, Vollset SE. Homocysteine and cardiovascular disease. Annu Rev Med. 1998; 49:31-62.

177. Hajjar KA. Homocysteine-induced modulation of tissue plasminogen activator binding to its endothelial cell membrane receptor. J Clin Invest. 1993;91:2873-2879.

178. Ling Q, Jacovina AT, Deora AB, et al. Annexin II is a key regulator of fibrin homeostasis and neoangiogenesis. J Clin Invest. 2004;113:38-48.

179. Ishii H, Yoshida M, Hiraoka M, et al. Recombinant annexin II modulates impaired fibrinolytic activity in vitro and in rat carotid artery. Circ Res. 2001;89:1240-1245.

180. Cesarman-Maus G, Rios-Luna NP, Deora AB, et al. Autoantibodies against the fibrinolytic receptor, annexin 2, in antiphospholipid syndrome. Blood. 2006;107:4375-4382.

181. Sebastiani P, Ramoni MF, Nolan V, et al. Genetic dissection and prognostic modeling of overt stroke in sickle cell anemia. Nat Genet. 2005;37:435-440.

182. Bu G, Warshawsky I, Schwartz AL. Cellular receptors for the plasminogen activators. Blood. 1994;83:3427-3436.

183. Beiseigel U, Weber W, Ihrke G, et al. The LDL-receptor–related protein, LRP, is an apolipoprotein E–binding protein. Nature. 1989;341:162-164.

184. Brown MS, Herz J, Kowal RC. The low-density lipoprotein receptor–related protein: double agent or decoy? Curr Opin Lipidol. 1991;2:65-72.

185. Orth K, Madison EL, Gething MJ, Sambrook JF. Complexes of tissue-type plasminogen activator and its serpin inhibitor plasminogen-activator inhibitor type 1 are internalized by means of the low density lipoprotein receptor–related protein/alpha-2-macroglobulin receptor. Proc Natl Acad Sci U S A. 1992;89:7422-7426.

186. Herz J, Goldstein JL, Strickland DK, et al. 39 kDa protein modulates binding of ligands to low density lipoprotein receptor–related protein/alpha-2-macroglobulin receptor. J Biol Chem. 1991;266:21232-21238.

187. Herz J, Clouthier DE, Hammer RE. LDL receptor–related protein internalizes and degrades uPA–PAI-1 complexes and is essential for embryo implantation. Cell. 1992;71:411-421.

188. Herz J, Clouthier DE, Hammer RE. Correction: LDL receptor–related protein internalizes and degrades uPA–PAI-1 complexes and is essential for embryo implantation. Cell. 1993;73:428.

189. Bu G, Morton PA, Schwartz AL. Identification and partial characterization by chemical cross-linking of a binding protein for tissue-type plasminogen activator (t-PA) on rat hepatoma cells. J Biol Chem. 1992;267:15595-15602.

190. Otter M, Barrett-Bergshoeff MM, Rijken DC. Binding of tissue type plasminogen activator by the mannose receptor. J Biol Chem. 1991;266:13931-13935.

191. Hajjar KA, Reynolds CM. α-Fucose–mediated binding and degradation of tissue plasminogen activator by HepG2 cells. J Clin Invest. 1994;93:703-710.

192. Bailey K, Bettelheim FR, Lorand L, Middlebrook WR. Action of thrombin in the clotting of fibrinogen. Nature. 1951;167:233-234.

193. Doolittle RF. The molecular biology of fibrin. In Stamatoyannopoulos G, Nienhuis AW, Majerus PW, Varmus H (eds). The Molecular Basis of Blood Diseases. Philadelphia, WB Saunders, 1994, pp 701-723.

194. Furlan M, Kemp G, Beck EA. Plasmic degradation of fibrinogen. Biochim Biophys Acta. 1975;400:95-111.

195. Gaffney PJ, Dobos P. A structural aspect of human fibrinogen suggested by its plasmin degradation. FEBS Lett. 1971;15:13-16.

196. Marder VJ, Budzinski AZ. Data for defining fibrinogen and its plasmic degradation products. Thromb Diath Haemorrh. 1975;33:199-207.

197. Latallo ZS, Flether AP, Alkjaersig N, Sherry S. Inhibition of fibrin polymerization by fibrinogen proteolysis products. Am J Physiol. 1962;202:681-686.

198. Pizzo SV, Schwartz ML, Hill RL, McKee PA. The effect of plasmin on the subunit structure of human fibrin. J Biol Chem. 1973;248:4574-4583.

199. Culasso DE, Donati MB, DeGaetano G, et al. Inhibition of human platelet aggregation by plasmin digests of human and bovine preparations: role of contaminating factor VIII–related material. Blood. 1974;44:169-175.

200. Buluk K, Malofiegen M. The pharmacologic properties of fibrinogen degradation products. Br J Pharmacol. 1969; 35:79-89.

201. Richardson DL, Pepper DS, Kay AB. Chemotaxis for human monocytes by fibrinogen degradation products. Br J Haematol. 1976;32:507-513.

202. Girmann G, Pees H, Schwarze G, Scheulen PG. Immunosuppression by micromolecular fibrin-fibrinogen degradation products in cancer. Nature. 1976;259:399-401.

203. Wiman B, Collen D. On the kinetics of the reaction between human antiplasmin and plasmin. Eur J Biochem. 1978;84:573-578.

204. Van Zonnefeld AJ, Veerman H, Pannekoek H. On the interaction of the finger and the kringle-2 domain of tissue-type plasminogen activator with fibrin: inhibition of kringle-1 binding to fibrin by epsilon-aminocaproic acid. J Biol Chem. 1986;261:14214-14218.

205. Camiolo SM, Thorsen S, Astrup T. Fibrinogenolysis and fibrinolysis with tissue plasminogen activator, urokinase, streptokinase-activated human globulin and plasmin. Proc Soc Exp Biol Med. 1971;138:277-280.

206. Lijnen HR, Zamarron C, Blaber M, et al. Activation of plasminogen by prourokinase: I. Mechanism. J Biol Chem. 1986;261:1253-1258.

207. Pannell R, Black J, Gurewich V. Complementary modes of action of tissue-type plasminogen activator and pro-urokinase by which their synergistic effect on clot lysis may be explained. J Clin Invest. 1988;81:853-859.

208. Bell W. Fibrinolytic therapy: indications and management. In Hoffman R, Benz EJ, Shattil SJ, et al (eds). Hematology: Basic Principles and Practice. New York, Churchill Livingstone, 1995, pp 1814-1829.

209. Aoki N, Moroi M, Sakata Y, et al. Abnormal plasminogen: a hereditary molecular abnormality found in a patient with recurrent thrombosis. J Clin Invest. 1978;61:1186-1195.

210. Ichinose A, Espling ES, Takamatsu J, et al. Two types of abnormal genes for plasminogen in families with a predisposition for thrombosis. Proc Natl Acad Sci U S A. 1991;88:115-119.

211. Sartori MT, Patrassi GM, Theodoridis P, et al. Heterozygous type I plasminogen deficiency is associated with an increased risk for thrombosis: a statistical analysis of 20 kindreds. Blood Coagul Fibrinolysis. 1994;5:889-893.

212. Robbins KC. Dysplasminogenemia. Prog Cardiovasc Dis. 1992;34:295-308.

213. Tefs K, Gueorguieva M, Klammt J, et al. Molecular and clinical spectrum of type I plasminogen deficiency. Blood. 2006;108:3021-3026.

214. Schott D, Dempfle CE, Beck P, et al. Therapy with a purified plasminogen concentrate in an infant with ligneous conjunctivitis and homozygous plasminogen deficiency. N Engl J Med. 1998;339:1679-1686.

215. Schuster V, Mingers AM, Seidenspinner S, et al. Homozygous mutations in the plasminogen gene of two unrelated girls with ligneous conjunctivitis. Blood. 1997;90:958-966.

216. Schuster V, Seidenspinner S, Zeitler P, et al. Compound-heterozygous mutations in the plasminogen gene predispose to the development of ligneous conjunctivitis. Blood. 1999;93:3457-3466.

217. Schwarz T, Siegert G, Oettler W, et al. Venous thrombosis after long-haul flights. Arch Intern Med. 2003;163:2759-2764.

218. Lisman T, De Groot PG, Meijers JCM, Rosendaal FR. Reduced plasma fibrinolytic potential is a risk factor for venous thrombosis. Blood. 2005;105:1102-1105.

219. Demarmels Biasiutti F, Sulzer I, Stucki B, et al. Is plasminogen deficiency a thrombotic risk factor? A study on 23 thrombophilic patients and their family members. Thromb Haemost. 1998;80:167-170.

220. Brandt JT. Plasminogen and tissue-type plasminogen activator deficiency as risk factors for thromboembolic disease. Arch Pathol Lab Med. 2002;126:1376-1381.

221. Francis CW. Plasminogen activator inhibitor-1 levels and polymorphisms: association with venous thromboembolism. Arch Pathol Lab Med. 2002;126:1401-1404.

222. Hamsten A, Wiman B, De Faire U, Blomback M. Increased plasma levels of a rapid inhibitor of tissue plasminogen activator in young survivors of myocardial infarction. N Engl J Med. 1985;313:1557-1563.

223. Tilburg NH, Rosendaal FR, Bertina RM. Thrombin activatable fibrinolysis inhibitor and the risk for deep vein thrombosis. Blood. 2000;95:2855-2859.

224. Fay WP, Shapiro AD, Shih JL, et al. Complete deficiency of plasminogen activator inhibitor type 1 due to a frameshift mutation. N Engl J Med. 1992;327:1729-1733.

225. Saito H. Alpha-2-plasmin inhibitor and its deficiency states. J Lab Clin Med. 1988;112:671-678.

226. Suh TT, Holmback K, Jensen NJ, et al. Resolution of spontaneous bleeding events but failure of pregnancy in fibrinogen-deficient mice. Genes Dev. 1995;9:2020-2033.

227. Bugge TH, Flick MJ, Daugherty CC, Degen JL. Plasminogen deficiency causes severe thrombosis but is compatible with development and reproduction. Genes Dev. 1995;9:794-807.

228. Ploplis VA, Carmeliet P, Vazirzadeh S, et al. Effects of disruption of the plasminogen gene on thrombosis, growth, and health in mice. Circulation. 1995;92:2585-2593.

229. Busuttil SJ, Drumm C, Ploplis VA, Plow EF. Endoluminal arterial injury in plasminogen-deficient mice. J Surg Res. 2000;91:159-164.

230. Lijnen HR, Carmeliet P, Bouche A, et al. Restoration of thrombolytic potential in plasminogen-deficient mice by bolus administration of plasminogen. Blood. 1996;88:870-876.

231. Bugge TH, Kombrinck KW, Flick MJ, et al. Loss of fibrinogen rescues mice from the pleiotropic effects of plasminogen deficiency. Cell. 1996;87:709-719.

232. Drew AF, Kaufman AH, Kombrinck KW, et al. Ligneous conjunctivitis in plasminogen-deficient mice. Blood. 1998;91:1616-1624.

233. Carmeliet P, Schoonjans L, Kieckens L, et al. Physiological consequences of loss of plasminogen activator gene function in mice. Nature. 1994;368:419-424.

234. Carmeliet P, Collen D. Gene targeting and gene transfer studies of the plasminogen/plasmin system: implications in thrombosis, hemostasis, neointima formation, and atherosclerosis. FASEB J. 1995;9:934-938.

235. Eitzman DT, Westrick RJ, Nabel EG, Ginsburg D. Plasminogen activator inhibitor-1 and vitronectin promote vascular thrombosis in mice. Blood. 2000;95:577-580.

236. Zhu Y, Carmeliet P, Fay WP. Plasminogen activator inhibitor-1 is a major determinant of arterial thrombolysis resistance. Circulation. 1999;99:3050-3055.

237. Erickson LA, Fici GJ, Lund JE, et al. Development of venous occlusions in transgenic mice for the plasminogen activator inhibitor-1 gene. Nature. 1990;346:74-76.

238. Eitzman DT, Krauss JC, Shen T, et al. Lack of plasminogen activator inhibitor-1 effect in a transgenic mouse model of metastatic melanoma. Blood. 1996;87:4718-4722.

239. Griffin GC, Mammen EF, Sokol RJ, et al. Alpha2-antiplasmin deficiency. Am J Pediatr Hematol Oncol. 1993;15:328-330.

240. Lijnen HR, Okada K, Matsuo O, et al. α_2-Antiplasmin gene deficiency in mice is associated with enhanced fibrinolytic potential without overt bleeding. Blood. 1999;93:2274-2281.

241. Dougherty KM, Pearson JM, Yang AY, et al. The plasminogen activator inhibitor-2 gene is not required for normal murine development or survival. Proc Natl Acad Sci U S A. 1999;96:686-691.

242. Nagashima M, Yin ZF, Zhao L, et al. Thrombin-activatable fibrinolysis inhibitor (TAFI) deficiency is compatible with murine life. J Clin Invest. 2002;109:101-110.

243. Palabrica TM, Liu AC, Aronovitz MJ, et al. Antifibrinolytic activity of apolipoprotein(a) in vivo: human apolipoprotein(a) transgenic mice are resistant to tissue plasminogen activator-mediated thrombolysis. Nat Med. 1995;1:256-259.

244. Lou XJ, Boonmark NW, Horrigan FT, et al. Fibrinogen deficiency reduces vascular accumulation of apolipoprotein(a) and development of atherosclerosis in apolipoprotein(a) transgenic mice. Proc Natl Acad Sci U S A. 1998;95:12591-12595.

245. Dewerchin M, Van Nuffelen A, Wallays G, et al. Generation and characterization of urokinase receptor–deficient mice. J Clin Invest. 1996;97:870-878.

246. Bugge TH, Flick MJ, Danton MJS, et al. Urokinase-type plasminogen activator is effective in fibrin clearance in the absence of its receptor or tissue-type plasminogen activator. Proc Natl Acad Sci U S A. 1996;93:5899-5904.

247. Romer J, Bugge TH, Pyke C, et al. Impaired wound healing in mice with a disrupted plasminogen gene. Nat Med. 1996;2:287-292.

248. Drew AF, Liu H, Davidson JM, et al. Wound-healing defects in mice lacking fibrinogen. Blood. 2001;97:3691-3698.

249. Kanno Y, Hirade K, Ishisaki A, et al. Lack of alpha2-antiplasmin improves cutaneous wound healing via over-released vascular endothelial growth factor–induced angiogenesis in wound lesions. J Thromb Haemost. 2006;4:1602-1610.

250. Chan JCY, Duszczyszyn DA, Castellino FJ, Ploplis VA. Accelerated skin wound healing in plasminogen activator inhibitor-1–deficient mice. Am J Pathol. 2001;159:1681-1688.

251. Akassoglou K, Kombrinck KW, Degen JL, Strickland S. Tissue plasminogen activator–mediated fibrinolysis protects against axonal degeneration and demyelination after sciatic nerve injury. J Cell Biol. 2000;149:1157-1166.

252. te Velde EA, Wagenaar GT, Reijerkerk A, et al. Impaired healing of cutaneous wounds and colonic anastomoses in mice lacking thrombin-activatable fibrinolysis inhibitor. J Thromb Haemost. 2003;1:2087-2096.

253. Ploplis VA, Wilberding J, McLennnan LC, et al. A total fibrinogen deficiency is compatible with the development of pulmonary fibrosis in mice. Am J Pathol. 2000;157:703-708.

254. Fujimoto H, Gabazza EC, Taguchi O, et al. Thrombin-activatable fibrinolysis inhibitor deficiency attenuates bleomycin-induced lung fibrosis. Am J Pathol. 2006;168:1086-1096.

255. Swaisgood CM, French EL, Noga C, et al. The development of bleomycin-induced pulmonary fibrosis in mice deficient for components of the fibrinolytic system. Am J Pathol. 2000;157:177-187.

256. Hattori N, Degen JL, Sisson TH, et al. Bleomycin-induced pulmonary fibrosis in fibrinogen-null mice. J Clin Invest. 2000;106:1341-1350.

257. Ross R. Atherosclerosis: an inflammatory disease. N Engl J Med. 1999;340:115-126.

258. Xiao Q, Danton MJS, Witte DP, et al. Plasminogen deficiency accelerates vessel wall disease in mice predisposed to atherosclerosis. Proc Natl Acad Sci U S A. 1997;94:10335-10340.

259. Xiao Q, Danton MJS, Witte DP, et al. Fibrinogen deficiency is compatible with the development of atherosclerosis in mice. J Clin Invest. 1998;101:1184-1194.

260. Moons L, Wi C, Ploplis V, et al. Reduced transplant arteriosclerosis in plasminogen-deficient mice. J Clin Invest. 1998;102:1788-1797.

261. Plow EF, Plow JH. The functions of plasminogen in cardiovascular disease. Trends Cardiovasc Med. 2004;14:180-186.

262. Creemers E, Cleutjens J, Smits J, et al. Disruption of the plasminogen gene in mice abolishes wound healing after myocardial infarction. Am J Pathol. 2000;156:1865-1873.

263. Carmeliet P, Moons L, Ploplis VA, et al. Impaired arterial neointima formation in mice with disruption of the plasminogen gene. J Clin Invest. 1997;99:200-208.

264. Drew AF, Tucker HL, Kombrinck KW, et al. Plasminogen is a critical determinant of vascular remodeling in mice. Circ Res. 2000;87:133-139.

265. Murphy G, Stanton H, Cowell S, et al. Mechanisms of promatrix metalloproteinase activation. APMIS. 1999;107:38-44.

266. Nagase H. Activation mechanisms of matrix metalloproteinases. Biol Chem. 1997;378:151-160.

267. Ramos-DeSimone N, Hahn-Dantona E, Sipley J, et al. Activation of matrix metalloproteinase-9 (MMP-9) via a converging plasmin/stromelysin-1 cascade enhances tumor cell invasion. J Biol Chem. 1999;274:13066-13076.

268. Falcone DJ, McCaffrey TA, Haimovitz-Friedman A, et al. Macrophage and foam cell release of matrix-bound growth factors. Role of plasminogen activation. J Biol Chem. 1993;268:11951-11958.

269. Sporn MB, Roberts AB, Wakefield LM, Assoian RK. Transforming growth factor-beta: biological function and chemical structure. Science. 1986;233:532-534.

270. Lyons RM, Gentry LE, Purchio AF, Moses HL. Mechanism of activation of latent recombinant transforming growth factor beta1 by plasmin. J Cell Biol. 1990;110:1361-1367.

271. Carmeliet P, Moons L, Herbert JM, et al. Urokinase but not tissue plasminogen activator mediates arterial neointima formation in mice. Circ Res. 1997;81:829-839.

272. Carmeliet P, Moons L, Dewerchin M, et al. Receptor-independent role of urokinase-type plasminogen activator in pericellular plasmin and matrix metalloproteinase proteolysis during vascular wound healing in mice. J Cell Biol. 1998;140:233-245.

273. Carmeliet P, Moons L, Lijnen R, et al. Urokinase-generated plasmin activates matrix metalloproteinases during aneurysm formation. Nat Genet. 1997;17:439-444.

274. Heymans S, Luttun A, Nuyens D, et al. Inhibition of plasminogen activators or matrix metalloproteinases prevents cardiac rupture but impairs therapeutic angiogenesis and causes cardiac failure. Nat Med. 2003;5:1135-1142.

275. Bugge TH, Konbrinck KW, Xiao Q, et al. Growth and dissemination of Lewis lung carcinoma in plasminogen-deficient mice. Blood. 1997;90:4522-4531.

276. Bugge TH, Lund LR, Kombrinck KW, et al. Reduced metastasis of polyoma virus middle T antigen–induced mammary cancer in plasminogen deficient mice. Oncogene. 1998;16:3097-3104.

277. Palumbo JS, Kombrinck KW, Drew AF, et al. Fibrinogen is an important determinant of the metastatic potential of circulating tumor cells. Blood. 2000;96:3302-3309.

278. Palumbo JS, Potter JM, Kaplan LS, et al. Spontaneous hematogenous and lymphatic metastases, but not primary tumor growth or angiogenesis, is diminished in fibrinogen-deficient mice. Cancer Res. 2002;62:6966-6972.

279. Gutierrez LS, Schulman A, Brito-Robinson T, et al. Tumor development is retarded in mice lacking the gene for urokinase-type plasminogen activator or its inhibitor, plasminogen activator inhibitor-1. Cancer Res. 2000;60:5839-5847.

280. Shapiro RL, Duquette JG, Roses DF, et al. Induction of primary cutaneous neoplasms in urokinase-type plasminogen activator (u-PA)-deficient and wild type mice: cellular blue nevi invade but do not progress to malignant melanoma in u-PA deficient animals. Cancer Res. 1996;56:3597-3604.

281. Sabapathy KT, Pepper MS, Kiefer F, et al. Polyoma middle T–induced vascular tumor formation: the role of the plasminogen activator/plasmin system. J Cell Biol. 1997;137:953-963.

282. Reijenkerk A, Meijers JCM, Havik SR, et al. Tumor growth and metastases are not affected in thrombin-activatable fibrinolysis inhibitor–deficient mice. J Thromb Haemost. 2004;2:769-779.

283. Bajou K, Noel A, Gerard RD, et al. Absence of host plasminogen activator inhibitor 1 prevents cancer invasion and vascularization. Nat Med. 1998;4:923-928.

284. Lahteenmaki K, Kukkonen M, Korhonen TK. The Pla surface protease/adhesin of *Yersinia pestis* mediates bacterial invasion into human endothelial cells. FEBS Lett. 2001;504:69-72.

285. Lahteenmaki K, Edelman S, Korhonen TK. Bacterial metastasis: the host plasminogen system in bacterial invasion. Trends Microbiol. 2005;13:79-85.

286. Coleman JL, Gebbia JA, Piesman J, et al. Plasminogen is required for efficient dissemination of *B. burgdorferi* in ticks and for enhancement of spirochetemia in mice. Cell. 1997;89:1111-1119.

287. Goguen JD, Bugge T, Degen JL. Role of the pleiotropic effects of plasminogen deficiency in infection experiments with plasminogen-deficient mice. Methods. 2000;21:179-183.

288. Lathem WW, Price PA, Miller VL, Goldman WE. A plasminogen-activating protease specifically controls the development of primary pneumonic plague. Science. 2007;315:509-513.

289. Li Z, Ploplis VA, French EL, Boyle MDP. Interaction between group A streptococci and the plasmin(ogen) system promotes virulence in a mouse skin infection. J Infect Dis. 1998;179:907-914.

290. Sun H, Ringdahl U, Homeister JW, et al. Plasminogen is a critical host pathogenicity factor for group A streptococcal infection. Science. 2004;305:1283-1286.

291. Ploplis VA, French EL, Carmeliet P, et al. Plasminogen deficiency differentially affects recruitment of inflammatory cell populations in mice. Blood. 1998;91:2005-2009.

292. Gyetko MR, Chen G-H, McDonald RA, et al. Urokinase is required for the pulmonary inflammatory response to *Cryptococcus neoformans*. J Clin Invest. 1996;97:1818-1826.

293. Beck JM, Preston AM, Gyetko MR. Urokinase-type plasminogen activator in inflammatory cell recruitment and host defense against *Pneumocystis carinii* in mice. Infect Immun. 1999;67:879-884.

294. Gyetko MR, Sud S, Kendall T, et al. Urokinase receptor–deficient mice have impaired neutrophil recruitment in response to pulmonary *Pseudomonas aeruginosa* infection. J Immunol. 2000;165:1513-1519.

295. Gualandris A, Jones T, Strickland S, Tsirka S. Membrane depolarization induces the Ca++-dependent release of tissue plasminogen activator. J Neurosci. 1996;16:2220-2225.

296. Qian Z, Gilbert ME, Colicos MA, et al. Tissue-plasminogen activator is induced as an immediate-early gene during seizure, kindling and long-term potentiation. Nature. 1993;361:453-457.

297. Seeds NW, Williams BL, Bickford PC. Tissue plasminogen activator induction in Purkinje neurons after cerebellar motor learning. Science. 1995;270:1992-1994.

298. Murtomaki S, Ekkhart T, Wright J, et al. Increased proteolytic activity of the granule neurons may contribute to neuronal death in the weaver mouse cerebellum. Dev Biol. 1995;168:635-648.

299. Frey U, Muller M, Kuhl D. A different form of long-lasting potentiation revealed in tissue plasminogen activator mutant mice. J Neurosci. 1996;16:2057-2063.

300. Huang Y, Bach M, Lipp H, et al. Mice lacking the gene encoding tissue-type plasminogen activator show a selective interference with late-phase long-term potentiation in both Schaffer collateral and mossy fiber pathways. Proc Natl Acad Sci U S A. 1996;93:8699-8704.

301. Chen ZL, Strickland SE. Neuronal death in the hippocampus is promoted by plasmin-catalyzed degradation of laminin. Cell. 1997;91:917-925.

302. Seeds NW, Basham ME, Haffke SP. Neuronal migration is retarded in mice lacking the tissue plasminogen activator gene. Proc Natl Acad Sci U S A. 1999;96:14118-14123.

303. Ripley TL, Rocha BA, Oglesby MW, Stephens DN. Increased sensitivity to cocaine, and over-responding during cocaine self-administration in tPA knockout mice. Brain Res. 1999;826:117-127.

304. Wu YP, Siao CJ, Lu W, et al. The tissue plasminogen activator (tPA)/plasmin extracellular proteolytic system regulates seizure-induced hippocampal mossy fiber outgrowth through a proteoglycan substrate. J Cell Biol. 2000;148:1295-1304.

305. Wang YF, Tsirka SE, Strickland S, et al. Tissue plasminogen activator (tPA) increases neuronal damage after focal cerebral ischemia in wild-type and tPA-deficient mice. Nat Med. 1998;4:228-231.

306. Nagai N, De Mol M, Lijnen HR, et al. Role of plasminogen system components in focal cerebral ischemic infarction. Circulation. 1999;99:2440-2444.

307. Tabrizi P, Wang L, Seeds N, et al. Tissue plasminogen activator (tPA) deficiency exacerbates cerebrovascular fibrin deposition and brain injury in a murine stroke model. Arterioscler Thromb Vasc Biol. 1999;19:2801-2806.

308. Cheng T, Petraglia AL, Li Z, et al. Activated protein C inhibits tissue plasminogen activator–induced brain hemorrhage. Nat Med. 2006;12:1278-1285.

309. Simon DI, Ezratty AM, Francis SA, et al. Fibrin(ogen) is internalized and degraded by activated human monocytoid cells via Mac-1 (CD11b/CD18): a nonplasmin fibrinolytic pathway. Blood. 1993;82:2414-2422.

310. Bini A, Wu D, Schnuer J, Kudryk BJ. Characterization of stromelysin 1 (MMP-3), matrilysin (MMP-7), and membrane type 1 matrix metalloproteinase (MT1-MMP) derived fibrin(ogen) fragments D-dimer and DF-like monomer: NH2-terminal sequences of late-stage digest fragments. Biochemistry. 1999;38:13928-13936.

311. Hiraoka N, Allen E, Apel IJ, et al. Matrix metalloproteinases regulate neovascularization by acting as pericellular fibrinolysins. Cell. 1998;95:365-377.

312. Vassalli JD, Pepper MS. Membrane proteases in focus. Nature. 1994;370:14-15.

28 Clinical and Laboratory Approach to the Patient with Bleeding

Madhvi Rajpurkar and Jeanne M. Lusher

HISTORY AND CLINICAL EVALUATION

Hemostasis involves a complex interplay between the vessel wall, platelets, coagulation factors, and fibrinolysis (see Chapters 25 to 27). A hematologist is often consulted to evaluate patients who have unusual, spontaneous, prolonged, or delayed bleeding. Occasionally, patients are referred because of abnormal coagulation test results obtained as a part of preoperative evaluation. As in any other field of medicine, when a clinician is confronted with a child who has a possible bleeding disorder, a detailed assessment of the patient's bleeding history and a physical examination should be performed before ordering a battery of laboratory studies. The art of history taking comes with experience and should guide the extent to which one investigates bleeding and requests laboratory tests. In view of the variability of patients' perception of bleeding, as well as the lack of a uniform clinical measure of bleeding severity, the history is most discriminatory when a standardized and validated questionnaire is used and a "bleeding score" is incorporated into the diagnosis.[1,2] Several such instruments currently exist, but there is no consensus on a single questionnaire that can quantitate bleeding optimally.[3-5]

Site of Bleeding

The observed pattern of bleeding is an important factor in establishing a differential diagnosis. The severity of bleeding may also aid the physician in differentiating between bruising after normal child play and pathologic bleeding. Persistent bleeding from a single site is generally suggestive of a local cause (e.g., unilateral epistaxis is often due to excoriation of a superficial vessel in the Kiesselbach triangle). Mucous membrane bleeding (epistaxis, excessive menorrhagia, bleeding from gums) is often the consequence of a problem with primary hemostasis, namely, a platelet disorder or von Willebrand disease (VWD).[6] Hereditary hemorrhagic telangiectasia may also be manifested as mucosal bleeding. Profuse bleeding into soft tissues or joints is suggestive of deficiency of a coagulation factor (such as factors VIII or IX). Umbilical stump bleeding is typically seen with factor XIII deficiency, but it may also occur with deficiencies of prothrombin, factor X, and fibrinogen.[7]

Clinical Manifestations

The immediate history often provides useful clues to the diagnosis (Table 28-1). A sick child with fever, shock, and mucocutaneous purpura frequently has disseminated intravascular coagulation (DIC) associated with bacteremia. A male toddler who has just started crawling and exhibits subcutaneous or joint bleeding frequently has hemophilia. A girl who has had severe menorrhagia since menarche may have VWD. A well-looking child covered with petechiae often has immune thrombocytopenia, or if the bruising is localized to the buttocks, ankles, and feet, Henoch-Schönlein purpura should be considered.

Age at Onset

Generally, early age at onset correlates with the severity of the bleeding disorder and also indicates its congenital nature. The development of bleeding later in childhood may indicate an acquired problem or be suggestive of a milder congenital disease. For example, mild hemophilia may be missed in early childhood and first be noted in an older adolescent at a time of increased hemostatic challenge from increased sports activities.[8,9] Diagnostic considerations in neonates with bleeding are quite different and often unique.

Past Medical History

Response to trauma is an excellent screening test. In eliciting the child's past history, it is important to inquire about past surgical procedures, serious injuries, and fractures that provide hemostatic challenges. Additional details that are often helpful include the bleeding outcome after invasive dentistry, transfusion requirement, or iron-responsive anemia. A history of surgical procedures or tooth extractions without any abnormal bleeding is good evidence against the presence of a congenital hemorrhagic disorder. A detailed menstrual history should be obtained when applicable. The prevalence of bleeding disorders in women with menorrhagia is as high as 20%. Conversely, menorrhagia is a common initial symptom in women with VWD and has been reported to occur in more than 90% of patients.[10-14]

TABLE 28-1	Differences in Clinical Manifestations of Primary Hemostatic Defects and Clotting Factor Deficiencies (Individual Patients May Vary)	
Clinical Characteristic	**Primary Hemostatic Defect**	**Clotting Factor Deficiency**
Site of bleeding	Skin, mucous membranes	Soft tissues, muscles, joints
Bleeding after minor cuts	Yes	Not usually
Petechiae	Present	Absent
Ecchymosis	Small, superficial	Larger, deeper, palpable
Hemarthrosis	Rare	Common
Bleeding after trauma/surgery	Immediate	Delayed

It is also important to note whether the patient has an underlying medical disorder that may affect hemostasis, such as hepatic or renal disease, malabsorption syndrome, or Ehlers-Danlos syndrome (Table 28-2).[15,16] Most of the coagulation proteins are synthesized in hepatocytes.[17,18] Certain metabolites that accumulate in individuals with uremia can interfere with platelet function,[19,20] whereas low-molecular-weight coagulation proteins (factors IX and XI) are lost through the kidney in children with nephrotic syndrome.[21] In malabsorption syndrome, levels of the vitamin K–dependent coagulation factors (II, VII, IX, and X) (see Chapter 26) may be depleted and lead to excessive bleeding.[22,23] A child with cyanotic congenital heart disease and polycythemia may have petechiae and excessive bleeding with surgery, in part as a result of thrombocytopenia and hypofibrinogenemia.[24] Reducing the red cell mass (by phlebotomy and replacement with normal saline solution) to lower the child's hematocrit will often lessen the hemostatic abnormalities associated with these conditions.

Family History

The child's family history may be very helpful in formulating a differential diagnosis. One should inquire about any known bleeding problems in other family members and whether a specific diagnosis has been made. If the family history is positive for bleeding, one should note the type and severity of bleeding (e.g., joint bleeding, epistaxis, or menorrhagia), age at onset, and the relationship of the affected family member or members to the patient. An X-linked recessive inheritance pattern suggests a diagnosis of hemophilia A or B,[25] whereas an autosomal dominant pattern would be more consistent with VWD or hereditary hemorrhagic telangiectasia. Most of the other clotting factor deficiencies are inherited in an autosomal recessive manner. In the latter group of disorders, the family history is frequently negative for bleeding, although consanguinity may be noted.

Approximately a third of infants and young children with newly diagnosed hemophilia have a negative family history, consistent with the Haldane hypothesis for the fraction of new mutations in all lethal X-linked recessive disorders.[26,27] For VWD, considerable variation in symptoms may be noted among affected family members. Bleeding manifestations may be very mild in some and give the impression of a "negative" family history. Factor XI deficiency, an autosomal trait most often (but not exclusively) seen in persons of Ashkenazi Jewish descent, may be associated with a very mild or a moderate tendency for bleeding. The degree of bleeding manifestations does not correlate well with the level of factor XI or the partial thromboplastin time, although the patient's specific mutation may be predictive.[28,29]

TABLE 28-2	Acquired Bleeding Disorders	
Underlying Bleeding Disorder	**Hemostatic Defect**	**Cause**
Overwhelming sepsis	Acute disseminated intravascular coagulation	Initiation of coagulation, damage to the endothelium; decrease in clotting and anticlotting factors
Liver disease	Multiple coagulation factor deficiency	Decreased hepatic synthesis
	Increased fibrinolysis	Decreased clearance of plasminogen activators
	Hypercoagulable state	Decreased production of natural anticoagulants
	Thrombocytopenia	Hypersplenism
Malabsorption syndrome	Decreased production of factors II, VII, IX, and X and proteins C and S	Vitamin K deficiency
Cyanotic congenital heart disease	Mild to moderate thrombocytopenia	Shortened platelet survival
	Abnormal platelet function	Acquired defects in platelet aggregation
Acyanotic congenital heart disease (e.g., ASD, PDA)	Decreased high-molecular-weight VWF multimers	Consumption
ECMO and CPB	Platelet dysfunction	Platelet activation in the oxygenator and physical damage to the platelet membrane
	Coagulation factor deficiency	Consumption of coagulation factors in the circuit
	Hyperfibrinolysis	Increase in tPA and decrease in α_2-antiplasmin
Acute promyelocytic leukemia	Thrombocytopenia	Decreased production in bone marrow and increased consumption
	Disseminated intravascular coagulation	Release of procoagulant material from the leukemic cells
	Hyperfibrinolysis	Increased synthesis of plasminogen activators

ASD, atrial septal defect; CPB, cardiopulmonary bypass; ECMO, extracorporeal membrane oxygenation; PDA, patent ductus arteriosus; tPA, tissue plasminogen activator; VWF, von Willebrand factor.

Medications

A careful history of medication use should be obtained, including prescribed medications, over-the-counter drugs, and herbal products.[30] A number of drugs are associated with bleeding diatheses, with mechanisms including induction of thrombocytopenia and platelet dysfunction.[31,32] Drug use may also exacerbate the bleeding symptoms of an underlying coagulation disorder. In addition, prolonged antibiotic use may lead to lower vitamin K levels and induce bleeding secondary to acquired deficiency of vitamin K–dependent factors.

PHYSICAL EXAMINATION

When examining a child with bleeding, the bleeding pattern should be noted. Petechiae are small capillary hemorrhages and characteristically develop in crops in areas of increased venous pressure, as in dependent parts of the body. Petechiae are nonpainful, nonpalpable, and nonblanching and need to be distinguished from small telangiectases and angiomas. In general, petechiae are indicative of problems with primary hemostasis (platelet number or function or vascular integrity). Ecchymotic lesions are palpable purplish lesions induced by subcutaneous bleeding and are usually indicative of deficiency of a coagulation factor. Additional note should be made of joint size, swelling, and limitation of motion, findings indicative of hemarthrosis. Identification of hepatomegaly and splenic enlargement may point toward coagulopathy associated with systemic disorders such as leukemia or hepatocellular disease.

APPROACH TO BLEEDING IN NEONATES

In the pediatric age group, the neonatal period, despite being a short 4 weeks, is quite unique. The neonate has physiologically decreased levels of most procoagulant and anticoagulant proteins (although factor VIII levels are normal), and thus the hemostatic system can be easily overwhelmed (see Chapter 5). Moreover, a neonate undergoes significant trauma to the head during labor and delivery. A recent study reported intracranial hemorrhage (ICH) after spontaneous vaginal delivery at a rate of 1 per 1900, whereas the rate of ICH in babies delivered by vacuum-assisted delivery was 1 in 860.[33] In addition, 15% to 30% of patients with inherited bleeding disorders have bleeding manifestations in the neonatal period.[34] Certain disorders, such as neonatal alloimmune thrombocytopenia (NAIT), are unique to the neonatal period. Furthermore, the neonate is significantly affected by the state of maternal health and medications used during labor. Blood volume in a neonate is small, and a relatively small degree of blood loss can have major consequences.

When evaluating bleeding in a neonate, the first step is to assess whether the baby is well or has medical conditions that may have precipitated hemorrhage. It is important to inquire about prolonged rupture of membranes, chorioamnionitis, and fetal distress during labor. Additional details about the maternal state of health, including infections, autoimmune disease, and maternal platelet count, should be obtained. Vitamin K administration to the baby should be confirmed. The neonate should be examined with particular attention directed to the presence of birth trauma, bruises and petechiae, and evidence of flank masses (renal vein thrombosis). The presence of hepatosplenomegaly may suggest disseminated intrauterine infection. When obtaining blood for various coagulation tests, particular attention should be paid to the hematocrit of the patient and the volume of the sample. Additionally, all laboratory results should be compared with normal values for different gestational ages (see Chapter 5).[35,36]

Isolated thrombocytopenia in a well infant may be seen in NAIT, in maternal autoimmune thrombocytopenia, or in cases of decreased platelet production such as amegakaryocytic thrombocytopenia or the syndrome of thrombocytopenia with absent radii (TAR). Rarely, type 2B VWD may be manifested as thrombocytopenia in a well infant. Thrombocytopenia in sick neonates is often due to the underlying cause, such as infection or DIC. Isolated prolongation of the prothrombin time (PT) or activated partial thromboplastin time (APTT) in a well baby may be due to a clotting factor deficiency, and prolongation of both the PT and APTT is suggestive of a clotting factor deficiency (in the common pathway) or vitamin K deficiency (hemorrhagic disease of the newborn). In sick babies, prolongation of clotting studies along with thrombocytopenia is suggestive of DIC.

LABORATORY ASSESSMENT

Sample Collection and Technique

A properly drawn blood sample is crucial for proper interpretation of the results of coagulation tests.[37] Blood for coagulation assays should be obtained by clean venipuncture without air bubbles and without contamination by tissue fluids. Drawing of samples from an indwelling catheter often results in sample contamination with heparin or intravenous fluids and spuriously abnormal values. Improper sample collection is one of the most common reasons for falsely elevated clotting times.[38]

Whole blood is collected into citrated anticoagulant in an evacuated sample tube containing a fixed amount of citrate (3.2% or 3.8%) as anticoagulant in the ratio of one part citrate to nine parts whole blood. If the patient is polycythemic (hematocrit >55%), the amount of plasma in the tube would be reduced in proportion to the citrate, thereby leading to falsely abnormal coagulation test results. In such circumstances, the amount of citrated anticoagulant should be reduced proportionate to the high hematocrit (Box 28-1).[39,40] Conversely, anemia

Box 28-1	Formula for Calculating the Amount of Citrate Appropriate for the Observed Hematocrit

$C = (1.85 \times 10^{-3})(100 - Hct)(V_{blood})$

where C = volume of citrate to be added
Hct = Observed hematocrit for the patient
V_{blood} = Volume of blood to be added

From Marlar RA, Potts RM, Marlar AA. Effect on routine and special coagulation testing values of citrate anticoagulant adjustment in patients with high hematocrit values. Am J Clin Pathol. 2006;126:400-405.

(hematocrit < 25%) does not seem to significantly affect the accuracy of coagulation tests, and adjustment of citrate need not be done.[41] For infants and children, small 3.0-mL tubes (2.7 mL blood to 0.3 mL citrate) are available. The tubes need to be filled to the appropriate mark on the tubes. It is recommended that the tubes be filled to at least 90% of the expected fill volume. Incompletely filled tubes often lead to falsely elevated clotting times.[38]

Once the tube is filled, the anticoagulated blood should be gently mixed by inversion three to four times and sent to the coagulation laboratory in an expeditious manner. Samples with visible hemolysis or clots should be discarded. Samples should be tested within 2 hours of collection if maintained at room temperature or within 4 hours if kept cold. Plasma samples must be frozen if not tested within this time frame. When they are to be analyzed, frozen samples should be rapidly thawed at 37° C and tested immediately. It is helpful to the laboratory to know whether the patient is taking a medication that may affect one or more coagulation tests. Normal values differ from one laboratory to another and between instruments and reagents. Thus, the values obtained should be compared with the normal range for that laboratory. It should also be kept in mind that normal values for coagulation and anticoagulant proteins in children differ with age (Chapter 5).[35,36]

Screening Tests

Often the child's history and physical examination will lead the physician to obtain certain assays immediately. However, if the initial evaluation is not suggestive of a specific disorder, a panel of screening tests should be ordered, including a complete blood count with evaluation of platelet number, morphology, PT, APTT, and thrombin time (TT) (Fig. 28-1).

Prothrombin Time

The PT is performed by adding a thromboplastin reagent that contains calcium chloride to the citrated plasma sample. The time required for clot formation is recorded with an automated instrument that signals the end point, as defined by optical or electromechanical change. The normal (reference) range varies depending on the laboratory (its instrumentation and the lot of thromboplastin), but it is generally 10 to 11 seconds. The PT measures the activities of factors I (fibrinogen), II (prothrombin), V, VII, and X. Prolongation of the PT beyond the reference range is not generally seen until the functional level of one of these factors is less than 30% or until fibrinogen is less than 100 mg/dL. Isolated prolongation of the PT may reflect factor VII deficiency. Though rare, the PT can also be prolonged by a circulating inhibitor or by the presence of abnormal fibrinogen molecules or fragments in the circulation.

The PT is also quite useful for monitoring the effect of coumarin-type anticoagulants. When the PT is used to monitor a patient taking warfarin, differences in the sensitivities of different thromboplastin preparations need to be taken into account. This consideration has led to the development of a standardized method of expressing the prolongation as an international normalized ratio (INR). The INR is calculated as INR = (patient's PT/control PT)$^{\text{International Sensitivity Index (ISI)}}$. The ISI should be determined for each thromboplastin reagent and instrument.

Activated Partial Thromboplastin Time

The APTT is performed by adding a "partial thromboplastin" reagent, which is a source of phospholipids without tissue factor, to the patient's citrated plasma sample, plus introducing controlled activation of the contact factors (factors XI and XII, prekallikrein, and high-molecular-weight kininogen) (Chapter 26) by preincubation with a surface-activating reagent (such as celite, kaolin, silica, or ellagic acid).[42] This mixture is incubated for 2 to 5 minutes before calcium chloride is added, and the time required for clot formation is recorded. As for the PT, automated instruments are generally used. The APTT measures factors I (fibrinogen), II (prothrombin), V, VIII, IX, X, XI, and XII; prekallikrein; and high-molecular-weight kininogen. Deficiency of any of the latter three factors can result in a markedly prolonged APTT in the absence of clinically significant bleeding. Isolated prolongation of the APTT in a patient with clinical bleeding is likely to result from a deficiency of factor VIII, IX, or XI. It should be noted that the sensitivity and reproducibility of the APTT are highly dependent on the specific reagents used (particularly the activator in the partial thromboplastin reagent).[43] With most APTT reagents, the APTT will not be prolonged until the amount of factor VIII is less than 35% (0.35 U/mL). The laboratory should establish a reference range for each new lot of reagent and each new method of clot detection. The reference range will generally be approximately 26 to 35 seconds for children and adults but longer (30 to 54 seconds) in term infants (and often even longer in premature infants).

The APTT is somewhat less sensitive than the PT to deficiency of the vitamin K–dependent factors, but it is more sensitive to the presence of circulating anticoagulants and heparin. The APTT can detect circulating

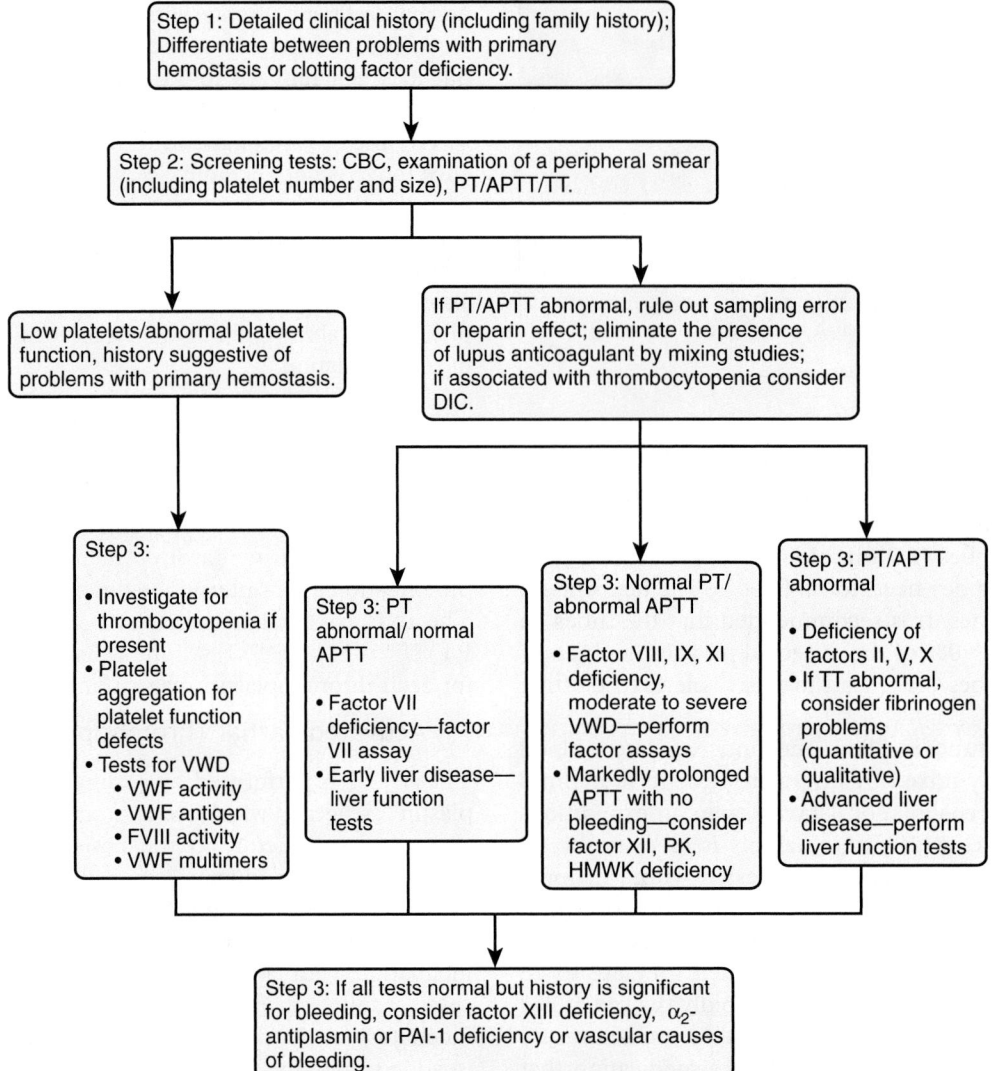

FIGURE 28-1. Stepwise approach to bleeding. APTT, activated partial thromboplastin time; CBC, complete blood count; DIC, disseminated intravascular coagulation; FVIII, factor VIII; HMWK, high-molecular-weight kininogen; PAI-1, plasminogen activator inhibitor 1; PK, prekallikrein; PT, prothrombin time; TT, thrombin time; VWD, von Willebrand's disease; VWF, von Willebrand factor.

anticoagulants (such as lupus anticoagulants [LAs]) and is routinely used to monitor standard heparin therapy.[44] Among hospitalized infants or children, unintentional contamination of patient samples with heparin is a common cause of an unexpected prolongation of the APTT that does not correct on mixing.

Thrombin Time

The TT measures the thrombin-induced conversion of fibrinogen to fibrin and is performed by adding bovine thrombin to the patient's citrated plasma and recording the clotting time. The TT measures the amount and the clotting function of fibrinogen and is also prolonged in the presence of heparin or circulating fibrin degradation products (FDPs). An extremely prolonged TT usually indicates a heparin effect. Reptilase, a snake venom protease, clots fibrinogen in the presence of heparin and thus can be used to identify heparin as the cause of a prolonged TT. Thus, in the presence of heparin the TT is prolonged, whereas the reptilase time is normal. Alternatively, one can test for heparin activity by its anti–factor Xa activity or with the use of commercial heparinase. The sensitivity of the TT can be increased by dilution of the thrombin to give a control TT of 16 to 18 seconds.

Platelet Count

The normal platelet count (for all ages) ranges from 150,000 to 450,000/μL. Platelets are counted with an electronic particle counter or (less often) by direct-phase microscopy. Review of the platelets on a well-prepared, stained blood smear should give a visual estimate that matches the laboratory's printed value. A spuriously low automated platelet count (pseudothrombocytopenia) may result from ethylenediaminetetraacetic acid (EDTA) anticoagulant plus an IgG or IgM platelet antibody, platelet cold agglutinins, or platelet clumping from a partially clotted sample. In the setting of thrombocytopenia, increased or decreased platelet size may suggest increased platelet turnover or decreased production, respectively. Large platelets are also seen in the hereditary giant platelet syndromes, and small platelets are characteristic of Wiskott-Aldrich syndrome. Electric particle counters also often provide a mean platelet volume and platelet volume (size) distribution.

Bleeding Time

The bleeding time (BT) is a measure of the interaction of platelets with the blood vessel wall. Although the BT can provide useful information, it does have significant limitations. It is no doubt the most difficult of the tests of hemostasis to standardize, and thus results may not be reliable. The most widely used method is the modified Ivy BT performed with a template. Although commercially available devices incorporate a spring-loaded blade that is designed to make a skin incision of standard depth and width, arm wiggling in young children, the amount of pressure applied to the arm, and operator experience are a few examples of details that can influence test results.

The BT is performed with a tourniquet maintained at 40 mm Hg and placement of the template device on an area of the forearm (just below the elbow) that is devoid of obvious superficial veins. By breaking off the small tab, the spring is activated and the blade or blades make a linear cut 1 to 2 mm deep (if done correctly, this superficial cut is above the pain fibers). With a stop watch and a piece of filter paper, the blood coming from the cut is gently blotted away while taking care to not touch the filter paper to the cut (which would remove the fragile platelet plug). A normal BT is 3 to 9 minutes. The BT is an approximate measure of the relationship between platelet number and function, as originally demonstrated by Harker and Slichter.[45] With normally functioning platelets, the BT begins to prolong at a platelet count of less than 100,000/μL. The BT can also be prolonged with congenital and acquired platelet function defects (the latter include acquired defects resulting from certain drugs, uremia, and cyanotic congenital heart disease), VWD, vasculitis (e.g., Henoch-Schönlein purpura), and connective tissue disorders such as Ehlers-Danlos syndrome.

PFA-100

Current platelet function tests are often viewed as inaccurate and unreliable (BT) or labor intensive and time consuming (platelet aggregation studies). Recently, a range of new instruments have been developed that attempt to simulate in vivo platelet adhesion and aggregation. The Platelet Functional Analyzer 100 (PFA-100; Dade Behring, Mahburg, Germany) is a commercially available instrument that uses test cartridges containing collagen/adenosine diphosphate (CADP)- or collagen/epinephrine (CEPI)-coated membranes with a small aperture (150 μm). Citrated blood is aspirated under high shear (5000 to 6000/sec) from the sample reservoir through a capillary tube onto the membrane, and blood flow is monitored through the aperture. Platelets begin to adhere and aggregate primarily through interactions of von Willebrand factor (VWF) with glycoprotein Ib and IIb/IIIa, thereby resulting in closure of the aperture. The instrument monitors the drop in flow rate with time as the aperture gradually occludes and records the final closure time (CT) with either cartridge. Although the test is reproducible between cartridge lots and instruments, each laboratory should establish normal control times. Citrate samples have been shown to be stable for up to 4 hours after sample collection, but transport through a pneumatic vacuum transport system ("tube system") is not recommended.[46]

The test is sensitive to the platelet count, hematocrit, platelet function, and VWF level and function. Generally, a platelet count of less than 80 to 100 × 10⁹/L and a hematocrit of less than 30% lead to a prolonged CT.[46] The PFA-100 CT is inversely proportional to the VWF level and has been used by some as a screening test for VWD.[47] Consumption of flavinoid-rich foods (red wine, cocoa, or chocolate) can prolong CEPI CT. Other dietary effects (e.g., fish oil consumption) on the PFA-100 CT have not been studied. In congenital platelet disorders, PFA-100 CT depends on the severity of the disorder. Severe platelet function defects in glycoprotein Ib/V/IX (Bernard-Soulier syndrome or platelet-type VWD) and glycoprotein IIb/IIIa (Glanzmann's thrombasthenia) result in a markedly prolonged CT (see Chapter 29). In platelet dense granule deficiency or secretion defects, the prolongation in CT is variable and is often seen in the CEPI cartridge. Thus, although the PFA-100 CT is abnormal in some forms of platelet disorders, the test does not have sufficient sensitivity or specificity to be used as a screening tool for platelet disorders in general.[48] Additionally, PFA-100 CT may be altered by drugs that affect platelet function. Aspirin and other nonsteroidal anti-inflammatory drugs (NSAIDs) prolong the CEPI CT by inhibition of thromboxane generation. The role of the PFA-100 in therapeutic monitoring is currently being investigated.[48]

Other Assays

Specific Coagulation Factors

Each of the coagulation factors of the intrinsic pathway (prekallikrein, high-molecular-weight kininogen, and factors VIII, IX, XI, and XII) can be measured by one-stage, APTT-based methods. A specific factor assay measures the clotting time of a mixture of diluted test plasma and a specific factor–deficient substrate plasma that supplies all factors except the one being measured.[49] Though

$^{1}/_{2}$

seldom performed in U.S. clinical laboratories, a chromogenic substrate assay kit for factor VIII (as well as chromogenic kits for certain other clotting factors) that is based on measuring the generation of factor Xa is also commercially available.

Each of the extrinsic and common pathway coagulation factors (V, VII, and X) can be measured by specific one-stage assays based on the PT. The patient's diluted test plasma is incubated with commercially available plasma that is deficient in either factor V, VII, or X; a mixture of tissue factor and calcium chloride is added, and the clotting time is determined.[49]

For each clotting factor assay based on the APTT or PT, the clotting times of serial dilutions of a plasma sample representing a pool obtained from a large number of normal individuals is used to construct a standard curve. The concentration of the specific factor in each of the several dilutions of patient plasma is determined from the standard curve and is used to calculate the level of that clotting factor in the patient's undiluted plasma.[49] In most laboratories, automated instruments are used to perform the assays, and many of these instruments are preprogrammed with a statistical package for plotting the data. The reference pooled plasma should be calibrated with a commercial or national standard that has been assayed against an international standard when available.[50]

Covalent stabilization of fibrin by factor XIIIa is essential for normal hemostasis (Chapter 26). Factor XIIIa catalyzes the formation of covalent cross-links between the γ and α chains of fibrin, which results in increased mechanical stability of the fibrin clot and resistance to its degradation by plasmin. Congenital deficiency of factor XIII is a rare hereditary (autosomal recessive) cause of moderate to severe hemorrhage, often with a characteristic pattern of delayed bleeding (see Chapter 31). None of the routine screening tests (PT, APTT, or BT) detect factor XIII deficiency.[51] A screening test for factor XIII deficiency can be done with the clot solubility test: solubility of the patient's recalcified plasma clot in 5 mol/L urea or monochloroacetic acid is assessed after 30 minutes and periodically at 1, 2, 4, and 24 hours. Clots from patients with less than 1% factor XIII activity are soluble. Quantitation of factor XIII can be done with specific amine incorporation assays, although these tests are generally performed only in specialized research laboratories.[51]

Recommended tests for VWD include APTT, factor VIII assay, ristocetin cofactor assay as a measure of VWF activity, VWF antigen assay, and ABO blood group typing. If these tests are suggestive of VWD, VWF multimer analysis should be performed. Treatment of VWD depends on accurate subtype diagnosis (see Chapter 30).

Antiphospholipid Antibodies

Antiphospholipid antibodies (APAs) include LAs, anticardiolipin antibodies, antiphosphatidylserine antibodies, and antiphosphatidylethanolamine antibodies. APAs are immunoglobulins (IgG, IgM, and IgA) directed against anionic phospholipids or phospholipid–plasma protein complexes. Approximately 30% of APAs are found in association with thromboembolic events, recurrent abortions, or thrombocytopenia (referred to as the APA syndrome).

APAs have been associated with autoimmune disorders, infectious disease processes, acquired immunodeficiency syndrome, hematologic malignancies, lymphoproliferative disorders, seizure disorders, migraine, stroke, and subdural hematomas. Anticardiolipin antibodies are distinct from LAs. The antigenic target for anticardiolipin antibodies is thought to be cardiolipin, β_2-glycoprotein I, or a complex of the two. Cardiolipin is an important lipid component of mammalian cell membranes. LAs are often seen in persons with no underlying disease and no history of abnormal bleeding. They may be detected in pediatric patients receiving certain drugs, particularly antibiotics. LAs are immunoglobulins that interfere with one or more phospholipid-dependent coagulation tests, such as the APTT, PT, dilute Russell viper venom time, and kaolin clotting time. Coagulation tests for LAs are based on their interference with reactions that depend on the phospholipid added to substitute for platelets when citrated plasma is recalcified in vitro. The presence of LAs may be chronic (as in autoimmune disorders) or transient.[52]

The APTT is the test generally used to screen for LAs, although the sensitivity of the APTT for LAs depends on the reagent and method used. Many modifications of the APTT have been recommended in an attempt to increase its sensitivity to LAs, including the addition of less phospholipid. The PT is often normal in the presence of LAs. The dilute Russell viper venom time performed with dilute phospholipid can also be used to detect LAs, as can the STACLOT LA.[52] LAs must be differentiated from inhibition caused by heparin, from a clotting factor deficiency, or from an acquired inhibitor to a clotting factor (usually factor VIII). LAs can also occur in patients with hemophilia A. In one study, 21% of subjects with hemophilia A were found to have LAs.[53] According to guidelines developed by the Scientific and Standardization Subcommittee on Lupus Anticoagulants of the International Society on Thrombosis and Hemostasis, the minimum diagnostic criteria for LAs are (1) an abnormal phospholipid-dependent coagulation assay, (2) demonstration of an inhibitor as a cause of the abnormality, and (3) demonstration that the inhibitor is directed against a phospholipid and not a specific coagulation factor.[52] Genetic determinants may play a role in the development of clinical manifestations related to APAs and the APA syndrome.[54]

If the APTT is prolonged, a mixing study is performed. Failure of the APTT to correct on mixing indicates an inhibitor, and confirmatory studies can then be performed. Such tests typically alter the phospholipid content of the assay, either increasing it, as in the platelet neutralization procedure, or decreasing it, as in the dilute Russell viper venom time.

Fibrinogen

Fibrinogen's concentration in plasma can be measured immunologically (fibrinogen antigen) or by a chemical method in which the ability of fibrinogen to clot does not influence the assay. Normal fibrinogen antigen levels are between 200 to 400 mg/dL. Fibrinogen is an acute phase reactant, and elevated levels are commonly seen in stress or acute illness.

The level of functional fibrinogen or fibrinogen activity can also be measured. The von Clauss kinetic assay uses a dilute solution of patient plasma and an excess of thrombin, which makes fibrinogen the rate-limiting step in the clotting reaction.[55] The resulting clotting time in seconds is compared with a standard dilution curve to determine the concentration of clottable fibrinogen. Fibrinogen is decreased in congenital afibrinogenemia, hypofibrinogenemia, and consumptive states such as DIC. The assay is also sensitive to abnormalities in fibrinogen function (dysfibrinogenemia) or the presence of inhibitors of fibrin formation such as FDPs.

Fibrin(ogen) Degradation Products and D-Dimer

FDPs are usually measured in serum samples because these degradation products consist predominantly of nonclottable derivatives that remain in solution after clot formation. These global tests involve the use of flocculation, tanned red cell hemagglutination, radioimmunoassay, or radioautograph analysis. Latex bead and enzyme-linked immunosorbent assays based on monoclonal antibodies specific to cross-linked D-dimer fragments are commercially available and in widespread use. The D-dimer assay will identify only cross-linked FDPs (indicating that fibrin has formed intravascularly, has been cross-linked, and has then been cleaved into D-dimers by plasmin; see Chapter 27). The patient's plasma or serum sample is serially diluted, and each dilution of the sample is mixed with latex beads coated with antibody to D-dimer. The end point of the assay is determined by the highest dilution of patient serum or plasma that produces visible agglutination. This titer is then used to calculate the D-dimer concentration in the patient's sample.[56,57]

Euglobulin Clot Lysis Time

The euglobulin clot lysis time (ECLT) is a screening test for excessive fibrinolysis. It is performed by using the plasma euglobulin fraction prepared from fresh, citrated, platelet-poor plasma. After clot formation, lysis is measured. The normal ECLT is 60 to 300 minutes. It is shortened in conditions characterized by increased fibrinolysis (e.g. α_2-antiplasmin deficiency, plasminogen activator inhibitor 1 deficiency, or systemic fibrinolysis).

Platelet Function Tests

When ordering tests of platelet function, one must be aware that a wide variety of drugs can affect the platelet count and alter test results. Drugs such as aspirin irreversibly affect platelet function for the entire life span of the platelet (10 to 11 days). Thus, tests of platelet function should be scheduled at a time when the individual has not taken any relevant drugs for at least 10 days.

The most common test of platelet function is platelet aggregometry. Platelet aggregation can be performed in whole blood by impedance technique or in platelet-rich plasma (PRP) by the turbidometric technique. Whole blood platelet aggregation can be combined with release of adenosine triphosphate (ATP) by using a lumi-aggregometer. A variety of platelet agonists (ristocetin, epinephrine, collagen, adenosine diphosphate, and arachidonic acid) can be added to an aliquot of the patient's sample. The rapidity and extent of platelet agglutination are detected by changes in optical density (PRP) or impedance (whole blood) and are graphically recorded for each agonist used.[58] In Glanzmann's thrombasthenia, the patient's platelets will agglutinate normally with ristocetin but not at all with the addition of adenosine diphosphate, epinephrine, collagen, or arachidonic acid. In Bernard-Soulier syndrome, platelet agglutination will occur normally on addition of each of these agonists except ristocetin.[58]

Global Tests for the Evaluation of Bleeding

As knowledge of the coagulation system developed in the 1950s, specific assays were devised to measure the individual clotting factors. However, it soon became apparent that individual clotting factor assays were inadequate to assess the true nature of the hemostatic system. It was obvious that static end point laboratory tests such as the PT or APTT were also not accurately reflective of the patient's overall hemostatic status and could not assess the dynamic clotting cascade. The common clinical observation that hemophilia patients have great phenotypic variation in bleeding despite identical factor levels stresses this point. This has led to a revival of interest in global clotting assays. In addition, the development of technical innovations and computer-assisted methods of analysis has improved the reliability and reproducibility of global assays. Two such techniques are described here: thromboelastography (TEG) and thrombin generation assays (TGAs). TEG is usually performed on whole blood and quantitatively measures the dynamics of fibrin formation. TGAs are generally performed on plasma and measure thrombin formation.

Thromboelastography

Hartert first described TEG as a global test for blood coagulation more than 50 years ago.[59] TEG monitors the whole dynamic process of hemostasis from clot formation to its dissolution and also provides information about platelet function. TEG produces a continuous profile of the overall rheologic changes occurring during coagulation while using a small amount of whole blood.

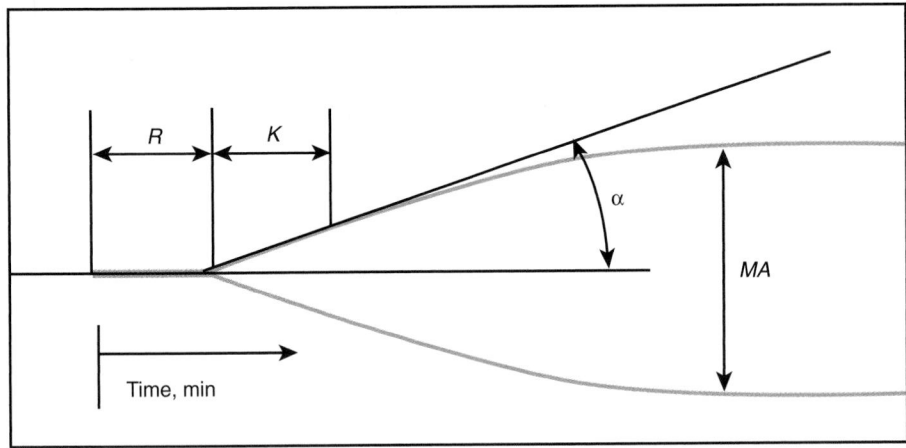

R: Time to initial clot formation.
K: Measure of the speed to reach a certain level of clot strength.
Alpha angle: Measure of rapidity of fibrin cross linking.
MA: Maximum amplitude, depends on function of fibrin and platelets, represents clot strength.

FIGURE 28-2. Tracing of a normal thromboelastogram.

By processing the data, the viscoelastic changes occurring during whole blood clot formation can be transformed into a dynamic velocity profile that is then recorded as a tracing (Fig. 28-2). Currently, reagent-modified TEG with various activators (tissue factor, kaolin) and inhibitors is used with the aim of accelerating the coagulation cascade and obtaining differential diagnostic information.[60] The two commonly used instruments are the TEG (Haemoscope Corp, Skokie, Illinois) and the rotating thromboelastometer ROTEM (Pentapharm, Munich).[61] Currently used primarily as a tool to decrease transfusion requirement during cardiac[62] and hepatic surgery, these instruments are also being investigated as a screening tool for bleeding disorders.[63,64]

Thrombin Generation Assays

TGAs have been used extensively in research laboratories but are cumbersome to perform.[65] A more recently developed test, calibrated automated thrombography (CAT), may be applicable to the routine clinical laboratory. CAT measures the concentration of thrombin in clotting plasma by monitoring the splitting of a fluorogenic substrate and comparing the results with known constant thrombin activity in a parallel nonclotting sample (control).[66] Application of TGAs is currently being investigated for monitoring of hemophilia treatment and anticoagulation therapy and to better understand the differing clinical patterns in bleeding disorders.[67]

Laboratory Findings in Disseminated Intravascular Coagulation

DIC is an acquired systemic disorder characterized by widespread activation of coagulation and deposition of fibrin leading to the formation of thrombi in the microcirculation accompanied by secondary activation of fibri-

Box 28-2	Conditions Associated with Disseminated Intravascular Coagulation

Sepsis (particularly gram-negative bacteremia)
Trauma
    Massive tissue injury
    Head injury
Fat embolism
Malignancy
    Acute promyelocytic leukemia
    Myeloproliferative disorders
Obstetric accidents
Vascular disorders
    Giant hemangiomas (Kasabach-Merritt syndrome)
    Aortic aneurysm
Toxins
    Snake venom
    Drug overdose
Immunologic reactions
    Severe anaphylaxis
    Acute hemolysis
    Acute transplant rejection

nolyis[68] (see Chapter 34). DIC can be acute or chronic, compensated or decompensated, and can be caused by a wide variety of conditions (Box 28-2). DIC should be suspected in children with shock and bleeding manifestations. In DIC, the PT and APTT are usually both prolonged, with decreased fibrinogen, factor VIII, and factor V. A concomitant decrease in natural anticoagulants (protein C, protein S, and antithrombin III) may also be seen. Examination of the peripheral smear usually reveals the presence of schistocytes and thrombocytopenia.[69] There is also an increase in D-dimer and FDPs secondary to the formation of plasmin (Fig. 28-3).

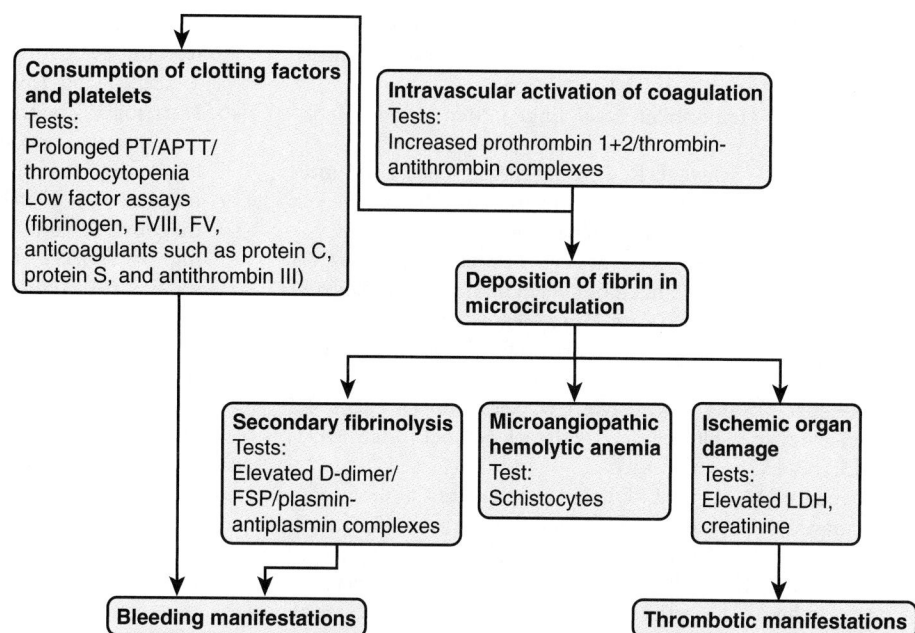

FIGURE 28-3. Pathophysiology of disseminated intravascular coagulation. APTT, activated partial thromboplastin time; FSP, fibrin split products; FVIII, factor VIII; LDH, lactate dehydrogenase; PT, prothrombin time.

REFERENCES

1. Sramek A, Eikenboom JC, Briet E, et al. Usefulness of patient interview in bleeding disorders. Arch Intern Med. 1995;155:1409-1415.

2. Koreth R, Weinert C, Weisdorf DJ, et al. Measurement of bleeding severity: a critical review. Transfusion. 2004;44: 605-617.

3. Hedlund-Treutiger I, Revel-Vilk S, Blanchette VS, et al. Reliability and reproducibility of classification of children as "bleeders" versus "non-bleeders" using a questionnaire for significant mucocutaneous bleeding. J Pediatr Hematol Oncol. 2004;26:488-491.

4. Buchanan GR, Adix L. Grading of hemorrhage in children with idiopathic thrombocytopenic purpura. J Pediatr. 2002;141:683-688.

5. Rodeghiero F, Castaman G, Tosetto A, et al. The discriminant power of bleeding history for the diagnosis of type 1 von Willebrand disease: an international, multicenter study. J Thromb Haemost. 2005;3:2619-2626.

6. Tosetto A, Rodeghiero F, Castaman G, et al. A quantitative analysis of bleeding symptoms in type 1 von Willebrand disease: results from a multicenter European study (MCMDM-1 VWD). J Thromb Haemost. 2006;4:766-773.

7. Mannucci PM, Duga S, Peyvandi F. Recessively inherited coagulation disorders. Blood. 2004;104:1243-1252.

8. Aledort LM, Green D, Teitel JM. Unexpected bleeding disorders. Hematol Am Soc Hematol Educ Program. 2001; 306-321.

9. Hayward CP. Diagnosis and management of mild bleeding disorders. Hematol Am Soc Hematol Educ Program. 2005; 423-428.

10. James AH, Ragni MV, Picozzi VJ. Bleeding disorders in premenopausal women: (another) public health crisis for hematology? Hematol Am Soc Hematol Educ Program. 2006;474-485.

11. Demers C, Derzko C, David M, Douglas J. Gynaecological and obstetric management of women with inherited bleeding disorders. Int J Gynaecol Obstet. 2006;95:75-87.

12. Kadir RA, Chi C. Women and von Willebrand disease: controversies in diagnosis and management. Semin Thromb Hemost. 2006;32:605-615.

13. Chi C, Shiltagh N, Kingman CE, et al. Identification and management of women with inherited bleeding disorders: a survey of obstetricians and gynaecologists in the United Kingdom. Haemophilia. 2006;12:405-412.

14. Friberg B, Orno AK, Lindgren A, Lethagen S. Bleeding disorders among young women: a population-based prevalence study. Acta Obstet Gynecol Scand. 2006;85: 200-206.

15. Holzberg M, Hewan-Lowe KO, Olansky AJ. The Ehlers-Danlos syndrome: recognition, characterization, and importance of a milder variant of the classic form. A preliminary study. J Am Acad Dermatol. 1988;19:656-666.

16. Oderich GS. Current concepts in the diagnosis and management of vascular Ehlers-Danlos syndrome. Perspect Vasc Surg Endovasc Ther. 2006;18:206-214.

17. Trotter JF. Coagulation abnormalities in patients who have liver disease. Clin Liver Dis. 2006;10:665-678.

18. Caldwell SH, Hoffman M, Lisman T, et al. Coagulation disorders and hemostasis in liver disease: pathophysiology and critical assessment of current management. Hepatology. 2006;44:1039-1046.

19. Brophy DF, Martin EJ, Carr SL, et al. The effect of uremia on platelet contractile force, clot elastic modulus and bleeding time in hemodialysis patients. Thromb Res. 2007;119: 723-729.

20. Hassan AA, Kroll MH. Acquired disorders of platelet function. Hematol Am Soc Hematol Educ Program. 2005; 403-408.

21. Kaysen GA. Plasma composition in the nephrotic syndrome. Am J Nephrol. 1993;13:347-359.

22. Ertekin V, Selimoglu MA. Prevalence of prolonged prothrombin time in children with coeliac disease. Eur J Gastroenterol Hepatol. 2006;18:579-580; author reply 580.

23. Vaynshtein G, Rosenbaum H, Groisman GM, et al. Celiac sprue presenting as severe hemorrhagic diathesis due to vitamin K deficiency. Isr Med Assoc J. 2004;6:781-783.

24. Tempe DK, Virmani S. Coagulation abnormalities in patients with cyanotic congenital heart disease. J Cardiothorac Vasc Anesth. 2002;16:752-765.

25. Hoyer LW. Hemophilia A. N Engl J Med. 1994;330:38-47.

26. Oldenburg J, Schwaab R, Grimm T, et al. Direct and indirect estimation of the sex ratio of mutation frequencies in hemophilia A. Am J Hum Genet. 1993;53:1229-1238.

27. Bell J, Haldane JB. The linkage between the genes for colour-blindness and haemophilia in man. By Julia Bell and J.B.S. Haldane, 1937. Ann Hum Genet. 1986;50:3-34.

28. Seligsohn U. Factor XI deficiency. Thromb Haemost. 1993;70:68-71.

29. Asakai R, Chung DW, Davie EW, Seligsohn U. Factor XI deficiency in Ashkenazi Jews in Israel. N Engl J Med. 1991;325:153-158.

30. Dinehart SM, Henry L. Dietary supplements: altered coagulation and effects on bruising. Dermatol Surg. 2005;31:819-826; discussion 826.

31. Winter SL, Kriel RL, Novacheck TF, et al. Perioperative blood loss: the effect of valproate. Pediatr Neurol. 1996;15:19-22.

32. Loiseau P. Sodium valproate, platelet dysfunction, and bleeding. Epilepsia. 1981;22:141-146.

33. Nuss R, Hathaway WE. Effect of mode of delivery on neonatal intracranial injury. N Engl J Med. 2000;342:892-893.

34. Kulkarni R, Ponder KP, James AH, et al. Unresolved issues in diagnosis and management of inherited bleeding disorders in the perinatal period: a White Paper of the Perinatal Task Force of the Medical and Scientific Advisory Council of the National Hemophilia Foundation, USA. Haemophilia. 2006;12:205-211.

35. Andrew M, Vegh P, Johnston M, et al. Maturation of the hemostatic system during childhood. Blood. 1992;80:1998-2005.

36. Reverdiau-Moalic P, Delahousse B, Body G, et al. Evolution of blood coagulation activators and inhibitors in the healthy human fetus. Blood. 1996;88:900-906.

37. Lippi G, Salvagno GL, Montagnana M, et al. Influence of the needle bore size on platelet count and routine coagulation testing. Blood Coagul Fibrinolysis. 2006;17:557-561.

38. Lippi G, Franchini M, Montagnana M, et al. Quality and reliability of routine coagulation testing: can we trust that sample? Blood Coagul Fibrinolysis. 2006;17:513-519.

39. Ingram GI, Hills M. The prothrombin time test: effect of varying citrate concentration. Thromb Haemost. 1976;36:230-236.

40. Marlar RA, Potts RM, Marlar AA. Effect on routine and special coagulation testing values of citrate anticoagulant adjustment in patients with high hematocrit values. Am J Clin Pathol. 2006;126:400-405.

41. Siegel JE, Swami VK, Glenn P, et al. Effect (or lack of it) of severe anemia on PT and APTT results. Am J Clin Pathol. 1998;110:106-110.

42. Koepke JA. Performance guidelines for the partial thromboplastin time test. Ric Clin Lab. 1989;19:359-362.

43. Hillman C, Lusher JM. Determining sensitivity of coagulation screening reagents: a simplified method. J Lab Med. 1982;13:162-165.

44. Adcock DM, Marlar RA. Activated partial thromboplastin time reagent sensitivity to the presence of the lupus anticoagulant. Arch Pathol Lab Med. 1992;116:837-840.

45. Harker LA, Slichter SJ. The bleeding time as a screening test for evaluation of platelet function. N Engl J Med. 1972;287:155-159.

46. Harrison P. The role of PFA-100 testing in the investigation and management of haemostatic defects in children and adults. Br J Haematol. 2005;130:3-10.

47. Favaloro EJ, Kershaw G, Bukuya M, et al. Laboratory diagnosis of von Willebrand disorder (vWD) and monitoring of DDAVP therapy: efficacy of the PFA-100 and vWF:CBA as combined diagnostic strategies. Haemophilia. 2001;7:180-189.

48. Hayward CP, Harrison P, Cattaneo M, et al. Platelet function analyzer (PFA)-100 closure time in the evaluation of platelet disorders and platelet function. J Thromb Haemost. 2006;4:312-319.

49. Hultin M. Coagulation factor assays. In Beutler E, Lichtman MA, Coller BS, et al (eds). Williams Hematology, 5th ed. New York, McGraw-Hill, 1995, pp 189-190.

50. Hubbard AR, Rigsby P, Barrowcliffe TW. Standardisation of factor VIII and von Willebrand factor in plasma: calibration of the 4th International Standard (97/586). Thromb Haemost. 2001;85:634-638.

51. Lorand L, Urayama T, De Kiewiet JW, et al. Diagnostic and genetic studies on fibrin-stabilizing factor with a new assay based on amine incorporation. J Clin Invest. 1969;48:1054-1064.

52. Miyakis S, Lockshin MD, Atsumi T, et al. International consensus statement on an update of the classification criteria for definite antiphospholipid syndrome (APS). J Thromb Haemost. 2006;4:295-306.

53. Blanco AN, Cardozo MA, Candela M, et al. Anti–factor VIII inhibitors and lupus anticoagulants in haemophilia A patients. Thromb Haemost. 1997;77:656-659.

54. Galli M. MHC class II and III polymorphisms and the antiphospholipid syndrome. Thromb Haemost. 2001;85:193-194.

55. Nieuwenhuizen W. Biochemistry and measurement of fibrinogen. Eur Heart J. 1995;16(Suppl A):6-10; discussion 10.

56. Carr JM, McKinney M, McDonagh J. Diagnosis of disseminated intravascular coagulation. Role of D-dimer. Am J Clin Pathol. 1989;91:280-287.

57. Dempfle CE. What role does the measurement of fibrinogen and its derivatives have in the diagnosis of disseminated intravascular coagulation? Blood Rev. 2002;16(Suppl 1):S23-28.

58. Kottke-Marchant K, Corcoran G. The laboratory diagnosis of platelet disorders. Arch Pathol Lab Med. 2002;126:133-146.

59. Hartert H. [Thromboelastography, a method for physical analysis of blood coagulation.] Z Gesamte Exp Med. 1951;117:189-203.

60. Nielsen VG, Audu P, Cankovic L, et al. Qualitative thromboelastographic detection of tissue factor in human plasma. Anesth Analg. 2007;104:59-64.

61. Lang T, Bauters A, Braun SL, et al. Multi-centre investigation on reference ranges for ROTEM thromboelastometry. Blood Coagul Fibrinolysis. 2005;16:301-310.

62. Nydegger UE, Gygax E, Carrel T. Point-of-care testing in the cardiovascular operating theatre. Clin Chem Lab Med. 2006;44:1060-1065.

63. Rugeri L, Levrat A, David JS, et al. Diagnosis of early coagulation abnormalities in trauma patients by rotation

thrombelastography. J Thromb Haemost. 2007;5:289-295.

64. Collins PW, Macchiavello LI, Lewis SJ, et al. Global tests of haemostasis in critically ill patients with severe sepsis syndrome compared to controls. Br J Haematol. 2006;135: 220-227.

65. Luddington R, Baglin T. Clinical measurement of thrombin generation by calibrated automated thrombography requires contact factor inhibition. J Thromb Haemost. 2004;2:1954-1959.

66. Hemker HC. Calibrated automated thrombinography (CAT). Thromb Res. 2005;115:255.

67. Hemker HC, Al Dieri R, Beguin S. Thrombin generation assays: accruing clinical relevance. Curr Opin Hematol. 2004;11:170-175.

68. Levi M, Ten Cate H. Disseminated intravascular coagulation. N Engl J Med. 1999;341:586-592.

69. Toh CH, Downey C. Back to the future: testing in disseminated intravascular coagulation. Blood Coagul Fibrinolysis. 2005;16:535-542.

29

Inherited Platelet Disorders

Michele P. Lambert and Mortimer Poncz

Platelets are small (1 to 4 µm in diameter) cells once thought to be fragments of other mature blood cells and dismissed as "blood dust." They are now known to be highly specialized and organized fragments released by a still poorly understood process from intramedullary megakaryocytes within the bone marrow. Platelets are a critical component for the first phase of hemostasis (formation of the platelet plug), which can halt the loss of blood from vessels whose endothelial integrity has been interrupted. If platelets are deficient in number or defective in function, excessive bleeding may occur. The clinical manifestations of platelet-type bleeding typically involve the skin or mucous membranes and include petechiae, ecchymosis, epistaxis, menorrhagia, and gastrointestinal hemorrhage (Box 29-1). Intracranial bleeding can occur, but it is infrequent. The deep muscle hematomas and hemarthrosis typically seen in patients with defects in the fluid-phrase (plasma) hemostatic system infrequently occur in platelet disorders.

Inherited platelet disorders can involve a qualitative or quantitive defect and can be broadly classified according to one of these two categories. In this chapter these disorders are classified by their predominant feature, although many involve defects in both platelet number and function. For example, Bernard-Soulier syndrome (BSS) results from defects in the platelet receptor glycoprotein Ibα/Ibβ/IX/V (GPIb/IX) complex, which binds von Willebrand factor (VWF) and is critical for adherence of platelets at sites of vascular injury. This receptor is anchored to the cytoskeleton and is critical in platelet formation from megakaryocytes. Thus, many of these patients have macrothrombocytes and low platelet counts, as well as a defect in platelet function. Furthermore, although many inherited platelet disorders have been described, most are extremely rare, and even the well-known disorders such as BSS and Glanzmann's thrombasthenia (GT) are uncommon, with a frequency in the general population of 10^{-5} to 10^{-6}, and are mostly seen in inbreeding populations or consanguineous relationships. In aggregate, however, these disorders are not uncommon and, given the diverse nature of the underlying defects, may pose a significant diagnostic challenge.

QUALITATIVE DISORDERS

Platelet Membrane

Sensing abnormalities in their microenvironment, adhering to damaged vascular wall, and aggregating to each other are central functions of circulating platelets. Over the past 20 years many of the membrane receptors in these processes have been cloned. Initially, many of these protein receptors were classified by their electrophoretic mobility and molecular mass and numbered sequentially. Now, it is clear that many of these proteins are members of several large families of receptors, including the integrin α/β heteroduplexes, the leucine-rich receptors, the G protein–coupled receptors (GPCRs), and the immunoglobulin superfamily. Such a classification takes advantage of the similar structure and function of members of these families. Frequently, family members share a common family of ligands or activate cells by a common pathway. Table 29-1 lists the members of these families of receptors that are found on platelets, as well as several receptors that do not belong to any of these families. Many of these receptors have other historical names, and these, as well as their cluster differentiation (CD) antigen nomenclature, are noted in the table. Many of the receptors involved in inherited platelet disorders are described in the following text.

Glanzmann's Thrombasthenia: Defective Platelet Integrin $\alpha_{IIb}\beta_3$

In 1918, a Swiss pediatrician named Glanzmann described a heterogeneous group of disorders that he termed "thrombasthenie" ("weak platelets"); these disorders were characterized by normal platelet counts but abnormal clot retraction.[1] In 1956 it was noted that these platelets failed to spread onto a surface or to stick to each other (aggregate).[2,3] GT is now known to be a rare, inherited, autosomal recessive bleeding disorder, the hallmark of which is failure of platelets to bind fibrinogen and aggregate after activation. The underlying defect is an abnormality in the genes encoding either chain of the integrin $\alpha_{IIb}\beta_3$ fibrinogen receptor (see Table 29-1). GT is the most common of the inherited platelet disorders.[4]

Biology of the $\alpha_{IIb}\beta_3$ Receptor

The α_{IIb} and β_3 subunits are encoded by separate genes that are closely linked on chromosome 17q21-23.[5] α_{IIb} is approximately 145 kd in size and contains 18 cysteine residues arranged into nine disulfide bonds that are rather evenly spaced throughout its length (Fig. 29-1). The α_{IIb} prochain complexes with the β_3 subunit in the endoplasmic reticulum. During maturation in the Golgi body, the α_{IIb} prochain is cleaved into the α_{IIb} heavy fragment and the α_{IIb} light fragment, with the two fragments remaining linked by a disulfide bond.[6] Like most other integrin α chains, α_{IIb} contains four calcium-binding domains near its N-terminal.[7] This region in all α subunits contains seven homologous repeats[8] that fold into a β-propeller structure[9,10]; portions of the surface loops of this structure are critical for ligand binding (in interaction with the βA domain of the β_3 subunit).[9,11]

TABLE 29-1 **Major Platelet Membrane Receptors**

Class of Receptor	Receptor	Other Names	Number of Receptors per Platelet	Ligand
Integrins	$\alpha_{IIb}\beta_3$	GPIIb/IIIa, CD41b	≈80,000	Fibrinogen, VWF, fibronectin
	$\alpha_V\beta_3$		≈500	Vitronectin, osteopontin
	$\alpha_2\beta_1$	CD49b	≈2,000	Collagen
	$\alpha_5\beta_1$	CD49e	≈4,000	Fibronectin
	$\alpha_6\beta_1$	CD49f		Laminin
Leucine-rich repeats receptor	GPIb-IX	CD42a, b, c	≈25,000	VWF, thrombin, P-selectin
G protein–coupled receptors	PAR-1		≈2,000	Thrombin
	PAR-4		Low	Thrombin
	P2Y1			ADP
	P2X1			ADP
	P2Y12			ADP
	α_{2A}		≈700	Epinephrine
	TP		≈1,000	Thromboxane
	IP			Prostaglandin I_2
	CXCR1 and CXCR2		≈2,000 each	Interleukin-8
	CXCR4		≈2,000	Stromal-derived factor 1
	CCR4		≈2,000	CCL22
Immunoglobulin superfamily receptors	GPVI		1,000-3,000	Collagen
	P-selectin	GMP-140, PADGEM, MARK		P-selectin, glycoprotein-1
	PECAM-1	CD31	≈10,000	PECAM-1
	FcγRIIA	CD32	1,000-5,000	Immune complexes
Others	GPIV	CD36	≈25,000	Collagen
	p65			Collagen

ADP, adenosine diphosphate; GPIIb, glycoprotein IIb; PADGEM, platelet activation-dependent granule-external membrane protein; MAPK, mitogen-activate protein kinase; PAR, protease-activated receptor; PECAM-1, platelet–endothelial cell adhesion molecule 1; VWF, von Willebrand factor.

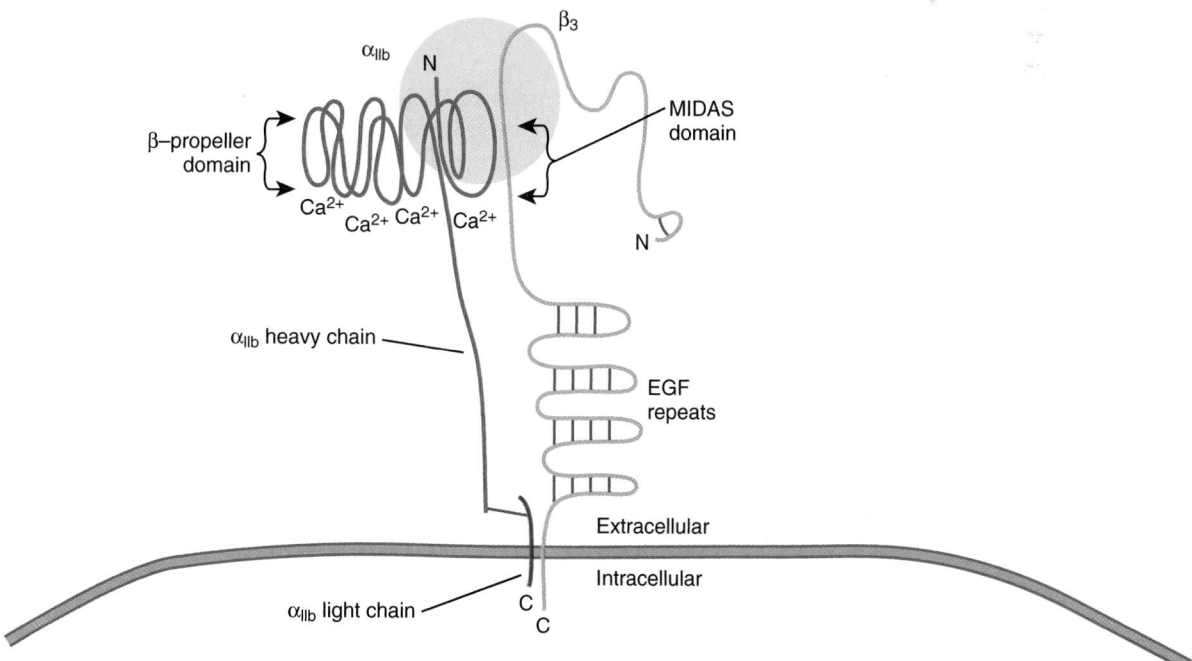

FIGURE 29-1. Structure of the $\alpha_{IIb}\beta_3$ receptor. Both units of the $\alpha_{IIb}\beta_3$ heteroduplex contain a transmembrane domain with short intracellular tails. The α_{IIb} extracellular domain is cleaved into two parts: the α_{IIb} heavy chain, which has the N-terminal β-propeller domain, and the α_{IIb} light chain, which spans from the extracellular to the intracellular compartment. The β_3 chain contains multiple cysteine disulfide bonds represented by the *gray lines*. The MIDAS (metal ion–dependent adhesion site) domain is indicated. The pocket on $\alpha_{IIb}\beta_3$ that may represent the ligand-binding domain is shown as a *gray ball*. EGF, epidermal growth factor.

Similar to other integrin β chains, $β_3$ is approximately 90 kd and contains 762 amino acid residues in its mature form (see Fig. 29-1).[12] $β_3$ contains five cysteine-rich regions for a total of 56 cysteine residues, including a large disulfide-bonded loop, termed the βA region, that extends from amino acids Cys5 to Cys435.[9] This loop participates in fibrinogen binding and contains three divalent cation-binding domains that appear to be important in ligand binding. One of these cation-binding sites (the βA MIDAS—metal ion–dependent adhesion site), interacts directly with ligand,[9] and binding of cations to the βA domain may stabilize the ligand-occupied conformation.

There are about 8×10^4 $α_{IIb}β_3$ receptors per platelet, the most abundant receptor on platelets (see Table 29-1).[12] Most of these receptors are located on the platelet surface, although a portion are found on the inner surface of alpha granules and are involved in the localization of fibrinogen to these granules.[13] On resting platelets, $α_{IIb}β_3$ exists in a folded, inactive state that does not interact with its ligand. However, upon platelet activation, an "inside-out" signaling event takes place in which the $α_{IIb}β_3$ complex is activated and unfolded like a switch blade,[9] thereby resulting in binding of fibrinogen at the N-terminals of the two proteins and platelet aggregation. After ligand binding, an "outside-in" signal mediates integrin-cytoskeleton interactions and platelet spreading.[14]

Many integrin ligands contain an arginine–glycine–aspartic acid (RGD) motif[15] that participates in integrin binding. Conversely, RGD-containing peptides act as competitive inhibitors of ligand binding.[15,16] For example, the RGD motif located in the C1 domain of VWF[17] appears to be necessary for binding of VWF to $α_{IIb}β_3$. In contrast, deletion of the two RGD sequences in the fibrinogen α chain does not impair its ability to bind to $α_{IIb}β_3$.[18] Rather, binding of fibrinogen to $α_{IIb}β_3$ requires a KQAGD sequence located at the carboxyl-terminal of the fibrinogen γ chain.[18]

Whereas expression of the $α_{IIb}$ chain is restricted to megakaryocytes, the $β_3$ subunit is expressed more widely as a component of the $α_Vβ_3$ (vitronectin) receptor. Mouse studies have shown that deletion of $α_Vβ_3$ function results in placental defects and osteosclerosis,[19] although to date no differences have been noted between patients with GT caused by an $α_{IIb}$ or $β_3$ defect.[4]

Clinical Features

Thrombasthenia is characterized by repeated mucocutaneous bleeding beginning at an early age (Fig. 29-2A). Epistaxis and gastrointestinal bleeding are frequent issues in early childhood that often require intervention, as well as iron supplementation. Menorrhagia is a critical problem in teenage girls.[21] The bleeding that normally accompanies pregnancy, surgical procedures, tooth extraction, or physical trauma can be excessive in GT patients. Unprovoked intracranial or gastrointestinal hemorrhage occurs and accounts for a significant portion of the observed 5% to 10% lifelong mortality rate. In addition, some patients experience joint bleeding or muscle hematomas more characteristic of the hemophilias.[21] Frequently, local compression strategies or topical application of thrombin is useful when bleeding occurs. DDAVP (1-deamino-8-D-arginine vasopressin) has been used as well, and oral contraceptive management of menorrhagia is generally sufficient. Platelet transfusions may be useful until resistance to platelet infusions develops, although patients do not necessarily form antibodies to the $α_{IIb}β_3$ receptor. Antibodies may be particularly problematic because they may not only result in increased platelet clearance or platelet refractoriness but may also directly interfere with platelet function.[22] Recent evidence suggests that recombinant activated factor VII may be a useful supplement to platelet transfusions.[23] We have also successfully used embolic block of arterioles feeding the nose and uterus in cases of recurrent, life-threatening hemorrhage.

Incidence

Though infrequent worldwide, GT is found at high incidence among certain isolated populations and in the setting of consanguineous relationships, particularly among Arab populations,[24] Iraqi Jews,[25] French gypsies,[26] and individuals from southern India.[27] Obligate heterozygotes for this disease have approximately 50% of the normal number of $α_{IIb}β_3$ receptors, but no evidence of platelet dysfunction or clinically significant bleeding.[21] Although most cases are observed in specific populations or in the setting of consanguinity and are thus homozygous for a shared mutation inherited from both parents, about a third of patients with identified mutations are compound heterozygotes.

Classification and Laboratory Diagnosis

In 1972, Caen classified GT according to platelet intracellular fibrinogen content and the ability of platelets to retract a fibrin clot.[28] Type I patients, representing 80% of those studied, lacked platelet fibrinogen and had an absence of clot retraction. Type II thrombasthenic platelets contained appreciable levels of platelet fibrinogen and maintained some clot retraction capability. Soon thereafter, the technique of sodium dodecyl sulfate–polyacrylamide gel electrophoresis (SDS-PAGE) became widespread, and it became clear that there were three different patterns seen with thrombasthenic platelet membrane glycoproteins.[29,30] Type I platelets lacked detectable levels of $α_{IIb}β_3$, whereas type II platelets expressed moderate (15% to 25%) levels of these glycoproteins. Adding to the complexity of this classification was the identification of variant forms of thrombasthenia characterized by normal to nearly normal levels of a dysfunctional form of $α_{IIb}β_3$.[31,32] Another integrin dysfunction syndrome in which $β_1$, $β_2$, and $β_3$ integrins are involved results in a GT-like syndrome with leukocyte adhesion deficiency type 1 and immune dysfunction.[33] All three groups fail to aggregate in response to physiologic agonists such as adenosine diphosphate (ADP),

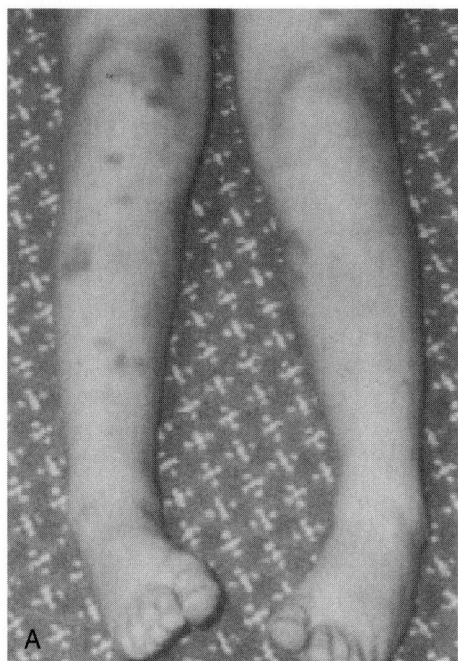

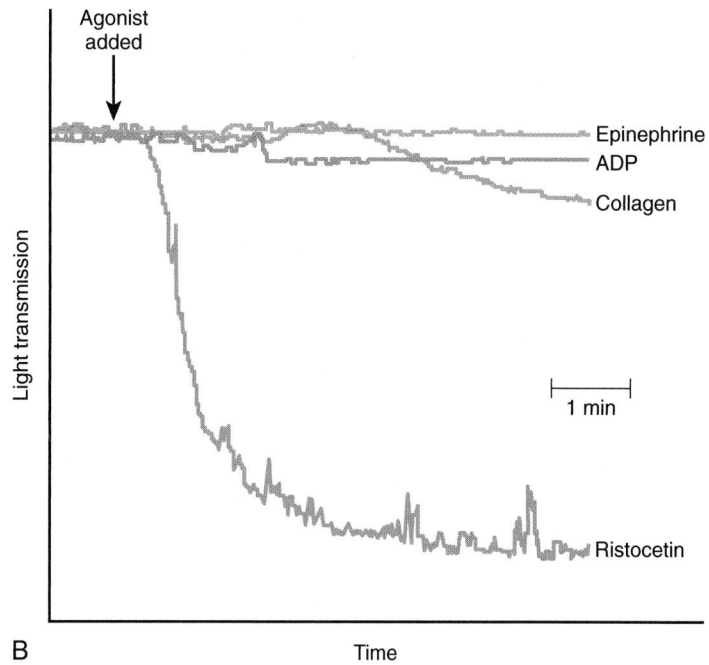

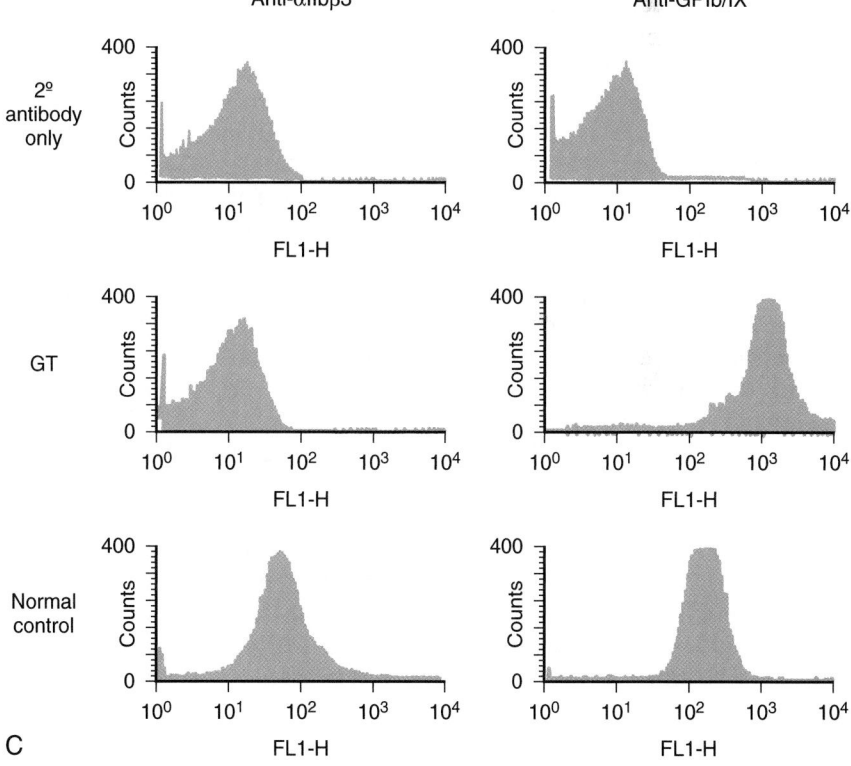

FIGURE 29-2. Glanzmann's thrombasthenia. The patient shown has a mutation in the fourth cysteine-binding domain of α_{IIb} secondary to a Gly273Asp substitution.[35] **A,** Representative ecchymosis seen in the patient at the age of 6 years. **B,** Platelet aggregation studies show an absence of secondary aggregation to adenosine diphosphate (ADP), epinephrine, and collagen but a normal response to ristocetin. **C,** Flow cytometric platelet analysis using an anti-$\alpha_{IIb}\beta_3$ primary antibody (*left*) or an anti-GPIb/IX antibody as a positive control (*right*), followed by a fluorescein isothiocyanate–labeled secondary antibody. Shown at the *top* is the fluorescence with the secondary antibody only on normal platelets. In the *middle* is a patient with primary followed by secondary antibody, and at the *bottom* is the same with normal platelets. The patient's platelets show little $\alpha_{IIb}\beta_3$ antibody binding when compared with the control. The patient's platelets do express high levels of glycoprotein Ib/IX (GPIb/IX).

thrombin, or epinephrine (see Fig. 29-2B) because they all have a functional deficiency of platelet surface $\alpha_{IIb}\beta_3$ receptors. The failure to bind fibrinogen and other adhesive ligands is the reason for the inability of platelets to cohere. No correlation exists between any of the proposed subtypes of GT and the severity of bleeding symptoms in patients.[21] Some patients with no $\alpha_{IIb}\beta_3$ have relatively mild clinical symptoms, whereas others with a full complement of $\alpha_{IIb}\beta_3$, albeit dysfunctional, can have

frequent bleeding episodes requiring repeated platelet transfusions.

Currently, the most common method used for determining levels of $\alpha_{IIb}\beta_3$ on thrombasthenic platelets involves flow cytometry[34] and immunoblot analysis.[35] Figure 29-2C illustrates flow cytometric analysis of the $\alpha_{IIb}\beta_3$ content of both a normal control and a GT patient with a severe deficiency of $\alpha_{IIb}\beta_3$ secondary to a mutation in one of the Ca^{2+}-binding domains of her α_{IIb} chain.[20]

This mutation blocks export of the $\alpha_{IIb}\beta_3$ receptor out of the endoplasmic reticulum and into the Golgi body for final processing, as indicated by failure to cleave the α_{IIb} prochain into an α_{IIb} heavy chain.

Several hundred individuals with GT have been described in the literature. To date, more than a hundred of these cases have been solved at the molecular level. As in most genetic disorders, the molecular abnormalities have been found to range from major deletions and inversions to single point mutations (for review, see elsewhere[36] and http://sinaicentral.mssm.edu/intranet/research/glanzmann). Some of the better-characterized subgroups of mutations are described in the following text.

The earliest and largest group of thrombasthenic mutations described failed to express $\alpha_{IIb}\beta_3$ on the cell surface. Several of these patients had major deletions or inversions in their α_{IIb} or β_3 genes. In addition, a number of point mutations or small deletions in the α_{IIb} or β_3 genes have been described with no surface expression of $\alpha_{IIb}\beta_3$; both chains are formed intracellularly and complex but fail to undergo intracellular processing or reach the cell surface. These defects result in a type 1 form of thrombasthenia. One major subgroup of these patients involves missense mutations in the N-terminal β-propeller repeats of α_{IIb} near the proposed Ca^{2+}-binding sites on its lower surface as exemplified by the patient in Figure 29-2.[20,37]

Another group of mutations occur in the same β-propeller region of α_{IIb} but take place on the upper surface and have a different phenotype. These mutations are located within three upper loops of β-propeller, the connecting loop between the second to the third blade, the loop in the middle of the third blade, and the loop connecting the third and fourth blade.[38] These mutations occur within the RGD ligand binding pocket of α_{IIb}.[9]

Another group of thrombasthenic defects with significant levels of $\alpha_{IIb}\beta_3$ surface expression (although the complex is not able to interact with its natural ligands) involve the β_3 chain. These mutations result in a surface $\alpha_{IIb}\beta_3$ that is easily dissociable by chelation of external calcium ions.[39] Many of these missense mutations have been identified within the cation-binding MIDAS domain.[9] The importance of these sites was reinforced by the identification of a group of in vitro–generated mutant $\alpha_{IIb}\beta_3$ receptors expressed in Chinese hamster ovary (CHO) cells, which provided independent support for the importance of the MIDAS domain in ligand binding.[40]

A second group of mutations with normal levels of surface $\alpha_{IIb}\beta_3$ receptors have mutations in the cytoplasmic domain of β_3, thus demonstrating the importance of this domain for integrin activation and regulation of ligand binding.[41,42] These mutations do not affect surface expression of platelet $\alpha_{IIb}\beta_3$ complexes, but mutant receptors are unresponsive to agonist stimulation. Mammalian cell expression studies show normal adhesion to immobilized fibrinogen but abnormal platelet spreading. These mutations provide compelling evidence for the role of the β_3 cytoplasmic tail in downstream platelet activation by $\alpha_{IIb}\beta_3$.

Other Integrins in Inherited Platelet Disorders

Integrin $\alpha_2\beta_1$ is an Mg^{2+}-dependent collagen receptor on many cells, including platelets.[43] In platelets, collagen not only serves as an adhesive substrate but also functions as an agonist for platelet aggregation. Two patients with histories of bleeding have been reported whose platelets failed to respond normally to collagen and lacked $\alpha_2\beta_1$, thus suggesting that binding of collagen to $\alpha_2\beta_1$ is a necessary component for collagen-induced signaling.[44] In addition, a recent report described several families with autosomal dominant thrombocytopenia and mild platelet dysfunction associated with mutations in the α_2 subunit.[45]

There is substantial variability in the density of $\alpha_2\beta_1$ on the surface of platelets from different individuals.[46] These differences in $\alpha_2\beta_1$ expression are associated with the inheritance of three different α_2 alleles. The higher the receptor density, the greater the attachment of platelets to type I collagen.[47] Some, but not all epidemiologic surveys suggest that increased $\alpha_2\beta_1$ density is a risk factor for cardiovascular disease in younger individuals.[48,49] An increased prevalence of the allele with lower $\alpha_2\beta_1$ density has been reported in patients with type 1 von Willebrand's disease (VWD), which suggests that this allele may contribute to bleeding symptoms in these patients.[50]

Bernard-Soulier Syndrome: Defective Glycoprotein Ib/IX Complex

BSS was first described in 1948 in a 5-month-old infant with a prolonged bleeding time, giant platelets on blood smear, and a sibling who had died of hemorrhage.[51] Over the following years, additional patients with the combination of mucocutaneous bleeding; enlarged platelets; normal platelet aggregation with ADP, collagen, and epinephrine with a delayed response to thrombin; and absent platelet aggregation with human VWF and ristocetin or with bovine VWF alone were described as having BSS, now the second most recognized inherited platelet disorder.

Biology of the Glycoprotein Ib/IX Complex

Adhesion through the GPIb/IX complex involves binding of VWF to the subendothelium. Platelet membranes contain two binding sites for VWF (see Table 29-1). One of these sites requires previous platelet activation and is located on the platelet membrane $\alpha_{IIb}\beta_3$ complex. The second binding site involves the GPIb/IX complex, and it is this membrane complex that is crucial for initial attachment and proper adhesion to the extracellular matrix of a damaged vessel wall. It should be pointed out

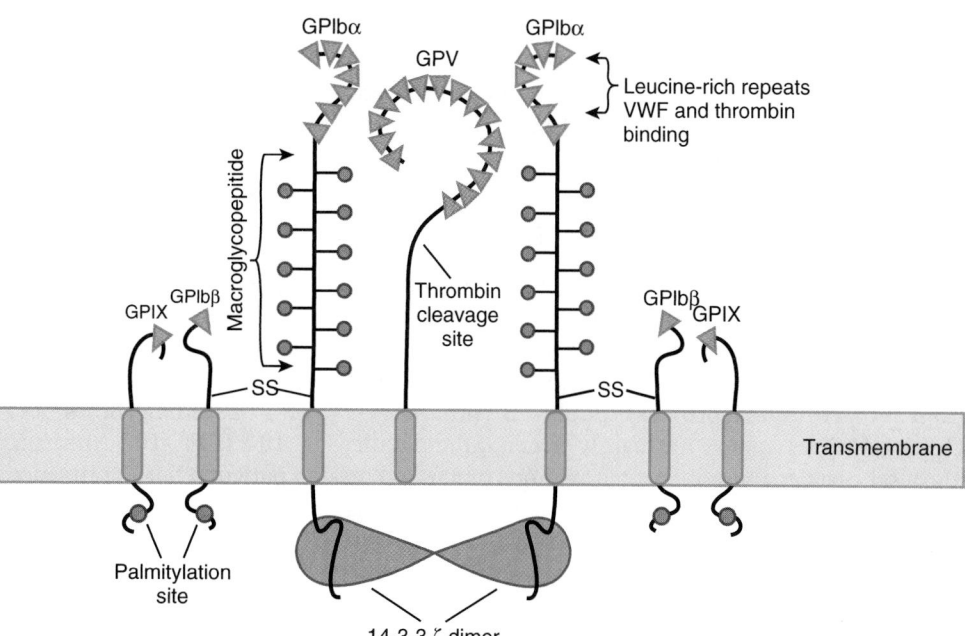

FIGURE 29-3. Structure of the glycoprotein Ib/IX (GPIb/IX) receptor. Each receptor consists of two GPIbα chains, each disulfide linked to a GPIbβ chain. There are two GPIX chains and one GPV chain in each complex as well. The leucine-rich repeats on all the chains are indicated, as are the sites for binding of von Willebrand factor (VWF) and thrombin. Known intracellular interactions or modification sites are also indicated. SS, cysteine disulfide bond.

that the GPIb/IX complex may also bind to other ligands, including P-selectin,[52] thrombospondin-1,[53] high-molecular-weight kininogen, and Mac-1.[54] Furthermore, GPIb/IX also binds thrombin, and its role in the activation of platelets by thrombin is discussed later.

The GPIb/IX complex is the second most abundant receptor on the platelet membrane surface, with approximately 25,000 copies per platelet.[55] This complex actually consists of four different proteins (Fig. 29-3), all of which have one or more leucine-rich repeats composed of a 24–amino acid motif with seven conserved leucine residues. Other proteins have been described with this leucine-rich repeat, and these regions mediate ligand binding.[56]

GPIbα is the largest subunit (135 kd, 610 amino acids, chromosome 17p12) and has seven leucine repeats.[57] It is susceptible to cleavage by trypsin or calpain, which gives rise to a heavily glycosylated 135-kd fragment known as "glycocalicin."[58] In addition to containing the binding site for VWF, the glycocalicin portion of GPIbα also binds thrombin.[59] In vivo, plasma VWF does not bind to the GPIb complex,[60] but under shear stress conditions, VWF simultaneously binds to collagen and the GPIb/IX complex.[60] In clinical assays, the antibiotic ristocetin or the venom-derived protein botrocetin are used to mimic this effect by inducing conformational changes in VWF that promote binding to GPIb/IX in stirred platelet-rich plasma.[61]

GPIbα is disulfide-bonded to GPIbβ (25 kd, 181 amino acids, chromosome 22q11.2)[57] through a single cysteine residue located in each subunit near the transmembrane domains of GPIbα and GPIbβ (see Fig. 29-3). This peptide has only one leucine repeat. The cytoplasmic tail of GPIbβ contains a filamin binding site that links the receptor complex to F-actin below the membrane[62] and a binding site for 14-3-3ζ.[63] The disul-

fide-bound GPIbα-β is noncovalently associated with platelet GPIX and GPV.[64] GPIX is the smallest member of the GPIb complex (22 kd, 160 amino acids, chromosome 3q29), with only one leucine repeat.[65] GPV (82 kd, 344 amino acids, chromosome 3q21) is a transmembrane protein with 15 leucine repeats.[66] This protein is a proteolytic substrate for thrombin and releases a 69-kd soluble fragment.[67] GPV is present in only a single copy per complex, whereas there are two copies of the other three subunits in a single receptor (see Fig. 29-3). Furthermore, cleavage of the GPV extracellular domain by thrombin bound to GPIbα activates platelets.[68] Consistent with this observation, the GPV-knockout mouse has a mild prothrombotic state.[69]

Binding of activated VWF to the GPIb/IX complex activates platelets through activation of phospholipase C (PLC) and mobilization of protein kinase C, which together with increases in [Ca^{2+}]$_i$, promotes platelet secretion and potentiates platelet aggregation.[70] The GPIb-IX complex also appears to activate the cell by binding to the cytoskeleton protein 14-3-3ζ[63] and by interacting with the FcγRIIA receptor on platelets, where it activates an intracellular tyrosine–based activation motif (ITAM) receptor[71] (see Fig. 29-3).

Clinical Features

The bleeding manifestations of patients with BSS are similar to those of other patients with severe platelet dysfunction and center on mucocutaneous bleeding with purpura, epistaxis, gastrointestinal hemorrhage, and menorrhagia.[72] Alloantibodies to components of the GPIb/IX complex can develop after platelet transfusions with resulting platelet refractoriness.[72] Care of bleeding in these patients is similar to that of patients with GT discussed earlier, including the use of DDAVP.[73] Studies evaluating DDAVP have demonstrated improved bleeding times, although the improvement did not correlate with the ability of DDAVP to increase the level of circulating VWF. Activated factor VIIa has also been reported to be useful in patients with BSS,[74] but we believe that this factor is best used as a supplement to platelet infusions.

Classification and Laboratory Diagnosis

BSS patients have a variable degree of thrombocytopenia. Most patients are thrombocytopenic to some degree, but some patients may have platelet counts as low as 20,000/μL.[72] The platelets have a mean diameter ranging from 3 to 20 times normal (Figs. 29-4B and 29-5A).[75] Other cell types appear normal. In general, the circulating total platelet mass in people is more precisely conserved than the platelet count is,[76] and part of the decrease in platelet count in BSS may well reflect this compensa-

tory mechanism. Megakaryocytes in this disorder appear normal in size and appearance by light microscopy. However, on electron microscopy, a striking feature in these cells is the variable and intermittent nature of the demarcation system, which is often vacuolar.[77] Absence of GPIbα results in an abnormal demarcation membrane in a mouse model of BSS, whereas restoration of the protein returns the electron microscopic structure of the megakaryocyte to normal.[78] Studies have shown that GPIb/IX contributes to platelet formation in that this complex lines up with the cytoskeleton during thrombopoiesis[79] and plays a role in cell cycle regulation.[80]

Bleeding times and Platelet Functional Analyzer 100 (PFA-100) measurements[81] are prolonged in these patients, but the distinctive abnormality of BSS platelets is the failure of agglutination in the presence of ristocetin, an abnormality that cannot be corrected by the addition

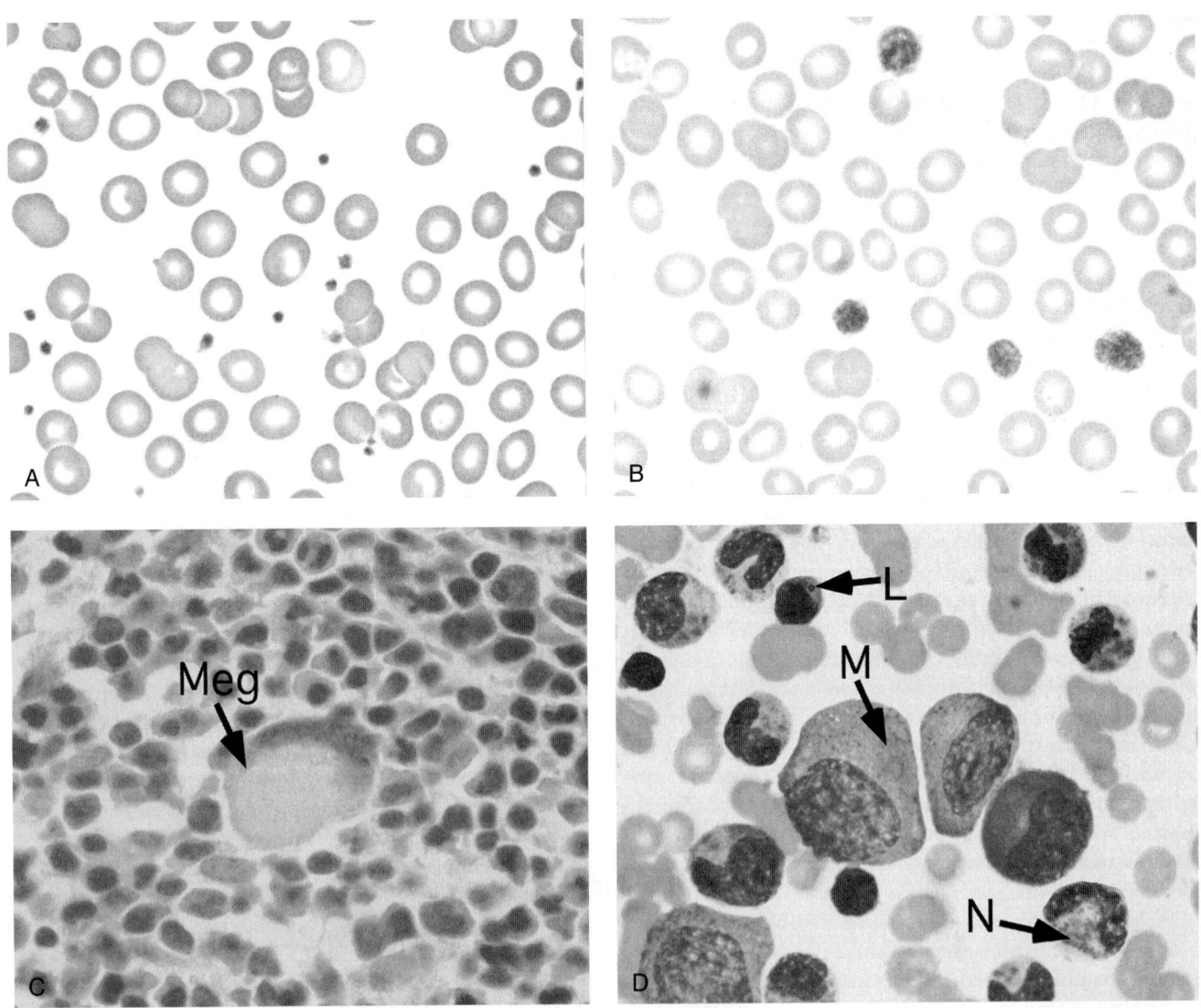

FIGURE 29-4. Light microscopy. **A,** Normal peripheral smear showing typical-size platelets (original magnification ×100). **B,** Peripheral smear of a patient with Bernard-Soulier syndrome showing a decreased number of enlarged platelets (original magnification ×100). **C,** Dysmorphic megakaryocyte (Meg) with the nuclei pushed to the side in a patient with a *GATA1* mutation (original magnification ×50). **D,** Bone marrow in a patient with Chédiak-Higashi syndrome showing inclusion bodies in a myelocyte (M), neutrophil (N), and lymphocyte (L) (original magnification ×100). *(Courtesy of Marybeth Helfrich, The Children's Hospital of Philadelphia.)*

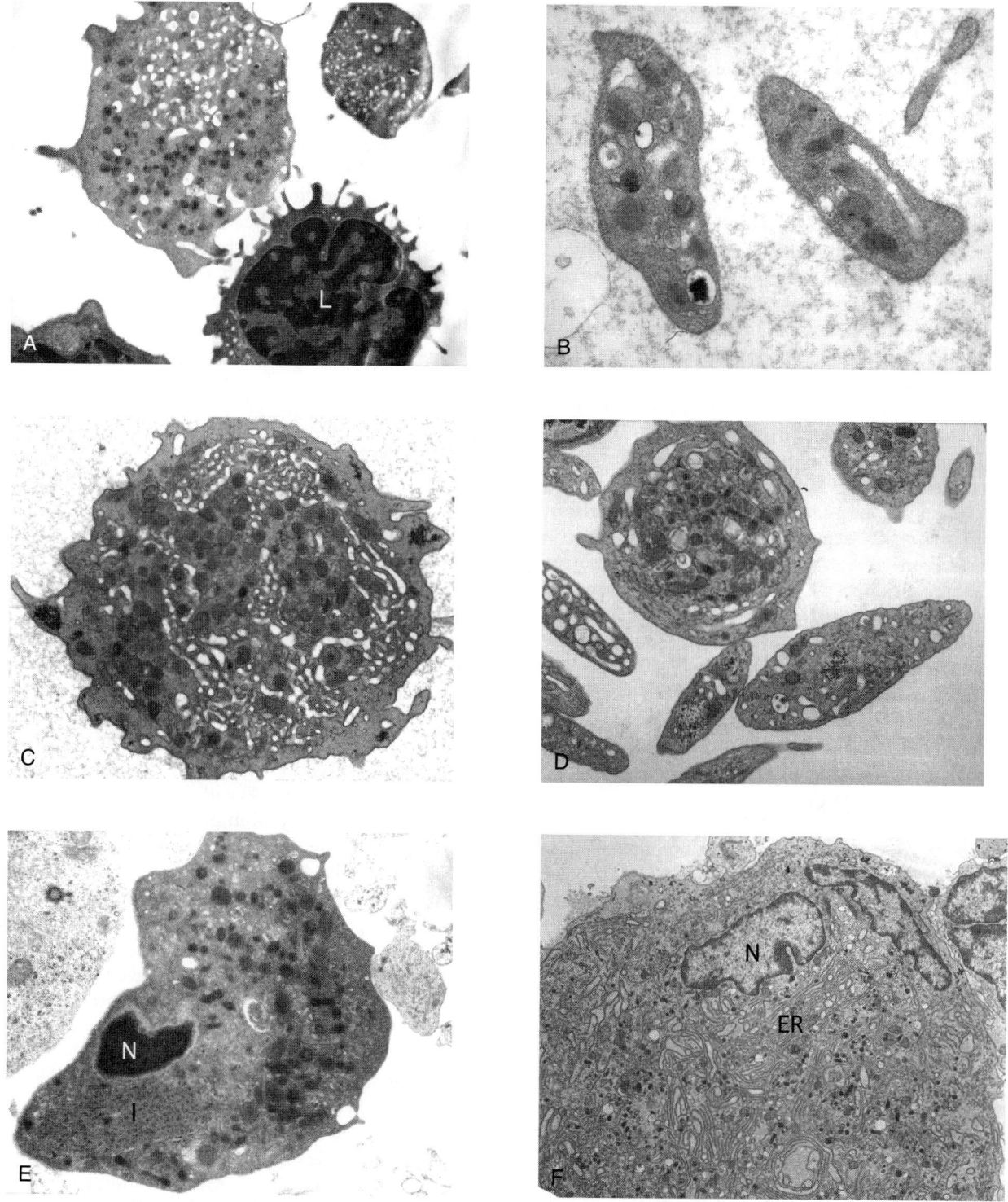

FIGURE 29-5. Electron microscopy. **A,** Platelet in a patient with Bernard-Soulier syndrome that is as large as a lymphocyte (L). Otherwise, platelet morphology is normal (original magnification ×18,000). **B,** Platelets in patients with Wiskott-Aldridge syndrome are half to two thirds the normal size but otherwise normal in appearance (original magnification ×38,500). **C,** Platelets in patients with Fechtner's syndrome are enlarged and the canalicular system is exuberant, but otherwise the platelets look normal (original magnification ×13,000). **D,** Platelets in patients with gray platelet syndrome vary in granule content. Most of the platelets seen have an absence of alpha granules, whereas others (such as the large platelet here) may have identifiable granules (original magnification ×16,500). **E,** Neutrophil in a patient with May-Hegglin anomaly showing an inclusion body (I) below the nucleus (N) forming longitudinally oriented filaments (original magnification ×14,000). **F,** Megakaryocyte from a patient with a *GATA1* mutation showing the nucleus (N) pushed to the side by exuberant endoplasmic reticulum (ER), which fills most of the cytoplasm (original magnification ×38,000). *(All electron micrographs courtesy of Dr. James White, University of Minnesota.)*

of normal plasma.[82] Aggregation by other agonists such as ADP, collagen, and epinephrine is normal, although the response to low-dose thrombin may be delayed.[82] Flow cytometric analysis of platelet glycoproteins may also aid in the diagnosis.[83]

Molecular Abnormalities

More than 30 molecular defects in BSS have been defined.[84] These disorders can be classified by whether any complex reaches the platelet membrane and by the specific subunit affected. The first described mutation was a chain termination mutation within GPIbα that results in a protein lacking a portion of the extracellular domain and the entire transmembrane and cytoplasmic domains.[85]

Mutations in the GPIbα chain are most common in patients with BSS[86]; however, mutations in GPIbβ and GPIX have also been described in patients with similar clinical phenotypes.[87,88] Most of the mutations described are missense or nonsense mutations. Deletions are uncommon but do occur, as in one patient who had partial deletion of the GPIbβ gene on chromosome 22q11.2 in association with velocardiofacial syndrome.[89] Compound heterozygotes have also been described.[90] The disease is most commonly autosomal recessive, but autosomal dominant mutations have likewise been reported.[91]

Platelet-Type (Pseudo-) von Willebrand Disease

Platelet-type VWD is an autosomal dominant bleeding disorder often associated with a prolonged bleeding time, mild thrombocytopenia, and decreased circulating levels of high-molecular-weight VWF multimers.[90,91] Patients with this disorder have a mild to moderate bleeding diathesis. Platelet-type VWD is very similar to type 2B VWD (see Chapter 30) in that both are characterized by platelet agglutination in the presence of low concentrations of ristocetin and by decreased circulating levels of high-molecular-weight VWF. Binding of VWF to circulating platelets results in the reduced levels of VWF seen in these patients, as well as some degree of platelet activation, mild thrombocytopenia, and an increased risk of clotting.

Unlike type 2B VWD, where mutations in VWF result in increased affinity for normal platelet GPIb/IX complex, pseudo-VWD is caused by an alteration in the platelet GPIb/IX complex that leads to increased affinity for normal VWF multimers. Platelet-type VWD can be distinguished from type 2B VWD by the addition of normal VWF to patient platelet-rich plasma, which results in spontaneous aggregation of pseudo-VWD platelets but not type 2B VWD platelets.[90,92] It is important to distinguish patients with platelet-type VWD from other VWD patients because care of patients with VWD often involves infusion of cryoprecipitate or DDAVP. This therapy can worsen the thrombocytopenia in patients with platelet-type VWD.[92] A patient with mild thrombocytopenia and a prolonged bleeding time should be evaluated for this disorder as described earlier.

The molecular basis of platelet-type VWD has been defined in several patients.[92,93] Mutations, such as Gly-233Val and Met239Val, occur in the region of GPIbα that has been previously shown to be important in VWF binding. It has been hypothesized that these mutations alter GPIbα such that it maintains an adhesive conformation much as wild-type GPIb/IX receptor becomes activated on exposure to components of the extracellular matrix at sites of vascular injury and flow.

Other Inherited Defects of Platelet Receptors

G Protein–Coupled Receptors

Many agonists that activate platelets, such as thrombin, ADP, and thromboxane A_2 (TxA_2), activate cells through a GPCR (see Table 29-1). These seven-transmembrane receptors are linked to a heterotriplex of intracellular guanosine diphosphate (GDP)/guanosine triphosphate (GTP)-binding proteins, Gα,β,γ. The strongest platelet agonist is thrombin. As mentioned previously, one receptor for thrombin is the GPIb/IX complex. However, thrombin appears to have its greatest effect on human platelets through two GPCRs, protease-activated receptor 1 (PAR-1) and PAR-4, with PAR-1 being the major human receptor.[94] Thrombin binds to PAR-1, releases an N-terminal peptide, and leaves a new N-terminal. An oligopeptide of this N-terminal sequence, SFLLRN, can mimic the effects of thrombin and activate platelets. Surprisingly, no patients with defects in PAR-1 have been described. In mice, PAR-1 is not important for platelet biology, although its absence does have in vitro consequence because it is expressed on other tissues.[95] Instead, on murine platelets PAR-3 and PAR-4 are biologically relevant.[96]

ADP is stored in platelet dense granules and released upon platelet activation. When added to platelets in vitro, ADP causes TxA_2 formation, protein phosphorylation, an increase in cytosolic Ca^{2+}, shape change, aggregation, and secretion. ADP also inhibits the formation of cyclic adenosine monophosphate (cAMP). Several patients with bleeding defects have been described whose platelets showed greatly diminished responsiveness to ADP and reduced numbers of binding sites for ADP analogues,[97,98] a phenotype not dissimilar from that produced by ADP antagonists such as ticlopidine or clopidogrel. ADP receptors on human platelets include P2Y1, P2Y12, and P2X1.[99-101] P2Y1 is a GPCR that activates PLC. P2Y12 inhibits cAMP formation by adenyl cyclase. P2X1 is a ligand-gated nonspecific cation channel that may contribute to the influx of extracellular Ca^{2+} that occurs in response to ADP. Mutations in each of these receptors have been reported in patients and have resulted in mild to moderate bleeding symptoms.[97]

In several respects, epinephrine is unique among human platelet agonists in that it causes aggregation and secretion, but not the cytoskeletal reorganization that underlies shape change. Activation of PLC by epinephrine appears to be dependent on TxA$_2$ formation and can be suppressed with aspirin.[102] Aspirin also blocks second-wave, or secretion-dependent, platelet aggregation in response to epinephrine. This gives rise to a characteristic aggregometer tracing in which epinephrine-induced primary aggregation is followed by disaggregation of the platelet clumps. Platelet responses to epinephrine are mediated by α_2-adrenergic receptors.[103] There are reports of families in which a mild bleeding disorder was associated with impaired epinephrine-induced aggregation and reduced numbers of α_2-adrenergic receptors.[104] However, platelets from up to 10% of apparently normal people may fail to aggregate when challenged with epinephrine, and the clinical significance of this finding is unclear.

TxA$_2$ is produced from arachidonate in platelets by the aspirin-sensitive cyclooxygenase pathway. When the stable thromboxane analogue U46619 is added to platelets in vitro, the platelets undergo shape change, aggregation, secretion, phosphoinositide hydrolysis, protein phosphorylation, and an increase in [Ca^{2+}]$_i$. Similar responses are seen when platelets are incubated with exogenous arachidonate.[105] Platelets express TP, a GPCR for TxA$_2$.[106] Platelets also contain a receptor for prostacyclin (PGI$_2$), an endothelial cell prostaglandin that is a potent platelet inhibitor. Binding of PGI$_2$ to this receptor stimulates adenylate cyclase activity and inhibits platelet function.[107] A few patients have been described who have a mild bleeding disorder caused by congenital absence of the TxA$_2$ receptor. Two Japanese patients have had their mutations defined and were found to have an R60L substitution in the first cytoplasmic loop of TxA$_2$.[108] In addition, three patients have been described who have normal TxA$_2$ binding but absent platelet aggregation in the presence of this agonist, thus suggesting uncoupling between the receptor and downstream signaling events.[109] There are as yet no known clinical disorders ascribed to the PGI$_2$ receptor, but deletion of the gene in mice increases their risk for thrombosis after arterial injury.[110]

Immunoglobulin Superfamily Receptors

GPVI, a 62-kd protein encoded by a gene on human chromosome 19q13.4,[111] is a member of the immunoglobulin superfamily of receptors. It is the platelet signaling receptor for collagen, and patients with a mild bleeding disorder have been described whose platelets could not be activated by fibrillar collagen types I and III and lacked GPVI despite having normal levels of the other platelet collagen receptor $\alpha_2\beta_1$.[112] Unlike $\alpha_2\beta_1$, GPVI's interaction with collagen initiates the intracellular signaling that results in platelet activation. GPVI exists on the platelet surface complexed with the FcR γ chain,[113] and

signaling seems to occur via phosphorylation of PLCγ2 and Syk through the FcR γ chain.[114,115] Fab antibodies derived from GPVI-deficient individuals who had received platelet transfusions recognize GPVI and are capable of blocking activation of platelets by collagen, thereby resulting in thrombocytopenia and internalization of surface GPVI.[116] Convulxin, a snake venom protein isolated from a South American rattlesnake, is also a potent activator of platelets that is capable of desensitizing platelets to collagen and has been demonstrated to bind specifically to GPVI.[117]

GPVI seems to be the major collagen receptor on platelets,[118] although a few patients[119,120] have been described who lack GPVI and show a mild bleeding tendency. These patients have some residual platelet aggregation to collagen, which is likely to be through the $\alpha_2\beta_1$ receptor.[121] In addition, autoantibodies to GPVI have been described in patients with immune thrombocytopenic purpura[116,122] and systemic lupus erythematosus.[123] These patients lack surface GPVI on their platelets and show a mild bleeding diathesis with abnormal platelet aggregation to collagen. Interestingly, several genetic polymorphisms affecting GPVI surface expression have been described and suggested to be a risk factor for myocardial infarction. Platelets with less GPVI showed less vigorous aggregation in vitro, although further study is ongoing on the true relevance of these findings.[124,125]

Scott's Syndrome

The platelet surface also functions as one of the principal sites for plasma coagulation reactions by providing a surface on which coagulation factor complexes assemble and accelerate these important reactions several thousand-fold. This property of activated platelets has been termed platelet factor 3 activity. In a resting platelet, there is little anionic phospholipid on the platelet's surface. Activation by agonists such as thrombin or collagen is thought to reorient membrane phospholipids and bring anionic phospholipids, chiefly phosphatidylserine, to the outer leaflet. Activation also induces membrane vesiculation and the production of platelet microparticles with procoagulant activity.[126]

Deficiency in platelet coagulant activity is a rare clinical event that has been termed Scott's syndrome, named after the propositus of a well-studied family.[126,127] The patient had prolonged bleeding after dental extractions, bleeding after surgical procedures, and a spontaneous retroperitoneal hematoma.[127] The patient secreted a normal quantity of factor V, a platelet alpha granule constituent, but had only 25% of the normal number of binding sites for factor Xa on activated platelets.[128] When her platelets were challenged with such agonists as thrombin and collagen, aggregation and secretion were normal, but fewer anionic phospholipid-binding sites were translocated to the platelet surface.[129] In addition, the formation of microparticles is defective in patients with Scott's syndrome.[126] Standard screening tests for plasma coagulation, such as the prothrombin time and partial thromboplastin time, which use artificial lipid micelles, are normal. A patient has been described who had aberrant expression of the adenosine triphosphate (ATP)-binding cassette transporter AI (ABCA1), which is important in translocation of phosphatidylserine.[130] This patient had a single–base pair substitution in exon 42 that was predicted to substitute R1925 with glutamine. The diagnostic abnormality is a shortened serum prothrombin time as a result of reduced consumption of prothrombin. Additionally, these patients have a prolonged dilute Russell viper venom time that corrects when the patient's plasma is added to normal platelets, but not when normal plasma is added to the patient's blood.[131] This is due to the inability to generate normal platelet procoagulant activity. Patients can be readily treated with platelet transfusions, which improves hemostasis and reduces postoperative blood loss.

Platelet Storage Granule Defects

Human platelets contain several types of intracellular granules that can be distinguished by electron microscopy, including dense granules, alpha granules, and lysosomes.[132] Dense granules are the most rapidly secreted granules after platelet activation and contain ADP, ATP, serotonin, and calcium.[133] Two thirds of platelet adenine nucleotides are stored in these granules, with an ADP/ATP ratio of 3:2, as opposed to 1:8 in the cytoplasm.[132] Platelet alpha granules contribute many of the proteins involved in the formation of a platelet plug. After platelet activation, the alpha granules centralize in the platelet and release their contents via membrane fusion with the open canalicular system.[134] Interestingly, not all proteins present in alpha granules have the same origin. Some, such as VWF, thrombospondin, and platelet factor 4 (PF4), are synthesized in and packaged by megakaryocytes,[135] whereas others, such as albumin, IgG, and fibrinogen, are endocytosed from plasma.[136]

Dense Granule Defects

Patients with defects in platelet dense granules have a form of storage pool deficiency (δ-SPD).[132,137] Patients with δ-SPD exhibit a mild to moderate bleeding diathesis, as well as abnormalities in platelet aggregation. The second wave of aggregation is absent in response to ADP and epinephrine and virtually absent in response to collagen. Bleeding times in these patients are often prolonged. In 1969 it was shown that these patients have a deficiency in total platelet ADP,[138] and this deficit was subsequently localized to the ADP pool of the dense granule.[139] The abnormalities in the ultrastructure of the dense granules are heterogeneous,[140] but most patients show a characteristic lack of dense granules by electron microscopy[141] (see Fig. 29-5).

Some individuals have other associated defects. The two most common SPDs are Hermansky-Pudlak syndrome (HPS)[142] and Chédiak-Higashi syndrome (CHS).[143,144] HPS is characterized by tyrosinase-positive, severe oculocutaneous albinism in association with photophobia, rotatory nystagmus, loss of visual acuity, excessive accumulation of ceroid-like material in reticuloendothelial cells, and a mild to moderate hemorrhagic diathesis. This disease is inherited as an autosomal recessive disorder, and although it occurs in many populations, it is seen with high frequency in people from the northwest part of Puerto Rico.[145,146] Patients exhibit bruising and epistaxis in early childhood. Fatal bleeding is rare, but a significant proportion of patients will have received packed red cell or platelet transfusions in their lifetime.[142,147] The major cause of death is progressive pulmonary fibrosis, which generally begins in their late twenties or early thirties,[142,148] perhaps secondary to higher plasma serotonin levels because of failure to package the serotonin into dense granules.[149] This disease is also associated with a 15% incidence of granulomatous colitis.[147] One of the genes involved is located at chromosome 10q23.1-23.3[150] and encodes a 700–amino acid protein termed HPS-1 that has one transmembrane domain but little homology with other known proteins, although the transcript appears to be present in multiple tissues. The northwest Puerto Rican mutation is a 16–base pair insert at codon Pro496 that results in a frameshift, and patients from northwest Puerto Rico with HPS are homozygous for the same mutation, thus suggesting a founder effect.[151] About a quarter of patients from other parts of Puerto Rico have other mutations in HPS-1.[152] Additionally, cases of HPS have been described throughout the world, and only 25% to 40% of these patients have disease caused by a mutation in a gene known to be associated with HPS. Mutations in other genes that have been described to cause HPS include changes in ADTB3A (HPS-2), which is important in vesicle formation from existing membrane.[153] To date, mutations in eight different genes (termed HPS-1 to HPS-8) have been described in patients with phenotypic HPS. Some genotype/phenotype associations have also been documented. For example, pulmonary fibrosis develops in patients with mutations in HPS-1 and HPS-4, whereas this lifethreatening complication does not develop in patients with HPS-3, HSP-5, and HSP-6 mutations. In addition, patients with HPS-2 mutations also have associated neutropenia and a predilection for infections, particularly in childhood.[154]

CHS is a rare autosomal disorder that has been described in approximately 200 affected individuals.[142] It is characterized by immune dysfunction, platelet storage pool defects, and partial albinism. Patients often have a white forelock or ashen hair secondary to abnormally large melanosomes.[137,142] Hematologic manifestations of this disease are characterized by the presence of large intracytoplasmic granules in leukocytes, lymphocytes, monocytes, and platelets (see Fig. 29-4D), with a concurrent defect in mobilization of the marrow leukocyte pool,[155] defective chemotaxis,[156] and decreased bactericidal activity.[157] Many other tissues also contain abnormal granules.[158,159] CHS patients often die in the first 2 decades of life of either overwhelming infections or an unusual lymphoproliferative disorder called the "accelerated phase," which involves fever, anemia, neutropenia, and occasionally, thrombocytopenia, hepatosplenomegaly, lymphadenopathy, and jaundice.[160] These patients are particularly susceptible to Epstein-Barr virus infections.[155] The gene involved in CHS is located on chromosome 1q42.1-42.2 and encodes a 3801–amino acid protein called LYST (lysosomal trafficking regulator).[160] This complex protein has several repeated series of hydrophobic helices interspersed with hydrophobic membrane association domains. The helical regions resemble the previously defined HEAT and ARM elements involved in vesicular transportation[161] and membrane associations,[160] respectively. Mutations have been defined in an increasing number of affected patients and involve truncated products,[162,163] although there is no correlation between residual protein length and clinical phenotype.[142]

Diagnosis of dense granule defects is difficult because it requires expertise in proper preparation of specimens for electron microscopy, as well as competence in interpretation of the findings. It is also complicated by the fact that a small percentage of these rare patients may have a prolonged bleeding time but normal platelet aggregation studies.[164] Recent studies have begun to use flow cytometry on quinacrine-loaded platelets to aid in the diagnosis because quinacrine is selectively taken up by dense granules.[165]

Alpha Granule Defects

Patients with alpha granule deficiencies have a bleeding phenotype similar to that of patients with dense granule deficiencies, with mild to moderate bleeding, mild thrombocytopenia, and a prolonged bleeding time. Because of the initial light microscopic observation of gray platelets in the peripheral blood smear of these patients after Romanovsky stain, this disorder was termed gray platelet syndrome.[166] On electron microscopy, these platelets are most notable for the absence or marked reduction of alpha granules (see Fig. 29-5D).[167] These platelets are also deficient in alpha granule–specific proteins such as PF4, VWF, factor V, and fibronectin.[168] Gray platelet aggregation to various agonists, especially thrombin, is impaired.[169] These platelets have a delayed and blunted Ca^{2+} mobilization response.[170] The vacuolar structures seen in gray platelets appear to be aborted alpha granules that contain both P-selection and $\alpha_{IIb}\beta_3$ in their membranes.[170] They also contain a significant amount of proteins, including immunoglobulin and albumin,[171] that are normally endocytosed into alpha granules. Endogenously synthesized alpha granule–specific proteins such as PF4 leak out.[172] This latter phenomenon may contribute to the observed myelofibrosis and pulmonary fibrosis associated with this disease.[172]

Other Granular Defects

A small number of patients have been described with a combined alpha/dense granule deficiency.[173] The dense granule deficiency was often much more severe than the alpha granule deficiency. These patients also have mild to moderate bleeding histories, and laboratory results are similar to those of dense granule–deficient patients, with a decreased platelet ADP/ATP ratio in the cells and low levels of serotonin. In one patient with a severe deficiency in both alpha and dense granules, there was a deficiency in total platelet P-selectin,[174] thus suggesting that unlike the gray platelet syndrome, in which there may be an alpha granule–targeting defect, platelet granule formation itself may be defective in this disorder.

Quebec platelet syndrome is a rare disorder that results from the degradation of alpha granule contents within the platelet because of expression of ectopic urokinase-type plasminogen activator in developing megakaryocytes.[175,176] This disorder, inherited in an autosomal dominant pattern within two large kindreds in Quebec,[175,177] was previously known as factor V Quebec because the initial observations in these patients revealed a relative intraplatelet deficiency of factor V.[177] These patients manifest moderate to severe *delayed* bleeding after surgery or trauma.[178] Bleeding can be controlled by antifibrinolytic therapy with tranexamic acid, but platelet transfusions are generally ineffective.[175,177] The molecular abnormality responsible for this disorder has not yet been defined.

Defects in Signal Transduction

With multiple overlapping pathways of platelet activation, it has been difficult to define specific defects in patients with inherited disorders of platelet signal transduction. Nonetheless, a small number of patients have been described with phenotypes and abnormal platelet aggregation patterns consistent with such a diagnosis.[179] One such group of patients lack the ability to liberate arachidonic acid.[180] This may be due to deficiency of phospholipase A_2.[181] Another patient appears to have difficulty with tyrosine phosphorylation through the ADP receptor system.[182]

Other patients have diminished cyclooxygenase enzyme activity that mimics an aspirin-like defect.[183,184] These patients have abnormal platelet aggregation in response to ADP, epinephrine, collagen, and arachidonic acid while responding normally to prostaglandin G_2, consistent with a defect in cyclooxygenase-1 and subsequent TxA_2 synthesis. Most patients with this disorder have normal antigen levels of a functionally abnormal prostaglandin synthetase.[185] Other patients have been described who have decreased protein expression.[186] Additionally, patients have been reported who appear to lack the thromboxane synthetase that converts prostaglandin H_2 to TxA_2.[187,188] Over the past few years, other models of platelet dysfunction secondary to a signaling defect have been recognized, including the Wiskott-Aldrich syndrome (WAS), which is described later under disorders of platelet size and numbers. For all these signaling disorders, platelet transfusions are effective in the management of bleeding.

QUANTITATIVE DISORDERS

General Comments

Megakaryocytes are large, polyploid, terminally differentiated hematopoietic cells that release platelets into the bloodstream.[189] These cells arise from self-regenerating pluripotent stem cells that also give rise to all other hematopoietic lineages. Megakaryocyte lineage commitment involves a number of precursor stages, including CFU-GEMM (colony-forming unit–granulocyte, erythrocyte, monocyte, megakaryocyte), which in culture results in a mix of granulocytes, erythrocytes, monocytes, and megakaryocytes; CFU-EMM, which gives rise to mixed colonies of erythrocytes, monocytes, and megakaryocytes; BFU-Meg (burst-forming unit–megakaryocyte), which gives rise to a burst of 10 to 20 megakaryocytes; and CFU-Meg, which gives rise to a smaller megakaryocyte colony.[190]

Various growth factors regulate megakaryocyte differentiation at different points of their development. Certain cytokines stimulate proliferation of megakaryocytic progenitors, such as interleukin-3 (IL-3), IL-6, IL-11, IL-12, granulocyte-macrophage colony-stimulating factor (GM-CSF), and erythropoietin (EPO)[191,192]; however, all the aforementioned growth factors and cytokines have very broad effects on all hematopoietic cell lines. The discovery and cloning of thrombopoietin (TPO), the ligand for the myeloproliferative ligand receptor (Mpl), opened a new perspective in megakaryocyte differentiation study. TPO was found to be a specific factor controlling megakaryocytic cell proliferation and maturation and platelet reactivity.[193,194] This 353–amino acid protein is homologous at its N-terminal with EPO. Either the full-length protein, a truncated N-terminal TPO, or even mimetic peptides can dimerize Mpl and stimulate megakaryocytopoiesis.[195] On immature progenitor cells, activation of Mpl stimulates proliferation, much like IL-11 or c-kit ligand. On megakaryocyte precursors and megakaryocytes it leads to increased megakaryocyte differentiation and platelet formation. Targeted disruption in murine models of either the Mpl or TPO genes results in a decrease in platelet count to approximately 20% of normal with normal-appearing megakaryocytes.[196-198] Thus, this cytokine pathway appears to be permissive for megakaryocytopoiesis but is not absolutely required for this differentiation process.

The end product of differentiation is the megakaryoblast, a small lymphocyte-like cell that undergoes the process of nuclear endoduplication, cytoplasmic enlargement, and differentiation to form the mature megakaryocyte with a cell volume of approximately 10^4 to 10^5 μm^3. Each of these huge cells eventually results in the formation of approximately 10^3 to 10^4 platelets. The finding of

naked megakaryocyte nuclei in marrow[199] and the presence of proplatelets in central venous blood[200] support the hypothesis that platelets are formed in bone marrow. It is also possible that platelets are, in part, released from megakaryocytes that have migrated to the pulmonary bed.[201,202] Studies have demonstrated that there are more circulating megakaryocytes in the pulmonary artery than in the pulmonary venous system and that the opposite is true for platelet numbers.[203]

The process by which platelets actually derive from megakaryocytes is beginning to be understood, but it does not appear to involve the extensive membrane system termed the "demarcation membrane system" (DMS) that may represent inverted membranes. Rather, extensive pseudopods form and re-form in a dynamic process that eventually leads to a beaded appearance that fragments to form particles with the size and ultrastructural appearance of platelets.[204] This process can be inhibited by agents that disrupt microtubules[205] and promoted by actin filament–depolymerizing agents,[205,206] thus suggesting involvement of the cytoskeleton in this process. Targeted disruption of the murine hematopoietic transcription factor NF-E2 results in severe thrombocytopenia and very large, bizarre megakaryocytes.[207] Loss of NF-E2 expression results in altered expression of multiple proteins, including the cytoskeletal protein β-tubulin.[208]

The normal range of platelet counts is 150 to 400 × 10^3/μL. Even more constant than the circulating platelet count is the circulating thrombocrit, which is the platelet count multiplied by the mean platelet volume, so there is an inverse relationship between platelet count and platelet size.[76] Regulation of megakaryocytopoiesis by TPO is in large part regulated by the platelet mass. TPO produced by the liver is secreted at a relatively constant level.[209] As platelet mass rises, the amount of bound TPO increases and less is available for stimulation of marrow megakaryocytes. The inverse situation would also be true: as platelet mass falls, there is more free TPO to stimulate marrow megakaryocyte development.

The molecular basis for the regulated expression of genes during megakaryocytopoiesis is only beginning to be understood. This understanding has grown with the development of targeted disruption of hematopoietic genes in mice, which has demonstrated the importance of the transcription factors GATA-1, NF-E2, and FOG-1 in megakaryocyte development.[208,210,211] Both GATA-1 knockdown and NF-E2 knockout result in viable mice with large and dysmorphic megakaryocytes and very low platelet counts.[212,213]

Disordered Platelet Production

Disorders involving platelet production include congenital amegakaryocytic thrombocytopenia (CAMT), characterized by a complete absence of megakaryocytes; thrombocytopenia with absent radii (TAR), in which there is a decrease in megakaryocytes in infancy; amegakaryocytic thrombocytopenia with radioulnar synostosis (ATRUS), characterized by skeletal anomalies and thrombocytopenia that improves with time; and disorders of hematopoietic transcription factors, often associated with an excess of dysmorphic megakaryocytes.

Thrombopoietin-Mpl Axis

CAMT is a rare disorder associated with very low platelet counts, absence of megakaryocytes in bone marrow, and risk for the development of aplastic anemia. These children have no skeletal abnormalities, and the platelet count does not improve with age and often necessitates bone marrow transplantation because of the severe bleeding.[214] CAMT results from mutations in the Mpl gene.[215] These patients demonstrate the importance of TPO in normal hematopoiesis in that patients who survive long enough exhibit pancytopenia during the first or second decade of life.[216] In addition, no TPO mutations have been found in this disorder or in other disorders associated with thrombocytopenia, including TAR (see later).

In contrast, excessively high platelet counts ($>600 \times 10^3/\mu L$) are seen in essential thrombocythemia, an acquired myelodysplastic disorder seen primarily in adults that in approximately 20% of cases is associated with a JAK2 V617F mutation.[217] A rare congenital form of familial thrombocytosis occurs in children that can be associated with enhancing mutations in the TPO promoter[218] or activating mutations in Mpl.[219] Unlike the adult form, myelodysplastic conversion is rare,[220] so it is unclear whether therapeutic intervention (suppression of the platelet count with hydroxyurea or anagrelide[221]) is necessary, although antithrombotic strategies are often still used in the management of these children.

Thrombocytopenia and Skeletal Abnormalities

TAR is one of the more common inherited disorder of platelet number and was first described in 1951.[222] This disorder involves hypomegakaryocytic thrombocytopenia and bilateral absence of the radii. Patients are born with platelet counts in the approximate $10^4/\mu L$ range, which improves slowly and reaches normal levels after the first year of life. During infancy, environmental stress, such as viral illness, can precipitate episodes of severe thrombocytopenia.[223] Several TAR patients have an associated storage pool defect and bleed out of proportion to their platelet count.[224] In addition, these patients have other hematologic changes, including leukemoid reactions to the approximate 30,000/μL range and anemia, partly as a result of blood loss.[223] In addition, 30% of patients have recurrent gastroenteritis and bleeding.[223] The major skeletal manifestation is complete absence of the radii, but with functional thumbs. Other orthopedic abnormalities are seen in about 50% of cases, and the more severe the upper limb deformity, the more likely the patient is to have a lower limb deformity. Approximately 30% of patients have cardiac anomalies, including the tetralogy of Fallot and atrial septal or neural defects.

The etiology of this disorder is unknown. Megakaryocytes are present in the bone marrow, although there may be some decrease in comparison to what one would see in thrombocytopenia secondary to increased peripheral destruction.[225] Serum levels of TPO in patients with TAR are elevated despite normal Mpl levels on hematopoietic cells.[226] Bone marrow cultures from these patients reveal reduced numbers of megakaryocytes,[227] and CFU-Meg do not grow in response to TPO.[228] Together, these findings suggest a disconnection between the TPO receptor and downstream signaling events. Certainly other disorders, such as Fanconi's anemia and Schwachman's syndrome, also have skeletal abnormalities and hematopoietic defects. Whether a common growth factor or shared environmental factors underlie these disorders is unknown.

ATRUS is an autosomal dominant disorder characterized by amegakaryocytic thrombocytopenia, skeletal anomalies (including radioulnar synostosis, hip dysplasia, and clinodactyly or syndactyly), and sensorineural hearing loss.[229] The thrombocytopenia in these patients occurs in the neonatal period and may be severe but will often resolve within the first few years of life.[230] Mutations of HOXA11 have been demonstrated as the molecular abnormality in most patients with ATRUS.[231] HOXA11 is a member of the homeobox group of regulatory proteins that play a role in hematopoietic proliferation and differentiation. Studies in animal models have shown the role of HOXA11 in forearm skeletal development. However, although bone marrow from HOXA11-overexpressing mice shows increased immature megakaryocyte colonies,[232] a clear role in megakaryocytopoiesis has not been defined.

Platelet Disorders Secondary to Transcription Factor Defects

X-linked anemia with severe thrombocytopenia secondary to defects in GATA-1 has been reported.[233,234] The first of these cases involved a site on GATA-1 in which GATA-1 binds to FOG, whereas the second case involved a mutation in one of the DNA-binding domains. The megakaryocytes in the marrow of these patients are similar to those described in GATA-1–knockdown mice[212] and were numerous and large with poorly organized granular content and nuclei pushed off to the side (see Figs. 29-4C and 29-5F).

Familial platelet deficiency/acute myelogenous leukemia (FPD/AML) is a dominantly inherited thrombocytopenia of approximately 100,000/μL that is often associated with a bleeding diathesis out of proportion to the decreased platelet count.[235,236] Platelet studies in some families show a classic and profound storage pool defect, but the precise defect can vary between families. There is about a 50% lifetime risk of AML developing in any affected family member, as well as an increased risk for other cancers. Recent studies have shown that in many of these extended families the defect resides in the *CBFA2* (AML-1) gene (chromosome 21q22.1-22.2).[237]

CBFA2 is a nuclear transcription factor often involved in translocations that results in AML or related cancers.[238] This gene is involved in early hematopoietic differentiation from endothelial cells and is also important for myeloid differentiation.[239] How CBFA2 haploinsufficiency results in a qualitative and quantitative platelet deficiency is not understood.

Thrombocytopenia Associated with Microthrombocytes or Macrothrombocytes

WAS patients have microthrombocytes and thrombocytopenia, but the phenotype involves multiple aspects of platelet and lymphocyte biology (Chapter 23). WAS was first recognized in two case reports as a sex-linked disorder with thrombocytopenia and eczema.[240,241] Platelets are small, usually half-normal volume, and the platelet mass is decreased.[242] There appears to be an associated platelet storage pool defect. The thrombocytopenia seen is severe and can be less than 10,000 platelets/μL. These patients also have a severe immune defect. Many die during the first decade of overwhelming infection or immune-based disorders such as immune thrombocytopenia or hemolytic anemia and from lymphoma-like illnesses during the second decade of life.[243] These patients have an impaired ability to form antibodies to carbohydrate antigens[244] and appear to have a defect in B and especially T lymphocytes.[245] Splenectomy, although it increases the risk for opportunistic infection, often alleviates the thrombocytopenia and bleeding diathesis in this disorder. Immune-related complications respond variably to steroids, intravenous immunoglobulin, vincristine, or plasmapheresis.[246] Bone marrow transplantation has been efficacious in treating this disorder.[247]

The gene involved in WAS (and X-linked thrombocytopenia) has been localized to the short arm of the X chromosome (Xp11.22), and the encoded protein WASP is 501 amino acids long, has no transmembrane domain, but has two highly charged C-terminal domains.[248] In addition, there is a potential nuclear localization signal. There is a pleckstrin homology domain and a cofilin domain by which WASP can depolymerize actin. WASP expression is limited to lymphocytes and platelets. WASP binds to a number of intracellular signaling proteins such as the Rho family member guanosine triphosphatase (GTPase) Cdc42.[249,250] Tyrosine phosphorylation signaling in the cell appears to cause WASP to become bound to cytoskeletal proteins such as PSTPIP (WIN)[251,252] and to be involved in megakaryocytopoiesis.[251,253]

Additional proof that WASP was involved in WAS came from the original description of the gene. One affected patient had a single base deletion, a second had a G→T transversion that led to an Arg86Leu substitution, and a third had a G→A transition of the same Arg leading to a His substitution.[248] Since then, the number of defined mutations has increased and their relationship to the genetic severity has been better defined.[254] Patients have been described with X-linked thrombocytopenia not associated with the severe immunologic defects of full-blown WAS.[254] In particular, patients have been described with isolated X-linked microthrombocytopenia, and these patients have missense mutations in the WASP gene, only some of which overlap with the mutations seen in WAS.[254] To complicate matters, the GATA-1 gene is closely linked to the WASP gene, and this may limit the usefulness of linkage studies for defining which of these two genes is affected in a patient with X-linked thrombocytopenia.[234]

There are also a number of inherited platelet disorders involving large platelets and thrombocytopenia. The most common of these is the autosomal dominant May-Hegglin anomaly (MHA), in which macrothrombocytes are associated with thrombocytopenia and normal coagulation studies.[255,256] In addition, leukocytes contain large spindle-shaped inclusions known as Döhle bodies[255] (see Fig. 29-5E). For a long time, MHA was known to overlap with Sebastian's syndrome, in which the inclusions were thought to be somewhat different in appearance[257]; with Epstein's syndrome associated with sensorineural deafness and nephritis[258]; and with Fechtner's syndrome (Fig. 29-5C) associated with sensorineural deafness, nephritis, and ocular abnormalities.[259] However, it is now clear that all are due to mutations in the cytoskeletal protein nonmuscle myosin heavy chain IIA (MYH9).[260] Another macrothrombocyte disorder, Montreal platelet syndrome (MPS), is characterized by macrothrombocytes, a prolonged bleeding time, and spontaneous aggregation of platelets at pH 7.4. The molecular basis of this abnormality is unknown, although there appears to be a defect in calpain metabolism in MPS.[261,262]

REFERENCES

1. Glanzmann E. Hereditare hamorrhagische Thrombasthenia: ein beitragzur Pathologie der blut Plattchen. J Kinderkr. 1918;88:113-141.
2. Braunsteiner H, Pakesch F. Thrombocytoasthenia and thrombocytopathia—old names and new diseases. Blood. 1956;11:965-976.
3. Hardisty RM, Dormandy KM, Hutton RA. Thrombasthenia. Studies on three cases. Br J Haematol. 1964;10:371-387.
4. Nurden AT, Nurden P. Inherited disorders of platelets: an update. Curr Opin Hematol. 2006;13:157-162.
5. Bray PF, Rosa JP, Lingappa VR, et al. Biogenesis of the platelet receptor for fibrinogen: evidence for separate precursors for glycoproteins IIb and IIIa. Proc Natl Acad Sci U S A. 1986;83:1480-1484.
6. O'Toole TE, Loftus JC, Plow EF, et al. Efficient surface expression of platelet GPIIb-IIIa requires both subunits. Blood. 1989;74:14-18.
7. Gulino D, Boudignon C, Zhang LY, et al. Ca(2+)-binding properties of the platelet glycoprotein IIb ligand–interacting domain. J Biol Chem. 1992;267:1001-1007.
8. Tuckwell DS, Humphries MJ, Brass A. A secondary structure model of the integrin alpha subunit N-terminal domain based on analysis of multiple alignments. Cell Adhes Commun. 1994;2:385-402.

9. Xiao T, Takagi J, Coller BS, et al. Structural basis for allostery in integrins and binding to fibrinogen-mimetic therapeutics. Nature. 2004;432:59-67.

10. Xiong JP, Stehle T, Diefenbach B, et al. Crystal structure of the extracellular segment of integrin alphaVbeta3. Science. 2001;294:339-345.

11. Xiong JP, Stehle T, Zhang R, et al. Crystal structure of the extracellular segment of integrin alphaVbeta3 in complex with an Arg-Gly-Asp ligand. Science. 2002; 296:151-155.

12. Wagner CL, Mascelli MA, Neblock DS, et al. Analysis of GPIIb/IIIa receptor number by quantification of 7E3 binding to human platelets. Blood. 1996;88:907-914.

13. Woods VL Jr, Wolff LE, Keller DM. Resting platelets contain a substantial centrally located pool of glycoprotein IIb-IIIa complex which may be accessible to some but not other extracellular proteins. J Biol Chem. 1986; 261:15242-15251.

14. Bennett JS. Structure and function of the platelet integrin $\alpha_{IIb}\beta_3$. J Clin Invest. 2005;115:3363-3369.

15. Plow EF, Marguerie G. Inhibition of fibrinogen binding to human platelets by the tetrapeptide glycyl-L-prolyl-L-arginyl-L-proline. Proc Natl Acad Sci U S A. 1982;79: 3711-3715.

16. Plow EF, Pierschbacher MD, Ruoslahti E, et al. The effect of Arg-Gly-Asp–containing peptides on fibrinogen and von Willebrand factor binding to platelets. Proc Natl Acad Sci U S A. 1985;82:8057-8061.

17. Sadler JE, Shelton-Inloes BB, Sorace JM, et al. Cloning and characterization of two cDNAs coding for human von Willebrand factor. Proc Natl Acad Sci U S A. 1985;82: 6394-6398.

18. Rooney MM, Farrell DH, van Hemel BM, et al. The contribution of the three hypothesized integrin-binding sites in fibrinogen to platelet-mediated clot retraction. Blood. 1998;92:2374-2381.

19. McCarty JH, Lacy-Hulbert A, Charest A, et al. Selective ablation of alphaV integrins in the central nervous system leads to cerebral hemorrhage, seizures, axonal degeneration and premature death. Development. 2005;132:165-176.

20. Poncz M, Rifat S, Coller BS, et al. Glanzmann thrombasthenia secondary to a Gly273→Asp mutation adjacent to the first calcium-binding domain of platelet glycoprotein IIb. J Clin Invest. 1994;93:172-179.

21. George JN, Caen JP, Nurden AT. Glanzmann's thrombasthenia: the spectrum of clinical disease. Blood. 1990;75: 1383-1395.

22. Jacobin MJ, Laroche-Traineau J, Little M, et al. Human IgG monoclonal anti-alpha(IIb)beta(3)-binding fragments derived from immunized donors using phage display. J Immunol. 2002;168:2035-2045.

23. Poon MC, Zotz R, Di Minno G, et al. Glanzmann's thrombasthenia treatment: a prospective observational registry on the use of recombinant human activated factor VII and other hemostatic agents. Semin Hematol. 2006;43: S33-S36.

24. Awidi AS. Inherited bleeding disorders in Jordan: an update of a 25 year registry. Pathophysiol Haemost Thromb. 2006;35:152.

25. Reichert N, Seligsohn U, Ramot B. Clinical and genetic aspects of Glanzmann's thrombasthenia in Israel: report of 22 cases. Thromb Diath Haemorrh. 1975;34:806-820.

26. Levy JM, Mayer G, Sacrez R, et al. [Glanzmann-Naegeli thrombasthenia. Study of a strongly endogamous ethnic group.] Ann Pediatr (Paris). 1971;18:129-137.

27. Peretz H, Rosenberg N, Landau M, et al. Molecular diversity of Glanzmann thrombasthenia in southern India: new insights into mRNA splicing and structure-function correlations of $\alpha_{IIb}\beta_3$ integrin (ITGA2B, ITGB3). Hum Mutat. 2006;27:359-369.

28. Caen JP. Glanzmann's thrombasthenia. Clin Haematol. 1972;1:383-392.

29. Nurden AT, Caen JP. An abnormal platelet glycoprotein pattern in three cases of Glanzmann's thrombasthenia. Br J Haematol. 1974;28:253-260.

30. Phillips DR, Agin PP. Platelet membrane defects in Glanzmann's thrombasthenia. Evidence for decreased amounts of two major glycoproteins. J Clin Invest. 1977;60:535-545.

31. Kunicki TJ, Aster RH. Deletion of the platelet-specific alloantigen PlA1 from platelets in Glanzmann's thrombasthenia. J Clin Invest. 1978;61:1225-1231.

32. Hagen I, Nurden A, Bjerrum OJ, et al. Immunochemical evidence for protein abnormalities in platelets from patients with Glanzmann's thrombasthenia and Bernard-Soulier syndrome. J Clin Invest. 1980;65:722-731.

33. McDowall A, Inwald D, Leitinger B, et al. A novel form of integrin dysfunction involving beta1, beta2, and beta3 integrins. J Clin Invest. 2003;111:51-60.

34. Jennings LK, Ashmun RA, Wang WC, Dockter ME. Analysis of human platelet glycoproteins IIb-IIIa and Glanzmann's thrombasthenia in whole blood by flow cytometry. Blood. 1986;68:173-179.

35. Nurden AT, Didry D, Kieffer N, McEver RP. Residual amounts of glycoproteins IIb and IIIa may be present in the platelets of most patients with Glanzmann's thrombasthenia. Blood. 1985;65:1021-1024.

36. The molecular genetics of Glanzmann's thrombasthenia. Platelets. 1998;9:5-20.

37. Basani RB, Vilaire G, Shattil SJ, et al. Glanzmann thrombasthenia due to a two amino acid deletion in the fourth calcium-binding domain of alpha IIb: demonstration of the importance of calcium-binding domains in the conformation of alpha IIb beta 3. Blood. 1996;88:167-173.

38. Basani RB, French DL, Vilaire G, et al. A naturally occurring mutation near the amino terminus of alphaIIb defines a new region involved in ligand binding to alphaIIbbeta3. Blood. 2000;95:180-188.

39. Loftus JC, O'Toole TE, Plow EF, et al. A beta 3 integrin mutation abolishes ligand binding and alters divalent cation-dependent conformation. Science. 1990;249:915-918.

40. Baker EK, Tozer EC, Pfaff M, et al. A genetic analysis of integrin function: Glanzmann thrombasthenia in vitro. Proc Natl Acad Sci U S A. 1997;94:1973-1978.

41. Chen YP, Djaffar I, Pidard D, et al. Ser-752→Pro mutation in the cytoplasmic domain of integrin beta 3 subunit and defective activation of platelet integrin alpha IIb beta 3 (glycoprotein IIb-IIIa) in a variant of Glanzmann thrombasthenia. Proc Natl Acad Sci U S A. 1992;89: 10169-10173.

42. Wang R, Shattil SJ, Ambruso DR, Newman PJ. Truncation of the cytoplasmic domain of beta3 in a variant form

of Glanzmann thrombasthenia abrogates signaling through the integrin alpha(IIb)beta3 complex. J Clin Invest. 1997; 100:2393-2403.

43. Staatz WD, Rajpara SM, Wayner EA, et al. The membrane glycoprotein Ia-IIa (VLA-2) complex mediates the Mg++-dependent adhesion of platelets to collagen. J Cell Biol. 1989;108:1917-1924.

44. Nieuwenhuis HK, Akkerman JW, Houdijk WP, Sixma JJ. Human blood platelets showing no response to collagen fail to express surface glycoprotein Ia. Nature. 1985;318:470-472.

45. Noris P, Guidetti GF, Conti V, et al. Autosomal dominant thrombocytopenias with reduced expression of glycoprotein Ia. Thromb Haemost. 2006;95:483-489.

46. Kunicki TJ, Orchekowski R, Annis D, Honda Y. Variability of integrin alpha 2 beta 1 activity on human platelets. Blood. 1993;82:2693-2703.

47. Kritzik M, Savage B, Nugent DJ, et al. Nucleotide polymorphisms in the alpha2 gene define multiple alleles that are associated with differences in platelet alpha2 beta1 density. Blood. 1998;92:2382-2388.

48. Alberio L, Dale GL. Review article: platelet-collagen interactions: membrane receptors and intracellular signaling pathways. Eur J Clin Invest. 1999;29:1066-1076.

49. Yee DL, Bray PF. Clinical and functional consequences of platelet membrane glycoprotein polymorphisms. Semin Thromb Hemost. 2004;30:591-600.

50. Di Paola J, Federici AB, Mannucci PM, et al. Low platelet alpha2beta1 levels in type I von Willebrand disease correlate with impaired platelet function in a high shear stress system. Blood. 1999;93:3578-3582.

51. Bernard J, Soulier JP. Sur une nouvelle variété de dystrophie thrombocytaire hémorragipare congénitale. Semin Hematol Paris. 1948;24:3217-3222.

52. Romo GM, Dong JF, Schade AJ, et al. The glycoprotein Ib-IX-V complex is a platelet counter receptor for P-selectin. J Exp Med. 1999;190:803-814.

53. Jurk K, Clemetson KJ, de Groot PG, et al. Thrombospondin-1 mediates platelet adhesion at high shear via glycoprotein Ib (GPIb): an alternative/backup mechanism to von Willebrand factor. FASEB J. 2003;17:1490-1492.

54. Chavakis T, Santoso S, Clemetson KJ, et al. High molecular weight kininogen regulates platelet-leukocyte interactions by bridging Mac-1 and glycoprotein Ib. J Biol Chem. 2003;278:45375-45381.

55. Coller BS, Peerschke EI, Scudder LE, Sullivan CA. Studies with a murine monoclonal antibody that abolishes ristocetin-induced binding of von Willebrand factor to platelets: additional evidence in support of GPIb as a platelet receptor for von Willebrand factor. Blood. 1983; 61:99-110.

56. Whisstock JC, Shen Y, Lopez JA, et al. Molecular modeling of the seven tandem leucine-rich repeats within the ligand-binding region of platelet glycoprotein Ib alpha. Thromb Haemost. 2002;87:329-333.

57. Lopez JA, Chung DW, Fujikawa K, et al. The alpha and beta chains of human platelet glycoprotein Ib are both transmembrane proteins containing a leucine-rich amino acid sequence. Proc Natl Acad Sci U S A. 1988;85:2135-2139.

58. Okumura I, Lombart C, Jamieson GA. Platelet glycocalicin. II. Purification and characterization. J Biol Chem. 1976;251:5950-5955.

59. Handa M, Titani K, Holland LZ, et al. The von Willebrand factor–binding domain of platelet membrane glycoprotein Ib. Characterization by monoclonal antibodies and partial amino acid sequence analysis of proteolytic fragments. J Biol Chem. 1986;261:12579-12585.

60. Ruggeri ZM. Mechanisms initiating platelet thrombus formation. Thromb Haemost. 1997;78:611-616.

61. Howard MA, Firkin BG. Ristocetin—a new tool in the investigation of platelet aggregation. Thromb Diath Haemorrh. 1971;26:362-369.

62. Englund GD, Bodnar RJ, Li Z, et al. Regulation of von Willebrand factor binding to the platelet glycoprotein Ib-IX by a membrane skeleton–dependent inside-out signal. J Biol Chem. 2001;276:16952-16959.

63. Du X, Harris SJ, Tetaz TJ, et al. Association of a phospholipase A2 (14-3-3 protein) with the platelet glycoprotein Ib-IX complex. J Biol Chem. 1994;269: 18287-18290.

64. Modderman PW, Admiraal LG, Sonnenberg A, von dem Borne AE. Glycoproteins V and Ib-IX form a noncovalent complex in the platelet membrane. J Biol Chem. 1992;267:364-369.

65. Hickey MJ, Williams SA, Roth GJ. Human platelet glycoprotein IX: an adhesive prototype of leucine-rich glycoproteins with flank-center-flank structures. Proc Natl Acad Sci U S A. 1989;86:6773-6777.

66. Lanza F, Morales M, de La Salle C, et al. Cloning and characterization of the gene encoding the human platelet glycoprotein V. A member of the leucine-rich glycoprotein family cleaved during thrombin-induced platelet activation. J Biol Chem. 1993;268:20801-20807.

67. Zafar RS, Walz DA. Platelet membrane glycoprotein V: characterization of the thrombin-sensitive glycoprotein from human platelets. Thromb Res. 1989;53:31-44.

68. Ramakrishnan V, DeGuzman F, Bao M, et al. A thrombin receptor function for platelet glycoprotein Ib-IX unmasked by cleavage of glycoprotein V. Proc Natl Acad Sci U S A. 2001;98:1823-1828.

69. Ni H, Ramakrishnan V, Ruggeri ZM, et al. Increased thrombogenesis and embolus formation in mice lacking glycoprotein V. Blood. 2001;98:368-373.

70. Yuan Y, Kulkarni S, Ulsemer P, et al. The von Willebrand factor–glycoprotein Ib/V/IX interaction induces actin polymerization and cytoskeletal reorganization in rolling platelets and glycoprotein Ib/V/IX–transfected cells. J Biol Chem. 1999;274:36241-36251.

71. Ozaki Y, Asazuma N, Suzuki-Inoue K, Berndt MC. Platelet GPIb-IX-V–dependent signaling. J Thromb Haemost. 2005;3:1745-1751.

72. Lanza F. Bernard-Soulier syndrome (hemorrhagiparous thrombocytic dystrophy). Orphanet J Rare Dis. 2006;1: 46.

73. Lozano M, Escolar G, Bellucci S, et al. 1-Deamino (8-D-arginine) vasopressin infusion partially corrects platelet deposition on subendothelium in Bernard-Soulier syndrome: the role of factor VIII. Platelets. 1999;10:141-145.

74. Ozelo MC, Svirin P, Larina L. Use of recombinant factor VIIa in the management of severe bleeding episodes in patients with Bernard-Soulier syndrome. Ann Hematol. 2005;84:816-822.

75. George JN, Reimann TA, Moake JL, et al. Bernard-Soulier disease: a study of four patients and their parents. Br J Haematol. 1981;48:459-467.

76. Bessman JD, Williams LJ, Gilmer PR Jr. Mean platelet volume. The inverse relation of platelet size and count in normal subjects, and an artifact of other particles. Am J Clin Pathol. 1981;76:289-293.

77. Hourdille P, Pico M, Jandrot-Perrus M, et al. Studies on the megakaryocytes of a patient with the Bernard-Soulier syndrome. Br J Haematol. 1990;76:521-530.

78. Poujol C, Ware J, Nieswandt B, et al. Absence of GPIbalpha is responsible for aberrant membrane development during megakaryocyte maturation: ultrastructural study using a transgenic model. Exp Hematol. 2002;30:352-360.

79. Meyer SC, Zuerbig S, Cunningham CC, et al. Identification of the region in actin-binding protein that binds to the cytoplasmic domain of glycoprotein IBalpha. J Biol Chem. 1997;272:2914-2919.

80. Feng S, Christodoulides N, Kroll MH. The glycoprotein Ib/IX complex regulates cell proliferation. Blood. 1999;93:4256-4263.

81. Harrison P, Robinson M, Liesner R, et al. The PFA-100: a potential rapid screening tool for the assessment of platelet dysfunction. Clin Lab Haematol. 2002;24:225-232.

82. de la Salle C, Lanza F, Cazenave JP. Biochemical and molecular basis of Bernard-Soulier syndrome: a review. Nouv Rev Fr Hematol. 1995;37:215-222.

83. Cohn RJ, Sherman GG, Glencross DK. Flow cytometric analysis of platelet surface glycoproteins in the diagnosis of Bernard-Soulier syndrome. Pediatr Hematol Oncol. 1997;14:43-50.

84. Balduini CL, Savoia A. Inherited thrombocytopenias: molecular mechanisms. Semin Thromb Hemost. 2004;30:513-523.

85. Ware J, Russell SR, Vicente V, et al. Nonsense mutation in the glycoprotein Ib alpha coding sequence associated with Bernard-Soulier syndrome. Proc Natl Acad Sci U S A. 1990;87:2026-2030.

86. Kunishima S, Kamiya T, Saito H. Genetic abnormalities of Bernard-Soulier syndrome. Int J Hematol. 2002;76:319-327.

87. Hillmann A, Nurden A, Nurden P, et al. A novel hemizygous Bernard-Soulier Syndrome (BSS) mutation in the amino terminal domain of glycoprotein (GP)Ibα—platelet characterization and transfection studies. Thromb Haemost. 2002;88:1026-1032.

88. Sachs UJ, Kroll H, Matzdorff AC, et al. Bernard-Soulier syndrome due to the homozygous Asn-45Ser mutation in GPIX: an unexpected, frequent finding in Germany. Br J Haematol. 2003;123:127-131.

89. Budarf ML, Konkle BA, Ludlow LB, et al. Identification of a patient with Bernard-Soulier syndrome and a deletion in the DiGeorge/velo-cardio-facial chromosomal region in 22q11.2. Hum Mol Genet. 1995;4:763-766.

90. Gonzalez-Manchon C, Larrucea S, Pastor AL, et al. Compound heterozygosity of the GPIbalpha gene associated with Bernard-Soulier syndrome. Thromb Haemost. 2001;86:1385-1391.

91. Miller JL, Lyle VA, Cunningham D. Mutation of leucine-57 to phenylalanine in a platelet glycoprotein Ib alpha leucine tandem repeat occurring in patients with an autosomal dominant variant of Bernard-Soulier disease. Blood. 1992;79:439-446.

90. Miller JL, Castella A. Platelet-type von Willebrand's disease: characterization of a new bleeding disorder. Blood. 1982;60:790-794.

91. Takahashi H. Studies on the pathophysiology and treatment of von Willebrand's disease. IV. Mechanism of increased ristocetin-induced platelet aggregation in von Willebrand's disease. Thromb Res. 1980;19:857-867.

92. Miller JL, Kupinski JM, Castella A, Ruggeri ZM. von Willebrand factor binds to platelets and induces aggregation in platelet-type but not type IIB von Willebrand disease. J Clin Invest. 1983;72:1532-1542.

93. Miller JL, Cunningham D, Lyle VA, Finch CN. Mutation in the gene encoding the alpha chain of platelet glycoprotein Ib in platelet-type von Willebrand disease. Proc Natl Acad Sci U S A. 1991;88:4761-4765.

94. Kahn ML, Nakanishi-Matsui M, Shapiro MJ, et al. Protease-activated receptors 1 and 4 mediate activation of human platelets by thrombin. J Clin Invest. 1999;103:879-887.

95. Connolly AJ, Ishihara H, Kahn ML, et al. Role of the thrombin receptor in development and evidence for a second receptor. Nature. 1996;381:516-519.

96. Kahn ML, Zheng YW, Huang W, et al. A dual thrombin receptor system for platelet activation. Nature. 1998;394:690-694.

97. Cattaneo M, Lecchi A, Randi AM, et al. Identification of a new congenital defect of platelet function characterized by severe impairment of platelet responses to adenosine diphosphate. Blood. 1992;80:2787-2796.

98. Nurden P, Savi P, Heilmann E, et al. An inherited bleeding disorder linked to a defective interaction between ADP and its receptor on platelets. Its influence on glycoprotein IIb-IIIa complex function. J Clin Invest. 1995;95:1612-1622.

99. Oury C, Toth-Zsamboki E, Van Geet C, et al. A natural dominant negative P2X1 receptor due to deletion of a single amino acid residue. J Biol Chem. 2000;275:22611-22614.

100. Hollopeter G, Jantzen HM, Vincent D, et al. Identification of the platelet ADP receptor targeted by antithrombotic drugs. Nature. 2001;409:202-207.

101. Leon C, Hechler B, Vial C, et al. The P2Y1 receptor is an ADP receptor antagonized by ATP and expressed in platelets and megakaryoblastic cells. FEBS Lett. 1997;403:26-30.

102. Siess W, Weber PC, Lapetina EG. Activation of phospholipase C is dissociated from arachidonate metabolism during platelet shape change induced by thrombin or platelet-activating factor. Epinephrine does not induce phospholipase C activation or platelet shape change. J Biol Chem. 1984;259:8286-8292.

103. Kaywin P, McDonough M, Insel PA, Shattil SJ. Platelet function in essential thrombocythemia. Decreased epinephrine responsiveness associated with a deficiency of platelet alpha-adrenergic receptors. N Engl J Med. 1978;299:505-509.

104. Saxena R, Gupta M, Gupta S, Choudhry VP. An unusual platelet function defect: report of 19 cases. Indian J Pathol Microbiol. 2003;46:576-578.

105. Gerrard JM, Carroll RC. Stimulation of platelet protein phosphorylation by arachidonic acid and endoperoxide analogs. Prostaglandins. 1981;22:81-94.

106. Hirata M, Hayashi Y, Ushikubi F, et al. Cloning and expression of cDNA for a human thromboxane A_2 receptor. Nature. 1991;349:617-620.

107. Schafer AI, Cooper B, O'Hara D, Handin RI. Identification of platelet receptors for prostaglandin I_2 and D_2. J Biol Chem. 1979;254:2914-2917.

108. Higuchi W, Fuse I, Hattori A, Aizawa Y. Mutations of the platelet thromboxane A_2 (TXA_2) receptor in patients characterized by the absence of TXA_2-induced platelet aggregation despite normal TXA_2 binding activity. Thromb Haemost. 1999;82:1528-1531.

109. Fuse I, Higuchi W, Aizawa Y. Pathogenesis of a bleeding disorder characterized by platelet unresponsiveness to thromboxane A_2. Semin Thromb Hemost. 2000;26:43-45.

110. Murata T, Ushikubi F, Matsuoka T, et al. Altered pain perception and inflammatory response in mice lacking prostacyclin receptor. Nature. 1997;388:678-682.

111. Ezumi Y, Uchiyama T, Takayama H. Molecular cloning, genomic structure, chromosomal localization, and alternative splice forms of the platelet collagen receptor glycoprotein VI. Biochem Biophys Res Commun. 2000;277:27-36.

112. Santoro SA. Identification of a 160,000 dalton platelet membrane protein that mediates the initial divalent cation–dependent adhesion of platelets to collagen. Cell. 1986;46:913-920.

113. Tsuji M, Ezumi Y, Arai M, Takayama H. A novel association of Fc receptor gamma-chain with glycoprotein VI and their co-expression as a collagen receptor in human platelets. J Biol Chem. 1997;272:23528-23531.

114. Blake RA, Schieven GL, Watson SP. Collagen stimulates tyrosine phosphorylation of phospholipase C-gamma 2 but not phospholipase C-gamma 1 in human platelets. FEBS Lett. 1994;353:212-216.

115. Yanaga F, Poole A, Asselin J, et al. Syk interacts with tyrosine-phosphorylated proteins in human platelets activated by collagen and cross-linking of the Fc gamma-IIA receptor. Biochem J. 1995;311:471-478.

116. Boylan B, Chen H, Rathore V, et al. Anti-GPVI–associated ITP: an acquired platelet disorder caused by autoantibody-mediated clearance of the GPVI/FcRγ-chain complex from the human platelet surface. Blood. 2004;104:1350-1355.

117. Jandrot-Perrus M, Lagrue AH, Okuma M, Bon C. Adhesion and activation of human platelets induced by convulxin involve glycoprotein VI and integrin alpha2beta1. J Biol Chem. 1997;272:27035-27041.

118. Watson SP, Auger JM, McCarty OJ, Pearce AC. GPVI and integrin alphaIIb beta3 signaling in platelets. J Thromb Haemost. 2005;3:1752-1762.

119. Moroi M, Jung SM, Okuma M, Shinmyozu K. A patient with platelets deficient in glycoprotein VI that lack both collagen-induced aggregation and adhesion. J Clin Invest. 1989;84:1440-1445.

120. Arai M, Yamamoto N, Moroi M, et al. Platelets with 10% of the normal amount of glycoprotein VI have an impaired response to collagen that results in a mild bleeding tendency. Br J Haematol. 1995;89:124-130.

121. Moroi M, Jung SM. Platelet glycoprotein VI: its structure and function. Thromb Res. 2004;114:221-233.

122. Sugiyama T, Ishibashi T, Okuma M. Functional role of the antigen recognized by an antiplatelet antibody specific for a putative collagen receptor in platelet-collagen interaction. Int J Hematol. 1993;58:99-104.

123. Takahashi H, Moroi M. Antibody against platelet membrane glycoprotein VI in a patient with systemic lupus erythematosus. Am J Hematol. 2001;67:262-267.

124. Croft SA, Samani NJ, Teare MD, et al. Novel platelet membrane glycoprotein VI dimorphism is a risk factor for myocardial infarction. Circulation. 2001;104:1459-1463.

125. Joutsi-Korhonen L, Smethurst PA, Rankin A, et al. The low-frequency allele of the platelet collagen signaling receptor glycoprotein VI is associated with reduced functional responses and expression. Blood. 2003;101:4372-4379.

126. Sims PJ, Wiedmer T, Esmon CT, et al. Assembly of the platelet prothrombinase complex is linked to vesiculation of the platelet plasma membrane. Studies in Scott syndrome: an isolated defect in platelet procoagulant activity. J Biol Chem. 1989;264:17049-17057.

127. Weiss HJ, Vicic WJ, Lages BA, Rogers J. Isolated deficiency of platelet procoagulant activity. Am J Med. 1979;67:206-213.

128. Miletich JP, Kane WH, Hofmann SL, et al. Deficiency of factor Xa–factor Va binding sites on the platelets of a patient with a bleeding disorder. Blood. 1979;54:1015-1022.

129. Rosing J, Bevers EM, Comfurius P, et al. Impaired factor X and prothrombin activation associated with decreased phospholipid exposure in platelets from a patient with a bleeding disorder. Blood. 1985;65:1557-1561.

130. Albrecht C, McVey JH, Elliott JI, et al. A novel missense mutation in ABCA1 results in altered protein trafficking and reduced phosphatidylserine translocation in a patient with Scott syndrome. Blood. 2005;106:542-549.

131. Zwaal RF, Comfurius P, Bevers EM. Scott syndrome, a bleeding disorder caused by defective scrambling of membrane phospholipids. Biochim Biophys Acta. 2004;1636:119-128.

132. Rao AK. Congenital disorders of platelet function. Hematol Oncol Clin North Am. 1990;4:65-86.

133. Meyers KM, Holmsen H, Seachord CL. Comparative study of platelet dense granule constituents. Am J Physiol. 1982;243:R454-R461.

134. White JG, Krumwiede M. Further studies of the secretory pathway in thrombin-stimulated human platelets. Blood. 1987;69:1196-1203.

135. Cramer EM, Debili N, Martin JF, et al. Uncoordinated expression of fibrinogen compared with thrombospondin and von Willebrand factor in maturing human megakaryocytes. Blood. 1989;73:1123-1129..

136. Handagama P, Rappolee DA, Werb Z, et al. Platelet alpha-granule fibrinogen, albumin, and immunoglobulin G are not synthesized by rat and mouse megakaryocytes. J Clin Invest. 1990;86:1364-1368.

137. White JG. Inherited abnormalities of the platelet membrane and secretory granules. Hum Pathol. 1987;18:123-139.

138. Weiss HJ, Chervenick PA, Zalusky R, Factor A. A familial defect in platelet function associated with impaired release of adenosine diphosphate. N Engl J Med. 1969;281:1264-1270.

139. Holmsen H, Weiss HJ. Hereditary defect in the platelet release reaction caused by a deficiency in the storage pool

of platelet adenine nucleotides. Br J Haematol. 1970;19: 643-649.

140. Weiss HJ, Lages B, Vicic W, et al. Heterogeneous abnormalities of platelet dense granule ultrastructure in 20 patients with congenital storage pool deficiency. Br J Haematol. 1993;83:282-295.

141. Rendu F, Brohard-Bohn B. The platelet release reaction: granules' constituents, secretion and functions. Platelets. 2001;12:261-273.

142. Huizing M, Anikster Y, Gahl WA. Hermansky-Pudlak syndrome and Chédiak-Higashi syndrome: disorders of vesicle formation and trafficking. Thromb Haemost. 2001;86:233-245.

143. Chediak MM. [New leukocyte anomaly of constitutional and familial character.] Rev Hematol. 1952;7:362-367.

144. Higashi O. Congenital gigantism of peroxidase granules; the first case ever reported of qualitative abnormity of peroxidase. Tohoku J Exp Med. 1954;59:315-332.

145. Witkop CJ, Almadovar C, Pineiro B, Nunez Babcock M. Hermansky-Pudlak syndrome (HPS). An epidemiologic study. Ophthalmic Paediatr Genet. 1990;11:245-250.

146. Mahadeo R, Markowitz J, Fisher S, Daum F. Hermansky-Pudlak syndrome with granulomatous colitis in children. J Pediatr. 1991;118:904-906.

147. Gahl WA, Brantly M, Kaiser-Kupfer MI, et al. Genetic defects and clinical characteristics of patients with a form of oculocutaneous albinism (Hermansky-Pudlak syndrome). N Engl J Med. 1998;338:1258-1264.

148. Brantly M, Avila NA, Shotelersuk V, et al. Pulmonary function and high-resolution CT findings in patients with an inherited form of pulmonary fibrosis, Hermansky-Pudlak syndrome, due to mutations in HPS-1. Chest. 2000;117:129-136.

149. Herve P, Drouet L, Dosquet C, et al. Primary pulmonary hypertension in a patient with a familial platelet storage pool disease: role of serotonin. Am J Med. 1990;89:117-120.

150. Wildenberg SC, Oetting WS, Almodovar C, et al. A gene causing Hermansky-Pudlak syndrome in a Puerto Rican population maps to chromosome 10q2. Am J Hum Genet. 1995;57:755-765.

151. Witkop CJ, Nunez Babcock M, Rao GH, et al. Albinism and Hermansky-Pudlak syndrome in Puerto Rico. Bol Asoc Med P R. 1990;82:333-339.

152. Oh J, Ho L, Ala-Mello S, et al. Mutation analysis of patients with Hermansky-Pudlak syndrome: a frameshift hot spot in the HPS gene and apparent locus heterogeneity. Am J Hum Genet. 1998;62:593-598.

153. Shotelersuk V, Dell'Angelica EC, Hartnell L, et al. A new variant of Hermansky-Pudlak syndrome due to mutations in a gene responsible for vesicle formation. Am J Med. 2000;108:423-427.

154. Wei ML. Hermansky-Pudlak syndrome: a disease of protein trafficking and organelle function. Pigment Cell Res. 2006;19:19-42.

155. Blume RS, Bennett JM, Yankee RA, Wolff SM. Defective granulocyte regulation in the Chédiak-Higashi syndrome. N Engl J Med. 1968;279:1009-1015.

156. Clark RA, Kimball HR. Defective granulocyte chemotaxis in the Chédiak-Higashi syndrome. J Clin Invest. 1971;50: 2645-2652.

157. Root RK, Rosenthal AS, Balestra DJ. Abnormal bactericidal, metabolic, and lysosomal functions of Chédiak-Higashi syndrome leukocytes. J Clin Invest. 1972;51: 649-665.

158. Valenzuela R, Morningstar WA. The ocular pigmentary disturbance of human Chédiak-Higashi syndrome. A comparative light- and electron-microscopic study and review of the literature. Am J Clin Pathol. 1981;75: 591-596.

159. Sung JH, Stadlan EM. Neuropathological changes in Chédiak-Higashi disease. J Neuropathol Exp Neurol. 1968;27:156-157.

160. Nagle DL, Karim MA, Woolf EA, et al. Identification and mutation analysis of the complete gene for Chédiak-Higashi syndrome. Nat Genet. 1996;14:307-311.

161. Andrade MA, Bork P. HEAT repeats in the Huntington's disease protein. Nat Genet. 1995;11:115-116.

162. Barbosa MD, Barrat FJ, Tchernev VT, et al. Identification of mutations in two major mRNA isoforms of the Chédiak-Higashi syndrome gene in human and mouse. Hum Mol Genet. 1997;6:1091-1098.

163. Certain S, Barrat F, Pastural E, et al. Protein truncation test of LYST reveals heterogenous mutations in patients with Chédiak-Higashi syndrome. Blood. 2000;95:979-983.

164. Israels SJ, McNicol A, Robertson C, Gerrard JM. Platelet storage pool deficiency: diagnosis in patients with prolonged bleeding times and normal platelet aggregation. Br J Haematol. 1990;75:118-121.

165. Ramstrom A, Fagerberg I, Lindahl T. A flow cytometric assay for the study of dense granule storage and release in human platelets. Platelets. 1999;10:153-158.

166. Raccuglia G. Gray platelet syndrome. A variety of qualitative platelet disorder. Am J Med. 1971;51:818-828.

167. White GC 2nd. Congenital and acquired platelet disorders: current dilemmas and treatment strategies. Semin Hematol. 2006;43:S37-S41.

168. Nurden AT, Kunicki TJ, Dupuis D, et al. Specific protein and glycoprotein deficiencies in platelets isolated from two patients with the gray platelet syndrome. Blood. 1982;59:709-718.

169. Levy-Toledano S, Caen JP, Breton-Gorius J, et al. Gray platelet syndrome: alpha-granule deficiency. Its influence on platelet function. J Lab Clin Med. 1981;98:831-848.

170. Srivastava PC, Powling MJ, Nokes TJ, et al. Grey platelet syndrome: studies on platelet alpha-granules, lysosomes and defective response to thrombin. Br J Haematol. 1987;65:441-446.

171. Rosa JP, George JN, Bainton DF, et al. Gray platelet syndrome. Demonstration of alpha granule membranes that can fuse with the cell surface. J Clin Invest. 1987;80: 1138-1146.

172. Caen JP, Deschamps JF, Bodevin E, et al. Megakaryocytes and myelofibrosis in gray platelet syndrome. Nouv Rev Fr Hematol. 1987;29:109-114.

173. Rao AK, Gabbeta J. Congenital disorders of platelet signal transduction. Arterioscler Thromb Vasc Biol. 2000;20:285-289.

174. Lages B, Shattil SJ, Bainton DF, Weiss HJ. Decreased content and surface expression of alpha-granule membrane protein GMP-140 in one of two types of platelet alpha delta storage pool deficiency. J Clin Invest. 1991; 87:919-929.

175. Hayward CP, Cramer EM, Kane WH, et al. Studies of a second family with the Quebec platelet disorder: evidence

that the degradation of the alpha-granule membrane and its soluble contents are not secondary to a defect in targeting proteins to alpha-granules. Blood. 1997;89:1243-1253.

176. Kahr WH, Zheng S, Sheth PM, et al. Platelets from patients with the Quebec platelet disorder contain and secrete abnormal amounts of urokinase-type plasminogen activator. Blood. 2001;98:257-265.

177. Hayward CP, Rivard GE, Kane WH, et al. An autosomal dominant, qualitative platelet disorder associated with multimerin deficiency, abnormalities in platelet factor V, thrombospondin, von Willebrand factor, and fibrinogen and an epinephrine aggregation defect. Blood. 1996;87:4967-4978.

178. McKay H, Derome F, Haq MA, et al. Bleeding risks associated with inheritance of the Quebec platelet disorder. Blood. 2004;104:159-165.

179. Rao AK. Inherited defects in platelet signaling mechanisms. J Thromb Haemost. 2003;1:671-681.

180. Rao AK, Koike K, Willis J, et al. Platelet secretion defect associated with impaired liberation of arachidonic acid and normal myosin light chain phosphorylation. Blood. 1984;64:914-921.

181. Rendu F, Breton-Gorius J, Trugnan G, et al. Studies on a new variant of the Hermansky-Pudlak syndrome: qualitative, ultrastructural, and functional abnormalities of the platelet dense bodies associated with a phospholipase A defect. Am J Hematol. 1978;4:387-399.

182. Levy-Toledano S, Maclouf J, Rosa JP, et al. Abnormal tyrosine phosphorylation linked to a defective interaction between ADP and its receptor on platelets. Thromb Haemost. 1998;80:463-468.

183. Lagarde M, Byron PA, Vargaftig BB, Dechavanne M. Impairment of platelet thromboxane A_2 generation and of the platelet release reaction in two patients with congenital deficiency of platelet cyclo-oxygenase. Br J Haematol. 1978;38:251-266.

184. Malmsten C, Hamberg M, Svensson J, Samuelsson B. Physiological role of an endoperoxide in human platelets: hemostatic defect due to platelet cyclo-oxygenase deficiency. Proc Natl Acad Sci U S A. 1975;72:1446-1450.

185. Roth GJ, Machuga ET. Radioimmune assay of human platelet prostaglandin synthetase. J Lab Clin Med. 1982;99:187-196.

186. Matijevic-Aleksic N, McPhedran P, Wu KK. Bleeding disorder due to platelet prostaglandin H synthase-1 (PGHS-1) deficiency. Br J Haematol. 1996;92:212-217.

187. Mestel F, Oetliker O, Beck E, et al. Severe bleeding associated with defective thromboxane synthetase. Lancet. 1980;1:157.

188. Defreyn G, Machin SJ, Carreras LO, et al. Familial bleeding tendency with partial platelet thromboxane synthetase deficiency: reorientation of cyclic endoperoxide metabolism. Br J Haematol. 1981;49:29-41.

189. Szalai G, LaRue AC, Watson DK. Molecular mechanisms of megakaryopoiesis. Cell Mol Life Sci. 2006;63:2460-2476.

190. Vainchenker W, Debili N, Mouthon MA, Wendling F. Megakaryocytopoiesis: cellular aspects and regulation. Crit Rev Oncol Hematol. 1995;20:165-192.

191. Deutsch VR, Tomer A. Megakaryocyte development and platelet production. Br J Haematol. 2006;134:453-466.

192. Gordon MS, Hoffman R. Growth factors affecting human thrombocytopoiesis: potential agents for the treatment of thrombocytopenia. Blood. 1992;80:302-307.

193. Souyri M, Vigon I, Penciolelli JF, et al. A putative truncated cytokine receptor gene transduced by the myeloproliferative leukemia virus immortalizes hematopoietic progenitors. Cell. 1990;63:1137-1147.

194. Lok S, Kaushansky K, Holly RD, et al. Cloning and expression of murine thrombopoietin cDNA and stimulation of platelet production in vivo. Nature. 1994;369:565-568.

195. Bussel JB, Kuter DJ, George JN, et al. AMG 531, a thrombopoiesis-stimulating protein, for chronic ITP. N Engl J Med. 2006;355:1672-1681.

196. Bunting S, Widmer R, Lipari T, et al. Normal platelets and megakaryocytes are produced in vivo in the absence of thrombopoietin. Blood. 1997;90:3423-3429.

197. Gurney AL, Carver-Moore K, de Sauvage FJ, Moore MW. Thrombocytopenia in c-mpl-deficient mice. Science. 1994;265:1445-1447.

198. Kimura S, Roberts AW, Metcalf D, Alexander WS. Hematopoietic stem cell deficiencies in mice lacking c-Mpl, the receptor for thrombopoietin. Proc Natl Acad Sci U S A. 1998;95:1195-1200.

199. Radley JM, Haller CJ. Fate of senescent megakaryocytes in the bone marrow. Br J Haematol. 1983;53:277-287.

200. Tong M, Seth P, Penington DG. Proplatelets and stress platelets. Blood. 1987;69:522-528.

201. Kaufman RM, Airo R, Pollack S, Crosby WH. Circulating megakaryocytes and platelet release in the lung. Blood. 1965;26:720-731.

202. Pedersen NT. Occurrence of megakaryocytes in various vessels and their retention in the pulmonary capillaries in man. Scand J Haematol. 1978;21:369-375.

203. Kallinikos-Maniatis A. Megakaryocytes and platelets in central venous and arterial blood. Acta Haematol. 1969;42:330-335.

204. Italiano JE Jr, Lecine P, Shivdasani RA, Hartwig JH. Blood platelets are assembled principally at the ends of proplatelet processes produced by differentiated megakaryocytes. J Cell Biol. 1999;147:1299-1312.

205. Handagama PJ, Feldman BF, Jain NC, et al. In vitro platelet release by rat megakaryocytes: effect of metabolic inhibitors and cytoskeletal disrupting agents. Am J Vet Res. 1987;48:1142-1146.

206. Radley JM, Scurfield G. The mechanism of platelet release. Blood. 1980;56:996-999.

207. Lecine P, Villeval JL, Vyas P, et al. Mice lacking transcription factor NF-E2 provide in vivo validation of the proplatelet model of thrombocytopoiesis and show a platelet production defect that is intrinsic to megakaryocytes. Blood. 1998;92:1608-1616.

208. Lecine P, Italiano JE Jr, Kim SW, et al. Hematopoietic-specific beta 1 tubulin participates in a pathway of platelet biogenesis dependent on the transcription factor NF-E2. Blood. 2000;96:1366-1373.

209. Wolber EM, Jelkmann W. Thrombopoietin: the novel hepatic hormone. News Physiol Sci. 2002;17:6-10.

210. Shivdasani RA, Fujiwara Y, McDevitt MA, Orkin SH. A lineage-selective knockout establishes the critical role of transcription factor GATA-1 in megakaryocyte growth and platelet development. EMBO J. 1997;16:3965-3973.

211. Tsang AP, Visvader JE, Turner CA, et al. FOG, a multi-type zinc finger protein, acts as a cofactor for transcription factor GATA-1 in erythroid and megakaryocytic differentiation. Cell. 1997;90:109-119.

212. McDevitt MA, Shivdasani RA, Fujiwara Y, et al. A "knockdown" mutation created by *cis*-element gene targeting reveals the dependence of erythroid cell maturation on the level of transcription factor GATA-1. Proc Natl Acad Sci U S A. 1997;94:6781-6785.

213. Levin J, Peng JP, Baker GR, et al. Pathophysiology of thrombocytopenia and anemia in mice lacking transcription factor NF-E2. Blood. 1999;94:3037-3047.

214. Henter JI, Winiarski J, Ljungman P, et al. Bone marrow transplantation in two children with congenital amegakaryocytic thrombocytopenia. Bone Marrow Transplant. 1995;15:799-801.

215. Ballmaier M, Germeshausen M, Schulze H, et al. c-mpl mutations are the cause of congenital amegakaryocytic thrombocytopenia. Blood. 2001;97:139-146.

216. Ballmaier M, Germeshausen M, Krukemeier S, Welte K. Thrombopoietin is essential for the maintenance of normal hematopoiesis in humans: development of aplastic anemia in patients with congenital amegakaryocytic thrombocytopenia. Ann N Y Acad Sci. 2003;996:17-25.

217. Campbell PJ, Green AR. The myeloproliferative disorders. N Engl J Med. 2006;355:2452-2466.

218. Ghilardi N, Skoda RC. A single-base deletion in the thrombopoietin (TPO) gene causes familial essential thrombocythemia through a mechanism of more efficient translation of TPO mRNA. Blood. 1999;94:1480-1482.

219. Ding J, Komatsu H, Wakita A, et al. Familial essential thrombocythemia associated with a dominant-positive activating mutation of the c-MPL gene, which encodes for the receptor for thrombopoietin. Blood. 2004;103:4198-200.

220. Dame C, Sutor AH. Primary and secondary thrombocytosis in childhood. Br J Haematol. 2005;129:165-177.

221. Schafer AI. Molecular basis of the diagnosis and treatment of polycythemia vera and essential thrombocythemia. Blood. 2006;107:4214-4222.

222. Bernhard WG, Gore I, Kilby RA. Congenital leukemia. Blood. 1951;6:990-1001.

223. Greenhalgh KL, Howell RT, Bottani A, et al. Thrombocytopenia–absent radius syndrome: a clinical genetic study. J Med Genet. 2002;39:876-881.

224. Day HJ, Holmsen H. Platelet adenine nucleotide "storage pool deficiency" in thrombocytopenic absent radii syndrome. JAMA. 1972;221:1053-1054.

225. de Alarcon PA, Graeve JA, Levine RF, et al. Thrombocytopenia and absent radii syndrome: defective megakaryocytopoiesis-thrombocytopoiesis. Am J Pediatr Hematol Oncol. 1991;13:77-83.

226. Ballmaier M, Schulze H, Strauss G, et al. Thrombopoietin in patients with congenital thrombocytopenia and absent radii: elevated serum levels, normal receptor expression, but defective reactivity to thrombopoietin. Blood. 1997;90:612-619.

227. al-Jefri AH, Dror Y, Bussel JB, Freedman MH. Thrombocytopenia with absent radii: frequency of marrow megakaryocyte progenitors, proliferative characteristics, and megakaryocyte growth and development factor responsiveness. Pediatr Hematol Oncol. 2000;17:299-306.

228. Letestu R, Vitrat N, Masse A, et al. Existence of a differentiation blockage at the stage of a megakaryocyte precursor in the thrombocytopenia and absent radii (TAR) syndrome. Blood. 2000;95:1633-1641.

229. Thompson AA, Woodruff K, Feig SA, et al. Congenital thrombocytopenia and radio-ulnar synostosis: a new familial syndrome. Br J Haematol. 2001;113:866-870.

230. Sola MC, Slayton WB, Rimsza LM, et al. A neonate with severe thrombocytopenia and radio-ulnar synostosis. J Perinatol. 2004;24:528-530.

231. Thompson AA, Nguyen LT. Amegakaryocytic thrombocytopenia and radio-ulnar synostosis are associated with HOXA11 mutation. Nat Genet. 2000;26:397-398.

232. Horvat-Switzer RD, Thompson AA. HOXA11 mutation in amegakaryocytic thrombocytopenia with radio-ulnar synostosis syndrome inhibits megakaryocytic differentiation in vitro. Blood Cells Mol Dis. 2006;37:55-63.

233. Nichols KE, Crispino JD, Poncz M, et al. Familial dyserythropoietic anaemia and thrombocytopenia due to an inherited mutation in GATA1. Nat Genet. 2000;24:266-270.

234. Raskind WH, Niakan KK, Wolff J, et al. Mapping of a syndrome of X-linked thrombocytopenia with thalassemia to band Xp11-12: further evidence of genetic heterogeneity of X-linked thrombocytopenia. Blood. 2000;95:2262-2268.

235. Dowton SB, Beardsley D, Jamison D, et al. Studies of a familial platelet disorder. Blood. 1985;65:557-563.

236. Gerrard JM, Israels ED, Bishop AJ, et al. Inherited platelet-storage pool deficiency associated with a high incidence of acute myeloid leukaemia. Br J Haematol. 1991;79:246-255.

237. Song WJ, Sullivan MG, Legare RD, et al. Haploinsufficiency of CBFA2 causes familial thrombocytopenia with propensity to develop acute myelogenous leukaemia. Nat Genet. 1999;23:166-175.

238. Lo Coco F, Pisegna S, Diverio D. The AML1 gene: a transcription factor involved in the pathogenesis of myeloid and lymphoid leukemias. Haematologica. 1997;82:364-370.

239. North T, Gu TL, Stacy T, et al. Cbfa2 is required for the formation of intra-aortic hematopoietic clusters. Development. 1999;126:2563-2575.

240. Aldrich RA, Steinberg AG, Campbell DC. Pedigree demonstrating a sex-linked recessive condition characterized by draining ears, eczematoid dermatitis and bloody diarrhea. Pediatrics. 1954;13:133-139.

241. Wiskott A. Familiarer angeborener Morbus Werlhofi? Monatsschr Kinderheilkd. 1937;68:212.

242. Grottum KA, Hovig T, Holmsen H, et al. Wiskott-Aldrich syndrome: qualitative platelet defects and short platelet survival. Br J Haematol. 1969;17:373-388.

243. Ochs HD. The Wiskott-Aldrich syndrome. Clin Rev Allergy Immunol. 2001;20:61-86.

244. Cooper MD, Chae HP, Lowman JT, et al. Wiskott-Aldrich syndrome. An immunologic deficiency disease involving the afferent limb of immunity. Am J Med. 1968;44:499-513.

245. Prchal JT, Carroll AJ, Prchal JF, et al. Wiskott-Aldrich syndrome: cellular impairments and their implication for carrier detection. Blood. 1980;56:1048-1054.

246. Srivastava A, Swaid HA, Kabra M, Verma IC. Management of Wiskott-Aldrich syndrome. Indian J Pediatr. 1996;63:709-712.

247. Kobayashi R, Ariga T, Nonoyama S, et al. Outcome in patients with Wiskott-Aldrich syndrome following stem cell transplantation: an analysis of 57 patients in Japan. Br J Haematol. 2006;135:362-366.

248. Derry JM, Ochs HD, Francke U. Isolation of a novel gene mutated in Wiskott-Aldrich syndrome. Cell. 1994;78:635-644.

249. Kolluri R, Tolias KF, Carpenter CL, et al. Direct interaction of the Wiskott-Aldrich syndrome protein with the GTPase Cdc42. Proc Natl Acad Sci U S A. 1996;93:5615-5618.

250. Symons M, Derry JM, Karlak B, et al. Wiskott-Aldrich syndrome protein, a novel effector for the GTPase CDC42Hs, is implicated in actin polymerization. Cell. 1996;84:723-734.

251. Wu Y, Spencer SD, Lasky LA. Tyrosine phosphorylation regulates the SH3-mediated binding of the Wiskott-Aldrich syndrome protein to PSTPIP, a cytoskeletal-associated protein. J Biol Chem. 1998;273:5765-5770.

252. de la Fuente MA, Sasahara Y, Calamito M, et al. WIP is a chaperone for Wiskott-Aldrich syndrome protein (WASP). Proc Natl Acad Sci U S A. 2007;104:926-931.

253. Miki H, Nonoyama S, Zhu Q, et al. Tyrosine kinase signaling regulates Wiskott-Aldrich syndrome protein function, which is essential for megakaryocyte differentiation. Cell Growth Differ. 1997;8:195-202.

254. Ochs HD, Notarangelo LD. Structure and function of the Wiskott-Aldrich syndrome protein. Curr Opin Hematol. 2005;12:284-291.

255. Wassmuth DR, Hamilton HE, Sheets RF. May-Hegglin anomaly. Hereditary affection of granulocytes and platelets. JAMA. 1963;183:737-740.

256. Seri M, Pecci A, Di Bari F, et al. MYH9-related disease: May-Hegglin anomaly, Sebastian syndrome, Fechtner syndrome, and Epstein syndrome are not distinct entities but represent a variable expression of a single illness. Medicine (Baltimore). 2003;82:203-215.

257. Tsurusawa M, Mamiya S. What is the difference between May-Hegglin anomaly and Sebastian platelet syndrome? Int J Hematol. 2000;71:400-401.

258. Epstein CJ, Sahud MA, Piel CF, et al. Hereditary macrothrombocytopathia, nephritis and deafness. Am J Med. 1972;52:299-310.

259. Peterson LC, Rao KV, Crosson JT, White JG. Fechtner syndrome—a variant of Alport's syndrome with leukocyte inclusions and macrothrombocytopenia. Blood. 1985;65:397-406.

260. Kunishima S, Kojima T, Matsushita T, et al. Mutations in the NMMHC-A gene cause autosomal dominant macrothrombocytopenia with leukocyte inclusions (May-Hegglin anomaly/Sebastian syndrome). Blood. 2001;97:1147-1149.

261. Milton JG, Frojmovic MM. Shape-changing agents produce abnormally large platelets in a hereditary "giant platelets syndrome (MPS)." J Lab Clin Med. 1979;93:154-161.

262. Okita JR, Frojmovic MM, Kristopeit S, et al. Montreal platelet syndrome: a defect in calcium-activated neutral proteinase (calpain). Blood. 1989;74:715-721.

30

Hemophilia and von Willebrand Disease

Robert R. Montgomery, Joan Cox Gill, and Jorge Di Paola

The clinical and laboratory features of the three most common hereditary bleeding disorders—hemophilia A (factor VIII deficiency), hemophilia B (factor IX deficiency), and von Willebrand disease (VWD)—are discussed in this chapter. Hemophilia A and hemophilia B are both caused by a functional deficiency of a plasma protein inherited in an X-linked manner. Because these two proteins, factor VIII and factor IX, form the complex that subsequently activates factor X, the clinical features and many of the diagnostic considerations for hemophilia A and B are similar. Thus, these two types of hemophilia are discussed together, although the treatment of each is presented separately. Factor XI deficiency, sometimes referred to as hemophilia C, is discussed in Chapter 31 because its clinical manifestations are markedly different from those of hemophilia A and hemophilia B. The last part of this chapter is devoted to VWD, which is the most common, albeit usually less symptomatic bleeding disorder. Because von Willebrand factor (VWF) and factor VIII exist as a circulating noncovalent complex in plasma, historically they copurified during plasma fractionation. Thus, for many years, severe VWD and hemophilia A were treated with the same plasma-derived therapeutic products. As the therapeutic product to treat hemophilia A became more pure, factor VIII was subfractionated away from its carrier protein VWF, thereby making high-purity factor VIII products unsatisfactory for the treatment of VWD. The most commonly used products to treat hemophilia A contain recombinant factor VIII and do not contain VWF. To treat severe VWD, intermediate-purity plasma-derived concentrate containing both VWF and factor VIII or, in some regions of the world, purified plasma-derived VWF concentrates are available to treat deficiency of VWF when replacement therapy is indicated. In the not too distant future, recombinant VWF will probably be available, but its formulation, either with or without factor VIII, is not yet known.

HEMOPHILIA A AND HEMOPHILIA B

Hemophilia A and hemophilia B are the most common severe inherited bleeding disorders. Historically, hemophilia has been recognized as an entity since biblical times.[1] Use of the term *hemophilia* was ascribed to Schönlein in the 1820s.[2] Progressive insight into the pathophysiologic course of the disease has led to the development of powerful tools for diagnosis and agents for improved therapy, as well as the need to minimize the primary and secondary complications of the disease and its therapy.[3] The prolonged clotting time of hemophilic blood was first noted in 1893,[4] and the associated decrease in factor VIII levels in hemophilia A was initially identified in 1947.[5,6] In 1952, levels of factor IX were found to be decreased in *Christmas disease*, which was the early term used to denote hemophilia B.[7]

Early therapy for hemophilia was primarily supportive, but after the observation in the 1930s that adminis-

tration of plasma corrected the clotting time of hemophilic blood, treatment evolved to include transfusion with whole blood and plasma to achieve improved clotting function.[8,9] The modern era of treatment began in 1964 with the discovery of cryoprecipitate[9] and plasma fractions containing factor IX[10] and their use to treat bleeding episodes in hemophilia. More purified products were introduced in 1965 and were referred to as factor VIII concentrates (containing both factor VIII and VWF).[11,12] The next major improvements in replacement therapy were the result of attempts to limit transfusion-related viral infections during the 1980s, which included improved donor selection, heat treatment of the product, and further refined purification schemes.[13-15]

In 1985 the genes for both factor VIII and factor IX were cloned,[16-19] and in 1989, recombinant factor VIII was first used clinically.[20,21] In recent years, more highly purified factor IX and recombinant factor IX products have been developed. With the advent of recombinant products, patients with hemophilia could more readily and safely be treated with primary[22-26] and secondary prophylactic therapy.[27] Such vigorous treatment programs markedly reduce the likelihood of spontaneous bleeding episodes and the progression of hemophilic arthropathy. Although much attention today is focused on gene therapy as a potential, efficient means of preventing a bleeding episode without the need for regular prophylactic therapy, there have been no major successes. Thus, prophylaxis continues to be the preferred approach to patients with severe hemophilia.

Pathophysiology

The structure and function of factors VIII and IX in the coagulation pathway were outlined in Chapter 26. Both factors are crucial for normal thrombin generation. The classic representation of hemostasis shows factor VII together with tissue factor activating factor X; however, recent studies suggest that the primary physiologic pathway of activation of factor X by tissue factor and factor VII is through the activation of factor IX.[28,29] Activated factor IX complexes with factor VIIIa, calcium, and phosphatidylserine on physiologic membranes to generate factor Xa, which subsequently participates in formation of the prothrombinase complex. Thus, physiologically, the tissue factor pathway of factor X activation requires factor VIII and factor IX for normal thrombin generation, and the absence of either protein severely impairs the ability to generate thrombin and fibrin. This absence is not identified by use of the classic prothrombin time; the prothrombin time is normal in patients with hemophilia A or hemophilia B.

After injury, the initial hemostatic event is formation of a platelet plug, and the subsequent generation of fibrin is crucial to prevent continued oozing. Because of the primary clotting factor deficiency in either hemophilia A or hemophilia B, clot formation is delayed and is not robust. Thus, patients with hemophilia do not bleed more rapidly; rather, there is delayed formation of an abnormal clot.[30] Thrombin is crucial for platelet aggregation, fibrin generation, clot retraction, and activation of factor XIII. Because thrombin generation in hemophilia is markedly delayed, hemorrhage may occur after minimal or unknown trauma. Deep bleeding into joints and muscles is characteristic of hemophilia. When bleeding occurs in a closed space such as a joint and is untreated, it ceases by tamponade, whereas open wounds in which tamponade cannot occur may bleed profusely with the potential for significant blood loss. In hemophilia, the clot formed is often friable, and rebleeding is a common observation in inadequately treated patients. Medications such as aspirin may alter platelet function and further impair hemostasis in affected individuals and are therefore contraindicated.[31]

Demographics and Classification

Hemophilia occurs in approximately 1 in 5000 males.[32-34] Of all patients with hemophilia, 80% to 85% have hemophilia A, and 10% to 15% have hemophilia B. Hemophilia shows no apparent racial predilection and appears in all ethnic groups.

The severity of hemophilia is classified on the basis of the patient's baseline level of factor VIII or factor IX. One unit of each factor is defined as the amount found in 1 mL of normal plasma. Factor levels are often expressed as a percentage of activity, with a 100% level (100 U/dL) being equal to the activity found in 1 mL of normal plasma. Severe hemophilia is characterized by a factor level of less than 1 U/dL (<1%). In moderate hemophilia, the clotting factor level is between 1 and 5 U/dL, and in mild hemophilia, factor VIII or IX levels are greater than 5 U/dL. This classification provides a rough guide for the patient's expected rate of occurrence of bleeding episodes. Patients with severe hemophilia often have bleeding episodes after minimal or unknown trauma, with children experiencing unprovoked muscle and joint bleeding between one and six times per month. With more aggressive prophylactic administration of factor VIII, instances of bleeding are markedly reduced. Patients with moderate hemophilia will have bleeding after mild to moderate injuries, whereas mild hemophilia may often be undiagnosed for many years and these patients may have bleeding only after significant trauma or at the time of surgery.

Clinical Manifestations

Approximately 30% of male infants with hemophilia have bleeding with circumcision.[35] In some reports as many as 1% to 2% of neonates with hemophilia may experience an intracranial hemorrhage.[36,37] It is important to avoid head trauma during delivery. Forceps or vacuum extraction should be avoided.[36,38] In the majority of patients hemophilia is diagnosed at birth because of a family history, although in approximately a third of patients the occurrence of hemophilia represents a new mutation.[39]

In these latter patients, the diagnosis is often made when the child begins to crawl and walk. The usual initial symptoms include easy bruising; oral bleeding, especially from a torn frenulum; hemarthrosis; and intramuscular hemorrhage. When the diagnosis of hemophilia is suspected on the basis of either clinical findings or a positive family history, the initial diagnostic studies should include determination of the prothrombin time, partial thromboplastin time (PTT), bleeding time, and fibrinogen or thrombin time; a platelet count; and studies to identify VWD (see Chapter 28). If the PTT is prolonged, assays for factor VIII and factor IX should be performed. The presence of an antibody inhibiting either factor VIII or IX can be ruled out by mixing normal plasma in equal volume with the test plasma, incubating the mixture for 30 to 60 minutes, and repeating the PTT to be sure that it has been normalized. The specific assays for factor VIII and factor IX are not as easily affected by difficult venipuncture and are therefore more reliable. Factor VIII and VWF levels may be elevated by stress and inflammation, however, and repeated studies may be necessary to establish the diagnosis and the severity of the disorder.

Specific types of bleeding are described in the following paragraphs. In general, the clinical bleeding episodes associated with deficiency of factor VIII or factor IX are identical.

Musculoskeletal Bleeding

Although patients with hemophilia may bleed in any area of the body, the hallmark of hemophilia is deep bleeding into joints and muscles.[40] The occurrence of such hemorrhage usually corresponds to the severity of the clotting factor deficiency in patients with either hemophilia A or hemophilia B. Patients with severe hemophilia may have a bleeding episode as often as once or twice per week. Bleeding occurs most commonly into the joint space, a condition referred to as *hemarthrosis*. These joint hemorrhages usually begin when the child reaches the toddler age. As the toddler attempts to maintain an upright position, the ankle becomes particularly prone to hemorrhage. Thus, in toddlers the ankle is the most common site of hemorrhage, with the knee being the second most common. As the child grows older, the most frequent bleeding sites are the knees and elbows.

Patients who sustain hemarthrosis usually first note an aura of tingling or warmth, followed shortly thereafter by increasing pain and decreased range of motion of the joint as the joint capsule becomes progressively distended.[41-43] As children get older, they are often able to tell their parents and the physician when a hemorrhage is beginning to occur, even in the absence of significant signs on physical examination. In young children who are unable to verbalize symptoms, severe pain and distention of the joint space often occur before the location of the hemorrhage can be easily determined. On examination, pain and limitation of range of motion of the joint are obvious and followed by the development of warmth, swelling, and tenderness. Prompt, early coagulation factor replacement therapy is the key to minimizing long-term complications of these hemorrhages. Patients with severe hemophilia are increasingly being treated prophylactically to prevent most bleeding episodes (see later). Prompt aspiration of hip hemarthrosis should be performed if joint distention is present to reduce the risk for avascular necrosis of the femoral head. As children and their parents become familiar with the early symptoms of bleeding, aggressive early treatment can be given to reduce the degree of joint damage. If the child experiences repeated hemorrhage within a joint, chronic effusion and hyperemia often occur, and an aggressive secondary prophylactic therapy program may be needed to return the joint to a more normal state of recovery.[27] Severe chronic arthropathy may develop in older children and adults who have not received aggressive early treatment. These individuals often experience pain very early with little swelling. The joints of younger children are usually more distensible, and massive joint swelling may be observed. Splinting and application of ice packs as auxiliary measures may provide a modicum of relief but are not substitutes for early coagulation factor replacement therapy. When one has doubts, treatment should be initiated; it is not appropriate to watch and wait.

The clinical diagnosis of intramuscular hematoma is often elusive. Such hemorrhage occurs deep within the body of the muscle and is associated with a vague feeling of pain on motion. Because the bleeding is not in a closed space, the mass may be difficult to palpate, although the circumference of the affected limb is generally increased. Muscle hemorrhage should be considered to be as severe as hemarthrosis because it may result in severe muscular contractures as a result of fibrosis and atrophy or even pseudotumor formation. Muscle weakness also predisposes patients to joint hemorrhage. Appropriate replacement therapy is critical for reducing the size of the hematoma, and physical therapy is important to restore normal range of motion and prevent fibrosis of the muscle.

Iliopsoas bleeding is a particularly troublesome form of intramuscular hemorrhage. A patient with an iliopsoas hemorrhage is generally seen with vague symptoms of lower abdominal or upper thigh discomfort. The patient may have a characteristic gait; the hip is flexed and inwardly rotated. On examination the patient is unable to extend the hip, but usually both internal and external rotation of the hip joint is normal; the latter finding often distinguishes an iliopsoas hemorrhage from a true hemarthrosis of the hip joint. The diagnosis is made clinically by these findings and should be confirmed by either ultrasonography or computed tomography.[44] Appropriate treatment is crucial; iliopsoas hemorrhages may be life threatening because large volumes of blood can be lost into the retroperitoneal space. Physical examination demonstrates loss of hyperextension of the hip. If an iliopsoas hemorrhage is identified, an aggressive infusion program should be initiated and maintained for at least

10 to 14 days or longer, followed by at least several months of prophylactic therapy until clinical and radiographic evidence demonstrates resolution.

Life-Threatening Hemorrhages

Bleeding episodes of the central nervous system (CNS), bleeding into and around the airway, and exsanguinating hemorrhage are the most common causes of life-threatening hemorrhage in hemophilia. The first element of treatment is prompt therapy with clotting factor concentrate to bring the plasma clotting factor level to normal. CNS hemorrhage may occur without known trauma, and early symptoms may be minimal. Thus, therapy should be initiated before radiologic evaluation or lumbar puncture. Rarely, an infant who has bloody cerebrospinal fluid on lumbar puncture is seen with "meningitis." If this is the initial finding, a markedly prolonged PTT will usually suggest the diagnosis.[45-47] Prompt performance of computed tomography is often critical in the early diagnosis of intracranial bleeding, although an astonishingly large volume of blood can be present within the cranium in infants with relatively few neurologic findings. Treatment of life-threatening hemorrhage involves replacement therapy to achieve a level of 100 U/dL for factor VIII and 80 U/dL for factor IX, maintenance of adequate hemostatic levels (>50 to 60 U/dL) for a minimum of 14 days, and a more prolonged period of prophylactic therapy for an additional 2 to 3 weeks or longer to ensure resolution of the underlying event (Table 30-1). Patients with intracranial hemorrhage should receive prophylaxis for at least 6 months after the more intense initial therapy.

Preparation for Surgery

Preparation of a hemophilic patient for surgery includes a careful history and physical examination, measurement of inhibitor titer, careful determination of the incremental recovery and half-life after infusion of the appropriate clotting factor (VIII or IX), and assurance that adequate amounts of coagulation factor replacement material and red cells are available for transfusion.[48] Before surgery, the replacement materials should be infused to achieve a level of 80 to 100 U/dL for factor IX and 100 to 150 U/dL for factor VIII; levels should be maintained at greater than 50 to 60 U/dL for 7 to 10 days postoperatively. Lower doses to maintain levels at greater than 20 to 30 U/dL for an additional 1 to 2 weeks may then be used and continued until healing has occurred (see Table 30-1). Because recovery of recombinant factor IX activity is less than that of therapeutic plasma-derived factor IX, 1.2 to 1.5 times the dose should be administered if using recombinant factor IX.[49,50]

Miscellaneous Hemorrhages

A common manifestation of hemophilia is oral bleeding, whether from a torn frenulum in a young child or after

TABLE 30-1 Treatment of Specific Hemorrhages in Hemophilia

Type of Hemorrhage	Hemophilia A	Hemophilia B*
Hemarthrosis†	*50 U/kg* factor VIII concentrate initially,‡ 20 U/kg the following day; consider additional treatment every other day, depending on response	*80 U/kg* factor IX concentrate initially, 40 U/kg the following day; consider additional treatment every other day, depending on response
Muscle or significant subcutaneous hematoma	*50 U/kg* factor VIII concentrate; may need 20 U/kg every other day until well resolved	*80 U/kg* factor IX concentrate; may need 40 U/kg every other day until well resolved
Mouth, deciduous tooth, or tooth extraction	*20 U/kg* factor VIII concentrate (40 U/kg if molar extraction), antifibrinolytic therapy; remove loose deciduous tooth	*40 U/kg* factor IX concentrate (80 U/kg if molar extraction), antifibrinolytic therapy; remove loose deciduous tooth
Epistaxis	*Apply pressure* for 15-20 min, Nosebleed QR, pack with petrolatum gauze, antifibrinolytic therapy; 20 U/kg factor VIII concentrate if above fails	*Apply pressure* for 15-20 min, Nosebleed QR, pack with petrolatum gauze, antifibrinolytic therapy§; 30 U/kg factor IX concentrate if above fails
Major surgery, life-threatening hemorrhage (e.g., central nervous system, gastrointestinal, airway)	*50-75 U/kg* factor VIII concentrate, then initiate continuous infusion of 3 U/kg/hr to maintain factor VIIII > 100 U/dL for 24 hr, and then give 2-3 U/kg/hr for 5-7 days to maintain the level greater than 50 U/dL and an additional 5-7 days at a level >30 U/dL (bolus dosing to maintain these levels is acceptable); monitor factor VIII levels	*80-100 U/kg* factor IX concentrate, then 20-40 U/kg every 12-24 hr to maintain factor IX > 40 U/dL for 5-7 days, and then >30 U/dL for 5-7 days‖; monitor factor IX levels
Iliopsoas hemorrhage	*50 U/kg* factor VIII concentrate, then 25 U/kg every 12 hr until asymptomatic, and then 20 U/kg every other day for a total of 10-14 days¶	*80 U/kg* factor IX concentrate, then 20-40 U/kg every 12-24 hr to maintain factor IX > 40 IU/dL until asymptomatic, and then 30 U/kg every other day for a total of 10-14 days‖,¶
Hematuria	*Bed rest*, 1.5 × maintenance fluids; if not controlled in 1-2 days, 20 U/kg factor VIII concentrate; if not controlled, prednisone if human immunodeficiency virus negative	*Bed rest*, 1.5 × maintenance fluids; if not controlled in 1-2 days, 30 U/kg factor IX concentrate; if not controlled, prednisone if human immunodeficiency virus negative

*Dosing of recombinant factor IX should be increased to 1.3 to 1.5 times the recommended doses or, preferably, be based on an individual in vivo recovery study.

†For hip hemarthrosis, orthopedic evaluation for possible aspiration is advisable.

‡For mild or moderate hemophilia, desmopressin, 0.3 µg/kg, should be used instead of factor VIII concentrate if patient is known to respond with a hemostatic level of factor VIII; if repeated doses are given, monitor factor VIII levels for tachyphylaxis.

§Do not give antifibrinolytic therapy until 4 to 6 hours after a dose of prothrombin complex concentrate.

‖If repeated doses of factor IX concentrate are required, use highly purified, specific factor IX concentrate.

¶Repeat radiologic assessment should be performed before discontinuation of therapy.

tooth extraction in an older patient. Replacement therapy to achieve a factor level of 30 to 40 U/dL is adequate for initial therapy. Because the oral cavity contains abundant fibrinolytic activity, therapy with antifibrinolytic agents (aminocaproic acid [Amicar] or tranexamic acid [Cyklokapron]) is useful to stabilize the clot until the wound has healed.[51-53]

Hematuria can be a particularly troublesome problem. Blood in the urine may arise spontaneously, and determination of an actual bleeding site is often difficult. Therapy is also controversial. Replacement therapy with 40 to 50 U/kg of factor VIII or IX followed by bed rest is generally advisable after other common causes of hematuria have been ruled out. Treatment with corticosteroids may be helpful.[54] Sudden abdominal or flank pain should be investigated for the possibility of ureteral obstruction and hydronephrosis secondary to bleeding.

Gastrointestinal bleeding is an occasional complication of hemophilia. All of the common causes of gastrointestinal bleeding can occur in patients with hemophilia, as well as spontaneous hemorrhage after no known insult. An initial episode of gastrointestinal hemorrhage requires that the patient receive a thorough gastrointestinal evaluation after the acute bleeding is controlled with replacement therapy. If substantial blood loss has occurred, patients should be treated with high doses of concentrate as though they were at risk for life-threatening hemorrhage.

Long-Term Complications of Joint Bleeding

Chronic arthropathy is the major long-term disabling complication of hemophilia. The articular surface of a normal joint is lined with cartilage that is lubricated by synovial fluid produced by the synovial lining of the joint. A thick fibrous capsule protects the joint. The natural history of hemophilic arthropathy is one of a cycle of recurrent hemorrhage into a "target" joint leading to synovial thickening and friability, followed by additional hemorrhage into the joint.[41,42,55] After a joint hemorrhage, proteolytic enzymes are released by granulocytes into the joint space.[56] In addition, heme iron is ingested by macrophages and may contribute to inflammation by the release of oxidative products. The synovium of the joint, originally the width of a single cell, proliferates in response to inflammation and develops frond-like projections into the joint. These projections are by nature friable and bleed with minimal trauma, thus setting up a vicious cycle of recurrent hemorrhage. With recurrence of hemorrhage, there is further release of substances injurious to the joint cartilage that causes it to develop a roughened, lunar landscape–like surface. As the cartilage erodes, the joint space becomes narrowed.

On examination, the clinical findings depend on the stage of arthropathy that has developed. The early stages are characterized by synovial thickening with little evidence of joint damage. With synovitis alone, the range of motion of the joint is nearly normal, although recurrent bleeding episodes usually result in weakness of the proximal muscles. With time, however, proliferative changes become associated with erosion of the cartilage. The patient at this stage may note the development of arthritic symptoms that are often difficult to distinguish from joint bleeding. Crepitus and decreased range of motion are prominent findings on physical examination. At this stage, proximal muscle weakness is accentuated because of inability of the joint to attain full range of motion. Finally, with progressive bleeding and further narrowing of the joint space, the joint fuses.

This progression of joint disease was once commonly seen in hemophilia centers throughout the United States and other countries. The most commonly affected joints were the knees, ankles, and elbows. With the development of modern concentrates for replacement therapy, home therapy, and prophylactic therapy, this cycle has now been disrupted in the vast majority of children with severe hemophilia. Primary prophylactic therapy and early diagnosis and treatment of joint hemorrhage have limited the number of "target joints" that develop. When a joint becomes a target, hemorrhage into that joint must be treated vigorously and the joint must be carefully watched for the cycle of rebleeding every 1 to 2 weeks that is characteristic of incompletely treated hemarthrosis. If evidence of early synovitis or loss of range of motion is present, a secondary prophylactic therapy program of every-other-day treatment for 30 to 90 days is often helpful for "cooling down" the affected joint and allowing healing to occur.[27,57] Alternatively, a lifelong prophylactic therapy program to prevent spontaneous, severe joint bleeding may be started in young infants (see later). If medical therapy fails, synovectomy frequently reduces the occurrence of bleeding and may prevent progression of the joint disease. With the advent of arthroscopic means to perform synovectomy, this procedure has been more readily performed with reduced morbidity; equally important, early mobilization of the affected joint allows more rapid return of range of motion.[58,59] Another procedure in which various radioisotopes are used to reduce the mass of inflamed synovium is termed *radioactive synovectomy.*[60] This approach is recommended for patients with inhibitors. Fewer radioactive synovectomies are now performed because of the development of acute lymphoblastic leukemia in two children who underwent this procedure.[61] When aggressive medical and "less" invasive surgical management fails to halt progression of the joint disease, some adults have benefited from joint replacement.[62-64] If pain and bleeding are severe in a joint with minimal range of motion, joint fusion may provide a significant decrease in pain and rebleeding. A critical element in the care of patients with chronic joint disease is the need for a team approach to the problem because the care of these children requires the combined expertise of an orthopedic surgeon, physical therapist, nurse, social worker, and hematologist to achieve optimal results.

Symptomatic Carriers

Although the usual patient with hemophilia A or hemophilia B is a male, carriers of a factor VIII gene mutation may also be symptomatic. Known carriers should have their levels of clotting factor measured at least once to determine whether they are at increased risk for clinical bleeding episodes. There are several potential explanations for the observation of a female with moderate or severe deficiency of factor VIII or factor IX.[65-68] Skewed lyonization of a carrier female is the most commonly accepted explanation. As predicted by the Lyon hypothesis, the X chromosome in each female cell is randomly inactivated early in embryonic development; by chance, some carriers of hemophilia will have a high percentage of inactivated normal X chromosomes. The active abnormal X chromosome will result in deficient synthesis of factor VIII or factor IX. Other explanations for the presence of hemophilia A or B in a phenotypic female include testicular feminization of a genotypic male,[69,70] Turner's syndrome with the genotype XO,[71-73] and a daughter of a maternal carrier and a father with hemophilia A. Factor VIII deficiency is also found in type 2N VWD as a result of mutations in the factor VIII–binding region of the VWF protein.[74]

Laboratory Evaluation

Severe hemophilia A or hemophilia B is easily identified by a markedly prolonged PTT and the absence of either factor VIII or factor IX. The diagnosis of mild hemophilia A or hemophilia B may be more difficult to make because the newborn has a slightly prolonged PTT secondary to a physiologic reduction in vitamin K–dependent factors such as factor IX. In addition, the stress of delivery and other neonatal problems may transiently elevate factor VIII levels into the normal or nearly normal range. Thus, in the absence of clinical bleeding, mild deficiencies may be identified only after repeated testing in the weeks or months after birth (see Chapter 28). VWF testing must be done to distinguish mild or moderate factor VIII deficiency secondary to hemophilia from deficiencies of factor VIII secondary to VWD.

Partial Thromboplastin Time

The PTT measures all of the procoagulant clotting factors except factor VII and factor XIII (see Chapters 26 and 28). In general, the PTT is most sensitive for deficiencies of the "intrinsic" pathway.[75] Deficiencies of factor XII, prekallikrein, and high-molecular-weight kininogen give the longest clotting times, although paradoxically, these deficiencies are not associated with clinical bleeding episodes. In general, commercial PTT reagents have good sensitivity for factor VIII deficiency, but their sensitivity for factor IX deficiency is more variable.[76-78] Use of some of these reagents will give normal PTTs even with factor IX levels of 15 to 20 U/dL. Because the hemostatic level of factor IX is approximately 30 U/dL, mild or moderate factor IX deficiency may be missed. Thus, if hemophilia is suspected, a factor IX assay should be performed even if the PTT is normal. The clinical laboratory should study the sensitivity of each lot of PTT reagent to be able to advise the clinician about the likelihood that a normal PTT implies normal clotting factor levels. In patients with severe hemophilia A or hemophilia B, the PTT is generally prolonged to two to three times the upper limit of the normal range. The prolonged PTT will correct to within the normal range when the reagent is mixed 1:1 with normal plasma. Failure of the PTT to correct on 1:1 mixing of the reagent with normal plasma implies the presence of an anticoagulant (e.g., lupus inhibitor, antibody to factor VIII or IX, or heparin). The presence of a specific anti–factor VIII or anti–factor IX inhibitory antibody is described in more detail later.

Specific Assays for Factor VIII and Factor IX

Functional assays for factor VIII and factor IX are performed on plasma samples that contain no factor VIII or factor IX, respectively (either hemophilia A or hemophilia B plasma); alternatively, normal plasma from which the respective clotting factor is selectively removed by a monoclonal antibody can be used.[79] If adsorbed plasma is used for factor VIII–deficient plasma, the VWF content of that plasma should be normal. A standard curve is constructed with the use of normal plasma, with the 100% point being a 1:10 dilution of normal plasma. Serial dilutions of this normal plasma should usually be linear through a dilution of 1:640 or 1:1280 when plotted semilogarithmically versus the clotting time. Serial dilutions of the patient's plasma are compared with this normal curve and expressed in units per deciliter.

One unit is the amount of factor VIII or factor IX present in 1 mL of normal plasma.

Immunoassays for factor VIII and factor IX are sometimes performed to identify dysfunctional proteins or dysproteinemias. The majority of patients with severe hemophilia A have undetectable levels of factor VIII protein, but some patients with mild or moderate hemophilia A possess levels of factor VIII protein that are detectable with an immunoassay.[80-82] In hemophilia B, about 50% of patients will have detectable or even normal levels of factor IX antigen and therefore have true dysproteinemias.[83,84] Immunoassays are not usually required for the clinical management of these disorders because the coagulant-based assays predict the functional concentration of these clotting factors.

Inhibitory Antibodies to Factor VIII or Factor IX

The presence of a factor VIII or factor IX inhibitory antibody is usually suspected when the PTT does not correct to normal after being mixed 1:1 with normal plasma. Because of the kinetics of the inhibitory antibody, this mixture should be incubated 60 minutes before the PTT is performed. When a low-titer inhibitory antibody is identified, the PTT performed on a 1:1 mixture with normal plasma may initially be prolonged only by several seconds, but when the mixture is incubated for 1 hour, the PTT may be as long as or even longer than the PTT when it was originally performed on the patient's plasma.

Specific assays for factor VIII or factor IX antibodies are performed with the Bethesda assay. Dilutions of the test plasma are mixed with normal plasma and incubated for 120 minutes. A standard factor VIII or factor IX assay is then performed. One Bethesda unit is defined as the amount of antibody that will inactivate 50% of the normal factor VIII or factor IX in 2 hours when the residual factor VIII or factor IX level is between 25 and 75 U/dL.[85] The dilution of the test plasma that inhibits this amount of factor VIII is determined. If a 1:10 dilution of test plasma has this effect, the inhibitor plasma is said to contain 10 Bethesda units.

Genetic Testing

The genes for both factor VIII and factor IX are located near the terminus of the long arm of the X chromosome.[86-89] Therefore, both hemophilia A and B are inherited as X-linked traits. Genetic testing for hemophilia A and hemophilia B is now widely available.[86-88,90-92] Such testing is usually performed on the propositus and potential carriers of hemophilia. Prenatal testing for hemophilia is performed by amniocentesis or chorionic villus biopsy[90] and may be useful for the perinatologist and neonatologist in the management of pregnancy, delivery, and immediate neonatal care. Databases of the known mutations causing hemophilia A are available on the Internet (http://europium.csc.mrc.ac.uk/WebPages/Main/main.htm). The most common genetic alteration is inversion. Gene inversion occurs in approximately 45% of patients with severe hemophilia A, with most inversions originating in male germ cells. In families in which the propositus has a known molecular abnormality, genetic screening and carrier detection are highly accurate. Direct DNA sequence analysis is available for families in which the results of testing for the factor VIII gene inversion are negative. If genetic testing is uninformative, a coagulation-based assay to detect the carrier state may be also useful[93,94] and is approximately 90% accurate.

In contrast to the complexity of the factor VIII gene, the factor IX gene is considerably smaller (≈33 versus 187 kilobases [kb]). More than 60% of factor IX gene defects are due to missense point mutations, and an identifiable defect in the gene can be found in nearly all patients[95] (http://www.kcl.ac.uk/ip/petergreen/haemBdatabase.html). In approximately 50% of patients with hemophilia B, a factor IX protein that is nonfunctional is produced, whereas in the other patients no factor IX protein is produced.

Other Laboratory Studies

Laboratory evaluation of a patient with hemophilia also includes a search for transfusion-transmissible diseases and their secondary complications, such as hepatitis and liver disease (see Chapter 34).

Fundamentals of Treatment

Knowledge of the half-life, volume of distribution, patient's inhibitor status, and appropriate replacement material is necessary to make intelligent decisions for the treatment of bleeding episodes.[96-98] Prompt and appropriate treatment of hemorrhage and prophylactic therapy are the key to excellent care of patients with hemophilia. The use of home therapy and prophylactic therapy has revolutionized the care of children and adults with hemophilia. Early or prophylactic treatment prevents the long-term morbidity of hemophilia. For mild to moderate hemorrhage, it is necessary that factor VIII levels of 30 to 50 U/dL or factor IX levels of 30 U/dL be achieved.

For patients with mild hemophilia A who have previously shown a satisfactory response to desmopressin acetate (DDAVP, 1-deamino-8-D-arginine vasopressin), this drug is the treatment of choice for bleeding episodes of mild to moderate severity.[99-101] For life-threatening hemorrhage, the immediate aim is to correct the patient's clotting factor level to normal (100 to 150 U/dL) and to maintain a nadir level between 50 and 60 U/dL for 5 to 7 days, followed by a vigorous maintenance treatment program.

Table 30-1 summarizes the treatment of specific types of hemorrhage in hemophilia A and hemophilia B. Calculation of the dose, recommendations concerning prophylaxis, and the specific treatment products for hemophilia A and hemophilia B are reviewed later.

Hemophilia A

Calculation of Dose

Calculation of the dose required to achieve a desired hemostatic level is based on a convenient formula derived from the work of Abildgaard and colleagues[11]:

$$\text{Dose factor VIII (units)} = \text{U/dL desired rise in plasma factor VIII} \times \text{Body weight (kg)} \times 0.5$$

Thus, for treatment of hemarthrosis in a 20-kg child with severe hemophilia A, to achieve a plasma level of 60 U/dL, the dose would be 60 U/dL × 20 kg × 0.5 = 600 units of factor VIII.

For patients undergoing major surgery or with serious hemorrhage, the plasma factor VIII level should be initially corrected to 100 to 150 U/dL (immediately before the procedure if given for surgery) and maintained at greater than 50 to 60 U/dL for 5 to 7 days and then at greater than 30 U/dL for an additional 5 to 7 days. This can be accomplished by infusion of intermittent doses of factor VIII based on a half-life of 12 hours (e.g., administration of 30 U/kg [60-U/dL correction] every 12 hours).

Alternatively, a level of 50 to 60 U/dL can be maintained by continuous infusion of factor VIII at a rate of 2 to 3 U/kg/hr.[102,103] The level of factor VIII should be monitored periodically to ensure that the expected levels are attained. Immediately after surgery, it is advisable to administer 25 U/kg of factor VIII concentrate to compensate for the loss of factor VIII by increased consumption and blood loss during the surgical procedure. For surgical procedures and limb- or life-threatening hemorrhage, factor VIII levels should be monitored at least every 24 hours. CNS bleeding should be treated for a 2- to 3-week course of therapy. Such patients have a risk of recurrence of CNS bleeding for approximately 6 months after an episode, and these patients often continue to receive prophylactic therapy. At the conclusion of therapy for CNS hemorrhage, computed tomography should be performed to provide a baseline scan for comparison if any subsequent CNS symptoms appear and to demonstrate resolution of the previous hemorrhage.

For treatment of more routine bleeding episodes, such as hemarthrosis, often only one to two doses of clotting factor replacement (plasma factor VIII level of 80 to 100 U/dL), initially followed by infusions as recommended in Table 30-1, are required to produce significant clinical improvement. Nevertheless, many centers are now using a more aggressive approach to managing severe joint hemorrhage by administering follow-up infusions daily until the signs and symptoms have resolved and then every other day for 7 to 10 days to limit the potential development of chronic joint disease.

For dental extractions, mouth lacerations, or recurrent epistaxis, adjuvant antifibrinolytic therapy is used (see later).

Prophylactic Factor VIII Therapy

Prophylactic therapy with plasma-derived factor VIII was not previously considered for all patients because of the cost, the limited amount of plasma and blood products donated by volunteer donors, and the inherent risk of transfusion-transmitted diseases. However, most centers are now routinely giving individuals factor VIII prophylactic replacement therapy with recombinant factor VIII.[27,104,105] Most centers initiate prophylactic therapy as soon as joint bleeding occurs. This therapy is usually administered through a subcutaneous access port after the insertion of a central venous line.[106,107] Insertion of such lines is often associated with catheter infections or thrombosis (or both), so patients and family members need to be aware of the signs and symptoms.[107] In general, a dose of 20 to 40 U/kg of factor VIII is administered every other day or three times a week. The dose and rate are adjusted to ensure that the nadir before the next infusion is greater than 1 U/dL. The levels attained by use of this regimen usually prevent spontaneous bleeding, although hemorrhage caused by trauma may still require additional replacement therapy. The goal is to prevent recurrent hemarthrosis and associated chronic hemophilic arthropathy and thereby promote a normal lifestyle. A number of centers throughout the world have initiated prophylactic therapy programs and have demonstrated their cost-effectiveness when productivity and lifestyle are used as indicators of success.[25,108] However, this long-term vision is not always shared by administrators of managed health care systems, and the most successful programs have been carried out in countries with nationalized health care.

Factor VIII Treatment Products

Clotting factor replacement products should be rendered as free as possible of transfusion-transmissible agents, but vigilance is still necessary. As a result, recombinant products are generally considered to be preferable to plasma-derived products. Because even recombinant products may contain human albumin added as a stabilizer, products have recently been developed that contain no human plasma–derived protein.[109,110] The question of which product to use, the rate of administration, and the potential use of prophylaxis are decisions that need to be made by the health care provider, the family, and the patient.

Recombinant Factor VIII Concentrates. The factor VIII gene has been cloned, sequenced, and used to successfully transfect mammalian cells to produce recombinant factor VIII,[111] and several recombinant factor VIII products have been licensed. Clinical trials have documented that the half-life, recovery, and efficacy of these recombinant factor VIII products are similar to those for plasma-derived factor VIII.[20,21] Advantages of these recombinant factor VIII products are their freedom from human viral contamination and their production by methods that do not require human blood or plasma

donors. There was initial concern that there may be an increase in the incidence of inhibitor development in previously untreated patients, but this appears to not be warranted.[112-117] Careful study of patients receiving recombinant products identified inhibitors in 20% to 25%, as opposed to the previously reported 14% prevalence of inhibitors.[118] The difference is now thought to be due to detection of transient inhibitors that subsequently disappear and not due to differences between the immunogenicity of recombinant factor VIII and plasma-derived factor VIII. Recent studies have revived interest in this issue, and a number of studies are re-evaluating whether factor VIII in the presence of VWF might be less immunogenic.[119-122] A recombinant factor VIII product missing the B domain has been licensed, which may require a different approach to laboratory monitoring because its activity differs between one- and two-stage factor VIII assays.[123,124] Recently developed products are formulated so that other human proteins are removed.[109,110]

Plasma-Derived Factor VIII Concentrates. Several commercial plasma-derived factor VIII concentrates are available. Intermediate-purity concentrates are produced from large pools of donor plasma by a combination of cryoprecipitation or precipitation with glycine, polyethylene glycol, or ethanol.[125] These intermediate-purity products contain 2 to 5 units of factor VIII per milligram of protein. Products of higher purity have also been developed and are produced by immunopurification of factor VIII with the use of monoclonal antibodies to factor VIII[126] or VWF.[127] All these products undergo multiple purification steps that involve heat treatment, as well as other modalities, to reduce the risk of viral transmission. As a result, the risk of human immunodeficiency virus (HIV) infection, hepatitis B, hepatitis C, and more recently, transmission of hepatitis A and parvovirus B19 has been markedly reduced or eliminated.[128-130] In the 1990s, one lot of plasma-derived product was found to be associated with a very high frequency of factor VIII inhibitors in patients who had previously been treated extensively with plasma-derived products. This was thought to be due to an alteration in the factor VIII product during fractionation and purification.[120]

With the improved purity of plasma-derived products, the incidence of complications has greatly diminished. Allergic reactions, isohemagglutinin-induced hemolytic anemia, immune complex–mediated hematuria, and granulocyte antibody–induced lung injury are rarely seen. The use of immunoaffinity-purified factor VIII concentrates and recombinant factor VIII concentrates appears to stabilize CD4+ counts in HIV-infected patients with hemophilia.[131,132]

To minimize the risk for hepatitis B and hepatitis A, unimmunized patients should be immunized at the time of diagnosis.[133,134] If clotting factor replacement therapy is needed at the time of diagnosis, hepatitis B immune globulin can be administered along with the first dose of vaccine to maintain passive protection until vaccine-induced antibodies are formed. Family members of patients with hemophilia who are chronic carriers of hepatitis B and those who assist in administration of clotting factor should be immunized as well.

Cryoprecipitate. The first widely used preparation of factor VIII was made by Judith Graham Poole in 1965 by a method called cryoprecipitation.[135] Each bag of cryoprecipitate contains only 100 units of factor VIII, and thus 10 to 20 donor units are required for the treatment of joint hemorrhage in an adult. Because cryoprecipitate lacks any active method of viral inactivation, possesses significant amounts of other human proteins, and is inconvenient to administer, it is no longer considered a viable alternative to purified factor VIII products, except in areas of the world where other forms of therapy are unavailable or in short supply.

Desmopressin. Desmopressin is a synthetic vasopressin analogue that increases plasma factor VIII and VWF levels, thereby allowing successful treatment of bleeding episodes associated with dental and surgical procedures in patients with mild and moderate hemophilia A and VWD.[136,137] Desmopressin is now considered the treatment of choice in patients with mild and moderate hemophilia A who have shown a response to the drug during a therapeutic trial. It is not effective in the treatment of severe hemophilia A, severe VWD, or any form of hemophilia B.

The individual response to desmopressin is varied,[138] with the range of increase in factor VIII level being between 2- and 15-fold over baseline in patients with mild or moderate hemophilia A. It is therefore recommended that patients undergo a therapeutic trial of desmopressin with laboratory measurement of response to factor VIII before it is used for the treatment of bleeding episodes or as prophylactic therapy before dental and other surgical procedures. A similar degree of response is generally seen in an individual patient with subsequent doses,[139] and thus the factor VIII level attained after a trial dose can be used to predict the response to future therapy. The level of response to factor VIII is not usually sufficient to treat life- or limb-threatening hemorrhage. Tachyphylaxis may occur with repeated doses of desmopressin, but this varies from patient to patient.[140] Consequently, if repeated doses of desmopressin are to be administered, factor VIII levels should be monitored, and if necessary, exogenous factor VIII should be administered. In general, if several days has elapsed between doses, a response similar to that for the baseline infusion can be expected. Side effects from the administration of desmopressin are minimal and include headache, flushing, a slight change in pulse rate or blood pressure, and rarely, hyponatremia. Because hyponatremia after the administration of desmopressin may cause a seizure in

rare instances,[141] fluid intake should be restricted to maintenance levels for at least 24 hours. If repeated doses of the drug are given, serum sodium levels should be monitored. Because of rare reports of thrombosis after the use of desmopressin,[142] the drug should be used with caution in patients with an increased risk for thrombosis.

The recommended intravenous dose of desmopressin is 0.3 μg/kg, and it is administered in 25 to 50 mL of normal saline over a period of 20 to 30 minutes.[100,136] If desmopressin is being given before a procedure such as a dental extraction, it should be administered as close to the procedure as possible because the maximal response occurs 30 to 60 minutes after administration. A concentrated form of desmopressin (Stimate) is available for intranasal administration to treat bleeding disorders. This preparation should not be confused with the far less concentrated formulation (brand name DDAVP) that is used to treat enuresis; the latter formulation is ineffective for the treatment of hemophilia and VWD. The appropriate dose of intranasal Stimate is 150 μg (1 puff) for persons weighing less than 50 kg and 300 μg (1 puff in each nostril) for persons weighing more than 50 kg.[143] It is particularly important to document the response to intranasal desmopressin before it is used for the treatment of bleeding.

Antifibrinolytic Therapy

Bleeding from mucosal surfaces in patients with hemophilia is often problematic because of the increased fibrinolytic activity associated with the mucosa. Antifibrinolytic therapy has been found to be effective in controlling mucosal bleeding, especially from the oral mucosa. Although hemostasis is generally achieved with either factor VIII replacement or desmopressin, the risk of recurrent bleeding from oral mucosal surfaces is dramatically reduced with the administration of antifibrinolytic agents. Use of these agents for nasal bleeding or for bleeding from the urinary tract or gastrointestinal surfaces has not been studied extensively. The clearest demonstration of their efficacy is with dental extractions, for which transfusion therapy was previously required for 10 to 12 days. With the use of antifibrinolytic therapy, a single infusion of factor VIII and 7 to 10 days of antifibrinolytic therapy are usually sufficient to prevent recurrent hemorrhage after dental extractions.[51,144] In addition, tranexamic acid has been shown to be effective when used topically as a mouthwash.[145] The intravenous form of ε-aminocaproic can also be used as an effective mouthwash.

Two antifibrinolytic agents, aminocaproic acid and tranexamic acid, are available. Aminocaproic acid is formulated in an intravenous form, oral tablets, and an elixir.[146,147] The tablets contains 500 or 1000 mg, and the elixir contains 250 mg/mL. Because the tablets are large and the usual dose is 5 g (5 to 10 tablets), most adult patients prefer taking the elixir. The oral dose of ε-aminocaproic acid is 100 to 200 mg/kg initially (maximum dose, 10 g), followed by 50 to 100 mg/kg per dose every 6 hours (maximum dose, 5 g). The second agent, tranexamic acid, is available in 500-mg capsules. The dose of tranexamic acid is 25 mg/kg every 6 to 8 hours. No elixir is available for tranexamic acid. Both tranexamic acid and aminocaproic acid are available in intravenous forms.

Treatment of Patients with Hemophilia A Who Have Inhibitory Antibodies to Factor VIII

In 14% to 25% of patients with severe hemophilia A, antibodies develop that inactivate the procoagulant activity of factor VIII; these antibodies are referred to as factor VIII inhibitors.[112-118] The clinical hallmark of inhibitor development is failure to respond to routine replacement therapy. Patients with factor VIII inhibitors can be divided into two general categories: high responders and low responders. High responders are those in whom high-titer antibody develops with exposure to factor VIII and in whom an anamnestic response usually occurs with subsequent exposure. The titer of their antibody is in excess of 5 Bethesda units and may increase to hundreds or thousands of Bethesda units after repeat exposure. In low responders, a titer of inhibitory antibody is maintained at less than 5 Bethesda units, even when they are exposed to repeated doses of factor VIII. The clinical approach is different for these two groups.

Low-Responding Factor VIII Inhibitors

Patients with inhibitor titers of less than 5 Bethesda units[148] can generally be treated with factor VIII concentrates at higher doses. Because the effect of hemophilic factor VIII inhibitor is usually time dependent, the Bethesda titer in plasma is determined after a 2-hour incubation period. As a result of this time delay, continuous administration of factor VIII is usually found to be effective.[149] For a serious limb- or life-threatening bleeding episode, a bolus infusion of 100 U/kg of factor VIII is administered, and the level is maintained by treatment at a rate of 20 U/kg/hr. An assay for factor VIII should be performed 1 hour after the bolus infusion and at least daily thereafter. As the antibody titer drops (caused by the formation of an immune complex with the high-dose factor VIII), the daily level of factor VIII may rise and thus require downward adjustment of the continuous infusion rate. For routine joint and muscle hemorrhage, patients can usually be managed[144] with infusions at twice the usual dosage. A survival study can be performed to determine the peak and half-life of the infused factor VIII. Routine inhibitor assays should be performed after exposure to factor VIII to determine whether an anamnestic response has occurred. Whether the patient remains a low responder or becomes a high responder will determine how the patient is treated for future bleeding episodes.

High-Responding Factor VIII Inhibitors

Treatment of patients with high-responding factor VIII inhibitors requires a much more aggressive approach with one of several alternative therapies. Such treatment is usually performed in sophisticated tertiary care centers by experts in the management of hemophilia.

Continuous Factor VIII Infusion. Most clinicians caring for patients with limb-threatening or life-threatening bleeding episodes prefer to use products for which therapeutic levels can be monitored. As described earlier, continuous administration of factor VIII is often effective because of the time delay in inhibition by the antibody. An initial dose of 100 to 200 U/kg can be administered, and factor VIII levels can be determined 1 hour after initiation of continuous infusion at a rate of 20 to 40 U/kg/hr. If a factor VIII level cannot be obtained (i.e., patients with Bethesda titers greater than 5 to 10 Bethesda units), alternative approaches are usually indicated.

Porcine Factor VIII Concentrate. In patients whose Bethesda titer is less than 50 Bethesda units, a therapeutic factor VIII level can usually be attained by using a porcine factor VIII concentrate. Porcine factor VIII is a highly purified material produced by polyelectrolyte ion exchange chromatography.[150,151] Because of contamination of porcine factor VIII with parvovirus, plasma-derived factor VIII is no longer available. Recombinant porcine factor VIII is being explored as a new therapeutic option for factor VIII inhibitor patients, but it is not yet licensed.[152] The recommended starting dose of porcine factor VIII is 100 to 150 U/kg, and the response is measured with a standard factor VIII assay. Alternatively, continuous infusion of porcine factor VIII can be initiated after the bolus infusion. Factor VIII levels should be monitored frequently (at least daily) with a standard one-stage PTT-based assay. The clinician should measure the antiporcine factor VIII titer with a Bethesda-type assay to determine the anamnestic response. Knowing that the porcine titer is low or undetectable permits the clinician to form a rational plan for using porcine factor VIII during future bleeding episodes.

Recombinant Factor VIIa. A recombinant factor VIIa (activated factor VII) concentrate has been developed and demonstrated to produce hemostasis in patients with high-responding inhibitors.[153,154] It is thought to interact with tissue factor and platelets at the site of vascular injury and thereby activate factor X and promote thrombin generation in a manner that bypasses the factor VIII–dependent steps.[155]

The initial dose is 90 to 120 μg/kg of factor VIIa, with additional doses administered every 2 hours. The subsequent rate of infusion and duration of therapy must then be individualized on the basis of the clinical response and severity of bleeding. Recently, the use of higher bolus doses of 180 to 270 µg/kg has been advocated to presumably establish a higher "thrombin burst" at the site of vascular injury.[156]

Prothrombin Complex Concentrate. Prothrombin complex concentrates may sometimes be used to treat routine joint and muscle hemorrhage in patients with hemophilia A and inhibitors. The exact mechanism by which the beneficial effects of these concentrates are produced is still not fully understood. A multicenter controlled study of hemarthrosis demonstrated that these concentrates promoted hemostasis in 50% of bleeding episodes. The initial dose is 75 U/kg of factor IX. If there is no response after two or three infusions given 12 hours apart, it is unlikely that additional treatments will be successful. If repeated doses of these concentrates are administered, consideration should be given to the addition of heparin.

Activated Prothrombin Complex Concentrates. There is currently one commercially available "activated" prothrombin complex concentrate, FEIBA (factor eight inhibitor–bypassing activity). This product has been purposefully activated during the fractionation process to achieve increased amounts of activated factor VII, factor X, or thrombin. Double-blind controlled trials have demonstrated that this product has small but significant advantages over standard prothrombin complex concentrates.[157] In contrast to porcine factor VIII or continuous-infusion factor VIII, these products are effective even in patients with high-titer inhibitors. The initial dose of 75 U/kg can be repeated in 6 to 12 hours. If multiple doses are administered, the patient should be monitored for the development of disseminated intravascular coagulation or even myocardial infarction, which has been reported with the use of these concentrates.[158] The simultaneous use of antifibrinolytic therapy should be avoided in these patients. If this treatment is not successful, recombinant factor VIIa treatment is usually considered.

Immune Tolerance to Factor VIII. Immune tolerance was first attempted in the 1970s and was achieved by the administration of high doses of factor VIII (100 to 150 U/kg) twice daily and the use of activated prothrombin complex concentrates for acute bleeding episodes.[159] After a period of months to even years, the titer of factor VIII antibodies was markedly reduced, and the dose could be decreased to a smaller daily dose or even doses given every other day. A less aggressive approach using lower doses of factor VIII has generally been demonstrated to be less effective.[160] Various reports have also described the use of intravenous gamma globulin, immunosuppressive therapy, removal of the antibody by extracorporeal immunoadsorption on *Staphylococcus* protein A columns, or a combination of these modalities.[161] Immune tolerance in four of five patients treated with porcine factor VIII on a home-based infusion program has also been reported.[162] Reports suggest that early treatment of patients with inhibitors to induce immune tolerance is more successful.[163-165]

Hemophilia B

Calculation of Dose

Because factor IX has a volume of distribution different from that of factor VIII, the amount of plasma-derived factor IX that is required to achieve a similar plasma level is approximately twice that for factor VIII:

$$\text{Dose of factor IX (units)} = \\ \text{U/dL (percent) desired rise} \times \\ \text{Body weight (kg)}$$

Thus, for the treatment of hemarthrosis in a 20-kg child in whom a level of 80 U/dL is desired, the dose would be 80 U/dL × 20 kg = 1600 units of factor IX.

If recombinant factor IX concentrate is used, the dose must be increased 1.2- to 1.5-fold because of the poorer recovery of recombinant factor IX.[166] Thus, in the example just presented, the dose of recombinant factor IX would be 1920 to 2400 units. It is recommended that the recovery of factor IX after an infusion be established for each patient to accurately determine subsequent therapeutic doses. The half-life of factor IX (18 to 24 hours) is much longer than that of factor VIII (10 to 12 hours), and therefore factor IX does not need to be administered as often. Whereas the minimal hemostatic level of factor VIII is 30 to 40 U/dL, that of factor IX appears to be 25 to 30 U/dL.[167]

Factor IX Concentrates

Plasma-Derived Factor IX Concentrates. Hemophilia B can now be treated with highly purified factor IX products derived from plasma through purification or monoclonal immunoaffinity.[168] These highly purified factor IX concentrates are preferred over prothrombin complex concentrates for the treatment of major bleeding episodes, especially in patients with impaired liver function, massive crush injury, or a history of thrombosis. As discussed later, prothrombin complex concentrates are much more likely to be thrombogenic because of the presence of activated vitamin K–dependent clotting factors. Anaphylaxis in association with inhibitor development has been reported in patients receiving high-purity factor IX concentrates.[169,170] It is therefore usually recommended that administration of the first several doses of factor IX be observed in an emergency department where anaphylaxis can be treated if necessary.

Recombinant Factor IX Concentrates. Recombinant factor IX is considered the preferred product for treating patients with hemophilia B. As mentioned earlier, there is reduced recovery of recombinant factor IX, so 20% to 50% more factor IX must be used to achieve the same plasma concentration as plasma-derived factor IX.[171,172]

Prothrombin Complex Concentrates

The vitamin K–dependent clotting factors are of similar size and have similar biochemical and physical chemical properties. Thus, fractionation procedures such as barium sulfate precipitation and column chromatography with various adsorbents purify many of the vitamin K–dependent clotting factors together.[173,174] This material is therefore called prothrombin complex concentrate. These concentrates have been found on rare occasion to cause life-threatening thrombotic complications, including deep venous thrombosis, myocardial infarction, pulmonary emboli, and disseminated intravascular coagulation.[175,176] The risk of thrombosis is increased in patients receiving high or repetitive doses, in patients with impaired fibrinolysis (liver disease or after treatment with antifibrinolytic agents), and in those with impaired ability to clear activated clotting factors (i.e., patients with liver disease). When prothrombin complex concentrates are used repetitively, especially in high doses, the International Society of Thrombosis and Hemostasis (ISTH) has recommended the addition of 100 units of heparin to each 500 units of factor IX concentrate.[177] When factor IX is replaced, this level of heparin is not a problem. Rather than adding heparin to the prothrombin complex concentrates, most physicians currently prefer to use the more purified factor IX products or recombinant factor IX to treat patients with factor IX deficiency when high or repetitive doses are required. Factor IX concentrates and prothrombin complex concentrates have undergone dry heating or vapor heating at high temperatures to reduce the risk of HIV infection and hepatitis C.[178]

Fresh Frozen Plasma

Although fresh frozen plasma was historically used to treat hemophilia B, its use today is limited to areas of the world where factor IX concentrates are unavailable or in emergency situations when factor IX concentrates are not available. If large amounts of fresh frozen plasma are used, the plasma should be ABO blood type compatible to avoid the complication of hemolytic anemia caused by the infusion of isohemagglutinins. Patients with a normal cardiovascular system can safely tolerate a dose of 15 to 20 mL/kg.[179]

Treatment of Hemophilia B Patients with Factor IX Inhibitors

The incidence of inhibitory antibodies to factor IX is much lower than that seen with factor VIII. When such antibodies are identified, activated prothrombin complex concentrates and factor VIIa have been found to be the most successful therapies. However, the use of activated prothrombin concentrates is contraindicated in patients in whom anaphylaxis has developed along with the inhibitor because they too contain factor IX. Recombinant factor VIIa does not contain any factor IX and is therefore the preferred therapeutic approach. The induction of immune tolerance has been disappointing in patients

with factor IX inhibitors. In several patients, nephrotic syndrome has developed when factor IX was given in high doses for induction of tolerance.[180,181]

Complications of Transfusion Therapy for Hemophilia A and Hemophilia B

Transfusion-transmitted infectious diseases are a complication of transfusion therapy with plasma-derived therapeutic products in patients with hemophilia A and hemophilia B. Such diseases include HIV infection, hepatitis B, hepatitis C, and more recently, hepatitis A (see Chapter 35). With the use of recombinant factor VIII and factor IX and the newer methods of viral attenuation, many of the secondary problems associated with these complications can be avoided or minimized. As discussed earlier, hepatitis B and hepatitis A vaccines should be administered to patients before or concomitant with initial therapy.

Comprehensive Care and Home Therapy

Care of patients with hemophilia requires a comprehensive team of health care providers that includes a hemophilia specialist, nurse coordinator, social worker, psychologist, physical therapist, dentist, orthopedic surgeon, financial counselor, primary care physician, and sometimes an infectious disease specialist.[182-184] This approach is considered to be the standard of care and is provided primarily through comprehensive hemophilia treatment centers. The occurrence of primary and secondary complications of hemophilia is reduced, and patient performance both at school and in the workplace is improved.[182]

A revolution occurred in hemophilia care with the development of factor concentrates and the potential for treatment of bleeding episodes at home. This has become the standard venue for the administration of replacement therapy for the majority of hemorrhages in patients with hemophilia. With home therapy, treatment can be administered sooner, which can reduce the long-term morbidity of hemophilia and thereby reduce the total cost of the disease. Home care programs should be monitored closely by the comprehensive hemophilia team and requires the physician, nurse coordinator, and patient and family to have a close working relationship.[185] Today, many patients receive routine primary prophylactic therapy at home administered through a subcutaneous port and a central venous access line.

Future Gene Therapy for Hemophilia A and Hemophilia B

Gene therapy for either hemophilia A or hemophilia B is not yet available.[172,186] Animal models of hemophilia A and hemophilia B have been developed or maintained in dogs and mice. Early success with gene therapy in these animal models has been achieved, but long-term maintenance of a satisfactory plasma level of clotting factor continues to be a problem. Human gene therapy trials have been carried out for both hemophilia A[187-189] and hemophilia B.[190-192] Although extensive preclinical studies have demonstrated the potential for gene therapy in hemophilia, the clinical trials to date are disappointing. Because inhibitory antibodies will develop in more than 25% of patients treated with clotting factor concentrates, it is not yet clear whether gene therapy will have a similar incidence or whether continuous release by the transgene will provide tolerance in these patients. One recent preclinical approach consists of directing factor VIII expression to platelets where the factor VIII is stored and can be released locally by platelets.[193-197] One group has demonstrated that this approach appears to be effective even in the presence of high-titer inhibitory antibodies.[196] Gene therapy is expected to be available in the next 5 to 10 years, but many problems remain, including selection of both appropriate vectors and the appropriate cell in which to express the gene. Control of potential deleterious side effects must still be solved.[186]

VON WILLEBRAND DISEASE

VWD is a disorder of VWF, a large multimeric glycoprotein that (1) contributes to the adherence of platelets to damaged endothelium and (2) serves as a carrier protein for plasma factor VIII. Deficiency of VWF results in mucocutaneous and post-traumatic or postsurgical bleeding, but if VWF is absent or markedly reduced, the secondary reduction in plasma factor VIII may also result in muscle and joint bleeding similar to hemophilia A. This disorder was first described by Erik von Willebrand in 1925 in persons living on the Åland Islands off the coast of Finland.[198-200] VWD is a very common, but heterogeneous disorder that is the result of a variety of genetic defects ranging from congenital absence of VWF to major dysproteinemias in which the structure and function of the molecule are markedly abnormal. It is inherited autosomally; thus, in contrast to hemophilia A and hemophilia B, the incidence of VWD in men and women is comparable, although more women may be assigned this diagnosis because of menorrhagia being a common symptom.

Pathophysiology

VWF is a large multimeric glycoprotein that is synthesized in megakaryocytes and endothelial cells and stored in specific cellular storage granules: the Weibel-Palade body in endothelial cells and the alpha granule in platelets.[201-204] It is present in plasma, but reduced levels can be significantly increased by administering drugs such as desmopressin that induce the release of VWF from endothelial storage sites into plasma.[136] Figure 30-1 depicts the role of VWF in localizing and facilitating the hemostatic process. After an injury to the endothelial cell wall of the blood vessel, the local concentration of VWF is increased by the interaction of VWF with components of the subendothelial matrix such as collagen.[205] This bound VWF changes conformation and binds to the platelet glycoprotein Ib (GPIb) receptor, thereby resulting in adherence of circulating platelets to the site of damaged endothelium.[206,207] VWF is also capable of interacting with the GPIIb-IIIa receptor on platelets, and this action may be promoted by shear stress.[208-210] Once VWF causes the platelet to adhere by means of its GPIb receptor, these platelets are activated, which causes the recruitment of additional platelets.[211] This is termed platelet aggregation and results in the formation of a platelet plug (see Fig. 30-1). Formation of the platelet plug also depends on the presence of plasma fibrinogen, the primary ligand for platelet aggregation. The surface of aggregated platelets is altered with the externalization of phosphatidylserine, which interacts with plasma clotting factors (prothrombinase and factor X-ase) that catalyze generation of the local fibrin clot (see Figs. 30-1). Thus, in the absence of VWF (or in the presence of VWF with abnormal structure), platelets are poorly targeted to the area of endothelial cell damage, and less than optimal hemostasis results.

VWF also serves as a carrier protein for the plasma factor VIII molecule and, in fact, is necessary for the normal recovery and survival of factor VIII.[212-214] In the absence of VWF, lack of the carrier molecule function results in a secondary deficiency of plasma factor VIII. This deficiency of factor VIII is the result of accelerated clearance.[74,215] Recombinant factor VIII is produced more efficiently within cells transfected with genes for both VWF and factor VIII.[216,217] Thus, patients with severe VWD (type 3) usually have a prolonged bleeding time and a prolonged PTT caused by a decrease in both VWF and factor VIII. Milder forms of this disorder can differ and are described in more detail later.

Variant forms of VWF have been characterized in patients with type 2 variants (see later) that cause reduced binding of VWF to factor VIII, reduced binding to platelets, and reduced size of VWF multimers. Each of these forms can therefore lead to abnormal hemostasis and clinical VWD.

Genetics

VWD is an autosomal disorder, but some patients exhibit a classic recessive inheritance (type 3 and type 2N VWD) and others exhibit dominant inheritance (type 2B and 2A VWD).[218-220] The most common form, type 1 VWD, has variable penetrance and symptoms even within the same family.[218,221] Studies have been carried out that suggest that VWD may occur in as many as 1% or 2% of the general population,[222,223] but this high frequency has been challenged recently and will be discussed later.[224-226] VWF gene defects are rare in individuals with VWF antigen (VWF:Ag) levels just below the normal range.[218,221,227-229]

The VWF gene spans 178 kb and contains 52 exons.[230-232] It results in an 8.5-kb message that directs the synthesis of a 22–amino acid signal peptide and a 2791–amino acid pro-VWF monomer that is subsequently cleaved into a 741–amino acid propeptide and a

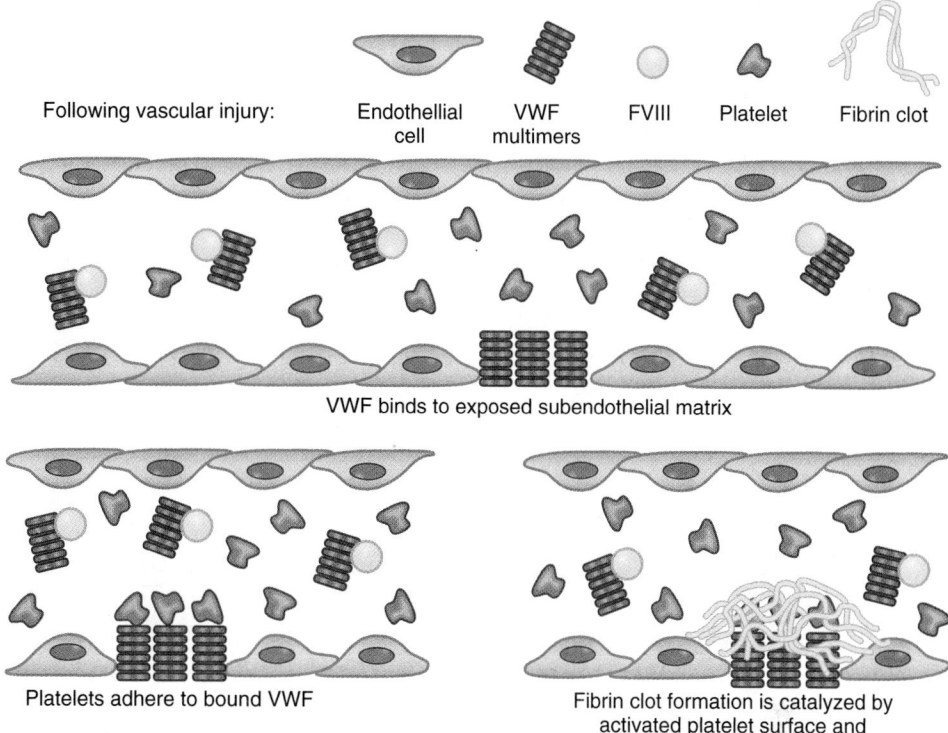

Following vascular injury: Endothelial cell   VWF multimers   FVIII   Platelet   Fibrin clot

VWF binds to exposed subendothelial matrix

Platelets adhere to bound VWF

Fibrin clot formation is catalyzed by activated platelet surface and phospholipid-bound FVIII

FIGURE 30-1. After vascular injury, plasma von Willebrand factor (VWF) binds to the subendothelial matrix. Under shear stress, VWF changes conformation, which enables the adherence of circulating platelets (platelet adhesion) through the glycoprotein receptor GPIb. Platelets are activated and recruit other platelets through platelet aggregation (platelet cohesion and aggregation). These activated platelets alter their surface phospholipids so that factor VIII (FVIII) binds, interacts with FIXa to activate the X-ase complex, and facilitates formation of the fibrin clot (coagulation). *(Courtesy of R. R. Montgomery.)*

2050–amino acid mature VWF monomer. The propeptide was initially termed von Willebrand antigen II,[233] but the VWF propeptide is currently referred to as VWFpp.[234,235] Figure 30-2 illustrates the relationship of the complementary DNA (8.5 kb) to structural and functional regions of the VWF protein. The areas of this gene that have been found to contain clusters of genetic defects that cause similar phenotypes are illustrated and include type 2A,[236,237] type 2B,[238,239] type 2N variants with abnormal interaction between VWF and factor VIII,[74,240,241] hereditary persistence of pro-VWF,[242] and a type 1 variant of VWD with accelerated clearance of VWF (Vicenza variant or type 1C VWD).[235,243,244] These genetic defects can be identified either by sequencing segments of the gene after amplification by polymerase chain reaction (PCR) or by reverse transcription of messenger RNA from circulating platelets and sequencing the "derived" complementary DNA after amplification by PCR.[236,239,240] Confirmation that these point mutations are responsible for the disease requires expression of the abnormal protein after transfection in vitro.[240] Many laboratories are now carrying out such DNA analysis on unusual variants. Three recent studies of relatively large cohorts of families have identified a number of VWF mutations associated with the most common type of VWD—type 1 VWD.[218,228,245-248] A summary of the mutations and polymorphisms in the VWF gene has been established by the VWF Subcommittee of the ISTH (maintained on http://www.vwf.group.shef.ac.uk/), and a summary of the variant types of VWF has been published by the VWF Subcommittee of the Scientific and Standardization Committee of the International Society of Thrombosis and Haemostasis (SSC/ISTH).[220] Genetic

diagnosis is complicated by a partial, unprocessed 25-kb pseudogene located at chromosome 22q11.2.[249] Because this duplication has greater than 96% homology with VWF and spans the A1 to A3 domains, PCR primers need to be designed to avoid amplification of this pseudogene for identification of mutations in this region of VWF.[250] In the mouse, extragenic causes of low VWF have been found and are the result of accelerated clearance of VWF because of abnormal glycosylation.[251] In humans, extragenic causes of VWD are being sought, but to date, the major modifier of plasma VWF is the ABO blood group,[252] thought to be the result of glycosylation differences in the ABH antigens that have been known for many years.[253] Additional modifiers of VWF:Ag levels or of clinical bleeding symptoms are being sought.

Low von Willebrand Factor Versus Type 1 von Willebrand Disease

As mentioned earlier, patients with VWF levels below 2 SD of normal VWF have historically been used to define the level for diagnosis of VWD. However, a 2-SD normal range by definition leaves 2.5% of the population above that range and 2.5% below that range. Some studies suggest that VWD is present in 1% to 2% of the general population.[222,223] The diagnosis of mild type 1 VWD has been challenged based on the argument that the plasma level of VWF is a continuous variable and may be a risk factor for bleeding and not necessarily a defined disease state.[224,225,254] Recently, guidelines have been published by the National Institutes of Health (www.nhlbi.nih.gov/guidelines/vwd) in which the suggested level for the designation of type 1 VWD was a VWF:Ag or plasma ristocetin cofactor (VWF:RCo) level of less than 30 IU/dL,

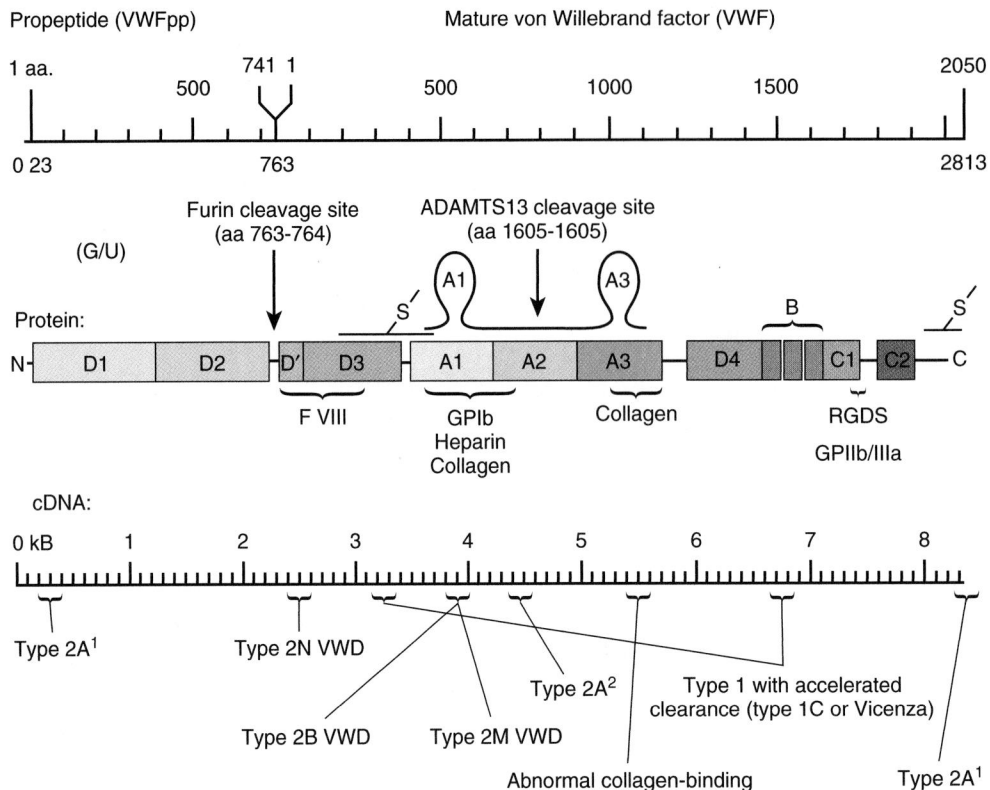

FIGURE 30-2. Protein structure and its relationship to von Willebrand disease (VWD) variant subtype mutation location. von Willebrand factor (VWF) contains specific domains that have been shown to have discrete functions, including (1) the interaction with factor VIII (FVIII; D′ and D3), glycoprotein Ib (GPIb; A1), collagen (A1 and A3), ADAMTS-13 (A2), platelet GPIIb/IIIa (C1), and furin (D2-D′). The *lower panel* localizes hot spots for DNA mutations that cause VWF variants that tend to correlate with the functional domains. The variants include type 2A¹ (2A variants that fail to multimerize properly), type 2N (decreased interaction with FVIII), type 2B (increased binding to platelet GPIb), type 2M (decreased binding to GPIb but with normal VWF multimers), type 2A² (2A variants caused by increased spontaneous proteolysis of VWF by ADAMTS-13), abnormal binding to collagen, and type 1C (type 1 VWD variant with accelerated VWF clearance). aa, amino acid. *(Courtesy of R. R. Montgomery.)*

but patients with bleeding and VWF levels below the normal range may still benefit from therapy such as DDAVP to raise the level of plasma VWF. Controversy therefore remains over this issue, and many clinicians still use the term "mild type 1 VWD" to refer to individuals with VWF:Ag levels between 30 and 50 IU/dL. Low VWF or even clinical bleeding symptoms are not always associated with a clearly identifiable VWF gene mutation. Conversely, not all patients inheriting a VWF gene mutation will manifest bleeding symptoms (referred to as variable penetrance),[255,256] and among those who do bleed, severity can vary widely (variable expressivity).[218,246,257] Alternatively, low VWF or clinical bleeding symptoms in the absence of a VWF gene mutation may result from the effects of mutations in another gene (or genes) (locus heterogeneity). Research is still necessary to characterize these complex genetic factors in greater detail.

Demographics and Classification

While males and females should have a similar prevalence; VWD is diagnosed more frequently in boys in childhood but then more commonly in teenage and adult females because of the frequent complication of menor-

rhagia. VWD occurs in all racial groups, although localized pockets with a very high incidence of VWD do exist, such as those in the Åland Islands of Finland and areas of Sweden, Israel, and Iran.[258-260] African Americans have been shown to have higher levels of plasma VWF:Ag, but their VWF:RCo level is not similarly increased.[261,262]

VWD has numerous subtypes that can be defined by structural, functional, and molecular genetic techniques. Of patients with VWD, 65% to 80% have type 1 VWD, characterized by a parallel reduction in both VWF antigen and VWF activity as measured by the ristocetin cofactor assay.[263-265] This assay is described in more detail later. The second most common variant is type 2A VWD, in which the multimeric structure of VWF is altered such that only the smallest VWF multimers are present in plasma.[266,267] This results in a marked reduction in ristocetin cofactor activity with a somewhat milder reduction in the level of VWF antigen. Figure 30-3 summarizes the more common variants of VWD and their relative prevalence. Descriptions of types 1, 2A, 2B, 2N, 2M, and 3 VWD and platelet-type pseudo-VWD are provided later.

Because VWD is common, the possibility of inheriting VWD from both parents is significant. These patients

VON WILLEBRAND DISEASE VARIANTS AND PLATELET DISORDERS AFFECTING VWF BINDING

	Normal	Type 1	Type 3	Type 2A	Type 2B	Type 2N	Type 2M	PT-VWD*	BSS*
VWF:Ag	N	↓	absent	↓	↓	N or ↓	↓ or N	↓	N
VWF:RCo	N	↓	absent	↓↓↓	↓↓	N or ↓	↓↓	↓↓	N
FVIII	N	↓ or N	1-6%	N or ↓	N or ↓	↓↓	N	N or ↓	N
RIPA	N	often N	absent	↓	often N	N	N or ↓	often N	absent
LD-RIPA	absent	absent	absent	absent	↑↑↑	absent	absent	↑↑↑	absent
PFA	N	N or ↑	↑↑↑	↑	↑	N	↑	↑	↑ ↑ ↑
BT	N	N or ↑	↑↑↑	↑	↑	N	↑	↑	↑↑↑
Platelet count	N	N	N	N	↓ (rarely N)	N	N	↓	↓
Usual Tx		DDAVP VWF conc	VWF conc	VWF conc (DDAVP)	VWF conc	VWF conc (DDAVP)	VWF conc	platelets	platelets
Response to DDAVP		good	none	poor	decreases platelets	poor	poor	decreases platelets	none or modest
Response to VWF Conc		good	good	good	good	good	good	decreases platelets	no response
Frequency in general population		reported as 1–2%	very rare 1:250,000	rare	rare	rare	rare	rare	rare
VWF multimers	N	N or ↓	absent	abnormal	abnormal	N but ↓	N but ↓	abnormal	normal

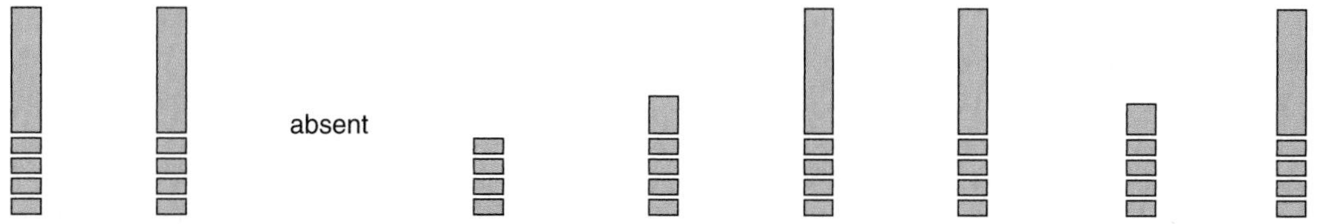

* Platelet disorders that affect VWF interaction with platelets.

FIGURE 30-3. Summary of types of von Willebrand disease (VWD types 1, 3, 2A, 2B, 2M, 2N) and absent or defective platelet glycoprotein Ib receptor for von Willebrand factor (VWF) (platelet-type VWD [PT-VWF]) or Bernard-Soulier syndrome (BSS). The *lower portion* illustrates the VWF multimers that are identified by sodium dodecyl sulfate–agarose gel electrophoresis of VWF for each of these variants. BT, bleeding time; Conc, concentrate; DDAVP, desmopressin (1-deamino-8-D-arginine vasopressin); LD-RIPA, ristocetin-induced platelet aggregation to low-dose ristocetin; N, normal; PFA, platelet function analyzer; Tx, treatment; VWF:Ag, von Willebrand factor antigen; VWF:RCo, VWF activity by ristocetin cofactor assay. *(Courtesy of R. R. Montgomery.)*

with severe homozygous or compound heterozygous or type 3 VWD have undetectable levels of VWF and a significant reduction in factor VIII (1 to 6 U/dL). Such patients have a much more severe bleeding tendency.

Clinical Screening Using a Semiquantitative Bleeding Assessment

Several recent studies have focused on the clinical symptoms associated with VWD and have attempted to quantify these symptoms in the hope of improving the specificity of the diagnosis.[268-270] These scoring systems evaluated epistaxis, skin bleeding, oral/dental bleeding, gastrointestinal bleeding, muscle/joint bleeding, and CNS bleeding. Even though the two reports are similar, the second one was modified to give weight to surgical, dental, or delivery procedures that were not treated and did not result in excessive bleeding. Although these scoring systems were extensive, they have not been validated or carried out in children. Currently, there is a great deal of interest in developing such an assessment for use in children, but increasing specificity and sensitivity may be difficult.

Laboratory Evaluation

Laboratory evaluation of VWD often requires multiple assays to quantitate VWF and characterize its function and structure. Because results of screening tests (bleeding time and PTT) may be normal in patients with mild or moderate VWD, more specific assays for VWF are performed to diagnose VWD in patients with a history of significant bleeding episodes. VWD cannot be ruled out on the basis of a normal PTT and bleeding time or even with a platelet function analyzer such as the PFA-100.[271,272]

Immunoassay for von Willebrand Factor Antigen

VWF can be measured by using a variety of quantitative immunoassays. The most widely used assays are the enzyme-linked immunosorbent assay (ELISA)[273-275] and the quantitative immunoelectrophoretic assay (Laurell assay).[276] Nearly all large laboratories use the ELISA assay. Despite a great deal of variability in the measurement of VWF:Ag, the problem is probably not due to the assay but to the standard that is used in the assay. The World Health Organization (WHO) and ISTH have established standards for these assays and recommend reporting of results in international units standardized by the WHO.[277]

Determination of von Willebrand Factor Activity by the Ristocetin Cofactor Assay

The activity of VWF is most commonly measured in vitro with the antibiotic ristocetin (VWF:RCo).[264,265] Ristocetin induces binding of VWF to the GPIb receptor on platelets.[208] This assay is usually carried out with formalin-fixed platelets. The amount of plasma VWF activity is proportional to the slope of the agglutination curve. Some laboratories perform ristocetin-induced platelet aggregation, which is a measure of both binding of VWF to the GPIb receptor and the ability of this binding to induce aggregation. This test is not nearly as sensitive as the ristocetin cofactor assay and should not be used to rule out the diagnosis of VWD. Various methods have been developed to automate the ristocetin cofactor assay.[278-280] Ristocetin is an antibiotic that induces a conformational change in VWF so that it agglutinates platelets. Because this is a nonphysiologic activity assay, a number of alternative assays attempt to use shear as the stimulus for platelet binding, but to date, VWF:RCo remains the most widely used assay for VWF function. Large multimers of VWF have more VWF:RCo activity than do the intermediate and small VWF multimers. Newer assays for ristocetin cofactor are being developed that use bound GPIb in an ELISA format to determine that amount of patient plasma VWF that binds in the presence of ristocetin.[281,282]

Low-Dose Ristocetin-Induced Platelet Aggregation

One specific use for the low-dose ristocetin-induced platelet aggregation (LD-RIPA) assay is to diagnose the hyperresponsiveness of VWF with platelets in either type 2B VWD or platelet-type, pseudo-VWD (see Fig. 30-3).[283,284] These variants are important to differentiate appropriately because their response to the administration of desmopressin may be suboptimal. Each variant requires specific treatment to correct the qualitative abnormality. Differentiation of these types from one another can be done by a method devised to use frozen plasma to identify the increased binding of plasma VWF to platelets in patients with type 2B VWD.[285]

Collagen-Binding Assay for von Willebrand Factor

Assays have been developed to measure the binding of plasma VWF to collagen. In general, large multimers of VWF bind preferentially, although the type of collagen may affect this specificity. Some have advocated replacement of the VWF:RCo assay with a collagen-binding assay (VWF:CB),[286,287] but the two assays measure different "activities"—one with platelets and the other with subendothelial matrix collagen. A few families have been identified who lack binding of VWF to collagen. This mutation has been identified in the D3 region of VWF.[288,289] Some patients with type 2M VWD will show low binding in ristocetin cofactor assays but normal results with collagen-binding assays.[290,291]

von Willebrand Factor Multimers

VWF is present in plasma in multimers ranging from dimers of approximately 600,000 daltons to very large multimers of up to 20 million daltons.[267] The full range of VWF multimers is best demonstrated through the use of low concentrations of agarose (0.65 percent) and staining the multimers with radiolabeled antibody to VWF. The multimers are visualized by luminography.[266,292,293] Figure 30-4 demonstrates the multimers in type 1 VWD, as well as in types 2A, 2B, and 3. Acquired alteration of VWF multimers may also occur in various clinical disorders, with the loss of high-molecular-weight multimers seen in patients with disseminated intravascular coagulation or ventricular septal defects.[294] Larger than normal multimers can be identified in patients with recurrent thrombotic thrombocytopenia purpura.[295,296] Figure 30-4 also illustrates an additional method for multimer analysis in which satellite bands of the lower-molecular-weight multimers are identified. The individual multimers are resolved into five discrete bands, but the overall multimeric structure is not so well depicted as with the lower-agarose–containing gels. Patients with some type 2 variants may have increased satellite bands (see Figure 30-4).[297] Because these assays are difficult to

LOW-RESOLUTION GEL HIGH-RESOLUTION GEL

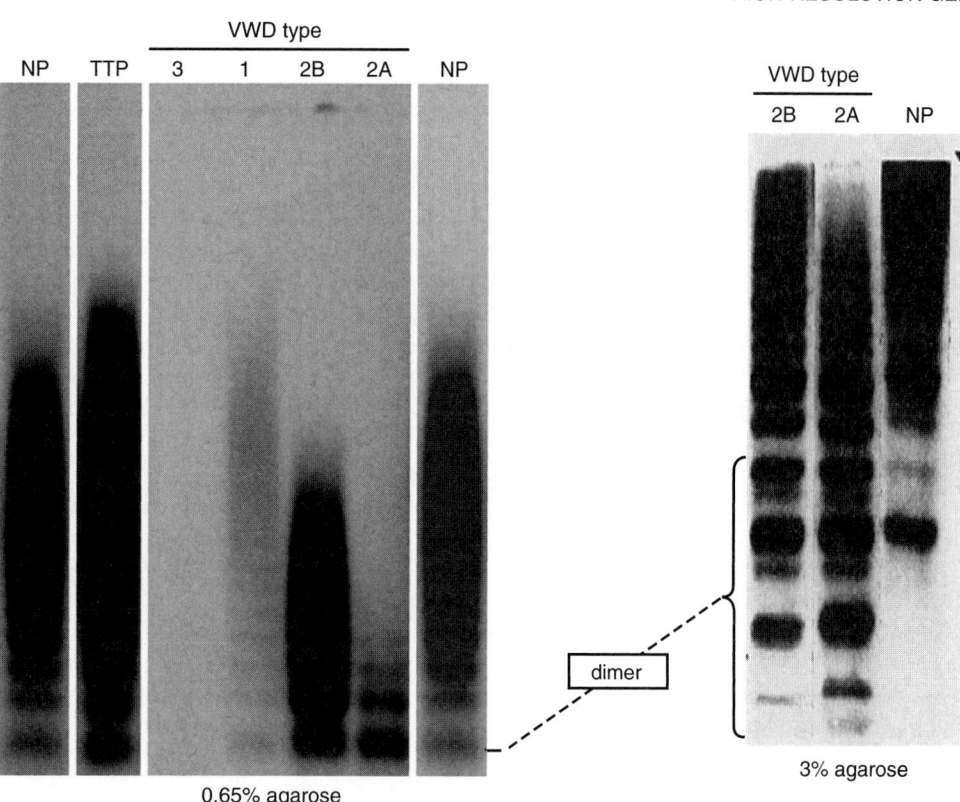

FIGURE 30-4. Multimeric analysis of von Willebrand factor (VWF) with low (0.65%) and high (3%) concentrations of agarose. Representative samples are compared and demonstrate that the low-agarose gels are preferable for detecting the loss of high-molecular-weight multimers, as seen in some VWF variants, and the increased size of VWF multimers seen in patients with thrombotic thrombocytopenic purpura (TTP). The gels with higher agarose concentration (*left*) demonstrate that single multimer bands (*left*) can be resolved into multiple satellite bands that may be selectively increased in plasma from patients with variant forms of VWD. NP, normal plasma. *(Courtesy of R. R. Montgomery.)*

perform, multimeric analysis is often performed at specialized centers.

Assay for von Willebrand Factor Propeptide

A number of laboratories now offer quantitation of VWFpp. Because this 741–amino acid propeptide of VWF is synthesized on a 1:1 basis with VWF monomer, quantitation of this protein is useful in characterizing clinical states in which VWF has accelerated clearance by identifying individuals whose plasma VWFpp/VWF:Ag ratio is markedly elevated. This is possible because the accelerated clearance affects only the VWF:Ag level and not the level of VWFpp. One recent study reported four families with accelerated clearance of VWF who had VWFpp/VWF:Ag ratios between 2.3 and 6.8.[298] This ratio is also markedly elevated in acquired VWD associated with an autoantibody that promotes rapid clearance of VWF.[299] Quantitation of VWFpp and VWF:Ag has also been suggested as a marker to differentiate acute and chronic endothelial purtubation.[300]

Other Assays to Define Variants of von Willebrand Disease

Several more assays are available at specialized centers to help classify variant forms of VWD. In type 2B VWD, the VWF spontaneously binds to platelets in the presence of low-dose ristocetin and is termed a *type 2B platelet-binding assay*.[239,301] In type 2N VWD, VWF has reduced affinity for factor VIII, and this is best studied with a *type 2N*

VWF factor VIII–binding assay.[240,302] The *VWF:RCo/ VWF:Ag ratio* has been studied and helps identify patients with type 2M VWD.[290] These latter two assays are depicted in Figure 30-5.

Approximately half of the patients with type 2A VWD have reduced VWF multimer size and VWF:Ag secondary to mutations in the VWF A2 domain that make the molecule more susceptible to spontaneous proteolysis by a metalloproteinase termed ADAMTS-13.[303-305] Such proteolysis results in cleavage of VWF between amino acids 1605 and 1606 in the A2 domain (see Fig. 30-2).[306] A number of assays have been developed for ADAMTS-13.[307-310]

Variables That Affect Laboratory Assays for von Willebrand Factor

A large number of preinstrument variables may affect the determination of VWF. Standardization of assays for VWF has only recently been initiated, and a number of clinical reference plasma samples may have altered ratios of VWF antigen to activity, as well as loss of the high-molecular-weight multimers; therefore, it is imperative that each laboratory establish its own normal range and perform careful quality control. Alternatively, samples can be sent to laboratories that specialize in testing for VWF. When frozen samples are shipped, meticulous attention must be paid to the presence of contaminating platelets in the frozen plasma. If plasma is centrifuged only at 1500g for 5 to 10 minutes, the residual

Ristocetin included platelet binding for type 2B VWD

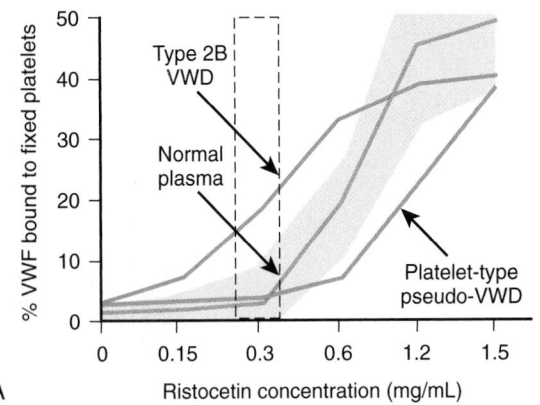

A

FVIII binding to VWF in type 2N VWD

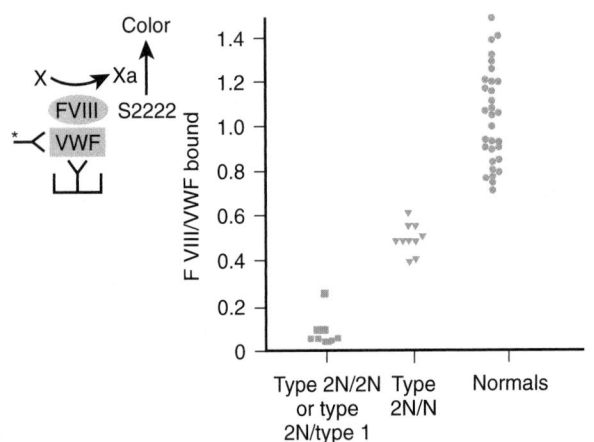

B

VWF:RCo / VWF:Ag ratio in type 2M VWD

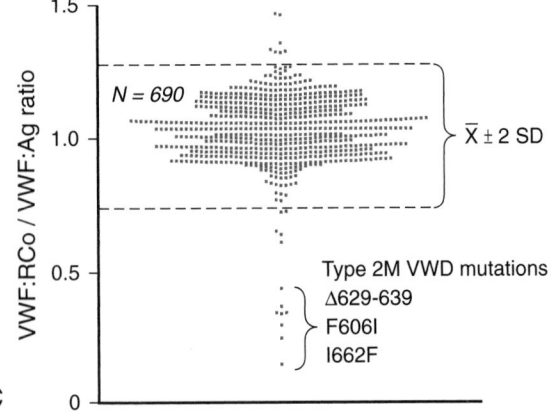

C

FIGURE 30-5. Variant forms of von Willebrand disease (VWD) can be identified by specialized phenotypic assays of patient plasma. **A,** A non-inhibitory, radiolabeled antibody is added to patient plasma, and binding to normal formalin-fixed platelets is determined with various concentrations of ristocetin. At a low concentration of ristocetin (0.3 mg/mL), normal von Willebrand factor (VWF) does not bind, but type 2B VWF exhibits increased binding that is due to a shift of the dose-response curve to the left. In contrast, plasma from a patient with platelet-type pseudo-VWD shifts to the right. Thus, if platelet aggregation with platelet-rich plasma (PRP) exhibits increased aggregation to low-dose ristocetin, type 2B VWD can be clearly differentiated from platelet-type pseudo-VWD with this dose-response curve. **B,** Patient VWF is bound to a microtiter well with a monoclonal antibody to VWF after patient factor VIII (FVIII) is removed. Recombinant FVIII is added and the activity of the bound FVIII determined by chromogenic (S2222) assay. The ratio of bound FVIII to captured VWF:Ag is determined and identifies heterozygous type 2N VWF (usually asymptomatic) and type 2N patients with absent FVIII binding (homozygous or compound heterozygous with a 2N allele and a "VWF-null" mutation allele). **C,** Ristocetin cofactor–antigen (VWF:RCo/VWF:Ag) ratio in a large group of patients evaluated with low-normal or abnormally low VWF levels. The ratios of eight patients with type 2M VWD are clearly below 2 SD of normal, and each of these patients has an identified point mutation (F1379I or I1425F) or a deletion (?1392-1402) in the A1 domain of VWF. Patients with ratios below 0.7 and normal VWF multimers are considered to have type 2M VWD. *(Courtesy of R. R. Montgomery.)*

platelet count in plasma may be as high as 30,000 to 40,000/mL. When this plasma containing platelets is frozen, platelet proteases are released, which alters the multimeric structure of VWF and results in an increase in the apparent amount of von Willebrand antigen and a decrease in the amount of activity.[311] Furthermore, refrigeration of samples of whole blood before separation of plasma at a central reference laboratory may result in reducing the amount of VWF in the plasma to be tested.[312]

Clinical Disorders That Affect Assays for von Willebrand Factor

A variety of clinical disorders may affect the level of VWF. VWF behaves as an acute phase reactant protein.[313-315] Its level is markedly elevated in collagen vascular disorders, after surgery, in pregnancy, and in conditions associated with marked endothelial stimulation, such as intravascular clotting or liver disease. The VWF level is reduced in hypothyroidism and increased in hyperthyroidism.[316-319] In hypothyroidism, VWF levels as low as 15 to 20 U/dL have been observed and therefore may be associated with clinical bleeding. The multimeric structure of plasma VWF from patients with disseminated intravascular coagulation, thrombotic thrombocytopenic purpura, hemolytic-uremic syndrome, or ventricular septal defects may be altered with the loss or gain of high-molecular-weight multimers. Pregnancy and even the clinical stress of a difficult phlebotomy, especially in anxious young children, may double or triple the level of VWF, thus making it impossible to rule out VWD without repeated testing. The stress of normal vaginal delivery has a marked stimulatory effect on levels of VWF in newborns,[320,321] hence making it difficult to rule out VWD in the neonatal period.

Clinical Manifestations and Medical History

The clinical manifestations of VWD are primarily epistaxis, ecchymoses, menorrhagia, and postoperative or postpartum bleeding.[322] Because this disorder is often mild, the initial manifestation may be bleeding after surgery such as tonsillectomy and adenoidectomy. Although both hemophilia and VWD may be accompanied by ecchymoses, large hematoma formation is more commonly associated with hemophilia, and it is rare to find hemarthrosis in VWD except in patients with severe (type 3) disease. In eliciting the patient's clinical history, it is important to determine whether the size and distribution of ecchymoses are proportional to the severity of the initiating trauma. Because both bruising and epistaxis are moderately common complaints in children and are usually a result of normal childhood trauma, identification of either severe recurrent epistaxis or bruising in unusual places (back and shoulders, upper part of the arms, and thighs) may be more suggestive of a hereditary bleeding disorder. In a normal active child, minor trauma to the anterior tibial region or the forearm may result in small ecchymoses. Recurrent epistaxis is a common complaint in childhood, but in an older child or adult it is an unusual symptom that may require further evaluation. Although screening for VWD is often performed in such patients, in the absence of ecchymoses, isolated epistaxis is not usually the result of VWD. Even though petechiae are more commonly associated with mild platelet function defects, occasional patients with VWD have petechiae.

A careful family history may identify symptoms in the parents or a sibling that are similar to the patient's. The presence of recurrent epistaxis and excessive bruising in an adult is more often abnormal and suggestive of a familial bleeding disorder. The clinician should determine whether either of the parents has experienced postoperative bleeding after major surgery, particularly tonsillectomy. Because VWD is often mild and some families learn to accept increased bruising as the norm

in their family, they may not seek medical attention until bleeding occurs in the postoperative state after either routine surgery or dental extractions. In teenagers, epistaxis or menorrhagia, when excessive, will sometimes lead to iron deficiency anemia; therefore, iron deficiency, particularly in menstruating teenage girls, may trigger evaluation for the presence of VWD. In a patient with severe (type 3) VWD, profuse epistaxis may occur and even result in shock,[323] although replacement therapy is generally needed less often in patients with type 3 VWD than in patients with hemophilia. In rare instances, VWD has been reported in association with congenital hemorrhagic telangiectasia (Osler-Weber-Rendu syndrome); telangiectases should be sought in a patient with recurrent epistaxis or significant gastrointestinal bleeding.[237,324,325] Gastrointestinal blood loss may result from either occult or overt bleeding. Although bleeding may be associated with telangiectasia, usually no such anatomic cause can be determined. Such gastrointestinal bleeding may be more common in elderly patients with VWD than in children.

In patients with mild VWD, the stress associated with certain operations (e.g., ruptured appendix) may minimize clinical bleeding symptoms, whereas relatively minor surgery, such as cosmetic or mucosal surgery, may induce a major hemorrhage in a nonstressed individual.

Fundamentals of Treatment

Appropriate treatment of VWD requires a specific diagnostic laboratory workup and correct classification of the type of VWF deficiency. If the patient produces normal VWF but its concentration is reduced, the plasma level can usually be increased by administering desmopressin (see later). If the protein that is present is abnormal (dysproteinemia), mild bleeding episodes might still be resolved with increased concentrations of the "abnormal" VWF (induced by desmopressin), but severe bleeding episodes may require the administration of or replacement with normal VWF from plasma-derived products.

Whereas in the past most products used to treat hemophilia A (factor VIII deficiency) could also be used to treat bleeding episodes in VWD, the factor VIII products most commonly used at present (recombinant factor VIII or monoclonal antibody–purified factor VIII) do not contain VWF. Today, physicians use licensed VWF/factor VIII concentrates to treat VWD because these products are labeled for both VWF and factor VIII content. Clinical trials have demonstrated their efficacy in the cessation of bleeding in patients with VWD.[326-329] It is important to emphasize that the ratio of VWF to factor VIII varies in the currently licensed VWF products Humate-P and Alphanate. The ratio of VWF to factor VIII varies from 2.0 to 0.5 and has an impact on the initial and maintenance treatment of patients with these products.[326-329] Cryoprecipitate contains substantial levels of VWF but is not used regularly because of the lack of viral attenuation treatment. The use of cryoprecipitate is reserved for areas of the world where VWF-containing concentrates are not available.

Treatment of VWD variants is discussed separately to emphasize their differences and how the molecular abnormality might affect the patient's clinical response to treatment.

Type 1 von Willebrand Disease

Type 1 VWD, the easiest and safest variant to treat, is also the most common variant (70% to 80% of all occurrences of VWD). Type 1 VWD is generally due to heterozygous deficiency of VWF. The VWF produced is structurally normal but its concentration is reduced. Most patients have levels of VWF antigen and ristocetin cofactor activity of between 20 and 40 U/dL, although the lower range of normal must be established in each individual laboratory. Patients with mild deficiencies of VWF generally do not experience spontaneous hemor-

rhage unless it is provoked by a major injury, surgical procedure, or dental extraction.

The safest therapy is to augment the patient's plasma VWF concentration by stimulating the endogenous release of VWF. This is achieved with desmopressin as described earlier in this chapter for treating mild hemophilia A.[136] More than 90% of patients with type 1 VWD have a twofold to fourfold increase in their plasma levels of VWF (Fig. 30-6) and factor VIII within 15 to 30 minutes of infusion, and they usually have the same half-life as transfused VWF or factor VIII (approximate half-life of 12 hours). Occasionally, patients are encountered who do not mount an adequate response to the infusion of desmopressin. This is particularly true for children younger than 1 to 1$\frac{1}{2}$ years of age, who may exhibit a diminished response or symptoms of hyponatremia, or both.[141] It is usually recommended that patients in whom VWD is diagnosed be given a therapeutic trial of desmopressin to determine their responsiveness to the drug so

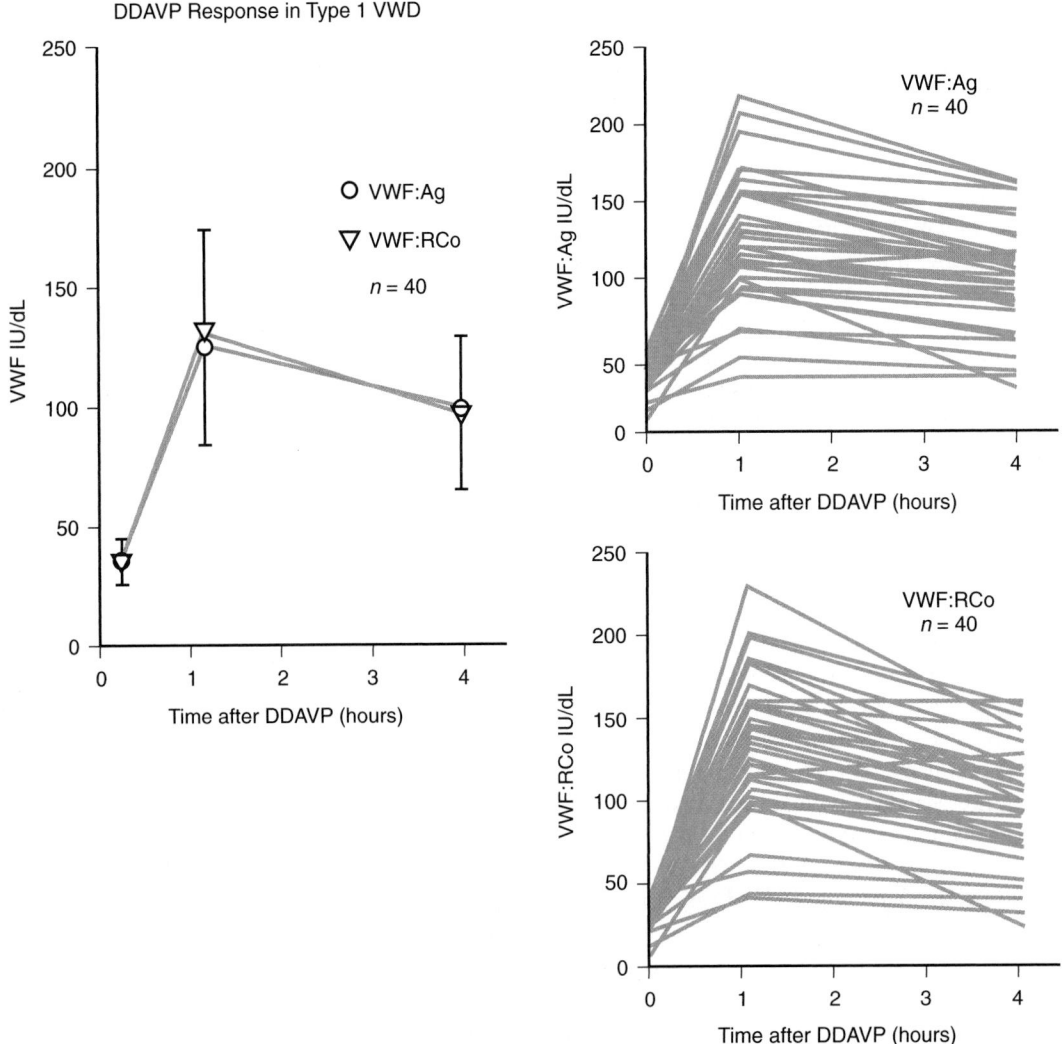

FIGURE 30-6. Desmopressin (DDAVP, 0.3 µg/kg intravenously) was administered to 40 patients with type 1 von Willebrand disease (VWD). Plasma samples were obtained before infusion and at 1 and 4 hours after infusion. The *left-hand* panel illustrates the mean and 1-SD range for these 40 individuals. The *right-hand* panels illustrate the consistency of the response in these 40 individuals for both von Willebrand factor antigen (VWF:Ag) and ristocetin cofactor (VWF:RCo) activity. *(Courtesy of J. P. Scott and R. R. Montgomery.)*

that when future therapy is required, the clinician knows that this form of treatment will be effective. The treatment of choice for type 1 VWD is the administration of desmopressin. The dose of desmopressin is 0.3 μg/kg of body weight administered intravenously in 25 to 50 mL of saline over a period of 20 to 30 minutes. This represents the most effective route of administration. Alternatively, subcutaneous injections of desmopressin at approximately the same dose have been used effectively.[330] Stimate (1.5 mg/mL DDAVP) is a concentrated form of desmopressin that has been shown to be effective.[331,332] The effective dose in teenagers and adults is 2 puffs—1 puff (150 μg) in each nostril for a total dose of 300 μg. Children weighing less than 50 kg should receive 1 puff containing 150 μg. For the drug to be effective, the child should be old enough to be able to cooperate with administration of the drug. The clinician should be aware that a diluted intranasal solution of desmopressin (100 μg/mL) (DDAVP) is available for patients with diabetes insipidus and enuresis. This latter dilute form is ineffective in patients with bleeding disorders.

Although one or two doses dose of desmopressin combined with either aminocaproic acid or tranexamic acid (see discussion under hemophilia A earlier) is generally effective for dental extractions, major surgery usually requires maintenance of increased levels of VWF and factor VIII until healing has occurred. For most patients, repeated infusions of desmopressin at 12- to 24-hour intervals are effective, but tachyphylaxis may develop.[140,333] Thus, preinfusion and 30- to 60-minute postinfusion measurements of either VWF:RCo or VWF:Ag should be performed to establish the continued clinical responsiveness of the patient to desmopressin if used repeatedly. If a patient with type 1 VWD has a very low level of VWF (15 to 20 U/dL) and is to undergo major surgery, the levels achieved after desmopressin may be insufficient even though a twofold increase is achieved. Such patients, like those who either show no response to desmopressin or have tachyphylaxis, must be treated with plasma-derived VWF/factor VIII.

The current Food and Drug Administration (FDA)-licensed products that contain both VWF and factor VIII for the treatment of VWD are Humate-P and Alphanate. Studies have compared these and other products for VWF and factor VIII content, as well as for VWF multimer content.[219] In these comparative studies, Humate-P usually has the larger forms of VWF multimers, similar to normal plasma. The two products also differ in their relative concentration of factor VIII, with Humate-P containing approximately 0.5 IU factor VIII per IU VWF:RCo and Alphanate containing 2.0 IU factor VIII per IU VWF:RCo. Currently, Humate-P is approved by the FDA for surgery and urgent bleeding in patients with types 1, 2, and 3 VWD, and Alphanate is approved for surgery in patient with types 1 and 2 VWD. Other intermediate-purity factor VIII and VWF concentrates are sometimes used off-label, but such use is not currently recommended.

The dose of VWF concentrate is calculated as follows:

Dose of VWF : RCo =
U/dL (percent) desired rise in plasma VWF ×
Body weight (kg) × 0.75

One unit per kilogram of VWF will increase the plasma level 1.5 U/dL. In preparing a patient for surgery, one usually tries to correct the plasma level to about 100 U/dL; plasma levels should be maintained at greater than 50 to 60 U/dL for 3 to 7 days after major surgery. For dental extractions or minor surgery, such as the procedure for a laceration, the patient can generally be treated with one or two infusions of VWF concentrate along with antifibrinolytic therapy.

Type 1C or the Vicenza Variant of von Willebrand Disease

Within the type 1 VWD group are individuals with accelerated clearance of their VWF who usually have plasma VWF:Ag and VWF:RCo levels below 12 to 20 IU/dL and factor VIII below 30 IU/dL. The initial prototype for this disorder was termed the Vicenza variant because of a number of families who were identified in Italy and subsequently shown to have a common mutation (R1205H in the VWF D3 domain).[244,334,335] These patients have also been shown to have larger than normal VWF multimers and normal levels of platelet VWF. Recently, four additional families were identified with this phenotype and different mutations in the D3 and D4 domains (W1144G and S2179F).[235] This group is now referred to collectively as type 1C because they have type 1 laboratory results secondary to increased clearance. This group of individuals has a normal level of VWF synthesis. When DDAVP is administered, they exhibit hyperresponsiveness, and their plasma VWF will increase 5- to 10-fold, but the half life is 2 to 3 hours rather than the normal 10 to 14 hours.[235,336] Furthermore, the half-life of factor VIII released by DDAVP is similarly accelerated.[235] Infused VWF and factor VIII have a normal half-life reflecting the origin of the clinical phenotype to the presence of endogenous abnormal VWF. Thus, treatment with DDAVP will normalize the plasma concentration of VWF and factor VIII, but not for the normal time period. Minor bleeding can be approached with DDAVP, but major bleeding or surgery may require VWF concentrates to maintain the level of VWF activity and factor VIII in the normal range. In this group, assays of VWFpp versus VWF:Ag are diagnostically elevated in the plasma of these patients and reflect the accelerated clearance of VWF but not VWFpp.[235]

Type 3 von Willebrand Disease

Type 3 VWD is usually due to autosomal recessive or compound (double) heterozygous inheritance of a null VWF allele. Thus, the level of plasma VWF is usually undetectable, but the factor VIII level is generally less than 6 U/dL. This plasma level of factor VIII is the steady-state level of factor VIII in the absence of its carrier protein VWF. Giving such patients desmopressin is not effective because their cells do not contain endogenous VWF and the DDAVP-induced release of factor VIII is dependent on endogenous synthesis of VWF.[215] Sometimes a therapeutic trial of desmopressin in these patients is worthwhile because it might identify patients with type 1C who might have VWF:Ag levels below the detection limit for VWF:Ag in some laboratories.[336] In patients with undetectable VWF or an inadequate response to desmopressin, bleeding symptoms must be managed with plasma-derived VWF or factor VIII/VWF concentrates. Patients with type 3 VWD may have spontaneous bleeding, including profound epistaxis, subcutaneous hemorrhage, or rarely, joint bleeding as seen in patients with hemophilia.[337,338] In such situations, management is similar to that for patients with severe hemophilia and consists of factor VIII concentrates that contain normal or nearly normal VWF. Survival of the transfused VWF is virtually identical to that for factor VIII (see earlier). Levels similar to those used for treatment of hemophilia, both preoperatively and postoperatively, should be maintained for adequate hemostasis. Because the licensed concentrates Humate-P and Alphanate have different ratios of factor VIII to VWF, care must be exercised to ensure adequate factor VIII levels with the first infusion and to avoid excessively high factor VIII levels after several days of intensive or postsurgical treatment.[339]

A number of centers are now using prophylaxis to prevent bleeding in type 3 VWD patients if clinically indicated because of the number or severity of recurrent bleeding.[340-343] Since the half-lives of VWF and factor VIII are comparable, the approach is similar to that used in hemophilia A.

In Europe a concentrate containing very little factor VIII is approved, but these products are not available in the United States.[344-348] Because synthesis of factor VIII is normal in a type 3 VWD patient, providing VWF alone avoids the problems of elevated factor VIII in patients treated with factor VIII containing VWF concentrates.[349,350] Figure 30-7 illustrates the delayed rise in endogenous factor VIII when a patient with severe type 3 VWD is administered a concentrate primarily containing just VWF. Currently, clinical trials using recombinant VWF are being initiated, and it is hoped that this product will be available in the near future.

In patients with type 3 VWD and large gene deletions, there is an increased likelihood of antibody development.[351,352] Recombinant VIIa has been reported to be effective in some patients with severe VWD with alloantibodies.[353-355]

Type 2 Variant Types of von Willebrand Disease

Type 2A von Willebrand Disease

In type 2A VWD, there is a loss of intermediate- and high-molecular-weight multimers as a result of two dif-

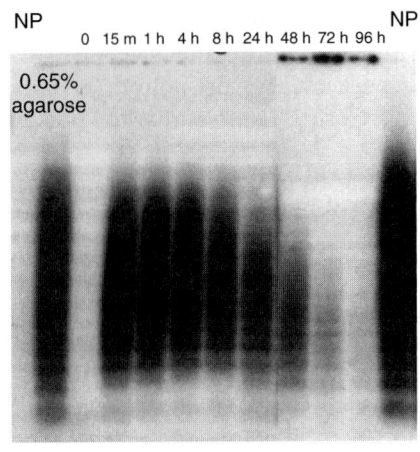

Sample	1	2	3	4	5	6	7	8	9
Time	0	15 m	1 h	4 h	8 h	24 h	48 h	72 h	96 h
VWF:Ag	<1	192	184	161	123	55	16	9	3
VWF:RCO	<3	180	160	140	110	53	14	8	<3
FVIII:C	3.1	8.7	14	28	46	71	55	34	20

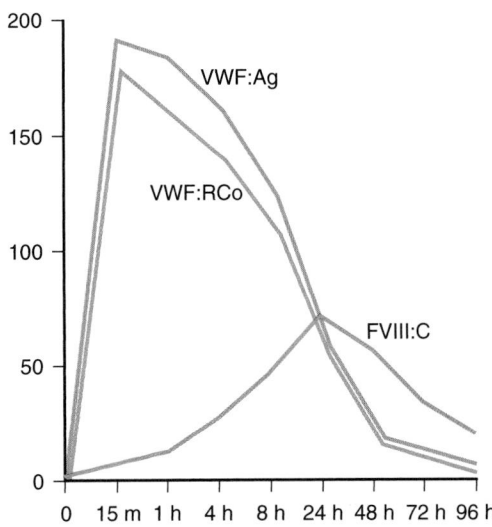

FIGURE 30-7. A patient with severe type 3 von Willebrand disease was infused with a von Willebrand factor (VWF) concentrate containing minimal amounts of factor VIII (FVIII). Within 15 minutes after infusion, VWF antigen (VWF:Ag) and ristocetin cofactor (VWF:RCo) are markedly increased. At 24 hours the factor VIII level in the patient has increased to 71 U/dL because of the endogenous production of factor VIII. NP, normal plasma. *(Courtesy of D. Menache-Aronson, J. C. Gill, and R. R. Montgomery.)*

ferent mechanisms that were defined in the first molecular report of VWF mutations in this variant form of VWD.[356] One group is characterized by failure to synthesize intermediate- and high-molecular-weight VWF multimers (referred to as type 2A[1] in Fig. 30-2); in the other group, full-length VWF is synthesized, stored, and released, but the VWF undergoes rapid proteolysis by ADAMTS-13 (referred to as 2A[2] in Fig. 30-2).[305,356] Thus, if desmopressin is administered, the correction of VWF multimers is transient, and the bleeding time may or may not shorten.[357] Therefore, patients with type 2A VWD may require treatment with plasma-derived factor VIII/VWF concentrate containing normal VWF multimers (see earlier). It may be possible to treat minor bleeding episodes and bleeding after dental extractions with the brief increase in plasma levels that follows desmopressin administration, but a trial of DDAVP and measurement of in vitro survival of VWF:RCo are required to determine potential efficacy.

Type 2B von Willebrand Disease

Type 2B VWD is due to a mutant VWF molecule that binds spontaneously to platelets under physiologic shear; it results in clearance of the highest-molecular-weight multimers and usually mild thrombocytopenia.[238,239,358-360] The thrombocytopenia is caused by spontaneous agglutination and clearance of platelets as a consequence of the abnormal VWF and results in loss of the high-molecular-weight multimers. Thus, stress, pregnancy, or surgery can trigger increased levels of VWF with resultant increased agglutination of platelets and enhanced thrombocytopenia.[361,362] Although one might assume that desmopressin would not be efficacious, studies have demonstrated its effectiveness in some patients.[363,364] Therefore, for mild bleeding, a trial of desmopressin can be initiated and the platelet count and bleeding monitored. For internal bleeding or major surgery, administration of VWF/factor VIII concentrate is generally required. Although thrombocytopenia is present, therapy should be focused on correcting the plasma VWF level. The dose is identical to that used for the treatment of severe type 1 or type 3 VWD. If profound thrombocytopenia is present, concomitant administration of platelets may be necessary. Administration of platelets alone without replacement of VWF is not usually effective. Sometimes, pseudothrombocytopenia may be present and cause the platelet count to be lower because of platelet clumping.[363,365,366]

Although *platelet-type pseudo-VWD* is due to a defect in the platelet GPIb receptor[367,368] (Chapter 29), it is considered in the differential diagnosis of type 2B VWD because of the loss of high-molecular-weight VWF multimers and reduced levels of VWF. The plasma assays of VWF are identical to those for patients with type 2B VWD, but these disorders must be distinguished because of the markedly different approaches to therapy (see Fig. 30-3). Platelet-type pseudo-VWD should be treated with platelets.[369] Although the plasma level of VWF is reduced and the distribution of multimers is abnormal, these findings are secondary to the abnormal GPIb receptor on platelets. Thus, as platelets are appropriately used to treat the bleeding disorder, the secondary VWF abnormalities will actually lessen. Standard doses of platelets should be used to treat hemorrhage. If the hemorrhage is severe or if bleeding persists, VWF/factor VIII concentrates may be needed to correct the secondary deficiency of VWF. Similar to the normal platelet counts found in patients with intrinsic platelet disorders, the increment in platelets is not necessarily a good measure of the response to

therapy because a nearly normal number of abnormal platelets will remain in the circulation. Improvement in the hemostatic abnormality may not become evident until a large proportion of the platelets are replaced by normal platelets from transfusion.

Type 2N von Willebrand Disease

Type 2N VWD is the result of an abnormal VWF molecule with reduced binding of factor VIII.[74,370,371] This leads to accelerated clearance of the unbound factor VIII and a resultant reduction in plasma factor VIII as compared with the level of VWF.[372] In fact, mild hemophilia A may be misdiagnosed in some of these patients. It appears that the phenotype is clinically expressed only in the presence of a second allele carrying a *null* allele or a second type 2N VWD allele (see Fig. 30-5). Therefore, if the plasma VWF level is reduced modestly and the factor VIII level is even more reduced or if a patient with mild hemophilia A is given factor VIII and the half-life is markedly shortened, type 2N VWD should be considered. A specific assay has been developed in which the patient's VWF is captured with a monoclonal antibody in a microtiter well, factor VIII is removed by changes in pH or salt concentration or the addition of thrombin, and binding of recombinant factor VIII is determined. Decreased affinity is the hallmark of type 2N VWD (see Fig. 30-5).[74,240,302] Because symptomatic patients are either homozygous or compound heterozygous, administration of desmopressin might have only a transient effect on factor VIII levels.[372] Administration of recombinant or monoclonal factor VIII would similarly have only transient effects. For a major bleeding episode or for preparation for surgery, the preferred treatment is a plasma-derived VWF/factor VIII concentrate.

Type 2M von Willebrand Disease

Type 2M VWD is the result of a mutation in VWF that decreases the interaction of VWF with the platelet GPIb receptor, thereby resulting in reduced VWF:RCo—the converse of that seen with type 2B VWD.[290,291,373,374] Similar to type 2A, plasma VWF exhibits discordance between VWF:Ag and VWF:RCo (see Fig. 30-3), but patients with type 2M VWD have normal VWF multimers, whereas those with type 2A VWD have abnormal multimers. If the VWF:Ag and VWF:RCo assays are carefully standardized, the ratio of VWF ristocetin cofactor to VWF antigen may be used to diagnose type 2M VWD. Figure 30-5 demonstrates the relationship of these two assays in 690 persons with normal VWF multimers and VWF:Ag or VWF:RCo levels of less than 55 IU/dL. The VWF protein can be released by DDAVP, but the released VWF exhibits abnormal interaction with platelets. Thus, for major bleeding episodes or in preparation for surgery, replacement therapy with VWF concentrates should be given. Recently, a study of type 1 VWD in two large cohorts has identified patients with mild type 2M VWD,[218,227,375] but whether clinical treatment is different in these patients will require additional study.

Acquired von Willebrand Disease

Acquired VWD may be caused by at least three pathophysiologic mechanisms: (1) an acquired clinical state such as hypothyroidism resulting in decreased VWF synthesis, (2) an acquired autoimmune state in which an autoantibody develops against VWF and results in accelerated clearance of VWF (and usually factor VIII), or (3) a clinical disease develops in which VWF structure and function may be altered.

Congenital or acquired hypothyroidism can result in reduced VWF and bleeding symptoms.[318,376-379] Treating these patients to make them euthyroid results in normalization of the VWF level. If acute bleeding is present, the patient can generally be managed as would a patient with type 1 VWD—by administration of DDAVP or VWF concentrate. In hypothyroid patients, the VWFpp level is usually reduced in parallel with the VWF level and suggests normal clearance of VWF.

Acquired VWD can also be the result of an isolated acquired autoantibody to VWF, autoantibody to VWF in autoimmune diseases (e.g., systemic lupus erythematosus), or monoclonal gammopathies.[380-382] Assays for an inhibitor of VWF:RCo activity are generally negative because the autoantibody is directed against other regions of VWF and promotes only clearance. An abnormal VWFpp/VWF:Ag ratio can be used to demonstrate increased clearance of VWF.[235,299,383] In monoclonal gammopathies, VWF multimers may demonstrate loss of high-molecular-weight multimers.[384-387] Either plasmapheresis or a trial of intravenous immunoglobulin, or both, may sometimes be beneficial.[388,389] Desmopressin may also induce a transient rise in the VWF level, but its survival may be markedly reduced. Recently, some success has been achieved with recombinant VIIa.[390-392]

Wilms' tumor has been reported to cause acquired VWD. In at least one case, synthesis of VWF was still present in endothelial cells in the removed kidney, and in another study, the elevated hyaluronidase resulted in a reduced amount of VWF by Laurell quantitative immunoelectrophoresis.[393-396] Acquired loss of high-molecular-weight VWF multimers has been identified in children with ventricular septal defects[294] and in others with pulmonary hypertension.[397-399]

Von Willebrand Disease without Known Subtyping

Occasionally, a clinician is called on to treat VWD when the appropriate subtype is not known and the patient's acute condition does not permit taking the time to collect appropriate samples to determine the subtype. In such instances, a blood sample should be obtained for appropriate subtyping of VWD, followed by a carefully monitored therapeutic trial of desmopressin, VWF concentrates, or both. The response to such treatment should be monitored by close observation of the platelet count and the response of VWF activity and its survival. In a patient with known but untyped VWD and major

hemorrhage, VWF/factor VIII concentrates are probably the preferred treatment. This therapeutic approach will appropriately treat all forms of VWD, with the exception of platelet-type pseudo-VWD. The use of desmopressin may be either ineffective or exacerbate thrombocytopenia in patients with type 2A or 2B VWD, respectively.

Thus, therapy for VWD must be closely integrated with the correct laboratory diagnosis and often requires intensive laboratory evaluation through one episode of the treatment. However, once an appropriate response is obtained with a given therapy, laboratory monitoring can be greatly curtailed.

General Comments on the Treatment of von Willebrand Disease

Although the previous section presents the current clinical approach to VWD, many unanswered questions remain. Our current clinical approach may overdiagnose type 1 VWD because of the presence of low plasma VWF levels (see the earlier section on low VWF versus type 1 VWD). Because these patients in general have a preexisting history of excessive bleeding, we do not always know the contribution of their low VWF to these symptoms. We therefore generally treat them as having VWD. However, in postsurgical states in normal individuals, it is not uncommon to have VWF and factor VIII levels in excess of 200 to 300 IU/dL, yet we usually focus our therapy only to achieve a hemostatic level above 60 to 100 IU/dL. Whether the normal postsurgical elevation is a pathologic state brought on by surgical stress or a physiologic response to adapt to the surgical stress remains unknown. Normally, VWF is present in plasma, endothelial cells, platelets, and subendothelial matrix. When we treat a patient with type 3 VWD, we normalize only plasma VWF; endothelial cells, platelets, and subendothelium remain abnormal and their relative contribution to hemostasis is not fully defined. If clinical bleeding continues in the absence of adequate plasma VWF and factor VIII, consideration should be given to platelet transfusion as a means of providing normal platelet VWF.[400]

Future of Gene Therapy for von Willebrand Disease

Although effective gene therapy for hemophilia has still not been realized, VWD gene transfer into endothelial cells ex vivo has been achieved.[401-403] Some of the early studies using chimeraplasty offered potential hope for bypassing some of the point mutations that result in VWD.[404] More recent studies have brought into question whether this approach will optimally be successful.[405]

In the porcine model of VWD, bone marrow transplantation has been demonstrated to be a successful means of replacing platelet VWF; however, platelet VWF does not result in a detectible level in plasma even thought there may be some benefit from platelet VWF alone.[406-409]

REFERENCES

1. Rosner F. Hemophilia in the Talmud and rabbinic writings. Ann Intern Med. 1969;70:833-837.
2. Hopff F. Uber die Haemophilie oder die Erbliche. Wurzburg, Germany, CW Becker, 1828.
3. Brinkhous K. A short history of hemophilia with some comments on the word "hemophilia." In Brinkhous K, Hemker HC (eds). Handbook of Hemophilia. New York, Elsevier, 2001, p 3.
4. Wright AE. On a method of determining the condition of blood coagulability for clinical and experimental purposes, and on the effect of administration of calcium salts in hemophilia and actual or threatened haemorrhage. Br Med J. 1893;2:223.
5. Brinkhous KM. Clotting defect in hemophilia: deficiency in a plasma factor required for platelet utilization. Proc Soc Exp Biol Med. 1947;66:117-120.
6. Quick AJ. Studies on the enigma of the haemostatic dysfunction of hemophilia. Am J Med Sci. 1947;214:272-280.
7. Biggs R, Douglas AS, MacFarlane RG, et al. Christmas disease: a condition previously mistaken for haemophilia. Br Med J. 1952;2:1378-1382.
8. Patek AJ. Hemophilia II: some properties of a substance obtained from normal plasma effective in accelerating the clotting of hemophilic blood. J Clin Invest. 1937;16:113-124.
9. Pool JG, Hershgold EJ, Papenhagen AR. High potency anti-haemophilic factor concentrate prepared from cryoglobulin precipitate. Nature. 1964;203:312.
10. Tullis JL, Melin M, Jurigian P. Clinical use of human prothrombin complexes. N Engl J Med. 1965;273:667-674.
11. Abildgaard CF, Simone JV, Corrigan JJ, et al. Treatment of hemophilia with glycine-precipitated factor 8. N Engl J Med. 1966;275:471-475.
12. McDougal JS, Martin LS, Cort SP, et al. Thermal inactivation of the acquired immunodeficiency syndrome virus, human T lymphotropic virus-III/lymphadenopathy-associated virus, with special reference to antihemophilic factor. J Clin Invest. 1985;76:875-877.
13. Mannucci PM, Zanetti AR, Colombo M. Prospective study of hepatitis after factor VIII concentrate exposed to hot vapour. Br J Haematol. 1988;68:427-430.
14. Mannucci PM, Schimpf K, Brettler DB, et al. Low risk for hepatitis C in hemophiliacs given a high-purity, pasteurized factor VIII concentrate. International Study Group. Ann Intern Med. 1990;113:27-32.
15. Graham JB, Buckwalter JA, Hartley LJ, Brinkhous KM. Canine hemophilia: observations on the course, the clotting anomaly, and the effect of blood transfusions. J Exp Med. 1949;90:97-111.
16. Gitschier J, Wood WI, Goralka TM, et al. Characterization of the human factor VIII gene. Nature. 1984;312:326-330.
17. Vehar GA, Keyt B, Eaton D, et al. Structure of human factor VIII. Nature. 1984;312:337-342.
18. Toole JJ, Knopf JL, Wozney JM, et al. Molecular cloning of a cDNA encoding human antihaemophilic factor. Nature. 1984;312:342-347.
19. Yoshitake S, Schach BG, Foster DC, et al. Nucleotide sequence of the gene for human factor IX (antihemophilic factor B). Biochemistry. 1985;24:3736-3750.
20. White GC, McMillan CW, Kingdon HS, Shoemaker CB. Use of recombinant antihemophilic factor in the treatment of two patients with classic hemophilia. N Engl J Med. 1989;320:166-170.
21. Schwartz RS, Abildgaard CF, Aledort LM, et al. Human recombinant DNA–derived antihemophilic factor (factor VIII) in the treatment of hemophilia A. recombinant Factor VIII Study Group. N Engl J Med. 1990;323:1800-1805.
22. Lusher JM. Prophylaxis in children with hemophilia: is it the optimal treatment? Thromb Haemost. 1997;78:726-729.
23. Lofqvist T, Nilsson IM, Berntorp E, Pettersson H. Haemophilia prophylaxis in young patients—a long-term follow-up. J Intern Med. 1997;241:395-400.
24. Brinkhous KM, Sigman JL, Read MS, et al. Recombinant human factor IX: replacement therapy, prophylaxis, and pharmacokinetics in canine hemophilia B. Blood. 1996;88:2603-2610.
25. Manco-Johnson MJ, Abshire TC, Shapiro AD, et al. Prophylaxis versus episodic treatment to prevent joint disease in boys with severe hemophilia. N Engl J Med. 2007;357:535-544.
26. Manco-Johnson M. Comparing prophylaxis with episodic treatment in haemophilia A: implications for clinical practice. Haemophilia. 2007;13(Suppl 2):4-9.
27. Manco-Johnson MJ, Nuss R, Geraghty S, et al. Results of secondary prophylaxis in children with severe hemophilia. Am J Hematol. 1994;47:113-117.
28. Lawson JH, Mann KG. Cooperative activation of human factor IX by the human extrinsic pathway of blood coagulation. J Biol Chem. 1991;266:11317-11327.
29. Repke D, Gemmell CH, Guha A, et al. Hemophilia as a defect of the tissue factor pathway of blood coagulation: effect of factors VIII and IX on factor X activation in a continuous-flow reactor. Proc Natl Acad Sci U S A. 1990;87:7623-7627.
30. Vander VP, Giles AR. A detailed morphological evaluation of the evolution of the haemostatic plug in normal, factor VII and factor VIII deficient dogs. Br J Haematol. 1988;70:345-355.
31. Kaneshiro MM, Mielke CH Jr, Kasper CK, Rapaport SI. Bleeding time after aspirin in disorders of intrinsic clotting. N Engl J Med. 1969;281:1039-1042.
32. Pilot Study of Hemophilia Treatment in the United States. National Heart, Lung, and Blood Institute Resource Studies. Washington, DC, US Government Printing Office, 1972.
33. Ramgren O. A clinical and medico-social study of haemophilia in Sweden. Acta Med Scand Suppl. 1962;379:111-190.
34. Study to Evaluate the Supply-Demand Relationships for AHF and PTC through 1980. National Heart, Lung and Blood Institute Study. Washington, DC, US Government Printing Office, 1977.
35. Schneider T. Circumcision and "uncircumcision." S Afr Med J. 1976;50:556-558.
36. Bray GL, Luban NL. Hemophilia presenting with intracranial hemorrhage. An approach to the infant with intracranial bleeding and coagulopathy. Am J Dis Child. 1987;141:1215-1217.

37. Kulkarni R, Lusher JM. Intracranial and extracranial hemorrhages in newborns with hemophilia: a review of the literature. J Pediatr Hematol Oncol. 1999;21:289-295.

38. Ljung R, Lindgren AC, Petrini P, Tengborn L. Normal vaginal delivery is to be recommended for haemophilia carrier gravidae. Acta Paediatr. 1994;83:609-611.

39. Ljung R, Petrini P, Nilsson IM. Diagnostic symptoms of severe and moderate haemophilia A and B. A survey of 140 cases. Acta Paediatr Scand. 1990;79:196-200.

40. Aronstam A, Rainsford SG, Painter MJ. Patterns of bleeding in adolescents with severe haemophilia A. Br Med J. 1979;1:469-470.

41. Gill JC, Thometz J, Scott JP, Montgomery RR. Musculoskeletal problems in hemophilia. In Hilgartner MV, Pochedly C (eds): Hemophilia in the Child and Adult, 3rd ed. New York, Raven Press, 1989.

42. Arnold WD, Hilgartner MW. Hemophilic arthropathy. Current concepts of pathogenesis and management. J Bone Joint Surg Am. 1977;59:287-305.

43. Gilbert MS. Musculoskeletal manifestations of hemophilia. Mt Sinai J Med. 1977;44:339-358.

44. McVerry BA, Voke J, Vicary FR, Dormandy KM. Ultrasonography in the management of haemophilia. Lancet. 1977;1:872-874.

45. Eyster ME, Gill FM, Blatt PM, et al. Central nervous system bleeding in hemophiliacs. Blood. 1978;51:1179-1188.

46. Andes WA, Wulff K, Smith WB. Head trauma in hemophilia. A prospective study. Arch Intern Med. 1984;144:1981-1983.

47. Martinowitz U, Heim M, Tadmor R, et al. Intracranial hemorrhage in patients with hemophilia. Neurosurgery. 1986;18:538-541.

48. Kasper CK, Boylen AL, Ewing NP, et al. Hematologic management of hemophilia A for surgery. JAMA. 1985;253:1279-1283.

49. White GC, Beebe A, Nielsen B. Recombinant factor IX. Thromb Haemost. 1997;78:261-265.

50. White G, Shapiro A, Ragni M, et al. Clinical evaluation of recombinant factor IX. Semin Hematol. 1998;35:33-38.

51. Forbes CD, Barr RD, Reid G, et al. Tranexamic acid in control of haemorrhage after dental extraction in haemophilia and Christmas disease. Br Med J. 1972;2:311-313.

52. Tavenner RW. Epsilon-aminocaproic acid in the treatment of haemophilia and Christmas disease with special reference to the extraction of teeth. Br Dent J. 1968;124:19-22.

53. Bjorlin G, Nilsson IM. Tooth extractions in hemophiliacs after administration of a single dose of factor VIII or factor IX concentrate supplemented with AMCA. Oral Surg Oral Med Oral Pathol. 1973;36:482-489.

54. Rizza CR, Kernoff PB, Matthews JM, et al. A comparison of coagulation factor replacement with and without prednisolone in the treatment of haematuria in haemophilia and Christmas disease. Thromb Haemost. 1977;37:86-90.

55. Harris ED Jr, Parker HG, Radin EL, Krane SM. Effects of proteolytic enzymes on structural and mechanical properties of cartilage. Arthritis Rheum. 1972;15:497-503.

56. Mainardi CL, Levine PH, Werb Z, Harris ED Jr. Proliferative synovitis in hemophilia: biochemical and morphologic observations. Arthritis Rheum. 1978;21:137-144.

57. Kasper CK, Dietrich SL, Rapaport SI. Hemophilia prophylaxis with factor VIII concentrate. Arch Intern Med. 1970;125:1004-1009.

58. Esser P, Weller M, Heimann K, Wiedemann P. [Thrombospondin and its importance in proliferative retinal diseases.] Fortschr Ophthalmol. 1991;88:337-340.

59. Wiedel JD. Arthroscopic synovectomy for chronic hemophilic synovitis of the knee. Arthroscopy. 1985;1:205-209.

60. Fernandez-Palazzi F, de Bosch NB, de Vargas AF. Radioactive synovectomy in haemophilic haemarthrosis. Follow-up of fifty cases. Scand J Haematol Suppl. 1984;40:291-300.

61. Dunn AL, Manco-Johnson M, Busch MT, et al. Leukemia and P32 radionuclide synovectomy for hemophilic arthropathy. J Thromb Haemost. 2005;3:1541-1542.

62. Rovere GD, Webb LX, Nicastro JF, et al. Total knee replacement in the adult hemophilic patient. Contemp Orthop. 1985;11:15-22.

63. Beeton K, Rodriguez-Merchan EC, Alltree J. Total joint arthroplasty in haemophilia. Haemophilia. 2000;6:474-481.

64. Kamineni S, Adams RA, O'Driscoll SW, Morrey BF. Hemophilic arthropathy of the elbow treated by total elbow replacement. A case series. J Bone Joint Surg Am. 2004;86:584-589.

65. Nisen P, Stamberg J, Ehrenpreis R, et al. The molecular basis of severe hemophilia B in a girl. N Engl J Med. 1986;315:1139-1142.

66. Gilchrist GS, Hammond D, Melnyk J. Hemophilia A in a phenotypically normal female with XX-XO mosaicism. N Engl J Med. 1965;273:1402-1406.

67. Lusher JM, Zuelzer WW, Evans RK. Hemophilia A in chromosomal female subjects. J Pediatr. 1969;74:265-271.

68. Lusher JM, McMillan CW. Severe factor VIII and factor IX deficiency in females. Am J Med. 1978;65:637-648.

69. Holmberg L. Genetic studies in a family with testicular feminization, haemophilia A and colour blindness. Clin Genet. 1972;3:253-257.

70. Andrejev NJ, Korenevskaya MI, Rutberg RA, et al. Haemophilia A in a patient with testicular feminization. Thromb Diath Haemorrh. 1975;33:208-216.

71. Bithell TC, Pizarro A, MacDiarmid WD. Variant of factor IX deficiency in female with 45, X Turner's syndrome. Blood. 1970;36:169-179.

72. Neuschatz J, Necheles TF. Hemophilia B in a phenotypically normal girl with XX (ring) XO mosaicism. Acta Haematol. 1973;49:108-113.

73. Chuansumrit A, Sasanakul W, Goodeve A, et al. Inversion of intron 22 of the factor VIII gene in a girl with severe hemophilia A and Turner's syndrome. Thromb Haemost. 1999;82:1379.

74. Montgomery RR, Hathaway WE, Johnson J, et al. A variant of von Willebrand disease with abnormal expression of factor VIII procoagulant activity. Blood. 1982;60:201-207.

75. Barna L, Triplett DA. Use of the activated partial thromboplastin time for the diagnosis of congenital coagulation

disorders: problems and possible solutions. Ric Clin Lab. 1989;19:345-354.

76. Hathaway WE, Assmus SL, Montgomery RR, Dubansky AS. Activated partial thromboplastin time and minor coagulopathies. Am J Clin Pathol. 1979;71:22-25.

77. Marlar RA, Bauer PJ, Endres-Brooks JL, et al. Comparison of the sensitivity of commercial APTT reagents in the detection of mild coagulopathies. Am J Clin Pathol. 1984;82:436-439.

78. Brandt JT, Arkin CF, Bovill EG, et al. Evaluation of APTT reagent sensitivity to factor IX and factor IX assay performance. Results from the College of American Pathologists Survey Program. Arch Pathol Lab Med. 1990;114:135-141.

79. Takase T, Rotblat F, Goodall AH, et al. Production of factor VIII deficient plasma by immunodepletion using three monoclonal antibodies. Br J Haematol. 1987;66:497-502.

80. Peake IR, Bloom AL, Giddings JC, Ludlam CA. An immunoradiometric assay for procoagulant factor VIII antigen: results in haemophilia, von Willebrand disease and fetal plasma and serum. Br J Haematol. 1979;42:269-281.

81. Girma JP, Lavergne JM, Meyer D, Larrieu MJ. Immunoradiometric assay of factor VIII: coagulant antigen using four human antibodies. Study of 27 cases of haemophilia A. Br J Haematol. 1981;47:269-282.

82. Lazarchick J, Hoyer LW. Immunoradiometric measurement of the factor VIII procoagulant antigen. J Clin Invest. 1978;62:1048-1052.

83. Kasper CK, Osterud B, Minami JY, et al. Hemophilia B: characterization of genetic variants and detection of carriers. Blood. 1977;50:351-366.

84. Pechet L, Tiarks CY, Stevens J, et al. Relationship of factor IX antigen and coagulant in hemophilia B patients and carriers. Thromb Haemost. 1979;40:465-477.

85. Giles AR, Verbruggen B, Rivard GE, et al. A detailed comparison of the performance of the standard versus the Nijmegen modification of the Bethesda assay in detecting factor VIII: C inhibitors in the haemophilia A population of Canada. Association of Hemophilia Centre Directors of Canada. Factor VIII/IX Subcommittee of Scientific and Standardization Committee of International Society on Thrombosis and Haemostasis. Thromb Haemost. 1998;79:872-875.

86. Gitschier J, Wood WI, Tuddenham EG, et al. Detection and sequence of mutations in the factor VIII gene of haemophiliacs. Nature. 1985;315:427-430.

87. Antonarakis SE, Waber PG, Kittur SD, et al. Hemophilia A. Detection of molecular defects and of carriers by DNA analysis. N Engl J Med. 1985;313:842-848.

88. Furie B, Furie BC. Molecular basis of hemophilia. Semin Hematol. 1990;27:270-285.

89. Lawn RM, Wood WI, Gitschier J, et al. Cloned factor VIII and the molecular genetics of hemophilia. Cold Spring Harbor Symp Quant Biol. 1986;51:365-369.

90. Antonarakis SE, Copeland KL, Carpenter RJ Jr, et al. Prenatal diagnosis of haemophilia A by factor VIII gene analysis. Lancet. 1985;1:1407-1409.

91. Antonarakis SE, Kazazian HH, Gitschier J, et al. Molecular etiology of factor VIII deficiency in hemophilia A. Adv Exp Med Biol. 1995;386:19-34.

92. Lawn RM, Vehar GA. The molecular genetics of hemophilia. Sci Am. 1986;254:48-54.

93. Graham JB, Rizza CR, Chediak J, et al. Carrier detection in hemophilia A: a cooperative international study. I. The carrier phenotype. Blood. 1986;67:1554-1559.

94. Zimmerman TS, Ratnoff OD, Littell AS. Detection of carriers of classic hemophilia using an immunologic assay for antihemophilic factor (factor 8). J Clin Invest. 1971;50:255-258.

95. Thompson AR. Molecular biology of the hemophilias. Prog Hemost Thromb. 1991;10:175-214.

96. Abildgaard, CF Cornet JA, Fort E, Schulman I. The in vivo longevity of antihaemophilia factor (factor VIII). Br J Haematol. 1964:10:225-237.

97. Over J, Bouma BN, Van Mourik JA, et al. Heterogeneity of human factor VIII. I. Characterization of factor VIII present in the supernatant of cryoprecipitate. J Lab Clin Med. 1978;91:32-46.

98. Hultin MB. Studies of factor IX concentrate therapy in hemophilia. Blood. 1983;62:677-684.

99. Mannucci PM, Ruggeri ZM, Pareti FI, Capitanio A. D.D.A.V.P. in haemophilia. Lancet. 1977;2:1171-1172.

100. Warrier AI, Lusher JM. DDAVP: a useful alternative to blood components in moderate hemophilia A and von Willebrand disease. J Pediatr. 1983;102:228-233.

101. Casonato A, Dannhauser D, Pontara E, et al. DDAVP infusion in haemophilia A carriers: different behaviour of plasma factor VIII and von Willebrand factor. Blood Coagul Fibrinolysis. 1996;7:549-553.

102. Hathaway WE, Christian MJ, Clarke SL, Hasiba U. Comparison of continuous and intermittent factor VIII concentrate therapy in hemophilia A. Am J Hematol. 1984;17:85-88.

103. Bona RD, Weinstein RA, Weisman SJ, et al. The use of continuous infusion of factor concentrates in the treatment of hemophilia. Am J Hematol. 1989;32:8-13.

104. Nilsson IM. Experience with prophylaxis in Sweden. Semin Hematol. 1993;30:16-19.

105. Gilbert MS. Prophylaxis: musculoskeletal evaluation. Semin Hematol. 1993;30:3-6.

106. Vidler V. Use of Port-a-Caths in the management of paediatric haemophilia. Prof Nurse. 1994;10:48-50.

107. Vidler V, Richards M, Vora A. Central venous catheter–associated thrombosis in severe haemophilia. Br J Haematol. 1999;104:461-464.

108. Nilsson IM. Is haemophilia prophylaxis achievable in the context of self-sufficiency? Blood Coagul Fibrinolysis. 1994;5(Suppl 4):S71-S75.

109. Meeks SL, Josephson CD. Should hemophilia treaters switch to albumin-free recombinant factor VIII concentrates. Curr Opin Hematol. 2006;13:457-461.

110. Josephson CD, Abshire T. The new albumin-free recombinant factor VIII concentrates for treatment of hemophilia: do they represent an actual incremental improvement? Clin Adv Hematol Oncol. 2004;2:441-446.

111. Wood WI, Capon DJ, Simonsen CC, et al. Expression of active human factor VIII from recombinant DNA clones. Nature. 1984;312:330-337.

112. Lusher JM, Arkin S, Abildgaard CF, Schwartz RS. Recombinant factor VIII for the treatment of previously untreated patients with hemophilia A. Safety, efficacy, and development of inhibitors. Kogenate Previously Untreated Patient Study Group. N Engl J Med. 1993;328:453-459.

113. Ehrenforth S, Kreuz W, Scharrer I, et al. Incidence of development of factor VIII and factor IX inhibitors in haemophiliacs. Lancet. 1992;339:594-598.

114. Kamiya T, Takahashi I, Saito H. Retrospective study of inhibitor formation in Japanese hemophiliacs. Int J Hematol. 1995;62:175-181.

115. Colvin BT, Hay CR, Hill FG, Preston FE. The incidence of factor VIII inhibitors in the United Kingdom, 1990-93. Inhibitor Working Party. United Kingdom Haemophilia Centre Directors Organization. Br J Haematol. 1995;89: 908-910.

116. Briet E, Rosendaal FR, Kreuz W, et al. High titer inhibitors in severe haemophilia A. A meta-analysis based on eight long-term follow-up studies concerning inhibitors associated with crude or intermediate purity factor VIII products. Thromb Haemost. 1994;72:162-164.

117. Aledort L. Inhibitors in hemophilia patients: current status and management. Am J Hematol. 1994;47: 208-217.

118. McMillan CW, Shapiro SS, Whitehurst D, et al. The natural history of factor VIII:C inhibitors in patients with hemophilia A: a national cooperative study. II. Observations on the initial development of factor VIII:C inhibitors. Blood. 1988;71:344-348.

119. Gouw SC, van der Bom JG, Auerswald G, et al. Recombinant versus plasma-derived factor VIII products and the development of inhibitors in previously untreated patients with severe hemophilia A: the CANAL cohort study. Blood. 2007;109:4693-4697.

120. Laub R, Di Giambattista M, Fondu P, et al. Inhibitors in German hemophilia A patients treated with a double virus inactivated factor VIII concentrate bind to the C2 domain of FVIII light chain. Thromb Haemost. 1999;81:39-44.

121. Gringeri A, Musso R, Mazzucconi MG, et al. Immune tolerance induction with a high purity von Willebrand factor/VIII complex concentrate in haemophilia A patients with inhibitors at high risk of a poor response. Haemophilia. 2007;13:373-379.

122. Ettingshausen CE, Kreuz W. Recombinant vs. plasma-derived products, especially those with intact VWF, regarding inhibitor development. Haemophilia. 2006; 12(Suppl 6):102-106.

123. Barrowcliffe TW, Raut S, Sands D, Hubbard AR. Coagulation and chromogenic assays of factor VIII activity: general aspects, standardization, and recommendations. Semin Thromb Hemost. 2002;28:247-256.

124. Mikaelsson M, Oswaldsson U, Jankowski MA. Measurement of factor VIII activity of B-domain deleted recombinant factor VIII. Semin Hematol. 2001;38:13-23.

125. Webster WP, Roberts HR, Thelin GM, et al. Clinical use of a new glycine-precipitated antihemophilic fraction. Am J Med Sci. 1965;250:643-651.

126. Piszkiewicz D, Sun CS, Tondreau SC. Inactivation and removal of human immunodeficiency virus in monoclonal purified antihemophilic factor (human) (Hemofil M). Thromb Res. 1989;55:627-634.

127. Brettler DB, Forsberg AD, Levine PH, et al. Factor VIII: C concentrate purified from plasma using monoclonal antibodies: human studies. Blood. 1989;73:1859-1863.

128. Mosley JW, Nowicki MJ, Kasper CK, et al. Hepatitis A virus transmission by blood products in the United States. Transfusion Safety Study Group. Vox Sang. 1994;67(Suppl 1):24-28.

129. Yee TT, Cohen BJ, Pasi KJ, Lee CA. Transmission of symptomatic parvovirus B19 infection by clotting factor concentrate. Br J Haematol. 1996;93:457-459.

130. Prowse C, Dow B, Pelly SJ, et al. Human parvovirus B19 infection in persons with haemophilia. Thromb Haemost. 1998;80:351.

131. Brettler DB, Levine PH. Factor concentrates for treatment of hemophilia: which one to choose? Blood. 1989;73: 2067-2073.

132. de Biasi R, Rocino A, Miraglia E, et al. The impact of a very high purity factor VIII concentrate on the immune system of human immunodeficiency virus–infected hemophiliacs: a randomized, prospective, two-year comparison with an intermediate purity concentrate. Blood. 1991;78: 1919-1922.

133. Hepatitis B vaccine. Health and Public Policy Committee, American College of Physicians. Ann Intern Med. 1984;100:149-150.

134. Ragni MV, Lusher JM, Koerper MA, et al. Safety and immunogenicity of subcutaneous hepatitis A vaccine in children with haemophilia. Haemophilia. 2000;6:98-103.

135. Pool JG, Shannon AE. Production of high-potency concentrates of antihemophilic globulin in a closed-bag system. N Engl J Med. 1965;273:1443-1447.

136. Mannucci PM, Canciani MT, Rota L, Donovan BS. Response of factor VIII/von Willebrand factor to DDAVP in healthy subjects and patients with haemophilia A and von Willebrand disease. Br J Haematol. 1981;47:283-293.

137. de la Fuente B, Kasper CK, Rickles FR, Hoyer LW. Response of patients with mild and moderate hemophilia A and von Willebrand disease to treatment with desmopressin. Ann Intern Med. 1985;103:6-14.

138. Prowse CV, Sas G, Gader AM, et al. Specificity in the factor VIII response to vasopressin infusion in man. Br J Haematol. 1979;41:437-447.

139. Rodeghiero F, Castaman G, Di Bona E, Ruggeri M. Consistency of responses to repeated DDAVP infusions in patients with von Willebrand disease and hemophilia A. Blood. 1989;74:1997-2000.

140. Mannucci PM. Desmopressin: a nontransfusional form of treatment for congenital and acquired bleeding disorders. Blood. 1988;72:1449-1455.

141. Smith TJ, Gill JC, Ambruso DR, Hathaway WE. Hyponatremia and seizures in young children given DDAVP. Am J Hematol. 1989;31:199-202.

142. Mannucci PM, Lusher JM. Desmopressin and thrombosis. Lancet. 1989;2:675-676.

143. Nilsson IM, Mikaelsson M, Vilhardt H. The effect of intranasal DDAVP on coagulation and fibrinolytic activity in normal persons. Scand J Haematol. 1982;29:70-74.

144. Walsh PN, Rizza CR, Matthews JM, et al. ε-Aminocaproic acid therapy for dental extractions in haemophilia and Christmas disease: a double blind controlled trial. Br J Haematol. 1971;20:463-475.

145. Sindet-Pedersen S, Ramstrom G, Bernvil S, Blomback M. Hemostatic effect of tranexamic acid mouthwash in anticoagulant-treated patients undergoing oral surgery. N Engl J Med. 1989;320:840-843.

146. Vinckier F, Vermylen J. Dental extractions in hemophilia: reflections on 10 years' experience. Oral Surg Oral Med Oral Pathol. 1985;59:6-9.

147. Evans BE. The use of epsilon-aminocaproic acid for the management of hemophilia in dental and oral surgery patients. J Am Dent Assoc. 1977;94:21.

148. Kasper CK, Aledort L, Aronson D, et al. Proceedings: a more uniform measurement of factor VIII inhibitors. Thromb Diath Haemorrh. 1975;34:612.

149. White GC, Taylor RE, Blatt PM, Roberts HR. Treatment of a high titer anti–factor-VIII antibody by continuous factor VIII administration: report of a case. Blood. 1983;62:141-145.

150. Brettler DB, Forsberg AD, Levine PH, et al. The use of porcine factor VIII concentrate (Hyate:C) in the treatment of patients with inhibitor antibodies to factor VIII. A multicenter US experience. Arch Intern Med. 1989;149:1381-1385.

151. Verroust F, Allain JP. Immune response induced by porcine factor VIII in severe hemophiliacs with antibody to F VIII. Thromb Haemost. 1982;48:238.

152. Parker ET, Craddock HN, Barrow RT, Lollar P. Comparative immunogenicity of recombinant B domain–deleted porcine factor VIII and Hyate:C in hemophilia A mice presensitized to human factor VIII. J Thromb Haemost. 2004;2:605-611.

153. Hedner U, Glazer S, Pingel K, et al. Successful use of recombinant factor VIIa in patient with severe haemophilia A during synovectomy. Lancet. 1988;2:1193.

154. Schmidt ML, Smith HE, Gamerman S, et al. Prolonged recombinant activated factor VII (rFVIIa) treatment for severe bleeding in a factor-IX–deficient patient with an inhibitor. Br J Haematol. 1991;78:460-463.

155. Rao LV, Rapaport SI. Factor VIIa–catalyzed activation of factor X independent of tissue factor: its possible significance for control of hemophilic bleeding by infused factor VIIa. Blood. 1990;75:1069-1073.

156. Kavakli K, Makris M, Zulfikar B, et al. Home treatment of haemarthroses using a single dose regimen of recombinant activated factor VII in patients with haemophilia and inhibitors. A multi-centre, randomised, double-blind, cross-over trial. Thromb Haemost. 2006;95:600-605.

157. Sjamsoedin LJ, Heijnen L, Mauser-Bunschoten EP, et al. The effect of activated prothrombin-complex concentrate (FEIBA) on joint and muscle bleeding in patients with hemophilia A and antibodies to factor VIII. A double-blind clinical trial. N Engl J Med. 1981;305:717-721.

158. Chavin SI, Siegel DM, Rocco TA Jr, Olson JP. Acute myocardial infarction during treatment with an activated prothrombin complex concentrate in a patient with factor VIII deficiency and a factor VIII inhibitor. Am J Med. 1988;85:245-249.

159. Brackmann HH, Gormsen J. Massive factor-VIII infusion in haemophiliac with factor-VIII inhibitor, high responder. Lancet. 1977;2:933.

160. Ewing NP, Sanders NL, Dietrich SL, Kasper CK. Induction of immune tolerance to factor VIII in hemophiliacs with inhibitors. JAMA. 1988;259:65-68.

161. Nilsson IM, Berntorp E, Zettervall O. Induction of immune tolerance in patients with hemophilia and antibodies to factor VIII by combined treatment with intravenous IgG, cyclophosphamide, and factor VIII. N Engl J Med. 1988;318:947-950.

162. Hay CR, Laurian Y, Verroust F, et al. Induction of immune tolerance in patients with hemophilia A and inhibitors treated with porcine VIIIC by home therapy. Blood. 1990;76:882-886.

163. Unuvar A, Warrier I, Lusher JM. Immune tolerance induction in the treatment of paediatric haemophilia A patients with factor VIII inhibitors. Haemophilia. 2000;6:150-157.

164. Berntorp E, Shapiro A, Astermark J, et al. Inhibitor treatment in haemophilias A and B: summary statement for the 2006 international consensus conference. Haemophilia. 2006;12(Suppl 6):1-7.

165. Feldman BM, Pai M, Rivard GE, et al. Tailored prophylaxis in severe hemophilia A: interim results from the first 5 years of the Canadian Hemophilia Primary Prophylaxis Study. J Thromb Haemost. 2006;4:1228-1236.

166. Kisker CT, Eisberg A, Schwartz B. Prophylaxis in factor IX deficiency product and patient variation. Haemophilia. 2003;9:279-284.

167. Smith KJ, Thompson AR. Labeled factor IX kinetics in patients with hemophilia-B. Blood. 1981;58:625-629.

168. Mannucci PM, Bauer KA, Gringeri A, et al. No activation of the common pathway of the coagulation cascade after a highly purified factor IX concentrate. Br J Haematol. 1991;79:606-611.

169. Barnes C, Rudzki Z, Ekert H. Induction of immune tolerance and suppression of anaphylaxis in a child with haemophilia B by simple plasmapheresis and antigen exposure. Haemophilia. 2000;6:693-695.

170. Warrier I. Factor IX antibody and immune tolerance. Vox Sang. 1999;77(Suppl 1):70-71.

171. Shapiro AD, Di PJ, Cohen A, et al. The safety and efficacy of recombinant human blood coagulation factor IX in previously untreated patients with severe or moderately severe hemophilia B. Blood. 2005;105:518-525.

172. Lambert T, Recht M, Valentino LA, et al. Reformulated BeneFix: efficacy and safety in previously treated patients with moderately severe to severe haemophilia B. Haemophilia. 2007;13:233-243.

173. Hoag MS, Johnson FF, Robinson JA, Aggeler PM. Treatment of hemophilia B with a new clotting-factor concentrate. N Engl J Med. 1969;280:581-586.

174. Gunay U, Choi HS, Maurer HS, et al. Commercial preparations of prothrombin complex. A clinical comparison. Am J Dis Child. 1973;126:775-777.

175. Kasper CK. Postoperative thromboses in hemophilia B. N Engl J Med. 1973;289:160.

176. Campbell EW, Neff S, Bowdler AJ. Therapy with factor IX concentrate resulting in DIC and thromboembolic phenomena. Transfusion. 1978;18:94-97.

177. Gobel U, von Voss H, Petrich C. Use of heparin in combination with factor-VII–rich prothrombin complex concentrate [letter]. Lancet. 1975;2:279.

178. Fricke WA, Lamb MA. Viral safety of clotting factor concentrates. Semin Thromb Hemost. 1993;19:54-61.

179. Urbaniak SJ, Cash JD. Blood replacement therapy. Br Med Bull. 1977;33:273-282.

180. Dharnidharka VR, Takemoto C, Ewenstein BM, et al. Membranous glomerulonephritis and nephrosis post factor IX infusions in hemophilia B. Pediatr Nephrol. 1998;12:654-657.

181. Ewenstein BM, Takemoto C, Warrier I, et al. Nephrotic syndrome as a complication of immune tolerance in hemophilia B. Blood. 1997;89:1115-1116.

182. Hoots WK. Comprehensive care for hemophilia and related inherited bleeding disorders: why it matters. Curr Hematol Rep. 2003;2:395-401.

183. Brettler DB. Comprehensive hemophilia care and home factor infusions. Southeast Asian J Trop Med Public Health. 1993;24(Suppl 1):41-42.

184. Soucie JM, Cianfrini C, Janco RL, et al. Joint range-of-motion limitations among young males with hemophilia: prevalence and risk factors. Blood. 2004;103:2467-2473.

185. Soucie JM, Symons J, Evatt B, et al. Home-based factor infusion therapy and hospitalization for bleeding complications among males with haemophilia. Haemophilia. 2001;7:198-206.

186. Dimichele D, Chuansumrit A, London AJ, et al. Ethical issues in haemophilia. Haemophilia. 2006;12(Suppl 3):30-35.

187. Powell JS, Ragni MV, White GC, et al. Phase 1 trial of FVIII gene transfer for severe hemophilia A using a retroviral construct administered by peripheral intravenous infusion. Blood. 2003;102:2038-2045.

188. VandenDriessche T, Collen D, Chuah MK. Viral vector–mediated gene therapy for hemophilia. Curr Gene Ther. 2001;1:301-315.

189. Roth DA, Tawa NE Jr, O'Brien JM, et al. Nonviral transfer of the gene encoding coagulation factor VIII in patients with severe hemophilia A. N Engl J Med. 2001;344:1735-1742.

190. Manno CS, Pierce GF, Arruda VR, et al. Successful transduction of liver in hemophilia by AAV–factor IX and limitations imposed by the host immune response. Nat Med. 2006;12:342-347.

191. High KA. Clinical gene transfer studies for hemophilia B. Semin Thromb Hemost. 2004;30:257-267.

192. Kay MA, Manno CS, Ragni MV, et al. Evidence for gene transfer and expression of factor IX in haemophilia B patients treated with an AAV vector. Nat Genet. 2000;24:257-261.

193. Yarovoi H, Nurden AT, Montgomery RR, et al. Intracellular interaction of von Willebrand factor and factor VIII depends on cellular context: lessons from platelet-expressed factor VIII. Blood. 2005;105:4674-4676.

194. Yarovoi HV, Kufrin D, Eslin DE, et al. Factor VIII ectopically expressed in platelets: efficacy in hemophilia A treatment. Blood. 2003;102:4006-4013.

195. Shi Q, Wilcox DA, Fahs SA, et al. Lentivirus-mediated platelet-derived factor VIII gene therapy in murine haemophilia A. J Thromb Haemost. 2007;5:352-361.

196. Shi Q, Wilcox DA, Fahs SA, et al. Factor VIII ectopically targeted to platelets is therapeutic in hemophilia A with high-titer inhibitory antibodies. J Clin Invest. 2006;116:1974-1982.

197. Wilcox DA, Shi Q, Nurden P, et al. Induction of megakaryocytes to synthesize and store a releasable pool of human factor VIII. J Thromb Haemost. 2003;1:2477-2489.

198. von Willebrand EA. Hereditary pseudohaemophilia. Haemophilia. 1999;5:223-231.

199. von Willebrand EA. Hereditar pseudohemofi. Finska Lak Handl. 1926;68:87.

200. Nilsson IM. Commentary to Erik von Willebrand's original paper from 1926 "Hereditar pseudohemofili." Haemophilia. 1999;5:220-221.

201. Ruggeri ZM, Zimmerman TS. von Willebrand factor and von Willebrand disease. Blood. 1987;70:895-904.

202. Sadler JE. New concepts in von Willebrand disease. Annu Rev Med. 2005;56:173-191.

203. Kawai Y, Montgomery RR. Endothelial cell processing of von Willebrand proteins. Ann N Y Acad Sci. 1987;509:60-70.

204. Montgomery RR, Scott JP. Homologous functions and interactions of platelets and endothelial cells. In Kunicki TJ, George JN (eds): Platelet Immunology. Philadelphia, JB Lippincott, 1989, p 255.

205. Baumgartner HR, Tschopp TB, Weiss HJ. Platelet interaction with collagen fibrils in flowing blood. II. Impaired adhesion-aggregation in bleeding disorders. A comparison with subendothelium. Thromb Haemost. 1977;37:17-28.

206. Miyata S, Goto S, Federici AB, et al. Conformational changes in the A1 domain of von Willebrand factor modulating the interaction with platelet glycoprotein Ibα. J Biol Chem. 1996;271:9046-9053.

207. Goto S, Salomon DR, Ikeda Y, Ruggeri ZM. Characterization of the unique mechanism mediating the shear-dependent binding of soluble von Willebrand factor to platelets. J Biol Chem. 1995;270:23352-23361.

208. Ruggeri ZM, De Marco L, Gatti L, et al. Platelets have more than one binding site for von Willebrand factor. J Clin Invest. 1983;72:1-12.

209. O'Brien JR, Salmon GP. Shear stress activation of platelet glycoprotein IIb/IIIa plus von Willebrand factor causes aggregation: filter blockage and the long bleeding time in von Willebrand disease. Blood. 1987;70:1354-1361.

210. Savage B, Saldivar E, Ruggeri ZM. Initiation of platelet adhesion by arrest onto fibrinogen or translocation on von Willebrand factor. Cell. 1996;84:289-297.

211. Ruggeri ZM. Platelet interactions with vessel wall components during thrombogenesis. Blood Cells Mol Dis. 2006;36:145-147.

212. Fay PJ, Cavallaro C, Marder VJ, et al. Comparison of the in vivo survival of human factor VIII with and without von Willebrand factor in the hemophilic dog. Thromb Res. 1986;41:425-429.

213. Muntean W, Hathaway WE, Montgomery RR. Influence of high molecular weight factor VIII on the measurement of low molecular weight factor VIII procoagulant in different assay systems. Br J Haematol. 1982;51:649-658.

214. Over J, Sixma JJ, Bouma BN, et al. Survival of iodine-125–labeled factor VIII in patients with von Willebrand disease. J Lab Clin Med. 1981;97:332-344.

215. Montgomery RR, Gill JC. Interactions between von Willebrand factor and factor VIII: where did they first meet. J Pediatr Hematol Oncol. 2000;22:269-275.

216. Kaufman RJ. Genetic engineering of factor VIII. Nature. 1989;342:207-208.

217. Kaufman RJ, Wasley LC, Davies MV, et al. Effect of von Willebrand factor coexpression on the synthesis and secretion of factor VIII in Chinese hamster ovary cells. Mol Cell Biol. 1989;9:1233-1242.

218. Goodeve A, Eikenboom J, Castaman G, et al. Phenotype and genotype of a cohort of families historically diagnosed with type 1 von Willebrand disease in the European study, Molecular and Clinical Markers for the Diagnosis and Management of Type 1 von Willebrand Disease (MCMDM-1VWD). Blood. 2007;109:112-121.

219. Budde U, Metzner HJ, Muller HG. Comparative analysis and classification of von Willebrand factor/factor VIII concentrates: impact on treatment of patients with von Willebrand disease. Semin Thromb Hemost. 2006;32:626-635.

220. Sadler JE, Budde U, Eikenboom JC, et al. Update on the pathophysiology and classification of von Willebrand disease: a report of the Subcommittee on von Willebrand Factor. J Thromb Haemost. 2006;4:2103-2114.

221. James PD, Paterson AD, Notley C, et al. Genetic linkage and association analysis in type 1 von Willebrand disease: results from the Canadian type 1 VWD study. J Thromb Haemost. 2006;4:783-792.

222. Rodeghiero F, Castaman G, Dini E. Epidemiological investigation of the prevalence of von Willebrand disease. Blood. 1987;69:454-459.

223. Werner EJ, Broxson EH, Tucker EL, et al. Prevalence of von Willebrand disease in children: a multiethnic study. J Pediatr. 1993;123:893-898.

224. Sadler JE. New concepts in von Willebrand disease. Annu Rev Med. 2005;56:173-191.

225. Sadler JE. Slippery criteria for von Willebrand disease type 1. J Thromb Haemost. 2004;2:1720-1723.

226. Sadler JE. Von Willebrand disease type 1: a diagnosis in search of a disease. Blood. 2003;101:2089-2093.

227. Peake I, Goodeve A. Type 1 von Willebrand disease. J Thromb Haemost. 2007;5(Suppl 1):7-11.

228. James PD, Notley C, Hegadorn C, et al. The mutational spectrum of type 1 von Willebrand disease: Results from a Canadian cohort study. Blood. 2007;109:145-154.

229. Lillicrap D. Von Willebrand disease—phenotype versus genotype: deficiency versus disease. Thromb Res. 2007;120(Suppl 1):S11-S16.

230. Ginsburg D, Handin RI, Bonthron DT, et al. Human von Willebrand factor (vWF): isolation of complementary DNA (cDNA) clones and chromosomal localization. Science. 1985;228:1401-1406.

231. Verweij CL, de Vries CJ, Distel B, et al. Construction of cDNA coding for human von Willebrand factor using antibody probes for colony-screening and mapping of the chromosomal gene. Nucleic Acids Res. 1985;13:4699-4717.

232. Sadler JE, Shelton-Inloes BB, Sorace JM, et al. Cloning and characterization of two cDNAs coding for human von Willebrand factor. Proc Natl Acad Sci U S A. 1985;82:6394-6398.

233. Montgomery RR, Zimmerman TS. von Willebrand disease antigen II. A new plasma and platelet antigen deficient in severe von Willebrand disease. J Clin Invest. 1978;61:1498-1507.

234. Fay PJ, Kawai Y, Wagner DD, et al. Propolypeptide of von Willebrand factor circulates in blood and is identical to von Willebrand antigen II. Science. 1986;232:995-998.

235. Haberichter SL, Balistreri M, Christopherson P, et al. Assay of the von Willebrand factor (VWF) propeptide to identify patients with type 1 von Willebrand disease with decreased VWF survival. Blood. 2006;108:3344-3351.

236. Ginsburg D, Konkle BA, Gill JC, et al. Molecular basis of human von Willebrand disease: analysis of platelet von Willebrand factor mRNA. Proc Natl Acad Sci U S A. 1989;86:3723-3727.

237. Iannuzzi MC, Hidaka N, Boehnke M, et al. Analysis of the relationship of von Willebrand disease (vWD) and hereditary hemorrhagic telangiectasia and identification of a potential type IIA vWD mutation (IIe865 to Thr). Am J Hum Genet. 1991;48:757-763.

238. Cooney KA, Nichols WC, Bruck ME, et al. The molecular defect in type IIB von Willebrand disease. Identification of four potential missense mutations within the putative GpIb binding domain. J Clin Invest. 1991;87:1227-1233.

239. Kroner PA, Kluessendorf ML, Scott JP, Montgomery RR. Expressed full-length von Willebrand factor containing missense mutations linked to type IIB von Willebrand disease shows enhanced binding to platelets. Blood. 1992;79:2048-2055.

240. Kroner PA, Friedman KD, Fahs SA, et al. Abnormal binding of factor VIII is linked with the substitution of glutamine for arginine 91 in von Willebrand factor in a variant form of von Willebrand disease. J Biol Chem. 1991;266:19146-19149.

241. Cacheris PM, Nichols WC, Ginsburg D. Molecular characterization of a unique von Willebrand disease variant. A novel mutation affecting von Willebrand factor/factor VIII interaction. J Biol Chem. 1991;266:13499-13502.

242. Rayner JC, Gill JC, Vokac E, et al. Genetic cause of hereditary persistence of pro-vWf. Clin Res. 1990:38:427a.

243. Randi AM, Sacchi E, Castaman GC, et al. The genetic defect of type I von Willebrand disease "Vicenza" is linked to the von Willebrand factor gene. Thromb Haemost. 1993;69:173-176.

244. Casonato A, Pontara E, Sartorello F, et al. Reduced von Willebrand factor survival in type Vicenza von Willebrand disease. Blood. 2002;99:180-184.

245. Hashemi SM, Peake IR, Marsden L, et al. Mutational analysis of the von Willebrand factor gene in type 1 von Willebrand disease using conformation sensitive gel electrophoresis: a comparison of fluorescent and manual techniques. Haematologica. 2007;92:550-553.

246. Eikenboom J, Van Marion V, Putter H, et al. Linkage analysis in families diagnosed with type 1 von Willebrand disease in the European study, molecular and clinical markers for the diagnosis and management of type 1 VWD. J Thromb Haemost. 2006;4:774-782.

247. James P, Lillicrap D. Genetic testing for von Willebrand disease: the Canadian experience. Semin Thromb Hemost. 2006;32:546-552.

248. Cumming A, Grundy P, Keeney S, et al. An investigation of the von Willebrand factor genotype in UK patients diagnosed to have type 1 von Willebrand disease. Thromb Haemost. 2006;96:630-641.

249. Mancuso DJ, Tuley EA, Westfield LA, et al. Human von Willebrand factor gene and pseudogene: structural analysis and differentiation by polymerase chain reaction. Biochemistry. 1991;30:253-269.

250. Sadler JE. von Willebrand factor. J Biol Chem. 1991;266:22777-22780.

251. Nichols WC, Cooney KA, Mohlke KL, et al. von Willebrand disease in the RIIIS/J mouse is caused by a defect outside of the von Willebrand factor gene. Blood. 1995;86:2461.

252. Gill JC, Endres-Brooks J, Bauer PJ, et al. The effect of ABO blood group on the diagnosis of von Willebrand disease. Blood. 1987;69:1691-1695.

253. Sodetz JM, Paulson JC, McKee PA. Carbohydrate composition and identification of blood group A, B, and H

oligosaccharide structures on human factor VIII/von Willebrand factor. J Biol Chem. 1979;254:10754-10760.

254. Sadler JE. von Willebrand factor: two sides of a coin. J Thromb Haemost. 2005;3:1702-1709.

255. Abildgaard CF, Suzuki Z, Harrison J, et al. Serial studies in von Willebrand disease: variability versus "variants." Blood. 1980;56:712-716.

256. Miller CH, Graham JB, Goldin LR, Elston RC. Genetics of classic von Willebrand disease. I. Phenotypic variation within families. Blood. 1979;54:117-136.

257. Levy G, Ginsburg D. Getting at the variable expressivity of von Willebrand disease. Thromb Haemost. 2001;86:144-148.

258. Larsson SA. Hemophilia in Sweden. Studies on demography of hemophilia and surgery in hemophilia and von Willebrand disease. Acta Med Scand Suppl. 1984;684:1-72.

259. Shoa'i I, Lavergne JM, Ardaillou N, et al. Heterogeneity of von Willebrand disease: study of 40 Iranian cases. Br J Haematol. 1977;37:67-83.

260. Berliner SA, Seligsohn U, Zivelin A, et al. A relatively high frequency of severe (type III) von Willebrand disease in Israel. Br J Haematol. 1986;62:535-543.

261. Miller CH, Haff E, Platt SJ, et al. Measurement of von Willebrand factor activity: relative effects of ABO blood type and race. J Thromb Haemost. 2003;1:2191-2197.

262. Miller CH, Dilley A, Richardson L, et al. Population differences in von Willebrand factor levels affect the diagnosis of von Willebrand disease in African-American women. Am J Hematol. 2001;67:125-129.

263. Howard MA, Firkin BG. Ristocetin—a new tool in the investigation of platelet aggregation. Thromb Diath Haemorrh. 1971;26:362-369.

264. Howard MA, Sawers RJ, Firkin BG. Ristocetin: a means of differentiating von Willebrand disease into two groups. Blood. 1973;41:687-690.

265. Weiss HJ, Hoyer LW, Rickles FR, et al. Quantitative assay of a plasma factor deficient in von Willebrand disease that is necessary for platelet aggregation. Relationship to factor VIII procoagulant activity and antigen content. J Clin Invest. 1973;52:2708-2716.

266. Ruggeri ZM, Zimmerman TS. The complex multimeric composition of factor VIII/von Willebrand factor. Blood. 1981;57:1140-1143.

267. Ruggeri ZM, Zimmerman TS. Classification of variant von Willebrand disease subtypes by analysis of functional characteristics and multimeric composition of factor VIII/von Willebrand factor. Ann N Y Acad Sci. 1981;370:205-209.

268. Rodeghiero F, Castaman G, Tosetto A, et al. The discriminant power of bleeding history for the diagnosis of type 1 von Willebrand disease: an international, multicenter study. J Thromb Haemost. 2005;3:2619-2626.

269. Tosetto A, Castaman G, Rodeghiero F. Assessing bleeding in von Willebrand disease with bleeding score. Blood Rev. 2007;21:89-97.

270. Tosetto A, Rodeghiero F, Castaman G, et al. A quantitative analysis of bleeding symptoms in type 1 von Willebrand disease: results from a multicenter European study (MCMDM-1 VWD). J Thromb Haemost. 2006;4:766-773.

271. Quiroga T, Goycoolea M, Munoz B, et al. Template bleeding time and PFA-100 have low sensitivity to screen patients with hereditary mucocutaneous hemorrhages: comparative study in 148 patients. J Thromb Haemost. 2004;2:892-898.

272. Podda GM, Bucciarelli P, Lussana F, et al. Usefulness of PFA-100((R)) testing in the diagnostic screening of patients with suspected abnormalities of hemostasis: comparison with the bleeding time. J Thromb Haemost. 2007;5:2393-2398.

273. Gilchrist M, Stewart MW, Etches WS, Gordon PA. Rapid diagnosis of von Willebrand disease using ELISA technology. Thromb Res. 1990;57:659-664.

274. Silveira AM, Yamamoto T, Adamson L, Hessel B, Blomback B. Application of an enzyme-linked immunosorbent assay (ELISA) to von Willebrand factor (vWF) and its derivatives. Thromb Res. 1986;43:91-102.

275. Ingerslev J. A sensitive ELISA for von Willebrand factor (vWf:Ag). Scand J Clin Lab Invest. 1987;47:143-149.

276. Zimmerman TS, Hoyer LW, Dickson L, Edgington TS. Determination of the von Willebrand disease antigen (factor VIII–related antigen) in plasma by quantitative immunoelectrophoresis. J Lab Clin Med. 1975;86:152-159.

277. Hubbard AR, Heath AB. Standardization of factor VIII and von Willebrand factor in plasma: calibration of the WHO 5th International Standard (02/150). J Thromb Haemost. 2004;2:1380-1384.

278. Miller CH, Platt SJ, Daniele C, Kaczor D. Evaluation of two automated methods for measurement of the ristocetin cofactor activity of von Willebrand factor. Thromb Haemost. 2002;88:56-59.

279. Lattuada A, Preda L, Sacchi E, et al. A rapid assay for ristocetin cofactor activity using an automated coagulometer (ACL 9000). Blood Coagul Fibrinolysis. 2004;15:505-511.

280. Strandberg K, Lethagen S, Andersson K, et al. Evaluation of a rapid automated assay for analysis of von Willebrand ristocetin cofactor activity. Clin Appl Thromb Hemost. 2006;12:61-67.

281. Federici AB, Canciani MT, Forza I, et al. A sensitive ristocetin co-factor activity assay with recombinant glycoprotein Ibα for the diagnosis of patients with low von Willebrand factor levels. Haematologica. 2004;89:77-85.

282. Caron C, Hilbert L, Vanhoorelbeke K, et al. Measurement of von Willebrand factor binding to a recombinant fragment of glycoprotein Ibα in an enzyme-linked immunosorbent assay–based method: performances in patients with type 2B von Willebrand disease. Br J Haematol. 2006;133:655-663.

283. Ruggeri ZM, Pareti FI, Mannucci PM, et al. Heightened interaction between platelets and factor VIII/von Willebrand factor in a new subtype of von Willebrand disease. N Engl J Med. 1980;302:1047-1051.

284. Miller JL, Kupinski JM, Castella A, Ruggeri ZM. von Willebrand factor binds to platelets and induces aggregation in platelet-type but not type IIB von Willebrand disease. J Clin Invest. 1983;72:1532-1542.

285. Scott JP, Montgomery RR. The rapid differentiation of type IIb von Willebrand disease from platelet-type (pseudo-) von Willebrand disease by the "neutral" monoclonal antibody binding assay. Am J Clin Pathol. 1991;96:723-728.

286. Favaloro EJ. Von Willebrand factor collagen-binding (activity) assay in the diagnosis of von Willebrand disease:

a 15-year journey. Semin Thromb Hemost. 2002;28: 191-202.

287. Favaloro EJ. Collagen binding assay for von Willebrand factor (VWF:CBA): detection of von Willebrands disease (VWD), and discrimination of VWD subtypes, depends on collagen source. Thromb Haemost. 2000;83: 127-135.

288. Ribba AS, Loisel I, Lavergne JM, et al. Ser968Thr mutation within the A3 domain of von Willebrand factor (VWF) in two related patients leads to a defective binding of VWF to collagen. Thromb Haemost. 2001;86:848-854.

289. Romijn RA, Bouma B, Wuyster W, et al. Identification of the collagen-binding site of the von Willebrand factor A3-domain. J Biol Chem. 2001;276:9985-9991.

290. Hillery CA, Mancuso DJ, Evan SJ, et al. Type 2M von Willebrand disease: F606I and I662F mutations in the glycoprotein Ib binding domain selectively impair ristocetin- but not botrocetin-mediated binding of von Willebrand factor to platelets. Blood. 1998;91:1572-1581.

291. Mancuso DJ, Kroner PA, Christopherson PA, et al. Type 2M:Milwaukee-1 von Willebrand disease: an in-frame deletion in the Cys509-Cys695 loop of the von Willebrand factor A1 domain causes deficient binding of von Willebrand factor to platelets. Blood. 1996;88:2559-2568.

292. Montgomery RR, Johnson J. Specific factor VIII–related antigen fragmentation: an in vivo and in vitro phenomenon. Blood. 1982;60:930-939.

293. Cumming AM, Wensley RT. Analysis of von Willebrand factor multimers using a commercially available enhanced chemiluminescence kit. J Clin Pathol. 1993;46:470-473.

294. Gill JC, Wilson AD, Endres-Brooks J, Montgomery RR. Loss of the largest von Willebrand factor multimers from the plasma of patients with congenital cardiac defects. Blood. 1986;67:758-761.

295. Moake JL, Rudy CK, Troll JH, et al. Unusually large plasma factor VIII:von Willebrand factor multimers in chronic relapsing thrombotic thrombocytopenic purpura. N Engl J Med. 1982;307:1432-1435.

296. Moake JL. Defective processing of unusually large von Willebrand factor multimers and thrombotic thrombocytopenic purpura. J Thromb Haemost. 2004;2:1515-1521.

297. Mannucci PM, Abildgaard CF, Gralnick HR, et al. Multicenter comparison of von Willebrand factor multimer sizing techniques. Report of the Factor VIII and von Willebrand Factor Subcommittee. Thromb Haemost. 1985;54:873-876.

298. Haberichter SL, Fahs SA, Montgomery RR. von Willebrand factor storage and multimerization: 2 independent intracellular processes. Blood. 2000;96:1808-1815.

299. van Genderen PJ, Boertjes RC, Van Mourik JA. Quantitative analysis of von Willebrand factor and its propeptide in plasma in acquired von Willebrand syndrome. Thromb Haemost. 1998;80:495-498.

300. Van Mourik JA, Boertjes R, Huisveld IA, et al. von Willebrand factor propeptide in vascular disorders: a tool to distinguish between acute and chronic endothelial cell perturbation. Blood. 1999;94:179-185.

301. Scott JP, Montgomery RR. The rapid differentiation of type IIb von Willebrand disease from platelet-type (pseudo-) von Willebrand disease by the "neutral" mono-

clonal antibody binding assay. Am J Clin Pathol. 1991;96:723-728.

302. Kroner PA, Foster PA, Fahs SA, Montgomery RR. The defective interaction between von Willebrand factor and factor VIII in a patient with type 1 von Willebrand disease is caused by substitution of Arg19 and His54 in mature von Willebrand factor. Blood. 1996;87:1013-1021.

303. Lankhof H, Damas C, Schiphorst ME, et al. Recombinant vWF type 2A mutants R834Q and R834W show a defect in mediating platelet adhesion to collagen, independent of enhanced sensitivity to a plasma protease. Thromb Haemost. 1999;81:976-983.

304. Furlan M, Robles R, Affolter D, et al. Triplet structure of von Willebrand factor reflects proteolytic degradation of high molecular weight multimers. Proc Natl Acad Sci U S A. 1993;90:7503-7507.

305. Zimmerman TS, Dent JA, Ruggeri ZM, Nannini LH. Subunit composition of plasma von Willebrand factor. Cleavage is present in normal individuals, increased in IIA and IIB von Willebrand disease, but minimal in variants with aberrant structure of individual oligomers (types IIC, IID, and IIE). J Clin Invest. 1986;77:947-951.

306. Lankhof H, Damas C, Schiphorst ME, et al. von Willebrand factor without the A2 domain is resistant to proteolysis. Thromb Haemost. 1997;77:1008-1013.

307. Studt JD, Bohm M, Budde U, et al. Measurement of von Willebrand factor–cleaving protease (ADAMTS-13) activity in plasma: a multicenter comparison of different assay methods. J Thromb Haemost. 2003;1:1882-1887.

308. Zhou W, Tsai HM. An enzyme immunoassay of ADAMTS13 distinguishes patients with thrombotic thrombocytopenic purpura from normal individuals and carriers of ADAMTS13 mutations. Thromb Haemost. 2004;91:806-811.

309. Kokame K, Nobe Y, Kokubo Y, et al. FRETS-VWF73, a first fluorogenic substrate for ADAMTS13 assay. Br J Haematol. 2005;129:93-100.

310. Kato S, Matsumoto M, Matsuyama T, et al. Novel monoclonal antibody–based enzyme immunoassay for determining plasma levels of ADAMTS13 activity. Transfusion. 2006;46:1444-1452.

311. Kunicki TJ, Montgomery RR, Schullek J. Cleavage of human von Willebrand factor by platelet calcium-activated protease. Blood. 1985;65:352-356.

312. Favaloro EJ. Effect of overnight 4 degrees C storage of whole blood on von Willebrand factor. Transfusion. 2006; 46:1057-1059.

313. Pottinger BE, Read RC, Paleolog EM, et al. von Willebrand factor is an acute phase reactant in man. Thromb Res. 1989;53:387-394.

314. Blann AD. von Willebrand factor antigen as an acute phase reactant and marker of endothelial cell injury in connective tissue diseases: a comparison with CRP, rheumatoid factor, and erythrocyte sedimentation rate. Z Rheumatol. 1991;50:320-322.

315. Zezos P, Papaioannou G, Nikolaidis N, et al. Elevated plasma von Willebrand factor levels in patients with active ulcerative colitis reflect endothelial perturbation due to systemic inflammation. World J Gastroenterol. 2005;11: 7639-7645.

316. Rogers JS, Shane SR. Factor VIII activity in normal volunteers receiving oral thyroid hormone. J Lab Clin Med. 1983;102:444-449.

317. Cuianu M, Nussbaum A, Cristea A, et al. High levels of plasma von Willebrand factor in hyperthyroidism. Med Interne. 1987;25:205-210.

318. Galli-Tsinopoulou A, Stylianou C, Papaioannou G, Nousia-Arvanitakis S. Acquired von Willebrand's syndrome resulting from untreated hypothyroidism in two prepubertal girls. Haemophilia. 2006;12:687-689.

319. Homoncik M, Gessl A, Ferlitsch A, et al. Altered platelet plug formation in hyperthyroidism and hypothyroidism. J Clin Endocrinol Metab. 2007;92:3006-3012.

320. Johnson SS, Montgomery RR, Hathaway WE. Newborn factor VIII complex: elevated activities in term infants and alterations in electrophoretic mobility related to illness and activated coagulation. Br J Haematol. 1981;47:597-606.

321. Weinger RS, Cecalupo AJ, Olson JD, Frankel L. Neonatal von Willebrand disease: diagnostic difficulty at birth. Am J Dis Child. 1980;134:793-794.

322. Sramek A, Eikenboom JC, Briet E, et al. Usefulness of patient interview in bleeding disorders. Arch Intern Med. 1995;155:1409-1415.

323. Josso F. [Severe epistaxis in hemorrhagic syndromes (excepting Rendu-Osler disease).] Ann Otolaryngol Chir Cervicofac. 1976;93:15-21.

324. Quick AJ. Telangiectasia: its relationship to the Minot–von Willebrand syndrome. Am J Med Sci. 1967;254:585-601.

325. Ahr DJ, Rickles FR, Hoyer LW, et al. von Willebrand disease and hemorrhagic telangiectasia: association of two complex disorders of hemostasis resulting in life-threatening hemorrhage. Am J Med. 1977;62:452-458.

326. Thompson AR, Gill JC, Ewenstein BM, et al. Successful treatment for patients with von Willebrand disease undergoing urgent surgery using factor VIII/VWF concentrate (Humate-P). Haemophilia. 2004;10:42-51.

327. Gill JC, Ewenstein BM, Thompson AR, et al. Successful treatment of urgent bleeding in von Willebrand disease with factor VIII/VWF concentrate (Humate-P): use of the ristocetin cofactor assay (VWF:RCo) to measure potency and to guide therapy. Haemophilia. 2003;9:688-695.

328. Dobrkovska A, Krzensk U, Chediak JR. Pharmacokinetics, efficacy and safety of Humate-P in von Willebrand disease. Haemophilia. 1998;4(Suppl 3):33-39.

329. Mannucci PM, Chediak J, Hanna W, et al. Treatment of von Willebrand disease with a high-purity factor VIII/von Willebrand factor concentrate: a prospective, multicenter study. Blood. 2002;99:450-456.

330. Rodeghiero F, Castaman G, Mannucci PM. Prospective multicenter study on subcutaneous concentrated desmopressin for home treatment of patients with von Willebrand disease and mild or moderate hemophilia A. Thromb Haemost. 1996;76:692-696.

331. Leissinger C, Becton D, Cornell C Jr, Cox GJ. High-dose DDAVP intranasal spray (Stimate) for the prevention and treatment of bleeding in patients with mild haemophilia A, mild or moderate type 1 von Willebrand disease and symptomatic carriers of haemophilia A. Haemophilia. 2001;7:258-266.

332. Kohler M, Hellstern P, Miyashita C, et al. Comparative study of intranasal, subcutaneous and intravenous administration of desamino-D-arginine vasopressin (DDAVP). Thromb Haemost. 1986;55:108-111.

333. Mannucci PM, Bettega D, Cattaneo M. Patterns of development of tachyphylaxis in patients with haemophilia and von Willebrand disease after repeated doses of desmopressin (DDAVP). Br J Haematol. 1992;82:87-93.

334. Castaman G, Federici AB, Bernardi M, et al. Factor VIII and von Willebrand factor changes after desmopressin and during pregnancy in type 2M von Willebrand disease Vicenza: a prospective study comparing patients with single (R1205H) and double (R1205H-M740I) defect. J Thromb Haemost. 2006;4:357-360.

335. Dini E, Barbui T, Chisesi T, et al. Von Willebrand's disease in Italy. A study of 13 families from a small area in the province of Vicenza. Acta Haematol. 1974;52:29-39.

336. Rodeghiero F, Castaman G, Di Bona E, et al. Hyper-responsiveness to DDAVP for patients with type I von Willebrand disease and normal intra-platelet von Willebrand factor. Eur J Haematol. 1988;40:163-167.

337. MacFarlane JD, Kroon HM, Caekebeke-Peerlinck KM. Arthropathy in von Willebrand disease. Clin Rheumatol. 1989;8:98-102.

338. Sankarankutty M, Evans DI. Chronic arthropathy in von Willebrand disease. Clin Lab Haematol. 1983;5:149-156.

339. Federici AB. Management of von Willebrand disease with factor VIII/von Willebrand factor concentrates: results from current studies and surveys. Blood Coagul Fibrinolysis. 2005;16(Suppl 1):S17-S21.

340. Abshire TC. Prophylaxis and von Willebrand disease (vWD). Thromb Res. 2006;118(Suppl 1):S3-S7.

341. Berntorp E. Prophylaxis and treatment of bleeding complications in von Willebrand disease type 3. Semin Thromb Hemost. 2006;32:621-625.

342. Coppola A, Cimino E, Conca P, et al. Long-term prophylaxis with intermediate-purity factor VIII concentrate (Haemate P) in a patient with type 3 von Willebrand disease and recurrent gastrointestinal bleeding. Haemophilia. 2006;12:90-94.

343. Berntorp E, Petrini P. Long-term prophylaxis in von Willebrand disease. Blood Coagul Fibrinolysis. 2005;16(Suppl 1):S23-S26.

344. Borel-Derlon A, Federici AB, Roussel-Robert V, et al. Treatment of severe von Willebrand disease with a high-purity von Willebrand factor concentrate (Wilfactin): a prospective study of 50 patients. J Thromb Haemost. 2007;5:1115-1124.

345. Chtourou S, Porte P, Nogre M, et al. A solvent/detergent-treated and 15-nm filtered factor VIII: a new safety standard for plasma-derived coagulation factor concentrates. Vox Sang. 2007;92:327-337.

346. Mazurier C, Poulle M, Samor B, et al. In vitro study of a triple-secured von Willebrand factor concentrate. Vox Sang. 2004;86:100-104.

347. Mazurier C. In vitro evaluation of the haemostatic value of the LFB–von Willebrand factor concentrate. Haemophilia. 1998;4(Suppl 3):40-43.

348. Goudemand J, Mazurier C, Marey A, et al. Clinical and biological evaluation in von Willebrand disease of a von Willebrand factor concentrate with low factor VIII activity. Br J Haematol. 1992;80:214-221.

349. Menache D, Aronson DL, Darr F, et al. Pharmacokinetics of von Willebrand factor and factor VIIIC in patients with severe von Willebrand disease (type 3 VWD): estimation

of the rate of factor VIIIC synthesis. Cooperative Study Groups. Br J Haematol. 1996;94:740-745.

350. Mannucci PM. Venous thromboembolism in von Willebrand disease. Thromb Haemost. 2002;88:378-379.

351. Mancuso DJ, Tuley EA, Castillo R, et al. Characterization of partial gene deletions in type III von Willebrand disease with alloantibody inhibitors. Thromb Haemost. 1994;72:180-185.

352. Shelton-Inloes BB, Chehab FF, Mannucci PM, et al. Gene deletions correlate with the development of alloantibodies in von Willebrand disease. J Clin Invest. 1987;79:1459-1465.

353. Meijer K, Peters FT, van der Meer J. Recurrent severe bleeding from gastrointestinal angiodysplasia in a patient with von Willebrand disease, controlled with recombinant factor VIIa. Blood Coagul Fibrinolysis. 2001;12:211-213.

354. Tarantino MD, Aberle R. Recombinant factor VIIa (NovoSeven) for post-prostatectomy hemorrhage in a patient with type I von Willebrand disease. Am J Hematol. 2001;68:62-63.

355. Grossmann RE, Geisen U, Schwender S, Keller F. Continuous infusion of recombinant factor VIIa (NovoSeven) in the treatment of a patient with type III von Willebrand disease and alloantibodies against von Willebrand factor. Thromb Haemost. 2000;83:633-634.

356. Lyons SE, Bruck ME, Bowie EJ, Ginsburg D. Impaired intracellular transport produced by a subset of type IIA von Willebrand disease mutations. J Biol Chem. 1992;267:4424-4430.

357. Gralnick HR, Williams SB, McKeown LP, et al. DDAVP in type IIa von Willebrand disease. Blood. 1986;67:465-468.

358. Cooney KA, Lyons SE, Ginsburg D. Functional analysis of a type IIB von Willebrand disease missense mutation: increased binding of large von Willebrand factor multimers to platelets. Proc Natl Acad Sci U S A. 1992;89:2869-2872.

359. Mathew P, Greist A, Maahs JA, et al. Type 2B vWD: the varied clinical manifestations in two kindreds. Haemophilia. 2003;9:137-144.

360. Rendal E, Penas N, Larrabeiti B, et al. Type 2B von Willebrand's disease due to Val1316Met mutation. Heterogeneity in the same sibship. Ann Hematol. 2001;80:354-360.

361. Casonato A, Steffan A, Pontara E, et al. Post-DDAVP thrombocytopenia in type 2B von Willebrand disease is not associated with platelet consumption: failure to demonstrate glycocalicin increase or platelet activation. Thromb Haemost. 1999;81:224-228.

362. Castaman G, Eikenboom JC, Rodeghiero F, et al. A novel candidate mutation (Arg611→His) in type I "platelet discordant" von Willebrand disease with desmopressin-induced thrombocytopenia. Br J Haematol. 1995;89:656-658.

363. Casonato A, Sartori MT, De Marco L, Girolami A. 1-Desamino-8-D-arginine vasopressin (DDAVP) infusion in type IIB von Willebrand disease: shortening of bleeding time and induction of a variable pseudothrombocytopenia. Thromb Haemost. 1990;64:117-120.

364. McKeown LP, Connaghan G, Wilson O, et al. 1-Desamino-8-arginine-vasopressin corrects the hemostatic

defects in type 2B von Willebrand disease. Am J Hematol. 1996;51:158-163.

365. Casonato A, Fabris F, Girolami A. Platelet aggregation and pseudothrombocytopenia induced by 1-desamino-8-D-arginine vasopressin (DDAVP) in type IIB von Willebrand disease patient. Eur J Haematol. 1990;45:36-42.

366. Lopez-Fernandez MF, Lopez-Berges C, Martin-Bernal JA, et al. Type IIB von Willebrand disease associated with a complex thrombocytopenic thrombocytopathy. Am J Hematol. 1988;27:291-298.

367. Weiss HJ, Meyer D, Rabinowitz R, et al. Pseudo–von Willebrand disease. An intrinsic platelet defect with aggregation by unmodified human factor VIII/von Willebrand factor and enhanced adsorption of its high-molecular-weight multimers. N Engl J Med. 1982;306:326-333.

368. Miller JL, Castella A. Platelet-type von Willebrand disease: characterization of a new bleeding disorder. Blood. 1982;60:790-794.

369. Miller JL. Platelet-type von Willebrand disease. Clin Lab Med. 1984;4:319-331.

370. Mazurier C, Gaucher C, Jorieux S, et al. Evidence for a von Willebrand factor defect in factor VIII binding in three members of a family previously misdiagnosed mild haemophilia A and haemophilia A carriers: consequences for therapy and genetic counselling. Br J Haematol. 1990;76:372-379.

371. Gaucher C, Jorieux S, Mercier B, et al. The "Normandy" variant of von Willebrand disease: characterization of a point mutation in the von Willebrand factor gene. Blood. 1991;77:1937-1941.

372. Mazurier C, Gaucher C, Jorieux S, Goudemand M. Biological effect of desmopressin in eight patients with type 2N ("Normandy") von Willebrand disease. Collaborative Group. Br J Haematol. 1994;88:849-854.

373. Howard MA, Salem HH, Thomas KB, et al. Variant von Willebrand disease type B—revisited. Blood. 1982;60:1420-1428.

374. Rabinowitz I, Tuley EA, Mancuso DJ, et al. von Willebrand disease type B: a missense mutation selectively abolishes ristocetin-induced von Willebrand factor binding to platelet glycoprotein Ib. Proc Natl Acad Sci U S A. 1992;89:9846-9849.

375. James PD, Notley C, Hegadorn C, et al. Challenges in defining type 2M von Willebrand disease: results from a Canadian cohort study. J Thromb Haemost. 2007;5:1914-1922.

376. Coccia MR, Barnes HV. Hypothyroidism and acquired von Willebrand disease. J Adolesc Health. 1991;12:152-154.

377. Dalton RG, Dewar MS, Savidge GF, et al. Hypothyroidism as a cause of acquired von Willebrand disease. Lancet. 1987;1:1007-1009.

378. Gullu S, Sav H, Kamel N. Effects of levothyroxine treatment on biochemical and hemostasis parameters in patients with hypothyroidism. Eur J Endocrinol. 2005;152:355-361.

379. Nitu-Whalley IC, Lee CA. Acquired von Willebrand syndrome—report of 10 cases and review of the literature. Haemophilia. 1999;5:318-326.

380. Michiels JJ, Berneman Z, Gadisseur A, et al. Immune-mediated etiology of acquired von Willebrand syndrome in systemic lupus erythematosus and in benign monoclo-

nal gammopathy: therapeutic implications. Semin Thromb Hemost. 2006;32:577-588.

381. Niiya M, Niiya K, Takazawa Y, et al. Acquired type 3–like von Willebrand syndrome preceded full-blown systemic lupus erythematosus. Blood Coagul Fibrinolysis. 2002;13: 361-365.

382. Michiels JJ, Schroyens W, van der Planken M, Berneman Z. Acquired von Willebrand syndrome in systemic lupus erythematosus. Clin Appl Thromb Hemost. 2001;7: 106-112.

383. Van Mourik JA, Romani DW. Von Willebrand factor propeptide in vascular disorders. Thromb Haemost. 2001;86: 164-171.

384. Lopez-Fernandez MF, Lopez-Berges C, Martin R, et al. Unique multimeric pattern of von Willebrand factor in a patient with a benign monoclonal gammopathy. Scand J Haematol. 1986;36:302-308.

385. Tatewaki W, Takahashi H, Hanano M, Shibata A. Multimeric composition of plasma von Willebrand factor in chronic myelocytic leukaemia. Thromb Res. 1988;52: 23-32.

386. Casonato A, Pontara E, Doria A, et al. Lack of multimer organization of von Willebrand factor in an acquired von Willebrand syndrome. Br J Haematol. 2002;116:899-904.

387. Kumar S, Pruthi RK, Nichols WL. Acquired von Willebrand's syndrome: a single institution experience. Am J Hematol. 2003;72:243-247.

388. Schwartz RS, Gabriel DA, Aledort LM, et al. A prospective study of treatment of acquired (autoimmune) factor VIII inhibitors with high-dose intravenous gammaglobulin. Blood. 1995;86:797-804.

389. Macik BG, Gabriel DA, White GC, et al. The use of high-dose intravenous gamma-globulin in acquired von Willebrand syndrome. Arch Pathol Lab Med. 1988; 112:143-146.

390. Smaradottir A, Bona R. A case of acquired von Willebrand syndrome successfully treated with recombinant Factor VIIa during thyroidectomy. Thromb Haemost. 2004;92: 666-667.

391. Friederich PW, Wever PC, Briet E, et al. Successful treatment with recombinant factor VIIa of therapy-resistant severe bleeding in a patient with acquired von Willebrand disease. Am J Hematol. 2001;66:292-294.

392. Majumdar G, Phillips JK, Lavallee H, Savidge GF. Acquired haemophilia in association with type III von Willebrand disease: successful treatment with high purity von Willebrand's factor and recombinant factor VIIa. Blood Coagul Fibrinolysis. 1993;4:1035-1037.

393. Scott JP, Montgomery RR, Tubergen DG, Hays T. Acquired von Willebrand disease in association with Wilm's tumor: regression following treatment. Blood. 1981;58:665-669.

394. Coppes MJ, Zandvoort SW, Sparling CR, et al. Acquired von Willebrand disease in Wilms' tumor patients. J Clin Oncol. 1992;10:422-427.

395. Bracey AW, Wu AH, Aceves J, et al. Platelet dysfunction associated with Wilms tumor and hyaluronic acid. Am J Hematol. 1987;24:247-257.

396. Michiels J, Schroyens W, Berneman Z, van der Planken M. Atypical variant of acquired von Willebrand syndrome in Wilms tumor: is hyaluronic acid secreted by nephroblastoma cells the cause? Clin Appl Thromb Hemost. 2001;7:102-105.

397. Caramuru LH, Soares RP, Maeda NY, Lopes AA. Hypoxia and altered platelet behavior influence von Willebrand factor multimeric composition in secondary pulmonary hypertension. Clin Appl Thromb Hemost. 2003;9:251-258.

398. Lopes AA, Maeda NY, Aiello VD, et al. Abnormal multimeric and oligomeric composition is associated with enhanced endothelial expression of von Willebrand factor in pulmonary hypertension. Chest. 1993;104:1455-1460.

399. Sucker C, Feindt P, Zotz RB, et al. Functional von Willebrand factor assays are not predictive for the absence of highest-molecular weight von Willebrand factor multimers in patients with aortic-valve stenosis. Thromb Haemost. 2005;94:465-466.

400. Castillo R, Escolar G, Monteagudo J, et al. Hemostasis in patients with severe von Willebrand disease improves after normal platelet transfusion and normalizes with further correction of the plasma defect. Transfusion. 1997;37: 785-790.

401. Haberichter SL, Merricks EP, Fahs SA, et al. Re-establishment of VWF-dependent Weibel-Palade bodies in VWD endothelial cells. Blood. 2005;105:145-152.

402. De Meyer SF, Vanhoorelbeke K, Chuah MK, et al. Phenotypic correction of von Willebrand disease type 3 blood-derived endothelial cells with lentiviral vectors expressing von Willebrand factor. Blood. 2006;107:4728-4736.

403. Pergolizzi RG, Jin G, Chan D, et al. Correction of a murine model of von Willebrand disease by gene transfer. Blood. 2006;108:862-869.

404. Blaese RM. Optimism regarding the use of RNA/DNA hybrids to repair genes at high efficiency. J Gene Med. 1999;1:144-147.

405. De Meyer SF, Pareyn I, Baert J, et al. False positive results in chimeraplasty for von Willebrand disease. Thromb Res. 2007;119:93-104.

406. Drouin J, Lillicrap DP, Izaguirre CA, et al. Absence of a bleeding tendency in severe acquired von Willebrand disease. The role of platelet von Willebrand factor in maintaining normal hemostasis. Am J Clin Pathol. 1989;92: 471-478.

407. Bowie EJ, Solberg LA Jr, Fass DN, et al. Transplantation of normal bone marrow into a pig with severe von Willebrand's disease. J Clin Invest. 1986;78:26-30.

408. Nichols TC, Samama CM, Bellinger DA, et al. Function of von Willebrand factor after crossed bone marrow transplantation between normal and von Willebrand disease pigs: effect on arterial thrombosis in chimeras. Proc Natl Acad Sci U S A. 1995;92:2455-2459.

409. Ware RE, Parker RI, McKeown LP, Graham ML. A human chimera for von Willebrand disease following bone marrow transplantation. Am J Pediatr Hematol Oncol. 1993;15:338-342.

31

Rare Hereditary Coagulation Factor Abnormalities

Kenneth A. Bauer

Although von Willebrand's disease, hemophilia A, and hemophilia B represent the majority of hereditary bleeding disorders caused by clotting factor deficiencies, hereditary abnormalities of other coagulation factors may occasionally be encountered. Each of these latter disorders is reviewed in the following chapter; however, the reader is referred to reviews or hemostasis texts in the references for a more complete description of these abnormalities.

FIBRINOGEN DISORDERS

Fibrinogen deficiency states (afibrinogenemia and hypofibrinogenemia) and hereditary functional abnormalities of fibrinogen (dysfibrinogenemias) are infrequently encountered but should be considered when a prolonged thrombin time (TT) is found in a patient with a bleeding history who is otherwise essentially healthy. Prolongations of the prothrombin time (PT) and activated partial thromboplastin time (APTT) are found in patients with afibrinogenemia, in severely hypofibrinogenemic patients, and in patients with some types of dysfibrinogenemia.

Hypofibrinogenemia and Afibrinogenemia

Genetic abnormalities causing decreased fibrinogen synthesis may occur either as a heterozygous deficiency (hypofibrinogenemia) or as a homozygous deficiency (afibrinogenemia).[1] Clinical findings include ecchymoses, hemarthroses, and subcutaneous hematomas. Patients with a virtual absence of fibrinogen are frequently seen in the neonatal period with gastrointestinal bleeding, hemorrhage, or major hematomas from delivery trauma. Surprisingly, symptoms in patients with afibrinogenemia are not as severe as those seen in the classic hemophilic disorders.

Laboratory evaluation of a patient with afibrinogenemia reveals prolongations of the TT, PT, and APTT (see Chapter 28). With automated clotting instruments, the amount of fibrin clot needed for clot detection is greater than that needed with manual methods. Thus, these tests are frequently prolonged to the limits of the instrument even though some fibrinogen may be present and a clot detected by manual methods. Because fibrinogen is the ligand for the glycoprotein IIb-IIIa receptor that enables platelet aggregation, both the bleeding time and platelet aggregation tests are usually abnormal. Interestingly, in the absence of fibrinogen, von Willebrand factor is able to bind to the glycoprotein IIb-IIIa complex on platelets and provides a backup mechanism for platelet aggregation.[2,3] This may result in a reduction in symptoms associated with this disorder. In many patients, a small amount of platelet fibrinogen might facilitate some of these interactions, although this fibrinogen is not believed to be derived from synthesis by megakaryocytes.

Thus, the presence of fibrinogen in platelets may result from the acquisition of a small amount of fibrinogen that is acquired from plasma by circulating platelets. The best screening tests to detect fibrinogen deficiency are the TT and reptilase time, which measure the time required for conversion of fibrinogen in plasma to a fibrin clot. Reptilase is a thrombin-like enzyme obtained from snake venom. Unlike the TT, the reptilase time is unaffected by heparin treatment. Thus, if one encounters a very prolonged TT, the possibility of heparinization must be considered, but marked prolongation of the reptilase time is suggestive of fibrinogen deficiency. Fibrinogen may be detected by functional, precipitation, or immunologic assays. However, patients with afibrinogenemia generally have undetectable levels of fibrinogen.

Clinical bleeding episodes in patients with afibrinogenemia, similar to those observed in hemophilia, require episodic replacement therapy. Because of the long plasma half-life of fibrinogen, prophylactic infusions of fibrinogen should be considered in patients with severe symptoms. The only readily available sources of fibrinogen are fresh frozen plasma and cryoprecipitate.[4] Cryoprecipitate is currently the most practical source for replacement and contains approximately 200 mg of fibrinogen per bag, or "unit," of cryoprecipitate. Hemorrhagic symptoms are usually controlled by initially achieving plasma levels of 80 to 100 mg/dL and maintaining this level above 50 to 60 mg/dL until the bleeding subsides. To raise the fibrinogen level in an afibrinogenemic patient to 100 mg/dL, approximately 0.17 unit of cryoprecipitate per kilogram of body weight must be infused. Because of the prolonged half-life of fibrinogen, replacement therapy can be given at intervals of 3 to 4 days.

Dysfibrinogenemia

Numerous dysfibrinogenemias have been reported and are named after the city in which they were originally identified.[1] Dysfibrinogenemias are associated either with no clinical symptoms or with hemorrhage, whereas others, interestingly, are associated with a predisposition to venous or arterial thrombosis (see Chapter 32). Functional abnormalities of fibrinogen are generally inherited in an autosomal dominant manner. Occasionally, however, index cases are associated with consanguinity and major hemorrhagic or thrombotic symptoms. Hereditary dysfibrinogenemia that is associated with hemorrhage usually results in a prolonged TT. Laboratory evaluation for dysfibrinogenemia includes functional and immunologic assays for fibrinogen, which should show a normal level of fibrinogen antigen with a reduction in fibrinogen when measured by functional coagulation assays. The reptilase time may also be prolonged. An occasional individual with dysfibrinogemia may have a prolonged PT or APTT. The inability of some abnormal fibrinogen to clot completely in vitro can result in false-positive results in fibrin(ogen) degradation product tests. Infusion of fibrinogen in the form of cryoprecipitate may be indicated in patients with clinical bleeding, and survival of this fibrinogen can be expected to be normal. Further evaluation usually requires the assistance of a specialized laboratory that studies fibrinogen at the molecular level.

A small number of variant fibrinogens have been reported in association with thrombotic complications.[1] These defects can be detected with the TT and reptilase time, which are often prolonged. Occasionally, the TT is substantially shortened.[5,6] Functional fibrinogen measurements are generally substantially lower than antigenic measurements in the plasma of these individuals, similar to those in patients with a hemorrhagic tendency. Severe liver disease is occasionally associated with acquired dysfunction of fibrinogen.[7] Studies usually demonstrate that this is not hereditary in nature, and the liver disease is generally overt.

PROTHROMBIN DEFICIENCY

Hereditary prothrombin deficiency, similar to congenital abnormalities of fibrinogen, may be present either as a markedly reduced prothrombin level (hypoprothrombinemia) or as an abnormal prothrombin (dysprothrombinemia).[8] Congenital hypoprothrombinemia results in levels of prothrombin as low 6 U/dL. A variety of dysprothrombinemias have been reported that are associated with abnormalities in calcium binding and γ-carboxylation, although specific abnormalities in the thrombin portion of the molecule have also been reported. Symptoms generally consist of post-traumatic hemorrhage and mild mucocutaneous bleeding. However, one child with a dysprothrombinemia lost approximately 20% of his blood volume into his thigh after a routine injection of diphtheria and tetanus toxoid and pertussis (DPT) vaccine given at 6 weeks of age.[9] Although the APTT may be slightly prolonged, the hallmark is usually a prolonged PT and a normal TT. In some cases of dysprothrombinemia, such as prothrombin Cardeza, the PT may be nearly normal (12 seconds) even though prothrombin activity is markedly reduced.[10] Thus, specific assays comparing the immunologic levels of prothrombin with the functional levels of prothrombin are required to diagnose dysprothrombinemias. The lack of deficiencies of other vitamin K–dependent factors (factors VII, IX, and X) and liver-dependent factors (factor V and fibrinogen) usually direct attention to the diagnosis of a hereditary deficiency of prothrombin. Immunoassays and assays of electrophoretic mobility help identify dysprothrombinemia.

Although prothrombin is contained in prothrombin complex concentrates, fresh frozen plasma is generally effective in decreasing hemorrhagic symptoms because of the 60-hour plasma half-life of prothrombin. Treatment can therefore be accomplished without significant volume overload. Achievement of plasma levels of prothrombin in excess of 20 to 30 U/dL is usually associated with cessation of symptoms.

Factor V Deficiency

Factor V deficiency, first reported by Owren in 1947 and termed parahemophilia, is associated with a mild to moderate bleeding disorder.[11] It is transmitted autosomally and is generally symptomatic only in the homozygous or doubly heterozygous state. Mucocutaneous bleeding and hematomas are the most common symptoms, and hemarthroses are rarely encountered. Menarche is frequently associated with severe menorrhagia. Both the PT and the APTT are prolonged, which usually prompts specific factor assays. Immunoassays for factor V are not readily available, and thus most cases are defined by functional deficiencies of factor V with the use of clotting assays.

Clinical bleeding can be controlled with fresh frozen plasma, the only currently available source of factor V. Normal hemostasis is achieved with levels above 25 U/dL. In a patient with severe factor V deficiency, hemostasis can be achieved with a loading dose of 20 mL of plasma per kilogram of body weight followed by infusions of approximately 6 mL/kg every 12 hours. Because factor V is more labile in frozen plasma than other hemostatic factors are, it is important to use fresh frozen plasma that is less than 1 to 2 months old.

Occasionally, one may encounter a patient with an acquired antibody to factor V who has a negative family history. Even though the PT is markedly prolonged, some of these patients do not have major hemorrhagic symptoms.[12] In rare instances, antibodies to factor V arise in patients with congenital absence of factor V. This latter group of patients is, of course, quite symptomatic but can generally be managed by infusing fresh platelets that contain normal platelet factor V.

Combined Deficiency of Factor V and Factor VIII

More than 50 pedigrees with an autosomal recessive bleeding disorder characterized by a combined deficiency of both factor V and factor VIII have been reported.[13-15] In some cases, the mutations responsible for this disorder are in the *LMAN1* gene (also known as endoplasmic reticulum [ER]-Golgi intermediate compartment protein or ERGIC-53), which functions as a molecular chaperone from the ER to the Golgi apparatus in the biosynthesis of both factor V and factor VIII.[16,17] In other kindreds, this disorder is associated with mutations in the multiple coagulation factor deficiency 2 gene.[18] *MCFD2* encodes a protein that forms a calcium-dependent stoichiometric complex with LMAN1 and acts as a cofactor in the intracellular trafficking of factors V and VIII. The disease is associated with a moderate bleeding tendency and plasma factor V and factor VIII levels of 5% to 30% of normal. Combined factor V and factor VIII deficiency is usually accompanied by fewer symptoms than hemophilia A is, but when required, hemostasis can generally be achieved with fresh frozen plasma.

Factor X Deficiency

Factor X deficiency is a rare autosomal disorder that results in mucocutaneous and post-traumatic bleeding.[8] Deficiency of factor X may be caused by either a deficiency of factor X antigen or a functionally abnormal factor X molecule. Both cause prolongation of the PT and APTT. A reduced factor X level is identified by a factor X clotting assay. In patients with dysfunctional factor X, the factor X clotting assay is prolonged, but results of the immunoassay are normal.[19,20] Russell viper venom contains a procoagulant enzyme that can activate factor X, thereby bypassing the need for clotting factors other than factor X, factor V, prothrombin, and fibrinogen. Some dysfunctional factor X molecules may be associated with normal Russell viper venom times and thus will be detected only by PT assay in affected family members.

The biologic half-life of factor X is about 40 hours. Infusion of approximately 20 mL of fresh frozen plasma per kilogram of body weight followed by 6 mL/kg every 12 hours increases the level of factor X sufficiently to achieve hemostasis for minor bleeding episodes. In instances when major surgery must be undertaken, prothrombin complex concentrates can be used to correct the factor X deficiency. However, the amount of factor X is not usually assayed in these products and they can be thrombogenic. If elective surgery is anticipated and it is decided to use prothrombin complex concentrate, several different preparations should be obtained and measured for their content of factor X. Although factor X is a vitamin K–dependent factor, vitamin K has no therapeutic effect on factor X in congenitally deficient patients. Factor X levels of 20 to 30 U/dL are generally associated with the cessation of hemorrhagic symptoms.

Though not usually a pediatric problem, amyloidosis may be associated with factor X deficiency because of adsorption of factor X to the amyloid material.[21,22] Therapeutic infusions are not generally efficacious in patients with acquired deficiency of factor X secondary to amyloidosis.

Factor VII Deficiency

Factor VII deficiency has an estimated incidence of 1 per 500,000 in the general population and an autosomal recessive pattern of inheritance. The hemorrhagic predisposition in affected patients is highly variable and correlates poorly with plasma factor VII activity levels.[23,24] Patients with levels that are less than 1% of normal can experience severe bleeding episodes, including hemarthroses and crippling arthropathy, comparable to patients with the classic hemophilias. Neonates with factor VII deficiency are at increased risk for the development of intracranial hemorrhage, which is attributable to trauma at the time of delivery.[23]

Hemostasis screening tests in patients with factor VII deficiency reveal a prolonged PT with a normal PTT and a normal TT. Heterozygotes typically have normal PTs and are identified only after specific factor VII assays are performed in family members of patients with homozygous or compound heterozygous factor VII deficiency. Heterozygous deficiency is not usually associated with hemorrhagic symptoms. Laboratory evaluation of factor VII deficiency relies on specific assay of plasma factor VII coagulant activity (VII:C) with the use of animal or human thromboplastin, as well as immunologic quantitation of factor VII antigen.[25,26] Patients have been categorized by their plasma level of factor VII antigen (VII:Ag) or cross-reacting material (CRM⁻, low or absent antigen; CRM^R, reduced antigen; CRM⁺, normal antigen). CRM⁻ defects result from defective factor VII biosynthesis or accelerated clearance in vivo, CRM⁺ defects are structurally abnormal factor VII molecules, and CRM^R defects may result from a combination of these mechanisms. Some CRM^R or CRM⁺ factor VII molecules give variable VII:C results when assayed with tissue factor from different animal species (e.g., rabbit brain, ox brain, simian brain, human brain).[24,27-29] As anticipated, the molecular basis of factor VII deficiency is heterogeneous, and several different types of mutations have been described in patients with factor VII deficiency.[30] Most have been missense mutations, but nonsense mutations, small deletions, splice site abnormalities, and promoter mutations have also been identified.

Factor VII is a vitamin K–dependent factor, but vitamin K administration is of no therapeutic benefit in the treatment of hereditary deficiencies. Although commercial prothrombin complex concentrates may contain some factor VII, the amount is highly variable among the different commercial preparations. The factor VII content also varies between different lots produced by a single manufacturer. Because the plasma half-life of factor VII is short (approximately 3 to 6 hours), plasma infusions may not achieve adequate levels for normal hemostasis. Factor VII concentrates have been available for patients with factor VII deficiency in clinical trials or on a compassionate-use basis.[31] The use of activated recombinant factor VII, which has a half-life similar to that of factor VII, has also been shown to provide effective hemostasis in patients with factor VII deficiency[32] and has received regulatory approval for this indication in the United States. Anecdotally, the therapeutic effect of factor VII infusions appears to be longer than the time during which measurable factor VII levels can be identified in plasma. In one patient treated with prothrombin complex concentrates on a regular basis, mucocutaneous bleeding was controlled for 3 to 4 days after a single infusion, even though factor VII was not measurable after 24 hours. Whether this results from surface binding of factor VII to endothelial cells or platelets, removal of it from plasma, or some nonspecific effect from the concentrate infusion was not clear.

Factor XI Deficiency

Factor XI deficiency is usually inherited as an autosomal recessive disorder. The APTT is prolonged in factor XI deficiency, whereas the PT is normal. A specific assay for factor XI coagulant activity is necessary to make the diagnosis. Factor XI assays are best performed on fresh plasma because the apparent factor XI level may be increased after freezing plasma.[33]

Although factor XI deficiency is most frequently encountered in Jewish persons of Ashkenazi descent, it is occasionally found in other ethnic groups, and the mutations have been characterized.[34-36] In Israel, 1 to 3 per 1000 Ashkenazi Jews are homozygous or doubly heterozygous for this deficiency, which calculates to a gene frequency of 4.3%.[37] Sephardic Jews, on the other hand, are rarely affected by factor XI deficiency. Three different point mutations in the factor XI gene account for nearly all cases of factor XI deficiency in Ashkenazi Jews: a splice site mutation at the last intron that disrupts normal mRNA processing (type I), a nonsense mutation in exon 5 resulting in a premature stop codon (type II), and a missense mutation in exon 9 resulting in substitution of Leu for Phe at amino acid 238.[38] Although the genotype correlates well with plasma factor XI levels, there is not good correlation with the hemorrhagic tendency.[39] In Ashkenazi Jewish patients who are homozygous or doubly heterozygous for factor XI deficiency, the APTT is often longer than it is in patients with either severe factor VIII or factor IX deficiency.

Although factor XI deficiency has been termed *hemophilia C*, the bleeding tendency is highly variable and bleeding almost always occurs in association with surgery or trauma. Epistaxis, soft tissue hemorrhage, and bleeding after dental extractions may occur, but hemarthroses and concomitant arthropathy are not seen. Affected women may experience menorrhagia. Even though low factor XI levels are not always associated with bleeding, patients with a significant personal or familial history of bleeding should probably receive fresh frozen plasma before major surgery. In the absence of such a history, prophylaxis with fresh frozen plasma should probably be administered for ear, nose, and throat (e.g., tonsillectomy), neurosurgical, cardiac, or urologic procedures. Patients who have previously undergone major surgery without bleeding or who are having minor procedures that can be controlled easily by local pressure (e.g., dental extraction) may be monitored closely and treatment initiated only if hemorrhage occurs. Heterozygous patients with factor XI levels greater than 20% of normal may also occasionally experience bleeding.[40]

Plasma infusions of 1 U/kg body weight can increase the circulating factor XI concentration by about 1.5 U/dL. A loading dose of 15 to 20 mL of plasma per kilogram will result in plasma levels of 20 to 30 U/dL, a level that is usually sufficient to control moderate hemorrhage. Additional plasma infusions of 7.5 to 10 mL/kg can be administered at 12- to 24-hour intervals until hemostasis is achieved. The half-life of factor XI is in excess of 48 hours. In factor XI–deficient patients deemed to be at risk for bleeding, antifibrinolytic agents such as ε-aminocaproic acid or tranexamic acid can be used to prevent hemorrhage after minor surgical procedures (e.g., dental extractions).

Factor XIII Deficiency

Factor XIII (fibrin-stabilizing factor) is responsible for clot stabilization and cross-linking of the fibrin polymer. Deficiency of this factor is associated with reduced clot stability.[41] Factor XIII deficiency is an autosomal recessive disorder that results in delayed hemorrhage. A typical patient will sustain trauma on one day, and a bruise or hematoma will develop on the following day. Other symptoms of factor XIII deficiency include delayed separation of the umbilical stump in the neonatal period (beyond 3.5 to 4 weeks), intracranial hemorrhage with little or no trauma, poor wound healing, and recurrent spontaneous abortions in women.

Laboratory evaluation reveals normal hemostasis screening test results, including bleeding time, APTT, PT, and TT. For a patient with normal screening test results but clinical symptoms of a bruising disorder, one should perform a factor XIII assay. Screening tests for factor XIII deficiency are based on the observation that there is increased solubility of the clot because of the lack of cross-linking. Thus, a normal clot remains insoluble in 5 mol/L urea, whereas a clot formed from a patient with factor XIII deficiency is soluble.

Because factor XIII has a very long half-life of 5 to 7 days and a hemostatic level of only 2 to 3 U/dL is required, infusion of 5 to 10 mL/kg of fresh frozen plasma is usually effective therapy. Cryoprecipitate may also be used. One bag of cryoprecipitate contains 75 units of factor XIII. If a patient is particularly symptomatic, prophylaxis is also easily achieved with infusions of plasma every 2 to 4 weeks.

Contact Factor Deficiencies

Although factor XI deficiency may be associated with bleeding symptoms, deficiency of the other contact factors (factor XII, prekallikrein, and high-molecular-weight kininogen) is not associated with bleeding symptoms.[42,43] Thus, these factors do not appear to play a major physiologic role in normal hemostasis (see Chapter 26). Because these contact factors function at the initiation step of the intrinsic system, the APTT in severely deficient individuals (contact factor activity less than 1% of normal) frequently demonstrates prolongations beyond those seen with hemophilia A and hemophilia B. As a result, one encounters the paradoxical situation in which an extremely prolonged PTT is not associated with a bleeding disorder.

The clinician usually encounters contact factor deficiency when asked to evaluate a patient without bleeding symptoms who has a markedly prolonged APTT obtained as a preoperative screening test. It is frequently advisable to carry out these same screening tests on other family members once the specific contact factor deficiency is determined to identify affected family members who could have future surgery inappropriately delayed because of such clotting studies.

Paradoxically, there have been a number of case reports of venous thromboembolism or myocardial infarction in factor XII–deficient patients,[44] including the initial patient described with the abnormality.[45] This thrombophilic tendency has been attributed to reduced plasma fibrinolytic activity.[46] A literature review of 121 patients with factor XII deficiency found an 8% incidence of thromboembolism, including several myocardial infarctions in relatively young individuals.[44] Interpretation of such data is difficult because these complications are likely to be reported in the literature, unlike asymptomatic patients with factor XII deficiency. This led some groups to perform cross-sectional analyses of thromboembolic events in larger numbers of unselected families with factor XII deficiency.[47,48] In Swiss families with factor XII deficiency, 2 of 18 homozygous or doubly heterozygous patients had sustained deep venous thrombosis, although each occurred at a time that other predisposing thrombotic risk factors were present.[47] Among heterozygotes with factor XII deficiency, only 1 in 45 had a possible history of venous thrombosis. These investigators concluded that heterozygous factor XII deficiency does not constitute a major thrombotic risk factor, although a severe deficiency may predispose some affected persons to venous thrombosis. Other groups have found a 10% to 20% incidence of thrombotic episodes in heterozygotes.[48,49] Thus, it remains uncertain whether an increased thrombotic risk is associated with factor XII deficiency.

ANTIPLASMIN DEFICIENCY

Antiplasmin is a major regulatory protein that controls the activity of plasmin, the pivotal enzyme in the fibrinolytic system that cleaves fibrin. In familial α_2-antiplasmin deficiency, the plasmin activity generated under physiologic conditions is poorly regulated and results in a bleeding disorder.[50] These patients have mucocutaneous bleeding as well as joint hemorrhage and must be differentiated from those with mild hemophilia. The usual hemostatic screening test results are normal, including the PT, APTT, and TT. The euglobulin clot lysis time, a measure of fibrinolytic activity, is generally shortened. Although fresh frozen plasma contains α_2-antiplasmin, this clinical disorder is most commonly treated with the intermittent administration of antifibrinolytic agents, including ε-aminocaproic acid and tranexamic acid.

Plasminogen Activator Inhibitor 1 Deficiency

Deficiency of plasminogen activator inhibitor 1 (PAI-1) has been shown to cause a hereditary bleeding disorder.[51,52] In one homozygous case, the genetic defect was shown to be a frameshift mutation.[53] Affected patients can experience recurrent bleeding, especially after surgery or trauma. The PT, APTT, and TT are normal in such patients. The euglobulin clot lysis time can be abnormally short. Specific assays for PAI-1 antigen and activity are required to make a diagnosis of PAI-1 deficiency. Treatment with antifibrinolytic agents, such as tranexamic acid and ε-aminocaproic acid, is effective in treating bleeding complications.

Antitrypsin Pittsburgh

Antitrypsin is not normally a significant regulatory protein of hemostasis. A family has been described, however, with an alteration in the α_1-antitrypsin molecule such that the protein has spontaneous antithrombin activity.[54] Continuous inactivation of thrombin results in delayed clot formation and a hemorrhagic syndrome that like α_2-antiplasmin deficiency, resembles mild hemophilia. Therapy for a disorder in which there is excessive activity is often more difficult than replacement of a protein in a patient with a familial deficiency.

MULTIPLE FACTOR DEFICIENCIES

Hereditary deficiencies of multiple factors are rare clinical disorders that are associated with a bleeding diathesis of variable severity. Combined deficiency of the vitamin K–dependent factors (i.e., factors II, VII, IX, and X) can result from deficient vitamin K–dependent γ-carboxylase activity, which mediates post-translational modifications of these proteins,[55,56] or defective vitamin K metabolism secondary to mutations in vitamin K 2,3-epoxide reductase (VKOR).[57] VKOR is the target of the oral anticoagulant warfarin. As mentioned earlier, factor V and factor VIII deficiency has been reported in more than 50 families. In general, when a patient with multiple factor deficiencies is identified, it is imperative to rule out acquired causes such as liver disease or vitamin K deficiency and to perform a family study before one assumes that such a defect is hereditary.

REFERENCES

1. Moen JL, Lord ST. Afibrinogenemias and dysfibrinogenemias. In Colman RW, Marder VJ, Clowes AW, et al (eds). Hemostasis and Thrombosis: Basic Principles and Clinical Practice, 5th ed. Philadelphia, Lippincott Williams & Wilkins, 2006, pp 939-952.

2. De Marco L, Girolami A, Zimmerman TS, Ruggeri ZM. von Willebrand factor interaction with the glycoprotein IIb/IIIa complex. Its role in platelet function as demonstrated in patients with congenital afibrinogenemia. J Clin Invest. 1986;77:1272-1277.

3. Weiss HJ, Hawiger J, Ruggeri ZM, et al. Fibrinogen-independent platelet adhesion and thrombus formation on subendothelium mediated by glycoprotein IIb-IIIa complex at high shear rate. J Clin Invest. 1989;83:288-297.

4. Rodriguez RC, Buchanan GR, Clanton MS. Prophylactic cryoprecipitate in congenital afibrinogenemia. Clin Pediatr (Phila). 1988;27:543-545.

5. Egeberg OP. Inherited fibrinogen abnormality causing thrombophilia. Thromb Diath Haemorrh. 1967;17:175-187.

6. Thorsen LI, Brosstad F, Solum NO, et al. Increased binding to ADP-stimulated platelets and aggregation effect of the dysfibrinogen Oslo I as compared with normal fibrinogen. Scand J Haematol. 1986;36:203-210.

7. Francis JL, Armstrong DJ. Acquired dysfibrinogenaemia in liver disease. J Clin Pathol. 1982;35:667-672.

8. Roberts HR, Escobar MA. Inherited disorders of prothrombin conversion. In Colman RW, Marder VJ, Clowes AW, et al (eds). Hemostasis and Thrombosis: Basic Principles and Clinical Practice, 5th ed. Philadelphia, Lippincott William & Wilkins, 2006, pp 923-937.

9. Montgomery RR, Corrigan JJ, Clarke S, Johnson M. Prothrombin Denver: A new dysprothrombinemia [abstract]. Circulation. 1980;62:279.

10. Shapiro SS, Martinez J, Holburn RR. Congenital dysprothrombinemia: an inherited structural disorder of human prothrombin. J Clin Invest. 1969;48:2251-2259.

11. Owren PA. Parahaemophilia: hemorrhagic diathesis due to absence of a previously unknown clotting factor. Lancet. 1947;1:446-448.

12. Kessler CM, Acs P, Mariani G. Acquired disorders of coagulation: the immune coagulopathies. In Colman RW, Marder VJ, Clowes AW, et al (eds). Hemostasis and Thrombosis: Basic Principles and Clinical Practice, 5th ed. Philadelphia, Lippincott Williams & Wilkins, 2006, pp 1061-1084.

13. Seibert RH, Margolius A, Ratnoff OD. Observation on hemophilia, parahemophilia and co-existent hemophilia and parahemophilia. J Lab Clin Med. 1958;52:449-462.

14. Seligsohn U, Ramot B. Combined factor V and factor VIII deficiency: report of four cases. Br J Haematol. 1969;16:475-486.

15. Seligsohn U, Zivelin A, Zwang E. Combined factor V and factor VIII deficiency among non-Ashkenazi Jews. N Engl J Med. 1982;307:1191-1195.

16. Nichols WC, Seligsohn U, Zivelin A, et al. Mutations in the ER-Golgi intermediate compartment protein ERGIC-53 cause combined deficiency of coagulation factors V and VIII. Cell. 1998;93:61-70.

17. Neerman-Arbez M, Johnson KM, Morris MA, et al. Molecular analysis of the ERGIC-53 gene in 35 families with combined factor V–factor VIII deficiency. Blood. 1999;93:2253-2260.

18. Zhang B, Cunningham MA, Nichols WC, et al. Bleeding due to disruption of a cargo-specific ER-to-Golgi transport complex. Nat Genet. 2003;34:220-225.

19. Fair DS, Revak DJ, Hubbard JG, Girolami A. Isolation and characterization of the factor X Friuli variant. Blood. 1989;73:2108-2116.

20. Watzke HH, Lechner K, Roberts HR, et al. Molecular defect (Gla+14→Lys) and its functional consequences in a hereditary factor X deficiency (factor X Vorarlberg). J Biol Chem. 1990;265:11982-11989.

21. Korsan-Bengsten K, Hjort PF, Ygge J. Acquired factor X deficiency in a patient with amyloidosis. Thromb Diath Haemorrh. 1962;7:558-566.

22. Furie B, Greene E, Furie BC. Syndrome of acquired factor X deficiency and systemic amyloidosis: in vivo studies of the metabolic fate of factor X. N Engl J Med. 1977;297:81-85.

23. Ragni MV, Lewis JH, Spero JA, et al. Factor VII deficiency. Am J Hematol. 1981;10:79-88.

24. Triplett DA, Brandt JT, McGann Batard MA, et al. Hereditary factor VII deficiency: heterogeneity defined by combined functional and immunochemical analysis. Blood. 1985;66:1284-1287.

25. Fair DS. Quantitation of factor VII in the plasma of normal and warfarin-treated individuals by radioimmunoassay. Blood. 1983;62:784-791.

26. Boyer C, Wolf M, Rothschild C, et al. An enzyme immunoassay (ELISA) for the quantitation of human factor VII. Thromb Haemost. 1986;56:250-255.

27. Girolami A, Falezza G, Patrassi G, et al. Factor VII Verona coagulation disorder: double heterozygosis with an abnormal factor VII and heterozygous factor-VII deficiency. Blood. 1977;50:603-610.

28. Girolami A, Fabris F, Dal Bo Zanon R, et al. Factor VII Padua: a coagulation disorder due to an abnormal factor VII with a peculiar activation pattern. J Lab Clin Med. 1978;91:387-395.

29. Girolami A, Cottarozzi G, Dal Bo Zanon R, et al. Factor VII Padua2: another factor VII abnormality with defective ox brain thromboplastin activation and a complex hereditary pattern. Blood. 1979;54:46-53.

30. Tuddenham EGD, Pemberton S, Cooper DN. Inherited factor VII deficiency: genetics and molecular pathology. Thromb Haemost. 1995;74:313-321.

31. Cohen LJ, McWilliams NB, Neuberg R, et al. Prophylaxis and therapy with factor VII concentrate (human) Immuno, vapor heated in patients with congenital factor VII deficiency: a summary of case reports. Am J Hematol. 1995;50:269-276.

32. Hunault MA, Bauer KA. Recombinant factor VIIa for the treatment of congenital factor VII deficiency. Semin Thromb Hemost. 2000;26:401-405.

33. Pearson RW, Triplett DA. Factor XI assay results in the CAP survey (1981). Am J Clin Pathol. 1982;78(4 Suppl):615-620.

34. O'Connell NM. Factor XI deficiency—from molecular genetics to clinical management. Blood Coagul Fibrinolysis. 2003;14(Suppl 1):S59-S64.

35. Kravtsov DV, Wu W, Meijers JC, et al. Dominant factor XI deficiency caused by mutations in the factor XI catalytic domain. Blood. 2004;104:128-134.

36. Kravtsov DV, Monahan PE, Gailani D. A classification system for cross-reactive material–negative factor XI deficiency. Blood. 2005;105:4671-4673.

37. Seligsohn U. High gene frequency of factor XI (PTA) deficiency in Ashkenazi Jews. Blood. 1978;51:1223-1228.

38. Asakai R, Chung DW, Ratnoff OD, et al. Factor XI (plasma thromboplastin antecedent) deficiency in Ashkenazi Jews is a bleeding disorder that can result from three types of point mutations. Proc Natl Acad Sci U S A. 1989;86:7667-7671.

39. Asakai R, Chung DW, Davie EW, et al. Factor XI deficiency in Ashkenazi Jews in Israel. N Engl J Med. 1991;325:153-158.

40. Bolton-Maggs PHB, Wan-Yin BY, McCraw AH, et al. Inheritance and bleeding in factor XI deficiency. Br J Haematol. 1988;69:521-528.

41. Greenberg CS, Sane DC, Lai TS. Factor XIII and fibrin stabilization. In Colman RW, Marder VJ, Clowes AW, et al (eds). Hemostasis and Thrombosis: Basic Principles and Clinical Practice, 5th ed. Philadelphia, Lippincott William & Wilkins, 2006, pp 317-334.

42. Ratnoff OD, Colopy JE. Familial hemorrhagic trait associated with deficiency of clot-promoting fraction of plasma. J Clin Invest. 1955;34:602-613.

43. Saito H. Contact factors in health and disease. Semin Thromb Hemost. 1987;13:36-49.

44. Goodnough LT, Saito H, Ratnoff OD. Thrombosis or myocardial infarction in congenital clotting factor abnormalities and chronic thrombocytopenias: a report of 21 patients and a review of 50 previously reported cases. Medicine (Baltimore). 1983;62:248-255.

45. Ratnoff OD, Busse RJ, Sheon RP. The demise of John Hageman. N Engl J Med. 1968;279:760-761.

46. Lodi S, Isa L, Pollini E, et al. Defective intrinsic fibrinolytic activity in a patient with severe factor XII deficiency and myocardial infarction. Scand J Haematol. 1984;33:80-82.

47. Lammle B, Wuillemin WA, Huber I, et al. Thromboembolism and bleeding tendency in congenital factor XII deficiency—a study on 74 subjects from 14 Swiss families. Thromb Haemost. 1991;65:117-121.

48. Rodeghiero F, Castaman G, Ruggeri M, et al. Thrombosis in subjects with homozygous and heterozygous factor XII deficiency [letter]. Thromb Haemost. 1992;67:590.

49. Mannhalter C, Fischer M, Hopmeier P, et al. Factor XII activity and antigen concentrations in patients suffering from recurrent thrombosis. Fibrinolysis. 1987;1:259-263.

50. Saito H. α_2-Plasmin inhibitor and its deficiency states. J Lab Clin Med. 1988;112:671-678.

51. Schleef RR, Higgins DL, Pillemer E, Levitt LJ. Bleeding diathesis due decreased functional activity of type I plasminogen activator inhibitor. J Clin Invest. 1989;83:1747-1752.

52. Dieval J, Nguyen G, Gross S, et al. A lifelong bleeding disorder associated with a deficiency of plasminogen activator inhibitor type I. Blood. 1991;77:528-532.

53. Fay WP, Shapiro AD, Shih JL, et al. Brief report: complete deficiency of plasminogen-activator inhibitor type I due to a frame-shift mutation. N Engl J Med. 1992;327:1729-1733.

54. Owen MC, Brennan SO, Lewis JH, Carrell RW. Mutation of antitrypsin to antithrombin: alpha 1-antitrypsin Pittsburgh (358 Met leads to Arg), a fatal bleeding disorder. N Engl J Med. 1983;309:694-698.

55. Wu SM, Stanley TB, Mutucamarana P, Stafford DW. Characterization of gamma-glutamyl carboxylase. Thromb Haemost. 1997;78:599-604.

56. Brenner B. Hereditary deficiency of vitamin K–dependent coagulation factors. Thromb Haemost. 2000;84:935-936.

57. Oldenburg J, Watzka M, Rost S, et al. VKORC1: molecular target of coumarins. J Thromb Haemost. 2007;5(Suppl 1):1-6.

32

Inherited Disorders of Thrombosis and Fibrinolysis

Kenneth A. Bauer

For many years, researchers suspected that hereditary coagulation defects underlie a large percentage of venous thromboembolic events that could not be attributed to identifiable acquired risk factors. Acquired risk factors for venous thrombosis consist of a heterogeneous group of conditions and clinical disorders with diverse and poorly understood prothrombotic mechanisms. With expanding scientific knowledge of the hemostatic mechanism and the regulatory role of natural anticoagulants, major advances have been made in identifying hereditary defects in the heparan sulfate–antithrombin and protein C pathways over the last 3 decades. This chapter reviews the hereditary disorders of thrombosis and fibrinolysis associated with an increased risk for thrombosis. Issues relating to diagnosis and treatment of the hereditary thrombophilias are also discussed.

HEREDITARY THROMBOTIC DISORDERS
(Box 32-1)

Before 1980, there were only isolated reports of thrombosis in the pediatric population. This paucity of thrombotic events might be related to the incompletely understood protection against thrombosis in young children through the mid-teen years, notwithstanding the fact that some of the physiologic inhibitors do not attain their full normal adult levels until mid-childhood (protein C and protein S) (see Chapters 5 and 28). Even patients with hereditary deficiencies of natural physiologic anticoagulants, such as antithrombin, protein C, and protein S, have few thrombotic symptoms during early childhood. Over the past 30 years, however, more vigorous supportive and specific treatment for sick preterm infants has resulted in a markedly improved survival rate of even very preterm infants. Because these infants are quite prone to thrombotic events, the physiologic "hypercoagulability" of the developing hemostatic system has received increased attention and is discussed elsewhere (see Chapter 5). Thus, the newborn infant can be expected to be at greater risk for thrombosis if there is also an underlying hereditary deficiency of an anticoagulant protein.

Box 32-1	Inherited Alterations of Coagulation Proteins That Have Been Clearly Associated with a Prethrombotic State

Antithrombin deficiency
Protein C deficiency
Protein S deficiency
Resistance to activated protein C because of the factor V Leiden mutation (factor V Arg506Gln)
Prothrombin G20210A mutation
Dysfibrinogenemias (rare)

Antithrombin Deficiency

Antithrombin is a plasma protein synthesized by the liver that binds and neutralizes the serine proteinases generated by the coagulation cascade, including thrombin, factor Xa, and factor IXa (see Chapter 26). Inhibition of these coagulation serine enzymes by antithrombin is relatively slow but is markedly enhanced by binding to heparin. Antithrombin has two major active functional sites: the reactive center toward the carboxyl end and the heparin-binding site located at the amino-terminal of the molecule. Thrombin cleaves the reactive site followed by the formation of an inactive complex, which is rapidly cleared from the circulation.

Antithrombin deficiency was the first hereditary hypercoagulable disorder identified. In 1965, Egeberg investigated a Norwegian family with a strong history of thrombosis and found that affected individuals had plasma antithrombin concentrations that were 40% to 50% of normal.[1] Subsequent studies described families with similar clinical and laboratory abnormalities.[2,3] Heterozygosity for antithrombin deficiency can be found in approximately 4% of families with inherited thrombophilia and in 1% of consecutive patients with a first episode of deep venous thrombosis.[4]

The thrombotic risk associated with antithrombin deficiency depends on the population selected. In older reviews of antithrombin deficiency that included families with a high penetrance of thrombosis, more than 50% of affected patients experienced venous thrombotic episodes.[5,6] The initial clinical manifestations occur spontaneously in about 42% of subjects but are related to pregnancy, parturition, ingestion of oral contraceptives, surgery, or trauma in 58% of patients.[5] The most common sites of disease are the deep veins of the leg and the mesenteric veins. Recurrent thrombotic episodes occur in approximately 60% of affected persons, and clinical signs of pulmonary embolism are evident in 40%.[5] Although cases have been reported in which antithrombin-deficient infants sustained cerebral venous thrombosis,[7-9] thrombotic episodes are rare in affected children before puberty, at which time thrombotic events start to occur with some frequency and the risk of thrombosis increases substantially with advancing age.[5] First-degree relatives of symptomatic individuals with antithrombin deficiency have an 8- to 10-fold increased risk for thrombosis over that in noncarriers.[10,11] In the Leiden Thrombophilia Study, a case-control study of 474 consecutive patients after an initial episode of deep venous thrombosis,[12] the prevalence of antithrombin deficiency was just 1.1%, and the odds ratio for thrombosis was 5.0.[13]

Antithrombin deficiency is inherited in an autosomal dominant fashion and thus affects both sexes equally. Two major types of inherited antithrombin deficiency have been delineated (Table 32-1). The type I deficiency state is a result of reduced synthesis of biologically normal protease inhibitor molecules.[14] In these cases the antigenic and functional activities of antithrombin in blood

TABLE 32-1	Assay Measurements in Heterozygous Antithrombin Deficiency		
			ACTIVITY
Types	**Antigen**	**Heparin Cofactor**	**Progressive Antithrombin**
I	Low	Low	Low
II			
Active-site defect	Normal	Low	Low
Heparin-binding site defect	Normal	Low	Normal

are reduced in parallel. The molecular basis of this disorder is either deletion of a major segment of the antithrombin gene or, more commonly, the occurrence of small deletions/insertions or single base substitutions. These mutations introduce a frameshift, a direct termination codon, a change in mRNA processing, or unstable translation products. The antithrombin mutation database includes more than 100 distinct mutations in patients with type I deficiency.[15]

The second type of antithrombin deficiency is produced by a discrete molecular defect within the protease inhibitor (type II). Plasma levels of antithrombin are greatly reduced as judged by functional activity, whereas antithrombin immunologic activity is essentially normal. The first family with type II antithrombin deficiency was described in 1974.[16] Many families with this type of deficiency state have been reported, and they have been further subcategorized on the basis of two different functional assays of antithrombin activity. The first is the antithrombin–heparin cofactor assay, which measures the ability of heparin to bind to lysyl residues on the inhibitor and catalyze the neutralization of coagulation enzymes such as thrombin and factor Xa. The second test is the progressive antithrombin activity assay, which quantitates the capacity of this inhibitor to neutralize the enzymatic activity of thrombin in the absence of heparin. Heterozygous type II patients with both diminished heparin cofactor activity and progressive antithrombin activity have mutations near the thrombin-binding site at the carboxy-terminal end of the molecule; those with reductions only in heparin cofactor activity have mutations in the heparin-binding domain at the amino-terminal end of the molecule. The distinction between type II defects is clinically relevant because variants with heparin–binding site defects are infrequently associated with thrombotic events, except when present in the homozygous state.[17] The latter patients with homozygous antithrombin deficiency were young children in whom severe venous or arterial thrombosis, or both, developed along with plasma antithrombin–heparin cofactor levels below 10%.[18,19] In each instance, there was a history of parental consanguinity and the parents had type II antithrombin deficiency with heparin–binding site defects.

The prevalence of type I antithrombin deficiency in the adult population is approximately 1 in 2000.[20,21] Studies of healthy blood donors with functional assays that measure heparin cofactor activity have found a prevalence of antithrombin deficiency in the general population of 1 in 250 to 1 in 500[22,23]; a substantial number, however, have a type II defect with mutations at the heparin-binding site.[21] The best single screening test for the disorder is the antithrombin–heparin cofactor assay, which measures inhibition of factor Xa; it is the functional antithrombin assay that is most widely used today.

The mean concentration of antithrombin in normal pooled plasma is approximately 140 µg/mL. Most laboratories report a normal range between 75% and 120% of normal pooled plasma for antithrombin–heparin cofactor determinations and a somewhat wider range for immunoassay results. A variety of pathophysiologic conditions can reduce the concentration of antithrombin in blood. Antithrombin levels can drop substantially in patients with disseminated intravascular coagulation (DIC), sepsis, burns, and severe trauma but less commonly in the setting of acute thrombosis.[24] Reduced levels can also be seen in liver disease as a result of decreased synthesis or in nephrotic syndrome as a result of urinary protein loss.[25,26] Modest reductions are also found in users of oral contraceptives or estrogens.[27,28] In addition, the administration of heparin decreases plasma antithrombin levels, presumably by accelerated clearance of the heparin-antithrombin complex.[29] Thus, evaluation of plasma samples from individuals during a period of heparinization can potentially lead to an erroneous diagnosis of antithrombin deficiency.

Healthy newborns have about half the normal adult concentration of antithrombin[30,31] and gradually reach the adult level by 6 months of age.[32] Levels may be considerably lower in infants born at 30 to 36 weeks of gestation[32] and are even further reduced in infants with respiratory distress, necrotizing enterocolitis, sepsis, or DIC.[33] Thromboembolic events are rare in children with hereditary antithrombin deficiency. In the absence of heparin, antithrombin contributes approximately 80% of the thrombin-neutralizing capacity of normal adult plasma.[34,35] The levels of a second thrombin inhibitor, α_2-macroglobulin, are higher during the first 2 decades of life than in adults, and this may lessen the risk for thromboembolic complications in antithrombin-deficient patients during childhood.[36]

A number of clinical disorders can be associated with reductions in the plasma concentration of antithrombin, thus often making a definitive diagnosis of the hereditary state difficult. Although an antithrombin level in the normal range is usually sufficient to exclude the disorder, low levels should be confirmed at a later date. This determination is ideally performed when the individual is no longer receiving warfarin because plasma antithrombin concentrations can occasionally be elevated into the normal range in individuals with the deficiency state. In such situations, clinical assessment of the individual's risk for recurrent thrombosis will determine whether discontinuation of warfarin is feasible. In most antithrombin-deficient subjects, however, this effect of oral anticoagulants is not of sufficient magnitude to obscure the diagnosis.[37] Confirmation of the hereditary nature of the disorder requires the investigation of other family members. Diagnosis of other affected family members also allows appropriate counseling regarding the need for prophylaxis against venous thrombosis.

Protein C Deficiency

Protein C is a vitamin K–dependent protein synthesized by the liver that circulates as a zymogen. It exerts its anticoagulant function after activation to the serine protease activated protein C (APC). This process can be mediated by thrombin alone but occurs more efficiently when thrombin is bound to thrombomodulin on endothelial cells (see Chapter 26).

In 1981, Griffin and associates[38] described low levels of protein C in a family with recurrent thrombotic events. Subsequently, many other families with heterozygous protein C deficiency were reported.[39-41] Heterozygous protein C deficiency is inherited in an autosomal dominant fashion; a more severe form of protein C deficiency is an autosomal recessive disorder. The phenotype of patients with heterozygous protein C deficiency is similar to that of persons with hereditary antithrombin deficiency. In severely affected families, approximately 75% of protein C–deficient individuals experienced one or more thrombotic events. The initial episode occurs spontaneously in approximately 70% of those experiencing such events. The remaining 30% have the usual associated risk factors (pregnancy, parturition, contraceptive pill use, surgery, or trauma) at the time that the acute thrombotic events take place. Patients are infrequently symptomatic until their early twenties, with increasing numbers experiencing thrombotic events as they reach the age of 50.

The most common sites of disease are the deep veins of the legs, the iliofemoral veins, and the mesenteric veins. Approximately 63% of affected patients experience recurrent venous thrombosis, and approximately 40% exhibit signs of pulmonary embolism.[42] Superficial thrombophlebitis of the leg veins, as well as cerebral venous thrombosis, can occur in protein C–deficient patients.[39] There have been reports of nonhemorrhagic arterial stroke in young adults with hereditary protein C deficiency, but a causal relationship is unproven.

The prevalence of protein C deficiency in outpatients who have experienced an initial episode of venous thromboembolism ranges from 0.5% to 4%.[4,13,43] In earlier reports of more selected patient populations, protein C deficiency was more frequently identified and occurred in 2% to 9%. Initial estimates placed the prevalence of protein C deficiency between 1 in 16,000 and 1 in 32,000 within the general population based on the assumption that protein C was an autosomal dominant disorder with high penetrance and that at least half the individuals with the deficiency would demonstrate symptomatic thrombosis. However, it was difficult to reconcile this figure with the infrequent history of thrombosis in the parents of infants with purpura fulminans, which is due to the homozygous or doubly heterozygous form of protein C deficiency. This disparity led to studies of healthy blood donors in which a much higher prevalence of heterozygosity for protein C deficiency was found than previously estimated, with a range of 1 in 200 to 1 in 500.[44,45]

The risk of thrombosis initially attributed to protein C deficiency was subject to selection bias in that it was overestimated from familial reports. Data from the Leiden Thrombophilia Study indicate that heterozygous protein C deficiency is associated with about a sevenfold increased risk for an initial episode of deep venous thrombosis over that in normal persons.[13] Among Italian patients, protein C deficiency is associated with a similar sevenfold increase in venous thrombotic risk.[10] In asymptomatic carriers of protein C deficiency, the incidence of thrombosis is fairly low at 0.4% to 1.0% annually.[46] Similar to other inherited thrombophilias, this variability in phenotypic expression of protein C deficiency is not explained by differences in the particular genetic defect alone and probably represents a complex interaction with other modulating factors.

Two major subtypes of heterozygous protein C deficiency have been identified with the use of immunologic and functional assays (Table 32-2). The type I deficiency state is the most common form and is characterized by a reduction in both the immunologic and biologic activity of protein C to approximately 50% of normal. More than 195 different mutations have been identified, most commonly missense or nonsense mutations.[47] The functional or type II deficiency state is characterized by normal

TABLE 32-2	Assay Measurements in Heterozygous Protein C Deficiency		
		ACTIVITY	
Types	**Antigen**	**Amidolytic**	**Coagulant**
I	Low	Low	Low
II	Normal	Low	Low
	Normal	Normal	Low

synthesis of an abnormal protein. The functional capacity of protein C is most often assessed by using a snake venom protease (Protac)-based assay to directly activate the protein. After activation, an amidolytic assay can assess the functionality of the catalytic site of the protein. A few individuals have been described with normal levels of protein C antigen and amidolytic activity but with substantial reductions in protein C anticoagulant activity.[48] In such cases, protein C anticoagulant activity can be measured with a clotting assay (based on prolongation of the activated partial thromboplastin time [APTT]), and abnormalities presumably reflect a reduced ability of activated protein C to interact with the platelet membrane or its substrates such as factor Va and factor VIIIa. The coagulant assay thus has the highest sensitivity in screening patients for hereditary protein C deficiency.

Levels of protein C antigen in the heterozygous deficiency state overlap with those in the normal population, thus making it difficult to define the diagnosis in some patients. In general, antigen levels of 60% to 70% of normal represent borderline values and warrant repeat testing. Protein C antigen levels can also vary with age. Protein C levels in newborns are 20% to 40% of normal adult levels,[49] and preterm infants have even lower levels.[50] Neonates with significant perinatal thrombosis can have levels suggestive of homozygous deficiency.[51] In adults, protein C levels typically increase 4% per decade.[44]

Acquired protein C deficiency is found in numerous disease states, including liver disease, DIC, and sepsis. A particularly severe form of acquired protein C deficiency has been reported in association with purpura fulminans and DIC in individuals with acute meningococcal infections.[52,53] In contrast to antithrombin, antigenic concentrations of vitamin K–dependent plasma proteins, including protein C, are often elevated in individuals with nephrotic syndrome.[54] Most individuals with uremia have low levels of protein C anticoagulant activity but normal levels of protein C amidolytic activity and antigen.[55] This is attributable to a dialyzable moiety in uremic plasma that interferes with most clotting assays for protein C activity.[56]

As for other γ-carboxylase coagulation proteins (see Chapter 26), warfarin therapy reduces functional and, to a lesser extent, immunologic measurements of protein C, thus complicating diagnosis of the deficiency state.[48] Several researchers have proposed that the diagnosis can still be made in this setting based on the ratios of protein C antigen to factor II or factor X antigen. This method, however, will not detect patients with type II deficiency, and it can be used only in subjects in a stable phase of oral anticoagulation.[57] Other groups have used protein C activity assays in conjunction with functional measurements of factor VII, a vitamin K–dependent zymogen with a similar plasma half-life.[58] In practice, it is preferable to investigate individuals suspected of having the deficiency state after oral anticoagulation has been discontinued for at least 1 week and to perform family studies. If it is not possible to discontinue warfarin because of the severity of the thrombotic diathesis, such individuals can be studied while receiving heparin therapy, which does not alter plasma protein C levels.

Warfarin-induced skin necrosis has been associated with the presence of heterozygous protein C deficiency.[59-61] This syndrome typically occurs during the first several days of warfarin therapy, often in association with the administration of large loading doses of the medication. Skin lesions occur on the extremities, breasts, and trunk, as well as on the penis, and marginate over a period of hours from an initial central erythematous macule. If a product containing protein C is not administered rapidly, the affected cutaneous areas become edematous, central purpuric zones develop, and the lesions ultimately become necrotic. Biopsies demonstrate fibrin thrombi within cutaneous vessels with interstitial hemorrhage. The dermal manifestations of warfarin-induced skin necrosis are clinically and pathologically similar to those seen in infants with purpura fulminans resulting from severe protein C deficiency (see later).

The pathogenesis of warfarin-induced skin necrosis is attributable to the emergence of a transient hypercoagulable state. Initiation of the drug at standard doses leads to a decrease in protein C anticoagulant activity to approximately 50% of normal within 1 day.[48] Although factor VII activity follows a pattern similar to that of protein C, levels of the other vitamin K–dependent factors decline at slower rates, consistent with their longer half-lives. Increased thrombin generation has been documented in patients during this early phase of warfarin therapy.[62] During this period the drug's suppressive effect on protein C has a greater influence on the hemostatic mechanism than its reduction of factor VII does. These effects are augmented when a large–loading dose schedule (i.e., >10 mg of warfarin daily) is used to initiate oral anticoagulation or the patient has an underlying hereditary deficiency of protein C. However, only about a third of patients with warfarin-induced skin necrosis have an inherited deficiency of protein C,[63] and this complication is a rather infrequently reported event in individuals with the heterozygous deficiency state. This syndrome has been reported in association with an acquired functional deficiency of protein C.[64] There are also reports of hereditary protein S deficiency and the factor V Leiden mutation in association with warfarin-induced skin necrosis.[65-68]

The long-established syndrome of purpura fulminans is classically described as a complication of meningococcal infection in children. However, newborns rarely exhibit a syndrome of purpura fulminans, which is associated with laboratory evidence of DIC and protein C antigen levels less than 1% of normal.[69-78] In some instances there is a history of consanguinity in the family, thus making it highly likely that the affected infants were homozygous for the deficiency state.[70,73,76] Such newborns can also be double heterozygotes, as was demonstrated in a Chinese patient[74] who had a five-nucleotide deletion in one protein C allele and a missense mutation in the other.[79] The heterozygous parents of infants with purpura fulminans in association with severe protein C deficiency only infrequently have thromboses, in contrast to patients with thrombotic histories and a hereditary partial deficiency of protein C. There are, however, numerous reports of older patients with homozygous or doubly heterozygous protein C deficiency in whom purpura fulminans was not present. These individuals generally have protein C levels under 20% of normal in the absence of oral anticoagulant therapy, and their clinical manifestations were similar to that of severely affected subjects from thrombophilic kindreds with the heterozygous deficiency state.[80,81]

Protein S Deficiency

Protein S is a vitamin K–dependent protein that enhances the anticoagulant effect of APC. Primarily synthesized by hepatocytes but also by endothelial cells, megakaryocytes, and brain cells, protein S serves as a cofactor for APC, which then inactivates factors Va and VIIIa. Factor Va inactivation occurs by an ordered series of peptide bond scissions in the molecule's heavy chain: first, rapid cleavage at Arg506 takes place, followed by slower cleavage at Arg306 and then Arg679 (see Chapter 26).[82] Interaction of protein S with APC results in both an increased affinity for negatively charged phospholipids and a 20-fold enhancement of the slower phase of factor Va inactivation. In plasma, only 40% of protein C is available in the "free" form, whereas the remainder is bound to C4b-binding protein and cannot interact with APC.

Protein S deficiency is an autosomal dominant disorder that was originally described in 1984 in several kindreds with low levels of protein S and a striking history of recurrent thrombosis.[83,84] There is a reported frequency of approximately 10% in families with inherited thrombophilia[10,85]; however, the prevalence is lower (between 1% and 7%) in consecutive outpatients with a first episode of deep venous thrombosis.[4,13] Protein S deficiency is generally considered to confer a risk of thrombosis similar to that in protein C deficiency, although the association has been complicated by considerable phenotypic variability.

The clinical findings in patients with heterozygous protein S deficiency are similar to those outlined for deficiencies of antithrombin and protein C. Among 71 protein S–deficient members from 12 Dutch pedigrees,[86] 74%, 72%, and 38% of the individuals sustained deep venous thrombosis, superficial thrombophlebitis, and pulmonary emboli, respectively. The mean age at the first thrombotic event was 28 years, with a range of 15 to 68; 56% of the episodes were apparently spontaneous, and the remainder were precipitated by an identifiable factor. Thrombosis has also been reported in the axillary, mesenteric, and cerebral veins. Although there have been case reports of young patients with arterial thrombosis and

TABLE 32-3	Assay Measurements in Heterozygous Protein S Deficiency		
	PROTEIN S ANTIGEN		
Types	Total	Free	Protein S Activity
I	Low	Low	Low
II	Normal	Normal	Low
III	Normal	Low	Low

protein S deficiency, current data do not support an association between hereditary protein S deficiency and an increased risk for arterial thrombosis.[87]

Three types of protein S deficiency states can be identified based on measurements of total and free antigen, as well as functional activity (Table 32-3). The type I deficiency state is associated with approximately 50% of the normal total protein S antigen level[84] and greater reductions in free protein S antigen and protein S functional activity.[88] This defect is most often secondary to missense mutations and base pair insertions or deletions. The type II qualitative deficiency state, characterized by normal total and free protein S levels but abnormal functional activity, has been identified infrequently, thus suggesting that current functional assays may not screen for all such defects. In type III deficiency, total protein S antigen levels are normal, with disproportionately decreased free protein S and functional activity.

The biologic basis of the type III protein S deficiency state is uncertain. Furthermore, coexistence of type I and type III deficiency has been reported in some protein S–deficient families, which has led to the proposal that the two types of protein S deficiency are phenotypic variants of the same genotype and are not the product of distinct genetic mutations.[89] In a follow-up analysis of one large family with a high prevalence of both type I and type III deficiency, total protein S antigen, but not free protein S antigen levels, were shown to directly correlate with age.[90] These findings were independent of gender and were also seen in nondeficient family members. The researchers concluded that a single point mutation in the protein S gene was responsible for the quantitative type I deficiency but that the type III phenotype was actually due to an age-dependent free protein S deficiency; with increasing age, the relative concentrations of free protein S to total protein S decreased. However, a Dutch cohort study of first-degree family members with protein S deficiency found that affected relatives of probands with type I deficiency were at increased risk for venous thromboembolism whereas affected relatives of probands with type III deficiency were not.[87]

There are multiple causes of acquired protein S deficiency, including pregnancy and oral contraceptive use. Protein S levels are commonly low in inflammatory states, including DIC and acute thrombosis, largely because of protein S interaction with C4b-binding protein. C4b-binding protein is an acute phase reactant and shifts protein S to the complexed, inactive form, which leads to decreased protein S activity.[91] Levels of total and free protein S are significantly reduced in men infected with human immunodeficiency virus (HIV).[92] Although total protein S antigen measurements are generally increased in individuals with nephrotic syndrome, functional assays are often reduced[54] because of loss of free protein S in urine and elevated C4b-binding protein levels.

The lower limit of normal total and free protein S in plasma is approximately 65%; however, there is considerable overlap between the heterozygous deficiency state and low normal. Such overlap is largely due to the influence of age, which leads to an increase in protein S levels, and the influence of sex, with females having a lower normal limit for plasma protein S levels than males do. Thus, it is difficult to diagnose heterozygous protein S deficiency by performing a single assay; repeat sampling and family studies are usually required to make the diagnosis.

Young patients with recurrent venous thromboembolic disease associated with doubly heterozygous or homozygous protein S deficiency have been identified.[83] The parents of these patients were asymptomatic and had laboratory studies consistent with type I protein S deficiency. Neonatal purpura fulminans has been described in association with homozygous protein S deficiency.[93,94]

Resistance to Activated Protein C and the Factor V Leiden Mutation

Before 1993, hereditary deficiencies were infrequently identified in patients with familial thromboembolic disease. Dahlbäck and colleagues[95] identified several probands with venous thrombosis that appeared to be resistant to APC in an APTT-based clotting assay. When compared with controls, many family members of the probands also had a blunted anticoagulant response to APC. The following year, Bertina and associates[96] identified the genotype underlying most cases of APC resistance as a single point mutation in the factor V gene leading to substitution of Arg506 by glutamine. This mutation at an APC cleavage site renders factor Va relatively resistant to inactivation by APC.[82,96]

After Dahlbäck and coworkers' description of APC resistance, several studies revealed that this defect was relatively common in individuals with venous thrombosis. Svensson and Dahlbäck[97] screened 104 consecutive Swedish individuals referred for evaluation of venous thrombosis and found that 33% of the subjects demonstrated APC resistance. In a U.S. referral population of individuals younger than 50 years with unexplained venous thromboembolic disease, Griffin and colleagues[98] found that approximately 50% exhibited APC resistance.

Dutch investigators had previously initiated the Leiden Thrombophilia Study to identify risk factors for a first episode of venous thrombosis. Excluding patients with known malignancies, 345 consecutive outpatients younger than 70 years with confirmed deep venous thrombosis were initially reported.[99] Using a screening APTT-based assay, APC resistance was identified in 21% of individuals with thrombosis and in 5% of age- and sex-matched healthy controls. The factor V Arg506Gln (or factor V Leiden) mutation was found in more than 80% of the patients who had been found to be APC resistant.[96] The lower frequency of APC resistance seen in the Leiden Thrombophilia Study than in previous studies is attributable to differences in selection criteria and referral cohorts.

The U.S. Physicians' Health Study has also provided valuable data regarding factor V Leiden as a risk factor for venous and arterial thrombosis. In a retrospective case-control study of 14,916 healthy men older than 40 with a mean follow-up period of 8.6 years, heterozygosity for the factor V Leiden mutation was identified in 12% of patients (14/121) with a first episode of deep venous thrombosis or pulmonary embolism and in 6% of controls.[100] The relative risk for venous thromboembolism was increased 3.5-fold in those with no other concomitant risk factors but was reduced to 1.7-fold in patients with preexistent cancer or recent surgery. This study also showed that elderly patients with venous thrombosis frequently have the mutation.[100] Among men older than 60 years with initial episodes of venous thrombosis and no identifiable triggering factors, 26% (8/31) were heterozygotes for factor V Leiden.

A cohort study of more than 9000 randomly selected adults in Denmark found that the simultaneous presence of smoking, obesity (body mass index > 30 kg/m^2), older age (>60 years), and the factor V Leiden mutation resulted in absolute 10-year venous thromboembolism rates of 10% in heterozygotes and 51% in homozygotes.[101]

A prospective cohort study determined the incidence of venous thromboembolism in asymptomatic carriers of the factor V Leiden mutation identified through family studies of symptomatic probands. Nine events occurred in 1564 observation-years, for an annual incidence of 0.58%. It was concluded that the absolute annual incidence of venous thromboembolism in asymptomatic carriers of the mutation is low.[102]

A number of studies have examined whether factor V Leiden, a prevalent abnormality in white populations, leads to an increased risk for arterial thrombotic events. There are no convincing data that other thrombophilic states such as deficiencies of antithrombin, protein C, and protein S confer an increased risk for arterial thrombosis, but evaluation of these associations is complicated by the relative infrequency of these defects. In a cohort of men older than 40 years with a low prevalence of smoking, the U.S. Physicians' Health Study did not find an association between the factor V Leiden mutation and myocardial infarction or stroke.[100] In a younger cohort of

Italian patients with myocardial infarction occurring before 45 years of age, an increased incidence of the factor V Leiden mutation relative to that in controls also was not found.[103]

Because of the frequency of heterozygosity for the factor V Leiden mutation in white individuals, homozygosity is not a particularly rare occurrence, and its presence is compatible with normal gestational survival. However, homozygotes for factor V Leiden are at significantly higher risk for venous thrombosis than heterozygotes are[104,105] and demonstrate heightened APC resistance in APTT assays.[96,104,106] Patients with heterozygosity for the factor V Leiden mutation along with deficiencies of protein C, antithrombin, or protein S[107-111] are also at significantly greater risk for venous thromboembolism than individuals with only a single genetic defect are. The genes for factor V and antithrombin are both located on the long arm of chromosome 1, thereby allowing coinheritance of the factor V Leiden mutation and an antithrombin mutation within all affected members of a family. This situation is expected to lead to an even more severe thrombotic diathesis.[109]

Obstetric complications, such as severe preeclampsia, abruptio placentae, fetal growth retardation, and stillbirth, are associated with intervillous or spiral artery thrombosis and consequent placental insufficiency. Factor V Leiden, as well as other hereditary thrombophilias, is associated with an approximate tripling of the risk for late fetal loss.[112,113] An increased incidence of factor V Leiden, as well as other thrombophilias, was also reported in women in association with other obstetric complications[114]; associations with preeclampsia and intrauterine growth restriction/retardation have, however, not been corroborated.[115,116]

The prevalence of heterozygosity for the factor V Leiden mutation in whites, including European, Jewish, Israeli Arab, and Indian populations, ranges between 1% and 8.5%. The mutation apparently is not present in African blacks or in Chinese, Japanese, or Native American populations.[117] In Europe, the mutation has been found to be more prevalent in northern countries such as Sweden than in southern countries such as Spain and Italy. By using dimorphic sites in the factor V gene to perform haplotype analysis, data have been provided that support the existence of a single founder allele among whites of differing ethnic background.[118] It was also estimated that the mutation originated approximately 30,000 years ago, which came after the evolutionary divergence of white, African, and Asian populations.

Two mutations at the Arg306 residue in factor V, the second APC cleavage site in the activated cofactor, have been described in patients with a history of thrombosis. These mutations are replacement of Arg306 with threonine (factor V Cambridge)[119] and with glycine (in Hong Kong Chinese).[120] The latter mutation, however, evidently has no clinical relevance because it is not associated with APC resistance and the mutation is as common in healthy Chinese blood donors as in patients with thrombosis (4.5% and 4.7%, respectively).[121] The factor V Cambridge mutation is extremely rare among whites with venous thromboembolic disease.

Cosegregation of heterozygous APC resistance as a result of the factor V Leiden mutation and type I factor V deficiency has been reported in some patients.[122-124] The plasma of these individuals manifests severe APC resistance in partial thromboplastin time (PTT) assays, as found in homozygous factor V Leiden patients (i.e., the patients with such cosegregation are pseudohomozygous). These patients were seemingly more prone to thrombosis than were heterozygous relatives with factor V Leiden alone, thus suggesting that their clinical phenotype is similar to that of homozygous factor V Leiden patients.

Several polymorphisms are present in the factor V gene.[125,126] An extended factor V gene haplotype (HR2) containing the R2 polymorphism (His1299Arg) is associated with mild APC resistance and occurs with increased frequency in heterozygous patients with the factor V Leiden mutation and the lowest APC resistance ratios.[126] Although one case-control study found that the R2 allele was a risk factor for venous thromboembolism with an odds ratio of 2.0 after excluding subjects with genetic defects such as factor V Leiden,[127] another case-control study found no significant increase in risk.[128]

The initial observations of Dahlbäck and associates[95] facilitated the development of a PTT-based assay that serves as a screening test for APC resistance. The PTT assay is performed in the presence or absence of a standardized amount of APC, and the two clotting times are converted to an APC ratio. Results can be interpreted by comparing the ratio with the normal range or by normalizing it to the APC resistance ratio obtained with normal pooled plasma. Although this first-generation APC resistance assay was conceptually quite simple and easy to perform in a coagulation laboratory, it required careful standardization and determination of the normal range in at least 50 controls. The level of APC, the PTT reagent, and the instrumentation used for clot detection affected the performance characteristics of the assay. Some assays using this format therefore had inadequate sensitivity and specificity for the factor V Leiden mutation. Moreover, patients who were receiving anticoagulants or had an abnormal PTT because of other coagulation defects could not be evaluated with this assay, and the test was not validated in patients with acute thrombosis or in pregnant women.

The discovery that factor V Leiden is the dominant genetic defect responsible for APC resistance facilitated the development of second-generation coagulation tests that with proper standardization can give nearly 100% sensitivity and 100% specificity for detection of the mutation. For these tests, patient plasma is diluted in a sufficient volume of factor V–deficient plasma, and then a PTT-based assay is performed. This modification also permits evaluation of the plasma of patients who are receiving anticoagulants or have abnormal PTT results because of coagulation factor deficiencies other than factor V.

The fact that the dominant mutation underlying APC resistance is factor V Leiden makes it attractive to diagnose this defect by analyzing genomic DNA in peripheral blood mononuclear cells. This can readily be accomplished by amplifying a DNA fragment containing the factor V mutation site by polymerase chain reaction (PCR) and analyzing the cleavage products on ethidium bromide–stained agarose gels after restriction enzyme digestion with MnlI.[96] The substitution of an A for a G at nucleotide 1691 in factor V cDNA (CGA to CAA) results in the Arg506Gln mutation and loss of a MnlI cleavage site. Other diagnostic approaches include hybridization with allele-specific oligonucleotide probes.

Prothrombin G20210A Mutation

In 1996, investigators from Leiden reported that a G-to-A substitution at nucleotide 20210 in the 3′-untranslated region of the prothrombin gene is associated with elevated plasma prothrombin levels and an increased risk for venous thrombosis.[129] This mutation, which was discovered by directly sequencing the prothrombin gene of selected patients with venous thrombosis, is located in the 3′-untranslated region at the cleavage site for polyadenylation of prothrombin mRNA. The prothrombin 20210A mutation changes the position of the 3′-cleavage/polyadenylation reaction in prothrombin mRNA, thereby leading to increased prothrombin biosynthesis by the liver[130]; this finding is in contrast to previous data that the mutation changes mRNA stability by increasing mRNA 3′-end formation.[131]

Investigation of a referral population with a personal and family history of venous thrombosis demonstrated that 18% had the mutation in the 3′-untranslated region of the prothrombin gene whereas it was present in only 1 of 100 healthy controls.[129] Among these thrombosis patients, 40% also carried the factor V Leiden mutation, thus emphasizing the current view of venous thrombosis as a multigene disorder.

In the Leiden Thrombophilia Study, 6.2% of venous thrombosis patients and 2.3% of healthy matched controls had the prothrombin gene mutation.[129] This mutation independently confers a 2.8-fold increased risk for venous thrombosis, and the effect is operative in both sexes and all age groups. Among heterozygotes with the prothrombin gene mutation, 87% of patients with thrombosis and controls in the study had prothrombin activity levels that were greater than 1.15 U/mL, whereas only

23% of those with a normal prothrombin genotype had levels elevated to this degree.

The prothrombin G20210A mutation has been documented in numerous studies to have a significantly higher incidence in patients with venous thrombosis than in healthy controls.[132-134] Large population studies have shown an overall prevalence of about 2% in the general white population, with significant geographic variation. In southern Europeans the prevalence is about 3%, but it was only very rarely identified in individuals of Asian or African descent.

PCR methods have been used to detect the prothrombin G20210A mutation in genomic DNA.[129] In addition, methods are available to detect both the prothrombin G20210A mutation and factor V Leiden in the same reaction.[135] Although plasma prothrombin activity and antigen levels are significantly higher in individuals with the prothrombin G20210A mutation, prothrombin concentrations cannot be used to screen for the defect because of significant overlap with the normal population.[129,136]

HYPERHOMOCYSTEINEMIA

Homocysteine is a sulfur-containing amino acid involved in metabolic pathways leading to the formation of other amino acids; methionine is generated through the remethylation of homocysteine or metabolized to cysteine via trans-sulfuration. The normal plasma homocysteine concentration is 5 to 16 μmol/L.

Homocystinuria is a rare autosomal recessive inborn error of metabolism that occurs in childhood. The most frequent cause is homozygous cystathionine β-synthase deficiency, which has a frequency in the general population of approximately 1 in 250,000. As a result of impaired intracellular metabolism of homocysteine, increased amounts of the amino acid accumulate in blood and are excreted in urine. Children with homocystinuria exhibit premature atherosclerosis and venous thromboembolism, along with mental retardation, ectopic lenses, and skeletal abnormalities. A small number of cases are due to homozygous defects in the gene encoding methylenetetrahydrofolate reductase (MTHFR), and persons so affected are similarly afflicted with premature vascular disease and thrombosis along with neurologic problems. The mechanisms by which hyperhomocysteinemia acts as an atherogenic and thrombogenic risk factor have been only partially elucidated.[137,138]

During the last 2 decades, mild or moderate hyperhomocysteinemia was identified as a seemingly independent risk factor for venous and arterial thrombotic events.[139-141] Mild (16 to 24 μmol/L) or moderate (25 to 100 μmol/L) hyperhomocysteinemia results from genetic and acquired abnormalities. Although heterozygous cystathionine β-synthase deficiency is found in only approximately 0.3% of the general population, a MTHFR variant with an alanine-to-valine substitution at amino acid 677 is common[142] and can be present in 1.4% to 15% of the population, depending on their origin.[141] This mutation causes thermolability of MTHFR and a 50% reduction in its specific activity. The most common causes of acquired hyperhomocysteinemia are deficiencies of vitamin B_{12}, folate, or vitamin B_6, which are cofactors in homocysteine metabolism. There is a strong inverse correlation between hyperhomocysteinemia and folate levels and, to a lesser extent, with vitamin B_{12} and B_6 concentrations. Elderly patients frequently have elevated plasma homocysteine concentrations, even in the absence of vitamin deficiencies, as do patients with renal failure. Cigarette smoking is also associated with acquired hyperhomocysteinemia.

Whereas patients with homocystinuria secondary to cystathionine β-synthase deficiency have levels higher than 100 μmol/L, individuals with heterozygous defects in this gene or inadequate vitamin B_6 levels may have normal or only slightly elevated levels of fasting homocysteine. Discrimination of such patients from normal individuals can be improved by demonstrating an abnormal increase in plasma homocysteine 4 hours after an oral methionine load. Defects in the remethylation pathway as a result of MTHFR gene defects or inadequate folate or vitamin B_{12} levels tend to cause elevated homocysteine levels under fasting conditions. The prevalence of hyperhomocysteinemia is almost twice as high when based on homocysteine measurements performed after methionine loading as when based on fasting levels. Genetic testing for the common Ala677Val mutation in MTHFR is also possible.

Because folic acid, vitamin B_6, and vitamin B_{12} supplementation can decrease plasma homocysteine levels, it was hypothesized that treatment with these supplements would reduce the risk for arterial and venous thrombosis. Large randomized placebo-controlled clinical trials, however, reported that clinical outcomes are not improved by providing supplements of these vitamins to patients with histories of ischemic stroke,[143] myocardial infarction,[144] vascular disease,[145] or venous thrombosis.[146]

Because there are currently no data that persons with mild hyperhomocysteinemia and a history of venous or arterial thrombosis should be managed any differently from those with normal homocysteine levels, there is no longer justification for routinely determining homocysteine levels in such patients. In addition, results from the Leiden MEGA (Multiple Environmental and Genetic Assessment of risk factors for venous thrombosis) study indicate that the presence of homozygosity for the MTHFR C6777T polymorphism, which mildly increases homocysteine levels, is not associated with an increased risk for venous thrombosis.[147] It should furthermore be noted that the prevalence of hyperhomocysteinemia in the U.S. population has declined since the wheat supply was fortified with folic acid in the late 1990s. Although there were previous reports that hyperhomocysteinemia significantly increased the risk for a first venous thrombotic event in patients with the factor V Leiden mutation,[148] a recent publication found no additive or multiplicative interaction between these abnormalities for the risk of venous thrombosis.[149]

DYSFIBRINOGENEMIAS

Qualitative fibrinogen abnormalities are inherited in an autosomal dominant manner. The dysfibrinogenemias are a heterogeneous group of disorders that may be asymptomatic or be manifested as a bleeding diathesis or recurrent venous or arterial thromboembolism. A small number of variant fibrinogens have been reported to be associated with thrombotic complications. These defects can be detected with thrombin and reptilase times, which are often prolonged. Functional fibrinogen measurements are usually substantially lower than antigenic measurements in the plasma of affected patients. An occasional patient with dysfibrinogenemia may have a prolonged prothrombin time or PTT, and the inability of some abnormal fibrinogens to clot completely in vitro can result in false-positive results in fibrin(ogen) degradation product tests.

The functional and biochemical defects of a number of abnormal fibrinogens associated with thromboembolic disease have been characterized.[150,151] The conversion of fibrinogen to fibrin by thrombin results in the proteolytic cleavage of fibrinopeptides A and B from the molecule. Defects in the release of these two peptides[152-155] or abnormalities in fibrin polymerization[156-159] have been reported. Such functional defects do not, however, offer a ready explanation for the thrombotic diathesis seen in these subjects. Abnormalities in the binding of thrombin to fibrin have also been found in some dysfibrinogenemias.[160-163] In one of these kindreds, three homozygous siblings with a Bβ-chain substitution of Ala by Thr at position 68 had a severe clinical phenotype and sustained both arterial and venous thrombosis at a young age.[162,164] It has been suggested that decreased binding of thrombin by this mutant fibrinogen may lead to the presence of excessive thrombin in the circulation and the occurrence of thrombosis.[164] Other fibrinogen mutants have been shown to cause abnormal fibrin polymerization.[156-158,161] Some abnormal fibrinogens have been evaluated for their ability to resist or promote fibrinolysis upon incorporation into a fibrin clot. The fibrin formed from fibrinogen "Chapel Hill III" has been demonstrated to be abnormally resistant to lysis by plasmin.[156] Activation of plasminogen is decreased in the presence of the fibrin formed from fibrinogen Dusart despite normal binding of tissue plasminogen activator to the substrate.[165-169] These abnormalities clearly have the potential for decreasing fibrinolytic activity in vivo, which results in a familial thrombotic diathesis in biochemically affected persons. The coexistence of factor V Leiden may predispose individuals with certain dysfibrinogenemias to thrombo-embolism.[170]

INHERITED ABNORMALITIES OF FIBRINOLYSIS

Although investigators have identified a few individuals with inherited abnormalities of the fibrinolytic mechanism and recurrent venous thromboembolism, the clinical association is considerably less striking than that in many kindreds with deficiencies of antithrombin, protein C, or protein S or with the prothrombin gene mutation or APC resistance as a result of the factor V Leiden mutation. Dysplasminogenemia or hypoplasminogenemia has been reported in a number of individuals with thromboembolic disease; the first case of an abnormal plasminogen was identified in Japan.[171] The propositus had a history of recurrent thrombosis, and family studies demonstrated that the biochemical abnormality followed an autosomal dominant inheritance pattern. Despite the hereditary nature of the defect, none of the other biochemically affected members of the kindred had experienced a thrombotic event. Other Japanese pedigrees without thrombosis have since been described with the same biochemical defect; the gene frequency of this variant in the Japanese population was 0.018.[172] Population studies in the United States have not uncovered any cases of this dysplasminogenemia. The non-Japanese cases of dysplasminogenemia and hypoplasminogenemia have also been characterized by the absence of thrombotic episodes in biochemically affected family members other than the propositi.

Severe type 1 plasminogen deficiency is associated with a rare chronic inflammatory disease of the mucous membranes. The disorder is characterized by the presence of fibrin-rich pseudomembranous lesions, and the most common clinical manifestations are ligneous conjunctivitis (80%) and ligneous gingivitis (34%); less common sites of involvement are the vagina, respiratory tract, ears, and gastrointestinal tract.[173] Patients with this disorder have been found to be homozygous or compound heterozygous for a number of different mutations in the plasminogen gene.[173] Although this disorder can occasionally be life threatening, venous thrombosis was not observed in these patients. A severely affected infant with ligneous conjunctivitis has been treated successfully with a purified plasminogen concentrate,[174] but this product is not generally commercially available.

There have been reports documenting the existence of thrombophilic families with impaired fibrinolysis.[175,176] Re-evaluation of several of these families demonstrated the presence of hereditary protein S deficiency and no association between elevations in plasminogen activator inhibitor 1 (PAI-1) activity and a history of thrombosis.[177,178]

MANAGEMENT OF PATIENTS WITH INHERITED THROMBOTIC DISORDERS

Acute Thrombosis and Long-Term Management

When a patient with one of the inherited thrombotic disorders is discovered, family studies should be conducted because approximately half the members of a given kindred may be affected. Institution of long-term anticoagulation is not generally recommended for individuals who have not yet sustained thrombotic episodes. Affected individuals, however, should receive counseling regarding the implications of the diagnosis and advice regarding the symptoms that require immediate medical attention. In women of childbearing age, oral contraceptives are generally contraindicated in view of the increased thrombotic risk associated with the use of these medications. All biochemically affected individuals should be carefully evaluated before surgical, medical, or obstetric procedures that carry an increased thrombotic risk. These subjects should then receive appropriate prophylactic anticoagulation regimens. If specific concentrates are available for a patient with a particular deficiency state, these concentrates can also be administered to raise plasma levels of the protein to the normal range during the perioperative period. All women with previous thrombotic episodes should receive prophylactic heparin throughout pregnancy, and asymptomatic women should also generally receive such treatment.

Management of an acute thrombotic event in patients with a hereditary thrombotic disorder is generally similar to that for patients without an identifiable risk factor. Anticoagulant therapy is initiated with appropriate doses of heparin, low-molecular-weight heparin, or fondaparinux for 5 to 10 days, and warfarin (or another vitamin K antagonist) is begun within 24 hours to produce an international normalized ratio (INR) of 2.0 to 3.0. The indications for thrombolytic therapy in patients with these disorders are similar to those in other patients with acute venous thrombosis or pulmonary embolism. Standard therapy for patients with deep venous thrombosis or pulmonary embolism typically includes anticoagulation with warfarin for 3 to 12 months at a target INR of between 2 and 3; this regimen results in more than a 90% reduction in risk of recurrence.

In patients with a first episode of symptomatic venous thromboembolism, Prandoni and colleagues[179] found the cumulative incidence of recurrent venous thrombosis after the cessation of anticoagulant therapy to be 24.8% at 5 years and 30.3% at 8 years. Other investigators have confirmed that this risk is about 5% to 15% per year for the first several years after a first or even a second episode of unprovoked venous thrombosis. Recurrences are less common when the initial event is associated with a transient risk factor (e.g., surgery, trauma, pregnancy). Despite the relatively high recurrence risk in patients with a first episode of unprovoked venous thrombosis, anticoagulation with warfarin has not proved to have sufficient benefit in terms of bleeding risk to support long-term prophylaxis for all patients at substantial risk for recurrence. For example, one controlled trial evaluated the efficacy of long-term warfarin therapy (INR of 2 to 2.85) for 6 months or indefinitely in 227 patients with a second venous thrombotic episode, but not specifically inherited thrombophilia.[180] Long-term warfarin was highly effective in preventing recurrences when compared with 6 months of therapy (2.6% versus 21% over a period of 4 years); this benefit was partially counterbalanced by a trend toward an increased incidence of major hemorrhage (8.6% versus 2.3%), and there was no difference in mortality rate between the two groups.

Because of the relatively high frequency of the factor V Leiden mutation in patients with a first episode of venous thromboembolism, there is a substantial amount of data on the risk of recurrence. Although two groups initially reported that patients with factor V Leiden who had a first venous thrombotic event were more than twice as likely to have a recurrent episode than those without the mutation were,[148,181] several other groups have not found that heterozygosity for this defect or the prothrombin G20210A mutation confers a higher risk for recurrence.[182-186] Thus, the consensus view is that neither of these defects alone is predictive of recurrence, and several studies have argued against the use of long-term warfarin therapy after a first thromboembolic episode in these patient populations. There is no increase in mortality among patients with the factor V Leiden mutation.[187] The recurrence risk appears to be significantly higher in the small subset of patients who are heterozygous for two hereditary prothrombotic defects or homozygous for factor V Leiden.[107-110,185,188]

As a result of the relatively low frequency of antithrombin, protein C, or protein S deficiency in unselected cohorts with an initial episode of venous thromboembolism, randomized clinical trials have included too few patients with these deficiencies to draw firm conclusions. A literature review and retrospective cohort study suggested that they have a high annual incidence of recurrent venous thromboembolism during the years immediately after a first episode and that this incidence declines thereafter.[189] Retrospective studies are unable to demonstrate an increase in mortality in patients with antithrombin[190] or protein C deficiency.

For the individual patient, the decision to continue anticoagulation indefinitely requires estimation of the quantitative risk over time for recurrent thrombosis (including fatal pulmonary embolism) and major bleeding (including fatal bleeding). Patient compliance has a major impact on the success of therapy, and patient preferences must be factored into the decision. Thus, given that future events in a patient with only one previous thrombotic episode cannot currently be accurately predicted and because there is a finite risk of bleeding associated with warfarin therapy, recommendations regarding long-term anticoagulation are individualized. The following clinical features should be considered in making this decision:

1. The number, sites, and severity of thrombosis. A patient who previously sustained massive pulmonary embolism is more likely to receive long-term warfarin than is a subject in whom deep venous thrombosis developed in a calf vein unless there are symptoms or signs of a significant postphlebitic syndrome.

2. Whether the thrombotic episodes were spontaneous or whether precipitating factors were present. If a precipitating event such as a major abdominal operation was present when the initial venous thrombotic event occurred, the risk of recurrence is substantially lower than if the event was spontaneous, and the patient does not require long-term oral anticoagulation after the initial episode is adequately treated.

3. The patient's risk of bleeding while receiving warfarin. A history of bleeding or difficulty accurately monitoring and controlling warfarin therapy because of altered gastrointestinal function will lead to an increased risk for bleeding.

4. The sex and lifestyle of the individual. Situations in which these factors may influence the decision to recommend long-term anticoagulation include women of childbearing age planning to conceive (warfarin is generally contraindicated in women bearing a fetus, especially during the 6th to 12th weeks of gestation because of the teratogenic risk), occupations that entail prolonged periods of immobilization and therefore might be associated with an increased risk for thromboembolism, and jobs with a higher than average chance of trauma that might lead to thrombotic or bleeding complications, or both.

5. A history of thromboembolism in other biochemically affected members of the family. Although marked intrafamilial and interfamilial heterogeneity has been observed in the phenotypic expression of inherited thrombotic disorders, it is reasonable for biochemically affected patients from severely affected kindreds with a single thrombotic episode to take oral anticoagulants indefinitely.

Antithrombin Deficiency

Patients with antithrombin deficiency can usually be treated successfully with intravenous heparin,[191] although in some situations unusually high doses of the drug are required to achieve adequate anticoagulation. In patients with antithrombin deficiency who are receiving heparin for the treatment of acute thrombosis, the adjunctive role of antithrombin concentrate purified from human plasma is not clearly defined because controlled trials have not been performed.[191] The latter product should probably be administered when difficulty is encountered in achieving adequate heparinization or recurrent thrombosis is observed despite adequate anticoagulation. It is also reasonable to treat subjects who are antithrombin deficient with concentrate before major surgery or in obstetric situations in which the risks of bleeding from anticoagulation are unacceptable. The manufacturing processes used to prepare antithrombin concentrate result in a product that is greater than 95% pure; they also inactivate hepatitis B virus and HIV type 1.[192,193] Hence, it is preferable to administer antithrombin concentrate rather than fresh frozen plasma. A human antithrombin concentrate has also been produced from the milk of transgenic goats by recombinant DNA technology[194] and is commercially available in Europe.

The biologic half-life of antithrombin is approximately 48 hours.[14] Infusion of 50 units of plasma-derived antithrombin concentrate per kilogram of body weight (1 unit is defined as the amount of antithrombin in 1 mL of pooled normal human plasma) will usually raise the plasma antithrombin level to approximately 120% in a congenitally deficient individual with a baseline level of 50%.[193,195-198] Plasma levels should be monitored to ensure that they remain above 80%; administration of 60% of the initial dose at 24-hour intervals is recommended to maintain inhibitor levels in the normal range.[198]

Coumarin-Induced Skin Necrosis

Because coumarin-induced skin necrosis is a rare complication, therapy has been guided primarily by knowledge regarding its pathogenesis. The diagnosis should be suspected in patients with painful, red skin lesions developing within a few days after initiation of the drug, and immediate intervention is required to prevent rapid progression and reduce complications. Therapy should consist of immediate discontinuation of warfarin, administration of vitamin K, and infusion of heparin at therapeutic doses. Lesions have been reported to progress, however, despite adequate anticoagulation with heparin. In patients with hereditary protein C deficiency, administration of a source of protein C should be seriously considered, and it may also be appropriate in other patients with coumarin-induced skin necrosis because they invariably have reduced plasma levels of functional protein C when the skin lesions first appear. Fresh frozen plasma has been used, but improved results can be expected after the administration of a highly purified protein C concentrate, which facilitates rapid and complete normalization of plasma protein C levels.[199]

Because of the infrequent occurrence of coumarin-induced skin necrosis, it may be advisable to take special precautions when initiating oral anticoagulant treatment in a patient who is previously known or likely to have protein C deficiency. Warfarin should be started only when the patient is fully heparinized, and the dose of the drug should be increased gradually, starting at a relatively low level (e.g., 2 mg for the first 3 days and then in increasing amounts of 2 to 3 mg until therapeutic anticoagulation is achieved). Patients with heterozygous protein C deficiency and a history of warfarin-induced skin necrosis have been successfully retreated with oral anticoagulants. Protein C administration either in the form of fresh frozen plasma or protein C concentrate provides protection against the development of recurrent skin necrosis until a stable level of anticoagulation is achieved.[60,200]

Homozygous or Doubly Heterozygous Protein C Deficiency and Neonatal Purpura Fulminans

Management of neonatal purpura fulminans in association with homozygous or doubly heterozygous protein C deficiency is complicated, and neither heparin therapy nor antiplatelet agents have been shown to be effective.[69,71-75] Administration of a protein C source appears to be critical in the initial treatment of these patients. Fresh frozen plasma has been used successfully to treat these infants. However, the half-life of protein C in the circulation is only about 6 to 16 hours,[48,201] and frequent administration of plasma is limited by the development of hyperproteinemia or hypertension, loss of venous access, and the potential for exposure to infectious viral agents. A highly purified concentrate of protein C has been developed and is efficacious in treating neonatal purpura fulminans.[202] Warfarin has been administered to these infants without the redevelopment of skin necrosis during the phased withdrawal of fresh frozen plasma infusions,[69,74,76,203,204] and this medication has been used chronically to control the thrombotic diathesis. A 20 month-old child with liver failure and homozygous protein C deficiency successfully underwent liver transplantation, which normalized his protein C levels and resolved the thrombotic diathesis.[205]

REFERENCES

1. Egeberg O. Inherited antithrombin deficiency causing thrombophilia. Thromb Diath Haemorrh. 1965;13:516-530.
2. Gruenberg JC, Smallridge RC, Rosenberg RD. Inherited antithrombin-III deficiency causing mesenteric venous infarction: a new clinical entity. Ann Surg. 1975;181:791-794.
3. Marciniak E, Farley CH, DeSimone PA. Familial thrombosis due to antithrombin III deficiency. Blood. 1974;43:219-231.
4. Heijboer H, Brandjes DPM, Büller HR, et al. Deficiencies of coagulation-inhibiting and fibrinolytic proteins in outpatients with deep venous thrombosis. N Engl J Med. 1990;323:1512-1516.
5. Thaler E, Lechner K. Antithrombin III deficiency and thromboembolism. In Prentice CRM (ed). Clinics in Haematology. London, WB Saunders, 1981, pp 369-380.

6. Demers C, Ginsberg JS, Hirsh J, et al. Thrombosis in antithrombin-III–deficient persons. Report of a large kindred and literature review. Ann Intern Med. 1992;116: 754-761.

7. Ambruso DR, Jacobson LJ, Hathaway WE. Inherited antithrombin III deficiency and cerebral thrombosis in a child. Pediatrics. 1980;65:125-131.

8. Winter JH, Bennett B, Watt JL, et al. Confirmation of linkage between antithrombin III and Duffy blood group and assignment of AT3 to 1q22-q25. Ann Hum Genet. 1982;46:29-34.

9. Brenner B, Fishman A, Goldsher D, et al. Cerebral thrombosis in a newborn with a congenital deficiency of antithrombin III. Am J Hematol. 1988;27:209-211.

10. Martinelli I, Mannucci PM, DeStefano V, et al. Different risks of thrombosis in four coagulation defects associated with inherited thrombophilia: a study of 150 families. Blood. 1998;92:2353-2358.

11. Simioni P, Sanson BJ, Prandoni P, et al. Incidence of venous thromboembolism in families with inherited thrombophilia. Thromb Haemost. 1999;81:198-202.

12. van der Meer FJM, Koster T, Vandenbroucke JP, et al. The Leiden Thrombophilia Study (LETS). Thromb Haemost. 1997;78:631-635.

13. Koster T, Rosendaal FR, Briët E, et al. Protein C deficiency in a controlled series of unselected outpatients: an infrequent but clear risk factor for venous thrombosis (Leiden Thrombophilia Study). Blood. 1995;85:2756-2761.

14. Ambruso DR, Leonard BD, Bies RD, et al. Antithrombin III deficiency: decreased synthesis of a biochemically normal molecule. Blood. 1982;60:78-83.

15. Bayston T, Lane D. Antithrombin Mutation Database. Department of Haematology, Imperial College London Website. Available at http://www1.imperial.ac.uk/medicine/about/divisions/is/haemo/coag/antithrombin/. Accessed April 4, 2008.

16. Sas G, Blasko G, Banhegyi D, et al. Abnormal antithrombin III (antithrombin III "Budapest") as a cause of familial thrombophilia. Thromb Diath Haemorrh. 1974;32: 105-115.

17. Finazzi G, Caccia R, Barbui T. Different prevalance of thromboembolism in the subtypes of congenital antithrombin deficiency: review of 404 cases [letter]. Thromb Haemost. 1987;58:1094.

18. Brunel F, Duchange N, Fischer AM, et al. Antithrombin III Alger: a new case of Arg47-Cys mutation. Am J Haematol. 1987;25:223-224.

19. Ueyama H, Murakami T, Nishiguchi S, et al. Antithrombin III Kumamoto: identification of a point mutation and genotype analysis of the family. Thromb Haemost. 1990;63:231-234.

20. Wells PS, Blajchman MA, Henderson P, et al. Prevalence of antithrombin deficiency in healthy blood donors: a cross-sectional study. Am J Hematol. 1994;45:321-324.

21. Tait RC, Walker ID, Perry DJ, et al. Prevalence of antithrombin deficiency in the healthy population. Br J Haematol. 1994;87:106-112.

22. Meade TW, Dyer S, Howarth DJ, et al. Antithrombin III and procoagulant activity; sex differences and effects of the menopause. Br J Haematol. 1990;74:77-81.

23. Tait RC, Walker ID, Davidson JF, et al. Antithrombin III activity in healthy blood donors: age and sex related changes and the prevalence of asymptomatic deficiency [letter]. Br J Haematol. 1990;75:141-142.

24. de Boer AC, van Riel LAM, den Ottolander GJH. Measurement of antithrombin III, α_2-macroglobulin and α_1-antitrypsin in patients with deep venous thrombosis and pulmonary embolism. Thromb Res. 1979;15:17-25.

25. von Kaulla E, von Kaulla KN. Antithrombin III and diseases. Am J Clin Pathol. 1967;48:69-80.

26. Kauffman RH, Veltkamp JJ, Van Tilburg NH, et al. Acquired antithrombin III deficiency and thrombosis in the nephrotic syndrome. Am J Med. 1978;65:607-613.

27. Weenink GH, Kahle LH, Lamping RJ, et al. Antithrombin III in oral contraceptive users and during normotensive pregnancy. Acta Obstet Gynecol Scand. 1984;63:57-61.

28. Caine YG, Bauer KA, Barzegar S, et al. Coagulation activation following estrogen administration to postmenopausal women. Thromb Haemost. 1992;68:392-395.

29. Marciniak E, Gockemen JP. Heparin-induced decrease in circulating antithrombin III. Lancet. 1978;2:581-584.

30. McDonald MM, Hathaway WE, Reeve EB, et al. Biochemical and functional study of antithrombin III in newborn infants. Thromb Haemost. 1982;47:56-58.

31. Andrew M, Paes B, Milner R, et al. Development of the human coagulation system in the full-term infant. Blood. 1987;70:165-172.

32. Andrew M, Paes B, Milner R, et al. Development of the human coagulation system in the healthy premature infant. Blood. 1988;72:1651-1657.

33. Manco-Johnson MJ. Neonatal antithrombin III deficiency. Am J Med. 1989;87(Suppl 3B):49S-52S.

34. Rosenberg RD, Damus PS. The purification and mechanism of action of human antithrombin–heparin cofactor. J Biol Chem. 1973;248:6490-6505.

35. Downing MR, Bloom JW, Mann KG. Comparison of the inhibition of thrombin by three plasma protease inhibitors. Biochemistry. 1978;17:2649-2653.

36. Mitchell L, Piovella F, Ofosu F, et al. α_2-Macroglobulin may provide protection from thromboembolic events in antithrombin III–deficient children. Blood. 1991;78:2299-2304.

37. Kitchens CS. Amelioration of antithrombin III deficiency by coumarin administration. Am J Med Sci. 1987;293: 403-406.

38. Griffin JH, Evatt B, Zimmerman TS, et al. Deficiency of protein C in congenital thrombotic disease. J Clin Invest. 1981;68:1370-1373.

39. Broekmans AW, Veltkamp JJ, Bertina RM. Congenital protein C deficiency and venous thromboembolism: a study of three Dutch families. N Engl J Med. 1983;309: 340-344.

40. Horellou MH, Conard J, Bertina RM, et al. Congenital protein C deficiency and thrombotic disease in nine French families. BMJ. 1984;289:1285-1287.

41. Bovill EG, Bauer KA, Dickerman JD, et al. The clinical spectrum of heterozygous protein C deficiency in a large New England kindred. Blood. 1989;73:712-717.

42. Broekmans AW, Bertina RM. Protein C. In Poller L (ed). Recent Advances in Blood Coagulation. IV. New York, Churchill Livingstone, 1985, pp 117-137.

43. Mateo J, Oliver A, Borrell M, et al. Laboratory evaluation and clinical characteristics of 2,132 consecutive unselected patients with venous thromboembolism—results of the

Spanish multicentric study on thrombophilia (EMET Study). Thromb Haemost. 1997;77:444-451.

44. Miletich JP, Sherman L, Broze GJ Jr. Absence of thrombosis in subjects with heterozygous protein C deficiency. N Engl J Med. 1987;317:991-996.

45. Tait RC, Walker ID, Reitsma PH, et al. Prevalence of protein C deficiency in the healthy population. Thromb Haemost. 1995;73:87-93.

46. Sanson BJ, Simioni P, Tormene D, et al. The incidence of venous thromboembolism in asymptomatic carriers of a deficiency of antithrombin, protein C, or protein S: a prospective cohort study. Blood. 1999;94:3702-3706.

47. D'Ursi P, Marino F, Caprera A, et al. ProCMD: a database and 3D web resource for protein C mutants. BMC Bioinformatics. 2007;8(Suppl 1):S11.

48. D'Angelo SV, Comp PC, Esmon CT, et al. Relationship between protein C antigen and anticoagulant activity during oral anticoagulation and in selected disease states. J Clin Invest. 1986;77:416-425.

49. Manco-Johnson MJ, Marlar RA, Jacobson LJ, et al. Severe protein C deficiency in newborn infants. J Pediatr. 1988;113:359-363.

50. Karpatkin M, Mannucci PM, Bhogal M, et al. Low protein C in the neonatal period. Br J Haematol. 1986;62:137-142.

51. Polack B, Pouzol P, Amiral J, et al. Protein C level at birth. Thromb Haemost. 1984;52:188-190.

52. Auletta MJ, Headington JT. Purpura fulminans. A cutaneous manifestation of severe protein C deficiency. Arch Dermatol. 1988;124:1387-1391.

53. Gerson WT, Dickerman JD, Bovill EG, et al. Severe acquired protein C deficiency in purpura fulminans associated with disseminated intravascular coagulation: treatment with protein C concentrate. Pediatrics. 1993;91:418-422.

54. Vigano-D'Angelo S, D'Angelo A, Kaufman CE Jr, et al. Protein S deficiency occurs in the nephrotic syndrome. Ann Intern Med. 1987;107:42-47.

55. Sorensen PJ, Knudsen F, Nielsen AH, et al. Protein C activity in renal disease. Thromb Res. 1985;38:243-249.

56. Faioni EM, Franchi F, Krachmalnicoff A, et al. Low levels of the anticoagulant activity of protein C in patients with chronic renal insufficiency: an inhibitor of protein C is present in uremic plasma. Thromb Haemost. 1991;66:420-425.

57. Pabinger I, Kyrle PA, Speiser W, et al. Diagnosis of protein C deficiency in patients on oral anticoagulant treatment: comparison of three different functional protein C assays. Thromb Haemost. 1990;63:407-412.

58. Jones DW, Mackie IJ, Winter M, et al. Detection of protein C deficiency during oral anticoagulant therapy—use of the protein C:factor VII ratio. Blood Coagul Fibrinolysis. 1991;2:407-411.

59. McGehee WG, Klotz TA, Epstein DJ, et al. Coumarin necrosis associated with hereditary protein C deficiency. Ann Intern Med. 1984;100:59-60.

60. Zauber NP, Stark MW. Successful warfarin anticoagulation despite protein C deficiency and a history of warfarin necrosis. Ann Intern Med. 1986;104:659-660.

61. Bauer KA. Coumarin-induced skin necrosis. Arch Dermatol. 1993;129:766-768.

62. Conway EM, Bauer KA, Barzegar S, et al. Suppression of hemostatic system activation by oral anticoagulants in the blood of patients with thrombotic diatheses. J Clin Invest. 1987;80:1535-1544.

63. Broekmans AW, Teepe RGC, van der Meer FJM, et al. Protein C (PC) and coumarin-induced skin necrosis [abstract]. Thromb Res. 1986;6:137.

64. Teepe RGC, Broekmans AW, Vermeer BJ, et al. Recurrent coumarin-induced skin necrosis in a patient with an acquired functional protein C deficiency. Arch Dermatol. 1986;122:1408-1422.

65. Sallah S, Abdallah JM, Gagnon GA. Recurrent warfarin-induced skin necrosis in kindreds with protein S deficiency. Haemostasis. 1998;28:25-30.

66. Gailani D, Reese EP Jr. Anticoagulant-induced skin necrosis in a patient with hereditary deficiency of protein S. Am J Hematol. 1999;60:231-236.

67. Makris M, Bardhan G, Preston FE. Warfarin induced skin necrosis associated with activated protein C resistance [letter]. Thromb Haemost. 1996;75:523-524.

68. Freeman BD, Schmieg RE Jr, McGrath S, et al. Factor V Leiden mutation in a patient with warfarin-associated skin necrosis. Surgery. 2000;127:595-596.

69. Branson HE, Katz J, Marble R, et al. Inherited protein C deficiency and coumarin-responsive chronic relapsing purpura fulminans in a newborn infant. Lancet. 1983;2:1165-1168.

70. Seligsohn U, Berger A, Abend M, et al. Homozygous protein C deficiency manifested by massive venous thrombosis in the newborn. N Engl J Med. 1984;310:559-562.

71. Sills RH, Marlar RA, Montgomery RR, et al. Severe homozygous protein C deficiency. J Pediatr. 1984;105:409-413.

72. Estelles A, Garcia-Plaza I, Dasi A, et al. Severe inherited 'homozygous' protein C deficiency in a newborn infant. Thromb Haemost. 1984;52:53-56.

73. Marciniak E, Wilson HD, Marlar RA. Neonatal purpura fulminans: a genetic disorder related to the absence of protein C in blood. Blood. 1985;65:15-20.

74. Yuen P, Cheung A, Lin HJ, et al. Purpura fulminans in a Chinese boy with congenital protein C deficiency. Pediatrics. 1986;77:670-676.

75. Rappaport ES, Speights VO, Helbert B, et al. Protein C deficiency. South Med J. 1987;80:240-242.

76. Peters C, Casella JF, Marlar RA, et al. Homozygous protein C deficiency: observations on the nature of the molecular abnormality and the effectiveness of warfarin therapy. Pediatrics. 1988;81:272-276.

77. Tarras S, Gadia C, Meister L, et al. Homozygous protein C deficiency in a newborn. Clinicopathologic correlation. Arch Neurol. 1988;45:214-216.

78. Pegelow CH, Curless R, Bradford B. Severe protein C deficiency in a newborn. Am J Pediatr Hematol Oncol. 1988;10:326-329.

79. Sugahara Y, Miura O, Yuen P, et al. Protein C deficiency Hong Kong 1 and 2: hereditary protein C deficiency caused by two mutant alleles, a 5-nucleotide deletion and a missense mutation. Blood. 1992;80:126-133.

80. Bauer KA, Broekmans AW, Bertina RM, et al. Hemostatic enzyme generation in the blood of patients with hereditary protein C deficiency. Blood. 1988;71:1418-1426.

81. Melissari E, Kakkar VV. Congenital severe protein C deficiency in adults. Br J Haematol. 1989;72:222-228.

82. Kalafatis M, Bertina RM, Rand MD, et al. Characterization of the molecular defect in factor VR506Q. J Biol Chem. 1995;270:4053-4057.

83. Comp PC, Nixon RR, Cooper MR, et al. Familial protein S deficiency is associated with recurrent thrombosis. J Clin Invest. 1984;74:2082-2088.

84. Schwarz HP, Fischer M, Hopmeier P, et al. Plasma protein S deficiency in familial thrombotic disease. Blood. 1984;64:1297-1300.

85. Gandrille S, Borgel D, Ireland H, et al. Protein S deficiency: a database of mutations. For the Plasma Coagulation Inhibitors Subcommittee of the Scientific and Standardization Committee of the International Society on Thrombosis and Haemostasis. Thromb Haemost. 1997;77:1201-1214.

86. Engesser L, Broekmans AW, Briet E, et al. Hereditary protein S deficiency: clinical manifestations. Ann Intern Med. 1987;106:677-682.

87. Brouwer JP, Veeger NJGM, van der Schaaf W, et al. Difference in absolute risk of venous and arterial thrombosis between familial protein S deficiency type I and type III. Results from a family cohort study to assess the clinical impact of a laboratory test–based classification. Br J Haematol. 2005;128:703-710.

88. Comp PC, Doray D, Patton D, et al. An abnormal plasma distribution of protein S occurs in functional protein S deficiency. Blood. 1986;67:504-508.

89. Zöller B, García de Frutos P, Dahlbäck B. Evaluation of the relationship between protein S and C4b-binding protein isoforms in hereditary protein S deficiency demonstrating type I and type III deficiencies to be phenotypic variants of the same genetic disease. Blood. 1995;85:3524-3531.

90. Simmonds RE, Zöller B, Ireland H, et al. Genetic and phenotypic analysis of a large (122-member) protein S–deficient kindred provides an explanation for the familial coexistence of type I and type III plasma phenotypes. Blood. 1997;89:4364-4370.

91. D'Angelo A, Vigano-D'Angelo S, Esmon CT, et al. Acquired deficiencies of protein S. Protein S activity during oral anticoagulation, in liver disease, and in disseminated intravascular coagulation. J Clin Invest. 1988;81:1445-1454.

92. Stahl CP, Wideman CS, Spira TJ, et al. Protein S deficiency in men with long-term human immunodeficiency virus infection. Blood. 1993;81:1801-1807.

93. Mahasandana C, Suvatte V, Chuansumrit A, et al. Homozygous protein S deficiency in an infant with purpura fulminans. J Pediatr. 1990;117:750-753.

94. Pegelow CH, Ledford M, Young J, et al. Severe protein S deficiency in a newborn. Pediatrics. 1992;89:674-676.

95. Dahlbäck B, Carlsson M, Svensson PJ. Familial thrombophilia due to a previously unrecognized mechanism characterized by poor anticoagulant response to activated protein C: prediction of a cofactor to activated protein C. Proc Natl Acad Sci U S A. 1993;90:1004-1008.

96. Bertina RM, Koeleman BPC, Koster T, et al. Mutation in blood coagulation factor V associated with resistance to activated protein C. Nature. 1994;369:64-67.

97. Svensson PJ, Dahlback B. Resistance to activated protein C as a basis for venous thrombosis. N Engl J Med. 1994;330:517-522.

98. Griffin JH, Evatt B, Wideman C, et al. Anticoagulant protein C pathway defective in majority of thrombophilic patients. Blood. 1993;82:1989-1993.

99. Koster T, Rosendaal FR, de Ronde H, et al. Venous thrombosis due to poor anticoagulant response to activated protein C: Leiden thrombophilia study. Lancet. 1993;342:1503-1506.

100. Ridker PM, Hennekens CH, Lindpaintner K, et al. Mutation in the gene coding for coagulation factor V and the risk of myocardial infarction, stroke, and venous thrombosis in apparently healthy men. N Engl J Med. 1995;332:912-917.

101. Juul K, Tybjaerg-Hansen A, Scshnohr P, et al. Factor V Leiden and the risk for venous thromboembolism in the adult Danish population. Ann Intern Med. 2004;140:330-337.

102. Middeldorp S, Meinardi JR, Koopman MM, et al. A prospective study of asymptomatic carriers of the factor V Leiden mutation to determine the incidence of venous thromboembolism. Ann Intern Med. 2001;135:322-327.

103. Ardissino D, Mannucci PM, Merlini PA, et al. Prothrombotic genetic risk factors in young survivors of myocardial infarction. Blood. 1999;94:46-51.

104. Zöller B, Svensson PJ, He X, et al. Identification of the same factor V gene mutation in 47 out of 50 thrombosis-prone families with inherited resistance to activated protein C. J Clin Invest. 1994;94:2521-2524.

105. Rosendaal FR, Koster T, Vandenbroucke JP, et al. High-risk of thrombosis in patients homozygous for factor V Leiden (APC-resistance). Blood. 1995;85:1504-1508.

106. Greengard JS, Sun X, Xu X, et al. Activated protein C resistance caused by Arg506Gln mutation in factor Va. Lancet. 1994;343:1361-1362.

107. Koeleman BPC, Reitsma PH, Allaart CF, et al. Activated protein C resistance as an additional risk factor for thrombosis in protein C–deficient families. Blood. 1994;84:1031-1035.

108. Gandrille S, Greengard JS, Alhenc-Gelas M, et al. Incidence of activated protein C resistance caused by ARG 506 GLN mutation in factor V in 113 unrelated symptomatic protein C–deficient patients. Blood. 1995;86:219-224.

109. van Boven HH, Reitsma PH, Rosendaal FR, et al. Factor V Leiden (R506Q) in families with inherited antithrombin deficiency. Thromb Haemost. 1996;75:417-421.

110. Zöller B, Berntsdotter A, de Frutos GP, et al. Resistance to activated protein C as an additional risk factor in hereditary deficiency of protein S. Blood. 1995;12:3518-3523.

111. Koeleman BPC, van Rumpt D, Hamulyak K, et al. Factor V Leiden: an additional risk factor for thrombosis in protein S deficient families? Thromb Haemost. 1995;74:580-583.

112. Preston FE, Rosendaal FR, Walker ID, et al. Increased fetal loss in women with heritable thrombophilia. Lancet. 1996;348:913-916.

113. Martinelli I, Taioli E, Cetin I, et al. Mutations in coagulation factors in women with unexplained late fetal loss. N Engl J Med. 2000;343:1015-1018.

114. Kupferminc MJ, Eldor A, Steinman N, et al. Increased frequency of genetic thrombophilia in women with complications of pregnancy. N Engl J Med. 1999;340:9-13.

115. de Groot CJ, Bloemenkamp KW, Duvekot EJ, et al. Pre-eclampsia and genetic risk factors for thrombosis: a case-control study. Am J Obstet Gynecol. 1999;181:975-980.

116. Infante-Rivard C, Rivard GE, Yotov WV, et al. Absence of association of thrombophilia polymorphisms with intrauterine growth restriction. N Engl J Med. 2002;347:19-25.

117. Rees DC, Cox M, Clegg JB. World distribution of factor V Leiden. Lancet. 1995;346:1133-1134.

118. Zivelin A, Griffin JH, Xu X, et al. A single genetic origin for a common Caucasian risk factor for venous thrombosis. Blood. 1997;89:397-402.

119. Williamson D, Brown K, Luddington R, et al. Factor V Cambridge: a new mutation (Arg306→Thr) associated with resistance to activated protein C. Blood. 1998;91:1140-1144.

120. Chan WP, Lee CK, Kwong YL, et al. A novel mutation of Arg306 of factor V gene in Hong Kong Chinese. Blood. 1998;91:1135-1139.

121. Liang R, Lee CK, Wat MS, et al. Clinical significance of Arg306 mutations of factor V gene. Blood. 1998;92:2599-2600.

122. Simione P, Soudeller A, Radossi P, et al. "Pseudo homozygous" activated protein C resistance due to double heterozygous factor V defects (factor V Leiden mutation and type I quantitative factor V defect) associated with thrombosis: report of two cases belonging to two unrelated kindreds. Thromb Haemost. 1996;75:422-426.

123. Guasch JF, Lensen RPM, Bertina RM. Molecular characterization of a type I quantitative factor V deficiency in a thrombosis patient that is "pseudo homozygous" for activated protein C resistance. Thromb Haemost. 1996;77:252-257.

124. Zehnder JL, Jain M. Recurrent thrombosis due to compound heterozygosity for the factor V Leiden mutation and factor V deficiency. Blood Coagul Fibrinolysis. 1996;7:361-362.

125. Lunghi B, Iacoviello L, Gemmati D, et al. Detection of new polymorphic markers in the factor V gene: association with factor V levels in plasma. Thromb Haemost. 1996;75:45-48.

126. Bernardi F, Faioni EM, Castoldi E, et al. A factor V genetic component differing from factor V R506Q contributes to the activated protein C resistance phenotype. Blood. 1997;90:1552-1557.

127. Alhenc-Gelas M, Nicaud V, Gandrille S, et al. The factor V gene A4070G mutation and the risk of venous thrombosis. Thromb Haemost. 1999;81:193-197.

128. Luddington R, Jackson A, Pannerselvam S, et al. The factor V R2 allele: risk of venous thromboembolism, factor V levels and resistance to activated protein C. Thromb Haemost. 2000;83:204-208.

129. Poort SR, Rosendaal FR, Reitsma PH, et al. A common genetic variation in the 3′-untranslated region of the prothrombin gene is associated with elevated prothrombin levels and an increase in venous thrombosis. Blood. 1996;88:3698-3703.

130. Pollak ES, Lam H, Russell JE. The G20210A mutation does not affect the stability of prothrombin mRNA in vivo. Blood. 2002;100:359-362.

131. Gehring NH, Frede U, Neu-Yilik G, et al. Increased efficiency of mRNA 3′ end formation: a new genetic mechanism contributing to hereditary thrombophilia. Nat Genet. 2001;28:389-392.

132. Hillarp A, Zöller B, Svensson P, et al. The 20210 A allele of the prothrombin gene is a common risk factor among Swedish outpatients with verified deep vein thrombosis. Thromb Haemost. 1997;78:990-992.

133. Kapur RK, Mills LA, Spitzer SG, et al. A prothrombin gene mutation is significantly associated with venous thrombosis. Arterioscler Thromb Vasc Biol. 1997;17:2875-2879.

134. Margaglione M, Brancaccio V, Giuliani N, et al. Increased risk for venous thrombosis in carriers of the prothrombin G→A20210 gene variant. Ann Intern Med. 1998;129:89-93.

135. Gomez E, van der Poel SC, Jansen JH, et al. Rapid simultaneous screening of factor V Leiden and G20210A prothrombin variant by multiplex polymerase chain reaction on whole blood [letter]. Blood. 1998;91:2208-2209.

136. Soria J, Almasy L, Souto J, et al. Linkage analysis demonstrates that the prothrombin G21210A mutation jointly influences plasma prothrombin levels and risk of thrombosis. Blood. 2000;95:2780-2785.

137. Welch GN, Loscalzo J. Homocysteine and atherothrombosis. N Engl J Med. 1998;1998:1042-1050.

138. Feinbloom D, Bauer KA. Assessment of hemostatic risk factors in predicting arterial thrombotic events. Arterioscler Thromb Vasc Biol. 2005;25:2043-2053.

139. Den Heijer M, Koster T, Blom HJ, et al. Hyperhomocysteinemia as a risk factor for deep-vein thrombosis. N Engl J Med. 1996;334:759-762.

140. De Stefano V, Finazzi G, Mannucci PM. Inherited thrombophilia: Pathogenesis, clinical syndromes, and management. Blood. 1996;87:3531-3544.

141. D'Angelo A, Selhub J. Homocysteine and thrombotic disease. Blood. 1997;90:1-11.

142. Frosst P, Blom HJ, Milos R, et al. A candidate genetic risk factor for vascular disease: a common mutation in methylenetetrahydrofolate reductase. Nat Genet. 1995;10:111-113.

143. Toole JF, Malinow MR, Chambless LE, et al. Lowering homocysteine in patients with ischemic stroke to prevent recurrent stroke, myocardial infarction, and death. The vitamin intervention for stroke prevention (VISP) randomized controlled trial. JAMA. 2004;291:565-575.

144. Bønaa KH, Njølstad I, Ueland PM, et al. Homocysteine lowering and cardiovascular events after acute myocardial infarction. N Engl J Med. 2006:354:1578-1588.

145. The Heart Outcomes Prevention Evaluation (HOPE) 2 Investigators. Homocysteine lowering with folic acid and B vitamins in vascular disease. N Engl J Med. 2006;354:1567-1577.

146. den Heijer M, Willems HP, Blom HJ, et al. Homocysteine lowering by B vitamins and the secondary prevention of deep vein thrombosis and pulmonary embolism: a randomized, placebo-controlled, double-blind trial. Blood. 2007;109:139-144.

147. Bezemer ID, Doggen CJ, Vos HL, Rosendaal FR. No association between the common MTHFR 677C→T polymorphism and venous thrombosis: results from the MEGA Study. Arch Intern Med. 2007;167:497-501.

148. Ridker PM, Miletich JP, Stampfer MJ, et al. Factor V Leiden and risks of recurrent idiopathic venous thromboembolism. Circulation. 1995;92:2800-2802.

149. Keijzer MB, Borm GF, Blom HJ, et al. No interaction between factor V Leiden and hyperhomocysteinemia or MTHFR C677T genotype in venous thrombosis. Results of a meta-analysis of published studies and a large case-control study. Thromb Haemost. 2007;97:32-37.

150. Mossesson MW. Dysfibrinogenemia and thrombosis. Semin Thromb Hemost. 1999;25:311-319.

151. Roberts HR, Stinchcombe TE, Gabriel DA. The dysfibrinogenemias. Br J Haematol. 2001;114:249-257.

152. Beck EA, Charache P, Jackson DP. A new inherited coagulation disorder caused by an abnormal fibrinogen (fibrinogen "Baltimore"). Nature. 1965;208:143-145.

153. Beck EA, Shainoff JR, Vogel A, et al. Functional evaluation of an inherited abnormal fibrinogen: fibrinogen Baltimore. J Clin Invest. 1971;50:1874-1884.

154. Sandbjerg-Hansen J, Clemmensen I, Wither D. Fibrinogen Copenhagen: an abnormal fibrinogen with defective polymerization and release of fibrinopeptide A, but normal absorption of plasminogen. Scand J Clin Lab Invest. 1980;40:221-226.

155. Henschen A, Kehl M, Southan C, et al. Genetically abnormal fibrinogens—some current characterization strategies. In Haverkate F, Henschen A, Nieuwenhuizen W, Straub PW (eds). Fibrinogen—Structure, Functional Aspects, Metabolism. Berlin, Walter de Gruyter, 1983, pp 125-144.

156. Carrell N, Gabriel DA, Blatt PM, et al. Hereditary dysfibrinogenemia in a patient with thrombotic disease. Blood. 1983;62:439-447.

157. Carrell N, McDonagh J. Functional defects in abnormal fibrinogens. In Henschen A, Hessel B, McDonagh J, Saldeen T (eds). Fibrinogen: Structural Variants and Interactions. Berlin, Walter de Gruyter, 1985, pp 155-164.

158. Soria J, Soria C, Samama M, et al. Fibrinogen Haifa: fibrinogen variant with absence of protective effect of calcium on plasmin degradation of gamma chains. Thromb Haemost. 1987;57:310-313.

159. Lounes KC, Soria C, Mirshahi SS, et al. Fibrinogen Ales: a homozygous case of dysfibrinogenemia (gamma-Asp(330)→Val) characterized by a defective fibrin polymerization site "a." Blood. 2000;96:3473-3479.

160. Al-Mondhiry HAB, Bilezikian SB, Nossel HL. Fibrinogen "New York"—an abnormal fibrinogen associated with thromboembolism: functional evaluation. Blood. 1975;45:607-619.

161. Soria J, Soria C, Samama M, et al. Study of 10 cases of congenital dysfibrinogenemia. Clinical and molecular biological aspects. In Henschen A, Hessel B, McDonagh J, Saldeen T (eds). Fibrinogen: Structural Variants and Interactions. Berlin, Walter de Gruyter, 1985, pp 165-183.

162. Haverkate F, Koopman J, Kluft C, et al. Fibrinogen Milano II: a congenital dysfibrinogenemia associated with juvenile arterial and venous thrombosis. Thromb Haemost. 1986;55:131-135.

163. Marchi R, Lundberg U, Grimbergen J, et al. Fibrinogen Caracas V, an abnormal fibrinogen with an Alpha 532 Ser→Cys substitution associated with thrombosis. Thromb Haemost. 2000;84:263-270.

164. Koopman J, Haverkate F, Lord ST, et al. The molecular basis of fibrinogen Naples associated with defective α-thrombin binding and congenital thrombophilia: homozygous substitution of Bb 68 Ala-Thr [abstract]. Thromb Haemostas. 1991;65:809.

165. Soria J, Soria C, Caen JP. A new type of congenital dysfibrinogenemia with defective fibrin lysis—Dusard syndrome: possible relation to thrombosis. Br J Haematol. 1983;53:575-586.

166. Lijnen HR, Soria J, Soria C, et al. Dysfibrinogenemia (fibrinogen Dusard) associated with impaired fibrin-enhanced plasminogen activation. Thromb Haemost. 1984;51:108-109.

167. Koopman J, Haverkate F, Grimbergen J, et al. Molecular basis for fibrinogen Dusart (Aa 554 Arg-Cys) and its association with abnormal fibrin polymerization and thrombophilia. J Clin Invest. 1993;91:1637-1643.

168. Collet J-P, Soria J, Mirshahi M, et al. Dusart syndrome: a new concept of the relationship between fibrin clot architecture and fibrin clot degradability: hypofibrinolysis related to an abnormal clot structure. Blood. 1993;82:2462-2469.

169. Tarumi T, Martincic D, Thomas A, et al. Familial thrombophilia associated with fibrinogen paris V: Dusart syndrome. Blood. 2000;96:1191-1193.

170. Siebenlist KR, Mosesson MW, Meh DA, et al. Coexisting dysfibrinogenemia (gammaR275C) and factor V Leiden deficiency associated with thromboembolic disease (fibrinogen Cedar Rapids). Blood Coagul Fibrinolysis. 2000;11:293-304.

171. Aoki N, Moroi M, Sakata Y, et al. Abnormal plasminogen. A hereditary abnormality found in a patient with recurrent thrombosis. J Clin Invest. 1978;61:1186-1195.

172. Aoki N, Tateno K, Sakata Y. Differences of frequency distributions of plasminogen phenotypes between Japanese and American populations: new methods for the detection of plasminogen variants. Biochem Genet. 1984;22:871-881.

173. Tefs K, Gueorguieva M, Klammt J, et al. Molecular and clinical spectrum of type I plasminogen deficiency: a series of 50 patients. Blood. 2006;108:3021-3026.

174. Schott D, Dempfle CE, Beck B, et al. Therapy with a purified plasminogen concentrate in an infant with ligneous conjunctivitis and homozygous plasminogen deficiency. N Engl J Med. 1998;339:1679-1686.

175. Johansson L, Hedner U, Nilsson IM. A family with thromboembolic disease associated with deficient fibrinolytic activity in vessel wall. Acta Med Scand. 1978;203:477-480.

176. Stead NW, Bauer KA, Kinney TR, et al. Venous thrombosis in a family with defective release of vascular plasminogen activator and elevated plasma factor VIII/von Willebrand factor. Am J Med. 1983;74:33-39.

177. Bolan CD, Krishnamurti C, Tang DB, et al. Association of protein S deficiency with thrombosis in a kindred with elevated levels of plasminogen activator-1. Ann Intern Med. 1993;119:779-785.

178. Zöller B, Dahlbäck B. Protein S deficiency in a large family with thrombophilia previously characterized as having an inherited fibrinolytic defect [abstract]. Thromb Haemost. 1993;69:1256.

179. Prandoni P, Lensing AWA, Cogo A, et al. The long-term clinical course of acute deep venous thrombosis. Ann Intern Med. 1996;125:1-7.

180. Schulman S, Granqvist S, Holmström M, et al. The duration of oral anticoagulant therapy after a second episode

of venous thromboembolism. N Engl J Med. 1997;336: 393-398.

181. Simioni P, Prandoni P, Lensing AWA, et al. The risk of recurrent venous thromboembolism in patients with an Arg506→Gln mutation in the gene for factor V (factor V Leiden). N Engl J Med. 1997;336:399-403.

182. Eichinger S, Minar E, Hirschl M, et al. The risk of early recurrent venous thromboembolism after oral anticoagulant therapy in patients with the G20210A transition in the prothrombin gene. Thromb Haemost. 1999;81: 14-17.

183. Lindmarker P, Schulman S, Sten-Linder M, et al. The risk of recurrent venous thromboembolism in carriers and non-carriers of the G1691A allele in the coagulation factor V gene and the G20210A allele in the prothrombin gene. Thromb Haemost. 1999;81:684-690.

184. Margaglione M, D'Andrea G, Colaizzo D, et al. Coexistence of factor V Leiden and factor II A20210 mutations and recurrent venous thromboembolism. Thromb Haemost. 1999;82:1583-1587.

185. De Stefano V, Martinelli I, Mannucci PM, et al. The risk of recurrent deep venous thrombosis among heterozygous carriers of both factor V Leiden and the G20210A prothrombin mutation. N Engl J Med. 1999;341:801-806.

186. Christiansen SC, Cannegieter SC, Koster T, et al. Thrombophilia, clinical factors, and recurrent venous thrombotic events. JAMA. 2005;293:2352-2361.

187. Hille ET, Westendorp RG, Vandenbroucke JP, et al. Mortality and causes of death in families with the factor V Leiden mutation (resistance to activated protein C). Blood. 1997;89:1963-1967.

188. Emmerich J, Rosendaal FR, Cattaneo M, et al. Combined effect of factor V Leiden and prothrombin 20210A on the risk of venous thromboembolism—pooled analysis of 8 case-control studies including 2310 cases and 3204 controls. Study Group for Pooled-Analysis in Venous Thromboembolism. Thromb Haemost. 2001;86:809-816.

189. van den Belt AG, Sanson BJ, Simioni P, et al. Recurrence of venous thromboembolism in patients with familial thrombophilia. Arch Intern Med. 1997;157:2227-2232.

190. van Boven HH, Vandenbroucke JP, Westendorp RG, et al. Mortality and causes of death in inherited antithrombin deficiency. Thromb Haemost. 1997;77:452-455.

191. Schulman S, Tengborn L. Treatment of venous thromboembolism in patients with congenital deficiency of antithrombin III. Thromb Haemost. 1992;68:634-636.

192. Hoffman DL. Purification and large-scale preparation of antithrombin III. Am J Med. 1989;87:23S-26S.

193. Menache D, O'Malley JP, Schorr JB, et al. Evaluation of the safety, recovery, half-life, and clinical efficacy of antithrombin III (human) in patients with hereditary antithrombin III deficiency. Blood. 1990;75:33-39.

194. Edmunds T, Van Patten SM, Pollock J, et al. Transgenically produced human antithrombin: structural and functional comparison to human plasma–derived antithrombin. Blood. 1998;91:4561-4571.

195. Mannucci PM, Boyer C, Wolf M, et al. Treatment of congenital antithrombin III deficiency with concentrates. Br J Haematol. 1982;50:531-535.

196. Winter JH. Transfusion studies in patients with familial antithrombin III deficiency: half disappearance time of infused antithrombin III and influence of such infusions on platelet life span. Br J Haematol. 1981;49:449-453.

197. Brandt P. Observations during the treatment of antithrombin III deficient women in heparin and antithrombin III during pregnancy, parturition, and abortion. Thromb Res. 1981;22:15-24.

198. Schwartz RS, Bauer KA, Rosenberg RD, et al. Clinical experience with antithrombin III concentrate in treatment to congenital and acquired deficiency of antithrombin. Am J Med. 1989;87:53S-60S.

199. Schramm W, Spannagl M, Bauer KA, et al. Treatment of coumarin-induced skin necrosis with a monoclonal antibody purified protein C concentrate. Arch Dermatol. 1993;129:753-756.

200. De Stefano V, Mastrangelo S, Schwarz HP, et al. Replacement therapy with a purified protein C concentrate during initiation of oral anticoagulation in severe protein C congenital deficiency. Thromb Haemost. 1993;70:247-249.

201. Vigano S, Mannucci PM, Solinas S, et al. Decrease in protein C antigen and formation of an abnormal protein soon after starting oral anticoagulant therapy. Br J Haematol. 1984;29:120-121.

202. Dreyfus M, Magny JF, Bridey F, et al. Treatment of homozygous protein C deficiency and neonatal purpura fulminans with a purified protein C concentrate. N Engl J Med. 1991;325:1565-1568.

203. Garcia-Plaza I, Jiminez-Astorga C, Borrego D, et al. Coumarin prophylaxis for fulminant purpura syndrome due to homozygous protein C deficiency [letter]. Lancet. 1985;1:634-635.

204. Hartman KR, Manco-Johnson M, Rawlings JS, et al. Homozygous protein C deficiency: early treatment with warfarin. Am J Pediatr Hematol Oncol. 1989;11: 395-401.

205. Casella JF, Lewis JH, Bontempo FA, et al. Successful treatment of homozygous protein C deficiency by hepatic transplantation. Lancet. 1988;1:435-438.

33 Acquired Platelet Defects

David B. Wilson

Platelets play a critical role in hemostasis. When the vascular endothelium is disrupted, platelets adhere to the subendothelium and initiate primary hemostasis. The details of normal platelet physiology and function are presented in Chapter 25. Excessive bleeding occurs if primary hemostasis is abnormal because platelets are either deficient in number or defective in function. Acquired platelet defects, both quantitative and qualitative in nature, are discussed in this chapter and the corresponding inherited disorders in Chapter 29.

The normal circulating platelet count for all ages ranges from 150,000 to 400,000/μL. Circulating platelets constitute two thirds of total body platelets; the remaining platelets are located within the spleen.[1] Platelets exhibit marked heterogeneity in size. Two factors have been proposed to account for this heterogeneity.[2] First, as platelets age, they may become smaller as a result of fragmentation or loss of granule contents or membrane proteins. Second, megakaryocytes produce platelets of varying size. In thrombolytic states, megakaryocytes preferentially produce large platelets, a phenomenon analogous to stress erythropoiesis.[2] The average life span of platelets is 7 to 10 days, although survival of transfused platelets in a thrombocytopenic recipient is reduced proportionately to the severity of the thrombocytopenia.[3] These findings suggest either that there is increased platelet utilization in thrombocytopenic states or that a fixed number of platelets are removed from the circulation each day, irrespective of the platelet count.[4]

QUANTITATIVE PLATELET ABNORMALITIES

Thrombocytopenia

The clinical manifestations of thrombocytopenia typically involve the skin or mucous membranes and include petechiae, ecchymoses, prolonged bleeding at incision or venipuncture sites, epistaxis, gastrointestinal hemorrhage, hematuria, and menorrhagia. Intracranial hemorrhage (ICH) can occur but is rare. As discussed in Chapter 28, the deep muscle hematomas and hemarthroses typically seen in individuals with deficiencies of factor VIII or factor IX generally do not occur with platelet disorders. Causes of thrombocytopenia fall into three broad categories: platelet sequestration (usually in the spleen), increased platelet destruction, or decreased platelet production. The differential diagnosis of thrombocytopenia in children is outlined in Box 33-1. Discriminating among these diagnoses is important because the cause of thrombocytopenia affects the choice of therapy.

When a patient with thrombocytopenia is assessed, the risk of bleeding episodes should be estimated. If the risk is significant, treatment is warranted. Unfortunately, there is a lack of direct correlation between the platelet count and the risk of bleeding episodes, which confounds treatment decisions. The risk of hemorrhage is affected by many factors, such as coexisting coagulation defects,

trauma, and surgery. In older children and adults, serious spontaneous bleeding does not occur until the platelet count is less than 20,000/μL. Many physicians use a platelet count of 10,000 to 20,000/μL as the threshold for intervention. This threshold was derived from a study of children with leukemia and may not be relevant for all cases of thrombocytopenia. For example, because of the increased risk for ICH in neonates, a threshold of 20,000 to 50,000/μL is often used. In addition, patients with a defect in production are more likely to have serious bleeding than those with a destructive platelet problem because in the latter patients, platelets tend to be larger and more functional.

Thrombocytopenia Reflecting Laboratory Artifact or Sequestration

Spurious Thrombocytopenia

Thrombocytopenia may be an incidental finding. If the history and physical examination do not suggest a defect in primary hemostasis, a low platelet count may represent a laboratory artifact. Potential causes of a falsely low platelet count include platelet activation during blood collection, undercounting of megathrombocytes,[5] or pseudothrombocytopenia as a result of in vitro agglutination by ethylenediaminetetraacetic acid (EDTA)-dependent antibodies.[6] In a patient with artifactual thrombocytopenia, large clumps of agglutinated platelets may be found at the periphery of the blood film, or platelets may be adherent to leukocytes and form platelet "satellites" (Fig. 33-1).[7]

Pseudothrombocytopenia secondary to EDTA-dependent antibodies can be confirmed by repeating the platelet count with another anticoagulant (e.g., citrate, oxalate, or heparin) or by preparing a blood film directly from a finger or heel puncture sample. The cause of EDTA-associated pseudothrombocytopenia is an IgG or IgM directed against a cryptic platelet antigen exposed only in the presence of this anticoagulant.[6] The phenom-

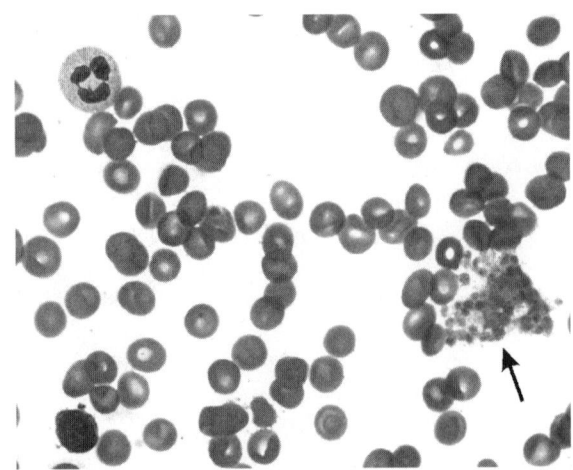

FIGURE 33-1. Pseudothrombocytopenia: photomicrograph of ethylenediaminetetraacetic acid–dependent platelet clumping (*arrow*).

Box 33-1	Differential Diagnosis of Thrombocytopenia in Children and Adolescents

DESTRUCTIVE THROMBOCYTOPENIAS

Primary Platelet Consumption Syndromes

Immune thrombocytopenias
  Acute and chronic ITP
  Autoimmune diseases with chronic ITP as a
  manifestation
    Cyclic thrombocytopenia
    ALPS and its variants
    SLE
    Evans' syndrome
    Antiphospholipid antibody syndrome
    Neoplasia-associated immune thrombocytopenia
  Thrombocytopenia associated with HIV
  Neonatal immune thrombocytopenia
    Alloimmune
    Autoimmune (e.g., maternal ITP)
  Drug-induced (including HIT)
  Post-transfusion purpura
  Allergy and anaphylaxis
Nonimmune thrombocytopenias
  Thrombocytopenia of infection
    Bacteremia or fungemia
    Viral infection
    Protozoan infection
  Thrombotic microangiopathic disorders
    TTP
    HUS
    BMT–associated microangiopathy

  Drug-induced
  Platelets in contact with foreign material
  Congenital heart disease
  Drug-induced via direct platelet effects (ristocetin,
    protamine)
  Type 2b VWD or platelet-type VWD

Combined Platelet and Fibrinogen Consumption Syndromes

DIC
Kasabach-Merritt syndrome
HLH

IMPAIRED PLATELET PRODUCTION

Hereditary disorders (see Chapter 29)
Acquired disorders
  Aplastic anemia
  MDS
  Marrow infiltrative process
  Nutritional deficiency states (Fe, folate, vitamin B_{12},
    anorexia nervosa)
  Drug- or radiation-induced thrombocytopenia
  Neonatal hypoxia or placental insufficiency

SEQUESTRATION

Hypersplenism
Hypothermia
Burns

ALPS, autoimmune lymphoproliferative syndrome; BMT, bone marrow transplant; DIC, disseminated intravascular coagulation; HLH, hemophagocytic lymphohistiocytosis; HIT, heparin-induced thrombocytopenia; HIV, human immunodeficiency virus; HUS, hemolytic-uremic syndrome; ITP, immune thrombocytopenic purpura; MDS, myelodysplastic syndrome; SLE, systemic lupus erythematosus; TTP, thrombotic thrombocytopenic purpura; VWD, von Willebrand's disease.

---

enon is not associated with any particular pathology and may be observed in both healthy subjects and patients with diseases. In some individuals the antibodies responsible persist indefinitely, whereas in others the antibodies are transient. No abnormalities in hemostasis or thrombosis have been reported in any of these patients.

Other causes of pseudothrombocytopenia include drugs[8] and EDTA-independent cold agglutinins.[9] The overall incidence of pseudothrombocytopenia in hospitalized adult patients is approximately 1%, but it is less common in pediatric patients.[6] No further evaluation or treatment is indicated for a patient documented as having a spuriously low platelet count.

Apparent Thrombocytopenia Caused by Hypersplenism

The spleen normally retains about a third of the body's platelets in an exchangeable pool.[1] The fraction of platelets sequestered in the spleen increases in proportion to spleen size. Thus, an apparent thrombocytopenia can result from increased pooling in an enlarged spleen—a condition referred to as *hypersplenism*. In patients with hypersplenism, recovery of transfused autologous platelets is only 10% to 30%, whereas in normal individual it is 60% to 80% and in asplenic patients it is 90% to 100%. Splenic blood flow is the major determinant of the size of the exchangeable splenic platelet pool in splenomegalic states.[10] Administration of intravenous epinephrine causes constriction of the splenic artery and results in passive emptying of platelets into the circulation. This increase in platelet count is proportionately greater in patients with splenomegaly than in normal subjects.

In general, the apparent thrombocytopenia that results from pooling in an enlarged spleen is mild (50,000 to 150,000/μL). Platelet counts of less than 50,000/μL should not be attributed to splenomegaly alone without further investigation. The degree of hypersplenism is proportional to spleen weight, whether the splenomegaly is due to congestion (e.g., cirrhosis with portal hypertension), hemolytic anemia (e.g., hemoglobin SC disease), or other causes. Because thrombocytopenia secondary to splenic pooling is not usually clinically important, no treatment is warranted, although splenectomy may be indicated for patients with severe thrombocytopenia, as can occur in Gaucher's disease or other storage diseases.

Apparent Thrombocytopenia Caused by Hypothermia

Platelets are transiently sequestered in the spleen, liver, and other organs of experimental animals subjected to hypothermia. Upon rewarming of the animal, these platelets return to the circulation. A similar phenomenon has been observed in hypothermic patients. Transient thrombocytopenia (platelet counts of 7000 to 62,000/μL) has been reported in hypothermic patients of various age.[11,12] Less significant thrombocytopenia has been observed in patients undergoing cardiac surgery with hypothermic perfusion. Treatment of the thrombocytopenia associated with hypothermia consists of rewarming and documentation of return of the platelet count to the normal range, which usually occurs in 4 to 10 days.

Thrombocytopenia Caused by Increased Platelet Destruction

A major etiologic classification of acquired thrombocytopenia of childhood is increased platelet destruction. Clinical conditions associated with increased platelet destruction are listed in Box 33-1. These conditions can be further subgrouped into immune and nonimmune causes.

Immune Thrombocytopenias

Autoantibodies, alloantibodies, or drug-dependent antibodies may associate with platelet membranes and target the cells for accelerated destruction by phagocytes of the reticuloendothelial system. An antibody mediating immune destruction of platelets may be directed against a platelet membrane antigen, or it may be part of an immune complex that binds Fc receptors on platelets.

Platelet antigens fall into two general classes. Glycoproteins that occur predominantly on platelets, such as the glycoprotein IIb/IIIa (GPIIb/IIIa) or GPIb/IX/V complexes, are often termed *platelet-specific antigens*. The glycoproteins (e.g., human leukocyte antigen [HLA] class I) and glycolipids (e.g., blood group ABH antigens) expressed on platelets, leukocytes, and other cell types are termed *platelet-nonspecific antigens*. Antibodies against platelet-specific and platelet-nonspecific antigens are responsible for a number of clinical syndromes, including autoimmune thrombocytopenia, neonatal alloimmune thrombocytopenia (NAIT), post-transfusion purpura (PTP), and platelet transfusion refractoriness. Antibodies directed against platelet integrins are common in immune thrombocytopenias. For example, autoantibodies directed against GPIIb/IIIa are seen in immune thrombocytopenic purpura (ITP)[13,14] and in drug-induced thrombocytopenia.[15,16] Several clinically significant alloantigens are

located on GPIIb/IIIa, including HPA-1a, the human platelet antigen most frequently implicated in NAIT (see later). Autoantibodies against GPIb or GPIX also have been reported in patients with ITP[13,14] and drug-induced thrombocytopenia.[15,17]

HLA class I antigens are expressed on a wide range of cells, including platelets, and are important for the recognition of self by cytotoxic T cells. HLA-A and HLA-B antigens are strongly expressed on platelets.[18] Alloantibodies against HLA-A or HLA-B antigens frequently form in multiparous women and multiply transfused patients, and these alloantibodies contribute to platelet transfusion refractoriness. HLA-C antigens are weakly expressed on platelets and are far less likely to induce alloantibodies, thus making it less necessary to match the HLA-C locus for donor-recipient compatibility in platelet transfusions. HLA class II antigens, which function in antigen presentation by macrophages and B lymphocytes, are not expressed on platelets.

ABH blood group antigens are carried on a number of platelet glycoproteins, including the GPIIb/IIIa and GPIb/IX/V complexes.[19] ABH antigens are also expressed on glycolipids.[19] In rare instances, these antigens have been implicated as the cause of immune-mediated platelet destruction, but in general, these platelet-nonspecific antigens play only a minor role in immune thrombocytopenias.

Platelet Antibody Testing. A large number of assays have been developed to detect antibodies directed against or associated with platelet membrane antigens.[20] These assays can be categorized into direct (detecting antibody associated with the patient's platelets) or indirect (detecting antibody in the patient's serum that binds to control platelets). Indirect tests may detect, in addition to autoantibodies, alloantibodies (e.g., HLA related), particularly in multiparous women and individuals who have received multiple transfusions, and thus give false-positive results. Autoantibodies tend to be associated with the patient's platelets and are usually present in low concentration in serum. Therefore, a direct test is the preferred test for autoimmune thrombocytopenias such as ITP.[20]

A number of direct assays measure immunoglobulin on platelets, regardless of whether the immunoglobulin is specifically or nonspecifically bound to the platelet surface. These assays generally detect platelet-associated IgG (PAIgG), but they can also be engineered to detect IgM or IgA. PAIgG is increased in immune disorders such as ITP and in nonimmune thrombocytopenic disorders such as leukemia and myelodysplastic syndrome. Thus, the specificity of these tests is limited. Moreover, the sensitivity of these tests is limited because autoantibodies, such as those responsible for ITP, represent only a small fraction of the total PAIgG. Megakaryocytes nonspecifically take up plasma proteins, including IgG and albumin, and incorporate these proteins into the alpha granules of platelets, especially in disease states associated with increased thrombopoiesis.[21] Therefore, increased

PAIgG can result from elevated antibody production for any reason.

More recent assays use antigen capture techniques to detect platelet glycoprotein–specific antibodies, such as those that recognize GPIIb/IIIa and GPIa/IX/V, and have high specificity. Unfortunately, the sensitivity is generally too low for these assays to be used for the routine serologic diagnosis of most immune thrombocytopenias.[20] A newly developed method is based on flow cytometric detection of autoantibodies reacting with specific platelet proteins immobilized on microbeads.[22]

Macrophage and Platelet Fcγ Receptors. Receptors for the Fc domain of IgG (Fcγ receptors) are found on a variety of cell types, including macrophages and platelets. These receptors have been shown to play a critical role in immune complex–mediated platelet destruction. Fcγ receptors are diverse in structure and function and fall into two major classes: those that activate effector functions, such as phagocytosis or platelet activation, and those that inhibit effector functions.[23]

Activating Fcγ receptors on macrophages include the low-affinity receptors FcγRIIA and FcγRIIIA and the high-affinity receptor FcγRI (Fig. 33-2).[23] As discussed later, cross-linking of the activating receptor FcγRIII promotes phagocytosis of antibody-coated platelets in certain disease states, including ITP. One of the drugs used to treat ITP, intravenous IgG (IVIG), acts by inducing expression of the inhibitory receptor FcγRIIB on phagocytes.[24]

The only Fcγ receptor expressed on platelets is the activating receptor FcγRIIA. Binding of IgG complexes to this receptor results in receptor cross-linking, which in turn initiates platelet aggregation and activation. This process is involved in heparin-induced thrombocytopenia (HIT), the most common drug-induced thrombocytopenia.

Immune Thrombocytopenic Purpura

ITP is a disorder characterized by accelerated destruction of antibody-sensitized platelets by phagocytic cells, especially those of the spleen. ITP is the most common autoimmune disorder affecting a blood element. The annual incidence is about 1 in 10,000 children. Two major forms are seen: acute ITP and chronic ITP. Acute ITP is usually a benign, self-limited condition that occurs in young children, typically those younger than 10 years Often a viral infection or vaccination precedes the onset of acute ITP. In the majority of these patients, the thrombocytopenia resolves within weeks or a few months of the original manifestation. Chronic ITP is defined arbitrarily as persistence of thrombocytopenia (platelet count >150,000/μL) for longer than 6 months after the initial manifestation, although some hematologists advocate a later cutoff point (Box 33-2).

Children in whom ITP is diagnosed have an excellent chance of spontaneous recovery, irrespective of therapy. The platelet count returns to normal in 4 to 8 weeks in approximately half of the patients and by 3 months after diagnosis in two thirds of children.[30] In a review[31] of 12 publications involving more than 1500 children with ITP, 76% achieved complete remission within 6 months of initial evaluation. Spontaneous recovery was documented in 37% of the remaining patients with thrombocytopenia persisting longer than 6 months. These findings have been confirmed in other large

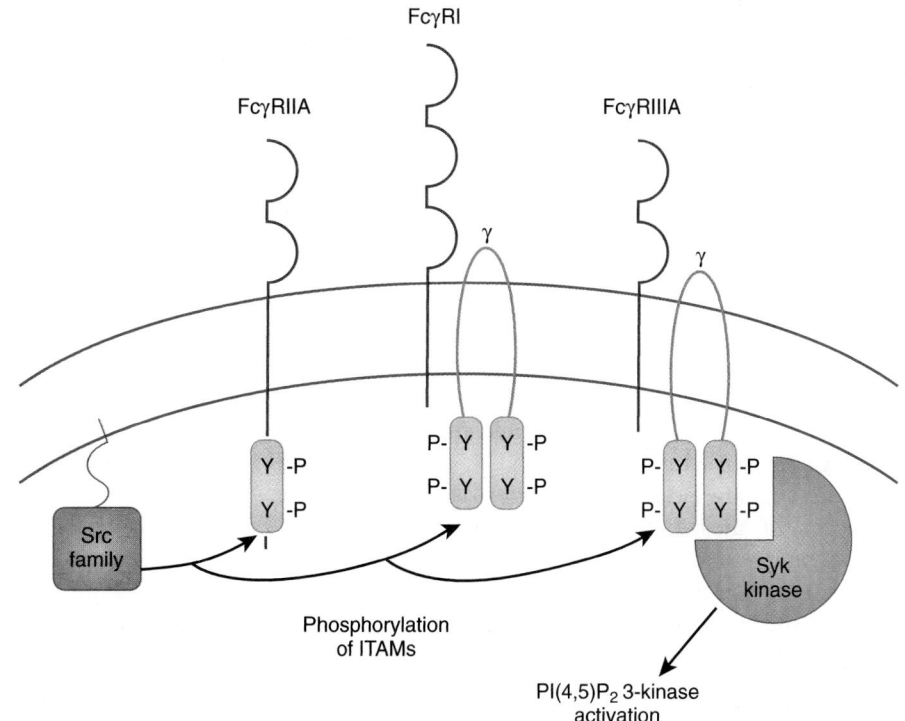

FIGURE 33-2. Activating Fcγ receptors on macrophages. Fcγ receptors signal phagocytosis via their phosphorylated ITAM (immunoglobulin gene–related tyrosine activation motif) domains. Receptor cross-linking stimulates src family kinases to phosphorylate tyrosine (Y) residues within the ITAM domain of FcγRIIA or within the dimerized γ subunits of FcγRI or FcγRIIIA. The tyrosine kinase syk is then recruited to the phosphorylated ITAM domains and activated. Syc mediates phagocytosis by activating phosphatidylinositol 3′-kinase and phospholipase C. PI(4,5)P₂, phosphatidylinositol 4,5-bisphosphate. *(Adapted with permission from Aderem A, Underhill DM. Mechanisms of phagocytosis in macrophages. Annu Rev Immunol. 1999;17:595 © 1999 by Annual Reviews. Available at www.AnnualReviews. org.)*

CONTROVERSIAL ISSUE 1

What is the definition of chronic ITP? Traditionally, chronic ITP has been defined as thrombocytopenia lasting longer than 6 months. Many pediatric hematologists take exception to this definition because a significant fraction of children with ITP recover in 6 to 12 months. The Intercontinental Childhood ITP Study Group has recommended that a 12-month rather than a 6-month cutoff point be used to define chronicity.[25]

CONTROVERSIAL ISSUE 2

Is it necessary to perform bone marrow aspiration in patients with suspected ITP before starting glucocorticoid therapy? Although the diagnosis of leukemia is extremely unlikely when the clinical history, physical examination, and peripheral smear are consistent with ITP, many hematologists routinely perform bone marrow aspiration before initiating glucocorticoid therapy. Retrospective studies[26-28] suggest that this may not be necessary. Bone marrow aspiration or biopsy is warranted for children with atypical laboratory features and for those in whom initial therapy fails.

CONTROVERSIAL ISSUE 3

Where does splenectomy belong in the therapeutic decision tree for chronic ITP? There is a consensus that splenectomy should be deferred as long as possible and be reserved for patients with severe, symptomatic thrombocytopenia. The favorable safety profile of rituximab and the possibility of a sustained response could justify its use instead of splenectomy in the decision tree, but this has yet to be demonstrated in a prospective clinical trial. Despite the invasive and irreversible nature of splenectomy, some pediatric hematologists[29] advocate the use of rituximab only after splenectomy has failed.

studies.[25,32] Factors associated with the development of chronic ITP include age older than 10 years, insidious onset, and female gender.[32]

Pathogenesis. ITP is caused by autoantibodies that interact with membrane glycoproteins on the surface of platelets and megakaryocytes. These antibodies result in accelerated platelet destruction and may also impair thrombopoiesis. More than a third of adults with ITP have inadequate platelet production despite increased numbers of megakaryocytes in their bone marrow.[33] Certain antiplatelet antibodies have been shown to inhibit megakaryocytopoiesis or egress of platelets from the marrow space.[34,35] The GPIIb/IIIa complex is the autoantigen implicated most often as the cause of childhood and adult ITP.[14,36] Autoantibodies directed against the GPIb/IX/V[36] and GPIa/IIa[37] complexes have also been

reported. In rare instances, platelet glycolipids have been implicated as autoantigen targets in chronic ITP.[38] Autoantibodies diminish or disappear when platelet levels are restored to normal.[39]

Factors that trigger platelet autoantibody formation in acute ITP are not well understood. Although various mechanisms by which viruses may induce autoimmune disease have been suggested, the link between the immune response initiated by infection (or vaccination) and the subsequent production of platelet autoantibodies has not been established. Proposed mechanisms include adsorption of virus to platelets, deposition of virus-containing immune complexes onto platelet membranes, or exposure of cryptic neoantigens on the platelet surface.[40] There are data to both support[41] and refute[42] the hypothesis that acute ITP is triggered by antiviral antibodies that cross-react with platelet antigens.

Recent studies suggest that T lymphocytes also play a role in the pathogenesis of ITP. Dysregulated helper T cells can promote the expansion of antiplatelet antibody–producing B-cell clones.[43] Cytotoxic T cells from some ITP patients have the capacity to destroy platelets ex vivo.[44] CD3$^+$ T lymphocytes from ITP patients are resistant to glucocorticoid-induced apoptosis, thus suggesting that disturbed apoptosis may contribute to defective clearance of autoreactive T lymphocytes.[45]

Genetic factors have been proposed to influence the development of ITP. Studies have failed to detect linkage of the disease to particular HLA genotypes. Polymorphisms in genes encoding phagocyte Fcγ receptors or proinflammatory cytokines may influence the development of ITP.[46] Immunodeficiency states, including inherited conditions, that have been associated with chronic ITP are discussed later.

Clinical and Laboratory Features. The typical manifestation of acute ITP is the abrupt onset of bruising and bleeding in an otherwise healthy child. Frequently, there is a history of a viral illness in the weeks preceding the onset of bruising. Seasonal fluctuation in the diagonsis of ITP has been noted, with a peak during spring and a nadir in the autumn.[47] Petechiae and ecchymoses are evident in most patients. Epistaxis and oral mucosal bleeding are seen in less than a third of patients. Hematuria, hematochezia, or melena is evident in less than 10%. Menorrhagia may be observed in adolescent girls with ITP. Although children with ITP may have extremely low platelet counts, bleeding episodes are less severe in these patients than in those with hypoproductive thrombocytopenia. This finding has been attributed to enhanced platelet production and young, large, hemostatically effective circulating platelets.[48] A palpable spleen is present in about 10% of reported cases of childhood ITP. Malaise, bone pain, and adenopathy are uncommon and should raise concern for another cause, such as acute leukemia.

The peak age at diagnosis is 2 to 6 years. Although acute ITP may be diagnosed in children of any age, ado-

TABLE 33-1	Characteristics of Childhood versus Adult Immune Thrombocytopenic Purpura
Childhood ITP	**Adult ITP**
Females = males	Females > males (2:1)
Abrupt onset	Insidious onset
Infectious prodrome common	Infectious prodrome uncommon
<20% chronic	>50% chronic

lescents and infants are more likely to have chronic ITP develop in combination with some other immune disorder. In children, ITP is seen equally in males and females, whereas in adults, ITP is seen predominantly in females by a 2:1 ratio (Table 33-1).

Roughly 80% of children have platelet counts below 20,000/μL, often less than 10,000/μL.[25,32] Leukocyte and red cell counts are usually normal, although anemia may be seen in as many as 15% of these children, especially those with a significant history of epistaxis, hematuria, or gastrointestinal bleeding. A review of the peripheral blood film is mandatory in every child suspected of having ITP; features inconsistent with a diagnosis of ITP should prompt further investigation. Bone marrow aspiration or biopsy reveals normal or increased numbers of megakaryocytes. Increased numbers of eosinophils and their precursors may be noted, although this is not predictive of outcome.

The need for bone marrow examination in children with typical features of acute ITP is a subject of debate. There is a consensus that bone marrow aspiration is not necessary if the initial management is observation alone or administration of IVIG or anti-D. Controversy exists regarding whether bone marrow aspiration needs to be performed in all children before glucocorticoid therapy is started to exclude the possibility of acute leukemia (see Box 33-2).

Additional tests that may be considered in the initial evaluation and management of suspected ITP include serologic testing for human immunodeficiency virus (HIV), a direct Coombs test, and antinuclear antibody testing. Retrospective studies have shown that the antinuclear antibody test is positive in approximately 30% of pediatric patients with otherwise uncomplicated ITP and may predict a subset of patients at risk for the development of further autoimmune symptoms.[49]

Options for the Initial Management of Immune Thrombocytopenic Purpura. Childhood acute ITP is usually a benign, self-limited disorder that requires minimal or no therapy in the majority of cases.[25,31,50] There is no convincing evidence that medical therapy alters the natural history of the disease. Indications for treatment vary among practitioners and are a source of debate.[31,50,51] One set of practice guidelines put forth by the American Society of Hematology (ASH)[31] recommends that chil-

dren with ITP and platelet counts less than 20,000/μL plus significant mucosal membrane bleeding or those with platelet counts less than 10,000/μL and minor purpura be treated with IVIG or a glucocorticoid. However, many pediatric hematologists take exception to this recommendation.[50,52] In treatment guidelines put forth by the British Paediatric Haematology Group,[53] a child's condition rather than the platelet count steers management; children with bruising but without mucosal or more severe hemorrhage may be treated by observation alone, irrespective of the platelet count.

At the heart of the treatment debate is the perceived risk for ICH, a rare but potentially life-threatening complication in children with ITP. In a review of 12 case series involving 1293 children, the incidence of ICH was 0.9%.[31] Other surveys[32,54,55] suggest that this may be an overestimate and that the true incidence of ICH in children with ITP is between 0.1% and 0.5%. The subgroup of children with ITP who appear to be at greatest risk for ICH are those with platelet counts less than 20,000/μL and additional risk factors such as a history of head trauma, aspirin use, or arteriovenous malformation.[31] However, the platelet count alone has never been shown to predict the severity of bleeding symptoms.[30]

There is no evidence that medical therapy, such as administration of a glucocorticoid or IVIG, reduces the incidence of ICH. Indeed, retrospective studies[54-56] have shown that ICH may occur despite previous or concomitant therapy with IVIG or a glucocorticoid. The low incidence of ICH in children with ITP precludes a randomized clinical trial to determine whether treatment reduces the risk.

The results of randomized trials for various treatment approaches have been summarized previously.[31] Regardless of whether pharmacologic therapy is used, detailed education and careful follow-up should be provided to the patient and family. The child's activities should be limited, and aspirin-containing medications should be avoided. Although hospitalization is appropriate for the treatment of a child with a severe bleeding episode, there is no evidence to support routine hospitalization of patients with otherwise uncomplicated ITP.

Observation Only. For a patient with ITP and only minor purpura, medical therapy may not be necessary. There is uniform consensus that patients with platelet counts greater than 20,000/μL and only minor purpura do not require therapy. As noted earlier, management of patients with platelet counts lower than 20,000/μL and minor bleeding is controversial.

First-Line Medical Therapies

GLUCOCORTICOIDS. Glucocorticoids are presumed to act through several mechanisms, including inhibition of both phagocytosis and antibody synthesis, improved platelet production, and increased microvascular endothelial stability.[57] The latter effect may explain why symptomatic bleeding episodes often subside before the platelet count increases.

In randomized trials, prednisone therapy has been shown to induce more prompt normalization of the platelet count than placebo does.[58-60] Although various doses have been used, the traditional glucocorticoid regimen is prednisone at 2 mg/kg/day (maximum of 60 to 80 mg) for approximately 21 days.[58] A regimen of 4 mg/kg/day for 7 days and then tapered to day 21 is equally effective and appears to have fewer side effects.[60] Prednisone at a dose of 4 mg/kg/day orally for 4 days with no tapering is also effective.[61] An alternative to these regimens is megadose pulse therapy (methylprednisolone, 30 mg/kg/day intravenously or orally for 3 days).[62] Side effects of glucocorticoid therapy include cushingoid facies, weight gain, fluid retention, acne, hyperglycemia, hypertension, moodiness, pseudotumor cerebri, cataracts, growth retardation, avascular necrosis, and osteoporosis.

INTRAVENOUS IMMUNOGLOBULIN. Imbach and associates[63] first reported the successful use of IVIG for the treatment of acute ITP in a small series of children. This was followed by many reports that documented the ability of IVIG to effect a rapid increase in the platelet count in patients with acute and chronic ITP.[64-66]

IVIG slows the clearance of antibody-coated blood cells from the circulation by inhibiting the phagocytic activity of cells of the reticuloendothelial system.[67] Studies in the early 1980s suggested that this effect is mediated primarily through the Fc portion of IgG. Specially treated preparations of intravenous IgG lacking the Fc portion of the molecule were inferior to unmodified IgG at increasing the platelet count in ITP patients. The proposed mechanism for this effect was Fc receptor blockade.[67] More recent studies in FcγR-deficient mice[24] suggest that IVIG elicits its effect via activation of inhibitory pathways and not simply receptor blockade (Fig. 33-3). Although there are some data to support the notion that anti-idiotypic antibodies may also be present in commercial preparations and contribute to the action of IVIG,[68] the clinical importance of this mechanism remains unproved.

The traditional dose of IVIG is 2 g/kg divided over a period of 2 to 5 days. However, several studies suggest that lower doses are effective. In a randomized trial,[65] pediatric patients who received 0.8 g/kg IVIG had at least as rapid a response rate as those who received 2 g/kg over a 2-day period. In more recent randomized trials,[66,69] favorable results have been seen with even lower doses of IVIG (250 mg/kg/day for 2 days). Among pediatric

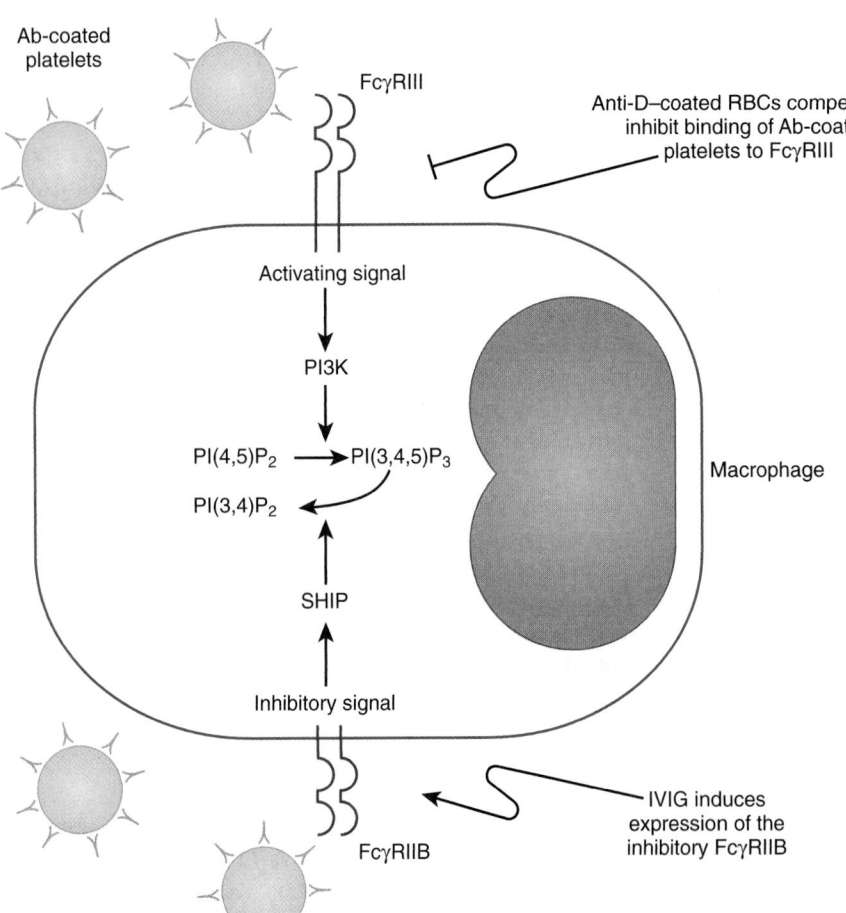

FIGURE 33-3. Mechanism of action of intravenous IgG (IVIG) in immune thrombocytopenia. Binding of antibody-coated platelets to activating Fcγ receptors (FcγRIII) on macrophages results in the production of phosphatidylinositol 3,4,5-triphosphate ($PI[3,4,5]P_3$) via the action of phosphatidylinositol 3′-kinase (PI3K). These activated macrophages phagocytose the platelet-antibody complexes. IVIG induces expression of the inhibitory Fc receptor (FcγRIIB) on macrophages. Stimulation of the inhibitory receptor results in recruitment of SHIP, a 5-phosphatase that degrades $PI(3,4,5)P_3$ into phosphatidylinositol 3,4-bisphosphate $PI(3,4)P_2$. *(Adapted with permission from Lin SY, Kinet JP. Immunology: giving inhibitory receptors a boost. Science. 2001; 291:446. © American Association for the Advancement of Science.)*

patients in whom a response is seen, IVIG produces a more rapid increase in platelet count than do traditional doses of a glucocorticoid (2 mg/kg/day of prednisone), as documented in controlled trials.[60,70]

Several other general conclusions have emerged from studies on IVIG in pediatric patients.[71] First, both splenectomized and nonsplenectomized patients may respond to IVIG. Second, responses to IVIG are generally reproducible. Third, the duration of the response is brief, approximately 2 to 4 weeks.

Enthusiasm for the use of IVIG is offset by cost considerations. IVIG is considerably more expensive than prednisone or anti-D.[72] One study concluded that IVIG may be cost-effective if it reduces hospital stay or if splenectomy is avoided.[64]

Complications associated with IVIG are common and occur in 15% to 75% of patients.[31] Frequent side effects include flu-like symptoms such as headache, nausea, lightheadedness, and fever. Some of these adverse effects can be alleviated by pretreatment with analgesics or antihistamines. Approximately 10% of patients treated with IVIG (2 g/kg) experience aseptic meningitis manifested as a severe, protracted headache and photophobia.[73] These symptoms, which can cause considerable anxiety in patients, parents, and physicians, may spur additional diagnostic studies (e.g., computed tomography) or result in prolonged hospitalization. A rare but serious side effect of IVIG infusion is anaphylaxis, which can occur in patients who are totally deficient in IgA.[74] Most preparations of IVIG contain small amounts of IgA, and IgE antibodies responsible for anaphylaxis form after an initial exposure to IgA in these preparations.

Anti-D. Anti-D is a plasma-derived immunoglobulin prepared from donors selected for a high titer of anti-$Rh_0(D)$ antibody. Anti-D elicits a rise in platelet count, along with mild to moderate anemia, in most patients with ITP.[65,72,75-78] A role for anti-D in the treatment of chronic ITP is now well established. Its utility in acute ITP has been studied less extensively, but it is also effective in this clinical setting.[76,78,79]

Anti-D can be used to treat only $Rh_0(D)$-positive patients with ITP because $Rh_0(D)$-negative patients do not show a response. The presumed mechanism of action is phagocytic cell blockade. Patients with intact spleens are more likely to respond to anti-D than splenectomized patients are.

The generally recommended dose is 50 to 75 µg/kg as a short intravenous infusion[76] or subcutaneous injection.[80] Uncontrolled studies have demonstrated that anti-D treatment increases the platelet count in approximately 80% of $Rh_0(D)$-positive children.[75,77] The therapeutic effect of anti-D lasts for 1 to 5 weeks. A controlled trial showed that anti-D therapy was less effective than IVIG or a glucocorticoid in terms of days required to attain a platelet count of 20,000/µL.[65] Anti-D is less expensive than IVIG, with an estimated cost savings of 35% per

episode of ITP.[72] The shorter administration time required for anti-D therapy also makes the medication more convenient to use than IVIG.

Adverse reactions of headache, nausea, chills, dizziness, and fever have been reported in 3% of infusions, and these adverse reactions were classified as severe in only a minority of cases.[75,81] Some degree of hemolysis, the main adverse reaction with anti-D, is inevitable because of binding of anti-D antibody to $Rh_0(D)$-positive erythrocytes. There is laboratory evidence of hemolysis in most patients. The average decline in hemoglobin ranges from 0.5 to 1 g/dL,[76-78] and most cases of hemolysis do not require medical intervention. In a small subset of patients, more significant hemolysis has been observed, which has tempered enthusiasm for use of the drug. Postmarketing surveillance by the U.S. Food and Drug Administration[82] documented 15 cases of hemoglobinemia or hemoglobinuria after anti-D therapy. Of these patients, six required transfusion, eight experienced an onset or exacerbation of renal insufficiency, and two underwent dialysis. The incidence of intravascular hemolysis was estimated to range from 0.1% to 1.5%. Why certain patients experience severe intravascular hemolysis after anti-D therapy is unclear. Subcutaneous delivery of anti-D may be associated with a lower incidence of severe hemolytic reactions.[80]

Relapses or Treatment Failures. Many patients treated with a glucocorticoid, IVIG, or anti-D will become thrombocytopenic again after a few weeks. These patients are likely to respond again to the therapy used initially. Patients who require therapy and whose thrombocytopenia does not respond to initial treatment with a glucocorticoid, IVIG, or anti-D are usually treated with one of the alternative front-line therapies. There are no clinical studies that document the response rate in these instances. Patients with persistent mild hemorrhage may benefit from low-dose glucocorticoid therapy.

Management of Chronic Immune Thrombocytopenic Purpura. In about 20% of children in whom ITP is diagnosed, thrombocytopenia persists for longer than 6 months. In adolescents and adults, chronic ITP is more common in females than in males. Chronic ITP sometimes occurs in association with other autoimmune diseases or in conjunction with an underlying condition known to predispose to disorders of autoimmunity, such as lymphoma (Box 33-3).

In up to a third of children with chronic ITP, spontaneous remission will occur months or years later. It is unclear why the condition resolves in these individuals. An estimated 5% of children have recurrent ITP characterized by intermittent episodes of thrombocytopenia followed by lengthy periods of remission. This is presumed to reflect a chronic compensated state of ITP. During periods of remission, increased platelet production balances the increased rate of platelet destruction. During exacerbations, platelet production by the marrow is sup-

Box 33-3	Conditions Associated with Chronic Immune Thrombocytopenic Purpura of Childhood

Immunodeficiency
    Hypogammaglobulinemia
    Common variable immunodeficiency
Lymphoproliferative disorders
    Autoimmune lymphoproliferative disorder
    Hodgkin's disease
Collagen vascular disorders
    Systemic lupus erythematosus
Infection
    Human immunodeficiency virus

pressed by viral infections or other factors and is unable to offset the rate of destruction.

Evaluation of patients with chronic ITP should include bone marrow aspiration, if not already done; screening tests for immunodeficiency (e.g., quantitative immunoglobulin levels/subsets, specific antibody titers, or lymphocyte subsets), systemic lupus erythematosus (SLE), and other autoimmune diseases (antinuclear antibody tests, direct Coombs test, antiphospholipid antibody tests, thyroid function tests); and serologic testing for HIV. Obtaining blood counts and peripheral blood smears from the parents may help exclude familial disorders.

The primary goal of treatment in patients with chronic ITP is to prevent bleeding, not cure the disease. As with acute ITP, therapy decisions should be based more on symptoms than on platelet count. In formulating a treatment plan, one must balance the potential side effects of treatment with the risk of bleeding episodes caused by the disease. Because the goal of treatment is a safe platelet count, not necessarily a normal platelet count, observation alone is an appropriate approach for many patients, especially those with minimal symptoms.[83]

Splenectomy. Splenectomy is thought to be effective because in most patients the spleen is the major site of both platelet destruction and autoantibody production. Platelet survival studies indicate improved platelet life span after splenectomy.[57]

Splenectomy should be considered in a pediatric patient with chronic ITP whose risk for hemorrhage precludes the use of observation alone. However, there is debate about where splenectomy belongs in the therapeutic decision tree for chronic ITP (see Box 33-2). Because remissions are often delayed in children and the risk of postsplenectomy sepsis is significant, especially in those younger than 5 years, splenectomy is deferred longer in children with ITP than in adults. ASH practice guidelines[31] recommend that splenectomy be considered for children in whom ITP has persisted for at least 1 year

and who have bleeding symptoms and a platelet count of less than 10,000/μL (ages 3 to 12) or 10,000 to 30,000/μL (ages 8 to 12 years). Practice guidelines in the United Kingdom are similar.[53]

Laparoscopic splenectomy is preferred over open splenectomy in children with chronic ITP.[84,85] Advantages of the laparoscopic procedure include less postoperative pain, earlier return of gastrointestinal function, shorter hospitalization, more rapid resumption of normal activities, and smaller incisions. To ensure adequate hemostasis, the platelet count can be raised preoperatively with a glucocorticoid, IVIG, or anti-D. Despite these interventions, many patients will still have thrombocytopenia at the time of splenectomy; however, most will not exhibit excess bleeding. Accordingly, prophylactic platelet transfusions are not warranted. Instead, platelet transfusions should be reserved for patients with intraoperative bleeding. Most experienced surgeons have become comfortable performing laparoscopic splenectomy on patients with platelet counts in the range of 50,000 to 100,000/μL. Overall perioperative mortality is less than 1%.

The majority of children with chronic ITP will have a response to splenectomy. In a review[31] of 16 case series involving 271 children undergoing elective splenectomy for chronic ITP, a complete remission rate of 72% was reported. The platelet count usually rises immediately after splenectomy and reaches a maximum 1 to 2 weeks postoperatively. If the peak platelet count achieved after splenectomy is greater than 500,000/μL, permanent remission is likely.[86] Certain patient characteristics are associated with a higher probability of response to splenectomy, including a previous response to glucocorticoid therapy.[87-89] However, there is no single factor or combination of factors that will predict the response to splenectomy in all cases.[90]

Relapse after an immediate response to splenectomy may be due to transient viral suppression of thrombopoiesis. If the thrombocytopenia persists, an accessory spleen should be considered. Approximately 40% of patients with persistent thrombocytopenia will have a residual accessory spleen that can be seen with sensitive imaging techniques such as ^{99m}Tc sulfur colloid scans (Fig. 33-4) or ^{111}In platelet localization studies.[91] Many of these patients will achieve complete remission after removal of the accessory spleen.[91] The presence of Howell-Jolly bodies on a peripheral blood smear does not rule out an accessory spleen.

The major risk after splenectomy is fatal sepsis caused by encapsulated organisms. The risk of septicemia in splenectomized patients is estimated to be 1 per 300 to 1000 patient-years.[92] To lessen the risk of future sepsis, patients should receive vaccinations for pneumococcus, *Haemophilus influenzae* type b, and meningococcus at least 2 weeks before surgery.[93] In addition, penicillin prophylaxis is indicated for splenectomized patients younger than 5 years. The benefit of penicillin prophylaxis in older asplenic children is controversial.[94]

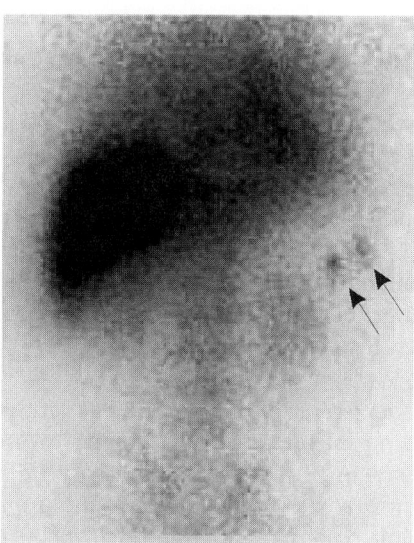

FIGURE 33-4. Detection of accessory spleens after splenectomy. A sulfur colloid scan shows accessory spleens (*arrows*) in a teenage girl with chronic immune thrombocytopenic purpura and persistent thrombocytopenia after splenectomy. (*Courtesy of Dr. Robert Minkes, Louisiana State University.*)

Phagocyte Blockade. Intermittent maintenance therapy with a glucocorticoid, IVIG, or anti-D can be used to delay splenectomy. These medications may also be useful in the management of patients with chronic ITP who experience symptomatic thrombocytopenia after splenectomy.

In some patients a safe platelet count can be maintained with low doses of prednisone. However, even low doses of prednisone, comparable to physiologic cortisol secretion, can cause osteoporosis.[95] In 1994, Andersen[96] reported a striking response rate in a series of 10 adults with chronic ITP treated with pulses of high-dose oral dexamethasone (adult dose, 40 mg/day for 4 sequential days per month for 6 months). These results have not been confirmed in subsequent studies of adults and children; the complete response rate in children at doses of approximately 20 mg/m^2 was approximately 17%.[97-99]

IVIG (1 to 2 g/kg total dose administered) elevates the platelet count in most children with chronic ITP.[63,64] Periodic doses of IVIG may be used as maintenance therapy to defer splenectomy in young children with chronic ITP.[64] This approach is cost-effective in young children.[100] In about 25% of children, ITP will become refractory to maintenance therapy with IVIG.[101] Low-dose alternate-day prednisone therapy can be used as an adjunct to maintenance IVIG therapy. Although repeated infusions of IVIG induce short-term platelet responses in most patients with chronic ITP, there is no evidence that such therapy will affect the natural history of the disease and induce a long-lasting remission.

Anti-D administration raises the platelet count in most Rh$_0$(D)-positive children with chronic ITP. However, the benefit is usually transient, with a median duration of 3 to 5 weeks.[102] Anti-D can be effective as maintenance therapy in patients who are not appropriate candidates for splenectomy or other therapies because of young age or other factors.[102,103] In Rh$_0$(D)-positive patients with chronic ITP, anti-D is preferred over IVIG because of ease of administration, comparable efficacy, and lower cost.

Monoclonal Antibodies That Target B Cells or T Cells

RITUXIMAB. Rituximab, a humanized monoclonal antibody directed against CD20, is now commonly used to treat chronic ITP despite limited clinical trial data documenting its efficacy in children with this condition (see Box 33-2).[104] Rituximab is generally administered in four weekly intravenous infusions of 375 mg/m^2 each. This agent causes rapid depletion of pre-B cells and B cells that lasts for 6 to 12 months. Pre-B cells efficiently present antigen to T cells, and disruption of this interaction may attenuate the autoimmune response. Approximately 30% to 60% of patients with chronic ITP respond to rituximab, and in many cases these responses are sustained.[105-110] The initial response may be immediate (within 1 week) or delayed (up to 3 months).[105-110] Side effects of rituximab include fever, urticaria, pruritus, throat tightness, and serum sickness.[110]

ALEMTUZUMAB. Alemtuzumab (Campath 1H) is a humanized monoclonal antibody that targets CD52, a protein on both B and T cells. There are anecdotal reports of its use in patients with chronic ITP.[111] Part of the effect of alemtuzumab can be attributed to B-cell depletion, analogous to rituximab, and part to depletion of T cells. Unlike rituximab, alemtuzumab induces profound generalized immunosuppression associated with opportunistic infections.[104]

Other Immunosuppressive Agents.
A large number of other immunosuppressive medications have been used to treat refractory ITP, as reviewed elsewhere.[49,112,113] No randomized studies have evaluated the effectiveness of these various therapies. The choice of therapy must be individualized to the patient.

AZATHIOPRINE. Azathioprine acts preferentially on lymphocytes and was one of the first drugs reported to be effective in the treatment of chronic refractory ITP.[114,115] Recommended doses range from 50 to 200 mg/m^2/day orally. Continuous therapy for 4 to 6 months is required before a patient is considered unresponsive. Once a response is obtained, the dose should be tapered to the lowest level that results in a hemostatic platelet count. In adults with refractory ITP treated with azathioprine, approximately 20% achieve a complete response and 45% exhibit a partial response. Relapse often occurs when the therapy is stopped. The combination of azathioprine and oral steroids may be synergistic, and azathioprine therapy may allow a reduction in the dose of glucocorticoids. Toxicities include dose-related leukopenia, opportunistic infection, and an increased risk for malignancy.

CYCLOPHOSPHAMIDE. The alkylating agent cyclophosphamide has also been used to treat chronic refractory ITP, with a response rate similar to that with azathioprine.[115] Greater risks are associated with the use of cyclophosphamide than with azathioprine. Side effects include myelosuppression, alopecia, nausea, infertility, teratogenecity, hemorrhagic cystitis, and an increased risk for malignancy.

CYCLOSPORINE. The potent immunosuppressive agent cyclosporine disrupts T-cell function through calcineurin inhibition. There are case reports of patients with refractory ITP who had increases in platelet counts after treatment with cyclosporine.[116] Response rates vary. A starting dose of 5 mg/kg/day given in divided oral doses is recommended, with the aim of maintaining a serum cyclosporine level of 200 to 400 ng/mL. The drug should be discontinued after 4 weeks if there is no response. Hypertension, renal insufficiency, hirsutism, and liver dysfunction are common side effects.

TACROLIMUS. Though not structurally related to cyclosporine, tacrolimus has a similar mechanism of action and has been used anectodally to treat chronic ITP.[43] Initial dosing recommendations for tacrolimus in children are 0.15 to 0.3 mg/kg/day given in divided oral doses. Doses should be adjusted to maintain trough tacrolimus concentrations of 5 to 20 ng/mL in whole blood. Common adverse effects associated with tacrolimus include hypertension, tremor, headache, and hyperglycemia.

MYCOPHENOLATE MOFETIL. There are reports showing the effectiveness of another immunomodulatory drug, mycophenolate mofetil (MMF), in patients with steroid-resistant chronic ITP.[117,118] MMF is a prodrug of mycophenolic acid, a noncompetitive inhibitor of inosine-5α-monophosphate dehydrogenase, a key enzyme in the purine biosynthetic pathway. MMF inhibits proliferation of both T cells and B cells. In one series,[118] a sustained platelet increase to a level greater than 50,000/μL was seen in 7 of 18 patients with refractory ITP. For adults, the usual starting dose is 250 mg orally twice daily, with an increase to 1 g twice daily by 3 weeks. MMF has few side effects and is generally well tolerated.

VINCA ALKALOIDS. The vinca alkaloids vincristine and vinblastine may induce a response in some patients with chronic refractory ITP.[119] These drugs bind tubulin and inhibit microtubule polymerization, which is presumed to disrupt phagocytosis. Either vincristine or vinblastine may be used; the efficacy of the two drugs is comparable. The usual dose of vincristine is 1.5 mg/m^2 (maximum of 2 mg) intravenously, whereas the dose of vinblastine is 6 mg/m^2 (maximum of 10 mg) intrave-

nously. These doses are repeated weekly for a month. If no response is seen, additional doses are unwarranted because subsequent improvement is unlikely. Patients who show a response often require repeated doses at 2- to 3-week intervals to maintain a safe platelet count. In adults, the response rate is approximately 12% and the partial response rate is 35%. The response rate in children is not established and varies considerably in the reports available. Adverse effects include peripheral neuropathy, constipation, and alopecia. Vinblastine causes dose-related myelosuppression.

DANAZOL. Danazol, an attenuated androgen with mild virilizing effects, has been shown to increase the platelet count in patients with refractory ITP, although the mechanism of action is uncertain. Approximately 40% of adult patients will respond to danazol with an increase in platelet count to greater than 50,000/μL.[120] A typical dose is 300 to 400 mg/m^2/day orally, although smaller doses (50 mg/m^2) have been reported to be effective.[121] In general, 2 months of therapy is required before a response is seen. Often the medication must be continued to maintain the platelet count, although effort should be made to minimize the dose. Danazol may be especially useful for the treatment of older adolescent or adult women with chronic, refractory ITP and uncontrollable menorrhagia. Side effects of danazol include acne, fluid retention, hirsutism, deepening of the voice in women, headache, nausea, rash, breast tenderness, and oligomenorrhea or amenorrhea. Patients should be monitored for the development of liver toxicity.

INTERFERON ALFA. Although the mechanism is unknown, 25% of adults with chronic ITP treated with interferon alfa display a significant, albeit transient increase in platelet count.[122] Interferon alfa has also been used to treat children with chronic ITP.[123] The recommended dose is 3 million U/m^2 subcutaneously three times per week for 4 weeks. Adverse effects of interferon alfa include flu-like symptoms and neutropenia.

COMBINATION CHEMOTHERAPY. Combination chemotherapy with or without autologous stem cell transplantation has been used successfully to treat some adults with chronic, refractory ITP, with an overall sustained remission rate of approximately 40%.[124,125]

Thrombopoiesis-Stimulating Agents. In ITP the rate of platelet production is inadequate to offset the increased rate of platelet destruction.[33] Two new drugs for the treatment of chronic ITP act by stimulating thrombopoiesis. AMG 531 is a recombinant protein that contains two domains: a peptide that binds to the thrombopoietin receptor c-Mpl and an antibody Fc domain that increases the half-life in circulation.[126] In a placebo-controlled, phase II study this agent was efficacious when administered subcutaneously on a weekly basis (1 to 3 μg/kg) to adults with chronic ITP.[127] Toxicity was minimal. Another small-molecule c-Mpl agonist in clinical testing for chronic ITP is eltrombopag.[126] This agent is given orally once daily. A phase II trial on adults with chronic ITP showed that eltrombopag at doses of 50 and 75 mg was significantly better than placebo at increasing platelet counts to greater than 50,000/μL. The drug appears to have few side effects.

Management of Life-Threatening Hemorrhage in Immune Thrombocytopenic Purpura.

ICH or another life-threatening form of bleeding mandates intervention with multiple therapeutic modalities, including IVIG (1 g/kg), anti-D (50 to 75 μg/kg), high-dose glucocorticoids (e.g., methylprednisolone, 30 mg/kg intravenously), platelet transfusions, or a combination of these interventions. Because IVIG and anti-D act to inhibit phagocytosis by distinct and potentially synergistic mechanisms (see Fig. 33-3), these two agents may be used together for instances of severe bleeding. Recombinant factor VIIa has also been used in the management of ICH in patients with thrombocytopenia refractory to platelet-enhancing agents.[128] If a craniotomy is required, consideration should be given to splenic artery embolization[129] or emergency splenectomy,[130] although most hematologists reserve splenectomy for patients in whom ITP does not respond rapidly to therapy with glucocorticoids, IVIG, anti-D, and platelet transfusions.[31,131] Optimal therapy for ICH also includes supportive care with mechanical ventilation and mannitol.

Thrombocytopenia Associated with Lymphoproliferative and Autoimmune Disorders

Chronic ITP may be a manifestation of an associated autoimmune disease or immunodeficiency state. This is especially true in young children in whom chronic, refractory ITP develops or in adolescent girls with systemic symptoms.

Autoimmune lymphoproliferative syndrome (ALPS) is a rare syndrome that occurs in early childhood and is characterized by massive, nonmalignant lymphadenopathy, splenomegaly, hypergammaglobulinemia, and autoimmune manifestations, including immune thrombocytopenia.[132] ALPS has been linked to inherited defects in *FAS* and other genes that regulate lymphocyte apoptosis. An abnormal accumulation of lymphocytes results in lymphadenopathy, hepatosplenomegaly, and hypersplenism. In young children the lymphadenopathy may be pronounced and then wane later in life. Impaired elimination of autoreactive lymphocytes also causes autoimmune manifestations, including autoantibody formation. Patients with ALPS commonly exhibit episodic autoimmune cytopenia, including thrombocytopenia, hemolytic anemia, neutropenia, or combined cytopenias.

A significant proportion of young children with chronic ITP may have a variant of ALPS.[133-135] For example, in one survey[134] of 20 pediatric patients with chronic cytopenia, 25% were found to have profound defects in Fas-mediated lymphocyte death. Two of these patients, aged 4 and 9 years, had chronic refractory ITP without other clinical manifestations of ALPS. Neither patient had an identifiable mutation in *FAS* or caspase-10, and it is presumed that they may have defects in one of the molecules involved in Fas signaling. Similar results have been reported in other studies,[133,135] thus suggesting that altered Fas signaling, independent of *FAS* mutations, is associated with and may precipitate chronic hematologic autoimmunity, including ITP. The lymphadenopathy and cytopenias associated with ALPS generally respond to glucocorticoid therapy.

Thrombocytopenia occurs at some time in approximately 25% of patients with SLE and may be the first manifestation of autoimmunity.[136] Both autoantibodies and complement-fixing immune complexes have been implicated in the pathogenesis of thrombocytopenia in SLE.[137] In addition, antiphospholipid antibodies are frequently observed in the sera of patients with SLE.[138] Antibodies against antigens nonspecifically adsorbed to the surface of platelets, such as DNA, have also been reported.[139]

The initial therapy for thrombocytopenia in patients with SLE is administration of a glucocorticoid, but there is a high incidence of recurrent thrombocytopenia when the steroid dose is tapered. Long-term use of low doses of glucocorticoids may be justified, especially if these drugs also control the other symptoms of SLE. Splenectomy can be used in the management of patients with SLE and chronic, symptomatic thrombocytopenia. In some case series,[140] splenectomy for SLE has been shown to yield response rates comparable to those for ITP, whereas in other series[141] the response rate has been lower.

Thrombocytopenia may be associated with an antiphospholipid antibody syndrome, whether the syndrome occurs as a primary disorder or in association with SLE or another autoimmune disorder. Patients with antiphospholipid antibody syndrome often experience recurrent venous or arterial thrombotic complications rather than bleeding (see Chapter 34). Autoantibodies against GPIIb/IIIa, GPIa/IIa, and GPIb/IX have been documented in this syndrome.[142] Enhancement of platelet activation by antiphospholipid antibodies may contribute to the prothrombotic state in these patients.[143] In general, the degree of thrombocytopenia is moderate. A variety of therapies have been used to treat antiphospholipid antibody syndrome and the accompanying thrombocytopenia, including glucocorticoids and other immunosuppressive agents.

Evans' syndrome is the coexistence of autoimmune hemolytic anemia and thrombocytopenia. Autoimmune neutropenia also develops in many of these patients.[144] Frequently, patients with Evans' syndrome have associated disorders, such as dysgammaglobulinemia. Distinct antiplatelet and antierythrocyte antibodies rather than cross-reactive antibodies are responsible for the association of autoimmune hemolytic anemia and thrombocytopenia. In many patients the course of the disorder is marked by exacerbations of thrombocytopenia, anemia, or neutropenia. Unlike the majority of patients with ITP or isolated autoimmune hemolytic anemia, therapy with glucocorticoids, IVIG, or splenectomy often fails in patients with Evans' syndrome.[144] Patients with Evans' syndrome have been treated with rituximab, which induces remission in the majority, although relapses tend to occur within 12 months.[144] For severe and refractory cases, hematopoietic stem cell transplantation is a consideration.

Immune thrombocytopenia can complicate other autoimmune diseases, including dermatomyositis, juvenile rheumatoid arthritis, Hashimoto's thyroiditis, Graves' disease, myasthenia gravis, inflammatory bowel disease, sarcoidosis, and protein-losing enteropathy.[145-148] Immune thrombocytopenia can also precede, accompany, or follow neoplastic disease, especially lymphoproliferative disorders such as Hodgkin's and non-Hodgkin's lymphoma.[149] Immune thrombocytopenia has also been seen in association with childhood acute lymphoblastic leukemia.[150] In some patients, the thrombocytopenia of neoplastic disease resolves in response to antineoplastic therapy, whereas in others the thrombocytopenia requires specific treatment.

Thrombocytopenia occurs in 5% to 10% of patients with HIV infection. Immune-mediated platelet destruction is a major contributor to the thrombocytopenia seen in patients with HIV. The antibodies in HIV-associated thrombocytopenia are directed against the same target epitopes commonly seen in idiopathic ITP, namely, epitopes on GPIIb/IIIa.[151] Immune complexes composed of anti-idiotype antibodies and antibodies directed against the HIV antigen gp160/120 may also induce platelet destruction.[151] Whereas half of patients with ITP have normal or increased platelet production, most patients with HIV-associated thrombocytopenia have decreased platelet production.[152] Infection of megakaryocytes or bone marrow stromal cells may account for the reduced platelet production noted in HIV-associated thrombocytopenia.

Thrombocytopenia may occur early in the course of HIV infection and is often seen within the first 2 years.[153] Platelet counts are rarely lower than 50,000/µL, and symptomatic bleeding is uncommon. However, in HIV-infected patients with hemophilia, the bleeding can be more severe, even life threatening. Therapy is similar to that for ITP, except that HIV-associated thrombocytopenia may respond to antiviral therapy. Patients with severe or symptomatic thrombocytopenia despite antiviral therapy should be managed in the same way as patients with severe ITP.

Neonatal Alloimmune Thrombocytopenia

NAIT is a syndrome in newborns characterized by transient, isolated, severe thrombocytopenia. The syndrome results from placental transfer of maternal alloantibodies directed against paternally inherited antigens present on fetal platelets but absent from maternal platelets. Hence, this condition is the platelet counterpart of hemolytic disease of the newborn.

Alloantigens. Platelet alloantigens and the platelet membrane glycoproteins on which they reside are listed in Table 33-2. Most of the antigens were originally named on the basis of the patient's surname. In many cases, duplicate names were assigned to the same alloantigens (e.g., Pl^A1 = Zw^a, Pen^a = Yuk^b). The HPA, or human platelet antigen, nomenclature was proposed in the 1990s to systemize platelet alloantigens.[156] Each HPA system represents a biallelic polymorphism caused by a single amino acid substitution (see Table 33-2).

TABLE 33-2	**Platelet Alloantigen Systems**					
					PHENOTYPE FREQUENCY	
Current Designation	Original Designation	Platelet Localization	Polymorphism		Whites	Japanese
HPA-1a	Pl^A1, Zw^a	GPIIIa	Leu33		0.98	0.99
-1b	Pl^A2, Zw^b		Pro33		0.027	0.037
HPA-2a	Ko^b	GPIb_α	Thr145		0.99	ND
-2b	Ko^a, Sib^a		Met145		0.017	0.25
HPA-3a	Bak^a, Lek^a	GPIIb_α	Ile843		0.85	0.79
-3b	Bak^b, Lek^b		Ser843		0.66	0.71
HPA-4a	Pen^a, Yuk^b	GPIIIa	Arg143		>0.999	>0.999
-4b	Pen^b, Yuk^a		Gln143		<0.0001	0.017
HPA-5a	Br^b, Zav^b	GPIa	Glu505		0.99	0.99
-5b	Br^a, Zav^a		Lys505		0.021	0.087
HPA-6b	Tu^a, Cu	GPIIIa	Gln489		<0.01	ND
HPA-7b	Mo^a	GPIIIa	Pro407		<0.01	ND
HPA-8b	Sr^a	GPIIIa	Cys636		<0.01	ND

Other low-frequency human platelet alloantigens exist but are not listed here. Comprehensive reviews are available.[154,155]
GPIb_α, glycoprotein Ib_α; GPIa, glycoprotein Ia; GPIIIa, glycoprotein IIIa; HPA, human platelet antigen; ND, not determined.

In white populations the most frequently implicated alloantigen in NAIT is HPA-1a (Pl^A1), which accounts for 78% of serologically confirmed cases.[157] Incompatibility for the HPA-5b alloantigen is the next most common cause. Approximately 98% of white individuals express the HPA-1a antigen on their platelets; most of the remaining 2% are homozygous for an alternative allele that encodes the HPA-1b (Pl^A2) antigen. The protein products of these two alleles differ only by a single amino acid (Leu33 versus Pro33). The incidence of NAIT is approximately 1 in 2000 births,[158] which is much lower than the predicted incidence based on distribution of the HPA-1a and HPA-1b alleles in the population. Other immune response genes appear to regulate HPA-1a alloantibody formation. Women with the HLA-DR3 antigen have about a 20-fold relative risk of forming HPA-1a alloantibodies. In the Asian population, incompatibility of the HPA-4 system is the most common cause of NAIT (80%), followed by incompatibility of the HPA-3 system.[159] HLA class I antigens are expressed on platelets, and maternal sensitization to HLA has been implicated as a cause of NAIT in a few patients.[160] HLA alloantibodies are present in 10% to 30% of pregnant women, especially multiparous women. The relative rarity of NAIT secondary to HLA alloantibodies may be due to binding of these antibodies to the placenta or other tissues. Blood group ABH alloantibodies have been found in a small number of patients with NAIT.[161]

Clinical and Laboratory Features. The degree of thrombocytopenia in NAIT can be severe, with platelet counts of less than 10,000/μL on the first day of life.[161] Common hemorrhagic manifestations include petechiae (90%), hematomas (66%), and gastrointestinal bleeding (30%). The maternal platelet count is normal, an important laboratory value for distinguishing this condition from neonatal thrombocytopenia secondary to maternal ITP[162] (see later). Unlike Rh disease of the newborn, NAIT can occur in both the first and subsequent pregnancies. A history of a previously affected infant provides strong supportive evidence for a diagnosis of NAIT.

Patients with NAIT are at increased risk for ICH, both prenatally and postnatally.[158,161] About 15% of affected neonates have ICH, and 50% of these cases occur antenatally. In utero bleeding can result in hydrocephalus, porencephaly, seizures, or fetal loss.[163] The pronounced bleeding diathesis associated with anti–HPA-1a alloimmune thrombocytopenia may reflect the combination of severe thrombocytopenia and antibody-mediated interference with the function of the GPIIb/IIIa complex on the few remaining platelets.

Treatment. The diagnosis of NAIT is confirmed by serologic or genotypic testing, including immunophenotyping of maternal, paternal, and occasionally neonatal platelets; maternal or fetal serum also can be examined for the presence of antiplatelet antibody. Several sensitive assays have been developed for platelet antigen typing and detection of alloantibody.[164] Despite the availability of sensitive tests, serologic evidence of alloantibodies is lacking in a least a third of cases identified by clinical criteria; therefore, NAIT is a clinical diagnosis. Because delays may be associated with serologic testing, therapy should be initiated as soon as the diagnosis is suspected.

The treatment of choice for severe NAIT (platelet count < 30,000/μL or clinically significant bleeding) is transfusion of washed, irradiated, maternal platelets (Fig. 33-5).[156] Irradiation prevents transfusion-associated graft-versus-host disease. In the interest of time, normal donor screening procedures may have to be abridged. Random-donor platelet infusions can be used in a neonate with active bleeding if maternal platelets are not immediately available.[165] However, only a modest and short-lived increase in the platelet count may be observed after the infusion of random-donor platelets. IVIG (1 g/kg daily for 2 days) or a glucocorticoid (methylprednisolone, 2 mg/kg/day) can also be used as a temporary measure, although these interventions may have limited benefit. If

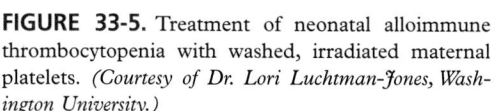

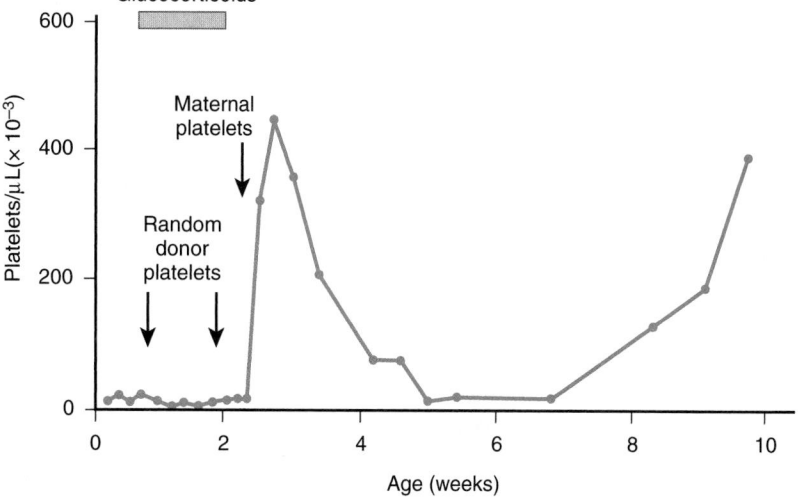

FIGURE 33-5. Treatment of neonatal alloimmune thrombocytopenia with washed, irradiated maternal platelets. *(Courtesy of Dr. Lori Luchtman-Jones, Washington University.)*

the offending alloantigen is known, platelets from an antigen-negative unrelated donor may be used. In white populations, the use of HPA-1a– and HPA-5b–negative donors has been advocated because these two antigens are responsible for more than 95% of cases of NAIT. To provide transfusion support for fetuses and neonates with NAIT, the National Blood Service of England has established an accredited platelet donor panel of HPA-1a–negative individuals with no antibodies to HLA, HPA, or red cell antigens.[166] The majority of these donors are HPA-5b negative.

Platelets produced by neonates with alloimmune thrombocytopenia may exhibit accelerated clearance for weeks, until antiplatelet antibody is removed from the circulation (see Fig. 33-5). Consequently, it is not unusual for additional transfusions of maternal (or an antigen-compatible unrelated donor) platelets to be required after the first few weeks of life.

Management of Future Pregnancies. The likelihood is high that subsequent infants born to mothers of infants with NAIT will be affected. Moreover, the severity of antenatal and postnatal hemorrhage tends to increase in later pregnancies.[167] Therefore, detailed counseling on the risk of recurrence should be provided to the family at the time that thrombocytopenia is diagnosed in the first infant. Although the neonate's thrombocytopenia may have resolved before completion of the full diagnostic laboratory evaluation, it is important that the diagnosis and presumed antigen incompatibility be confirmed by formal serologic and genotypic testing to guide the management of future pregnancies. Antibody titers begin to decline after delivery; thus, the evaluation should ideally be initiated in the postpartum period. Because the likelihood of thrombocytopenia in subsequent infants depends on whether the father is HPA-1a homozygous or HPA-1a/1b heterozygous, performance of DNA-based genotyping is desirable.

Fetuses at risk for ICH should be monitored with serial ultrasound examinations, although fetal ICH may not always be detected by this method. In some centers, prenatal diagnosis of the platelet alloantigen genotype has been performed with DNA obtained by chorionic villus sampling or amniocentesis. More commonly, percutaneous umbilical blood sampling is performed at 20 to 22 weeks of gestation to obtain a fetal platelet count and perform platelet antigen typing. However, this procedure may be associated with fetal loss because of exsanguination; thus, compatible antigen-negative (e.g., maternal) platelets should be available when percutaneous umbilical blood sampling is performed and should be infused if the fetus is severely thrombocytopenic.[158]

When the diagnosis of alloimmune thrombocytopenia is confirmed in the fetus, two treatment approaches are available. In most North American centers, the favored approach is weekly maternal infusion of IVIG.[168,169] In some European centers, the preferred approach for severe cases of alloimmune thrombocytopenia is repeated in utero platelet transfusions; administration of IVIG and a glucocorticoid is reserved for mildly affected fetuses.[164]

Neonatal Autoimmune Thrombocytopenia

This condition can occur in infants of mothers with immune thrombocytopenia as a result of ITP, SLE, or other autoimmune disorders and is caused by placental transfer of maternal autoantibodies.[162] Antigens implicated as causes of neonatal autoimmune thrombocytopenia mirror those seen in ITP. In general, this condition is less serious than NAIT.

This diagnosis should be considered when both the neonate and the mother have evidence of thrombocytopenia or in infants of mothers with a previous history of immune thrombocytopenia. Neonatal thrombocytopenia has been observed in infants of mothers rendered asymptomatic for chronic ITP by splenectomy. Maternal ITP must be distinguished from the mild decrease in platelets that frequently accompanies pregnancy at term, presumably because of plasma volume expansion.[170]

The thrombocytopenia associated with maternal immune thrombocytopenia is generally milder than NAIT. The incidence of cord platelet counts lower than 50,000/μL is only about 3%,[171] and the incidence of ICH is only about 1%.[162] Although clinically significant bleeding episodes are rare, newborns with this condition should be monitored closely because platelet counts often decrease in the days after birth. The threshold for medical intervention in neonates with thrombocytopenia differs from that in older children with ITP because of concern about ICH in the newborn. A platelet count of less than 40,000 to 50,000/μL in a neonate is considered by many to be a useful indicator for starting therapy. IVIG (1 g/kg daily for 2 days) elevates the platelet count in most patients.[172] A glucocorticoid (methylprednisolone, 2 mg/kg/day) may be used in addition to or in lieu of IVIG therapy.

Perinatal management of mothers with immune thrombocytopenia, including the mode of delivery of a thrombocytopenic fetus, is controversial. Because the cord platelet count rarely is below 50,000/μL, perinatal ICH is uncommon and not necessarily related to delivery. The degree of maternal thrombocytopenia is a poor predictor of the degree of neonatal thrombocytopenia, although the clinical course of thrombocytopenia in the first sibling does predict that of the next sibling.[162] Otherwise, there are no reliable predictors of severe thrombocytopenia in the newborn. Direct determination of the fetal platelet count by percutaneous umbilical venous sampling can be performed, but this procedure is rarely justified for this condition.

Post-transfusion Purpura

PTP is a very rare syndrome in childhood. Typically, this syndrome affects a multiparious woman with HPA-1a–negative platelets who is reimmunized with that alloantigen via blood transfusion.[173] Severe, acute thrombocytopenia ensues 1 week later, presumably reflecting an anamnestic response to the platelet alloantigen. PTP has been reported to develop in males and in nulligravida females as a result of initial exposure to the alloantigen through a previous blood transfusion. HPA-1a is the alloantigen found in 90% of occurrences of PTP.

Alloantibodies cause PTP, but the mechanism of platelet destruction is unclear. A variety of hypotheses[173] have been put forward to explain how alloantibody promotes destruction of autologous platelets, including immune complex–mediated platelet destruction; adsorption of allogeneic platelet antigens onto autologous platelets, which renders them susceptible to alloimmune destruction; and transient induction of autoantibodies. Because on average 2% of transfusion recipients have an HPA-1a incompatibility and PTP is very rare, other factors probably influence the development of this syndrome. Thrombocytopenia is usually severe (platelet count <10,000/μL), and hemorrhage is common. A high-titer alloantibody is often detectable. Patients generally recover in a few weeks. However, life-threatening bleeding, including ICH, may occur. Prednisone and plasma exchange have been used, but IVIG is probably the treatment of choice for severe occurrences.[174] Random-donor platelet infusions are ineffective and should not be administered. The efficacy of compatible, alloantigen-negative platelet transfusions is controversial.

Severe, transient thrombocytopenia has been associated with passive transfusion of plasma-containing products that have high-titer alloantibodies against HPA-1a or HPA-5b.[175] This condition has been reported in neonates.[176] The thrombocytopenia occurs within hours of transfusion. Most patients recover spontaneously, but treatment with IVIG or a glucocorticoid should be considered for severely affected patients.[176]

Drug-Induced Immune Thrombocyopenia

Numerous drugs have been implicated as causes of antibody-mediated thrombocytopenia.[177] In general, the risk associated with any drug is low, but some drugs cause immune thrombocytopenia more commonly than others do. The thrombocytopenia generally resolves when use of the drug is discontinued, but the severity of bleeding symptoms and the duration of thrombocytopenia vary widely among patients. In some instances, the sensitizing drug induces a second, drug-independent antibody (autoantibody) in addition to a drug-dependent one.[178] Usually, these drug-induced autoantibodies are transient and disappear when treatment with the drug is discontinued. Occasionally, however, autoantibody production may be sustained and lead to a clinical picture indistinguishable from that of ITP.[178] Once established, sensitivity to a drug generally persists indefinitely.[177]

Pathogenesis. Several mechanisms have been implicated in drug-induced immune thrombocytopenia.[177]

Hapten Formation. Small compounds can become covalently linked to blood cell membrane proteins and stimulate the production of antibodies specific for the hapten-protein complex. This mechanism is responsible for the hemolytic anemia seen in some patients treated with penicillin (see Chapter 14). Similarly, antibodies directed against hapten-protein complexes appear to be responsible for cases of penicillin-induced thrombocytopenia.[179]

Compound Epitope Formation. In patients with quinine-induced thrombocytopenia, antibodies that bind to normal platelets can be detected only when quinine is present in the soluble phase. These antibodies are usually specific for GPIIb/IIIa[180,181] or GPIb/IX.[182] The mechanism by which quinine promotes binding of antibody to platelets is not well understood. It is postulated that this agent binds noncovalently to one or more platelet membrane proteins and creates a "compound epitope" recognized by an antibody. Alternatively, the drug may interact with the target protein and cause a conformational change elsewhere in the molecule for which antibody is specific.[183] In addition to quinine, sulfonamide antibiotics and certain other drugs have been shown to induce antibodies that bind to platelets only when the sensitizing drug or one of its metabolites is present in the soluble state.[177] Among children, sulfamethoxazole is one of the more common causes of drug-induced immune thrombocytopenia.

Drug-Induced Autoantibodies. Certain drugs, such as gold salts, procainamide, levodopa, and interferon alfa, induce true autoantibodies that bind to platelet membrane targets in the absence of the drug.[177,184] The mechanisms by which these drugs induce autoantibodies is poorly understood.[178]

Clinical Features. Severe thrombocytopenia generally develops within 1 day of ingestion of quinine in a previously sensitized individual. A minimum of 1 week is required for initiation of the primary immune response in individuals taking this drug for the first time. Prodromal symptoms such as fever and chills may be observed. Bleeding may be severe, and its onset is abrupt. Hemorrhagic vesicles are common in the oral mucosa. The presence of a platelet antibody may be verified by a variety of techniques. Readministration of a suspected drug in an attempt to confirm an etiologic relationship is not recommended as a routine diagnostic measure.

Treatment. Discontinuation of treatment with the offending drug is the main therapy. With quinine, the thrombocytopenia usually begins to abate in 1 day if no additional drug is taken, and a normal platelet count is restored within 1 week. In patients with severe drug-induced thrombocytopenia, IVIG or glucocorticoid has been used to ameliorate bleeding.[185] However, there is little evidence that these medications are effective in this clinical setting. For life-threatening hemorrhage, platelet transfusion may be used, although this may be of limited value because of the persistence of slowly dissociating drug-antibody complexes. A sensitized individual is presumed to remain at lifelong risk for additional episodes of drug-induced thrombocytopenia, so further use of the offending drug is contraindicated.

Heparin-Induced Thrombocytopenia/Thrombosis

HIT is a complex clinical syndrome with an overall estimated incidence of 1% to 5% in adult patients exposed to heparin; the incidence in children is probably less.[186,187] The thrombocytopenia usually begins 5 to 10 days after heparin therapy is started, but it can occur within hours if the patient previously received heparin. The risk of HIT is higher for therapeutic than for low drug doses, for bovine than for porcine heparin, and for unfractionated than for low-molecular-weight heparin (LMWH).[188] In contrast to drug-induced thrombocytopenia caused by quinine or sulfonamides, severe thrombocytopenia (platelet count < 10,000/μL) is rare in HIT. Typically, platelet counts range from 20,000 to 150,000/μL, with a median of 50,000/μL.[177,189] The thrombocytopenia itself is rarely severe enough to cause bleeding symptoms and resolves after heparin therapy is discontinued. However, as many as 30% of patients with HIT experience arterial or venous thromboses. The development of thrombosis in patients with HIT is known as thrombocytopenia with thrombosis syndrome (HITTS), and this condition is associated with significant morbidity and mortality.

Pathogenesis. The antibodies responsible for HIT recognize the complex of heparin and platelet factor 4 (PF4), an alpha granule constituent.[190] After treatment with heparin, PF4 is released into the circulation and binds with heparin to form a reactive antigen on the platelet surface.[189] The heparin-PF4 complex is immunogenic in some patients. IgG against this complex triggers platelet activation by binding to FcγRIIA receptors on the surface membrane. The activated platelets release substances that stimulate other platelets and result in thrombin generation.[191] PF4 bound to glycosaminoglycans on the surface of endothelial cells may also serve as a target for antibody binding and lead to antibody-mediated injury to the endothelium and a predisposition to thrombosis.[192]

Approximately 50% of patients exposed to heparin during cardiac catheterization and subsequently during cardiac surgery form antibodies against heparin-PF4 complexes, but HITTS develops in only a small percentage.[193] It is unclear why heparin-PF4 complexes, which are composed of two substances normally present in the body, are so immunogenic. Moreover, it is not known why thrombocytopenia or thrombosis develops in some patients and not in others.

Diagnosis. The diagnosis of HIT is based on the interpretation of clinical findings together with labora-tory confirmation of heparin-PF4 antibodies. A scoring system has been proposed to assess the pretest probability of HIT,[194] although this system has not been validated for pediatric patients. The gold standard laboratory test for diagnosing HIT is a platelet [14C]serotonin release assay. Unfortunately, the complexity and availability of this assay limit its usefulness. An enzyme-linked immunosorbent assay (ELISA) for detection of antibodies against heparin-PF4 complexes is available, and results obtained with the serotonin release assay and ELISA are generally in agreement in patients with a clinical diagnosis of HIT.[188,195] However, ELISA has a more limited specificity and therefore produces false-positive results.

Treatment. It is standard practice to discontinue heparin in patients in whom HIT is suspected, but many of these patients will have thrombotic complications over the subsequent days. Therefore, ongoing antithrombotic therapy is indicated. Patients with HIT should not be given warfarin as a substitute for heparin during the acute episode because this can cause an abrupt decrease in the level of protein C and put the patient at greater risk for thromboembolic complications such as warfarin-induced limb gangrene.[196] LMWH is not recommended for the treatment of HIT because unfractionalted heparin and LMWH preparations display significant platelet aggregation cross-reactivity in vitro and in vivo.[188,197] Danaparoid, a low-molecular-weight heparinoid consisting of a mixture of heparan sulfate, dermatan sulfate, and small amounts of chondroitin sulfate, has been used for more than a decade to treat patients with HIT.[198] For pediatric patients with HIT, the recommended dosing scheme for danaparoid is an intravenous bolus of 30 IU/kg followed by an infusion of 1.2 to 2.0 IU/kg/hr to obtain anti–factor Xa levels of 0.4 to 0.8 IU/mL.[186] Hirudin, a compound originally purified from the leech salivary gland, inactivates thrombin by forming a 1:1 complex. A recombinant hirudin, lepirudin, is effective in the treatment of HIT or HITTS.[199] In children, lepirudin should be started as a continuous infusion at 0.1 mg/kg/hr without a preceding bolus, with a target activated partial thromboplastin time (APTT) of 1.5 to 2.5 times the patient's baseline value (first assessed 4 hours after infusion).[186] Other agents that are effective in this clinical setting are the synthetic antithrombin argatroban[200] and the synthetic pentasaccharide fondaparinux.[201]

Thrombotic Microangiopathic Disorders

This spectrum of disorders is characterized by destructive thrombocytopenia, disseminated capillary thrombosis, and microangiopathic hemolytic anemia (Box 33-4). Often there is organ dysfunction because of microvascular thrombosis and ischemic necrosis. Thrombotic microangiopathic disorders may be primary or secondary. There are both acute and chronic (familial) relapsing forms.

Box 33-4	Causes of Schistiocytic Hemolysis and Thrombocytopenia

Thrombotic thrombocytopenic purpura
Hemolytic-uremic syndrome
Disseminated intravascular coagulation
Vasculitis, including systemic lupus erythematosus and sclerodermal kidney
Drug-induced (cyclosporine, mitomycin C, etc.)
Dysfunctional prosthetic heart valves
Endocarditis
Bone marrow transplant–associated microangiopathy

TABLE 33-3 Clinical Manifestations of Thrombotic Thrombocytopenic Purpura

Symptoms	Cases	%
Fever	237/243	98
Pallor or anemia	246/256	96
Hemorrhage	241/251	96
Neurologic abnormalities	250/271	92
Renal abnormalities	191/217	88
Jaundice	113/271	42
Fatigue, malaise	92/271	34
Nausea and vomiting	69/271	25
Abdominal pain	36/271	13
Chest pain or arrhythmias	21/271	8
Arthralgia or myalgia	18/271	7

Adapted from Amorosi EL, Ultman JE. Thrombotic thrombocytopenic purpura. Medicine (Baltimore). 1966;25:139.

The two major thrombotic microangiopathic disorders affecting children and adolescents are thrombotic thrombocytopenic purpura (TTP), a classic disease of hematology, and hemolytic-uremic syndrome (HUS), a classic disease of nephrology. Patients with TTP always have thrombocytopenia and schistiocytic hemolysis, frequently with central nervous system and renal impairment. In HUS, the microangiopathic process is usually, but not always limited to the kidneys. However, the boundary between these two clinical syndromes may be nebulous. Renal impairment can be prominent in TTP, and neurologic injury can occur in HUS. In adults, these two microangiopathic syndromes are often viewed as a joint entity termed TTP-HUS.[202] In pediatrics, however, the two syndromes are generally considered to be distinct, albeit overlapping entities. In addition to TTP and HUS, other conditions can produce shistocytic hemolysis and thrombocytopenia, including bone marrow transplant–associated microangiopathy (see Box 33-4).

Thrombotic Thrombocytopenic Purpura. TTP is a syndrome characterized by reversible aggregation of platelets in the microvasculature that results in waxing and waning ischemia in various organs.[203-205] The defining clinical features of TTP are listed in Table 33-3. The pentad of thrombocytopenia, microangiopathic hemolytic anemia, neurologic abnormalities, fever, and renal abnormalities is present in many patients. Before the development of an effective therapy, the risk of mortality associated with the disease was greater than 90%. With the advent of plasma infusion/exchange therapy, TTP has become a curable disease. There are two major forms of TTP: an acute, acquired form and a rare, inherited, chronic relapsing form. Acute TTP can be further subcategorized into primary (idiopathic) and secondary forms. Drugs, infections, and other factors have been associated with secondary TTP.

Pathophysiology. The characteristic pathologic lesion of TTP is a hyaline thrombus composed of aggregated platelets in the absence of a perivascular inflammatory response. The thrombotic lesions of TTP typically involve terminal arterioles and capillaries and are most commonly seen in the brain, abdominal viscera, and heart, but not the lungs. Red blood cells are damaged as a result of interactions with microthrombi in the small vessels.

Immunohistochemistry of early lesions of TTP reveals an abundance of von Willebrand factor (VWF) but little fibrin.[206,207] VWF within these thrombi is thought to be critical in pathogenesis. In 1982, unusually large multimers of VWF (UL-VWF) were observed in the plasma of patients with chronic relapsing TTP (Fig. 33-6).[208,209] UL-VWF multimers are most prominent in plasma samples taken from these patients during remission and decrease at the time of relapse. These UL-VWF multimers, which are synthesized by endothelial cells, are composed of increased numbers of mature VWF subunits. Under conditions of shear stress, the UL-VWF forms are more efficient than other VWF multimers at binding to the GPIb/IX/V and GPIIb/IIIa complexes on platelets and inducing aggregation.[208,210,211] These findings, coupled with the observation that VWF was abundant in the early thrombotic lesions of TTP, led to the hypothesis that intravascular platelet aggregation in TTP was due to either excessive release of UL-VWF multimers into plasma or impaired degradation of these UL-VWF multimers into smaller, nonaggregating forms.

Under ordinary circumstances, UL-VWF multimers are processed into multimers of normal size through the action of ADAMTS13, a VWF-cleaving metalloproteinase in normal plasma.[212,213] This protease cleaves a specific Tyr-Met bond in the second of the three A domains in VWF subunits (Fig. 33-7).[214] Physiologically, UL-VWF multimers are thought to be cleaved by ADAMTS13 under conditions of high shear stress, which partially unfolds the molecules. In vitro this partial denaturation can be mimicked by guanidinium or urea treatment.

Acquired or constitutional deficiency of the VWF-cleaving protease predisposes individuals to TTP. Chronic relapsing TTP, which usually begins in early childhood, is due to loss-of-function mutations in the ADAMTS13 gene.[215-219] The acute TTP more commonly seen in adults

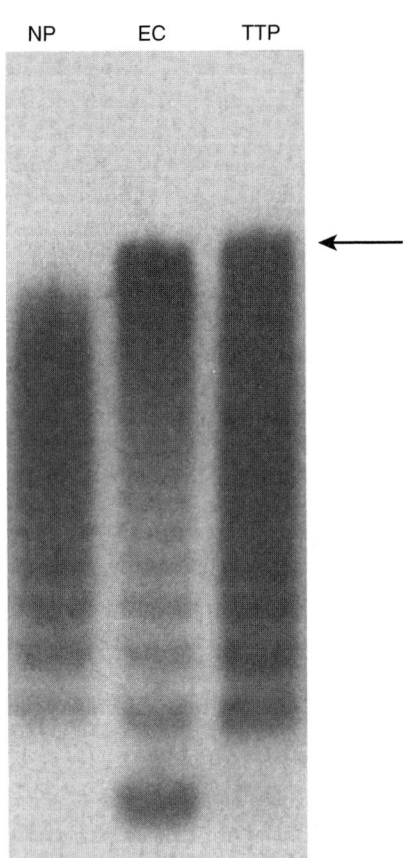

FIGURE 33-6. Autoradiogram demonstrating unusually large multimers of von Willebrand factor (VWF) near the top of the gel (*arrow*) in the plasma of a patient (thrombotic thrombocytopenic purpura [TTP]) obtained early during a single episode of TTP. Normal pooled plasma (NP) and the culture supernatant from human umbilical vein endothelial cells (EC) are shown for comparison. Ethylenediaminetetraacetic acid (EDTA)-anticoagulated samples were subjected to agarose gel electrophoresis in sodium dodecyl sulfate–urea-EDTA. VWF multimers were visualized by incubation with ^{125}I-labeled rabbit antihuman VWF antibody followed by autoradiography. (*From Moake JL, Chow TW. Thrombotic thrombocytopenic purpura: understanding a disease no longer rare. Am J Med Sci. 1998;316:108.*)

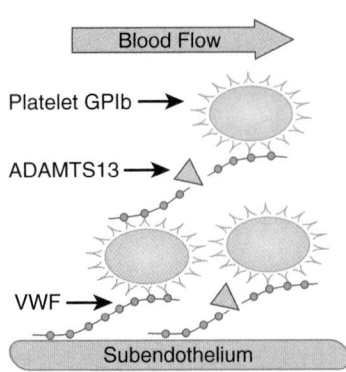

FIGURE 33-7. Pathogenesis of thrombotic thrombocytopenic purpura (TTP). von Willebrand factor (VWF) multimers facilitate platelet adhesion to the subendothelium by binding to exposed connective tissue and then to platelet glycoprotein Ib (GPIb). In flowing blood, shear stress unfolds ultralarge VWF multimers in the platelet-rich thrombus and enables ADAMTS13 to cleave a specific Tyr-Met bond in the second of the three A domains in VWF subunits. Cleavage reduces VWF multimer size and limits thrombus growth. In the absence of ADAMTS13, VWF-dependent platelet accumulation continues and eventually results in microvascular thrombosis and TTP. (*Courtesy of Dr. Evan Sadler, Washington University.*)

is usually due to an acquired deficiency in VWF-cleaving protease activity resulting from an IgG autoantibody against ADAMTS13.[220,221] The reasons for this transient immune dysregulation and for the selective antigenic targeting of ADAMTS13 are unknown. Fresh frozen plasma, cryoprecipitate-poor plasma (cryosupernatant), and plasma treated with solvent or detergent all contain the VWF-cleaving protease activity, which presumably accounts for the efficacy of plasma exchange therapy (see later).

Clinical Features. TTP is a relatively rare disorder with an estimated annual incidence of 1 to 4 per million population.[222,223] TTP is more common in women than in men (ratio of 3:2) and has a peak incidence in persons between the ages of 30 and 40 years. The condition has been reported in adolescents; indeed, the first instance reported in the literature was a teenage female.[204] The incidence of the disease is increasing, in part because of increased awareness of the condition and the availability of effective therapy.[202,224]

TTP usually develops in previously healthy individuals (idiopathic TTP). In approximately 15% of patients, the syndrome is associated with an underlying condition (secondary TTP), such as bacterial or viral infection,[225,226] pregnancy,[227] collagen vascular disorders,[228] or pancreatitis.[229] Several drugs[230] have been associated with the development of secondary TTP, including ticlopidine, clopidogrel, lopidogrel, quinine, mitomycin C, cyclosporine, and tacrolimus. The mechanisms by which these drugs promote TTP are not well understood. Inhibitory antibodies against ADAMTS13 have been observed in ticlopidine- and clopidogrel-associated TTP.[231]

In the usual occurrence of TTP, the onset of symptoms is abrupt. The most common initial manifestations are bleeding and neurologic abnormalities. The neurologic symptoms can progress rapidly and may include headache, confusion, stupor, coma, hemiparesis, cranial nerve palsies, and seizures. Fever is uncommon initially but invariably develops during the course of the disease. TTP is a clinical diagnosis that rests on the signs and symptoms presented in Table 33-3. The primary diagnostic criteria are thrombocytopenia and microangiopathic hemolytic anemia. Some patients may not be anemic initially, although their hematocrit levels may fall sharply afterward, and in some patients red cell fragmentation may not be apparent.[232] Therefore, the diagnosis of TTP initially is often provisional. Serum lactate dehydrogenase (LDH) levels are increased, frequently to very high levels, because of not only hemolysis but also diffuse tissue ischemia. If considerable tissue ischemia and necrosis are present, disseminated intravascular coagulation (DIC) may ensue.

The diagnosis of TTP can be confirmed by measuring ADAMTS13 activity and by screening for inhibitory antibodies against this enzyme.[219] These tests may also provide prognostic information in cases of idopathic TTP. In one prospective study,[233] 6 of 14 patients (43%) with severe ADAMTS13 deficiency later relapsed, whereas only 2 of 25 patients (8%) without severe ADAMTS13 deficiency relapsed. In two other series,[234,235] patients with detectable anti-ADAMTS13 antibodies had a higher mortality rate than patients without detectable antibodies did. More recently, the presence of high-titer anti-ADAMTS13 IgA has been associated with a higher mortality rate.[236]

Though less common than acquired TTP secondary to autoantibodies, TTP caused by mutations in the ADAMTS13 gene is an autosomal recessive disease (also referred to as Upshaw-Schulman syndrome) that can be manifested at birth or in early childhood, with rare patients remaining asymptomatic until adulthood. The age at onset and severity can be highly variable, even among patients in the same family (carrying the same ADAMTS13 mutation).[214-219] Congenital TTP occurring in early childhood may be misdiagnosed as chronic ITP or Evans' syndrome.[219]

Treatment. Congenital TTP typically exhibits a chronic relapsing course that usually requires long-term treatment with fresh frozen plasma to replace the deficient ADAMTS13 protein. The regimen is determined empirically, and stable remission can generally be maintained with plasma infusions as infrequently as once every few weeks to months.[208,209,214-217]

Plasma exchange is the mainstay of therapy for acquired TTP (secondary to anti-ADAMTS13 autoantibodies). At least 50% to 80% of patients recover with this therapy. A randomized trial demonstrated the superiority of plasma exchange over plasma infusion.[237] This finding has been attributed to removal of antibody against VWF-cleaving protease. Another randomized study showed that fresh frozen plasma and cryoprecipitate-poor plasma were equally effective in the initial treatment of adults with TTP.[238] Glucocorticoid therapy is often used as an adjunct to plasma exchange therapy, but there is no direct evidence that the addition of glucocorticoids produces results that are superior to those of plasma therapy alone.[202]

Although TTP in most patients responds to plasma exchange therapy, the response is varied. Mental status changes may resolve immediately. Typically, the initial recovery from thrombocytopenia requires several days. Serum LDH levels may improve promptly, but patients often remain dependent on red cell transfusion for days. Recovery from renal failure is generally slow. Chronic renal insufficiency, defined as creatinine clearance of less than 40 mL/min/1.73 m^2 at 1 year after diagnosis, occurs in about 25% of patients.

Preliminary studies[239-241] suggest that rituximab can induce a complete response in patients with idiopathic TPP who are refractory to plasma exchange. This agent may also be beneficial as prophylatic therapy in patients with idiopathic TTP who are at high risk for relapse.[239-241]

Patients with secondary TTP caused by dose-related drug toxicity (e.g., mitomycin C) or allogeneic marrow transplantation may not benefit from plasma exchange treatment. Likewise, the course in a patient who has a clinically apparent additional condition, such as SLE, is unpredictable. Management of plasma exchange treatment is often dictated by the activity of the associated condition.

Hemolytic-Uremic Syndrome. HUS is another microangiopathic hemolytic anemia characterized by capillary thrombosis and ischemic necrosis. The kidneys are the end organs most severely affected, but ischemic injury of the intestines, central nervous system, or other organs may occur. HUS typically follows a diarrheal illness (mainly *Escherichia coli* O157:H7 infection) but also occurs in nonenteropathic settings. HUS occurs most often in infants and young children and is the most common cause of acute renal failure in this age group. The annual incidence is approximately 1 in 100,000 and may be increasing.[242] HUS can also occur in adults, particularly in the elderly, thus suggesting that susceptibility to HUS is greatest at the extremes of age.

Enteropathic Hemolytic-Uremic Syndrome
PATHOGENESIS. Certain strains of enteric bacteria produce a toxin that is cytopathic to Vero cells, a monkey kidney cell line. In the early 1980s, Karmali and associates[243] reported that 75% of children with HUS had evidence of gastrointestinal infection by verotoxin-producing *E. coli.* Subsequent studies showed that strains of other enteric pathogens, including *Shigella*, *Salmonella*, and *Campylobacter*, produce verotoxin and can cause HUS.

The term *verotoxin* has been replaced by the term *Shiga toxin* or *Shiga-like toxin* (Stx). This toxin is the key factor that differentiates infection with enterohemorrhagic *E. coli* (EHEC), which is associated with watery diarrhea, hemorrhagic colitis, and HUS, from enteropathogenic *E. coli* (EPEC), which is associated only with watery diarrhea and vomiting. Stx1 and Stx2, the two most prevalent forms of the toxin found in EHEC strains, are encoded by bacteriophages. Stx1 is identical to Shiga toxin produced by *Shigella dysenteriae* type I. Stx2 is immunologically distinct from Stx1.[244]

Stx is structurally related to ricin and cholera toxin. Each of these toxins is composed of a single A subunit noncovalently associated with a pentamer of identical B subunits.[244] The enzymatic activity of the toxin resides in the A subunit, whereas the B subunits are required for cellular uptake. Stx is taken up via endocytosis and transported to the endoplasmic reticulum via retrograde trafficking through the secretory pathway.[245] The A subunit enters the cytosol and targets 28S ribosomal RNA, which is depurinated by the toxin at a specific adenine residue and causes protein synthesis to cease and the infected cells to die by apoptosis. Renal microvascular endothelial cells appear to be particularly sensitive to Stx.[246,247] Hemorrhagic enterocolitis has been ascribed to the action of Stx on endothelial cells in vessels of the intestinal submucosa. The toxin also inhibits protein synthesis in certain nonendothelial cells, including renal mesangial and cortical tubular cells.[248,249] Because EHEC is not invasive, it has long been assumed that HUS-related tissue damage results from the spread of bacterial products from the intestine to the kidney and other target organs. It is thought that Stx enters the systemic circulation after translocation across the intestinal epithelium.[250]

CLINICAL AND LABORATORY FEATURES. Approximately 50% of cases of acquired HUS appear after gastrointestinal infection with *E. coli* O157:H7. For unclear reasons, in only 9% to 30% of persons with *E. coli* O157:H7 colitis does HUS develop. Elevated leukocyte counts and C-reactive protein levels have been identified as risk factors for progression to HUS.[251,252] Other risk factors are the extremes of age, the presence of bloody diarrhea, and the use of antimotility drugs.[253]

Gastrointestinal symptoms can range from mild to severe. The colonic mucosa is hemorrhagic and edematous; ischemic infarcts can occur in the colon, and perforations have been reported. Stool cultures may be positive for the pathogenic organism.[254] Other diagnostic techniques include demonstration of Stx or specific bacterial DNA in stool samples or a rise in the titer of specific antibodies.

The anemia and thrombocytopenia associated with HUS tend to be less severe than those associated with TTP. The platelet count is greater than 100,000/μL in half of the patients, and bleeding is uncommon. Laboratory evidence of DIC is not usually present, but it can occur, especially in HUS associated with *Shigella*. The serum LDH level is less elevated than in TTP. A study of 16 children in whom HUS developed after *E. coli* O157:H7 infection showed normal levels of VWF-cleaving protease activity in plasma.[255] This finding has been confirmed by other investigators.[213]

Acute renal failure with oliguria, hypertension, and proteinuria usually develops in affected patients. Renal histopathologic examination reveals a preglomerular and glomerular thrombotic microangiopathy.[256] Mental status changes attributable to uremia are common. More rarely, focal neurologic signs are evident.

TREATMENT. Supportive care is the mainstay of therapy. Parenteral volume expansion with isotonic fluid during acute *E. coli* O157:H7 enteritis may attenuate the renal injury.[257] Dialysis and renal transplantation are performed when necessary. Independent trials have shown that antimotility agents increase the risk for HUS after *E. coli* O157:H7 infection.[253]

The role of antimicrobial agents in the treatment of HUS is controversial. There is no compelling evidence that antibiotics are beneficial, and there is some indirect evidence that the use of antimicrobials may be dangerous. Antibiotics increase the amount of Stx released from EHEC in vitro, so antibiotic therapy might paradoxically increase the risk for HUS in vivo. A prospective, controlled study[258] evaluated the effect of trimethoprim-sulfamethoxazole in children with *E. coli* O157:H7 enteritis. There was no statistically significant effect of treatment on progression of symptoms, fecal pathogen excretion, or the incidence of HUS. A prospective study of 71 children with diarrhea caused by *E. coli* O157:H7 suggested that antibiotic therapy was associated with an increased risk for HUS.[252]

Other treatments that have been tried without obvious benefit include infusion of fresh frozen plasma, glucocorticoids, heparin, thrombolytic agents, and prostacyclin.[259,260] Although plasma infusion or exchange has no proven role in the management of diarrhea-associated HUS in children, this therapy may be beneficial in adults with HUS or children with nonenteropathic HUS (see later).[196] Despite treatment, approximately 5% of children with HUS die of the disease and 10% have severe, chronic renal impairment.[261,262]

Atypical Hemolytic-Uremic Syndrome. Approximately 10% of pediatric patients seen with an HUS-like illness do not have antecedent bloody diarrhea and are classified as having atypical HUS (aHUS). There are both familial and sporatic forms of aHUS. The associated mortality rate is higher than that of enteropathic HUS. About half of survivors have a relapse, and a third require chronic dialysis.[263]

PATHOGENESIS. Deficiency of complement regulators is a major risk factor for the development of aHUS. More than 50% of patients with aHUS have a mutation in one of three complement control proteins: factor H (fH), membrane cofactor protein (MCP; CD46), or factor I (fI).[264,265] Additionally, autoantibodies against fI have been described in patients with sporatic aHUS.[265] MCP and fH serve as cofactors for fI, a serine protease that inactivates C3b (and C4b) through limited proteolytic cleavage (Fig. 33-8). Deficiency of fH, MCP, or fI results in excessive complement deposition, which promotes the development of microthrombi in the kidneys and other tissues.[266]

Invasive infection with certain strains of pneumococcus can also cause aHUS.[267] These strains produce neuraminidase, which exposes the normally hidden Thomsen-Freidenreich antigen on erythrocytes, platelets, and renal glomerular cells. Naturally occuring IgM antibodies in human plasma bind the exposed antigen, promote complement fixation, and trigger anemia, thrombocytopenia, and uremia.[267] Other nondiarrheal infections have also been linked to aHUS.[268]

TREATMENT. Although plasma therapy is often used in the management of aHUS secondary to complement

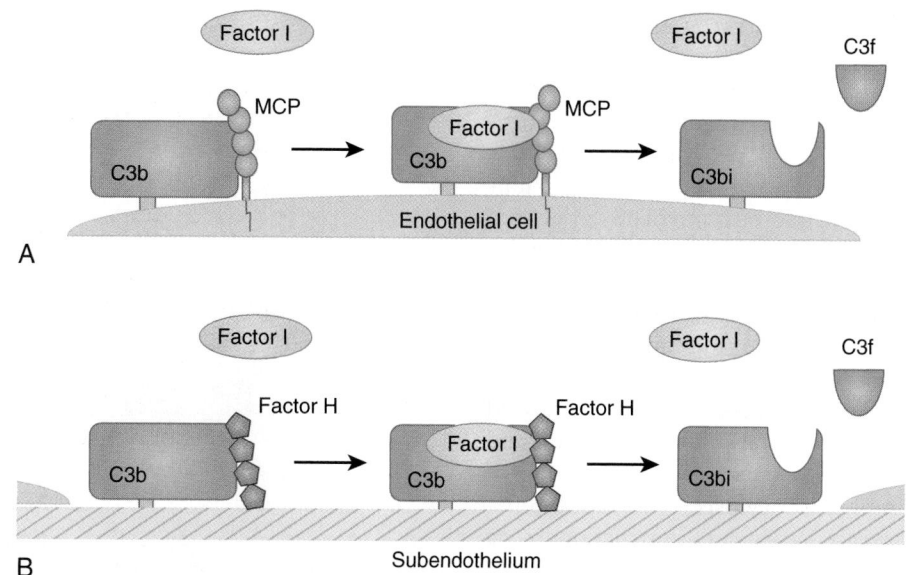

FIGURE 33-8. Role of complement regulatory proteins in the pathogenesis of atypical hemolytic-uremic syndrome. **A,** Membrane cofactor protein (MCP), a complement regulatory protein, is expressed on the surface of endothelial cells and other cell types and binds to C3b that has been deposited on the cell surface either spontaneously or in response to injury. In cooperation with MCP, the plasma serine protease factor I then cleaves C3b into its inactive form C3bi, thereby preventing further complement activation via the alternative pathway. In patients with MCP or factor I deficiency, excessive complement deposition occurs and leads to further cellular injury, endothelial cell necrosis, and ultimately thrombosis. **B,** Endothelial cell necrosis exposes basement membranes that are devoid of complement regulators. Factor H, a plasma-derived complement regulatory protein, binds to exposed basement membranes and, in cooperation with factor I, inactivates C3b that is deposited at these sites. Factor H deficiency leads to excess complement deposition on basement membranes. *(Courtesy of Dr. J. P. Atkinson, Washington University.)*

regulator deficiency, its benefit in preventing progression to end-stage renal disease or relapse is questionable.[269-271] Patients with an MCP mutation have a satisfactory outcome after renal transplantation because MCP is a transmembrane protein and the allografts are protected by wild-type MCP.[264] In contrast, recurrent aHUS develops in patients with a deficiency of fH or fI after renal transplantation because the allograft cannot compensate for deficiency of these plasma proteins, which are produced primarily in the liver. Therapeutic complement inhibition with monoclonal antibodies or recombinant regulators may be the treatment of choice in the future.[272]

Patients with aHUS caused by neuraminidase-producing pneumococcus should receive only washed red blood cells or platelets if transfusion is required.[267] Plasma products should be avoided in these patients.

Bone Marrow Transplant–Associated Thrombotic Microangiopathy

Thrombotic microangiopathy has emerged as one of the major complications of bone marrow transplantation (BMT).[273] The incidence ranges from 6% to 21%.[274] It is seen after allogeneic and less commonly after autologous BMT. The diagnosis may be difficult to make because of the presence of coexisting complications of BMT, such as graft-versus-host disease, cytomegalovirus infection, and hepatic veno-occlusive disease. Although BMT-associated microangiopathy (BMT-MA) shares features with other microangiopathies such as TTP and

HUS, it has a distinctive clinical course and response to therapy. The pathogenesis of BMT-MA is unknown but appears to be distinct from that of primary TTP.

The condition ranges in severity from self-limited microangiopathic hemolytic anemia to a fulminant, usually fatal disorder. The fulminant form of the disease is more common in adults than children. In one adult series,[275] the incidence of BMT-MA was 2% with matched sibling donor transplants and 6% with unrelated donor transplants. Risk factors for the development of BMT-MA in adults include the use of unrelated or mismatched donors, grade II through IV acute graft-versus-host disease, and systemic bacterial or fungal infection.[274] In contrast to primary TTP, plasma exchange therapy appears to be of limited benefit in BMT-MA.[274] Most pediatric patients primarily exhibit signs of renal insufficiency. The mainstay of management is supportive care and, if feasible, a reduction of the dose of cyclosporine or tacrolimus. If the patient's clinical condition deteriorates (worsening hemolysis, progressive renal insufficiency, or neurologic symptoms), plasma exchange should be considered.[273]

Other Causes of Increased Platelet Destruction

Systemic bacterial or fungal infections are also commonly associated with thrombocytopenia. The degree of thrombocytopenia may range from moderate to severe. Thrombocytopenia associated with systemic bacterial or fungal infection is usually due to increased platelet destruction. A variety of mechanisms contribute to this destruction, including immune mediated, direct effects of bacterial toxins, DIC, and hypersplenism.

Acute viral infections in children are commonly complicated by thrombocytopenia. For example, thrombocytopenia develops in about 75% of patients with infectious mononucleosis caused by Epstein-Barr virus.[276] Viral-induced thrombocytopenia may be immediate or delayed, and the decrease in platelet count may range from mild to severe. Thrombocytopenia can follow immunization with live virus vaccines. Viruses may cause thrombocytopenia through both nonimmune and immune mechanisms, including cytotoxic effects on megakaryocytes, direct injury to platelets, immune complex–mediated destruction (see earlier discussion of ITP and HIV), and hyperspenism. Thrombocytopenia is a manifestation of hemophagocytic lymphohistiocytosis. Thrombocytopenia caused by increased platelet destruction is a uniformly seen complication of malaria and African trypanosomiasis.[277]

Thrombocytopenia commonly accompanies extracorporeal membranous oxygenation, cardiopulmonary bypass, hemodialysis, and apheresis.[278] There are many causes, including adherence of platelets to synthetic materials in the perfusion device, hemodilution, hemorrhage, and drug effects (e.g., heparin). The thrombocytopenia associated with hemodialysis or apheresis is generally mild, but more severe thrombocytopenia may be seen in association with extracorporeal membranous oxygenation.

A healthy fetus has a platelet count of greater than 150,000/μL by the second trimester of pregnancy, and only 2% of term infants are thrombocytopenic at birth.[279] Severe thrombocytopenia, defined as a platelet count lower than 50,000/μL, is evident in fewer than 3 of 1000 term infants, the most important cause being NAIT. In contrast, thrombocytopenia is common among patients in neonatal intensive care units. Thrombocytopenia is also common in patients with intrauterine growth retardation and has been ascribed to placental insufficiency or chronic hypoxia. Thrombocytopenia is seen in preterm neonates with respiratory distress syndrome. Neonatal viral infections, including rubella, herpes, cytomegalovirus, and enterovirus, have also been associated with thrombocytopenia. Acute thrombocytopenia commonly accompanies necrotizing enterocolitis and is often an early sign of the disease. Thrombocytopenia is commonly seen in neonates with polycythemia, especially if they have associated cyanotic heart disease, although this phenomenon is probably multifactorial.[280] Infants with severe Rh hemolytic disease of the newborn may exhibit thrombocytopenia along with neutropenia.[281]

Kasabach-Merritt Syndrome. Kasabach-Merritt syndrome is the association between thrombocytopenia and a giant hemangioma of infancy. Most patients are seen in the first few weeks of life, although rare occurrences have been described in later childhood.[282] The vascular lesions are usually solitary and involve the extremities,

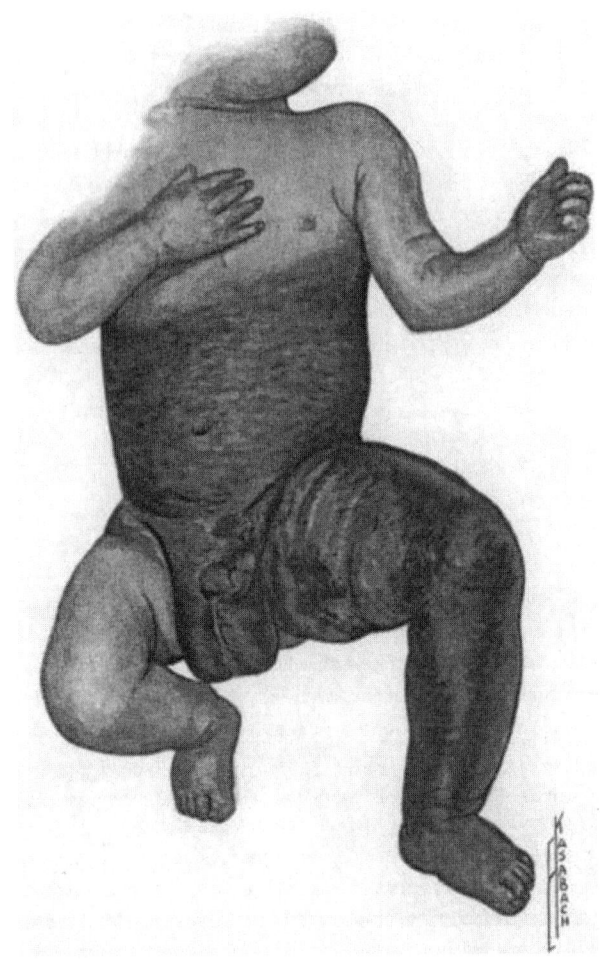

FIGURE 33-9. Drawing of an affected infant in the original article by Kasabach and Merritt. *(From Kasabach HHM, Merritt KK. Capillary hemangioma with extensive purpura. Report of a case. Am J Dis Child. 1940;59:1063-1070.)*

neck, or trunk (Fig. 33-9). Sometimes the lesions are located in the viscera, including the retroperitoneum. The possibility of an occult hemangioma should be considered in a neonate with unexplained thrombocytopenia. Detection may require radiographic imaging of the brain, liver, spleen, or gastrointestinal tract.

The hemangiomas associated with Kasabach-Merritt syndrome have a natural history of rapid growth for several months, followed by spontaneous regression. The thrombocytopenia subsides as the hemangioma regresses. Kasabach-Merritt syndrome, which is marked by severe thrombocytopenia and spontaneous regression in the first few years of life, is distinct from the mild, chronic thrombocytopenia associated with venous malformations, which are lifelong lesions (Box 33-5).

The pathogenesis is poorly understood, but platelets are thought to be trapped by abnormal endothelium within the hemangioma. Usually, the platelet count is less than 50,000/μL, and schistocytes are frequently present on the peripheral blood film. In a majority of cases there is laboratory evidence of DIC. These tumors grow rapidly

to a large size and are often characterized by cutaneous
purpura, edema, and an advancing ecchymotic margin.
Imaging studies are essential in delineating the extent of
the lesion and determining whether it is surgically resectable.
In contrast to common hemangiomas, magnetic
resonance imaging shows diffuse enhancement with ill-defined
margins, cutaneous thickening, stranding of subcutaneous
fat, hemosiderin deposits, and small feeding
and draining vessels.[282]

The mortality rate is as high as 40%,[287] and the
development of a life-threatening consumptive coagulopathy
warrants aggressive treatment. Surgical removal
may be effective, but most lesions are not able to be
resected. Radiation therapy can be effective but carries
serious long-term risks for a young infant[288] and is not
appropriate for most patients. Vascular ligation or embolization
has been used to promote regression of a large
hemangioma, especially in patients in whom a solitary,
major feeding vessel can be obliterated.[282] Glucocorticoid
therapy may be beneficial in some patients.[282] Interferon
alfa has been shown to be effective if no response to glucocorticoid
therapy is seen.[289] Vincristine is another treatment
option in the management of patients with
Kasabach-Merritt syndrome.[290]

Thrombocytopenia Caused by Decreased Platelet Production

The second major etiologic classification of acquired
thrombocytopenia of childhood is impaired platelet production.
Box 33-1 lists clinical conditions associated with
decreased platelet production. Patients with thrombocytopenia
caused by a production defect are more likely to
have serious bleeding than patients with destructive
thrombocytopenia are.

A common cause of thrombocytopenia in patients
with cancer is chemotherapy-induced bone marrow suppression.
This is an expected complication of therapy and
rarely poses a diagnostic problem. Traditional management
is straightforward and relies on transfusion of platelet
concentrates and adjustment of chemotherapy doses.
Considerable effort has also been put into the clinical
study of cytokines that promote thrombopoiesis (see
Chapter 35).

Valproic acid is commonly used in the treatment of
childhood epilepsy, bipolar disorder, and other conditions.
Hematologic toxicity, including thrombocytopenia,
is often seen in patients treated with valproate.[291] Valproate
causes direct bone marrow suppression that may vary
in onset and severity and is more common in patients
with serum valproate levels greater than 100 µg/mL.[291]
In addition to bone marrow suppression, valproate
may have other effects on platelets, including immune-mediated
destruction and impaired function.[291]

Thrombocytopenia can result from replacement of
normal marrow elements by abnormal cells, as seen in
leukemia, solid tumors (neuroblastoma, rhabdomyosarcoma,
Ewing's sarcoma), storage diseases, and disseminated
Langerhans cell histiocytosis. Other acquired
disorders of hematopoietic cells that are associated with
thrombocytopenia include myelodysplastic syndrome,
aplastic anemia, paroxysmal nocturnal hemoglobinuria,
and osteopetrosis. In osteopetrosis, the bone marrow
space is obliterated by new bone formation. This condition
can be diagnosed by x-ray studies but may not be
clinically obvious in a neonate with thrombocytopenia.
Peripheral smear findings include teardrop cells and
nucleated erythrocytes.

Although iron deficiency is usually associated with
thrombocytosis, thrombocytopenia may accompany
severe iron deficiency in children and adults[292] (see
Chapter 12). Anemia caused by folate or vitamin B_{12}
deficiency (see Chapter 11) is also often associated with
thrombocytopenia. Severe thrombocytopenia secondary
to impaired hematopoiesis has been reported in association
with anorexia nervosa.[293] The thrombocytopenia
reverses with improved nutrition.

Thrombocytosis

Thrombocytosis is defined as a platelet count greater
than 2 SD above the mean. Conditions associated with
thrombocytosis in childhood are listed in Box 33-6.

When the platelet count is elevated, the clinician
must determine whether the patient has a true increase
in total body platelet mass. Under normal circumstances,
a third of the body's platelets are sequestered in the
spleen. Individuals with surgical or functional asplenia
who have a normal total body platelet mass will have
an elevated platelet count. This situation is normal for
an asplenic individual and no therapy is warranted.
Spuriously elevated automated platelet counts may
be caused by the presence of microspherocytes,
Pappenheimer bodies, red cell and leukocyte fragments,
or bacteria.

Causes of true thrombocytosis fall into two categories:
autonomous (or primary) thrombocytosis and

Box 33-6	Causes of Thrombocytosis in Childhood

PRIMARY OR AUTONOMOUS THROMBOCYTOSIS

Myeloproliferative disorders
   Essential thrombocythemia
      Nonfamilial
      Familial
   Polycythemia vera
   Chronic myelogenous leukemia
   Agnogenic myeloid metaplasia
   M7 acute myelogenous leukemia
   5q– syndrome

SECONDARY OR REACTIVE THROMBOCYTOSIS

Inflammatory diseases
   Infection
      Acute
      Chronic (tuberculosis, hepatitis, osteomyelitis)
   Rheumatoid arthritis
   Inflammatory bowel disease
   Ankylosing spondylitis
   Sarcoidosis
   Acute rheumatic fever
   Kawasaki's syndrome
Hematologic disorders
   Iron deficiency
   Chronic hemolytic anemias
   Vitamin E deficiency
   Acute hemorrhage
   "Rebound" following thrombocytopenia

Drug-induced
   Vinca alkaloids
   Corticosteroids
Neoplastic diseases
   Lymphoma
   Neuroblastoma
   Other childhood solid tumors
Miscellaneous
   After exercise
   Following surgery
   Caffey's disease

RELATIVE THROMBOCYTOSIS DUE TO DECREASED SPLENIC POOLING

Asplenia
   Surgical
   Congenital
   Afunctional
Drug-induced
   Epinepherine

SPURIOUS THROMBOCYTOSIS

Microspherocytes
Pappenheimer bodies
Red cell and leukocyte fragments
Bacteria

reactive (or secondary) thrombocytosis. In primary thrombocytosis, platelet production is unresponsive to normal regulatory processes.[294] The decrease in megakaryocyte size that normally results from an increase in platelet mass is not seen. In childhood, most occurrences of thrombocytosis are secondary. In general, occurrences of reactive thrombocytosis are moderate in degree and asymptomatic and respond with treatment of the underlying disorder. Reactive thrombocytosis is often seen in association with inflammatory disorders (see Box 33-6). In these situations, the degree of thrombocytosis usually parallels the activity of the underlying condition. Therapy to decrease the platelet count is not indicated. Iron deficiency is often associated with an increase in the platelet count (see Chapter 12). Moderate thrombocytosis that persists for 1 to 2 weeks occurs commonly after major trauma or surgery.[295]

Rarely, a child with thrombocytosis will have a primary myeloproliferative disorder such as essential thrombocythemia or chronic myelogenous leukemia. These patients may be predisposed to thrombosis or hemorrhage.

ACQUIRED DEFECTS IN PLATELET FUNCTION

Drug-Induced Platelet Dysfunction

Many substances have been shown to inhibit platelet function, including both prescription drugs and medicinals such as garlic and various Chinese herbs.[296,297] In otherwise normal individuals, the impairment in platelet function produced by these substances is of no clinical significance. On the other hand, these agents may cause serious hemorrhage in patients with underlying coagulopathies, such as uremia, hemophilia, or thrombocytopenia, or in patients taking anticoagulants such as heparin or warfarin.[298]

Oxygenated metabolites of arachidonic acid, collectively termed eicosanoids, are involved in a variety of processes, including thrombosis, inflammation, and allergy. Eicosanoids include prostaglandins, thromboxanes, and other compounds. Interference with eicosanoid synthesis is the basis for the action of many therapeutic agents, including analgesics, anti-inflammatory agents, and antithrombotic drugs. The first enzyme in the synthetic pathway of prostaglandins and thromboxanes is cyclooxygenase (COX). There are two isoforms of his enzyme, COX-1 and COX-2. The former is constitutively expressed in most cells, including platelets. The latter is not normally present but may be induced in certain cells after stimulation with cytokines or other factors. In platelets, thromboxane X_2 (TxA_2) is the major product of COX. TxA_2 induces platelet aggregation and vasoconstriction. Aspirin blocks production of TxA_2 by covalently acetylating a serine residue near the active site of COX.[299] Because platelets do not synthesize new proteins, the action of aspirin is permanent and lasts the life of the platelet. Complete inactivation of platelet COX-1 is achieved when adults take 160 mg of aspirin daily. In pregnant women, aspirin may cross the placenta and impair platelet function in the fetus.[300,301] Aspirin prolongs the bleeding time but seldom produces values above the normal range.

Most other anti-inflammatory drugs act on platelets in a manner similar to that of aspirin, although the majority are less potent. Such agents include ibuprofen, naproxen, phenylbutazone, indomethacin, sodium salicylate, and related drugs. In contrast to those of aspirin, the effects of these medications are reversible.

Dipyridamole is a vasodilator that interferes with platelet function by increasing the intracellular concentration of cyclic adenosine monophophate (cAMP). This effect is mediated by inhibition of cyclic nucleotide phosphodiesterase.[302] In combination with warfarin, dipyridamole is used to inhibit embolization from prosthetic heart valves. Other drugs that raise cAMP levels by inhibiting phosphodiesterase, such as methylxanthines, also inhibit platelet function.

The thienopyridine derivative class of drug, including ticlopidine, inhibits platelet activation[303] and prolongs the bleeding time by blocking signaling through the $P2Y_{12}$ platelet adenosine diphosphate (ADP) receptor. Abnormal platelet function continues for several days after use of the drug is discontinued. A newer member of this class, clopidogrel, has supplanted ticlopidine because of its efficacy and better safety profile.[304-306]

Though used sparingly in pediatrics, GPIIb/IIIa antagonists are now widely used as anticoagulants in adult patients with heart disease.[307,308] These agents inhibit the final common pathway of platelet aggregation mediated by fibrinogen or VWF binding to GPIIb/IIIa. Therefore, GPIIb/IIIa antagonists more completely inhibit platelet aggregation than aspirin or clopidogrel does, each of which inhibits only one initiating pathway of platelet activation (COX and ADP receptors, respectively). Several GPIIb/IIIa inhibitors are commercially available for use in coronary intervention procedures or unstable angina.[307,308]

A number of antibiotics inhibit platelet aggregation and the release reaction,[309] although the mechanisms are not well understood. Penicillin causes platelet dysfunction when administered at high doses, but this effect is usually clinically insignificant. However, certain semisynthetic penicillins, notably carbenicillin, may cause clinically significant bleeding when administered at the usual therapeutic doses.[310-313] Bleeding times are prolonged in patients receiving carbenicillin therapy, and serious episodes of hemorrhage have been reported.

Calcium channel blockers, such as verapamil and nifedipine, interfere with both adrenergic receptors and TxA_2 receptors in the platelet membrane[314] but do not prolong the bleeding time. Some antidepressants, including amitriptyline, imipramine, and chlorpromazine, interfere with platelet function through ill-defined effects on platelet membranes.[315] Propranolol and other β-adrenergic receptor antagonists mildly inhibit platelet function through effects on the cell membrane and serotonin transport.[316] Sulfonylureas used in the management of hyperglycemia have been associated with mild qualitative platelet defects.[317] Valproic acid, in addition to causing thrombocytopenia, can directly inhibit platelet function.[291]

Platelet Abnormalities Associated with Systemic Diseases

Uremia

Platelet dysfunction is a well-recognized and potentially serious complication of uremia. Patients with severe renal insufficiency may experience petechiae, purpura, gastrointestinal hemorrhage, and other forms of bleeding. Dialysis can correct the platelet dysfunction associated with uremia.[318] The precise cause of the platelet defect in uremia is unknown. A dialyzable substance in plasma causes platelet dysfunction, but the identity of this factor (or factors) remains controversial.

Bleeding may be severe, although the incidence of serious hemorrhage has declined in recent years because of more intensive dialysis and avoidance of drugs that further impair platelet function. If there is symptomatic bleeding or surgery is planned, patients should be treated with dialysis or desmopressin. Typically, only partial correction is achieved. The anemia of chronic renal insufficiency should be treated with erythropoietin because this has been shown to reduce the risk of serious bleeding.[318-323] If these approaches are not effective, cryoprecipitate may be added.

Liver Disease

Patients with liver disease have a multifactorial bleeding disorder. A reduction in plasma coagulation factors synthesized by the liver contributes to the increased risk of bleeding in these patients. Moderate thrombocytopenia is a common finding in liver disease and is well tolerated in most instances. Thrombocytopenia in cirrhotic liver disease has long been ascribed to portal hypertension and concomitant hypersplenism. Recent studies suggest that altered thrombopoietin production may contribute to the thrombocytopenia in liver disease. Qualitative platelet

Box 33-7	Vascular Purpuras of Childhood

Vasculitis
  Henoch-Schönlein purpura
  Kawasaki's syndrome
  Polyarteritis nodosa
Purpura fulminans
Connective tissue diseases
  Ehlers-Danlos syndrome
  Marfan's syndrome
  Osteogenesis imperfecta
  Minkes' disease
  Pseudoxanthoma elasticum
Hereditary hemorrhagic telangiectasia (Osler-Weber-Rendu syndrome)

defects have also been reported to occur in adult patients with liver failure,[324-327] although the mechanisms responsible are not well understood.

Vascular Purpuras

The vascular purpuras, also termed the nonthrombocytopenic purpuras, are mentioned in this chapter because these diseases share features with ITP. These conditions often follow acute infection. A list of childhood vascular purpuras is presented in Box 33-7.

Henoch-Schönlein Purpura

Henoch-Schönlein purpura (HSP), also known as allergic purpura or anaphylactoid purpura, is a vasculitis affecting capillaries of the skin, synovial membranes, renal mesangium, and small intestine. The purpuric manifestations of the disease are usually self-limited.

HSP is presumably the result of an autoimmune process. The basic lesion is a microvasculitis with endothelial cell injury. Deposits of IgA are evident on capillary endothelial cells of the skin, kidney, and gastrointestinal tract. The renal manifestations of HSP are indistinguishable from those of so-called IgA nephropathy.[328]

The median age at diagnosis is 5 years (range, 0.4 to 15 years). Males predominate at a ratio of 3:2. An acute febrile illness precedes the syndrome in a majority of cases. In about 50% of patients, raised purpuric papules (palpable purpura) are evident over the lower extremities and buttocks, whereas in the remainder of patients the purpuric rash is more extensive.[329] Bullae, urticaria, diffuse erythema, and ulceration may also be seen. Joint pain or swelling is evident in about 80% of cases. Two thirds of patients exhibit abdominal signs or symptoms, including pain, hematemesis, or melena. Intussusception occurs in about 4% of patients with HSP. Edema, including scrotal swelling, is common. Renal involvement is evident in 40% of patients, many of whom exhibit severe proteinuria. The manifestations of this syndrome resolve within 1 to 6 weeks in the vast majority of patients. In a small subset of patients, permanent renal or joint damage may ensue.[330]

Glucocorticoid therapy can reduce the skin, joint, and gastrointestinal manifestations of the disease but should be reserved for those with severe symptoms. There is little evidence that glucocorticoids prevent renal involvement[331,332] or intussusception.

Purpura Fulminans

Purpura fulminans is a potentially fatal disorder that follows infection with meningococcus, streptococcus, varicella, and rubella. Thrombosis of small arterioles leads to infarction and hemorrhage of skin, subcutaneous tissues, and muscle. The disease occurs suddenly 2 to 4 weeks after a relatively mild infection such as varicella or scarlet fever. It begins with purpuric lesions on the skin that coalesce and then become necrotic. Patients become extremely ill with fever, hypotension, and laboratory evidence of DIC. The disease resembles pupura fulminans neonatalis, a disorder associated with homozygous protein C or protein S deficiency (see Chapter 32).

REFERENCES

1. Aster RH. Pooling of platelets in the spleen: role in the pathogenesis of "hypersplenic" thrombocytopenia. J Clin Invest. 1966;45:645-657.
2. Paulus JM. Platelet size in man. Blood. 1975;46:321-336.
3. Shulman NR, Jordan JV Jr, Falchuk S. A normal fixed-loss component of platelet utilization accounting for short survival of transfused platelets. Ann N Y Acad Sci. 1985;459:367-374.
4. Hanson SR, Slichter SJ. Platelet kinetics in patients with bone marrow hypoplasia: evidence for a fixed platelet requirement. Blood. 1985;66:1105-1109.
5. Racchi O, Rapezzi D. Megathrombocytes and spurious thrombocytopenia. Eur J Haematol. 2001;66:140-141.
6. Bizzaro N. EDTA-dependent pseudothrombocytopenia: a clinical and epidemiological study of 112 cases, with 10-year follow-up. Am J Hematol. 1995;50:103-109.
7. Morselli M, Longo G, Bonacorsi G, et al. Anticoagulant pseudothrombocytopenia with platelet satellitism. Haematologica. 1999;84:655.
8. Yoshikawa H. EDTA-dependent pseudothrombocytopenia induced by valproic acid. Neurology. 2003;61:579-580.
9. Cunningham VL, Brandt JT. Spurious thrombocytopenia due to EDTA-independent cold-reactive agglutinins. Am J Clin Pathol. 1992;97:359-362.
10. Wadenvik H, Denfors I, Kutti J. Splenic blood flow and intrasplenic platelet kinetics in relation to spleen volume. Br J Haematol. 1987;67:181-185.
11. Gunn AJ, Gluckman PD, Gunn TR. Selective head cooling in newborn infants after perinatal asphyxia: a safety study. Pediatrics. 1998;102:885-892.
12. Chan KM, Beard K. A patient with recurrent hypothermia associated with thrombocytopenia. Postgrad Med J. 1993;69:227-229.
13. Fujisawa K, Tani P, O'Toole TE, et al. Different specificities of platelet-associated and plasma autoantibodies to platelet GPIIb-IIIa in patients with chronic immune

thrombocytopenic purpura. Blood. 1992;79:1441-1446.

14. Beardsley DS, Spiegel JE, Jacobs MM, et al. Platelet membrane glycoprotein IIIa contains target antigens that bind anti-platelet antibodies in immune thrombocytopenias. J Clin Invest. 1984;74:1701-1707.

15. Pfueller SL, Bilston RA, Logan D, et al. Heterogeneity of drug-dependent platelet antigens and their antibodies in quinine- and quinidine-induced thrombocytopenia: involvement of glycoproteins Ib, IIb, IIIa, and IX. Blood. 1988;72:1155-1162.

16. Curtis BR, McFarland JG, Wu GG, et al. Antibodies in sulfonamide-induced immune thrombocytopenia recognize calcium-dependent epitopes on the glycoprotein IIb/IIIa complex. Blood. 1994;84:176-183.

17. Gentilini G, Curtis BR, Aster RH. An antibody from a patient with ranitidine-induced thrombocytopenia recognizes a site on glycoprotein IX that is a favored target for drug-induced antibodies. Blood. 1998;92:2359-2365.

18. Pereira J, Cretney C, Aster RH. Variation of class I HLA antigen expression among platelet density cohorts: a possible index of platelet age? Blood. 1988;71:516-519.

19. Ogasawara K, Ueki J, Takenaka M, Furihata K. Study on the expression of ABH antigens on platelets. Blood. 1993;82:993-999.

20. Chong BH, Keng TB. Advances in the diagnosis of idiopathic thrombocytopenic purpura. Semin Hematol. 2000;37:249-260.

21. George JN. Platelet immunoglobulin G: its significance for the evaluation of thrombocytopenia and for understanding the origin of alpha-granule proteins. Blood. 1990;76:859-870.

22. Tomer A, Koziol J, McMillan R. Autoimmune thrombocytopenia: flow cytometric determination of platelet-associated autoantibodies against platelet-specific receptors. J Thromb Haemost. 2005;3:74-78.

23. Aderem A, Underhill DM. Mechanisms of phagocytosis in macrophages. Annu Rev Immunol. 1999;17:593-623.

24. Samuelsson A, Towers TL, Ravetch JV. Anti-inflammatory activity of IVIG mediated through the inhibitory Fc receptor. Science. 2001;291:484-486.

25. Imbach P, Kühne T, Muller D, et al. Childhood ITP: 12 months follow-up data from the prospective registry I of the Intercontinental Childhood ITP Study Group (ICIS). Pediatr Blood Cancer. 2006;46:351-356.

26. Calpin C, Dick P, Poon A, Feldman W. Is bone marrow aspiration needed in acute childhood idiopathic thrombocytopenic purpura to rule out leukemia? Arch Pediatr Adolesc Med. 1998;152:345-347.

27. Halperin DS, Doyle JJ. Is bone marrow examination justified in idiopathic thrombocytopenic purpura? Am J Dis Child. 1988;142:508-511.

28. Westerman DA, Grigg AP. The diagnosis of idiopathic thrombocytopenic purpura in adults: does bone marrow biopsy have a place? Med J Aust. 1999;170:216-217.

29. Roganovic J. Rituximab treatment in refractory idiopathic thrombocytopenic purpura in children. Eur J Pediatr. 2005;164:334.

30. Medeiros D, Buchanan GR. Idiopathic thrombocytopenic purpura: beyond consensus. Curr Opin Pediatr. 2000;12:4-9.

31. George JN, Woolf SH, Raskob GE et al. Idiopathic thrombocytopenic purpura: a practice guideline developed by explicit methods for the American Society of Hematology. Blood. 1996;88:3-40.

32. Kühne T, Buchanan GR, Zimmerman S, et al. A prospective comparative study of 2540 infants and children with newly diagnosed idiopathic thrombocytopenic purpura (ITP) from the Intercontinental Childhood ITP Study Group. J Pediatr. 2003;143:605-608.

33. Gernsheimer T. Pathophysiology and thrombokinetics in autoimmune thrombocytopenia. Blood Rev. 2002;16:7-8.

34. Chang M, Nakagawa PA, Williams SA, et al. Immune thrombocytopenic purpura (ITP) plasma and purified ITP monoclonal autoantibodies inhibit megakaryocytopoiesis in vitro. Blood. 2003;102:887-895.

35. McMillan R, Wang L, Tomer A, et al. Suppression of in vitro megakaryocyte production by antiplatelet autoantibodies from adult patients with chronic ITP. Blood. 2004;103:1364-1369.

37. McMillan R. Autoantibodies and autoantigens in chronic immune thrombocytopenic purpura. Semin Hematol. 2000;37:239-248.

38. Szatkowski NS, Kunicki TJ, Aster RH. Identification of glycoprotein Ib as a target for autoantibody in idiopathic (autoimmune) thrombocytopenic purpura. Blood. 1986;67:310-315.

39. Koerner TA, Weinfeld HM, Bullard LS, Williams LC. Antibodies against platelet glycosphingolipids: detection in serum by quantitative HPTLC-autoradiography and association with autoimmune and alloimmune processes. Blood. 1989;74:274-284.

39. Berchtold P, Wenger M. Autoantibodies against platelet glycoproteins in autoimmune thrombocytopenic purpura: their clinical significance and response to treatment. Blood. 1993;81:1246-1250.

40. Kazatchkine MD, Lambre CR, Kieffer N, et al. Membrane-bound hemagglutinin mediates antibody and complement-dependent lysis of influenza virus–treated human platelets in autologous serum. J Clin Invest. 1984;74:976-984.

41. Wright JF, Blanchette VS, Wang H, et al. Characterization of platelet-reactive antibodies in children with varicella-associated acute immune thrombocytopenic purpura (ITP). Br J Haematol. 1996;95:145-152.

42. Mayer JL, Beardsley DS. Varicella-associated thrombocytopenia: autoantibodies against platelet surface glycoprotein V. Pediatr Res. 1996;40:615-619.

43. Bennett CM, de Jong JL, Neufeld EJ. Targeted ITP strategies: do they elucidate the biology of ITP and related disorders? Pediatr Blood Cancer. 2006;47:706-709.

44. Olsson B, Andersson PO, Jernas M, et al. T-cell–mediated cytotoxicity toward platelets in chronic idiopathic thrombocytopenic purpura. Nat Med. 2003;9:1123-1124.

45. Olsson B, Andersson PO, Jacobsson S, et al. Disturbed apoptosis of T-cells in patients with active idiopathic thrombocytopenic purpura. Thromb Haemost. 2005;93:139-144.

46. Foster CB, Zhu S, Erichsen HC, et al. Polymorphisms in inflammatory cytokines and Fcgamma receptors in childhood chronic immune thrombocytopenic purpura: a pilot study. Br J Haematol. 2001;113:596-599.

47. Kuhne T, Imbach P, Bolton-Maggs PH, et al. Newly diagnosed idiopathic thrombocytopenic purpura in childhood: an observational study. Lancet. 2001;358:2122-2125.

48. Kenet G, Lubetsky A, Shenkman B, et al. Cone and platelet analyser (CPA): a new test for the prediction of bleeding among thrombocytopenic patients. Br J Haematol. 1998;101:255-259.

49. Blanchette V, Carcao M. Approach to the investigation and management of immune thrombocytopenic purpura in children. Semin Hematol. 2000;37:299-314.

50. Buchanan GR, de Alarcon PA, Feig SA, et al. Acute idiopathic thrombocytopenic purpura—management in childhood. Blood. 1997;89:1464-1465.

51. Tarantino MD. On the conservative management of acute immune thrombocytopenia in children. J Pediatr. 2001;138:787-788.

52. Sutor AH. Acute immune thrombocytopenia in childhood. Are we treating the platelet count? Semin Thromb Hemost. 1998;24:545-548.

53. Eden OB, Lilleyman JS. Guidelines for management of idiopathic thrombocytopenic purpura. The British Paediatric Haematology Group. Arch Dis Child. 1992;67:1056-1058.

54. Lilleyman JS. Intracranial hemorrhage in chronic childhood ITP. Pediatr Hematol Oncol. 1997;14:iii-iiv.

55. Iyori H, Bessho F, Ookawa H, et al. Intracranial hemorrhage in children with immune thrombocytopenic purpura. Japanese Study Group on childhood ITP. Ann Hematol. 2000;79:691-695.

56. Medeiros D, Buchanan GR. Major hemorrhage in children with idiopathic thrombocytopenic purpura: immediate response to therapy and long-term outcome. J Pediatr. 1998;133:334-339.

57. Gernsheimer T, Stratton J, Ballem PJ, Slichter SJ. Mechanisms of response to treatment in autoimmune thrombocytopenic purpura. N Engl J Med. 1989;320:974-980.

58. Sartorius JA. Steroid treatment of idiopathic thrombocytopenic purpura in children. Preliminary results of a randomized cooperative study. Am J Pediatr Hematol Oncol. 1984;6:165-169.

59. Buchanan GR, Holtkamp CA. Prednisone therapy for children with newly diagnosed idiopathic thrombocytopenic purpura. A randomized clinical trial. Am J Pediatr Hematol Oncol. 1984;6:355-361.

60. Blanchette VS, Luke B, Andrew M, et al. A prospective, randomized trial of high-dose intravenous immune globulin G therapy, oral prednisone therapy, and no therapy in childhood acute immune thrombocytopenic purpura. J Pediatr. 1993;123:989-995.

61. Carcao MD, Zipursky A, Butchart S, et al. Short-course oral prednisone therapy in children presenting with acute immune thrombocytopenic purpura (ITP). Acta Paediatr Suppl. 1998;424:71-74.

62. Yetgin S, Yenicesu IC, Ersoy F. The effects of megadose methylprednisolone therapy on the immune system in childhood immune thrombocytopenia. Pediatr Hematol Oncol. 2005;22:401-407.

63. Imbach P, Barandun S, d'Apuzzo V, et al. High-dose intravenous gammaglobulin for idiopathic thrombocytopenic purpura in childhood. Lancet. 1981;1:1228-1231.

64. Bussel JB, Schulman I, Hilgartner MW, Barandun S. Intravenous use of gammaglobulin in the treatment of chronic immune thrombocytopenic purpura as a means to defer splenectomy. J Pediatr. 1983;103:651-654.

65. Blanchette V, Imbach P, Andrew M, et al. Randomised trial of intravenous immunoglobulin G, intravenous anti-D, and oral prednisone in childhood acute immune thrombocytopenic purpura. Lancet. 1994;344:703-707.

66. Warrier I, Bussel JB, Valdez L, et al. Safety and efficacy of low-dose intravenous immune globulin (IVIG) treatment for infants and children with immune thrombocytopenic purpura. Low-Dose IVIG Study Group. J Pediatr Hematol Oncol. 1997;19:197-201.

67. Bussel JB. Fc receptor blockade and immune thrombocytopenic purpura. Semin Hematol. 2000;37:261-266.

68. Rossi F, Dietrich G, Kazatchkine MD. Antiidiotypic suppression of autoantibodies with normal polyspecific immunoglobulins. Res Immunol. 1989;140:19-31.

69. Benesch M, Kerbl R, Lackner H, et al. Low-dose versus high-dose immunoglobulin for primary treatment of acute immune thrombocytopenic purpura in children: results of a prospective, randomized single-center trial. J Pediatr Hematol Oncol. 2003;25:797-800.

70. Imbach P. A multicenter European trial of intravenous immune globulin in immune thrombocytopenic purpura in childhood. Vox Sang. 1985;49(Suppl 1):25-31.

71. Blanchette M, Freedman J. The history of idiopathic thrombocytopenic purpura (ITP). Transfus Sci. 1998;19:231-236.

72. Simpson KN, Coughlin CM, Eron J, Bussel JB. Idiopathic thrombocytopenia purpura: treatment patterns and an analysis of cost associated with intravenous immunoglobulin and anti-D therapy. Semin Hematol. 1998;35:58-64.

73. Sekul EA, Cupler EJ, Dalakas MC. Aseptic meningitis associated with high-dose intravenous immunoglobulin therapy: frequency and risk factors. Ann Intern Med. 1994;121:259-262.

74. Chapel HM, Spickett GP, Ericson D, et al. The comparison of the efficacy and safety of intravenous versus subcutaneous immunoglobulin replacement therapy. J Clin Immunol. 2000;20:94-100.

75. Scaradavou A, Woo B, Woloski BM, et al. Intravenous anti-D treatment of immune thrombocytopenic purpura: experience in 272 patients. Blood. 1997;89:2689-2700.

76. Tarantino MD, Madden RM, Fennewald DL, et al. Treatment of childhood acute immune thrombocytopenic purpura with anti-D immune globulin or pooled immune globulin. J Pediatr. 1999;134:21-26.

77. Bussel JB, Graziano JN, Kimberly RP, et al. Intravenous anti-D treatment of immune thrombocytopenic purpura: analysis of efficacy, toxicity, and mechanism of effect. Blood. 1991;77:1884-1893.

78. Zunich KM, Harkonen WS, Woloski M, Kingsbury L. Intravenous anti-D immunoglobulin for childhood acute immune thrombocytopenic purpura. Lancet. 1995;346:1363-1365.

79. Smith N. Intravenous anti-D immunoglobulin in the management of immune thrombocytopenic purpura. Curr Opin Hematol. 1996;3:498-503.

80. Meyer O, Kiesewetter H, Hermsen M, Salama A. Efficacy and safety of anti-D given by subcutaneous injection to patients with autoimmune thrombocytopenia. Eur J Haematol. 2004;73:71-72.

81. Imbach P, Kuhne T. Sequelae of treatment of ITP with anti-D (Rho) immunoglobulin. Lancet. 2000;356:447-448.

82. Gaines AR. Acute onset hemoglobinemia and/or hemoglobinuria and sequelae following Rh(0)(D) immune

globulin intravenous administration in immune thrombocytopenic purpura patients. Blood. 2000;95:2523-2529.

83. George JN, Kojouri K, Perdue JJ, Vesely SK. Management of patients with chronic, refractory idiopathic thrombocytopenic purpura. Semin Hematol. 2000;37:290-298.

84. Minkes RK, Lagzdins M, Langer JC. Laparoscopic versus open splenectomy in children. J Pediatr Surg. 2000;35:699-701.

85. Brunt LM, Langer JC, Quasebarth MA, Whitman ED. Comparative analysis of laparoscopic versus open splenectomy. Am J Surg. 1996;172:596-599.

86. Katkhouda N, Grant SW, Mavor E, et al. Predictors of response after laparoscopic splenectomy for immune thrombocytopenic purpura. Surg Endosc. 2001;15:484-488.

87. Coon WW. Splenectomy for idiopathic thrombocytopenic purpura. Surg Gynecol Obstet. 1987;164:225-229.

88. Brennan MF, Rappeport JM, Moloney WC, Wilson RE. Correlation between response to corticosteroids and splenectomy for adult idiopathic thrombocytopenic purpura. Am J Surg. 1975;129:490-492.

89. Mintz SJ, Petersen SR, Cheson B, et al. Splenectomy for immune thrombocytopenic purpura. Arch Surg. 1981;116:645-650.

90. Law C, Marcaccio M, Tam P, et al. High-dose intravenous immune globulin and the response to splenectomy in patients with idiopathic thrombocytopenic purpura. N Engl J Med. 1997;336:1494-1498.

91. DiFino SM, Lachant NA, Kirshner JJ, Gottlieb AJ. Adult idiopathic thrombocytopenic purpura. Clinical findings and response to therapy. Am J Med. 1980;69:430-442.

92. Lortan JE. Management of asplenic patients. Br J Haematol. 1993;84:566-569.

93. Davies JM, Barnes R, Milligan D. Update of guidelines for the prevention and treatment of infection in patients with an absent or dysfunctional spleen. Clin Med. 2002;2:440-443.

94. Kaplinsky C, Spirer Z. Post-splenectomy antibiotic prophylaxis–unfinished story: to treat or not to treat? Pediatr Blood Cancer. 2006;47:740-741.

95. Lukert BP, Raisz LG. Glucocorticoid-induced osteoporosis: pathogenesis and management. Ann Intern Med. 1990;112:352-364.

96. Andersen JC. Response of resistant idiopathic thrombocytopenic purpura to pulsed high-dose dexamethasone therapy. N Engl J Med. 1994;330:1560-1564.

97. Chen JS, Wu JM, Chen YJ, Yeh TF. Pulsed high-dose dexamethasone therapy in children with chronic idiopathic thrombocytopenic purpura. J Pediatr Hematol Oncol. 1997;19:526-529.

98. Borgna-Pignatti C, Rugolotto S, Nobili B, et al. A trial of high-dose dexamethasone therapy for chronic idiopathic thrombocytopenic purpura in childhood. J Pediatr. 1997;130:13-16.

99. Demiroglu H, Dundar S. High-dose pulsed dexamethasone for immune thrombocytopenia. N Engl J Med. 1997;337:425-427.

100. Hollenberg JP, Subak LL, Ferry JJ Jr, Bussel JB. Cost-effectiveness of splenectomy versus intravenous gamma globulin in treatment of chronic immune thrombocytopenic purpura in childhood. J Pediatr. 1988;112:530-539.

101. Bussel JB, Kimberly RP, Inman RD, et al. Intravenous gammaglobulin treatment of chronic idiopathic thrombocytopenic purpura. Blood. 1983;62:480-486.

102. Becker T, Kuenzlen E, Salama A, et al. Treatment of childhood idiopathic thrombocytopenic purpura with Rhesus antibodies (anti-D). Eur J Pediatr. 1986;145:166-169.

103. Andrew M, Blanchette VS, Adams M, et al. A multicenter study of the treatment of childhood chronic idiopathic thrombocytopenic purpura with anti-D. J Pediatr. 1992;120:522-527.

104. Andersson PO, Wadenvik H. Chronic idiopathic thrombocytopenic purpura (ITP): molecular mechanisms and implications for therapy. Expert Rev Mol Med. 2004;6:1-17.

105. Bennett CM, Rogers ZR, Kinnamon DD, et al. Prospective phase 1/2 study of rituximab in childhood and adolescent chronic immune thrombocytopenic purpura. Blood. 2006;107:2639-2642.

106. Stasi R, Pagano A, Stipa E, Amadori S. Rituximab chimeric anti-CD20 monoclonal antibody treatment for adults with chronic idiopathic thrombocytopenic purpura. Blood. 2001;98:952-957.

107. Stasi R, Stipa E, Forte V, et al. Variable patterns of response to rituximab treatment in adults with chronic idiopathic thrombocytopenic purpura. Blood. 2002;99:3872-3873.

108. Cooper N, Stasi R, Cunningham-Rundles S, et al. The efficacy and safety of B-cell depletion with anti-CD20 monoclonal antibody in adults with chronic immune thrombocytopenic purpura. Br J Haematol. 2004;125:232-239.

109. Parodi E, Nobili B, Perrotta S, et al. Rituximab (anti-CD20 monoclonal antibody) in children with chronic refractory symptomatic immune thrombocytopenic purpura: efficacy and safety of treatment. Int J Hematol. 2006;84:48-53.

110. Wang J, Wiley JM, Luddy R, et al. Chronic immune thrombocytopenic purpura in children: assessment of rituximab treatment. J Pediatr. 2005;146:217-221.

111. Willis F, Marsh JC, Bevan DH, et al. The effect of treatment with Campath-1H in patients with autoimmune cytopenias. Br J Haematol. 2001;114:891-898.

112. George JN. Treatment options for chronic idiopathic (immune) thrombocytopenic purpura. Semin Hematol. 2000;37:31-34.

113. Imbach P. Refractory idiopathic immune thrombocytopenic purpura in children: current and future treatment options. Paediatr Drugs. 2003;5:795-801.

114. Bouroncle BA, Doan CA. Refractory idiopathic thrombocytopenic purpura treated with azathioprine. N Engl J Med. 1966;275:630-635.

115. Pizzuto J, Ambriz R. Therapeutic experience on 934 adults with idiopathic thrombocytopenic purpura: Multicentric Trial of the Cooperative Latin American group on Hemostasis and Thrombosis. Blood. 1984;64:1179-1183.

116. Emilia G, Messora C, Longo G, Bertesi M. Long-term salvage treatment by cyclosporin in refractory autoimmune haematological disorders. Br J Haematol. 1996;93:341-344.

117. Hou M, Peng J, Shi Y, et al. Mycophenolate mofetil (MMF) for the treatment of steroid-resistant idiopathic thrombocytopenic purpura. Eur J Haematol. 2003;70:353-357.

118. Provan D, Moss AJ, Newland AC, Bussel JB. Efficacy of mycophenolate mofetil as single-agent therapy for refractory immune thrombocytopenic purpura. Am J Hematol. 2006;81:19-25.

119. Ahn YS, Harrington WJ, Mylvaganam R, et al. Slow infusion of vinca alkaloids in the treatment of idiopathic thrombocytopenic purpura. Ann Intern Med. 1984;100: 192-196.

120. Schreiber AD, Chien P, Tomaski A, Cines DB. Effect of danazol in immune thrombocytopenic purpura. N Engl J Med. 1987;316:503-508.

121. Ahn YS, Mylvaganam R, Garcia RO, et al. Low-dose danazol therapy in idiopathic thrombocytopenic purpura. Ann Intern Med. 1987;107:177-181.

122. Proctor SJ, Jackson G, Carey P, et al. Improvement of platelet counts in steroid-unresponsive idiopathic immune thrombocytopenic purpura after short-course therapy with recombinant alpha 2b interferon. Blood. 1989;74: 1894-1897.

123. Donato H, Kohan R, Picon A, et al. Alpha-interferon therapy induces improvement of platelet counts in children with chronic idiopathic thrombocytopenic purpura. J Pediatr Hematol Oncol. 2001;23:598-603.

124. Figueroa M, Gehlsen J, Hammond D, et al. Combination chemotherapy in refractory immune thrombocytopenic purpura. N Engl J Med. 1993;328:1226-1229.

125. McMillan R. Long-term outcomes after treatment for refractory immune thrombocytopenic purpura. N Engl J Med. 2001;344:1402-1403.

126. Nichol JL. AMG 531: an investigational thrombopoiesis-stimulating peptibody. Pediatr Blood Cancer. 2006;47:723-725.

127. Bussel JB, Kuter DJ, George JN, et al. AMG 531, a thrombopoiesis-stimulating protein, for chronic ITP. N Engl J Med. 2006;355:1672-1681.

128. Barnes C, Blanchette V, Canning P, Carcao M. Recombinant FVIIa in the management of intracerebral haemorrhage in severe thrombocytopenia unresponsive to platelet-enhancing treatment. Transfus Med. 2005;15: 145-150.

129. Puapong D, Terasaki K, Lacerna M, Applebaum H. Splenic artery embolization in the management of an acute immune thrombocytopenic purpura–related intracranial hemorrhage. J Pediatr Surg. 2005;40:869-871.

130. Woerner SJ, Abildgaard CF, French BN. Intracranial hemorrhage in children with idiopathic thrombocytopenic purpura. Pediatrics. 1981;67:453-460.

131. Lightsey AL Jr, McMillan R, Koenig HM. Childhood idiopathic thrombocytopenic purpura. Aggressive management of life-threatening complications. JAMA. 1975; 232:734-736.

132. Rao VK, Straus SE. Causes and consequences of the autoimmune lymphoproliferative syndrome. Hematology. 2006;11:15-23.

133. Van Der Werff Ten Bosch J, Otten J, Thielemans K. Autoimmune lymphoproliferative syndrome type III: an indefinite disorder. Leuk Lymphoma. 2001;41:55-65.

134. Shenoy S, Mohanakumar T, Chatila T, et al. Defective apoptosis in lymphocytes and the role of IL-2 in autoimmune hematologic cytopenias. Clin Immunol. 2001;99: 246-255.

135. Dianzani U, Bragardo M, DiFranco D, et al. Deficiency of the Fas apoptosis pathway without Fas gene mutations in pediatric patients with autoimmunity/lymphoproliferation. Blood. 1997;89:2871-2879.

136. Mestanza-Peralta M, Ariza-Ariza R, Cardiel MH, Alcocer-Varela J. Thrombocytopenic purpura as initial manifestation of systemic lupus erythematosus. J Rheumatol. 1997; 24:867-870.

137. Kurata Y, Hayashi S, Kosugi S, et al. Elevated platelet-associated IgG in SLE patients due to anti-platelet autoantibody: differentiation between autoantibodies and immune complexes by ether elution. Br J Haematol. 1993;85:723-728.

138. Alarcon-Segovia D, Deleze M, Oria CV, et al. Antiphospholipid antibodies and the antiphospholipid syndrome in systemic lupus erythematosus. A prospective analysis of 500 consecutive patients. Medicine (Baltimore). 1989;68: 353-365.

139. Rauch J, Meng QH, Tannenbaum H. Lupus anticoagulant and antiplatelet properties of human hybridoma autoantibodies. J Immunol. 1987;139:2598-2604.

140. Jacobs P, Wood L, Dent DM. Splenectomy and the thrombocytopenia of systemic lupus erythematosus. Ann Intern Med. 1986;105:971-972.

141. Hall S, McCormick JL Jr, Greipp PR, et al. Splenectomy does not cure the thrombocytopenia of systemic lupus erythematosus. Ann Intern Med. 1985;102:325-328.

142. Godeau B, Piette JC, Fromont P, et al. Specific antiplatelet glycoprotein autoantibodies are associated with the thrombocytopenia of primary antiphospholipid syndrome. Br J Haematol. 1997;98:873-879.

143. Martinuzzo ME, Maclouf J, Carreras LO, Levy-Toledano S. Antiphospholipid antibodies enhance thrombin-induced platelet activation and thromboxane formation. Thromb Haemost. 1993;70:667-671.

144. Norton A, Roberts I. Management of Evans syndrome. Br J Haematol. 2006;132:125-137.

145. Lin SJ, Jaing TH. Thrombocytopenia in systemic-onset juvenile chronic arthritis: report of two cases with unusual bone marrow features. Clin Rheumatol. 1999;18: 241-243.

146. Chintu C, McClure P. Idiopathic thrombocytopenic purpura in two children with Graves disease. Am J Dis Child. 1975;129:101-102.

147. Jansen PH, Renier WO, de Vaan G, et al. Effect of thymectomy on myasthenia gravis and autoimmune thrombocytopenic purpura in a 13-year-old girl. Eur J Pediatr. 1987;146:587-589.

148. Zlatanic J, Korelitz BI, Wisch N, et al. Inflammatory bowel disease and immune thrombocytopenic purpura: is there a correlation? Am J Gastroenterol. 1997;92:2285-2288.

149. Xiros N, Binder T, Anger B, et al. Idiopathic thrombocytopenic purpura and autoimmune hemolytic anemia in Hodgkin's disease. Eur J Haematol. 1988;40:437-441.

150. Rao S, Pang EJ. Idiopathic thrombocytopenic purpura in acute lymphoblastic leukemia. J Pediatr. 1979;94:408-409.

151. Nardi M, Karpatkin S. Antiidiotype antibody against platelet anti-GPIIIa contributes to the regulation of thrombocytopenia in HIV-1–ITP patients. J Exp Med. 2000;191:2093-2100.

152. Ballem PJ, Belzberg A, Devine DV, et al. Kinetic studies of the mechanism of thrombocytopenia in patients with

human immunodeficiency virus infection. N Engl J Med. 1992;327:1779-1784.

153. Peltier JY, Lambin P, Doinel C, et al. Frequency and prognostic importance of thrombocytopenia in symptom-free HIV-infected individuals: a 5-year prospective study. AIDS 1991;5:381-384.

154. Valentin N, Newman PJ. Human platelet alloantigens. Curr Opin Hematol. 1994;1:381-387.

155. Newman PJ, Valentin N. Human platelet alloantigens: recent findings, new perspectives. Thromb Haemost. 1995;74:234-239.

156. Blanchette VS, Kühne T, Hume H, Hellmann J. Platelet transfusion therapy in newborn infants. Transfus Med Rev. 1995;9:215-230.

157. Davoren A, Curtis BR, Aster RH, McFarland JG. Human platelet antigen–specific alloantibodies implicated in 1162 cases of neonatal alloimmune thrombocytopenia. Transfusion. 2004;44:1220-1225.

158. Blanchette VS, Johnson J, Rand M. The management of alloimmune neonatal thrombocytopenia. Baillieres Best Pract Res Clin Haematol. 2000;13:365-390.

159. Seo DH, Park SS, Kim DW, et al. Gene frequencies of eight human platelet-specific antigens in Koreans. Transfus Med. 1998;8:129-132.

160. Chow MP, Sun KJ, Yung CH, et al. Neonatal alloimmune thrombocytopenia due to HLA-A2 antibody. Acta Haematol. 1992;87:153-155.

161. Bussel JB, Skupski DW, MacFarland JG. Fetal alloimmune thrombocytopenia: consensus and controversy. J Matern Fetal Med. 1996;5:281-292.

162. Bussel JB. Immune thrombocytopenia in pregnancy: autoimmune and alloimmune. J Reprod Immunol. 1997; 37:35-61.

163. Radder CM, Brand A, Kanhai HH. Will it ever be possible to balance the risk of intracranial haemorrhage in fetal or neonatal alloimmune thrombocytopenia against the risk of treatment strategies to prevent it? Vox Sang. 2003; 84:318-325.

164. Letsky EA, Greaves M. Guidelines on the investigation and management of thrombocytopenia in pregnancy and neonatal alloimmune thrombocytopenia. Maternal and Neonatal Haemostasis Working Party of the Haemostasis and Thrombosis Task Force of the British Society for Haematology. Br J Haematol. 1996;95:21-26.

165. Kiefel V, Bassler D, Kroll H, et al. Antigen-positive platelet transfusion in neonatal alloimmune thrombocytopenia (NAIT). Blood. 2006;107:3761-3763.

166. Ranasinghe E, Walton JD, Hurd CM, et al. Provision of platelet support for fetuses and neonates affected by severe fetomaternal alloimmune thrombocytopenia. Br J Haematol. 2001;113:40-42.

167. Bussel JB, Zabusky MR, Berkowitz RL, McFarland JG. Fetal alloimmune thrombocytopenia. N Engl J Med. 1997;337:22-26.

168. Bussel JB, Berkowitz RL, Lynch L, et al. Antenatal management of alloimmune thrombocytopenia with intravenous gamma-globulin: a randomized trial of the addition of low-dose steroid to intravenous gamma-globulin. Am J Obstet Gynecol. 1996;174:1414-1423.

169. Thung SF, Grobman WA. The cost effectiveness of empiric intravenous immunoglobulin for the antepartum treatment of fetal and neonatal alloimmune thrombocytopenia. Am J Obstet Gynecol. 2005;193:1094-1099.

170. Crowther MA, Burrows RF, Ginsberg J, Kelton JG. Thrombocytopenia in pregnancy: diagnosis, pathogenesis and management. Blood Rev. 1996;10:8-16.

171. Burrows RF, Kelton JG. Incidentally detected thrombocytopenia in healthy mothers and their infants. N Engl J Med. 1988;319:142-145.

172. Ballin A, Andrew M, Ling E, et al. High-dose intravenous gammaglobulin therapy for neonatal autoimmune thrombocytopenia. J Pediatr. 1988;112:789-792.

173. Kickler TS, Ness PM, Herman JH, Bell WR. Studies on the pathophysiology of posttransfusion purpura. Blood. 1986;68:347-350.

174. Becker T, Panzer S, Maas D, et al. High-dose intravenous immunoglobulin for post-transfusion purpura. Br J Haematol. 1985;61:149-155.

175. Warkentin TE, Smith JW, Hayward CP, et al. Thrombocytopenia caused by passive transfusion of anti-glycoprotein Ia/IIa alloantibody (anti–HPA-5b). Blood. 1992;79: 2480-2484.

176. Marzich C, Strohm PL, Ayas M, Cochran RK. Neonatal thrombocytopenia caused by passive transfer of anti-PLA1 antibody by blood transfusion. J Pediatr. 1996;128: 137-139.

177. Aster RH. Drug-induced immune thrombocytopenia: an overview of pathogenesis. Semin Hematol. 1999;36:2-6.

178. Aster RH. Can drugs cause autoimmune thrombocytopenic purpura? Semin Hematol. 2000;37:229-238.

179. Salamon DJ, Nusbacher J, Stroupe T, et al. Red cell and platelet-bound IgG penicillin antibodies in a patient with thrombocytopenia. Transfusion. 1984;24:395-398.

180. Visentin GP, Newman PJ, Aster RH. Characteristics of quinine- and quinidine-induced antibodies specific for platelet glycoproteins IIb and IIIa. Blood. 1991;77:2668-2676.

181. Chong BH, Du XP, Berndt MC, et al. Characterization of the binding domains on platelet glycoproteins Ib-IX and IIb/IIIa complexes for the quinine/quinidine-dependent antibodies. Blood. 1991;77:2190-2199.

182. Lopez JA, Li CQ, Weisman S, Chambers M. The glycoprotein Ib-IX complex–specific monoclonal antibody SZ1 binds to a conformation-sensitive epitope on glycoprotein IX: implications for the target antigen of quinine/quinidine-dependent autoantibodies. Blood. 1995;85: 1254-1258.

183. Bougie DW, Wilker PR, Aster RH. Patients with quinine-induced immune thrombocytopenia have both "drug-dependent" and "drug-specific" antibodies. Blood. 2006; 108:922-927.

184. Zuffa E, Vianelli N, Martinelli G, et al. Autoimmune mediated thrombocytopenia associated with the use of interferon-alpha in chronic myeloid leukemia. Haematologica. 1996;81:533-535.

185. Chute JP, Frame JN, Ganey JT, et al. Intravenous immunoglobulin followed by platelet transfusion in the acute treatment of trimethoprim/sulfamethoxazole-induced immune thrombocytopenia. Am J Hematol. 1993;43:329-330.

186. Risch L, Huber AR, Schmugge M. Diagnosis and treatment of heparin-induced thrombocytopenia in neonates and children. Thromb Res. 2006;118:123-135.

187. Girolami B, Girolami A. Heparin-induced thrombocytopenia: a review. Semin Thromb Hemost. 2006;32:803-809.

188. Kelton JG. The clinical management of heparin-induced thrombocytopenia. Semin Hematol. 1999;36:17-21.

189. Amiral J. Antigens involved in heparin-induced thrombocytopenia. Semin Hematol. 1999;36:7-11.

190. Greinacher A, Potzsch B, Amiral J, et al. Heparin-associated thrombocytopenia: isolation of the antibody and characterization of a multimolecular PF4-heparin complex as the major antigen. Thromb Haemost. 1994;71:247-251.

191. Warkentin TE, Hayward CP, Boshkov LK, et al. Sera from patients with heparin-induced thrombocytopenia generate platelet-derived microparticles with procoagulant activity: an explanation for the thrombotic complications of heparin-induced thrombocytopenia. Blood. 1994;84:3691-3699.

192. Visentin GP, Ford SE, Scott JP, Aster RH. Antibodies from patients with heparin-induced thrombocytopenia/thrombosis are specific for platelet factor 4 complexed with heparin or bound to endothelial cells. J Clin Invest. 1994;93:81-88.

193. Visentin GP, Malik M, Cyganiak KA, Aster RH. Patients treated with unfractionated heparin during open heart surgery are at high risk to form antibodies reactive with heparin:platelet factor 4 complexes. J Lab Clin Med. 1996;128:376-383.

194. Lo GK, Juhl D, Warkentin TE, et al. Evaluation of pretest clinical score (4 T's) for the diagnosis of heparin-induced thrombocytopenia in two clinical settings. J Thromb Haemost. 2006;4:759-765.

195. Arepally G, Reynolds C, Tomaski A, et al. Comparison of PF4/heparin ELISA assay with the ^{14}C-serotonin release assay in the diagnosis of heparin-induced thrombocytopenia. Am J Clin Pathol. 1995;104:648-654.

196. Warkentin TE, Elavathil LJ, Hayward CP, et al. The pathogenesis of venous limb gangrene associated with heparin-induced thrombocytopenia. Ann Intern Med. 1997;127:804-812.

197. Warkentin TE, Levine MN, Hirsh J, et al. Heparin-induced thrombocytopenia in patients treated with low-molecular-weight heparin or unfractionated heparin. N Engl J Med. 1995;332:1330-1335.

198. Acostamadiedo JM, Iyer UG, Owen J. Danaparoid sodium. Expert Opin Pharmacother 2000;1:803-814.

199. Greinacher A, Lubenow N. Recombinant hirudin in clinical practice: focus on lepirudin. Circulation. 2001;103:1479-1484.

200. Argatroban for treatment of heparin-induced thrombocytopenia. Med Lett Drugs Ther. 2001;43:11-12.

201. Efird LE, Kockler DR. Fondaparinux for thromboembolic treatment and prophylaxis of heparin-induced thrombocytopenia. Ann Pharmacother. 2006;40:1383-1387.

202. George JN. How I treat patients with thrombotic thrombocytopenic purpura–hemolytic uremic syndrome. Blood. 2000;96:1223-1229.

203. Moake JL, Chow TW. Thrombotic thrombocytopenic purpura: understanding a disease no longer rare. Am J Med Sci. 1998;316:105-119.

204. Moake JL. Moschcowitz, multimers, and metalloprotease. N Engl J Med. 1998;339:1629-1631.

205. Baker KR, Moake JL. Thrombotic thrombocytopenic purpura and the hemolytic-uremic syndrome. Curr Opin Pediatr. 2000;12:23-28.

206. Asada Y, Sumiyoshi A. [Histopathology of thrombotic thrombocytopenic purpura.] Nippon Rinsho. 1993;51:159-162.

207. Asada Y, Sumiyoshi A, Hayashi T, et al. Immunohistochemistry of vascular lesion in thrombotic thrombocytopenic purpura, with special reference to factor VIII related antigen. Thromb Res. 1985;38:469-479.

208. Moake JL, Rudy CK, Troll JH, et al. Unusually large plasma factor VIII:von Willebrand factor multimers in chronic relapsing thrombotic thrombocytopenic purpura. N Engl J Med. 1982;307:1432-1435.

209. Moake JL, Chow TW. Thrombotic thrombocytopenic purpura: understanding a disease no longer rare. Am J Med Sci. 1998;316:105-119.

210. Moake JL, Turner NA, Stathopoulos NA, et al. Involvement of large plasma von Willebrand factor (vWF) multimers and unusually large vWF forms derived from endothelial cells in shear stress–induced platelet aggregation. J Clin Invest. 1986;78:1456-1461.

211. Moake JL, Turner NA, Stathopoulos NA, et al. Shear-induced platelet aggregation can be mediated by vWF released from platelets, as well as by exogenous large or unusually large vWF multimers, requires adenosine diphosphate, and is resistant to aspirin. Blood. 1988;71:1366-1374.

212. Gerritsen HE, Robles R, Lammle B, Furlan M. Partial amino acid sequence of purified von Willebrand factor–cleaving protease. Blood. 2001;98:1654-1661.

213. Fujikawa K, Suzuki H, McMullen B, Chung D. Purification of human von Willebrand factor–cleaving protease and its identification as a new member of the metalloproteinase family. Blood. 2001;98:1662-1666.

214. Zheng X, Majerus EM, Sadler JE. ADAMTS13 and TTP. Curr Opin Hematol. 2002;9:389-394.

215. Furlan M, Lammle B. Deficiency of von Willebrand factor–cleaving protease in familial and acquired thrombotic thrombocytopenic purpura. Baillieres Clin Haematol. 1998;11:509-514.

216. Barbot J, Costa E, Guerra M, et al. Ten years of prophylactic treatment with fresh-frozen plasma in a child with chronic relapsing thrombotic thrombocytopenic purpura as a result of a congenital deficiency of von Willebrand factor–cleaving protease. Br J Haematol. 2001;113:649-651.

217. te Loo DM, Levtchenko E, Furlan M, et al. Autosomal recessive inheritance of von Willebrand factor–cleaving protease deficiency. Pediatr Nephrol. 2000;14:762-765.

218. Levy GG, Nichols WC, Lian EC, et al. Mutations in a member of the ADAMTS gene family cause thrombotic thrombocytopenic purpura. Nature. 2001;413:488-494.

219. Schneppenheim R, Budde U, Oyen F, et al. von Willebrand factor cleaving protease and ADAMTS13 mutations in childhood TTP. Blood. 2003;101:1845-1850.

220. Tsai HM, Lian EC. Antibodies to von Willebrand factor-cleaving protease in acute thrombotic thrombocytopenic purpura. N Engl J Med. 1998;339:1585-1594.

221. Furlan M, Robles R, Solenthaler M, Lammle B. Acquired deficiency of von Willebrand factor–cleaving protease in a patient with thrombotic thrombocytopenic purpura. Blood. 1998;91:2839-2846.

222. Kwaan HC. Clinicopathologic features of thrombotic thrombocytopenic purpura. Semin Hematol. 1987;24:71-81.

223. Petitt RM. Thrombotic thrombocytopenic purpura: a thirty year review. Semin Thromb Hemost. 1980;6:350-355.

224. Clark WF, Rock GA, Buskard N, et al. Therapeutic plasma exchange: an update from the Canadian Apheresis Group. Ann Intern Med. 1999;131:453-462.

225. Satoh K, Takahashi H, Nagai K, Shibata A. Thrombotic thrombocytopenic purpura and herpes zoster infection. Ann Intern Med. 1988;108:154-155.

226. Leaf AN, Laubenstein LJ, Raphael B, et al. Thrombotic thrombocytopenic purpura associated with human immunodeficiency virus type 1 (HIV-1) infection. Ann Intern Med. 1988;109:194-197.

227. Weiner CP. Thrombotic microangiopathy in pregnancy and the postpartum period. Semin Hematol. 1987;24:119-129.

228. Brunner HI, Freedman M, Silverman ED. Close relationship between systemic lupus erythematosus and thrombotic thrombocytopenic purpura in childhood. Arthritis Rheum. 1999;42:2346-2355.

229. Vergara M, Modolell I, Puig-Divi V, et al. Acute pancreatitis as a triggering factor for thrombotic thrombocytopenic purpura. Am J Gastroenterol. 1998;93:2215-2218.

230. Moake JL, Byrnes JJ. Thrombotic microangiopathies associated with drugs and bone marrow transplantation. Hematol Oncol Clin North Am. 1996;10:485-497.

231. Tsai HM, Rice L, Sarode R, et al. Antibody inhibitors to von Willebrand factor metalloproteinase and increased binding of von Willebrand factor to platelets in ticlopidine-associated thrombotic thrombocytopenic purpura. Ann Intern Med. 2000;132:794-799.

232. Fava S, Galizia AC. Thrombotic thrombocytopenic purpura–like syndrome in the absence of schistocytes. Br J Haematol. 1995;89:643-644.

233. Vesely SK, George JN, Lammle B, et al. ADAMTS13 activity in thrombotic thrombocytopenic purpura–hemolytic uremic syndrome: relation to presenting features and clinical outcomes in a prospective cohort of 142 patients. Blood. 2003;102:60-68.

234. Zheng XL, Kaufman RM, Goodnough LT, Sadler JE. Effect of plasma exchange on plasma ADAMTS13 metalloprotease activity, inhibitor level, and clinical outcome in patients with idiopathic and nonidiopathic thrombotic thrombocytopenic purpura. Blood. 2004;103:4043-4049.

235. Coppo P, Wolf M, Veyradier A, et al. Prognostic value of inhibitory anti-ADAMTS13 antibodies in adult-acquired thrombotic thrombocytopenic purpura. Br J Haematol. 2006;132:66-74.

236. Ferrari S, Scheiflinger F, Rieger M, et al. Prognostic value of anti-ADAMTS13 antibodies features (Ig isotype, titer and inhibitory effect) in a cohort of 35 adult French patients undergoing a first episode of thrombotic microangiopathy with an undetectable ADAMTS13 activity. Blood. 2007;109:2815-2822.

237. Rock GA, Shumak KH, Buskard NA, et al. Comparison of plasma exchange with plasma infusion in the treatment of thrombotic thrombocytopenic purpura. Canadian Apheresis Study Group. N Engl J Med. 1991;325:393-397.

238. Zeigler ZR, Shadduck RK, Gryn JF, et al. Cryoprecipitate poor plasma does not improve early response in primary adult thrombotic thrombocytopenic purpura (TTP). J Clin Apheresis. 2001;16:19-22.

239. Yomtovian R, Niklinski W, Silver B, et al. Rituximab for chronic recurring thrombotic thrombocytopenic purpura: a case report and review of the literature. Br J Haematol. 2004;124:787-795.

240. Fakhouri F, Vernant JP, Veyradier A, et al. Efficiency of curative and prophylactic treatment with rituximab in ADAMTS13-deficient thrombotic thrombocytopenic purpura: a study of 11 cases. Blood. 2005;106:1932-1937.

241. George JN, Woodson RD, Kiss JE, et al. Rituximab therapy for thrombotic thrombocytopenic purpura: a proposed study of the Transfusion Medicine/Hemostasis Clinical Trials Network with a systematic review of rituximab therapy for immune-mediated disorders. J Clin Apheresis. 2006;21:49-56.

242. Tarr PI, Neill MA, Allen J, et al. The increasing incidence of the hemolytic-uremic syndrome in King County, Washington: lack of evidence for ascertainment bias. Am J Epidemiol. 1989;129:582-586.

243. Karmali MA, Steele BT, Petric M, Lim C. Sporadic cases of haemolytic-uraemic syndrome associated with faecal cytotoxin and cytotoxin-producing *Escherichia coli* in stools. Lancet. 1983;1:619-620.

244. Nakao H, Takeda T. *Escherichia coli* Shiga toxin. J Nat Toxins. 2000;9:299-313.

245. Yu M, Haslam DB. Shiga toxin is transported from the endoplasmic reticulum following interaction with the luminal chaperone HEDJ/ERdj3. Infect Immun 2005;73:2524-2532.

246. Yoshida T, Fukada M, Koide N, et al. Primary cultures of human endothelial cells are susceptible to low doses of Shiga toxins and undergo apoptosis. J Infect Dis. 1999;180:2048-2052.

247. Morigi M, Galbusera M, Binda E, et al. Verotoxin-1–induced up-regulation of adhesive molecules renders microvascular endothelial cells thrombogenic at high shear stress. Blood. 2001;98:1828-1835.

248. Taguchi T, Uchida H, Kiyokawa N, et al. Verotoxins induce apoptosis in human renal tubular epithelium derived cells. Kidney Int. 1998;53:1681-1688.

249. Karpman D, Hakansson A, Perez MT, et al. Apoptosis of renal cortical cells in the hemolytic-uremic syndrome: in vivo and in vitro studies. Infect Immun. 1998;66:636-644.

250. Nataro JP, Kaper JB. Diarrheagenic *Escherichia coli*. Clin Microbiol Rev. 1998;11:142-201.

251. Dundas S, Todd WT. Clinical presentation, complications and treatment of infection with verocytotoxin-producing *Escherichia coli*. Challenges for the clinician. Symp Ser Soc Appl Microbiol. 2000;29:24S-30S.

252. Wong CS, Jelacic S, Habeeb RL, et al. The risk of the hemolytic-uremic syndrome after antibiotic treatment of *Escherichia coli* O157:H7 infections. N Engl J Med. 2000;342:1930-1936.

253. Bell BP, Griffin PM, Lozano P, et al. Predictors of hemolytic uremic syndrome in children during a large outbreak of *Escherichia coli* O157:H7 infections. Pediatrics. 1997;100:E12.

254. Tarr PI, Neill MA, Clausen CR, et al. *Escherichia coli* O157:H7 and the hemolytic uremic syndrome: impor-

tance of early cultures in establishing the etiology. J Infect Dis. 1990;162:553-556.

255. Tsai HM, Chandler WL, Sarode R, et al. von Willebrand factor and von Willebrand factor–cleaving metalloprotease activity in *Escherichia coli* O157:H7–associated hemolytic uremic syndrome. Pediatr Res. 2001;49:653-659.

256. Richardson SE, Karmali MA, Becker LE, Smith CR. The histopathology of the hemolytic uremic syndrome associated with verocytotoxin-producing *Escherichia coli* infections. Hum Pathol. 1988;19:1102-1108.

257. Ake JA, Jelacic S, Ciol MA, et al. Relative nephroprotection during *Escherichia coli* O157:H7 infections: association with intravenous volume expansion. Pediatrics. 2005;115:e673-e680.

258. Proulx F, Turgeon JP, Delage G, et al. Randomized, controlled trial of antibiotic therapy for *Escherichia coli* O157:H7 enteritis. J Pediatr. 1992;121:299-303.

259. Rizzoni G, Claris-Appiani A, Edefonti A, et al. Plasma infusion for hemolytic-uremic syndrome in children: results of a multicenter controlled trial. J Pediatr. 1988;112:284-290.

260. Loirat C, Sonsino E, Hinglais N, et al. Treatment of the childhood haemolytic uraemic syndrome with plasma. A multicentre randomized controlled trial. The French Society of Paediatric Nephrology. Pediatr Nephrol. 1988;2:279-285.

261. Van Dyck M, Proesmans W, Depraetere M. Hemolytic uremic syndrome in childhood: renal function ten years later. Clin Nephrol. 1988;29:109-112.

262. Kelles A, Van Dyck M, Proesmans W. Childhood haemolytic uraemic syndrome: long-term outcome and prognostic features. Eur J Pediatr. 1994;153:38-42.

263. Noris M, Ruggenenti P, Perna A, et al. Hypocomplementemia discloses genetic predisposition to hemolytic uremic syndrome and thrombotic thrombocytopenic purpura: role of factor H abnormalities. Italian Registry of Familial and Recurrent Hemolytic Uremic Syndrome/Thrombotic Thrombocytopenic Purpura. J Am Soc Nephrol. 1999;10:281-293.

264. Caprioli J, Noris M, Brioschi S, et al. Genetics of HUS: the impact of MCP, CFH, and IF mutations on clinical presentation, response to treatment, and outcome. Blood. 2006;108:1267-1279.

265. Tsai HM. The molecular biology of thrombotic microangiopathy. Kidney Int. 2006;70:16-23.

266. Liszewski MK, Leung MK, Schraml B, et al. Modeling how CD46 deficiency predisposes to atypical hemolytic uremic syndrome. Mol Immunol. 2007;44:1570-1579.

267. Huang DT, Chi H, Lee HC, et al. T-antigen activation for prediction of pneumococcus-induced hemolytic uremic syndrome and hemolytic anemia. Pediatr Infect Dis J. 2006;25:608-610.

268. Chand DH, Brady RC, Bissler JJ. Hemolytic uremic syndrome in an adolescent with *Fusobacterium necrophorum* bacteremia. Am J Kidney Dis. 2001;37:E22.

269. Warwicker P, Goodship TH, Donne RL, et al. Genetic studies into inherited and sporadic hemolytic uremic syndrome. Kidney Int. 1998;53:836-844.

270. Ohali M, Shalev H, Schlesinger M, et al. Hypocomplementemic autosomal recessive hemolytic uremic syndrome with decreased factor H. Pediatr Nephrol. 1998;12:619-624.

271. Rougier N, Kazatchkine MD, Rougier JP, et al. Human complement factor H deficiency associated with hemolytic uremic syndrome. J Am Soc Nephrol. 1998;9:2318-2326.

272. Mollnes TE, Kirschfink M. Strategies of therapeutic complement inhibition. Mol Immunol. 2006;43:107-121.

273. Schriber JR, Herzig GP. Transplantation-associated thrombotic thrombocytopenic purpura and hemolytic uremic syndrome. Semin Hematol. 1997;34:126-133.

274. George JN, Li X, McMinn JR, et al. Thrombotic thrombocytopenic purpura–hemolytic uremic syndrome following allogeneic HPC transplantation: a diagnostic dilemma. Transfusion. 2004;44:294-304.

275. Fuge R, Bird JM, Fraser A, et al. The clinical features, risk factors and outcome of thrombotic thrombocytopenic purpura occurring after bone marrow transplantation. Br J Haematol. 2001;113:58-64.

276. Jenson HB. Acute complications of Epstein-Barr virus infectious mononucleosis. Curr Opin Pediatr. 2000;12:263-268.

277. Conrad ME. Hematologic manifestations of parasitic infections. Semin Hematol. 1971;8:267-303.

278. Bick RL. Hemostasis defects associated with cardiac surgery, prosthetic devices, and other extracorporeal circuits. Semin Thromb Hemost. 1985;11:249-280.

279. Roberts IA, Murray NA. Neonatal thrombocytopenia: new insights into pathogenesis and implications for clinical management. Curr Opin Pediatr. 2001;13:16-21.

280. Gross S, Keefer V, Liebman J. The platelets in cyanotic congenital heart disease. Pediatrics. 1968;42:651-658.

281. Koenig JM, Christensen RD. Neutropenia and thrombocytopenia in infants with Rh hemolytic disease. J Pediatr. 1989;114:625-631.

282. Hall GW. Kasabach-Merritt syndrome: pathogenesis and management. Br J Haematol. 2001;112:851-862.

283. Shim WK. Hemangiomas of infancy complicated by thrombocytopenia. Am J Surg. 1968;116:896-906.

284. Enjolras O. Classification and management of the various superficial vascular anomalies: hemangiomas and vascular malformations. J Dermatol. 1997;24:701-710.

285. Enjolras O, Mulliken JB, Wassef M, et al. Residual lesions after Kasabach-Merritt phenomenon in 41 patients. J Am Acad Dermatol. 2000;42:225-235.

286. Enjolras O, Wassef M, Mazoyer E, et al. Infants with Kasabach-Merritt syndrome do not have "true" hemangiomas. J Pediatr. 1997;130:631-640.

287. el Dessouky M, Azmy AF, Raine PA, Young DG. Kasabach-Merritt syndrome. J Pediatr Surg. 1988;23:109-111.

288. Mitsuhashi N, Furuta M, Sakurai H, et al. Outcome of radiation therapy for patients with Kasabach-Merritt syndrome. Int J Radiat Oncol Biol Phys. 1997;39:467-473.

289. Ezekowitz RA, Mulliken JB, Folkman J. Interferon alfa-2a therapy for life-threatening hemangiomas of infancy. N Engl J Med. 1992;326:1456-1463.

290. Haisley-Royster C, Enjolras O, Frieden IJ, et al. Kasabach-Merritt phenomenon: a retrospective study of treatment with vincristine. J Pediatr Hematol Oncol. 2002;24:459-462.

291. Acharya S, Bussel JB. Hematologic toxicity of sodium valproate. J Pediatr Hematol Oncol. 2000;22:62-65.

292. Lopas H, Rabiner SF. Thrombocytopenia associated with iron deficiency anemia. A report of five cases. Clin Pediatr (Phila). 1966;5:609-616.

293. Devuyst O, Lambert M, Rodhain J, et al. Haematological changes and infectious complications in anorexia nervosa: a case-control study. Q J Med. 1993;86:791-799.

294. Dror Y, Blanchette VS. Essential thrombocythaemia in children. Br J Haematol. 1999;107:691-698.

295. Breslow A, Kaufman RM, Lawsky AR. The effect of surgery on the concentration of circulating megakaryocytes and platelets. Blood. 1968;32:393-401.

296. Hammerschmidt DE. Szechwan purpura. N Engl J Med. 1980;302:1191-1193.

297. Wang Z, Roberts JM, Grant PG, et al. The effect of a medicinal Chinese herb on platelet function. Thromb Haemost. 1982;48:301-306.

298. Kaneshiro MM, Mielke CH Jr, Kasper CK, Rapaport SI. Bleeding time after aspirin in disorders of intrinsic clotting. N Engl J Med. 1969;281:1039-1042.

299. Roth GJ, Stanford N, Majerus PW. Acetylation of prostaglandin synthase by aspirin. Proc Natl Acad Sci U S A. 1975;72:3073-3076.

300. Harker LA, Slichter SJ. The bleeding time as a screening test for evaluation of platelet function. N Engl J Med. 1972;287:155-159.

301. Stuart MJ, Gross SJ, Elrad H, Graeber JE. Effects of acetylsalicylic-acid ingestion on maternal and neonatal hemostasis. N Engl J Med. 1982;307:909-912.

302. McElroy FA, Philip RB. Relative potencies of dipyridamole and related agents as inhibitors of cyclic nucleotide phosphodiesterases: possible explanation of mechanism of inhibition of platelet function. Life Sci. 1975;17:1479-1493.

303. Pengo V, Boschello M, Marzari A, et al. Adenosine diphosphate (ADP)-induced alpha-granules release from platelets of native whole blood is reduced by ticlopidine but not by aspirin or dipyridamole. Thromb Haemost. 1986;56:147-150.

304. Bhatt DL, Chew DP, Hirsch AT, et al. Superiority of clopidogrel versus aspirin in patients with prior cardiac surgery. Circulation. 2001;103:363-368.

305. Bhatt DL, Hirsch AT, Ringleb PA, et al. Reduction in the need for hospitalization for recurrent ischemic events and bleeding with clopidogrel instead of aspirin. CAPRIE investigators. Am Heart J. 2000;140:67-73.

306. Easton JD. Clinical aspects of the use of clopidogrel, a new antiplatelet agent. Semin Thromb Hemost. 1999;25(Suppl 2):77-82.

307. Nguyen-Ho P, Lakkis NM. Platelet glycoprotein IIb/IIIa receptor antagonists and coronary artery disease. Curr Atheroscler Rep. 2001;3:139-148.

308. Bhatt DL, Topol EJ. Current role of platelet glycoprotein IIb/IIIa inhibitors in acute coronary syndromes. JAMA. 2000;284:1549-1558.

309. Johnsson H, Niklasson PM. Effects of some antibiotics of platelet function in vitro and in vivo. Thromb Res. 1977;11:237-251.

310. Brown CH III, Natelson EA, Bradshaw W, et al. The hemostatic defect produced by carbenicillin. N Engl J Med. 1974;291:265-270.

311. Shattil SJ, Bennett JS, McDonough M, Turnbull J. Carbenicillin and penicillin G inhibit platelet function in vitro

312. by impairing the interaction of agonists with the platelet surface. J Clin Invest. 1980;65:329-337.

312. Brown CH III, Bradshaw MJ, Natelson EA, et al. Defective platelet function following the administration of penicillin compounds. Blood. 1976;47:949-956.

313. Brown CH III, Natelson EA, Bradshaw MW, et al. Study of the effects of ticarcillin on blood coagulation and platelet function. Antimicrob Agents Chemother. 1975;7:652-657.

314. Barnathan ES, Addonizio VP, Shattil SJ. Interaction of verapamil with human platelet alpha-adrenergic receptors. Am J Physiol. 1982;242:H19-H23.

315. Jain MK, Eskow K, Kuchibhotla J, Colman RW. Correlation of inhibition of platelet aggregation by phenothiazines and local anesthetics with their effects on a phospholipid bilayer. Thromb Res. 1978;13:1067-1075.

316. Rudnick G, Bencuya R, Nelson PJ, Zito RA Jr. Inhibition of platelet serotonin transport by propranolol. Mol Pharmacol. 1981;20:118-123.

317. Qi R, Ozaki Y, Satoh K, et al. Sulphonylurea agents inhibit platelet aggregation and $[Ca^{2+}]i$ elevation induced by arachidonic acid. Biochem Pharmacol. 1995;49:1735-1739.

318. Stewart JH, Castaldi PA. Uraemic bleeding: a reversible platelet defect corrected by dialysis. Q J Med. 1967;36:409-423.

319. Remuzzi G, Benigni A, Dodesini P, et al. Reduced platelet thromboxane formation in uremia. Evidence for a functional cyclooxygenase defect. J Clin Invest. 1983;71:762-768.

320. Castaldi PA, Rozenberg MC, Stewart JH. The bleeding disorder of uraemia. A qualitative platelet defect. Lancet. 1966;2:66-69.

321. Vigano G, Benigni A, Mendogni D, et al. Recombinant human erythropoietin to correct uremic bleeding. Am J Kidney Dis. 1991;18:44-49.

322. Fabris F, Cordiano I, Randi ML, et al. Effect of human recombinant erythropoietin on bleeding time, platelet number and function in children with end-stage renal disease maintained by haemodialysis. Pediatr Nephrol. 1991;5:225-228.

323. Montini G, Zacchello G, Baraldi E, et al. Benefits and risks of anemia correction with recombinant human erythropoietin in children maintained by hemodialysis. J Pediatr. 1990;117:556-560.

324. Thomas DP, Ream VJ, Stuart RK. Platelet aggregation in patients with Laennec's cirrhosis of the liver. N Engl J Med. 1967;276:1344-1348.

325. Hillbom M, Muuronen A, Neiman J. Liver disease and platelet function in alcoholics. Br Med J (Clin Res Ed). 1987;295:581.

326. Ingeberg S, Jacobsen P, Fischer E, Bentsen KD. Platelet aggregation and release of ATP in patients with hepatic cirrhosis. Scand J Gastroenterol. 1985;20:285-288.

327. Krauss JS, Jonah MH. Platelet dysfunction (thrombocytopathy) in extrahepatic biliary obstruction. South Med J. 1982;75:506-507.

328. Andreoli SP. Chronic glomerulonephritis in childhood. Membranoproliferative glomerulonephritis, Henoch-Schönlein purpura nephritis, and IgA nephropathy. Pediatr Clin North Am. 1995;42:1487-1503.

329. Al Sheyyab M, El Shanti H, Ajlouni S, et al. The clinical spectrum of Henoch-Schönlein purpura in infants and young children. Eur J Pediatr. 1995;154:969-972.

330. Mitsuhashi H, Mitsuhashi M, Tsukada Y, et al. Henoch-Schönlein purpura in rheumatoid arthritis. J Rheumatol. 1994;21:1138-1140.

331. Saulsbury FT. Corticosteroid therapy does not prevent nephritis in Henoch-Schönlein purpura. Pediatr Nephrol. 1993;7:69-71.

332. Rosenblum ND, Winter HS. Steroid effects on the course of abdominal pain in children with Henoch-Schönlein purpura. Pediatrics. 1987;79:1018-1021.

34 Acquired Disorders of Hemostasis

Steven W. Pipe and Neil A. Goldenberg

The application of clinical skills forms the cornerstone for assessment of a potential bleeding disorder. After confirming that a bleeding disorder is present through a comprehensive medical history and physical examination, the clinician should next address whether the condition is probably familial or acquired, which is sometimes difficult because some patients with mild underlying heritable hemostatic defects (e.g., mild von Willebrand's disease or platelet function defects) may not demonstrate suspicious clinical symptoms until faced with a traumatic injury or a surgical challenge at a later age. Nevertheless, acquired bleeding disorders remain a frequent clinical scenario with findings varying between acute unexpected bleeding during or immediately after surgery to unusual or excessive clinical manifestations of bruising, petechiae, epistaxis, gum bleeding, or hematoma formation that occur over a period of weeks to months. Distinguishing whether the bleeding most likely represents an abnormality in primary hemostasis, fibrin formation, or fibrinolysis provides a framework for the generation of a differential diagnosis (see Chapter 28). For example, petechiae are seen almost exclusively with defects in platelet number or function, whereas deep tissue hematomas are more likely to be associated with defects in fibrin formation, as would occur with clotting factor deficiencies. Standard laboratory screening tests such as the prothrombin time (PT) and activated partial thromboplastin time (APTT) are most often used in the initial evaluation but are insensitive to mild but clinically significant reductions in hemostatic capacity.[1] In addition, a platelet count does not provide any assessment of platelet function. Therefore, the clinician must rely on the history and physical findings to guide the extent of additional coagulation studies. The most common causes of acquired hemorrhagic disorders include drug-induced bleeding (e.g., anticoagulants), disseminated intravascular coagulation (DIC), liver disease, vitamin K (VK) deficiency, massive transfusion, renal disease, and rarely, acquired inhibitors to coagulation proteins.

ACQUIRED HEMORRHAGIC DISORDERS

Drug-Induced Bleeding

Many drugs have been associated with abnormal platelet function, although not all result in bleeding manifestations. The major classes include anti-inflammatory agents, antibiotics, cardiovascular drugs, psychotropic drugs, anticonvulsants, and anticoagulants. Aspirin is the most common example; it acts by irreversibly acetylating a serine residue at the active site of cyclooxygenase,[2] whereas other nonsteroidal anti-inflammatories (e.g., ibuprofen, naproxen) are reversible inhibitors.[3] β-Lactam antibiotics can interfere with platelet function through binding to the platelet membrane.[4,5] Calcium channel blockers, such as nifedipine,[6] and tricyclic antidepressants, such as amytriptyline,[7] can give rise to decreased

platelet aggregation responses but are unlikely to result in clinical bleeding. Valproic acid has become one of the most commonly used anticonvulsants in children. Interestingly, several mechanisms of relevant valproate-induced coagulopathy have been described, including thrombocytopenia and platelet dysfunction, acquired von Willebrand's disease, decreased VK-dependent clotting factors, hypofibrinogenemia, and decreased factor XIII levels.[8] Therapeutic anticoagulants (heparin, low-molecular-weight-heparin [LMWH], warfarin) should be the most readily apparent cause of drug-induced bleeding and in most patients can be correlated with laboratory monitoring. Platelet receptor antagonists (IIb/IIIa inhibitors, e.g., abciximab, eptifibatide, tirofiban; adenosine diphosphate receptor antagonists, e.g., clopidogrel) are increasingly being used in patients with congenital heart disease and those undergoing interventional studies.[9]

In most cases, discontinuation of the offending drug should resolve the hemorrhagic manifestations, but resolution will depend on the reversibility and half-life of the drug. Administration of VK will in most cases rapidly reverse warfarin-induced bleeding. Alternatively, fresh frozen plasma (FFP) can be used to replace VK-dependent clotting factors rapidly. Recently, recombinant factor VIIa (rVIIa) has proved effective at rapidly reversing warfarin-induced coagulopathy.[10] Transfusions of fresh platelets are indicated in patients with life-threatening or unremitting bleeding as a result of drug-induced platelet dysfunction. In cases of minor bleeding in which the drug cannot readily be discontinued (e.g., anticonvulsants), desmopressin has been used with some success.[11]

Disseminated Intravascular Coagulation

DIC is a pathologic syndrome in which the normal physiology of coagulation is disturbed by the simultaneous action of four mechanisms: increased thrombin generation, suppressed physiologic anticoagulant pathways, activation and subsequent impairment of fibrinolysis, and activation of the inflammatory pathway.[12] It leads to widespread intravascular deposition of fibrin with resultant thrombotic end-organ complications and consumption of platelets and coagulation proteins, all of which combine to result in severe bleeding. Associated damage to the microvasculature can contribute to organ dysfunction, capillary leak, and shock.

Etiology

DIC is always a secondary phenomenon and not a disease entity in its own right. Thus, recognition of it should prompt the clinician to identify and treat the underlying cause rather than merely react to the bleeding manifestations. It most frequently occurs in the settings of sepsis, trauma, and systemic inflammatory syndrome at an approximate frequency of 0.4% to 1% in hospitalized children, with sepsis accounting for approximately 95% of cases.[13,14] It is primarily a clinical diagnosis based on the evaluation of laboratory results in patients with a clinical condition known to be associated with DIC (Box 34-1).

Clinical Manifestations

The clinical manifestations of DIC include bleeding, thrombosis, or both, although bleeding typically predominates. Early indicators are bleeding from venipuncture sites, intravascular access, and surgical wounds. Mucocutaneous bleeding may be manifested as bruising, petechiae, epistaxis, gum bleeding, blood from tracheal aspirates, gastrointestinal bleeding, and hematuria. In fulminant cases, DIC may lead to bleeding into vital organs. However, with increasingly sensitive diagnostic tests that can detect endogenous activation of the hemostatic process, the clinical spectrum of DIC is broad. Nonovert DIC describes a stressed but compensated hemostatic system in which laboratory test results are abnormal but there are no clinical manifestations.[15] Overt DIC is described as a stressed and decompensated hemostatic system in which laboratory test results are abnormal and clinical bleeding or microvascular thrombosis and organ dysfunction are noted. Overt DIC may be controlled or uncontrolled, depending on whether the process will resolve when the underlying stimulus is removed.

Diagnosis

The clinical findings of a profoundly ill child with bleeding believed to be secondary to DIC can be supported by laboratory tests showing evidence of a consumptive coagulopathy with activation of the fibrinolytic cascade. Moderate to severe thrombocytopenia with or without anemia will be evident from the complete blood count. Thrombocytopenia is present in approximately 50% of patients and suggests consumption of platelets.[16] Anemia could be caused by bleeding or, when accompanied by schistocytes on the blood smear, by microangiopathic hemolysis. The PT and APTT are prolonged in 50% to 60% of patients[17] as a result of consumption of many coagulation proteins, including prothrombin, factors V, VII, and VIII, and fibrinogen. Fibrinogen/fibrin degradation products and D-dimers are both increased in most patients with DIC, thus suggesting activation of the fibrinolytic process.[18] Marked reductions in plasma anticoagulants, including proteins C and S and antithrombin, have also been described.[12,19] The most sensitive tests for the diagnosis of DIC are markers of endogenous thrombin generation: prothrombin fragment 1.2 and thrombin-antithrombin complexes (TATs).[20] Prothrombin fragment 1.2 is released when thrombin is generated from prothrombin. TATs are generated by binding of thrombin

---

Box 34-1	**Causes of Disseminated Intravascular Coagulation**

INFECTIOUS

Meningococcemia (purpura fulminans)
Other gram-negative bacteria (*Haemophilus*, *Salmonella*)
Gram-positive bacteria (group B streptococci)
Rickettsia (Rocky Mountain spotted fever)
Viruses
Malaria
Fungi

TISSUE INJURY

Central nervous system trauma (massive head injury)
Multiple fractures with fat emboli
Crush injury
Profound shock or asphyxia
Hypothermia or hyperthermia
Massive burns

MALIGNANCY

Acute promyelocytic leukemia
Acute monoblastic or myelocytic leukemia
Widespread malignancies (neuroblastoma)

VENOM OR TOXIN

Snake bites
Insect bites

MICROANGIOPATHIC DISORDERS

"Severe" thrombotic thrombocytopenic purpura
Hemolytic-uremic syndrome
Giant hemangioma (Kasabach-Merritt syndrome)

GASTROINTESTINAL DISORDERS

Fulminant hepatitis
Severe inflammation bowel disease
Reye's syndrome

HEREDITARY THROMBOTIC DISORDERS

Homozygous protein C deficiency

MISCELLANEOUS

Severe graft rejection
Acute hemolytic transfusion reaction
Severe collagen vascular disease
Kawasaki's disease
Heparin-induced thrombosis
Infusion of "activated" prothrombin complex concentrates
Hyperpyrexia/encephalopathy, hemorrhagic shock
   syndrome

Reproduced from Colman R, Marder V. Disseminated intravascular coagulation (DIC): pathogenesis, pathophysiology, and laboratory abnormalities. In Colman R, Marder V, Salzman E (eds). Hemostasis and Thrombosis: Basic Principles and Clinical Practice. Philadelphia, JB Lippincott, 1982, p 654.

with its inhibitor antithrombin. The standard assays (PT, APTT, platelet count, and D-dimers) are relatively rapid and simple to perform. However, changes in these test results do not always occur at the same time, and laboratory values can change rapidly, depending on the patient's clinical status. This may create confusion in patient management and make the diagnosis of DIC at an early stage particularly difficult. The International Society on Thrombosis and Haemostasis Scientific Standardization Subcommittee on DIC proposed a scoring system developed from a previously described set of diagnostic criteria.[15] The five-step algorithm assigns a score based on the severity of abnormality of each of the following: platelet count ($>100 \times 10^9$/L = 0; $<100 \times 10^9$/L = 1; $<50 \times 10^9$/L = 2), elevated fibrin-related markers (no increase = 0; moderate increase = 2; strong increase = 3), prolonged PT (<3 seconds = 0; >3 seconds but <6 seconds = 1; >6 seconds = 2), and fibrinogen level (>1 g/L = 0; <1 g/L = 1). A total score of 5 or more is considered compatible with overt DIC. The sensitivity and specificity of this scoring system are greater than 90%. However, the algorithm should be applied only in the presence of an underlying disorder known to be associated with DIC. A modified algorithm that scores for rates of change in the PT, platelet count, and D-dimer and incorporation of antithrombin, protein C, and TAT complexes may help identify nonovert DIC in its early stages.[15]

Treatment

The fundamental principle of treatment of DIC is specific and vigorous management of the underlying disorder. In some cases, DIC will completely resolve within hours after resolution of the underlying condition (e.g., appropriate control of sepsis with antimicrobials). However, in other cases, supportive measures are required to control the DIC until the underlying condition is resolved (e.g., the use of all-*trans*-retinoic acid and chemotherapy for the treatment of acute promyelocytic leukemia and DIC[21]). Therapeutic interventions remain controversial and need to be individualized according to the underlying basis of the DIC and the severity of the clinical symptoms. For example, in nonovert DIC, children do not usually require therapy for the DIC itself. However, in the presence of uncontrolled overt DIC, therapeutic intervention, including administration of blood replacement products, may be indicated to improve hemostasis while waiting for effective therapy for the underlying condition. Treatment modalities investigated include blood component therapy, anticoagulants, restoration of the natural anticoagulant pathways, and other agents.

Blood Component Therapy. In general, the more severe the laboratory abnormalities, in particular, the degree of thrombocytopenia and depletion of coagulation factors, the greater the risk of bleeding complications with DIC. Hence, treatment with FFP, fibrinogen, cryoprecipitate, platelets, or any combination of these components appears to be a rational therapy in bleeding patients or those at risk for bleeding because of significant depletion of these hemostatic factors. However, blood component therapy should not be instituted on the basis of laboratory results alone and is indicated only for patients with active bleeding, those who require an invasive procedure, or those who are otherwise at risk for bleeding complications.[22] Large volumes of plasma may be necessary to correct the coagulation defect. Reasonable goals are to maintain platelet counts above 50×10^9/L, fibrinogen concentrations greater than 1 g/L, and PT values less than double the normal range.

Anticoagulant Therapy. In view of the central role played by thrombin in DIC, the use of heparin or other anticoagulants to inhibit thrombin generation appears reasonable. Heparin can at least partly inhibit the activation of coagulation in sepsis and other causes of DIC.[23] However, a beneficial effect of heparin on clinically important outcome events in patients with DIC has never been demonstrated in controlled clinical trials and is not a standard of care in overt cases of DIC. Nonetheless, therapeutic doses of heparin may be indicated in patients with clinically overt thromboembolism (TE), chronic DIC, or extensive fibrin deposition, such as seen in purpura fulminans or acral ischemia.[24]

Replacement of Natural Anticoagulant Pathways. Depleted levels of antithrombin, protein C, and protein S cannot be effectively replaced with FFP alone because of the short plasma half-life of these proteins. Antithrombin and protein C concentrates have been extensively evaluated in patients with DIC.[25-29] Trials of antithrombin therapy have not yet provided conclusive evidence sufficient to make treatment recommendations.[30] However, the double-blind, placebo-controlled, phase III trial of recombinant human activated Protein C Worldwide Evaluation in Severe Sepsis (PROWESS) demonstrated a significant decrease in mortality in the protein C–treated group when compared with placebo.[28] The dose of recombinant activated protein C is 24 μg/kg/hr.[31] Bleeding is the only recognized adverse effect with this therapy, so maintaining the platelet count above 30×10^9/L is prudent. Interestingly, activated protein C was equally effective in patients with reduced or normal plasma levels of protein C, thus suggesting that activation of protein C may be a limiting factor in sepsis.

Other Agents. Recently, rVIIa has become an attractive strategy to control bleeding in various scenarios.[32] In situations in which volume overload is an issue or bleeding persists despite adequate blood component support, use of rVIIa has been shown to be effective.[33] However, these data have been generated mostly from anecdotal reports, and given the potential adverse thrombotic complications with this agent, controlled randomized trials are required to address its safety and efficacy in the setting of DIC. Newer anticoagulants directed against the tissue factor/factor VIIa complex, such as recombinant nematode anticoagulant protein c2 (rNAPc2), are currently being evaluated in phase II/III clinical studies.[34-36]

Liver Disease

Pathophysiology

The liver is the main site of synthesis for most hemostatic components. However, the hemostatic impairment in liver disease involves a variety of mechanisms, including impaired hepatic synthesis, activation of the coagulation and fibrinolytic systems, poor clearance of activated hemostatic components, loss of hemostatic proteins into ascitic fluid, concurrent VK deficiency, thrombocytopenia, and impaired platelet function.[37,38] When both procoagulant and anticoagulant levels are reduced, the resulting hemostatic dysregulation can lead to pathologic hemorrhage, as well as thrombosis. Along with reduced synthesis, abnormal forms of the hemostatic proteins may be secreted that might function as inhibitors of coagulation. For example, abnormal fibrinogens (dysfibrinogenemia) are very common in liver disease.[39] Similarly, VK-dependent proteins (factors II, VII, IX, and X and proteins C, S, and Z) decrease in liver disease. However, they may also be secreted as forms with incomplete γ-carboxylation (see Chapter 26), thereby leading to reduced functional activity.[40]

Clinical Manifestations

Clinical symptoms are variable and depend, to some extent, on the etiology of the liver failure. Symptoms include ecchymosis and petechiae, mucous membrane bleeding, hemorrhage from gastrointestinal varices, and hemorrhage into the abdomen or central nervous system (CNS). Coagulation screening tests (APTT, PT, thrombin clotting time) are usually prolonged, platelet counts are reduced, and the bleeding time is increased. Plasma concentrations of factors VII and V and, less commonly, fibrinogen are decreased.[37] Levels of factor VIII may be normal or elevated, possibly reflecting reduced clearance via low-density lipoprotein receptor–related protein,[41] and can be helpful in distinguishing severe liver disease from DIC. However, both conditions may occur simultaneously.[42] Fibrin degradation products or D-dimer levels are often increased in hepatic failure and contribute to prolongation of the thrombin clotting time and impaired platelet function.[43] Dysfibrinogenemia will contribute to prolongation of the PT and APTT, but the thrombin time and reptilase assays are more sensitive. Dysfibrinogenemia may be confirmed by demonstrating an abnormal ratio of clot-table fibrinogen (functional assay) to fibrinogen antigen (immunoassay).

Treatment

Treatment of the hemostatic manifestations of severe hepatic failure is difficult. The enhanced hemostasis after replacement therapy is usually transient because adequate volumes of FFP cannot be infused as a result of the associated hypervolemia. In addition, many coagulation proteins are cleared rapidly, thereby limiting any beneficial effect. Usually, therapy specifically directed at the coagulopathy is reserved for active bleeding or to facilitate invasive procedures. A common indication for FFP is an international normalized ratio (INR) higher than 2 or PT prolongation greater than 4 seconds.[44] Desmopressin can induce the release of factor VIII and von Willebrand factor and thereby result in a shortened bleeding time. However, in randomized trials, desmopressin failed to control bleeding from acute variceal hemorrhage[45] or decrease blood loss with hepatectomy.[46] Cryoprecipitate can be administered to increase plasma fibrinogen concentrations if necessary. Secondary VK deficiency caused by impaired VK utilization or absorption, the latter often resulting from intrahepatic and extrahepatic biliary atresia, requires treatment with VK.[47] rVIIa has been shown to correct the prolonged PT in nonbleeding cirrhotic patients, but randomized trials in the setting of liver biopsy or variceal bleeding have shown either no difference in hemostasis or only early, modest reductions in the rebleeding rate with no difference in overall bleeding or transfusion requirements.[40] Larger studies are still required to evaluate the efficacy and safety of this agent in liver disease.

Patients requiring liver transplantation invariably have severe, end-stage hepatic failure with its associated hemorrhagic complications. Additional risk factors that contribute to bleeding in children during transplantation include extensive scar tissue from previous surgery, prolonged duration of the surgery, downsizing the donor organ to fit the small patient, dilutional coagulopathy, and excessive activation of the fibrinolytic system during the anhepatic phase.[48-50] Although treatment with antifibrinolytic agents is an attractive option, this approach should be used with caution because either hemorrhagic or thrombotic complications may develop in children after liver transplantation. The prophylactic use of rVIIa to reduce blood loss and transfusion requirements in patients undergoing liver transplantation has been studied in two multicenter randomized controlled trials.[51,52] These trials failed to demonstrate a benefit to support its use as a universal preemptive therapy for liver transplantation. rVIIa could be considered in individual cases as "rescue therapy" for patients with life-threatening coagulopathy and bleeding during transplantation or in situations in which blood products are unavailable or unacceptable (e.g., Jehovah witnesses).[53]

Vitamin K Deficiency

The role of VK in coagulation is detailed in Chapter 26, and bleeding as a result of VK deficiency in newborns is discussed in Chapter 5.

Clinical Manifestations

Symptoms of VK deficiency include mild to moderate bleeding, ecchymoses, oozing from intravenous puncture sites, and rarely, internal bleeding. Primary VK deficiency in healthy children is uncommon because of a relatively low VK requirement and the widespread distribution of VK in plant and animal tissues. In plants, the only important molecular form is phylloquinone (VK_1). Bacteria synthesize a family of vitamin K compounds called menaquinones (VK_2). The contribution of microbiologic flora of the gut to VK dietary intake is unknown but may be as high as 50%.[54] Although broad-spectrum antibiotics may reduce VK_2 production by intestinal bacteria, VK deficiency is rare in individuals consuming a normal diet.

Groups of children at high risk for VK deficiency include breast-fed newborns, chronically ill children with inadequate dietary intake of VK, children with disorders that interfere with the absorption of VK (diarrhea, cystic fibrosis, cholestatic liver disease, celiac disease), and children with poor nutrition who are receiving broad-spectrum antibiotics.[55-58] Cystic fibrosis, biliary atresia, and obstructive jaundice interfere with the absorption of fat-soluble vitamins and transport to the liver, with resultant VK deficiency. Therapeutic drugs can interfere with vitamin K metabolism (e.g., phenytoin and warfarin). However, at least in the case of warfarin, this side effect is expected. Accidental exposure to toxic doses may occur in small children with access to warfarin in the home. Anticoagulant rodenticides can be another source of accidental exposure. Because of the emergence of warfarin-resistant strains of rats, newer "long-acting" second-generation compounds have been used. These so-called "superwarfarins" have higher affinity for VK_1-2,3-epoxide reductase, are able to disrupt the VK_1-epoxide cycle at more than one point, exhibit hepatic accumulation, and have unusually long biologic half-lives because of high lipid solubility and enterohepatic circulation. Upon accidental ingestion, these compounds can cause anticoagulation for several days or even weeks. However, in most cases involving small children, the exposure is low and bleeding manifestations are rare.[59,60]

VK deficiency has been described in bone marrow transplant and oncology patients, in whom the cause is multifactorial as a result of drug antagonism, liver dysfunction, fat malabsorption, anorexia, or inadequate dietary intake (or any combination of such causes). A study of children evaluated before bone marrow transplantation identified 31% (8 of 26) with evidence of VK deficiency (as detected by circulating abnormally carboxylated forms of prothrombin), although only 1 patient had a prolonged PT, thus highlighting that PT alone is an insensitive marker of VK deficiency. Six of the eight affected patients exhibited peritransplant bleeding.[61]

Laboratory Diagnosis

The PT and APTT may both be abnormal in VK deficiency but should correct in a 1 : 1 mix with normal plasma. Other acquired or congenital coagulopathies can result in similar screening test abnormalities, and thus specific coagulation factor assays need to be performed. Decreased levels of more than one VK-dependent factor should raise suspicion of VK deficiency. A normal factor V level together with normal liver function study results would argue against significant liver disease as the underlying explanation. Normal factor VIII and fibrinogen levels and absence of elevated D-dimers would make DIC unlikely. However, VK deficiency can complicate other coagulopathies, such as DIC or liver disease. If there is any doubt about the diagnosis, the patient should receive VK therapy in conjunction with other supportive care.

Treatment

The route and specific type of therapy are dictated by the urgency of the clinical situation and the potential side effects of treatment. For example, severe anaphylactoid reactions, though rare, have complicated intravenous VK administration, even when the solution is diluted and infused slowly. Therefore, intravenous administration of VK, at a rate no faster than 1 mg/min, should be restricted to situations in which other routes are not feasible and the risk is justified. Intramuscular VK should be avoided because it can result in pain, swelling, and hematoma formation. The preferred systemic route is subcutaneous injection because it is safe and effective. Oral VK is effective if absorption is unimpaired. Although oral administration is generally thought to produce slower correction of the PT (6 to 8 hours) than achieved with parenteral VK (2 to 6 hours), a study in adults suggested that the oral route may actually be faster, at least in reversing the effect of warfarin.[62]

Asymptomatic patients with mildly abnormal coagulation results that are presumed secondary to VK deficiency should be given VK subcutaneously (1 to 5 mg, depending on size). This approach is both therapeutic and diagnostic, with correction of coagulation abnormality generally expected within 2 to 6 hours. A patient bleeding because of VK deficiency should receive 2 to 10 mg of VK subcutaneously. FFP (10 to 20 mL/kg) is particularly useful when the precise nature of the coagulopathy is unknown and the bleeding is severe. However, the amount of plasma needed for total correction of severe VK deficiency is so great that it may result in volume overload. A patient with life-threatening hemorrhage or an intracranial hemorrhage would probably benefit from administration of prothrombin complex concentrates at a minimum dose of 50 U/kg, in addition to systemic VK (5 to 20 mg). Prothrombin complex concentrates contain relatively uniform amounts of factors

II, IX, and X, with amounts of factor VII/VIIa varying.[63] rVIIa has been used anecdotally.[64,65]

Prevention

Prophylactic VK should be given to patients at risk, such as patients with inadequate nutrition and those receiving broad-spectrum antibiotics. Most patients requiring total parenteral nutrition (TPN) are supplemented with VK. There has been concern in the past that maternal anticonvulsant therapy may be associated with an increased risk of neonatal bleeding related to enzymatic degradation of vitamin K.[66] This suggestion has prompted recommendations that VK prophylaxis be given to pregnant mothers taking anticonvulsants. However, recent studies have demonstrated that the incidence of bleeding in infants exposed to these drugs antenatally is no higher than in controls,[67] with no benefit seen for routine VK prophylaxis in this setting.[68]

Massive Transfusion Coagulopathy

Uncontrolled bleeding can be a clinical problem associated with the management of trauma and surgical patients and often necessitates transfusion of large amounts of blood and blood derivatives. Massive transfusion has commonly been defined as replacing at least one blood volume in 24 hours.[69] Patients with this degree of bleeding are at risk for defective hemostasis related to the transfusions, in addition to the underlying precipitating trauma or surgical insult. The resulting bleeding diathesis may be complex and include evidence of DIC, depletion of hemostatic factors through blood loss, tissue injury, and consumption of factors, dilutional coagulopathy secondary to aggressive blood component resuscitation, hypothermia, platelet dysfunction, and excessive fibrinolysis.[69] In surgical procedures with a high risk for blood loss, aprotinin has been used because it inhibits multiple protease targets.[70-73] Prospective studies in adults have shown that it reduces the proportion of patients who require blood transfusion.[74] A meta-analysis of prospective trials in children undergoing cardiac surgery involving cardiopulmonary bypass showed that aprotinin reduced the proportion of children requiring transfusion by 33% but did not have an effect on the volume of blood transfused or the volume of chest tube drainage.[75] rVIIa has demonstrated effectiveness in patients with bleeding associated with massive transfusion who were refractory to conventional treatments.[76] The limited experience with rVIIa in pediatric patients undergoing cardiopulmonary bypass and extracorporeal membrane oxygenation suggests efficacy as rescue therapy, but it has not been studied prospectively.[77-80]

Acquired Inhibitors of Coagulation Proteins

Acquired inhibitors directed against coagulation factors are either circulating alloantibodies or autoantibodies that specifically neutralize procoagulant activity or increase clearance and thereby lead to deficiency of plasma coagulation factors, often accompanied by bleeding.[81] Examples of alloantibodies include those directed against infused factor VIII, as observed in 15% to 25% of patients with hemophilia A (discussed in Chapter 30). Autoantibodies directed against endogenous factor VIII have also been observed in individuals without hemophilia and typically occur in postpartum women, elderly individuals, or those with autoimmune disorders. However, autoantibodies to other coagulation proteins have been described as well, including factors II, V, VII, IX, and XI and von Willebrand factor. Antiphospholipid antibodies (APAs), including lupus anticoagulants (LAs), are a heterogeneous group of antibodies that react with proteins bound to phospholipids. Though primarily functioning as inhibitors of in vitro phospholipid-dependent clotting assays, these antibodies paradoxically predispose to thrombosis rather than hemorrhage. However, a unique LA coagulopathy has been observed as a hemorrhagic syndrome associated with hypoprothrombinemia (see later).

Acquired Inhibitors to Factor VIII

Anti–factor VIII autoantibodies are rare in children but can result in severe bleeding and significant morbidity. These antibodies are associated with underlying medical conditions in half of those affected, including malignancy, autoimmune disease, lymphoproliferative disorders, or drugs (e.g., penicillin).[82] Patients can exhibit bleeding symptoms ranging from easy bruising to intracranial hemorrhage. In one patient, the clinical course was also complicated by nephrotic syndrome.[83] Laboratory screening studies will show a prolonged APTT that does not fully correct upon mixing with normal plasma in a 1 : 1 mix ("inhibitor screen"). Factor VIII inhibitors can also be distinguished from LAs by performing the APTT 1 : 1 mix again with an incubation phase (typically 30 minutes at 37° C). The latter study will show further prolongation of the APTT, indicative of progressive neutralization of factor VIII provided by the normal plasma mixing. This additional prolongation will not be seen with incubation in the presence of an LA.

Treatment is two-pronged and directed at stopping the bleeding and eradicating the inhibitor. Hemostasis can be achieved with high doses of factor VIII concentrates, activated prothrombin complex concentrates, and rVIIa. Immunosuppression may be accomplished with cytotoxic agents such as cyclophosphamide or prednisone or with gamma globulin. Inhibitors have also been eradicated by extracorporeal immunoadsorption and immune tolerance through regular exposure to high-dose factor VIII infusions. Review of the available literature suggests that in contrast to adults, anti–factor VIII autoantibodies in children may resolve more quickly and easily and do not necessarily require steroids and cytotoxic agents.[82,84] Recombinant factor VIII should be considered in the initial treatment and additional hemostatic support with activated prothrombin complex concentrates and rVIIa administered as needed. Withdrawal of instigating drugs such as penicillin may also facilitate resolution.

Acquired Inhibitors to Factor IX

Few cases of spontaneous factor IX inhibitors have been reported in nonhemophiliacs, and most adult cases have been related to underlying systemic disorders such as systemic lupus erythematosus (SLE), hepatitis, multiple sclerosis, rheumatic fever, collagen vascular disease, postpartum status, and prostatectomy. Descriptions in children are limited to a few case reports.[85-87] Bleeding manifestations have included cutaneous ecchymoses and soft tissue hematomas. Diagnostic studies are similar to those for anti–factor VIII inhibitors. Treatment has included any combination of corticosteroids, gamma globulin, or cyclophosphamide, with rapid resolution of the inhibitor. One child underwent spontaneous resolution.[86] Recombinant factor IX and rVIIa can be considered for the acute management of bleeding.

Acquired Inhibitors As a Result of Exposure to Bovine Thrombin

Topical preparations of bovine thrombin are widely used for surgical hemostasis and contain fibrinogen, as well as small amounts of factor V and other proteins. The development of acquired inhibitors to coagulation factors as a consequence of exposure to this highly immunogenic agent is a frequent occurrence, though often unrecognized. In this context, antibodies directed against factor V are most frequent, although antiprothrombin and anti–factor X antibodies have also been described.[88,89] The incidence of symptomatic inhibitors is not known. In a study of 151 adult patients exposed to bovine thrombin during cardiac surgery, antibodies directed against human coagulation proteins developed in 56% of the patients.[88] However, adverse clinical outcomes did not correlate with antibody formation. A literature review identified 12 cases of inhibitors in pediatric patients after exposure to thrombin.[89] In eight cases, the antibodies were directed against human coagulation proteins, with hemorrhagic complications developing in five patients. Bleeding manifestations included cutaneous, gastrointestinal, pulmonary, and cerebral hemorrhages. Patients exhibited prolongation of both the PT and APTT and mixing studies consistent with an inhibitor. Specific factor activity assays revealed the target for the inhibitor, but there was no correlation between laboratory studies and clinical bleeding. Corticosteroids and gamma globulin have been used, with resolution of the inhibitor over a period of days to weeks. Platelet transfusions are another option inasmuch as approximately 20% of factor V activity is present in platelet granules, which are shielded from circulating antibodies.[90] Coagulation factor inhibitors should be suspected in any postoperative patient who is exposed to topical bovine thrombin and has a prolonged PT and APTT.

Acquired von Willebrand's Syndrome

Acquired von Willebrand's syndrome (AVWS) is a rare bleeding disorder with clinical and laboratory findings similar to those of inherited von Willebrand's disease. Since its original description in 1968 in a patient with SLE, more than 300 cases have been reported.[91] AVWS usually occurs in individuals with no personal or family history of von Willebrand's disease and is accompanied by bleeding symptoms in about three quarters of patients. Diagnosis in the remaining patients is based on abnormalities found during routine hemostasis screening tests.[92] As would be expected, mucocutaneous bleeding symptoms predominate. Underlying disorders are identified frequently and fall into six main categories: lymphoproliferative and myeloproliferative disorders, solid tumors, immunologic and cardiovascular disorders, and other miscellaneous conditions, including drug associations. Though typically a syndrome of advanced age, AVWS has also been reported in children, primarily associated with congenital heart disease, collagen vascular diseases, Wilms' tumor, hypothyroidism, and certain drugs. Drug-associated AVWS has been described in up to 20% of pediatric patients taking valproic acid, although bleeding manifestations were mild and did not require discontinuation of the anticonvulsant.[93]

Four main pathogenic mechanisms can lead to AVWS: (1) specific or nonspecific autoantibodies that form immune complexes with von Willebrand factor leading to inactivation and increased clearance of this factor, (2) absorption of von Willebrand factor onto malignant cell clones, (3) loss of high-molecular-weight von Willebrand factor multimers because of high shear stress, and (4) increased proteolytic degradation of von Willebrand factor by circulating proteases.[91] Laboratory studies can include a prolonged bleeding time, reduced functional von Willebrand factor (ristocetin cofactor activity, collagen-binding assay), and reduced high-molecular-weight multimers (see Chapter 30). A search for evidence of an inhibitor should be performed by measuring von Willebrand factor activity after mixing experiments involving patient plasma and normal plasma incubated at 37° C.

The three goals of treatment should be control of active bleeding, prevention of bleeding with invasive procedures as needed, and treatment of the underlying disease. Desmopressin and factor VIII/von Willebrand factor concentrates have provided only short-term control of bleeding in the presence of autoantibodies,[91] and gamma globulin, corticosteroids, or other immunosuppressive agents have been used. rVIIa may also be effective in this situation.[94] In non–inhibitor-associated AVWS, desmopressin is the preferred therapy, with factor VIII/von Willebrand factor concentrates being reserved for those who do not achieve sufficient control with desmopressin alone. Ultimately, normalization of hemostasis may not be seen until the underlying precipitating condition is treated effectively (e.g., surgery or chemotherapy, or both, for Wilms' tumor).

Acquired Inhibitors to Prothrombin—Hemorrhagic Lupus Anticoagulant Syndrome

LAs represent a diverse group of antibodies directed against proteins bound to phospholipids. They may be found in patients with SLE and other autoimmune disorders, as well as in otherwise healthy individuals, and have been implicated in thrombotic complications. However, in children, LAs are most often identified after investigation of a prolonged APTT noted during presurgical evaluation or associated with a history of infection.[95] In the vast majority of cases, the patients are asymptomatic (including no bleeding manifestations), and the LA usually resolves spontaneously over a period of days to weeks, without interfering with any required invasive procedure.

However, a rare hemorrhagic LA syndrome (ecchymoses, epistaxis, gastrointestinal bleeding, hematomas, and even hemarthroses) has been observed with associated low prothrombin levels.[96-101] Such patients exhibit concurrent prolongation of the PT (unusual for uncomplicated LA), which is thought to be caused by antiprothrombin antibodies. These antibodies are not typically neutralizing, and mixing studies may thus not indicate the presence of an inhibitor. Instead, the reduced prothrombin level is thought to result from the formation of immune complexes and subsequent increased plasma clearance.[102] Antibodies directed against the carboxyterminal portion of the prothrombin molecule have been detected.[103] Bleeding symptoms usually resolve without therapy, although patients with significant bleeding may be treated with prothrombin complex concentrates. Corticosteroids and other immunosuppressants have been used in some cases.

ACQUIRED THROMBOEMBOLIC DISEASE

TE has been diagnosed increasingly in children in recent years because of enhanced survival from serious underlying illnesses, heightened use of invasive vascular procedures and devices, and a growing (albeit still suboptimal) awareness that TE does indeed occur in children. The remainder of this chapter summarizes the clinical spectrum and characterization of pediatric TE, key considerations for diagnostic evaluation and antithrombotic management, and long-term outcomes. Emphasis is also placed on unresolved and emerging clinical/investigative issues in the field.

Characterization of Thromboembolism in Children

TE is anatomically classified by vascular type (i.e., venous versus arterial), distribution (e.g., distal, proximal, or central part of the lower extremity; superficial versus deep vasculature), and organ system affected, if applicable (e.g., renal vein thrombosis [RVT], cerebral sinovenous thrombosis [CSVT], pulmonary embolism [PE]). TE is also distinguished by the additional clinically relevant factors of first-episode versus recurrent, symptomatic versus asymptomatic, acute versus chronic (a distinction that can be difficult at times), veno-occlusive versus nonocclusive, and idiopathic versus risk associated. This last category includes both clinical prothrombotic risk factors (e.g., exogenous estrogen administration, indwelling central venous catheter, reduced mobility) and blood-based thrombophilic conditions (e.g., transient or persistent APAs, acquired or congenital anticoagulant deficiencies, factor V Leiden or prothrombin 20210 mutations), as discussed in greater detail later under "Etiology." Because of the frequency of indwelling central venous catheters as a clinical risk factor for TE in children, TE is also often classified as catheter related versus non–catheter related.

Venous Thromboembolism

Epidemiology

Several national and international registries have evaluated the incidence of venous thromboembolism (VTE) in children over the past 13 years. From these data a cumulative incidence of 0.07 per 10,000 (5.3 per 10,000 hospitalizations) was estimated for extremity deep venous thrombosis (DVT) or PE (or both) in non-neonatal Canadian children,[104] and an incidence rate of 0.14 per 10,000 children per year was reported for all forms of VTE in the Netherlands.[105] More recently, evaluation of the National Hospital Discharge Survey and census data for all forms of VTE in the United States disclosed an overall incidence rate of 0.49 per 10,000 per year.[106]

Closer examination of the epidemiologic data reveals that the age distribution of VTE in children is bimodal, with a peak incidence in the neonatal period and adolescence. With regard to the newborn period, the cumulative incidence of venous or arterial TE (or both) was reported to be 0.51 per 10,000 births in Germany[107] and 24 per 10,000 admissions to neonatal intensive care units in southern Ontario.[108] The Dutch registry indicated a VTE-specific incidence rate of 14.5 per 10,000 per year in the neonatal period, approximately 100 times greater than the overall rate in childhood.[105] Among adolescents 15 to 17 years of age, the VTE-specific incidence rate in the United States was determined to be 1.1 per 10,000 per year, a rate nearly threefold that observed overall in childhood.[106]

Although differing selection criteria have contributed to the considerable variability in incidence estimates just presented, it is clear that the incidence of VTE in children is lower than that in middle-aged and elderly adults. Nevertheless, as discussed later in this chapter, the sequelae of VTE in children, particularly with regard to

Etiology

The pathogenesis of VTE can be readily appreciated by considering Virchow's triad, which consists of venous stasis, endothelial damage, and the hypercoagulable state. In children, more than 90% of VTE episodes are associated with risk factors[105,109,110] (versus approximately 60% in adults), with risk factors often being derived from more than one component of this triad. Specific examples of VTE risk factors in children are shown in Figure 34-1. Among the most common clinical prothrombotic risk factors in childhood is an indwelling central venous catheter. More than 50% of DVT cases in children and more than 80% of cases in newborns occur in association with central venous catheters.[104,108] The reported cumulative incidence or prevalence of catheter-related thrombosis (CRT) in children receiving home TPN ranges widely from 1% to 80%[111-116]; this broad variation is largely influenced by differing study designs, selection criteria, and diagnostic imaging modalities. Indwelling central venous catheters, an underlying malignancy or disorder for which bone marrow transplantation was undertaken, and congenital cardiac disease and its corrective surgery were all highly prevalent in the Canadian pediatric thrombosis registry,[110] whereas underlying infectious illness and the presence of an indwelling central venous catheter were identified as pervasive clinical risk factors in a recent cohort study analysis from the United States.[109] It is likely that differences in the composition of referral populations strongly contribute to differences in observed causes of VTE across major pediatric thrombosis centers.

With regard to blood-based risk factors for VTE, potent thrombophilic conditions (e.g., anticoagulant deficiencies such as protein C deficiency, APAs) in chil-dren are frequently acquired and, more rarely, may be congenital. By contrast, mild congenital thrombophilic traits (e.g., the factor V Leiden and prothrombin 20210 mutations, see Chapter 32) are common in white children, as in adults. Thrombophilia can potentially be caused by any alteration in hemostatic balance that increases thrombin production, enhances platelet activation/aggregation, mediates endothelial activation/damage, or inhibits fibrinolysis. Common examples of acquired thrombophilia in children include increased factor VIII activity with significant infection and inflammatory states, anticoagulant deficiencies as a result of consumption in bacterial sepsis and DIC, production of inhibitory antibodies in acute viral infection, and para-infectious development of APAs. A panel of thrombophilia traits and markers that have been identified as risk factors for VTE in pediatric studies, and as such are recommended by the Subcommittee for Perinatal and Pediatric Thrombosis of the Scientific and Standardization Committee of the International Society of Thrombosis and Haemostasis for the diagnostic laboratory evaluation of acute VTE in children,[117] is presented in Table 34-1. To provide an appreciation of the magnitude of the increase in risk for VTE associated with several congenital/genetically influenced thrombophilia traits, population-based estimates of risk for VTE derived from the adult literature are presented in Table 34-2 (also see Chapter 32).

Clinical Manifestations

The degree of clinical suspicion for acute VTE in children should be influenced principally by clinical prothrombotic risk factors and a family history of early VTE or other vascular disease elicited by thorough interview, known thrombophilia traits and risk factors, and clinical signs and symptoms. The signs and symptoms of VTE depend on the anatomic location and organ systems affected and are influenced by the characteristics of veno-

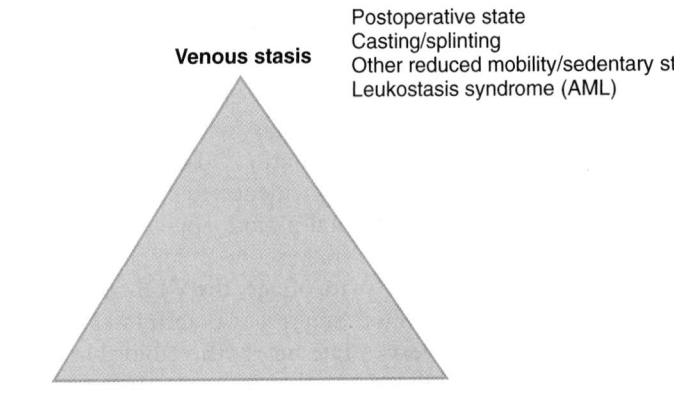

FIGURE 34-1. Clinical prothrombotic risk factors: Virchow's triad applied to venous thromboembolism in children. APA, antiphospholipid antibody.

TABLE 34-1	Pediatric Thrombophilia Traits, Conditions, and Markers: Comprehensive Diagnostic Laboratory Evaluation
Trait/Condition/Marker	**Testing Method(s)**
GENETIC	
Factor V Leiden mutation	PCR
Prothrombin 20210 mutation	PCR
Elevated plasma lipoprotein(a) concentration	ELISA
ACQUIRED AND/OR GENETIC	
Antithrombin deficiency	Chromogenic assay
Protein C deficiency	Chromogenic assay
Protein S deficiency	ELISA (for free protein S antigen)
Elevated plasma factor VIII activity*	One-stage clotting assay (APTT based)
Hyperhomocysteinemia	Mass spectroscopy
Antiphospholipid antibodies	ELISA for anticardiolipin and anti–β_2-glycoprotein-I IgG and IgM; clotting assay (dilute Russel viper venom time or APTT-based phospholipid neutralization method for lupus anticoagulant)
Disseminated intravascular coagulation	Includes platelet count, fibrinogen by clotting method (Clauss), and D-dimer by semiquantitative or quantitative latex agglutination assay
Activated protein C resistance	Clotting assay (APTT based)

*Noted as worthy of consideration in the original International Society on Thrombosis and Haemostasis recommendations.[14] Also noted as worthy of consideration is other testing involving the fibrinolytic system and the systemic inflammatory response.

APPT, activated partial thromboplastin time; ELISA, enzyme-linked immunosorbent assay; PCR, polymerase chain reaction.

TABLE 34-2	Estimate of Risk for Venous Thromboembolism with Selected Thrombophilia Traits and Conditions
Trait/Condition	**VTE Risk Estimate**
Hyperhomocysteinemia	2.5×
Prothrombin 20210 mutation, heterozygous	3×
Oral contraceptive pill (standard-dose estrogen)	4×
Factor V Leiden mutation, heterozygous	2-7×
Factor V Leiden mutation, heterozygous, plus oral contraceptive pill use	35×
Factor V Leiden mutation, homozygous	80×

occlusiveness and chronicity. The classic manifestation of *acute extremity DVT* is painful unilateral limb swelling. The lack of other findings on physical examination (e.g., Homan's sign or the presence of a palpable cord in the popliteal fossa) should not reduce clinical suspicion for DVT. In upper extremity DVT with extension into and occlusion of the superior vena cava (SVC), signs and symptoms may include swelling of the neck and face, bilateral periorbital edema, and headache.

PE is classically manifested by sudden-onset, unexplained shortness of breath and pleuritic chest pain. When PE is proximal or bilaterally extensive in the distal pulmonary arterial tree, hypoxemia is often present. Associated right heart failure may be manifested as hepatomegaly, peripheral edema, or both. Proximal PE and especially saddle emboli can be accompanied by cyanosis or sudden collapse. However, in many cases, PE may be asymptomatic or produce only subtle symptoms in children,[118-121] especially when involving limited segmental branches of the pulmonary arteries. In one retrospective series, only 50% of affected children had clinical symptoms attributable to PE.[119]

Acute *CSVT* may cause unusually severe and persistent headache, blurred vision, neurologic signs (e.g., cranial nerve palsy, papilledema), or seizures. The classic findings in *RVT* are hematuria and thrombocytopenia, sometimes associated with uremia (especially when bilateral). Initial signs include oliguria (especially when bilateral), and in the neonatal period (the time at which RVT is most common during childhood) a flank mass is often palpable on examination.[122] RVT in older children is frequently associated with nephrotic syndrome (a risk factor for VTE in general because of loss of anticoagulant proteins) and hence may be accompanied by stigmata of peripheral and periorbital edema when diagnosed in conjunction with nephrosis.[120] Thrombocytopenia may be an initial manifestation not only of RVT but also of *intracardiac* (e.g., right atrial) *thrombosis*, particularly CRT associated with sepsis.[123] Isolated intracardiac thrombosis in association with cardiac surgery or central venous catheter placement is most often asymptomatic.[124] *Portal vein thrombosis* is one of the most common causes of portal hypertension in children and is characteristically manifested as splenomegaly in association with findings of hypersplenism (anemia, neutropenia, and thrombocytopenia); gastrointestinal bleeding typically signals the presence of gastroesophageal varices.[125,126] *Internal jugular vein thrombosis* may be manifested as neck pain or swelling and, when part of Lemierre's syndrome, is classically also associated with fever, trismus, pain on lateral rotation of the neck, and a palpable mass in the lateral triangle of the neck.[127]

Chronic VTE may be diagnosed incidentally without signs or symptoms (as sometimes occurs for CSVT during unrelated brain imaging) or may be accompanied by signs and symptoms of chronic venous obstruction or PTS, including pain and edema of the dependent extremities, dilated superficial collateral veins, venous stasis dermatitis, frank ulceration of the skin, or any combination of these findings.

Diagnosis

Although venography has historically been the gold standard for diagnosis of venous thrombosis, this modality is invasive and has experienced a diminishing role in recent years with the development of effective noninvasive or minimally invasive radiologic imaging technologies. Radiologic imaging is used not only to confirm the clinical diagnosis of VTE but also to define both the extent and occlusiveness of the thrombosis. For suspected DVT of the distal or proximal end of the lower extremity, compression ultrasound with Doppler is typically used for objective confirmation. When the thrombus may affect or extend into deep pelvic or abdominal veins, computed tomography (CT) is often necessary. For circumstances in which radiation exposure is a significant concern or alternative diagnoses (e.g., myositis) are being evaluated, magnetic resonance imaging (MRI) may be performed instead. MR venography may be useful in documenting May-Thurner syndrome, an uncommon cause of lower extremity DVT in which the iliac vein is compressed by an overriding right common iliac artery.[128] In suspected DVT of the upper extremity, compression ultrasound with Doppler effectively evaluates the limb, but echocardiography or CT (or both) is required to disclose involvement of more central vasculature (e.g., right atrial thrombosis). In the case of asymptomatic nonocclusive extremity DVT, venography may be used as an alternative to CT. It is important to recognize that venography (in which radiographic contrast material is administered into a vein in the limb) should not be confused with "line-o-grams" (in which radiographic contrast material is instilled into a central venous catheter). The latter studies are useful for delineating catheter tip thrombi but cannot reliably detect DVT along the intravascular length of a central venous catheter.[129] MR venography has replaced traditional venography in most centers. However, dynamic venography may be required to evaluate patients for thoracic outlet syndrome (mechanical compression and entrapment of the subclavian vessels in the region of the first rib).[130] To establish a diagnosis of DVT of the jugular venous system, compression ultrasound with Doppler is typically sufficient.

PE in children is commonly diagnosed by spiral CT or, alternatively, by ventilation-perfusion scanning. The latter is generally suboptimal in the presence of other lung pathology or at centers with limited availability or expertise in this modality. CSVT is typically diagnosed by standard CT or CT venography and, alternatively, by MRI or MR venography. The diagnosis of RVT is most often made clinically in neonates and is supported by Doppler ultrasound findings of intrarenal vascular resistive indices; however, in some cases a discrete thrombus may be suggested by Doppler ultrasound, especially when extending into the inferior vena cava (IVC). When RVT occurs in older children, Doppler ultrasound or CT is often diagnostic. Similarly, portal vein thrombosis is typically visualized by Doppler ultrasound or CT.

When new-onset venous thrombosis is being evaluated in patients with areas of anatomic abnormality of the venous system (e.g., extensive collateral venous circulation because of a previous VTE episode, May-Thurner anomaly, atretic IVC with azygous continuation), more sensitive methods such as CT or MR venography are frequently required to adequately delineate the vascular anatomy, as well as the presence, extent, and occlusiveness of the thrombosis.

Diagnostic laboratory evaluation for pediatric acute VTE includes a complete blood count, comprehensive thrombophilia panel (see "Etiology," earlier), and β-human chorionic gonadotropin (β-HCG) in postmenarchal females. Additional laboratory studies may be warranted depending on associated medical conditions and involvement of specific organ systems by VTE.

Treatment

A summary of conventional antithrombotic agents and corresponding target anticoagulant levels, based on recent pediatric recommendations,[131] is provided in Table 34-3 for both initial (i.e., acute phase) and extended (i.e., subacute phase) treatment. Conventional anticoagulants attenuate hypercoagulability, thereby decreasing the risk for progression of thrombosis and embolism, and rely on intrinsic fibrinolytic mechanisms to break the thrombus up over time. The most commonly used conventional anticoagulants in children are heparins and warfarin. Heparins, including unfractionated heparin and LMWH, enhance the activity of antithrombin III, an intrinsic anticoagulant that serves as a key inhibitor of thrombin (Chapter 26). Warfarin acts through antagonism of VK, thereby interfering with γ-carboxylation of the VK-dependent procoagulant factors II, VII, IX, and X.

Initial Anticoagulation. Initial anticoagulant therapy (i.e., acute phase) for VTE in children uses unfractionated heparin or LMWH. LMWH has become increasingly used as a first-line agent for initial anticoagulant therapy in children given the relative ease of subcutaneous over intravenous administration, the decreased need for blood monitoring of anticoagulant efficacy, and decreased risk for the development of heparin-induced thrombocytopenia. Unfractionated heparin is typically preferred in circumstances of heightened bleeding risk or labile acute clinical status as a result of rapid extinction of anticoagulant effect after cessation of the drug. In addition, because of renal excretion of LMWH, unfrac-

TABLE 34-3	Recommended Intensities and Durations of Conventional Antithrombotic Therapy in Children, by Etiology and Treatment Agent		
	Agents and Target Anticoagulant Activity		
Episode	**Initial Treatment**	**Extended Treatment**	**Duration of Therapy, by Etiology**
First	UFH, 0.3-0.7 anti-Xa U/mL LMWH, 0.5-1.0 anti-Xa U/mL	Warfarin, INR of 2.0-3.0 LMWH, 0.5-1.0 anti-Xa U/mL	Resolved risk factor: 3-6 months No known clinical risk factor: 6-12 months Chronic clinical risk factor: 12 months Potent congenital thrombophilia: indefinite
Recurrent	UFH, 0.3-0.7 anti-Xa U/mL LMWH, 0.5-1.0 anti-Xa U/mL	Warfarin, INR of 2.0-3.0 LMWH, 0.5-1.0 anti-Xa U/mL	Resolved risk factor: 6-12 months No known clinical risk factor: 12 months Chronic clinical risk factor: indefinite Potent congenital thrombophilia: indefinite

INR, international normalized ratio; LMWH, low-molecular-weight heparin; UFH, unfractionated heparin.

tionated heparin is used for acute VTE therapy in patients with renal insufficiency.

Common initial maintenance dosing for unfractionated heparin in non-neonatal children ranges from 15 to 25 U/kg/hr preceded by a loading dose of 50 to 75 U/kg. In full-term neonates, a maintenance dose of up to 50 U/kg/hr may be required, especially if the clinical condition is complicated by antithrombin consumption. The starting dose for the LMWH enoxaparin in non-neonatal children commonly ranges between 1.0 and 1.25 mg/kg; no bolus dose is given. In full-term neonates, an enoxaparin starting dose of 1.5 mg/kg is typically necessary.[132] For the LMWH dalteparin, initial maintenance dosing of 1.0 to 1.5 mg/kg (100 to 150 anti-Xa U/kg) appears appropriate based upon available pediatric data.[133] Heparin therapy is monitored most accurately by anti-factor Xa activity. It is essential that the clinical laboratory be made aware of the type of heparin being administered so that the appropriate assay standard (unfractionated heparin versus LMWH) is used. For unfractionated heparin, the therapeutic range is 0.3 to 0.7 anti-Xa activity U/mL, whereas for LMWH, the therapeutic range is 0.5 to 1.0 U/mL. When anti-Xa assay is not available, the APTT may be used, but it is distinctly suboptimal in the pediatric age group, in whom APAs may interfere with or artifactually prolong the clotting end point; indeed, one study of pediatric heparin monitoring demonstrated inaccuracy of the APTT approximately 30% of the time.[134] When dosed by weight in childhood, LMWH does not require frequent monitoring, but anti-Xa activity should be evaluated with changes in renal function. In addition, in cases of acute VTE in which acquired antithrombin deficiency is related to consumption in acute infection or inflammation, anti-Xa activity may rise as antithrombin levels normalize with resolution of the acute illness; in this circumstance, follow-up evaluation of anti-Xa activity is warranted in the subacute period.

The recommended duration of initial heparin therapy for acute VTE, 5 to 10 days, has been extrapolated from

adult data.[135] Unfractionated heparin treatment is rarely maintained beyond the acute period given the risk of osteoporosis with extended administration[131] and the inconvenience of continuous intravenous administration. Although adult data suggest efficacy of subcutaneous administration of unfractionated heparin for acute VTE,[136] this route has been evaluated only for the acute therapy period before extended therapy with warfarin, and the appropriateness of such an approach in children has not been established.

Extended Anticoagulation. Extended anticoagulant therapy (i.e., subacute phase) for VTE in children may be achieved with LMWH or warfarin. Warfarin may be started during the acute phase; however, because severe congenital deficiencies involving the protein C pathway can be manifested as VTE in early childhood and are associated with warfarin-related skin necrosis,[137] warfarin should ideally be initiated only after therapeutic anticoagulation has been achieved with heparin-based treatment. Warfarin is monitored by the INR, which is derived from the measured PT. The therapeutic INR range for warfarin anticoagulation in patients with VTE is 2.0 to 3.0.[131] Recent adult data do not agree with the historical evidence for maintaining a higher INR (2.5 to 3.5) in the presence of APA[138,139]; however, maintaining an INR of 2.5 to 3.0, when feasible, satisfies both the older and the more recent literature with regard to appropriate safety and efficacy in this subset of patients.

Duration of Therapy. Pediatric recommendations for the duration of antithrombotic therapy in acute VTE[131] are largely derived from evidence from adult trials. For first-episode VTE in children in the absence of potent chronic thrombophilia (e.g., APA syndrome, homozygous anticoagulant deficiency, or homozygous factor V Leiden), the recommended duration of anticoagulant therapy is 3 to 6 months in the presence of an underlying reversible risk factor (e.g., postoperative VTE), 6 to 12 months when idiopathic, and 12 months to lifelong when a chronic risk factor persists (e.g., SLE). Recurrent VTE is treated for 6 to 12 months in the patients with an underlying reversible risk factor, 12 months to lifelong when idiopathic, and lifelong when a chronic risk factor persists. In the setting of APA syndrome or potent congenital thrombophilia, the duration of treatment for first-episode VTE is often indefinite. Children with SLE and persistence of an LA have a 16- to 25-fold greater risk for TE than do children with SLE and no LA.[140] However, in children with primary (i.e., idiopathic) or secondary (i.e., associated with SLE or other underlying chronic inflammatory condition) VTE, it is possible that the auto-immune disease will become quiescent in later years such that the benefit of continued VTE prophylaxis may be re-evaluated. Some experts have recommended consideration of low-dose anticoagulation as secondary VTE prophylaxis after a conventional 3- to 6-month course of therapeutic anticoagulation for VTE in children with SLE who have APA syndrome.[141] However, further study to optimize the intensity and duration of therapy/secondary prophylaxis for VTE in children with APA syndrome is urgently needed, especially given the recent evidence in adult VTE that secondary prophylaxis with low-dose warfarin may not only offer little risk reduction beyond no anticoagulation but also is associated with bleeding complications despite a reduced warfarin dose.[142,143]

Thrombolytics. Although the aforementioned anticoagulant therapies are conventional in acute pediatric VTE, thrombolytic approaches are gaining increasing attention and use during acute VTE therapy in children with hemodynamically significant PE or extensive limb-threatening VTE. Unlike conventional anticoagulants, thrombolytics directly promote fibrinolysis. Tissue-type plasminogen activator is an intrinsic activator of the fibrinolytic system (Chapter 27) and has been administered exogenously as a systemic bolus or short-duration infusion, a systemic low-dose continuous infusion, or a local catheter-directed infusion with or without interventional mechanical thrombectomy/thrombolysis. A recent cohort study analysis of children with acute lower extremity DVT who had an a priori high risk for poor post-thrombotic outcomes (by virtue of a completely veno-occlusive thrombus and plasma factor VIII activity >150 U/dL or D-dimer concentration >500 ng/mL) revealed that a thrombolysis regimen followed by standard anticoagulation may substantially reduce the risk for PTS when compared with standard anticoagulation alone.[144] Further investigation via a randomized controlled trial of the efficacy and safety of the thrombolytic regimen versus standard anticoagulation for high-risk acute lower extremity DVT in children will be necessary to confirm these findings.

Other Anticoagulants. Other antithrombotic agents include factor Xa inhibitors and direct thrombin inhibitors. Fondaparinux is a selective factor Xa inhibitor. It is a synthetic pentasaccharide that rapidly binds to anti-

thrombin in the blood and potentiates the natural inhibitory effect of antithrombin against factor Xa, thus indirectly inhibiting thrombin.[145] Fondaparinux is administered once daily as a subcutaneous injection. Dosing is based on weight and generally does not require monitoring, although anti-Xa assays have been used by some investigators.[146]

A variety of modified factor Xa inhibitors are under evaluation in clinical trials or are in preclinical development with enhancements in half-life[147] and oral bioavailability.[148] Direct thrombin inhibitors, by contrast, inhibit thrombin directly by binding to exosite I or the active site of thrombin, or both.[149] These drugs include hirudin and recombinant hirudins such as lepirudin. Argatroban is a synthetic small molecule derived from L-arginine that functions as a reversible direct thrombin inhibitor.[150] All of the currently available direct thrombin inhibitors are administered intravenously and are routinely monitored by the APTT, with the therapeutic goal ranging from a 1.5- to 3.0-fold prolongation of the APTT. Oral direct thrombin inhibitors have been developed as a possible alternative to warfarin. They have the advantage of oral bioavailability, low intersubject variation, no metabolism by the hepatic cytochrome P-450 system, a low incidence of drug-drug interactions, and no dietary influence. However, an early candidate was not approved by the U.S. Food and Drug Administration for clinical use because of concerns of potential liver toxicity and failure to prove noninferiority to warfarin in clinical trials.[149] Other such agents are under ongoing development and investigation. At present, intravenous direct thrombin inhibitors are indicated for the treatment of heparin-induced thrombocytopenia, particularly when associated with acute thrombosis.

Other Therapeutic Agents. Other products may have antithrombotic roles in selected circumstances but await demonstration of efficacy in clinical trials. For example, plasma replacement with protein C concentrate is a useful adjunctive therapy for VTE or purpura fulminans secondary to microvascular thrombosis in severe congenital protein C deficiency[151-153] and may play a beneficial role in the treatment of microvascular thrombosis–related purpura fulminans in children with sepsis, particularly those with meningococcemia.[154-156] In addition, case series have suggested a role for antithrombin replacement in prevention of VTE in children and young adults with congenital severe antithrombin deficiency,[157] for the prevention of L-asparaginase–associated VTE in pediatric acute lymphoblastic leukemia (ALL),[158,159] and as combination therapy with defibrotide for the prevention and treatment of hepatic sinusoidal obstruction syndrome (formerly termed veno-occlusive disease) in children undergoing hematopoietic stem cell transplantation.[160] The potential benefit of a regimen of antithrombin replacement combined with daily prophylactic LMWH in reducing the risk for VTE during the induction and consolidation phases of therapy for ALL has now also been suggested by a historically controlled cohort study of the BFM 2000 protocol experience in Europe.[161] Antithrombin replacement may also be worthy of consideration in patients with acute VTE undergoing heparinization in whom significant antithrombin deficiency prevents the achievement of therapeutic anti-Xa levels (i.e., heparin "resistance"). This may be seen in neonates with clinical conditions complicated by antithrombin consumption superimposed on the physiologic relative deficiency of this key intrinsic thrombin inhibitor in the newborn period. However, antithrombin replacement in preterm neonates has been investigated as a means of improving the outcome of respiratory distress syndrome, intracranial hemorrhage, and sepsis but has failed to demonstrate benefit and may contribute to adverse events.[162]

Vena Cava Filters. Vena cava filters may serve an adjunctive role in the antithrombotic management of children in selected circumstances. The use of vena cava filters should be considered in children of appropriate size in whom contraindications to anticoagulation exist or in whom recurrent VTE (especially PE) has occurred despite therapeutic anticoagulation and in the absence of a reversible risk factor. In addition, "temporary" or retrievable vena cava filters may be considered during times of especially heightened risk for PE or at times when therapeutic anticoagulation is thought to transiently engender a heightened risk for hemorrhagic complications (e.g., recent neurosurgery). The presence of the filter alone is not an indication for long-term anticoagulation because the risk for vena cava thrombosis related to the device is low. Long-term outcomes in adult series have shown a failure rate (clinically relevant, symptomatic PE) of 3.3% to 5.6%.[163-165] Major complications were infrequent (<1%) and included rare cases of caudal migration, filter fracture, or perforation of the cava wall.[165] A retrospective review of 15 children 18 years or younger suggested efficacy of long-standing vena cava filters with regard to primary and secondary prevention of PE.[166] Follow-up was a mean of 9.2 years (range, 19 months to 16 years), and there were no significant complications, thus complementing similar findings in other small case series.[167,168] However, until the impact of such nonretrievable devices on the vena cava of a developing child has been studied better, use of such filters in preadolescents should be undertaken with caution. Experience with surgical removal of retrievable vena cava filters is quite limited in children, with unknown risks and costs of extraction. Surgical removal of permanent vena cava filters should be strongly discouraged because vena cava ligation is frequently required.[169]

Outcomes

Complications of VTE can occur both acutely and over the long term and are germane to both CRT and non-CRT. *Short-term adverse outcomes* include the major hemorrhagic complications of antithrombotic interventions,

as well as complications of the thrombotic event itself, such as post-thrombotic hemorrhage in the brain or adrenal gland; early recurrent VTE, including DVT and PE[170]; SVC syndrome in DVT of the upper venous system[170,171]; acute renal insufficiency in RVT[172]; catheter-related sepsis[173], PE,[174,175] and catheter malfunction (sometimes necessitating surgical replacement) in CRT; severe acute venous insufficiency leading to venous infarction with limb gangrene in rare cases of occlusive DVT involving the extremities; and death from hemodynamic instability in patients with extensive intracardiac thrombosis or proximal PE.[104] *Long-term adverse outcomes* in pediatric VTE have recently been reviewed[176] and include recurrent VTE, chronic hypertension and renal insufficiency in RVT, variceal hemorrhage in portal vein thrombosis,[104] chronic SVC syndrome in CRT involving SVC occlusion, loss of availability of venous access in recurrent or extensive CRT of the upper venous system, and development of PTS, a condition of chronic venous insufficiency after DVT. Manifestations of PTS (in order of increasing severity) include edema, visibly dilated superficial collateral veins, venous stasis dermatitis, and venous stasis ulcers (Fig. 34-2). Given the long-term and sometimes lifelong risk of disease sequelae as in RVT and functional impairment as in PTS, venous thrombosis is best considered a chronic disorder in children.

Long-term Outcomes. The long-term outcomes of VTE in children, with specific regard to recurrent VTE, PTS, major hemorrhage, and death, are summarized in Table 34-4. Registry[104,110,179] and cohort study[109] data in pediatric VTE of all types indicate that children appear to have a lower risk for recurrent thromboembolism than adults do (cumulative incidence at 1 to 2 years of 6% to 11% versus 12% to 22%,[181,182] respectively). However, the risk for PTS in children with DVT of the limbs appears to be at least as great as that in adults (cumulative incidence at 1 to 2 years of 33% to 70%[105,109] versus 29%, respectively[182]). In addition, in a German cohort study of children with spontaneous VTE[177] (i.e., VTE in the absence of identified clinical risk factors), the cumulative incidence of VTE at a median follow-up of 7 years was 21%, thus suggesting that in this subgroup of pediatric VTE, the risk for recurrent VTE is long-lived. Although VTE-specific mortality in children is quite low, ranging from 0% to 2% in these and other[181,182] studies, a considerably higher all-cause mortality is indicative of the severity of the underlying conditions (e.g., sepsis, cancer, congenital cardiac disease) in pediatric VTE. Neonate-specific outcomes data in pediatric non-RVT VTE reflect an all-cause mortality of 12% to 18%,[107,108,183] including one series of premature infants with CRT treated with enoxaparin.[183] The frequency of major bleeding complications during the anticoagulation period in children range from 0% to 9% in recent studies.[109]

Outcomes by Anatomic Site. Outcomes of VTE in children may differ depending on the specific anatomic

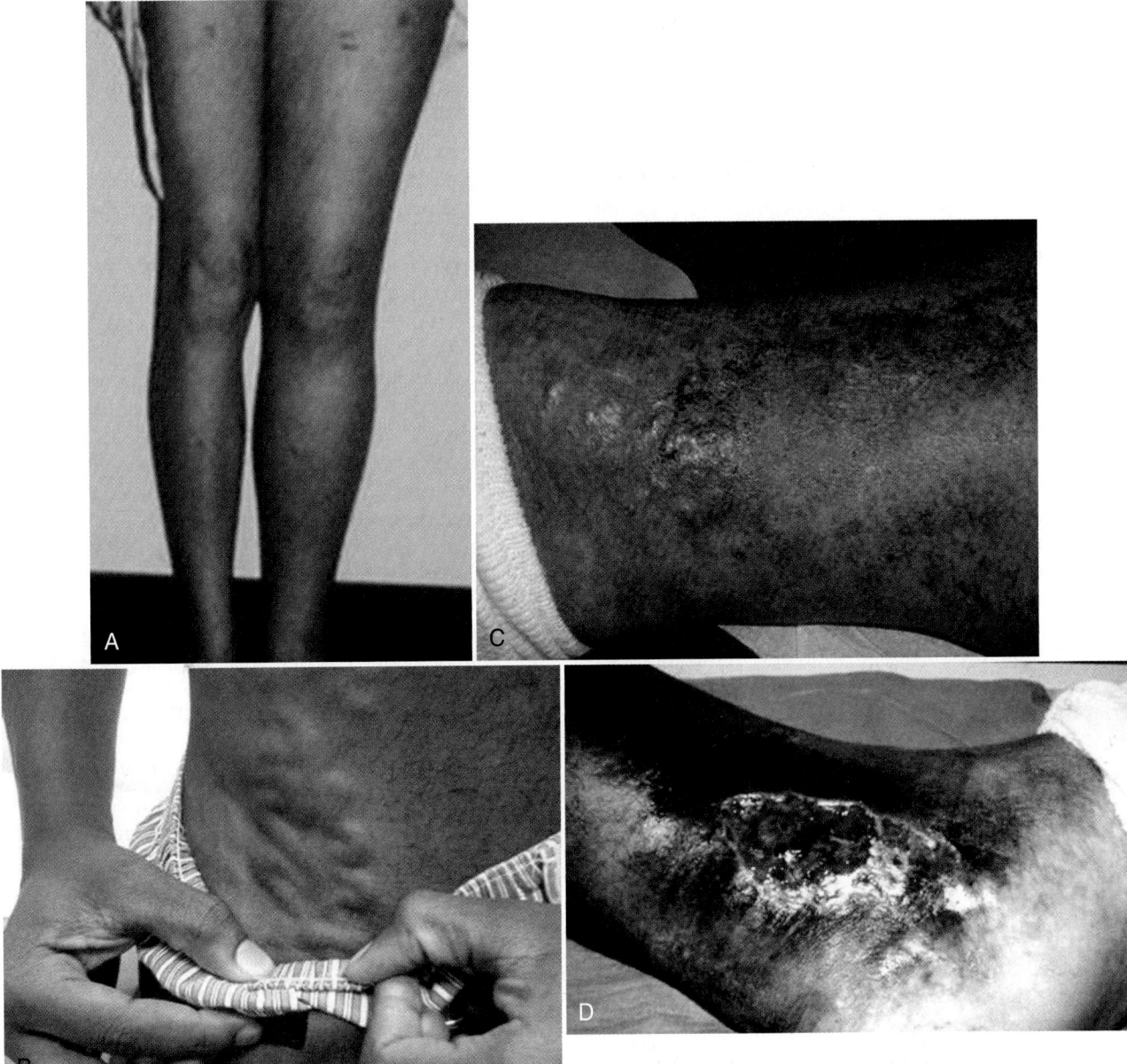

FIGURE 34-2. Manifestations of post-thrombotic syndrome (PTS) in children. **A,** Stage 1: chronic edema with iliofemoral deep venous thrombosis (DVT) at 16 years of age. The patient was heterozygous for factor V Leiden and was taking oral contraceptive pills. **B,** Stage 2: dilated superficial venous collateral circulation in a 14-year-old adolescent with inferior vena cava (IVC) DVT as a result of antiphospholipid antibody (APA) and prolonged travel. **C,** Stage 3: chronic venous stasis dermatitis in a 13-year-old with IVC DVT who was heterozygous for factor V Leiden and exhibited APA. **D,** Stage 4: chronic venous ulceration in a 10-year-old with femoral-popliteal DVT, homozygous protein C deficiency, and a tibial fracture.

sites and organ systems affected, as well as the presence/absence of a central venous catheter. Analyses devoted specifically to CRT in children are limited; however, given the high prevalence of CRT in registries and cohort studies of pediatric VTE, outcomes of CRT are likely to considerably influence the data discussed earlier for VTE in general. In a Canadian study of CRT in children from 1990 to 1996,[175] VTE-specific mortality was 4% and, in PE cases, 20%. No major bleeding episodes were observed. At a median follow-up duration of 2 years, the cumulative incidence of symptomatic recurrent VTE was

6.5%, and PTS developed in 9% of the children. In published series of RVT[122,172,184-186] (primarily in neonates), VTE-related death has been very rare, and the cumulative incidence of recurrent VTE has ranged from 0% to 4%, albeit with wide variation in duration of follow-up across studies. The cumulative incidence of chronic hypertension in RVT in these studies was reported to be 22% to 33%. The pediatric literature devoted to CSVT[187-190] is somewhat smaller than that for RVT and suggests a broad range of VTE-specific mortality of 4% to 20%, with a cumulative 8% incidence of recurrent

TABLE 34-4		**Outcomes of Venous Thromboembolism in Children**						
Author	Year of Publication	Country	# VTE Cases	Mean/Median Duration of Follow-up	Major Bleeding	Recurrent VTE	PTS	VTE-Related Mortality
Monagle et al.[110]	2000	Canada	405	3 yr	N/A	8%	12%	2%
Nowak-Göttl et al.[177]	2001	Germany	301	7 yr	N/A	21%	N/A	0%
Massicotte et al.[178]	2003	Canada	76	6 mo	9%	9%	N/A	0%
Van Ommen et al.[179]	2003	Netherlands	100	4 yr	N/A	9% (3 yr)	70%	1%
Ören et al.[180]	2004	Turkey	186	N/A	N/A	9%	N/A	2%
Goldenberg et al.[109]	2004	USA	74	1 yr	0%	6%	33%	0%

N/A, not available; PTS, post-thrombotic syndrome; VTE, venous thromboembolism.

VTE for neonatal CSVT cases and 17% for CSVT occurring in older children.[189] Long-term neurologic sequelae were noted in 17% to 26% of CSVT cases diagnosed in the neonatal period and 8% to 47% of those occurring later in childhood. It is worthy of note that in the aforementioned pediatric series of RVT and CSVT, both the proportion of children who received anticoagulation and the duration of the anticoagulation course varied considerably across studies. Few pediatric series reporting outcomes of portal vein thrombosis have been published; however, it appears that the risk for recurrent gastrovariceal bleeding in this population is substantial, often despite surgical interventions to reduce portal hypertension.[191] The long-term outcomes of PE in childhood, including the prevalence of chronic pulmonary hypertension and pulmonary function, remain to be determined.

An additional outcome of interest to patients and families of children with VTE is persistence versus resolution of thrombosis. Data to date, largely from adult VTE populations, suggest that persistence of thrombosis after a therapeutic course of anticoagulation of appropriate duration does not appreciably increase the risk for recurrent VTE, including PE. However, some evidence[192] indicates that persistent thrombosis is associated with the development of venous valvular insufficiency, an important risk factor for the development (albeit an imperfect correlate[193]) of PTS. The prevalence of persistence of thrombosis despite adequate anticoagulation in neonatal VTE has ranged from 12% in premature newborns with CRT[175] (representing one of eight patients with VTE in whom extension of thrombosis led to progressive SVC syndrome and death) to 62% in full-term neonatal VTE survivors.[110] Among primarily older children, the prevalence of persistent thrombosis has ranged broadly from 37% to 68% in the few longitudinal studies to date that have systematically evaluated thrombus evolution radiologically.[109,133]

Prognostic Indicators. The ability to predict clinically relevant long-term outcomes of VTE at diagnosis and during the acute phase of treatment is essential for implementation of a future risk-stratified approach to anti-

thrombotic management in children. Historically, few prognostic indicators have been defined in pediatric VTE. The presence of homozygous anticoagulant deficiencies and the persistence of APAs after the diagnosis of VTE have been associated with an increased risk for recurrent VTE. More recently, the presence of multiple thrombophilia traits has been associated with an increased risk for recurrent VTE. In addition, the radiologic finding of complete veno-occlusion at diagnosis of DVT has been linked to an increased risk for persistent thrombosis[194] (which in turn has been associated with the development of venous valvular insufficiency,[193] as noted earlier). Most recently, plasma factor VIII activity greater than 150 U/dL and a D-dimer concentration higher than 500 ng/mL at the time of diagnosis of VTE in children, as well as after 3 to 6 months of standard anticoagulation, have been defined as markers of a composite adverse thrombotic outcome characterized by persistent thrombosis, recurrent VTE, or the development of PTS[109]; similar prognostic findings have been observed in adult VTE.[195-197]

Ischemic Arterial Stroke

Epidemiology

The incidence of perinatal and neonatal ischemic arterial stroke (IAS) has recently been estimated from U.S. National Hospital Discharge Survey data to be approximately 18 per 100,000 per year or 1 in 5000 live births annually.[198] The rate of stroke in later childhood is about a 10th of that for the neonatal period, approximately 2 in 100,000 children per year in the United States.[199] Similar estimates have been provided by the Canadian and Swiss pediatric stroke registries.[200] An early Mayo Clinic retrospective analysis of cases in Rochester, Minnesota, in the late 1970s yielded an equivalent incidence rate for all pediatric IAS of 2.5 per 100,000 per year.[201] However, just as for VTE in children, these epidemiologic data for pediatric IAS probably represent underestimates because of the relatively low index of suspicion for cardiovascular and cerebrovascular events in children as opposed to adults, as well as inaccuracies engendered by

International Classification of Diseases, 9th revision (ICD-9), coding.[202]

Etiology

Causes of IAS in children are less well characterized than in adults, largely as a result of challenges posed by the lower incidence of the disorder in the pediatric population. Whereas in adults, hypertension, diabetes, smoking, and hypercholesterolemia are prominent risk factors for cerebrovascular disease, in children, sickle cell disease, infection, cerebral arteriopathy,[203-205] head/neck trauma (with or without identified arterial dissection),[206-208] congenital cardiac disease, previous transient ischemic attack (TIA),[209] and thrombophilia[209-213] appear to be the most prevalent identified risk factors for IAS. Whether anemia and polycythemia are independent risk factors for pediatric IAS or instead constitute epiphenomena of underlying acute and chronic diseases remains unclear. The subsequent discussion focuses principally on IAS in children without sickle cell disease; for a detailed discussion of IAS in children with sickle cell disease, see Chapter 19.

Vasculopathy in pediatric IAS may be characterized by arterial dissection, narrowing, thrombosis, and an irregular arterial contour (suggestive of possible arteritis). Overall, vasculopathy may be identified in as many as half of non-neonatal IAS cases.[214] Dissection has been demonstrated in 7% to 20% of children with acute IAS.[209,214] Distinction between dissective and nondissective causes of arterial narrowing and thrombosis may be difficult, with variables including the imaging technology used (e.g., CT with angiography, MR angiography, cerebral angiography), the timing in relation to the event, and the experience of the neuroradiologist. Dissection may be due to head/neck trauma or may be spontaneous; limited data suggest that the prevalence of underlying connective tissue disorders may be increased in IAS cases associated with spontaneous dissection, but further controlled studies are needed.[215] Although some studies have indicated that antecedent head trauma appears to be prevalent in pediatric IAS cases, minor head trauma is not infrequent in active children, and there is also considerable potential for recall bias in such studies. A minority of cases of childhood IAS with vasculopathy represent moyamoya syndrome (defined as stenosis in the terminal portion of the internal carotid arteries bilaterally with the formation of collateral arteries, which produces the classic angiographic "puff of smoke") or possible moyamoya syndrome (recently characterized as either unilateral stenosis in the terminal segment of an internal carotid artery with collaterals or the presence of bilateral stenosis of the terminal portion of the internal carotid arteries without collaterals[205]). Other causes of nondissective cerebral arteriopathy in children include a history of recent varicella-zoster infection (i.e., within the previous year),[189] neurofibromatosis type 1, and cranial irradiation for malignancy.[205,216] Despite the high prevalence of vasculopathy in IAS, its etiology in most cases

remains unclear and cannot be attributed to moyamoya, dissection, or defined infections such as varicella. Efforts to further define the causes and natural history of vasculopathy-associated IAS will be fundamental to determining optimal therapeutic interventions in the future.

Infection as an underlying cause of pediatric IAS has been classically associated with tuberculous meningitis, human immunodeficiency virus infection, and primary herpes simplex and varicella virus infection, as well as secondary herpes zoster and varicella-zoster infections. Local bacterial and fungal infections of the head and neck may also contribute to the development of IAS in some pediatric patients. The pathophysiologic mechanisms of infection-associated IAS in children may include direct angioinvasion by the pathogen, local arteritis without direct angioinvasion, and systemic inflammatory and hypercoagulative responses. It is likely that in many instances more than one process contributes to the genesis of IAS. To what extent vasculopathy in pediatric IAS is para-infectious in nature remains poorly understood.

Thrombophilia Risk Factors. Thrombophilia may contribute to risk for IAS by arterial thrombosis or by cerebral embolism of a venous thrombus via a cardiac lesion with a right-to-left shunt. Thrombophilia risk factors in children with IAS include anticoagulant deficiencies (particularly deficiency of protein C[210]), APAs (particularly anticardiolipin antibodies[211,213]), and hyperhomocysteinemia.[217,218] In some cases of IAS developing after acute varicella infection, antibody-mediated acquired protein S deficiency has been demonstrated.[219] It is likely that as is the case for VTE in children, anticoagulant deficiencies are most commonly acquired in the setting of pediatric IAS and are most often para-infectious in nature. However, as in VTE, severe congenital anticoagulant deficiencies may be most likely to be manifested as IAS at an early age. Although homozygosity for the factor V Leiden or prothrombin 20210 mutation is a strong risk factor for VTE in children and hence is probably a risk factor for thromboembolic IAS, it remains unclear whether heterozygosity for the factor V Leiden or prothrombin 20210 mutation confers a meaningful increase in the risk for pediatric IAS.[210-213] Markedly elevated levels of homocysteine are classically associated with metabolic disorders such as homocysteinuria (secondary to cystathionine β-synthase deficiency) and appear to be rare in individuals possessing the thermolabile variant of methylenetetrahydrofolate reductase (MTHFR C677T) in countries in which routine folate supplementation of the diet is undertaken. Therefore, most evidence suggests that this highly prevalent polymorphism is not an independent risk factor for IAS. Although a recent single-institutional U.S. study[220] may contradict this evidence, no contemporaneous control group was used, and further study is therefore necessary. It remains possible that an alternative mechanism other than hyperhomocysteinemia may mediate the risk for IAS, if substantiated.

Another thrombophilia trait, an elevated lipoprotein(a) concentration, has been associated with increased odds for spontaneous IAS (i.e., IAS occurring in the absence of identified clinical risk factors) in non-neonatal German children[212] when a conventional lipoprotein(a) threshold of the 75th percentile derived from previous data in healthy adults was used. This work was recently supported by findings in a U.S. case-control study of porencephaly and IAS in children in which the same lipoprotein(a) threshold was used.[221] However, the magnitude of risk for acute neonatal and childhood IAS (both in the majority of cases with and in the minority without identified clinical risk factors) conferred by elevated levels of lipoprotein(a) remains unclear. In addition, it is unknown whether the adult-derived threshold for lipoprotein(a) concentration historically used clinically and in case-control and cohort studies is appropriate for children. These are key clinically relevant issues that warrant further study.

Clinical Manifestations

The clinical findings in neonates and older children with IAS are largely dependent on the territory and extent of the CNS affected by ischemia/infarction. The most common manifestation of perinatal and neonatal IAS is seizure, sometimes associated with subtle hemiparesis when IAS involves a unilateral middle cerebral artery distribution. Apnea and poor feeding in a term infant should also raise concern for possible perinatal/neonatal IAS. Prenatal IAS in the distribution of the middle cerebral artery, by contrast, is frequently asymptomatic until noted by parents as one-sided weakness, spasticity, or disuse as development of motor activity progresses, frequently with asymmetric reaching for objects or gross motor delay between 4 and 12 months of age.

Manifestations of acute IAS occurring after the neonatal period (i.e., later childhood) include acute- or subacute-onset focal neurologic deficit (e.g., hemiparesis, cranial nerve palsy, dysphasia, incoordination), severe headache, or unexplained new-onset seizure, sometimes accompanied by altered mental status. In cases of dissection-associated IAS in children, a recent history of head/neck trauma is common (see also "Etiology," earlier). Interestingly, a recent single-center retrospective series of IAS in non-neonatal children found that a "nonabrupt" pattern of neurologic symptoms/signs (including those in whom the maximum severity of symptoms/signs in acute IAS developed more than 30 minutes after the onset of symptoms, the symptoms/signs were waxing and waning or were preceded by recurrent transient symptoms/signs with intercurrent resolution) was significantly associated with findings of arteriopathy on diagnostic neuroimaging.[222] Ischemic stroke that is not clearly arterial in distribution (i.e., is not AIS) may be due to global hypoxic-ischemic injury (e.g., with a watershed distribution), may be a regional complication of CNS venous thrombosis, or might be metabolic in etiology.

A classic example of ischemic stroke of metabolic etiology occurs in the syndrome of mitochondrial myopathy, encephalopathy, lactic acidosis, and stroke-like episodes (MELAS). MELAS is caused by mitochondrial DNA defects encoding tRNA involved in the generation of adenosine triphosphate via the electronic transport chain in the mitochondrion. The clinical manifestation of MELAS is ischemic stroke, often recurrent in nature, in preschool or school-age children. Imaging most often reveals persistent ischemia or an infarct in the posterior cerebral hemispheres, with relative sparing of the deep white matter; the affected territory often results in hemianopia.[223] Unlike the cerebral lesions in patients with acute IAS, acute abnormalities at the time of stroke in those with MELAS are bright on apparent diffusion coefficient (ADC) maps of diffusion-weighted MRI.[224] Associated symptoms and signs in MELAS, which are of varying severity and penetrance in affected individuals because of a threshold effect and heteroplasmy in mitochondrial DNA disorders,[225] include short stature, hearing loss, recurrent seizure, proximal muscle weakness, and optic atrophy.[223]

Diagnosis

Imaging Studies. Diagnostic evaluation for suspected acute IAS in children involves either urgent CT of the head with CT angiography of the head and neck or, alternatively, MRI of the brain with diffusion-weighted imaging and MR angiography of the head and neck. Although routine CT and MRI studies evaluate for ischemia, hemorrhage, mass/mass effect, and other non-IAS pathologies, the addition of angiography permits evaluation for arteriopathy, including dissection, stenosis, irregular contour, or intra-arterial thrombosis. CT is often more readily available on an urgent basis than MRI is; however, CT engenders greater radiation exposure than MRI does (especially if angiography is performed) and is less sensitive for the diagnosis of IAS, especially in the acute phase. For the latter reason, if CT is performed initially and is unremarkable in the setting of an acute focal neurologic deficit of unclear etiology, it should be followed by MRI of the brain with diffusion-weighted imaging and MR angiography of the head and neck. In circumstances in which the presence or extent of vasculopathy is unclear or in cases of moyamoya syndrome, the more invasive approach of cerebral angiography is warranted to establish a definitive diagnosis and guide subsequent management.

The pattern of ischemia/infarction may be informative with respect to etiology and consequent management of IAS. For example, multifocal infarction may suggest a thromboembolic cause. A subcortical distribution of ischemia/infarction may suggest disease of small arteries. A watershed distribution of ischemia/infarction may suggest an alternative diagnosis of hypoxic-ischemic injury related to hypotension and other global causes of poor perfusion.

An additional important component of diagnostic imaging in pediatric IAS is echocardiography (either transthoracic, with peripheral intravenous saline injection, or transesophageal) to evaluate for a right-to-left shunting cardiac lesion, with potential implications for management.

Laboratory Studies. Diagnostic laboratory evaluation in children with acute IAS involves a complete blood count, toxicology screen, complete metabolic panel, erythrocyte sedimentation rate/C-reactive protein, β-HCG testing in postmenarchal females, fasting lipid profile, and a comprehensive thrombophilia panel (see the section on VTE diagnosis, earlier). Given that TE is a mechanism for IA and that the cause and pathogenesis of IAS in children are often unclear at the time of diagnosis, thrombophilia testing during diagnostic evaluation for IAS should probably consist of the same comprehensive assessment recommended for acute VTE in children by the Subcommittee for Perinatal and Pediatric Thrombosis of the Scientific and Standardization Committee of the International Society of Thrombosis and Haemostasis (see Table 34-1). As clinical/translational research studies demonstrate the validity of additional IAS-specific thrombophilia risk factors, these should be included as well.

A particularly important issue of thrombophilia testing specific to perinatal IAS involves APA testing. When APA is positive in a neonate with IAS, it is informative to evaluate for APA in the mother to establish a possible cause of vertical (i.e., transplacental) transmission of IgG APA. It is plausible that in some instances APA may be induced by an inflammatory response to IAS rather than representing the cause of the IAS; in such instances, the APA may persist longer than observed for a vertically acquired APA. In IAS with vasculopathy, consideration should be given to investigation for infectious diseases, including serology for viral infections such as varicella-zoster virus, herpes simplex virus, Epstein-Barr virus, parvovirus, and enterovirus; a thorough workup may also include enteroviral cultures of the mouth and rectum and blood testing for *Helicobacter pylori*. If there is associated meningitis or relevant clinical risk factors, testing for tuberculosis should also be undertaken. In the setting of arteritis, rheumatologic evaluation should be considered, including testing for antinuclear antibodies and other markers as warranted. In certain circumstances, additional studies may be warranted, including evaluation for metabolic (including mitochondrial DNA–based) disorders, particularly in IAS with encephalopathy of unclear etiology, nonarterial distribution, lactic acidosis, or other multisystem disorders of unclear cause (e.g., hearing loss, myalgia, endocrinopathy).

The role of lumbar puncture, especially when weighed against the need to withhold anticoagulation periprocedurally, is controversial. Unfortunately, the circumstances in which risk for progression or early recurrence of IAS is among the greatest (e.g., acute/subacute period of IAS with vasculopathy) and therefore in which maintenance of effective anticoagulation may be most critical are also the same circumstances in which lumbar puncture for investigation of infectious diseases would be among the most informative (yet requires suspension of anticoagulation).

Treatment

Initial management of IAS in children must emphasize appropriate control of blood pressure, temperature, glycemia, oxygenation, and hydration. Unfortunately, there is no evidence from clinical trials on which to base specific interventions for acute IAS in children who do not have sickle cell disease. Nevertheless, pediatric IAS treatment recommendations[131,226] have been developed on the basis of registry and cohort study data in neonates and older children, as well as to some extent on evidence extrapolated from studies in adult IAS.

In the absence of a thromboembolic etiology, underlying vasculopathy, or potent thrombophilia, antithrombotic therapy is rarely used for perinatal/neonatal IAS, as appropriate for the low risk (cumulative incidence of approximately 3% at a median follow-up duration of 3.5 years[227]) for recurrent IAS/VTE. Therefore, for most cases of perinatal IAS, an emphasis on future treatments directed toward minimization of infarction during the acute and subacute period of IAS is likely to be more beneficial than reduction in risk for recurrent IAS.

In contrast to neonates, antithrombotic intervention in older children with acute IAS is generally recommended as secondary IAS prophylaxis, given the relatively high recurrence rate (cumulative incidence of approximately 40% at 5 years[209]). A nonrandomized prospective cohort-based study of LMWH versus aspirin as secondary IAS prophylaxis detected no significant difference in the cumulative incidence of recurrent IAS between the these two therapies.[228] The optimal type of antithrombotic strategy and duration of antithrombotic therapy for a given IAS subtype in this age group remain unclear in the absence of evidence from randomized controlled trials. Antiplatelet therapy with daily aspirin is widely used in childhood IAS, with variable intensity (e.g., 1 to 5 mg/kg per dose) and duration (3 months, 1 year, indefinitely). In the setting of childhood IAS with non–moyamoya-associated vasculopathy, either antiplatelet therapy or therapeutic anticoagulation with LMWH or warfarin (often initially with unfractionated heparin in the acute period given its rapid reversibility should bleeding complications arise) is often considered for a period of at least 3 months, especially in the presence of thrombophilia. Patients who experience recurrent IAS while maintained on antiplatelet therapy should be considered for therapeutic anticoagulation.

Pediatric IAS with moyamoya syndrome presents a particular challenge in optimal management. Anticoagulation and antiplatelet agents have been considered possible therapies. However, in view of the heightened risk for recurrent IAS, neurosurgical approaches at revascularization (including indirect means, such as encephaloduroarteriomyosynangiosis [EDAMS],[229] and direct means, such as superficial temporal artery branch–to–middle cerebral artery branch or anterior cerebral artery branch bypass[230]) are generally preferred, and anticoagulation or antiplatelet therapy is perhaps best reserved for children with appropriately defined "possible moyamoya" in the absence of recurrent symptoms or recurrent IAS/TIA events.

Thrombolytic approaches have been used in isolated cases of pediatric IAS.[231] Because only a minute proportion of cases of acute IAS in children are diagnosed within the first few hours of symptomatic onset, a multicenter collaborative clinical trial approach with stringent uniform exclusion criteria will be required to address whether adult evidence for a beneficial role of systemic administration of tissue plasminogen activator in the immediate period after onset of IAS may also apply to children. Other thrombolytic approaches include interventional pharmacomechanical thrombolysis/thrombectomy for acute IAS associated with arterial thrombosis. However, technical limitations (i.e., size constraints) are posed by the small-caliber pediatric cerebral vasculature, and the safety and efficacy of this approach warrant formal study.

In the subacute period after IAS in children and over the long term, treatment to optimize outcomes includes rehabilitation services (physical therapy, occupational therapy, speech therapy) and neuropsychological interventions (educational, vocational, and mental health services). The need for these services should be assessed on a case-by-case basis and provided in accordance with the findings of comprehensive multidisciplinary assessment involving the expertise of pediatric neurology, rehabilitation medicine, and neuropsychology. Furthermore, the impact of rehabilitative and neuropsychological interventions on the progress and future need of pediatric IAS

patients should be regularly reassessed in extended follow-up.

Outcomes

Complications. Complications of IAS can occur both acutely and over the long term. Short-term adverse outcomes include death from uncontrolled increased intracranial pressure with uncal herniation, status epilepticus, or hemodynamic instability in patients with extensive intracardiac thrombosis associated with cardioembolic IAS and major hemorrhagic complications, including those related to antithrombotic interventions, as well as postischemic CNS hemorrhage, acute neurologic deficits, and early recurrence of IAS or VTE. Long-term sequelae of IAS in children include residual neurologic deficits, cognitive impairments, and recurrent IAS or VTE.

The outcomes of pediatric IAS, stratified by diagnosis in the neonatal period versus older childhood, are summarized in Tables 34-5 and 34-6.[189,200,209,214,227,232-236] In brief, death as a result of perinatal/neonatal IAS is quite rare, and for childhood IAS the case fatality rate (i.e., cumulative incidence) ranges between 2% and 16% in various analyses, although the time period over which death was attributable to IAS has not been well delineated in most studies. The risk (i.e., cumulative incidence) of recurrent IAS/VTE in perinatal/neonatal IAS is approximately 3% at a median follow-up duration of 3.5 years,[227] whereas the risk for recurrence after nonneonatal IAS varies widely between 19% and 40% at a fixed follow-up duration of 5 years. With regard to neurologic and rehabilitative (neuromotor, speech) outcomes, the prevalence of neuromotor deficits after perinatal/neonatal IAS varies widely between 36% at a median follow-up of 19 months and approximately 60% at average follow-up times of 2 to 6 years across studies. Furthermore, the prevalence of either hemiplegia or asymmetric tone without hemiplegia has been shown in

TABLE 34-5	Outcomes of Neonatal Ischemic Arterial Stroke							
Author	Year of Publication	Country	# Cases	Average Duration of Follow-up	Recurrent IAS	Persistent Neuromotor Deficits	Persistent Cognitive Deficits	IAS-Related Mortality
deVeber et al.[189]	2000	Canada	33	2 yr	N/A	64%	3%	0%
Kurnik et al.[227]	2003	Germany	215	3.5 yr	2%	N/A	N/A	N/A
Mercuri et al.[232]	2004	UK	22	≈6 yr	N/A	59%	14%	2%
Steinlin et al.[200]	2005	Switzerland	19	6 mo	N/A	58%	N/A	0%
Kirton et al.[233]	2007	Canada	14	19 mo	N/A	36%	N/A	N/A
Fullerton et al.[234]	2007	USA	84	6 yr	0%	N/A	N/A	2%

Note: Expressive speech deficits were evaluated in one study,[62] with a defined prevalence of 12%.
IAS, ischemic arterial stroke; N/A, not available.

TABLE 34-6   Outcomes of Non-neonatal Childhood Ischemic Arterial Stroke

Author	Year of Publication	Country	# Cases	Average Duration of Follow-up	Recurrent IAS	Persistent Neuromotor Deficits	Persistent Cognitive Deficits	IAS-Related Mortality
deVeber et al.[189]	2000	Canada	90	2 yr	11%	67%	17%	0%
Lanthier et al.[235]	2000	Canada	46	N/A	17%	41%	N/A	N/A
Chabrier et al.[214]	2000	France	59	2.5 yr	22%	73%	N/A	N/A
Sträter et al.[236]	2002	Germany	301	3.7 yr	7%	N/A	N/A	2%
Steinlin et al.[200]	2005	Switzerland	38	6 mo	N/A	74%	N/A	3%
Ganesan et al.[209]	2006	UK	212	2.2 yr	41% (5 yr)	N/A	N/A	2%
Fullerton et al.[234]	2007	USA	92	5 yr	19% (5 yr)	N/A	N/A	4%

Note: Expressive speech deficits were evaluated in one study,[62] with a defined prevalence of 18%.
IAS, ischemic arterial stroke; N/A, not available.

one study to be 30% at approximately 5 to 7 years of age.[236] By comparison, the prevalence of persistent neuromotor deficits for IAS diagnosed in later childhood is approximately 70% at average follow-up durations ranging from 6 months to 2.5 years across studies. Expressive speech impairments have been noted in 12% of perinatal/neonatal and 18% of non-neonatal IAS cases in one study.[189] As for neuropsychological outcomes, cognitive or behavioral deficits have been discerned in a few studies in 3% to 14% of children with perinatal/neonatal IAS at 2 to 6 years' average follow-up and in 17% of children at 2 years' follow-up in whom IAS occurred later in childhood.

Long-Term Outcomes. As in pediatric VTE, the ability to predict clinically relevant long-term outcomes of IAS at diagnosis and during the acute phase of treatment is essential to the development of appropriate management paradigms in children. However, such efforts have been particularly challenged by the relative infrequency of pediatric IAS cases and the heterogeneity in causes and IAS subtypes in this complex disorder. In perinatal/neonatal ischemic stroke, a cohort study[237] of 24 neonates with ischemic stroke, including IAS mostly in the middle cerebral artery territory but some with primarily watershed area involvement, suggested that an abnormal background on early neonatal encephalography (as opposed to focal epileptiform discharges) and a distribution that includes a cerebral hemisphere along with both the internal capsule and basal ganglia (as opposed to only one or two of these regions) serve as factors that are each associated with the development of a persistent neurologic deficit. The deficits consisted of either hemiplegia or asymmetry of tone without hemiplegia. These data were subsequently substantiated at later follow-up in early childhood.[232] In a smaller series, the presence of signal abnormalities in the posterior limb of the internal capsule

or in the cerebral peduncles on MRI with diffusion-weighted imaging and ADC mapping in acute perinatal/neonatal IAS was recently found to be associated with the development of either hemiplegia or asymmetry of tone without hemiplegia at a median follow-up of longer than 18 months[238] and is supported by similar findings in a separate cohort at a median follow-up of 5.5 years. Most recently, the use of computer-assisted quantitation of the degree of descending corticospinal tract signal abnormality on MRI with diffusion-weighted imaging in a series of 14 neonates with IAS demonstrated that the proportion of the cerebral peduncle affected and the total length of the descending corticospinal tract involved correlate with the development of hemiparesis.[233] Whereas correlates of neuromotor outcome in perinatal/neonatal IAS are becoming better defined, predictors of recurrent stroke in this group have been elusive, particularly given the infrequency of recurrent IAS after perinatal/neonatal IAS.

Prognostic Indicators. A single-center retrospective study in the 1990s demonstrated a statistically significant increase in the odds of recurrent IAS in patients with more than one IAS risk factor (e.g., vasculopathy, thrombophilia traits, cardiac disorders, infection) identified at the time of the acute event as opposed to children with one or no risk factors.[232] In addition, patients with moyamoya are at greatly increased risk for recurrent IAS and persistent neurologic deficits.[209,214,239] In a large single-center cohort study of mixed prospective-retrospective design,[209] moyamoya was one of only two independent risk factors for recurrent ischemic events (consisting of IAS, TIA, or death with reinfarction). The association of vasculopathy with increased risk for recurrent IAS in children has recently been demonstrated in a U.S. population-based cohort,[234] thus confirming previous findings from a large multicenter German prospective cohort study of childhood IAS.[227] In the German study, elevated serum levels of lipoprotein(a), congenital protein C deficiency, and vasculopathy were each found to be independent risk factors for recurrent IAS. Although APAs were not evaluated in the multivariate model of the German cohort study, a two-center British-Canadian cohort study of non-neonatal IAS in 185 children reported that no increased risk for recurrent IAS appears to exist with respect to persistently positive IgG-type anticardiolipin antibody titers.[240] Although the statistically nonsignificant unadjusted difference in 3-year recurrence rates between groups positive and negative for anticardiolipin IgG, 38% versus 26%, might nevertheless be considered clinically meaningful, the difference in proportional hazard functions for recurrence of IAS between the two groups was also not statistically significant after adjustment for covariates of IAS causes and treatment types. However, few cases of high-titer antibodies were represented in the cohort. Clearly, further basic and translational research is needed to discern which subtypes of anticardiolipin antibodies may be most vasculopathic and thrombogenic, and such research will probably involve secondary characterization of APAs with functional assays.

Future studies should seek to validate the predictive capacity of these potentially quite meaningful associations in pediatric IAS cohorts distinct from those in which these associations have been derived. Collaborative multicenter cohort studies and trials groups, such as the International Pediatric Stroke Study Group, offer optimism for the establishment of more robust evidence of predictors of outcome in neonatal and childhood IAS according to common causes and vascular pathologies so that risk-stratified approaches to the management of pediatric IAS in future years can be optimized.

REFERENCES

1. Baglin T. Acquired bleeding disorders. Clin Med. 2005;5:326-328.
2. Smith WL, Garavito RM, DeWitt DL. Prostaglandin endoperoxide H synthases (cyclooxygenases)-1 and -2. J Biol Chem. 1996;271:33157-33160.
3. Catella-Lawson F, Reilly MP, Kapoor SC, et al. Cyclooxygenase inhibitors and the antiplatelet effects of aspirin. N Engl J Med. 2001;345:1809-1817.
4. Pastakia KB, Terle D, Prodouz KN. Penicillin-induced dysfunction of platelet membrane glycoproteins. J Lab Clin Med. 1993;121:546-554.
5. Pastakia KB, Terle D, Prodouz KN. Penicillin inhibits agonist-induced expression of platelet surface membrane glycoproteins. Ann N Y Acad Sci. 1993;677:437-439.
6. Dale J, Landmark KH, Myhre E. The effects of nifedipine, a calcium antagonist, on platelet function. Am Heart J. 1983;105:103-105.
7. Svehla C, Spankova H, Mlejnkova M. The effect of tricyclic antidepressive drugs on adrenaline and adenosine diphosphate induced platelet aggregation. J Pharm Pharmacol. 1966;18:616-617.
8. Gerstner T, Teich M, Bell N, et al. Valproate-associated coagulopathies are frequent and variable in children. Epilepsia. 2006;47:1136-1143.
9. Lefkovits J, Plow EF, Topol EJ. Platelet glycoprotein IIb/IIIa receptors in cardiovascular medicine. N Engl J Med. 1995;332:1553-1559.
10. Ingerslev J, Vanek T, Culic S. Use of recombinant factor VIIa for emergency reversal of anticoagulation. J Postgrad Med. 2007;53:17-22.
11. Koscielny J, von Tempelhoff GF, Ziemer S, et al. A practical concept for preoperative management of patients with impaired primary hemostasis. Clin Appl Thromb Hemost. 2004;10:155-166.
12. Levi M, de Jonge E, van der Poll T. New treatment strategies for disseminated intravascular coagulation based on current understanding of the pathophysiology. Ann Med. 2004;36:41-49.
13. Oren H, Cingoz I, Duman M, et al. Disseminated intravascular coagulation in pediatric patients: clinical and laboratory features and prognostic factors influencing the survival. Pediatr Hematol Oncol. 2005;22:679-688.
14. Manco-Johnson MJ. Disseminated intravascular coagulation. In Hoekelmann RA, Adam HM, Nelson NM, et al (eds). Primary Pediatric Care, 4th ed. St. Louis, CV Mosby, 2001.
15. Taylor FB Jr, Toh CH, Hoots WK, et al. Towards definition, clinical and laboratory criteria, and a scoring system for disseminated intravascular coagulation. Thromb Haemost. 2001;86:1327-1330.
16. Toh CH, Downey C. Back to the future: testing in disseminated intravascular coagulation. Blood Coagul Fibrinolysis. 2005;16:535-542.
17. Bick RL. Disseminated intravascular coagulation: pathophysiological mechanisms and manifestations. Semin Thromb Hemost. 1998;24:3-18.
18. Toh CH. Laboratory testing in disseminated intravascular coagulation. Semin Thromb Hemost. 2001;27:653-656.
19. Esmon CT. Possible involvement of cytokines in diffuse intravascular coagulation and thrombosis. Baillieres Best Pract Res Clin Haematol. 1999;12:343-359.
20. Asakura H, Wada H, Okamoto K, et al. Evaluation of haemostatic molecular markers for diagnosis of disseminated intravascular coagulation in patients with infections. Thromb Haemost. 2006;95:282-287.
21. Falanga A, Rickles FR. Pathogenesis and management of the bleeding diathesis in acute promyelocytic leukaemia. Best Pract Res Clin Haematol. 2003;16:463-482.
22. Levi M, de Jonge E, van der Poll T. Plasma and plasma components in the management of disseminated intravascular coagulation. Best Pract Res Clin Haematol. 2006;19:127-142.
23. Pernerstorfer T, Hollenstein U, Hansen J, et al. Heparin blunts endotoxin-induced coagulation activation. Circulation. 1999;100:2485-2490.
24. Feinstein DI. Diagnosis and management of disseminated intravascular coagulation: the role of heparin therapy. Blood. 1982;60:284-287.
25. Wiedermann CJ, Hoffmann JN, Juers M, et al. High-dose antithrombin III in the treatment of severe sepsis in patients with a high risk of death: efficacy and safety. Crit Care Med. 2006;34:285-292.
26. Kienast J, Juers M, Wiedermann CJ, et al. Treatment effects of high-dose antithrombin without concomitant

heparin in patients with severe sepsis with or without disseminated intravascular coagulation. J Thromb Haemost. 2006;4:90-97.

27. Hoffmann JN, Muhlbayer D, Jochum M, Inthorn D. Effect of long-term and high-dose antithrombin supplementation on coagulation and fibrinolysis in patients with severe sepsis. Crit Care Med. 2004;32:1851-1859.

28. Dhainaut JF, Yan SB, Joyce DE, et al. Treatment effects of drotrecogin alfa (activated) in patients with severe sepsis with or without overt disseminated intravascular coagulation. J Thromb Haemost. 2004;2:1924-1933.

29. Fourrier F, Chopin C, Huart JJ, et al. Double-blind, placebo-controlled trial of antithrombin III concentrates in septic shock with disseminated intravascular coagulation. Chest. 1993;104:882-888.

30. Wiedermann CJ, Kaneider NC. A systematic review of antithrombin concentrate use in patients with disseminated intravascular coagulation of severe sepsis. Blood Coagul Fibrinolysis. 2006;17:521-526.

31. Sajan I, Da-Silva SS, Dellinger RP. Drotrecogin alfa (activated) in an infant with gram-negative septic shock. J Intensive Care Med. 2004;19:51-55.

32. Hedner U. Mechanism of action of factor VIIa in the treatment of coagulopathies. Semin Thromb Hemost. 2006;32(Suppl 1):77-85.

33. Franchini M, Zaffanello M, Veneri D. Recombinant factor VIIa. An update on its clinical use. Thromb Haemost. 2005;93:1027-1035.

34. de Pont AC, Moons AH, de Jonge E, et al. Recombinant nematode anticoagulant protein c2, an inhibitor of tissue factor/factor VIIa, attenuates coagulation and the interleukin-10 response in human endotoxemia. J Thromb Haemost. 2004;2:65-70.

35. Lee AY, Vlasuk GP. Recombinant nematode anticoagulant protein c2 and other inhibitors targeting blood coagulation factor VIIa/tissue factor. J Intern Med. 2003;254:313-321.

36. Moons AH, Peters RJ, Bijsterveld NR, et al. Recombinant nematode anticoagulant protein c2, an inhibitor of the tissue factor/factor VIIa complex, in patients undergoing elective coronary angioplasty. J Am Coll Cardiol. 2003;41:2147-2153.

37. Senzolo M, Burra P, Cholongitas E, Burroughs AK. New insights into the coagulopathy of liver disease and liver transplantation. World J Gastroenterol. 2006;12:7725-7736.

38. Kerr R. New insights into haemostasis in liver failure. Blood Coagul Fibrinolysis. 2003;14(Suppl 1):S43-S45.

39. Green G, Thomson JM, Dymock IW, Poller L. Abnormal fibrin polymerization in liver disease. Br J Haematol. 1976;34:427-439.

40. Caldwell SH, Chang C, Macik BG. Recombinant activated factor VII (rFVIIa) as a hemostatic agent in liver disease: a break from convention in need of controlled trials. Hepatology. 2004;39:592-598.

41. Sarafanov AG, Ananyeva NM, Shima M, Saenko EL. Cell surface heparan sulfate proteoglycans participate in factor VIII catabolism mediated by low density lipoprotein receptor–related protein. J Biol Chem. 2001;276:11970-11979.

42. Carr JM. Disseminated intravascular coagulation in cirrhosis. Hepatology. 1989;10:103-110.

43. Paramo JA, Rocha E. Hemostasis in advanced liver disease. Semin Thromb Hemost. 1993;19:184-190.

44. Everson GT. A hepatologist's perspective on the management of coagulation disorders before liver transplantation. Liver Transpl Surg. 1997;3:646-652.

45. de Franchis R, Arcidiacono PG, Carpinelli L, et al. Randomized controlled trial of desmopressin plus terlipressin vs. terlipressin alone for the treatment of acute variceal hemorrhage in cirrhotic patients: a multicenter, double-blind study. New Italian Endoscopic Club. Hepatology. 1993;18:1102-1107.

46. Wong AY, Irwin MG, Hui TW, et al. Desmopressin does not decrease blood loss and transfusion requirements in patients undergoing hepatectomy. Can J Anaesth. 2003;50:14-20.

47. Pereira SP, Rowbotham D, Fitt S, et al. Pharmacokinetics and efficacy of oral versus intravenous mixed-micellar phylloquinone (vitamin K_1) in severe acute liver disease. J Hepatol. 2005;42:365-370.

48. Carlier M, Van Obbergh LJ, Veyckemans F, et al. Hemostasis in children undergoing liver transplantation. Semin Thromb Hemost. 1993;19:218-222.

49. Grosse H, Lobbes W, Sato M, et al. Systemic fibrinogenolysis in liver transplantation. Transplant Proc. 1990;22:2303-2304.

50. Superina RA, Pearl RH, Roberts EA, et al. Liver transplantation in children: the initial Toronto experience. J Pediatr Surg. 1989;24:1013-1019.

51. Planinsic RM, van der Meer J, Testa G, et al. Safety and efficacy of a single bolus administration of recombinant factor VIIa in liver transplantation due to chronic liver disease. Liver Transpl. 2005;11:895-900.

52. Lodge JP, Jonas S, Jones RM, et al. Efficacy and safety of repeated perioperative doses of recombinant factor VIIa in liver transplantation. Liver Transpl. 2005;11:973-979.

53. Gibbs NM. The place of recombinant activated factor VII in liver transplantation. Int Anesthesiol Clin. 2006;44:99-110.

54. Paiva SA, Sepe TE, Booth SL, et al. Interaction between vitamin K nutriture and bacterial overgrowth in hypochlorhydria induced by omeprazole. Am J Clin Nutr. 1998;68:699-704.

55. Bay A, Oner AF, Celebi V, Uner A. Evaluation of vitamin K deficiency in children with acute and intractable diarrhea. Adv Ther. 2006;23:469-474.

56. Kumar R, Marwaha N, Marwaha RK, Garewal G. Vitamin K deficiency in diarrhoea. Indian J Pediatr. 2001;68:235-238.

57. Rashid M, Durie P, Andrew M, et al. Prevalence of vitamin K deficiency in cystic fibrosis. Am J Clin Nutr. 1999;70:378-382.

58. Mager DR, McGee PL, Furuya KN, Roberts EA. Prevalence of vitamin K deficiency in children with mild to moderate chronic liver disease. J Pediatr Gastroenterol Nutr. 2006;42:71-76.

59. Ingels M, Lai C, Tai W, et al. A prospective study of acute, unintentional, pediatric superwarfarin ingestions managed without decontamination. Ann Emerg Med. 2002;40:73-78.

60. Watt BE, Proudfoot AT, Bradberry SM, Vale JA. Anticoagulant rodenticides. Toxicol Rev. 2005;24:259-269.

61. Barron MA, Doyle J, Zlotkin S. Vitamin K deficiency in children pre–bone marrow transplantation. Bone Marrow Transplant. 2006;37:151-154.

62. Crowther MA, Douketis JD, Schnurr T, et al. Oral vitamin K lowers the international normalized ratio more rapidly than subcutaneous vitamin K in the treatment of warfarin-associated coagulopathy. A randomized, controlled trial. Ann Intern Med. 2002;137:251-254.

63. Hellstern P. Production and composition of prothrombin complex concentrates: correlation between composition and therapeutic efficiency. Thromb Res. 1999;95: S7-S12.

64. Brady KM, Easley RB, Tobias JD. Recombinant activated factor VII (rFVIIa) treatment in infants with hemorrhage. Paediatr Anaesth. 2006;16:1042-1046.

65. Hubbard D, Tobias JD. Intracerebral hemorrhage due to hemorrhagic disease of the newborn and failure to administer vitamin K at birth. South Med J. 2006;99: 1216-1220.

66. Kaaja E, Kaaja R, Matila R, Hiilesmaa V. Enzyme-inducing antiepileptic drugs in pregnancy and the risk of bleeding in the neonate. Neurology. 2002;58:549-553.

67. Choulika S, Grabowski E, Holmes LB. Is antenatal vitamin K prophylaxis needed for pregnant women taking anticonvulsants? Am J Obstet Gynecol. 2004;190: 882-883.

68. Yamasmit W, Chaithongwongwatthana S, Tolosa JE. Prenatal vitamin K_1 administration in epileptic women to prevent neonatal hemorrhage: is it effective? J Reprod Med. 2006;51:463-466.

69. Levy JH. Massive transfusion coagulopathy. Semin Hematol. 2006;43:S59-S63.

70. Kokoszka A, Kuflik P, Bitan F, et al. Evidence-based review of the role of aprotinin in blood conservation during orthopaedic surgery. J Bone Joint Surg Am. 2005; 87:1129-1136.

71. Kinzel V, Shakespeare D, Derbyshire D. The effect of aprotinin on blood loss in bilateral total knee arthroplasty. Knee. 2005;12:107-111.

72. Levy JH. Efficacy and safety of aprotinin in cardiac surgery. Orthopedics. 2004;27:s659-s662.

73. Xia VW, Steadman RH. Antifibrinolytics in orthotopic liver transplantation: current status and controversies. Liver Transpl. 2005;11:10-18.

74. Levy JH, Pifarre R, Schaff HV, et al. A multicenter, double-blind, placebo-controlled trial of aprotinin for reducing blood loss and the requirement for donor-blood transfusion in patients undergoing repeat coronary artery bypass grafting. Circulation. 1995;92:2236-2244.

75. Arnold DM, Fergusson DA, Chan AK, et al. Avoiding transfusions in children undergoing cardiac surgery: a meta-analysis of randomized trials of aprotinin. Anesth Analg. 2006;102:731-737.

76. Gowers CJ, Parr MJ. Recombinant activated factor VIIa use in massive transfusion and coagulopathy unresponsive to conventional therapy. Anaesth Intensive Care. 2005;33: 196-200.

77. Tobias JD, Simsic JM, Weinstein S, et al. Recombinant factor VIIa to control excessive bleeding following surgery for congenital heart disease in pediatric patients. J Intensive Care Med. 2004;19:270-273.

78. Pychynska-Pokorska M, Moll JJ, Krajewski W, Jarosik P. The use of recombinant coagulation factor VIIa in uncontrolled postoperative bleeding in children undergoing cardiac surgery with cardiopulmonary bypass. Pediatr Crit Care Med. 2004;5:246-250.

79. Dominguez TE, Mitchell M, Friess SH, et al. Use of recombinant factor VIIa for refractory hemorrhage during extracorporeal membrane oxygenation. Pediatr Crit Care Med. 2005;6:348-351.

80. Razon Y, Erez E, Vidne B, et al. Recombinant factor VIIa (NovoSeven) as a hemostatic agent after surgery for congenital heart disease. Paediatr Anaesth. 2005;15: 235-240.

81. DiMichele DM. Acquired coagulation factor inhibitors. In Goodnight SH, Hathaway WE (eds). Disorders of Hemostasis and Thrombosis: A Clinical Guide, 2nd ed. New York, McGraw-Hill, 2001, pp 192-206.

82. Moraca RJ, Ragni MV. Acquired anti-FVIII inhibitors in children. Haemophilia. 2002;8:28-32.

83. Sakai M, Shima M, Shirahata A. Successful steroid pulse treatment in childhood acquired haemophilia with nephrotic syndrome. Haemophilia. 2005;11:285-289.

84. Green D, Lechner K. A survey of 215 non-hemophilic patients with inhibitors to factor VIII. Thromb Haemost. 1981;45:200-203.

85. Miller K, Neely JE, Krivit W, Edson JR. Spontaneously acquired factor IX inhibitor in a nonhemophiliac child. J Pediatr. 1978;93:232-234.

86. Berman BW, McIntosh S, Clyne LP, et al. Spontaneously acquired factor IX inhibitors in childhood. Am J Pediatr Hematol Oncol. 1981;3:77-81.

87. Mazzucconi MG, Peraino M, Bizzoni L, et al. Acquired inhibitor against factor IX in a child: successful treatment with high-dose immunoglobulin and dexamethasone. Haemophilia. 1999;5:132-134.

88. Ortel TL, Mercer MC, Thames EH, et al. Immunologic impact and clinical outcomes after surgical exposure to bovine thrombin. Ann Surg. 2001;233:88-96.

89. Savage WJ, Kickler TS, Takemoto CM. Acquired coagulation factor inhibitors in children after topical bovine thrombin exposure. Pediatr Blood Cancer. 2007;49: 1025-1029.

90. Chediak J, Ashenhurst JB, Garlick I, Desser RK. Successful management of bleeding in a patient with factor V inhibitor by platelet transfusions. Blood. 1980;56: 835-841.

91. Federici AB. Acquired von Willebrand syndrome: an underdiagnosed and misdiagnosed bleeding complication in patients with lymphoproliferative and myeloproliferative disorders. Semin Hematol. 2006;43:S48-S58.

92. Federici AB, Rand JH, Bucciarelli P, et al. Acquired von Willebrand syndrome: data from an international registry. Thromb Haemost. 2000;84:345-349.

93. Serdaroglu G, Tutuncuoglu S, Kavakli K, Tekgul H. Coagulation abnormalities and acquired von Willebrand's disease type 1 in children receiving valproic acid. J Child Neurol. 2002;17:41-43.

94. Friederich PW, Wever PC, Briet E, et al. Successful treatment with recombinant factor VIIa of therapy-resistant severe bleeding in a patient with acquired von Willebrand disease. Am J Hematol. 2001;66:292-294.

95. Casais P, Meschengieser SS, Gennari LC, et al. Morbidity of lupus anticoagulants in children: a single institution experience. Thromb Res. 2004;114:245-249.

96. Bernstein ML, Salusinsky-Sternbach M, Bellefleur M, Esseltine DW. Thrombotic and hemorrhagic complications in children with the lupus anticoagulant. Am J Dis Child. 1984;138:1132-1135.

97. Jaeger U, Kapiotis S, Pabinger I, et al. Transient lupus anticoagulant associated with hypoprothrombinemia and factor XII deficiency following adenovirus infection. Ann Hematol. 1993;67:95-99.

98. Bernini JC, Buchanan GR, Ashcraft J. Hypoprothrombinemia and severe hemorrhage associated with a lupus anticoagulant. J Pediatr. 1993;123:937-939.

99. Humphries JE, Acker MN, Pinkston JE, Ruddy S. Transient lupus anticoagulant associated with prothrombin deficiency: unusual cause of bleeding in a 5-year-old girl. Am J Pediatr Hematol Oncol. 1994;16:372-376.

100. Lee MT, Nardi MA, Hadzi-Nesic J, Karpatkin M. Transient hemorrhagic diathesis associated with an inhibitor of prothrombin with lupus anticoagulant in a $1\frac{1}{2}$-year-old girl: report of a case and review of the literature. Am J Hematol. 1996;51:307-314.

101. Becton DL, Stine KC. Transient lupus anticoagulants associated with hemorrhage rather than thrombosis: the hemorrhagic lupus anticoagulant syndrome. J Pediatr. 1997;130:998-1000.

102. Vivaldi P, Rossetti G, Galli M, Finazzi G. Severe bleeding due to acquired hypoprothrombinemia–lupus anticoagulant syndrome. Case report and review of literature. Haematologica. 1997;82:345-347.

103. Bajaj SP, Rapaport SI, Fierer DS, et al. A mechanism for the hypoprothrombinemia of the acquired hypoprothrombinemia–lupus anticoagulant syndrome. Blood. 1983;61:684-692.

104. Andrew M, David M, Adams M, et al. Venous thromboembolic complications (VTE) in children: first analyses of the Canadian Registry of VTE. Blood. 1994;83:1251-1257.

105. van Ommen CH, Heijboer H, Buller HR, et al. Venous thromboembolism in childhood: a prospective two-year registry in The Netherlands. J Pediatr. 2001;139:676-681.

106. Stein PD, Kayali F, Olson RE. Incidence of venous thromboembolism in infants and children: data from the National Hospital Discharge Survey. J Pediatr. 2004;145:563-565.

107. Nowak-Gottl U, von Kries R, Gobel U. Neonatal symptomatic thromboembolism in Germany: two year survey. Arch Dis Child Fetal Neonatal Ed. 1997;76:F163-F167.

108. Schmidt B, Andrew M. Neonatal thrombosis: report of a prospective Canadian and international registry. Pediatrics. 1995;96:939-943.

109. Goldenberg NA, Knapp-Clevenger R, Manco-Johnson MJ. Elevated plasma factor VIII and D-dimer levels as predictors of poor outcomes of thrombosis in children. N Engl J Med. 2004;351:1081-1088.

110. Monagle P, Adams M, Mahoney M, et al. Outcome of pediatric thromboembolic disease: a report from the Canadian Childhood Thrombophilia Registry. Pediatr Res. 2000;47:763-766.

111. Andrew M, Marzinotto V, Pencharz P, et al. A cross-sectional study of catheter-related thrombosis in children receiving total parenteral nutrition at home. J Pediatr. 1995;126:358-363.

112. Bagnall HA, Gomperts E, Atkinson JB. Continuous infusion of low-dose urokinase in the treatment of central venous catheter thrombosis in infants and children. Pediatrics. 1989;83:963-966.

113. Bern MM, Lokich JJ, Wallach SR, et al. Very low doses of warfarin can prevent thrombosis in central venous catheters. A randomized prospective trial. Ann Intern Med. 1990;112:423-428.

114. Mehta S, Connors AF Jr, Danish EH, Grisoni E. Incidence of thrombosis during central venous catheterization of newborns: a prospective study. J Pediatr Surg. 1992;27:18-22.

115. Mirro J Jr, Rao BN, Stokes DC, et al. A prospective study of Hickman/Broviac catheters and implantable ports in pediatric oncology patients. J Clin Oncol. 1989;7:214-222.

116. Moukarzel A, Azancot-Benisty A, Brun P, et al. M-mode and two-dimensional echocardiography in the routine follow-up of central venous catheters in children receiving total parenteral nutrition. JPEN J Parenter Enteral Nutr. 1991;15:551-555.

117. Manco-Johnson MJ, Grabowski EF, Hellgreen M, et al. Laboratory testing for thrombophilia in pediatric patients. On behalf of the Subcommittee for Perinatal and Pediatric Thrombosis of the Scientific and Standardization Committee of the International Society of Thrombosis and Haemostasis (ISTH). Thromb Haemost. 2002;88:155-156.

118. Buck JR, Connors RH, Coon WW, et al. Pulmonary embolism in children. J Pediatr Surg. 1981;16:385-391.

119. David M, Andrew M. Venous thromboembolic complications in children. J Pediatr. 1993;123:337-346.

120. Hoyer PF, Gonda S, Barthels M, et al. Thromboembolic complications in children with nephrotic syndrome. Risk and incidence. Acta Paediatr Scand. 1986;75:804-810.

121. van Ommen CH, Monagle P, Peters M. Pulmonary embolism in children. In van Beek E, Oudkerk M, ten Cate JW (eds). Pulmonary Embolism: Epidemiology, Diagnosis and Treatment. Oxford, Blackwell Scientific, 1999.

122. Kuhle S, Massicotte P, Chan A, Mitchell L. A case series of 72 neonates with renal vein thrombosis. Data from the 1-800-NO-CLOTS Registry. Thromb Haemost. 2004;92:729-733.

123. Berman W Jr, Fripp RR, Yabek SM, et al. Great vein and right atrial thrombosis in critically ill infants and children with central venous lines. Chest. 1991;99:963-967.

124. Ross P Jr, Ehrenkranz R, Kleinman CS, Seashore JH. Thrombus associated with central venous catheters in infants and children. J Pediatr Surg. 1989;24:253-256.

125. Schettino GC, Fagundes ED, Roquete ML, et al. Portal vein thrombosis in children and adolescents. J Pediatr (Rio J). 2006;82:171-178.

126. Greenway A, Massicotte MP, Monagle P. Neonatal thrombosis and its treatment. Blood Rev. 2004;18:75-84.

127. Goldenberg NA, Knapp-Clevenger R, Hays T, Manco-Johnson MJ. Lemierre's and Lemierre's-like syndromes in children: survival and thromboembolic outcomes. Pediatrics. 2005;116:e543-e548.

128. Raffini L, Raybagkar D, Cahill AM, et al. May-Thurner syndrome (iliac vein compression) and thrombosis in adolescents. Pediatr Blood Cancer. 2006;47:834-838.

129. Andrew M, Monagle P, Brooker LA. Epidemiology of venous thromboembolic events. In Andrew M, Monagle P, Brooker LA (eds). Thromboembolic Complications during Infancy and Childhood. Hamilton, Ontario, Canada, BC Decker, 2000, pp 111-146.

130. Vercellio G, Baraldini V, Gatti C, et al. Thoracic outlet syndrome in paediatrics: clinical presentation, surgical treatment, and outcome in a series of eight children. J Pediatr Surg. 2003;38:58-61.

131. Monagle P, Chan A, Massicotte P, et al. Antithrombotic therapy in children: the Seventh ACCP Conference on Antithrombotic and Thrombolytic Therapy. Chest. 2004;126:645S-687S.

132. Manco-Johnson MJ. How I treat venous thrombosis in children. Blood. 2006;107:21-29.

133. Nohe N, Flemmer A, Rumler R, et al. The low molecular weight heparin dalteparin for prophylaxis and therapy of thrombosis in childhood: a report on 48 cases. Eur J Pediatr. 1999;158(Suppl 3):S134-S139.

134. Andrew M, Marzinotto V, Massicotte P, et al. Heparin therapy in pediatric patients: a prospective cohort study. Pediatr Res. 1994;35:78-83.

135. Hull RD, Raskob GE, Rosenbloom D, et al. Heparin for 5 days as compared with 10 days in the initial treatment of proximal venous thrombosis. N Engl J Med. 1990;322:1260-1264.

136. Kearon C, Ginsberg JS, Julian JA, et al. Comparison of fixed-dose weight-adjusted unfractionated heparin and low-molecular-weight heparin for acute treatment of venous thromboembolism. JAMA. 2006;296:935-942.

137. Chan YC, Valenti D, Mansfield AO, Stansby G. Warfarin induced skin necrosis. Br J Surg. 2000;87:266-272.

138. Lim W, Crowther MA, Eikelboom JW. Management of antiphospholipid antibody syndrome: a systematic review. JAMA. 2006;295:1050-1057.

139. Finazzi G, Marchioli R, Brancaccio V, et al. A randomized clinical trial of high-intensity warfarin vs. conventional antithrombotic therapy for the prevention of recurrent thrombosis in patients with the antiphospholipid syndrome (WAPS). J Thromb Haemost. 2005;3:848-853.

140. Berube C, Mitchell L, Silverman E, et al. The relationship of antiphospholipid antibodies to thromboembolic events in pediatric patients with systemic lupus erythematosus: a cross-sectional study. Pediatr Res. 1998;44:351-356.

141. Monagle P, Andrew M. Acquired disorders of hemostasis. In Nathan DG, Orkin SH, Ginsburg D, Look AT (eds). Nathan and Oski's Hematology of Infancy and Childhood, 6th ed. Philadelphia, WB Saunders, 2003, pp 1631-1667.

142. Kearon C, Ginsberg JS, Kovacs MJ, et al. Comparison of low-intensity warfarin therapy with conventional-intensity warfarin therapy for long-term prevention of recurrent venous thromboembolism. N Engl J Med. 2003;349:631-639.

143. Kovacs MJ. Long-term low-dose warfarin use is effective in the prevention of recurrent venous thromboembolism: no. J Thromb Haemost. 2004;2:1041-1043.

144. Goldenberg NA, Durham JD, Knapp-Clevenger R, Manco-Johnson MJ. A thrombolytic regimen for high-risk deep venous thrombosis may substantially reduce the risk of post-thrombotic syndrome in children. Blood. 2007;110:45-53.

145. Petitou M, Lormeau JC, Choay J. Chemical synthesis of glycosaminoglycans: new approaches to antithrombotic drugs. Nature. 1991;350:30-33.

146. Depasse F, Gerotziafas GT, Busson J, et al. Assessment of three chromogenic and one clotting assays for the measurement of synthetic pentasaccharide fondaparinux (Arixtra) anti-Xa activity. J Thromb Haemost. 2004;2:346-348.

147. Investigators P. A novel long-acting synthetic factor Xa inhibitor (SanOrg34006) to replace warfarin for secondary prevention in deep vein thrombosis. A phase II evaluation. J Thromb Haemost. 2004;2:47-53.

148. Eriksson BI, Borris L, Dahl OE, et al. Oral, direct factor Xa inhibition with BAY 59-7939 for the prevention of venous thromboembolism after total hip replacement. J Thromb Haemost. 2006;4:121-128.

149. Schwienhorst A. Direct thrombin inhibitors—a survey of recent developments. Cell Mol Life Sci. 2006;63:2773-2791.

150. Walenga JM. An overview of the direct thrombin inhibitor argatroban. Pathophysiol Haemost Thromb. 2002;32(Suppl 3):9-14.

151. Dreyfus M, Magny JF, Bridey F, et al. Treatment of homozygous protein C deficiency and neonatal purpura fulminans with a purified protein C concentrate. N Engl J Med. 1991;325:1565-1568.

152. Dreyfus M, Masterson M, David M, et al. Replacement therapy with a monoclonal antibody purified protein C concentrate in newborns with severe congenital protein C deficiency. Semin Thromb Hemost. 1995;21:371-381.

153. Vukovich T, Auberger K, Weil J, et al. Replacement therapy for a homozygous protein C deficiency-state using a concentrate of human protein C and S. Br J Haematol. 1988;70:435-440.

154. de Kleijn ED, de Groot R, Hack CE, et al. Activation of protein C following infusion of protein C concentrate in children with severe meningococcal sepsis and purpura fulminans: a randomized, double-blinded, placebo-controlled, dose-finding study. Crit Care Med. 2003;31:1839-1847.

155. Ettingshausen CE, Veldmann A, Beeg T, et al. Replacement therapy with protein C concentrate in infants and adolescents with meningococcal sepsis and purpura fulminans. Semin Thromb Hemost. 1999;25:537-541.

156. Rivard GE, David M, Farrell C, Schwarz HP. Treatment of purpura fulminans in meningococcemia with protein C concentrate. J Pediatr. 1995;126:646-652.

157. Konkle BA, Bauer KA, Weinstein R, et al. Use of recombinant human antithrombin in patients with congenital antithrombin deficiency undergoing surgical procedures. Transfusion. 2003;43:390-394.

158. Mitchell L, Andrew M, Hanna K, et al. Trend to efficacy and safety using antithrombin concentrate in prevention of thrombosis in children receiving L-asparaginase for acute lymphoblastic leukemia. Results of the PAARKA study. Thromb Haemost. 2003;90:235-244.

159. Zaunschirm A, Muntean W. Correction of hemostatic imbalances induced by L-asparaginase therapy in children with acute lymphoblastic leukemia. Pediatr Hematol Oncol. 1986;3:19-25.

160. Haussmann U, Fischer J, Eber S, et al. Hepatic veno-occlusive disease in pediatric stem cell transplantation: impact of pre-emptive antithrombin III replacement and

combined antithrombin III/defibrotide therapy. Haematologica. 2006;91:795-800.

161. Meister B, Kropshofer G, Klein-Franke A, et al. Comparison of low-molecular-weight heparin and antithrombin versus antithrombin alone for the prevention of thrombosis in children with acute lymphoblastic leukemia. Pediatr Blood Cancer. 2008;50:298-303.

162. Bassler D, Schmidt B. Antithrombin replacement in neonates: is there any indication? Thromb Res. 2006;118:107-111.

163. Ferris EJ, McCowan TC, Carver DK, McFarland DR. Percutaneous inferior vena caval filters: follow-up of seven designs in 320 patients. Radiology. 1993;188:851-856.

164. Greenfield LJ, Proctor MC. Twenty-year clinical experience with the Greenfield filter. Cardiovasc Surg. 1995;3:199-205.

165. Athanasoulis CA, Kaufman JA, Halpern EF, et al. Inferior vena caval filters: review of a 26-year single-center clinical experience. Radiology. 2000;216:54-66.

166. Cahn MD, Rohrer MJ, Martella MB, Cutler BS. Long-term follow-up of Greenfield inferior vena cava filter placement in children. J Vasc Surg. 2001;34:820-825.

167. Reed RA, Teitelbaum GP, Stanley P, et al. The use of inferior vena cava filters in pediatric patients for pulmonary embolus prophylaxis. Cardiovasc Intervent Radiol. 1996;19:401-405.

168. Tracy T Jr, Posner MP, Drucker DE, et al. Use of the Greenfield filter in adolescents for deep vein thrombosis and pulmonary embolism. J Pediatr Surg. 1988;23:529-532.

169. Dentali F, Ageno W, Imberti D. Retrievable vena cava filters: clinical experience. Curr Opin Pulm Med. 2006;12:304-309.

170. Mollitt DL, Golladay ES. Complications of TPN catheter–induced vena caval thrombosis in children less than one year of age. J Pediatr Surg. 1983;18:462-467.

171. Graham L Jr, Gumbiner CH. Right atrial thrombus and superior vena cava syndrome in a child. Pediatrics. 1984;73:225-229.

172. Nuss R, Hays T, Manco-Johnson M. Efficacy and safety of heparin anticoagulation for neonatal renal vein thrombosis. Am J Pediatr Hematol Oncol. 1994;16:127-131.

173. Randolph AG, Cook DJ, Gonzales CA, Andrew M. Benefit of heparin in central venous and pulmonary artery catheters: a meta-analysis of randomized controlled trials. Chest. 1998;113:165-171.

174. Derish MT, Smith DW, Frankel LR. Venous catheter thrombus formation and pulmonary embolism in children. Pediatr Pulmonol. 1995;20:349-354.

175. Massicotte MP, Dix D, Monagle P, et al. Central venous catheter related thrombosis in children: analysis of the Canadian Registry of Venous Thromboembolic Complications. J Pediatr. 1998;133:770-776.

176. Goldenberg NA. Long-term outcomes of venous thrombosis in children. Curr Opin Hematol. 2005;12:370-376.

177. Nowak-Gottl U, Junker R, Kreuz W, et al. Risk of recurrent venous thrombosis in children with combined prothrombotic risk factors. Blood. 2001;97:858-862.

178. Massicotte P, Julian JA, Gent M, et al. An open-label randomized controlled trial of low molecular weight heparin compared to heparin and Coumadin for the treatment of venous thromboembolic events in children: the REVIVE trial. Thromb Res. 2003;109:85-92.

179. van Ommen CH, Heijboer H, van den Dool EJ, et al. Pediatric venous thromboembolic disease in one single center: congenital prothrombotic disorders and the clinical outcome. J Thromb Haemost. 2003;1:2516-2522.

180. Oren H, Devecioglu O, Ertem M, et al. Analysis of pediatric thrombotic patients in Turkey. Pediatr Hematol Oncol. 2004;21:573-583.

181. Bick RL. Prothrombin G20210A mutation, antithrombin, heparin cofactor II, protein C, and protein S defects. Hematol Oncol Clin North Am. 2003;17:9-36.

182. Prandoni P, Lensing AW, Cogo A, et al. The long-term clinical course of acute deep venous thrombosis. Ann Intern Med. 1996;125:1-7.

183. Michaels LA, Gurian M, Hegyi T, Drachtman RA. Low molecular weight heparin in the treatment of venous and arterial thromboses in the premature infant. Pediatrics. 2004;114:703-707.

184. Keidan I, Lotan D, Gazit G, et al. Early neonatal renal venous thrombosis: long-term outcome. Acta Paediatr. 1994;83:1225-1227.

185. Kosch A, Kuwertz-Broking E, Heller C, et al. Renal venous thrombosis in neonates: prothrombotic risk factors and long-term follow-up. Blood. 2004;104:1356-1360.

186. Mocan H, Beattie TJ, Murphy AV. Renal venous thrombosis in infancy: long-term follow-up. Pediatr Nephrol. 1991;5:45-49.

187. De Schryver EL, Blom I, Braun KP, et al. Long-term prognosis of cerebral venous sinus thrombosis in childhood. Dev Med Child Neurol. 2004;46:514-519.

188. deVeber G, Andrew M, Adams C, et al. Cerebral sinovenous thrombosis in children. N Engl J Med. 2001;345:417-423.

189. deVeber GA, MacGregor D, Curtis R, Mayank S. Neurologic outcome in survivors of childhood arterial ischemic stroke and sinovenous thrombosis. J Child Neurol. 2000;15:316-324.

190. Kenet G, Waldman D, Lubetsky A, et al. Paediatric cerebral sinus vein thrombosis. A multi-center, case-controlled study. Thromb Haemost. 2004;92:713-718.

191. Gurakan F, Eren M, Kocak N, et al. Extrahepatic portal vein thrombosis in children: etiology and long-term follow-up. J Clin Gastroenterol. 2004;38:368-372.

192. Meissner MH, Manzo RA, Bergelin RO, et al. Deep venous insufficiency: the relationship between lysis and subsequent reflux. J Vasc Surg. 1993;18:596-605.

193. Kahn SR, Desmarais S, Ducruet T, et al. Comparison of the Villalta and Ginsberg clinical scales to diagnose the post-thrombotic syndrome: correlation with patient-reported disease burden and venous valvular reflux. J Thromb Haemost. 2006;4:907-908.

194. Revel-Vilk S, Sharathkumar A, Massicotte P, et al. Natural history of arterial and venous thrombosis in children treated with low molecular weight heparin: a longitudinal study by ultrasound. J Thromb Haemost. 2004;2:42-46.

195. Eichinger S, Minar E, Bialonczyk C, et al. D-dimer levels and risk of recurrent venous thromboembolism. JAMA. 2003;290:1071-1074.

196. Kyrle PA, Minar E, Hirschl M, et al. High plasma levels of factor VIII and the risk of recurrent venous thromboembolism. N Engl J Med. 2000;343:457-462.

197. Palareti G, Legnani C, Cosmi B, et al. Risk of venous thromboembolism recurrence: high negative predictive value of D-dimer performed after oral anticoagulation is stopped. Thromb Haemost. 2002;87:7-12.

198. Lynch JK, Hirtz DG, DeVeber G, Nelson KB. Report of the National Institute of Neurological Disorders and Stroke workshop on perinatal and childhood stroke. Pediatrics. 2002;109:116-123.

199. Kittner SJ, Adams RJ. Stroke in children and young adults. Curr Opin Neurol. 1996;9:53-56.

200. Steinlin M, Pfister I, Pavlovic J, et al. The first three years of the Swiss Neuropaediatric Stroke Registry (SNPSR): a population-based study of incidence, symptoms and risk factors. Neuropediatrics. 2005;36:90-97.

201. Schoenberg BS, Mellinger JF, Schoenberg DG. Cerebrovascular disease in infants and children: a study of incidence, clinical features, and survival. Neurology. 1978;28:763-768.

202. Golomb MR, Garg BP, Saha C, Williams LS. Accuracy and yield of ICD-9 codes for identifying children with ischemic stroke. Neurology. 2006;67:2053-2055.

203. Chabrier S, Lasjaunias P, Husson B, et al. Ischaemic stroke from dissection of the craniocervical arteries in childhood: report of 12 patients. Eur J Paediatr Neurol. 2003;7:39-42.

204. Danchaivijitr N, Cox TC, Saunders DE, Ganesan V. Evolution of cerebral arteriopathies in childhood arterial ischemic stroke. Ann Neurol. 2006;59:620-626.

205. Sebire G, Fullerton H, Riou E, deVeber G. Toward the definition of cerebral arteriopathies of childhood. Curr Opin Pediatr. 2004;16:617-622.

206. Ganesan V, Prengler M, McShane MA, et al. Investigation of risk factors in children with arterial ischemic stroke. Ann Neurol. 2003;53:167-173.

207. Kieslich M, Fiedler A, Heller C, et al. Minor head injury as cause and co-factor in the aetiology of stroke in childhood: a report of eight cases. J Neurol Neurosurg Psychiatry. 2002;73:13-16.

208. Shaffer L, Rich PM, Pohl KR, Ganesan V. Can mild head injury cause ischaemic stroke? Arch Dis Child. 2003;88:267-269.

209. Ganesan V, Prengler M, Wade A, Kirkham FJ. Clinical and radiological recurrence after childhood arterial ischemic stroke. Circulation. 2006;114:2170-2177.

210. Haywood S, Liesner R, Pindora S, Ganesan V. Thrombophilia and first arterial ischaemic stroke: a systematic review. Arch Dis Child. 2005;90:402-405.

211. Kenet G, Sadetzki S, Murad H, et al. Factor V Leiden and antiphospholipid antibodies are significant risk factors for ischemic stroke in children. Stroke. 2000;31:1283-1288.

212. Nowak-Gottl U, Strater R, Heinecke A, et al. Lipoprotein (a) and genetic polymorphisms of clotting factor V, prothrombin, and methylenetetrahydrofolate reductase are risk factors of spontaneous ischemic stroke in childhood. Blood. 1999;94:3678-3682.

213. Strater R, Vielhaber H, Kassenbohmer R, et al. Genetic risk factors of thrombophilia in ischaemic childhood stroke of cardiac origin. A prospective ESPED survey. Eur J Pediatr. 1999;158(Suppl 3):S122-S125.

214. Chabrier S, Husson B, Lasjaunias P et al. Stroke in childhood: outcome and recurrence risk by mechanism in 59 patients. J Child Neurol. 2000;15:290-294.

215. Brandt T, Orberk E, Weber R, et al. Pathogenesis of cervical artery dissections: association with connective tissue abnormalities. Neurology. 2001;57:24-30.

216. Bowers DC, Liu Y, Leisenring W, et al. Late-occurring stroke among long-term survivors of childhood leukemia and brain tumors: a report from the Childhood Cancer Survivor Study. J Clin Oncol. 2006;24:5277-5282.

217. Cardo E, Vilaseca MA, Campistol J, et al. Evaluation of hyperhomocysteinaemia in children with stroke. Eur J Paediatr Neurol. 1999;3:113-117.

218. van Beynum IM, Smeitink JA, den Heijer M, et al. Hyperhomocysteinemia: a risk factor for ischemic stroke in children. Circulation. 1999;99:2070-2072.

219. Josephson C, Nuss R, Jacobson L, et al. The varicella-autoantibody syndrome. Pediatr Res. 2001;50:345-352.

220. Rook JL, Nugent DJ, Young G. Pediatric stroke and methylenetetrahydrofolate reductase polymorphisms: an examination of C677T and A1298C mutations. J Pediatr Hematol Oncol. 2005;27:590-593.

221. Lynch JK, Han CJ, Nee LE, Nelson KB. Prothrombotic factors in children with stroke or porencephaly. Pediatrics. 2005;116:447-453.

222. Braun KP, Rafay MF, Uiterwaal CS, et al. Mode of onset predicts etiological diagnosis of arterial ischemic stroke in children. Stroke. 2007;38:298-302.

223. Hirano M, Pavlakis SG. Mitochondrial myopathy, encephalopathy, lactic acidosis, and strokelike episodes (MELAS): current concepts. J Child Neurol. 1994;9:4-13.

224. Yoneda M, Maeda M, Kimura H, et al. Vasogenic edema on MELAS: a serial study with diffusion-weighted MR imaging. Neurology. 1999;53:2182-2184.

225. Wallace DC. Mitochondrial diseases in man and mouse. Science. 1999;283:1482-1488.

226. Royal College of Physicians, London. Paediatric Stroke Working Group. Stroke in Childhood. Clinical Guidelines for Diagnosis, Management and Rehabilitation. November 2004. Royal College of Physicians website. Available at www.rcplondon.ac.uk/pubs/books/childstroke/childstroke_guidelines.pdf. Accessed May 24, 2008.

227. Kurnik K, Kosch A, Strater R, et al. Recurrent thromboembolism in infants and children suffering from symptomatic neonatal arterial stroke: a prospective follow-up study. Stroke. 2003;34:2887-2892.

228. Strater R, Kurnik K, Heller C, et al. Aspirin versus low-dose low-molecular-weight heparin: antithrombotic therapy in pediatric ischemic stroke patients: a prospective follow-up study. Stroke. 2001;32:2554-2558.

229. Ozgur BM, Aryan HE, Levy ML. Indirect revascularisation for paediatric moyamoya disease: the EDAMS technique. J Clin Neurosci. 2006;13:105-108.

230. Khan N, Schuknecht B, Boltshauser E, et al. Moyamoya disease and moyamoya syndrome: experience in Europe; choice of revascularisation procedures. Acta Neurochir (Wien). 2003;145:1061-1071.

231. Amlie-Lefond C, Benedict SL, Benard T, et al. Thrombolysis in children with arterial ischemic stroke: initial results from the International Paediatric Stroke Study. Stroke. 2007;38:485a.

232. Mercuri E, Barnett A, Rutherford M, et al. Neonatal cerebral infarction and neuromotor outcome at school age. Pediatrics. 2004;113:95-100.

233. Kirton A, Shroff M, Visvanathan T, deVeber G. Quantified corticospinal tract diffusion restriction predicts neonatal stroke outcome. Stroke. 2007;38:974-980.

234. Fullerton HJ, Wu YW, Sidney S, Johnston SC. Risk of recurrent childhood arterial ischemic stroke in a population-based cohort: the importance of cerebrovascular imaging. Pediatrics. 2007;119:495-501.

235. Lanthier S, Carmant L, David M, et al. Stroke in children: the coexistence of multiple risk factors predicts poor outcome. Neurology. 2000;54:371-378.

236. Sträter R, Becker S, von Eckardstein A, et al. Prospective assessment of risk factors for recurrent stroke during childhood—a 5-year follow-up study. Lancet. 2002;360: 1540-1545.

237. Mercuri E, Rutherford M, Cowan F, et al. Early prognostic indicators of outcome in infants with neonatal cerebral infarction: a clinical, electroencephalogram, and magnetic resonance imaging study. Pediatrics. 1999;103:39-46.

238. De Vries LS, Van der Grond J, Van Haastert IC, Groenendaal F. Prediction of outcome in new-born infants with arterial ischaemic stroke using diffusion-weighted magnetic resonance imaging. Neuropediatrics. 2005;36:12-20.

239. Nagata S, Matsushima T, Morioka T, et al. Unilaterally symptomatic moyamoya disease in children: long-term follow-up of 20 patients. Neurosurgery. 2006;59: 830-836.

240. Lanthier S, Kirkham FJ, Mitchell LG, et al. Increased anticardiolipin antibody IgG titers do not predict recurrent stroke or TIA in children. Neurology. 2004;62:194-200.

XI Supportive Therapy

Transfusion Medicine

35 Transfusion Medicine

Steven R. Sloan, David F. Friedman, Grace Kao, Richard M. Kaufman, and Leslie Silberstein

Transfusion medicine focuses on the administration of blood, blood components, and purified blood proteins to patients for therapeutic purposes. Red blood cells (RBCs) are the most frequently used blood component, and RBC transfusions have been studied extensively. In this chapter, RBC transfusions are discussed first and issues that pertain to all transfusions, such as transfusion reactions and transfusion-transmitted diseases, are discussed in this section. Platelets are often transfused to some patients such as oncology patients and are discussed in the next section of this chapter. Hematopoietic progenitor cells (HPCs) are the most recently blood-derived component to be developed for transfusion. Although these cells are often said to be transplanted rather than transfused, they are also discussed in this chapter. Finally, granulocyte components collected by apheresis for transfusion and other apheresis procedures that allow simultaneous removal and transfusion of blood components are discussed at the end of the chapter.

RED BLOOD CELL TRANSFUSIONS

Indications for Transfusion

The primary function of RBCs is to bind oxygen as they circulate through the pulmonary bed and to release oxygen in the capillaries at a pressure high enough for diffusion into tissues. The configuration of the oxyhemoglobin dissociation curve provides proper diffusion as long as only part of the oxygen is released during capillary transit. The oxygen tension of fully oxygenated blood in the arteries is approximately 100 mm Hg; release of 20% of the oxygen in the capillaries maintains a pressure of 40 mm Hg, which is sufficient to propel oxygen to all cells within a truncated cone segment around the capillary.[1] RBCs compensate for a loss in oxygen-carrying capacity relatively rapidly by a shift in the oxyhemoglobin dissociation curve to the right, which decreases oxygen's affinity for hemoglobin. In addition, cardiac output increases. On a more chronic basis, blood volume, the size of the vascular bed, and the rate of production of RBCs increases. These compensatory mechanisms permit states of mild to moderate anemia without significant symptoms.

For most patients the only indication for RBC transfusion is to provide a patient with sufficient RBCs to prevent or reverse tissue hypoxia as a result of insufficient compensation. One large multicenter randomized controlled study of adult critically ill patients is probably applicable to some pediatric patients, especially adolescents.[2] That trial compared a liberal transfusion strategy, in which patients received RBC transfusions when their hemoglobin level was less than 10.0 g/dL, with a restrictive transfusion strategy, in which patients were transfused when their hemoglobin was less than 7.0 g/dL. Among patients younger than 55 years, those who were transfused according to the more restrictive strategy had significantly lower 30-day mortality. A similar study of stable critically ill pediatric patients in intensive care units found similar outcomes in patients transfused at a hemoglobin level of 7 g/dL or less and patients transfused at level of 9.5 g/dL or less.[3] Additionally, experience with sickle cell patients undergoing surgery in Jamaica suggests that otherwise healthy young people can tolerate a hematocrit of 20% without experiencing short-term adverse consequences.[4]

Two prospective randomized controlled studies have compared transfusion strategies for low-weight premature infants. The triggers used for transfusion depended on the oxygen support requirements in both studies,[5,6] as well as the baby's age in one of the studies.[6] One study by Bell and colleagues found in that neonates on the liberal transfusion strategy, intraventricular hemorrhage or periventricular leukomalacia was less likely to develop and the neonates were less likely to have more than one apnea episode per day.[5] Patients randomized to the liberal transfusion strategy were transfused when their hematocrit was less than 46% if they were tracheally intubated for assisted ventilation. They received transfusions when their hematocrit was less than 38% if they were receiving nasal continuous positive airway pressure or supplemental oxygen, and transfusions were administered when their hematocrit was less than 30% if they required no oxygen support. The other study by Kirpalani and associates used different liberal and restrictive transfusion algorithms and found no differences in outcomes between patients assigned to liberal and restrictive groups.[6] Because neonates often receive multiple aliquots from the same RBC unit, there was no statistically significant difference in donor exposure between the liberal and restrictive transfusion groups in either study. As no harm has been seen with a more liberal transfusion strategy in premature infants, some have argued that it is safer to transfuse more liberally for premature infants, especially since one study found a neurologic risk associated with undertransfusion.[7]

Children who are chronically anemic from thalassemia may also benefit from a more liberal transfusion policy. These patients benefit from a hypertransfusion program that maintains their hemoglobin level higher than 9 to 10 g/dL. Hypertransfusion of these patients allows them to attain normal height and weight and improves hepatosplenomegaly, osteoporosis, and cardiac dilation.[8-12] Transfusions benefit these patients by increasing tissue oxygenation and particularly by suppressing endogenous erythropoiesis.

Acute Blood Loss

RBC transfusions are frequently used to replace blood lost either in the operating room or after trauma. In practice, diagnosis of the presence and degree of blood loss is quite difficult, especially in a young, otherwise healthy child. In fact, a child may sustain a relatively large hemorrhage with few external signs of distress. Signs of impending shock, such as pallor, anxiety, and tachypnea, are frequently subtle and easily overlooked or attributed

Box 35-1 **Diseases Requiring Intermittent or Chronic Red Cell Transfusion in Childhood**

Chronic renal failure
Thalassemia
Sickle cell disease
Aplastic anemia
  Constitutional
  Acquired
  Oncologic (leukemia, solid tumors)
  Diamond-Blackfan anemia
  Transient erythroblastopenia

to other causes. By the time that signs of cardiovascular compromise become evident (i.e., stupor, tachycardia or bradycardia, hypotension, coolness of the extremities, weak peripheral pulses, and decreased capillary filling), the patient has most probably lost at least 25% of total blood volume. Hypotension is one useful clinical sign of moderate to severe blood loss. Patients who have lost more than 25% of their blood volume frequently manifest age-related systolic hypotension: less than 65 mm Hg in children younger than 4 years, less than 75 mm Hg in children 5 to 8 years of age, less than 85 mm Hg in children 9 to 12 years of age, and less than 95 mm Hg in adolescents and adults.

Chronic Transfusion Therapy

In chronic anemia, the body is deficient in RBCs, whereas plasma volume is normal or increased. Box 35-1 lists the childhood conditions that are likely to require intermittent or long-term transfusion therapy.

The following guidelines apply when planning for chronic transfusions (months to years):

1. If possible, transfusion should be avoided or minimized by aggressive treatment of the underlying disorder (e.g., administration of recombinant human erythropoietin to patients maintained on dialysis or with chronic renal failure).
2. Leukocyte-reduced RBCs should be used to avert or delay sensitization to leukocyte alloantigens, the most common cause of febrile nonhemolytic transfusion reactions.
3. RBCs should be administered in an amount sufficient to prevent symptomatic anemia and allow normal growth.
4. The patient's iron status should be monitored by determination of serum ferritin, iron, and iron-binding capacity and liver iron stores.

Packed Red Blood Cells

A packed cell product is the component of choice for replacement during surgery, red cell loss, and chronic transfusion therapy. The hematocrit of the cells varies

with the preservative solution used by the collection facility. Blood collected in citrate-phosphate-dextrose-adenosine (CPDA-1) and stored as red cells has an average hematocrit of approximately 75%.[13] Red cells stored in an additive nutrient solution such as Adsol or Nutricel have a hematocrit of 50% to 60%. Adsol contains mannitol. Some institutions avoid units containing Adsol for large transfusions to neonates because of concerns about the effects of mannitol. However, mannitol has no adverse consequences with standard simple transfusions of 5 to 20 mL/kg per dose in premature infants.[14]

Blood Storage

During storage, red cell metabolism continues and some leakage through red cell membranes occurs. This results in changes such as decreasing plasma dextrose and increasing plasma potassium. These changes are acceptable for most transfusions, but in some situations the increased potassium in solution may cause problems. In such cases, fresh blood (<7 to 10 days old) may be beneficial and is indicated when small patients receive large amounts of blood, such as neonates undergoing exchange transfusion or infants receiving large transfusions rapidly during surgery. However, neonates can tolerate 5- to 20-mL/kg transfusions of older units of RBCs, and some blood banks dedicate a unit of blood for repeated transfusions to one infant to minimize the number of donors to which the infant is exposed.[14]

Leukoreduction of Red Cells

Transfusion of allogeneic cellular blood products is associated with deleterious effects caused by the presence of residual leukocytes, including alloimmunization to histocompatibility antigens, transmission of viruses, febrile reactions, and graft-versus-host disease (GVHD).[15,16] Filters are used to reduce the number of leukocytes in whole blood, red cells, and platelets.[17,18] Routine leukoreduction of red cells to less than 5×10^6 leukocytes per unit reduces the frequency of febrile nonhemolytic transfusion reactions in patients who are transfusion dependent.[19,20] Removal of leukocytes from blood also reduces the risk of leukocyte-associated transmission of viruses such as cytomegalovirus (CMV). Leukoreduction of red cells and platelets to a level less than 5×10^6 has been demonstrated to substantially reduce CMV transmission in neonates and transplant patients.[21,22]

In addition, allogeneic lymphocytes may modulate the immune system and be immunosuppressive.[23] The use of leukoreduction has been recommended to prevent immune modulation in neonates and surgical patients, especially those undergoing surgery for a malignancy. Until more definitive studies have been performed, these situations can be considered only possible indications.[24,25]

Irradiation of Red Cells

Transfusion-associated GVHD is a rare complication after the transfusion of cellular products. Patients most susceptible to GVHD include premature neonates, some patients with congenital immunodeficiency syndromes, immunosuppressed oncology patients undergoing chemotherapy or radiation therapy (or both), and patients receiving certain immunosuppressive drugs after solid organ transplantation and some other indications.[26-28] In addition, normal recipients who are heterozygous for HLA antigens do not reject lymphocytes that are transfused from a donor who is homozygous for one of the recipient's haplotypes.[29] This is not merely theoretical because transfusion-associated GVHD has developed in normal recipients undergoing surgery who received unirradiated directed donor blood from a first-order relative.[30,31] Because of the wide variety of patients at risk for GVHD, some transfusion services have chosen to irradiate all cellular blood products to ensure that this life-threatening complication does not develop in any patient.

Immunologic Considerations

Multiple antigens expressed on erythrocyte cell surfaces can be recognized by the immune system of a transfusion recipient. Before an RBC transfusion, erythrocytes that are immunologically compatible with the patient must be identified. Erythrocyte antigens are polymorphic inherited structural characteristics located on proteins, glycoproteins, or glycolipids on the outside surface of the RBC membrane. Erythrocyte antigens are clinically important in the immune destruction of RBCs in allogeneic blood transfusions, maternal-fetal blood group incompatibility, autoimmune hemolytic anemia, and organ transplantation. Our ability to detect and identify antibodies to erythrocyte antigens and identify compatible donor RBCs lacking the specific antigens has contributed significantly to the safe supportive blood transfusion practices used today.

The ABO and H System

The H Antigen

A and B antigens on RBCs are defined by a terminal sugar attached to a carbohydrate chain on membrane glycosphingolipids. The H antigen is the precursor molecule on which A and B antigens are built. The H antigen on RBCs is defined by fucose at the terminus of carbohydrate chains.[32] Expression of the H antigen is determined by a fucosyltransferase that transfers a fucose to an oligosaccharide side chain attached to integral membrane proteins on red cells. This fucoslytransferase is encoded by a gene on chromosome 19.[33,34] The fucosyltransferase and thus the H antigen are present in all persons except those with the rare Bombay (O$_h$) phenotype.[35]

The A and B Antigens

Transferases responsible for the A or B antigens add N-acetylgalactosamine or galactose, respectively, to the

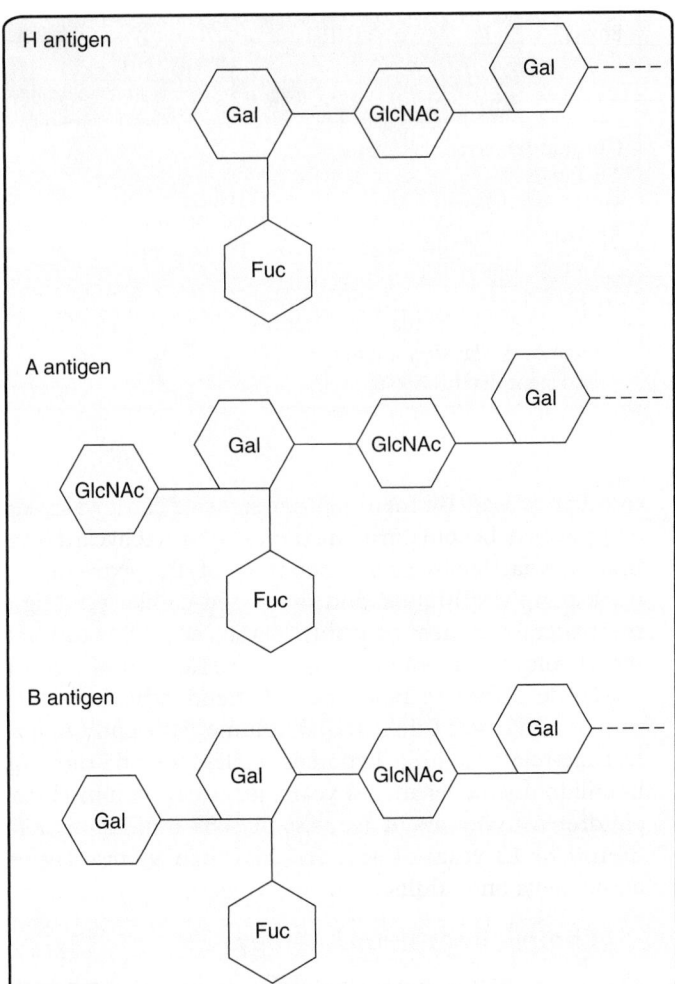

FIGURE 35-1. Structure of the precursor H structure and the A and B antigens. GlcNAc, *N*-acetylglucosamine.

precursor chain carrying the H antigen (Fig. 35-1).[32,36-40] The genes encoding these transferases reside on chromosome 9.[41] The genes for the A and B blood group antigens are codominant because people with both transferases will transfer galactosamine and galactose and thus express A and B antigens. Group O is the amorph of the ABO blood group system. RBCs from group O persons have H antigens but lack A and B antigens.[42] It is likely that falciparum malaria has shaped the distribution of the ABO blood groups in humans.[43]

Although ABO antigens are detectable on the RBCs of 5- to 6-week-old embryos, these antigens are not fully developed until 2 to 4 years of age.[44-47] RBCs from infants carry A, B, and H antigens on linear oligosaccharide chains that have only one terminus to which the A, B, and H sugars can be added.[32,36,38,48-50] The fact that the A and B antigens are not fully developed at birth may be a reason why ABO hemolytic disease of the newborn (HDN) is usually a mild disease.[50,51] As the infants grow older, the oligosaccharides branch and create additional termini to which the A, B, and H sugars can be added.[39]

After 2 to 4 years of age, expression of A and B antigens remains fairly constant throughout life.

Antibodies to A and B antigens, also known as isohemagglutinins, may develop as a result of environmental stimulants, such as bacteria that carry similar antigens.[52] Because isohemagglutinins are naturally occurring, it is essential to select ABO-compatible blood for transfusion.[53] Indeed, ABO incompatibility is the most frequent cause of fatal hemolytic transfusion reactions.

Isohemagglutinin production begins several months after birth, reaches a peak at 5 to 10 years of age, and declines with increasing age.[54] Thus, infants younger than 4 months who have isohemagglutinins will have acquired them through placental transfer of maternal IgG anti-A, anti-B, or anti-A,B.[50]

Isohemagglutinins from group A and B individuals are predominantly IgM and do not usually cross the placenta and cause HDN.[55] However, because group O serum contains IgG isohemagglutinins, ABO HDN is most frequently seen in non–group O infants of group O mothers.

The Lewis System

The Lewis antigens, Le^a and Le^b, are not intrinsic to RBCs but instead are carried on plasma glycosphingolipids that are adsorbed onto the red cell membrane.[56] These antigens are structurally related, with the Le^b antigen containing an additional fucose that is not present on the Le^a antigen. Furthermore, the one additional fucose present on the Le^b antigen is not very different from the Le^a antigen. Thus, Le^a individuals rarely make anti-Le^b. Hence, in most cases Lewis antibodies are made only in individuals who are Le(a–b–).[50]

In most cases, Lewis antibodies do not cause hemolysis, and donor RBCs lacking the Lewis antigens do not usually need to be selected.[50] However, rare hemolytic transfusion reactions have been reported when Le(a+) RBCs were transfused to recipients with anti-Le^a.[57] This may occur when the antibody reacts at 37° C. In such cases it is not difficult to identify Le(a–) donor units because the RBCs in almost 80% of donors are Le(a–).[58] Anti-Le^a and anti-Le^b are not known to cause HDN; they are usually IgM, and fetal RBCs have the phenotype Le(a–b–).[50] Interestingly, Lewis antigens are also expressed on *Helicobacter pylori*, a causative agent of gastric ulcers, and play a role in adhesion and colonization of the bacteria in the gastric mucosa.[59,60]

The Ii Collection

The I and i antigens reside in the subterminal portions of carbohydrate chains on glycolipids or glycoproteins of the RBC membrane. The i antigen appears on fetal RBCs when disaccharide units are linked in a straight chain.[61] In the first 2 years of life, many of these linear chains are modified into branched chains.[39] I specificity results at the expense of i antigens when the branched structures appear. Adults have RBCs with predominantly I antigen and little or no i antigen, whereas newborns have RBCs

with strong expression of i antigen and small amounts of I antigen.[62]

Anti-I is a common autoantibody that is reactive at room temperature and below and generally produces no hemolysis.[63,64] In cold agglutinin disease, anti-I causes in vivo hemolysis, and such pathologic autoantibodies often react at 30° C in albumin.[65] Adult I-negative RBCs are not readily available for transfusion, and patients with cold agglutinin disease secondary to anti-I are transfused with I-positive RBCs through a blood warmer.[50] The titer and thermal range of anti-I are often increased after infection with *Mycoplasma pneumoniae*.[50] The presence of a cold agglutinin secondary to an anti-I antibody frequently occurs in *M. pneumoniae* infection, but this finding is neither a specific nor a sensitive test for this infection.[66]

Analogously, cold agglutinins caused by anti-i antibodies are sometimes present in Epstein-Barr virus (EBV) infection, but this is also neither a sensitive nor a specific test for this infection.[67]

Levels of the i antigen can aid in differentiating Diamond-Blackfan anemia from transient erythroblastopenia of childhood. The i antigen is enhanced on RBCs from patients with Diamond-Blackfan anemia and is absent or of reduced strength on RBCs from children with transient erythroblastopenia of childhood.[68-70] However, the enhanced i antigen associated with Diamond-Blackfan anemia reflects stress hematopoiesis[71] and is not a specific aspect of the disease. In transient erythroblastopenia of childhood, the reduced levels of I antigen reflect the selective suppression of erythropoiesis secondary to infection, but during recovery from this disorder, the patient's marrow is active and the I antigen may be enhanced as a result of hematopoietic stress.[70]

The P System

Like the A, B, and H antigens, the P blood group antigens are defined by sugars added to precursor glycosphingolipids. Antigens in this group include P1, P, and P^k. Among whites, 21% have the P1-negative phenotype and they commonly produce anti-P1. This cold reactive IgM antibody does not cross the placenta and has rarely been reported to cause hemolysis in vivo.[72] An autoantibody, autoanti-P, is found in patients with paroxysmal cold hemoglobinuria and in some patients with acquired immune hemolytic anemia. It is called the Donath-Landsteiner antibody and is most frequently seen in children.[73] This IgG autoantibody is a biphasic hemolysin that binds to RBCs in the cold and then hemolyzes them when warmed. The patient's serum causes hemolysis of RBCs that have been incubated first in melting ice and then at 37° C.[74] This antibody should be considered when the patient has hemoglobinuria and C3 alone is present on the RBCs.

The P antigen serves as a receptor for parvovirus B19[75] and pyelonephritic *Escherichia coli*.[76,77] Persons with the very rare p phenotype lack the antigens P1, P, and P^k and are not susceptible to infection by parvovirus B19.

People with the rare p phenotype may produce anti-P1+P+P^k, a potent hemolytic IgM antibody that can cause immediate hemolytic transfusion reactions.[50,78] This antibody has also been associated with HDN, fetal death, and miscarriages during early pregnancy in women whose RBCs have the p phenotype.[79]

The Rh System

The Rh blood group system includes D, C, c, E, e, and 40 other antigens.[80] The terms *Rh positive* and *Rh negative* refer to the presence and absence of the D antigen, respectively. The D antigen is, after A and B, the most important RBC antigen in transfusion practice. Persons who lack the D antigen do not have anti-D unless exposed to D antigen by pregnancy or transfusion. In more than 80% of persons who lack the D antigen, anti-D will develop after transfusion of a unit of D-positive donor blood.[81,82] Although this statistic probably does not apply to infants younger than 4 months, some young infants can probably respond to the Rh(D) antigen.[83]

The RBCs of 0.2% to 1% of white individuals and a greater percentage of African Americans carry reduced expression of the D antigen known as weak D. Weak D that is not detected by routine anti-D reagents can be identified by a more sensitive test, the indirect antiglobulin test. There is no hard and fast line between D and weak D; weak D RBCs are merely ones with a relatively smaller number of D antigen sites[84] that is usually due to point mutations in the gene encoding the Rh(D) antigen, the *RHD* gene.[85,86] Most patients with the weak D phenotype can safely receive blood transfusions from individuals who are Rh(D) positive. However, there are different types of weak D based on the specific genetic polymorphisms that are present, and patients with two weak D types can make anti-D antibodies.[87] Often only reference laboratories can determine the specific type of weak D that is present; sometimes molecular testing that is not yet widely available is necessary to determine the weak D type. All D-negative donor blood is tested for weak D by the antiglobulin test.[52] Donor RBCs that are agglutinated by this test are labeled Rh(D)+, and RBCs that are not agglutinated by this test are labeled Rh– for transfusion.

There are rare reports of fetuses with weak D having HDN when born to a mother with anti-D formed during an earlier pregnancy.[50] In practice, an infant at birth is designated Rh(D) negative when negative results are obtained with the routine anti-D test, as well as anti-globulin tests.[51] Similarly, during and after pregnancy, a woman is designated Rh negative only if negative results are obtained with the routine anti-D test, as well as by the indirect antiglobulin test.[53] This is to prevent possible misinterpretation of the D typing result in the event of fetal-maternal hemorrhage.[42,50]

Rh antigens are carried on Rh proteins that pass through the RBC membrane 12 times and are encoded by at least two genes on chromosome 1.[88-91] These Rh proteins associate with the RhAG protein required for cell surface expression of the Rh antigens D, C, c, E, and e, which are associated with specific amino acid substitutions on the Rh proteins.[90,91] Erythrocytes totally deficient in Rh proteins exhibit spherocytosis and stomatocytosis and have a diminished life span that results in a mildly hemolytic state known as Rh deficiency syndrome.[92,93] Although the function of the Rh proteins is unknown, RhAG may play a role in ammonium transport.[94]

The MNS System

The M, N, S, s, and U antigens are carried on sialoglycoproteins on the RBC membrane. M and N are encoded by paired allelic forms of the glycophorin A gene (*GPA*) and are the result of amino acid substitutions at residues 1 and 5 of GPA.[95-97] Human RBCs type as M+N–, M–N+, or M+N+, which represents homozygosity for M, homozygosity for N, and heterozygosity for both genes, respectively. S and s antigens are encoded by alternative forms of the glycophorin B gene (*GPB*). GPA and GPB are encoded by homologous genes on chromosome 4q28-q31.[98] GPA binds *E. coli*[99] and plays a role in malarial invasion of RBCs. RBCs lacking glycophorin A, B, or C are resistant to invasion by *Plasmodium falciparum* to varying degrees.[100]

Anti-M and anti-N can be IgG, IgM, or a mixture of both. These antibodies are usually clinically insignificant and are often present in persons who have not previously been transfused or pregnant. Antibodies that react at 37° C may cause hemolysis of transfused cells. Antibodies to S, s, and U usually occur after stimulation and are capable of causing hemolytic transfusion reactions and HDN.[50]

The Kell System

The Kell system antigens reside on two transmembrane proteins, the Kell protein and the XK protein, that are linked by a single disulfide bond. The Kell protein is a 93-kd glycoprotein that carries more than 20 antigens, and the XK protein is a 440–amino acid protein that carries just one antigen known as Kx.

The major antigen of the Kell blood group system resides on the Kell protein. This antigen is the K antigen, which is present in 9% of white donors.[78] Anti-K is the most common immune RBC antibody after those in the ABO and Rh systems. However, because more than 90% of donors are K–, it is not difficult to find compatible blood for patients with anti-K antibodies. The molecular basis of antithetical K and k antigens has been shown to be an amino acid substitution of methionine to threonine at residue 193 of the Kell protein.[101] This allows prenatal testing for K and k antigens on amniocytes from a mother whose fetus is at risk for HDN because of anti-K or anti-k. Antibodies to other antigens on the Kell protein, such as Kp^a, Kp^b, Js^a, and Js^b, are less common but are also clinically significant.[78,102] The Kell protein is a member of a large family of zinc-dependent endopeptidases.[103]

The other protein of the Kell system, the XK protein, carries one antigen, the Kx antigen.[104] The function of the XK protein is unknown, but its absence, known as the McLeod phenotype, is associated with a variety of abnormalities. Absence of membrane XK protein results in diminished expression of Kell protein on the membrane and reduced expression of all antigens in the Kell blood group system. In addition, these patients have acanthocytotic erythrocytes and hemolytic anemia. The McLeod phenotype is X-linked because the gene for the XK protein resides on the X gene. Some patients with the X-linked McLeod phenotype have concomitant chronic granulomatous disease (CGD) as a result of deletion of a region of the X chromosome that includes genes encoding XK and the gene associated with CGD.[102] Patients with CGD and McLeod's syndrome usually make antibodies to the XK and Kell proteins if they are transfused with RBCs containing the XK and Kell proteins. This can lead to major problems in transfusing these patients.[105] To avoid this problem, patients with McLeod's syndrome should be transfused with blood of the McLeod phenotype. Ko blood that lacks the Kell protein is not appropriate because such RBCs have increased expression of the Kx antigen that is expressed on the XK protein. However, males with the McLeod phenotype and no concomitant CGD (non-CGD McLeod's syndrome) do not make anti-Kx and can be transfused with McLeod- or Ko-type blood.[102,106]

The Duffy System

The Duffy antigens are epitopes present on a cell surface glycoprotein. The Duffy glycoprotein is a chemokine receptor that is expressed on many cell types and can bind a variety of chemokines.[107] Although the Duffy chemokine receptor can bind chemokines, its function is unknown and people lacking the receptor on their red cells, or on all cells, are totally healthy.[108]

The two most common alleles in people of European or Asian descent are Fy^a and Fy^b, which differ by a single amino acid substitution. Anti-Fy^a and anti-Fy^b have been implicated in transfusion reactions.[50] Anti-Fy^a has caused mild HDN, but anti-Fy^b has not been implicated.[50] Anti-Fy^a is commonly encountered, but because a third of donors are Fy(a–), compatible blood is not difficult to find.

The red cells of many people of African descent lack the Fy^a and Fy^b antigens (Fy[a–b–]) on their erythrocytes. However, the Fy^b allele is usually expressed in the lung, colon, and spleen of these individuals.[109] Thus, these individuals cannot mount an immune response to the Fy^b antigen but can produce anti-Fy^a.[50,78] In West Africa, most blacks are Fy(a–b–) because of natural selection; these RBCs are resistant to *Plasmodium vivax* malaria because the Duffy protein is a receptor for *P. vivax*.[107,109-111]

The Kidd System

The Kidd gene encodes two antigens, Jk^a and Jk^b, that represent a single amino acid substitution (Asp280Asn)

in the Kidd glycoprotein.[112] They are usually expressed in one of three phenotypes: Jk(a+b–), Jk(a–b+), or Jk(a+b+). The fourth phenotype, Jk(a–b–), is exceedingly rare.[78] Antibodies to both Kidd antigens can cause delayed hemolytic transfusion reactions. Because these antibodies are often weak and may become undetectable over time, they may escape detection in a sensitized patient's serum before transfusion. If the patient is then transfused with antigen-positive RBCs, the anamnestic response causes an increase in titer of the antibody and hemolysis of the transfused antigen-positive RBCs.[50] Once the antibody is identified, compatible blood is not difficult to find because a fourth of donors are negative for each antigen.

The Kidd glycoprotein is a urea transporter that prevents red cells from shrinking and swelling as they pass into and out of the high urea concentration of the renal medulla.[113-115] The Kidd urea transporter also prevents red cells from carrying urea away from the renal medulla and decreasing the urea-concentrating efficiency of the kidney.[115] Individuals who have RBCs with the Jk(a–b–) phenotype are unable to concentrate urine as efficiently as those who have the Kidd glycoprotein.[116-118]

The Lutheran System

The Lutheran blood group antigens are carried on a cell surface glycoprotein. The Lu^a antigen is present on the RBCs of 8% of people, whereas the antithetical antigen, Lu^b, is present in more than 99% of random blood samples. Antibodies in this system are variable and rarely encountered.[50] The glycoprotein carrying these antigens has five extracellular immunoglobulin superfamily domains that serve as laminin-binding receptors.[119,120] The Lu(a–b–) phenotype of the dominant type is associated with acanthocytosis.[121]

Other Systems

Other systems are included in Table 35-1.[80] Antibodies to antigens in these systems are less common than those just described, and information regarding their clinical significance is summarized in Table 35-2.

Maturation of Blood Group Antigens

Several blood group antigens are not expressed or are only weakly expressed on cord RBCs and have usually reached adult levels in children 2 years of age. Antibodies to these antigens are unlikely to cause HDN. Cord RBCs do not express Le^a, Sd^a, Ch, Rg, or AnWj antigens. Cord RBCs express the following antigens more weakly than RBCs from adults do: A, B, H, I, Le^b, P1, Lu^a (but not Lu^b), Yt^a, Vel, Do^a, Do^b, Gy^a, Hy, Jo^a, Xg^a, and Bg.[50,78,122]

Clinical Significance of Blood Group Antibodies

A blood group antigen has no immediate untoward effect on blood transfusion. It is the corresponding antibody that has clinical relevance and dictates the need for tests

TABLE 35-1	Blood Group Systems with Associated Gene Product
Blood Group System	**Gene Product**
CARBOHYDRATE ANTIGENS	
ABO	Glycosyltransferase
P	Glycosyltransferase
Lewis	Glycosyltransferase
Hh	Glycosyltransferase
PROTEIN ANTIGENS	
MNS	Glycophorin A, glycophorin B
Rh	D polypeptide
	RHCE polypeptide
	CcEe polypeptide
Lutheran	Lutheran glycoprotein
Kell	Kell glycoprotein
Kx	Xk glycoprotein
Duffy	Fy glycoprotein
Kidd	Jk glycoprotein
Diego	Band 3 (AE1)
Yt	Acetylcholinesterase
Xg	Xg^a glycoprotein
Scianna	Sc glycoprotein
Dombrock	Glycoprotein (possibly adenosine 5′-diphosphate [ADP]-ribosyltransferase)
Colton	Channel-forming integral protein
LW	Glycoprotein
Chido/Rodgers	C′ component 4 (C4)
Gerbich	Glycophorin C, glycophorin D
Cromer	CD55 (DAF)
Knops	CD35 (CRI)
Indian	CD44

in a transfusion service to detect blood group antibodies.

Antibodies recognizing antigens in the ABO blood group system are by far the most clinically significant. With antibodies in the other blood group systems, as a general rule, the more immunogenic an antigen, the more clinically significant its corresponding alloantibody. Other clinically significant antibodies occur in the following order, from most to least commonly encountered in transfusion practice: anti-D, anti-K, anti-E, anti-c, anti-Fy^a, anti-C, anti-Jk^a, anti-S, anti-Jk^b.[123,124] All other clinically significant antibodies occur at an incidence of less than 1% of serum-containing antibodies,[123,124] which explains why orders for blood lacking different combinations of the aforementioned antigens are by far the most common. Anti-P1, anti-M, anti-N, anti-Lu^a (Lutheran), anti-Le^a, anti-Le^b, and anti-Sd^a are all considered clinically insignificant unless the alloantibodies are reactive in tests performed strictly at 37° C.[50,122] Clinically insignificant antibodies that react at 37° C by the indirect antiglobulin test are those of the Knops and Ch/Rg systems and anti-JMH.[50,123] Other alloantibodies are clinically significant in some patients but not in others; examples

are anti-Vel, anti-Ge (Gerbich), anti-Yt^a, and anti-Co^a (Colton).[50] Table 35-2 summarizes the clinical significance of antibodies to RBC blood group antigens.

The clinical significance of an antibody to a low-incidence antigen depends on whether it was found during crossmatching or prenatal testing. Such an antibody detected during compatibility testing need not be identified to locate antigen-negative blood with which to transfuse that patient because the full crossmatch will be positive in the rare event that another unit of donor blood from the stock supply carries the low-incidence antigen. In contrast, if an antibody to an uncommon antigen is detected in the serum of a pregnant woman, identification of the antibody or determination of the antigen carried by fetal or paternal RBCs can be used as a predictor of the likelihood and severity of HDN. Blood for exchange transfusion will not be hard to find.[50]

If a patient's serum contains alloantibodies to a high-incidence antigen, blood may be hard to find. Examples are anti-U, anti-Kp^b, anti-Js^b, anti-Lu^b, and all antigens in the high series recognized by the International Society for Blood Transfusion (ISBT) working party.[80] Regardless of whether the investigation is for transfusion purposes or prediction of HDN, the antibody should be identified to aid in both assessing its clinical significance and locating appropriate blood for transfusion.

Blood group antibodies in donor plasma present almost no hazard to an antigen-positive recipient. Donor blood is always tested for the presence of blood group antibodies in plasma.

Sera from some patients contain autoantibodies that recognize antigenic determinants on RBCs from the majority of individuals, as well as their own. In such cases it may be impossible to locate compatible blood and only incompatible blood will be available. Instances in which this situation may arise include autoimmune hemolytic anemia, cold agglutinin disease, and paroxysmal cold hemoglobinuria, and these scenarios are discussed later in this chapter.[50]

Testing Donor Blood

Donor blood is routinely tested for its ABO and Rh blood group status. More extensive typing for other antigens is performed either when antigen-negative RBCs are required for a recipient whose serum contains clinically significant antibodies or when building an inventory of donors with certain antigenic profiles for future use, such as in the transfusion management of sickle cell disease (see later). In a patient with multiple alloantibodies, it is useful to estimate the time needed to locate compatible blood. The more alloantibodies present, especially to high-frequency antigens, the longer the time needed to locate compatible units.

Compatibility Procedures

The routine approaches used involve testing a blood sample from a prospective recipient for ABO and Rh

TABLE 35-2	Clinical Significance of Selected Alloantibodies to Antigens in Blood Group Systems				
Antibody	**IgG**	**IgM**	**Complement**	**Transfusion Reaction Binding**	**HDN***
ABO	Some	Most	Common	Mild to severe; immediate	Moderate
MNS					
MN	Some	Some	Rare	Extremely rare	Extremely rare
SsU	Most	Some	Rare	Immediate or delayed	Rare
P1	Rare	Most	Rare	None	None
RH	Most	Some	No	Immediate or delayed	Mild/severe
Lutheran					
Lu^a	Most	Some	No	None	None
Lu^b	Most	Rare	No	Mild; delayed	Mild/rare
Kell	Most	Some	Some	Immediate or delayed	Mild/severe
Lewis					
Le^a	Some	Most	Some	Rare; immediate	None
Le^b	Rare	Most		None	None
Duffy					
Fy^a	Most	Rare	Rare	Delayed	Mild
Fy^b	Most		No	Mild; delayed	None
Kidd	Most	Few	Common	Immediate or delayed	Mild/rare
Diego	Most			Delayed	Mild/severe
Yt	Most			Some; mild	None
Xg	Most		Some	None	None
Scianna	Most			None	None
Dombrock	Most			Delayed	Mild
Colton	Most			Mild; delayed	Mild/rare
LW	Most			Mild; delayed	Mild
Ch/RG	Most			None	None
H	Rare	Most		None (except in O$_h$)	None
XK	Most		None known	Delayed	None
Gerbich	Most	Some	Some	Immediate or delayed	None
Cromer	Most			Delayed	Mild
Knops	Most			None	None
Indian	Most			None	None

*The most severe form of hemolytic disease of the newborn (HDN) that has been reported is indicated. Remember that exceptions exist.

blood groups and for detection of blood group antibodies.[53] In most cases no unexpected antibodies are detected, and donor RBCs of the appropriate ABO and Rh blood type will be selected for transfusion. A sample of this blood may be crossmatched with the patient's serum by an immediate spin procedure or an "electronic crossmatch" in which a validated computer system verifies that the patient is receiving an RBC unit that is ABO and Rh(D) compatible with the patient's blood group.

When an antibody is detected, it should be identified if possible. Knowing the specificity of an antibody will establish whether it is likely to be clinically significant and the approach that will be necessary to provide an adequate supply of compatible blood.

Compatibility in ABO and Rh

Determination of the ABO and Rh(D) type of the patient is the first step in compatibility testing. In neonates, the ABO group is determined by testing the neonate's RBCs only because the plasma may contain maternal antibodies and young neonates' immune systems do not make isohemaglutinins. In patients older than 4 months, the ABO group is determined by testing both the patient's RBCs (forward group) and the plasma or serum (reverse group). The forward and reverse groups should correspond, except that infants younger than 9 months may not yet be making isohemaglutinins. In all other patients, until any discrepancy is resolved, only group O RBCs and AB plasma should be given.

Blood and blood components must be selected to be ABO and Rh compatible (Table 35-3). In general, for patients older than 4 months, type-specific RBCs and whole blood are selected, which means that the donor and recipient have the same ABO and Rh type; it is acceptable to transfuse ABO- and Rh-compatible but not identical RBCs. For transfusion of a fetus, group O Rh(D–), irradiated, CMV antibody–negative or leukoreduced RBCs (or both) are usually given regardless of the ABO group of the recipient. For neonates, some centers transfuse type-specific whereas others transfuse group O RBCs to all infants. If the RBCs selected for transfusion are not group O, the neonate's serum or plasma should be tested for anti-A and anti-B.[53] If anti-A or anti-B is detected, ABO-compatible RBCs should be transfused.[53]

Patients ABO/D	COMPATIBLE DONORS*							
	O Positive	O Negative	A Positive	A Negative	B Positive	B Negative	AB Positive	AB Negative
O positive	+	+						
O negative		+						
A positive	+	+	+	+				
A negative		+		+				
B positive	+	+			+	+		
B negative		+				+		
AB positive	+	+	+	+	+	+	+	+
AB negative		+		+		+		+

TABLE 35-3   Compatible Donors for Red Blood Cell Transfusion

*For massive transfusions and directed donor transfusions, compatible red blood cells (RBCs) may be used when type-specific RBCs are unavailable. Crossmatch-compatible group O Rh(D–) donor RBCs can be given to any recipient. Group AB Rh(D+) patients can receive RBCs of any ABO and Rh type.

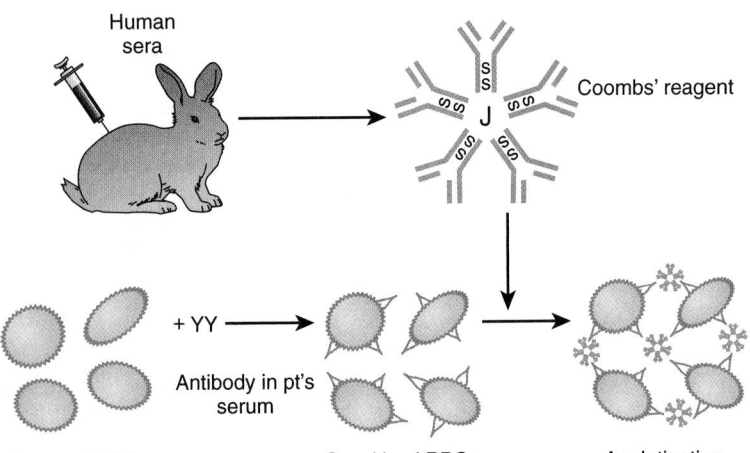

FIGURE 35-2. Antibody screen. Reagent red blood cells (RBCs) of known antigenic phenotypes are mixed with a patient's serum and Coombs' reagent. If the patient's cells agglutinate, the patient has an antibody to an antigen present on the reagent cells.

Treatment with Rh immune globulin for prevention of immunization to D may be appropriate for a Rh(D–) patient who has received Rh(D+) RBCs, including those transfused with platelet or granulocyte products because these products contain RBCs.[53]

Compatibility in Other Blood Groups

Compatibility testing for blood groups other than ABO is achieved by antibody screen and crossmatch (Figs. 35-2 and 35-3). These tests detect unexpected RBC antibodies in the patient's serum. The patient's serum or plasma or, in the case of a neonate, maternal serum or plasma may be used for the antibody screen.[53] In the antibody screen, the patient's serum is mixed with group O reagent RBCs, which have most of the important blood group antigens. Because neonates are unlikely to produce new antibodies, the antibody screen needs to be performed only once per admission if the initial antibody screen is negative.[53] In the crossmatch, the patient's serum is mixed with donor RBCs or "electronically" crossmatched with a validated computer system.[53] In patients older than 4 months, crossmatch is performed for every unit of RBCs or whole blood transfused. In neonates, if the initial antibody screen is negative, it is unnecessary to crossmatch donor RBCs.[53]

If a blood group alloantibody is detected in the recipient's serum, every attempt should be made to identify the antibody. The clinical significance of an antibody is based on knowledge of the specificity of the alloantibody and the reported experience in other patients whose serum contains the same antibody specificity (see Table 35-2).[50] If the antibody has potential clinical significance, antigen-negative blood should be selected and crossmatched by a procedure that includes the antiglobulin phase.[42,53]

Selection of Blood for Transfusion to Patients with Blood Group Alloantibodies

Many alloantibodies detected in vitro in human sera do not have the potential to induce in vivo destruction of incompatible RBCs. No technical procedure is able to differentiate, with certainty, between clinically benign and clinically significant antibodies. Although the in vitro characteristics of an antibody may not reflect its behavior

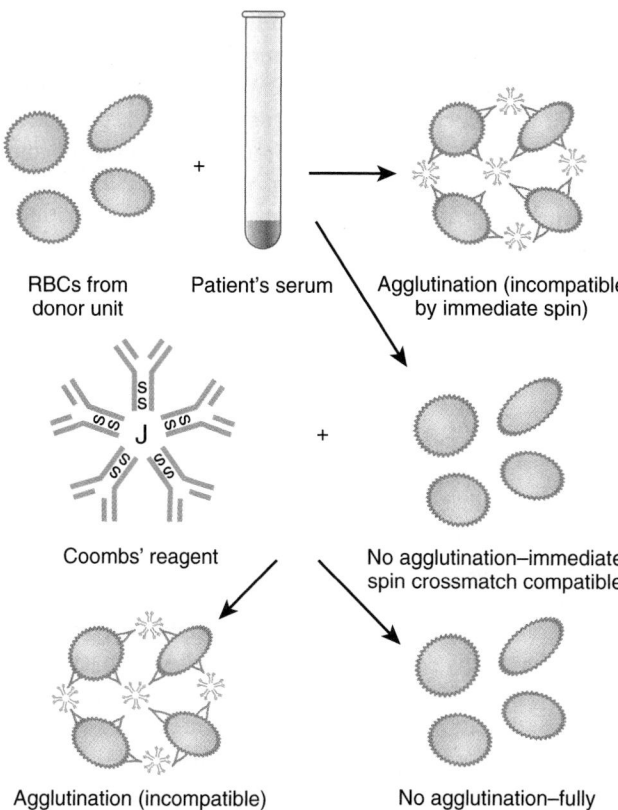

RBCs from donor unit

Patient's serum

Agglutination (incompatible by immediate spin)

Coombs' reagent

No agglutination–immediate spin crossmatch compatible

Agglutination (incompatible)

No agglutination–fully crossmatch compatible

FIGURE 35-3. Compatibility procedures. Red blood cells (RBCs) from a donor unit are mixed with a patient's serum. If agglutination of the cells occurs, the cells are incompatible by the immediate spin technique. If a full crossmatch is performed, Coombs' reagent is added to the cells and serum and the cells are examined for agglutination.

in vivo, the following features can be used to help establish its potential significance in that patient. In general, antibodies of the IgG class are more clinically significant than those of the IgM class.[50] In addition, the higher the titer of an antibody, the more likely it is to destroy antigen-positive RBCs in vivo. An antibody that causes in vitro hemolysis because of complement activation (see Table 35-2) of antigen-positive RBCs is likely to be clinically significant. Antibodies that react at 37° C are more likely to be clinically significant than those that do not.[50] For cold-reacting IgM antibodies, the wider the thermal range of reactivity in vitro, the more clinically significant it is likely to be. Alloantibodies that react in the cold and are not usually clinically significant include antibodies to M, N, P1, Le[a], and Le[b] antigens.[123] In difficult cases, a few reference laboratories can also perform a monocyte monolayer assay, which has some value in predicting whether an antibody will cause a hemolytic transfusion reaction.[125]

Once a patient is actively immunized to an RBC antigen and produces a clinically significant alloantibody, the patient is considered immunized for life and must be transfused with antigen-negative RBCs for life. Neonates with passively acquired maternal antibody are not actively

immunized and thus need to be transfused with antigen-negative RBCs only while the antibody is still present.

Emergency Need

When RBC transfusion is urgently needed in a rapidly bleeding patient, compatibility testing should be abbreviated so that transfusion is not delayed. The clinician should indicate the need for emergency release of blood. A pretransfusion sample is obtained from the patient, the blood bank rapidly determines the ABO and D type on this sample, and the patient receives type-specific blood. However, if time is not available, the blood bank will issue group O Rh(D–) RBCs and AB plasma. In some cases of severe inventory shortages, these patients, especially males, may receive group O Rh(D+) RBCs. In cases of emergency transfusion, the antibody screen and crossmatch may be performed after the blood has been transfused, and the clinician is notified if any antibodies are identified.[53]

Massive Transfusion

When a child or neonate is massively transfused (i.e., one blood volume or more within 24 hours), the usual guidelines for selection of compatible blood may not apply. For alloimmunized patients, blood not tested for antigen may be used during an acute bleeding period and antigen-negative blood reserved for the late transfusion period.[53] If the supply of Rh(D–) blood is very limited, the patient's clinical situation should be assessed. If the expected amount of further bleeding is small, such as at the end of a surgical procedure, every effort should be made to avoid transfusion of Rh(D+) blood. However, in some cases the expected amount of further bleeding is large and the patient's transfusion needs clearly cannot be met by the limited amount of Rh(D–) blood available. In such cases it may be better for the Rh(D–) patient to switch to Rh(D+) RBCs early during the period of bleeding and reserve the Rh(D–) RBCs for the end of the bleeding episode.

Autologous Blood

Autologous blood transfusion is possible for some children who undergo elective surgery for which transfusion is anticipated. Transfusion of such blood reduces the risk of transfusion-transmitted viral diseases, but no blood transfusion is without risk. For example, autologous blood transfusions can be contaminated with bacteria or can cause volume overload, and there is always the risk that an incorrect unit could be transfused. Intraoperative RBC salvage can be used if tumor cells or bacteria are not expected to contaminate the surgical field.

To donate autologous blood before surgery, a child must meet the size or age requirements of the blood donor center, have adequate venous access, and have a hemoglobin concentration of 11 g/dL or greater and a hematocrit of 33% or greater.[53] Some blood donor centers will collect small units that are proportional to the child's size. Donation should begin 4 to 5 weeks before surgery to allow time for RBC regeneration. Oral iron supplementation should be given. Recombinant erythropoietin is not routinely recommended for autologous blood donors and has not been licensed by the Food and Drug Administration (FDA) for autologous donation. However, it may be useful in selected circumstances.[126-129]

Directed Donations

Some institutions allow family and friends to direct their blood donations to be used for a child or infant. This is no safer than random banked blood and adds additional administrative expense. GVHD can occur when the patient shares an HLA haplotype with an HLA homozygous blood donor, and it is more likely to occur if a patient receive blood from a relative.[30,31,130] Hence, directed donations from blood relatives should be irradiated, and most institutions irradiate all blood donated by directed donors.

Choice of Blood for the Fetus

For intrauterine transfusions, group O Rh(D–) (and antigen negative if mother has an alloantibody) blood should be used. To prevent graft-versus-fetus disease, the blood is irradiated. To prevent CMV infection, CMV antibody–negative blood or leukocyte-reduced blood, or both, should be used.

Choice of Blood for the Neonate

Cellular components should be selected from CMV antibody–negative donors for neonate recipients weighing less than 1200 g at birth if their mothers are CMV antibody negative.[131] Alternatively, leukocyte-reduced blood can also be used to prevent CMV infection if the blood product has less than 5×10^6 donor leukocytes.[132] Cellular blood components should be irradiated to prevent GVHD in these low-weight premature infants.[133]

In exchange transfusions for a neonate with HDN, the RBCs used must be negative for the implicated antibody (e.g., Rh[D–] RBCs when hemolysis is due to anti-Rh[D]). In terms of ABO group selection, group O RBCs and plasma of the infant's ABO group are often used. Group-compatible RBCs and plasma can likewise be used if the RBCs are also compatible with any maternal antibodies that are present in the infant's circulation.[50]

Choice of Blood for Patients with Sickle Cell Anemia

Two important principles must be followed in the transfusion of sickle cell patients: (1) avoidance of excessive viscosity and (2) prevention of sensitization to red cell antigens.

Sickle cells are intrinsically less deformable than normal cells; thus, elevating the hematocrit without significantly reducing the proportion of sickle cells may raise blood viscosity to dangerous levels.[134] Simple transfusion must be used with caution, particularly in children with hematocrits greater than 30%.

The question of what to use for transfusion of patients with sickle cell anemia has been the subject of many heated debates.[135-137] There is still no consensus regarding the best and most practical approach. Sickle cell patients, like all patients, are at risk for the development of alloantibodies, and alloantibodies may pose specific hazards to patients with sickle cell disease. Sickle cell patients usually need many transfusions throughout their lives, and an antibody to a blood group alloantigen that develops in childhood may be undetectable later in their lives. If they are then transfused with blood expressing that antigen, an anamnestic response to the antigen and a delayed hemolytic transfusion reaction are likely to develop. Sickle cell patients have been reported to suffer painful crises secondary to delayed hemolytic transfusion reactions. Additionally, a sickle cell patient in whom red cell alloantibodies develop may be at increased risk for the development of red cell autoantibodies, which can significantly complicate the disease.[137] For these reasons, some transfusion services provide phenotype-matched blood for sickle cell patients. Approaches that are used include those described in Table 35-4. Note that none of these approaches will prevent the production of antibodies to high-incidence antigens, such as U, Js[b], Cr[a], hr[S], and hr[B]. African Americans tend to be null for antigens commonly expressed in the general donor population, which consists of mostly whites in the United States. For this reason, some blood donor facilities have programs to recruit African Americans to donate blood to support the transfusion needs of sickle cell patients.

Choice of Blood for Patients with Thalassemia

In thalassemia, the goals of transfusion therapy are prevention of anemia and maintenance of a circulating hemoglobin level that is sufficient to suppress endogenous erythropoiesis. For most patients, maintenance of a pretransfusion hemoglobin level of 9 to 10 g/100 mL is sufficient.[138] Red cell alloantibodies are not a significant problem in most thalassemia patients, probably because transfusions are usually initiated at an early age when tolerance may develop. Therefore, most institutions in the United States do not provide red cells that are phenotypically matched to the patient's red cells.[139,140]

Choice of Blood for Allogeneic Hematopoietic Progenitor Cell Transplants

Because an HLA-identical donor is usually required for allogeneic HPC transplantation, the donor may not have the same ABO and Rh type as the patient.[42] In major ABO incompatibility, the recipient has antibodies against donor RBCs (e.g., the recipient is group O and has anti-A and anti-B; the donor is group A). In minor ABO incompatibility, the donor has antibodies against the recipient's RBCs (e.g., the donor is group O and has anti-A and anti-B; the recipient is group A). These incompatibilities may produce hemolysis,[50] but the hemolysis is often minimized by proper selection of blood products for transfusion.

TABLE 35-4   Approaches to Antigen Typing of Blood for Patients with Sickle Cell Disease

Approach	Advantages	Disadvantages
Treat like other patients (i.e., avoid antigens to which the patient has made antibodies)	Simple. Avoids unnecessary work	Some patients will make antibodies that can result in serious transfusion reactions that may be especially dangerous in these patients Patients are probably at increased risk for the development of autoantibodies
Provide fully antigen-matched blood before the patient makes antibodies (i.e., matched for D, C, E, c, e, K, Fy^a, Fy^b, Jk^a, and Jk^b antigens). Note that antigen matching for Fy^b is not needed for patients of African descent who are Fy(a–b–) because they have the *FYB* gene, which is expressed in the lung and colon, and do not mount an immune response to the Fy^b antigen on transfusion of Fy(b+) RBCs	Reduces the risk of alloantibody and autoantibody formation and the risks associated with these antibodies	Significant work to reduce the risk for an antibody that may never develop There may be difficulty identifying units with extended phenotype matches
Provide antigen-matched blood after the first antibody is made	Reduces the chance of multiple antibodies with less work than extended phenotype matching for all patients	Some patients will make multiple antibodies quickly
Provide partially antigen-matched blood (i.e., matched for D, C, E, and K antigens)	Reduces the chance of multiple antibodies with less work than extended phenotype matching that includes antigens that are not very immunogenic	Some patients will make antibodies against unmatched antigens

In major ABO incompatibility (e.g., the donor is group A; the recipient is group O), host-versus-graft reactions can cause delayed erythropoiesis and even RBC aplasia.[141] To prevent recipient destruction of donor RBCs at the time of HPC infusion, donor RBCs are removed from the HPC preparation before infusion. A group O recipient may continue to produce anti-A and anti-B after transplantation, which can cause hemolysis of the newly produced donor group A RBCs. If transfusions are necessary during this period, group O RBCs can be given (Table 35-5). Before transplantation, the group O recipient has anti-A and anti-B. After engraftment of group A donor marrow, the anti-B will persist but the anti-A will become undetectable. Donor group A RBCs are given only after the recipient stops producing anti-A, that is, when the recipient's group O blood type changes to the donor group A and anti-A is not detected in the patient's serum.

In minor ABO incompatibility, hemolysis of recipient RBCs by donor antibody is usually preventable. To prevent hemolysis of recipient RBCs by passively transfused donor antibody during HPC infusion, plasma is removed from the HPC preparation before infusion. In addition, passenger B lymphocytes in the donor HPC unit may produce antibodies that could destroy the recipient RBCs. To prevent hemolysis of transfused RBCs, group O RBCs are used for transfusion during the post-transplant period if the antibody is detected. If the donor or recipient has a clinically significant antibody to an erythrocyte antigen, blood lacking the antigen should be given after transplantation.[53]

TABLE 35-5   Choice of Blood for Bone Marrow Transplant Patients

Recipient	Donor	Red Cells
A	O	O
A	B	O
A	AB	A or O
B	O	O
B	A	O
B	AB	B or O
AB	O	O
AB	B	B or O
AB	A	A or O
O	A	O
O	B	O
O	AB	O

Choice of Blood for Organ Transplantation

The ABO antigens are strong histocompatibility antigens and thus are of major importance in organ transplantation. Because ABO antigens are expressed on vascular endothelium, the recipient can reject and damage the vascular endothelium of a donor organ that is a major ABO mismatch. For this reason, major ABO-incompatible vascular organ transplants (liver, kidney, heart, lungs, pancreas) are not usually performed. However, ABO-incompatible heart transplants may be performed in infants and young children who have not yet produced isohemagglutinins or who have produced only low levels of isohemagglutinins.[142]

When organ transplants are performed in the presence of minor ABO incompatibility, the same hemolytic problems as in HPC transplantation may occur.[143] Passenger B lymphocytes may produce antibodies against the recipient's RBCs. Hemolysis of transfused RBCs can usually be prevented when an antibody is detected by transfusion of group O RBCs for ABO incompatibility and transfusion of antigen-negative RBCs for incompatibility caused by other blood groups.

Selection of Blood for Transfusion to Patients with Blood Group Autoantibodies

Autoimmune hemolytic anemia is described in detail in Chapter 14. In hemolytic anemia secondary to warm-reactive autoantibodies, no compatible blood can usually be found. The direct antiglobulin test (DAT, Fig. 35-4) will almost always be positive in autoimmune hemolytic anemia. Blood bank serologic testing is aimed at determining whether any underlying clinically significant alloantibodies are present and identifying the specificity of any such antibodies that are detected. This can be determined, with time, at a hospital transfusion service, which may need to have the testing performed at an immunohematology reference laboratory. Patients without a history of immunization are unlikely to have underlying alloantibodies. Transfused RBC units should be compatible with any underlying clinically significant alloantibodies. However, the blood is still usually incompatible with the patient's serum, and the clinically necessary amount of red cells should be transfused with careful monitoring but without delay. In some patients, the warm autoantibody has a clear-cut specificity for an antigen, and antigen-negative RBCs may be compatible in the crossmatch test.[144]

In paroxysmal cold hemoglobinuria associated with the Donath-Landsteiner antibody, transfusion is rarely necessary. The antibody binds RBCs only at cold temperatures (<20° C). In theory, it is reasonable to transfuse blood through a blood warmer; however, in practice, crossmatch-compatible, unwarmed random RBCs have been given without problem.[145] Only rarely is transfusion of RBCs of the rare phenotype p needed.[146,147] Most cases of paroxysmal cold hemoglobinuria in children are transient and occur after viral infection.

In cold agglutinin disease, a rare condition in children, RBCs should be transfused through a blood warmer. As described previously, the same issue of testing for underlying alloantibodies pertains here.

Adverse Effects of Transfusion

All reactions other than mild allergic (urticarial) reactions require immediate cessation of the transfusion and delivery of a fresh blood sample from the patient to the blood bank for serologic evaluation.

Allergic Reactions

The typical urticarial reaction is characterized by itching and hives. Localized urticaria simply requires interrupting the transfusion and administering an antihistamine. If the symptoms resolve within 30 minutes, the transfusion can be continued. Recurrent allergic reactions may require pretreatment with antihistamine.

Some children exhibit more severe allergic reactions, such as laryngospasm and bronchospasm. These patients may require steroids or epinephrine, or both (Table 35-6). The same unit of blood should not be restarted, even after the symptoms have responded to treatment. Saline-washed blood products may be helpful in patients with severe or recurrent allergic reactions. Anaphylactic reactions may occur if the patient is IgA deficient and has formed an IgE anti-IgA antibody. In these cases, either washed blood products or products drawn from rare IgA-deficient donors are indicated.

Febrile Nonhemolytic Reactions

The occurrence of fever, chills, or diaphoresis is usually due to cytokines released from leukocytes. Cytokines can be released from leukocytes during storage or on infusion in a patient who has antibodies that react with antigens on foreign white blood cells. Febrile nonhemolytic transfusion reactions are not associated with serious sequelae and may be treated with antipyretics. Of note, fever during a transfusion may represent another, more serious type of transfusion reaction: acute hemolysis, sepsis from a bacterially contaminated unit, or transfusion-related acute lung injury.

Acute Hemolytic Transfusion Reactions

Acute hemolytic transfusion reactions are most often due to donor-recipient ABO incompatibility. These reactions are generally caused by managerial errors, such as misidentification of a transfusion recipient.[148,149] The clinical manifestations of acute hemolytic transfusion reactions vary. Signs and symptoms may include any or all of the

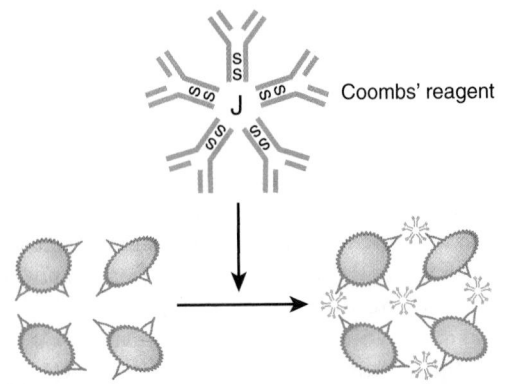

FIGURE 35-4. Direct antiglobulin test (DAT). Red blood cells (RBCs) are incubated with Coombs' reagent; if the cells agglutinate after incubation, the DAT is positive.

Coombs' reagent

Sensitized patient's RBCs   Agglutination

TABLE 35-6   Guidelines for the Management of Transfusion Reactions

Agent	Use	Dose	Comment
Diphenhydramine	Treating pruritus and rash (hives)	6.25-25 mg IV over period of 10-20 min	Diphenhydramine cannot prevent and has no place in the treatment of severe transfusion reactions
Epinephrine	Severe reactions characterized by bronchospasm, hypotension, and shock	0.1-0.4 mg SC (or IV if the patient is hypotensive)	For patients in shock not responding to epinephrine, treatment with an initial fluid bolus should be initiated. As in patients with shock from other causes, fluids, vasopressors, airway protection, and oxygenation should also be used
1:20 Aqueous suspension of epinephrine	After stabilization with epinephrine	0.05-0.2 mg SC	
Fluids			For hypotensive patients, a bolus of 20 mL/kg of normal saline should be administered simultaneously with epinephrine and steroids
Narcotics	Specific and effective treatment of rigors	0.1 mg/kg of morphine IV (or equivalent dose of meperidine hydrochloride)	
Acetaminophen (Tylenol)	Prevention or reversal of elevations in temperature in mild to moderate febrile reactions	Appropriate for age	
Steroids	In moderate to severe reactions; may occasionally be required for severe urticaria; indicated in all reactions characterized by fever, shaking chills, diaphoresis, and pallor	1-2 mg/kg of methylprednisolone (or equivalent dose of dexamethasone or hydrocortisone by IV push)	

IV, intravenously; SC, subcutaneously.

following: fever, chills, dyspnea, tachycardia, hypotension, flank pain, abdominal pain, pain at the infusion site, apprehension, nausea, vomiting, and hemoglobinuria. Other serious sequelae may include acute renal failure, shock, or disseminated intravascular coagulation (DIC), which may be manifested as bleeding. Some acute hemolytic reactions are characterized by only minor initial symptoms. In anesthetized recipients, the only findings may be diffuse bleeding (secondary to DIC) or red urine (hemoglobinuria). When an acute hemolytic transfusion reaction is suspected, the transfusion should be stopped immediately and an investigation initiated. The identity of the patient and unit should be reconfirmed. The remainder of the unit and a fresh blood sample should be sent to the blood bank, where the required workup includes (1) a clerical check, (2) visual inspection of the recipient's plasma for hemolysis, and (3) a DAT. If there is no visible hemolysis in the patient's plasma and the DAT result is negative, immune-mediated hemolysis can be excluded. A fresh urine specimen should be tested for hemoglobinuria.

Therapy for an acute hemolytic reaction is supportive. Depending on the size of the child, urine output of 40 to 100 mL/hr should be maintained. Early consultation with a nephrologist is warranted. Intravenous administration of furosemide or mannitol, which increase renal blood flow, may be required.

Delayed Hemolytic Transfusion Reactions

Delayed hemolytic transfusion reactions consist of two types: primary immunization and anamnestic response. Primary immunization is mild and occurs weeks after transfusion. It rarely causes significant hemolysis and may be suspected after an unexplained decrease in the patient's hemoglobin level 2 to 3 weeks after transfusion.

Secondary immune responses occur in patients who have been sensitized to one or more non-ABO blood group antigens during a previous transfusion or pregnancy. When a patient is re-exposed to the antigen, an anamnestic response occurs and results in a rapid rise in antibody level and accelerated clearance of the transfused antigen-positive red cells. These patients experience some of the symptoms of a hemolytic reaction 3 to 10 days after transfusion. The clinical syndrome is generally mild, but delayed transfusion reactions can result in profound anemia. These reactions should be suspected in patients who have received multiple transfusions and unexplained anemia, bilirubinemia, or both develop 3 to 10 days after transfusion. The diagnosis is confirmed by a positive DAT result and identification of red cell alloantibodies in the patient's serum or on the patient's RBCs, or both.

Transfusion-Transmitted Diseases

Because of improvements in both donor screening and product testing, blood products are currently extremely safe. However, although the risks of transfusion-transmitted disease have been greatly reduced, they have not been eliminated entirely. Currently, all blood donations in the United States are tested for the presence of human immunodeficiency virus 1 and 2 (HIV-1/2), hepatitis B virus (HBV), hepatitis C virus (HCV), human T-cell lymphotropic virus 1 and 2 (HTLV-1/2), West Nile virus (WNV), and syphilis, and testing for Chagas' disease (*Trypanosoma cruzi*) is initiated. The battery of tests performed includes a combination of serologic testing and nucleic acid testing (NAT). The tests are exquisitely sensitive. However, very recent infections may be missed (so-called window period donations). The risks listed in the following sections and summarized in Table 35-7 are based on mathematical models estimating the number of infectious donors whose blood tests negative for a disease because they are in the window period.

Post-transfusion Hepatitis

Hepatitis B Virus. The estimated risk of post-transfusion HBV infection is presently 1 in 200,000 to 1 in 500,000 units transfused.[150] Acute HBV infection is symptomatic in about 50% of adults, and 5% to 10% of those infected become chronic carriers. In contrast, HBV infection acquired in early childhood is usually asymptomatic and leads to a chronic carrier state in more than 70% of those infected.[151]

Hepatitis C Virus. With the routine use of screening by NAT, the per-unit risk for HCV infection is currently

estimated to be about 1 in 2,000,000.[150] Children who receive HCV-infected blood products have a 30% to 50% chance of spontaneously clearing their infection.[152] Most others become chronically infected. In approximately 20% of children who have been infected with HCV, signs of cirrhosis develop after 18 years of age.[153,154]

Human Immunodeficiency Virus

All units are tested for HIV-1/2 by immunoassay, as well as by NAT. With NAT, the window period for HIV has been reduced to about 10 days. The per-unit risk of HIV infection is currently estimated to be 1 in 2,000,000.[150]

Human T-Cell Lymphotropic Virus

HTLV is the causative agent of both adult T-cell leukemia and endemic spastic myelopathy.[155,156] Most cases have been reported in residents of or emigrants from Japan, Africa, and the Caribbean region. The most comprehensive report of transfusion-transmitted HTLV indicated that 65% of patients who received whole blood or cellular products from HTLV antibody–positive donors seroconverted. Blood from all donations is tested for HTLV-1/2; the current per-unit risk is estimated to be 1 in 641,000.[157]

West Nile Virus

West Nile virus (WNV) is a flavivirus common in Africa, western Asia, and the Middle East. A febrile illness will develop in approximately 20% of infected individuals. Rarely, WNV infection causes an encephalitis syndrome; elderly and immunocompromised individuals are those primarily at risk. WNV has recently become established in North America. The vast majority of cases are transmitted by mosquito bites, but transfusion-related transmission does occur rarely. In 2003, nationwide routine screening for WNV by NAT was begun. As with HIV and HCV, NAT has almost completely eliminated WNV from the U.S. blood supply.

Cytomegalovirus

CMV is carried in and transmitted via lymphocytes. In most patients, transfusion-associated CMV infection causes no symptoms, although it may induce a mild mononucleosis-type illness 3 to 4 weeks after transfusion. Transfusion of CMV-containing blood products into an immunocompromised host with no serologic evidence of previous exposure to CMV can result in a lethal systemic infection. Patients at risk for severe CMV infection include bone marrow transplant patients, organ transplant candidates and recipients, and high-risk neonates. Therefore, patients who have never been infected with CMV and have an inherited or acquired immunodeficiency states should receive CMV-negative or leukoreduced red cells.[158]

Bacteria (Platelet Units)

Platelets are associated with the same range of infectious pathogens as any other blood component, but septic

TABLE 35-7	Estimated Risk of Transfusion-Transmitted Diseases
Agent	**Number of Infections/Million Units**
HIV	0.5
HCV	0.5
HBV	2-5
HTLV	0.5-4

HBV, hepatitis B virus; HCV, hepatitis C virus; HIV, human immunodeficiency virus; HTLV, human T-cell lymphotropic virus.

transfusion reactions, caused by bacterially contaminated units, are a unique risk of platelet transfusion. In contrast to all other blood components, which are either stored at 4° C or frozen, platelets are stored at room temperature. The reason is that if platelets are chilled before transfusion, they are cleared rapidly from the recipient's circulation.[159] Although room-temperature storage dramatically improves platelet survival in vivo, it also tends to promote bacterial growth. Currently, bacteria can be cultured from approximately 1 in 5000 apheresis platelet units.[160] In the United States, large donor centers generally use culture methods to screen for bacteria in all platelet products. With current screening methods, the per-unit risk of a clinically apparent septic transfusion reaction is estimated to be 1 in 75,000 platelet transfusions.[150]

PLATELET TRANSFUSION

Platelets are prepared for transfusion from a single unit of freshly collected whole blood (a platelet concentrate) or from apheresis by means of continuous-flow centrifugation (single-donor platelets). Regardless of the technique used, platelets must always be collected and stored at 20° C to 24° C and in anticoagulant containing citrate-phosphate-dextrose (CPD) or CPDA-1. Citrate anticoagulates the blood by binding plasma calcium, whereas dextrose is a nutrient source for actively metabolizing platelets.

Random-Donor Platelet Concentrates

In the United States, platelet concentrates are prepared from whole blood by the platelet-rich plasma (PRP) method. PRP is separated from packed RBCs by centrifugation of whole blood ("soft spin"). The PRP is then centrifuged again ("hard spin"). All but 50 to 70 mL of the platelet-poor plasma is transferred to an adjoining bag to be used for the production of fresh frozen plasma or other blood components such as cryoprecipitate or albumin. When optimal centrifugation techniques are used, approximately 85% of the platelets (5.0 to 7.0 × 10^{10} platelets) are recovered from a unit of whole blood.[161-163] In Canada and Europe, the alternative "buffy coat" method is used to generate platelet concentrates from whole blood.

Single-Donor Apheresis Platelets

Automated blood collection for the production of apheresis platelets may be accomplished with either continuous or discontinuous flow centrifugation.[164,165] Apheresis platelets from one individual should yield more than 3.0 × 10^{11} platelets in 200 to 300 mL of plasma. This preparation may also be called single-donor apheresis platelets as opposed to pooled platelet concentrates from random donors. Modern apheresis equipment is often able to yield more than 6.5 × 10^{11} platelets per procedure and

typically incorporates a leukoreduction step that leaves fewer than $1 × 10^6$ leukocytes per product. This allows units to be split into two doses, each with six platelet concentrate equivalents.

Once they are processed, platelet units are stored on elliptical, circular, or flat-bed agitators.[166,167] This constant mild agitation prevents platelet clumping or activation as platelets settle to the bottom of the bag.[168,169] Constant agitation also facilitates gas exchange, which is important for maintaining an optimal pH range for platelet metabolism and function at 20° C.[170] Because of the risk of bacterial growth associated with room-temperature storage, platelet units are generally stored for only 5 days. In some settings, the FDA has allowed bacterially tested platelets to be stored for up to 7 days.[171]

Prophylactic Platelet Transfusion

Today, the vast majority of platelet transfusions are given prophylactically to prevent bleeding in nonbleeding patients, as opposed to therapeutically to treat active bleeding. If there is no evidence of platelet dysfunction, patients do not usually experience active bleeding if the platelet count is greater than 10,000/mm³ and have minimal risk for spontaneous life-threatening hemorrhage until the count is 5000/mm³ or less.[172-176] However, additional coagulation abnormalities, such as acquired or congenital platelet dysfunction, clotting protein deficiencies, or vascular or tissue defects, require more aggressive platelet support to decrease the risk for hemorrhage.

Risk assessment for surgical patients is somewhat more difficult. Retrospective data suggest that a platelet count of 50,000/mm³ or greater is acceptable for a patient to undergo major surgery.[177] Certain circumstances may warrant more aggressive correction of thrombocytopenia before or after surgery. In areas in which even a small amount of bleeding might cause permanent deficits, such as the eye or central nervous system, it is traditional to aim for a platelet count of greater than 100,000/mm³. During prolonged procedures in which the patient will be maintained on cardiopulmonary bypass or extracorporeal membrane oxygenation (ECMO), platelets may be dysfunctional because of activation after passage through the extracorporeal perfusion equipment. In general, there is no need to administer platelets to patients after extracorporeal circulation if there is no evidence of bleeding and the platelet count is at least 50,000/mm³.[178-180] When bleeding is present, it is more commonly due to heparin, inadequate protamine correction, fibrinolysis, or problems with surgical closure.

Minor procedures such as liver biopsy have been performed safely with platelet counts greater than 25,000/mm³.[181] Similarly, lumbar puncture has been shown to be safe in the setting of thrombocytopenia. Howard and co-workers[182] reported a series of 956 consecutive pediatric patients with newly diagnosed acute lymphoblastic leukemia who underwent lumbar puncture. No serious bleeding complications occurred in 5223 lumbar punctures, including 170 performed when the platelet count was 11,000 to 20,000/μL. The authors concluded that prophylactic platelet transfusion was unnecessary in patients with platelet counts above 10,000/μL. These procedures were performed in only 29 patients with platelet counts of 10,000/μL or less, so it was not possible to assess the risk of bleeding in patients with extremely low platelet counts with confidence.

Platelet Dosing

Guidelines for determining the platelet dose have been published in a number of reviews.[183-185] In general, 1 unit of random-donor platelets (5.0 to 7.0 × 10^10 platelets) per 10 kg of body weight should increase the platelet count by 40,000 to 50,000/mm^3 within 1 hour after the infusion. In an average-sized adolescent or adult, 6 units of platelet concentrate, or 1 single-donor apheresis unit (3 to 5 × 10^11), will increase the platelet count by 50,000/mm^3 or greater.

To determine the effectiveness of platelet transfusion, a platelet count should be obtained before infusion, at 1 hour, and at 24 hours after infusion. There is no significant difference in the post-transfusion platelet count when measured 10 minutes versus 60 minutes after transfusion.[186] These estimates assume normal spleen function and size; approximately 30% of transfused platelets are removed from circulation in the spleen.[185,187]

Normally, a third of the platelets released into circulation from the bone marrow are stored in the spleen. This platelet pool is mobilized when patients are treated with corticosteroids, which results in an increase in circulating platelet number. Hypersplenism causes a larger percentage of transfused platelets to be sequestered in the spleen. This condition results in a decrease in platelet recovery immediately after platelet infusion but does not have an effect on platelet survival once a steady state has been achieved.[188]

Since the mid-1950s, clinicians have recognized that fever may reduce platelet recovery by 20% to 40%.[189,190] In one study, decreased platelet recovery was documented in bone marrow transplant patients with fever and negative blood cultures. Although occult infection cannot be ruled out, fever alone was the only change associated with poor platelet increment in these patients.[190]

Consumptive coagulopathy (DIC) refers to excessive activation of thrombin resulting in accelerated conversion of fibrinogen to fibrin. This process may be acute and accompanied by rapid consumption of procoagulant factors and platelets in association with extensive bleeding, as in sepsis, shock, or certain forms of malignancy.[191,192] A chronic form of DIC may occur if the procoagulant consumption is slow enough for the liver to compensate for limited consumption, as found in hemangiomas or a necrotic lesion in the lung or brain, for example. In either form of DIC, recovery plus survival of transfused platelets is shortened.[193-195] Diseases associated with primary endothelial cell damage, such as hemolytic-uremic syndrome (HUS) and thrombotic thrombocytopenic purpura (TTP), are also associated with decreased platelet recovery because of the formation of microaggregates in areas of vascular damage.[196] Additional bleeding may be seen with these syndromes as result of the acquired platelet dysfunction associated with renal failure and uremia.[184,197]

Errors in calculating the expected increment in platelet count may occur if one overestimates the number of platelets in a platelet concentrate or single-donor unit. Local manipulation in hospital pharmacies or blood services, such as filtering, concentrating, or washing of platelets, results in a variable amount of platelet loss, thus making calculations of platelet increment difficult.

Older platelets may not remain in circulation as long as freshly collected platelet concentrates because of excessive activation during storage or the metabolic effects of acidosis.[170] Platelets also express small amounts of ABO antigens, which makes ABO-incompatible transfusions less effective than ABO-matched transfusions. Finally, analysis of multiply transfused patients shows that there is a tendency for decreased average count increments with successive transfusions. A patient's 1st platelet transfusion may result in a 30% higher count increment than their 15th transfusion despite equal numbers of platelets being transfused and the absence of other factors. No definitive cause of this decrease has been discerned other than the hypothesis that patients subjected to multiple rounds of chemotherapy may sustain subtle endothelial damage that consumes transfused platelets.[198]

To compare the effectiveness of platelet transfusion on different occasions or with different donors and recipients, a commonly used ratio is the corrected count increment (CCI):

$$CCI = \frac{(\text{Post-transfusion count} - \text{Pretransfusion count})(\text{Body surface area}[m^2])}{\text{Number of platelets given }(\times 10^{11})}$$

With this equation one can correct for the variations in number of platelets infused and for differences in patient size.[184,185] For example, if the platelet count is increased from 5000 to 65,000/mm^3 after the transfusion of 3 × 10^11 platelets in a child with a body surface area of 1.2 m^2,

$$CCI = \frac{60,000 \times 1.2}{3.0} = 24,000$$

This formula is most commonly used to define platelet refractoriness (CCI < 5000 at 1 hour), but it has limited use in comparing single transfusions directly because it does not factor in the multitude of other issues that may affect platelet count increments, as outlined earlier (Table 35-8).

TABLE 35-8	Variables Resulting in Decreased Post-transfusion Platelet Counts
Platelet Component	**Clinical Condition**
Donor platelet count	Fever
Technique of platelet collection	Sepsis
	Amphotericin B therapy
Temperature of storage	Disseminated intravascular coagulation
Platelet component age	
Storage conditions	Hepatosplenomegaly
Infusion time	Alloantibodies
Blood filter type	Autoantibodies
Leukocyte removal	Massive blood loss
Reducing platelet plasma volume	Hemolytic-uremic syndrome
	Thrombotic thrombocytopenic purpura
Washing platelets	Necrotizing enterocolitis
ABO match	Multiple previous platelet transfusions

Clinical Indications for Transfusion

Bone Marrow Failure

Bone marrow failure resulting in thrombocytopenia is the major reason for patients to receive platelet transfusions. Iatrogenic induction of bone marrow failure, secondary to chemotherapy or irradiation, is the most common cause of bone marrow failure in all age groups. Patients with malignancies involving the bone marrow (e.g., leukemia, lymphoma, neuroblastoma, metastatic disease from solid tumors, or myelofibrosis) may also require platelet support. The decreased marrow production in these diseases is due to displacement of megakaryocytes by malignant elements. In some cases, the tumor cells produce substances (e.g., tumor necrosis factor) that inhibit the growth of normal marrow cells. In the absence of other coagulation deficiencies, uremia, or vascular disease, patients do not have significant spontaneous bleeding until the platelet count is less than 20,000/mm³.[172,173] The original studies that examined the utility of prophylactic platelet transfusion in children with thrombocytopenia secondary to chemotherapy were published in 1962. During this period, aspirin was used routinely for management of pain and fever in all thrombocytopenic patients. Similarly, blood donors were not aware of the detrimental effects of aspirin ingestion on platelet function. Now that aspirin use is less prevalent in both patients and donors, it should be possible to lower the level for prophylactic infusion to 10,000/mm³.[175,200]

Patients with primary bone marrow failure caused by a constitutional defect such as Fanconi's anemia will also be thrombocytopenic. However, platelets are usually withheld from these patients unless they are actively bleeding because they are rapidly alloimmunized, which in turn will significantly reduce the success of future transfusions. The incidence of sensitization to platelets is higher in patients with aplastic anemia because prior to

definitive treatment these patients are not receiving immunosuppressive chemotherapy concurrent with platelet transfusions, as is the case with oncology patients. Furthermore, long-term cure for aplastic anemia, regardless of the cause, is best achieved with bone marrow transplantation.[200] Studies before the introduction of modern leukoreduction filters found that exposure to more than five platelet donors results in a significant reduction in successful transplantation because of rejection of donor bone marrow.[201] Although it is unclear whether this finding applies to current leukoreduced platelets, it is still recommended that if these patients do require therapy for bleeding, it is best to use irradiated, single-donor, filtered platelets in an attempt to minimize sensitization. The decision to transfuse a patient with newly diagnosed aplastic anemia should not be taken lightly because even a single exposure to transfused platelets may adversely affect long-term survival if bone marrow transplantation fails. Once the patient has become refractory to single-donor and HLA-matched platelets, family donors might also undergo plateletpheresis if these patients are *not* candidates for bone marrow transplantation.

Platelet Destruction

Shortened platelet survival may be due to immune-mediated destruction or nonimmune mechanisms that result in accelerated platelet consumption. In general, prophylactic platelet transfusions are contraindicated in these patients because the infused platelets are rapidly destroyed and thus a "safe" platelet count cannot be maintained. Therefore, platelet transfusions are reserved for episodes of active bleeding or in preparation for surgical procedures.

Nonimmune Mechanisms

Nonimmune mechanisms include the consumption of platelets in areas of endothelial damage, such as occurs with HUS, TTP, or necrotizing enterocolitis. DIC results in decreased platelet life span as a result of consumption of platelets and activated clotting factors, such as fibrinogen in the formation of microthrombi in association with sepsis, shock, acidosis, or severe head trauma. In these syndromes it is essential to assess the risk for bleeding when determining the need for transfusion. Infants with necrotizing enterocolitis are transfused more aggressively because many demonstrate marked gastrointestinal blood loss and may have a preexisting central nervous system hemorrhage associated with prematurity. Similarly, even though their counts may not be less than 10,000/mm³, patients with DIC are often given platelets because of consumption of clotting factors and evidence of ongoing bleeding. Successful outcomes for these patients depend on elimination of the underlying disease, for example, treating sepsis with antibiotics, restoration of organ perfusion in states of shock, or removal of necrotic tissue. Patients with large cavernous sinus hemangiomas (Kasabach-Merritt syndrome) have a localized consumption of platelets and clotting factors that results in a laboratory picture of DIC.[193-195] Until the lesion is removed or begins to involve, the platelet and clotting factor consumption will continue. These patients do not usually require transfusion for thrombocytopenia because the high rate of platelet turnover results in younger and more hemostatically effective platelets in the circulation. Finally, in TTP and HUS, platelet infusions are withheld as long as possible because it is thought that the infused platelets would lead to further hemolysis and organ damage by contributing to the formation of microthrombi in areas of endothelial damage.[196] Many of these patients have renal involvement and may be uremic with secondary platelet dysfunction. In this setting, patients undergoing peritoneal catheter placement often require platelet transfusions to control active bleeding.

Hypersplenism may result in poor platelet survival as a result of trapping of platelets in the expanded splenic bed. A more complex clinical situation arises with acute or chronic liver disease.[192] Splenic pooling, DIC, and poor platelet production may all contribute to the thrombocytopenia of hepatic disease. The presence of portal hypertension and esophageal varices from cirrhosis may push clinicians to consider platelet transfusion in the presence of gastrointestinal bleeding or when the platelet count falls below 20,000/mm³.[181,202] Acquired platelet dysfunction is associated with both acute and chronic liver disease secondary to decreased hepatic clearance of circulating fibrin degradation products. When platelet transfusion is required, splenomegaly may affect initial platelet recovery measured in the first hour after transfusion, but not platelet survival as determined by the platelet count 24 hours later.[181,188,197,202]

Immune-Mediated Thrombocytopenia

Immune thrombocytopenia is mediated by antibodies that bind to epitopes on the platelet membrane and result in their rapid removal from the circulation. These antibodies are either "self-reactive" autoantibodies or specific for alloantigens, polymorphic epitopes expressed on platelet membrane receptors. Alloantibodies cause thrombocytopenia in neonatal alloimmune thrombocytopenia (NATP) and post-transfusion purpura (PTP), both of which are discussed later in this chapter. Alloantibodies responsible for poor response to platelet transfusion are discussed in the section on the platelet refractory state.

Autoantibody-Mediated Thrombocytopenia

Autoantibody to platelets may be present in association with other diseases such as systemic lupus erythematosus, EBV infection, CMV infection, varicella virus infection, multiple sclerosis, diabetes, thyroid disease, or drug-induced autoantibody as seen with valproic acid. It may also be present without other disease associations, as in idiopathic thrombocytopenic purpura. In either setting there is rapid removal of antibody-coated platelets in the spleen and, to a lesser extent, in the liver. Immune complexes may nonspecifically adhere or bind by means of Fc receptors on the platelet surface. A particularly interesting example of the latter is the entity heparin-induced thrombocytopenia.[203] In this case patients exposed to heparin therapy produce antibodies directed to platelet factor 4 (PF4) bound to heparin. Immune complexes of PF4-heparin and antibody bind via Fc receptors to platelets and cause platelet activation and a prothrombotic state in which platelets are consumed. This could be a devastating complication of heparin therapy that may be suspected in patients with falling platelet counts a few days after initiating heparin therapy. Platelet transfusions are generally contraindicated because they may exacerbate the prothrombotic state.

In states that increase platelet turnover, bone marrow responds by increasing megakaryocyte number, size, and ploidy. This, in turn, results in fresher platelets that are slightly larger in size and represent a younger population than normal because of the rapid turnover of thrombocytes. Thus, the bleeding time in patients with immune-mediated thrombocytopenia is shortened relative to the absolute number of platelets, and they rarely experience major bleeding even though the platelet count may fall below 10,000/mm³.[204] Autoantibodies that interfere with functional epitopes on platelet glycoprotein receptors, such as in acquired Glanzmann's thrombasthenia, are a notable exception to this rule. In this setting, patients manifest bleeding even with platelet counts greater than 20,000/mm³.

In patients with rapid consumption of platelets by autoantibody, physicians withhold transfusions until there is evidence of bleeding, regardless of the platelet count. Central nervous system and gastrointestinal bleeding may be the initial feature of autoantibody-mediated thrombocytopenia and requires immediate aggressive therapy, including platelet transfusion. Although the platelets are consumed rapidly, active bleeding may stop or decrease significantly. Platelet transfusions should be used judiciously in combination with therapy aimed at reducing autoantibody production and blocking reticuloendothelial cell clearance of antibody-coated cells. Therapy for immune-mediated thrombocytopenia is discussed at length elsewhere in this textbook.

When medical management fails, splenectomy may be required to decrease platelet destruction and autoantibody production. Administration of intravenous immunoglobulin (IVIG) before surgery may obviate the need for platelet transfusion; however, in patients who are profoundly thrombocytopenic, platelets may be given to decrease the risk for major bleeding. If possible, platelets should be given after clamping of the splenic pedicle because survival of the transfused platelets is markedly improved once the splenic circulation is blocked.

Alloantibody-Mediated Thrombocytopenia

Neonatal Alloimmune Thrombocytopenic Purpura

In NATP, maternal antiplatelet alloantibody has crossed the placenta and caused thrombocytopenia in the fetus

TABLE 35-9　Platelet Alloantigen Phenotype and Frequency

Alloantigen System	Glycoprotein Location	Allelic Forms	Phenotypic Frequency
HPA-1 (Pl^A, Zw)	GPIIIa Leu–Pro33	HPA-1a (Pl^{A1})/HPA-1b (Pl^{A2})	72% a/a 26% a/b 2% b/b
HPA-2 (Ko, Sib)	GP1b Thr–Met145	HPA-2a (Ko^b)/HPA-2b (Ko^a)	85% a/a 14% a/b 1% b/b
HPA-3 (Bak, Lek)	GPIIb Ile–Ser843	HPA-3a (Bak^a)/HPA-3b(Bak^b)	37% a/a 48% b/b 15% b/b
HPA-4 (Pen, Yuk)	GPIIIa Arg–Gln143	HPA-4a (Pen^a)/HPA-4b(Pen^b)	99% a/a <0.1% a/b <0.1% b/b
HPA-5 (Br, Hc, Zav)	GPIa Glu–Lys505	HPA-5a (Br^b)/HPA-5b (Br^a)	80% a/a 19% a/b 1% b/b
HPA-6 (Ca, Tu)	GPIIIa Arg–Gln489	HPA-6a (Ca^b)/HPA-6b (Ca^a)	99% a/a <1% a/b <1% b/b
HPA-7 (Mo)	GPIIIa Pro–Ala407	HPA-7a (Mo^b)/HPA-7b (Mo^a)	99% a/a <1% a/b <1% b/b
HPA-8 (Sr^a)	GPIIIa Arg–Cys636	HPA-8a (Sr^b)/HPA-8b (Sr^a)	99% a/a <1% a/b <1% b/b

or neonate. Harrington and associates first reported the observation that pregnant women may become alloimmunized to antigens expressed on fetal platelets.[205] Even during the first pregnancy, maternal antiplatelet alloantibodies can cross the placenta and cause profound thrombocytopenia in the fetus and newborn. In North America, the alloantibodies identified are most commonly directed against Pl^{A1}. A complete list of platelet alloantigens and their frequency in populations that have been studied thus far are listed in Table 35-9. The finding of thrombocytopenia in a healthy infant whose mother has a normal platelet count is often due to maternal alloantibodies.

The diagnosis of NATP is made with the demonstration of antiplatelet antibody in maternal plasma that is reactive with *paternal* platelets. Maternal plasma is also screened to rule out the presence of autoantibody. More than 50% of the platelet-specific alloantibodies in NATP are reactive with the Pl^{A1} epitope on glycoprotein IIIa, which is also known as human platelet antigen 1 (HPA-1).[206] The predominance of Pl^{A1} alloantibodies in reported cases of NATP suggest that this epitope is more immunogenic than other platelet alloantigens. Based on the high probability that these Pl^{A1}-negative women, who constitute less than 2% of the population, would marry Pl^{A1}-positive men, it is surprising that the actual incidence of NATP is so low at 1 to 4 per 10,000 live births.[207,208] Perhaps mild cases of NATP are missed in the absence of routine screening of newborn platelet counts. Healthy infants may not bleed or exhibit petechiae until the platelet count drops below 20,000/mm^3.

Reports suggest that immune response genes may also play a role in platelet alloimmunization.[209-211] Based on these studies, there appears to be an increased incidence of alloimmunization against Pl^{A1} in mothers positive for HLA-B8 and HLA-DR3.

The diagnosis of maternal alloimmunization is usually made after the birth of her first thrombocytopenic infant. Women who are then identified as being sensitized to a platelet-specific alloantigen should be monitored very closely throughout subsequent pregnancies. Intermittent screening of maternal serum should be performed similar to prenatal Coombs' testing in women who are Rh negative. All women in the mother's family should also be evaluated before or during their pregnancies to determine whether they might likewise be at risk for alloimmunization. If a Pl^{A1}-negative woman is also positive for HLA-DR3 (DRw52), she has a greatly increased risk of alloimmunization, even during her first pregnancy.[211-213]

To determine whether the infant is at risk for thrombocytopenia secondary to maternal alloantibody, it is advantageous to establish the platelet phenotype of the fetus early in pregnancy. As early as the eighth week of gestation, DNA from nucleated cells obtained from chorionic villus sampling can be amplified through the use of polymerase chain reaction. DNA typing is then determined with glycoprotein-specific oligonucleotide primers and probes unique for each alloantigen sequence or phenotype.[213-215] A prospective study reported 100% correlation between DNA typing and subsequent serologic response in mothers with alloantibodies to Pl^{A1} or Bak.[216] This technique is useful only when the nucleotide sequences that define the polymorphisms are known, as listed in Table 35-9.[214] This is an important technologic advance because if the obstetrician knows that the fetal phenotype is negative for these alloantigens, it is *not* necessary to obtain cord blood samples to monitor fetal thrombocytopenia, a procedure that is associated with risks for both the mother and child.

Because of the high frequency of these alloantigens, random-donor platelets are usually ineffective in treating alloimmune thrombocytopenia in the neonate. When platelets are given, it is best to use washed, irradiated *maternal* apheresis platelets because they lack the alloantigen. Washing is required to remove maternal plasma that contains the alloantibody. *Irradiation is routinely performed on all blood products from first-degree relatives when there is an increased risk for GVHD, particularly in neonates.* When severe thrombocytopenia is anticipated in the newborn, maternal platelets may be harvested before elective delivery and made available for transfusion shortly after birth to infants with NATP diagnosed prenatally. Alternatively, many blood donor centers maintain lists of Pl^A1-negative donors who may be called on at short notice to donate. IVIG has also been used successfully in the newborn and is particularly helpful in areas in which plateletpheresis and washing are unavailable.[217-220] In families with a history of prenatal intracranial hemorrhage, the fetal platelet count should be monitored closely and ultrasonography performed to rule out bleeding before delivery.[221]

Post-transfusion Purpura

PTP occurs 7 to 10 days after blood product infusion in a patient who has previously been transfused or pregnant.[207] Paradoxically, alloantibodies are produced that destroy not only any transfused platelets but also the patient's own platelets. Though extremely rare, PTP occurs most commonly in the less than 2% of the population who are Pl^A1 negative.[206] The post-transfusion plasma usually has high-titer anti-Pl^A1 activity, but the mechanism of autologous platelet destruction is unclear. Hypotheses suggesting the presence of a cross-reactive alloantibody that binds to autoepitopes in close proximity to the Pl^A1 site have yet to be proved. There are individual cases reported of PTP secondary to alloantibody to Bak^a and Pen^a and two cases of anti-Pl^A2 antibody.[222-224] Of the approximately 100 cases reported since its description in 1959, only four men have been described as having PTP.[206] A series of PTP patients with anti-Pl^A1 alloantibody were HLA-typed, and more than 90% were HLA-DR3 positive, with the supertype HLA-DRw52 predominating in these individuals.[210,211] Patients are usually in their late forties or older, but PTP has been reported in a 16-year-old girl not previously pregnant.[224]

Platelet transfusions are contraindicated in PTP patients, in whom the treatment of choice is IVIG or plasmapheresis, or both.[225] The frequency of transfusion reactions in these patients is quite high, with 46% experiencing chills and fever during blood product infusion.

Therefore, red cells should be washed and filtered whenever possible. If platelets must be given for life-threatening hemorrhage, they should be Pl^A1 negative, washed, and filtered. Further discussion of therapy and possible mechanisms of autologous platelet destruction in PTP is more thoroughly addressed in two extensive reviews of this disorder.[207,214]

Platelet Transfusion in Selected Clinical Situations

Patients with congenital platelet dysfunction, such as Glanzmann's thrombocytopathy or Bernard-Soulier syndrome, may experience episodes of profuse bleeding. In this setting, platelets may be administered to control massive hemorrhage. Because normal platelets express proteins that these individuals lack, isoantibodies to these receptors develop in some patients and they eventually become refractory to all platelet transfusions. Efforts to minimize menstrual bleeding by hormonal suppression may decrease the number of platelet infusions in women. Bleeding in patients with congenital platelet dysfunction secondary to abnormal platelet secretion may respond to desmopressin, thereby avoiding exposure to blood.[226,227]

Acquired platelet dysfunction in children is most commonly due to drugs, chronic renal failure, or antiplatelet antibodies. Rarely, children exhibit platelet dysfunction as a manifestation of myelodysplastic syndrome or chronic leukemia. Platelet transfusions may be used if the patient is actively bleeding, but eventually the transfused platelets will be affected by exposure to drug, uremia, or antiplatelet antibodies, which limits their survival and function. For this reason, platelets are not given prophylactically to these patients. Every effort should be made to ameliorate the platelet dysfunction so that exposure to blood product is avoided. Patients with uremia may respond to infusion of desmopressin, and those with antiplatelet autoantibodies may respond to immunoglobulin infusion or corticosteroid therapy. When possible, alternative medications should replace those known to cause platelet dysfunction.

Neonatal Thrombocytopenia

Platelet transfusions in the neonatal unit are a common event. In acutely ill premature infants, DIC or platelet consumption often develops in association with perinatal asphyxia, respiratory distress syndrome, sepsis, intracranial hemorrhage, necrotizing enterocolitis, and acidosis. A chronically ill newborn with poor caloric intake and growth may also require platelet support because of inadequate platelet production. Platelets are often given after double-volume exchange transfusion if dilutional thrombocytopenia occurs. To minimize the problems of blood-borne infection and possible GVHD from transfused lymphocytes in an immunocompromised host, platelets given to newborns are CMV negative and irradiated. In centers in which single-donor platelets are available, units can be split, similar to packed RBCs, and transfused over a period of 4 days to minimize exposure to multiple donors.

Platelet Refractory State

When a patient no longer achieves the expected rise in platelet count after a platelet transfusion, one must first assess whether the shortened platelet recovery and survival are due to immune or nonimmune mechanisms. Examples of nonimmune mechanisms are listed in Table 35-8; they are responsible for the majority of cases in which post-transfusion count increments are lower than expected. The most notable of these mechanisms includes splenomegaly, DIC, and fever.

Alloimmune Mechanisms

Alloimmunization is characterized by increasingly poor recovery and survival of platelets in a multiply transfused patient. The majority of alloantibodies react to determinants on HLA class I molecules, ABO blood group antigens, and platelet-specific antigens expressed primarily on membrane glycoproteins.[228] Although alloantibody does not not develop in every patient exposed to platelets, those who eventually become refractory present a very serious challenge to the skills of physicians and blood centers. Production of antiplatelet alloantibodies does not depend on the number of exposures or transfusions. However, there is an association with the underlying disease state. For example, only 30% to 60% of patients with leukemia become alloimmunized, in contrast to 80% to 90% of aplastic anemia patients.[29,230] This suggests that the aggressive chemotherapy used to eliminate the malignant cells also plays a role in prevention of alloimmunization. Thus, it would appear that the true rate of alloimmunization is further influenced by the individual's immune responsiveness and competence.

Unlike RBCs, it is not practical or efficient to cross-match platelet donors and recipients in most blood centers or hospitals. The antigens known to elicit an immune response on platelets are allelic molecules. Such antigens include a variety of class I HLA alloantigens, platelet-specific alloepitopes such as PlA1, and blood group antigens. There is rarely any problem in providing ABO-compatible platelets in most blood centers. However, it is not reasonable to match all donors and recipients for HLA or platelet-specific alloantigens. As seen in Table 35-9, the platelet-specific alloepitopes are diallelic with a high frequency of expression of one allele in the general population. Therefore, the incidence of alloimmunization to platelet-specific antigens after a single transfusion may be a serious problem for only a very small percentage of the population, depending on which epitope is involved.[185,230] An algorithm for dealing with patients who appear to be refractory to platelet transfusions is presented in Figure 35-5. The role of

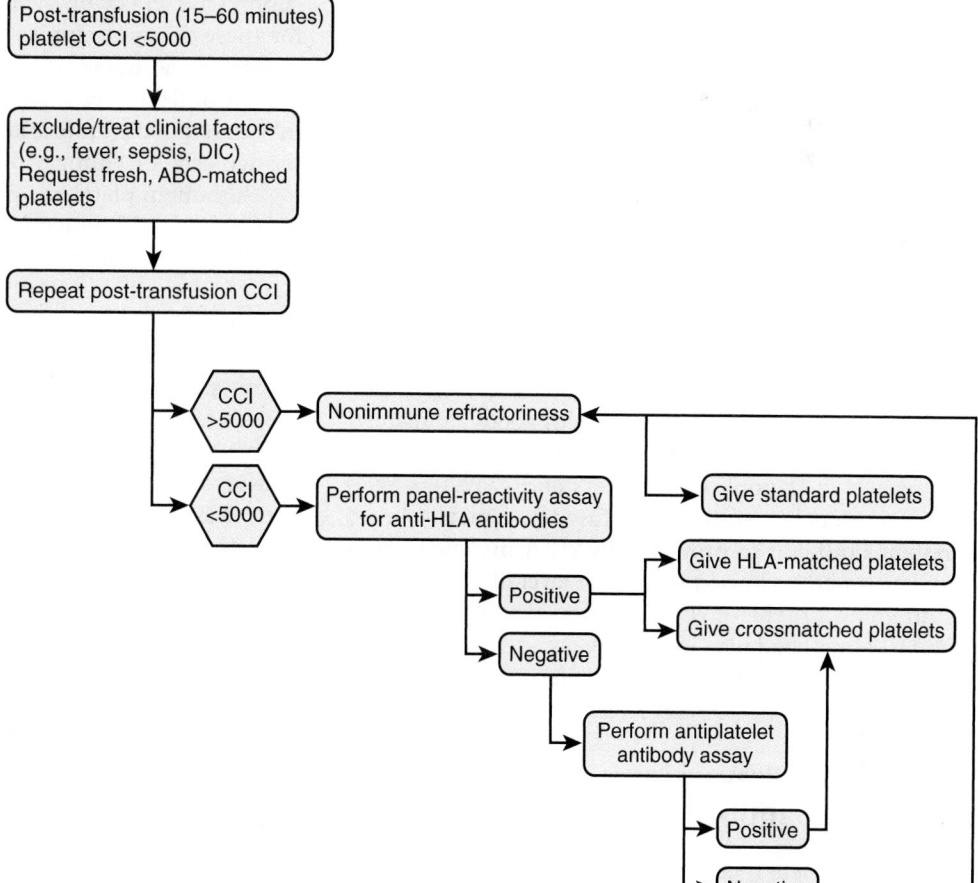

FIGURE 35-5. Algorithm for the management of patients refractory to platelet transfusion. CCI, corrected count increment; DIC, disseminated intravascular coagulation.

platelet-specific alloantibodies in NATP was discussed in the section on clinical indications for platelet transfusions.

The majority of alloantibodies that mediate rapid clearance of transfused platelets in a refractory patient bind to epitopes on class I HLA molecules. Platelets express the class I (HLA-A, -B, and -C) gene products,[231] but class II molecules (HLA-DR, -DP, -DQ) have been shown only on platelets in a high-turnover state, such as immune thrombocytopenic purpura, in which the majority of circulating platelets have just been released from the bone marrow.[232] As with other precursor cells, early megakaryoblasts express HLA-DR in normal individuals[233,234]; however, this antigen is not generally detectable on circulating platelets.

Initially, class I HLA alloantigens were defined serologically, that is, with plasma from patients or postpartum women with high-titer alloantibodies. Subsequently, molecular typing and monoclonal antibodies (MoAbs) helped clarify the number and types of epitopes associated with the HLA-A, HLA-B, and HLA-C loci. Interestingly, it is the serologic definitions that are important in platelet refractoriness. In categorizing the alloantigens serologically, it became clear that two categories of epitopes were expressed. The first group of alloantibodies recognizes private epitopes, or antigens that are uniquely associated with only one HLA gene product. The second category contains alloantibodies that recognize public epitopes, or those expressed on more than one class I HLA gene product. The broad reactivity associated with the platelet refractory state is most commonly caused by alloantibodies that recognize *public* epitopes shared by many HLA gene products.[235,236] By categorizing HLA-A and HLA-B loci according to these public epitopes or cross-reactive groups (CREGs), blood centers may be able to provide single-donor platelets based on reactivity to CREG subsets. Blood centers take advantage of this observation to provide "HLA-compatible" platelets (type B matches) when HLA-identical donors are limited in number.[237] Although the platelets may not be identical at the HLA-A or HLA-B loci, if the CREGs shared by a subset of class I allotypes can be avoided, non–HLA-identical product can still be used with adequate platelet recovery and survival. By using this system, blood centers can expand their pool of volunteers and provide single-donor platelets for multiply transfused patients; however, it remains difficult to provide fully HLA-matched platelets consistently. Consequently, the overall success rate for attaining suitable post-transfusion count increments with HLA-matched platelets is only about 50% in alloimmunized patients, even in major centers.[237]

Methods for Preventing Platelet Alloantibodies

When a physician can anticipate that an individual will be multiply transfused, every effort to prevent alloimmunization will ultimately result in better recovery and survival of later platelet transfusions and may delay the onset of platelet refractoriness. Three blood procedures have been introduced to reduce alloimmunization: (1) single-donor pheresis platelets, (2) leukocyte-poor platelets, and (3) ultraviolet (UV)-irradiated platelets. Although UV irradiation has been shown to be effective in preventing alloimmunization, it is no more effective than the use of leukocyte-reduced products and has not been introduced into widespread clinical practice.[238]

Supported by a huge network of community volunteers, many centers can provide single-donor platelets to patients who have not been previously transfused. As single-donor platelets became more readily available, prospective trials were initiated to assess relative rates of alloimmunization. These studies demonstrated that in patients receiving ABO-matched, single-donor platelets, lymphocytotoxic antibodies were less likely to develop than in individuals receiving pooled platelet concentrates.[239] This seems inherently obvious because the exposure rate to alloantigens with single-donor platelets would be roughly a sixth to an eighth that seen in patients receiving pooled platelet concentrates.[240] However, these studies were performed in patients with acute leukemia in Europe, where patients receive very few platelet transfusions in comparison to practice in the United States. Additionally, the rate of alloimmunization is relatively low in acute leukemia patients because of the immunosuppressive effect of their chemotherapy.[241,242] Probably for these reasons, similar results have not been demonstrated in the United States; nevertheless, the additional benefit of decreased exposure to blood-borne pathogens in single-donor units makes this a preferred product, particularly for younger patients.

Although platelets express class I gene products, it is the class II molecules expressed on contaminating leukocytes that are primarily responsible for the induction of alloantibodies.[243,244] With the use of washed platelets devoid of white cells, lymphocytotoxic antibodies failed to develop in multiply transfused animals.[245,246] These studies were eventually repeated in patients with the use of pooled random-donor platelets, with or without leukocyte depletion. At least 90% of the contaminating leukocytes had to be removed (<10^6 remaining), but there was a striking decrease in the rate of alloimmunization from 93% to 24%.[247-251] Prospective studies in humans suggest that the leukocyte threshold for alloimmunization is 5.0×10^6 cells or less per infusion. As outlined earlier, the Trial to Reduce Alloimmunization to Platelets (TRAP)[238] has conclusively demonstrated in a randomized, prospective study that the use of leukocyte-reduced products can effectively decrease but not eliminate the risk of alloimmunization. Most centers recommend leukoreduction in the blood center during collection,[252] which may also decrease the accumulation of cytokines produced by white cells during storage.[253,254]

PRINCIPLES OF HEMATOPOIETIC CELLULAR THERAPY

With advancement of molecular technology, better understanding of human immunology, and increased interest in regenerative medicine, the use of cellular therapy is no longer limited to HPC transplantation. Current applications have expanded to include the use of cells as adoptive immunotherapy and cancer vaccines. Future applications may also include the use of cells as drug delivery vehicles or as source of tissue engineering for regenerative medicine.[255] However, HPC transplantation is still the best-established type of hematopoietic-based cellular therapy. In this section, the sources, processing, and complications associated with hematopoietic cell–based therapy are reviewed.

Hematopoietic Cell Sources

Donors of therapeutic hematopoietic cells can be autologous or allogeneic. Autologous donors are usually patients who will be undergoing HPC transplantation. These donors have their own cells collected and cryopreserved, and their own cells are infused during transplantation. Because the donor and recipient are the same, complications from major histocompatibility complex (MHC) or human leukocyte antigens (HLA) disparities are negligible for autologous cell infusion. The MHC/HLA molecules are displayed on cell surfaces and are responsible for lymphocyte recognition and "antigen presentation." They control the immune responses through recognition of "self" and "nonself" and, consequently, serve as targets in transplantation. However, during allogeneic transplantation, the degree of HLA disparity is extremely important for donor selection because large numbers of lymphocytes are transfused. These donor lymphocytes can recognize the recipient's tissue as foreign or "nonself" and mediate GVHD. In humans, HLA molecules are located on chromosome 6. There are two classes of HLA antigens, class I and class II. The class I antigens HLA-A and HLA-B and the class II antigen HLA-DR are the three most important molecules contributing to GVHD. Given that each person has two alleles of chromosomes, a minimum

of six out of six HLA antigen matches are often required for transplantation. Donors of allogeneic HPCs are often siblings of the recipients and are referred to as related donors. For patients who do not have related donors, cells from HLA-matched unrelated donors are used frequently. These donors are obtained from international donor registries such as the National Marrow and Donor Program (NMDP), and the amount of time spent searching for appropriate and available donors can be unpredictable. Because only 50% to 60% of patients have an HLA-matched sibling or unrelated donor, not all patients who may benefit from an HPC transplant can proceed to transplantation. Timely search for an appropriate donor is essential for successful allogeneic HPC transplantation.[256] A prolonged donor search period can lead to death, increased risk, or ineligibility of patients. The incidence of GVHD is also significantly increased when HPC transplantation is performed with unrelated donors.[257,258]

Bone marrow, cytokine-stimulated peripheral blood, and umbilical cord blood (UCB) are the sources of HPCs for transplantations. Unstimulated peripheral blood cells are either used in an unmanipulated state or can be further processed to be used as adoptive immunotherapy. Characteristic differences between various HPC sources will be discussed individually in detail.

HPC transplants can be performed with unmanipulated bone marrow, peripheral blood, or UCB. Depending on the source of cellular products used, they can be contaminated with different degrees of RBCs and leukocytes. When compared with peripheral blood–derived HPCs, bone marrow products have higher RBC contamination and lower T-cell and CD34⁺ HPC content. The original HPC transplants were performed with bone marrow. In recent years, investigators have routinely use mobilized peripheral blood for transplantation[259-261] because of a higher CD34⁺ HPC content and faster post-transplant hematopoietic recovery (Table 35-10).

Mobilized peripheral blood collected by leukapheresis has become the most commonly used HPC component for both autologous and allogeneic HPC transplantation because of the ease of collection and ample number of CD34⁺ stem cells.[262] In the autologous setting, the benefits of peripheral blood over bone marrow

TABLE 35-10	Differences in Transplanted Cell Dose and Hematopoietic Recovery between Cell Sources				
	TOTAL CELL DOSE TRANSPLANTED		**DAYS TO HEMATOPOIETIC RECOVERY**	
Hematopoietic Stem Cell Source	**Mononuclear Cells/kg (×10⁸)**	**CD34⁺ Cells/kg (×10⁶)**	**Neutrophil**	**Platelets**
G-CSF–stimulated peripheral blood	9.6 ± 6.1	9.3 ± 7.0	13 ± 4	17 ± 15
Bone marrow	2.6 ± 1.5	1.8 ± 1.2	19 ± 5	23 ± 12
Umbilical cord blood	0.44 ± 0.12	0.23 ± 0.14	29 ± 16	52 ± 23

G-CSF, granulocyte colony-stimulating factor.
From Dana-Farber Cancer Institute adult hematopoietic stem cell data, 2005.

have been well documented[263] and include more rapid engraftment, decreased need for transfusions, decreased incidence of infection and antibiotic use, and shorter hospital stay. To mobilize stem cells into the peripheral blood, patients are treated with cytokines such as granulocyte colony-stimulating factor (G-CSF) or granulocyte-macrophage colony-stimulating factor (GM-CSF), in many cases after receiving chemotherapy, and the cells are collected in the outpatient setting. After chemotherapy, patients undergo leukapheresis when their cell counts recover from the nadir. Circulating peripheral blood CD34$^+$ cell levels may be used to predict yield.[264,265] If cytokines are used in patients without previous chemotherapy, collection is begun on a predetermined day during the course of administration. In approximately 10% of autologous donors, peripheral blood stem cell cannot be mobilized successfully. Risk factors for poor mobilization include patients' disease status, nonconducive marrow environment secondary to a history of heavy chemotherapy, and radiation therapy.[266-269] In these patients the risks for delayed engraftment is higher, and they are often deferred from autologous HPC transplantation.

If peripheral blood collections are used for allogeneic transplantation, collection is begun on the fourth or fifth day of G-CSF administration. As in the autologous setting, engraftment may be more rapid with allogeneic peripheral blood than with bone marrow. However, peripheral blood components typically contain at least 1 log more T cells than bone marrow components do, thus potentially increasing the risk for GVHD. Nonetheless, the incidence of acute GVHD has not been found to be significantly elevated.[270] This may be due in part to effects of the G-CSF used for mobilization on the T cells. However, reports have suggested that chronic GVHD may be more frequent in recipients of peripheral blood components.[271]

The biology of CD34$^+$ stem cell mobilization is now better understood. The bone marrow environment heavily regulates the movement of these CD34$^+$ HPCs. Cytokines such as G-CSF stimulate the generation of granulocytes in both bone marrow and peripheral blood.[272,273] These granulocytes release serum proteases such as cathepsin G and neutrophil elastase. Studies have reported that accumulation of these serum proteases coincides with increased inhibition of adhesion molecule interaction between the very late antigen 4 (VLA-4) on the CD34$^+$ HPCs and the vascular cell adhesion molecule 1 (VCAM-1) on the surface of bone marrow stromal cells.[274] This adhesion molecule disruption allows the CD34$^+$ HPCs to float free within the bone marrow environment, and their movement can then be influenced by chemokines. Interestingly, proteolysis of the chemokine receptor CXCR4 on the CD34$^+$ cell surface and the chemokine stromal cell–derived factor 1 (SDF-1), also known as CXCL12, was also observed to coincide with accumulation of serum proteases during G-CSF treatment and chemotherapy such as cyclophosphamide

in human bone marrow.[275] With decreased chemotaxis signals within the marrow, the free-floating CD34$^+$ HPCs can traffic toward the peripheral blood compartment.[276] With G-CSF and chemotherapy mobilization, peripheral blood circulating CD34$^+$ HPCs can be increased to approximately 10- to 100-fold.

Many centers are also evaluating the use of UCB as a source of allogeneic HPCs. The use of UCB as an alternate source of allogeneic HPCs was first reported by Gluckman and co-authors in 1989.[277] Since that time, hundreds of UCB transplants have been performed in North America and Europe.[278] Because of the success of UCB transplantation in both related and unrelated donor settings, many cord blood banks (CBBs) have been established worldwide. UCB is collected from the umbilical cord or placental veins (or both) after delivery of the infant and is therefore a readily available component. Parents/mothers have the option of banking the cells for their own use in a private CBB or donate to a public CBB. If the UCB samples are donated to public CBBs, these cells will undergo stringent quality control evaluation and only qualified products will be processed and cryopreserved for use. The UCB products stored in public CBBs will be available for public use when requested and prescribed by appropriate transplantation physicians. As UCB transplantation becomes more widely accepted, the number of CBBs and the size of the inventory within the CBBs have been increasing.[279] There are at least 15 public CBBs in the United States. UBC transplantation offers many advantages, and various reports have suggested that UCB is less immunogenic and transplants may be performed across HLA barriers with less GVHD than would be anticipated if a bone marrow donor with the same HLA type were used.[280] The low dose of UCB may contribute to the decreased incidence of GVHD. Therefore, UCB transplantation is an attractive alternative for patients requiring allogeneic transplantation who do not have an HLA-matched donor. From a donor's point of view, when compared with mobilized peripheral blood stem cells and bone marrow, collection of UCB after birth carries no risk for the donor. The collected UCB is HLA-typed, tested for infectious agents, and banked for use; it is therefore available immediately on request and can be shipped to any transplant center in the world. Despite the ease of availability and safety of the donation procedure, UCB transplants have their limitations. Studies continue to show that an appropriate stem cell infusion dose is essential for speedy hematopoietic cell engraftment and successful transplantation.[280-283] The limited cell dose in the UCB products poses problems, especially for large adult recipients. In the case of disease progression or relapse, it is also impossible to go back to the original UCB donor for lymphocyte or additional stem cell collections. Research working on expansion of cord blood stem cells is ongoing.[284,285] Most recently, the successful use of double UCB transplantation in adult patients may overcome the dosing limitation issues.[286]

Infusion-Related Toxicities

Infusion of HSC products can be associated with either immediate reactions or long-term side effects. The immediate infusion toxicities are similar to blood transfusion reactions and include febrile reactions from the infusion of a large number of leukocytes and related cytokines, allergic reactions secondary to plasma protein content, and occasional hemolytic reactions as a result of donor-recipient erythrocyte ABO incompatibility. To reduce the occurrence of febrile and allergic reactions, patients are always premedicated with antipyretic medication and antihistamines before HSC infusion. Special manipulation to reduce the erythrocyte contents can be performed to prevent hemolytic reactions. The type of manipulations used to reduce the erythrocyte content is described in detail later. For HSC products or lymphocytes that are cryopreserved in dimethyl sulfoxide (DMSO) for storage in liquid nitrogen, infusion of thawed products can lead to frequent DMSO-related toxicities. In the Dana-Farber Cancer Institute, DMSO-related toxicity is a frequently described reaction related to HSC infusion. Common symptoms attributed to DMSO include nausea, vomiting, flushing, and headaches. Anaphylactoid symptoms caused by the release of histamine are also common. Embolic events associated with the infusion of bone marrow and apheresed HSC products have been reported. Most of the cases described involved infusion of products with particulate matter secondary to cell clumps or bone débridement in recipients with congenital cardiac septal defects.[287,288]

GVHD is the most common long-term toxicity associated with allogeneic HSC transplantation. Approximately 30% to 70% of patients undergoing allogeneic HSC transplantation can anticipate experiencing GVHD.[289] GVHD is mediated primarily through donor graft lymphocytes (T-cell population). Graft lymphocytes target tissues with alloantigens and cause alloimmune reactions in recipient organs.[290,291] Severe GVHD is observed when donors are not fully identical with the recipient at MHC antigens (HLA-A, -B, -DR). However, most allogeneic HSC transplantations are conducted with donors and recipients who are identical at MHC antigens. In these recipients, minor histocompatibility antigens (mHAs) are thought to be the primary targets of donor alloimmunity.[292-294] Studies have shown that mHAs can be expressed on hematopoietic tumor cells. When donor T cells target leukemia mHAs, alloimmunity results in a graft-versus-leukemia effect and can contribute to eradication of leukemia cells.[295,296] The use of donor lymphocytes as adoptive immunotherapy for patients with relapse of chronic myelogenic leukemia has shown to be successful in a population of patients with cytogenetic relapse after allogeneic HSC transplantation.[297-299] Conversely, depletion of T-cell content in the graft has been shown to reduce the incidence of GVHD, but at the expense of losing the graft-versus-leukemia effect.[291]

Component Assessment

For customized cell therapy such as HSC transplantation, each product is donor-patient specific. The quality of the product can vary for different donors and even changes daily for a product that came from the same donor. As mentioned earlier, the content of the product can lead to various types of infusion reactions, immunologic effects, and time to hematopoietic cell engraftment. Most importantly, like any blood product, infusion of products with microbial or viral contamination can lead to transmission of infectious diseases.

Achieving rapid hematopoietic cell engraftment is essential for successful HSC transplantation. Insufficient infusion of HSCs is linked to prolonged hematopoietic cell recovery. Patients who experienced delayed hematopoietic engraftment will require long-term blood component support and are more likely to contract severe bacterial, fungal, and other opportunistic infectious diseases because of prolonged neutropenia and lack of proper immune function. Functional assays such as granulocyte-macrophage colony-forming unit (CFU-GM), granulocyte-erythrocyte-macrophage-megakaryocyte colony-forming unit (CFU-GEMM), and long-term culture–initiating cell (LTC-IC) content have been described as measures of HSC quality and content. The results of these assays correlate well with post-transplantation hematopoietic recovery. However, these culture-based assays have a long turnaround time and are unable to rapidly quantify the number of stem cells. Enumeration of CD34+ cells via flow cytometry analysis is now commonly performed as a measure of HSC content because of its fast turnaround time and proven correlation with clinical engraftment data. As with other assays, CD34+ cell enumeration methods vary between centers, thus making characterization of an HSC component adequate to achieve hematologic engraftment difficult.[300,301] Standardized protocols for CD34+ cell enumeration have been proposed in an attempt to limit variability and permit comparison of the HSC content of components collected and infused at different centers.[302] Methodologies to determine absolute cell concentrations instead of percentages may further improve the accuracy of the CD34+ cell enumeration procedure.[303] Analysis of graft T-cell content by flow cytometry in HSC or donor lymphocyte products is now also used to correlate with GVHD outcome.

In addition to quantifying HPC content, components must be tested for contaminants. Contamination rate increases with component manipulation, such as ex vivo cell isolation or depletion and long-term cell culture, and may be associated with adverse clinical sequelae. This emphasizes the need to include bacterial cultures as a component of quality control of hematopoietic cell collection, processing, cryopreservation, thawing, and reinfusion procedures.[304]

Finally, critical evaluation of the donor of the product is also an essential quality assessment of the product. All allogeneic and autologous donors should be tested for infectious disease markers just like routine blood donors. Donor who are positive for certain viral markers can still donate their cells for transplantation if the transplantation was deemed to be the only lifesaving procedure and the patient was informed of the risk by the transplant physicians. However, the practice of using high-risk allogeneic donors for transplantation should be discouraged.

Processing and Storage of Hematopoietic Progenitor Cell Components

Autologous and, occasionally, allogeneic HPC components are collected before the patient receives myeloablative therapy and are cryopreserved. Cells are suspended in a mixture of an electrolyte solution, a protein source, and a cryoprotectant such as DMSO or hydroxyethyl starch.[305] Cryopreserved cells are infused rapidly when thawed, with the freezing solution being infused along with the cells. Premedication is required to minimize toxicity.[306-308]

In the allogeneic setting, processing may be performed to avoid acute hemolysis associated with the infusion of an ABO-incompatible component.[309] If there is a major ABO incompatibility, defined as the recipient's plasma containing antibodies against donor red cells, many centers will deplete the donor component of RBCs. If there is a minor ABO incompatibility in which the donor plasma contains antibodies against recipient red cells, the component will be washed or volume-reduced to remove plasma. Alternatives to these procedures include plasma or red cell exchange in the recipient, as well as the infusion of sources of donor blood group antigens to absorb recipient antibodies.[310,311]

Laboratories are increasingly performing more extensive procedures in an attempt to deplete unwanted cell populations from the HSC component. Tumor cells are removed from autologous components in an effort to decrease the risk of relapse, whereas T lymphocytes are removed from allogeneic components to abrogate acute GVHD. The majority of these procedures are performed with either negative or positive selection methods.

Negative selection targets the cells to be removed from the component while preserving other cell populations.[312] Methods for negative selection that have been used include attempts to separate cells based on physical characteristics, in vitro sensitivity to chemotherapeutic agents, and MoAb-mediated separation or damage. Density gradient centrifugation and centrifugal elutriation have been used to separate cells based on size. Trials have used 4-hydroxycyclophosphamide or mafosfamide to kill tumor cells. Cells can bind to MoAbs conjugated to magnetic beads, dense particles, or surfaces and be physically separated from the other cell populations within a component. In addition, MoAbs may be used to destroy tumor cells or T cells by conjugation with toxins or complement-mediated lysis.[313]

In contrast, positive selection enriches the cell population to be retained while nonspecifically depleting all other cell populations. The systems currently available for positive selection use MoAbs directed against various hematopoietic cell surface antigens. Cells are incubated with the MoAbs, and separation is achieved by biotin-avidin, magnetic bead, or high-speed cell sorting methods.[314-317] Most of these cell manipulation techniques were initially designed to reduce the incidence of GVHD or disease relapse associated with HSC transplantation. Recently, some of these techniques have also been applied to the development of cell-based immunotherapy. For example, monocytes or CD34+ cells from peripheral blood can be isolated by selection techniques and educated ex vivo into potent antigen-presenting cells called dendritic cells. Animal models have shown that dendritic cells can act as tumor vaccines to stimulate and enhance cell-mediated immunity in patients who may have defective tumor immunity.[318-320] Specialized lymphocytes can also be isolated and expanded with appropriate growth factors and antigen stimulation to target specific tumor cells or infectious agents. Most of the cell-based immunotherapies are still under investigation and considered experimental. Encouragingly, early clinical data on dendritic cell therapy in melanoma, prostate cancer, and EBV-specific T cells targeting post-transplant lymphoproliferative diseases have shown immunologic responses with potential clinical effects.[321-324]

Standards and Regulations

The use of various types of cellular therapy has increased over the last few decades as a result of abundant research findings, the development of novel technologies, and interest in innovative therapeutic modalities. Consequently, the regulations associated with processing and administration of cell-based therapy are in evolution. Principles of current good manufacturing practice (cGMP) and total quality management should be applied to the production of therapeutic cellular products. In 1991, the 14th edition of *Standards for Blood Banks and Transfusion Services* by the American Association of Blood Banks (AABB) was extended to include HPCs. In 1996, the AABB published a separate *Standards for Hematopoietic Progenitor Cells*.[325,326] These standards include sections concerning donor selection, component collection, processing, testing, labeling, storage, transportation, issue, infusion, and record keeping for HPCs, including autologous as well as allogeneic bone marrow, peripheral blood progenitor cells, and cord blood. Furthermore, the Foundation for the Accreditation of Cell Therapy (FACT) was formed in 1993 and created programs for inspection and accreditation of HSC collection and processing facilities, as well as transplantation programs. The FACT standards represent a consensus document of several organizations working together in the field of clinical conduct of HPC transplantation, including the International Society for Hematotherapy and Graft Engineering (ISHAGE), the American Society for Blood and Marrow Transplantation (ASBMT), and nine others.[327] The U.S. FDA has been recognizing the need for regulatory oversight of these products and finally published, in the *Federal Register* on November 24, 2004, a document that represents a comprehensive system for regulating human cells and cellular and tissue-based products referred to as the Current Good Tissue Practice for Human Cell, Tissue and Cellular and Tissue-based Product Establishments; Inspection and Enforcement; Final Rule (cGTP rule). The purpose of the cGTP rule is to prevent documented evidence of transmission of communicable disease to recipients of infected donor tissue through tissue and organ transplantation, as well as bacterial and fungal infections. Second, this regulation will provide more oversight for a therapeutic cell-based industry with its increased demand for international commerce and increased risk of intercontinental transmission of disease. Finally, the cGTP rule will legally enforce the voluntary standards established by cell therapy organizations not uniformly followed by all cell-processing facilities.[327-329]

Future Directions

Several areas regarding the use of hematopoietic stem cells are actively being investigated. First, definitive trials are necessary to clarify whether there is any clinical benefit associated with CD34+ cell selection or tumor cell or T-cell depletion. Second, by building on platforms in which cells have been expanded but differentiated,[330] it may be possible to expand primitive hematopoietic stem cells as new cytokines are identified and new systems are developed. Expanded populations of primitive cells would be useful for infusion in patients whose autologous graft contains insufficient numbers for transplantation. In addition, the ability to expand HSCs could make UCB components available to larger recipients with less perceived risk. Furthermore, expanded cells may be useful for gene therapy approaches.

Much effort has taken place in recent years to use HPCs as a strategy for clinical gene therapy or to use other cells therapeutically. Stable expression of a transgene in a primitive HPC would, in theory, be an ideal method to replace missing gene products in a patient. However, despite numerous attempts, until very recently there were no durable results. Consequently, when Cavazzana-Calvo and co-workers reported successful treatment of severe combined immune deficiency (SCID) with gene therapy,[331] interest was renewed. Unfortunately, some SCID patients who received genetically engineered autologous HPCs later suffered leukemia because of insertional mutagenesis of CD34+ cells. The occurrence of these adverse events raises the safety concern of gene therapy.[332]

APHERESIS

Apheresis (from the Greek *aphairesis*, meaning "removal") refers to a technique of drawing peripheral blood, separating it, and selectively removing one or more of the components while returning the remainder. Apheresis techniques may be manual or automated, and the phases of drawing, separating, removing, and returning blood and components may be continuous or discontinuous. The technique of apheresis may be used for collecting transfusable blood components from donors, and it may be used to treat patients with conditions for which removal or replacement of a portion of the blood may be therapeutic. The terms cytapheresis, erythrocytapheresis, leukapheresis, plateletpheresis, and plasmapheresis refer to the use of apheresis to remove, respectively, cells, RBCs, white cells, platelets, and plasma. The terms plasma exchange and RBC exchange imply that the component removed is replaced in like amount with normal plasma or RBCs. In practice, nearly all donor and therapeutic apheresis is performed via automated techniques with specialized programmable separation devices designed for this purpose.

The principle by which most apheresis instruments fractionate the components of whole blood is simple density centrifugation. The instrument contains a sterile, closed, and disposable centrifugation chamber in which whole blood is separated into RBC, plasma, and buffy coat layers. The densest component (RBCs) is segregated to the bottom of the centrifugal field, the least dense component (plasma) is pushed to the top, and the other layer of cellular components remains in between, as shown in Figure 35-6. The efficiency of separation depends not only on the density of the components but also on the geometry and rotational speed of the centrifugal chamber, as well as the specific technique for isolating the separated layers. Pure separation of plasma from RBCs and concentrated suspensions of platelets nearly devoid of RBCs can be achieved reliably. Because the

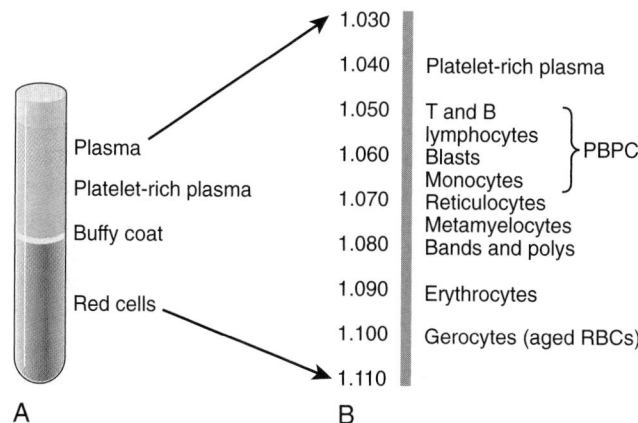

FIGURE 35-6. A, Separation of anticoagulated whole blood. **B,** Specific gravity of blood components. PBPC, peripheral blood progenitor cells; Polys, polymorphonuclear leukocytes; RBCs, red blood cells.

white cell layer is much smaller than either the RBC or plasma layer and close in density to the RBC layer, both the RBC and the platelet components will contain leukocytes. For the same reason, although it is possible to use apheresis to isolate leukocyte fractions that are enriched in granulocytes or mononuclear cells, these fractions will also contain other types of white cells, as well as RBCs and platelets.

Apheresis instruments also exist that separate blood by filtration rather than centrifugation. Because this technique cannot separate cellular elements, it is used primarily in donor applications for collection of plasma.

Donor Apheresis

Overall, the most common medical use of automated apheresis technology is for donor procedures, that is, collection of platelet concentrates or plasma from individual volunteer donors. The principal reason to use apheresis techniques to collect these products, rather than deriving them from whole blood donations, is that the yield per donation is much higher. Six to eight times the number of platelets can be harvested in one apheresis donation than can be isolated from 1 unit of whole blood. Automated systems can be programmed to collect two or even three separate blood components (i.e., units of packed cells, plasma, or single-donor platelets) from one donor during a single apheresis procedure. The same advantage applies to these apheresis collection techniques—a much larger yield is obtained per donation, with little or no compromise in donor safety. The blood products derived from these donor procedures have slightly different quality control characteristics from whole blood–derived components, but in clinical use they are as efficacious as those derived from whole blood donations.

Granulocyte concentrates drawn by apheresis technology to treat refractory fungal or bacterial infections in patients with profound neutropenia are once again being evaluated.[333] Studies in the 1970s showed that granulocyte transfusions had limited efficacy and considerable toxicity. However, the advent of a granulocyte-specific hematopoietic cytokine (G-CSF) in concert with apheresis technology has made it possible to collect up to 10-fold more granulocytes for transfusion than were available for the older studies.[334] Unlike products from unstimulated donors, granulocyte concentrates collected with cytokine stimulation of the donor can yield substantial increments in peripheral granulocyte counts in the recipient.[335,336] Whether these greater increments correspond to greater efficacy has yet to be proved.[337-340]

Apheresis technology can also facilitate obtaining multiple units of plasma from the same donor to provide single-donor plasma support to a recipient with a congenital coagulation factor deficiency treatable with plasma, such as factor X or XIII deficiency.

Although adult donor apheresis, especially for platelet collection, has a large impact on the blood banks that supply blood products for pediatric patients, child donor

apheresis is rarely used. The one exception is donor apheresis collections of peripheral blood progenitor cells, described later.

Therapeutic Apheresis

A broad spectrum of indications exist for automated apheresis used for therapeutic effect in children. For some indications, the mechanism of the therapeutic benefit is readily apparent and the efficacy of the treatment well substantiated. For many other indications, the rationale for the use of apheresis to treat a disease condition is less clear and based on extrapolation from studies in adults or on anecdotal evidence. It is important to remember that the therapeutic value may be derived from removal of a portion of the patient's blood, from administration of a fluid to replace what was removed, or from both. In some cases, the therapeutic value of an apheresis procedure is derived from the ability to control the patient's blood volume independent of the rate and total volume of blood product administered, as with complete exchange of the RBC mass or plasma volume.

Manual Apheresis

Although it is theoretically possible to carry out most apheresis procedures by entirely manual techniques, with steps analogous to those used to derive blood components from donated whole blood, in practice, manual methods are usually reserved for situations in which the automatic equipment is not available or the volume of blood to be processed is too small to warrant use of the automated cell separator. For example, for a newborn with isoimmune thrombocytopenia, it might be possible to obtain an adequate dose of platelets by drawing 1 unit of whole blood from the mother, isolating the platelets manually, and transfusing the residual RBCs and plasma back into the mother rather than subjecting the mother to an automated plateletpheresis procedure. Another manual apheresis procedure is whole blood exchange for neonatal hyperbilirubinemia, typically performed in a discontinuous fashion with reconstituted whole blood, an empty blood collection bag, a three-way stopcock, and a syringe to remove and replace blood in 10-mL cycles. Occasionally, manual exchange of red cells or plasma may be the only alternative in a patient whose venous access is inadequate for automated exchange and for whom a simple transfusion is not an alternative.

Automated Apheresis

The development of mechanical devices to perform selective collections and blood component exchanges was truly an individual inspiration. The son of IBM engineer George Jackson contracted leukemia and was treated at the National Cancer Institute. Recognizing the need for a better way to produce the large number of platelet concentrates required by oncology patients, Jackson developed the first mechanical blood cell separator. Over the subsequent 3 decades, numerous improvements have led to the automated units found in every blood center today.[341] Modern blood separators offer the advantages of a sterile, closed, single-use system, automated control of volume balance, traps to prevent air embolism, and other safety features. Each machine can perform several types of apheresis procedures, with highly automatic modes as well as the capacity to modify procedure parameters for individual patient needs. By comparison, manual exchanges are more awkward to perform, generally use open systems, involve manual tracking of intake and output, and are therefore potentially less safe.

Apheresis devices may be either continuous or discontinuous. A discontinuous device withdraws a volume of blood, separates it, removes the selected component, and returns the remainder, all in serial steps. The sole advantage of a discontinuous device is that it requires only a single site of vascular access. In the donor setting, this is often reason enough to use a discontinuous device. However, when compared with a continuous device, the discontinuous apheresis technique requires longer processing time and involves larger volume shifts in the donor or patient. The latter consideration may be critically important in pediatric patients and imposes a practical limitation on the use of these devices in children. In contrast, continuous devices withdraw, separate, and return blood simultaneously, thus permitting apheresis procedures that affect the patient's intravascular volume only minimally. Separators that operate in a continuous mode include the COBE Spectra, the Baxter-Fenwal CS 3000, the Fresenius AS104, and the Amicus. The COBE Spectra and the Amicus can be operated in either continuous or discontinuous mode.

For any apheresis procedure, there is a fixed extracorporeal blood volume and extracorporeal RBC mass that must be taken into account in planning the procedure. The extracorporeal blood volume depends on the specific make and model, as well as the type of procedure planned, but all devices fall into a range of 200 to 400 mL. A detailed comparison of the features of each automated cell separator is beyond the scope of this chapter.

Unique Aspects of Apheresis in Pediatrics

Performing apheresis procedures in pediatric patients is often more challenging than performing analogous procedures in adults. Specific challenges include vascular access, anticoagulation, volume shifts, hypothermia, and patient cooperation.

Vascular Access

The vessel used for the apheresis draw line, through which whole blood is drawn into the extracorporeal system, must be large and resilient enough to accommodate a large catheter and sustain the required flow rate without collapsing. When peripheral veins are used, a rigid needle, 18 gauge or larger, is used for drawing the blood. In adults and older children, it is usually possible to find veins in the antecubital fossae large enough to accommodate this needle, but children younger than 7 years often do not have adequate access. Because access requirements for returning blood are less demanding, a smaller-gauge (20- to 22-gauge) flexible catheter may be used. Although every child undergoing apheresis should be evaluated first for peripheral access, it is often necessary to obtain access to a larger central vessel. Such access may be accomplished in several ways: a single-lumen central venous catheter or an arterial line to draw the blood and a peripheral vein to return it, or a double-lumen venous catheter. The catheters, often referred to as "dialysis catheters" because the same access issues apply in hemodialysis, may be designed either for temporary placement (usually stiff, straight catheters intended for bedside percutaneous placement) or for permanent placement (softer, tunneled catheters with cuffs that require placement in the operating room).[342] Temporary polyurethane catheters as small as 7 French are available for patients as small as 5 to 10 kg. Permanent catheters designed for apheresis are available in sizes as small as 8 French for children as small as 10 to 12 kg.[343] It is important to realize that most of the double- and triple-lumen catheters available for general purpose central access in children may fail under the draw pressure of an apheresis procedure because the lumen is too small or the catheter wall too soft. Some multiple-lumen catheters also have inadequate separation of the openings of the lumens, thereby permitting recirculation and decreasing the efficiency of apheresis.[343] Hence, it is imperative to consider the possibility that apheresis will be required before placement of a central catheter. Finally, there is growing experience with successful use of implanted access devices (ports) to support chronic apheresis therapy in children.[344,345]

Anticoagulation

Because the blood is exposed to artificial surfaces, apheresis procedures usually require an anticoagulant to prevent activation of platelets, initiation of the coagulation cascade, and the formation of clots within the extracorporeal circuit. The standard anticoagulants used in apheresis are sodium citrate, heparin, or combinations of these two. The anticoagulant is added to the circuit at a controlled rate just at the point where the blood is drawn, and a portion of the anticoagulant is eventually returned to the patient. The amount of anticoagulant that the patient receives depends on the type of procedure, the replacement fluid, and the rates of blood drawing and replacement.

Citrate chelates the available calcium, a necessary cofactor for the clotting cascade, and also prevents platelet aggregation. The infusion of citrated plasma or blood does not cause systemic anticoagulation in the donor or patient, but it may reduce the ionized calcium level in plasma. Pediatric patients are particularly subject to citrate toxicity, in part because the flow rates used during apheresis procedures—and therefore the citrate doses—are often higher on a per-kilogram basis than for adults. Citrate toxicity is first manifested as tingling around the mouth and fingers and sometimes nausea and abdominal discomfort. More serious citrate toxicity includes hypotension and cardiac rhythm disturbances.[346] Because a young or critically ill child may be unable to inform the operator about the earlier warning signs of citrate toxicity, the use of citrate as an anticoagulant requires careful attention to ionized calcium levels, calcium replacement by mouth or intravenous infusion,[95] and cardiac monitoring.

Alternatively, citrate may be either replaced or supplemented with heparin anticoagulation, which may be monitored by the activated clotting time, a crude measure of whole blood clotting time.[347,348] Heparin anticoagulation may be achieved with a bolus, with or without subsequent continuous infusion. The dose of heparin used for an apheresis procedure is similar to those used for therapeutic anticoagulation, and the patient may be expected to have a systemic anticoagulation effect lasting 4 to 6 hours after the end of the procedure, a side effect that may be significant in a patient who has recently undergone surgery or is otherwise at risk for bleeding.

Volume Considerations

The extracorporeal volume for an apheresis procedure, including the centrifugation chamber, tubing, filters, air traps, and possibly a blood warmer, may exceed 400 mL, depending on the machine and tubing configuration. Because the majority of this extracorporeal volume will consist of whole blood or packed cells within the centrifugation chamber, there is also an obligate extracorporeal RBC mass. Discontinuous machines carry out stepwise cycles of removal and return of extracorporeal volume. In a continuous apheresis machine, extracorporeal volume is filled at the start by drawing blood from the patient and remains fixed through the duration of the procedure. An older child or an adult with a blood volume of around 5000 mL can generally tolerate the temporary loss of 300 to 400 mL of blood in either a discontinuous or a continuous technique. At the other extreme, for a child of 12 kg with a blood volume of about 800 mL, the extracorporeal volume represents roughly half the patient's blood. Thus, for younger children, the discontinuous apheresis technique is not feasible, and continuous apheresis procedures may require priming with exogenous RBCs to compensate for the extracorporeal volume and RBC mass.

Many apheresis devices have automated modes that at completion of the procedure return the RBCs in the circuit to the patient by flushing with saline. This return cycle results in the rapid reinfusion of up to 450 mL over a period of several minutes. An older child or adult who was able to tolerate the temporary loss of volume and RBC mass incurred during a discontinuous or unprimed continuous apheresis procedure will usually tolerate rapid return of the volume. However, a younger patient may not tolerate the return cycle, so some or all of the obligate extracorporeal RBC mass must be left in the machine. This loss of RBC mass must be compensated for by using packed RBCs as the priming fluid at the start of the procedure.

Beyond the principles that have been described here, there are also strategies to avoid fluid overload without the use of RBC priming, to administer or remove intravascular fluid, and to administer blood products during the course of an apheresis procedure. The apheresis physician must take into consideration the patient's size, the extracorporeal volume of the apparatus in use, the patient's RBC mass and volume status, and disease factors that may affect the patient's ability to tolerate rapid changes in blood volume and RBC mass. Management of volume and RBC balance during apheresis procedures in children requires careful, individualized planning and thorough understanding of the operation and programming of the automated cell separator.

Hypothermia

Because a portion of the patient's blood volume circulates outside the body during apheresis, considerable heat loss to the environment can occur. Adult platelet donors may lose enough heat to require blankets by the end of a 90-minute collection. For children undergoing apheresis, the physiologic impact of this heat loss is much greater, and the use of a blood warmer may be required to prevent life-threatening hypothermia. The amount of heat loss is a function of (1) the ratio of extracorporeal volume to the patient's blood volume, (2) the rate of blood removal or replacement, and (3) the thermal properties of the system. A blood warmer reduces this heat loss at the expense of increasing the extracorporeal volume, albeit modestly. Only approved devices should be used to warm the blood.

Other hazards of therapeutic apheresis are rare. Some severe complications can occur, but they appear to be largely related to the underlying disorder as opposed to the apheresis itself.[3489,349] This is consistent with the rarity of serious complications in apheresis platelet donors. Pediatric series have also reported complications. However, more were related to the need for vascular access than the procedure itself.[347,350]

Cooperation

The staff of a pediatric apheresis unit must be facile with age-appropriate communication and psychosocial support. The aspects of the apheresis procedure that are most upsetting to children are needle sticks, the need to remain seated, immobilization of one or both arms, frequent squeezing of the blood pressure cuff, and boredom with a prolonged procedure. Expertise in phlebotomy and intravenous line placement is a basic requirement for the staff. The other issues can usually be managed with age-appropriate explanations, parental involvement, and distracting entertainment. Sedation is almost never necessary, except for extremely uncooperative patients, such as those with a significant psychiatric diagnosis or movement disorder.

Indications

Every 7 years a consensus committee of the American Society for Apheresis has reviewed the apheresis literature supporting and refuting the use of apheresis-based therapies in a variety of disorders in which it has been tried (Table 35-11).[351-353] For each disorder, the strength of the evidence supporting the efficacy of apheresis was evaluated and the indication placed into one of five categories. Category I means that efficacy is well documented and the use of therapeutic apheresis is "standard and acceptable"; in category II, apheresis is probably efficacious and its use is "generally accepted," but as an adjunct to primary therapy; in category III, efficacy is debatable, and the evidence is mostly anecdotal or conflicting; in category IV, apheresis has been shown to be ineffective and use of apheresis should be "discouraged"; and in category P (for pending), an apheresis device is not approved for use in the United States, although trials may be under way. Table 35-11 is excerpted from the consensus review, with only diagnoses listed that are usually encountered in the practice of pediatric apheresis.[354]

Erythrocytapheresis: Red Cell Exchange

Sickle Cell Disease

In sickle cell disease, small vessels become occluded when RBCs deformed (sickled) by polymerized hemoglobin S obstruct blood flow in capillaries. If the percentage of cells that can be deformed in this way is reduced below 30% to 50% by transfusion with normal RBCs, there is usually a substantial decrease in many of the clinical manifestations of sickling. Such reduction can be accomplished either by serial simple transfusion or by erythrocytapheresis. When rapid reduction in the percentage of hemoglobin S–containing cells is desirable, such as in the acute management of stroke or chest syndrome or in preparation for emergency surgery, erythrocytapheresis is the method of choice. A series of two to four simple transfusions given over a period of 2 to 3 weeks can also reduce the percentage of hemoglobin S–containing cells to less than 30%, an approach suitable for preparation for elective surgery.

Acute Chest Syndrome

Acute chest syndrome is a leading cause of premature death in patients with sickle cell disease. Transfusion with

TABLE 35-11	Indications for Therapeutic Apheresis in Pediatrics	
Disorders	**Therapeutic Procedure**	**Category***
AUTOIMMUNE		
Catastrophic antiphospholipid syndrome	Plasma exchange	III
Systemic lupus erythematosus, nephritis	Plasma exchange	IV
Systemic lupus erythematosus, other	Plasma exchange	III
Polymyositis-dermatomyositis	Plasma exchange	IV
Rheumatoid arthritis	Lymphocytapheresis	II
	Immunoadsorption	II
HEMATOLOGY AND ONCOLOGY		
ABO-incompatible stem cell transplant	Plasma exchange (recipient)	II
Aplastic anemia/red cell aplasia	Plasma exchange	III
Autoimmune hemolytic anemia	Plasma exchange	III
Babesiosis, severe	Erythrocytapheresis	II
Coagulation factor inhibitors	Plasma exchange	III
	Immunoadsorption	III
Erythrocytosis/polycythemia vera	Erythrocytapheresis	II
Graft-versus-host disease, skin	Extracorporeal photopheresis	II
Graft-versus-host disease, nonskin	Extracorporeal photopheresis	III
Hyperleukocytosis, leukostasis	Leukapheresis	I
Hyperleukocytosis, prophylaxis	Leukapheresis	III
Idiopathic thrombocytopenic purpura, refractory	Immunoadsorption	II
Idiopathic thrombocytopenic purpura, any	Plasma exchange	IV
Malaria, severe	Erythrocytapheresis	II
Sickle cell disease, life or organ threatening	Erythrocytapheresis	I
Sickle cell disease, stroke prophylaxis	Erythrocytapheresis	II
Sickle cell disease, prevention of iron overload	Erythrocytapheresis	II
Thrombocytosis, symptomatic	Thrombocytapheresis	II
Thrombocytosis, prophylactic or secondary	Thrombocytapheresis	III
Thrombotic thrombocytopenic purpura	Plasma exchange	I
Platelet refractoriness	Plasma exchange	III
	Staphylococcal protein A adsorption	III

Continues

TABLE 35-11   Indications for Therapeutic Apheresis in Pediatrics—cont'd

Disorders	Therapeutic Procedure	Category*
METABOLIC		
Acute liver failure	Plasma exchange	III
Familial hypercholesterolemia, homozygotes	Selective removal	I
Familial hypercholesterolemia, heterozygotes	Plasma exchange, selective removal	II
Hypertriglyceridemic pancreatitis	Plasma exchange	III
Mushroom poisoning	Plasma exchange	II
Other poisoning and overdoses	Plasma exchange	III
Phytanic acid storage disease (Refsum's)	Plasma exchange	II
Sepsis	Plasma exchange	III
Thyrotoxicosis	Plasma exchange	III
Miscellaneous		
Dilated cardiomyopathy	Immunoadsorption	P
Inflammatory bowel disease	Adoptive cytapheresis	P
NEUROLOGY		
Acute disseminated encephalomyelitis	Plasma exchange	III
Acute Guillain-Barré syndrome	Plasma exchange	I
Chronic inflammatory demyelinating polyneuropathy	Plasma exchange	I
Lambert-Eaton myasthenic syndrome	Plasma exchange	II
Multiple sclerosis, Devic's syndrome	Plasma exchange	III
Myasthenia gravis	Plasma exchange	I
PANDAS, severe	Plasma exchange	I
Sydenham's chorea, severe	Plasma exchange	I
Rasmussen's encephalitis	Plasma exchange	II
RENAL		
ANCA-associated RPGN (Wegener's)	Plasma exchange	II
Focal segmental glomerulosclerosis	Plasma exchange	III
Goodpasture's disease (anti-GBM)	Plasma exchange	I
Hemolytic-uremic syndrome, diarrhea associated	Plasma exchange	IV
Hemolytic-uremic syndrome, other	Plasma exchange	III
Rapidly progressive nephritis (without anti-GBM)	Plasma exchange	III
Renal allograft rejection, antibody mediated	Plasma exchange	II
Renal allograft HLA desensitization	Plasma exchange	II
RHEUMATIC		
Scleroderma	Plasma exchange	III
Scleroderma	Extracorporeal photopheresis	IV
TRANSPLANTATION		
ABO-incompatible solid organ transplant		
Kidney	Plasma exchange	II
Heart (infants)	Plasma exchange	II
Liver	Plasma exchange	III
Heart allograft rejection, prophylaxis	Extracorporeal photopheresis	I
Heart allograft rejection, treatment	Extracorporeal photopheresis	II
Heart allograft rejection, treatment	Plasma exchange	III
Lung transplant	Extracorporeal photopheresis	III

*I: Therapeutic apheresis is standard and acceptable, either as primary therapy or as a valuable first-line adjunct to other initial therapies. Efficacy is documented by controlled clinical trials and published experience.

II: Therapeutic apheresis is generally accepted as supportive to other more definitive treatments; there is some literature support of its efficacy.

III: Anecdotal reports may suggest the use of therapeutic apheresis; however, no controlled trials have documented its efficacy. No consensus can be reached regarding its risk-benefit ratio.

IV: Controlled trials show lack of efficacy of therapeutic apheresis. Anecdotal studies suggesting efficacy have not been reproduced.

P: Pending.

ANCA, antineutrophil cytoplasmic antibody; GBM, glomerular basement membrane; NS, not specified; PANDAS, pediatric autoimmune neuropsychiatric disorders associated with streptococcal infections; RPGN, rapidly progressive glomerulonephritis.

From Shaz BH, Linenberger ML, Bandarenko N, et al. Category IV indications for therapeutic apheresis: ASFA fourth special issue. J Clin Apheresis. 2007;22:176-180.

RBCs is commonly used to treat acute chest syndrome both to increase the oxygen-carrying capacity of the blood and to reduce the percentage of hemoglobin S. Although controversy exists about the advantages of exchange transfusion over simple transfusion (see Chapter 19), their efficacy in acute chest syndrome is probably similar.[355] In practice, exchange transfusion by automated apheresis is often performed in patients with severe acute chest syndrome to reduce the hemoglobin S percentage in a shorter time than possible with simple transfusion or manual exchange and without the accompanying fluid loading.[135]

Stroke

The observed incidence of stroke in sickle cell patients varies from 6% to 34%. Although transfusion therapy is not thought to affect the neurologic outcome of completed strokes, it remains the mainstay of acute management as a measure to halt progression of cerebral vasculopathy. Considerable evidence exists that long-term transfusion after a central nervous system event is effective prophylaxis against progression of central nervous system disease and against recurrence of clinical stroke (secondary stroke prevention).[356] Transfusion has also been shown to be effective in primary prevention of stroke in patients with sickle cell disease who have been identified as high risk based on transcranial Doppler ultrasound studies of blood flow velocity in the circle of Willis.[357] Although the standard target hemoglobin S percentage for prevention of stroke is less than 30%, for secondary stroke prevention, some neurologically stable patients may be maintained safely at a target hemoglobin S of less than 50%, which is generally easily achievable with a program of chronic erythrocytapheresis.[358] For primary stroke prevention, the standard approach is to maintain the hemoglobin S percentage at less than 30%, which is also achievable with erythrocytapheresis. Very recent published evidence suggests that hydroxyurea treratment may reduce the risk for stroke, as well as the need for chronic apheresis or chronic simple RBC transfusion.[359]

Priapism

Although prepubescent priapism has a good prognosis for eventual potency, episodes of postpubescent priapism are associated with eventual impotence. In addition, there is some correlation with the duration of the episode of priapism and loss of erectile function. Whether this is due to efficacious therapeutic intervention or simply because the worst cases last longer and are more likely to cause irreversible damage remains unclear. Some authors advocate RBC exchange for severe cases,[360] but the efficacy of exchange transfusion for priapism in patients with sickle cell disease is unclear.

Transfusion before General Anesthesia

Although it has been a widely accepted practice to perform RBC transfusions or exchanges in patients with sickle cell anemia before most surgical procedures that require general anesthesia, it is increasingly apparent that not all procedures warrant such large exposure to blood. In one study that examined postoperative complications in patients subjected to surgery without prior transfusion, the complications tended to occur after procedures that adversely affected postoperative oxygenation, specifically, procedures affecting the airway (e.g., tonsillectomy/adenoidectomy) or major abdominal surgery.[361] Investigators in one study prospectively randomized patients with sickle cell disease undergoing surgery either to aggressive transfusion, with a therapeutic goal of a hemoglobin S content of less than 30%, or to simple transfusion, with a therapeutic goal of a hemoglobin level above 10 g/dL. They observed no benefit with the more aggressive transfusion regimen, which was complicated by a higher rate of alloimmunization and hemolytic transfusion reaction (acute and delayed).[362]

Red Cell Exchange for Chronic Transfusion

Erythrocytapheresis has an important role to play in chronic transfusion therapy for patients with sickle cell disease. Children with sickle cell disease in whom complications develop for which chronic, lifelong RBC transfusion is indicated are at risk for the development of transfusional iron overload. Although this can be successfully managed by chelation therapy with deferoxamine, compliance with nightly infusions of the chelator must be high to achieve negative iron balance. Compliance with the oral iron chelator deferasirox may prove to be better. Even though the efficacy and safety of this agent in sickle cell disease have not yet been well established, it is likely that this orally active drug will largely replace deferoxamine. The iron overloading of long-term simple transfusion therapy can be substantially reduced or eliminated by a program of erythrocytapheresis.[363] This approach involves removal and replacement of approximately half of the patient's RBC mass every 3 to 4 weeks. Transfusion by erythrocytapheresis will generally require 23% to 73% more donor units and exposure than is the case with simple transfusion. Because the general risk for transmission of infectious disease and for transfusion reactions is low, the additional risk of these donor exposures may be outweighed by the benefit of reducing or avoiding iron overload and chelation therapy. Of greater concern is the relatively high risk for RBC alloantibody formation in patients with sickle cell disease. It is not clear whether patients chronically transfused by erythrocytapheresis have a greater risk for alloimmunization than do those treated by simple transfusion because both populations will eventually be exposed to a large number of donors.

Normovolemic Red Cell Transfusion. RBC transfusion in hemodynamically unstable patients may be accomplished in a normovolemic fashion with apheresis technology. For example, thalassemia patients with end-stage cardiac failure secondary to transfusional iron overload may better tolerate transfusion to raise the hemoglobin level if the blood volume is not increased rapidly. Exchange transfusion in the setting of overwhelming hemolysis has also been advocated when transfusion requirements would exceed the patient's ability to handle the volume to be transfused. This may occur in autoimmune hemolytic processes (especially IgM mediated), as well as in infectious hemolytic processes, including malaria and babesiosis.[364,365]

Erythrocytapheresis may also be used to remove RBCs from a patient or donor. Patients with polycythemia secondary to chronic cyanotic congenital heart disease complicated by Eisenmenger's syndrome may have improved hemodynamic function and symptomatic relief after phlebotomy, which is well tolerated with apheresis technology.[366] Finally, more than 1 unit of RBCs at a time can be drawn safely from a donor if normovolemia is maintained.[367] This technique is being used increasingly in routine red cell collection[368,369] and autologous red cell collection[160] and is especially useful when obtaining rare blood from donors or from a single donor to support a specific recipient.

Leukapheresis

Leukocytosis is a negative prognostic indicator in childhood leukemia, especially when the initial white cell count exceeds 200,000/μL. In many centers it is standard practice to perform leukapheresis or whole blood exchange in patients who have extremely high counts with the goal of treating or preventing symptoms related to hyperviscosity and tumor lysis syndrome.[370] Although the leukocyte count can be reduced rapidly, typically dropping by 50% to 75% immediately after the procedure, a long-term survival advantage for patients treated by leukapheresis for hyperleukocytosis has not been demonstrated. The value of this intervention may depend in part on the initial immunophenotype. Specifically, complications of hyperleukocytosis, such as cerebral thrombosis and hemorrhage, may be more common in acute myeloblastic leukemia than in acute lymphoblastic leukemia.[371] Furthermore, in one retrospective study, electrolyte abnormalities during induction chemotherapy were reduced in the group of patients with acute lymphoblastic leukemia and hyperleukocytosis who underwent leukapheresis or exchange transfusion, thus suggesting that leukapheresis may reduce the severity of tumor lysis syndrome.[372] Some authors propose that all patients with acute myeloblastic leukemia or acute undifferentiated leukemia with initial white blood cell counts in excess of 200,000/μL undergo exchange or leukapheresis and that only selective patients with acute lymphoblastic leukemia require this intervention.[373] Technically, leukapheresis may be performed either by using specific tubing sets designed to remove the buffy coat layer or by using the tubing set for plasmapheresis and collecting down into the RBC interface. It is often desirable to maintain a relatively low hematocrit during therapeutic leukapheresis because the RBC mass contributes to viscosity of the blood.

PERIPHERAL BLOOD PROGENITOR CELLS

Peripheral blood progenitor cells, or stem cells, are hematopoietic progenitors with potential for self-renewal that circulate in the blood. At steady state they are present in very low numbers, but during the early phase of recovery from chemotherapy-induced myelosuppression or as a result of exogenous hematopoietic cytokine mobilization (e.g., G-CSF), their relative numbers may increase 10- to 100-fold. This observation has made it possible to collect sufficient numbers of progenitor cells by apheresis to allow autologous hematopoietic rescue after high-dose chemotherapy and to serve as the sole source of stem cells, in lieu of bone marrow, for allogeneic transplantation.[374-377] Collection of peripheral progenitor cells for autologous transplantation in children has been reported by several centers.[375-378] Early engraftment of granulocytes and platelets after high-dose chemotherapy was observed, similar to the findings in adult trials.[378] (See Chapter 9 for discussion of the role of HSC transplants and evaluation of progenitor harvests.) Growth in the number of clinical protocols involving their use has had a profound effect on most clinical apheresis units.[379] Hence, some discussion of the unique aspects of pediatric peripheral progenitor cell apheresis is warranted.

Because almost all pediatric peripheral blood progenitor protocols are directed toward treatment of aggressive cancer with a high risk of relapse (advanced-stage neuroblastoma, leukemia, relapsed lymphoma, high-risk brain tumors), the protocols have most commonly timed the collection of cells to occur during the initial rise in white blood cell count after chemotherapy-induced myelosuppression. Most protocols also use mobilization with a hematopoietic cytokine (GM-CSF or G-CSF).[380-384] The general considerations for access for progenitor cell collections are the same as have previously been described. Because many of the candidates for peripheral blood progenitor cell collections will have central lines for their chemotherapy and supportive care placed at the time of diagnosis or relapse, it is important to select a catheter stiff enough to use for leukapheresis. As with large-volume leukapheresis collections in adults, four to seven blood volumes may be processed by the cell separator in a single 4-hour apheresis collection. More prolonged collections are technically feasible and do increase the net yield, but they may tax the patience of the child and apheresis staff. The adequacy and quality of collections are usually monitored with a complete blood cell count and a measure of progenitor content consisting of tissue culture assays for CFU-GM or, more commonly, counts of CD34$^+$ cells by fluorescence-activated cell sorter analysis, or both. A typical yield from a single collection might be 2.5×10^6 CD34$^+$ cells per kilogram of recipient body weight. Actual yields vary widely, depending on factors such as a history of previous chemotherapy, timing of collections, intercurrent illness, precollection counts, and other factors.[381-384] Cytopenias, especially thrombocytopenia, have been reported after progenitor cell collections,[385] but catheter-related problems such as mechanical obstruction, thrombosis, and infection are the most common difficulties.[386]

Extracorporeal Photopheresis

Extracorporeal photopheresis is a therapeutic use of apheresis technology that takes advantage of the conversion by UVA light (spectrum, 320 to 400 nm) of

8-methoxypsoralen from an inactive molecule to an agent that can induce irreversible lesions in the DNA of leukocytes. The intended target for this DNA damage is T cells that may have a role in pathogenesis. Disorders mediated by excessive autoreactivity or alloreactivity might theoretically be treated by this approach. Some photopheresis protocols involve performing leukapheresis to collect mononuclear cells, ex vivo psoralen treatment and UV irradiation of the cells, and reinfusion of the treated cells. In other protocols, the patient is treated with the psoralen systemically before leukapheresis and UV irradiation of the product. The best-documented therapeutic effect of photopheresis is in the treatment of cutaneous T-cell lymphomas (Sezary's syndrome found exclusively in adults), in which response rates greater than 60% and cure rates of 10% to 15% have been achieved.[387]

More recently, photopheresis has been applied to treat rejection of solid organ grafts in which immunosuppressive interventions have failed and to treat chronic GVHD, especially skin GVHD, after bone marrow transplantation, including treatment in children.[388-393] Anecdotal reports have described striking responses in patients with cardiac rejection refractory to standard treatment, and a randomized pilot study demonstrated the efficacy of photopheresis in preventing cardiac allograft rejection.[394] Controlled trials are needed before the efficacy of this application can be evaluated.[395] Additional reports of control of rejection of other solid organ transplants (including lung transplants) by extracorporeal photopheresis have emerged.[396,397] Wider application of this technology in pediatrics is currently limited in the United States by the lack of an approved photopheresis instrument that uses continuous-flow cell separation.

PLASMA EXCHANGE

Plasma exchange is performed either to remove harmful constituents of plasma (such as autoantibodies or excess cholesterol) or to replace missing plasma proteins, such as coagulation factors in liver failure. The extent of removal of a particular molecule or compound by plasmapheresis is a function of the amount of plasma removed and the distribution of the molecule in the body. The most efficient clearance is achieved for substances (such as IgM) that are limited to the intravascular compartment. If the molecule is distributed within the compartment defined by extracellular water (such as IgG), the efficiency of removal is also affected by the rate of re-equilibration between the extravascular and the intravascular space. Plasmapheresis is least efficient when the molecule targeted for removal is distributed over the entire body (many drugs and toxins). Similarly, the efficiency of replacement of missing plasma factors is a function of the factors' distribution and ongoing rate of consumption.[345]

For some indications, the underlying mechanism of an observed therapeutic effect of plasmapheresis may be unknown. For example, in TTP, controlled clinical trials[387] have documented the superiority of plasma exchange over simple plasma transfusion well before the pathogenesis of the disease was understood. This result was commonly extrapolated to the treatment of HUS because it shares certain clinical features with TTP, even though the empirical evidence supporting the use of plasma exchange in adult HUS[398] and pediatric HUS[347,399,400] was not well founded. In light of the demonstration in patients with TTP (but not HUS) of an autoantibody that removes the activity of a serum metalloproteinase responsible for cleaving von Willebrand factor,[401-403] it appears that plasma exchange treats TTP by removal of the autoantibody, as well as by replacement of the serum metalloproteinase and normal von Willebrand factor. Although this discovery has provided a sound explanation of how plasma exchange helps in TTP, it has invalidated the previous assumption that HUS and TTP represent a spectrum of a single disease process that will respond to plasma exchange.

The role of plasma exchange in liver failure is controversial. In acute severe liver failure, metabolic toxins (the so-called middle molecules, which are not effectively removed by conventional dialysis) accumulate and lead to hepatic encephalopathy, coma, and death. Furthermore, failure of production of intravascular proteins, including albumin and coagulation factors, leads to ascites, edema, and bleeding. Plasma exchange can offer temporizing supportive care by providing the missing plasma components in larger doses than could be delivered by simple transfusion. However, plasmapheresis is inefficient for removal of the toxins that accumulate in liver failure and has not been shown to prevent or forestall the development of hepatic encephalopathy. The use of plasma exchange to provide a bridge to support patients awaiting liver transplantation or to normalize coagulation parameters immediately before transplant surgery is well documented.[404]

Autoimmune Disorders

Guillain-Barré Syndrome

Several controlled studies comparing plasmapheresis with conventional therapy for Guillain-Barré syndrome (GBS) have documented a therapeutic benefit from plasmapheresis, especially when initiated early in the course of the illness.[405] Lack of a uniform response to plasmapheresis had led some researchers to speculate whether the syndrome may be a common outcome of diverse causes.[406] Because children with GBS have a somewhat better prognosis than adults do, plasmapheresis is generally reserved for those who deteriorate rapidly or who require ventilator assistance.[407] High-dose IVIG has also been shown to have efficacy in treatment of GBS, and a randomized trial in adults demonstrated that IVIG may be slightly superior to plasma exchange for GBS.[408] This result has led neurologists to treat with IVIG first and reserve plasmapheresis for refractory or especially severe cases. Both IVIG and plasmapheresis have efficacy in childhood GBS but have not been compared in a randomized trial.[409,410] Patients with chronic inflammatory demyelinating polyradiculopathy, an insidious peripheral neuropathy with a waxing and waning course and some similarities to GBS, may also benefit from plasmapheresis.[411,412]

Myasthenia Gravis

Myasthenia gravis is a neuromuscular disorder characterized by progressive proximal muscle weakness. It follows damage to motor end plates caused by an autoantibody directed against postsynaptic acetylcholine receptors. Plasmapheresis has been shown to provide acute temporary relief of myasthenic crises and to be a useful adjunct along with immunosuppressive therapies for longer-term treatment.[413,414]

Systemic Lupus Erythematosus

Systemic lupus erythematosus is an autoimmune disorder with protean manifestations that may affect many organ systems, especially the skin, kidney, central nervous system, and blood. Controlled trials of plasmapheresis in systemic lupus erythematosus have generally failed to show long-term benefit.[415] Nonetheless, some authors advocate the use of plasmapheresis to treat certain acute flares of the disease, especially when they are severe or threaten the function of vital organs (kidney, central nervous system). Flares during pregnancy, for example, when other more toxic treatments might be contraindicated, have been proposed as appropriate indications for apheresis.[416]

Immune Hemolysis

Cold agglutinin disease, a form of autoimmune hemolytic anemia mediated by an RBC antibody of the IgM isotype, may be effectively treated in the acute phase by plasmapheresis because IgM antibodies are efficiently removed by plasmapheresis.[417] Plasmapheresis has also been used in life-threatening IgG-mediated autoimmune hemolysis, even though removal of IgG is much less efficient. The reduction in hemolysis is transient in either case, and in general, apheresis is warranted only to buy time until other treatments, such as splenectomy, can be performed or to treat disease refractory to other therapies.[418]

Other Autoimmune Disorders

Rasmussen's encephalitis, a rare disease resulting in an intractable seizure disorder previously treated by hemispherectomy, has been shown to result from autoantibodies directed against the glutamate receptor (GluR3) in the brain.[419] The antibodies reportedly act as constitutive agonists and result in excessive neuronal activation and subsequent seizures.[420,421] Case reports suggest that plasmapheresis has a role in acute treatment. A syndrome called pediatric autoimmune neuropsy-

chiatric disorders associated with streptococcal infections (PANDAS) consists of a movement disorder with involuntary tics and a behavioral disorder with obsessive-compulsive features.[422] The pathophysiology is thought to involve group A β-hemolytic streptococci triggering antibodies that cross-react with the basal ganglia of genetically susceptible individuals, a mechanism parallel to the pathophysiology of Sydenham's chorea.[423] One randomized trial has demonstrated that both IVIG and plasma exchange have efficacy in treating the symptoms of PANDAS,[424] and another trial suggested that plasmapheresis and IVIG may have efficacy in Sydenham's chorea.[425]

Hyper-IgE syndrome (Job's syndrome) is a rare autosomal recessive disorder characterized by extremely high IgE levels, recurrent infections (typically with *Staphylococcus*), and chronic dermatitis. Plasmapheresis results in a reduction in IgE levels and correspondingly decreases inflammatory lesions. It is generally reserved for patients who have failed to respond to other therapies, including antibiotics and IVIG replacement.[426] An unusual complication of hyper-IgE syndrome is keratoconjunctivitis, which may threaten vision; it has reportedly been improved with apheresis.[427]

Other Coagulopathies

A preexisting coagulopathy has historically been a contraindication to managing a patient by ECMO because of the additional anticoagulation required to prevent clotting in the membrane oxygenation circuit and the high risk of intracranial hemorrhage. Several centers have observed that it is possible to perform plasmapheresis via the ECMO circuit itself, thereby replacing the missing coagulation factors in the hope of decreasing the risk for hemorrhage.[428,429]

Renal Disease. Cryoglobulinemia, a disorder rare in pediatrics, involves the pathologic production of proteins that reversibly precipitate or gel on exposure to cold. In general, they are antibodies, although they are not necessarily limited to the IgM class. These immune complexes may be deposited in the kidney and result in end-organ damage. Because immune complexes are largely intravascular, they are efficiently cleared by apheresis.[430] Apheresis has also been advocated in Goodpasture's syndrome, an autoimmune disorder caused by antibodies against glomerular basement membranes. Controlled trials to measure the efficacy of plasmapheresis, often as an adjunct to other immunosuppressive agents, have yielded conflicting results. Some appear to show clear benefit,[431] whereas the benefit in other studies appears to be marginal.[432]

Although plasmapheresis has not been shown to prevent renal allograft rejection, it may prove useful as an adjunctive therapy in preventing recurrence of corticosteroid-resistant nephrotic syndrome with focal sclerosing glomerulosclerosis (FSGS) in the transplanted kidney when used in conjunction with cyclophosphamide and pulse corticosteroids.[433,434] The mechanism of this therapeutic effect is thought to be removal of a protein permeability factor in plasma that mediates the renal injury in FSGS.

Hypercholesterolemia. Genetic absence of the low-density lipoprotein receptor results in extreme hypercholesterolemia and the development of severe atherosclerotic complications within the first several decades. Cholesterol-lowering drugs are largely ineffective in patients with completely absent of receptors or nonfunctional receptors. Hence, plasmapheresis is the treatment of first choice. It may be performed by simply removing plasma and replacing it with albumin or by selective lipid absorption columns. The reported advantages of the latter treatment are the greater volumes that may be processed with less depletion of coagulation factors, immunoglobulins, and high-density lipoproteins. Columns come in many varieties, and the most commonly used are disposable dextran sulfate columns. A dual-column method has been developed that cannot be saturated; the lipid collected is eluted from one column while the second is collecting. This system has been shown to be effective in pediatric patients.[435] Disadvantages of using columns include additional extracorporeal volume (150 to 400 mL) added to the system and some reports of adverse side effects.

Transplantation

ABO-incompatible bone marrow or solid organ transplantation is most problematic when the recipient has IgM antibodies against the donor ABO type.[436] Apheresis can be used to deplete isohemagglutinins (naturally occurring anti-A, anti-B antibodies).[437] Although this approach is effective in reducing IgM titers, the requirement for several daily procedures often results in a large number of donor exposures.[438] Most bone marrow transplant programs have switched to depleting the donor marrow of RBCs, a one-time procedure that has not been shown to compromise engraftment. For ABO-incompatible cardiac transplantation in neonates, however, plasmapheresis, either as a separate procedure or incorporated into cardiopulmonary bypass, may be used immediately before or after transplant surgery to remove isohemagglutinins.[142] Plasmapheresis has also been used to reduce HLA antibodies in patients who are candidates for renal transplantation but who have high degrees of HLA sensitization that restrict the availability of compatible organs and increase the risk of hyperacute rejection.[439]

Disseminated Intravascular Coagulation/Purpura Fulminans

Plasmapheresis may be used in desperate situations. Specifically, the dramatic coagulopathy of purpura fulminans associated with meningococcal sepsis can be treated by plasmapheresis. In trials using historical controls, improved survival and correction of coagulopathy have been documented, but because the trials had no concurrent controls, it is impossible to be sure that plasmapheresis contributed to the improvement.[440]

Special Applications and Selective Adsorption

Plasmapheresis allows the selective removal of components within plasma by additional processing of the separated plasma. Various devices such as immunoadsorbent columns may be incorporated in series into the plasma flow. For example, the plasma can be exposed to beads coated with antigen to remove a specific antibody or with staphylococcal protein A to remove IgG. Therapeutic protein A immunoadsorption has been applied to an array of hematologic disorders, including autoimmune thrombocytopenic purpura and alloimmune platelet transfusion refractoriness.[441] Coagulation factor VIII alloantibodies have also been treated extensively with this technique.

Types of Columns

Two general types of staphylococcal protein A columns for clinical use exist: disposable columns intended for single use and renewable columns that are part of a system to remove IgG continuously.[441] Both techniques use staphylococcal protein A attached to a solid matrix to permit selective removal of IgG antibodies, including subclasses IgG1, IgG2, and IgG4, either as free antibody or as immune complexes. IgG3 and immunoglobulins of other classes are less avidly bound to protein A and hence are less efficiently removed by these devices.[442]

An inherent limitation of this adsorption chromatography is saturation of the staphylococcal protein A binding sites. For example, the disposable column is saturated after 200 to 250 mL of plasma has passed over the column. A method to circumvent this problem of rapid saturation has been developed whereby two columns are used alternatively, collecting on one while eluting (flushing with a low pH solution) from the other column. Clinical studies using each of these systems have been performed, but only the disposable column is licensed for use in idiopathic thrombocytopenic purpura and the two-column system is available only for research protocols.[443]

Both types of staphylococcal protein A columns have been used to treat platelet refractoriness (platelet alloimmunization), but the clinical value of such intervention is not well established.

Use in Congenital Hemophilia with Inhibitors

The two-column immunoabsorption system has demonstrated efficacy for removal of coagulation factor inhibitors, either acquired or secondary to congenital deficiency (hemophilia A or B). One study of 22 patients used staphylococcal protein A adsorption to treat patients with a wide array of starting inhibitor titers. A majority achieved greater than 90% reduction in inhibitor titer;

however, a starting titer of greater than 200 Bethesda units (BU) typically resulted in postadsorption titers greater than 5.[444] Below this level one can overwhelm an inhibitor simply by giving larger doses of factor concentrate. For short-term removal of coagulation factor inhibitors, the technique has documented efficacy. In the Malmö protocol, staphylococcal protein A adsorption is used as the initial stage of inhibitor ablation therapy to reduce the initial titer to less than 10 BU, followed by the administration of IVIG, cyclophosphamide, and high doses of the missing coagulation factor (VIII or IX). In a published series, 8 of 11 inhibitor patients achieved durable responses to this inhibitor ablation protocol.[445] Limiting factors for generalized application of this protocol include both unavailability of the two-column system and the large quantities of factor concentrates used, issues that result in considerable expense when carrying out the protocol.

Other Autoimmune Diseases

Staphylococcal protein A columns have been applied to numerous different autoimmune disorders.[446] The common finding is that antibody can be removed with the system, but conclusions regarding whether staphylococcal protein A apheresis is warranted in each of these disorders must await prospective clinical trials.

Another selective-removal apheresis methodology has been developed to target the removal of some populations of granulocytes and monocytes based on their adherence to cellulose acetate beads. There are several reports from Japan of the efficacy and safety of this form of granulocytapheresis in the treatment of ulcerative colitis, but the device is not currently available in the United States.[447-449]

CONCLUSION

The addition of mechanical apheresis devices to the therapeutic armamentarium of transfusion medicine specialists has allowed dramatic interventions in both acute and chronic disorders. The complexity of the clinical settings in which apheresis is sometimes used often makes it difficult to assess the value of apheresis-based therapies. As economic constraints increasingly encroach on the application of medical technologies, it is imperative to design well-controlled studies to document the efficacy of the intervention. Consensus statements provide an opportunity to pose testable questions for interventions in multicenter trials. The involvement of pediatric transfusion medicine specialists early in the design of such trials is warranted because of the technical complexity of the procedures and the unique requirements of pediatric patients. Producers of apheresis devices must also be mindful of these unique requirements lest protocols designed for adults not be applicable for children. Reduction of extracorporeal volume, for example, may be beneficial to adults as well as pediatric patients.

REFERENCES

1. Erslev AJ, Caro J, Schuster SJ. Is there an optimal hemoglobin level? Transfus Med Rev. 1989;3:237-242.
2. Hebert PC, Wells G, Blajchman MA, et al. A multicenter, randomized, controlled clinical trial of transfusion requirements in critical care. Transfusion Requirements in Critical Care Investigators, Canadian Critical Care Trials Group. N Engl J Med. 1999;340:409-417.
3. Lacroix J, Hebert PC, Hutchison JS, et al. Transfusion strategies for patients in pediatric intensive care units. N Engl J Med. 2007;356:1609-1619.
4. Homi J, Reynolds J, Skinner A, et al. General anaesthesia in sickle-cell disease. BMJ. 1979;1:1599-601.
5. Bell EF, Strauss RG, Widness JA, et al. Randomized trial of liberal versus restrictive guidelines for red blood cell transfusion in preterm infants. Pediatrics. 2005;115:1685-1691.
6. Kirpalani H, Whyte RK, Andersen C, et al. The Premature Infants in Need of Transfusion (PINT) study: a randomized, controlled trial of a restrictive (low) versus liberal (high) transfusion threshold for extremely low birth weight infants. J Pediatr. 2006;149:301-307.
7. Bell EF. Transfusion thresholds for preterm infants: how low should we go? J Pediatr. 2006;149:287-289.
8. Kattamis C, Touliatos N, Haidas S, et al. Growth of children with thalassaemia: effect of different transfusion regimens. Arch Dis Child. 1970;45:502-509.
9. Piomelli S, Danoff SJ, Becker MH, et al. Prevention of bone malformations and cardiomegaly in Cooley's anemia by early hypertransfusion regimen. Ann N Y Acad Sci. 1969;165:427-436.
10. Piomelli S, Karpatkin MH, Arzanian M, et al. Hypertransfusion regimen in patients with Cooley's anemia. Ann N Y Acad Sci. 1974;232:186-192.
11. Cazzola M, Borgna-Pignatti C, Locatelli F, et al. A moderate transfusion regimen may reduce iron loading in beta-thalassemia major without producing excessive expansion of erythropoiesis. Transfusion. 1997;37:135-140.
12. Olivieri NF. The beta-thalassemias. N Engl J Med. 1999;341:99-109.
13. Beutler E, West C. The storage of hard-packed red blood cells in citrate-phosphate-dextrose (CPD) and CPD-adenine (CPDA-1). Blood. 1979;54:280-284.
14. Strauss RG, Burmeister LF, Johnson K, et al. AS-1 red cells for neonatal transfusions: a randomized trial assessing donor exposure and safety. Transfusion. 1996;36:873-878.
15. Snyder EL. Clinical use of white cell–poor blood components. Transfusion. 1989;29:568-571.
16. Freedman JJ, Blajchman MA, McCombie N. Canadian Red Cross Society symposium on leukodepletion: report of proceedings. Transfus Med Rev. 1994;8:1-14.
17. Ciavarella D, Snyder E. Clinical use of blood transfusion devices. Transfus Med Rev. 1988;2:95-111.
18. Wenz B. Clinical and laboratory precautions that reduce the adverse reactions, alloimmunization, infectivity, and possibly immunomodulation associated with homologous transfusions. Transfus Med Rev. 1990;4:3-7.
19. Brubaker DB. Clinical significance of white cell antibodies in febrile nonhemolytic transfusion reactions. Transfusion. 1990;30:733-737.

20. Wenz B. Microaggregate blood filtration and the febrile transfusion reaction. A comparative study. Transfusion. 1983;23:95-98.

21. de Graan-Hentzen YC, Gratama JW, Mudde GC, et al. Prevention of primary cytomegalovirus infection in patients with hematologic malignancies by intensive white cell depletion of blood products. Transfusion. 1989;29:757-760.

22. Gilbert GL, Hayes K, Hudson IL, et al. Prevention of transfusion-acquired cytomegalovirus infection in infants by blood filtration to remove leucocytes. Neonatal Cytomegalovirus Infection Study Group. Lancet. 1989;1:1228-1231.

23. Roelen DL, van Rood JJ, Brand A, et al. Immunomodulation by blood transfusions. Vox Sang. 2000;78:273-275.

24. Vamvakas E, Moore SB. Perioperative blood transfusion and colorectal cancer recurrence: a qualitative statistical overview and meta-analysis. Transfusion. 1993;33:754-765.

25. Shirwadkar S, Blajchman MA, Frame B, et al. Effect of blood transfusions on experimental pulmonary metastases in mice. Transfusion. 1990;30:188-190.

26. Roberts JP, Ascher NL, Lake J, et al. Graft vs. host disease after liver transplantation in humans: a report of four cases. Hepatology. 1991;14:274-281.

27. Wisecarver JL, Cattral MS, Langnas AN, et al. Transfusion-induced graft-versus-host disease after liver transplantation. Documentation using polymerase chain reaction with HLA-DR sequence–specific primers. Transplantation. 1994;58:269-271.

28. Anderson KC, Goodnough LT, Sayers M, et al. Variation in blood component irradiation practice: implications for prevention of transfusion-associated graft-versus-host disease. Blood. 1991;77:2096-2102.

29. Anderson KC, Weinstein HJ. Transfusion-associated graft-versus-host disease. N Engl J Med. 1990;323:315-321.

30. Thaler M, Shamiss A, Orgad S, et al. The role of blood from HLA-homozygous donors in fatal transfusion-associated graft-versus-host disease after open-heart surgery. N Engl J Med. 1989;321:25-28.

31. Juji T, Takahashi K, Shibata Y, et al. Post-transfusion graft-versus-host disease in immunocompetent patients after cardiac surgery in Japan. N Engl J Med. 1989;321:56.

32. Watkins WM. Biochemistry and genetics of the ABO, Lewis, and P blood group systems. Adv Hum Genet. 1980;10:1-136.

33. Ball SP, Tongue N, Gibaud A, et al. The human chromosome 19 linkage group FUT1 (H), FUT2 (SE), LE, LU, PEPD, C3, APOC2, D19S7 and D19S9. Ann Hum Genet. 1991;55:225-233.

34. Oriol R, Danilovs J, Hawkins BR. A new genetic model proposing that the Se gene is a structural gene closely linked to the H gene. Am J Hum Genet. 1981;33:421-431.

35. Bhende YM, Deshpande CK, Bhatia HM, et al. A "new" blood-group character related to the ABO system. Lancet. 1951;1:903-904.

36. Clausen H, Hakomori S. ABH and related histo-blood group antigens; immunochemical differences in carrier isotypes and their distribution. Vox Sang. 1989;56:1-20.

37. Oriol R, Le Pendu J, Mollicone R. Genetics of ABO, H, Lewis, X and related antigens. Vox Sang. 1986;51:161-171.

38. Watkins WM, Greenwell P, Yates AD, et al. Regulation of expression of carbohydrate blood group antigens. Biochimie. 1988;70:1597-611.

39. Hakomori S. Blood group ABH and Ii antigens of human erythrocytes: chemistry, polymorphism, and their developmental change. Semin Hematol. 1981;18:39-62.

40. Watkins W. Blood-group substances. Science. 1966;152:172-181.

41. Povey S, Goudie D. Report of the committee on the genetic constitution of chromosome 9. Cytogenet Cell Genet. 1990;55:136-141.

42. Vengelen-Tyler V. Technical Manual, 13th ed. Bethesda, MD, American Association of Blood Banks, 1999, p 798.

43. Cserti CM, Dzik WH. The ABO blood group system and *Plasmodium falciparum* malaria. Blood. 2007;110:2250-2258.

44. Grundbacher F. Changes in the human A antigen of erythrocytes with the individual's age. Nature. 1964;204:192-194.

45. Witebsky E, Engasser LM. Blood groups and subgroups of the newborn. I. The A factor of the newborn. J Immunol. 1949;61:171-178.

46. Giles CM, Parkin DM. Observations of the A_2 gene and H antigen in foetal life. Br J Haematol. 1963;9:63-67.

47. Crawford H, Cutbush M, Mollison PL. Hemolytic disease of the newborn due to anti-A. Blood. 1953;8:620-639.

48. Watanabe K, Hakomori SI. Status of blood group carbohydrate chains in ontogenesis and in oncogenesis. J Exp Med. 1976;144:645-653.

49. Fukuda M, Fukuda MN, Hakomori S. Developmental change and genetic defect in the carbohydrate structure of band 3 glycoprotein of human erythrocyte membrane. J Biol Chem. 1979;254:3700-3703.

50. Mollison PL, Engelfriet CP, Contreras M (eds). Blood Transfusion in Clinical Medicine, 10th ed. Oxford, Blackwell Science, 1997.

51. Romans DG, Tilley CA, Dorrington KJ. Monogamous bivalency of IgG antibodies. I. Deficiency of branched ABHI-active oligosaccharide chains on red cells of infants causes the weak antiglobulin reactions in hemolytic disease of the newborn due to ABO incompatibility. J Immunol. 1980;124:2807-2811.

52. Springer GF, Horton RE. Blood group isoantibody stimulation in man by feeding blood group–active bacteria. J Clin Invest. 1969;48:1280-1291.

53. AABB Standards Committee. Standards for Blood Banks and Transfusion Services, vol 24. Bethesda, MD, American Association of Blood Banks, 2006.

54. Baumgarten A, Kruchok AH, Weirich F. High frequency of IgG anti-A and -B antibody in old age. Vox Sang. 1976;30:253-260.

55. Kochwa S, Rosenfield RE, Tallal L, Wasserman RL. Isoagglutinins associated with erythroblastosis. J Clin Invest. 1961;40:874-883.

56. Grubb R. Observations of the human group system Lewis. Acta Pathol Microbiol Scand. 1951;28:61-81.

57. Waheed A, Kennedy MS, Gerhan S, et al. Transfusion significance of Lewis system antibodies. Success in transfusion with crossmatch-compatible blood. Am J Clin Pathol. 1981;76:294-298.

58. Waheed A, Kennedy MS, Gerhan S. Transfusion significance of Lewis system antibodies. Report on a nationwide survey. Transfusion. 1981;21:542-545.

59. Boren T, Falk P, Roth KA, et al. Attachment of *Helicobacter pylori* to human gastric epithelium mediated by blood group antigens. Science. 1993;262:1892-1895.

60. Appelmelk BJ, Monteiro MA, Martin SL, et al. Why *Helicobacter pylori* has Lewis antigens. Trends Microbiol. 2000;8:565-570.

61. Feizi T. The blood group Ii system: a carbohydrate antigen system defined by naturally monoclonal or oligoclonal autoantibodies of man. Immunol Commun. 1981;10:127-156.

62. Marsh WL. Anti-i: a cold antibody defining the Ii relationship in human red cells. Br J Haematol. 1961;7:200-209.

63. van Loghem JJ, van der Hart M, Veenhoven-Van Riesz E, et al. Cold auto-agglutinins and haemolysins of anti-I and anti-i specificity. Vox Sang. 1962;7:214-221.

64. Tippett P, Noades J, Sanger J, et al. Further studies of the I antigen and antibody. Vox Sang. 1960;5:107-121.

65. Garratty G, Petz LD, Hoops JK. The correlation of cold agglutinin titrations in saline and albumin with haemolytic anaemia. Br J Haematol. 1977;35:587-95.

66. Janney FA, Lee LT, Howe C. Cold hemagglutinin cross-reactivity with *Mycoplasma pneumoniae*. Infect Immun. 1978;22:29-33.

67. Horwitz CA, Moulds J, Henle W, et al. Cold agglutinins in infectious mononucleosis and heterophil-antibody–negative mononucleosis-like syndromes. Blood. 1977;50:195-202.

68. Wang WC, Mentzer WC. Differentiation of transient erythroblastopenia of childhood from congenital hypoplastic anemia. J Pediatr. 1976;88:784-789.

69. Ware RE, Kinney TR. Transient erythroblastopenia in the first year of life. Am J Hematol. 1991;37:156-158.

70. Link MP, Alter BP. Fetal-like erythropoiesis during recovery from transient erythroblastopenia of childhood (TEC). Pediatr Res. 1981;15:1036-1039.

71. Hillman RS, Giblett ER. Red cell membrane alteration associated with "marrow stress." J Clin Invest. 1965;44:1730-1736.

72. Chandeysson PL, Flye MW, Simpkins SM, et al. Delayed hemolytic transfusion reaction caused by anti-P1 antibody. Transfusion. 1981;21:77-82.

73. Levine P, Celano MJ, Falkowski F. The specificity of the antibody in paroxysmal cold hemoglobinuria. Transfusion. 1963;3:278-328.

74. Petz LD, Garratty G. Acquired Immune Hemolytic Anemias. New York, Churchill Livingstone, 1980.

75. Brown KE, Anderson SM, Young NS. Erythrocyte P antigen: cellular receptor for B19 parvovirus. Science. 1993;262:114-117.

76. Lomberg H, Cedergren B, Leffler H, et al. Influence of blood group on the availability of receptors for attachment of uropathogenic *Escherichia coli*. Infect Immun. 1986;51:919-926.

77. Leffler H, Svanborg-Eden C. Glycolipid receptors for uropathogenic *Escherichia coli* on human erythrocytes and uroepithelial cells. Infect Immun. 1981;34:920-929.

78. Race RR, Sanger R. Blood Groups in Man, 6th ed. Oxford, Blackwell Science, 1975.

79. Levine P. Comments on hemolytic disease of newborn due to anti-PP1 P k (anti-Tj a). Transfusion. 1977;17:573-578.

80. Daniels GL, Anstee DJ, Cartron JP, et al. Blood group terminology 1995. ISBT Working Party on terminology for red cell surface antigens. Vox Sang. 1995;69:265-279.

81. Bowman HS. Effectiveness of prophylactic Rh immunosuppression after transfusion with D-positive blood. Am J Obstet Gynecol. 1976;124:80-84.

82. Pollack W, Ascari WQ, Crispen JF, et al. Studies on Rh prophylaxis. II. Rh immune prophylaxis after transfusion with Rh-positive blood. Transfusion. 1971;11:340-344.

83. Haspel RL, Walsh L, Sloan SR. Platelet transfusion in an infant leading to formation of anti-D: implications for immunoprophylaxis. Transfusion. 2004;44:747-749.

84. Hughes-Jones NC, Gardner B, Lincoln PJ. Observations of the number of available c, D, and E antigen sites on red cells. Vox Sang. 1971;21:210-216.

85. Blumenfeld OO, Patnaik SK. Allelic genes of blood group antigens: a source of human mutations and cSNPs documented in the Blood Group Antigen Gene Mutation Database. Hum Mutat. 2004;23:8-16.

86. Wagner FF, Gassner C, Muller TH, et al. Molecular basis of weak D phenotypes. Blood. 1999;93:385-393.

87. Wagner FF, Frohmajer A, Ladewig B, et al. Weak D alleles express distinct phenotypes. Blood. 2000;95:2699-2708.

88. Avent ND, Ridgwell K, Tanner MJ, et al. cDNA cloning of a 30 kDa erythrocyte membrane protein associated with Rh (Rhesus)-blood-group-antigen expression. Biochem J. 1990;271:821-825.

89. Le van Kim C, Mouro I, Cherif-Zahar B, et al. Molecular cloning and primary structure of the human blood group RhD polypeptide. Proc Natl Acad Sci U S A. 1992;89:10925-10929.

90. Mouro I, Colin Y, Cherif-Zahar B, et al. Molecular genetic basis of the human Rhesus blood group system. Nat Genet. 1993;5:62-65.

91. Cartron JP. Defining the Rh blood group antigens. Biochemistry and molecular genetics. Blood Rev. 1994;8:199-212.

92. Nash R, Shojania AM. Hematological aspect of Rh deficiency syndrome: a case report and a review of the literature. Am J Hematol. 1987;24:267-275.

93. Schmidt PJ, Vos GH. Multiple phenotypic abnormalities associated with Rh-null (–/–). Vox Sang. 1967;13:18-20.

94. Marini AM, Matassi G, Raynal V, et al. The human Rhesus-associated RhAG protein and a kidney homologue promote ammonium transport in yeast. Nat Genet. 2000;26:341-344.

95. Blanchard D. Human red cell glycophorins: biochemical and antigenic properties. Transfus Med Rev. 1990;4:170-186.

96. Reid ME. Some concepts relating to the molecular genetic basis of certain MNS blood group antigens. Transfus Med. 1994;4:99-111.

97. Fukuda M. Molecular genetics of the glycophorin A gene cluster. Semin Hematol. 1993;30:138-151.

98. Rahuel C, London J, d'Auriol L, et al. Characterization of cDNA clones for human glycophorin A. Use for gene localization and for analysis of normal of glycophorin-A–deficient (Finnish type) genomic DNA. Eur J Biochem. 1988;172:147-153.

99. Parkkinen J, Rogers GN, Korhonen T, et al. Identification of the O-linked sialyloligosaccharides of glycophorin A as the erythrocyte receptors for S-fimbriated *Escherichia coli*. Infect Immun. 1986;54:37-42.

100. Hadley TJ, Miller LH, Haynes JD. Recognition of red cells by malaria parasites: the role of erythrocyte-binding proteins. Transfus Med Rev. 1991;5:108-122.

101. Lee S, Wu X, Reid M, et al. Molecular basis of the Kell (K1) phenotype. Blood. 1995;85:912-916.

102. Marsh WL, Redman CM. Recent developments in the Kell blood group system. Transfus Med Rev. 1987; 1:4-20.

103. Turner AJ, Tanzawa K. Mammalian membrane metallo-peptidases: NEP, ECE, KELL, and PEX. FASEB J. 1997;11:355-364.

104. Lee S, Russo D, Redman CM. The Kell blood group system: Kell and XK membrane proteins. Semin Hematol. 2000;37:113-121.

105. Reid ME. Associations of red blood cell membrane abnormalities with blood group phenotype. In Garratty G (ed). Immunobiology of Transfusion Medicine. New York, Marcel Dekker, 1994, p 256.

106. Marsh WL, Redman CM. The Kell blood group system: a review. Transfusion. 1990;30:158-167.

107. Neote K, Mak JY, Kolakowski LF Jr, et al. Functional and biochemical analysis of the cloned Duffy antigen: identity with the red blood cell chemokine receptor. Blood. 1994;84:44-52.

108. Mallinson G, Soo KS, Schall TJ, et al. Mutations in the erythrocyte chemokine receptor (Duffy) gene: the molecular basis of the Fy^a/Fy^b antigens and identification of a deletion in the Duffy gene of an apparently healthy individual with the Fy(a–b–) phenotype. Br J Haematol. 1995;90:823-829.

109. Chaudhuri A, Polyakova J, Zbrzezna V, et al. The coding sequence of Duffy blood group gene in humans and simians: restriction fragment length polymorphism, antibody and malarial parasite specificities, and expression in nonerythroid tissues in Duffy-negative individuals. Blood. 1995;85:615-621.

110. Horuk R, Chitnis CE, Darbonne WC, et al. A receptor for the malarial parasite *Plasmodium vivax*: the erythrocyte chemokine receptor. Science. 1993;261:1182-1184.

111. Miller LH, Mason SJ, Clyde DF, et al. The resistance factor to *Plasmodium vivax* in blacks. The Duffy-blood-group genotype, FyFy. N Engl J Med. 1976;295: 302-304.

112. Olives B, Neau P, Bailly P, et al. Cloning and functional expression of a urea transporter from human bone marrow cells. J Biol Chem. 1994;269:31649-31652.

113. Olives B, Mattei MG, Huet M, et al. Kidd blood group and urea transport function of human erythrocytes are carried by the same protein. J Biol Chem. 1995;270: 15607-15610.

114. Macey RI, Yousef LW. Osmotic stability of red cells in renal circulation requires rapid urea transport. Am J Physiol. 1988;254:C669-C674.

115. Olives B, Merriman M, Bailly P, et al. The molecular basis of the Kidd blood group polymorphism and its lack of association with type 1 diabetes susceptibility. Hum Mol Genet. 1997;6:1017-1020.

116. Heaton DC, McLoughlin K. Jk(a–b–) red blood cells resist urea lysis. Transfusion. 1982;22:70-71.

117. Frohlich O, Macey RI, Edwards-Moulds J, et al. Urea transport deficiency in Jk(a–b–) erythrocytes. Am J Physiol. 1991;260:C778-C783.

118. Sands JM, Gargus JJ, Frohlich O, et al. Urinary concentrating ability in patients with Jk(a–b–) blood type who lack carrier-mediated urea transport. J Am Soc Nephrol. 1992;2:1689-1696.

119. Anstee DJ. Blood group antigens defined by the amino acid sequences of red cell surface proteins. Transfus Med. 1995;5:1-13.

120. El Nemer W, Gane P, Colin Y, et al. The Lutheran blood group glycoproteins, the erythroid receptors for laminin, are adhesion molecules. J Biol Chem. 1998;273: 16686-16693.

121. Udden MM, Umeda M, Hirano Y, et al. New abnormalities in the morphology, cell surface receptors, and electrolyte metabolism of In(Lu) erythrocytes. Blood. 1987;69:52-57.

122. Issitt PD, Issitt CH: Applied Blood Group Serology, 2nd ed. Oxnard, CA, Biologicals, 1975.

123. Giblett ER. Blood group alloantibodies: an assessment of some laboratory practices. Transfusion. 1977;17:299-308.

124. Hoeltge GA, Domen RE, Rybicki LA, et al. Multiple red cell transfusions and alloimmunization. Experience with 6996 antibodies detected in a total of 159,262 patients from 1985 to 1993. Arch Pathol Lab Med. 1995;119: 42-45.

125. Arndt PA, Garratty G. A retrospective analysis of the value of monocyte monolayer assay results for predicting the clinical significance of blood group alloantibodies. Transfusion. 2004;44:1273-1281.

126. Thompson FL, Powers JS, Graber SE, et al. Use of recombinant human erythropoietin to enhance autologous blood donation in a patient with multiple red cell allo-antibodies and the anemia of chronic disease. Am J Med. 1991;90:398-400.

127. Gaudiani VA, Mason HD. Preoperative erythropoietin in Jehovah's Witnesses who require cardiac procedures. Ann Thorac Surg. 1991;51:823-824.

128. Fullerton DA, Campbell DN, Whitman GJ. Use of human recombinant erythropoietin to correct severe preoperative anemia. Ann Thorac Surg. 1991;51:825-826.

129. Kiyama H, Ohshima N, Imazeki T, et al. Autologous blood donation with recombinant human erythropoietin in anemic patients. Ann Thorac Surg. 1999;68: 1652-1656.

130. Arsura EL, Bertelle A, Minkowitz S, et al. Transfusion-associated graft-vs-host disease in a presumed immuno-competent patient. Arch Intern Med. 1988;148: 1941-1944.

131. Yeager AS, Grumet FC, Hafleigh EB, et al. Prevention of transfusion-acquired cytomegalovirus infections in newborn infants. J Pediatr. 1981;98:281-287.

132. Pamphilon DH, Rider JR, Barbara JA, et al. Prevention of transfusion-transmitted cytomegalovirus infection. Transfus Med. 1999;9:115-123.

133. Funkhouser AW, Vogelsang G, Zehnbauer B, et al. Graft versus host disease after blood transfusions in a premature infant. Pediatrics. 1991;87:247-250.

134. Schmalzer EA, Lee JO, Brown AK, et al. Viscosity of mixtures of sickle and normal red cells at varying

hematocrit levels. Implications for transfusion. Transfusion. 1987;27:228-233.

135. Wayne AS, Kevy SV, Nathan DG. Transfusion management of sickle cell disease. Blood. 1993;81:1109-1023.

136. Ness PM. To match or not to match: the question for chronically transfused patients with sickle cell anemia. Transfusion. 1994;34:558-560.

137. Rosse WF, Telen MJ, Ware RE. Transfusion Support for Patients With Sickle Cell Disease. Bethesda, MD, AABB Press, 1998.

138. Fosburg MT, Nathan DG. Treatment of Cooley's anemia. Blood. 1990;76:435-444.

139. Sirchia G, Zanella A, Parravicini A, et al. Red cell alloantibodies in thalassemia major. Results of an Italian cooperative study. Transfusion. 1985;25:110-112.

140. Rosse WF, Gallagher D, Kinney TR, et al. Transfusion and alloimmunization in sickle cell disease. The Cooperative Study of Sickle Cell Disease. Blood. 1990;76:1431-1437.

141. Heyll A, Aul C, Runde V, et al. Treatment of pure red cell aplasia after major ABO-incompatible bone marrow transplantation with recombinant erythropoietin. Blood. 1991;77:906.

142. West LJ, Pollock-Barziv SM, Dipchand AI, et al. ABO-incompatible heart transplantation in infants. N Engl J Med. 2001;344:793-800.

143. Triulzi DJ, Shirey RS, Ness PM, et al. Immunohematologic complications of ABO-unmatched liver transplants. Transfusion. 1992;32:829-833.

144. Sloan SR, Silberstein LE. Transfusion in the face of autoantibodies. In Reid ME, Nance SJ (eds). Red Cell Transfusion: A Practical Guide. Totowa, NJ, Humana Press, 1998, pp 55-70.

145. Wolach B, Heddle N, Barr RD, et al. Transient Donath-Landsteiner haemolytic anaemia. Br J Haematol. 1981;48:425-434.

146. Rausen AR, LeVine R, Hsu TC, et al. Compatible transfusion therapy for paroxysmal cold hemoglobinuria. Pediatrics. 1975;55:275-278.

147. Silvergleid AJ, Wells RF, Hafleigh EB, et al. Compatibility test using ^{51}chromium-labeled red blood cells in crossmatch positive patients. Transfusion. 1978;18:8-14.

148. Sazama K. Reports of 355 transfusion-associated deaths: 1976 through 1985. Transfusion. 1990;30:583-590.

149. Linden JV, Wagner K, Voytovich AE, et al. Transfusion errors in New York State: an analysis of 10 years' experience. Transfusion. 2000;40:1207-1213.

150. Stramer SL. Current risks of transfusion-transmitted agents: a review. Arch Pathol Lab Med. 2007;131:702-707.

151. Maynard JE. Hepatitis B: global importance and need for control. Vaccine. 1990;8(Suppl):S18-S20; discussion S1-S3.

152. Schwimmer JB, Balistreri WF. Transmission, natural history, and treatment of hepatitis C virus infection in the pediatric population. Semin Liver Dis. 2000;20:37-46.

153. Seeff LB, Buskell-Bales Z, Wright EC, et al. Long-term mortality after transfusion-associated non-A, non-B hepatitis. The National Heart, Lung, and Blood Institute Study Group. N Engl J Med. 1992;327:1906-1911.

154. Koretz RL, Abbey H, Coleman E, et al. Non-A, non-B post-transfusion hepatitis. Looking back in the second decade. Ann Intern Med. 1993;119:110-115.

155. Poiesz BJ, Ruscetti FW, Gazdar AF, et al. Detection and isolation of type C retrovirus particles from fresh and cultured lymphocytes of a patient with cutaneous T-cell lymphoma. Proc Natl Acad Sci U S A. 1980;77:7415-7419.

156. Uchiyama T, Yodoi J, Sagawa K, et al. Adult T-cell leukemia: clinical and hematologic features of 16 cases. Blood. 1977;50:481-492.

157. Schreiber GB, Busch MP, Kleinman SH, et al. The risk of transfusion-transmitted viral infections. The Retrovirus Epidemiology Donor Study. N Engl J Med. 1996;334:1685-1690.

158. Bowden RA, Slichter SJ, Sayers M, et al. A comparison of filtered leukocyte-reduced and cytomegalovirus (CMV) seronegative blood products for the prevention of transfusion-associated CMV infection after marrow transplant. Blood. 1995;86:3598-3603.

159. Murphy S, Gardner FH. Platelet preservation: effect of storage temperature on maintenance of platelet viability; the deleterious effect of refrigerated storage. N Engl J Med. 1969;280:1094-1098.

160. Fang CT, Chambers LA, Kennedy J, et al. Detection of bacterial contamination in apheresis platelet products: American Red Cross experience, 2004. Transfusion. 2005;45:1845-1852.

161. Murphy S, Kahn RA, Holme S, et al. Improved storage of platelets for transfusion in a new container. Blood. 1982;60:194-200.

162. Murphy S, Gardner FH. Improved storage of platelets for transfusion in a new container. Blood. 1975;46:209-218.

163. Aster RH. The effect of anticoagulant and ABO incompatibility on recovery of transfused human platelets. Blood. 1965;26:732-743.

164. Simon TL. The collection of platelets by apheresis procedures. Trans Med Rev. 1994;8:132-145.

165. Parkman PD. Guideline for the Collection of Platelets, Pheresis Prepared by Automated Methods. Bethesda, MD, Food and Drug Administration, 1988.

166. Snyder EL, Koermer TAW Jr, Kakaiya R, et al. Effect of mode of agitation on storage of platelet concentrates in PL-732 containers for 5 days. Vox Sang. 1983;44:300-304.

167. Simon TL, Nelson EJ, Murphy S. Extension of platelet concentrate storage to 7 days in second-generation bags. Transfusion. 1987;27:6-9.

168. Fijnheer R, Modderman PW, Veldman H, et al. Detection of platelet activation with monoclonal antibodies and flow cytometry. Change during platelet storage. Transfusion. 1990;30:20-25.

169. Frantantoni JC, Poindexter BJ, Bonner RF. Quantitative assessment of platelet morphology by light scattering: a potential method for the evaluation of platelets for transfusion. J Lab Clin Med. 1984;103:620-631.

170. Murphy S. Platelet storage for transfusion. Semin Hematol. 1985;22:165-177.

171. Post Approval Surveillance Study of Platelet Outcomes, Release Tested (PASSPORT) Study. Available at www.passportstudy.com. Accessed August 31, 2007.

172. Murphy S, Litwin S, Herring LM, et al. Indications for platelet transfusion in children with acute leukemia. Am J Hematol. 1982;12:347-356.

173. Gaydos LA, Freireich EJ, Mantel N. The quantitative relation between platelet count and hemorrhage in patients with acute leukemia. N Engl J Med. 1962;266:905-909.

174. Schiffer CA, Anderson KC, Bennett CL, et al. Platelet transfusion for patients with cancer: clinical practice guidelines of the American Society of Clinical Oncology. J Clin Oncol. 2001;9:1519-1538.

175. Beutler E. Platelet transfusion: the 20,000/μL trigger. Blood. 1993;81:1411-1413.

176. Consensus Conference: Platelet transfusions. JAMA. 1987;257:1777-1780.

177. Bishop JF, Schiffer CA, Aisner J, et al. Surgery in acute leukemia: a review of 167 operations in thrombocytopenic patients. Am J Hematol. 1987;26:147-155.

178. George JN, Pickett EB, Saucerman S, et al. Platelet surface glycoproteins. Studies on resting and activated platelets and platelet membrane microparticles in normal subjects, and observations in patients during adult respiratory distress syndrome and cardiac surgery. J Clin Invest. 1986;78:340-348.

179. Harker LA, Maplass TW, Branson HE, et al. Mechanism of abnormal bleeding in patients undergoing cardiopulmonary bypass: acquired transient platelet dysfunction assciated with selective alpha-granule release. Blood. 1980;56:824-834.

180. Simon TL, Akl BF, Murphy W. Controlled trial of routine administration platelet concentrates in cardiopulmonary bypass surgery. Ann Thorac Surg. 1984;37:359-364.

181. Losowsky MS, Walker BE. Liver biopsy and splenoportography in patients with thrombocytopenia. Gastroenterology. 1968;54:241-245.

182. Howard SC, Gajjar A, Ribeiro RC, et al. Safety of lumbar puncture for children with acute lymphoblastic leukemia and thrombocytopenia. JAMA. 2000;284:2222-2224.

183. Herman JH, Kamel HT. Platelet transfusion. Current techniques, remaining problems, and future prospects. Am J Pediatr Hematol Oncol. 1987;9:272-286.

184. Simpson MB. Platelet transfusion in selected clinical situations. In Smith DM, Summers SH (eds). Platelets. Arlington, VA, American Association of Blood Banks; 1988, pp 129-166.

185. Slichter SJ. Mechanisms and management of platelet refractoriness. In Transfusion Medicine in the 1990's. Arlington, VA, American Association of Blood Banks, 1990.

186. Gorgone BC, Anderson JW, Anderson KC. Comparison of 15 min and 1 hour post platelet counts in pediatric patients. Transfusion. 1986;26:555.

187. Slichter SJ. Controversies in platelet transfusion therapy. Annu Rev Med. 1980;31:509.

188. Hill-Zobel RL, McCandless B, Kang SA, et al. Organ distribution and fate of human platelets: studies of asplenic and splenomegalic patients. Am J Hematol. 1986;23:231-238.

189. McFarland JG, Anderson AJ, Slichter SJ. Factors influencing the transfusion response to HLA-selected apheresis donor platelets in patients refractory to random platelet concentrates. Br J Haematol. 1989;73:380-386.

190. Yam P, Petz LD, Scott EP, Santos S. Platelet crossmatch tests using radiolabelled staphylococcal protein A or peroxidase anti-peroxidase in alloimmunized patients. Br J Haematol. 1984;57:337-347.

191. Ratnoff OD. Disseminated intravascular coagulation. In Ratnoff OD, Forbes CD (eds). Disorders of Hemostasis. New York, Grune & Stratton, p 1984.

192. Bick RL. Disseminated intravascular coagulation and related syndromes: a clinical review. Semin Thromb Hemost. 1988;14:299-338.

193. Shim WK. Hemangiomas of infancy complicated by thrombocytopenia. Am J Hematol. 1968;116:896-906.

194. Straubb PW, Kessler S, Schreiber A, Frick PG. Chronic intravascular coagulation in Kasabach-Merritt syndrome: preferential accumulation of fibrinogen 131 I in a giant hemangioma. Arch Intern Med. 1972;129:475-478.

195. Schmidt RP, Lentle BC. Hemangioma with consumptive coagulopathy (Kasabach-Merritt syndrome): detection by indium-111 oxine-labeled platelets. Clin Nucl Med. 1984;9:389-391.

196. Byrnes JJ, Moake JL. Thrombocytopenic purpura and the haemolytic-uraemic syndrome; evolving concepts of pathogenesis and therapy. Clin Haematol. 1986;15:413-442.

197. Eberst ME, Berkowitz LR. Hemostasis in renal disease: pathophysiology and management. Am J Med. 1994;96:168-179.

198. Davis KB, Slichter SJ, Corash L. Corrected count increment and percent platelet recovery as measures of postransfusion platelet response; problems and a solution. Transfusion. 1999;39:586-592.

199. Beutler E. Prophylactic platelet transfusion, In Abstracts of the NIH Consensus Development Conference of Platelet Transfusion Therapy. Bethesda, MD, Office of Medical Application of Research, National Heart, Lung, and Blood and Biologics, Food and Drug Administration, and U.S. Department of Health and Human Services, 1986, pp 47-48.

200. Storb R, Prentice RL, Thomas ED. Marrow transplantation for the treatment of aplastic anemia. An analysis of factors associated with graft rejection. N Engl J Med. 1977;296:61-66.

201. Storb R, Thomas ED, Buckner CD, et al. Marrow transplantation in thirty untransfused patients with severe aplastic anemia. Ann Intern Med. 1980;92:30-31.

202. Aster RH. Pooling of platelets in the spleen: role in the pathogenesis of "hypersplenic" thrombocytopenia. J Clin Invest. 1966;45:645-657.

203. Warkentin TE, Levine MN, Hirsh J, et al. Heparin-induced thrombocytopenia in patients treated with low-molecular-weight heparin or unfractionated heparin. N Engl J Med. 1995;332:1330-1335.

204. Slichter SJ. Controversies in platelet transfusion. Annu Rev Med. 1980;31:509-540.

205. Harrington WJ, Sprague CC, Minnich V, et al. Immunologic mechanisms in neonatal and thrombocytopenic purpura. Ann Intern Med. 1953;38:433-469.

206. Kunicki TJ, Bearsley DS. The alloimmune thrombocytopenias: neonatal alloimmune thrombocytopenic purpura and post-transfusion purpura. Prog Hemost Thromb. 1989;9:203-232.

207. Shulman NR, Marder V, Hiller MC, Collier EM. Platelet and leukocyte isoantigens and their antibodies serologic, physiologic and clinical. Prog Hematol. 1964;4:222-304.

208. Blanchette VS, Peters MA, Pegg-Feige K. Alloimmune thrombocytopenia. Review from a neonatal intensive care

unit. Curr Stud Hematol Blood Transfus. 1986;52: 87-96.

209. Reznikoff-Etievant MF, Dangu C, Lobet RJ. HLA-B8 antigens and PIA 1 alloimmunization. Tissue Antigens. 1981;18:66-68.

210. Mueller-Eckhardt C, Mueller-Eckhardt G, Willen-Ohff H, et al. Immunogenicity of and immune response to the human platelet antigen Zwᵃ is strongly associated with HLA-B8 and DR3. Tissue Antigens. 1985;26:71-76.

211. deWaal LP, van Dalen CM, Engelfreit CP, von dem Borne AE. Alloimmunization against the platelet-specific Zwᵃ antigen, resulting in neonatal alloimmune throbocytopenia or post-transfusion purpura, is associated with the supertypic DRw52 antigen including DR3. Hum Immunol. 1986;17:45-53.

212. Daffos F, Forestier F, Kaplan C, Cox W. Prenatal diagnosis and management of bleeding disorders with fetal blood sampling. Am J Obstet Gynecol. 1988;158:939-946.

213. Newman PJ, Derbes RS, Aster RH. The human platelet alloantigens, PIA1 and PIA2 are associated with a leucine 33/proline 33 amino acid polymorphism in membrane glycoprotein IIIa, and are distinguishable by DNA typing. J Clin Invest. 1989;83:1778-1781.

214. McFarland JG. Platelet immunology and alloimmunization. Semin Hematol. 1996;33:315-328.

215. Lyman S, Aster RH, Visentin GP, Newman PJ. Polymorphism of human platelet membrane glycoprotein IIb associated with the Bakᵃ/Bakᵇ alloantigen system. Blood. 1990;75:2343-2348.

216. McFarland JG, Aster RH, Bussel JB, et al. Prenatal diagnosis of neonatal alloimmune thrombocytopenia using allele-specific oligonucleotide probes. Blood. 1991;78: 2276-2282.

217. Massey GV, McWilliams NB, Mueller DG, et al. Intravenous immunoglobulin in treatment of neonatal isoimmune thrombocytopenia. J Pediatr. 1987;111:133-135.

218. Bussel JB, Berkowitz T, McFarland JG, et al. Antenatal treatment of neonatal alloimmune thrombocytopenia. N Engl J Med. 1988;319:1374-1378.

219. Kaplan C, Daffos F, Forestier F, et al. Management of alloimmune thrombocytopenia: antenatal diagnosis and in utero transfusion of maternal platelets. Blood. 1988;72: 340-343.

220. Bizzaro N, Dianses G. Neonatal alloimmune amegakaryocytosis. Vox Sang. 1988;54:112-114.

221. Lynch L, Bussel JB, McFarland JG, et al. Antenatal treatment of alloimmune thrombocytopenia. Obstet Gynecol. 1992;80:67-71.

222. Taaning E, Morling N, Ovesen H, Svejgaard A. Post transfusion purpura an anti-Zwᵇ (-P1A2). Tissue antigens. 1985;26:143-146.

223. Furihata K, Nugent DJ, Bissonette A, et al. On the association of the platelet-specific alloantigen, Pen, with glycoprotein IIIa. Evidence for heterogeneity of glycoprotein IIIa. J Clin Invest. 1987;80:1624-1630.

224. Chapman JF, Murphy MF, Berney SE, et al. Post-transfusion purpura associated with anti-Bakᵃ and anti-P1ᴬ² platelet antibodies and delayed haemolytic transfusion reaction. Vox Sang. 1987;52:313-317.

225. Mueller-Eckhardt C. Post-transfusion purpura. Br J Haematol. 1986;64:419-424.

226. Kobrinsky NL, Israels ED, Gerrard JM, et al. Shortening of bleeding time by I-deamino-8-arginine vasopressin in various bleeding disorders. Lancet. 1984;1:1145-1148.

227. Schulman S, Johnson H, Egberg N, Blombäck M. DDAVP-induced correction of prolonged bleeding time in patients with congenital platelet function defects. Thromb Res. 1987;45:165-174.

228. Rodey GE. Prevention of Alloimmunization in Thrombocytopenic Patients. Bethesda, MD, American Association of Blood Banks 1988, pp 93-114.

229. Lee EJ, Norris D, Schiffer CA. Intravenous immune globulin for patients alloimmunized to random donor platelet transfusion. Transfusion. 1987;27:245-247.

230. Schiffer CA, Hogge DE, Aisner J. High-dose intravenous gammaglobulin in alloimmunized platelet transfusion recipients. Blood. 1984;64:937-940.

231. Sontoso S, Kalb R, Kiefel V, Mueller-Eckhardt C. The presence of messenger RNA for HLA class in human platelets and its capability for protein biosynthesis. Br J Haematol. 1993;84:451-456.

232. Boshkov LK, Kelton JG, Halloran PF. HLA-DR expression by platelets in acute idiopatic thrombocytopenic purpura. Br J Haematol. 1992;81:552-557.

233. Koike T, Aoki S, Maruyama S, et al. Cell surface phenotyping of megakaryoblasts. Blood. 1987;69:957-960.

234. Briddell RA, Bandt JE, Straneva JE. Characterization of the human burst forming unit megakaryocyte. Blood. 1989;74:145-151.

235. Oldfather J, Anderson CB, Phelan DL, et al. Prediction of crossmatch outcome in highly sensitized patients based on the identification of serum HLA antibodies. Transplantation. 1986;42:267-270.

236. MacPherson BR, Hammond PB, Maniscalco CA. Alloimmunization to public HLA antigens in multi-transfused platelet recipients. Am Clin Lab Sci. 1986;16:38-44.

237. Friedberg RC, Donnelly SF, Mintz PD. Independent roles for platelet crossmatching and HLA in the selection of platelets for alloimunized patients. Transfusion. 1994;34: 215-220.

238. Leukocyte reduction and ultraviolet B irradiation of platelets to prevent alloimmuniztion and refractoriness to platelet transfusions. The Trial to Reduce Alloimmunization to Platelets Study Group. N Engl J Med. 1997;337: 1861-1869.

239. Gmür J, von Felton A, Osterwalder B, et al. Delayed alloimmunization using random single donor platelet transfusions: a prospective study in thrombocytopenic patients with acute leukemia. Blood. 1983;62:473-479.

240. Sintnicolaas K, Sizoo W, Haije WG, et al. Delayed alloimmunization by random single donor platelet transfusions. Lancet. 1981;1:750-754.

241. Dutcher JP, Schiffer CA, Aisner J, Wiernik PH. Long-term follow-up of patients with leukemia receiving platelet transfusion: identification of a large group of patients who do not become alloimmunized. Blood. 1981;58: 1007-1011.

242. Lee EJ, Schiffer CA. Serial measurement of lymphocytotoxic antibody and response to non-matched platelet transfusions in alloimmnized patients. Blood. 1987;70: 1727-1729.

243. Fuller TC, Delmonico FL, Cosimi AB, et al. Effects of various transfusions on HLA alloimmunization and renal allograft survival. Transplant Proc. 1977;9:117-119.

244. Meryman HT. Transfusion-induced alloimmunization and immunosuppression and the effects of leukocyte depletion. Trans Med Rev. 1989;3:180.

245. Claas FHJ, Smeenk RJT, Schmidt R, et al. Allimmunization against the MHC antigens after platelet transfusions is due to contaminating leukocytes in the platelet suspension. Exp Hematol. 1981;9:84-89.

246. Braine HG, Kickler TS, Charache P, et al. Bacterial sepsis secondary to platelet transfusion: an adverse effect of extended storage at room temperature. Transfusion. 1986;2: 391-393.

247. Eernisse JG, Brand A. Prevention of platelet refractoriness due to HLA antibodies by adminstration of leukocyte-poor blood components. Exp Hematol. 1981;9:77-83.

248. Murphy MF, Metcalfe P, Thomas H, et al. Use of leucocyte-poor blood components and HLA matched-platelet donors to prevent HLA alloimmunization. Br J Haematol. 1986;62:529-534.

249. Sniecinski I, O'Donnell MR, Nowixki B, Hill LR. Prevention of refractoriness and HLA-alloimmunization using filtered blood products. Blood. 1988;71:1402-1407.

250. Saarinen UM, Koskimes, Myllylä F. Systemic use of leukocyte free blood components to prevent alloimmunization and platelet refractoriness in multitransfused children with cancer. Vox Sang. 1993;65:286-292.

251. Heddle NM, Blajchman MA. The leukodepletion of cellular blood products in the prevention of HLA-alloimmunization and refractoriness to allogeneic platelet transfusions. Blood. 1995;85:60-6063.

252. Williamson LM, Wimperis JZ, Williamson P, et al. Bedside filtration of blood products in the prevention of HLA alloimmunization: a prospective randomized study. Blood. 1994;83:3028-3035.

253. Popovsky MA. Quality of blood components filtered before storage and at the bedside; implications for transfusion practice. Transfusion. 1996;36:470-474.

254. Slack G, Snyder EL. Cytokine generation in stored platelet concentrates. Transfusion. 1994;34:20-25.

255. Dove A. Cell-based therapies go live. Nat Biotech. 2002;20:339-343.

256. Barker JN, Krepski TP, DeFor TE, et al. Searching for unrelated donor hematopoietic stem cells: availability and speed of umbilical cord blood versus bone marrow. Biol Blood Marrow Transplant. 2002;8:257-260.

257. Beatty PG, Clift RA, Mickelson EM, et al. Marrow transplantation from related donors other than HLA-identical siblings. N Engl J Med. 1985;313:765-771.

258. Kernan NA, Bartsch G, Ash RC, et al. Analysis of 462 transplantations from unrelated donors facilitated by the National Marrow Donor Program. N Engl J Med. 1993; 328:593-602.

259. Hartmann O, Le Corroller AG, Blaise D, et al. Peripheral blood stem cell and bone marrow transplantation for solid tumors and lymphomas: hematologic recovery and costs. A randomized, controlled trial. Ann Intern Med. 1997; 126:600-607.

260. Faucher C, le Corroller AG, Blaise D, et al. Comparison of G-CSF–primed peripheral blood progenitor cells and bone marrow auto transplantation: clinical assessment and cost-effectiveness. Bone Marrow Transplant. 1994;14: 895-901.

261. Jerjis S, Croockewit S, Muus P, et al. Cost analysis of autologous peripheral stem cell transplantation versus autologous bone marrow transplantation for patients with non Hodgkin's lymphoma and acute lymphoblastic leukaemia. Leuk Lymphoma. 1999;36:33-43.

262. Cutler C, Antin JH. Peripheral blood stem cells for allogeneic transplantation: a review. Stem Cells. 2001;19: 108-117.

263. Gillespie TW, Hillyer CD. Peripheral blood progenitor cells for marrow reconstitution: mobilization and collection strategies. Transfusion. 1996;36:611-624.

264. Fontao-Wendel R, Lazar A, Melges S, et al. The absolute number of circulating CD34(+) cells as the best predictor of peripheral hematopoietic stem cell yield. J Hematother. 1999;8:255-262.

265. Remes K, Matinlauri I, Grenman S, et al. Daily measurements of blood CD34+ cells after stem cell mobilization predict stem cell yield and posttransplant hematopoietic recovery. J Hematother. 1997;6:13-19.

266. Bensinger W, Appelbaum F, Rowley S, et al. Factors that influence collection and engraftment of autologous peripheral-blood stem cells. J Clin Oncol. 1995;13: 2547-2555.

267. Tricot G, Jagannath S, Vesole D, et al. Peripheral blood stem cell transplants for multiple myeloma: identification of favorable variables for rapid engraftment in 225 patients. Blood. 1995;85:588-596.

268. Dreger P, Kloss M, Petersen B, et al. Autologous progenitor cell transplantation: prior exposure to stem cell-toxic drugs determines yield and engraftment of peripheral blood progenitor cell but not of bone marrow grafts. Blood. 1995;86:3970-3978.

269. Moskowitz CH, Stiff P, Gordon MS, et al. Recombinant methionyl human stem cell factor and filgrastim for peripheral blood progenitor cell mobilization and transplantation in non-Hodgkin's lymphoma patients—results of a phase I/II trial. Blood. 1997;89:3136-3147.

270. Bensinger WI, Martin PJ, Storer B, et al. Transplantation of bone marrow as compared with peripheral-blood cells from HLA-identical relatives in patients with hematologic cancers. N Engl J Med. 2001;344:175-181.

271. Storek J, Gooley T, Siadak M, et al. Allogeneic peripheral blood stem cell transplantation may be associated with a high risk of chronic graft-versus-host disease. Blood. 1997;90:4705-4709.

272. Liu F, Poursine-Laurent J, Link DC. The granulocyte colony-stimulating factor receptor is required for the mobilization of murine hematopoietic progenitors into peripheral blood by cyclophosphamide or interleukin-8 but not flt-3 ligand. Blood. 1997;90:2522-2528.

273. Pruijt JF, van Kooyk Y, Figdor CG, et al. Anti–LFA-1 blocking antibodies prevent mobilization of hematopoietic progenitor cells induced by interleukin-8. Blood. 1998;91:4099-4105.

274. Levesque JP, Takamatsu Y, Nilsson SK, et al. Vascular cell adhesion molecule-1 (CD106) is cleaved by neutrophil proteases in the bone marrow following hematopoietic progenitor cell mobilization by granulocyte colony-stimulating factor. Blood. 2001;98:1289-1297.

275. Levesque JP, Hendy J, Takamatsu Y, et al. Disruption of the CXCR4/CXCL12 chemotactic interaction during hematopoietic stem cell mobilization induced by GCSF or cyclophosphamide. J Clin Invest. 2003;111:187-196.

276. Aiuti A, Webb IJ, Bleul C, et al. The chemokine SDF-1 is a chemoattractant for human CD34+ hematopoietic

progenitor cells and provides a new mechanism to explain the mobilization of CD34$^+$ progenitors to peripheral blood. J Exp Med. 1997;185:111-120.

277. Gluckman E, Broxmeyer HA, Auerbach AD, et al. Hematopoietic reconstitution in a patient with Fanconi's anemia by means of umbilical-cord blood from an HLA-identical sibling. N Engl J Med. 1989;321:1174-1178.

278. Rubinstein P, Carrier C, Scaradavou A, et al. Outcomes among 562 recipients of placental-blood transplants from unrelated donors]. N Engl J Med. 1998;339:1565-1577.

279. Schoemans H, Theunissen K, Maertens J, et al. Adult umbilical cord blood transplantation: a comprehensive review. Bone Marrow Transplant. 2006;38:83-93.

280. Rocha V, Wagner JE Jr, Sobocinski KA, et al. Graft-versus-host disease in children who have received a cord-blood or bone marrow transplant from an HLA-identical sibling. Eurocord and International Bone Marrow Transplant Registry Working Committee on Alternative Donor and Stem Cell Sources. N Engl J Med. 2000;342: 1846-1854.

281. Migliaccio AR, Adamson JW, Stevens CE, et al. Cell dose and speed of engraftment in placental/umbilical cord blood transplantation: graft progenitor cell content is a better predictor than nucleated cell quantity. Blood. 2000; 96:2717-2722.

282. Locatelli F, Rocha V, Chastang C, et al. Factors associated with outcome after cord blood transplantation in children with acute leukemia. Eurocord-Cord Blood Transplant Group. Blood. 1999;93:3662-3671.

283. Wagner JE, Barker JN, DeFor TE, et al. Transplantation of unrelated donor umbilical cord blood in 102 patients with malignant and nonmalignant diseases: influence of CD34 cell dose and HLA disparity on treatment-related mortality and survival. Blood. 2002;100:1611-1618.

284. Jaroscak J, Goltry K, Smith A, et al. Augmentation of umbilical cord blood (UCB) transplantation with ex vivo–expanded UCB cells: results of a phase 1 trial using the AastromReplicell System. Blood. 2003;101:5061-5067.

285. Shpall EJ, Quinones R, Giller R, et al. Transplantation of ex vivo expanded cord blood. Biol Blood Marrow Transplant. 2002;8:368-376.

286. Barker JN, Weisdorf DJ, DeFor TE, et al. Rapid and complete donor chimerism in adult recipients of unrelated donor umbilical cord blood transplantation after reduced-intensity conditioning. Blood. 2003;102:1915-1919.

287. Darabi K, Brown JR, Kao GS. Paradoxical embolism after peripheral blood stem cell infusion. Bone Marrow Transplant. 2005;36:561-562.

288. Moore TB, Chow VJ, Ferry D, et al. Intracardiac right-to-left shunting and the risk of stroke during bone marrow infusion. Bone Marrow Transplant. 1997;19:855-856.

289. Lee SJ, Vogelsang G, Flowers ME. Chronic graft-versus-host disease. Biol Blood Marrow Transplant. 2003;9:215-233.

290. Ferrara JL, Levy R, Chao NJ. Pathophysiologic mechanisms of acute graft-vs.-host disease. Biol Blood Marrow Transplant. 1999;5:347-356.

291. Marmont AM, Horowitz MM, Gale RP, et al. T-cell depletion of HLA-identical transplants in leukemia. Blood. 1991;78:2120-2130.

292. Goulmy E, Schipper R, Pool J, et al. Mismatches of minor histocompatibility antigens between HLA-identical donors and recipients and the development of graft-versus-host disease after bone marrow transplantation. N Engl J Med. 1996;334:281-285.

293. Falkenburg JH, van de Corput L, Marijt EW, et al. Minor histocompatibility antigens in human stem cell transplantation. Exp Hematol. 2003;31:743-751.

294. Miklos DB, Kim HT, Miller KH, et al. Antibody responses to H-Y minor histocompatibility antigens correlate with chronic graft-versus-host disease and disease remission. Blood. 2005;105:2973-2978.

295. Marijt WA, Heemskerk MH, Kloosterboer FM, et al. Hematopoiesis-restricted minor histocompatibility antigens HA-1– or HA-2–specific T cells can induce complete remissions of relapsed leukemia. Proc Natl Acad Sci U S A. 2003;100:2742-2747.

296. Bonnet D, Warren EH, Greenberg PD, et al. CD8(+) minor histocompatibility antigen–specific cytotoxic T lymphocyte clones eliminate human acute myeloid leukemia stem cells. Proc Natl Acad Sci U S A. 1999;96: 8639-8644.

297. Kolb HJ, Mittermuller J, Clemm C, et al. Donor leukocyte transfusions for treatment of recurrent chronic myelogenous leukemia in marrow transplant patients. Blood. 1990;76:2462-2465.

298. van Rhee F, Lin F, Cullis JO, et al. Relapse of chronic myeloid leukemia after allogeneic bone marrow transplant: the case for giving donor leukocyte transfusions before the onset of hematologic relapse. Blood. 1994;83: 3377-3383.

299. Porter DL, Roth MS, McGarigle C, et al. Induction of graft-versus-host disease as immunotherapy for relapsed chronic myeloid leukemia. N Engl J Med. 1994;330: 100-106.

300. Brecher ME, Sims L, Schmitz J, et al. North American multicenter study on flow cytometric enumeration of CD34$^+$ hematopoietic stem cells. J Hematother. 1996;5: 227-236.

301. Johnsen HE, Knudsen LM. Nordic flow cytometry standards for CD34$^+$ cell enumeration in blood and leukapheresis products: report from the second Nordic workshop. J Hematother. 1996;5:237-245.

302. Sutherland DR, Anderson L, Keeney M, et al. The ISHAGE guidelines for CD34$^+$ cell determination by flow cytometry. J Hematother. 1996;5:213-226.

303. Keeney M, Chin-Yee I, Weir K, et al. Single platform flow cytometric absolute CD34$^+$ cell counts based on the ISHAGE guidelines. Cytometry. 1998;34:61-70.

304. Webb IJ, Coral FS, Andersen JW, et al. Sources and sequelae of bacterial contamination of hematopoietic stem cell components: implications for the safety of hematotherapy and graft engineering. Transfusion. 1996;36: 782-788.

305. Rowley SD. Hematopoietic stem cell processing and cryopreservation. J Clin Apheresis. 1992;7:132-134.

306. Davis J, Rowley SD, Santos GW. Toxicity of autologous bone marrow graft infusion. Prog Clin Biol Res. 1990;333: 531-540.

307. Dhodapkar M, Goldberg SL, Tefferi A, et al. Reversible encephalopathy after cryopreserved peripheral blood stem cell infusion. Am J Hematol. 1994;45:187-188.

308. Stroncek DF, Fautsch SK, Lasky LC, et al. Adverse reactions in patients transfused with cryopreserved marrow. Transfusion. 1991;31:521-526.

309. Greeno EW, Perry EH, Ilstrup SJ, et al. Exchange transfusion the hard way: massive hemolysis following transplantation of bone marrow with minor ABO incompatibility. Transfusion. 1996;36:71-74.

310. Nussbaumer W, Schwaighofer H, Gratwohl A, et al. Transfusion of donor-type red cells as a single preparative treatment for bone marrow transplants with major ABO incompatibility. Transfusion. 1995;35:592-595.

311. Webb IJ, Soiffer RJ, Andersen JW, et al. In vivo adsorption of isohemagglutinins with fresh frozen plasma in major ABO-incompatible bone marrow transplantation. Biol Blood Marrow Transplant. 1997;3:267-272.

312. Champlin R. Purging: the separation of normal from malignant cells for autologous transplantation. Transfusion. 1996;36:910-918.

313. Freedman AS, Neuberg D, Mauch P, et al. Long-term follow-up of autologous bone marrow transplantation in patients with relapsed follicular lymphoma. Blood. 1999;94:3325-3333.

314. Webb IJ, Schlossman RL, Jiroutek M, et al. Predictors of high yield and purity of CD34$^+$ cell selected peripheral blood progenitor cells, collected from patients with multiple myeloma. Cytotherapy. 1999;1:175-182.

315. McNiece I, Briddell R, Stoney G, et al. Large-scale isolation of CD34$^+$ cells using the Amgen cell selection device results in high levels of purity and recovery. J Hematother. 1997;6:5-11.

316. Tricot G, Gazitt Y, Leemhuis T, et al. Collection, tumor contamination, and engraftment kinetics of highly purified hematopoietic progenitor cells to support high dose therapy in multiple myeloma. Blood. 1998;91:4489-4495.

317. Shpall EJ, Jones RB, Bearman SI, et al. Transplantation of enriched CD34-positive autologous marrow into breast cancer patients following high-dose chemotherapy: influence of CD34-positive peripheral-blood progenitors and growth factors on engraftment. J Clin Oncol. 1994;12:28-36.

318. Mayordomo JI, Zorina T, Storkus WJ, et al. Bone marrow–derived dendritic cells pulsed with synthetic tumour peptides elicit protective and therapeutic antitumour immunity. Nat Med. 1995;1:1297-1302.

319. Paglia P, Chiodoni C, Rodolfo M, et al. Murine dendritic cells loaded in vitro with soluble protein prime cytotoxic T lymphocytes against tumor antigen in vivo. J Exp Med. 1996;183:317-322.

320. Celluzzi CM, Falo LD Jr. Epidermal dendritic cells induce potent antigen-specific CTL-mediated immunity. J Invest Dermatol. 1997;108:716-720.

321. Waeckerle-Men Y, Uetz-von Allmen E, Fopp M, et al. Dendritic cell–based multi-epitope immunotherapy of hormone-refractory prostate carcinoma. Cancer Immunol Immunother. 2006;55:1524-1533.

322. Savoldo B, Goss JA, Hammer MM, et al. Treatment of solid organ transplant recipients with autologous Epstein Barr virus–specific cytotoxic T lymphocytes (CTLs). Blood. 2006;108:2942-2949.

323. Nestle FO, Alijagic S, Gilliet M, et al. Vaccination of melanoma patients with peptide- or tumor lysate–pulsed dendritic cells. Nat Med. 1998;4:328-332.

324. Banchereau J, Palucka AK, Dhodapkar M, et al. Immune and clinical responses in patients with metastatic melanoma to CD34(+) progenitor-derived dendritic cell vaccine. Cancer Res. 2001;61:6451-6458.

325. Menitove JE. Standards for Hematopoietic Progenitor Cells. Bethesda, MD, American Association of Blood Banks Press, 1996.

326. Klein H. Standards for Blood Banks and Transfusion Services. Bethesda, MD, American Association of Blood Banks, 1996.

327. Foundation for the Accreditation of Hematopoietic Cell Therapy (FAHCT). Standards for Hematopoietic Progenitor Cell Collection, Processing, and Transplantation. Omaha, NE, FAHCT, 1996.

328. Halme DG, Kessler DA. FDA regulation of stem-cell–based therapies. N Engl J Med. 2006;355:1730-1735.

329. Food and Drug Administration, Department of Health and Human Services. Current good tissue practice for manufacturers of human cellular tissue-based products; inspection and enforcement. Final rule. Fed Regist. 2004;69:68611-68688.

330. Stiff P, Chen B, Franklin W, et al. Autologous transplantation of ex vivo expanded bone marrow cells grown from small aliquots after high-dose chemotherapy for breast cancer. Blood. 2000;95:2169-2174.

331. Cavazzana-Calvo M, Hacein-Bey S, de Saint Basile G, et al. Gene therapy of human severe combined immunodeficiency (SCID)-X1 disease. Science. 2000;288:669-672.

332. Hacein-Bey-Abina S, Von Kalle C, Schmidt M, et al. LMO2-associated clonal T cell proliferation in two patients after gene therapy for SCID-X1. Science. 2003;302:415-419.

333. Freireich EJ. White cell transfusions born-again. Leuk Lymphoma. 1994;11(Suppl 1):161-165.

334. Bensinger WI, Price TH, Dale DC, et al. The effects of daily recombinant human granulocyte colony-stimulating factor administration on normal granulocyte donors undergoing leukapheresis. Blood. 1993;81:1883-1838.

335. Strauss RG. Therapeutic granulocyte transfusions in 1993. Blood. 1993;81:1675-1678.

336. Price TH, Bowden RA, Boeckh M, et al. Phase I/II trial of neutrophil transfusions from donors stimulated with G-CSF and dexamethasone for treatment of patients with infections in hematopoietic stem cell transplantation. Blood. 2000;95:3302-3309.

337. Grigull L, Pulver N, Goudeva L, et al. G-CSF mobilised granulocyte transfusions in 32 paediatric patients with neutropenic sepsis. Support Care Cancer. 2006;14:910-916.

338. Hubel K, Rodger E, Gaviria JM, et al. Effective storage of granulocytes collected by centrifugation leukapheresis from donors stimulated with granulocyte-colony-stimulating factor. Transfusion. 2005;45:1876-1889.

339. Price TH. Granulocyte transfusion: current status. Semin Hematol. 2007;44:15-23.

340. Sachs UJ, Reiter A, Walter T, et al. Safety and efficacy of therapeutic early onset granulocyte transfusions in pediatric patients with neutropenia and severe infections. Transfusion. 2006;46:1909-1914.

341. Jones AL. The IBM blood cell separator and blood cell processor: a personal perspective. J Clin Apheresis. 1988;4:171-182.

342. Thompson L. Central venous catheters for apheresis access. J Clin Apheresis. 1992;7:154-157.

343. Grishaber JE, Cunningham MC, Rohret PA, et al. Analysis of venous access for therapeutic plasma exchange in patients with neurological disease. J Clin Apheresis. 1992;7:119-123.

344. Gonzalez A, Sodano D, Flanagan J, et al. Long-term therapeutic plasma exchange in the outpatient setting using an implantable central venous access device. J Clin Apheresis. 2004;19:180-184.

345. Raj A, Bertolone S, Bond S, et al. Cathlink 20: a subcutaneous implanted central venous access device used in children with sickle cell disease on long-term erythrocytapheresis—a report of low complication rates. Pediatr Blood Cancer. 2005;44:669-672.

346. Dzik WH, Kirkley SA. Citrate toxicity during massive blood transfusion. Transfus Med Rev. 1988;2:76-94.

347. Fosburg M, Dolan M, Propper R, et al. Intensive plasma exchange in small and critically ill pediatric patients: techniques and clinical outcome. J Clin Apheresis. 1983;1:215-224.

348. Huestis D. Complications of therapeutic apheresis. In Kasprisin DO, MacPherson JL (eds). Therapeutic Hemapheresis. Boca Raton, FL, CRC Press, 1986, p 179.

349. Sutton DM, Nair RC, Rock G. Complications of plasma exchange. Transfusion. 1989;29:124-127.

350. Stefanutti C, Lanti A, Di Giacomo S, et al. Therapeutic apheresis in low weight patients: technical feasibility, tolerance, compliance, and risks. Transfus Apheresis Sci. 2004;31:3-10.

351. Shaz BH, Linenberger ML, Bandarenko N, et al. Category IV indications for therapeutic apheresis: ASFA fourth special issue. J Clin Apheresis. 2007;22:176-180.

352. Szczepiorkowski ZM, Bandarenko N, Kim HC, et al. Guidelines on the use of therapeutic apheresis in clinical practice: evidence-based approach from the Apheresis Applications Committee of the American Society for Apheresis. J Clin Apheresis. 2007;22:106-175.

353. Szczepiorkowski ZM, Shaz BH, Bandarenko N, et al. The new approach to assignment of ASFA categories—introduction to the fourth special issue: clinical applications of therapeutic apheresis. J Clin Apheresis. 2007;22:96-105.

354. McCloud B. Introduction to the third special issue: clinical applications of therapeutic apheresis. J Clin Apheresis. 2000;15:1-5.

355. Vichinsky EP, Neumayr LD, Earles AN, et al. Causes and outcomes of the acute chest syndrome in sickle cell disease. National Acute Chest Syndrome Study Group. N Engl J Med. 2000;342:1855-1865.

356. Russell MO, Goldberg HI, Hodson A, et al. Effect of transfusion therapy on arteriographic abnormalities and on recurrence of stroke in sickle cell disease. Blood. 1984;63:162-169.

357. Adams RJ, McKie VC, Hsu L, et al. Prevention of a first stroke by transfusions in children with sickle cell anemia and abnormal results on transcranial Doppler ultrasonography. N Engl J Med. 1998;339:5-11.

358. Cohen AR, Martin MB, Silber JH, et al. A modified transfusion program for prevention of stroke in sickle cell disease. Blood. 1992;79:1657-1661.

359. Zimmerman SA, Schultz WH, Burgett S, et al. Hydroxyurea therapy lowers transcranial Doppler flow velocities in children with sickle cell anemia. Blood. 2007;110:1043-1047.

360. Hamre MR, Harmon EP, Kirkpatrick DV, et al. Priapism as a complication of sickle cell disease. J Urol. 1991;145:1-5.

361. Griffin TC, Buchanan GR. Elective surgery in children with sickle cell disease without preoperative blood transfusion. J Pediatr Surg. 1993;28:681-685.

362. Vichinsky EP, Haberkern CM, Neumayr L, et al. A comparison of conservative and aggressive transfusion regimens in the perioperative management of sickle cell disease. The Preoperative Transfusion in Sickle Cell Disease Study Group. N Engl J Med. 1995;333:206-213.

363. Kim HC, Dugan NP, Silber JH, et al. Erythrocytapheresis therapy to reduce iron overload in chronically transfused patients with sickle cell disease. Blood. 1994;83:1136-1142.

364. Eisenman A, Baruch Y, Shechter Y, et al. Blood exchange [correction of exchance]—a rescue procedure for complicated falciparum malaria. Vox Sang. 1995;68:19-21.

365. Lercari G, Paganini G, Malfanti L, et al. Apheresis for severe malaria complicated by cerebral malaria, acute respiratory distress syndrome, acute renal failure, and disseminated intravascular coagulation. J Clin Apheresis. 1992;7:93-96.

366. Oldershaw P, Sutton MG. Haemodynamic effects of haematocrit reduction in patients with polycythemia secondary to cyanotic congenital heart disease. Br Heart J. 1980;44:584-588.

367. Meyer D, Bolgiano DC, Sayers M, et al. Red cell collection by apheresis technology. Transfusion. 1993;33:819-824.

368. Elfath MD, Whitley P, Jacobson MS, et al. Evaluation of an automated system for the collection of packed RBCs, platelets, and plasma. Transfusion. 2000;40:1214-1222.

369. Valbonesi M, Bruni R, Florio G, et al. Evaluation of dosed red blood cell units collected with Gambro BCT—TRIMA. Transfus Apheresis Sci. 2001;24:65-70.

370. Eguiguren JM, Schell MJ, Crist WM, et al. Complications and outcome in childhood acute lymphoblastic leukemia with hyperleukocytosis. Blood. 1992;79:871-875.

371. Wald BR, Heisel MA, Ortega JA. Frequency of early death in children with acute leukemia presenting with hyperleukocytosis. Cancer. 1982;50:150-153.

372. Maurer HS, Steinherz PG, Gaynon PS, et al. The effect of initial management of hyperleukocytosis on early complications and outcome of children with acute lymphoblastic leukemia. J Clin Oncol. 1988;6:1425-1432.

373. Bunin NJ, Pui CH. Differing complications of hyperleukocytosis in children with acute lymphoblastic or acute nonlymphoblastic leukemia. J Clin Oncol. 1985;3:1590-1595.

374. Dunbar CE, Cottler-Fox M, O'Shaughnessy JA, et al. Retrovirally marked CD34-enriched peripheral blood and bone marrow cells contribute to long-term engraftment after autologous transplantation. Blood. 1995;85:3048-3057.

375. Bensinger WI, Weaver CH, Appelbaum FR, et al. Transplantation of allogeneic peripheral blood stem cells mobilized by recombinant human granulocyte colony-stimulating factor. Blood. 1995;85:1655-1658.

376. Bensinger W, Singer J, Appelbaum F, et al. Autologous transplantation with peripheral blood mononuclear cells

collected after administration of recombinant granulocyte stimulating factor. Blood. 1993;81:3158-3163.

377. Takaue Y, Watanabe T, Abe T, et al. Experience with peripheral blood stem cell collection for autografts in children with active cancer. Bone Marrow Transplant. 1992;10:241-248.

378. Lasky LC, Bostrom B, Smith J, et al. Clinical collection and use of peripheral blood stem cells in pediatric patients. Transplantation. 1989;47:613-616.

379. Snyder EL. Hematopoietic cell therapy and transfusion medicine—carpe diem? Transfusion. 1995;35:371-373.

380. Fernandez JM, Shepherd V, Millar J, et al. When is the optimum time to harvest peripheral blood stem cells in children following standard dose chemotherapy? Med Pediatr Oncol. 1993;21:465-469.

381. Cecyn KZ, Seber A, Ginani VC, et al. Large-volume leukapheresis for peripheral blood progenitor cell collection in low body weight pediatric patients: a single center experience. Transfus Apheresis Sci. 2005;32:269-274.

382. Diaz MA, Sevilla J, de la Rubia J, et al. Factors predicting peripheral blood progenitor cell collection from pediatric donors for allogeneic transplantation. Haematologica. 2003;88:919-922.

383. Pulsipher MA, Levine JE, Hayashi RJ, et al. Safety and efficacy of allogeneic PBSC collection in normal pediatric donors: the pediatric blood and marrow transplant consortium experience (PBMTC) 1996-2003. Bone Marrow Transplant. 2005;35:361-367.

384. Sevilla J, Diaz MA, Fernandez-Plaza S, et al. Risks and methods for peripheral blood progenitor cell collection in small children. Transfus Apheresis Sci. 2004;31:221-231.

385. Takaue Y, Watanabe T, Kawano Y, et al. Sustained cytopenia after leukapheresis for collection of peripheral blood stem cells in small children. Vox Sang. 1989;57:168-171.

386. Goldberg SL, Mangan KF, Klumpp TR, et al. Complications of peripheral blood stem cell harvesting: review of 554 PBSC leukaphereses. J Hematother. 1995;4:85-90.

387. Rock GA, Shumak KH, Buskard NA, et al. Comparison of plasma exchange with plasma infusion in the treatment of thrombotic thrombocytopenic purpura. Canadian Apheresis Study Group. N Engl J Med. 1991;325:393-397.

388. Salvaneschi L, Perotti C, Zecca M, et al. Extracorporeal photochemotherapy for treatment of acute and chronic GVHD in childhood. Transfusion. 2001;41:1299-1305.

389. Chan KW. Extracorporeal photopheresis in children with graft-versus-host disease. J Clin Apheresis. 2006;21:60-64.

390. Dall'Amico R, Messina C. Extracorporeal photochemotherapy for the treatment of graft-versus-host disease. Ther Apheresis. 2002;6:296-304.

391. Halle P, Paillard C, D'Incan M, et al. Successful extracorporeal photochemotherapy for chronic graft-versus-host disease in pediatric patients. J Hematother Stem Cell Res. 2002;11:501-512.

392. Kanold J, Messina C, Halle P, et al. Update on extracorporeal photochemotherapy for graft-versus-host disease treatment. Bone Marrow Transplant. 2005;35(Suppl 1):S69-S71.

393. Kanold J, Paillard C, Halle P, et al. Extracorporeal photochemotherapy for graft versus host disease in pediatric patients. Transfus Apheresis Sci. 2003;28:71-80.

394. Barr ML, Meiser BM, Eisen HJ, et al. Photopheresis for the prevention of rejection in cardiac transplantation. Photopheresis Transplantation Study Group. N Engl J Med. 1998;339:1744-1751.

395. Wieland M, Thiede VL, Strauss RG, et al. Treatment of severe cardiac allograft rejection with extracorporeal photochemotherapy. J Clin Apheresis. 1994;9:171-175.

396. Dall'Amico R, Montini G, Murer L, et al. Extracorporeal photochemotherapy after cardiac transplantation: a new therapeutic approach to allograft rejection. Int J Artif Organs. 2000;23:49-54.

397. Dall'Amico R, Murer L: Extracorporeal photochemotherapy: a new therapeutic approach for allograft rejection. Transfus Apheresis Sci. 2002;26:197-204.

398. Bell WR, Braine HG, Ness PM, et al. Improved survival in thrombotic thrombocytopenic purpura–hemolytic uremic syndrome. Clinical experience in 108 patients. N Engl J Med. 1991;325:398-403.

399. Beattie TJ, Murphy AV, Willoughby ML, et al. Plasmapheresis in the haemolytic-uraemic syndrome in children. Br Med J (Clin Res Ed). 1981;282:1667-1668.

400. Misiani R, Appiani AC, Edefonti A, et al. Haemolytic uraemic syndrome: therapeutic effect of plasma infusion. Br Med J (Clin Res Ed). 1982;285:1304-1306.

401. Fulan M. von Willebrand factor proteolysis in thrombotic thrombocytopenic purpura. Blood. 1999;94:3611-3612.

402. Tsai HM, Lian EC. Antibodies to von Willebrand factor–cleaving protease in acute thrombotic thrombocytopenic purpura. N Engl J Med. 1998;339:1585-1594.

403. Furlan M, Robles R, Galbusera M, et al. von Willebrand factor–cleaving protease in thrombotic thrombocytopenic purpura and the hemolytic-uremic syndrome. N Engl J Med. 1998;339:1578-1584.

404. Vacanti JP, Lillehei CW, Jenkins RL, et al. Liver transplantation in children: the Boston Center experience in the first 30 months. Transplant Proc. 1987;19:3261-3266.

405. The Guillain-Barré Syndrome Study Group. Plasmapheresis and acute Guillain-Barré syndrome. Neurology. 1985;35:1096-1104.

406. Mendell JR, Kissel JT, Kennedy MS, et al. Plasma exchange and prednisone in Guillain-Barré syndrome: a controlled randomized trial. Neurology. 1985;35:1551-1555.

407. Evans OB. Guillain-Barré syndrome in children. Pediatr Rev. 1986;8:69-74.

408. van der Meche FG, Schmitz PI. A randomized trial comparing intravenous immune globulin and plasma exchange in Guillain-Barré syndrome. Dutch Guillain-Barré Study Group. N Engl J Med. 1992;326:1123-1129.

409. Sladky JT. Guillain-Barré syndrome in children. J Child Neurol. 2004;19:191-200.

410. Dyck PJ, Daube J, O'Brien P, et al. Plasma exchange in chronic inflammatory demyelinating polyradiculoneuropathy. N Engl J Med. 1986;314:461-465.

411. Dyck PJ, Litchy WJ, Kratz KM, et al. A plasma exchange versus immune globulin infusion trial in chronic inflammatory demyelinating polyradiculoneuropathy. Ann Neurol. 1994;36:838-845.

412. Koller H, Kieseier BC, Jander S, et al. Chronic inflammatory demyelinating polyneuropathy. N Engl J Med. 2005;352:1343-1356.

413. Seybold ME. Plasmapheresis in myasthenia gravis. Ann N Y Acad Sci. 1987;505:584-587.

414. Newsom-Davis J, Wilson SG, Vincent A, et al. Long-term effects of repeated plasma exchange in myasthenia gravis. Lancet. 1979;1:464-468.

415. Lewis EJ. Plasmapheresis therapy is ineffective in SLE. Lupus Nephritis Collaborative Study Group. J Clin Apheresis. 1992;7:153.

416. Thomson BJ, Watson ML, Liston WA, et al. Plasmapheresis in a pregnancy complicated by acute systemic lupus erythematosis. Case report. Br J Obstet Gynaecol. 1985;92:532-534.

417. Geurs F, Ritter K, Mast A, et al. Successful plasmapheresis in corticosteroid-resistant hemolysis in infectious mononucleosis: role of autoantibodies against triosephosphate isomerase. Acta Haematol. 1992;88:142-146.

418. McConnell ME, Atchison JA, Kohaut E, et al. Successful use of plasma exchange in a child with refractory immune hemolytic anemia. Am J Pediatr Hematol Oncol. 1987; 9:158-160.

419. Rogers SW, Andrews PI, Gahring LC, et al. Autoantibodies to glutamate receptor GluR3 in Rasmussen's encephalitis. Science. 1994;265:648-651.

420. Barinaga M. Antibodies linked to rare epilepsy. Science. 1995;268:362-363.

421. Twyman RE, Gahring LC, Spiess J, et al. Glutamate receptor antibodies activate a subset of receptors and reveal an agonist binding site. Neuron. 1995;14: 755-762.

422. Swedo SE, Leonard HL, Garvey M, et al. Pediatric autoimmune neuropsychiatric disorders associated with streptococcal infections: clinical description of the first 50 cases. Am J Psychiatry. 1998;155:264-271.

423. Trifiletti RR, Packard AM. Immune mechanisms in pediatric neuropsychiatric disorders. Tourette's syndrome, OCD, and PANDAS. Child Adolesc Psychiatr Clin N Am. 1999;8:767-775.

424. Perlmutter SJ, Leitman SF, Garvey MA, et al. Therapeutic plasma exchange and intravenous immunoglobulin for obsessive-compulsive disorder and tic disorders in childhood. Lancet. 1999;354:1153-1158.

425. Garvey MA, Snider LA, Leitman SF, et al. Treatment of Sydenham's chorea with intravenous immunoglobulin, plasma exchange, or prednisone. J Child Neurol. 2005;20: 424-429.

426. Geha RS, Leung DY. Hyper immunoglobulin E syndrome. Immunodefic Rev. 1989;1:155-172.

427. Aswad MI, Tauber J, Baum J. Plasmapheresis treatment in patients with severe atopic keratoconjunctivitis. Ophthalmology. 1988;95:444-447.

428. Hernandez ME, Lovrekovic G, Schears G, et al. Acute onset of Wegener's granulomatosis and diffuse alveolar hemorrhage treated successfully by extracorporeal membrane oxygenation. Pediatr Crit Care Med. 2002;3: 63-66.

429. Humphreys D, Galacki D. Automated plasma exchange for the coagulopathic neonate on extracorporeal membrane oxygenation. Paper presented at a meeting of the American Society for Clinical Apheresis, Boston, 1993.

430. Ferri C, Gremignai G, Bombardieri S, Moriconi L. Plasma-exchange in mixed cryoglobulinemia. Effects on renal, liver and neurologic involvement. Ric Clin Lab. 1986;16:403-411.

431. Lockwood CM, Boulton-Jones JM, Lowenthal RM, et al. Recovery from Goodpasture's syndrome after immunosuppressive treatment and plasmapheresis. BMJ. 1975;2: 252-254.

432. Glockner WM, Sieberth HG, Wichmann HE, et al. Plasma exchange and immunosuppression in rapidly progressive glomerulonephritis: a controlled, multi-center study. Clin Nephrol. 1988;29:1-8.

433. Pradhan M, Petro J, Palmer J, et al. Early use of plasmapheresis for recurrent post-transplant FSGS. Pediatr Nephrol. 2003;18:934-938.

434. Cochat P, Kassir A, Colon S, et al. Recurrent nephrotic syndrome after transplantation: early treatment with plasmaphaeresis and cyclophosphamide. Pediatr Nephrol. 1993;7:50-54.

435. Zwiener R, Uauy R, Petruska ML, Huet BA. Low-density lipoprotein apheresis as long-term treatment for children with homozygous familial hypercholesterolemia. J Pediatr. 1995;126:728-735.

436. Sniecinski IJ, Oien L, Petz LD, et al. Immunohematologic consequences of major ABO-mismatched bone marrow transplantation. Transplantation. 1988;45:530-534.

437. Bensinger WI, Buckner CD, Thomas ED, et al. ABO-incompatible marrow transplants. Transplantation. 1982; 33:427-429.

438. Braine HG, Sensenbrenner LL, Wright SK, et al. Bone marrow transplantation with major ABO blood group incompatibility using erythrocyte depletion of marrow prior to infusion. Blood. 1982;60:420-425.

439. Beimler JH, Susal C, Zeier M. Desensitization strategies enabling successful renal transplantation in highly sensitized patients. Clin Transplant. 2006;20(Suppl 17):7-12.

440. van Deuren M, Santman FW, van Dalen R, et al. Plasma and whole blood exchange in meningococcal sepsis. Clin Infect Dis. 1992;15:424-430.

441. Howe RB, Christie DJ. Protein A immunoadsorption treatment in hematology: an overview. J Clin Apheresis. 1994;9:31-32.

442. Jones FR, Baliant JP Jr, Snyder HW Jr. Selective extracorporeal removal of immunoglobulin G and circulating immune complexes: a review. Plasma Ther Transfus Technol. 1986;7:333-349.

443. Gjörstrup P, Watt RM. Therapeutic protein A immunoadsorption. Transfus Sci. 1990;11:281-323.

444. Watt RM, Bunitsky K, Faulkner EB, et al. Treatment of congenital and acquired hemophilia patients by extracorporeal removal of antibodies to coagulation factors: a review of US clinical studies 1987-1990. Hemophilia Study Group. Transfus Sci. 1992;13:233-253.

445. Nilsson IM, Berntorp E, Zettervall O. Induction of immune tolerance in patients with hemophilia and antibodies to factor VIII by combined treatment with intravenous IgG, cyclophosphamide, and factor VIII. N Engl J Med. 1988;318:947-950.

446. Freiburghaus C, Larsson LA. A summary of five years' clinical experience with extensive removal of immunoglobulins. Plasma Therapeutics Transfus Technol. 1986;7: 545-550.

447. Naganuma M, Funakoshi S, Sakuraba A, et al. Granulocytapheresis is useful as an alternative therapy in patients with steroid-refractory or -dependent ulcerative colitis. Inflamm Bowel Dis. 2004;10:251-257.

448. Shimoyama T, Sawada K, Hiwatashi N, et al. Safety and efficacy of granulocyte and monocyte adsorption apheresis in patients with active ulcerative colitis: a multicenter study. J Clin Apheresis. 2001;16:1-9.

449. Tomomasa T, Kobayashi A, Kaneko H, et al. Granulocyte adsorptive apheresis for pediatric patients with ulcerative colitis. Dig Dis Sci. 2003;48:750-754.

XII Hematologic Manifestations of Systemic Diseases

Hematologic Manifestations of Systemic Diseases

Hematologic Manifestations of Systemic Diseases in Children of the Developing World

36 Hematologic Manifestations of Systemic Diseases

R. Alan B. Ezekowitz

Evaluation of almost any patient who seeks medical attention, particularly in a hospital setting, includes the obligatory complete white blood cell count. In fact, the vast majority of patients do not have a primary hematologic problem. So the question is what information can be gleaned from this test and how can it inform the clinician about systemic diseases? There are many pathophysiologic paradigms that have secondary effects on hematopoiesis and many ways to approach the problem. The most satisfying is to dissect the mechanism whereby a systemic disease affects the complete blood count or results in a defect in coagulation. In this chapter an organ system approach is used, together with identification of certain diseases in which the diagnostic clue may lie in examination of the peripheral blood smear. In addition, some common infections, usually viral, that result in characteristic hematologic responses are discussed. Finally, the newly recognized application of a class of serum proteins as markers of systemic disease that play a role in host defense and serve as modulators of inflammation is addressed. A chapter on the hematologic manifestations of systemic diseases includes information that overlaps other sections of this book, and thus readers are encouraged to refer to other relevant chapters.

CARDIAC DISEASE

The focus of this section is on the three major hematologic complications of cardiac disease—hemolytic anemia, coagulopathy, and increased platelet turnover.

Hemolysis

A number of instances of continuing hemolysis and progressive anemia have been reported after the insertion of prosthetic valves, particularly in the aortic area.[1,2] These conditions may also occur postoperatively when intracardiac patches have been placed (the "Waring blender" syndrome). They are also being recognized as an increasing problem after endoluminal closure of the ductus arteriosus[3,4] and occasionally after repair of a ventriculoseptal defect.[5] The mechanism of such erythrocyte destruction has been related to failure of endothelialization of patches, thrombosis or perforation of prosthetic valves, and improper placement of prosthetic valves, especially when insufficiency develops at the suture lines. Erythrocyte destruction and ensuing hemolysis, however, have been described in the absence of these complications and been attributed to red blood cell mechanical trauma associated with apparently normal function of the prosthetic valve.[6,7]

Red cell survival studies have clearly shown that prosthetic valve and patch hemolysis is due to an extracorpuscular defect.[8] In general, hemolytic anemia results from fragmentation of the red cells as they are mechanically "battered" against a distorted vascular surface.[9] In some instances it has been postulated that the red cell fragmentation may be caused by contact with fibrin deposited in small blood vessels as a result of localized intravascular coagulation.[10] Most times, however, hemolysis is the result of direct mechanical trauma. Nevaril and associates[9] demonstrated that a shearing stress of 300 dynes/cm^2 causes hemolysis in vitro whereas less stress may result in deformed red cell morphologically similar in appearance to cells in cardiac hemolytic anemia and microangiopathic hemolytic anemia.[9]

The consequence of the process is hemolytic anemia of the intravascular type associated with hemoglobinemia and often hemoglobinuria. Iron deficiency develops quickly in patients with this disorder as a result of increased loss of body iron in the form of hemosiderin, which is shed within the renal tubular cells into urine.[11,12]

The onset of iron deficiency may be of clinical importance. The microcytic hypochromic cell in iron deficiency is more rigid, thereby leading to an accelerated rate of hemolysis from mechanical shearing in the microvasculature.[13] Plasma haptoglobin and hemopexin levels fall. Large quantities of red cell lactate dehydrogenase are released into serum, and a close correlation exists between the logarithm of serum lactate dehydrogenase and the half-life of chromium-labeled erythrocytes.[14] The rate of hemolysis may or may not result in anemia. If surgical correction of the defect causing hemolysis is not possible, the patient should be treated with both iron and folate, as well as red cell transfusion. The latter is intended to correct anemia, reduce stroke volume, and presumably reduce shear force. Sears and Crosby[15] observed that the severity of hemolysis is directly related to physical activity. This finding has been used as a test to determine whether the hemolysis is of cardiac origin because if it is, rest also diminishes the rate of hemolysis. If the source of the problem cannot be corrected surgically, propranolol, which reduces the shearing stress between red blood cells and the vascular wall by slowing the velocity of the circulation, may be given.[16]

Mechanical injury to red cells may result in loss of pieces of cell membrane, with or without loss of hemoglobin. Such loss will lead to the formation of spherocytes. Consequently, in many patients with heart valve hemolysis, results of the red cell osmotic fragility test may be abnormal.[16] Mechanical destruction of red blood cells on abnormal surfaces of the vasculature can result in hyperkalemia. This has been reported to cause ventricular arrhythmias.[17]

Occasionally, autoimmune hemolytic anemia is observed after cardiac surgery involving the placement of foreign material within the vascular system.[18] This condition may also occur in association with subacute bacterial endocarditis.

Erythrocyte disturbances in children with cardiac disease must be understood in the context of compensatory states or the context of iron deficiency as a complication. For example, infants with cyanotic congenital heart disease have erythropoietin-induced compensatory polycythemia. Aortic oxygen saturation higher than 80% is usually associated with low erythropoietin titers and hemoglobin levels that will not cause hyperviscosity. Even with moderate degrees of hypoxemia, elevated erythropoietin levels are not seen; presumably, the modest elevation in hemoglobin levels provides adequate tissue oxygenation.[19-21] Infants with cyanotic congenital heart disease have higher iron requirements because of the greater hemoglobin mass. Diminished iron stores in patients with cyanotic congenital heart disease are associated with a more right-shifted oxyhemoglobin dissociation curve.[22] Most children with cyanotic congenital heart disease have evidence of mild macrocytosis. A mean corpuscular volume greater than the 90th percentile for age and sex nearly eliminates the possibility of iron deficiency.[22]

Coagulation Abnormalities

Many investigations have suggested that a coagulopathy exists in some patients with cyanotic congenital heart disease. Newborns with protein C activity at or below the lower limit of the normal neonatal range may have a greater risk for either consumptive coagulopathy or major thrombosis.[23] Thrombocytopenia, low plasma fibrinogen levels, defective clot retraction, hypoprothrombinemia, factor V and VIII deficiency, and evidence of fibrin degradation products in serum have been reported.[24-28] Marked derangements in coagulation often accompany surgery involving cardiopulmonary bypass.[29] Management of the coagulation problems with heparin requires very careful and regular monitoring.[30]

Dennis and associates[31] were the first to report five patients with cyanotic congenital heart disease associated with coagulation abnormalities that were correctable by heparin.[31] Consumptive coagulopathy was thought to be responsible, but technical problems cast doubt on that interpretation.[32]

It is now generally thought that the presence of coagulation abnormalities correlates best with the extent of polycythemia.[33] The exact mechanism producing the coagulopathy, when present, is not known.

Hyperviscosity may lead to tissue hypoxemia, which then triggers a consumptive process.[34] Conflicting data suggest that the coagulation defects associated with cyanotic congenital heart disease must be multifactorial in origin. Therefore, each child should be studied individually. Data suggest that certain forms of heart disease may be associated with specific abnormalities. For example, subjects with mitral valve prolapse may experience factor VIII complex abnormalities.[35]

Platelet Abnormalities

Quantitative and qualitative platelet abnormalities are commonly associated with cardiac disease. In one series, the mean platelet count in cyanotic patients with an arterial oxygen saturation of less than 60% was 185,000 cells/mm^3 as compared with 315,000 cells/mm^3 in patients with an arterial oxygen saturation greater than 60%.[36,37] These abnormalities are readily noted on preoperative evaluation of the coagulation status of individuals about to undergo surgery.[38] Examination of bone marrow has failed to demonstrate any quantitative changes in megakaryocytes to account for these platelet differences.[36] This, together with the finding of shortened platelet survival in many patients, has suggested that the mechanism of the thrombocytopenia is destructive. Some patients, especially those with minimal cyanosis, may have elevated platelet counts. It should be noted that although iron deficiency is commonly associated with cyanotic congenital heart disease, the quantitative platelet abnormalities are not related to iron status.

Qualitative platelet defects associated with cyanotic congenital heart disease may include prolonged bleeding times and abnormal aggregation in response to adenosine diphosphate, epinephrine, and collagen.[39] In as many as 70% of patients, either a delayed or no second wave of platelet aggregation and disaggregation is observed.[40] These platelet functional abnormalities appear to be due to a defective platelet release mechanism because diminished release of [^{14}C]serotonin occurs in response to adenosine diphosphate whereas uptake of [^{14}C]serotonin is normal.[41] Platelet release abnormalities are more common in patients older than 4 years, in those with a hematocrit greater than 60%, and in those with platelet counts less than 175,000 cells/mm^3. There is no correlation between abnormalities in platelet aggregation and release and the abnormal bleeding time.

Treatment

Management of these hemostatic defects is not settled. It is agreed that they may predispose patients to postoperative hemorrhage, but they are rarely associated with preoperative clinical bleeding tendencies. Suggested management procedures have included the use of heparin[31] to lower viscosity, erythrocytapheresis with plasma exchange,[34,42] and ε-aminocaproic acid to inhibit fibrinolysis.[43] Whether any of these modalities are indicated and, indeed, whether they might be uniformly effective is speculative. If erythrocytapheresis is chosen, the procedure should be done with great care in cyanotic patients. Withdrawal of red cells must be accompanied by infusion of an equal volume of fresh frozen plasma. Simple removal of red cells without volume replacement in polycythemic individuals may cause an acute increase in viscosity, vascular collapse, seizures, and even stroke.[44] Because of the high incidence of cerebrovascular accidents in children with cyanotic congenital heart disease, some workers have thought that a "hypercoagulable" state exists. Hyperviscosity alone may account for some ischemic infarctions. The clinician should be alert to the possibility of iron deficiency predisposing patients to stroke in the presence of polycythemia. Several children in whom neurologic deficits developed after the onset of iron deficiency in the presence of polycythemia have been described.[45,46] Card and Weintraub[47] showed that red blood cells from animals with iron deficiency have decreased deformability. Altered deformability in the presence of increased blood viscosity could theoretically result in vascular ischemia.

Shortening of platelet survival with or without thrombocytopenia has been observed in both children and adults with prosthetic heart valves.[48] The increased platelet turnover may result from a combination of mechanical damage to the platelet and adhesion to the foreign material. The use of anti–platelet-aggregating agents may correct this shortened survival, although clinical benefit of the use of this class of drug has not been established. Drugs such as acetylsalicylic acid, dipyridamole, and sulfinpyrazone have been used either singly or in combination.[49-51]

Miscellaneous Hematologic Manifestations of Heart Disease

Subacute bacterial endocarditis may be associated with a variety of hematologic manifestations. Anemia is often present and is usually the result of chronic infection. The white blood cell count is generally normal, although marked leukocytosis or leukopenia may occur. A 25-year review of the evolving pattern of pediatric endocarditis shows that anemia is present in 40% of children with endocarditis and leukocytosis in 30% of such patients.[52] Pancytopenia has been reported,[53] and thrombocytopenia has been noted in a few patients.[54,55]

Congestive heart failure may result in sufficient hypoxia to cause nucleated red blood cells to appear in the peripheral blood in association with mild reticulocytosis.[56] Thrombocytopenia may be present but is almost exclusively the result of hypersplenism.[57]

Cyanotic heart disease may result in poor perfusion of the spleen and subsequent functional hyposplenism manifested by Howell-Jolly bodies in peripheral blood.[58] This finding is likely to lead to the mistaken conclusion that a child may have the asplenia syndrome (absence of the spleen, cardiovascular malformations, abdominal situs inversus, and other anatomic malformations), which is associated with a poor prognosis.

GASTROINTESTINAL DISEASE

Hematologic complications of gastrointestinal disease appear in many disorders. This section does not include the wide range of situations in which blood loss from the gastrointestinal tract occurs but rather focuses on specific diseases and their hematologic complications.

Diseases of the Upper Gastrointestinal Tract

Esophagus

Plummer-Vinson syndrome (dysphagia, postcricoid webs, and iron deficiency)[59] occurs in older individuals. It is rarely seen in young adults. Iron deficiency anemia may be the only manifestation of gastroesophageal reflux; thus, endoscopy is important in the evaluation of unexplained iron deficiency anemia.[60] Chronic gastroesophageal reflux may cause Barrett's esophagus with its attendant risk for the development of adenocarcinoma.[61]

Stomach

The gastric mucosa is important in both vitamin B_{12} and iron absorption, and disorders of the gastric mucosa may cause defective absorption of either of these nutrients.

Chronic atrophic gastritis is usually a disorder of older adults but occasionally is seen in young adults. The accompanying iron deficiency results from a combination of blood loss and iron malabsorption secondary to achlorhydria.[62] Vitamin B_{12} absorption defects may occur in association with chronic atrophic gastritis.[63]

Gastric resection may also result in iron or vitamin B_{12} deficiency—the former from bleeding at sites of anastomosis and the latter, years later, from lack of intrinsic factor. Vitamin B_{12} deficiency may develop in infants breast-fed by women who have undergone gastric or intestinal bypass procedures.[64] Macrocytic, megaloblastic anemia resulting from vitamin B_{12} deficiency has been reported in association with gastric trichobezoars.[65] This is presumed to be due to bacterial overgrowth of the upper gastrointestinal tract.

In congenital intrinsic factor deficiency, gastric biopsy results are normal, and no antibodies to parietal cells or intrinsic factor are present.[66]

Zollinger-Ellison syndrome is a disorder associated with increased parietal cell production of hydrochloric acid. This excess acid may cause iron deficiency as a result of mucosal ulceration. Carcinoid syndrome may cause a similar problem. In both conditions, vitamin B_{12} malabsorption may occur because of reduced pH in the ileum.

Small Bowel

Celiac disease may cause a panmalabsorption syndrome. Isolated iron deficiency results from blood loss secondary to ulcerations at the origins of the loop, and vitamin B_{12} deficiency may be due to consumption of this vitamin by stagnant intestinal bacteria.[67] Iron deficiency is quite common in patients with celiac disease.[68] It may be the sole initial manifestation of celiac disease.[69] The iron deficiency is generally mild and is readily corrected with a gluten-free diet.[70,71] Separate from iron deficiency, pica may be a symptom of childhood celiac disease.[72] Folate deficiency may also be seen.[73] Blind loops created surgically for the treatment of obesity have been reported to cause an unusual autoimmune disorder in young adults[74] characterized by immune intravascular hemolysis, neutropenia, and thrombocytopenia. Immune complex–mediated complement activation apparently accounts for the blood cell destruction, perhaps as a result of bacterial antigens that enter the blood and initiate immune complex formation. Hyposplenism is also associated with celiac disease.[75,76] The incidence of carcinoma and lymphoma is increased in adult patients with celiac disease.[77] Before the onset of lymphoma, elevations in placental ferritin, a tumor-associated antigen, may be found.[78]

Ileal resection may result in vitamin B_{12} deficiency if receptors for the vitamin B_{12}–intrinsic factor complex have been removed.

Regional enteritis may cause iron deficiency from blood loss, as well as vitamin B_{12} deficiency from inflammatory disease of the terminal ileum or from development of the blind loop syndrome as small bowel fistulas form. Low factor XIII levels have been observed in active disease associated with regional enteritis.[79] An abnormality in arachidonic acid metabolism may occur in patients with chronic inflammatory bowel disease, including regional enteritis. This may result in alterations in platelet function.[80] Diminished neutrophil function may be seen in both regional enteritis and other forms of inflammatory bowel disease. The condition may be identified by decreased oxidative metabolism and low superoxide dismutase content of neutrophils.[81] Perinuclear antineutrophil cytoplasmic antibodies are commonly found in patients with inflammatory bowel disease.[82,83]

Disorders such as tropical sprue, dermatitis herpetiformis, bowel lymphoma, amyloidosis, and connective tissue disturbances (including Ehlers-Danlos syndrome and pseudoxanthoma elasticum) may produce panselective or selective malabsorption. Certain disorders such as intestinal lymphangiectasia may cause protein loss of a magnitude sufficient to impair globin chain synthesis. Protein loss may also be associated with selective loss of thymic-dependent (T) lymphocytes into the bowel lumen, which causes lymphopenia and altered delayed-type hypersensitivity. This lymphopenia may be associated with hypogammaglobulinemia.[84]

Eosinophilic gastroenteritis is a disorder most often characterized by recurrent bouts of abdominal pain, nausea, vomiting, diarrhea, and an elevated peripheral blood eosinophil count for which there is no other explanation.[85] The gut wall may be infiltrated by eosinophils.[85]

Common diarrheal illnesses during infancy may result in life-threatening methemoglobinemia, especially if the diet has been high in nitrates.[86-89]

Diseases of the Lower Gastrointestinal Tract

Ulcerative colitis is often associated with iron deficiency anemia as a result of blood loss. Immune hemolytic anemia is also observed. Autoimmune hemolytic anemia identified by positive results on a Coombs test is a relatively rare complication of ulcerative colitis, however, and develops in less than 1% of patients.[90] Occasionally, vitamin B_{12} deficiency occurs after many years if a "backwash" ileitis is present. Polymorphonuclear leukocytosis is common. Occasionally, an increase in plasma fibrinolytic activity will be observed. A significant decrease in antithrombin III levels may be found.[91] Some clinicians have treated this complication with ε-aminocaproic acid.[92] Platelet functional abnormalities may exist and are discussed elsewhere. Alterations in T-cell subsets may also be seen in children with inflammatory bowel disease.[93]

Constipation has been reported to cause an increase in sulfmethemoglobin levels.[94] It has been suggested that excess nitrite absorption from the gut may be present in some patients as a result of abnormal bowel function.[95]

Symptoms of Peutz-Jeghers syndrome (gastrointestinal polyposis and mucocutaneous pigmentation) may occur in early childhood.[96] The increased risk for intestinal cancer associated with this syndrome may also be manifested in childhood.[97]

Hereditary hemorrhagic telangiectasia (Osler-Weber-Rendu disease) may result in iron deficiency from gastrointestinal bleeding. Alterations in hemostasis (disseminated intravascular coagulation [DIC], platelet dysfunction, and factor XI deficiency) have been reported.[98] An association between this disorder and von Willebrand disease may exist.[99]

PANCREATIC DISEASE

Acute hemorrhagic pancreatitis may cause acute anemia during the first week of the illness as a result of hemodilution, intravascular coagulation, and blood loss.[100] Anemia may also be seen with pancreatic insufficiency in association with the Shwachman syndrome (congenital exocrine pancreatic insufficiency and neutropenia). Defects in neutrophil chemotaxis are likewise seen in the Shwachman syndrome,[101] as well as anemia and abnormalities of the ribs and metaphyses of long bones.[102] Leukocytosis with neutrophilia is a usual finding. Markedly elevated levels of fibrin split products usually suggest that a consumptive coagulopathy is present. A concomitant decrease in platelet count is also common.[103] High levels of methemalbumin are common in the ascitic fluid of individuals with hemorrhagic pancreatitis[104] and can be used to distinguish this disorder from nonhemorrhagic pancreatitis. Patients with ascitic fluid are the ones most likely to have evidence of consumptive coagulopathy. For example, fibrin degradation products are seen in 40% of subjects with fulminant pancreatitis without ascites but in 100% of patients with clinically apparent peritoneal fluid.[105]

Cystic fibrosis may cause malabsorption, which produces the expected hematologic abnormalities. A specific pattern of anemia in association with edema and hypoproteinemia may be observed in some children with cystic fibrosis. It is found most commonly in children who have low dietary intake of nitrogen, such as those who receive their protein primarily from breast milk or soybean formula.[106] The edema is caused by hypoalbuminemia. The anemia responds to adequate dietary protein enrichment and pancreatic enzyme supplementation but not to iron administration. Cystic fibrosis may also be associated with malabsorption of fat-soluble vitamins, and the consequent coagulopathy is related to vitamin K deficiency. Vitamin E deficiency may also occur and is manifested by mild hemolytic anemia and abnormal red cell peroxide hemolysis, as well as by hyperaggregation of platelets.[107]

In 1979, Pearson described a syndrome in which the main symptoms were severe sideroblastic anemia and exocrine pancreatic dysfunction.[108] Pearson's syndrome is not confined to the bone marrow and pancreas but is a multiorgan disorder associated with deletions in mitochondrial DNA.[109-111]

LIVER DISEASE

Red Blood Cell Disturbances

Anemia is common in acute and chronic liver disease and apparently has a diverse etiology.[112] Erythropoietin levels are elevated in the anemia associated with liver disease.[113]

The red blood cells in liver disease are often macrocytic, with mean corpuscular volumes in the range of 100 to $110/m^3$. Target cells and acanthocytes or spur cells are commonly observed.[114,115] Stomatocytosis has been reported in alcoholic liver disease.[116] These morphologic abnormalities appear to be in direct proportion to the increase in red cell membrane phospholipid and cholesterol that may accompany liver disease whenever any obstructive component is present.[117-119] Such membrane lipid alterations result in an increase in red cell membrane area, which accounts for the target and spur cells. Increased osmotic resistance is a consequence of this increased surface area.

Shortened red cell survival may be observed in some patients with no evidence of blood loss.[120,121] Acute hemolysis has also been observed in patients with acute liver disease who have glucose-6-phosphate dehydrogenase deficiency as well.

The exact mechanism by which red blood cell survival is shortened is unclear. Erythrocytes from patients with active liver disease have an increased tendency to form Heinz bodies after incubation with an oxidant chemical such as acetylphenylhydrazine or sodium ascorbate. This increase in Heinz body formation is associated with increased instability of red cell reduced glutathione, decreased hexose monophosphate shunt activity, and reduced glucose recycling through the hexose monophosphate shunt.[122] It has not been possible to demonstrate any decreased activity of red cell glutathione reductase, glutathione peroxidase, glucose-6-phosphate dehydrogenase, 6-phosphogluconate dehydrogenase, or transketolase.[123] Activation of superoxide dismutase and glutathione reductase may be observed in the red blood cells of patients with profound liver disease. This may partially explain the alterations in the antioxidant system noted with these disorders.[124] The hemolytic anemia associated with liver disease secondary to Wilson's disease is especially severe.[125] The same is true of the hemolytic anemia related to protoporphyria.[126]

The exact significance of these metabolic alterations has not yet been determined. Red cell metabolism appears to return to normal within a few weeks after an insult to the liver. All of the metabolic consequences of liver disease can be reproduced in normal intact red cells by prolonged incubation in plasma from patients with active liver disease.

In patients with active liver disease, it may be wise to withhold any drug that has the potential to present an oxidant challenge to the red blood cell. Similar acquired abnormalities in hexose monophosphate shunt activity have been associated with drug-induced hemolysis in patients with uremia. Yawata and associates[127] have reported that primaquine therapy results in accelerated hemolysis in such patients.

Coagulation Abnormalities

Because the liver is involved to some extent in the synthesis of most of the coagulation factors, it is not unexpected that liver dysfunction would be associated with the presence of abnormal clotting studies. In most instances these abnormalities are a laboratory finding only. Less commonly, severe aberrations in clotting are seen and result in a serious risk of bleeding. The coagulation abnormalities common in patients with fulminant hepatic failure have been reviewed in detail.[128,129]

Factor I (Fibrinogen)

Fibrinogen levels are usually normal in liver disease. This may be accounted for by the fact that although fibrinogen synthesis has been demonstrated in liver cells, it is also produced in extrahepatic sites.[130]

Low levels of fibrinogen may be observed in fulminant acute liver failure. In these circumstances it has been speculated that intravascular coagulation contributes to the coagulation disturbance by depletion of some of the clotting factors.

An increased catabolic rate of labeled fibrinogen has been noted in acute and chronic active hepatitis despite normal levels of plasma fibrinogen.[131] In chronic active hepatitis, the rate of fibrinogen catabolism appears to correlate with the activity of the disease as assessed by variations in plasma aminotransferase levels.[131] This situation is less clear in acute hepatitis. Altered rates of fibrinogen catabolism may be the result of primary fibrinogenolysis or intravascular coagulation. In 1949, Ratnoff[132] documented primary fibrinolysis in cirrhosis of the liver, although more recent studies have failed to note this finding consistently. DIC in patients with liver disease is a complex and controversial area that is discussed later.

High levels of fibrinogen are occasionally observed in liver disease, mainly because fibrinogen is an acute phase reactant. Elevated levels of fibrinogen commonly accompany obstructive jaundice, biliary cirrhosis, and hepatoma.[133]

An abnormal fibrin monomer aggregate has been described in a number of patients with liver dysfunction.[134] The appearance of clotting defects involving prolongation of reptilase and thrombin clotting times, despite a normal fibrinogen concentration, should suggest that dysfibrinogenemia is present. Examination by sodium dodecyl sulfate–polyacrylamide gel electrophoresis of isolated fibrin from patients with liver disease failed to detect any molecular or structural defect associated with the polypeptide chains of fibrinogen.[135] An increase in sialic acid in the carbohydrate moiety of fibrinogen has been noted.[136]

Factors II, VII, IX, and X (Vitamin K–Dependent Factors)

Levels of vitamin K–dependent factors are often reduced in patients with liver disease.[137] This appears to result primarily from impaired synthesis. When hepatocellular damage is minimal (e.g., in mild acute or chronic hepatitis, obstructive jaundice, or biliary cirrhosis), these factors may be normal or increased.[138,139]

In acute and chronic liver disease, factor VII activity is generally reduced first and factor IX activity last.[140]

Of all the factors that may reflect hepatocellular damage, factor VII appears to be the most sensitive. Factor VII is synthesized almost exclusively in the liver and has the most rapid half-life (about 2 hours) of all the liver-dependent factors. In a study of patients with acute liver failure, it appeared that all those with factor VII activity exceeding 8% survived whereas the others died.[141] It is unfortunate that a direct factor VII assay is not available in many clinical laboratories, although some indication of factor VII activity is implied from the prothrombin time.

Factor V

Factor V activity usually parallels the activity of factors II and X in liver disease when the defect appears to be solely one of hepatic synthesis.[142] If DIC occurs in association with liver disease, the factor V level may be significantly depressed. Markedly elevated levels of factor V may be seen in obstructive liver disease, again as an acute phase reactant phenomenon.[138]

Factor VIII

Factor VIII procoagulant activity is generally normal or elevated in liver disease of all types.[143] Factor VIII antigen activity follows a similar pattern, except that antigenic activity will often exceed procoagulant activity by severalfold.[144] The explanation for this finding is not known.

Factors XI and XII

Factor XI activity is usually normal in hepatocellular disease but may be decreased.[145] The same is true of factor XII activity. The activity of both these factors may be elevated when the primary insult is obstructive.[138]

Factor XIII (Fibrin-Stabilizing Factor)

There are conflicting reports concerning factor XIII levels in liver disease. Reports of low activity have been based primarily on results of clot solubility tests[146]; however, when immunologic or radioisotopic techniques are used, more varied results are found.[147]

Plasminogen

Plasminogen levels are commonly decreased in liver disease. In one study, such levels were depressed in 45%

of patients with liver disease but without hepatic failure, whereas all patients with hepatic failure had diminished plasminogen levels.[142]

Antithrombin III

Antithrombin III levels are often decreased in patients with acute and chronic liver disease, whereas elevations may be observed in those with obstructive disease.[138,148]

α_2-Macroglobulin

Levels of this inhibitor of thrombin and plasmin have been found to be elevated in liver cirrhosis.

Tests for Coagulation Disturbances

Screening tests for coagulation disturbances often fail to give any indication that liver dysfunction exists. The sensitivity of both the prothrombin time and partial thromboplastin time for detecting mild to moderate depressions of factor levels varies markedly from laboratory to laboratory.

Although most studies have failed to show good correlation between clotting tests and cholesterol, transaminase, or γ-globulin levels, the prothrombin time still appears to be the most convenient clotting test for monitoring liver function.

As noted earlier, factor VIII antigen activity increases to very high levels with hepatocellular dysfunction. The level of factor VIII antigen can therefore be used to determine whether chronic active hepatitis is present because in uncomplicated acute hepatitis, antigen activity returns to normal within a few months.

Disseminated Intravascular Coagulation

Patients with liver disease commonly manifest a spectrum of coagulation abnormalities that are highly suggestive of DIC.[149,150] Findings consistent with DIC include hypofibrinogenemia, thrombocytopenia, increased fibrinogen catabolism, increased levels of fibrin degradation products, and depressed levels of other coagulation factors. This pattern of abnormalities is not specific for DIC and may simply reflect the severity of the hepatocellular disease process. For example, fibrinogen levels may be depressed on a synthetic basis alone. Increased catabolism of fibrinogen may reflect distribution in extravascular spaces, such as the formation of ascitic fluid or proteolysis by enzymes other than thrombin. Thrombocytopenia may occur for a variety of reasons and frequently is not present when other signs of DIC are seen. Changes in levels of factors V and VIII are varied and nonspecific. Because fibrin degradation products are cleared by the liver, severe liver dysfunction itself may cause elevations of these products without implicating DIC.[129] Studies reporting that heparin corrects DIC in liver disease are also open to some criticism because there is no evidence that the conditions of the patients studied were in a steady state at the time of heparin therapy.

Whether true DIC occurs in liver disease will probably remain a controversial subject for some time to come. As yet, no general recommendation for the use of heparin can be made. In the only controlled trial of heparin therapy in acute hepatic necrosis to date, no difference was found in recovery rates with or without heparin.[151] Fresh frozen plasma factor concentrates and platelet transfusions remain the treatment of choice. Care must be taken when factor concentrates are used because if contaminated by activated factor X, they may cause diffuse thrombosis.[152]

RENAL DISEASE

Renal disease may produce disturbances in red cells, white cells, platelets, and coagulation factors. In many instances the abnormalities that are found do not parallel the status of renal function but rather reflect the activity of the disease process that results in renal dysfunction. The hematologic aspects of renal insufficiency have been reviewed in detail.[153]

The Red Blood Cell

Anemia

Anemia is a common finding in renal disease. The erythrocytes of patients with renal disease are generally normochromic and normocytic without any distinguishing morphologic characteristics. Occasionally, scalloped or burr cells are observed, usually in association with uremia secondary to specific causes or related to specific syndrome complexes such as hemolytic-uremic syndrome.[154] In diseases associated with microangiopathic hemolytic anemia, red cell fragmentation is common. It may be observed in patients with malignant hypertension, renal cortical necrosis, polyarteritis nodosa, hemolytic-uremic syndrome, systemic lupus erythematosus, and thrombotic thrombocytopenic purpura.

The anemia of renal disease can have many causes, including a decreased rate of red blood cell production (the "anemia of chronic disorders"), shortened red blood cell survival, and nutritional factors.

In renal disease, unlike many other chronic disease states, close correlation exists between erythrocyte mass and erythrocyte survival.[155] This implies that shortening of red cell survival has an important role in the development of anemia in these patients. About 70% of patients with renal disease have shortened red cell survival related to a host of potential alterations. These cells demonstrate increased mechanical fragility, autohemolysis, diminished deformability, and a variety of metabolic defects.[156,157]

Decreased red cell production is, however, the major cause of the anemia of chronic renal failure. A deficiency in erythropoietin production is probably the primary cause,[158,159] but toxic suppression of hematopoiesis is also a contributing factor. In patients with acute or chronic renal failure as a result of nephrectomy, normal or even increased erythropoietin production can be maintained.[160]

The red cells of patients with uremia have either a normal or an increased rate of glucose utilization. The increased glycolytic rate appears to be primarily a result of the associated hyperphosphatemia because inorganic phosphorus is a well-recognized stimulant of red cell glucose utilization.[161]

In uremic states, the level of hemoglobin A_1 (HbA$_1$) is elevated.[162] The increased HbA$_1$ level in uremia correlates with the level of blood urea nitrogen and results from carbamylation of hemoglobin by urea-derived cyanate. Most interestingly, the carbamylated hemoglobin level integrates the average blood urea nitrogen levels—a situation analogous to that seen in glycosylation of hemoglobin in diabetes.[162]

A circulating inhibitor of red cell metabolism accumulates in some, but not all uremic patients. This inhibitor diminishes recycling of glucose through the hexose monophosphate shunt,[156] a defect that may be clinically important. There are several reports of severe hemolytic disease in uremic patients given sulfa drugs. In patients with renal disease who have undergone splenectomy, Heinz bodies are commonly observed. Because of this problem, caution in the use of oxidant drugs is advised in those with azotemia.[163] The decreased shunt activity may be secondary to a metabolic defect within the shunt itself or due to a block within the main glycolytic pathway. When erythrocytes from patients with renal insufficiency are stressed with oxidant compounds such as sodium ascorbate, glucose consumption and lactate formation are abnormally increased, whereas lactate-to-pyruvate ratios are abnormally diminished. Red cell glycolytic intermediates—including fructose 1,6-diphosphate, glyceraldehyde 3-phosphate, 3-phosphoglycerate, phosphoenolpyruvate, and pyruvate—markedly accumulate. No increase in 2-phosphoglycerate occurs, thus suggesting that inefficient phosphoglyceromutase activity may underlie this defective glucose reutilization.[156]

Adenosine triphosphate levels are significantly increased in uremic red blood cells. This increase may not result solely from elevated serum phosphorus levels because red cells from uremic patients incubated in medium with an artificially low phosphate concentration demonstrate increased adenosine triphosphate synthesis activity.[164] Pyruvate kinase activity is significantly increased in uremic as opposed to normal red cells, thus suggesting the presence of a younger red blood cell population.[164]

Red blood cell 2,3-diphosphoglycerate (2,3-DPG) levels are increased as well for similar reasons.[165] This increase results in a significant shift to the right in the hemoglobin-oxygen dissociation curve, which favors oxygen release. After dialysis with correction of acidosis and hyperphosphatemia, there is a sharp increase in arterial pH and a decrease in red cell 2,3-DPG levels. Both these changes result in an acute change in the oxygen dissociation characteristics of red cells. Whether this produces any physiologic impairment after dialysis is unclear.[164] Recombinant human erythropoietin administered two to three times weekly is extremely effective in eliminating the need for transfusion in subjects with chronic renal failure.[166] This has been shown in children as well as adults.[167]

Other incidental causes of hemolysis may be observed during hemodialysis. Contaminants such as copper, nitrate, and chloramines in hemodialysis baths may cause varying degrees of hemolysis.[168-170]

Anemia associated with megaloblastic changes in bone marrow is not uncommon in chronic renal failure. This anemia is usually due to folate deficiency[171] caused by poor dietary intake, hemodialysis, peritoneal dialysis, or the effects of immunosuppressive drugs. In addition, defective protein-mediated folate transport may be present.[172] Serum from uremic patients may contain an increased concentration of folic acid–binding protein.[172] Folate deficiency is usually suspected when large numbers of macro-ovalocytes are seen in association with hypersegmentation of polymorphonuclear leukocytes on the peripheral blood smear.

Treatment may be needed for the anemia associated with renal disease. In chronic renal disease, anemia is partially compensated for by improved oxygen unloading as a result of the high red cell content of 2,3-DPG. The treatment of choice for the anemia of chronic renal failure is the use of recombinant erythropoietin.[173,174] Recent studies, however, have challenged its efficacy in stage 3 and 4 chronic kidney disease. A randomized controlled trial enrolled 603 patients with chronic kidney disease and found that raising the hemoglobin to 14 g and higher did not improved cardiovascular outcomes.[175] In fact, a meta-analysis revealed that hemoglobin concentrations higher than 12 g/L place patients at increased risk for death, and thus the guidelines have been modified accordingly.[176] Iron therapy may be required as well.[177] The possible benefits of androgen therapy must be weighed against the side effects of this class of drugs.

Polycythemia

Erythrocytosis is a well-recognized complication of hydronephrosis[178] and has occasionally been noted in association with chronic glomerulonephritis, pyelonephritis, nephrosclerosis, and nephrotic syndrome in adults.[179] Erythrocytosis is a common finding after renal transplantation.[180] The cause of the elevated red cell mass in most patients appears to be mediated by erythropoietin.

The White Blood Cell

Azotemia and uremia per se appear to have relatively little effect on white blood cell function. Granulocytopenia is common during hemodialysis[181] and appears to be due to transient sequestration of granulocytes in the pulmonary vascular bed followed by later release back into the circulation. After hemodialysis, a transient augmentation in granulocyte adherence coincides with the time of sequestration of the pulmonary vascular bed.[182] The adherence-augmenting factor in the plasma of patients undergoing dialysis is heat stable. Craddock and co-workers[183] believe that this factor is complement activated by contact with the dialysis coil. However, the use of 5-hydroxyindole-3-acetic acid, a complement inhibitor, fails to block the granulocytopenia associated with dialysis.[184]

Neutropenia as a result of folate deficiency may be present in patients with renal failure. The cause of the neutrophil nuclear hypersegmentation associated with uremia is unknown and should not be attributed to folate deficiency.

Coagulation Abnormalities

Patients with uremia may have varied changes in some coagulation factors. Among the most common abnormalities observed are mild to moderate depressions in factors V, VII, IX, and X.[185,186] These abnormalities are related to the high incidence of hepatic dysfunction in patients with uremia or vitamin K deficiency.[39] The level of fibrinogen is regularly elevated because it is an acute phase reactant.[187-189] Increased fibrinogen turnover has been demonstrated in experimental models,[190] and excessive fibrin degradation products have been found in the urine and serum of uremic patients.[191] When a decrease in one or more consumable clotting factors (factors I, II, V, or VIII) is also present, it may signify the existence of consumptive coagulopathy.[185,186,192] Because fibrin deposition may occur in the absence of such a coagulopathy, it is often helpful to determine whether high-molecular-weight fibrin degradation products are present in the urine and serum. If found only in the urine, such products are probably derived from the dissolution of fibrin deposits in the kidneys. If demonstrable simultaneously in urine and serum, their presence indicates renal injury because such degradation products cannot be demonstrated in the urine of patients with streptokinase-induced fibrinolysis who have no renal disease.[193,194] Fibrin degradation products in the urine and serum usually indicate active renal disease, although other reasons for this finding may be seen in patients with renal disease. Fibrin degradation products may also result from concomitant liver disease or from an external shunt used for hemodialysis.[47] Urinary fibrinolytic activity is either diminished or absent in renal failure, and inhibitors of urokinase-induced plasminogen activation are demonstrable.[193]

Nephrotic syndrome is often accompanied by changes in a number of coagulation factors.[195] Increased levels of fibrinogen, factor VIII, and the factor VII-X complex are commonly present.[196] A prolonged partial thromboplastin time is often observed and is usually due to a decrease in the plasma level of factor IX.[197] Factor IX is consistently found in urine containing more than 10 g of protein per 24 hours in patients with nephrotic syndrome.[198] Plasma levels of factor IX rarely decrease to less than 10%, and clinical bleeding episodes are unusual. With resolution of the proteinuria in patients receiving corticosteroid therapy, levels of factor IX increase. Factors II and VII have also been identified in considerable quantity in the urine of patients with nephrotic syndrome despite normal levels of these factors in plasma.[199] This finding suggests that loss of some coagulation factors into urine can be fully compensated for by an increased rate of synthesis. A prolonged partial thromboplastin time may also be due to a low level of Hageman factor (factor XII).[200] Hageman factor has a molecular mass of approximately 75,000 kd, similar to that of albumin, and losses in urine are to be expected.[201] Although factor XII levels may decrease to less than 10%, as with congenital deficiency of this factor, bleeding is not a problem. Patients with nephrotic syndrome appear to have a substantially higher risk for thromboembolic complications,[193] although the exact reasons are still mainly unknown. Enhanced platelet function characterized by hyperaggregability has been observed.[202] An identical defect is seen in diabetics[203] and many patients with advanced cirrhosis of the liver.[204] Such changes may relate to alterations in plasma lipid fractions and are discussed in detail in Chapter 29. The coagulation defects associated with nephrotic syndrome have been reviewed by Kaufmann and colleagues.[205]

The hypercoagulable state seen in many forms of renal disease may be compounded by the occurrence of lupus-like anticoagulants. This is common in a variety of end-stage renal diseases, with a rate of occurrence as high as 22%.[206] Whether therapy focused on prevention of fibrin deposition within the kidney is of benefit to patients with certain forms of glomerulonephritis remains uncertain. Kincaid-Smith[207,208] used a combination of an anticoagulant, dipyridamole, and cyclophosphamide in a series of patients with membranoproliferative glomerulonephritis. A similar approach was reported by Robson and associates,[209] but with azathioprine substituted for cyclophosphamide. In both studies it was suggested that these therapies produced improvement in the patients' clinical course. The concept of anticoagulation therapy for these disorders has been reviewed.[210] The pathophysiology and management of hemolytic-uremic syndrome are discussed in Chapter 29.

Platelet Abnormalities

Mild thrombocytopenia occurs in approximately 25% of patients with acute renal failure and 10% of those with chronic renal disease.[211] The thrombocytopenia is most likely due to impaired production because platelet life span in uremia is generally normal.[188] Platelet function is abnormal in patients with renal failure. The standardized Ivy bleeding time is usually prolonged and generally correlates with the clinical tendency for bleeding in these patients.[212] Platelet adhesion and platelet factor 3 availability are diminished in acute and chronic uremia.[213] Impaired aggregation of platelet-rich plasma in the presence of adenosine diphosphate,[214] epinephrine,[215] thrombin,[215] and collagen[215] has been observed by various workers. Clinical bleeding episodes related to these platelet abnormalities can usually be managed with 1-deamino-8-D-arginine vasopressin given intravenously.[216] Long-term administration of recombinant erythropoietin also improves the biochemical and functional changes in the platelets of uremic patients.[217]

Platelet functional abnormalities are not due to an intrinsic platelet defect because dialysis quickly reverses these changes and incubation of normal platelets in plasma from uremic patients promptly induces functional aberrations. Rather, platelet dysfunction appears to be due to the interaction of intrinsically normal platelets with various abnormal dialyzable metabolites found in the plasma of uremic patients.[218] If urea and creatinine levels are elevated, some of these findings can be reproduced.[218] Phenols[187] and guanidinosuccinic acid,[219] which accumulate in the plasma of uremic patients, can also account for platelet functional abnormalities. These findings are discussed in detail in Chapter 29.

Several hereditary disorders have been reported in which quantitative or qualitative platelet abnormalities occur in association with nephritis. In 1972, Epstein and associates[220] described a family with hereditary macrothrombopathia, nephritis, and deafness. The renal pathologic findings are identical to those described in patients with classic hereditary nephritis and nerve deafness (Alport's syndrome) and consist of sclerosing and proliferative glomerulonephritis and interstitial nephritis with fibrosis. Members of these families have large platelets, prolonged bleeding times, defective platelet factor 3 activity, and defective platelet aggregation in the presence of adenosine diphosphate, collagen, and epinephrine. Coexpression of May-Hegglin anomaly and hereditary nephritis has been described in several families.[221] Thrombocytopenia is also present in this autosomal dominant disorder.[222] A similar disorder, but with normal platelet function, has been described by Eckstein and associates.[223] In these families, platelet survival studies have been normal.

Vascular occlusion of the kidney may result in eosinophilia. Approximately 80% of adult subjects with embolic renal disease have eosinophil counts ranging from 540 to 2000 cells/mm³.[224]

ENDOCRINE DISORDERS

Disturbances in endocrine balance tend to produce real, but relatively mild hematologic abnormalities. The most thoroughly evaluated of these abnormalities are those caused by thyroid disorders.

Thyroid Gland

Thyroid hormone appears to have many hematologic effects (Table 36-1), with the most impressive being its

TABLE 36-1	Hematologic Effects of Thyroid Hormone	
↑ Thyroid Hormone	**↓ Thyroid Hormone**
↑ PRBC volume	↓ PRBC volume
Variable effect on RBCs	↑ Or normal MCV;
↑ Glucose utilization and	spiculated RBCs
hexose monophosphate	↑ O₂ affinity
shunt activity	↓ 2,3-Diphosphoglycerate
↓ RBC glutathione,	↓ RBC Na⁺
reduced	↓ Platelet adhesion
↑ Red cell	↓ (Slight) platelet
2,3-diphosphoglycerate	aggregability
↓ O₂ affinity	↓ Factor VIII activity
↑ Diphosphoglycerate	↑ Fibrinolytic activity
mutase activity	↑ Plasminogen
↑ Glyceraldehyde-3-	↑ Plasminogen activation
phosphate	↓ Plasminogen activation
dehydrogenase	↓ Capillary fragility
↑ Glucose 6-phosphate	↑ Factors VIII, VII, IX,
activity	XI activity
↓ RBC carbonic anhydrase	
↓ RBC zinc	
↑ RBC Na²⁺	
↑ (Slight) platelet turnover	
↑ Platelet adhesion	
↑ Platelet aggregability	
↑ Factor VIII activity	
↓ Plasminogen activation	
↑ Capillary fragility	

MCV, mean corpuscular volume; PRBC, packed red blood cell; RBC, red blood cell.

effect on erythropoiesis. Although thyroid hormone slightly stimulates erythropoiesis in vitro,[225] the anemia caused by thyroid hormone deficiency is a secondary finding. Autoimmune hemolytic anemia may be seen in association with Graves' disease.[226] Most workers have correlated the erythropoietic effects of thyroid hormones with their calorigenic properties. Thyroid hormone increases oxygen consumption, which results in increased renal production of erythropoietin and stimulation of erythropoiesis. However, the erythropoietic stimulatory effect may, in fact, occur independently of erythropoietin. Administration of triiodothyronine and thyroxine to nephrectomized rats produces an increase in bone marrow erythroid precursors.[227]

The anemia of hypothyroidism is usually normochromic and normocytic and occasionally mildly macrocytic.[228] Small numbers of irregularly contracted red blood cells may be noted on the peripheral blood smear (Fig. 36-1).[229] Red cell survival is normal, and ferrokinetic studies demonstrate a decreased rate of iron clearance. In adults with hypothyroidism, an unusually high incidence of iron deficiency[230] and pernicious anemia is found.[231] A single confounding occurrence of erythrocytosis in association with hypothyroidism has been described.[232] Subsequent to this case report, a series of 23 patients with congenital hypothyroidism have been

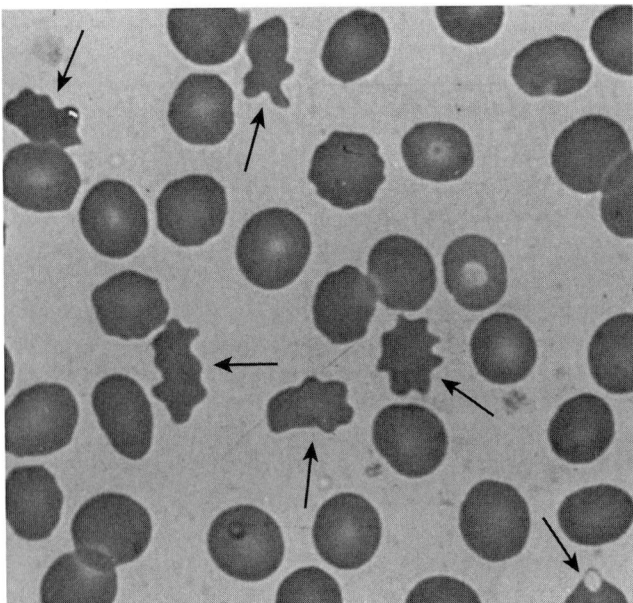

FIGURE 36-1. Red blood cell morphologic features in hypothyroidism. *(From Wardrop C, Hutchinson HE. Red cell shape in hypothyroidism. Lancet. 1969;2:1243.)*

evaluated for the presence of anemia. Of these infants, 26% had elevated hemoglobin levels, some of which were marked.[233]

Somewhat opposite findings are noted in uncomplicated hyperthyroidism. Anemia is rare, and red blood cell indices are normal. There is usually an increase in red blood cell mass that does not result in significant increases in hemoglobin concentration because a similar elevation in plasma volume also occurs.[234] Erythrocyte survival is normal or mildly diminished, especially in thyrotoxic children.[235] Peripheral blood and bone marrow lymphocyte counts may be increased.

Thyroid hormone may play a role in the regulation of red cell metabolism. Thyroxine has been reported to increase red cell glycolysis.[236] It helps regulate red cell carbonic anhydrase I concentrations.[237] Hexose monophosphate shunt activity may increase in the presence of triiodothyronine.[238] The activity of glucose-6-phosphate dehydrogenase is consistently elevated in thyrotoxicosis, whereas normal levels are found in most patients with mild hyperthyroidism.[239] Glutathione levels are usually depressed in hyperthyroidism. Thyroid hormone may affect the activities of several other red cell enzymes. This hormone stimulates diphosphoglycerate mutase and glyceraldehyde-3-phosphate dehydrogenase.[240] These effects may be the cause of the elevated levels of red cell 2,3-DPG that are seen in patients with hyperthyroidism and that result in decreased whole blood oxygen affinity and a shift to the right in the hemoglobin-oxygen dissociation curve.[241] Opposite effects are seen in hypothyroidism. The carbonic anhydrase activity of erythrocytes is diminished in hyperthyroidism and increased in hypothyroidism. Because red cell zinc is almost exclusively con-

tained in carbonic anhydrase, hyperthyroidism will result in a decrease in total red cell zinc levels.[242]

The red blood cells of patients with hyperthyroidism may have increased osmotic resistance.[243] The red cell sodium concentration is significantly increased in hyperthyroidism, and decreased sodium pump activity may be present.[244]

Neutropenia may occur in approximately 5% of children with hyperthyroidism.[245] The mechanism of this abnormality is unclear, although some patients will have antineutrophil antibodies.[246]

Multiple effects on platelets and blood coagulation factors may occur in thyroid disease states. Marked hyperthyroidism may reduce platelet survival.[247] Egeberg[248] reported on a patient with hypothyroidism who had a prolonged bleeding time and low factor VIII activity, similar to findings in von Willebrand's disease. Autoimmune thrombocytopenia has been observed in association with hyperthyroidism[249] and is related to increases in mean platelet volume.[250]

Simone and associates[251] reported on patients with hypothyroidism who had multiple coagulation factor deficiencies. Diminished platelet responsiveness to epinephrine and low platelet adhesiveness may be present as well.[252] Impressively low levels of factor VIII occur occasionally, with milder depression of factors VII, IX, and XI being found either alone or in combination.[253] In hypothyroidism, increased plasma fibrinolytic activity may result from an elevation in plasma plasminogen and a decrease in an inhibitor of plasminogen activation.[253,254] This may account for the mild to moderate increase in levels of fibrinogen and fibrin split products occasionally found in patients with hypothyroidism.[253] Menorrhagia secondary to acquired hypothyroidism-related von Willebrand's disease has been reported.[255]

Adrenal Gland

Adrenal cortical steroid hormones appear to have a stimulatory effect on erythropoiesis. In Addison's disease, the adrenal insufficiency may cause mild to moderate anemia, probably as a result of reduced basal metabolism. In most patients, a decrease in plasma volume masks the decreased red cell mass. After treatment of adrenal insufficiency, the plasma volume corrects quickly, whereas the red cell mass responds over a period of several weeks. The usual effect of treatment is therefore a prompt decrease in hemoglobin concentration followed by a gradual increase.[256]

Erythrocytosis may occur in Cushing's syndrome, but in most patients the reported increase has been slight.

A variety of effects on leukocytes occur after steroid administration or endogenous overproduction of a steroid, including granulocytosis, a reduced lymphocyte count, involution of lymphatic tissue, and a decrease in peripheral blood eosinophils and monocytes. In Addison's disease, neutropenia, eosinophilia, and lymphocytosis appear.[257] Coagulation abnormalities suggesting a hypercoagulable state may be seen in patients with Cushing's syndrome.[258]

Glucocorticosteroids affect lymphoid cells in many ways. The effects, however, are species specific. The mouse, rat, hamster, and rabbit are steroid sensitive; many of their lymphoid cells are easily lysed by steroids, and in these species, steroids inhibit antibody production. Human, simian, and guinea pig lymphoid cells are not easily lysed by steroids; in these species, it is difficult to demonstrate profound steroid inhibition of antibody production.[259] Cellular metabolism, including nucleic acid synthesis and glucose uptake, is inhibited.

The mechanism by which endogenous or exogenous steroids lower the number of circulating eosinophils is unknown.

Testes and Ovaries

Hematologic abnormalities are rare in association with gonadal dysfunction. This does not mean that the gonadal hormones play no role in hematopoiesis. Androgens stimulate erythropoiesis, whereas estrogens, in general, depress red cell production. Castration of the adult male results in a definite decrease in red cell mass.[260] In disorders associated with androgen excess, such as Cushing's syndrome and congenital adrenal hyperplasia, the hemoglobin concentration may exceed normal values. Exogenous androgen administration may cause polycythemia and may also increase red cell 2,3-DPG.[261] Androgens appear to stimulate erythropoiesis by increasing erythropoietin production, as well as by having a direct effect on bone marrow stem cells.

The normal menstrual cycle is associated with hematologic variations. Delivoria-Papadopoulos and colleagues[262] described cyclic variations in endogenous carbon monoxide production during the menstrual cycle of fertile women and suggested that heme catabolism was increased during the progesterone phase. It has been known for some time that reticulocyte counts are increased during the progesterone phase.[263] A cyclic variation in erythrocyte deformability also occurs during the menstrual cycle.[264] The relationship between decreased red cell deformability, reticulocytosis, and increased heme catabolism is speculative. A similar decrease in deformability occurs during the last trimester of pregnancy and with the use of oral contraceptives.[265,266]

Pregnancy causes increases in levels of several coagulation factors, including factors I, VII, VIII, IX, and X.[267] Carriers of genes for classic hemophilia and von Willebrand's disease may have significantly increased factor VIII activity during pregnancy.[267] Plasma fibrinolytic activity diminishes during pregnancy.

Pituitary Gland

The hematologic effects of pituitary disease are usually a consequence of the action of trophic hormone on target endocrine organ function. For example, anemia is common in patients with hypopituitarism.[268] This normochromic, normocytic anemia is associated with findings of lymphocytosis and eosinophilia, which indicate that this effect of hypopituitarism results from adrenal insufficiency. Erythropoietin production may be diminished as a consequence of a lower metabolic rate.

Growth hormone may play an important role in erythropoiesis.[269] This hormone stimulates erythropoiesis directly and indirectly by increased production of erythropoietin. The red blood cell count may decrease with isolated growth hormone deficiency.[270] Erythrocyte glucose-6-phosphate dehydrogenase activity is low in hypopituitarism and increases with growth hormone administration.[271] Growth hormone depresses erythrocyte glycolysis.[272]

Megaloblastic and sideroblastic anemia, neutropenia, and thrombocytopenia have been reported in children with the DIDMOAD syndrome (diabetes insipidus, diabetes mellitus, optic atrophy, and deafness). It is thought to be an inherited abnormality of thiamine metabolism.[273]

PULMONARY DISEASE

Hypoxia may be caused by a wide variety of pulmonary disorders and, in turn, results in a form of secondary polycythemia and compensatory shifts in the hemoglobin-oxygen dissociation curve that can be attributed to an increase in the red cell content of 2,3-DPG. Rarely, the polycythemia results in a state of extreme hyperviscosity and decreased tissue blood flow. Other than polycythemia, the hematologic findings of specific pulmonary disorders tend to be unique to those disorders.

Idiopathic Pulmonary Hemosiderosis

Idiopathic pulmonary hemosiderosis (IPH) is an uncommon chronic disease that usually affects children and young adults. However, the age at onset may be as early as the newborn period.[274] IPH is characterized by recurrent intrapulmonary hemorrhage and may result in hemoptysis and pulmonary insufficiency. The hematologic manifestation of this disorder is iron deficiency anemia.

The etiology of IPH is not known. A hereditary or familial tendency has been suggested. An immunologic cause seems likely because other occasional findings include positive Coombs' test results, the presence of cold agglutinins, and an increased number of mast and plasma cells in the lungs. Various etiologic hypotheses such as congenital weakness or fragility of the capillaries, milk allergy, and abnormal growth and function of alveolar epithelial cells have all been suggested.[275] Cow's milk pulmonary vasculitis as the cause of pulmonary hemosiderosis remains a popular theory.[276]

The most helpful clinical signs for identifying IPH are iron deficiency anemia and recurrent or chronic cough, hemoptysis, dyspnea, wheezing, and frequently cyanosis. Any single feature may be present without the others. For example, occasionally the only clinical sign is iron deficiency anemia.[277] Pulmonary symptoms may be present without radiologic findings and vice versa. When pulmonary symptoms are predominant, there may be associated fever, tachycardia, tachypnea, leukocytosis, an elevated sedimentation rate, and occasionally, abdominal pain.[278] Roentgenographic abnormalities vary from minimal transient infiltrates to massive parenchymal involvement with atelectasis, emphysema, and hilar adenopathy.[279,280]

The anemia reflects an iron deficiency state resulting from excessive accumulation of iron in the lungs. This iron is usually sequestered in alveolar macrophages and is largely unavailable for new red cell formation. With time, however, the iron is eventually lost from the lungs.[281] In some patients, iron administration fails to correct the anemia. This is usually a reflection of inadequate heme synthesis resulting from the anemia of chronic disorders. Immune hemolytic anemia may occur, and cold agglutinins are often present. Eosinophilia is found in 15% to 20% of children with IPH.

A diagnosis of IPH may be made by the finding of siderophages in the gastric aspirate. Siderophages will stain positive with Prussian blue dye. If the diagnosis of IPH is seriously being considered, it may be necessary to perform a lung biopsy. Typical findings include alveolar epithelial hyperplasia, degeneration with excessive shedding of cells, large numbers of siderocytes, varying amounts of interstitial fibrosis and mast cell accumulation, elastic fiber degeneration, and sclerotic vascular changes.[282] Electron microscopic examination shows no evidence of subendothelial deposits or basement membrane lesions.[283] No evidence for localization of immunoglobulin G (IgG), IgM, B_{1c}, C1q, or fibrinogen has been found.[281] The results of needle aspiration or needle biopsy may also provide a diagnosis,[284] although some workers have considered these procedures to be hazardous.

Treatment of IPH continues to be a controversial subject. Corticosteroid therapy will sometimes produce a remission of disease activity.[285,286] Immunosuppressive therapy may be useful, but the results of such treatment are unpredictable.[287,288] In 1962, Heiner and associates[289] reported the presence of precipitating antibodies to a small number of cow's milk antigens in the sera of several children with IPH. Reversal of symptoms followed withdrawal of cow's milk, and recurrence was noted with reinstitution of cow's milk in the diet. Although many, if not most children with IPH fail to show these responses, a trial of removal of cow's milk from the diet is appropriate in most instances.[290] Abstinence should be continued for 2 to 3 months.

Pulmonary Hemosiderosis from Other Causes

Clinical findings of hypochromic and microcytic anemia and pulmonary infiltrates may be seen in association with glomerulonephritis (Goodpasture's syndrome), collagen vascular disease (especially periarteritis nodosa), Wegener's granulomatosis, and occasionally, systemic lupus erythematosus.[291-294] Similar findings in association with anaphylactoid purpura have been noted. Episodes of pulmonary hemosiderosis have been described in subjects with cystic fibrosis and celiac disease.[295,296]

Hematologic Findings in Other Pulmonary Disorders

Sarcoidosis does not usually cause specific hematologic disturbances, although a higher than average incidence of blood group antigen A has been reported in this disorder.[297,298] Anemia and leukopenia have been reported in sarcoidosis. One study has suggested that 87% of affected patients will have hematologic abnormalities, the most common of which is anemia (28%). Bone marrow granulomas are noted occasionally.[299] The significance of this finding is not known, but the altered immune response of these patients[300] and an association of sarcoidosis with hemolytic anemia[301] and immune thrombocytopenia[302-304] suggest that sarcoidosis represents a generalized autoimmune disorder and that it may be related to abnormal balance of T-cell subset production. Severe thrombocytopenia may occur in subjects with sarcoidosis.[305]

Eosinophilia may be observed in a variety of pulmonary disorders, including asthma, Löffler's syndrome, tropical pulmonary eosinophilia, polyarteritis nodosa, and sarcoidosis.

Patients with cystic fibrosis demonstrate a significant impairment in erythropoietic response to hypoxemia.[306] There is neither an appropriate increase in hemoglobin level nor an adequate shift in the red cell–oxygen affinity curve. Failure of the hemoglobin-oxygen dissociation curve to compensate means that such patients may be more symptomatic at any given hemoglobin level than patients who have anemia and other disorders. Disturbances in erythropoietin regulation, as seen in the anemia of chronic disorders and iron deficiency, appear to be the principal cause of the relative anemia in children with cystic fibrosis.[307] If a severe hemolytic anemia is observed in a subject with cystic fibrosis, it may be related to vitamin E deficiency.[308]

COLLAGEN VASCULAR DISEASES AND THE ANEMIA OF CHRONIC DISORDERS

The anemia of chronic disorders and its concomitant reticuloendothelial siderosis are associated with a wide

TABLE 36-2	Findings in the Anemia of Chronic Disorders and Iron Deficiency	
Factor	Chronic Disease	Iron Deficiency
Plasma iron	↓	↓
Iron-binding capacity	↓	↑
Transferrin saturation	↓	↓
Marrow sideroblasts	↓	↓
Reticuloendothelial iron	Normal or ↑	↓
Free erythrocyte protoporphyrin	↑	↑
Serum ferritin	Normal	↓

variety of illnesses, including cancer, lymphoma, collagen vascular disease, severe tissue injuries, renal failure, and infectious processes.[309] Unfortunately, each of these disorders may be associated with multiple sources of anemia, including blood loss, hemolysis, and drug suppression. A diagnosis of anemia of chronic disorders should not be made without consideration of other potential causes.

The anemia of chronic disorders is usually mild. It is characterized by decreased plasma iron levels, decreased total iron-binding capacity of plasma, decreased saturation of transferrin by iron, reduced numbers of bone marrow sideroblasts, and normal or increased levels of reticuloendothelial iron (Table 36-2).[310]

The anemia, when it occurs, develops slowly over a period of a month or longer until a plateau is reached. The hematocrit rarely decreases to less than 30% in adults and the low 20% range in children. The anemia is most often normochromic and normocytic with a low or normal percentage of reticulocytes. Occasionally, hypochromic and normocytic anemia is observed; less often, hypochromia and microcytosis are found.[309] In contrast to the situation in iron deficiency anemia, the uncommon microcytosis of chronic disorders is rarely proportional to the degree of anemia associated with these conditions.

The pathophysiologic processes that cause the anemia of chronic disorders are complex. At least three factors are commonly operating: shortened red cell survival, impaired marrow response to anemia, and impaired flow of iron from reticuloendothelial cells to the bone marrow.

The shortening of red cell survival is not seen in the anemia of all chronic disorders.[311] Autologous survival may be mildly shortened, but when the red blood cells of an affected individual are transfused into normal recipients, survival is normal.[312] The nature of the extracorpuscular defect has not been defined.

Bone marrow fails to develop an erythropoietic response to the anemia. Although normal bone marrow can increase red blood cell production sixfold to eightfold, the maximum response in the anemia of chronic disorders is one to two times normal.

Studies of the release of erythropoietin have produced conflicting results. In some cases there appears to be defective production or release of erythropoietin.[313]

Response to erythropoietin has been noted in rats with chronic inflammatory reactions.[314] Cobalt, which acts by means of the production of cellular hypoxia and release of erythropoietin, improves the anemia of infection in dogs and humans.[315,316] However, some resistance to the effects of erythropoietin is seen that probably relates to the block of iron release to transferrin.[317]

An impairment in iron release from the reticuloendothelial system accounts for the iron-deficient type of erythropoiesis seen in these disorders. This block in iron utilization is most easily demonstrated by iron kinetic studies in which plasma iron clearance is normal but the presence of iron in circulating red blood cells (utilization) is markedly diminished.[318,319] The consequences of this blockage are a decrease in plasma iron levels, a decrease in marrow sideroblasts, and an increase in red cell protoporphyrin concentration, all in the presence of normal or increased reticuloendothelial iron.

Iron absorption in the anemia of chronic disorders may be either normal or diminished. Diminished absorption is not due to defective uptake of iron into intestinal cells but rather results from an inability to release intracellular iron.[320] In any event, sufficient iron is absorbed to maintain adequate reticuloendothelial stores.

The reduced levels of plasma transferrin so commonly noted may be due to diminished production or to increased binding to iron-overloaded reticuloendothelial cells.[309] The latter cause may, in fact, be more important because transferrin levels tend to increase in the anemia of chronic disorders if iron deficiency develops.

There has been a common clinical impression that the degree of anemia associated with inflammation may vary with the specific cause of the inflammation. If the cause of the inflammation is infectious, this impression may not be true. Subjects with meningitis, cellulitis, mastoiditis, septic arthritis, osteomyelitis, bacterial endocarditis, and streptococcal pharyngitis all experience a mean decrease in hemoglobin concentration of 1.8 g/dL during active inflammation over a 6-day period.[321] The anemia of mild viral infection is associated with a decrease in hemoglobin of 1.0 g/dL in 9% of individuals and greater than 0.6 g/dL in 24%. After the administration of live attenuated measles vaccine, 22% of infants overall are expected to be anemic. This anemia persists for 14 to 31 days.[322]

Diagnosis of the anemia of chronic disorders is based on the typical findings of a low plasma iron level, low plasma transferrin concentration, and a low percentage of marrow sideroblasts despite normal or increased reticuloendothelial iron levels (see Table 36-2). Bone marrow examination is not critical in establishing the diagnosis if a serum ferritin determination is obtained because the serum ferritin level is normal or increased in the anemia of chronic disorders,[323] even in the presence of hypoferremia. Plasma copper levels are usually increased.

No specific therapy is available for this anemia other than treatment of the basic disease. Iron therapy is of no value because when given either orally or by intramuscular injection, the iron is first cleared in the reticuloendothelial system. Intravenous iron infusions would most probably improve marrow iron delivery but are neither practical nor therapeutically indicated for this problem. Occasionally, a patient with the anemia of chronic disorders is also iron deficient, particularly one with rheumatoid arthritis,[324] in whom gastrointestinal bleeding caused by aspirin therapy is common. Such a patient may respond partially to iron therapy.

Readers interested in a comprehensive review of the anemia of chronic disorders are referred to Hansen's 1983 report[325] and Chapter 12.

Hematologic Aspects of Collagen Vascular Disease

Many of the hematologic manifestations of the various collagen vascular diseases are similar. However, the characteristics that are unique to each syndrome are emphasized in this section.

Rheumatoid Arthritis

The most common causes of anemia in rheumatoid arthritis are the anemia of chronic disorders and iron deficiency. These two causes can be difficult to distinguish because of overlap in many of the laboratory findings. In both instances, the serum iron level is depressed, and free erythrocyte protoporphyrin levels are elevated. The serum ferritin level may be normal in the iron deficiency associated with rheumatoid arthritis.[324] In the absence of iron deficiency, the anemia of rheumatoid arthritis can be corrected with recombinant erythropoietin therapy.[326]

A high incidence of iron deficiency is seen in children with rheumatoid arthritis, possibly secondary to the ingestion of large quantities of aspirin or in part to defective iron absorption. Koerper and co-workers[324] found that a serum ferritin concentration less than 25 ng/mL was useful in predicting a response to oral iron, but a value greater than 25 ng/mL does not preclude a response.[325] Laboratory tests often fail to distinguish between iron deficiency and the anemia of chronic disorders, so a clinical trial of iron therapy may be necessary. Because medicinal iron may be absorbed poorly in subjects with chronic inflammatory states, low-dose intravenous iron may be used effectively.[327]

Microcytosis is very common in juvenile chronic forms of arthritis, with a rate of occurrence of about 40%. The degree of microcytosis relates directly to disease activity.[328] Occasionally, macrocytic anemia develops in patients with juvenile rheumatoid arthritis.[329] Although abnormal vitamin B_{12} metabolism has been suggested as a cause, this is not seen in children. Folate metabolism may, however, be abnormal. Some children with rheumatoid arthritis have diminished plasma and red cell folate levels.[330] Increased folic acid plasma clearance and reduced protein binding have also been observed.[331]

A few patients have had mild shortening of red cell survival as a result of an extracorpuscular defect.[332] More severe hemolytic anemia is much less common than in other collagen vascular diseases. Erythroid aplasia responsive to corticosteroid therapy has been reported in a child with juvenile rheumatoid arthritis.[333] Circulating inhibitors of erythropoiesis have also been noted.[334]

Leukocytosis and neutrophilia are common during acute flare-ups of juvenile rheumatoid arthritis; however, this is uncommon in the adult form of the disorder. Neutrophil chemotaxis may be mildly diminished.[335] Phagocytosis is normal or mildly impaired.[336] Nitroblue tetrazolium dye reduction may be increased during active phases of this disease.[337] These minimal alterations in white cell function do not produce any clinical disturbances. Wound healing, for example, is normal even after surgery in patients who have not been receiving high-dose corticosteroid therapy.[338] A peripheral blood eosinophil count greater than 5% has been noted in slightly more than 50% of children with juvenile rheumatoid arthritis.[339] Some will also demonstrate basophilia and plasmacytoid lymphocytes.[340,341]

A consumptive coagulopathy may be seen in association with systemic juvenile rheumatoid arthritis.[342-344] Acquired circulating inhibitor to factor VIII has been described in juvenile rheumatoid arthritis and may cause bleeding.[343] Clinical problems related to coagulation abnormalities in this disorder are rare, however.[344]

Transient thrombocytopenia may be observed in systemic-onset juvenile rheumatoid arthritis. It need not be an autoimmune form of thrombocytopenia.[345]

The symptoms and signs of rheumatoid arthritis can be very similar to those of acute lymphatic leukemia and include fever, joint pain, and anemia. Therefore, the diagnosis of acute lymphatic leukemia should be excluded before treatment of rheumatoid arthritis is instituted.

Elevated platelet counts occur in many patients with juvenile rheumatoid arthritis. No consistent functional defects have been described.

Felty's Syndrome

Felty[346] originally described the triad of rheumatoid arthritis, splenomegaly, and neutropenia in 1924. Whether Felty's syndrome occurs with juvenile rheumatoid arthritis is unclear. Splenomegaly is seen in about 20% of all children with rheumatoid arthritis and especially in those with the acute extra-articular exacerbations of this disease. However, splenomegaly alone does not suggest Felty's syndrome.

The neutropenia of Felty's syndrome is not a consequence of hypersplenism per se because only 60% of adults who undergo splenectomy experience resolution of their neutropenia.[347] In some patients, bone marrow demonstrates granulocyte arrest. Neutropenia in association with cytotoxic lymphocytes directed against granulocyte progenitors has also been reported.[348] Lower than normal levels of granulocyte colony-stimulating activity have been reported rarely.[349] The neutropenia of Felty's syndrome may represent, in part, an immunologic phenomenon because IgG antibodies directed against neutrophils have been observed in the sera of patients with rheumatoid arthritis.[350,351]

The neutropenia may be associated with serious infections. Splenectomy may be indicated in these circumstances because a favorable response may be observed, but the response is variable. The most consistent result is a reduction in serum granulocyte-binding immunoglobulin.[352] An alternative to splenectomy is the use of granulocyte colony-stimulating factor, which has been effective in some patients.[353-355]

Systemic Lupus Erythematosus

Anemia is the most common hematologic abnormality in systemic lupus erythematosus.[356,357] There are multiple causes of anemia in this disease, although the anemia of chronic disorders is probably the most common.

Acquired immune hemolytic anemia may precede the onset of active lupus. Although positive results on an antiglobulin test are common (either to γ-globulin, complement, or both), true hemolysis is seen in less than 10% of patients.[358]

Aplastic anemia has been reported in association with lupus but appears to be more common in scleroderma.[359]

A reduction in the total white blood cell count is seen in most patients but is more common in adults than children. The leukopenia is usually caused by a combination of decreased numbers of granulocytes and lymphocytes.[360] Antibodies to granulocytes have been proposed as one mechanism for the granulocytopenia. Granulocyte antibodies and peripheral granulocyte destruction have been observed.[361] Bone marrow depression of granulocyte formation may also occur. Sera from patients with systemic lupus erythematosus can inhibit mouse bone marrow colony-forming units.[362] Qualitative abnormalities in granulocyte function have also been noted. Although several investigators have found no abnormalities in chemotaxis,[335,363] others have observed abnormal migration by the skin window technique and diminished in vitro phagocytosis.[364,365] These defects parallel the observed depressions in complement. The qualitative defects in granulocyte function may be the result of altered humoral factors rather than defects in the phagocytic cells themselves.

Lymphopenia may be severe in lupus[366] and is sometimes due to IgG or IgM antilymphocyte antibodies.[367-369] In contrast to the depression of T and B cells, the percentage and absolute number of null cells increase.[370] The magnitude of the reduction in T cells parallels disease activity and is associated with defects in cellular immunity as measured by skin tests of delayed hypersensitivity, blast transformation in response to mitogen (phytohemagglutinin and concanavalin A), and macrophage-

inhibiting factor production.[366,371] Unlike T-cell function, B-cell function is increased despite the decrease in the absolute number of B cells.[372,373] There is actually an increase in IgG-synthesizing peripheral blood lymphocytes, as well as elevated numbers of cells capable of binding native DNA and elevated numbers of IgM- and IgG-producing cells with antibody specificity against DNA antigen.[374,375] These changes in peripheral blood lymphocytes are associated with certain morphologic alterations. A strongly basophilic cytoplasm and a high nuclear-to-cytoplasmic ratio are noted in many lymphocytes thought to be "immunoblasts."[376] On electron microscopic examination, inclusions are identified within lymphocytes that appear as undulating tubules characteristically associated with the endoplasmic reticulum.

Platelet survival is shortened, and there are increased numbers of bone marrow megakaryocytes. The platelet antibody is an IgG with a molecular mass of 150,000 to 330,000 daltons, and it binds complement.[377] The latter feature distinguishes the immune thrombocytopenia of systemic lupus erythematosus from that of idiopathic thrombocytopenic purpura.[378,379] Danazol may have several serologic effects in patients with systemic lupus erythematosus, including a decrease in DNA antibodies and antiplatelet antibodies. This drug has shown some therapeutic effectiveness in patients with this disease who have immune complex–mediated thrombocytopenia.[380] A qualitative defect in platelet function may also be present.[381] Patients with systemic lupus erythematosus may have a serum inhibitor of platelet aggregation.[382] Thrombocytopenia may be seen in association with systemic lupus erythematosus and the lupus anticoagulant.[383]

Patients with systemic lupus erythematosus may also have a circulating anticoagulant in their plasma.[384,385] The incidence of this anticoagulant in children is unknown, but it is seen in 5% to 10% of adults with this disease.[386] The prevalence of thrombosis in children with lupus anticoagulant is not known. In adults, the prevalence of thrombosis is about 30%, with the predominant site being the legs in 66%, followed by the peripheral arteries in 10% and the cerebral arteries in 2%.[387] The anticoagulant inhibits the interaction between the prothrombin activator (factor V, factor Xa, phospholipid, and calcium complex) and prothrombin, but the exact molecular substrate against which it is directed is not known.[388] Most investigators have reported that lupus anticoagulant is an immunoglobulin that may be of the IgG, IgM, or mixed IgG-IgM class.[389-392] In addition to the inhibitor itself, a cofactor in normal plasma is necessary for maximal action of the lupus anticoagulant. This cofactor, which may be a γ-globulin, potentiates the inhibitory action of lupus anticoagulant.[393]

The partial thromboplastin time is invariably prolonged in patients with the lupus anticoagulant and is considered to be the most sensitive screening test.[386] The inhibitor is suspected when the addition of normal plasma to the patient's plasma fails to correct the defect.[389]

The prothrombin time in patients with the lupus anticoagulant is often normal or minimally prolonged because of the influence of the inhibitor. True prothrombin deficiency may occur in patients with the inhibitor, but it is rare.[394,395]

Prolonged thrombin times in the absence of elevated levels of fibrin split products may occasionally be seen.[396] The exact significance of this finding is unclear.

Lupus anticoagulant is usually found coincidentally on routine coagulation screening.[397] Bleeding is a rare manifestation, and patients have undergone surgery without unusual postoperative bleeding.[398] In fact, some patients with lupus anticoagulant may manifest thrombotic events, a situation observed with other inhibitors,[399] particularly if the inhibitor has activity against antithrombin III.

Renal involvement with some types of microangiopathy has been associated with the presence of antiphospholipid antibodies in patients with systemic lupus erythematosus and in those with other types of connective tissue disorders.[400]

Because bleeding is rarely a problem as a consequence of the presence of the inhibitor, specific therapy is not generally indicated.

Polyarteritis Nodosa

Anemia resulting from a chronic disease state is seen occasionally in patients with polyarteritis nodosa. A more common occurrence is microangiopathic hemolytic anemia in association with renal disease or hypertensive crises. The hemolytic process in these circumstances parallels disease activity. Neutropenia occurs and is associated with the presence of antineutrophil cytoplasmic antibodies.[401]

Neutrophilia and eosinophilia are also common. The eosinophilia may be extensive, with levels suggesting eosinophilic leukemia or Löffler's endocarditis often being reached. Marked eosinophilia is generally restricted to patients with clinically apparent pulmonary involvement.

Wegener's Granulomatosis

Wegener's granulomatosis, characterized by necrotizing vasculitis (particularly in the lungs and kidneys), is rare but can affect children.[402,403] The disease can also occur in the newborn period.[404] The course of the disease is marked by fever, cough, hemoptysis, epistaxis, nasal discharge, obliteration of the nasal sinuses, and nodular pulmonary infiltrates. Renal failure may occur. As with most chronic disease states, normochromic, normocytic anemia develops.[405] The peripheral blood smear may demonstrate anisocytosis, poikilocytosis, and marked fragmentation reflective of a microangiopathic process associated with vasculitis.[406] Hemolytic anemia with splenomegaly that gives negative Coombs' test results may be present.[405] The white blood cell count is elevated, and eosinophilia can occur.[407] The disease is characterized by marked thrombocytosis.[405] Various immunosuppressive

therapies have been attempted. Cyclophosphamide is occasionally effective in the management of children with Wegener's granulomatosis.[408] Autoantibodies directed against cytoplasmic components of neutrophil granulocytes and monocytes have been described as a disease-specific marker for Wegener's granulomatosis.[409,410]

The hematologic manifestations of these disorders are relatively nonspecific. No consistent hematologic abnormalities are recorded in polymyositis and dermatomyositis. Scleroderma may result in malabsorption of vitamin B_{12}, but this disease is rare in children. Coagulation abnormalities may be seen with scleroderma. Elevations in levels of factor VIII–related antigen and β-thromboglobulin are often noted. Additionally, about half of subjects with active disease show elevations in levels of fibrin degradation products.[411] Autoimmune hemolytic anemia and thrombocytopenia may also be seen in patients with scleroderma,[412] and some will have autoimmune neutropenia.[413] The hematologic manifestations of scleroderma, particularly the magnitude of elevated factor VIII–related antigen levels, may be used as a marker for disease activity.[414]

INFECTIONS

General Hematologic Signs of Infection

Red Blood Cell Disturbances

The pathophysiologic findings of the anemia of chronic infection are similar to those of the anemia of chronic disorders. Although some infections, particularly viral ones, cause transient bone marrow aplasia or selective erythroid aplasia, anemia from this cause is rare because of the long life span of red blood cells. In contrast, patients with hemolytic anemia may experience a rapid decrease in hemoglobin concentration during viral and some bacterial infections. This is especially common in association with infectious episodes caused by parvovirus. Such infections should be considered in any child with a congenital hemolytic anemia who experiences an "aplastic" crisis.

Even common childhood infections, especially those associated with inflammation, will cause a decline in hemoglobin concentration. During active inflammation, the hemoglobin concentration declines about 13%, usually within 1 week, followed by an increase of nearly 25% during resolution of the active inflammation.[321]

Severe hemolytic anemia may be observed in certain types of infections. Clostridial infections may result in a high titer of hemolysins and cause severe anemia with hemoglobinemia and hemoglobinuria.[415] A similar severe anemia may result from sepsis related to other bacterial organisms, including staphylococci, streptococci, pneumococci, and *Haemophilus influenzae*.[416] Immune hemolytic anemia mediated by a cold agglutinin may be observed with *Listeria* and *Mycoplasma* infections[417] and occasionally with infections by other organisms such as Epstein-Barr virus (EBV).

Many viral illnesses may be associated with what appears to be a mild hemolytic anemia for which no pathologic mechanism has been defined. The most common morphologic finding in these circumstances is poikilocytosis. Certain viruses, such as most strains of influenza virus, contain neuraminidase activity, which is, at least theoretically, capable of affecting the sialic acid content of the red cell membrane. Whether this plays any significant role in the hemolysis associated with some viral diseases is not known.

Many congenital infections, including cytomegalovirus, herpes simplex, rubella, toxoplasmosis, and syphilis, produce profound hemolytic anemia in the newborn period, even though these same agents may not significantly alter red cell survival at other times of life. The explanation for this finding is also unclear.

Finally, anemia may result from blood loss associated with intestinal parasitic infestation.

White Blood Cell Disturbances

The white blood cell count may be normal, low, or high with infection. Viral illnesses may be associated with leukocyte counts lower than 5000 cells/mm^3, although bacterial diseases of certain types or overwhelming sepsis of any type may also cause leukopenia. The most common viral illnesses associated with leukopenia are infectious hepatitis, infectious mononucleosis, rubella, measles, and occasionally, influenza. Of the bacterial infections, shigellosis may produce leukopenia with a marked increase in band cell forms. Sepsis caused by meningococci, pneumococci, staphylococci, and a few other bacterial pathogens may also cause leukopenia.

Neutrophilia, with or without an increase in band cell count, is a common result of bacterial infection. White blood cell counts do not differ between white and black children with bacteremia, and the total white blood cell count and neutrophil counts may be interpreted without regard to race.[418] Occasionally, viral illness will also initially be manifested as neutrophilia. A variety of morphologic changes may appear in the neutrophils of patients with infection. Döhle bodies, pale blue cyst-like inclusion bodies usually located in the periphery of the cytoplasm of neutrophils, may appear in bacterial infections.[419] They are occasionally associated with viral illness but are also commonly seen in patients with burns, massive trauma, and cancer, as well as in pregnancy and after the use of cyclophosphamide.[419] In addition, Döhle bodies are seen in the May-Hegglin anomaly.[420] Increased size of neutrophil granules ("toxic granulation") may be seen in both bacterial and viral illnesses, as well as in many of the other disorders associated with the presence of Döhle bodies. Vacuolization of the cytoplasm of neutrophils is the next most common morphologic abnormality of neutrophils in patients with significant bacteremia. In a study of the neutrophils of patients with bacteremia, Zipursky and associates[421] found toxic granulation, Döhle bodies,

and vacuolization in 75%, 29%, and 24%, respectively, of the patients studied.

Increased neutrophil alkaline phosphatase activity and nitroblue tetrazolium dye reduction may also occur,[422,423] but neither of these characteristics is specific for bacterial infection. Infections may be associated with development of the Pelger-Huët anomaly, in which granulocytes and eosinophils have one or two lobes per nucleus and assume a round, dumbbell, or peanut shape.[424] This is most commonly observed with tuberculosis. The Pelger-Huët anomaly is seen in 1 in 6000 people as an autosomal disorder and is also occasionally observed in patients with preleukemia, leukemia, and other cancers and in those taking colchicine and sulfonamide medications.[424]

In newborns, especially those born prematurely, an increase in total white cell or mature neutrophil counts may not be seen in the presence of infection. In fact, a decrease in the neutrophil count often occurs. The most helpful signs of septicemia in this age group are an increase in the band cell count and the presence of toxic granulations and Döhle bodies.[421,425]

Leukocytosis may result from lymphocytosis. The most common infections producing the greatest increases in lymphocyte counts are infectious mononucleosis, cat-scratch disease, "acute infectious lymphocytosis of childhood," and pertussis. Many other viral illnesses such as cytomegalovirus, rubella, mumps, and hepatitis may also cause an increase in the lymphocyte count. T lymphopenia is a common finding after measles infection. It is predominantly due to suppression of OKT4$^+$ lymphocytes.[426]

Eosinophilia may reflect the presence of parasitic infections. In the United States, the most common cause of marked elevations in eosinophil counts is *Toxocara* infestation, which is often accompanied by high titers of isohemagglutinins. Other parasites commonly causing eosinophilia include organisms belonging to *Trichinella*, *Echinococcus*, *Filaria*, *Strongyloides*, *Schistosoma*, *Enterobius*, and *Ancylostoma* and tapeworms other than *Echinococcus*. Allergic sensitization to mites may cause eosinophilia, as well as fungal infections, especially aspergillosis.[427] Eosinophilia is, of course, not specific for infestation. Marked degrees of eosinophilia may occur in association with prematurity. An absolute eosinophilia may be expected in about 75% of low-birth-weight infants.[428] In some, the eosinophilia is marked (>3000 cells/mm^3), and the maximal increase seems to occur at about the time that birth weight is regained, although this is not true in all infants.[429]

Monocytosis is occasionally seen with specific infections, especially tuberculosis, syphilis, and subacute bacterial endocarditis. Monocytosis is often noted early in the course of many infections and again on recovery, particularly if it is associated with granulocytopenia.

Basophilia is rarely seen in infection but has been reported with tuberculosis, influenza, and hookworm infestation.[430]

Clotting Abnormalities and Thrombocytopenia

DIC may be triggered by infectious processes. Of the infectious causes, gram-negative septicemia is probably most common. *Meningococcus, Escherichia coli, Proteus, Pseudomonas, Aerobacter,* and *Klebsiella* are among the most common etiologic agents recovered from the bloodstream.[431,432] Gram-positive septicemia can cause a similar picture. The most common offender is *Diplococcus pneumoniae*, especially in asplenic individuals. Other gram-positive agents causing DIC include *Staphylococcus aureus, Streptococcus,* and *Clostridium*. A wide range of viral infections may cause a consumptive coagulopathy that often leads to purpura fulminans. Among the most common agents are those that cause infectious hepatitis, measles, rubella, varicella, and infectious mononucleosis. Less common causes of DIC are severe mycoplasmal, rickettsial, and malarial infections.

Thrombocytopenia occurring separately from a true disseminated consumptive process is quite common in many infectious processes, especially in association with infectious mononucleosis, cytomegalovirus infection, rubella, measles, gram-negative bacteria, and rickettsial diseases. Congenital viral infections and congenital syphilis and toxoplasmosis, if clinically apparent, are almost invariably associated with increased platelet turnover with or without thrombocytopenia. Thrombocytopenia may occur after immunization with live viral vaccines, particularly measles vaccines.[433] Corrigan[434] found that thrombocytopenia without consumptive coagulopathy is an extremely common finding in infants and children with septicemia. In contrast, thrombocytosis is often present during the active phases of infectious processes. The platelet distribution width and mean platelet volume may be helpful in predicting whether the thrombocytopenia is due to infection. In the late neonatal period, thrombocytopenia associated with an infection dramatically increases the mean platelet volume and platelet distribution width as determined by electronic counting equipment.[435]

Immune complex–mediated thrombocytopenia is commonly associated with a variety of infectious agents.[436]

Hematologic Aspects of Selected Specific Infections

Certain infectious processes are associated with specific or unique hematologic findings distinct from those described in the preceding section. Such infections include *Bordetella pertussis* (pertussis or whooping cough), *Salmonella typhi* (typhoid fever), *Mycobacterium tuberculosis* (tuberculosis), *Plasmodium falciparum* (malaria), *Clostridium perfringens,* and *Bartonella bacilliformis* (bartonellosis or Carrión's disease).

Typhoid fever produces remarkable leukopenia and neutropenia early in the course of the illness. The number of bone marrow precursor cells is increased. A high white blood cell count in this disease usually suggests a secondary bacterial infection. The leukopenia of typhoid fever is often associated with thrombocytopenia. Shigellosis may also be associated with leukopenia. The hallmark of *Shigella* infection, however, is a sharp increase in the band cell count.

In the pediatric age group, *C. perfringens* infections are most common in adolescent girls who have undergone septic abortion. This organism has a potent exotoxin, a lecithinase, that disrupts cell membranes and liberates hemolytic material such as lysolecithins. Such disruption may result in fatal intravascular hemolytic anemia with spherocytosis.[415]

Pertussis may cause a marked increase in the white blood cell count, with elevations to 40,000 cells/mm³ or higher, most of which is due to an increase in the lymphocyte count.

Tuberculosis produces a variety of hematologic abnormalities. Leukemoid reactions mimicking myeloproliferative disorders are common.[437] Bone marrow involvement in miliary tuberculosis may result in a leukoerythroblastic pattern with teardrop-shaped red cells, nucleated red cells, and myeloblasts apparent on the peripheral blood smear.[438] In this respect, the manifestation of tuberculosis is similar to some occurrences of sarcoidosis. Bone marrow biopsy may show evidence of granulomas. Monocytosis is common, and thrombocytopenia and pancytopenia have been reported.[439]

Bartonellosis is a disease transmitted by the sandfly and is associated with potentially severe hemolytic anemia. It was first recognized in 1885 when a medical student inoculated himself with the *Bartonella* organism. The student, Daniel Carrión, died of severe hemolytic anemia. For this reason, human bartonellosis caused by *B. bacilliformis* is still called Carrión's disease.[440] This organism infects red blood cells, coats them (Fig. 36-2), and causes them to be rapidly removed from the circula-

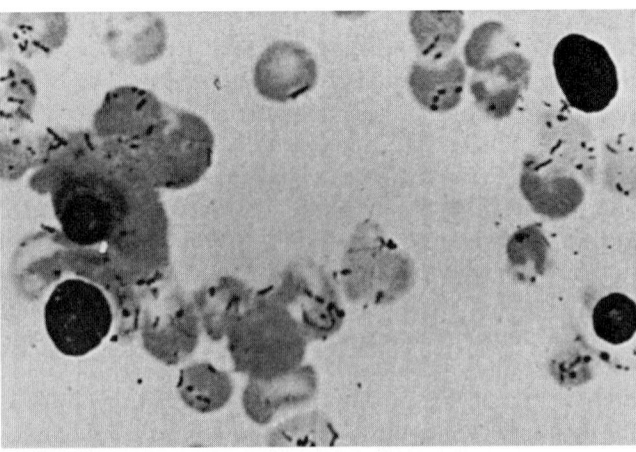

FIGURE 36-2. Parasitism of red blood cells in human *Bartonella* infection. *(From Ricketts WE. Bartonella bacilliformis anemia [Oroya fever]: a study of thirty cases. Blood. 1948;3:1025-1049.)*

tion. Unlike malarial organisms, *Bartonella* organisms do not invade the red blood cell.[441]

Hemolysis is common in malaria, especially with infection by *P. falciparum*.[442] This disease, transmitted by *Anopheles* mosquitoes, results in parasitization with organisms at the merozoite stage within the red cell. The parasitization causes altered permeability and increased osmotic fragility.[443] The presence of the organism within the cell is also reflected in a defect in red cell membrane shape. Hemolysis in malaria has been attributed to direct damage to the red cell by the parasite, to autoimmune destruction, to hypersplenism, to splenic pitting with the formation of microspherocytes, and to loss of the cell surface negative charge resulting from alteration of the cell's metabolic function by the parasite.[444-446] In addition to destroying infected cells, the spleen may merely remove the offending organisms and leave membrane pits or cavities that may be seen on scanning electron microscopic examination.[447] A particularly severe form of hemolysis called blackwater fever may occur with *P. falciparum* infection. The basis of the massive hemolysis is unknown. *Babesia* and *Babesia*-like infections produce intraerythrocytic merozoite forms similar to those seen in malaria. These infections may also cause hemolytic anemia and DIC.[448]

Infectious Mononucleosis

There is unequivocal evidence that links infectious mononucleosis to EBV. Before etiologic evidence was established, the diagnosis of infectious mononucleosis was based on the triad of (1) a classic clinical picture, (2) atypical lymphocytosis, and (3) positive results on a heterophil antibody test.[449] It was maintained that absence of any one of these three would negate the diagnosis. Serologic testing for EBV has helped explain certain puzzling diagnostic features. For example, it was previously not recognized that children younger than 5 years often contract infectious mononucleosis. The results of a heterophil antibody test are usually negative in this age group, but antibody to EBV is seen. This specific serologic test also explains some occurrences in adults who seem to have a typical clinical picture of infectious mononucleosis and demonstrate atypical lymphocytosis but whose heterophil test results are negative. The masquerading disease is cytomegalovirus infection in most instances.

History

The major landmarks in the diagnosis of infectious mononucleosis have occurred in three areas. The first was the emergence of this disease as a separate clinical entity. The second was establishment of a diagnostic test, the heterophil antibody test, and the third was identification of EBV as an etiologic agent.

The history spans about 100 years. The earliest clinical descriptions are found in writings of Filatov[450] in 1885 and Pfeiffer[451] in 1889. The disease was initially termed

glandular fever until 1920, when Sprunt and Evans,[452] appreciating the presence of the now well-known atypical lymphocytosis, coined the name infectious mononucleosis.

The serendipitous discovery of the heterophil antibody was surpassed only by that of EBV as an etiologic agent. By the 1920s, the occurrence of sheep cell antibodies in serum sickness was well known. Because of similarities in the symptomatology of serum sickness and rheumatic fever, Paul[453] began to look for these antibodies in patients with rheumatic fever. Little came of the primary purpose of this study, but one day, as part of this investigation, Paul and Bunnell[454] found that a control serum sample had an extraordinarily high titer of heterophil antibody. This control serum was from a medical student who had typical infectious mononucleosis. Davidsohn and Lee[455] completed this phase of the story in 1937 when they organized the differential absorption procedures.

The etiologic agent of infectious mononucleosis eluded investigators for half a century. In 1958, Burkitt[456] described African children with the lymphoma now bearing his name. Because the distribution pattern of the disease coincided with the African mosquito belt, many investigators believed that a viral agent might be the cause of this lymphoma. After successful culturing of this tumor tissue in 1964, Epstein and associates[457] noted herpes-like virus particles in the tissues of patients with this lymphoma. By 1966, the Henles and their associates[458,459] had developed an indirect immunofluorescence test to detect this viral particle, which was already called the Epstein-Barr virus. With this test, EBV antibody was found to be present in many healthy American children. A fortunate chance occurrence was observed when infectious mononucleosis developed in a technician in the Henles' laboratory. Her white cells, which previously could not be grown in culture, now grew in continuous culture, and demonstrable EBV antibody was noted. With sera that had been obtained previously from Yale University students, a clear correlation linking EBV with the clinical appearance of infectious mononucleosis was found.[460]

Epidemiology

EBV infection is acquired at an early age in lower socioeconomic groups. In economically privileged children, infection is often delayed until adolescence and young adulthood. About 40% of American children are seropositive for EBV by 5 years of age.[461-463] In a report from the U.S. Military Academy at West Point, 63.5% of entering cadets had EBV antibody, indicative of previous infection.[464] During the college years, the infection rate among susceptible individuals is 12% to 15% per year. The pattern of infection in different groups of susceptible persons is probably best explained by transmission of this virus in throat secretions. Low titers of infectious virus in throat specimens account for the moderate contagiousness of this infection and the requirement of intimate contact for transmission. Thus, infection might be more common at younger ages in lower socioeconomic groups because of a greater opportunity for oral or oral/fecal transmission.

Another possible route of transmission of EBV is transfusion. EBV is carried in circulating white blood cells. In 1942, Wising[465] suggested that infectious mononucleosis could be transferred by blood transfusions. Subsequently, it was demonstrated that in approximately 8% of individuals undergoing cardiopulmonary bypass, EBV antibody developed in the postoperative period.[466] EBV does not appear, however, to be the cause of postperfusion syndrome, which is most likely due to cytomegalovirus. Except for a rare instance in which a clinical manifestation of infectious mononucleosis appeared after transfusion of blood from a donor with this disorder, clinical disease from transfusion-transmitted EBV is largely unknown.

EBV is present in the saliva of most patients with infectious mononucleosis, in up to 20% of healthy persons with EBV antibodies, and in 50% or more of seropositive patients receiving immunosuppressive drugs. The ease with which EBV is recovered from the oral secretions of persons with primary or reactivated EBV infection suggests that a cell type that freely permits EBV replication exists in the oropharynx. The oropharyngeal epithelial cell may be the target cell type that is productively infected in infectious mononucleosis.[467] Transmission requires intimate contact, so there is no significant spread of EBV in the school setting. Intrafamilial spread, however, does occur frequently, and in this setting an incubation period of 4 to 6 weeks has been demonstrated.[468]

It has been suggested that EBV infection may be transmitted congenitally.[469,470] A fatal illness in a 2-week-old infant in whom EBV genomes were detected in a lymph node biopsy specimen has been described.[471] Such occurrences, if representative of true congenital EBV infection, must be rare. A study of 4063 pregnant women showed that only 1.1% were susceptible to infection early in gestation and less than 0.1% showed seroconversion. Two of three infants born of women who seroconverted were normal, but one had tricuspid atresia. None of the infants could be demonstrated to be actively infected.[472,473] Similar findings have been found by others.[474]

The relationship of infectious mononucleosis to other disorders known to be associated with EBV infection or virus isolation is unclear. Such disorders include nasopharyngeal carcinoma, in addition to Burkitt's African lymphoma.[475] A higher than anticipated association of EBV with sarcoidosis,[476] leprosy,[477] and systemic lupus erythematosus[478] has been observed, although any specific relationship to these disorders remains speculative.[479]

In patients who undergo renal transplantation, a spectrum of lymphoproliferative diseases may occur as a result of activation of EBV. These diseases may vary from an infectious mononucleosis–like polyclonal B-cell proliferation to a monoclonal B-cell lymphoma. Therapeutic approaches to this problem usually fail.[480] Acyclovir therapy may be helpful early in the course of illness. When frank malignancy has developed, chemotherapy is suggested.

Clinical Features

The classic clinical manifestation of infectious mononucleosis is generally seen only in adolescents and young adults. Younger children rarely exhibit the typical findings of this disease, and most generally have only a mild viral respiratory illness.[461-463]

The onset of typical illness is usually a subtle prodrome consisting of fatigue, malaise, sweating, feverishness, and anorexia. As with infectious hepatitis, a distaste for cigarettes is common. Headache, nausea, and vomiting are seen frequently. The most common symptom during this period is a sore throat, which begins slowly and increases in intensity over a 1-week period. The usual findings of infectious mononucleosis then follow (Table 36-3). The course of fever often follows a specific pattern, with no temperature elevation in the morning but daily

TABLE 36-3	Infectious Mononucleosis—Approximate Rate of Occurrence of Various Signs and Symptoms in Young Adults
Symptom or Sign	**%**
Adenopathy	100
Malaise and fatigue	90-100
Fever	80-95
Sweats	80-95
Sore throat, dysphagia	80-95
Pharyngitis	65-85
Anorexia	50-80
Nausea	50-70
Splenomegaly	50-60
Headache	40-70
Chills	40-60
Bradycardia	35-50
Cough	30-50
Periorbital edema	25-40
Palatal enanthema	25-35
Liver or splenic tenderness	15-30
Myalgia	12-30
Hepatomegaly	15-25
Rhinitis	10-25
Ocular muscle pain	10-20
Chest pain	5-20
Jaundice	5-10
Arthralgia	5-10
Diarrhea or soft stools	5-10
Photophobia	5-10
Rash	3-6
Conjunctivitis	5
Abdominal pain	5
Gingivitis	3
Pneumonitis	3
Epistaxis	3

From Finch SC. Clinical symptoms and signs of infectious mononucleosis. In Carter RL, Penman HG (eds). Infectious Mononucleosis. Oxford, Blackwell Scientific, 1969, p 35.

afternoon or evening peaks of 38.3° C to 39.4° C (101° F to 103° F). Occasionally, higher temperatures are observed. The fever usually lasts about 2 weeks.

Lymphadenopathy is seen in all patients. Symmetrical, moderately enlarged, discrete, slightly tender nodes, especially in the posterior cervical region, are most characteristic. Adenopathy is common in the axillary, epitrochlear, and inguinal areas. The nodes are not matted and do not show signs of heat, redness, or fluctuation. Rarely, enlargement of the mediastinal glands constitutes the only evidence of adenopathy and may be confused with a lymphomatous process.

Splenomegaly occurs in more than 50% of patients with infectious mononucleosis. The spleen is usually just barely palpable but on rare occasion may be quite large. It is smooth, soft to firm, and sometimes slightly tender. In a few patients, splenomegaly persists for months, but the most common situation is resolution by 2 to 3 weeks after onset of the illness.

Hepatomegaly occurs in about 20% of patients, and clinical jaundice is seen in 10%. The jaundice is invariably mild. Despite the low rate of occurrence of apparent hepatic dysfunction, virtually all patients with infectious mononucleosis demonstrate abnormal liver enzyme levels. Except in rare patients with acute liver failure, the hepatitis associated with this illness is self-limited. There is no evidence that chronic liver disease or cirrhosis results from infectious mononucleosis. Reye's syndrome has been reported in a child with infectious mononucleosis.[481]

Rashes occur occasionally, and their manifestation follows no particular pattern. The rash may be a diffuse, faint, erythematous or maculopapular eruption, or it may be urticarial, scarlatiniform, petechial, or herpetiform. In general, the rashes of infectious mononucleosis have no unique features and are of little or no help for diagnosis. Circulating immune complexes and complement sequence activation occur only when rashes are present.[482] If ampicillin is administered to patients with infectious mononucleosis, a rash will develop in 69% to 100%.[483] Other penicillins may cause this response, but less often. This rash is not a reagin-mediated allergic reaction, and these antibiotics may be administered subsequently without ill effect.

Only a few patients with infectious mononucleosis have no pharyngitis. Almost all demonstrate hyperplasia of the pharyngeal lymphoid follicles. The presence of an exudate is common, and membrane formation occurs frequently. The inflammation may be severe enough to cause respiratory obstruction. Peritonsillar abscesses may complicate the course of the illness.[484] A palatal enanthema is seen in about a third of patients and consists of crops of sharply circumscribed petechiae, symmetrically distributed at the junction of the soft palate. Unfortunately, such petechiae are not specific for infectious mononucleosis and have been described in rubella and other viral disorders. In fact, the entire pharyngeal manifestation of infectious mononucleosis is clinically indistinguishable from that of streptococcal disease.

Periorbital edema is not rare and occasionally leads to the erroneous suspicion that renal disease or hypoproteinemia is present. The edema is self-limited and lasts only a few days.

Complications

Much attention is paid to the complications associated with infectious mononucleosis, although their overall occurrence is low (Table 36-4).

The incidence of the neurologic complications reported varies from 0.37% to 7.3%, depending on the

TABLE 36-4	Infectious Mononucleosis—Reported Complications
Type of Complication	**Diagnosis or Description of Abnormalities**
Neurologic	Bell's palsy, cerebellar syndrome, encephalitis, encephalomyelitis, encephalomyelopathy, Guillain-Barré syndrome, meningitis, meningoencephalitis, myelitis, optic neuritis, peripheral neuritis, psychosis, radiculoneuritis
	Ataxia, positive Babinski's sign, coma, convulsions, diplopia, extraocular palsy, facial diplegia, hemiplegia, hyperesthesia, meningismus, mental confusion, nystagmus, papilledema, psychotic reaction, ptosis, respiratory paralysis, positive Romberg's sign, seizure, status epilepticus, scotomas
Cardiac	Electrocardiographic changes, myocarditis, pericarditis
Ocular	Conjunctivitis, diplopia, cyclic edema, hemianopia, lacrimal pericyclitis, nystagmus, optic neuritis, ptosis, retinal edema, retinal hemorrhage, retro-orbital pain, scotomas, uveitis
Respiratory	Laryngeal obstruction, peritonsillar abscess, pharyngeal edema, pleural effusion, pleuritis, pneumonitis
Hematologic	Acquired hemolytic anemia, agranulocytosis, eosinophilia, fibrinolysis, pancytopenia, splenic rupture, thrombocytopenia
Digestive	Esophageal varices, gingivitis, hepatic dysfunction, hepatic necrosis, jaundice, melena
Renal	Hematuria, hemoglobinuria, nephritis, nephrotic syndrome, porphyrinuria, proteinuria
Other	Bullous myringitis, endocervicitis, orchitis, otitis media, pancreatitis, porphyria, rashes

From Finch SC. Clinical symptoms and signs of infectious mononucleosis. In Carter RL, Penman HG (eds). Infectious Mononucleosis. Oxford, Blackwell Scientific, 1969, p 35.

series.[485] A not rare occurrence in adolescence is the "Alice in Wonderland" phenomenon in which objects are visualized in a very distorted fashion, with exaggerations in size, being either too large or too small.[486,487] A transverse myelopathy characterized by a sudden onset of profound weakness of the lower extremities and urinary retention may complicate the clinical course of infectious mononucleosis.[488] A list of the neurologic complications appears in Table 36-4.

Cardiac complications are rare and occur in 1% to 6% of reported series. They usually consist of only nonspecific T-wave changes or minor conduction abnormalities. Myocarditis and pericarditis are also rare.

Liver function abnormalities are rarely severe, although enzyme changes are common. Primary EBV infection has been associated with a Reye syndrome–like illness.[489] Severe liver dysfunction causing death is a common complication of EBV infection in the X-linked lymphoproliferative syndrome. Hepatic dysfunction is uniformly present with this disorder at the time of death and is the cause of death in about a third of such patients.[490] An unusual manifestation of infectious mononucleosis may be intense jaundice. It generally results from a combination of hemolysis and mild hepatitis.[491] Spontaneous rupture of the spleen may occur.[492] Respiratory difficulties usually consist of upper airway obstruction. Transient interstitial infiltrations, some with effusions, have been recorded. Infectious mononucleosis should be considered in the differential diagnosis of any child with pleural effusions.[493] Renal complications of infectious mononucleosis generally consist of hematuria associated with a mild nephritis. Not all occurrences have been clearly separated from poststreptococcal glomerulonephritis. Severe rhabdomyolysis can be associated on rare occasion with EBV infection.[494] Eye findings in infectious mononucleosis are unusual but may be significant when they do occur. Severe retinochoroiditis is such an ocular complication.[495] In some patients with infectious mononucleosis, a chronic fatigue syndrome will develop in which lethargy, particularly daytime lethargy, is seen for prolonged periods, often longer than a year.[496] The mechanism is not known, but the lethargy is often associated with serologic evidence of persistent infection.[497,498] Hematologic complications of infectious mononucleosis include disturbances resulting in anemia, granulocytopenia, thrombocytopenia, and occasional coagulation defects.

Anemia is rare. In approximately 3% of West Point cadets with infectious mononucleosis, anemia of the immune hemolytic type developed.[464] When hemolysis does occur, it usually begins 1 to 2 weeks into the course of the illness. The majority of occurrences terminate in less than 1 month, and chronic hemolysis is rare. Though usually mild, hemolysis occasionally occurs rapidly and can then result in severe anemia. Jenkins and associates in 1965[499] reported the first instance of hemolytic anemia in infectious mononucleosis that was mediated by the temporary induction of a high–thermal amplitude cold

agglutinin of anti-i specificity.[500] Since then, several series have verified the high incidence of anti-i antibody as the cause of hemolysis in infectious mononucleosis. It should be noted that although hemolysis is not common in infectious mononucleosis, the presence of anti-i in serum is seen in as many as 50% of all patients. Not all instances of immune hemolysis in infectious mononucleosis are caused by anti-i antibodies. Anti-N antibodies have also been reported, and in some patients the nature of the antibody has not been identified.[501]

Aplastic anemia has been reported to follow the onset of infectious mononucleosis.[502] Aplastic anemia caused by EBV infection has also been reported after bone marrow transplantation.[503] Localization of EBV in the bone marrow of some patients with aplastic anemia supports a causative role of the virus in this disorder.[504]

Granulocytopenia is common during the acute phase of infectious mononucleosis. It is rarely severe but on occasion is a cause of secondary bacterial infection.[505] Bone marrow myeloid hyperplasia with myeloid arrest is the most typical finding.[506] Spontaneous resolution is the rule.

Immune thrombocytopenia occurs rarely in infectious mononucleosis.[507] The peak age at incidence is between 10 and 30 years with a male preponderance. Most occurrences of thrombocytopenia are mild.[508] The signs and symptoms of severe occurrences are similar to those of idiopathic thrombocytopenic purpura, except that in infectious mononucleosis hemorrhagic bullae may develop in the mouth. Platelet counts as low as 3000/L have been reported in association with EBV infection.[509] This is a rare finding in idiopathic thrombocytopenic purpura. The usual duration of thrombocytopenia is 4 to 8 weeks. Severe hemorrhagic complications are rare.[510]

The thrombocytopenia of infectious mononucleosis appears to be immune in nature and has been associated with the presence of antiplatelet antibodies in several patients.

Treatment of the thrombocytopenia of infectious mononucleosis should be expectant. Severe occurrences may be treated with corticosteroid therapy, which generally increases the platelet count promptly.[511] The rate of occurrence of these hematologic abnormalities is shown in Table 36-5.

The total spectrum of the rare complications and unusual syndromes associated with EBV infection have been reviewed by Timár and colleagues.[512]

Laboratory Diagnosis

Atypical lymphocytosis is the hallmark of infectious mononucleosis (Fig. 36-3). Several attempts have been made to classify these abnormal cells on morphologic grounds, the best known method being that of Downey and McKinlay.[513] However, it is clear that atypical lymphocytes cannot be easily classified into separate categories and that a spectrum of cell types exists. Undue emphasis on minor morphologic detail in stained films is not very rewarding. In general, the atypical lymphocytes of infectious mononucleosis are large, but they vary in size considerably. Their outlines are irregular, and many cells show a characteristic tendency to flow around adjacent erythrocytes. Nuclei are large and usually eccentrically located and pleomorphic, with abundant coarse chromatin and occasional nucleoli. The cytoplasm is generally abundant and typically basophilic. Cytoplasmic vacuoles may be seen. These types of cells are not morphologically specific for infectious mononucleosis. Morphologic characteristics similar to these are associated with infections such as cytomegalovirus, infectious hepatitis, rubella, rubeola, and herpes simplex; after the administration of certain drugs such as phenytoin and *p*-aminosalicylic acid; and after a number of chemical intoxications.[514]

TABLE 36-5 Infectious Mononucleosis—Laboratory Features

Findings	% Positive
Lymphocytosis, relative and absolute	100
Atypical lymphocytes, definite*	100
Epstein-Barr virus antibody in serum	100
Heterophile antibody	80-100
Liver enzyme abnormalities	80-100
Leukocytosis	60-80
Neutropenia	60-80
Hyperbilirubinemia	30-50
Bone marrow granulomas	50
Slight thrombocytopenia	25-50
Increased cold agglutinins	10-50
Occult hemolysis	20-40
Hyperuricemia	15-20
Leukopenia	10-20
Severe thrombocytopenia with bleeding	Rare
Positive direct Coombs' test results	Rare
Significant anemia (usually caused by hemolysis)	Rare

*Twenty percent or more of white blood cells in peripheral blood.

The vast majority of atypical lymphocytes from patients with infectious mononucleosis are thymus derived.[515,516] These atypical cells possess human T-lymphocyte–specific antigens, as well as sheep erythrocyte receptors.[515] T lymphocytes appear to lack receptors for EBV, and it would appear that only B lymphocytes are infected by this virus.[516,517] A possible unifying interpretation of the role of T lymphocytes is that these cells represent an immune reaction that protects against this potentially oncogenic virus. Increased numbers of B cells are found during the first week of illness and decline to normal levels in 3 weeks. T lymphocytes reach their peak later, usually 10 to 14 days after the onset of symptoms, and remain elevated for 5 weeks.[518] There may be an early reversal of the ratio of T to B lymphocytes, with a subsequent increase in the percentage of T cells during the second through fifth weeks of illness. It is possible that both T and B cells may be "transformed" into atypical lymphocytes—B cells by infection with EBV and T cells by an immunologic response to viral antigen itself—or the B cells may respond to altered antigens on their surface. EBV-infected B lymphocytes account for only a minority of the atypical lymphocytes found in peripheral blood. In the very early stages of symptomatic illness, however, nearly 20% of all B cells in the circulation may be infected with the virus. The majority of atypical lymphocytes are T lymphocytes. Natural killer (NK) cell activity has been shown to be present during the acute phase of infectious mononucleosis. Interferons, which are inducers of NK cell activity, may have an inhibitory effect on the outgrowth of EBV-infected B lymphocytes in vitro. Significant anergy and diminished lymphocyte responsiveness in vitro to mitogens and antigens exist during the first week of illness. These lymphocyte changes are reflected in a great increase in uric acid turnover, with 55% of infected patients having serum uric acid levels of 8 mg/dL or higher.[519]

Patients with infectious mononucleosis have lymph node pathologic findings that are easily confused with

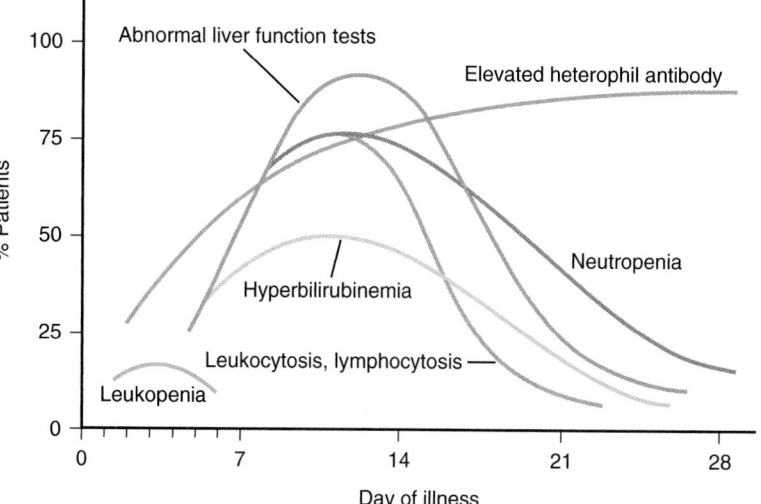

FIGURE 36-3. Major laboratory findings in infectious mononucleosis. (*Redrawn from Finch SC. Laboratory findings in infectious mononucleosis. In Carter RL, Penman HG [eds]. Infectious Mononucleosis. Oxford, Blackwell Scientific, 1969, p 47.*)

lymphoma. The nodal architecture is distorted by large, dark lymphoid cells, and the capsule may be infiltrated. Reed-Sternberg cells have been reported on several occasions.[520,521] Pathologic changes are not confined to lymphoid tissue, however. Perivascular cuffing of the brain vasculature, inflammation of the liver, and inflammatory infiltration of the kidney and bone marrow have been repeatedly observed.

The heterophil antibody is so named because the antigen to which the antibody reacts is found in more than one species. The antibody, like anti-i, is an IgM macroglobulin. It agglutinates sheep red cells and can be removed completely from serum by preincubation with beef red cells but not with guinea pig kidney. Heterophil antibody titers usually increase after the third day of illness, peak at 2 weeks, and may remain positive for several months before ultimately becoming negative (unlike the antibody specific for EBV).[522] This traditional Paul-Bunnell serologic agglutination method has been largely replaced for screening purposes by the spot test, in which finely ground guinea pig kidney or beef red cell stroma is added to serum on a slide, followed by a drop of horse cells.[523] Results of the test are considered positive if agglutination occurs in the presence of guinea pig kidney (which absorbs out Forssman antibody but not heterophil antibody) but are negative with beef red cell stroma. The spot test requires only 2 minutes and is 96% to 99% accurate. Results of both the Paul-Bunnell test and the spot test are usually negative in preschool-aged children, in whom heterophil antibody production is limited.[524] This age group does produce diagnostic levels of EBV-specific antibody.

EBV is a herpes-like DNA virus. It is a relatively complex virus, and a variety of virus-associated antigens have been described.[525] Antibodies to viral capsid antigen (VCA) and early antigen (EA) are detected early after the onset of EBV-associated infectious mononucleosis.[526] Levels of antibodies to VCA reach their peak at about 3 weeks after the onset of clinical illness. Their levels decline somewhat thereafter, but they remain for life.[527] Antibodies to EA usually last 2 to 4 months. EA has two components that are differentiated by their immunofluorescent staining: "D" for diffuse and "R" for restricted staining. A technique for determining EBV-specific IgM has been described.[528] EBV-specific IgM almost always occurs in the acute phase of infectious mononucleosis. It rarely persists more than 2 to 3 months. During this period, virus shedding from the oropharynx is easily demonstrable.[529]

Figure 36-4 shows the characteristic antibody patterns observed in young adults with EBV-induced infectious mononucleosis.[530] Before infection, no antibodies are present. During the acute phase of illness, high titers of IgM and IgG antibodies to VCA are seen. IgM antibodies are transient and disappear after 1 to 2 months. Antibodies appearing against EA disappear after a few weeks to months. Antibodies against Epstein-Barr nuclear antigen are the last to appear and are seen 1 to 2 months after the illness. In young infants, VCA IgM is found in only 60% of patients, and EA antibody is identified in

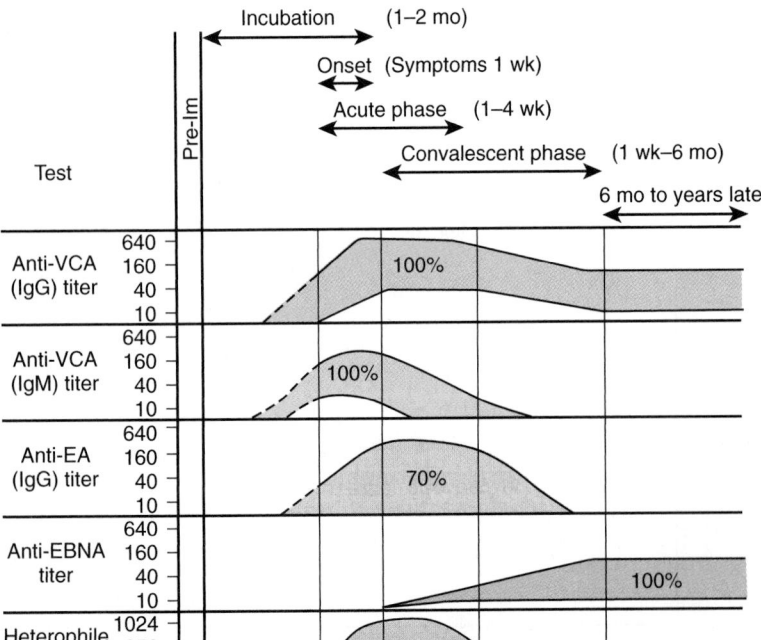

FIGURE 36-4. Characteristic Epstein-Barr virus (EBV)-specific antibody responses observed in young adults with acute infectious mononucleosis. (*Adapted from Henle W, Henle GE, Howwitz CA. Epstein-Barr virus specific diagnostic tests in infectious mononucleosis. Hum Pathol. 1974; 5:551-565; and Sullivan JL. Epstein-Barr virus and the X-linked lymphoproliferative syndrome. Adv Pediatr. 1984;30: 365-399.*)

only 50%. The only persistent antibody response should be VCA IgG and antibodies to Epstein-Barr nuclear antigen. Polymerase chain reaction (PCR) analysis for the EBV genome in peripheral blood is a more sensitive test than heterophile antibody in children, but it is more costly and it is wise to perform the serologic erythropoietin tests as a screen.[531]

Association with Malignancy

In 1974 and 1975, three families were described in whom fatal infectious mononucleosis caused by EBV occurred in young male members of these kindreds.[532-534] Subsequently, many families have been described. Acquired immunodeficiency and lymphoproliferative disorders occur at a higher than expected incidence in susceptible males. Of males who become affected, approximately 70% die of fatal infectious mononucleosis. Of those who survive the initial infection, a lymphoproliferative disorder will develop in up to 40%. Virtually all patients who survive are immunocompromised. Sullivan and colleagues[535] have found that those with common variable immunodeficiency demonstrate hypogammaglobulinemia and abnormal immune responses to in vivo immunization with various phage types of *Staphylococcus*.[535] NK cell activity is diminished and unresponsive to interferon therapy. This presumably leaves affected individuals with little defense against lymphoproliferative disorders characterized by multiplication of malignant cells containing the EBV genome. Of males who survive the initial infection, 80% have absent or abnormal humoral immune responses to EBV.[536] Before EBV infection, susceptible males usually had no history of recurrent infections or difficulty in limiting infections.

Recognition of X-linked lymphoproliferative syndrome has led to wider understanding of the effect of EBV infection and its immunologic consequences in other states. Transient immunodeficiency during asymptomatic EBV infection may occur in otherwise healthy children.[537] A non–X-linked susceptibility to severe EBV infection has now been described.[538-540] X-linked lymphoproliferative syndrome was first described in 1975. Fatal or severe infectious mononucleosis, acquired hypogammaglobulinemia, and malignant lymphoma are the three major phenotypes in X-linked lymphoproliferative syndrome. Fatal infectious mononucleosis occurs in two thirds of these individuals, with an overall mortality rate of 85%.

Recently, three different groups independently identified mutations in a novel gene in families with X-linked lymphoproliferative syndrome. The gene encodes for a cytoplasmic protein that has a 128–amino acid intracytoplasmic domain termed Src homology 2 domain–containing protein (SH2D1A) or signaling lymphocyte activation molecule (SLAM)-associated molecule.[541-543] It appears that this molecule acts as a regulator of at least two CD2-like lymphocyte receptors, in particular, 2B4. The 2B4 receptor is expressed primarily on NK cells and a subset of CD8⁺ T cells. Ligation of 2B4 in NK cells by its natural ligand CD48 on target cells results in selective activation of NK cells. SH2D1A seems to be required for activation of 2B4. It appears that NK cells from patients with X-linked lymphoproliferative syndrome have abnormal 2B4 activation and are unable to lyse EBV-infected targets.[544]

As noted, the outcome in susceptible individuals with the infection is extremely guarded.[545] Acyclovir treatment of two subjects with life-threatening EBV infection (one of whom had X-linked lymphoproliferative syndrome) produced no apparent improvement.[546] There may be a role for acyclovir very early in the course of serious complications of infectious mononucleosis when EBV induces polyclonal B-cell activation. Treatment subsequently is not likely to be effective.[547] Trials with interferon are under way. Bone marrow transplantation has been used successfully in the management of X-linked lymphoproliferative syndrome.[548]

A variety of other malignancies have been linked to EBV, including clonal T-cell proliferations.[549] EBV infection can also result in a hemophagocytic syndrome.[550] The interaction between EBV and human immunodeficiency virus (HIV) is discussed elsewhere in this chapter.

Management

There is no evidence that bed rest or rest in general shortens the clinical course of infectious mononucleosis. Patients will determine their own level of activity. The most significant risk during acute illness is splenic rupture, but its incidence is extremely low.

Corticosteroid therapy is often used for infectious mononucleosis. Although these agents may produce improvement of symptoms, enhancement of general well-being, and reduction of fever, their use for these purposes should be restricted.[532] Less controversial is the use of corticosteroid therapy for patients with airway obstruction secondary to tonsillar hypertrophy, severe hemolytic anemia, and hemorrhagic thrombocytopenia.[551]★

The hematologic and oncologic consequences of EBV-host interactions have been reviewed.[552]

METABOLIC DISEASES

Discussion in this section is restricted to the hematologic consequences of diabetes mellitus, some of the lipid

---

★*Editor's comment*: Young adolescents with persistent but non–life-threatening viral infections may be seen with symptoms and signs suggesting serious systemic diseases, such as tuberculosis or lymphoma. The symptoms may persist for weeks and include sweating, weight loss, fatigue, anorexia, low-grade fever, lymphadenopathy, and splenomegaly. There may be mild microcytic anemia, particularly in young women. Thrombocytosis with an elevated sedimentation rate and rare lymphoblasts with basophilic cytoplasm may be detected in peripheral blood, particularly in smokers.

disorders of metabolic origin, and methylmalonic and orotic aciduria.

Diabetes Mellitus

That diabetic patients are prone to anemia,[553] infection,[554] and thrombotic episodes with macrovascular and microvascular sequelae[555] has long been recognized.

An unusual hemoglobin component in hemolysates prepared from the blood of some diabetic patients was first noted by Rahbar.[556] A component that migrated near the position of fetal hemoglobin was described on agar gel electrophoresis at pH 6.2 in citrate buffers. This hemoglobin is present in normal individuals; it constitutes 5% to 7% of total hemoglobin[557] and is called HbA_{1c}. Rahbar's group observed a twofold increase in this hemoglobin fraction in some diabetic patients.[558] Structurally, HbA_{1c} is a condensation product, by means of a Schiff base, between 1 molecule of HbA and 1 molecule of an aldehyde or ketone, linked at the N-terminals of β chains. The aldehyde or ketone group appears to be one or more hexoses, thus making HbA_{1c} a glycohemoglobin. Bunn and Briehl[559] have shown that the oxygen affinity of HbA_{1c} is little affected by the addition of 2,3-DPG, which leads to decreased oxygen affinity when added to HbA. Although an early study failed to demonstrate any correlation between the degree of elevation in HbA_{1c} and clinical parameters of disease activity,[557] other investigations have shown highly significant relationships between the percentage of HbA_{1c} and the response to an oral glucose tolerance test and overall diabetic control, as reflected in quantitative urinary glucose determinations.[560,561] In this sense, measurement of the glycohemoglobin provides an insight into diabetic control over many days. Although HbA_{1c} is a glycohemoglobin and an unusual glycoprotein has been found in the basement membrane material of kidneys of diabetic patients, correlation between these findings has yet to be found.[560]

Red blood cell survival, as measured by chromium (^{51}Cr) labeling, may be mildly impaired during periods of poor diabetic control (mean erythrocyte half-life of 27 days). With improvement of diabetic control, red cell survival will increase (mean half-life of 31 days).[562] During episodes of ketoacidosis, rapid shifts in the oxygen affinity of hemoglobin may also occur. A decrease in pH causes a shift to the right with an increase in oxygen unloading. Very rapid correction of pH may impede oxygen delivery. A prompt decrease in red cell 2,3-DPG levels occurs at these times.[563] This decrease is probably compensatory—an attempt to correct the oxygen affinity disturbances caused by the acidosis. A decrease in red cell 2,3-DPG levels may also result from hypophosphatemia, if it occurs during insulin treatment.

Other red cell abnormalities have been found in diabetic subjects. The red blood cells of such individuals show evidence of lipid peroxidation and antiperoxidative enzyme changes when compared with those of healthy subjects.[564] An increase in the glycosylated form of erythrocyte superoxide dismutase has been found in diabetic subjects and is related to nonenzymatic glycosylation of this enzyme.[565] Erythrocytes from diabetic subjects also show sodium influx.[566] Red blood cell sorbitol concentrations will increase in subject with poorly controlled diabetes; the amount of red blood cell sorbitol is related to the degree of diabetic control.[567] Finally, if electronic counting equipment is used to determine the mean corpuscular volume of red cells, artifactual elevations in mean corpuscular volume may be seen in subjects with hyperglycemia.[568]

Anemia in diabetes is usually an example of the anemia of chronic disorders (discussed earlier). Adult diabetic patients have a higher incidence of pernicious anemia than normal individuals do. A thiamine-responsive anemia, neutropenia, and thrombocytopenia have been reported in the DIDMOAD syndrome.[569]

Polymorphonuclear cell function may be disturbed in diabetic patients. Leukocyte adherence is diminished in individuals with poor control of diabetes, as is phagocytic capacity.[570] Chemotaxis may also be abnormal, but this does not correlate with the status of diabetic control.[571] Impaired cellular metabolism and DNA synthesis have been reported in the lymphocytes of some patients with diabetes.[572] Increased superoxide production by mononuclear cells is observed in patients with diabetes and hypertriglyceridemia.[573]

A variety of coagulation and platelet abnormalities have been described in diabetic patients. A state of hypercoagulability associated with changes in clotting factors and platelet function has been postulated to be important in the increased thrombotic complications in diabetic patients. Approximately a third of patients with diabetes will show abnormally increased factor VIII coagulant activity and diminished antithrombin III levels. Abnormalities in fibrinolysis do not appear to be common.[574] In addition to this, factor XI and factor XII levels are higher in some diabetic patients with evidence that the kallikrein-prekallikrein system has been activated.[575] Ketoacidosis may be associated with DIC.[576] Altered levels of factors V and VIII and diminished fibrinolytic activity have been reported in a few patients.[577]

Many studies have emphasized the abnormalities in platelet adhesion and aggregation in patients with diabetes. The finding that enhanced platelet aggregation occurs before clinical evidence of diabetic vascular disease suggested that this defect may be acquired early in the natural history of diabetes and could underlie the vascular disease.[578] Platelet aggregation in diabetic subjects is characterized by a shortened adenosine diphosphate–induced aggregation time.[579] Increased platelet adhesiveness and platelet factor 3 and 4 activity also occur.[562,580] Normal platelets incubated in the plasma of diabetic patients will become abnormal. This aggregation-enhancing activity is present in both plasma and serum and is nondialyzable and heat resistant.[579] In patients with this plasma factor, von Willebrand factor activity is also increased, thus suggesting that the two are related.[581] The enhanced in vitro responsiveness of platelets from diabetic patients can be decreased by prostaglandin synthetase inhibitors.[578,582] Platelets from diabetic patients demonstrate increased activity of the prostaglandin synthetase system, which results in increased synthesis of prostaglandin endoperoxides and, therefore, of prostaglandin E_2.[583] When induced to aggregate with arachidonic acid, the platelets of diabetic patients with vascular disease tend to produce more thromboxane A_2 than those of normal subjects do.[584] A lower prevalence and severity of diabetic retinopathy have been observed in a group of diabetic patients with concurrent rheumatoid arthritis who were taking high doses of aspirin. This finding suggests that inhibition of platelet aggregation and prostaglandin synthesis may be desirable in the management of diabetic patients.[585] The increased glycosylation of connective tissue proteins in diabetic patients has been suggested to increase their aggregation potency.[586]

The hematologic consequences of diabetes also extend to infants born of diabetic mothers. An increased incidence of thrombosis or thromboembolic phenomena is well recognized in these infants.[587] Complications such as renal vein thrombosis, peripheral gangrene secondary to vascular occlusion, and cerebral thrombosis may occur.[588]

It may be difficult to resist the urge to perform lymph node biopsy or abdominal exploration in such patients. However, most of them should be treated expectantly with simple home remedies, such as white meat of chicken or chicken soup.[589]

Abnormalities in Lipid Metabolism

Abetalipoproteinemia is an autosomal recessive disorder that results in abnormalities in plasma lipids. Plasma levels of triglycerides, cholesterol, and phospholipids are diminished.[590] These findings are associated with the presence of acanthocytic red blood cells. The cholesterol content of the red cell is normal or slightly increased, whereas the phospholipid content reflects that of serum.[590] Autohemolysis[591] and peroxidative hemolysis[592] may be increased, but osmotic fragility[591] and rates of glycolysis[591] are normal. Anemia, if present, is mild.

Patients with familial hyperbetalipoproteinemia (type II hyperlipoproteinemia) have abnormal platelet function[593] characterized by increased sensitivity to aggregating agents and release of increased amounts of nucleotides in response to aggregating agents. These changes are associated with platelet plasma membrane ultrastructural changes, particularly in type IIa hypercholesterolemia.[594] Such subjects may truly demonstrate a "hypercoagulable state." The latter has been demonstrated in severely hypertriglyceridemic conditions.[595] These findings suggest the possibility that platelet function may be involved in the thrombotic complications of familial hyperbetalipoproteinemia. Erythrocytes from

patients with various disorders in lipoprotein metabolism have abnormal red blood cell morphologic characteristics, including acanthocytes, stomatocytes, and crenated cells.[596,597]

Essential fatty acid deficiency will result in a variety of characteristic changes in plasma lipids. Decreased prostaglandin formation in in vitro platelet studies involving animals with essential fatty acid deficiency has been reported.[598] This results in a thrombocytopathy with impaired platelet aggregation and may reflect a deficiency of arachidonic acid necessary for the formation of thromboxane A_2.[598] Clinically, essential fatty acid deficiency is being recognized more often as a result of prolonged fat-free parenteral nutrition.[599] Several infants have been described with hemorrhagic complications from this disorder.[598]

Other Metabolic Disorders

A single infant with methylmalonic aciduria was found to have neutropenia.[600] The mechanism of neutropenia in this child is unclear. More commonly, excessive urinary excretion of methylmalonic acid occurs as a result of vitamin B_{12} deficiency.[601]

A child has been described with altered vitamin B_{12} metabolism in association with megaloblastic anemia and homocystinuria secondary to a defect in methionine biosynthesis.[602] Homocystinuria and megaloblastic anemia responsive to vitamin B_{12} therapy have also been reported as an inborn error of metabolism caused by a defect in cobalamin metabolism.[603] Infants and children with orotic aciduria, hyperglycinemia, and hyperglycinuria may have neutropenia.[604] Patients with orotic aciduria may exhibit megaloblastic changes in bone marrow and have macrocytic indices.

NEUROLOGIC AND PSYCHIATRIC DISORDERS

Muscular Dystrophy

Roses and Appel[605] reported decreased levels of red cell membrane protein phosphorylation in patients with myotonic muscular dystrophy. As a further example of the usefulness of red cells as biopsy tissue and also as possible additional evidence for the clinical importance of membrane protein phosphorylation, increased phosphorylation of red cell spectrin has been reported to occur in patients with Duchenne's muscular dystrophy.[606] These observations have prompted the hypothesis that the muscular defects in dystrophic patients may represent specific manifestations of a generalized membrane disorder.[607] In addition, the red cells of patients with muscular dystrophy may demonstrate decreased deformability.[608,609] Increased osmotic fragility is seen in almost 85% of patients.[610] It has been suggested that analysis of intramembrane particles in freeze-fractured erythrocyte plasma membranes will show the same abnormalities in carriers of human Duchenne's muscular dystrophy as in affected subjects and may be used as a rapid, simple, and highly accurate diagnostic tool for such carrier detection.[611] The Pelger-Huët anomaly has been associated with the autosomal dominant form of muscular dystrophy in one family,[612] as has the Jordan anomaly.[613] All these findings are subtle and require careful evaluation and confirmation. Structural platelet membrane abnormalities have also been described in subjects with muscular dystrophy, although this finding is not universal.[614,615]

Myasthenia Gravis

Because both myasthenia gravis and acquired pure red cell aplasia have been associated with the presence of thymoma, occasional reports of patients with myasthenia gravis and concomitant pure red cell aplasia have appeared.[616] Pancytopenia may also occur. Such occurrences in children are rare. In addition, there is a higher than average incidence of autoimmune hemolytic anemia in patients with myasthenia gravis.[617] Antibody-mediated pure neutrophil aplasia may result from recurrent myasthenia gravis and thymoma.[618]

Lesch-Nyhan Syndrome

The Lesch-Nyhan syndrome is an X-linked recessive disorder characterized by mental retardation, choreoathetosis, hyperuricemia, and self-mutilation. Cells from affected individuals are unable to convert hypoxanthine and guanine to the corresponding nucleotides because of an inactive phosphoribosyltransferase. A patient with this syndrome has been described in whom megaloblastic anemia developed, presumably as a result of deficient nucleic acid synthesis because the administration of large amounts of adenine reversed the process.[619] The enzyme is present in red cells, but its deficiency does not generally alter the function or survival of mature red cells.[620] On an experimental basis, erythrocyte transfusions have been used as a source of enzyme replacement in Lesch-Nyhan syndrome.[621]

Rivard and associates[622] have shown that in patients with Lesch-Nyhan syndrome, radioactive hypoxanthine cannot be incorporated into platelet nucleotides. This results in a significantly lower adenosine triphosphate platelet content. Nonetheless, platelet function and number are normal in Lesch-Nyhan syndrome.

Brain Trauma

Brain tissue from all mammalian species is rich in thromboplastin activity. Severe injury to the brain that disrupts the brain architecture may release this material into the circulation. This most commonly occurs after gunshot wounds or crush injury to the head and has resulted in acute DIC.

Anorexia Nervosa

Patients with anorexia nervosa may demonstrate many of the hematologic manifestations of severe malnutrition. In one patient with anorexia nervosa, the total amount of red cell lipids was normal, but there was an increased proportion of the long-chain polyunsaturated fatty acids associated with starvation.[623] Small numbers of irregularly shaped red blood cells are often seen.[624] The sedimentation rate is low. About a third of subjects will have a normochromic, normocytic anemia.[625] Slight to moderate leukopenia and neutropenia develop in about half of the patients who are severely malnourished. This may be associated with an increased risk for infection.[626] The bone marrow may become hypoplastic and filled with gelatinous material and fat.[627] Leukocyte response to bacterial infection may be suboptimal. Several months may be needed for the white cell abnormalities in anorexia nervosa to resolve after adequate caloric intake. Platelet counts are generally normal, but mild depressions and occasionally severe depressions are observed.[628] A marked increase in platelet hyperaggregability may be found.[629]

SKIN DISEASES

Skin diseases are only rarely a direct cause of hematologic disturbances. More often than not, the hematologic alterations reflect a simultaneous disturbance in more than one developmental system, such as the skin and blood. Certain disorders that affect the hematologic system in a major way, such as Wiskott-Aldrich syndrome, are described in Chapter 23.

Eczema and Psoriasis

Patients with extensive eczema or psoriasis commonly have a mild anemia.[630] The anemia is usually normochromic and normocytic, although microcytosis may occur. Typically, this anemia is associated with a low serum iron level and normal or decreased iron-binding capacity. Because the level of iron in bone marrow is not diminished, the anemia is best classified as an anemia of chronic disorders.[630] A defect in red blood cell deformability resulting in decreased deformability in eczematous patients has been reported.[631] Some individuals with extensive rash will have greatly expanded whole blood and plasma volumes, which may result in a dilutional anemia.[621,633] In rare patients with eczema or psoriasis, long-standing steatorrhea may develop and cause folate malabsorption and macrocytic anemia.[634] Psoriasis may be a widespread membrane disorder. Alterations in red blood cell sodium and potassium fluxes are seen, as well as alterations in membrane lipid composition (an increase in arachidonic acid and unsaturated fatty acid content).[635,636] The increased erythrocyte membrane arachidonate and platelet malondialdehyde production noted in patients with psoriasis may normalize after treatment with fish oil.[637]

Dermatitis Herpetiformis

Anemia may result from the malabsorption syndrome found in many individuals with dermatitis herpetiformis. It usually causes a megaloblastic anemia.[638] Splenic hypofunction and atrophy may also occur[639] and are detectable by the presence of Howell-Jolly bodies on the peripheral blood smear. This lymphoreticular dysfunction probably relates to the high incidence of celiac disease found in association with dermatitis herpetiformis. Hyposplenism is also common in children and adults with celiac disease.[640] In any event, it is generally held that the hematologic consequences of dermatitis herpetiformis are simply a result of the nutritional problems produced by this disease.[641]

Dyskeratosis Congenita

An illness resembling Fanconi's aplastic anemia may occur in patients with dyskeratosis congenita.[642] Before onset of the skin problem, thrombocytopenia, macrocytosis, and elevations in fetal hemoglobin may be seen.[643] These abnormalities, which result in hypoplastic anemia, appear to be a stem cell defect because they are preceded by a prolonged period characterized by a decrease in the number of precursor cells in both the bone marrow and peripheral blood of such patients.[644] Interested readers are referred to Chapter 8 for recent findings in this disorder.

Hereditary Hemorrhagic Telangiectasia

This inherited structural abnormality of the vasculature is characterized by mucocutaneous telangiectases caused by localized dilation and convolution of venules and capillaries. It is an autosomal dominant disorder that results in a bleeding tendency because of the friable blood vessels. Telangiectases predominate on the lips, buccal mucosa, gingivae, palate, tongue, and skin of the face and upper parts of the body and may be present in visceral organs as well. Pulmonary arteriovenous fistulas are not rare but tend to appear later in life. Easy bruisability, epistaxis, and respiratory and gastrointestinal bleeding may be caused by these telangiectases.

Ehlers-Danlos Syndrome and Other Connective Tissue Disorders

The elastic tissue defects seen in Ehlers-Danlos syndrome may result in an increased bleeding tendency. A somewhat similar problem occurs in association with pseudoxanthoma elasticum and Marfan's syndrome. Platelet dysfunction in the form of reduced aggregation in the presence of adenosine diphosphate, collagen, and norepinephrine has been described in both Ehlers-Danlos and Marfan's syndrome. A defective fibronectin has been proposed as the cause of the hypermobility and platelet dysfunction.[645] An unusual sensitivity to aspirin has been noted in one family with Ehlers-Danlos type IV syndrome.[646]

Mast Cell Disease

In this disorder, large numbers of mast cells are found, often diffusely located in the skin or the gastrointestinal tract.[647] These cells periodically release histamine and heparin-like substances.[647,648] Trauma to involved areas may trigger release of these substances and may also cause urticaria and blistering of affected parts of the body. A coagulation defect is the hematologic manifestation of mast cell disease. Laboratory testing demonstrates a heparin-like effect. Because fatal hemorrhage may result from this excessive anticoagulant effect, treatment with protamine sulfate may be necessary.

Urticaria pigmentosa is one form of mast cell disease. On rare occasion, mast cell disease and urticaria pigmentosa precede the onset of mast cell leukemia.[649]

LEUKOCYTE VARIATIONS IN DISEASE STATES

Since the recognition by Huët[650] in 1931 that a nuclear segmentation defect, now called the Pelger-Huët anomaly, was inherited, a wide variety of morphologic variations in leukocytes have been found. Many of these alterations are discussed in detail in other chapters.

Nuclear Changes

Pelger-Huët Anomaly

In this anomaly, segmentation of lobes in neutrophilic leukocytes is limited (Fig. 36-5). The anomaly was described first by Pelger in 1928, who thought that the finding was a manifestation of tuberculosis.[651] Huët[650] recognized that it appeared to be inherited as an autosomal dominant trait. Individuals with this disorder rarely have neutrophils or eosinophils with more than two lobes. In heterozygotes, the neutrophils are unsegmented, dumbbell shaped, or bilobed in the nuclei. In homozygotes, the vast majority of neutrophils have round nuclei.

This anomaly affects 1 in 6000 individuals. Although neutrophil migration may be minimally impaired, granulocyte function is otherwise normal, and individuals with this inherited anomaly suffer no adverse effects. The Pelger-Huët anomaly is inherited in an autosomal dominant fashion and is due to mutations within the lamin B receptor, a member of the sterol reductase family.[652] Expression of the lamin B receptor affects neutrophil nuclear shape and chromatin distribution.

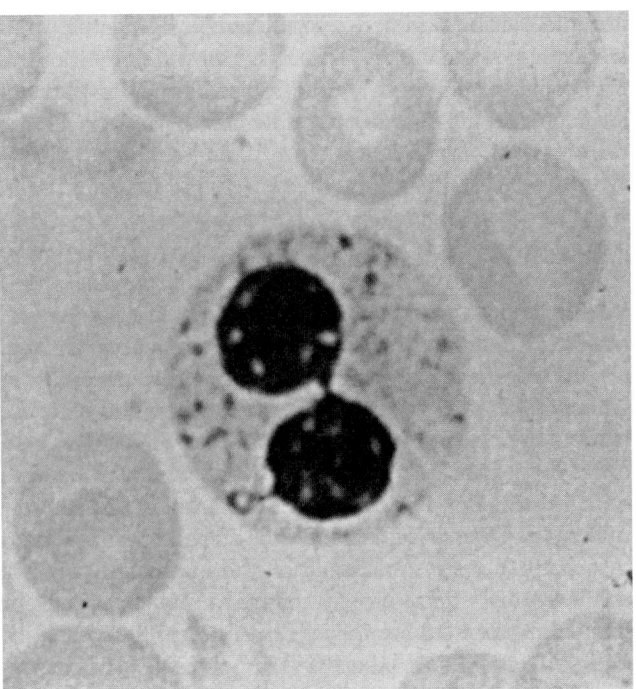

FIGURE 36-5. Pelger-Huët anomaly.

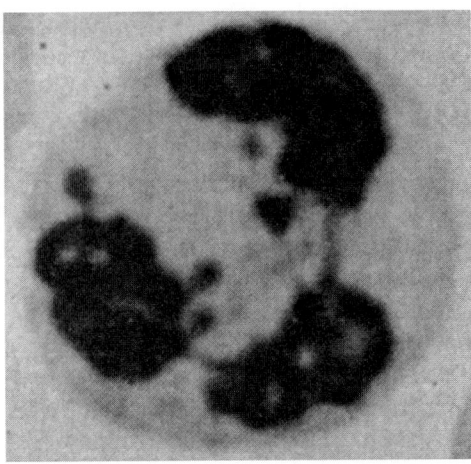

FIGURE 36-6. Increased nuclear appendages in a neutrophil of a patient with trisomy 13-15. *(From Huehns ER, Lutzner M, Hechte F. Nuclear abnormalities of the neutrophils in D-(13-15)-trisomy syndrome. Lancet. 1964;1:589-590.)*

A Pelger-Huët–like change in granulocyte morphologic characteristics may occur as an acquired condition in several disease states, such as chronic infections of the bowel, glandular fever, malaria, leukemia, and diffuse metastatic disease.[653,654] This same finding may be produced by toxins and certain drugs such as colchicine.[655] A reversible Pelger-Huët anomaly has been seen with acute gastroenteritis caused by *Salmonella* group D.[656] Not only does leukemia potentially result in a Pelger-Huët anomaly, but non-Hodgkin's lymphoma may as well.[657] Pelger-Huët anomaly has been reported in association with Sjögren's syndrome.[658] It has also been found in some patients with trisomy 18 syndrome.[659] A transient acquired Pelger-Huët anomaly may be observed with *Mycoplasma pneumoniae* infection.[660] Valproic acid toxicity may be associated with the anomaly.[661] Bilobed nuclei are common in many other animal species, most notably in the rabbit.

Hereditary Constitutional Hypersegmentation of Neutrophils

In this autosomal dominant condition, the mean number of neutrophil nuclear lobes is approximately four as compared with the approximately three lobes found in normal neutrophils.[662] This hereditary form of neutrophil hypersegmentation is not associated with any adverse effects and appears to be more common than previously thought. It must be distinguished from more significant disorders such as vitamin B_{12} and folate deficiency and myeloproliferative states.

Hereditary Constitutional Hypersegmentation of Eosinophils

This is probably an autosomal disorder in which the mean lobe count of eosinophils is between 3 and 4, unlike the mean lobe count of normal eosinophils, which is 2.3. Affected individuals are otherwise normal.[663]

Hereditary Giant Neutrophils

Normal neutrophils have an average cell size of 12.7 μm. In this hereditary autosomal dominant disorder, neutrophil diameter is about 17 μm, which represents an approximate doubling of white cell size.[664] There are usually 6 to 10 nuclear lobes. In actuality, only relatively few neutrophils demonstrate these morphologic abnormalities in affected individuals, but they are clearly distinguished from the normal population because these findings never occur otherwise.

Hereditary Prevalence of Nuclear Appendages

In general, thread-like and other small projections from the nucleus of neutrophils are relatively nonspecific. Excessive numbers of projections may be seen in various forms of carcinoma, in trisomy 13-15, and as a hereditary phenomenon (Fig. 36-6).[665]

These disorders must be distinguished from those that increase the number of neutrophil drumsticks, which are female-specific nuclear appendages. In normal women, drumsticks are present in 2% to 10% of mature neutrophils.[666] At least six drumsticks per 500 neutrophils must be present for the sex to be determined as female. Pseudodrumsticks in males generally occur, if at all, in fewer than 6 of 500 neutrophils. Drumstick number is increased in any condition with an increased average number of lobes per cell—for example, in the hypersegmentation anomaly, when there are multiple X chromosomes in the karyotype, and when there is an isochromosome of the long arms of an X chromosome (X-iso X). The presence of a Y chromosome reduces the drumstick number when there are supernumerary X chromosomes (XXY, XXXY, or XXXXY). The normal drumstick head is 1.5 μm in diameter. The diameter is increased in females with a long-arm isochromosome.

Cytoplasmic Abnormalities

Granulation Disturbances

Alder-Reilly Anomaly

This anomaly, described independently by Alder and Reilly, is discussed in detail in Chapter 24.[667] It is a hematologic manifestation of Hurler's syndrome in which prominent granules (often called Reilly bodies) are found in neutrophils that stain positively with metachromatic stains (Fig. 36-7). Increased numbers of dense cytoplasmic granules may also be seen in other mucopolysaccharidoses. Lymphocytes, monocytes, and plasma cells may also be affected.

May-Hegglin Anomaly

In this rare autosomal dominant disorder, large (up to 5 μm) pale blue–staining inclusions are found in the cytoplasm of neutrophils, eosinophils, basophils, and monocytes.[668] Thrombocytopenia and giant platelets are also observed. The inclusions consist of material derived from the endoplasmic reticulum, and their gross appearance is similar to that of Döhle bodies. Ultrastructural and functional abnormalities of platelets may be observed in patients with the May-Hegglin anomaly.[669]

The May-Hegglin anomaly is only one of three forms of hereditary thrombocytopenia seen in association with giant platelets and inclusion bodies in leukocytes. Fechtner's syndrome is a variant of Alport's syndrome with inclusion bodies consisting of dispersed filaments, ribosomes, and a few segments of rough and smooth endoplasmic reticulum. The Sebastian platelet syndrome shows the same platelet and leukocyte morphologic characteristics observed in Fechtner's syndrome, but the anomalies of Alport's syndrome are lacking.[670]

Chédiak-Higashi Syndrome

This disorder is discussed in detail in Chapter 21. Giant granules give the cytoplasm of the neutrophil a bizarre appearance. The granules seen in the neutrophils of patients with Chédiak-Higashi syndrome are not specifically isolated to the neutrophil. The granule abnormality is due to a defect in the *LYST1* gene, which predisposes these patients to hemophagocytosis.[671] Giant membrane-bound cytoplasmic granules have been observed in the epidermal Langerhans cells of a patient with Chédiak-Higashi syndrome.[672]

Batten-Spielmeyer-Vogt Disease

This degenerative neurologic disease was noted by Strouth and colleagues[673] in 1966 to be associated with coarse azurophilic granulation in neutrophils. Because these granules do not exhibit metachromasia, they can be easily differentiated from those observed in the mucopolysaccharidoses.

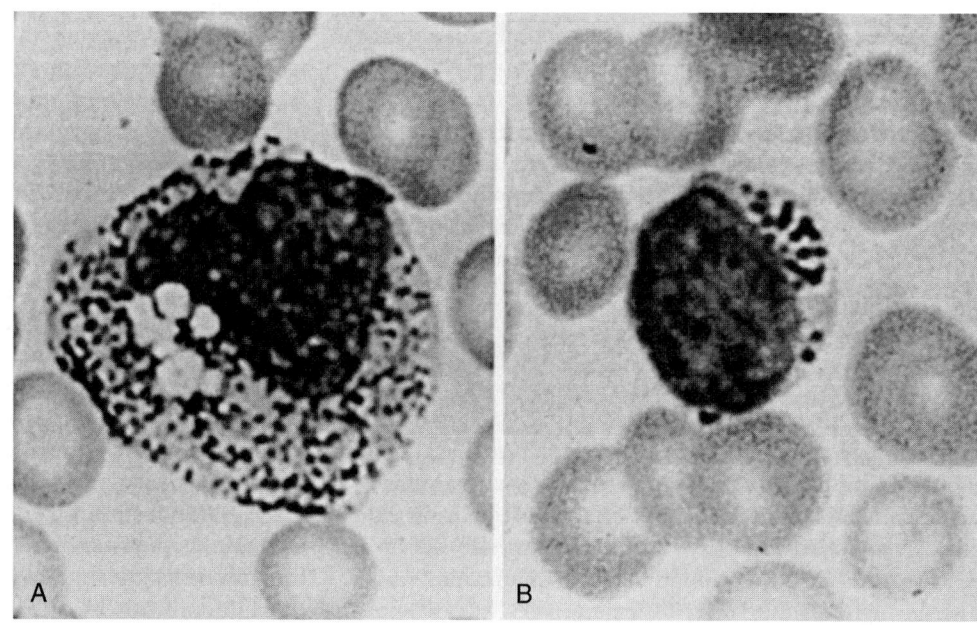

FIGURE 36-7. Reilly bodies in the cytoplasm of neutrophils (**A**) and lymphocytes (**B**) in a patient with Hurler's syndrome. Vacuoles are also present in the cytoplasm of the neutrophil.

A

B

Hereditary Dense Granulation of Neutrophils

It should be emphasized that several normal individuals have been described who demonstrate dense granulation of neutrophils.

Hermansky-Pudlak Syndrome

Hermansky-Pudlak syndrome (HPS) is a rare familial disorder characterized by albinism, a bleeding problem related to platelet dysfunction and accumulation of ceroid-like pigment in bone marrow macrophages, and the presence of lipopigment bodies, as well as other dense inclusions.[674,675] Similar ceroid deposition may be found within dermal macrophages.[676] The bleeding time abnormality seen in HPS may be correctable by the administration of 1-desamino-8-D-arginine vasopressin. HPS is a heterogeneous group of disorders that result from defective lysosome-related organelle formation. Lysosome-related organelles are found in melanosomes, platelets, and cytotoxic T cells, and defects in seven genes in humans disrupt the function of protein complexes such as BLOC-1, BLOC-2, BLOC-3, and AP3. This disorder has been important in defining key components of intracellular organelle trafficking.[677]

Vacuolization

Small vacuoles are not uncommonly associated with granules in the cytoplasm of normal lymphocytes. Large vacuoles in both lymphocytes and neutrophils develop rapidly in specimens collected in anticoagulants, especially ethylenediaminetetraacetic acid. Cytoplasmic vacuolization may occur in response to certain stresses, such as burns and infections. Vacuolization of lymphocytes is noted in a variety of inherited disorders, including Tay-Sachs disease, Niemann-Pick disease, and some instances of Hurler's syndrome, possibly after the disappearance of specific granules.[678-680] Some patients with type II glycogen storage disease (Pompe's disease) have vacuolated lymphocytes. In this disease, a high percentage of the vacuoles stain with the periodic acid–Schiff reaction.

A familial vacuolization of leukocytes (Jordan's anomaly) has been described in which vacuoles are present in the cytoplasm of granulocytes, monocytes, and occasionally lymphocytes and plasma cells.[681] These vacuoles contain lipids and range in size from 2 to 5 µm. Members of some affected families have had ichthyosis, whereas others have had a progressive form of muscular dystrophy.[682]

Eosinopenia and Eosinophilia

The lowest normal eosinophil counts are found in the immediate newborn period, after which such values in infants, children, and adults are remarkably similar.[683] The mean absolute eosinophil count of children and adults is 150 cells/mm³, with values of up to 700 cells/mm³.[684] A diurnal variation in the eosinophil count exists, and the highest value is seen in the evening. These changes

Box 36-1	Causes of Eosinophilia

Allergic disorders: Asthma, urticaria, hay fever, angioneurotic edema, occasional drug sensitivity, or simple exposure

Parasitic infections: Usual in invasive helminthic infections such as *Toxocara* infections, trichinosis, echinococcal infections, and ascariasis and less common in intestinal parasitism; rare in protozoal infection except for malaria

Skin disorders: Pemphigus, dermatitis herpetiformis

Hematologic and oncologic disorders: Hodgkin's disease, acute lymphatic leukemia, chronic myelogenous leukemia, pernicious anemia, postsplenectomy effects, immunodeficiency syndromes, polycythemia vera and other chronic myeloproliferative states, some solid tumors

Infectious disorders other than parasitism: Scarlet fever, chorea, erythema multiforme, chlamydial infections

Inherited eosinophilia

Miscellaneous disorders: Rheumatoid arthritis, periarteritis nodosa, sarcoidosis, radiation therapy, peritoneal dialysis, cirrhosis, Löffler's syndrome (including pulmonary infiltration with eosinophilia syndrome)

probably reflect varying activity in the production of adrenal corticosteroids. Premature infants commonly demonstrate eosinophilia.[428,429] Infection with falciparum malaria can result in eosinopenia.[685]

Eosinopenia may occur as a result of adrenocortical hyperfunction or after the administration of pharmacologic doses of corticosteroids.[686] Some children with Down syndrome also have eosinopenia.

There are many causes of eosinophilia (Box 36-1). In the United States, allergy is the single most common cause of this finding. All types of allergy may result in eosinophilia, including asthma, hay fever, urticaria, eczema, serum sickness, and angioneurotic edema.

Drug exposure is frequently a cause of eosinophilia. In most instances, no specific signs of drug allergy are present, and eosinophilia is noted coincidentally. Although some drugs are associated with a higher incidence of associated eosinophilia, any drug may potentially cause this finding.

Parasitic infections are the most common causes of eosinophilia on a worldwide basis. A general rule is that whereas helminthic infections often cause eosinophilia, protozoal infections (with the exception of malaria) do not. Of the helminthic infections, those associated with tissue invasion rather than those remaining within the bowel lumen cause the greatest degree of eosinophilia. Among the infectious causes of eosinophilia, visceral larva migrans produces the most profound elevations in eosinophil counts, with white blood cell counts greater than 100,000 cells/mm³ not being uncommon. Parasitic infection as a cause of eosinophilia cannot be excluded because of failure to demonstrate larvae or eggs in feces. In children with blood groups other than type AB, a marked increase in isohemagglutinin titer is highly suggestive of infection with *Toxocara* organisms.

Hypereosinophilic syndrome, which is characterized by pulmonary infiltrates, cardiomegaly, congestive heart failure, and an elevated eosinophil count, is a well-described but poorly understood entity.[687] The eosinophilia in this disorder is marked. Hypereosinophilic syndrome is a term that encompasses disorders such as Löffler's syndrome, eosinophilic leukemoid reaction, endocarditis parietalis fibroplastica, pulmonary infiltrates with eosinophilia, disseminated eosinophilic collagen disease, and eosinophilic leukemia. The etiology of these syndromes is controversial, and the possibility exists that these disorders represent a spectrum of a similar pathologic process. Eosinophilia has been noted in association with acute lymphoblastic leukemia.[688] In several of the patients described, an illness similar to Löffler's syndrome preceded the onset of leukemia.[689] The eosinophilia in these patients is an interesting finding because it is thought to be mediated by interleukin-5 (IL-5) released by thymus-dependent lymphocytes, which in turn stimulates eosinophil proliferation.[690,691] In the last 5 years great progress has been made in recognizing that fusion of tyrosine kinases FIPIL1-PDGFRA leads to the proliferation of T cells that secrete IL-5. This understanding has opened the way for targeted therapy with anti–IL-5 antibody or kinase inhibitors.[692]

There are many other causes of eosinophilia, including collagen vascular disease, malignancy, cirrhosis, and certain skin disorders. Eosinophilia may also be observed as an autosomal dominant familial trait in some families.[693]

Basophilia

Basophilia is usually said to occur when the basophil count exceeds 100 to 150 cells/mm^3.[694] Adrenocorticosteroids, infection, hyperthyroidism, and irradiation will decrease the basophil count. A wide variety of disorders may increase the basophil count, including ulcerative colitis, smallpox, varicella, and some occurrences of nephrosis.[695] Basophilia is extremely common in association with myeloproliferative disorders such as chronic myelogenous leukemia, polycythemia vera, and myeloid metaplasia.[696] Basophilia is occasionally seen in Hodgkin's disease and some hemolytic anemias (Box 36-2).[697]

Although increased numbers of basophils in the bone marrow and certain other tissues are found in urticaria pigmentosa and mast cell disease, numbers of blood basophils are not usually increased.

Monocytosis

Monocytosis is common in many protozoal and rickettsial infections and is one of the hematologic hallmarks of certain bacterial infections, especially tuberculosis, subacute bacterial endocarditis, and syphilis.[698] In any process

---

Box 36-2	Causes of Basophilia

Hematologic and oncologic disorders: Some hemolytic anemias, Hodgkin's disease, many chronic myeloproliferative disorders, including chronic myelogenous leukemia and polycythemia vera
Infections: Chronic sinusitis, smallpox, varicella
Endocrine disorders: Hypothyroidism, ovulation, pregnancy
Drugs: Estrogens, antithyroid medications
Miscellaneous: Stress, nephrosis, radiation (may also decrease the basophil count)

Box 36-3	Causes of Monocytosis

Bacterial infections: Syphilis, tuberculosis, subacute bacterial endocarditis, brucellosis
Nonbacterial infections: Rocky Mountain spotted fever, typhus, malaria, kala-azar, trypanosomiasis
Hematologic and oncologic disorders: Hodgkin's disease, preleukemia, leukemia, non-Hodgkin's lymphomas, myeloproliferative disorders, congenital and acquired neutropenia, some hemolytic anemias, metastatic solid tumors, splenectomy
Collagen vascular diseases: Systemic lupus erythematosus, rheumatoid arthritis, polyarteritis nodosa
Miscellaneous: Ulcerative colitis, regional enteritis, sarcoidosis, tetrachlorethane poisoning, Hand-Schüller-Christian syndrome

---

that is associated with granulocytopenia, monocytosis will usually precede and herald recovery. Monocytosis parallels disease activity in some patients with systemic lupus erythematosus and rheumatoid arthritis.[699] Several hematologic malignancies may be associated with peripheral blood monocytosis (Box 36-3).

Lymphocytosis

Except for pertussis, acute bacterial infections are rarely associated with lymphocytosis. Lymphocytosis should not be expected to be uniformly present in infants younger than 6 months who have pertussis.[700] Only 25% of these infants will have an elevated lymphocyte count suggestive of pertussis. Chronic bacterial infections such as tuberculosis and brucellosis may cause a sustained lymphocytosis. Although many nonspecific viral infections may cause a mild lymphocytosis with the presence of transient atypical lymphocytes, infectious mononucleosis and cytomegalovirus infection are the only probable causes of persistent atypical lymphocytosis. Markedly increased lymphocyte counts are sometimes seen in association with a disorder known as "acute infectious lymphocytosis." Marker analysis of the blood of such individuals has shown that the increased lymphocytes are predominantly T cells associated with a rise in the helper-inducer

Box 36-4	Causes of Lymphocytosis

Infection: Pertussis, infectious mononucleosis, infectious lymphocytosis, infectious hepatitis, cytomegalovirus (including postperfusion syndrome), toxoplasmosis, syphilis, brucellosis, many common viral illnesses
Hematologic disorders: Lymphocytic leukemias, neutropenia (a relative lymphocytosis)
Miscellaneous: Thyrotoxicosis, Addison's disease (a relative lymphocytosis)

Box 36-5	Causes of Lymphocytopenia

Infection: Active tuberculosis, malaria (sometimes)
Collagen vascular disease: Systemic lupus erythematosus, regional enteritis
Certain immunodeficiency syndromes
Endocrine disorders: Hyperadrenalism and adrenal corticosteroid administration
Hematologic and oncologic disorders: Hodgkin's disease, solid tumors (some), aplastic anemia
Excessive loss: Thoracic duct drainage, intestinal lymphangiectasia

phenotype (CD4$^+$) population of lymphocytes.[701] Thyrotoxicosis in both children and adults will also cause lymphocytosis (Box 36-4).[702]

Causes of lymphocytopenia are summarized in Box 36-5.

ACQUIRED IMMUNODEFICIENCY SYNDROME

In the early 1980s a newly described constellation of symptoms that resulted from immune compromise and led to death from opportunistic infections and unusual malignancies was recognized in a cluster of homosexual males.[703-705] These early descriptions of what is now known as acquired immunodeficiency syndrome (AIDS) heralded the beginning of what has become one of the major medical, public health, and social issues of our time. Identification of the retrovirus HIV as the etiologic agent that transmits the disease[706,707] has led to major advances in understanding the pathogenesis of AIDS. At least two types of HIV, HIV-1[706,707] and HIV-2,[708] exist; both are considered lentiviruses based on similarities in genetic composition, mechanisms of replication, and interaction with their hosts.[709] A characteristic of lentivirus infections is that they cause slowly progressive disease with an incubation period of months to years before clinical symptoms appear. Although this concept is new with respect to human viral diseases, it is well established in lentivirus infections of domestic animals such as sheep, in which maedi-visna develops, or in goats infected with caprine-arthritis-encephalitis virus.[710] The worldwide spread of AIDS has led to a plethora of information

about the biology of the virus and its epidemiology and incidence projections in different countries, as well as a concerted search for effective means of prevention and treatment. Increasing numbers of infected adults, in particular women of childbearing age, have highlighted a rapidly growing pediatric population with AIDS. A discussion of the hematologic complications and manifestations of this disorder must include comments about the epidemiology, biology, and transmission of HIV infection because all are germane to the clinical findings, diagnosis, and treatment in children.

Epidemiology

The first occurrences of AIDS in the pediatric population in the United States took place in children born to mothers infected with HIV or in children, especially neonates, who had received blood products contaminated with HIV.[711] The actual number of children infected with HIV in the United States is unknown, but increasing spread into the pediatric population reflects a change in the demographics of the adult infection. Greater numbers of women of childbearing age are at risk of being infected, either from illicit drug use and direct contact from contaminated needles or from sexual relations with an infected person.[712,713] A 1988 study examining HIV infection in the United States reported 737 occurrences of AIDS in children younger than 13 years, a 64% increase over the number found in the previous year. In 75% of these patients the disease was acquired perinatally, in 13% it was associated with transfusions, and in 5% it occurred in children with hemophilia.[714] More than 70% of cases of AIDS acquired perinatally were related to intravenous drug use by the child's mother or the mother's sexual partner.[714] In July 1989, 1600 cases of perinatal AIDS in the United States had been reported to the Centers for Disease Control and Prevention, and a rise to 10,000 to 20,000 cases was predicted for the next few years.[715] The findings of the HIV Survey in Childbearing Women[716] estimated that 7000 HIV-infected women gave birth to infants in the United States in 1993. If a perinatal transmission rate of 15% to 30% is assumed, approximately 1000 to 2000 infants were infected with HIV perinatally in 1993.[717] HIV infection is increasing in urban women throughout Europe and is having a dramatic impact in central and eastern Africa and Haiti. In Zaire, 5% to 10% of women of childbearing age are seropositive for HIV, and heterosexual transmission unrelated to drug abuse accounts for nearly all of the reported cases.[718] Of interest is the fact that initially the western Africa population seemed to be relatively free of AIDS until reports of patients with typical symptoms started to appear.[719-721] Unexpectedly, these patients were seronegative for HIV-1 antigens but were found to be infected with a related virus termed HIV-2. The sequence of HIV-2 differs significantly from that of HIV-1 and is remarkably similar to that of a virus isolated from captive macaques, termed simian immunodeficiency virus (SIV) mac.[722,723] This noted similarity has led to an interesting discourse on the origins of HIV, and debate still continues on whether HIV-1 and HIV-2 could indeed have a common ancestor that resided in the genome of nonhuman primates or whether the related viruses evolved from two separate horizontal infections in humans.[724] Although the origins of HIV are not known, certain routes of transmission are understood, and it is anticipated that with control of the blood supply in most developed countries, vertical transmission from mother to child will be the sole route of pediatric HIV infection in the future.

The AIDS pandemic in Africa and, in particular, southern Africa has reached catastrophic proportions. The rising incidence of the disease in eastern Europe, India, and Thailand and throughout most of the Third World poses many political, social, and medical challenges that are beyond the scope of this chapter.

Transmission

Transmitted primarily through contact with infected lymphocytes and monocytes, HIV may be found in blood, semen, and vaginal secretions.[725,726] Isolation of the virus from 13- and 15-week abortuses, placenta, and cord blood provides strong support for intrauterine infection.[711,727-729] AIDS has developed in children born by cesarean section who were never again in contact with their mothers,[730] and the fact that life-threatening illness is often manifested within the first few months of life favors vertical transmission in utero. Maternal-fetal transfusion at delivery remains another possible route of infection.[731] Postpartum transmission via breast milk, though possible, appears to be rare. Accordingly, in countries in which safe feeding substitutes are not readily available, breast-feeding should not be curtailed; however, in developed countries where alternatives exist, breast-feeding by HIV-infected women is discouraged.

The rate of transmission from mother to child is estimated to be about 25% based on several studies from the United States and Europe.[732-735] Factors that influence transmission are related to maternal health, with asymptomatic mothers experiencing a lower rate of infected children. Transmission from mother to child can be reduced from 25% to 2% by the use of antiretroviral therapy during pregnancy, labor, and the neonatal period. Although it is clear that breast milk may be a source of maternal transfer of virus from mother to child, the risk-benefit ratio is dependent on the socioeconomic status of the mother and child.[731]

Major advances in screening and testing of the blood supply in the United States after 1985 led to a reduction in the risk of receiving a contaminated single transfusion in 1988 to 1 in 250,000.[736] The first screening test is a questionnaire to exclude people who engage in high-risk activities. The next step is an enzyme-linked immunosorbent assay for detection of antibodies to HIV antigens. In rare individuals who are infected but seronegative, HIV can escape detection, but newer, sensitive screening tests detect the viral genome by PCR.[737] In addition, routine screening for cytomegalovirus antibody serves as a surrogate screening test for HIV because it is also present in 95% of HIV-infected donors.[738]

Tragically, individuals with bleeding disorders such as hemophilia A and B who received clotting factors from a large donor pool for a single infusion have had an increased likelihood of acquiring AIDS. In large metropolitan areas, the number of these patients who are affected approaches 90%. Recognition of the problem and the availability of heat-pasteurized preparations of factor concentrates and recombinant factor preparations should eliminate the risk in patients with newly diagnosed AIDS.

Sexually active adolescents are at risk to the same degree as adults, and younger children have been infected as a result of sexual abuse.[711]

Biology

The genome of HIV encodes the structural proteins GAG, POL, and ENV, which are common to all replication-competent retroviruses.[738] The life cycle of the virus begins with entry into a susceptible cell. Infection by HIV appears to be initiated by binding of gp120 of the viral envelope protein (encoded by the *ENV* gene) to the CD4 antigen.[739-741] Cell surface expression of CD4 is necessary and sufficient for viral infection of human cells in vitro.[742] Interaction between CD4 and HIV envelope proteins mediates the formation of syncytia, which are multinucleate collections of fused infected and uninfected cells.[743] The interaction between gp120 and CD4 triggers a conformational change in gp120 that promotes engagement of the HIV coreceptors CCR5 or CXCR4. These events result in gp41 envelope protein–mediated fusion of viral and cellular membranes. Fusion then allows the HIV capsid component to be inserted into the cell. Viral entry appears to occur through coated pit–dependent and coated pit–independent pathways; however, the precise subcellular compartments of viral uncoating remain unresolved. After uncoating is complete, the HIV preintegration complex is formed with the loss of some viral core proteins. The preintegration complex components include the double-stranded DNA version of the viral genome, as well as the reverse transcriptase, matrix, integrase, and Vpr proteins.[744] It was initially thought that G_0 cells lacked the cellular factors necessary for complete synthesis of the DNA provirus and were probably unable to support effective DNA provirus integration into the host genome.[745,746] Recent work has shown that both nondividing macrophages and naïve T cells serve as important targets for HIV infection in vivo. It now appears that nuclear import signals in the viral integrase, matrix, and Vpr proteins, as well as a DNA flap produced during reverse transcription, play a key role in allowing the HIV preintegration complex to enter the nucleus. It also appears that activation of HIV-1 provirus in dividing cells is influenced by the action of constitutively expressed host transcription factors, such as Sp1, TDFII, CTF/NFI, and LBP-1,[747] and inducible cellular transcription factors, such as NFκB and NFAT-1.[748] The HIV-1 long terminal repeat (LTR) contains *cis*-acting motifs that act as signatures to which these *trans*-acting proteins can bind. In particular, the LTR has a duplicated NFκB site to which NFκB, which is induced by T-cell activation, is able to *trans*-activate the expression of viral genes. In this way, the HIV LTR acts like a T-cell activation gene.[748]

The HIV genome also codes for two different proteins required for viral morphogenesis and maturation (VF and VPU) and three nonstructural regulatory proteins (TAT, REV, and NEF).[749] The TAT protein is a very effective *trans*-activator of all genes linked to the LTR, including the *TAT* gene itself.[750,751] The target sequence for TAT recognition coincides with a predicted RNA secondary structure,[7525] and the so-called *trans*-activation response element appears to be present within all HIV transcripts. The *REV* gene product is a 19-kd phosphorylated protein[753] that appears to regulate nuclear export of the incompletely spliced viral RNA that is normally excluded from the cell cytoplasm.[754] During the initial course of infection only spliced viral RNA is transported to the cytoplasm for the translation of TAT, REV, and NEF proteins. The TAT protein induces a positive feedback on transcription, whereas the REV protein recognizes a REV response element that enhances the transport of singly spliced or unspliced RNA to the cytoplasm. These latter transcripts encode structural proteins, and it has been proposed that the action of REV restricts the expression of viral structural protein to a relatively short period, thereby diminishing the host's ability to recognize infected cells.[748] The critical roles of these regulatory proteins in the HIV life cycle may provide targets for future antiviral agents, and in this regard, *trans*-dominant mutants of REV have been shown to be effective in vitro.[755]

Mononuclear phagocytes harbor HIV-1, and it has been suggested that their tropism contributes to the latency of the infection.[756] Megakaryocytes also harbor the virus.[757,758] Indeed, tropism of macrophages is via CCR5 tropic strains, and CXCR4 tropic virus predominately infects nondividing T cells. Direct in vitro infection of microglia cells[759] and epithelial cells, especially in the gut, may partly explain some of the clinical manifestations of HIV infection, which are most likely a result of a direct cytopathic effect of the virus and the consequences of immune suppression.

Work has focused on the biologic and immunologic characterization of long-term survivors of patients infected with HIV-1.[760,7661] These studies have to be viewed in the context of a new understanding that has modified thought pertaining to the dynamics of HIV replication and host responses during the early phases of the disease.[762] It was previously assumed that the latent phase of HIV infection involved less extensive viral turnover. Two articles have indicated that HIV viremia is a balance between continuous rounds of de novo viral infection and replication and vigorous induction of CD4+

and CD8+ lymphocytes that attempt to induce sterilizing immunity.[763,764] Mathematical modeling has allowed a projection that billions of virions escape; however, when they do, they rapidly acquire resistance to single-drug therapy. These studies raise the hope for combination antiviral therapy and the possibility that sterilization immunity may occur. In fact, Bryson and colleagues[765] described an infant who was infected with HIV perinatally, but the infection subsequently resolved. HIV infection was not detectable in this child 5 years later. The authors of this study convincingly demonstrated that the child was indeed infected, but it is not clear how the infection was resolved.[766] The question of effective immunity to HIV infection has also been studied in a subgroup of patients who remain asymptomatic despite HIV infection. In one study it appeared that asymptomatic long-term survivors have a decreased viral load in their plasma and low levels of HIV in their lymphoid tissue.[761] Furthermore, lymphoid architecture and immune function appeared to be intact in 15 subjects with nonprogressive HIV infection as compared with 18 subjects who had progressive disease. The implication of these findings is that therapies focused on induction of some degree of viral attenuation in combination with stimulation of immune responses may offer the best hope for curtailing HIV infection.

The idea that a reduction in viral load is an important hallmark of therapy is further bolstered by a study that showed a reduction in maternal-infant transmission of HIV with zidovudine treatment.[767] In a study of 363 HIV-positive pregnant women, 180 were randomly assigned to receive zidovudine and 183 to receive placebo; 13 infants in the zidovudine group and 40 in the placebo group were infected with HIV. The results strongly suggest that a regimen of antepartum zidovudine treatment reduces the risk of maternal-infant HIV transmission by approximately two thirds.[767] More recent studies involving protease inhibitors used with other agents strongly suggest that combination therapy is the appropriate approach to the treatment of this pernicious disease.[768] The latest study revealed that combination therapy with protease inhibitors has reduced the mortality from 5.3% in 1996 to 0.7% in 1999 in a cohort of HIV-infected children from 0 to 20 years of age in the United States. Furthermore, the combination of HIV screening in pregnancy and the use of antiviral therapy has reduced the risk of vertical transmission in the United States from 25% to 1.4% such that the incidence of HIV infection in infants is 300 per year.[768] This should be contrasted to the situation in Third World countries, where it is estimated that 1700 new pediatric infections occur per day.[770]

Clinical Features

General

Infection with HIV results in a spectrum of disease from an asymptomatic state to severe immunodeficiency involving multiple organ systems. The heterogeneity of symptoms is explained by the underlying pathophysiologic course in that (1) the incubation period may be weeks, months, or years; (2) the direct cytopathic effect on target cells, predominantly CD4+ lymphocytes, monocytes, and accessory cells, results in dysregulation of the immune system; and (3) the viral elimination phase that is accompanied by a host response to infection varies with the immune competence of the host. Because many children are infected congenitally, they show signs early in life and often have constitutional symptoms such as unexplained diarrhea, fever, night sweats, generalized lymphadenopathy, and hepatosplenomegaly. Failure to thrive and developmental delay are often prominent early manifestations of HIV infection in children. Susceptibility to recurrent infections by common bacterial and viral pathogens, as well as to opportunistic infections, increases the index of suspicion that the underlying disorder is in fact AIDS. These and other manifestations of HIV infection are summarized in Box 36-6.

Hematologic Findings

The hematopoietic dysfunction that is invariably associated with HIV infection results from global dysregulation of the physiologic cascades of antibody formation, coagulation and complement, and direct infection of key regulatory cells. Acute and chronic infections and therapies for the underlying disorder also affect hematopoiesis. Although for the purposes of discussion it is simpler to view these changes according to cell lineage, it should be stressed that these events rarely occur in isolation. Examination of the peripheral blood smear from the majority of AIDS patients reveals anemia and granulocytopenia and, in a third of patients, associated thrombocytopenia.[771]

Box 36-6	**Clinical Manifestations**

PRIMARY MANIFESTATIONS OF HIV INFECTION

Hematologic and Immune Abnormalities

Hypergammaglobulinemia
Lymphopenia (CD4+ cells decrease)
Decreased CD4/CD8 ratio
Thrombocytopenia
Anemia
Neutropenia
Drug allergies (e.g., trimethoprim in 40% to 60% of patients)

Nonspecific Findings (includes children with two or more unexplained findings for more than 2 months)

Failure to thrive
Hepatosplenomegaly
Generalized lymphadenopathy
Parotitis
Diarrhea (three or more loose stools per day)

Neurologic Disease

Loss of intellectual ability or developmental milestones
Impaired brain growth (acquired microcephaly, brain atrophy, or both)
Progressive systemic motor defects
  Paresis
  Abnormal tone
  Pathologic reflexes
  Ataxia or gait disturbance

Cardiovascular Disease

Cardiomyopathy
Arrhythmias

Other Diseases

Hepatitis
Nephropathy (sclerosing glomerulonephritis)
Dermatologic diseases (most commonly seborrheic dermatitis)

SECONDARY MANIFESTATIONS OF HIV INFECTION

Secondary Infections

Pneumocystis carinii pneumonia
Chronic cryptosporidiosis
Disseminated toxoplasmosis (onset after 1 month of age)
Extraintestinal strongyloidiasis
Chronic isosporiasis
Candidiasis (esophageal, bronchial, and pulmonary)
Extrapulmonary cryptococcosis
Disseminated histoplasmosis
Mycobacterial infection
Cytomegalovirus infection (onset after 1 month of age)
Coccidioidomycosis
Nocardiosis
Progressive multifocal leukoencephalopathy
Lymphocytic interstitial pneumonitis

Secondary Cancers

Kaposi's sarcoma
B-cell non-Hodgkin's lymphoma
Primary lymphoma of the brain

HIV, human immunodeficiency virus.
From Centers for Disease Control and Prevention (CDC). Classification systems for human immunodeficiency virus (HIV) in children under 13 years of age. MMWR Morbid Mortal Wkly Rep. 1987;36(15):225-230, 235-236.

Bone Marrow Findings

In several studies, the bone marrow morphologic changes in patients with AIDS were reported.[772] The most common findings were hypercellularity, lymphoid aggregates, plasmacytosis, and dysplasia. When thrombocytopenia is present, the marrow often contains adequate megakaryocytes, thus suggesting an immune mechanism of platelet destruction (see later). The anemia and granulocytopenia appear to be related to the dysplastic bone marrow and result from ineffective hematopoiesis. Increases in reticulum and fibrosis have been reported in association with *Mycobacterium avium* infection.

Thrombocytopenia

The underlying mechanism of thrombocytopenia, which can be the initial finding of HIV infection in children, appears to be immune destruction of platelets. Several studies have identified a high incidence of cytophilic antibodies[773,774] and have highlighted concomitant complement deposition on the platelet.[775] In addition, a 25-kd platelet-associated antigen has been detected in thrombocytopenic adults and children with AIDS[776]; however, the presence of the antibody in serum does not invariably lead to thrombocytopenia because 15 of 16 nonthrombocytopenic patients with AIDS and generalized adenopathy also had this antibody. Purified platelet eluates from homosexuals and narcotic addicts with AIDS and thrombocytopenia contain anti-HIV antibodies; however, no viral antigens were detected on the platelet surface, and PCR failed to detect provirus.[777] In 1983, an idiopathic thrombocytopenic purpura syndrome in patients with hemophilia was reported,[778] and it was subsequently recognized that these patients, like many older patients with hemophilia, had AIDS. The mechanisms of platelet destruction in hemophilia, as with that in other AIDS populations, remain an open question and as such pose a challenge in the design of rational treatment regimens. Spontaneous recovery from thrombocytopenia does occur; for instance, in one study, 8 of 25 patients with thrombocytopenia recovered.[779] Treatment is often considered when the platelet count decreases to less than 20,000/mL or a clinical bleeding episode is encountered. The question whether prednisone therapy worsens the underlying disease remains unanswered, but prednisone has been used as the initial therapy for thrombocytopenia in homosexual men. In 16 of 17 patients with a mean platelet count of 21,000/mL who were treated with 60 to 100 mg/day of prednisone, platelet counts increased to greater than 50,000/mL. However, platelet counts decreased to pretreatment levels with a reduction of the prednisone dose.[780] Similar findings were observed in another study in which 19 of 24 patients responded initially to prednisone treatment, but the improvement was sustained in only 2 when prednisone therapy was stopped.[781] Several studies have indicated that splenectomy is effective in most patients whose platelet counts decline after prednisone therapy, and it is often considered in patients with hemophilia and thrombocytopenia.[775]

High-dose intravenous immunoglobulin, 1 g/kg on days 1, 2, and 15 and every 3 weeks, resulted in a transient increase in platelet count.[781] However, all patients experienced relapse during the 3-week maintenance therapy period. Other modalities include danazol anti-Rh immunoglobulin[782] and zidovudine, which has been used in patients who are asymptomatic and have mild thrombocytopenia (50,000/mL),[783-785] as well as in patients with lower platelet counts who are asymptomatic.

Some consensus can be drawn from these studies. Immediate treatment of patients with platelet counts below 20,000/mL or clinical bleeding appears to be prednisone, 30 to 40 mg daily, and possibly high-dose intravenous gamma globulin, with splenectomy being a good option for long-term control. Zidovudine and other new treatment modalities should also be considered as maintenance therapy.

Anemia and Granulocytopenia

Anemia and granulocytopenia are found in most patients with AIDS and reflect, in large part, ineffective hematopoiesis. The anemia is typically normochromic and normocytic, with a low reticulocyte count and mild to severe anisocytosis and poikilocytosis. Up to 40% of patients with AIDS may have positive findings on a direct Coombs test as a result of absorbed immunoglobulin. Although antibodies have been detected on the surface of granulocytes,[786,787] the mechanism for granulocytopenia appears to be suppression of bone marrow progenitors. Bone marrow from patients with HIV infection exhibits colony formation (colony-forming units–granulocyte-macrophage and burst forming units–erythroid) similar to that in HIV-seronegative control subjects when cultivated in serum from an HIV-seronegative donor. However, there is selective suppression of colony formation in bone marrow derived from a patient with HIV infection versus bone marrow from seronegative donors when cultivated in seropositive sera. This suggests that progenitor cells and progeny are able to be infected with HIV and express HIV antigens on their surface that are recognized by HIV antibodies, thus accounting for the suppression. Further support for this hypothesis comes from the demonstration of provirus in megakaryocytes from the bone marrow of patients with AIDS.[788,789]

Alloantibodies are detected in 30% to 60% of patients with AIDS in different series, with anti-i and anti-I being the most common.[786] Anti-i has also been associated with EBV and cytomegalovirus infections, both of which often coexist with HIV infection and may account for the presence of specific red cell antibodies. Antibodies to Le, PL, E, K, Lu, and Sd all have been found, although their relationship to the pathophysiologic course of the anemia in HIV, which in large part does not appear to be hemolytic, remains an open question.

Zidovudine is now widely used in pediatric patients with AIDS,[790] and therefore treatment often causes anemia and neutropenia. Macrocytosis with 25- to 40-unit increases in mean corpuscular volume is observed in 74% of patients receiving zidovudine. The macrocytosis is not usually accompanied by anemia, but when it does occur, the anemia is usually mild and dose related. In a subgroup of patients, anemia caused by bone marrow suppression is observed. A depressed reticulocyte count is an early sign of toxicity and is accompanied by normal to elevated serum folate and vitamin B_{12} levels. In patients with advanced disease, maintenance of zidovudine therapy requires regular blood transfusions.[791]

Neutropenia (absolute neutrophil count of 750 to 1000) is seen early in zidovudine treatment and is often dose limiting. More severe neutropenia is observed in patients with advanced disease and can be reversed by cessation of therapy. Pancytopenia has also been described but does not seem to resolve after withdrawal of treatment.[791]

Mitochondrial myopathy may result from long-term treatment.[792]

Coagulation Defects

In 1984, four homosexual patients with AIDS were reported to have prolonged partial thromboplastin times in the absence of any factor deficiency.[793] Because these defects were not correctable with kaolin or normal serum and were accompanied by a prolonged Russell viper venom time, they appeared to be due to the presence of lupus anticoagulant. Although one of these patients had documented deep venous thrombosis and pulmonary embolism, no other sequelae related to lupus anticoagulant have been reported. The lupus anticoagulant is a member of a family of antiphospholipid antibodies that includes anticardiolipin antibody and the Venereal Disease Research Laboratory (VDRL) test for syphilis. The antibody may be an IgG or an IgM and may be directed against the phospholipid components of the prothrombin activator complex and hence is capable of prolonging the lipid-dependent coagulation tests. Although it has been proposed that the presence of antiphospholipid antibodies is strongly associated with *Pneumocystis* infection, the significance of this claim remains open to doubt.[772] In short, therefore, coagulopathies do not appear to be of great clinical importance in AIDS, but they can be part of DIC in an associated superinfection.

Diagnosis in Infants and Children

Detection of antibodies to HIV antigens is a standard approach to the diagnosis of HIV infection. The first screen is an enzyme-linked immunosorbent assay; positive results may be confirmed by a specific immunoblot. However, the presence of anti-HIV immunoglobulin of the IgG subclass in an infant does not necessarily indicate that the infant is infected with HIV because maternal IgG crosses the placenta and has a half-life of 28 days. In fact, persistence of maternal IgG has been detected beyond 15 months of age.[733] In contrast, several seronegative HIV-infected children have been reported.[794-796] Although IgM or IgA anti-HIV antibodies are better indicators of active infection in children because these subclasses of antibody do not cross the placenta, the sensitivity and specificity of the enzyme-linked immunosorbent assays for these antibody isotypes are much lower than those for IgG anti-HIV. Definitive proof of HIV infection rests with viral culture and demonstration of the provirus via the very sensitive PCR.[796] The importance of early diagnosis, which combines laboratory tests and clinical findings, lies in the possibility and hope that early antiviral therapy may alter the natural history of the disease in children. Thus, the search for novel therapies is being actively pursued, and it appears that the newer nucleoside analogues may be associated with less bone marrow toxicity than seen with zidovudine. Current U.S. treatment guidelines for pediatric HIV infection advocate aggressive therapy with a combination of antiretroviral regimens. The goal is durable suppression of viral replication with preservation of immune function. A combination of a protease inhibitor and dual nucleoside reverse transcriptase inhibitors (NRTIs) is the most commonly used form of highly active antiretroviral therapy (HAART) in children.[797] The expense and difficulty of adhering to this regimen limit access to the vast majority of infected children in the world. Prevention and education remain the most effective short-term modes of limiting the spread of AIDS.[798]

REFERENCES

1. Dale J, Myhre R. Mechanical fragility of erythrocytes in normals and patients with heart valve prostheses. Acta Med Scand. 1971;190:127-131.
2. Indeglia RA, Shea MA, Varco RL, Bernstein EF. Erythrocyte destruction by prosthetic heart valves. Circulation. 1968;37(4 Suppl):II86-II93.
3. Okita Y, Miki S, Ueda Y, et al. Propranolol for intractable hemolysis after open heart operation. Ann Thorac Surg. 1991;52:1158-1160.
4. Hayze AM, Redington AN, Rigby ML. Severe haemolysis after transcatheter duct occlusion: a non-surgical remedy. Br Heart J. 1992;67:321-322.
5. de Geeter B. [Severe hemolysis after endoluminal closure of the ductus arteriosus and recovery following implantation of a second obturator.] Arch Mal Coeur Vaiss. 1993; 86:629-630.
6. Kastor JA, Akbarian M, Buckley MJ, et al. Paravalvular leaks and haemolytic anaemia following insertion of Starr-Edwards aortic and mitral valves. J Thorac Cardiovasc Surg. 1968;56:279-288.
7. Baird RJ, Lipton IH, Labrosse CH, et al. An evaluation of the late results of aortic valve repair. J Thorac Cardiovasc Surg. 1965;49:562-573.
8. Brodeur MTH, Sutherland DW, Koler RD, et al. Red blood cell survival in patients with aortic valvular disease and ball-valve prosthesis. Circulation. 1965;32: 570-581.

9. Nevaril GG, Lynd EC, Alfrey CP Jr, Hellums JD. Erythrocyte damage and destruction induced by shearing stress. J Lab Clin Med. 1968;71:784-790.

10. Steele P, Weitz H, Davies H, et al. Platelet survival time following aortic valve replacement. Circulation. 1975;51:358-362.

11. Eyster E, Rothchild J, Mychajliw O. Chronic intravascular hemolysis after aortic valve replacement. Long-term study comparing different types of ball-valve prosthesis. Circulation. 1971;44:657-665.

12. Slater SD, Fell GS. Intravascular hemolysis and urinary iron losses after replacement of heart valves by a prosthesis. Clin Sci. 1972;42:545-553.

13. Linderkamp O, Klose HJ, Betke K, et al. Increased blood viscosity in patients with cyanotic congenital heart disease and iron deficiency. J Pediatr. 1979;95:567-569.

14. Myhre E, Rasmussen K, Andersen A. Serum lactate dehydrogenase activity in patients with prosthetic heart valves: a parameter of intravascular hemolysis. Am Heart J. 1970;80:463-468.

15. Sears DA, Crosby WH. Intravascular hemolysis due to intracardiac prosthetic devices. Am J Med. 1965;39:341-354.

16. Meguro A, Kuribayashi R, Sakurada T, et al. [Intravascular hemolysis due to residual shunt after patch closure of VSD: a case report.] Kyobu Geka. 1992;45:537-540.

17. Vellodi A, Bini RM. Malignant ventricular arrhythmias caused by hyperkalemia complicating the Kasabach-Merritt syndrome. J R Soc Med. 1988;81:167-168.

18. Pirofsky B, Sutherland DW, Starr A, Griswold HE. Haemolytic anemia complicating aortic valve surgery. An autoimmune syndrome. N Engl J Med. 1965;272:235-239.

19. Tyndall MR, Teitel TF, Lutin WA, et al. Serum erythropoietin levels in patients with cyanotic congenital heart disease. J Pediatr. 1987;110:538-544.

20. Haga P, Cotes P, Till JA, et al. Is oxygen supply the only regulator of erythropoietin levels? Serum immunoreactive erythropoietin during the first four months of life in term infants with different levels of arterial oxygenation. Acta Paediatr Scand. 1987;76:907-913.

21. Gidding S, Stockman JA 3rd. Erythropoietin in cyanotic congenital heart disease. Am Heart J. 1988;116:128-132.

22. Gidding SS, Stockman JA 3rd. The effect of iron deficiency on tissue oxygen delivery in cyanotic congenital heart disease. Am J Cardiol. 1988;61:605-607.

23. Macdonald PD, Gibson BE, Brownlee J, et al. Protein C activity in severely ill newborns with congenital heart disease. J Perinat Med. 1992;20:421-427.

24. Bahnson HT, Siegler RF. A consideration of the causes of death following operation for congenital heart disease of the cyanotic type. Surg Gynecol Obstet. 1950;90:60-76.

25. Hartmann RC. A hemorrhagic disorder occurring in patients with cyanotic congenital heart disease. Bull Johns Hopkins Hosp. 1952;91:49-67.

26. Kontras SB, Sirak HD, Newton WA Jr. Hematologic abnormalities in children with congenital heart disease. JAMA. 1966;195:611-615.

27. Ekert H, Gilchrist GS. Coagulation studies in congenital heart disease. Lancet. 1968;2:280.

28. Ekert H, Gilchrist GS, Stanton R, Hammond D. Hematostasis and cyanotic congenital heart disease. J Pediatr. 1970;76:221-230.

29. Kern FH, Morana NJ, Sears JJ, Hickey PR. Coagulation defects in neonates during cardiopulmonary bypass. Ann Thorac Surg. 1992;54:541-546.

30. Andrew M, Marzinotto V, Massicotte P, et al. Heparin therapy in pediatric patients: a prospective cohort study. Pediatr Res. 1994;35:78-83.

31. Dennis LH, Stewart JL, Conrad ME. Heparin treatment of hemorrhagic diathesis in cyanotic congenital heart disease. Lancet. 1967;1:1088-1089.

32. Johnson CA, Abelgaard CF, Schulman I. Absence of coagulation abnormalities in children with cyanotic congenital heart disease. Lancet. 1968;2:660-662.

33. Komp DM, Sparrow AW. Polycythemia in cyanotic heart disease—a study of altered coagulation. J Pediatr. 1970;76:231-236.

34. Kontras SB, Bodenbender JG, Craenen J, Hosier DM. Hyperviscosity in congenital heart disease. J Pediatr. 1970;76:214-220.

35. Gamba G, Venco A, Grandi A, et al. Mitral valve prolapse and factor VIII complex abnormalities. Haematologica. 1984;69:549-555.

36. Gross S, Keefer V, Liebman J. The platelet in cyanotic congenital heart disease. Pediatrics. 1968;42:651-658.

37. Colon-Ontero G, Gilchrist G, Holcomb GR, et al. Preoperative evaluation of hemostasis in patients with congenital heart disease. Mayo Clin Proc. 1987;62:379-385.

38. Hara T, Mizuno Y, Akeda H, et al. Thrombocytopenia: a complication of Kawasaki disease. Eur J Paediatr. 1988;147:51-53.

39. Mauer HM, McCue CM, Caul J, Still WJ. Impairment in platelet aggregation in congenital heart disease. Blood. 1972;40:207-216.

40. Ekert H, Sheers M. Preoperative and postoperative platelet function in cyanotic congenital heart disease. J Thorac Cardiovasc Surg. 1974;67:184-190.

41. Ekert H, Dowling SV. Platelet release abnormality and reduced prothrombin levels in children with cyanotic congenital heart disease. Aust Paediatr J. 1977;13:17-21.

42. Rosenthal A, Nathan DG, Marty AT, et al. Acute hemodynamic effects of red cell volume reduction in polycythemia of cyanotic congenital heart disease. Circulation. 1970;13:297-308.

43. Gralnick HR. ε-Aminocaproic acid in preoperative correction of haemostatic defect in cyanotic congenital heart disease. Lancet. 1970;1:1204-1205.

44. Maurer HM. Hematologic effects of cardiac disease. Pediatr Clin North Am. 1972;19:1083-1093.

45. Martelle RR, Linde LM. Cerebrovascular accidents with tetralogy of Fallot. Am J Dis Child. 1961;101:206-209.

46. Cottrill CM, Kaplan S. Cerebrovascular accidents in cyanotic congenital heart disease. Am J Dis Child. 1973;125:484-487.

47. Card RT, Weintraub LR. Metabolic abnormalities of erythrocytes in severe iron deficiency. Blood. 1971;37:725-732.

48. Stuart RK, McDonald JW, Ahuja SP, Coles JC. Platelet survival times in patients with prosthetic heart valves. Am J Cardiol. 1974;33:840-844.

49. Steele P, Weitz H, Davies H, et al. Platelet survival time following aortic valve replacement. Circulation. 1975;35: 358-362.

50. Bonchek LI, Starr A. Ball valve prostheses: current appraisal of late results. Am J Cardiol. 1975;35:843-854.

51. Harker LA, Slichter SJ. Studies of platelet and fibrinogen kinetics in patients with prosthetic heart valves. N Engl J Med. 1970;283:1302-1305.

52. Coultée F, Carceller AM, Deschamps L, et al. The evolving pattern of pediatric endocarditis from 1960 to 1985. Can J Cardiol. 1990;6:164-170.

53. Lerner PI, Weinstein L. Infective endocarditis in the antibiotic era. N Engl J Med. 1966;274:199-206.

54. Mandell GL, Douglas RG, et al. Principles and Practice of Infectious Diseases. New York, John Wiley, 1979.

55. Pacheco-Ríos A, Araujo-Hernández L, Cashat-Cruz M, et al. *Candida* endocarditis in the first year of life. Bol Med Hosp Infant Mex. 1993;50:157-161.

56. Ward HP, Holman J. The association of nucleated red cells in the peripheral smear with hypoxemia. Ann Intern Med. 1967;67:1190-1194.

57. Palva IP, Salokannel SJ, Takkunen JT. Thrombocytopenia in heart failure: preliminary report. Acta Med Scand. 1970;187:429-430.

58. Pearson HA, Schiebler GL, Spencer RP. Functional hyposplenia in cyanotic congenital heart disease. Pediatrics. 1971;48:277-280.

59. Chisholm M, Ardran GM, Callender ST, Wright R. Iron deficiency and auto-immunity in postcricoid webs. Q J Med. 1971;40:421-433.

60. Fisher M, Katz S, Katzka I. Silent erosive esophagitis with severe iron deficiency anemia. N Y State J Med. 1980; 1:1740-1742.

61. Cheu HW, Grosfeld JL, Heifetz SA, et al. Persistence of Barrett's esophagus in children after antireflux surgery: influence on follow-up care. J Pediatr Surg. 1992;27:260-264; discussion 265-266.

62. Delamore IW, Shearman DJC. Chronic iron deficiency anemia and atrophic gastritis. Lancet. 1965;1:889-891.

63. Wood IJ, Ralston M, Ungar B, Cowling DC. Vitamin B_{12} deficiency in chronic gastritis. Gut. 1964;5:27-37.

64. Grange DK, Finlay JL. Nutritional vitamin B_{12} deficiency in a breastfed infant following maternal gastric bypass. Pediatr Hematol Oncol. 1994;11:311-318.

65. Bernstein LH, Gutstein S, Efron G, et al. Trichobezoar: an unusual cause of megaloblastic anemia and hypoproteinemia in childhood. Dig Dis. 1973;18:67-71.

66. McIntyre OR, Sullivan LW, Jeffries GH, Silver RH. Pernicious anemia in childhood. N Engl J Med. 1965;272: 981-986.

67. Grady M, Madoff MA, Duhamel RC, et al. Intestinal absorption in the contaminated small bowel syndrome. Gut. 1971;12:403-410.

68. Bouguerra L, Ben-Ammar B, Bibi D, et al. Incidence of iron deficiency anemia in celiac disease. Tunis Med. 1990;68:131-133.

69. Encinas Sotillos A, Romero Ganuza FJ, Hernández Navarrete C. Iron deficiency as the first manifestation of celiac disease. Rev Esp Enferm Dig. 1991;79:163-164.

70. Ståhlberg MR, Savilahti E, Siimes MA. Iron deficiency in coeliac disease is mild and it is detected and corrected by gluten-free diet. Acta Paediatr Scand. 1991;80:190-193.

71. Hjelt K, Krasilnikoff PA. The impact of gluten on haematological status, dietary intakes of haematopoietic nutrients and vitamin B_{12} and folic acid absorption in children with coeliac disease. Acta Paediatr Scand. 1990;79: 911-919.

72. Korman SH. Pica as a presenting symptom in childhood celiac disease. Am J Clin Nutr. 1990;51:139-141.

73. Zittoun J. Celiac disease revealed by an acute folate deficiency. CESA. Committee of experts for specific investigations in complex anemias. Nouv Rev Fr Hematol. 1989;31:379-382.

74. Moake JL, Kageler WV, Cimo PL, et al. Intravascular hemolysis, thrombocytopenia, leukopenia and circulatory immune complexes after jejunal-ileal bypass surgery. Ann Intern Med. 1977;86:576-578.

75. O'Grady JG, Harding B, Stevens FM, et al. Influence of splenectomy and the functional hyposplenism of coeliac disease on platelet count and volume. Scand J Haematol. 1985;34:425-428.

76. O'Grady JG, Stevens FM, McCarthy CF. Celiac disease: does hyposplenism predispose to the development of malignant disease? Am J Gastroenterol. 1985;80:27-29.

77. Katz AJ, Falchuk ZM. Current concepts in gluten sensitive enteropathy (celiac sprue). Pediatr Clin North Am. 1975;22:767-785.

78. Dinari G, Zahavi I, Marcus H, Moroz C. Placental ferritin in coeliac disease: Relation to clinical stage, origin, and possible role in pathogenesis of malignancy. Gut. 1991; 32:999-1003.

79. Wisén O, Gardlund B. Hemostasis in Crohn's disease: low factor XIII levels in active disease. Scand J Gastroenterol. 1988;23:961-966.

80. Nielsen OH, Ahnfelt-Rønne I, Elmgreen J, et al. Abnormal metabolism of arachidonic acid in chronic inflammatory bowel disease: enhanced release of leukotriene B_4 from activated neutrophils. Gut. 1987;28: 181-185.

81. Verspaget HW, Peña AS, Weterman IT, Lamers CB. Neutrophil function in Crohn's disease and ulcerative colitis identified by decreased oxidative metabolism and low superoxide dismutase content. Gut. 1988;29:223-228.

82. Patel RT, Stokes R, Birch D, et al. Influence of total colectomy on serum antineutrophil cytoplasmic antibodies in inflammatory bowel disease. Br J Surg. 1994;81: 724-726.

83. Broekroelofs J, Mulder AH, Nelis GF, et al. Anti-neutrophil cytoplasmic antibodies (ANCA) in sera from patients with inflammatory bowel disease (IBD). Relation to disease pattern and disease activity. Dig Dis Sci. 1994; 39:545-549.

84. Heresbach D, Raoul JL, Genetet N, et al. Immunological study in primary intestinal lymphangiectasia. Digestion. 1994;55:59-64.

85. Kravis LP, South MA, Rosenlund ML. Eosinophilic gastroenteritis in the pediatric patient. Clin Pediatr (Phila). 1982;21:713-717.

86. Kay MA, O'Brien W, Kessler B, et al. Transient organic aciduria and methemoglobinemia with acute gastroenteritis. Pediatrics. 1990;85:589-592.

87. Gebara BM, Goetting MG. Life-threatening methemoglobinemia in infants with diarrhea and acidosis. Clin Pediatr (Phila). 1994;33:370-373.

88. Lebby T, Roco JJ, Arcinue EL. Infantile methemoglobinemia associated with acute diarrheal illness. Am J Emerg Med. 1993;11:471-472.

89. Centers for Disease Control and Prevention (CDC). Methemoglobinemia in an infant—Wisconsin, 1992. MMWR Morbid Mortal Wkly Rep. 1993;42(12):217-219.

90. Gumaste V, Greenstein AJ, Meyers R, Sachar DB. Coombs' positive autoimmune hemolytic anemia and ulcerative colitis. Dig Dis Sci. 1989;34:1457-1461.

91. Stadnicki A, Kloczko J, Nowak A, et al. Factor XIII subunits in relation to some other hemostatic parameters in ulcerative colitis. Am J Gastroenterol. 1991;86:690-693.

92. Salter RH, Read AE. Epsilon aminocaproic acid therapy in ulcerative colitis. Gut. 1970;11:585-587.

93. Qiao L, Golling M, Autschbach F, et al. T-cell receptor repertoire and mitotic responses of lamina propria T lymphocytes in inflammatory bowel disease. Clin Exp Immunol. 1994;97:303-308.

94. Discombe G. Sulphaemoglobinemia and gluthathione. Lancet. 1962;2:371.

95. Finch CA. Methemoglobinemia and sulfhemoglobinemia. N Engl J Med. 1948;239:470-478.

96. Yosovitz P, Hobson R, Ruymann F. Sporadic Peutz-Jeghers syndrome in early childhood: a diagnostic dilemma. Am J Dis Child. 1974;128:709-712.

97. Reid JD. Intestinal carcinoma in the Peutz-Jeghers syndrome. JAMA. 1974;229:833-834.

98. Bick RL, Fekete LF. Hereditary hemorrhagic telangiectasia and associated thrombohemorrhagic defects. Blood. 1979;54:745.

99. Conlon CL, Weinger RS, Cimo PL, et al. Telangiectasia and von Willebrand's disease in two families. Ann Intern Med. 1978;89:921-924.

100. Murphy D, Imrie CW, Davidson JF. Haematological abnormalities in acute pancreatitis. A prospective study. Postgrad Med. 1977;53:310-314.

101. Goeteyn M, Oranje AP, Vuzevski VD, et al. Ichthyosis, exocrine pancreatic insufficiency, impaired neutrophil chemotaxis, growth retardation, and metaphyseal dysplasia (Shwachman syndrome). Report of a case with extensive skin lesions (clinical, histological, and ultrastructural findings). Arch Dermatol. 1991;127:225-230.

102. Paterson CR, Wormsley KG. Hypothesis: Shwachman's syndrome of pancreatic exocrine insufficiency may be caused by neonatal copper deficiency. Ann Nutr Metab. 1988;32:127-132.

103. Shinowara GY, Stutman LJ, Walters MI, et al. Hypercoagulability in acute pancreatitis. Am J Surg. 1963;105:714-719.

104. Geokas MC, Rinderknecht H, Walberg CB, Weissman R. Methemalbumin in the diagnosis of acute hemorrhagic pancreatitis. Ann Intern Med. 1974;81:483-486.

105. Lasson A, Ohlsson K. Consumptive coagulopathy, fibrinolysis, and protease-antiprotease interactions during acute human pancreatitis. Thromb Res. 1986;1:167-183.

106. Bass HN, Miller AA. Cystic fibrosis presenting with anemia and hypoproteinemia in identical twins. J Pediatr. 1977;59:126-127.

107. Farrell PM, Bieri JG, Fratantoni JF, et al. The occurrence and effects of human vitamin E deficiency. A study in patients with cystic fibrosis. J Clin Invest. 1972;60:233-241.

108. Danse PW, Jakobs C, Rötig A, et al. Pearson's syndrome: a multi-system disorder based on a mt-DNA deletion. Tijdschr Kindergeneeskd. 1991;59:196-202.

109. Superti-Furga A, Schoenle E, Tuchschmid P, et al. Pearson bone marrow–pancreas syndrome with insulin-dependent diabetes, progressive renal tubulopathy, organic aciduria and elevated fetal haemoglobin caused by deletion and duplication of mitochondrial DNA. Eur J Pediatr. 1993;152:44-50.

110. Bernes SM, Bacino C, Prezant TR, et al. Identical mitochondrial DNA deletion in mother with progressive external ophthalmoplegia and son with Pearson marrow-pancreas syndrome. J Pediatr. 1993;123:598-602.

111. Rötig A, Cormier V, Koll F, et al. Site-specific deletions of the mitochondrial genome in the Pearson marrow-pancreas syndrome. Genomics. 1991;10:502-504.

112. Kimber C, Deller DJ, Ibbotson RN, Lander H. The mechanism of anemia in chronic liver disease. Q J Med. 1965;34:33-64.

113. Spivak JL. Serum immunoreactive erythropoietin in health and disease. Int J Cell Cloning. 1990;8(Suppl 1):211-224; discussion 224-226.

114. Smith JA, Lonergan ET, Sterling K. Spur-cell anemia: henolytic anemia with red cells resembling acanthocytes in alcoholic cirrhosis. N Engl J Med. 1966;275:639-643.

115. Silber R, Amorosi E, Lhowe J, Kayden HJ. Spur-shaped erythrocytes in Laennec's cirrhosis. N Engl J Med. 1966;275:639-643.

116. Douglass CC, Twomey JJ. Transient stomatocytosis with hemolysis: a previously unrecognized complication of alcoholism. Ann Intern Med. 1970;72:159-164.

117. Neerhout RC. Abnormalities of erythrocyte stromal lipids in hepatic disease. J Lab Clin Med. 1968;71:438-447.

118. Cooper RA, Diloy-Purray M, Lando P, Greenverg MS. An analysis of lipoproteins, bile acids and red cell membranes associated with target cells and spur cells in patients with liver disease. J Clin Invest. 1972;51:3182-3192.

119. Balistreri WF, Leslie MH, Cooper RA. Increased cholesterol and decreased fluidity of red cell membranes (spur cell anemia) in progressive intrahepatic cholestasis. Pediatrics. 1981;67:461-466.

120. Jandl JH. The anemia of liver disease: observations on its mechanisms. J Clin Invest. 1953;34:390-404.

121. Cooper RA. Hemolytic syndromes and red cell membrane abnormalities in liver disease. Semin Hematol. 1980;17:103-112.

122. Smith JR, Kay NE, Gottlieb AJ, Oski FA. Abnormal erythrocyte metabolism in hepatic disease. Blood. 1975;46:955-964.

123. Yawata Y, Kitajima K, Koresawa S, et al. Abnormal red cell metabolism in patients with hepato-biliary disorders: increased susceptibility to oxidative stress. Acta Haematol Jpn. 1977;40:9-15.

124. Makarenko EV, Kozlovskii IV. [The erythrocyte antioxidant system in chronic liver disease.] Ter Arkh. 1989;61:115-118.

125. Zudenigo D, Relja M. Hepatolenticular degeneration. Neurologija. 1990;39:115-127.

126. Key NS, Rank JM, Freese D, et al. Hemolytic anemia in protoporphyria: possible precipitating role of liver failure and photic stress. Am J Hematol. 1992;39:202-207.

127. Yawata Y, Howe R, Jacobs HS. Abnormal red cell metabolism causing hemolysis in uremia. Ann Intern Med. 1973;79:362-367.

128. O'Grady JG, Langley PG, Isola LM, et al. The coagulopathy of fulminant hepatic failure. Semin Liver Dis. 1986; 6:159-163.

129. Iwabuchi S, Takatori M, Okabe K. [Adequate parameters for the diagnosis of disseminated intravascular coagulation (DIC) in patients with liver diseases.] Nippon Rinsho. 1993;51:67-73.

130. Deutsch E. Blood coagulation changes in liver disease. In Popper H, Schaffner F (eds). Progress in Liver Disease. New York, Grune & Stratton, 1965, p 69.

131. Clark RD, Gazzard BG, Lewis ML, et al. Fibrinogen metabolism in acute hepatitis and active chronic hepatitis. Br J Haematol. 1975;30:95-102.

132. Ratnoff OD. Studies on proteolytic enzyme in human plasma. IV. The rate of lysis of plasma clots in normal and diseased individuals with particular reference to hepatic disease. Bull Johns Hopkins Hosp. 1949;84: 29.

133. Jedrychowski A, Hillenbrand P, Ajdukiewicz AB, et al. Fibrinolysis in cholestatic jaundice. BMJ. 1973;1: 640-642.

134. Lane DA, Scully MF, Thomas DP, et al. Acquired dysfibrinogenemia in acute and chronic liver disease. Br J Haematol. 1977;35:301-308.

135. Mester L, Szabados L. Structure défecteuse et biosynthese des fractions glucidiques dans les variantes pathologiques du fibrinogène. Nouv Rev Fr Hematol. 1970;10: 679-693.

136. Mester L, Szabados J, Soria J. Les modifications de la composition glucidique du fibrinogène dans les cas de dysfibrinogénémie acquisé. CR Acad Sci Hebd Seances Acad Sci D. 1970;271:1813-1815.

137. Rapaport SI, Ames SB, Mikkelsen S, Goodman JR. Plasma clotting factors in chronic hepatocellular disease. N Engl J Med. 1960;263:278-282.

138. Cederblad G, Korsan-Bengtsen K, Olssen R. Observations of increased levels of blood coagulation factors and other plasma proteins in cholestatic liver disease. Scand J Gastroenterol. 1976;11:391-396.

139. Ganrot PO, Niléhn JE. Synthesis of an abnormal prothrombin in malnutrition and biliary obstruction and during dicumarol treatment. Scand J Clin Lab Invest. 1971;28:245-249.

140. Lechner K, Niessner H, Thaler E. Coagulation abnormalities in liver disease. Semin Thromb Hemost. 1977;4: 40-56.

141. Dymock IW, Tucker JS, Wolf IL, et al. Coagulation studies as a prognostic index in acute liver failure. Br J Haematol. 1974;29:385-391.

142. Gallus AS, Lucas CR, Hirsh J. Coagulation studies in patients with acute infectious hepatitis. Br J Haematol. 1972;22:761-771.

143. Kupfer HG, Gee W, Ewald AT, Turner ME. Statistical correlation of liver function tests with coagulation factor deficiencies in Laennec's cirrhosis. Thromb Diath Haemorrh. 1964;10:317-331.

144. Green AJ, Ratnoff OD. Elevated antihemophiliac factor (AHF, factor VIII) procoagulant activity and AHF-like antigen in alcoholic cirrhosis of the liver. J Lab Clin Med. 1974;83:189-197.

145. Rapaport SI. Plasma thromboplastin antecedent levels in patients receiving Coumarin anticoagulants and in patients with Laennec's cirrhosis. Proc Soc Exp Biol Med. 1961; 108:115-116.

146. Gerhold WM, Tiongson T, Mandell EE. Studies of fibrin stabilizing factor. Fed Proc. 1966;25:446.

147. Hedner U, Henriksson P, Nilsson IM. Factor XIII in a clinical material. Scand J Haematol. 1975;14:114-119.

148. Abildgaard U, Fagerhol MK, Egeberg O. Comparison of progressive antithrombin activity and the concentrations of three thrombin inhibitors in human plasma. Scand J Clin Lab Invest. 1970;26:349-354.

149. Straub PW. Diffuse intravascular coagulation in liver disease. Semin Thromb Hemost. 1977;4:29-39.

150. Langley PG, Forbes A, Hughes RD, Williams R. Thrombin–antithrombin III complex in fulminant hepatic failure: evidence for disseminated intravascular coagulation and relationship to outcome. Eur J Clin Invest. 1990;20: 627-631.

151. Gazzard BG, Clark R, Borirakchanyavat V, Williams R. A controlled trial of heparin therapy in the coagulation defect of paracetamol induced hepatic necrosis. Gut. 1974;15:89-93.

152. Marassi A, Manzullo U, di Carlo V, Mannucci PM. Thromboembolism following prothrombin complex concentrates in major surgery in severe liver disease. Thromb Haemost. 1978;39:248-249.

153. Schiller GJ, Berkman SA. Hematologic aspects of renal insufficiency. Blood Rev. 1989;3:141-146.

154. Rowe PC, Walop W, Lior H, Mackenzie AM. Haemolytic anaemia after childhood *Escherichia coli* O 157 H7 infection: are females at increased risk? Epidemiol Infect. 1991;106:523-530.

155. Rosenmund A, Binswanger U, Struab PW. Oxidative injury to erythrocytes, cell rigidity and splenic hemolysis in hemodialyzed uremic patients. Ann Intern Med. 1975;82:460-465.

156. Yawata Y, Jacob HS. Abnormal red cell metabolism in patients with chronic uremia: nature of the defect and its persistence despite adequate hemodialysis. Blood. 1975; 45:231-239.

157. Forman S, Bischel M, Hochstein P. Erythrocyte deformability in uremic hemodialyzed patients. Ann Intern Med. 1973;79:841-843.

158. Anagnostou A, Vercellotti G, Barone J, Fried W. Factors which affect erythropoiesis in partially nephrectomized and sham-operated rats. Blood. 1976;48:425-433.

159. Anagnostou A, Barone J, Kedo A, Fried W. Effect of erythropoietin therapy on the red cell volume of uraemic and non-uraemic rats. Br J Haematol. 1977;37:85-91.

160. Nathan DG, Schupak E, Stohlman F Jr, Merrill JP. Erythropoiesis in anephric man. J Clin Invest. 1964;43:2158-2165.

161. Lichtman MA, Miller DR. Erythrocyte glycolysis, 2,3 diphosphoglycerate, and adenosine triphosphate concentration in uremic subjects: relationship to extracellular phosphate concentration. J Lab Clin Med. 1970;76: 267-279.

162. Fluckiger R, Harmon W, Meier W, et al. Hemoglobin carbamylation in uremia. N Engl J Med. 1981;304:823-827.

163. Yawata Y, Howe R, Jacobs HS. Abnormal red cell metabolism during hemolysis in uremia. A defect potentiated by

tap water hemodialysis. Ann Intern Med. 1973;79:362-367.

164. Chillar RK, Desferges JF. Red-cell organic phosphates in patients with chronic renal failure on maintenance haemodialysis. Br J Haematol. 1974;26:549-556.

165. Hurt GA, Chanutin A. Organic phosphate compounds of erythrocytes from individuals with uremia. J Lab Clin Med. 1964;64:675-684.

166. Eschbach JW, Abdulhadi MH, Browne JK, et al. Recombinant human erythropoietin in anemic subjects with end-stage renal disease. Results of a phase III multicenter clinical trial. Ann Intern Med. 1989;111:992-1000.

167. Sinai-Trieman L, Salusky IB, Fine RN. The use of subcutaneous recombinant erythropoietin in children undergoing continuous cycling peritoneal dialysis. J Pediatr. 1989;114:550-554.

168. Matter BJ, Pederson J, Psimenos G, et al. Lethal copper intoxication in hemodialysis. Trans Am Soc Artif Intern Organs 1969;15:309-315.

169. Carlson DJ, Shapiro FL. Methemoglobin from well water nitrates: a complication of hemodialysis. Ann Intern Med. 1970;73:757-759.

170. Eaton JW, Kolpin CF, Swofford HS, et al. Chlorinated urban water. A cause of dialysis-induced hemolytic anemia. Science. 1973;181:463-464.

171. Retief FP, Heyns AP, Oosthuizen M, Reenen OR. Aspects of folate metabolism in renal failure. Br J Haematol. 1977;36:405-415.

172. Waxman S, Schreiber C. Characteristics of folic acid–binding protein in folate deficient serum. Blood. 1973;42:291-301.

173. Goldraich I, Goldraich N. Once weekly subcutaneous administration of recombinant erythropoietin in children treated with CAPD. Adv Perit Dial. 1992;8:440-443.

174. Moynot A, Zins B, Naret C, et al. [One year treatment of 43 chronic hemodialysis patients with recombinant human erythropoietin.] Presse Med. 1990;19:111-115.

175. Drüeke TB, Locatelli F, Clyne N, et al. Normalization of hemoglobin level in patients with chronic kidney disease and anemia. N Engl J Med. 2006;355:2071-2084.

176. Phrommintikul A, Haas SJ, Elsik M, Krum H. Mortality and target haemoglobin concentrations in anaemic patients with chronic kidney disease treated with erythropoietin: a meta-analysis. Lancet. 2007;369:381-388.

177. Kooistra MP, van Es A, Struyvenberg A, Marx JJ. Iron metabolism in patients with the anaemia of end-stage renal disease during treatment with recombinant human erythropoietin. Br J Haematol. 1991;79:634-639.

178. Ways P, Huff JW, Kosmaler CH, Young LE. Polycythemia and histologically proven renal disease. Arch Intern Med. 1961;107:154-162.

179. Hoppin EC, Depner T, Yanuchi H, Hopper J Jr. Erythrocytosis associated with diffuse parenchymal lesions of the kidney. Br J Haematol. 1976;32:557-563.

180. Wong KC, Bandler NS, Kerr PG, Atkins RC. Control of post-transplant erythrocytosis by enalapril. Med J Aust. 1994;161:544-546.

181. Kaplow LS, Goffinit JA. Profound neutropenia during the early phase of hemodialysis. JAMA. 1968;203:1135-1137.

182. Mac Gregor RR. Granulocyte adherence changes induced by hemodialysis, endotoxin, epinephrine, and glucocorticoids. Ann Intern Med. 1977;86:35-39.

183. Craddock PR, Fehr J, Dalmasso AP, et al. Hemodialysis leukopenia. Pulmonary vascular leukostasis resulting from complement activation by dialyzer cellophane membranes. J Clin Invest. 1977;59:879-888.

184. Woodward J, Brubaker LH. Production of neutropenia-over-shoot cycle in sheep by reinfusion of cellophane exposed blood [abstract]. Clin Res. 1973;21:56.

185. Lewis JH, Tucker MB, Zucker MB. Bleeding tendency in uremia. Blood. 1956;11:1073-1076.

186. Singh G, Hussain SK, Matthai TP, et al. Hemostatic mechanism in uremia. Indian J Med Sci. 1969;23:387-394.

187. Rabiner SF. Bleeding in uremia. Med Clin North Am. 1972;56:221-233.

188. Kendall AG, Lowenstein L, Morgen RO. The hemorrhagic diathesis in renal disease (with special reference to acute uremia). Can Med Assoc J. 1961;85:405-411.

189. Wardle EN, Taylor G. Fibrin breakdown products and fibrinolysis in renal disease. J Clin Pathol. 1968;21:140-146.

190. Galasinski W, Worowski K, Niewiarowski S, Franecki G. Turnover of ^{131}I-fibrinogen in mercury chloride intoxicated dogs. Thromb Diath Haemorrh. 1967;18:268-275.

191. Larsson SO. On coagulation and fibrinolysis in renal failure. Scand J Haematol Suppl. 1971;15:1-59.

192. Vaziri ND, Branson HE, Ness R. Changes of coagulation factors IX, VIII, VII, X, V in nephrotic syndrome. Am J Med Sci. 1980;280:167-171.

193. Bouma BN, Hedner U, Nilsson IM. Typing of fibrinogen degradation products in urine in various clinical disorders. Scand J Clin Lab Invest. 1971;27:331-335.

194. Salem HH, Whitworth JA, Koutts J, et al. Hypercoagulation in glomerulonephritis. Br Med J (Clin Res Ed). 1981;282:2083-2085.

195. Erickson RV, Williams M, Pendras JP. A true hypercoagulability state in patients on chronic hemodialysis. Trans Am Soc Artif Intern Organs. 1966;12:205-206.

196. Dossetor JB, Gutelius JR, Kendall AC. The thromboembolic potential of the nephrotic syndrome [abstract]. In Proceedings of the International Congress of Nephrology. Paris, International Congress of Nephrology, 1966, p 184.

197. Handley DA, Lawrence JR. Factor IX deficiency in the nephrotic syndrome. Lancet. 1967;1:1079-1081.

198. Natelson E, Lynch EC, Hettig RA, Alfrey CP Jr. Acquired factor IX deficiency in the nephrotic syndrome. Ann Intern Med. 1970;73:373-378.

199. Lewis JH. Separation and molecular weight estimation of coagulation and fibrinolytic proteins by Sephadex gel filtration. Proc Soc Exp Biol Med. 1964;116:120-122.

200. Honig GR, Lindley A. Deficiency of Hageman factor (factor XIII) in patients with the nephrotic syndrome. J Pediatr. 1971;78:633-637.

201. Donaldson VH, Ratnoff OD. Hageman factor: alterations in physical properties during activation. Science. 1965;150:754-756.

202. Bang NU, Trygstad CW, Schroeder JE, et al. Enhanced platelet function in glomerular renal disease. J Lab Clin Med. 1973;81:651-660.

203. Kwaan HC, Colwell JA, Cruz S, et al. Increased platelet aggregation in diabetes mellitus. J Lab Clin Med. 1972;80:236-246.

204. Thomas DP. Abnormalities of platelet aggregation in cirrhosis. Ann N Y Acad Sci. 1972;201:243-250.

205. Kauffmann RH, Veltkamp JJ, Van Tilburg NH, Van Es LA. Acquired antithrombin III deficiency and thrombosis in the nephrotic syndrome. Am J Med. 1978;65:607-613.

206. Quereda C, Pardo A, Lamas S, et al. Lupus-like in vitro anticoagulant activity in end-stage renal disease. Nephron. 1988;49:39-44.

207. Kincaid-Smith P. The natural history and treatment of mesangiocapillary glomerulonephritis. In Kincaid-Smith P, Matthew TH, et al (eds). Glomerulonephritis: Morphology, Natural History and Treatment. New York, John Wiley, 1973, p 515.

208. Kincaid-Smith P. The treatment of chronic mesangiocapillary (membranoproliferative) glomerulonephritis with impaired renal function. Med J Aust. 1972;2:587-592.

209. Robson AM, Cole BR, Kienstra RA, et al. Severe glomerulonephritis complicated by coagulopathy: treatment with anticoagulant and immunosuppressive drugs. J Pediatr. 1977;90:881-892.

210. West CD. Anticoagulant and immunosuppressive drugs in the treatment of severe glomerulonephritis with coagulopathy. J Pediatr. 1977;90:1051-1052.

211. Stewart JH. Platelet numbers and lifespan in acute and chronic renal failure. Thromb Diath Haemorrh. 1967;17:532-542.

212. Willoughby MCN, Crouch SJ. An investigation of the hemorrhagic tendency in renal failure. Br J Haematol. 1961;7:315-326.

213. Salzman EW, Neri LL. Adhesiveness of blood platelets in uremia. Thromb Diath Haemorrh. 1966;15:84-92.

214. Castaldi PA, Rozenberg MC, Stewart JH. The bleeding disorder of uremia. A qualitative platelet defect. Lancet. 1966;2:66-69.

215. Joist JH, Pechan J, Schikowski U, et al. Studies on the nature and etiology of uremic thrombocytopathy. Verh Dtsch Ges Inn Med. 1969;75:476-479.

216. DiMichele DM, Hathaway WE. Use of DDAVP in inherited and acquired platelet dysfunction. Am J Hematol. 1990;33:39-45.

217. Turi S, Soos J, Torday C, et al. The effect of erythropoietin on platelet function in uraemic children on haemodialysis. Pediatr Nephrol. 1994;8:727-732.

218. Hellem AJ, Odegaard AE, et al. Platelet adhesiveness in chronic renal failure [abstract]. Paper presented before the Xth Congress International Society of Haematology. Stockholm, 1964, p K1.

219. Horowitz HI. Uremic toxins and platelet function. Arch Intern Med. 1970;126:823-826.

220. Epstein CJ, Sahud MA, Piel CF, et al. Hereditary macrothrombocytopathia, nephritis, and deafness. Am J Med. 1972;52:299-310.

221. Bepler G, Melhus O, Gunnells JC. Coexpression of May-Hegglin anomaly and hereditary nephritis in a family. South Med J. 1994;87:202-205.

222. Gubler M, Levy M, Broyer M, et al. Alport's syndrome: a report of 58 cases and a review of the literature. Am J Med. 1981;70:493-505.

223. Eckstein JD, Filip DJ, Watts JC. Hereditary thrombocytopenia, deafness and renal disease. Ann Intern Med. 1975;82:639-645.

224. Kasinath BS, Corwin HL, Bidani AK, et al. Eosinophilia in the diagnosis of atheroembolic renal disease. Am J Nephrol. 1987;7:173-177.

225. Golde DW, Bersch N, Chopra IJ, Cline MJ. Thyroid hormones stimulate erythropoiesis in vitro. Br J Haematol. 1977;37:173-177.

226. O'Brien D, Lyons DJ, Fielding JF. A case of Graves' disease associated with autoimmune hemolytic anemia. Ir J Med Sci. 1989;158:155.

227. Malgor LA, Blanc CC, Klainer E, et al. Direct effects of thyroid hormones on bone marrow erythroid cells of rats. Blood. 1975;45:671-679.

228. Chu JY, Monteleone JA, Peden VH, et al. Anemia in children and adolescents with hypothyroidism. Clin Pediatr (Phila). 1981;20:696-699.

229. Wardrop C, Hutchinson HE. Red cell shape in hypothyroidism. Lancet. 1969;2:1243.

230. Tudhope GR, Wilson GM. Anemia in hypothyroidism. Q J Med. 1960;29:513-537.

231. Tudhope GR, Wilson GM. Deficiency of vitamin B_{12} in hypothyroidism. Lancet. 1962;1:703-706.

232. Falko JM, Cohen JR. Erythrocytosis and hypothyroidism. Ann Intern Med. 1976;84:446-447.

233. Weinblatt ME, Fort P, Kochen J, DiMayio M. Polycythemia in hyperthyroid infants. Am J Dis Child. 1987;141:1121-1123.

234. Das KC, Mukherjee M, Sarkar TJ, et al. Erythropoiesis and erythropoietin in hypo- and hyperthyroidism. J Clin Endocrinol. 1975;40:211-220.

235. Rodman GP, Jensen WN. A study of red blood cell survival in hypo- and hyperthyroidism. Clin Res Proc. 1957;5:8.

236. Macho L. The effect of thyroid hormone on the glycolytic activity of blood. Clin Chim Acta. 1957;2:345-347.

237. Kiso Y, Yoshida K, Kaise K, et al. Erythrocyte carbonic anhydrase-I concentrations in patients with Graves' disease and subacute thyroiditis reflect integrated thyroid hormone levels over the previous few months. J Clin Endocrinol Metab. 1991;72:515-518.

238. Necheles TF, Beutler E. The effect of triiodothyronine on the oxidative metabolism of erythrocytes. I. Cellular studies. J Clin Invest. 1959;38:788-797.

239. Pearson HA, Druyan R. Erythrocyte glucose-6-phosphate dehydrogenase activity related to thyroid activity. J Lab Clin Med. 1961;57:343-349.

240. Pangaro JA, Weinstein M, Devetak MC, Soto RJ. Red cell zinc and red cell zinc metalloenzymes in hyperthyroidism. Acta Endocrinol. 1974;76:645-650.

241. Synder LM, Reddy WJ. Mechanism of action of thyroid hormones on erythrocyte 2,3 diphosphoglycerate. J Clin Invest. 1970;49:1993-1998.

242. Lie-Injo LE, Lopez CG, Hart PL. Erythrocyte carbonic anhydrase activity in health and disease. Clin Chim Acta. 1970;29:541-550.

243. Matsuda Y. [Studies on osmotic abnormalities of erythrocytes in thyrotoxicosis.] Nippon Ketsueki Gakkai Zasshi. 1966;29:717-726.

244. Goolden AWG, Bateman D, Torr S. Red cell sodium in hyperthyroidism. BMJ. 1971;2:552-554.

245. Barnes HV, Blizzard RM. Antithyroid drug therapy for toxic diffuse goiter (Graves disease): 30 years experience in children and adolescents. J Pediatr. 1977;91:313-320.

246. Lightsey AL, Chapman RM, McMillan R, et al. Immune neutropenia. Ann Intern Med. 1977;86:60-62.

247. Lamberg BA, Kivikangas V, Pelkonen R, Vuopio P. Thrombocytopenia and decreased life span of thrombocytes in hyperthyroidism. Ann Clin Res. 1971;3:98-102.

248. Egeberg O. Thyroid function and hemostasis. Scand J Clin Lab Invest. 1964;16:511-512.

249. Mogucheva EI, Idel'son LI, Granovskaia-Tsvetkova AM, et al. Autoimmune thrombocytopenia and diffuse-toxic goiter. Ter Arkh. 1985;57:79-84.

250. Panzer S, Haubenstock A, Minar E. Platelets in hyperthyroidism: studies on platelet counts, mean platelet volume, 111-indium–labeled platelet kinetics, and platelet-associated immunoglobulins G and M. J Clin Endocrinol Metab. 1990;70:491-496.

251. Simone JV, Abildgaard CT, Schulman I. Blood coagulation in thyroid dysfunction. N Engl J Med. 1965;27:1057-1061.

252. Edson JR, Fecher DR, Doe RP. Low platelet adhesiveness and other hemostatic abnormalities in hypothyroidism. Ann Intern Med. 1975;82:342-346.

253. Hume R. Fibrinolytic activity and thyroid function. BMJ. 1965;1:686-688.

254. Ardeman S, Boralessa H, Sale RF. Coagulation inhibitor in hypothyroidism. BMJ. 1981;282:1508.

255. Blesing NE, Hambley H, McDonald GA. Acquired von Willebrand's disease and hypothyroidism: report of a case presenting with menorrhagia. Postgrad Med J. 1990;66:474-476.

256. Báez Villaseñor J, Rath CE, Finch CA. The blood picture in Addison's disease. Blood. 1948;3:769-773.

257. Plotz CM, Knowlton AI, Ragan C. The natural history of Cushing's syndrome. Am J Med. 1952;13:597-614.

258. Patrassi GM, Dal Bo Zannon R, Boscaro M, et al. Further studies on the hypercoagulable state of patients with Cushing's syndrome. Thromb Haemost. 1985;54:518-520.

259. Claman HN. Corticosteroids and lymphoid cells. N Engl J Med. 1972;287:388-397.

260. Van Dyke DC, Contopoulos AN, Williams BS, et al. Hormonal factors influencing erythropoiesis. Acta Haematol. 1954;11:203-222.

261. Parker JP, Beirne GJ, Desai JN, et al. Androgen-induced increase in red cell 2,3-diphosphoglycerate. N Engl J Med. 1972;287:381-383.

262. Delivoria-Papadopoulos M, Coburn CF, Foster RE. Cyclic variations of rate of carbon monoxide production in normal women. J Appl Physiol. 1974;36:49-51.

263. Berlin R. Red cell survival studies in normal and leukemic subjects. Acta Med Scand. 1951;252:1-141.

264. Mercke C, Lundh B. Erythrocyte filterability and heme catabolism during the menstrual cycle. Ann Intern Med. 1976;85:322-324.

265. Durocher JR, Weir MS, Lundblad EG, et al. Effect of oral contraceptives and pregnancy on red cell deformability and surface charge. Proc Soc Exp Biol Med. 1975;150:368-370.

266. Oski FA, Lubin B, Buchert ED. Reduced red cell filterability with oral contraceptive agents. Ann Intern Med. 1972;77:417-419.

267. Pechet L, Alexander B. Increased clotting factors in pregnancy. N Engl J Med. 1961;265:1093-1097.

268. Escamilla RF, Lisser VH. Simmond's disease. J Clin Endocrinol. 1942;2:65-96.

269. Ardizzi A, Guzzaloni G, Grugni G, et al. The effect of growth hormone on erythropoiesis in vivo. Minerva Endocrinol. 1993;18:83-85.

270. Rodriguez JM, Shahidi NT. Red cell 2,3-DPG in adaptive red-cell-volume deficiency. N Engl J Med. 1971;285:479-482.

271. Root AW, Oski FA, Bongiovanni AM, Eberlein WR. Red cell G-6-PD activity in children with hypothyroidism and hypopituitarism. J Pediatr. 1967;70:369-375.

272. Oski FA, Root AW, Winegrad AI. In vitro inhibition of RBC glucose consumption by human growth hormone. Nature. 1967;215:81-82.

273. Borgna-Pignatti C, Marradi P, Pinelli L, et al. Thiamine-responsive anemia in the DIDMOAD syndrome. J Pediatr. 1989;114:405-410.

274. Livingstone CS, Boczarow B. Idiopathic pulmonary hemosiderosis in a newborn. Arch Dis Child. 1967;42:543.

275. Soergel KM, Sommers SC. Idiopathic pulmonary hemosiderosis and related syndromes. Am J Med. 1962;32:499-509.

276. Fossati G, Perri M, Careddu G, et al. Pulmonary hemosiderosis induced by cow's milk proteins: a discussion of a clinical case. Pediatr Med Chir. 1992;14:203-207.

277. Gilman PA, Zinkham WH. Severe idiopathic pulmonary hemosiderosis in the absence of clinical or radiologic evidence of pulmonary disease. J Pediatr. 1969;75:118-121.

278. Matsaniotis N, Karpousas J, Apostolopoulou E, Messaritakis J. Idiopathic pulmonary hemosiderosis in children. Arch Dis Child. 1968;43:307-309.

279. Elgenmark O, Kjellberg SR. Hemosiderosis of the lungs—typical roentgenological findings. Acta Radiol. 1948;29:32.

280. Fleischner FG, Berenberg AL. Idiopathic pulmonary hemosiderosis. Radiology. 1954;62:522-526.

281. Hammond D, Crane J. Sequestration of iron in the lungs in idiopathic pulmonary hemosiderosis [abstract]. Am J Dis Child. 1958;96:503.

282. Hyatt RW, Edelstein ER, Halazun JF, Lukens JN. Ultrastructure of the lung in idiopathic pulmonary hemosiderosis. Am J Med. 1972;58:822-829.

283. Irwin RS, Cottrell TS, Hsu KC, et al. Idiopathic pulmonary hemosiderosis: an electron microscopic and immunofluorescent study. Chest. 1974;65:41-45.

284. Gellis SS, Reinhold JL, Green S. Use of aspiration lung puncture in diagnosis of idiopathic pulmonary hemosiderosis. Am J Dis Child. 1953;85:303-307.

285. Halvorsen S. Cortisone treatment of idiopathic pulmonary hemosiderosis. Acta Paediatr. 1956;45:139-146.

286. Saha V, Ravikumar E, Khanduri U, et al. Long-term prednisolone therapy in children with idiopathic pulmonary hemosiderosis. Pediatr Hematol Oncol. 1993;10:89-91.

287. Byrd RB, Gracey DR. Immunosuppressive treatment of idiopathic pulmonary hemosiderosis. JAMA. 1973;226:458-459.

288. Colombo JL, Stolz SM. Treatment of life-threatening primary pulmonary hemosiderosis with cyclophosphamide. Chest. 1992;102:959-960.

289. Heiner DC, Sears JW, Kniker WT. Multiple precipitins to cow's milk in chronic respiratory disease. A syndrome

including poor growth, gastrointestinal symptoms, evidence of allergy, iron deficiency anemia and pulmonary hemosiderosis. Am J Dis Child. 1962;103:634-654.

290. Matthews TS, Soothill JF. Complement activation after milk feeding in children with cow's milk allergy. Lancet. 1970;2:893-895.

291. Rose GA, Spencer H. Polyarteritis nodosa. Q J Med. 1957;26:43-81.

292. DeGowin RL, Oda Y, Evans RH. Nephritis and lung hemorrhage. Goodpasture's syndrome. Arch Intern Med. 1963;111:16-22.

293. Byrd RB, Trunk G. Systemic lupus erythematosus presenting as pulmonary hemosiderosis. Chest. 1973;64:128-129.

294. Thomas AM. A case of Wegener's granulomatosis. J Clin Pathol. 1958;11:146-154.

295. Valletta EA, Cipolli M, Cazzola G, Mastella G. Pulmonary hemosiderosis in a child with cystic fibrosis. Helv Paediatr Acta. 1989;43:487-490.

296. Perelman S, Dupuy C, Bourrillon A. The association of pulmonary hemosiderosis and celiac disease. Apropos of a new case in a child. Ann Pediatr. 1992;39:185-188.

297. Jorgensen G, Wurm K. The ABO blood group in sarcoidosis. Proceedings of the International Conference on Sarcoidosis. Stockholm, 1963.

298. Lewis JG, Woods AC. The ABO and rhesus blood groups in patients with respiratory disease. Tubercle. 1961;42:362-365.

299. Lower EE, Smith JT, Martelo OJ, Baughman RP. The anemia of sarcoidosis. Sarcoidosis. 1988;5:51-55.

300. Mathur A, Kremer JM. Immunopathology, rheumatic features, and therapy of sarcoidoses. Curr Opin Rheumatol. 1992;4:76-80.

301. Hirschman RJ, Johns CJ. Hemoglobin studies in sarcoidosis. Ann Intern Med. 1965;62:129-132.

302. Edwards MH, Wagner JA, Krause LA. Sarcoidosis with thrombocytopenia. Ann Intern Med 1952;37:803-812.

303. Scully RE, Galdabini JJ, McNeeley BU. Case records of the Massachusetts General Hospital. N Engl J Med. 1978;299:765.

304. Dickerman JD, Holbrook PR, Zinkham WH. Etiology and therapy of thrombocytopenia associated with sarcoidosis. J Pediatr. 1972;81:758-764.

305. Knodel AR, Beekman RF. Severe thromboyctopenia in sarcoidosis. JAMA. 1980;243:258-259.

306. Vichinsky EP, Pennathur-Das R, Nickerson B, et al. Inadequate erythroid response to hypoxia in cystic fibrosis. J Pediatr. 1984;105:15-21.

307. Ater JL, Herbst JJ, Landaw SA, O'Brien RT. Relative anemia and iron deficiency in cystic fibrosis. Pediatrics. 1983;71:810-814.

308. Wilfond BS, Farrell PM, Laxova A, Mischler E. Severe hemolytic anemia associated with vitamin E deficiency in infants with cystic fibrosis. Implications for neonatal screening. Clin Pediatr (Phila). 1994;33:2-7.

309. Cartwright GE. The anemia of chronic disorders. Semin Hematol. 1966;3:351-375.

310. Cartwright GE, Wintrobe MM. The anemia of infection. Adv Intern Med. 1952;5:165.

311. Freireich EJ, Ross JF, Bayles TB, Finch SC. Radioactive iron metabolism and erythrocyte survival studies of the mechanisms of the anemia associated with rheumatoid arthritis. J Clin Invest. 1951;36:1043.

312. Ebaugh FG. The anemia of rheumatoid arthritis. In Wallerstein M, Methier G (eds). Iron in Clinical Medicine. Berkeley, CA, University of California Press, 1958, p 261.

313. Ward HP, Kurnick JE, Pisarczyk MJ. Serum level of erythropoietin in anemias associated with chronic infection, malignancies and hematopoietic disease. J Clin Invest. 1971;50:332-335.

314. Lukens JN. Control of erythropoiesis in rats with adjuvant-induced chronic inflammation. Blood. 1973;41:37-44.

315. Wintrobe MM, Grinstein M, Dubash JJ, et al. The anemia of infection. VI. The influence of cobalt on the anemia associated with inflammation. Blood. 1947;2:323-331.

316. Robinson JC, James GW III, Kark RM. The effect of oral therapy with cobaltous chloride on the blood of patients suffering with chronic suppurative infection. N Engl J Med. 1949;240:749-753.

317. Hillman RA, Henderson DA. The control of marrow production by the level of iron supply. J Clin Invest. 1969;48:454-460.

318. Haurani FI, Burke W, Martinez EJ. Defective reutilization of iron in the anemia of inflammation. J Lab Clin Med. 1965;65:560-570.

319. Wells DA, Dargneault-Creech CA, Simrell CR. Effect of iron status on reticulocyte mean channel fluorescence. Am J Clin Pathol. 1992;97:130-134.

320. Shade SG. Normal incorporation of iron into intestinal ferritin in inflammation. Proc Soc Exp Biol Med. 1972;139:620-622.

321. Abshire TC, Reeves JD. Anemia of inflammation in children. J Pediatr. 1983;103:868-871.

322. Olivares M, Walter T, Osorio M, et al. Anemia of mild viral infection: the measles vaccine as a model. Pediatrics. 1989;84:851-855.

323. Lipschitz DA, Cook JD, Finch CA. A clinical evaluation of serum ferritin as an index of iron stores. N Engl J Med. 1974;290:1213-1216.

324. Koerper MA, Stempel DA, Dallman PR. Anemia in patients with juvenile rheumatoid arthritis. J Pediatr. 1978;92:930-933.

325. Hansen NE. The anaemia of chronic disorders: a bag of unsolved questions. Scand J Haematol. 1983;31:397-402.

326. Murphy EA, Bell AL, Wojtulewski J, et al. Study of erythropoietin in treatment of anaemia in patients with rheumatoid arthritis. BMJ. 1994;309:1337-1338.

327. Montecucco C, Caporali R, Invernizzi R. Iron status in Still's disease. Lancet. 1994;345:58-59.

328. Harvey AR, Pippard MJ, Ansell BM. Microcytic anaemia in juvenile rheumatoid arthritis. Scand J Rheumatol. 1987;16:53-59.

329. Partridge REH, Duthie JJR. Incidence of macrocytic anemia in rheumatoid arthritis. BMJ. 1963;1:89-91.

330. Omer A, Mowat AG. Nature of anemia in rheumatoid arthritis. IX. Folate metabolism in patients with rheumatoid arthritis. Ann Rheum Dis. 1968;27:414-424.

331. Alter HJ, Zvaifler NJ, Rath CE. Interrelationship of rheumatoid arthritis, folic acid and aspirin. Blood. 1971;38:405-416.

332. Richmond J, Alexander WRM, Potter JL, Duthie JJ. Nature of anemia in rheumatoid arthritis. V. Red cell sur-

vival measured by radioactive chromium. Ann Rheum Dis. 1961;20:133-137.

333. Rubin RN, Walker BK, Ballas SK, Travis SF. Erythroid aplasia in juvenile rheumatoid arthritis. Am J Dis Child. 198;132:760-762.

334. Dainiak N, Hardin J, Floyd V, et al. Humoral suppression of erythropoiesis in SLE and rheumatoid arthritis. Am J Med. 1980;69:537-544.

335. Mowat AG, Baum J. Chemotaxis of polymorphonuclear leukocytes from patients with rheumatoid arthritis. J Clin Invest. 1971;50:2541-2549.

336. Turner RA, Schumacker HR, Myers AR. Phagocytic function of polymorphonuclear leukocytes in rheumatic diseases. J Clin Invest. 1973;52:1632-1635.

337. Segal AW. Nitroblue-tetrazolium tests. Lancet. 1974;2: 1248-1252.

338. Garner RW, Mowat AG, Hazleman BL. Wound healing after operations on patients with rheumatoid arthritis. J Bone Joint Surg Br. 1973;55:134-144.

339. Brewer EJ Jr. Juvenile Rheumatoid Arthritis. Philadelphia, WB Saunders, 1980.

340. Athreya BH, Moser G, Raghavan TE. Increased circulating basophils in juvenile rheumatoid arthritis: A preliminary report. Am J Dis Child. 1975;129:935-937.

341. Debarre F, Le Gô A, Kahan A. Hyperbasophilic immunoblasts in circulating blood in chronic inflammatory, rheumatic and collagen diseases. Ann Rheum Dis. 1975; 34:422-430.

342. Silverman ED, Miller JJ 3rd, Bernstein B, Shafai T. Consumptive coagulopathy associated with systemic juvenile rheumatoid arthritis. J Pediatr. 1983;103:872-876.

343. De Inocencio J, Lovell DJ, Gabriel CA. Acquired factor VII inhibitor in juvenile rheumatoid arthritis. Pediatrics. 1994;94:550-553.

344. Mukamel M, Bernstein BH, Brik R, Lehman TJ. The prevalence of coagulation abnormalities in juvenile rheumatoid arthritis. Rheumatology. 1987;14:1147-1149.

345. Sherry DD, Redich DD. Transient thrombocytopenia and systemic onset juvenile rheumatoid arthritis. Pediatrics. 1985;76:600-603.

346. Felty AR. Chronic arthritis in the adult associated with splenomegaly and leukopenia. Bull Johns Hopkins Hosp. 1924;35:16-20.

347. Collier RL, Brush BE. Hematologic disorders in Felty's syndrome. Prolonged benefits of splenectomy. Am J Surg. 1966;112:869-873.

348. Berliner N, Duby AD, Linch DC, et al. T cell receptor gene rearrangements define a monoclonal T cell proliferation in patients with T cell lymphocytosis and cytopenia. Blood. 1986;67:914-918.

349. Gupta R, Robinson WA, Albrecht D. Granulopoietic activity in Felty's syndrome. Ann Rheum Dis. 1975;34: 156-161.

350. Rosenthal FD, Beeley JM, Gelsthorpe K, Doughty RW. White cell antibodies and the etiology of Felty's syndrome. Q J Med. 1974;43:187-203.

351. Hartman KR. Anti-neutrophil antibodies of immunoglobulin M class in autoimmune neutropenia. Am J Med Sci. 1994;308:102-105.

352. Blumfelder TM, Logue GL, Shimm DS. Felty's syndrome: effects of splenectomy upon granulocyte count and granulocyte-associated IgG. Ann Intern Med. 1981; 94:623-628.

353. Toshioka K. Combined therapy of G-CSF and prednisolone for neutropenia in a patient with Felty's syndrome. Am J Hematol. 1995;48:130-131.

354. Choi MF, Mant MJ, Turner AR, et al. Successful reversal of neutropenia in Felty's syndrome with recombinant granulocyte colony stimulating factor. Br J Haematol. 1994;86:663-664.

355. Pixley JS, Yoneda KY, Manalo PB. Sequential administration of cyclophosphamide and granulocyte-colony stimulating factor relieves impaired myeloid maturation in Felty's syndrome. Am J Hematol. 1993;43:304-306.

356. DuBois EZ, Tuffanelli DL. Clinical manifestations of systemic lupus erythematosus. Computer analysis of 520 cases. JAMA. 1964;190:104-111.

357. Fries JF, Holman HH. Systemic Lupus Erythematosus, Clinical Analyses. Philadelphia, WB Saunders, 1975, p 79.

358. Weens JH, Schwartz RS. Etiologic factors in hemolytic anemia. Semin Hematol. 1974;7:303-327.

359. Westerman MP, Martinez RC, Medsger TA Jr, et al. Anemia and scleroderma: frequency, causes, marrow findings. Arch Intern Med. 1968;122:39-42.

360. Michael SR, Vural IL, Bassen FA, Schaefer L. The hematological aspects of systemic lupus erythematosus. Blood. 1951;6:1059-1072.

361. Boxer LA, Greenberg MS, Boxer GJ, Stossel TP. Autoimmune neutropenia. N Engl J Med. 1975;293:748-753.

362. Duckham DJ, Rhyne RL, Smith FE, Williams RC Jr. Retardation of colony growth of in vitro bone marrow culture using sera from patients with Felty's syndrome, disseminated lupus erythematosus (SLE), rheumatoid arthritis, and other disease states. Arthritis Rheum. 1975; 18:323-333.

363. Zivkovic M, Baum J. Chemotaxis of polymorphonuclear leukocytes from patients with systemic lupus erythematosus and Felty's syndrome. Immunol Commun. 1972;1: 39-49.

364. Gewurz H, Page AR, Pickering RJ, Good RA. Complement activation and inflammatory neutrophil exudation in man. Int Arch Allergy Appl Immunol. 1967;32:64-90.

365. Orozco JH, Jasin HE, et al. Defective phagocytosis in patients with systemic lupus erythematosus (SLE) [abstract]. Arthritis Rheum. 1970;13:342.

366. Messner RP, Lindstrom FD, Williams RC Jr. Peripheral blood lymphocyte cell surface markers during the course of systemic lupus erythematosus. J Clin Invest. 1973;52: 3046-3056.

367. Winfield JB, Winchester RJ, et al. Different types of anti-lymphocyte antibodies in the sera of systemic lupus erythematosus (SLE) patients [abstract]. Clin Res. 1974; 22:432a.

368. Williams RC Jr, Emmons JD, Yunis EJ. Studies of human sera with cytotoxic activity. J Clin Invest. 1971;50: 1514-1524.

369. Stastny P, Ziff M. Lymphocyte and platelet autoantibodies in S.L.E. Lancet. 1971;1:1239-1240.

370. Glinski W, Gershwin ME, Steinberg AD. Fractionation of cells on a discontinuous Ficoll gradient. Study of peripheral blood lymphocyte subpopulations in normal humans and patients with systemic lupus erythematosus. J Clin Invest. 1976;57:604-614.

371. Lockshin MD, Eisenhauer AC, Kohn R, et al. Cell-mediated immunity in rheumatic diseases. II. Mitogen

responses in systemic lupus erythematosus and other illnesses: correlation with T- and B-lymphocyte populations. Arthritis Rheum. 1975;18:245-250.

372. Jasin HE, Ziff M. Immunoglobulin synthesis by peripheral blood cells in systemic lupus erythematosus. Arthritis Rheum. 1975;18:219-228.

373. Vaughan JH, Chihara T. Lymphocyte function in rheumatic disorders. Arch Intern Med. 1975;135:1324-1328.

374. Bankhurst AD, Williams RC Jr. Identification of DNA binding lymphocytes in patients with systemic lupus erythematosus. J Clin Invest. 1975;56:1378-1385.

375. Bell DA, Clark C, Blomgren SE, Vaughan JH. Anti DNA antibody production by lymphoid cells of NZB/W mice and human systemic lupus erythematosus (SLE). Clin Immunol Immunopathol. 1973;1:293-303.

376. Delbarre F, Le Gô A, Hahan A. Hyperbasophilic immunoblasts in the circulating blood in chronic inflammatory rheumatic and collagen diseases. Ann Rheum Dis. 1975;34:422-430.

377. Karpatkin S, Strick N, Karpartkin MB, Siskind GW. Cumulative experience in the detection of antiplatelet antibody in 234 patients with idiopathic thrombocytopenic purpura, systemic lupus erythematosus and other clinical disorders. Am J Med. 1972;52:776-785.

378. Rabinowitz Y, Dameshek W. Systemic lupus erythematosus after idiopathic thrombocytopenia purpura: a review. Ann Intern Med. 1960;52:1-28.

379. Dixon R, Rosse W, Ebbert L. Quantitative determination of antibody in idiopathic thrombocytopenic purpura. Correlation of serum and platelet bound antibody with clinical response. N Engl J Med. 1975;292:230-236.

380. Agnello V, Pariser K, Gell J, et al. Preliminary observations on danazol therapy of systemic lupus erythematosus: effects on DNA antibodies, thrombocytopenia and complement. J Rheumatol. 1983;10:682-687.

381. Clancy R, Jenkins E, Firkin B. Qualitative platelet abnormalities in idiopathic thrombocytopenic purpura. N Engl J Med. 1972;286:622-626.

382. Karpatkin S, Lackner HL. Association of antiplatelet antibody with functional platelet disorders. Am J Med. 1975;59:599-604.

383. Averbuch M, Koifman B, Levo Y. Lupus anticoagulant, thrombosis, and thrombocytopenia in systemic lupus erythematosus. Am J Med Sci. 1987;293:2-5.

384. Conley CL, Hartman RC. A haemorrhagic disorder caused by circulating anticoagulant in patients with disseminated lupus erythematosus. J Clin Invest. 1952;31:621-622.

385. Farrugia E, Torres VE, Gastineau D, et al. Lupus anticoagulant in systemic lupus erythematosus: a clinical and renal pathological study. Am J Kidney Dis. 1992;20:463-471.

386. Feinstein DI, Rapaport SI. Acquired inhibitors of blood coagulation. Prog Hemost Thromb. 1972;1:75-95.

387. Lechner K, Pabinger-Fasching I. Lupus anticoagulants and thrombosis. A study of 25 cases and a review of the literature. Haemostasis. 1985;15:254-262.

388. Lechner K. Acquired inhibitors in nonhemophiliac patients. Haemostasis. 1974;3:65-93.

389. Lechner K. A new type of coagulation inhibitor. Thromb Diath Haemorrh. 1969;21:482-499.

390. Regan MG, Lachner H, Karpatkin S. Platelet function and coagulation profile in lupus erythematosus. Studies in 50 patients. Ann Intern Med. 1974;81:462-468.

391. Green D. Circulating anticoagulants. Med Clin North Am. 1972;56:145-151.

392. Gonyea L, Herdman R, Bridges RA. The coagulation abnormalities in systemic lupus erythematosus. Thromb Diath Haemorrh. 1968;20:455-464.

393. Rivard GE, Schiffman S, Rapaport SI. Co-factor of the lupus anticoagulant. Thromb Diath Haemorrh. 1974;32:554-563.

394. Corrigan J, Patterson JH, May NE. Incoagulability of the blood in systemic lupus erythematosus. Am J Dis Child. 1970;119:365-369.

395. Rapaport SI, Ames SB, Duvall BJ. A plasma coagulation defect in systemic lupus erythematosus arising from hypoprothrombinemia combined with anti-prothrombinase activity. Blood. 1960;15:212-227.

396. Ratnoff OD. An accelerating property of plasma for the coagulation of fibrinogen by thrombin. J Clin Invest. 1954;33:1175-1182.

397. Lupus anticoagulant [editorial]. Lancet. 1984;1:1157.

398. Veltkamp JJ, Kerkhoven P, Loeliger EA. Circulating anticoagulant in disseminated lupus erythematosus. Haemostasis. 1973-1974;2:253-259.

399. Green D, Rezza CR. Myocardial infarction in a patient with a circulating anticoagulant. Lancet. 1967;2:434-436.

400. Roberti I, Reisman L, Churg J. Vasculitis in childhood. Pediatr Nephrol. 1993;7:479-481.

401. Quereda C, Otero GG, Pardo A, et al. Prevalence of antiphospholipid antibodies in nephropathies not due to systemic lupus erythematosus. Am J Kidney Dis. 1994;23:555-561.

402. Chyu JY, Hagstrom WJ, Soltani K, et al. Wegener's granulomatosis in childhood: cutaneous manifestations as the presenting signs. J Am Acad Dermatol. 1984;10:341-346.

403. Hansen LP, Jacobsen J, Skytte H. Wegener's granulomatosis in a child. Eur J Respir Dis. 1983;64:620-624.

404. Teiselkötter W, Müller KM. Infantile Wegener's granulomatosis. Arch Anat Cytol Pathol. 1977;25:273-276.

405. Fauci AS, Wolff SM. Wegener's granulomatosis: studies in eighteen patients and a review of the literature. Medicine (Baltimore). 1973;52:535-561.

406. Crummy CS, Perlin E, Moquin RB. Microangiopathic hemolytic anemia in Wegener's granulomatosis. Am J Med. 1971;51:544-548.

407. DeRemee RA, McDonald TJ, Harrison EG Jr, Coles DT. Wegener's granulomatosis: anatomic correlates, a proposed classification. Mayo Clin Proc. 1976;51:777-781.

408. Moorthy AY, Chesney RW, Segar WE, Groshong T. Wegener granulomatosis in childhood: prolonged survival following cytotoxic therapy. J Pediatr. 1977;91:616-618.

409. Lüdemann J, Utecht B, Gross WL. Detection and quantitation of anti-neutrophil cytoplasmic antibodies in Wegener's granulomatosis by ELISA using affinity-purified antigen. J Immunol Methods. 1988;114:167-174.

410. Markey BA, Warren JS. Use of anti-neutrophil cytoplasmic antibody assay to distinguish between vasculitic disease activity and complications of cytotoxic therapy. Am J Clin Pathol. 1994;102:589-594.

411. Lee P, Norman CS, Sukenik S, Alderdice CA. Clinical significance of coagulation abnormalities in systemic sclerosis (scleroderma). J Rheumatol. 1985;12:514-517.

412. Pettersson T, von Bonsdorff M. Autoimmune hemolytic anemia and thrombocytopenia in scleroderma. Acta Haematol. 1988;80:179-180.

413. Sipos A, Sonkoly I, Czirják L, et al. Anti-granulocyte antibodies in immune neutropenia and autoimmune disorders. Acta Paediatr Hung. 1988;29:97-100.

414. Lee P, Norman CS, Sukenik S, Alderdice CA. The clinical significance of coagulation abnormalities in systemic sclerosis scleroderma. J Rheumatol. 1985;12:514-517.

415. Mahn HE, Dantuono LM. Postabortal septicotoxemia due to *Clostridium welchii*. Am J Obstet Gynecol. 1955;70: 604-610.

416. Neter E. Bacterial hemagglutination and hemolysis. Bacteriol Rev. 1956;20:166-188.

417. Rytel MW. Primary atypical pneumonia: current concepts. Am J Med Sci. 1964;247:84-104.

418. Kline MW, Lorin MI. Similarity in white blood cell counts between white and black children with bacteremia. Pediatr Infect Dis. 1986;5:636-639.

419. Itoga T, Laszlo J. Dohle bodies and other granulocytic alterations with cyclophosphamide. Blood. 1962;20: 668-674.

420. Jordan SW, Larsen WE. Ultrastructure studies of the May-Hegglin anomaly. Blood. 1965;250:921-932.

421. Zipursky A, Palko J, Milner R, Akenzua GI. The hematology of bacterial infections in premature infants. Pediatrics. 1976;57:839-853.

422. Segal AW. Nitroblue-tetrazolium tests. Lancet. 1974;2: 1248-1252.

423. Steigbigel RT, Johnson PK, Remington JS. The nitroblue tetrazolium blue test versus conventional hematology in the diagnosis of bacterial infections. N Engl J Med. 1974; 290:235-238.

424. Dorr AD, Moloney WC. Acquired pseudo–Pelger anomaly of granulocytic leukocytes. N Engl J Med. 1959;261: 742-746.

425. Faden HS. Early diagnosis of neonatal bacteremia by buffy coat examination. J Pediatr. 1976;88:1032-1034.

426. Kiepiela P, Coovadia HM, Coward P. T helper cell defect related to severity in measles. Scand J Infect Dis. 1987; 19:185-192.

427. Crofton JW, Livingstone JL, Oswald NC, Roberts AT. Pulmonary eosinophilia. Thorax. 1952;7:1-35.

428. Gibson EL, Vaucher Y, Corrigan JJ Jr. Eosinophilia in premature infants: relationship to weight gain. J Pediatr. 1979;95:99-101.

429. Bhat AM, Scanlon JW. The pattern of eosinophilia in premature infants. J Pediatr. 1981;98:612.

430. Paar JA, Steinman MM, Weaver RA. Disseminated nonreactive tuberculosis with basophilia, leukemoid reaction and terminal pancytopenia. N Engl J Med. 1966;274: 335.

431. Corrigan JJ Jr, Jordan CM. Heparin therapy in septicemia with disseminated intravascular coagulation. N Engl J Med. 1970;233:778-782.

432. Corrian JJ Jr, Walker LR, Ray WL, May N. Changes in the blood coagulation system associated with septicemia. N Engl J Med. 1968;279:851-856.

433. Oski FA, Naiman JL. Effect of live measles vaccine on the platelet count. N Engl J Med. 1966;275:352-356.

434. Corrigan JJ Jr. Thrombocytopenia: a laboratory sign of septicemia in infants and children. J Pediatr. 1974;85: 219-221.

435. Patrick CH, Lazarchick J. The effect of bacteremia on automated platelet measurements in the neonate. Am J Clin Pathol. 1990;93:391-394.

436. Murray JC, Kelley PK, Hogrefe WR, McClain KL. Childhood idiopathic thrombocytopenic purpura: association with human parvovirus B19 infection. Am J Pediatr Hematol Oncol. 1994;16:314-319.

437. Proudfoot AT. Cryptic disseminated tuberculosis. Br J Hosp Med. 1971;5:773-780.

438. Glasser RM, Walker RI, Herion JC. The significance of hematologic abnormalities in patients with tuberculosis. Arch Intern Med. 1970;125:691-695.

439. Medd WE, Hayhoe FGJ. Tuberculous miliary necrosis with pancytopenia. Q J Med. 1955;24:351-364.

440. Ricketts WE. *Bartonella bacilliformis* anemia (Oroya fever): a study of thirty cases. Blood. 1948;3:1025-1049.

441. Clark KGA. A basophilic, micro-organism infecting human red cells. Br J Haematol. 1975;29:301-304.

442. George JN, Wicker DJ, Fogel BJ, et al. Erythrocytic abnormalities in experimental malaria. Soc Exp Biol Med. 1967;124:1086-1090.

443. Overman RR. Reversible cellular permeability alterations in disease: in vivo studies on sodium, potassium and chloride concentrations in erythrocytes of the malarious monkey. Am J Physiol. 1948;152:113-121.

444. George JN, Stokes EF, Wicker DJ, Conrad ME. Studies of the mechanism of hemolysis in experimental malaria. Mil Med. 1966;131:1217-1224.

445. Conrad ME. Pathophysiology of malaria. Hematologic observation in human and animal studies. Ann Intern Med. 1969;70:134-141.

446. Woodruff AW, Ansdell VE, Pettitt LE. Cause of anaemia in malaria. Lancet. 1979;2:1055-1057.

447. Balcerzak SP, Arnold JD, martin DC. Anatomy of red cell damage by *Plasmodium falciparum* in man. Blood. 1972; 40:98-104.

448. Persing DH, Herwaldt BL, Glaser C, et al. Infection with a *Babesia*-like organism in northern California. N Engl J Med. 1995;332:298-303.

449. Hoagland RJ. Infectious Mononucleosis. New York, Grune & Stratton, 1967, p 3.

450. Filatov NF. Lektsii ob ostrych infektsionnykh boleznyakh u detei (Lectures on Acute Infectious Diseases of Children). Moscow, 1885.

451. Pfeiffer E. Drüsenfieber. Jahrb Kinderheilkd. 1889;29: 257-264.

452. Sprunt TP, Evans FA. Mononucleosis leukocytosis in reaction to acute infections (infectious mononucleosis). Bull Johns Hopkins Hosp. 1920;31:409-417.

453. Paul JR. From the notebook of John Rodman Paul. In Horstman DM (ed). Virology and Epidemiology. Hamden, CT, Archon Books, 1971, p 2.

454. Paul JR, Bunnell WW. The presence of heterophile antibodies in infectious mononucleosis. Am J Med Sci. 1932;183:90-104.

455. Davidsohn I, Lee CL. The laboratory diagnosis of infectious mononucleosis, with additional notes on epidemiology, etiology and pathogenesis. Med Clin North Am. 1962;46:225-244.

456. Burkitt D. A sarcoma involving the jaws in African children. Br J Surg. 1958;46:218-223.

457. Epstein MA, Achong BG, Barr YM. Virus particles in cultured lymphoblasts from Burkitt's lymphoma. Lancet. 1964;1:702-703.

458. Henle G, Henle W. Immunofluorescence in cells derived from Burkitt's lymphoma. J Bacteriol. 1966;91:1248-1256.

459. Henle G, Henle W, Clifford P, et al. Antibodies to Epstein-Barr virus in Burkitt's lymphoma and control groups. J Natl Cancer Inst. 1969;43:1147-1157.

460. Niederman JC, McCollum RW, Henle G, Henle W. Infectious mononucleosis. Clinical manifestations in relation to EB virus antibodies. JAMA. 1968;203:205-209.

461. Pereira MS, Blake JM, Macrae AD. EB virus antibody at different ages. BMJ. 1969;4:526-527.

462. Joncas JH, Boucher J, Granger-Julian M, Filion C. Epstein-Barr virus infection in the neonatal period and in childhood. Can Med Assoc J. 1974;110:33-37.

463. Shapiro LR, Hirshaut Y, Kanef DM, Glade P. Epstein-Barr virus in infancy. J Pediatr. 1972;80:1025-1026.

464. Hallee TJ, Evans AS, Niederman JC, et al. Infectious mononucleosis at the United States Military Academy. A prospective study of a single class over four years. Yale J Biol Med. 1974;3:182-195.

465. Wising PJ. A study of infectious mononucleosis (Pfeiffer's disease) from the etiological point of view. Acta Med Scand. 1942;133(Suppl):1.

466. Henle W, Henle GE, Scriba M, et al. Antibody responses to Epstein-Barr virus and cytomegaloviruses after open-heart and other surgery. N Engl J Med. 1970;282:1068-1074.

467. Sixbey JW, Nedrud JG, Raab-Traub N, et al. Epstein-Barr virus replication in oropharyngeal epithelial cells. N Engl J Med. 1984;310:1225-1230.

468. Fleisher GR, Pasquariello PS, Warren WS, et al. Intrafamilial transmission of Epstein-Barr virus infections. J Pediatr. 1981;98:16-19.

469. Joncas JH, Alfieri C, Leyritz-Wills M, et al. Simultaneous congenital infection with Epstein-Barr virus and cytomegalovirus. N Engl J Med. 1981;304:1399-1403.

470. Goldberg GN, Fulginiti VA, Ray CG, et al. In utero Epstein-Barr virus (infectious mononucleosis) infection. JAMA. 1981;246:1579-1581.

471. Horwitz CA, McClain K, Henle W, et al. Fatal illness in a 2-week-old infant: diagnosis by detection of Epstein-Barr virus genomes from a lymph node biopsy. J Pediatr. 1983;103:752-755.

472. Fleisher G, Bolognese R. Epstein-Barr virus infections in pregnancy: a prospective study. J Pediatr. 1984;104:374-379.

473. Fleisher G, Bolognese R. Infectious mononucleosis during gestation: report of three women and their infants studied prospectively. Pediatr Infect Dis. 1984;3:308-311.

474. Le CT, Chang RS, Lipson MH. Epstein-Barr virus infections during pregnancy. A prospective study and review of the literature. Am J Dis Child. 1983;137:466-468.

475. Henle W, Ho HC, Henle G, Kwan HC. Antibodies to Epstein-Barr virus–related antigens in nasopharyngeal carcinoma. Comparison of active cases with long-term survivors. J Natl Cancer Inst. 1973;510:361-369.

476. Hirshaut Y, Glade P, Vieira BD, et al. Sarcoidosis, another disease associated with serologic evidence for herpes-like virus infection. N Engl J Med. 1970;283:502-506.

477. Papageorgiou PS, Sorokin C, Kouzoutzakoglou K, Glade PR. Herpes-like virus in leprosy. Nature. 1971;231:47-49.

478. Evans AS, Rothfield NF, Niederman JC. Raised antibody titres to EB virus in systemic lupus erythematosus. Lancet. 1971;1:167-168.

479. Evans AS. Clinical syndromes associated with EB virus infection. Adv Intern Med. 1972;18:77-93.

480. Hanto DW, Gajl-Peczalska KJ, Frizzera G, et al. Epstein-Barr virus (E.B.V.) induced polyclonal and monoclonal B-cell lymphoproliferative diseases occurring after renal transplantation. Ann Surg. 1983;198:356-369.

481. Rahal JJ Jr, Henle G. Infectious mononucleosis and Reye's syndrome. A fatal case with studies for Epstein-Barr virus. Pediatrics. 1970;46:776-780.

482. Wands JR, Perrotto JL, Isselbacher KJ. Circulating immune complexes and complement sequence activation in infectious mononucleosis. Am J Med. 1976;60:269-272.

483. Kerns D, Shira JE, Go S, et al. Ampicillin rash in children. Relationship to penicillin allergy and infectious mononucleosis. Am J Dis Child. 1973;125:187-190.

484. Portman M, Ingall D, Wentenfelder G, Yogev R. Peritonsillar abscess complicating infectious mononucleosis. J Pediatr. 1984;104:742-744.

485. Connelly KP, DeWitt LD. Neurologic complications of infectious mononucleosis. Pediatr Neurol. 1994;10:181-184.

486. Copperman SM. "Alice in Wonderland" syndrome as a presenting symptom of infectious mononucleosis in children: a description of three affected young people. Clin Pediatr (Phila). 1977;16:143-146.

487. Cinbis M, Aysun S. Alice-in-Wonderland syndrome as an initial manifestation of Epstein-Barr virus infection. Br J Opthalmol. 1992;76:316.

488. Silber MH. Acute transverse myelopathy in Epstein-Barr virus infection. Case reports. S Afr Med J. 1983;64:753-754.

489. Fleisher G, Schwartz J. Primary Epstein-Barr virus infection in association with Reye syndrome. J Pediatr. 1980;97:935-937.

490. Markin RS, Linder J, Zuerlein K, et al. Hepatitis and fatal infectious mononucleosis. Gastroenterology. 1987;93:1210-1217.

491. Chambers CV, Irwin CE Jr. Intense jaundice in an adolescent. An unusual presentation of infectious mononucleosis. J Adolesc Health Care. 1986;7:195-197.

492. Johnson MA. Spontaneous rupture of the spleen in infectious mononucleosis. AJR Am J Roentgenol. 1981;136:111-114.

493. Cloney DL, Kugler JA, Donowitz LG, Lohr JA. Infectious mononucleosis with pleural effusion. South Med J. 1988;81:1441-1442.

494. Poels PJ, Ewals JA, Joosten EM, Van Loon AM. Rhabdomyolysis associated with simultaneous Epstein-Barr virus infection and isolation of echovirus 6 from muscle: a dual infection. J Neurol Neurosurg Psychiatry. 1989;52:412-414.

495. Kelly SP, Rosenthal AR, Nicholson KG, Woodward CG. Retinochoroiditis, a complication of infectious mononucleosis. Br J Ophthalmol. 1989;73:1002-1003.

496. Linde A, Anderssen B, Svensen SB, et al. Serum levels of lymphokines and soluble cellular receptors in primary Epstein-Barr virus infection and in patients with chronic fatigue syndrome. J Infect Dis. 1992;165:994-1000.

497. Schooley RT. Chronic fatigue syndrome: a manifestation of Epstein-Barr virus infection? Curr Clin Top Infect Dis. 1988;9:126-146.

498. Guilleminault C, Mondini S. Mononucleosis and chronic daytime sleepiness. A long-term follow-up study. Arch Intern Med. 1986;146:1333-1335.

499. Jenkins WJ, Koster HG, Marsh WL, Carter RL. Infectious mononucleosis: an unsuspected source of anti-i. Br J Haematol. 1965;11:480-483.

500. Chapman CJ, Spellerberg MB, Smith GA, et al. Auto-anti–red cell antibodies synthesized by patients with infectious mononucleosis. J Immunol. 1993;151:1051-1061.

501. Wilkinson LS, Petz LD, Garraty G. Preappraisal of the role of anti-i in haemolytic anemia in infectious mononucleosis. Br J Haematol. 1973;25:715-722.

502. Mir MA, Delamore IW. Aplastic anemia complicating infectious mononucleosis. Scand J Haematol. 1973;11:314-318.

503. Inoue H, Shinohara K, Nomiyama J, Oeda E. Fatal aplastic anemia caused by Epstein-Barr virus infection after autologous bone marrow transplantation. Intern Med. 1994;33:303-307.

504. Baranski B, Armstrong G, Truman JT, et al. Epstein-Barr virus in the bone marrow of patients with aplastic anemia. Ann Intern Med. 1988;109:695-704.

505. Neel EU: Infectious mononucleosis. Death due to agranulocytosis and pneumonia. JAMA. 1976;236:1493-1494.

506. Sumimoto S, Kasajima Y, Hamamoto T, et al. Agranulocytosis following infectious mononucleosis. Eur J Pediatr. 1990;149:691-694.

507. Kanegane T, Miyawaki T, Iwai K, et al. Acute thrombocytopenic purpura associated with primary Epstein-Barr virus infection. Acta Paediatr Jpn. 1994;36:523-526.

508. Radel EGL, Schorr JB. Thrombocytopenic purpura with infectious mononucleosis. J Pediatr. 1963;63:46-60.

509. Steeper TA, Horwitz CA, Moore SB, et al. Severe thrombocytopenia in Epstein-Barr virus induced mononucleosis. West J Med. 1989;150:170-173.

510. Carter RL, Penman HG. Infectious Mononucleosis. Oxford, Blackwell Scientific, 1969.

511. Carter RL. Platelet levels in infectious mononucleosis. Blood. 1965;25:817-821.

512. Timár L, Budai J, Gerö A, et al. Rare complications and unusual syndromes associated with Epstein-Barr virus. Pediatr Infect Dis. 1985;4:212-213.

513. Downey H, McKinlay CA. Acute lymphadenosis compared with acute lymphatic leukemia. Arch Intern Med. 1923;32:82-112.

514. Litwins J, Leibowitz S. Abnormal lymphocytes (virocytes) in virus diseases other than infectious mononucleosis. Acta Haematol. 1951;5:223-231.

515. Pattengale PK, Smith RW, Perlin E. Atypical lymphocytes in acute infectious mononucleosis. Identification by multiple T and B lymphocyte markers. N Engl J Med. 1974; 291:1145-1148.

516. Enberg RN, Eberle BJ, Williams RC Jr. T and B cells in peripheral blood during infectious mononucleosis. J Infect Dis. 1974;130:104-111.

517. Pattengale PK, Smith RW, Gerber P. B-cell characteristics of human peripheral and cord blood lymphocytes transformed by Epstein-Barr virus. J Natl Cancer Inst. 1974; 52:1081-1086.

518. Mangi RJ, Neiderman JC, Kelleher JE Jr, et al. Depression of cell-mediated immunity during acute infectious mononucleosis. N Engl J Med. 1974;291:1149-1153.

519. Nessan VJ, Geerken RC, Ulvilla J. Uric acid excretion in infectious mononucleosis: a function of increased purine turnover. J Clin Endocrinol Metab. 1974;38:652-654.

520. Lukes RJ, Tindle BH, Parker JW. Reed-Sternberg–like cells in infectious mononucleosis. Lancet. 1969;2:1003-1004.

521. Agliozzo CM, Rheingold IM. Infectious mononucleosis simulating Hodgkin's disease. Am J Clin Pathol. 1971; 56:730-735.

522. Hoagland RJ. Infectious mononucleosis. Am J Med. 1952;13:158-171.

523. Lee CL, Davidsohn I, Panczyszun O. Horse agglutinins in infectious mononucleosis. II. The spot test. Am J Clin Pathol. 1968;49:12-18.

524. Tamir D, Benderly A, Levy J, et al. Infectious mononucleosis and Epstein-Barr virus in childhood. Pediatrics. 1974;53:330-335.

525. Henle W, Henle GE, Howwitz CA. Epstein-Barr virus specific diagnostic tests in infectious mononucleosis. Hum Pathol. 1974;5:551-565.

526. Sumaya CV. Primary Epstein-Barr virus infections in children. Pediatrics. 1977;59:16-21.

527. Tischendorf P, Shramek GJ, Panczyszyn RC, et al. Development and persistence of immunity to Epstein-Barr virus in man. J Infect Dis. 1970;122:401-409.

528. Schmitz H, Scherer M. IgM antibodies to Epstein-Barr virus in infections. Arch Gesamte Virusforsch. 1972;37:332-339.

529. Miller G, Niederman JC, Andrews LL. Prolonged oropharyngeal excretion of Epstein-Barr virus after infectious mononucleosis. N Engl J Med. 1973;288:229-232.

530. Sullivan JL. Epstein-Barr virus and the X-linked lymphoproliferative syndrome. Adv Pediatr 1984;30:365-399.

531. Bell AT, Fortune B, Sheeler R. Clinical inquiries. What test is the best for diagnosing infectious mononucleosis? J Fam Pract. 2006;55:799-802.

532. Purtilo DT, DeFlorio D Jr, Hutt LM, et al. Variable phenotypic expression of an X-linked recessive lymphoproliferative syndrome. N Engl J Med. 1977;297:1077-1080.

533. Bar RS, Delor CJ, clausen KP, et al. Fatal infectious mononucleosis in a family. N Engl J Med. 1974;290:363-367.

534. Provisor AJ, Iacuone JJ, Chilcote RR, et al. Acquired agammaglobulinemia after a life-threatening illness with clinical and laboratory features of infectious mononucleosis in three related male children. N Engl J Med. 1975; 243:62-65.

535. Sullivan JL, Byron KS, Brewster FE, Purtilo DT. Deficient natural killer cell activity in the X-linked lymphoproliferative syndrome. Science. 1980;105:543-545.

536. Sakamoto K, Freed H, Purtilo DT. Antibody responses to Epstein-Barr virus in families with the X-linked lymphoproliferative syndrome. J Immunol. 1980;125:921-925.

537. Bowen TJ, Wedgwood RJ, Ochs HD, Henle W. Transient immunodeficiency during asymptomatic Epstein-Barr virus infection. Pediatrics. 1983;71:964-967.

538. Purtilo DT, Sakamoto K, Barnabei V, et al. Epstein-Barr virus induced diseases in boys with the X-linked lymphoproliferative syndrome (XLP): update on studies of the registry. Am J Med. 1982;73:49-56.

539. Fleisher G, Starr S, Koven N, et al. A non–X-linked syndrome with susceptibility to severe Epstein-Barr virus infections. J Pediatr. 1982;100:727-730.

540. Tatsumi E, Purtilo DT. Epstein-Barr virus (EBV) and the X-linked lymphoproliferative syndrome (XLP). AIDS Res. 1986;2:S109-S113.

541. Coffey AJ, Brooksbank RA, Brandau O, et al. Host response to EBV infection in X-linked lymphoproliferative disease results from mutations in an SH2-domain encoding gene. Nat Genet. 1998;20:129-135.

542. Sayos J, Wu C, Morra M, et al. The X-linked lymphoproliferative-disease gene product SAP regulates signals induced through the co-receptor SLAM. Nature. 1998; 395:462-469.

543. Nichols KE, Harkin DP, Levitz S, et al. Inactivating mutations in an SH2 domain–encoding gene in X-linked lymphoproliferative syndrome. Proc Natl Acad Sci U S A. 1998;95:13765-13770.

544. Parolini S, Bottino C, Falco M, et al. X-linked lymphoproliferative disease. 2B4 molecules displaying inhibitory rather than activating function are responsible for the inability of natural killer cells to kill Epstein-Barr virus–infected cells. J Exp Med. 2000;192:337-346.

545. Sullivan JL, Byron KS, Brewster FE, et al. X-linked lymphoproliferative syndrome. J Clin Invest. 1983;71: 1765-1778.

546. Sullivan JL, Byron KS, Brewster FE, et al. Treatment of life-threatening Epstein-Barr infections with acyclovir. Am J Med. 1982;73:262-266.

547. Andersson J, Erenberg I. Management of Epstein-Barr virus infections. Am J Med. 1988;85:107-115.

548. Pracher E, Panzer-Grümayer ER, Zoubek A, et al. Successful bone marrow transplantation in a boy with X-linked lymphoproliferative syndrome and acute severe infectious mononucleosis. Bone Marrow Transplant. 1994;13:655-658.

549. Gaillard F, Mechinaud-Lacroix F, Papin S, et al. Primary Epstein-Barr virus infection with clonal T cell lympho-proliferation. Am J Clin Pathol. 1992;98:324-333.

550. Chen RL, Su IJ, Lin KH, et al. Fulminant childhood hemophagocytic syndrome mimicking histiocytic medullary reticulosis. An atypical form of Epstein-Barr virus infection. Am J Clin Pathol. 1991;96:171-176.

551. Muthuswamy K, Lee CK, Dosik H, et al. Infectious mononucleosis and severe thrombocytopenia. Am J Med Sci. 1976;272:221-224.

552. Giller RH, Grose C. Epstein-Barr virus: the hematologic and oncologic consequences of virus-host interaction. Crit Rev Oncol Hematol. 1989;9:149-195.

553. Goldstein HH. Disorders of the blood. In Marble A, White P, et al (eds). Joslin's Diabetes Mellitus. Philadelphia, Lea & Febiger, 1971, p 637.

554. Westlund K. Mortality of diabetes: Life Insurance Companies Institute for Medical Statistics at the Oslo City Hospital. Report 13. Oslo, Univeritelsforlaget, 1969.

555. Bensoussan D, Levy Toledano S, Passa P, et al. Platelets hyperaggregation and increased plasma level of von Willebrand's factor in diabetics with retinopathy. Diabetologia. 1975;11:307-312.

556. Rahbar S. An abnormal hemoglobin in red cells of diabetics. Clin Chim Acta. 1968;22:296-298.

557. Trivelli LA, Ranney HM, Lai HT. Hemoglobin components in patients with diabetes mellitus. N Engl J Med. 1971;284:353-357.

558. Rahbar S, Blumenfeld O, Ranney HM. Studies of an unusual hemoglobin in patients with diabetes mellitus. Biochem Biophys Res Commun. 1969;36:838-848.

559. Bunn HF, Briehl RW. The interaction of 2,3-diphosphoglycerate with various human hemoglobins. J Clin Invest. 1970;49:1088-1095.

560. Koenig RJ, Peterson CM, Kilo C, et al. Hemoglobin A_k as an indicator of the degree of glucose intolerance in diabetes. Diabetes. 1976;25:230-232.

561. Lanoe R, Soria J, Thibult N, et al. Glycosylated haemoglobin concentrations and Clinitest results in insulin-dependent diabetes. Lancet. 1977;1:1156-1157.

562. Peterson CM, Jones RL, Koenig RJ, et al. Reversible hematologic sequelae of diabetes mellitus. Ann Intern Med. 1977;86:425-429.

563. Alberti KGM, Emerson PM, Darley JH, Hockaday TD. 2,3-Diphosphoglycerate and tissue oxygenation in uncontrolled diabetes mellitus. Lancet. 1972;2:391-395.

564. Selvam R, Anuradha CV. Red blood cell lipid peroxidation in diabetes mellitus. Indian J Biochem Biophys. 1988;25:268-272.

565. Arai K, Iizuka S, Tada Y, et al. Increase in the glucosylated form of erythrocyte Cu-Zn-superoxide dismutase in diabetes and close association of the nonenzymatic glucosylation with the enzyme activity. Biochem Biophys Acta. 1987;924:292-296.

566. Chimori K, Miyazaki S, Kosada K, et al. Erythrocyte membrane cation flux in diabetics. Clin Exp Hypertens. 1986;8:185-199.

567. Vertommen J, Rillaerts E, Gysels M, De Leeuw I. Red blood cell sorbitol in poorly controlled diabetics. Diabetes Metab. 1987;13:182-186.

568. Bock HA, Fluckinger R, Berger W. Mean corpuscular volume artifactual changes resulting from hyperglycemia. Diabetologia. 1985;28:335-338.

569. Borgna-Pignatti C, Marradi P, Pinelli L, et al. Thiamine-responsive anemia in DIDMOAD syndrome. J Pediatr. 1989;115:405-410.

570. Bybee JD, Rodgers DE. The phagocytic activity of polymorphonuclear leukocytes obtained from patients with diabetes mellitus. J Lab Clin Med. 1964;64:1-13.

571. Miller ME, Baker L. Leukocyte functions in juvenile diabetes mellitus: humoral and cellular aspects. J Pediatr. 1972;81:979-982.

572. Brody JI, Merlie K. Metabolic and biosynthetic features of lymphocytes from patients with diabetes mellitus: similarities to lymphocytes in chronic lymphocytic leukemia. Br J Haematol. 1970;19:193-201.

573. Hiramatsu K, Arimori S. Monocyte superoxide formation in diabetics with hypertriglyceridemia. Diabetes. 1988;37: 832-837.

574. Hughes A, McVerry BA, Wilkinson L, et al. Diabetes, a hypercoagulable state? Hemostatic variables in newly

diagnosed type 2 diabetic patients. Acta Haematol. 1983;69:254-259.

575. Patrassi GM, Vettor R, Padovan D, Girolami K. Contact phase of blood coagulation in diabetes mellitus. Eur J Clin Invest. 1982;12:307-311.

576. Egeberg O. The blood coagulability in diabetic patients. Scand J Clin Lab Invest. 1963;15:533-538.

577. Mayne EE, Bridges JM, Weaver JA. Platelet adhesiveness, plasma fibrinogen and factor VIII level in diabetes mellitus. Diabetologia. 1970;6:436-440.

578. Sagel J, Colwell JA, Crook L, Laimins M. Increased platelet aggregation in early diabetes mellitus. Ann Intern Med. 1975;82:733-738.

579. Kwaan HC, Colwell JA, Cruz S, et al. Increased platelet aggregation in diabetes mellitus. J Lab Clin Med. 1972;80:236-246.

580. Nordoy A, Rodset JM. Platelet phospholipids and their function in patients with juvenile diabetes mellitus. Diabetes. 1970;19:698-702.

581. Colwell JA, Halushka PV, Sarji K, et al. Altered platelet function in diabetes mellitus. Diabetes. 1976;25(2 Suppl):826-831.

582. Born GVR. Aggregation of blood platelets by adenosine diphosphate and its reversal. Nature. 1962;194:927-929.

583. Halushka PV, Lurie D, Colwell JA. Increased synthesis of prostaglandin-E–like material by platelets from patients with diabetes mellitus. N Engl J Med. 1977;297:1306-1310.

584. Butkus A, Shirey EK, Schumacher OP. Thromboxane biosynthesis in platelets of diabetic and coronary artery disease patients. Artery. 1982;11:238-251.

585. Powell EDU, Field RA. Diabetic retinopathy and rheumatoid arthritis. Lancet. 1964;2:17-18.

586. Viinikka L. Platelet function and thrombosis in diabetes. Acta Endocrinol. 1985;272:31-34.

587. Grupe W. Renal vascular thrombosis. In Schaffer AJ, Avery ME (eds). Diseases of the Newborn. Philadelphia, WB Saunders, 1977, p 456.

588. Ward TF. Multiple thromboses in an infant of a diabetic mother. J Pediatr. 1977;90:982-984.

589. Caroline NL, Schwartz H. Chicken soup rebound and relapse of pneumonia: report of a case. Chest. 1975;67:215-216.

590. Ways P, Reed CF, Hanahan DJ. Red cell and plasma lipids in acanthocytosis. J Clin Invest. 1963;42:1248-1260.

591. Simon ER, Ways R. Incubation hemolysis and red cell metabolism in acanthocytosis. J Clin Invest. 1964;43:1311-1321.

592. Dodge JT, Cohen G, Kayden HJ, Phillips GB. Peroxidative hemolysis of red blood cells from patients with abetalipoproteinemia (acanthocytosis). J Clin Invest. 1967;46:357-368.

593. Carvalho ACA, Coleman RW, Lees RS. Platelet function in hyperlipoproteinemia. N Engl J Med. 1974;290:434-438.

594. Bianciardi G, Weber G, Toti P, et al. Platelet plasma membrane changes in human type IIa hypercholesterolemia. Appl Pathol. 1986;4:253-259.

595. Simpson HC, Mann JI, Meade TW, et al. Hypertriglyceridemia and hypercoagulability. Lancet. 1983;1:786-790.

596. Atkinson JB, Stacpoole PW, Swift LL. Red blood cell morphology in the hyperlipidemias. Biochim Biophys Acta. 1982;712:211-216.

597. Stewart GW, O'Brien H, Morris SA, et al. Stomatocytosis, abnormal platelets, and pseudo-homozygous hypercholesterolemia. Eur J Haematol. 1987;38:376-380.

598. Friedman Z, Lamberth EL, Stahlman MT, Oates JA. Platelet dysfunction in the neonate with essential fatty acid deficiency. J Pediatr. 1977;90:439-443.

599. Vincent JE, Melai A. Comparison of the effect of prostaglandin E on platelet aggregation in normal and essential fatty acid–deficient rats. Prostaglandins. 1974;5:369-373.

600. Rosenberg LE, Lilljeqvist A, Hsia YE. Methylmalonic aciduria: an inborn error leading to metabolic-acidosis, long chain ketonuria and intermittent hyperglycinemia. N Engl J Med. 1968;278:1319-1322.

601. Cox EV, White AM. Methylmalonic acid excretion: a sensitive indicator of vitamin B_{12} deficiency in man. Lancet. 1962;2:853-856.

602. Rosenblatt DS, Cooper BA, Pottier A, et al. Altered B_{12} metabolism in fibroblasts from a patient with megaloblastic anemia and homocystinuria due to a new defect in methionine biosynthesis. J Clin Invest. 1984;74:2149-2156.

603. Schuh S, Rosenblatt DS, Cooper BA, et al. Abnormal cobalamin metabolism and megaloblastic anemia. N Engl J Med. 1984;310:386-390.

604. Huguley CM, Bain JA, Rivers SL, Scoggins RB. Refractory megaloblastic anemia associated with excretion of orotic acid. Blood. 1959;14:615-634.

605. Roses AD, Appel SH. Protein kinase activity in erythrocyte ghosts of patients with myotonic muscular dystrophy. Proc Natl Acad Sci U S A. 1973;70:1855-1859.

606. Roses AD, Herbstreith MH, Appel SH, et al. Membrane protein kinase alteration in Duchenne muscular dystrophy. Nature. 1975;254:350-351.

607. Shohet SB, Layzer RB. Editorial: the "muscle" of the red cell. N Engl J Med. 1976;294:221-222.

608. Matheson DW, Howland JL. Erythrocyte deformation in human muscular dystrophy. Science. 1974;181:165-166.

609. Percy AK, Miller ME. Reduced deformability of erythrocyte membranes from patients with Duchenne muscular dystrophy. Nature. 1975;258:147-148.

610. Kim HD, Luthra MG, Watts RP, Stern LZ. Factors influencing osmotic fragility of red blood cells in Duchenne muscular dystrophy. Neurology. 1980;30:726-731.

611. Shivers RR, Martin K, Atkinson BG: Detection of carriers of Duchenne muscular dystrophy by freez fracture analysis of plasmalemmal intramembrane particles. Am J Clin Pathol. 1986;85:131-134.

612. Scheneiderman LJ, Sampson WI, Schoene WC, Haydon GB. Genetic studies of a family with two unusual autosomal conditions: muscular dystrophy and Pelger-Huët anomaly. Clinical, pathologic and linkage considerations. Am J Med. 1969;46:380-393.

613. Jordans GHW. The familial occurrence of fat-containing vacuoles in the leukocytes diagnosed in two brothers suffering from dystrophia musculorum progressiva (ERB). Acta Med Scand. 1953;145:419-423.

614. Yarom R, Meyer S, More R, et al. Platelet abnormalities in muscular dystrophy. Thromb Haemost. 1983;49:168-172.

615. Nicholson GA, McLeoid JG, Sugars JW. A study of platelet protein phosphorylation in Duchenne muscular dystrophy. Further evidence against the generalized membrane defect theory. J Neurol Sci. 1984;64:21-32.

616. Schmid JR, Kiely JM, Harrison EG Jr, et al. Thymoma associated with pure red cell agenesis. Review of the literature and report of 4 cases. Cancer. 1965;18:216-230.

617. Cohen SM, Waxman S. Myasthenia gravis, chronic lymphocytic leukemia and autoimmune hemolytic anemia. A spectrum of thymic abnormalities? Arch Intern Med. 1967;110:717-720.

618. Mathieson PW, O'Neill JH, Durrant ST, et al. Antibody-mediated pure red cell neutrophil aplasia, recurrent myasthenia gravis and previous thymoma: a case reported in literature review. Q J Med. 1990;74:57-61.

619. van der Zee SP, Schretlen ED, Monnens LA. Megaloblastic anemia in the Lesch-Nyhan syndrome. Lancet. 1968;1:1427.

620. Seegmiller JE, Rosenbloom FM, Kelley WN. An enzyme defect associated with a sex-linked human neurological disorder and excessive purine synthesis. Science. 1967;155:1682-1684.

621. Edwards NL, Jeryc W, Fox IH. Enzyme replacement in the Lesch-Nyhan syndrome with long-term erythrocyte transfusions. Adv Exp Med Biol. 1984;165:23-26.

622. Rivard GF, Izadi E, Lazerson J, et al. Functional and metabolic studies of platelets from patients with Lesch-Nyhan syndrome. Br J Haematol. 1975;31:245-253.

623. Cooper RA, Jandl JH. Acanthocytosis. In Williams WJ (ed). Hematology. New York, McGraw-Hill, 1977, p 464.

624. Mant MJ, Faragher BS. The hematology of anorexia nervosa. Br J Haematol. 1972;23:737-749.

625. Kay J, Strickler RB. Hematologic and immunologic abnormalities in anorexia nervosa. South Med J. 1983;76:1008-1010.

626. Devuyst O, Lambert M, Rodhain J, et al. Haematological changes and infectious complications in anorexia nervosa: a case-control study. Q J Med. 1993;86:791-799.

627. Pearson HA. Marrow hypoplasia in anorexia nervosa. J Pediatr. 1967;71:211-215.

628. Amrein PC, Friedman R, Kosinski K, Ellman L. Hematologic changes in anorexia nervosa. JAMA. 1979;241:2190-2191.

629. Luck P, Mikhailidis DP, Dashwood MR, et al. Platelet hyperaggregability and increased adrenoceptor density in anorexia nervosa. J Clin Endocrinol Metab. 1983;57:911-914.

630. Marks J, Shuster S. Iron metabolism and skin disease. Arch Dermatol. 1968;98:469-475.

631. el-Saaiee L, Meky N. Deformability of red blood cells in eczema. J Med. 1986;17:273-283.

632. Fox RH, Shuster S, Williams R, et al. Cardiovascular metabolic and thermoregulatory disturbances in patients with erythrodermic skin diseases. BMJ. 1965;1:619-622.

633. Marks J, Shuster S. Method for measuring capillary permeability and its use in patients with skin disease. BMJ. 1966;2:88-90.

634. Summerly R, Giles C. Question of psoriatic enteropathy. Arch Dermatol. 1971;103:678-679.

635. Semplicini A, Mozzato MG, Rigon E, et al. Red blood cell sodium and potassium fluxes in psoriatic patients. Eur J Clin Invest. 1988;18:47-51.

636. Corrocher R, Bassi A, Gandini A, et al. Transmembrane cation fluxes and fatty acid composition of erythrocytes in psoriatic patients. Clin Chim Acta. 1990;186:335-344.

637. Schena D, Chieregato GC, de Gironcoli M, et al. Increased erythrocyte membrane arachidonic and platelet malondialdehyde (MDA) production in psoriasis: normalization after fish oil. Acta Derm Venereol. 1989;146:42-44.

638. Fry L, Keir P, McMinn RM, et al. Small intestinal structure and function and haematological manifestations of dermatitis herpetiformis. Lancet. 1967;2:729-733.

639. Pettit JE, Hoffbrand AV, Seah PP, Fry L. Splenic atrophy in dermatitis herpetiformis. BMJ. 1972;2:438-440.

640. McCarthy CF, Fraser ID, Evans KT, Read AE. Lymphoreticular dysfunction in idiopathic steatorrhea. Gut. 1966;7:140-148.

641. Magnusson B. Is dermatitis herpetiformis a nutritional disease with hematologic consequences? Int J Dermatol. 1984;23:316-317.

642. Trowbridge AA, Sirinavin C, Linman JW. Dyskeratosis congenita: hematologic evaluation of a sibship and review of the literature. Am J Hematol. 1977;3:143-153.

643. De Boeck K, Degreef H, Verwilghen R, et al. Thrombocytopenia: first symptom in a patient with dyskeratosis congenita. Pediatrics. 1981;67:898-903.

644. Friedland M, Lutton JD, Spitzer R, Levere RD. Dyskeratosis congenita with hypoplastic anemia: a stem cell defect. Am J Hematol. 1985;20:85-87.

645. Arneson MA, Hammerschmidt DE, Furcht LT, King RA. A new form of Ehlers-Danlos syndrome: fibronectin corrects platelet dysfunction. JAMA. 1980;244:144-147.

646. Grenko RT, Burns SL, Golden EA, et al. Type IV Ehlers-Danlos syndrome with aspirin sensitivity. A family study. Arch Pathol Lab Med. 1993;117:989-992.

647. Brett EM, Ong BH, Friedmann T. Mast-cell disease in children. Br J Dermatol. 1967;79:197-209.

648. Griffith GC, Nichols G Jr, Asher JD, Hanagan B. Heparin osteoporosis. JAMA. 1965;193:91-94.

649. Waters WJ, Lacson PS. Mast cell leukemia presenting as urticaria pigmentosa. Pediatrics. 1957;19:1033-1042.

650. Huët GJ. Familial anomaly of leukocytes. Discuss Med Tijdschr Geeneesk. 1931;75:5956.

651. Pelger K. Demonstratie van een paar zeldzaam voorkomende typhen van bloedlichaampjes en bespreking der patienten. Discuss Med Tijdschr Geneesk. 1928;72:1178.

652. Hoffmann K, Dreger CK, Olins AL, et al. Mutations in the gene encoding the lamin B receptor produce an altered nuclear morphology in granulocytes (Pelger-Huët anomaly). Nat Genet. 2002;31:410-414.

653. Dorr AD, Moloney WC. Acquired pseudo–Pelger anomaly of granulocytic leukocytes. N Engl J Med. 1959;261:742-746.

654. Linman JW, Saarni MI. The preleukemic syndrome. Semin Hematol. 1974;11:93-100.

655. Laszlo J, Rundles RW. Morphology of granulocytes and their precursors. In Williams WJ, Beutler E, et al (eds). Hematology. New York, McGraw-Hill, 1977, p 665.

656. Rosell A, Rodriquez M, et al. Reversible Pelger-Huët anomaly associated with acute gastroenteritis caused by *Salmonella* group D. An Esp Pediatr. 1989;30:143.

657. Liesveld J, Smith BD. Acquired Pelger-Huët anomaly in a case of non-Hodgkin's lymphoma. Acta Haematol. 1988;79:46-49.

658. Kashida H, Yabe H, Yoshida T, et al. Sjögren's syndrome in a patient with familial Pelger-Huët anomaly. Rinsho Ketsueki. 1985;26:1306-1310.

659. Irken G, Olgun N, Oren H, et al. Pelger-Huët anomaly with trisomy 18 syndrome. Am J Hematol. 1993;43:328-329.

660. van Hook L, Spivack C, Duncanson FP. A transient acquired Pelger-Huët anomaly may be observed with *Mycoplasma pneumoniae* infections. Am J Clin Pathol. 1985;84:248-251.

661. Ganick DJ, Sunder T, Finley JL. Severe hematologic toxicity of valproic acid. A report of four patients. Am J Pediatr Hematol Oncol. 1990;12:80-85.

662. Undritz E. Eine neue Sippe mit erblichkonstitutioneller Hochsegmentierung der Neutrophilenkerne. Schweiz Med Wochenschr. 1958;88:1000-1001.

663. Presentey B. A new anomaly of eosinophilic granulocytes. Tech Bull Regist Med Technol. 1968;38:131-134.

664. Davidson WM, Milner RDG, Lawler SD, Warner W. Giant neutrophil leucocytes: an inherited anomaly. Br J Haematol. 1960;6:339-343.

665. Huehns ER, Lutzner M, Hechte F. Nuclear abnormalities of the neutrophils in D-(13-15)-trisomy syndrome. Lancet. 1964;1:589-590.

666. Davidson WM. Sexing the blood leucocytes in abnormalities of the sex chromosomes. Minerva Pediatr. 1965;17:585-587.

667. Reilly WA. The granules in the leukocytes in gargoylism. Am J Dis Child. 1941;62:489-491.

668. Davidson WM. Inherited variations in leukocytes. Br Med Bull. 1960;17:190-195.

669. Djaldetti M, Creter D, Bujanover Y, Elian E. Ultrastructural abnormalities of platelets in the May-Hegglin anomaly. Haematologica. 1982;67:535-538.

670. Greinacher A, Mueller-Eckhardt C. Hereditary types of thrombocytopenia with giant platelets and inclusion bodies in the leukocytes. Blut. 1990;60:53-56.

671. Filipovich AH. Hemophagocytic lymphohistiocytosis and related disorders. Curr Opin Allergy Clin Immunol. 2006;6:410-415.

672. Carrillo-Farga J, Gutiérrez-Palomera G, Ruiz-Maldonado R, et al. Giant cytoplasmic granules in Langerhans' cells of the Chédiak-Higashi syndrome. Am J Dermatopathol. 1990;12:81-87.

673. Strouth JC, Zeman W, Merritt AD, et al. Leukocyte abnormalities in familial amaurotic idiocy. N Engl J Med. 1966;274:36-38.

674. Halon PJ, Mitus WJ. Ceroid storage in albinism [abstract]. Paper presented ath the 13th Congress of the International Society of Hematology, 1970, Munich, p 322.

675. White JG, Witkop CJ Jr, Gerritsen SM. The Hermansky-Pudlak syndrome: inclusions in circulating leucocytes. Br J Haematol. 1973;24:761-765.

676. Schachne JP, Glaser N, Lee SH, et al. Ceroid and dermal macrophages. J Am Acad Dermatol. 1990;22:926-932.

677. Bonifacino JS. Insights into the biogenesis of lysosome-related organelles from the study of the Hermansky-Pudlak syndrome. Ann N Y Acad Sci. 2004;1038:103-114.

678. Plum CM. Lymphocyte degeneration in amaurotic familial idiocy. Dan Med Bull. 1957;4:156.

679. Mittwoch U. Nuclear segmentation of the neutrophils in heterozygous carriers of gargoylism. Nature. 1962;193:1209-1210.

680. Bowman JE, Mittwoch U, Schneiderman LJ. Persistence of mucopolysaccharide inclusions in culture of lymphocytes from patients with gargoylism. Nature. 1962;195:612-613.

681. Jordan GH. The familial occurrence of fat-containing vacuoles in leukocytes. Acta Med Scand. 1953;145:419-424.

682. Rozenszajn L. Jordan's anomaly in the white blood cells. Blood. 1966;28:258-265.

683. Lukens JN. Eosinophilia in children. Pediatr Clin North Am. 1972;19:969-981.

684. Orfanakis NG, Ostlund RE, Bishop CR, Athens JW. Normal blood leukocyte concentration values. Am J Clin Pathol. 1970;53:647-651.

685. el-Shoura SM. Falciparum malaria in naturally infected human patients: IV—Ultrastructural changes in peripheral white blood cells. Ann Parasitol Hum Comp. 1993;68:169-175.

686. Archer RK. Regulatory mechanisms in eosinophil leukocyte production, release and distribution. In Gordon AS (ed). Regulation of Hematopoiesis, vol 2. New York, Appleton-Century-Crofts, 1972.

687. Hardy WR, Anderson RE. The hypereosinophilic syndromes. Ann Intern Med. 1968;68:1120-1129.

688. Nelken RP, Stockman JA III. The hypereosinophilic syndrome in association with acute lymphoblastic leukemia. J Pediatr. 1976;89:771-773.

689. Spitzer G, Garson OM. Lymphoblastic leukemia with marked eosinophilia: a report of two cases. Blood. 1973;42:377-384.

689. Basten A, Boyer MH, Beeson PB. Mechanisms of eosinophilia. I. Factors affecting the eosinophil response of rats to *Trichinella spirilis*. J Exp Med. 1970;131:1271-1287.

690. Yamaguchi Y, Suda J, Suda M, et al. Purified interleukin 5 supports the terminal differentiation and proliferation of murine eosinophil precursors. J Exp Med. 1988;167:43-46.

691. Basten A, Beeson PB. Mechanism of eosinophilia. II. Role of the lymphocyte. J Exp Med. 1970;131:1288-1305.

692. Gotlib J, Cross NC, Gilliland DG. Eosinophilic disorders: molecular pathogenesis, new classification, and modern therapy. Best Pract Res Clin Haematol. 2006;19:535-569.

693. Naiman JL, Oski FA, Allen FH Jr, Diamond LK. Hereditary eosinophilia: report of a family and review of the literature. Am J Hum Genet. 1964;16:195-203.

694. Braunsteiner H, Thumb N. Quantitative Veränderungen der Blutbasophilen und ihre klinische Bedeutung. Acta Haematol. 1958;20:339.

695. Dvorak HF, Mihm MC Jr. Basophilic leukocytes in allergic contact dermatitis. J Exp Med. 1972;135:235-254.

696. Juhlin L. Basophilic leukocyte differential in blood and bone marrow. Acta Haematol. 1963;29:89-95.

697. Mitchell RG. Basophilic leukocytes in children in health and disease. Arch Dis Child. 1958;33:193-207.

698. Hill RW, Bayrd ED. Phagocytic reticuloendothelial cells in subacute bacterial endocarditis with negative cultures. Ann Intern Med. 1960;52:310.

699. Michael SR, Vural IL. The hematological aspects of disseminated (systemic) lupus erythematosus: review of the literature and clinical analysis of 138 cases. Medicine (Baltimore). 1954;33:291-437.

700. Lagergren J. The white blood cell count and the erythrocyte sedimentation rate of pertussis. Acta Pediatr. 1963;50:405-409.

701. Bertotto A, de Felicis Arcangeli C, Spinozzi F, et al. Acute infectious lymphocytosis: phenotype of the proliferating cell. Acta Paediatr Scand. 1985;74:633-635.

702. Daughaday WH, Williams RH, Daland G. The effect of endocrinopathies on the blood. Blood. 1948;3:1342-1366.

703. Gottlieb MS, Schroff R, Schanker HM. *Pneumocystis carinii* pneumonia and mucosal candidiasis in previously healthy homosexual men: evidence of a new acquired cellular immunodeficiency. N Engl J Med. 1981;305:1425-1431.

704. Masur H, Michelis MA, Greene JB, et al. An outbreak of community-acquired *Pneumocystis carinii* pneumonia: initial manifestation of cellular immune dysfunction. N Engl J Med. 1981;305:1431-1438.

705. Siegal FP, Lopez C, Hammer GS, et al. Severe acquired immunodeficiency in male homosexuals, manifested by chronic perianal ulcerative herpes simplex lesions. N Engl J Med. 1981;305:1439-1444.

706. Barré-Sinoussi F, Chermann JC, Rey F, et al. Isolation of a T-lymphotropic retrovirus from a patient at risk for acquired immune deficiency syndrome (AIDS). Science. 1983;220:868-871.

707. Gallo RC, Salahuddin SZ, Popovic M, et al. Frequent detection and isolation of cytopathic retroviruses (HTLV-III) from patients with AIDS and at risk for AIDS. Science. 1984;224:500-503.

708. Clavel F, Guértard D, Brun-Vézinet F, et al. Isolation of new human retrovirus from West African patients with AIDS. Science. 1986;233:343-346.

709. Guyader M, Emerman M, Sonigo P, et al. Genome organization and transactivation of the human immunodeficiency virus type 2. Nature. 1987;326:662-669.

710. Narayan O, Clements JE. Biology and pathogenesis of lentiviruses. J Gen Virol. 1989;70:1617-1639.

711. Rubinstein A. Pediatric AIDS. Curr Probl Pediatr. 1986;16:361-409.

712. Guinan ME, Hardy A. Epidemiology of AIDS in women in the United States. JAMA. 1987;257:2039-2076.

713. Piot P, Kreiss JK, Ndinya-Achola JO, et al. Heterosexual transmission of HIV. AIDS. 1987;1:199-206.

714. Curran JW, Jaffe HW, Hardy AM, et al. Epidemiology of HIV infection and AIDS in the United States. Science. 1988;239:610-616.

715. Falloon J, Eddy J, Wiener L, Pizzo PA. Human immunodeficiency virus infection in children. J Pediatr. 1989;114:1-30.

716. Gwinn M, Pappaioanou M, George JR, et al. Prevalence of HIV infection in childbearing women in the United States. Surveillance using newborn blood samples. JAMA. 1991;265:1704-1708.

717. Centers for Disease Control and Prevention (CDC). Update: AIDS among women—United States, 1994. MMWR Morbid Mortal Wkly Rep. 1995;44(5):81-84.

718. Ryder RW, Nsa W, Hassig SE, et al. Perinatal transmission of the human immunodeficiency virus type I to infants to seropositive women in Zaire. N Engl J Med. 1989;320:1637-1642.

719. Clavel F, Mansinho K, Chamaret S, et al. Human immunodeficiency virus type 2 infection associated with AIDS in West Africa. N Engl J Med. 1987;316:1180-1185.

720. Brun-Vezinet F, Rey MA, Katalama C, et al. Lymphadenopathy-associated virustype 2 in AIDS and AIDS-related complex. Clinical and virological features in four patients. Lancet. 1987;1:128-132.

721. Denis F, Barin F, Gershy-Damet G, et al. Prevalence of human T-lymphotrophic retrovirus type III and type IV in Ivory Coast. Lancet. 1987;1:408-411.

722. Kanki PJ, Alroy J, Essex M. Isolation of T-lymphotropic retrovirus related to HTLV-III/LAV from wild-caught African green monkeys. Science. 1985;230:951-954.

723. Franchini G, Gurgo C, Guo HG, et al. Sequence of simian immunodeficiency virus and its relationship to the human immunodeficiency viruses. Nature. 1987;328:539-543.

724. Doolittle RF. Immunodeficiency viruses: the simian-human connection. Nature. 1989;339:338-339.

725. Curran JW, Jaffe HW, Hardy AM, et al. Epidemiology of HIV infection and AIDS in the United States. Science. 1988;239:610-616.

726. Fauci AS. The human immunodeficiency virus: infectivity and mechanisms of pathogenesis. Science. 1988;239:617-622.

727. Rogers MF. AIDS in children: a review of the clinical, epidemiologic and public health aspects. Pediatr Infect Dis. 1986;4:230-236.

728. Novick BE, Rubinstein A. AIDS—the pediatric perspective. AIDS. 1987;1:3-7.

729. Luciw PA, Shacklett BL. Molecular biology of the human and simian immunodeficiency viruses. In Morrow WJW, Haigwood NI (eds). HIV Molecular Organization, Pathogenicity and Treatment. New York, Elsevier; 1993.

730. Scott GB, Fischl MA, Klimas N, et al. Mothers of infants with the acquired immunodeficiency syndrome: evidence for both symptomatic and asymptomatic carriers. JAMA. 1985;253:363-366.

731. Gardillo B, Preti E, Zanchi S, et al. [Perinatal transmission of HIV.] Minerva Ginecol. 2007;59:139-149.

732. Blanche S, Rouziou C, Moscato ML, et al. A prospective study of infants born to women seropositive for human immunodeficiency virus type I. N Engl J Med. 1989;320:1643-1648.

733. Mother-to-child transmission of HIV infection. The European Collaborative Study. Lancet. 1988;2:1038-1043.

734. Epidemiology, clinical features and prognostic factors of pediatric HIV infection. Italian Multicenter Study. Lancet. 1988;1:1043-1046.

735. Barton JJ, O'Connor TM, Cannon MJ, Weldon-Linne CM. Prevalence of human immunodeficiency virus in a general perinatal population. Am J Obstet Gynecol. 1989;160:1316-1320; discussion 1320-1324.

736. Bove JR. Transfusion-associated hepatitis and AIDS: what is the risk? N Engl J Med. 1987;317:242-245.

737. Chanock SJ, McIntosh K. Pediatric infection with the human immunodeficiency virus: issues for the otolaryngologist. Otolaryngol Clin North Am. 1989;22:637-660.

738. Greene WC. The molecular biology of human immunodeficiency virus type 1 infection. N Engl J Med. 1991;324:308-317.

739. Dalgleish AG, Beverley PC, Clapham PR, et al. The CD4 (T4) antigen is an essential component of the receptor for the AIDS retrovirus. Nature. 1984;312:763-767.

740. Klatzmann D, Champagne E, Chamaret S, et al. T-lymphocyte T4 molecule behaves as the receptor for human retrovirus LAV. Nature. 1984;312:767-768.

741. McDougal JS, Kennedy MS, Sligh JM, et al. Binding of HTLV-III/LAV to T4 + T cells by a complex of the 110K viral protein and the T4 molecule. Science. 1986;231: 382-385.

742. Maddon PJ, Dalgleish AG, McDougla JS, et al. The T4 gene encodes the AIDS virus receptor and is expressed in the immune system and the brain. Cell. 1986;47: 333-348.

743. Lifson J, Coutré S, Huang E, Engleman E. Role of envelope glycoprotein carbohydrate in human immunodeficiency virus (HIV) infectivity and virus-induced cell fusion. J Exp Med. 1986;164:2101-2106.

744. Sherman MP, Greene WC. Slipping through the door: HIV entry into the nucleus. Microbes Infect. 2002;4: 67-73.

745. Varmus HE, Padgett T, Heasley S, et al. Cellular functions are required for the synthesis and integration of avian sarcoma virus–specific DNA. Cell. 1977;11:307-319.

746. Fritsch EF, Temin HM. Inhibition of viral DNA synthesis in stationary chicken embryo fibroblasts infected with avian retroviruses. J Virol. 1977;24:461-469.

747. Toohey MG, Jones KA. In vitro formation of short RNA polymerase II transcripts that terminate within the HIV-1 and HIV-2 promoter proximal downstream regions. Genes Dev. 1989;3:265-282.

748. Cullen BR, Greene WC. Regulatory pathways governing HIV-1 replication. Cell. 1990;58:423-426.

749. Gallo R, Wong-Staal F, et al. HIV/HTLV gene nomenclature [letter]. Nature. 1988;333:504.

750. Arya SK, Guo C, Josephs SF, Wong-Staal F. Trans-activator gene of human T-lymphotropic virus type III (HTLV-III). Science. 1985;229:69-73.

751. Sodroski J, Patarca R, Rosen C, et al. Location of the trans-activating region on the genome of human T-cell lymphotrophic virus type III. Science. 1985;229:74-77.

752. Feng S, Holland EC. HIV TAT trans-activation requires the loop sequence within TAR. Nature. 1988;334: 165-167.

753. Felber BK, Hadzopoulou-Cladaras M, Cladaras C, et al. Rev protein of the human immunodeficiency virus-I affects the stability and transport of the viral mRNA. Proc Natl Acad Sci U S A. 1989;86:1495-1499.

754. Malim MH, Hauber J, Le SY, et al. The HIV-1 rev trans-activator acts through a structured target sequence to activate nuclear export of unspliced viral mRNA. Nature. 1989;338:254-257.

755. Malim MH, Böhnlein S, Hauber J, Cullen BR. Functional dissection of HIV-I Rev trans-activator—derivation of a trans-dominant repression of Rev function. Cell. 1989;58: 205-214.

756. Gendelman HE, Orenstein JM, Martin MA, et al. Efficient isolation and propagation of human immunodeficiency virus on recombinant colony-stimulating factor 1–treated monocytes. J Exp Med. 1988;167:1428-1441.

757. Zucker-Franklin D, Cao YZ. Megakaryocytes of human immunodeficiency virus–infected individuals express viral RNA. Proc Natl Acad Sci U S A. 1989;86:5595-5599.

758. Zucker-Franklin D, Termin CS, Cooper MC. Structural changes in the megakaryocytes of patients infected with the human immunodeficiency virus (HIV-1). Am J Pathol. 1989;134:1295-1303.

759. Watkins BA, Dorn HH, Kelly WB, et al. Specific tropism of HIV-I for microglial cells in primary human brain cultures. Science. 1990;249:549-553.

760. Cao Y, Qin L, Zhang L, et al. Virologic and immunologic characterization of long-term survivors of human immunodeficiency virus type 1 infection. N Engl J Med. 1995;332:201-208.

761. Pantaleo G, Menzo S, Vaccarezza M, et al. Studies in subjects with long-term nonprogressive human immunodeficiency virus infection. N Engl J Med. 1995;332: 209-216.

762. Baltimore D. Lessons from people with nonprogressive HIV infection [editorial]. N Engl J Med. 1995;332:259-260.

763. Ho DD, Neumann AU, Perelson AS, et al. Rapid turnover of plasma virions and CD4 lymphocytes in HIV-1 infection. Nature. 1995;373:123-126.

764. Wei X, Ghosh SK, Taylor ME, et al. Viral dynamics in human immunodeficiency virus type 1 infection. Nature. 1995;373:117-122.

765. Bryson YJ, Pang S, Wei LS, et al. Clearance of HIV infection in a perinatally infected infant. N Engl J Med. 1995;332:833-838.

766. McIntosh K, Burchett SK. Clearance of HIV—lessons from newborns [editorial]. N Engl J Med. 1995;332: 883-884.

767. Connor EM, Sperling RS, Gelber R, et al. Reduction of maternal-infant transmission of human immunodeficiency virus type 1 with zidovudine treatment. Pediatric AIDS Clinical Trials Group Protocol 076 Study Group. N Engl J Med. 1994;331:1173-1180.

768. Ho DD. Time to hit HIV, early and hard [editorial]. N Engl J Med. 1995;333:450-451.

769. Gortmaker SL, Hughes M, Cervia J, et al. Effect of combination therapy including protease inhibitors on mortality among children and adolescents infected with HIV-1. N Engl J Med. 2001;345:1522-1528.

770. Sullivan JL, Luzuriaga K. The changing face of pediatric HIV-1 infection [editorial]. N Engl J Med. 2001;345: 1568-1569.

771. Zon LI, Arkin C, Groopman JE. Hematological manifestations of the human immunodeficiency virus. Br J Haematol. 1987;66:251-256.

772. Zon LI, Groopman JE. Hematological manifestations of the human immunodeficiency virus. Semin Hematol. 1988;25:208-218.

773. Walsh CM, Nardi MA, Karpatkin S. On the mechanism of thrombocytopenic purpura in sexually active homosexual men. N Engl J Med. 1984;311:635-639.

774. Savona S, Nardi MA, Lennette ET, Karpatkin S. Thrombocytopenic purpura in narcotics addicts. Ann Intern Med. 1985;102:737-741.

775. Walsh C, Karpatkin S. Thrombocytopenia and human immunodeficiency virus-I infection. Semin Oncol. 1990;17:367-374.

776. Schneider DR, Picker LJ. Myelodysplasia in the acquired immune deficiency syndrome. Am J Clin Pathol. 1985;84: 144-152.

777. Karpatkin S, Nardi M, Lennette ET, et al. Anti HIV-I antibody complexes on platelets of seropositive thrombocytopenic homosexuals and narcotic addicts. Proc Natl Acad Sci U S A. 1988;85:9763-9767.

778. Ratnoff OD, Menitove JE, Aster RH, Ledermann MM. Coincident classic hemophilia andidiopathic thrombocytopenic purpura in patients under treatment with concentrations of AHF. N Engl J Med. 1983;308:439-442.

779. Walsh K, Krigel R, Lennette E, Karpatkin S. Thrombocytopenia in homosexual patients. Prognosis, response to therapy, and prevalence of antibody to the retrovirus associated with the acquired immune deficiency syndrome. Ann Intern Med. 1985;103:542-545.

780. Abrams DI, Kiprov DP, Goedert JJ, et al. Antibodies to HTLV-III and development of AIDS in homosexual men presenting with immune thrombocytopenia. Ann Intern Med. 1986;104:47-50.

781. Rarick M, Loureiro C, et al. IGIV in treatment of HIV-related thrombocytopenia [abstract]. Proc Am Soc Hematol. 1986;72:359a.

782. Oksenhendler E, Bierling P, Brossary Y, et al. Anti Rh immunoglobulin therapy for hjuman immunodeficiency virus–related immune thrombocytopenic purpura. Blood. 1988;71:1499-1502.

783. Hymes KB, Greene J, Karpatkin S. The effect of azidothymidine on HIV-related thrombocytopenia. N Engl J Med. 1988;318:516-517.

784. Zidovudine for the treatment of thrombocytopenia associated with HIV. A prospective study. The Swiss Group for Clinical Studies in AIDS. Ann Intern Med. 1988;109:718-721.

785. Oksenhendler E, Bierling P, Ferchal F, et al. Zidovudine for thrombocytopenic purpura related to HIV infection. Ann Intern Med. 1989;110:365-368.

786. Mayer K. Transfusion of the patient with acquired immunodeficiency syndrome. Arch Pathol Lab Med. 1990;114:295-297.

787. Murphy MF, Metcalfe P, Waters AH, Linch DC. Immune neutropenia in homosexual men [letter]. Lancet. 1985;1:217-218.

788. Zucker-Franklin D, Seremetis S, Zheng ZY. Internalization of human immunodeficiency virus type I and other retroviruses by megakaryocytes and platelets. Blood. 1990;75:1920-1923.

789. Zucker-Franklin D, Cao Y. Megakaryocytes of human immunodeficiency virus–infected individuals express viral RNA. Proc Natl Acad Sci U S A. 1989;86:5595-5599.

790. Pizzo PA. Emerging concepts in the treatment of HIV infection in children. JAMA. 1989;262:1989-1992.

791. Fischl MA. Zidovudine: clinical experience in symptomatic HIV disease. In Voldberdingm P, Jacobson M (eds). AIDS Clinical Review. New York, Marcel Dekker, 1989, p 221.

792. Dalakas MC, Illa I, Pezeshkpour GH, et al. Mitochondrial myopathy caused by long-term zidovudine therapy. N Engl J Med. 1990;322:1089-1105.

793. Bloom EJ, Abrams DI, et al. Lupus anticoagulant in acquired immunodeficiency syndrome [abstract]. Blood. 1984;64:93a.

794. Blanche S, Rouzioux C, Moscato ML, et al. A prospective study of infants born to women seropositive for human immunodeficiency virus type I. HIV Infection in Newborns French Collaborative Study Group. N Engl J Med. 1989;320:1643-1648.

795. Borkowsky W, Krasinski K, Paul D, et al. Human immunodeficiency virus infections in infants negative for anti-HIV by enzyme-linked immunoassay. Lancet. 1987;1:1168-1171.

796. Goetz DW, Hall SE, Harbison RW, Reid MJ. Pediatric acquired immunodeficiency syndrome with negative human immunodeficiency virus antibody response by enzyme-linked immunosorbent assay and Western blot. Pediatrics. 1988;81:356-359.

797. Gaum PJ, Yogen R. The role of protease inhibitor therapy in children with HIV. Pediatr Drugs. 2002;4:581-607.

798. Centers for Disease Control and Prevention (CDC). Classification systems for human immunodeficiency virus (HIV) in children under 13 years of age. MMWR Morbid Mortal Wkly Rep. 1987;36(15):225-230, 235-236.

37 Hematologic Manifestations of Systemic Diseases in Children of the Developing World

David J. Weatherall, Dominic P. Kwiatkowski, and David J. Roberts

Diagnosis and management of hematologic disorders in children in developing countries pose a number of problems that are not encountered in advanced Western societies.[1,2] Although all the conditions that have been described in this book are seen in these populations, their clinical features may be modified to a varying degree by the coexistence of malnutrition, chronic bacterial infection, or parasitic illness. Furthermore, many of the common killers, particularly in tropical climates, produce their own complicated hematologic manifestations.

It therefore follows that the study of hematologic disease in these populations presents a particular challenge to hematologists. It is often very difficult to define the clinical features and pathophysiology of a single hematologic disorder in this setting. Sickle cell anemia is a good example. This disorder, as described in Chapter 19, usually produces a well-defined clinical and hematologic picture in North American or European children. However, the disease may be different in the rural populations of Africa, where its course is generally complicated by diarrheal illness, malnutrition, endemic malaria, and as yet ill-defined climatic effects on the clinical phenotype. It is very difficult to separate the environmental and genetic factors that must underlie the extraordinarily varied severity of this condition in different parts of the world.

The same problems are posed when attempts are made to define the hematologic manifestations of disorders that are peculiar to tropical climates. For example, despite many years of intensive investigation it is still not possible to provide a clear picture of the pathophysiologic cause of the anemia of malaria caused by *Plasmodium falciparum* infection. Although there are many reasons, the major one for those who wish to study this important problem is finding patients with malaria who do not have other diseases that may cloud the clinical picture, such as chronic bacterial infection, human immunodeficiency virus (HIV) infection, malnutrition, hemoglobinopathies, or red cell glucose-6-phosphate dehydrogenase (G6PD) deficiency (see Chapter 17).

Despite these difficulties, in recent years it has been possible to start to understand the pathogenesis of some of the hematologic manifestations of systemic disease in children in the Third World. In this chapter some of the

progress that has been made in this extremely important area of childhood hematology is reviewed.

PREVALENCE AND MULTIPLE CAUSES OF ANEMIA IN THE THIRD WORLD

Numerous surveys have been conducted to determine the prevalence of anemia in tropical populations.[3-6] However, because of differences in methodology and demographic design, it is very difficult to interpret the results and compare one study with another. Representative data from several countries, using the World Health Organization definition of anemia (Table 37-1),[7] are shown in Table 37-2. It is clear that in many populations the prevalence of anemia in preschool children is extremely high, and in some locations almost 100% of the population is affected. Although the data shown in Table 37-2 were compiled more than 20 years ago, the situation does not seem to have improved. In 2002, the World Health Organization reported that 0.8 million (1.5%) deaths worldwide are attributable to iron deficiency, 1.3% of male deaths and 1.8% of female deaths. Attributable disability-adjusted life years (DALYs), the current measure of health burden, is even greater and amounts to the loss of about 35 million healthy life years.[8]

It is equally difficult to determine the relative importance of different causes of anemia in the tropics. Most

TABLE 37-1	World Health Organization Criteria for Hemoglobin Concentrations below Which Anemia Is Considered to Be Present in Populations at Sea Level
Age	**Hemoglobin Concentration (g/dL)**
Children, 6 mo-6 yr	11
Children, 6-14 yr	12
Adult males	13
Adult females (nonpregnant)	12
Adult females (pregnant)	11

From World Health Organization: Nutritional anemias. Report of a WHO group of experts. World Health Organ Tech Rep Ser 1972;503:1-29.

TABLE 37-2	Prevalence (%) of Anemia (World Health Organization Criteria) in Different Populations			
Geographic Area	**Preschool Children**	**Nonpregnant Women**	**Pregnant Women**	**Adult Males**
Latin America (7 countries)	—	17	24	4
Chile	35	—	—	—
Nigeria	63	46	52	36
Northern India	90	84	80	48
Southern India	76	81	88	56
Burma	3-27	5-15	82	1-5
Philippines	42	37	72	7

From Weatherall DJ, Ledingham (eds). The Oxford Textbook of Medicine. Oxford, Oxford University Press, 1987. Copyright © 1987 by D. J. Weatherall, J. G. G. Ledingham, and D. A. Warell, Used by permission of Oxford University Press, Inc.

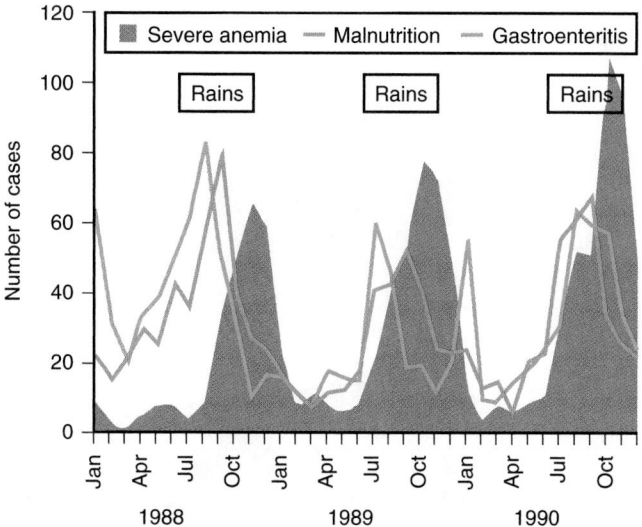

FIGURE 37-1. Admissions to the children's ward of a hospital in Gambia, where malaria transmission is confined to the rainy season. The incidence of severe malarial anemia corresponds to seasonal epidemics of malaria fever and cerebral malaria. Gastroenteritis and malnutrition also reach a peak incidence in the early part of the rainy season and thus contribute to the multifactorial etiology of the anemia. *(Data from Brewster DR, Greenwood BM. Seasonal variation of paediatric diseases in The Gambia, West Africa. Ann Trop Paediatr. 1993;13:133-146.)*

surveys have concentrated on only one mechanism, such as iron or folate deficiency. However, to get a true picture of the cause of anemia in a particular population it is necessary to obtain consecutive data over a substantial period. For example, studies in Gambia have shown that mean hemoglobin levels in children vary significantly at different times of the year; anemia is much more common in the wet season when malaria transmission it at its highest (Fig. 37-1).[5] This is also the time when diarrhea and malnutrition are most common because heavy rains after many dry months have profound effects on the community, sanitation measures are disrupted, and food stores are at a low point in the annual cycle.[9] Although these observations emphasize the multifactorial etiology of anemia, it is clear that iron deficiency, which affects at least 20% of the world's population, is the major factor and that the numerous other diseases that may exacerbate anemia are often operating in the setting of low body iron stores.

Iron deficiency and anemia are less common in groups that have persisted as hunter-gatherers, for example, the Hadza in Tanzania and the pastoralists who eat blood and meat, such as the Masai in Kenya.[2] On the other hand, absorption of nonheme iron, except from breast milk, is comparatively restricted, and the content of iron in breast milk is very low. Therefore, iron deficiency is common in communities whose food is predominantly of vegetable origin.[10] The three great staples in these populations are rice, wheat, and maize. Sorghum and millet are also important in some areas of Africa and Asia. Soy and similar legumes are major sources of protein

in many countries. The iron content of these diets is generally low and absorption is inhibited by fiber, phytates, phosphates, and polyphenols, which are all found at high levels in these largely vegetarian diets.[10] Loss of iron from chronic hemorrhage secondary to hookworm infection or schistosomiasis further contributes to the high incidence of iron deficiency anemia in the developing world.

The infants of mothers with iron deficiency have low iron stores, their folate status at birth reflects that of their mother, and the folate content of breast milk is diminished by maternal deficiency and maternal malaria.[11-13]

In many populations anemia may be associated with folate deficiency.[3,4,13] Again, the reasons are complex and multifactorial. Although intake of folate varies widely among different populations, depending on the way in which food is prepared and the temperature at which it is cooked, it is clear that low intake is not necessarily the result of lack of folate in the diet. Work in Africa suggests that the continuous anorexia associated with recurrent infections such as malaria or tuberculosis is the most important cause of folate deficiency in children.[2] As discussed later, postinfective malabsorption is a particularly common cause of folate deficiency, especially in the Indian subcontinent. Folate deficiency may be exacerbated by erythroid hyperplasia associated with chronic malarial infection or hemoglobinopathy.[14]

Although nutritional vitamin B_{12} deficiency is uncommon, Indian infants born to mothers with sprue (see later) who are fed breast milk or goat milk containing insufficient vitamin B_{12} may be susceptible to megaloblastic anemia with locomotor complications during the early months of life.[2] This syndrome, which is often fatal, appears to be complicated by a marked predisposition to infection.

Although many of the population surveys on the prevalence of anemia in tropical countries have concentrated on one particular cause and intercurrent illness has not been assessed, studies in Africa, in which attempts have been made to assess body iron stores, folate levels, and the presence of intercurrent infection, indicate that chronic recurrent malaria, without other important complicating factors, is the major cause of anemia in these populations.

A major issue is whether iron supplementation is the most effective way to prevent anemia in regions where malaria is highly endemic. For example, a study in Tanzania showed that either iron supplementation or malaria chemoprophylaxis could be used to reduce the incidence of anemia in the first year of life but that the benefits of malaria prophylaxis were outweighed by increased risk for both malaria and anemia after the prophylaxis was stopped, thus suggesting that iron supplementation is the better option.[15] Then again, a reduction in iron levels is part of natural host defense against infection, and there is long-standing debate about whether supplementation has adverse consequences, particularly on mortality from infectious diseases.

Studies with a large sample size are needed to address this issue, and two have recently been published. On Pemba Island, Zanzibar, where malaria is endemic, an initial study found that iron supplementation improved motor and language development,[16] but a subsequent larger study involving 24,000 children found that deaths and hospital admissions were significantly higher in those who received iron and folate supplementation than in those who did not.[17] Although the cause of increased deaths in those receiving supplementation was not precisely defined, malaria appeared to play a major role. In contrast, a study of 25,000 preschool children in southern Nepal found that children who received iron and folic acid had no significant difference in mortality from those who did not, but there was a suggestion of modest protective effects against diarrhea, dysentery, and acute respiratory illness.[18]

Iannotti and colleagues[19] reviewed 26 randomized controlled trials of preventive oral iron supplementation in children younger than 5 years. Their general conclusion is that iron-deficient children may need to be identified to ensure that iron supplementation programs are effectively targeted to improve hemoglobin levels and cognitive and motor development. Although most studies found no effect on morbidity, few had adequate sample size or study design to resolve this issue. The outcome of a supplementation program may depend greatly on the pattern of endemic disease in the population.

HEMATOLOGIC CHANGES ASSOCIATED WITH SPECIFIC INFECTIONS IN THE TROPICS

Malaria

Malaria is the most important parasitic illness of humans.[20] The total burden of disease has recently been estimated to be 515 million episodes annually, and malaria is responsible for 18% of all childhood deaths in sub-Saharan Africa, equivalent to 800,000 deaths each year.[21,22] With increasing drug resistance of the malarial parasite, the problems of both treatment and control are becoming more complex, and this disease remains one of the major unsolved world health problems, although the widespread use of insecticide and bed nets appears to be reducing the incidence of severe malaria in many parts of Africa.

Life Cycle and Species

Because of its peculiar life cycle (Fig. 37-2), the malarial parasite is particularly prone to cause hematologic manifestations. Female anopheline mosquitos, during a blood meal, inject sporozoites that disappear from the circulation after about 1 hour and enter liver parenchymal cells, where they proliferate into thousands of merozoites. The period of development in liver cells varies between species. Merozoites rupture from liver cells, pour into the blood-

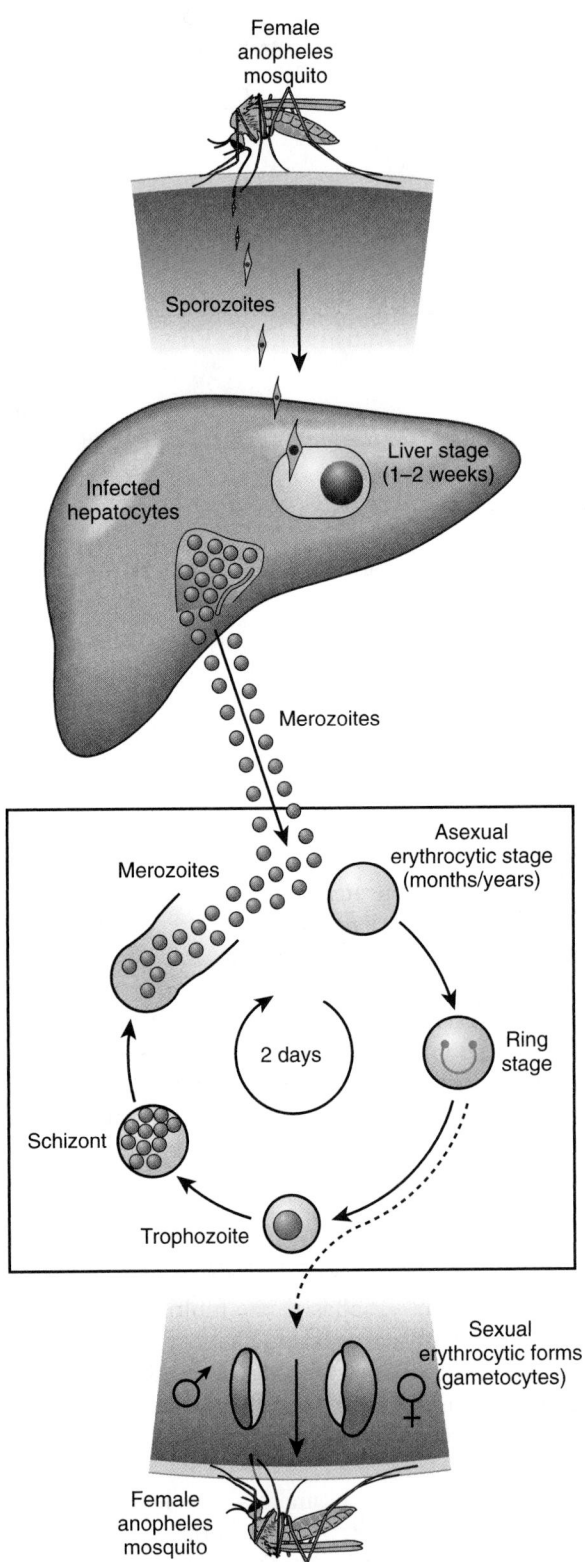

FIGURE 37-2. The life cycle of malarial parasites. The duration of the erythrocyte cycle is 48 hours for all human malaria parasites except *Plasmodium malariae*, which has a 72-hour cycle.

stream, and invade erythrocytes. Further development of the intraerythrocytic parasite follows one of two pathways: asexual differentiation or differentiation into sexual parasites called gametocytes. The latter continue their development within anopheline mosquitos. Asexual parasites develop from young ring forms through trophozoites to dividing forms called schizonts. On rupture of infected erythrocytes, forms called merozoites are released, invade other erythrocytes, and thus continue the erythrocyte cycle. When billions of schizonts rupture simultaneously and release cytokine-inducing toxins, they cause paroxysms of malarial fever.

When a child is infected with malaria for the first time, the result is usually an intermittent febrile illness lasting a few weeks, but complete eradication of malarial parasites from the bloodstream may take months or years. In the phase between cessation of the fever and final resolution of the infection, the child may appear well, but the destruction of red cells continues. From a hematologic viewpoint, the major question is how soon will the child be reinfected, for in some communities reinfection occurs almost every day, and immunity to malaria is slowly acquired and never complete. In regions of high transmission, children eventually acquire the ability to maintain a parasite density below the level that causes fever, but chronic or repeated infections cause a state of chronic anemia.

Four species of *Plasmodium* infect humans—*P. falciparum*, *P. vivax*, *P. ovale*, and *P. malariae*—and a fifth species, *P. knowlesi*, normally restricted to macaque monkeys, has recently been discovered in the human population in Borneo.[23] Each has particular morphologic and biologic properties and clinical manifestations. *P. falciparum* is the predominant cause of clinical malaria in Africa and much of Southeast Asia, whereas *P. vivax* tends to predominate in Central America and the Indian subcontinent, but their distribution overlaps considerably and multiple infections are not uncommon. *P. vivax* is essentially absent in populations of Central and West Africa because their erythrocytes fail to express the Duffy antigen or interleukin-8 (IL-8) receptor, to which the merozoites of this species attach during invasion.[24,25]

Another peculiarity of *P. vivax*, shared also with *P. ovale*, is the ability to form hypnozoites, which can remain dormant in cells for months or years. This ability results in relapsing infections that are often associated with mild chronic anemia. However, profound anemia and other grave complications are almost always seen with *P. falciparum* malaria, and the following sections apply mainly to this particular species.

Severe Malaria

Life-threatening complications are estimated to occur in about 1% of episodes of *P. falciparum* infection in African children, and it has been estimated that a child in rural Africa has a 15% lifetime risk of a malaria infection requiring hospital admission as a result of complications.[26] Such complications include profound anemia, cerebral malaria (a syndrome of unrousable coma, often accompanied by severe convulsions), hypoglycemia, jaundice, renal failure, pulmonary edema, and coagulation abnormalities. There are important and as yet largely unexplained differences in the clinical spectrum of severe

P. falciparum malaria in different parts of the world.[27] In Southeast Asia, all the aforementioned complications are commonly seen, whereas in Africa, where cerebral malaria and severe malarial anemia together account for about 1 million deaths per year and hypoglycemia is also common, the other complications of *P. falciparum* malaria are surprisingly rare. Malarial illness affects mostly children in Africa, whereas adults are more commonly affected in some other parts of the world; it has been suggested that much of the variation in clinical symptomatology is related to age. However, this does not provide a full explanation. Even among African children there are regional differences, and there is a growing impression that higher rates of malarial transmission lead to a greater prevalence of anemia but, paradoxically, a low incidence of cerebral malaria.[28]

The lethality of *P. falciparum* as compared with other species of *Plasmodium* probably stems from two biologic properties. First, the parasite density that it achieves is typically a hundred times higher than that of other species before its growth is curtailed by host defense mechanisms.[29] Second, mature intraerythrocytic forms of *P. falciparum* adhere to the endothelium of postcapillary venules and thus sequester in tissues. Because these properties are common to all strains of *P. falciparum*, the greater puzzle is why lethal complications arise in only a minority of infected individuals. Some important clues have emerged recently. Parasite sequestration is mediated by a parasite-derived molecule known as PfEMP1 that is expressed on the surface of a mature infected erythrocyte and binds to a variety of endothelial adhesion molecules, including CD36, intracellular adhesion molecule 1, E-selectin, and vascular cell adhesion molecule.[30] Whether a parasite will bind to a specific endothelial adhesion molecule is determined by its PfEMP1 type, and this shows an extraordinary degree of phenotypic variability.[31] Expression of endothelial adhesion molecules varies between organs and is regulated by cytokines released by the host in response to the infection, such as tumor necrosis factor (TNF). There is evidence that genetic variation in the host TNF response influences susceptibility to cerebral malaria.[32] Another potentially important pathophysiologic mechanism is vascular sludging, which results from the clumping of parasitized erythrocytes, either with platelets ("autoagglutination" or "clumps") or with unparasitized erythrocytes ("rosettes"). Both phenomena are strain specific and have been associated with the severity of malaria. As usual, the parasite uses diverse adhesive mechanisms; complement receptor-1 is a key binding target for some rosetting parasites,[33] whereas the platelet glycoprotein CD36 and other as yet unknown proteins are used in the formation of autoagglutinates or clumps.[34]

There is an association between salmonellosis and malarial infection.[35] This association goes beyond the growing recognition that a significant proportion of cases of severe malaria in the tropics are bacteremic[36] in that salmonellosis in Africa seems to be specifically associated with malarial anemia.[37] It remains open to speculation whether *Salmonella* infection aggravates malarial anemia, anemia is a marker of chronic malarial infections that favor salmonellosis, or there is some other explanation for this curious and striking relationship.[38]

Malarial Anemia

The pattern of hematologic changes in malaria varies considerably, depending on the type of patient. During an acute attack of *P. falciparum* malaria in a nonimmune person, the hematocrit starts to decrease after 1 or 2 days and continues to decrease for about 1 week after antimalarial treatment.[39,40] Subsequently, there is usually a steady increase in the hematocrit, although it may take several weeks before the hematologic picture is back to normal. The anemia, which is not usually life threatening, is characterized by both hemolysis and an ineffective marrow response,[39,40] features that have also been documented in acute *P. vivax* infection. When profound anemia occurs with acute *P. falciparum* malaria, it is often associated with multiorgan failure, although it can also occur as an isolated complication.

From the perspective of tropical child health, the most important hematologic problem is seen in a child chronically infected with *P. falciparum*, whose anemia is debilitating and sometimes fatal. Although this problem most commonly occurs in areas of high malarial transmission, it is a growing problem in regions of lower transmission because of the increase in resistance to antimalarial drugs, which has served to prolong the average duration of infection. Attempts to investigate the problem of chronic malarial anemia are often hampered by the coexistence of iron or folate deficiency and hemoglobinopathies. In a study in which patients with these conditions were carefully excluded, the most striking pathophysiologic findings were hemolysis, hypersplenism, and a suboptimal bone marrow response.[40] In the sections that follow, some of the mechanisms for these components of the anemia of malaria are discussed in more detail.

Role of Hemolysis

Normal children living in rural Africa typically have extremely low levels of haptoglobin that increase significantly after malaria prevention programs,[40,41] thus providing some indication of the burden of chronic hemolysis that malaria causes in many tropical communities. The mechanisms of red cell destruction in *P. falciparum* malaria are complex and not fully understood.[42] Clearly, erythrocytes are destroyed when schizonts rupture and release their progeny, and depending on the state of immunity, a proportion of the parasitized erythrocytes are destroyed by the host before schizont rupture can take place. Both mechanisms can have devastating consequences if the patient is hyperparasitemic (sometimes more than 50% of erythrocytes are infected), but such patients are rare. In most infections, less than 1% of erythrocytes are infected, a loss that is important in the context of chronic

infection but would not account for the severity of anemia that is commonly observed. Both mathematical modeling and clinical observation suggest that 10 times as many uninfected erythrocytes are removed from the circulation for each infected erythrocyte.[43] Indeed, cross-transfusion experiments clearly indicate that erythrocyte survival is shortened both in the acute phase of malaria and during convalescence.[44,45]

Role of the Spleen

Some degree of splenomegaly is a normal feature of malarial infection, and the prevalence of splenomegaly in regions of malarial transmission is used as a major indicator of the level of malarial endemicity. The importance of the spleen in host defense against malaria has been demonstrated in experimental systems, and individuals whose spleens have been surgically removed are thought to be more susceptible to severe infection (see later). The phenomenon of parasitic sequestration, discussed earlier, is thought to have evolved primarily as an immune evasion strategy whereby the mature parasite can avoid passing through the spleen.[46]

Several studies have attempted to define the pathophysiologic changes in the spleen during acute malaria. In animal models, malaria is accompanied by increased intravascular clearance of infected or rigid heat-treated cells by the spleen,[47] alterations in the splenic microcirculation,[48] and recruitment of myelomonocytes to the spleen and liver.[49] In studies of human malaria it has been found that increased splenic clearance of heated red cells occurs during acute attacks.[50] Reduced deformability of uninfected red cells is observed in *P. falciparum* malaria and is a significant predictor of the severity of anemia, consistent with the notion that these cells are being removed by the spleen[51] (see later). It has also been found that immunoglobulin G (IgG)-sensitized red cells are rapidly removed from the circulation by the spleen and that unusually rapid clearance persists well into the convalescent phase.[52] Undoubtedly, the activity and number of macrophages are increased during human malarial infection, and this may therefore contribute to the increased removal of uninfected cells.[53-55]

In rodent malaria, a model of chronic anemia has been developed in which *Plasmodium berghei*–infected semi-immune mice show a 5- to 10-fold increase in the clearance of uninfected erythrocytes, although the extent of parasitemia remains below 1%.[56] In this study, clearance of uninfected red cells was delayed in mice depleted of macrophages, thus supporting the view that removal of uninfected erythrocytes is an important factor in anemia.

All the available evidence, therefore, points to increased reticuloendothelial clearance in *P. falciparum* malaria that persists long after recovery. These changes are presumably a host defense mechanism to maximize the clearance of parasitized erythrocytes. Clinical studies have also uncovered a curious phenomenon whereby some erythrocytes appear to be returned to the circulation after having had their parasites removed,[57] but killing parasites usually means destroying erythrocytes, and it appears that the survival of uninfected red cells is reduced in the process.

These observations in patients are consistent with findings at the cellular level. Active erythrophagocytosis is a conspicuous feature within the bone marrow during *P. vivax* and *P. falciparum* malaria,[58,59] and it is highly probable that it also occurs within the spleen. Children with acute *P. falciparum* malaria have high circulating levels of interferon-γ and TNF,[60] a synergistic combination of cytokines that activate macrophages.[61] Transgenic mice that constitutively overexpress human TNF are anemic and show enhanced clearance of autologous erythrocytes, which is presumed (though not proved) to be due to erythrophagocytosis.[62] When infected with *Plasmodium yoelii* or *P. berghei*, transgenic mice suppress parasite density much more effectively than their littermates do. This finding supports the notion that with relatively nonspecific effector mechanisms such as erythrophagocytosis within the spleen, anemia is part of the price that the host has to pay for protection against overwhelming parasitemia.

Massive Intravascular Hemolysis

A peculiar example of malaria-associated hemolysis is blackwater fever.[42,63] The classic form of this syndrome, often reported in colonial times among Europeans living in Africa, was characterized by fever and massive intravascular hemolysis associated with low or no parasitemia; it led to renal failure and was associated with high mortality. It was suspected that intermittent quinine ingestion might have led to a drug-induced immune hemolysis, although this mechanism was never proved and recent reports have implicated newer antimalarial drugs such as halofantrine and mefloquine/artemisinin combinations.[64,65] Classic blackwater fever is now much less common, but it is important to remember that massive intravascular hemolysis with hemoglobinuria remains an important complication of *P. falciparum* malaria in Southeast Asia in both children and adults.[39] Blackwater fever is sometimes associated with high parasitemia or destruction of G6PD-deficient red cells by oxidant antimalarial drugs. A survey of cases in Vietnam found considerable overlap of quinine ingestion, G6PD deficiency, and concurrent malaria, thus suggesting that these different factors may interact but certainly do not all have to be present for blackwater fever to occur.[66] It is conceivable that hemolysis is caused by the rupture of a large number of sequestered parasites, but the possibility of another hemolytic process has yet to be ruled out.

Decreased Erythrocyte Deformability

The increased clearance of uninfected erythrocytes is due not only to the activation of splenic macrophages but also to extrinsic and intrinsic factors that enhance their recognition and phagocytosis. Uninfected erythrocytes have reduced deformability, which leads to enhanced clear-

ance in the spleen. The mechanism responsible for the loss of deformability is not completely understood, however. Increased oxidation of membranes in uninfected erythrocytes has been demonstrated in children with severe *P. falciparum* malaria, and the ongoing inflammatory insults associated with acute malaria (proinflammatory cytokines) or the direct effects of parasite products have been shown to cause loss of red cell deformability.[54,67,68] Intriguingly, a severe reduction in red cell deformability measured on admission is also a strong predictor not just for anemia but also for mortality, both in adults and children with severe malaria.[51,69]

Immune Complex–Mediated Hemolysis

It is also possible that at least part of the hemolysis in *P. falciparum* malaria might have an immune basis. A positive direct Coombs antiglobulin test (DAT) is seen in some patients with malaria.[40,70-76] Like all studies on malaria, there seem to be considerable differences in the incidence of positive DAT results in malarial infection in different populations and at different ages. For example, in Thai children or adults during their first attack or with subsequent attacks in those who live in areas where a degree of immunity has not developed, DAT results are invariably negative.[75] Furthermore, studies using labeled immunoglobulin have shown that the number of antibodies bound to the red cells of patients with malaria of this type is no different from that in uninfected control patients of the same age and in the same location.[75]

The position is different in African children who have suffered repeated attacks of malaria. Positive DAT results have been found in up to 50% of these children, and the incidence is significantly higher in children with active malarial infection than in those who are not infected.[71-74,76] The phenomenon is age related and is more common in young children. DAT results may remain positive for several weeks after an acute infection. With specific antisera it has been found that the most common type of red cell sensitization occurs with C3; other specificities include IgG alone, IgG plus C3, IgG plus C3 and C4, and various other combinations of IgG with complement components.[71-75] The IgG that can be eluted from these cells has specific activity against *P. falciparum* schizont antigen.[71] This suggests that the erythrocyte coating results from passive attachment of circulating complement-fixing malarial antigen-antibody complexes. It is therefore likely that the development of positive DAT results is part of the immune response to *P. falciparum*.

Recent studies have suggested that the *P. falciparum* ring surface protein 2 (RSP-2) may be one component of the immunoglobulin-antigen complexes deposited on uninfected erythrocytes. This protein is expressed on infected erythrocytes shortly after merozoite invasion and may mediate some adhesion of infected erythrocytes to endothelial cells. RSP-2 is also deposited on uninfected erythrocytes and forms immune complexes that contribute to the phagocytosis of uninfected erythrocytes. Limited clinical studies have shown that high levels of anti–RSP-2 antibodies are found in the sera of immune adults and children with severe anemia.[77] This antigen is also present on the surface of erythroblasts in the bone marrow of *P. falciparum*–infected patients, thus indicating that clearance or damage to developing erythroid cells by RSP-2 and anti–RSP-2 could contribute to the development of anemia.

However, it is far from clear whether the presence of positive DAT results indicates that immune destruction of red cells occurs in African children with malaria. Several studies have shown that there is no correlation between the degree of anemia and positive DAT results,[75,76] and other measured parameters of hemolysis have not correlated with coating of red cells. Nonetheless, immune destruction may occasionally be of importance. A small number of patients have been described with severe anemia and positive DAT results who had active C3 components on their red cells.[72] In these patients, striking monocyte erythrophagocytosis of nonparasitized erythrocytes was seen.

In some patients with *P. falciparum* infection, IgM antibodies have been reported to develop against triose-phosphate isomerase, and disappearance of the antibodies coincides with disappearance of the hemolysis. Because these antibodies can induce erythrocyte lysis and complement activation in vitro, it has been postulated that they may contribute to a hemolytic process in vivo.[78]

In short, there is little evidence for immune destruction of red cells in *P. falciparum* malarial infections in nonimmune adults. Although a varying proportion of children with chronic malaria in Africa have positive DAT results, only occasionally is evidence of genuine immune destruction of red cells seen. It is possible, of course, that a sensitized red cell population is very rapidly destroyed and subsequent serologic studies have missed this event. However, the persistence of shortened red cell survival of nonparasitized cells in the absence of any consistent serologic abnormalities suggests that there must be another factor involved in the shortened red cell survival in malaria. This factor appears to be nonspecific "overactivity" of the monocyte/macrophage populations of the spleen and liver, as discussed earlier.

Defective Marrow Response

In addition to the hemolytic components of the anemia of *P. falciparum* malaria, there is undoubtedly an inappropriate marrow response.[39,40,42,79,80] That the reticulocytosis in response to the decrease in hematocrit is often inappropriately low and delayed has been noted for many years (Fig. 37-3). It remains unclear whether defective erythropoietin production is a significant cause, with some studies suggesting an appropriate rise[81] or even enhanced response[80] and others observing a blunted response,[82,83] but there is no question that significant dysfunction of marrow takes place and appears to have a complex multifactorial basis.

Some of the features of iron metabolism and bone marrow morphology and function in acute malaria resemble those of other acute infections. Thus, the serum iron level rapidly decreases and iron appears to be sequestrated into the storage compartments of the marrow.[39,40] Serum ferritin levels are extremely high during the acute phase, although studies of isoferritins suggest a complex source; in many instances it appears that much of the ferritin is released as a consequence of liver damage.[39]

During acute malarial infections there may be marked dyserythropoietic changes in the bone marrow.[39,40] Although changes are most marked in African children with chronic relapsing malaria,[40] they have also been observed in nonimmune Thais[39] and in travelers returning to the United Kingdom.[42] These morphologic abnor-

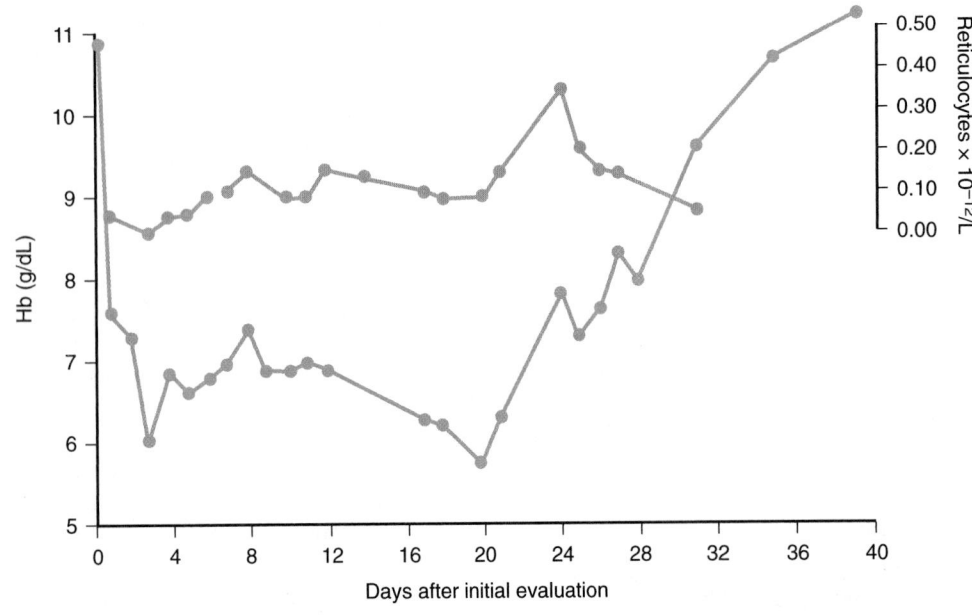

FIGURE 37-3. Hemoglobin level and reticulocyte response in a non-immune patient with *Plasmodium falciparum* malaria.

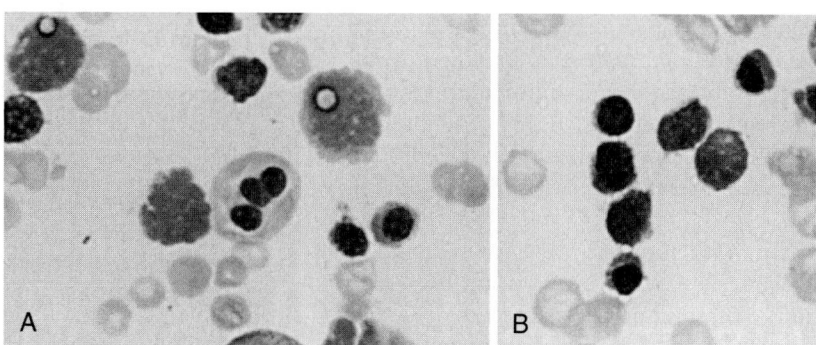

FIGURE 37-4. Bone marrow in *Plasmodium falciparum* malaria. **A**, Multinucleate red cell precursors. **B**, Intercytoplasmic bridging (Leishman stain, magnification ×500).

malities, which have been studied by both light and electron microscopy, consist of erythroblast multinuclearity, karyorrhexis, incomplete and unequal amitotic nuclear divisions, and cytoplasmic bridging (Fig. 37-4).[40] On electron microscopic examination, binucleate or multinucleate erythroblasts, bizarre myelination with loss of parts of the nuclear membrane, and widening of the space between the two layers of the nuclear membrane have been observed.[40,59] There appears to be some degree of iron loading of the mitochondria and a reduction in electron density of the cytoplasmic matrix, together with a paucity of ribosomes. In addition, in acute infection there is widespread sequestration of erythrocytes in the sinuses of the bone marrow.[59]

With [³H]thymidine autoradiography and Feulgen microspectrophotometry it is clear that a significant abnormality of red cell proliferation in the bone marrow occurs in acute malaria. Changes include an increased proportion of red cell precursors in the G_2 phase and arrest in progress of cells in the S phase. These findings are nonspecific and have been observed in other conditions associated with ineffective erythropoiesis.[79]

In addition to these dyserythropoietic changes, erythrophagocytosis is particularly common in the bone marrow in *P. falciparum* malaria.[40] This phenomenon is not restricted to the marrow and may be seen in the spleen and other organs and, as mentioned earlier, may play a role in the hemolytic component of the disease.

Although the mechanism of these dyserythropoietic changes is unknown, it is possible that they are an exaggerated example of the bone marrow suppression that occurs in other situations of chronic infection. An important factor may be the high levels of TNF production that occur during malarial infection because this cytokine has been strongly implicated in the anemia of chronic infection and severe malarial anemia has been associated with certain TNF promoter polymorphisms.[84] TNF suppresses the proliferation of erythroid progenitor cells in human marrow culture, although the effect declines as the cells differentiate.[85] On the other hand, TNF stimulates fibroblasts to secrete growth factors for colony-forming unit (CFU)–granulocyte-erythrocyte-monocyte-macrophage and burst-forming unit–erythrocyte (BFU-E).[86] In nude mice implanted with transfected Chinese hamster ovary cells that can constitutively express the human TNF

gene, erythropoiesis is preferentially suppressed, with a marked reduction of CFU-E and BFU-E in the marrow and spleen.[87] Chronic malaria has specific features that might augment these effects because huge numbers of pigment particles are ingested by the resident macrophages of the spleen and marrow, thereby providing a sustained stimulus for TNF production at the site of erythropoiesis.[88] Furthermore, experimental findings in mice are consistent with a role for TNF in the dyserythropoietic changes of malaria.[89]

Other cytokines have also been implicated. IL-10 is an anti-inflammatory cytokine that inhibits TNF, and two clinical studies in African children with severe malarial anemia have found a low ratio of IL-10 to TNF in plasma, thus leading the investigators to propose that defective IL-10 production may pave the way to marrow suppression by TNF.[90,91] IL-12 protects against severe anemia in experimental murine malaria,[92] which might reflect both its antiparasitic actions and effects on erythropoiesis.[93]

Several studies have suggested that a parasite byproduct of hemoglobin digestion, hemozoin, may have an indirect or direct role in impaired erythroid development.[80] Hemozoin stimulates the secretion of biologically active endoperoxides from monocytes, such as 15(*S*)-hydroxyeicosatetraenoic acid (HETE) and hydroxynonenal (HNE), via oxidation of membrane lipids,[94,95] which may affect erythroid growth.[96]

Hemozoin and TNF-α also have additive effects on erythropoiesis in vitro, and in a clinical study hemozoin-containing macrophages and plasma hemozoin were associated with anemia and reticulocyte suppression.[80] Moreover, bone marrow sections from children who died with severe malaria show a significant association between the quantity of hemozoin (located in erythroid precursors and macrophages) and the proportion of erythroid cells that were abnormal. These findings are consistent with a direct inhibitory effect of hemozoin on erythropoiesis.

Coagulation Abnormalities

Modest thrombocytopenia is not uncommon during acute *P. falciparum* attacks, and occasionally the platelet count decreases to as low as 10,000 to 20,000/mL.[39] The mechanisms have not been determined but probably involve platelet activation and adhesion of infected erythrocytes to platelets, and experimental studies in mice suggest that platelets sequester in venules during malarial infection.[97] Adherence of platelets to epithelium appears to be mediated through a specific receptor-ligand interaction involving lymphocyte function antigen-1. There is also evidence to indicate reduced thrombopoiesis during acute infection.

In some patients with severe *P. falciparum* malaria, a severe bleeding diathesis may develop during the acute phase of the illness. Although it has been suggested that the diathesis results from disseminated intravascular coagulation, studies in Thailand have not substantiated this supposition.[39] Rather, the bleeding appears to reflect gross thrombocytopenia together with liver damage. However, it is becoming apparent that approximately 10% of African children with severe malaria also have bacteremia,[36] so when disseminated intravascular coagulation occurs, the etiology may be complex.

Malaria in Pregnancy

In endemic regions, malaria in pregnancy is extremely common. The placenta provides a favorable environment for parasite replication, and specific pathways of adhesion of infected erythrocytes to the surface of syncytiotrophoblasts have now been unraveled. A specific variant antigen, PfEMP1, expressed on the surface of infected erythrocytes (varCSA-2), mediates adhesion of infected erythrocytes to chondroitin sulfate. Primigravidae are particularly susceptible to malarial infection and may become systemically unwell, but immunity to this variant antigen modulates the duration and severity of infection in subsequent confinements. These observations suggest that varCSA-2 may be an excellent candidate antigen for a pregnancy-specific malaria vaccine. Apart from effects on the mother, it is an important cause of low birth weight and increased perinatal mortality. Studies of cord hemoglobin levels indicate that it is also a significant cause of fetal anemia. Because the severity of the fetal anemia is out of proportion to the degree of maternal anemia, it has been suggested that intrauterine hemolysis may be involved.[98] Malaria in pregnancy is a preventable illness, although it has become more difficult to control with the rise of resistance to antimalarial drugs. Studies in different parts of Africa have found placental malaria to be an important risk factor for anemia in the first 6 months of life.[99,100]

Given the high prevalence of malaria in pregnancy and the strong association of placental malaria with infantile anemia, it is surprising how few infants have overt symptoms of congenital malaria in the tropics. On the rare occasions when it does occur, it can result in a perplexing hematologic disorder. The manifestations of malaria may not be seen until several months after birth, presumably because of passive immunization from the mother and possibly the fact that *P. falciparum* tends to grow less effectively in cells containing relatively large amounts of fetal hemoglobin. The disease is characterized by a febrile illness associated with anemia that may

often be profound.[98] As in conventionally acquired malaria, the pathophysiologic course of the anemia is a complex combination of hemolysis and marrow suppression. Thus, it is important to obtain a careful travel history from the parents of any infant with unexplained hemolysis. This condition is commonly misdiagnosed because it is not considered.

Malaria in Splenectomized Patients

Although it is generally believed that malaria may be associated with particularly severe infections in individuals who have been splenectomized, in a review[101] of this important question no clear evidence was found. Until this problem is resolved, it is wise to advise visitors to the tropics who have had their spleens removed and splenectomized patients who live in regions where malaria is endemic to be particularly careful about continuing to maintain malaria prophylaxis.

Hyperreactive Malarial Splenomegaly Syndrome

Although splenomegaly is a feature of many tropical disorders, there is increasing evidence, particularly from work in East and West Africa and Papua New Guinea, that a specific entity, formerly known as tropical splenomegaly syndrome, occurs widely throughout Africa, India, and Southeast Asia.[1,102,103] This condition is characterized by gross splenomegaly, high malarial antibody titer, and serum IgM levels at least 2 SD above the local mean. The classic syndrome regresses after prolonged antimalarial prophylaxis with proguanil, a dihydrofolate reductase inhibitor marketed outside the United States as Paludrine.

Etiology and Pathophysiology

Evidence that malaria plays an important role in this syndrome is increasing. Epidemiologic studies indicate that its prevalence is related to patterns of malarial transmission and that affected individuals have higher malarial antibody titer than do those who live in the same environment and are unaffected; this seems to involve IgM rather than IgG. These observations, together with the partial clinical response to treatment with antimalarial drugs and the fact that individuals with sickle cell trait seem to be partially protected, suggest that the condition probably results from an unusual form of immune response to chronic malarial infection. For this reason it is now commonly referred to as hyperreactive malarial splenomegaly (HMS).

With progressive splenomegaly, there is pooling of the formed elements of blood; in patients with particularly large spleens, a third to half of the total circulating red cell mass may be sequestered. Such sequestration produces a dilutional anemia that is made worse by an absolute increase in plasma volume. There is also pooling of neutrophils and platelets, so the hematologic picture is characterized by pancytopenia. No characteristic changes in bone marrow are seen.

Some evidence of a genetic predisposition to HMS exists.[104] A recent study in Ghana found that splenomegaly, high IgM levels, and anemia were more common in relatives of HMS patients than in the general population, but there was no clear pattern of mendelian segregation, thus suggesting that the etiology in this population is likely to be complex and involve multiple genetic and environmental factors.[105] For some years researchers have debated about whether HMS is premalignant because it sometimes becomes refractory to antimalarial treatment, and it can also be associated with a lymphocytosis resembling chronic lymphocytic leukemia (CLL). Clonal rearrangements of the J_H region of the immunoglobulin gene have been noted in some patients whose clinical syndrome appears to be intermediate between HMS and CLL, thus suggesting that HMS has premalignant potential.[106]

Clinical Features

The clinical picture of HMS is typical and consists of massive splenomegaly, weight loss, and a variable degree of anemia.[102,103] Serum IgM levels are high, and a relative increase in T lymphocytes in peripheral blood may be seen. Serum may also show increased cold agglutinin titers and an increase in rheumatoid factor, antibodies to thyroglobulin and antinuclear factor, and circulating immune complexes.

The prognosis for patients with this condition is remarkably poor in parts of Africa, with up to 50% mortality in some populations. It is managed by long-term antimalarial prophylaxis, most commonly with proguanil.

Visceral Leishmaniasis (Kala-azar)

Leishmaniasis is an infection caused by intracellular protozoan parasites transmitted by various species of sandflies.[107,108] Human infections can result in three main forms of disease: cutaneous, mucocutaneous, and visceral (kala-azar). The important hematologic manifestations of leishmanial infection are found in the visceral forms.

The generalized form of leishmanial disease involves the liver, spleen, bone marrow, and lymph nodes and is caused by organisms belonging to the *Leishmania donovani* complex. The parent species, *L. donovani*, is found throughout Asia and Africa and can affect individuals of all ages. However, the parasite that causes kala-azar in countries bordering the Mediterranean, in southern Europe, and in North Africa affects primarily young children and infants. It differs from *L. donovani* to such an extent that it warrants the designation of a special species and is called *Leishmania infantum*. Similarly, in the Western Hemisphere, kala-azar is also a disease of very young children; the causative organism is *Leishmania chagasi*.

Although visceral leishmaniasis is primarily a disease of indigenous populations, it may be contracted on short-term visits. For example, in the United Kingdom it is being recognized increasingly after return from Mediterranean holidays, and particularly in young children, it can cause considerable diagnostic difficulty; occurrences have been mislabeled as leukemia when the diagnosis of leishmaniasis was not considered. The risk for leishmaniasis is greatly increased in individuals infected with HIV.[109]

Although the incubation period is usually 1 to 3 months, it can be as short as a few weeks. The onset is usually insidious and consists of fever, sweating, malaise, and anorexia, although a much more acute onset may be seen. As the disease progresses, the acute symptoms abate, but there is gradual enlargement of the spleen and liver for several months. By this time there may be marked splenomegaly, cachexia, and anorexia. Generalized lymphadenopathy is also present.

Hematologic findings in later stages of the illness include anemia, neutropenia, and thrombocytopenia, manifestations characteristic of hypersplenism. The bone marrow is hyperplastic with dyserythropoietic changes, and the diagnosis can usually be made by finding Leishman-Donovan bodies—macrophages containing intracellular organisms with characteristic staining properties. The diagnosis can also be made by splenic or lymph node puncture.

Red cell survival studies and ferrokinetic analyses have suggested that hemolysis is the major cause of anemia in leishmaniasis[110-112] but that there may also be plasma volume expansion associated with the massively enlarged spleen.[112] Surprisingly, ferrokinetic studies have shown very little evidence of ineffective erythropoiesis, but a reduced plasma iron level in the presence of greatly increased iron stores suggests that the reticuloendothelial hyperplasia is accompanied by abnormal iron retention by macrophages, typical of the anemia of chronic disorders.[112] This may limit the marrow response to hemolysis.

In babies or young children with acute visceral leishmaniasis, the clinical and hematologic findings may differ from those described earlier. For example, in Mediterranean populations a very rapid onset of anemia with severe hemolysis is commonly observed.[113] Occasionally, both IgG and complement components are found on the red cells, but this finding is not consistent and its significance remains to be determined. In most instances there is no evidence of immune hemolysis, and it appears that nonsensitized red cells are destroyed by macrophages recruited to the spleen and liver as part of the inflammatory response to the parasite. Severe neutropenia may also occur in young children, and this, together with dyserythropoietic changes in the marrow, marked erythrophagocytosis, and bizarre mononuclear infiltrates, may cause confusion with leukemia.

Schistosomiasis

The schistosomes are a group of trematodes that cause major health problems in many parts of the developing world.[114] The major human parasites include *Schistosoma haematobium*, *Schistosoma mansoni*, and *Schistosoma japonicum*. Schistosomiasis affects mainly children and young adults. Two hundred million people worldwide are estimated to have schistosomiasis, 80% in sub-Saharan Africa.[115]

The location of adult worms in the human host varies with the parasite species: *S. hematobium* in the veins of the bladder, *S. mansoni* in the superior mesenteric veins, and *S. japonicum* in the inferior mesenteric veins. Sexual maturity of female schistosomes depends on their interaction with living male worms. Egg deposition occurs in the small venules of the bladder or portal venous system. When freshly deposited, the ova are partially developed. Hatching of the eggs leads to the liberation of miracidia. Further development occurs when miracidia penetrate a snail intermediate host. After two generations, cercariae are released that are capable of penetrating intact skin and migrating through tissues to reach their final home.

S. haematobium infections occur in Africa and the Middle East, whereas *S. mansoni* is found in Africa, the Middle East, and parts of South America. *S. japonicum* occurs in Japan, the Philippines, and together with the related species *Schistosoma mekongi*, in mainland Indochina.

The most consistent hematologic changes are found in association with *S. mansoni* infection. The acute phase is characterized by fever, myalgia, and progressive hepatosplenomegaly. At this time the most common finding in peripheral blood is eosinophilia. As the disease progresses, there may be massive hepatosplenomegaly associated with anemia, neutropenia, and thrombocytopenia.[116] Good descriptions of the appearance of bone marrow in this condition are few, and the data available suggest that the anemia is predominantly due to hypersplenism and hemodilution from the massive splenomegaly.

S. haematobium infection leads to urinary tract symptoms, in particular, hematuria and dysuria. The hematuria may be gross and persistent and lead to iron deficiency anemia. In addition, affected children have typical features of the anemia of chronic disorders.

A major advance in control of schistosomiasis is the availability of a highly effective drug, praziquantel, which is safe in both children and pregnant women. The cost of control programs may be reduced by combination therapy for schistosomiasis, gastrointestinal helminths, and filariasis; in 2001 the World Health Assembly resolved that at least 75% of school-aged children in high-burden areas should be treated for schistosomiasis and soil-transmitted helminth infections by 2010 to reduce morbidity.[115]

Trypanosomiasis

Trypanosomal infections are a major cause of ill health throughout the world. The disease syndromes produced by these infections vary widely but, in general, are divided into the American and African forms.[117-119]

American Trypanosomiasis (Chagas' Disease)

American trypanosomiasis is a zoonosis caused by *Trypanosoma cruzi*, which is transmitted to humans by blood-sucking insects. It was first described by Carlos Chagas in 1909.

In its invertebrate host, *T. cruzi* grows extracellularly. Epimastigotes divide in the insect gut and differentiate into metacyclic trypomastigotes, which are the infective form for mammalian hosts. They are released close to the site of a bite and enter the host via the skin or mucous membranes. After invasion they enter cells, where they replicate as rounded amastigote forms that differentiate into trypomastigotes, which are released into the circulation and tissues. A variety of organs are involved, but the most important pathophysiologic result is a chronic cardiomyopathy.

There are characteristic clinical findings at each of these different stages of infection. After penetration of the skin, a local cutaneous lesion called an inoculation chagoma develops and is accompanied by swelling of the local lymph glands. Occasionally, the route of inoculation is through the eye, where the initial lesion is characterized by unilateral conjunctivitis with edema of the eyelids. Invasion may or may not be followed by an acute phase consisting of fever, generalized lymphadenopathy, hepatosplenomegaly, and acute myocarditis.

The chronic phase of Chagas' disease takes several forms. If cardiac involvement is predominant, a slowly progressive cardiomyopathy with heart failure, arrhythmias, and embolic complications is seen. In other patients, gastrointestinal symptoms predominate as a result of denervation and destruction of the myenteric plexus, which may give rise to megaesophagus or megacolon.

A congenital form of Chagas' disease may occur. The organism can traverse the placental villi and from there be released into the fetal circulation. The most common findings include growth retardation; hepatosplenomegaly; acute myocarditis; neurologic lesions, including a meningoencephalitic picture with tremors and convulsions; and occasionally, a generalized hemorrhagic tendency with purpura or more widespread bleeding. The prognosis for patients with congenital Chagas' disease is poor, and most infants die during the first week of life.

The hematologic changes in Chagas' disease are nonspecific. In the acute phase, mild anemia and lymphocytosis may occur. At this stage the parasite can be found in the blood or in leukocyte concentrates. Parasites may be concentrated by sedimentation of heparinized blood cells with the addition of phytohemagglutinin. Similarly, it is possible to find amastigote forms of *T. cruzi* in muscle or lymph node biopsy samples. The results of serologic tests for anti–*T. cruzi* IgM antibodies typically become positive about 20 to 40 days after the onset of symptoms.

African Trypanosomiasis

In Africa these conditions are caused by subspecies of the hemoflagellate *Trypanosoma brucei* known as *T. brucei gambiense*, which causes a chronic illness called sleeping sickness, and *T. brucei rhodesiense*, which is associated with a more acute illness. *T. brucei* is transmitted by the tsetse fly *Glossina*, in which it undergoes a variety of developmental changes.

At the site of the tsetse bite a small nodule called a trypanosomal chancre forms from which organisms may be isolated. After this self-limited lesion subsides, the parasite invades and multiplies extracellularly in the blood, which leads to the systemic phase of the illness characterized by fever, lymphadenopathy, and splenomegaly. In the later phase of African trypanosomiasis, invasion of the central nervous system takes place and results in meningoencephalitis.

During the acute phase, normochromic normocytic anemia associated with hypoalbuminemia may be present. Occasionally, patients have hemorrhagic manifestations and evidence of disseminated intravascular coagulation. The total white blood cell count is either normal or elevated with relative lymphocytosis. The sedimentation rate is markedly elevated, and circulating immune complexes may be present together with rheumatoid factor.

The parasite can often be demonstrated in thin or thick blood films stained with Giemsa or Field stain. Several concentration techniques have been developed to increase the likelihood of finding the parasite. A variety of immunodiagnostic tests are available, notably indirect immunofluorescence and enzyme-linked immunosorbent assay, but visualization of the parasite is necessary for a confident diagnosis. In the more chronic stage, it is important to examine cerebrospinal fluid, which often shows lymphocytosis, an elevated protein level, and the presence of morular cells of Mott or motile trypanosomes. High levels of IgM in cerebrospinal fluid may suggest the diagnosis in advanced disease if trypanosomes have not been found.

A novel test for African trypanosomiasis involves analysis of serum samples by mass spectrometry to detect distinct proteomic signatures; this test appears to provide more sensitive and specific detection than other diagnostic tests.[120]

Hookworm

It has been estimated that more than 900 million people are infected with hookworms.[121] There are two main species, *Ancylostoma duodenale* and *Necator americanus*, sometimes called the Old World and the New World hookworms, respectively. Both species are widely distributed in tropical and subtropical Asia and Africa. The prevalence of infection ranges from 80% to 90% in rural areas in the moist parts of the tropics, such as west Bengal, to 10% to 20% in relatively dry countries, such as those of the Middle East and Pakistan.

Both species of hookworm produce enormous numbers of eggs—approximately 20,000 per day per female. The eggs are discharged into the intestinal lumen, where they undergo a number of cell divisions before being passed in stool. Given appropriate conditions, the eggs develop further and hatch, with liberation of larvae. These free-living stages go through a series of developments designated L1 to L3, after which they penetrate the skin and the infective filarial larval forms migrate to the intestinal tract via the circulation, lungs, and respiratory tract. The final larval stage, L4, and the adult worms are found in the small intestine.

Hookworms attach to the mucosa of the upper intestine by their buccal capsules. Although they are found mainly in the jejunum, in very heavy infections they may be distributed as low as the ileum. Attachment of the worm results in bleeding into the gastrointestinal tract.

The worms change their attachment site every few hours. Continuous or intermittent suction causes tissue and blood to be drawn into the worm's intestinal tract.[122] Only about 50% of the iron lost as hemoglobin into the gut may be reabsorbed. Therefore, there is a marked increase in fecal iron concentration that is related directly to the worm load, which can be assessed by the fecal egg count. Direct recordings of blood loss have given values on the order of 0.03 mL/day per worm for *N. americanus* and up to 0.26 mL/day per worm for *A. duodenale*,[122] and the latter species tends to cause more profound levels of iron deficiency in the community.[123]

The hematologic findings in children or adults with heavy hookworm infections are characteristic. Because the condition is usually chronic, anemia is the major clinical feature. In severe cases, hemoglobin values of 2 to 5 g/dL are common.[124] The blood film shows the typical changes of iron deficiency anemia, such as microcytosis, hypochromia, and a normal reticulocyte count. The serum iron level is low, and iron is absent from bone marrow stores. Because of associated protein loss, these children often have hypoalbuminemia.[124-127] Mild eosinophilia may be present[124] in patients with established illness, although very high eosinophil counts may occur during the phase of the illness in which the worms are migrating from the skin to the gastrointestinal tract (see later).

The diagnosis is made by analysis of stool for eggs. In heavy infections, a fecal film can be examined directly after the sample is mounted in saline or iodine solution. In lighter infections, concentration by zinc sulfate flotation is required.

Affected children require oral iron treatment to restore the iron stores, as well as treatment with anthelmintic drugs. Although many of these children are severely anemic, they have had chronic anemia for many years, and rapid restoration of the hemoglobin level is not usually required. However, in profoundly anemic children with high-output failure and associated hypoalbuminemia, it may be necessary to administer red cells slowly, together with appropriate diuretics. These children may have greatly increased blood volume, and it is easy to precipitate circulatory overload and cardiac failure. For patients with severe heart failure, an exchange transfusion consisting of removal of blood from one arm while infusing red cells into the other may be helpful. Whatever method is chosen, monitoring of the patient's central venous pressure is essential.

In recent years a growing number of tropical countries have made concerted efforts to reduce the effects of hookworm infection by anthelmintic strategies in the community. For example, mass administration of mebendazole to 30,000 schoolchildren in Zanzibar was estimated to prevent 1260 cases of moderate to severe anemia and 276 cases of severe anemia in 1 year, although it appeared that at least two doses per year would be necessary to maintain this level of protection, thus raising the issue of long-term sustainability.[128]

Bartonellosis

Bartonellosis (Carrión's disease, Oroya fever) is an infectious disease that is endemic in the western Andes of Peru and is seen occasionally in Colombia and Ecuador.[129] It results from infection by an aerobic, gram-negative bacillus, *Bartonella bacilliformis*. It is usually transmitted through a sandfly bite. After inoculation, the organism multiplies in endothelial and red blood cells. In severe disease, almost 100% of red cells are infected with numerous bacteria. Hence the major feature of the disease is profound anemia resulting from the infection and subsequent phagocytosis of red cells. Although the precise mechanisms of the anemia are not fully understood, it seems to have many of the features of anemia of acute malarial infection. Survival of infected and noninfected red cells is shortened, and a limited response to the hemolysis associated with dyserythropoietic changes in the bone marrow is seen.

The disease has two stages, anemic and eruptive, with an asymptomatic period between the stages. After an incubation period of approximately 60 days, the onset of the condition is acute and consists of malaise, chills, fever, and headache. The clinical picture is then dominated by severe hemolytic anemia associated with hepatosplenomegaly, lymphadenopathy, and occasionally a fine petechial rash. In the later eruptive stage, nodule lesions of varying size appear on the face, trunk, and limbs. Arthralgia and fever may also be present. The lesions, which are widespread on the arms and legs, may be confused with leprosy, yaws, or even Kaposi's sarcoma. Although the infection is often present for a prolonged period, the eruptive phase tends to regress spontaneously.

During the anemic stage, moderate to severe hemolytic anemia is seen with reticulocyte counts in the 5% to 10% range. The organisms can be seen on thick and thin blood films stained with Giemsa, Wright, or related stains. The bone marrow is hyperactive with dyserythropoietic changes. The white blood cell count is not usually elevated, but thrombocytopenia is common.

The principal complication of this disease, apart from profound anemia, is superinfection with other organisms, particularly *Salmonella typhi* and *Mycobacterium tuberculosis*. Fortunately, *B. bacilliformis* is extremely sensitive to chloramphenicol, penicillin, and tetracyclines. Supportive treatment includes regular transfusion through the anemic phase of the illness.

Complex Hematology of Childhood Human Immunodeficiency Virus Infection in the Developing Countries

The devastating impact of perinatally acquired HIV infection in an increasing number of developing countries is mirrored by the complexity of the hematologic complications of this disease in these populations. In some central African countries, seroprevalence rates in pregnant mothers in 1990 ranged from 20% to 30%, and in several others they exceeded 10%.[130] In India and Southeast Asia, the figures are presently much lower than this but are rapidly rising. Perinatal transmission rates have been difficult to establish with certainty but seem to be considerably higher than in the West. In 1989, an estimated figure in Zaire was 39%.[131] Although some children are infected through breast-feeding, the current consensus is that the benefits of breast-feeding probably outweigh the risk in countries where infectious diseases are the major cause of infant mortality.

The clinical picture of childhood HIV infection in the tropics does not differ greatly from that seen elsewhere, except that protein-energy malnutrition occurs much earlier. Tuberculosis and measles, both major causes of mortality by themselves, are more severe in HIV-infected children, but surprisingly, the severity of malaria does not seem to be affected. In Malawi, it is estimated that approximately half of perinatally infected infants die in the first year of life,[132] a considerably earlier mortality than seen in the West.[133]

HIV infection provides yet another example of the complex pathogenesis of hematologic problems in the tropics. The virus can infect hematopoietic precursors,[134,135] as well as bone marrow macrophages and stromal fibroblasts, an observation that may explain the marked dyserythropoiesis that is commonly observed in the bone marrow of affected children, but these changes may also be complicated by opportunistic infection, malnutrition, and drug toxicity. Anemia with a low reticulocyte count and a microcytic hypochromic blood picture is common and may reflect both coexistent iron deficiency and the anemia of chronic disorders.[133,136,137] HIV may cause immune thrombocytopenia early in the course of the disease, but this is not regarded as an adverse prognostic feature. Thrombocytopenia may also be accompanied by microangiopathic hemolytic anemia as part of thrombotic thrombocytopenic purpura, which in the context of HIV infection responds well to plasma infusion. Later, in addition to the progressive lymphopenia that characterizes acquired immunodeficiency syndrome, both reduced production and increased cellular clearance may contribute to neutropenia and thrombocytopenia.[137,138] Finally, advancing immunodeficiency contributes to a greatly increased risk for lymphoid neoplasms, particularly lymphoma.

The wide spectrum of hematologic complications associated with HIV and the high prevalence of infection make HIV testing an essential part of the investigation of cytopenia in most tropical areas. One of the most difficult dilemmas that HIV infection poses for pediatricians in the tropics is management of a child with life-threatening anemia. The conventional approach would be blood transfusion, but in many regions this is now a major risk factor for HIV infection that is not adequately prevented by the available screening programs.[139,140] This problem is discussed further in a later section.

TROPICAL EOSINOPHILIA

The structure and function of eosinophils are described in Chapter 21. Here the importance of eosinophilia in the tropics is discussed.

After anemia, eosinophilia is probably the next most common hematologic abnormality in children in the tropics.[141] An increase in eosinophils in bone marrow and peripheral blood, as well as in tissues, is a major feature of infections caused by worms that migrate through extraintestinal organs. There is a strong association between eosinophilia and infection with tissue nematodes, trematodes, or cestodes. In contrast, however, there is no well-documented evidence that worms that do not invade tissues or protozoal infections are associated with elevated eosinophil counts.

Some common causes of eosinophilia in the tropics are summarized in Box 37-1. A functional role for eosinophils in host protection against some invasive helminths has been demonstrated. For example, incubation of human eosinophils with the larval forms of *S. mansoni* or *Trichinella spiralis*, together with specific antibodies or complement, causes the destruction of these organisms. These in vitro studies have been confirmed by in vivo experiments in mice depleted of eosinophils; animals treated in this manner lose resistance to these helminths. It appears that killing of these organisms is initiated by attachment of eosinophils to the parasite surface, followed by extracellular degranulation and deposition of electron-dense material.

An absolute elevation in the peripheral blood reticulocyte count may occur in any of the conditions listed in Box 37-1. However, the term *tropical eosinophilic syndrome* was first used in the 1940s to describe patients with a paroxysmal cough and wheezing, particularly at night, scanty sputum production, weight loss, low-grade fever, lymphadenopathy, and extreme blood eosinophilia (>3000/μL). Later, this syndrome was discovered to be due to filarial infection.

Hypereosinophilic syndrome is seen in children or young adults and is found most commonly in India,

Box 37-1	Causes of Eosinophilia in Tropical Populations

TISSUE NEMATODES

Wuchereria bancrofti
Loa loa
Onchocerca volvulus
Ankylostoma braziliense
Strongyloides
Ascaris lumbricoides
Necator americanus
Toxocara
Trichinella spiralis

TISSUE TREMATODES

Schistosoma
Fasciola hepaticum

TISSUE CESTODES

Echinococcus granulosus

Indonesia, Sri Lanka, Pakistan, and Southeast Asia, although it may occur in any area where human filariasis is common.[142-145] In addition to typical clinical and hematologic findings, these patients have very high levels of serum IgE together with increased levels of specific antifilarial antibodies. Although it is usually easy to make this diagnosis in a tropical setting, if patients with these symptoms return to nontropical countries, other conditions that cause eosinophilia have to be considered, including chronic eosinophilic pneumonia, allergic aspergillosis, vasculitic syndromes, and idiopathic hypereosinophilic syndrome. The major distinguishing features of tropical hypereosinophilic syndrome are a marked elevation in antifilarial antibody and very high IgE levels. It may be possible to identify filaria on blood films. Traditionally, better results have been obtained with films prepared from blood samples taken at night, although some studies suggest that this may not be necessary.[145]

What is the best approach to determine a diagnosis in a child who has spent time in the tropics and who has persistent eosinophilia? It is important to determine which parts of the tropics have been visited. A careful respiratory history should be taken. Detailed studies of stool for cysts and ova should be performed several times by an experienced observer. Serologic studies for *Filaria*, *Toxocara*, and *Trichinella* infection should be carried out, and immunoglobulin levels should be determined. If a diagnosis has not been determined after these investigations, it is important to exclude nontropical causes of eosinophilia, including collagen vascular disease, allergy, drug reactions, lymphoma, and leukemia associated with an eosinophil response. It may be necessary to initiate a trial of the antifilarial drug diethylcarbamazine under careful medical supervision as part of the diagnostic workup.

HEMATOLOGIC ASPECTS OF MALABSORPTION IN THE TROPICS

One of the major difficulties in discussing the problem of malabsorption in the tropics is definition.[146] A large proportion of people in tropical climates, both indigenous populations and expatriates who have lived and worked in rural areas, have mild abnormalities of the intestinal mucosa, often associated with impairment of absorption. These structural and functional alterations of the gut have been called tropical enteropathy.[147-149] It is likely that they reflect an adaptation to life in the contaminated environment of the tropics with its recurrent enteric infections and peculiarities of diet. Interestingly, similar morphologic lesions have been demonstrated in the colon of otherwise healthy residents of southern India. After expatriates return to temperate climates, these changes in the gut revert to normal.[150]

The more severe malabsorption syndromes, sprue and postinfective malabsorption, are associated with chronic diarrhea, wasting, and a variety of hematologic changes.

The term *sprue* was first coined by the English physician Manson while working in China; it is an Anglicization of the Dutch term *indische sprouw*. During the 19th and 20th centuries, tropical sprue was thought to be a disease of expatriates, but during World War II it became apparent that similar syndromes commonly occur in indigenous populations. The occurrence of severe malabsorption syndromes is not distributed evenly in the tropical world.[150-152] They are particularly common in the Indian subcontinent, Burma, Malaysia, Vietnam, Borneo, Indonesia, and the Philippines. They are also seen in the West Indies, in parts of Central America (particularly Puerto Rico, Cuba, and the Dominican Republic), and in northern parts of South America. There are a few reports from the Middle East and temperate areas. Tropical Africa seems to be spared.

These syndromes are believed to originate from an infection.[153,154] They usually start as an acute attack of diarrhea, which then becomes chronic. Many well-documented epidemics of sprue have been reported both in southern India and in the Philippines among American military personnel. However, despite a vast amount of work and the establishment of units specifically assigned to study the problem, no organism has been isolated that could even approach meeting Koch's postulates. It may be that these disorders can follow infection with a variety of agents, but the reason for the peculiar geographic distribution remains unexplained. Remarkably, genetic factors have been almost totally ignored in the investigation of this disease.

Tropical malabsorption syndromes can occur in individuals of any age. They are characterized by intermittent diarrhea, weight loss, and anemia. Varying degrees of mucosal damage are found on biopsy of the small intestine, although an absolutely flat mucosa, as seen in gluten-induced enteropathy, is rare. Hematologic findings in patients with tropical malabsorption syndromes vary considerably. In more advanced disease, megaloblastic anemia is common. It is usually caused by folate deficiency but may also be complicated by vitamin B_{12} deficiency. Frequently, bizarre mixed pictures of iron and folic acid deficiency are found.

Interestingly, although much of the data derive from uncontrolled studies, many of the symptoms and hematologic changes associated with these syndromes can be reversed by a course of oral tetracycline. However, recovery is much more rapid if folate or vitamin B_{12} treatment is given as well.

In a tropical setting, malabsorption can also result from colonization of the small bowel by specific parasites, including *Giardia lamblia*, *Strongyloides stercoralis*, *Cryptosporidium*, and others. Furthermore, abdominal tuberculosis with malabsorption is particularly common, and in Africa, HIV infection may be an important cause of malabsorption.[155,156] The local name "slim disease" acknowledges the severe wasting that can occur with HIV infection.[155]

Hematologists without experience in the tropics should be aware that the clinical and hematologic findings of tropical malabsorption syndromes can be extreme. In young children particularly, a good history of diarrheal illness may not always be available, and in many tropical populations recurrent diarrheal illness is the norm anyway. Folate deficiency, as well as producing anemia, may give rise to severe neutropenia and thrombocytopenia with associated infection or bleeding. If intercurrent infection is present, as is often seen in severely affected children, the bone marrow appearance may be deceiving, although there is nearly always some megaloblastic change even if overall the bone marrow is much less hyperplastic than usually observed with folate or B_{12} deficiency in Western settings.

A major diagnostic problem that is often encountered in children returning from the tropics with persistent diarrhea and malabsorption is determining whether they have postinfective malabsorption or celiac disease. If symptoms do not resolve, it may be necessary to initiate a trial of a gluten-free diet and then reintroduce gluten at a later date while monitoring progress with repeated small bowel biopsies.

HEMOSTATIC FAILURE AS A MANIFESTATION OF SYSTEMIC DISEASE IN THE TROPICS

Many tropical infections or other hazards produce serious bleeding disorders. Malaria was considered in an earlier section. Here, a few other causes of bleeding disorders that are seen in the tropics are discussed.

Dengue

The dengue viruses are four antigenically related but distinct organisms that are transmitted to humans by mosquitos of the species *Aedes aegypti*.[157] The clinical manifestations of this very common infection vary in different parts of the world. In American, African, and Indian populations the disease is characterized by classic dengue fever, but in Southeast Asia a much more serious condition develops in many children, dengue hemorrhagic fever (DHF)/dengue shock syndrome (DSS). The latter develops in infants born to dengue-immune mothers during initial infections or in children older than 1 year during secondary infections. It appears that this curious paradox reflects enhancement of dengue viral infection in mononuclear phagocytes mediated by subneutralizing concentrations of dengue antibody.

The pathophysiologic course of DHF/DSS is quite remarkable.[157,158] Dengue viruses appear to be parasites of mononuclear phagocytes. Furthermore, they use antibody as a specific receptor for gaining entry to these cells. Such antibodies are known as infection-enhancing antibodies. Epidemiologic studies have shown that children 1 year or older always have detectable dengue antibody before acquiring a subsequent infection that results in DHF/DSS. Infants who acquire dengue antibody passively from their mothers are also at risk for development of the syndrome. DHF/DSS is characterized by simultaneous activation of the complement and hemostatic systems, together with a marked increase in vascular permeability.[158-160] It appears that complement activation follows both the classical and alternative pathways. The hemostatic abnormalities include gross thrombocytopenia, prolonged bleeding time, elevated prothrombin time, and a reduction in the levels of factors II, V, VII, and IX, together with marked hypofibrinogenemia and an increase in fibrin degradation products. The abnormalities in vascular permeability are characterized by an elevated hematocrit, normal or low serum protein levels because of selective loss of albumin, and variable serous effusions.

Precisely what triggers these remarkable events is not clear. However, it seems likely that the mediators are the product of dengue virus–infected mononuclear phagocytes. Studies in Thailand have suggested that low levels of heterotypic neutralizing antibody from a single previous infection prevent the illness in those who acquire dengue 2 infections.[157,160] On the other hand, children with circulating dengue-enhancing antibodies but no neutralizing antibodies are at high risk.

Once DHF has been triggered, however, the immune disturbance is not confined to antibodies. Both the CD4+ and CD8+ subpopulations of T lymphocytes are more intensively activated in DHF than in uncomplicated dengue fever.[161] High levels of TNF and other procoagulant cytokines may also contribute to the pathologic changes.[162] A further factor might be antibodies to plasminogen, which are found in a significant proportion of dengue infections, particularly if hemorrhage is present.[163] These antibodies are thought to arise because of structural homology between plasminogen and the dengue envelope glycoprotein.[164] Findings in Vietnamese children with DSS suggest that rather than causing true

disseminated intravascular coagulation, the virus may act to directly degrade fibrinogen and thereby result in secondary activation of procoagulant homeostatic mechanisms.[165]

The clinical findings of DHF/DSS consist of fever, malaise, and anorexia, and about 2 to 5 days later a second phase occurs in which there are widespread hemorrhagic phenomena, including purpura, large spontaneous ecchymoses, and bleeding from previous venipuncture sites. These children then enter a phase of profound shock. The hematologic findings are characterized by a normal or even high hematocrit associated with gross thrombocytopenia and evidence of disseminated intravascular coagulation.

The fact that the most serious pathophysiologic mechanism in this disease is fluid loss rather than hemorrhage has focused attention on the development of treatment regimens similar to those used for the management of severe diarrheal illnesses in children in the tropics. A study in Vietnamese children concluded that initial resuscitation with lactated Ringer's solution was appropriate for moderately severe DSS whereas hydroxyethyl starch had fewer adverse reactions than dextran for colloid treatment of severe DSS.[166] Clinical trials of heparin treatment to counteract disseminated intravascular coagulation have not produced impressive results.

Other Viral Hemorrhagic Fevers

Severe hemorrhagic fevers caused by viruses occur throughout the tropical world and are encountered on every continent except Australia and North America.[167] They are the result of RNA viruses of four distinct families, each of which is a zoonosis with typical epidemiologic features. They are transmitted by a variety of agents, including tics and mosquitos. In many instances the reservoirs and vectors are unknown. These diseases are associated with specific clinical entities in different parts of the world, such are Rift Valley fever, Lassa fever, Argentine hemorrhagic fever, Bolivian hemorrhagic fever, and others.

Many of these conditions are accompanied by hemorrhagic diatheses of varying severity ranging from mild purpura to severe hemostatic failure.[168] As with dengue, shock is a major feature and is often associated with an elevated hematocrit. The bleeding manifestations reflect both increased vascular permeability and consumptive coagulopathy. There have been few extensive coagulation studies performed in patients with these disorders, although disseminated intravascular coagulation has been implicated as the basis for the hemostatic failure.

Snake Bite

Snake bite is an important and neglected problem in the rural tropics; its incidence is underestimated because of the lack of reliable epidemiologic data.[169] In northern Ghana, the carpet viper (*Echis* complex of species) is responsible for some 86 bites per 100,000 population per year, with 28% mortality. This particular snake, whose geographic range extends throughout the northern half of Africa and the Middle East to India, probably bites and kills more people than any other species. In the Indian subcontinent, the most important species are the cobra (*Naja naja*), the common krait (*Bungarus caeruleus*), Russell's viper (*Vipera russelli*), and *Echis* species. In Sri Lanka there are about 60,000 bites and 900 deaths (6 per 10,000 population) each year. In Southeast Asia, the Malayan pit viper (*Calloselasma rhodostoma*), *D. russelli*, and green pit vipers cause most bites and deaths. In Burma, Russell's viper bite has been the fifth major cause of death, with an annual mortality of about 15 per 100,000 population. Snake bite is also a common public health problem in Central and South America.

The hematologic complications of snake bite are a reflection of the complex chemistry of venoms.[170-172] Although much work remains to be done, at least some components of snake venom have been well defined. Venom may contain 20 or more different components. More than 90% of the dry weight of venom is protein in the form of enzymes, nonenzymatic polypeptide toxins, and nontoxic proteins. The mechanisms of envenomation have been most clearly defined for some of the venom procoagulants. For example, *V. russelli* venom contains a glycoprotein that activates factor X and an arginine ester hydrolase that activates factor V. *Echis* venom contains a zinc metalloprotein called ecarin that activates prothrombin. Many crotaline venoms contain proteases that cleave fibrinogen (e.g., arvin and reptilase). Some venoms contain phospholipase A_2 (lecithinase), which probably contributes to their neurotoxicity, cardiotoxicity, and hemolysis and is also responsible for increasing vascular permeability.

After a snake bite, swelling and bruising of the limb result from increased permeability induced by proteases, phospholipase, polypeptide toxins, and hyaluronidase, as well as by endogenous activators released by the venom such as histamine, 5-hydroxytryptamine, and kinins. The acute hemostatic failure that may follow envenomation is mediated in several ways.[173,174] Bites from snakes that produce procoagulants that activate factors V or X or prothrombin are associated with a rapid consumptive coagulopathy. In other instances there may be rapid defibrinogenation that is due to either direct attack on fibrinogen or activation of the endogenous fibrinolytic system. Thrombocytopenia results from either aggregation or consumption. The bleeding is potentiated by damage to vascular endothelium. The combination of defibrination, thrombocytopenia, and increased vessel wall permeability leads to massive bleeding, which is a common cause of death.

Although as mentioned earlier, many venoms are hemolytic in vitro, massive intravascular hemolysis is seen rarely and usually in association with bites by *V. russelli*.

Management of snake bite includes supportive treatment, careful correction of the coagulation abnormali-

ties, appropriate respiratory support if the venom is associated with neurotoxins, and judicious use of appropriate antivenin. Hemostatic disturbances usually respond well to antivenin treatment, and replacement therapy with fresh whole blood, fresh frozen plasma, specific factors, or platelet concentrates is not generally required. Even though a theoretical case can be made for the use of heparin in patients bitten by Russell's viper, particularly if there is definite evidence of disseminated intravascular coagulation, thus far clinical trials have not shown any benefit.

Although the long-term prognosis for those who recover from a snake bite is good, work in Burma has shown that chronic pituitary failure and renal failure may develop later. These conditions are believed to be caused by infarction of the pituitary gland during the phase of intravascular coagulation, similar in pathophysiology to that observed after childbirth and called, in this setting, Sheehan's syndrome.[175] It may be accompanied by a mild normochromic anemia.

GEOGRAPHIC VARIABILITY IN THE DISTRIBUTION AND EXPRESSION OF HEMATOLOGIC DISEASE

In addition to the unique hematologic problems caused by disorders that are specific to the tropics or other parts of the developing world, the pattern of distribution of primary disorders of the blood varies considerably among different populations. Furthermore, there are some hematologic syndromes, as yet ill defined, that are unique to certain parts of the developing world.

Lymphoma and Leukemia

The pathophysiologic and clinical features of the lymphomas and childhood leukemias[176,177] are described elsewhere in this book. Burkitt's lymphoma is endemic throughout large regions of sub-Saharan Africa and in Papua New Guinea. In Burkitt's classic descriptions of the tumor, he pointed out that its occurrence is related closely to altitude, temperature, and rainfall, features that are similar in sub-Saharan Africa and Papua New Guinea. Although this distribution, together with work relating this B-cell tumor to infection with Epstein-Barr virus and evidence for loss of immunologic control of Epstein-Barr virus during acute attacks of malaria,[168,178] relates the prevalence of the tumor to malaria, this is certainly not the whole story. For example, it is not found in Zanzibar, although it is very common in the coastal regions of neighboring Tanzania.

The T-cell leukemia/lymphoma syndrome, first recognized in southern Japan and now known to be due to infection with human T-cell leukemia/lymphoma virus type 1 (HTLV-1), has a very restricted distribution in southern Japan and the Caribbean.[177] It is not yet clear which particular lymphocyte populations are involved in the very common histiocytic lymphomas that occur throughout the Middle East and across parts of Central and South America.

The curious syndrome of primary upper intestinal lymphoma (Mediterranean lymphoma) and immunoproliferative disease of the small intestine has to be distinguished from the rare primary intestinal lymphomas that occur sporadically throughout the world, usually in elderly patients.[179,180] In endemic regions, primary upper intestinal lymphoma and immunoproliferative disease of the small intestine occur in much younger age groups, usually of poor socioeconomic background. The pathologic lesions are found predominantly in the upper part of the small intestine and are associated with a clinical picture characterized by malabsorption, which often precedes development of the tumor.

Although this condition is still known as Mediterranean lymphoma, it was first described in Peru. However, the largest epidemic area is the region of the Mediterranean and the Middle East, and many cases have now been reported from Israel, Lebanon, Iraq, Syria, and Iran, as well as Greece.

Studies of the population distribution of classic Hodgkin's disease have also shown some discrepancies.[176,181] High rates are found in most affluent westernized countries and lower rates in poorer countries and the tropics; this does not seem to be due entirely to ascertainment bias. Interestingly, particularly low rates are seen in Japan and also in China, India, and Malaysia. In addition, there are considerable variations in age distribution and histologic subtype in different parts of the world. In poorer or lesser developed countries, Hodgkin's disease occurs at a younger age and is usually the histologic type with a poorer prognosis.

Some interesting differences in rate of occurrence and type of acute leukemia throughout the world are also seen.[176,182] In North America and Europe and in all other westernized populations, acute lymphoblastic leukemia (ALL) accounts for a high proportion of acute leukemia in children between the ages of 2 and 5. In contrast, ALL is uncommon in the tropics, particularly in sub-Saharan Africa, where Burkitt's lymphoma is the predominant childhood tumor. On the other hand, in older children the incidence of acute myeloid leukemia and various subtypes of ALL is similar to that in Western societies.

Hereditary Blood Disorders

The distribution of hemoglobin disorders in the world is described elsewhere in this book. Particularly as developing countries pass through the epidemiologic transition toward a reduction in childhood mortality secondary to malnutrition and infection, children with these conditions tend to survive long enough to be evaluated for treatment. Hence they are producing an increasingly serious burden on health care resources in many of the developing countries. For environmental and cultural reasons, their diagnosis, management, and control raise problems in many developing countries completely different from those encountered in developed countries. A full description of these complex issues is beyond the scope of this chapter; they have been covered in detail in two recent monographs.[183,184]

The manifestations of G6PD deficiency in some developing countries also differ from those seen in the West. The problems of drug-induced hemolysis and favism are discussed elsewhere in this book. It is important to point out, however, that in parts of Southeast Asia, Greece, and Africa, G6PD deficiency appears to be associated with neonatal jaundice.[185-187] This is not a common problem in G6PD deficiency in advanced Western societies. Although this observation was first made more than 30 years ago, the precise mechanism of the neonatal jaundice is not clear. In Singapore it is enough of a public health problem to have led to routine screening of all newborn babies for G6PD levels.

The high frequency of the hemoglobin disorders and G6PD deficiency reflects relative protection of carriers against malaria. This mechanism is also responsible for the unusually high frequency of ovalocytosis in Melanesia, a condition that is relatively rare in Western populations. Melanesian ovalocytosis is asymptomatic in heterozygotes, although the absence of reported homozygotes suggests that it may have a much more severe phenotype. There is clear evidence that it has reached high frequencies in Melanesia by protection against malaria, particularly cerebral malaria.[188]

Aplastic Anemia

Although more data are needed for confirmation, there is growing evidence that aplastic anemia, particularly in childhood, is much more common in parts of Southeast Asia and South America than in developed Western countries.[189] The ease of availability of potentially toxic agents such as chloramphenicol may be reflected by this finding, but this is probably not the whole story. The possibility exists that that it reflects the action of an as yet unidentified infectious agent. This challenging question certainly requires further detailed prospective studies because a full hematologic workup, including bone marrow trephine biopsy, is rarely available in many parts of the world, even at tertiary referral hospitals.

Hematologic Disorders Unique to Certain Countries

A number of ill-defined hematologic disorders appear to be common to particular countries. In Thailand, for example, there is a well-recognized disorder called acquired prothrombin complex deficiency, a condition seen mainly in infants who have been breast-fed.[190] Despite a great deal of work, the etiology is not yet known, although it is suspected that mothers may have ingested substances antagonistic to prothrombin.

Also in Thailand, a very curious condition called acquired platelet dysfunction with eosinophilia is seen.[191] It is a pediatric disorder characterized by bleeding and ecchymoses. There is associated eosinophilia and abnormal platelet function test results. The etiology is unknown, and current efforts are focused on trying to define a parasitic cause.

In India an increase has been seen in hemolytic disease of the newborn, which appears to be due to fetomaternal ABO incompatibility.[192] Evidence showing that this may be related to the administration of tetanus toxoids to pregnant women to prevent the major problem of tetanus neonatorum in that population is increasing; there is a marked increase in the maternal titer of anti-A/anti-B antibodies after the injection of tetanus toxoid.

ASPECTS OF CLINICAL MANAGEMENT

Treatment of Severe Anemia in the Tropics

The definition of severe anemia depends on the clinical context, and the normal level of hemoglobin in the community has to be considered. In an African child with malaria, a hemoglobin level of approximately 5 g/dL is commonly used as the criterion for transfusion, although a transfusion would normally be given sooner if the parasitemia were extremely high. The fatality rate for severe malarial anemia varies widely between clinics, but a typical figure is approximately 7%.[193] Until recently, most tropical pediatricians have endeavored to improve survival by improving the availability of transfusion.

The situation has altered dramatically as a result of the significant risk of HIV infection that now accompanies blood transfusion in many tropical regions.[139,194] Apart from the logistic and financial difficulties of screening blood donations, these screening procedures are an unreliable means of preventing transfusion-associated HIV infection in the developing world[140] (see later). There are also other problems with blood transfusion that tend to be ignored. Cross-matching can be erratic in a clinic with inadequate resources, and the infusion is often unsupervised. Occasionally, the consciousness level of a child with malaria deteriorates dramatically after the transfusion. Such occurrences are rare, but there are theoretical reasons why transfusion might worsen sequestration, such as the blood group favoring the formation of erythrocyte rosettes.[195]

An urgent need exists to define the clinical criteria that make transfusion absolutely essential. Decision trees have been devised,[196] but the underlying risk-benefit equation may vary from place to place, and a meta-analysis found no clear evidence of benefit for transfusion in anemic children whose conditions are clinically stable.[197] One issue that has become clear is the prognostic importance of respiratory distress. For example, in Kenyan children, malarial anemia rarely causes death unless respiratory distress is present,[198] and the only clear evidence that blood transfusion is beneficial is seen in the group of children who have both anemia and respiratory distress.[199]

Investigations into the clinical physiologic course of severe malarial anemia in African children have yielded important insight into the management of this condition. Lactic acidosis appears to be the main cause of the relationship between anemia and respiratory distress,[200] and there is a substantial oxygen debt.[201] Rapid transfusion may be lifesaving, not only because it increases hemoglobin but also because volume repletion reduces acidosis,[200] and a careful study in Kenya showed no evidence that it was likely to cause fluid overload. This is contrary to the notion that a severely anemic child is likely to be in high-output failure and should therefore be depleted of fluids or undergo diuresis before transfusion. However, before rewriting the textbook on the management of severe anemia, we need data from other parts of the tropics, where different pathophysiologic factors may be operative.[202]

With the steady increase in levels of resistance to antimalarial drugs worldwide, the incidence of severe childhood anemia in the tropics is expected to increase. As the criteria for transfusion become stricter, there is a need for more data on optimal hematinic therapy for children with malarial anemia. The practices of pediatricians vary, but many prescribe both iron and folic acid in addition to antimalarial therapy. One concern has been that iron deficiency may help suppress parasite growth, and in some studies[203,204] but not others,[15] iron repletion has been found to increase the risk for subsequent infection. Another concern has been that folic acid supplements might reduce the efficacy of the antifolate drugs that are increasingly being used to treat chloroquine-resistant malaria in the community.[205] These issues were addressed in a study of moderately anemic Gambian children with *P. falciparum* infection.[206] Supplementary iron therapy was found to result in a small, but significant improvement in hemoglobin levels after 1 month and did not increase the risk for reinfection within this period. Folic acid supplements failed to improve hemoglobin levels and increased the risk for parasite recrudescence if sulfadoxine-pyrimethamine was used to treat the infection. However, it cannot be assumed that these findings would necessarily apply to regions with different rates of malarial transmission and different nutritional problems, and the need for locally based research into this type of problem cannot be overemphasized.

Problems with Blood-Borne Infection and Blood Transfusion

The risk of contracting an infection after blood transfusion is increasing and becoming a major economic burden for developing countries. Whereas the most important infections are those resulting from blood-borne HIV and hepatitis B and C viruses, the incidence of other infections is increasing. As mentioned earlier, although donor screening has had a major effect in reducing the occurrence of HIV infection in patients who are receiving regular blood transfusions, such as those with thalassemia, even if blood is screened adequately, the risk for infection remains. Hepatitis C is becoming a major problem throughout the southern Mediterranean region, the Indian subcontinent, and Southeast Asia, whereas hepatitis B remains a problem in many of the poorer countries. With the reappearance of malaria as a major problem in parts of the Indian subcontinent and Southeast Asia, post-transfusion malarial infection is increasing. Indeed, in many clinics it is becoming standard practice to treat recipients of transfusions with antimalarial drugs prophylactically.

In addition to these common viral and parasitic infections, the risk of blood-borne disease caused by other bacteria and parasites must always be considered, particularly in places where these infectious diseases are endemic. For example, Chagas' disease is often transmitted through blood transfusion, although remarkably, pretreatment of blood with gentian violet seems to result in a major reduction of this complication. In parts of South America, transfusion-borne infections with *Bartonella* may occur. Diseases associated with HTLV-1 and HTLV-2, notably tropical spastic paraparesis and adult T-cell leukemia, which seem to be restricted mainly to the Caribbean and certain Japanese populations, can also be transmitted by blood transfusion.

Clearly, screening programs must be tailored to the particular infections that are common in individual communities, and blood should be administered only when absolutely necessary in these populations.

Management of Imported Malaria

The most important part of the management of malaria is to be constantly aware of the possibility of the diagnosis.[207] Obtaining an accurate travel history is critical. Children who have flown from one nonmalarious region to another may have had a brief stopover during which they could have been infected. It is vital to obtain a detailed account of all countries visited and the use of malaria prophylaxis. Clinical symptoms are usually seen within a month of infection, but they can occasionally appear after several months if the infection has been partially suppressed by a prophylactic drug with a long half-life such as mefloquine. In a child who has previously been infected with *P. vivax* or *P. malariae* and parasites in the dormant stage in the liver have not been eradicated, symptoms may recur years after the initial infection. If malaria is suspected, it is important to not discard the diagnosis if parasites are not found at first, and thick blood film stains may have to be repeated several times, ideally during episodes of fever. Results with thin films are unreliable for diagnostic screening, but they can be useful for determining the species of parasite when infection has been confirmed. Dipstick assays based on detection of *P. falciparum* antigens in serum are now available. The most commonly used is based on *P. falciparum* lactate dehydrogenase, which is present in blood at the time of infection but is cleared rapidly.[208] An alternative is based on *P. falciparum* histidine-rich protein 2, which persists for some time after infection.[209] A positive result with this test may be helpful in a medical emergency, but the thick blood film remains the diagnostic "gold standard."

A child with malaria may lack the classic symptoms of paroxysmal fever and body pain. The presence of vomiting, diarrhea, cough, or tachypnea can be particularly misleading. Febrile convulsions are common and need to be distinguished from the seizures that accompany cerebral malaria, the defining feature of which is coma secondary to *P. falciparum* from which patients cannot be aroused. Hypoglycemia sometimes contributes to the coma and must be immediately excluded. Other potential problems include severe anemia, jaundice, circulatory collapse, pulmonary edema, renal failure, and coagulation abnormalities. Vigilance is needed because although these potentially lethal complications occur in only a minority of infections, they can arise after treatment has commenced.

The choice of antimalarial treatment depends on the species of parasite, the geographic source of infection, the age of child, and the severity of infection. Here it is only possible to outline the general principles involved, and specific recommendations should be sought from an up-to-date formulary or reference center. Oral chloroquine is generally the drug of choice for all species other than *P. falciparum*, although it is important to be aware of the increasing prevalence of chloroquine-resistant *P. vivax* in Papua New Guinea and Indonesia.[210] With *P. vivax* or *P. ovale* infection, it is also necessary to destroy the dormant liver forms with primaquine. The child's G6PD activity should be checked before giving this drug; if it is deficient, a lower dose of primaquine may be given over a longer period. If the infective species is not known, treatment should initially be the same as for falciparum malaria because this is the most dangerous form.

The presence of chloroquine-resistant forms of *P. falciparum* is now so widespread that chloroquine can no longer be recommended for imported infections with this species. For uncomplicated infection, several alternative treatments are available. The most convenient are combination therapies: proguanil with atovaquone (Malarone) or artemether with lumefantrine (Riamet). The alternative and classic method is a course of oral quinine, but this needs to be followed by a course of either pyrimethamine-sulfadoxine (Fansidar) if from an area where the parasites are likely to be sensitive, doxycycline if older than 12 years, or clindamycin.

For severe malaria, the standard therapy is quinine or quinidine given by carefully controlled intravenous infusion. The use of intravenous infusion is impractical for many pediatric wards in the tropics because of nursing shortages and inadequate infusion equipment. In this situation, quinine is commonly given intramuscularly (diluted to reduce the likelihood of abscess formation),[211] and there is increasing use of artemisinin (qinqhaosu) derivatives because of their rapid antimalarial action.[212,213]

The principles of intensive management for complications of *P. falciparum* infection are the same as those for any other serious systemic infection. Dextrose infusion is often required to maintain blood glucose levels, which may be suppressed by quinine or by the infection.[214] Renal function and hemoglobin levels need to be closely monitored. In a child with cerebral malaria, overt seizures are usually controlled by diazepam and phenobarbital, but subclinical seizures are common and may be highly refractory to treatment. If high doses of anticonvulsant are necessary, it is important to recognize that the child's system is often trying to compensate for metabolic acidosis and that respiratory arrest is the most common mode of death[215]; indeed, high doses of phenobarbital have been shown to increase mortality.[216]

Fluid management of a child with severe malaria has been the focus of considerable recent debate. Studies in Kenyan children with severe malaria have concluded that overall volume status is generally low and that relatively aggressive fluid replacement may be beneficial,[200] with preliminary evidence that volume replacement with albumin results in lower fatality rates than replacement with saline does.[217] In contrast, studies of Gabonese children with severe malaria found no evidence of significant hypovolemia,[218] and these authors recommend that fluid replacement regimens be relatively conservative because intracranial pressure tends to be moderately elevated.[219] Use of steroids does not improve the outcome for adult cerebral malaria; whether this is true for children remains unknown. There is no conclusive evidence that any other form of adjunctive therapy is beneficial in childhood cerebral malaria. Exchange transfusion is sometimes used in patients with very high parasitemia, although its efficacy has not been evaluated in a controlled trial. More effective forms of treatment of severe malaria are badly needed.

Leishmaniasis

Leishmaniasis may be contracted on short visits to countries where the condition is endemic. It is a disease that may cause considerable diagnostic difficulty when seen in the setting of a hospital in the developed world. In children with this disorder, a primary hematologic disorder such as leukemia may be misdiagnosed if the diagnosis of visceral leishmaniasis is not considered. It may be manifested as an acute disorder with fever, hepatosplenomegaly, and hemolysis or as a more chronic condition characterized by increasing hepatosplenomegaly, lymphadenopathy, and pancytopenia. The hematologic and diagnostic features were mentioned earlier in this chapter.

Treatment remains difficult, with several different drugs to chose from, all of which have potential toxic effects, so expert advice should be sought.[220-222] For many years pentavalent antimony has been the drug of choice; the preparation that is available in the United States, stibogluconate (Pentostam), is classified as an investigational drug and is obtained from the Centers for Disease Control and Prevention in Atlanta, Georgia, which provides advice on dosage schedules for particular preparations. However, significant resistance is emerging, particularly in patients with kala-azar in India, and even in patients who show a good response to treatment, relapses may occur. Pentamidine has long been used as alternative for antimonial-resistant visceral leishmaniasis, but it is relatively toxic.

The past decade has seen the introduction of new therapies, including liposomal amphotericin, oral miltefosine, and paromomycin.[222] Although these are significant advances, they are not ideal drugs, and cheaper and less toxic therapies are still needed. Liposomal amphotericin has been shown to be is at least as effective and less toxic than antimony-containing compounds for the treatment of visceral leishmaniasis, and it is now licensed in the United States for that purpose, although its high cost is a significant impediment to use in the developing world. It has been used successfully for the treatment of visceral leishmaniasis in children.[223] Miltefosine, an alkyl phospholipid developed for use in cancer treatment, has been demonstrated to be an effective oral treatment of visceral leishmaniasis, including antimony-resistant infection.[224] A recent comparison of the different regimens for visceral leishmaniasis concluded that sodium stibogluconate is the most cost-effective option in areas with high response rates to antimonials; in other areas, miltefosine is most cost-effective, but its use as a first-line drug is limited by teratogenicity and the rapid development of resistance; and liposomal amphotericin remains an expensive option for poor countries where the disease is endemic.[225]

REFERENCES

1. Weatherall DJ, Wasi P. Anemia. In Warren KS, Mahmoud AAF (eds). Tropical and Geographic Medicine. New York, McGraw Hill, 1989, pp 55-65.
2. Weatherall DJ. Anaemia as a world health problem. In Warrell Dam Cox TM, Firth JD (eds). Oxford Textbook of Medicine, 4th ed. Oxford, Oxford University Press, 2003, pp 644-648.
3. Baker SJ. Nutritional anaemias: Part 2: tropical Asia. Clin Haematol. 1981;10:843-871.
4. Stoltzfus RJ, Dreyfuss ML. Guidelines for the Use of Iron Supplements to Prevent and Treat Iron Deficiency. Washington DC, ILSI Press, 1998.
5. McGregor IA, Williams K, Billewicz WZ, Thompson AM. Haemoglobin concentration and anaemia in young West African (Gambian) children. Trans R Soc Trop Med Hyg. 1966;60:650-667.
6. Baker SJ, DeMaeyer EM. Nutritional anemia: its understanding and control with special reference to the work of

the World Health Organization. Am J Clin Nutr. 1979; 32:368-417.

7. World Health Organization. Nutritional Aanaemias, Technical Report Series. Geneva, WHO, 1972, p 503.

8. World Health Report 2002. Geneva, World Health Organization, 2002.

9. Brewster DR, Greenwood BM. Seasonal variation of paediatric diseases in The Gambia, West Africa. Ann Trop Paediatr 1993;13:133-146.

10. Bothwell TH, Clydesdale FM, Cook JD, et al. The effects of cereals and legumes on iron availability. Washington, DC, International Nutritional Anemia Consultative Group (INACG), 1982.

11. World Health Report 2005. Geneva, World Health Organization, 2005, p 45.

12. Fleming AF. Iron deficiency in the tropics. Clin Haematol. 1982;11:365-388.

13. Fleming AF, Ghatoura GBS, Harrison KA, et al. The prevention of anaemia in pregnancy in primigravidae in the guinea savanna of Nigeria. Ann Trop Med Parasitol. 1985;80:212-233.

14. Pitney WR. Anaemia in the tropics. In Goldberg A, Brain MC (eds). Recent Advances in Haematology. Edinburgh, Churchill Livingstone, 1971, pp 337-356.

15. Menendez C, Kahigwa E, Hirt R, et al. Randomised placebo-controlled trial of iron supplementation and malaria chemoprophylaxis for prevention of severe anaemia and malaria in Tanzanian infants. Lancet. 1997; 350:844-850.

16. Stoltzfus RJ, Kvalsvig JD, Chwaya HM, et al. Effects of iron supplementation and anthelmintic treatment on motor and language development of preschool children in Zanzibar: double blind, placebo controlled study. BMJ. 2001;323:1389-1393.

17. Sazawal S, Black RE, Ramsan M, et al. Effects of routine prophylactic supplementation with iron and folic acid on admission to hospital and mortality in preschool children in a high malaria transmission setting: community-based, randomised, placebo-controlled trial. Lancet. 2006;467: 133-143.

18. Tielsch JM, Khatry SK, Stoltzfus RJ, et al. Effect of routine prophylactic supplementation with iron and folic acid on preschool child mortality in southern Nepal: community-based, cluster-randomised, placebo-controlled trial. Lancet. 2006;367:144-152.

19. Iannotti LL, Tielsch JM, Black MM, et al. Iron supplementation in early childhood: health benefits and risks. Am J Clin Nutr. 2006;84:1261-1276.

20. Miller LH, Warrell DA. Malaria. In Warren KS, Mahmood AAF (eds). Tropical and Geographic Medicine. New York, McGraw-Hill, 1989, pp 245-264.

21. Rowe AK, Rowe SY, Snow RW, et al. The burden of malaria mortality among African children in the year 2000. Int J Epidemiol. 2006;35:691-704.

22. Snow RW, Guerra CA, Noor AM, et al. The global distribution of clinical episodes of *Plasmodium falciparum* malaria. Nature. 2005;434:214-217.

23. Singh B, Kim Sung L, Matusop A, et al. A large focus of naturally acquired *Plasmodium knowlesi* infections in human beings. Lancet. 2004;363:1017-1024.

24. Miller LH, Mason SJ, Clyde DF, et al. The resistance factor to *Plasmodium vivax* in blacks. The Duffy-blood-group genotype F$_y$F$_y$. N Engl J Med. 1976;295:302-304.

25. Horuk R, Chitnis CE, Darbonne WC, et al. A receptor for the malarial parasite *Plasmodium vivax*: the erythrocyte chemokine receptor. Science. 1993; 61:1182-1184.

26. Greenwood BM, Bradley AK, Greenwood AM, et al. Mortality and morbidity from malaria among children in a rural area of The Gambia, West Africa. Trans R Soc Trop Med Hyg. 1987;81:478-486.

27. Warrell DA, Molyneux ME, Beales P. Severe and complicated malaria. Trans R Soc Trop Med Hyg. 1990;84(Suppl 2):1-65.

28. Slutsker L, Taylor TE, Wirima JJ, et al. In-hospital morbidity and mortality due to malaria-associated severe anaemia in two areas of Malawi with different patterns of malaria infection. Trans R Soc Trop Med Hyg. 1994;88: 548-551.

29. Kitchen SF. Symptomatology. In Boyd MF (ed). Malariology, vol 2. Philadelphia, WB Saunders, 1949, pp 966-994.

30. Berendt AR, Ferguson DJP, Newbold CI. Sequestration in *Plasmodium falciparum* malaria: sticky cells and sticky problems. Parasitol Today. 1990;6:247-254.

31. Roberts DJ, Craig AG, Berendt AR, et al. Rapid switching to multiple antigenic and adhesive phenotypes in malaria. Nature. 1992;357:689-692.

32. McGuire W, Hill AVS, Allsopp CEM, et al. Variation in the TNF-α promoter region is associated with susceptibility to cerebral malaria. Nature. 1994;371:508-511.

33. Rowe JA, Moulds JM, Newbold CI, et al. *P. falciparum* rosetting mediated by a parasite-variant erythrocyte membrane protein and complement-receptor 1. Nature. 1997; 388:292-295.

34. Pain A, Ferguson DJ, Kai O, et al. Platelet-mediated clumping of *Plasmodium falciparum*–infected erythrocytes is a common adhesive phenotype and is associated with severe malaria. Proc Natl Acad Sci U S A. 2001;98: 1805-1810.

35. Mabey DC, Brown A, Greenwood BM. *Plasmodium falciparum* malaria and *Salmonella* infections in Gambian children. J Infect Dis. 1987;155:1319-1321.

36. Berkley J, Mwarumba S, Bramham K, et al. Bacteraemia complicating severe malaria in children. Trans R Soc Trop Med Hyg. 1999;93:283-286.

37. Graham SM, Walsh AL, Molyneux EM, et al. Clinical presentation of non-typhoidal *Salmonella* bacteraemia in Malawian children. Trans R Soc Trop Med Hyg. 2000;94: 310-314.

38. Graham SM, Hart CA, Molyneux EM, et al. Malaria and *Salmonella* infections: cause or coincidence? Trans R Soc Trop Med Hyg. 2000;94:227.

39. Phillips RE, Looareesuwan S, Warrell DA, et al. The importance of anaemia in cerebral and uncomplicated falciparum malaria: role of complications, dyserythropoiesis and iron sequestration. Q J Med. 1986;58:305-323.

40. Abdalla S, Weatherall DJ, Wickramasinghe SN, Hughes M. The anaemia of *P. falciparum* malaria. Br J Haematol. 1980;46:171-183.

41. McGuire W, D'Alessandro U, Olaleye BO, et al. C-reactive protein and haptoglobin in the evaluation of a community-based malaria control programme. Trans R Soc Trop Med Hyg, 1996;90:10-14.

42. Weatherall DJ. The anaemia of malaria. In Wernsdorfer WH, McGregor IA (eds). Malaria: Principles and Practice

of Malariology. Edinburgh, Churchill Livingstone, 1988, pp 735-751.

43. Jakeman GN, Saul A, Hogarth WL, et al. Anaemia of acute malaria infections in non-immune patients primarily results from destruction of uninfected erythrocytes. Parasitology. 1999;119:127-133.

44. Looareesuwan S, Merry AH, Phillips RE, et al. Reduced erythrocyte survival following clearance of malarial parasitaemia in Thai patients. Br J Haematol. 1987;67:473-478.

45. Rosenberg EB, Strickland GT, Yang SL, Whalin GE. IgM antibodies to red cells and autoimmune anemia in patients with malaria. Am J Trop Med Hyg. 1973;22:146-152.

46. Allred D. Immune evasion by *Babesia bovis* and *Plasmodium falciparum*: cliff-dwellers of the parasite world. Parasitol Today. 1995;11:100-105.

47. Wyler DJ. The spleen in malaria. Ciba Found Symp. 1983;94:98-116.

48. Weiss L, Geduldig U, Weidanz W. Mechanisms of splenic control of murine malaria: reticular cell activation and the development of a blood-spleen barrier. Am J Anat. 1986;176:251-285.

49. Lee SH, Crocker PR, Gordon S. Macrophage plasma membrane and secretory properties in murine malaria. J Exp Med. 1986;163:54-74.

50. Looareesuwan S, Ho M, Wattanagoon Y, et al. Dynamic alterations in splenic function during acute falciparum malaria. N Engl J Med. 1987;317:675-679.

51. Dondorp AM, Angus BJ, Chotivanich K, et al. Red blood cell deformability as a predictor of anemia in severe falciparum malaria. Am J Trop Med Hyg. 1999;60:733-737.

52. Lee SH, Looareesuwan S, Wattanagoon Y, et al. Antibody-dependent red cell removal during *P. falciparum* malaria: the clearance of red cells sensitised with an IgG anti-D. Br J Haematol. 1989;73:396-402.

53. Bron AE, Webster HK, Teja-Isavadharm P, et al. Macrophage activation in falciparum malaria as measured by neopterin and interferon-gamma. Clin Exp Immunol. 1990;82:97-101.

54. Mohan K, Dubey ML, Ganguly NK, et al. *Plasmodium falciparum*: role of activated blood monocytes in erythrocyte membrane damage and red cell loss during malaria. Exp Parasitol. 1995;80:54-63.

55. Ladhani S, Lowe B, Cole AO, et al. Changes in white blood cells and platelets in children with falciparum malaria: relationship to disease outcome. Br J Haematol. 2002;119:839-847.

56. Evans KJ, Hansen DS, van Rooijen N, et al. Severe malarial anemia of low parasite burden in rodent models results from accelerated clearance of uninfected erythrocytes. Blood. 2006;107:1192-1199.

57. Angus BJ, Chotivanich K, Udomsangpetch R, et al. In vivo removal of malaria parasites from red blood cells without their destruction in acute falciparum malaria. Blood. 1997;90:2037-2040.

58. Wickramasinghe SN, Looareesuwan S, Nagachinta B, White NJ. Dyserythropoiesis and ineffective erythropoiesis in *Plasmodium vivax* malaria. Br J Haematol. 1989;72:91-99.

59. Wickramasinghe SN, Phillips RE, Looareesuwan S, et al. The bone marrow in human cerebral malaria: parasite sequestration within sinusoids. Br J Haematol. 1987;66:295-306.

60. Kwiatkowski D, Hill AVS, Sambou I, et al. TNF concentration in fatal cerebral, non-fatal cerebral, and uncomplicated *Plasmodium falciparum* malaria. Lancet. 1990;336:1201-1204.

61. Adams DO, Hamilton TA. Macrophages as destructive cells in host defence. In Gallin JI, Goldstein IM, Snyderman R (eds). Inflammation: Basic Principles and Clinical Correlates. New York, Raven Press, 1992, pp 637-662.

62. Taverne J, Sheikh N, de Souza JB, et al. Anaemia and resistance to malaria in transgenic mice expressing human tumour necrosis factor. Immunology. 1994;82:397-403.

63. Manson-Bahr PEC, Bell DR. Manson's Tropical Diseases. London, Bailliere Tindall, 1987, pp 19-22.

64. Price R, van Vugt M, Phaipun L, et al. Adverse effects in patients with acute falciparum malaria treated with artemisinin derivatives. Am J Trop Med Hyg. 1999;60:547-555.

65. Mojon M, Wallon M, Gravey A, et al. Intravascular haemolysis following halofantrine intake. Trans R Soc Trop Med Hyg. 1994;88:91.

66. Tran TH, Day NP, Ly VC, et al. Blackwater fever in southern Vietnam: a prospective descriptive study of 50 cases. Clin Infect Dis. 1996;23:1274-1281.

67. Dondorp AM, Omodeo-Sale F, Chotivanich K, et al. Oxidative stress and rheology in severe malaria. Redox Rep. 2003;8:292-294.

68. Omodeo-Sale F, Motti A, Dondorp A, et al. Destabilisation and subsequent lysis of human erythrocytes induced by *Plasmodium falciparum* haem products. Eur J Haematol. 2005;74:324-332.

69. Dondorp AM, Nyanoti M, Kager PA, et al. The role of reduced red cell deformability in the pathogenesis of severe falciparum malaria and its restoration by blood transfusion. Trans R Soc Trop Med Hyg. 2002;96:282-286.

70. Zuckerman A. Recent studies on factors involved in malarial anaemia. Mil Med. 1966;131(Suppl):1201.

71. Facer CA: Direct Coombs antiglobulin reactions in Gambian children with *Plasmodium falciparum* malaria. II: Specificity of erythrocyte bound IgG. Clin Exp Immunol. 1980;39:279-288.

72. Facer CA. Direct antiglobulin reactions in Gambian children with *P. falciparum* malaria. III. Expression of IgG subclass determinants and genetic markers and association with anaemia. Clin Exp Immunol. 1980;41:81-90.

73. Facer CA, Bray RS, Brown J. Direct Coombs' antiglobulin reactions in Gambian children with *Plasmodium falciparum* malaria. I. Incidence and class specificity. Clin Exp Immunol. 1979;35:119-127.

74. Abdalla SH, Kasili FG, Weatherall DJ. The Coombs direct antiglobulin test in Kenyans. Trans R Soc Trop Med Hyg. 1983;77:99-102.

75. Merry AH, Looareesuwan S, Phillips RE, et al. Evidence against immune haemolysis in falciparum malaria in Thailand. Br J Haematol. 1986;64:187-194.

76. Abdalla S, Weatherall DJ. The direct antiglobulin test in *P. falciparum* malaria. Br J Haematol. 1982;51:415-425.

77. Layez C, Nogueira P, Combes V, et al. *Plasmodium falciparum* rhoptry protein RSP2 triggers destruction of the erythroid lineage. Blood 2005;106:3632-3638.

78. Ritter K, Kuhlencord A, Thomssen R, Brommer W. Prolonged haemolytic anaemia in malaria and autoantibodies

against triosephosphate isomerase. Lancet. 1993;342: 1333-1334.

79. Wickramasinghe SN, Abdalla A, Weatherall DJ. Cell cycle distribution of erythroblasts in *P. falciparum* malaria. Scand J Haematol. 1982;29:83-88.

80. Casals-Pascual C, Kai O, Cheung O, et al. Suppression of erythropoiesis in malarial anemia is associated with hemozoin in vitro and in vivo. Blood. 2006;108:2569-2577.

81. Burchard GD, Radloff P, Philipps J, et al. Increased erythropoietin production in children with severe malarial anemia. Am J Trop Med Hyg. 1995;53:547-551.

82. el Hassan AM, Saeed AM, Fandrey J, et al. Decreased erythropoietin response in *Plasmodium falciparum* malaria–associated anaemia. Eur J Haematol. 1997;59:299-304.

83. Burgmann H, Looareesuwan S, Kapiotis S, et al. Serum levels of erythropoietin in acute *Plasmodium falciparum* malaria. Am J Trop Med Hyg. 1996;54:280-283.

84. McGuire W, Knight JC, Hill AV, et al. Severe malarial anemia and cerebral malaria are associated with different tumor necrosis factor promoter alleles. J Infect Dis. 1999;179:287-290.

85. Roodman GD, Bird A, Hutzler D, Montgomery W. Tumor necrosis factor-α and hematopoietic progenitors: Effects of tumor necrosis factor on the growth of erythroid progenitors CFU-E and BFU-E and the hematopoietic cell lines K562, HL60, HEL cells. Exp Hematol. 1987; 15:928-935.

86. Zucali JR, Broxmeyer HE, Gross MA, Dinarello CA. Recombinant human tumor necrosis factors α and β stimulate fibroblasts to produce hemopoietic growth factors in vitro. J Immunol. 1988;140:840-844.

87. Johnson RA, Waddelow TA, Caro J, et al. Chronic exposure to tumor necrosis factor in vivo preferentially inhibits erythropoiesis in nude mice. Blood. 1989;74: 130-138.

88. Pichangkul S, Saengkrai P, Webster HK. *Plasmodium falciparum* pigment induces monocytes to release high levels of tumor necrosis factor alpha and interleukin 1-beta. Am J Trop Med Hyg. 1994;51:430-435.

89. Miller KL, Silverman PH, Kullgren B, Mahlmann LJ. Tumor necrosis factor alpha and the anemia associated with murine malaria. Infect Immunol. 1989;19: 1542-1546.

90. Othoro C, Lal AA, Nahlen B, et al. A low interleukin-10 tumor necrosis factor-alpha ratio is associated with malaria anemia in children residing in a holoendemic malaria region in Western Kenya. J Infect Dis. 1999;179: 279-282.

91. Kurtzhals JA, Adabayeri V, Goka BQ, et al. Low plasma concentrations of interleukin 10 in severe malarial anaemia compared with cerebral and uncomplicated malaria [published erratum appears in Lancet 1998; 352:242]. Lancet. 1998;351:1768-1772.

92. Mohan K, Stevenson MM. Interleukin-12 corrects severe anemia during blood-stage *Plasmodium chabaudi* AS in susceptible A/J mice. Exp Hematol 1998;26:45-52.

93. Mohan K, Stevenson MM. Dyserythropoiesis and severe anaemia associated with malaria correlate with deficient interleukin-12 production. Br J Haematol. 1998;103:942-949.

94. Schwarzer E, Ludwig P, Valente E, et al. 15(S)-hydroxye-icosatetraenoic acid (15-HETE), a product of arachidonic

acid peroxidation, is an active component of hemozoin toxicity to monocytes. Parassitologia. 1999;41:199-202.

95. Schwarzer E, Kuhn H, Valente E, et al. Malaria-parasitized erythrocytes and hemozoin nonenzymatically generate large amounts of hydroxy fatty acids that inhibit monocyte functions. Blood. 2003;101:722-728.

96. Giribaldi G, Ulliers D, Schwarzer E, et al. Hemozoin- and 4-hydroxynonenal–mediated inhibition of erythropoiesis. Possible role in malarial dyserythropoiesis and anemia. Haematologica. 2004;89:492-493.

97. Grau GE, Tacchini-Cottier F, Vesin C, et al. TNF-induced microvascular pathology: active role for platelets and importance of the LFA-1/ICAM-1 interaction. Eur Cytokine Netw. 1993;4:415-419.

98. Brabin B. Fetal anaemia in malarious areas: its causes and significance. Ann Trop Paediatr. 1992;12:303.

99. Reed SC, Wirima JJ, Steketee RW. Risk factors for anemia in young children in rural Malawi. Am J Trop Med Hyg. 1994;51:170-174.

100. Cornet M, Le Hesran JY, Fievet N, et al. Prevalence of and risk factors for anemia in young children in southern Cameroon. Am J Trop Med Hyg. 1998;58:606-611.

101. Looareesuwan S, Suntharasamai P, Webster HK, et al. Malaria in splenectomized patients: report of four cases and review. Clin Infect Dis. 1993;16:361-366.

102. Fakunle YM. Tropical splenomegaly. Part I: tropical Africa. Clin Haematol. 1981;10:963-975.

103. Crane GG. Tropical splenomegaly. Part 2: Oceania. Clin Haematol. 1981;10:976-982.

104. Ziegler JL, Stuiver PC. Tropical splenomegaly syndrome in a Rwandan kindred in Uganda. BMJ. 1972;3:79-82.

105. Martin-Peprah R, Bates I, Bedu-Addo G, et al. Investigation of familial segregation of hyperreactive malarial splenomegaly in Kumasi, Ghana. Trans R Soc Trop Med Hyg. 2006;100:68-73.

106. Bates I, Bedu-Addo G, Bevan DH, et al. Use of immunoglobulin gene rearrangements to show clonal lymphoproliferation in hyper-reactive malarial splenomegaly. Lancet. 1991;337:505-507.

107. Neva F, Sacks D. Leishmaniasis. In Warren KS, Mahmoud AAF (eds). Tropical and Geographic Medicine. New York, McGraw-Hill, 1989, pp 296-308.

108. Herwaldt BL. Leishmaniasis. Lancet. 1999;354:1191-1199.

109. Alvar J, Canavate C, Gutierrez-Solar B, et al. *Leishmania* and human immunodeficiency virus coinfection: the first 10 years. Clin Microbiol Rev. 1997;10:298-319.

110. Musumeci S, Romeo M, D'Agata A. Red cell survival and iron kinetics in kala-azar. J Trop Med Hyg. 1974;77:106-110.

111. Woodruff AW, Topley E, Knight R, Downie CG. The anaemia of kala-azar. Br J Haematol. 1972;22:319-329.

112. Pippard MJ, Moir D, Weatherall DJ, Lenicker HM. Mechanism of anaemia in resistant visceral leishmaniasis. Ann Trop Med Parasitol. 1986;80:317-323.

113. Li Volti S, Fischer A, Musumeci S. Hematological and serological aspects of Mediterranean kala-azar in infancy and childhood. Acta Trop. 1980;37:351-365.

114. Mahmoud AAF, Wahab MFA. Schistosomiasis. In Warren KS, Mahmoud AAF (eds). Tropical and Geographic Medicine. New York, McGraw-Hill, 1989, pp 458-473.

115. Southgate VR, Rollinson D, Tchuem Tchuenté LA, Hagan P. Towards control of schistosomiasis in sub-Saharan Africa. J Helminthol. 2005;79:181-185.

116. World Health Organization: Progress in Assessment of Morbidity Due to *Schistosoma haematobium* Infection: A Review of Recent Literature, WHO/Schisto/87.91. Geneva, World Health Organization, 1987.

117. Englund PT, Smith DH. African trypanosomiasis. In Warren KS, Mahmoud AAF (eds). Tropical and Geographic Medicine. New York, McGraw-Hill, 1989, pp 268-281.

118. Nogueira N, Coura JR. American trypanosomiasis (Chagas' disease). In Warren KS, Mahmoud AAF (eds). Tropical and Geographic Medicine. New York, McGraw-Hill, 1989, pp 281-296.

119. Barrett MP, Burchmore RJ, Stich A et al. The trypanosomiases. Lancet. 2003;362:1469-1480.

120. Papadopoulos MC, Abel PM, Agranoff D, et al. A novel and accurate diagnostic test for human African trypanosomiasis. Lancet. 2004;363:1358-1363.

121. Schad GA, Banwell JG. Hookworms. In Warren KS, Mahmoud AAF (eds). Tropical and Geographic Medicine. New York, McGraw-Hill, 1989, pp 379-393.

122. Roche M, Layrisse M. The nature and causes of "hookworm anemia." Am J Trop Med Hyg. 1966;15:1029-1102.

123. Albonico M, Stoltzfus RJ, Savioli L, et al. Epidemiological evidence for a differential effect of hookworm species, *Ancylostoma duodenale* or *Necator americanus*, on iron status of children. Int J Epidemiol. 1998;27:530-537.

124. Gilles HM, Watson-Williams EJ, Ball PA. Hookworm infection and anaemia. Q J Med. 1964;33:1-24.

125. Tripathy K, Garcia FT, Lotero H. Effect of nutritional repletion on human hookworm infection. Am J Trop Med Hyg. 1971;20:219-223.

126. Banwell JG, Marsden PD, Blackman V, et al. Hookworm infection and intestinal absorption amongst Africans in Uganda. Am J Trop Med Hyg. 1967;16:304-308.

127. Variyam EP, Banwell JG: Nutrition implications of hookworm infection. Rev Infect Dis. 1982;4:830-835.

128. Stoltzfus RJ, Albonico M, Chwaya HM, et al. Effects of the Zanzibar school–based deworming program on iron status of children. Am J Clin Nutr. 1998;68:179-186.

129. Blackman V, Marsden P, Banwell J, Craggs MH. Albumin metabolism in hookworm anemia. Trans R Soc Trop Med Hyg. 1965;59:472-482.

130. Quinn TC, Ruff A, Halsey N. Special considerations for developing nations. In Pizzo PA, Wilfert CM (eds). Pediatric AIDS: The Challenge of HIV Infection in Infants, Children and Adolescents. Baltimore, Williams & Wilkins, 1994, pp 31-49.

131. Ryder RW, Nsa W, Hassig SE, et al. Perinatal transmission of the human immunodeficiency virus type 1 to infants of seropositive women in Zaire. N Engl J Med. 1989;320:1637-1642.

132. Semba RD, Miotti PG, Chiphangwi JD, et al. Maternal vitamin A deficiency and mother-to-child transmission of HIV-1. Lancet. 1994;343:1593-1597.

133. Tovo PA, De Martino M, Gabiano C, et al. Prognostic factors and survival in children with perinatal HIV-1 infection. The Italian Register for HIV Infection in Children. Lancet. 1992;339:1249-1253.

134. Folks TM, Kessler SW, Orenstein JM, et al. Infection and replication of HIV-1 in purified progenitor cells of normal human bone marrow. Science. 1988;242:919-922.

135. Zucker-Franklin D, Cao Y: Megakaryocytes of human immunodeficiency virus–infected individuals express viral RNA. Proc Natl Acad Sci U S A. 1989;86:5595-5599.

136. Ellaurie M, Burns ER, Rubinstein A. Hematologic manifestations in pediatric HIV infection: severe anemia as a prognostic factor. Am J Pediatr Hematol Oncol. 1990;12:449-453.

137. Perkocha LA, Rodgers GM. Hematologic aspects of human immunodeficiency virus infection: laboratory and clinical considerations. Am J Hematol. 1988;29:94-105.

138. Labrune P, Blanche S, Catherine N, et al. Human immunodeficiency virus–associated thrombocytopenia in infants. Acta Paediatr Scand. 1989;78:811-814.

139. Mann JM, Francis H, Davachi F, et al. Risk factors for human immunodeficiency virus seropositivity among children 1-24 months old in Kinshasa, Zaire. Lancet. 1986;2:654-647.

140. Jäger H, N'Galy B, Perriens J, et al. Prevention of transfusion-associated HIV transmission in Kinshasa, Zaire: HIV screening is not enough. AIDS. 1990;4:571-574.

141. Mahmoud AAF. Eosinophilia. In Warren KS, Mahmoud AAF (eds). Tropical and Geographic Medicine. New York, McGraw-Hill, 1989, pp 65-70.

142. Ottesen EA. The filariases and tropical eosinophilia. In Warren KS, Mahmoud AAF (eds). Tropical and Geographic Medicine. New York, McGraw-Hill, 1989, pp 407-429.

143. Danaraj TJ, Pacheco G, Shanmugaratnam K, Beaver PC. The etiology and pathology of eosinophilic lung (tropical eosinophilia). Am J Trop Med Hyg. 1966;15:183-189.

144. Joe LK. Occult filariasis: its relationship with tropical pulmonary eosinophilia. Am J Trop Med Hyg. 1962;11:646-651.

145. Dennis DT, McConnell E, White GB. Bancroftian filariasis and membrane filters: are night surveys necessary? Am J Trop Med Hyg. 1976;25:257-262.

146. Mathan VI. Gastrointestinal manifestations. In Warren KS, Mahmoud AAF (eds). Tropical and Geographic Medicine. New York, McGraw-Hill, 1989, pp 8-15.

147. Baker SJ, Mathan VI. Tropical enteropathy and tropical sprue. Am J Clin Nutr. 1972;25:1047-1055.

148. Mathan M, Mathan VI: Rectal mucosal morphologic abnormalities in normal subjects in southern India. A tropical colonopathy. Gut. 1985;26:710-717.

149. Farthing MJG. Malabsorption in the tropics. In Weatherall DJ, Ledingham JGG, Warrell DA (eds). Oxford Textbook of Medicine. Oxford, Oxford University Press, 1995, pp 14.112-14.118.

150. Lindenbaum J, Gerson CD, Kent TH. Recovery of small intestinal structure and function after residence in the tropics. I. Studies of Peace Corps volunteers. Ann Intern Med. 1971;74:218-222.

151. Klipstein FA. Tropical sprue in travelers and expatriates living abroad. Gastroenterology. 1981;80:590-600.

152. Klipstein FA, Samloff MI, Schenk EA. Tropical sprue in Haiti. Ann Intern Med. 1966;64:575-594.

153. Klipstein FA, Holdeman LV, Corcino JJ, Moore WE. Enterotoxigenic intestinal bacteria in tropical sprue. Ann Intern Med. 1973;79:632-641.

154. Bhat P, Shanthakumari S, Rajan D, et al. Bacterial flora of the gastrointestinal tract in southern Indian control subjects and patients with tropical sprue. Gastroenterology. 1972;62:11-21.

155. Serwadda D, Mugerwa RD, Sewankambo NK, et al. Slim disease: a new disease in Uganda and its association with HTLV-III infection. Lancet. 1985;2:849-852.

156. Sewankambo N, Mugerwa RD, Goodgame R, et al. Enteropathic AIDS in Uganda: an endoscopic, histological and microbiological study. AIDS. 1987;1:9-13.

157. Halstead SB. Dengue. In Warren KS, Mahmoud AAF (eds). Tropical and Geographic Medicine. New York, McGraw-Hill, 1989, pp 675-685.

158. World Health Organization: Dengue Hemorrhagic Fever: Diagnosis, Treatment and Control. Geneva, World Health Organization, 1986.

159. Bhamarapravati N, Tuchinda P, Boonyapaknavik V. Pathology of Thailand, haemorrhagic fever: A study of 100 autopsy cases. Ann Tropical Med Parasitol. 1967;61: 500-510.

160. Pathogenetic mechanisms in dengue haemorrhagic fever. Report of an internal collaborative study. Bull World Health Organ. 1973;48:117-133.

161. Kurane I, Innis BL, Nimmannitya S, et al. Activation of T lymphocytes in dengue virus infections. High levels of soluble interleukin 2 receptor, soluble CD4, soluble CD8, interleukin 2 and interferon-gamma in sera of children with dengue. J Clin Invest. 1991;88:1473-1480.

162. Bethell DB, Flobbe K, Cao XT, et al. Pathophysiologic and prognostic role of cytokines in dengue hemorrhagic fever. J Infect Dis. 1998;177:778-782.

163. Chungue E, Poli L, Roche C, et al. Correlation between detection of plasminogen cross-reactive antibodies and hemorrhage in dengue virus infection. J Infect Dis. 1994;170:1304-1307.

164. Markoff LJ, Innis BL, Houghten R, Henchal LS. Development of cross-reactive antibodies to plasminogen during the immune response to dengue virus infection. J Infect Dis. 1991;164:294-301.

165. Wills BA, Oragui EE, Stephens AC, et al. Coagulation abnormalities in dengue hemorrhagic fever: serial investigations in 167 Vietnamese children with dengue shock syndrome. Clin Infect Dis. 2002;35:277-285.

166. Wills BA, Nguyen MD, Ha TL, et al. Comparison of three fluid solutions for resuscitation in dengue shock syndrome. N Engl J Med. 2005;353:877-889.

167. McCormick JB, Fisher-Hoch S. Viral hemorrhagic fevers. In Warren KS, Mahmoud AAF (eds). Tropical and Geographic Medicine. New York, McGraw-Hill, 1989, pp 700-728.

168. Cosgriff TM. Viruses and hemostasis. Rev Infect Dis. 1989;11:S672-S688.

169. Warrell DA. Venomous and poisonous animals. In Warren KS, Mahmoud AAF (eds). Tropical and Geographic Medicine. New York, McGraw-Hill, 1989, pp 533-556.

170. Mebs D. Pharmacology of reptilian venoms. In Gans C, Gans KA (eds). Biology of the Reptilia, vol 8. London, Academic Press, 1978, pp 437-560.

171. Ménez A. Molecular immunology of snake toxins. Pharmacol Ther. 1985;30:91-113.

172. Kornalík F. The influence of snake venom enzymes on blood coagulation. Pharmacol Ther. 1985;29:353-405.

173. Warrell DA, Greenwood BM, Davidson NM, et al. Necrosis, haemorrhage and complement depletion following bites by the spitting cobra (*Naja nigricollis*). Q J Med. 1976;45:1-22.

174. Malasit P, Warrell DA, Chanthavanich P, et al. Prediction, prevention and mechanism of early (anaphylactic) antivenom reactions in victims of snake bites. BMJ. 1986;292: 17-20.

175. Tun-Pe, Phillips RE, Warrell DA, et al. Acute and chronic pituitary failure resembling Sheehen's syndrome following bites by Russell's viper in Burma. Lancet. 1987;2: 763-767.

176. Hutt MSR, Burkitt DP. The Geography of Non-Infectious Disease. Oxford, Oxford University Press, 1986, pp 98-107.

177. Blattner WA, Blayney DW, Robert-Guroff M, et al. Epidemiology of human T-cell leukaemia/lymphoma virus. J Infect Dis. 1983;147:406-416.

178. Whittle HC, Brown J, Marsh K, et al. T-cell control of Epstein-Barr virus–infected B cells is lost during *P. falciparum* malaria. Nature. 1984 312:449-450.

179. Ramot B, Hulu N. Primary intestinal lymphoma and its relation to alpha chain disease. Br J Cancer. 1975;11: 343-349.

180. Dutz W, Borochovitz D, et al. The two basic forms of primary intestinal lymphoma. In Proceedings of the Symposium on Prevention and Detection of Cancer. New York, Marcel Dekker, 1980.

181. Burn C, Davies JNP, Dodge OG, Nias BC. Hodgkin's disease in English and African children. J Natl Cancer Inst. 1971;46:37-41.

182. Williams CKO, Folami AO, Laditan AA, Ukaljiofo EO. Childhood acute leukaemia in a tropical population. Br J Cancer. 1982;46:89-94.

183. Weatherall DJ, Clegg JB. The Thalassaemia Syndromes. Oxford, Blackwell Science, 2001.

184. Weatherall D, Akinyanju O, Fucharoen S, et al. Inherited disorders of hemoglobin. In Jamison DT, Breman JG, Measham AR, et al (eds). Disease Control Priorities in Developing Countries. New York, Oxford University Press and the World Bank, 2006, pp 663-680.

185. Bienzle U. Glucose-6-phosphate dehydrogenase deficiency. Part I: tropical Africa. Clin Haematol. 1981;10: 785-799.

186. Panich V: Glucose-6-phosphate dehydrogenase deficiency. Part 2: tropical Asia. Clin Haematol. 1981;10:800-814.

187. Chan MCK. Neonatal jaundice. In Hendrickse RG (ed). Paediatrics in the Tropics. Oxford, Oxford Medical, 1981, pp 13-26.

188. Allen SJ, O'Donnell A, Alexander NDE, et al. Prevention of cerebral malaria in children in Papua New Guinea by Southeast Asian ovalocytosis band 3. Am J Trop Med Hyg. 1999;60:1056-1060.

189. Wasi P, Piankijagum A, et al. Geographical variation in blood disease: Southeast Asia. In Weatherall DJ, Ledingham JGG, Warrell DA (eds). Oxford Textbook of Medicine. Oxford, Oxford University Press, 1987, pp 19.266-19.268.

190. Bhanchet-Isarangkura P. The pathogenesis of acquired prothrombin complex deficiency syndrome (APCD syndrome) in infants. Southeast Asian J Trop Med Public Health. 1979;10:350-352.

191. Suvatte V, Mahasandana C, Tanphaichitr V, Tuchinda S. Acquired platelet dysfunction with eosinophilia: study of platelet function in 62 cases. Southeast Asian J Trop Med Public Health. 1979;10:358-367.

192. Mehta BC. Geographical variation in blood disease: India. In Weatherall DJ, Ledingham JGG, Warrell DA (eds). Oxford Textbook of Medicine. Oxford, Oxford University Press, 1987, pp 19.270-19.273.

193. Brewster DR, Kwiatkowski D, White NJ. Neurological sequelae of cerebral malaria in children. Lancet. 1990;336:1039-1043.

194. Greenberg AE, Nguyen-Dinh P, Mann JM, et al. The association between malaria, blood transfusion and HIV seropositivity in a pediatric population in Kinshasa, Zaire. JAMA. 1988;259:545-549.

195. Carlson J, Wahlgren M: *Plasmodium falciparum* erythrocyte rosetting is mediated by promiscuous lectin-like interactions. J Exp Med. 1992;176:1311-1317.

196. Obonyo CO, Steyerberg EW, Oloo AJ, et al. Blood transfusions for severe malaria-related anemia in Africa: A decision analysis. Am J Trop Med Hyg. 1998;59:808-812.

197. Meremikwu M, Smith HJ. Blood transfusion for treating malarial anaemia. Cochrane Database Syst Rev 2000;2:CD001475.

198. Marsh K, Forster D, Waruiru C, et al. Indicators of life-threatening malaria in African children. N Engl J Med. 1995;332:1399-1404.

199. Lackritz EM, Campbell CC, Ruebush TKD, et al. Effect of blood transfusion on survival among children in a Kenyan hospital. Lancet. 1992;340:524-528.

200. English M, Waruiru C, Marsh K. Transfusion for respiratory distress in life-threatening childhood malaria. Am J Trop Med Hyg 1996;55:525-530.

201. English M, Muambi B, Mithwani S, et al. Lactic acidosis and oxygen debt in African children with severe anaemia. Q J Med. 1997;90:563-569.

202. English M. Life-threatening severe malarial anaemia. Trans R Soc Trop Med Hyg. 2000;94:585-588.

203. Murray MJ, Murray AB, Murray NJ, Murray CJ. The adverse effect of iron repletion on the course of certain infections. BMJ. 1978;2:1113-1115.

204. Oppenheimer SJ, Gibson FD, Macfarlane SB, et al. Iron supplementation increases prevalence and effects of malaria: Report on clinical studies in Papua New Guinea. Trans R Soc Trop Med Hyg. 1986;80:603-612.

205. Watkins WM, Sixsmith DG, Chulay JD, Spencer HC. Antagonism of sulfadoxine and pyrimethamine antimalarial activity in vitro by *p*-aminobenzoic acid, *p*-aminobenzoylglutamic acid and folic acid. Mol Biochem Parasitol. 1985;14:55-61.

206. van Hensbroek MB, Morris-Jones S, Meisner S, et al. Iron, but not folic acid, combined with effective antimalarial therapy promotes haematological recovery after acute falciparum malaria. Trans R Soc Trop Med Hyg. 1995;89:672-676.

207. Lynk A, Gold R. Review of 40 children with imported malaria. Pediatr Infect Dis. 1989;8:745-750.

208. Pattanasin S, Proux S, Chompasuk D, et al. Evaluation of a new *Plasmodium* lactate dehydrogenase assay (OptiMAL-IT) for the detection of malaria. Trans R Soc Trop Med Hyg. 2003;97:672-674.

209. Beadle C, Long GW, Weiss WR, et al. Diagnosis of malaria by detection of *Plasmodium falciparum* HRP-2 antigen with a rapid dipstick antigen-capture assay. Lancet. 1994;343:564-568.

210. Murphy GS, Basri H, Purnomo, et al. Vivax malaria resistant to treatment and prophylaxis with chloroquine. Lancet. 1993;341:96-100.

211. Waller D, Krishna S, Craddock C, et al. The pharmacokinetic properties of intramuscular quinine in Gambian children with severe falciparum malaria. Trans R Soc Trop Med Hyg. 1990;84:488-491.

212. Hien TT, White NJ. Qinghaosu. Lancet. 1993;341:603-608.

213. Wyler DJ. Bark, weeds, and iron chelators—drugs for malaria. N Engl J Med. 1992;327:1519-1521.

214. Taylor TE, Molyneux ME, Wirima JJ, et al. Blood glucose levels in Malawian children before and during the administration of intravenous quinine for severe falciparum malaria. N Engl J Med. 1988;319:1040-1046.

215. Taylor TE, Borgstein A, Molyneux ME. Acid-base status in paediatric *Plasmodium falciparum* malaria. Q J Med. 1993;86:99-109.

216. Crawley J, Waruiru C, Mithwani S, et al. Effect of phenobarbital on seizure frequency and mortality in childhood cerebral malaria: a randomised, controlled intervention study. Lancet. 2000;355:701-706.

217. Maitland K, Pamba A, English M, et al. Randomized trial of volume expansion with albumin or saline in children with severe malaria: preliminary evidence of albumin benefit. Clin Infect Dis. 2005;40:538-545.

218. Planche T, Onanga M, Schwenk A, et al. Assessment of volume depletion in children with malaria. PLoS Med 2004;1:e18.

219. Newton CRJC, Kirkham FJ, Winstanley PA, et al. Intracranial pressure in African children with cerebral malaria. Lancet. 1991;337:573-576.

220. Davidson RN. Practical guide for the treatment of leishmaniasis. Drugs. 1998;56:1009-1018.

221. Murray HW. Treatment of visceral leishmaniasis (kala-azar): a decade of progress and future approaches. Int J Infect Dis. 2000;4:158-177.

222. Alvar J, Croft S, Olliaro P. Chemotherapy in the treatment and control of leishmaniasis. Adv Parasitol. 2006;61:223-274.

223. di Martino L, Davidson RN, Giacchino R, et al. Treatment of visceral leishmaniasis in children with liposomal amphotericin B. J Pediatr. 1997;131:271-277.

224. Sundar S, Rosenkaimer F, Makharia MK, et al. Trial of oral miltefosine for visceral leishmaniasis. Lancet. 1998;352:1821-1823.

225. Vanlerberghe V, Diap G, Guerin PJ, et al. Drug policy for visceral leishmaniasis: a cost-effectiveness analysis. Trop Med Int Health. 2007;12:274-283.

Appendices

Reference Values in Infancy and Childhood

Carlo Brugnara

APPENDIX 1	Hematologic Values in Normal Fetuses at Different Gestational Ages						
Week of Gestation	Hemoglobin (g/dL)	RBCs (×10⁶/mL)	Hematocrit (%)	Mean Corpuscular Volume (fL)	Total WBCs (×10⁶/μL)	Corrected WBCs (×10⁶/μL)	Platelets (×10⁶/μL)
18-21 (n = 760)	11.69 ± 1.27	2.85 ± 0.36	37.3 ± 4.32	131.1 ± 11.0	4.68 ± 2.96	2.57 ± 0.42	234 ± 57
22-25 (n = 1200)	12.2 ± 1.6	3.09 ± 0.34	38.59 ± 3.94	125.1 ± 7.8	4.72 ± 2.82	3.73 ± 2.17	247 ± 59
26-29 (n = 460)	12.91 ± 1.38	3.46 ± 0.41	40.88 ± 4.4	118.5 ± 8.0	5.16 ± 2.53	4.08 ± 0.84	242 ± 69
>30 (n = 440)	13.64 ± 2.21	3.82 ± 0.64	43.55 ± 7.2	114.4 ± 9.3	7.71 ± 4.99	6.4 ± 2.99	232 ± 87

Hematologic data obtained with a Coulter S plus II instrument. Total WBC count included nucleated red blood cells. Corrected WBC count included only WBCs, after subtracting the nucleated red cell component, based on a 100-cell manual differential.

From Forestier F, Daffos F, Catherine N, et al: Developmental hematopoiesis in normal human fetal blood. Blood 1991; 77:2360.

APPENDIX 2	White Cell Manual Differential Counts in Normal Fetuses at Different Gestational Ages					
Week of Gestation	Lymphocytes (%)	Neutrophils (%)	Eosinophils (%)	Basophils (%)	Monocytes (%)	Nucleated Red Cells (% of WBC)
18-21 (n = 186)	88 ± 7	6 ± 4	2 ± 3	0.5 ± 1	3.5 ± 2	45 ± 86
22-25 (n = 230)	87 ± 6	6.5 ± 3.5	3 ± 3	0.5 ± 1	3.5 ± 2.5	21 ± 23
26-29 (n = 144)	85 ± 6	8.5 ± 4	4 ± 3	0.5 ± 1	3.5 ± 2.5	21 ± 67
>30 (n = 172)	68.5 ± 15	23 ± 15	5 ± 3	0.5 ± 1	3.5 ± 2	17 ± 40

From Forestier F, Daffos F, Catherine N, et al: Developmental hematopoiesis in normal human fetal blood. Blood 1991; 77:2360.

APPENDIX 3	Hematologic Parameters in Normal, Full-Term Cord Blood		
	Paterakis et al. (1993)*	Diagne et al. (1995)†	Boulot et al. (1993)‡
Hemoglobin (g/dL)	15.6 ± 1.2	15.3 ± 1.3	13.9 ± 1.6
RBCs (×10⁶/μL)	4.42 ± 0.35	4.30 ± 0.4	—
Hematocrit (%)	51.0 ± 4.5	49 ± 5	41.3 ± 4.9
Mean Corpuscular Volume (fL)	119.1 ± 4.8	112 ± 6	109 ± 9.8
Mean Corpuscular Hemoglobin (pg)	36.4 ± 1.6	36.2 ± 2.2	38.7 ± 4.0
Mean Corpuscular Hemoglobin Concentration (g/dL)	30.6 ± 1.3	30.9 ± 1.3	33.3 ± 1.4

Data are expressed as mean ± SD.

*Paterakis GS, Lykopoulou L, Papassotiriou J, et al: Flow-cytometric analysis of reticulocytes in normal cord blood. Acta Haematol 1993; 90:182. Data obtained in 35 specimens with H*1 Technicon analyzer.

†Diagne I, Archambeaud MP, Diallo D, et al: Parametres erythrocytaires et reservés en fer dans le sang du cordon. Arch Fr Pediatr 1995; 2:208. Data obtained in 142 specimens with H*2 Technicon analyzer.

‡Boulot P, Cattaneo A, Taib J, et al: Hematologic values of fetal blood obtained by means of cordocentesis. Fetal Diagn Ther 1993; 8:309.

APPENDIX 4	Erythroblast and Leukocyte Counts in Umbilical Cord Blood	
Type of Delivery	Erythroblast Count (×10⁹/L)	Leukocyte Count (×10⁹/L)
Spontaneous, vaginal (n = 55)	0.75 (0.0-5.3)	13.8 (7.25-48.0)
Elective cesarean section (n = 39)	0.30 (0.0-0.49)	10.6 (6.2-17.7)
Emergency cesarean section (n = 55)	1.10 (0.0-15.9)	13.5 (4.2-40.3)

Values are expressed as mean (range). Erythroblast counts were significantly higher in the spontaneous vaginal and emergency cesarean section groups compared with the elective cesarean delivery group.

From Thilaganathan B, Athanasiou S, Ozmen S, et al: Umbilical cord blood erythroblast count as an index of intrauterine hypoxia. Arch Dis Child 1994; 70: F192.

APPENDIX 5   Hematologic Values for Normal Cord Blood

	Mean ± SD
RED BLOOD CELLS	
Hb (g/dL)	15.3 ± 1.3
Hct (%)	49 ± 5
RBC (×10⁶/μL)	4.3 ± 0.4
MCV (fL)	112 ± 6
MCH (pg)	36.2 ± 2.2
MCHC (g/dL)	30.9 ± 1.3
CHCM (g/dL)	30.4 ± 1.2
% HYPO (MCHC < 28 g/dL)	17.3 ± 11.9
% HYPER (MCHC > 41 g/dL)	0.6 ± 0.3
% MICRO (MCV < 61 fL)	0.8 ± 0.3
% MACRO (MCV > 120 fL)	31.8 ± 9.7
RETICULOCYTES	
%	3.63 ± 1.11
Absolute reticulocytes (×10⁹/L)	156.1 ± 47.7
MCVr (fL)	125.8 ± 7.3
CHCMr (g/dL)	25.6 ± 1.2
CHr (pg)	31.3 ± 1.4

MCV = mean corpuscular volume; MCHC = mean corpuscular hemoglobin concentration; MCH = mean corpuscular hemoglobin; CHCM = cell hemoglobin concentration mean; % HYPO = % hypochromic red cells; % HYPER = % hyperchromic red cells; % MICRO = % microcytic red cells; % MACRO = % macrocytic red cells; MCVr = reticulocyte mean corpuscular volume; CHCMr = reticulocyte cell hemoglobin concentration mean; CHr = reticulocyte hemoglobin content. Values obtained with Technicon H˙2 and H˙3 Hematology analyzers (Bayer Diagnostics) in neonates delivered at term with weight ≥ 2500 g.

Adapted from Diagne I, Archambeaud MP, Diallo D, et al: Parametres erythrocytaires et reservés en fer dans le sang du cordon. Arch Fr Pediatr 1995; 2:208, and from G Tchernia, personal communication. Data obtained in 142 specimens with H˙2 Technicon analyzer.

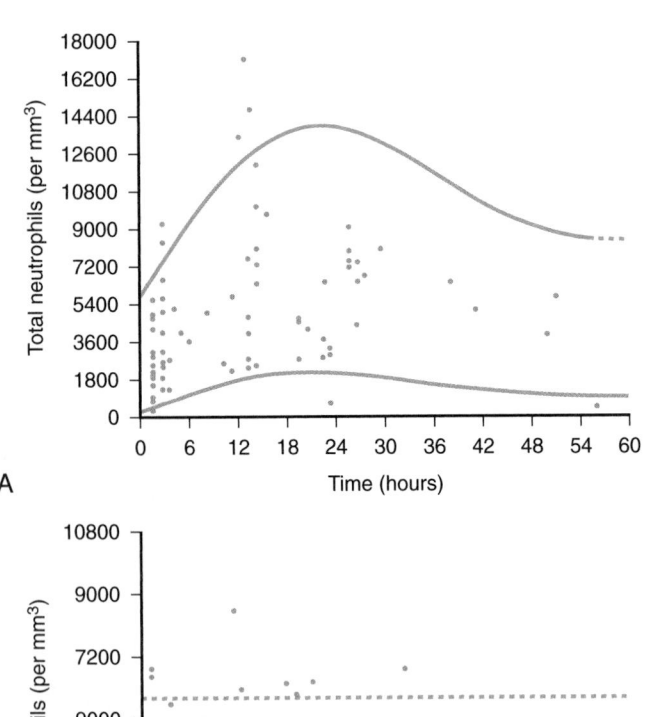

A

B

APPENDIX 6.   Reference range for circulating neutrophil counts in healthy very-low-birth-weight neonates. Based on 160 neutrophil counts obtained in 63 infants without perinatal complications at 0 to 60 hours of age. Birth weight was 1220 ± 203 g, gestational age 29.9 ± 2.3 weeks (± SD). **A,** Neutrophil count at birth to 60 hours of life. **B,** Neutrophil count at 61 hours to 28 days of life. Bold (*A*) and dotted (*B*) lines represent the envelopes bounding these data, respectively. (Redrawn from Mouzinho A, Rosenfeld CR, Sanchez PJ, et al: Revised reference ranges for circulating neutrophils in very-low-birth-weight neonates. Pediatrics 1994; 94:76. Reproduced by permission of Pediatrics, Copyright 1994.)

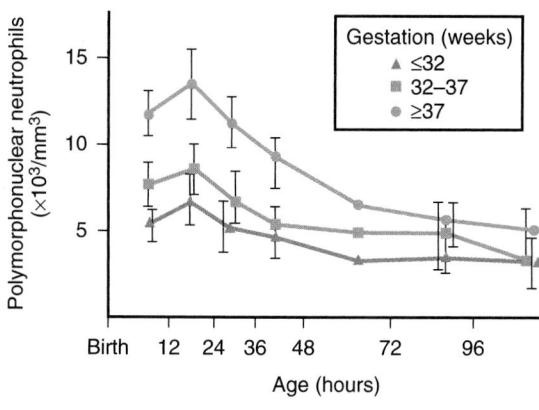

APPENDIX 7.   Changes in polymorphonuclear neutrophils after birth in three groups with different gestational ages. Total WBC counts were obtained with a Coulter S analyzer; manual differential counts were performed on 200 nucleated cells. (Redrawn from Coulombel L, Dehan M, Tchernia G, et al: The number of polymorphonuclear leukocytes in relation to gestational age in the newborn. Acta Paediatr Scand 1979; 68:709.)

APPENDIX 8	Normal Hematologic Values During the First 2 Weeks of Life in the Term Infant*				
Value	**Cord Blood**	**Day 1**	**Day 3**	**Day 7**	**Day 14**
Hemoglobin (g/dL)	16.8	18.4	17.8	17.0	16.8
Hematocrit (%)	53.0	58.0	55.0	54.0	52.0
Red cells (mm³)	5.25	5.8	5.6	5.2	5.1
MCV (fL)	107	108	99.0	98.0	96.0
MCH (pg)	34	35	33	32.5	31.5
MCHC (g/dL)	31.7	32.5	33	33	33
Reticulocytes (%)	3-7	3-7	1-3	0-1	0-1
Nucleated RBCs (/mm³)	500	200	0-5	0	0
Platelets (1000's/mm³)	290	192	213	248	252

MCV = mean corpuscular volume; MCH = mean corpuscular hemoglobin; MCHC = mean corpuscular hemoglobin concentration.

*During the first 2 weeks of life a venous hemoglobin value below 13.0 g/dL or a capillary hemoglobin value below 14.5 g/dL should be regarded as anemic.

From Oski FA, Naiman JL: Hematologic Problems in the Newborn. 2nd ed. Philadelphia, W.B. Saunders Co., 1972, p 13.

APPENDIX 9	Normal Hematologic Values During the First Year of Life in Healthy Term Infants*						
	AGE (mo)						
n	**0.5 (n = 232)**	**1 (n = 240)**	**2 (n = 241)**	**4 (n = 52)**	**6 (n = 52)**	**9 (n = 56)**	**12 (n = 56)**
Hemoglobin (mean ± SE)	16.6 ± 0.11	13.9 ± 0.10	11.2 ± 0.06	12.2 ± 0.14	12.6 ± 0.10	12.7 ± 0.09	12.7 ± 0.09
−2 SD	13.4	10.7	9.4	10.3	11.1	11.4	11.3
Hematocrit (mean ± SE)	53 ± 0.4	44 ± 0.3	35 ± 0.2	38 ± 0.4	36 ± 0.3	36 ± 0.3	37 ± 0.3
−2 SD	41	33	28	32	31	32	33
RBC count (mean ± SE)	4.9 ± 0.03	4.3 ± 0.03	3.7 ± 0.02	4.3 ± 0.06	4.7 ± 0.05	4.7 ± 0.04	4.7 ± 0.04
−2 SD +2 SD	3.9-5.9	3.3-5.3	3.1-4.3	3.5-5.1	3.9-5.5	4.0-5.3	4.1-5.3
MCH (mean ± SE)	33.6 ± 0.1	32.5 ± 0.1	30.4 ± 0.1	28.6 ± 0.2	26.8 ± 0.2	27.3 ± 0.2	26.8 ± 0.2
−2 SD	30	29	27	25	24	25	24
MCV (mean ± SE)	105.3 ± 0.6	101.3 ± 0.3	94.8 ± 0.3	86.7 ± 0.8	76.3 ± 0.6	77.7 ± 0.5	77.7 ± 0.5
−2 SD	88	91	84	76	68	70	71
MCHC (mean ± SE)	314 ± 1.1	318 ± 1.2	318 ± 1.1	327 ± 2.7	350 ± 1.7	349 ± 1.6	343 ± 1.5
−2 SD	281	281	283	288	327	324	321

MCH = mean corpuscular hemoglobin; MCV = mean corpuscular volume; MCHC = mean corpuscular hemoglobin concentration.

*These values were obtained from a selected group of 256 healthy term infants followed at the Helsinki University Central Hospital who were receiving continuous iron supplementation and who had normal values for transferrin saturation and serum ferritin.

Values at the ages of 0.5, 1, and 2 months were obtained from the entire group, and those at the later ages were obtained from the iron-supplemented infant group after exclusion of iron deficiency.

From Saarinen UM, Siimes MA: Developmental changes in red blood cell counts and indices of infants after exclusion of iron deficiency by laboratory criteria and continuous iron supplementation. J Pediatr 1978; 92:414.

APPENDIX 10 Hemoglobin Concentration During the First 6 Months of Life in Iron-Sufficient Preterm Infants*

		BIRTH WEIGHT	
Age	No.	1000-1500 g	1501-2000 g
2 wk	17, 39	16.3 (11.7-18.4)	14.8 (11.8-19.6)
1 mo	15, 42	10.9 (8.7-15.2)	11.5 (8.2-15.0)
2 mo	17, 47	8.8 (7.1-11.5)	9.4 (8.0-11.4)
3 mo	16, 41	9.8 (8.9-11.2)	10.2 (9.3-11.8)
4 mo	13, 37	11.3 (9.1-13.1)	11.3 (9.1-13.1)
5 mo	8, 21	11.6 (10.2-14.3)	11.8 (10.4-13.0)
6 mo	9, 21	12.0 (9.4-13.8)	11.8 (10.7-12.6)

*These infants were admitted to the Helsinki Children's Hospital during a 15-month period. None had a complicated course during the first 2 weeks of life or had undergone an exchange transfusion. All infants were iron sufficient, as indicated by a serum ferritin ≥ 10 ng/mL.

From Lundstrom U, Siimes MA, Dallman PR: At what age does iron supplementation become necessary in low birth weight infants? J Pediatr 1977; 91:882.

APPENDIX 11 Normal Hematologic Values in Children*

Age	HEMOGLOBIN (g/dL)		HEMATOCRIT (%)		RED CELL COUNT (10^{12}/L)		MCV (fL)		MCH (pg)		MCHC (g/dL)	
	Mean	−2 SD	Mean	−2 SD	Mean	−2 SD	Mean	−2 SD	Mean	−2 SD	Mean	−2 SD
Birth (cord blood)	16.5	13.5	51	42	4.7	3.9	108	98	34	31	33	30
1 to 3 days (capillary)	18.5	14.5	56	45	5.3	4.0	108	95	34	31	33	29
1 week	17.5	13.5	54	42	5.1	3.9	107	88	34	28	33	28
2 weeks	16.5	12.5	51	39	4.9	3.6	105	86	34	28	33	28
1 month	14.0	10.0	43	31	4.2	3.0	104	85	34	28	33	29
2 months	11.5	9.0	35	28	3.8	2.7	96	77	30	26	33	29
3 to 6 months	11.5	9.5	35	29	3.8	3.1	91	74	30	25	33	30
0.5 to 2 years	12.0	10.5	36	33	4.5	3.7	78	70	27	23	33	30
2 to 6 years	12.5	11.5	37	34	4.6	3.9	81	75	27	24	34	31
6 to 12 years	13.5	11.5	40	35	4.6	4.0	86	77	29	25	34	31
12 to 18 years												
Female	14.0	12.0	41	36	4.6	4.1	90	78	30	25	34	31
Male	14.5	13.0	43	37	4.9	4.5	88	78	30	25	34	31
18 to 49 years												
Female	14.0	12.0	41	36	4.6	4.0	90	80	30	26	34	31
Male	15.5	13.5	47	41	5.2	4.5	90	80	30	26	34	31

*These data have been compiled from several sources. Emphasis is given to studies employing electronic counters and to the selection of populations that are likely to exclude individuals with iron deficiency. The mean ±2 SD can be expected to include 95% of the observations in a normal population.

From Dallman PR: In Rudolph A (ed): Pediatrics, 16th ed. New York, Appleton-Century-Crofts, 1977, p 1111.

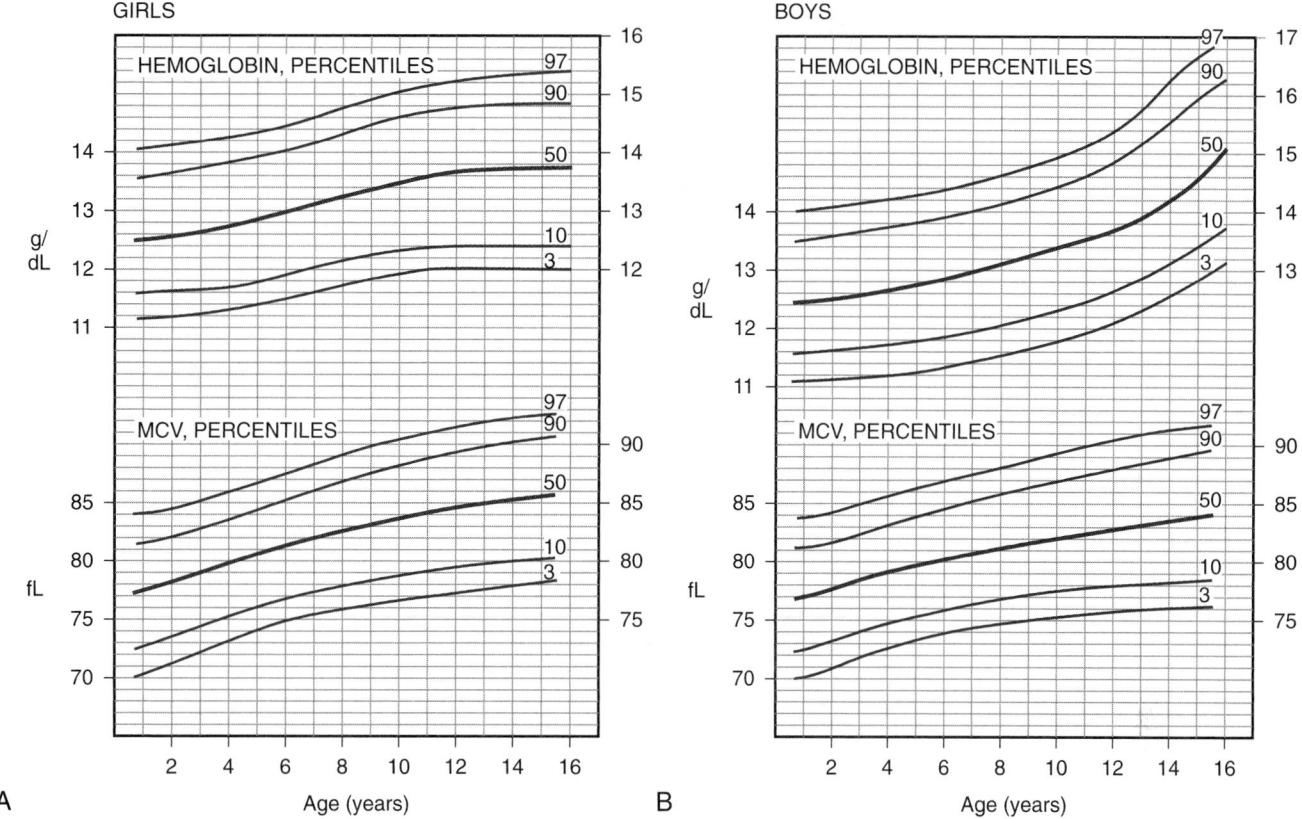

APPENDIX 12. **Hemoglobin and mean conpuscular volume (MCV) percentile curves for girls and boys. A,** Hemoglobin and MCV percentile curves for girls. **B,** Hemoglobin and MCV percentile curves for boys. These figures were obtained from populations of nonindigent white children residing in either northern California or Finland. Hemoglobin values were derived from a total of 9946 children and MCV values from 2314 children. The reference population excluded subjects with laboratory evidence of iron deficiency, thalassemia minor, and hemoglobinopathy. (Redrawn from Dallman PR, Siimes MA: Percentile curves for hemoglobin and red cell volume in infancy and childhood. J Pediatr 1979; 94:28.)

APPENDIX 13	Hemoglobin Concentration in White, Black, and East Asian Children*					
	MALES			**FEMALES**		
Age	No.	Median	2.5 to 97.5 Percentile Range	No.	Median	2.5 to 97.5 Percentile Range
5 to 9 years						
White	305	13.0	11.6-14.3	291	12.9	11.5-14.4
Black	87	12.6	11.1-14.1	104	12.5	11.2-13.6
East Asian	50	13.1	11.9-14.4	64	13.0	11.6-14.2
10 to 14 weeks						
White	447	13.7	12.3-15.5	484	13.4	12.0-14.9
Black	143	13.1	11.5-15.2	150	12.9	11.2-14.3
East Asian	87	13.7	12.1-15.6	79	13.5	12.2-14.7

*Hemoglobin concentration in subjects with hemoglobin AA, normal glucose-6-phosphate-dehydrogenase screen, and mean corpuscular volume 95% or more of median value for whites of same age and sex. The data strengthen the impression that blacks normally have a concentration of hemoglobin averaging about 0.5 g/dL less than whites.

From Dallman PR, Barr GD, Allen CM, et al: Hemoglobin concentration in white, black, and Oriental children: is there a need for separate criteria in screening for anemia? Am J Clin Nutr 1978; 31:379. © Am J Clin Nutr, American Society for Clinical Nutrition.

APPENDIX 14   Activities of Red Cell Enzymes

Enzyme	Activity at 37° C (mean ± SD)
Acetylcholinesterase	36.93 ± 3.83
Adenosine deaminase	1.11 ± 0.23
Adenylate kinase	258 ± 29.3
Aldolase	3.19 ± 0.86
Bisphosphoglyceromutase (2,3-diphosphoglyceromutase)	4.78 ± 0.65
Catalase	$15.3 ± 2.4 × 10^4$
Enolase	5.39 ± 0.83
Epimerase	0.23 ± 0.06
Galactokinase	0.029 ± 0.004
Galactose-1-phosphate uridyl transferase	28.4 ± 6.94
Glucose phosphate isomerase	60.8 ± 11.0
Glucose-6-phosphate dehydrogenase	8.34 ± 1.59
WHO method	12.1 ± 2.09
Glutamic oxaloacetic transaminase without PLP	3.02 ± 0.67
Glutamic oxaloacetic transaminase with PLP	5.04 ± 0.90
γ-Glutamyl-cysteine synthetase	0.43 ± 0.04
Glutathione peroxidase★	30.82 ± 4.65
Glutathione reductase without FAD	7.18 ± 1.09
Glutathione reductase with FAD	10.4 ± 1.50
Glutathione-S-transferase	6.66 ± 1.81
Glyceraldehyde phosphate dehydrogenase	226 ± 41.9
Hexokinase	1.78 ± 0.38
Hypoxanthine phosphoribosyl-transferase	1.72 ± 0.30
Lactate dehydrogenase	200 ± 26.5
Methemoglobin reductase	2.60 ± 0.71
Monophosphoglyceromutase	37.71 ± 5.56
NADH-methemoglobin reductase	19.2 ± 3.85 (30°)
NADPH diaphorase	2.26 ± 0.16
Phosphofructokinase	11.01 ± 2.33
Phosphoglucomutase	5.50 ± 0.62
Phosphoglycerate kinase	320 ± 36.1
Phosphoglycolate phosphatase	1.23 ± 0.10
Pyrimidine 5' nucleotidase	0.11 ± 0.03
Pyruvate kinase	15.0 ± 1.99
6-Phosphogluconate dehydrogenase	8.78 ± 0.78
Triose phosphate isomerase	2111 ± 397

★From Beutler E, Blum KG: In Altman PL, Dittmer DS (eds): Human Health and Disease. Bethesda, MD, Federation of American Societies for Experimental Biology, 1977, p 156; and Beutler E. Red cell metabolism: a manual of biochemical methods. 3rd ed. Orlando, FL, Grune & Stratton, 1984.

APPENDIX 15   Levels of Intermediate Metabolites in Normal Adult Erythrocytes

Metabolite	Abbreviation	CONCENTRATION (mean ± 1 SD)		
		nmol/g Hb	nmol/mL Red Cells	μmol/L in Whole Blood
Adenosine-5'-diphosphate	ADP	6635 ± 105	216 ± 36	—
Adenosine-5'-monophosphate	AMP	62 ± 10	21.1 ± 3.4	—
Adenosine-5'-triphosphate	ATP	4230 ± 290 (whites)	1438 ± 99	—
		3530 ± 301 (blacks)	1200 ± 102	—
2,3-Diphosphoglycerate	2,3-DPG	1227 ± 1870	4171 ± 636	—
Glutathione	GSH	6570 ± 1040	2234 ± 354	—
Glutathione (oxidized)	GSSG	12.3 ± 4.5	4.2 ± 1.53	—
Glucose-6-phosphate	G6P	82 ± 22	27.8 ± 7.5	—
Fructose-6-phosphate	F6P	27 ± 5.8	9.3 ± 2.0	—
Fructose-6-diphosphate	FDP	5.6 ± 1.8	1.9 ± 0.6	—
Dihydroxyacetone phosphate	DHAP	27.6 ± 8.2	9.4 ± 2.8	—
3-Phosphoglyceric acid	3-PGA	132 ± 15.0	44.9 ± 5.1	—
2-Phosphoglyceric acid	2-PGA	21.5 ± 7.35	7.3 ± 2.5	—
Phosphoenolpyruvate	PEP	35.9 ± 6.47	12.2 ± 2.2	—
Creatine		1310 ± 310 (male)	445 ± 105	—
		1500 ± 250 (female)	510 ± 85	—
Lactate		—	—	932 ± 211
Pyruvate		—	—	53.3 ± 21.5

From Beutler E: Red Cell Metabolism: A Manual of Biochemical Methods. 3rd ed. Orlando, FL, Grune & Stratton, 1984.

APPENDIX 16 Red Cell Enzyme Activity in Adults and Term Infants*

Enzyme	Adults (20)	Infants (10)
Hexokinase	12.9 ± 2.1	34.0 ± 6.0
Phosphoglucose isomerase	406 ± 37	560 ± 112
Phosphofructokinase	148 ± 24.5	84.5 ± 24
Aldolase	24.5 ± 3.7	42.0 ± 10.0
Glyceraldehyde-3-phosphate dehydrogenase	885 ± 127	884 ± 245
Triosephosphate isomerase	26,323 ± 3240	29,111 ± 4100
Phosphoglycerate kinase	2795 ± 144	3926 ± 528
Phosphoglycerate mutase	751 ± 99	1049 ± 160
Enolase	252 ± 54	517 ± 121
Pyruvate kinase	179 ± 16	256 ± 50
Lactic dehydrogenase	2033 ± 287	2756 ± 425
Glucose-6-phosphate dehydrogenase	215 ± 18	328 ± 40

*Infant samples were obtained from newborns weighing more than 2800 g whose gestational age was 39 weeks or greater. Blood was drawn within 24 hours of birth. All the newborns were clinically healthy. Adult samples were obtained from healthy, normal volunteers.

From Oski FA: Red cell metabolism in the newborn infant: V. Glycolytic intermediates and glycolytic enzymes. Pediatrics 1969; 44:89. Reproduced by permission of Pediatrics, Copyright 1969.

APPENDIX 17 Red Cell Glycolytic Intermediate Metabolites in Normal Adults, Term Infants, and Premature Infants*

Metabolite	Normal Adults (10)	Term Infants (10)	Premature Infants (11)	Normals (5)
Glucose-6-phosphate	24.8 ± 9.8	45.2 ± 8.7	66.8 ± 34.8	27 ± 2.4
Fructose-6-phosphate	5.4 ± 1.0	9.9 ± 2.3	20.5 ± 8.9	11 ± 2.5
Fructose, 1,6-diphosphate	4.6 ± 1.0	3.8 ± 0.7	3.6 ± 0.8	5 ± 0.9
Dihydroxyacetone phosphate	4.9 ± 3.5	11.9 ± 5.0	18.6 ± 10.7	12 ± 3.7
Glyceraldehyde-3-phosphate	2.6 ± 0.7	1.9 ± 1.6	6.5 ± 3.2	4 ± 1.5
3-Phosphoglycerate	61.6 ± 12.4	58.2 ± 14.4	47.5 ± 14.2	48 ± 16.1
2-Phosphoglycerate	4.3 ± 1.8	4.9 ± 1.6	4.4 ± 2.5	7 ± 1.7
Phosphoenolpyruvate	8.8 ± 2.6	7.6 ± 2.9	7.4 ± 3.0	12 ± 0.9
Pyruvate	73.5 ± 33.1	70.4 ± 32.3	78.4 ± 4.15	71 ± 17.7
2,3-Diphosphoglycerate	4423 ± 1907	3609 ± 800	3152 ± 2133	4000

*Samples from normal adults and term infants were identical to those described in Appendix 18. Premature infants had birth weights below 2200 g and gestational age less than 37 weeks. These premature infants were healthy at the time of investigation.

From Oski FA: Red cell metabolism in the newborn infant: V. Glycolytic intermediates and glycolytic enzymes. Pediatrics 1969; 44:87. Reproduced with permission of Pediatrics, Copyright 1969.

APPENDIX 18 Red Cell Enzyme Activity Levels in Cord Blood and 4th-Day Blood

	Cord	4th Day	P
Glucose-6-phosphate dehydrogenase	8.51 ± 1.20	6.23 ± 1.45	.005
Glutathione peroxidase	12.73 ± 1.32	14.01 ± 1.10	.001
Glutathione reductase	5.27 ± 1.21	6.49 ± 1.15	.004
Catalase	11.36 ± 1.28	12.73 ± 1.12	.025
Superoxide dismutase	1.21 ± 0.09	1.20 ± 0.08	NS

Data expressed in IU/g Hb as mean ± SD; n = 36.

From Buonocore G, Berni S, Gioia D, et al: Characteristics and functional properties of red cells during the first days of life. Biol Neonate 1991; 60:137. Reproduced with permission of S. Karger AG, Basel.

APPENDIX 19 Hemoglobin A Content (%) in Blood of Male and Female Newborns According to Birth Weight		
Birth Weight (g)	**Males Hb A (%)**	**Females Hb A (%)**
<1501	7.1 ± 1.3 (9)	13.2 ± 11.3 (14)
1501-2000	12.2 ± 8.2 (36)	13.1 ± 10.4 (44)
2001-2500	12.6 ± 5.2 (139)	14.9 ± 6.5 (206)*
2501-3000	15.8 ± 6.4 (635)	17.8 ± 6.2 (776)*
3001-3500	18.2 ± 6.5 (1289)	19.9 ± 6.8 (1204)*
3501-4000	20.0 ± 6.6 (803)	20.9 ± 7.2 (590)*
4001-4500	19.7 ± 6.3 (200)	22.6 ± 8.6 (94)*
>4500	21.7 ± 7.0 (45)	20.9 ± 7.2 (20)

*$P < .05$ between males and females.

From Galacteros F, Guilloud-Bataille M, Feingold J: Sex, gestational age, and weight dependency of adult hemoglobin concentration in normal newborns. Blood 1991; 78:1121.

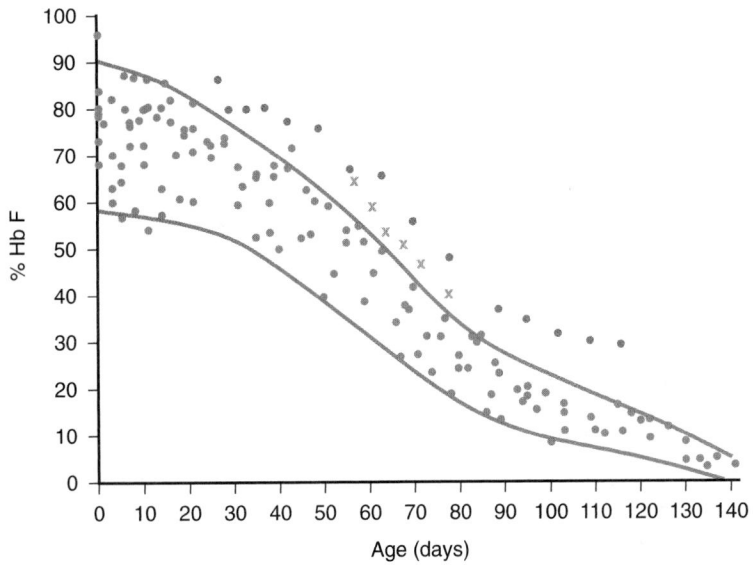

APPENDIX 20.   Relative concentration of hemoglobin F in infants and its variation with age. The region between the curved lines contains 120 observations in 17 normal children. (Redrawn from Garby L, Sjolin S: Development of erythropoiesis. Acta Paediatr 1962; 51:245.)

APPENDIX 21 Percentage of Hemoglobins F and A2 in the Newborn and Adult*		
	% Hb F (Gα:Aα ratio)	**% Hb A2**
Newborn	60-90 (3:1)	<1.0
Adult	<1.0 (2:3)	1.6-3.5

*The α chains of fetal hemoglobin contain either a glycyl residue or an alanyl residue at position 136. The Gα:Aα ratio in the newborn undergoes a considerable change between the third and fourth months of life, at which time it approximates that of the Hb F of adults.

From Charache S: In Altman PL, Dittmer DS (eds): Human Health and Disease. Bethesda, MD, Federation of American Societies for Experimental Biology, 1977, p 159.

APPENDIX 22 Methemoglobin Levels in Normal Children*

	No. Cases	No. Det.	METHEMOGLOBIN (g/dL)				No. Cases	No. Det.	METHEMOGLOBIN AS PERCENTAGE OF TOTAL HEMOGLOBIN		
			Mean	Range	Standard Dev.				Mean	Range	Standard Dev.
Prematures (birth-7 days)	29	34	0.43	(0.02-0.83)	±0.07		24	28	2.3	(0.08-4.4)	±1.26
Prematures (7-72 days)	21	29	0.31	(0.02-0.78)	±0.19		18	23	2.2	(0.02-4.7)	±1.07
Prematures (total)	50	63	0.38	(0.02-0.83)	±0.10		42	51	2.2	(0.08-4.7)	±1.10
Cook County Hospital, prematures (1-14 days)	8	8	0.52	(0.18-0.83)	±0.08		—	—	—	—	—
Newborns (1-10 days)	39	39	0.22	(0.00-0.58)	±0.17		25	30	1.5	(0.00-2.8)	±0.81
Infants (1 month-1 year)	8	8	0.14	(0.02-0.29)	±0.09		8	8	1.2	(0.17-2.4)	±0.78
Children (1-14 years)	35	35	0.11	(0.00-0.33)	±0.09		35	35	0.79	(0.00-2.4)	±0.62
Adults (14-78 years)	30	30	0.11	(0.00-0.28)	±0.09		27	27	0.82	(0.00-1.9)	±0.63

*The premature and full-term infants were free of known disease. None had respiratory distress or cyanosis. Analysis of milk and water ingested by these infants revealed a nitrate level less than 0.027 ppm. The premature infants routinely received vitamin C orally each day from the seventh day of life.

From Kravitz H, Elegant LD, Kaiser E, et al: Methemoglobin values in premature and mature infants and children. Am J Dis Child 1956; 91:2. Copyright 1956, American Medical Association.

APPENDIX 23 Membrane Lipid Composition of Fetal Erythrocytes

	G1 20-25 wk (n = 8)	G2 28-35 wk (n = 7)	G3 38-41 wk (n = 7)	G4 Adults (n = 10)
Cholesterol (µg/µg prot.)	0.22 ± 0.01	0.23 ± 0.01	0.22 ± 0.01	0.23 ± 0.01
Phospholipids (µg/µg prot.)	0.70 ± 0.14	0.81 ± 0.07	0.89 ± 0.16	0.93 ± 0.11
CH/PL	0.36 ± 0.05	0.30 ± 0.03	0.26 ± 0.02	0.27 ± 0.02
PHOSPHOLIPIDS				
Sphingomyelin (%)	30.11 ± 0.91	30.64 ± 0.65	31.97 ± 0.62	30.83 ± 0.3
Phosphatidylcholine (%)	30.30 ± 0.48	30.17 ± 1.0	26.78 ± 0.30*	26.88 ± 0.4*
Phosphatidylinositol (%)	3.76 ± 0.29	3.70 ± 0.24	3.39 ± 0.2	3.38 ± 0.21
Phosphatidylserine (%)	11.75 ± 1.24	11.87 ± 0.8	12.73 ± 0.31	12.02 ± 0.81
Phosphatidic acid (%)	2.98 ± 0.11	2.99 ± 0.22	2.79 ± 0.12	2.81 ± 0.18
Phosphatidylethanolamine (%)	20.93 ± 0.6	20.68 ± 1.33	22.25 ± 0.63	21.82 ± 0.43
FATTY ACIDS				
16:0 (%)	22.51 ± 0.92	25.31 ± 0.78*	22.95 ± 0.73	23.02 ± 0.79
18:0 (%)	17.74 ± 0.92	17.52 ± 0.51	18.18 ± 0.33	17.92 ± 0.46
18:1w9 (%)	13.03 ± 0.21	11.74 ± 0.38*	10.70 ± 0.30*	10.57 ± 0.33*
18:1bw7 (%)	1.75 ± 0.12	1.57 ± 0.07	1.73 ± 0.08	1.59 ± 0.07
18:2w6 (%)	4.81 ± 0.36	4.85 ± 0.42	4.38 ± 0.31	4.18 ± 0.32
20:3w6 (%)	2.40 ± 0.14	2.79 ± 0.11	3.42 ± 0.11*†	3.59 ± 0.11*
20:4w6 (%)	21.95 ± 0.5	23.13 ± 0.4	22.36 ± 0.46	22.47 ± 0.48
22:4w6 (%)	3.76 ± 0.34	4.28 ± 0.19	4.98 ± 0.23*	5.31 ± 0.40*
22:5w3 (%)	1.29 ± 0.19	1.45 ± 0.04	1.76 ± 0.17	1.63 ± 0.15
22:6w3 (%)	9.41 ± 0.71	8.79 ± 0.26	9.49 ± 0.46	9.48 ± 0.52
FATTY ACIDS OF PHOSPHATIDYLCHOLINE				
16:0 (%)	40.40 ± 2.10	40.78 ± 1.74	35.75 ± 2.76	32.12 ± 2.58
18:0 (%)	9.36 ± 0.48	9.32 ± 0.53	12.27 ± 0.57*	13.07 ± 0.51*
18:1w9 (%)	20.10 ± 0.82	15.96 ± 0.65*	14.63 ± 0.56*	12.23 ± 0.88*
18:1bw7 (%)	3.51 ± 0.15	3.05 ± 0.15	3.62 ± 0.21	3.45 ± 0.18
18:2w6 (%)	6.37 ± 0.47	6.94 ± 0.5	8.71 ± 0.78*	10.42 ± 0.9*
20:3w6 (%)	1.97 ± 0.15	2.92 ± 0.20*	4.89 ± 0.28*	6.05 ± 0.21*
20:4w6 (%)	16.23 ± 0.98	17.18 ± 14.2	14.21 ± 1.17	14.12 ± 1.74
22:4w6 (%)	0.54 ± 0.06	0.57 ± 0.07	0.73 ± 0.09	0.73 ± 0.08
22:5w3 (%)	0	0.35 ± 0.07	0.42 ± 0.03	0.22 ± 0.03
22:6w3 (%)	1.93 ± 0.16	2.6 ± 0.47	3.73 ± 0.43*	4.37 ± 0.49*

Continues

APPENDIX 23	Membrane Lipid Composition of Fetal Erythrocytes—cont'd			
	G1 20-25 wk (n = 8)	G2 28-35 wk (n = 7)	G3 38-41 wk (n = 7)	G4 Adults (n = 10)
FATTY ACIDS OF PHOSPHATIDYLETHANOLAMINE				
16:0 (%)	29.83 ± 0.83	30.19 ± 1.71	30.20 ± 1.44	28.55 ± 1.23
18:0 (%)	11.62 ± 0.68	10.36 ± 0.64	9.16 ± 0.57★	7.63 ± 0.58★
18:1w9 (%)	17.25 ± 1.20	16.44 ± 0.22	17.36 ± 0.33	16.17 ± 0.62
18:1bw7 (%)	1.63 ± 0.08	1.22 ± 0.05	1.59 ± 0.15	1.28 ± 0.13
18:2w6 (%)	3.01 ± 0.2	2.71 ± 0.15	3.11 ± 0.20	4.52 ± 0.26★
20:3w6 (%)	1.61 ± 0.11	1.82 ± 0.16	2.16 ± 0.14★	2.4 ± 0.12★
20:4w6 (%)	22.85 ± 0.68	24.22 ± 1.4	21.60 ± 0.98	23.6 ± 1.5
22:4w6 (%)	3.95 ± 0.29	4.92 ± 0.52	5.14 ± 0.27★	5.5 ± 0.43★
22:5w3 (%)	1.52 ± 0.16	1.37 ± 0.09	1.65 ± 0.17	1.72 ± 0.12
22:6w3 (%)	7.81 ± 0.30	7.27 ± 0.45	8.01 ± 0.42	9.00 ± 0.88

Results are expressed as mean ± SEM; $P < .05$ versus G1 (★) or G2 (†).
From Colin FC, Gallois Y, Rapid D, et al: Impaired fetal erythrocytes' filterability: relationship with cell size, membrane fluidity, and membrane lipid composition. Blood 1992; 79:2148.

APPENDIX 24	Geometric Data for Unfractionated, Top, and Bottom Neonatal and Adult Erythrocytes	
	Neonatal	**Adult**
Volume (fL)		
Unfractionated	107.3 ± 5.6★†	90.5 ± 4.4†
Top	130.8 ± 13.1★†	99.2 ± 6.3†
Bottom	89.4 ± 5.9★	80.3 ± 4.0
Surface Area (μm²)		
Unfractionated	153.5 ± 7.0★†	137.1 ± 6.7†
Top	186.1 ± 10.6★†	150.6 ± 8.4†
Bottom	108.5 ± 8.2★	118.6 ± 6.2
Surface area/volume		
Unfractionated	1.43 ± 0.04★†	1.51 ± 0.04
Top	1.43 ± 0.05★	1.51 ± 0.03
Bottom	1.21 ± 0.05★	1.49 ± 0.04
Diameter (μm)		
Unfractionated	8.8 ± 0.4†	7.9 ± 0.4
Top	9.8 ± 0.4★†	8.6 ± 0.5†
Bottom	6.9 ± 0.5	7.5 ± 0.4
Mean thickness (μm)		
Unfractionated	1.76 ± 0.10†	1.84 ± 0.13
Top	1.70 ± 0.11	1.71 ± 0.11†
Bottom	2.39 ± 0.13★	1.83 ± 0.14
Surface area index		
Unfractionated	1.40 ± 0.05†	1.41 ± 0.04†
Top	1.49 ± 0.07†	1.46 ± 0.05†
Bottom	1.12 ± 0.04★	1.33 ± 0.04

Data are presented as mean ± SD for 10 neonatal and 10 adult samples.
★Significant difference ($P < .05$, unpaired † test) between adult and neonatal erythrocytes.
†Significant difference ($P < .05$, paired † test) between top or bottom fraction and unfractionated erythrocytes.
From Linderkamp O, Friederichs E, Meiselman HJ: Mechanical and geometrical properties of density-separated neonatal and adult erythrocytes. Pediatr Res 1993; 34:688.

APPENDIX 25 Estimated Blood Volumes

Age	Plasma Volume (mL/kg) (PV)	Red Cell Mass (mL/kg) (RCM)	TOTAL BLOOD VOLUME (mL/kg)	
			From PV	From RCM
Newborn	41.3	43.1	82.1	86.1
	46.0			84.7
1-7 days	51-54	37.9	78.0	77.8
			82-86	
1-12 months	46.1	25.5	78.1	72.8
1-3 years	44.4	24.9	73.8	69.1
	47.2		81.8	
4-6 years	48.5	25.5	80.0	67.5
	49.6		85.6	
7-9 years	52.2	24.3	87.6	67.5
	49.0		86.1	
10-12 years	51.9	26.3	87.6	67.4
	46.2		83.2	
13-15 years	51.2		88.3	
16-18 years	50.1		90.2	
Adults	39-44	25-30	68-88	55-75

From Price DC, Ries C: In Handmaker H, Lowenstein JM (eds): Nuclear Medicine in Clinical Pediatrics. New York, Society of Nuclear Medicine, 1975, p 279.

APPENDIX 26 Reference Ranges for Leukocyte Counts in Children*

Age	TOTAL LEUKOCYTES		NEUTROPHILS			LYMPHOCYTES			MONOCYTES		EOSINOPHILS	
	Mean	Range	Mean	Range	%	Mean	Range	%	Mean	%	Mean	%
Birth	18.1	9.0-30.0	11.0	6.0-26.0	61	5.5	2.0-11.0	31	1.1	6	0.4	2
12 hours	22.8	13.0-38.0	15.5	6.0-28.0	68	5.5	2.0-11.0	24	1.2	5	0.5	2
24 hours	18.9	9.4-34.0	11.5	5.0-21.0	61	5.8	2.0-11.5	31	1.1	6	0.5	2
1 week	12.2	5.0-21.0	5.5	1.5-10.0	45	5.0	2.0-17.0	41	1.1	9	0.5	4
2 weeks	11.4	5.0-20.0	4.5	1.0-9.5	40	5.5	2.0-17.0	48	1.0	9	0.4	3
1 month	10.8	5.0-19.5	3.8	1.0-9.0	35	6.0	2.5-16.5	56	0.7	7	0.3	3
6 months	11.9	6.0-17.5	3.8	1.0-8.5	32	7.3	4.0-13.5	61	0.6	5	0.3	3
1 year	11.4	6.0-17.5	3.5	1.5-8.5	31	7.0	4.0-10.5	61	0.6	5	0.3	3
2 years	10.6	6.0-17.0	3.5	1.5-8.5	33	6.3	3.0-9.5	59	0.5	5	0.3	3
4 years	9.1	5.5-15.5	3.8	1.5-8.5	42	4.5	2.0-8.0	50	0.5	5	0.3	3
6 years	8.5	5.0-14.5	4.3	1.5-8.0	51	3.5	1.5-7.0	42	0.4	5	0.2	3
8 years	8.3	4.5-13.5	4.4	1.5-8.0	53	3.3	1.5-6.8	39	0.4	4	0.2	2
10 years	8.1	4.5-13.5	4.4	1.8-8.0	54	3.1	1.5-6.5	38	0.4	4	0.2	2
16 years	7.8	4.5-13.0	4.4	1.8-8.0	57	2.8	1.2-5.2	35	0.4	5	0.2	3
21 years	7.4	4.5-11.0	4.4	1.8-7.7	59	2.5	1.0-4.8	34	0.3	4	0.2	3

*Numbers of leukocytes are in thousands per mm^3, ranges are estimates of 95% confidence limits, and percentages refer to differential counts. Neutrophils include band cells at all ages and a small number of metamyelocytes and myelocytes in the first few days of life.
From Dallman PR: In Rudolph AM (ed): Pediatrics, 16th ed. New York, Appleton-Century-Crofts, 1977, p 1178.

APPENDIX 27   Reference Ranges for Pediatric Lymphocyte Subsets at Different Ages

Age		Total Lymphocytes	CD4	CD8	CD2	CD3	CD19	Helper/ Suppressor Ratio
0-6 mo	%	0.62-0.72	0.50-0.57	0.08-0.31	0.55-0.88	0.55-0.82	0.11-0.45	1.17
(n = 10)	A	5.4-7.2	2.8-3.9	0.35-2.5	3.9-5.3	3.5-5.0	0.43-3.3	6.22
6-12 mo	%	0.60-0.69	0.49-0.55	0.08-0.31	0.55-0.88	0.55-0.82	0.11-0.45	1.17
(n = 9)	A	5.3-6.7	2.6-3.5	0.35-2.5	3.8-4.9	3.4-4.6	0.43-3.3	6.22
12-18 mo	%	0.56-0.63	0.46-0.51	0.08-0.31	0.55-0.88	0.55-0.82	0.11-0.45	1.17
(n = 9)	A	4.9-5.9	2.3-2.9	0.35-2.5	3.5-4.2	3.2-3.9	0.43-3.3	6.22
18-24 mo	%	0.52-0.59	0.42-0.48	0.08-0.31	0.55-0.88	0.55-0.82	0.11-0.45	1.17
(n = 10)	A	4.4-5.5	1.9-2.5	0.35-2.5	3.1-3.9	2.8-3.5	0.43-3.3	6.22
24-30 mo	%	0.45-0.57	0.38-0.46	0.08-0.31	0.55-0.88	0.55-0.82	0.11-0.45	1.17
(n = 9)	A	3.9-5.2	1.5-2.2	0.35-2.5	2.6-3.6	2.3-3.3	0.43-3.3	6.22
30-36 mo	%	0.39-0.53	0.33-0.44	0.08-0.31	0.55-0.88	0.55-0.82	0.11-0.45	1.17
(n = 10)	A	3.3-5.1	1.2-2.0	0.35-2.5	2.2-3.5	1.9-3.1	0.43-3.3	6.22
3 years	%	0.22-0.69	0.27-0.57	0.14-0.34	0.65-0.84	0.55-0.82	0.09-0.29	0.98
(n = 73)	A	1.6-5.4	0.56-2.7	0.33-1.4	1.2-4.1	1.0-3.9	0.20-1.3	3.24

Values are expressed as 95th percentile reference range; %, relative %; A, Absolute cell count $\times 10^9$/L.

From Kotylo PK, Finenberg NS, Freeman KS, et al: Reference ranges for lymphocyte subsets in pediatric patients. Am J Clin Pathol 1993; 100:111. See also Denny T, Yogev R, Gelman R, et al: Lymphocyte subsets in healthy children during the first 5 years of life. JAMA 1992; 267:1484.

APPENDIX 28   Lymphocyte Subsets in Term and Premature Neonates in the First Week of Life

		Term (n = 21)	Premature (n = 104)	Healthy Premature (n = 36)	Sick Premature (n = 68)
Total leukocytes	—	15.44 ± 1.42	13.63 ± 0.94	13.81 ± 1.12	13.54 ± 1.32
Lymphocytes	—	3.51 ± 0.38	5.47 ± 0.23	6.04 ± 0.36	5.18 ± 0.28
CD2	%	67 ± 4	72 ± 1.5	77 ± 3	70 ± 2
	A	2.65 ± 0.34	3.97 ± 0.20	4.61 ± 0.33	3.63 ± 0.24
CD4	%	45 ± 2	47 ± 1.5	52 ± 2	45 ± 2
	A	1.56 ± 0.20	2.58 ± 0.14	3.16 ± 0.14	2.29 ± 0.17
CD8	%	13 ± 1	12 ± 0.5	12.6 ± 0.7	12 ± 0.6
	A	0.57 ± 0.13	0.67 ± 0.04	0.73 ± 0.07	0.64 ± 0.05
CD20	%	5.3 ± 0.4	6.4 ± 0.4	5.6 ± 0.4	6.8 ± 0.6
	A	0.18 ± 0.03	0.34 ± 0.03	0.34 ± 0.04	0.34 ± 0.03
CD21	%	9.1 ± 0.6	8.6 ± 0.5	6.8 ± 0.6	9.5 ± 0.7
	A	0.33 ± 0.06	0.44 ± 0.03	0.39 ± 0.04	0.47 ± 0.05

Values are expressed as mean ± SEM; %, relative %; A, Absolute cell count $\times 10^9$/L.

From Series IM, Pichette J, Carrier C, et al: Quantitative analysis of T and B cell subsets in healthy and sick premature infants. Early Hum Develop 1991; 26:143.

APPENDIX 29 Bone Marrow Cell Populations of Normal Infants*

Cell Type	MONTH										
	0 (n = 57)†	1 (n = 71)	2 (n = 48)	3 (n = 24)	4 (n = 19)	5 (n = 22)	6 (n = 22)	9 (n = 16)	12 (n = 18)	15 (n = 12)	18 (n = 19)
Small lymphocytes	14.42 ± 5.54	47.05 ± 9.24	42.68 ± 7.90	43.63 ± 11.83	47.06 ± 8.77	47.19 ± 9.93	47.55 ± 7.88	48.76 ± 8.11	47.11 ± 11.32	42.77 ± 8.94	43.55 ± 8.56
Transitional cells	1.18 ± 1.13	1.95 ± 0.94	2.38 ± 1.35	2.17 ± 1.64	1.64 ± 1.01	1.83 ± 0.89	2.31 ± 1.16	1.92 ± 1.39	2.32 ± 1.90	1.70 ± 0.82	1.99 ± 1.00
Proerythroblasts	0.02 ± 0.06	0.10 ± 0.14	0.13 ± 0.19	0.10 ± 0.13	0.05 ± 0.10	0.07 ± 0.10	0.09 ± 0.12	0.07 ± 0.09	0.02 ± 0.04	0.07 ± 0.12	0.08 ± 0.13
Basophilic erythroblasts	0.24 ± 0.25	0.34 ± 0.33	0.57 ± 0.41	0.40 ± 0.33	0.24 ± 0.24	0.47 ± 0.33	0.32 ± 0.24	0.31 ± 0.24	0.30 ± 0.25	0.38 ± 0.37	0.50 ± 0.34
Early erythroblasts	0.27 ± 0.26	0.44 ± 0.42	0.71 ± 0.51	0.50 ± 0.38	0.28 ± 0.30	0.55 ± 0.36	0.41 ± 0.30	0.39 ± 0.28	0.39 ± 0.27	0.46 ± 0.36	0.59 ± 0.34
Polychromatic erythroblasts	13.06 ± 6.78	6.90 ± 4.45	13.06 ± 3.48	10.51 ± 3.39	6.84 ± 2.58	7.55 ± 2.35	7.30 ± 3.60	7.73 ± 3.39	6.83 ± 3.75	6.04 ± 1.56	6.97 ± 3.56
Orthochromatic erythroblasts	0.69 ± 0.73	0.54 ± 1.88	0.66 ± 0.82	0.70 ± 0.87	0.34 ± 0.30	0.46 ± 0.51	0.38 ± 0.56	0.39 ± 0.48	0.37 ± 0.51	0.50 ± 0.65	0.44 ± 0.49
Extruded nuclei	0.47 ± 0.46	0.16 ± 0.17	0.26 ± 0.22	0.19 ± 0.12	0.16 ± 0.17	0.14 ± 0.11	0.16 ± 0.22	0.22 ± 0.25	0.23 ± 0.25	0.17 ± 0.12	0.21 ± 0.19
Late erythroblasts	14.22 ± 7.14	7.60 ± 4.84	13.99 ± 3.82	11.40 ± 3.43	7.34 ± 2.54	8.16 ± 2.58	7.85 ± 4.11	8.34 ± 3.31	7.42 ± 4.11	6.72 ± 1.80	7.62 ± 3.63
Early/late erythroblasts ratio‡	1:50	1:15	1:18	1:22	1:23	1:15	1:17	1:19	1:17	1:15	1:10
Fetal erythroblasts	14.48 ± 7.24	8.04 ± 5.00	14.70 ± 3.86	11.90 ± 3.52	7.62 ± 2.56	8.70 ± 2.69	8.25 ± 4.31	8.72 ± 3.34	7.81 ± 4.26	7.18 ± 1.95	8.21 ± 37.1
Blood reticulocytes	4.18 ± 1.46	1.06 ± 1.13	3.39 ± 1.22	2.90 ± 0.91	1.65 ± 0.73	1.38 ± 0.65	1.74 ± 0.80	1.67 ± 0.52	1.79 ± 0.79	2.10 ± 0.91	1.84 ± 0.46
Neutrophils											
Promyelocytes	0.79 ± 0.91	0.76 ± 0.65	0.78 ± 0.68	0.76 ± 0.80	0.59 ± 0.51	0.87 ± 0.80	0.67 ± 0.66	0.41 ± 0.34	0.69 ± 0.71	0.67 ± 0.58	0.64 ± 0.59
Myelocytes	3.95 ± 2.93	2.50 ± 1.48	2.03 ± 1.14	2.24 ± 1.70	2.32 ± 1.59	2.73 ± 1.82	2.22 ± 1.25	2.07 ± 1.20	2.32 ± 1.14	2.48 ± 0.94	2.49 ± 1.39
Early neutrophils	4.74 ± 3.43	3.27 ± 1.94	2.81 ± 1.62	3.00 ± 2.18	2.91 ± 2.01	3.60 ± 2.50	2.89 ± 1.71	2.48 ± 1.46	3.02 ± 1.52	3.16 ± 1.19	3.14 ± 1.75
Metamyelocytes	19.37 ± 4.84	11.34 ± 3.59	11.27 ± 3.38	11.93 ± 13.09	6.04 ± 3.63	11.89 ± 3.24	11.02 ± 3.12	11.80 ± 3.90	11.10 ± 3.82	12.48 ± 7.45	12.42 ± 4.15
Bands	28.89 ± 7.56	14.10 ± 4.63	13.15 ± 4.71	14.60 ± 7.54	13.93 ± 6.13	14.07 ± 5.48	14.00 ± 4.58	14.08 ± 4.53	14.02 ± 4.88	15.17 ± 4.20	14.20 ± 5.23
Mature neutrophils	7.37 ± 4.64	3.64 ± 2.97	3.07 ± 2.45	3.48 ± 1.62	4.27 ± 2.69	3.77 ± 2.44	4.85 ± 2.69	3.97 ± 2.29	5.65 ± 3.92	6.94 ± 3.88	6.31 ± 3.91
Late neutrophils	55.63 ± 7.98	29.08 ± 6.79	27.50 ± 6.88	31.00 ± 11.17	31.30 ± 7.80	29.73 ± 7.19	29.86 ± 6.74	29.86 ± 7.36	30.77 ± 8.69	34.60 ± 7.35	32.93 ± 7.01
Early/late neutrophil ratio	1:12	1:9	1:9	1:9	1:11	1:8	1:10	1:12	1:10	1:10	1:10
Total neutrophils	60.37 ± 8.66	32.35 ± 7.68	30.31 ± 7.27	34.01 ± 11.95	34.21 ± 8.61	33.12 ± 8.34	32.75 ± 7.03	32.33 ± 7.75	33.79 ± 8.76	37.76 ± 7.32	36.06 ± 7.40
Total eosinophils	2.70 ± 1.27	2.61 ± 1.40	2.50 ± 1.22	2.54 ± 1.46	2.37 ± 4.13	1.98 ± 0.86	2.08 ± 1.16	1.74 ± 1.08	1.92 ± 1.09	3.39 ± 1.93	2.70 ± 2.16
Total basophils	0.12 ± 0.20	0.07 ± 0.16	0.08 ± 0.10	0.09 ± 0.09	0.11 ± 0.14	0.09 ± 0.13	0.10 ± 0.13	0.11 ± 0.13	0.13 ± 0.15	0.27 ± 0.37	0.10 ± 0.12
Total myeloid cells	63.19 ± 9.10	35.03 ± 8.09	32.90 ± 7.85	36.64 ± 2.26	36.69 ± 8.91	35.40 ± 8.54	34.93 ± 7.52	34.18 ± 8.13	35.83 ± 8.84	41.42 ± 7.43	38.86 ± 7.92
Monocytes	0.88 ± 0.85	1.01 ± 0.89	0.91 ± 0.83	0.68 ± 0.56	0.75 ± 0.75	1.29 ± 1.06	1.21 ± 1.01	1.17 ± 0.97	1.46 ± 1.52	1.68 ± 1.09	2.12 ± 1.59
Miscellaneous											
Megakaryocytes	0.06 ± 0.15	0.05 ± 0.09	0.10 ± 0.13	0.06 ± 0.09	0.06 ± 0.06	0.08 ± 0.09	0.04 ± 0.07	0.09 ± 0.12	0.05 ± 0.08	0.00 ± 0.00	0.07 ± 0.12
Plasma cells	0.00 ± 0.02	0.02 ± 0.06	0.02 ± 0.05	0.00 ± 0.02	0.01 ± 0.03	0.05 ± 0.11	0.03 ± 0.07	0.01 ± 0.03	0.03 ± 0.07	0.07 ± 0.12	0.06 ± 0.08
Unknown blasts	0.31 ± 0.31	0.62 ± 0.50	0.58 ± 0.50	0.63 ± 0.60	0.56 ± 0.53	0.50 ± 0.37	0.56 ± 0.48	0.42 ± 0.50	0.37 ± 0.33	0.46 ± 0.32	0.43 ± 0.45
Unknown cells	0.22 ± 0.34	0.21 ± 0.25	0.16 ± 0.24	0.19 ± 0.21	0.23 ± 0.25	0.17 ± 0.22	0.10 ± 0.15	0.14 ± 0.17	0.11 ± 0.14	0.13 ± 0.18	0.20 ± 0.23
Damaged cells	5.79 ± 2.78	5.50 ± 2.46	5.09 ± 1.78	4.75 ± 2.30	4.80 ± 2.29	4.86 ± 1.25	5.04 ± 1.08	4.89 ± 1.60	5.34 ± 2.19	4.99 ± 1.96	5.05 ± 2.15
Total	6.38 ± 2.84	6.39 ± 2.63	5.94 ± 1.94	5.63 ± 2.36	5.66 ± 2.30	5.66 ± 1.41	5.78 ± 1.16	5.55 ± 1.74	5.90 ± 2.03	5.65 ± 2.02	5.81 ± 2.16

*Percentages of cell types (means ± standard deviation) in tibial bone marrow of infants from birth to 18 months of age. Data were obtained from normal American infants of black, white, and Asian racial origin. The changes in the marrow during the first 18 months of postnatal life are based on differential counts of 1000 cells classified on stained smears on each of 10 serial marrow samples aspirated from the same population of infants. Criteria for including bone marrow data in this study consisted of absence of any clinical evidence of disease, normal rate of growth, and normal serum proteins and transferrin saturations.

†n = number of infants studied at each stage.

‡Expressed in round figures for facilitating comparison. Means ± SD were calculated from values obtained in individual infants, and statistical comparisons were performed.

From Rosse C, Kraemer MJ, Dillon TL, et al: Bone marrow cell populations of normal infants: the predominance of lymphocytes. J Lab Clin Med 1977; 89:1228.

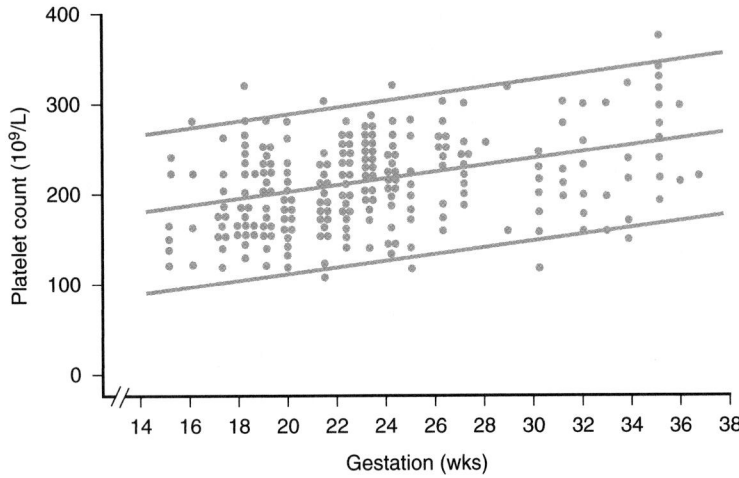

APPENDIX 30.   Platelet counts as a function of gestational age. Reference range (mean ± 2SD) for fetal platelet counts as a function of gestational age in 229 pregnancies. (Redrawn from Van den Hof MC, Nicolaides KH: Platelet count in normal, small and anemic fetuses. Am J Obstet Gynecol 1990; 162:735.)

APPENDIX 31	Circulating Platelet Counts and Serum Thrombopoietin (TPO) Levels at Different Ages	
Age Categories	**Platelet Count (10⁹/L)**	**Serum TPO (fmol/L)**
Cord blood	288 ± 53	3.73 ± 1.48 (1.44-6.74)
2 days	303 ± 48	5.92 ± 1.4 (4.33-9.18)
5 days	338 ± 59	4.32 ± 0.94 (2.38-5.76)
1 month	343 ± 72	3.77 ± 1.45 (2.25-7.60)
2-11 months	365 ± 49	2.10 ± 0.69 (1.04-4.24)
1-2 years	314 ± 78	2.23 ± 0.89 (0.43-4.54)
3-4 years	304 ± 66	1.97 ± 0.67 (0.98-3.73)
5-6 years	303 ± 65	1.67 ± 0.66 (0.58-3.14)
7-10 years	295 ± 58	1.39 ± 0.63 (0.53-2.94)
11-15 years	251 ± 40	1.24 ± 0.40 (0.49-1.99)
Adult	234 ± 48	0.83 ± 0.36 (0.25-1.72)

Data are expressed as mean ± SD. The range of values for TPO is reported in ( ).
All children values are significantly different (*P* < 0.001, Mann-Whitney U test) from adult values.
From Ishiguro, A, Nakahata T, Matsubara K, et al. (1999). Age-related changes in thrombopoietin in children: reference interval for serum thrombopoietin levels. Br J Haematol 106(4):884-888.

APPENDIX 32	Comparison of Selected Coagulation Factor Values in Newborns						
Age	**Fibrinogen (mg/dL)**	**F II (U/mL)**	**F VIII (U/mL)**	**F IX (U/mL)**	**F XII (U/mL)**	**Antithrombin (U/mL)**	**Protein C (U/mL)**
TERM							
Hathaway and Bonnar (1987) and Manco-Johnson et al. (1988)*	240 (150)	0.52 (0.25)	1.5 (0.55)	0.35 (0.15)	0.44 (0.16)	0.56 (0.32)	0.32 (0.16)
Andrew et al. (1987, 1988)†	283 (177)	0.48 (0.26)	1.0 (0.50)	0.53 (0.25)	0.53 (0.20)	0.63 (0.25)	0.35 (0.17)
Corrigan (1992)‡	246 (150)	0.45 (0.22)	1.68 (0.50)	0.40 (0.20)	0.44 (0.16)	0.52 (0.20)	0.31 (0.17)
PRETERM							
Hathaway and Bonnar (1987) and Manco-Johnson et al. (1988)*	300 (120)	0.45 (0.26)	0.93 (0.54)	0.41 (0.20)	0.33 (0.23)	0.40 (0.25)	0.24 (0.18)
Andrew et al. (1987, 1988)†	243 (150)	0.45 (0.20)	1.1 (0.50)	0.35 (0.19)	0.38 (0.10)	0.38 (0.14)	0.28 (0.12)
Corrigan (1992)‡	240 (150)	0.35 (0.21)	1.36 (0.21)	0.35 (0.10)	0.22 (0.09)	0.35 (0.10)	0.28 (0.12)

Data are expressed as mean and lower limits of normal. Preterm, 30-36 wk gestational age.
From Hathaway W, Corrigan J: Report of scientific and standardization subcommittee on neonatal hemostasis. Thromb Haemost 1991; 65:323.
*Hathaway W, Bonnar J: Hemostatic Disorders of the Pregnant Woman and Newborn Infant. New York, Elsevier Science Publishing Co., 1987; Manco-Johnson M, Marlar R, et al: Severe protein C deficiency in newborn infants. J Pediatr 1988; 113:359.
†Andrew M, Paes B, Milner R, et al: Development of the human coagulation system in the full-term infant. Blood 1987; 70:165; Andrew M, Paes B, Milner R, et al: Development of the human coagulation system in the healthy premature infant. Blood 1988; 72:1651.
‡Corrigan JJ Jr: Normal hemostasis in fetus and newborn. Coagulation. In Polin RA, Fox WW (eds): Fetal and Neonatal Physiology. Philadelphia, WB Saunders, 1992, pp 1368-1371.

APPENDIX 33	Changes in Prothrombin Time, Activated Partial Thromboplastin Time, and Thrombin Time in Term and Premature Infants		
	Prothrombin Time	**Activated Partial Thromboplastin Time**	**Thrombin Time**
Normal control	1	1	1
Term infants (ratio)	1.15-1.3	1.2-1.5	1.16-1.4
(increase in sec)	(3-4 sec)		
Small preterm (ratio)	1.30	1.4-2.4	1.31-1.50
(increase in sec)	(4-5 sec)		

Due to the variability of normal values for these tests, the results are expressed as a ratio of the newborn clotting times to the mean value for adult controls. Small preterm, less than 32 weeks of gestational age.

From Hathaway W, Corrigan J: Report of scientific and standardization subcommittee on neonatal hemostasis. Thromb Haemost 1991; 65:323.

APPENDIX 34	Reference Values for Coagulation Tests in Healthy, Full-Term Newborns Compared with Normal Adults		
Test	**Newborns**	**Adults**	**P<**
PT (sec)	13.1 ± 0.9	11.9 ± 0.6	.0001
aPTT (sec)	35 ± 4.5	28.8 ± 2.7	.0001
Platelets ($\times 10^9$/L)	214 ± 55	258 ± 66	.0001
Fibrinogen (mg/dL)	251 ± 51	262 ± 44	NS
Factor II (%)	73 ± 7	100 ± 15	.0001
Factor V (%)	93 ± 13	98 ± 19	NS
Factor VII (%)	88 ± 12	95 ± 18	.005
Factor VIII (%)	113 ± 38	92 ± 21	.0001
Factor IX (%)	86 ± 18	94 ± 16	.003
Factor X (%)	72 ± 10	97 ± 15	.0001
Hematocrit (%)	59 ± 3.0	44 ± 2.5	.0001

Data were obtained in 71 newborns and 100 adults and expressed as mean ± SD. Samples were collected with a constant anticoagulant-to-blood ratio, based on a previous determination of hematocrit.

From Cerneca F, de Vonderweid U, Simeone R, et al: The importance of hematocrit in the interpretation of coagulation tests in the full-term newborn infant. Haematologica 1994; 79:25.

APPENDIX 35	Bleeding Time in Children	
Age (y)	**Number of Subjects**	**Bleeding Time (s)**
0-2	33	180 ± 30
2-4	33	240 ± 60
4-9	75	300 ± 60
9-18	66	300 ± 70
0-18	201	270 ± 60
Adults	90	320 ± 90

Values are expressed as mean ± SD, using a Disposable Simplate method.

From Aversa LA, Vázquez A, Peñalver JA, et al: Bleeding time in normal children. J Pediatr Hematol Oncol 1995; 17:25.

APPENDIX 36	Reference Values for Coagulation Tests in Healthy Children Aged 1 to 16 Years Compared with Adults

	AGE			
	1 to 5 y	**6 to 10 y**	**11 to 16 y**	**Adult**
Coagulation Tests	*Mean (Boundary)*	*Mean (Boundary)*	*Mean (Boundary)*	*Mean (Boundary)*
PT (s)	11 (10.6-11.4)	11.1 (10.1-12.1)	11.2 (10.2-12.0)	12 (11.0-14.0)
INR	1.0 (0.96-1.04)	1.01 (0.91-1.11)	1.02 (0.93-1.10)	1.10 (1.0-1.3)
APTT (s)	30 (24-36)	31 (26-36)	32 (26-37)	33 (27-40)
Fibrinogen (g/L)	2.76 (1.70-4.05)	2.79 (1.57-4.0)	3.0 (1.54-4.48)	2.78 (1.56-4.0)
Bleeding time (min)	6 (2.5-10)*	7 (2.5-13)*	5 (3-8)*	4 (1-7)
II (U/mL)	0.94 (0.71-1.16)*	0.88 (0.67-1.07)*	0.83 (0.61-1.04)*	1.08 (0.70-1.46)
V (U/mL)	1.03 (0.79-1.27)	0.90 (0.63-1.16)*	0.77 (0.55-0.99)*	1.06 (0.62-1.50)
VII (U/mL)	0.82 (0.55-1.16)*	0.85 (0.52-1.20)*	0.83 (0.58-1.15)*	1.05 (0.67-1.43)
VIII (U/mL)	0.90 (0.59-1.42)	0.95 (0.58-1.32)	0.92 (0.53-1.31)	0.99 (0.50-1.49)
vWF (U/mL)	0.82 (0.60-1.20)	0.95 (0.44-1.44)	1.00 (0.46-1.53)	0.92 (0.50-1.58)
IX (U/mL)	0.73 (0.47-1.04)*	0.75 (0.63-0.89)*	0.82 (0.59-1.22)*	1.09 (0.5-1.63)
X (U/mL)	0.88 (0.58-1.16)*	0.75 (0.55-1.01)*	0.79 (0.50-1.17)*	1.06 (0.70-1.52)
XI (U/mL)	0.97 (0.56-1.50)	0.86 (0.52-1.20)	0.74 (0.50-0.97)*	0.97 (0.67-1.27)
XII (U/mL)	0.93 (0.64-1.29)	0.92 (0.60-1.40)	0.81 (0.34-1.37)*	1.08 (0.52-1.64)
PK (U/mL)	0.95 (0.65-1.30)	0.99 (0.66-1.31)	0.99 (0.53-1.45)	1.12 (0.62-1.62)
HMWK (U/mL)	0.98 (0.64-1.32)	0.93 (0.60-1.30)	0.91 (0.63-1.19)	0.92 (0.50-1.36)
XIIIa (U/mL)	1.08 (0.72-1.43)*	1.09 (0.65-1.51)*	0.99 (0.57-1.40)	1.05 (0.55-1.55)
XIIIs (U/mL)	1.13 (0.69-1.56)*	1.16 (0.77-1.54)*	1.02 (0.60-1.43)	0.97 (0.57-1.37)

All factors except fibrinogen are expressed as units per milliliter, where pooled plasma contains 1.0 U/mL. All data are expressed as the mean, followed by the upper and lower boundary encompassing 95% of the population. Between 20 and 50 samples were assayed for each value for each age-group. Some measurements were skewed due to a disproportionate number of high values. The lower limit, which excludes the lower 2.5% of the population, is given.

PT = prothrombin time; APTT = activated partial thromboplastin time; VIII = factor VIII procoagulant; vWF = von Willebrand factor; PK = prekallikrein; HMWK = high molecular weight kininogen.

*Values that are significantly different from adults.

From Andrew M, Vegh P, Johnston M, et al: Maturation of the hemostatic system during childhood. Blood 1992; 80:1998.

APPENDIX 37	Reference Values for the Inhibitors of Coagulation in Healthy Children Aged 1 to 16 Years Compared with Adults

	AGE			
	1 to 5 y	**6 to 10 y**	**11 to 16 y**	**Adult**
Coagulation Inhibitors	*Mean (Boundary)*	*Mean (Boundary)*	*Mean (Boundary)*	*Mean (Boundary)*
ATIII (U/mL)	1.11 (0.82-1.39)	1.11 (0.90-1.31)	1.05 (0.77-1.32)	1.0 (0.74-1.26)
α_2M (U/mL)	1.69 (1.14-2.23)*	1.69 (1.28-2.09)*	1.56 (0.98-2.12)*	0.86 (0.52-1.20)
C_1-Inh (U/mL)	1.35 (0.85-1.83)*	1.14 (0.88-1.54)	1.03 (0.68-1.50)	1.0 (0.71-1.31)
α_1AT (U/mL)	0.93 (0.39-1.47)	1.00 (0.69-1.30)	1.01 (0.65-1.37)	0.93 (0.55-1.30)
HCII (U/mL)	0.88 (0.48-1.28)*	0.86 (0.40-1.32)*	0.91 (0.53-1.29)*	1.08 (0.66-1.26)
Protein C (U/mL)	0.66 (0.40-0.92)*	0.69 (0.45-0.93)*	0.83 (0.55-1.11)*	0.96 (0.64-1.28)
Protein S				
Total (U/mL)	0.86 (0.54-1.18)	0.78 (0.41-1.14)	0.72 (0.52-0.92)	0.81 (0.60-1.13)
Free (U/mL)	0.45 (0.21-0.69)	0.42 (0.22-0.62)	0.38 (0.26-0.55)	0.45 (0.27-0.61)

All values are expressed in units per milliliter, where for all factors pooled plasma contains 1.0 U/mL, with the exception of free protein S, which contains a mean of 0.4 U/mL. All values are given as a mean, followed by the lower and upper boundary encompassing 95% of the population. Between 20 and 30 samples were assayed for each value for each age-group. Some measurements were skewed due to a disproportionate number of high values. The lower limits, which exclude the lower 2.5% of the population, are given.

*Values that are significantly different from adults.

From Andrew M, Vegh P, Johnston M, et al: Maturation of the hemostatic system during childhood. Blood 1992; 80:1998.

APPENDIX 38	Reference Values for the Fibrinolytic System in Healthy Children Aged 1 to 16 Years Compared with Adults

	AGE			
	1 to 5 y	**6 to 10 y**	**11 to 16 y**	**Adult**
	Mean (Boundary)	*Mean (Boundary)*	*Mean (Boundary)*	*Mean (Boundary)*
Plasminogen (U/mL)	0.98 (0.78-1.18)	0.92 (0.75-1.08)	0.86 (0.68-1.03)★	0.99 (0.77-1.22)
Tissue plasminogen activator (TPA) (ng/mL)	2.15 (1.0-4.5)★	2.42 (1.0-5.0)★	2.16 (1.0-4.0)★	4.90 (1.40-8.40)
Alpha$_2$-antiplasmin (α_2-AP) (U/mL)	1.05 (0.93-1.17)	0.99 (0.89-1.10)	0.98 (0.78-1.18)	1.02 (0.68-1.36)
Plasminogen activator inhibitor (PAI) (U/mL)	5.42 (1.0-10.0)	6.79 (2.0-12.0)★	6.07 (2.0-10.0)★	3.60 (0-11.0)

For α_2-AP, values are expressed as units per milliliter, where pooled plasma contains 1.0 U/mL. Values for TPA are given as nanograms per milliliter. Values for PAI are given as U/mL, where 1 U of PAI activity is defined as the amount of PAI that inhibits 1 IU of human single-chain TPA. All values are given as the mean, followed by the lower and upper boundary encompassing 95% of the population (boundary).
★Values that are significantly different from adults.
From Andrew M, Vegh P, Johnston M, et al: Maturation of the hemostatic system during childhood. Blood 1992; 80:1998.

APPENDIX 39	Endogenous Plasma Concentrations of Thrombin–Antithrombin Complexes (TATs) and Prothrombin Fragment 1.2 (F1.2) in Children and Adults

	1-5 years	**6-10 years**	**11-16 years**	**20-45 years**
TAT (μg/L)	2.30 ± 0.08	2.38 ± 0.13	2.80 ± 0.18	2.15 ± 0.09
F1.2 (nm/L)	1.04 ± 0.06	0.87 ± 0.07	0.82 ± 0.06	0.83 ± 0.06

Data are expressed as mean ± SEM.
From Andrew M, Mitchell L, Vegh P, et al: Thrombin regulation in children differs from adults in the absence and presence of heparin. Thromb Haemost 1994; 72:836.

APPENDIX 40	Coagulation Screening Tests and Factor Levels in Fetuses and Full-Term Newborns

	FETUSES (WEEKS' GESTATION)				
Parameter	**19-23 (n = 20)**	**24-29 (n = 22)**	**30-38 (n = 22)**	**Newborns (n = 60)**	**Adults (n = 40)**
PT (s)	32.5 (19-45)	32.2 (19-44)†	22.6 (16-30)†	16.7 (12.0-23.5)★	13.5 (11.4-14.0)
PT (INR)	6.4 (1.7-11.1)	6.2 (2.1-10.6)†	3.0 (1.5-5.0)★	1.7 (0.9-2.7)★	1.1 (0.8-1.2)
APTT (s)	168.8 (83-250)	154.0 (87-210)†	104.8 (76-128)†	44.3 (35-52)★	33.0 (25-39)
TCT (s)	34.2 (24-44)★	26.2 (24-28)★	21.4 (17.0-23.3)	20.4 (15.2-25.0)†	14.0 (12-16)
Factor					
I (g/L Von Clauss)	0.85 (0.57-1.50)	1.12 (0.65-1.65)	1.35 (1.25-1.65)	1.68 (0.95-2.45)†	3.0 (1.78-4.50)
I Ag (g/L)	1.08 (0.75-1.50)	1.93 (1.56-2.40)	1.94 (1.30-2.40)	2.65 (1.68-3.60)†	3.5 (2.50-5.20)
IIc (%)	16.9 (10-24)	19.9 (11-30)★	27.9 (15-50)†	43.5 (27-64)†	98.7 (70-125)
VIIc (%)	27.4 (17-37)	33.8 (18-48)★	45.9 (31-62)	52.5 (28-78)†	101.3 (68-130)
IXc (%)	10.1 (6-14)	9.9 (5-15)	12.3 (5-24)†	31.8 (15-50)†	104.8 (70-142)
Xc (%)	20.5 (14-29)	24.9 (16-35)	28.0 (16-36)†	39.6 (21-65)†	99.2 (75-125)
Vc (%)	32.1 (21-44)	36.8 (25-50)	48.9 (23-70)†	89.9 (50-140)	99.8 (65-140)
VIIIc (%)	34.5 (18-50)	35.5 (20-52)	50.1 (27-78)†	94.3 (38-150)	101.8 (55-170)
XIc (%)	13.2 (8-19)	12.1 (6-22)	14.8 (6-26)†	37.2 (13-62)†	100.2 (70-135)
XIIc (%)	14.9 (6-25)	22.7 (6-40)	25.8 (11-50)†	69.8 (25-105)†	101.4 (65-144)
PK (%)	12.8 (8-19)	15.4 (8-26)	18.1 (8-28)†	35.4 (21-53)†	99.8 (65-135)
HMWK (%)	15.4 (10-22)	19.3 (10-26)	23.6 (12-34)†	38.9 (28-53)†	98.8 (68-135)

Values are the mean, followed in parentheses by the lower and upper boundaries including 95% of the population.
Abbreviations: Ag, antigenic value; c, coagulant activity.
★$P < .05$.
†$P < .01$.
From Reverdiau Moalic P, Delahousse B, Body G, et al: Evaluation of blood coagulation activators and inhibitors in the healthy human fetus. Blood 1996; 88:900.

APPENDIX 41   Coagulation Inhibitors in Fetuses and Full-Term Newborns

Parameter	FETUSES (WEEKS' GESTATION)			Newborns (n = 60)	Adults (n = 40)
	19-23 (n = 20)	24-29 (n = 22)	30-38 (n = 22)		
ATIII (%)	20.2 (12-31)*	30.0 (20-39)	37.1 (24-55)†	59.4 (42-80)†	99.8 (65-130)
HCII (%)	10.3 (6-16)	12.9 (5.5-20)	21.1 (11-33)†	52.1 (19-99)†	101.4 (70-128)
TFPI (ng/mL)‡	21.0 (16.0-29.2)	20.6 (13.4-33.2)	20.7 (10.4-31.5)†	38.1 (22.7-55.8)†	73.0 (50.9-90.1)
PC Ag (%)	9.5 (6-14)	12.1 (8-16)	15.9 (8-30)†	32.5 (21-47)†	100.8 (68-125)
PC Act (%)	9.6 (7-13)	10.4 (8-13)	14.1 (8-18)*	28.2 (14-42)†	98.8 (68-129)
Total PS (%)	15.1 (11-21)	17.4 (14-25)	21.0 (15-30)†	38.5 (22-55)†	99.6 (72-118)
Free PS (%)	21.7 (13-32)	27.9 (19-40)	27.1 (18-40)†	49.3 (33-67)†	98.7 (72-128)
Ratio of free PS to total PS	0.82 (0.75-0.92)	0.83 (0.76-0.95)	0.79 (0.70-0.89)†	0.64 (0.59-0.98)†	0.41 (0.38-0.43)
C4b-BP (%)	1.8 (0.6)	6.1 (0-12.5)	9.3 (5-14)	18.6 (3-40)†	100.3 (70-124)

Values are the mean, followed in parentheses by the lower and upper boundaries including 95% of the population.
Abbreviations: Ag, antigen; Act, activity.
*$P < .05$.
†$P < .01$.
‡Twenty samples were assayed for each group, but only 10 for 19- to 23-week-old fetuses.
From Reverdiau Moalic P, Delahousse B, Body G, et al: Evaluation of blood coagulation activators and inhibitors in the healthy human fetus. Blood 1996; 88:900.

APPENDIX 42   Hemoglobin, Serum Transferrin Saturation, Serum Ferritin, and Red Cell Indices in Adolescents (15-16 Years of Age)

	Mean ± SD	PERCENTILE				
		10th	25th	50th	75th	90th
BOYS						
Hb (g/dL)	14.7 ± 0.831	135	14.2	14.7	15.2	15.7
Transferrin saturation (%)	32.7 ± 10.25	21.2	25.7	31.7	38.6	46.3
Serum ferritin (μg/L)	26.4 ± 17.71	13.2	22	29	40.8	52
MCV (fL)	88.4 ± 3.87	83.5	85.5	88.1	90.9	93.2
RDW (%)	13.0 ± 0.95	12.3	12.5	12.9	13.2	13.5
MCH (pg)	29.4 ± 1.43	27.7	28.6	29.2	30.2	31.0
GIRLS						
Hb (g/dL)	13.4 ± 0.763	12.3	12.9	13.4	13.9	14.3
Transferrin saturation (%)	29.9 ± 10.7	17.2	22.8	29	35.2	43.4
Serum ferritin (μg/L)	18.2 ± 1.98	7.5	12	18.2	28.5	41.5
MCV (fL)	90.1 ± 3.86	84.8	87.6	90.3	92.8	94.8
RDW (%)	12.8 ± 0.71	12.1	12.4	12.7	13.2	13.6
MCH (pg)	29.6 ± 1.43	27.8	28.8	29.5	30.6	31.3

Data for serum ferritin are presented as geometric means ± antilog of logarithmic values. Data collected in 197 to 207 boys and 215 to 220 girls, aged 15-16.
From Hallberg L, Hultén L, Lindstedt G, et al: Prevalence of iron deficiency in Swedish adolescents. Pediatr Res 1993; 34:680-687.

APPENDIX 43   Values of Serum Iron (SI), Total Iron-Binding Capacity (TIBC), and Transferrin Saturation (S%) from Infants During the First Year of Life*

			AGE (mo)						
			0.5	1	2	4	6	9	12
SI	Median	μmol/L	22	22	16	15	14	15	14
	95% range		11-36	10-31	3-29	3-29	5-24	6-24	6-28
		μg/dL	120	125	87	84	77	84	78
			63-201	58-172	15-159	18-164	28-135	34-135	35-155
TIBC	(mean ± SD)	μmol/L	34 ± 8	36 ± 8	44 ± 10	54 ± 7	58 ± 9	61 ± 7	64 ± 7
		μg/dL	191 ± 43	199 ± 43	246 ± 55	300 ± 39	321 ± 51	341 ± 42	358 ± 38
S%	Median		68	63	34	27	23	25	23
	95% range		30-99	35-94	21-63	7-53	10-43	10-39	10-47

*These data were obtained from a group of healthy, full-term infants who were born at the Helsinki University Central Hospital. Infants received iron supplementation in formula and cereal throughout the 12-month period. Infants with hemoglobin below 110 g/dL, mean corpuscular volume of red blood cells below 71 μ³, or serum ferritin below 10 ng/mL, were excluded from the study. The 95% range of the transferrin saturation values indicates that the lower limit of normal is about 10% after 4 months of age.
From Saarinen UM, Siimes MA: Serum iron and transferrin in iron deficiency. J Pediatr 1977; 91:876.

APPENDIX 44 Serum Ferritin, Iron, Total Iron-Binding Capacity, and Transferrin Saturation

Age	Male Subjects		Female Subjects	
FERRITIN	ng/mL	µg/L	ng/mL	µg/L
1-30 d[†]	6-400	6-400	6-515	6-515
1-6 mo[†]	6-410	6-410	6-340	6-340
7-12 m[†]	6-80	6-80	6-45	6-45
1-5 y[*‡]	6-24	6-24	6-24	6-24
6-9 y[*‡]	10-55	10-55	10-55	10-55
10-14 y[‡]	23-70	23-70	6-40	6-40
14-19 y[‡]	23-70	23-70	6-40	6-40
IRON	µg/dL	µmol/L	µg/dL	µmol/L
1-5 y[*‡]	22-136	4-25	22-136	4-25
6-9 y[*‡]	39-136	7-25	39-136	7-25
10-14 y[‡]	28-134	5-24	45-145	8-26
14-19 y[‡]	34-162	6-29	28-184	5-33
IRON-BINDING CAPACITY				
1-5 y[*‡]	268-441	48-79	268-441	48-79
6-9 y[*‡]	240-508	43-91	240-508	43-91
10-14 y[‡]	302-508	54-91	318-575	57-103
14-19 y[‡]	290-570	52-102	302-564	52-101
TRANSFERRIN SATURATION				
1-5 y[*‡]	0.07-0.44		0.07-0.44	
6-9 y[*‡]	0.17-0.42		0.17-0.42	
10-14 y[‡]	0.11-0.36		0.02-0.40	
14-19 y[‡]	0.06-0.33		0.06-0.33	
TRANSFERRIN		U/L (males and females)		
0-5 d[§]		1.43-4.46		
1-3 y[§]		2.18-3.47		
4-6 y[§]		2.08-3.78		
7-9 y[§]		2.25-3.61		
10-13 y[§]		2.24-4.42		
14-19 y[§]		2.33-4.44		

[*]No significant differences between males and females; range derived from combined data.

[†]Soldin SJ, Morales A, Albalos F, et al: Pediatric reference ranges on the Abbott IMx for FSH, LH, prolactin, TSH, T4, T3, free T3, T-uptake, IgE, and ferritin. Clin Biochem 1995; 28:603. Study based on hospitalized patients; values represent 2.5 and 97.5th percentiles.

[‡]Lockitch G, Halstead AC, Wadsworth L, et al: Age- and sex-specific pediatric reference intervals for zinc, copper, selenium, iron, vitamins A and E and related proteins. Clin Chem 1988; 34:1625. Study based on healthy children; values represent the 0.025 and 0.975 fractiles. Transferrin saturation calculated from iron (µmol/L)/TIBC. Note that the lower reference limits for serum iron and transferrin saturation in this study are below the limits used to define acceptable levels for these two analytes (see O'Neal RM, Johnson OC, Schaefer AE: Guidelines for the classification and interpretation of group blood and urine data collected as part of the National Nutritional Survey. Pediatr Res 1970; 4:103).

[§]Lockitch G, Halstead AC, Quigley G, et al: Age- and sex-specific pediatric reference intervals: study design and methods illustrated by measurement of serum proteins with the Behring LN nephelometer. Clin Chem 1988; 34:1618. Results are 2.5-97.5 percentiles.

APPENDIX 45 Reference Limits for Serum Transferrin Receptor in Children

Age Groups	2.5% Reference Limit mg/L	97.5% Reference Limit mg/L
6 months to 4 years	1.5 (1.4-1.5)	3.3 (3.1-3.4)
4 to 10 years	1.3 (1.3-1.4)	3.0 (2.9-3.2)
10 to 16 years	1.1 (1.1-1.2)	2.7 (2.7-2.8)
>16 years	0.9 (0.9-1.0)	2.3 (2.2-2.4)

The 95% confidence interval for each limit is given in parentheses.

From Suominen, P, Virtanen A, Lehtonen-Veromaa M, et al. Regression-based reference limits for serum transferrin receptor in children 6 months to 16 years of age. Clin Chem 2001;47(5):935-937.

APPENDIX 46   Plasma Levels of Folic Acid and Vitamin B₁₂ in Children

	Males	Females
FOLIC ACID	nmol/L	nmol/L
0-1 y	16.3-50.8	14.3-51.5
2-3 y	5.7-34.0	3.9-35.6
4-6 y	1.1-29.4	6.1-31.9
7-9 y	5.2-27.0	5.4-30.4
10-12 y	3.4-24.5	2.3-23.1
13-18 y	2.7-19.9	2.7-16.3
VITAMIN B₁₂	pmol/L	pmol/L
0-1 y	216-891	168-1117
2-3 y	195-897	307-892
4-6 y	181-795	231-1038
7-9 y	200-863	182-866
10-12 y	135-803	145-752
13-18 y	158-638	134-605

Hicks JM, Cook J, Godwin ID, et al: Vitamin B₁₂ and folate: pediatric reference ranges. Arch Pathol Lab Med 1993; 117:704. Data collected from hospitalized patients; 2.5-97.5th percentile values obtained with the Hoffman technique.

APPENDIX 47   Plasma Levels of Vitamin E (α-Tocopherol) in Children

Age	MALES AND FEMALES	
	μmol/L	μg/mL
Prematures★	1-8	0.5-3.5
Full term★	2-8	1.0-3.5
2-5 mo★	5-14	2.0-6.0
6-24 mo★	8-19	3.5-8.0
2-12 y★	13-21	5.5-9.0
1-6 y†	7-21	3.0-9.0
7-12 y†	10-21	4.0-9.0
13-19 y†	13-24	6.0-10.1

★Meites S (ed): Pediatric Clinical Chemistry. 3rd ed. Washington, DC, AACC Press, 1989, pp 295-296.

†Lockitch G, Halstead AC, Wadsworth L, et al: Age- and sex-specific pediatric reference intervals for zinc, copper, selenium, iron, vitamins A and E and related proteins. Clin Chem 1988; 34:1625. Study based on healthy children; values represent the 0.025 and 0.975 fractiles.

APPENDIX 48   Serum Erythropoietin Levels During the First Year of Life

Days After Birth	Erythropoietin (mU/mL)	Hemoglobin (g/dL)	RBC (×10⁶/μL)
0-6	33.0 ± 31.4 (11)	15.6 ± 2.2 (11)	4.51 ± 0.74 (11)
7-50	11.7 ± 3.6 (7)	12.8 ± 1.1 (5)	3.92 ± 0.35 (5)
51-100	21.1 ± 5.5 (13)	11.4 ± 1.0 (10)	4.09 ± 0.51 (10)
101-150	15.1 ± 3.9 (5)	11.2 ± 1.1 (3)	4.21 ± 0.31 (3)
151-200	17.8 ± 6.3 (6)	—	—
>201	23.1 ± 9.7 (10)	11.8 ± 0.8 (9)	4.57 ± 0.24 (9)

Values are expressed as mean ± SD; ( ), number of specimens.

From Yamashita H, Kukita J, Ohga S. Serum erythropoietin levels in term and preterm infants during the first year of life. Am J Pediatr Hematol Oncol 1994; 16:213.

APPENDIX 49   Plasma Erythropoietin Reference Ranges in Children

Age (y)	MALE SUBJECTS		FEMALE SUBJECTS	
	2.5%	97.5%	2.5%	97.5%
1-3	1.7	17.9	2.1	15.9
4-6	3.5	21.9	2.9	8.5
7-9	1.0	13.5	2.1	8.2
10-12	1.0	14.0	1.1	9.1
13-15	2.2	14.4	3.8	20.5
16-18	1.5	15.2	2.0	14.2

Values expressed in mIU/mL. Data obtained from a total of 1122 hospitalized and outpatient children age 1-18 years.

Levels found in anemic patients cannot be compared with normal values. In fact, as long as the erythropoietin-generating apparatus in the kidney is efficient, serum levels increase exponentially as the hematocrit decreases. Serum erythropoietin must therefore be evaluated in relation to the degree of anemia, and every single laboratory should determine the exponential regression of serum erythropoietin versus hematocrit (or hemoglobin) in a home-made reference population of anemic subjects and define the 95% confidence limits. The patients gathered to calculate a reference regression equation should have an anemia with a single simple mechanism and no evidence of either renal failure or excessive cytokine production (i.e., normal values for C-reactive protein and α₂-globulins). Chronic iron deficiency anemia patients due to non-neoplastic and noninflammatory chronic blood loss have the advantages of being easily found, unequivocally defined, and homogeneous. They could become the universal reference population, although patients with hemolytic anemia or thalassemia intermedia also may be studied as reference subjects. Serum erythropoietin levels are also much higher for hemoglobin concentration in hypoplastic than in hyperplastic states. Thus, for the same hemoglobin concentration, serum erythropoietin levels are lower in thalassemia intermedia than in Diamond-Blackfan anemia.

From Krafte-Jacobs B, Williams J, Soldin SJ: Plasma erythropoietin reference ranges in children. J Pediatr 1995; 126:601.

APPENDIX 50	Complement Fractions C3 and C4 in Males and Females		
		AGE	**g/L**
C3			
Zilow et al (1993)*		Healthy infants	0.30-0.98
Lockitch et al (1988)†		0-5 day	0.26-1.04
		1-19 yr	0.51-0.95
		Adult	0.45-0.83
C4			
Lockitch et al (1988)†		0-5 day	0.06-0.37
		1-19 yr	0.08-0.44
		Adult	0.11-0.41

*Zilow G, Zilow EP, Burger R, et al: Complement activation in newborn infants with early onset infection. Pediatr Res 1993; 34:199. Results are 0-100th percentiles.

†Lockitch G, Halstead AC, Quigley G, et al: Age- and sex-specific pediatric reference intervals: study design and methods illustrated by measurement of serum proteins with the Behring LN nephelometer. Clin Chem 1988; 34:1618. Results are 0.025-0.975 fractiles.

APPENDIX 51	Acute Phase Proteins and Complement Activation Products in Healthy Newborns	
	Median	**Range**
C3a-desArg (μg/L)	157	19-494
C3 (g/L)	0.67	0.30-0.98
C3bBbP (U/mL)	9.5	1.0-33.9
C1rsC1-inactivator (U/mL)	5.8	0.1-25.7
C-reactive protein (mg/L)	2	0-4

From Zilow G, Zilow EP, Burger R, et al: Complement activation in newborn infants with early onset infection. Pediatr Res 1993; 34:199.

APPENDIX 52	Reference Values for Serum C-Reactive Protein (CRP) and Interleukin-6 (IL-6) in Newborns		
	Geometric Mean (95% confidence interval)	**90th Percentile**	**95th Percentile**
CRP (mg/L)			
Mothers	4.3 (3.9-4.8)	—	—
Newborns			
At birth	3.3 (3.1-3.5)	4.1	5.0
At 24 hours	4.1 (3.7-4.5)	7.8	14.0
At 48 hours	4.0 (3.7-4.4)	8.0	9.7
IL-6 (ng/L)			
Term Mothers	2.87 (2.17-3.79)	—	—
Term Newborns			
At birth	1.69 (1.28-2.23)	15.7	24.8
At 24 hours	4.09 (3.13-5.33)	25.3	40.9
At 48 hours	3.45 (2.70-4.43)	20.0	27.0
Near-term Mothers	7.0 (4.59-18.4)	—	—
Near-term Newborns			
At birth	10.9 (6.53-18.4)	136.8	262.2
At 24 hours	9.3 (6.2-14.1)	36.2	55.4
At 48 hours	8.4 (5.97-11.9)	21.5	28.0

Undetectable CRP values (below 4 mg/L) were given the arbitrary value of 3 mg/L.

Undetectable IL-6 values (below 1 ng/L) were given the arbitrary value of 0.5 ng/L.

From Chiesa C, Signore F, Assoma M, et al. Serial measurements of C-reactive protein and interleukin-6 in the immediate postnatal period: reference intervals and analysis of maternal and perinatal confounders. Clin Chem 2001;47:1016-1022.

APPENDIX 53   Serum Acid Glycoprotein (AGP), α1-Antitrypsin (α1-AT) and Haptoglobin Levels Reference Ranges at Different Ages

Age (Years)	ACID GLYCOPROTEIN (g/L)			α₁-ANTITRYPSIN (g/L)			HAPTOGLOBIN (g/L)		
	2.5th	50th	97.5th	2.5th	50th	97.5th	2.5th	50th	97.5th
MALES									
1	0.52	0.88	1.47	0.87	1.40	1.91	0.07	1.11	3.1
4	0.50	0.84	1.42	0.89	1.44	1.96	0.05	0.83	2.31
7	0.49	0.83	1.39	0.90	1.45	1.98	0.04	0.74	2.05
10	0.47	0.80	1.34	0.91	1.46	1.99	0.04	0.68	1.90
14	0.44	0.74	1.25	0.86	1.38	1.88	0.27	0.81	1.63
18	0.46	0.78	1.31	0.83	1.34	1.83	0.31	0.93	1.87
20	0.47	0.80	1.34	0.83	1.33	1.82	0.32	0.98	1.97
30	0.51	0.87	1.46	0.82	1.31	1.79	0.38	1.15	2.31
FEMALES									
1	0.63	1.07	1.80	0.92	1.48	2.02	0.08	1.38	3.84
4	0.54	0.92	1.55	0.90	1.44	1.97	0.06	0.95	2.63
7	0.51	0.86	1.45	0.89	1.43	1.95	0.05	0.81	2.26
10	0.49	0.83	1.40	0.88	1.42	1.94	0.04	0.74	2.05
14	0.48	0.80	1.35	0.88	1.41	1.93	0.31	0.95	1.90
18	0.46	0.78	1.31	0.92	1.48	2.02	0.35	1.07	2.14
20	0.46	0.77	1.31	0.92	1.49	2.03	0.37	1.11	2.23
30	0.50	0.83	1.40	0.90	1.45	1.98	0.40	1.22	2.45

From Ritchie, RF, Palomaki GE, Neveux LM, et al: Reference distributions for the positive acute phase proteins, alpha1-acid glycoprotein (orosomucoid), alpha1-antitrypsin, and haptoglobin: a comparison of a large cohort to the world's literature. J Clin Lab Anal. 2000;14(6):265-270; see also Ritchie, RF, Palomaki GE, Neveux LM, et al: Reference distributions for the positive acute phase serum proteins, alpha1-acid glycoprotein (orosomucoid), alpha1-antitrypsin, and haptoglobin: a practical, simple, and clinically relevant approach in a large cohort. J Clin Lab Anal. 2000;14(6):284-292.

APPENDIX 54   Plasma Levels of Immunoglobulin A in Males and Females

Age	g/L	mg/dL
Lockitch et al (1988)*		
0-12 mo	0.00-1.00	0-100
1-3 y	0.24-1.21	24-121
4-6 y	0.33-2.35	33-235
7-9 y	0.41-3.68	41-368
10-11 y	0.64-2.46	64-246
12-13 y	0.70-4.32	70-432
14-15 y	0.57-3.00	57-300
16-19 y	0.74-4.19	74-419
Children's Hospital†		
Newborn	0.00-0.11	0-11
1-3 mo	0.06-0.05	6-50
4-6 mo	0.08-0.90	8-90
7-12 mo	0.16-1.00	16-100
1-3 y	0.20-2.30	20-230
3-6 y	0.50-1.50	50-150
Adult	0.50-2.00	50-200

*Lockitch G, Halstead AC, Quigley G, et al: Age- and sex-specific pediatric reference intervals: study design and methods illustrated by measurement of serum proteins with the Behring LN nephelometer. Clin Chem 1988; 34:1618. Results are 0.025-0.975 percentiles.

†Children's Hospital, Boston, Massachusetts, by laser nephelometry (Dade-Behring BN2).

APPENDIX 55   Serum Levels of Immunoglobulin D in Males and Females

Age	mg/L
Cord blood*	0.04-1.02
Adult†	2.0-173

*Ownby DR, Johnson CC, Peterson EL: Maternal smoking does not influence cord serum IgE or IgD concentrations. J Allergy Clin Immunol 1991; 88:555. Values constitute 95% of the measured samples.

†Tozawa T, Nakata N, Adachi K: Serum IgD concentrations in normal individuals 20-39 years of age. Rinsho Byori Jpn J Clin Pathol 1994; 42:656.

APPENDIX 56	Serum Levels of Immunoglobulin E in Males and Females

Age	IU/mL
Cord blood*	0.02-2.08
<1 y[†]	0-6.6
1-2 y[†]	0-20.0
2-3 y[†]	0.1-15.8
3-4 y[†]	0-29.2
4-5 y[†]	0.3-25.0
5-6 y[†]	0.2-17.6
6-7 y[†]	0.2-13.1
7-8 y[†]	0.3-46.1
8-9 y[†]	1.8-60.1
9-10 y[†]	3.6-81.0
10-11 y[†]	8.0-95.0
11-12 y[†]	1.5-99.7
12-13 y[†]	3.9-83.5
13-16 y[†]	3.3-188.0
<3 y[‡]	<30
<10 y[‡]	<200
10-14 y[‡]	<500
Adult[‡]	<120

	Females (KIU/L)	Males (KIU/L)
0-12 mo[§]	0-20	2-24
1-3 y[§]	2-55	2-149
4-10 y[§]	8-279	4-249
11-15 y[§]	5-295	7-280
16-18 y[§]	7-698	5-268

*Ownby DR, Johnson CC, Peterson EL: Maternal smoking does not influence cord serum IgE or IgD concentrations. J Allergy Clin Immunol 1991; 88:555. Values constitute 95% of the measured samples.

[†]Lindenberg RE, Arroyave C: Levels of IgE in serum from normal children and allergic children as measured by an enzyme immunoassay. J Allergy Clin Immunol 1986; 78:614.

[‡]Children's Hospital, Boston, Massachusetts.

[§]Soldin SJ, Morales A, Albalos F, et al: Pediatric reference ranges on the Abbott IMx for FSH, LH, prolactin, TSH, T4, T3, free T3, T-uptake, IgE, and ferritin. Clin Biochem 1995; 28:603. Study based on hospitalized patients; values represent 2.5 and 97.5th percentiles.

APPENDIX 57	Plasma Levels of Immunoglobulin M in Males and Females

Age	g/L	mg/dL
Lockitch et al (1988)*		
0-12 mo	0.0-2.16	0-216
1-3 y	0.28-2.18	28-218
4-6 y	0.36-3.14	36-314
7-9 y	0.47-3.11	47-311
10-11 y	0.46-2.68	46-268
12-13 y	0.52-3.57	52-357
14-15 y	0.23-2.81	23-281
16-19 y	0.35-3.87	35-387
Children's Hospital[†]		
Newborn	0.05-0.30	5-30
1-3 mo	0.15-0.70	15-70
4-6 mo	0.10-0.90	10-90
7-12 mo	0.25-1.15	25-115
1-3 y	0.30-1.20	30-120
3-6 y	0.22-1.0	22-100
Adult	0.50-2.0	50-200

*Lockitch G, Halstead AC, Quigley G, et al: Age- and sex-specific pediatric reference intervals: study design and methods illustrated by measurement of serum proteins with the Behring LN nephelometer. Clin Chem 1988; 34:1618. Results are 0.025-0.975 percentiles.

[†]Children's Hospital, Boston, Massachusetts, by laser nephelometry (Dade-Behring BN2).

APPENDIX 58	Plasma Levels of Immunoglobulin G in Males and Females

Age	g/L	mg/dL
Lockitch et al (1988)*		
0-12 mo	2.73-16.60	273-1660
1-3 y	5.33-10.78	533-1078
4-6 y	5.93-17.23	593-1723
7-9 y	6.73-17.34	673-1734
10-11 y	8.21-18.35	821-1835
12-13 y	8.93-18.23	893-1823
14-15 y	8.42-20.13	842-2013
16-19 y	6.46-18.64	646-1864
Children's Hospital[†]		
Newborn	7.0-1.30	700-1300
1-3 mo	2.80-7.50	280-750
4-6 mo	2.0-12.0	200-1200
7-12 mo	3.0-15.0	300-1500
1-3 y	4.0-13.0	400-1300
3-6 y	6.0-15.0	600-1500
Adult	6.0-13.4	600-1344

*Lockitch G, Halstead AC, Quigley G, et al: Age- and sex-specific pediatric reference intervals: study design and methods illustrated by measurement of serum proteins with the Behring LN nephelometer. Clin Chem 1988; 34:1618. Results are 0.025-0.975 percentiles.

[†]Children's Hospital, Boston, Massachusetts, by laser nephelometry (Dade-Behring BN2).

APPENDIX 59   Serum Levels of Immunoglobulin G Subclasses (IgG$_1$, IgG$_2$, IgG$_3$, IgG$_4$)*

Age	IgG$_1$	IgG$_2$	IgG$_3$	IgG$_4$
Miles and Riches (1994)[†]				
Cord blood, preterm	3.4-9.7	0.7-1.7	0.2-0.5	0.2-0.7
Cord blood, term	5.8-13.7	0.6-5.2	0.2-1.2	0.2-1.0
5 y	5.6-12.7	0.4-4.4	0.3-1.0	0.1-0.8
6 y	6.2-11.3	0.5-4.0	0.3-0.8	0.2-0.9
7 y	5.4-10.5	0.9-3.5	0.3-1.1	0.2-1.1
8 y	5.6-10.5	0.7-4.5	0.2-1.1	0.1-0.8
9 y	3.9-11.4	0.7-4.7	0.4-1.2	0.2-1.0
10 y	4.4-10.8	0.6-4.0	0.3-1.2	0.1-0.9
11 y	6.4-10.9	0.9-4.3	0.3-0.9	0.2-1.0
12 y	6.0-11.5	0.9-4.8	0.4-1.0	0.2-0.9
13 y	6.1-11.5	0.9-7.9	0.2-1.1	0.1-0.8
Adults	4.8-9.5	1.1-6.9	0.3-0.8	0.2-1.1
Children's Hospital[‡]				
Cord	4.35-10.84	1.43-4.53	0.27-1.46	0.01-0.47
0-2 mo	2.18-4.96	0.40-1.67	0.04-0.23	<0.01-1.20
3-5 mo	1.43-3.94	0.23-1.47	0.04-1.0	<0.01-1.20
6-8 mo	1.90-3.88	0.37-0.60	0.12-0.62	<0.01-1.20
9 mo-2 y	2.86-6.80	0.30-3.27	0.13-0.82	<0.01-1.20
2-4 y	3.81-8.84	0.70-4.43	0.17-0.90	<0.01-1.20
4-6 y	2.92-8.16	0.83-5.13	0.08-1.11	0.02-1.12
6-8 y	4.22-8.02	1.13-4.80	0.15-1.33	<0.01-1.38
8-10 y	4.56-9.38	1.63-5.13	0.26-1.13	0.01-0.95
10-12 y	4.56-9.52	1.47-4.93	0.12-1.79	0.01-1.53
12-14 y	3.47-9.93	1.40-4.40	0.23-1.17	0.01-1.43
Adults	4.22-12.92	1.17-7.47	0.41-1.29	0.01-0.67

*Values for males and females, expressed in g/L.
[†]Miles J, Riches P: The determination of IgG subclass concentrations in serum by enzyme linked immunosorbent assay: establishment of age-related reference ranges for cord blood samples, children aged 5-13 years and adults. Ann Clin Biochem 1994; 31:245.
[‡]Children's Hospital, Boston, Massachusetts, by laser nephelometry (Dade-Behring BN2).

APPENDIX 60   Serum Levels of Immunoglobulin Light Chains in Males and Females

Age	(Kappa) g/L	(Lambda) g/L
Newborn	7.7-8.7	1.7-1.9
Premature	3.1-4.9	1.6-1.9
1 mo	3.6-4.8	1.6-2.0
2 mo	2.4-2.7	1.6-1.7
3 mo	1.7-2.5	1.0-1.3
4 mo	1.9-2.4	0.8-1.0
5 mo	2.0-3.2	1.0-1.1
1 y	3.0-5.3	0.9-1.2
2 y	3.6-6.4	1.3-1.5
3 y	4.1-5.4	1.1-1.4
4 y	4.8-8.3	1.2-1.7
5 y	5.4-7.1	1.3-1.7
6 y	6.0-8.5	1.6-1.7
7 y	4.6-7.5	1.4-1.8
8 y	7.3-9.1	1.4-1.7
9 y	7.1-9.6	1.5-1.8
10 y	8.2-9.6	1.3-1.9
11 y	6.0-8.3	1.4-1.8
12 y	8.2-9.6	1.7-2.0
13 y	8.2-10.5	1.4-1.7
14 y	8.0-10.8	1.9-2.2
15 y	7.2-11.0	1.7-2.3
16 y	7.0-11.2	1.5-2.2

From Herkner KR, Salzer H, Bock A, et al: Pediatric and perinatal reference intervals for immunoglobulin light chains kappa and lambda. Clin Chem 1992; 38:548. Ranges are for 10th-90th percentiles.

APPENDIX 61   Conjugated Bilirubin in Males and Females

	μmol/L	mg/dL
Neonates*	<10	<0.6
>Neonates*	<7	<0.4
Preterm infants[†]	<10	<0.6

*Children's Hospital, Boston, Massachusetts.
[†]Lockitch G, Halstead AC, Albersheim S, et al: Age- and sex-specific pediatric reference intervals for biochemistry analytes as measured with the Ektachem 700 analyzer. Clin Chem 1988; 34:1622.

APPENDIX 62   Total Bilirubin in Males and Females

	μmol/L	mg/dL
Birth-1 d*	<103	<6.0
1-3 d*	<137	<8.0
3-7 d*	<205	<12.0
7 d-1 mo	<120	<7.0
1 mo-adult*	<21	<1.2
Bottle-fed infants[†]	<212	<12.4
Breast-fed infants[†]	<253	<14.8

*Children's Hospital, Boston, Massachusetts.
[†]Maisels MJ, Gifford K: Normal serum bilirubin levels in the newborn and the effect of breast feeding. Pediatrics 1986; 78:837.

APPENDIX 63	Selected Biochemical Parameters in Cord Blood		
	Cord Blood (Term)	**Cord Blood (Preterm)**	**Adult or Maternal Blood**
ERYTHROCYTES			
Magnesium (mmol/L)[*]	1.76 ± 0.15 (44)	—	—
Copper (μmol/L)[*]	12.9 ± 3.0 (39)	—	—
Zinc (μmol/L)[*]	40.4 ± 13.6 (44)	—	—
Ferritin (ag/cell)[†]	265 (47)	92.7 (47)	
SERUM/PLASMA			
Ferritin (μg/L)[†]	56.8 (47)	17.7 (47)	—
Free riboflavin (nM)[‡]	20.2 (31)[‖]	25.0[‖]	4.7 (31)
Flavocoenzymes (nM)[‡]	55.8 (31)[‖]	71.8[‖]	90.7 (31)
Vitamin B$_2$ (nM)[‡]	77.2 (31)[‖]	92.6	94.9 (31)
Flavocoenzymes uptake (nmol/min per kg)[‡]	0.4	1.5[¶]	—
Free riboflavin release (nmol/min per kg)[‡]	0.2	0.4[¶]	—
Selenium (μmol/L)[§]	1.04 ± 0.21[‖]	0.89 ± 0.27[‖]	1.56 ± 0.27
Retinol (μmol/L)[§]	0.66 ± 0.22[‖]	0.52 ± 0.12[‖]	1.26 ± 0.45
Alpha-Tocopherol (μmol/L)[§]	7.10 ± 2.1[‖]	8.81 ± 2.8[‖]	32.4 ± 9.2
Glutathione peroxidase (U/L)[§]	456 ± 108[‖]	305 ± 89[‖]	873 ± 176

[*]Speich M. Murat A, Acget JC, et al: Magnesium, total calcium, phosphorus, copper and zinc in plasma and erythrocytes of venous cord blood from infants of diabetic mothers: comparison with a reference group by logist discriminant analysis. Clin Chem 1992; 38:2002. Values expressed as mean ± SD; ( ), n of samples.

[†]Carpani G, Marini F, Ghisoni C, et al: Red cell and plasma ferritin in a group of normal fetuses at different ages of gestation. Eur J Haematol 1992; 49:260. Values expressed as mean geometrical value; ( ), n of samples.

[‡]Zempleni J, Link G, Bitsch I: Intrauterine vitamin B$_2$ uptake of preterm and full-term infants. Pediatr Res 1995; 38:585. Concentrations measured in the umbilical vein are reported in this table; values for umbilical artery are reported in the chapter text as well.

[§]Dison PJ, Lockitch G, Halstead AC, et al: Influence of maternal factors on cord and neonatal plasma micronutrient levels. Am J Perinatol 1993; 10:30. Data obtained in 107 term, 23 preterm (<32 wk), and 58 maternal samples.

[‖]P < .05 compared with full term.

[¶]P < .05 compared with adult/maternal.

APPENDIX 64	Relationship of Serum Protein Levels to Age					
	Total Proteins (g/dL) Mean ± 1 SD and Range	**Albumin (g/dL) Mean ± 1 SD and Range**	**Alpha-1 (g/dL) Mean ± 1 SD and Range**	**Alpha-2 (g/dL) Mean ± 1 SD and Range**	**Beta (g/dL) Mean ± 1 SD and Range**	**Gamma (g/dL) Mean ± 1 SD and Range**
Cord blood	6.22 ± 1.21 (4.78-8.04)	3.23 ± 0.82 (2.17-4.04)	0.41 ± 0.10 (0.25-0.66)	0.68 ± 0.14 (0.44-0.94)	0.74 ± 0.30 (0.42-1.56)	1.28 ± 0.23 (0.81-1.16)
1-3 mo	5.64 ± 1.04 (3.64-7.38)	3.41 ± 0.72 (2.05-4.46)	0.24 ± 0.09 (0.08-0.43)	0.74 ± 0.24 (0.40-1.13)	0.59 ± 0.20 (0.39-1.14)	0.66 ± 0.24 (0.25-1.05)
4-6 mo	5.43 ± 0.84 (4.29-6.10)	3.46 ± 0.36 (3.17-3.88)	0.17 ± 0.04 (0.12-0.25)	0.67 ± 0.11 (0.52-0.84)	0.61 ± 0.14 (0.44-0.76)	0.61 ± 0.26 (0.24-0.90)
7-12 mo	6.54 ± 0.76 (5.10-7.31)	3.62 ± 0.60 (3.22-4.31)	0.35 ± 0.15 (0.15-0.55)	0.99 ± 0.30 (0.78-1.46)	0.79 ± 0.16 (0.63-0.91)	0.84 ± 0.36 (0.32-1.18)
13-24 mo	6.66 ± 0.93 (3.69-7.50)	3.63 ± 0.80 (1.89-5.03)	0.31 ± 0.15 (0.09-0.58)	0.88 ± 0.42 (0.41-1.36)	0.77 ± 0.31 (0.36-1.41)	1.09 ± 0.32 (0.36-1.62)
25-36 mo	6.98 ± 0.66 (6.38-8.06)	4.11 ± 0.78 (3.57-5.50)	0.23 ± 0.09 (0.19-0.26)	0.89 ± 0.14 (0.68-1.09)	0.67 ± 0.14 (0.47-0.91)	1.08 ± 0.28 (0.73-1.46)
3-5 y	6.65 ± 0.85 (4.88-8.06)	3.95 ± 0.57 (2.93-5.21)	0.21 ± 0.08 (0.08-0.40)	0.70 ± 0.15 (0.43-0.99)	0.67 ± 0.11 (0.47-1.01)	1.13 ± 0.31 (0.54-1.66)
6-8 y	6.95 ± 0.55 (5.97-7.94)	4.03 ± 0.45 (3.26-4.95)	0.22 ± 0.09 (0.09-0.45)	0.67 ± 0.10 (0.50-0.83)	0.72 ± 0.11 (0.45-0.93)	1.21 ± 0.32 (0.70-1.95)
9-11 y	7.43 ± 0.84 (6.32-9.00)	4.24 ± 0.79 (3.16-4.97)	0.30 ± 0.07 (0.12-0.38)	0.75 ± 0.27 (0.67-0.87)	0.84 ± 0.16 (0.63-1.02)	1.46 ± 0.41 (0.79-2.03)
12-16 y	7.25 ± 0.85 (6.25-8.75)	4.26 ± 0.64 (3.19-5.13)	0.19 ± 0.07 (0.09-0.32)	0.71 ± 0.15 (0.50-0.97)	0.68 ± 0.15 (0.48-0.88)	1.40 ± 0.31 (1.08-1.96)
Adult	7.41 ± 0.96 (6.44-8.32)	4.31 ± 0.59 (3.46-4.78)	0.23 ± 0.06 (0.16-0.30)	0.61 ± 0.14 (0.51-0.86)	0.81 ± 0.22 (0.59-1.06)	1.45 ± 0.46 (0.68-2.11)

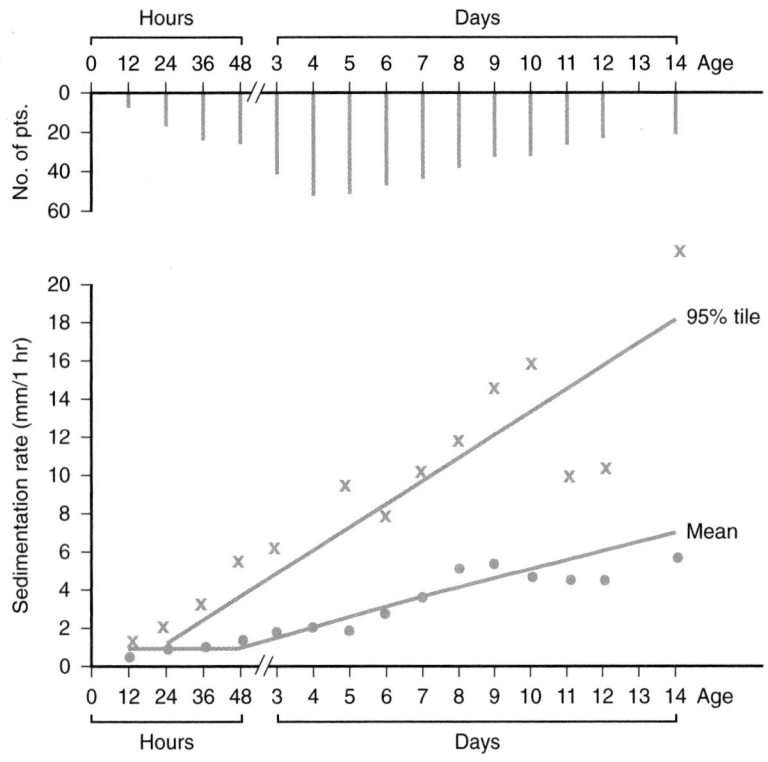

APPENDIX 65. Sedimentation rate in the newborn period. The erythrocyte sedimentation rate was measured in capillary blood in healthy full-term and low-birth-weight newborns. Normal values ranged from 1 mm/h at 12 hours of age to 17 mm/h at 14 days of age. All values of neonates with hematocrit values less than 40% were corrected to 40%. (Redrawn from Adler SM, Denton RL: The erythrocyte sedimentation rate in the newborn period. J Pediatr 1975; 86:942.)

Index

Note: Page numbers followed by f, t, or b denote figures, tables, or boxes, respectively.

A

A antigens, 1626-1627, 1626f
Aase's syndrome, Diamond-Blackfan anemia and, 356-357
Abdominal pain
  in acute intermittent porphyria, 579, 580t
  in sickle cell crisis, 967
Abetalipoproteinemia (Bassen-Kornzweig syndrome), 773-774
ABO blood group
  antigens of, 1626-1627, 1626f
  compatibility procedures for, in red blood cell transfusion, 1631-1632, 1631t, 1632t
  incompatibility of, 114-115
    neonatal, vs. hereditary spherocytosis, 735
    transplant-related, 415-416
ABO hemolytic disease, 91-92. *See also* Hemolytic disease of newborn.
  historical perspective on, 4
Absorption
  cobalamin, 472-473
    tests of, 477
  folate, 490-491
Acanthocytes
  disorders associated with, 773-779
  morphology of, 773, 773f
Acetaminophen, for transfusion reactions, 1637t
Acid glycoprotein, reference ranges for, 1792
Acid lipase deficiency, 1349-1351. *See also* Cholesteryl ester storage disease; Wolman's disease.
  low cholesterol and triglyceride diets for, 1350
Acidified glycerol lysis test, for hereditary spherocytosis, 715, 733
Aciduria, methylmalonic, 488-489, 1707
Acquired immunodeficiency syndrome. *See* AIDS/HIV.
Acquired pure red cell aplasia, 293-296. *See also* Pure red cell aplasia, acquired.
Acrodermatitis enteropathica, 1071-1072
Actin, 690-691
  adducin binding of, 696
  neutrophil, dysfunction of, 1164
Activated partial thromboplastin time (aPTT)
  changes in, in term and premature infants, 1785
  in bleeding evaluation, 1453-1454, 1454f
  in clotting, 1400
  in disseminated intravascular coagulation evaluation, 1593
Activated prothrombin complex concentrates, for hemophilia A, 1498
Activation receptors, in fibrinolysis, 1431-1433
Acute abdominal pain, in sickle cell crisis, 967

Acute chest syndrome
  erythrocytapheresis for, 1655-1656
  in sickle cell crisis, 965-967
Acute intermittent porphyria, 579-583. *See also* Porphyria(s).
  clinical manifestations of, 579-580, 580t
  frequency of, 579
  gene mutations in, 574t, 579
  laboratory diagnosis of, 581-582
  pathogenesis of, 580-581, 581b
  pregnancy and, 583
  treatment of, 582-583
Acute iron poisoning, 546-547
Acute lymphoblastic leukemia
  geographic variability of, 1759
  Philadelphia chromosome in, 419
  recurrence of, 420
  treatment of, stem cell transplantation in, 419-420
Acute megakaryoblastic leukemia, in Down syndrome, 157, 169, 350-351
Acute myelogenous leukemia
  development of, platelet disorder in, 170
  familial platelet deficiency with, 1477-1478
  in dyskeratosis congenita, 332
  in Fanconi's anemia, 317
    management of, 328
  in Shwachman-Diamond syndrome, 345
  relapse rates in, 421
  risk of, severe congenital neutropenia and, 1141, 1142
  treatment of, stem cell transplantation in, 420-421
Acyl side chains, lipid, 667-668
ADAMTS13 enzyme
  in thrombotic thrombocytopenic purpura, 641, 1571-1572
  von Willebrand factor cleavage by, 157, 642
ADAMTS13 gene, 641
  mutations of, in thrombotic thrombocytopenic purpura, 1573
Addison's disease, 1690
Adducin, 695-697, 696f
  β
    mice lacking, 746
    red cell lacking, 697
  cell-cell contact of, in nonerythroid cells, 697
  genes for, polymorphism of, 697
  red cells lacking, 697
  spectrin interaction with, 688
Adenosine deaminase
  deficiency of, in severe combined immunodeficiency, 1257-1259
  overproduction of, 866
Adenosine diphosphate (ADP), storage of, 1472
Adenosine monophosphate (AMP), cyclic, 957, 1383, 1389

Adenosine triphosphate (ATP)
  depletion of, 858-860
    in xerocytosis, 769
  glycolytic production of, 840
  in uremic red blood cells, 1687
  P-5'-N deficiency and, 864
Adenosylcobalamin
  and methylcobalamin, combined deficiency of, 486-488
  deficiency of, 488-489
  synthesis of, 475
Adenylate kinase (AK) deficiency, 865-866
Adhesion
  disorders of, 1157-1161, 1158t
  platelet, 1384, 1385f
Adhesion molecules. *See also specific type.*
  selectin family of, 1123, 1123f
Adhesive interactions, during phagocyte emigration, 1122, 1122f
Adolescent(s)
  cobalamin deficiency in, 483-484
  folate deficiency in, 496
  hemoglobin, serum transferrin, serum ferritin, and red cell indices in, 1788
Adrenal gland(s)
  congenital hyperplasia of, 1691
  disorders of, 1690-1691
  iron deposition in, 1064
Adrenocorticotropic hormone (ACTH) levels, in thalassemia major, 1064
Adult(s)
  coagulation factor levels in, 148t
  coagulation inhibitor levels in, 153t
  coagulation tests in, reference values for, 1785
  hemoglobin A2 in, 1778
  hemoglobin F in, 1778
  red cell enzyme activity in, 1777
  red cell metabolites in, 1776, 1777
  thrombin-antithrombin complexes in, endogenous plasma concentrations of, 1787t
  unfractionated erythrocytes in, geometric data for, 1780
Afibrinogenemia, 1526
African iron overload syndrome, 544
African trypanosomiasis, 1752-1753
Agammaglobulinemia
  autosomal recessive, 1274
  X-linked (Bruton's), 1273-1274
    neutropenia associated with, 1149
Age, gestational. *See* Gestational age.
Age of onset
  of bleeding, 1450
  of storage diseases, 1304t
Agglutinins, 618
Agonist receptors, in platelet activation, 1387-1388, 1387f
AIDS/HIV, 1714-1719
  alloantibodies in, 1718
  anemia in, 279, 1718-1719

O